Clinical Laboratory Medicine

Clinical Laboratory Medicine

Edited by

Kenneth D. McClatchey, M.D., D.D.S.
Professor
Department of Pathology and Otolaryngology
University of Michigan Hospitals and Medical School
Ann Arbor, Michigan

SANS TACHE

Williams & Wilkins

BALTIMORE • PHILADELPHIA • HONG KONG
LONDON • MUNICH • SYDNEY • TOKYO

A WAVERLY COMPANY

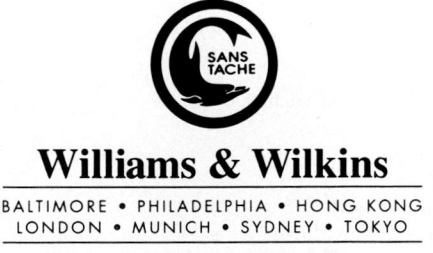

Editor: Charles M. Mitchell
Project Manager: Victoria M. Vaughn
Copy Editors: Thomas Lehr, Judith Minkove
Designer: Wilma E. Rosenberger
Illustration Planner: Lorraine Wrzosek

Printed in the United States of America

Chapter reprints are available from the publisher.

Library of Congress Cataloging-in-Publication Data

Clinical laboratory medicine / edited by Kenneth D. McClatchey.
p. cm.
Includes bibliographical references and index.
ISBN 0-683-05755-3
1. Diagnosis, Laboratory. I. McClatchey, Kenneth D.
[DNLM: 1. Diagnosis, Laboratory. QY 4 C6414 1994]
RB37.C5897 1994
616.07'56—dc20
DNLM/DLC
for Library of Congress 93-29335
CIP

93 94 95 96 97
1 2 3 4 5 6 7 8 9 10

To my wife, Martha, and our children:
Sean, Suki, Suni, and Stephen,
all of whom provide constant support
yet remind me of the balance that must be maintained in one's life
—no matter what the venture.

Preface

It is an honor to be the editor of this new comprehensive textbook devoted to clinical laboratory medicine. This textbook should ultimately educate a wide variety of users from medical laboratory technicians, medical technologists, medical students, residents in pathology and internal medicine, to clinical laboratory scientists, pathologists, and other physicians with an interest in clinical laboratory medicine.

This textbook, from beginning to end, is devoted to providing the reader with the latest in clinical laboratory medicine in an organized, well-illustrated manner. The general outline of every chapter in the text is as follows:

I. Introduction
II. Disease status (including pathophysiology)
III. Diagnostic methods
IV. Interpretation (including sensitivity, specificity, precision, and accuracy issues, where applicable)

Since the late 1950s, with the rapid increase in clinical laboratory "automation" and the emergence of quality management issues, textbooks in clinical pathology and clinical laboratory medicine have had great difficulty in keeping up with the advancement of this diverse science. There was even difficulty in defining the new technologies. This textbook has been designed to include as many of the "new" technologies as is humanly possible at this time. For example, the "new" technologies in the text include cytogenetics, HLA, molecular biology, and even such areas in the general section as quality management, cost accounting, and informatics.

The eleven sections of this textbook start with a beautiful color plate and short introduction, and are subsequently illustrated with an easily identifiable color composition that allows the reader to focus on necessary information quickly and efficiently. Finally, we the section editors and chapter authors feel that this text provides a relevant, comprehensive, scientific, and artful approach to the ever-widening scope of clinical laboratory medicine. We welcome the readers' input regarding this edition so that future editions will be even better.

Acknowledgments

It is with deep satisfaction and gratitude that I acknowledge the collaboration of my esteemed colleagues as section editors. Each section editor has performed his or her tasks in a diligent and professional manner. In addition, the chapter authors have completed, in a timely and professional manner, chapters that bring to the reader the latest science from the ever-widening universe of clinical laboratory medicine. They have accomplished their task using a format that allows both students and practicing health professionals to efficiently learn the many disciplines of clinical laboratory medicine. The textbook would not have been designed and written if I had not been influenced during my career by laboratory professionals such as John G. Batsakis, M.D., and Adam J. French, M.D. Their inspiration to pursue a career in clinical laboratory medicine was immeasurable.

I would also like to thank the staff of Williams & Wilkins, specifically Timothy S. Satterfield, Charles M. Mitchell, and Victoria M. Vaughn for their advice and counsel during the long ordeal of "text writing." A special thank you is in order for Lydia Kibiuk for the superb artwork prepared for the text.

Finally, and most importantly, *Clinical Laboratory Medicine* is written to acknowledge the many laboratory professionals who have devoted their lives to better patient care by constantly striving to improve the art and science of clinical laboratory medicine.

Contributors

Thomas M. Annesley, Ph.D.
Associate Professor of Pathology, Director of Drug Analysis and Toxicology Laboratory, University of Michigan Hospitals and Medical School, Ann Arbor, Michigan

Joseph D. Artiss, Ph.D.
Associate Professor, Department of Pathology, Wayne State University School of Medicine, Detroit, Michigan

V. Ramesh Babu, Ph.D.
Scientific Director, Cytogenetics, Nichols Institute, San Juan Capistrano, California; Adjunct Associate Professor of Urology, University of Southern California School of Medicine, Los Angeles, California

Miriam G. Blitzer, Ph.D.
Director of Biochemical Genetics and α-Fetoprotein Laboratories, Assistant Professor of Pediatrics, University of Maryland School of Medicine, Baltimore, Maryland

Jeffrey Bonadio, M.D.
Assistant Professor, Department of Pathology, University of Michigan Hospitals and Medical School, Ann Arbor, Michigan

Bruce F. Bower, M.D.
Chief of Endocrinology, Hartford Hospital, Hartford, Connecticut; Clinical Professor of Medicine, University of Connecticut School of Medicine, Farmington, Connecticut

John T. Brandt, M.D.
Director of Clinical Pathology, Department of Pathology, The Ohio State University, Columbus, Ohio

Eric Brestel, M.D.
Associate Professor of Medicine, Department of Medicine, East Carolina University School of Medicine, Greenville, North Carolina

Robert W. Burnett, Ph.D.
Department of Pathology and Laboratory Medicine, Hartford Hospital, Hartford, Connecticut; Assistant Professor of Laboratory Medicine, University of Connecticut School of Medicine, Farmington, Connecticut

Thomas E. Carey, Ph.D.
Research Scientist, Director of Head and Neck Cancer Biology Laboratory, Department of Otolaryngology/Head and Neck Surgery, University of Michigan Hospitals and Medical School, Ann Arbor, Michigan

John L. Carey III, M.D.
Director of Immunopathology Laboratory, Department of Pathology, Henry Ford Hospital and Health Care Corporation, Detroit, Michigan

Maimon M. Cohen, Ph.D.
Division of Human Genetics, Departments of Obstetrics and Gynecology and Pediatrics, University of Maryland School of Medicine, and The Medical Biotechnology Center, Baltimore, Maryland

Tina M. Cowan, Ph.D.
Co-Director of Biochemical Genetics Laboratory, Associate Professor of Pediatrics, University of Maryland School of Medicine, Baltimore, Maryland

Gordon W. Dewald, Ph.D.
Professor of Laboratory Medicine and Medical Genetics, Director of Cytogenetics Laboratory, Chair, Division of Laboratory Genetics, Mayo Clinic and Mayo Foundation, Rochester, Minnesota

Fred R. Dick, M.D.
Professor of Pathology, Director of Hematopathology, Department of Pathology, University of Iowa, Iowa City, Iowa

Stephen G. Emerson, M.D., Ph.D.
Associate Professor, Internal Medicine and Pediatrics; Chief of Hematology; Associate Chief, Division of Hematology/Oncology, University of Michigan Hospitals and Medical School, Ann Arbor, Michigan

Barry G. England, Ph.D.
Associate Professor, Department of Pathology, University of Michigan Hospitals and Medical School, Ann Arbor, Michigan

John P. Farnen, M.D.
Fellow, Internal Medicine, Hemeoncology, University of Michigan Hospitals and Medical School, Ann Arbor, Michigan

Annette W. Fothergill, B.S., M.T. (ASCP), C.L.S. (NCA)
Technical Supervisor, Fungus Testing Laboratory, Department of Pathology, University of Texas Health Science Center, San Antonio, Texas

Alfred J. Grindon, M.D.
Senior Principal Officer, American Red Cross Blood Services, Norcross, Georgia; Professor, Department of Pathology and Laboratory Medicine, Emory University School of Medicine, Atlanta, Georgia

Meryl H. Haber, M.D.
Borland Professor and Chairman, Department of Pathology; Assistant Dean for Continuing Medical Education, Rush Medical College and Rush-Presbyterian–St. Luke's Medical Center, Chicago, Illinois

Emanuel Hackel, Ph.D.
Professor of Medicine and Zoology, Michigan State University, East Lansing, Michigan

DeVon Hale, M.D.
University of Utah, Salt Lake City, Utah

Curtis A. Hanson, M.D.
Director of Hematology, Mayo Clinic, Rochester, Minnesota

Alfred E. Hartmann, M.D.
Clinical Assistant Professor, Department of Laboratory Medicine, University of South Dakota School of Medicine; Medical Director, Department of Pathology, McKennan Hospital, Sioux Falls, South Dakota

Gordon N. Hoag, Ph.D., M.D.
Director of Clinical Chemistry, Island Medical Laboratories, Ltd., Victoria, British Columbia, Canada

Gerald A. Hoeltge, M.D.
Head, Section of Blood Banking and Transfusion Medicine, Department of Clinical Pathology, The Cleveland Clinic Foundation, Cleveland, Ohio

George C. Hoffman, M.B., B.Chir., F.R.C. Path.
Emeritus Staff, The Cleveland Clinic Foundation, Cleveland, Ohio

Charles A. Horwitz, M.D.
Professor of Pathology and Laboratory Medicine, University of Minnesota Medical School; Pathologist, Abbott-Northwestern Hospital, Minneapolis, Minnesota

Karen James, Ph.D.
Immunology Consultant, Boone, North Carolina

Stephen G. Jenkins, Ph.D.
Director of Clinical Microbiology, University Medical Center, Jacksonville, Florida

W. John Judd, F.I.M.L.S., M.I.Biol.
Professor of Immunohematology; Director, Blood Bank Reference Laboratory, Department of Pathology, University of Michigan Hospitals and Medical School, Ann Arbor, Michigan

David F. Keren, M.D.
Medical Director, Warde Medical Laboratory, Department of Pathology, Catherine McAuley Health System, Ann Arbor, Michigan

Thomas R. Koch, Ph.D.
Director, Clinical Chemistry and Toxicology; Associate Professor of Pathology; University of Maryland School of Medicine, Baltimore, Maryland

Franklin P. Koontz, Ph.D.
Director of Clinical Microbiology, University of Iowa Hospitals and Clinics, Iowa City, Iowa

Brian D. Kueck, M.D.
Pathologist, Franciscan Shared Laboratory, Inc., Milwaukee, Wisconsin

Tai C. Kwong, Ph.D.
Associate Professor, Department of Pathology and Laboratory Medicine, University of Rochester Medical Center, Rochester, New York

George M. Lawson, Ph.D.
Section of Clinical Biochemistry, Department of Laboratory Medicine and Pathology, Mayo Clinic, Rochester, Minnesota

Elizabeth Lee-Lewandrowski, Ph.D., M.P.H.
Clinical Chemistry Fellow, Hartford Hospital, Hartford, Connecticut

Kent Lewandrowski, M.D.
Assistant Professor, Harvard Medical School, Boston, Massachusetts; Department of Pathology, Massachusetts General Hospital, Boston, Massachusetts

Virginia C. Lilla, C.T. (ASCP), C.L.Sp. (CG)
Laboratory Technologist, Cytogenetics Laboratory, Mayo Clinic and Mayo Foundation, Rochester, Minnesota

John B. Lowe, M.D.
Associate Investigator, Howard Hughes Medical Institute; Associate Professor of Pathology, University of Michigan Hospitals and Medical School, Ann Arbor, Michigan

Naomi L. C. Luban, M.D.
Director, Blood Bank Hematology, Department of Laboratory Medicine, Children's Hospital, Washington, D.C.

Kenneth D. McClatchey, M.D., D.D.S.
Professor, Department of Pathology and Otolaryngology, University of Michigan Hospitals and Medical School, Ann Arbor, Michigan

J. Philip McCoy, Jr., Ph.D.
Director, Flow Cytometry Laboratory, Division of Pediatric Hematology/Oncology, Cooper Hospital, University of Medicine and Dentistry of New Jersey; Robert Wood Johnson Medical School at Camden, Camden, New Jersey

Deanna A. McGough, M.T., S.M. (ASCP), R.M., S.M. (AAM)
Instructor, Department of Pathology; Administrative Director of Fungus Testing Laboratory, University of Texas Health Science Center, San Antonio, Texas

Michael D. D. McNeely, M.D., F.R.C.P.C.
Chairman and Chief Executive Officer, Island Medical Laboratories, Ltd., Victoria, British Columbia, Canada

Jay E. Menitove, M.D.
Professor of Internal Medicine, University of Cincinnati College of Medicine; Deputy Director, Medical Services, Hoxworth Blood Center, Cincinnati, Ohio

Robert E. Moore, Ph.D., D.A.B.C.C.
Associate Director, Clinical Chemistry, Hartford Hospital; Professor, Department of Pathology, University of Connecticut, Storrs, Connecticut

S. Breanndan Moore, M.B., B.Ch., F.R.C.P.I.
Chairman, Division of Transfusion Medicine; Professor of Laboratory Medicine and Pathology, Mayo Medical School, Mayo Graduate School of Medicine, Rochester, Minnesota

Mary Ann Morris, C.L.S. (NCA)
Supervisor, Hematopathology Laboratory, Mayo Clinic and Mayo Foundation, Rochester, Minnesota

Thomas P. Moyer, Ph.D.
Chairman, Division of Clinical Biochemistry, Mayo Clinic, Rochester, Minnesota

Harold A. Oberman, M.D.
Professor of Pathology; Director of Blood Bank and Transfusion Service, University of Michigan Hospitals and Medical School, Ann Arbor, Michigan

James C. Overall, Jr., M.D.
Professor of Pediatrics and Pathology, University of Utah School of Medicine, Salt Lake City, Utah

Catherine G. Palmer, Ph.D.
Director, Cytogenetics; Professor of Medical and Molecular Genetics, Indiana University School of Medicine, Indianapolis, Indiana

Powers Peterson, M.D.
Associate Professor of Pathology; Director, Laboratory of Clinical Hematology, Department of Pathology, The New York Hospital, Cornell University Medical Center, New York, New York

Thomas Peterson, M.T. (ASCP)
Computer System Consultant III, Pathology Data Systems, Department of Pathology, University of Michigan Hospitals and Medical School, Ann Arbor, Michigan

Marie Pezzlo, M.A., F(AAM)
Senior Supervisor, Medical Microbiology Division, University of California, Irvine Medical Center, Orange, California

Michael A. Pfaller, M.D.
Professor and Co-Director, Clinical Microbiology, Department of Pathology, University of Iowa College of Medicine, Iowa City, Iowa

Carl L. Pierson, M.D.
Associate Director of Microbiology, Department of Pathology, University of Michigan Hospitals and Medical School, Ann Arbor, Michigan

Michael Pins, M.D.
Chief Resident, Clinical Pathology, Massachusetts General Hospital; Clinical Fellow in Pathology, Harvard Medical School, Boston, Massachusetts

Larry G. Reimer, M.D.
Associate Professor of Pathology; Adjunct Associate Professor of Medicine, Division of Clinical Microbiology, University of Utah School of Medicine, Salt Lake City, Utah

Daniel G. Remick, M.D.
Associate Professor of Pathology, Department of Pathology, University of Michigan Hospitals and Medical School, Ann Arbor, Michigan

Mary J. Reznicek, M.D.
Associate Pathologist, Department of Pathology, West Allis Memorial Hospital, West Allis, Wisconsin

Roger S. Riley, M.D., Ph.D.
Associate Professor of Pathology; Director of Hematopathology, West Virginia University School of Medicine, Morgantown, West Virginia

Michael G. Rinaldi, Ph.D.
Director of Fungus Testing Laboratory, Professor of Pathology and Medicine, University of Texas Health Science Center; Chief of Clinical Microbiology Laboratory, Director of VA Microbiology Reference Laboratory, Audie L. Murphy Memorial Veterans Hospital, San Antonio, Texas

Jacquelyn R. Roberson, M.D.
Director, Prenatal Diagnosis, Medical Genetics and Birth Defects Center, Henry Ford Hospital, Detroit, Michigan

Charles W. Ross, M.D.
Assistant Professor of Pathology; Director, Flow Cytometry, University of Michigan, Ann Arbor, Michigan

Michael A. Saubolle, Ph.D.
Director, Microbiology Sections, Department of Pathology, Good Samaritan Regional Medical Center, Phoenix, Arizona

Ron B. Schifman, M.D.
Associate Professor, Pathology, University of Arizona; Director, Clinical Pathology, Tucson VA Medical Center, Tucson, Arizona

David L. Sewell, Ph.D.
Chief, Microbiology Section, Veterans Affairs Medical Center; Associate Professor, Pathology Department, Oregon Health Sciences University, Portland, Oregon

James B. Smart, Ph.D.
Senior Research Associate, Department of Pathology, University of Michigan Hospitals and Medical School, Ann Arbor, Michigan

Edward L. Snyder, M.D.
Director, Blood Bank, Yale–New Haven Hospital; Professor and Vice-Chairman, Department of Laboratory Medicine, Yale University School of Medicine, New Haven, Connecticut

Gary Stack, M.D., Ph.D.
Assistant Professor, Department of Laboratory Medicine, Yale University School of Medicine, New Haven, Connecticut; Chief, Pathology and Laboratory Medicine Service, Veterans Affairs Medical Center, West Haven, Connecticut

Theresa A. Steeper, M.D.
Assistant Professor of Pathology and Laboratory Medicine, University of Minneapolis Medical School; Pathologist, Abbott-Northwestern Hospital, Minneapolis, Minnesota

Fred Tenover, Ph.D.
Nosocomial Pathogens Laboratory Branch, Centers for Disease Control and Prevention, Atlanta, Georgia

Karl S. Thiel, M.D.
Associate Professor of Clinical Pathology, Department of Pathology, The Ohio State University, Columbus, Ohio

John G. Toffaletti, Ph.D.
Associate Professor of Pathology, Director of Blood Gas Laboratory, Duke University Medical Center, Durham, North Carolina

Eleanor M. Travers, M.D.
Associate Clinical Professor, Pathology & Laboratory Medicine, Georgetown University School of Medicine, Washington, D.C.

Douglas A. Triplett, M.D., F.A.C.P., F.C.A.P.
Professor of Pathology and Assistant Dean, Indiana University School of Medicine; Director of Hematology, Ball Memorial Hospital, Muncie, Indiana

Daniel L. Van Dyke, Ph.D.
Director of Cytogenetics, Henry Ford Hospital, Detroit, Michigan

Jeffrey S. Warren, M.D.
Associate Professor; Director, Division of Clinical Pathology/Clinical Laboratories, Department of Pathology, University of Michigan Hospitals and Medical School, Ann Arbor, Michigan

Richard P. Wenzel, M.D., M.Sc.
Professor of Medicine and Preventive Medicine; Director, Division of General Medicine; Director, Hospital Epidemiology Program, The University of Iowa Hospitals and Clinics, Iowa City, Iowa

Donald A. Wiebe, Ph.D.
Associate Professor, Department of Pathology and Laboratory Medicine, University of Wisconsin Medical School, Madison, Wisconsin

Anne Wiktor, B.S. M.T. (ASCP)
Senior Laboratory Technologist, The Medical Genetics and Birth Defects Center, Henry Ford Hospital, Detroit, Michigan

Alan H. B. Wu, Ph.D., D.A.B.C.C.
Director, Clinical Chemistry Laboratory, Hartford Hospital, Hartford, Connecticut; Associate Professor, Department of Laboratory Medicine, University of Connecticut Health Center, Farmington, Connecticut

Chester M. Zmijewski, Ph.D., C.L.D.
Professor of Pathology and Laboratory Medicine; Associate Director, William Pepper Laboratory; Director, Histocompatibility Laboratory, University of Pennsylvania Medical Center, Philadelphia, Pennsylvania

Contents

Section I

Section Chief: *Kenneth D. McClatchey*

Management in the clinical laboratory consists of the many processes of planning and organizing, leading the efforts of staff, and using other laboratory and hospital resources to achieve stated goals. As clinical laboratory medicine continues to grow as a service industry, modern management theory and practice have become more and more a part of our lives. At the same time, patients, faced with escalating medical costs, are insisting that they receive value for their health insurance dollar. Such requirements are vividly reflected in the actions of hospital and laboratory accrediting agencies, as well as payors such as insurance companies. It is no longer satisfactory to ignore the business aspects of our practices. Now we must know the language of quality assurance, quality improvement, utilization management, cost analysis, billing, collecting, etc. In addition, to be a responsible manager requires a solid foundation in risk management and laboratory safety. Furthermore, the manager, as a health professional, must provide accurate laboratory data for his or her patients, knowing full well that variability is a part of the preanalytic and analytic test process. This variability must be kept to a minimum, yet it should be clearly explained, when necessary, to colleagues.

In the laboratory of today and tomorrow, laboratory information systems are the backbone of success. The ability to communicate accurately in the high-volume environment of a clinical laboratory is a prerequisite for successful management of a clinical laboratory. Knowing the basic requirements of laboratory information systems (as well as having a basic knowledge of contract negotiation for information systems) allows the health professional an opportunity to control his or her destiny in result reporting, order entry, archiving, test menu selection, etc.

This section is intended to acquaint the reader with selected basic management skills that will hold him or her in good stead as quality management becomes more and more a part of the laboratory professional's life.

GENERAL LABORATORY

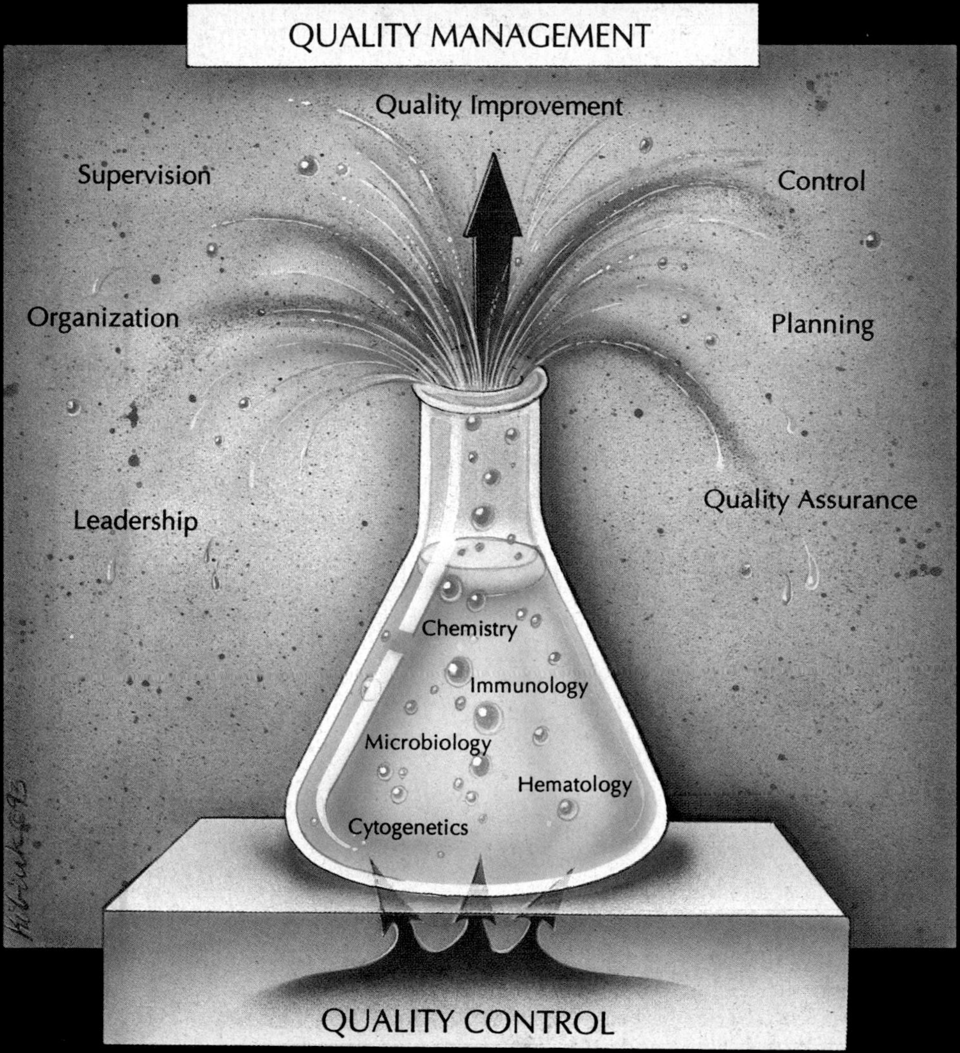

1 Laboratory Management

Eleanor M. Travers and Kenneth D. McClatchey

GENERAL MANAGEMENT ISSUES

The pathologist of the 1990s must be a medical scientist, a manager of people, a clinical consultant, and business manager. Without the integration of these attributes, and the active participation of the pathologist, the profession of laboratory medicine is likely to be drawn into increasing conflict with other health professions and health administrative agencies. Patients, clinical laboratories, and clinicians will not be well served by such divisions (1, 2).

After World War II, clinical laboratory medicine grew rapidly with a primary focus on only quality control (1, 2). Quality control is defined as procedures that, when applied to analysis of patient specimens, provide assurance that a laboratory functions properly for the benefit of the patient. Daily or run-to-run data points are plotted over time using charts (3). However, there has been a major paradigm shift in the philosophy and the role of the laboratory in medical practice.

With the advent of clinical laboratory automation, "fee for service" funding arrangements, and increasing scientific ethic in medical practice in the 1950s, the 1960s produced a logarithmic growth in clinical laboratory services. By the late 1970s, the spiraling growth of laboratory medicine was increasingly viewed as a fiscal problem by reimbursement agencies.

In reality, the health care industry, including laboratory medicine, is speeding toward a *trillion* dollar price tag by the turn of the century despite continued efforts to control costs.

On the other hand, financing mechanisms for overall health services and laboratory services have developed in a plodding, intermittent fashion over the years. Health policy emerged with the development of Blue Cross and Blue Shield health insurance in the 1930s and the Hill Burton Hospital Construction Program of the 1940s and 1950s. The subsequent decades were filled with health care delivery issues, the latest of which have strong impacts on laboratory management and practice (1, 4):

1960s
- Medicare—Publicly funded health insurance for all citizens over age 65.
- Medicaid—Health insurance for citizens receiving public assistance.

1970s
- Health maintenance organizations (HMOs) are established.
- Professional standard review organizations (PSROs) are established.

1980s
- Diagnosis-related group (DRG) system of reimbursement is introduced.
- Deficit Reduction Act (DRA) developed to control outpatient fees, including laboratory fees.
- Health maintenance organizations (HMOs) begin to flourish, with enrollment of over 30 million.
- Preferred provider organizations (PPOs) (physicians and hospitals contracted with agencies for discounted services) develop rapidly.
- Independent practice associations (IPAs) (loosely structured groups of physicians and hospitals contracted to provide discounted services) become established.
- Exclusive provider organizations (EPOs) (strict contracts with physicians and hospitals to provide discounted services to a select group of patients) make their appearance.

1990s
- Resource-based relative value units (RBRVUs)—a complex reimbursement program for physicians that is based on overall work effort and includes the correlation of multiple disciplines of medicine—are established to replace DRGs.
- Clinical Laboratory Improvement Amendments of 1988 (CLIA '88)—applies to laboratories licensed for interstate commerce under the Clinical Laboratory Improvement Act of 1967 as well as laboratories certified to receive reimbursement from Medicare and Medicaid—will be implemented through the publication of final regulations in 1993.

Major provisions of the proposed final regulations include:

- Laboratory administration
- Proficiency testing
- Patient test management
- Quality control
- Personnel standards
- Quality assurance
- Laboratory accreditation
- Enforcement and sanctions

Basic Management Concepts

Today there are four basic economic problems in the United States: money, machines, management, and manpower. Economists refer to the same four topics as capital, technology, management, and labor. If one thinks about the problems facing laboratory medicine today, the same broad areas are applicable.

Management is probably the world's oldest unheralded profession. In *The History of Management Thought*, Claude S. George, Jr., traces the profession of management from the ancient Egyptians, who engaged in *planning, organizing, and controlling* the activities of their numerous workers, to China, where planning and control systems were established around 1100 BC; to the United States, where Joseph Wharton established college courses in business management at the University of Pennsylvania in 1881 (5). George also notes that in 400 BC Socrates stated the universality of the management function in human behavior. In 350 BC, Plato established the principle of specialization for human efficiency. In 1436 the Arsenal of Venice employed over 1000 people. They used accounting systems, planning, inventory control, assembly line techniques, interchangeable parts, and a formal system of personnel management to build ships and armament.

The first "clinical" manager was probably Robert Owen, an industrialist in Scotland who, in the 1820s, first tackled the problems of productivity and motivation, of the relationship of worker to work, of worker to enterprise, and of worker to management. Such problems are obviously legitimate today.

The science of management in the United States began in the late 1800s with the efforts of Frederick W. Taylor. Taylor defined his work on scientific management as a systematic or scientific investigation of all the facts and elements of the work being managed. It was the antithesis of "management by tradition" that was the rule prior to his work (and incidentally used widely today in medicine in teaching clinical skills). Beginning with the industrial revolution to today's explosion of science and technology, management theory has evolved, bringing with it the involvement of the tools of the behavioral sciences. As a discipline, it is young—barely a century old (5, 6).

Certainly management is a science, but more importantly, it is people interacting with one another. As Peter F. Drucker states, "Every achievement of management is the achievement of a manager. Every failure is the failure of a manager. People manage, rather than forces or facts. The vision, dedication, and integrity of managers determines whether there is management or mismanagement. Management must always be done in an organization—that is, with a web of human relations." Interestingly, Drucker further compares a manager to a teacher: "Only a teacher has the same twofold dimension, the dimension of *skill* and *performance* and the dimension of personality, example, and integrity (7).

Managers come in different forms and with different labels: administrator, commander, executive, for example. They have evolved with the growth of institutions in the industrialized world. Drucker states that in the early 1900s, people asked, "What do you do?" Today they tend to ask, "Whom do you work for?" (7)

The "science" of management in this country that has been practiced for decades is being challenged. The traditional scientific approach to management is changing; learning to look on people as *resources* and *opportunities* rather than problems, costs, and threats. In such approaches, the "art" of leadership is critical (8–11).

According to Max DePree, leadership is "liberating people to do what is required of them in the most effective and humane way possible" (11). A leader, according to DePree, has the following attributes:

- Has consistent and dependable integrity
- Cherishes heterogeneity and diversity
- Searches out competence
- Is open to contrary opinion
- Communicates easily at all levels
- Understands the concept of equity and consistently advocates it
- Leads through serving
- Is open to the skills and talents of others
- Is intimate with the organization and its work
- Is able to see the broad picture (beyond his or her own area of focus)
- Is a spokesperson and diplomat
- Can be a tribal storyteller (an important way of transmitting corporate culture)
- Tells why rather than how

DePree goes on to state that the measure of leadership is "not the quality of the head, but the tone of the body." The sign of outstanding leadership appears primarily among the followers. It is fundamental that leaders endorse a concept of persons, thus an understanding of the diversity of people's gifts, talents, and skills.

There are two types of relationships in our industrialized society that influence the management of people: contractual relationships and convenantal relationships.

Contractual relationships cover the quid pro quo of working together. Contractual relationships break down during the demands of conflict and change. Alexander Solzhenitsyn stated that whenever the tissue of life is woven of legalistic relationships, this creates an atmosphere of spiritual mediocrity that paralyzes men's noblest impulses (11).

Covenantal relationships induce freedom, not paralysis. A covenantal relationship rests on shared commitment to ideas, to issues, to values, to goals, and to management processes. Covenantal relationships are open to influence (11).

A good manager studies management as a daily practice. A good manager is an entrepreneur; one who tends to accept change as part of the business of managing. A good manager is a "high-performance" manager (6). The high-performance manager is:

A strategist. One who looks to the future, makes educated guesses about the major forces and trends he or she can see, and interprets them in terms of opportunities for growth and progress.

A problem solver. One who clearly perceives the differences between the anticipated future and the unfolding present, and who decides what must be done with those factors under his or her control to influence the environment or to adapt to it most effectively.

A leader. One who offers those who answer to him or her a clear course of action, which will gain their commitment and serve their individual objectives as well as the higher objectives of the organization.

A teacher. One who guides others and helps them to identify and solve problems, so that they can perform their tasks effectively and can develop themselves as individuals as well as workers.

It is of utmost importance in the management process to realize that the human resources of an organization make the organization what it is. Human resource management is an art form. The basic components of human resource management are motivation, delegation, and supervision. Motivation is a basic psychological need of any employee, thus an important task of any manager. Delegation is the critical ability to place tasks and responsibilities at the level at which they can best be accomplished. Supervision is the combination of technical and human relations skills that ensures that organizational goals are met and policies followed.

The management process has been artfully diagrammed by Hartwick to delineate the tasks associated with the basic elements of management: ideas, things, and people (Fig. 1.1).

Management

Elements	Ideas	Things	People	
Tasks	Conceptual thinking	Administration	Leadership	
Continuous Functions	Analyze problems	Make decisions	Communicate	
Definitions of continuous functions	Gather facts, ascertain causes, develop alternatives	Arrive at conclusions and judgements	Ensure understanding	
Sequential functions	Plan	Organize and staff	Direct	Control
Activities	Set objectives Define performance standards Develop strategies Prepare budgets	Organize work-flow and tasks Establish organizational structure Select and schedule staff	Monitor performance against established standards Take actions to bring system under control	

Figure 1.1. The management process. (From Hartwick DF. Directing the clinical laboratory. New York: Field and Wood, 1990:2.)

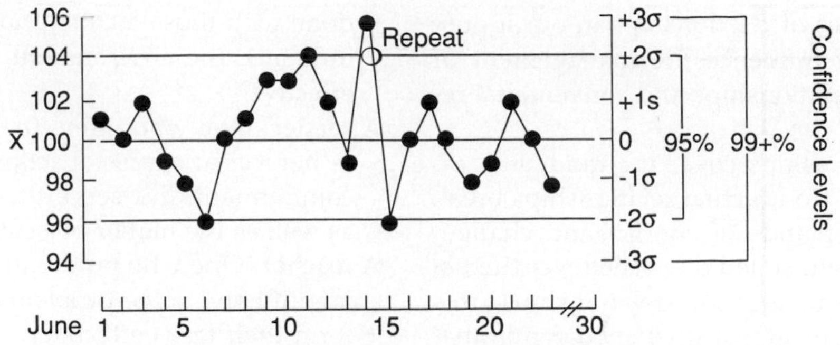

Figure 1.2. Levey-Jennings or Shewhart process control chart. (From Weisbrot IM. Statistics for the clinical laboratory. Philadelphia: JB Lippincott, 1885:64.)

The Evolution of Quality Management Concepts

The evolution of quality concepts begins with the publication of Shewhart's *Economic Control of Quality of Manufactured Product* in 1931 (8, 12). This publication put quality on a scientific footing. Shewhart developed the concept of statistical control, and describes it as follows:

> A phenomenon will be said to be controlled when through the use of past experience we can predict, at least within limits, how the phenomenon may be expected to vary in the future. Here it is understood that prediction means that we can state, at least approximately, the probability that the observed phenomenon will fall within the given limits (12).

An outgrowth of such a method was the process control chart, well known in every clinical laboratory in this country (Fig. 1.2).

Joseph Juran worked with Shewhart at Bell Laboratories and eventually played a prominent role in the evolution of quality management from the 1960s through the 1980s. In 1951 Juran published a book entitled *Quality Control Handbook* (13). He subsequently developed a system of management called "Managing for Quality" (14). His system is based on what he calls the Juran trilogy:

- Quality Planning
- Quality Control
- Quality Improvement

Quality planning includes:

- Determining who the customers are;
- Determining the needs of the customers;
- Developing product features that respond to customer needs;
- Developing processes able to produce the product features; and
- Transferring the plans to the operating forces.

Quality control includes:

- Evaluating actual product performance;
- Comparing actual performance to product goals; and
- Acting on the difference

Quality improvement includes:

- Establishing the infrastructure;
- Identifying the improvement projects;
- Establishing project teams; and
- Providing the teams with resources, training and motivation to:
  Diagnose the causes,
  Stimulate remedies, and
  Establish controls to hold the gains.

The Juran trilogy can be diagrammed to demonstrate how beneficial change can be used to develop improved levels of performance (Fig. 1.3). There is no question that improved levels of performance place an increased workload on all levels of the management team. An example of workload allocation is demonstrated with the Itoh model. In the Itoh model, time is allocated to (*a*) development, (*b*) improvement, and (*c*) control and maintenance throughout the management structure (Fig. 1.4) (14).

After World War II, W. Edwards Deming, another associate of Dr. Walter Shewhart, also espoused a philosophy of management that calls for organizations to produce products and services that help people live better. Deming believes that real profits are generated by loyal customers. In addition, Deming radically departs from the classic relationships among quality, costs, productivity, and profit. According to Deming, as quality is increased, cost decreases due to elimination of repeats and waste. Improved quality leads to lower costs and higher productivity. Lower costs and higher productivity lead to lower prices. A competitive edge is hopefully established (15).

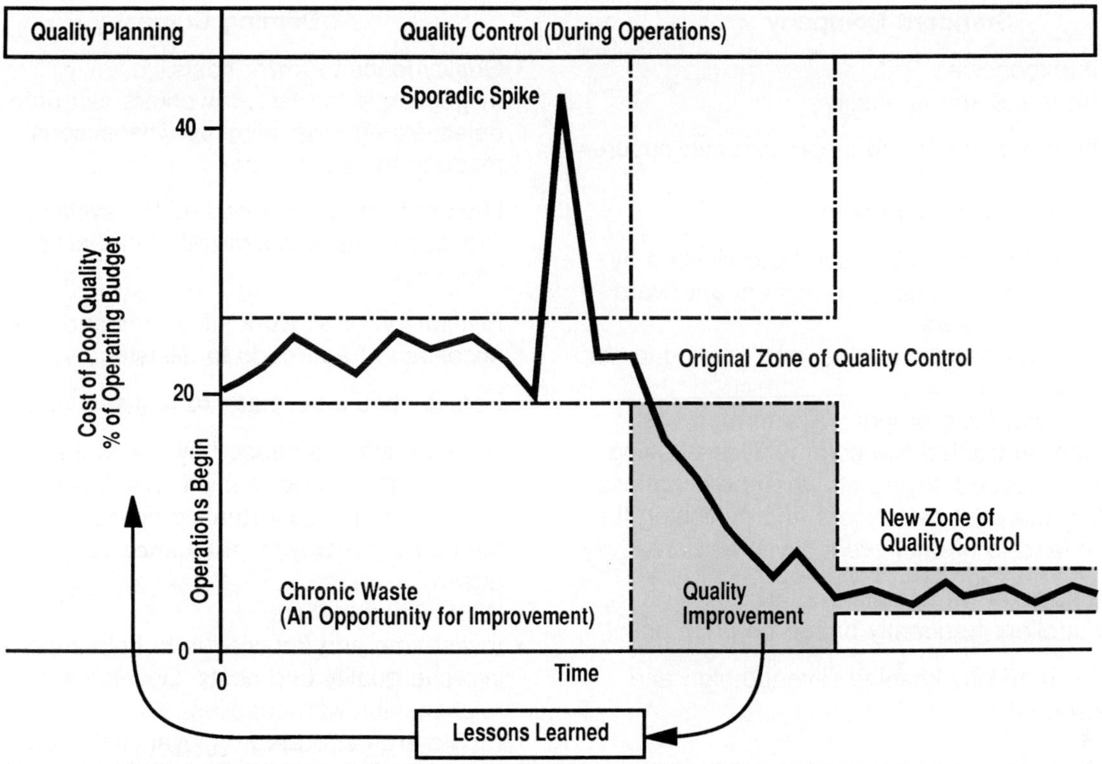

Figure 1.3. The Juran trilogy. (From Juran JM. Juran on planning for quality. New York: The Free Press, 1988:12.)

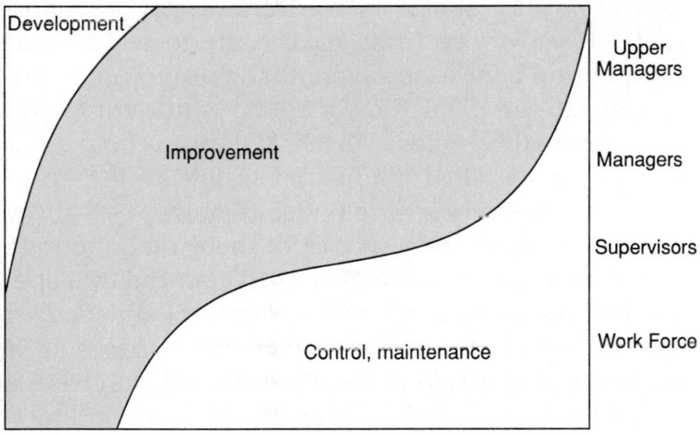

Figure 1.4. The Itoh model. (From Juran JM. Making quality happen: upper management's role. Wilton, CT: The Juran Institute, 1993.)

"Companies," including hospitals and clinical laboratories, that follow Deming's philosophy have some distinct differences from the "standard" company (Fig. 1.5). Advocates of Deming's quality management philosophy believe that it is workers who pay for management errors. They also believe that quality is difficult to define, yet the lack of quality is easy to define. The Deming philosophy ultimately describes quality as "anything that enhances the product from the viewpoint of the customer." In laboratory practice, there are two customers: the physician (the patient's advocate), who orders tests, and the hospital/corporation that uses the services provided by laboratories to make revenue and measure contribution (non-profit) or profit (for-profit).

Development of a Service Economy

Integrated with the evolution of management in this country is the transition from an industrial economy to a more predominant "service economy." The evolution of a service economy in the United States parallels the increasing importance of quality improvement programs (16–18). In addition and most importantly, the service economy is also directly related to the purchasing power of the populace. The health industry has grown because the consumers (patients, with health insurance) have no information on the true costs of health care. John Naisbitt noted that in 1956 for the first time in American history, white-collar workers in technical, managerial, and clerical positions outnumbered blue-collar workers (19). He called such a change the "era of the information society" (Fig. 1.6). The "information society," throughout its evolution and maturation, has required a service economy. The "classic" management pyramid structure (Fig. 1.7), therefore, is now an inverted pyramid (Fig. 1.8).

A service economy meets customer expectations in the course of selling and post-sales activity as well as providing a series of functions that match or better the competition in a way that provides an incremen-

Standard Company

- Quality is expensive.
- Inspection is the key to quality.
- Quality control experts and inspectors can ensure quality.
- Defects are caused by workers.
- The manufacturing process can be optimized by outside experts. No change in system afterward.
- No input from workers.
- Use of work standards, quotas, and goals can help productivity.
- Fear and reward are proper ways to motivate.
- People can be treated like commodities—buying more when needed, laying off when needing less.
- Rewarding the best performers and punishing the worst will lead to greater productivity and creativity.
- Buy one supplier off against another.
- Switch suppliers frequently based on price only.
- Profits are made by keeping revenue high and costs down.

Deming Company

- Quality leads to lower costs.
- Inspection is too late. If workers can produce defect-free goods, eliminate inspections. Quality is made in the boardroom.
- Most defects are caused by the system.
- Process is never optimized; it can always be improved.
- Elimination of all work standards and quotas is necessary. Fear leads to disaster.
- People should be made to feel secure in their jobs.
- Most variation is caused by the system. Review systems that judge, punish, and reward above, or below-average performance destroy teamwork and the company. Buy from vendors committed to quality.
- Work with suppliers.
- Invest time and knowledge to help supplier improve quality and costs. Develop long-term relationships with suppliers.
- Profits are generated by loyal customers.

Figure 1.5. Comparison between Deming management principles and traditional management principles.

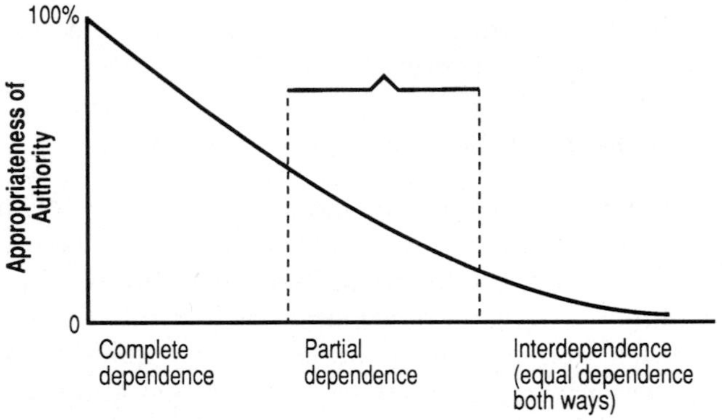

Figure 1.6. Dependence of subordinates in U.S. industry today. (From Naisbitt J. Megatrends: ten new directions transforming our lives. New York: Warner Books, 1982.)

tal profit for the supplier. For most services, four basic characteristics can be identified:

1. Services are more or less intangible.
2. Services are activities or a series of activities rather than things.
3. Services are at least to some extent produced and consumed simultaneously.
4. The customer participates in the production process at least to some extent.

In 1990 Christian Gronroos described the "hidden service sector" and the "official service sector" in our economy (18). Such service sectors have direct relationships with laboratory medicine. Gronroos states that today, service firms have come to realize that competition is now so severe that mere technical solutions offered to customers are not sufficient to create a competitive edge. Further, Gronroos points out that in the so-called "industrial sector" of the economy, manufacturing firms offer customers a variety of services as an integral part of their total offering.

If one analyzes laboratory medicine today, especially in the outpatient environment, the outcome of the analysis is the same; performing a package of tests at a reasonable price is not enough to create a competitive edge. The array of "hidden (indirect) costs" required in the outpatient environment include information services (i.e., computerized order entry, line connects, printers, and CRTs), couriers, specimen containers, laboratory consultation, costs of marketing and advertising, and many other costs to run the business (see Fig. 1.14).

Another way to address the issue is that the clinical laboratory "test" in today's service economy, especially in the ambulatory care setting, is not simply a number or a brief statement; it is a cluster of issues surrounding the laboratory test, such as:

- The seller (the laboratory or its representative);
- The organization represented by the laboratory (private corporation, university, clinic, etc.);
- The service reputation;
- The service personnel;

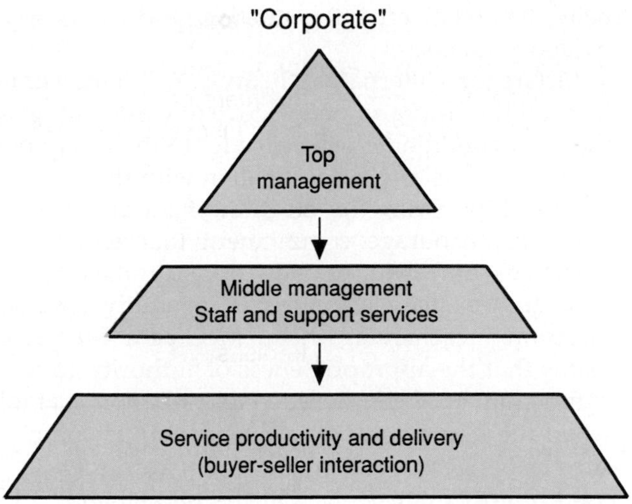

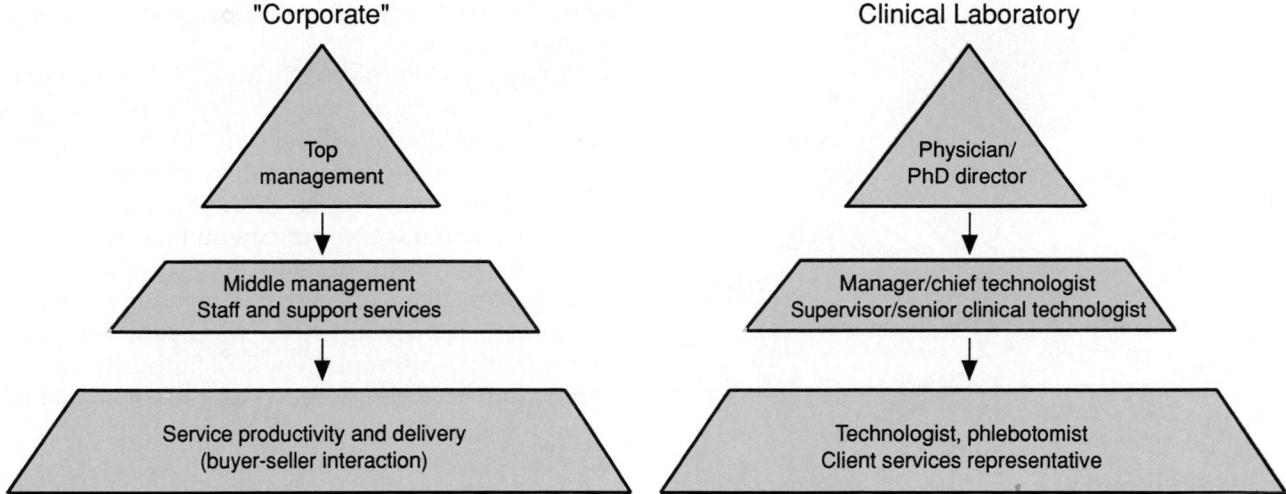

Figure 1.7. Classic management structure.

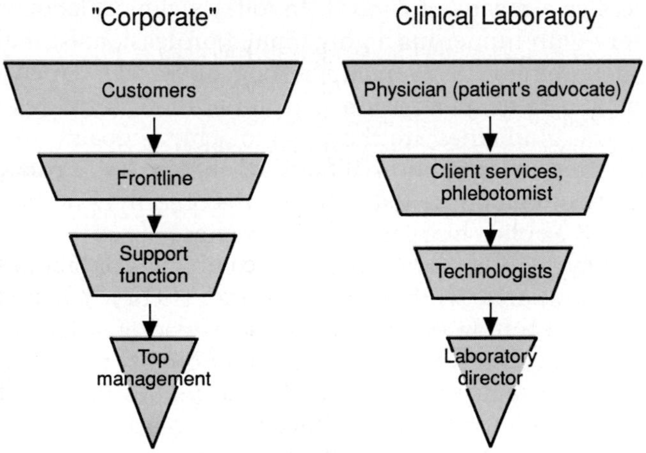

Figure 1.8. Service-oriented management structure.

- The buyer (patient, physician);
- The organization represented by the buyer; and
- The image of both organizations in the marketplace.

It is argued that ultimately the intangibles—the service activities that companies or laboratories offer their customers or patients—may be the most important source of value added in the service economy. It has been noted by Albrecht and Zemke that the marketplace prefers to do business with those who serve, and is declining involvement with those who only supply (17).

It is noteworthy that the interest in service quality increased exponentially in the 1980s. During the same time, interest in quality assurance in laboratory medicine grew very rapidly. In the 1960s and 1970s, there was a steady drift away from the classic quality control mentality to the applications of quality assurance. Quality assurance applications are well defined by the Joint Commission on Accreditation of Healthcare Organizations (JCAHO) (20, 21).

At the core of a successful service economy and, coincidentally, at the core of a successful quality improvement program, are four basic entities:

- *Involvement*: Recognition by management that a situation exists.
- *Measurement*: Necessary, but cannot be used alone as a measurement of success or failure.
- *Reward*: The success of employee-owned companies demonstrates the need for rewards.
- *Follow-through*: Successful service economies or successful quality improvement programs become a way of life.

The overall success of these entities is incumbent on the leadership of management. Service and quality improvement require management's personal, visible involvement.

In discussing service management and marketing, Gronroos has observed that "far too often people in an organization view customers as an abstract phenomenon or a mass that is present somewhere. Customers are seen in terms of numbers. When someone stops being a customer there are always new potential customers to take their place. Customers, individuals and organization alike are numbers only. In reality this is, of course, not true. Every single customer forms a customer relationship with the seller, which the firm has to develop and maintain" (18). This applies to laboratory practice in its managerial sense, i.e., the pathologist must make his or her customers happy with the laboratory's services.

If one were to substitute physician (the patient's advocate) for customer, and hospital (or corporation) for organization, the above discussion could not be

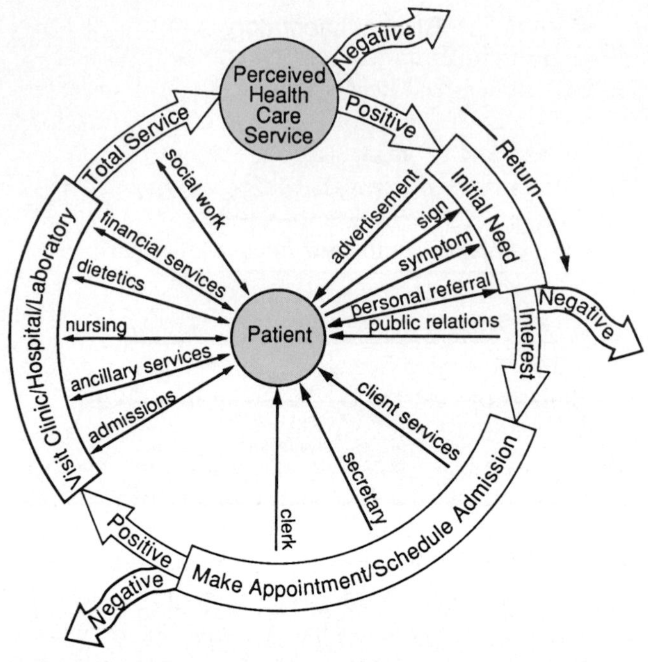

Figure 1.9. Patient-health care provider "life cycle." (Modified from Gronroos C. Service management and marketing. Lexington, MA: DC Heath, 1990:130.)

more timely, as health care and clinical laboratory medicine head for the next century.

Gronroos developed a "customer relationship life cycle" (CRLC) that can be modified or adopted to health care and clinical laboratory medicine. In the CRLC the initial stage is when the customer establishes a need that a firm may be able to satisfy. The customer subsequently makes himself or herself aware of a firm's services. A first purchase follows if all is viewed positively. Subsequent purchases follow if a positive relationship continues. "During this process the customer may observe the firm's ability to take care of his or her problems and provide services which the customer determines to have an acceptable technical and functional quality." Such a service certainly fits the patient's health care provider "life cycle" (Fig. 1.9).

Theory X, Theory Y

In 1960, Douglas McGregor contrasted two types of companies (22). The first, "X," was organized to demonstrate that no one works unless they have to or are made to work. Because of this human characteristic of dislike of work, most people must be coerced, controlled, directed, or threatened with punishment to get them to put forth adequate effort toward the achievement of organizational objectives. Thus, theory X assumes that the average human being prefers to be directed, wishes to avoid responsibility, has relatively little ambition, and wants security above all else.

McGregor's alternative theory, "Y," demonstrates that, on the contrary, people love to work and, given the right conditions, will strive to do their very best. Theory Y leads to a preoccupation with the nature of relationships, with the creation of an environment that will encourage commitment to organizational objectives and will provide opportunities for the maximum exercise of initiative, ingenuity, and self-direction in achieving them. McGregor further explains that the appropriateness of authority varies as a function of dependence (Fig 1.6). For example, when the dependence in a relationship is complete, such as between a parent and child, authority can be used almost exclusively. On the other hand, when dependence is almost equal, such as two staff physicians working on the same patient, authority is useless as a means of control. In today's clinical laboratory with numerous highly trained professionals, the predominant relationship is one of partial dependence; thus, persuasion and application of professional guidelines are the ways to achieve goals.

Toughness is the hallmark of theory X. A company or laboratory that relies on the objectives of theory X applies hire-and-fire techniques.

On the other hand, theory Y companies or laboratories operate with a velvet glove. Theory Y gives people room to exercise initiative instead of strict supervision. With the development of quality management systems such as continuous quality improvement and total quality, theory Y companies and laboratories are in vogue.

Further evidence for promoting quality management programs is provided by the widely accepted Need-Hierarchy theory developed by Abraham Maslow (23). Maslow describes an ascending hierarchy of human needs, which each individual strives to achieve in his or her personal and work environments (Fig. 1.10):

1. Physiologic or survival needs
2. Safety or security needs
3. Social needs
4. Esteem or ego needs
5. Self-actualization or self-fulfillment needs

Modern methods of quality management address these needs.

Continuous Quality Improvement

As quality assurance has matured, there has been a shift to a more consumer-oriented, more positive approach to health care management. Such an approach is called continuous quality improvement

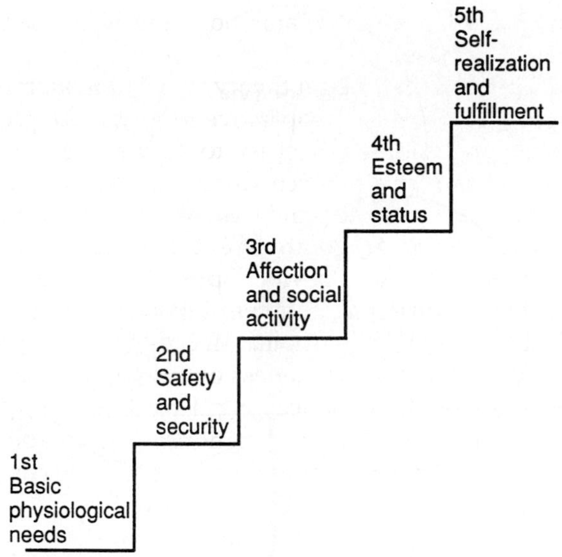

Figure 1.10. Hierarchy of human needs. (From Maslow A. Psychol Rev 1943;50:370–396.)

(CQI). CQI is a consumer-oriented, proactive response to negative public perceptions of the health care business. (Fig. 1.11).

As described by Richard E. Thompson, M.D., there are eleven essential points that differentiate quality assurance from continuous quality improvement (24).

1. The goal of CQI is to *improve* the norm of practice and behavior rather than to strive to comply with a standard based on normative behavior.
2. CQI uses supportive, positive approaches to change behavior rather than more investigative techniques.
3. In CQI, individual and corporate attitudes are as critical and as valid and/or useful as QA data.
4. In CQI, performance indicators rather than quality criteria may be easier to define and implement.
5. CQI, using a cooperative effort, avoids the separatist approach to quality assurance, utilization review, and risk management that is often seen in hospital management settings.
6. CQI, because of the overall approach, is open to applications research.
7. CQI methods appear to be less complex than quality assurance methods simply because many quality assurance methods are developed by committee.
8. CQI changes traditional medical staff functions such as credentialing and peer review to a patient-protective methodology.
9. In contrast to the absolute confidentiality of quality assurance, CQI allows for public comparison of physicians and/or hospitals without providing litigious information to anyone.
10. CQI affects medical staff bylaws and organization structure by allowing physicians to feel comfortable about "taking responsibility for yourself."
11. CQI provides a system that the Joint Commission on Accreditation of Healthcare Organizations (JCAHO) will find *functionally* useful.

JCAHO—The Agenda for Change

In 1975, the Joint Commission on Accreditation of Hospitals (now called the Joint Commission on Accreditation of Healthcare Organizations) published in their *Accreditation Manual for Hospitals* a requirement "to demonstrate that the quality of care was consistently optimal by *continually evaluating care* through reliable and valid measures." Subsequently, in 1980 the Joint Commission adopted the quality assurance standard for hospitals. The 1980 quality assurance standard (*a*) emphasized the value of a coordinated hospital-wide quality assurance program; (*b*) allowed greater flexibility in approaches to problem identification assessment and resolution; and (*c*) emphasized the importance of focusing quality assurance activity on areas where demonstrable problem resolution is possible (20, 21, 25).

In addition, the Joint Commission launched the Agenda for Change in 1986 to focus health care organizations and the general public on the quality of patient care. The goals of the Agenda for Change are:

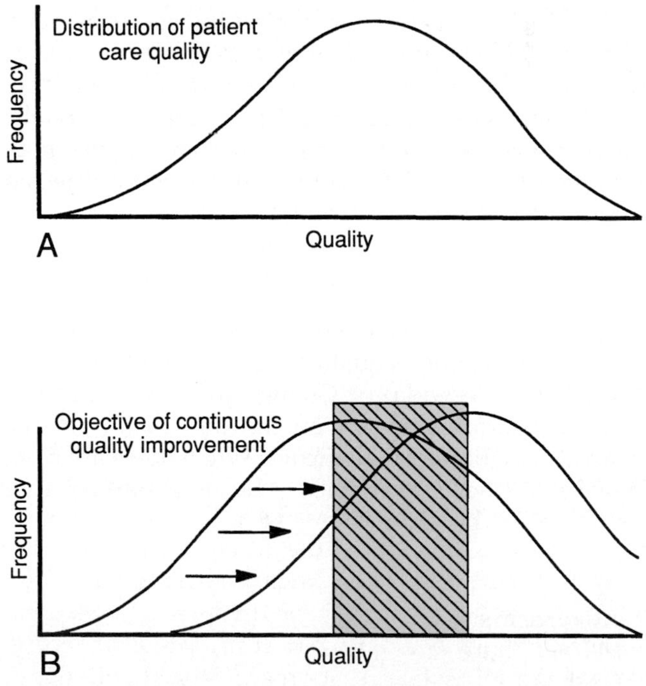

Figure 1.11. Shifting the mean: QA to QI. **A**, Quality assurance. **B**, Continuous quality improvement.

1. Use valid and reliable clinical indicators as screening devices to identify potential problems in the organization, provision, or monitoring of care;
2. Apply more relevant organizational standards and related indicator measures in evaluating the effectiveness of organizations' governance and management; and
3. Render accreditation decisions that reflect more accurately the adequacy of an organization's attention to providing high-quality care.

The quality assurance activities of the Agenda for Change must follow a monitoring and evaluation process. The monitoring and evaluation process has 10 basic steps:

1. Assign responsibility;
2. Delineate the scope of care (inventory clinical activities);
3. Identify important aspects of care (e.g., high risk, high volume, and/or problem prone);
4. Identify indicators (e.g., variables related to outcome of care);
5. Establish thresholds for evaluation;
6. Collect and organize data;
7. Evaluate care;
8. Take action to solve problems;
9. Assess the actions and document improvement; and
10. Communicate relevant information to the organization-wide quality assurance program.

The 10-step process for monitoring and evaluation can also be used for such hospital-wide programs as infection control, utilization review, risk management, and safety management. In many hospitals, such programs are under the governance of the quality assurance administrative team, usually directed by a physician.

Conclusion and Summary

The quality management issues of quality assurance and continuous quality improvement, including the JCAHO Agenda for Change have had, and will have a profound impact on the bottom line of the practice of laboratory medicine. When these are combined with the key variables of business performance as described by Gavin (9):

- Price
- Advertising
- Market share
- Cost
- Productivity
- Profitability

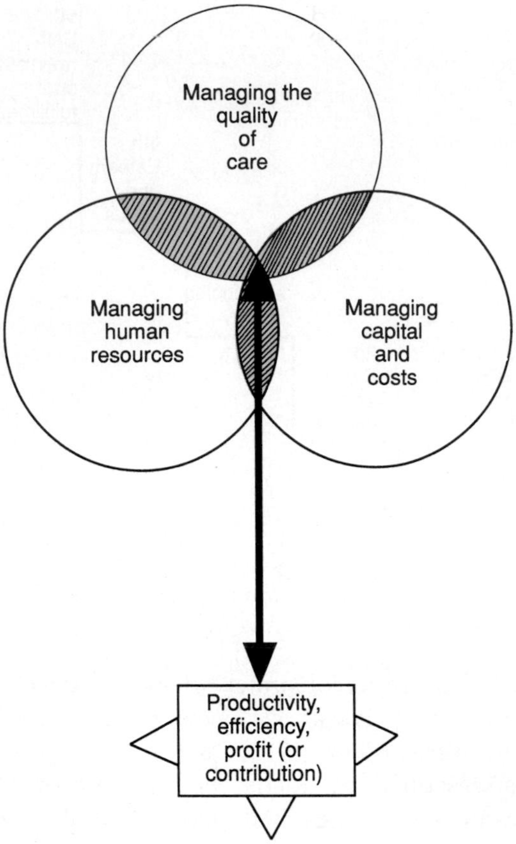

Figure 1.12. Key elements for success in laboratory management.

the laboratory of the future will be assured of success, both in quality of care and in management. However, unless quality management is practiced assiduously, such entities as quality assurance, continuous quality improvement, and even the Agenda for Change certainly will lose their impact.

An understanding of the principles of managing laboratory costs is vital to the business success of the laboratory. The section that follows provides the tools needed to successfully manage a cost-effective laboratory. A balance between the principles described in the preceding section and those contained in the next section is the secret to management of a productive, efficient, cost-effective, and profitable (or contributory) laboratory. (Fig. 1.12)

MANAGING LABORATORY COSTS

Strategies, Problems, and Principal Areas of Laboratory Expenditure

STRATEGIES

Establishing strategies for cost-effective laboratory management begins with an assessment of the laboratory's *external* and *internal* fiscal environ-

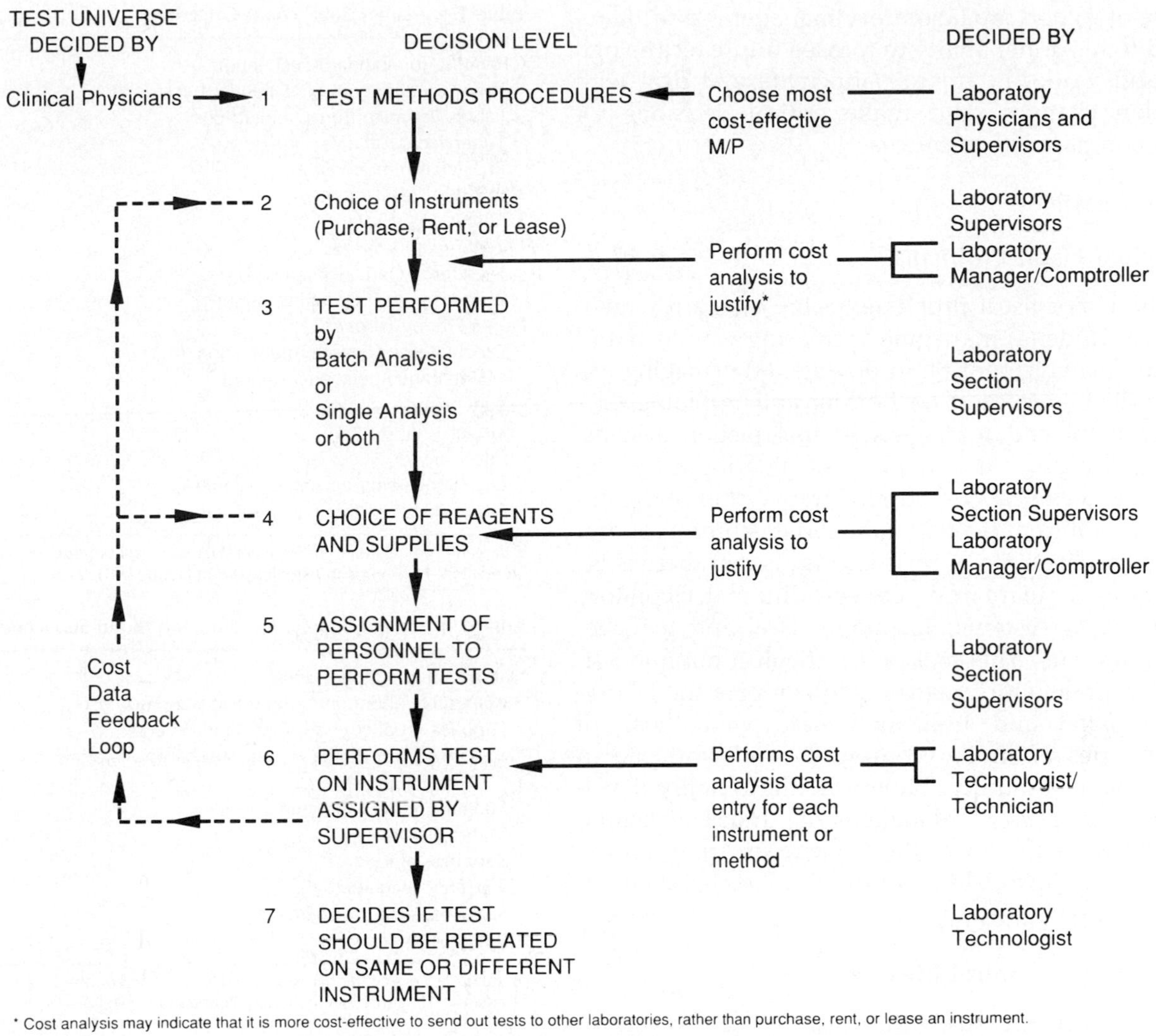

Figure 1.13. Laboratory financial decision flowchart. (From Travers EM. Managing costs in clinical laboratories. New York: McGraw-Hill Information Systems, 1989:5.)

ments. In the *external* environment the laboratory director must understand the laboratory's strategic plan, its market share and product line, its financial goals, its role in the local medical community, its administrative responsibility to its source of operating capital (i.e., a hospital, corporation, multihospital group, HMO, or federal, state, or municipal government), its capital asset structure (where applicable), and the limitations on current operating capital. In the *internal* environment the laboratory director must assess the age and condition of equipment, staffing adequacy and balance, salary structure, and types of reimbursement received and their sources, and must analyze the volume and complexity of the laboratory's input (workload). If the laboratory is engaged in teaching resident physicians or laboratory professionals or is performing research and development, the impact of these resource-consuming programs must also be assessed.

The Fiscal Management Team

Accomplishing this comprehensive fiscal assessment is impossible without the cooperation and interaction of a management team in the laboratory that works closely with hospital, corporate, or institutional management. Although the overall responsibility for cost-effective management rests with the laboratory director, the task ultimately requires an integrated effort between top management, middle management/supervisory personnel, and laboratory technical staff (Fig. 1.13).

The Pathologist's Role in Laboratory Fiscal Management

The pathologist's role is critical to success in fiscal management, and rests on good planning, excellent control, and recognition of the major differences in managing anatomic and clinical pathology. The value of a good top laboratory manager is directly related to his or her ability to foresee future technological and workload trends, anticipate and deal with sudden changes, and make critical decisions for managing limited resources.

PROBLEMS

Principal Fiscal Problems

The major fiscal problems facing laboratory managers include (*a*) managing increasing workload and quality management requirements, (*b*) managing uncontrolled costs, and (*c*) finding and installing adequate fiscal and management information systems that will capture the majority of data input and relieve the technical and administrative staff of the onerous, inefficient task of manual data entry. A subset of this problem (as of this writing) is that there is little or no compatibility between different laboratory information systems, let alone fiscal and management systems. This makes it difficult if not impossible for a laboratory manager to compare the laboratory's fiscal and utilization data with those of laboratories of similar complexity and workload in the same community. However, the recently developed Laboratory Management Index Program (LMIP) (available from the College of American Pathologists, Northfield, IL) provides a comprehensive peer grouping system.

Lack of Cost Control Measures

Additional measures that can be used to control costs include (*a*) controlling automation, primarily by avoiding additional or excessive labor costs associated with the acquisition and operation of unnecessary and excessive automated equipment; (*b*) avoiding the additional costs for reagents and supplies associated with excessive automation (and workload/QC demands); (*c*) providing more efficiency in chemistry (50 to 70% of total laboratory workload); and finally (*d*) controlling the *total* laboratory budget more closely (especially labor costs) by consolidating groups of tests and convincing clinicians to reduce unnecessary routine, daily testing practices.

PRINCIPAL AREAS OF LABORATORY EXPENDITURE

Direct Costs

Labor Costs. Of all costs in laboratories, the most difficult to control are labor costs. Labor costs account for the majority of expenditures, regardless of the complexity and size of the laboratory (50 to 70%, depending on seniority, benefits, and number and size of the staff). A categorization of labor costs appears in Table 1.1.

Table 1.1. Labor Subaccount Categories[a]

Operating (or standard cost) labor
Labor, quality control at standard cost
Labor, variance from standard cost
Supervisors' salaries
Physician remuneration
Doctoral level salaries
Technologist salaries
Technician salaries
Secretarial/clerical salaries
Aide and other operating salaries
Nonoperating labor
Executive personnel remuneration
Maintenance personnel salaries
Supervisors' salaries
Driver salaries
Pilot salaries
Data processing personnel salaries
Other nonoperating personnel salaries

[a]Adapted from Gaither JF, Resinger HE. Cost accounting in the laboratory. Mundelein, IL: American Pathology Foundation, 1981:V–20.

Table 1.2. Major Supply, Reagent, and Blood Subaccounts[a]

Materials and supplies, total
Materials, laboratory, total (or at standard cost)
Supplies, quality control, at standard cost
Variance from standard cost, laboratory materials, and quality control supplies
Supplies, other laboratory
Materials, other
Supplies, office
Supplies, teaching
Supplies, data processing
Supplies, other

[a]Adapted from Gaither JF, Resinger HE. Cost accounting in the laboratory. Mundelein, IL: American Pathology Foundation, 1981:V–20.

Reagent Costs. The second major category of laboratory expenditure is for reagents and supplies (consumables). These usually account for 10 to 15% of total laboratory expenditures, depending on how carefully discounts are obtained and how efficiently reagents are used. In fact, the inefficient and excessive use of quality control and standards, especially in chemistry, can accumulate to 30 to 35% of chemistry costs if not carefully monitored (Table 1.2).

Costs for Blood and Components. Costs for blood and components are far more difficult to control, based on the cyclical and unpredictable nature of patients' illnesses and the need for emergency or operative treatment. One of the most difficult areas of cost to control is the blood bank's transfusion service, since the clinical factors noted above will have a profound influence on the type and volume of blood and components utilized. Furthermore, laboratories that do not collect and process their own blood are dependent on outside sources and have limited ability to control their costs and/or optimally set their annual charges for blood and components.

A major factor that has escalated the cost of collecting and processing blood is the cost of testing for transmissible diseases. Human immunodeficiency virus, the hepatitides, and new viruses to be detected in the future make the transfusion service a costly operation. Again, one must not forget that the cost of the testing reagents may not be the major source of cost. The major cost is dependent on the skill level and the amount of labor required to perform the tests.

Fee Basis Testing Costs. Fee basis tests are send-out tests that cannot be performed in-house due to lack of equipment, technical expertise, or personnel or for other reasons. This category of expenditure may be a major source of additional expense for laboratories that do not have a large, highly trained staff with special testing expertise and/or state-of-the-art equipment. Also, fee basis testing may be necessary if the type and complexity of tests ordered is of a tertiary nature, i.e., those ordered in teaching or tertiary care settings.

Large increases in fee basis testing expense can be avoided by controlling the test-ordering process at the clinical level and by choosing the lowest cost for the desired tests through competitive bidding and comparison of prices. It is also important for laboratory management to advise clinicians of test costs and turnaround time using published lists of tests with this information.

Capital Equipment Acquisition Costs. There are several ways to acquire equipment, each of which has its advantages and disadvantages. The principal methods are purchase, lease, rental, and special rental contracts (e.g., cost per test, reagent rental, and other customized contracts). Without consideration of the cash flow requirements of each method, appropriate planning is necessary to ensure that the laboratory's budget can accommodate the acquisition, since additional equipment may escalate operational costs.

The criteria for choosing among the different alternatives are the minimization of the cost of acquiring the equipment and the yearly net cash outflow associated with each alternative. These subjects are usually best handled by an accountant who understands laboratory operations and who will perform the required analyses to compare purchase with a time-sale contract, financial lease arrangement, rental, or other contractual method.

However, the difficulties with availability of money for investment in capital equipment make it imperative that hospital laboratory managers present a complete and convincing presentation to hospital or corporate management when requesting *purchase* of new or replacement equipment. The process itself is segmented into five distinct categories:

1. Development of depreciable costs;
2. Estimation of appropriate depreciation life and timing;
3. Isolation of related cash flow variables;
4. Forecast of production volume and revenue; and
5. Measurement and comparison with hospital criteria.

The laboratory manager should realize that other equally important factors must be considered in the capital acquisition process, viz., turnaround time, rapid response, precision, accuracy, reproducibility, and availability of service.

A combination of the two processes discussed above should result in a smooth final acquisition determination. A detailed description of the elements of this process is beyond the scope of this chapter, but can be reviewed in an article by Oszustowicz (26) and a textbook by Travers (27), which provides a format for a marketing opportunity package for capital equipment (see Methods for Acquiring Equipment, below).

Indirect Costs

Indirect costs are all costs of test production that cannot be directly traced to test production. A list of typical items used in estimating indirect costs for tests is included in Figure 1.14. A detailed explanation of indirect costs using formulas and examples can be found in "Cost Accounting in the Clinical Laboratory," published by the National Committee for Clinical Laboratory Standards (28).

Indirect costs are assigned to total cost based on a multitude of factors that are part of hospital or corporate operations. They are added to the cost of tests as a percentage rather than as actual amounts for each item.

Total indirect costs to operate an organization or department must be recovered through the pricing of products or services. The total cost of performing a test or procedure is the sum of the direct cost plus a proportionate share of indirect costs.

The indirect cost percentage will vary in each laboratory based on the total number of factors that are used to calculate indirect costs. These are considered as principal expenditures in this section, since in some private sector settings, indirect costs may be as high as 148% of total cost (27).

The Laboratory Fiscal System

Every organization—regardless of its size or complexity, profit or nonprofit status—must maintain a system for financial data collection and coding for recording in journals and ledgers. The prerequisite for accomplishing these tasks is a properly established account structure. This fiscal system is known as the chart of accounts.

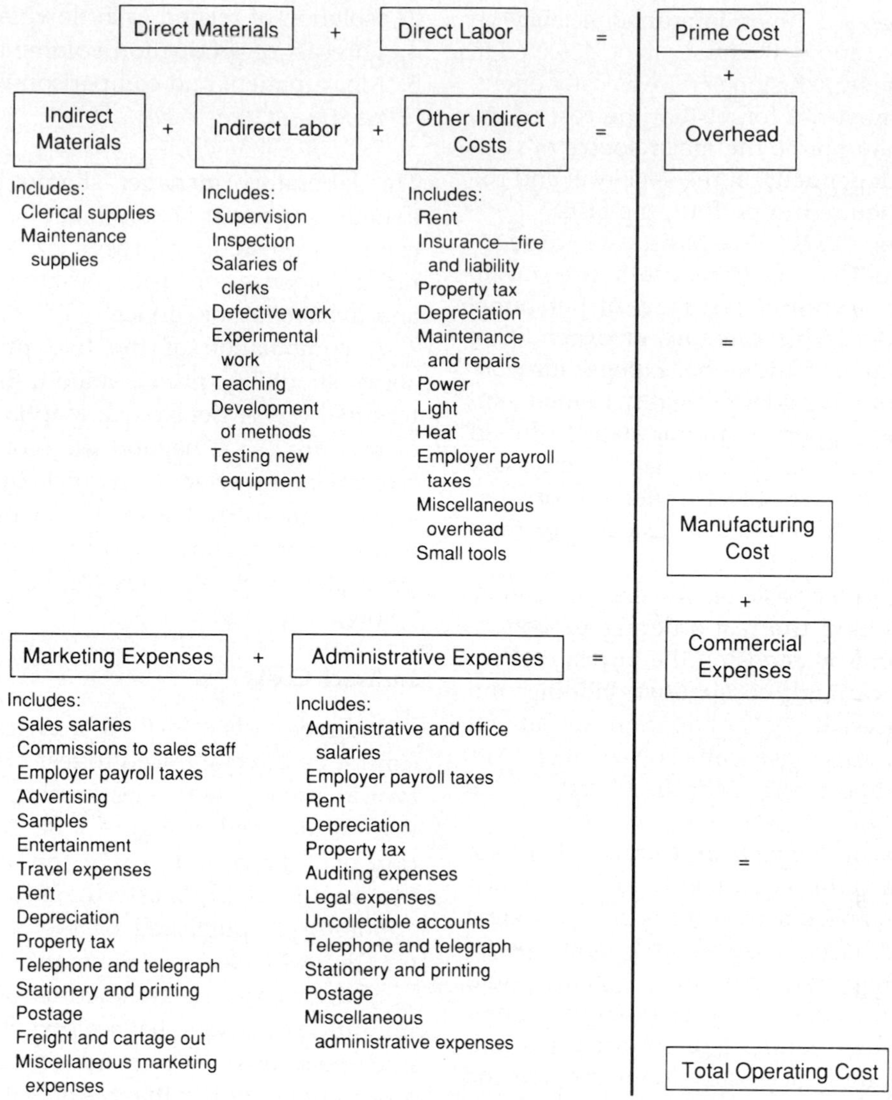

Figure 1.14. Analysis of total operating cost. (Adapted from Matz A, Usry MF. Cost accounting: planning and control, 7th ed. Cincinnati, OH: Southwestern Publishing Co., 1980:45.)

THE CHART OF ACCOUNTS

The organization's chart of accounts is the fundamental means for budgetary and control accounting. It provides control accounts for the recognized elements of cost, and it segregates and details all expenses not included in prime cost (the total cost of direct materials and labor in test production). The chart of accounts is the foundation of the financial management system for the laboratory. It includes information on the historic financial data base and current financial information about the laboratory, and is a future financial planning aid. It also allows consistency of financial data collection for planning and control. The comprehensive chart of accounts (Fig. 1.15) provides management data breakdown in categories needed by management, namely, assets, liabilities/equity, revenues, and costs (expenses).

The chart of accounts has two major sections: (*a*) the *balance sheet* and (*b*) the *operating statement (income statement)*. The balance sheet is divided into three major sections: *assets, liabilities,* and *equity*. The operating statement is divided into *revenues* and *expenses*. Since laboratories vary in their activities and complexity, the chart of accounts will also vary, according to the information the managers believe they need to accomplish the task of sound fiscal management. Not even a large, independent laboratory will use more than a small fraction of the available accounts, but the accounts they need are available, since the fine structure of the chart of accounts meets virtually every conceivable need for detail (27).

THE BALANCE SHEET

The purpose of the balance sheet is to report the financial position of the laboratory at a particular

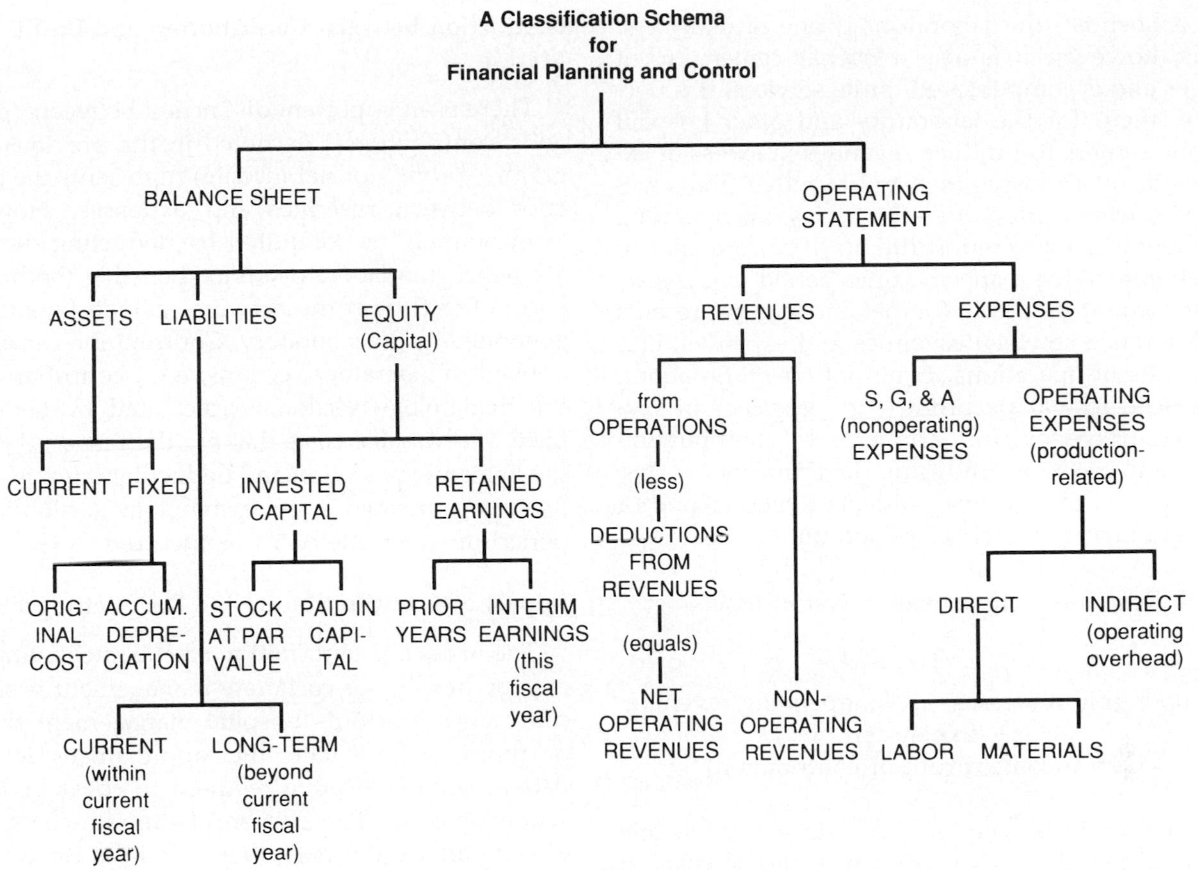

Figure 1.15. The chart of accounts for laboratories. (From Travers EM. Managing costs in clinical laboratories. New York: McGraw-Hill Information Systems, 1989:36.)

time. Financial position refers to the amount of resources (i.e., assets) and liabilities of the laboratory on a specific date. The balance sheet provides the laboratory manager with a recorded, systematic statement of each transaction involving assets, liabilities, or equity. The accounting process provides the raw data for each subaccount, whether it be handwritten, mechanized, or computerized. Each transaction is recorded in one of the major sections of the balance sheet and is ultimately used to construct the laboratory's financial statements.

The basic formula for the fundamental accounting model is:

$$\text{Assets} = \text{Liabilities} + \text{Equity}$$

This formula leads to an understanding of the basic and broad perspective of accounting as it relates to overall fiscal management. *The basic objective of cost-effective laboratory management is to balance this equation.* In situations where improved profit is desired, the need to minimize and reduce liabilities is even greater, while maximizing assets and equity. In not-for-profit situations, where assets or profit are not desired, minimizing liabilities becomes even more important to preserve operating capital (27, 29). Major categories of liabilities are listed in Figure 1.15.

THE OPERATING (INCOME) STATEMENT

The section of the chart of accounts includes a format for determining the laboratory's revenues, expenses, and profit (or losses).[a] Revenues are obtained from operations or from non-operating sources. Operating revenues are characterized by type of payment agreement and type of guarantor. Non-operating revenues are obtained from categories such as technical school operations, grants, investments, rent, and miscellaneous revenue-generating activities other than laboratory operations.

[a] Profit is defined as relative efficiencies of scale for government-operated laboratories and other not-for-profit laboratories; relative efficiencies of scale include cost avoidance and cost savings produced as a result of efficient management of personnel (most costly aspect of operational costs) and operational resources; these "saved" resources are usually recorded by the not-for-profit hospital's finance department and are redistributed by hospital management during the current fiscal year in which they were "saved."

In a hospital, the laboratory is one of many *cost centers;* however, it is also a *revenue* center; i.e., it charges and is compensated for its services. It is necessary, then, for the laboratory and other hospital revenue centers to produce revenues in excess of expenses to offset losses incurred by other non–revenue producing centers. In laboratories, the operating statement is used to report the profit performance of the laboratory for a specific time period (e.g., year, quarter, month). Profit (or net income) represents the difference between revenues and expenses, i.e., the results of operations. Even not-for-profit laboratories need to make a profit (e.g., efficiency or savings) to survive, expand, and make a "contribution" to the non–revenue producing departments.

Therefore, the income statement reflects one of the fundamental principles of accounting, i.e.,

$$\text{Revenue} - \text{Expenses} = \text{Net income}$$

or

$$(\text{Net operating revenues} + \text{Nonoperating revenues} - \text{Expenses}) = \text{Net income (Profit or contribution)}$$

Revenues include sales of laboratory tests, while expenses include the general categories of costs of test performance, marketing and selling expenses, general and administrative expenses, financial expenses, and income tax expenses.[b] More detailed information and a listing of income statement categories can be found in the books of Gaither (29) and Travers (27).

DETERMINING PROFIT OR LOSS

One of the techniques used to establish profit or loss is known as cost-volume-profit (CVP) analysis, also known as marginal analysis in general industry. It is used to provide relevant information for selecting product lines, pricing individual products, and developing market strategies. It is a valuable method for analyzing profitability in many firms. CVP analysis permits the study of the relationships between prices, variable costs, fixed costs, and workload volume to aid in management decision making. In laboratory use, the key relationship is the difference between test price and variable costs per test, otherwise known as the *contribution margin*.

[b] Publicly funded laboratories will not use these categories unless they generate "revenue" for the hospital by performing tests for other laboratories using "sharing" agreements that specify that a fee will be collected for a service shared between hospitals. Ordinarily, the revenue collected will only cover costs incurred for tests performed for the duration of the sharing agreement.

Distinction between Contribution and Profit Margin

There is an important distinction between "profit" and "contribution." As noted in the previous paragraph, "profit" (or net income) represents the difference between revenues and expenses. However, "contribution" is computed by deducting the costs for which the laboratory is responsible (both direct and indirect) from the revenues gained for the tests generated by the laboratory. Contribution can also be applied to laboratory sections; e.g., contribution for the hematology section is calculated by taking all fixed and variable costs that are the responsibility of the hematology section and deducting them from the revenue generated in the hematology section for the period in which the cost was incurred.

Impact of Contribution on the Rate-Setting Process

The impact of contribution on the rate-setting process by hospital or corporate management is significant, since it affords hospital management the opportunity to calculate the approximate level of patient service revenue required to cover budgeted economic costs. The portion of the rate charge that directly affects the operating margin is the *contribution factor*.

There are both internal and external reasons for placing minimum and maximum limitations on departmental rate increases and decreases. Among these factors are competition, governing board policy, limitations imposed by rate-setting authorities, and contractual arrangements. Each of these factors is reviewed as applicable, and upper and lower limits are established within which rates may be charged. For example, suppose the hospital has determined that the room rate is well below that of neighboring hospitals and a room rate increase of 5% to 25% would be acceptable. However, emergency room charges are slightly higher than acceptable. A survey has shown that laboratory rates could be increased by as much as 20% but the hospital's governing board has indicated that a 10% reduction would be desirable. Finally, the radiologist's contract provides that there be no reduction in departmental rates while the contract is in effect. Based on this information, the hospital establishes the following rate change limitations:

	Lower Limit	Upper Limit
Routine Care	+5%	+25%
Emergency Room	−5%	0%
Laboratory	−10%	+20%
Radiology	0%	+10%

By applying rate increases to the departments with the highest contribution factors and rate decreases to those with the lowest contribution factors until the target profit contribution factor is reached, the aggregate rate change will be minimized (30).

Management Responsibilities and Contribution Margin

During times of unrestrained resource availability, profit-maximizing decision-makers will elect to produce all the products they can as long as their marginal revenue (MR) (the price or charge) exceeds marginal cost. However, in times of limited resource availability, profit-maximizing decision-makers should (and will only) select those tests for market expansion that will have the greatest effect on producing a high contribution margin.

BUDGETING

Principles

A budget is generally defined as a comprehensive plan or guide for some future period of time, usually, by convention, a year, a quarter, or a month. Budget plans can be expressed in a variety of ways; in manhours, dollars, outputs, etc. A budget, however, is primarily a financial plan and is therefore expressed in dollars. Thus, the term budget might be defined more explicitly as a comprehensive financial plan, based on anticipated outputs and predetermined hospital goals and policies for future operations, that is expressed in dollars of expense and corresponding dollars of revenue.

For purposes of understanding and discussion, the budget translation process can be viewed as consisting of two primary steps: (*a*) converting the hospital's or corporation's strategy into an operating plan for the laboratory, and (*b*) expressing the operating plan as a budget for the laboratory. The first step involves defining the specific workloads, projects, and other operating activities that must be undertaken to transform the corporate strategy into reality. The second step focuses on expressing the operating plan in financial terms, for example, dollars of expense, revenues, capital purchases, etc. Therefore, there are four basic types of budgets: statistical (workload, etc.), expense, revenue, and capital budgets.

Before constructing the budget, an additional element is necessary: a budget preparation procedure. This includes the technical, mechanical aspect, as well as the management of the entire process. The technical part focuses on (31)

- Projecting workload (volume);
- Converting volume estimates into resource requirements and revenue estimates;
- Converting resource requirements into direct cost estimates;
- Calculating indirect costs; and
- Adjusting revenues and total costs to obtain the necessary equality.

Sectional Budget Analysis

Once the basic concepts of budgeting are understood, the actual construction of budgets for laboratory-specific elements can begin. A general sectional analysis format (Fig. 1.16) is adaptable for all laboratory sections and includes entries for all major areas of laboratory instrumentation and manual methods. Costs are established first, using a microcost analysis method (see Appendix A), then these data are entered into the appropriate section for instrument-based or manual methods. The cost is then multiplied by the raw test count for each category for the period in which the budget is constructed. The final product for each instrument or method is added to produce the total direct cost for test production. Added to this figure are other major sectional costs, viz., professional salaries and fees, blood and component costs, transportation, fee-basis (send-out) costs, costs for operations, administration, travel, etc., depending on the laboratory's organizational structure and fiscal control points.

Departmental Budget Analysis and Allocating Costs Across Sections

An important concept is the allocation of costs to a budget format that includes the costs for the time of general employees who are not specifically assigned to a laboratory section but whose work helps to produce or interpret tests (e.g., secretaries, couriers, computer personnel, maintenance personnel). Some laboratories use formulas for allocation; however, there is no uniform set of formulas that will apply to every laboratory. A good manager should be able to create accurate formulas for each production area and the department. The only requirement is that the formulas must realistically reflect the section's or department's use of that function. Examples of allocation within a laboratory section budget are given in Figure 1.17 and within a departmental budget in Figure 1.18. Figure 1.19 further illustrates budgeted expenses for a total laboratory, by breaking major cost categories into their cost accounting subcomponents.

	Instrument Name	Cost/Test†	Test/Year	Cost/Instrument
Chemistry				
Instrument	1________	$________	________	$________
	2________	________	________	________
	3________	________	________	________
	4________	________	________	________
	5________	________	________	________
Manual Tests	1________	________	________	________
	2________	________	________	________
	3________	________	________	________
		TOTALS:	1. Instrument Costs	________
			2. Cost Professional Salaries/ Administrative Salaries	________
			3. Cost Blood/Components	N.A.
			4. Cost Transportation/Travel	________
			5. Cost Fee Basis	________
			6. Cost Operations/Administration	________
		TOTAL COST	Operations/Laboratory/Year for Chemistry	$________

*This format can be utilized for all laboratory sections. Chemistry is used here as an example. For instance, if used for the blood bank section, item 3 in TOTALS would be applicable.

† Cost/Test Includes:
- Direct Costs
  - Labor (Technical/Clerical/Phlebotomy)
  - Reagents and Supplies
- Indirect Costs
  - Amortization
  - Depreciation
  - Maintenance
  - Site Preparation
  - All Other Costs

Figure 1.16. Worksheet for sectional analysis of chemistry costs based on equipment configuration manual procedures. (From Travers EM. Managing costs in clinical laboratories. New York: McGraw-Hill Information Systems, 1989:130.)

		A (Demand)	B (Astra)	C (ACA)	G (ABL Blood Gas)	H (Centrifichem)	
Example 1:	General Function That Varies per Instrument						Total Chemistry Tes
	Total Billable* Procedures	39,232	65,068	23,922	5,052	6,890	140,164
	Percent of Total Chemistry Tests	27.9	46.4	17.1	3.6	4.9	
		x	x	x	x	x	
	Phlebotomy Salaries† for Chemistry	$100,128	$100,128	$100,128	$100,128	$100,128	
		=	=	=	=	=	
	Cost of Phlebotomy per Instrument	$ 27,936	$ 46,459	$ 17,122	$ 3,605	$ 4,906	
Example 2:	General Function That Applies Equally to All Instruments/Sections						Total Professional Salaries for Chemistr
	Pathologist's Salaries (Professional Fees)‡	12,500	12,500	12,500	12,500	12,500	62,500

*Test result actually billed to patient. Example: a chemistry profile with 18 determinations counts as one billable procedure, not 18 tests.

†Determined by the following ratio:

1. $\frac{\text{Total Billable Procedures/Chem}}{\text{Total Billable Procedures/Lab}} = \frac{175{,}999}{394{,}000} = .447 = 44.7\%$

2. 44.7% × Total Phlebotomy Salaries/Lab = .447 × $224,000 = $100,128

‡Pathologist's time in this lab is allocated as follows:

50% Histology/Surgical Pathology	10% Hematology
10% Chemistry	10% Immunology
10% Microbiology	10% Blood Bank

¶For Chemistry:
a. 10% × Total Prof. Fees/Lab = 10% × $625,000 = $62,500/Chem
b. 62,500/5 (instruments) = $12,500 Prof. Fees/Instrument

Figure 1.17. Allocating costs for general functions among chemistry workstations. (Adapted from Sharp JW. A cost accounting system targeted to DRGs. Medical Laboratory Observer 1985; September: 2–8.)

	Chemistry	Serology	Histology	Microbiology	Total Laboratory
Billable procedures	176,000	17,000	21,000	42,000	415,000
Technical FTEs	21	3	8	9	64
Revenue	$ 2,640,000	$ 230,000	$ 1,050,000	$ 756,000	$ 6,716,000
Expenses					
Salaries (technical)	$ 595,000	$ 75,000	$ 200,000	$ 225,000	$ 1,600,000
Supplies	600,000	75,000	40,000	155,000	1,035,000
Allocated expenses					
Phlebotomy[1]	$ 100,061	$ 9,655	$ 0	$ 23,870	$ 223,992
Path. secretaries[2]	7,500	1,875	60,000	1,075	74,200
Professional fees[2]	62,500	62,500	312,500	62,500	625,000
Lab receptionists[1]	67,005	6,472	0	15,990	150,000
Reference lab fees[3]	227,500	32,500	16,250	16,250	325,000
Cost of blood[3]	0	0	0	0	310,000
Equip. maintenance[3]	65,000	2,500	5,000	15,000	128,500
Depreciation[4]	75,063	3,146	11,438	21,161	169,995
Travel[5]	3,333	3,333	3,333	3,333	19,998
Other[3]	19,167	19,167	19,167	19,167	115,002
Direct expense	$ 1,752,129	$ 291,158	$ 667,688	$ 558,346	$ 4,776,687
Indirect expense[6]	$ 506,530	$ 48,926	$ 60,438	$ 120,877	$ 1,194,375
Total expense	$ 2,258,659	$ 340,084	$ 728,126	$ 679,223	$ 5,971,062
Net income(loss)	$ 381,341	($ 110,084)	$ 321,874	$ 76,777	$ 744,938

[1]Allocation based on section's percentage of all nonhistology billable procedures (394,000).
[2]Based on estimated work done for each section.
[3]Based on utilization by each section.
[4]Depreciation over seven years; zero salvage value.
[5]Total expense shared equally by all six sections.
[6]Based on section's percentage of 415,000 procedures.

Figure 1.18. Example of a department laboratory budget. (Adapted from Sharp JW. A cost accounting system targeted to DRGs. Medical Laboratory Observer 1985; September:2–8.)

Cost Behavior

Traceability	Variable	Fixed	Semifixed	Total
Direct	Salaries (part-time) $4,000 Supplies 5,000 $9,000	Salaries (full-time) $1,000	Salaries (other) $10,000	$20,000
Indrect	Employee Benefits $150 Housekeeping 100 $250	Depreciation $160 Administration 500 Housekeeping 100 $760	Maintenance $250 Laundry 100 $350	$1,360
Total	$9,250	$1,760	10,350	$21,360

Figure 1.19. Laboratory cost example. (Modified from Cleverly WO. Handbook of health care accounting and finance. Rockville, MD: Aspen Publishers, 1982;1:146.)

Cost Accounting

DEFINITIONS

Accounting focuses on measuring and reporting the input and output of resources in an organization, and the resources controlled by the organization. It provides an information base that allows decision makers to assess the potential financial implications and potentials of various alternatives being considered. Horngren points out that "the essential strength of the managerial cost accounting process is that it links 'promises' made during the budget process back to the responsibility center" (32).

The subject of accounting can be divided into two distinct major specialties: *financial accounting*, or external financial reporting to shareholders, creditors, the IRS, and regulatory and other external bodies; and *managerial accounting*, which deals with internal reporting. Within managerial accounting (also known as responsibility accounting), the subject of *cost accounting* defines, measures, reports, and analyzes the elements of costs associated with providing a unit of output—in the specific case of laboratories, a test.

Cost Accounting

In the past, cost accounting referred to the ways of accumulating and assigning historical costs to units of products and departments, primarily for purposes of inventory valuation and income determination. Cost accounting is now indistinguishable from management accounting because it serves multiple purposes. Fundamentally, cost accounting now refers to the gathering and providing of information for decision needs (which range from the management of recurring operations to the making of nonrecurring strategic management decisions) and for the formulation of major organizational policies.

Cost Categories Used to Determine Operational Expenses

Figure 1.19 lists the categories of costs that encompass both the *traceability* of costs (*direct* or *indirect*) and the *behavior* of costs (*fixed* or *variable*). Figure 1.19 also illustrates how laboratory costs fall into both traceable and behavior categories, and breaks down total costs for each major laboratory expense into direct or indirect, fixed or variable costs. *Direct costs* are test-specific costs that can be directly traced to the production of tests. These include all costs for labor and supplies needed to produce a test. *Indirect costs* (common or joint costs) cannot be traced to a particular test; however, they contribute to the provision of an adequate work environment. Examples are section-specific and general supervisory salaries, general quality control, miscellaneous supplies, education, travel, and global costs such as administrative costs, computers, maintenance, and security (Fig. 1.14). Ultimately all indirect costs must be allocated to each laboratory section and to each test. *Variable costs* are costs related to changes in the volume of tests produced. Examples are reagents, supplies, and labor that can be controlled by the laboratory by obtaining the best discounts, purchasing only when necessary, and using the instrument and method that uses the least labor and materials. *Fixed costs* are costs that remain constant regardless of the volume of tests produced. They buy the capacity to do business—space, equipment, and administrative and other general personnel (e.g., preventive maintenance contracts, equipment depreciation, insurance policies, automobiles for courier service).

Cost Accounting for Laboratory Tests

Accounting for the cost of a laboratory test considers three *prime cost* aspects of analysis: (*a*) labor costs, (*b*) materials (reagent, supply) costs, and (*c*) instrument-related costs. The interrelationship of these three areas is illustrated in Figure 1.14, which also shows the additional elements of test cost that must be added if the test is produced in a corporate setting, e.g., marketing and administrative expenses.

In 1989, Travers published a generic cost accounting method (27) (Appendix A) that can be used in any section of the laboratory to derive a total cost for any test produced, using any instrument or method. Known as the Instrument Cost Accounting Technique (ICAT), the method utilizes generally accepted accounting principles (GAAP) to construct actual total test costs. If charges or prices need to be established, ICAT provides the basis for identifying actual costs for labor, reagents, supplies, and instrument-related (and other indirect) costs incurred with the performance of the test. Using the total actual cost as a base, laboratory managers can realistically project test charges and prices by adding desired profit or contribution margin elements (see Setting Test Prices and Charges, below). Standard laboratory cost management texts and guidelines provide worksheets that can be used to develop test costs (27, 28).

Cost Accounting for Disease Categories

In the future, laboratory medicine will become even more dependent on accurate and realistic total reimbursement to survive financially. Therefore, the value of the ICAT becomes more important, since it can be used to calculate the actual laboratory costs for all tests performed for a patient's hospitalization by disease category. Once the cost per test for each

ajor Diagnostic Related Group
4.MDC 10M. Diabetes $\geq$36

incipal Diagnosis: 250.40 Adult-Onset Type
abetes Mellitus with Renal Manifestations/Noninsulin Dependent

tient Status: New Admission—Stable

equency of Test(s) Ordered: Order Once on Admission Only

			Cost Per Test					
			Direct			Indirect		
est	Value of Test(s)	Equipment	Reagents/ Supplies	Instrument	Labor GS-9 GS-7	Indirect	Frequency	Total Cost
JN	Highly Valuable	Demand	$ .13					
tassium	Highly Valuable	"	.22					
O_2	Highly Valuable	"	.21					
loride	Highly Valuable	"	.22					
eatinine	Highly Valuable	"	.09	$ .04	$ 7.01	$ .79	1	$ 9.45
dium	Highly Valuable	"	.13					
ucose	Highly Valuable	"	.13					
-Hour Creatinine	Highly Valuable	"	.09					
otein	Highly Valuable	"	.15					
olesterol	Moderate Value	"	.24					
ine Microscopic	Highly Valuable	Manual	.15	.03	1.55	.19	1	1.92
ematocrit	Moderate Value	Coulter }	.27	.36	2.09	.30	1	3.02
emoglobin	Moderate Value	S + IV }						
TAL COST/LDRG/NEW ADMISSION			$2.03	$ .43	$10.65	$1.28		$14.39

Figure 1.20. Example of a cost analysis worksheet. (From Travers EM. Laboratory diagnostic related groups. Department of Academic Affairs, Continuing Education Workshop, Washington, DC, May 1984.)

type of test (Na, K, glucose, etc.) is determined for the instrument or method used, the cost of a particular pattern of tests ordered can be established (Fig. 1.20). This technique will become more important as cost accounting software is developed that will rapidly accumulate costs as tests are produced.

The Role of Cost Accounting in Variance Analysis

Variance analysis is the comparison of the deviation of actual costs from budgeted or expected standard costs. Cost accounting provides the tools to develop actual costs, and over time, the averaging of actual costs provides the expected or standard cost figure. In times of shrinking economic resources, variance analysis provides a tool to monitor the financial performance of an operating department. The significance of variance analysis is its ability to break the total difference into elements such that the causes of the differences are revealed. This allows the manager to decide what action should be taken, by constructing an explanation work sheet to use as a basis for mutual resolution of variance problems (Fig. 1.21).

For example, if the department chairperson claims that the purchase of a certain analyzer will result in labor savings, but no labor savings are experienced, then this shortfall in performance needs to be either (*a*) explained by exogenous circumstances beyond the manager's control or (*b*) utilized annually to discount the judgment and the budget of the manager in question (33). More detailed explanations of variance analysis can be found in standard laboratory cost management references (27, 29).

Setting Test Prices and Charges; "Make or Buy" Decisions

One of the ultimate goals of a for-profit institution is to provide a profit or contribution through the production of a product. The preceding section has developed the rationale for deciding if a test (product) is profitable to perform, using cost accounting techniques and variance analysis. Both the complex, active tertiary care laboratory and the less active laboratory must manage critically short resources by establishing actual cost and determining if their prices or charges are adequate to cover costs and provide a profit (or contribution) margin to satisfy hospital or corporate management. Similarly, decisions must be made to determine if certain tests should be discon-

Expense Item	Amount	Explanation of Variance	Current Corrective Action
Direct Materials Material Usage	(380)	Poor reagent handling-outdating.	Variance should be eliminated with new plan for handling.
Direct Labor Labor Efficiency	(8855)	Lost three experienced workers. New replacements need training on equipment and upset routine of entire department.	New replacements not envisioned in setting standar last year. Expect training to be completed soon. Wil included next year. No standard revision believed necessary now.
Labor Rate	(150)	New union contract rate for workers at higher rates than used in planning standards.	No standard revision believed necessary. Will set u separate action for rate variance.
Overhead Efficiency	(4679)	Caused by 1519 excess hours of labor.	See Labor Efficiency above.
Overhead Spending Supervisor	300	Budgeted as fixed expense with provision for salary increase at midyear.	Not required, since variance will disappear by year
Indirect Labor	(752)	Cost of working every Saturday during quarter for extra volume.	Short-term contract completed.
Employee Benefits	200	Budgeted as fixed expense with provision for rate increase at midyear.	Not required since variance should disappear by ye end.
Supplies	50	Actual supplies used less than anticipated.	Not required. Year-to-date excess use has been reduced.
Maintenance & Repair	(884)	Repair of equipment causing down-time.	Temporary situation, now corrected.
Power & Light	(30)	Additional power requirements based on Saturday work.	Not required.
Taxes & Insurance	(20)	Not controllable.	Not required.

Figure 1.21. Example of a variance explanation work sheet. (Adapted from Gaither J. Cost accounting in the laboratory. Half Day, IL: American Pathology Foundation, 1981:10–14.)

tinued in-house and sent to other laboratories on a fee basis. The latter analysis is known as "make or buy" analysis.

PRICING STRATEGIES

There are a variety of ways to arrive at a price or charge for a test, which range in complexity from using the price charged by neighboring hospitals or commercial laboratories, to elaborate computerized systems. The most widely used method is comparison pricing, using rates from competing healthcare organizations in the community. Price or rate-setting is not often considered until hospital or corporate management asks for additional revenue from the laboratory. Frequently, increasing the price or charge still may not generate sufficient revenue; therefore laboratory managers may take the initiative to raise prices or charges on certain high-volume tests higher than the competitor's price or charge, regardless of how inaccurately the test prices or charges reflect the laboratory's cost.

The latter approach is not recommended, but is widely used. However, the only justifiable way to set prices or charges is on the basis of actual direct and indirect costs incurred in test performance, using the microcosting approach discussed above under Cost Accounting. However, *pricing tests does not consist of the mechanical task of adding up costs and tacking on a percentage that represents the desired profit margin*. Price-setting is one of the most difficult fields of business, since the manager's intuition; ability to understand the marketplace, reimbursement regulations, legal and government regulations (such as the Robinson-Patman Act); and awareness of the competition's prices (in the case of commercial laboratories) are all parts of the process.

It is interesting to note that many laboratories do not have a problem with pricing tests. This is especially true for commercial laboratories. If a market price exists, customers will usually not pay more than this price, and there is little reason for the test to be sold at a lower price. This is especially true for small laboratories that must compete in an industry where one or a few large companies exercise price leadership. In this case, the laboratory makes no pricing calculations; it simply charges the market price.

There are situations, however, where ethics must prevail. In some laboratories that offer the market price, or lower than the market price, there is always the chance that management may decide to "cut corners" on the quality of service to obtain more business. Examples of "corner cutting" include failure to spend adequate time screening cytology slides (labor costs are the highest costs for any test), or similar activities that might reduce the quality of a test result. Making the decision to charge more for a test is diffi-

Unit Selling Price	Estimated Quantity Sold	Total Revenue	Fixed Cost	Variable Cost (at $100 per unit)	Total Cost	Profit
$250	500	$125,000	$50,000	$ 50,000	$100,000	$25,000
200	1,000	200,000	50,000	100,000	150,000	50,000*
150	1,500	225,000	50,000	150,000	200,000	25,000
125	2,000	250,000	50,000	200,000	250,000	0

*Preferred alternative

Figure 1.22. Pricing analysis example. (From Anthony RN, Welsch GA. Fundamentals of management accounting. Homewood, IL: Richard D. Irvin, 1974:134–140.)

cult, especially if the costs for labor are higher, but the ethical laboratory manager should be able to explain to customers why the added cost will make a difference in the quality of patient care.

THE ECONOMIC BASIS FOR SETTING PRICES OR CHARGES

The description of pricing in standard economics textbooks is stated in the "law of supply and demand"; i.e., the demand for a test is determined by how many customers want to buy it. It is only reasonable to assume that the lower the price, the more customers will be attracted to use that laboratory. The "supply" part of the law refers to the test's cost. Similarly, the supply curve reflects the fact that unit costs decrease as test volume increases. This is because the fixed costs of a laboratory are distributed over more tests as test volume increases. (See example of fixed costs in Figure 1.19.) Figure 1.22 demonstrates the general rule that the most commonly utilized way to arrive at the best selling price is to estimate revenue and costs at several possible selling prices and select the price at which the difference between revenue and costs is the largest (34).

THE SELLING PRICE

The selling price or charge for a test should be high enough to (*a*) recover direct costs, (*b*) recover a fair share of all applicable indirect costs, and (*c*) yield a satisfactory profit for the corporation or provide contribution to the hospital (or, stated another way, profit for the "for profit" organization and efficiency for the "not-for-profit" organization). This must be understood as a statement of general tendency, rather than a prescription for setting the selling price for each and every test. There are some situations however, where the process works in reverse; i.e., the selling price that must be charged to meet competition is taken as a given; the problem then is to determine how much cost the laboratory can afford to incur if it is to earn a satisfactory profit at the given price. The laboratory manager must then design methods to "fit" the desired price. If the test cannot be produced at the desired price, then it may have to be dropped or the calculations should be redone, taking the next higher price point as a given (34).

THE BILLABLE TEST

Billable tests are defined as those that are charged to a patient or physician account and will generate revenues. Repeats performed to achieve a billable test are not counted, provided that the original test was counted. Typically, billable test records can be obtained through many sources; the source chosen will vary based on the accuracy of the data in a given institution. Potential data sources include (*a*) actual manual test counts, (*b*) instrument meter readings, (*c*) College of American Pathologists workload summaries, (*d*) laboratory information system workload information summaries, and (*e*) hospital information system billable summaries. Whichever method is used, an audit should be performed prior to or during the data collection to ensure the accuracy of the information being compiled.

METHODS FOR COMPUTATION OF PRICES OR CHARGES

Price-setting procedures are difficult and there are many methods for price-setting, which vary in complexity. The reader should consult standard accounting and laboratory cost management references if more detail is needed on the individual techniques noted below, which are beyond the scope of this text (27, 30, 32, 34). The method of choice discussed in this chapter is full cost pricing, since it includes all resources expended for a test.

1. *Profit maximization* relates total revenue to total cost; the objective of this method is to obtain a price that contributes the largest amount to profit.
2. Pricing based on *return of capital employed* is based on a percentage markup on cost.
3. *Conversion cost* pricing attempts to direct the manager's attention to the amount of labor and indirect costs required to produce tests.

4. The *contribution margin* approach to pricing indicates a laboratory's contribution to the recovery of fixed costs and to profit; this method sets the price below full cost (see method 7) but above the variable cost, where the difference between price and variable cost per test is the contribution margin.
5. *Standard cost* pricing represents the cost that should be attained in an efficiently operated laboratory at normal capacity.
6. *Direct cost* pricing sets prices at a certain percentage above the direct cost incurred in producing a test; it is used by those who feel that the results of using indirect costs are not sufficiently valid to be useful; they prefer to base pricing decisions on direct costs because these costs can be measured with a high degree of accuracy, using microcosting methods.
7. **Full cost pricing (total cost method)** includes all of the resources expended for a test; it is nearly identical to the Instrument Cost Accounting Techniques discussed above. Appendix A provides worksheets for this technique.
8. *Relative value* pricing assigns a weighting factor to each and every test, based on the labor effort required to perform the test or procedure; it is lengthy and time-consuming and requires that detailed, up-to-date information be included for all techniques, instruments, and methods; its weakness is the use of average values for each procedure, since it is known that some laboratories produce the same test faster and more efficiently than others.

MAKE-OR-BUY DECISIONS

Laboratory managers have the responsibility to decide where it is most expedient to perform tests—in-house or in another laboratory. This problem arises particularly in connection with the use of idle equipment, idle space, or idle labor or with not enough equipment, space, or labor to perform tests. Faced with a make-or-buy decision, the manager should (*a*) consider the quality of the tests offered, (*b*) compare the cost of buying the test with performing it in-house, (*c*) determine the medically necessary turnaround time, (*d*) evaluate consultation and clinician review capabilities, and (*e*) estimate the problems with the logistics of sample transport.

If the decision is made to send tests to another laboratory, the laboratory's financial manager should prepare a statement that compares the laboratory's cost of performing needed tests with the potential vendor's price. The statement should present the differential costs of the tests as well as a share of existing fixed expenses and a profit figure that compares the cost on a comparable basis. The laboratory's budget should also be revised to indicate the effect of the change once the transfer of tests is effected. A worksheet for calculating in-house test costs and pricing to aid in making make-or-buy decisions can be found in Appendix B.

THE BREAK-EVEN POINT

The break-even point (BEP) is the point at which there is no profit or loss, or in other words, the point at which total revenues and total expenses are equal and profit is zero. The most useful purpose of break-even analysis in the laboratory is for making decisions on pricing tests. It is calculated by dividing the laboratory's total fixed costs plus desired profit by the difference between revenue per test and variable cost per test.

The general formula for the break-even point is as follows:

$$\text{Break-even point} = \frac{\text{Fixed expenses} + \text{Desired profit}}{\text{Revenues} - \text{Variable expenses}}$$

Using the graphic technique, the break-even point can be plotted with dollars of revenue on the y axis and test volume on the x axis. The graph is a composite of (*a*) the revenue in dollars plotted against test volume, (*b*) total variable expense plotted against test volume, and (*c*) total fixed expense plotted against test volume (Fig. 1.23). More detailed examples and techniques for determining BEP are presented in Gaither (28) and Travers (27). Figure 1.23 shows not only the BEP but, as revenues increase beyond the BEP, it also shows the development of net income (profit). The break-even volume is useful for determining whether a procedure should be performed in-house or sent to a reference facility. If the calculated break-even volume is higher than current volume, it is not economically feasible to perform the test in-house (27, 28, 32, 34).

Cost Control and Cost Avoidance

CAUSES

When *all* problems and sources of difficulty in managing laboratories have been considered, there are several general conclusions that can be drawn and easily recognized by experienced managers who have long struggled with the dynamics of workload and budget. These basic assumptions are (27):

- *The supply (output) of tests is directly proportional to clinical demand;*
- *Costs are directly proportional to laboratory test output, until the maximum point of efficiency is exceeded, and*

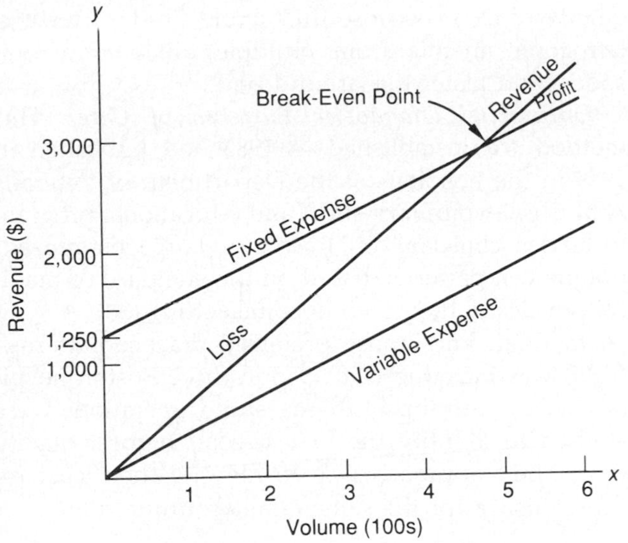

Figure 1.23. Break-even chart. (Adapted from Gaither J. Cost accounting in the laboratory. Half Day, IL: American Pathology Foundation, 1981:10–14.)

compliance with regulatory actions and quality control requires more procedures; and

- *Continuous test order input, without reduction in output, will escalate costs.*

As previously noted (see Strategies, Problems, and Principal Areas of Laboratory Expenditure above), there are three basic areas that need correction before any improvement can be made in reducing or avoiding costs. These are (*a*) *lack of information about clinical user needs;* (*b*) *lack of medical education in diagnostic procedures;* and (*c*) *increasing workload and quality control, inspection, and accreditation requirements.* Problems with uncontrolled costs in laboratories arise from the inefficient use of automated equipment, primarily from the acquisition and operation of too many analyzers in the automated sections of the laboratory without first performing a workflow and configuration analysis to determine the actual need for each analyzer based on the input (demand) from clinical services. The problems with operating too much automated equipment are (*a*) it generates too many labor costs; (*b*) optimum discounts are not always available unless test volume per instrument is very large; (*c*) it causes a requirement for additional QC and maintenance; and (*d*) it is usually not used to full capacity (35). Furthermore, if excessive or additional equipment is operated when staffing is not optimal, the staff will be overstressed, will exceed its "point of maximum efficiency," will produce errors, and may increase expenditures by using more reagents and supplies to keep up with the unchecked demand (Fig. 1.24).

SOLUTIONS

Finding solutions to the combined clinical-laboratory problems noted above is not an easy task. In the preceding section, only a few of the most significant problems were outlined. In fact there is little evidence that clinicians have made any attempt to alter their test-ordering behavior. The only way to begin to reduce unnecessary demand is for the laboratory physician to take the lead in promoting test appropriateness in the healthcare environment.

Test Appropriateness Education

In 1990, the Joint Commission on Accreditation of Healthcare Organizations (JCAHO) published a new standard that provides laboratory physicians with a strong policy to support education of clinical physicians in test appropriateness. The standard (PA 1.2.7), part of the Pathology and Medical Laboratory standards in JCAHO's annually published *Accreditation Manual for Hospitals* (36), states:

> Within the hospital's overall assurance program, the director of the pathology and medical laboratory services assures that the department/service participates in the monitoring and evaluation of the quality and appropriateness of the services provided.

Furthermore, the standard is a key factor in the decision-making process that is part of a new, streamlined "matrix" of factors that JCAHO inspectors consider vital for a laboratory to pass the inspection. The standard allows the laboratory physician to set up guidelines, working in conjunction with clinical physicians, for all tests.

The Pareto Principle (80/20 Rule). The task of deciding appropriateness for *all* tests in the laboratory's armamentarium would be impossible to accomplish. Therefore, the Pareto principle (the 80/20 rule) must

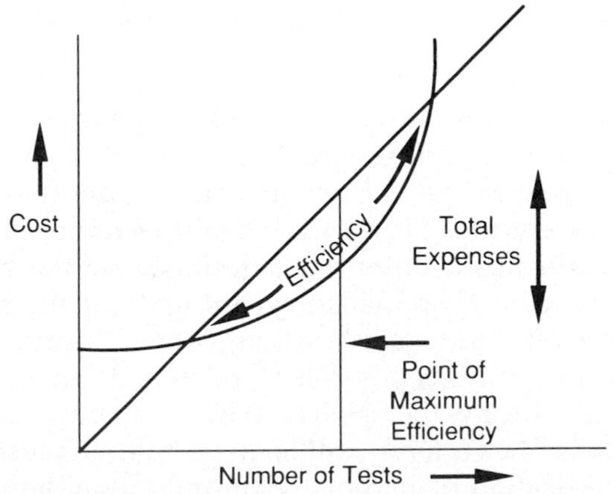

Figure 1.24. Effect of exceeding the point of maximum efficiency in the clinical laboratory. (From Craig TM. Dupont Insight, 1983.)

be applied to decide appropriateness for only the most commonly performed tests that account for the major portion of the laboratory's resource expenditure. The application of this concept is discussed in *Cost Accounting Guidelines* published by the National Committee on Clinical Laboratory Standards (28), which describes a method for selecting tests that are responsible for the laboratory's principal expenditures.

Management Control through Interpretive Reporting

Proceeding hand-in-hand with test appropriateness education for clinicians, the laboratory physician must again take the lead by providing consultations and providing interpretive reporting of laboratory test results, especially for abnormal values, since these are the only areas considered for reimbursement under Medicare. It is imperative that laboratory physicians network with clinical colleagues to encourage them to ask for consultations, and provide written educational information, improved cumulative laboratory reports with narrative statements, and other information about tests so that they will be used more judiciously. Fruitful areas to begin this exercise are therapeutic drug monitoring for antibiotics, cardiac, pulmonary, and other commonly used therapeutics (37), immunologic tests, DNA probes, and other newer tests as they emerge.

The philosophy is to convince the clinician that in inpatient practice, the hospital is prospectively reimbursed at a fixed rate for diagnosis-related groups (DRGs), which includes laboratory tests. If the tests ordered are excessive or inappropriate, the laboratory spends valuable resources that could be used for other tests. As of this writing, the outpatient reimbursement for the top 25 laboratory tests is also being cut back by the Health Care Financing Administration. The need for interpretive reporting is obvious.

Management Control Using Optimized Test Groupings

This method allows the laboratory physician to establish a clinician-designed, optimized set of diagnostic criteria that is "customized" for the hospital's practice setting. Using the Delphi technique, minimum diagnostic criteria are designed by the hospital's top clinical specialist, agreed upon by the physician staff and medical executive board. The laboratory physician's role is to provide the survey forms, educate the clinical staff by identifying the loss functions (money, utilities, personnel) caused by overutilization or inappropriate utilization, and convince clinicians that smaller, optimized test groupings for diseases and conditions provide greater quality of care, because they avoid "reflex" testing, iatrogenic anemia from multiple phlebotomy episodes, and faster turnaround time.

Optimizing Diagnostic Patterns of Care. This method was established in 1985 and published in 1989 in the hospitals of the Department of Veterans Affairs as a voluntary effort and educational program to advise clinicians on how to set up customized, unique test patterns, based on the standard of medical practice in their own hospital setting (38). A similar method, known as "preferred practice patterns" (PPP) was introduced in 1985 in three Boston hospitals where a group of diseases and operations were studied to identify the lowest cost, highest quality PPP. Their approach was to identify the "least resource usage for the same quality output" (39).

Management Control by Clinical Service Leaders

In 1980, Martin emphasized that clinical service leaders have the greatest amount of control and influence over the test-ordering behavior of their house staff in teaching hospitals (40). This factor can help to reduce unnecessary testing if the laboratory physician interfaces with clinical service leaders to provide them with computerized information about the frequency and volume of testing by clinical service and subspecialty. Again, the importance of interpersonal relationships, communication, and networking cannot be emphasized enough in this setting. It is a management control system of great importance for controlling test costs in daily hospital practice.

Deemphasizing the Use of Multitest Profiles

The wasteful practice of multitest profiling, a vestige of past "brainwashing" from the early days of laboratory automation in the 1960s, has created a "shotgun" approach to testing, since most clinicians believe that it is faster and cheaper to perform large groups of tests simultaneously. "Shotgun" testing is wasteful since it perpetuates "reflex" testing (repeat profiles with larger numbers of tests to verify one previously abnormal test result), causes workload increases, promotes iatrogenic anemia, and gives the false impression that "screening" for diseases gives highly specific diagnostic information about a patient's disease state. In fact, automated multiphasic health testing (AMHT) has failed to demonstrate an improved health yield through the use of screening tests, because most programs conducted for AMHT have lacked the continuing channel for long-term patient follow-up (41). It is the laboratory physician's responsibility to make these facts known to clinical physicians and recommend smaller, more specific test patterns for diseases.

Providing More Efficiency in Automated Areas of the Laboratory

As emphasized in the first paragraph of this section, the injudicious selection of automated equipment and its inefficient operation cause costs to escalate, especially labor costs, which account for 55 to 75% of all costs. Workflow and optimum configuration studies must be performed before additional equipment is added. Personnel must be utilized more efficiently to perform highly complex, manually oriented tasks, while instruments should be chosen to perform high-volume tests at the lowest possible cost per test for tests that are not labor intensive.

Monitoring Laboratory Budgets More Closely

Bulk discounts must be obtained, based on high-volume test needs. Unnecessary testing must be discouraged, and microcost analysis must be performed on the high-volume tests that account for 80% of the laboratory's expenditures (see Cost Accounting, above). If a test cost is high, and there is insufficient test volume ordered in-house to "break even" or make a profit, then the test should be sent to another laboratory. Labor scheduling should be seriously looked at, and wasted time must be identified. In situations where part-time staff can be utilized, this option should be exercised to reduce salary costs and provide optimum staffing for the peak periods of workload.

Justifying Capital Equipment Acquisition

The difficulties with availability of capital dollars for investment in laboratory equipment have made it imperative that laboratory managers present a complete, convincing presentation to hospital or corporate managers when requesting additional or replacement equipment.

There are basically four ways to acquire equipment: purchase, rental, lease, or special contractual arrangements with vendors for a cost-per-test fee, in which the equipment is owned by the vendor, who charges a set fee for each test performed.

Regardless of the type of acquisition, the laboratory manager's task is made more complex because of the need to justify the acquisition based on the presentation of cost data to hospital or corporate management, the promise of improved service, and the presentation of data on revenue impact (42). Failure of existing equipment or failure of management strategies to expand the laboratory's market share can further complicate the matter.

WORKFLOW IMPROVEMENT

It has already been noted that improving laboratory workflow is probably the most important consideration in acquiring a new analyzer. An instrument should not be selected because of its technology unless the technology has a direct positive impact on workflow. It is essential that there must be a workflow and configuration analysis performed prior to any acquisition to ensure that the laboratory's workload and menu justify additional equipment and that the new equipment's throughput is matched to the laboratory's workload volume (35). The goal of acquiring new instrumentation should be to improve workflow by integrating the analyzer into a newly organized system. An analyzer that is forced to be incorporated into an old workflow pattern rarely makes use of all of its capabilities. Broader test menus on an instrument are also important because they reduce the total number of pieces of equipment in the laboratory by consolidating workstations, eliminating or reducing batching, replacing existing equipment, and, if possible, reducing staff (10).

COST ANALYSIS

In addition, a microcost analysis should be performed to compare the cost of performing a test (or tests) on the existing equipment with the cost on the new equipment (see Cost Accounting, above). Appendix C provides a worksheet for comparing cost alternatives for the acquisition of laboratory equipment.

METHODS FOR ACQUIRING EQUIPMENT

Purchase

Purchase of equipment requires the performance of complicated analytical techniques to provide hospital or corporate management with information to assess several aspects of financial burden for the hospital or corporation. These include (*a*) development of depreciable costs, (*b*) estimation of appropriate depreciation life and timing, (*c*) isolation of related cash flow variables, (*d*) forecast of production volume and revenue, and (*e*) measurement and comparison with hospital corporate criteria. Appendix D provides a guideline for the recommended steps in a capital acquisition process for laboratory equipment. A format for deriving labor management indicators for instrument selection can be found in standard laboratory cost management texts (43).

If purchase is the desired method of acquisition, then the following key factors should be considered:

- The merits of each capital expenditure

- Future net increases in cash inflows or net savings in cash outflows
- Required total or lifetime investment

Economic or cost-benefit ratios are not the only quantitative considerations to be used in evaluating capital expenditures. The following are also very important:

- The number of patients who benefit
- The degree to which the patients will benefit
- Demographic characteristics of the patients who will benefit

The following factors are also key elements to analyze cost benefits:

- Anticipated time span (years) of project
- Original capital investment
- Annual operating expenses
- Present value of all expenditures
- Average annual savings or net earnings
- Number of patients served
- Age of patients served
- Average cost per patient served
- Intangible health care benefits, short and long term

Leasing/Rental Arrangements

Many hospitals that have entered into leasing or rental arrangements have done so out of necessity, rather than choice. Lease financing has turned into an important source of financing for hospitals, due to the scarcity of capital and the financial squeeze in which many hospitals have found themselves. Leasing, if used properly, can offer advantages. However, financial losses can also occur as a result of not fully understanding the factors involved in a lease arrangement and not properly evaluating the cost of a lease versus other alternatives. The principal advantage of leasing is that it serves as a protection against technological obsolescence and gives the laboratory greater flexibility in the replacement of equipment. With the purchase of equipment, private sector hospitals will ordinarily be reimbursed only for depreciation and operating costs. Depreciation is calculated on the basis of the original cost of the equipment, and may be estimated according to an unrealistic depreciation schedule.

With a lease, the private sector hospital avoids tying up capital. It can use the equipment and (in the private sector) still be reimbursed for the full cost of ownership and the net worth of the equipment is not affected by acquiring the services of the equipment. Federal and state hospitals also avoid the expenditure of capital but will also incur the additional cost for reagents, supplies, and incidentals required for test performance. The vendor also profits by deducting the lease (or rental) costs over time from corporate taxes.

The disadvantages associated with leasing result from the fact that the hospital does not own the asset. Therefore, the residual value at the end of the lease period belongs to the lessor. Second, the failure of the hospital to correctly estimate the technological life of the equipment might result in significant costs.

Cost-per-Test Contracting (Reagent Rental)

This type of acquisition is beneficial in that the vendor provides all reagents, supplies, disposables, ADP, training, installation, maintenance, and all other needs except labor. The hospital or corporation incurs the burden of labor expense (which encourages the optimal use of the equipment, as well the more efficient use of labor). The vendor charges a set cost per test, and provides quality controls, standards, and calibrators. Therefore, it behooves the laboratory to utilize the analyzer judiciously and to perform tests only in the most efficient way, avoiding unnecessary tests, repeats, duplicates, wastage, and all other tests that ordinarily would be charged (since they are billed for all reportable results). This arrangement is commonly found in multihospital corporations, and in 1990 was established for federal and military hospitals by a contract negotiated with laboratory equipment vendors through the General Services Administration.

The advantages of this type of contracting include vendor ownership of equipment, thus avoiding depreciation, maintenance costs, shipping costs, and training costs. Reagents and supplies are provided at the lowest possible cost for the duration of the contract between the hospital or corporation and the vendor. An additional advantage for federal and military hospital laboratories is the fixed reagent and supply costs that are negotiated, for instance, for a 5-year period.

CONCLUSION

In summary, before prospective payment, the purchase of an instrument could be justified on the basis of its technology alone. Currently, a good cost-benefit analysis has to be performed as well as sensitivity analysis, computations of net present value, break-even analysis, internal rate of return, and reduction in variable production costs. These tools are applied to alternative products and alternative ways of acquiring them (purchase, rental, lease, cost-per-test [reagent rental]) to determine the true acquisition cost over the lifetime of each instrument under study (42).

Table 1.3. Types of Productivity[a]

Major Type	Measures	Subtype	Components	Methods of Measurement	Measurement Tools
Operational	Timeliness of services provided	Labor	Technical staff Clerical staff	Industrial engineering time standards	Task list List of test times per instrument or method times Analysis sheets Personnel utilization report
	Quality and timeliness of services provided	Automation	Instruments Computers	Maintenance standards Temperature standards	Maintenance checklists Manufacturer's tolerance limits
	Quality and timeliness of agency	Clinical	Test turnaround time Precision Accuracy Reproducibility	Quality control standards	Quality control reagents Reference standards
	Quantity of services provided	Workload	Tests Quality control standards	Raw test count Relative value per test	Manual recording Computerized recording
Fiscal	Economic efficiency	Departmental Sectional Inpatient Outpatient	Laboratory work stations Laboratory sections	Cost accounting Cost allocation	Standard costs Operating expenses = actual costs Operating revenues Ratios

[a]From Travers EM. Managing costs in clinical laboratories. New York: McGraw-Hill Information Systems, 1989:204.

Measuring Laboratory Productivity

Managing laboratory costs is impossible without managing laboratory productivity. As the cost of hospital care has increased, the pressure for higher levels of productivity in the provision of services has also increased. One of the interesting aspects of laboratory operations is the potential for substantial improvements in productivity. An increase in productivity will have occurred if (*a*) the quality of tests provided increases for a given level of technical effort, (*b*) the quantity of technical effort used to produce a given quality of tests decreases, or (*c*) given amounts of tests and technical effort remain constant but the quality of tests increases (44).

An assessment of laboratory productivity implies that many factors must be included in an analytical process that determines the relative productivity of one laboratory compared to another or to determine total laboratory productivity (Table 1.3). For the purpose of this discussion, the concepts of work units and standard test times, usually thought of as "productivity" standards for laboratories, are considered only as one of several factors required for the total assessment of laboratory productivity. The shortcomings and limitations of using work units or standard times for tests as measures of planning and controlling labor activity are discussed in standard laboratory management references (27, 28). More important, however, is the fact that relative value work units and standard test times *by themselves* lack the basic ingredients necessary to enhance the improvement of productivity in a laboratory (45).

Instead, it is more important as a whole that laboratory productivity, rather than the workload of individual technical and clerical workers, must be the center of management's concern.

TYPES OF LABORATORY PRODUCTIVITY

There are four types of *operational* productivity: labor, automation, clinical, and workload productivity; and four types of *fiscal* productivity: departmental, sectional, inpatient, and outpatient productivity (Table 1.3). While all are important and must be integrated to achieve successful laboratory operations and financial performance, the most important of all eight types is labor productivity, for all other categories of productivity depend on the efficient utilization of labor resources.

Labor Productivity

The growing importance of the role of management in improving labor productivity in hospital clinical laboratories is especially pertinent in times of economic constraint. In fact, increasing labor productivity is a critical survival element in modern laboratory management practice.

The basic concepts underlying productivity and productivity measurement are quite clear and simple. However, in a laboratory environment, measur-

Table 1.4. Steps for Improving the Productivity of Automation[a]

Consolidate priority tests.
- Multichannel vs. discrete test costs should be determined.

Optimize test groupings (laboratory disease related groups).
- Interact with clinicians to prioritize/consolidate test/disease profiles.

Utilize cost accounting techniques for instruments, sections, and departments.

Utilize ADP to decrease turnaround time—decrease telephone/clerical/billing time.

Improve capital productivity.
- Use cost accounting.
  - Determine most/least expensive procedures.
  - Evaluate cost of lease/purchase or rent vs. capital purchase.

[a]From Travers EM. Managing costs in clinical laboratories. New York: 1989: 213.

Table 1.5. Recommendations for Improving Clinical Productivity[a]

Develop laboratory disease related test groups.
Interact with clinical physicians to prioritize and consolidate tests/disease.
Integrate test groups into laboratory's quality assurance plan.
Interact with clinical staff to determine their optimum test choices.
Provide interpretive reporting for clinicians.
Interact with hospital management to demonstrate cost avoidance and encourage administrative decisions that discourage unnecessary testing.

[a]From Travers EM. Managing costs in clinical laboratories. New York: McGraw-Hill Information Systems, 1989:213.

ing output in terms of number of tests is not always simple. Laboratory tests are subject to technological changes in methodology, and their performance times vary greatly. Furthermore, the laboratory manager is not always equipped with the knowledge or the time to apply workload measurement criteria precisely and must employ specialists to perform the studies properly and draw realistic conclusions.

Consequently, a more global approach is required to assess the laboratory's labor productivity. Appendix E provides a checklist/score sheet and a list of solutions for managers to assess their own causes of low labor productivity, as well as solutions for low labor productivity.

The Productivity of Automation

This subtype of productivity is difficult to separate from labor productivity, but it does have distinctly different characteristics that can be improved to enhance the quality and timeliness of services provided and provide more cost-effective utilization of equipment. Unfortunately, automation is purchased and utilized in this generation based on empirical needs, and is not matched to workload volume or test complexity, which causes under- or over-utilization. Table 1.4 provides suggestions for improving the productivity of automation.

Table 1.6. Causes of High Nonlabor Expenses[a]

Waste
Too many dollars spent on research, development, and nonpatient care
Excessive controls, standards, and repeat tests
Nonlab-related expenses charged against lab by the hospital or corporation
Too little spent on capital equipment, too much on reagent rental
Poor purchasing practices, poorly negotiated deals
An inconsistent definition of capital equipment (capital vs. noncapital expenses threshold is high)
Excessive inventory and/or poor inventory control
Excessive send-outs or too little send-outs, with no emphasis on true cost analysis
Excessive preventive maintenance
Poor preventive maintenance practices resulting in high equipment failure
Excessive travel and education expenses
Poor monitoring of long-distance telephone costs
Courier services are not cost-controlled
Inappropriate use of substitution products (such as in blood bank, the use of more expensive, but clinically equivalent blood products)
Capital equipment not properly sized for the laboratory workload flow
Stat equipment has high reagent cost, yet fast turnaround time is used for routine testing
Excessive accrediting agency fees
Excessive proficiency testing fees
Excessive dues to organizations
Excessive, unnecessary subscriptions
Excessive, unnecessary consulting fees
An unusual laboratory test mix, based on the hospital patient population
Lack of instrument standardization, resulting in excessive repeats
Need for backup instrumentation
Computer paper wastage

[a]Adapted from Travers EM. Managing costs in clinical laboratories. New York: McGraw-Hill Information Systems, 1989:217.

Clinical and Workload Productivity

Clinical productivity is synonymous with quality. The importance of producing a product (test) of the highest quality is especially important in view of increasing regulations from private sector accrediting bodies (JCAHO, CAP) and federal regulatory actions (CLIA 88). A laboratory manager's greatest concern is balancing quality with economic productivity, and there is no room for a trade-off of one or the other. However, there is some concern in today's highly computerized laboratory that there is too much quality control, especially when analyzers have been programmed to recognize errors instantaneously. This can be an additional area of unnecessary expense, and, if carefully reviewed, might result in considerable savings without reducing the quality of test results.

The other aspect of clinical productivity is the need to perform more cogent, specific test patterns, as discussed in the previous section on Test Appropriateness Education. Table 1.5 provides recommendations for improving clinical productivity. These recommendations, if implemented, can improve workload productivity by reducing unnecessary testing.

Improving Fiscal Productivity

Improving the economic efficiency of a laboratory can be applied to an entire department, a laboratory section or workstation(s), or to a hospital component to which services are directed, viz., inpatient or outpatient services. The causes of inefficient fiscal operations are most commonly related to salaries that are too high and/or being paid to too many laboratory staff members. Other nonlabor expenses can be inordinately high (Table 1.6) but should be considered for review after labor costs have been streamlined, since labor costs account for 55 to 70% (or more) of total costs.

References

1. Hardwick DF, Morrison JI. Directing the clinical laboratory. New York: Field and Wood, 1990:1–45.
2. Snyder JR, Senhauser DA. Administration and supervision in laboratory medicine. Philadelphia: JB Lippincott, 1989:1–20.
3. Westgard JO, Klee GG. Quality assurance. In: Tietz NW, ed. Textbook of clinical chemistry. Philadelphia: WB Saunders, 1986:424–458.
4. Gray BH, Field MJ. Controlling costs and changing patient care, the role of utilization management. Washington, DC: National Academy Press, 1989:27–58.
5. George CS Jr. The history of management thought. Englewood Cliffs, NJ: Prentice-Hall, 1965:13–17.
6. Albrecht K. Successful management by objectives. New York: Prentice Hall Press, 1988:1–40.
7. Drucker PF. Managing for results. New York: Harper & Row, 1964:1–50.
8. Drucker PF. Management—tasks, responsibilities, practices. New York: Harper & Row, 1974:1–48.
9. Garvin DA. Managing quality. New York: The Free Press, 1988:1–20.
10. Couch JB. Health care quality, management for the 21st century. Tampa, FL: The American College of Physician Executives, 1991:1–22.
11. DePree M. Leadership is an art. New York: Bantam/Doubleday/Dell Publishing Group, 1989.
12. Shewhart WA. Economic control of quality of manufactured product. New York: D. Van Nostrand, 1931.
13. Juran JM. Juran's quality control handbook. 4th ed. New York: McGraw Hill, 1988.
14. Juran JM. Juran on leadership for quality: an executive handbook. New York: Collier MacMillan, 1989:1–80.
15. DeAguayo R. Deming: the American who taught the Japanese about quality. New York: Simon and Schuster, 1990:1–66.
16. Davidow WH, Uttal B. Total customer service, the ultimate weapon. New York: Harper & Row, 1989.
17. Albrecht K, Zemke R. Service America. Homewood, IL: Warner Books, 1985:1–191.
18. Gronroos C. Service management and marketing. Lexington, MA: Lexington Books, 1990:1–257.
19. Naisbitt J. Megatrends: ten new directions transforming our lives. New York: Warner Books, 1982.
20. Clark GB. Quality assurance, an administrative means to a managerial end, Part I. a historical overview. Clinical Laboratory Management Review 1990;17:7–15.
21. Clark GB. Quality assurance, an administrative means to a managerial end, part II. The JCAHO ten step process selecting indicators of quality. Clinical Laboratory Management Review 1990;17:224–257.
22. McGregor D. The human side of enterprise. New York: McGraw-Hill, 1960:1–58.
23. Maslow A. Motivation and personality. New York: Harper and Bros, 1954.
24. Thompson RE. From quality assurance to continuous quality improvement. Physician Executive. 1991;17:3–8.
25. Fromberg R. The joint commission guide to quality assurance. Chicago: Joint Commission on Accreditation of Healthcare Organizations, 1988.
26. Oszustowicz RJ. A capital equipment acquisition process. Journal of the Healthcare Financial Management Association, April 1982.
27. Travers EM. Managing costs in clinical laboratories. New York: McGraw-Hill Information Services, 1989.
28. Cost Accounting in the Clinical Laboratory (GP11-P). Vol. 10, No. 13 Villanova, PA: National Committee for Clinical Laboratory Standards, December 1990.
29. Gaither J, Resinger H. Cost accounting in the laboratory. Mundelein, IL: The American Pathology Foundation, 1981:56.
30. Cleverley WO. Handbook of healthcare accounting and finance. Vol. I. Rockville, MD: Aspen Systems, 1982;1:295.
31. Berman HJ, Weeks LE, Kukla SF. The financial management of hospitals. 6th ed. Ann Arbor, MI: Health Administration Press, 1986:457–458.
32. Horngren C. Cost accounting: a managerial emphasis. 6th ed. Englewood Cliffs, NJ: Prentice-Hall, 1982.
33. Eastaugh R. Financing health care: economic efficiency and equity. Dover, MA: Auburn House, 1987:111.
34. Anthony RN, Welsch GA. Fundamentals of management accounting. Homewood, IL: Richard D. Irvin, 1974:134–140.
35. Lifshitz MS, DeCresce RP. Clinical laboratory instrument selection. Laboratory Medicine 1990;21:367–370.
36. Accreditation Manual for Hospitals. Chicago: Joint Commission on Accreditation of Healthcare Organizations, 1990:137–138.
37. Travers EM. Misuse of therapeutic drug monitoring. Clin Lab Med 1987;7.
38. Travers EM. Optimizing diagnostic patterns of care. Washington, DC: Department of Veterans Affairs, Veterans Health Services and Research Administration, Publication IB 11 82, November 1989.
39. McNeil B. Hospital response to DRG-based prospective payment. Medical Decision-Making 1985;5(1):15–21.
40. Martin AR, Wolf MA, Thibodeau LA, Dzau M, Braunwald E. A trial of two strategies to modify the test-ordering behavior of medical residents. N Engl J Med 1980;303:130–136.
41. Home HF. Application of AMHT in clinical medicine. JAMA, 1972;219:885.
42. Benezra N. Re-equipping the laboratory: how to win approval for acquisitions. Medical Laboratory Observer, August 1989: 33.
43. Travers EM. Workbook for managing costs in clinical laboratories. New York: McGraw-Hill Information Systems, 1989:117–124.
44. Hadley J. Research on health manpower productivity: a general overview. In: Rafferty J, ed. Health Manpower and Productivity. Lexington, MA: D.C. Heath, 1974.
45. Ozan TM. Productivity measures for the improvement of productivity in clinical laboratories. Examination of case studies of productivity improvements in clinical laboratories. Chicago: Center for Hospital Management Engineering of the American Hospital Association, 1974:243–261.
46. Sharp JW. A cost accounting system targeted to DRG's. Medical Laboratory Observer, September 1985:2–8.

Appendix A—Instrument Cost Accounting Technique[a]

If one component of laboratory operations can be identified as the controlling influence, it is the instrument configuration of the laboratory. It determines the major portion of costs (labor) for any laboratory and determines actual costs for the next largest component—reagents and supplies. The information and formats in this section provide laboratory managers with a microcosting "bottom-up" method for determining cost per test per instrument. This is the basic starting point in any laboratory cost accounting technique (Fig. A.1).

No standard cost accounting format has been developed for use in laboratories, and standard accounting texts are not suitable for most medical applications. The examples in

[a]Text adapted from Travers EM. Cost analysis in the toxicology laboratory. Clin Lab Med 1990;10(3):591–623.

I. TEST INSTRUMENT

Name:	GC/MS	Life Expectancy in Years:	5
Model Number:	5970B	Annual Maintenance Cost:	9442
Manufacturer:	H-P	Site-Preparation Cost:	2000
Purchase Price:	90000	Evaluation Period in Days:	1
		Starting Date:	9/15/89
		Completion Date:	9/15/89

II. DIRECT TEST MATERIALS

Name of Test/Profile A	Total No. Tests/Profiles B	Per Test/Profile in Evaluation Period $ Reagents C	$ Test-Related Supplies and Parts D	$ Equipment-Related Disposables E
1. Benzoylecgonine	30	$27.57	$12.56 (supplies)	$1.89
2.			$9.00 (parts)	
3.				
4. Controls	10	$190.00	included above	.63
5. Calibrators	10	$190.00	" "	.63
6.				
7.				
8.				
9.				
10.				
Totals	30 tests	$407.57	$21.56	$3.15

III. TEST LABOR

Time Segment per Test/Profile	Total FTE Minutes/ Procedure	Annual Salary + Benefits
Preanalytical	21 min.	$33880 + 4404 = $38284
Analytical	180 min.	38284
Postanalytical	120 min.	38284
Totals	321 min. x 1.15 PFD FACTOR = 369.2	

Figure A.1. Completed ICAT worksheet showing cost accumulation for gas chromatography/mass spectrometry procedure. See Figure A.2 for instructions. (Adapted from Travers EM: Workbook for Managing Costs in Clinical Laboratories. New York, McGraw-Hill Information Services Company, 1989, appendix; with permission.)

IN THE FIRST PART (I):

1. Enter the trade name of the instrument.
2. Enter the instrument model number, if applicable.
3. Enter the manufacturer's name.
4. Enter the purchase price of the equipment.
5. Enter the anticipated life expectancy of the equipment in years.
6. Enter the annual maintenance cost of the equipment.
7. Enter the site-preparation cost.
8. Enter the evaluation period (in whole days) and the starting date of the evaluation period.

IN THE GRID PORTIONS (II AND III):

9. Enter the name or designation for each test or panel that will be performed on the instrument. If the instrument performs both discrete and batch testing, do this analysis for both modes of operation and duplicate this form if necessary (Part A).
10. Enter the total number of tests or profiles performed on this instrument during the evaluation period (Part B).
11. Based on reagent costs incurred during the evaluation period, enter the reagent cost per test profile (Part C).
12. Based on cost of disposables used during the evaluation period, estimate the test-associated disposable cost per test/profile (Part D).
13. Enter the cost of any other equipment-related disposables per test/profile used during the evaluation period (Part E).
14. Continue with the labor analysis section and enter:
15. *Preanalytical time*—Include *time* to collect specimens from patients and laboratory central receiving. This includes all steps up to the actual testing procedure, such as work-list gathering, start-up, sample cup preparation, and preparation of daily quality controls and standards for this instrument. Phlebotomy or centrifugation is included.
16. *Analytical time*—Include labor to analyze the specimen(s) and to perform all routine procedures up to reporting of results. This includes calculation(s) and checking *but does not include* repeats.
17. *Postanalytical time*—Include labor to manually report results or to enter results into a computer system. This includes sorting, filing, and telephone calls related to the final report(s). Routine, daily maintenance normally performed and shut-down time must also be included.

When all blocks have been completed, provide totals where indicated and proceed to Figure A.9 (Formulas for ICAT).

Figure A.2. Instructions for completing ICAT worksheet. (From Travers EM: Managing Costs in Clinical Laboratories. New York, McGraw-Hill Information Company, 1989, p 112; with permission.)

the texts are not pertinent to laboratories and many of the problems are irrelevant. Therefore, the Instrument Cost Accounting Technique (ICAT) was developed as a method and in a form that managers can use in any laboratory for any instrument or combination of instruments to calculate the cost of tests or test profiles.

ICAT is based on standard cost accounting techniques and is derived from standard literature and generally accepted accounting principles (GAAP) in the field of accounting. These cover direct labor, materials, and instrument-related costs. Indirect expenses are usually estimated in each individual setting and will vary considerably from laboratory to laboratory, based on hospital or laboratory reimbursement. Indirect expenses will be discussed in a later section, because this important component of total cost is not considered in the overall determination of direct test production costs.

Instrument Cost Accounting Technique Format

The ICAT method considers the three prime cost aspects of analysis: (1) instrument-related costs, (2) direct materials cost, and (3) labor costs. No two laboratories are alike in their instrumentation configuration; therefore, ICAT was designed to be generic so that it could be used in each section of any laboratory to profile costs associated with every instrument or test method. Direct material expenses on the ICAT form include expenditures for supplies and reagents required to produce tests. Direct labor costs comprise total compensation required for preanalytic, analytic, and postanalytic personnel necessary to perform tests. By dividing all test production activities into the three major work effort segments, ICAT allows managers to estimate which segment of the test production process has the greatest impact on manpower and, subsequently, on compensation costs.

SAMPLE ICAT WORKSHEET

The reader should know that the ICAT method is universal and generic and can be used for any test performed in the laboratory. Regardless of whether or not an instrument is used, the method will be the same. If no instrument is used, then the section on indirect instrument costs (Section 1 of the ICAT) is left out, and the remaining sections are completed. The ICAT work sheet is used to accumulate costs (Fig. A.1); instructions for completing each major section of the ICAT appear in Figure A.2.

1. TEST INSTRUMENT

Name: ____________________ Life Expectancy in Years: ____________

Model Number: ____________________ Annual Maintenance Costs: ____________

Manufacturer: ____________________ Site-preparation Cost: ____________

Purchase Price: ____________________ Evaluation Period in Days: ____________

Starting Date: ____________

Completion Date: ____________

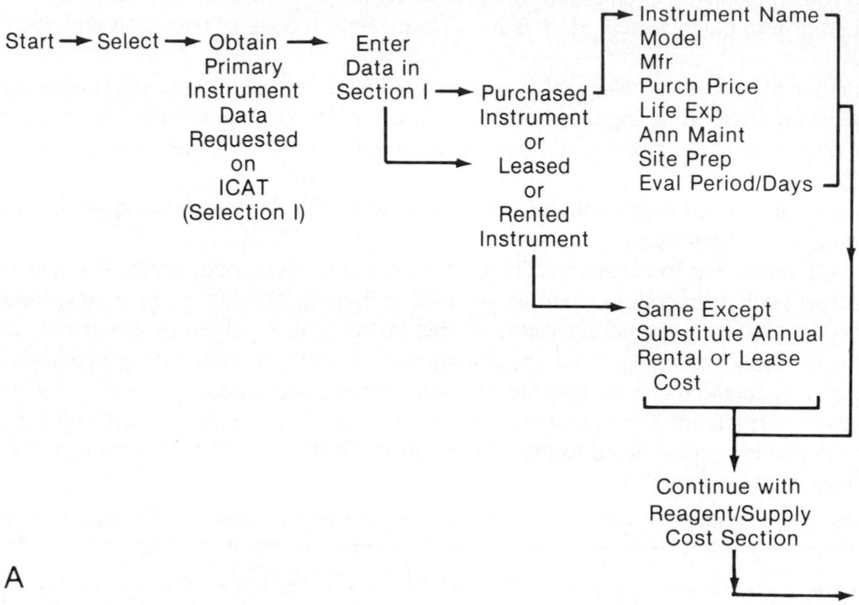

A

Figure A.3. Phase II: Data entry. **A**, Indirect instrument costs. **B**, Direct materials costs. (Adapted from Travers EM: Workbook for Managing Costs in Clinical Laboratories. New York, McGraw-Hill Information Services Company, 1989, appendix; and Travers EM: Managing Costs in Clinical Laboratories. New York, McGraw-Hill Information Services Company, 1989, p 126; with permission.)

Examples and algorithms for actual cost analysis for GC/MS are presented in Figures A.3 to A.14.

Section I—Indirect Costs of Test Production for Test Instrument

Indirect costs are all costs of test production not traceable to a test (unit of output) or to a segment of the equipment or operational requirements for test production. Indirect costs include those of materials, indirect labor, and all other expenses of test production that cannot conveniently be charged directly to laboratory sections, jobs, or products (Fig. A.2). They are assigned to the total cost based on a multitude of factors that are part of the hospital or corporate operations. These are commonly added into the cost of tests as a percentage rather than as actual amounts for each item (see Formula 6, in Fig. A.9 and Fig. A.10.)

Depreciation, Maintenance, and Site-Preparation Costs. Ten entries in part I of the ICAT form (Figs. A.1 and A.3) provide the format for indirect instrument-related cost calculations. They include the instrument's name, model number, manufacturer's name, purchase price, life expectancy in years, annual maintenance cost, cost of site preparation, length of the evaluation period in days, and dates that the evaluation was started and completed. A cost accumulation worksheet is provided in Figure A.4, which is coded to the formulas that follow. From this information three different equations are used to calculate each instrument's depreciation, maintenance expenses, and site-preparation costs per test or profile. They are as follows:

1. Depreciation costs =

$$\frac{\text{purchase \$}}{\text{years life}} \times \frac{\text{1 year}}{365} \times \frac{\text{\# evaluation days}}{\text{\# total tests}}$$

2. Maintenance costs =

$$\frac{\text{total maintenance \$}}{\text{years life}} \times \frac{\text{1 year}}{365} \times \frac{\text{\# evaluation days}}{\text{\# total tests}}$$

3. Site-preparation costs =

$$\frac{\text{site \$}}{\text{years life}} \times \frac{\text{1 year}}{365} \times \frac{\text{\# evaluation days}}{\text{\# total tests}}$$

DIRECT TEST MATERIALS

Name of Test/Profile	Total No. Tests/Profiles	Per Test/Profile in Evaluation Period:		
		$ Reagents	$ Test-Related Disposables	$ Equipment-Related Disposables
A	B	C	D	E
otals				

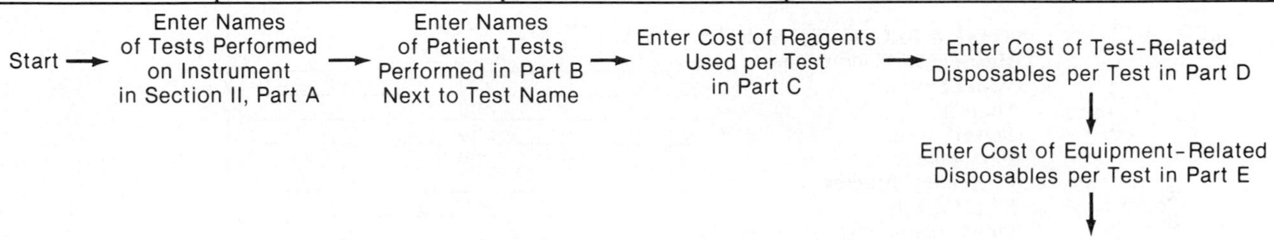
Start
Enter Names of Tests Performed on Instrument in Section II, Part A
Enter Names of Patient Tests Performed in Part B Next to Test Name
Enter Cost of Reagents Used per Test in Part C
Enter Cost of Test-Related Disposables per Test in Part D
Enter Cost of Equipment-Related Disposables per Test in Part E

Figure A.3. (continued)

Section II—Test-Performance Analysis: Direct Materials Costs

It is important to analyze the cost of direct materials used in test production for each test or panel that will be performed. If an instrument performs both discrete and batch testing, the analysis should be done on separate ICAT forms as required for both modes of testing. After the name of every test or panel, direct test-performance costs are divided into four segments (see Fig. A.1, section II; Figure A.3*B* provides a data entry algorithm for direct materials costs):

a. The total number of patient tests or profiles performed during the evaluation period (Fig. A.3*B* part IIB)
b. The cost of reagents per test or profile during the evaluation period (Fig. A.3*B*, part IIC) (use Fig. A.5 to accumulate materials costs)
c. The estimated cost of test-associated disposables used per test or profile based on the total cost of disposables used during the evaluation period (Fig. A.3*B*, part IID) (See Fig. A.5)
d. The cost of any other equipment-related disposables per test or profile used during the evaluation period (Fig. A.3*B*, part IIE) (see Fig. A.5)

Laboratory activity and consumables to be considered in test-performance analysis include some or all of the following components, depending on whether kits, containerized reagents, or batch or discrete (single) tests are performed: (1) the price per kit, or total reagent costs; (2) the number of tests per kit, or total reagent volume; (3) the number of controls run per test or profile; (4) the number of standards run per test or profile; (5) single or replicate analysis, as done during each test or profile performance; (6) the price for expendable items used to perform the test per batch or specimen; (7) the expense of specimen collection and processing; and (8) the total number of tests or profiles performed during the evaluation period. A flow diagram accumulation of test materials cost can be found in Figure A.6.

To calculate direct materials test costs per test or profile, use the formula that follows:

$$\text{Materials costs} = \frac{\$\text{ reagents} + \$\text{ test-associated disposables} + \text{equipment related disposables}}{\#\text{ of tests or profiles}}$$

Section III—Labor Costs

Labor costs are divided into three labor-intensive segments of test performance: preanalytic, analytic, and postanalytic time. The total full-time equivalent (FTE) required to produce a test must be measured in minutes using a stop watch, and the total compensation (annual salary plus cost of benefits) in dollars of the staff person or persons performing the test are entered for each segment. Figure A.7 provides a flow diagram for cumulating labor costs. Figure A.8 is a labor time accumulation worksheet that is

1. Depreciation costs[a] $= \frac{\$90000}{5\text{ yrs}} \times \frac{1\text{ year}}{365\text{ days/yr}} \times \frac{1\text{ d.}}{30\text{ tests/pd.}} = \frac{90000}{54750} = \$1.64\text{/test}$

2. Maintenance costs[b] $= \frac{\$47210}{5\text{ yrs}} \times \frac{1\text{ year}}{365} \times \frac{1\text{ d.}}{30\text{ tests/pd}} = \frac{47210}{54750} = \$0.86\text{/test}$

3. Site-preparation costs[c] $= \frac{\$2000}{5\text{ yrs}} \times \frac{1\text{ year}}{365} \times \frac{1\text{ d.}}{30\text{ tests/pd.}} = \frac{2000}{54750} = \$0.04\text{/test}$

	ANNUAL COST
EQUIPMENT	
Depreciation[a]	$90000/5 yr; 18000/yr
Lease Fee	—
Rental Fee	—
Maintenance[b]	9000 svc contract; $442 tech labor (2 hr/mo) = $9442/yr
Service Parts Kit[b]	—
Service Contract[b]	incl. in maintenance cost
Interface	—
Accessory Equipment[b]	—
Other	—
Subtotal	$27442/yr
INITIAL & RELOCATION SETUP COSTS	
Heating/Air Conditioning	$—
Water System[c]	500
Drain[c]	500
Power[c]	500
Remodeling[c]	500
Correlation Studies	—
Start-Up Kit[c]	—
Other	$—
Subtotal	$2000/5 yr; $400/yr
LAB INDIRECT COST TOTAL	$27,842

Figure A.4. Equipment indirect cost worksheet summary. (Adapted from Travers EM: Managing Costs in Clinical Laboratories. New York. McGraw-Hill Information Systems Company, 1989, pp 112–115; and Travers EM: Workbook for Managing Costs in Clinical Laboratories. New York, McGraw-Hill Information Systems Company, 1989, p 56.

used to outline specific labor tasks, which are divided into the following times:

1. *Preanalytic time* includes the time to gather specimens from laboratory central receiving and time for all the steps up to the actual testing procedure, such as work—list gathering, startup, sample-cup preparation, preparation of daily quality controls, and standards for this instrument. Preanalytic time includes phlebotomy and centrifugation.
2. *Analytic time* includes time for the labor effort required to analyze the specimen or specimens and to perform all routine procedures up to reporting of results. It includes calculation(s) and checking but does not include test repeats. Detailed instructions on analytic time-study performance are given.
3. *Postanalytic time* includes time for the labor effort required to report result manually or to enter results into a computer system as well as the sorting, filing, and telephoning related to final reports. Routine, daily maintenance time, and shut-down times are also postanalytic efforts.

After the minutes of time for each task are entered in column D of Figure A.8, they are divided into the categories noted above. The cumulative time for each category (preanalytic, analytic, and postanalytic) is then entered in section III of the ICAT Cost Accumulation Worksheet (see Fig. A.1).

Formulas Used for Test Cost Determination. There are six basic formulas that must be used to calculate materials, labor, and indirect costs for test production (Fig. A.9). The information accumulated on the ICAT work sheet (see Fig. A.1) is transferred to each of the formulas that appear in Figure A.9.

When all the formulas have been solved, their totals are entered on the test cost determination summary sheet (Fig. A.10) and added to a subtotal. The subtotal is multiplied by the indirect cost percentage for the hospital or corporation to provide a cost per test total (Fig. A.11).

Phase IV—Synthesis of Test Costs for Laboratory Instruments by Laboratory Section

When the total cost for each instrument selected for analysis in each laboratory section has been calculated, the manager can synthesize costs for all instruments in that section. The format appears in Figure A.12. Managers of laboratories should determine which instruments account for the major workload (Fig. A.13) and then proceed to the next phase to perform sectional cost analysis.

CONSUMABLES	QUANTITY PER 30 TESTS	COST PER RUN
FLUIDS		
Reagents	1	$27.57
Diluents	—	—
Calibration material	1	190
Reference fluids	—	—
Linearity standards	—	—
Control fluids	1	190
Rinse/wash solutions	—	—
Cleaning solutions	—	—
Deionized water	—	—
Analyzer specific solutions	—	—
Other		
Subtotal		$407.57/run
SUPPLIES*		
Chemicals	1	$10.46
Gasses	—	—
Paper	1	$50/yr.; ($0.02/test × 30) = $.60/run
Labels	—	—
Ribbons	1	$60/yr.; ($0.03/test × 30) = $.90/run
Water	—	—
Cartridges, filters, etc	1	$56/yr.; ($0.03/test × 30) = $.90/run
Other	—	—
Subtotal		$12.56/run
PARTS*		
Syringes	1	$600/yr.; ($0.29/test × 30) = $8.70/run
Tubing	—	—
Membranes	1	20.80/yr.; ($0.01/test × 30) = $.30/run
Valves	—	—
Reagent Caps	—	—
Seals	—	—
Reagent vessels	—	—
Cuvettes	—	—
Vials	—	—
Lamps	—	—
Needles	—	—
Probes	—	—
Electrodes	—	—
Filters	—	—
Detectors	—	—
Reaction Chambers	—	—
Other	—	—
Subtotal		$9.00/run
DISPOSABLES*		
Sample cups (Test Tubes)	50	$80/yr.; ($0.04/test × 30) = $1.20/run
Sample caps	50	$30/yr.; ($0.01/test × 30) = $0.30/run
Pipette tips	50	$30/yr.; ($0.01/test × 30) = $0.30/run
Glass tubes	50	$75/yr.; ($0.04/test × 30) = $1.20/run
Bar code labels		
Micro inserts/cups		
Cuvettes		
Other		$10/yr.; ($0.005/test × 30) = $0.15/run
Subtotal		$3.15/run
TOTAL		$432.28/run

* Cost estimates for supplies and parts based on 2080 tests/yr.

Figure A.5. Laboratory material cost worksheet summary. (Adapted from Travers EM: Managing Costs in Clinical Laboratories. New York, McGraw-Hill Information Systems Company, 1989, pp 237–238; with permission.)

The algorithm presented in Figure A.13 allows the manager to apply the 80/20 rule and to select instruments and methods that account for the highest volume (and highest costs) of test production.

Phase V—Sectional Cost Analysis

The generic sectional analysis format is adaptable for all laboratories and includes entries for all major areas of laboratory instrumentation and manual methods. It is assumed that the user will first establish the cost for an instrument's operation using the ICAT and then enter these data into the appropriate category in Figure A.12. A category is also included for entry of manually performed test costs for smaller laboratories that rely on the latter for a significant number of tests.

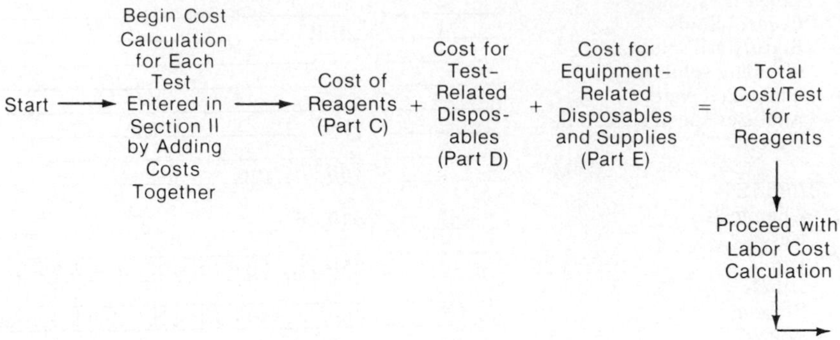
Start
Begin Cost Calculation for Each Test Entered in Section II by Adding Costs Together
Cost of Reagents (Part C)
+
Cost for Test-Related Dispos-ables (Part D)
+
Cost for Equipment-Related Disposables and Supplies (Part E)
=
Total Cost/Test for Reagents
Proceed with Labor Cost Calculation

Figure A.6. Phase II: Calculation of direct individual costs for reagents and supplies and equipment-related disposables. Part 1. Calculation of reagent and supply costs. (Adapted from Travers EM: Managing Costs in Clinical Laboratories. New York, McGraw-Hill Information Services Company, 1989, p 128; with permission.)

III. TEST LABOR

Time Segment per Test/Profile	Total FTE Minutes/ Procedure	Annual Salary + Benefits
Preanalytical		
Analytical		
Postanalytical		

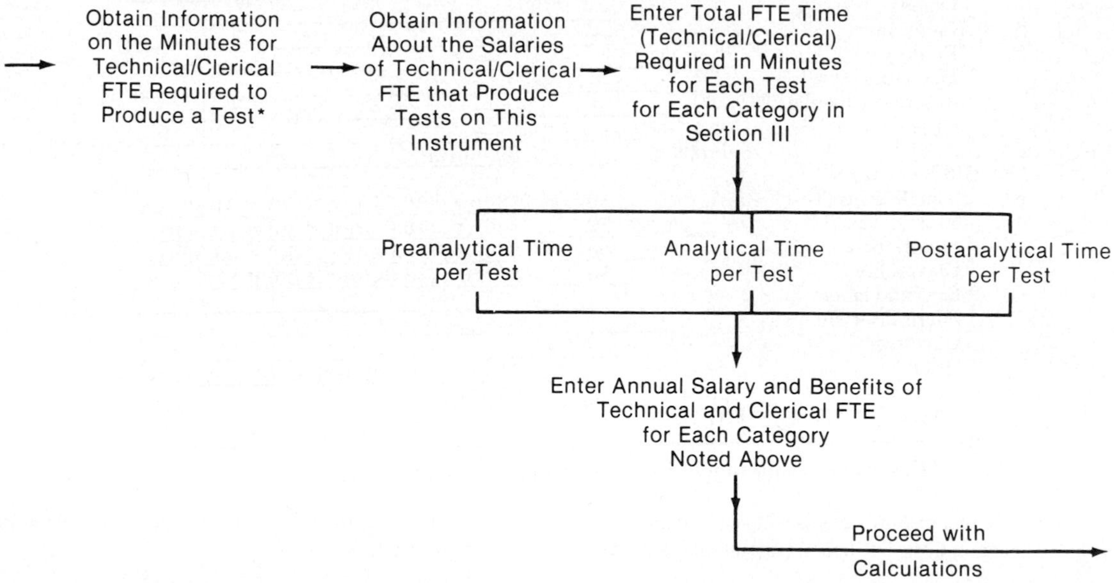
Obtain Information on the Minutes for Technical/Clerical FTE Required to Produce a Test*
Obtain Information About the Salaries of Technical/Clerical FTE that Produce Tests on This Instrument
Enter Total FTE Time (Technical/Clerical) Required in Minutes for Each Test for Each Category in Section III
Preanalytical Time per Test
Analytical Time per Test
Postanalytical Time per Test
Enter Annual Salary and Benefits of Technical and Clerical FTE for Each Category Noted Above
Proceed with Calculations

Figure A.7. Phase III Data entry (continued)—direct labor costs. *Involves all phases of production, starting with specimen collection and ending with delivery of test results to user. (Adapted from Travers EM: Workbook for Managing Costs in Clinical Laboratories. New York, McGraw-Hill Information Services Company, 1989, appendix and p 127; with permission.)

LABOR COST ACCUMULATION WORK SHEET

WORK MEASUREMENT PROJECT NONREPETITIVE TIME STUDY	1. Study Number 1
2. Operation Clinical Laboratory	3. Organization University Hospital
4. Test Name and Type Gas Chromatography/Mass Spectrometry; Benzoylecgonine	
5. Location Toxicology section	
6. Operator's Name Nancy Broderick	
7. Date 9/15/89	
8. Start Time 8:00 a.m. 9. Stop Time 2:09 p.m.	10. Elapsed Time 6 hrs, 9 min.

	11. A	Element Description B	Readings C	Time D	Level Factor E	Normal Time F	Occr. Factor G	Base Time H
Pre-Analytical Time (21 min.)	1	Make work list (computer)		5 min.				
	2	Get controls		2				
	3	Label tubes		4				
	4	Tune MS		10				
Analytical Time (180 min)	5	Pipette samples		20				
	6	Add internal std to buffer, mix soln.		2				
	7	Shake 20 min		2				
	8	Aspirate top layer		20				
	9	Transfer bottom layer		20				
	10	Evaporate		2				
	11	Add derivatizing reagent		10				
	12	Vortex; incubate		20				
	13	Wash		30				
	14	Centrifuge		4				
	15	Aspirate		20				
	16	Transfer upper layer to another tube		20				
	17	Evaporate		2				
	18	Inject into GC/MS		8				
Post Analytical Time (120 min)	19	Evaluate results		80				
	20	Enter results into computer and controls into log book		30				
	21	Copy data file on to tape		10				

12. Remarks Run of 30, including 10 standards, 10 controls	13. Total Base Time	321
	14. PF&D * Allowance 15 %	48.15
	15. Standard Time for One Test	Min. 369.2 for 30 tests
16. Approved Signature — 17. Date 9/15/89	369.2 / 30 = 12.3 min.	Hrs. 6.15 for 30 tests

Figure A.8. Labor time accumulation worksheet. PF&D, Personnel fatigue and delay. (From Travers EM: Workbook for Managing Costs in Clinical Laboratories. New York, McGraw-Hill Information Services Company, 1989, appendix; with permission.)

1. $$\text{Materials Costs/(Test or Profile)} = \frac{\text{Cost of Reagents + Cost of Test-Associated Supplies \& Parts + Cost of Equipment-Related Disposables}}{\text{\# of Tests or Profiles}}$$

$$= \frac{407.57 + 21.56 + 3.15}{30 \text{ tests}} = \frac{\$432.28 \text{ run}}{30 \text{ tests}} = \boxed{\$14.40/\text{test}}$$

2. $$\text{Labor Costs/(Test or Profile)} = \frac{\text{Salary Cost*}}{\text{year}} \times \frac{1 \text{ year}}{2080 \text{ hours}} \times \frac{1 \text{ hr}}{60 \text{ min}} \times \text{\# min. per test or run}$$

$$= \frac{\$38284 \times 1 \text{ yr} \times 1 \text{ hr}}{1 \text{ yr} \times 2080 \text{ hrs} \times 60 \text{ min}} \times 369.2 \text{ min per run} = \$0.31 \times 369.2 = \boxed{\$114.45/\text{run}}$$

$$\text{or} \div 30 \text{ tests} = \boxed{\$3.82/\text{test}}$$

3. $$\text{Instrument Depreciation Costs/(Test or Profile)} = \frac{\text{Instrument Purchase Price}}{\text{Anticipated Instrument Life Expectancy (in years)}} \times \frac{1 \text{ year}}{365 \text{ days}} \times \frac{\text{\# Days in Evaluation Period}}{\text{\# Tests in Evaluation Period}}$$

$$= \frac{\$90000 \times 1 \text{ yr} \times 1 \text{ day}}{5 \text{ yrs} \times 365 \text{ days } 30 \text{ tests/pd.}} = \frac{\$90000}{54750} = \boxed{\$1.64/\text{test}}$$

4. $$\text{Maintenance Costs/(Test or Profile)} = \frac{\text{Total Cost for Maintenance, Service, and Repairs}}{\text{Anticipated Instrument Life Expectancy (in years)}} \times \frac{1 \text{ year}}{365 \text{ days}} \times \frac{\text{\# Days in Evaluation Period}}{\text{\# Tests in Evaluation Period}}$$

$$= \frac{\$47210 \times 1 \text{ yr} \times 1 \text{ day}}{5 \text{ yrs} \times 365 \text{ days } 30 \text{ tests/pd.}} = \frac{\$47210}{54750} = \boxed{\$0.86/\text{test}}$$

5. $$\text{Site-Preparation Costs/(Test or Profile)} = \frac{\text{Costs to Install Instrument (Elec., Plumb., A/C, Constr., etc.)}}{\text{Anticipated Instrument Life Expectancy (in years)}} \times \frac{1 \text{ year}}{365 \text{ days}} \times \frac{\text{\# Days in Evaluation Period}}{\text{\# Tests in Evaluation Period}}$$

$$= \frac{\$2000 \times 1 \text{ yr} \times 1 \text{ day}}{5 \text{ yrs} \times 365 \text{ days } 30 \text{ test/pd.}} = \frac{\$2000}{54750} = \boxed{\$0.04/\text{test}}$$

6. $$\text{Indirect Costs} = (\text{Materials + Labor + Instrument Costs}) \times 60\%^{\dagger}$$

$$= (\$14.40 + 3.82 + 1.64 + .86 + .04) \times .60 = \boxed{\$12.46}$$

* Benefits at 13% rate included in salary cost (see Fig. 6); if benefits are not included in salary cost, then a factor must be added to this equatior multiply the result by 1.13 if the benefits are 13%.

† Percentage will vary in each laboratory/hospital; see Fiscal Service for rates.

Figure A.9. Formulas used for test cost determination for laboratory tests. (Adapted from Travers EM: Managing Costs in Clinical Laboratories. New York, McGraw-Hill Book Company, 1989, pp 227–228.)

DIRECT COSTS		
1. Materials (Reagents/Supplies) Cost	$14.40	Formula 1, Table 9
2. Labor Costs		
a. Preanalytical		
b. Analytical	$ 3.82	Formula 2, Table 9
c. Postanalytical		
INDIRECT INSTRUMENT COSTS		
1. Depreciation Costs	$ 1.64	Formula 3, Table 9
2. Maintenance Costs	.86	Formula 4, Table 9
3. Site-Preparation Costs	.04	Formula 5, Table 9
SUBTOTAL	$	
× (11%) Indirect Costs*	$12.46	Formula 6, Table 9
= Total cost per test	$33.22	

* Excludes all other indirect costs other than instrument-related indirect costs, e.g., rent, insurance, power, heat, lights, taxes, etc.; 11% is only an example since indirect costs are different for each hospital or corporate laboratory; private sector indirect costs may be as high as 148%

Figure A.10. Summary sheet—test cost determination. (Adapted from Travers EM: Workbook for Managing Costs in Clinical Laboratories. New York, McGraw-Hill Information Systems Company, 1989, p 57.)

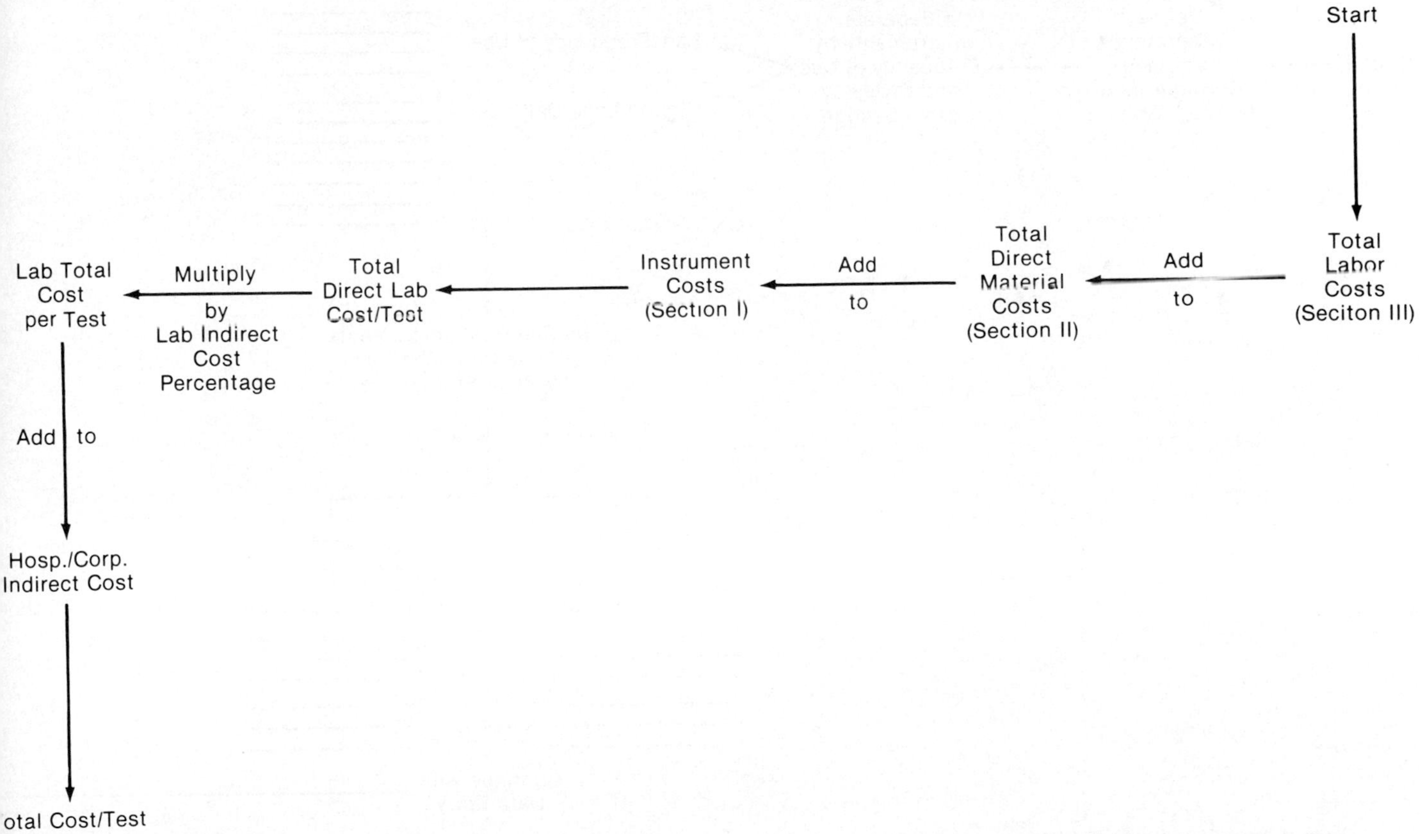

Figure A.11. Phase III, Part 2: Calculation of direct labor cost and summary sheet. (Adapted from Travers EM: Managing Costs in Clinical Laboratories. New York, McGraw-Hill Information Services Company, 1989, p 128; with permission).

	INSTRUMENT NAME	COST/TEST	TEST/YEAR	COST/INSTRUMENT
Chemistry Instrument	1.______	$______	______	$______
	2.______	______	______	______
	3.______	______	______	______
	4.______	______	______	______
	5.______	______	______	______
Manual Tests	1.______	______	______	______
	2.______	______	______	______
	3.______	______	______	______
TOTALS:	1. Instrument Costs			______
	2. Cost Professional Salaries/ Administrative Salaries			______
	3. Cost Blood/Components			N.A.
	4. Cost Transportation/Travel			______
	5. Cost Fee Basis			______
	6. Cost Operations/Administration			______
TOTAL COST	Operations/Laboratory/Year for Chemistry			$______

Figure A.12. Worksheet for sectional analysis of chemistry costs based on equipment configuration/manual procedures. This format can be used for all laboratory sections. (Adapted from Travers EM: Managing Costs in Clinical Laboratories. New York, McGraw-Hill Information Services Company, 1989, p 130; with permission.)

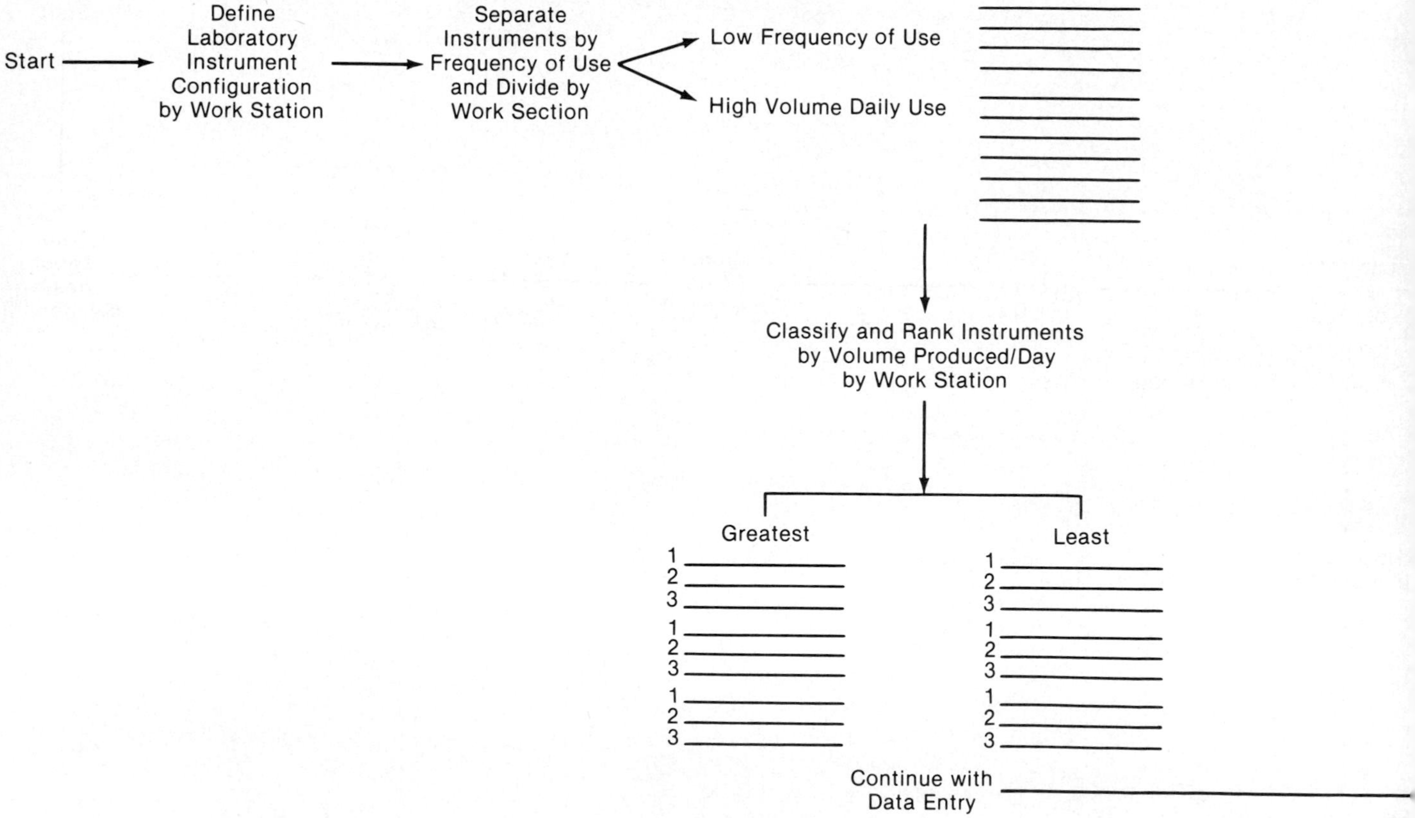
Start
Define Laboratory Instrument Configuration by Work Station
Separate Instruments by Frequency of Use and Divide by Work Section
Low Frequency of Use
High Volume Daily Use
Classify and Rank Instruments by Volume Produced/Day by Work Station
Greatest
Least
1
2
3
1
2
3
1
2
3
Continue with Data Entry

Figure A.13. Classification of laboratory's configuration by volume. Algorithm for identification of high-volume instruments. (Adapted from Travers EM: Managing Costs in Clinical Laboratories. New York, McGraw-Hill Information Services Company, 1989, p 125; with permission.)

INSTRUMENT	A	B	G	H	
Example 1: General Function That Varies per Instrument					**Total Chemistry Tests**
Total Billable* Procedures	39,232	65,068	5,052	6,890	116,242
Percent of Total Chemistry Tests	27.9	46.4	3.6	4.9	
	×	×	×	×	
Phlebotomy Salaries† for Chemistry	$100,128	$100,128	$100,128	$100,128	
	=	=	=	=	
Cost of Phlebotomy per Instrument	$ 27,936	$ 46,459	$ 3,605	$ 4,906	
Example 2: General Function That Applies Equally to All Instruments/Sections					**Total Professional Salaries for Chemistry¶**
Pathologist's Salaries (Professional Fees)‡	12,500	12,500	12,500	12,500	50,000

* Test result actually billed to patient. Example: a chemistry profile with 18 determinations counts as one billable procedure, not 18 tests.

† Determined by the following ratio:

1. $\frac{\text{Total Billable Procedures/Chem}}{\text{Total Billable Procedures/Lab}} = \frac{175{,}999}{394{,}000} = .447 = 44.7\%$
2. 44.7% × Total Phlebotomy Salaries/Lab = .447 × $224,000 = $100,128

‡ Pathologist's time in this lab is allocated as follows:

50% Histology/Surgical Pathology	10% Hematology
10% Chemistry	10% Immunology
10% Microbiology	10% Blood Bank

¶ For Chemistry:
a. 10% × Total Prof. Fees/Lab = 10% × $625,000 = $62,500/Chem
b. 62,500/5 (instruments) = $12,500 Prof. Fees/Instrument

Figure A.14. Allocating costs for general functions among chemistry workstations (Modified from Sharp JW. A cost accounting system targeted to DRGs. Medical Laboratory Observer 1985; September 2–8.)

Once the cost per test for each instrument is established using the ICAT, the laboratory manager must then determine the raw count of tests and profiles per year that have been (or will be) performed on each instrument, and multiply this by the cost per test. The final product for each instrument in each section is added together to produce the cost for the equipment configuration of the laboratory.

The format can also be used to cumulate other sectional major costs, namely professional salaries (professional fees), blood and component costs, transportation costs, fee-basis (send-out) costs, costs for operations, administration, travel, etc, depending on the organizational structure and fiscal control points of the laboratory.

Many cost accounting techniques are concerned only with direct costs for technical and clerical labor and materials for test production, and others use an estimation cost allocation technique for each laboratory section to include nontechnical and professional functions. These functions are not usually assigned to a particular workstation, or even to a section, and they are part of the cost of test production, interpretation, and reporting. This approach is used to distribute the total costs of the laboratory section equally among the total number of workstations. When all costs have been allocated, the total cost of each type of test in the section can be calculated.

ALLOCATING COSTS ACROSS LABORATORY SECTIONS FOR ALL COSTS

If physicians, clinical scientists, and technical, managerial, and general employees such as secretaries and other clerical workers are not specifically assigned to a laboratory section, yet their work helps to produce or interpret tests, then an allocation schedule that spans all departments should be developed. For instance, Sharp uses allocation schedule formulas to assign the costs of nontechnical personnel, professional functions, and other miscellaneous functions to each production center. The formulas may differ for each group or item allocated—and there is no uniform set of allocation formulas that will apply to every laboratory. A good manager should be able to create accurate formulas for each production area and the department based on his or her familiarity with laboratory operations. The only requirement is that the formulas realistically reflect the section's or department's use of that function. For example, allocation of expenses for phlebotomy and for clerical, reception, professional, and other miscellaneous functions allocated to each workstation in chemistry is presented in Figure A.14.

Appendix B—Price Setting Format

Name of procedure or test ______________________

Laboratory section ______________________

Date ______________ Prepared by ______________________

A. Direct costs

1. Labor costs

a. Performance of test

Number of minutes/test × average technical salary per minute

__________ × __________ __________

Labor to perform test

b. Specimen procurement (select probable method)

Venipuncture = 8 minutes

Fingerstick = 1 minute

Number of minutes/test × average salary per minute

__________ × __________ __________

Labor for specimen procurement

2. Supplies for specimen procurement

Item	*Cost*	×	*Number Used/Test*	=	*Cost/Test*
1.		×		=	
2.		×		=	
3.		×		=	
4.		×		=	
5.		×		=	

____

Supplies for specimen procurement

3. Supplies for performing test

Item	*Cost*	×	*Number Used/Test*	=	*Cost/Test*
1.		×		=	
2.		×		=	
3.		×		=	
4.		×		=	
5.		×		=	
6.		×		=	

____

Supplies for performing test

4. Reagents for performing test

Reagent	*Cost/Each*	÷	*Tests/Each*	=	*Cost/Test*
1.		÷		=	
2.		÷		=	
3.		÷		=	
4.		÷		=	
5.		÷		=	
6.		÷		=	
7.		÷		=	
8.		÷		=	

____

Reagents for performing test

Total direct costs __________

5. Labor for running standards and controls

[Standards (12 months) ÷ patient tests (12 months)] × minutes/test × average salary/min] =

[__________ ÷ __________] × [__________ × __________]

= __________

Labor for standards

[Controls (12 months) ÷ patient tests (12 months) × [Minutes/test × average salary/min] =

[__________ ÷ __________] × [__________ × __________]

= __________

Labor for controls

Figure B.1. An example of a format used for single test price setting using the full costing (total cost) method. (Modified from Perryman M. Cost accounting of test procedures. In: Karni KR, Viskochil KR, Amos PA, eds. Clinical laboratory management. Boston: Little, Brown, 1982:348–349.)

6. Reagents and supplies for standards and controls

[Standards (12 months) ÷ patient tests (12 months)] × [Supplies + reagents] =

[________ ÷ ________] × [______ + ______]

= ________

Reagents and supplies for standards

[Controls (12 months) ÷ patient tests (12 months) × [Supplies + reagents] =

[________ ÷ ________] × [______ + ______]

= ________

Reagents and supplies for controls

7. Costs of standards and controls

Standards (12 months) ÷ number of patient tests (12 months) = cost/test

1. ÷ =
2. ÷ =
3. ÷ =

____

Cost of standards

Controls (12 months) ÷ number of patient tests (12 months) = cost/test

1. ÷ =
2. ÷ =
3. ÷ =

____

Cost of controls

B. Indirect costs

1. Overhead

Allocated overhead (year) ÷ total laboratory tests (year) =

________ ÷ ________ = ________

Allocated overhead

Laboratory overhead (year) ÷ total laboratory tests (year) =

________ ÷ ________ = ________

Laboratory overhead

2. Depreciation of capital equipment

Equipment Used Depreciation/Year ÷ Tests/Year = Depreciation/Test

1. ÷ =
2. ÷ =
3. ÷ =
4. ÷ =

____

Capital equipment depreciation

3. Building depreciation

Depreciation allocated ÷ total laboratory tests (year) =

________ ÷ ________ = ________

Building depreciation

4. Contribution (15%) of direct and indirect costs

$$\frac{\text{Test Cost (Direct)}}{\text{Total from A.1}} + \frac{\text{\% Overhead}}{\text{Total B.1}} + \frac{\text{Equipment Depreciation}}{\text{Total B.2}} = \underline{\qquad\qquad}$$

Subtotal

Subtotal × 15% = ________

Contribution

†5. Professional overhead equivalent to 20% of test price

Contribution × 20% = ________

Suggested Price

† Professional Overhead is the addition to price for compensation of physicians on the laboratory staff by adjusting the percentage of overhead to cover the required amount. If the compensation is by some form of percentage of the gross arrangement, then a percentage amount must be added to the total of all other costs to give the required percentage of the total price.

Figure B.1. *(continued)*

Appendix C—Comparative Laboratory Equipment Cost Worksheet

Billable Tests______	Alternative A		Alternative B		Alternative C		Alternative D	
Consumables	Quantity per______	Annual Cost	Quantity per______	Annual Cost	Quantity per______	Annual Cost	Quantity per______	Annual Cost
FLUIDS								
Reagents		$		$		$		$
Diluents		$		$		$		$
Calibration Material		$		$		$		$
Reference Fluids		$		$		$		$
Linearity Standards		$		$		$		$
Control Fluids		$		$		$		$
Rinse/Wash Solutions		$		$		$		$
Cleaning Solutions		$		$		$		$
Deionized Water		$		$		$		$
Analyzer Specific Solutions		$		$		$		$
Other		$		$		$		$
Subtotal		$		$		$		$
SUPPLIES								
Chemicals		$		$		$		$
Gases		$		$		$		$
Paper		$		$		$		$
Labels		$		$		$		$
Ribbons		$		$		$		$
Water		$		$		$		$
Cartridges, Filters, etc.		$		$		$		$
Other		$		$		$		$
Subtotal		$		$		$		$
PARTS								
Syringes		$		$		$		$
Tubing		$		$		$		$
Membranes		$		$		$		$
Valves		$		$		$		$
Reagent Caps		$		$		$		$
Seals		$		$		$		$
Reagent Vessels		$		$		$		$
Cuvettes		$		$		$		$
Vials		$		$		$		$
Lamps		$		$		$		$
Needles		$		$		$		$
Probes		$		$		$		$
Electrodes		$		$		$		$
Filters		$		$		$		$
Detectors		$		$		$		$
Reaction Chambers		$		$		$		$
Other		$		$		$		$
Subtotal		$		$		$		$

Figure C.1. Comparative laboratory equipment cost worksheet. (Adapted from Travers EM. Managing costs in clinical laboratories. New York: McGraw-Hill Information Systems, 1989:237–238.)

Billable Tests________	Alternative A		Alternative B		Alternative C		Alternative D	
Consumables	Quantity per____	Annual Cost	Quantity per____	Annual Cost	Quantity per____	Annual Cost	Quantity per____	Annual Cost
DISPOSABLES								
Sample Cups	____	$____	____	$____	____	$____	____	$____
Sample Caps	____	$____	____	$____	____	$____	____	$____
Pipette Tips	____	$____	____	$____	____	$____	____	$____
Glass Tubes	____	$____	____	$____	____	$____	____	$____
Bar Code Labels	____	$____	____	$____	____	$____	____	$____
Micro Inserts/Cups	____	$____	____	$____	____	$____	____	$____
Cuvettes	____	$____	____	$____	____	$____	____	$____
Other	____	$____	____	$____	____	$____	____	$____
Subtotals	____	$____	____	$____	____	$____	____	$____
TOTALS								
1. Material Cost per Billable Test	____	$____	____	$____	____	$____	____	$____
2. Labor Costs (see Appendix I)	N.A.	$____	N.A.	$____	N.A.	$____	N.A.	$____
3. Indirect Costs (see Appendix I)	N.A.	$____	N.A.	$____	N.A.	$____	N.A.	$____
TOTAL COST (Sum of 1, 2 & 3)		$____		$____		$____		$____

Figure C.1. *(continued)*

Depreciation Costs

1. Provide generic and trade name of equipment; provide operating description
2. Provide total capital acquisition cost
3. Provide cost of first-year service contract
4. Provide cost of service arrangement included in the total cost, which extends beyond the first year
5. Provide installation cost
6. Provide shipping costs
7. Provide training cost
8. Calculate supply and other costs included in the price of the equipment; which items will be consumed less than the equipment's depreciable life and/or less than the financing term
9. Subtotal items 3–8
10. Calculate value of cash payment discount
11. Subtotal items 9 and 10
12. Calculate the pure capital equipment value (item 11 minus line 2)

Depreciation Life and Timing

13. Assign the equipment's proposed depreciable life
14. Project equipment arrival date
15. Forecast date of equipment acceptance
16. Forecast date of first use of equipment for testing

Related Cash Flow Variables

17. Provide other costs from outside vendors/contractors not included in equipment price
    a. Remodeling costs (outside contractor)
    b. Moving costs (outside contractor)
    c. Other costs (detailed list)
18. Calculate undepreciated value of equipment being replaced on date of first testing use for patient care
19. Provide trade-in value, if any, on the equipment being replaced
20. Calculate the value of departmental depreciation expense recorded for the last time during the year prior to the year of new equipment acquisition
21. Provide manufacturer's payment terms
    a. Amounts to be paid
        1. At signing of purchase order
        2. At time of equipment production
    b. Payments to be financed through internal and/or external sources
        1. At time of delivery
        2. At time of acceptance
    c. Total to be internally/externally financed

Production Volume and Revenues

22. Calculate production forecast data
    a. Test procedures—expected annual average
    b. Relative Value (minutes/test)
    c. Total Relative Values (a × b)
23. Calculate average test market price
24. Forecast gross patient revenue (item 22a × item 23)
25. Determine cost payers
    a. Medicare
    b. Medicaid
    c. Other third-party payers
26. Bad debts and charity expenses
27. Convert production forecast into man-hours

$$\frac{(22b \times 22a)}{60}$$

Figure D.1. Recommended steps in a capital acquisition process for laboratory equipment. (Modified from Oszustowicz RJ. A capital equipment acquisition process. Journal of the Healthcare Financial Management Association, April 1982.)

28. Annualize gross patient revenue per full-time equivalent employee forecast

$$\frac{\text{Actual full-time employee man-hours}}{\text{Annualized FTE man-hours}} = \frac{\text{1500 man-hours}}{\text{2080 man-hours}}$$

Raw tests for full-time equivalent employee

$$\frac{\text{Raw tests produced}}{\text{Actual FTE}} = \frac{\text{30,000 tests}}{.72}$$

$$= \text{41,667 tests/FTE}$$

29. Calculate hospital planned rate of return (%)
30. Calculate department planned rate of return (%)
31. Calculate net present value
32. Calculate internal rate of return
33. Determine payback period

Financial Profile Summary

Equipment cost	$82,194
Depreciable life	5 years
Date of return	15%
Tests/year	30,000
Total relative values (weighted workload units)	90,000
Average price/test	$10
Estimated cost payer adjustments	
Medicare	25%
Medicaid	5%
Bad debts/charity care	5%
Forecast net income	$59,319
Forecast depreciation/year	$16,439
Annual cash flow (income − depreciation)	$75,758
Net present value	$157,923
Internal rate of return	74%
Payback period	460 days

Figure D.1. *(continued)*

Appendix E—Causes of and Solutions for Low Labor Productivity

	Condition Present In This Laboratory YES	NO
1. There is inadequate automation.	____	____
2. There is poor skill level.	____	____
3. Consistency of reporting CAP WLUs needs to be assessed.	____	____
4. There is poor work flow caused by poor facility design.	____	____
5. There is poor information flow; computerization is lacking or is a problem.	____	____
6. Infrequently ordered tests are performed in-house	____	____
7. There is inappropriate batching of tests (tests are run seven times per week when three times per week are adequate.	____	____
8. Tests are performed in lab when they should be sent out.	____	____
9. There is inappropriate service level demands by physician staff.	____	____
10. There is a high percentage of stat testing.	____	____
11. There are inappropriate test turnaround time standards.	____	____
12. There are inappropriate quality control programs, resulting in test repeats.	____	____
13. There is excessive machine breakdown, resulting in repeat testing.	____	____
14. There is poor distribution of work between shifts, departments, and benches (could more tests be done during night shift?).	____	____
15. There is excessive paid time off due to staff longevity.	____	____
16. There are dollars spent on medical/technical schools or training programs that are not properly assigned to that function.	____	____
17. There is excessive orientation due to staff turnover or poor hiring practices.	____	____
18. The specialization and generalization of technical staff is not properly balanced.	____	____
19. There is an incorrect assessment of workload units.	____	____
20. There is unnecessary quality conytrolling.	____	____
Note: A predominance of "Yes" answers implies low labor productivity may exist in this laboratory; recommended solutions appear in Table 9–4. TOTAL SCORE		

Figure E.1. Self-analysis checklist for causes of low labor productivity. (From American Hospital Association. Assessing laboratory operations. Chicago: Clinical Services Division, 1987.)

Table E.1. Solutions for Low Labor Productivity[a]

1. Evaluate lab consolidation opportunities.
2. Increase work volume and batch sizes by marketing services.
3. Shift routine work to other shifts.
4. Make sure there is adequate space and design so that work flows smoothly.
5. Investigate flexible vs. fixed staffing.
6. Increase automation using low cost/test, nonlabor intensive equipment.
7. Computerize laboratory.
8. Increase personnel expectations and performance with consistent hiring, training, and reward practices.
9. Improve relationships with medical staff, i.e., strengthen pathologist's role in developing appropriate service levels and control inappropriate stat testing orders.
10. Investigate increasing test batching; relax turnaround time requirements.
11. Combine sections and/or consolidate workstations for maximum efficiency.
12. Reduce any duplication of services.
13. Cross-train staff—generalists vs. specialists.
14. Evaluate use of satellite labs.
15. Improve preventive maintenance and trouble-shooting skills of all staff.
16. Send out infrequently performed tests when staff efficiency remains low.
17. Investigate staff reduction.
18. Motivate staff to give 100% when at work.
19. Evaluate organizational chart and restructure if appropriate, i.e., flatten staffing if too "top heavy" in management personnel.
20. Evaluate appropriateness of research and development time.
21. Improve accuracy of workload.
22. Determine point of maximum efficiency for major automated equipment items.
23. Remove labor-intensive equipment.
24. Avoid highly specialized staff and use cross-trained staff.
25. Determine cost of manual vs. automated tests.
26. Determine "make vs. buy" cost.
27. Avoid too many high-salaried staff.

[a]From Travers EM. Managing costs in clinical laboratories. New York: McGraw-Hill Information Systems, 1989:212.

2 Laboratory Safety

Gerald A. Hoeltge

Clinical laboratories are complex environments. People are surrounded by chemicals, specimens, equipment, and technology. The chemicals may be toxic, the specimens infectious, the equipment malfunctioning, or the technology misunderstood. Some of the people immersed in this environment are technical experts, but others are patients, visitors, and nontechnical employees. Most technological processes and laboratory procedures expose the operator to the risk of injury. Every laboratory hazard can be contained. The foresightful laboratory manager will be cognizant of the hazards and responsive to ideas and suggestions for their control. No clinical laboratory can afford to operate without a safety program, and the best laboratories encourage a strong and comprehensive effort that promotes safe work practices.

The safety program must be organized. Writing a plan that defines the scope of the program and its goals is a start. The individuals who will be responsible for the program should be identified. The administration must provide these individuals with adequate resources—including time, equipment, and personnel—to accomplish the task. Most laboratories have a written safety policies manual that itemizes the requirements for that facility. All personnel should be familiar with the contents of this manual. This should be a comprehensive document that summarizes all of the laboratory's current safety policies within one volume (1). The technical procedures manuals that are used throughout the laboratory should articulate the specific safety precautions that are relevant to each analytic procedure contained therein (2). For example, the procedure for the preparation of bacteriologic media should cross-reference the portions of the safety manual that describe the operation of the autoclave and specify the types of gloves and face protection needed during the sterilization of culture media. The phlebotomy manual should be specific about the use of gloves and the discarding of used needles. The measures for the control of hazards associated with flammable and caustic reagents that are handled may be usefully expressed within the chemistry laboratory's analytic procedures manual. All documents that list safety policies and procedures should be reviewed on a regular basis. Annual review is suggested.

One of the most practical ways to ensure regular review of one's safety program is through the establishment of a laboratory safety committee. Representatives from each major analytic discipline should be included. Membership should reflect the degree of experience and involvement of the average worker in the facility; that is, the committee should be composed primarily of bench-level technologists. All members of the committee should promote the principles of safe work practices and lead by example. The most effective safety programs are found in institutions that value and reward safe work practice.

The appointment of a safety officer (SO) may be appropriate for larger laboratories and is required by some regulations (3). This individual helps administer safety policy and serves as an advisor on the management of safety-related matters. The SO may be responsible for maintaining accident records, conducting or coordinating the safety training program, and surveying the workplace for hazards. The SO or another official in the organization must ensure that the facility is in compliance with federal, state, and local regulations.

Definitions

Hazard containment is the system of routine control processes that keeps the incidence of accident and injury within reasonable expectations. Compliance with the appropriate and established safety policies of the facility should limit the risks that are associated with clinical laboratory practice. A determination of the potential dangers that require containment is part of a *hazard assessment* program. After a safety audit has identified opportunities for improvement in existing safety policies, new controls may be instituted as part of a *hazard abatement* program. Many efforts toward hazard abatement are instituted following investigation of a reported accident or after the external review of the facility by an accrediting or licensing agency. A *hazard minimization* program is a continuous and regular effort that has been instituted to reduce risk to a level as low as can reasonably be attained. Among the best examples are hazardous waste minimization programs that seek to reduce the volume and hazardous potential of the laboratory's toxic wastes to levels that are less than those of the previous year. Programs such as these should not be confused with *risk management* activities, which are focused attempts to reduce a facility's indemnity expenses and liability. Hazard containment, abatement, and minimization programs are directed toward the goal of laboratory safety; risk management strives to mitigate the consequences of unsafe action.

Control systems can be grouped into three broad categories. *Engineering controls* include all of the features and systems that are built into the design of the facility and its fixed equipment. Examples include fume hoods, biosafety cabinets, stream pressure regulators, and electrical circuit breaking switches. Also subsumed within this category are safety devices that are part of the design of technical tools and movable equipment. Sheaths to protect lancets and phlebotomy needles, centrifuge lids that lock when the motor is energized, immobilizing chains for storage of compressed gas cylinders, and double-walled containers for shipment of etiological agents are examples. *Personal protective devices* are barriers from potential hazards that the employee must select for use. Gloves, respirators, and mechanical pipetting aids are obvious examples. *Safe work practices* encompass techniques such as the avoidance of aerosol formation, segregation of hazardous wastes, and the proper operation of hazardous equipment. Engineering controls are preferred methods of hazard containment over approaches that require a deliberate choice on the part of the worker. The categories are not mutually exclusive.

PATIENT AND VISITOR SAFETY

Reagent chemicals, infectious agents, and laboratory equipment can be dangerous. Access to hazardous areas should be limited to individuals who have been trained to avoid injury. Patients and visitors to the laboratory should not be allowed free access to technical areas. The laboratory design should incorporate a reception and waiting area that protects nonemployees from the appliances, fumes, and aerosols that may harm them.

The phlebotomy area must be designated with patient safety in mind. The patient arriving in the laboratory for a blood specimen collection should be escorted to a comfortable chair designed specifically for phlebotomy. The chair should include an arm rest and a passive restraint system to protect against falls from syncopal attack. Spirits of ammonia inhalants should be within easy reach of the phlebotomist.

The patient should be asked about preexistent iodine allergies if iodophors are used as skin antiseptics. Each step of the procedure must be announced to prevent the patient from making involuntary, jerking movements. All needles, lancets, and capillary tubes should be kept out of the reach of patients. Needles and syringes must be kept under lock and key whenever unattended.

Gloves must be worn at all times during the phlebotomy and when handling the resultant specimen. A secondary container, such as a sealed plastic bag, is indicated when the exterior of the container is soiled with blood. All used materials must be properly discarded: Items soiled with blood must be considered contaminated and biohazardous. Such items are to be placed in an appropriately labeled container. All discarded sharps (whether or not soiled with blood) must be secured in an appropriately labeled, puncture-resistant container. The container for sharps must be conveniently located so that there is no need to transport an exposed needle even for a short distance.

As a general rule, used needles are never to be broken nor recapped. Clipping or breaking of needles can spatter blood and spread the area of contamination. Resheathing risks puncture injury of the hand that holds the cap. Although there may be acceptable alternatives, such as specially engineered caps (4) or a "one-handed" recapping technique (5), the simplest option is to drop the entire collection device into the waste container that is reserved for sharps. (Overfilling of such containers is also dangerous; the phlebotomist must never have to force the needle device into the container.) In addition, all spills and spatters that may have occurred must be cleaned with aqueous detergent and then disinfected. Papers that may have become bloodstained must be replaced with clean copy. Gloves are to be changed regularly and whenever visibly contaminated with blood. Washing hands between every glove change reduces the risk further and is strongly encouraged.

ATTIRE

The proper attire for laboratory work minimizes exposure to infectious and chemical agents. A distinction is made between personal attire (including uniforms and cloth lab coats) and *personal protective equipment (PPE)*. Personal attire may be worn in all areas of the facility and outside of the building. PPE is designed to protect the employee and his or her personal attire from harmful exposure. Each item of PPE (whether gloves, face protectors, gowns, aprons, or shoe covers) must be constructed of a material through which the infectious or chemical agent of concern may not penetrate. Protective equipment that is damaged and that may permit harmful materials to penetrate should be replaced immediately. All items of PPE are customarily removed prior to leaving the laboratory.

Attire should be matched to the task. For example, phlebotomists must be recognizable as laboratory professionals. This suggests a clean, neat uniform and proper identification. Such an appearance can help reduce a patient's anxiety. At the same time, the technician must protect himself or herself from the chance that blood might spray or leak from the collection device. A long-sleeved, buttoned lab coat worn with disposable gloves is appropriate.

The performance of a necropsy demands a higher level of containment and therefore more effective personal barrier protection. Water-resistant gowns that extend from the neck to below the level of the table are needed. The sleeves should be tight at the wrist and tucked inside vinyl or latex gloves. Facial protection (goggles and mask or full face shield) and shoe covers are appropriate. Slash-resistant gloves made of steel mesh or a specially selected polymer may be needed (6).

Most tasks in the clinical chemistry laboratory can be safely performed while wearing laboratory attire that protects the worker from common infectious hazards. A fluid-resistant lab coat, gown, tunic, or apron with disposable gloves is appropriate. Face protection must be provided whenever splashing or spraying with droplets of blood or other potentially infectious fluids is a risk. Some tasks will require additional protection. The handling of caustics and corrosives obligates the use of gloves, aprons, and face protectors that are made of materials known to be resistant to the liquid being manipulated. The handling of even small amounts of carcinogenic substances requires the use of gloves and forearm protection (as well as facial protection if splashing or spattering can be anticipated).

Shoes should be rubber-soled for effective traction and to decrease the shock hazard precipitated by an electrical accident. Shoe covers made from appropriately resistant materials are needed if splashing is a risk. In particular, individuals who must transport or decant corrosive liquids must not do so wearing unprotected cloth or porous shoes.

All outer clothing worn during the performance of laboratory tasks should be considered contaminated. It is for this reason that it is inappropriate to continue to wear such clothing outside of the laboratory and into public areas such as cafeterias and meeting rooms. All PPE are to be removed when leaving the laboratory. In contrast, phlebotomists who make rounds in patients' rooms may need to wear protective items outside of the laboratory. Some laboratories have adopted the use of color-coded outer wear—one color for use within the laboratory and a different color outside.

Between uses, reusable protective clothing should be hung away from sources of heat and potential ignition. Uncontaminated garments (such as street clothes) should be stored separately from laboratory wear. All items of personal barrier protection should be changed immediately if they are found to be contaminated with blood or toxic chemicals. Because of the chance of insensible contamination, protective clothing should be changed regularly. Obviously contaminated, single-use (disposable) gear should be discarded in properly marked containers. Reusable lab coats and gowns should be placed in leak-resistant bags to be laundered in a manner that ensures decontamination. To contain the hazards as much as possible, the laundering of contaminated clothing at home should be prohibited.

The principle of hazard containment also applies to hair styles and to personal adornments. Hair should be worn behind the head and off the shoulders to preclude its contact with contaminated surfaces. (Such an arrangement may also reduce the inevitable shedding of microorganisms onto work surfaces as well.) Disposable hair covers may be indicated for some activities. Hair, beards, and jewelry should not be allowed to overhang into contaminated areas nor risk entanglement in moving equipment like centrifuges.

GOOD LABORATORY HYGIENE

Handwashing is one of the most effective means to minimize personal exposure. Thorough lavage with a good detergent removes external bacteria and chemicals before they can be ingested or absorbed. Antibacterial agents are not required for a good laboratory hand detergent. Hands should be washed frequently throughout the day. Washing is especially important after removing gloves, before and after contact with patients, before leaving the laboratory, and preceding dining, applying cosmetics, and using lavatory facilities or smoking materials. The well-designed handwashing sink is operable with elbow blades or foot pedals. Paper towels can be disposed of with the general refuse.

All areas of the laboratory should enforce absolute proscriptions against eating, drinking, and manipulating items that may contact mucous membranes (such as contact lenses, cosmetics, and lip balm) within the technical work areas. Smoking is especially improper because it is a source of ignition and a fire hazard, but any activity of this kind risks exposure to both infectious agents and toxic substances.

Food and drink should never be brought into the technical work area. Refrigerators that are used for storage of reagents and specimens should never be used for food items. If refrigerated food storage is provided, the designated location should be reserved exclusively for food items.

Individuals who wear contact lenses must take special precautions. Any activity that might splash a toxic, irritating, or infectious fluid into the eyes presents a special hazard to contact lens wearers. Tightly fitting contact lenses can inhibit the naturally protective effects of tearing so that exogenous substances remain in contact with the corneal conjunctivae for longer periods of time. Irritants can induce immediate inflammation and swelling, rendering the contact lens difficult to remove. Scleral injection can hasten the absorption of toxic substances. Although some managers may prohibit the wearing of contact lenses in the laboratory altogether, goggles or face shields can provide an acceptable level of protection. Special precautions also need to be taken by lens wearers who are manipulating solvents that are capable of dissolving the plastic of the corrective lens. In formulating a contact lens policy, it must be remembered that individuals who do not wear such lenses are also at risk; the safest strategy is to encourage the wearing of full facial protection for all employees engaged in tasks that chance splashing or spraying.

Mechanical devices should be always used for pipetting tasks. The pipetting of fluids by mouth is to be strictly prohibited throughout the laboratory. Even innocuous fluids such as water should be pipetted mechanically for consistency.

HOUSEKEEPING

Cleanliness and good housekeeping are attributes of the best laboratories. Litter should not accumulate. Storage of laboratory implements between uses keeps work areas clear, and this facilitates disinfection, decontamination, and hazard containment. Cluttered aisles are a nuisance that can lead to trips, falls, and lower-leg injuries. Accumulations of chairs, equipment, and boxes that block exits or otherwise interfere with emergency egress must be forbidden. Smoke doors must remain completely unobstructed so that they will close automatically in the event of fire. Free access to all emergency equipment (such as portable fire extinguishers, showers, and eyewash fixtures) must be ensured at all times. Clothing, signs, and decorations should never be hung over doorways or safety windows in any manner that obstructs the view. Floors and walls should be cleaned on a regular schedule. All cabinetry—including refrigerators, freezers, incubators, and water baths—should be cleaned and disinfected regularly and of course immediately after spills.

PERSONAL BARRIER PROTECTION

Gloves

Gloves, the most commonly used personal protective device, protect the wearer from contact with noxious substances and dangerous materials. All gloves should be fitted as comfortably as possible. Glove length must be sufficient to extend over the cuffs of the sleeves to protect the wrists.

Heavy rubber gloves, made of neoprene, nitrile, or butyl rubber, are designed for chemical protection. The gloves should be made of a material known to resist the chemicals to which the worker will be exposed. Glove materials are rated (in hours) as to the duration of protection provided and/or the rate of chemical permeation through the fabric.

Thin latex or vinyl gloves provide short-term protection against dusts and contaminated aqueous solutions. Minute and insensible defects can develop easily in such gloves, and viruses can slowly penetrate intact glovewear. Such gloves must be changed and discarded regularly to be effective (7).

Heat-reflective and insulated gloves protect against thermal injury when handling items at blistering temperatures or when working in frigid conditions.

Stainless-steel mesh gloves provide shielding when handling sharp items such as knife blades or broken glass.

Outer Wear

Laboratory coats (lab coats) are long-sleeved jackets of sufficient length to extend below the level of the work bench when the worker is standing and to fully cover the individual's lap as he or she sits at the work station. Lab coats should always be worn fully buttoned, and should be made of water-resistant fabric. Coats that are constructed of absorbent cloth must usually be overlaid with a plastic apron or tunic. *Gowns* provide a greater measure of protection. Gowns fit snugly at the wrists and neck and have either no frontal openings or a fully fastened frontal opening. *Jumpsuits* are fitted to the ankles as well as the wrist; they are appropriate in areas where hazardous dusts or liquids may contaminate stockings or trousers. *Water-resistant* garments are to be used when performing tasks that risk splashing with infectious or otherwise potentially infectious fluids. When chemical exposure is anticipated, outer wear must be constructed of a material that is resistant to the chemical that is handled. All single-use, protective outer wear should be changed as soon as possible after contamination; PPE designed for reuse should be cleaned or decontaminated as soon as possible after soiling.

Eye and Face Protection

Safety glasses are spectacles made of high-impact plastic; imperforate side shields at the temples are standard. Safety glasses usually provide a minimal and usually inadequate level of protection. *Goggles,* which fit snugly around the face, are preferred, and should be combined with masks that protect one's mouth and nose. More complete protection is provided by a *face shield,* a shatterproof plastic device that wraps around the face to safeguard all exposed facial skin (including the neck). Small, freestanding *area shields* rest on or are suspended over the work space, allowing the technologist to manipulate hazardous fluids with an acceptable level of eye and face protection. Activities that risk splashing or spraying with infectious materials or fluids that may irritate mucous membranes should be performed behind shields or while wearing goggles and a mask. Corrosive liquids should be manipulated with shield protection.

Respiratory Protection

Many types of devices are manufactured for respiratory protection. Such devices must be used to prevent the inhalation of fumes, dusts, or aerosols that may be harmful. The use of properly designed air-handling cabinetry (such as chemical fume hoods) is preferable, but personal protective equipment must be used whenever engineering controls provide inadequate protection.

The choice of a device for respiratory protection is based on the nature of the hazard that is targeted for control. *Dust masks* are simple cloth or paper devices that are nonetheless effective at preventing the inhalation of aerosols and particulates when properly fitted. *Fume masks* cover half the face and employ replaceable cartridges that contain absorbent chemicals. Each cartridge, chosen to reduce the exposure level of a specific group of noxious fumes, must be changed periodically. An *air-line* or *self-contained breathing apparatus* (SCBA) offers the greatest level of protection because all inspired air is delivered from an uncontaminated source. Each device must be used in accordance with its manufacturer's directions.

Respirators that fit tightly around the mouth and nose impede ventilation. Although their use is sometimes necessary, only employees who are physically able to breathe properly through the device should be allowed in a work environment in which their use is required. Safe use of the more complicated devices may depend on proper fit and training.

An SCBA is required whenever the use of a simpler device would result in levels of toxic vapors in inspired air that exceed safe limits, whenever the nature of the hazard is unknown, whenever the concentration of oxygen in ambient air is less than 19.5%, and whenever there is an acute hazard to life or health (8).

Chemical fume hoods that are ducted to the roof of the building provide an engineering alternative that is usually preferable to the wearing of personal protective equipment. The rating of the device is based on the airflow velocity at the face of the work area. Airflow is typically controlled by means of a sash made of laminated safety glass. A face velocity airflow of 125 feet per minute (fpm) is recommended (9). A *perchloric acid hood* is a special type of chemical fume hood and ducting system that is constructed of corrosion-resistant stainless steel. Some limited tasks that generate minimally hazardous but noxious fumes may safely be performed on a *down-draft platform* or at a *rear-plenum exhaust* work station; both systems draw vapors away from the face of the operator. The absorbent chemical filters of such devices are similar to those in portable fume masks.

WARNING SIGNAGE

Regulatory and Advisory Systems

A number of placarding systems have been devised to warn individuals of hazards and potential injury. Each addresses a specific target audience, and a combination of several systems will be necessary for most laboratories.

The Occupational Safety and Health Administration (OSHA) has defined one system for area signs (10). The signs are simple, direct, and textual. Red letters indicate a dangerous location, the nature of which is identified with black letters on a white background. A yellow background with black letters prompts one to use caution. Green signs are advisory and display helpful safety information. By virtue of their clarity and simplicity, OSHA-style signs convey minimal detail. They are intended to alert an individual who is approaching the area. Additional information (such as emergency procedures) may need to be posted nearby.

The National Fire Protection Association (NFPA) has developed a hazard identification system specifically for fire fighting (11) (Fig. 2.1). A diamond-shaped emblem is divided into four fields that are color coded to distinguish the type of hazard. Three of the fields display a numeral from zero (negligible hazard) to four (severe hazard). At the pinnacle is a

Identification of Health Hazard Color Code: BLUE		Identification of Flammability Color Code: RED		Identification of Reactivity (Stability) Color Code: YELLOW	
Signal	Type of Possible Injury	Signal	Susceptibility of Materials to Burning	Signal	Susceptibility to Release of Energy
4	Materials that on very short exposure could cause death or major residual injury.	4	Materials that will rapidly or completely vaporize at atmospheric pressure and normal ambient temperature, or that are readily dispersed in air and that will burn readily.	4	Materials that in themselves are readily capable of detonation or of explosive decomposition or reaction at normal temperatures and pressures.
3	Materials that on short exposure could cause serious temporary or residual injury.	3	Liquids and solids that can be ignited under almost all ambient temperature conditions.	3	Materials that in themselves are capable of detonation or explosive decomposition or reaction but require a strong initiating source or that must be heated under confinement before initiation or that react explosively with water.
2	Materials that on intense or continued but not chronic exposure could cause temporary incapacitation or possible residual injury.	2	Materials that must be moderately heated or exposed to relatively high ambient temperatures before ignition can occur.	2	Materials that readily undergo violent chemical change at elevated temperatures and pressures or that react violently with water or may form explosive mixtures with water.
1	Materials that on exposure would cause irritation but only minor residual injury.	1	Materials that must be preheated before ignition can occur.	1	Materials that in themselves are normally stable but can become unstable at elevated temperatures and pressures.
0	Materials that on exposure under fire conditions would offer no hazard beyond that of ordinary combustible material.	0	Materials that will not burn.	0	Materials that in themselves are normally stable, even under fire exposure conditions, and are not reactive with water.

Figure 2.1. Standard definitions for hazard levels. (Reprinted with permission from NFPA 704-1985, *Identification of the Fire Hazards of Materials,* Copyright © 1985, National Fire Protection Association, Quincy, MA 02269. This reprinted material is not the complete and official position of the National Fire Protection Association on the referenced subject, which is represented only by the standard in its entirety.)

red diamond that indicates the flammability risk of the chemicals stored in the room or cabinet. On the left is a blue diamond for health hazard posed by acute exposure through inhalation or dermal contact to those chemicals or to their combustion products. On the right a yellow diamond reflects the reactivity risk. The white diamond at the low point on the emblem may be emblazoned with the insignia ₩ (do not use water), OX (oxidizers present), or the international radiation symbol. It is important to understand that NFPA 704 is designed for the protection of fire fighters. It is an appropriate system to post at eye level on entryways and on cabinet doors. It is not the ideal system for individual reagent vessels, because the effects of chronic exposure to a chemical are not considered. NFPA 704 symbology should be used only with the consent and cooperation of the fire brigade and local fire department.

The United States Department of Transportation (DOT) requires the use of a different signage system. Partly pictorial and partly numeric, DOT signs are usually found on cartage vessels and containers. The signs can be very useful to the laboratorian who must choose the proper response to contain and decontaminate an otherwise unidentified but leaking shipping container.

Additional emblems have been promoted for specific tasks. Figure 2.2 displays standardized symbols for radiation hazards, biological hazards, carcinogenic agents, and laser devices.

The labels on reagent vessels should clearly delineate the hazards of the contents and their adverse effects on specific target organs. The identity of the chemical(s) contained therein is best specified in accordance with the International Union of Pure and Applied Chemistry (IUPAC) or the Chemical Abstracts Service (CAS) rules of nomenclature. The label may also specify the personal protective equipment required. Commercially labeled reagent containers often display additional information such as advice on first aid and spill cleanup. Secondary containers into which the contents are transferred should always be labeled with the key safety information (unless the sole user is the individual who made the transfer).

These labels are not to be removed nor obscured unless a proper label is to be immediately applied. Unlabeled containers should never be opened but

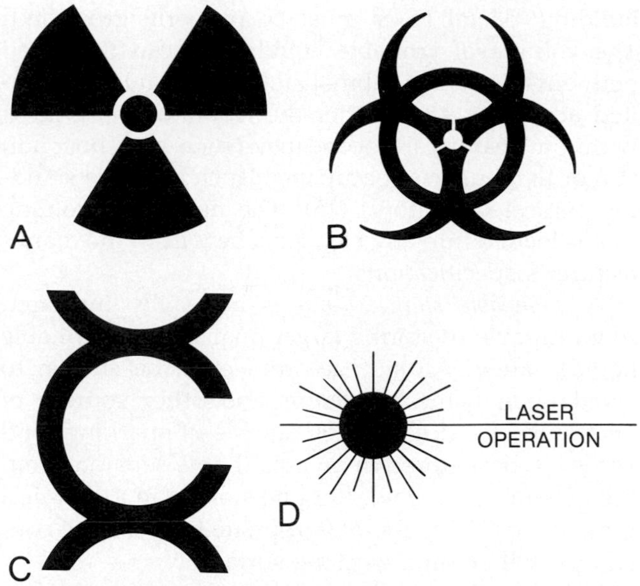

Figure 2.2. Standard symbols for radiation hazards (**A**), biohazards (**B**), carcinogens (**C**), and laser devices (**D**).

rather must be discarded as an unknown chemical that is presumed to be hazardous.

It is good laboratory practice to indicate on the label the date that each container was opened. Such a practice is a safety consideration when dealing with chemicals for which the hazard level increases with exposure to air. For example, diethyl ether slowly but spontaneously can form explosive peroxides when mixed with atmospheric oxygen; such a potential mandates limited storage after opening.

CHEMICAL HAZARDS

The smaller the quantity of hazardous materials that a laboratory has on hand, the better. The hazards of a laboratory chemical can be described in terms of ignitability, corrosivity, reactivity, and toxicity. The characteristics of many chemicals belong to more than one hazard class. Containment strategies are based on the nature of the hazards involved. A chemical hygiene plan (CHP) is a strategic approach to reagent and waste chemical hazard control (3). The CHP specifies the safety precautions appropriate for each class of chemicals that are in use in the laboratory. The goal is to promote the combination of engineering controls and safe work practices that best protects employees from the hazards of the chemicals they are using.

Exposures to fumes must be kept within permissible limits (see below). The CHP will identify (*a*) the criteria that will be used to determine the need for special control measures (such as personal protective equipment); (*b*) the exigencies for chemical exposure monitoring (i.e., anticipation of circumstances during which permissible exposure limits may be exceeded); and (*c*) the provision for medical attention when dangerous exposures do occur.

Corrosivity

The U.S. Environmental Protection Agency (EPA) has defined corrosive wastes on the basis of pH or the ability to corrode steel. Any aqueous waste that is extremely acidic (pH below 2.1), or extremely alkaline (pH above 12.5), or that can corrode SAE 1020 steel more than 0.250 inch/year at 55°C is corrosive (12). As a warning on a reagent label, however, the term may be used to refer to any substance that can cause visible destruction or irreversible alteration in human tissues at the site of contact.

Corrosives should always be stored near the floor and below eye level. A catchment basin on the floor near the point of use and the regular use of protective bottle carriers minimizes contact with a spilled chemical. Mutually incompatible chemicals (e.g., hydrocarbons [including organic acids] and strong oxidizers [such as sulfuric, nitric, or perchloric acid]) must be stored separately. Personnel must wear the proper equipment when handling corrosives. Gloves, aprons, and other protective garments should be constructed of materials that are known to be resistant to the corrosives in use. Vapors of corrosives are often highly irritating, and the pouring and pipetting of concentrated corrosive liquids within a chemical fume hood is highly recommended. The area of the laboratory in which corrosives are used must have an adequate source of water, such as an emergency shower and eyewash station, for rapid decontamination.

Ignitability

The NFPA has developed a useful classification system based on hazard potential (13). *Flammable* liquids are those with a very low flash point (the temperature at which a liquid gives off vapors in sufficient concentration to form an ignitable mixture with air) or boiling point (at normal atmospheric pressure) or both. Flammable liquids are divided into three groups. "Class IA" designates the most flammable liquids:

Class IA: flash point < 22.8°C and boiling point $<$ 37.8°C

Class IB: flash point < 22.8°C and boiling point $\geq$ 37.8°C

Class IC: flash point ≥ 22.8°C and boiling point $<$ 37.8°C

For example, diethyl ether (with a flash point of −45°C) and benzene (with a flash point of −11.1°C)

Table 2.1. Maximum Allowable Sizes of Containers of Ignitable Liquids[a]

Ignitability Class	Glass	Metal or Polyethylene	Safety Can
IA	1 pt (0.473 liter)	1 gal (3.8 liter)	2 gal (7.9 liter)
IB	1 gal (3.8 liter)	5 gal (19.0 liter)	5 gal (19.0 liter)
IC	1 gal (3.8 liter)	5 gal (19.0 liter)	5 gal (19.0 liter)
II	1 gal (3.8 liter)	5 gal (19.0 liter)	5 gal (19.0 liter)
III	5 gal (19.0 liter)	5 gal (19.0 liter)	5 gal (19.0 liter)

[a]Adapted with permission from NFPA 30-1987, *Flammable and Combustible Liquids Code*, Copyright © 1987, National Fire Protection Association, Quincy, MA 02269. This reprinted material is not the complete and official position of the National Fire Protection Association on the referenced subject, which is represented only by the standard in its entirety.

are Class IA liquids. Absolute ethanol has a flash point of 12.8° C and is a Class IB liquid.

Combustible liquids have a flash point that is greater than 37.8°C. Combustible liquids are also classified into three groups:

Class II: flash point ≥ 37.8°C and < 60°C
Class IIIA: flash point ≥ 60°C and < 93.3°C
Class IIIB: flash point ≥ 93.3°C

As an example, 37% aqueous formaldehyde (the solution usually referred to as "formalin") has a flash point of 85°C and is therefore grouped within NFPA Class IIIA.

The value of this classification system can be seen in Table 2.1. The ignitability risk of a stored chemical is a function of the nature of the substance, the type of storage vessel that contains it, and its shielding from sources of ignition. Specially designed flammable solvent containers are safer storage vessels than glass bottles. A *safety can* is made of metal or polymer. It has a spring-closing cap, a pressure-release valve, and a flame arrestor within the spout. Storing flammable liquids in an ordinary glass vessel is a greater hazard than storing the same amount of material in a safety can.

These definitions are derived from the National Fire Code. Regulatory agencies may use slightly different definitions. For example, the EPA uses the term "ignitable" to refer to liquids that have a flash point less than 60°C, are strong oxidizers, or have some other property that contributes significantly to a fire hazard (such as the capability to cause a fire through friction, absorption of moisture, or spontaneous chemical change) (14).

A *flammable storage cabinet* (FSC) is designed to sequester its contents from heat during a conflagration. The purpose is to allow personnel a short amount of time (about 10 minutes) to evacuate the laboratory before the liquids inside ignite. An FSC can be constructed of metal or wood. The door should fit tightly and preferably be self-closing. An FSC may be either entirely enclosed or vented to the exterior of the building. Metal FSCs must be properly grounded. The volume of ignitable liquids that can be stored both outside such a cabinet and within an FSC is limited according to whether the laboratory is located within a health care occupancy (such as a hospital) (15) or in a business occupancy (such as a free-standing clinical laboratory) (16). The maximum volume that is loaded into any FSC must be within the manufacturer's specifications.

A *flammable storage vault* is a heavily insulated room capable of storing larger quantities of ignitable liquids safely. All storage areas must be chosen to avoid open flames, radiators and other sources of heat, and electrical devices capable of sparking. Solvents are best stored in an area that is separate from the general work flow. Routine storage in a chemical fume hood is usually inappropriate because the containers will be on a working surface.

Cold liquids are less hazardous than warm liquids of the same composition because the vapor pressure is lower. Storage of volatile solvents in refrigerators and freezers is best avoided, however, because of the possibility of accumulation of vapors: when the door is opened, the concentrated vapors are released and may travel considerable distances along the floor to a point of ignition. Refrigerators that must be used for storage of flammable liquids must be "explosion proof"; i.e., be devoid of interior electrical switches and have specially shielded motors that prevent ignition of the vapors by the refrigerator unit itself.

Reactivity

Chemicals capable of violent decomposition at normal temperatures and pressures form a separate hazard class. This term is reserved for chemicals that are unstable or that can undergo violent change without detonation. It also applies to substances that react violently or form a potentially violent mixture in water, or that are capable of explosive decomposition (17). Examples are hydrazines and elemental sodium.

Toxicity

This term can refer to almost any substance in quantity. Aspirin, vitamin preparations, and other commonly encountered substances have all caused fatal poisonings. Even water can cause an acute intoxication if sufficient quantities are ingested over a short interval. In a safety context, the term is generally applied if a substance that is inhaled, ingested, or contacted in small amounts can cause serious biological effects. Toxicity may be short-term or long-term. *Irritants* cause a local inflammatory effect on living tissues at the site of contact. Irritants may be identified as either "primary skin irritants" or as "primary eye irritants" or both. A *sensitizer* is a chemical that can elicit an allergic reaction in a susceptible individual after repeated exposure. *Asphyxiants* are chemicals that exert an adverse effect by displacing atmospheric oxygen or by preventing the metabolic use of available oxygen. Many gases are asphyxiating in large quantity.

Among the long-term toxins, *mutagens* are chemicals that can cause a hereditable change in genetic material. There are many different test systems to detect mutagenic potential. Those that employ living organisms usually measure the effect of the substance on lower organisms such as bacteria, fungi, or insects. Because of this, the term "mutagen" is frequently applied to substances that have not been shown to cause genetic changes in mammalian species. *Reproductive effects* are those that affect fertility, that cause developmental abnormalities during gestation, or that can have adverse effects on newborns. *Tumorigens* are substances that have been reported to be associated with benign or malignant tumors. *Carcinogens* are substances that have been shown to cause malignant neoplasms in valid animal tests (using control animals and appropriate statistical methods) or that have conclusively been shown to cause malignant neoplasms in humans. Authoritative sources include the International Agency for Research on Cancer and the United States National Toxicology Program. *Neoplastinogens* cause tumors that cannot definitely be classified as either benign or malignant.

The mode of contact is an important variable in estimating the toxicity of a substance. Some chemicals may produce serious biological effects after only short-term exposure; such chemicals are termed *acutely toxic*. Standard tests have been developed to measure and define such acute toxins. The toxicity is usually defined by the dose required to kill 50% of test animals (LD_{50}). The route of administration and the stated dosage must be provided, followed by the species of animal in which the substance was tested. The lower the concentration at which toxic effects can be measured, the more toxic the chemical. For example, "LD_{50}(oral)<50 mg/kg," "LD_{50}(oral)<15 ml/kg," and "LD_{50}(inhalation)<100 ppm" are descriptions of extremely toxic chemicals.

Restrictions should be applied to the use of chemicals that precipitate the most serious consequences. Chemicals of special concern include acutely toxic chemicals as well as carcinogens and reproductive toxins.

Access to areas in which such chemicals can be found should be strictly limited to those who have specifically been trained to contain the hazards. Mandatory apparel may include gloves, tightly fitting goggles, dust masks, and jumpsuits. Disposable items are preferred. All personnel must thoroughly wash their hands and any areas of skin exposure thoroughly following accidental contact with restricted chemicals.

The American Conference of Governmental Industrial Hygienists (ACGIH) is one useful source for recommendations on chemical exposure limits (18). Sources used by the ACGIH include industrial experience as well as human and animal studies. Two major types of *permissible exposure limits* (PELs), designated as *threshold limits values* (TLVs), are recognized by the ACGIH. "TLV-TWAs" (TLVs based on 8-hour, time-weighted averages) are used to denote the permissible exposures for substances to which workers are exposed repeatedly, day after day and week after week, without adverse effect. "TLV-STELs" (TLVs based on *short-term exposure limits*) are the concentrations of vapors to which workers can be exposed continuously for brief periods (15 minutes) without suffering irritation, tissue damage, or narcosis. The OSHA has defined an *action level* (AL) for selected substances. ALs, generally set at one-half of the 8-hour PEL, are administrative decision points that trigger environmental monitoring or other occupational health undertakings.

Chemical spill control materials should be located strategically throughout the laboratory. The simplest material is sand (often mixed with soda ash) that can be applied around a spill as a dike to contain the hazard. The CHP should specify the appropriate decontamination procedure for each class of hazardous chemical. Only emergency response personnel should be allowed in the vicinity. If the vapor level of the spilled substance is dangerous, the proper respirators must be worn by everyone in the room.

An important source of information about the hazards of a chemical substance is the Material Safety Data Sheet (MSDS). These are OSHA-required documents that must be supplied by the vendor in the United States. MSDS information includes the chemical name and synonyms, its hazards, proper PPE, suggested medical intervention following acute exposure, and spill cleanup details. The MSDS may be the only source of information for some mixtures and proprietary formulations, but MSDSs should not be construed as the sole sources of authoritative data. Other sources are the Registry of Toxic Effects of Chemical Substances (National Institute of Occupational Safety and Health, Washington, DC), TOXLINE (National Library of Medicine, Bethesda, MD), and Chemical Abstracts Service (Columbus, OH).

COMPRESSED GASES

All compressed gases are hazardous because of the potential of rupture of the container; many are also toxic or ignitable. The breakage of the regulating valve of a compressed gas cylinder can propel the cylinder like a missile. A heated cylinder will explode when its ability to contain the growing internal pressure is exceeded.

All but the smallest cylinders should be secured upright. Each cylinder should be labeled indelibly as to its contents. Additional, temporary labels that read "in use" or "empty" may be applied. Cylinders should be moved only with hand carts to which they have been secured. The rolling or dragging of cylinders must be strictly forbidden.

Both gas cylinders and piped systems have pressure regulating devices. These valve systems are designed separately for each family of gases and must not be interchanged. Valve safety covers must be in place until pressure regulators are attached. Threaded fittings must be tightened carefully with the properly sized wrench. Cylinders and connections should always be tested with a soap solution for leaks after attaching, adjusting, or disconnecting the system. Valves should never be lubricated.

The typical valve system has two components: a high-pressure valve at or near the tank to release the contents and a low-pressure valve at the point of use to regulate the flow. Valves should be opened slowly, and personnel should stand to the side of the gauge as a precaution against blowout. Valves should be maintained in the closed position when the cylinder is not in active use.

Flammable gases must be used with special caution. Supplies should be minimal. Only cylinders in active use should be in the work area. The storage facility should be a secured room or enclosure reserved exclusively for that purpose. The location should be away from combustible materials, elevators, stairs, and passageways. Oxidizing gases must be separated from flammable gases. Sources of ignition should be carefully insulated from the emplacement of the cylinders.

"Empty" cylinders awaiting return to the vendor should be treated with respect, since considerable pressure may remain within.

MICROBIOLOGICAL HAZARDS

All clinical specimens are potential sources of infection. Human blood and body fluids may carry viruses such as the hepatitis B virus, hepatitis C virus, and the human immunodeficiency viruses. Control of hazards of this type is a concern throughout the clinical laboratory. Workers in microbiology laboratories face the additional risks of the pathogens that are isolated and cultured.

Development of an exposure control plan (ECP) (19) designed to contain the infectious hazards of the laboratory is highly recommended. Each task or procedure that involves the potential for exposure to infectious agents is to be identified in the ECP. Engineering controls should be introduced wherever feasible to minimize the hazards. Work practice controls should be specified. Required PPE should be clearly identified in the ECP for each hazardous task.

Containment systems must be designed with an understanding of the virulence and the route of introduction of the agent into the body. *Ingestion* of agents may complicate mouth pipetting. Failure to wash one's hands thoroughly when leaving the laboratory but before eating or smoking may introduce agents into the mouth. *Parenteral exposure* can result from direct inoculation or absorption through the mucous membranes of the eyes, nose, or mouth. Even small scratches and abrasions can allow entry of agents that would otherwise be excluded by intact skin. Contact leading to ingestion of agents or parenteral exposure may be either direct or indirect. *Direct contact* includes splashes and sprays of infectious fluids. The inadvertent transfer of contaminants from inanimate surfaces such as telephones or keyboards to the face or eyes is an example of *indirect contact*. Scrupulous attention to good work practices and consistent use of personal barrier protection minimizes the risk of ingestion and contact exposure.

Inhalation of aqueous aerosols and fomites can cause respiratory infections. Aerosols may be formed by dropping solutions onto hard surfaces, by the rapid heating of liquids (including moisture on inoculation loops), and by many other inadvertent motions. Containment is possible with careful technique and by performing all operations that predictably generate aerosols (such as centrifugation and sonication) within a biological safety cabinet.

Biological Safety Cabinetry

Microbiological hazards are best contained within a properly engineered biological safety cabinet (BSC) (20). *Class I* cabinets operate at negative pressure with a minimum face airflow velocity of 75 feet/minute. The air in the chamber is exhausted through a high efficiency particulate air (HEPA) filter. The front of the Class I BSC may be either open or fitted with arm-length rubber gloves. A *Class II* BSC features vertical airflow and interior air that is recirculated through HEPA filters. The chamber operates at a negative pressure with respect to the room identical to an open-front Class I cabinet, but the purified air within minimizes contamination of the cultures under study. Class I and Class II cabinets provide a similar level of personnel safety. *Class III* cabinetry must be used for the most virulent agents. The chamber is entirely enclosed. The contents must be manipulated by means of arm-length rubber gloves fitted to the chamber wall. All materials entering and exiting the Class III BSC must be autoclaved or decontaminated.

Class I and II cabinets are commonly found in clinical laboratories. Class III BSCs are needed in specialized facilities that culture agents such as *Mycobacterium tuberculosis* or systemic fungi and when production-level quantities of less infectious agents such as human immunodeficiency virus are involved.

Biosafety Levels

The Centers for Disease Control (CDC) and the National Institutes of Health have codified a system of increasing levels of containment for microbiological and clinical laboratories (20). *Biosafety Level (BSL) I* is designed for student laboratories using agents not ordinarily infectious for humans. Work may be conducted on open benchtops. Good laboratory practices include use of pipetting devices, prompt spill cleanup, daily disinfection, and proper waste disposal. Clinical laboratories should routinely follow *Biosafety Level II* precautions. BSL II differs from BSL I in that access to the area should be restricted to exclude untrained individuals and that certain procedures such as those that generate infectious aerosols are to be conducted in BSCs. BSL II is effective at containing the infectious hazards of blood-borne agents in clinical laboratory specimens. Routine bacteriological procedures such as plating and preparing smears for staining may be conducted at BSL II. Parasitic investigations, most bacterial studies, and some fungal and viral culture manipulations may safely be contained with BSL II precautions. *Biosafety Level III* is appropriate for laboratories that work with agents that may cause fatal disease following inhalation. Access to the laboratory and airflow are carefully controlled. All procedures must be performed in BSCs or similar devices. Personnel must wear fully protective laboratory clothing. Few clinical laboratories other than those culturing systemic fungi and tubercle bacilli need to follow BSL III containment.

Universal Precautions

Most clinical laboratory activities require the handling of blood or body fluids (5, 21, 22). The CDC and the National Committee for Clinical Laboratory Standards (NCCLS) have developed a system for worker protection commonly referred to as *universal precautions* (UP). This set of engineering controls, work practice controls, and use of personal protective equipment collectively shields the laboratory worker from the potential of exposure to blood-borne infectious agents.

The primary agents of concern are the human hepatitis and immunodeficiency viruses. The hepatitis B virus (HBV) is a DNA virus that causes approximately 12,000 infections in health care workers each year. During acute hepatitis B, the virus is in high concentration in the blood and serous fluids—10^8 to 10^9 infectious units/ml (5). One percent (or more) of hospitalized patients are chronic carriers of the virus (23). The virus can survive dried on work surfaces. Any procedure or material identified by the EPA as a sterilant or high-level disinfectant can inactivate HBV when used as directed.

The human immunodeficiency viruses (HIV-1 and HIV-2) are RNA retroviruses. HIV has been shown to spread by means of blood, semen, vaginal secretions, cerebrospinal fluid, serous fluids, and breast milk. The concentration of HIV in clinical specimens is far lower than that of HBV (10^0 to 10^2 infectious doses per milliliter (5). The virus is slowly inactivated by drying (24). Any disinfectant that is capable of inactivating HBV will be effective against HIV because the latter agent is far more susceptible to such treatment.

Other agents are transmissible in blood and body fluids. The viremia associated with hepatitis A is brief and precedes symptoms by several days. There is no chronic carrier state associated with hepatitis A. Hepatitis C virus (HCV) has not been fully characterized, although its proteins have. The degree of risk of occupational illness from HCV is unknown. HCV is the primary agent for transfusion-transmitted hepatitis (25) and it is therefore known to be blood-borne. Delta agent or hepatitis D virus is an incomplete virus found only in the blood of chronic carriers of HBV. Epidemiologic studies suggest that other, uncharacterized hepatitis viruses exist. Other blood-borne illnesses that could be transmitted through exposure to clinical blood specimens that contain viable agents include malaria, syphilis, babesiosis, brucellosis, leptospirosis, arboviral infections, borelliosis, Creutzfeld-Jacob disease, human T-lymphotropic virus type I, viral hemorrhagic fevers, and cytomegalovirus infection.

The concepts of universal precautions apply to all human blood and tissues. Serous fluids such as pleural, peritoneal, pericardial, amniotic, cerebrospinal, and synovial fluids are included. Semen and vaginal secretions are equally hazardous. All other clinical specimens (such as sputum, stool, sweat, urine, tears, gastric contents, and saliva) are of less concern; UP need apply only if such substances contain visible amounts of blood (5).

The elements of good general laboratory safety practice are part of universal precautions. Personnel must use proper barrier precautions when handling clinical specimens. Latex or vinyl gloves should be worn and changed regularly. Water-resistant gowns, aprons, or smocks and face protection should be added when there is the possibility of splashing or splatters. Additional, water-tight, occlusive dressings should be worn over any area of nonintact skin of the hands or forearms. Frequent handwashing throughout the day (especially whenever gloves are changed) is fundamental. All specimens of blood and body fluids should be collected and transported in containers that prevent leakage; any such container that has the potential for exterior contamination must be transported in a leak-resistant secondary container such as a plastic bag. Workers should be careful not to contaminate work surfaces, containers, requisitions, and reports. Visibly blood-tinged stains and spills must be decontaminated as soon as they occur or are discovered. All work surfaces must be decontaminated at the end of each work shift as well. Techniques that avoid the formation of spatters and droplets should be a regular part of new-employee training and continuing education programs. All pipetting tasks must be performed with the use of mechanical devices. Biohazard warning labels should be applied to all containers that contain contaminated items. Infectious wastes must be packaged and properly destroyed. All sharps must be handled with respect and discarded in puncture-resistant containers. Selection of technologies that employ less hazardous alternatives (such as avoiding the use of sharp implements or substitution of automated for manual methods) is also part of universal precautions.

Human tissues require special handling. All surgical specimens should be sealed in leakproof containers within the operating room. Containers with contaminated exterior surfaces must be placed in plastic bags prior to transport to the laboratory. Frozen sectioning of unfixed tissue requires special care. Most of the infectious agents of concern are not inactivated by freezing. Freezing of tissue must be performed cautiously; the spraying of tissue with freezing gases under pressure should be prohibited because it may spatter infectious materials. The interior of the tissue cryostat must be decontaminated regularly.

The entire autopsy suite should be considered to be a biohazardous area. Only those individuals essential to the performance of the examination should be allowed in the area. The individuals at the prosection table should wear full-barrier PPE including face and eye protection, masks, water-repellent clothing, aprons, shoe covers, and two sets of rubber gloves. Steel mesh gloves are highly desirable. An assistant whose clothing remains uncontaminated should be assigned to circulate in the clean areas of the morgue. All procedures that may spray or spatter blood or tissue must be performed carefully. Electric bone saws, for example, naturally generate aerosols and particulates; the connection of vacuum exhaust to the saws or the performance of such procedures under plastic shrouds help to contain the hazard. All tissues should be fixed at the autopsy table to limit the number of work surfaces that will inevitably be contaminated with blood.

Special precautions apply to the handling of tissues derived from patients with Creutzfeld-Jakob disease. The agent(s) are resistant to inactivation by formalin and other aldehyde fixative, alcohols, and heat (up to 100°C) (26). Strict adherence to UP is required. 5.25% aqueous sodium hypochlorite or 1 N sodium hydroxide is effective for inactivating the agents on surfaces. Discarded fluids and contaminated instruments may be treated by soaking in 5.25% sodium hypochlorite for 1 hour or by autoclaving at 132°C for 1 hour (27).

Decontamination

Any procedure or technology that reduces the infectivity of a substance or material to a safe (noninfectious) level is a *decontaminant*. *Germicide* is a general term for any substance that can kill pathogenic agents. The EPA registers germicides in three general categories. A *sterilant* completely destroys all infectious agents (including mycobacteria and bacterial spores). A *disinfectant* is effective against selected microorganisms. The spectrum of activity of commercial disinfectants can be found on the product label or in the accompanying literature. Disinfectants may not be effective against bacterial spores or mycobacteria. The effective action of all disinfectants requires adequate contact time; therefore, the manufacturer's instructions should always be followed. An *antiseptic* is a chemical germicide appropriate for use on skin, tissue, or mucous membranes. Antiseptics should not be used as laboratory disinfectants. Table 2.2 lists some common disinfectants and their spectra of activity.

Spilled blood or tissue samples must be cleaned up and the area decontaminated. Cleaning personnel must wear and use proper PPE. Forceps or scoops should be employed to remove broken glass without the need for manual contact. The bulk of the spill is absorbed onto paper towels, and the towels are properly discarded as infectious waste. Proteins and lipids in the stain can inactivate chemical disinfectants or form a barrier around infectious agents. Therefore, the residuum is next cleaned with detergent and water. After all visible blood has been removed, an appropriate disinfectant is applied. A freshly diluted, 1:10 solution of household bleach (5.25% aqueous sodium hypochlorite) suffices. Iodophors formulated as hard-surface disinfectants

Table 2.2. Decontaminants and Their Spectra of Activity[a]

Decontaminant	Concentration of Active Ingredient	Temperature °C	Contact Time (*min*)	Vegetative Bacteria	Lipo Viruses	Tubercle Bacilli	Hydrophilic Viruses	Bacterial Spores
Autoclave (saturated steam)	(15 lb/in^2)	121	50–90	+	+	+	+	+
Autoclave (saturated steam)	(27 lb/in^2)	132	10–20	+	+	+	+	+
Dry heat oven		160–180	180–240	+	+	+	+	+
UV irradiation	40 mW/cm^2		10–30	+	+	+	±	
Ethylene oxide	400–800 mg/liter	35–60	105–240	+	+	+	+	+
Paraformaldehyde (gas)	0.3 g/ft^3	>23	60–180	+	+	+	+	+
Quaternary ammonium compounds	0.1–2%		10–30	+	+			
Phenolic compounds	0.2–3%		10–30	+	+	±		
Chlorine compounds	0.1–5%		10–30	+	+	+	+	±
Iodophor compounds	0.47%		10–30	+	+	+	±	
Alcohol (ethyl or isopropyl)	75–85%		10–30	+	+		±	
Formaldehyde (liquid)	4–8%	75–85%	10–30	+	+	+	+	±
Glutaraldehyde	2%		10–600	+	+	+	+	+

[a]Adapted from Vesley D, Lauer J. Decontamination, sterilization, disinfection, and antisepsis in the microbiology laboratory. In: BM Miller, ed. Laboratory Safety: Principles and Practice. Washington, DC: American Society for Microbiology, 1986:188–189.
[b]+, very positive response; ±, less positive response; a blank denotes a negative response or not applicable.

may also be used. Aldehydes (as aqueous glutaraldehyde or formaldehyde) and phenols are also effective but are toxic; such substances should only be used in areas of adequate ventilation or with the aid of a chemical fume mask.

The decontamination of laboratory instruments should be a regular event. The frequency of application depends on the intensity of use. Maintenance personnel should wear gloves during all such activities. Additional equipment should be donned for special tasks. Steel mesh gloves are needed for cleaning microtome knives, and facial protection is important when working with pressurized devices. Accidental spills within instruments must be cleaned and disinfected promptly. Exposure potential can be minimized by sensible technique. Breakage of sample tubes within a centrifuge is an example. The rotor must be allowed to come to a full stop and 30 minutes or more should elapse before opening the lid; this allows airborne droplets to settle. Glass shards are removed with forceps. The interior may then be wiped down with detergent and disinfectant. The preferable routine is to use centrifuge cups that are equipped with tightly fitted lids; broken glass and blood will be confined to a single cup.

Accidental Exposures and Immunizations

All susceptible clinical laboratory workers who frequently come into contact with blood or tissue should be vaccinated against HBV (28). HBV vaccine is synthesized from recombinant DNA. Three intradeltoid injections are required, the second and third after 1 month and 6 months, respectively. The vaccine is not required for individuals who are known to have adequate titers of antibodies to the hepatitis B surface antigen.

Vaccines for immunoprophylaxis are available for workers who are regularly exposed to specific agents of virulence (29). Inactivated or live, attenuated vaccines may be considered for veterinary laboratory workers (e.g., anthrax, tularemia, Q-fever) or for workers in specialized public health laboratories (e.g., polio, yellow fever, equine encephalitis). All susceptible women of childbearing age who work with rubella should be vaccinated against this virus.

Plans for medical treatment following accidental exposures should be written in the laboratory's policy manual. Immediate treatment can prevent or mitigate an infection. The infectivity of the source and the susceptibility of the injured worker determine the type of therapy and the dosage schedule. For example, an unvaccinated individual exposed to HBV would be treated immediately with hepatitis B immune globulin and then begun on the HBV vaccine series.

There is no commercially available vaccine for HIV, but immediate prophylaxis with zidovudine (AZT) may be effective (5). (For this and all prophylactic and therapeutic decisions, the current recommendations of the Centers for Disease Control should be consulted. These are available through hospital departments of infection control and public health clinics.) Following acute exposure, the infectivity for HIV should be determined by testing the source material for HIV antibodies (or HIV antigen or

HIV DNA). Testing the exposed worker for antibodies to HIV at the time of exposure will allow detection of postexposure seroconversion. Subsequent antibody studies in seronegative workers should be performed at 6 weeks, 12 weeks, and 6 months. The results of all such studies must be accompanied by knowledgeable counseling.

RADIATION HAZARDS

Ionizing radiation can be one of the most toxic sources of exposure to personnel in the laboratory. Acute exposures can lead to lymphocytolysis, bone marrow suppression, and damage to enteric epithelia. Low-level exposure can produce genetic damage to germinal and somatic tissues with the potential for birth defects and neoplasms. Sources of radiation hazards in the laboratory include both medical devices and reagent materials.

Medical devices that generate ionizing radiation must always be used according to the manufacturers' instructions. Policies should be established to restrict the access of untrained individuals to the areas of radiation hazard. If the source is potent, continuous monitoring of the room to ensure that the shielding is intact is advisable. Moving or repairing the device must be done under the guidance of expert technicians who are skilled in radiation containment.

The radionuclides found in laboratories are generally limited to tracer chemicals that are of insignificant hazard unless ingested or absorbed. The same good laboratory techniques that effectively contain infectious hazards will limit personal exposure to soluble radionuclides. Gloves should be worn when handling radioactive materials, and handwashing after glove removal is to be emphasized. Any manipulation that might lead to hand-to-mouth or hand-to-mucous membrane transfer must be prohibited. Workbenches should always be covered with an absorbent paper toweling, to be changed at the end of each shift (or after overt contamination) and properly discarded.

Reagent nuclides include beta emitters (e.g., ^{3}H, ^{14}C, ^{32}P, and ^{35}S) and gamma emitters (e.g., ^{51}Cr, ^{125}I). Alpha particles are emitted by heavy elements and are unlikely to be found in clinical laboratories. Low-energy beta emitters such as ^{3}H or ^{14}C will produce adverse health effects only if ingested or absorbed; higher-energy beta emitters such as ^{32}P can produce significant skin exposure. Gamma and x-ray emissions are penetrating and can cause biological damage without contact. The amount of radiation to which an employee may be exposed is specified by law (30), but the general principle is that exposures be maintained "as low as reasonably achievable" (ALARA) (31). The U.S. Nuclear Regulatory Commission expects employers to have an operational ALARA program.

Warning signs that indicate the presence of radioactivity should be posted in all areas where radionuclides are stored, used, or discarded.

Regulations of the U.S. Nuclear Regulatory Commission and the Canadian Atomic Energy Commission specify procedures that must be followed when shipping and receiving radioactive materials. The individuals responsible for radiation safety in the clinical laboratory must be aware of the applicable regulations and incorporate them into the policies and procedures. Recommendations of this chapter for this reason may be superseded by governmental requirements. All shipments received should have the date and time received, the method of shipment, the condition of the package upon receipt, and the amount and type of radionuclide contained within recorded. Damaged packaging should be checked for contaminating radiation. A leaking package should be sealed in a plastic bag and secured. All areas that may have been contaminated should be surveyed and decontaminated as necessary.

Thermoluminescent dosimetry badges or film-badge dosimeters are suggested for all laboratory workers who are exposed to gamma irradiation, although their use with the usual low-level amounts of tracers found in clinical laboratories is optional. The type of badge device should be chosen by a knowledgeable radiation physicist or safety officer and should be based on the specific type of exposure anticipated.

All workbenches, refrigerators, and other storage areas should be checked regularly for signs of contamination. The most useful surveys are performed immediately after completion of a task; this allows estimation of maximal exposure. Surface activity should be below 200 disintegrations per minute (dpm) per 100 cm^2 (32). Work areas should be surveyed for contamination regularly. This may be performed with a typical survey rate meter. Acceptable levels are usually 2 to 3 times background. An alternative is to wipe the work areas with sponges soaked in alcohol or aqueous detergent. The sponges are wiped vigorously over a 100-cm^2 area of the contaminated surface, placed in a counting vial, and read on the usual analytic instrument.

Spills and Cleanup

Decontamination personnel must wear gown or coat, apron, gloves, and eye protection. Disposable items are strongly preferred over clothing that requires laundering. The contaminated area should be scrubbed with water and detergent (preferably using a cleaning compound designed for radiation decontamination). After the area is cleansed it should be checked for residual radioactivity. The process must be repeated if the radioactivity is greater than 3 times the background or more than 200 dpm. All disposable materials involved in the cleanup must be discarded as radioactive waste unless survey measurements have indicated the amount of radiation remaining in the materials to be less than twice background. Each spill incident and decontamination episode should be carefully documented. Personnel involved should be advised to seek medical evaluation if the exposure was significant.

FIRE PREVENTION AND CONTROL

There are multiple sources of combustible materials in the clinical laboratory. These include ignitable liquids and flammable gases, as well as paper and wood construction materials. The laboratory must be designed to minimize these hazards. It is prudent to train personnel to intercede as soon as possible in a fire emergency because fires are most easily extinguished when still small. Emergency evacuation may be necessary to prevent injury to personnel; therefore, plans to clear each location within the laboratory should be made beforehand and explained to the staff. Laboratories located within hospitals are potential sources of ignition that may place bedridden patients and visitors at risk.

The working supplies of all ignitable materials should be minimal. Only modest amounts of reserve supplies should be kept, and these should be stored in proper flammable liquid storage cabinets or vaults. Safety cans should be used for all bulk storage of 5 gallons or less in which the purity of the solvent will not be compromised by the steel or polyethylene container.

All potential ignition sources should be identified and controlled. Obvious sources include open flames and heating elements, but sparking may occur within any electrical switch or motor. Static discharges are preventable sources of ignition; grounding of metal containers during transfer of combustible liquids will prevent sparking. Exothermic chemical reactions may also generate sufficient heat to ignite a fuel source. Clear separation of flammable materials from such ignition points is indicated.

The laboratory should be designed for fire protection. Walls and doors should be constructed to contain a conflagration until fire fighting equipment and personnel can be mustered. (In general, this specifies that walls be rated at 1 hour and door assemblies at 45 minutes.) Fire exits must be provided for emergency evacuation of personnel. Rooms that have an area larger than 1000 ft^2 and all rooms in which flammability concerns are present must have at least two doors that open to exit corridors or to the outdoors.

A *fire alarm system* should be located in or near the laboratory. This may be a bell or public address system, but it must be audible in all areas of the facility, including storage areas, darkrooms, and lavatories.

Portable fire extinguishers should be located wherever significant fire hazards exist. Class A devices are appropriate for wood and paper fires, Class B devices for ignitable solvents, and Class C devices for electrical fires (33). Three types are commonly found in clinical laboratories: Halon 1211, carbon dioxide, and dry chemical. All are effective against solvent and electrical fires; the label on the device will specify the rating of the unit. *Halon* extinguishers are rapidly effective. They are most commonly found in electrical applications such as computer rooms because their vapor will not damage delicate equipment. *Carbon dioxide* acts by smothering and cooling a fire. Devices of this type are equally rapid but may cause thermal damage to instruments in the vicinity of use. Both types should be used only in well-ventilated areas or by a person wearing self-contained breathing apparatus. *Dry chemical* types are the least expensive. They are particularly effective against oil and grease fires, but cleanup is laborious and equipment damage can be expected. Water-based extinguishers are effective only against Class A fires, and should not be used in clinical laboratories.

Laboratory personnel should practice their responses to fire situations. Training sessions should emphasize sounding the alarm as the first action. Attempts to extinguish the fire should follow, but only if the proper devices are immediately available and the fire appears small enough to manage. Evacuation of the area may be necessary. Employees should be trained to close doors and windows as they leave by the designated exits.

All personnel working in hazardous areas should be trained to use the types of portable fire extinguishers chosen. There is no substitute for "hands-on" experience. Fire exit drills should be held regularly. Each employee should know the preferred and the alternate exit route for his or her work station well enough to be able to find them in a darkened, smoke-filled atmosphere. Exit drills should be held at least once a year for the benefit of all employees.

ELECTRICAL SAFETY

Electrical hazards are among the most difficult to detect in clinical laboratories. Shock hazards can develop in any electrical instrument or appliance. The laboratory should be surveyed at least once a year as part of an electrical safety inspection. All new instruments should be thoroughly inspected before being placed into service.

The *preventive maintenance* program should include regular safety inspections of all electrical devices by a qualified individual. The power supply cable must be checked for frayed or cracked insulation and for broken wires. Electrical equipment must be properly grounded, i.e., the power cable must be of three-wire construction and the neutral (green) wire must be in electrical continuity from the power supply chassis to the plug. (An exception may be made for a device that is doubly insulated or totally encased in plastic.) Grounding of electrical appliances to cold-water plumbing is not recommended, but if used, the adequacy should be verified annually.

Instruments should be checked by a qualified electrician for current leakage with the ground open. The manufacturer's specifications should be used to determine the maximum allowable current for this test. When such specifications are not provided, a 100-mA current may be used to test most devices.

Electrical receptacles should be checked for ganged plugs, loose fittings, and broken faceplates. Electrical tests for polarity and ground continuity should be performed annually. Ground fault circuit interrupters must be installed in "wet" locations.

Electrical equipment used in areas wherein ignitable vapors might accumulate should be designed and approved for such uses. Examples include flammable liquid storage vaults and applications that require heating of flammable and combustible solvents.

The safety training program should anticipate electrical accidents. All personnel should know that the first response is to disconnect power to the arcing or burning equipment *if it can be done without personal risk*. This is especially important for individuals working in the vicinity of high-voltage devices, such as those used for electrophoresis.

SPECIALIZED EQUIPMENT

Hazards may accompany any new item of laboratory equipment. Items that have moving parts, thermal elements, pressurized components, or radiant energy may be of particular concern. The procedures manuals that accompany such devices must describe the particular risk and make recommendations for worker protection.

Centrifuges that have large rotors are mechanical hazards. Hair or clothing can become entangled in the mechanism if the centrifuge is allowed to operate with its cover open. Unbalanced cups and broken glass can be especially dangerous. All centrifuges should be fitted with a lid that is connected to a power-interruption switch to prevent operation with the rotor exposed. Spinning rotors must never be slowed or stopped by manual means.

Autoclaves must be operated by trained and knowledgeable individuals. Steam under pressure and heated to temperatures above the normal boiling point of water presents risks of scalding and explosion. The installation and fittings should be examined periodically by a stationary engineer. The pumps and valves should be inoperable when the door is unsecured. The door latch should be automatically disabled after operation until the interior temperature and pressure conditions permit safe access. The personnel who unload the chamber should wear heat-resistant gloves, aprons, and face protection.

Laser devices may require the operators to wear special eye protection. *Electrothermal heating devices* may introduce radio frequency wave hazards to pacemaker wearers. *Microtome blades* should be changed only by individuals wearing cut-resistant gloves. It is not possible to list all of the possible hazards within this chapter. No piece of equipment should be placed into service until the special hazards have been defined, appropriate engineering controls have been installed, and the requisite personal protective equipment provided.

HAZARDOUS WASTE DISPOSAL

Nearly all laboratory processes result in discarded solutions or materials. Much of it is hazardous (about 80 pounds/1000 ft^2 of chemical wastes and about 1 ton/1000 ft^2 of biohazardous waste per year) (34), but all of it must be disposed of safely. Proper disposal implies protection of the workers who will handle the waste as well as consideration of the environment (35).

Waste may be discharged into water, buried, burned (or otherwise destroyed), or transformed for reuse. By U.S. law, the containment or destruction of a hazardous solid waste forever remains the responsibility of the generator regardless of any assistance in handling, transporting, treatment, or disposal of the waste (32).

Chemical Wastes

According to EPA regulations, chemical wastes may be hazardous because of the properties of ignitability, corrosivity, reactivity, or toxicity. Ignitable wastes include liquids (e.g., acetone, alcohols, toluene, xylene), gases (e.g., hydrogen, propane, butane), or solids (e.g., nitrate salts, peroxides). Corrosives include strong acids and alkalis. Examples of reactive wastes are dry picric acid and aged diethyl ether that contains peroxides. Toxicity is currently defined by the ability to generate dangerous leachates that can contaminate ground or surface water and by lists of specific chemicals.

Hazardous chemical wastes (HCWs) should not be mixed with each other unless one knows the compounds to be compatible. Likewise, they should not be mixed with nonhazardous wastes, radioactive wastes, or infectious wastes. Each HCW should remain segregated throughout transport, storage, and disposal. All workers must use appropriate personal protective equipment when handling HCWs.

A safe area for accumulation of HCW materials prior to transport will be well ventilated, secure from unauthorized access, surrounded by a berm or catchment basin, and provided with proper fire protection. HCWs should not be allowed to accumulate onsite for longer periods than necessary or in excessive amounts. The same principles of safe storage that are appropriate for the parent reagents apply to discarded chemicals: incompatible chemicals must be separated, and all waste containers must be properly labeled as to content and initial date of accumulation. Unlabeled containers of hazardous waste must be treated as hazardous.

Some HCWs may be treatable onsite. Examples include neutralization of acids and bases or precipitation of inorganic metal cations as sulfides. Such activities should only be performed under the direction of a knowledgeable chemist. Other HCWs may be reclaimed for reuse: organic solvents may be distilled; silver may be extracted from photographic darkroom wastes, etc. HCWs should never be discarded into ground water nor in natural waterways. All chemicals introduced into the sanitary sewerage system must be compatible with the treatment processes of the local publicly owned treatment works.

Infectious Wastes

Wastes capable of transmitting an infectious disease may come from (*a*) cultures and other discards from microbiologic laboratories; (*b*) human blood, body fluids and tissues, and items contaminated with blood; and (*c*) contaminated animal carcasses and bedding. Control of the hazards of infectious waste is an occupational health issue.

In microbiological laboratories, infectious wastes (IWs) should be handled according to the biosafety level appropriate for the etiologic agents under study. In all clinical laboratories handling blood and body substances, universal precautions apply.

Packaging materials must be of sufficient strength and integrity to protect all who must handle the containers. Bags should be red or orange or display the Universal Biohazard Symbol. Contaminated sharps must be in puncture-resistant containers; liquid wastes must be in leak-resistant packaging.

Most IWs will be accumulated prior to disposal. The storage site should have limited access and be protected from rodents or other vermin that could become disease vectors. Steps should be taken to prevent putrefaction, including temperature control and short storage duration. Handling and transport methods must maintain the integrity of the packaging.

Some IWs, such as microbiological cultures, must be treated prior to disposal. Steam sterilization is preferred. The adequacy of decontamination depends on the exposure time; the temperature; the size, density, and water content of the load; and the penetrability of the containers. Autoclaving operations must be monitored periodically with a biological indicator (or chemical equivalent) that is placed inside a sealed package near the center of the load. Other treatment methods include dry heat sterilization, gas vapor sterilization, and chemical disinfection. The method chosen must be one that is effective against the agents known to be included in the IW.

Radioactive Wastes

All radioactive waste handling must be consistent with the regulations and license under which the laboratory operates. General principles include segregation of such wastes from the normal trash in a properly labeled, designated area. Radionuclides with a short half-life, such as ^{32}P and ^{125}I, may be allowed to decay in a protected area onsite and be discarded as nonhazardous refuse. Materials that cannot be allowed to decay in storage, such as ^{3}H, ^{14}C, and ^{35}S, may be released into the sanitary sewer system or into the atmosphere (as a gas or via incineration) in limited quantities as prescribed by law. Transfer of radioactive materials to offsite locations for burial or long-term storage is discouraged.

Sharps

Discarded needles, lancets, scalpel blades, Pasteur pipettes, capillary tubes, and shards of glass and plastic can cause penetrating injury. Infectious agents contaminating waste sharps can gain a portal of entry into the body through a puncture wound.

All sharps should be discarded immediately into a rigid, leak-resistant, puncture-resistant vessel. Such containers should be located in every work area in which waste sharps may be generated. (This encourages proper disposal and precludes the need to carry pointed items any distance.) Containers must not be allowed to overfill; injury can result from forceful insertion. Infectious sharps should be treated prior to disposal. All sharps should be destroyed to prevent injury to waste handlers. Destruction methods include incineration, grinding, shredding, crushing, and melting.

Waste Disposal

The laboratory director must be aware of the disposal processes that are used for all wastes generated by the facility. The methods must comply with all federal, state, and local regulations. With regards to HCWs, federal law identifies the generator as responsible for all personal and environmental injury that may ultimately develop, i.e., transfer of the waste does not transfer the generator's liability.

Incineration may be a proper disposal method for all types of waste. The incinerator must be able to accommodate the materials in the waste mixture. HCWs should be burned only by appropriately licensed facilities. Incineration is both a treatment and a disposal method for IWs and sharps, but the large proportion of chlorine-containing plastic in the typical IW mix may require special incinerator design. *Burial in a landfill* should be considered only for nonhazardous wastes. *Sewer disposal* is appropriate for most aqueous liquid wastes, but not for any materials that might interfere with processes in the water treatment facility.

Waste Minimization

All laboratories should develop a program for reducing the generation of hazardous waste. Waste minimization can be achieved either by reducing the volume of hazardous wastes generated or by reducing the degree of hazard of the waste generated. The volume of HCWs can be reduced by (*a*) substituting less-hazardous chemicals in laboratory operations, (*b*) decreasing the amounts of reagents required by adopting micromethods, (*c*) recovering spent materials for recycling, and (*d*) redistributing surplus or unwanted chemicals to laboratories that can use them.

Reduction in the amount of IW generated is best achieved through proper *segregation* of such waste. The mixture of a small quantity of an IW with a large quantity of noninfectious waste generates a large quantity of IW. Segregation must be performed at the point of generation. All IW must be inserted into the proper packaging, and noninfectious refuse should be kept physically separated to focus the waste handlers' attention on the materials of greatest concern.

Contingency Planning

Spill containment and cleanup procedures must be defined and specified for each type of hazardous waste generated by the laboratory. Fires, explosions, or other unexpected releases that may involve the health of individuals outside the facility or that may contaminate surface water in the vicinity must be included in the plan.

Recordkeeping

Hazardous waste manifests must be completed and maintained as required by law. Injuries involving wastes must be reported as required to governmental agencies and to the facility's safety program for quality assessment and improvement.

EMERGENCY PLANNING

The laboratory's safety policies manual should define the appropriate actions and responses in the event of unforeseen emergency. The types of situations that must be included in the planning will vary with the nature of the laboratory, its equipment, and the materials that it stores.

Power Failure

Loss of electrical power incapacitates a modern clinical laboratory. Emergency lighting must be provided to enable workers to move about the premises safely and to facilitate egress if unsafe conditions prevail. Air-handling devices require electrical power. The exhaust fans in chemical fume hoods and biological safety cabinets may shut down in a power failure; all processes that must be performed in such cabinets must cease until power is restored. Laboratory policy should prohibit the use of any equipment that cannot be manipulated safely under conditions of emergency power.

Fires

Fire emergency preparedness is discussed in the section on Fire Prevention and Control.

Natural Disasters

Tornadoes, floods, and similar disasters may devastate the facility. Clinical operations must not be restarted until the safety of the workers has been ensured by qualified inspectors. Unauthorized individuals must not be allowed premature access to the premises. The building must be structurally sound. Electrical equipment that is not designed for wet locations must be disconnected until all water has been removed. Damaged containers of chemicals must be properly gathered and removed. Potentially infectious materials must be bagged, decontaminated, and safely discarded.

Spill Cleanup

All hazardous materials can be spilled, and appropriate provisions must be made for each. All individuals who work in an area should have sufficient understanding of the basic medical, chemical, radiation-related, or infectious problems that can occur there to be able to recognize an emergency and to call for help. Small spills can often be safely cleaned by the spiller. Larger spills require the intervention of specially trained personnel.

Medical Emergencies

Laboratories that deal directly with patients must be prepared for clinical crises. Individuals trained in basic cardiopulmonary resuscitation (CPR) should be immediately available. If emergency supplies of drugs and equipment are maintained onsite, a program to ensure the freshness of the medications and the proper functioning of the gear must be provided. If all emergency medical care is provided at or by remote facilities, the response time should be brief enough to minimize clinical complications.

Electrical shock injury may result in loss of consciousness. First responders should be trained to approach the victim with caution. The source of the electrical discharge must be inactivated if it can be identified. Power to the defective appliance should be cut, preferably at the junction box, or the device can be pushed away with a wooden broom or another nonconductive implement. CPR should be initiated if the individual is not breathing, and emergency response personnel should be called.

The laboratory's CHP includes the assessment of the health effects of all hazardous chemicals. Spills or other acute releases may expose workers to toxic vapors. The CHP should specify the criteria for medical intervention. Such criteria may be based on signs or symptoms of overexposure or on environmental measurements. Splashes or sprays of toxic chemicals may result in exposure by absorption through the skin or mucous membranes. All such incidents should be documented, and medical treatment should be provided according to the CHP.

Similarly, the laboratory's infection control plan should specify the criteria for referral of employees who have been accidentally exposed to infectious agents.

Bomb Threat

Telephoned threats of bombing or other malicious acts should be included among the facility's emergency planning. All such calls should be taken seriously. The police or security services should be notified immediately. The caller should be kept on the line, and all details of the call recorded. The police may direct evacuation of the facility, and if so, the exit should proceed in an orderly manner.

EMPLOYEE TRAINING

All personnel must have the information and skills to control the hazards in their environment. Training programs are required under many governmental regulations and for accreditation by various voluntary agencies. The basic elements of a training program are (*a*) content, (*b*) target audience, (*c*) educational methodology, (*d*) documentation, and (*e*) monitoring for effectiveness.

Content

All safety policies should be included in the training program. The program for each employee should include the particular hazards applicable to his or her job. The program must give the employee sufficient information to understand the hazards. The controls provided by the laboratory director to contain those hazards must be included, and the requisite work practices must be emphasized. Employees must know how and when to use personal protective devices. Chemical handling, infectious exposures, waste disposal, and emergency preparedness are requisite subjects. The material should be presented in a manner consistent with the educational level, literacy, and language background of the people to whom it is presented.

Employee right-to-know regulations are exemplified at the federal level in OSHA's Hazard Communication Standard (36). Such regulations typically require the employer to provide the employees access to copies of the regulations and to the facility's safety plans. Chemical hazards may be summarized in the CHP, referencing Material Safety Data Sheets and other suitable sources. Training that accompanies a comprehensive ECP will provide employees with information on infectious hazards, methods to contain those hazards, and emergency medical intervention to be initiated in the event of an exposure.

Target Audience

All employees who handle or are exposed to hazardous materials must be included. Training is necessary for newly hired employees, for individuals assigned to new work areas, and periodically to familiarize all employees with technological and policy developments. Training must be implemented when new hazards are introduced into the workplace and when policies or programs are changed. Periodic refresher briefings of existing policies for all employees is strongly recommended.

Methods

Most safety training will be in lecture format, but consideration of "hands-on" activities is suggested. The operation of portable fire extinguishers, tight-fitting respirators, and spill containment is best presented in safety workshops. Some of the most effective programs are those that encourage workers to suggest safer alternatives to current practice.

Documentation

The date, title, and a summary of each safety presentation should be recorded. Attendance should be documented in the individuals' employment records.

Monitoring and Evaluation

The educational plan should provide assurance that all important aspects of the safety program are included. Attendance by the individuals in the targeted audience must be recorded to ensure that no one is inadvertently excluded. The effectiveness of the program should be tested in an objective manner. Although this may be provided by a multiple-choice test or other academic tool, the best feedback is provided by assessment of resultant on-the-job behavior.

QUALITY ASSESSMENT AND IMPROVEMENT

There is probably no clinical laboratory that is so safe that it cannot be made safer. A periodic safety audit should be undertaken by the safety committee to assess the needs of the personnel. A checklist should be constructed from the facility's safety manual to provide a useful tool for this audit. The audit should provide a description of the physical facility—including housekeeping, warning signs, fire prevention and preparedness, electrical safety, storage of compressed gases and chemicals, and containment of infectious and radioactive hazards. The condition of the equipment and its maintenance should be assessed. It is equally important, although perhaps more difficult, to determine the prevailing attitudes of the employees toward safe work practices and their compliance with existing policies. Required documents of the program should be evaluated for completeness.

The role and function of the safety committee should be reviewed annually. Minutes of the meetings should reflect a comprehensive and investigational program. The review of incident and accident reports, whether required by OSHA or not, should be documented. Formal inquiry and follow-up of serious accidents or repetitive problems are essential. Reports prepared for governmental agencies, such as hazardous waste manifests, should be monitored by the safety committee or the administration for adequacy and timeliness.

Reports of external reviewers can be especially helpful in assessing the safety program. Safety audits may be provided by governmental inspectors (e.g., OSHA, NRC, licensing agencies, fire departments) and by voluntary programs (e.g., College of American Pathologists, Joint Commission on Accreditation of Healthcare Organizations, industrial risk insurers). Each itemized area of concern or recommendation is a potential opportunity to improve the safety program.

The program's action plan should prioritize the identified issues of concern according to the types of problems uncovered, their frequency and severity, and the probability of their recurrence. The effectiveness of all measures taken as a result should be assessed after a suitable period of follow-up.

A successful safety program is the result of the combined efforts of everyone in the laboratory. Each individual in the laboratory should contribute to the total effort. The administration of the facility must make a statement of commitment to the goal of a safe workplace. The authority for implementing the program must be vested in the responsible supervisory personnel. The employees' responsibilities for complying with the safety policies should be stated within their job descriptions. The administration must provide a proper training program for all of its employees, both those new to the organization and those whose formal training preceded the introduction of current technology. Employees must bring to the attention of the management any identified but unsafe working condition as well as perceived opportunities to improve general safety conditions. Senior managers must be responsive to suggestions for improving the safety program. The attitudes of laboratory workers toward safety practices should be positive. Work groups inevitably set their own safety standards; management cannot force employees to work safely (37). An ongoing program of audit for compliance with defined policy is important. This is a function that can (and should) be integrated with other quality assessment and improvement activities within the organization.

References

1. Hawk WA, Hoeltge GA. Safety in the medical laboratory. Clin Lab Med 1983;3:467–484.
2. Hoeltge GA. Documentation of safe work practices in the clinical laboratory. Clin Lab Med 1986;6:787–798.
3. 29 CFR §1910.1045.
4. Goldwater PN, Law R, Nixon AD, Officer JA, Clelend JF. Impact of a recapping device on venipuncture-related needlestick injury. Infect Control Hosp Epidemiol 1989;10:21–25.

5. Protection of laboratory workers from infectious disease transmitted by blood, body fluids, and tissue. NCCLS Document M29-T. Villanova, PA: National Committee for Clinical Laboratory Standards, 1988.
6. Geller SA. The autopsy in acquired immunodeficiency syndrome: how and why. Arch Pathol Lab Med 1990;114:324–330.
7. Korniewicz DM, Laughon BE, Butz A, Larson E. Integrity of vinyl and latex procedure gloves. Nurs Res 1989;36:144–146.
8. 29 CFR §1910.134.
9. Furr AK, ed. CRC handbook of laboratory safety. 3rd ed. Boca Raton, FL: CRC Press, 1990.
10. 29 CFR §1910.145.
11. NFPA 704: Standard system for the identification of the fire hazards of materials. Quincy, MA: National Fire Protection Association, 1990.
12. 40 CFR §261.22.
13. NFPA 30: Hazardous and Combustible Liquids Code. Quincy, MA: National Fire Protection Association, 1990.
14. 40 CFR §261.21.
15. NFPA 99: Health Care Facilities. Quincy, MA: National Fire Protection Association, 1993.
16. NFPA 45: Laboratories Using Chemicals. Quincy, MA: National Fire Protection Association, 1991.
17. 40 CFR §261.23.
18. TLVs: threshold limit values and biological exposure indices for 1985–86. Cincinnati: American Conference of Government Industrial Hygienists, 1986.
19. 29 CFR §1910.1030.
20. Richardson JH, Barkley WE, eds. Biosafety in microbiological and biomedical laboratories. HHS Publication No. (NIH) 88-8395. Washington: U.S. Government Printing Office, 1988.
21. Recommendations for prevention of HIV transmissions in health care settings and update: universal precautions for prevention of transmission of human immunodeficiency virus, hepatitis B virus, and other bloodborne pathogens in health care settings. MMWR 1987;36(suppl 12s).
22. 1988 Agent summary statement for human immunodeficiency virus and report on laboratory-acquired infection with human immunodeficiency virus. MMWR 1988;37(suppl S-4):1–17.
23. Gordin FM, Gibert C, Hawley HP, Willoughby A. Prevalence of human immunodeficiency virus and hepatitis B virus in unselected hospital admissions: implications for mandatory testing and universal precautions. J Infect Dis 1990;161:14–17.
24. Resnick L, Veren K, Salahuddin SZ, Tondreau S, Markham PD. Stability and inactivation of HTLV-III/LAV under clinical and laboratory environments. JAMA 1986;255:1887–1891.
25. Alter HJ, Purcell RH, Shih JW, Melpolder JC, Houghton M, Choo QL, Kuo G. Detection of antibody to hepatitis C virus in prospectively followed transfusion recipients with acute and chronic non-A, non-B hepatitis. N Engl J Med 1989;321:1494–1500.
26. Titford M, Bastian FO. Handling Creutzfeld-Jakob disease tissues in the histology laboratory. J Histotechnol 1989;12:214–216.
27. Asher DM, Gibbs CJ, Gajdusek DC. Slow viral infections: Safe handling of the agents of subacute spongiform encephalopathies. In: Miller BM, ed. Laboratory safety: principles and practices. Washington, DC: American Society for Microbiology, 1986.
28. Protection against viral hepatitis: recommendations of the Immunization Practices Advisory Committee (ACIP). MMWR 1990;39(No. RR-2):1–26.
29. Sullivan JF. Employee health and surveillance programs. In: Miller BM, ed. Laboratory safety: principles and practices. Washington, DC: American Society for Microbiology, 1986.
30. 10 CFR §20.101.
31. ALARA at medical institutions. Regulatory Guide 8.18. Washington, DC: Nuclear Regulatory Commission, 1982.
32. Staiger JW. Techniques for safe handling of radioactive materials. In Miller BM, ed. Laboratory safety: principles and practices. Washington, DC: American Society for Microbiology, 1986.
33. NFPA 10: Portable fire extinguishers. Quincy, MA: National Fire Protection Association, 1990.
34. Hoeltge GA. Managing hazardous waste in the clinical laboratory. Clin Lab Med 1989;9:573–586.
35. Hazardous waste disposal. NCCLS Document GP5-T. Villanova, PA: National Committee for Clinical Laboratory Standards, 1991.
36. 29 CFR §1910.1200.
37. Songer JR. Laboratory safety program organization. In: Miller BM, ed. Laboratory safety: principles and practices. Washington, DC: American Society for Microbiology, 1986.

Suggested Readings

Chaff LF. Safety guide for health care institutions. Chicago: American Hospital Publishing, 1989.

Guidelines for laboratory safety. Northfield, IL: College of American Pathologists, 1989.

National Research Council. Prudent practices for handling hazardous chemicals in the laboratory. Washington, DC: National Academy Press, 1981.

National Research Council. Prudent practices for disposal of chemicals from laboratories. Washington, DC: National Academy Press, 1983.

National Research Council. Prudent practices for disposal of infectious wastes. Washington, DC: National Academy Press, 1989.

NFPA 101: Life safety code. Quincy, MA: National Fire Protection Association.

Pipitone DA, ed. Safe storage of laboratory chemicals. New York: John Wiley & Sons, 1984.

Richardson JH, Schoenfeld E, Tulis JJ, Wagner WM, eds. Safety management in the public health laboratory. Wilmington, DE: The DuPont Company, 1986.

So you're going to collect a blood specimen: an introduction to phlebotomy. Northfield, IL: College of American Pathologists, 1989.

3 Analytical Test Variables

Thomas M. Annesley

As part of the decision process for diagnosing, confirming, treating, or monitoring diseases, physicians rely heavily on the results of clinical laboratory tests. Physicians now have a greater menu of diagnostic tests available than ever before, and these tests can be performed more rapidly than ever before. Advances in biochemical research and medical technology have allowed diagnostic testing to reach a sophistication inconceivable 20 years ago. Instead of relying solely on total cholesterol concentrations in blood, we now measure high-density lipoprotein (HDL) cholesterol and HDL/total cholesterol ratios. Even HDL cholesterol is being fractionated. Assays for δ-bilirubin and isoenzyme subtypes are common, and chiral separations of drugs are performed for therapeutic drug monitoring.

Unfortunately, with the availability of a greater selection of laboratory tests, there is also an increased potential for misuse and misinterpretation. Physicians often look on the results of laboratory tests as providing a definitive answer; i.e., the presence of disease will result in an abnormal test result, or the receipt of a normal result will exclude a presumptive diagnosis. It would be wonderful if this were always true, but unfortunately it is not. Factors other than the presence or absence of a disease process may affect the results obtained from a laboratory test. Many of these factors are physiological and have nothing to do with the quality or performance of the selected laboratory test. Others are direct analytical problems that the physician can neither predict nor control. Whatever their source, it is important to understand that these variables do exist and must be identified or controlled whenever possible.

The diagnostic testing process can be separated into three phases: (*a*) the preparation of the patient and collection of a specimen, usually blood or urine; (*b*) the analytical measurement by the laboratory; and (*c*) the reporting of the testing results to the physician. Variables that may affect the proper interpretation of test results are present in each of these three areas and can be classified accordingly as preanalytical, analytical, and postanalytical variables.

PREANALYTICAL VARIABLES—INDIVIDUAL EFFECTS

Intraindividual Variation

One factor not controllable by either physician or laboratory is the degree of normal diurnal, day-to-day, and seasonal variation in the concentration of measured components in biological fluids. While the intraindividual variation of analytes such as electrolytes and serum proteins is generally considered to be small, the serum or urinary content of other biological components such as enzymes, lipids, hormones, and iron may change considerably over both shorter and longer time intervals.

Many hormones show both a diurnal variation and random biological variation during each 24-hour period. The diurnal cycles are often regulated by day/night and wake/sleep cycles, and having a knowledge of the daily habits of the patient will help in the proper interpretation of results as well as guide in the decision of when to obtain a specimen for testing. Insulin levels in blood are higher in the morning than later in the day. The serum levels of growth hormone (GH) are normally low during the daytime, although short bursts of GH may be observed 3 to 4 hours after meals. The secretion of growth hormone increases significantly during the first 2 hours of sleep, and concentrations of GH are highest during the initial period of deep sleep. Adrenocorticotropic hormone (ACTH) (corticotropin) and cortisol secretion curves also show diurnal variation, with peak blood concentrations normally observed between 6 and 8 AM (1). Levels gradually fall throughout the day, reaching a nadir between 9 PM and 3 AM. As with many hormones, secretory spikes occur throughout the day, introducing another component to specimen timing and the interpretation of results. Stress will also cause a sharp rise in the secretion of ACTH and cortisol.

Thyroid-stimulating hormone (TSH) shows a circadian variation in which serum levels are highest around or after midnight and lowest at midday. TSH is also secreted in multiple pulses that occur throughout the 24-hour period (Fig. 3.1) (2). These pulses

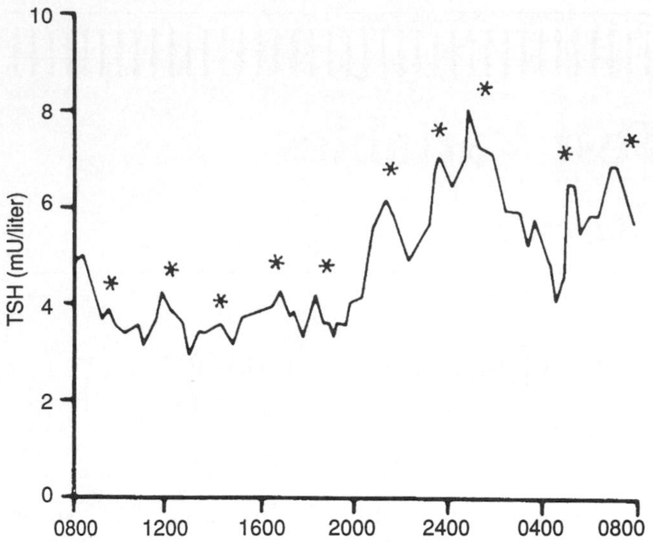

Figure 3.1. Serum TSH concentrations over 24 hours in a normal individual. *Asterisks* indicate TSH pulses. (From Samuels MH, Wood WM, Gordon DF, Kleinschmidt-DeMasters BK, Lillihei K, Ridgway EC. Clinical and molecular studies of a thyrotropin-secreting pituitary adenoma. J Clin Endocrinol Metab 1989;68:1211–1215.)

may result in measured TSH levels that are slightly outside of the reference range, especially if blood samples are obtained at night when the amplitude of these pulses tends to be greater. A recognition that such hormone pulses occur allows a more cautious interpretation of borderline abnormal results.

A diurnal variation can be observed for serum iron and potassium. Iron and potassium levels are higher during the morning hours than during the afternoon and evening hours. For serum iron, the difference can be as great as 30 to 50%. Serum iron levels also show intraindividual day-to-day variation of the same magnitude (3).

Seasonal changes in the concentrations of serum analytes may be observed. Vitamin D (cholecalciferol), whose dihydro-metabolite is an important regulator of calcium metabolism, is produced in the skin via ultraviolet radiation from sunlight. Seasonal changes in exposure to sunlight (winter vs. summer) may theoretically cause a reduction in the level of vitamin D. However, with the widespread enrichment of dietary components and food products, especially milk, this is unlikely to occur.

In some cases, diurnal and seasonal variations can coexist. The pineal gland hormone melatonin is purported to play a role in both sexual development and the etiology of affective disorders. The production of this hormone is regulated by light-dark cycles, with secretion occurring principally during the hours of darkness. The length of seasonal daily light exposure, which differs between winter and summer seasons, creates an additional circannual variation in the production of melatonin. Melatonin levels have been shown to be higher in patients suffering from a psychological depression called seasonal affective disorder (4).

In medical treatment, it is often necessary to follow the course of disease and to judge the progress or efficacy of a chosen mode of therapy. This is accomplished in part by evaluating the results of laboratory tests designed to monitor specific physiological parameters. Some changes may be the result of the analytical variation of the test (discussed later). Additionally, proper interpretation of a change between two consecutive determinations requires a consideration of the contribution that intraindividual day-to-day variation may play in the observed magnitude of the observed change. In other words, the patient is used as his or her own referent.

The actual day-to-day variation in any single patient can be accurately assessed only if a great many values are obtained. This is an impractical goal under normal circumstances. However, studies of the average variation for a group of individuals representative of the selected population have been performed. Although not universally applicable, these can be used as an estimate of expected biological intraindividual variation. For many analytes such as serum electrolytes and albumin, the day-to-day variation in healthy individuals is fairly small (Table 3.1) (5–9). Other serum constituents, including triglycerides, bilirubin, iron, TSH, and serum enzymes show considerable day-to-day variation. In some disease states, the day-to-day variation, even during periods in which the disease process is stationary, is greater than in healthy individuals (Table 3.1). For common serum analytes, the short-term intraindividual variation is similar to variation over longer periods of time (up to 40 weeks) (10).

Any decision-making process based on observed differences between two serial laboratory results obtained at separate times should include a consideration of what constitutes a significant change. Total intraindividual variation represents the combined contribution of biological variation and analytical variation and is estimated by use of the formula

$$CV_i = \sqrt{CV^2_{bi} + CV^2_a} \qquad (3.1)$$

where CV_i is the total coefficient of variation for the intraindividual variation, CV_{bi} is the biological intraindividual coefficient of variation, and CV_a is the analytical coefficient of variation. For changes in two serial laboratory results to be statistically significant ($P \leq 0.05$), the observed difference between the two results must exceed $2.77 \times CV_i$.

Serum cholesterol measurements are a good example for illustrating the magnitude of the changes required to produce statistically significant differ-

Table 3.1. Intraindividual Biological Coefficient of Variation (%) for Serum Analytes in Selected Patient Populations

	Mean Value of Combined Male and Female Groups			
	Normal Patients[a]	Chronic Renal Failure[b]	Chronic Liver Disease[a]	Insulin-Dependent Diabetes Mellitus[c]
Sodium	0.6	0.8	0.9	1.0
Potassium	3.7	5.7	7.0	5.9
Chloride	1.2	1.7	3.3	1.9
Calcium	1.4	2.8	—	—
Protein	2.5	3.5	4.4	3.9
Albumin	2.4	3.3	4.3	3.5
Urea	10.4	11.7	—	14.3
Creatinine	2.7	5.3	—	6.2
Uric acid	7.2	10.1	—	10.7
Cholesterol	4.6	6.0	5.2	7.3
Triglycerides	18.3	15.4	—	20.9
Alkaline phosphatase	6.9	7.0	6.6	—
Amylase	6.0	8.2	8.4	12.4
ALT	15.0	—	11.0	13.5
AST	10.1	—	10.6	13.4
Hemoglobin	2.6	3.6	4.0	3.7
Bilirubin	19.2[d]	—	—	—
Iron	29.3[e]	—	—	—
T_4	5.1[f]	—	—	—
Free T_4	9.5[f]	—	—	—
TSH	16.2[f]	—	—	—

[a]Data from Holzel WGE. Intra-individual variation of analytes in serum from patients with chronic liver disease. Clin Chem 1987;33:1133–1136.
[b]Data from Holzel WGE. Intra-individual variation of some analytes in serum of patients with chronic renal failure. Clin Chem 1987;33:670–673.
[c]Data from Holzel WGE. Intra-individual variation of some analytes in serum of patients with insulin-dependent diabetes mellitus. Clin Chem 1987;33:57–61.
[d]Data from Fraser CG, Cummings ST, Wilkinson SP, et al. Biologic variability of 26 clinical chemistry analytes in elderly people. Clin Chem 1989;35:783–786.
[e]Data from Statland BE, Winkel P. The relationship of the day-to-day variation of serum iron concentration values to the iron binding capacity values in a group of healthy young women. Am J Clin Pathol 1977;67:84–90.
[f]Data from Browning MCK, Ford RP, Callaghan SJ, Fraser CG. Intra- and interindividual biologic variation of five analytes used in assessing thyroid function: implications for necessary standards of performance and the interpretation of results. Clin Chem 1986;32:962–966.

ences between values. If the day-to-day analytical variation for a cholesterol assay in a particular laboratory is 5%, and the mean intraindividual variation (Table 3.1) of 4.6% is applied, then the change between two separately obtained laboratory results that can be confidently considered as statistically significant (Equation 3.1) will be $2.77 \times \sqrt{5^2 + 4.6^2} = 18.8\%$. Even if all serum samples obtained from an individual were analyzed at a single time and the analytical variation could be reduced to zero, the percent change that could be attributed to biological variation (Equation 3.1) would be nearly 13%. This emphasizes the fact that changes that physicians may consider to be clinically significant may result to a greater or lesser extent from normal intraindividual variation.

Effects of Gender

Sex-related differences in the mean serum concentrations of lipids, enzymes, and other analytes do exist. With several exceptions, these differences are not significant from a clinical point of view. Blood hemoglobin and ferritin concentrations are lower in adult females. Serum iron is lower in females, generally attributable to blood loss during menstruation. The serum concentrations of creatinine, urea nitrogen, and uric acid, as well as the enzyme activities of aldolase, aspartate aminotransferase, and creatine kinase are all greater in males than in females. Many of these differences result from the greater muscle mass in the male group. Alkaline phosphatase activities are lower in the younger adult female population, but they increase after menopause to levels equal to or greater than those for men.

Prior to age 50, males have higher serum levels of calcium, phosphorus, triglycerides, and cholesterol. However, after this age, females generally have higher serum levels for calcium, phosphorus, and cholesterol. Sex-specific hormone levels will quite naturally differ between males and females. Postpubertal testosterone levels are higher in males, while higher levels of estrogens, follicle-stimulating hormone, and luteinizing hormone can be expected in females.

Age-Related Variations

Historically, biological age groups have consisted of at least four categories—newborns, children (prepubertal), adults, and the elderly or geriatric population. The distinction between any two groups is never exact because chronological age and biological age do not run parallel throughout the population. The normal adult population is the age group to which the pediatric and geriatric groups are referenced, and any age-related effects are considered as differences relative to values attained during adulthood. The following material addresses some of the common biochemical changes that are observed between birth and puberty, followed by a review of changes that take place during the normal adult aging process.

In neonates, both albumin and total protein are low. The concentrations increase rapidly during the first 20 to 40 days of life and then continue to increase gradually until adult levels are attained. Albumin concentrations are generally close to adult levels by the age of 2 to 3 years, while total protein does not approach adult levels until approximately 7 years of age.

Serum bilirubin concentrations are significantly higher in neonates. Total bilirubin declines sharply during the first 2 weeks of life, reaching adult concentrations within 30 days. After this, no further age-related changes occur. Mean serum calcium concentrations in neonates are slightly less than adult levels during the first week, but stabilize at adult levels thereafter. Inorganic phosphorus may be 50 to 90% higher in neonates. The serum concentrations of phosphorus decline gradually over the next 15 years or so until adult concentrations are achieved.

Neonatal sodium and chloride concentrations approach adult values very rapidly, and there are essentially no age-related variations of these two electrolytes. Potassium concentrations are higher in newborns, and the serum potassium gradually declines until adult concentrations are reached by the age of approximately 3 years. Mean total CO_2 is lower in neonates and remains so for the first 24 months (11).

Creatinine concentrations are initially higher in newborns, but they decline during the first several weeks of life. From infancy throughout adolescence, creatinine concentrations gradually rise until the adult reference range is attained. The upper reference concentration will be approximately 0.6 mg/dl at age 1 to 2 years, 0.8 mg/dl at age 4 to 7, and 1.3 mg/dl after age 13. Blood urea nitrogen decreases shortly after birth, but it approaches adult concentrations within several years, after which no large age-related changes occur. Uric acid concentrations may be elevated above the adult reference range at birth, but after an initial transient drop, they rebound to adult-level concentrations. However, a divergence in uric acid values between males and females begins to develop at puberty. While the plasma urate concentrations in females remain at prior levels, the reference range for males becomes much higher (12). Hematocrit values are significantly higher at birth and decline to adult reference ranges within the first 1 to 2 months (13). The practical effect of this higher hematocrit is that, when laboratory testing is performed on neonates, the yield of serum that can be expected from drawing blood is less.

The normal range of serum activities of lactate dehydrogenase, creatine kinase, and γ-glutamyltransferase are higher in neonates. Shortly after birth, the serum activities of these enzymes undergo a progressive decrease that continues throughout childhood until adult levels are reached after approximately 10 years of age. Elevations in serum alkaline phosphatase activity are also observed, but the activity of this enzyme continues to remain high during the growing years. Alkaline phosphatase activity does not decrease to adult values until well after puberty.

Thyroid-stimulating hormone (TSH) concentrations increase very rapidly within 1 hour of birth, which subsequently results in an increase in both thyroxine (T_4) and triiodothyronine (T_3) (14). TSH then drops quickly to the normally expected low concentrations by the end of the first week. The mean serum concentration of T_4 is approximately twice adult values during the first week, and unlike TSH, it does not decrease rapidly. Rather, it gradually declines to adult concentrations during the next 5 to 10 years. T_3 concentrations follow a similar pattern. Other hormones, such as testosterone, estradiol, luteinizing hormone, follicle-stimulating hormone, dehydroepiandrosterone, and dehydroepiandrosterone sulfate, show rapid changes in serum levels. Somatomedin C levels are slightly lower than adult values at birth, rise gradually, peak at age 8 to 18 years when growth occurs, and then decrease to final adult concentrations.

Age-related biochemical changes in the pediatric population may affect drug therapy and the interpretation of therapeutic drug monitoring results. The hepatic microsomal enzymes responsible for drug metabolism are present and active at birth, but their levels are only approximately 50% of those of adults. Compared to adults, microsomal enzyme activity is low in premature infants and neonates. It increases to much higher levels during the period from age 5 to 12 and then decreases to the final intermediate activity present in adults and postpubertal adolescents.

During mid-adult years, age-related slow decreases in both albumin and total protein are observed in both men and women. A significant, continued decrease in serum inorganic phosphorus occurs in men beyond age 20. A decrease in serum phosphorus between ages 20 and 40 occurs in women, which is then followed by a subsequent rise throughout the remaining years (15). In addition to the rise in phosphorus, the serum activity of alkaline phosphatase increases after age 40. Decreases in serum calcium have been reported, but whether the effect is more prominent in men or women is not clear.

The median reference values for total cholesterol, triglycerides, and low-density lipoprotein (LDL) cholesterol gradually increase during the middle years. Recognition of this "normal," age-related physiological change in lipid concentrations has prompted many laboratories to develop reference ranges that are specific for sex and age. For both sexes, the median cholesterol values increase by approximately 50 mg/dl between the ages of 20 and 50 years and level off after this age (16). Median values for LDL-cholesterol and triglycerides also stabilize after age 50. Serum HDL-cholesterol levels also show age-related changes, although these are less pronounced than the changes in triglycerides and total cholesterol.

Serum glucose concentrations, both postprandial and after glucose tolerance test, increase with age, more significantly so in later adulthood. Postprandial glucose values change by an average of 4 mg/dl per decade (17). Two-hour post-challenge glucose concentrations increase by as much as 10 mg/dl per decade beyond age 40, and age must therefore be considered if an "abnormal" value greater than 200 mg/dl is observed.

During the middle to later years, there is a reduction in renal size and in the number of functional nephrons. Both the glomerular filtration rate (GFR) and tubular secretory capacity decline steadily after age 30. Creatinine clearance values decrease with age in a manner paralleling changes in the GFR. The accurate determination of creatinine clearance relies on the proper collection of a 24-hour urine specimen, and this may be difficult to control in the elderly patient. Formulas such as the one given in Equation 3.2 are often used to estimate creatinine clearance based on a single measurement of serum creatinine, with correction for age and weight (18):

$$\text{Creatinine clearance} = \frac{[140 - \text{age (years)}] \times \text{body weight (kg)}}{72 \times \text{serum creatinine (mg/dl)}} \qquad (3.2)$$

Serum albumin levels continue to decline with age even after the concentrations of other analytes stabilize. By the age of 80, serum albumin values will often have decreased by 15% or more. The presence of decreased albumin concentrations in the elderly requires a more careful interpretation of results for laboratory tests such as thyroxine, calcium, and many therapeutic drug levels. The measurement of total analyte concentration may not provide an accurate reflection of the free (active) concentration of the analyte.

Effects of Race

The effects of race or nationality on the basal concentrations of blood analytes can be considered small. More important are the effects of environmental and socioeconomic factors (e.g., diet, nutrition, exercise, habits) and the known higher incidence of genetic diseases (e.g., sickle cell anemia, thallasemia) in certain ethnic groups.

The amount of muscle mass is generally greater in black individuals. As a result, the observed activity of the muscle enzymes creatine kinase and lactate dehydrogenase are often higher in this group. Blacks also have higher concentrations of total protein. This can be attributed to the higher concentration of immunoglobulins present in the black population (19). A higher lgG/albumin ratio may also be observed.

PREANALYTICAL VARIABLES—EXTERNAL FACTORS

Exercise and Physical Training

Physical activity and exercise can have both short-term and long-term effects on the concentrations of biomolecules in blood and urine. Following episodes of physical exertion, transient hematologic changes may be observed, along with changes in the concentrations of trace elements, enzymes, lipids, hormones, and other blood constituents. The added demand for energy and the corresponding increase in metabolic activity during exercise result in some rapid changes in several analytes in blood. Lactate concentrations increase significantly during exercise, as does the level of the amino acid alanine. The concentration of free fatty acids falls rapidly and then subsequently increases (20). During physical exertion, the plasma concentrations of catecholamines, growth hormone, aldosterone, prolactin, and renin increase, as does the urinary excretion of cortisol and catecholamines.

After strenuous exercise, there is an increase in serum chromium concentration, and the serum levels of zinc and copper may rise to a lesser extent (21). These changes presumably result from the release of these substances from tissue stores for transport to areas of increased energy demand. Vigorous exercise causes a temporary, short-lasting activation of blood coagulation, platelet function, and the prostaglandin system. Coagulation factors VIII and Xa show pronounced increases during exercise, while platelet factor IV decreases (22).

During brief periods of strenuous physical exercise, renal blood flow and glomerular filtration decrease, and mild renal ischemia may develop. Both hematuria and proteinuria may be observed during the 24-hour period following physical activity. The degree of proteinuria is related to the strenuousness, not the extent, of the exercise. The magnitude of this effect decreases if a regular exercise program is followed, and proteinuria is not significant in well-trained individuals (23).

Likewise, transient changes in serum enzyme activities occur with exercise (24, 25). Glutathione reductase and γ-glutamyltransferase activities are not influenced. Alanine aminotransferase and alkaline phosphatase activities increase slightly but usually only after prolonged or strenuous exercise. However, the activities of enzymes of muscular origin, such as creatine kinase, lactate dehydrogenase, aldolase, and aspartate aminotranferase, rise significantly following physical exertion and may result in levels that are well outside of normal reference limits. Serum enzyme activities generally return to baseline levels within a 24- to 36-hour period. During exercise, muscles also release potassium, resulting in a rise in blood levels of potassium.

Long-term physical training and exercise programs will produce changes in the serum levels of a number of constituents. Compared to normal controls, well-trained individuals have lower mean levels for mean cell hemoglobin, creatinine, glucose, and WBC count (26, 27). Higher mean levels of bilirubin and urea nitrogen have been observed. Basal serum enzyme activities of the muscle enzymes creatine kinase and lactate dehydrogenase are often elevated in athletes. This probably represents a small, chronic release from muscle resulting from the more constant physical activity. The creatine kinase (CK) isoenzyme content of the muscle tissue of avid runners or marathoners differs from that of normal individuals in that significant percentages of the MB isoenzyme may be present. As a result, the serum isoenzyme pattern for these individuals may show elevated activity of CK-MB, which is normally considered diagnostic for myocardial damage. In these cases, however, these increases are due to post-marathon release of CK-MB from muscle.

Blood lipid concentrations change with improved body conditioning. Total serum cholesterol, LDL cholesterol, and triglyceride concentrations decrease, and HDL cholesterol values tend to increase.

Pregnancy

Numerous endocrinologic, hematologic, and biochemical changes are observed during pregnancy. The increased concentrations of estrogens and progesterone during pregnancy result in an increased secretion of prolactin (PRL) (28), but they also cause a suppression of the secretion of luteinizing hormone and follicle-stimulating hormone. Increased concentrations of estrogens during pregnancy or with the use of birth control pills contribute to higher levels of thyroxine binding globulin, thereby raising the concentrations of total T_4 and T_3. The free concentrations of these two thyroid hormones are not affected.

Changes in renal function, especially an increase in the glomerular filtration rate (GFR), lead to a greater excretion of glucose, urea nitrogen, creatinine, and protein in urine. Decreases in serum creatinine, urea, glucose, albumin, and total protein will be observed. Serum lipids are elevated, as are the serum activities of the enzymes lactate dehydrogenase, leucine aminopeptidase, and alkaline phosphatase. The increased activity of alkaline phosphatase results mainly from the presence of placental isoenzyme during pregnancy.

Changes in hematologic parameters often occur during pregnancy. Hematocrit and hemoglobin concentrations commonly decrease. Platelets may also show a slight progressive decrease. Coagulation factors VII and X commonly increase during pregnancy, and factor IX may also increase slightly (29). Plasma fibrinogen increases by 50%, contributing to an increase in the erythrocyte sedimentation rate (ESR). The ESR increases by the end of the first trimester and remains higher until shortly after delivery.

Diet and Food Ingestion

Following ingestion of a meal, the concentrations of several plasma constituents change noticeably. Potassium and phosphorus may increase or decrease depending on the type of meal ingested. Plasma glucose and triglycerides rise after the ingestion of food. The postprandial elevation in triglycerides may be present for up to 8 hours. The increased triglycerides may produce a lactescent serum, which has the potential to interfere with some clinical assays. Plasma alkaline phosphatase activities may increase in some individuals, especially after eating a meal high in fat content. The increase in alkaline phosphatase results primarily from an increase in the intestinal isoenzyme and is dependent on the blood group of the individual as well as the substrate used in the selected assay (30).

Tobacco, Caffeine, and Alcohol Use

The casual use of alcohol has not been reported to have any significant effect on most laboratory tests. Following ethanol intestion, increases in the serum concentrations of lactate, uric acid, and triglycerides are observed. The increase in serum triglycerides can be substantial (40%) during periods of more frequent ingestion of ethanol.

Changes in the concentration or serum activity of sodium, potassium, aspartate aminotransferase, alanine aminotransferase, creatine kinase, and lactate dehydrogenase following multiday challenges with ethanol have been studied. The reported changes have not been consistent in all studies, and even when statistically significant, they have not been considered to be clinically significant (31). Alcohol consumption, moderate and chronic, is associated with an increased serum activity of the enzyme γ-glutamyltransferase. The increase in serum activity of this enzyme is believed to result from induction of hepatic microsomal enzymes and is sometimes monitored as a predictor of chronic alcoholism.

Smoking of tobacco (nicotine) is associated with changes in a number of laboratory tests. Acute changes following tobacco smoking may include increases in plasma catecholamines, glucose, free fatty acids, and cortisol. Sustained exposure to carbon monoxide via tobacco smoke may lead to distinct elevations in carboxyhemoglobin and a left shift in the oxygen dissociation curve, which are compensated for by an increased hematocrit. Other observable hematologic changes include an increased white cell count and a decreased Po_2.

Caffeine ingestion will produce an increased release of catecholamines via stimulation of the adrenal medulla. Consumption of caffeine beverages will also result in an increase in serum free fatty acids. Habitual consumption of caffeine may lead to changes in serum concentrations of cholesterol and triglycerides.

Posture

When blood is obtained from patients, they may be in the supine, sitting, or standing position. Changes in posture can profoundly alter the concentration of components in the peripheral blood; therefore, it is important to know the physical circumstances under which the specimen was obtained. Hospitalized patients are often in the supine position, while outpatients are more active and have been in a sitting or standing position prior to blood collection. Mean reference values for many analytes are statistically different between inpatient and outpatient groups because of this postural effect.

When a patient changes from a lying to a more erect posture, the rise in hydrostatic pressure will result in a loss or efflux of water and small, filterable molecules from the intravascular compartment to the interstital spaces. This reduction in plasma volume will increase the concentration of substances of greater molecular weight such as proteins, as well as the concentration of other protein-bound analytes such as calcium, lipids, bilirubin, and even therapeutic drugs. The concentration of other small, readily diffusable blood analytes is largely unchanged by alterations in posture. A change in posture from the supine to the erect position increases the secretion of norepinephrine and epinephrine, resulting in levels nearly twice those observed in a relaxed, recumbent position. Plasma aldosterone and renin activity increase following a change from a supine to a standing position. Some of the observed changes in serum constituents on changing from a supine to a standing position are listed in Table 3.2.

Table 3.2. Approximate Differences in the Concentration of Serum Analytes after Change from Supine to Standing Position (32–35)

Analyte	Percent Increase
Acid phosphatase	5
Albumin	8–12
Alkaline phosphatase	7–12
Amylase	6
Aspartate aminotransferase	5
Bilirubin	17
Calcium	3–5
Cholesterol	7–13
Creatinine	4
Hemoglobin	5
Iron	7
IgA	7
IgG	7
IgM	5
Phosphate	3
Potassium	3–5
Protein	9–11
Thyroxine	11
Triglycerides	6
Red blood cells	5
White blood cells	3
Platelets	7

Effects of Blood Collection Technique, Evacuated Blood Collection Tubes, Anticoagulants, and Separator Gels

Blood specimens are most commonly procured via venipuncture using evacuated collection devices. Serum specimens are obtained from plain evacuated tubes or tubes containing a separator gel. When whole blood or plasma is required, a variety of anticoagulated tubes can be used. Multiple biochemical or analytical abnormalities may result from exposure of the blood specimen to anticoagulants and separator gels; therefore, it is crucial that the correct tube for the selected laboratory test be used.

HEPARIN

Heparin, available as the lithium, sodium, or ammonium salt, is recommended for the determination of potassium in plasma. Although the results of several studies have produced varied observations on the effects of heparin on the concentration of analytes in plasma versus serum (36–38), and some of these may be method dependent, it is well accepted that the use of heparinized plasma versus serum for potassium determinations will yield differing results. Because potassium is released from platelets during the normal clotting process, serum potassium concentrations will be approximately 0.3 mmol/liter higher than plasma values. The use of the lithium salt of heparin is preferred over the potassium or sodium salts because any interference with the measurement of these electrolytes should be avoided. Heparin has also been reported to invalidate coagulation testing results.

OXALATE/FLUORIDE

Oxalate will cause water to be transported from erythrocytes, thereby producing both a dilution of plasma (39) and a reduction in hematocrit. Additionally, there is the potential for disruptive effects on cell membranes and a change in the morphology of cells. Oxalate will bind calcium and will produce a low calcium result when colorimetric methods are employed for the analysis. The enzymes amylase, alkaline phosphatase, and lactate dehydrogenase are inhabited by oxalate.

Sodium fluoride is a urease inhibitor and should not be used when urease methods are chosen for the determination of urea nitrogen. Fluoride will increase the measured activity of amylase, diminish acid phosphatase activity, and inhibit glucose oxidase when this enzyme is used for the determination of glucose.

ETHYLENEDIAMINETETRAACETIC ACID

Ethylenediaminetetraacetic acid (EDTA) is the optimal anticoagulant for hematology testing because it does not produce changes in erythrocyte volume. However, EDTA binds calcium and will cause a decrease in the observed calcium value when colorimetric methods are used. The potassium or sodium salts of EDTA will produce a positive interference when assaying the same electrolyte. EDTA is an effective chelator of magnesium, which is purported to account for the inhibitory effect on enzymes such as creatine kinase and alkaline phosphatase.

CITRATE

Citrate is the preferred anticoagulant for coagulation studies because it appears to preserve labile procoagulants. Like EDTA, this anticoagulant also binds calcium and will have a similar effect on calcium assays. Citrate has been reported to produce a significant osmotic redistribution of fluid between plasma and blood cells, resulting in a decrease in the concentration of multiple analytes (37).

Table 3.3. Analyte Inaccuracy Associated with Gel Separator Blood Collection Devices[a]

Analyte	Problem
Lactate dehydrogenase	Increased
Cholesterol	Decreased
Triglyceride	Decreased
Ionized calcium	Increased
Progesterone	Decreased
Carbamazepine	Decreased
Digoxin	Increased
Lidocaine	Decreased
Phenobarbital	Decreased
Phenytoin	Decreased
Tricyclic antidepressants	Decreased

[a]Adapted from Calam RR. Specimen processing separator gels. An update. J Clin Immunoassay 1988;11:86–90.
[b]Observation of effect may depend on the device used.

GEL SEPARATION TUBES

Extended contact of serum with blood cells can alter the concentration of numerous analytes (discussed later). Specimen separator gel tubes have become widely used because of the barrier created between serum and cells after centrifugation. However, it is essential to understand that the properties of the different commercial materials do differ and that in vitro inaccuracies may be caused by one of the gel types and not by others (Table 3.3) (40). Moreover, laboratory professionals must be sensitive to the fact that, during the evaluation of new analytes or analytical procedures, it is necessary to validate any prior assumption that gel separation collection devices can be used for the procedure.

ORDER OF DRAW FOR BLOOD COLLECTION

In addition to the use of the proper type of evacuated tubes for specific testing purposes, it is also necessary to minimize cross-contamination between blood collection tubes. It is possible for contaminant problems to arise when blood is collected into tubes containing anticoagulant prior to use of a plain tube, as well as when anticoagulant tubes are used in an improper order. This is especially true for difficult blood draws. For example, use of tubes containing potassium-EDTA prior to an immediate draw with a nonadditive tube has been reported to cause spurious increases in serum potassium and a decrease in serum calcium due to cross-contamination by the potassium-EDTA present in the first collection tube (40).

Because tissue thromboplastin can contaminate a blood collection tube, tubes containing citrate should never be the first blood collection device used. Collection devices containing heparin may also contaminate a subsequent citrate tube, thus invalidating coagulation testing. Ideally, a nonadditive tube should be filled prior to the use of the tube containing citrate (41). Contamination of a heparinized tube drawn for electrolyte measurement may result if a potassium-EDTA tube is used immediately before the heparin tube. Hematologic testing may be invalidated if an oxalate/fluoride tube is used just prior to the intended EDTA collection tube.

Because of these types of potential contaminations, specific collection protocols have been recommended when several blood specimens are required for different purposes. The generally recommended order of collection is (*a*) collection of sterile culture tubes, (*b*) nonadditive tubes, (*c*) coagulation tubes, (*d*) anticoagulant/additive-containing tubes. In addition, an extended recommendation for the proper order of collection with additive-containing tubes has been provided (42). This recommended order is (*a*) citrate-containing tubes, (*b*) heparin tubes, (*c*) EDTA-K_3 tubes, and (*d*) oxalate/fluoride tubes.

TIME OF COLLECTION

Although blood specimens for a majority of laboratory tests can be randomly obtained, some specimens must be drawn at specified intervals or at specific times. Intraindividual and circadian variations, which are discussed above, may dictate that specimens be obtained at specific times of the day or night. Specimens for therapeutic drug monitoring must be obtained at specific intervals that are dictated by the mechanism of drug delivery (intravenous vs. oral), the dosage interval, absorption characteristics of the drug, or the half-life of the drug. It is most common for "trough" drug levels to be monitored. In some cases, however, both "peak" and "trough" levels may be required. Metabolic challenge studies, such as xylose absorption or glucose tolerance tests, also require specimen collection at specified timed intervals. The proper analysis of urine may require collection at a specific time, such as first morning excretion, or collection of a 24-hour specimen, to minimize any influence of diurnal variation or the varying osmolality of randomly voided urine specimens.

INCORRECT PATIENT AND SPECIMEN IDENTIFICATION

Laboratory results are valueless if they are reported on the wrong patient. Nonetheless, identification errors do infrequently occur in any hospital or clinic setting, and proper practices must be followed to minimize patient or sample misidentification. Verification of patient identity should be accomplished by visual inspection of identification badges or wristbands. Because many names are common within the population, identification using unique patient registration numbers is more accurate than verification by name alone. Wristbands found beside the patient should not be considered as positive proof of identification. The patient should be verbally questioned for his or her name and/or other unique identifiers such as Social Security number or birthdate. Collection tubes must be accurately labeled with patient name, identification number, and the date and time of collection. Proper labeling of specimen containers is important because the specimen may be part of a series of timed samples, such as a glucose tolerance test, or may be one of numerous specimens drawn from the same patient during a 24-hour period. Many medical centers identify every specimen with a unique accession number.

All necessary information must be included on the requisition accompanying the specimen. The required information may include the type of sample (blood, saliva, fluid, urine, etc.), the tissue site from which a biopsy was obtained, a preliminary history or diagnosis, pertinent medications, the date and time of specimen acquisition, and the name of the person obtaining the specimen. The name and patient identification number on the requisition must match the information listed on the specimen container. It is critical that the ward or clinic location in which the patient is located, as well as the name or number of the ordering physician, be clearly listed on the requisition. Valuable time may be lost if a physician or nurse cannot be identified and rapidly notified should a "critical" or "panic" result be found by the laboratory.

Transport and Processing of Specimens

Alterations in the concentration of chemical components are possible prior to analysis by the laboratory. Sources of these changes include delays in delivery of the sample and processing by the laboratory. Instability of bioanalytes during storage or evaporation of fluid specimens can also contribute to changes from the original concentration in the specimen. For blood specimens, it is recommended that serum be separated within 2 hours of collection, although special, immediate handling is required for numerous analytes such as cortisol, lactate, or pyruvate. Many serum hormones are unstable and require freezing of the serum if analysis is not to be performed immediately.

For the case of commonly measured serum constituents, delays in separating blood or prolonged contact of the serum with the clot will have a rapid effect on the observed concentration of potassium, glucose, and ammonia. Glycolysis occurring in the erythrocyte will cause glucose concentration to drop, while proteolytic reactions will cause the con-

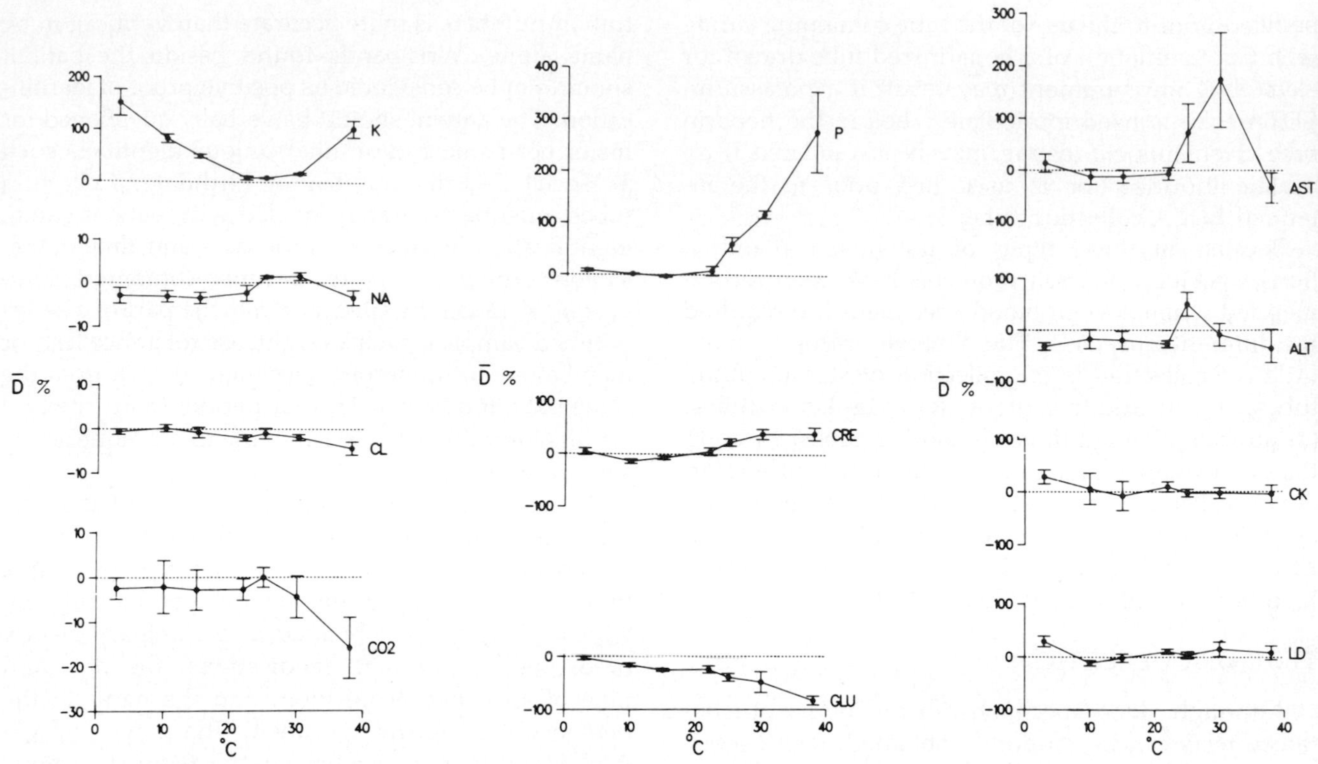

Figure 3.2. Percentage change from control value of serum analytes in blood samples stored for 24 hours at different temperatures. K, potassium; NA, sodium; CL, chloride; CO2, total carbon dioxide; P, phosphorus; CRE, creatinine; GLU, glucose; AST, aspartate aminotransferase; ALT, alanine aminotransferase; CK, creatine kinase; LD, lactate dehydrogenase. (From Rehak NN, Chiang BT. Storage of whole blood: effect of temperature on the measured concentration of analytes in serum. Clin Chem 1988;34:2111–2114.)

centration of ammonia to increase. Changes in the permeability of erythrocyte membranes or temperature-related changes in the activity of the sodium-potassium pump will result in increases in serum potassium. Although the loss of glucose in whole blood can be minimized by storage at 4°C, the greatest loss of potassium from erythrocytes into the serum occurs under these conditions, illustrating the fact that changes in the concentration of serum analytes may be temperature dependent (Fig. 3.2) (43, 44).

Serum specimens must often be sent from physicians' offices or small hospitals by mail or special courier. As a result, delays of 24 hours may occur prior to analysis of the serum sample. It is also common for laboratories to save previously analyzed serum specimens for 24 hours to be able to verify discrepant results. In each of these circumstances, the stability of the requested serum constituents becomes an important consideration. Rossing (45) has demonstrated that five commonly measured serum analytes—alkaline phosphatase, phosphate, bilirubin, cholesterol, and CO_2—undergo statistically significant changes in concentration during refrigerated storage for 24 hours. However, the only analyte that shows a medically significant change is CO_2 (45).

ANALYTICAL VARIABLES

Analytical Variation, Sensitivity, and Specificity

The analytical determinations performed within the diagnostic laboratory are subject to a variety of internal factors. The potential sources of the analytical variation are numerous, but they can typically be classified as resulting from either a *random* or a *systematic* variation. The underlying factors that contribute to both of these kinds of variation overlap, and therefore they may coexist at any given time.

Systematic variation is the degree of deviation or shifting away from a mean or true target value. Although they are not completely equivalent, systematic variation can be thought of as a reflection of the accuracy (or inaccuracy) of the diagnostic test. Systematic variation can have numerous origins. The manual or analytical technique of the members of the technical staff can differ widely. For interpretive or graded tests, the distinction points or cutoff criteria will very often be individual. Using the same reagents and instruments, one individual may consistently produce results that are higher or lower than those of the rest of the staff due to very subtle differences in pipetting, vortexing, staining technique, etc.

Incorrect preparation or assignment of standards will produce results that show a bias from expected values. Factors that may contribute to a systematic variation are the use of aged, outdated, or improperly stored reagents; nonlinearity of analytical response; inadequate calibration; and lack of reagent or solvent blanks. Due to stability or cost problems, artificial and animal-based standards are often used, and the differing matrix composition of such standards may not always react equivalently to fresh human sera in the analytical system employed. The presence of stabilizers, solubilizers, or other artificial components may also be a source of systematic bias.

Performing a test on two different instruments is a source of systematic variation that is often overlooked. It is common for different instruments or methodologies to be used for different situations. A small benchtop instrument may be used in an outpatient clinic; a different instrument may be used for stat work in the main laboratory; and a large, multichannel instrument may be used for performing daily profiles on inpatients. As a patient is chronologically followed from preadmission to discharge and outpatient follow-up, serial testing may have been performed using different instruments and different methodologies. Subtle biases or variation among these instrumental methods may be unknowingly interpreted as clinical changes by the physician. For a nephrologist or a transplant surgeon, a serial change in creatinine of 0.2 mg/dl may signal a change in renal function, although the change may have been solely due to an instrumental bias. To alleviate such problems, many medical centers set protocols whereby specimens and requisitions are specially labeled or "flagged" so that laboratory testing can be performed consistently on the same instrument.

Systematic variation can also result from the methods or mathematical models used to calculate results. A common example of this is the different methods used to derive results when using immunoassays. A majority of these are based on the principle of competitive binding, and these produce dose-response curves that are sigmoidal in character. To linearize the data, logit transformations are performed. Because the precision of the assay is not uniform across the standard curve (termed heteroscedasticity), a mathematical approach that utilizes a weighted regression is necessary. Different equations or computer models can be chosen for this purpose, which results in some variation in the mathematically assigned calibration curve and therefore in the results obtained.

Random variation results from the contribution of elements that produce fluctuation within an individual analytical run or between serial analyses performed on the same specimen. Random variation can be equated to the reproducibility or precision of an assay. Factors that are both within operator control and beyond routine control contribute to random variation. Instrument-related elements that contribute to random variation include normal fluctuations in electrical and optical sensors, variation in pipetting and dispensing systems, and other types of preset hardware configurations. These are often difficult to predict and control. Other causes of random variation include reagent stability, mixing or dissolution inconsistencies, temperature fluctuation, timing variation, unstable reagent or sample blanks, and evaporation of specimens and reagents.

Other properties of an analytical method that must be considered include the sensitivity and the specificity of the method. The analytical sensitivity and specificity are not the same as the diagnostic sensitivity and specificity of the clinical test. Analytical sensitivity, which is directly related to precision, is the ability of the assay to detect low concentrations, or small changes in concentration, of the compound of interest.

Analytical specificity is the ability of an assay to selectively measure only the analyte of interest. Although analytical specificity is achieved by minimizing interference from similarly structured, cross-reacting substances, chemical interference from other compounds such as lipids, bilirubin, proteins, and hemoglobin must also be circumvented. Poor analytical specificity will result in poor accuracy.

Interference

The accuracy of analytical methods is subject to the effects of interferents. Commonly encountered sources of analytical interference include the presence of drugs or metabolites, hemolysis, lipemia, turbidity, bilirubin, dietary components, improper anticoagulants, physical contaminants such as disinfectants or handcreams, bacterial contamination of the sample or reagents, contrast dyes and imaging agents, preservatives, stabilizers, and plasticizers. It is beyond the scope of this chapter to provide a comprehensive list of the many analytical interferents that have been described. It should be noted that published resources do exist that describe the effects of drugs, diseases, and other factors on laboratory tests (46, 47). Valuable information related to known interferents for individual analytical procedures can also be obtained from sources such as technical brochures provided by commercial companies and from published independent evaluations of instruments and kits.

Positive interference (falsely elevated answers) can result from the added contribution of biological components (e.g., bilirubin, hemoglobin, lipids, or proteins) that scatter light or absorb it at the desired wavelength. Other causes include the presence of turbidity, cross-reactivity with a similarly structured analyte or prescribed drug, or contamination of glassware and pipettes. Negative interference (falsely reduced answers) can also be encountered. Compounds may be present that delay color formation in a reaction, chemically reoxidize or reduce a colored end product, or competitively inhibit an enzyme reaction. Depletion or chelation of chemical reactants, including the desired analyte or a required cofactor, will produce a falsely low result. Contamination of enzyme reagents with trace amounts of other enzymes with similar substrate requirements may result in simultaneous competition for cofactors or may actually deplete the measured end product of the monitored reaction.

POSTANALYTICAL VARIABLES

An accurate test result is useless in patient care if it is transcribed incorrectly, not reported in a timely manner, reported in a format that is confusing or uninterpretable, or is delivered to the wrong medical record. The computerization of laboratories has helped to solve some of these difficulties, but as discussed below, it has also created a unique set of potential problems. Tests are often performed in a batch or sequence, utilizing a worklist containing the names or identification of the patient specimens to be analyzed. Errors are possible when analytical results must be transcribed from a raw data sheet or instrument printout onto a corresponding worklist. These errors may occur if numbers are transposed or the results are transcribed onto the wrong location on the worklist. Direct interfacing of instruments to laboratory information systems decreases the amount of written transfer of data, but a verification system is still needed to review patient results prior to electronic transmission or permanent storage. A review of all results, whether manually produced or automated, is valuable for catching mathematical or analytical problems. For example, if the reference range for albumin is 3.5 to 5.0 g/100 ml and an unrealistic patient value of 0.35 g/100 ml is identified, this may alert the analyst to an instrumental, mathematical, or decimal positioning error, which may have caused a 10-fold error from an expected value of 3.5 g/100 ml.

Computerization of reporting has its own variables that affect the proper utilization of laboratory results. In most circumstances, computerized report generation is under the control of the laboratories; therefore, it becomes a source of postanalytical variation. The format in which results are presented to clinicians can influence the ease with which abnormal results are identified by the ordering physician. Information that is inherently obvious to the laboratory staff or computer programmers may be foreign to the clinical staff. The lack of reference ranges, especially age- and sex-specific changes, on a printed report may make a result uninterpretable to a clinician who infrequently orders the test. Other items that become important in the proper presentation of results include the placement of results, reporting units, and reference ranges on the report; the placement of comments; the use of acronyms to name the test; and the inclusion of any necessary interpretive data.

The presentation of serial results for tests for which trends in values may be important may be more easily followed if the results are listed in a vertical rather than a horizontal format. If important observations, such as the fact that a serum specimen was hemolyzed, are not printed in an obvious location on the report or are not properly identified as belonging to that specimen, then abnormally high or low values for a test may be interpreted as true physiological changes and not as potentially due to an analytical artifact. Comments must be standardized and precise to avoid any misunderstanding of the information being conveyed. If one technologist enters the comment "specimen moderately hemolyzed" while a second individual enters "bad specimen" under the same circumstances, the clinician will receive different information from each of the two comments.

Acronyms are often used to shorten the test names listed on reports or computer monitor screens. If this is the case, these code names become another variable that must be considered in reporting test results. For example, the acronym "LAP" can stand for "leucine amino peptidase" and also for "leukocyte alkaline phosphatase." The computer code "ALDO" could be applied to both aldolase and aldosterone. Such names must be carefully chosen so as to avoid any confusion.

Proper reporting of a "panic value" or "critical result" can be an important postanalytical variable. It is important that the ordering physician's name and the patient's hospital location be listed on requisitions so that results can be called back as rapidly as possible. If panic values are called to a physician or nurse, then verification of such notification must be properly documented. Putting into a computer or on the medical chart a comment such as "Pat notified about glucose value at 10:00 by John" does not provide enough information about the handling of the panic value. Should a legal question arise 1 to 2 years later, this record may not provide sufficient information to properly review or to defend the treatment of a patient. Who was Pat? Does Pat work here anymore? Was Pat a nurse, a clerk, or a resident? Is there more than one technologist named John?

STATISTICAL EVALUATIONS OF POPULATIONS AND THE ESTABLISHMENT OF NORMAL REFERENCE RANGES

Both laboratorians and clinicians commonly use statistics as part of the evaluation of analytical methods, the establishment and review of reference ranges, and the interpretation of laboratory test results. The information that is normally sought through statistical review is a general description of the characteristics of a population or set of data points. Most commonly, this is some numerical reflection of the "typical" value (mean, median, mode) in the population, the dispersion or random variation of values within the population (standard deviation, coefficient of variation), and a description of how the values are distributed (gaussian, nongaussian). The most common practical applications of statistics to laboratory medicine are in the establishment of reference ranges and the evaluation of the performance of analytical methods.

When establishing reference ranges, it is not generally possible to test all members of the desired population. A more realistic approach is to obtain data from a selected subset of the larger group. It is important that (*a*) the number of data points be large enough and (*b*) the subset from which data are to be obtained approximates the overall population to be tested. For example, the reference range for serum creatine kinase values obtained from female nurses may not be applicable to elderly males being evaluated for myocardial damage. When establishing reference ranges, it is also necessary to account for the biological and environmental variables described earlier in this chapter.

For a large number of laboratory tests the distinction between normal and abnormal values has been based on a range within which approximately 95% of the healthy population will fall. Assuming that both abnormal low and high results will be observed, the ranges are set so that 2% of the levels will fall above the upper limit and 2% of values will fall below the lower reference limit. The simplest calculation for a reference range is based upon the presence of a gaussian distribution, for which the frequency patterns of results above and below the mean (symbolized $\bar{x}$) are identical. In this type of distribution, the interval between the arithmetic mean ± 1 standard deviation ($\bar{x}$ ± 1 SD) will contain 68% of the reference values, and the interval $\bar{x}$ ± 2 SD will contain 95% of reference values. Typically, the normal reference range for a set of results that closely follows a gaussian distribution would be estimated from the calculated mean and standard deviation ($\bar{x}$ ± 2 SD).

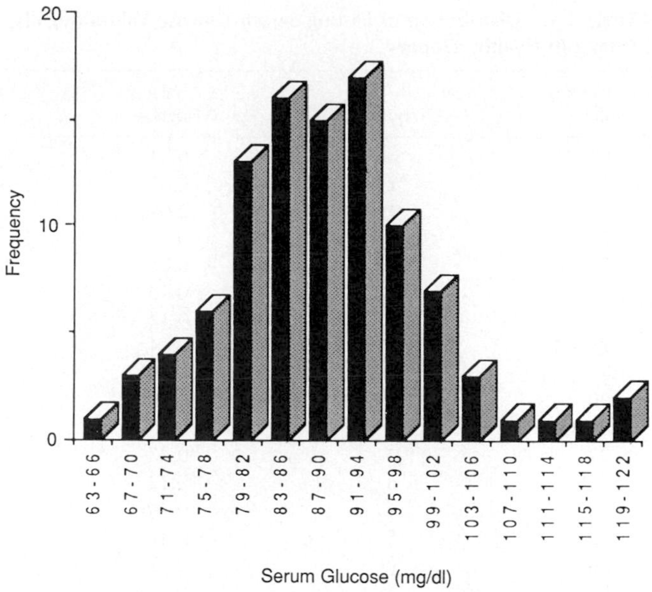

Figure 3.3. Histogram of serum glucose values from 100 healthy donors. Individual values are listed in Table 3.4.

Three parameters are used to describe the centrality of results; the arithmetic mean, median, and mode. The *arithmetic mean* $\bar{x}$ is the sum of the values divided by the number of values or observations. The arithmetic mean can be influenced by a single extremely high or low outlier value. The *median* is the value associated with the middle position (50th percentile) if all the results are listed in descending or ascending order. Unlike the mean, it is less affected by extremely high or low values. The *mode* is the value that occurs with the greatest frequency. Like the median, it is less influenced by outliers in the data group, but it is possible that within any group of data two or more values may occur with the same frequency. In a true gaussian distribution, the mean, median, and mode coincide due to the symmetrical nature of the distribution.

When establishing reference ranges, it is important to first determine whether the distribution of data follows a gaussian pattern. This is accomplished by creating a histogram (Fig. 3.3) that illustrates the frequency distribution of values. The range of values is plotted on the horizontal axis, and the frequency of occurrence of each value is plotted on the vertical axis. The data points are often grouped into intervals or clusters (e.g., serum glucose of 66 to 70, 71 to 75, 76 to 80, etc.) so that a better visualization of the distribution can be achieved. From the frequency distribution it is possible to determine whether (*a*) there are wild outliers that may require special considera-

Table 3.4. Distribution of Fasting Serum Glucose Values (mg/dl) from 100 Healthy Donors

Glucose Value	Frequency	Cumulative Fraction
63	1	0.01
67	2	0.03
69	1	0.04
71	2	0.06
73	2	0.08
75	2	0.10
77	2	0.12
78	2	0.14
79	4	0.18
80	2	0.20
81	3	0.23
82	4	0.27
83	5	0.32
84	4	0.36
85	5	0.41
86	2	0.43
87	4	0.47
88	5	0.52
89	2	0.54
90	4	0.58
91	4	0.62
92	6	0.68
93	5	0.73
94	2	0.75
95	3	0.78
96	2	0.80
97	2	0.82
98	3	0.85
99	1	0.86
100	4	0.90
101	2	0.92
103	1	0.93
104	1	0.94
105	1	0.95
110	1	0.96
112	1	0.97
115	1	0.98
119	1	0.99
120	1	1.00

tion, (*b*) the distribution is symmetrical or skewed, and (*c*) more than one population of values exists, such as in the case of a bimodal distribution. If the distribution is not gaussian, estimates of centrality may not hold true, and calculations of reference limits based on multiples of the standard deviation may be incorrect. The following examples illustrate these points.

Table 3.4 lists sample values for fasting serum glucose values that may be obtained from 100 volunteers. If an interval frequency distribution of the serum glucose values is plotted, as shown in Figure 3.3, the pattern approximates a gaussian distribution. Because of this, a calculation of reference limits based on the mean value plus and minus two standard deviations (2.5 to 97.5 percentiles) should be valid. For the values listed in Table 3.4, the arithmetic mean and the standard deviation are calculated to be 88.6 mg/dl and 10.7 mg/dl, respectively. From this, a normal range would be established as lying between 67 and 110 mg/dl ($\bar{x} \pm 2$ SD). For the data in Table 3.4, the median value was 88 mg/dl and the mode 92 mg/dl. The values for all three measures of centrality are very similar because the distribution of fasting glucose values is basically gaussian.

Another way to obtain the percentile distribution from a set of values is to make use of normal probability graph paper. In this case, the cumulative frequencies are plotted on the vertical axis, and the corresponding values, or highest value in each selected interval, are plotted on the horizontal axis (Fig. 3.4). If the distribution of values is gaussian, then the plot will yield a straight line. In real situations, such as the 100 glucose values in Table 3.4, a straight line is drawn to provide the best fit through the plotted points. Lines are then drawn from the 2.5 and 97.5 percentiles on the vertical axis until they intersect this line. From this intersection point, lines are dropped, and the corresponding glucose values are obtained.

When the same data for serum glucose values are evaluated using probability graph paper, as shown in Figure 3.4, the reference range established using

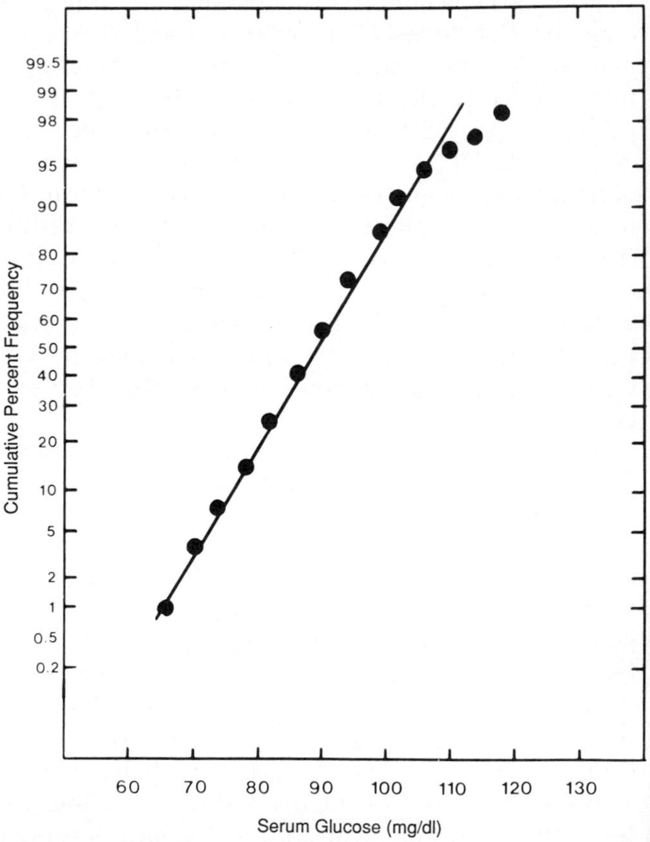

Figure 3.4. Cumulative frequency distribution of serum glucose values plotted on probability graph paper.

Table 3.5. Distribution of Serum Creatine Kinase Values (U/liter) from 100 Healthy Donors

CK Value	Frequency	Cumulative Fraction	CK Value	Frequency	Cumulative Fraction
31	1	0.01	99	1	0.58
32	1	0.02	101	1	0.59
33	1	0.03	102	1	0.60
36	1	0.04	105	1	0.61
37	1	0.05	108	1	0.62
40	1	0.06	111	2	0.64
41	1	0.07	112	1	0.65
44	1	0.08	114	1	0.66
45	2	0.10	115	1	0.67
46	2	0.12	118	1	0.68
47	3	0.15	120	3	0.71
50	1	0.16	121	1	0.72
51	4	0.20	123	1	0.73
55	2	0.22	124	1	0.74
57	2	0.24	128	1	0.75
58	1	0.25	131	1	0.76
60	2	0.27	140	1	0.77
62	1	0.28	141	1	0.78
64	1	0.29	145	1	0.79
65	1	0.30	154	1	0.80
66	1	0.31	155	1	0.81
68	2	0.33	162	1	0.82
69	3	0.36	163	1	0.83
70	1	0.37	171	1	0.84
72	1	0.38	178	1	0.85
74	2	0.40	179	1	0.86
75	3	0.43	183	1	0.87
77	1	0.44	185	1	0.88
78	1	0.45	192	1	0.89
80	1	0.46	193	1	0.90
83	1	0.47	194	1	0.91
84	1	0.48	199	1	0.92
87	1	0.49	201	1	0.93
90	1	0.50	211	1	0.94
91	1	0.51	216	1	0.95
92	1	0.52	220	1	0.96
94	1	0.53	248	1	0.97
95	1	0.54	258	1	0.98
96	2	0.56	261	1	0.99
97	1	0.57	268	1	1.00

the 2.5 and 97.5 percentiles is 68 to 109 mg/dl, which agrees well with the range that was established using the calculated arithmetic mean and the standard deviation. The observed median (50th percentile) for the line of best fit is 88 mg/dl, which also agrees with the actual median value in Table 3.4.

Frequently, the distribution of biological values among the normal healthy population is not gaussian. Table 3.5 lists the creatine kinase enzyme activities in serum samples from 100 donors. When a histogram of the frequency pattern of these values is drawn (Fig. 3.5), it becomes clear that the distribution of values in the normal population is skewed. This skewed pattern is also referred to as a log normal distribution because a normal distribution pattern can be achieved if the data are plotted logarithmically instead of on a linear scale. For these data, the three measures of centrality are widely different; the arithmetic mean value is 104 U/liter, the median value 90 U/liter, and the mode 51 U/liter. If the 95% reference limits for data from Table 3.5 were to be estimated using the arithmetic mean and standard deviation, the reference range ($\bar{x} \pm 2$ SD) would be calculated as −12 U/liter to +220 U/liter. This range would be quickly labeled as peculiar because values less than zero are not observed in the healthy or diseased population.

If the values are plotted on normal probability paper, as shown in Figure 3.6, the cumulative frequency demonstrates a line that curves to the right. Because any number of best-fit straight lines could be drawn through selected portions of the plot, it would be difficult to establish a reference range with a high degree of confidence. However, by plotting the cu-

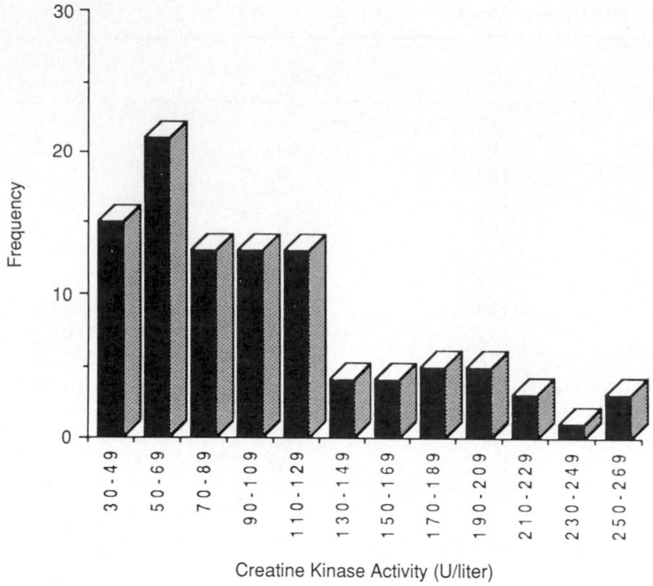

Figure 3.5. Histogram of serum creatine kinase values from 100 healthy donors. Individual values are listed in Table 3.5.

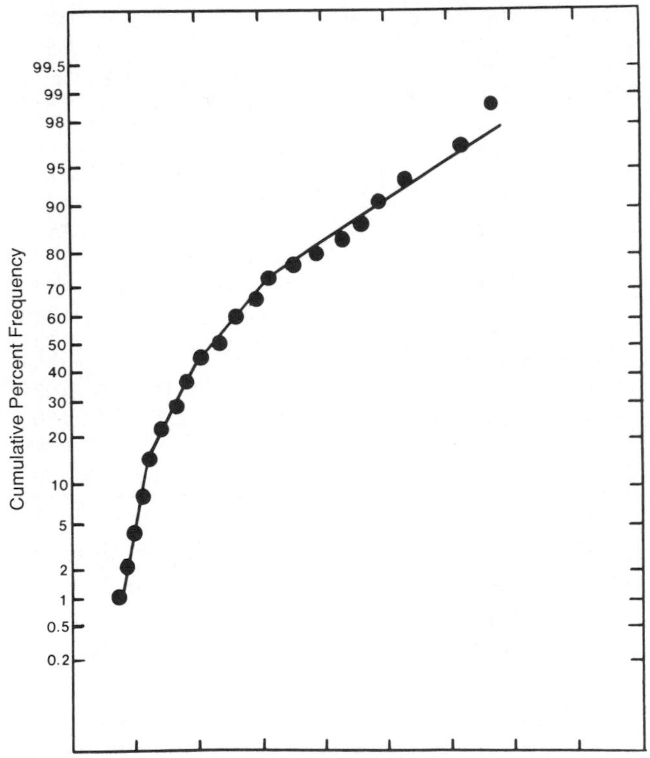

Figure 3.6. Cumulative frequency distribution of serum creatine kinase values plotted on probability graph paper.

mulative frequency on log probability paper (Fig. 3.7), it is possible to obtain a straight line. By connecting the ordinate and abscissa at the 2.5 and 97.5 percentiles, as was done for the previous glucose values in Figure 3.4, it is possible to determine that the

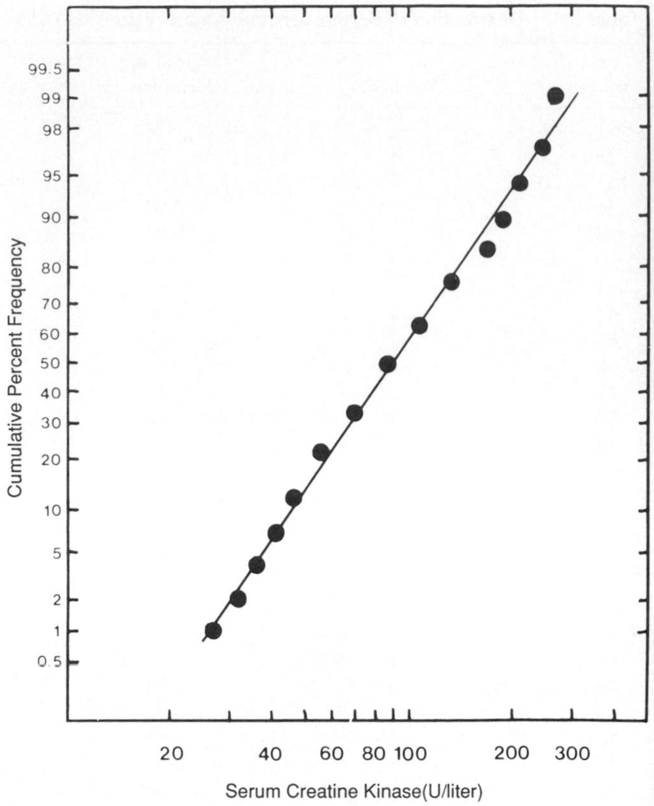

Figure 3.7. Cumulative frequency distribution of serum creatine kinase values plotted on logarithmic probability graph paper.

reference range is 32 to 260 U/liter. This range differs significantly from the one calculated from the mean and standard deviations, but it corresponds well with the actual creatine kinase values for the 2.5 percentile and 97.5 percentile positions (32 and 253 U/liter, respectively) in the raw data in Table 3.5.

PREDICTIVE VALUE THEORY

In addition to the analytical variability of a laboratory test, clinicians must also be concerned with weighing the diagnostic value of a test result. In an ideal situation, the populations of diseased and healthy individuals could be easily distinguished if the distribution of test results for the two groups were widely different and did not overlap. Unfortunately, this is never the case. The reference ranges for the two categories of patients overlap (Fig. 3.8); some nondiseased individuals will have abnormal results, and some patients with the particular disease will have normal test values.

The diagnostic utility or accuracy of a laboratory test is defined by the test's specificity, sensitivity, predictive value, and efficiency. The diagnostic sensitivity and specificity should not be confused with the analytical sensitivity and specificity, which were defined earlier. In the context of this discussion, the sensitivity is the frequency of abnormal or positive

Table 3.6. Predictive Value Model

	Patients with Positive Result	Patients with Negative Result	Total
Patients with selected disease	TP	FN	TP + FN
Patients without selected disease	FP	TN	FP + TN
Total	TP + FP	FN + TN	TP + FP + TN + FN

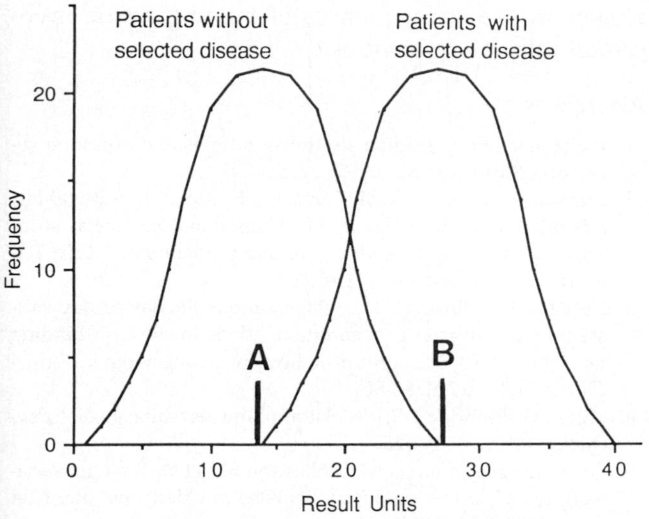

Figure 3.8. Example of distribution of results in populations of patients with and without disease. At setpoint *A* the sensitivity of the test is maximized. At setpoint *B* the specificity of the test is maximized.

test results in individuals who have a selected disease. The specificity is the frequency with which a normal or negative test result is observed in individuals free of the disease. Both the sensitivity and specificity are numerically expressed as percentages, and they are derived by using the values obtained from a predictive value model or table (Table 3.6).

Sensitivity is expressed as the percentage:

$$\frac{TP}{TP + FN} \times 100 \qquad (3.3)$$

where TP denotes the number of diseased patients having a positive test result (true positives), and FN denotes the number of diseased patients with a negative test result (false negatives).

Specificity is expressed as the percentage:

$$\frac{TN}{FP + TN} \times 100 \qquad (3.4)$$

where TN denotes the number of nondiseased patients with a negative test result (true negatives), and FP denotes the number of nondiseased patients with a positive test result (false positives).

In the actual clinical setting, a physician is often more interested in answering the question of whether an abnormal test result really indicates that the patient has a particular disease or whether a normal test result correctly excludes the existence of a disease in the patient. Expressed another way, what is the predictive value of the test? The predictive value of a positive (abnormal) result is obtained by dividing the number of true positives by the total number of patients, both true and false, with a positive test result. Conversely, the predictive value of a negative (normal) test result is calculated by dividing the number of true negatives by the total number of patients, both true and false, with a negative test result.

Predictive value of positive test result:

$$\frac{TP}{TP + FP} \times 100 \qquad (3.5)$$

Predictive value of negative test result:

$$\frac{TN}{TN + FN} \times 100 \qquad (3.6)$$

One additional characteristic that is often used to describe the diagnostic usefulness of a clinical test is the "efficiency" of the test. The efficiency can be described as the probability that a test result, whether positive or negative, correctly classifies the presence or absence of disease. This is calculated as the sum of the true results (positive and negative) divided by the sum of all test results.

Efficiency of test:

$$\frac{TP + TN}{TP + FP + FN + TN} \times 100 \qquad (3.7)$$

The prevalence of the disease within the selected population has a significant effect on the predictive value of a test, even when the sensitivity and specificity of the test may seem very high. Table 3.7 illustrates the effect of disease prevalence on the predictive value for a test with a sensitivity and specificity of 95%. When disease prevalence is low, the frequency that positive test results are correct is small. For a disease that occurs in 1% of the selected population, the predictive value of the test is only 16%. Because the prevalence of most diseases is low in the general population, the predictive value of a single test would also be expected to be low. This is one reason why it is important to select tests judiciously.

Table 3.7. Relationship of Disease Prevalence and Predictive Value of a Positive Test Result[a]

Prevalence of Disease within Population (%)	Predictive Value of Positive Test Result (%)
1	16.1
2	27.9
5	50.0
10	67.9
25	86.4
50	95.0

[a] Sensitivity 95%, specificity 95%.

If the test is performed on patients who have an appropriate medical history or symptoms consistent with a suspected disease, then the value of a positive test result will be much greater. In other words, the prevalence of the disease has been increased through selection of an appropriate subset of the general population for evaluation.

Sensitivity and specificity have an inverse relationship. Any attempts to improve one of these parameters will result in some negative change in the value of the other. It is not possible to maximize sensitivity and specificity at the same time. Because of this limitation, it is necessary to consider the consequences of setting the cut-off points, which are used to discriminate normal from abnormal test results, at any particular levels (Fig. 3.8). For a particular situation, is it more important to maximize the diagnostic sensitivity or specificity of the test?

If a test is the primary tool used to screen for a serious but treatable disease, it is important that the sensitivity of the test be maximized. It is also important that the consequences of a false-positive result not result in unnecessary harm, socially or medically, to a patient. It is common for a simple or cost-effective screening test to be used in conjunction with a secondary confirmatory test that has a high specificity. Examples of screening tests that have been adapted to the requirements of a high diagnostic sensitivity are neonatal screening tests for phenylketonuria and other metabolic disorders.

Alternatively, the circumstances surrounding the test may require that the specificity of the test be maximized. This is the case if the disease in question is serious but has no effective treatment, if the incidence of a false positive result will cause unnecessary harm to the patient, or if the test is used to confirm the results of another screening test. For example, tests used to evaluate genetic problems must be very specific. In most cases, the hereditary genetic abnormality cannot be cured in an affected family member. Nonetheless, an accurate identification of a genetic abnormality may be of importance for proper counseling purposes. A false-positive diagnosis may result in unnecessary psychological harm to the parents or may incorrectly influence a decision regarding future parenting.

It may be that a false positive or false negative result may induce unnecessary economic, psychological, or physical harm. In this situation, the efficiency of the test should be maximized. An example of this is the diagnosis of a myocardial infarct. A false positive diagnosis will produce a potentially inappropriate hospitalization and future anxiety for the patient. However, the consequences of missing a true myocardial infarct are obvious.

References

1. Weitzman ED. Circadian rhythms and episodic hormone secretion. Annu Rev Med 1976;27:225–243.
2. Samuels MH, Wood WM, Gordon DF, Kleinschmidt-DeMasters BK, Lillihei K, Ridgway EC. Clinical and molecular studies of a thyrotropin-secreting pituitary adenoma. J Clin Endocrinol Metab 1989;68:1211–1215.
3. Statland BE, Winkel P. The relationship of the day-to-day variation of serum iron concentration values to the iron binding capacity values in a group of healthy young women. Am J Clin Pathol 1977;67:84–90.
4. Miles A, Philbrick DRS. Melatonin and psychiatry. Biol Psychiatry 1988;23:405–425.
5. Fraser CG, Cummings ST, Wilkinson SP, et al. Biologic variability of 26 clinical chemistry analytes in elderly people. Clin Chem 1989;35:783–786.
6. Browning MCK, Ford RP, Callaghan SJ, Fraser CG. Intra- and interindividual biologic variation of five analytes used in assessing thyroid function: implications for necessary standards of performance and the interpretation of results. Clin Chem 1986;32:962–966.
7. Holzel WGE. Intra-individual variation of analytes in serum from patients with chronic liver disease. Clin Chem 1987;33:1133–1136.
8. Holzel WGE. Intra-individual variation of some analytes in serum of patients with chronic renal failure. Clin Chem 1987;33:670–673.
9. Holzel WGE. Intra-individual variation of some analytes in serum of patients with insulin-dependent diabetes mellitus. Clin Chem 1987;33:57–61.
10. Gowens EMS, Fraser CG. Longer-term biological variation of commonly analyzed serum constituents. Clin Chem 1987;33:717.
11. Gomez P, Coca C, Vargas C, Acebillo J, Martinez A. Normal reference intervals for 20 biochemical variables in healthy infants, children, and adolescents. Clin Chem 1984;30:407–412.
12. Lockitch G, Halstead AC, Albersheim S, MacCallum C, Quigley G. Age- and sex-specific pediatric reference intervals for biochemistry analytes as measured with the Ektachem-700 analyzer. Clin Chem 1988;34:1622–1625.
13. Matoth Y, Zaizov R, Varsano I. Postnatal changes in some red cell parameters. Acta Paediatr Scand 1971;60:317–323.
14. Fisher DA, Klein AH. Thyroid development and disorders of thyroid function in the newborn. N Engl J Med 1981;304:702–712.
15. Keating FP, Jones JD, Elveback LR, Randall RV. The relationship of age and sex to distribution of values in healthy adults of serum calcium, inorganic phosphorus, magnesium, alkaline phosphatase, total proteins, albumin, and blood urea. J Lab Clin Med 1969;73:825–834.
16. Lipid Research Clinics Program Epidemiology Committee. Plasma lipid distributions in selected North American popula-

tions. The Lipid Research Clinics Program prevalence study. Circulation 1979;60:427–439.
17. O'Sullivan JB. Age gradient in blood glucose. Diabetes 1974;23:713–715.
18. Cockcroft DW, Gault MH. Prediction of creatinine clearance from serum creatinine. Nephron 1976;16:31–41.
19. Buckley CE, Dorsey FC. Serum immunoglobulin levels throughout the life-span of healthy men. Ann Intern Med 1971;75:673–682.
20. Carlsten A, Hallgren B, Jagenburg R, Svanborg A, Werko L. Arterial concentration of free fatty acids and free amino acids in healthy individuals at rest and at different workloads. Scand J Clin Lab Invest 1962;14:185–191.
21. Campbell WW, Anderson RA. Effects of aerobic exercise and training on the trace minerals chromium, zinc, and copper. Sports Med 1987;4:9–18.
22. Sinzinger H, Virgolini I. Effects of exercise on parameters of blood coagulation, platelet function and the prostaglandin system. Sports Med 1988;6:238–245.
23. Poortmans JR. Exercise and renal function. Sports Med 1984;1:125–153.
24. King SW, Statland BE, Savory J. The effects of a short burst of exercise on activity values of enzymes in sera of healthy subjects. Clin Chim Acta 1976;72:211–218.
25. Noakes TD. Effect of exercise on serum enzyme activities in humans. Sports Med 1987;4:245–267.
26. Shideler CE, Stumphauser L. Effects of physical training on selected biochemical and physiological parameters. Clin Chem 1984;30:1005–1006.
27. Martin RP, Haskell WI, Wood PD. Blood chemistry and lipid profiles of elite distance runners. Ann NY Acad Sci 1977;301:346–360.
28. Green MF, Fencl M, Tulchinsky D. Biochemical aspects of pregnancy. In: Tietz N, ed. Textbook of clinical chemistry. Philadelphia: WB Saunders, 1986:1745–1787.
29. Todd ME, Thompson JH, Bowie EJW, Owen CA. Changes in blood coagulation during pregnancy. Mayo Clin Proc 1965;40:370–383.
30. Statland BE, Winkel P, Bokelund H. Serum alkaline phosphatase after fatty meals: the effect of substrate on the assay procedure. Clin Chim Acta 1973;49:299–300.
31. Leppanen EA, Grasbeck R. Experimental basis of standardized specimen collection: the effect of moderate ethanol consumption on some serum components (K, Na, ASAT, ALAT, CK, LD, total protein). Scand J Clin Lab Invest 1987;47:337–343.
32. Leppanen EA, Grasbeck R. Experimental basis of standardized blood collection: effect of posture on blood picture. Eur J Haematol 1988;40:222–226.
33. Felding P, Tryding N, Hyloft-Petersen P, Horder M. Effects of posture on concentrations of blood constituents in healthy adults: practical application of blood specimen collection procedures recommended by the Scandinavian Committee on Reference Values. Scand J Clin Lab Invest 1980;40:615–621.
34. Statland BE, Bokelund H, Winkel P. Factors contributing to intra-individual variation of serum constituents. 4. Effects of posture and tourniquet application on variation of serum constituents in healthy subjects. Clin Chem 1974;20:1513–1519.
35. Dixon M, Paterson CR. Posture and the composition of plasma. Clin Chem 1978;24:824–826.
36. Doumas BT, Hause LL, Simuncak DM, Breitenfeld D. Differences between values for serum and plasma in tests performed in the Ektachem 700 XR analyzer, and evaluation of "plasma separator tubes" (PST). Clin Chem 1989;35:151–153.
37. Smith JC, Lewis S, Holbrook J, Seidel K, Rose A. Effects of heparin and citrate on measured concentrations of various analytes in plasma. Clin Chem 1987;33:814–816.
38. Ladenson JH, Tsai LMB, Michael JM, et al. Serum versus heparinized plasma for eighteen common chemistry tests. Am J Clin Pathol 1974;62:545–552.
39. Schmidt LH. The nature of the difference in phospholipid content of oxalated and heparinized plasma. J Biol Chem 1935;109:449–453.
40. Calam RR. Specimen processing separator gels. An update. J Clin Immunoassay 1988;11:86–90.
41. McPhredan P, Clyne LP, Ortoli NA, et al. Prolongation of the activated partial thromboplastin time associated with poor venipuncture technique. Am J Clin Pathol 1974;62:16–20.
42. Calam RR, Cooper MH. Recommended order of draw for collecting blood specimens into additive-containing tubes. Clin Chem 1982;28:1399.
43. Rehak NN, Chiang BT. Storage of whole blood: effect of temperature on the measured concentration of analytes in serum. Clin Chem 1988;34(10):2111–2114.
44. Ono T, Kitaguchi K, Takehara M, Shiiba M, Hayami K. Serum-constituent analyses: effect of duration and temperature of storage of clotted blood. Clin Chem 1981;27:35–38.
45. Rossing RG, Foster DM. The stability of clinical chemistry specimens during refrigerated storage for 24 hours. Am J Clin Pathol 1980;73:91–95.
46. Young DS, Pestaner LC, Gibberman V. Effects of drugs on clinical laboratory tests. Clin Chem 1975;21:1D–432D.
47. Friedman RB, Anderson RE, Entine SB, Hirshberg SB. Effects of diseases on clinical laboratory tests. Clin Chem 1980;26:1D–476D.

4 Laboratory Information Systems

Kenneth D. McClatchey and Thomas Peterson

HISTORY OF HOSPITAL/LABORATORY INFORMATION SYSTEMS

Digital computers became available for general use in the late 1950s (1–3). Early computers provided few user-oriented features and required considerable knowledge and skill to operate. They ran batch-oriented programs and supported "single-tasking" only. FORTRAN and COBOL were the only high-level languages available. Typically, mainframe computer systems were encased in rooms with glass walls and were tended by computer specialists who spoke their own language and were often far removed from normal hospital activities. This specialization and remoteness often resulted in the development of applications that were ill-suited to the workaday departmental information processing needs of hospitals.

Most major computer manufacturers such as IBM, Burroughs, Honeywell, and NCR, understanding the potential for sales in the health care market, were active in their support of hospital information systems early in the development of the field. Corporations such as Lockheed and McDonnell-Douglas, which were experienced in using computers to manage complex management tasks, also decided to enter health care computing as business ventures. For example, Lockheed supported the early development of the Technicon Hospital Information System.

The Technicon system, begun by Lockheed in the 1960s, installed at the El Camino Hospital in Mountain View, California, became the best known and most successful patient management system of its time. The ultimate success of the system at El Camino led to the spread of this and other systems into other hospitals. The Technicon system is still being marketed today, which is unusual since many of the early software and hardware vendors have gone out of business or are no longer active in the hospital market.

In 1987, Hammond (4) listed five factors that have driven the development of hospital information systems:

1. *Hardware and software technological factors:* During the development period, computers evolved from single-tasking "untouchable" and "unfriendly" mainframe computers to highly interactive and multiuser minicomputers;
2. *Increasing technological expertise* on the part of system developers and users;
3. *Economic factors:* As the cost of delivering health care increased, computers seemed to offer at least the opportunity to operate in a more efficient manner;
4. *An increase in the amount of laboratory data generated,* which necessitated more automated procedures; and
5. *Increased influence of external organizations:* Information requirements of federal and state governments and third-party payers forced hospitals to turn to automated systems for financial and patient management applications.

An interesting phenomenon is taking place in hospitals in such places as hospital information systems, laboratory information systems, and other "computer foci." Physicians, Ph.Ds, medical technologists and other health professionals are taking a supreme interest in "their" information systems (5–7). No longer are "insiders" such as suppliers, consulting firms, and those in the computer department the only ones dealing with the complex issues of medical computing. Probably the biggest reason for such "outside" interest in hospital computing is the rapid evolution of personal computing. When, as described by Gunton, the insiders (health care providers) see the relationship between computing systems, success is the outcome (8).

The clinical laboratory is one of the most technologically advanced departments within a hospital. It requires sophisticated computer technology. Laboratory computer technology must, in addition, keep up with increasingly sophisticated diagnostic laboratory equipment. There are computer functions that are considered basic to clinical laboratory "computing";

- on-line order entry interface;
- results reporting interface;

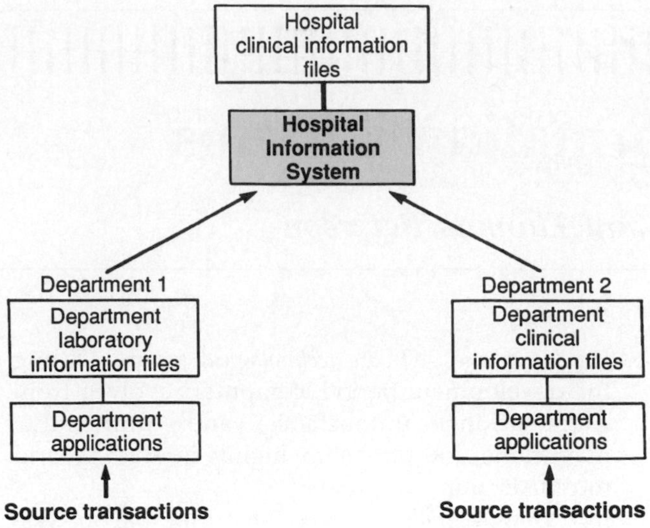

Figure 4.1. Distributed hospital information processing. (Modified from Gunton T. Inside information technology: a practical guide to management issues. Cambridge, United Kingdom: Prentice-Hall, 1990.)

- on-line admission, discharge, transfer interface;
- on-line instrument data acquisition;
- batch work lists; and
- batch reports.

Since the 1970s, information technology has become one of the most successful professions. The profession has developed, for example, ways to store vast quantities of information, to eliminate cumbersome laborious administrative work, and improve the operation of complex organizational systems by expediting the flow of information (8). With decentralized processing power brought on by personal computers, Grosch's law has ceased to operate. Grosch's law states that "processing power increases according to the square of its cost" (8). The legitimacy of such a statement no longer exists. Such theory has given way to distributed processing (Fig. 4.1).

Another important concept in the overall development of information systems is the concept of an integrated database—or a collection of interrelated items of data that not only holds the data itself (e.g., patient orders), but also records the relationships between the items it contains (Fig. 4.2).

As described by Elevitch and Aller (2, 3), management of the clinical laboratory (in the present customer service revolution that medicine finds itself) requires that laboratory management understand the "business" of the clinical laboratory. Some factors to consider include patient demographics, diagnostic case mix, patient therapeutic requirements, test ordering patterns, test mix, staffing patterns, and personnel and material costs.

TERMS USED IN CONNECTION WITH INFORMATION PROCESSING

The term *mainframe computer* is used to refer to the large and powerful computers that run the hospital financial and patient management applications. *Patient management software* provides the administrative support for hospital patients with applications such as admission-discharge-transfer (ADT) or appointment scheduling. Control of the mainframe computer resides with hospital administration. The mainframe computing group in a hospital is often referred to as *HIS*s, which stands for *hospital information systems* or *hospital information services*. The HIS group in the hospital should be distinguished from *HIS vendors*, who are the commercial providers of the software that runs on the mainframe computers. HIS applications increasingly can be found running on minicomputers rather than mainframe devices as minicomputers become more "powerful."

Departmental systems such as pathology, radiology, or cardiology generally run as stand-alone systems on minicomputers. *Stand-alone* refers to the capability of such a system to run independently of other systems. However, departmental systems are rarely totally autonomous and truly stand-alone; to run efficiently, interfaces that link departmental systems with a hospital mainframe computer for exchange of admission-discharge-transfer, patient management, and billing information must be installed. Departmental systems are often physically located in the departments they serve.

Another fairly common option is to locate the computer physically in an environmentally controlled mainframe computer room and allocate control for hardware and system software support to the HIS. In such a situation, clinical laboratory personnel retain control over the application software supplied by the laboratory information systems (LIS) vendor. Such a cost-saving measure avoids the duplication of computer rooms throughout the hospital.

A wide variety of discipline-specific departmental-type systems are installed in hospitals today. *Laboratory information systems (LISs)* are the most common type, which is undoubtedly because LISs were the first departmental systems to be developed commercially. Radiology information systems (RISs) are becoming increasing popular. RISs, which run applications like radiology report generation, patient scheduling, and film tracking, must be distinguished from picture archiving computer systems (PACS) which store and retrieve radiological images. Such systems are on the drawing board for clinical laboratory applications. Other rapidly evolving departmental systems include pharmacy systems and operating room information systems.

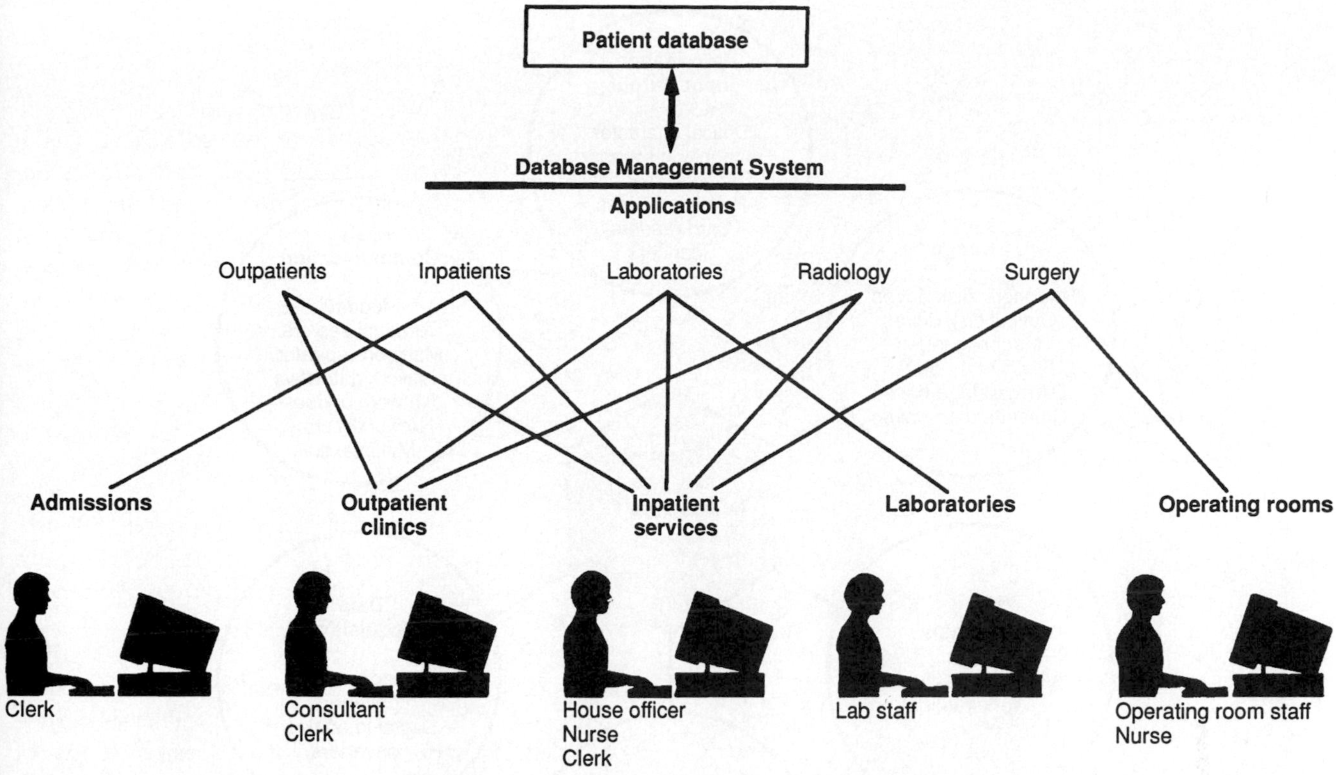

Figure 4.2. Applications sharing an integrated database.

LISs are often sold as so-called *turnkey systems,* which means that the software and hardware can be purchased as a single package from the software vendor. In such a case, the software vendor acts as a value-added reseller (VAR) for the computer hardware manufacturer by packaging the software with the hardware as a single unit. A hospital client often has the additional option of purchasing only software from a LIS vendor, and then negotiating separately with the hardware manufacturer for hardware. Turnkey, in relation to a LIS, implies that laboratory personnel need only turn such systems on after installation, and the system will then proceed to run all applications and provide the expected broad support. Given the sophistication of systems in today's marketplace, this term is a gross oversimplification and is quite misleading. However, the use of the term persists in the clinical laboratory environment.

A relatively new phenomenon in the medical computing marketplace has been the emergence of vendors of *clinical information systems (CISs).* These systems combine multiple clinical modules such as laboratory, pharmacy, and nursing, plus software to support order-entry, result-reporting, and archiving of patient care information. Such systems also generate and pass billing information to the financial system. CISs are now being developed by the vendors of LISs who are trying to increase their market share by developing products with greater breadth. HIS vendors are also crossovers from financial and patient management software development, and add clinical modules to their products to create what is called "a single-vendor solution" to offer hospital clients.

Laboratory Information Systems Hardware

One of the more exciting aspects of the field of laboratory information systems is the rapid advances in its technology. Hardware technology changes so rapidly, it causes significant changes to computer terminology. For example, what used to be a term used to benchmark hard disk storage capacity, the megabyte or MB (1,000,000 bytes), has been superseded by gigabyte (GB) (1,000 megabytes) and terabyte (TB) (10,000 megabytes). What is useful in this example of terms is the concept of byte as a storage unit (one byte is equivalent to one character). The laboratorian should simply expect the prefix to change as technology advances.

Most personal computer (PC) users are already familiar with disk drives, printers, modems, kilobytes, etc. Although knowledge of the personal computer is helpful in the understanding of information processing, it does not transfer as expertise regarding the concepts of information technology in the clinical laboratory. The reverse is equally true, that LIS experts are not necessarily experts at personal com-

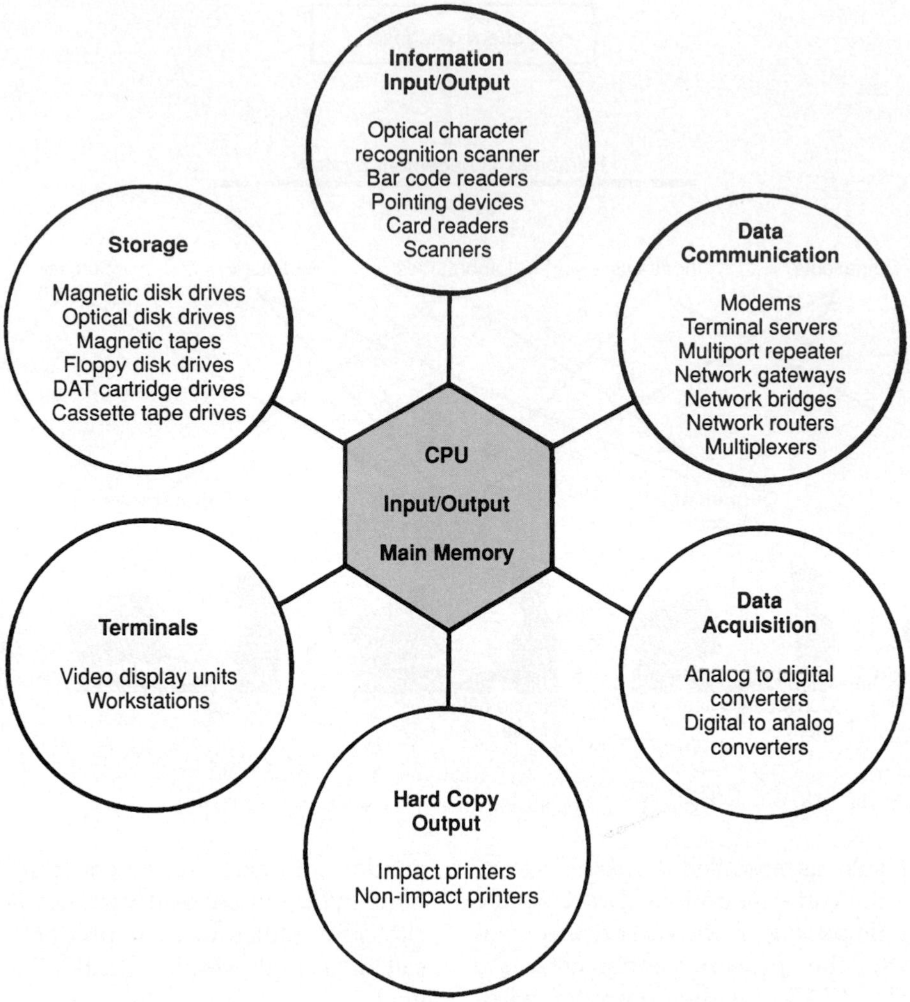

Figure 4.3. The hardware of a general computer system.

puter technology. Both "experts" are specialists in each of their fields, sharing a common subset of terminology. The purpose of this section is to review the terminology of computers and advise the reader on the current strategies of the use of this technology in laboratory information systems (LISs).

The basic hardware of a computer system includes (*a*) central processor unit; (*b*) main memory; (*c*) input/output processor; and (*d*) peripheral devices such as disk and tape drives, printers, and terminals (Fig. 4.3). The following section will discuss the devices and explain their operation and the problems associated with selecting and managing these components.

Central Processor Unit

The central processor unit (CPU) executes instructions and interacts with the main memory and various input/output (I/O) devices such as disk, tape drives, and printers. The executed instructions are in the form of machine language usually derived from higher level languages such as Pascal, FORTRAN, and COBOL. The I/O devices perform tasks as dictated by the CPU, and the information flows as a read or write instruction from main memory to disk, tape, terminals, or printers, or vice versa. The CPU is the single most important entity that determines the performance characteristics of a computer system. A common benchmark for computer systems is the number of million instructions per second (MIPS) that the CPU can perform. There is a wide variance in the speed rating of CPUs. The CPU is not the only factor that determines which computer system is the fastest. The overall I/O and main memory architecture of the computer's system will also affect the overall "efficiency" of a computer system.

One big difference between computers is the capacity and management of main memory. Minicomputers handle memory using a 32-bit (or better) architecture. The larger the size of the processor architecture, the more speed for information to be exchanged in and out of main memory. For comparison, look at PC technology; the IBM PC or XT has an 8-bit architecture, and the IBM AT has a 16-bit architecture. Another factor that optimizes the performance of a CPU is the use of virtual memory. Virtual memory is a memory management technique that effectively allows a computer system to appear to have nearly unlimited amounts of main memory. With virtual memory, the computer can run out of physical main memory blocks because the CPU will swap out inactive blocks of main memory to disk, allowing for additional loading of information into physical main memory. This permits the execution of programs that are larger than the available main memory.

Storage Devices

An important part of a computer system is the external storage devices such as hard disk drives. Hard disk drives serve as the primary storage device for information. The capacity and performance of these drives are always increasing while the cost per byte of such devices is decreasing. Capacities greater than 1 gigabyte per drive are now common. The lower cost per byte trend allows an LIS to keep more and more information on line at a lower direct cost. It is common to have 6 months to 1 year of general laboratory information on line. This lower cost per byte is also allowing LIS to shadow important drives. A shadow drive is a drive that is dedicated to maintain an exact copy of information stored on a primary drive. As the primary drive receives a write instruction, the shadow drive also receives a duplicate write instruction. If the primary drive fails to operate, the shadow drive becomes the active drive and continues servicing the mass storage needs of the LIS. This technique decreases recovery time in the event a drive fails. Using shadow drive techniques, recovery time from a drive failure is measured in terms of minutes. Without this technique, recovery time is measured in terms of hours.

A new technology for information storage that has emerged is optical drives. In optical drives information is written and read by a laser beam. There are two types of optical drives, the write once read many (WORM) drives, and the magnetic-optical (MO) drives. Both drive types write and read information on a removable media. Storage capacities for optical drives are 600 MB to 2 GB on one disk. Because the media in optical drives are removable, there is unlimited capacity for storage of information. Optical disks can be changed in the drive as the need arises. The WORM technology is gaining popularity as an alternative to tape storage for archivial purposes. Storage of the purged information from an LIS to a WORM drive gives the LIS system an additional option of "random accession" of archived data. In contrast, the purging of data to tape does not allow continued random access to the data unless the tape is reloaded and the information is copied to disk. The proliferation of WORM drives in LIS systems will extend the lifetime of information available on line. Archiving of purged data to a WORM drive allows the data to be randomly available yet on a medium for ready eventual archiving when full.

Another use for optical drives is the archiving of reports. An LIS system will generate many daily, weekly, or monthly reports that in the past were laboriously typed and printed. For example, daily activity reports by department are printed by most LIS systems. They are used for troubleshooting problems and clinical laboratory department statistics. Quite often these reports are shelved unless needed for one of the previously mentioned uses. Instead of printing these reports on paper, the reports are printed to a file on an optical disk. A report that is stored in this fashion saves paper, printing time, printer usage, and "people time." The report is actually in a more convenient electronic media that allows the reader to use electronic tools to find information imbedded in that report. A simple electronic viewer with "search for text capabilities" will allow the reader to find the information in a large report many times faster than a manual paper search. Also, an electronic search will be more accurate and thorough compared with performing a manual search using paper copy. Another advantage of this technique for storing reports is the ability to take the information from these electronic reports and use it for purposes not originally anticipated. In the past, laboratory professionals might use a paper report and realize if the report was compiled differently it would make a statistic report easier to accomplish. Electronic reports can ultimately be stripped, parsed, and transferred into a PC database to create new reports.

A new development in optical drive technology is magnetic-optical drives. These drives differ from the WORM drives in that they are erasable. They offer nearly the same capacity of WORM drives but the information can be erased; therefore, the disk can be reused. Considering that optical disks cost in the hundreds of dollars, being able to reuse a disk is most cost effective. MO drives can be used in the same fashion as the WORM drives.

Magnetic tape is typically used for backup of the information stored on the computer system. Backup is a procedure where a copy of all important information and programs used by the LIS are copied. Backup is performed daily by most systems and its sole purpose is to keep a copy of the information in another form in case a malfunction destroys the "on-line" active information. Important considerations when setting up a backup procedure is the frequency of backup. In some laboratory information systems, backup of important files are performed hourly. The frequency of backup usually determines the ease at which you can recover from a malfunction. The more frequent a backup procedure is performed, the easier it is to restore that loss of information. The low media costs and readily available tape units make the magnetic tape a standard tool in backup procedures.

A new type of magnetic tape drive using an 8-mm DAT cartridge is becoming very popular. This new technology offers greater storage capacity on a smaller-sized media and faster recording speed. A tape cartridge the size of an audio cassette can store 2 gigabytes of information, which is equivalent to 12 to 13 nine-track half-inch magnetic tapes.

Floppy disk drives that are found on most PCs can store only 360 KB to 1.44 MB of information, whereas hard disk and optical drives can store in the MB to GB range. Floppy disks are used to quickly transfer information from one computer to another, an auxiliary storage device, or for backup of important files. They are routinely used for workstation support only. Floppy disk drives are not routinely used for backup of LIS systems because of the limited storage capacity per disk.

Hard Copy Output (Printers)

The most common dedicated output device is a printer. A printer produces a paper copy of information stored in a computer system (patient reports, department logs, invoices, etc.). Most LIS printers can be categorized into two types: impact printers and nonimpact printers. Impact printers create images on paper by striking the paper (usually through a ribbon) using a mechanical device. Impact printer devices include dot matrix (most common), daisy wheel, and band line printers. Their speed ranges from 10 characters per second to 2,000 lines per minute. They are ideal for printing multipart forms. Their disadvantages arise from their very mechanical nature. Impact printers are noisy and require more maintenance than other types of printers. In a hospital setting where patients are in close proximity to the printers, the noise factor makes impact printers unacceptable. The main advantage of impact printers is the cost of the printer. Dot matrix printers are the cheapest of the impact printers and account for the majority of printers in clinical laboratories today.

Nonimpact printers are quiet printers compared with impact printers. They include laser, inkjet, and thermal printers. These printers all have different printing speeds and printing quality. Laser printers have the highest quality output, usually 300 dots per inch (DPI). Laser printers are very popular for producing a high-quality output for patient reports. The cost of laser printers is slowly declining. The laser printer has become the printer of choice for single-copy output. Thermal printers require special paper, and the images over long periods of time (years) may degrade. Thermal printers should be used only for temporary reports and summaries. Inkjet printers shoot electrostatically charged ink focused by magnetic fields onto paper. The problems with inkjet printers are that they tend to "clog" if not used frequently, and they usually require more expensive polished paper for a good, sharp image.

Terminals—Video Display Units

There are two main types of video display units (VDUs), smart and dumb terminals. Dumb terminals are terminals that cannot process any information locally. They do not have the capability of executing any programs locally. They serve as a slave communication device to a host. An example of a dumb terminal is a VT 220 VDU from DEC. A smart terminal is typically a personal computer that uses a communication program to communicate with the host LIS. The PC, of course, is capable of performing more than terminal emulation, and if properly configured, it is more appropriately termed a workstation. The cost of a PC workstation vs. a dumb terminal is becoming less every year, and more institutions are buying PCs to replace dumb VDUs. The LIS manager should be aware that there are hidden costs in supporting large numbers of PCs. Such costs are not necessary for the support of dumb VDUs. The PC does require software purchases for communicating with the host and expertise to configure the software. The PC requires additional training of users beyond the scope of LIS applications training. All of these costs can be minimized by standardizing the hardware and software platforms that are supported. The trend in today's laboratory informations systems is to use dumb terminals for routine data entry, patient inquiry, and "dedicated" LIS support functions and to use PCs for areas where additional functions are desired (word processing, graphics, data analysis, etc.).

New Input and Output Devices

Many I/O devices that were popular several years ago have gone through an "innovation revolution." Many devices improved in reliability and performance, but some devices did not survive the revolution. For example, card readers are becoming a rarely used technology in clinical laboratories. Card readers have suffered through the years from being very mechanical devices prone to failures. Accordingly, more technologically sophisticated alternative choices have become preferable. One such advanced alternative is the use of bar codes in concert with creative LIS software.

BAR CODE READERS

Bar code technology has been used successfully in discount stores and supermarkets for years to identify stock items customers buy. This technology was first introduced in the clinical laboratory incorporated into high-speed, high-volume "chemistry analyzers" such as Technicon analyzers. In these analyzers, the specimen cups have been tagged with bar codes that identify the specimen as the specimen is being sampled in the instrument. Bar coding of information as part of a laboratory information system has become a state-of-the-art technique. Bar coding allows easy identification of items without any keyboarding of any information. Typically, the accession number and/or the patient registration number is bar coded on each specimen label. This allows for efficient tracking of the specimen throughout its lifetime in the clinical laboratory. Both accuracy and speed of specimen handling are improved using bar coding techniques.

Bar codes can also be used to aid in result reporting. In areas where data input is limited to a series of coded phrases, a bar coded summary sheet becomes a handy tool. A summary sheet can contain 50 to 60 bar coded mnemonics or phrases on the coded summary sheet. This procedure eliminates the need of alternating from keyboard input to hand wand for each specimen processed.

For the new trainee, a customized coded summary sheet can be easily constructed to aid the computer LIS novice. This customized summary sheet amounts to a cheat sheet for the appropriate choices during a conversation with the LIS, thereby minimizing menu navigational and form entry problems. This type of bar coded sheet decreases training time for laboratory staff by supplementing the staff conversation with the LIS software.

Another use of a customized coded summary sheet is in the result entry process. For example, cytology results may have over 60 canned phrases that can be used to report a cytology result. In most LIS, these phrases are already coded into a result dictionary that can be referenced by a number or mnemonic. But because of the sheer number of possible choices, the recall of the appropriate number or mnemonic becomes challenging. Typically in those situations the users produce a table of codes and their phrases, then post this sheet next to all terminals used for result entry. These sheets serve as a quick look-up tool for the not so commonly used phrases. Instead of a simple listing of codes and their phrases, the addition of a bar code to each listing becomes the ideal result entry supplement.

DATA COMMUNICATION—MODEMS

Access of LIS data from a remote location (i.e., home or physician's office) can be accomplished efficiently using modems. A modem is a device that allows a user to gain access to information at computer centers using telephone lines (Fig. 4.4). The term modem is short for modulator-demodulator, a device that translates digital impulses from a computer or terminal into analog sound waves that are transmitted over phone lines. In turn, a receiving modem reverses the translation to digital impulses, thus allowing the user to access requested information. In practice, the process is not that simple.

For a data link to be complete, both modems must be compatible with each other. The first parameter to consider is the baud rate of the modems. Baud rate is the speed at which the modem can transfer information. The baud rate is measured in terms of change of audio signal per second and is usually equated to bits per second. The current baud rate standard is 2400, but baud rates of 9600 are now gaining popularity. If the remote modem does not match the baud rate of the host modem, no communication between the computers is possible. Most host modems are autobauding within a range of speeds (from 1200 to 2400 baud) and will try to match the remote modem's speed.

ERROR CORRECTION PROTOCOLS

The next parameter to consider is error correction protocols. The use of error correction protocols is very important to clinical applications. If an error correction protocol is not used, there is no assurance that the data received are 100% accurate. Voice quality phone lines have an average error rate of 6.5 errors per 10,000 characters at a 1,200 baud rate. At higher baud rates these error rates are even greater. A popular error correction protocol is Microcom's networking protocol (MNP), developed by Microcom, Inc. This protocol will package the data being sent with a data packet and a trailing verification packet. The trailing packet is derived from a calculation done on the preceding data packet. If both modems are using the same type of protocol, the receiving modem will read the data packet, perform the same calculation, and check to see if the verification packet agrees with its calculation. If the calculation agrees, the receiving modem acknowledges the acceptance of the packet to the sending modem and sends another set of packets. If the calculation does not agree (i.e., the signal was scrambled while being transmitted through the telephone line), then the receiving modem will send a request for retransmission of that data. The use of this type of error correction scheme will assure data integrity acceptable for

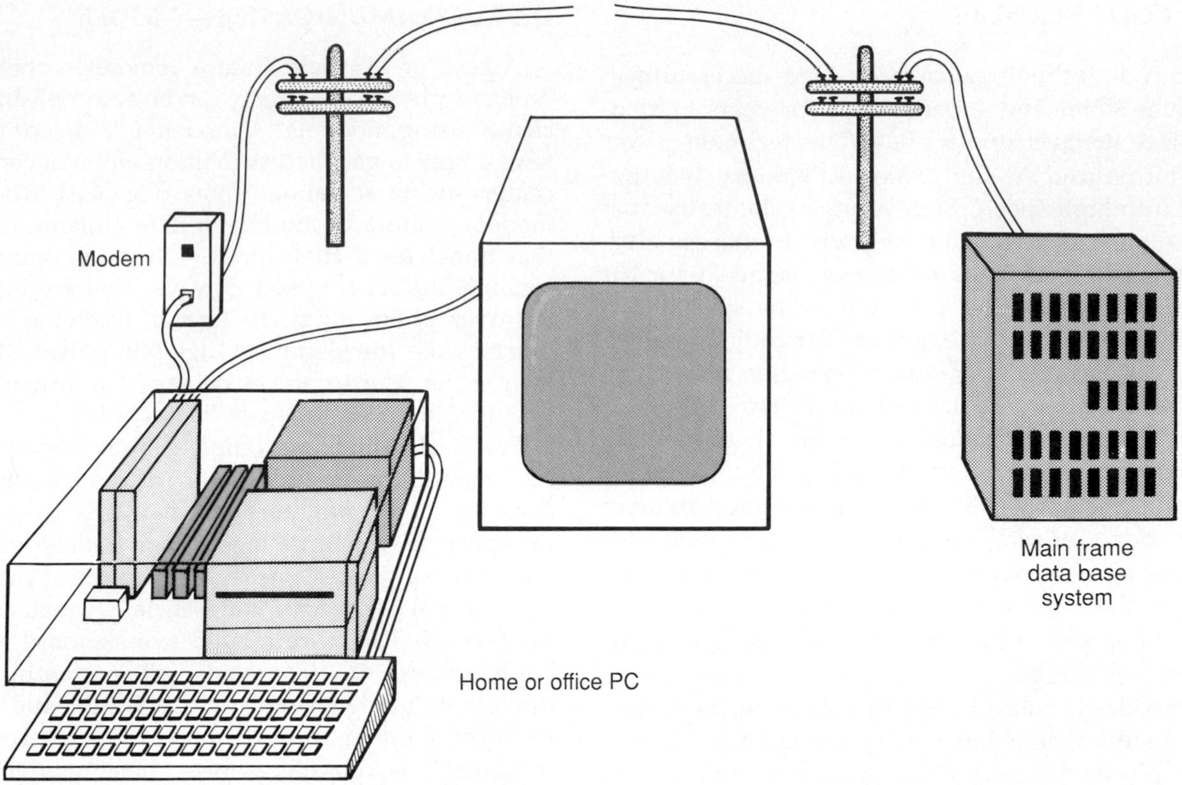

Figure 4.4. A modem provides a cost-effective way to distribute information.

clinical applications. Some protocols also incorporate data compression into their routine. Data compression serves to increase the effective rate of data transmission. As with error correction protocols, it is necessary for both the remote and host modems to employ the same data compression scheme.

Regardless of the types of modems used, the data must cross phone lines. The quality of the phone line will affect the reliability and speed of transmission. Voice quality lines are good for regular voice transmission but are sometimes not acceptable for data transmission. Conditioned lines that have been balanced by a phone company offer greater reliability in data transmission. For critical communication lines, a leased dedicated line can be purchased from a phone company. These leased lines are expensive and are used for high-traffic volumes or to support critical applications.

DATA COMMUNICATION—NETWORKS

One of the most significant advances in computer technology is the development of local area networks (LANs) (Fig. 4.5). LANs are high-speed highways used by computers to communicate with each other. LANs link computers and peripheral devices to one another, allowing the devices to share a common communication highway. Before LANs, computer devices such as terminals, printers, card readers, etc. were often connected by point-to-point cables that relied on RS-232 communication standards. Each device had its individual cable that extended back to a central communication cabinet located next to the central computer. These cables were expensive to install and maintain besides being difficult to expand the cable plan to accommodate additional peripheral devices. In point-to-point cabling, each device would communicate over shielded twisted pair wiring at typical baud rates of 2,400 to 9,600 bits/second. This rate of transmission is slow in comparison with today's LAN technology. There are various types of LANs but all offer data transfer rates that are approximately 10 to 16 megabits per second. Some of the most popular network standards are Ethernet and Token Ring networks. These two standards account for the majority of high-speed LANs on the market today. They rely on an advance wiring platform to carry information at high speeds. The physical connection is made using thick coaxial, thin coaxial, fiber-optical, or twisted pair cable. Each media has its advantages and disadvantages, and the types of cable used are usually determined by individual site requirements and budgets. Cabling a LAN is one of the more expensive parts of implementing and maintaining a LAN. The choice of cabling can make a big difference on the overall cost of implementing a LAN and how much it is going to cost to maintain it.

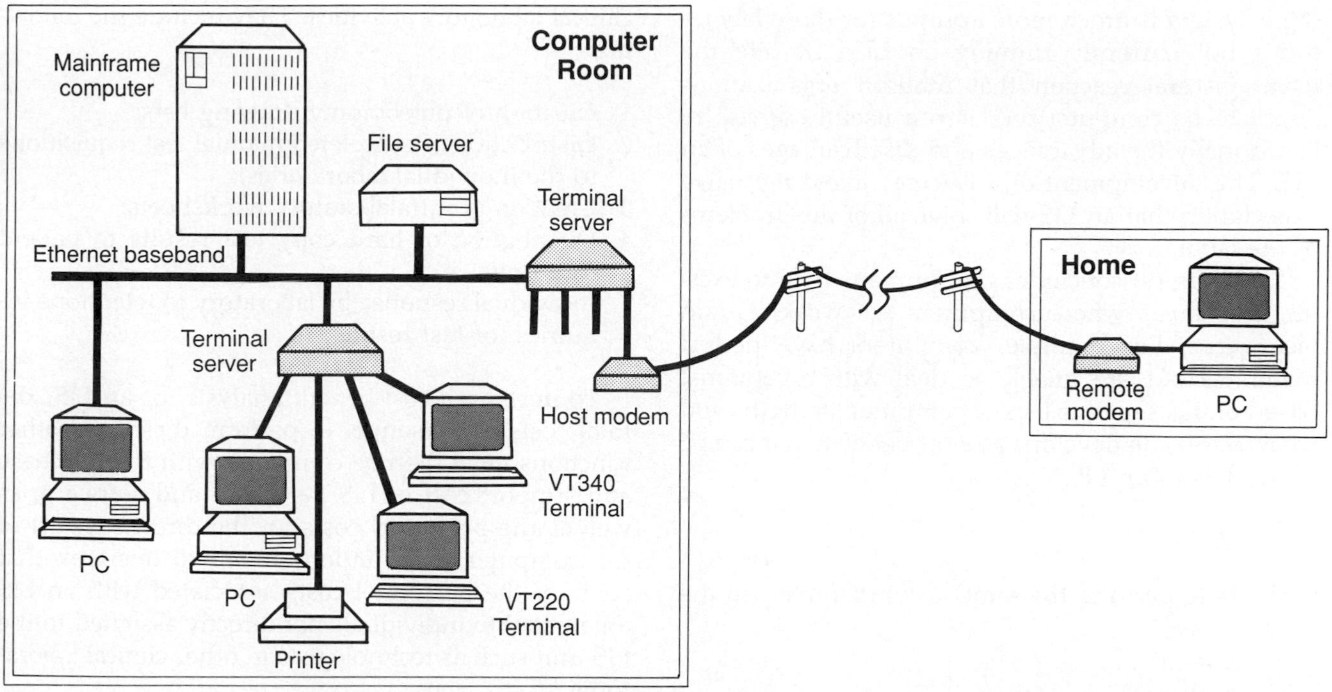

Figure 4.5. Remote access to a laboratory information system and local area network.

Whatever the cable plan strategy, a cable must be run between buildings, within buildings, between offices and laboratories, and within offices and laboratories between computer devices. The current strategy in local area networks is to use a coaxial cable system between adjacent buildings and between floors within buildings. Subsequently, twisted pairs that exist in most modern buildings are used to connect each device to the LAN. The use of any existing wire reduces the cost of implementing a cable plan. An alternative to coaxial cable is optical fiber backbones. This is expected to be a standard in the future. It is expensive to install but does offer a significant increase in performance (100 megabits/second). Another important aspect of implementing a cable system is careful planning for today's and the future's needs. Any installation must be followed by complete documentation of the cable plan. This is important for future expansion of the LAN and troubleshooting problems within the LAN. A carefully controlled installation of the network cable plan is very important. Too often a cable is hastily installed, not checked for quality, and/or poorly documented. Such an installation propagates network gremlins.

There seem to be unlimited options available in selecting networking hardware. Usually your choice in network hardware is dictated by what LIS system you are running. For example, your LIS may run on a DEC or IBM platform; therefore, your LAN architecture would be Ethernet or Token Ring, respectively. Choosing to purchase only DEC or IBM equipment because your LIS runs on those platforms simplifies the institutional support issues. Only one vendor needs to be contacted to correct a problem, to be consulted to expand the system, or to negotiate a maintenance contract. Clearly the easiest way to manage a system is to minimize the number of hardware vendors. This strategy minimizes the personnel costs needed to support a multivendor LIS/network platform usually at the expense of greater capital equipment cost. The purchase of hardware and software from other vendors may cost less initially, but additional in-house computer expertise can be a hidden cost for support of "cheaper" hardware or software network products.

There are many vendors for "networking products" including the computer giants. The networking market has become very competitive, and many vendors have mature network offerings. Network experts find it a challenge to keep current with the best purchasing strategy for networking products. The best guide for the selection networking products is to consult with your LIS vendor and to rely most importantly on proven installations in peer institutions.

PURCHASE OF A LABORATORY INFORMATION SYSTEM

For those clinical laboratories that are already computerized, the rationale for upgrading an existing LIS is relatively simple: it would be unthinkable to return to a manual information processing system. The need to develop a rationale for purchasing a system is much more apropos for those laboratories not currently running an LIS. Despite the usual visceral reaction that modern organizations ought to be computerized, it is a useful exercise to list formally the advantages and disadvantages of an LIS. The development of a list may avoid the naive expectation that an LIS will solve all of the problems of the laboratory.

Korpman (9) concludes that humans tend to excel in those areas where computers are weakest, and vice versa. For example, computers have perfect memories but are unable to deal with exceptions. Based on his separate lists of computer strengths and weaknesses, he develops a set of benefits that can be derived from an LIS:

Strengths:

- Ability to perform the same task indefinitely in the same way;
- Speed; and
- Perfect memory.

Weaknesses:

- Stupidity;
- Inability to make inferences;
- Inability to deal with exceptions; and
- Inability to deal with broad constructs.

Benefits with proper man/machine interface:

- Laboratory professionals acquire "perfect memory";
- The computer's ability to perform repetitive tasks relieves the laboratory staff of onerous aspects of work;
- Laboratory professionals deal with exceptions; and
- Laboratory professionals increase their capabilities and shift their emphasis toward the tasks for which they are trained.

The realization of these benefits assumes that the man/machine interface is properly designed. The basic thrust of Korpman's reasoning is that an LIS will shift much of the drudgery of routine repetitive "rote" tasks to the computer, allowing laboratory personnel to exercise their intellect by dealing primarily with exceptions (9). This is a very praiseworthy objective.

Although Korpman is undoubtedly correct in his analysis, the pathologist seeking to justify the purchase of an LIS to hospital administrators may sometimes require a more tangible/exact list of reasons for the purchase of such an expensive item (5, 9).

A number of data-handling activities must be performed manually if there is no LIS support for the clinical laboratory activities. They include the following:

1. Creation of phlebotomy drawing lists;
2. Distribution of completed manual test requisitions to the individual laboratories;
3. Creation of intralaboratory worksheets;
4. Distribution of hard copy test results to patient care units; and
5. Individual response by laboratory to telephone inquiries for test results.

To develop a cost-benefit analysis for an LIS, the total costs of personnel to perform these and other functions must then be compared with the purchase and support cost of LIS hardware and software, as well as the personnel costs for the direct support of the computer. It is important not to overlook that some of the personnel costs associated with an LIS are related to individuals not directly assigned to the LIS unit such as technologists in other clinical laboratories.

Hendricks and Langhofer in 1982 evaluated the impact of the acquisition of a laboratory information system upon a community hospital (10, 11). The acquisition produced a decrease in inflation-adjusted labor costs per unit of work, a decrease in inflation-adjusted direct cost per unit of work, a decline in the ratio of clerical to technical labor force, and an increase in overall laboratory productivity. Comparison of the average College of American Pathologists Manual for Laboratory Workload Recording Method (12) units per laboratory FTE for the 3 years before and 4 years after the LIS installation showed a 12% increase in productivity in comparison with a 5% increase in automated tests. The authors concluded that productivity in their laboratory rose by about 7% (overall productivity increase less the increase in automation) as the result of computerization.

Hendricks and Langhofer stress that there are a number of nonquantifiable effects of computerization that must be factored into any cost-benefit analysis. An example is the development of ad hoc reports by extraction of information from the laboratory database for quality assurance, utilization review, or risk management (10). With manual systems, such reports are the result of many man-hours of work.

Justifying the cost of an LIS is most interesting from the perspective of increasing the efficiency of physicians and providing a better patient outcome (11). Few would deny that the creation of a hard copy test interim, organized by laboratory with a moving 4-day window of current and previous results, makes physicians more efficient. They are also made more efficient by remote stat delivery of test results to critical care units immediately following test verification. Access to a long-term on-line archive of test results becomes critical when handling and transport of the paper record is difficult.

Ultimately, the necessity to computerize the clinical laboratories in a hospital is driven by two factors: (*a*) high labor costs in a hospital makes the automation of manual processes attractive from a financial point of view; and (*b*) reports and quality assurance activities, which simply cannot be provided by manual systems, are being demanded with increasing frequency in all hospitals regardless of the resource implications.

There are 13 major steps in the selection and installation of an LIS (13–15):

1. Creating an LIS project team;
2. Gathering information;
3. Reviewing and analyzing the information collected;
4. Developing and distributing a request for a proposal;
5. Evaluating vendor responses;
6. Selecting a vendor;
7. Negotiating with a vendor and developing a contract;
8. Training and site preparation;
9. Installing the hardware;
10. Making parallel runs;
11. Going live;
12. Fully operating; and
13. Evaluating and monitoring.

THE LIS PROJECT TEAM

Once the decision has been made to purchase an LIS, or to upgrade an existing system, it is necessary to assign a task force of hospital personnel to coordinate the project from its inception until the system is turned over to personnel in the LIS unit after the go-live date. The working core of the project team *must be* clinical laboratory personnel. They are the natural leaders of the project team because a successful LIS implementation is critical for them. On the other hand, the participation of personnel from outside the clinical laboratories can also be critical to the success of the project, and their participation should be encouraged. For example, a clinician who can speak to the needs of physicians in terms of test reporting formats and locations of terminals for data retrieval should be represented on the project team. Gunton describes the design process using a diagram. He explains the initial process as trying to close the "information gap." Ultimately, maintenance programmers and users will attempt to close the "maintenance gap" throughout the life of the system (8) (Fig. 4.6).

INFORMATION GATHERING

There are four general sources of information about laboratory information systems: casual conversations among professional colleagues, written publications by professional societies, vendor-generated print materials, and vendor displays at national and regional meetings. Even with written material from multiple sources at hand, it may be difficult to isolate the essential pieces of information (e.g., what language is the system written in, are all laboratory modules up and running, how many sites were installed in the last calendar year?).

In most instances, it is possible to reduce the large number of possible LIS vendors down to a half-dozen or fewer on the basis of the initial needs analysis of the clinical laboratories and information about the various systems garnered from both informal discussions and formal sources. Generally, hospital personnel should not feel the need for hands-on demonstrations of systems until they have pared their list down to a small number of vendors. Under such conditions, the competing vendors will be delighted to visit the hospital and set up a formal demonstration of the system under controlled conditions.

DEVELOPING A REQUEST FOR A PROPOSAL

A request for proposal (RFP) is a document developed by an LIS project team in which the information processing needs of the clinical laboratories and the hospital are delineated (15–19). This document is distributed to those LIS vendors with a reasonable chance of being successful bidders in the competition, some of whom will choose to issue a written response to the request for proposal (RFP). A successful vendor will then be chosen from the responders.

The key elements of a request for proposal are:

- Hospital and laboratory profile;
- Functional system requirements;
- Technical systems requirements;
- Training requirements;
- Implementation requirements;
- Financial considerations;
- Vendor profile;
- Conditions of bidding;
- Evaluation criteria; and
- Decision timetable.

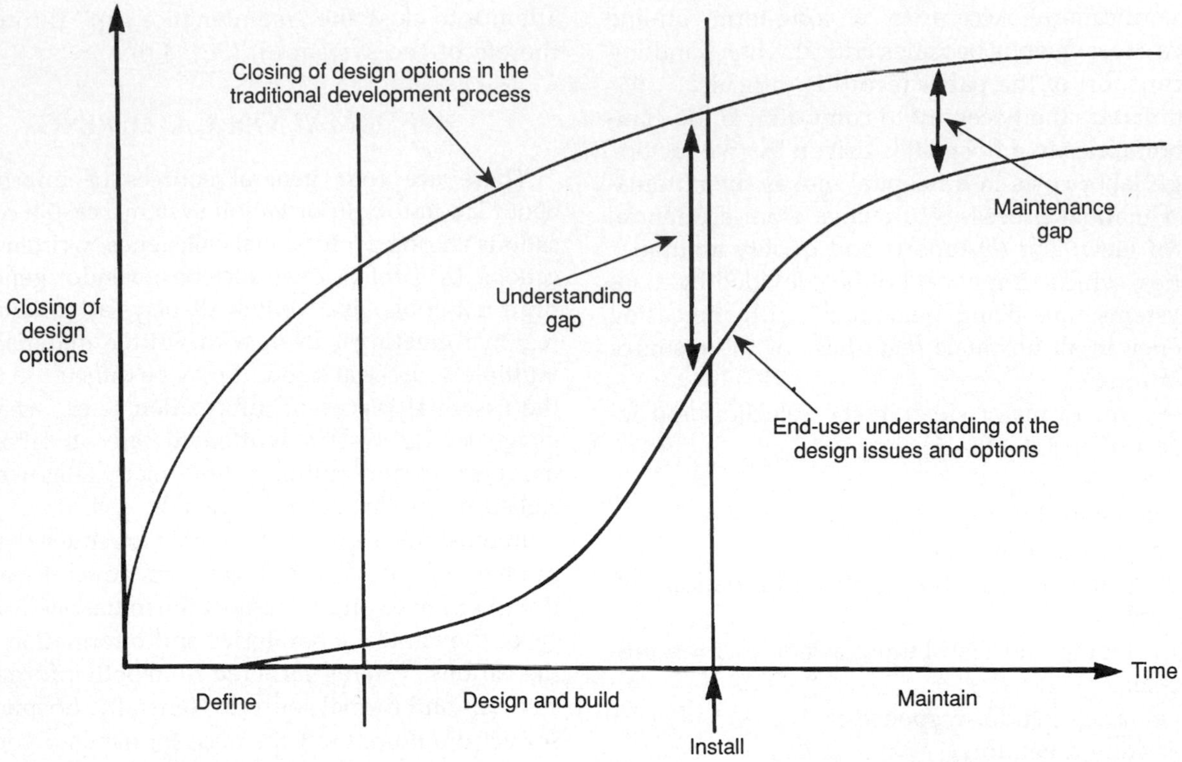

Figure 4.6. Laboratory information system design process and end-user learning curve.

The key goals during the development of a request for proposal are to:

1. Gather information about all potential LIS vendors and then develop a basis for comparison among those responding;
2. Analyze current laboratory operations to assist in vendor selection and to ensure successful system installation;
3. Create a long-term strategic plan for the automation of the clinical laboratories, including a prioritization among all available computer applications if funds are limited;
4. Develop a justification for the purchase and configuration of the LIS to ensure current and continuing resource support;
5. Build a consensus among the members of the LIS project team; and
6. Develop a formal plan for staffing the LIS unit and daily operations after implementation.

Analysis of Current Laboratory Operations

An important first step in the development of an RFP is a "systems analysis" of the various clinical laboratories (14–19). There are three primary objectives for systems analysis in the clinical laboratories as part of the RFP process: (*a*) to evaluate the information handling systems currently operating within the laboratories; (*b*) to document specific responsibility for "loop closure" in laboratory testing requests and recording procedures; and (*c*) to analyze the laboratories in terms of input, output, processing, and control. Loop closure means addressing the fundamental cause of a recurring problem, rather than continuing to treat it symptomatically.

Krieg and colleagues use several techniques for performing systems analysis including logic flow charts, data flow diagrams, and wall chart displays (20). Logic flow charts, also called system flow charts, are the most useful for planning and documenting laboratory operations, whereas data flow diagrams are especially useful for planning and documenting computer programs. The wall chart display is used to visualize forms and documents used in a particular data processing system.

The reason for proceeding with the systems analysis step is to take a hard look at current laboratory operations and information flow. An attempt should be made to correct any problems encountered *prior* to the installation of an LIS.

The installation of an LIS often requires that certain operational changes be made in laboratory operations. Although not always the case, such changes frequently serve to enhance the efficiency of information processing within the laboratories. Veteran laboratory personnel may balk at the implementation of changes mandated by an LIS installation, preferring to continue with the "tried and true." Such employees may be uncomfortable with change or may have instituted procedures scheduled to be discarded and therefore may have a vested interest in their continuation. Friedman (21) calls the persistence to use familiar procedures that appear to be more efficient than they actually are, the "competency trap."

Having completed a systems analysis, it becomes much easier to make informed judgments about the efficiency of current laboratory operations. Systems analysis will ultimately provide an inside look into current operations and suggest ways in which the LIS can be customized to meet the information needs of local users.

A fairly typical question that arises during the time that systems analysis is being performed on laboratory operations and vendor offerings are being reviewed in a preliminary way is whether all laboratory modules should be brought up simultaneously on the "go live" day.

The classic process has been to bring up the "numerical production" laboratories such as chemical pathology and hematology at one time, and then other laboratories with more complex applications such as microbiology and blood bank at a later time. With the sophistication of today's systems, the strategy is "all laboratories go live at the same time." Such a method hastens the return to normality from what is perceived to be an awkward transition state.

Purchasing an LIS with Sufficient Capacity

The proper sizing of an LIS for a hospital is a complex issue with major implications for the hospital. It is important to have a sufficiently powerful central processor and disk storage with the response time of the system and the number of months of test results on line being satisfactory to users.

To design a system of sufficient size, vendor personnel start with hospital volume statistics provided in the RFP including the (*a*) current laboratory workload; (*b*) the number of yearly inpatient discharges; (*c*) the number of yearly ambulatory care and emergency department visits; (*d*) workload measurement; and (*e*) the anticipated growth in laboratory activity.

Using these data plus the anticipated software configuration of the LIS, including the number of applications running and the requirements for on-line order entry and test results, the vendor will make recommendations about system size. The cost of the hardware will then be rolled up in the quotation for the system.

Vendors know that they are competing with other vendors on the basis of cost as well as system functionality. On the one hand, they will design a system with adequate capacity for near-term requirements. On the other, they will not build in excessive system capacity for the long term. LIS performance for the future will depend on the increase in the laboratory workload and increasing use of the system. Moreover, the vendor will undoubtedly release software upgrades with new features that may increase the system functionality, but will also require more computer power.

In the final analysis, the sizing of a LIS depends on the following:

1. The recommendation of the vendor in the RFP;
2. The hardware configuration of comparable hospitals in terms of complexity and workload, which will be analyzed during site visits; and
3. Some "fudge factor," taking into consideration local hospital resources and the interest and willingness of the hospital to invest in a state-of-the-art system.

Whenever possible, it is wise to buy more system capacity than will be necessary to run the LIS software on day one and then grow into the system.

Several questions pertaining to hardware "upgrades" should be addressed after vendors submit recommendations for a particular system configuration. For example, what is the relationship of the recommended system capacity to the maximum capacity of that configuration? What are the increments of growth when the recommended hardware configuration is deemed inadequate? What is the recommended hardware (and software) upgrade path from the recommended configuration, and is it smooth or complicated?

VENDOR SELECTION

Extreme care should always be taken when selecting a vendor. The importance of this decision rests in part with the large amount of money required for the initial system purchase, as well as for continuing software and hardware support. Equally important is the fact that the installation of an LIS requires a major investment in training. Having made such an investment, laboratory professionals are generally loathe to switch to another vendor at some later point. The status quo is often the path of least resistance, even when the current vendor may be providing an inferior product and service. LIS vendors understand that the switching costs for their current clients are high, and will try to maximize them to the extent feasible. For example, one major issue in switching from one LIS vendor to another is file conversion from the old to the new system, particularly for anatomic pathology and blood bank files. The LIS vendor being abandoned will do little to facilitate this process. The new LIS vendor may also be wary of actively participating in the file conversion for fear of charges of copyright infringement by the previous vendor. The scenario goes on and on.

Criteria for Vendor Selection

Some general criteria (13, 15) to use in the search process are:

1. Is the system designed to meet needs in multiple settings, such as a multihospital group with laboratories in geographically distributed sites?
2. Is the company adequately capitalized and financially healthy?
3. Is the system well documented, well designed, and written in a language such that software support could be obtained, in the event of vendor failure?
4. Will the vendor place and maintain, on site or in escrow, a copy of the source code and complete documentation?
5. Is the vendor investing sufficient resources in product development, as judged by the number of assigned personnel in the area and the frequency of major new product announcements?
6. Are contracted or purchased software modules clearly identified with their origin acknowledged, and do they integrate well into the total system?
7. Has the development cycle for the entire system been completed, and has it been running in test or prototype sites for at least a year?
8. Are all planned interfaces (instrument, hospital mainframe computer) running successfully at other sites?
9. Is the system, with all of the desired laboratory modules and applications, running successfully in another site of equal complexity?
10. Has the vendor shown continued and steady growth, as measured by the number of clients installed per year, or is the number of installations declining, indicating decreasing acceptance in the market?
11. Does the vendor's support and training staff meet local needs, and does the staff appear to be adequate for anticipated installations?
12. Does the hardware vendor have a major position in the market and a close collaborative relationship with the LIS vendor?

The installation of an LIS commits the clinical laboratories and the LIS vendor to a long-term and close relationship. It is extremely important that the "chemistry" is right between the two organizations in order to foster a positive and productive relationship.

Connelly, Glaser, and Chou provide an informative discussion of both formal and informal methods for sorting through the enormous amount of data about vendors generated through the RFP process (15). The subjective viewpoint holds that the large number of qualitative factors inherent in the LIS selection process make rigid and elaborate procedures for quantifying differences between favored vendors impractical. Such thinking favors either the *educated guess method*, wherein an overall impression of the system is garnered by the decision makers, the *cost only method*, or the *easy way out method*, whereby the most prominent vendor or the current vendor is selected.

According to Connelly and colleagues, there are two formal or structured approaches to vendor selection (15). In the first, the *elimination by aspect method*, key features that serve as mandatory requirements are identified. Systems not meeting these mandatory requirements are dropped from consideration. The approach that Connelly and colleagues favor is the *multiattribute utility model (weighted scoring model)*. This approach consists of nothing more than developing a set of major and subattributes for the desired system and values for each. Evaluators from the LIS project team score each subattribute for each vendor. Some simple calculations provide a performance score for each vendor. The leader of the LIS project team should review the scores of the anonymous evaluators carefully to make sure that no one is "gaming" the process by assigning highest scores to the favored vendor and zeros to all others. This could seriously skew the mean scores for the whole set of evaluators.

The Site Visit in Vendor Selection

The site visit is often omitted or given short shrift, perhaps because of the expense, coordination, and effort in transporting a large number of personnel to multiple hospitals. For either the first-time buyer or the department-switching vendors, it is necessary to view LISs in a production environment prior to final selection. Be sure to choose hospitals for site visits of equal size and complexity to the home institution, even though this may increase the travel costs. Vendors have a small cadre of "show" sites for visits where personnel are generally happy with the product. It may be worthwhile to attempt to schedule through the vendor a visit to a hospital other than a standard "show" site. Not all clients of a particular vendor will be equally satisfied with the product, so don't be surprised if some criticism is aired during site visits.

Variables that enter into the pricing equation for a laboratory information system are:

- Workload;
- Complexity of the system (e.g., multihospital cluster, large outreach program);
- Number of laboratory modules installed (e.g., blood bank, blood bank donor, anatomic pathology, microbiology);
- Discretionary products installed such as ad hoc report generator or decision-support software;
- Number of instrument interfaces;
- Complexity and function of the interface to the hospital mainframe computer (e.g., ADT, order entry-result reporting, test status);
- Processor power;
- Disk storage and archive storage requirements;
- System redundancy; and
- Scheduled down-time requirements.

Some possible reasons for a low bid from a vendor in response to an RFP are:

1. A reliable company with a good product, but anxious for the hospital as a client (e.g., prestigious hospital, first hospital in a region);
2. A relatively new company anxious to develop a client list;
3. A very new company that wants to use the hospital as an alpha-test site;
4. An established company that has already amortized the cost of its current software product and is not investing resources in research and development at present;
5. An underpowered or undersized system;
6. The bid is for a microcomputer-based LIS, which will always be cheaper by a substantial margin than a minicomputer-based system; and
7. The HIS vendor already has the hospital as a client and will bid low on the LIS software to maintain its position in the hospital.

It is important to write language into the contract guaranteeing system response time under specified system load conditions. Some vendors will balk at such contract language, calling it unrealistic or unnecessary, whereas others may actually insist on the inclusion of performance criteria in the contract to protect themselves. One of the most important reasons to include specifications about system performance in the contract is to discourage a vendor from "undersizing" a system recommendation in order to underbid competitors by keeping hardware costs low.

The advantages and disadvantages (13, 14) in the use of an outside consultant in the selection of an LIS are:

Advantages:

1. Saves work for the laboratory director and staff;
2. Provides special expertise and a potentially large repertoire of solutions;
3. Identifies problems that may be easier for an outsider to recognize;
4. Allows the arbitration of disputes between the various hospital factions; and
5. Lends an air of credibility to the process.

Disadvantages:

1. Consulting services have a cost, which may be high or perceived as high;
2. Selecting an effective consultant may be difficult;
3. Some organizations do not readily accept outside advice;
4. Consultants are not forced to "live" with their bad decisions;
5. Consultants may be tempted to apply a previous successful solution to all future problems;
6. Frequent use of consultants may stifle the development of local expertise or local "buy-in" to a system; and
7. Consultants may be unwilling to share the decision-making process with hospital personnel.

The major reasons for the failure of an LIS are:

1. Poor fit between the LIS and the laboratory/hospital environment;
2. Poor design of the LIS such that the replaced manual systems were actually superior;
3. Lack of acceptance or sabotage of the newly installed LIS by various user groups such as medical technologists and hospital physicians;
4. Unacceptable system response time;
5. Inadequate leadership during a politically complex and technically challenging process;
6. Inadequate training of the various user groups;
7. Inadequate system support from the vendor;
8. Belief that purchasing a turnkey system can create unrealistically low expectations about resources necessary to support the system;
9. Because it is difficult to hire skilled personnel to run a newly installed LIS, inexperienced personnel must be rapidly trained on top of other duties; and
10. Overambitious implementation schedule.

MANAGING A LABORATORY INFORMATION SYSTEM

One of the most important elements for the management of a high-quality LIS is a "test system" that consists of a copy of the production software and a patient test result database that can be used to simulate live runs. The basic idea of the test system is that new releases of software can be tested in the local environment before being brought up live on the production system. This is important because no software, even from the most reputable vendor, is bug-free. Moreover, no vendor can exactly replicate the various computing environments of all of their hospital clients when writing new software.

Even though no test system can exactly mimic the production environment of the hospital, it is always preferable to run new software on the test system, rather than immediately installing on the production system. If a hospital does not have a test system and new software must be immediately installed on the production system, the only alternative is to fall back to an audit approach where the system output is monitored closely for a period of time for errors.

Routine Operation

Each LIS unit needs to develop a written set of guidelines pertaining to some important aspects of routine operations. The following issues should be addressed:

- Physical site security;
- Backup and recovery;
- Software and database security; and
- Power outages and fluctuation of current.

Because the LIS plays such a critical role in laboratory operations and because it is relatively vulnerable to both vandalism and adverse changes in its operating environment, care must be taken to protect the hardware and software from harm. Many of the systems for protecting the LIS will be put in place when the system is installed such as door locks, fire protection system, an adequate air conditioning unit, and an uninterruptible power supply (UPS). Limiting access to the computer room and surveillance for the presence of unauthorized personnel is the best means for guarding against vandalism of the system.

Backup and Recovery

Backup and recovery are the means to restore an LIS to perfect working order after the system goes down, either on a scheduled or unscheduled basis. Of course, coming up after a scheduled down should present no problems in terms of restoring the systems because the system should be taken down on an orderly, regular basis. Unscheduled downs can occur on the basis of either a hardware or software problem. It is possible to build hardware redundancy into a system to minimize the risk of a hardware failure through the use of parallel processors or use of a hardware architecture with more than one CPU in a cluster. Such hardware redundancy, of course, does not guard against software defects creeping into the system and corrupting the database. The insidious aspect of software failure is that the system may continue to function on an apparently normal basis. Even if shadowing is in place to protect the database with simultaneous writing of data to two drives, both copies of the files may be corrupted by a software defect.

After an unscheduled down, the patient database must be reconstituted assuming that an up-to-date copy of system software is readily available. There are three components of the patient database: active on-line patient files, historical on-line patents files, and purge tapes of patient data. Although backup strategies will vary from vendor to vendor, a typical approach is to write test results to both purge tapes and to the on-line historical file when they are purged from the active files. Therefore, reconstituting lost data after an unscheduled down will usually involve asking the individual laboratories to reenter lost test results from active files plus recovering historical patient data from purge tapes.

Reentry of results from the individual laboratories may be simple if data are maintained for a short period of time in the memory of automated laboratory instruments. Manual data entry may also be required on occasion, if results are not maintained in electronic form in the laboratories. The extent to which data are maintained in an electronic format in the laboratories in the event of an unscheduled down is a trade-off question, comparing the resources necessary to maintain such files versus the cost of manual data entry at the time of system failure.

System Security

For the most part, turnkey LISs will come equipped with adequate security systems. The lowest level of security, commonly assigned to hospital physicians, is the ability to read test results only. Higher levels of security involving the ability to write to files will be assigned to bench-level medical technologists. Higher levels of security would be assigned to shift supervisors or chief technologists and involves the ability to modify test methodologies and generate management reports. High-level LIS managers in larger hospitals, of course, are assigned the highest security levels.

Most LISs are run as true turnkey operations after the system is installed and stable. This means that a small number of clinical laboratory personnel are trained to supervise and troubleshoot the system, but that it frequently runs unattended. The LIS vendors respond to software problems via dial-in modem. Hardware problems are handled in two different ways. If the equipment has been purchased directly from the hardware vendor, LIS personnel will summon field engineers under contract to attend to hardware problems. If both software and hardware have been purchased from the LIS vendor, apparent hardware problems may also be routed through the LIS vendor. Larger and more complex hospitals may not be content to run LIS operations on a true turnkey basis and will establish a management structure within the clinical laboratories to provide leadership to the clinical laboratory information system operation.

References

1. Blum BI, Duncan K. A history of medical informatics: Association for Computing Machinery Inc (ACM). New York: Addison Wesley, 1990:267–277.
2. Aller RD, Elevitch FR. Clinics in laboratory medicine, computers in the clinical laboratory. Philadelphia: WB Saunders 1983;3:1.
3. Elevitch FR, Aller RD. The ABCs of LIS, computerizing your laboratory information system. Chicago: American Society of Clinical Pathologists, 1989.
4. Hammond WE. Patient management systems: the early years, The Association for Computing Machinery Conferences on the history of medical informatics. New York: The Association for Computing Machinery, 1987:153–164.
5. Korpman RA. Using the computer to optimize human performance in health care delivery. Arch Pathol Lab Med 1987;111: 637–645.
6. Bull BS, Korpman RA. The clinical laboratory computer system: who is it for? Arch Pathol Lab Med 1980;104:449–451.
7. Hardwick DF, Morrison JI, Cassidy PA. Clinical laboratory—past, present and future: an opinion. Hum Pathol 1985;16:206–211.
8. Gunton T. Inside information technology: a practical guide to management issues. Cambridge: Prentice-Hall International Ltd. 1990.
9. Korpman RA. Laboratory computerization. A new analysis of workflow and reporting. Clin Lab Med 1983;3:79–100.
10. Hendricks EJ, Langhofer LA. A community hospital laboratory computer system: an eight-year longitudinal study of economic impact. Am J Clin Pathol 1982;77:297–304.
11. Nussbaum B, Mickler T, Roby R, Ackerman E. Economic impact of a computer-based centralized organization in a clinical laboratory. Amer J Clin Pathol 1977;67:149–158.
12. College of American Pathologists. Manual for laboratory workload recording method (1991 edition). Northfield, Illinois: College of American Pathologists, 1990.
13. Friedman BA. Personal communication, 1991.
14. Marquardt VC, Wertz RK, Wertman BG, et al. Relating to consultants. Pathologist 1982;36:89–91.
15. Connelly DP, Glaser JP, Chou D. A structured approach to evaluating and selecting clinical laboratory information systems. Pathologist 1984;38:714–720.
16. Hospital Computer System Planning. Preparation of the request for proposal. Chicago: American Hospital Publishing, Inc., 1984.
17. Mandell SF. The request for proposal (RFP). The key document in successful systems acquisition. J Med Syst 1986;10:31–39.
18. Ciotti V. The request for proposal: is it just a paper chase? Healthcare Financial Management 1988;42:48–50.
19. Walker K. Selecting computer applications using the RFP process. Dimens Health Serv 1987;64:18–20.
20. Krieg A, Marquardt VC, Lundberg GD, et al. Systems analysis and planning. Pathologist 1982;36:30–35.
21. Friedman BA. Laboratory information systems and the competency trap. In: Greenes RA, ed. Proceedings of the twelfth annual symposium on computer applications in medical care. New York: IEEE Computer Society Press, 1988:659–662.

Section II

Section Chiefs: *John Lowe and Kenneth D. McClatchey*

The diagnosis and characterization of genetic disease and of malignancy are increasingly dependent on analysis of specific genetic sequences that determine the pathologic processes in such disorders. This type of molecular genetic analysis is technology intensive; as with other, more established diagnostic methods, proper design and interpretation of these new diagnostic approaches requires understanding of the concepts behind the techniques and of the biological processes and molecular structures that are being examined. Chapter 5 addresses these issues by first providing fundamental information about the chemical basis for heredity and the organization of genes. This is followed in Chapter 6 by an overview of techniques used to detect specific genetic sequences and their RNA products, to clone these molecules, and to determine their overall structure and sequence.

Chapter 7 outlines the clinical and molecular pathogenesis of osteogenesis imperfecta, a dominantly inherited disorder that typically involves defects in the pro 1(I) and pro 2(I) collagen loci. This disease serves as a focus for illustrating the application of powerful molecular methods in the analysis of single-gene disorders in which small mutational events (single base pair changes, insertions, or deletions) are pathogenic.

Chapter 8 describes molecular techniques that are used to detect and characterize genetic abnormalities associated with hematopoietic malignancies and to characterize pathogenic mutations in the hemoglobinopathies and in hemophilia A. Molecular characterization of lymphoid and myeloid malignancies represents a major focus of this chapter, as it is increasingly clear that this type of analysis can yield important therapeutic and prognostic information.

MOLECULAR PATHOLOGY

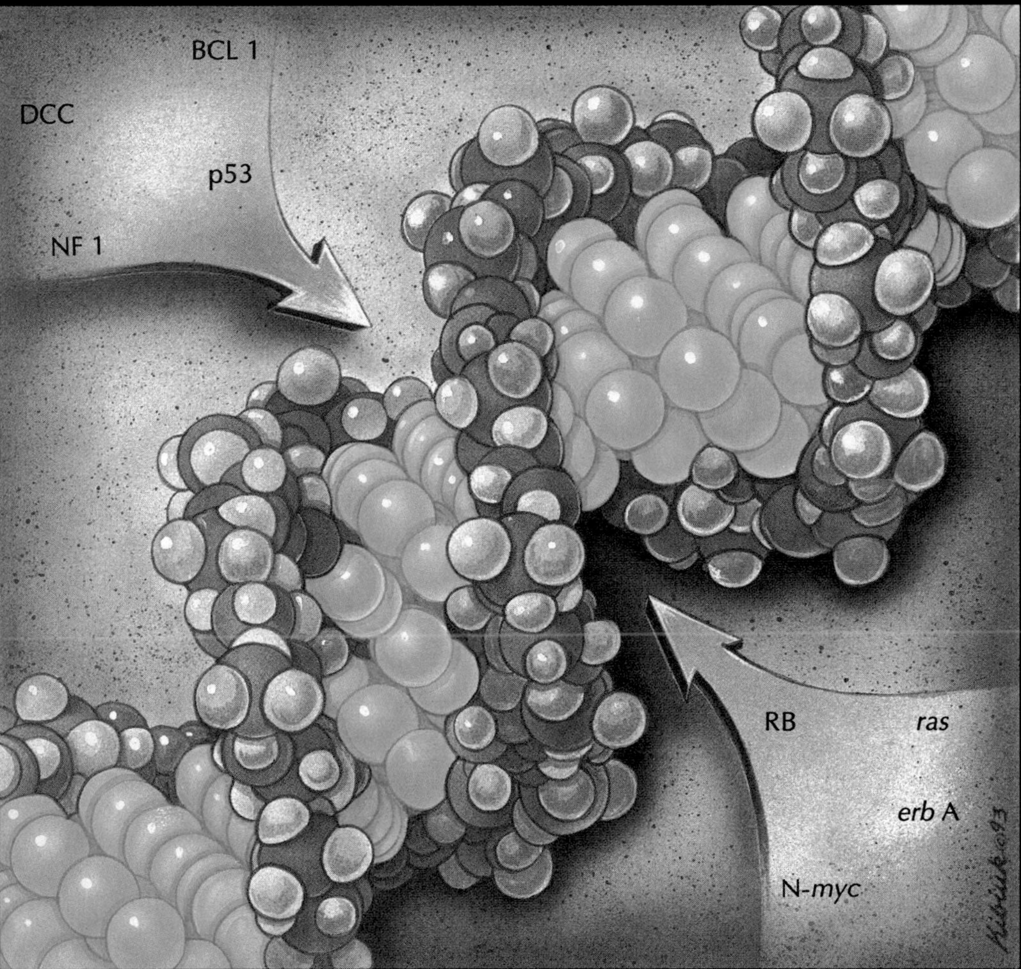

5 Basic Concepts in Molecular Biology

John B. Lowe

Since the classic study of Avery, MacLeod, and McCarty (1) demonstrated that DNA represents the "transforming principle," it has been known that nucleic acid molecules constitute the chemical basis for heredity. At the time of those studies, however, the structures of such molecules were just a matter of speculation. The ensuing years have seen an accelerating quest for a detailed understanding of the molecular basis of heredity. This venture has spawned a remarkable array of tools to allow the isolation and manipulation of DNA and RNA molecules. These tools have in turn enabled a rather precise understanding of gene structure, and a less complete but nonetheless remarkable comprehension of the mechanisms and accessory molecules that allow genes to be replicated, inherited, expressed, and mutated. Many of these insights have resulted from analyses of pathological circumstances, wherein genetic mutation, or other corruption of a gene or its context, have been instructive. These developments have already deeply enriched our understanding of the pathological basis for many diseases. There is every reason to expect substantial further progress in this area, especially given recent prospects for a concerted effort to map and sequence the entire human genome (2). Moreover, this quest has provided the clinical laboratory scientist with a spectacular new array of techniques that allow pre- and postnatal diagnosis of genetic disease. In addition, there are now sensitive and specific tests to detect infectious agents, and methods to complement or supersede conventional morphologic and histochemical approaches to the diagnosis and classification of malignancy. This chapter focuses primarily on the basic concepts behind these molecular techniques. A more extensive treatment of the use of molecular genetic approaches for pathological diagnosis may be found in Chapters 6–8 of this book and in Fenoglio-Preiser's and Willman's book (3).

STRUCTURE AND ORGANIZATION OF GENETIC MATERIAL

Deoxyribonucleic acid, or DNA, represents the genetic material in nearly all organisms, save those few animal and bacterial viruses whose genomes consist of ribonucleic acid, or RNA. DNA exists in mammals as a double-stranded, antiparallel polymer of deoxyribonucleotide phosphate molecules. The component nucleotides of each antiparallel strand are joined together through phosphodiester bonds formed between the 5′ and 3′ hydroxyl moieties of the pentose rings of the adjacent nucleotides (Fig. 5.1). The backbone of each strand thus consists of alternating deoxyribose and phosphate residues. The component purine (adenine, A or guanine, G) and pyrimidine (cytosine, C or thymine, T) bases, attached to the de-

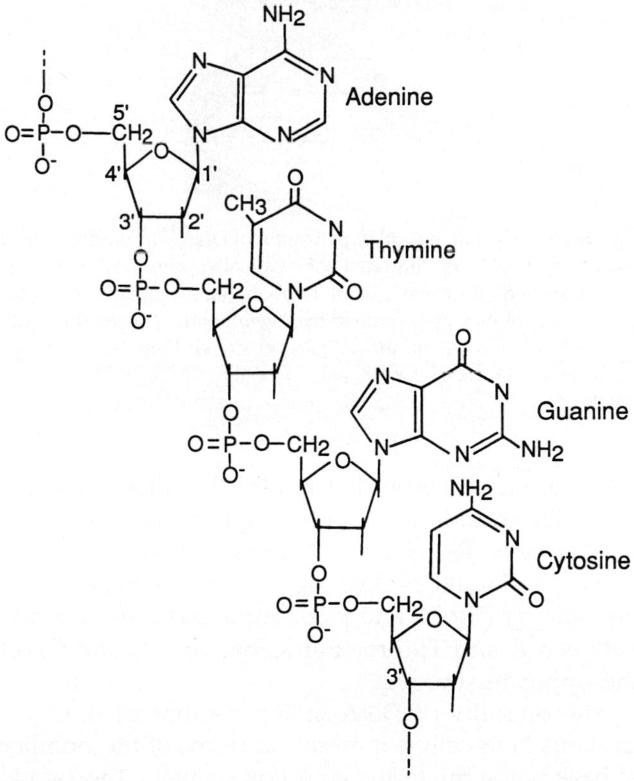

Figure 5.1. The chemical structure of DNA. The chemical structure of a segment of single-stranded DNA, showing the sequence 5′-ATGC-3′. Each deoxynucleotide ("A," "T," "G," or "C") is composed of a sugar (deoxyribose), a phosphate, and a base (the purines adenine and guanine, or the pyrimidines thymine and cytosine). Polarity in nucleic acid molecules is generally designated by referring to the 5′ or 3′ "end," which correspond to the numbering of the carbon substituents on the deoxyribose molecule.

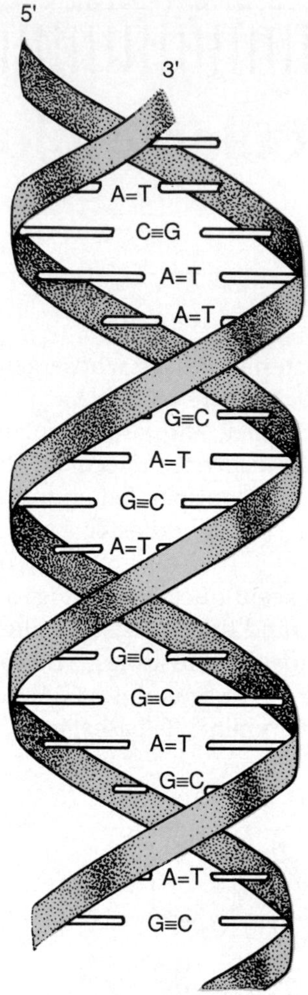

Figure 5.2. Double-helical organization of DNA. The double-helical character of DNA is illustrated schematically, with the sugar-phosphate backbone shown as a shaded ribbon. Bases protrude toward the middle, where they participate in hydrogen bonding interactions with complementary bases on the antiparallel strand. Complementary bases interact via either two (A and T) or three (G and C) hydrogen bonds.

oxyribose rings, protude from this backbone. The antiparallel strands are intertwined in the form of a double helix (Fig. 5.2). The stability of the double helix is maintained by hydrogen bonds between complementary purine and pyrimidine bases (two bonds between A and T; three bonds between G and C) on the opposite strands.

The quantity of DNA in the genome of most organisms is usually expressed in terms of the number of base pairs; the terms kb (kilobase pairs; thousands of base pairs), and mb (megabase pairs; millions of base pairs) are also commonly used to refer to nucleic acid size (length). The human genome is rather large; it contains an estimated 10^5 genes, interspersed within the roughly 3×10^9 base pairs of the haploid genome (Fig. 5.3). By contrast, the genome of the bacterium *Escherichia coli* is roughly 4×10^6 base pairs in size, and the human papilloma viruses maintain genomes of approximately 8×10^3 base pairs.

While the base pair may be considered the fundamental structural unit of genetic material in organisms with DNA genomes, the gene corresponds to the fundamental functional unit. A gene, or genetic locus, refers to a specific location on a chromosome. Generally, genes represent segments of genetic material that encode proteins with specific functions, or that encode RNA molecules with inherent functional properties.

In mammalian organisms, genes serve as templates for the process of transcription (Fig. 5.4). This occurs in the nucleus of the cell, and generates single-stranded RNA molecules whose sequences are initially colinear with the corresponding gene. These transcripts initiate at promoter sequences at the beginning, or 5′ end, of the gene, and terminate at the gene's 3′ end. These nuclear transcripts are then subjected to a series of complex processing events, known as splicing, that may precisely remove one or more specific segments of the transcript. The DNA segments corresponding to the segments of the transcript removed by the splicing process are known as intervening sequences, or introns, whereas the segments that remain after splicing, and are joined together, are termed exons. Nuclear transcripts are also subject to other processing events that truncate the transcript at its 3′ end, append a polyadenylate "tail" to the transcript, and transport the mature messenger RNA, or mRNA, to the cell's cytoplasm. This process thus yields mRNA molecules that are not continuously linear with their corresponding gene. These discontinuities, at intron-exon boundaries, may be found within the protein coding portion of the gene, or within sequences 5′ and/or 3′ to the coding sequence.

Mature, cytosolic polyadenylated messenger RNA (mRNA) is then a substrate for protein synthesis via the action of the cell's translational machinery. The portion of the mRNA that corresponds to its protein sequence, or translated portion, may be divided into coding units, or codons, consisting of three nucleotide bases. Each codon corresponds to a specific amino acid, or to a signal for termination of protein synthesis known as a termination codon (stop) (Table 5.1). Protein synthesis, directed by mRNA, is accomplished by complex mechanisms that convert the linear nucleic acid sequence into a linear polymer of amino acids. This "decoding" process involves transfer RNA molecules (tRNAs) and ribosomes. One or more transferase RNAs exists for each amino acid. These tRNAs become covalently bound to their cognate

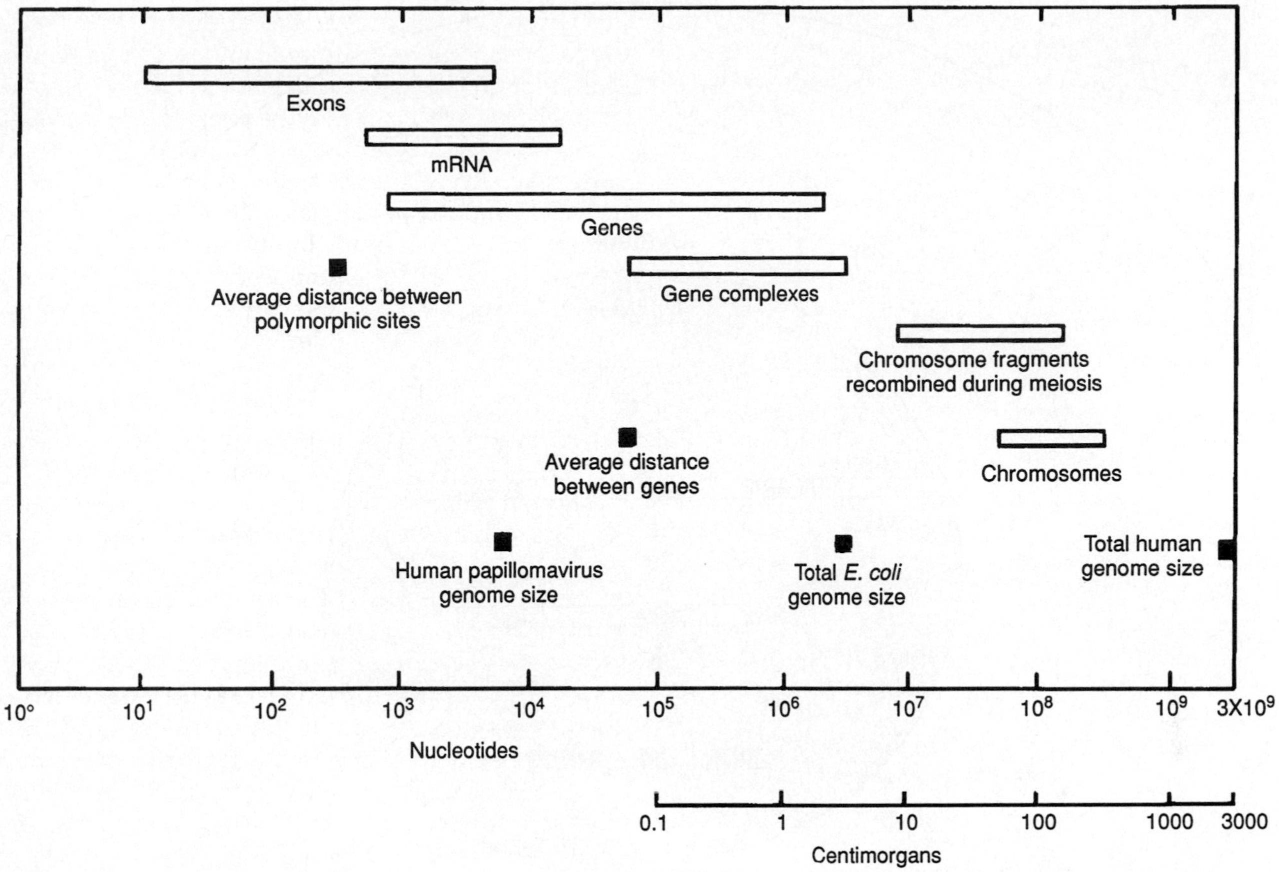

Figure 5.3. Size relationships between the structural and functional units of the human genome. Sizes are given in nucleotides and centimorgans. The sizes of the genomes of *E. coli* and human papilloma viruses are included for comparison. (Modified with permission from Landegren U, Kaiser R, Caskey CT, Hood L. DNA diagnostics—molecular techniques and automation. Science 1988;244:229–237.

amino acid, and then serve as substrates for the translational machinery. With the aid of ribosomes and other accessory proteins and nucleic acids, the 3-base anticodon portion of an aminoacyl tRNA recognizes its corresponding codon within the translated mRNA. The translational machinery initiates translation at the first initiation codon (AUG) with a methionyl tRNA, and then adds subsequent amino acids to the growing polypeptide chain, while releasing the tRNA component of each aminoacyl tRNA translational substrate. This process continues until a termination codon is reached, at which point the completed protein is released from the ribosome.

The 10^5 genes within the human genome are encoded by approximately 5% of the total amount of genomic DNA. Human genes are quite heterogeneous in size, the largest ones having spans exceeding 1 mb. In some instances, genes with similar function may exist as a cluster of adjacent sequences (like the human globin gene clusters, for example). Such clusters may span regions of a chromosome encompassing up to several mb. It is more common, however, to find genes existing as distinct entities located tens of kilobase pairs apart from adjacent genes.

It is useful to note that the units used to denote physical distance between genes differ from the units used to describe genetic distance. Genetic distance is defined in terms of the probability of recombination between two genes or loci as they are passed from a parent to a child (ie., during one meiotic event). The term centimorgan is used to define genetic distance; two loci are separated by a genetic distance of one centimorgan if there is a 1% probability of recombination between them through one generation. On the average, one centimorgan in genetic distance corresponds to 1 mb in physical distance. This relationship is not exactly linear, however, since recombination frequency can vary dramatically in a region-dependent manner.

Chromosomes represent the largest organizational unit of DNA. Human genes are distributed on 24 different chromosomes (22 autosomes, and the X and Y sex chromosomes). The 22 human autosomal chromosomes are of course each represented twice, each set inherited from one parent and accompanied by a

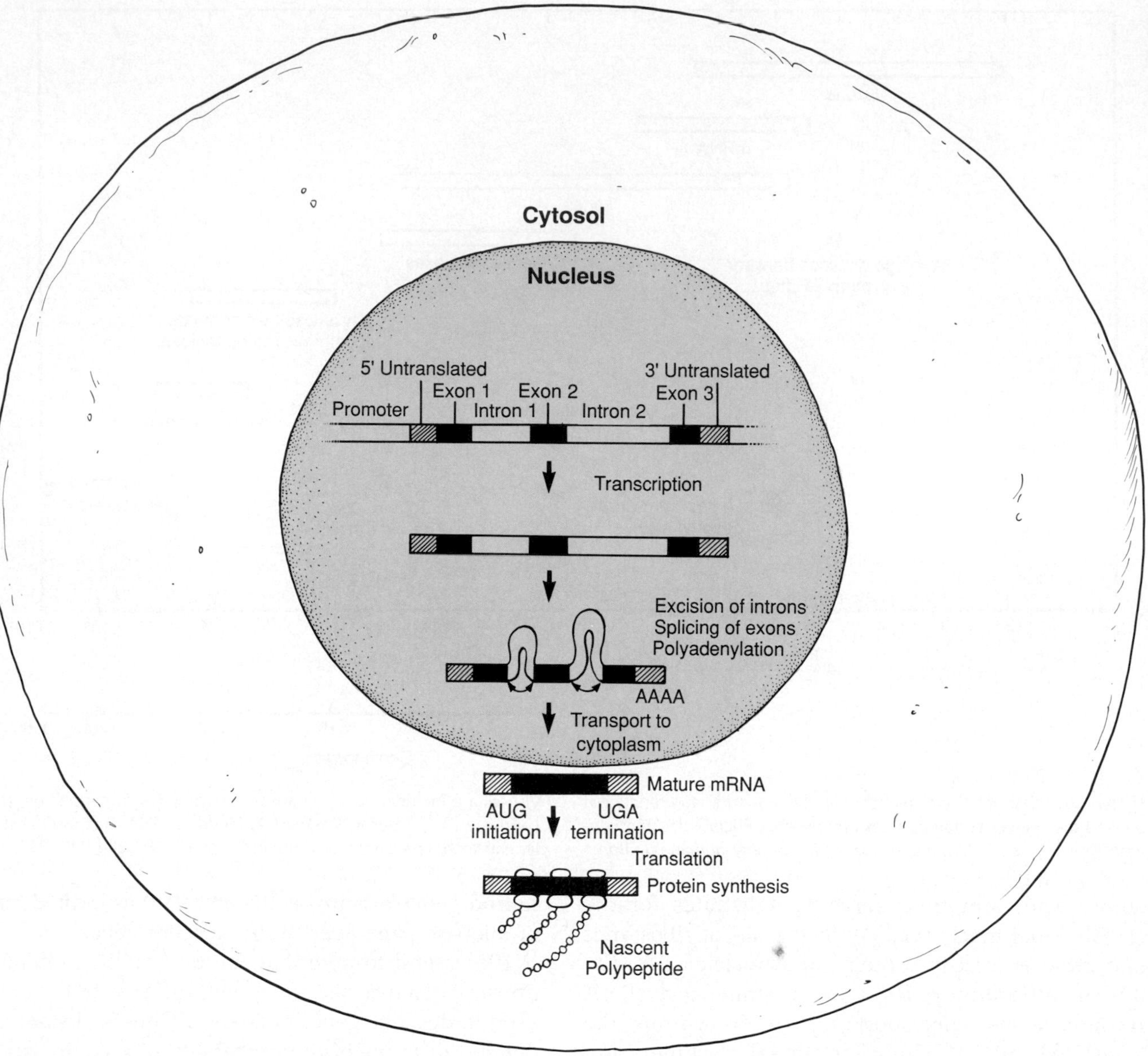

Figure 5.4. Structural and functional organization of a typical mammalian gene. Mammalian genes are transcribed from promoter sequences located 5′ to the beginning of the coding sequence (*solid areas*). Transcription yields a nuclear RNA molecule that undergoes splicing and polyadenylation, followed by transport to the cytoplasm. This processed messenger RNA (mRNA) contains 5′ and 3′ untranslated segments (*striped areas*), as well as a coding region. The mature mRNA is translated in the cytosol to yield protein molecules.

single sex chromosome. Each chromosome is composed of a single linear, double-stranded DNA polymer with a length of between tens of millions and hundreds of millions of base pairs. Within the chromosome, this DNA is associated with protein and RNA molecules in such a manner as to condense it into a compact, yet highly organized structure. Isolation of pure genomic DNA from cells or tissues typically involves procedures like phenol extraction and ethanol precipitation that remove these proteins and RNAs (4). Operationally, the pure DNA remaining may then be considered as a linear, double-stranded sequence of nucleotide bases.

APPROACHES TO THE ANALYSIS OF DNA AND RNA SEQUENCES

Hybridization

Molecular examination of particular DNA sequences, or their corresponding transcripts, is fundamental to diagnostic approaches involving nucleic acids. The considerable size and complexity of the human genome requires sensitive methods that also provide for highly specific identification of these molecules. Such sequence specificity is typically enabled by nucleic acid hybridization procedures,

Table 5.1. The Genetic Code[a]

First Position	Second Position U	C	A	G	Third Position
U	phe (F)	ser (S)	tyr (Y)	cys (C)	U
	phe (F)	ser (S)	tyr (Y)	cys (C)	C
	leu (L)	ser (S)	**STOP**	**STOP**	A
	leu (L)	ser (S)	**STOP**	trp (W)	G
C	leu (L)	pro (P)	his (H)	arg (R)	U
	leu (L)	pro (P)	his (H)	arg (R)	C
	leu (L)	pro (P)	gln (Q)	arg (R)	A
	leu (L)	pro (P)	gln (Q)	arg (R)	G
A	ile (I)	thr (T)	asn (N)	ser (S)	U
	ile (I)	thr (T)	asn (N)	ser (S)	C
	ile (I)	thr (T)	lys (K)	arg (R)	A
	met (M)	thr (T)	lys (K)	arg (R)	G
G	val (V)	ala (A)	asp (D)	gly (G)	U
	val (V)	ala (A)	asp (D)	gly (G)	C
	val (V)	ala (A)	glu (E)	gly (G)	A
	val (V)	ala (A)	glu (E)	gly (G)	G

[a]Amino acid abbreviations are shown in parentheses.

whereby a single-stranded nucleic acid "probe" is allowed to "find" its target nucleic acid sequence. Under appropriate conditions, a single-stranded DNA (or RNA) "probe" molecule will hydrogen bond, or hybridize, to single-stranded DNA (or RNA) molecules whose sequence is complementary to that of the probe. The stability of the double-stranded complex formed between the probe and its target is directly proportional to the degree of sequence complementarity between the two molecules as well as to the length of the complementarity between the molecules. Duplex stability is also strongly influenced by the temperature, pH, and ionic strength of the hybridization solution. Under "low stringency" hybridization conditions, duplex formation with less than perfect sequence complementarity is promoted, usually by lowering the hybridization temperature, or by increasing the buffer's ionic strength. By contrast, imperfectly matched duplexes are destabilized under "stringent" hybridization conditions of increased pH or temperature, or decreased buffer ionic strength. Stringent conditions will sustain only perfectly matched probe-target duplexes. Compounds like formamide that disrupt hydrogen bonding between strands of nucleic acid duplexes are also used to adjust hybridization stringencies. Identification and analysis of genes, gene fragments, specific DNA sequences, and RNA molecules may be accomplished by allowing a gene probe to hybridize to test nucleic acids under the appropriate hybridization stringency, and then detecting stable duplexes that form. Duplex detection is typically accomplished under circumstances where the target sequence is present in unamplified form, by procedures whereby the target sequence is enzymatically amplified immediately after the probe sequence is allowed to hybridize to the probe sequence(s) (i.e., via the polymerase chain reaction, or PCR), or with combinations and permutations of these two approaches.

Probe Labeling Methods for Detecting Unamplified Target Sequences

Gene probes are usually generated from double-stranded DNA restriction fragments, single-stranded synthetic DNA molecules, or RNA molecules synthesized in vitro. Most methods that detect stable probe-target duplexes generated with unamplified target sequences rely on the use of labeled probe molecules. The typically low concentration of target sequence in unamplified genetic material (approximately 10^{-2} fmol of a 10 kb segment of DNA in about 10 μg of human genomic DNA, for example) requires analytical methods that rely on probes that may be detected with high sensitivity (5). To achieve a high degree of sensitivity, nucleic acid probes have historically been most commonly labeled with radioisotopes, typically using one of several enzymatic techniques. Radioisotopes commonly used include ^{32}P, ^{35}S, and ^{3}H. These radionuclides are typically used as components of nucleoside triphosphate substrates for in vitro enzymatic reactions that can incorporate the radioactive portion of the substrate into a DNA segment corresponding to the probe segment.

One commonly used procedure of this type (Fig. 5.5) first employs heat denaturation to render a double-stranded DNA fragment single stranded (6). The single-stranded fragments are then hybridized to hexadeoxynucleotides of random sequence. Hexanucleotides that have hybridized to the two complementary single strands of the DNA segment then function to prime enzymatic synthesis of complementary DNA strands, in the presence of appropri-

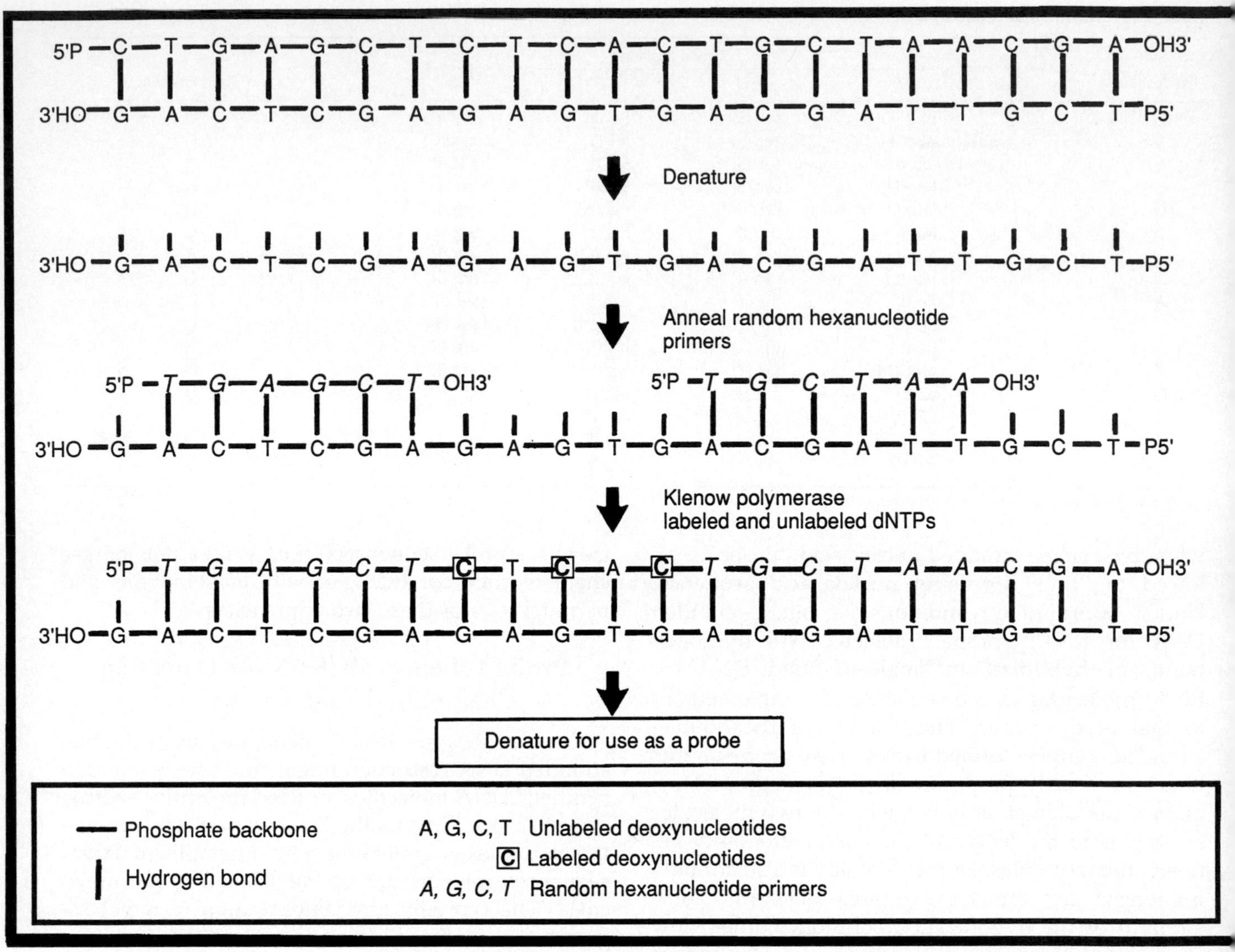

Figure 5.5. DNA labeling by the random hexamer method. A double-stranded DNA probe template is denatured, and mixed with random hexanucleotide primers. These primers hybridize or anneal to the single stranded components of the template DNA. The annealed primers serve to allow synthesis of a radiolabeled complementary strand, via the action of the Klenow fragment of *E. coli* DNA polymerase I operating with radiolabeled and unlabeled deoxynucleoside triphosphates that are incorporated into the synthesized strands. The radiolabeled double-stranded DNA molecules formed in this reaction are then denatured and used as a hybridization probe.

ate concentrations of one α^{32}P-labeled deoxynucleoside triphosphate, and the other three unlabeled deoxynucleoside triphosphate substrates. This synthesis is catalyzed by the DNA polymerase activity manifested by the Klenow fragment of *E. coli* DNA polymerase I, a proteolytic fragment of this enzyme that lacks one of the holoenzyme's exonucleolytic activities but retains its 3′→5′ polymerase activity. The sequences of the two complementary, newly synthesized radiolabeled DNA strands are essentially identical to those of their unlabeled counterparts. However, the incorporated ^{32}P molecules represent components of a significant fraction of the newly constructed phosphodiester bonds in these strands, allowing probes to be synthesized with specific activities in excess of 10^9 cpms per microgram of input template DNA. The nick-translation method (Fig. 5.6) embodies an approach similar to the random primed approach described above, wherein enzymatic incorporation of α^{32}P-labeled deoxynucleoside triphosphate molecules into a nicked, double-stranded template is accomplished via the combined exonucleolytic and polymerase activities of *E. coli* DNA polymerase I (7). In either instance, double-stranded radiolabeled heteroduplexes constructed by this approach may then be rendered single stranded by heating, and used to "find" their single-stranded, complementary target sequence(s) by hybridization. The necessary reagents for each of these labeling approaches are available in kit form from several commercial suppliers.

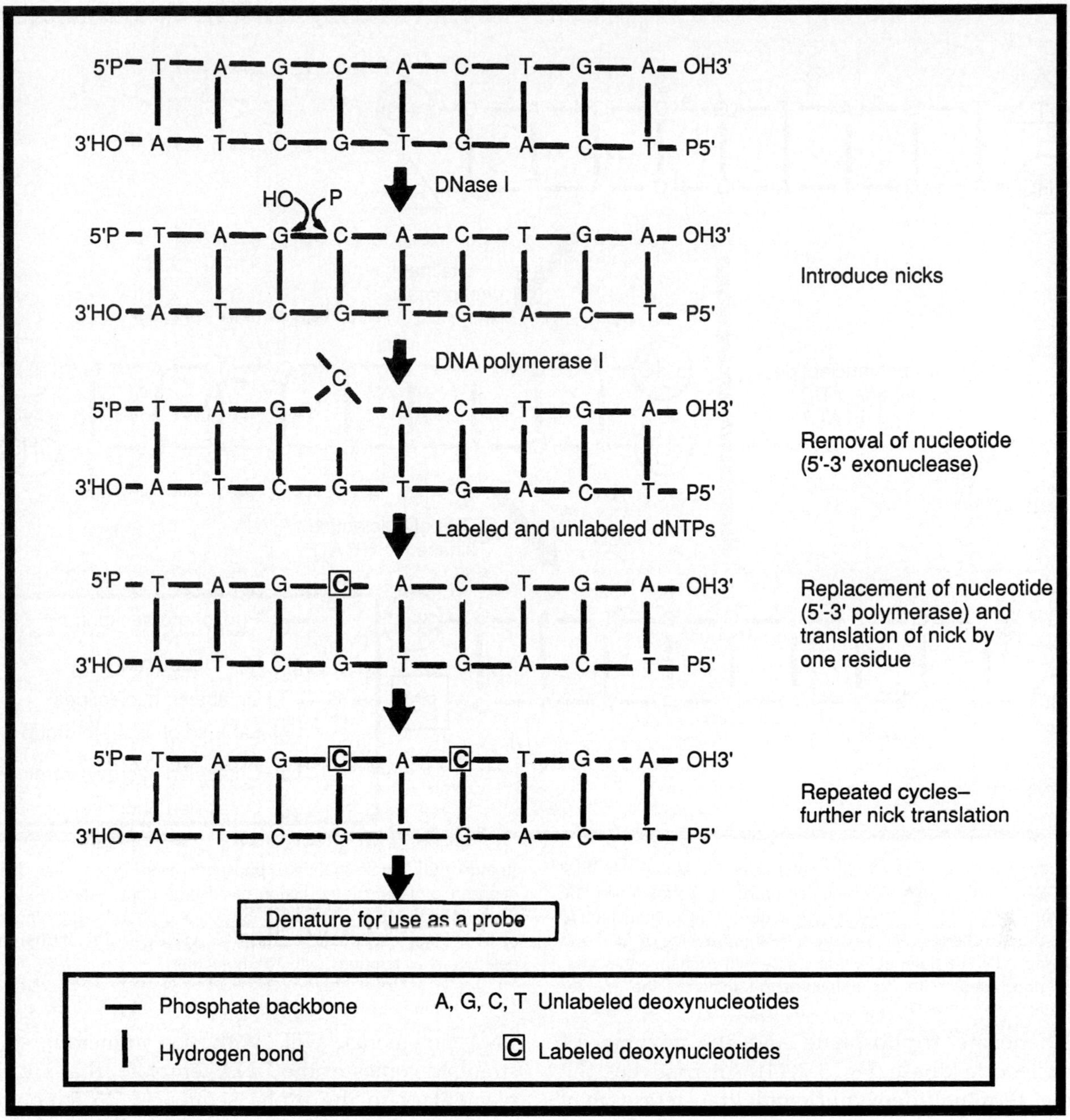

Figure 5.6. Labeling of DNA by nick translation. A double-stranded probe molecule is nicked (breakage of single phosphodiester bonds between nucleotides) by limited DNAase I digestion. These nicks serve to allow the 5′-3′ exonuclease activity of DNA polymerase I to processively remove nucleotides. The 5′-3′ polymerase activity of the DNA polymerase then replaces the excised nucleotides in a primer and template-dependent DNA synthesis reaction that incorporates radiolabeled and nonlabeled nucleotides into the probe molecule. This radiolabeled double-stranded molecule is then denatured and used as a hybridization probe.

These labeling approaches that utilize ^{32}P, when used with solution or solid-phase hybridization methods (see below), can reproducibly allow the detection of less than 100 pg of target sequence (i.e., about 10^{-2} fmol of a 10-kb restriction fragment). Because of this sensitivity, and because the cost of generating ^{32}P-labeled probes with those approaches is relatively low, these methods are in wide use in research and diagnostic laboratories.

Synthetic oligodeoxynucleotide hybridization probes are typically too short to be labeled by the random hexamer or nick translation methods. These single-stranded molecules, of lengths less than 50, are instead usually labeled with enzymatic processes that incorporate reporter molecules onto one or the other end of the probe. It is usually sufficient, and convenient, to incorporate a single ^{32}P atom at the 5′ OH terminus of a synthetic oligonucleotide, using

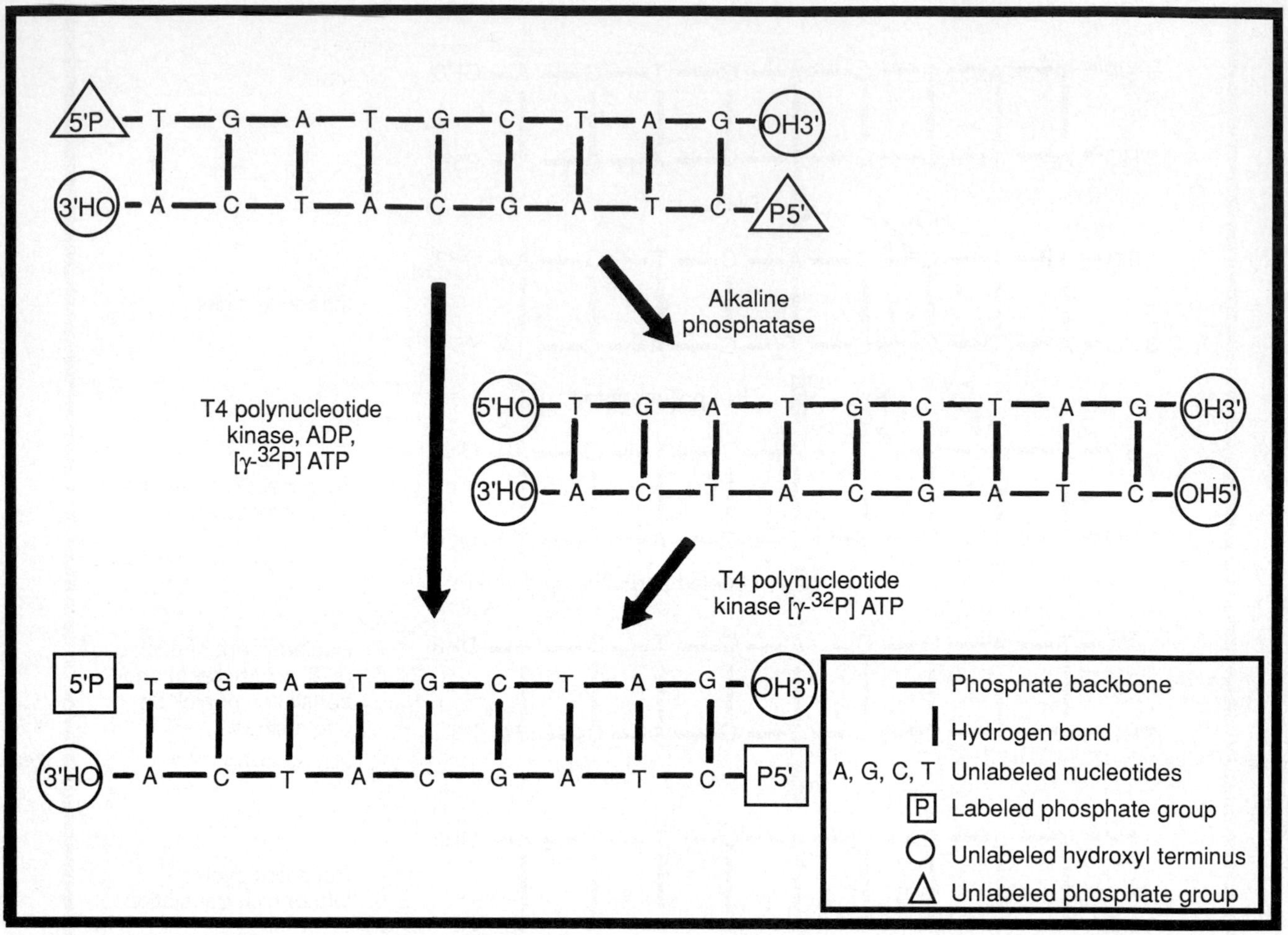

Figure 5.7. Labeling of DNA with polynucleotide kinase. Double-stranded DNA probes (or single-stranded probes, not shown) may be labeled directly at their 5′ ends by the action of T4 polynucleotide kinase in the "exchange reaction" (*left*). In the presence of ADP and γ^{32}P-labeled ATP, T4 polynucleotide kinase will exchange the unlabeled 5′ phosphates with ^{32}P molecules. Alternatively, the double-stranded (or single-stranded) phosphorylated probe may be first dephosphorylated by the action of alkaline phosphatase (*right*). The dephosphorylated probe may then be rephosphorylated by the action of T4 polynucleotide kinase and [γ^{32}P]ATP to yield a DNA probe labeled at its 5′ terminus with ^{32}P molecules.

[γ^{32}P]adenosine triphosphate and the enzyme T4 polynucleotide kinase (Fig. 5.7) (4). Alternatively, the enzyme terminal deoxynucleotidyltransferase may be utilized to incorporate one or many radiolabeled nucleotides onto the 3′ terminus of a short, single-stranded synthetic DNA molecule (Fig. 5.8) (4).

RNA molecules are also in wide use as hybridization probes. These probes are usually generated by RNA polymerase-catalyzed synthesis of single-stranded RNA molecules complementary to a probe sequence (Fig. 5.9). Typically, a DNA segment corresponding to the probe is first cloned into a plasmid vector adjacent to DNA sequences that serve as initiation sites for the action of RNA polymerases. This plasmid DNA template is then reacted with a recombinant RNA polymerase that recognizes its cognate DNA initiation sequence adjacent to the cloned probe sequence. In the presence of (α^{32}P-labeled) ribonucleoside triphosphate substrates, the added RNA polymerase will synthesize numerous single-stranded copies of the DNA template, that are complementary to the probe sequence. RNA polymerases typically used in this application include those encoded by the SP6, T7, or T3 phages that infect prokaryotic cells. Recombinant RNA polymerases from these phages are commercially available, and efficiently promote transcription from specific short DNA sequences distinct from those recognized by endogenous *E. coli* RNA polymerase. Depending upon the relative proportions of radioactive and unlabeled ribonucleoside triphosphates that are available to the added phage polymerase, probes with specific activities upwards of 10^9 cpm per μg may be generated (8). Subsequent to the synthesis of such RNA probes, the reaction is treated with RNAase-free DNAase to eliminate the plasmid DNA template, and may then be used to detect complementary target RNA or DNA sequences.

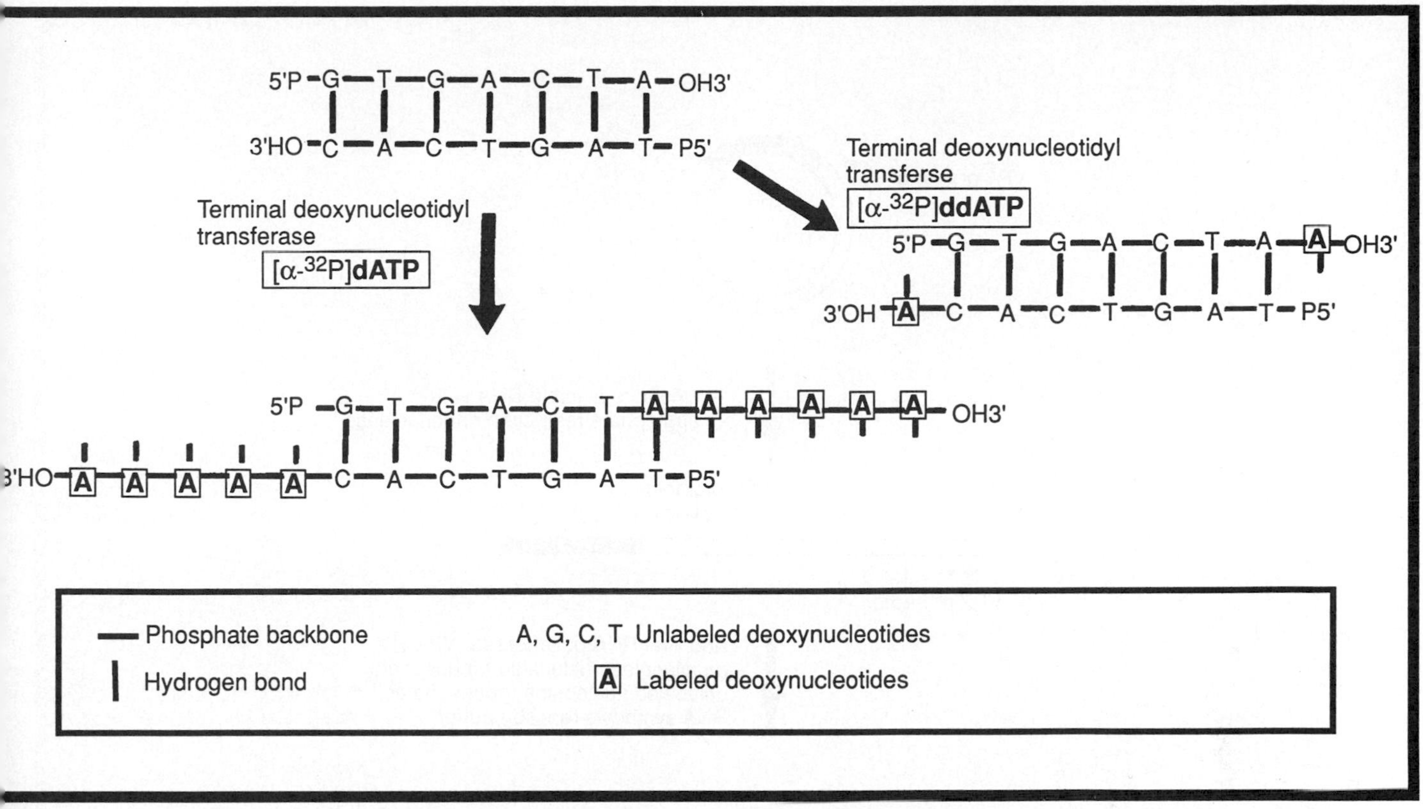

Figure 5.8. Labeling of DNA with terminal transferase. A double-stranded DNA probe (or single-stranded, not shown) may be labeled at its 3′ hydroxylated termini by the action of terminal deoxynucleotidyltransferase. Terminal transferase will catalyze the addition of multiple radiolabeled nucleotides to the 3′ hydroxyl termini when provided with α-labeled nucleoside triphosphates (*left*). Alternatively, a single radiolabeled nucleotide may be added to the 3′ hydroxyl terminus when terminal transferase is provided with an α-labeled dideoxynucleoside triphosphate (*right*).

Methods to prepare ^{32}P-labeled probes are convenient, relatively inexpensive, and provide for the sensitive detection of target DNA or RNA molecules. Nonetheless, the use of ^{32}P entails a number of significant drawbacks. First, the half-life of ^{32}P is rather short (14.31 days). Moreover, ^{32}P-labeled probes with high specific activities tend to undergo radiolysis within days. When considered together, these properties require that ^{32}P-labeled probes be used promptly after preparation, and thus may require the preparation of fresh probe at frequent intervals. An additional and significant factor to be considered when using ^{32}P for probe labeling is the radiation hazard associated with the use of this radionuclide. Laboratory personnel must be instructed in the proper use of the isotope. Procedures involving the preparation and use of ^{32}P-labeled probes must be performed with gloves behind cumbersome plexiglass shielding, and strict attention must be paid to disposal protocols designed for radioactive wastes. The use of ^{35}S-labeled nucleotide substrates for probe labeling lessens the requirement for cumbersome shielding procedures, and its longer half-life (87.2 days) can allow for less frequent probe preparation. Nonetheless, its use again requires implementation of careful waste disposal protocols and monitoring procedures. And, like ^{32}P-labeled probes, ^{35}S-labeled molecules require detection by autoradiographic or scintillation-counting methods. Because of these somewhat problematic characteristics associated with radiolabeled probes, numerous efforts have been made to develop sensitive and specific nonradioactive methods for labeling and detecting nucleic acids, especially in the context of use for Southern blotting and Northern blotting (see below).

Approaches that make use of nonradioactive detection methods involve the incorporation of chemically modified nucleotides into DNA or RNA probes. Such chemical modifications are typically designed to allow enzymatic incorporation of the modified nucleotide into the probe, and to result in a probe whose hybridization characteristics are not significantly altered, relative to a native probe. Finally, the chemical modification is engineered to allow its specific detection as incorporated into a probe molecule that will ultimately become a component of a stable probe-target duplex. The prototype chemical modification utilized for this approach is represented by the

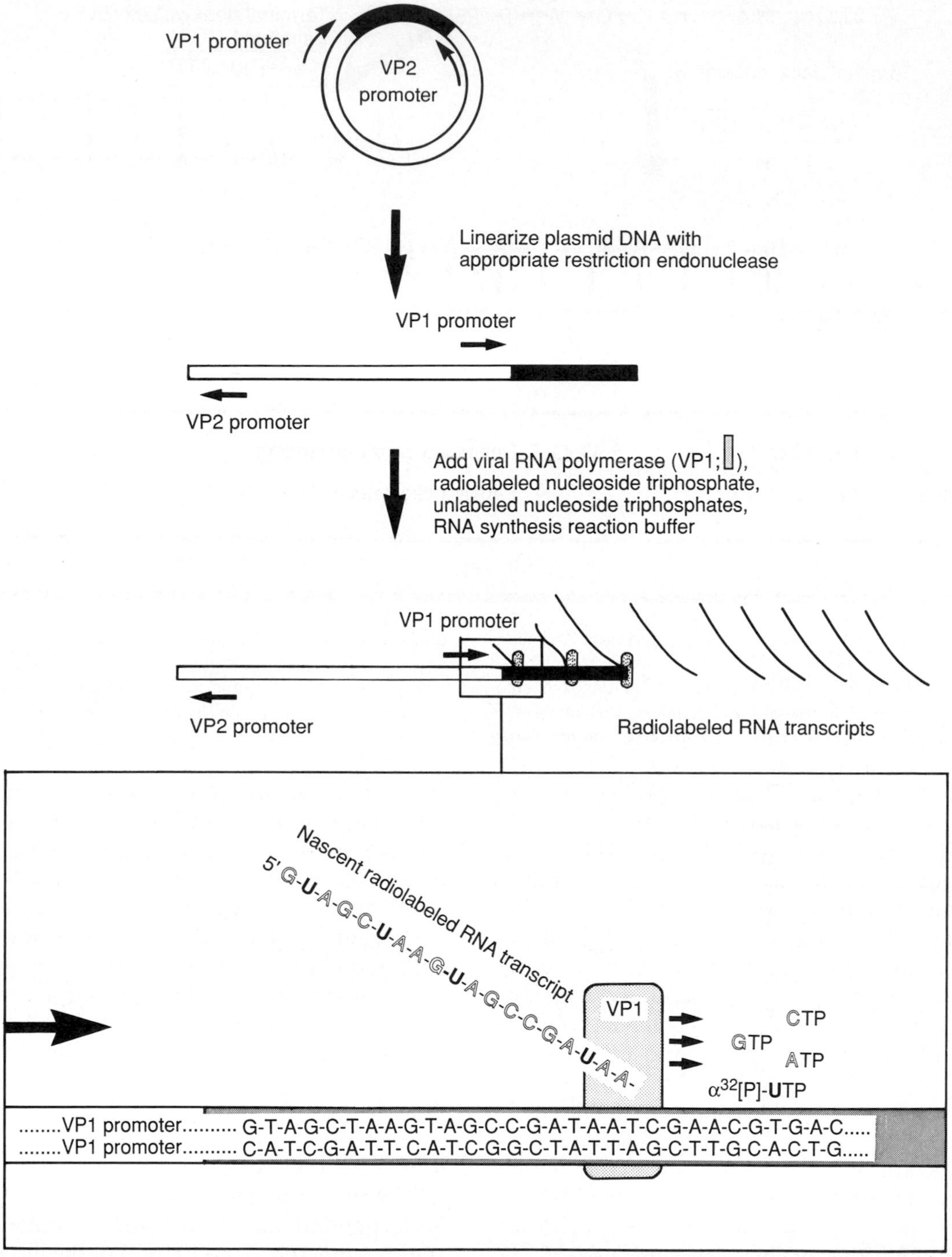

Figure 5.9. Preparation of radiolabeled RNA probes. A segment of DNA corresponding to the probe is cloned into a double-stranded circular plasmid DNA molecule between paired and oppositely oriented viral RNA polymerase promoter sequences VP1 and VP2 (*top*). The plasmid is linearized and then used as the template substrate in an RNA polymerase reaction catalyzed by the addition of the viral RNA polymerase VP1, buffer, and nucleoside triphosphates. Radiolabeled nucleoside triphosphates (^{35}S- or ^{32}P-labeled) are also included. The VP1 polymerase specifically initiates transcription at its promoter sequences adjacent to the cloned probe segment and generates RNA transcripts complementary to the DNA template. Ribonucleotide substrates labeled at the α position are incorporated into the nascent transcripts (*inset*).

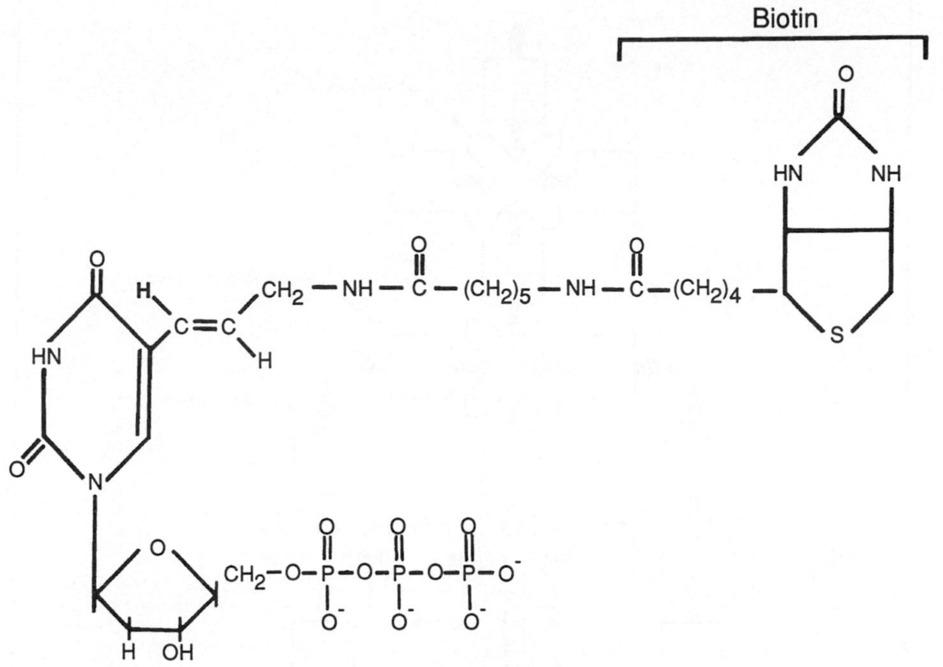

Figure 5.10. Structure of Bio-11 dUTP.

biotinylated nucleotide derivative deoxyuridine triphosphate (dUTP, or TTP) (9) (Fig. 5.10.). This derivative contains a biotin moiety covalently linked to the 5 position of the pyrimidine ring. Biotinylated derivatives of uridine triphosphate, deoxycytidine triphosphate, and deoxyadenine triphosphate have also been described. The biotin moiety is usually linked to the purine or pyrimidine ring via a spacer of 11, 16, or 21 atoms. Such modified deoxynucleotides can be incorporated into DNA probe molecules by nick translation or random priming methods in virtually the same way as that of natural deoxynucleotides. Moreover, the hybridization kinetics of probes that are highly substituted with biotinylated nucleotide derivatives are essentially identical to those displayed by unsubstituted probes. Similarly, biotinylated derivatives of ribonucleotides may be incorporated into single-stranded RNA probes using the phage RNA polymerases and in vitro transcription approaches outlined above.

Following hybridization, detection of stable probe-target duplexes is accomplished by a series of signal generation steps that utilize conjugates consisting of various enzymes coupled to streptavidin or avidin (Fig. 5.11). Such conjugates bind specifically and essentially irreversibly to probe-target duplexes by virtue of their interaction with biotin moieties incorporated into the probe. Probe-bound conjugates are then typically detected by enzymatic reactions in which the enzyme component of the conjugate is allowed to react with a soluble chromogenic substrate to produce an insoluble, colored product. Enzyme components of such conjugates include alkaline phosphatase, horseradish peroxidase, acid phosphatase, and β-galactosidase. In a typical scheme, alkaline phosphatase within the conjugate and bound to target molecules via its association with the probe, operates upon the substrate 5-bromo-4-chloro-3-indolyl phosphate (BCIP), in the presence of nitro blue tetrazolium (NBT). Alkaline phosphatase-catalyzed removal of the phosphate moiety from BCIP generates a compound that oxidizes and then dimerizes to produce an insoluble blue product. Simultaneously, NBT is reduced to yield the insoluble purple compound diformazan. These insoluble accumulated chromogens are directly visualized, at positions where stable probe-target heteroduplexes have accumulated.

A modification of this approach involves the use of a nucleotide analog in which the plant steroid digoxigenin is coupled via an 11-atom spacer to the pyrimidine ring of UTP (Fig. 5.12). Like the biotinylated derivatives, this chemically modified nucleotide can be enzymatically incorporated into RNA probes, and does not significantly affect the hybridization properties of the probe molecule. The digoxigenin moiety in stable probe-target duplexes is detected via methods involving antibodies specific for the digoxigenin portion of the nucleotide analogue and the use of enzyme-coupled conjugates to generate colored reaction products from chromogenic substrates.

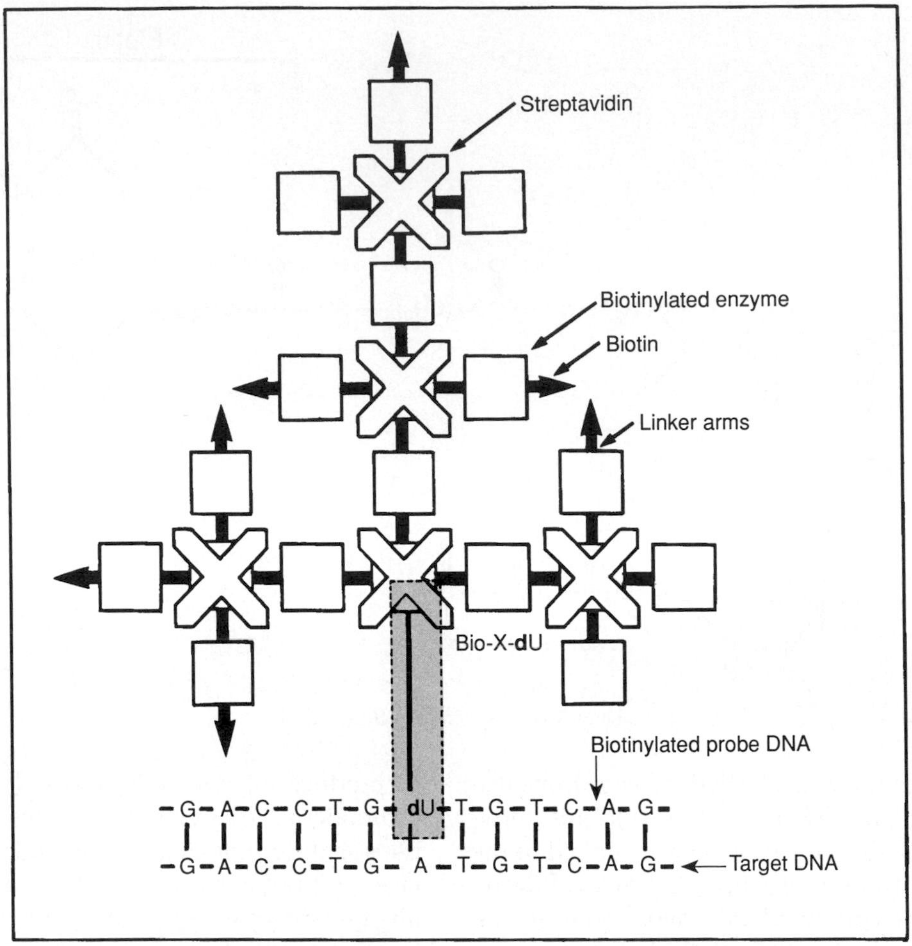

Figure 5.11. Detection of biotinylated DNA by streptavidin-alkaline phosphatase complexes. A biotinylated DNA probe that has formed a stable duplex with its target sequence may be detected by preformed streptavidin-alkaline phosphate complexes. Such complexes interact with the biotin moiety of the bio-X-dU previously incorporated into the probe DNA. Macromolecular complexes of the streptavidin-biotinylated alkaline phosphatase molecules form, and can serve to efficiently catalyze the hydrolysis of chromogenic or chemiluminescent substrates for alkaline phosphatase. The physical location of the chromogen or the emitted visible light corresponds to the location of the stable probe-target DNA duplexes, and to their concentration.

Such approaches are attractive alternatives to radioactive probe labeling procedures as they require no special radioactive shielding, licensing, monitoring, or disposal protocols. Probes prepared with the nonradioactive methods described earlier are quite stable and thus may be stored for prolonged periods of time. Detection by enzymatic conversion of chromogenic substrates may be accomplished within hours, versus much longer times that may be required for autoradiographic detection of ^{32}P-labeled probes. Nonetheless, there are drawbacks associated with these methods. In particular, the color of insoluble compounds generated from chromogenic substrates typically fades over time. Thus, in order to maintain experimental data in stable, hard copy form, blots must be photographed soon after color development. In addition, the chromogenic substrates yield colored products that cannot generally be removed from nitrocellulose blotting support, thus preventing reuse of the blot for subsequent hybridizations. Also of some concern is the sensitivity of these nonradioactive methods, in comparison with approaches involving the use of ^{32}P-labeled probes. Lower sensitivity is especially problematic when attempting to detect single-copy sequences in mammalian genomic DNA, or low abundance target sequences. In this regard, one of the major limitations to sensitivity encountered with coupled enzyme detection schemes involves inhibition of enzyme activity by accumulation of the insoluble product. While it has been demonstrated that the use of such methods can sometimes yield sensitivities that approach those exhibited by probes labeled with ^{32}P (see reference 9, for example), these nonradioactive approaches are not yet widely used for detecting low abundance target sequences.

A chemiluminescent approach has been developed recently, with a sensitivity that may equal that

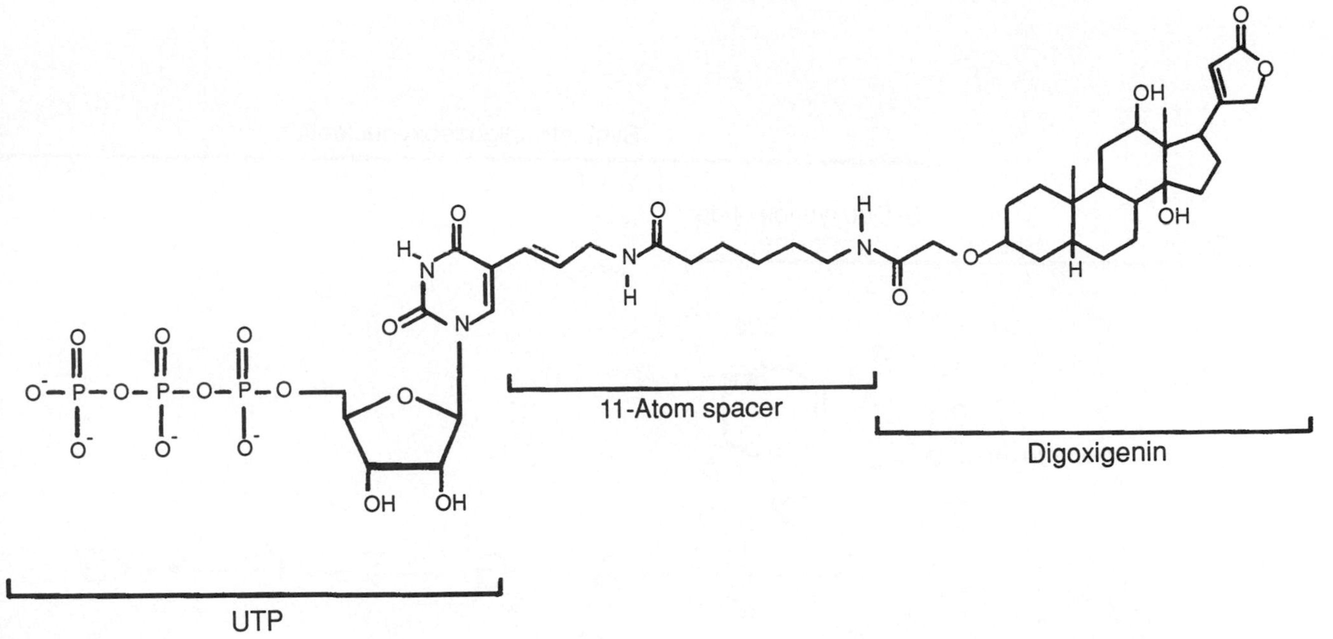

Figure 5.12. Digoxigenin-11-UTP. The steroid hapten digoxigenin is linked to UTP via an 11 atom spacer. This substance is commercially available (Boehringer-Mannheim), and may be enzymatically incorporated into RNA probes.

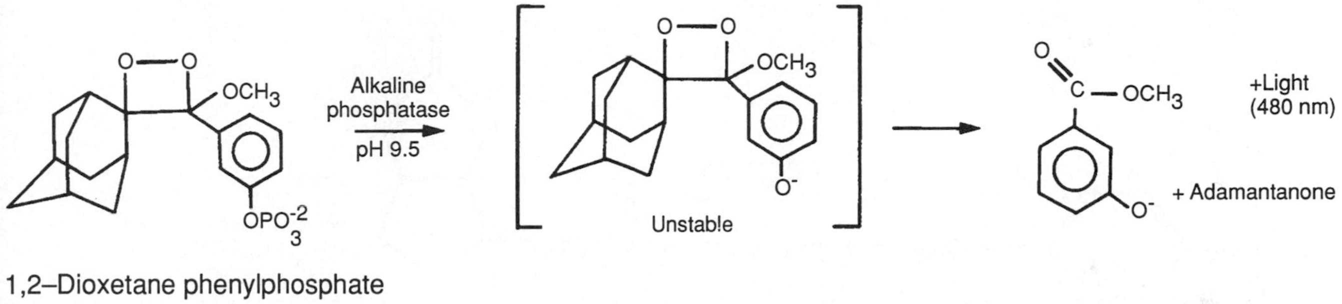

Figure 5.13. Alkaline phosphatase-generated chemiluminescence for probe detection. A phenylphosphate derivative of 1,2-dioxetane may be hydrolyzed by alkaline phosphate to yield an unstable derivative, which in turn decomposes to stable compounds. Decomposition is accompanied by the emission of light at a wavelength of 480 nanometers. Emitted light is detected by autoradiography and/or fluorescence methods.

exhibited by methods that utilize ^{32}P-labeled probes (10). This approach involves alkaline phosphatase-catalyzed conversion of a chemical substrate (a phenyl phosphate-substituted 1,2-dioxetane) to an unstable product (dephosphorylated phenyl 1,2-dioxetane). This compound in turn spontaneously decomposes to a stable product (adamantanone) and simultaneously yields light at a wavelength of 480 nm (Fig. 5.13). When used with a fluorescein derivative to increase the quantum yield, light emission is said to reach a steady state level in approximately 1 hour, and a signal is continuously generated for up to several days. Signal is detected by standard autoradiography. Sensitivity is enhanced, relative to approaches involving chromogenic substrates in that there is little, if any, product inhibition with the chemiluminescent substrate. Moreover, the low rate of spontaneous hydrolysis of the phenyl phosphate-substituted 1,2-dioxetane ensures that luminescent background remains low.

Numerous modifications of the aforementioned nonradioactive probe labeling approaches have been implemented, in which modified nucleotide substrates are enzymatically incorporated into probes, or in which the probe is chemically modified in a way that allows its detection. For example, short synthetic oligonucleotides may be labeled at their 3′ termini with biotinylated or digoxigenin modified deoxynucleotides using terminal deoxynucleotidyltransferase (Fig. 5.8). Oligonucleotides may also be labeled with biotin derivatives like biotin-*N*-hydroxysuccinimide ester (Fig. 5.14), in chemical reactions that link such components to a reactive 5′ amino group on the synthetic oligonucleotide probe (11). Double-stranded and single-stranded DNA probes, including synthetic oligonucleotides, as well as RNA

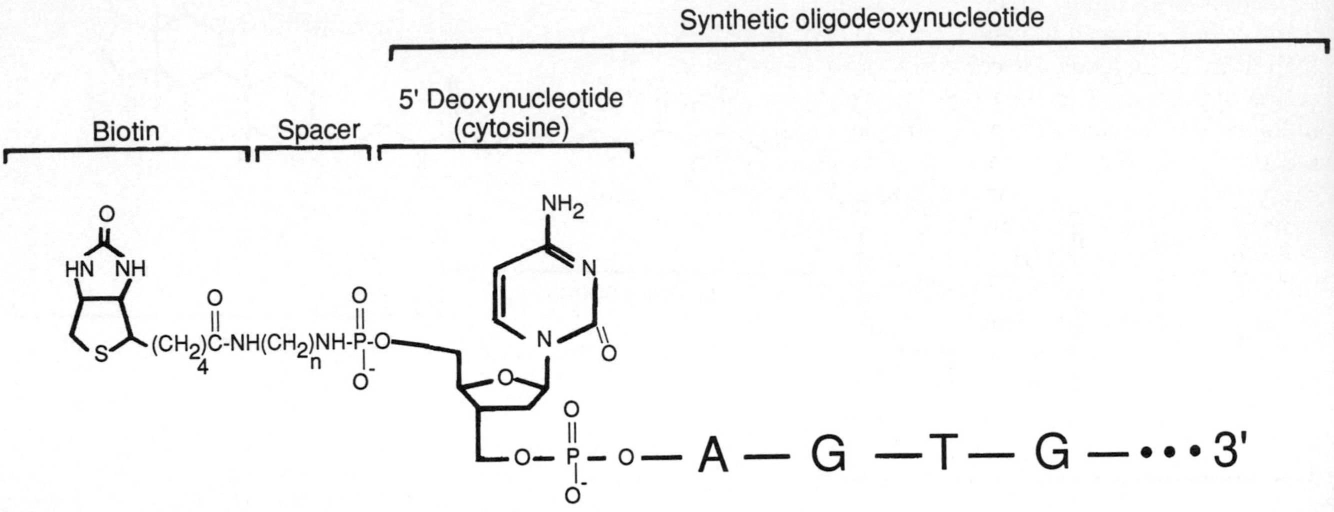

Figure 5.14. Biotinylated synthetic oligodeoxynucleotide. The 5′ deoxynucleotide (C, here) of a synthetic deoxyoligonucleotide has been chemically derivatized with biotin via biotin-*N*-hydroxysuccinimide ester.

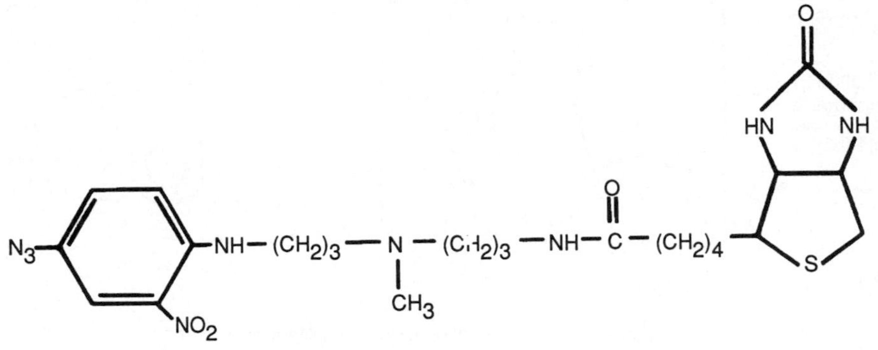

Photobiotin

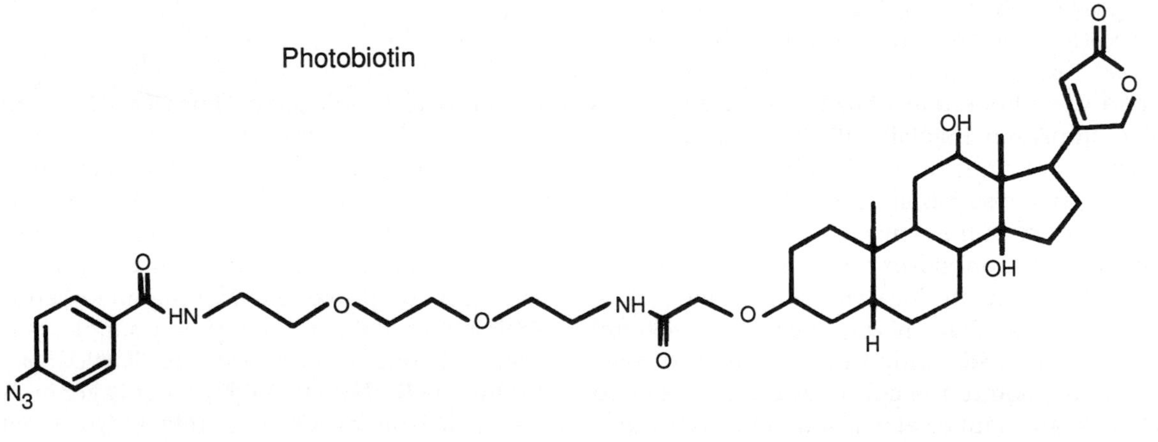

Photodigoxigenin

Figure 5.15. Photoactivatable aryl azide-derivatized biotin and digoxigenin compounds. Visible light converts the N_3^- on the aromatic ring to a reactive nitrene, which is then capable of forming a covalent bond with nucleic acid probes. Stable probe-target duplexes formed with such biotinylated or digoxigenylated probes may be detected by streptavidin-enzyme complexes, or by enzyme-derivatized antidigoxigenin antibodies.

probes, may also be chemically labeled with aryl azide-derivatized compounds like Photobiotin (12) (Biotechnology Research Enterprises S.A. Pty. Ltd.) or photodigoxigenin (Boehringer-Mannheim) (Fig. 5.15). When exposed to visible light, the azido group (N_3^-) in these molecules is converted into a highly reactive nitrene, that in turn can form stable covalent linkages with nucleic acid probes present in the same reaction. In each such instance, the chemical modifications serve as a mechanism whereby the probe may be detected after hybridization to its target, via coupling to systems involving antibody- or avidin-linked enzymes that operate on chromogenic or chemiluminescent substrates.

Fluorophores have also been used to label nucleic acids, by chemical or enzymatic incorporation methods. Typical organic fluorophores, however, do not engender sensitivity sufficient for diagnostic applications. By contrast, fluorescent chelates of rare earth metals such as terbium or europium exhibit long fluorescent lifetimes, relative to organic fluorophores, and when used with time-resolved fluorimetry, may yield detection sensitivities approaching those possible with ^{32}P-labeled probes (13, 14).

Enzymatic Amplification of Target Sequence: The Polymerase Chain Reaction

Historically, hybridization analyses of nucleic acid sequences have been performed directly after their extraction from a biological source. This often yields material with a relatively low concentration of the nucleic acid analyte, thus requiring rather sensitive analytical procedures. In some instances, however, direct extraction of biological material yields a relatively high concentration of the relevant target sequence, with a commensurate decrease in the need for extraordinarily sensitive detection methods; multiple copies of cloned DNA segments or pure cultures of pathogenic organisms represent two such examples of such "biological" nucleic sequence amplification. In the final analysis, biological amplification is the end result of enzymatic amplification of DNA sequences, performed by the DNA replication machinery of the host organism to maintain appropriate equivalency between the number of organisms and their nucleic acid genomes.

The introduction of the polymerase chain reaction procedure in 1985 (15) recapitulated, in vitro, the biological amplification of nucleic acid polymers, and has revolutionized the technologies used to analyze and detect DNA and RNA molecules. The PCR utilizes in vitro enzymatic synthesis procedures to create millions of identical copies of a target DNA or RNA sequence (Fig. 5.16). This process depends upon two synthetic oligonucleotides whose sequences are complementary to areas of the target that flank the region of the target to be amplified. The PCR is initiated when these two oligonucleotides are allowed to hybridize, or "anneal" to the component strands of a denatured target DNA molecule. The oligonucleotides are constructed such that their 3′OH termini are oriented towards each other. After annealing to the target, the oligonucleotides can thus serve as primers for enzymatic extension from the 3′

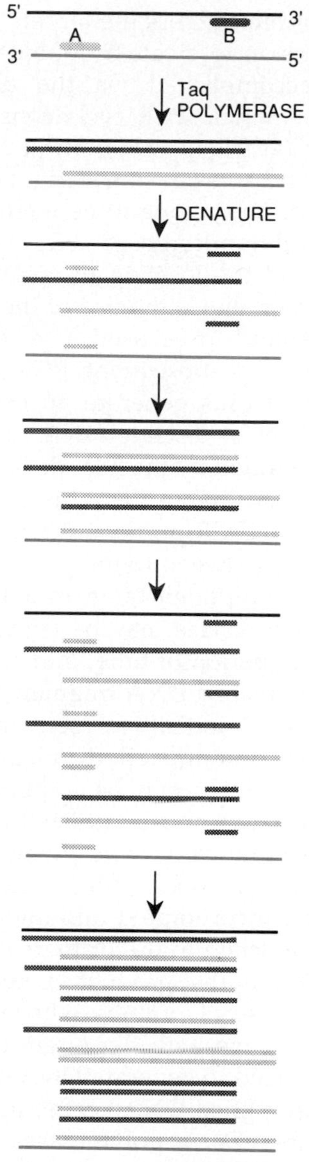

Figure 5.16. The polymerase chain reaction. A double-stranded DNA segment is denatured and annealed to oligonucleotide primers A and B. These serve to allow synthesis of DNA strands by the action of *Taq* polymerase and deoxynucleoside triphosphates. Subsequent pairs of synthesized double-stranded DNA molecules are again denatured and annealed to primers A and B, and serve as templates for another round of *Taq* polymerase-catalyzed DNA synthesis. Multiple cycles of this procedure yield a DNA product that begins precisely at the 5′ end of the A primer and ends precisely at the 5′ end of the B primer, as shown by the third and sixth double-stranded molecules in the bottom panel.

ends of the primers across the target "template." Enzymatic extension to create a double-stranded DNA product is accomplished via the use of a DNA polymerase. A single PCR cycle consists of a denaturation step (at 94° to 98°C), an annealing step (at 37° to 65°C), and an extension step (at 72°C) that typically lasts sufficiently long to generate a product exceeding several hundred base pairs. Extension of the product beyond the location of complementarity of the other primer allows the use of the newly synthesized DNA strand to be used as a template by the other primer in a subsequent PCR cycle. Iterative PCR cycles will thus generate an exponentially increasing number of discrete DNA fragments whose termini are bounded by the 5′ ends of the oligonucleotide primers, and whose lengths equal the sum of the length of the PCR primers plus the length of the target molecule between them.

Since each component step in a PCR cycle lasts minutes, tens of cycles may be completed within a relatively short period of time, and can generate microgram amounts of a DNA fragment amplified from a target sequence initially present in nanogram or even picogram amounts. Both single-stranded and double-stranded DNA may be amplified by the PCR. RNA molecules can also be utilized as templates by the PCR, after first converting them into cDNA, using reverse transcriptase. Since the PCR primers themselves are incorporated into the product, a variety of labels attached to the primers can thus also be incorporated into the product. Likewise, the PCR will allow the use of primers whose sequences are slightly mismatched with the target DNA sequence, which can be used to generate DNA sequence alterations in the amplified DNA segment.

Thermostable DNA polymerases, isolated from thermophilic bacteria, are used in the PCR extension step. These enzymes can withstand higher annealing and extension temperatures than the *E. coli* DNA polymerase Klenow fragment used initially for the PCR. These higher temperatures (noted previously) appear to promote a reduction in DNA secondary structure, and thus allow the amplification of relatively long fragments (up to several kb). The prototype thermostable polymerase is known as *Taq* DNA polymerase, isolated from *Thermus aquaticus*. This enzyme lacks the 3′ to 5′ exonuclease activity found with other DNA polymerases; absence of this "proofreading" activity is apparently responsible for the relatively high rate of misincorporation of nucleotides into amplified DNA fragments (10^{-5} aberrant nucleotides per cycle). Since for most applications, it is a population of amplified fragments that are subsequently analyzed, a rare misincorporation event will not normally be detected. These errors, and others, including in vitro recombination that may occur as a consequence of template strand switching, are detectable, and distinguishable as PCR artifacts from the correct template sequence, by DNA sequence analysis of multiple independently isolated cloned PCR products.

Recently, other naturally occurring polymerases (VENT polymerase from *Thermococcus litoralis*, *Tth* polymerase from *Thermus thermophilus*) and recombinant Taq polymerases have been described with altered and potentially useful enzymatic properties. VENT polymerase does exhibit the 3′ to 5′ exonuclease activity missing from Taq polymerase, and thus has the potential to yield a lower misincorporation rate. Truncated (Stoeffel fragment) or mutant Taq polymerases lacking the 5′ to 3′ exonuclease activity may allow more efficient synthesis of longer products. *Tth* polymerase exhibits RNA-dependent DNA polymerase activity (reverse transcriptase activity) and can be used for single-tube, single-enzyme PCR starting with RNA.

A large and growing list of research and clinical applications have been described for the PCR (16). Clinical diagnostic uses for this procedure have focused largely on the detection of specific mutations or DNA sequence polymorphisms, on the identification of specific chromosome abnormalities, and the detection and identification of specific viral, bacterial, fungal, and parasitic pathogens. Examples of these approaches are outlined in references 16 and 17 presented in detail in Chapters 6 and 7.

Restriction Endonucleases

Labeled DNA and RNA probes, when used with appropriate hybridization conditions, allow sensitive and specific detection of DNA and RNA target sequences. However, molecular analysis of such target sequences may be facilitated substantially by procedures that allow their structural manipulation, or in ways that allow their isolation and amplification by molecular cloning. Such sequence manipulations can involve the use of enzymes that cleave nucleic acids in a sequence-specific manner, often in conjunction with procedures and reagents that can synthesize and join these molecules. Enzymes that divide DNA sequences at specific sites are known as restriction endonucleases, and can fragment double-stranded DNA molecules into lengths amenable to further manipulation and analysis. Restriction endonucleases are isolated from diverse species of microorganisms, and many types are commercially available. Each restriction enzyme recognizes a specific DNA sequence of 4 or more nucleotides, and cuts the DNA by breaking a phosphodiester bond on both strands typically at or near this restriction "site." Examples of commonly used restriction enzymes and their corre-

Table 5.2. Four Examples of Commonly Used Restriction Endonucleases

Enzyme	Recognition Sequence	Cleavage Products	
EcoRI	GAATTC	—G	AATTC—
	CTTAAG	—CTTAA	G—
BamHI	GGATCC	—G	GATCC—
	CCTAGG	—CCTAG	G—
NotI	GCGGCCGC	—GC	GGCCGC—
	CGCCGGCG	—CGCCGG	CG—
HinfI	GANTC	—G	ANTC—
	CTNAG	—CTNA	G—

sponding recognition sequences are illustrated in Table 5.2. Such restriction sites are found distributed in a roughly random manner along the length of DNA molecules, but their locations are generally invariant within identical DNA molecules. Thus, the locations of such sites within a specific human gene will be generally independent of the origin of the DNA containing the gene (be it human tissue, a human cell line, or a recombinant microorganism containing a cloned copy of the gene, for example) and may be used to divide the gene, as well as its flanking DNA sequences, into discrete DNA fragments of predictable sizes.

The locations of such restriction sites are not always invariant, however. Differences in the DNA sequence at restriction site locations can exist between otherwise identical DNA segments isolated from different individuals (or between the two copies of an autosomal gene in a single individual). These structural differences, or sequence polymorphisms, can occur without altering the function of the sequence in which they are found, or they may correspond precisely to the DNA sequence alteration responsible for creating a genetic disease. In either event, however, detection of such polymorphic sites may be used for carrier detection and prenatal diagnosis in genetic disease by detecting DNA sequence alterations, or mutations, within or adjacent to specific genes (5).

Preparation of DNA

Many methods have been described for preparing human genomic DNA for analysis by restriction endonuclease cleavage (4). Cells or tissues are generally lysed directly with buffered solutions containing a detergent such as sodium dodecyl sulfate, or after disruption by freezing and pulverization. Solutions for DNA preparation are generally supplemented with ethylamine diamine tetraacetate (EDTA) at millimolar concentrations to prevent DNA degradation by divalent cation-dependent endogenous nucleases. This cell or tissue lysate is then subjected to digestion with pancreatic RNAase (to reduce endogenous RNA molecules to oligoribonucleotides), and then with a proteinase (proteinase K, for example). The digested lysate is extracted with phenol, and low molecular weight contaminants are removed by dialysis or by precipitation of the DNA from an ethanolic salt solution. Genomic DNA is susceptible to shearing during its preparation, but with a moderate amount of care, it is possible with such methods to isolate genomic DNA with fragment sizes ranging between 100 kb and 200 kb. Keep in mind, however, that this statement applies to DNA prepared from freshly isolated cells or tissues. By contrast, isolation of genomic DNA from formalin-fixed, paraffin-embedded specimens is problematic in that a large proportion of this DNA can be significantly degraded (18, 19).

Electrophoretic Fractionation of DNA

When digested with most restriction enzymes, mammalian genomic DNA isolated in the aforementioned manner will generate millions of discrete fragments with modal sizes ranging from a few hundred base pairs to tens of kb. Such fragments then may be fractionated according to size by standard electrophoretic methods that utilize agarose gels and Tris-borate or Tris-acetate buffers (Figs. 5.17–5.19). Detailed protocols for such methods are found in a number of molecular cloning laboratory manuals (4, 20). It is necessary in some circumstances, however, to generate and fractionate DNA molecules whose sizes exceed 25 kb. A few restriction endonucleases have been identified with sites that are either nonrandomly distributed within mammalian genomes, or that are present at relatively low frequency. These enzymes, including the few that recognize a specific sequence of 8 base pairs (NotI, Table 5.2, for example), tend to generate large DNA fragments whose sizes may exceed several hundred kilobase pairs. These enzymes can thus be useful for determining physical relationships between genetically linked sequences (21).

Such large molecules present special analytical problems, however. Firstly, since the DNA molecules in genomic DNA prepared in the usual manner are typically less than 200 kb in size, such DNA samples are not suitable for digestion and analysis by this subset of enzymes. Genomic DNA for such analyses is therefore typically prepared by first embedding intact cells in an agarose block, and then incubating the block in solutions containing detergent, RNAase, and proteinase K (22). These reagents reach the cells by diffusion, and operate to lyse the embedded cells, and then hydrolyze proteins and RNA molecules. Contaminating peptides, lipids, oligoribonucleotides, and other small molecules remaining after such treatment diffuse out of the block,

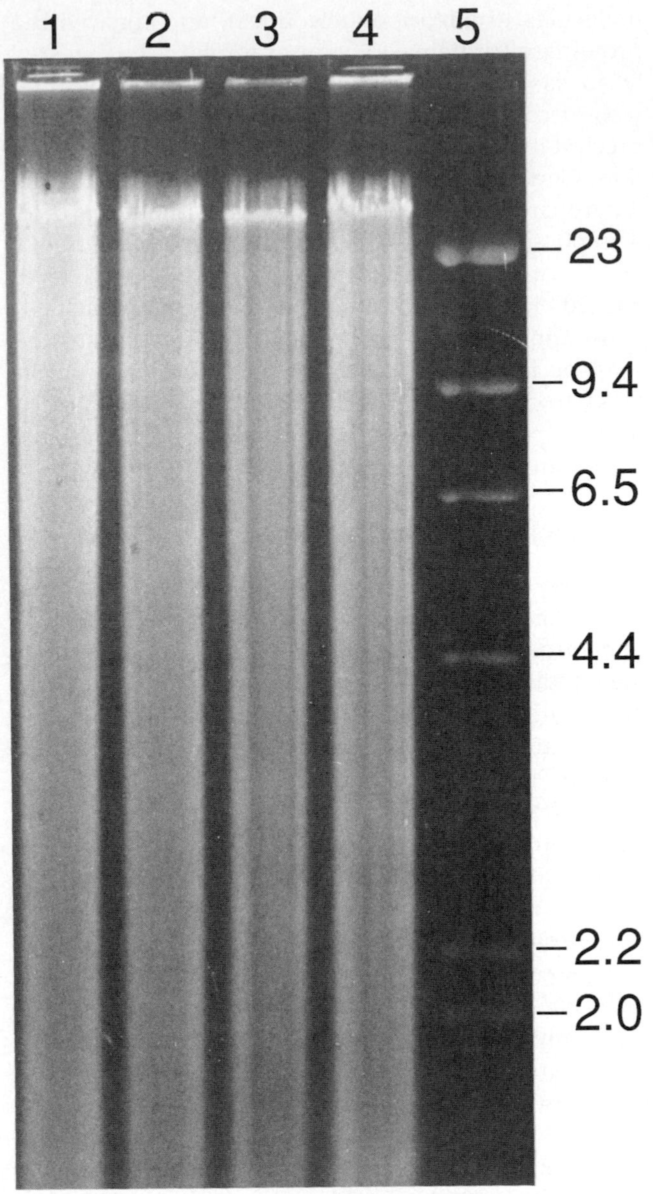

Figure 5.17. Gel electrophoresis of digested genomic DNA. Human genomic DNA was digested with four different restriction endonucleases (lanes 1–4), fractionated by standard agarose gel electrophoresis (see Fig. 5.18), and the gel was stained with ethidium bromide. Size markers (lane 5) were generated by a *Hind*III digestion of phage λ-DNA; sizes are given in kilobase pairs.

leaving behind genomic DNA molecules, with sizes that generally exceed several 1000 kb. DNA prepared in this manner may then be digested in situ by placing the agarose block into a buffered solution containing the appropriate restriction enzyme. After the digestion is completed, the intact block will contain DNA restriction fragments whose sizes may range upwards of 800 kb or more.

Since standard agarose gel electrophoresis methods are unable to adequately resolve linear DNA molecules whose sizes exceed approximately 25 kb, a number of approaches have been developed to separate the larger molecules generated by this approach (23). These methods, known generically as pulsed field gel electrophoresis, have in common the use of two or more alternating electric fields. They make use of the observation that large DNA molecules, in solution within the agarose gel matrix, are conformationally distorted by a voltage gradient and tend to elongate in the direction of the electric field to migrate through the gel. With these methods, the first electric field is removed, and a second one is applied at an angle to the first. The DNA molecules must reorient in response to this second field before they can migrate in the new direction. Longer DNA molecules spend proportionately more time reorienting rather than migrating, relative to smaller DNA molecules, thus allowing size-dependent separations. Numerous different types of pulsed field gel electrophoresis methods have been described, and the technology continues to evolve (23). These approaches differ according to their particular electric field geometries, and depending on fields being homogeneous or nonhomogeneous. Early configurations that relied on nonhomogeneous electric fields (pulsed field gel electrophoresis, PFGE; orthogonal field alternating field gel electrophoresis, OFAGE) yield adequate separation but produce "bent" lanes that make lane-to-lane comparisons difficult. The field inversion gel electrophoresis (FIGE) method makes use of an electrode geometry that allows a simple, 180° reorientation angle. The switching interval used for FIGE is typically changed in a progressive manner during the fractionation to minimize the tendency for this approach to yield anomalous, disproportional relationships between migration distance and molecular size. One of the more advanced types of pulsed field electrophoresis is the contour-clamped homogeneous electric field (CHEF) gel (Fig. 5.18). Multiple electrodes are arranged in a hexagonal array around a closed contour, and are used to generate homogeneous electric fields with reorientation angles of 60° or 120° (Fig. 5.18). DNA molecules migrate in a straight line through such gels, and sizes ranging up to several thousand kilobase pairs may be separated (Fig. 5.19). A more recent elaboration incorporates the capabilities of many of these types of apparatuses, and allows virtually unlimited variation of field angle and field pulsing configurations, with the capability to fractionate DNA molecules between 100 bp to more than 6,000,000 bp (programmable, autonomously-controlled electrodes—PACE) (24). Power switching units and companion gel boxes for several of these configurations are commercially available.

Agarose blocks containing large DNA fragments to be separated by pulsed field electrophoresis are placed directly into the sample wells of the agarose gel. Samples containing fragments smaller that 25

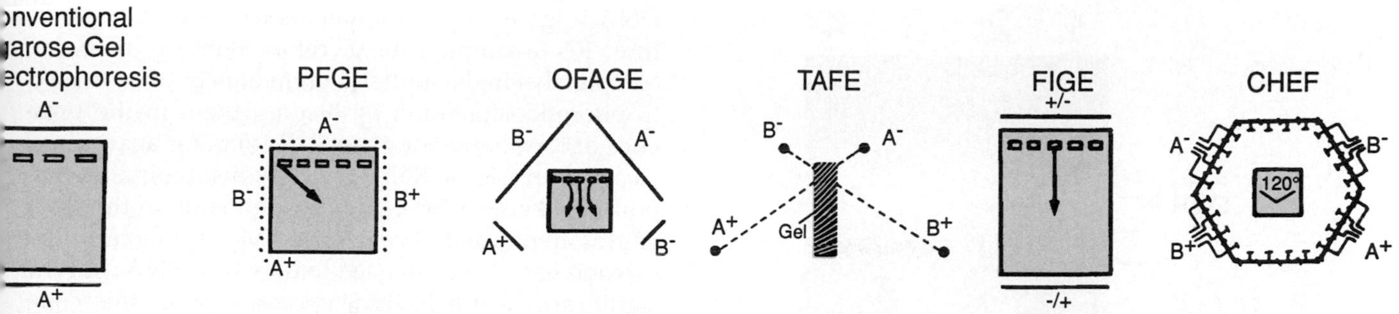

Figure 5.18. Schematic diagram of different configurations used to fractionate nucleic acid fragments by gel electrophoresis. A conventional agarose gel electrophoresis configuration is shown at the left. DNA samples are applied to the wells within the agarose gel and subjected to electrophoresis under the influence of a simple electrical field. Pulsed field gel electrophoresis (PFGE) separates DNA by using two alternative electrical fields (A−, A+:B−, B+). One of the alternating electrical fields is homogeneous, and the other is nonhomogeneous. Orthogonal field-alternation-gel electrophoresis (OFAGE) is similar to PFGE except that both electrical fields are nonhomogeneous. Transverse alternating field electrophoresis (TAFE) is similar to PFGE except that both fields are homogeneous across the width of the gel. Field inversion gel electrophoresis (FIGE) fractionates large DNA molecules by inverting a uniform electrical field in one dimension (i.e., a 180° reorientation angle). The forward and reverse electrical fields differ with respect to their duration and/or voltage, to achieve a net forward migration. The contour clamped homogenous electrical field method (CHEF) generates homogenous electrical fields around a closed contour using multiple electrodes.

kb, which will be fractionated by conventional electrophoretic methods, are pipetted as solutions directly into sample wells. Parallel separation of DNA molecules of known sizes is an important part of the electrophoretic fractionation of restriction endonuclease digests. Size markers for conventional electrophoresis typically consist of a set of DNA fragments of known, defined size, generated by restriction endonuclease digestion of phage-λ (Fig. 5.17). By contrast, size markers often used for pulsed field gel electrophoresis include concatamers of phage λ DNA (Fig. 5.19). These markers are comprised of polymerized units of the approximately 50-kb λ phage DNA genome, with molecular sizes ranging from 50 kb to 1000 kb or more, that consist of 1 to 20 or more 50 kb units. Chromosomes isolated from *Saccharomyces cerevisiae* and other yeasts are also commercially available for use as markers.

Preparation and Electrophoretic Fractionation of RNA

Isolation of RNA from mammalian cells or tissues has historically been a time-consuming and rather tedious procedure. Most approaches (4, 20) extract nucleic acids from pulverized cells or tissues with buffers containing phenol or chaotropic agents like guanidine isothiocyanate. These agents are used to inactivate virtually ubiquitous RNAases present in cells that would otherwise partially or completely degrade the RNA. Following extraction, the RNA is separated from DNA and other cellular components by differential precipitation methods or by ultracentrifugation procedures. Total cellular RNA isolated in this manner contains ribosomal and transfer RNAs as well as messenger RNA. Total cellular RNA may be used for many procedures for detection and analysis of RNA transcripts, including Northern blot, slot blot, and RNA-PCR methods. It is sometimes necessary, however, to further purify the messenger RNA transcripts from the total cellular RNA. Purified messenger RNA is the preferred substrate for preparing cDNA libraries (see below), for example. And since messenger RNA represents just 1 to 3% of total cellular RNA, analysis of relative nonabundant mRNA transcripts by Northern blot or slot blot analysis may be facilitated by the use of purified mRNA (*see* Fig. 5.20).

Methods used to purify mRNA rely on the observation that the majority of messenger RNA species are polyadenylated, containing upwards of 100 or more A residues at their 3′ ends, whereas ribosomal and transfer RNAs are not polyadenylated. Polyadenylated mRNA may be efficiently isolated by affinity chromatography on solid phase matrices containing oligodeoxythymidylate or polyuridine (4, 20). The polyA tract at the 3′ end of the messenger RNA molecules interacts with oligo dT or poly U matrices via stable hydrogen-bonded base pairing, whereas nonpolyadenylated RNA is not bound. The purified polyadenylated messenger RNA is eluted by disrupting the hydrogen bonded base pairing with low-salt buffers. At nearly all steps of an RNA isolation procedure, care must be taken to prevent contamination by RNAases. Buffers, containers, and equipment are all potential sources of such contamination. Buffers are typically treated when possible with diethylpyrocarbonate (DEPC), a reagent that inactivates RNAases. Disposable single-use plastic containers and pipettes are typically free from RNAase contamination; glass pipettes, bottles, beakers, and the like must be rendered RNAase-free by baking or

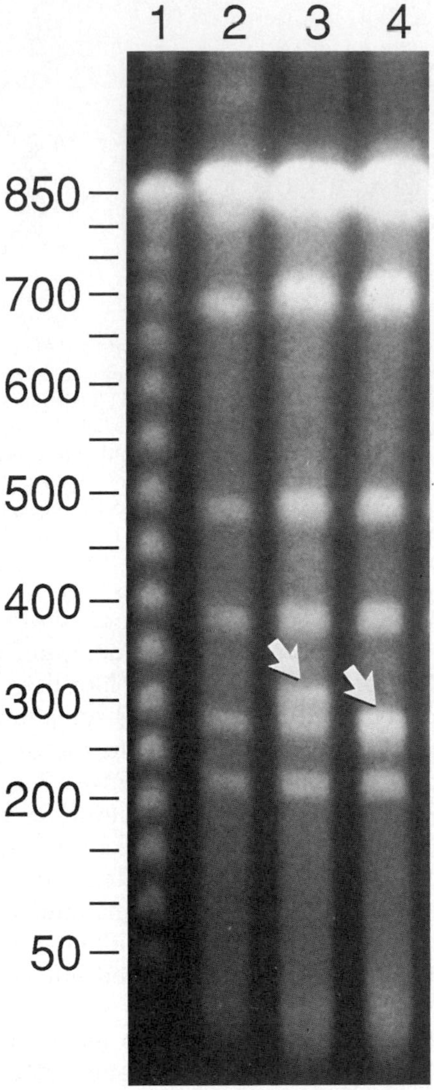

Figure 5.19. Electrophoretic separation of yeast chromosomes by pulsed field gel electrophoresis. A contour-clamped homogeneous electric field device (CHEF) was used to separate yeast chromosomes by gel electrophoresis. Chromosomal DNA was isolated from a laboratory strain of *Saccharomyces cerevisiae* (lane 2), or from this strain carrying two different yeast artificial chromosomes (YACs) (lanes 3 and 4). The arrows in lane 3 and 4 indicate the locations of the YACs. Size markers (lane 1) were generated by concatamerizing the 50 kb phage λ genome; sizes of the concatamers are given kilobase pairs.

DEPC treatment. Much of the inconvenience associated with preparing and testing these reagents may be avoided with the use of commercially available kits that allow the isolation of both total cellular RNA and polyadenylated RNA.

Total cellular RNA, or purified messenger RNA, may be fractionated by size via modifications of agarose gel electrophoresis procedures used for DNA fragment separations (4, 20). "Native" RNA molecules tend to assume secondary structure conformations that yield anomalous electrophoretic mobilities under conditions used to separate double-stranded DNA fragments. To eliminate such secondary structure, RNA samples are therefore typically rendered completely single-stranded immediately prior to electrophoretic separation by heating them in the presence of formamide or glyoxal. Buffers for agarose gel electrophoresis of RNA typically also contain compounds like formaldehyde, which maintain the RNA in this denatured, linear form. Methylmercuric hydroxide has also been used to denature RNA, but the significant health hazard associated with this compound, coupled with the reliability of the other methods described previously, has made this approach obsolete. Following electrophoresis, fractionated, single-stranded RNA molecules may be visualized by staining the gel with ethidium bromide (Fig. 5.20).

Blot Hybridization Procedures

It is readily apparent from Figures 5.17, 5.19, and 5.20 that electrophoretic separation of genomic DNA restriction fragments or RNA molecules cannot by itself allow a determination of the location of any particular molecular species that corresponds to a gene segment or transcript, for example. For DNA molecules, this may be accomplished, however, by the Southern blot procedure (25), which uses nucleic acid hybridization for the detection of specific DNA fragments amongst a large number of irrelevant fragments (Fig. 5.21). With this method, DNA restriction fragments are first fractionated by conventional or pulsed field agarose gel electrophoresis, and are then denatured in situ by incubating the gel with a salt solution of basic pH. The fragments are then transferred to a thin membrane that serves as a blotting support. This is generally accomplished by capillary action, although electrophoretic and vacuum methods are also in use. Transfer is accomplished in a manner that maintains the spatial relationships between the fragments, as generated by agarose gel electrophoresis.

The blotting support is typically a charged nylon membrane, or nitrocellulose. Following transfer, the fragments are tightly bound to the support by ultraviolet cross-linking (nylon supports), or with heat (nitrocellulose). The blot, which now displays the single-stranded DNA fragments arrayed according to their sizes, is then bathed for 6 to 24 hours, or longer, in a hybridization solution containing the single-stranded probe. The probe consists of a single-stranded DNA or RNA molecule that has been previously "labeled" with radioactive molecules, or by other methods, as outlined above. Following hybridization, the blot is washed free of unhybridized probe, and is subjected to procedures (autoradiography with radiolabeled probes, for example) that al-

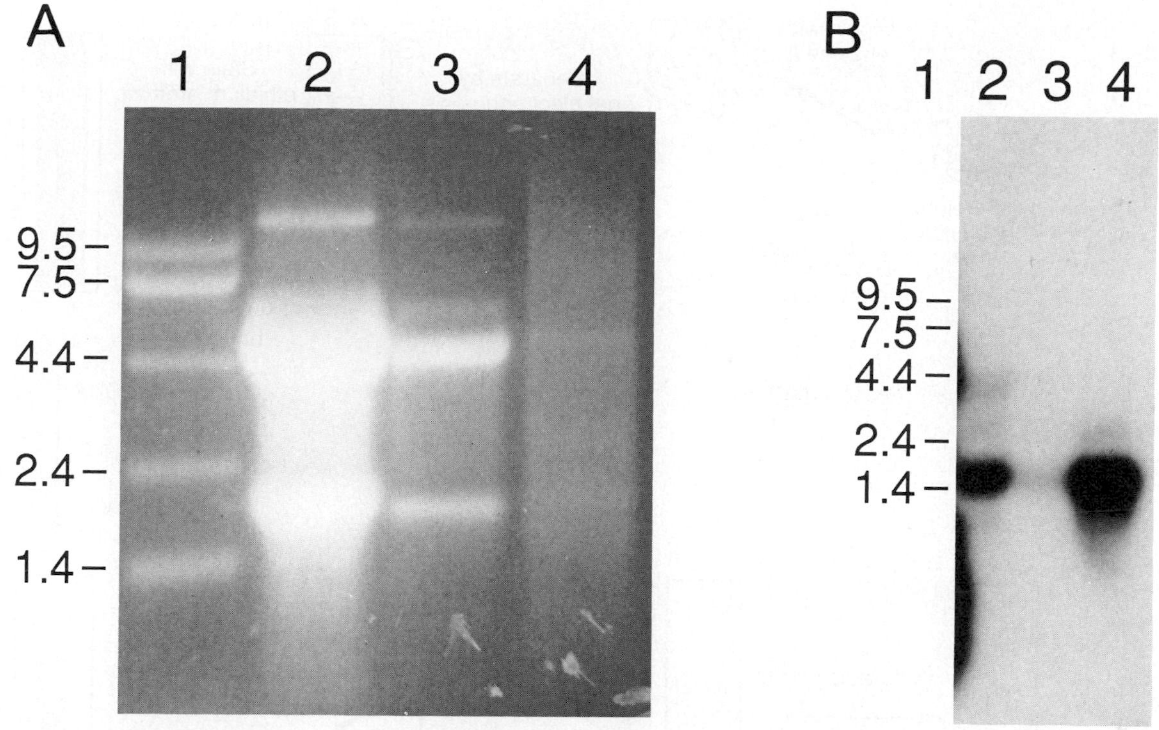

Figure 5.20. Electrophoretic fractionation and Northern blot analysis of RNA. **A**, Ethidium bromide–stained formaldehyde-agarose gel after electrophoretic fractionation of human RNA. Lanes 2 and 3 contain 10 μg and 1.0 μg, respectively, of total cellular RNA. Lane 4 contains 1.2 μg of oligo dT-selected human RNA corresponding to the RNA sample in lanes 2 and 3. The bands evident in lanes 2 and 3, which migrate at 2.2 and 4.4 kb respectively, are 28S and 18S ribosomal RNAs. **B**, Northern blot analysis of the gel shown in panel A. The blot was probed with a radiolabeled cDNA corresponding to about a 1.6-kb transcript, washed, and subjected to autoradiography. Note the signal intensity enhancement achieved by analysis of oligo dT-selected RNA, consisting largely of polyadenylated mRNA. Single-stranded RNA size markers are shown in lane 1 of **A**, and their sizes in **A** and **B** are given in kilobase pairs.

low detection of stable hybrids between the probe and its target sequence(s). DNA restriction fragments possessing sequence complementarity with the probe are identified as discrete bands after duplex detection, and the sizes of these complementary fragments can be determined from their positions on the blot.

Southern blot analyses of genomic DNA represents a relatively time-consuming procedure (4, 20). DNA extraction for standard gel electroporesis requires about 1 day to complete, whereas preparation of genomic DNA for pulsed field gel electrophoresis will take 2 days or longer. Gel electrophoresis, blotting, and hybridization also each require about 1 day to complete. Duplex detection may require 1 to several days. Thus, starting with a sample of cells or tissues, the entire procedure may require 5 or more days to complete. Southern blot analysis of DNA samples with sequence complexities less than human genomic DNA (such as DNA obtained from most microorganisms, or cloned DNA segments) may be completed much faster. This is because the effective concentration of the target sequence in these circumstances will generally be several orders of magnitude greater than in mammalian genomic DNA. For example, Southern blot analysis of cloned DNA segments, starting with restriction digestion, may be completed within 24 hours.

RNA molecules can be similarly analyzed with the Northern blot procedure (Fig. 5.20) (4, 20). Following electrophoresis, fractionated, single-stranded RNA molecules are directly transferred and bound to blotting support using approaches virtually identical to Southern blot transfers. Hybridization and probe-target duplex detection are also performed in a similar fashion.

"Dot blot" or "slot blot" hybridization procedures are also in use for analysis of genes and their transcripts, and for evaluation of clinical samples for pathogens. Denatured DNA samples are directly applied to blotting support, usually with the use of vacuum manifolds that pull the DNA solution through the support, via individual small round or slot-like, templated holes. Prior restriction digestion or size fractionation is not required. Likewise, RNA samples may also be applied to blotting support in this manner. The applied nucleic acid molecules are then bound to the support, and the blot is probed in a manner analogous to Southern or Northern blots. While absence of prior electrophoretic fractionation does not allow size-based confirmation that the target sequence is the only one detected with this

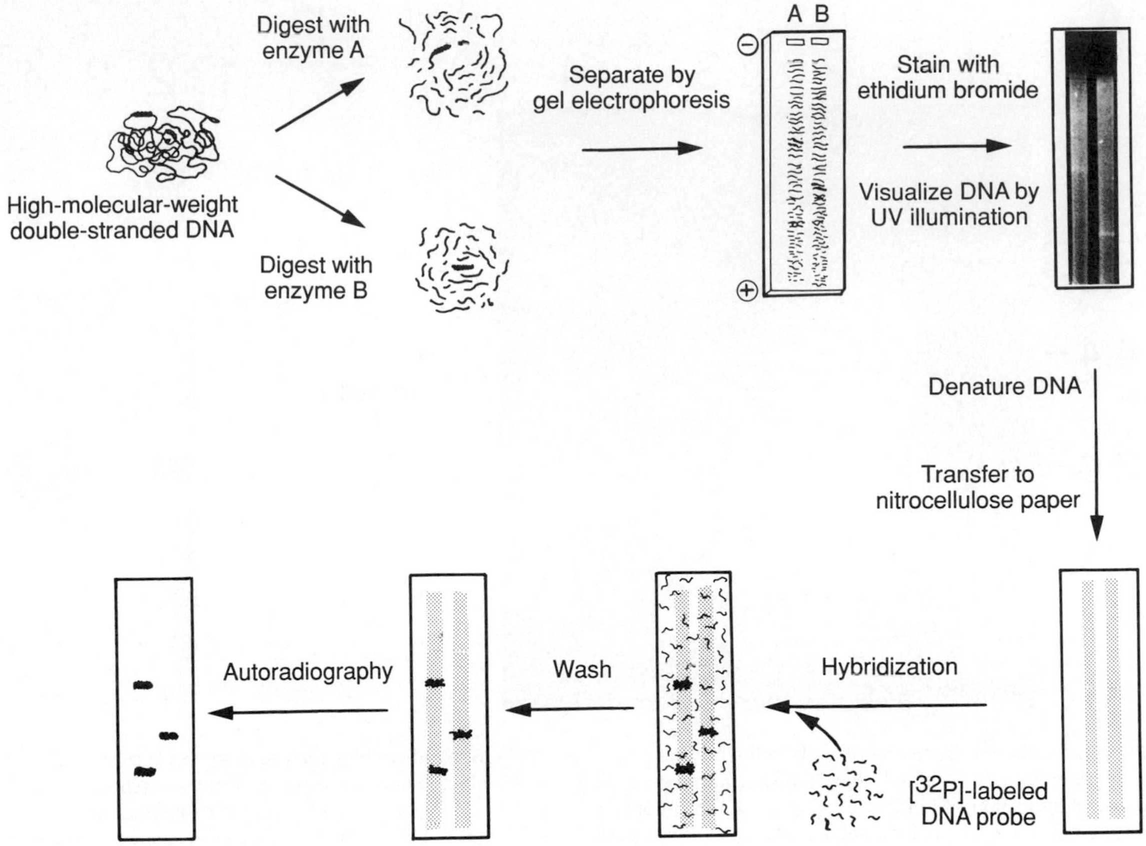

Figure 5.21. The Southern blot procedure. High molecular weight genomic DNA is digested by restriction endonucleases. The fragments in each digest are fractionated by agarose gel electrophoresis, and the DNA is visualized with ultraviolet light after staining with ethidium bromide. The DNA fragments are denatured within the gel by treatment with base, and are then transferred to nitrocellulose paper (shown here) or to a nylon-based blotting support. The transferred DNA is fixed to the blotting support, and the resulting blot is hybridized with a ^{32}P-labeled gene probe. Nonhybridized probe molecules are removed by washing, and fragments in the test DNA that have formed stable complexes with probe molecules are detected by autoradiography. (Reprinted with permission from Lowe JB. Clinical applications of gene probes in human genetic disease, malignancy, and infectious disease. Clin Chim Acta 1986;157:5.)

method, specificity is maintained by adjusting hybridization stringencies to yield a signal only when there is perfect complementarity between the probe and its target.

Molecular Cloning

Segments of nucleic acids to be used as labeled probes for diagnostic purposes must be available in pure form. Oligodeoxynucleotides with lengths of up to nearly 100 bases are available via automated synthetic procedures; these are typically supplied in pure form, and in quantities sufficient for direct use in the PCR, or for labeling and subsequent hybridization. By contrast, larger segments of DNA for direct or indirect use (i.e., as templates for the preparation of RNA probes; Fig. 5.9) must first be "cloned" in order to provide numerous identical copies, in amounts (hundreds of nanograms to a few micrograms) sufficient for labeling and hybridization procedures. Again, in vitro "cloning" of a DNA segment may be accomplished via the PCR. Traditionally, however, DNA segments are cloned by propagating them in a host microorganism. This is accomplished by replicating the DNA segment as a part of a vector, which is an accessory DNA molecule that contains other DNA sequences necessary to allow its maintenance in the host microorganism.

Plasmid Vectors

The bacterial plasmid may be considered the prototypical cloning vector (4, 20). Plasmids used for standard cloning methods are generally circular, double-stranded DNA molecules that replicate in *E. coli*. They are usually less than 10 kb in size, contain one or more genes that allow genetic selection for host cells that contain the plasmid (usually antibiotic resistance genes), and typically generate many tens or hundreds of copies within each host cell. Unique restriction endonuclease cleavage sites are located in plasmid vectors. These serve to allow the introduction of exogenous segments of DNA in the form of restriction fragments (Fig. 5.22). A plasmid molecule,

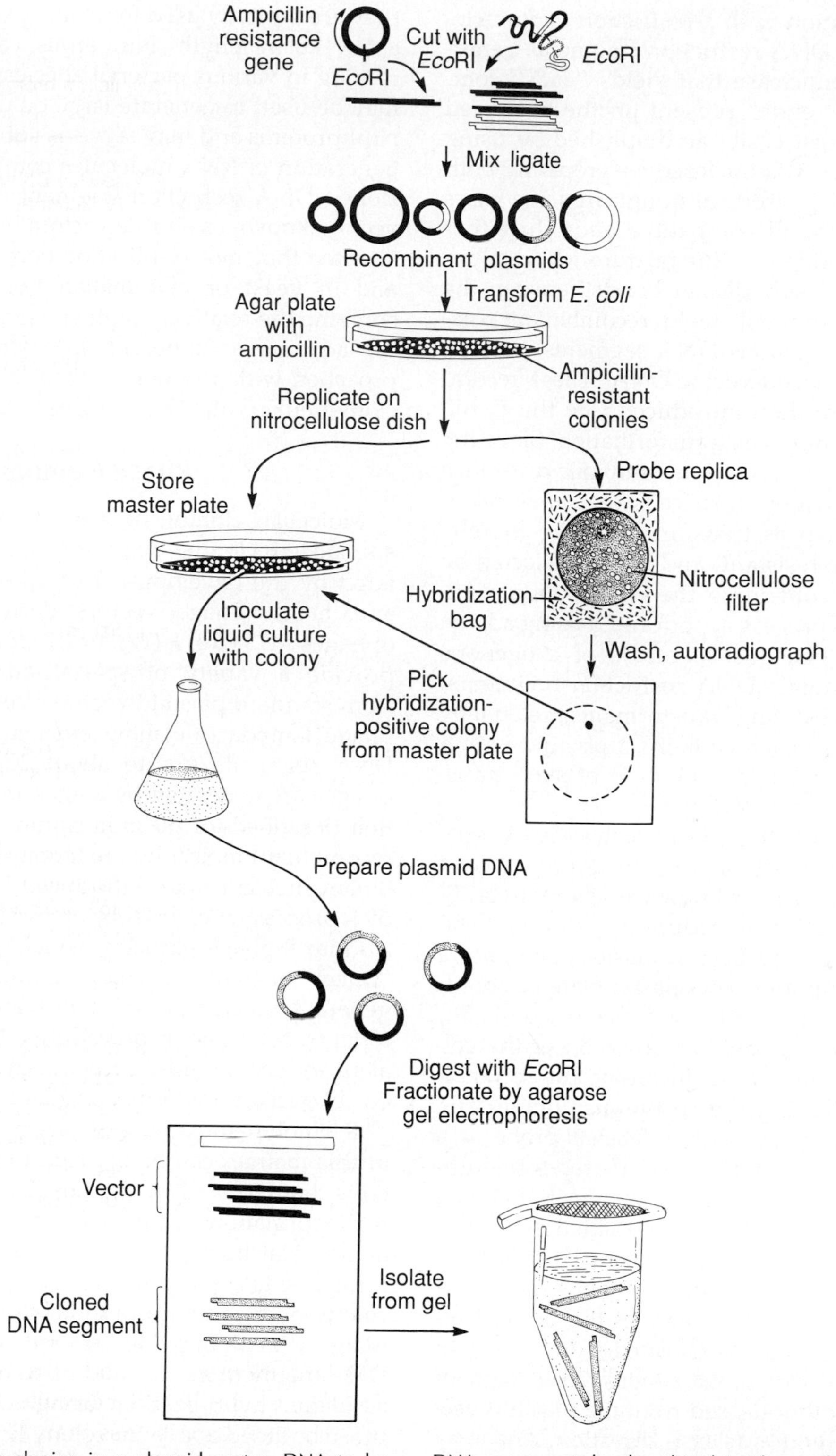

Figure 5.22. Molecular cloning in a plasmid vector. DNA to be cloned (*right*) and a plasmid vector (*left*) are separately digested with the enzyme restriction endonuclease *Eco*RI. The resulting *Eco*RI restriction fragments are mixed, ligated with T4 DNA ligase, and introduce into *E. coli* by transformation. *E. coli* transformants containing recombinant plasmids are selected by plating on an agar plate containing ampicillin. A replica is made of the ampicillin-resistant colonies on a flat nitrocellulose disk. The master agarose plate containing the ampicillin resistant colonies is stored (*left*). The nitrocellulose replica of the colonies is hybridized with a probe specific for the DNA sequence to be cloned (*right*). After washing, the hybridized nitrocellulose filter is subjected to autoradiography. A hybridization positive colony identified by autoradiography is picked from the stored master plate, and used to inoculate a large liquid culture. This culture is then used to prepare plasmid DNA. The recombinant plasmid DNA is digested with *Eco*RI to release the cloned fragment, and the vector and insert DNA fragments are separated by agarose gel electrophoresis. The cloned DNA segment, migrating at a position distinct from the vector sequence, is isolated from the gel, and is stored as a solution of DNA molecules for subsequent use.

linearized by digestion with a restriction endonuclease, is mixed with DNA restriction fragments generated with an endonuclease that yields "ends" complementary to the "ends" present on the linearized plasmid. This is most easily accomplished by using the same restriction endonuclease for preparing both the plasmid and the insert, although in some cases different enzymes yield compatible ends. In either case, DNA ligase added to this mixture will catalyze the synthesis of phosphodiester bonds between the compatible ends, and will yield recombinant plasmids containing exogenous DNA segments inserted within the recircularized vector DNA. These recombinant plasmids are then introduced into the *E. coli* host by a process known as transformation. Since the recombinant plasmids encode an antibiotic resistance gene, antibiotic-sensitive host cells that have taken up plasmids (known as transformants) are thereby rendered antibiotic-resistant, and may be selected by growth on media containing the corresponding antibiotic. When this process is performed using a large number of heterogeneous segments of exogenous DNA (as with genomic DNA restriction fragments, for example), the resulting transformants are equally heterogeneous since each contains a plasmid with a relatively unique insert. A collection of such transformants is known as a library.

It is possible to identify, within such a library, specific transformants that contain the desired cloned DNA segment by a process known as colony hybridization (4, 20). With this procedure, transformant colonies are first replicated from a master plate onto a nitrocellulose membrane. The master plate is stored, and the colonies on the replica are then lysed in situ, with virtually simultaneous denaturation of the colony DNA. The colony DNA, including the recombinant plasmid DNA, is fixed to the membrane, and probed by hybridization with a labeled probe in a manner conceptually identical to that used for Southern blotting. Colonies containing the desired cloned DNA fragment are identified by a positive hybridization signal. The transformant colony is retrieved from the master plate, and may be grown in liquid culture. Up to several milligrams of the desired recombinant plasmid may be isolated from a liter of such a culture. The cloned exogenous DNA segment may be subsequently released from the plasmid vector by restriction endonuclease digestion, and may be purified via agarose gel electrophoresis. Gene fragments isolated in this manner may be obtained in microgram amounts, are suitable as substrates for virtually all of the labeling procedures outline above, and are stable indefinitely when stored at −20°C or below.

Plasmid vectors allow the cloning of DNA fragments with sizes ranging up to tens of kb, although they are typically used for cloning segments less than a few kb in length. Numerous varieties that allow cloning in various bacterial species now exist, which may be used to generate large quantities of recombinant proteins and may serve as substrates for in vitro generation of RNA molecules complementary to the cloned DNA restriction fragment (Fig. 5.9). Plasmid vectors known as shuttle vectors have also been constructed that allow replication both in bacterial hosts, and in yeast or mammalian hosts. These vectors combine the relatively high efficiency and the technical advantages inherent in bacterial cloning approaches with the ability to test the function of a cloned eukaryotic DNA segment in its native host.

Phage Vectors

Molecular cloning of larger fragments, and other specialized cloning requirements have been facilitated by the development of other types of vectors and hosts. Phage vectors derived from bacteriophages M13 (26), λ (27), or P1 (28), for example, can provide a variety of specialized functions absent from standard plasmid vectors. Vectors derived from phage lambda can allow efficient cloning of larger DNA segments (up to about 20 kb); recombinant phages are generated by a ligation process similar to that described for plasmid cloning, but the resulting recombinant molecules are largely linear. The recombinant molecules are introduced into an *E. coli* host by a process whereby they are first "packaged" in vitro into λ phage particles, which in turn are used to "infect" or transduce the *E. coli* host. This process is generally much more efficient than the standard bacterial transformation procedures, but roughly equivalent to recently introduced electroporation-dependent bacterial transformation methods (29).

Recombinant λ-phage DNA molecules generated in this manner can be induced to form λ-phage proteins that in turn lyse the host bacterium. The result is the formation of a plaque, or clear area, on a lawn of bacterial host cells. Each recombinant phage can form a single plaque, analogous to a transformant colony obtained with plasmid cloning. Recombinant phage containing the desired cloned exogenous DNA fragment may be identified by a process known as plaque hybridization, using concepts identical to those outlined above for colony hybridization (4, 20). In plaque hybridization, however, plaques (containing recombinant phage) are transferred to a hybridization support, and the phage DNA in the plaques is denatured in situ, bound to the support, and probed with a labeled probe. Probe-positive recombinant phages are grown, and the phage DNA is isolated, using procedures that generally are more tedious than those used to isolate plasmid DNA. Indeed, recombinant restriction fragments present in such phages may be subsequently cloned into a plasmid vector for further analysis.

Cosmid and Phagemid Vectors

Cosmids are a hybrid of λ-phage and plasmid vectors (30). These vectors are approximately 3 to 8 kb in size; they contain small segments of phage-λ, known as cos sites, an antibiotic resistance gene, and a plasmid-type origin of replication. Exogenous DNA restriction fragments are ligated into the cosmid in such a way as to flank them with cos sites on both sides, and with a single plasmid replication origin and antibiotic resistance gene. This configuration allows the recombinant molecule to be packaged in vitro within a λ-phage particle. Such phage particles are capable of introducing the packaged DNA into an *E. coli* host by transduction. Once inside the host, circular recombinant DNA molecules replicate from the vector's plasmid-type replication origin; under selection by the antibiotic resistance gene, the transduced host forms colonies. Since the λ-phage genes necessary for phage replication and coat protein assembly are absent from cosmid vectors, plaques do not form. Moreover, absence of these phage genes allows the cloning of relatively large (about 30 to 40 kb) segments of DNA; such large fragments are in fact a virtual requirement since the phage packaging machinery will operate only upon cos-containing recombinant DNA molecules with sizes within the roughly 35 to 50 kb size range. Isolation of desired recombinant cosmids is accomplished by colony hybridization approaches.

Phagemids represent another type of plasmid-phage hybrid vector. Phagemids based upon the *E. coli* M13 or fd phage, for example, are in wide use for cloning and DNA sequencing purposes (31). These vectors can replicate to high copy number as a plasmid in *E. coli*, and can also be induced to give rise to single-stranded circular DNA molecules that become packaged within a phage coat. These latter single-stranded molecules can be isolated from purified phage particles (4, 20), and are useful as templates for DNA sequencing.

Isolation of Gene Probes

Isolation of recombinant plasmids, phages, or cosmids by the hybridization approaches outlined earlier assumes that a probe is already available for this purpose. Isolation of a new probe in essence represents the isolation of a new gene, generally a difficult process. Numerous approaches have been developed for gene isolation; these typically require specific information about the gene (amino acid sequence of its protein product; location in relation to other genes; function) or reagents that can detect the gene's protein product (antibodies directed against the protein product; ligands for receptor proteins). It is possible to use some of these approaches to directly isolate a segment of the new gene from a library of genomic DNA fragments. Such libraries are typically constructed in λ-phage or cosmid vectors, using random and heterogeneous genomic DNA fragments generated by partial restriction endonuclease digestion of genomic DNA. The DNA segments in a genomic library may contain exons, introns, and gene-flanking sequences, as well as repetitive DNA sequences and other "junk" DNA. Each such DNA sequence is, on the average, represented equally within the genomic DNA library. Based upon the average insert sizes in phage (about 12 to 20 kb) or cosmid (about 30 to 40 kb), one haploid human genome equivalent will be represented by roughly 200,000 independent phages, or by 100,000 independent cosmids (4, 20).

It is often more useful, however, to use a cDNA library to first isolate a cloned cDNA corresponding to the gene (Fig. 5.23). cDNA libraries contain a cloned representation of the mRNA transcripts in a tissue or cell. The relative abundance of a desired sequence in a cDNA library is therefore typically substantially higher than in a genomic DNA library. cDNA libraries are constructed by first isolating mRNA from a tissue or cell that transcribes the desired gene (Fig. 5.23). This mRNA serves as a substrate for the action of reverse transcriptase, which catalyzes the synthesis of a double-stranded copy of each mRNA molecule in the reaction. These double-stranded cDNAs are then cloned in a plasmid or phage vector.

Screening of cDNA libraries for a novel gene sequence may be accomplished with knowledge of a portion of its amino acid sequence. "Reverse translation" of the protein sequence will allow the design of a pool of synthetic oligonucleotides containing one that will hybridize to the corresponding gene (Fig. 5.24). These may be used to screen cDNA (or genomic DNA) libraries by hybridization. Alternatively, if two or more distinct segments of protein sequence are known, pairs of oligonucleotide pools corresponding to these segments may be used as PCR primers to generate a PCR product corresponding to the gene. cDNA is typically used as a template with this method, known as the mixed oligonucleotide primed amplification of cDNA, or MOPAC procedure (32). The product may then be used as a probe for hybridization screening.

If antibodies are available that can detect the protein product of a gene, these may be used to screen cDNA libraries constructed in the *E. coli* phage vector

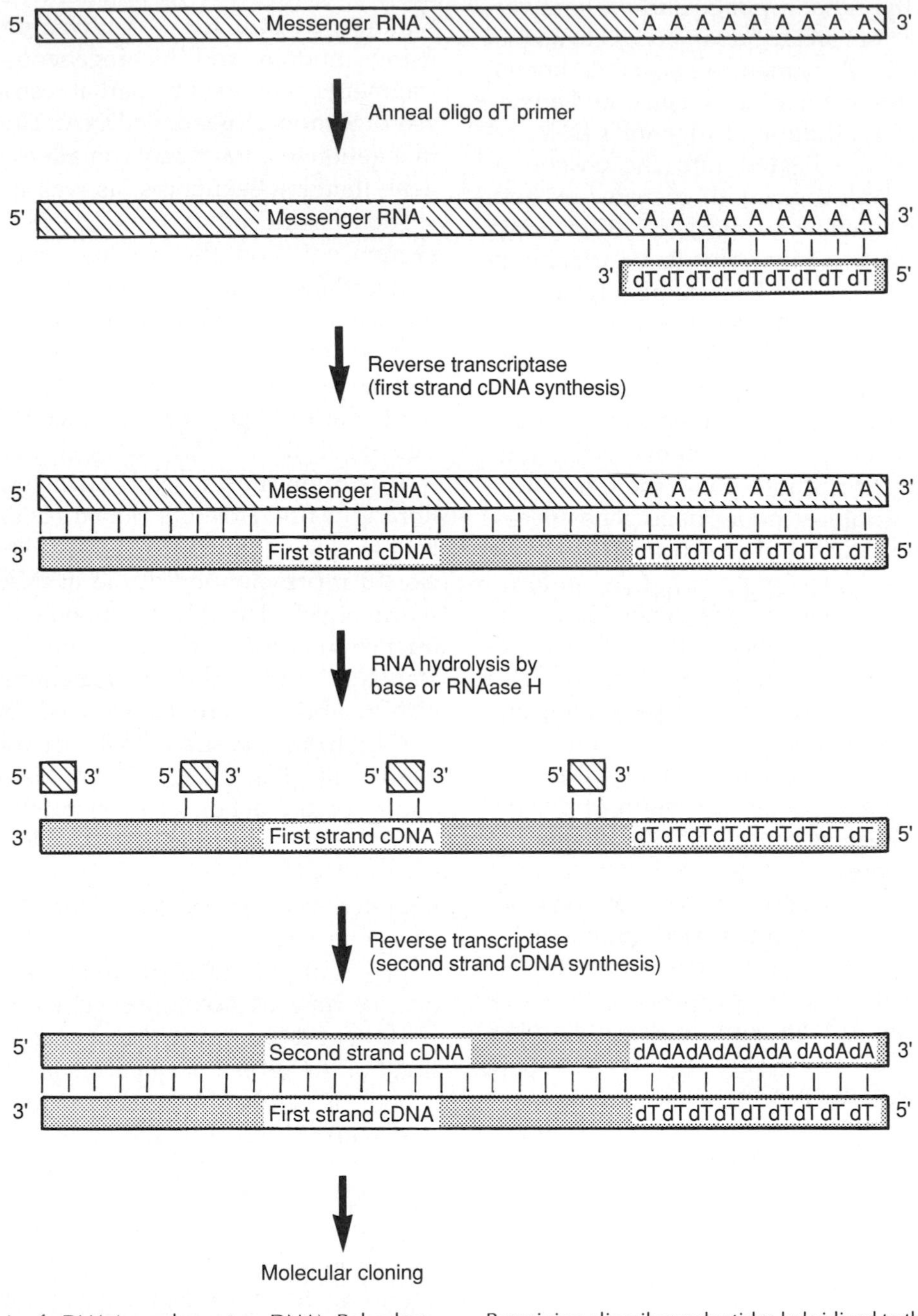

Figure 5.23. Synthesis of cDNA (complementary DNA). Polyadenylated messenger RNA is annealed to oligo dT primer molecules. Reverse transcriptase and deoxynucleoside triphosphates are added, catalyzing the synthesis of a segment of DNA complementary to the mRNA (first strand of cDNA synthesis). The RNA portion of this DNA-RNA hybrid is partially hydrolyzed by the action of base or RNAse H. Remaining oligoribonucleotides hybridized to the first strand of cDNA serve as primers for the synthesis of the second strand of cDNA, catalyzed again by the action of reverse transcriptase operating with deoxynucleoside triphosphates. The resulting double-stranded cDNA is then cloned into an appropriate or plasmid or phage vector.

Amino acid sequence	-Trp-Met-Glu-Asp-Cys-Met-
Oligonucleotides	TGG-ATG-GA$^{A}_{G}$-GA$^{T}_{C}$-TG$^{T}_{C}$-ATG

Figure 5.24. Design of a set of oligonucleotide hybridization probes using known amino acid sequence. When one or more portions of the amino acid sequence of a protein are known, a set of oligonucleotides corresponding to that protein sequence may be designed, using knowledge of amino acid codons (Table 5.1). Because of the degeneracy of the genetic code, some amino acids may be encoded by more than one codon. Consequently, some stretches of amino acid sequence have the potential to be encoded by many possible different DNA sequences. A pool of oligonucleotide containing each of these possibilities is therefore synthesized, radiolabeled, and used as a hybridization probe to isolate the corresponding gene or cDNA.

λ gt11 (27) (Fig. 5.25). If the desired gene encodes a surface-localized mammalian protein, such a gene may be isolated by using antibodies to screen a cDNA library constructed in a mammalian expression vector (33) (Fig. 5.26).

Novel gene sequences may also be isolated by genetic complementation in prokaryotic or eukaryotic hosts (34), as well as by virtue of physical and/or genetic linkage to previously isolated DNA segments in a process known as "reverse genetics" (35, 36).

Cloning with Yeast Artificial Chromosomes

From a simple consideration of the sizes of the DNA fragments that are capable of being cloned by the phage and cosmid vectors just outlined (less than 40 kb), these tools are clearly less than optimal for the isolation of some intact genes and gene clusters (Fig. 5.3). They are also generally inadequate for physically connecting genes spaced by genetic distances exceeding a few tenths of a centimorgan (Fig. 5.3). Other substantial technical obstacles exist with these host-vector systems, including the fact that many eukaryotic DNA sequences are rather unstable and prone to rearrangement when propagated in the usual *E. coli* hosts. These inadequacies have spawned the development of a new generation of vectors and allied technology capable of isolating—intact—segments of mammalian genomic DNA spanning upwards of 1000 kb, and propagating them in eukaryotic hosts. Yeast artificial chromosome, or YAC, vectors represent the prototype for these approaches (37). These vectors contain one or more genes for selection in yeast, as well as segments representing the ends of a yeast chromosome (telomeres), a centromere, and a replication origin, known as an autonomous replication sequence (ARS). Collectively, these segments allow replication of the vector, and inserted DNA, in the yeast *Saccharomyces cerevisiae* (Fig. 5.27).

Formidable technical modifications of standard molecular cloning procedures have enabled the isolation of large (many hundreds of kb) intact segments of human genomic DNA, and their cloning into YAC vectors. These procedures allow the propagation of segments of human genomic DNA with spans of several hundred kb (Fig. 5.19). Such segments are generally (though not always) colinear with their counterpart in a mammalian chromosome, and are usually (but not always) replicated within the yeast without rearrangements. Considering the size of the human genome (Fig. 5.3), and the average genomic DNA insert size in YAC human genomic DNA libraries (large sets of independently isolated YACs containing human genomic DNA), the entire human genome may be represented by roughly several thousand to tens of thousands of independently isolated YACs. Retrieving YACs from YAC libraries has presented special technical problems that have been overcome by the use of the PCR for screening purposes (38). To facilitate this screening, YAC libraries are stored frozen in arrays in 96-well microtiter plates. To screen such libraries by the PCR, a pair of PCR primers corresponding to the gene of interest is used in a series of reactions containing YAC DNA as a template. Initially, each of these reactions contains DNA corresponding to many independent YACs, generally prepared by pooling the DNA from multiple 96-well plates. In aggregate, such pools will completely represent the YAC library. The products of the PCR reaction from each reaction are analyzed by gel electrophoresis. The component DNAs corresponding to the pool or pools of YACs that yield the predicted product are then individually analyzed by the PCR. PCR-positive 96-well pools are further subdivided into their component YAC DNAs and analyzed again in this manner. Each iteration reduces the size of the pools analyzed, making it possible to ultimately identify single YACs containing the gene of interest. Following the identification of the desired YACs, their inserts may be analyzed by Southern blotting, and segments may be isolated and subcloned in cosmid, phages, or plasmid vectors. This approach has been used recently to isolate and map a number of human genetic loci including, for example, a segment of human chromosome 17 that corresponds to the cystic fibrosis gene (39).

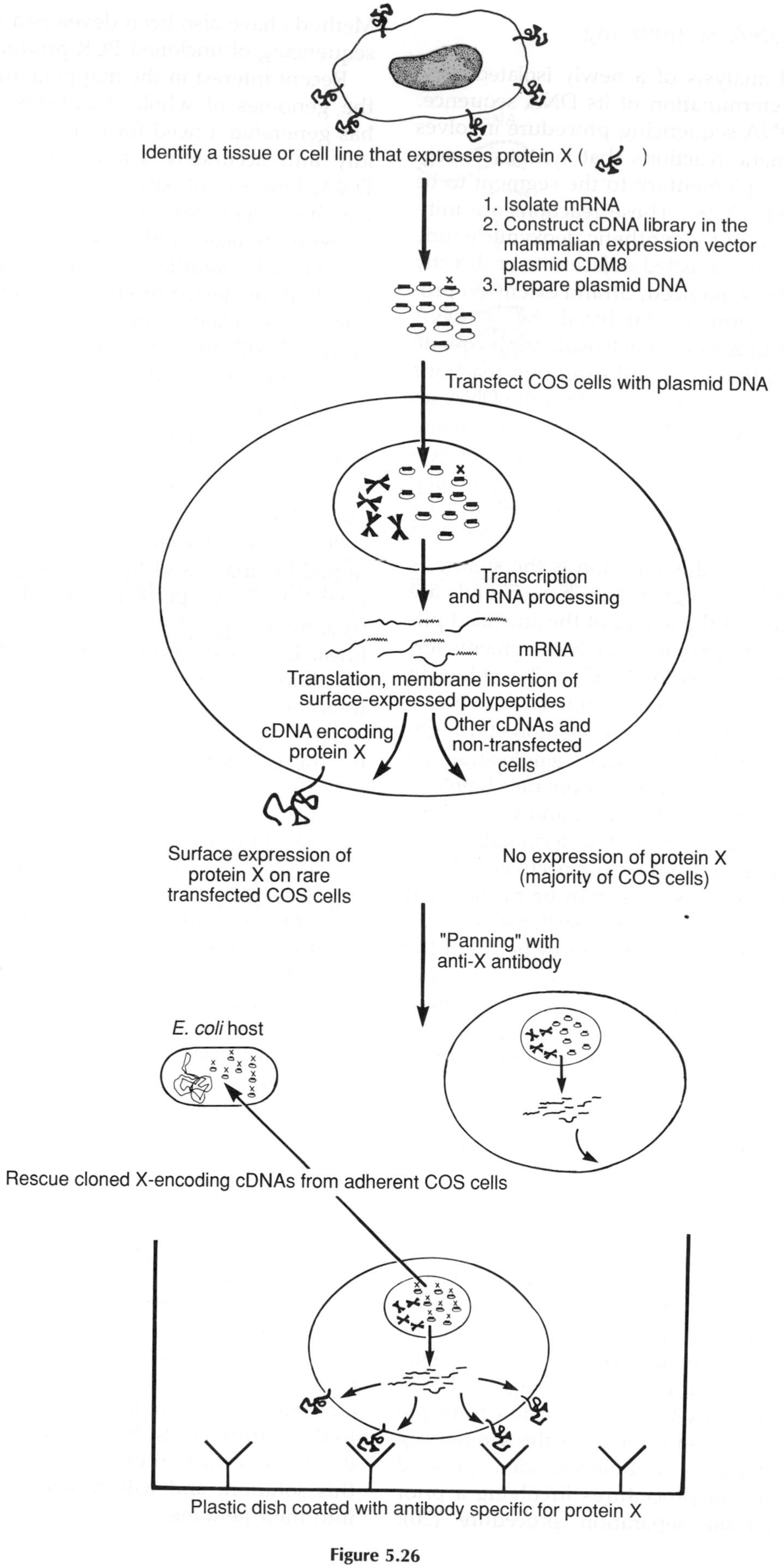
Identify a tissue or cell line that expresses protein X ( )
1. Isolate mRNA
2. Construct cDNA library in the mammalian expression vector plasmid CDM8
3. Prepare plasmid DNA
Transfect COS cells with plasmid DNA
Transcription and RNA processing
mRNA
Translation, membrane insertion of surface-expressed polypeptides
cDNA encoding protein X
Other cDNAs and non-transfected cells
Surface expression of protein X on rare transfected COS cells
No expression of protein X (majority of COS cells)
"Panning" with anti-X antibody
E. coli host
Rescue cloned X-encoding cDNAs from adherent COS cells
Plastic dish coated with antibody specific for protein X

Figure 5.26

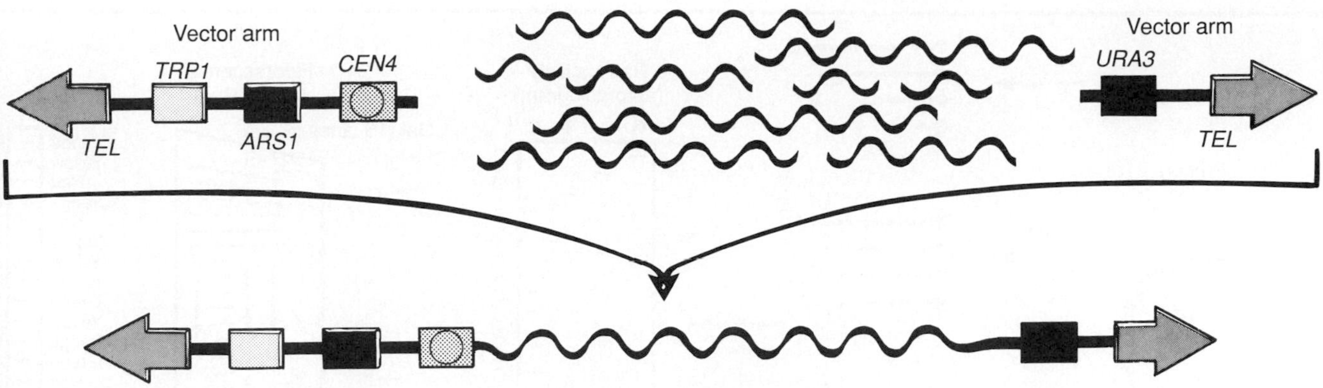

Figure 5.27. Cloning with yeast artificial chromosomes (YACs). Large segments of genomic DNA (hundreds of kilobase pairs) are isolated as restriction endonuclease fragments. These are ligated between the two arms of the yeast artificial chromosome vector. The vector arms are substantially smaller than the genomic DNA they flank (together, less than 10 kb). The YAC arms contain segments to allow propagation in yeast (telomers, TEL; centromeres, CEN; replication origin, ARS; and selectable markers, TRP1 and URA3). The resulting recombinant molecules propagate as linear chromosomes in yeast, and maintain sizes of several hundred kilobase pairs (see Fig. 5.19). (From Schlesinger D. Yeast artificial chromosome: tools for mapping and analysis of complex genomes. Trends Genet 1990;6:248–258.)

Transfectants are selected with the use of selection genes and corresponding antibiotics that function in mammalian cells. A commonly used mammalian selectable marker is the "Neo" gene segment, derived from a bacterial neomycin resistance gene encoding a neomycin phosphotransferase (45). In mammalian cells, this enzyme can also inactivate the neomycin analogue G418, a compound that is normally toxic to mammalian cells. When transfecting a vector containing a Neo segment physically linked to the gene to be tested, selection for G418 resistance will ensure that virtually all such transfectants will contain the desired test gene. Alternatively, the neo segment on one DNA molecule may be mixed with the test gene on another molecule, and cotransfected. If the test gene molecules are in molar excess over the G418 selection molecules, most or all of the G418-resistant transfectant will contain the test gene. The calcium phosphate method also allows the transient introduction of cloned DNA segments into mammalian cells. Numerous other approaches have been developed to introduce cloned DNA segments into mammalian cells. DNA complexes formed with DEAE-dextran (20) are taken up efficiently by a number of cultured mammalian cells. DNA may also be delivered to cells via encapsulation within liposomes (46). DNA may also be delivered to cells by electroporation (47). In this latter process, cells are incubated in a solution of cloned DNA segments, and are subjected to a carefully controlled high-voltage pulse of electrical current. It is thought that this creates transient discontinuities in the cell membranes, allowing the DNA molecules in the surrounding solution to enter the cell cytosol and/or nucleus.

Cloned DNA segments may also be introduced into mammalian cells with the use of viral vectors. These vectors are similar in concept to the bacteriophage vectors alluded to earlier for prokaryotic cloning purposes. Exogenous gene segments introduced into the genomes of mammalian viruses may be encapsulated within the viral coat. These recombinant viral particles may then be used to efficiently "infect" or transduce the appropriate mammalian host cell.

Figure 5.26. Expression cloning of a cDNA encoding a surface-localized mammalian protein when antibodies are available (33). To isolate a cDNA that encodes a mammalian protein X expressed at the cell surface, messenger RNA is prepared from a cell line or tissue that expresses the protein. This mRNA is used to prepare a cDNA library in a mammalian expression vector. Such vectors contain transcriptional control sequences that efficiently transcribe the cloned cDNAs after introduction into mammalian hosts by transfection. The library is initially propagated in *E. coli*; plasmid DNA prepared from the library is subsequently introduced by transfection into the primate-derived COS-1 or COS-7 cell lines. A significant proportion of the COS cells take up the transfected DNA. The transfected plasmids containing cDNA inserts replicate to high copy number in the COS cell nucleus. (COS cells stably express the large T antigen of the SV40 virus. This protein functions in *trans* to promote nuclear replication of the transfected vector-cDNA plasmid molecules from their SV40 viral origin of replication). The high copy number of the vector, its extrachromosomal location, and its highly active transcriptional control sequences yield substantial amounts of mRNA molecules corresponding to the transfected cDNAs. COS cells that have taken up cDNAs encoding protein X will in turn express large quantities of protein X on their surfaces (*middle, left*). Untransfected COS cells, and COS cells expressing other cDNAs will remain protein X-negative (*middle, right*). Protein X–expressing transfectants are isolated by "panning" on plastic dishes coated with an antibody directed against the surface-expressed portion of protein X (*bottom, left*). Protein X-negative cells are washed away (*bottom, right*). Vector molecules containing the protein X-encoding cDNA insert may be rescued from protein X-positive adherent COS cells and reintroduced into *E. coli* for subsequent amplification and analysis. Successful implementation of this system typically requires two or more sequential screens by panning, and requires that the COS cell host not express protein X.

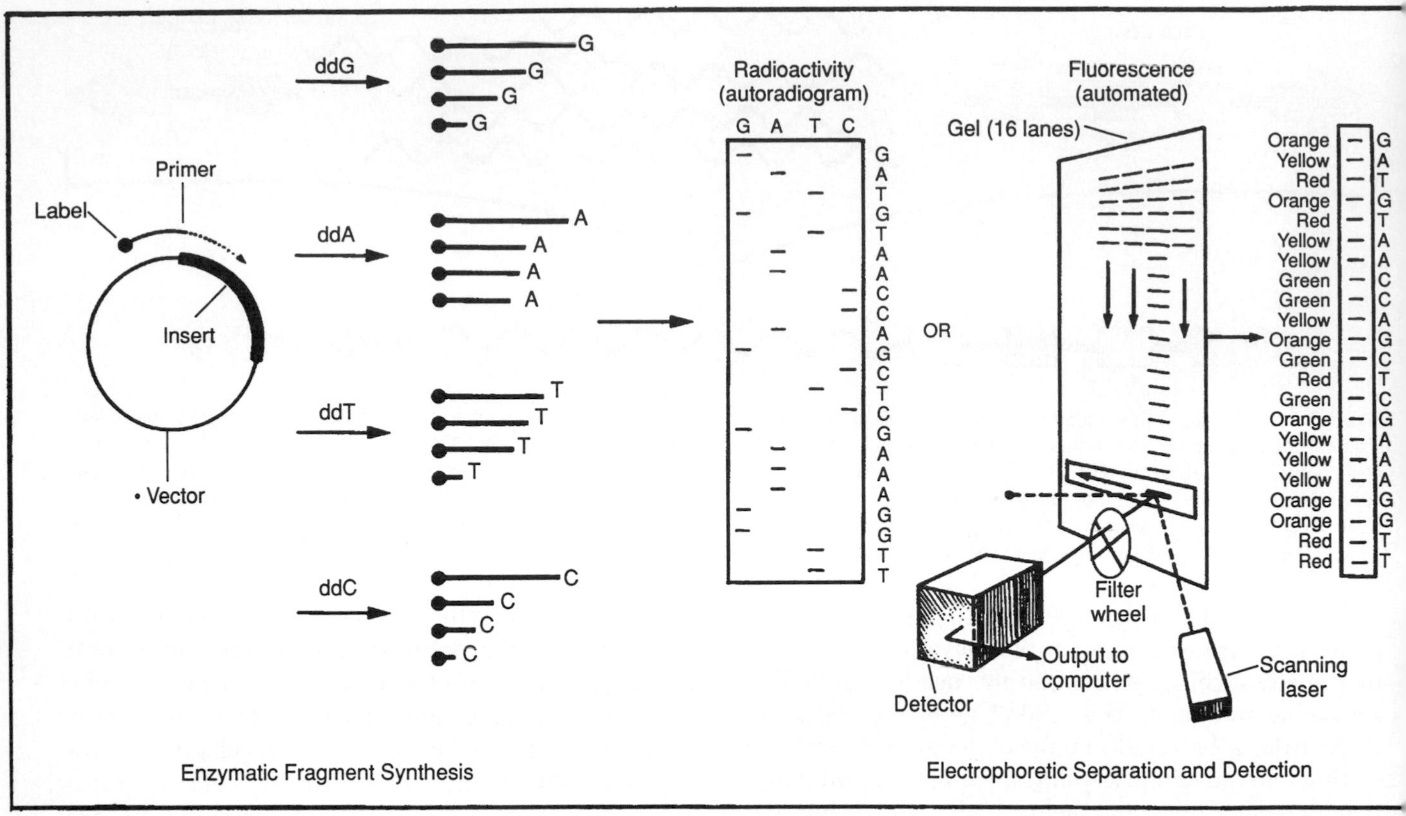

Figure 5.28. DNA sequencing. DNA sequence analysis by chain termination. A synthetic oligonucleotide is used to prime the enzymatic synthesis of a complementary DNA strand for a single-stranded template (16). Four different strand extension reactions are performed in the presence of deoxynucleotides mixed with one of the chain-terminating nucleotide analogs (dideoxynucleotides ddG, ddA, ddT, or ddC). This produces four sets of nested reaction products, all beginning at the same point and ending at every G, A, T, and C residue, respectively, over a 600-nucleotide stretch. Radioactivity labeled fragments are then separated according to size by electrophoresis in four adjacent lanes, one for each nucleotide, of a polyacrylamide gel. An image of the resolved fragments is obtained by autoradiography. The nucleotide sequence of the DNA segment is deduced from the size order of the resolved DNA fragments in the four different lanes. Alternatively, each of the four reactions may be color-coded by using sequencing primers labeled with a different fluorophore for each of the four sequencing reactions. The products of the reactions may then be combined and separated in a single lane of a polyacrylamide gel. The beam of an argon laser mechanically scans a horizontal segment at the bottom of the gel. As the fluorophore-labeled fragments undergoing electrophoresis pass through this region, they are excited to fluorescence. The emitted light is collected and focused onto a detector after passing through four different filters on a rotating wheel. The identity of the terminating nucleotide analog of each passing fragment is identified because of the unique fluorophore associated with it. The temporal order of passing fluorescent molecules is automatically translated into linear DNA sequence and stored by the computer. (Modified with permission from Landegren U, Kaiser R, Caskey CT, Hood L. DNA diagnostics—molecular techniques and automation. Science 1988;242:229–237.)

This approach can be extremely efficient, and can allow the introduction of exogenous DNA molecules into cells that are refractory to the usual transfection approaches.

The prototypical mammalian viral vectors are ones derived from retroviruses (48). In addition to the advantages noted above, retroviral vectors can promote the stable integration of the exogenous gene into the host chromosome. Retroviral vectors in common use have been derived from their parent retroviral genome by deletion of the viral structural genes required for viral replication. The portion of the viral genome required for packaging into the viral coat molecules is retained, however. Exogenous DNA molecules are cloned into this defective viral genome remnant, and the resulting recombinant molecule is introduced into a specialized mammalian host cell line by transfection. This host cell, known as a packaging line (49), expresses the viral structural genes deleted from the vector sequences. The products of the structural genes expressed by the packaging line operate in *trans* to allow packaging of the transfected retroviral vector into a transduction-competent retroviral particle. These defective viral particles do not normally contain complete, functional retroviral genomes and thus are not capable of transmitting an intact retroviral genome. These recombinant, defective viral particles are competent, however, to introduce the packaged recombinant sequences into a host cell. Cells infected with particles harvested from the transfected packaging line stably incorporate the recombinant DNA sequences into random locations

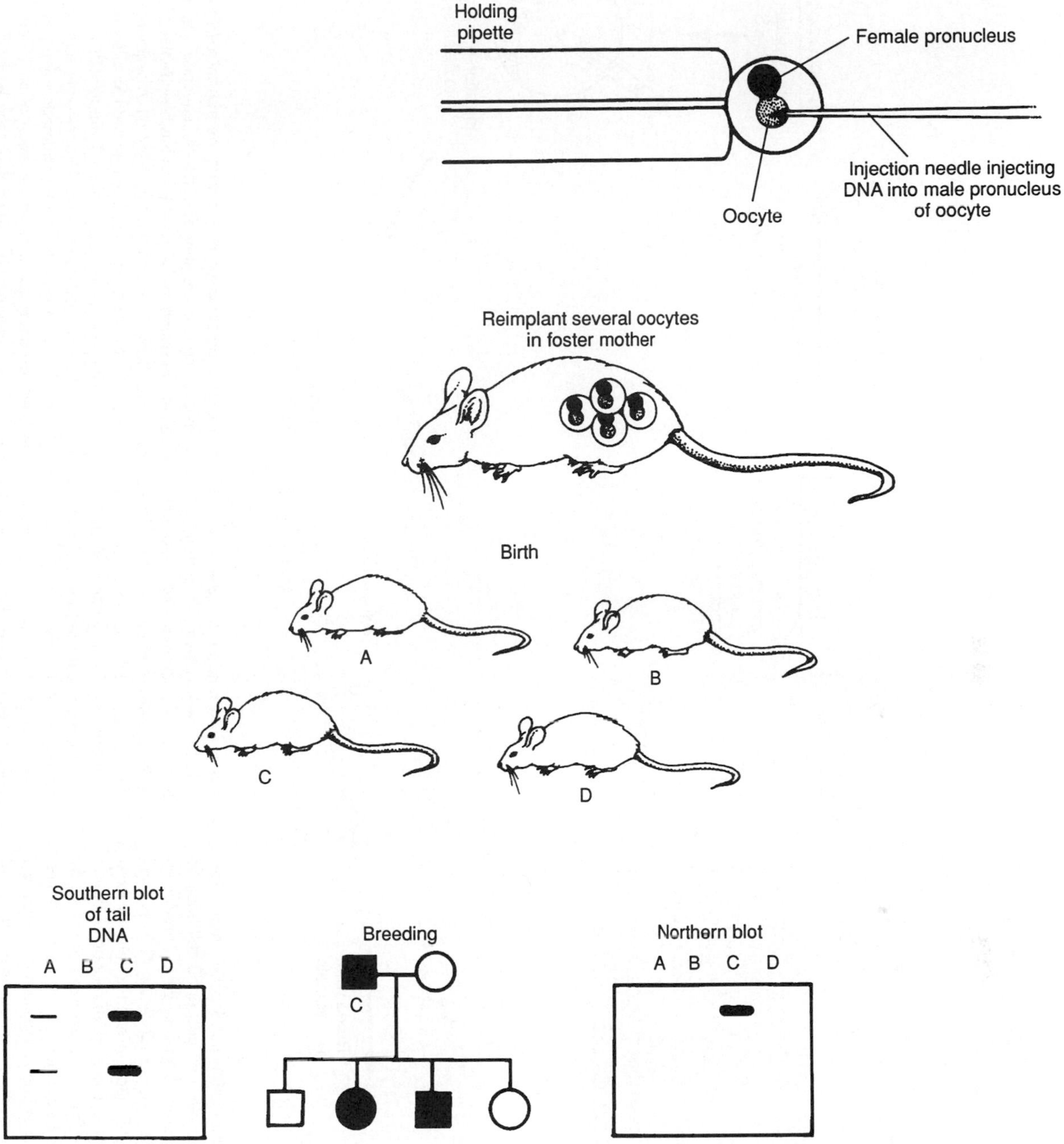

Figure 5.29. Construction of transgenic mice. Construction of transgenic mice begins with the isolation of fertilized oocytes from an ovulating mouse immediately after fertilization. A vector DNA sequence is injected into the male pronucleus of the oocytes. In a fraction of the injected oocytes, the injected vector DNA will integrate within the genome of the resulting preimplantation embryo. Multiple injected oocytes are reimplanted in pseudopregnant foster mothers. Some fraction of the injected oocytes will not have any vector sequences integrated into the genomes of the resulting mice (mice B and D). In some instances, a mouse may be transgenic (stable chromosomal integration the vector sequence) but does not express the integrated sequence (mouse A). Some transgenic mice will express the integrated DNA (mouse C), and will transmit the DNA to their progeny in a Mendelian fashion.

within their genome. Retroviral vectors have been used to introduce exogenous DNA sequences into cultured mammalian cell lines, into primary cell lines, and into specific tissues within whole animals (50, 51).

In each of these approaches, expression of the cloned test gene segment is dependent upon a number of factors. Mammalian promoter and other control sequences are necessary for efficient expression of the transfected foreign DNA segment. Stable incorporation into the host genome does not ensure its expression since it has been observed that the position of such integration events has a strong influence upon the functionality of gene expression control sequences. Expression levels may also vary dramatically depending upon the number of copies of the ex-

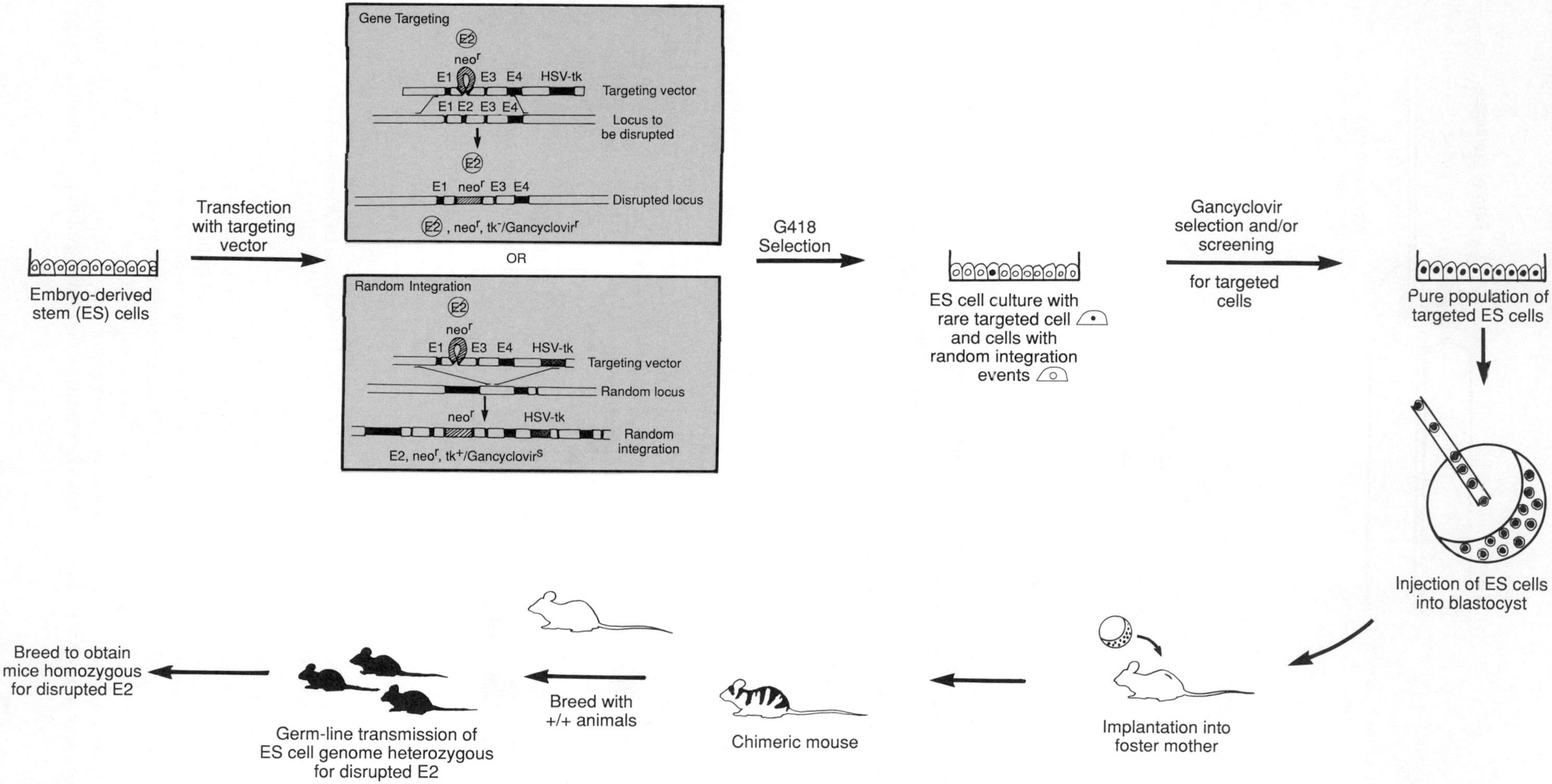

Figure 5.30. Targeted gene disruption by homologous recombination in ES cells. Embryo-derived stem cells (ES cells) are capable of participating in the formation of most or all cell lineages when injected into the cavity of a blastocyst stage embryo. Such cells may serve to introduce a gene deletion into the mouse by genetically modifying them with a targeting vector. The targeting vector generally contains a selectable marker (G418 resistance, neo^r) inserted within an exon (exon E2, *solid areas*) of a cloned representation of the gene to be inactivated; disruption of exon 2 in this manner will functionally inactivate the gene. Introduction of this targeting vector DNA by transfection into the ES cells, followed by G418 selection, yields ES transfectants containing targeting vector DNA that has stably integrated into the ES cell chromosome. Integration can occur via homologous recombination (gene targeting) or by random integration. Random integration will typically also incorporate a segment of the herpes simplex virus thymidine kinase gene (HSV-tk) that flanks the genomic sequences in the targeting vector. By contrast, the HSV-tk sequences will not be incorporated when chromosomal integration by homologous recombination occurs. Selection against random integration events can therefore be achieved by growing the transfected ES cells in gangcyclovir, an antibiotic that is toxic to cells expressing the HSV-tk sequence. This allows the isolation of a pure population of ES cells in which the relevant locus has been replaced by its targeting vector homolog, where exon 2 has been interrupted by the neo^r DNA segment. These targeted ES cells are then injected into a blastocyst-stage embryo. The injected ES cells will contribute to the formation of an intact mouse, after the injected blastocyst is implanted in a pseudopregnant foster mother. When ES cell lines and blastocysts are isolated from strains of mice differing in their coat colors, coat color chimerism can be used to identify chimeric mice produced with this method. Chimeric mice are bred to obtain germline transmission of an ES cell genome heterozygous for the disrupted exon 2. Such heterozygous mice may then be bred to obtain mice homozygous for the inactivated allele. (Modified from Capecchi MR. Altering the genome by homologous recombination Science 1989;244:1288–1292.)

ogenous sequence that have been introduced into the transfected host. Vector-host systems exist that address many or all of these considerations to allow efficient expression of heterologous test genes. One such commonly used system is nearly identical to the one described in Figure 5.26 for cDNA library screening (33). Expression of a desired cDNA sequence is accomplished by cloning it into a vector that replicates as an episome in COS cells, and that places it under the transcriptional control of a strong promoter. Since the expressed sequences undergo extrachromosomal replication, they are free from the position-dependent restraints on expression imposed upon stably transfected foreign DNA sequences. Moreover, their high copy number also ensures efficient gene expression.

Genetic Modification of Mammalian Organisms

For many genes, a complete understanding of function requires an analysis of its product in the context of an intact organism. Several of the gene transfer approaches already outlined have been used to genetically modify animal cells ex vivo, followed by their reintroduction into the animal (50, 51). A powerful alternative to these methods involves the permanent modification of an animal genome via transgenesis, a process extensively refined in the mouse (52). With this technique, it is possible to arrange overexpression of a test gene in a tissue where it is normally expressed at moderate levels, or to orchestrate its expression in tissues where it is normally not expressed. These circumstances are established within the background of the intact animal, which can facilitate an understanding of the function of the gene in a context more physiological than an in vitro culture system.

Transgenesis is accomplished by introducing a test gene into the murine genome at the oocyte stage (53) (Fig. 5.29). In a proportion of the injected oocytes, the foreign DNA sequences stably integrate into the murine chromosome. These are generally propagated in a Mendelian manner, and are transcribed in some fraction of the mice generated. This approach has found utility for the study of control sequences that confer tissue-specific expression patterns upon genes, for the analysis of tissue-specific effects upon the ability of transforming genes to yield tumors, and in the analysis of genetic events that generate antibody diversity, for example (52).

Techniques have recently been developed to allow targeted gene disruption in mice (54) (Fig. 5.30). The starting point for this approach is an embryonic stem cell line capable of contributing to the germ line when made part of a chimeric murine embryo. These cells are transfected with a recombinant exogenous gene into which an inactivating mutation has been introduced. By processes that remain poorly understood, such constructs may stably integrate into the ES genome by homologous recombination with one of its endogenous wild-type counterparts. The result is an ES cell line with one mutant and one wild-type allele of the test gene. This line may then be used to create a chimeric mouse containing cell lineages derived from the altered ES line. Should the germ cell lineage be derived from the ES line, the altered allele will be transmitted to the progeny, creating mice heterozygous for the inactivated allele. Mating of heterozygous progeny may produce embryos that are homozygous for the null allele. In principle, such embryos will develop into mice that are genetically deficient in the ability to express the product of the test gene (in the absence of embryonic lethality due to the deficiency). Correlation of genetic deficiency with the phenotype of the deficient mouse can provide important clues to the function(s) of genes whose purpose is otherwise unknown. This approach has been used recently to investigate genes whose precise functions were not known (55, 56), and is likely to become a commonly used technique in the armamentarium of contemporary molecular geneticists.

References

1. Avery OT, MacLeod CM, McCarty M. Studies on the chemical nature of the substance inducing transformation of pneumococcal types. Induction of transformation by a deoxyribonucleic acid fraction isolated from pneumococcus Type III. J Exp Med 1944;79:137–158
2. Watson JD. The human genome project: past, present and future. Science 1990;248:44–49.
3. Fenoglio-Preiser CM, Willman CL, eds. Molecular diagnostics in pathology. Baltimore: Williams & Wilkins, 1991.
4. Maniatis T. Molecular cloning: a laboratory manual. New York: Cold Spring Harbor Laboratory, 1982.
5. Lowe JB. Clinical applications of gene probes in human genetic disease, malignancy, and infectious disease. Clin Chim Acta 1986; 157:1–32.
6. Feinberg AP, Vogelstein, BA. Technique for radiolabeling DNA restriction endonuclease fragments to high specific activity. Anal Biochem 1983;132:6–13.
7. Rigby PW, Dieckmann M, Rhodes C, Berg P. Labeling deoxyribonucleic acid to high specific activity in vitro by nick translation with DNA polymerase I. J Mol Biol 1977;113:237–251.
8. Melton DA, Krieg PA, Rebagliati MR, Maniatis T, Zinn K, Green MR. Efficient in vitro synthesis of biologically active RNA and RNA hybridization probes from plasmids containing a bacteriophage SP6 promoter. Nucl Acids Res 1984;12:7035–7056.
9. Leary JJ, Brigati DJ, Ward DC. Rapid and sensitive colorimetric method for visualizing biotin-labeled DNA probes hybridized to DNA or RNA immobilized on nitrocellulose: Bio-blots. Proc Natl Acad Sci USA 1983;80:4045–4049.
10. Schaap AP, Akhavan H, Romano LJ. Chemiluminescent substrates for alkaline phosphatase: application to ultrasensitive enzyme-linked immunoassays and DNA probes. Clin Chem 1989;35:1863–1864.

11. Chollet A, Kawashima EH. Biotin-labeled synthetic oligodeoxyribonucleotides: chemical synthesis and uses as hybridization probes. Nucl Acids Res 1985;13:1529–1541.
12. Forster AC, McInnes JL, Skingle DC, Symons RH. Nonradioactive hybridization probes prepared by the chemical labelling of DNA and RNA with a novel reagent, photobiotin. Nucl Acids Res 1985;13:745–761.
13. Hurskainen P, Dahlen P, Siitari H, Lovgren T. Time-resolved fluorometry: principles and application to clinical microbiology and DNA probe technology. Adv Exp Med Biol 1990;263:123–130.
14. Oser A, Roth WK, Valet G. Sensitive non-radioactive dot-blot hybridization using DNA probes labelled with chelate group substituted psoralen and quantitative detection by europium ion fluorescence. Nucl Acids Res 1988;16:1181–1196.
15. Saiki RK, Scharf S, Faloona F, et al. Enzymatic amplification of beta-globin genomic sequences and restriction site analysis for diagnosis of sickle cell anemia. Science 1985;230:1350–1354.
16. Erlich HA, Gelfand D, Sninsky JJ. Recent advances in the polymerase chain reaction. Science 1991;252:1643–1651.
17. Rose EA. Applications of the polymerase chain reaction to genome analysis. FASEB J 1991;5:46–54.
18. Goelz SE, Hamilton SR, Vogelstein B. Purification of DNA from formaldehyde fixed and paraffin embedded human tissue. Biochem Biophys Res Commun 1985;130:118–126.
19. Dubeau L, Chandler LA, Gralow JR, Nichols PW, Jones PA. Southern blot analysis of DNA extracted from formalin-fixed pathology specimens. Cancer Res 1986;46:2964–2969.
20. Ausubel FM, Brent R, Kingston RE, et al., eds. Current protocols in molecular biology. New York: John Wiley & Sons, 1987.
21. Drumm ML, Smith CL, Dean M, Cole JL, Iannuzzi MC, Collins FS. Physical mapping of the cystic fibrosis region by pulsed-field gel electrophoresis. Genomics 1988;2:346–354.
22. Schwartz DC, Cantor CR. Separation of yeast chromosome-sized DNAs by pulsed field gradient gel electrophoresis. Cell 1984;37:67–75.
23. Lai E, Birren BW, Clark SM, Simon MI, Hood L. Pulsed field electrophoresis. Biotechniques 1989;7:34–42.
24. Clark SM, Lai E, Birren BW, Hood L. A novel instrument for separating large DNA molecules with pulsed homogeneous electric fields. Science 1988;241:1203–1205.
25. Southern EM. Detection of specific sequences among DNA fragments separated by gel electrophoresis. J Mol Biol 1975;98: 503–517.
26. Messing J. Cloning in M13 phage or how to use biology at its best. Gene 1991;100:3–12.
27. Young RA, Davis RW. Gene isolation with lambda gt11 system. Methods Enzymol 1991;194:230–238.
28. Sternberg N, Coulby J. Cleavage of the bacteriophage P1 packaging site (pac) is regulated by adenine methylation. Proc Natl Acad Sci USA 1990;87:8070–8074.
29. Dower WJ, Miller JF, Ragsdale CW. High efficiency transformation of *E. coli* by high voltage electroporation. Nucl Acids Res 1988;16:6127–6145.
30. Hohn B, Koukolikova-Nicola Z, Lindenmaier W, Collins J. Cosmids. Biotechnology 1988;10:113–127.
31. McClary JA, Witney F, Geisselsoder J. Efficient site-directed in vitro mutagenesis using phagemid vectors. Biotechniques 1989;7:282–289.
32. Schuchman EH, Jackson CE, Desnick RJ. Human arylsulfatase B: MOPAC cloning, nucleotide sequence of a full-length cDNA, and regions of amino acid identity with arylsulfatases A and C. Genomics 1990;6:149–158.
33. Seed B, Aruffo A. Molecular cloning of the CD2 antigen, the T-cell erythrocyte receptor, by a rapid immunoselection procedure. Proc Natl Acad Sci USA 1987;84:3365–3369.
34. Rajan VP, Larsen RD, Ajmera S, Ernst LK, Lowe JB. A cloned human DNA restriction fragment determines expression of a GDP-L-fucose:β-D-galactoside 2-α-L-fucosyltransferase in transfected cells. Evidence for isolation and transfer of the human H blood group locus. J Biol Chem 1989;264:11158–11167.
35. Rommens JM, Iannuzzi MC, Kerem B, et al. Identification of the cystic fibrosis gene: chromosome walking and jumping. Science 1989;245:1059–1065.
36. Wallace MR, Marchuk DA, Andersen LB, et al. Type 1 neurofibromatosis gene: identification of a large transcript disrupted in three NF1 patients. Science 1990;249:181–186.
37. Schlesinger D. Yeast artificial chromosome: tools for mapping and analysis of complex genomes. Trends Genet 1990;6:248–258.
38. Green ED, Olson MV. Systematic screening of yeast artificial-chromosome libraries by use of the polymerase chain reaction. Proc Natl Acad Sci USA 1990;87:1213–1217.
39. Green ED, Olson MV. Chromosomal region of the cystic fibrosis gene in yeast artificial chromosomes: a model for human genome mapping. Science 1990;250:94–98.
40. Sanger F, Nicklen S, Coulson AR. DNA sequencing with chain-terminating inhibitors. Proc Natl Acad Sci USA 1977;74: 5463–5467.
41. Ruano G, Kidd KK. Coupled amplification and sequencing of genomic DNA. Proc Natl Acad Sci USA 1991;88:2815–2819.
42. Landegren U, Kaiser R, Caskey CT, Hood L. DNA diagnostics—molecular techniques and automation. Science 1988;242: 229–237.
43. Smith LM, Sanders JZ, Kaiser RJ, et al. Fluorescence detection in automated DNA sequence analysis. Nature 1986;321:674–679.
44. Chen C, Okayama H. High-efficiency transformation of mammalian cells by plasmid DNA. Mol Cell Biol 1987;7:2745–2752.
45. Southern PJ, Berg P. Transformation of mammalian cells to antibiotic resistance with a bacterial gene under control of the SV40 early region promoter. J Mol Appl Genet 1982;1:327–341.
46. Felgner Pl, Gaedek TR, Holmm M. Lipofection: a highly efficient, lipid-mediated DNA-transfection procedure. Proc Natl Acad Sci USA 1987;84:7413–7417.
47. Neumann E, Schaefer-Ridder M, Wang V, Hofchneider PH. Gene transfer into mouse lyoma cells by electroporation in high electrical fields. EMBO J 1982;1:841–845.
48. Varmus H. Retroviruses. Science 1988;240:1427–1435.
49. Danos O, Mulligan RC. Safe and efficient generation of retroviruses with amphotropic and ecotropic host ranges. Proc Natl Acad Sci USA 1988;85:6460–6464.
50. Wilson JM, Johnston DE, Jefferson DM, Mulligan RC. Correction of the genetic defect in hepatocytes from the Watanabe heritable hyperlipidemic rabbit. Proc Natl Acad Sci USA 1988;85:4421–4425.
51. Nabel EG, Plautz, G, Nabel GJ. Site-specific gene expression in vivo by direct gene transfer into the arterial wall. Science 1990;249:1285–1288.
52. Hanahan D. Transgenic mice as probes into complex systems. Science 1989;246:1265–1275.
53. Palmiter RD, Brinster RL. Germ-line transformation of mice. Ann Rev Genet 1986;20:465–499.
54. Capecchi MR. Altering the genome by homologous recombination. Science 1989;244:1288–1292.
55. Thomas KR, Capecchi MR. Targeted disruption of the murine int-1 proto-oncogene resulting in severe abnormalities in midbrain and cerebellar development. Nature 1990;346:847–850.
56. Schwartzberg PL, Stall AM, Hardin JD, et al. Mice homozygous for the ablm1 mutation show poor viability and depletion of selected B and T cell populations. Cell 1991;65:1165–1175.

6 Investigation of the Pathogenesis of Single-Gene Disorders by Molecular Methods

Jeffrey Bonadio

Spectacular progress has been made in human genetics and molecular medicine during the past decade. Inherited diseases—including the hemoglobinopathies, familial hypercholesterolemia, certain connective tissue diseases, certain forms of cancer, cystic fibrosis, muscular dystrophy, and neurofibromatosis—are now much better understood. This progress has resulted from advances in molecular cloning techniques and the ability to efficiently characterize cloned fragments of DNA at the sequence level. A second important development has been the ability to prepare specific fragments of DNA by the polymerase chain reaction method.

One goal of the chapter is to show that the progress of characterizing a human disease mutation typically has four steps. These steps are (*a*) identifying the genetic locus of disease, (*b*) mapping mutations within the locus, (*c*) preparing relatively large amounts of the fragment of DNA targeted by the map, and (*d*) determining the sequence of the DNA fragment (and thus the sequence of the mutation). Rather than describe a series of techniques, the chapter describes the process of mutation analysis in two heritable disorders of connective tissue: osteogenesis imperfecta and Marfan's syndrome. These diseases were chosen because they allow for a discussion of the two major approaches to the first step in mutation analysis (identifying the genetic locus of disease), namely, functional cloning and positional cloning.

OSTEOGENESIS IMPERFECTA

Bone and soft connective tissue fragility are the hallmarks of osteogenesis imperfecta (OI). The disease occurs with equal frequency in males and females, and the overall incidence is one in 5,000 to 14,000 live births. All known cases of OI have resulted from mutations in the extracellular matrix molecule type I collagen, which is a prominent constituent of bone, tendon, ligament, tooth, skin dermis, the wall of large blood vessels, and sclera.

Mapping the OI Genetic Locus

In 1975, McKusick, Martin, and coworkers mapped the disease locus responsible for OI. Their hypothesis—that type I collagen genes harbored the mutations that cause OI—was based partly on the previous demonstration of morphological abnormalities in the collagen of affected individuals. The hypothesis was also based in part on the knowledge that normal type I collagen was a major structural protein in bone tissue. To establish this hypothesis, the investigators chose to examine procollagen biosynthesis in vitro. The OI cell strains they chose to examine were segregated into three groups (1). The first group secreted an abnormal ratio of collagen types I and III because of a defect in type I collagen production. The second group consisted of cell strains that secreted structurally abnormal collagen molecules. The third group consisted of cell strains for which no detectable biosynthetic abnormality could be demonstrated.

Clinical Classification

Sillence established a clinical classification scheme that divided OI patients according to natural history and mode of inheritance (2). Sillence recognized four types of OI. OI type I is a mild disorder characterized by bone fracture without deformity, blue sclerae, normal or nearly normal stature, and autosomal dominant inheritance. The incidence of OI type I is one in 5,000 to 20,000 live births. Affected individuals often show an increased rate of long bone fracture after the first year of life (i.e., upon ambulation). For reasons only beginning to be understood, the fracture frequently decreases dramatically at puberty and during young adult life, only to increase once again in late middle age. Hearing loss, often beginning in the second or third decade, is a feature of this disease in about half the families. Conductive or mixed hearing loss is most commonly observed, and deafness can progress despite the general decline in fracture frequency. Given its mild manifestations, OI type I may go undetected in many families; in several cases, this had led to the unfortunate misdiagnosis of child abuse.

In contrast, OI types II through IV represent a spectrum of more severe disorders associated with a shortened life span. Individuals with OI type II (perinatal lethal OI) have short stature, a soft calvarium, blue sclerae, fragile skin, a small chest, floppy-appearing lower extremities (due to external rotation and abduction of the femurs), fragile tendons and ligaments, and bone fracture with severe deformity. These infants typically die in the first few weeks of life because of respiratory insufficiency (3). Radiographic signs of bone weakness include compression of the femurs, bowing of the tibiae, broad and beaded ribs, and calvarial thinning. Individuals with OI type III have short stature, a triangular facies, severe scoliosis, and bone fracture with moderate deformity. Scoliosis in particular can lead to emphysema and a shortened life span due to respiratory insufficiency. Individuals with OI type IV have normal sclerae, bone fracture with mild to moderate deformity, tooth defects, and a natural history essentially intermediate between OI types II and I.

Evidence of Genetic Heterogeneity

Byers and coworkers at the University of Washington established the genetic heterogeneity of OI by providing evidence of structural and null mutations in collagen genes. Barsh and Byers initially demonstrated an association between OI type II and structural mutations in type I procollagen (4). In one OI cell strain, they found a population of proα1(I) chains that migrated faster than normal on SDS-PAGE. As shown by cyanogen bromide (CNBr) peptide mapping, the abnormal proα1(I) chain had a relatively large amino acid deletion that accounted for its abnormal electrophoretic mobility. The mutation also delayed the intracellular transport of type I procollagen that, in turn, led to a delay in procollagen secretion and a reduction in procollagen production.

Barsh et al. then demonstrated an association between OI type I and null mutations in type I procollagen (5). They studied primary fibroblast cell lines from three unrelated individuals with OI type I. Total collagen production by all three cell lines was nearly 50% of normal. The investigators presented evidence that the decrease in type I collagen production resulted from a decrease in proα1(I) chain synthesis. In contrast to what was found for OI type II, Barsh et al. showed that the rate of type I procollagen secretion by OI type I cells and the structure of proα1(I) and proα2(I) chains were both normal.

Characterization of the First Mutation in a Collagen Gene

The OI type II structural mutation described by Barsh and Byers was the first to be characterized at the DNA sequence level. Ramirez, Prockop, and coworkers used Southern blot hybridization and an S1 nuclease protection assay to demonstrate that the proband carried a heterozygous deletion of ~500 bp from one proα1(I) collagen gene (6). Two groups then sequenced across the deletion breakpoints (7, 8). The deletion removed three exons encoding a total of 84 amino acids within the triple helical domain. Cultured cells were able to synthesize a mutant proα1(I) chain because the mutation did not shift the frame of the coding sequence.

Mapping Structural Mutations Associated with OI Types II-IV

Large deletions and insertions of amino acid sequence were soon recognized to be an uncommon cause of OI. Investigators therefore turned their attention to their classes of structural mutation that could have been associated with OI type II. Because a majority of collagen gene exons encode perfect Gly-X-Y amino acid repeats (e.g., consisting of either 18 or 36 amino acids), small deletions or insertions could have resulted from the loss or gain, respectively, of a few exons. Alternatively, single amino acid substitutions could have been the cause of most cases of OI type II.

To discriminate between these possibilities, mutations had to be characterized at the sequence level. An important first step, therefore, was the development of a system to map subtle structural alterations in the type I procollagen molecule. To understand the mapping system that was developed initially, one must understand certain basic aspects of normal procollagen biosynthesis.

Translated in a 2:1 ratio, the initial translation products (i.e., proα1 and proα2 chains) of type I collagen have amino-terminal signal sequences that allow for their transport into the lumen of the rough endoplasmic reticulum (9). In contrast to many globular proteins, nascent procollagen chains assemble and achieve a stable quaternary structure only after translation is completed. Proα1(I) and proα2(I) chains associate in a 2:1 ratio through amino acid sequences within the carboxy-terminal propeptides. Assembly of the triple-stranded helix takes place soon thereafter. Several important cotranslational

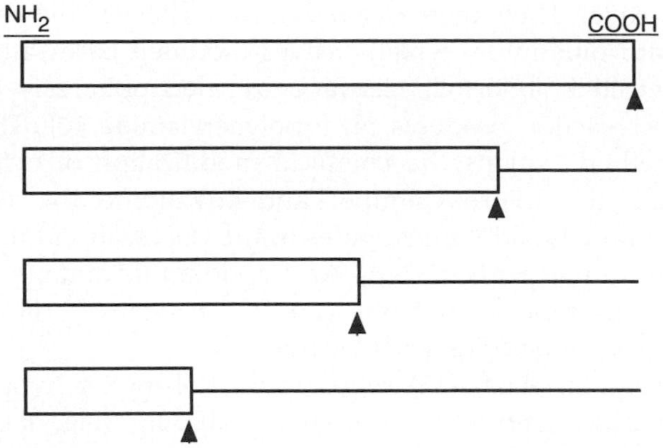

Figure 6.1. Schematic diagram depicting the pattern of excessive posttranslational modification of the collagen triple helix. Excessive posttranslational modification is shown as a box. Normally modified regions are shown as a single line. The arrowhead points to the predicted site of mutation.

and posttranslational modifications occur before the molecule achieves a stable triple helical conformation. These events occur in the rough endoplasmic reticulum of connective tissue cells, and they are regulated in part by the rate of stable triple helical formation.

An important initial observation was that mutant procollagen molecules were excessively modified (i.e., hydroxylated and glycosylated) in the rough endoplasmic reticulum. This result implied that structural mutations were able to delay the formation of the procollagen triple helix. CNBr peptide mapping was then used to ascertain the extent of overmodification in the abnormal procollagen produced by about 20 OI cell strains. Overmodification often occurred in an asymmetrical fashion, which suggested that the location of mutations could be correlated with the overmodified region of the molecule. Specifically, the prediction was that mutations could be localized to one end (the carboxy terminus) of the overmodified region (Fig. 6.1). This prediction was independently confirmed by many groups. To map OI mutations, therefore, investigators simply used peptide cleavage techniques to map the overmodified region of abnormal procollagen molecules.

With a mapping technique in hand, investigators next turned to the problem of cloning and sequencing structural mutations. Given the accumulated evidence regarding the abnormal structure of procollagen in vitro, it was assumed that a majority of structural collagen mutations would occur within exons. It was therefore desirable to sequence mutations at the level of mRNA. This strategy became possible with the availability of the polymerase chain reaction technique.

Polymerase Chain Reaction

Since its introduction, the polymerase chain reaction (PCR) has transformed the analysis of DNA (10). Developed by K. Mullis at the Cetus Corp., PCR involves the synthesis of several million copies of a specific DNA segment in 5 hours or less (Fig. 6.2). The reaction relies on the annealing and extension of two oligonucleotide primers that flank a target region in double-stranded DNA. After denaturation, each primer hybridizes to one of the separated strands and extends from one 3′ hydroxyl end. Extension of the annealed primers occurs on the template strand by the action of a DNA polymerase. These three steps (denaturation, primer binding, and DNA synthesis) represent a single PCR cycle. Repeated cycles of denaturation, primer annealing, and primer extension result in the exponential accumulation of a discrete fragment of DNA, i.e., the 5′ ends of the primers define the termini of the amplified fragment. Exponential amplification results because, under the appropriate conditions, the primer extension products synthesized in cycle n function as templates in cycle $n+1$. The length of the products generated during the PCR is equal to the sum of the lengths of the two primers plus the distance in the target DNA between the primers.

Patterson et al. (11) applied the polymerase chain reaction to the problem of analyzing a single amino

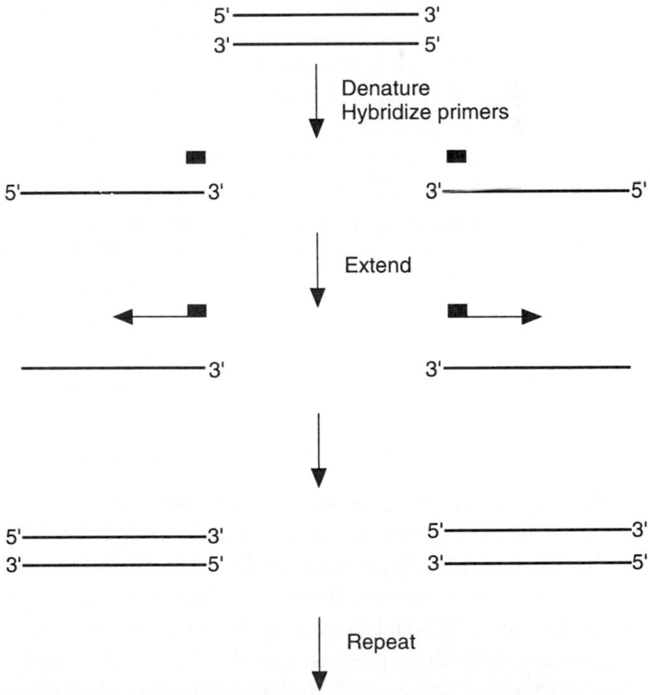

Figure 6.2. Schematic diagram depicting one PCR cycle. The steps include denaturation of double-stranded DNA, oligonucleotide primer annealing, and primer extension.

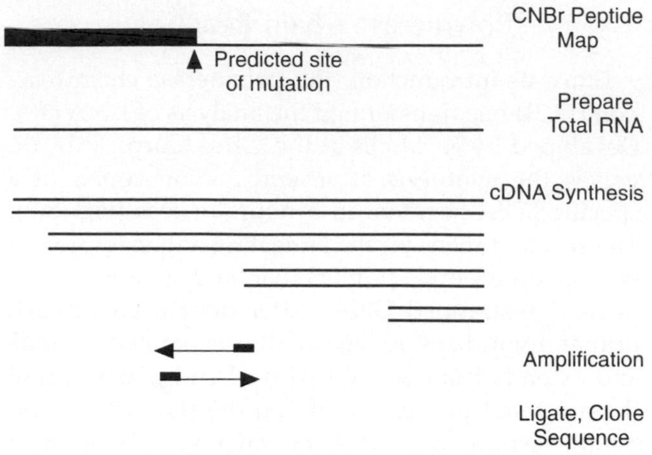

Figure 6.3. Schematic diagram depicting the strategy developed by Patterson et al. (11) to characterize OI mutations. The steps include mutation mapping in procollagen molecules, RNA preparation, cDNA synthesis, PCR, and sequence analysis of the PCR product.

acid substitution in the triple helical domain of a procollagen α chain (Fig. 6.3). These investigators isolated total RNA from a small number of OI cells in culture, synthesized cDNA from mRNA, and amplified and sequenced short cDNA fragments that were predicted to contain the OI mutation. Sequence analysis of the amplified cDNA revealed a heterozygous Gly→Val substitution at residue 256 in a population of proα1(I) collagen chains. The investigators confirmed the heterozygous nature of the Gly→Val substitution by allele-specific oligonucleotide hybridization, in which oligonucleotide probes consisting of the normal or the mutant sequence were used to probe an amplified fragment of genomic DNA. The normal probe hybridized with the normal DNA fragment and a fragment prepared from the proband, while the mutant probe hybridized only with the proband's DNA fragment. The general approach taken by Patterson et al. was used by other laboratories to analyze a relatively large number of OI mutations. This work has shown that the great majority of OI structural mutations result in single amino acid substitutions in the collagen triple helix rather than deletions or insertions of amino acid sequence.

Newer Mutation Mapping Techniques

New and more accessible techniques next allowed investigators to map collagen mutations at the level of mRNA and DNA. Lamande et al. (12) used a chemical cleavage method to detect single base changes in mRNA:cDNA hybrids in vitro (Fig. 6.4). These investigators prepared mRNA from the cells of an individual suspected to have OI type II, hybridized the mRNA with a complementary strand of normal cDNA, and incubated separate portions of the hybrid sample with hydroxylamine and osmium tetroxide. They then cleaved mismatches in hybrids with piperidine, which cleaves modified bases, and detected abnormal cleavage by electrophoresis of the reaction products on a polyacrylamide gel. The method exploits the chemical modification of cytosine (by hydroxylamine) and thymidine (by osmium tetroxide) nucleotides in the cDNA strand that fail to pair with mRNA. An important advantage of this method is that one can screen relatively large mRNA molecules with facility.

Marini et al. (13) reported an RNA:RNA hybrid analysis method of mutation mapping (Fig. 6.5). Here, total RNA was prepared from an individual suspected of having OI, and the sample was mixed with fragments of normal collagen RNA to form RNA:RNA hybrids. (More precisely, the latter consisted of complementary DNA synthesized and radiolabeled in vitro.) They digested the reaction mixture with RNase, which digested the hybrids at points of base pair mismatch. They then denatured and size fractionated the samples on a polyacrylamide gel. In this assay, heterozygous mutations give rise to one full-length radiolabeled digestion product and two short digestion products. The relative size of the

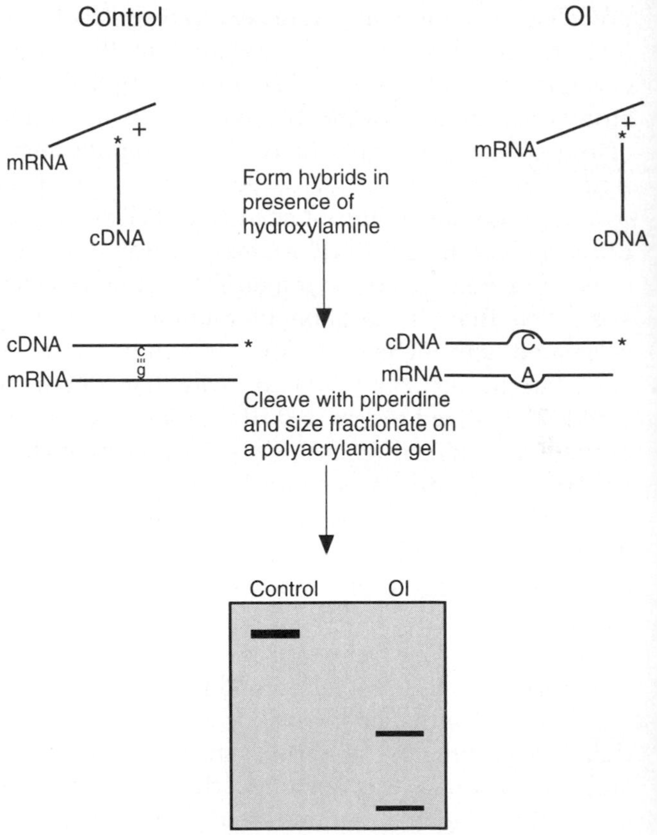

Figure 6.4. Schematic diagram depicting the chemical cleavage method of detecting mismatched bases in mRNA:cDNA hybrids. The radiolabeled cDNA probe is indicated by an asterisk. The behavior of the mutant allele (only) is shown.

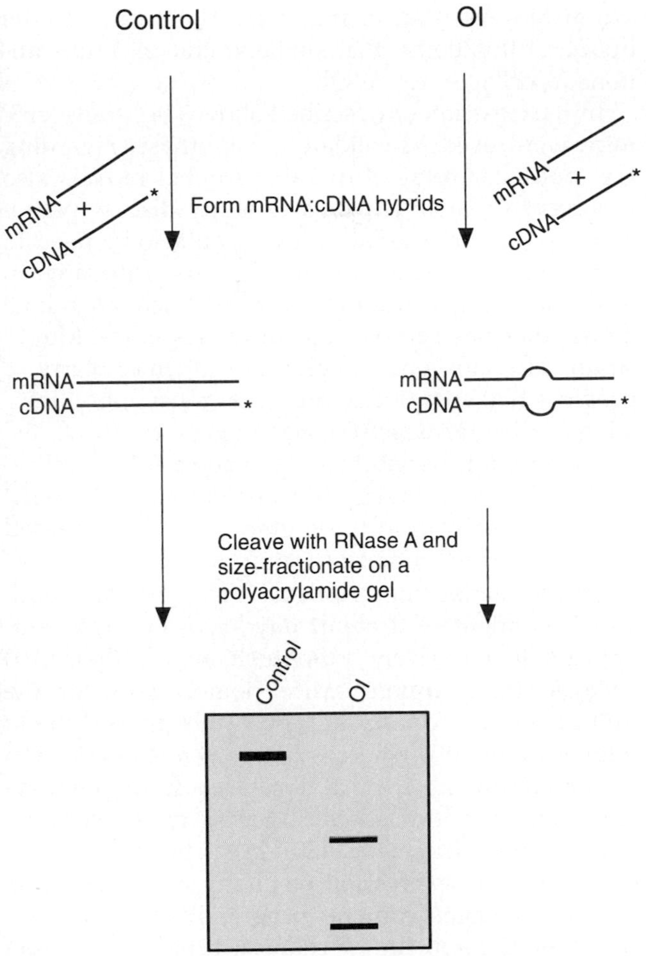

Figure 6.5. Schematic diagram depicting the RNA:RNA hybrid analysis of base pair mismatches. The radiolabeled cDNA probe is indicated by an asterisk. The behavior of the mutant allele (only) is shown.

short fragments is used to localize mismatches within a defined segment of the mRNA strand.

A final method of detection (used to identify OI mutations) is PCR single-strand conformation polymorphism (SSCP) analysis (Fig. 6.6). A target sequence—either genomic DNA or cDNA—is synthesized by PCR using labeled substrates. The PCR product is denatured and resolved by polyacrylamide gel electrophoresis. The electrophoretic mobility of a DNA single strand is determined by both size and shape. Under non-denaturing electrophoresis conditions, single-stranded DNA assumes a folded structure that depends in part on the DNA sequence. In SSCP analysis, a heterozygous mutation appears as two distinct bands, both of which migrate with altered mobility. The altered mobility indicates an alteration in folding and thus an alteration in sequence.

Although each of these methods localizes the mutation, none actually defines its sequence. Typically, this has been accomplished by PCR amplification of a targeted region of a gene followed by DNA sequence analysis. Automated sequencing technologies have facilitated this process. The convergence of powerful methods to map mutations, the polymerase chain reaction, and the automated sequencing technology has in many instances shortened the process of mutation analysis from several months to a few weeks. The latter has resulted in an explosive growth in our understanding of the structural mutations that cause OI.

Summary of the Molecular Basis of OI

More than 100 OI mutations have been characterized since 1989. The vast majority are heterozygous, single–amino acid substitutions for conserved glycine residues in the type I collagen triple helical domain. OI types II to IV result from structural mutations within the proα1(I) and proα2(I) collagen chains. A small number of deletions and insertions

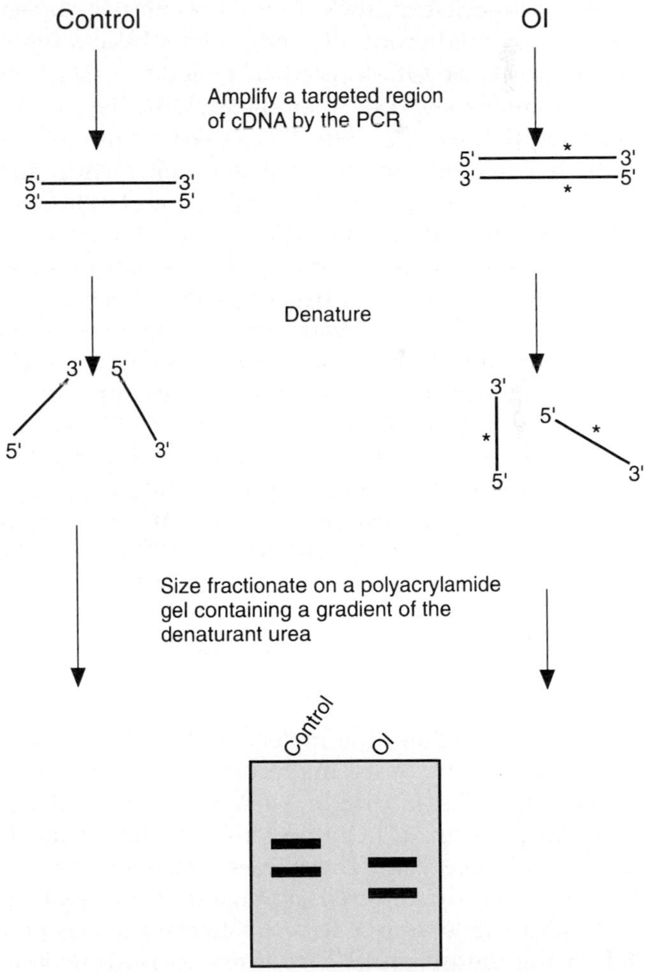

Figure 6.6. Schematic diagram depicting the PCR-single stranded polymorphism conformation (SSCP) analysis. The asterisks indicate the position of the mutation in one population of PCR products. The behavior of the mutant allele (only) is shown.

(recombinatorial errors or mRNA processing defects) have also produced the phenotype. About half of the latter leave the frame of the coding sequence intact, while the other half result in a frameshift. On the other hand, most cases of OI type I appear to result from heterozygous mutations that decrease collagen production but do not alter primary structure.

The sequence analysis has provided new insight into the inheritance of collagen mutations. The majority of OI mutations behave as heterozygous alleles that act in a dominant fashion. Four modes of inheritance are now recognized. First, inheritance of a dominant collagen mutation can be a consequence of germ cell mosaicism in one parent. Germ cell mosaicism implies that one parent has two populations of germ cells, i.e., normal and mutant. Since the somatic tissues of this parent do not contain cells harboring the mutant gene, he or she has a normal phenotype. Second, the dominant collagen mutation can be "handed down" from one generation to the next in a predictable (Mendelian) manner. For the third mode of inheritance, the OI mutation fails to "breed true," i.e., children of affected parents have a more severe form of OI. Molecular genetic analysis of these families suggests that the somatic as well as germinal tissues of the affected parent are mosaic for cells that harbor a mutant collagen gene. Thus, the phenotype of the parent carrying the mutation may vary from normal to moderate form of OI depending on the extent of mosaicism in the somatic tissues. However, all cells in all tissues of the affected children of this parent will carry the mutant allele, thus accounting for the more severe phenotypic manifestations. Fourth, there is one bona fide example of recessive inheritance producing a case of OI type III. Thus, the phenotypic expression of OI depends on the nature of the collagen mutation, the relative number of cells expressing the mutant procollagen molecule, and the tissue distribution of the mutant cells.

Animal Models—Pathogenesis and Development of Rational Therapies

While compelling, the molecular genetic evidence does not formally prove that mutations in type I collagen cause OI. Jaenisch, Bateman, Cole, and coworkers performed an important experiment using transgenic mice (14). These investigators used the technique of site-directed mutagenesis to create a Gly→Cys single amino acid substitution at position 988 of the mouse proα1(I) collagen chain. (Previous studies demonstrated that $Gly{\rightarrow}Cys_{988}$ caused OI type II.) Mice expressing the collagen transgene had a lethal phenotype, showed a reduced amount of type I collagen in tissues, and suffered from an astonishing number of fractures. There can be little doubt, at this point, that single amino acid substitutions in collagen cause OI.

In the experiment described above (14), transgenic mice were used to validate a hypothesis regarding the molecular basis of disease. Animal models also represent valuable reagents to study disease pathogenesis at the tissue level. They can also be used to develop and implement rational forms of therapy. In terms of osteogenesis imperfecta research, an animal model that has served both purposes is the Mov13 strain of transgenic mice. Mov13 mice carry a provirus that completely prevents transcription initiation of the murine α1(I) collagen gene in all cells except embryonic odontoblasts and about 5% of embryonic osteoblasts (15–18). (Regarding the latter, α1(I) collagen mRNA from the mutant allele is expressed only for a short period of time prior to the onset of retroviral gene transcription. Virus transcription, which is initiated at about day 16 of development, appears to effectively extinguish any further α1(I) collagen transcription.) Mice homozygous for the null mutation produce no type I collagen and die in midgestation (19), whereas heterozygotes survive to young adulthood. Dermal fibroblasts from heterozygous mice produce about 50% less type I collagen than normal littermates (20, 21). The partial deficiency in gene expression results in a 50% decrease in tissue collagen content, progressive hearing loss, and alterations in the mechanical properties of long bone (21). The heterozygous Mov13 mouse therefore serves as a model of OI type I.

It was recently hypothesized that the addition of a single functioning α1(I) collagen gene to the Mov13 genetic background would rescue the demonstrated defect in the mechanical properties of Mov13 long bone specimens A rescue experiment was feasible because of the availability of the HucII transgenic strain of mice, in which microinjection techniques were used to add a single α1(I) collagen gene to the X chromosome. A cohort of Mov13 mice with the desired change in genetic background (i.e., Mov13,HucII mice) were generated and the predicted result—the restoration of mechanical properties to wild type levels—was achieved (22). This experiment represents the first successful attempt to genetically rescue a heritable skeletal defect.

More recently, a natural adaptive response was identified in Mov13 mice that significantly improves the mechanical function of mutant bone (23). The adaptive response occurred over a 2-month period, during which time a small number of newly proliferated osteogenic cells produced a significant amount of matrix components and thus generated new bone along periosteal surfaces. New bone deposition resulted in a measurable increase in cross-sectional ge-

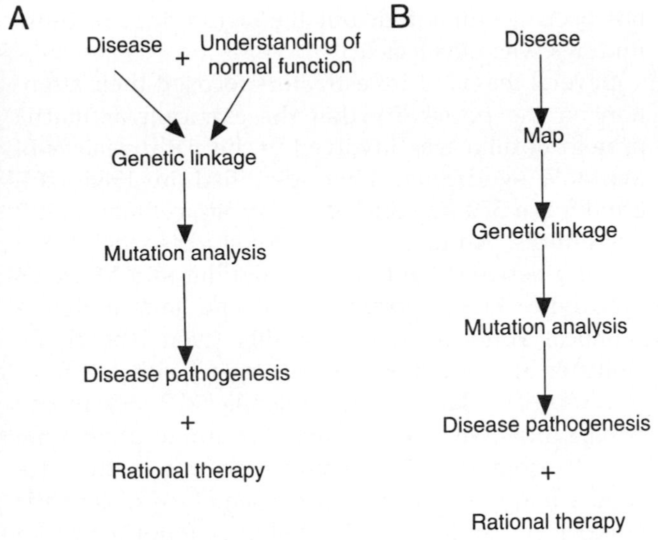

Figure 6.7. Schematic diagram depicting the steps associated with functional (**A**) and positional (**B**) cloning.

ometry, which in turn led to a dramatic increase in long bone bending strength.

The Mov13 adaptation suggests a general strategy to make weak bone stronger. The cellular target of this strategy is the osteoblast on the periosteal surface of bone. The goal is to induce these cells to synthesize, deposit, and mineralize new bone matrix, thereby increasing the cross-sectional radius. This strategy could be implemented by (*a*) increasing bone cell number but keeping the metabolic activity per cell constant, (*b*) keeping bone cell number constant but increasing the metabolic activity of each cell, or (*c*) both. The prediction is that small increases in cross-section will significantly increase the mechanical properties of bone. A principal goal of future studies will be to identify anabolic agents that stimulate periosteal new bone formation. An alternative would be to identify a gene or group of genes that, when overexpressed, achieve the same effect. The goal of these efforts is to decrease the fracture rate of individuals with heritable forms of skeletal fragility.

FUNCTIONAL VERSUS POSITIONAL CLONING

Functional and positional cloning are relatively new terms (24). Functional cloning refers to the identification of a disease gene based on pre-existing knowledge about the biochemical basis of the disease phenotype (Fig. 6.7). Prior knowledge could mean an understanding of a protein's primary sequence or anatomical location or physiological role. Positional cloning, on the other hand, refers to the identification of a disease gene in the absence of direct information about the biochemical defect. This process is initiated by mapping the disease gene to a chromosome (usually by a process known as linkage analysis). Linkage analysis depends on the collection of pedigrees in which the responsible gene segregates, and polymorphic DNA markers are often used in an effort to link a fragment of a chromosome with the disease phenotype. Additional fine mapping can then be used to further narrow down the region of interest. When no more information is available, the responsible region of DNA is cloned, and transcripts issued from the region are identified. Finally, alterations in the structure or expression of one of the transcripts are sought. The process can be arduous and long, but the tools for positional cloning have continued to be refined over the last few years, especially as a consequence of the Human Genome Project. The availability of probands that have cytogenetic rearrangements in genomic DNA can greatly speed up the process of disease gene identification.

Clearly, then, a functional cloning approach was taken to determine the molecular basis of OI, i.e., the disease gene was mapped on the basis of prior information about the pathological appearance of collagen in tissues of individuals with the disorder and on the basis of an understanding of the normal function of collagen in bone tissue (1). As discussed below, in the case of Marfan's syndrome, positional and functional cloning approaches were used to identify the disease gene.

MARFAN'S SYNDROME

Marfan's syndrome is a pleiotropic disorder of connective tissue with cardinal manifestations in the ocular, skeletal, and cardiovascular systems (25). The syndrome was first described nearly a century ago. Males and females are affected equally, and the incidence in the United States is reported to be around 1.5 per 100,000 of the general population.

Phenotypic Manifestations

In the absence of a specific laboratory test, the diagnosis of Marfan's syndrome has been based on family history, physical examination, and results of ophthalmologic and echocardiographic tests. For the individual with a classic case, the musculoskeletal findings characteristically include tall stature, long thin extremities (dolichostenomelia), long thin fingers (arachnodactyly), joint laxity, chest deformity (pectus excavatum and/or carinatum), spine deformity (scoliosis, lordosis, or kyphosis), and congenital contractures. The ocular manifestations include subluxation of the lens (ectopia lentis), retinal detachment, and myopia. The cardiovascular manifestations include mitral valve prolapse leading to aortic regurgitation, mitral regurgitation due to a floppy mitral valve, progressive dilatation of the aortic root and ascending aorta, and aneurysms. A large number of other phenotypic manifestations have been noted by various investigators.

Marfan's syndrome is one of the leading causes of dissecting aneurysm of the aorta in the younger decades. The life expectancy of Marfan's syndrome patients is reduced by one-third, and about 85% of these individuals die from cardiovascular manifestations of disease, typically heart failure or aortic dissection. Aortic dilatation may occur as early as the first year of life or as late as the sixth decade; it is usually confined to the ascending aorta proximal to the innominate artery. The aortic ring or the intrapericardial portion of the ascending aorta usually dilate first, stretching the aortic cusps and causing aortic regurgitation. A separate mechanism by which aortic regurgitation may occur is myxomatous degeneration of the aortic valve leaflets. Aortic dilatation by either mechanism is said to be progressive, and the clinical course generally follows a rapid downhill pattern once significant sequelae such as angina pectoris or left ventricular failure occur. The aortic wall ultimately degenerates as a consequence of progressive dilatation, with cystic medial necrosis, aneurysm, and mural dissection as the end result. Calcification of the aortic wall is not commonly associated with these pathological changes. Dissection has occurred as early as the first decade of life and as late as the seventh decade and may involve both the abdominal and thoracic aorta. Finally, involvement of the mitral and possibly the tricuspid valve with regurgitation may be the predominant cardiovascular manifestation of Marfan's syndrome, and may lead to death. Mitral regurgitation has especially been observed in infants with severe manifestations of Marfan's syndrome.

Mapping the Genetic Locus of Marfan's Syndrome

Although identification of the disease locus of Marfan's syndrome remained elusive until recently, most investigators remained convinced that a dominant mutation that disrupted connective tissue metabolism would be linked to the disorder. Elastin fiber abnormalities were associated with the disorder, but it could not be determined if these changes were primary or secondary. Early attempts to link the disease to a genetic marker by analysis of restriction fragment length polymorphisms were uninformative. An intense search for the disease locus based on genetic linkage studies effectively excluded several candidate extracellular matrix genes, including elastin and collagen types I, II, III, V, and VI. Reproducibly elevated glycosaminoglycan biosynthesis in vitro has been documented, but the significance of these findings was never clear.

Several teams of investigators focused their attention on the possibility that the extracellular matrix protein fibrillin was involved in the pathogenesis of Marfan's syndrome. First identified in 1986 (26), fibrillin is a 350-kd component of extracellular matrix microfibrils. An elegant series of studies established the link between mutations in fibrillin and Marfan's syndrome. First, morphological and immunohistochemical abnormalities in fibrillin were shown by Hollister and coworkers to segregate with Marfan's syndrome in a large series of families (27, 28). In one remarkable case, the Marfan's syndrome phenotype was distributed exclusively on one side of the proband's body, perhaps as a consequence of somatic mosaicism, and the morphologic abnormality in fibrillin segregated only to the phenotypically affected side (29). Second, Byers and coworkers reported abnormalities in fibrillin biosynthesis by cultured fibroblasts derived from Marfan's syndrome patients (30). Third, the fibrillin gene (designated FBN1) was localized to the same region on chromosome 15 that had been linked to the Marfan's syndrome phenotype, genetic linkage between Marfan's syndrome and FBN1 was established, and the first mutations were characterized using a combination of methods described earlier in the chapter (31–36). Cloning experiments further revealed the existence of a second fibrillin-like gene, designated FBN2, on chromosome 5 (31), and genetic linkage was established between FBN2 and congenital contractual arachnodactyly, a rare disorder that shares some of the skeletal manifestations of Marfan's syndrome (31, 37).

Elastic Fibers, 10- to 12-nm Microfibrils, and Fibrillin

Elastic fibers consist of two different morphologic components: elastin (the dominant protein of each fiber) and 10- to 12-nm microfibrils (38). Elastin is an unusual protein in that it contains few polar amino acids but is rich in hydrophobic amino acids such as valine. Molecular cloning studies have shown that tropoelastin, which is the secreted form of the elastin, consists of alternating hydrophobic domains and lysine-rich domains. Biochemical studies have shown that the latter are able to form pyridinium crosslinks. Elastic fibers are amorphous when viewed in the electron microscope. Although still controversial, elastic fibers derive their name from their resilient behavior when stretched—it appears that elastin molecules can change from a "randomly aggregated to aligned to randomly aggregated" configuration as they are stretched and then relaxed.

Elastic fibers are common constituents of tendon, elastic ligaments, certain cartilages, and many types of blood vessel. Arterial smooth muscle cells, tendon and ligament fibroblasts, and cartilage chondroblasts are thought to be responsible for the biosynthesis of elastic fibers in these tissues, and the fibers show tissue-specific patterns of organization. For example, the fibers are small, rope-like, and variable in length in tissues such as the lung, skin, and elastic ligaments. In major arteries such as the aorta, elastic fibers form concentric sheets or lamellae. In elastic cartilage, a three-dimensional honeycomb arrangement of relatively large anastomosing fibers has been identified. These differences in organization may result from differences in the usual mechanical forces experienced by the cells of these normal tissues.

Unlike elastin, 10- to 12-nm microfibrils are high in polar amino acids and have been known for some time to have a high cysteine content (39). Early attempts to purify the molecular constituents of microfibrils relied on extraction in strong denaturants followed by extraction in denaturant solutions containing strong reducing agents. Cleary and coworkers subsequently showed that many components can be extracted in NaCl, urea, or guanidine hydrochloride solutions as long as a strong reducing agent was present (40). These efforts led to the identification of protein bands of 340, 78, 70, 31, and 25 kd plus the cross-linking enzyme lysyl oxidase. Cleary and coworkers concluded from this work that disulfide bonding is important for the molecular integrity of microfibrils, a conclusion that is consistent with the high cysteine content of microfibrils.

Native microfibrils appear in the electron microscope as unbranched tubular filaments. Under denaturing conditions, however, regular variations in diameter have suggested a "beads on a string" appearance. Immunoelectron microscopy studies indicate that microfibrils consist of multiple thread-like filaments of the FBN1 gene product (41). Moreover, recent studies have shown that epitopes of the FBN1 and FBN2 gene products co-localize to the same microfibril (42). The discovery of two fibrillins and their association with the same structure and overlapping human phenotypes has led to the hypothesis that the fibrillins may have related extracellular matrix functions (43).

The Fibrillin Gene

The primary structure of the FBN1 gene product (referred to as Fib15), the organization of the FBN1 gene, and a physical map of the genetic locus were recently reported (43). The Fib15 transcript encodes a molecule consisting of 2871 amino acids that are arranged into five structurally distinct regions plus a signal peptide. The largest region (region D) comprises about 75% of the molecule and consists of 42 cysteine-rich repeats homologous to the epidermal growth factor (EGF) or to a cysteine-rich motif initially identified in the transforming growth factor-β1-binding protein (TGF-bp). Overall, 43 of the 46 EGF-like repeats encoded by the full-length Fib15 transcript contain the calcium binding consensus sequence:

$$\mathbf{D}X(\mathbf{N/D})ECX_{(6)}CX_{(4)}CX\mathbf{N}X_{(2)}GX(\mathbf{Y/F})XCXCX_{(2)}GX_{(9)}CX$$

As described by Pereira et al. (43), numbers in parentheses indicate an average number of residues and the amino acids of the calcium binding consensus sequence are shown in bold. EGF-like repeats that bind calcium (EGF-CB repeats) may mediate protein-protein interactions relevant to microfibril assembly and, in some instances, to organogenesis. Fibrillin also exhibits a few unique cysteine-rich repeats that may represent evolutionary variants of the EGF-CB and TGF-bp repeats. Almost all of the Fib15 cysteine-rich repeats are encoded by single exons; consequently, the FBN1 locus is relatively large (110 kb) and highly interrupted (65 exons). This effort to characterize the structure of FBN1 is expected to greatly facilitate the analysis of Marfan's syndrome mutations.

SUMMARY

The goal of this chapter has been to describe the process of determining the molecular basis of osteogenesis imperfecta and Marfan's syndrome, two of the inherited disorders of connective tissue. The process typically has four steps, which are (*a*) identifying the genetic locus of disease, (*b*) mapping mutations within the locus, (*c*) preparing relatively large amounts of the fragment of DNA targeted by the map, and (*d*) determining the sequence of the DNA fragment (and thus the sequence of the mutation). The chapter specifically has illustrated several molecular genetic methods of mutation analysis, including the use of animal models such as transgenic mice. It has also discussed the two major approaches to the first step in mutation analysis (identifying the genetic locus of disease), namely, functional cloning and positional cloning.

Acknowledgment

This work was supported in part by grants from the National Institutes of Health.

References

1. Penttinen RP, Lichtenstein JR, Martin GR, McKusick VA. Abnormal collagen metabolism in cultured cells in osteogenesis imperfecta. Proc Natl Acad Sci USA 1975;72:586–589.

2. Sillence DO, Senn A, Danks DM. Genetic heterogeneity in osteogenesis imperfecta. J Med Genet 1979;16:101–106.
3. Sillence DO, Barlow KK, Garber AP, Hall JG, Rimoin DL. Osteogenesis imperfecta type II: delineation of the phenotype with reference to genetic heterogeneity. Am J Med Genet 1984;17:407–423.
4. Barsh GS, Byers PH. Reduced secretion of structurally abnormal type I procollagen in a form of osteogenesis imperfecta. Proc Natl Acad Sci USA 1981;78:5142–5146.
5. Barsh GS, David KE, Byers PH. Type I osteogenesis imperfecta: a nonfunctional allele for proα1(I) chains of type I collagen. Proc Natl Acad Sci USA 1982;79:3838–3842.
6. Chu M-L, Williams CJ, Pepe G, Hirsch JL, Prockop DJ, Ramirez F. Internal deletion in a collagen gene in a perinatal lethal form of osteogenesis imperfecta. Nature 1983;304:78–80.
7. Chu M-L, Gargiulo V, Williams CJ, Ramirez F. Multiexon deletion in an osteogenesis imperfecta variant with increased type III collagen mRNA. J Biol Chem 1985;260:691–694.
8. Barsh GS, Roush CL, Bonadio J, Byers PH, Gelinas RE. Proc Natl Acad Sci USA 1985;82:2870–2874.
9. Kuhn K. The classical collagens: types I, II, and III. In: Mayne R, Burgeson RE, eds. Structure and function of collagen types. Orlando, FL: Academic Press, 1987:1–42.
10. Saiki RK, Scharf S, Faloona F, Mullis KB, Horn GT, Erlich HA, Arnheim N. Enzymatic amplification of β-globin genomic sequences and restriction site analysis for diagnosis of sickle cell anemia. Science 1985;230:1350–1354.
11. Patterson E, Smiley E, Bonadio J. RNA sequence analysis of a perinatal lethal osteogenesis imperfecta mutation. J Biol Chem 1989;264:10083–10087.
12. Lamande SR, Dahl HH, Cole WG, Bateman JF. Characterization of point mutations in the collagen COL1A1 and COL1A2 genes causing lethal perinatal osteogenesis imperfecta. J Biol Chem 1989;264:15809–15812.
13. Marini JC, Grange DK, Gottesman GS, Lewis MB, Koeplin DA. Osteogenesis imperfecta type IV. Detection of a point mutation in one α1(I) collagen allele (COL1A1) by RNA/RNA hybrid analysis. J Biol Chem 1989;264:11893–11900.
14. Stacey A, Bateman J, Choi T, Mascara T, Cole W, Jaenisch R. Perinatal lethal osteogenesis imperfecta in transgenic mice bearing an engineered mutant proα1(I) collagen gene. Nature 1988;332:131–136.
15. Schnieke A, Harbers K, Jaenisch R. Embryonic lethal mutation in mice induced by retrovirus insertion into the α1(I) collagen gene. Nature 1983;304:315–320.
16. Harbers K, Kuehn M, Delius H, Jaenisch R. Insertion of retrovirus into first intron of α1(I) collagen gene leads to embryonic lethal mutation in mice. Proc Natl Acad Sci USA 1984;81:1504–1508.
17. Kratochwil K, von der Mark K, Kollar EJ, Jaenisch R, Mooslehner K, Schwarz M, Haase K, Gmachl I, Harbers K. Retrovirus-induced insertional mutation in Mov13 mice affects collagen I expression in a tissue-specific manner. Cell 1989;57:807.
18. Schwarz M, Harbers K, Kratochwil K. Development 1990;108: 717–726.
19. Lohler J, Timpl R, Jaenisch R. Embryonic lethal mutation in mouse collagen I gene causes rupture of blood vessels and is associated with erythropoietic and mesenchymal cell death. Cell 1984;38:597–607.
20. Dziadek M, Timpl R, Jaenisch R. Collagen synthesis by cell lines derived from Mov13 mouse embryos which have a lethal mutation in the collagen α1(I) gene. Biochem J 1987;244:375–379.
21. Bonadio J, Saunders TL, Tsai E, Goldstein SA, Morris-Wiman J, Brinkley L, Dolan DF, Altschuler RA, Hawkins JE, Bateman JF, Mascara T, Jaenisch R. A transgenic mouse model of osteogenesis imperfecta type I. Proc Natl Acad Sci USA 1990;87: 7145–7149.
22. Jepsen K, Mansoura M, Kuhn JL, Jaenisch R, Bonadio J, Goldstein SA. An in vivo assessment of the contribution of type I collagen to the mechanical properties of cortical bone. Ortho Trans 1992;17(1):93.
23. Bonadio J, Jepsen K, Mansoura MK, Kuhn JL, Goldstein SA, Jaenisch R. An adaptive response by murine skeletal tissues that significantly increases the mechanical properties of cortical bone: implications for the treatment of skeletal fragility. J Clin Invest, in press.
24. Collins F. Positional cloning: let's not call it reverse anymore. Nature Genetics 1992;1:3–6.
25. Pyeritz RE, McKusick VA. The Marfan syndrome: diagnosis and management. N Engl J Med 1979;300:772–777.
26. Sakai LY, Keene DR, Engvall E. Fibrillin, a new 350-kd glycoprotein is a component of extracellular matrix microfibrils. J Cell Biol 1986;103:2499–2509.
27. Godfrey M, Menashe V, Weleber RG, Koler RD, Bigley RH, Lovrien E, Zonana J, Hollister DW. Cosegregation of elastin-associated microfibrillar abnormalities with the Marfan phenotype in families Am J Hum Genet 1990;46:652–660.
28. Hollister DW, Godfrey M, Sakai LY, Pyeritz RE. Immunohistological abnormalities of the microfibrillar-fiber system in the Marfan syndrome. N Engl J Med 1990;323:152–159.
29. Godfrey M, Olson S, Burgio RG, Martini A, Valli M, Cetta G, Hori H, Hollister DW. Unilateral microfibrillar abnormalities in a case of asymmetric Marfan syndrome. Am J Hum Genet 1990;46:661–671.
30. Milewicz DM, Pyeritz RE, Crawford ES, Byers PH. Marfan syndrome: defective synthesis, secretion and extracellular matrix formation of fibrillin by cultured dermal fibroblasts. J Clin Invest 1992;89:79–86.
31. Lee B, Godfrey M, Vitale E, Hori H, Mattei M-G, Sarfarazi M, Tsipoursas P, Ramirez F, Hollister DW. Linkage of Marfan syndrome and a phenotypically related disorder to two different fibrillin genes. Nature 1991;353:330–333.
32. Dietz HC, Cutting GR, Pyeritz RE, Maslen CL, Sakai LY, Corson GM, Puffenberger EG, Hamosh A, Nanthakumar EJ, Curristin SM, Stetten G, Meyers DA, Francomanno CA. Marfan syndrome caused by a recurrent de novo missense mutation in the fibrillin gene. Nature 1991;353:337–339.
33. Maslen C, Corson GM, Maddox BK, Glanville RW, Sakai LY. Partial sequence of a candidate gene for the Marfan syndrome. Nature 1991;353:334–337.
34. Kainulainen K, Sakai LY, Child A, Pope FM, Puhakka L, Ryhanen L, Palotie A, Kaitila I, Peltonen L. Two unique mutations in Marfan syndrome resulting in truncated polypeptide chains of fibrillin. Proc Natl Acad Sci USA 1992;88:5917–5921.
35. Dietz HC, Pyeritz RE, Puffenberger EG, Kendzior RJ, Corson GM, Maslen CL, Sakai LY, Francomano CA, Cutting GR. Marfan phenotype variability in a family segregating a missense mutation in the EGF-like motif of the fibrillin gene. J Clin Invest 1992;89:1647–1680.
36. Dietz HC, Valle D, Francomano CA, Kendzior RJ, Pyeritz RE, Cutting GR. The skipping of constitutive exons in vivo induced by nonsense mutations. Science 1993;259:680–683.
37. Tsipouras P, Del Mastro R, Sarfarazi M, Lee B, Vitale E, Child A, Godfrey M, Devereux RB, Hewett D, Steinmann B, Viljoen D, Sykes BC, Kilpatrick M, Ramirez F and the International Marfan syndrome Collaborative Study. Linkage of Marfan syndrome, dominant ectopia lentis, and congenital contractural arachnodactyly to the fibrillin genes on chromosomes 15 and 5. N Engl J Med 1992;326:905–909.
38. Low FN. Microfibrils: fine filamentous components of the tissue space. Anat Rec 1962;142:131–137.

39. Cleary EG, Gibson MA. Elastin-associated microfibrils and microfibrillar proteins. Int Rev Connect Tissue Res 1983;10:97–209.
40. Gibson MA, Kumaratilake JS, Cleary EG. The protein components of the 12-nanometer microfibrils of elastic and nonelastic tissues. J Biol Chem 1989;264:4590–4598.
41. Keene DR, Maddox K, Kuo H, Sakai LY, Glanville RW. Extraction of extendible beaded structures and their identification as fibrillin-containing matrix microfibrils. J Histochem Cytochem 1991;39:441–449.
42. Zhang H, Apfelroth SD, Davis EC, Sanguineti C, Bonadio J, Mecham RP, Ramirez F. Characterization of Fib5, the product of the fibrillin-like gene on human chromosome 5, reveals that this 350-kd protein is a component of extracellular microfibrils. Submitted for publication.
43. Pereira L, D'Alessio M, Ramirez F, Lynch JR, Sykes B, Pangilinan T, Bonadio J. Genomic organization of the sequences coding for fibrillin, the defective gene product in Marfan syndrome. Human Mol Genet 1993;2:961–968.

7 Clinical Applications of Molecular Biology

Daniel G. Remick

The powerful techniques of molecular biology are gaining rapid acceptance within the clinical laboratories. The transition of this sophisticated technology from the basic science laboratory into applied pathology has been rapid, and most pathology training programs provide experience for their residents in this methodology. The reasons for these rapid developments are several, but primarily it is due to the ability of molecular pathology to provide information where classical techniques are insufficient.

Understanding and applying the tools of molecular biology are not difficult, and the basic principles of protein and nucleic acid chemistry have already been described. There are stringent requirements with regard to sample processing and controls, and careful attention is critical to obtain accurate results.

Multiple molecular biology techniques may be used in the clinical laboratory. This chapter focuses only on two that have been most widely applied: in situ hybridization and the polymerase chain reaction (PCR). In situ hybridization is being applied in surgical pathology as both a research and a diagnostic tool, while PCR has had wide applications in several diagnostic areas, including hematology, forensic pathology, microbiology, and genetics, to name a few.

IN SITU HYBRIDIZATION

In situ hybridization applies the basic techniques of nucleic acid hybridization to tissue or cytologic specimens mounted on glass slides. It therefore couples the power of probing for specific sequences of nucleic acid with the exquisite specificity of microscopic localization. This allows the pathologist to evaluate the staining pattern with his or her assessment of the cells and provides a measure of "quality control." As an example, if the tissue is being probed for expression of a particular oncogene, yet all the normal tissue is as positive as the neoplastic tissue, then that particular probe is not a useful marker for malignant transformation of the cells. This cellular localization allows in situ hybridization to offer greater specificity compared to solution hybridization reactions, in which the nucleic acid from all cells in the tissue are combined and subjected to either Northern or Southern blot analysis. The basic protocol is shown in Figure 7.1, and essentially consists of labeling the nucleic acid probe, preparing the tissue, performing the hybridization, and finally detecting the bound, labeled probe. However, there are several technical pitfalls at each step that may jeopardize the quality of the preparation and make interpretation of the slides difficult, if not impossible.

Basic Concepts

In situ hybridization requires that tissue sections or cytologic preparations are placed on glass slides, deparaffinized if required, and the presence of a specific nucleic acid determined, using either radioactive or nonradioactive probes (1). An investigator may search for either specific DNA sequences or mRNA. It is also possible to combine in situ hybridization with immunohistochemistry for even more specific analysis (2). This combination permits searching for both the nucleic acid and the protein on the same slide.

In situ hybridization has been used extensively by researchers in the neurological sciences, and much of our present understanding of the basic concepts and practical approaches is based on their pioneering work (3). These early investigators used this methodology to explore the precise anatomic location of specific mRNAs within portions of the nervous system, and then used this information as a guide to cell function. It is logical to assume that if a normal cell has transcribed its DNA into an mRNA coding for a specific protein, then it probably intended to continue the process to its usual conclusion and translate the mRNA into protein. More recently, endocrine pathologists have followed a similar line of reasoning to search for both the mRNA coding for a hormone by in situ hybridization (4, 5), as well as the protein itself by conventional immunohistochemical methods. In situ hybridization has found particularly useful applications in the diagnosis of infectious diseases, especially in biopsy material (5–7).

The discovery that nucleic acids are preserved by routine formalin fixation and paraffin embedding

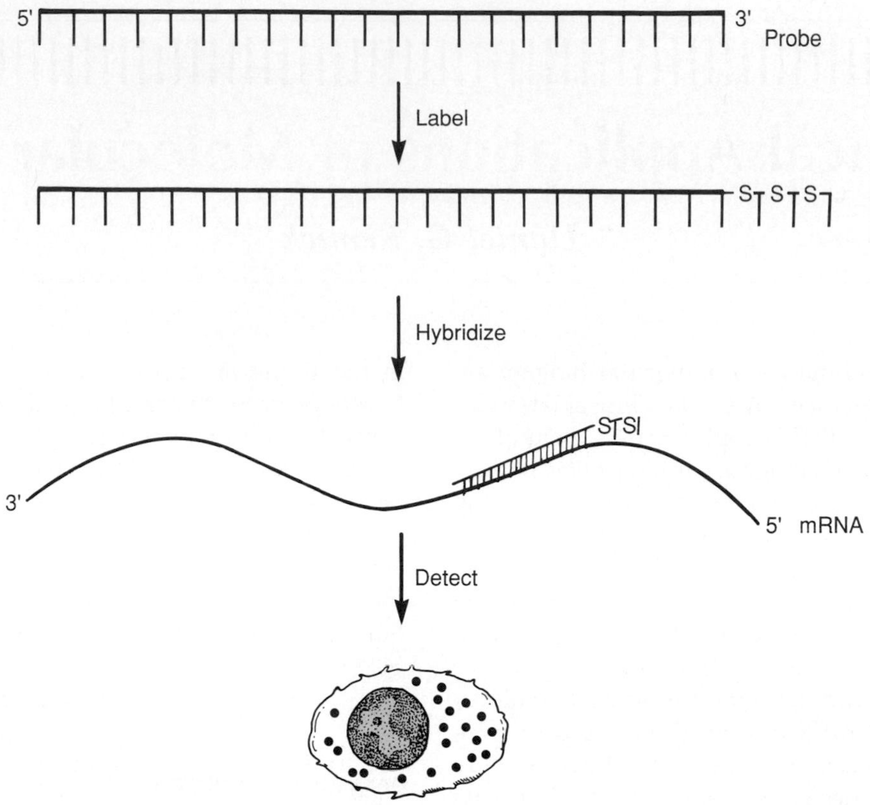

Figure 7.1. Schematic of a radioactive in situ hybridization. In the first step the oligonucleotide probe is labeled by adding ^{35}S-dATP sequentially to the 3′ end. This probe is then hybridized to the specific mRNA of interest. To detect the presence of hybridized probe, the cells are overlaid with a photographic emulsion. As the radioactivity decays it reduces the silver, which is then seen as black grains overlying the cells.

provided a boon for the field of in situ hybridization, since archival material is now available for study. Use of paraffin-embedded material, rather than frozen sections, offers the additional advantage of the superb cellular detail most pathologists require of diagnostic material (8). The same block may be used to cut slides for both in situ hybridization and routine slides, and the in situ slides may be evaluated for both the presence of the disease and the nucleic acid. In situ hybridization has an advantage over immunohistochemistry since one is probing for nucleic acid, while immunohistochemistry assesses the presence of antigenic material. The fixation of the tissues may render the antigen in such a form that it is no longer recognized by the antibody. Alternatively, the antigen may be rapidly exported, and thus no longer present within either the cytoplasm or the membrane for detection. Both of these conditions could result in false-negative reactions using immunohistochemistry but not with in situ hybridization. A false-positive reaction could occur with immunohistochemistry if a protein were made by one cell and then phagocytized by a neighboring cell. But again, in situ hybridization would provide the correct result. In situ hybridization, by probing for nucleic acids, has the potential to detect positive cells in situations where the antigen has been exported or is no longer transcribed. However, many mRNAs are extremely short-lived, especially in inflammatory conditions. Thus, it is quite possible that the protein may be present and not the nucleic acid, or that the nucleic acid is present but not the protein. In situ hybridization and immunohistochemistry may often be complementary.

Methods

One of the first considerations for performing an optimal in situ hybridization is the proper selection of probes (1, 3). There are three basic types of probes: cDNA, RNA (riboprobes), and oligonucleotide probes. Each probe has its advantages and disadvantages, which are summarized in Table 7.1. With the increasing use of molecular techniques, commercial vendors have entered the marketplace with reagents. Thus, it is now possible to purchase cDNA probes without first developing the expertise necessary to grow the bacteria and isolate plasmids. Some vendors offer probes prelabeled for use in nonradioactive detection systems. The American Type Culture Collection (Rockville, MD) also represents a source of DNA probes, and serves as a National Institutes of

Table 7.1. Types of Probes for In Situ Hybridization

Probe	Advantages	Disadvantages
cDNA	Several commercially available	May need to isolate plasmids
	Networking	Nonspecific interaction of vector sequences
	High specific activity	
RNA (Riboprobe)	Single-stranded probe	Increased nonspecific binding
	Increased stability of hybrids	Requires knowledge of molecular biology
	High specific activity	
Oligonucleotides	May be custom made	Requires prior knowledge of published sequences
	Good tissue penetration	Decreased stability of hybrids

Health repository for both human and mouse DNA probes. This is a nonprofit organization that can provide both probes and technical advice. Commercial vendors will also synthesize custom-designed oligonucleotide probes, so laboratories do not need to purchase the expensive nucleotide synthesizers (9).

Several factors need to be considered in the selection of probes; one of the most important of these is availability. As noted in the preceding paragraph, the availability of probes is becoming less of a problem, especially if viral DNAs are being sought. Historically, most in situ hybridization work has been performed with cDNAs since these were the most readily available probes. The cDNA probes may serve to amplify the signal if the coding insert is not cut from the plasmid. This increased sensitivity is apparently due to "networking," whereby fragments of the unannealed plasmid bind to other fragments of unannealed plasmids to form a network and result in a stronger signal. RNA:RNA and RNA:DNA interactions are stronger than DNA:DNA interactions. Thus, RNA probes will bind to the nucleic acid more strongly than DNA probes, and have the potential for additional sensitivity. However, RNA probes are not as widely available as the cDNA probes, and in most instances synthesizing an RNA probe would require growing the bacteria containing the plasmids, and then isolating and purifying the riboprobe. Oligonucleotide probes may be custom designed based on the known structure of the nucleic acid (9). Therefore, any published nucleic acid sequence may be used to construct an appropriate probe. Most oligonucleotide probes are 20 to 30 bases long and may be generated against any portion of the nucleic acid. Since only a portion of the nucleic acid is recognized by the short oligonucleotide, the entire nucleic acid sequence does not need to be known. Their smaller size also allows better tissue penetration. To increase the sensitivity, it is possible to generate more than one probe directed against different portions of the nucleic acid to be probed, and potentially enhance the signal.

Prior to hybridizing, it is necessary to label the probe so that it may be subsequently detected. The particular method of labeling depends on the type of probe that is used. Many of the methods use either radioisotopes (^{3}H, ^{32}P, ^{35}S), or nonradioactive means. cDNAs are usually labeled either by nick-translation or by random-prime labeling (10, 11). Both of these are enzymatic reactions in which the radioisotope is part of a nucleotide that is incorporated into a newly synthesized strand of DNA. Kits for these labeling procedures are commercially available, and may be followed in a straightforward manner. RNA probes may be labeled by enzymatically incorporating labeled bases into the RNA probe as it is transcribed, which results in a high specific activity. Oligonucleotides may be labeled at either the 5′ end or at the 3′ end. Labeling at the 3′ end is usually more advantageous, since multiple bases may be sequentially added, resulting in a higher specific activity and increasing the sensitivity (9).

A general protocol for performing in situ hybridization is given in Table 7.2. This protocol has worked very well in our laboratory for detecting mRNAs for inflammatory proteins, and results in a very low background (12). While this methodology may work well for this application, each laboratory needs to establish the optimal conditions for detecting the nucleic acids of their choice in their tissue. Brief mention should be made of the reagents, and the rationale for their use. Standard saline-citrate (SSC) is the usual salt/buffer system used (3, 10, 11). Formamide decreases the temperature to the optimal level for annealing. By using a lower temperature, typically 37° to 42°C, there is less disruption of the tissue architecture, and the sections are more likely to remain adherent to the slides. Dextran sulfate increases the speed of annealing and allows for optimal hybridization to occur in a shorter time. Many of the other reagents, including Denhardt's, tRNA, and DNA, are included to block nonspecific binding of the labeled probe (3).

In situ hybridization is a time-consuming procedure, but each of the steps is critical to ensure superior results. Fixation of the tissue must be optimal, to ensure both preservation of the nucleic acid and a good histologic appearance (13). If the fixation is too harsh there is the potential that precipitated proteins

Table 7.2. Basic Protocol for In Situ Hybridization

General Precautions

It is critical to prevent degradation of the nucleic acids, particularly if one is probing for mRNA. The following precautions should be used:

1. Wear gloves at all times.
2. Use molecular biology grade reagents.
3. Autoclave all glassware, or use tissue culture plasticware.

Recipes for most of the solutions may be found in standard molecular biology texts (10, 11).

Tissue Preparation

1. Promptly fix tissue, or prepare cell preparations and fix. The choice of fixative may need to be determined empirically.
2. Embed tissue in paraffin, and place cut sections on slides coated with poly-L-lysine or gelatin.
3. Dewax and rehydrate tissue sections.

When using cytospin preparations or cultured cells, begin the protocol here.

4. Wash in 0.5 × SSC for 10 minutes.
5. Treat cells with 5 μg/ml of protease K in 2 × SSC for 10 minutes.
6. Post fix cells in 4% paraformaldehyde, then wash in 0.5 × SSC.
7. Treat cells with 0.25% (v/v) acetic anhydride in 0.1 M triethanolamine, prepared fresh, for 5 minutes.
8. Wash in 0.5 × SSC for 10 minutes.

Hybridization

The prehybridization solutions and hybridization solutions are as follows:

Formamide	20%
SSC	5 ×
Dextran sulfate	10% (v/v)
DNA	100 μg/ml
tRNA	100 μg/ml
Denhardt's	1 ×
Dithiothrietol	10 mM

1. Apply 100 μl of prehybridization solution and incubate at 42°C for 1–2 hours. Place the slides in a sealed container on top of racks overlying paper towels soaked in 4 × SSC, 50% formamide.
2. Add the hybridization solution, which contains the labeled probe. Place a small amount (~15–100 μl) on the slide and place a coverslip so that the solution uniformly covers the tissue section.
3. If probing for DNA, seal the coverslip to the slide and denature the DNA by heating to 90°C for 15 minutes.
4. Hybridize at 42°C overnight.
5. Perform stringency washes by removing the coverslips and washing the slides 2 times in 2 × SSC at room temperature, and once at 1 × SSC at 42°C.

Detection

The detection system used depends on how the probe has been labeled. If a nonradioactive label has been used, then the detection system is usually a standard avidin-biotin complex procedure. The protocol below is for detecting radioactive probes.

1. Dehydrate the slides through graded alcohols.
2. Prepare a photographic emulsion by melting the emulsion to 42°–45°C. The choice of emulsion depends on the type of radioactivity used.
3. Carefully dip the slides in the emulsion, and allow the slides to dry vertically.
4. Place the slides in a lightproof container with desiccant and store at 4°C for 1 to 30 days, depending on the radioactive probe.
5. Develop the slides in D-19 developer (Eastman Kodak, Rochester NY) for 3 minutes, stop the reaction in water and then fix for 3 minutes in Kodak Rapid Fix.
6. Counterstain with hematoxylin and eosin, and coverslip.

will block the nucleic acid, such that the probe no longer binds. Routine formalin fixed tissue is usually adequate, if prior to hybridization a mild protease digestion is performed. Alcohol and paraformaldehyde fixation are also acceptable. Following paraffin embedding, sections are placed on slides coated to optimize tissue adherence without increasing the background binding of the probe (13). Poly-L-lysine solutions used routinely in immunohistochemistry have been found to work well. The sections are then dewaxed, rehydrated, and treated with a protease. After the protease treatment, the slides are refixed, usually in 4% paraformaldehyde in phosphate buffered saline. This both stops the protease activity and decreases the background. To further decrease the background by neutralizing electrostatic charge, the slides may be acetylated by treatment with acetic anhydride. The slides are prehybridized for 1 to 2 hours, then covered with the hybridization solution containing the labeled probe, and usually allowed to incubate overnight. The following day the slides are subjected to stringency washes to remove unbound probe, and the labeled probe is detected.

The method for detecting the probe obviously depends on the method used to initially label the probe, and may be generally placed into two categories: radioactive and nonradioactive. Radioactive probes are almost invariably detected by their ability to reduce silver in a photographic emulsion. The slides are coated with an emulsion of silver, and as the radioactive probe decays, the energy from the radioactivity will reduce the silver. The slides are then developed, and the presence of the probe is determined by microscopic examination for the presence of silver grains. This method may also be used for quantitation, by counting the number of silver grains overlying the individual cells. Figure 7.2 shows cells that are negative (panel *A*) and cells that are positive (panel *B*) for the presence of mRNA coding for the inflammatory mediator tumor necrosis factor. Nonradioactive detection systems are generally variations of immunoperoxidase techniques (6–8, 13). In many systems, the probe is labeled with UTP that has previously been coupled to biotin. The biotin is usually linked via a spacer so that it is further removed from the nucleic acid and less subject to steric hindrance. The biotinylated probe is then detected with an avidin-peroxidase technique.

No discussion of in situ hybridization would be complete without mentioning the need for controls. There are several different controls that are possible, and each tests a specific step. One of the first controls for in situ hybridization is determining which cells are positive. Usually, based on knowledge of the system being tested, the pathologist knows which types of cells should be positive, and if other

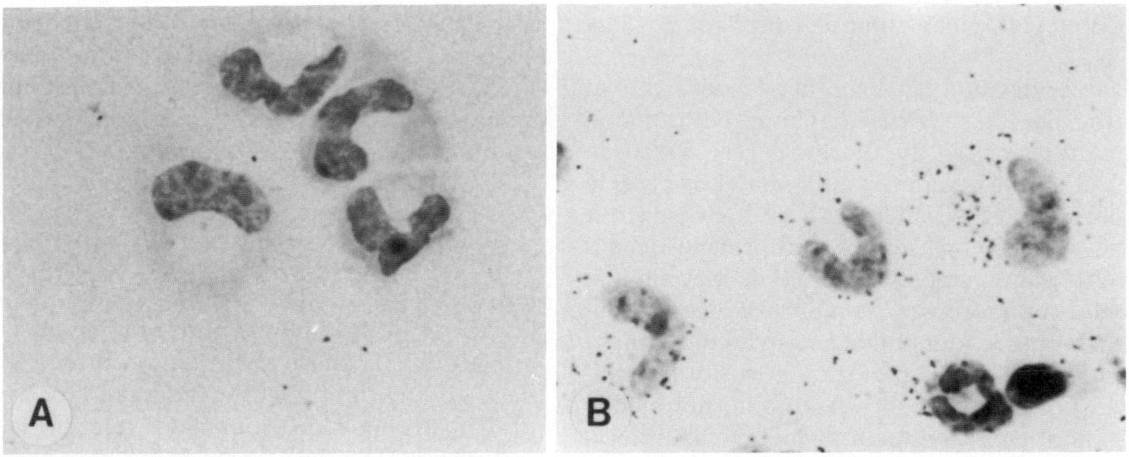

Figure 7.2. Photomicrographs of actual in situ hybridization. A macrophage population was stimulated to induce expression of mRNA coding for tumor necrosis factor. **A** is from unstimulated cells, and has essentially no grains overlying the cells. In contrast, **B**, from stimulated cells, has several grains, indicating the presence of mRNA. (Both pictures are the same magnification.)

cells are also positive then the reaction needs to be more carefully evaluated. As an example, if a thyroid lesion is being probed for calcitonin (8), and the follicular lining cells, endothelial cells, lymphocytes, and fibroblasts are all positive, then the results must be questioned.

As stated previously, in situ hybridization may be combined with immunohistochemistry, and this can serve as another control. While the nucleic acid and protein will not always be present together in the same cell, in many situations the protein and nucleic acid are expressed together.

Other controls are similar to those employed in standard immunohistochemistry. These controls do not include the probe, yet continue with the rest of the reaction. A very useful control is to compare "sense" to "antisense" binding. For this control, a sense probe is prepared that is not complementary to the nucleic acid in question but is, in fact, complementary to the antisense probe that represents the positive control. The sense probe has the same G-C content as the antisense probe and may be used to decipher nonspecific binding of the probe. Another control consists of treating the slide with excess unlabeled probe to compete with the labeled probe. Usually, nonspecific interactions cannot be competed away with excess unlabeled probe. Hybridization with irrelevant labeled probes also provide information concerning the level of background, and nonspecific binding. The tissue may also be predigested with ribonuclease (if looking for mRNA) or DNase (if looking for DNA) prior to performing the in situ hybridization. All of these controls do not need to be done for every study, and probably the best overall control is to compare "sense" to "antisense" probes on serial sections.

Uses in Diagnostic Pathology

In situ hybridization has widespread applications in the research laboratory, but its present clinical application is primarily restricted to endocrine (4, 5) and infectious diseases (6, 7). For endocrine disorders, the tissue is usually examined for the presence of mRNA encoding for a specific hormone. This information could be used to determine the status of a thyroid neoplasm that has produced a negative immunoperoxidase staining reaction but is suspected to be a medullary carcinoma. In situ hybridization for calcitonin mRNA may be positive, indicating the underlying nature of the neoplasm. It may also provide further insight into pituitary lesions to better define so-called "null cell adenomas."

Most of the recent literature on the application of in situ hybridization has focused on its utility for the diagnosis of infectious diseases, particularly viral infections. Compared to bacterial cultures, viral cultures are generally more difficult to perform and require longer incubation times. In situ hybridization offers an attractive alternative that is generally less expensive to perform and provides faster answers (14). This technique also provides information that is not always available using routine immunoperoxidase. As an example, in a latent viral infection, fragments of the viral DNA may be incorporated into the host genomic DNA such that there are no viral proteins present. Immunohistochemical analysis would be negative, but in situ hybridization would reveal the presence of the virus. The sensitivity of in situ hybridization compared to immunohistochemistry remains to be fully determined, since some reports indicate it is more sensitive for detecting cytomegalovirus infection (14), while other reports claim it is less effective (15).

In situ hybridization has been used extensively to subtype the papilloma virus that may be found in premalignant lesions in the uterine cervix. Based on a number of studies, human papilloma virus type 16 (16) appears to be associated with an increased risk of progression to neoplasm. This information could be of clinical utility, since such patients may require more careful monitoring. Commercial kits are available from several vendors that contain all the components necessary to begin performing in situ hybridization. Most of the materials not supplied are readily available in a well-equipped histology laboratory. These kits almost always use nonradioactively labeled probes and a variation of the avidin-biotin peroxidase technique. As mentioned previously, a number of vendors also supply specific probes. Presently, the greatest variety of probes are aimed at detecting viruses.

POLYMERASE CHAIN REACTION

The polymerase chain reaction (PCR) was first unveiled in 1985, and the uses for this powerful technology have rapidly grown (17). The PCR provides a rapid, yet specific, method of tremendous amplification of nucleic acid sequences. This amplification allows the direct detection of fragments of nucleic acid, and thus the identification of infectious agents, mRNAs for specific proteins, or DNA to identify individuals. The phenomenal sensitivity of PCR is illustrated by the fact that it allows detection of a specific DNA from a single cell. The development of automated instrumentation coupled with the discovery of heat-stable DNA polymerases has resulted in several applications for PCR in both research and clinical laboratories.

Basic Concepts

The basic principle of the polymerase chain reaction, and the power behind the technique, is the enzymatic amplification of a specific fragment of DNA. The specificity is provided by oligonucleotide primers that bind only to the DNA in question, and the amplification is performed by a heat-stable DNA polymerase. To perform PCR it is necessary to have a source of crudely purified nucleic acid, the heat-stable DNA polymerase (the enzyme), the necessary buffers and reagents, and specific oligonucleotide primers. The reaction is virtually always performed in an automated instrument, and while this is not an absolute requirement, the instruments are not very expensive and they are much more efficient than manual methods. After amplification of the DNA it must be detected in an appropriate detection system, usually an agarose gel followed by staining or a variation of Southern blotting. A technical restriction of the PCR is the length of the nucleic acid that may be amplified. The efficiency of PCR is reduced if amplification is attempted over more than 2000 base pairs.

Methods

The polymerase chain reaction is based on repeating cycles of amplification (18). Each cycle is composed of three sequential, independent steps (shown in Figure 7.3). These steps are performed in a cyclic manner, one right after the other, and for this reason PCR instruments are sometimes referred to as thermal cyclers. The three steps of the cycle are (*a*) denaturation of the double-stranded nucleic acid, (*b*) annealing of the primers, and (*c*) subsequent primer extension using a heat-stable DNA polymerase. In the first step, the isolated DNA is denatured by raising the temperature above 90°C. The separated strands of DNA stay free in solution until the temperature is lowered. During the second step, the temperature is lowered, and the oligonucleotide primers anneal to the DNA. These oligonucleotide primers are present in vast excess compared to the original, native DNA, and thus the formation of DNA:primer hybrids is stoichiometrically favored over reannealing and formation of DNA:DNA hybrids. The oligonucleotide primers are synthetic fragments of DNA, usually 15 to 25 nucleotides long. These will bind to DNA sequences that flank the portion of DNA that is being amplified. The specificity of the reaction is determined by the selection of primers, because only the DNA between the primers will be amplified. The choice of primers is critical, since inappropriate primers may not yield amplification of the desired end product. In other words, if primers are designed that bind to other portions of nucleic acid, then the portion of DNA spanned by both the nonspecific as well as the specific primers will be amplified. The detection of the amplified material may be important to differentiate between the desired product and the nonspecific DNA.

Primer extension is the final step in a PCR, and during this step a complementary DNA strand is synthesized. This synthesis is performed by a heat-stable DNA polymerase, the *Thermus aquaticus* (Taq) DNA polymerase (19). This DNA polymerase will only bind to stretches of double-stranded DNA, i.e. the DNA:primer hybrids, and proceed to extend the DNA in the 5′ to 3′ direction. This enzyme has the distinct advantage of being heat stable up to 98°C, and therefore will not degrade when the temperature is raised for the denaturation step. Use of the Taq polymerase has eliminated the need to add new enzyme for each round of amplification, and has

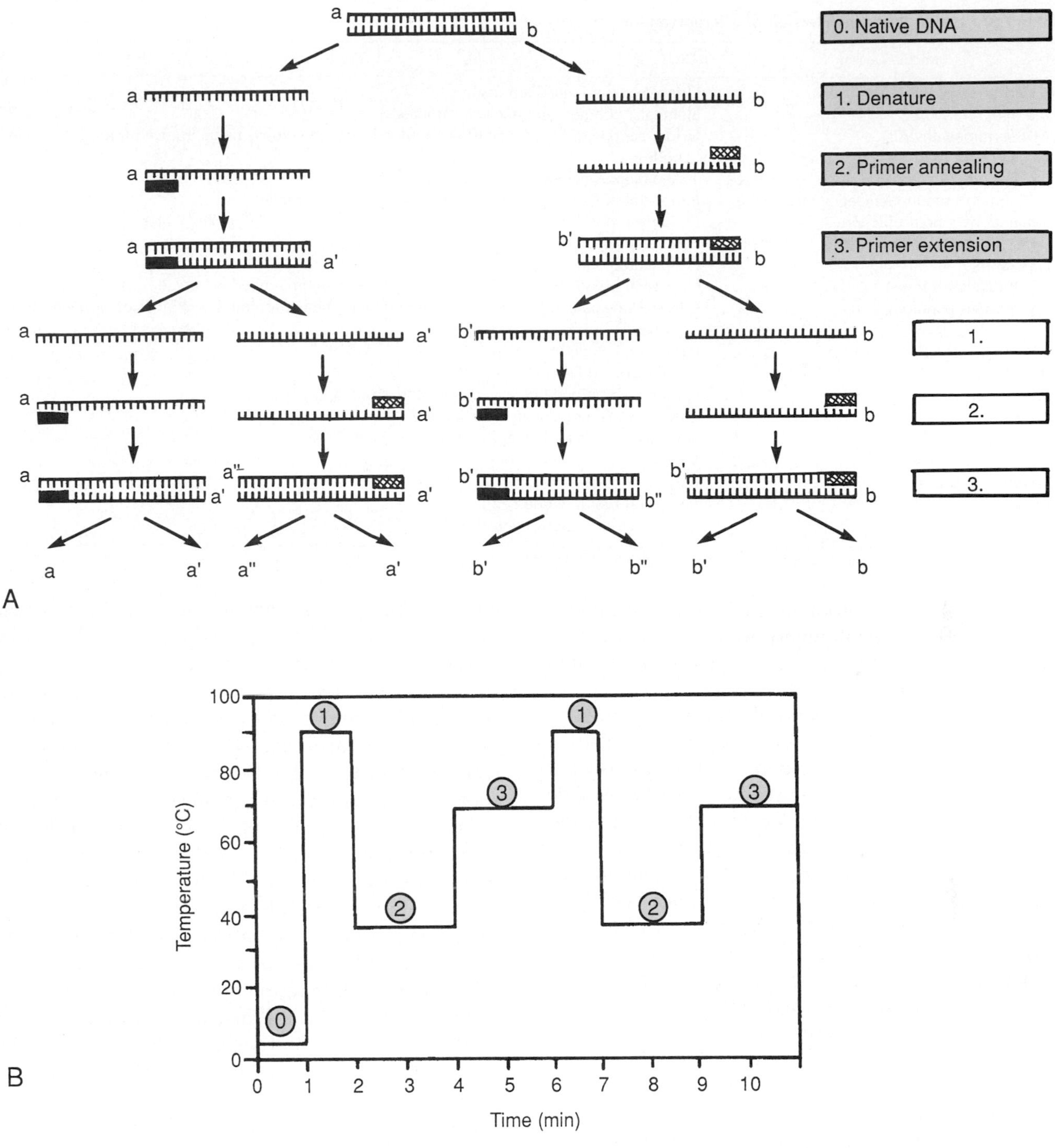

Figure 7.3. The theory of polymerase chain reaction. **A**, The sequence of enzymatic steps. In the first step both strands of the native DNA are annealed to each other in the usual double-stranded state. During step 1 the DNA denatures into independent a and b strands. The temperature is lowered and the primers anneal in step 2. The *black box* indicates the specific primer for strand a and the *shaded box* the primer for strand b. Primer extension occurs in step 3, in the 5′ to 3′ direction along both strands. The newly synthesized strands, labeled a′ and b′, represent the "long product." These steps are repeated in each cycle, that is, 1, denaturation; 2, primer annealing; and 3, primer extension. However, during the second and subsequent rounds, primer extension of the newly synthesized strands terminates at the site of the original primer. To illustrate, strand a′ is the same as the original strand b, except that the 5′ end terminates at the site of the black box primer. During annealing (step 2 of round 2), the shaded box primer will anneal as indicated, but as the primer extends in step 3 the reaction will terminate where the strand of DNA terminates. Therefore, at each enzymatic step this "short product" (a″ and b″) doubles and increases exponentially. In contrast, only the two original strands of DNA are capable of generating "long products" and only one copy of long product is generated with each cycle. **B**, This is a thermal histogram showing the temperature and length of time at each step. The numbers correspond to the enzymatic steps in **A**. This is only one example of a temperature profile; many different profiles may be used with varying times and temperatures for the different steps, depending on the system being studied. (From Remick DG, Kunkel SL, Holbook EA, Hanson CA. Theory and application of the polymerase chain reaction. Am J Clin Pathol 1990;93:S49–S54.)

Table 7.3. Use of PCR for Detection of Microorganisms[a]

Microorganism	Tissues
BK and JC virus	Urine, paraffin-embedded tissue
Chlamydia trachoma	Elementary bodies, conjunctival samples
CMV (cytomegalovirus)	Urine, peripheral blood, paraffin-embedded tissue, necropsy tissue from skin, lung, and lymph nodes
EBV (Epstein-Barr virus)	Tissue biopsy, necropsy tissue, throat swabs
HIV (human immunodeficiency virus)	Peripheral blood, endoscopy swabs, various tissue samples
Human B-lymphotrophic virus	Peripheral blood, tumor tissue
HTLV-I (human T-cell leukemia virus type 1)	Peripheral blood, tumor tissue
HTLV-II	Peripheral blood
HBV (hepatitis B virus)	Peripheral blood, cord blood, colostrum, liver, paraffin-embedded tissue
HPV (human papillomavirus)	Cervical smears and lavages, paraffin-embedded tissue, aspirates and biopsies of numerous tissues
HSV (herpes simplex virus)	Paraffin-embedded skin punch biopsies
Measles	Paraffin-embedded material
Mycobacteria	Sputum, lymph node biopsy, gastric and abscess aspirates
Mycoplasma	Throat swabs, bronchoalveolar lavages
Parvovirus B19	Sera, placenta, fetal tissue, paraffin-embedded tissue
Rhinovirus	Various
Rickettsia rickettsii	Purified rRNA
Toxoplasma	Peripheral blood, crude cell lysates
Trypanosoma cruzi	Insect vectors, various clinical isolates

[a]Adapted with permission Wright PA, Wynford-Thomas D, J Pathol 1990;162:99.

thereby facilitated automation of the entire process. A typical PCR run will incorporate 20 to 40 cycles of amplification, which may yield a final amplification of over 1 million-fold.

For the first cycle of amplification, the length of the newly synthesized DNA is dependent solely on the time of the reaction. The longer the Taq polymerase is functional, the longer the gene product will be. This piece of DNA is referred to as the "long product." However, the following cycles will result in shorter fragments of DNA, since the Taq polymerase will initiate at the site of the DNA:primer hybrid, but will terminate at the end of the piece of DNA. This termination point will be the initiation site of the previous cycle, i.e. where the DNA:primer hybrid was present. These smaller fragments of DNA are referred to as the "short product," and this short product is the DNA that is of interest. Since there is only one piece of original, template DNA, the long product will only increase arithmetically, while the short product will increase exponentially. The PCR may also be used to amplify mRNA; however, it is first necessary to generate DNA from the mRNA, since the Taq enzyme is a DNA and not an RNA polymerase. The DNA is generated by preparing a complementary DNA (cDNA) using reverse transcriptase, and the newly synthesized cDNA is then amplified using the basic methodology described above (20).

After the nucleic acid has been sufficiently amplified it is necessary to determine if the desired fragment of DNA was amplified. To achieve this, the products of the PCR reaction may be separated on electrophoresis gels and stained with ethidium bromide, yielding bands that should be the correct molecular weight of the amplified stretch of DNA. For further specificity, the PCR products may also be analyzed via Southern blot analysis. Alternatively, the short product may be cut with restriction endonucleases, and the resulting DNA fragments either directly analyzed on ethidium bromide–stained gels, or subjected to Southern blot analysis.

While the sensitivity of the PCR reaction is truly astonishing, it is possible to even further amplify the final product by using "nested primers." In this method, the initial PCR amplification product, i.e., the short product, is specifically synthesized so that it is sufficiently long to allow using another set of primers that will bind to regions lying within the sequence spanned by the first set of primers. At the completion of the first set of PCR reaction cycles, these new primers are added, and the entire process is repeated. Both sets of primers may be added at the start. This will still result in an increase in the final product and does not require two independent rounds of PCR.

Controls must be mentioned, as failure to adhere to strict procedures may yield false-positive results. Contamination is a very real problem, since one is effectively synthesizing new DNA with each cycle. Contamination at an early stage, with even trace quantities of DNA, will result in amplification and generation of a positive end product. Many laboratories have "detected" viral DNA in double distilled water or empty paraffin blocks, which is merely a false-positive reaction.

Table 7.4. Genetic Diseases Studied by PCR[a]

Disease	Defective Gene
α_1-Antitrypsin deficiency	α_1-Antitrypsin
Angioneurotic edema (hereditary type I)	C1 inhibitor
ApoC-II deficiency	Apolipoprotein C-II
Chronic granulomatous disease (X-linked)	Neutrophil NADPH oxidase
Cystic fibrosis (CF)	CF transmembrane regulator
Drug-induced hemolytic anemia	Glucose-6-phosphate dehydrogenase
Duchenne's muscular dystrophy	Dystrophin
Ehlers-Danlos syndrome type VIII	Pro-alpha 1 (I) collagen
Fabry's disease	Lysosomal α-galactosidase
Familial hypercholesterolemia	LDL receptor
Gerstmann-Straussler syndrome	Prion protein gene
Gyrate atrophy (chorioretinal)	Ornithine γ-amino-transferase
Hemophilia A	Factor VIII
Hemophilia B	Factor IX
Hereditary elliptocytosis	RBC spectrin
Hereditary fructose intolerance	Aldolase B
Huntington's disease	HD locus
Hyperinsulinemic syndrome	Insulin
Hypophosphatasia	Alkaline phosphatase
Lesch-Nyhan syndrome	HPRT
Leukocyte adhesion deficiency	Leukocyte integrins
Mitochondrial myopathy	Various
Osteogenesis imperfecta	Type I collagen
Pelizaeus-Mezbacher disease	Proteolipid protein
Phenylketonuria	Phenylalanine hydroxylase
Porphyria (acute intermittent)	Porphobilinogen deaminase
Pyruvate dehydrogenase deficiency	Pyruvate dehydrogenase
Retinoblastoma	RB1
Rickets (vitamin D resistant)	Vitamin D receptor
Sandhof's disease	β-Hexosaminidose
Sickle cell anemia	β-Globulin
Spondyloepiphyseal dysplasia	Type II collagen
Tay-Sachs disease	β-*N*-acetylhexosaminidase
Thalassaemia	α- and β-Globin
von Willebrand's disease	von Willebrand factor

[a]Adapted with permission from Wright PA, Wynford-Thomas D. J Pathol 1990;162:99.

Use in Diagnostic Pathology

A number of clinical applications have been found for the PCR, and one of the most useful is the detection of microorganism in tissues and fluids. A partial listing of where PCR has been successfully applied is found in Table 7.3. This methodology has tremendous advantage for diagnosing infectious diseases in cases where culture is difficult and time consuming, or if increased sensitivity is required. PCR offers a unique advantage in the diagnosis of acquired immune deficiency syndrome, where it is possible to detect PCR-amplified HIV-1 genomes from the peripheral blood of seropositive individuals (21). The PCR may be used to help resolve indeterminate Western blots, and may be useful in the diagnosis of HIV infections in infants born to seropositive mothers (22). The infants will have potentially false-positive Western blots, because of placental passage of the maternal antibody. PCR amplification has been used to detect a number of viruses, including human T-cell lymphoma/leukemia viruses, human immunodeficiency virus, Epstein-Barr virus, hepatitis B virus, enteroviruses, cytomegalovirus (23), and human papillomaviruses (24). The latter two viruses have been detected in paraffin-embedded tissue from archival material. The PCR could therefore be used to help resolve equivocal in situ hybridizations. PCR may be used to study genetic diseases. Table 7.4 provides a listing of diseases for which primers have been designed and used to help with the diagnosis. Since the genes are present in all tissues, it is possible to examine archival material, i.e., paraffin blocks. The PCR technology has additional advantages in prenatal diagnosis, neonatal screening, and carrier testing. Chorionic villus biopsy may be done, and virtually any amount of tissue that may be recovered will be adequate for PCR amplification and diagnosis. Because of the sensitivity, however, there is an increased risk of contamination with maternal tissue.

PCR has specific applications in the forensic sciences, since it is possible to generate DNA sequences from extremely small samples. As an example, sufficient DNA for analysis has been generated from a single human hair (25) or a spot of blood (26). After amplification, these sequences may then be used for analysis. These samples may be used to determine genetic individuality, and have been admitted into court as evidence. The correlation of the DNA from a spot of blood or a hair fragment with the DNA of the suspect can be made with an extraordinarily high degree of certainty.

Two recent publications describe combining the powerful amplification ability of the PCR with in situ hybridization to provide increased ability to localize human papillomavirus (HPV) DNA in cervical squamous epithelium (27, 28). In the first report, the reaction was performed on paraffin sections that had been placed on glass slides. The tissue was digested, and the reagents were added to the sections. The sections were then coverslipped, placed in aluminum foil "boats," and put directly on the heating block of the thermocycler. Detection was then performed using a biotin-labeled probe. This protocol worked very well, and showed enhanced detection over conventional in situ hybridization methods.

Modifications were made to the original protocol to improve both the sensitivity and specificity (28). This was done by utilizing the "hot start" technique. With this methodology, all reagents except the primers and Taq polymerase were added to the slides, which were then placed on the thermocycler and heated to 82°C. By withholding these essential components, nonspecific reactions that may occur prior to the initiation of the reaction are prevented. Biotin-labeled probes were used, as well as digoxigenin-labeled probes. Using the modifications, it was possible to show specific detection of HPV within individual cells. The "hot start" method also allowed the detection of smaller amplified products. Previously, it had been suggested that larger products were required, since smaller fragments would diffuse and not allow precise localization. Additionally, only one set of primers is required, as opposed to previous reports in which multiple sets of primers were required in order to have sufficient product to detect (27).

The marriage of PCR and in situ hybridization will allow studies to be performed on archival material. This is especially exciting, since formalin fixation has already been shown to represent a satisfactory fixative for PCR (29). Investigations may now be carried out to begin to document the presence of specific nucleic acids with specific disease states.

References

1. Myerson D. In situ hybridization. In: Colvin RB, Bhan AK, McCluskey RT, eds. Diagnostic immunopathology. New York: Raven Press, 1988:475–498.
2. Lloyd RV, Iacangelo A, Eiden LE, Cano M, Jin L, Grimes M. Chromogranin A and B messenger ribonucleic acids in pituitary and other normal and neoplastic human endocrine tissues. Lab Invest 1989;60:548–556.
3. Valentino KL, Eberwine JH, Barchas JD, eds. In situ hybridization: applications to neurobiology. New York: Oxford University Press, 1987.
4. Lloyd RV. Use of molecular probes in the study of endocrine diseases. Hum Pathol 1987;18:1199–1211.
5. Wolfe HJ. DNA probes in diagnostic pathology. Am J Clin Pathol 1988;90:340–344.
6. Brigati DJ, Myerson D, Leary JJ, et al. Detection of viral genomes in cultured cells and paraffin-embedded tissue sections using biotin-labeled hybridization probes. Virology 1983;126: 32–50.
7. Unger ER, Budgeon LR, Myerson D, Brigati DJ. Viral diagnosis by in situ hybridization. Description of a rapid simplified colorimetric method. Am J Surg Pathol 1986;10:1–8.
8. Hankin RC, Lloyd RV. Detection of messenger RNA in routinely processed tissue sections with biotinylated oligonucleotide probes. Am J Clin Pathol 1989;92:166–171.
9. Lewis ME, Sherman TG, Watson SJ. In situ hybridization histochemistry with synthetic oligonucleotides: strategies and methods. Peptides 1985;6:75–87.
10. Davis LG, Dibner MD, Battey JF, eds. Basic methods in molecular biology. New York: Elsevier, 1986.
11. Sambrook J, Fritsch EF, Maniatis T, eds. Molecular cloning: a laboratory manual. 2nd ed. Cold Spring Harbor, NY: Cold Spring Harbor Laboratory Press, 1989.
12. Remick DG, Scales WE, May MA, Spengler M, Nguyen D, Kunkel SL. In situ hybridization analysis of macrophage-derived tumor necrosis factor and interleukin-1 mRNA. Lab Invest 1988;59:809–816.
13. Singer RH, Lawrence JB, Villnave C. Optimization of in situ hybridization using isotopic and non-isotopic detection methods. Biotechniques 1986;4:230–249.
14. Grody WW, Cheng L, Lewin KJ. Application of in situ DNA hybridization technology to diagnostic surgical pathology. Pathol Annu 1987;22:151–175.
15. Robey SS, Gage WR, Kuhajda FP. Comparison of immunoperoxidase and DNA in situ hybridization techniques in the diagnosis of cytomegalovirus colitis. Am J Clin Pathol 1988;89:666–671.
16. Pilotti S, Gupta J, Stefanon B, De Palo G, Shah KV, Rilke F. Study of multiple human papillomavirus-related lesions of the lower female genital tract by in situ hybridization. Hum Pathol 1989;20:118–123.
17. Innis MA, Gelfand DH, Sninsky JJ, White TJ, eds. PCR protocols: a guide to methods and applications. New York: Academic Press, 1990.
18. Remick DG, Kunkel SL, Holbrook EA, Hanson CA. Theory and applications of the polymerase chain reaction. Am J Clin Pathol 1990:549–554.
19. Saiki RK, Gelfand DH, Stoffel S, et al. Primer-directed enzymatic amplification of DNA with a thermostable DNA polymerase. Science 1988;239:487–491.
20. Newman PJ, Gorski J, White GC 2d, Gidwitz S, Cretney CJ, Aster RH. Enzymatic amplification of platelet-specific messenger RNA using the polymerase chain reaction. J Clin Invest 1988;82:739–743.
21. Hart C, Schochetman G, Spira T, et al. Direct detection of HIV RNA expression in seropositive subjects. Lancet 1988;2:596–599.
22. Rogers MF, Ou CY, Rayfield M, et al. Use of the polymerase chain reaction for early detection of the proviral sequences of human immunodeficiency virus in infants born to seropositive mothers. New York City Collaborative Study of Maternal HIV Transmission and Montefiore Medical Center HIV Perinatal Transmission Study Group. N Engl J Med 1989;320:1649–1654.
23. Cassol SA, Poon MC, Pal R, et al. Primer-mediated enzymatic amplification of cytomegalovirus (CMV) DNA application to the early diagnosis of CMV infection in marrow transplant recipients. J Clin Invest 1989;83:1109–1115.
24. Shibata DK, Arnheim N, Martin WJ. Detection of human papilloma virus in paraffin-embedded tissue using the polymerase chain reaction. J Exp Med 1988;167:225–230.
25. Higuchi R, von Beroldingen CH, Sensabaugh GF, Erlich HA. DNA typing from single hairs. Nature 1988;332:543–546.
26. Witt M, Erickson RP. A rapid method for detection of Y-chromosomal DNA from dried blood specimens by the polymerase chain reaction. Hum Genet 1989;82:271–274.
27. Nuovo GJ, MacConnell P, Forde A, Delvenne P. Detection of human papillomavirus DNA in formalin-fixed tissues by in situ hybridization after amplification by polymerase chain reaction. Am J Pathol 1991;139:847–854.
28. Nuovo GJ, Gallery F, MacConnell P, Becker J, Bloch W. An improved technique for the in situ detection of DNA after polymerase chain reaction amplification. Am J Pathol 1991;139:1239–1244.
29. Nuovo GJ, Richart RM. Buffered formalin is the superior fixative for the detection of HPV DNA by in situ hybridization analysis. Am J Pathol 1989;134:837–842.

8 Hematopoietic Disorders

Curtis A. Hanson and Charles W. Ross

Molecular biological techniques have evolved into important diagnostic modalities in the clinical laboratory (1, 2). Hematopathology has often been at the forefront in adapting these advances in molecular biology to clinical application. This role has been fostered by the relative ease with which one can acquire diagnostic specimens (such as blood, bone marrow, and lymph nodes), the ability to make single-cell suspensions for further analysis, and the relative frequency of hematologic disease. As molecular biological techniques become further embedded into clinical laboratories, pathologists must understand both the technology and the clinical applications of these diagnostic modalities. To accomplish this, this chapter provides a basic background in the structure and function of the various immunoglobulin and T-cell receptor genes and how they are involved in the general immune response. In the second part, the applications and limitations of immunoglobulin and T-cell receptor hybridization studies as diagnostic markers of lymphoproliferations are discussed. The final section summarizes the various applications of other molecular diagnostic techniques that have had increasing importance in diagnostic hematology (Table 8.1).

IMMUNOGLOBULIN AND T-CELL RECEPTOR STRUCTURE AND FUNCTION

Lymphocytes play a key role in the human immune system and, together with macrophages, function as the "gatekeepers" of the immune system. This system must be capable of recognizing and reacting to all types of foreign antigens and, importantly, must also be capable of self-recognition to avoid autoimmune reactivity. Following antigen binding to either the immunoglobulin or T-cell receptor, the lymphocyte responds by producing and secreting various lymphokines and cytokines, which continue the immune response against the foreign antigen (3–5).

Both the immunoglobulin and T-cell receptors are heterodimers composed of two distinct disulfide-linked chains. These receptors are part of the so-called immunoglobulin supergene family. This family of related genes all have a similar molecular structure, and encode their genetic material through a process of DNA recombination before a functional protein can be produced (6, 7). The immunoglobulin genes (heavy chain, κ light chain, and λ light chain genes) and the T-cell receptor genes (α, β, γ, and δ chain genes) are each composed of three or four basic gene regions: variable (V), diversity (D), joining (J), and constant (C) regions (8, 9) (Fig. 8.1). As noted later, one segment from each of these regions recombine to encode for a particular immunoglobulin or T-cell receptor protein. Both receptor proteins are composed of a constant region and a variable region. The constant region confers a common characteristic structure, and the variable region is the site responsible for unique antigen recognition. The vast diversity of variable region structure is attributable to gene rearrangement, a process that is replayed uniquely in every developing B and T lymphocyte. To fully appreciate the applications of molecular techniques in the clinical laboratory, one must first understand this gene rearrangement process.

Table 8.1. Diagnostic Molecular Biology in Hematopoietic Disorders

Immunoglobulin/T-Cell Receptor Gene Rearrangement Studies
1. Determination of clonality
2. Lineage assessment
3. Detection of minimal or residual disease

Restriction Fragment Length Polymorphism (RFLP) Analysis in Bone Marrow Transplantation

Oncogenes in the Diagnosis of Hematopoietic Malignancies
1. t(9;22)(q34;q11): *bcr-abl* in chronic myelogenous leukemia/acute lymphoblastic leukemia
2. t(8;14)(q24;q32): *c-myc*/IgH in Burkitt's lymphoma/leukemia
3. t(11;14)(q13;q32): *bcl-1*/IgH in chronic lymphocytic leukemia/small lymphocytic lymphoma/intermediate differentiated lymphoma
4. t(14;18)(q32;q21): *bcl-2*/IgH in follicular center cell lymphoma

Evaluation of Hemoglobin Disorders
1. Sickle cell anemia
2. β-thalassemia

Evaluation of Hereditary Coagulation Disorders
1. Hemophilia A (Factor VIII deficiency)

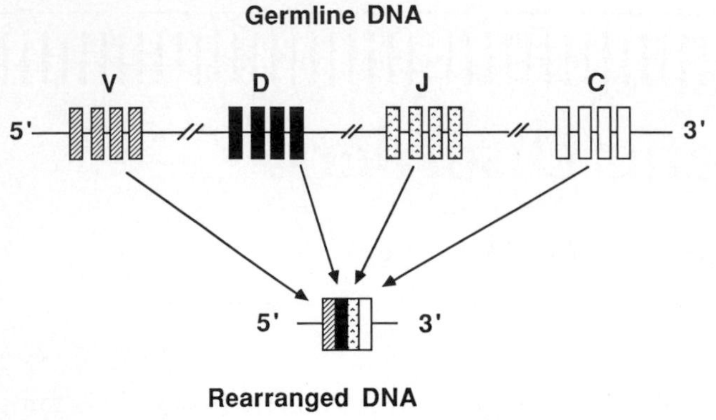

Figure 8.1. General structure of the Ig and T-cell receptor genes. One gene segment from each of the variable (V), diverse (D), joining (J), and constant (C) regions from the germline DNA recombine during the rearrangement process to form a unique gene sequence.

Immunoglobulin Genes

The production of immunoglobulin by B-lineage cells is the end result of exposure to a foreign antigen. The immunoglobulin, whether on the surface of the mature B lymphocyte or secreted into the serum by a plasma cell, binds to the foreign antigen and is subsequently cleared by the reticuloendothelial system. Immunologists were puzzled for years trying to explain how immunoglobulin-producing progenitor cells could be preprogrammed to recognize the vast array of foreign antigens to which an individual would be exposed. This puzzle was solved when Tonegawa and others (10) recognized that the construction of an intact immunoglobulin molecule was the result of rearrangements involving multiple regions within each of the immunoglobulin heavy and light chain genes.

Developmental Sequence. The normal development and differentiation sequence of B cells begins with the hematopoietic stem cell. The hematopoietic stem cell goes through the early stages of B-cell differentiation while still in the bone marrow, acquires surface immunoglobulin as a mature B lymphocyte, and finally ends with the plasma cell production of cytoplasmic immunoglobulin (Fig. 8.2). The earliest B-precursor cells in the bone marrow acquire cytoplasmic immunoglobulin heavy chain at the so-called pre-B cell stage of development. As these B-precursor cells mature, the immunoglobulin heavy chain fuses with an immunoglobulin light chain on the surface of the cell to form an intact immunoglobulin molecule (8).

Immunoglobulin Heavy Chain Gene. Although the immunoglobulin heavy and light chain genes are located at different chromosomal loci, all undergo a similar rearrangement process of their different gene regions. The immunoglobulin heavy chain gene is located on chromosome 14q32, the κ light chain gene on chromosome 2p12, and the λ light chain gene on chromosome 22q11 (11). The first rearrangement step in the early B-precursor cell begins with the heavy chain gene locus. The heavy chain gene contains approximately 100 variable (V) region genes, 15 to 20 diversity (D) region genes, and 6 joining (J) region genes (8, 12). The nine constant (C) region genes in this locus encode the immunoglobulin constant region and correspond to the particular immunoglobulin isotype: Cμ (IgM), Cδ (IgD), $C\gamma_{1\text{-}4}$ ($IgG_{1\text{-}4}$), $C\alpha_{1\text{-}2}$ ($IgA_{1\text{-}2}$), or Cε (IgE). Heavy chain rearrangement begins with one D region gene recombining with one J region gene, followed by recombination with a V region gene; the intervening sequences of DNA between the rearranged V, D, and J exons are then deleted (Fig. 8.3). The resulting rearranged DNA is transcribed and undergoes RNA splicing, which involves removing any intervening intron material and splicing the V, D, J, and Cμ exons together. The resulting mRNA product can then be translated into an immunoglobulin heavy chain molecule, which can be identified in the cytoplasm at the so-called "pre-B cell" stage of development. If, however, the initial D-J or V-D-J rearrangement mistakenly encodes for a termination or nonsense codon, then transcription or translation of the gene becomes "nonproductive." Subsequently, the same recombination process will begin on the second heavy chain gene located on the other chromosome 14. This control process prevents the simultaneous transcription and translation of two unique heavy chains from the same cell. If the second attempt at heavy chain rearrangement is unsuccessful, the B-precursor cell will die within the bone marrow (Fig. 8.4).

Immunoglobulin Light Chain Gene. The next step in the rearrangement process occurs in the late pre-B cell stage with attempts to rearrange one of the κ immunoglobulin light chain genes, located on chromosome 2p12 (13). The κ light chain gene structure differs slightly from the heavy chain gene: first, the κ gene lacks any known D regions, and second,

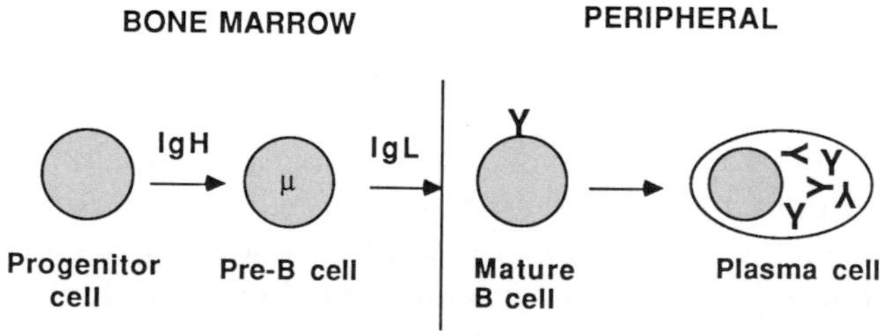

Figure 8.2. B-cell differentiation. The first step of B-cell maturation involves rearrangement of the immunoglobulin heavy chain gene (IgH). This is followed by the detection of cytoplasmic μ heavy chain at the pre-B cell stage of differentiation. Following heavy chain rearrangement, either κ or λ immunoglobulin light chain (IgL) gene rearrangement occurs. This leads to the deposition of surface Ig (Y) on the mature B cell and cytoplasmic Ig (Y) in the plasma cell.

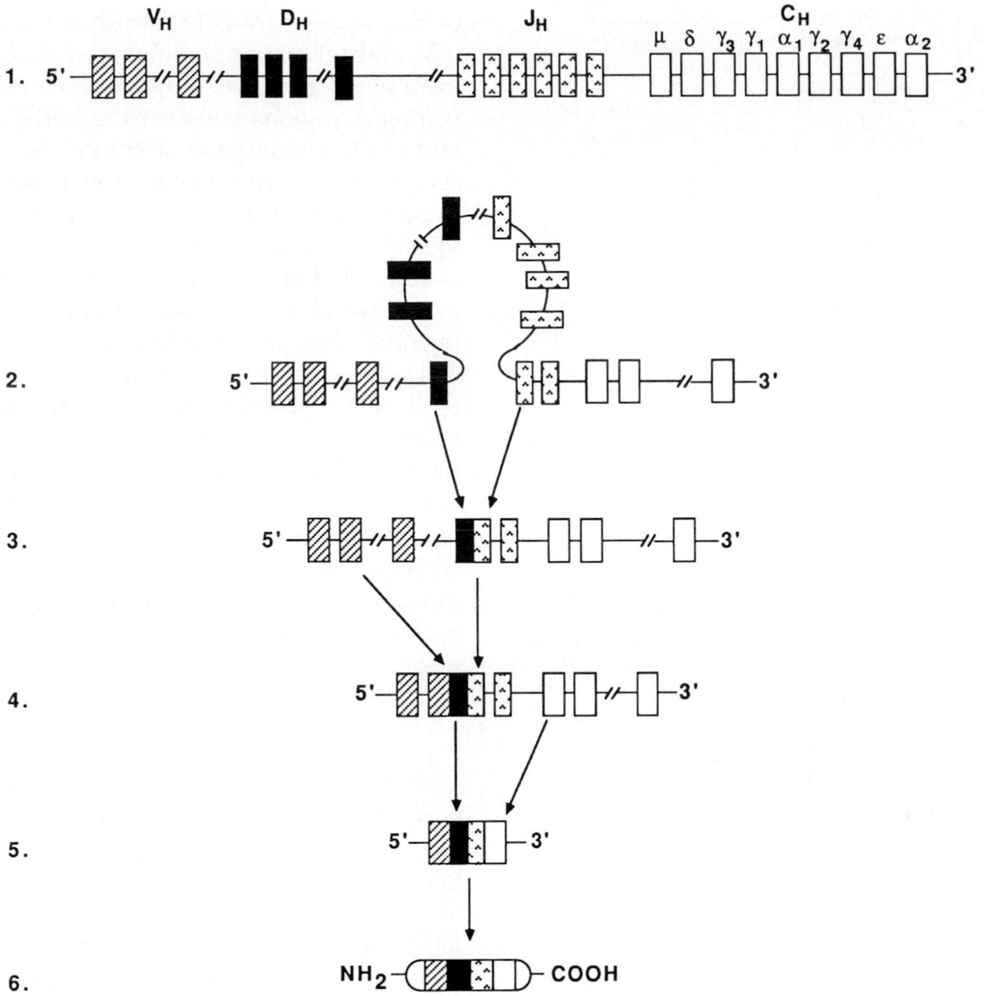

Figure 8.3. Rearrangement of the IgH gene. The hatched boxes [variable (V)], solid boxes [diversity (D)], stippled boxes [joining (J)], and open boxes [constant (C)] represent the exons of the respective gene regions. (1) Germline configurations; (2) The initial step in D-J rearrangement with "looping out" of intervening DNA, and (3) Eventual D-J recombination; (4) V-D-J rearrangement; (5) RNA transcription and splicing step; and (6) IgH chain production.

there is only one C region gene (Fig. 8.5). If the initial κ V-J rearrangement is a "productive" rearrangement, the transcription and translation process will lead to the formation of a complete immunoglobulin light chain. This light chain will then combine with the heavy chain to form an intact immunoglobulin molecule. If, however, the first V-J rearrangement is nonproductive, another V-J rearrangement is attempted on the second κ light chain gene on the other chromosome 2p12. If both κ rearrangements are nonproductive, the light chain gene rearrangement process begins anew with the λ light chain gene on chromosome 22q11. Like the κ gene, the λ light chain gene structure lacks any known D regions. In contrast to the κ gene, the λ gene includes six C regions, each having a high degree of homology to one another (Fig. 8.5). If the light chain gene rearrangement process fails with both λ genes, immunoglobulin differentiation cannot proceed, and the cell is destined to die in the bone marrow. The sequential rearrangement of κ before λ accounts for the normal 2:1 ratio of κ-to-λ positive B cells in peripheral blood (Fig. 8.4).

Completion of Immunoglobulin Synthesis. Once there is a successful light chain gene rearrangement and productive protein synthesis, the immunoglobulin light chain will bind to the immunoglobulin heavy chain within the endoplasmic reticulum and then be transported to the cell surface. This entire process of immunoglobulin heavy and light chain gene recombination can yield literally millions of unique B cell clones. This diversity results from the multitude of V, D, J, and C regions in the immunoglobulin heavy chain and light chain genes, with millions of unique recombinational possibilities among them.

Up to this point, we have described an IgM surface immunoglobulin-positive B cell. After transcrip-

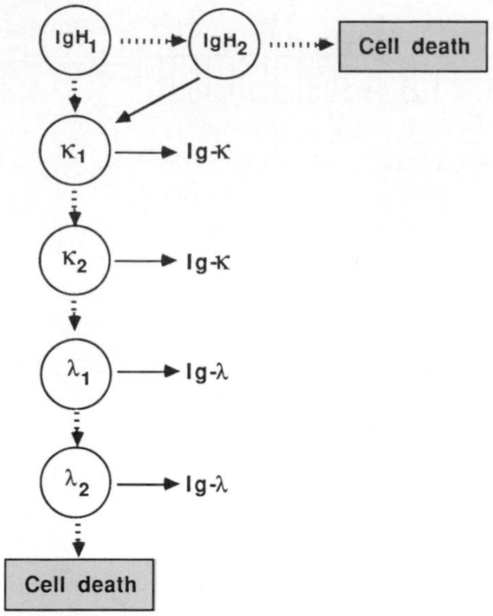

Figure 8.4. Hierarchy of Ig gene rearrangement. IgH genes are rearranged first, followed by sequential attempts at rearranging the κ and λ light chains. Solid lines indicate a successful rearrangement; dashed lines indicate a failed rearrangement.

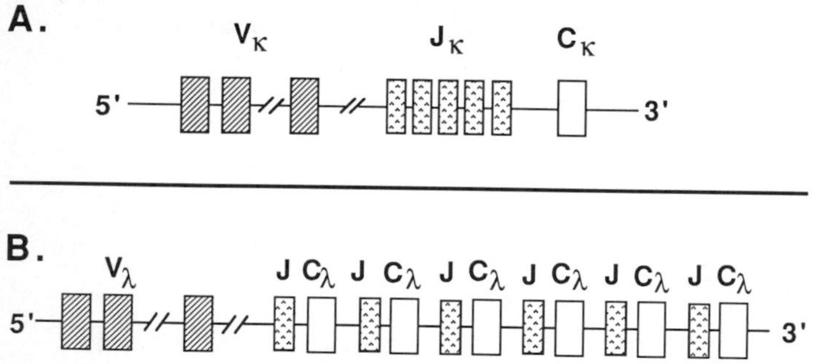

Figure 8.5. Structure of the Ig κ (**A**) and λ (**B**) light chain genes. (See Figs. 8.1 and 8.3 for general explanation of figure characters.)

tion, the rearranged V-D-J or V-J segments undergo RNA splicing, juxtaposing the V-D-J or V-J segments with the C region. The $C\mu$ gene is initially juxtaposed with the rearranged V-D-J sequence, since it is the first 5′ constant region exon. Only $C\mu$ will be spliced into this V-D-J sequence, and the remaining constant regions will be "ignored" during transcription. Therefore, the μ heavy chain constant region, i.e., IgM, will be the initial immunoglobulin expressed by the B lymphocyte.

Isotype Switching. The process by which B cells acquire other surface immunoglobulin isotypes is called isotype switching. Although these cells have different heavy chain constant regions, they still maintain the same antigen binding specificity because there has been no change in the variable region of the antibody. One mechanism of isotype switching involves the transcription of a long V-D-J-$C\mu$-$C\delta$ transcript; this results in the formation of a mixture of V-D-J-$C\mu$ and V-D-J-$C\delta$ mRNA and, consequently, IgM and IgD immunoglobulin (14). Another mechanism of isotype switching involves deletion of intervening C regions between the V-D-J rearrangement and the C region gene of choice. For example, for a rearrangement to result in the production of IgG_4, there must be a deletion of the intervening constant region genes, $C\mu$, $C\delta$, $C\gamma_3$, $C\gamma_1$, $C\alpha$, and $C\gamma_2$, between V-D-J and $C\gamma_4$ (Fig. 8.6). This splicing occurs in the switch regions located between the various C regions. The simultaneous expression of multiple heavy chain isotypes that may occasionally be found on B cells is probably due to the transient expression of multiple constant regions, which are spliced into the respective heavy chains in varying proportions. For example, a V-D-J-$C\mu$-$C\delta$-$C\gamma_3$ rearrangement may transiently produce a mixture of V-D-J-$C\mu$, V-D-J-$C\delta$, and V-D-J-$C\gamma_3$ RNA transcripts. This in turn, will transiently yield a mixture of IgM, IgD, and IgG_3 before the isotype switching to $C\gamma_3$ (IgG_3) is complete.

T-Cell Receptor Genes

Our understanding of the role and function of T lymphocytes has greatly expanded as a result of molecular biology-based studies. Immunologists have known for a long time that T lymphocytes play an important role in cellular immunity. Recent studies have shown that this process results from a close interaction with antigen-presenting macrophages (Fig.

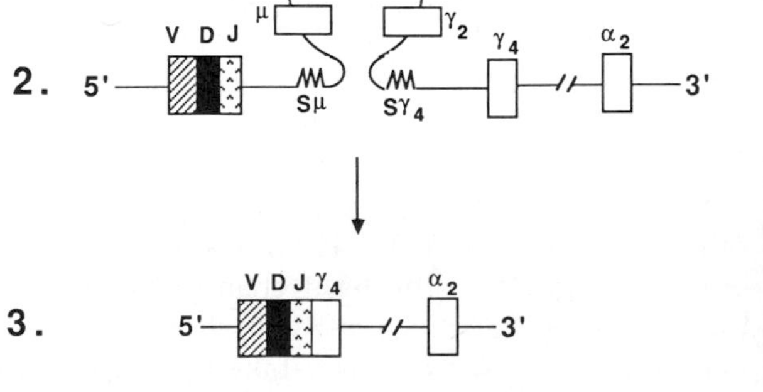

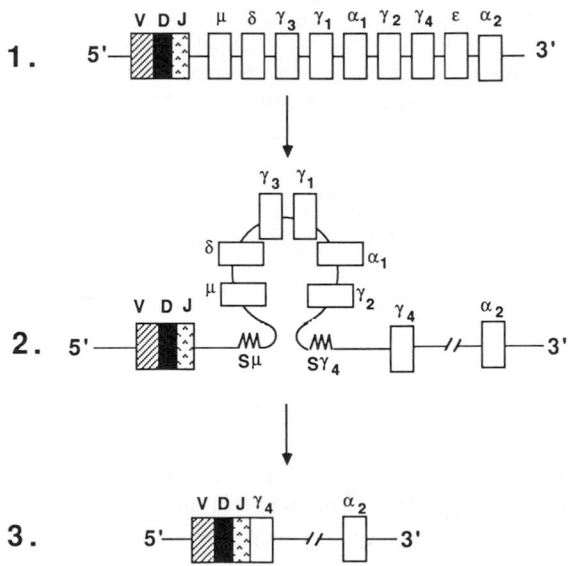

Figure 8.6. Isotype switching in the IgH gene. (See Figs. 8.1 and 8.3 for general explanation of characters.) (1) Gene structure following V-D-J recombination. Open boxes represent the various constant region isotypes. (2) An example of isotype switching where the switch regions (S) and μ (Sμ) and γ4 ($S\gamma_4$) are aligned, followed by (3) recombination of V-D-J with the $C\gamma_4$ exon. This will "switch" the cell production to an IgG_4 immunoglobulin.

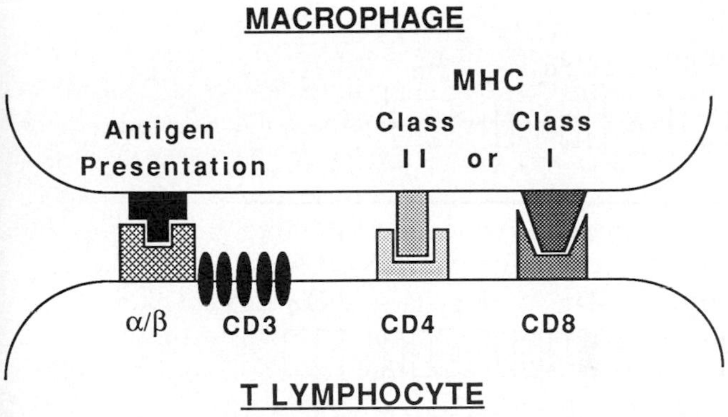

Figure 8.7. Schematic drawing of macrophage/T-cell interaction. The foreign antigen is presented by the macrophage to the T cell via the T-cell heterodimer α/β receptor. The associated CD3 complex is responsible for cell modulation following receptor binding. This is all done in context with major histocompatibility complex (MHC) antigens, which are thought to be recognized by CD8 and CD4 for class I and II antigens, respectively.

8.7). The foreign antigen presented by the macrophage is bound by the T-cell receptor. This sophisticated process involves interaction of the T-cell receptor with only cellular antigens. T cells appear to interact with MHC proteins to determine whether the cell in question is "foreign" or "self" (7, 8). Self-recognition through the MHC thus prevents autoimmune-type phenomena. Once the binding has occurred through the T-cell receptor/MHC complex, the T cell transmits its information internally through the CD3-complex of glycoproteins (5). This begins the cascade of protein kinase C production, calcium ion flux, and eventually "activation" of the cell with lymphokine production, etc. It is important to realize that the T-cell receptor is always associated with the CD3-complex in a one-to-one, noncovalently linked fashion.

The development of the mature T cell begins as a bone marrow-derived thymocyte precursor, which migrates to the thymus where subsequent maturation occurs. Immunologically, various stages in thymocyte development have been characterized and reviewed in detail elsewhere (15). It is in the thymus that T cell selection occurs, a process whereby cells that would react with "self" are removed and cells that express the preferred T-cell receptors and have appropriate MHC recognition are selected for further differentiation.

Just as understanding the immunoglobulin gene molecular structure is important for comprehending B-cell function, so is understanding the molecular structure of the T cell receptor system important for comprehending T cell function. All four T-cell receptor genes undergo a recombination process involving multiple gene regions, similar to that described for the immunoglobulin gene family. However, some important differences must be understood.

All four T-cell receptor genes (α, β, γ, and δ) undergo a recombination process involving V, D, J, and C regions, similar to the immunoglobulin heavy and light chain genes (16). We know from these molecular studies that there are at least two types of T-cell receptors expressed by T lymphocytes. A given T lymphocyte will express one type or the other. The most common T-cell receptor is composed of α and β chains, while the second type of T-cell receptor is composed of a γ/δ heterodimer (17). α/β-positive T cells predominate within the peripheral blood and lymph nodes, while γ/δ-positive T cells predominate in epithelial and epidermal locations (18–20). This differential localization suggests that each type of T-cell receptor serves a different role in the immune system. Both the α and δ chain genes are located on chromosome 14q11, with the δ chain gene located entirely within the α gene (21). The β chain gene is located on chromosome 7q34, and the γ chain gene is located on chromosome 7p15 (9). The β and δ genes consist of V, D, J, and C regions, while the α and γ genes are composed of V, J, and C regions. Each of these T-cell receptor genes undergoes recombination in a fashion similar to the immunoglobulin genes, leading to the production of an intact, heterodimeric, T-cell receptor protein (Fig. 8.8).

T-α Gene. The α gene consists of approximately 100 V regions and over 100 J regions, which are spread over a 1000-kb portion of chromosome 14 (Fig. 8.8). The large gene size and the numerous J regions have contributed to the difficulty in studying the α chain gene. The V-J recombination subsequently rearranges with the single α constant region, Cα, to form a complete α transcript.

T-β Gene. In constrast to the other members of the immunoglobulin supergene family, the β chain gene consists of two separate loci, β_1 and β_2, each composed of its own D, J, and C regions (Fig. 8.8). The β_1 and β_2 regions recombine only within their own groups, i.e., $D\beta_1$-$J\beta_1$-$C\beta_1$ or $D\beta_2$-$J\beta_2$-$C\beta_2$. The two constant regions, $C\beta_1$ and $C\beta_2$, are highly homologous, suggesting that the constant region of the β-receptor protein is functionally similar regardless of whether $C\beta_1$ or $C\beta_2$ is expressed (16). Rearrangement of Vβ within the β_2 locus is associated with deletion of the $D\beta_1$-$J\beta_1$-$C\beta_1$ locus. As with the immunoglobulin family, if the initial V-D-J rearrangement of the β chain gene is unsuccessful, an attempt will be made to rearrange the β chain gene on the other chromosomal allele.

T-γ Gene. The γ chain gene was initially discovered in a small subset of circulating T cells which were CD3-positive, but which lacked CD4, CD8 and the α/β T-cell receptor (17). The CD3-associated T-cell

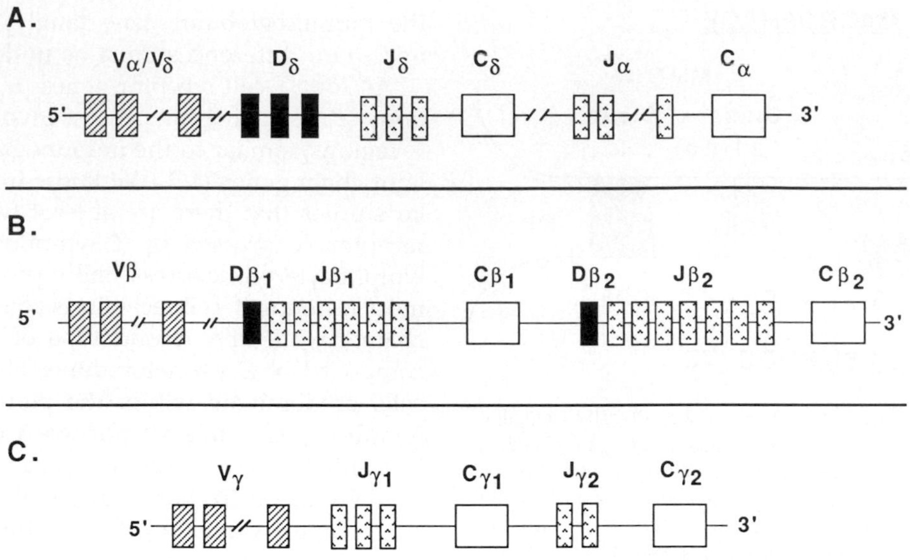

Figure 8.8. Structure of the T-cell receptor genes. (See Figs. 8.1 and 8.3 for explanation of figure characters.) **A** shows the structure of the Tα/δ gene on chromosome 14q11. **B** shows the germline configuration of the Tβ gene. **C** shows the Tγ gene structure.

receptor from this group of cells was found to have some similarities to the β chain gene, but offered less diversity, suggesting that it was based on a more primitive recognition system. The γ gene contains fewer than 10 V regions and only two J loci (17), which leads to a limited diversity in this gene subset (Fig. 8.8). Thus, a polyclonal mixture of T lymphocytes can demonstrate what appears to be oligoclonal rearrangements of the Tγ gene, as only seven or eight possible gene combinations can form (22, 23). Consequently, gene rearrangement analysis of the Tγ gene must be interpreted with great caution.

T-δ Gene. The δ gene has a unique structure, as it is located entirely within the α chain gene; the V, D, and J, regions of the δ locus are situated between the V and J regions of the α gene (21) (Fig. 8.8). Similar to the γ chain gene, only 10 Vδ regions have been identified. The δ gene locus contains only one C region, which is structurally similar to Cα. Obviously, based on the genomic structure of the α/δ locus, a V-Jα rearrangement will delete the entire δ gene. Thus, it would be impossible to express the δ receptor in a cell that has a functional α/β receptor. Because of their location and similar structure, it has been hypothesized that the α gene evolved as a result of a δ gene duplication (9).

Developmental Sequence. The precise sequential hierarchy of T-cell receptor gene rearrangements has not been definitively determined. It is thought that the δ locus is the first to undergo rearrangement in the early thymocyte. If that rearrangement is productive, then the cell is obligated to become a γ/δ receptor T cell with a higher propensity toward epidermal or epithelial recirculation. This δ rearrangement appears to be the critical step in determining whether a γ/δ or an α/β T cell develops (24). Shortly after rearrangement of the δ gene, the γ and/or β genes undergo rearrangement (Fig. 8.9). If the δ rearrangement is successful, then a γ/δ T cell will be the result; only exceedingly rare examples of cells expressing a δ/β receptor have been identified. If the initial δ rearrangement is unsuccessful or nonproductive, attempts are then made to rearrange the α locus (21). If successful, the α chain combines with the previously rearranged β chain to form an α/β T cell. In γ/δ T cells that contain a rearranged β chain gene, the β chain gene rearrangement is nonproductive and is not expressed by the cell. Likewise, a rearranged γ chain gene remains nonproductive in an α/β-positive T cell. From these and other studies, it is theorized that the γ/δ-positive T cells arise earlier in T cell ontogeny than those cells bearing the α/β heterodimer receptor.

Clonality

Clonality is an essential concept to understand before interpreting Southern blot hybridization studies. A clonal process is defined as a proliferation of daughter cells originating from a single precursor cell, each having identical phenotypes and growth characteristics as that original precursor cell. Normal B and T lymphocytes are polyclonal proliferations, with each lymphocyte having its own structure and functional characteristics. Theoretically, each lymphocyte within an individual should have a unique molecular structure and thus be capable of responding to a different antigenic stimulation.

Tonegawa's recognition that the immunoglobulin molecule was the result of recombining various re-

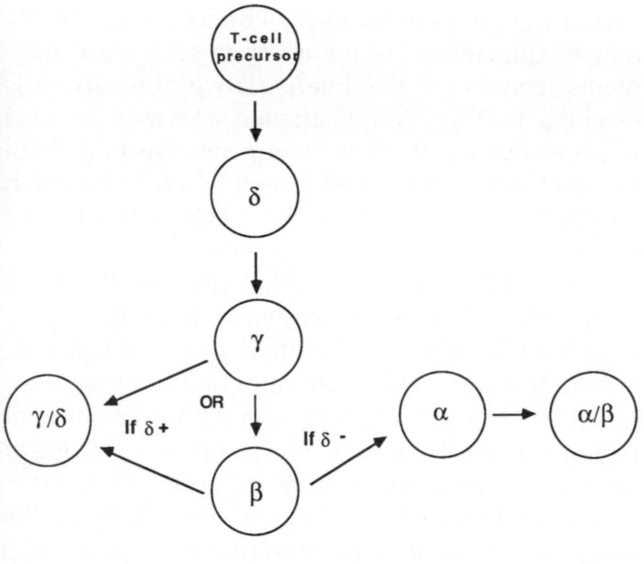

Figure 8.9. Presumptive hierarchy of T-cell gene rearrangement. The δ gene appears to undergo the initial T-cell rearrangement; this is most likely followed by rearrangement of the γ and/or β genes. If the δ rearrangement is successful, a γ/δ cell results. This cell may or may not have a concomitant rearrangement of the β chain gene. If the δ rearrangement fails, rearrangement of the α chain gene will be attempted. The presence of an intact α chain will then result in an α/β T cell.

gions within the gene was a startling concept which finally could account for the incredible diversity of the immunoglobulin system (7). As we previously stated in the immunoglobulin and T cell receptor section, there are millions of different potential recombinations that can occur among the V, D, and J regions in a gene. In addition to these random associations among V-D-J, so-called N-region diversification and somatic gene mutations can occur which further add to the tremendous diversity of the system (25). N-region diversification is a terminal deoxynucleotidyl transferase (TdT)-dependent process that results in additions of deletions of nucleotides at the V-J or V-D-J junctions (26).

Clonality is not a new concept in hematopoietic biology (Table 8.2). Monoclonal immunoglobulin has been used for years as the classic clonal marker of B-cell proliferations, such as multiple myeloma, chronic lymphocytic leukemia, hairy cell leukemia, non-Hodgkin's lymphoma, and Waldenstrom's macroglobulinemia. In 1977, Fialkow and colleagues demonstrated that chronic myelogenous leukemia (CML) was a clonal disorder by using glucose-6-phosphate dehydrogenase (G6PD) isoenzymes (27). The X-linked gene for G6PD may encode for either a G6PD-A or -B isoenzyme. By evaluating heterozygous females (each with two X chromosomes and thus having one G6PD-A and one G6PD-B isoenzyme gene), Fialkow showed that malignant cells of CML expressed only one of the isoenzymes as opposed to the normal mixture of both isoenzymes. Cytogenetic analysis of chromosomes has also been used to demonstrate clonality (28).

Table 8.2. Detection of Clonality

Monoclonal immunoglobulin protein
Glucose-6-phosphate dehydrogenase (G6PD) isoenzymes
Chromosomal karyotyping
Immunoglobulin/T-cell receptor gene rearrangement studies

Molecular gene rearrangement studies by Southern blot hybridization are the most recently developed assay for the detection of clonal proliferations, based on detecting clonal rearrangements of either the immunoglobulin or T-cell receptor genes. This technique is quite sensitive and is capable of detecting a clonal proliferation, if the specimen being studied contains as few as 1 to 5% monoclonal cells (29). Although this level of sensitivity may sound desirable, gene rearrangement studies may at times be too sensitive. Indeed, Southern blot hybridization studies have detected clonal rearrangements in several diseases that clinically do not behave in a "malignant" fashion. Thus, as we improve our ability to detect monoclonality, we must modify our concept that a clonal process is equivalent to a clinically malignant process. Several such disorders will be discussed in a later section to further illustrate this point.

Laboratory Analysis of DNA

Chapter 6 outlines the procedures used for DNA extraction, restriction endonuclease digestion, and Southern blot transfer and hybridization studies. Two important concepts that must be reviewed thoroughly before interpreting gene rearrangement studies are (*a*) probe structure and location, and (*b*) the restriction enzyme map of the gene.

Probes. Gene probes are specific sequences of DNA that are complementary to a portion of the gene being studied. These probes usually are not complementary to an entire gene, but are directed to a region of the gene which will always be present following a rearrangement. The most commonly used immunoglobulin heavy chain gene probe is complementary to the J_H region. Thus, when a clonal V-D-J rearrangement has occurred, the J_H probe will bind to the J_H segment; the J_H probe will recognize any or all of the six J_H exons. Other immunoglobulin gene probes that are commonly used include those directed against Cμ, Cκ, or Cλ. The Cμ and Cκ probes bind only to their complementary sequences, respectively. The Cλ probe, however, will bind to any of the six Cλ exons, as each constant region of the λ gene is relatively homologous to each other.

The T-cell receptor gene probes work in a fashion similar to their immunoglobulin gene equivalents. Both Jβ and Cβ probes have been used in the evaluation of the β chain gene. Since the two Jβ regions and the two Cβ regions each have a high degree of homology, the Jβ and Cβ probes will bind to both Jβ and both Cβ regions, respectively. Likewise, the Jγ and Cγ probes for the Tγ gene and the Jδ and Cδ probes for the Tδ gene recognize all the J and C regions for the γ and δ genes, respectively, due to the high degree of homology present within each gene.

Immunoglobulin Gene Rearrangement. Before a Southern blot study can be interpreted, the researcher must understand the restriction enzyme map of the desired gene. These maps localize various restriction enzyme sites relative to the gene of interest as well as to each other. The whole concept of gene rearrangement refers to the process by which a restriction enzyme site is "rearranged" relative to its previous location, thus changing the size and blot location of a particular hybridization fragment. For example, the immunoglobulin heavy chain gene contains a *Bam*H1 restriction enzyme site, located 5′ upstream from the joining region, and another *Bam*H1 site, located 3′ downstream from the Cμ constant region; this results in a germline 17-kilobase (kb) fragment after digestion with *Bam*H1. During the process of D-J or V-D-J rearrangement, the recombination into the J region removes the intervening sequences 5′ to the J region area, thus eliminating the initial 5′ *Bam*H1 restriction site (Fig. 8.10). Consequently, the germline 17 kb fragment seen with *Bam*H1-cut DNA would then be rearranged to either a larger or smaller fragment, depending on where the next random 5′ *Bam*H1 site is located. Because of its different size, the rearranged fragment will migrate to a different location in the blot and is thus referred to as a rearranged immunoglobulin heavy chain gene.

T-Cell Receptor Gene Rearrangement. In the T-cell receptor gene system, a similar rearrangement process occurs. The most commonly used gene probe for T-cell receptor gene rearrangement studies are those complementary to the T-cell receptor β chain gene. In this gene, there is a *Bam*H1 restriction enzyme site 5′ of the $J\beta_1$ region and 3′ of $C\beta_2$; this *Bam*H1 fragment, therefore, surrounds both Jβ-Cβ loci. Similar to the process described with the immunoglobulin heavy chain gene, the 5′ upstream *Bam*H1 enzyme site is eliminated during either a D-J or V-D-J rearrangement. Consequently, the germline fragment seen with *Bam*H1-cut DNA would be rearranged to either a larger or smaller fragment. Although this enzyme would appear ideal, the large size of the germline band (23 kb) seen with *Bam*H1 may be difficult to distinguish from rearranged fragments. Because of this interpretative difficulty, it is essential that multiple restriction enzymes be used when evaluating the T-β chain gene. Most laboratories will use *Bam*H1, *Eco*R1, and *Hind*III restriction enzymes when evaluating for T-cell receptor gene rearrangements.

The *Eco*R1 restriction enzyme sites for the T-cell receptor β chain gene are located 5′ of the $J\beta_1$ region, 3′ of the $C\beta_1$ region, and both 5′ and 3′ of $C\beta_2$ (Fig. 8.11*A*); this will yield a germline configuration of 11-kb and 4-kb bands when probed with a Tβ constant region probe (Fig. 8.11*B*). When either a $D\beta_1$-$J\beta_1$ or Vβ-$D\beta_1$-$J\beta_1$ rearrangement has occurred, the most 5′ *Eco*R1 restriction site is removed, thus changing the size of the germline 11-kb band (Fig. 8.11*C*). The 4 kb band is not changed, as the *Eco*R1 sites around β_2 are not disrupted following either $D\beta_1$-$J\beta_1$ or V-$D\beta_1$-$J\beta_1$ rearrangement.

The limitation of using *Eco*R1 for T-cell receptor β chain analysis is its inability to detect rearrangements involving the β_2 locus. When a $D\beta_2$-$J\beta_2$ or Vβ-$D\beta_2$-$J\beta_2$ rearrangement has occurred, the β_1 locus and, thus, the *Eco*R1 restriction sites around the β_1 locus, is deleted, including the germline 11 kb band. However, this D-J or V-D-J rearrangement into the β_2 locus will not disrupt either of the *Eco*R1 restriction sites surrounding the $C\beta_2$ region. Thus, with a β_2 rearrangement, the 4-kb band is not changed, and one is left with an allelic deletion of the 11-kb band. This deletion will not be evident with rearrangement studies if the other allele remains in germline configuration or if there are significant numbers of non-T lymphocytes in the specimen being analyzed which could contribute to the germline band.

To overcome this limitation, *Hind*III is usually used as an additional restriction enzyme for T-cell receptor β chain gene analysis (Fig. 8.11*D*). The *Hind*III restriction enzyme sites are located immediately 5′ and 3′ of $C\beta_1$, within the $C\beta_2$ segment, and 3′ of $C\beta_2$; this will yield germline bands of 3.5 kb, 6.5 kb, and 8 kb when probed with a Tβ constant region probe. If a rearrangement into the β1 locus has occurred, none of the *Hind*III restriction enzyme sites are affected, thus giving a germline configuration on Southern blot. However, rearrangement into the β2 locus will remove the *Hind*III site between $C\beta_1$ and $D\beta_2$, thus changing the size of the germline 8-kb band (Fig. 8.11*E*). The 3.5-kb band will be deleted along with the β_1 locus; the 6.5-kb band will be unchanged as the *Hind*III sites surrounding $C\beta_2$ are unaffected by the rearrangement process.

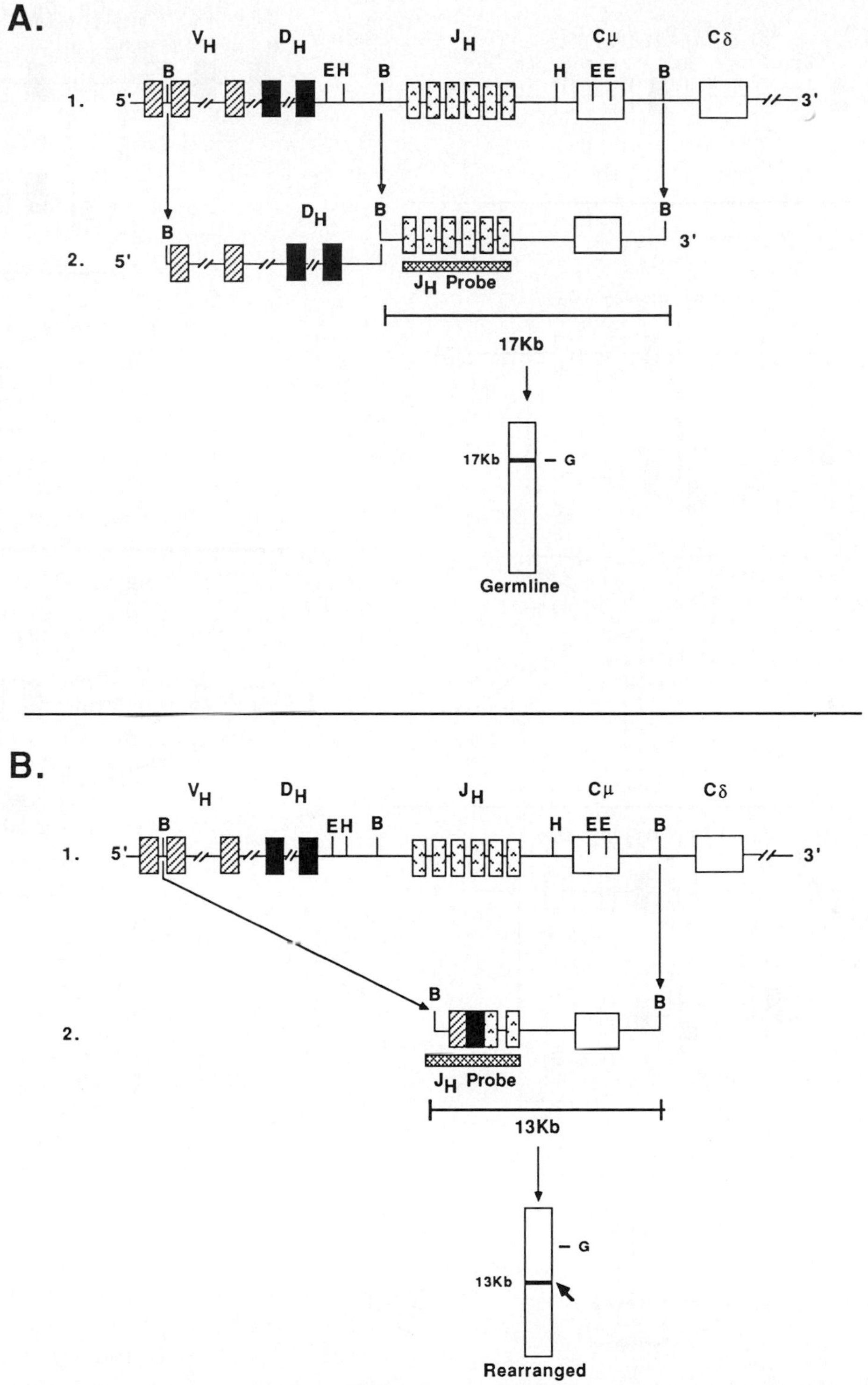

Figure 8.10. Restriction enzyme map of the immunoglobulin heavy chain gene. The thin vertical lines represent recognition sites for *Bam*H1 (*B*), *Eco*R1 (*E*), or *Hind*III (*H*). (See Figs. 8.1 and 8.3 for explanation of other characters.) **A**, The heavily stippled box represents the J_H probe. When cut with *Bam*H1, the unrearranged IgH gene leads to a germline 17-kb band. **B**, Following V-D-J rearrangement, the original 5′ *Bam*H1 site disappears and is replaced by the next random *Bam*H1 site, leading in this example to a rearranged 13-kb fragment as detected by the J_H gene probe. Other rearrangements might yield *Bam*H1 fragments of smaller or larger size.

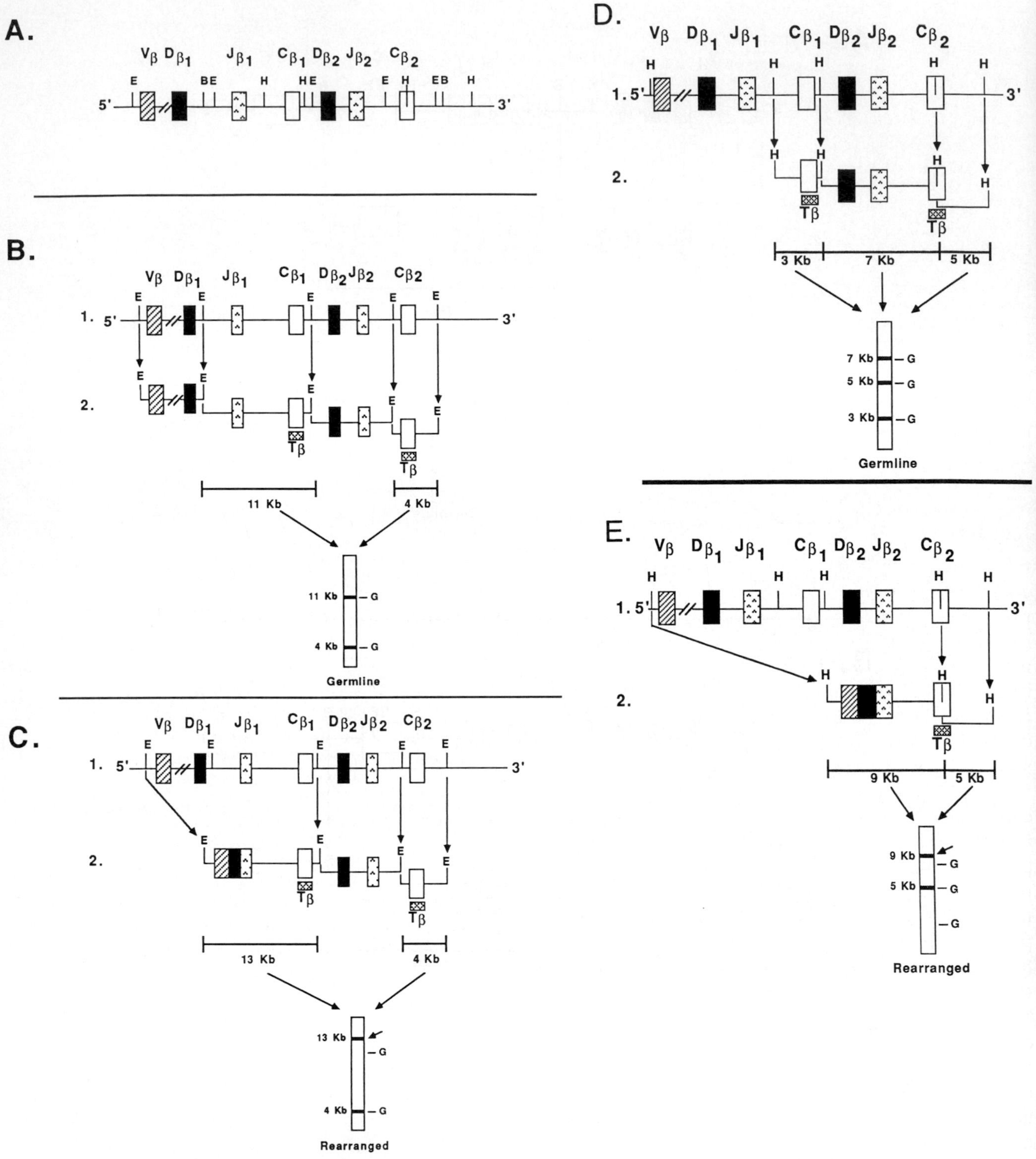

Figure 8.11. **A**, Restriction enzyme map of the Tβ chain gene. (See Figs. 8.1 and 8.3 for explanation of characters. See Fig. 8.12 for description of abbreviations.) **B**, The heavy stippled box represents the Tβ constant region probe. The germline configuration shows two bands following *Eco*R1 enzymatic digestion, as the probe will bind to both Cβ regions. **C**, Following Vβ-$D\beta_1$-$J\beta_1$ rearrangement, the 5′ *Eco*R1 site disappears and is replaced by the next random *Eco*R1 site. This leads to a rearranged 13-kb fragment (*arrow*). The 4-kb fragment of $C\beta_2$ has not been affected by this rearrangement process. **D**, The germline configuration shows three bands following *Hind*III enzymatic digestion, as the probe will bind to both Cβ regions. **E**, Following Vβ-$D\beta_2$-$J\beta_2$ rearrangement, the *Hind*III site 3′ of $C\beta_1$ is deleted and is replaced by the next random *Hind*III site. This leads to a rearranged fragment (*arrow*) and deletion of the 3.5-kb band. The 6.5-kb fragment surrounding $C\beta_2$ has not been affected by this rearrangement process.

Table 8.3. Gene Rearrangements in Lymphoma/Leukemia

	Immunoglobulin (%)			T-cell Receptor (%)		
	IgH[a]	κ	λ	Tβ	Tγ	Tδ
Lymphomas						
B-NHL	95	95	30	5–10	0[b]	0
T-NHL	5–10	0[b]	0	90	95	95
HD	15	10	5	15	—[c]	—[c]
Ki-1 anaplastic	10	10	0	60	60	—[c]
THL	20	10	0	40	40	—[c]
Leukemias						
B-precursor ALL	95	30	15	20	40–50	—[c]
T-ALL	10–20	0[b]	0	90	95	95
AML	5	0	0	10	10	—[c]
Lymphoproliferative disorders						
B-CLL	99	95	30	7	0	0
TγLPD	0	0	0	60	60	—[c]
HCL	100	95	30	5	0	0
MM	100	100	30	5	0	0

[a]IgH, immunoglobulin heavy chain; NHL, non-Hodgkin's lymphoma; HD, Hodgkin's disease; Ki-1 anaplastic, Ki-1-positive, large-cell, anaplastic lymphoma; THL, true histiocytic lymphoma; ALL, acute lymphoblastic leukemia; AML, acute myeloblastic leukemia; CLL, chronic lymphocytic leukemia; TγLPD, T-γ lymphoproliferative disorder; HCL, hairy cell leukemia; MM, multiple myeloma.
[b]Rare case report.
[c]Too few cases studied.

Thus, for T-cell receptor β chain gene analysis, *Bam*H1 restriction enzyme analysis will show rearrangements involving either the β_1 or β_2 locus. However, the large, germline band seen with *Bam*H1 presents its own unique problem. Analysis with *Eco*R1 restriction enzyme will demonstrate rearrangements of the β_1 locus, but will not show a rearranged band if the β_2 locus is involved. This is in contrast to *Hind*III restriction enzyme analysis, which will demonstrate β_2 loci rearrangements, but fail to demonstrate β_1 rearrangements.

The Rearrangement Process. An important concept to understand is that this technique is not sensitive enough to detect individual rearrangements in a polyclonal mixture of cells, as each cell has its own unique immunoglobulin or T-cell receptor rearrangement. Thus, by Southern blot hybridization, a clonal process will not be detected until at least 1 to 5% of the cells have an identical clonal rearrangement of the immunoglobulin or T-cell receptor genes. Nevertheless, this level of sensitivity is remarkably high, and has made gene rearrangement analysis a powerful tool for the detection of monoclonal processes. Figures 8.12 and 8.13 demonstrate a schematic to illustrate the rearrangement process in a normal and malignant lymph node, respectively.

APPLICATIONS OF GENE REARRANGEMENT STUDIES IN DIAGNOSTIC HEMATOPATHOLOGY

The utilization of gene rearrangement studies in diagnostic hematopathology has centered on two important concepts: first, as sensitive indicators of clonality, and second, to help determine the cellular lineage of a particular proliferation. Although rearrangement studies can often provide helpful information regarding lineage, certain limitations and problems exist in using gene rearrangement studies to determine the cellular lineage of lymphoproliferative processes. Table 8.3 summarizes the gene rearrangement findings in the various lymphomas and leukemias. Table 8.4 provides loose guidelines for interpretation of gene rearrangement studies from a clinical diagnostic viewpoint.

Table 8.4. Interpretation of Gene Rearrangement Studies

Gene Probes			
IgH[a]	IgL	TCR	Interpretation
G	G	G	Germline versus nonhematopoietic versus unusual or early lymphoid disorder
R	G	G	Clonal disorder; suggestive of B lineage
R	R	G	B-lineage disorder
R	G	R	Clonal disorder; cannot determine lineage
G	R	G	Probable B-lineage disorder; unusual
G	G	R	Clonal disorder; suggestive of T lineage
G	R	R	B- versus T-lineage disorder; unusual
R	R	R	B-lineage disorder

[a]IgH, immunoglobulin heavy chain; IgL, immunoglobulin light chain; TCR, T-cell receptor; G, germline; R, rearranged.

Malignant Lymphoma and Benign Lymphoid Hyperplasia

Molecular gene rearrangement studies have had the biggest diagnostic impact in non-Hodgkin's lymphoma (1, 29, 30). In particular, these studies have been used in (*a*) identifying clonal proliferations, especially in peripheral T-cell lymphoma; (*b*) confirming the cellular lineage of a lymphoproliferation; (*c*) analyzing for residual or recurrent disease, post-

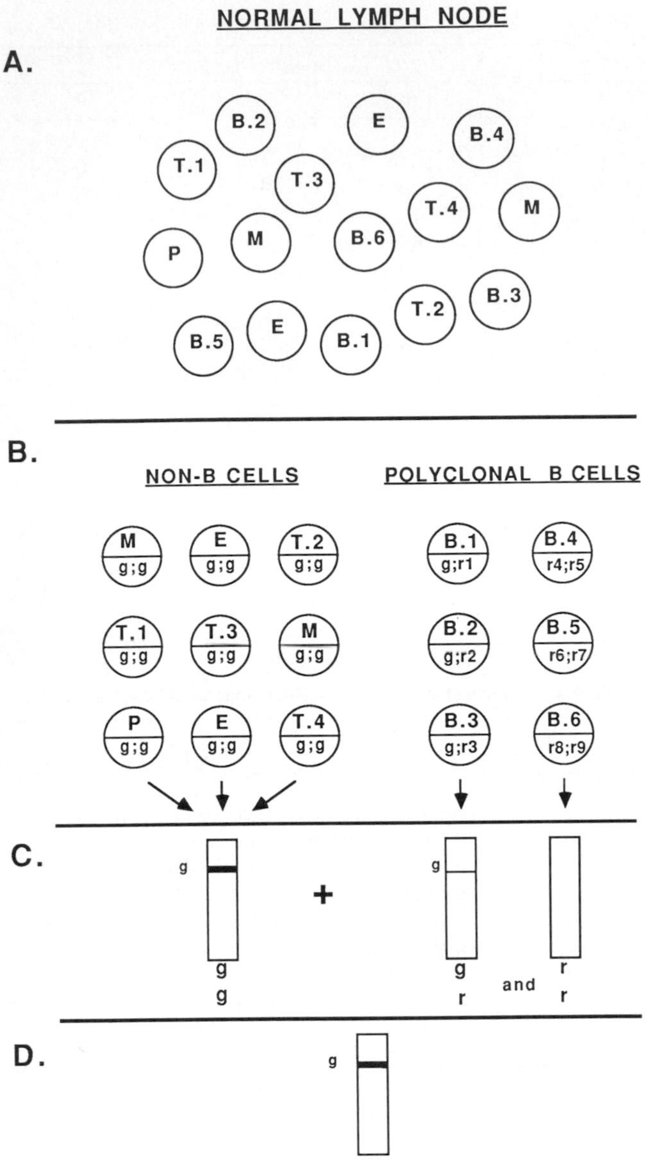

Figure 8.12. Schematic drawing of a normal lymph node and resulting Ig gene rearrangement studies. **A**, A normal lymph node consists of a mixture of polyclonal B cells (B.1–B.6), polyclonal T cells (T.1–T.4), macrophage/histiocytes (M), polymorphonuclear granulocytes (P), and endothelial cells (E). **B**, Schematic depiction of gene rearrangement analysis applied to cells from a normal lymph node. The non-B lymphocytes are shown on the left side and consist of T cells, macrophages, neutrophils, and endothelial cells. These cells retain their Ig genes in germline configuration. The polyclonal B cells, depicted on the right side, consist of a mixture of B cells (B.1–B.3) that retain one Ig gene allele in germline configuration while rearranging the other allele in a unique recombination (r1–r3). The remaining B cells (B.4–B.6) have attempted to rearrange both Ig alleles (r4–r9), with only one allele per cell exhibiting a "productive" rearrangement. **C**, This schematic of a Southern blot audioradiograph shows that the non-B cells contribute to the formation of one germline band since both alleles remain in germline configuration. Some polyclonal B cells have one germline allele and one uniquely rearranged allele; the germline alleles will contribute to the formation of a germline band on Southern blotting, while the single-copy rearranged alleles are undetectable by this method. The remaining B cells with two rearranged alleles also exhibit no detectable bands, as each rearrangement is again a unique recombination. **D**, Final Southern blot resulting from the combination of the non-B cell component and polyclonal B cells, therefore, leads to a single germline configuration with no rearranged bands identified.

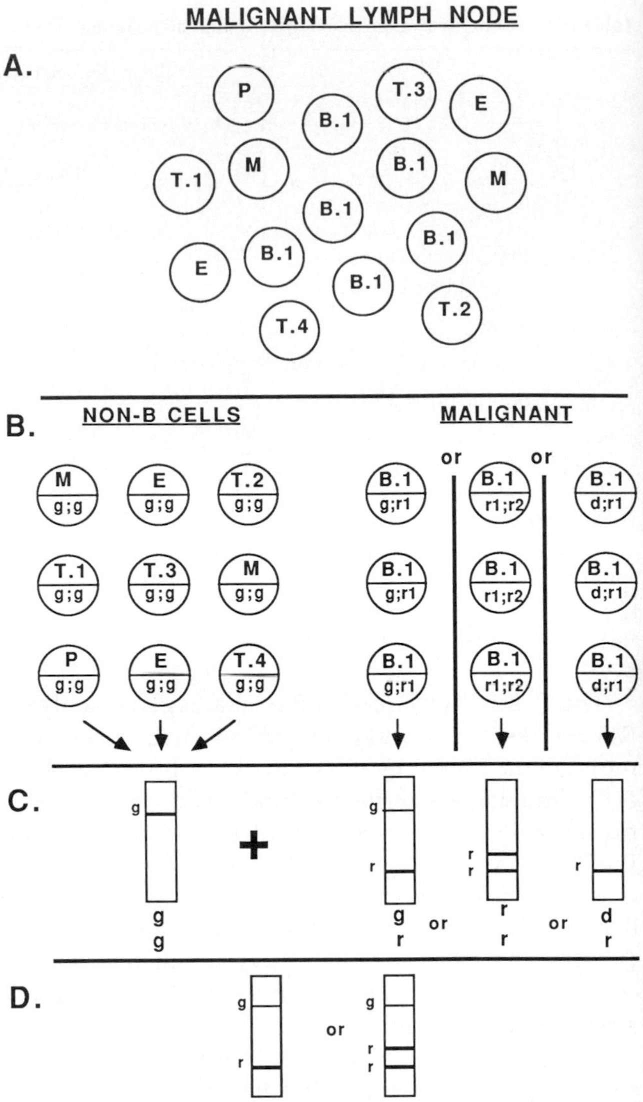

Figure 8.13. Schematic drawing of a malignant lymph node and resulting Ig gene rearrangement studies. **A**, A malignant lymph node consists of a mixture of monoclonal B cells (B.1), polyclonal T cells (T.1–T.4), macrophage/histiocytes (M), polymorphonuclear granulocytes (P), and endothelial cells (E). **B**, Schematic depiction of gene rearrangement analysis applied to cells from a neoplastic lymph node. The nonmalignant cells are shown on the left side; these cells retain their Ig genes in germline configuration. The monoclonal B cells depicted on the right side consist of monoclonal B cells that may be in one of three possible configurations: (1) the cells may have one rearranged Ig allele and the other allele in germline configuration; (2) the cells may have both Ig alleles rearranged, with only one productive rearrangement; or (3) one allele may be deleted and the other Ig locus rearranged. **C**, This schematic of a Southern blot audioradiograph shows that the few reactive cells contribute to the presence of a germline band. The monoclonal B cells will have one of three possible configurations depending on the status of both Ig alleles. **D**, Final Southern blot resulting from combination of the reactive cells and monoclonal B cells lead to a faint germline band, contributed from the few background normal cells and possibly a germline allele in the monoclonal B cells. The dominant band, however, appears rearranged.

Table 8.5. Utility of Gene Rearrangement Studies in Diagnostic Hematopathology

Peripheral T-cell lymphoma (PTCL) versus Hodgkin's disease: presence of a clonal T-cell rearrangement strongly favors PTCL diagnosis
Non-Hodgkin's lymphoma (NHL) versus reactive hyperplasia
Confirming clonality in a PTCL
Confirming clonality in surface immunoglobulin-negative NHL
Detection of recurrent/residual hematologic disease
Confirming clonality in Tγ lymphoproliferative disorder (TγLPD)

Table 8.6. Limitations of Gene Rearrangement Studies in Diagnostic Hematopathology

Detection of clonality in lymphoproliferations without clinical evidence of malignancy
Occasional cases of benign hyperplasia with clonal rearrangements
Fails to provide a clonal marker for Hodgkin's disease
Lack of lineage-specific rearrangements in acute leukemia.

chemotherapy or posttransplantation; and (*d*) evaluating "atypical" hyperplasias for the presence or absence of a clonal population when routine morphology or immunologic methods are equivocal (Table 8.5). The limitations of gene rearrangement studies must be considered equally when evaluating clinical specimens. Some of these limitations are listed in Table 8.6.

B-cell, Non-Hodgkin's Lymphoma. Molecular rearrangement studies in B-cell, non-Hodgkin's lymphoma have shown that 90 to 100% of cases will have demonstrable immunoglobulin heavy and light chain gene rearrangements (1, 31–36). Why haven't all B-cell lymphomas had detectable gene rearrangements? It is always possible that the tissue being studied does not contain malignant cells. As such, it is imperative to cut a frozen section of the study specimen for morphologic evaluation to confirm that a representative piece of the tumor is being evaluated. Secondly, there are rare B-cell, non-Hodgkin's lymphomas which may have rearrangements that comigrate with the germline band. These comigrating bands, however, can be distinguished from germline bands by using other restriction enzyme combinations. Thus, the use of at least two restriction enzymes for each sample has become a standard for evaluating clinical specimens.

As opposed to immunoglobulin heavy chain gene rearrangements, immunoglobulin light chain gene rearrangements have been considered highly specific for B cell processes. However, rare cases of T-cell malignancies with κ light chain gene rearrangements have been identified (37, 38). In spite of these rare reports, detection of an immunoglobulin light chain gene rearrangement is very strong evidence for a monoclonal B-cell process. If lineage determination by Southern blot analysis is a serious consideration, immunoglobulin light chain gene probes must be used and interpreted in conjunction with other laboratory and morphological data.

In most instances, immunophenotyping by frozen section studies or by flow cytometry will be sufficient to establish the monoclonal nature of a B-cell, non-Hodgkin's lymphoma. However, 10 to 20% of B-cell, non-Hodgkin's lymphoma cases will lack a convincing monoclonal surface immunoglobulin, thus complicating the immunophenotypic interpretation. Several studies have shown that rearrangements of the immunoglobulin heavy and light chain genes can be detected in nearly all of these surface immunoglobulin-negative cases, thus providing confirmatory evidence for a B-cell monoclonal process (33, 39, 40).

Nonlineage-specific gene rearrangements can be found in all types of lymphoreticular malignancies, with T-cell receptor rearrangements being found in some B lineage malignancies and immunoglobulin gene rearrangements found in some T-cell malignancies (41, 42). In the B-cell, non-Hodgkin's lymphomas, simultaneous T-cell receptor β chain and immunoglobulin gene rearrangements may be found in up to 10% of cases (29, 33–35, 42, 43). Studies that have looked at mRNA expression have consistently failed to show a complete Tβ transcript in those B-cell lymphomas. Most studies have not found rearrangements of the Tγ gene in B-cell, non-Hodgkin's lymphoma. The status of the Tδ gene in B-cell, non-Hodgkin's lymphoma has not been evaluated sufficiently at this time to draw any conclusion. These nonspecific T-cell rearrangements underline the importance of interpreting genotypic studies in the context of morphological and immunophenotypic data. If a sample has rearrangements of both immunoglobulin heavy and Tβ chain genes, the cellular lineage cannot be determined purely from the molecular studies. If, however, an immunoglobulin light chain gene rearrangement is found in addition to the aforementioned rearrangements, then the diagnosis of monoclonal B-cell process is very likely.

T-cell, Non-Hodgkin's Lymphoma. Molecular hybridization studies have also been useful in analyzing the peripheral T-cell lymphoma subgroup of non-Hodgkin's lymphoma. The diagnosis of T-cell lymphoma cannot always be made on morphological grounds and is often dependent on additional confirmatory evidence at the immunologic or molecular level. Immunologically, the evaluation of T-cell lymphomas has been made more difficult by the lack of a specific clonal marker. Several studies have demonstrated immunophenotypic aberrancy in T-cell lymphomas, that is, the lack of expression of one or more pan-T cell antigens; this has been used as indirect immunologic evidence of a T-cell malignancy (30). The ability to demonstrate clonal T-cell receptor gene rearrangements, however, provides for direct laboratory evidence of monoclonality and, thus, useful diagnostic information in this subset of lymphomas (44–47).

Most cases of peripheral T-cell lymphoma will exhibit rearrangements of the Tδ, Tγ, and Tβ chain genes; anywhere from 5 to 10% of peripheral T-cell lymphoma cases, however, will have germline T-cell receptor genes (30, 34, 40). Weiss and colleagues have published a series of seven such cases of peripheral T-cell lymphoma that lacked both Tβ and Tγ chain gene rearrangements (48). All seven of these patients had aberrant immunophenotypes and primarily expressed the CD2 (T11) antigen. Approximately 5 to 10% of peripheral T-cell lymphomas will have simultaneous rearrangement of the immunoglobulin heavy chain gene and a T-cell receptor gene (33, 42). To reiterate, these findings further confirm the necessity of evaluating and correlating all laboratory, morphological, and clinical data before a final diagnosis is determined.

Mycosis Fungoides/Sézary's Syndrome. Virtually all cases of mycosis fungoides and Sézary's syndrome will have rearrangement of the T-cell receptor genes (30, 35, 46). As with the other mature, T-cell malignancies, a low percentage of cases appear to have simultaneous rearrangement of both the Tβ gene and immunoglobulin heavy chain gene (49). From these data, it would appear that this subset of T-cell lymphomas has characteristics similar to the other T-cell lymphomas in that non–lineage-specific rearrangements can be identified.

Hodgkin's Disease. The origin and lineage of the Reed-Sternberg (R-S) cell and its variants in Hodgkin's disease have remained an enigma and a source of continuing controversy. Immunophenotypic studies have not been conclusive, and immunogenotypic studies have not clarified the issue. Estimates of gene rearrangement frequency in Hodgkin's disease have ranged from near zero to upwards of 75% of cases. However, to summarize the data from the most representative studies in the literature, T cell receptor gene rearrangements have been found in approximately 15% of cases, immunoglobulin heavy chain rearrangements in another 15% of cases, and immunoglobulin light chain rearrangements in 10% of cases (50–59). Only one case has been reported to have simultaneous T-cell receptor and immunoglobulin gene rearrangements.

Molecular analysis of Hodgkin's disease has been complicated by the usual paucity of neoplastic cells in the involved tissues. In fact, the number of R-S cells or R-S variants in a specimen is often less than 5%, falling at or below the sensitivity limits of the Southern blot technique. Some studies have tried to overcome this by analyzing specimens enriched in R-S cells or by studying cell culture lines derived from patients with Hodgkin's disease (56, 58, 60). Such studies have given some support to the postulate that Hodgkin's is a disease of lymphoid lineage. These findings are far from conclusive, and valid criticisms remain to be answered. Currently, gene rearrangement analysis may confuse rather than aid in the routine evaluation of Hodgkin's disease.

Ki-1 (CD30)-Positive, Large-Cell Anaplastic Lymphoma. Ki-1-positive, large-cell anaplastic lymphomas constitute a distinctive subset of non-Hodgkin's lymphoma and are defined by the presence of membrane-bound, Ki-1 (CD30) antigen on the neoplastic cells; a T cell immunophenotype has been identified in most cases (61–63). These lymphomas can occur in children or adults and usually present with skin lesions and/or peripheral lymphadenopathy. A histologic pattern of sinus infiltration is typical, with the neoplastic cells characteristically having abundant cytoplasm and pleomorphic nuclei.

Genotyping data from the three largest series of Ki-1 lymphomas support the concept that most of these tumors are of T cell origin (54, 63, 64). The majority of cases appear to exhibit T-cell receptor β chain gene rearrangements; estimates of the frequency of Tβ rearrangements range from 50 to 70% of cases in these studies. Correlation of genotype and immunophenotype is by no means perfect, however, as some cases with T cell immunophenotypes have both T-cell receptor and immunoglobulin heavy chain gene rearrangements. Occasionally, some Ki-1-positive large cell, anaplastic lymphomas have had a B cell immunophenotype with either immunoglobulin and/or Tβ gene rearrangements. Finally, up to one-third of Ki-1-positive lymphomas have been reported to have germline T-cell receptor and immunoglobulin gene configurations, suggesting the possibility that some cases may either be of early lymphoid or even nonlymphoid origin (54).

True Histiocytic Lymphoma/Malignant Histiocytosis. True histiocytic lymphomas are an uncommon type of non-Hodgkin's lymphoma composed of malignant cells with enzymatic and immunologic features of histiocytes. Three of seven well-documented cases of true histiocytic lymphoma have had T-cell receptor and/or immunoglobulin gene rearrangements, again emphasizing the point that molecular studies are sensitive indicators of clonality, but are not specific indicators of cellular lineage (65). Other studies have also reported histiocytic neoplasms with rearrangements of the Tβ gene (66); the findings in these studies suggest two possibilities: first, these cases might truly represent clonal T or B cell processes, or alternatively, certain subsets of the histiocytic/reticulum cell system are inherently capable of rearranging T cell and/or immunoglobulin chain genes. This information, together with the immunophenotypic data, strongly support the argument that cells of nonlymphoid origin are capable of rearranging lymphoid genes, but most likely do so in a nonproductive fashion.

Benign Lymphoid Hyperplasia. Gene rearrangement techniques have been utilized by various investigators who have examined histologically borderline lymphoid proliferations for evidence of monoclonality. Knowles and colleagues evaluated 16 extranodal, extracutaneous lymphoid hyperplasias occurring in the ocular region, salivary gland, breast, and thyroid. All cases were considered morphologically benign (67). All 16 cases had demonstrable rearrangements of the immunoglobulin genes. However, only two of the 16 progressed to bona fide malignant lymphomas. In a similar fashion, Wood and others evaluated 14 cases of cutaneous lymphoid hyperplasia for immunoglobulin rearrangements (68). Five of these 14 cases had such rearrangements, but only one progressed to a bona fide malignant lymphoma. Both of these studies are classic examples of how gene rearrangement studies offer exquisite sensitivity in the detection of monoclonality. However, from that same perspective, it must be realized that monoclonality in these cases did not always equate with the presence of malignancy or even the potential development of a clinically malignant process. These studies again emphasize the necessity of interpreting molecular rearrangement studies in the context of clinical findings, morphological features, and immunologic data. As our level of sensitivity in detecting clonality increases, we must modify our concept of clonality and malignancy. It is no longer safe to assume that monoclonality equates with clinical malignancy.

Acute Leukemia

Analysis of the immunoglobulin and T-cell receptor genes in the acute leukemias has provided a tremendous amount of data concerning the development of both normal lymphoid precursor cells and their leukemic counterparts. The initial studies using this technology were quite optimistic that gene rearrangement studies would lead to a new gold standard in the clinical evaluation of acute leukemia (34, 35, 44, 69). However, as with most new diagnostic tests, further studies have tempered this enthusiasm.

B-Lineage, Acute Lymphoblastic Leukemia. The B-lineage acute lymphoblastic leukemias (ALL) provide a classic example of both the sensitivity of gene rearrangement studies and the lack of absolute lineage specificity. Greater than 95% of all B-lineage ALL will have rearrangements of the immunoglobulin heavy chain gene, indicating that the heavy chain rearrangement occurs shortly after a cell becomes committed to the B-cell lineage (41, 70). Immunoglobulin light chain gene rearrangement appears to occur in the latter period of pre-B cell development, with approximately 30 to 40% of B-lineage ALL having rearranged light chain genes.

In addition to the immunoglobulin rearrangements, simultaneous T-cell receptor gene rearrangements can be identified in B-lineage ALL. The Tβ gene, as shown in multiple studies, may be rearranged in up to 20% of B-lineage ALL; Tγ gene rearrangements are found in 40 to 50% of B-lineage ALL cases (41, 42, 70). Interestingly, the Tγ gene rearrangements in B-lineage ALL almost exclusively involve the $C\gamma_1$ locus as opposed to predominant $C\gamma_2$ involvement in T cell ALL. Tδ rearrangements are also frequently found in B-lineage ALL (71). These non–lineage-specific rearrangements were initially quite puzzling. However, it is now felt that a putative "recombinase" process is active during early lymphoid development. It is theorized that this recombinase will initially "latch on" to any gene with the appropriate structure, like the immunoglobulin or T-cell receptor genes, and begin the D-J or V-J rearrangement process (72). An important question that has not been answered relates to the functionality of normal B cells that have these nonspecific rearrangements. Goorha and colleagues (73) have suggested, based on a detailed molecular and immunologic study, that the majority of functional B-cells are derived from cells that have immunoglobulin gene rearrangements, but lack any T-cell receptor gene rearrangements.

T-cell, Acute Lymphoblastic Leukemia. Molecular studies have shown similar findings in T-cell ALL. The great majority of T-ALL have rearrangements of the Tδ, Tγ, and Tβ genes (30, 47, 71, 74). Tγ or Tδ rearrangements alone may be found in some cases; in fact, Tδ together with Tγ rearrangements may be the earliest molecular markers of T-cell lineage (75). T-cell ALL that express the γ/δ protein receptor have also been identified (76). These cases have rearrangements of the Tγ and Tδ genes without rearrangements of the Tβ gene. As mentioned earlier, rearrangements involving the Tγ gene preferentially involve the $C\gamma_2$ locus in T-ALL (76a), supporting the concept that the locus of rearrangement may be predetermined by how the cell has been "programmed." Non–lineage-specific rearrangements can also be identified in T-ALL, although not as frequently as in β-lineage ALL. The immunoglobulin heavy chain gene is rearranged in approximately 10 to 20% of T-ALL (41, 42, 77). A rearranged light chain gene, however, is virtually diagnostic of a B-cell process; a single case has been reported of a κ gene rearrangement in a T-cell ALL (38). A small subset of early prethymic T cells may lack rearrangements of any of the T-cell receptor genes; these cells characteristically express a very early immunophenotype, including CD7, cytoplasmic CD3, and occasionally CD5 and/or CD2.

Infant Acute Lymphoblastic Leukemia. Gene rearrangements in infant ALL have also provided some interesting data. These ALL are immunophenotypically at a very early stage of lymphoid development and frequently have an 11q23 chromosomal translocation that may characterize a stem cell-like proliferation. These cases of ALL will occasionally lack any lymphoid gene rearrangements. In those 11q23 cases with rearrangements, immunoglobulin light chain gene rearrangements are usually absent, and they usually lack the non–lineage-specific rearrangements that have characterized typical childhood ALL (78–80). Gene rearrangement studies, in conjunction with immunophenotyping data, suggest that infant ALL cases arise very early in lymphoid development.

In summary, gene rearrangement analysis of ALL has provided us with a tremendous amount of data about how lymphoid cells develop. However, utilization of this technique as a clinical diagnostic tool has been limited by its lack of absolute lineage-specificity. As with any diagnostic modality, the information gleaned from molecular studies must be correlated with clinical, morphological, and immunologic data.

Acute Myelogenous Leukemia. The issue of immunoglobulin and T-cell receptor gene rearrangements in acute myeloid leukemia (AML) is fraught with controversy. Estimates of the frequency of gene rearrangements in AML vary widely, from extremes of approximately 0 to 70% (81–87). In most series, however, it would appear that immunoglobulin and T-cell receptor gene rearrangements occur in approximately 5 to 10% of AML. The wide variation in results raises questions about the diagnostic criteria used to classify the leukemias in these studies. A corollary of these findings has been the frequent presence of gene rearrangements in cases of terminal deoxynucleotidyl transferase (TdT)-positive AML (84, 85, 87). These results suggest that this TdT activity might be associated with an active, cellular recombination process resulting in rearranged, lymphoid-associated genes. In any case, it is apparent that much remains to be learned about the lymphoid gene rearrangements in AML. As these studies indicate, the presence of lymphoid gene rearrangements in an acute leukemia is by no means definitive in establishing a lymphoid lineage.

Chronic Lymphoproliferative Disorders

Chronic Lymphocytic Leukemia. Chronic lymphocytic leukemia (CLL) is a hematopoietic disorder that usually does not create a diagnostic dilemma and is easily recognized morphologically and clinically. Immunophenotyping studies are quite useful in this disorder and have shown that CLL has a characteristic staining pattern of weak, monoclonal surface immunoglobulin, expression of pan-B cell markers, and staining with CD5, an otherwise typical pan-T cell marker. At the genotypic level, CLL will almost uniformly have rearrangements of the immunoglobulin heavy and light chain genes, as would be expected for a mature B-cell malignancy (88, 89). $T\beta$ gene rearrangements can be found, however, in fewer than 10% of B-CLL cases; $T\gamma$ gene rearrangements have not been identified in CLL. The $T\beta$ rearrangements appear to be nonproductive and lead to a truncated RNA transcript.

T-γ Lymphoproliferative Disorder. Gene rearrangement and flow cytometric studies in T-γ lymphoproliferative disorder (TγLPD), sometimes called large granular lymphocytosis, have shown that probably two general subsets exist both genotypically and immunophenotypically. Immunophenotypic expression of CD2, CD3, CD8, and CD57 (Leu 7) has characterized the most common group of TγLPD. These cells correspond to the cytotoxic/suppressor subset of T cells and exhibit rearrangements of the $T\beta$ and $T\gamma$ genes in 80 to 90% of cases (90–92). Gene rearrangement studies are quite useful in confirming the clonal nature of this disorder and can be used to differentiate this subset of TγLPD from a benign, reactive condition. The remaining cases of TγLPD have what some have called a "true" natural killer cell immunophenotype with expression of CD2, CD16, and CD56 (NKH-1), while lacking CD3, CD8, and CD57. This group of granular lymphocytes typically lacks any rearrangements of the $T\beta$ or $T\gamma$ genes (91, 92). Clinically, both subsets of TγLPD are characterized by an indolent course and seldom progress to a full-blown "malignancy." Correlation with immunophenotyping is essential; if a true NK immunophenotype is found, then finding a germline T cell receptor gene does not rule out a TγLPD.

Hairy Cell Leukemia. The cell of origin in hairy cell leukemia (HCL) remained an enigma for many years. Some laboratory evidence, such as latex bead phagocytic activity, glass adherence, and ultrastructural morphology, favored a monocyte-derived process. Monoclonal antibody studies, however, have since showed monoclonal surface immunoglobulin expression by these leukemic cells; this finding strongly supported the B-lymphocyte origin of HCL (93). Molecular gene rearrangement studies have also confirmed its B-cell origin, with immunoglobulin heavy and light chain gene rearrangements present in virtually all cases of HCL (94–97). Only a few cases have had simultaneous rearrangement of the Tβ gene. The occasional finding of a T-cell receptor rearrangement in HCL should not be too surprising given the large number of other B-cell malignancies that have T-cell gene rearrangements.

Multiple Myeloma. Multiple myeloma has long been known to be a monoclonal B-cell process by serum protein and immunoelectrophoresis studies. All cases of multiple myeloma that have been studied have exhibited immunoglobulin heavy and light chain gene rearrangements (98). A single case of an IgA-positive multiple myeloma with simultaneous rearrangement of the Tβ gene has been reported. No Tβ transcript could be detected by RNA studies, indicating that this was most likely a nonproductive D-J rearrangement of the Tβ locus.

Clonal Lymphoproliferations without Clinical Evidence of Malignancy

The detection of clonality in lymphoproliferative disorders was once tantamount to the diagnosis of malignancy. It is now clear, however, that not all processes with a monoclonal population are clinically progressive diseases. Monoclonal gammopathy of undetermined significance (MGUS) is a classic example of a monoclonal disease that seldom progresses to its malignant counterpart, multiple myeloma. Molecular genetic analysis is the most recent and advanced approach for the assessment of clonality in hematopoietic disorders. With the advent of these studies, several diseases considered to be clinically benign have exhibited clonal gene rearrangements.

Sjögren's Disease. One of the first "borderline" entities studied by molecular gene rearrangement analysis was the benign lymphoepithelial lesion associated with Sjögren's disease. Fishleder and coworkers described clonal rearrangements of the immunoglobulin genes in 10 patients with Sjögren's disease despite its relatively benign clinical course (99). These results suggested that clonality at the molecular level could not always be equated with a malignant clinical course.

Dermatologic Disorders. Clonal T-cell rearrangements have been described in the majority of patients with lymphomatoid papulosis (100, 101); clinically, less than one-fourth of patients with this disease progress to malignant lymphoma. Several other dermatologic conditions have also been associated with T-cell receptor gene rearrangements. Pityriasis lichenoides et varioliformis acuta (PLEVA or Mucha-Habermann disease) (102), erythrodermic follicular mucinosis (103), granulomatous slack skin (104), and pagetoid reticulosis (Woringer-Kolopp disease) (105) are all relatively uncommon skin disorders that have been associated with T-cell, β-chain gene rearrangements. These findings raise the possibility that these conditions may in fact be unusual variants of mycosis fungoides from the outset. This will remain unknown until larger numbers of these dermatologic variants are studied by immunologic and molecular techniques.

Castleman's Disease. Molecular studies of the classic, hyaline-vascular variant of Castleman's disease have shown no gene rearrangements. However, the majority of cases of Castleman's disease with widespread, systemic disease have demonstrated immunoglobulin gene rearrangements; some have had simultaneous T-cell receptor gene rearrangements (106, 107). Interestingly, some of these cases with rearrangements also have had evidence of incorporated Epstein-Barr virus (EBV) genomes at the molecular level (106). Clinically, this disorder is felt to be a nonmalignant process, with only a small number of patients subsequently developing malignant lymphoma. Based on current information, one may speculate that these patients have some type of an immunologic deficit. If so, it is conceivable that in patients with Castleman's disease, clonal proliferations of EBV-infected B-cells could escape immunologic detection and become "immortalized," yet not represent truly malignant clones.

HIV-Lymphadenopathy. Clonal rearrangements of immunoglobulin genes have been detected in about 20% of morphologically benign lymph nodes from patients with HIV-lymphadenopathy syndrome (108). It is likely that many of these cases have ongoing viral-associated proliferations, such as associated with EBV, as a result of the underlying deficient immune response. The abnormal immune response could allow an EBV-infected cell to "escape" normal cellular control and potentially lead to cellular transformation and a clonal proliferation.

Angioimmunoblastic Lymphadenopathy with Dysproteinemia (AILD). AILD is a lymphoproliferative disorder of uncertain etiology that may progress to a non-Hodgkin's lymphoma. Genotypic analysis of AILD has identified clonal Tβ rearrangements in about 70% of cases (109–112). The rearranged bands in these cases are typically much fainter in intensity than the germline band, suggesting that the clonal population of cells accounts for only a small percentage of the overall cellular content. Frizzera (113) has summarized these findings by concluding that AILD probably consists of multiple subtypes including (*a*) cases having clonal T-cell populations and histologic features consistent with peripheral T-cell lymphoma; (*b*) cases that lack detectable rearrangements, favoring the existence of a nonmalignant AILD proliferation; and (*c*) cases with or without rearrangements that are clinically, morphologically, and immunologically intermediate between the benign and malignant AILD category. Further prospective studies will be needed to determine whether or not these molecular studies, in combination with other laboratory findings, have important clinical relevance in AILD.

Conclusion. The ability to detect clonal rearrangements of genes has appreciably increased the ability to find cellular clonal proliferations. All the disorders that we have described in this section are clinically borderline disorders, which are not uniformly considered to be malignant. Indeed, some patients with the above diseases do progress into clearly malignant processes. However, the mere presence of clonal, rearranged bands in a lymphoproliferative process may not have any clinical significance. If a clonal gene rearrangement can be demonstrated in a morphologically or clinically benign situation, then it is in the best interest of the patient that this not be interpreted as malignancy. Instead, the patient should be followed at close intervals until the biology of the particular lesion has declared itself as clinically benign or malignant. Prospective studies, correlating clinical data, immunologic findings, cytogenetic data, and molecular rearrangement studies, are all needed to appropriately evaluate the biological significance of clonal gene rearrangements in these disorders.

Detection of Minimal or Residual Disease by Gene Rearrangement Analysis

The detection of minimal or residual disease in hematologic disorders has typically been based on a combination of morphologic and immunologic findings. The ability of Southern blot hybridization studies to detect small numbers of clonal cells has enabled patients to be evaluated for either minimal disease or residual disease following chemotherapy or bone marrow transplantation. Some studies have utilized immunoglobulin gene rearrangement analysis for the evaluation of minimal disease in the peripheral blood of patients with non-Hodgkin's lymphomas (114, 115). All these studies have demonstrated the ability of molecular studies to detect small clonal populations and suggest that rearrangements may be a more sensitive indicator of clonality than either morphology or immunophenotyping. It is essential in all these studies that the rearrangements in the original diagnostic specimens be well characterized so as to allow for accurate comparison of follow-up material.

MISCELLANEOUS APPLICATIONS OF MOLECULAR DIAGNOSTIC TECHNIQUES IN HEMATOLOGIC DISEASE

Restriction Fragment Length Polymorphism Analysis in Bone Marrow Transplant Patients

Bone marrow transplantation has become an important therapeutic option for numerous hematologic disorders and malignancies. Bone marrow transplants may be either autologous or allogeneic, depending on the underlying malignancy and/or availability of bone marrow donors. In both types of transplants, the patient undergoes an intensive course of chemotherapy and/or radiotherapy, which aim to ablate the bone marrow and the malignant cells; normal bone marrow is then infused into the patient, which should engraft in the host marrow. Autologous transplants involve reinfusing the patient's own previously harvested bone marrow. Allogeneic bone marrow transplantations are commonly used in patients with acute or chronic leukemias who have failed standard therapy or are at high risk for relapse. Allogeneic transplantation involves ablating the patient's marrow, followed by infusion of normal donor bone marrow from an HLA-matched individual, usually a sibling of the patient. This latter procedure involves complex interactions between the donor and host immune systems and leads to a cascade of events posttransplantation in which the donor cells eventually become engrafted. Although the bulk of the host's tumor cells are destroyed in the pretransplantation ablative therapy, recent studies have shown that donor T lymphocytes have an important role in suppressing the few host tumor cells that may remain and, thus, appear to be important in preventing recurrence of malignancy.

Analysis of this posttransplantation system for the presence of engraftment or recurrence of disease is obviously critical in determining whether the transplant has been a success. Morphology has been the quickest and perhaps easiest method to evaluate a patient for recurrence of disease. However, morphological analysis has a low sensitivity and cannot determine whether differentiating marrow cells are of host or donor origin based on morphology. Chromosomal karyotyping, red cell antigen determination, and HLA-typing have also been used as markers of engraftment. However, because of the profound leukopenia, transfusion dependence, and marked immunologic suppression commonly found in these patients, these assays have not been routinely utilized in post–bone marrow transplant patients.

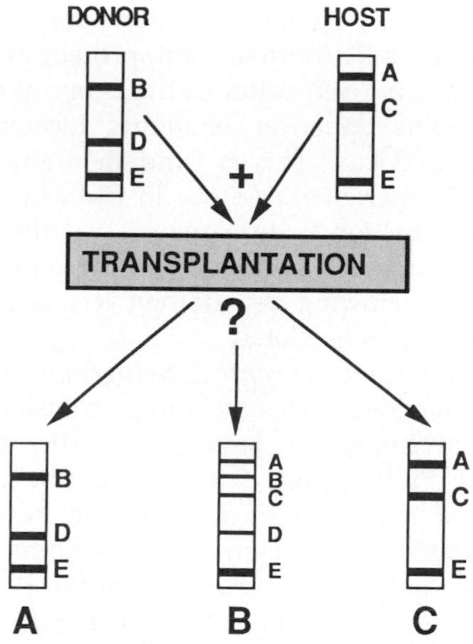

Figure 8.14. Southern blot hybridization schematic of an RFLP study in a bone marrow transplant patient. An appropriate probe/restriction enzyme combination is chosen, which allows for the unique distinction between the donor and host DNA. As depicted in this schematic, the donor and host both have two unique bands (donor: bands *B* and *D*; host: bands *A* and *C*), while sharing a single common band (*E*). Following transplantation, one of three possible scenarios may be detected by Southern blot hybridization studies using the same pretransplant RFLP probe/enzyme combination. **A**, The host bone marrow cells may have a donor RFLP pattern, consistent with total engraftment of donor cells. **B**, The host contains a chimeric population of both donor and host cells, indicating the presence of at least some host cells. **C**, The host may have an RFLP pattern identical to the original host configuration, consistent with the lack of any donor engraftment.

The use of molecular genetic probes in post–bone marrow transplant patients has become the new standard in evaluating these patients for evidence of engraftment or early recurrence of disease. These molecular studies are based on finding DNA restriction fragment length polymorphisms (RFLPs). Among different individuals, segments of DNA, or restriction fragments, can be detected that differ in length because of either mutations in restriction enzyme cleavage sites or variations in the length of DNA between such enzymatic sites as the result of insertions and/or deletions; these variations are quite normal and are referred to as RFLPs. RFLPs become inherited as part of an individual's DNA and constitute a reliable set of markers that are characteristic of a particular individual and are not reflective of any underlying disease process. RFLP analysis can be performed on all types of nucleated hematopoietic cells and, in contrast to cytogenetics, does not require dividing cells. The success of such genotypic analysis depends solely on finding informative DNA polymorphisms that distinguish the host from the donor, i.e., detecting distinctly different DNA fragments when using the same DNA probe and enzyme combination (Fig. 8.14). The likelihood that a particular probe will reveal distinct alleles depends totally on the frequency of the allelic distribution in the overall population. One particularly useful probe recognizes distinct DNA segments from the Y chromosome and can be used to detect the host, male genotypic pattern in sex mismatched (female-to-male) transplantation cases.

From a practical standpoint, the first step in this RFLP analysis involves extracting DNA from the donor and patient (host) prior to transplantation. Various restriction endonucleases are used to digest the DNA and then, following Southern blot transfer, are hybridized with a variety of probes that recognize highly polymorphic DNA sites; a Y chromosome-specific probe would also be used in sex-mismatched (female-to-male) cases. After hybridization and autoradiography, a restriction endonuclease/probe combination is chosen that detects DNA fragments that are distinctly different in the donor as compared with the host. In cases where host and donor cells are both present, rough quantification of host and donor components can be accomplished based on the relative intensity of the hybridization bands. Using such an analysis, the molecular diagnostics laboratory is capable of distinguishing (*a*) patients with stable engraftment of donor cells; (*b*) patients with chimeric donor and host cell populations, which may be associated with either a stable clinical condition or recurrence of disease; and (*c*) patients with host cells only, consistent with the lack of any donor engraftment (Fig. 8.14). The significance of finding small chimeric populations in clinically stable patients is unknown and may not necessarily herald the recurrence of disease.

Oncogenes in the Diagnosis of Hematopoietic Malignancies

The discovery of the Philadelphia chromosome in patients with chronic myelogenous leukemia (CML) by Nowell and Hungerford in 1960 heralded the beginning of modern-day cytogenetics (116). This finding led to the hypothesis that specific chromosomal abnormalities are associated with, and perhaps even responsible for, malignant transformation. Developments during the 1980s in the field of molecular biology led to the realization that these cytogenetic translocations involved genes responsible for the oncogenesis of these tumors. An essential part of these discoveries was the identification and characterization of cellular protooncogenes at the sites of various chromosomal breakpoints. These protooncogenes exhibit significant homology to retroviruses; these retroviruses are capable of tumor induction in

Table 8.7. Oncogenes in the Diagnosis of Hematopoietic Malignancies

Chronic Myelogenous Leukemia: t(9;22)(q34;q11)	
	9q34: *c-abl*
	22q11: BCR (*phl*)
Acute Lymphocytic Leukemia: t(9;22)(q34;q11)-(5-20% of cases)	
	9q34; *c-abl*
	22q11: BCR (*phl*)
Burkitt's Lymphoma/Leukemia: t(8;14)(q24;q32)/t(2;8)(p12;q24)/t(8;22)(q24;q11)	
	8q24: *c-myc*
	14q32: Ig heavy chain locus
	2p12: κ Ig light chain locus
	22q11:λ Ig light chain locus
Intermediate Differentiated Lymphoma/Chronic Lymphocytic Leukemia/Small Lymphocytic Lymphoma (some): t(11;14)(q13;q32)	
	11q13: *bcl-1* gene
	14q32: Ig heavy chain locus
Follicular Center Cell Lymphomas: t(14;18)(q32;q21)	
	14q32: Ig heavy chain locus
	18q21: *bcl-2* gene

experimental models. Subsequent observations that these protooncogenes were located at sites of tumor-specific chromosomal translocations demonstrated that these protooncogenes were clearly associated with, if not responsible for, the respective hematopoietic neoplasms.

Cytogenetic studies of hematopoietic malignancies have demonstrated a myriad of reciprocal translocations, inversions, deletions, insertions, and duplications that are associated with unique subtypes of leukemia or lymphoma. Currently, however, only a few chromosomal translocations have been clearly elucidated at the molecular level (Table 8.7); the actual molecular mechanisms of tumorigenesis for most chromosomal translocations have not yet been determined. It is likely that many of these translocations will be characterized in the near future.

Two different mechanisms of oncogenic activation have been commonly described in leukemias and lymphomas. These prototypes have enhanced our understanding of tumorigenesis and have led to the development of diagnostic applications for hematologic diseases. The first prototype is exemplified by the t(9;22)(q34;q11) of chronic myelogenous leukemia (CML), involving the *c-abl* oncogene on chromosome 9q34 and the *BCR* (or *phl*) gene on chromosome 22q11. In this translocation, a chimeric *bcr-abl* gene is formed which leads to an abnormal *bcr-abl* fusion protein. The second oncogenic prototype is represented by the t(8;14)(q24;q34) found in Burkitt's lymphoma/leukemia and, occasionally, in other B cell, non-Hodgkin's lymphomas. In this scenario, the *c-myc* oncogene on chromosome 8q24 becomes juxtaposed to the immunoglobulin heavy chain gene locus at chromosome 14q32. By physically moving these two genes together, the translocation leads to deregulation of the normal *c-myc* protein production; this results from activation of the *c-myc* gene by immunoglobulin enhancer elements located in the heavy chain locus. This is fundamentally different from the chimeric *bcr-abl* story in CML in that *c-myc* protein production is deregulated, yet the molecule remains structurally normal. With these examples as a basis, the following hematologic translocations are described in greater detail.

t(9;22)(q34;q11): Chronic Myelogenous Leukemia. The characteristic chromosomal translocation in chronic myelogenous leukemia (CML) has been called the Philadelphia chromosome (Ph′). The Ph′ consists of a reciprocal translocation between the *c-abl* protooncogene region of chromosome 9q34 and the breakpoint cluster region (*bcr*) of the *BCR* (or *phl*) oncogene of chromosome 22q11 (Fig. 8.15*A-B*). This chromosomal marker is found in the leukemic cells of greater than 95% of patients with CML, approximately 25% of adults with acute lymphocytic leukemia (ALL), about 5% of childhood ALL patients, and less than 1% of acute myelogenous leukemia (AML) patients.

The translocation breakpoint in CML almost invariably lies within a 5.8-kb region of the *BCR* (or *phl*) gene; this region has been termed *bcr*. Detailed mapping of the breakpoints in the *c-abl* gene has shown that virtually all translocations occur 5′ of the *c-abl* exon 2; the actual molecular breakpoint varies tremendously from case to case and is spread over a 100-kb segment of the 5′ region. The majority of *bcr* breakpoints in Ph′-positive CML cases are between either exons 2 and 3 or exons 3 and 4; only rare cases of CML have breakpoints between exons 1 and 2 or 3′ of the *bcr* region. Transcription of the chimeric *bcr-abl* gene in CML gives rise to an 8.5-kb mRNA, consisting of *bcr* sequences at the 5′ end and *abl* sequences at the 3′ end. Compared with the normal *c-abl* gene product of 145 kd, the fusion *bcr-abl* protein is 210 kd and has elevated tyrosine kinase activity.

Southern Blot Studies for bcr-abl. Since this translocation consistently involves a remarkably narrow region of chromosome 22, DNA hybridization studies were developed to detect rearrangements into the *bcr* locus. These gene probe studies have been remarkably successful in CML patients due to the *bcr-abl* rearrangement phenomenon. In these probe studies, the translocation of the *c-abl* oncogene into the *bcr* region disrupts a restriction enzyme site on the normal chromosome 22, thus changing the normal germline banding pattern of the *bcr* locus (Fig. 8.15*C-D*). Several clinical studies have shown that 90 to 95% of CML patients will exhibit rearrangement of the *bcr* region. These studies have required the use of multiple restriction enzymes and occasionally more than a single probe because of the occasional failure of the most commonly used 1.2-kb, *Hind*III/*Bgl*II probe to detect rearrangements in CML cells. This failure to detect a rearrangement may be due to (*a*) rearrangements occurring outside the region covered by the particular enzyme-probe combination; (*b*) *bcr-abl* rearrangements occurring within the enzyme-probe region, but giving rise to DNA fragments that comigrate with the germline DNA band; or (*c*) deletion of the *bcr-abl* region which is homologous to the probe used, despite the successful rearrangement of *bcr-abl*. This latter situation is the most likely explanation for many of the cases that have not had detectable rearrangements with the 1.2-kb, *Hind*III/*Bgl*II probe.

Several studies have attempted to correlate the distribution of *bcr* breakpoints with clinical outcome. Some investigators have looked for possible differences in breakpoint locations between CML in chronic phase and CML in blast crisis. Several studies have suggested that the more aggressive CML cases are more likely to have 3′ involvement of the *bcr* region; likewise, 3′ breakpoints have been more frequently identified in CML in blast crisis. Nonetheless, the results from these studies are preliminary at the time of this writing and cannot be used for providing reliable prognostic information.

t(9;22)(q34;q11): Acute Lymphoblastic Leukemia. The biological relationship between CML and Ph′-positive ALL has been an enigma for many years. Questions have been raised as to whether these are two distinct diseases or just different manifestations of the same disease. Molecular studies have been very helpful in this regard and have provided important data concerning the similarities and differences between CML and Ph′-positive ALL. Molecular analysis of Ph′-positive ALL has revealed two basic types of rearrangements, both involving the *BCR* (or *phl*) and *c-abl* genes. Approximately one-half of cases have exhibited a translocation identical to that found in patients with CML. In other words, these patients have a translocation of *c-abl* into the 5.8-kb *bcr* region, followed by transcription of an 8.5 kb mRNA and synthesis of a 210-kd phosphoprotein. Since the DNA breakpoint is the same as seen in patients with CML, this group of ALL patients can be analyzed successfully with the same DNA hybridization procedure described above for CML.

The second group of Ph′-positive ALL, however, has a DNA translocation into an entirely different region of the *BCR* (or *phl*) gene. This second breakpoint region, which has been tentatively termed *bcr-2*, is located within a 10-kb region of the first 5′ intron of the *BCR* (or *phl*) gene. This 5′ rearrangement leads to the expression of a 7.0-kb chimeric mRNA and a resulting 190-kd phosphoprotein with enhanced tyrosine kinase activity. The 190-kd and 210-kd fusion proteins differ only in the amount of *BCR*-derived sequences. It is not known whether these two proteins have different functions or different levels of functional activity in the leukemic process. Since the *bcr-2* DNA breakpoint is outside the *bcr-1* region, DNA hybridization studies with a *bcr-1* probe (as used for CML cases) will not be successful. Moreover, DNA hybridization studies have been fraught with difficulties in analyzing this 5′ breakpoint region because of the variable location of breakpoints within this large intron area.

PCR Studies for bcr-abl. The newest molecular methodology to be adapted to the detection of *BCR* rearrangements is the polymerase chain reaction (PCR). The PCR is a technique that uses a DNA polymerase to amplify short segments of either DNA or cDNA. Because the breakpoint on chromosome 9 (*c-abl* oncogene) in patients with the Ph′ may occur over a 100-kb region, PCR detection based on DNA has not been successful as PCR is best suited to amplify segments less than 2 kb. This problem, however, has been easily overcome in CML by using mRNA as the template for PCR. The *bcr-abl* mRNA encompasses a much shorter molecular distance and gives a very consistent *bcr-abl* junction. The specimen is readied for PCR amplification by converting the *bcr-abl* mRNA to cDNA by a reverse transcriptase reaction. With the use of appropriate oligonucleotide primers, one can amplify the *bcr-abl* segment and then determine which exon of the *bcr* region is involved in the 9;22 translocation (Fig. 8.16). Preliminary studies have also successfully used PCR to detect the 5′ *bcr-abl* translocations seen in Ph′-positive ALL. Since this translocation occurs in the first 5′ intron, the first exon of the *BCR* gene will always be translocated next to the second exon of the *c-abl* gene. This consistent translocation makes it amenable for PCR studies based on an mRNA template.

Overall, these PCR studies have been quite successful in detecting the *bcr-abl* translocation for diagnostic purposes in patients with CML or Ph′-positive ALL. Though these PCR studies and the DNA hybridization studies previously described are quite effective in detecting the *bcr-abl* translocation, traditional cytogenetic studies still remain the gold standard. Cytogenetic studies, in addition to detecting the Ph′, can also identify other karyotypic abnormalities that have prognostic importance in these patients. These molecular studies are best utilized for evaluating (*a*) those cases suspected of being CML, but lacking a Ph′ (the so-called Ph′-negative CML);

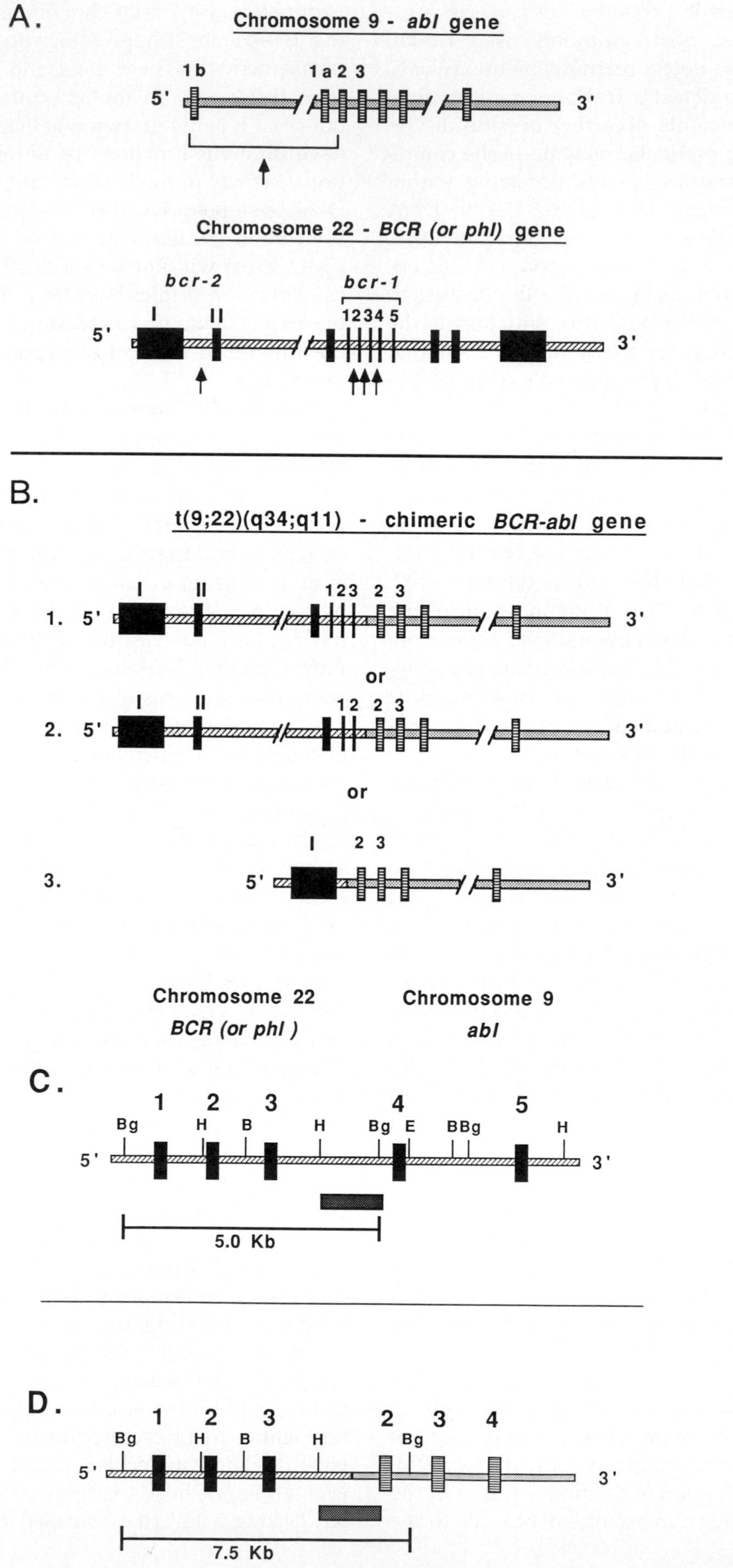
A.
Chromosome 9 - abl gene
1b
1a 2 3
5'
3'
Chromosome 22 - BCR (or phl) gene
bcr-2
bcr-1
I
II
1 2 3 4 5
5'
3'
B.
t(9;22)(q34;q11) - chimeric BCR-abl gene
1.
I
II
1 2 3
2
3
5'
3'
or
2.
I
II
1 2
2
3
5'
3'
or
3.
I
2
3
5'
3'
Chromosome 22
BCR (or phl)
Chromosome 9
abl
C.
1
2
3
4
5
Bg
H
B
H
Bg
E
BBg
H
5'
3'
5.0 Kb
D.
1
2
3
2
3
4
Bg
H
B
H
Bg
5'
3'
7.5 Kb

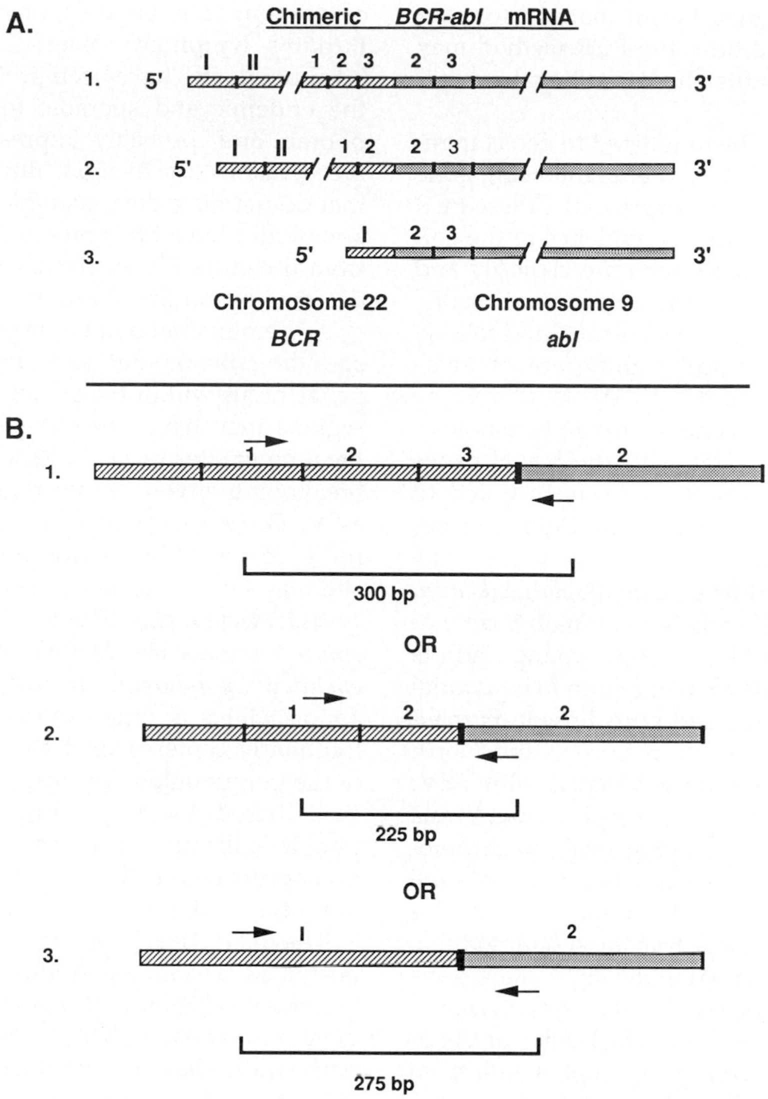

Figure 8.16. Gene structure of the chimeric *BCR-abl* mRNA and polymerase chain reaction (PCR) analysis. (See Figure 8.15 for explanation of characters.) **A**, (1) and (2) represent the *bcr-abl* mRNA that is formed after translocation into *bcr-1*. (3) represents translocation of *c-abl* into the 5′ intron (*bcr-2*) that is associated with Philadelphia chromosome-positive ALL. **B**, Schematic of PCR analysis for *BCR-abl* mRNA. The horizontal arrows represent the locations for oligonucleotide primers. (1) and (2). A 300-bp fragment is amplified if an exon 3 (*bcr-1*) rearrangement has occurred or a 225-bp is amplified if an exon 2 (*bcr-1*) rearrangement has occurred. (3) PCR amplification of a 5′ intron (*bcr-2*)-*abl* translocation.

Figure 8.15. Molecular gene structure and schematic of the Philadelphia chromosome. The drawings do not accurately reflect distances and are drawn for schematic purposes only. **A**, Structure of the normal chromosome 9, *c-abl* protooncogene, and chromosome 22, the *BCR* or *phl* gene. Boxes represent exons. Arrows indicate breakpoint regions. The large bracket with the arrow at the *c-abl* gene represents a 100-kb region where virtually all translocations occur. *bcr-1* and *bcr-2* represent the breakpoint cluster regions in the *BCR* gene. Numbers and roman numerals indicate the given nomenclature for the *abl* and *BCR* exons. **B**, As a result of the reciprocal translocation between chromosome 9 and chromosome 22, a chimeric *BCR-abl* gene is formed. (1) and (2) represent over 95% of the translocations occurring in the *bcr-1* region with breakpoints occurring between exons 3 and 4 or exons 2 and 3, respectively; (3) represents the reciprocal translocation of chromosome 9 into the first 5′ intron (*bcr-2*) of the *BCR* gene. **C**, The germline configuration of the *bcr-1* region (Bg = *Bgl*II restriction enzyme) shows a 5.0-kb, *Bgl*II fragment with the *bcr* probe. **D**, Rearrangement of *c-abl* into the *bcr* region replaces the 3′ *Bgl*II restriction enzyme site, leading to the formation of a larger, 7.5-kb band.

or (*b*) those cases with insufficient material for routine cytogenetics. In addition, the PCR method may provide more rapid results than traditional cytogenetic studies.

PCR studies have also been utilized to detect minimal residual disease in CML patients following bone marrow transplantation. Not surprisingly, these PCR studies have been able to detect evidence of the chimeric *bcr-abl* gene in patients who are clinically and morphologically engrafted without evidence of disease. Because these studies are so recent, and follow-up time is short, the clinical significance of these findings is not yet known.

The revolution of oncogene testing in hematology was ignited by these studies with the *bcr-abl* genes (117–120). These initial studies subsequently led to further investigations of other translocations in hematologic malignancies.

t(8;14)(q24;q32): Burkitt's Lymphoma/Leukemia. Burkitt's lymphoma/leukemia is a common B-cell neoplasm involving children and young adults throughout the world; its endemic form in equatorial Africa is commonly associated with Epstein-Barr virus (EBV). The sporadic form in Europe and North America is only occasionally associated with EBV. Approximately 80% of Burkitt's lymphoma/leukemia have the t(8;14)(q24;q32) involving *c-myc* on chromosome 8 and the immunoglobulin heavy chain gene locus on chromosome 14. The remaining 20% of Burkitt's cases exhibit a *c-myc* translocation into the κ (2p12) or λ(22q11) immunoglobulin light chain gene loci: t(2;8)(p12;q24) or t(8;22)(q24;q11), respectively.

The expression of *c-myc* in normal cells correlates with transition in the cell cycle from a quiescent phase to active cell division. Normally, the expression of the *c-myc* protein is tightly controlled by transcriptional promoters on chromosome 8, and also by *c-myc* mRNA instability. As described earlier, the translocation process brings the *c-myc* gene into contact with one of the immunoglobulin gene loci and separates *c-myc* from its normal self-controlling elements. This leads to deregulation of *c-myc* transcription and results in constitutive expression of the *c-myc* gene at a level similar to that found in proliferating cells. Activation of *c-myc* also occurs as a result of its proximation to immunoglobulin enhancer segments in the immunoglobulin heavy or light chain genes. Thus, the continued activation of the *c-myc* gene within the immunoglobulin loci leads to enhanced production of *c-myc* proteins and subsequent cellular proliferation.

Chromosomal breakpoints in Burkitt's lymphoma/leukemia have been localized to particular segments of both the *c-myc* and the immunoglobulin heavy chain gene and are shown in Figure 8.17. By using molecular probes for *c-myc*, rearrangements of the *c-myc* gene can be demonstrated in over 50% of Burkitt's lymphoma cases. Different chromosomal breakpoint sites have been preferentially identified in the endemic and sporadic forms of Burkitt's lymphoma and probably represent different genetic mechanisms of activation. Burkitt's lymphoma cases that do not have demonstrable *c-myc* rearrangements apparently have breakpoints that are located too far from the currently available *c-myc* gene probes to be detected by routine Southern blotting methods.

As demonstrated in Figure 8.17, most of the corresponding breakpoint sites in the immunoglobulin genes occur within the switch regions. These switch regions may have some sequence homology to the breakpoint sites in *c-myc*. When the immunoglobulin breakpoints involve other regions of the gene, such as V, D, or J segments, *c-myc* rearrangements may not be detected by routine probes as the breakpoint site may be 5′ of available gene probes.

t(11;14)(q13;q32): Chronic Lymphocytic Leukemia/small Lymphocytic Lymphoma/Intermediate Differentiated Lymphoma. Investigations of cytogenetic abnormalities in other hematologic neoplasms have frequently centered on translocations involving loci of the immunoglobulin supergene family. This premise is based on the paradigm of the Burkitt's lymphoma/leukemia model, in which oncogenic activation occurs by translocating a protooncogene into the immunoglobulin heavy chain gene locus.

The t(11;14)(q13;q32) translocation has been reported as a common finding in small lymphocytic lymphoma/chronic lymphocytic leukemia or intermediate differentiation lymphocytic lymphoma. Cytogenetic studies have shown the breakpoint site on chromosome 14 involves the immunoglobulin heavy chain gene locus, 14q32, and, in particular, the joining region (J_H). By analogy to the *c-myc* and immunoglobulin heavy chain gene involvement in the Burkitt's lymphoma model, it was initially hypothesized that an oncogene must be localized to the 11q13 segment involved in this translocation. This proposed oncogenic site has been called *bcl-1*(B-cell leukemia/lymphoma-1); no true transcriptional or functional unit (i.e., protooncogene) has been isolated near this breakpoint site. Thus, no protooncogene has been definitively identified at 11q13 and has only been hypothesized to exist.

Gene rearrangement studies using the *bcl-1* gene have found good concordance with cytogenetic studies in demonstrating the t(11;14)(q13;q32). However, it appears that less than 10% of all small lymphocytic lymphomas/chronic lymphocytic leukemias contain a rearranged *bcl-1* gene (121–123). Recent studies, however, have shown that the majority of intermediate differentiated lymphoma or mantle zone lymphomas have a *bcl-1* rearrangement. Thus, a *bcl-1* rearrange-

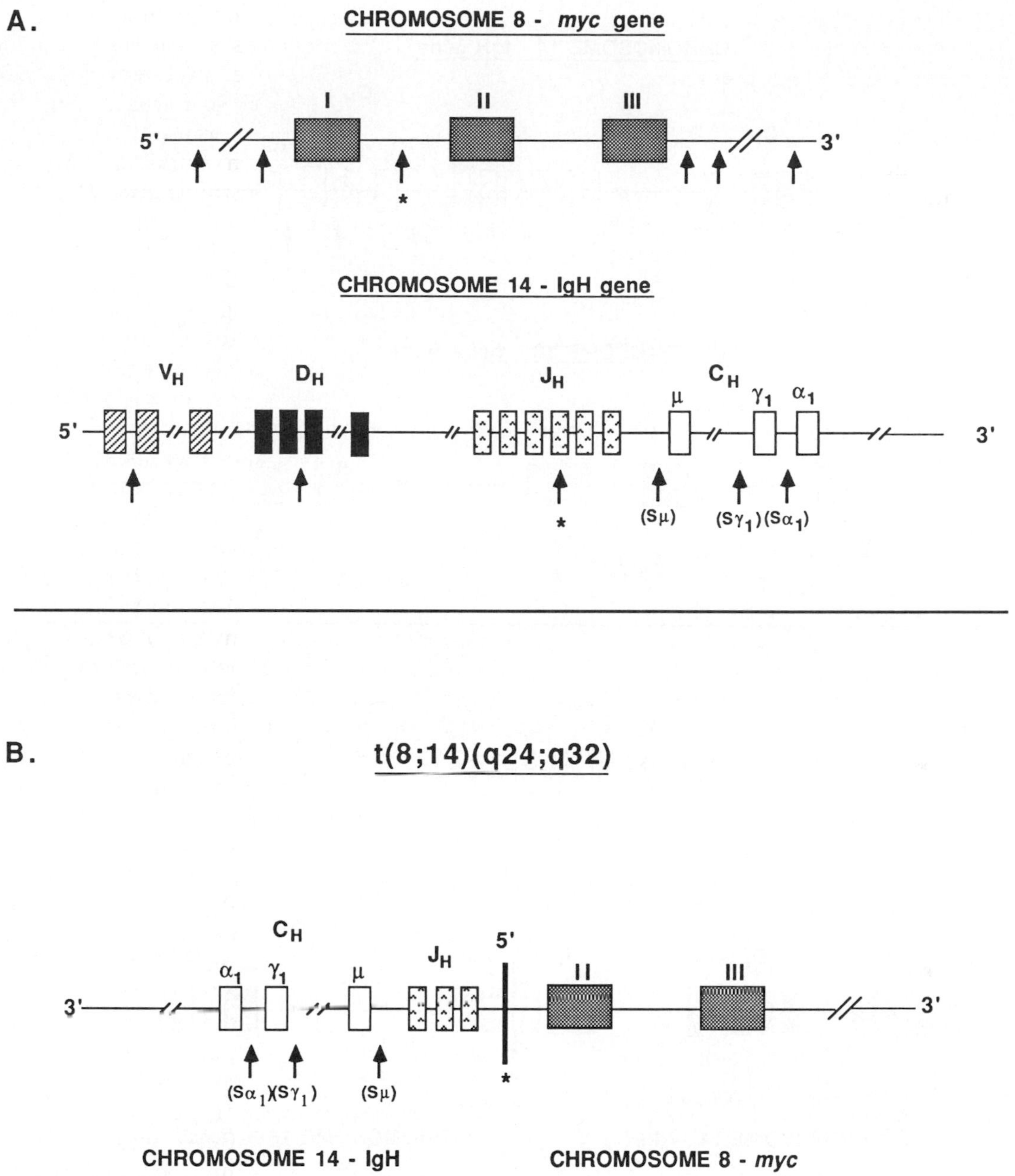

Figure 8.17. Molecular gene structure of chromosomes 8 and 14. **A**, The arrows indicate preferential locations of breakpoint sites in the t(8;14) translocations. The Sμ, Sγ, and Sα, represent the respective switch regions for particular constant region exons. (See Figs. 8.1 and 8.3 for explanation of characters.) **B**, This is one example of a reciprocal translocation between the *myc* oncogene and the IgH gene. The breakpoint on chromosome 8q24 has occurred between *c-myc* exons I and II (*). The breakpoint on chromosome 14q32 has occurred within the middle of the J_H region and has joined in a 5′ to 5′ fashion with the *c-myc* oncogene.

ment, although specific for a t(11;14), cannot presently be used as a sensitive diagnostic marker for these low-grade lymphoproliferative disorders.

t(14;18)(q32;q21): Follicular Center Cell Lymphoma. The t(14;18)(q32;q21) translocation is a commonly identified translocation in B cell, non-Hodgkin's lymphoma of follicular center cell origin. Cytogenetic studies have shown that virtually all follicular, small cleaved cell lymphomas contain the t(14;18) translocation. A smaller percentage of diffuse large-cell lymphomas also contain such a translocation, suggesting that these large-cell lymphomas may have transformed from an underlying follicular center cell process. The breakpoint in this translocation clusters in the J_H region of the immunoglobulin heavy chain gene locus at 14q32, similar to the *bcl-1* rearrangement in the t(11;14) translocation and many of the t(8;14) translocations of Burkitt's lymphoma/leukemia. The corresponding translocation site on chromosome 18q21 has been termed *bcl-2* and has

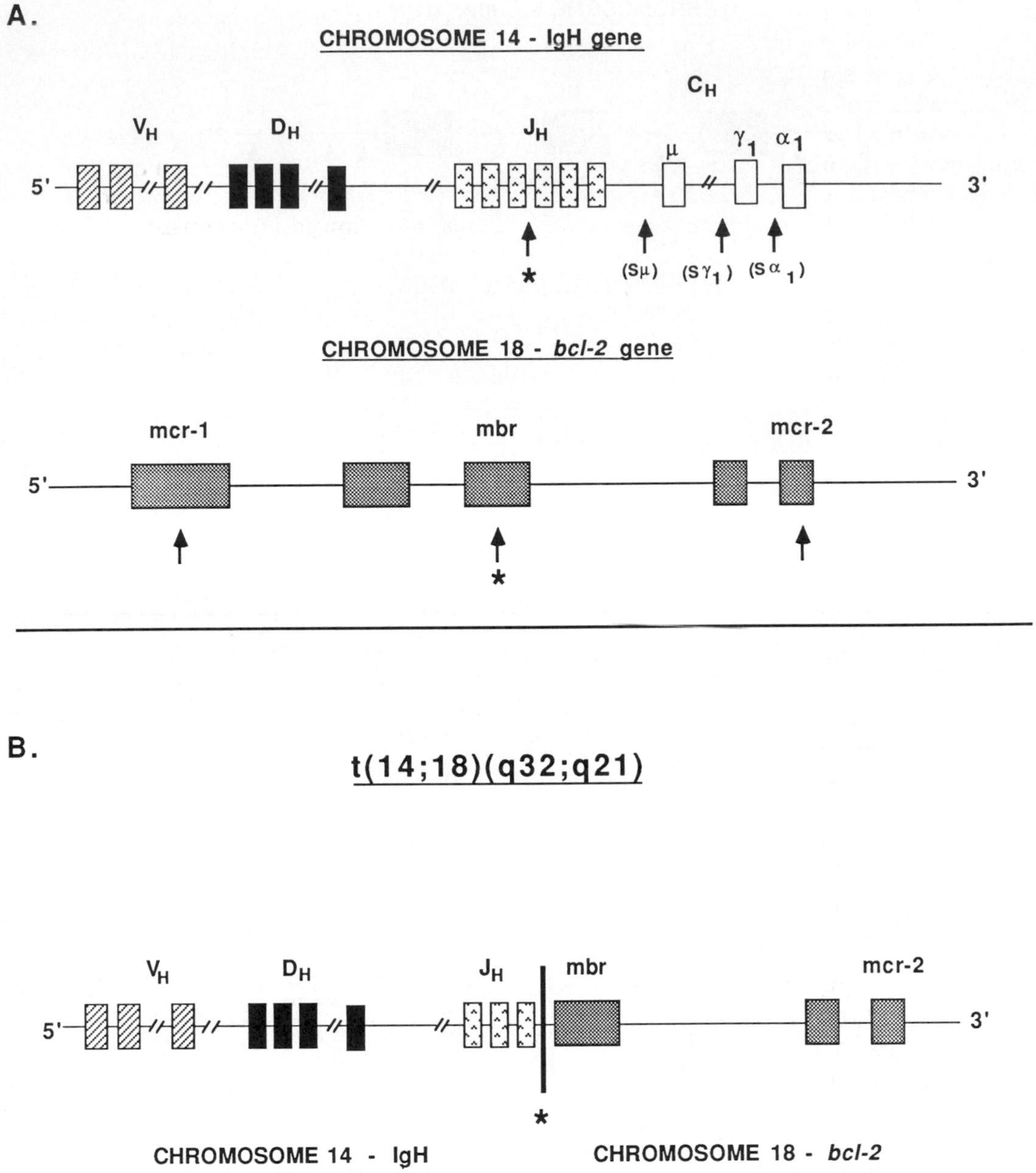

Figure 8.18. Molecular gene structure of chromosomes 14 and 18. (See Figures 8.1, 8.3, and 8.17 for explanation of characters.) **A**, Normal gene structure of chromosomes 14 and 18. Arrows indicate locations of the most common breakpoint sites. *mcr* stands for minor cluster regions, and *mbr* represents the major breakpoint region of the *bcl-2* gene. **B**, Schematic of the t(14;18) translocation between the IgH chain gene and the *bcl-2* gene. The breakpoint on chromosome 18 has occurred at the *mbr* site; the breakpoint on chromosome 14 is within the joining region.

been found to be a transcriptionally active gene. The breakpoint site on the *bcl-2* gene varies, as shown in Fig. 8.18. The majority of rearrangements occur in a very narrow area in *bcl-2*, which has been called the major breakpoint region, or *mbr*. By using appropriate restriction endonucleases located around this breakpoint site, routine Southern blotting will detect a rearranged *bcl-2* gene in approximately 60% of follicular center cell lymphomas with the t(14;18) translocation. Another 30% of cases will have a demonstrable rearrangement in the so-called minor cluster region, or *mcr*, which is located 50 kb upstream of the *mbr* site. Finally, a small percentage of cases have cytogenetic evidence of the t(14;18) translocation, but apparently have breakpoint sites outside the *mbr* and *mcr* sites. These breakpoints are not detectable with currently available probes.

Structurally, *bcl-2* consists of two exons and generates three RNA transcripts. Two *bcl-2* proteins are encoded by these messages and are similar to each other in structure. Preliminary studies have suggested that *bcl-2* has a major role in hematopoietic cell proliferation and differentiation and, in particular, B-cell growth. The molecular mechanism of activation appears to be quite similar to that described in Burkitt's lymphoma/leukemia, where translocation of a normally well-controlled and regulated gene (*bcl-2*) is placed within the environment of an active enhancer site of the immunoglobulin gene. This deregulation subsequently leads to constitutive expression of the *bcl-2* gene and over-production of the *bcl-2* protein.

The polymerase chain reaction (PCR) is an ideal technique to detect the t(14;18) because virtually all the breakpoint sites are clustered in relatively narrow DNA regions on both the immunoglobulin heavy chain gene (chromosome 14) and the *bcl-2* gene (chromosome 18). This is in contrast to the *c-myc* and immunoglobulin heavy chain gene rearrangement in Burkitt's lymphoma/leukemia, where the breakpoint sites in the *c-myc* gene vary over several hundred kb and can occur in multiple breakpoint sites within the immunoglobulin heavy chain gene locus. The use of PCR requires both an oligonucleotide probe complementary to the 5′ portion of the immunoglobulin heavy chain gene, J_H region, and another oligonucleotide primer corresponding to the anti-sense strand of the *mbr* or *mcr* region of *bcl-2*. A junctional, J_H-*bcl-2* oligonucleotide probe is then used for hybridization studies to confirm the presence of the chimeric, immunoglobulin heavy chain/*bcl-2* gene. Several studies have shown the applicability of PCR to detect the t(14;18) in cases of follicular center cell lymphoma. Routinely fixed, paraffin-embedded material has also been successfully used as a source of DNA for such PCR procedures. The PCR technique can also detect very small numbers of circulating lymphoma cells in the peripheral blood of patients with follicular center cell lymphomas; this method, thus, is much more sensitive than morphological examination.

Despite this ability to detect *bcl-2* by PCR, it must still be remembered that there are probably various breakpoint sites in the *bcl-2* gene that will not be detected by using *mbr* or *mcr* region primers. At the very least, it appears that PCR detection of *bcl-2* rearrangements in malignant lymphoma requires that at least two sets of primers be used to determine if there is *mbr* or *mcr* involvement.

Evaluation of Hemoglobin Disorders by Molecular Studies

Sickle Cell Anemia. The hereditary hemoglobin disorders, including α and β thalassemia and sickle cell anemia, are the most common genetic disorders in man. The World Health Organization has estimated that up to 7% of the world population are carriers for significant hemoglobinopathies. Since none of these diseases can be cured, the best hope for treatment is often centered on carrier detection and prenatal diagnosis. Two important developments have led to improvements in carrier evaluation and prenatal detection. First, recombinant DNA technology, together with advances in our understanding of the molecular genetic structure of the hemoglobin genes, has allowed for a consistent and highly sensitive method of detecting hemoglobin gene mutations. Second, the development of simpler methods to obtain fetal tissue has obviously been just as important in aiding the transition to DNA-based diagnosis. Despite the inherent advantages of DNA technology, several problems and limitations have prevented its widespread incorporation into diagnostic laboratories. However, it seems inevitable that analysis of hemoglobin disorders will become one of the major clinical applications of molecular diagnostic studies.

Sickle cell anemia results from homozygous expression of an abnormal hemoglobin β-gene that causes a β6 substitution of valine for glutamic acid. The amino acid change is a result of a single nucleotide base substitution, with an adenine being replaced by a thymine. Historically, detection of sickle cell anemia has been based on electrophoretic detection of an abnormally migrating hemoglobin. Subsequently, newer technologies of restriction endonuclease mapping of genes have been applied to detecting structural gene deletions in fetal DNA. By using these technologies, it was discovered that the normal β-globin gene contains a recognition sequence for the restriction enzymes, *Mst II* and *Cvn I*, located at the site of the sickle cell nucleotide mutation. These enzymes cleave DNA at the sequence of CCTNAGG (C = cytosine, T = thymine, A = adenine, G = guanine, and N = any of the four nucleotide bases) and will cut the normal β-globin gene in the region corresponding to amino acids 5, 6, and 7 (CCT-GAG-GAG) (Fig. 8.19). In contrast, the sickle cell gene mutation at codon 6 (CCT-GTG-GAG) abolishes this *Mst II* recognition site; digestion of the mutant gene yields a 1.35 kb fragment around the sickle cell gene mutation, as opposed to the normal 1.15 kb and .20 kb fragments (Fig. 8.19). This technique can detect sickle cell carriers as well as individuals homozygous for hemoglobin S.

Although this technique offers the advantage of high sensitivity and specificity, it comes with the burden of being a labor-intensive procedure with expensive costs, the need for highly purified DNA, and long turnaround time for results. All of these problems have prevented its development as a routine screening assay for sickle cell anemia or sickle cell carriers; any delay in prenatal diagnosis can lead to increased risk and uncertainty in therapeutic deci-

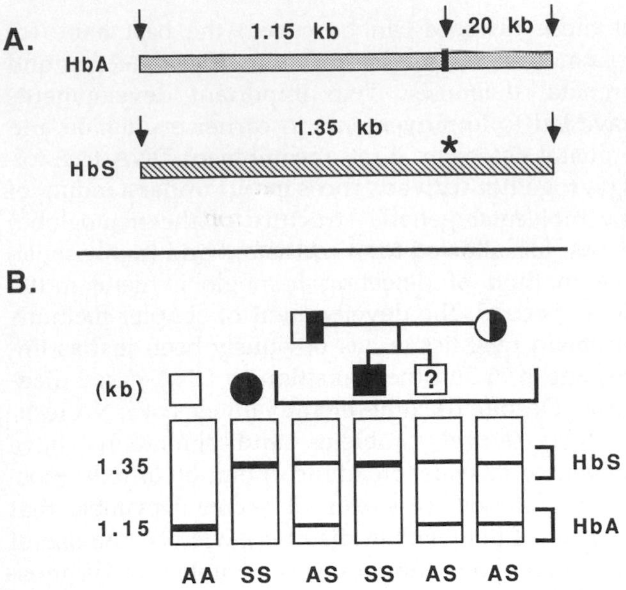

Figure 8.19. Molecular gene structure and schematic of Southern blot hybridization of the sickle cell gene. **A**, The stippled box represents a normal β-globin gene leading to the formation of hemoglobin A (HbA). The striped box represents the abnormal β-globin gene which leads to the formation of hemoglobin S (HbS). The arrows (↓) indicate the locations of the *Mst*II restriction enzyme sites. Digestion of normal β-globin gene leads to the formation of 1.15-kb and 0.20-kb fragments. A *Mst*II site is deleted in the sickle cell gene due to the codon 6 mutation (*). This leads to the formation of a 1.15-kb and 0.20-kb *Mst*II digestion fragment in a normal β-globin gene and a combined 1.35-kb *Mst*II fragment from the sickle cell gene. **B**, This Southern blot hybridization schematic shows a hypothetical family study of the sickle cell gene. Open boxes represent patients with the normal β-globin gene (HbA); solid circle/squares represent patients with sickle cell anemia (HbS): half-filled boxes or circles represent carriers of the sickle cell gene. Following digestion with *Mst*II and probing with a β-globin gene probe, three possible band combinations can be seen. The first two lanes represent controls for HbA (AA) and sickle cell anemia (SS), respectively. The parents, represented in lanes 3 and 6, are sickle cell carriers (AS), having both the 1.15-kb and 1.35-kb *Mst*II fragments, and a son (lane 4) has sickle cell anemia (SS). The fetus in question contains both the 1.15-kb and 1.35-kb *MstII* fragments, consistent with the diagnosis of a sickle cell carrier (AS).

sionmaking. Thus, the problems inherent with this procedure have limited its utilization to those troublesome cases not clearly identified by routine hemoglobin electrophoresis.

The polymerase chain reaction (PCR), however, may eventually overcome some of these problems common to Southern blotting methods. By amplifying the region of the hemoglobin gene involved with the sickle cell mutation (Fig. 8.20), the restriction enzyme digestion and gel analysis can be performed in a few hours as opposed to 7 to 14 days for routine DNA studies. Furthermore, PCR can be performed on miniscule amounts of tissue (less than 1 μg) and can be directly visualized on ethidium bromide-stained gels, thus eliminating the need for radiolabeled probes. The only word of caution is that the exquisite sensitivity of PCR can also lead to contamination problems, such as could happen if there is maternal or other exogenous tissue that is amplified during the PCR process. In the coming decade, it will be most interesting to observe the role of PCR in evaluating amniocentesis or chorionic villi samples for hemoglobin abnormalities.

β-Thalassemia. β-thalassemia major is an autosomal recessive disease characterized by a chronic, transfusion-dependent anemia. While the β-thalassemia carriers have only mild clinical symptoms, those individuals with homozygous β-thalassemia suffer from all the problems of a chronic hemolytic process and, as a result, have a shortened life expectancy. It has been estimated that up to 3% of the world's population are carriers of a β-thalassemia gene. β-thalassemia is primarily located in equatorial regions around the world including southern Europe, northern Africa, Black Africa, the Middle East, the Asian subcontinent, and China/Southeast Asia.

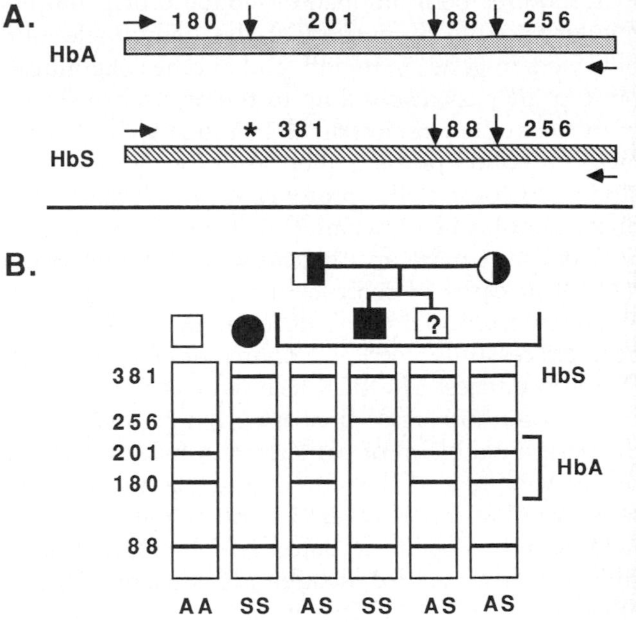

Figure 8.20. Schematic of a polymerase chain reaction (PCR) study for the sickle cell gene. **A**, This is a more "microscopic" view of Figure 8.19. (See Fig. 8.19 for explanation of figure characters.) The down arrows represent the enzyme recognition sites for *Mst*II; the horizontal arrows represent the locations of the oligonucleotide primers used for the PCR reaction. The sickle cell gene mutation destroys any *MstII* restriction enzyme site (*) leading to the amplification of a larger 381-bp fragment. All numbers refer to the length of the *Mst*II products in base pairs. **B**, This drawing shows a gel electrophoresis study of the PCR products from *A* following *Mst*II digestion; controls for hemoglobin A (HbA) and hemoglobin S (HbS) are in lanes 1 and 2, respectively. The 180-bp and 201-bp bands are unique to HbA while the 381-bp fragment is characteristic of HbS. The 256-bp and 88-bp fragments are found in both genes. As shown in lanes 3 and 6, the parents are sickle cell carriers exhibiting both HbA and HbS bands (AS). The son has sickle cell anemia, while the fetus in question is a sickle cell gene carrier, having both the HbA and HbS genes (AS).

Obviously, through the process of immigration, β-thalassemia is now distributed throughout the world and is not restricted to the aforementioned geographic areas. This common hemoglobinopathy is concentrated in areas of the world endemic for malaria; affected individuals are thought to have a selective advantage over normal individuals with regard to surviving a malarial infection.

The genetic defect in β-thalassemia was poorly understood for decades as it is a clinically heterogeneous disorder. The diagnosis of β-thalassemia was based on indirect diagnostic laboratory tests, such as red blood cell indices and/or hemoglobin electrophoresis. These common tests are usually quite adequate to diagnose most cases of β-thalassemia. However, they do not detect the actual genetic defect in patients with this hemoglobinopathy. Furthermore, since hemoglobin electrophoretic diagnoses are based on abnormal distributions of hemoglobin F and hemoglobin A_2 relative to hemoglobin A_1, the traditional approach to diagnosing β-thalassemia cannot be employed as a prenatal screening test. The reason for this is that the distribution of hemoglobin subtypes is much different in a first trimester fetus than in an adult.

Unlike sickle cell anemia and other hemoglobinopathies that have unique nucleotide mutations which lead to an amino acid substitution, β-thalassemia is an incredibly heterogeneous disorder both clinically and at the molecular level. During the molecular biology explosion of the last decade, many of the molecular defects of the β-globin gene in β-thalassemia were elucidated. The genotypic abnormalities leading to β-thalassemia are characterized by multiple types of molecular abnormalities, primarily involving point mutations in the β-globin gene. These point mutations, which number over 50 according to reviews published in 1988, result in a spectrum of β-globin abnormalities ranging from severe to only mild impairment of hemoglobin synthesis. The most severe types are the result of nonfunctional mRNA mutants or deletions/insertions that affect mRNA splicing. β-thalassemias with mild to moderate globin abnormalities result from other mutations that do not totally disrupt the transcription and/or translation process. The multiplicity of mutations accounts for the clinical and laboratory heterogeneity in β-thalassemia and conceptually points to the great difficulty scientists have had in characterizing and diagnosing this common hemoglobinopathy.

At first glance, this heterogeneity appears to be an overwhelming obstacle to the utilization of molecular diagnostic techniques in evaluating β-thalassemias, It turns out, however, that most ethnic group populations have only a limited number of allelic mutations that account for over 90% of the β-globin abnormalities in a given population group. This analysis becomes more complicated in countries such as the United States, Canada, and the United Kingdom which have large immigrant populations, each having large indigenous populations of β-thalassemia. Thus, in countries that have patients with varied ethnic backgrounds originating from multiple "hot spots" of β-thalassemia, detection of the molecular defects in the β-globin gene may become quite complex. Molecular analysis can be accomplished only by having a thorough knowledge of the spectrum of mutations in those respective ethnic groups.

Historically, the prenatal diagnosis of β-thalassemia by molecular diagnostic techniques was first carried out in the early 1980s by using RFLP studies. This is an indirect method and depends on identifying a DNA marker linked to the β-thalassemia gene; this marker is polymorphic and has a different DNA sequence in the affected individual as compared with the normal one. If the fetus carries the linked marker similar to the affected parent, then a prenatal diagnosis of β-thalassemia can be made.

Direct detection of β-globin mutations has now become reality because of our growing knowledge of the molecular abnormalities in β-thalassemia, as just described. This may be accomplished by using either radioactive or nonradioactive probes, or by using a polymerase chain reaction (PCR)-based method. This latter method is ideal for analyzing small samples such as those obtained from chorionic villi biopsies or amniocentesis.

One method of detecting a mutant allele is based on hybridization with an allele-specific oligonucleotide that detects only that specific point mutation (Fig. 8.21). Another common detection method is based on the fact that many mutations alter a known restriction endonuclease site; this technique is similar to that described for detection of the sickle cell gene mutation. The mutation may either cause a loss of such an enzymatic site by the changing of a single nucleotide (as in the sickle cell gene mutation) or create a new restriction endonuclease site (Fig. 8.22). Such changes can then be detected by gel electrophoretic procedures. Since only a few (usually 4 to 9) allelic mutations account for over 90% of abnormalities in a particular ethnic group, the laboratory need only screen for those representative mutations in a patient or fetus at risk.

The polymerase chain reaction has greatly enhanced the ability to evaluate for β-globin mutations in the following ways: (*a*) it is an automated procedure; (*b*) it allows for rapid turnaround time for results; and (*c*) it requires only a minimal amount of specimen (for fetal diagnosis). The major drawback of PCR evaluation for β-thalassemia includes the potential risk of amplifying contaminating maternal

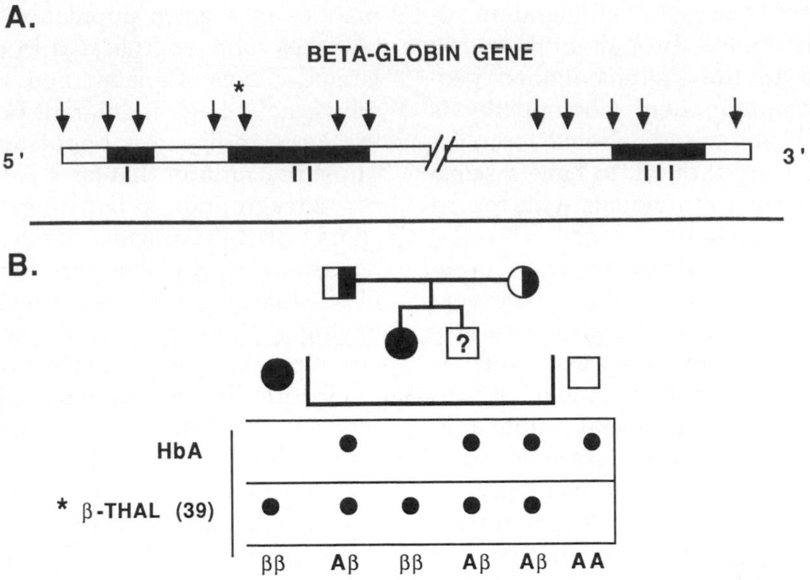

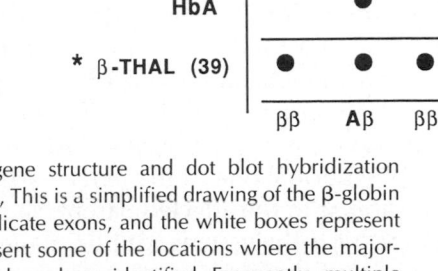

Figure 8.21. β-globin gene structure and dot blot hybridization study for β-thalassemia. **A**, This is a simplified drawing of the β-globin gene. The solid boxes indicate exons, and the white boxes represent introns. The arrows represent some of the locations where the majority of β-globin mutations have been identified. Frequently, multiple mutations have been identified in each of these "hot-spots." The asterisked arrow (*) represents the 39th codon, which is one of the most frequently deleted mutations in β-thalassemia. **B**, This dot blot hybridization schematic shows the results of using both an oligonucleotide probe for the normal β-globin sequence (HbA) and a probe for the abnormal codon 39 mutation seen in β-thalassemia (*). Positive controls are seen in lane 1 for a homozygous B-thalassemia mutation (ββ) and lane 6 for the normal β-globin gene (AA). The parents, represented in lanes 2 and 5, are carriers for this thalassemia mutation having evidence of both the hemoglobin A and β-thalassemia sequences (Aβ). One daughter (lane 3) is homozygous for β-thalassemia (ββ). The fetus in question (lane 4) is a carrier, showing evidence of both the hemoglobin A and β-thalassemia gene (Aβ).

cells/DNA obtained with the fetal sample. Like all other molecular diagnostic techniques, these results must be interpreted in conjunction with other clinical and laboratory data. By using only these molecular screening assays for β-globin or hemoglobin S abnormalities, complex hemoglobinopathies (such as hemoglobin SC, hemoglobin S/thalassemia, hemoglobin E/thalassemia, etc.) may be missed. Therefore, current molecular diagnostic techniques can supplement but do not replace the standard hemoglobin electrophoretic methods. While the current data suggest that over 90% of all thalassemia mutations are known, it seems unlikely that a screening lab will be able to evaluate for all such possibilities. In other words, some false-negative results have to be expected. These studies, therefore, can provide useful screening information in high-risk populations if the limitations are known and considered.

Education about the inheritance patterns of hemoglobin disorders continues to be the main tool in reducing high-risk pregnancies. The implementation of prenatal testing requires that adequate obstetric services be available to those population groups undergoing hemoglobin screening. Awareness of these social issues is indeeed a prerequisite to successful implementation of hemoglobin screening procedures and cannot be ignored by those wishing to become involved with such testing.

Coagulation Abnormalities: Hemophilia A

Hemophilia A is one of the most common inherited bleeding disorders in humans and is due to a defect in the coagulation factor VIII gene. This X-linked disorder affects approximately one out of every 5,000 males throughout the world. Clinical manifestations of hemophilia A are quite diverse, ranging from onset of severe bleeding in early childhood to occasional milder cases that do not present with clinical bleeding problems until early adulthood. This heterogeneity of clinical severity reflects to the underlying spectrum of molecular defects and is inversely related to the degree of activity of the mutated Factor VIII gene.

Over the past 20 years, scientific advances have led to the development of physiological and immunologic bioassays for the prenatal and postnatal diagnosis of hemophilia. The diagnostic error rate of these assays has been estimated to be less than 1%. The test has excellent sensitivity and specificity for diagnosing affected males. For purposes of genetic counseling, however, there is a need to detect female carriers of this X-linked gene. Current non–DNA-based techniques for carrier detection may accurately identify anywhere from 70 to 95% of all carriers. The large potential error rate in carrier detection is due to the broad range of factor VIII activity in the normal

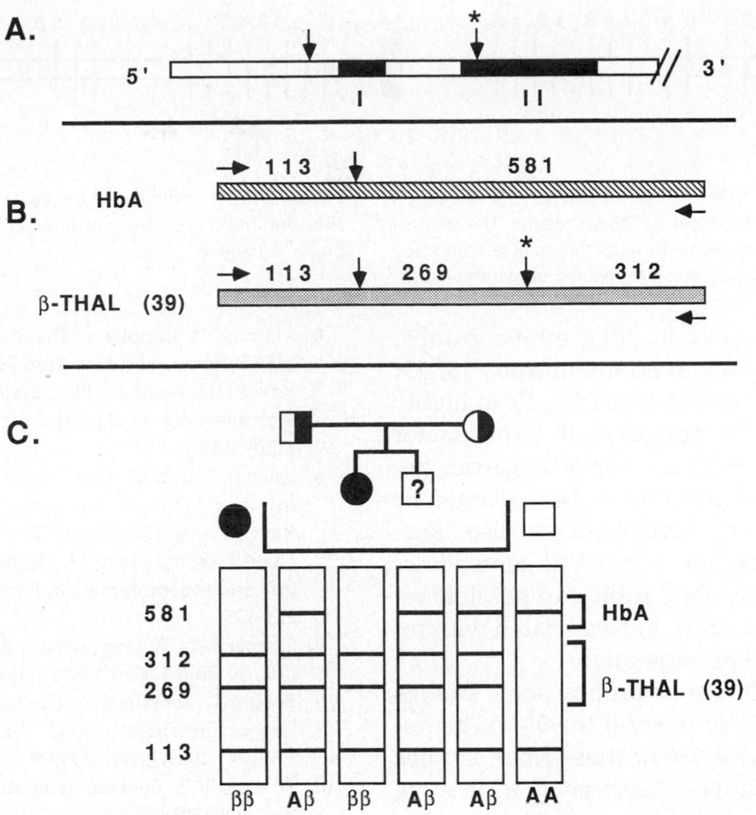

Figure 8.22. Polymerase chain reaction (PCR) study of the β-globin gene in β-thalassemia. **A**, Partial structure of the β-globin gene. The arrows represent the recognition sites for the *MspI* restriction enzyme site. The * marks the *MspI* restriction enzyme site that is formed with the codon 39 mutation. **B**, PCR schematic for the codon 39 mutation in β-thalassemia. The vertical arrows represent the *MspI* restriction enzyme sites. The horizontal arrows represent the locations of the oligonucleotide primers used for PCR. Amplification of the normal β-globin gene results in two fragments following *MspI* digestion: 113 and 581 base pairs. The codon 39 mutation in the β-thalassemia gene leads to the formation of three amplified, *MspI* fragments of 113, 269, and 312 base pairs. **C**, The PCR studies are shown in this family study. Controls for the β-thalassemia mutation (ββ) (lane 1) and the normal β-globin allele (AA) (lane 6) are shown. The parents, shown in lanes 2 and 5, are heterozygous for this mutation, showing both the hemoglobin A and β-thalassemia fragments (Aβ). One daughter (lane 3) is homozygous for β-thalassemia (ββ). The fetus in question is a carrier, showing both the 581 (hemoglobin A) and 269/312 (β-thalassemia) base pair fragments (Aβ).

population and the random inactivation, or lyonization, of the X chromosomes in females. Furthermore, prenatal diagnosis has been limited to examination of peripheral blood, which means that fetal diagnosis cannot be performed until about the 16th to 18th week of gestation. Molecular DNA methods, in contrast, examine the genotype and can be accomplished as early as the 10th week of gestation.

The X-linked factor VIII gene has been cloned and characterized. It is one of the largest genes identified to date; this large size has slowed the evolution of molecular analytic techniques in the evaluation of hemophiliacs. The entire gene is 186 kb in length and contains 26 exons; these exons, however, account for less than 5% of the total gene length. Large introns account for the majority of the genetic material (Fig. 8.23). The cDNA from this gene encodes a protein with a molecular weight of about 300 kd. As would be expected from such a large and complex gene, no single mutation is held responsible for all cases of hemophilia A. Indeed, both single nucleotide mutations and larger gene deletions have been described in cases of hemophilia A. Not unexpectedly, these mutations and deletions tend to occur in "hot-spots" in the gene, which has provided important information in understanding the pathogenesis of this disease. The existence of "hot-spots" suggests that spontaneous mutations may occur, leading to sporadic cases of hemophilia. Indeed, these spontaneous, mutations are thought to be responsible for up to 30% of hemophilia cases, accounting for the large number of hemophiliacs with no definite family history of disease.

Current techniques in carrier detection and prenatal diagnosis of hemophilia by DNA analysis are based on the identification of DNA polymorphisms (RFLP) associated with the factor VIII gene. Four well-characterized RFLPs are intragenic and are associated with a high frequency of informative polymorphisms in the Caucasian population. These

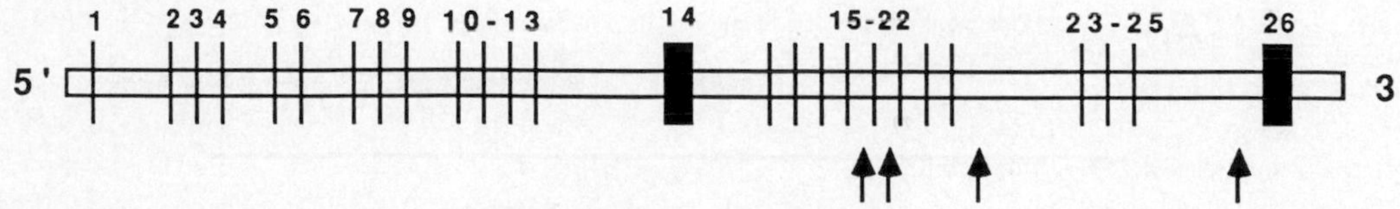

Figure 8.23. Structure of the factor VIII gene. This gene is located on the X chromosome and stretches over a 186-kb region. The vertical lines and solid boxes represent exons; most of the gene is composed of intronic material. The exon numbers are located above the exons. The arrows (↑) indicate the locations of four well-characterized RFLP sites that have been used as intragenic probes in the study of hemophilia A patients.

may not be as polymorphic in other ethnic groups. Because of their intragenic locations (introns 18, 19, 22, and 26) (Fig. 8.23), use of these RFLPs is highly specific as a marker of the normal or abnormal factor VIII gene, with only a negligible error in carrier detection or in pre-natal diagnosis. Two extragenic RFLPs, termed ST14 and DXS52, have also been widely used in evaluating the factor VIII gene. However, these extragenic sites are subject to possible recombination events and, thus, are associated with up to a 5% false-positive diagnosis rate.

By using multiple DNA gene probes, some studies have reported detection of over 90 to 95% of hemophilia gene carriers. Since use of these RFLP studies for carrier detection has been associated with some false-positive diagnoses (when using extragenic RFLPs), DNA results must be interpreted in conjunction with conventional factor VIII assays. As with all DNA tests, the molecular diagnosis of hemophilia A is labor-intensive and expensive to perform. In addition, since current methods are based on RFLPs, the pedigree information must be accurate and the paternity status well documented. Finally, it is important to remember that up to 30% of hemophilia cases are sporadic and may not have any associated family history of disease. In conclusion, the initial enthusiasm for using DNA analysis to evaluate carrier status in hemophiliac families has been tempered by an appreciation of its limitations. Indeed, the small increase in carrier identification may be offset by the potential for misdiagnosis or by the complications associated with obtaining samples of fetal DNA.

Acknowledgments

The authors wish to thank Shannon Fitzgerald for her help in the preparation of this manuscript and Robin Kunkel for her artistic assistance. Their patience and dedication are greatly appreciated.

References

1. Cossman J, Uppenkamp M, Sundeen J, Coupland R, Raffeld M. Molecular genetics and the diagnosis of lymphoma. Arch Pathol Lab Med 1988;112:117–127.
2. Fenoglio-Preiser CM, Willman CL. Molecular biology and the pathologist: general principles and applications. Arch Pathol Lab Med 1987;111:601–619.
3. Marrack P, Kappler J. The T cell receptor. Science 1987;238: 1073–1079.
4. Marrack P, Kappler J. The T-cell repertoire for antigen and MHC. Immunol Today 1988;9:308–315.
5. Royer HD, Reinherz EL: T lymphocytes: ontogeny, function, and relevance to clinical disorders. N Engl J Med 1987;317: 1136–1142.
6. Jeske JJ, Capra JD. Immunoglobulins: structure and function. In: Paul WE, ed. Fundamental immunology. New York: Raven Press, 1984:131–165.
7. Hood L, Kronenberg M, Hunkapiller T. T cell antigen receptors and the immunoglobulin supergene family. Cell 1985;40: 225–229.
8. Cooper MD. B lymphocytes: normal development and function. N Engl J Med 1987;317:1452–1456.
9. Boehm T, Rabbitts TH. The human T cell receptor genes are targets for chromosomal abnormalities in T cell tumors. FASEB J 1989;3:2344–2359.
10. Tonegawa S. Somatic generation of antibody diversity. Nature 1983;302:575–581.
11. Korsmeyer SJ, Hieter PA, Ravetch JV, et al. Developmental hierarchy of immunoglobulin gene rearrangements in human leukemic pre-B-cells. Proc Natl Acad Sci USA 1981;78:7096–7100.
12. Paige CJ, Wu GE. The B cell repertoire. FASEB 1989;3:1818–1824.
13. Hieter PA, Korsmeyer SJ, Waldmann TA, et al. Human immunoglobulin κ light-chain genes are deleted or rearranged in γ-producing B cells. Nature 1981;290:369–372.
14. Gritzmacher CA. Molecular aspects of heavy-chain class switching. Crit Rev Immunol 1989;9:173–200.
15. Reinherz EL, Kung PC, Goldstein G, Levey RH, Schlossman SF. Discrete stages of human intrathymic differentiation: analysis of normal thymocytes and leukemic lymphoblasts of T-cell lineage. Proc Natl Acad Sci USA 1980;77:1588–1592.
16. Toyonaga B, Yoshikai Y, Vadasz V, et al. Organization and sequences of the diversity, joining and constant region genes of the human T cell receptor β chain. Proc Natl Acad Sci USA 1985;82:8624–8628.
17. Brenner MB, McLean J, Dialynas DP, et al. Identification of a putative second T cell receptor. Nature 1986;322:145–149.
18. Brandzaeg P, Halstensen TS, Scott H, Sollid LM, Valnes K: Epithelial homing of δγ T cells? Nature 1989;341:113–114.
19. Augustin A, Kubo RT, Sim GK. Resident pulmonary lymphocytes expressing the δγ T-cell receptor. Nature 1989;340: 239–241.
20. Triebel F, Hercend T. Subpopulations of human peripheral T gamma delta lymphocytes. Immunol Today 1989;10:186–188.
21. Satyanarayana K, Hata S, Devlin P, et al. Genomic organization of the human T-cell antigen-receptor α/δ locus. Proc Natl Acad Sci USA 1988;85:8166–8170.
22. Uppenkamp M, Andrade R, Sundeen J, Raffeld M, Coupland R, Cossman J. Diagnostic interpretation of Tγ gene rearrangement: effect of polyclonal T cells. Hematol Pathol 1988;2:15–24.

23. Macintyre EA, Sigaux F. T cell receptor γδ:current state of knowledge and potential clinical applications in haematology. Br J Haematol 1989;73:2–5.
24. Havran WL, Allison JP. Developmentally ordered appearance of thymocytes expressing different T-cell antigen receptors. Nature (London) 1988;335:443–445.
25. Desiderio SV, Yancopoulos GD, Paskinl M, et al. Insertion of N regions into heavy-chain genes is correlated with expression of terminal deoxytransferase in B-cells. Nature 1984;311: 752–755.
26. Leiden JM and Strominger JL. Generation of diversity of the β chain of the human T-lymphocyte receptor for antigen. Proc Natl Acad Sci USA 1986;83:4456–4460.
27. Fialkow PJ, Jacobson RJ, Papayannopoulou T. Chronic myelocytic leukemia: clonal origin in a stem cell common to the granulocyte, erythrocyte, platelet and monocyte/macrophage. Am J Med 1977;63:125–130.
28. Yunis JJ. The chromosomal basis of human neoplasia. Science 1988;221:227–236.
29. Cleary ML, Sklar J. DNA rearrangements in non-Hodgkin's lymphomas. Cancer Surv 1985;4:331–348.
30. Knowles DM. Immunophenotypic and antigen receptor gene rearrangement analysis in T cell neoplasia. Am J Pathol 1989;134:761–785.
31. Arnold A, Cossman J, Bakhshi A, et al. Immunoglobulin-gene rearrangements as unique clonal markers in human lymphoid neoplasms. N Engl J Med 1983;309:1593–1600.
32. Cleary ML, Warnke R, Sklar J. Monoclonality of lymphoproliferative lesions in cardiac-transplant recipients; clonal analysis based on immunoglobulin-gene rearrangements. N Engl J Med 1984;310:477–482.
33. Henni T, Gaulard P, Divine M, et al. Comparison of genetic probe with immunophenotype analysis in lymphoproliferative disorders: a study of 87 cases. Blood 1988;72:1937–1943.
34. O'Connor NTJ, Weatherall DJ, Feller AC, et al. Rearrangement of the T-cell receptor β-chain gene in the diagnosis of lymphoproliferative disorders. Lancet 1985;1:1295–1297.
35. Griesser H, Feller A, Lennert K, Minden M, Mak TW. Rearrangement of the β chain of the T cell antigen receptor and immunoglobulin genes in lymphoproliferative disorders. J Clin Invest 1986;78:1179–1184.
36. Krolewski JJ, Dalla-Favera R. Molecular genetic approaches in the diagnosis and classification of lymphoid malignancies. Hematol Pathol 1989;3:45–61.
37. Sheibani K, Wu A, Ben-Ezra J, Stroup R, Rappaport H, Winberg C. Rearrangement of κ-chain and T-cell receptor β-chain genes in malignant lymphomas of "T-cell" phenotype. Am J Pathol 1987;129:201–207.
38. Hanson CA, Thamilarasan M, Ross CW, Stoolman LM, Schnitzer B. Kappa light chain gene rearrangement in T-cell acute lymphoblastic leukemia. Am J Clin Pathol 1990;93(4): 563–568.
39. Siminovitch KA, Jensen JP, Epstein AL, Korsmeyer SJ. Immunoglobulin gene rearrangements and expression in diffuse histiocytic lymphomas reveal cellular lineage, molecular defects, and sites of chromosomal translocation. Blood 1986;67:391–397.
40. Weiss LM, Picker LJ, Copenhaver CM, Warnke RA, Sklar J. Large-cell hematolymphoid neoplasms of uncertain lineage. Hum Pathol 1988;19:967–973.
41. Tawa K, Hozumi N, Minden M, Mak TW, Gelfand EW. Rearrangement of the T-cell receptor β-chain gene in non-T-cell, non-B-cell acute lymphoblastic leukemia of childhood. N Engl J Med 1985;313:1033–1037.
42. Pelicci PG, Knowles DM, Dalla-Favera RD. Lymphoid tumors displaying rearrangements of both immunoglobulin and T cell receptor genes. J Exp Med 1985;162:1015–1024.
43. Leber BF, Amlot P, Hoffbrand AV, Norton JD. T-cell receptor gene rearrangement in B-cell non-Hodgkin's lympoma: correlation with methylation and expression. Leuk Res 1989;13: 473–481.
44. Waldmann TA, Davis MM, Bongiovanni KF, Korsmeyer SJ. Rearrangements of genes for the antigen receptor on T cells as markers of lineage and colonality in human lymphoid neoplasms. N Engl J Med 1985;313:776–783.
45. Aisenberg AC, Krontiris TG, Mak TW, Wilkes BM. Rearrangement of the gene for the beta chain of the T-cell receptor in T-cell chronic lymphocytic leukemia and related disorders. N Engl J Med 1985;313:529–533.
46. Weiss LM, Hu E, Wood GS, et al. Clonal rearrangements of T-cell receptor genes in mycosis fungoides and dermatopathic lymphadenopathy. N Eng J Med 1985;313:539–544.
47. Minden MD, Mak TW. The structure of the T cell antigen receptor genes in normal and malignant T cells. Blood 1986;68: 327–336.
48. Weiss LM, Picker LJ, Grogan TM, Warnke RA, Sklar J. Absence of clonal beta and gamma T-cell receptor gene rearrangements in a subset of peripheral T-cell lymphomas. Am J Pathol 1988;130:436–442.
49. Bignon YJ, Souteyrand P, Roger H, Bernard D. Dual genotype in cutaneous T cell lymphoma: immunoglobulin gene rearrangement in clonal T cell malignancy. J Invest Dermatol 1989;92:775.
50. Anastasi J, Variakojis D. Heterogenity in Hodgkin's disease: no simple answer for a complex disorder. Hum Pathol 1988;19:1251–1254.
51. Drexler HG, Jones DB, Diehl V, Minowada J. Is the Hodgkin cell a T- or B-lymphocyte? Recent evidence from geno- and immunophenotypic analysis and in-vitro cell lines. Hematol Oncol 1989;7:95–113.
52. O'Connor NTJ, Crick JA, Gatter KC, Mason DY, Falini B, Stein HS. Cell lineage in Hodgkin's disease. Lancet 1987;1: 158.
53. Raghavachar A, Binder T, Bartram CR. Immunoglobulin and T-cell receptor gene rearrangements in Hodgkin's disease. Cancer Res 1988;48:3591–3594.
54. Herbst H, Tippelmann G, Anagnostopoulos I, et al. Immunoglobulin and T-cell receptor gene rearrangements in Hodgkin's disease Ki-1-positive anaplastic large cell lymphoma: dissociation between phenotype and genotype. Leuk Res 1989;13:103–116.
55. Roth MS, Schnitzer B, Bingham EL, Harnden CE, Hyder DM, Ginsburg D. Rearrangement of immunoglobulin and T-cell receptor genes in Hodgkin's disease. Am J Pathol 1988;131:331–338.
56. Weiss LM, Strickler JG, Hu E, Warnke RA, Sklar J. Immunoglobulin gene rearrangements in Hodgkin's disease. Hum Pathol 1986;17:1009–1014.
57. Brinker MGL, Poppema S, Buys CHCM, Timens W, Osinga J, Visser L. Clonal immunoglobulin gene rearrangements in tissues involved by Hodgkin's disease. Blood 1987;70:186–191.
58. Sundeen J, Lipford E, Uppenkamp M, et al. Rearranged antigen receptor genes in Hodgkin's disease. Blood 1987;70:96–103.
59. Griesser H, Feller AC, Mak TW, Lennert K. Clonal rearrangements of T-cell receptor and immunoglobulin genes and immunophenotypic antigen expression in different subclasses of Hodgkin's disease. Int J Cancer 1987;40:157–160.
60. Falk MH, Tesch H, Stein H, et al. Phenotype versus immunoglobulin and T-cell receptor genotype of Hodgkin-derived cell lines: activation of immature lymphoid cells in Hodgkin's disease. Int J Cancer 1987;40:262–269.

61. Kadin ME, Sako D, Berliner N, et al. Childhood Ki-1 lymphoma presenting with skin lesions and peripheral lymphadenopathy. Blood 1986;68:1042–1049.
62. Schnitzer B, Roth MS, Hyder DM, Ginsburg D. Ki-1 lymphomas in children. Cancer 1988;1213–1221.
63. O'Connor NTJ, Stein H, Gatter KC, et al. Genotypic analysis of large cell lymphomas which express the Ki-1 antigen. Histopathology 1987;11:773–740.
64. Griesser H, Feller A, Lennert K, Minden M, Mak TW. Rearrangement of the β chain of the T cell antigen receptor and immunoglobulin genes in lymphoproliferative disorders. J Clin Invest 1986;78:1179–1184.
65. Hanson CA, Jaszcz W, Kersey JH, et al. True histiocytic lymphoma: histopathologic immunophenotypic and genetypic analysis. Br J Haematol 1989;73(2):187–198.
66. Weiss LM, Trela MJ, Cleary ML, Turner RR, Warnke RA, Sklar J. Frequent immunoglobulin and T-cell receptor gene rearrangements in "histiocytic" neoplasms. Am J Pathol 1985;121:369–373.
67. Knowles DM, Athan E, Ubriaco A, et al. Extranodal noncutaneous lymphoid hyperplasias represent a continuous spectrum of B-cell neoplasia: demonstration by molecular genetic analysis. Blood 1989;73:1635–1645.
68. Wood GS, Ngan BY, Tung R, et al. Clonal rearrangements of immunoglobulin genes and progression of B cell lymphoma in cutaneous lymphoid hyperplasia. Am J Pathol 1989;135: 13–19.
69. Bakhshi A, Minowada J, Arnold A, et al. Lymphoid blast crises of chronic myelogenous leukemia represent stages in the development of B-cell precursors. N Engl J Med 1983;309: 826–831.
70. Aisenberg AC, Wilkes BM. The genotype and phenotype of T cell and non-T, non-B acute lymphoblastic leukemia. Blood 1985;66:1215–1218.
71. Greenberg JM, Quertermous T, Seidman JG, Kersey JH. Human T cell γ-chain gene rearrangements in acute lymphoid and nonlymphoid leukemia: comparison with the T cell receptor β-chain gene. J Immunol 1986;137:2043–2049.
72. Yancopoulos GD, Blackwell TK, Suh H, Hood L, Alt FW. Introduced T cell receptor variable region gene segments recombine in pre-B cells: evidence that B and T cells use a common recombinase. Cell 1986;44:251–559.
73. Goorha R, Bunin N, Mirro J, et al. Provocative pattern of rearrangements of the genes for the γ and β chains of the T-cell receptor in human leukemias. Proc Natl Acad Sci USA 1987;84:4547–4551.
74. Foroni L, Foldi J, Matutes E, et al. α, β and γ T-cell receptor genes: rearrangements correlate with haematological phenotype in T cell leukaemias. Br J Haematol 1987;67:307–318.
75. Raghavachar A, Thiel E, Hansen-Hagge TE, Kranz B, Bartram CR. Rearrangement of T cell receptor β, γ, and δ gene loci in human pre-T cell acute lymphoblastic leukemia. Leukemia 1989;3:413–418.
76. Gonzalez-Sarmiento R, LeBien TW, Bradley JG, et al. Acute leukemia expressing the gamma gene product of the putative second T cell receptor. J Clin Invest 1987;79:1281–1284.
76a. Subar M, Pelicci PG, Neri A, Allavena P, Littman DR, Knowles DM, Dalla-Favera R. Patterns of T cell receptor gamma gene rearrangements and expression in B and T lymphoid malignancies. Leukemia 1988;2:19–26.
77. Kitchingman GR, Rovigatti U, Mauer AM, Melvin S, Murphy SB, Stass S. Rearrangement of immunoglobulin heavy chain genes in T cell acute lymphoblastic leukemia. Blood 1985;65: 725–729.
78. Katz F, Malcolm S, Gibbons B, et al. Cellular and molecular studies on infant null acute lymphoblastic leukemia. Blood 1988;71:1438–1447.
79. Felix CA, Reaman GH, Korsmeyer SJ, et al. Immunoglobulin and T cell receptor gene configuration in acute lymphoblastic leukemia of infancy. Blood 1987;70:536–541.
80. Ludwig WD, Bartram CR, Harbott J, et al. Phenotypic and genotypic heterogeneity in infant acute leukemia I. Acute lymphoblastic leukemia. Leukemia 1989;3:431–439.
81. Ha K, Minden M, Hozumi N, Gelfand EW. Immunoglobulin gene rearrangement in acute myelogenous leukemia. Cancer Res 1984;44:4658–4660.
82. Rovigatti U, Mirro J, Kitchingman G, et al. Heavy chain immunoglobulin gene rearrangement in acute nonlymphocytic leukemia. Blood 1984;63:1023–1027.
83. Cheng GY, Minden MD, Toyonaga B, Mak TW, McCulloch EA. T cell receptor and immunoglobulin gene rearrangements in acute myeloblastic leukemia. J Exp Med 1986;163: 414–424.
84. Seremetis SV, Pelicci PG, Tabilio A, et al. High frequency of clonal immunoglobulin or T cell receptor gene rearrangements in acute myelogenous leukemia expressing terminal deoxyribonucleotidyl transferase. J Exp Med 1987;165:1703–1712.
85. Parreira A, De Oliveira P, Matutes E, Foroni L, Morilla R, Catovsky D. Terminal deoxynucleotidyl transferase positive acute myeloid leukaemia: an association with immature myeloblastic leukaemia. Br J Haematol 1988;69:219–224.
86. Norton JD, Campana D, Hoffbrand AV, et al. Rearrangement of immunoglobulin and T cell receptor genes in acute myeloid leukemia with lymphoid-associated markers. Leukemia 1987;1:757–761.
87. Foa R, Casorati G, Giubellino MC, et al. Rearrangements of immunoglobulin and T cell receptor β and γ genes are associated with terminal deoxynucleotidyl transferase expression in acute myeloid leukemia. J Exp Med 1987;165:879–890.
88. Soper L, Bernhardt B, Eisenberg A, et al. Clonal immunoglobulin gene rearrangements in chronic lymphocytic leukemia: a correlative study. Am J Hematol 1988;27:257–264.
89. Norton JD, Pattinson J, Hoffbrand AV, Jani H, Yaxley JC, Leber BF. Rearrangement and expression of T cell antigen receptor genes in B cell chronic lymphocytic leukemia. Blood 1988;71:178–185.
90. Foroni L, Matutes E, Foldi J. T-cell leukemias with rearrangement of the γ but not β T-cell receptor genes. Blood 1988;71: 356–362.
91. Loughran TP, Starkebaum G, Aprile JA. Rearrangement and expression of T-cell receptor genes in large granular lymphocyte leukemia. Blood 1988;71:822–824.
92. Loiseau P, Divine M, LePaslier D, et al. Phenotypic and genotypic heterogeneity in large granular lymphocyte expansion. Leukemia 1987;1:205–209.
93. Naeim F. Hairy cell leukemia: characteristics of the neoplastic cells. Hum Pathol 1988;19:375–388.
94. Korsmeyer SJ, Greene WC, Cossman J, et al. Rearrangement and expression of immunoglobulin genes and expression of Tac antigen in hairy cell leukemia. Proc Natl Acad Sci USA 1983;80:4522–4526.
95. Cleary ML, Wood GS, Warnke R, Chao J, Sklar J. Immunoglobulin gene rearrangements in hairy cell leukemia. Blood 1984;64:99–104.
96. Foroni L, Catovsky D, Luzzatto L. Immunoglobulin gene rearrangements in hairy cell leukemia and other chronic B cell lymphoproliferative disorders. Leukemia 1987;1:389–392.
97. Migone N, Giubellino MC, Casorati G, Tassinari A, Laurie F, Foa R. Configuration of the immunoglobulin and T cell receptor gene regions in hairy cell leukemia and B-chronic lymphocytic leukemia. Leukemia 1987;1:393–394.

98. Berenson J, Lichtenstein A. Clonal rearrangement of the β-T cell receptor gene in multiple myeloma. Leukemia 1989;3: 133–136.
99. Fishleder A, Tubbs R, Hesse DO, Levine H. Uniform detection of immunoglobulin-gene rearrangement in benign lymphoepithelial lesions. N Engl J Med 1987;316:1118–1121.
100. Weiss LM, Wood GS, Trela M, Warnke RA, Sklar J. Clonal T-cell populations in lymphomatoid papulosis: evidence of a lymphoproliferative origin for a clinically benign disease. N Engl J Med 1986;315:475–479.
101. Kadin ME, Vonderheid EC, Sako D, Clayton LK, Olbricht S. Clonal composition of T cells in lymphomatoid papulosis. Am J Pathol 1987;126:13–17.
102. Weiss LM, Wood GS, Ellisen LW, Reynolds TC, Sklar J. Clonal T-cell populations in pityriasis lichenoides et varioliformis acuta (Mucha-Habermann disease). Am J Pathol 1987;126:417–421.
103. LeBoit PE, Abel EA, Cleary ML, et al. Clonal rearrangement of the T cell receptor β gene in the circulating lymphocytes of erythrodermic follicular mucinosis. Blood 1988;71:1329–1333.
104. LeBoit PE, Beckstead JH, Bond B, Epstein WL, Frieden IJ, Parslow TG. Granulomatous slack skin: clonal rearrangement of the T-cell receptor β gene is evidence for the lymphoproliferative nature of a cutaneous elastolytic disorder. J Invest Dermatol 1987;89:183–186.
105. Wood GS, Weiss LM, Hu CH, Abel EA, et al. T-cell antigen deficiencies and clonal rearrangements of T-cell receptor genes in pagetoid reticulosis (Woringer-Kolopp disease). N Engl J Med 1988;318:164–168.
106. Hanson CA, Frizzera G, Patton DF, et al. Clonal rearrangement for immunoglobulin and T-cell receptor genes in systemic Castleman's disease: association with Epstein-Barr virus. Am J Pathol 1988;131:84–91.
107. Levison DA, Hall PA, Cotter FE, Donaghy M, Stansfeld AG. An immunohistological study of the plasma cell form of Castleman's disease. Proceedings of the 157th Meeting of the Pathological Society of Great Britain and Ireland, July 1988. J Pathol 1988;155:340(A).
108. Pelicci PG, Knowles DM II, Arlin ZA, et al. Multiple monoclonal B cell expansions and c-myc oncogene rearrangements in acquired immune deficiency syndrome-related lymphoproliferative disorders: Implications for lymphomagenesis. J Exp Med 1986;164:2049–2060.
109. Lipford EH, Smith HR, Pittaluga S, Jaffe ES, Steinberg AD, Cossman J. Clonality of angioimmunoblastic lymphadenopathy and implications for its evolution to malignant lymphoma. J Clin Invest 1987;79:637–642.
110. Feller AC, Griesser H, Schilling CV, et al. Clonal gene rearrangement patterns correlate with immunophenotype and clinical parameters in patients with angioimmunoblastic lymphadenopathy. Am J Pathol 1988;133:549–556.
111. Weiss LM, Strickler JG, Dorfman RF, Horning SJ, Warnke RA, Sklar J. Clonal T-cell populations in angioimmunoblastic lymphadenopathy and angioimmunoblastic lymphadenopathy-like lymphoma. Am J Pathol 1986;122:392–397.
112. O'Connor NTJ, Crick JA, Wainscoat JS, et al. Evidence for monoclonal T lymphocyte proliferation in angioimmunoblastic lymphadenopathy. J Clin Pathol 1986;39:1229–1232.
113. Frizzera G, Kaneko Y, Sakurai M. Angioimmunoblastic lymphadenpathy and related disorders: a retrospective look in search of definitions. Leukemia 1989;3:1–5.
114. Lindh J, Lindstrom A, Lenner P, Lundgren E, Roos G. Immunoglobulin heavy-chain gene rearrangement in peripheral blood mononuclear cells in non-Hodgkin's lymphomas—correlation with kappa:lambda analysis and clinical features. Eur J Haematol 1989;42:134–142.
115. Berliner N, Ault KA, Martin P, Weinberg DS. Detection of clonal excess in lymphoproliferative disease by kappa/lambda analysis: correlation with immunoglobulin gene DNA rearrangement. Blood 1986;67:80–85.
116. Nowell PC, Hungerford DA. A minute chromosome in human granulocytic leukemia. Science 1960;132:1497–1503.
117. Campbell ML, Arlinghaus RB. Current status of the BCR gene and its involvement with human leukemia. Adv Cancer Res 1991;57:227–256.
118. Daley GQ, Ben-Neriah Y. Implicating the bcr/abl gene in the pathogenesis of Philadelphia chromosome-positive human leukemia. Adv Cancer Res 1991;57:151–184.
119. Berger R, Chen SJ, Chen Z. Philadelphia-positive acute leukemia. Cytogenetic and molecular aspects. Cancer Genet Cytogenet 1990;44:143–152.
120. Hughes TP, Ambrosetti A, Barbu V, Bartram C, Battista R, Biondi A, Chiamenti A, Cimino G, Ernst P, Frassoni F, et al. Clinical value of PCR in diagnosis and follow-up of leukaemia and lymphoma: report of the third Workshop of the Molecular Biology/BMT study group. Leukemia 1991;5:448–451.
121. Medeiros LJ, Van Krieken JH, Jaffe ES, Raffeld M. Association of bcl-1 rearrangements with lymphocytic lymphoma of intermediate differentiation. Blood 1990;76:2086–2090.
122. Williams ME, Meeker TC, Swerdlow SH. Rearrangement of the chromosome 11 bcl-1 locus in centrocytic lymphoma: analysis with multiple breakpoint probes. Blood 1991;78:493–498.
123. Raffeld M, Jaffe ES. bcl-1, t(11;14), and mantle cell-derived lymphomas [editorial]. Blood 1991;78:259–263.

Section III

Section Chiefs: *Robert W. Burnett, Kent Lewandrowski, and Elizabeth Lee-Lewandrowski*

Most illnesses either have a primary biochemical origin or result in a secondary disturbance to the intricate biochemical equilibria that characterize the healthy human organism. It follows that careful measurement of selected compounds in blood or other body fluids can provide information useful in diagnosis, and such measurements are also useful in monitoring disease processes and the response to therapy.

Although clinical chemistry is sometimes viewed as a narrow subspecialty, it is also a very broad field encompassing a huge variety of quantitative and qualitative analytical techniques. Analytes range from simple ionic species and small organic molecules to proteins, hormones, and drugs. The range of concentrations of the various species of interest spans more than nine orders of magnitude. Methodologies range from difficult and labor-intensive manual methods to highly automated instrumental methods.

This section is intended to cover the most important analytes of interest in clinical chemistry. Where applicable, chapters include normal biochemistry and physiology, an outline of laboratory techniques for measuring the analyte, and the clinical relevance of the laboratory results. It is hoped that this section will serve as a reference for the most commonly used information about clinical chemistry, as well as an introduction to the more detailed discussions found in specialized textbooks and journal articles.

CLINICAL CHEMISTRY

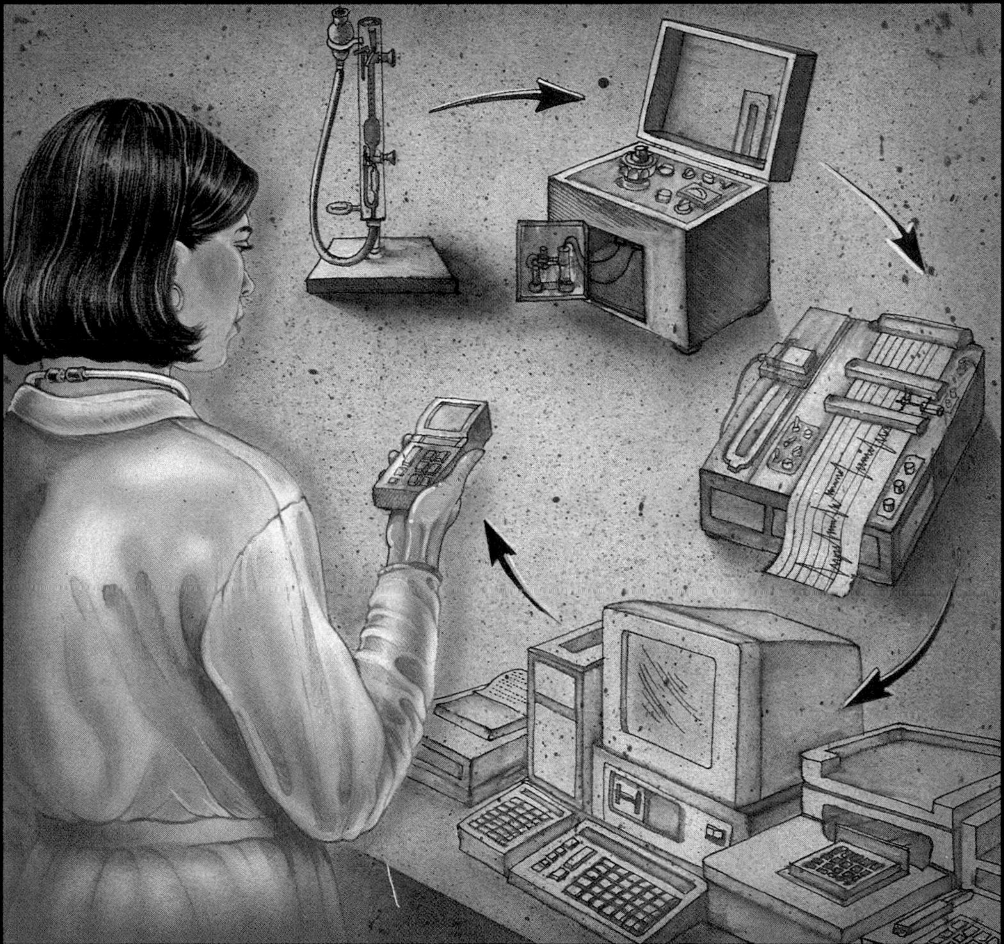

9 Immunochemical Methods

Robert E. Moore

Immunoassay, as a diagnostic tool, originates with the much older clinical discipline of serology. Approximately 100 years ago it was demonstrated that certain types of bacteria could be agglutinated by antiserum. It was also suggested at that time that this could be an aid in the diagnosis of typhoid fever, and the procedure was given the name Grüber-Widal test. From this modest beginning, immunoassay has developed into the fastest-growing methodology in the clinical laboratory. The transition, however, has not been easy. Numerous recent advances have allowed immunoassay to achieve its present popularity. The first of these came in the late 1950s when Drs. Berson and Yalow published a series of studies on ^{131}I-labeled insulin to detect antibodies to insulin and later to measure the insulin itself. These studies demonstrated beyond any doubt that a new analytical technique with exquisite sensitivity and specificity was possible. There were, however, some practical problems that kept the technique from being an instant success. First, iodine-131 is a high-energy nuclide that requires nuclear counting instrumentation equipped with a large sodium iodide crystal for efficient measurement. At the time, this represented a new type of equipment for clinical laboratories, and institutions were reluctant to make a significant capital investment in such instrumentation until the technique had wider applicability. Second, antibodies were primarily responsible for the specificity and to a lesser extent the sensitivity of the assay. These reagent antibodies were not commonly available, and investigators had to produce and characterize their own antibodies for each analyte that was to be measured. Antibody production was not a technique common to the clinical laboratory, and laboratories that were capable of undertaking antibody production found it to be a labor-intensive effort. Third, these early assays were based on competitive binding, a technique that depends on a labeled antigen competing equivalently with the natural antigen for a fixed number of sites, which meant most antigens had to be labeled in the laboratory. The short half-life of ^{131}I, and the difficulty in controlling the organic reactions required to attach this radioactive atom to the analyte, made this a very inefficient and expensive procedure. The instability of the labeled compounds required this labeling procedure to be done just prior to performing the analysis. Generally, these early radioimmunoassay (RIA) methods were long and tedious. In addition, if the results were unacceptable, the process had to be repeated, including the labeling procedure.

The next significant improvement was the regular availability of ^{125}I. The longer half-life—60 days for ^{125}I compared with 8 days for ^{131}I—and the lower energy associated with ^{125}I had several advantages for the clinical laboratory. First there was the impact on laboratory equipment. The lower energy of ^{125}I meant that smaller, less expensive crystals could be used to count the nuclide with reasonable efficiency. Second, the preparation and labeling of the antigens or antibodies done with ^{125}I were more stable, and repeat analyses could be performed using the originally prepared label if there was a problem with the assay. There was still the inconvenience of having to produce your own antibodies, and you still had to do your own labeling, which meant having large quantities of ^{125}I in the laboratory with all the incumbent regulatory and safety requirements. It was apparent that the analytical potential of the immunoassay with a radioactive label was virtually unlimited and had allowed the quantitation of hormones and peptides for the first time. It was also evident that this potential would be sufficient to stimulate commercial vendors to begin supply assay materials in a more convenient form, thereby giving smaller laboratories access to this technology. By the late 1960s and early 1970s antibodies were being prepared commercially. Investigators could pick from an ever-increasing menu of prepared antibodies and prelabeled antigens. It was a small step from antibody and antigen availability to the appearance of kit packaging. These kits contained all the reagents that the researcher would need to perform a specific assay. This also made the immunoassay available to significantly more laboratories. With this proliferation came demands for higher quality and standardized reagents.

A parallel development occurred with small organic molecules such as steroids, thyroid hormones, and drugs. These molecules had been synthesized for some time with tritium or carbon-14 atoms at specific structural sites. Antibodies for these materials were not readily available. One problem with this type of molecule is that it is not immunogenic by itself. That is, these compounds will bind with antibodies but are not capable of evoking an immunologic response in an animal to produce an antibody. This was an additional problem that was not encountered with the larger peptide hormones or proteins. The solution to this problem was to covalently attach these small molecules to much larger immunogenic molecules. As investigators began to couple these haptens to proteins, it became apparent that the stereochemistry of the coupling reactions was extremely important. Since there is a great deal of homology among steroids, drugs, and thyroid hormones, judicious choice of coupling site was required to improve the specificity of antibodies. As with the peptide hormones, it soon became apparent that the commercial vendors would be supplying antibodies and prepackaged reagent systems for these assays.

These assays were dependent upon liquid scintillation methods for detection, and although this equipment was more common than γ counting equipment, it was not common to the clinical laboratory. In addition, liquid scintillation has unique methodological problems of quenching, low efficiency, added expense for special solvents and counting vials, and limited throughput.

As more investigators became interested in the RIA, it was inevitable that some effort would be invested in finding alternative methods. Because the specificity of these reactions is due to the antibody, and the sensitivity is mainly due to the amplification system (i.e., multiple radioactive atoms per molecule of analyte), any chemical method that had amplification potential became a candidate to replace the radioactive label. The only limitation seems to be the imagination as multiple types of labels are combined with detection systems and methodologies to produce the wide spectrum of immunoassays currently available.

All immunoassays share one common feature. These assays use one or more antibodies to effect the analytic measurement. They owe their specificity and to some extent their sensitivity to the quality of the antibody used in the assay.

ANTIGENS

To try to define antigen in a chapter on immunoassay would be quite problematic. Immunologists and practitioners of the immunologic sciences have struggled, with limited success, to provide a precise and all-inclusive meaning for antigen. For purposes of this discussion the functional definition will be used: antigens are substances capable of binding to an antibody. This is in contrast to immunogens, which are substances capable of eliciting a humoral antibody response when presented to a host. The definitions in this chapter are not refined, but they are attempts to minimize confusion.

IMMUNOGENS

Immunogens have several qualities that have been determined empirically. Good immunogens are usually large, complex molecules that differ significantly from normal molecular species found in the host. Although the term large is difficult to describe, molecules with molecular weights greater than 10,000 are usually good immunogens, while, conversely, molecules with molecular weights below 10,000 are poorer.

Molecular size is not the only requirement. Structure is a significant characteristic in determining the efficacy of the immunogen. If the overall structure has incorporated in it lipids, glycoproteins, polysaccharides, or nucleic acids, these will generate a better antibody response in the host than will synthetic peptides composed of one or two simple amino acids. In addition to primary structure, there is also a relationship between immunogenicity and tertiary structure. The more complex spatial relationships found in biomolecules tend to be more immunogenic than less complex synthetic linear peptides and proteins.

The quality of the immune response of the host improves dramatically as the host is able to identify the immunogen as a foreign substance. When the host animal is challenged, there is an attempt to categorize the material as self or nonself. For obvious reasons, materials that are identified as nonself elicit a much more vigorous response. If the origin of the nonself material is from an evolutionally divergent species, the immune response is expected to be far greater than if the nonself is from a closely related species or the same species.

Finally, the route of administration has some effect on the quality of the immune response. All immunogens are not equal in their ability to elicit antibody formation independent of administrative routes. Intradermal, subcutaneous, and intramuscular approaches seem to be the most convenient and effective routes commonly employed.

For biomolecules of clinical interest that are not immunogenic in and of themselves, i.e., steroids, thyroid hormones, drugs, and small peptides, they can be made effective immunogens by covalently coupling them to a much larger protein backbone. Multiple moles of a small molecule can be covalently linked per mole of large protein to produce a very

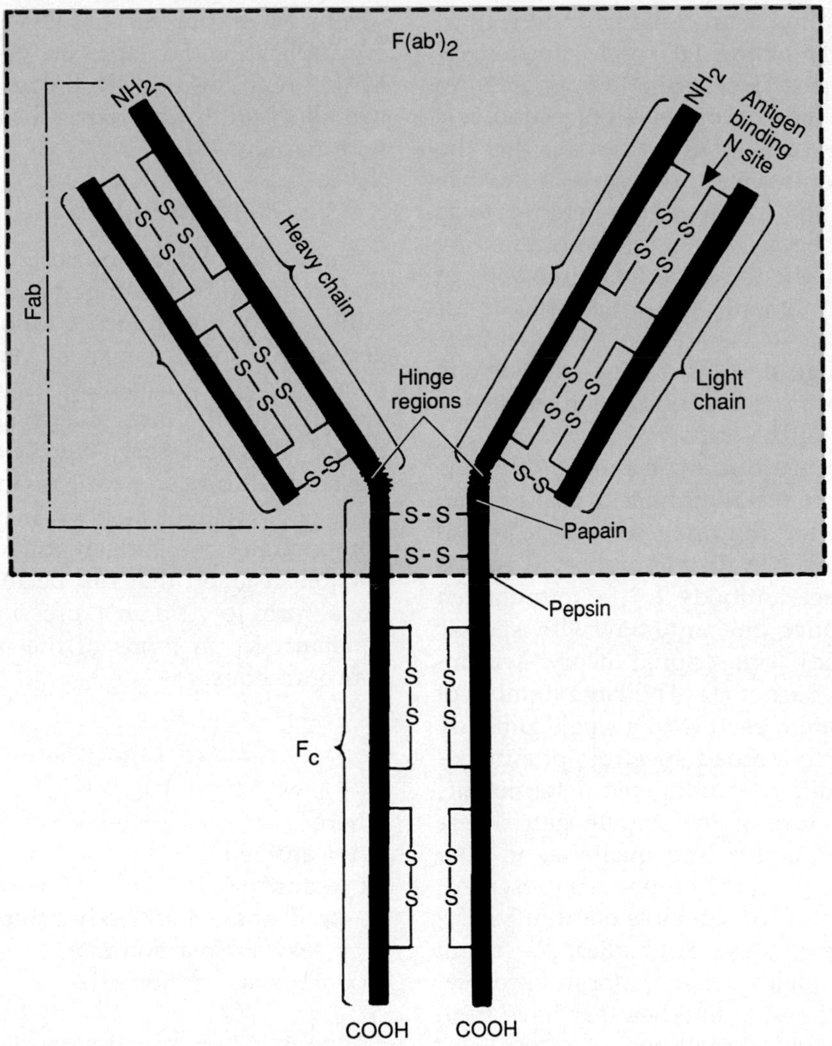

Figure 9.1. Schematic representation of IgG antibody. Papain digestion releases two Fab fragments and one Fc fragment. Pepsin digestion releases one $F(ab')_2$ fragment. Both enzyme digestions conserve antigen binding sites.

effective immunogen. Molecules that require coupling to other molecules to produce immunogenicity are referred to as haptens. Because many of these small molecules share similar structure, as in the case of steroids, it is possible to select the organic coupling reaction so that the common portion of the structure is used for attachment to the protein backbone, while the unique portion of the structure is left exposed to the environment. This process increases the probability that antibodies will be generated against this unique structure.

ANTIBODIES

Once the immunogen has been presented to an appropriate host, a type of lymphocyte called a "B cell" will begin to produce antibody against the immunogen. These antibodies are immunoglobulin class proteins predominantly of the IgG and IgM type, with the IgG making up most of the analytic antibodies in use today. As shown in Figure 9.1, IgG is composed of two identical heavy and two identical light chains held together by a series of interdisulfide and intradisulfide bonds. The heavy chains are designated (H) and the light chains (L). The specific heavy chain associated with IgG is designated as a γ chain, while the light chains are either κ or λ, but both do not occur on the same molecule. There are two binding sites on each IgG molecule, and these are located at the ends of the "arms" at the juncture of the heavy and light chains.

Enzymatic digestion of the IgG molecule yields some interesting structural characteristics. Pepsin digestion cleaves the two arms of the "Y" from the body of the molecule and these arms remain attached to each other and retain the divalent antibody binding characteristics. The body of the IgG is digested to small fragments. If papain is used to digest the IgG molecule, three fragments are obtained. The two arms are cleaved as independent fragments, each with its antibody binding characteristic, and the third fragment is the body of the IgG molecule that remains intact. When the two antibody fragments remain together, as in the case of pepsin digestion, it is referred to as a Fab′$_2$ fragment, indicating that the two antibody fragments remain together. In the case of papain, the antibody fragments are referred to as Fab, since they have been cleaved into single binding sites by the enzyme. The third fragment, the body of the IgG, is the Fc fragment. The *c* here stands for crystallizable, referring to a characteristic of that fragment after papain digestion. The actual binding site on the IgG molecule is at the amino end, with one binding site in each of the arms.

It is possible to generate analytic antibodies in one of two ways. The historical method is to challenge an animal species with an immunogen to elicit an immune response. Each B cell or lymphocyte that is stimulated to produce antibody to the immunogen will ultimately produce one antibody with specific binding characteristics. This "clonal theory" was introduced in 1957 by Burnet (1). The large number of lymphocytes stimulated, each with a single antibody response, gives rise to a broad spectrum of antibodies that recognize different antigenic determinants over the entire structure of the immunogen. These antibodies differ in quantity and quality as to their ability to identify the specific immunogen presented, but with some luck and considerable effort in purifying and characterizing these antibodies, the result can yield very high-quality reagents for in vitro use. These are the polyclonal antibodies that have been used for years in analytical methods.

The second and more recent approach is to generate monoclonal antibodies. Köhler and Milstein exploited the fact that each lymphocyte clone would produce only one type antibody. They developed a technique to continuously produce a selected antibody from cultured lymphocytes (2). This method produces very specific antibodies that recognize a single antigenic determinant on a given molecule, and the clone can be cultured virtually forever. The procedure requires inoculating mice, taking the spleen cells from responsive animals, and fusing them with a myeloma cell line. The fusion products are cultured and screened for the clone that generates the desired antibody. In theory this approach should have produced the ideal analytic antibody. Practice has demonstrated that monoclonal antibodies (MAbs) have some deficiencies. The affinity of MAbs is often less than that required for analytic procedures resulting in low limits of detection, and the specificity for small molecules is difficult to achieve (3). Some of these drawbacks can be overcome by combining multiple clones from a given fusion—in essence producing a polyclonal serum from several MAb sources—but this is not effective for every application. For large analytes the combination of MAbs with differing affinities has improved the overall affinity. This effect has not been observed with haptens (4).

Antigen-Antibody Interactions

Immunoassays can be designed to measure either the formation of an antigen-antibody complex or the inhibition of that complex formation. Individual investigators and commercial vendors design immunoassays to take advantage of a particular detection system or to maximize analytical sensitivity, if that is critical. It is necessary, therefore, to understand the basic qualities of the antigen-antibody complex that yield good analytic assays. As equations 9.1 and 9.2 demonstrate, the antigen-antibody reaction is a reversible reaction that can be rearranged in conventional form to yield an expression for the association constant, K_a, in terms of the reactant and product concentrations.

$$A_g + A_b \underset{k_2}{\overset{k_1}{\rightleftharpoons}} A_g{\cdot}A_b \qquad (9.1)$$

where
A_g = antigen
A_b = antibody
$A_g{\cdot}A_b$ = antigen-antibody complex
k_1 = forward reaction rate
k_2 = reverse reaction rate

$$\frac{[A_g{\cdot}A_b]}{[A_g]\,[A_b]} = \frac{k_1}{k_2} = K_a \text{ association constant} \qquad (9.2A)$$

$$\frac{[A_g]\,[A_b]}{[A_g{\cdot}A_b]} = \frac{k_2}{k_1} = K_d \text{ dissociation constant} \qquad (9.2B)$$

Good antibodies, and consequently good assays, are characterized by large K_a values. The interpretation of this is that the equilibrium reaction lies far to the right and there is minimal dissociation of the antigen-antibody complex once it has formed. A small dissociation constant (K_d) is interpreted to mean the antibody is bound very tightly to the specific antigen. In other words, the fit between the antigen and the antibody is optimal and the binding forces have been maximized; therefore, the dissociation rate constant, k_2, is minimized. The practical implication of this is that assays designed around antigen-antibody complexes of this quality are called "robust" and tend to be less sensitive to minor changes in assay conditions such as pH, reaction time, temperature, and ionic strength. If the K_a were small, then the dissociation of the complex would become appreciable and the assay would be insensitive due to a low concentration of complexes at any given time.

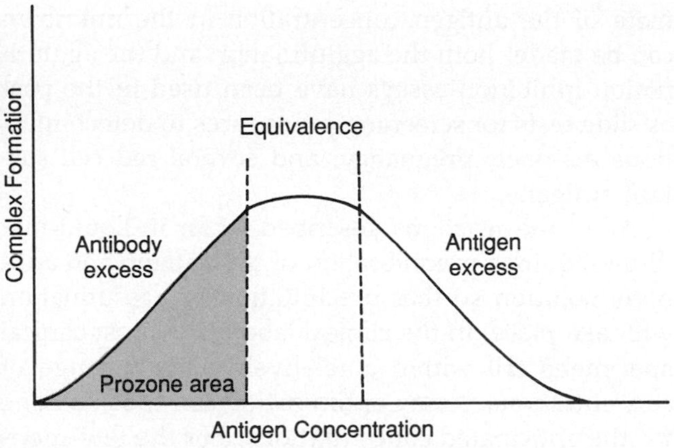

Figure 9.2. Titration curve for a constant quantity of antibody. In antibody excess (prozone region) there are insufficient antigen molecules to produce maximum complex formation. At equivalence, the complex formation is optimized. If the complexes are separated from the liquid phase, no free antigen or antibody is detected in the remaining solution. In antigen excess, each antibody is saturated with antigen, and complex formation is reduced.

The forces that determine the antigen-antibody complex are all of the intermolecular forces with the exception of covalent bonding. Ionic bonds, hydrogen bonds, van der Walls' forces, and hydrophobic-hydrophilic repulsion constitute the forces that are responsible for maintaining the integrity of the complex. These forces act over short molecular distances. As the fit between the antigen and the antibody improves, more and more of these noncovalent bonds are formed and the rate of dissociation of the complex is reduced. This property is called antibody affinity for a single site, for complexes that are formed using multiple antibodies on multiple antigenic sites, the sum of these forces is referred to as antibody avidity. It is an interesting property of these bonds that the total adhesive force in the complex exceeds the sum of the individual forces (5).

The stoichiometry of the antigen-antibody reaction plays a critical role in assays that are dependent on maximum precipitation. As Figure 9.2 illustrates, when a polyvalent antibody reacts with an antigen with multiple determinants, the precipitation increases gradually to a maximum and then begins to decrease. Initially there is excess antibody for the amount of antigen in the solution. In this situation each antigen molecule has the maximum complement of antibodies but each epitope has a different antibody bound. With excess antibody available there is little opportunity for cross-linking antigens and forming large molecular complexes. As the concentration of antigen increases, a point is reached where the antigen and antibody concentrations are balanced so that a macromolecular lattice can be formed. These lattice structures are so large that precipitation is at a maximum. The point at which maximum precipitation occurs is called the equivalence point. At this point if one were to analyze the solution after precipitation of the antigen-antibody complex, there would be very little antigen or antibody remaining. If antigen continues to increase to a concentration where it is in excess, then each antibody becomes saturated with antigen molecules. In the case of IgG this is two antigens per antibody molecule. Similar to the case of antibody excess, antigen excess results in different antigens binding to the antibody, again limiting the possibility for cross-linking. The complexes formed under conditions of antigen excess are not large enough to affect total precipitation, and so considerable complex is left in solution. Note also that the x-axis calibrated in concentration and the y-axis calibrated for a response to complex formation, there is a low and a high concentration that will yield the same response. Assays that depend on measuring complex formation—particularly if they are fully automated assays—must take this effect into account and be prepared to test for antigen excess conditions.

PRECIPITATION TECHNIQUES

Immunodiffusion Liquid Systems

The formation of precipitates between antigens and antibodies in liquid media are the simplest and oldest precipitation reactions conducted in the laboratory. This approach takes advantage of the diffusive property of molecules and the precipitation of antigen-antibody complexes. The reaction is carried out in either small test tubes, small-diameter capillary tubes, or microtiter wells. A mixture of antigen and antibody is allowed to incubate for several hours. At the end of this time a precipitant will have formed and will have settled to the bottom of the reaction vessel. If this reaction is carried out with a constant amount of antigen and varying dilutions of antibody, a qualitative assessment of the equivalence point can be determined by evaluating the amount of precipitate that has formed in each of the tubes. The equivalence point will be equal to the concentration that formed the greatest amount of precipitant.

Another way to perform this reaction is to add the antibody solution to the tube and then very carefully layer the antigen solution on top, trying to avoid actual mixing of the solutions. At the interface, a ring will form as the antigen-antibody complex is formed.

In each of the aforementioned cases, the antigen and antibody were soluble and multivalent so that a macromolecular species could form that would eventually precipitate out of solution. Techniques have been developed for small antigens that do not have multiple binding sites and therefore tend to form

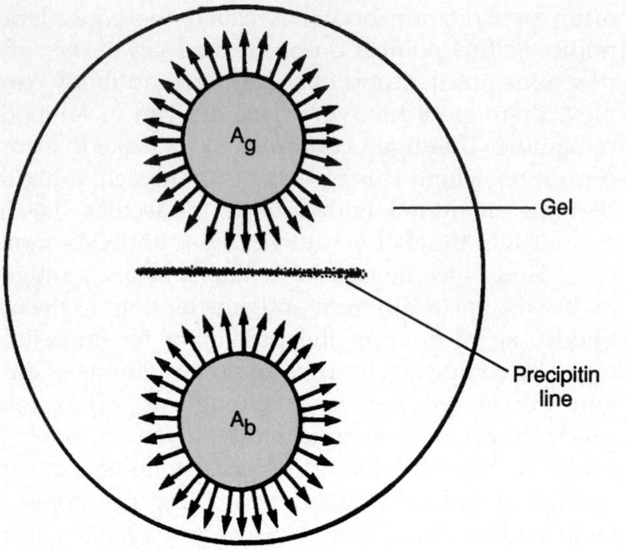

Figure 9.3. Immunodiffusion. Two wells are punched out of gel. Antigen (*Ag*) is placed in one well and antibody (*Ab*) is placed in the other. As the solutions diffuse through the gel, antigen-antibody complexes form and a precipitin line results. If antigen and antibody are not pure, a precipitin line will form for each antigen-antibody pair of complexes generated.

complexes that remain soluble. One approach is to coat larger particles with the antigen before exposing it to the specific antibody. A typical support would be sheep erythrocytes or latex particles coated with the antigen of interest. Once these large support particles contain many antigens, multiple antibodies will bind and the particles will become aggregated in solution. The term aggregation generally applies to reactions in which the antigen or antibody is coated on the surface of a cell or synthetic particle used as a support medium. In this reaction, the aggregation of particles indicates the presence of the analyte. When these reactions are carried out in a series of increasing dilutions, a qualitative assessment of the concentration of analyte can be determined.

A variation on the aggregation reaction is the aggregation inhibition reaction. Like the aggregation reaction, antigens or antibodies are coated on a support such as animal erythrocytes or latex beads. The first step of the reaction is to incubate the solution to be analyzed with free antibody. This reaction proceeds to form soluble antigen-antibody complexes. At the end of this initial incubation period the support particles with the antigens coated on the surface are incubated with the preformed soluble antigen-antibody complexes. The quantity of antigen in the test solution will determine the number of free antibodies available for agglutinating the support particles. In this case the concentration of analyte is inversely proportional to the amount of agglutination. If a series of standard solutions is run concurrently, an estimate of the antigen concentration in the unknown can be made. Both the agglutination and the agglutination inhibition assays have been used in the past as slide tests for screening procedures to detect infectious diseases, pregnancy, and several red cell surface antigens.

All of the reactions described so far in liquid medium require a precalibration of the antigen and antibody solution so that precipitation or agglutination will take place. In the clinical laboratory most clinical specimens fall within a relatively narrow range of concentrations. Assay optimization can thus be done for the anticipated concentrations. For the few specimens that have concentrations outside the expected range, adjustments to those samples in terms of concentration or dilution can be made. In any case, it is important to check the analytic reagents periodically, and especially as new lots of reagent are incorporated into the procedure.

GEL SYSTEMS

These reactions are carried out in a gel support, usually an agar or agarose gel, that has been heated to liquid state and then poured onto a solid support and allowed to solidify. This solid support can be glass, acetate sheets, plastic, or any appropriate transparent material. It is important that the seal between the gel and the solid support is intact to prevent the solutions from wicking along the interface. As shown in Figure 9.3, two wells are cut in the gel. An antigen solution is placed in one and an antibody solution in the other. The solutions are allowed to incubate at room temperature, during which time the solutions diffuse through the gel in a radial fashion. The rate of diffusion is dependent on several conditions: the concentration of the respective solutions, the molecular size of the antigens and antibody, and the lattice structure of the gel. As these solutions diffuse, their fronts will meet and at a point where the antigen and antibody are in equivalence, a precipitation line will be formed. Some characteristics of the precipitin line are quite useful in interpretation. First, the solution of higher concentration will diffuse more rapidly, and so the precipitin arc will be closer to the lower-concentration solution. Larger molecules will diffuse more slowly than smaller molecules, and if the antibody molecular weight is known, the molecular weight of the antigen can be approximated, assuming the two concentrations are similar. If there are multiple antigens or multiple antibodies, a separate line will be formed for each antigen-antibody pair. When this technique is set up in a circular fashion with multiple wells so that the antibody solution is in the center well and the circumference has sev-

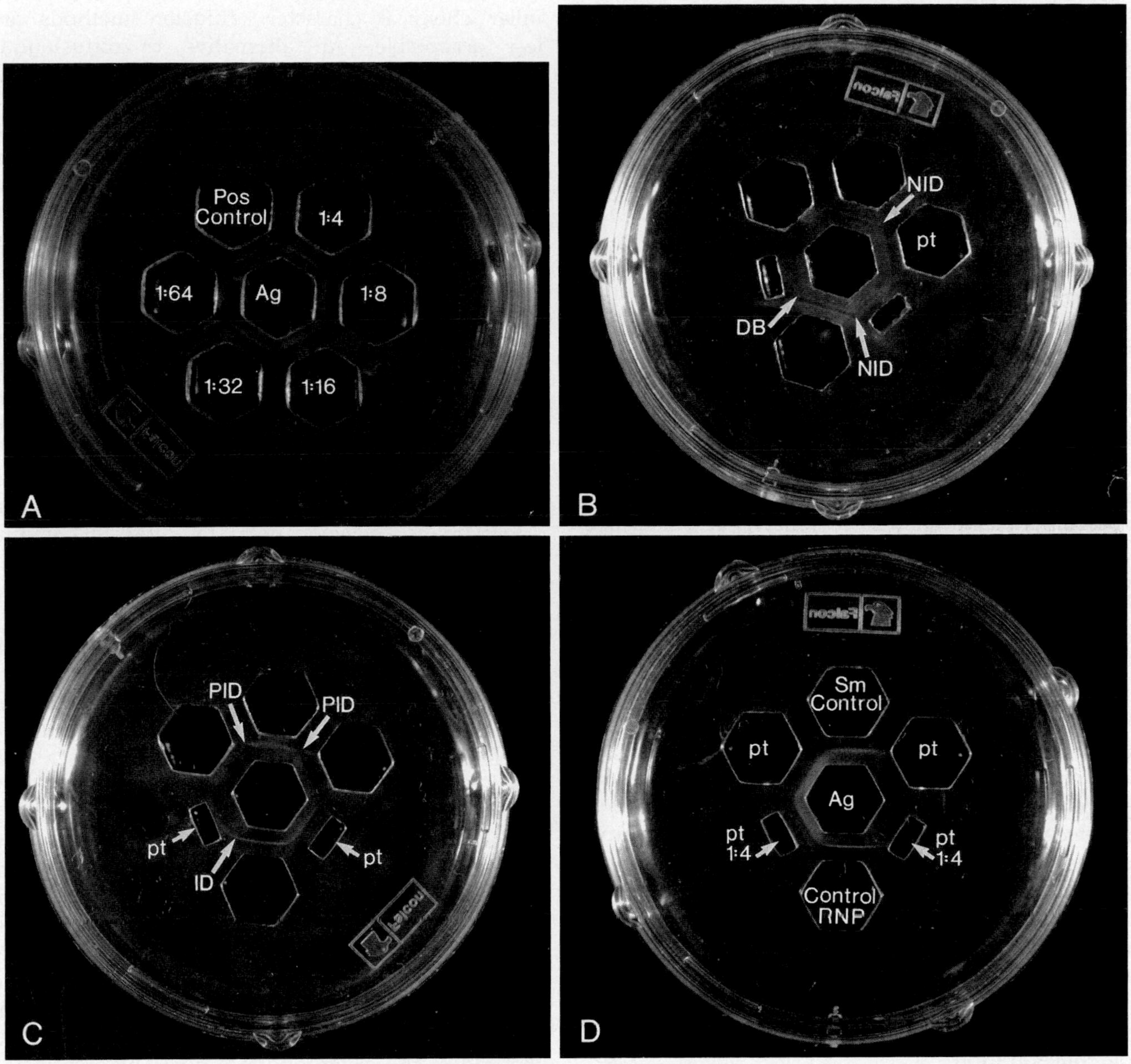

Figure 9.4. **A**, Radial immunodiffusion plate. Antigen (Ag) is placed in the center well. Positive control for antigen is placed in the well marked *Pos Control*. Patient serum dilutions are made clockwise from 1:4 to 1:64. Notice that the precipitin line migrates closer to the patient wells that contain the more dilute specimen. The precipitin line forms a circle with positive control and no "spurs" or cross lines are observed. These are arcs of identity. **B**, Immunodiffusion plate with arc of nonidentity (*NID*). Precipitin lines cross at the point of the *arrow*. Also visible is a double precipitin line (*DB*). This occurs when multiple antigens and antibodies are present in the sample and reagents. **C**, Radial immunodiffusion plate with lines of partial identity (*PID*) and identity (*ID*). PID lines have a "spur" at the *arrows* unlike the smooth arc of identity. The precipitin line moves closer to the wells with higher dilution of specimen. **D**, Immunodiffusion plate showing multiple precipitin lines. Patient sample (*pt*) on the left demonstrates antibodies for both Sm control and RNP control. The small rectangular well contains patient serum equivalent to 1:4 dilution.

eral wells with different antigen solutions, the precipitin lines can be quite telling about the antigen-antibody complexes formed. As seen in Figure 9.4*A*, if the antigen is similar in two adjacent wells, the precipitin line is a continuous arc. If the antigens in adjacent wells are dissimilar, there are two separate arcs that cross (Fig. 9.4*B*), and if the antigens are similar but not identical, the precipitin line will have a single spur on one of the arcs (Fig. 9.4C). The terminology applied to these precipitin lines is "arc of identity," "arc of nonidentity," and "arc of partial identity," respectively. This is known as the Ouchterlony technique. Figure 9.4*D* demonstrates a real case with multiple precipitin lines showing positivity for the antibody controls, with additional unknown precipitin lines.

This procedure is relatively simple and inexpensive but lacks sensitivity for quantitative applications. It is useful for applications that either identify an antigen or antibody or determine their relative purities. Some experimentation has to be done to ensure that there is a reasonable relationship between the concentration of antigen and the concentration of antibody, or no preciptin line will form. If the starting protein solutions must be adjusted to achieve an acceptable concentration, adjustment of the final ionic strength and pH may also be required.

Another common diffusion technique is referred to as the Mancini technique. This procedure incorporates antibody into the agarose gel. The gel is heated to 50° to 55°C and the antibody is dispersed in this liquefied gel. If the temperature of the gel is not allowed to exceed 55°C, significant antibody denaturation will not take place. The gel is then poured onto a solid support and allowed to solidify, at which time small wells are cut into the gel. Each of these wells will hold a solution to be analyzed, and on a single slide a range of standard solutions as well as unknown samples may be assayed. The antigen in the well diffuses radially and precipitates as it encounters antibody in the gel. The antigen creates a concentration gradient as it diffuses from the well, and at the diffusion front when the antigen and antibody are at equivalence, a precipitate forms. As more antigen flows to the front, this precipitate redissolves because of antigen excess, and a precipitate forms farther away from the well. After several hours of incubation this process stabilizes. Quantitative results can be obtained by plotting the diameter of the ring formed around the antigen well versus the concentration of the standards. Unknown concentrations can then be extrapolated from the curve by finding the diameter of the ring and reading the corresponding concentration.

This technique is dependent on a well-characterized monospecific antibody and reasonably simple antibody solutions. The formation of multiple rings generally means that the antibody is recognizing more than one antigen in the antigen solution, while the formation of asymmetrical rings is usually traced to a defect in the gel formation. With a little practice this can be a moderately sensitive, simple, and cost-effective approach to analyzing some clinically important antigenic proteins.

ELECTROPHORESIS

The previously described diffusion methods are quite adequate for solutions that have relatively few components. In situations where the solution being analyzed is complex due to the number of components, or if it has multiple components of very similar chemical character, diffusion methods are less acceptable. An alternative to diffusion is electrophoresis. With this method, the components of a solution are separated based on size and charge in an electric field, and efficient separations can be effected on very similar molecules. Once the components of the solution have been separated, immunotechniques can be combined with the electrophoretic results to produce a quantitative analytical method.

Laurell Rocket Immunoelectrophoresis

This particular technique is named for the originator of the procedure, C. B. Laurell, and the rocket or triangular shape that the antigen-antibody complexes form at the end of the analysis (6). In this method the antibody is dispersed in the agarose gel and the pH of the gel is adjusted to 8.6. This is an approximate isoelectric point for most IgG immunoglobulins, meaning that in the electrophoresis phase of the analysis the antibodies will not migrate through the gel. When the gel is cool, wells are punched at the bottom of the gel and are filled with the antigen solution to be analyzed. Electrode wicks are carefully applied to the top and bottom of the gel plate as illustrated in Figure 9.5. The wicks must be carefully attached to the gel so that there is a constant current per cross-sectional areas of the gel. It is preferable to have a cooling device to keep the gel cool during the electrophoresis so there is no "drying and cooking" of the gel. As the antigens are electrophoresed from the well, they encounter the antibody that has been dispersed through the gel, and the antigen-antibody complex forms at the electrophoresis front. As the antigen concentration changes, the complex dissolves and reforms, eventually forming a triangular or rocket-shaped pattern at the end of the electrophoresis run. The area inside these triangular patterns is directly proportional to the concentration of antigen that was placed in the well. If the triangular shapes are symmetrical, peak height can be substituted for the area in determining the concentration of unknowns.

This technique is particularly sensitive to antigen-antibody concentrations and electric field strengths. It is important to use as low an antibody concentration as possible in the gel, and one indication of too high an antibody concentration would be the formation of excessive precipitant within the outline of the rocket.

Crossed Immunoelectrophoresis

This variation on rocket immunoelectrophoresis is also referred to as double-crossed immunoelectrophoresis or two-dimensional immunoelectro-

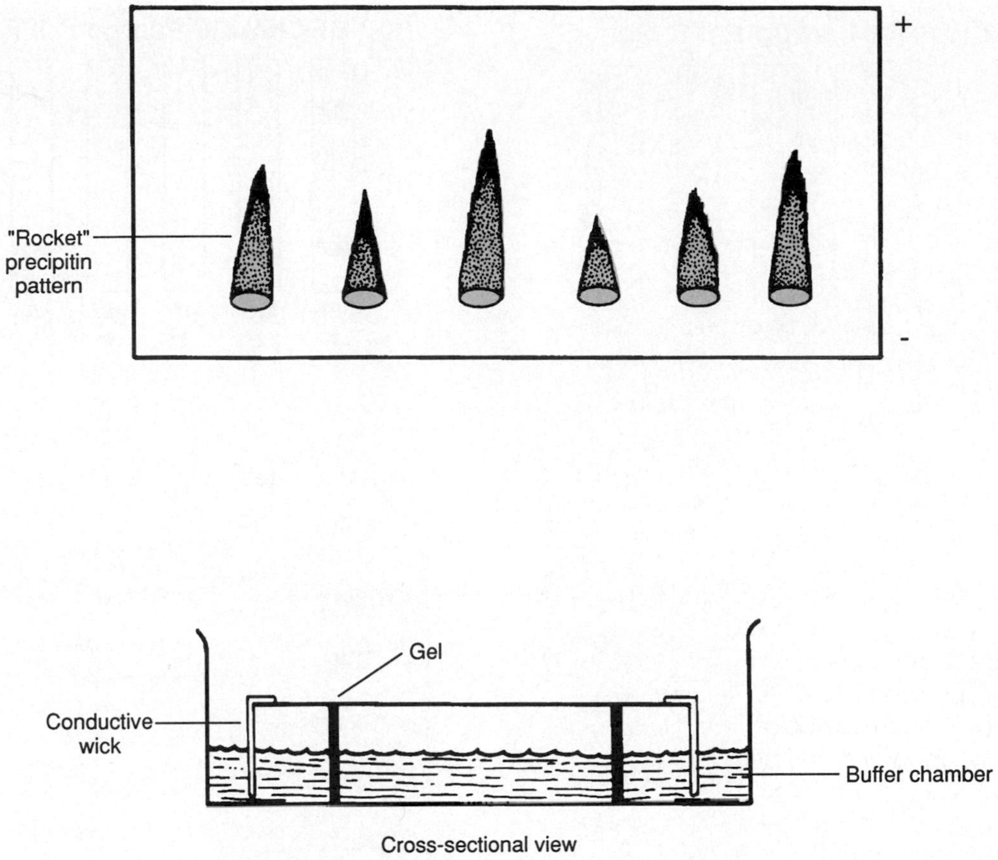

Figure 9.5. Laurell rocket electrophoresis. Antibody is mixed with gel and allowed to cool on a plate, forming a conductive surface. Small wells are punched at the cathode (–) side of the gel. The antigen forms, dissolves, and reforms the complexes at the electrophoresis front until the patterns are stabilized. The triangular shape of the precipitation front gives rise to the name rocket immunoelectrophoresis.

phoresis. The technique starts by electrophoresing the antigen solution on standard agarose gel under any set of electrophoretic conditions that will effect the separation of the antigens of interest. Once these antigens have been separated, the gel is sliced so that the separated antigens are contained in a long thin strip of agarose. This gel strip of separated antigens is then placed in or up against a second gel that has antibody dispersed through it. A second electrophoresis is conducted with the field at right angles to the original separation. From this point the procedure is very similar to rocket immunoelectrophoresis in that, as the antigens enter and migrate through the antibody-containing gel, a precipitant forms, dissolves, and reforms, ultimately yielding triangular or triangular-like patterns of precipitation. Because several antigens can be analyzed at the same time, this technique is quite useful for metabolic studies, enzyme studies, and kinetic studies where there is interconversion of initial reactant and product.

The technique is susceptible to the same errors as Laurell rocket immunoelectrophoresis. The same conditions of low antibody concentration and low electric field strength should be observed.

Immunoelectrophoresis

One of the more common techniques used in the clinical laboratory is immunoelectrophoresis (IEP). This technique is relatively straightforward, is cost-effective, and is amenable to processing large numbers of specimens as well as having the potential for being automated. The technique finds its primary application in the identification of serum proteins, and particularly in identifying pathological conditions such as monoclonal gammopathies, light chains, and general protein deficiencies.

The technique consists of preparing or purchasing a special gel plate for electrophoresis of the specimen containing the antigens. The special preparation of the plate requires cutting a trough in the gel and punching two small wells on either side of the trough. This is most easily accomplished by using a commercially available template and gel punch or by purchasing the prepared gel from one of several manufacturers. The antigen solutions are placed in the small punched-out wells and electrophoresed long enough to separate the components of the antigen solution. Once the electrophoresis is complete,

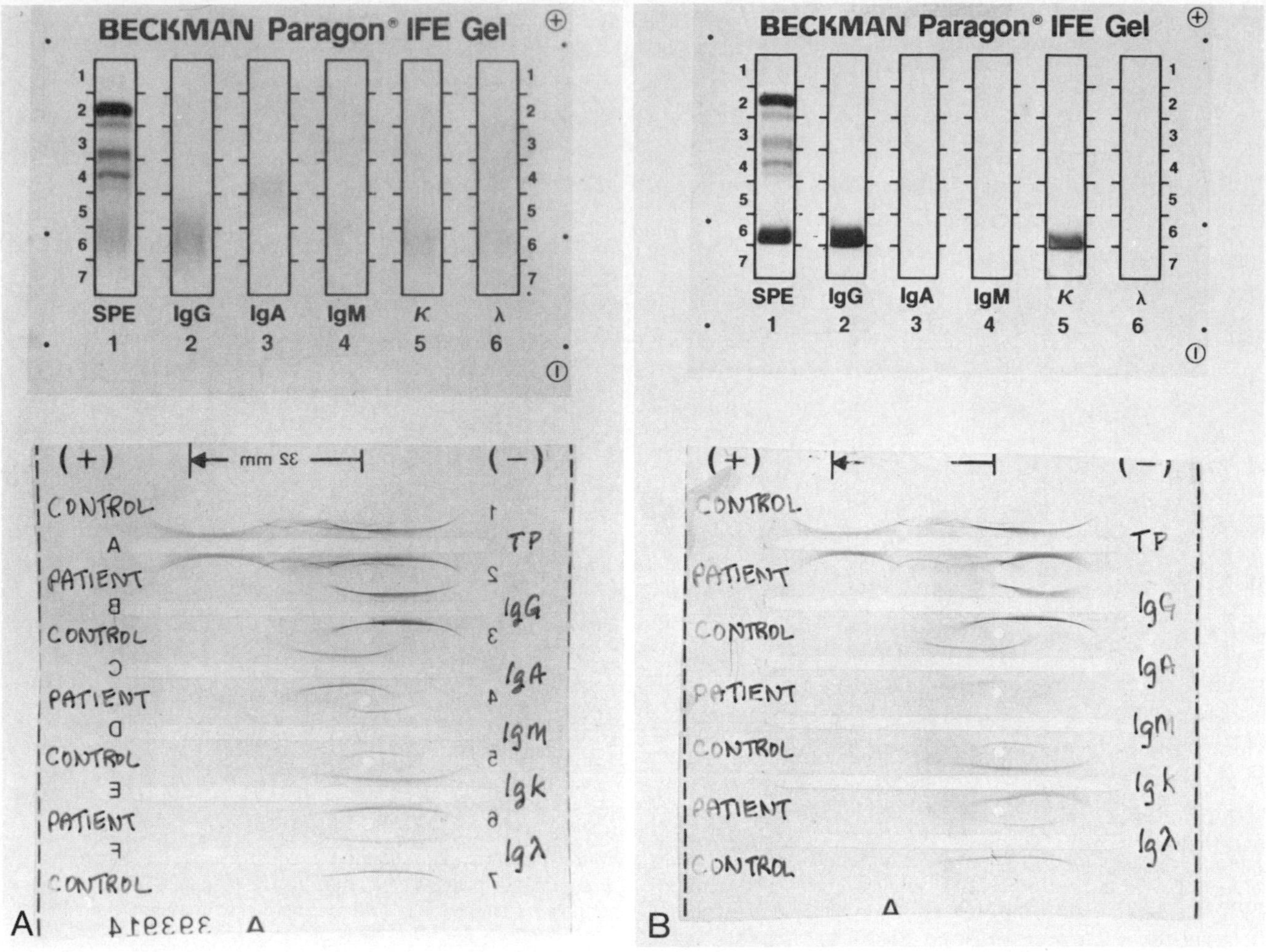

Figure 9.6. **A**, Normal immunofixation electrophoresis (IFE) (*top*) and the same serum on immunoelectrophoresis (IEP) (*bottom*). Dark bands on IFE indicate the presence of a serum protein precipitated with antibody. Diffuse bands are indicative of polyclonal production of protein. IEP develops serum proteins as arcs with antibody. Control and patient serum are alternated in the gel wells so arcs can be compared directly. Antisera is placed in the trough between the wells. **B**, Monoclonal gammopathies of the IgG κ type. Dark bands in the serum lane and the IgG lane indicate increased concentration of IgG. The sharp band in the κ lane indicates a monoclonal increase in IgG with a κ light chain. This is also observed in the IEP (bottom) with a broad, thickened arc above the IgG trough. The arc below the κ trough demonstrates a nonsmooth arc resembling a spoon shape. All other arcs compare well with the normal control serum.

antiserum is placed in the trough and allowed to diffuse into the gel. This antiserum can either be directed against numerous proteins, as in the case of antiserum directed against human serum, or it can be specific for a single protein. In either case the diffusion of the antiserum forms precipitin arcs where it intercepts the antigen previously separated by the electrophoresis. These plates can then be read by looking at the opacity due to the precipitation of the antigen-antibody complexes, or the gel can be stained with one of the commercially available blue, red, or black protein stains. The arcs in the specimen can then be compared to controls and an interpretation can be made as to the presence or absence or proteins as well as the presence of unusual or pathological forms. Figure 9.6*A* depicts the gel plate with the trough and wells properly positioned and demonstrates the stained protein bands on a normal serum specimen. Figure 9.6*B* is an IgG myeloma.

Immunofixation Electrophoresis

A modification of the immunoelectrophoresis technique was first described in the early 1960s by Alfonso and later refined by Alper and Johnson (7). The technique, known as immunofixation electrophoresis (IFE), has the advantages of rapidity and ease of interpretation over immunoelectrophoresis but suffers the disadvantages of being a technique-dependent procedure as well as a more costly procedure. Commercial materials are available, and the need for investigators to pour and generate their own electrophoresis plates is no longer necessary. Figure 9.6*A* depicts a normal serum specimen on an IFE plate with six lanes labeled serum proteins, IgG,

IgA, IgM, κ and λ. The clinical specimen, be it serum, cerebral spinal fluid, or urine, is placed at the indicated origin on each side of the lanes. Total sample volume is approximately 5 μl. The specimens are then electrophoresed to separate the individual proteins in the sample. At the end of the electrophoresis time, a template is placed over the gel and pressed gently but firmly into the gel to create a seal around each of the lanes. For the lane marked serum protein, a protein fixative is added to denature and immobilize the serum proteins. For each of the other lanes, a specific antiserum is placed over the lane. The plate is covered and allowed to incubate for approximately 30 minutes. At the end of this time, the plate is washed in saline several times to remove all the proteins that have not been complexed or fixed. Therefore, the only proteins remaining in the individual lanes will be those that were denatured with the fixative and those that formed complexes with the specific antiserum placed on the lane. Once the plate has been washed thoroughly, it is stained with a standard protein stain and the bands are visualized. Lanes marked G, A, and M indicate G, A, and M antisera and the presence of a band. A diffuse area of stain is indicative of a monoclonal protein complexing with the antisera. The lanes marked κ and λ will indicate the type of light chain associated with the heavy-chain globulin or will indicate the presence of free light chains. A more detailed discussion of immunoglobulin gammopathies and protein band interpretation is available elsewhere in this edition. The main advantage of IFE is that the individual globulins and the light chains can be compared directly to the band staining of the whole sample serum proteins. If there are unusual intensities or the presence of abnormal bands in the whole serum sample, they can be compared directly to bands that are generated with specific antisera on the same plate. Figure 9.6*B* is an IgG monoclonal gammopathy of the κ light chain type.

INSTRUMENTAL METHODS

As immunoassays began to develop, there was an evolution from early qualitative observations of precipitant to techniques that attempted to separate the antigen and antibody and isolate the complex on a gel, stain it, and quantify the stain densitometrically. The work by Drs. Berson and Yalow opened the door to a new era of instrumental techniques that had the requisite precision and sensitivity to make immunoassays a more controllable and routine analytical technique in the clinical laboratory (8). The original work of these investigators used a labeled technique whereby a molecule with a different physical characteristic was linked to the antigen-antibody reaction so that a quantitative measurement could be made. From this, investigators began to pursue alternative methods. One approach took advantage of the formation of the antigen-antibody complex without the introduction of additional molecules or atoms. In another method, investigators sought alternative labels that would have the same characteristics as the radioactive label but not share some of the disadvantages. The next sections describe these instrumental techniques. They have been arbitrarily divided into those that do not employ a label or marker for the measurement of the antigen-antibody complex and those that do.

Nonlabeled Methods

LIGHT SCATTERING

Light scattering is the result of the interaction of electromagnetic radiation on particles as it passes through a sample. Light, being electromagnetic radiation, has both an electric field and a magnetic field component. As the particles in solution come under the influence of the electric field, the electrons move in one direction and the nuclei in the other, causing a relative separation. Since the electric field is sinusoidal in nature, the particle oscillates or resonates in synchrony with the electric component. This oscillation results in the re-emission of energy with the same frequency as the incidence light. This re-emission phenomenon is spherical in nature; that is, with reference to the specimen it can be measured in all directions. There are several characteristics of both the incident light and the particles that will affect the nature of the scattered signal. Among these are the wavelength of the incident light, whether or not the incident light is polarized, the size of the particle, the molecular weight, the concentration of particles, and the distance at which the observation or measurement is made.

Particle size is generally divided into two categories: one in which the particle is less than one-tenth the wavelength of the incident light, and the other in which the particles are greater than one-tenth the wavelength of light. In the first instance the particle is small enough to be totally within the influence of the electric field. In this case the particle sees the field strength equally and becomes a point source of re-radiation of the incident light. This phenomenon was first described by Lord Rayleigh and is described by the Rayleigh equation for small particle scattering.

$$I_s = I_i \left[\frac{16\pi^2 a \sin^2\theta}{\lambda^4 r^2} \right] \quad (9.3)$$

In this expression, I_s is the intensity of the scattered light; I_i is the intensity of the incident light; a is the polarizability of the small molecule (i.e., the ability of the electric field to separate the electronic and the nuclear components of the particle); θ is the angle of observation measured from the line of the incident light; λ is the wavelength of the incident light; and r is the distance of the observation. Although several important relationships can be taken from this equation, it is important to remember that this was derived for particles suspended in a gaseous medium and requires some corrections for solutions. The main characteristics of this expression are:

- The intensity of the scattered light is a function of the fourth power of the wavelength of the incident light; that is, short wavelengths will scatter more intensely than longer wavelengths;
- The intensity of the scattered light will be reduced by the square of the distance of the obstruction. Therefore, the collectors or the measurement device should be as close to the source of scatter as is physically possible;
- As this equation is written, the right-hand side has essentially two components. The first is the intensity of the incident light, and the second is the combination of factors and constants that describe a given system. Therefore, for any given system, the scattered intensity will increase directly as the intensity of the incidence light is increased. This is the rationale for the use of high-intensity sources such as lasers to yield higher scatter intensities.

The corresponding equation for liquid systems with particles in suspension and a nonpolarized source of incident radiation is given below:

$$I_s = I_i \left[\frac{4\pi^2 \, ({}^{dn}/_{dc})^2 \, Mc \, (1+\cos\theta)}{N \, \lambda^4 r^2} \right] \qquad (9.4)$$

The symbols remain the same as in the previous equation, with the addition of the dn/dc, a correction factor for the incremental change in refractive index of the solution with an incremental change in the concentration of particles; M is the molecular weight of the particles in question; c is the concentration; N is Avogadro's number. This expression now relates the concentration and the molecular weight of particles to the intensity of the scattered light. This is the more useful form for solution chemistry and the one that has been utilized in immunoassay systems.

There are other considerations in using light scattering for immunoassay. Among these is whether or not the source is polarized. Other sections in this text give a detailed description of the difference between polarized and nonpolarized light. Suffice it to say that for the nonpolarized source, the scattering intensity is generally greater. Looking at the scattering intensity diagram associated with small molecules, one realizes that the scattering envelope is symmetrical about a 90° axis to the particle. The scattering envelope has a remote resemblance to a figure eight. This is in contrast to the scattering envelope of large molecules, which is asymmetrical with the greatest intensity in the forward direction and minimal intensity in the backward direction. Figure 9.7 depicts these differences. By comparing these two diagrams, it is clear that, when using scattered intensity as a measure of the presence of small molecules in a sample composed of both large and small molecules, it would be most advantageous to measure the backward scatter, since this would be least affected by large particles.

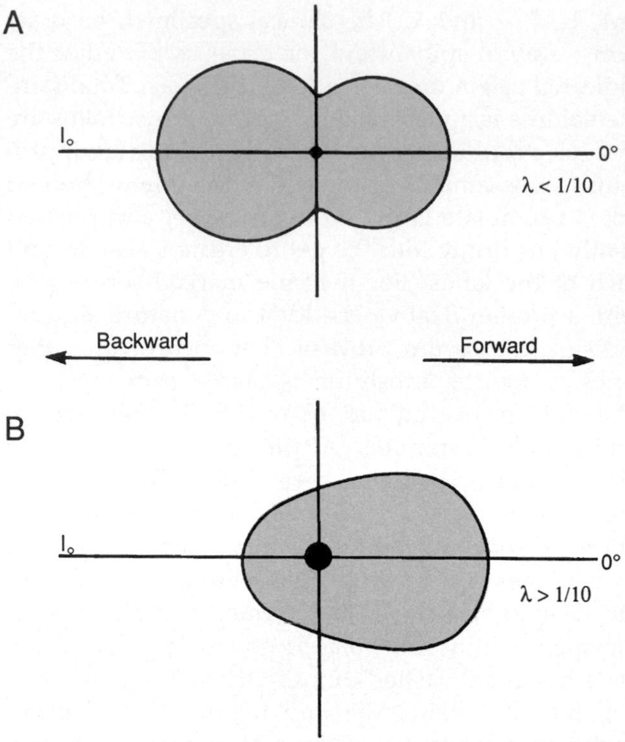

Figure 9.7. Light scattering as a function of particle size and angle. **A**, Small particles (particle size less than one-tenth wavelength) scatter in a symmetrical envelope about the center of the particle. **B**, Large particles (greater than one-tenth λ) scatter asymmetrically about the particle center, with greater intensity in the forward direction. The light source is unpolarized in both diagrams.

Large-particle scattering differs from small-particle scattering in that the particle is generally considered to be larger than one-tenth the wavelength of incident light. This larger particle size means that as the electric fields impinge on the particle, different portions of the particle will respond to differences in the electric field strength. Therefore, a large molecule can have several points of oscillation and re-emission of light that will constructively and destructively interfere with each other. The net result of multiple points of scattering is that the strongest intensity is in the forward direction and the weakest in the backward direction.

The molecular weight characteristic that is measured in light scattering is a weight average molecular weight. In immunoassay measurements this means any reaction that takes place must increase the average molecular weight of the particles in solution. The greater this average molecular weight change, the greater the changes in intensity of the scattered signal. This last point is one of the reasons that light scattering techniques have not enjoyed the popularity that was initially expected. The principle of light scattering should allow the direct measurement of the complex formation. There is no requirement for additional labels or secondary indicator molecules. The problem arises when one tries to measure steroids, drugs, or other low–molecular weight compounds in moderate to low concentrations in a matrix made up of serum proteins and lipids. The combination of an antibody to these monovalent antigens does not shift the average molecular weight sufficiently to generate a strong signal above background. Many things have been done to decrease the background signal and improve the scattered signal from the solution being investigated, but once additional steps are required, light scattering methodologies begin to have practical limitations. When an immunoassay system is set up to measure high–molecular weight proteins in moderate to large concentrations, light scattering is very effective. If the concentration of large molecules is too high, the macromolecular complexes that form begin to take on the appearance of aggregates. Aggregate formation does one of several things. First, the *number* of molecules present in the solution changes. Aggregates are seen as a single particle, thereby effectively reducing the number of particles in solution. Second, the average molecular weight changes by a very significant amount. Third, the physical size of these complexes exceeds the limitations of the Rayleigh-Debye scattering theory. A much more complex physical-chemical model must be employed to describe the scattering phenomenon as associated with aggregates in solution. Because of these multiple changes in the solution, the results are nonlinear. Fortunately, this nonlinearity of response can be handled by the conventional data handling techniques employed in other immunoassay procedures. These are discussed under Data Reduction.

TURBIDIMETRY AND NEPHELOMETRY

Light scattering can be measured in the laboratory by one of two methods, turbidimetry or nephelometry. The difference is in the angle at which the analytic signal is measured. For turbidimetry, the detector is in line with the incident source and is usually referred to as either zero angle or 180°. For nephelometry, any other angle is used to measure the scattered signal. Turbidimetry measures a decrease in signal due to the scattering of incident light by particles in the solution. This means that you are measuring a small difference between large numbers. Nephelometry, on the other hand, measures scattered signal against no signal since it is out of line from the incident radiation. The sophistication of modern spectrophotometers is such that turbidimetric measurements are adequate for many laboratories procedures when the antigen or antibody of interest is in moderate to high concentration. Nephelometry, however, is suited to making those measurements when the antibody or antigen is in low concentration. The much smaller signal generated by these molecules will be more easily detected against a very low background.

The sample preparation for light scattering measurements is the same whether one uses a turbidimetric or a nephelometric approach. Samples must be free of any material that is capable of scattering light such as chylomycra, dust, or other particulates introduced from the collection and preparation process. It is also important that the wavelength of light used to measure the scattering is chosen so that it is not in a transition band of one of the components of the solution. This means that radiating a specimen with a wavelength of light that will be absorbed by any of the components in the serum will reduce the emitted light. Turbidimetric measurements will interpret this as high scattering due to a high concentration of analyte, while nephelometric measurements will be made with an extremely weak signal. Interference from phosphorescence and fluorescence can be controlled with good optic design or by using polarizing filters. A potential problem for scattering and all methods that measure antigen-antibody reactions is that of antigen excess. Instrumentation that relies on endpoint determination—that is, takes a measurement at the beginning of the reaction and one at a later time—must be capable of detecting antigen excess. This becomes less of a problem in automated instruments that use a kinetic approach, because algorithms are available for the microprocessor to determine whether the kinetics are taking place in the antigen-deficient, the equivalent, or the antigen excess zone of the curve.

Several instruments are currently on the market that are capable of doing turbidimetric or nephelometric measurements in either an endpoint or kinetic mode or both. The computer processing power within these instruments is significant, and most have complex data handling routines that allow analysis of complex curves.

Labeled Methods

It is obvious from the previous sections that there is no single immunoassay system that is suited for all the analytic measurements in the clinical laboratory. To increase the sensitivity of immunoassays, labels or markers were introduced. The first of these was the radioactive label, but that has been followed by enzymes; fluorescent, luminescent, and phosphorescent compounds; as well as metals and particle labels. The objective in using labels in immunoassay is to improve the sensitivity so that heretofore unmeasurable analytes can be quantitated. A second objective, particularly of more recent labels, is to make the methodology simple and straightforward so increasing numbers of laboratorians would have access to the technology using standard clinical laboratory equipment. The second objective has been somewhat amended because some of the newer labels employ technologies that are quite complex, rely on equipment that has not historically been in the clinical laboratory, and necessitate the use of powerful on-board computers for data reduction. Most of this complexity has been hidden from the technologists with the "black box" design. In addition, although the objectives are somewhat universal, the types, methods, and approaches to labeling are diverse. Labels have been covalently linked to antigens and antibodies, both the primary antibody used to detect an analyte, and secondary antibodies used for the detection of the antigen-antibody complex. Also, molecules such as enzyme inhibitors, cofactors, and fluorescent quenchers have been used as the covalently linked molecule but are there to affect the action of another molecule that is monitored for analyte quantitation. The current laboratory and research literature is replete with methods and variations on methods dealing with new labels, the chemistry of label analyte attachment, and system design. Although the details of these methods differ, they can be grouped into broad classifications based on conceptual similarities.

LABELED ANTIGEN

There are several points to consider when selecting labels to be covalently attached to an antigen. One is the size of the antigen. For small antigens such as drugs, vitamins, and steroids, the antigenic binding site may comprise a significant portion of the molecule. If a very large label, such as an enzyme, were to be linked to this antigen, it must be done in a manner that will not sterically block the epitope on the antigen. Small labels such as isotopes, spin labels, and fluorophores must be attached at sites other than the binding site and should not significantly alter the electronic environment of the binding site. In all cases the label must be attached so that it remains an efficient monitor of the antigen-antibody interaction but must not destabilize or significantly alter that antigen-antibody interaction.

Some successful approaches to these problems have been the use of carbon spacer arms, that is, long carbon chains that attach the antigen on one end and the label on the other. This spatially separates the label and the antigen so that steric and electronic interference are minimized. Synthesizing the antigen with carbon-14 or tritium atoms, so that it is radioactive, has the advantage of providing a true label that is structurally indistinguishable from the natural antigen. If the antigen is large, such as proteins, then the labels can be added much more easily and with less probability of interfering with the antigen-antibody interaction. Fortunately, except for research and very specialized applications, the antigens of clinical interest have been prepared with various types of labels and are commercially available. If an investigator elected to label his or her own antigen, a first approach would be to investigate using derivatives of carbodiimide, succinimide, isothiocyanate, or other organic reactions that would be appropriate for the reactive groups available on the antigen.

Antibody labeling is similar to labeling peptide or protein antigens. Most of the antibodies used in clinical chemistry are commercially available with a wide selection of labels.

ASSAY DESIGN

Once the reagents have been assembled, there are several possible configurations for the ultimate assay system. These include competitive, noncompetitive, homogeneous, and heterogeneous systems. Each of these has its specific advantages and disadvantages. The choice of an essay system is generally a function of the type and quality of label and antibody available.

COMPETITIVE ASSAY

In this type of assay the labeled antigen and native antigen compete directly for a limited number of binding sites in the reaction mixture. These binding sites are usually present as a fixed concentration of primary antibody. The reaction follows the law of mass action. Equations 9.1 and 9.2 illustrate the relationship between labeled and unlabeled antigen in the final antigen-antibody complex. To achieve maximum sensitivity in this assay system, it is imperative that the labeled antigen have the same binding characteristics to the antibody as the unlabeled antigen.

Labels that are very large compared with the native antigen or that significantly alter the electronic environment of the antigen can alter the binding characteristics of the antigen with the antibody. This would make one of the antigens a favored binding partner, and, although the assay may work, it could have several technical difficulties, including a lack of sensitivity. The favored binding partner here is not always the native antigen.

When the antibodies are generated against an antigen with a covalently linked carrier, one of the epitopes recognized by the antibody is the organic linkage. When the antigen is labeled, if that same organic linkage is used, the antibody could bind most strongly to that epitope. In this case the native antigen would have difficulty in displacing the labeled antigen, and a serious reduction in sensitivity would result. These competitive designs are sometimes referred to as limited reagent systems because the concentration of antibody is held constant at a level that is insufficient to bind all antigen present. This was the predominant assay design of the original RIA methodologies.

NONCOMPETITIVE ASSAY

In noncompetitive methods there is sufficient reagent to bind the antigen present in the specimen. One very popular approach to this technique is to fix an antibody to a solid support. That support can be a microtiter well, test tube, bead, or other appropriate solid support. Sample containing the antigen is added with the appropriate buffer to the solid support and allowed to incubate. During the incubation time, the antigen binds to the fixed antibody. The support material is then washed and incubated with a second antibody, which may be labeled. This second antibody then binds to a different epitope on the antigen and forms what is commonly referred to as a "sandwich." The support is washed a second time to remove all the unbound antibody, and, if the second antibody had been labeled, the measurement is made. If the second antibody is not labeled, a third antibody that will recognize the second antibody is added. This third antibody carries the label. The requisite reactants are added, and the measurement is made.

HETEROGENEOUS AND HOMOGENEOUS ASSAY SYSTEMS

In heterogeneous assay systems the physical characteristic of the label is unchanged by the binding process. The label that indicates the presence of the antigen-antibody complex must be separated from the extraneous label to make the quantitative measurement. An obvious example would be the radioimmunoassay system, in which the bound radioactive label emits the same signal as the unbound radioactive label. Techniques have been developed that will allow the separation of these two forms of label, allowing the measurement of either fraction. Separation techniques such as precipitation with other antibodies or chemicals, adsorption onto solid surfaces, chromatography, electrophoresis, and some innovative approaches such as coated magnetic particles, have all been successfully employed. The choice of the separation technique used in a heterogeneous assay is primarily dependent on the label used and the clinical application. For example, if the application is one that requires processing large numbers of specimens in a short period of time, then a precipitation, adsorption, or decanting technique would be most appropriate. Conversely, in some research applications, one may be able to process small numbers of specimens by using chromatographic or electrophoretic separation.

In homogeneous assays the physical characteristic of the label changes upon binding; therefore no separation technique is required. If enzymes are used as labels, the enzymatic activity can either increase or decrease when the antigen-antibody complex formation takes place. Likewise, fluorophores can be either activated or quenched upon formation of the complex. These assay methods are generally thought to be simpler and more straightforward since the analytic measurement can be made in the presence of all the reactants.

Immunoassays designed around any of these techniques require a significant number of controls. It is important to monitor antibody characteristics, background signals, nonspecific signals, and potential interference.

SPECIFIC ASSAY TYPES

Radioimmunoassay

Radioimmunoassays take advantage of a radioactive atom being incorporated into one of the reactants as a label. The most common clinical atoms used are ^{125}I, ^{57}Co, ^{3}H, and ^{14}C. The γ-emitting nuclides ^{125}I and ^{57}Co can be incorporated directly into the structure of the antigen, as in the case of the thyroid hormones (^{125}I) and vitamin B_{12} (^{57}Co). The ^{125}I can also be inserted through organic reactions into the ring structure of the amino acids of peptides and proteins. These γ emitters decay at a rate that is characteristic of the atom itself. This decay is unaffected by the environment of the immunoassay reaction and can be counted with reasonable efficiency with standard γ-counting instrumentation.

The β emitters ^{14}C and tritium are generally reserved for small molecules such as drugs and steroids and are usually substituted for "cold" atoms in the structure. As with the γ emitters, the physical decay of β emitters is unaffected by the environment of the assay. However, the energy of the β emission is such that it is easily absorbed by many naturally occurring compounds, making it impossible to measure β emission directly. In order to detect β emission, the samples are counted in a scintillation cocktail. This cocktail contains a carefully chosen solvent and organic flurophore that absorb the β energy and reemit it as a flash of light. This flash is then counted in a scintillation counter that detects these flashes as individual events. Because energy transfer is involved, the efficiency of the detection of events is much lower than with γ emitters.

Because of the characteristics of radioactive labels, all RIAs are heterogeneous assays. The separation step in RIA is generally designed to fit the type of label employed. For labels that are small, like drugs and steroids, an adsorbent such as activated charcoal can be used to adsorb out the unbound label. This is a carefully timed process so that the charcoal does not strip away the label from the antibody, thus destroying the antigen-antibody complex. At the end of the incubation time the samples are centrifuged and the supernatant is decanted into a second tube. The investigator has the choice of counting the supernatant that contains the bound complexes, the charcoal precipitant that contains free label, or both fractions so that a total and percent bound can be calculated on each specimen. This is older technology that has generally been replaced by simpler methods.

Another procedure is to precipitate the antigen-antibody complex with agents such as ammonium sulfate, polyethylene glycol, or additional antibodies that recognize the first antibody used to form the antigen-antibody complex. Here the second antibody is used to make a large lattice of the antigen-antibody complex in solution. All of these methods require centrifugation to pellet the precipitant. The supernatant is decanted, and the pelleted material can be counted as the antigen-antibody complex.

Other methods use a first antibody that is fixed to a solid surface. The solutions containing the antigen and the label are added, and at the end of the incubation time, the solution is decanted. The bound antigen being fixed to the surface of the reaction vessel is then counted directly.

RIAs are capable of precise and accurate quantitation of antigen-antibody complexes if sufficient controls are included in each assay. Obviously, standard concentrations of unlabeled antigen must be used to construct a dose-response or standard curve. In addition, controls must be added to monitor the total amount of radiation added to each tube, the nonspecific binding of the radioactive label to other proteins and surfaces in the reaction medium, and—in the case of β emitters—quench controls that monitor the energy transfer process in the specimen matrix under investigation. It is not unusual in an RIA to find a large percentage of the samples being processed to be control or calibration specimens.

The advantages of RIA are its exquisite sensitivity and the ease with which multiple specimens can be processed. With a little experience, a laboratorian can batch process 100 or more specimens in duplicate with all the requisite controls. This makes it an attractive technology for the medium to large clinical laboratory.

The disadvantages of RIA are the short shelf-life of the labeled reagents due to the short half-life of the radioactive nuclides themselves and the damage that the nuclides do to the proteins in the reagent. In addition, there is a requirement for strict record keeping and personnel monitoring. This makes RIA somewhat more costly than other immunoassay methods, although in recent years, competition from nonisotopic methods has forced the price of prepackaged materials to a more affordable level.

ENZYME IMMUNOASSAY

Enzyme immunoassay (EIA) is a generic term that encompasses all assays that fulfill the following criteria. First, they employ immunologic elements to detect the analyte of interest, and second, enzyme activity is used to quantitate the analyte. It will become obvious that although these two criteria are relatively straightforward, some of the chemistry and assay designs are not. There are many reasons that can account for this. There is the general attractiveness of monitoring immunoassays with enzymes. Enzyme reactions are well-defined, familiar measurements that have been made in the clinical laboratory for decades. The enzymes themselves have been isolated, purified, and characterized and are made available by commercial suppliers at relatively low cost. The enzyme preparations are stable with long shelf lives, and they represent a minimal hazard to the laboratorian. Theoretical sensitivities range from 10^{-14} to 10^{-16} mol/liter, giving these assays the sensitivity required for many clinical assays (9, 10). Measurements can either be made on standard spectrophotometers or be automated on high-throughput instrumentation. In addition, unlike the RIAs, EIAs require no extra licensing, record keeping, or expensive disposal procedures that ultimately contribute to the cost of laboratory analysis.

When laboratorians and researchers are left to their own devices they tend to "tinker." This inherent inquisitiveness, coupled with the almost unlimited number of combinations and permutations of reactions that can be put together, has led to some very ingenious and complicated assay systems. Obviously, only the most reliable and useful of these techniques will find their way to the clinical laboratory for routine use.

The function of the enzyme in the EIA is to act as an amplifier. Each enzyme linked to the antigen-antibody complex will operate on the substrate and produce products that can be measured to quantitate the formation of the antigen-antibody complex. Enzymes will continue to turn over substrate, so a few bound enzymes will result in multiple moles of product formed, resulting in an amplified signal. The assay can be designed so that there is maximum activity when no free analyte is present or there can be maximum activity when maximum free analyte is present. The following sections provide the basic requirements of the enzyme and the substrate that must be considered when designing an assay.

Enzyme Availability

Enzymes can be of plant or animal origin as long as they are abundant and isolated without difficulty. The enzymes should be robust in the sense that they can be subjected to mild organic reactions without losing appreciable activity, and they should have significant activity in the environment in which they will ultimately be used to make analytic measurements. Enzyme activity can be defined as the quantity (micromole, nanomole, picomole) of product formed (or substrate consumed) per unit time under a given set of reaction conditions. The more product formed per unit time, the greater the potential sensitivity of the assay. The enzymes should be inexpensive and available in virtually unlimited quantity. These criteria have essentially limited commercial assays to the use of horseradish peroxidase and animal source alkaline phosphatase.

Substrate

The substrate should share some of the characteristics of the preferred enzymes in that it should be available at reasonable cost in a purified form. There should be a significant difference in the measured characteristic of the substrate compared with the products formed in the enzyme reaction. This means that if the substrate is colorless, the generated product should be colored or fluorescent or should possess any other characteristic that allows confident measurement of the products in the presence of the substrate and other potential interferents. The substrate should also be stable so that it undergoes minimal nonenzymatic conversion to products. As with other reagents, biological hazards should be minimized.

One very popular type of EIA, known as the enzyme-multiplied immunoassay technique (EMIT) assay, has been developed commercially. This is a homogeneous type assay in which the enzyme has been conjugated to the analyte in such a way that the enzyme retains its activity in the absence of analyte binding antibody. When free analyte is added as either a control or a specimen with a fixed amount of antianalyte antibody, the free analyte and the enzyme conjugated analyte compete for the limited number of binding sites on the antibody. When the antibody binds with an analyte that has been conjugated to an enzyme, the enzyme activity is inhibited. Consequently, the inhibition of the enzyme activity is directly proportional to the concentration of free analyte in the solution. This approach has been used very successfully in the therapeutic drug monitoring area. This is a particularly good example of a homogeneous assay because no separation step is required to measure enzyme activity. The final activity measurement can be made in the presence of all the components in the reaction.

A second type of EIA that has been popularized by researchers and commercial vendors is the enzyme-linked immunosorbent assay (ELISA). Although the term ELISA is used interchangeably with EIA, it is more appropriately applied to assays of the heterogeneous solid-phase type. Any solid material can be a candidate for the support component in an ELISA as long as it is capable of irreversibly adsorbing protein to its surface, or the surface can react chemically to covalently bond protein to the surface. Materials that have been used successfully in the past include membranes, microtiter plates, plastic test tubes, plastic beads, various polymers, and coated metal particles. These solid surfaces all perform the same function in the ELISA—to fix one of the components so that the bound enzyme can be separated from the free enzyme. In this assay the enzyme usually retains its activity independent of its bound or free state.

In the competitive ELISA, controlled quantities of the analytic antibody are fixed to the solid phase. Then, the analyte from the specimen is mixed with the enzyme and conjugated analyte, and these are allowed to compete for the limited number of antibody binding sites on the solid surface. After a sufficient incubation time, substrate is added, and the amount of conjugated analyte bound to the fixed antibody will generate measurable product. The concentration of the substrate product is inversely proportional to the concentration of free analyte in the test specimen.

Table 9.1. Enzymes Commonly Used in EIA

Enzyme	Some Substrates
Alkaline phosphatase	4-Methylumbelliferone phosphate *p*-nitrophenyl phosphate
Glucose-6-phosphate dehydrogenase	Glucose-6-phosphate + $NADP^+$
Glucose oxidase	Glucose
Peroxidase	H_2O_2
β-Galactosidase	β-Galactosides

Another approach to an ELISA system is the "sandwich" or capture design. In this procedure an analytic antibody is fixed to the solid phase. The analyte from the test specimen standard or control is added and allowed to react with the antibody on the fixed surface. After a sufficient incubation period, the surface is washed and a second analytic antibody conjugated to an enzyme is added and allowed to incubate. The second antibody recognized a different epitope on the antigen; therefore, this system works best with analytes or antigens that are large enough to have epitopes separated on the molecule so that the two antibodies can bind freely. After the second enzyme-conjugated antibody has incubated, the surface is washed and substrate is added. The generated product is directly proportional to the concentration of analyte in the test specimens.

ELISAs may also be designed to determine antibody concentrations. Applications to screen cultures for antibody production or measure antibody in the serum of patients suffering from various autoimmune diseases have been used in the clinical laboratory. In these assays the antigen is fixed to the solid surface and the test specimen is added so that the antibody will bind to the fixed antigen. The surfaces are washed, as in the other assays, and a second antibody—directed against the IgG of the species generating the first antibody, e.g., human IgG in the case of autoimmune disease—which has been conjugated to an enzyme, is added. After incubation, the surfaces are washed, the substrate is added, and the concentration of the generated chromogen is directly proportional to the antibody concentration in the test specimen.

It should be obvious that there are numerous combinations of antigen-antibody, enzyme, cofactor, and substrate that can be combined in various ways to detect antigen-antibody interaction. The more complex the assay design and the more steps involved, the more difficult it will be to maintain a consistent and reproducible assay over a long period of time. In the simplest of these assays one still has to be concerned about maintaining an optimum environment for both the antigen-antibody binding and the enzyme activity. As more steps are added, the potential for poisoning the enzyme, reducing the antigen-antibody interaction, or just generally increasing the background signal, becomes greater. Some of the more common enzyme reactions are listed in Table 9.1.

FLUORESCENT IMMUNOASSAY

Fluorescence is a phenomenon exhibited by molecules that have the ability to absorb light energy and then dissipate that energy, with some of its being re-emitted as light of a longer wavelength. Fluorescence lifetimes are on the order of 10^{-9} to 10^{-5} seconds, which means there is a delay between the absorption of the exciting light and the emission of the fluorescent light (11). Figure 9.8 depicts the relationship between the wavelength of the absorbed light and the wavelength of the emitted light. The difference between these two wavelengths is referred to as Stokes' shift. Fluorometers have been designed to take advantage of both of these characteristics. Excitation sources can be pulsed, i.e., turned on and off very quickly, so that measurement of the emitted light is less encumbered with the more intense exciting light. The delay between absorption and emission makes this possible. This can be combined with detectors chosen to be more sensitive to the emitted light than the exciting light for increased performance. In addition, fluorescence is emitted in all directions, so detectors can be placed anywhere around the sample and are not in direct line with the exciting light, as is the case in most adsorption spectrophotometers.

Molecules that fluoresce generally have some common characteristics. First, they are usually ring compounds that exhibit extensive conjugation. The greater the number of alternating single and double

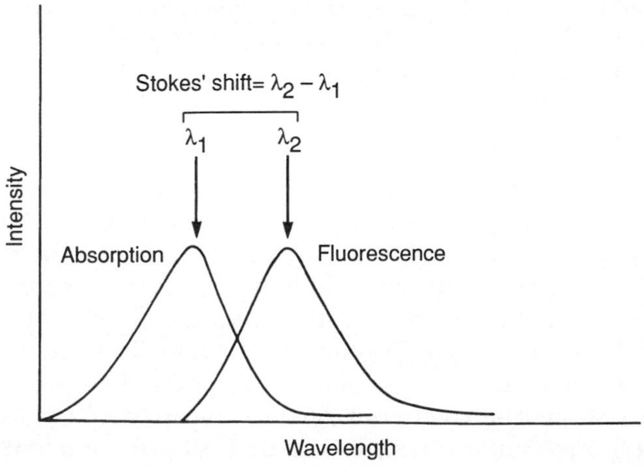

Figure 9.8. Relationship of absorption spectrum to emission spectrum of fluorescent molecule. Peak absorption is indicated by λ, and peak emission by λ_2. Stokes' shift is the difference between the wavelengths at the spectral peaks.

bonds the greater the stability of the excited molecule, which leads to enhanced fluorescence. It is also observed that the greater the molecular planarity and the molecular rigidity, the greater the tendency to fluoresce. Some molecules, particularly chelaters, can be made strong fluorophores by adding the metal ion for chelation (11). It is also known that concentration, temperature, pH, and ionic strength among other things have a significant effect on the fluorescent efficiency of a molecule.

Fluorescent efficiency is termed quantum yield and is a number between 0 and 1 that expresses the amount of emitted light compared with the amount of absorbed light. Any condition that will allow an excited molecule to dissipate its excess energy through processes other than light emission will decrease the quantum yield. Conditions that are commonly encountered allowing a molecule to dissipate its energy are intermolecular collisions caused by high concentrations of fluorophore, elevated temperatures of reaction mixtures, and destabilization of resident structures by other components in the reaction mixture.

Very dilute solutions of fluorophores, in the range of micromolar to picomolar concentrations, are generally used at room temperature or cooler. Fluorescence can be measured with common clinical laboratory instrumentation and present relatively inexpensive, nonhazardous methodologies. It should be noted that fluorescence is a complex process usually dealt with in advanced chemistry and physics textbooks. The observations outlined here are presented as broad concepts so the reader has an appreciation for the requirements of a usable fluorescent immunoassay.

Assay designs in fluoroimmunoassay are very similar to the EIA designs. A fluorescent molecule can be conjugated to an antibody or an analyte and the reaction can be monitored by the presence or absence of fluorescence. The concentration of analyte in the specimen is determined by comparison to standards. The assays can be designed to be heterogeneous, homogeneous, competitive, or any other design that satisifies basic analytical principles. The more interesting uses of fluorescence are in the techniques of fluorescence polarization and time-resolved fluorescence.

Fluorescence Polarization

Fluorescence and fluorescence polarization measurements take advantage of three of the characteristics of fluorescent molecules. These are quantum yield, the time differential between adsorption and emission, and emitted light of a different wavelength than exciting light. The specific nature of the interaction of electromagnetic radiation and matter can be found elsewhere in this book and in other texts. Suffice it to say that a molecule must have a specific orientation in relation to the exciting light for the molecule to absorb energy and be elevated to an excited state. Normal light has a mixture of orientations of electric and magnetic fields. If a polarizing filter were placed between the light source and the sample, the sample would see only one orientation of the electric and magnetic component. Samples with the appropriate orientation would then absorb this light and be elevated to an excited state. If this system were frozen in time, the fluorescence emission would have the same orientation as the exciting light. However, due to the molecular rotation and the length of time required for a molecule to go from exited state to ground state, the resulting fluorescence is a mixture of electric and magnetic orientations. By imposing another polarizing filter between the sample and the detector only the fluorescent light with the appropriate orientation will be detected. Therefore, the intensity of the polarized fluorescent signal is related to molecular orientation. Conceptually, this means if something can be done to decrease the velocity of the rotation of fluorescent molecules so they retain their original orientation until they fluoresce, the intensity of the fluorescence signal will increase. In fluorescent immunoassays employing polarized signals, the rationale is that the analyte is labeled with a small fluorophore and it will rotate rapidly. In addition, relatively few molecules will emit the appropriate plain polarized light for detection. Once these analyte molecules are bound to an antibody, however, their hydrodynamic radius increases significantly. This reduces the rotational velocity, increasing the number of molecules that have the appropriate orientation. The fluorescent signal is thus increased. Under these conditions, a competitive fluorescent immunoassay (FIA) may be set up so that maximum fluorescence signal is obtained in the absence of any unlabeled analyte. When unlabeled analyte is added, competition between the labeled and unlabeled species will reduce the fluorescent signal. The concentration of analyte is inversely proportional to the fluorescent signal. Quantitation is achieved by comparison to a standard response curve.

It was mentioned earlier that the quantum yield is also taken advantage of by fluorescent and fluorescent polarization methodologies. Remembering that quantum yield is defined as the number of photons emitted divided by the number of photons absorbed and starting with the Beer-Lambert equation, one can make a series of substitutions and algebraic rearrangements to demonstrate that the intensity of the fluorescent signal is directly proportional to the intensity of the exciting signal. That means for a given system, if the intensity of the exciting light is increased (i.e., through high-intensity lamps and/or lasers), the intensity of the fluorescent signal can be increased. This is one of the reasons that fluorescence measurements are intrinsically more sensitive than absorbence measurements. Absorbence is dependent on the concentration of absorbing species and independent of incident light. Fluorescence is dependent on the intensity of the exciting signal, which can be changed in any given system. High-intensity sources coupled with polarization techniques and photon counting detectors give fluorescence immunoassay a sensitivity that is adequate for many assays. The best fluorescent polarization assays appear to be those dealing with small to medium-sized analytes.

Time-Resolved Fluorescence

Another innovative technique employing fluorescence is time-resolved fluorescence. Again, the basic design of the immunoassay is similar to the other immunoassay designs discussed. The unique feature about time-resolved fluorescence is the selection of a fluorophore that has a large Stokes' shift and an extended decay time. The large Stokes' shift means that the emitted light is separated from the exciting light, reducing the contributions from the excitation source in analyzing the signal. It is, however, from the time-resolved feature of this system that significant advantages are realized.

When a fluorophore has an extended decay time, it means that the fluorescence from a single excitation is extended over a long period of time. One of the characteristics of the lanthanide chelate complexes is that the fluorescence decay extends into the microsecond range, compared with nanoseconds for conventional fluorophores (11). For assays employing this type of fluorescent detection, the instrumentation would excite the fluorophore with a high-intensity pulsed excitation, then allow the passage of time for the background and nonspecific fluorescence to decay and then make a measurement of the analytic fluorescence due to the lanthanide chelate complex. If this process is repeated several times over the course of a few seconds, a significant number of measurements can be made, and a statistically reliable value can be generated for the complex being measured. Since all of the background and nonspecific fluorescence is separated (resolved) from the specific analytic measurement based on time, the process is called time-resolved fluorescence. The analytic measurement is separated from the nonanalytic measurements by the passage of time. Coupled with the fact that there is a large Stokes' shift, and the emission wavelength is very sharp, only a very small correction has to be made for the nonspecific signal of the lanthanide chelate complex. In principle, this methodology can potentially have sensitivity equal to or beyond that of radioimmunoassays. There are at least two commercial systems that take advantage of lanthanide chelate time-resolved fluorescence.

All fluorescent techniques suffer from several limiting factors. First, fluorescence is sensitive to temperature and viscosity. Reaction conditions must accordingly be held within very narrow tolerances. In addition, most biological specimens contain materials that have natural fluorescence. In the serum or plasma specimen commonly found in the clinical laboratory, serum proteins as well as molecules such as bilirubin have considerable fluorescence that contributes to a significant background signal. In these cases extensive controls or corrections must be applied to separate the analytic measurement from the background signal. Time-resolved fluorescence tends to minimize these problems but does not do away with them totally. Additional interference can be due to the internal filter effect. This internal filtering occurs when there are molecules in the measurement system that absorb light of the same wavelength as the light being emitted by the fluorescent molecule. One can try to minimize these internal filter effects by choosing fluorescent labels that emit at longer wavelengths. Biological specimens absorb the shorter visible wavelengths more often than the longer wavelengths of light.

Bioluminescence and Chemiluminescence

Chemiluminescent and bioluminescent reactions are similar to fluorescent reactions in that the measured signal is emitted light generated by the relaxation of an excited molecule. The difference between fluorescence and chemiluminescent or bioluminescent reactions is the method by which the molecule becomes excited. In fluorescence, adsorbed light energy raises the molecules to the excited state. In chemiluminescent and bioluminescent reactions, the energy is supplied by a chemical reaction. If the reaction occurs in vivo it is classified as a bioluminescent reaction. Reactions that require reactants or conditions not found in biological systems are referred to as chemiluminescent reactions.

Although many organisms produce bioluminescent reactions, probably the best known is the firefly reaction. In that reaction the substrate, firefly luciferin, is oxidized by the enzyme luciferase in the presence of magnesium ion and oxygen ATP, yielding a photon. This is an extremely sensitive reaction and can be used to measure ATP at the femtomole level. The quantum efficiency of this reaction approaches unity since each molecule will emit 1 photon of light for each photon absorbed. This and other bioluminescent reactions have found limited applicability in the immunoassay field because the reagents are expensive and the reaction works best with small molecules.

Chemiluminescent reactions have been far more successful in immunoassay applications because they are less expensive and easier to work with in assay systems. Chemiluminescent reactions never approach the efficiency of the firefly reaction, but modern photon counting equipment has been able to compensate for this deficiency. The most commonly used chemiluminescent molecules are the luminals, acridinium esters, and dioxetanes.

Luminal

Luminal, its isomer, and derivatives belong to the class of compounds known as aromatic hydrazides. When these compounds are oxidized, they emit light. This reaction is usually carried out with a catalytic agent such as peroxidase in an alkaline medium. When luminal is conjugated to one of the reactants in the immunoassay, the efficiency of the light production decreases significantly. Therefore, one of the more successful designs has been to conjugate the peroxidase to one of the reagents and then use luminal as an indicator of the peroxidase. Competitive and noncompetitive solid-phase systems are the most commonly employed designs using luminal.

Acridinium Esters

Acridinium esters are perhaps the most common of the chemiluminescent labels in use today. These compounds can be oxidized without the requirement of a catalyst. The efficiency of this reaction is greater than that of luminal. For these reasons, acridinium esters form the basis of many of today's automated immunoassay systems. Acridinium esters can be conjugated to large or small molecules without significant loss of light-emitting efficiency. They work equally well in most assay system designs; thus, instrument considerations usually dictate the type of assay system.

Dioxetanes

Dioxetanes are thermally unstable molecules that stabilize by thermal cleavage with the emission of light. These compounds can be made stable by adding a phosphate group to the phenyl ring. Under these conditions an immunoassay can be designed that uses alkaline phosphatase conjugated to one of the reactants. Then, the phosphorylated dioxetane can be added as an indicator. Once the phosphate group is removed from the dioxetane by the alkaline phosphatase, the compound reverts to its thermally unstable condition and will emit light. Enhancers, which are essentially carefully chosen inner filters, can be used to lengthen the time that the light is emitted from the reaction.

The instrumentation required for chemiluminescence is a photometer with special adaptations. Generally there is a reagent injection system so that reagents can be added while the reaction cuvette is in front of the detector. The detector is usually a high-efficiency photomultiplier tube that counts photons for a prescribed time and then employs some type of averaging algorithm to quantitate the signal. If enhancers or other types of chemistry are used to extend the light emission, less stringent requirements are placed on the photomultiplier tube.

Data Reduction

In the early days of radioimmunoassay, data reduction was a do-it-yourself project. Investigators did what they thought was appropriate to calibrate an assay and in turn to calculate results on unknown specimens. In addition, an effort was made to glean appropriate quality control indicators from these numerical procedures. There was a flurry of activity in the literature as each data reduction scheme was proposed, followed by discussions of the strengths and primarily weaknesses of the proposed system. The evolution of both immunoassays and data reduction systems has evolved to a point where there is more agreement on the approaches that should be used as well as significant improvement in instrumentation, desktop computers, and software. That is not to say, however, that the procedure for data reduction and quality control should be accepted from the vendor without a thorough understanding of the procedures and approaches used. All data reduction packages share a similar objective, which is to make an accurate and precise estimate of the concentration of an analyte in a given solution. Some of the more common approaches to achieving this objective are described below.

One of the first questions asked about an assay is, "What is its limit of detection or sensitivity?" Because of the number of steps in most assays and the imprecision associated with any physical measurement process, there is a degree of uncertainty associated with each result calculated. The appropriate way to determine the limit of detection or sensitivity is to evaluate that uncertainty at zero concentration, and this becomes the level that is indistinguishable from zero. A simple and practical approach to accomplishing this is to make multiple measurements on several concentrations of analyte within the range of interest, calculate the mean and standard deviations

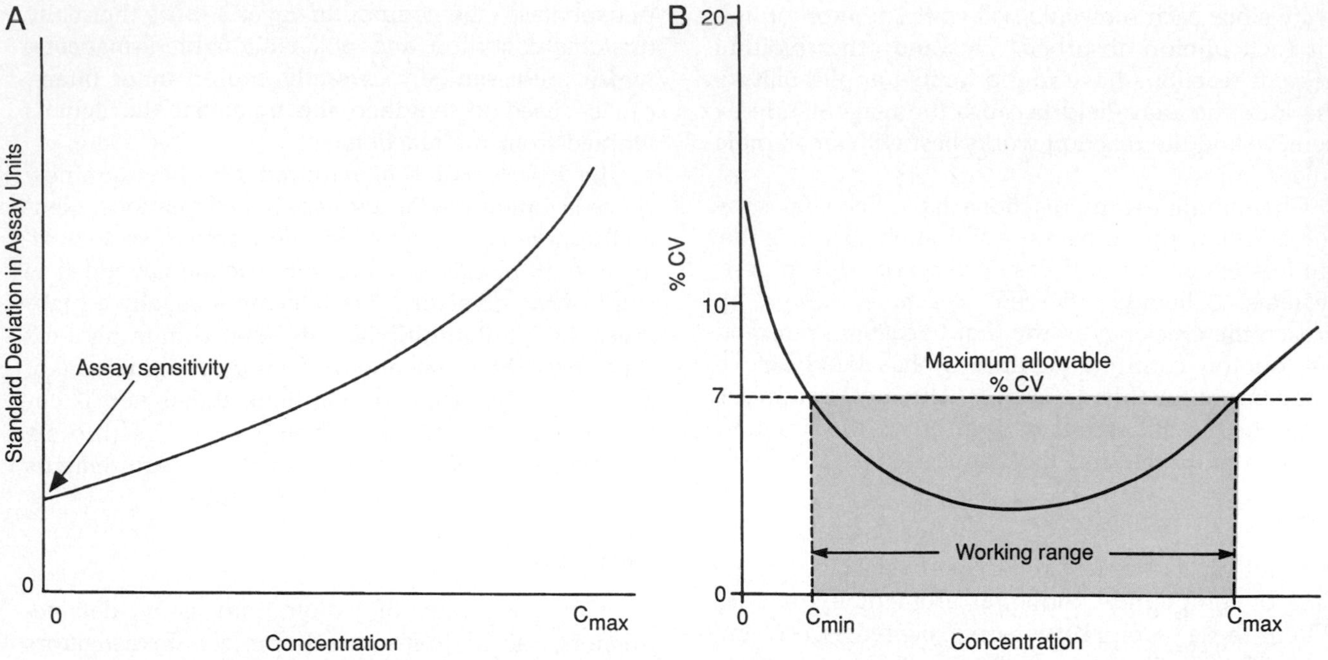

Figure 9.9. Precision profile diagrams. **A**, The standard deviation for several analyte concentrations has been plotted versus the analyte concentration. The units are the same as the analyte units. The line is extrapolated to zero analyte concentration and yields the level of analyte that does not differ from zero concentration in the assay. If 1 SD is used for the plot, the actual sensitivity will be 2 or 3 times the intercept value, depending on the level of confidence required. **B**, A slightly different plot is presented to determine the working range of the assay based on the maximum allowable %CV. The *y* axis is calibrated in %CV. The *x* axis is analyte concentration. One possible plot is presented. A line drawn parallel to the *x* axis at a level of the maximum allowable %CV for the assay intersects the original line. These intersections then determine the minimum and maximum concentrations in the working range of the assay.

for each of these concentrations, and plot the standard deviations versus the concentration. Extrapolation of this line to zero concentration gives an appreciation for the smallest detectable analyte concentration that differs from zero (Fig. 9.9*A*). This plot, also referred to as a precision profile, can be informative in terms of the working range of the assay. An effective approach is to plot %CV versus several analyte concentrations. Then decide on the maximum allowable %CV the procedure can tolerate. Draw a line parallel to the *x* axis at this point. The intersection with the original plot yields the working range (Fig. 9.9*B*). By evaluating the precision profile, an investigator can determine if at any concentration the standard deviation of the measurement exceeds an acceptable limit.

Once a series of measurements has been made under the assay conditions, the investigator is faced with the dilemma of selecting the best approach for using this information to calculate the concentration of analyte in other specimens. This calculation procedure is generally a part of automated methodologies, most of which present the user with a menu of data reduction choices. Manual calculations and plotting of data for the purposes of calculating the concentration of analyte in specimens is less common in the modern laboratory than it was at the time of the original radioimmunoassay. Manual plotting of data and the subsequent extrapolation of concentration for unknowns is an error-prone process. Each individual will connect the points in a slightly different manner and will read the resultant concentrations for unknowns the same way. In addition, manual data reduction is a slow and expensive process that is more important as a teaching procedure than as a daily analytic procedure.

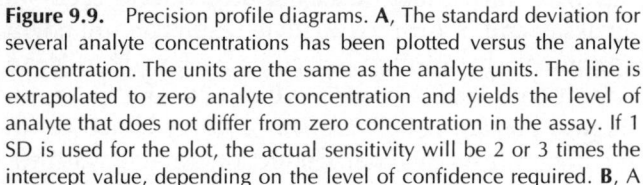

Data reduction methods can be grossly divided into two types. The first are the point-to-point methods in which an attempt is made to draw a smooth line through the data points progressing from one point to the next. Approaches that utilize this method are point-to-point, methods in which an attempt is made to draw a smooth line through the data points progressing from one point to the next. Approaches that utilize this method are point-to-point, spline, and polynomial interpolative methods. Computers can be programmed to generate these lines very quickly, but the computer does not correct the underlying weakness of these approaches. That weakness is that there are errors inherent in the values assigned to each concentration and the assumption that all concentrations throughout the working range behave identically. Once a line has been generated through these concentration points, it is as-

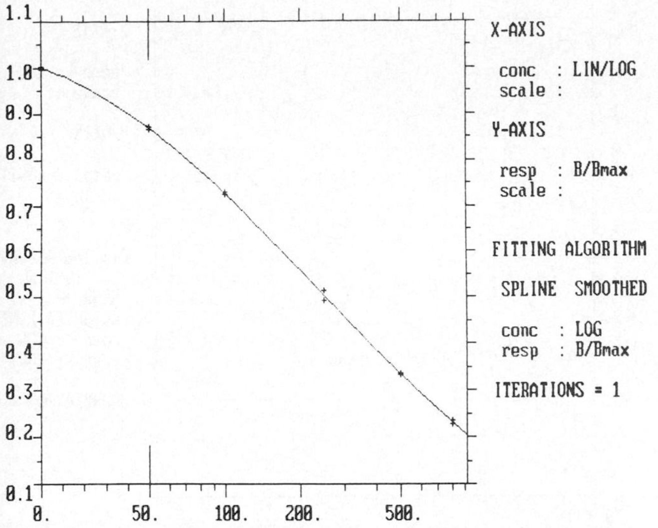

Figure 9.10. Spline fit to assay data. The data represent a spline fit to actual laboratory data. The x axis is Lin/Log due to a zero concentration of analyte that does not have a log value. The response plotted on the y axis is percent of maximum response. In this example the spline fit required one iteration to develop an acceptable curve.

sumed that the intervening concentrations, which have not been measured, will fall on that line. It is also possible, as in the case of polynomial and spline fits, that if the data are "noisy," it is possible to generate a line that has so-called "hooks" where the computer has generated multiple inflection points to go through all of the data. If this situation is severe enough, a single response on an unknown can generate multiple potential concentrations from the curve. If this type of plot is used, it is essential that the curve be visualized to ensure that the standard concentrations are following an anticipated response line. Figure 9.10 illustrates a spline fit to actual assay data.

Regression methods are the other approach to data reduction. Regression methods fit a line through the data points in such a way that each data point is a minimum distance from the line. In other words, if you were to measure the distance from each data point to the line, that would be a minimum compared with any other line that could be drawn in relation to those data points. The potential problem with this approach is that it treats every data point equally. Therefore, if the method has greater imprecision at the ends of the curve or if there are outliers, the standard regression analysis fails to recognize this and treats all points equally. The method most software packages use to overcome this weakness is that of weighting. In a weighted regression, each point is adjusted by a weighting factor in accordance with its reliability. The points in a region of the curve where the error is greater and the reliability of the measurement is lower are given less influence in the calculation than those points that lie in regions of the curve where the certainty of the measurement is greater. These weighting factors can be determined by calculating the variance of multiple measurements or can be generated from mathematical models if there is sufficient information known about the behavior of the curve under study. Figures 9.11 shows a regression and a weighted regression.

A popular family of algorithms for fitting data are the logistic fit equations. These are derived from statistical functions that have been adapted to immunoassay data. Equation 9.5 shows several parameters that are related to the analyte concentration, represented by x, and the response measured, represented by y.

$$y = \frac{a-d}{1+(x/c)^b} + d \tag{9.5}$$

The four parameters a, b, c, and d have interesting interpretation in terms of the curve generated. Parameter a is the predicted response at zero analyte concentration; d is the predicted response at infinite analyte concentration; c is the inflection point on the sigmoidal curve; and b is the slope at that inflection point. Using this equation places no demand on any of the equation parameters. Only the concentration of the solutions and the response associated with those concentrations are required. The computer then assigns a first estimate to the value of the parameters and begins solving the equation in an iterative process. This means that the computer solves the equation, evaluates the results, makes a small change in the parameters, and continues this process until successive solutions begin to converge on the same line through the data points. This is a very effective approach to fitting a curve to experimental data, and in principle, there should be only one best-fit line that goes through a given set of data points. Because of the differences in assumptions, approaches, and software programs, it is possible to have variations from program to program. However, once it has been determined that a four-parameter logistic fit procedure is appropriate, this approach yields some additional advantages. First, there are the four parameters that can be used as quality control points for the long-term performance of the assay. Significant changes in endpoints or slopes indicate that the assay should be reviewed. In addition, concentrations can be read from the curve at 20, 50, and 80% as another quality control monitor. The one precaution that should be kept in mind when employing four-parameter logistic fit equations is that you are at high risk once you exceed your calibrating solutions. That is, to extrapolate the concentration of an analyte in an unknown solution beyond the high-

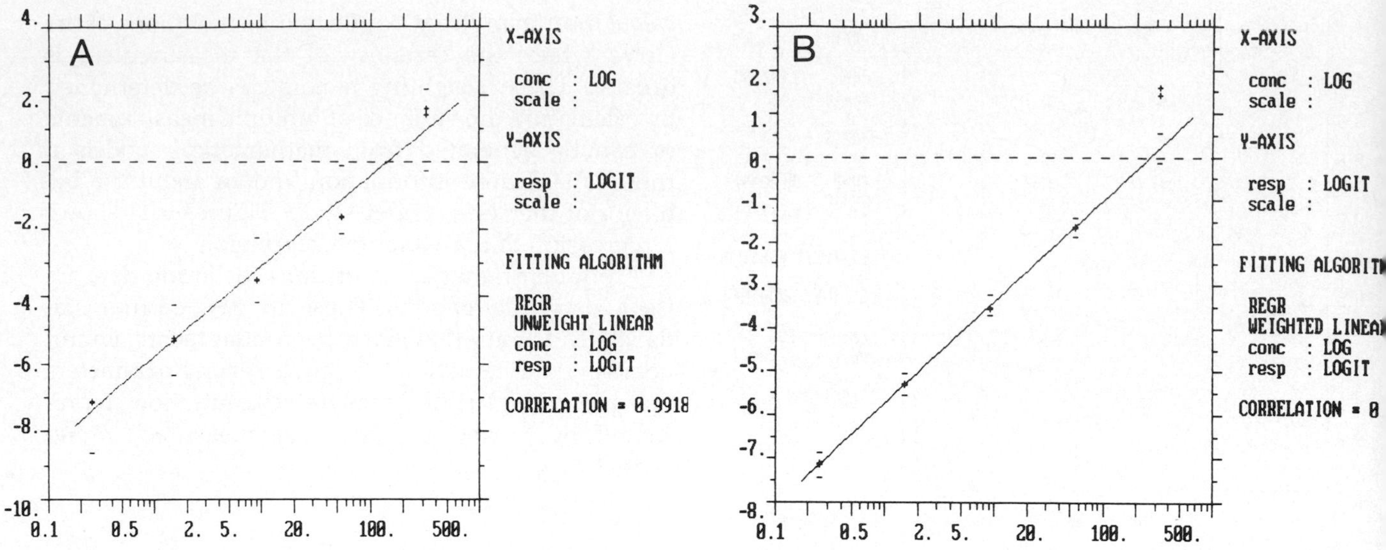

Figure 9.11. The figure presents an unweighted (**A**) and a weighted (**B**) linear regression. The *x* axis is in log of concentration, and the *y* axis is in logit of the response. Notice the relative error around the line is smaller in the weighted regression, and the point at a concentration of 200 units has less effect on the line due to the unreliability of the measurement at that concentration.

est or lowest concentration of a calibrator leaves the analysis vulnerable to significant error. The reason for this is the four-parameter logistic fit sacrifices the ends of the curves, where the variance or error may be considerable.

Even in this day of computerized calculations, it is critical that the operator know the algorithm and assumptions used to calculate calibration curves. This information should not only be logical but should employ basic statistical concepts wherever possible. Once this information is known to the researchers, they should process their laboratory data, control specimens, and previous assays and evaluate the quality of the calculation in their hands. There are numerous software packages, both stand-alone and incorporated into instrumentation, that will calculate results for any given immunoassay. The process of choosing the correct software is primarily one of evaluating the candidate products and being comfortable with the assumptions and procedures used.

Automation in Immunoassay

As might be expected, immunoassay is following a course close to classic clinical chemistry; that is, initially there were laborious manual methods designed to measure one analyte at a time in batch fashion. This was followed by assisted manual procedures in which dilutors, pumps, and spectrophotometers took over some of the steps in the assay system. Nevertheless, it remained essentially a manual procedure. Next came automation wherein specimens were prepared and presented to the system at one end and completed results were returned at the other, with relatively little hands-on intervention. In the past several years, immunoassay has reached the point of full automation. Several companies are now marketing instrumentation that takes advantage of the nonisotopic methodologies. These instruments are complete with bar-code readers, reagent monitors, and total software packages for calculating results, monitoring quality control, and generating management reports. In addition, most have the capability of being interfaced with the main laboratory computer for bidirectional communication. Companies such as Ciba Corning, Cirrus Diagnostics, Becton Dickinson, Technicon, Boehringer Mannheim, Biotrol, Abbott, and Baxter. along with several others, have marketed instruments described as automated immunoassay systems. Each of these instruments takes advantage of a slightly different technique and solves a particular problem. It is not evident at this time that there is a single approach or a single instrument that can solve all of the immunoassay problems in a modern clinical laboratory.

References

1. Burnet FM. A modification of Jerne's theory of antibody production using the concept of clonal selecton. Aust J Sci 1957;20:67–69.
2. Köhler G, Milstein C. Continuous cultures of fused cells secreting antibody of predetermined specificity. Nature 1975;256:495–497.
3. Chappey ON, Sandouk P, Scherrmann JMG. Monoclonal antibodies in hapten immunoassays. Pharm Res 1992;9(11):1375–1379.
4. Moyle WR, Lin C, Corson RL and Erlich PH. Quantitative explanation for increased affinity shown by mixtures of monoclonal antibodies: importance of circular complex. Mol Immunol 1983;20:439–452.
5. Tedford MC, Stimson WH. Molecular recognition in antibodies and its application. Experientia 1991;47:1129–1138.

6. Laurell CB. Quantitative estimation of proteins by electrophoresis in agarose gel containing antibodies. Anal Biochem 1966;15:45.
7. Apler CC, Johnson AM. Immunofixation electrophoresis: a technique for the study of protein polymorphism. Vox Sang 1969;17:445.
8. Yalow RS, Berson SA. Immunoassay of endogenous plasma insulin in man. J Clin Invest 1960;39:1157–1175.
9. Ekins R. Merits and disadvantages of different labels and methods of immunoassay. In: Voller A, Bartlett A, Bidwell D, eds. Immunoassay for the 80's. Baltimore: University Park Press, 1981.
10. Jackson T, Marshall N, Ekins R. Optimization of immunoradiometric (labelled antibody) assays. In: Hunter WM, Corrie JET, eds. Immunoassays for Clinical Chemistery. Edinburgh: Churchill Livingstone, 1983.
11. Diamandis EP. Immunoassays with time-resolved fluorescence spectroscopy: principles and applications. Clin Biochem 1988;21:139–150.

Suggested Readings

Bioluminescence and Chemiluminescence

Abelson JN, et al., eds. Methods in enzymology, volume 184. New York: Academic Press, 1990.

Bonini PA, Banfi G, Murone M. Enhanced chemiluminescence in the measurement of proteins and haptens: evaluation of choriogonadotropin (hCG) and free thyroxin. J Bioluminescence and Chemiluminescence 1990;5:193–195.

Colowick SP, ed. Methods in enzymology, volume 133. New York: Academic Press, 1986.

De Boever J, Kohen F, Leyseele D, et al. Isolaminol as a marker in direct chemiluminescence immunoassays for steroid hormones. J Bioluminescence and chemiluminescence 1990;5:5–10.

Fert V, Baret A. Preparation and characterization of xanthine oxidase-antibody and -hapten conjugates for use in sensitive chemiluminescent immunoassays. J Immunol Methods 1990;131: 237–247.

Gorus F, Schram E. Applications of bio- and chemiluminescence in the clinical laboratory. Clin Chem 1979;25(4):512–519.

Roche D, Susini de Luca H, Tugendhaft N. Chemiluminescence and radioimmunology compared for 10 allergens. Clin Chem 1991;37(3):474–475.

Woodhead JS, Weeks I. Immunochemiluminometric assays based on acridinium labels with a microtiter plate luminometer. Clin Chem 1991;37(3):472.

Data Analysis

Ezan E, Tiberghien C, Dray F. Practical methods for optimizing radioimmunoassay detection and precision limits. Clin Chem 1991;37(2):226–230.

Haven MC, Orsulak PJ, Arnold LL, et al. Data-reduction methods for immunoradiometric assays of thyrotropin compared. Clin Chem 1987;33(7):1207–1210.

Klee GG, Post G. Effect of counting errors on immunoassay precision. Clin Chem 1989;35(7):1362–1366.

Miller JJ, Valdes R Jr. Approaches to minimizing interference by cross-reacting molecules in immunoassays. Clin Chem 1991;37(2):144–153.

Sadler WA, Smith MH, Legge HM. A method for direct estimation of imprecision profiles, with reference to immunoassay data. Clin Chem 1988;34(6):1058–1061.

Seth J. Estimation of sensitivity of immunoassays. Clin Chem 1990;36(1):178.

Fluorescence

Calvin J, Burling K, Blow C, et al. Evaluation of fluorescence excitation transfer immunoassay for measurement of specific proteins. J Immunol Methods 1986;86:249–256.

Diamandis EP. Immunoassays with time-resolved fluorescence spectroscopy: principles and applications. Clin Biochem 1988;21: 139–150.

Hemmilä I. Fluoroimmunoassays and immunofluorometric assays. Clin Chem 1985;31(1):359–370.

Schwan WR, Waltenbaugh C, Duncan JL. Bacteria as solid phase in a concentration fluorescence immunoassay analysis of antibodies to surface antigens. J Immunol Methods 1990;126:247–252.

Immunoassay

Abelson JN, Simon MI, eds. Methods in enzymology, volume 182. New York: Academic Press, 1990.

Gosling JP. A decade of development in immunoassay methodology. Clin Chem 1990;36(8):1408–1427.

Latner AL, Schwartz MK, eds. Advances in clinical chemistry, volume 24. New York: Academic Press, 1985.

Miscellaneous

Azimzadeh A, Van Regenmortel MHV. Antibody affinity measurements. J Mol Recognition 1990;3(3):108–116.

Demers LM. Monoclonal antibodies to lutropin: are our immunoassays too specific? Clin Chem 1991;37(3):311–312.

Pfund WP, Bourdage JS. The confirmation-sensitive immunoassay: a membrane based ELISA system for identifying antibodies sensitive to alterations of protein conformation. Mol Immunol 1990;27(6):495–502.

Sorensen K, Brodbeck U. Assessment of coating-efficiency in ELISA plates by direct protein determination. J Immunolog Methods 1986;95:291–293.

Vilja P. Flexibility of noncompetitive avidin-biotin immunoassay: immunoassay of Lutropin applied to different signal detection systems. Clin Chem 1990;36(11):1897–1901.

Nephelometry

Cuilliere ML, Montagne P, Bessou TH, et al. Microparticle-enhanced nephelometric immunoassay (Nephelia®) for immunoglobulins G, A, and M. Clin Chem 1991;37(1):20–25.

Appendix—Glossary

Affinity—Describes the strength of binding of a single binding site on an antigen with its corresponding antibody. For well-defined systems, this can be equated to the association constant of the reaction.

Antibody—An immunoglobulin class protein that is produced by a special class of lymphocyte in response to its stimulation by foreign material.

Antigen—Any material capable of reacting with an antibody to produce an antibody-antigen complex.

Avidity—Describes the stability of antigen-antibody complexes. It is the net of all the forces of all the binding sites on an antigen and is generally greater than the simple sum of these forces.

Bioluminescence—A special category of chemiluminescence that takes place in living organisms. Photons are emitted as a result of biologically mediated reactions. Characteristically, these reactions have very high quantum yields.

Chemiluminescence—A reaction in which the product molecules are in an excited state due to the engery released by the reaction. Relaxation of these excited molecules results in the emission of a photon. Generally, quantum yields are low.

Detection limit—The smallest amount of analyte that is measurable above zero. Usually arrived at by measuring a zero response and taking the mean of that response plus three standard deviations.

Fluorescence—The emission of a photon from a molecule that was raised to an excited state by external radiation.

Hapten—A small organic molecule that represents a single antigenic determinant. Usually is not capable of generating an immune response by itself.

Heterogeneous assay—Assay that requires the separation of bound and free species before the analytic measurement is made.

Homogeneous assay—Assay that is designed to have the analytic measurement made in the presence of both bound and free species.

Immunogen—Any substance capable of stimulating lymphocytes to produce antibodies.

Nephelometry—A technique that measures the amount of scattered light from a sample at angles other than 0°.

Sensitivity—Synonymous with detection limit.

Specificity—A characteristic of antibodies that denotes the antibody's ability to recognize a specific antigenic determinant in the presence of similar structures. The greater the specificity the less cross-reactivity.

Turbidimetry—A technique that measures the reduction in incident light after the incident light passes through a sample. Angle of measurement is 0°.

10 The Plasma Proteins

Elizabeth Lee-Lewandrowski and Kent Lewandrowski

The plasma proteins are a diverse group of molecules that perform a wide variety of functions. Over 500 plasma proteins have been identified, and new ones continue to be discovered. Some plasma proteins such as albumin and transferrin are routinely measured in the clinical laboratory, while others are of interest only in specialized situations. Although it is assumed that all proteins perform some function in the body, in many cases the precise role has not been defined. With the growth of more sophisticated and sensitive methods to study these molecules, new applications for protein analysis in clinical practice will surely arise.

Some of the plasma proteins can be conveniently grouped as related molecules that collectively carry out a specific function. Examples include the immunoglobulins, the complement proteins, the coagulation cascade, lipoproteins, and a variety of protein hormones and hormone binding globulins. These are covered in other chapters and will be mentioned only briefly here. This chapter is concerned with the physiology, pathology, and laboratory assessment of the remaining plasma proteins with an emphasis on those that are important in clinical medicine.

True plasma proteins should be distinguished from proteins that occur only incidentally in the blood. For example, a number of enzymes may be released from damaged cells and appear in plasma but perform no known function outside of the cell. Other proteins are found in plasma only during certain pathological states. In contrast, true plasma proteins are specifically synthesized for release into the blood, where they carry out their respective functions.

In spite of their name, most of the plasma proteins are not confined to the vascular compartment (1). In the capillary vessels, proteins escape from the blood either by active transport mechanisms or by diffusion through the junctions between endothelial cells. In some cases the extravascular fraction exceeds the amount in the intravascular pool. Many of these proteins carry out part of their function in the interstitial space, ultimately returning to the vascular compartment by the lymphatics. Some plasma proteins cross the blood-brain barrier and thus enter the cerebrospinal fluid. Small amounts are found in virtually all other extracellular fluids.

A number of systems have been used to classify the plasma proteins. Historically albumin was distinguished from the globulins (nonalbumin proteins) on the basis of its greater solubility in water (1). However, this distinction is not absolute since some other proteins are also soluble in low–ionic strength solutions. Alternatively, proteins may be classified according to function (Table 10.1). For example, some proteins perform mainly transport functions for metals (transferrin), lipids (lipoproteins), or hormones (thyroid-binding globulin). Others are involved in

Table 10.1. Functional Classification of Selected Plasma Proteins

Proteinase inhibitors
α_1-Antitrypsin
Antithrombin III
α_1-Antichymotrypsin
α_2-Macroglobulin
Antiplasmin
Inter-alpha-trypsin inhibitor
Carrier/transport proteins
Retinol binding protein
Gc-globulin (Vitamin D binding protein)
Lipoproteins
Hormone binding globulins
Prealbumin
Iron transport and metabolism
Transferrin
Haptoglobin
Hemopexin
Mixed function proteins
Albumin
Immune function and host defense
Immunoglobulins
Complement proteins
C-Reactive protein
Blood clotting
Clotting factors
Fibrinogen
Fetal proteins
α-Fetoprotein
Carcinoembryonic antigen
Unknown or controversial
Ceruloplasmin
α_1-Acid glycoprotein (Orosomucoid)
β_2-Microglobulin

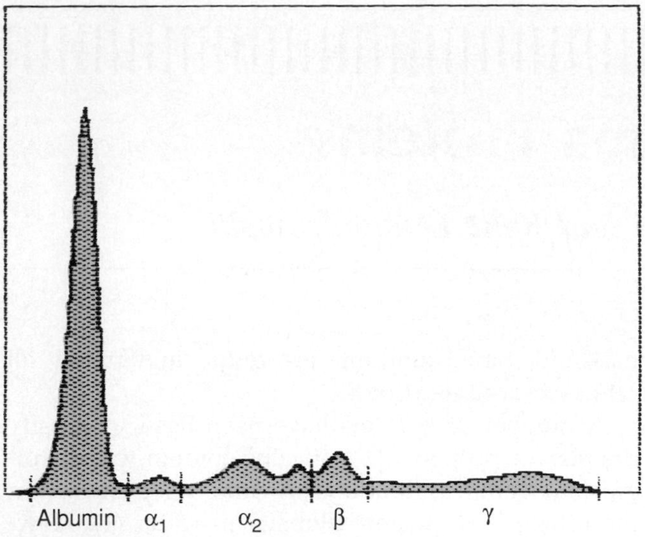

Figure 10.1. Densitometric scan of a normal serum protein electrophoresis pattern showing the relative position of the albumin, α_1, α_2, β, and γ regions.

Table 10.2. Classification of Selected Major *(Boldface)* and Minor Plasma Proteins by Electrophoretic Mobility

1. Albumin zone
Albumin
Prealbumin
2. α_1 zone
α_1-Antitrypsin
HDL (α-lipoproteins)
α_1-Antichymotrypsin
Orosomucoid
α-fetoprotein
3. α_2 zone
α_2-Macroglobulin
Haptoglobin
Ceruloplasmin
GC-Globulin
4. β zone
LDL (β-lipoproteins)
Transferrin
C3
β_2-Microglobulin
Hemopexin
Fibrinogen (may be in γ zone)
5. γ zone
Immunoglobulins
C-Reactive protein
Fibrinogen
Lysozyme

the clotting cascade (fibrinogen) or function as enzyme inhibitors (α_1-antitrypsin). Some proteins perform more than one function. Albumin, for example, serves as a carrier protein for bilirubin, some hormones, and inorganic ions. It also provides a protein source for cells and contributes the major portion of the plasma colloid oncotic pressure, which is essential for normal hemodynamics.

Plasma proteins are often classified on the basis of their electrophoretic mobility on cellulose acetate or agarose gel. Electrophoresis separates proteins into five regions designated albumin, α_1, α_2, β, and γ (Fig. 10.1). Individual proteins characteristically migrate in one of these regions (Table 10.2). The albumin band is relatively homogeneous, while the remaining regions contain many different proteins and are simply groups of proteins with similar mobilities.

With some exceptions (e.g., immunoglobulins, protein hormones, and some clotting factors), most of the plasma proteins are synthesized in the liver. The liver is also the major site of plasma protein catabolism. Most of the plasma proteins are synthesized on the rough endoplasmic reticulum of the liver hepatocytes. Following assembly of the amino acid backbone, a variety of posttranslational modifications may occur, including proteolytic removal of proprotein fragments, phosphorylation, and the addition of sugars and other prosthetic groups. Ultimately the proteins pass through the Golgi apparatus and are packed into secretory vesicles for release into the blood. Further details of protein structure and synthesis may be found in standard biochemistry textbooks.

Hepatocytes are capable of synthesizing more than one protein simultaneously. The balance between synthesis and degradation maintains the level of plasma proteins within a relatively narrow range. Each protein is regulated independently of the others. The level of the individual protein in plasma serves as the signal for regulation, and the rates of synthesis and catabolism are the mechanism for modulating its concentration (1). Details of the regulatory steps for specific proteins are provided under separate headings later in this chapter.

Given the diversity of the plasma proteins, it is not surprising that a wide variety of diseases and physiological alterations may affect protein levels. Plasma protein abnormalities arise from one or more of the following:

- Congenital abnormalities affecting a specific protein (e.g., analbuminemia, α_1-antitrypsin deficiency).
- Acquired abnormalities affecting a specific protein (e.g., transferrin in anemia, haptoglobin in hemolysis).
- Alterations affecting multiple proteins reflecting variations in the physiological state (e.g., age, race, sex, and pregnancy).
- Alterations affecting multiple proteins secondary to disease (e.g., cirrhosis, acute phase response, and protein-losing syndromes).

In this chapter we begin with a discussion of the total plasma protein followed by a description of the acute phase response. Then the individual plasma proteins are considered. In the final section of the chapter, a number of methods for protein separation, identification, and quantitation are described. Assays of specific proteins are described under individual headings.

TOTAL PROTEIN

The total serum protein concentration is one of the more common measurements in the clinical laboratory. A number of factors affect the protein concentration, including alterations in fluid balance, changes in synthesis or catabolism, and protein losses. Measurement of total protein is therefore a relatively sensitive but nonspecific screening test of overall health status.

The total protein may be measured on either serum or plasma. Serum samples are generally preferred since they are more convenient to use on automated equipment (2). If plasma is used, the total protein is 3 to 5% higher owing to the contribution of fibrinogen. A number of preanalytic errors may alter the serum protein value (2). Prolonged tourniquet application during venipuncture results in hemoconcentration, which can increase the total protein by up to 5 g/liter. Values in recumbent subjects may be 10% lower than in ambulatory individuals. There is also a normal diurnal variation of 4 g/liter and a seasonal fluctuation with peak levels in November and lowest values in June. Exercise increases the serum protein concentration by up to 10%, but this effect is transient.

The total serum protein includes both albumin (60%) and the globulins (40%). All contribute some fraction to the colloid oncotic pressure (COP) of plasma, which is essential for normal hemodynamics. Unlike sodium salts and glucose, the movement of proteins from plasma to interstitial fluid is limited (3). The contribution of proteins to the plasma osmotic pressure tends to retain water in the vascular space. The osmotic pressure generated by the plasma proteins is called the colloid oncotic pressure, or simply oncotic pressure. Due to its abundance and small size, albumin is responsible for 80% of the total COP.

The movement of fluid from the capillaries to the interstitial space is governed by the balance between four forces. The plasma oncotic pressure acts to hold fluid in the vascular space. This force is counterbalanced by the capillary hydrostatic (hydraulic) pressure, which tends to force water out of the vascular compartment. The interstitial oncotic pressure is derived from the proteins and proteoglycans of the interstitial space and acts to draw fluid out of the capillary vessels. The small interstitial hydrostatic pressure is usually negative and thus it also pulls fluid out of the vascular compartment. The sum of these four forces varies in different tissues (3), and water may move either into or out of the plasma compartment depending on the balance between the forces. Ordinarily the net effect is a 0.3 to 0.5 mm Hg gradient favoring movement out of the capillaries. On the other hand, in the postcapillary venules the forces normally allow return of some of the water to the circulation. The remainder is returned to the vascular space by the lymphatics. A decrease in the total protein concentration will decrease the plasma colloid oncotic pressure, which may result in edema. However, since hypoproteinemia will also decrease the amount of protein in the interstitial space, the decrease in plasma oncotic pressure will be partially offset by a decrease in the interstitial oncotic pressure. In general, hypoproteinemia must be severe to result in edema.

The total protein concentration may be altered by changes in fluid balance (plasma water). Dehydration causes a proportional increase in all of the serum proteins. This occurs with decreased water intake or with increased water losses such as excessive sweating, diarrhea, vomiting, salt-losing syndromes, and osmotic or drug-induced diuresis. Conversely, volume expansion causes a proportional decrease in serum proteins. Examples include the administration of volume expanders (such as dextran), excessive administration of intravenous fluids, pregnancy, and salt retention syndromes. These changes do not affect the actual body pools of serum proteins, and correction of the underlying fluid imbalance will correct the total protein concentration.

Changes in the amounts of plasma proteins may result from alterations in synthesis or catabolism, or from protein losses. Increased synthesis of some proteins is seen in the "acute phase" response to infection or tissue injury, but this is offset to some degree by a concomitant decrease in albumin synthesis. The use of steroids, including oral contraceptives, will increase protein synthesis and may increase the total protein concentration (2). Marked hyperproteinemia in the absence of dehydration usually reflects increased synthesis of γ-globulins. Hyperproteinemia due to increased albumin synthesis is quite rare if it occurs at all.

Hypoproteinemia can be caused by decreased protein synthesis and is seen in malnutrition and in chronic liver disease. Protein calorie malnutrition deprives the liver of the necessary substrates to make plasma proteins and is a common problem in hospitalized patients (4). In chronic liver disease the protein synthetic machinery is disturbed, which also results in hypoproteinemia. However, this is often accompanied by increased (extrahepatic) synthesis of γ-globulins, which may normalize or occasionally even increase the total protein value. Increased protein catabolism is seen in a variety of inflammatory and neoplastic conditions.

Excessive protein losses can occur through the kidney, the gastrointestinal tract, or the skin. Examples include the nephrotic syndrome, inflammatory bowel disease, extensive burns, and any severe exudative process. The most severe losses are seen in the nephrotic syndrome, in which a number of plasma proteins, especially albumin, are passed through the glomerulus into the urine. In severe cases of nephrotic syndrome the serum albumin level may fall to less than 5 g/liter (2).

Changes in the total serum protein may result from changes in albumin, globulins, or both. As mentioned earlier, a change in one protein may be offset by a change in the opposite direction of another. For this reason it may be useful to determine the ratio of the albumin concentration to the globulin concentration (A:G ratio). The ratio may be markedly abnormal in spite of a normal total protein, such as in the acute phase response, in which increased globulins are associated with a decreased albumin concentration.

Methods for measuring the total protein are discussed at the end of this chapter.

ACUTE PHASE REACTANTS

The acute phase reactants (APRs) are a group of proteins whose plasma concentration changes in response to a variety of inflammatory states including infection, postsurgery, trauma, post–myocardial infarction, malignancy, and any condition associated with tissue necrosis. Collectively, the changes in plasma proteins are referred to as the acute phase response. Some of these proteins are called positive APRs, meaning that their plasma levels increase, while others are designated negative APRs to indicate that their levels decrease (Table 10.3). Measurement of APRs, especially C-reactive protein (CRP), may be useful to detect and follow patients with acute inflammatory disorders. However, these changes are nonspecific and provide no information on the cause or source of the inflammation. Elevations in the white blood cell count and erythrocyte sedimentation rate (ESR) provide similar information and have been considered more practical since they are easier to measure and are more readily available. However, it should be noted that the increase in the ESR seen in inflammatory states directly results from changes in the APRs, most notably an increase in fibrinogen.

Table 10.3. Major Acute Phase Reactants

Positive APRs	Negative APRs
α_1-Antitrypsin	Albumin
α_1-Antichymotrypsin	Prealbumin
Haptoglobin	Transferrin (rises in late acute phase)
Ceruloplasmin	Retinol binding protein
Fibrinogen	
C3	
C-Reactive protein	
Hemopexin	
Serum amyloid A protein	

The advent of more sensitive assays for CRP has aroused new interest in the potential applications of APRs to clinical practice. Recent reports suggest that assay of CRP may be superior to the ESR in a variety of clinical situations (5). Serial measurements may provide an index of disease activity and are useful to assess the response to therapy. Potential applications of APRs include monitoring postoperative patients for infectious complications, detection of occult infections, monitoring disease activity in patients with rheumatic diseases and inflammatory bowel disease, and detecting renal allograft transplant rejection. Further studies are needed to more fully define the role of APRs in clinical practice.

The changes in plasma proteins seen during the acute phase response potentially serve a variety of functions. Among the positive APRs are the protease inhibitors α_1-antitrypsin and α_1-antichymotrypsin. These proteins protect the body from indiscriminant proteolysis by proteases released from leukocytes and macrophages at sites of tissue injury and repair. Other proteins such as haptoglobin and hemopexin function as salvage molecules to preserve body iron stores (1). CRP appears to function as an immunomodulator by activating the complement system as well as neutrophils and monocyte-macrophages (5). On the other hand, transferrin is a late APR, its level rising in plasma only after the other APRs have reached their maximum. It is thought that the elevation in transferrin is probably a secondary event brought about by the decrease in plasma iron associated with inflammation. The function of some APRs such as α_1-acid glycoprotein is not known. The role of the negative APRs is more difficult to conceptualize. The decrease in albumin during the acute phase response may serve to divert the protein synthetic machinery of the liver away from production of this nonessential protein. In theory, this would facilitate the synthesis of critical elements needed for the inflammatory response.

The individual APRs respond at different rates, and the factor by which their concentration changes in plasma varies. Within hours, CRP and α_1-an-

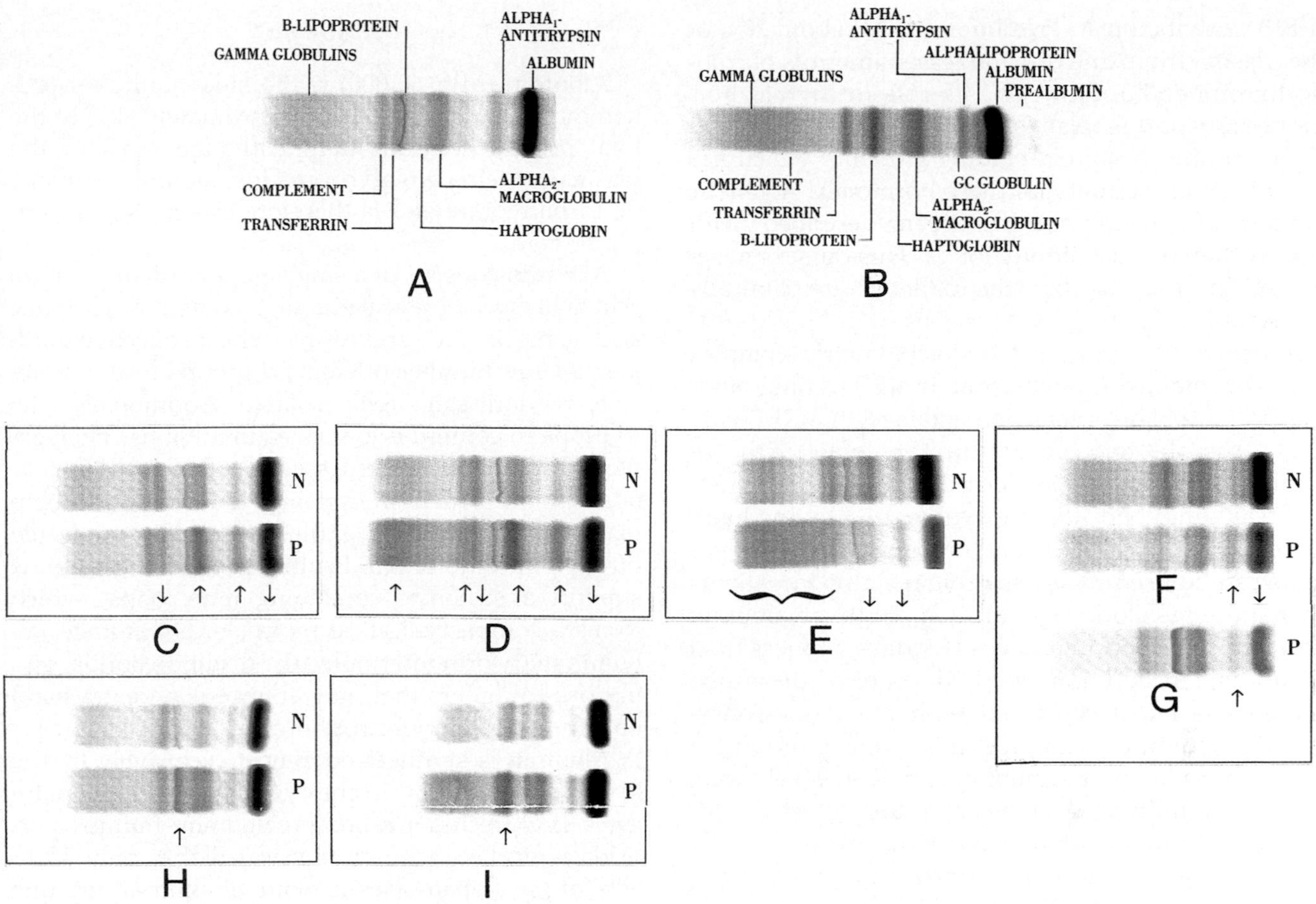

Figure 10.2. Representative patterns of serum proteins seen on serum protein electrophoresis. **A**, Normal pattern. **B**, Normal pattern on high-resolution electrophoresis. **C**, Acute inflammatory pattern. **D**, Chronic inflammatory pattern. **E**, Cirrhotic pattern. **F**, Nonselective protein loss. **G**, Nephrotic syndrome. **H**, Hyperbetalipoproteinemic pattern. **I**, Iron deficiency anemia. (Courtesy of Michael Burke, Beckman Instruments, Inc., Beckman Paragon Serum Protein Electrophoresis Patterns.)

tichymotrypsin rise. Soon thereafter, α_1-acid glycoprotein increases, followed by α_1-antitrypsin, haptoglobin, C4, and fibrinogen. Later C3, ceruloplasmin, and transferrin become elevated. Within 2 to 5 days most of the APRs have reached their maximum (6). Quantitatively, the most striking elevation is seen with CRP, which may increase by a factor of 3000. The other APRs generally show much more modest increases (factors of 2 to 4). The early rise in CRP together with the large factor by which it increases makes it the most useful APR to measure in the clinical laboratory.

Although APRs may be measured individually, the overall pattern of the acute phase response is most easily appreciated on serum protein electrophoresis (Fig. 10.2*C* and *D*). The total protein is usually normal, owing to a decrease in albumin with a concomitant marked increase in the α_1 and α_2 globulins. CRP may appear as a distinct band in the slow γ to mid-β region. The γ-globulin fraction is often normal during the early acute phase. In the course of an infectious process, oligoclonal bands may be seen, followed later by a diffuse polyclonal increase in the γ-globulins.

Patients with severe liver disease, malnutrition, or protein-losing syndromes often show an absent or blunted acute phase response. Individuals with congenital protein deficiencies may fail to increase a specific protein or may exhibit only a partial response. This can have the effect of normalizing the level of the deficient protein and masking the underlying congenital defect.

INDIVIDUAL PROTEINS AND DISEASE STATES

Prealbumin

Prealbumin (MW 54,000) is a tryptophan-rich tetrameric glycoprotein named for its anodal migration relative to albumin on protein electrophoresis. Synonyms for prealbumin include transthyretin and thyroid-binding prealbumin. The only known functions of prealbumin are as a carrier protein for thyroid hormone, and, together with retinol binding protein

(RBP), for vitamin A. Prealbumin binds about 20% of the plasma thyroxine (T_4) and lesser amounts of triiodothyronine (T_3). However, its role in thyroid hormone transport is relatively minor since most T_4 and T_3 are bound to thyroid-binding globulin, which has a much greater affinity for these hormones. A genetic variant of prealbumin has been described with higher than normal affinity for T_4. This causes an elevation in total T_4, but the patients are clinically euthyroid.

Prealbumin forms a 1:1 stoichiometric complex with the vitamin A carrier protein RBP (retinol-binding protein). This interaction stabilizes the RBP-vitamin A complex and prevents urinary losses of the vitamin (since free RBP is filtered by the glomerulus).

Prealbumin and RBP are synthesized by the liver. Together with albumin and transferrin, these proteins can be used to assess protein status in patients with protein-calorie malnutrition. Both prealbumin and RBP have short half-lives (1.9 days and less than 12 hours). In addition, the body pool of these two proteins is small compared with albumin. Consequently, a deficiency in protein intake will produce a noticeable fall in prealbumin and RBP levels long before albumin and transferrin are affected. Although albumin and transferrin have traditionally been used to assess protein status, measurement of prealbumin and RBP may provide a better index of acute changes. For this reason, they are also useful in monitoring the adequacy of protein replacement therapy (4, 7).

Prealbumin levels are significantly decreased in a number of liver diseases due to impaired synthesis. Unlike serum enzymes, which primarily indicate hepatocellular damage, prealbumin levels reflect hepatic synthesis and can serve as an index of liver function (8). However, prealbumin is also a negative acute phase reactant and is thus not a specific indicator of liver function.

Prealbumin may be increased in patients receiving steroids, in pregnancy, and in chronic renal failure.

Because of the low level of prealbumin in serum, this protein is often not visualized on serum protein electrophoresis. However, prealbumin is a compact molecule that can cross the blood-brain barrier, and may also be synthesized by cells of the choroid plexus. This results in about a 40-fold increase in the prealbumin to albumin ratio in cerebrospinal fluid (CSF). Consequently, on CSF electrophoresis, prealbumin appears as a distinct band slightly anodal to albumin. Prealbumin can also be measured by a variety of immunoassays, including RID, EID, and nephelometry. The normal reference range is somewhat method dependent but is about 150 to 360 mg/liter.

Albumin

Albumin (MW 60,000) is the most abundant protein in plasma, comprising approximately 60% of the total protein concentration. Although most of the plasma proteins are glycoproteins, albumin contains no carbohydrate and is therefore classified as a simple protein.

Albumin consists of a single peptide chain. Amino acid analysis has revealed a high content of glutamic acid, aspartic acid, and lysine, which collectively impart a large number of charged groups to the molecule, rendering it highly soluble. Additionally, the tryptophan content is low, a feature that has been exploited in some albumin assays. Albumin also contains a high content of cysteine residues, which help maintain the tertiary structure of the molecule through intramolecular disulfide bonds. These bonds support a structure containing nine loops, which forms a compact elliptical molecule. On storage, albumin may form intermolecular disulfide bonds, giving rise to dimers that may appear as an extra band on serum protein electrophoresis.

Albumin is synthesized almost exclusively by the liver, appearing first in the cytoplasm of the hepatocytes as a precursor called proalbumin. Immunoperoxidase studies have demonstrated that only 10 to 35% of the hepatocytes contain albumin at any one time, suggesting that synthesis is either restricted to a limited population of cells or occurs in a cyclical fashion throughout the liver (9). Fasting decreases the rate of synthesis up to 60%, whereas refeeding results in a prompt increase in synthesis. Regulation of synthesis is accomplished by a negative feedback effect exerted on the hepatocytes by the plasma albumin level (6) and possibly by the plasma colloid oncotic pressure (9). The biological half-life of albumin is about 19 days.

Albumin has several important and diverse functions, including contributing nearly 80% of the plasma colloid oncotic pressure. Albumin serves as an amino acid source to a variety of cells and functions as a major transport protein because the large number of negatively charged groups on the molecule are potential binding sites. Bilirubin binds to albumin, and this is the major mechanism for sequestering and transporting bilirubin to the liver from sites of hemoglobin catabolism. Albumin is intimately involved in lipid metabolism, accepting free fatty acids from lipoprotein lipase and transporting them between the liver and peripheral tissues. A number of hormones bind to albumin, including thyroxine, triiodothyronine, cortisol, aldosterone, estradiol, and progesterone. Since these hormones preferentially bind to their respective hormone binding globulins, albumin serves mainly as a high-capacity, low-affinity overflow reservoir (9). Many drugs bind to albumin, including warfarin (97%), phenylbutazone (99%), salicylate (40%), penicillin (65%), and chlorothiazide (89%), among many others. Significant amounts of calcium and lesser quantities of magnesium are also bound.

Only 40% of total body albumin is in the plasma at any one time. The remaining 60% is distributed among virtually every other body fluid compartment, forming an exchangeable pool with plasma (9). Hyperalbuminemia generally results from dehydration and is otherwise quite rare. Artifactual increases may occur after prolonged tourniquet application during venipuncture. Conversely, hypoalbuminemia is common. Decreased albumin levels may result from a variety of mechanisms, including impaired synthesis (liver disease), increased catabolism (acute phase response), excessive losses (nephrotic syndrome), or "third-spacing" (ascites, effusions). The most severe states of hypoalbuminemia occur in protein-losing syndromes such as the nephrotic syndrome or protein-losing enteropathy. Excessive losses may also occur in hemorrhage, burns, or exudative processes, especially of the skin and gastrointestinal tract. In the acute phase response, albumin levels begin to fall within 12 to 36 hours, presumably as a result of increased catabolism. In chronic wasting diseases such as tuberculosis and malignancy, however, both increased catabolism and decreased synthesis are contributing factors. Malnutrition results in decreased synthesis by denying the liver the necessary amino acid substrates needed to make albumin but may also impair liver function by other mechanisms. Malabsorption syndromes produce hypoalbuminemia by mechanisms similar to those in malnutrition. Chronic liver disease of any cause impairs albumin synthesis, although in alcoholic patients this is often accompanied by poor nutritional status. Hypoalbuminemia is also a common finding in pregnancy.

Whatever the cause, hypoalbuminemia decreases the plasma colloid oncotic pressure. Severe decreases may result in edema. In addition, the binding and transport of a number of substances are correspondingly impaired.

Over 20 genetic variants of albumin have been described (6). The most common type is called albumin A. Variant albumins may result in a wide albumin band on serum protein electrophoresis or may give rise to two distinct bands (bisalbuminemia) (6). None of these variants has yet been associated with human disease, although one variant has an increased affinity for thyroxine (10). In the rare syndrome analbuminemia, there is a congenital absence of albumin. These patients may have mild edema but are otherwise spared the hemodynamic consequences of severe hypoalbuminemia due to compensatory mechanisms, including an increase in plasma globulins, which take over some of the functions of albumin. The major biochemical problem in these patients is a disturbance in lipid metabolism including hypercholesterolemia, increased plasma phospholipids, and lipoproteins (11).

A variety of methods are available to measure albumin, including electrophoretic, immunochemical, and dye-binding techniques. Albumin may be estimated indirectly by subtracting the measured total globulins from the total protein value. This method exploits the fact that plasma globulins contain substantially more tryptophan residues per gram of protein than does albumin. To estimate albumin, the total protein is first measured by standard methods. Then the globulins are assayed by reaction of their tryptophan residues with glycoxylic acid, forming a purple color which is measured spectrophotometrically. The value for the globulins is then subtracted from the total protein.

Albumin may also be estimated by quantitative densitometric scanning of the albumin band on serum protein electrophoresis. The scan is integrated to provide an estimate of albumin as a percentage of the total electrophoretic protein. Separate measurement of the total serum protein permits the estimate to be converted to mass units. Specificity can be improved by using immunochemical techniques, including radial immunoassay, nephelometry, enzyme-linked immunoassay, and radioimmunoassay, although these methods are relatively expensive to perform (6).

A variety of dye-binding methods are available to measure albumin (12), and these methods have been widely used. The assays are based on the ability of albumin to bind a number of organic anionic dyes. Binding results in a shift in the absorption maximum of the dye, which can be quantitated spectrophotometrically despite the presence of unbound excess dye. Plasma globulins either do not bind the dyes or do so only showly. The two most popular dyes are bromocresol green and bromocresol purple. Bromocresol green is not specific for albumin and also binds to globulins, but this occurs slowly and is not a problem if the sample is assayed promptly. On the other hand, bromocresol purple does not bind to globulins.

Urine or CSF samples may contain only small amounts of albumin. Traditionally these samples were therefore concentrated prior to measurement, but some of the newer assays are sufficiently sensitive to permit elimination of the concentration step. Urinary albumin may also be estimated by a screening dipstick method (Albustix) that exploits the change in visible color of bromophenol blue from yellow to green to blue with increasing albumin concentration (12). This method is relatively nonspecific.

The reference range for serum albumin varies slightly with age, sex, posture, and the method of assay. Values may be 5 g/liter greater in supine versus recumbent patients and are slightly higher in adults than in children. The adult reference range is 35 to 50 g/liter.

α_1-Antitrypsin

α_1-Antitrypsin (AAT) is one of the major plasma proteins, comprising nearly 90% of the α_1 globulin region on serum protein electrophoresis. Deficiency of AAT has been associated with pulmonary emphysema and hepatic cirrhosis. The molecule consists of an MW 52,000 glycoprotein that is synthesized by the liver and released into the plasma. It is also found in a number of other body fluids, including tears, lymph, bile, semen, and amniotic fluid (13). AAT is one of the acute phase reactants. Plasma levels may double in states of acute and chronic inflammation, in malignancy, after trauma or surgery, and during pregnancy or estrogen therapy.

AAT belongs to a family of serum proteins collectively known as proteinase inhibitors. Other proteins in this group include α_2-macroglobulin, α_1-antichymotrypsin, antithrombin III, antiplasmin, C1 inhibitor, and a variety of lesser-known proteins. Although 90% of the serum antitrypsin activity is attributable to AAT, significant amounts of trypsin are not found in plasma. Consequently, AAT functions mainly to inhibit nontrypsin proteinases, especially elastase and collagenase in tissues and body fluids. These enzymes are released by leukocytes and macrophages at sites of inflammation. Thus, AAT is an important component of the body's mechanism to control endogenous proteolysis. Left unchecked, these enzymes would ultimately destroy normal tissues.

AAT exerts its effect by forming a covalent complex with serine-type proteinases. Complex formation inhibits the enzyme, and the complex is subsequently removed by the reticuloendothelial system, primarily in the liver. The genes encoding the AAT protein comprise an autosomal allelic system containing at least 75 codominant genes (14) inherited on a single locus called Pi for proteinase inhibitor. The resultant AAT variant proteins are immunologically similar but can be distinguished on the basis of their electrophoretic mobility (13). A number of the alleles give rise to normal variants of AAT, while others produce abnormal molecules and are associated with AAT deficiency. The most common normal allele is PiM, which encodes for the M protein variant of AAT. In the United States, 95% of the population have the homozygous PiMM genotype. The alleles PiZ and PiF are also relatively common in Caucasian populations (15). The PiZ and PiS alleles produce an abnormal AAT protein. The rare null allele, Pi−, produces no protein product. Non-PiM alleles are rare in black Africans (13).

The PiZ allele is the most common variant associated with AAT deficiency. The heterozygote gene frequency of PiZ in the United States is 2 to 3%, while homozygotes comprise one in 3630 individuals. In homozygous PiZZ subjects the plasma AAT level is reduced to 10 to 15% of normal, while heterozygotes with the PiMZ phenotype are reduced to 60% of normal. The phenotypes PiSS and PiMS have levels 63 and 83% of normal, respectively (15).

Deficiency of AAT may be congenital or acquired. Acquired decreases are seen in protein-losing syndromes, in malnutrition, in severe liver damage, and in some respiratory diseases, including neonatal RDS. Congenital deficiency is associated with pulmonary emphysema and with hepatic cirrhosis. Nearly 70 to 80% of homozygous PiZZ individuals develop chronic obstructive pulmonary disease (COPD) (16), often by the age of 20 to 30 years. The spectrum of COPD in AAT deficiency includes patients with chronic bronchitis and bronchectasis in addition to those with emphysema. It is currently unclear whether heterozygotes for the Z allele (PiMZ) are also at increased risk for pulmonary disease, but some studies have suggested that this may be the case. Cigarette smoking rapidly accelerates the progression of pulmonary disease in homozygous PiZZ individuals and appears also to increase the risk of heterozygotes. Not all subjects with severe AAT deficiency develop lung disease, and most patients with COPD are not AAT deficient. Possibly as few as 1% of patients with emphysema have AAT deficiency (16).

The phenotypes PiZZ, MZ and SZ have also been associated with liver disease (17). Fifty percent of homozygous PiZZ patients exhibit intermittent abnormalities in liver function tests, and 10 to 20% develop permanent abnormalities. Nonetheless, most patients with AAT deficiency do not develop chronic liver disease. Patients may present during the neonatal period with jaundice or with neonatal hepatitis. The latter entity may appear similar clinically and morphologically to viral hepatitis or chronic active hepatitis. AAT deficiency should be considered in all infants with jaundice and in all children with liver disease (17). Some patients with AAT deficiency develop cirrhosis by 2 to 3 years of age, while in others the onset is delayed until adulthood.

Homozygous PiZZ AAT deficiency can usually be detected on serum protein electrophoresis by noting a marked decrease in the α_1 region. This region is never completely empty since 10% of the α_1 zone is comprised of other proteins. Heterozygotes often have a normal-appearing α_1 zone. A semiquantitative estimate of AAT may obtained by densitometric scanning of the serum electrophoretogram. Traditionally, AAT activity was assessed in a functional assay that measured its ability to inhibit the catalytic activity of trypsin on certain synthetic substrates (trypsin inhibitory activity). Recently, immunochemical methods, including nephelometric assays, have replaced older methods (6).

Quantitative assays are useful to detect patients with AAT deficiency, but they do not provide information about the Pi phenotype. The normal reference range of AAT is 200 to 400 mg/dl. Caution should be exercised in interpreting AAT levels in patients exhibiting an acute phase response since heterozygotes and some homozygotes can increase their AAT level in this situation. In patients with M protein levels below 50 mg/dl, AAT phenotyping should be performed (6). Methods for phenotyping include isoelectric focusing, starch gel electrophoresis, and two-dimensional immunoelectrophoresis. Recently, monoclonal antibodies against the Z protein have been developed. For an excellent review of AAT deficiency the reader is referred to Brantly et al. (14).

α_2-Macroglobulin

α_2-Macroglobulin (AMG), haptoglobin, and ceruloplasmin together make up the α_2 region on serum protein electrophoresis. AMG is one of the largest serum proteins (MW 725,000) and functions as an inhibitor of a variety of endopeptidases, including serine proteinases (trypsin, plasmin, elastase, collagenase), thiol proteases, metal proteases, and the carboxy protease cathepsin D. Unlike AAT, in which inhibition occurs by formation of a covalent bound with the active site of the proteinase, AMG irreversibly binds proteinases without affecting the active center of the enzyme (18). Once bound, the AMG-proteinase complex is rapidly cleared from the circulation by the reticuloendothelial system of the liver, spleen, and bone marrow.

AMG is synthesized by the liver with a half-life in serum of 5 days. The half-life of AMG-proteinase complexes is about 8 minutes (19). Owing to the wide spectrum of activity of AMG against a variety of proteinases, it has been difficult to ascribe a specific function to this protein. Although it appears important in defense against proteolytic enzymes, AMG is present in plasma at only one-tenth the concentration (on a molar basis) of α_1-antitrypsin.

AMG levels are greatly increased in the nephrotic syndrome and may attain levels greater than 1000 mg/dl. This occurs because the large size of AMG prevents its loss in the urine through the damaged glomeruli, while the smaller plasma proteins are selectively lost. AMG may also be increased up to 70% in cirrhosis despite significant loss of the liver cell mass. This finding is opposite that of most other plasma proteins, although the immunoglobulins may also be elevated in liver disease. Minor increases are seen in diabetes mellitus. Unlike AAT, which behaves as an acute phase reactant, AMG levels are not altered in states of inflammation. A very rare human deficiency of AMG has been reported (autosomal dominant), but the patients are asymptomatic. No other disease has yet been identified in which measurement of AMG is of clinical value, although nephelometric and immunochemical assays exist. The reference range is 125 to 215 mg/dl. Values are slightly higher in women, and are age dependent.

Ceruloplasmin

Ceruloplasmin (CER) (MW 132,000) is a glycoprotein synthesized by the liver as a single polypeptide chain to which six copper atoms are attached (20). CER migrates as an α_2-globulin on protein electrophoresis but is not normally visible on routine gels except in situations where it is significantly increased. The pure protein is blue because of its high copper content. Increased levels may impart a green tinge to plasma samples. Although CER is one of the APRs, its precise role in the acute phase response has not been defined.

The principal importance of CER in laboratory medicine is in the diagnosis of Wilson's disease, which typically is associated with low plasma CER levels. Despite intensive investigation, the function of this protein remains an enigma. Historically it was thought that CER played a central role in copper transport since CER-bound copper normally constitutes 90% of the total plasma copper. However, radioisotope studies have shown a negligible turnover of CER-bound copper, indicating that copper is neither lost nor gained from the molecule in the circulation (6). Furthermore, the protein deficiency state of hypoceruloplasminemia, which is dominantly inherited, produces no symptoms of copper deficiency. It is now thought that CER may play a role in copper metabolism by acting as a donor of copper to certain key copper-containing enzymes. This is accomplished through uptake and degradation of CER by a number of cells but does not involve transfer of copper from intact CER molecules. However, the precise role of this protein in copper metabolism still remains poorly defined.

Both CER and transferrin are antioxidants, together accounting for most of the antioxidant activity of plasma. In this capacity CER may play a role in preventing lipid oxidation and free radical formation, both of which are damaging to cells.

While copper is an essential nutrient, it is also highly toxic to cells. Consequently, efficient means of maintaining copper homeostasis are required. After absorption in the intestine, dietary copper is bound to albumin and then is taken up by the liver and to a lesser extent by all cells. The liver functions as a storage site. Copper is incorporated into the CER apoprotein in the liver and is released into the plasma. Roughly 90% of plasma copper is bound to CER, the remainder being found in a dialyzable fraction bound to albumin and histidine. However, the mechanism by which copper is transported to cells is unknown. The principal route of copper excretion is through the biliary tract, with a small amount being excreted in the urine. Copper homeostasis reflects the balance between intestinal absorption and biliary excretion. The liver is the main recipient of dietary copper and the primary route of excretion.

Wilson's disease (hepatolenticular degeneration) is an autosomal recessive disorder associated with toxic accumulation of copper, particularly in the liver and brain. Although the incidence is low (one in 50,000 to 100,000) it may be the most common cause of chronic liver disease in childhood. It was once believed that Wilson's disease resulted from a heritable defect in CER, but this concept has subsequently been refuted (21). It has been shown that the gene responsible for Wilson's disease resides on chromosome 13, while the gene for CER is on chromosome 3. The defect in Wilson's disease appears to involve both an impairment in biliary copper excretion and a decreased incorporation of copper into CER. These defects cause a progressive accumulation of copper in the liver, resulting in chronic liver disease. Ultimately, copper may overflow from the liver and deposit in other tissues, most notably in the basal ganglia of the brain (lenticular degeneration) and in the cornea of the eye. Deposition in the brain causes neurological symptoms, including dysarthria and loss of coordination of voluntary movements. Corneal deposits produce the classic appearance known as Kayser-Fleischer rings. Copper deposition in other tissues may result in renal tubular damage, kidney stones, osteoporosis, arthropathy, cardiomyopathy, and hypoparathyroidism (21).

Hepatic involvement in Wilson's disease produces variable degrees of liver dysfunction. Some patients exhibit only minor impairment in liver function, while others develop severe liver damage as early as age 8. The onset of hepatic failure may be abrupt or may result from progressive cirrhosis over many years. Fortunately, patients with Wilson's disease can be effectively treated with penicillamine, which chelates body copper and promotes its excretion in the urine. If patients are diagnosed before the onset of cirrhosis and neurological symptoms, a normal life span can be expected. For this reason, early diagnosis and treatment are essential, as is the evaluation of the patients siblings who have a 1 in 4 chance of developing the disease. However, the majority of cases go undetected and ultimately present with advanced disease (6). Consequently, Wilson's disease should be considered in all patients with chronic liver disease and in all patients above 12 years of age with relevant neurological findings (21). Heterozygotes for the Wilson's gene do not develop manifestations of the disease.

The majority of patients with Wilson's disease exhibit decreased levels of plasma CER (less than 10 mg/dl) with a concomitant decrease in the total serum copper concentration. However, the nonceruloplasmin copper is increased, with a resultant increase in urinary copper excretion. Administration of pencillamine augments urinary copper excretion and may be helpful in establishing the diagnosis. While all patients with neurological disease exhibit the classic laboratory findings in addition to the Kayser-Fleischer rings, perhaps as many as 20% of patients with disease limited to hepatic involvement have normal CER levels. Liver biopsy with measurement of the hepatic copper content by atomic absorption is a fairly reliable test for Wilson's disease when the level is greater than 300 mg/g dry weight. However, the hepatic copper content may also be increased in some other types of liver disease. The best test for the diagnosis of Wilson's disease is the demonstration of a negligible incorporation of radioactive copper into ceruloplasmin. In this test either ^{64}Cu or ^{67}Cu is administered intravenously and the plasma radioactivity counted periodically for 48 hours. Since free radiolabeled copper is rapidly assimilated by the liver, the residual plasma radioactivity reflects copper incorporation into CER (21).

Low levels of plasma CER are not specific for Wilson's disease. Any condition associated with severe liver dysfunction (particularly primary biliary cirrhosis) will impair CER synthesis. Decreased levels are also seen in malnutrition and protein-losing states (6). Conversely, plasma CER levels are increased in pregnancy, with oral contraceptive use, and in the acute phase response. Biliary tract obstruction may also result in an elevated plasma CER.

The reference range for CER varies with age, being highest in young children and somewhat lower in both infants and adults. Values less than 10 mg/dl are suggestive of Wilson's disease, but normal levels do not exclude the diagnosis. The adult range varies with the method of assay but is approximately 27 to 37 mg/dl. Most CER assays are based on immunochemical methods, including nephelometry and

RID. Alternatively, the oxidase activity of CER can be measured using the substrate *p*-phenylenediamine in a colorimetric assay.

Haptoglobin

Haptoglobin (MW 100,000) is a glycoprotein synthesized by the liver that migrates as an α_2 globulin. Its function is to bind free hemoglobin released by intravascular red blood cell destruction, thus conserving body iron and preventing renal filtration of potentially nephrotoxic hemoglobin. Free hemoglobin dissociates into α-β dimers that are bound by haptoglobin. The complexes are subsequently removed by the reticuloendothelial system, which degrades the heme groups to iron and bilirubin. Complex formation occurs through the α chain of the hemoglobin dimers. Consequently, haptoglobin can bind hemoglobin A, F, S, and D but not hemoglobin types that lack an α chain. Methemoglobin and free heme moieties do not bind haptoglobin. The total plasma binding capacity of haptoglobin is about 3 g of hemoglobin.

Normally, intravascular destruction accounts for less than 10% of the total red cell turnover. Continued synthesis of haptoglobin by the liver prevents it from being depleted under normal circumstances. In states of accelerated intravascular hemolysis, haptoglobin may become depleted, resulting in free hemoglobin dimers, which are filtered by the kidney. Once filtered, free hemoglobin is degraded by the renal tubular epithelial cells, with heme-iron ultimately being converted to hemosiderin. The kidney can process up to 5 g of hemoglobin per day, but above this level free hemoglobin appears in the urine. Free hemoglobin that has not been bound by haptoglobin or processed by the kidneys is oxidized in the plasma to methemoglobin and the heme groups are subsequently released. The free heme groups are taken up by another binding protein, hemopexin, which carries them to the liver, where they are degraded. Like haptoglobin, hemopexin may also become depleted in states of accelerated hemolysis.

Three distinct phenotypes of haptoglobin have been identified by electrophoresis and designated HP1-1, Hp1-2, Hp2-2. These phenotypes have not been associated with human disease and are of no significance. Rare individuals with congenital anhaptoglobinemia have no detectable haptoglobin.

Haptoglobin is an acute phase reactant and may therefore be elevated in the acute phase response. Elevated haptoglobin levels are also seen in the nephrotic syndrome where other proteins are preferentially lost.

Haptoglobin is decreased in diseases associated with intravascular hemolysis, including hemolytic anemias, hemoglobinopathies, hemolytic transfusion reactions, extensive burns, malaria, disseminated intravascular coagulation, and exercise-induced hemolysis. In severe hemolysis, haptoglobin may be totally depleted, requiring up to 1 week to return to normal. In chronic hemolytic states such as are seen with mechanical heart valves or hemoglobinopathies, there may be a steady decline in haptoglobin. In these conditions, serial measurements are a better index of ongoing hemolysis than single haptoglobin values. Haptoglobin may also be depressed in ineffective erythropoiesis associated with intramarrow red cell destruction and in liver disease due to decreased synthesis.

Historically, haptoglobin was measured by determining the hemoglobin binding capacity of serum. In this assay, a patient sample is first saturated with hemoglobin followed by electrophoretic separation of the free from the bound hemoglobin. The haptoglobin-hemoglobin complex is then quantified by its reaction with benzidine and expressed as milligrams of hemoglobin binding capacity per deciliter of serum. This cumbersome procedure has now been replaced by immunochemical methods, including nephelometry and RID. The reference range is 40 to 336 mg/dl.

Transferrin

Transferrin (siderophilin) appears as a distinct band on serum protein electrophoresis and constitutes the major component of the β-globulin fraction. It functions as the principal plasma protein responsible for the transport of iron. Transferrin is a glycoprotein (MW 79,550) containing two iron binding sites on a single polypeptide chain. Most of the transferrin in plasma is synthesized by the liver, although small amounts are made in a variety of other sites, including the reticuloendothelial system, the gonads, and the submaxillary gland (22). Transferrin binds ferric iron in a reversible ionic bond accompanied by the uptake of one bicarbonate anion per atom of iron. The complex is stable at physiological pH, but dissociation occurs in acidic solution. Transferrin is also capable of loosely binding a variety of other metal ions, including copper, zinc, cobalt, and calcium, but with the exception of copper this is not of physiological significance (22).

The body contains about 3 to 5 g of iron, but only 3 to 5 mg of iron is found in plasma. Almost all of this iron is bound to transferrin, with a small amount bound to other proteins such as albumin. The level of free iron is very low (less than 1 μg/dl). Consequently, the serum iron concentration refers mainly to iron bound to transferrin, whereas the total iron binding capacity (TIBC), which is also commonly measured, is simply an approximation of the transferrin concentration. Normally only about 33% of the iron binding sites on transferrin are occupied. This is sometimes reported as the percent saturation of transferrin.

Transferrin is responsible for the transport of iron from its site of absorption in the intestine (or from sites of hemoglobin catabolism) to red cell precursors in the bone marrow or to sites of iron storage in the reticuloendothelial system of the bone marrow, liver, and spleen. After unloading its iron, transferrin returns to the plasma and is recycled. Radiolabel tracer studies have demonstrated a biological half-life of about 8 days. In addition to its transport function, transferrin minimizes the level of free iron in plasma, thus reducing urinary iron losses and preventing the potentially toxic effects of high free iron levels.

The transferrin protein exhibits extensive genetic polymorphism arising largely from amino acid substitutions in the peptide chain. A number of variants have been identified on protein electrophoresis. They are named according to their relative electrophoretic mobility when compared to the most common transferrin type, known as transferrin C. For example, transferrin D was the first variant protein discovered. Transferrin D is found in certain American blacks and Australian aborigines. Although none of the electrophoretic variants has been associated with human disease, they will occasionally masquerade as M components on serum electrophoresis. Heterozygotes exhibit two transferrin bands, one with a normal mobility and reduced concentration (C protein) and the second migrating either above or below the normal band. Immunofixation techniques will distinguish these variants from true M components. Rarely, congenital atransferrinemia results in very low levels of plasma transferrin in association with iron overload and severe anemia due to the inability to mobilize the body's iron stores (6).

Decreased levels of serum transferrin may be seen in liver disease and in protein-losing disorders such as the nephrotic syndrome and protein-losing enteropathy. Transferrin levels are depressed in starvation and are a useful marker of protein malnutrition in hospitalized patients (4). Like albumin and β-lipoprotein, transferrin behaves as a negative acute phase reactant (6). Consequently, low levels are seen in a variety of acute and chronic inflammatory states and in malignancy. Transferrin levels may rise during the late stages of the acute phase response (see APRs).

Assay of serum transferrin is most commonly performed in the evaluation of anemia. In iron deficiency anemia, the transferrin level is elevated but the percent saturation is low. In the anemia of chronic disease, transferrin is normal and the percent saturation increased. Transferrin levels may also be increased in the early stages of acute hepatitis, in pregnancy, and with estrogen administration. In idiopathic hemochromatosis and in hemosiderosis due to excessive blood transfusions, the serum transferrin is normal but the percent saturation is markedly elevated (up to 90%).

The normal serum transferrin level is 200 to 400 mg/dl (2.0 to 4.0 g/liter). Increases or decreases in transferrin may be detected on serum protein electrophoresis, and marked increases may simulate a paraprotein band.

A variety of immunochemical assays are available, including radial immunodiffusion and rate nephelometry, and transferrin may also be estimated indirectly by determination of the TIBC. The TIBC in (mg/dl) is then multiplied by 0.70 to give an estimated transferrin value in mg/dl (6).

β-Lipoprotein

Lipoproteins constitute a family of molecules composed of lipids and proteins whose function is to transport cholesterol, triglycerides, and phospholipids in the blood. Lipoproteins have been subclassified into four categories designed chylomicrons, very low density (VLDL), low density (LDL) and high density (HDL) lipoproteins.

On serum protein electrophoresis HDLs migrate between the albumin zone and the α region (α-lipoproteins), forming a diffuse background pattern that is not readily discernible. Likewise, the VLDLs migrate in the pre-β region but are not resolved from other proteins. However, the β-lipoproteins (LDLs) appear in the slow α_2 or β region as a wavy, broad band with a sharp leading edge and a trailing anodal tail.

Increases or decreases in the β-lipoproteins can often be recognized on serum protein electrophoresis (SPE). Elevations may occur in the nephrotic syndrome, hepatobiliary disease, hypothyroidism, diabetes mellitus, and some of the familial hyperlipidemia syndromes.

An increase produces a high-intensity band that may be cathodally displaced; this finding should prompt further investigation. Decreased β-lipoproteins are associated with a faint band of faster mobility (23).

β_2-Microglobulin

β_2-Microglobulin (B2M) is a small protein (MW 11,818) comprising the common light chain of the class I MHC antigen on the surfaces of all nucleated cells (24). It consists of a single polypeptide chain that is noncovalently linked to the HLA heavy chain. B2M may be necessary for insertion of the HLA molecule into the cell membrane, and its presence appears to stabilize the HLA heavy chain. It also plays a role (currently poorly defined) in the regulation of some lymphocyte functions.

A small amount of B2M is normally present in the plasma, urine, and CSF, presumably because the protein is shed from cell surfaces into the blood (6). Its function in these fluids, if any, is unknown.

Due to its small size, B2M is filtered by the renal glomerulus, but most is resorbed and degraded by the renal tubular epithelial cells. The plasma level of B2M is a good index of the glomerular filtration rate. Only trace amounts of the protein are normally present in urine. Elevated levels of urinary B2M may be seen in patients with renal tubulointerstitial disorders, including heavy metal toxicity, anticancer drug toxicity, aminoglycoside toxicity, upper urinary tract infections, and renal allograft rejection. In contrast, patients with renal failure on the basis of glomerular dysfunction typically show elevated plasma B2M levels. Plasma B2M may also be increased in a number of inflammatory diseases (e.g., hepatitis, rheumatoid arthritis, SLE, the acquired immune deficiency syndrome, and sarcoidosis) and in patients with leukemia, lymphoma, and some solid tumors. A recent report has indicated that serum B2M is the best available predictor of survival duration in patients with multiple myeloma (25). In some of these disorders, the elevation in the plasma B2M may reflect increased lymphocyte turnover.

B2M may sometimes be seen on high-resolution electrophoresis. However, because of its low concentration it is usually measured by immunoassay. The normal upper reference limit is 2.4 mg/liter in serum and 0.3 mg/liter in urine.

C-Reactive Protein

C-Reactive protein (CRP) (MW 115,000 to 140,000) was first identified in 1930 as a substance present in the sera of patients with pneumococcal pneumonia that could bind to C-polysaccharide isolated from *Streptococcus pneumoniae*, producing a flocculation reaction. Subsequently it was found that CRP is elevated in a variety of other acute inflammatory diseases. Thus, CRP was the first recognized acute phase reactant. CRP can bind to a number of molecules, including phosphate esters, lipids, polyanions (DNA, polylysine), polycations (histones, protamine), and a variety of polysaccharides (6, 26).

CRP is synthesized by the liver and released into the plasma. Small amounts are also made by a subset of peripheral lymphocytes, but this remains bound to the surface of the cells (26). The intact molecule is a pentameric protein with five identical subunits arranged in a doughnut-shaped polymer.

A number of functions have been ascribed to CRP, including initiation of opsinization and phagocytosis (6) and activation of complement, neutrophils, and monocyte-macrophages (5). Collectively these properties imply an important role for CRP in the recognition of microbial organisms and as an immunomodulator in host defense. CRP may also be important to the recognition of necrotic tissues.

Small amounts of CRP are normally found in plasma at levels less than 0.8 mg/dl. Levels may increase markedly during the acute phase response. Although CRP is not ordinarily seen on serum protein electrophoresis, it may appear as a distinct band in the mid-β to slow γ region when levels are elevated. This can be confused with a monoclonal M component.

Traditional methods for measuring CRP included precipitation and agglutination assays. These had low sensitivity and provided only qualitative results. The lack of a satisfactory assay caused a loss in popularity of CRP testing in favor of the ESR for detecting patients with inflammatory diseases. Recently, highly specific antibodies to CRP have become available. These antibodies permit the development of rapid, specific, and very sensitive assays for this protein. These newer immunoassays include laser nephelometry (the most popular method), RIA, and enzyme immunoassays (5) and have created a renewed interest in CRP testing in a variety of clinical settings. These were mentioned in the section on acute phase reactants and were recently reviewed by Hart (5). Measurement of CRP may be superior to the erythrocyte sedimentation rate and may someday replace it.

METHODS OF PROTEIN ANALYSIS

Measurement of Total Protein

A variety of methods are available to measure the total protein in serum or plasma. Most methods are based on the assumption that protein molecules are pure polypeptides, and that different proteins react with chemical reagents in the same way (6). Neither of these assumptions is strictly true. For example, many proteins contain carbohydrates substituents that may constitute a significant part of the molecule but might not be included in the total protein value as measured by standard methods. In addition, the reactivity of different proteins depends on the structure and amino acid composition of the molecule and is not the same for all proteins. The fact that biological fluids are composed of mixtures of proteins in varying proportions complicates the quantification of proteins in serum, urine, and CSF.

Historically, the Kjeldahl procedure for measuring total nitrogen has been considered a reference method against which other methods for protein could be compared. In this procedure the sample is first subjected to acid hydrolysis, which converts protein nitrogen to ammonium ions. The ammonia nitrogen is then determined by titration or by nesslerization. Because nitrogen contained in nonprotein compounds is also detected by this procedure, a deproteinized sample must be tested in parallel and the value subtracted from the total nitrogen content of the original specimen. The nitrogen content of proteins varies between 15.1 and 16.8% (2), which imparts a slight error when different proteins or protein mixtures of varying proportions are analyzed. The Kjeldahl procedure is too time-consuming and complex for routine use.

The biuret method is the most widely used procedure for the measurement of total protein in the clinical laboratory. It is both simple and easily automated but lacks sufficient sensitivity for use on low-concentration samples such as CSF or urine. The method is based on the reaction of peptide bonds with copper ions (Cu^{2+}) in alkaline solution, forming a pink to violet complex that is measured spectrophotometrically at 540 nm. The intensity of the color is proportional to the protein concentration. A similar reaction occurs between copper ions and the organic compound biuret from which this method derives its name (6). The biuret reaction will occur with any peptide with three or more amino acids. Common causes of interference are lipemia, hemolysis, bilirubinemia, and turbidity, all of which may contribute to the total absorbance at 540 nm. The appropriate use of serum blanks will correct for these sources of interference.

The Lowry method employs a two-stage reaction sequence and is one of the most sensitive (but not specific) procedures for the measurement of total protein. Proteins are first allowed to undergo the biuret reaction. This is followed by reaction of the tryptophan and tyrosine residues with the Folin-Ciocalteu reagent (phosphotungstic-phosphomolybdic acid), yielding a blue color. Histidine and cysteine residues also react but produce weaker chromogens. The combined absorbance of the copper-peptide bond complexes and the reduced Folin-Ciocalteu chromogens is measured at 650 to 750 nm. The copper-peptide bond complexes account for most of the absorbance.

The Lowry method has not been widely used in clinical laboratories for several reasons. First, a variety of nonprotein compounds and drugs react, causing a positive interference. Second, the tyrosine and tryptophan content of proteins varies widely, which complicates the analysis of mixed protein samples. For example, albumin contains only 0.2% tryptophan by weight, whereas the tryptophan content of the globulins is generally between 2 and 3% (6). The method is best for measuring pure proteins of known composition. The major advantage of the Lowry method is that it is nearly 100 times more sensitive than the biuret reaction. It has been used extensively in research to measure samples of low protein concentration.

The absorption of ultraviolet light by proteins at either 280 nm or at 200 to 225 nm provides a simple method to estimate the concentration of proteins in solution. The absorbance at 280 nm is caused mainly by the aromatic rings of tyrosine and tryptophan. The content of these amino acids varies in different proteins, and free tryptophan and tyrosine cause a positive interference. The peptide bonds of proteins are largely responsible for the absorbance at 200 to 225 nm, but measurements this low in the ultraviolet region are also subject to a number of interferences. Again, the problem of poor specificity limits the usefulness of methods based on UV-light absorption.

A very rapid estimate of the total protein in serum may be obtained by refractometry. This method is based on the principle that dissolved solutes increase the refractive index of water. Although serum contains a number of nonprotein compounds, these normally contribute very little to the refractive index of serum. The total protein value is simply read from a precalibrated scale on the refractometer. A positive interference is seen with azotemia, hyperglycemia, hyperbilirubinemia, and lipemia.

A number of dye-binding procedures are available to measure the total protein in clinical specimens. The principle of these assays is similar to the dye-binding methods used for albumin. The most widely used dyes are Coomassie brilliant blue and amido black. Dye-binding methods are limited by the fact that different proteins exhibit different dye-binding characteristics.

Finally, a number of turbidimetric and nephelometric methods are available for measuring proteins in serum or other fluids. These involve precipitation of the proteins with sulfosalicylic acid or trichloracetic acid. The resulting precipitate will scatter a beam of incident light, which forms the basis of the assay.

The normal reference range for serum proteins is 60 to 84 g/liter (6.0 to 8.4 g/dl) (2). The level in infants is somewhat lower than in adults, with adult levels being achieved by 3 years of age. Values in women may be slightly lower than in men.

The measurement of protein in urine or CSF is more difficult than in serum because protein is present in much lower concentrations in these fluids. The most commonly used procedures employ modifications of turbidimetric and dye-binding assays. Among the latter group, Coomassie brilliant blue and Ponceau S are currently popular. A number of immunoassays are also available. All methods suffer from the types of problems described previously, and no assay is totally satisfactory.

Serum Protein Electrophoresis

Serum protein electrophoresis (SPE) is a common laboratory screening test that may be used to evaluate a variety of disease processes. The most common indication for SPE is the detection of monoclonal paraproteins, although the technique has value in a number of other clinical situations. Electrophoretic methods have also been applied to the analysis of isoenzymes, lipoproteins, and hemoglobinopathies, and to the detection of genetic variants of various proteins.

Principles of Electrophoresis

Electrophoresis is a method of separating charged molecules on the basis of their relative mobilities in an electric field. A number of different support media may be used as the stationary phase (e.g., paper, agarose gel, cellulose acetate), while the mobile phase is composed of buffer ions moving under the influence of an electric field. When an electric field is applied, the negatively charged species migrate toward the anode (positive electrode), and positively charged species toward the cathode (negative electrode). Proteins contain both carboxylic acid groups (COOH), which can deprotonate to form negative charges, and amino groups ($-NH_2$), which can accept protons to form positive charges. The net charge on the protein molecule thus depends on its amino acid composition, the presence of charged substituent groups such as carbohydrates, and the pH of the electrophoresis buffer.

The direction of migration of a protein in an electric field depends on the pH of the buffer and the isoelectric point of the protein. The isoelectric point (PI) is defined as the pH at which the sum of all positive and negative charges on the molecule add up to zero. Thus, a protein at its isoelectric point has no net charge and will not migrate in an electric field. At a pH below the isoelectric point, the protein has a net positive charge and the protein will therefore migrate toward the cathode. At a pH above the isoelectric point, the protein will migrate toward the anode.

Other factors that influence the migration of proteins in an electric field are the size and shape of the molecule, the strength of the electric field, the temperature, the effects of convection and diffusion, and the ionic and pore properties of the electrophoresis medium (27).

The first electrophoresis system was described by Tiselius in 1937. This method used a U-shaped tube filled with an electrolyte solution. The sample was then placed at the bottom of the tube. When a current was run through the system, the proteins were separated into four fractions designated albumin, α, β, and γ. The fractions could be identified by observing a change in the refractive index of the electrolyte at the boundaries between the fractions. The Tiselius procedure has been called the moving boundary method.

A number of technical innovations have occurred since the original description of Tiselius. Modern electrophoresis methods utilize a solid supporting medium such as cellulose acetate, agarose gel, or polyacrylamide that is saturated with buffer. The supporting medium is connected to two electrodes by wicks that are also saturated with buffer. A power supply capable of delivering a constant voltage or current is connected to the electrodes. When a protein mixture is placed on the supporting medium, it migrates through the electric field and separates into individual components. Methods that utilize a solid supporting medium are referred to as zone electrophoresis.

The choice of electrophoresis buffer is one of the most important factors affecting the resolution of the system. The buffer defines the pH, which determines the net charge on the protein. This influences both the speed and direction of movement. In addition, the ionic strength of the buffer affects the rate of protein migration. Increasing the ionic strength increases the ionic association between buffer ions and exposed charge groups on the protein molecule. This has the effect of slowing the rate of movement of the protein through the support medium, producing sharper bands on the electrophoretogram. However, as the ionic strength is increased, so too are the current and heat generated during electrophoresis. This effect may denature heat-labile proteins and cause evaporation of buffer from the support medium. The effects of heating can be minimized by incorporating a cooling unit into the electrophoresis apparatus and by performing the procedure in a closed chamber to reduce evaporation.

A variety of support media are available for protein electrophoresis. These can be divided into two types. One type separates proteins solely on the basis of net molecular charge. Examples of this type include paper, cellulose acetate, and agarose gel. The second type separates proteins on the basis of both charge and molecular size. The use of two parameters to separate proteins greatly increases the resolution of the system. Examples of the latter category are starch gel and polyacrylamide (28). Both of these media contain minute pores through which the proteins must travel when migrating under the influence of the electric field. Small molecules traverse the pores more easily than larger ones, producing a molecular sieve effect. The rate of migration of proteins through these media is therefore inversely proportional to their molecular size. Proteins of different sizes but with similar size to charge ratios are not separated on cellulose acetate or agarose, whereas separation may be achieved on starch gel and polyacrylamide.

Some electrophoretic support media adsorb hydroxyl ions from the buffer, creating fixed negative charges. This property is responsible for an effect called electroendosmosis. The fixed charges are surrounded by a cloud of mobile positive ions in the buffer. When a current is applied to the system, the ionic cloud is free to move toward the cathode while the fixed negative charges are immobilized on the support medium. The migrating positive ions are hydrated and therefore carry a shell of solvent molecules with them. The movement of positive ions and solvent toward the cathode creates the endosmotic effect. Proteins migrating toward the anode must move against this force. At the usual pH of electrophoretic buffers most proteins contain enough negative charges to overcome electroendosmosis. However, proteins that bear relatively few negative charges, such as the γ-globulins, may remain still during electrophoresis or be swept backwards toward the cathode by the force of endosmosis. This is the reason why most of the γ-globulins are found cathodal to the origin on standard electrophoretograms. Endosmosis is most pronounced with support media containing a large number of fixed negative charges (paper, cellulose acetate, and conventional agarose) but is less important with systems utilizing polyacrylamide or purified agarose gels.

Serum protein electrophoresis on paper was once popular but has been largely replaced by methods using cellulose acetate or agarose gels. Polyacrylamide and starch gel electrophoresis provide the greatest resolution of protein bands but are generally used only in specialized situations or in research, where high resolution is desirable.

Some laboratories have begun to run an improved method for SPE known as high-resolution electrophoresis (HRE). HRE separates serum into 13 zones instead of the usual five. In addition, a number of protein bands are detected on HRE that are not well resolved by conventional SPE. HRE may be particularly useful to detect faint monoclonal paraproteins but is of limited benefit for analyzing other serum protein patterns.

Agarose Gel Electrophoresis

Both cellulose acetate and agarose have been widely used in the clinical laboratory. The use of agarose gels for serum protein electrophoresis is becoming increasingly popular. A comparison of the two methods was reported by Aguzzi and coworkers (29). The remainder of this section is devoted to a discussion of agarose gel electrophoresis.

A distinction should be made between agar and agarose. Agar contains both agarose and agaropectin. Agaropectin is a highly charged substance with both carboxylic and acid sulfate groups, which create a significant endosmotic effect. In addition, agar tends to retain protein stains, which decreases the clarity of the electrophoresis pattern. Agarose is a purified form of agar in which most of the agaropectin has been removed. Partially purified agarose preparations showing moderate endosmosis are now commercially available and provide a virtually transparent gel. This facilitates visualization and quantitation of the protein bands.

A standard method for serum protein agarose gel electrophoresis was described as a proposed selected method in 1979 (23). A number of variations of this procedure have been used. Electrophoresis kits containing premade gels, staining solutions, and all of the necessary apparatus are available from several suppliers. Most systems utilize a 0.5 to 1.0% gel with either a barbital or tris-boric acid–EDTA buffer at pH 8.6. Fully automated electrophoresis systems have been developed that eliminate many of the manual manipulations normally required in the procedure.

For a detailed description of a standard agarose gel electrophoresis method, the reader is referred to Jeppsson et al. (23). In this method, a serum sample is first spotted on the surface of the agarose support medium and allowed to absorb into the gel. The gel is then connected to two electrodes by filter paper wicks saturated with buffer. The electrodes are attached to a constant-voltage power supply. A current is then passed through the gel to separate the proteins. When electrophoresis is complete, the gel is removed from the electrode apparatus and placed in a bath of fixing solution. The fixing solution usually contains acetic acid, which denatures the proteins and immobilizes them in the gel. This prevents diffusion of the protein bands in the support medium. Proteins in an agarose gel are invisible. Therefore, a staining solution is needed to visualize the bands. A variety of stains have been used, including Coomassie brilliant blue (CBB), amido black, and Ponceau S, which differ in their protein-binding affinities, sensitivity, and absorbence spectra. CBB is the most sensitive of the commonly used stains. Highly sensitive silver staining methods are available but are seldom necessary in routine practice. Once the proteins have been stained, the gel is placed in a destaining solution (usually a mixture of methanol, acetic acid, and water) that clears the excess stain from the gel, pro-

Table 10.4. Typical Serum Protein Electrophoresis Reference Pattern

Zone	Percent of Total Protein
Albumin	45.8–68.2 (mean 57.0)
α_1	2.1– 6.1 (mean 4.1)
α_2	8.8–18.0 (mean 13.4)
β	7.8–13.0 (mean 10.4)
γ	7.8–22.6 (mean 15.2)

ducing sharp protein bands on a transparent background. The finished gel is quite fragile and is not suitable as a permanent record. However, the gel may be dried on a sheet of clear plastic, creating a durable record that can be stored for subsequent review.

Standard agarose gel electrophoresis systems separate serum into five zones designated albumin, α_1, α_2, β, and γ (Fig. 10.2). The albumin band is relatively homogeneous, whereas the other zones are composed of mixtures of different proteins. Interpretation of electrophoretograms requires practice and a thorough understanding of the disease processes that may affect the protein pattern. The most useful information is obtained by careful visual inspection of the stained gel. In addition, the individual fractions can be quantitated by scanning the electrophoretogram with a densitometer. Most commercial kits are equipped with a scanning densitometer that produces a two-dimensional tracing of the electrophoresis pattern. (Fig. 10.1). An integrator is used to calculate the area under each of the zones, which can then be expressed as a percentage of the total area under the tracing. If the total protein concentration is known, the results can be converted into grams per liter, since the area under each zone is proportional to its concentration. The reference range for each of the five zones depends on the electrophoresis method and also varies somewhat with the age, sex, and race of the reference population and a variety of other minor factors. A typical reference range is shown in Table 10.4.

Quantitative densitometric scanning provides a good measurement of the total serum albumin and a crude estimate of the γ-globulin fraction. It is not reliable for measuring other serum proteins because each zone is composed of a mixture of proteins that are not easily resolved by the densitometer. For this reason, densitometric scanning is of limited value. Most laboratories rely primarily on visual interpretation of the overall electrophoresis pattern.

The proteins that make up each of the five electrophoretic zones are listed in Table 10.2. Most of these have been discussed in the preceding pages.

Albumin migrates to the far anodal region of the gel. The mobility of the albumin band may be affected by both congenital and acquired alterations in the molecule. Individuals who are heterozygotes for genetic albumin variants may show a widening of the band, or it may be split into two separate bands (bisalbuminemia). Hyperbilirubinemia, bound fatty acids, and some drugs (aspirin, penicillin) may increase the mobility of albumin (24). The significance of increases and decreases in the serum albumin has been discussed previously. Sometimes a faint prealbumin band may be seen anodal to albumin.

The α_1 zone contains mostly α_1-antitrypsin with minor contributions from several other proteins (Table 10.2). Although AAT cannot be reliably quantitated on serum electrophoretograms, a marked decrease in the AAT band or a band with altered mobility may suggest AAT deficiency and prompt further investigation.

The principal components of the α_2 zone are AMG and haptoglobin. The β-lipoprotein band (LDL) may be found in the α_2 region on some systems but more commonly appears in the β zone. AMG and haptoglobin usually merge into a composite fraction but are sometimes resolved into two separate bands. In patients with hemolytic anemia, haptoglobin may be noticeably decreased.

The major components of the β zone are transferrin, the third component of complement (C3), and the β-liporoteins. In iron deficiency anemia the transferrin band may be increased, although this finding is not specific. The C3 band is quite labile and is often absent unless fresh serum is used. The conversion product of C3 (C3c) sometimes appears in the fast β region. A true decrease in C3 may occur in a variety of inflammatory disorders, including systemic lupus erythematosus. The β-lipoproteins appear as a wavy band with a sharp leading edge and a smudgy tail. Increases in this band are seen in a number of conditions, including liver diseases, the nephrotic syndrome, malnutrition, and some familial hyperlipidemia syndromes.

The immunoglobulins are found in the γ region. This heterogeneous group of proteins is distributed throughout the entire region, and they do not ordinarily produce discrete bands. The finding of a band in the γ region should alert the observer to the possibility of a monoclonal paraprotein. Other proteins—including CRP, lysozyme, and traces of fibrinogen—may also produce bands in this zone. Normally, fibrinogen is not seen on serum protein electrophoresis, but occasionally a faint band appears in patients receiving anticoagulant therapy. Marked elevations in CRP occur in the acute phase response, which may produce a faint band in the γ region.

The most important use of serum protein electrophoresis is for the detection of monoclonal paraproteins.

In addition to the abnormalities in the individual aforementioned proteins, certain diseases produce alterations in more than one protein, which affect the overall electrophoretic pattern. These patterns may be recognized on visual examination of the electrophoretogram (Fig. 10.2) or by quantitative densitometric scanning.

The acute inflammatory pattern produces predictable changes based on the behavior of the positive and negative APRs. The albumin band is normal or decreased, while the α_1 and α_2 globulins show a marked increase. The transferrin band is usually decreased, and the γ-globulins, at least initially, appear normal. The acute phase response may in time evolve into a chronic inflammatory pattern. Albumin continues to be decreased, and the α-globulins remain elevated. In addition, a diffuse polyclonal increase in γ-globulins appears, reflecting increased antibody synthesis. This feature serves to distinguish the acute from the chronic inflammatory pattern.

Cirrhosis produces a decrease in both albumin and the α-globulins due to defective hepatocellular synthesis. This is associated with an increase in the β-lipoprotein band and a polyclonal hypergammaglobulinemia. The increase in γ-globulins may result in fusion of the β and γ globulin zones, which has been called β-γ bridging.

The electrophoretic pattern in patients with acute liver disease is quite variable. The most common pattern is a decrease in albumin with increases in the α- and γ-globulins. However, other patterns may be seen, including an isolated decrease in albumin, diffuse hypergammaglobulinemia, or a normal pattern.

Patients with nonselective protein-losing syndromes such as burns or exudative disorders of the skin, lung, and gastrointestinal tract may have decreases in all of the serum proteins. This pattern may be superimposed on acute or chronic inflammatory changes, which cause an increase in some bands in the α and γ regions. Malnutrition and malabsorption result in generalized hypoproteinemia.

In the nephrotic syndrome there is a selective protein loss. The α_2 region is often noticeably increased due to the increase in AMG. The β-lipoprotein band may be prominent, reflecting the hyperlipidemia seen in nephrotic syndrome. However, albumin is markedly decreased, as are most of the other fractions. The large increase in AMG differentiates this pattern from that seen with nonselective protein losses.

An alteration in the electrophoretic pattern is often seen in pregnancy and in some patients taking oral contraceptives. Pregnancy is associated with an increase in the plasma volume, which causes a dilutional decrease in albumin. In late pregnancy an increase in α_1-glycoprotein may elevate the α_1 globulins, while the α_2 and β-globulins are elevated by increases in ceruloplasmin, β-lipoprotein, and transferrin. The γ-globulins may also be slightly elevated.

Immunochemical Methods

Immunochemical methods are becoming increasingly important in the clinical laboratory for the separation, quantitation, and identification of proteins.

Other Methods

A wide variety of methods are available for the study of proteins. These include methods that separate proteins on the basis of molecular size (ultrafiltration, density gradient centrifugation, molecular exclusion chromatography), solubility (isoelectric precipitation, salt precipitation, solvent fractionation), electric charge (electrophoresis, isoelectric focusing, ion exchange chromatography), and selective adsorption (affinity chromatography). A number of these methods have been used extensively in research. For further details, the reader is referred to standard biochemistry texts. Only a few of these techniques are used with any frequency in the clinical laboratory and are described briefly below.

ION EXCHANGE CHROMATOGRAPHY

All forms of chromatography contain a stationary phase and a mobile phase. The mobile phase provides the driving force to separate molecules, while the stationary phase may partially or completely retard their movement, thus permitting separation. Molecules that differ in their size, charge, or other physical parameters can be resolved by selecting appropriate stationary and mobile phases.

Ion exchange chromatography utilizes a charged supporting medium to separate molecules based on their acid-base properties. The supporting medium consists of minute particles ("beads") to which fixed charges are attached. The beads are loaded in a plastic or glass column. The sample is then placed on top of the column and allowed to percolate through the medium. Some molecules bind tightly to the fixed charges, some bind only weakly, while others do not bind at all. Those that do not bind pass unhindered through the column and are collected in a fraction tube. Molecules that remain bound to the beads are then sequentially eluted with buffers of increasing ionic strength or varying pH, which displace the bound molecules from the column.

Ion exchange resins are often derivatives of cellulose. Carboxymethylcellulose (CM-cellulose) contains fixed negative charges at pH 7.0 and thus is called a cation exchange resin because cationic molecules bind by exchanging for Na ions bound to the negative charges on the resin. In contrast, diethylaminocellulose (DEAE-cellulose) contains fixed positive charges at neutral pH and is used as an anion exchange resin. By selecting an appropriate resin, sample pH, and elution buffers (pH and ionic strength), complex protein mixtures can be separated for further study.

Ion exchange methods have been used to separate isoenzymes, glycosylated hemoglobins, and genetic variants of some proteins. Minicolumns for separating certain proteins are available in kit form.

AFFINITY CHROMATOGRAPHY

Affinity chromatography is based on the principle that some proteins will bind by noncovalent forces to specific ligands. Examples of protein ligand combinations include hormone-receptor pairs, enzyme-coenzyme pairs, and antigen-antibody pairs. Since the ligand may be highly specific to a particular protein, affinity chromatography permits a high degree of purification of the protein, often in a single step.

The method of affinity chromatography is similar to other column methods. The ligand is first immobilized to an inert supporting medium. This is then loaded into a column and the sample added to the top of the column. As the sample percolates through, the protein binds to its specific ligand. Other proteins flow through the column and are collected in a fraction tube. Then an eluting buffer is added to the top of the column. The eluting buffer may be a high–ionic strength salt solution or a solution containing a high concentration of some other compound that competes with the bound protein for the ligand. The protein is thus displaced from its ligand binding site and is eluted from the column.

Affinity chromatography is one of the most powerful techniques used to purify proteins but has as yet received only limited use in the clinical laboratory.

ISOELECTRIC FOCUSING

Isoelectric focusing (IEF) or electrofusing is a type of electrophoresis that separates proteins on the basis of their isoelectric point (PI) (see earlier discussion). A protein at its isoelectric point will not migrate in an electric field, and this feature has been exploited in IEF. IEF is performed in a glass tube filled with a gel supporting medium that contains a pH gradient extending from the top to the bottom of the tube. The sample is loaded on the top of the column and a current is applied to the apparatus. The proteins in the sample migrate through the pH gradient until they reach their isoelectric point, where they stop ("focus"). Because the isoelectric point of proteins changes with even minor changes in amino acid composition, complex mixtures of proteins can be separated by IEF.

Like affinity chromatography, IEF is a powerful method to separate protein. However, its use in the clinical laboratory is currently restricted to specialized situations (such as detecting AAT variants), and most laboratories are not equipped to perform this technique.

References

1. Schreiber G. Synthesis, processing and secretion of plasma proteins by the liver and other organs and their regulation. In: Putman FW, ed. The plasma proteins. New York: Academic Press, 1987:293–349.
2. DeCresce R. Total serum protein: review of methods. American Society of Clinical Pathologists Check Sample, Core Chemistry Series 1988;4(8):1–7.
3. Rose B. The total body water and the plasma sodium concentration. In: Rose B. Clinical physiology of acid base and electrolyte disorders. 3rd ed. New York: McGraw-Hill, 1989: 211–247.
4. Haider M, Haider S. Assessment of protein calorie malnutrition. Clin Chem 1984;30:1286–1299.
5. Hart W. C-reactive protein: the best laboratory indicator for monitoring disease activity. Clev Clin J Med 1989;56:126–130.
6. Silverman L, Christenson R, Grant G. Amino acids and proteins. In: Tietz N, ed. Textbook of clinical chemistry. Philadelphia: WB Saunders, 1986:519–618.
7. Moskowitz S, Pereira G, Spitzer A, Heaf L, Amsel J, Watkins J. Prealbumin as a biochemical marker of nutritional adequacy in premature infants. J Pediatr 1983;102:749–753.
8. Hutchinson D, Halliwell M, Smith M, Parke D. Serum prealbumin as an index of liver function in human hepatobiliary disease. Clin Chim Acta 1981;114:69–74.
9. Peters T. Serum albumin. In: Putnam FW, ed. The plasma proteins. New York: Academic Press, 1975;1:133–173.
10. Ruiz M, Rajatanavin R, Young R, et al. Familial dysalbuminemic hyperthyroxinemia. N Engl J Med 1982;306:635.
11. Keller H, Morrell A, Noseda G, Riva G. Analbuminamie Pathephysiologische Untersuchunge an einem Fall. Schweiz Med Wochenschr 1972;102:71–78.
12. Gendler S. Proteins. In: Kaplan L, Pesce A, eds. Clinical chemistry: theory, analysis, and correlation. St. Louis: CV Mosby, 1989:1029–1065.
13. Moore J. Alpha-1-antitrypsin deficiency. N Engl J Med 1978;299:1045–1099.
14. Brantly M, Nukiwa T, Crystal R. Molecular basis of alpha-1-antitrypsin deficiency. Am J Med 1988;84(suppl 6A):13–27.
15. Bearn A, Hartwig C. Genetic variations of plasma proteins. In: Stanbury J, Wyngaarden J, Fredickson D, eds. The metabolic basis of inherited disease. 3rd ed. New York: McGraw-Hill, 1972:1629–1641.
16. Robbins S. The respiratory system. In: Robbins S, Cotran R, eds. Pathologic basis of disease. 2nd ed. Philadelphia: WB Saunders, 1979:814–885.
17. Ruebner B, Cox K. Liver disease in infancy. In: Peters R, Craig J, eds. Liver pathology. New York: Churchill Livingstone. 1986:37–60.
18. Laurell C, Jeppsson J. Protease inhibitors in plasma. In: Putnam FW, ed. The plasma proteins. 2nd ed. New York: Academic Press, 1975:229–263.
19. Ohlsson K. Elimination of 125-I-trypsin alpha-macroglobulin complexes from blood by reticuloendothelial cells in dogs. Acta Physiol Scand 1971;81:269–272.

20. Czaja M, Weiner F, Schwarzenberg S, et al. Molecular studies of ceruloplasmin deficiency in Wilson's disease. J Clin Invest 1987;80:1200–1204.
21. Danks D. Disorders of copper transport. In: Jeffers J, Gavert G, eds. The metabolic basis of inherited disease, 6th ed. New York: McGraw-Hill, 1989:1411–1424.
22. Putnam F. Transferrin. In: Putnam FW, ed. The plasma proteins. 2nd ed. Vol. 1 New York: Academic Press, 1975;1: 265–315.
23. Jeppsson J, Laurell C, Franzen B. Agarose gel electrophoresis. Clin Chem 1979;25:629–638.
24. Messner R. Beta-2-Microglobulin: an old molecule assumes a new look. J Lab Clin Med 1984;104:141–145.
25. Durie B, Stock-Novack D, Salmon S, et al. Prognostic value of pretreatment serum beta-2-microglobulin in myeloma. Blood 1990;75(4):823–830.
26. Gotschlich E. C-Reactive Protein. Ann NY Acad Sci 1988;553: 9–15.
27. Harrison H, Levitt M. Serum protein electrophoresis: basis principles, interpretations, and practical considerations. ASCP Core Chemistry Check Sample Series. 1987;3(7):1–16.
28. McManamon T, Lott J. Serum protein electrophoresis. In: Kaplan L, Pesce A, eds. Clin chem 2nd ed. St. Louis: CV Mosby, 1989:1054–1057.
29. Aguzzi F, Jayakar S, Merlini G, Petrini C. Electrophoresis: cellulose acetate versus agarose gel, visual inspection versus densitometry. Clin Chem 1981;27:1944.

11 Diagnostic Enzymology

Alan H. B. Wu

Enzymes play a vital role in catalyzing the biochemical reactions necessary for normal human growth, maturation, and reproduction. Diagnostic enzymology involves the measurement of enzymes in body fluids for the diagnosis of disease. In most cases, serum or blood levels are the most useful, although urine, cerebrospinal, and extracellular fluid levels are sometimes important.

This chapter focuses on the analytical aspects and clinical significance of important enzymes that are measured for diagnostic purposes. The major emphasis is on the use of these enzymes for the diagnosis of cancer and of diseases involving the liver, myocardium, skeletal muscle, pancreas, prostate, and bone. In the case of myocardial infarction, non-enzyme markers such as myoglobin and troponin are also discussed.

BASIC CONCEPTS FOR DIAGNOSTIC ENZYMOLOGY

Pathologic Role of Enzymes in Blood

Most enzymes that are used for diagnostic purposes have no direct physiologic role in the blood. Their presence under normal circumstances is the result of natural aging and turnover of cells. Enzymes released into the blood are usually cleared from the circulation by metabolism within the reticuloendothelial system, although some are cleared by the kidneys (e.g., amylase). The normal level of activity of these enzymes in the serum is a function of the rate of release and clearance. The half-lives of these enzymes vary greatly from an estimated 2 hours for the BB isoenzyme of creatine kinase to 170 hours for placental alkaline phosphatase.

High levels of enzymes in the blood can indicate increased cellular turnover and tissue necrosis caused by disease. This was first demonstrated by LaDue et al. in 1954, when they observed that aspartate aminotransferase activity increased following acute myocardial infarction (1). In subsequent studies using carbon tetrachloride–induced liver injury in rats, these investigators showed that high serum enzyme levels were caused by leakage from the damaged hepatocytes. Once released from cells, enzymes can either pass directly into the blood (if the tissue is highly vascular and there is no obstruction to flow) or reach the bloodstream through slower lymphatic drainage. The subcellular origin plays a role in how readily an enzyme will appear in the blood. Soluble cytoplasmic enzymes pass through one set of membranes, while mitochondrial enzymes must also pass through a second set of membranes.

An equally important and largely overlooked cause of high enzyme levels in blood is tissue synthesis of new enzymes that occurs in response to disease, induction by various drugs, and carcinogenesis (2). For example, in obstructive liver disease, hepatic alkaline phosphatase is increased largely because of increased synthesis due to abnormal intracanalicular pressure. Phenobarbital and several other drugs induce microsomal enzyme production that leads to increased synthesis of γ-glutamyltransferase. Also, enzymes normally absent in serum can appear as the result of a neoplastic process.

Factors in Enzyme Assay Development

ENZYME KINETICS AND SUBSTRATE CONCENTRATION

Enzymes (E) are biological catalysts that combine with substrates (S) to form intermediate complexes (ES) leading to the formation of product (P) and restoration of the original enzyme (3). Reactions involving one substrate exhibit the following kinetics:

$$S + E \rightarrow [ES] \rightarrow P + E$$

Amylase and lipase are examples of enzymes of this scheme. But most other enzymes catalyze more complex reactions in which there are two or more substrates that form multiple products.

The reaction rate is a function of several factors, including substrate and enzyme concentration, temperature, pH, and the presence of cofactors, coenzymes, activators, and inhibitors. The rate equations for enzyme-catalyzed reactions were first developed by Michaelis and Menten in 1913 following the em-

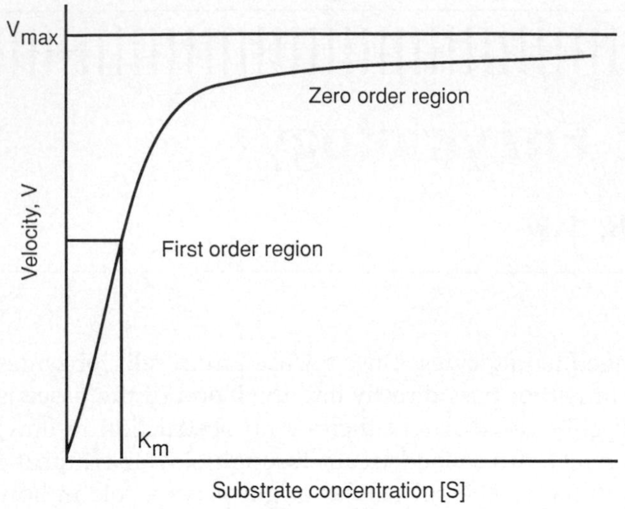

Figure 11.1. General form of the relation between substrate concentration and the velocity of an enzyme-catalyzed reaction. V_{max} denotes maximum velocity and K_m denotes the Michaelis-Menten constant (see text).

pirical observation that reaction velocity is proportional to substrate concentration at relatively low values (3). At high concentrations, the reaction rate is maximized. This behavior is shown in Figure 11.1. In the region where reaction velocity is directly proportional to substrate concentration, the reaction is termed first-order with respect to substrate. At high substrate concentration, the velocity is independent of substrate concentration, and the reaction is termed zero-order with respect to substrate. The Michaelis-Menten constant, K_m, is defined as the substrate concentration that corresponds to one-half the maximum reaction rate.

In diagnostic enzymology, the goal is the measurement of the activity or concentration of the enzyme itself. Therefore, test conditions are chosen such that the reaction rate will depend only on the amount of enzyme present in the sample to be measured. The substrate concentration should be in the zero-order region, and all other factors that influence the reaction rate should be optimized and controlled.

SELECTION OF OTHER REACTION CONDITIONS

Many parameters must be considered when developing a reagent formulation for measuring enzymes. Most enzymes operate optimally within a narrow pH range. Values above or below this range can inactivate enzymes by altering the tertiary structure of the active site or by denaturing the protein. The pH can also influence the direction of the reaction, such as for lactate dehydrogenase, for which the conversion of lactate to pyruvate is favored at alkaline pH, while the reverse reaction is favored at physiologic pH. The specific buffer chosen to maintain pH can also be important, as some buffers participate in the reaction and increase its rate. For example, for alkaline phosphatase, the reagent 2-amino-2-methyl-1-propanol acts both as a buffer and as a phosphate group acceptor.

Cofactors and coenzymes not present in the sample or supplied by the buffer must also be added to the reaction mixture to ensure optimum activity. Pyridoxal phosphate is a necessary coenzyme for both aspartate and alanine aminotransferase, while magnesium is a cofactor needed for alkaline phosphatase. Other substances that are needed to enhance activity are called activators and are also added to the reaction mixture. For example, *N*-acetyl cysteine is used to activate creatine kinase.

The temperature used for the reaction must be tightly controlled because reaction rates generally double with every 10°C that the temperature increases. High temperatures can denature many proteins and enzymes. By convention, most enzymes are assayed at 37°C. Although this choice is somewhat arbitrary, having a standard temperature facilitates the comparison of test results from one laboratory to another.

INHIBITORS

Inhibitors are substances that can decrease the rate of enzyme-catalyzed reaction. They interact with the enzyme in a number of ways. *Competitive* inhibitors compete with substrate for binding to the active site on the enzyme. The effect of a competitive inhibitor is to increase K_m while not affecting the maximum velocity, V_{max}. Increasing the substrate concentration counteracts the effect of a competitive inhibitor. *Noncompetitive* inhibitors decrease the reaction rate by interacting with the enzyme without directly affecting the enzyme-substrate binding. V_{max} is decreased with no effect on K_m. In this case, the effect cannot be counteracted by increasing the substrate concentration. *Uncompetitive* inhibitors interact with the enzyme-substrate complex, prohibiting the formation of product. Both V_{max} and K_m are altered.

Inhibitors play an important role in diagnostic enzymology. Inhibitors are used to selectively eliminate activity from specific isoenzymes, providing a means for detecting other isoenzymes. Tartrate, for example, is used to inhibit some acid phosphatase isoenzymes, while dibucaine is used to detect the presence of genetic variants of serum cholinesterase.

Enzyme Assay Procedures

Enzyme measurements have traditionally used kinetic assays to determine activity. Newer assays have been developed, however, that measure protein (mass) concentrations. Both types of assays are discussed in this section.

SINGLE-REAGENT KINETIC ASSAYS

Figure 11.2 illustrates a typical enzyme-catalyzed reaction for a single-reagent kinetic assay. The reaction is monitored at a wavelength at which the reaction product absorbs light. The initial lag phase is caused by the time necessary for the enzyme to be fully activated by cofactors and coenzymes added to the reagent. A delay of 30 to 120 seconds is usually necessary before absorbance readings become meaningful. After the lag phase, the reaction begins the linear phase, characterized by a constant rate of change in absorbance. The reaction is monitored by taking readings at regular intervals for 2 to 5 minutes after the lag phase.

If the reaction proceeds long enough, the substrate concentration becomes limiting, and the reaction enters a first-order phase. When the substrate is used up the reaction stops. Samples with very high enzyme activity can deplete the substrate even before the first analytical reading is taken. In this case, falsely low results may be obtained (Fig. 11.3A), and the sample may appear the same as one with little or no enzyme activity (Fig. 11.3B). Enzyme analyzers must be able to detect samples with high enzyme activity. As shown in Figure 11.3, a large difference in absorbance between the zero time point and the first reading may be used to detect the presence of a sample that has depleted the substrate. When this has occurred, the enzyme activity in these samples is obtained by dilution.

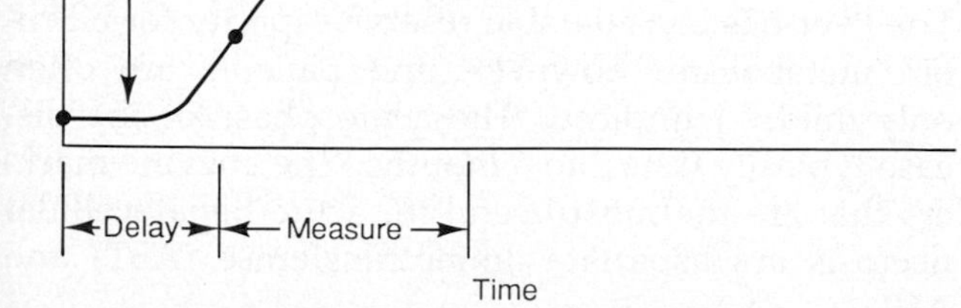

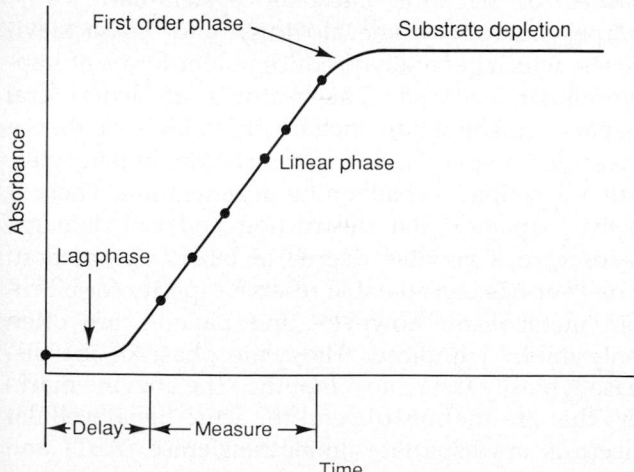

Figure 11.2. Absorbance versus time curve for a single-reagent assay system. The lag phase is the time necessary for activation of the enzyme. The linear phase (zero-order kinetics) is where the reaction rate is proportional to enzyme activity. The end of the first-order phase is where the substrate is depleted and the reaction ends.

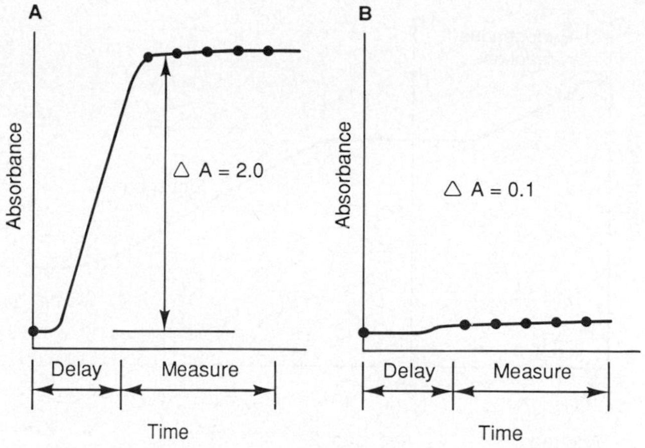

Figure 11.3. Absorbance versus time curves for samples with very high (**A**) and very low (**B**) enzyme activity. Since the measurement window is fixed, both samples appear to have low activity. Calculation of the difference in absorbance between the baseline and the first reading permits the distinction between samples with high enzyme activity (curve **A**) and those with low activity (curve **B**).

START REAGENT ACTIVITY ASSAYS

Certain enzyme assay designs require the sequential addition of two reagents. The first includes the serum sample, which contains all reagents except one of the substrates. Incubation of this reagent allows both for the activation of the enzyme and for substrate-independent side reactions to occur, which, when present, erroneously contribute to the apparent activity of the enzyme. The analytical reaction of interest is triggered by the addition of the substrate (sometimes termed the "start reagent") after an appropriate incubation period, usually 5 minutes. Figure 11.4 illustrates the reaction rate versus time profile for a start reagent assay. The analysis of alanine aminotransferase (ALT), for example, is improved by use of the start reagent system, because high concentrations of pyruvate (which may occur in some serum specimens) will produce an apparent consumption of NADH that is not dependent on ALT activity. Note that in Figure 11.4, absorbance is shown decreasing as the reaction proceeds, indicating that the rate of consumption of a reactant is being followed.

ENZYME ACTIVITY CALCULATIONS

Enzyme activity can be expressed in either units per liter or nanokatals per liter. An International Unit is defined as the amount of enzyme necessary to catalyze the conversion of one micromole of substrate per minute. The corresponding SI unit is the amount of enzyme that will catalyze the conversion of one nanomole of substrate per second (nanokatal). Because Beer's law states that concentration is proportional to absorbance, enzyme activity can be deter-

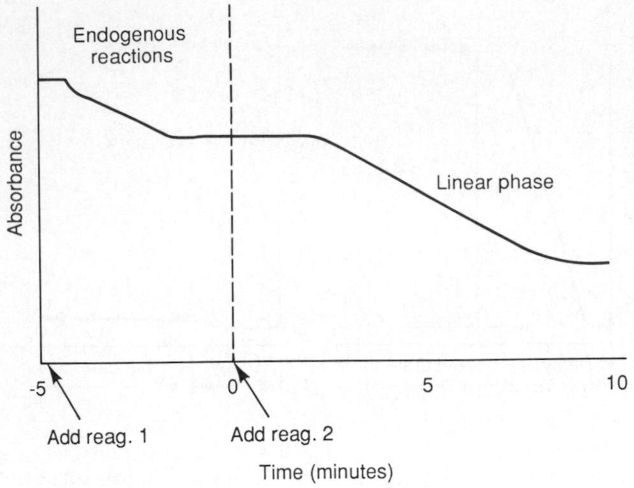

Figure 11.4. Absorbance versus time curve for the two-addition reagent assay system. The first reagent contains all reagents minus the substrate. The second reagent, the start or trigger reagent, initiates the reaction of interest, which is measured following a delay period.

mined from the change in absorbance per unit of time. The rate of change in absorbance is multiplied by factors to account for the molar absorptivity of the product or substrate that is being monitored, the cell path length, and the dilution of the sample by the reagents in the reaction mixture:

$$\text{activity (U/liter)} = \frac{\Delta A/\text{min} \times TV}{\epsilon \times b \times SV} \times 1000$$

where ΔA/min is the change in absorbance versus time,
TV = total volume (in μl),
SV = sample volume (in μl),
ϵ = micromolar absorptivity (in liters/millimol · cm),
and b = path length (in cm).

As an example, if an enzyme produces NADH (millimolar absorptivity = 6.3) with a ΔA/min of 0.046, and if the total and sample volumes are 300 and 5 μl, respectively, and a 1-cm pathlength is used, the activity (in U/L) is calculated as:

$$\text{activity} = \frac{0.046 \times 300}{6.3 \times 1 \times 5} \times 1000 = 438 \text{ U/liter}$$

MASS MEASUREMENTS

The development of immunoassays has permitted the measurement of enzyme concentration rather than activity. These assays are particularly useful for isoenzyme analysis, as antisera can be directed toward specific isoenzymes, isoforms, or subunits. Studies have shown that for the detection of diseases, enzymes do not need to be present in an active form in blood, and mass measurements are equivalent to enzyme activity assays in diagnostic efficiency and are sometimes preferred. The enzyme concentration is determined from a calibration curve. Mass measurements are also used to measure the concentration of protein markers (e.g., myoglobin) that do not possess enzymatic activities. Specific immunoassays for enzymes are discussed in more detail under specific examples.

LIVER DISEASES

The enzymes alanine and aspartate aminotransferase, alkaline phosphatase, lactate dehydrogenase, γ-glutamyltransferase, and 5′-nucleotidase are commonly measured for the assessment of liver function. The first four of these are typically included in comprehensive chemistry profiles. None of these markers is specific for any single liver disorder. This section covers liver dysfunction, describes individual liver enzymes and their laboratory measurement, and explains how patterns of liver enzyme data can be used to aid in the diagnosis of liver diseases.

Acute Hepatocellular Injury

VIRAL HEPATITIS

Acute viral hepatitis is a common cause of hepatocellular injury. The isolation and characterization of specific viral agents in recent years, coupled with the development of specific serologic markers, has resulted in the definitive diagnosis of these infections. A more complete description of the virology, etiology, epidemiology, and relevant serology of hepatitis types A, B, C, and D can be found in Chapter 54. Also described in this section are the other viral causes of hepatitis such as Epstein-Barr virus, herpesviruses, cytomegalovirus, and coxsackieviruses, which generally produce milder forms of hepatocellular necrosis. The features of acute viral hepatic inflammation include infiltration of monocytes and hyperplasia of parenchymal hepatocytes, often described as ballooning degeneration. There is active hepatocellular destruction and cell damage, leading to a variable degree of biliary obstruction. The liver has considerable reserve capacity for bilirubin metabolism, however, and patients are often only mildly jaundiced. The acute phase of the disease typically lasts 3 to 6 months. The enzyme markers that are the most useful for acute hepatocellular necrosis are aspartate aminotransferase (AST) and ALT.

ACUTE LIVER FAILURE

Acute liver failure is characterized by extensive hepatocellular necrosis and a very high mortality; it

Table 11.1. Causes of Toxic Hepatitis

Solvents	Carbon tetrachloride
	Trichloroethylene
Mushrooms	*Amanita phalloides*
Metals	Yellow phosphorus
Drugs	Acetaminophen
	Halothane
	Isoniazid
	Rifampicin
Metabolic	Reye's syndrome
	Wilson's disease
	Galactosemia
	α_1-Antitrypsin deficiency
	Liver metastasis

has a number of etiologies. One is the progression to fulminant hepatitis, most frequently seen with hepatitis B. Toxic hepatitis is also a major cause. Table 11.1 lists various substances that can produce acute liver failure. Clinical manifestations include metabolic dysfunctions such as encephalopathy and water and electrolyte imbalance, coagulation abnormalities, hypoglycemia, respiratory failure, and renal failure. As with hepatocellular disease, acute liver failure is characterized by large increases in serum AST and ALT.

Cholestatic Liver Diseases

Cholestasis is suppression of bile flow and can be either extrahepatic or intrahepatic in origin. Delineation between these types is not possible solely on the basis of enzyme testing, although certain patterns of enzyme activities favor one form over the other. Morphologically, the presence of bile pigments in hepatocytes defines this condition. Serum levels of liver enzymes and bilirubin are abnormal in cholestasis. Because of the reserve capacity of the liver for metabolism and excretion, however, these enzymes and salts increase in the serum only when more than 80% of the hepatocellular functional capacity has become impaired. Chapter 8 describes the role of conjugated and unconjugated bilirubin in cholestatic disease. Enzyme markers of obstruction include alkaline phosphatase, γ-glutamyltransferase, 5′-nucleotidase, and leucine aminopeptidase.

INTRAHEPATIC OBSTRUCTION

Intrahepatic cholestasis often results from cirrhosis or hepatitis, but administration of certain drugs such as chlorpromazine, estrogens, and anabolic steroids can also induce cholestasis. The mechanism may include the precipitation of bile salts which impairs the flow of bile. Idiopathic familial intrahepatic jaundice is also seen in the third trimester of some otherwise uncomplicated pregnancies. This condition is relatively benign but may recur in future pregnancies. Other congenital disorders associated with intrahepatic obstruction include Dubin-Johnson syndrome and Rotor's syndrome.

EXTRAHEPATIC OBSTRUCTION

Extrahepatic cholestasis is usually the result of mechanical obstruction of the common bile duct or hepatic duct. Common etiologies of this disorder include cholelithiasis and carcinoma of the tip of the pancreas, papilla of Vater, or common bile duct. These processes lead to dilatation of the ductal tree immediately above the obstruction. Inflammatory processes such as pancreatitis, and bile duct lesions seen in sclerosing cholangitis can also produce extrahepatic cholestasis.

Chronic Liver Diseases

CHRONIC HEPATITIS

Chronic hepatitis is a disease with diverse etiologies, including viral, autoimmune, and lupoid causes. In viral causes, some 5 to 10% of hepatitis B patients and up to 50% of hepatitis C patients develop this recurring disease. The active form is characterized by monocyte infiltration and hepatic necrosis. Chronic active hepatitis commonly leads to disruption of lobular architecture and fibrosis and can progress to liver cirrhosis. In contrast, chronic persistent hepatitis is a milder disorder that rarely progresses to cirrhosis and fibrosis. The liver enzyme results tend to be more elevated in the active form; however, differentiation is best made by performing a liver biopsy.

CIRRHOSIS

Chronic liver disease that leads to an increase in diffuse fibrosis and progression toward a nodular architecture defines cirrhosis. Some of the etiologic factors for cirrhosis are liver damage secondary to drug use, chronic hepatitis infections, biliary obstruction, and metabolic disease (such as Wilson's disease, hemochromatosis and α_1-antitrypsin deficiency). Alcoholic cirrhosis is very prevalent in the United States and western Europe, while cirrhosis due to chronic active hepatitis B infections is more common in Asia and Africa. Liver enzyme levels in cirrhosis are variably elevated, and can be normal during the terminal stages of the disease.

Primary biliary cirrhosis is characterized by impairment of bile excretion and has been linked to an autoimmune process. It affects women more often than men. Inflammation and destruction of bile ducts are observed in this disorder. Elevations in alkaline phosphatase and aminotransferases are expected along with high titers of antimitochondrial antibody.

LIVER CANCER

Primary hepatocellular and cholangiocellular carcinomas often occur in patients with longstanding hepatitis B infections and liver cirrhosis. The diagnosis is aided by computed tomography, ultrasound, nuclear scans, and α-fetoprotein levels in blood. Primary liver cancer is especially prevalent among Oriental and black African males. Metastatic liver disease is very common in the United States, particularly from tumors that originate in the colon, lung, breast, and skin. Enzyme levels in primary and secondary cancer are usually elevated; this is caused by the destruction of surrounding normal tissue and obstruction of normal architecture by these "space-occupying" tumors.

Enzymes Useful in Liver Disease

ALKALINE PHOSPHATASE (EC 3.1.3.1)

The phosphatases are a collection of sialoproteins located mostly within the cell membrane. They function to transport inorganic phosphate from donor to receptor molecules. Phosphatases with catalytic activity at a pH of 10.0 and higher make up the collection of alkaline phosphatase (ALP, orthophosphoric acid monoester phosphohydrolase).

Measurement of Total ALP Activity

Because of the heterogeneous nature of the enzyme, and because a single physiologic substrate has not been identified, all analytical methods for ALP make use of synthetic substrates. The most common substrate is *p*-nitrophenylphosphate (*p*-NPP), which is converted to *p*-nitrophenoxide (*p*-NP) and inorganic phosphate:

$$p\text{-NPP} + H_2O \xrightarrow{\text{ALP}} PO_4^{-3} + p\text{-nitrophenoxide}$$

Since *p*-NPP is colorless, the reaction is monitored by the increasing absorbance of *p*-NP at 404 nm. The pH of the reaction is controlled at 10.3 by 2-amino-2-methyl-1-propanol (AMP) buffer, which also acts as a phosphate acceptor to facilitate the phosphatase action of the enzyme. A magnesium salt is also part of the reagent formulation and acts as an activator of the enzyme. In other procedures, such as that recommended by the International Federation of Clinical Chemistry, zinc ions are added along with *N*-hydroxy-EDTA to maintain the precise ratio of Mg^{2+}/Zn^{2+} necessary for optimum activation. The millimolar absorptivity of *p*-NP is 18.75 liters/mmol·cm.

The reference range for alkaline phosphatase is dependent on age, and relates to different stages of bone growth and demineralization during life. Figure 11.5 illustrates this dependency. Children have higher reference ranges than adults, particularly during adolescence. Older populations have increasing alkaline phosphatase reference ranges, reflecting increases in the incidence of osteoporosis in this population.

ALP Isoenzymes

Alkaline phosphatase is widely distributed throughout the tissues of the body. Among those with the highest relative activity are the adrenals, placenta, gastrointestinal tract, bone, kidney, and liver. In normal nonpregnant adults, however, most of the serum ALP originates from the bone and liver. For patients with high ALP levels, measurement of alkaline phosphatase isoenzymes is useful for differentiating between bone and liver sources. However, because of technical difficulties with zonal electrophoresis and the increasing use of more specific enzyme markers for hepatic obstruction, such as γ-glutamyltransferase, the clinical need for ALP isoenzymes is rare, and most laboratories do not offer routine fractionation.

Analytical methods for ALP isoenzymes include selective chemical inhibition, such as with phenylalanine, heat inactivation, electrophoresis, and isoelectric focusing. Incubation of serum at 56°C for 15 minutes can provide an estimate of the ALP isoenzyme content. The placental isoenzyme and placental-like forms such as the Regan isoenzyme are very stable and will remain active following incubation at this temperature. The liver fraction will retain 25 to 50% of residual activity, while the bone fraction will be largely inactive after this incubation.

Zonal electrophoresis has been extensively studied and will produce bands for the (*a*) placental, (*b*) intestinal, and (*c*) bone, liver, and kidney fractions. There are varying degrees of overlapping between ALP isoenzymes from tissues of the last group, depending on the electrophoresis support medium. ALP isoenzymes from bone, liver, and kidney originate from a single gene expression that has been post-synthetically modified. Improvement in resolution between the bone and liver fractions is possible by treating either of the electrophoresis supports with wheat-germ lectin, or by treating the samples themselves with neuraminidase. Electrophoretic studies have also demonstrated a new isoenzyme fraction migrating anodic to the liver fraction. The isoenzyme, termed the "α" or fast liver fraction, is seen in hepatobiliary disorders and may be a useful marker for liver cancer.

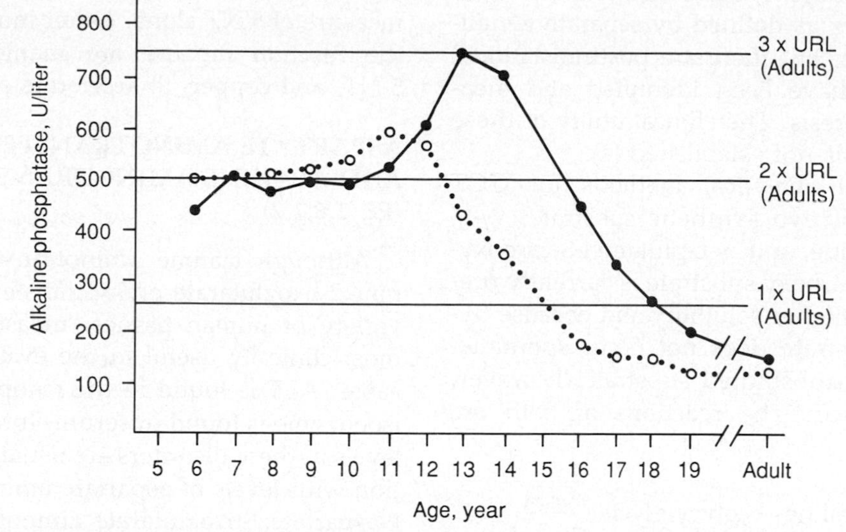

Figure 11.5. Plasma alkaline phosphatase activity as a function of age and sex (•–•, males; o–o females). Horizontal lines refer to multiples of the adult upper reference limit (URL). (From McComb RB, Bowers CN Jr, Posen S. Alkaline phosphatase. New York: Plenum Press, 1979:532.)

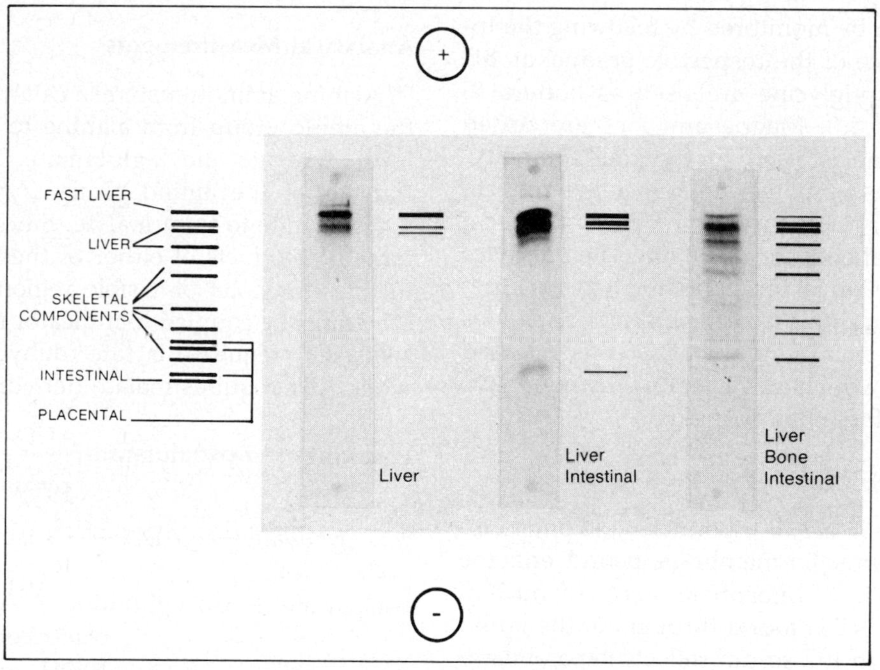

Figure 11.6. Isoenzyme fractions of alkaline phosphatase by isoelectric focusing. (Resolve-ALP, Isolab Inc., Akron, OH).

More definitive assessment of ALP isoenzymes is possible with isoelectric focusing (IEF). Figure 11.6 illustrates a commercially available alkaline phosphatase isoenzyme assay by IEF. At least 12 distinct ALP bands can be identified with pI's ranging from 3.01 for the fast liver fraction to 4.86 for the intestinal ALP. Prior to the development of this assay, routine use of isoelectric focusing has been largely limited to research applications because of the complexity of the analytical procedure.

γ-GLUTAMYLTRANSFERASE (EC 2.3.2.2)

γ-Glutamyltransferase (GGT, γ-glutamyl-peptide: amino acid γ-glutamyltransferase) catalyzes the transfer of γ-glutamyl groups between donor and acceptor molecules. GGT is located in the cell membrane of nearly all human cells and tissues, and functions to transport amino acids into the cell. GGT has two subunits: a light hydrophilic fraction, where the active site is located, and a heavy hydrophobic site, which anchors the enzyme to the membrane. It does not have isoenzymes as defined by separate genetically encoded forms, but there are posttranslational modifications that have been identified and measured by electrophoresis. The clinical utility of these isoforms, however, is not established (4).

Most commercial analytical methods for GGT make use of one of two synthetic substrates: γ-L-glutamyl-*p*-nitroanilide and γ-L-glutamyl-3-carboxy-4-nitroanilide. The carboxy substrate is currently preferred because of a higher solubility and because hydrolysis of the substrate does not occur spontaneously. The older unsubstituted substrate, however, is more widely used. The reactions of both are shown below:

$$\gamma\text{-glutamyl-}p\text{-nitroaniline} + \text{glycylglycine} \xrightarrow{\text{GGT}} \gamma\text{-glutamylglycylglycine} + p\text{-nitroaniline}$$

$$\gamma\text{-glutamyl-3-carboxy-4-nitroanilide} + \text{glycylglycine} \xrightarrow{\text{GGT}} p\text{-nitroaniline} + \text{5-amino-2-nitrobenzoate}$$

Either reaction can be monitored by following the increasing absorbance of the respective product at 405 nm. Tris and glycylglycine are used as buffers to maintain a pH of 8.0. Magnesium ions are added when γ-nitroaniline is used to facilitate solubility. The millimolar absorptivites are 9.9 liters/mmol•cm for *p*-nitroaniline at 405 nm and 7.9 liters/mmol•cm for 5-amino-2-nitrobenzoate at 410 nm. The reference ranges at 37°C are 9 to 50 for males and 8 to 40 U/liter for females. Although most of the enzyme originates from the liver, a small amount of GGT is released from the prostate, which may explain why men have slightly higher values than women.

5′-NUCLEOTIDASE (EC 3.1.3.5)

5′-Nucleotidase (5′NT, 5′-ribonucleotide phosphohydrolase) is a cytosolic membrane-bound enzyme that hydrolyzes the 5′-phosphate esters of nucleotides. Although 5′NT is found throughout the body, increased activity in the serum reflects hepatobiliary diseases. Methods for 5′NT analysis involve the use of adenosine-5′-monophosphate as a substrate:

$$\text{adenosine-5}'\text{-monophosphate} + H_2O \xrightarrow{5'\text{NT}} \text{adenosine} + \text{phosphate}$$

The reaction is monitored by measuring phosphate, using conventional methods. Because the substrate is also hydrolyzed by alkaline phosphatase in the serum sample, the total activity observed is the sum of 5′NT and ALP activities. The reaction is repeated with the addition of nickel ions, which selectively inhibit 5′NT, thus measuring only ALP activity. This number is then subtracted from the total to give a measure of 5′NT alone. Other inorganic ions used in the reaction mixture are manganese, to activate 5′NT, and copper, to accelerate color development.

ASPARTATE AMINOTRANSFERASE (EC 2.6.1.1) AND ALANINE AMINOTRANSFERASE (EC 2.6.1.2)

Although alanine aminotransferase (ALT, L-alanine:2-oxoglutarate aminotransferase) is found in a variety of human tissues, measurement of ALT is most clinically useful in the evaluation of liver diseases. ALT is found in the cytoplasm and only one isoenzyme is found in serum. Interpretations of ALT levels in these disorders are usually made in conjunction with levels of aspartate aminotransferase (AST, L-aspartate:2-oxoglutarate aminotransferase). Unlike ALT however, AST is also useful in the evaluation of acute myocardial infarction and skeletal muscle diseases. AST has cytosolic and mitochondrial isoenzymes that appear in the serum.

Analytical Measurements

Alanine aminotransferase catalyses the transfer of the amino group from alanine to α-ketoglutarate to form pyruvate and L-glutamate. AST catalyzes the transfer of the amino group from aspartate to α-ketoglutarate to form malate. Since none of the reactants or products of either of these reactions absorb in the ultraviolet or visible region of the spectrum, they must be coupled to indicator reactions for analysis. ALT requires lactate dehydrogenase (LDH), while AST requires malate dehydrogenase (MDH):

$$\text{L-alanine} + \alpha\text{-oxoglutarate} \xrightarrow{\text{ALT}} \text{pyruvate} + \text{L-glutamate}$$

$$\text{pyruvate} + \text{NADH} \xrightarrow{\text{LDH}} \text{lactate} + \text{NAD}^+$$

$$\text{L-aspartate} + \alpha\text{-oxoglutarate} \xrightarrow{\text{AST}} \text{oxaloacetate} + \text{L-glutamate}$$

$$\text{oxaloacetate} + \text{NADH} \xrightarrow{\text{MDH}} \text{L-malate} + \text{NAD}^+$$

The reactions are monitored by following the decrease in the absorbance at 340 nm as NADH is consumed in the reaction. Pyridoxal-5′-phosphate (P5′P) is needed as a coenzyme for both the ALT and AST reactions. Normally, serum contains adequate amounts of P5′P and additional coenzyme is not necessary. However, patients with a vitamin B_6 deficiency or those undergoing renal dialysis have decreased P5′P concentration, which will produce falsely low serum aminotransferase levels unless P5′P is added to the reagent formulation.

Table 11.2. Markers for Liver Function and Disease

Disease or Function	Markers
Functional evaluation	
Normal synthesis capacity	Albumin, retinol binding protein, prealbumin, prothrombin time, cholinesterase
Excretory function	Bilirubin, bile acids, rose bengal and sulfobromophthalein excretion
Metabolic function	Ammonia, amino acids, lipids, serum protein electrophoresis, globulins
Drug metabolism	Antipyrine breath and clearance test $^{14}CO_2$ breath test
Pathologic evaluation	
Hepatocellular injury	AST, ALT, LDH
Obstruction	Bilirubin, ALP, GGT, 5′NT, bile acids
Infections	Viral and autoimmune serologies
Malignancies	CEA, α-fetoprotein

Reference Ranges

The adult reference range for both AST and ALT is roughly 10 to 40 U/liter when measured at 37°C. Although males have slightly higher values than females, most laboratories use a single range for both sexes.

Aspartate Aminotransferase Isoenzymes

The major AST activity in serum is due to the cytosolic isoenzyme. Studies of patients with acute myocardial infarction have shown that mitochondrial AST (mAST) is more slowly released into the circulation than the cytosolic form, presumably because it has to pass through two sets of membranes. Measurement of mAST may be most useful in the diagnosis of chronic alcoholism. Although it is not in routine use in clinical laboratories, mitochondrial AST can be measured by electrophoresis and by selective immunoprecipitation techniques.

Patterns of Liver Enzymes for Interpretation of Disease

Unlike some disorders such as acute pancreatitis and myocardial infarction, for which there are enzyme markers that are primarily used for one disorder and have high diagnostic efficiencies, there are no enzyme markers that are specific for any single liver disease. When evaluating these disorders, therefore, it is appropriate to consider a panel of markers, sometimes called liver function tests (LFTs). Through common usage, this term has come to mean a group of tests that usually includes bilirubin, AST, ALT, ALP, and sometimes GGT and 5′NT. However, the term is a misnomer, because while these tests can reflect various disease processes in the liver, they do not reflect hepatic reserve for synthesis and metabolic functions. Table 11.2 lists some markers for both liver function and disease.

HEPATOCELLULAR VERSUS OBSTRUCTIVE LIVER DISEASES

Acute Injury

The most useful enzyme markers of acute hepatocellular injury are ALT and AST. Other markers—such as lactate, glutamate, isocitrate, and malate dehydrogenases—do exhibit elevations secondary to hepatocellular necrosis, but they are neither as sensitive nor as specific as the combination of AST and ALT and are therefore rarely used for diagnostic purposes.

The highest absolute levels of ALT and AST are seen following acute hepatitis, either viral or toxic. Values exceeding 1000 U/liter are commonly seen during the early phases of these diseases. In toxic hepatitis, such as with acetaminophen overdoses, levels of ALT and AST rise within a few hours after exposure and remain high for many days or weeks. Unfortunately, the extent of ALT and AST elevations do not reflect the severity of the disease, nor can they be correlated to patient prognosis. In acute hepatitis A, ALT is one of the first markers to be elevated, usually 3 to 4 weeks after infection. Levels return to normal within 8 to 12 weeks. In acute hepatitis B, the preclinical incubation phase is longer and ALT and AST may remain normal for 2 to 6 months. In acute hepatitis B, ALT and AST return to normal within 2 to 3 months, and a similar course is observed in hepatitis C. In chronic active hepatitis, enzyme levels are elevated 5 to 10 fold, depending on the stage of the disease. Similar elevations are also seen in acute hepatocellular injury secondary to mononucleosis. In end-stage liver disease, enzyme levels return to normal or subnormal levels as hepatocytes become depleted of enzyme content.

In contrast, levels of ALP, GGT, and 5′NT are not as markedly elevated in these disorders. Levels of these enzymes generally do not exceed 2 to 3 times the upper limit of normal. Therefore, a disproportionate increase in ALT and AST relative to ALP and GGT favors a diagnosis of hepatocellular necrosis rather than liver obstruction. The relationship of these enzymes in hepatocellular liver disease is summarized in Figure 11.7 (5).

Cholestasis

The best markers for intrahepatic and extrahepatic cholestasis are ALP, GGT, and 5′NT. The largest elevations (4 to 10 fold) of ALP are typically seen in obstruction due to gallstones or malignancy, and in biliary cirrhosis. The source of ALP in malignancy may

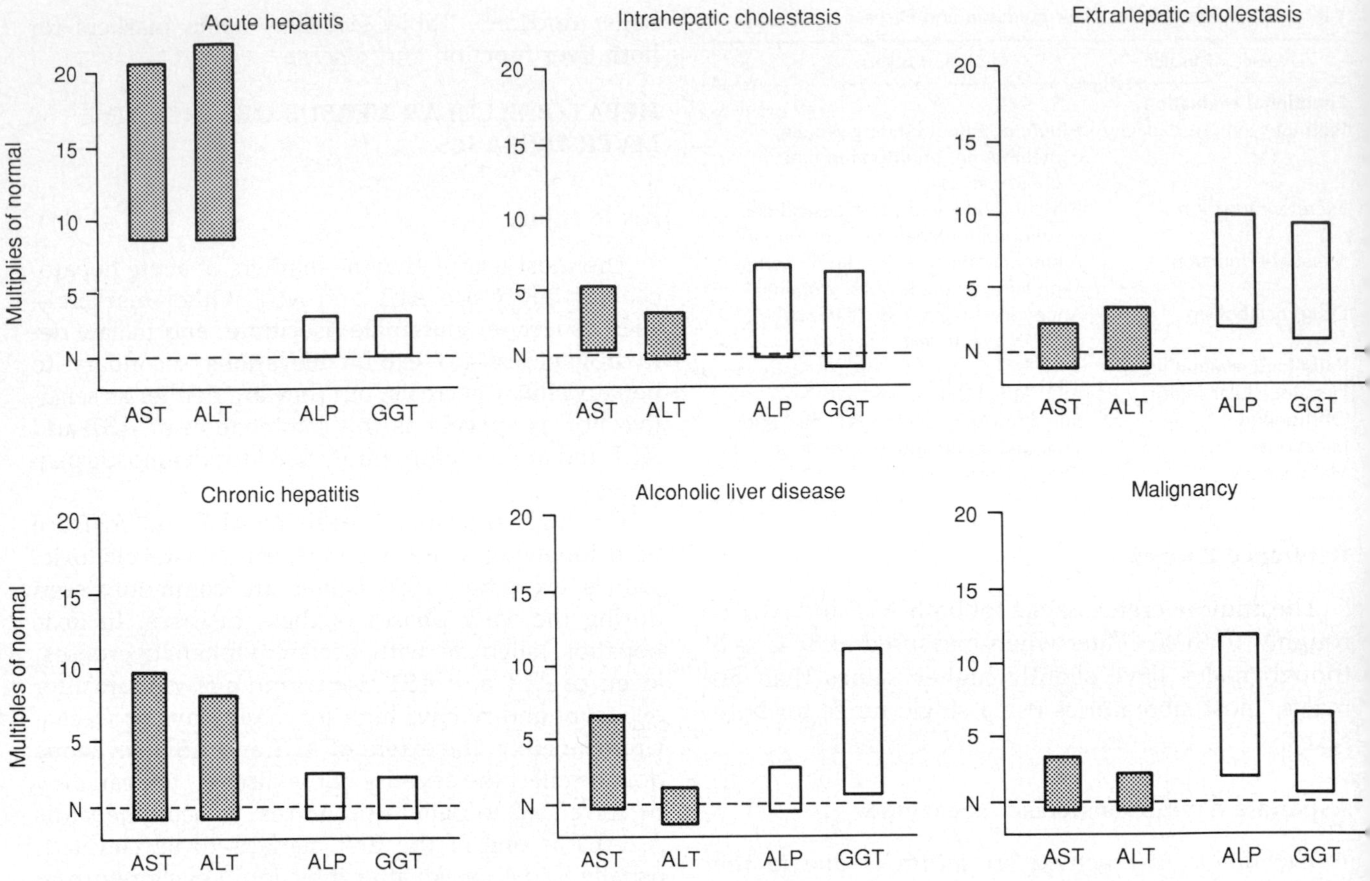

Figure 11.7. Relationship of ALT and AST to ALP and GGT in a variety of liver diseases. (Adapted from Zimmerman HJ. Function and integrity of the liver. In: Henry JB, ed. Clinical diagnosis and management. 17th ed. Philadelphia: WB Saunders, 1984.)

be obstruction of hepatic architecture in either primary or secondary liver cancers but other causes of ALP elevations must be ruled out (see Osseous Alkaline Phosphatase, below). Obstructive liver disease as a cause of ALP elevations can be confirmed by measurement of either GGT or 5′NT. Increases in these enzymes are also expected in cholestasis, but these assays are more specific because, while bone disease can produce elevations of ALP in the same range expected for obstructive liver disease, GGT and 5′NT are not found in the bone. Measurement of total and direct bilirubin are also important in making the diagnosis of obstructive jaundice.

Cholestasis can be readily distinguished from hepatocellular injury on the basis of a disproportionate increase of ALP and GGT relative to AST and ALT (Fig. 11.7). The latter two enzymes are generally only slightly elevated in cholestasis, rarely more than 500 U/liter.

THE DE RITIS RATIO (AST/ALT)

Further differentiation of specific liver diseases is aided by calculating the ratio of AST to ALT levels (6). Although there is considerable overlapping of values within a given diagnosis, the de Ritis ratio can give a general indication of whether a disorder is acute or chronic, and whether it is intrahepatic or extrahepatic in origin. Values for these ratios are most useful when standard AST and ALT assays are used. When using the assays recommended by the International Federation of Clinical Chemistry, the de Ritis ratio is normally about 1.15. Figure 11.8 illustrates results of the de Ritis ratio from patients with a variety of liver diseases.

Acute versus Chronic Liver Diseases

Acute disorders of the liver, such as acute viral hepatitis and infectious mononucleosis, generally have higher values of ALT relative to AST, and the de Ritis ratio is less than 1.0. In Reye's syndrome, in which there is an acute onset of encephalopathy, the de Ritis ratio is also less than 1 in most cases. It has been postulated that elevations in ALT are seen before elevations in AST in acute liver processes because AST includes mitochondrial isoenzymes, and more time is needed for these enzymes to pass through a second set of membranes to reach the circulation. Indeed, chronic disorders such as alcoholic liver disease, postnecrotic cirrhosis, and chronic active hepatitis have de Ritis ratios that are greater than

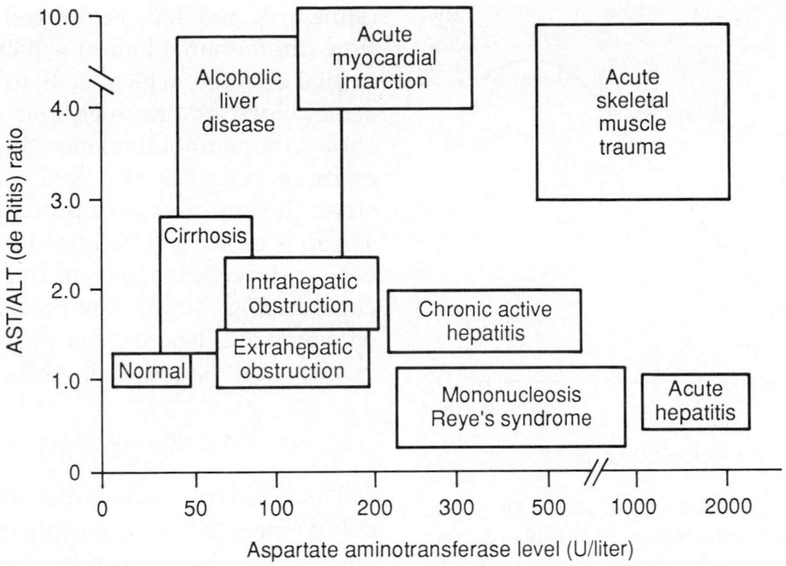

Figure 11.8. Ratio of AST:ALT versus aspartate aminotransferase levels in various liver diseases.

1. Although this is a convenient way of remembering this relationship, the mitochondrial fraction of AST actually contributes only a small percentage of the total AST and is insufficient to significantly lower the de Ritis ratio (Fig. 11.8). Patients with chronic persistent hepatitis will have a normal or slightly elevated aminotransferase level, reflecting the mild clinical course of this disease.

Intrahepatic versus Extrahepatic Obstruction

The de Ritis ratio may be helpful in differentiating between intrahepatic and extrahepatic cholestasis (Fig. 11.8). Ratios of 1.5 or greater suggest intrahepatic cholestasis, while values less than 1.5 suggest an extrahepatic process. This difference is also consistent with the notion of acute versus chronic liver disorders. Extrahepatic obstruction is often caused by the acute passage of a stone, whereas intrahepatic causes such as biliary cirrhosis and malignancy develop over a period of time. Other laboratory test results such as high conjugated bilirubin (above 75%), high amylase, and the presence of occult blood in the stool favor extrahepatic rather than intrahepatic obstruction. In addition, alkaline phosphatase is more often elevated in extrahepatic than in intrahepatic obstruction.

Alcoholic Liver Disease

Disproportionate increases of AST relative to ALT are observed in alcoholic liver disease, and the de Ritis ratio can exceed 6.0 (Fig. 11.8). Decreased levels of ALT relative to AST are caused in part by deficiencies of dietary pyridoxal phosphate in alcoholics, a component that is more important for normal hepatic ALT synthesis than for AST. Other markers of alcoholism include GGT and mAST. GGT is highly sensitive to recent alcohol intake, in part because ethanol is a potent inducer of GGT synthesis by the microsomal P-450 enzyme system. Significant elevations of GGT are also observed following prolonged drinking episodes of several months or more. Recent data suggest that mitochondrial AST may be a more powerful discriminator for chronic alcoholism than GGT (7). High levels of mAST in the absence of other causes of liver disease indicate repeated ethanol abuse.

Muscle Disease

The largest increases of AST relative to ALT are seen in myocardial and skeletal muscle diseases, because of the different distribution of the enzymes in these tissues. A ratio greater than 10 can be seen in these disorders (Fig. 11.8), which are discussed more fully in the following section.

MYOCARDIAL AND SKELETAL MUSCLE DISEASES

Unstable Angina and Acute Myocardial Infarction

The development of acute myocardial infarction (AMI) is the result of a sequence of events that takes place over many years. The process begins with atherosclerosis, which is characterized by the narrowing of coronary arteries by plaque formation. The syndrome that immediately precedes an AMI is unstable angina, which occurs when there is disruption of lipid-filled atherosclerotic plaques. This produces chest pain at rest and formation of a thrombotic clot.

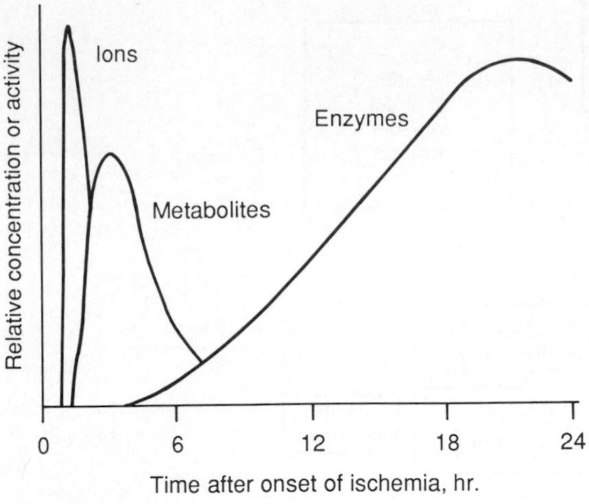

Figure 11.9. Release of ions, metabolites, and proteins after acute myocardial infarction. (Adapted from Hearse DJ. Cellular damage during myocardial ischaemia: metabolic changes leading to enzyme leakage. In: Hearse DJ. Enzymes in cardiology. Diagnosis and research. New York: John Wiley, 1979.)

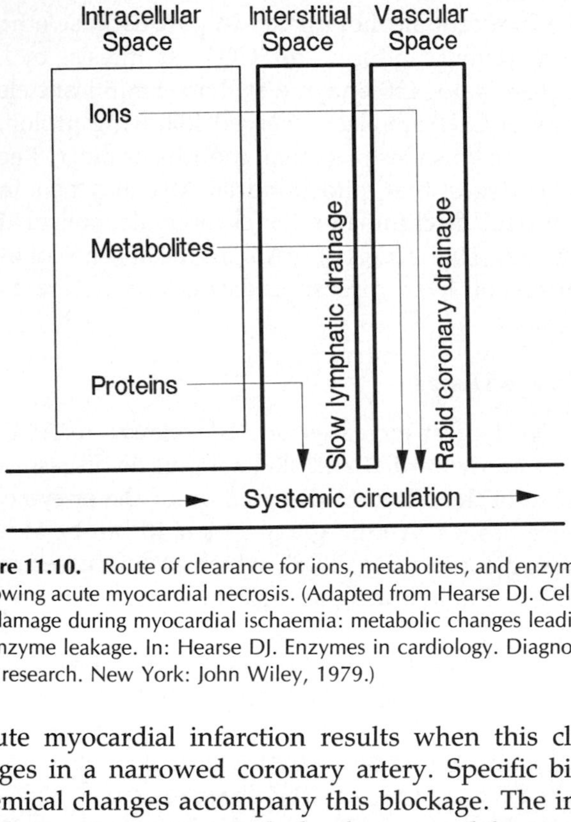

Figure 11.10. Route of clearance for ions, metabolites, and enzymes following acute myocardial necrosis. (Adapted from Hearse DJ. Cellular damage during myocardial ischaemia: metabolic changes leading to enzyme leakage. In: Hearse DJ. Enzymes in cardiology. Diagnosis and research. New York: John Wiley, 1979.)

Acute myocardial infarction results when this clot lodges in a narrowed coronary artery. Specific biochemical changes accompany this blockage. The immediate consequence is lack of oxygen delivery to the myocardium and tissue anoxia. This leads to an energy deficit and a shift toward anaerobic metabolism. Electrolytes are released into the interstitial space as the result of ATP-dependent ion pump failure. If coronary circulation is restored before the onset of irreversible damage, either spontaneously or by therapeutic intervention, jeopardized myocardial tissue may be salvaged and substantial irreversible damage is avoided. Prolonged deprivation of blood flow (more than 4 hours) will cause irreversible myocardial damage, which leads to leakage of macromolecules such as enzymes and proteins. Figure 11.9 shows the temporal relationship between the release of these materials as a function of disease progression. The appearance of proteins and enzymes in the serum is prolonged because this clearance is dependent on slow drainage from the cardiac lymphatic circulation (Fig. 11.10). The presence of cardiac-specific enzymes and isoenzymes provides the basis for the biochemical diagnosis of AMI (8).

Congestive Heart Failure

Heart failure results when the myocardium is unable to meet the blood supply demands of the tissues and organs. Failure can be classified as either acute or chronic. Primary acute failure can be caused by massive AMI or valve rupture. Chronic congestive heart failure (CHF) is seen in cardiomyopathies and valve disease. Factors that can precipitate CHF include infections, hypertension, endocarditis and myocarditis, arrhythmias, and pulmonary embolism. Physical exertion, emotional stress, and increased blood volume secondary to excessive sodium intake or discontinuation of diuretics can also cause CHF. Serum enzyme measurements are important in the evaluation of changes in myocardial and liver status as a result of heart failure.

Skeletal Muscle Disorders

Evidence of high creatine kinase activity in the serum is useful for the diagnosis and evaluation of both acute and chronic skeletal muscle diseases. Acute release of muscle enzymes occurs in surgery, trauma, crush injuries, excessive muscular contractions (as in long-distance running or uncontrolled convulsions), hyperthermia, viral myositis, and exposure to toxins. Chronic progressive muscular fiber dystrophies include Duchenne's, Becker's, limb-girdle, and myotonic dystrophy. These genetic disorders generally affect young children. Inflammatory disorders of skeletal muscle include dermatomyositis and polymyositis, which are also associated with progressive muscle weakness. Neurogenic disorders of the lower motor neurons include amyotropic lateral sclerosis and spinal muscular atrophies, while myasthenia gravis is caused by a disorder at the neuromuscular junction. The measurement of enzymes and isoenzymes is useful in the diagnosis of muscle disorders and, in the case of Duchenne's muscular dystrophy, for detection of the carrier state in women (9).

Enzymes and Proteins Useful in Myocardial Disease

CREATINE KINASE (EC 2.7.3.2)

The mitochondrial isoenzyme of creatine kinase (CK, ATP:creatine *N*-phosphotransferase) functions in muscle cells to catalyze the transfer of a high-energy phosphate bond from ATP to creatine to form creatine phosphate. During active muscle contractions, cytoplasmic CK catalyzes the reverse reaction, thereby providing myocytes an immediate source of ATP. Cytoplasmic CK consists of dimeric combinations of two subunits, M and B. This enables three possible isoenzymes, MM, MB, and BB. In addition, posttranslational modifications of isoenzymes will produce three MM and two MB isoforms. Each of these forms has a combined molecular weight of about 80 kd.

Measurement of Total CK Activity

Nearly all analytical methods for total creatine kinase enzyme activity make use of the formulation involving creatine phosphate and ADP. The product of the reverse reaction, ATP, is coupled with hexokinase and glucose-6-phosphate dehydrogenase (G+6+PD) to form NADH:

$$\text{creatine phosphate} + \text{ADP} \xrightarrow{\text{CK}} \text{creatine} + \text{ATP}$$

$$\text{ATP} + \text{glucose} \xrightarrow{\text{hexokinase}} \text{glucose-6-phosphate} + \text{ADP}$$

$$\text{glucose-6-phosphate} + \text{NAD}^+ \xrightarrow{\text{G6PD}} \text{6-phosphogluconate} + \text{NADH} + \text{H}^+$$

The reaction is monitored by the increase in absorbance of NADH measured at 340 nm. A lag phase of 90 to 120 seconds is required for CK before a linear reaction rate is initiated. The pH of the reaction is maintained at 7.0 with imidazole buffer. *N*-Acetylcysteine is added as an activator to maintain a supply of reduced sulfhydryl groups necessary for the complete activation of CK. The presence of adenylate kinase (AK) in the serum will produce a positive interference in this assay. AK catalyzes the production of ATP from ADP alone, which will falsely increase the apparent CK activity:

$$2\ \text{ADP} \xrightarrow{\text{AK}} \text{ATP} + \text{AMP}$$

Adenylate kinase originates from skeletal muscle, red cells, liver and kidney. Most commercial assay systems utilize adenosine monophosphate and diadenosine pentaphosphate to inhibit AK activity. Alternatively, a blank can be used by measuring AK

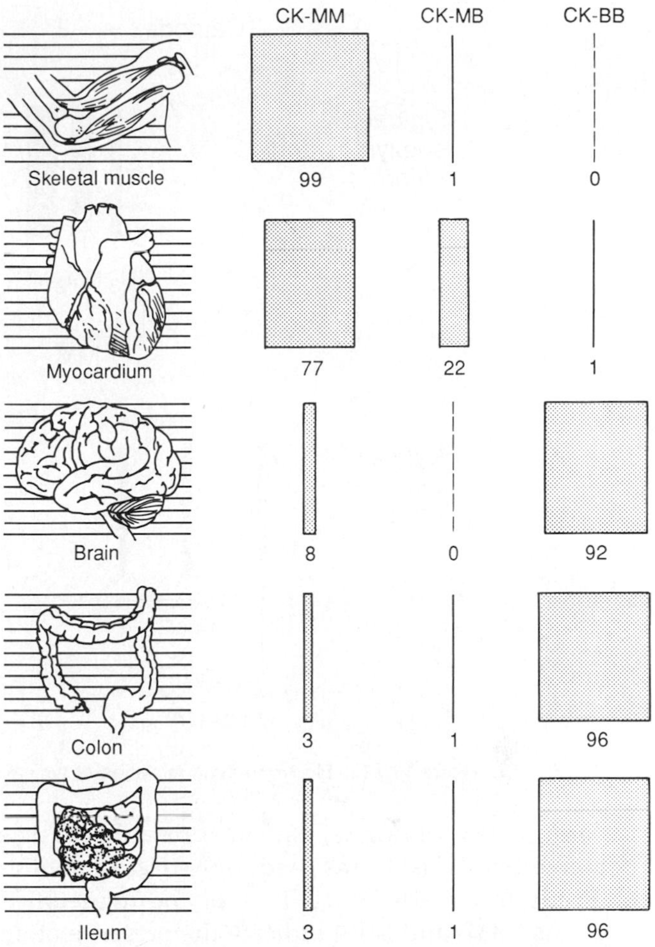

Figure 11.11. Tissue distribution of CK isoenzymes. (Adapted from Lott JA, Wolf PL. Clinical enzymology. A case-oriented approach. New York: Year Book, 1986.)

activity with creatine phosphate omitted. The reference range at 37°C for total CK is 38 to 174 U/liter for adult males and 96 to 140 U/liter for adult females.

CK Isoenzymes, Isoforms, and Variants

Isoenzyme Tissue Distribution. The clinical utility of CK isoenzyme measurements stems from the fact that skeletal and myocardial muscle tissue have different distributions of CK isoenzymes. As shown in Figure 11.11, CK-MM is the predominant isoenzyme in both tissues (10), but in skeletal muscle, only trace levels of CK-MB are present. In contrast, the myocardium contains a much higher percentage of CK-MB. CK-BB is found throughout the brain and smooth muscle.

CK Isoforms. Examination of human muscle tissue isoenzymes reveals the presence of single pure gene products for CK-MM and MB. However, when released from the tissues these enzymes are slowly converted to multiple CK isoforms (MM_1, MM_2, and MB_1) through the successive cleavage of the C-terminal amino acids by serum carboxypeptidase. The

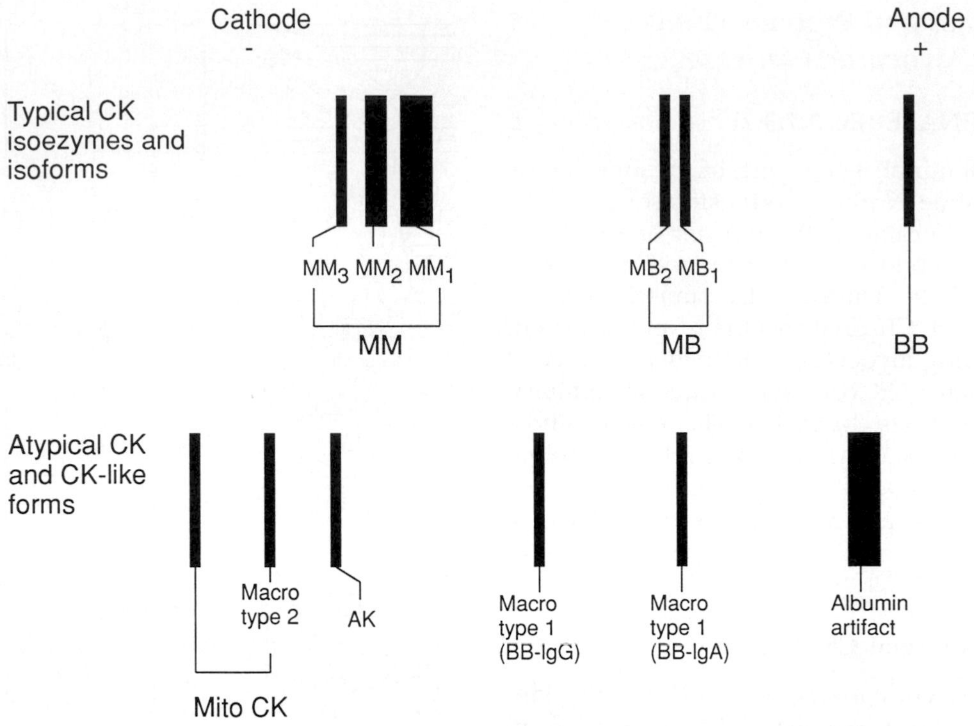

Figure 11.12. Electrophoretic migration of typical and atypical isoenzymes and isoforms of creatine kinase.

isoform pattern of normal patients primarily consists of converted CK isoforms, with only trace quantities of tissue forms. High activities of the unmodified isoforms (MM_3 and MB_2) indicate the presence of an acute process.

CK Variants. Besides the CK isoenzymes and isoforms that are present in normal sera, two atypical isoenzymes have been identified in about 2% of hospitalized patients. Macro CK type 1 has been identified to be CK-BB linked with an immunoglobulin. The IgG form migrates between CK-MM and MG by electrophoresis, while the IgA form migrates with MB. Macro CK type 2 is a polymeric aggregate of mitochondrial CK. Macro CK type 1 had no clinical significance, while type 2 is seen in metastatic cancer. Assays such as immunoinhibition and electrophoresis (especially with the type 1 IgA form) will produce false-positive results for CK-MB in the presence of macro CK.

Analytical Measurements. There are several analytical methods currently in use for CK isoenzyme analysis, including ion-exchange chromatography, electrophoresis, immunoinhibition, radioimmunoassay, and enzyme immunoassay (11). The column chromatographic method is not extensively used any longer except in the automated DuPont ACA method.

Electrophoresis for isoenzymes and isoforms is widely used. Isoenzymes are resolved on agarose gel following electrophoresis at 100 V for 20 minutes. Bands are observed fluorometrically after incubating the gels with CK reagents. The CK activity attributed to each band can be determined by scanning densitometry. Figure 11.12 illustrates the electrophoretic migration of CK isoenzymes, isoforms, and all known CK variants. Most normal samples will exhibit a single band due to CK-MM. Patients with acute myocardial infarction will have high concentrations of CK-MM and MB. Increasing the electrophoresis time or the applied voltage permits the resolution and analysis of CK isoforms. Figure 11.13 illustrates the major CK-MM and MB isoforms. Electrophoresis is less sensitive than immunoassay methods, yet it has remained popular because it permits visualization of all CK isoenzymes, and because of the development of automated electrophoresis instrumentation.

In the immunoinhibition method, serum is analyzed for CK after the addition of specific antibodies. The technique, illustrated in Figure 11.14, involves inhibiting CK-M subunit activity with anti-M antibodies and measuring the residual B-subunit activity. If CK-BB and atypical CK forms are absent, the MB content of the sample can be determined by multiplying the B-subunit activity by 2. However, if CK-BB or macro CK is present, an usually high percentage of CK-MB/total CK will occur and the analysis should be confirmed by a more specific CK-MB assay. The immunoinhibition technique is very useful for screening, because it is inexpensive and can be linked to automated chemistry analyzers.

The latest class of analytical methods for CK-MB are nonisotopic immunoassays, which measure enzyme concentration instead of enzyme activity. All commercial immunoassays make use of a two-site sandwich technique. The first antibody recognizes a particular determinant on the CK-MB molecule and is linked to a solid phase such as a tube, bead, magnetic particle, or fibrous surface. Monoclonal antibodies to CK-MB have been used to capture MB from the sample in this first step. The second antibody recognizes a different MB determinant and is conjugated to a label, such as an enzyme, fluorophore, or chemoluminescent tag. The concentration of CK-MB from the sample is determined from a standard curve. Figure 11.15 illustrates the Dade Stratus II method as one example. Immunoassays are very sensitive and rapid. Improvements in analytical precision and clinical performance have been reported over enzyme-activity assays, particularly when total CK levels are low.

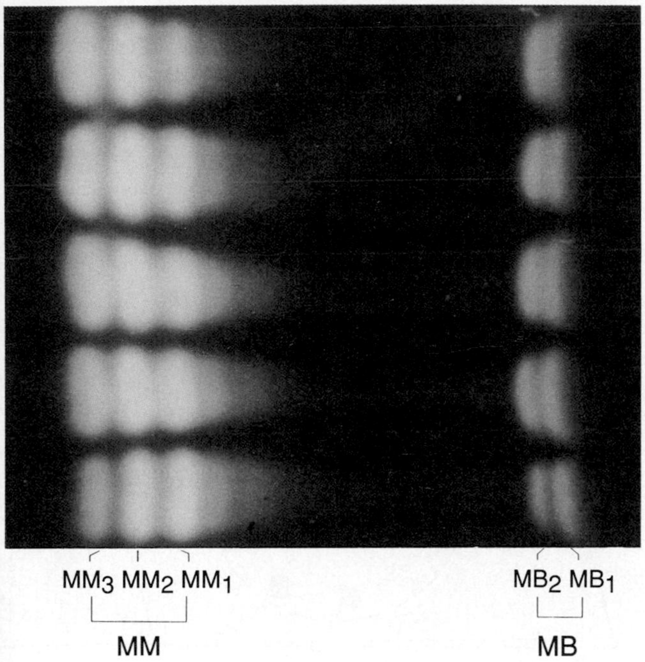

Figure 11.13. CK isoforms as measured by agarose electrophoresis. (CK-isoforms, Helena Labs., Beaumont, TX.)

Reference Values. Reference values for CK-MB are dependent on the analytical method used and are often expressed as a fraction of total CK activity. Reference values from a healthy population should not be used as decision limits for the diagnosis of AMI however, because there would not be adequate discrimination between the AMI and non-AMI patient (e.g., unstable angina). Cutoff values for electrophoresis and immunoinhibition are usually set around 5% of total CK or 10 U/liter. For immunoassays, decision limits are expressed in mass quantities and are approximately 5 to 10 ng/ml. CK-BB is normally absent in adult serum. CK-MB and CK-BB levels are higher in children but there are no established reference ranges, as CK isoenzyme analysis is not usually performed for this population.

There are two ways by which CK-MB results can be expressed: absolute activity (U/liter) or mass concentration (ng/ml), and a percentage of total CK (relative index). The relative index is defined as:

$$\text{relative index: } \frac{\text{CK-MB (activity or mass)}}{\text{total CK (activity)}} \times 100$$

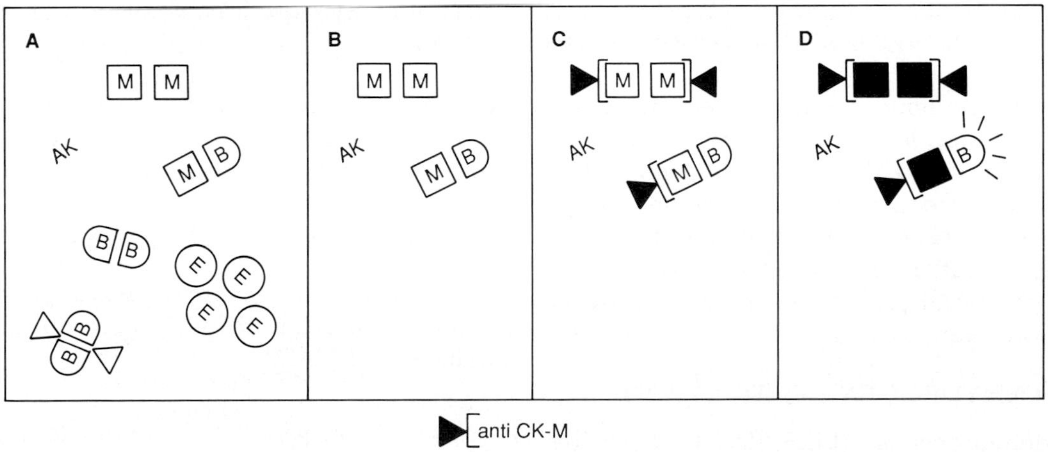

Figure 11.14. The immunoinhibition technique for CK-B. **A**, Normal and atypical isoenzymes of CK and adenylate kinase. **B**, Only CK-MM, MB, and adenylate kinase are assumed to be present. **C**, Addition of anti-CK-M antibodies. **D**, Measurement of residual B-subunit activity after M-subunit inactivation (*blackened symbols*). Inhibitors to adenylate kinase minimize the contribution of this interferant. The CK-MB activity is calculated by multiplying the residual activity by 2. (Reproduced with permission from Wu AHB. Clinical chemistry. Bethesda, MD: Health Education Resources, 1991.)

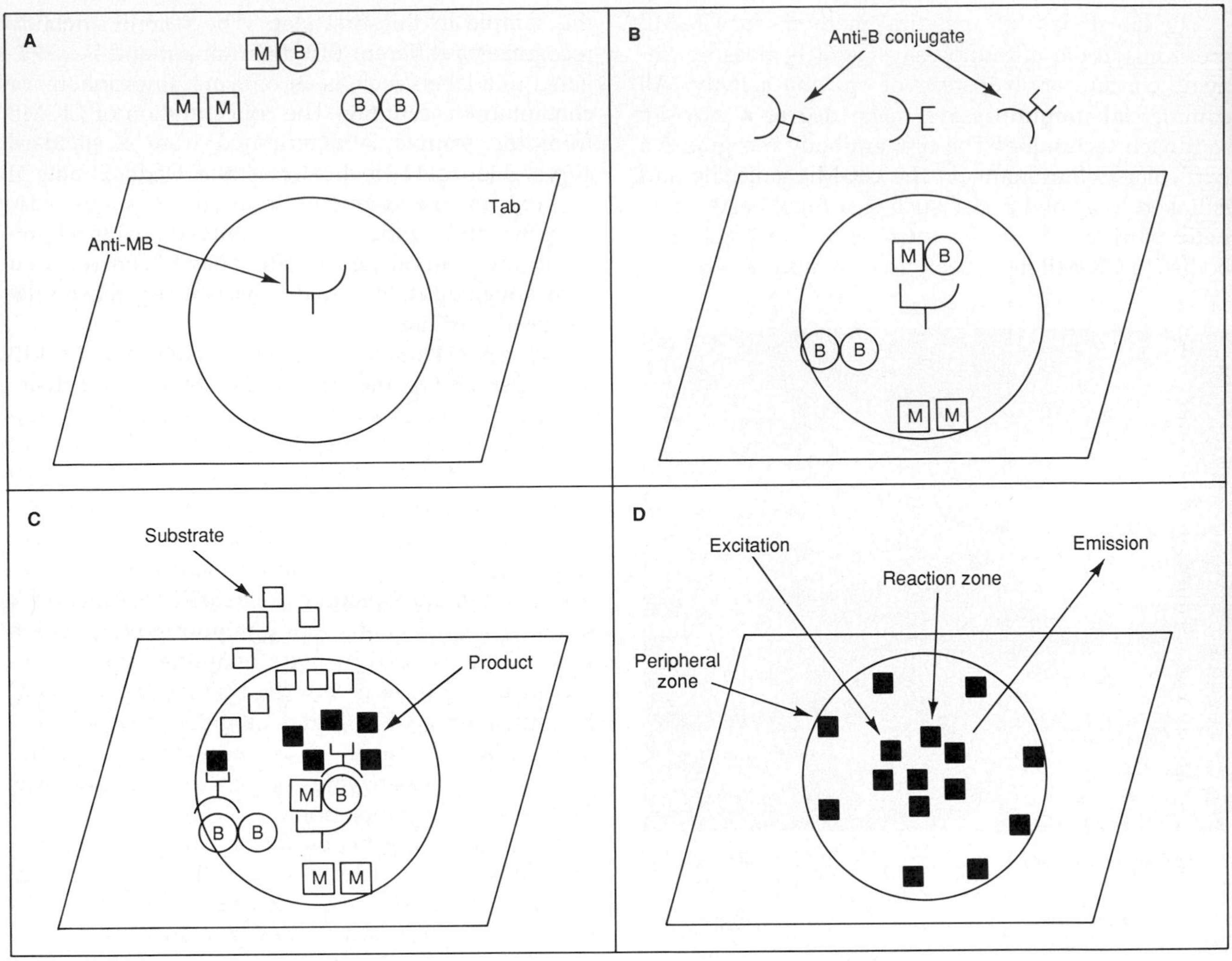

Figure 11.15. Radial partition immunoassay for CK-MB. **A**, A serum sample with CK isoenzymes is added to the center of a tab containing anti-CK-MB antibodies linked to glass fiber paper. The MB isoenzyme becomes immobilized. **B**, Anti-CK-B antibodies linked to alkaline phosphatase are added. These bind both to the immobilized CK-MB isoenzymes and to BB. **C**, Substrate to ALP is added to the center of the tab to produce a fluorescent product. CK-MM and BB are not bound to anti-MB and are washed outward from the reaction zone. **D**, The fluorescence intensity is proportional to [MB] measured at the center of the front surface of the tab. The fluorescence of conjugate (of CK-BB) migrating outward from the periphery of the reaction zone is not measured.

As a rule, absolute limits are most useful when the total CK is low (e.g., less than 1000 U/liter). Because CK-MB is found in skeletal muscles, however, CK-MB levels will exceed absolute reference limits in patients with severe skeletal muscle injury or disease. In this case, a relative limit (CK-MB expressed as a percentage of total CK) is more useful when the total exceeds 1000 U/liter.

LACTATE DEHYDROGENASE (EC 1.1.1.27)

Lactate dehydrogenase (LDH,I-lactate:NAD$^+$ oxidoreductase) is a ubiquitous enzyme found in the cytoplasm of nearly all cells; it catalyzes an important step in glycolysis. LDH has a molecular weight of about 134 kd and is a tetramer of H and M subunits. There are five possible isoenzyme results from these combinations. Measurement of LDH is useful for a variety of different diseases involving the blood, liver, kidneys, skeletal muscle, and myocardium.

Measurement of Total LDH Activity

Lactate dehydrogenase catalyzes the reversible oxidation of L-lactate to pyruvate, with simultaneous reduction of NAD$^+$:

$$\text{lactate} + \text{NAD}^+ \xrightarrow{\text{LDH}} \text{pyruvate} + \text{NADH}$$

Both the "forward" (lactate-to-pyruvate) and "reverse" (pyruvate-to-lactate) reactions are currently in use in clinical laboratories. In the United States, the forward assay is most widely used. The advantage of

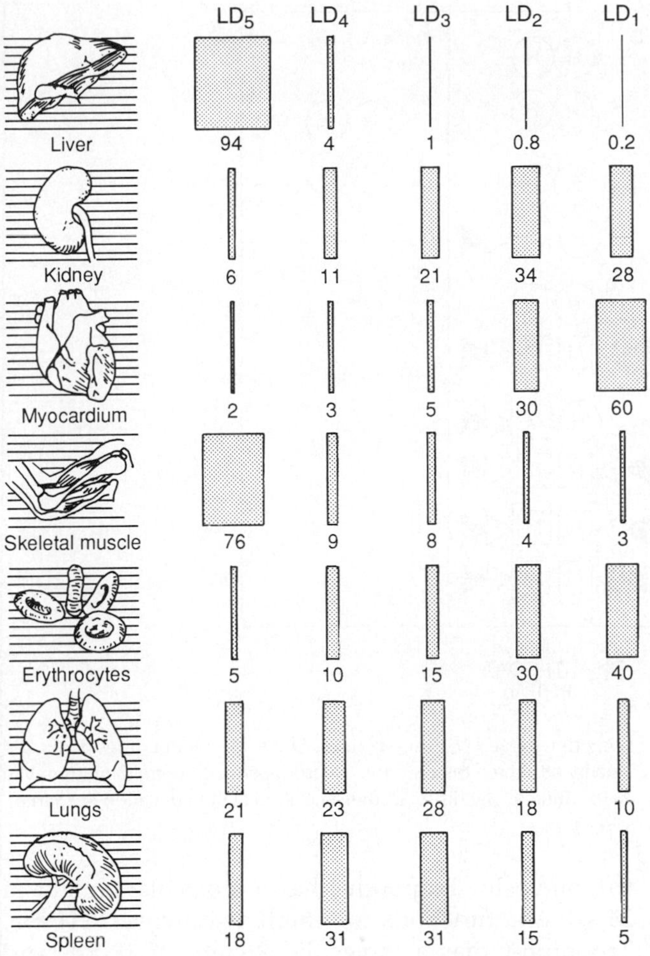

Figure 11.16. Tissue distribution of LDH isoenzymes. (From Lott JA, Wolf PL. Clinical enzymology. A case-oriented approach. New York: Year Book, 1986.)

this method is that the reaction rate is slower and is held more constant than for the reverse assay. The reaction is monitored by measuring the absorbance of NADH at 340 nm. The optimum pH range for this reaction is 8.8 to 9.8. The reaction rate for the reverse assay is higher than for the forward, and the precision is therefore somewhat improved. The pH range for the reverse reaction is 7.4 to 7.8. The reference interval for the forward reaction is about 80 to 200 U/liter at 37°C, and about 200 to 400 U/liter for the reverse reaction.

LDH Isoenzymes

Tissue Distribution. The LDH isoenzyme distribution of various tissues is shown in Figure 11.16 (10). Requests for LDH isoenzymes are most frequently made in conjunction with the diagnosis of acute myocardial infarction, although measuring LDH isoenzymes can be used to determine other sources of tissue injury. Since the heart is richest in LD_1, newer analytical methods have focused on this isoenzyme alone. The decision limit most widely used is that LD_1 activity in excess of 40% of total LDH activity supports the diagnosis of AMI. LDH isoenzyme fractionation is rarely of any value in the diagnosis of other conditions (e.g., liver disease) because there are other more specific markers available, and there is overlap in the tissue distribution of LDH isoenzymes from other organs.

Analytical Methods. *Electrophoresis:* The only routinely used procedure that allows analysis of all LDH isoenzymes is electrophoresis. Bands are visualized by densitometrically scanning the fluorescence of the NADH product, or reacting NADH with a tetrazolium salt to form a colored product that can be measured at 600 nm. Normal serum contains all five LDH isoenzymes. The serum of some patients will exhibit the presence of other LDH forms such as macro-LD (immunoglobulin bound), but the significance of these other forms is unknown.

Immunoprecipitation: The LD_1 isoenzyme can be measured directly by the Roche immunoprecipitation method described in Figure 11.17. A goat antibody directed toward the M subunit is added to serum samples and binds to LDH isoenzymes LD_2 through LD_5. This is followed by the addition of a second precipitating (donkey anti-goat) antibody, which recognizes and binds with the first antibody. After centrifugation, only the LD_1 isoenzyme remains, as it does not contain any M subunits. The extracted sample is then measured for residual LDH activity.

Chemical inhibition: The newest procedure for measuring LD_1 isoenzymes involves the use of selective chemical inhibition. The Boehringer Mannheim Corporation LD_1 assay makes use of guanidine thiocyanate, which acts as a competitive inhibitor for LD_1 and a noncompetitive inhibitor for LD_5. The degree of inhibition is greatest for LD_5; intermediate for LD_4, LD_3, and LD_2; and least for LD_1. The reagent is formulated to optimize recovery of LD_1 activity. The chemical inhibition method gives results that are equivalent to immunoprecipitation and has the advantage that it does not require a centrifugation step to isolate LD_1; therefore the assay can be automated to high-volume clinical chemistry analyzers.

ALDOLASE (EC 4.1.2.13)

Aldolase (D-fructose-1,6-diphosphate D-glyceraldehyde-3-phosphate-lyase) is an important enzyme in glycolysis and catalyzes the conversion of fructose-1,6-diphosphate to dihydroxyacetone phosphate and glyceraldehyde-3-phosphate. Although it is found in nearly all tissues, elevated serum levels usually reflect skeletal muscle or myocardial tissue necrosis. However, since serum aldolase is also ele-

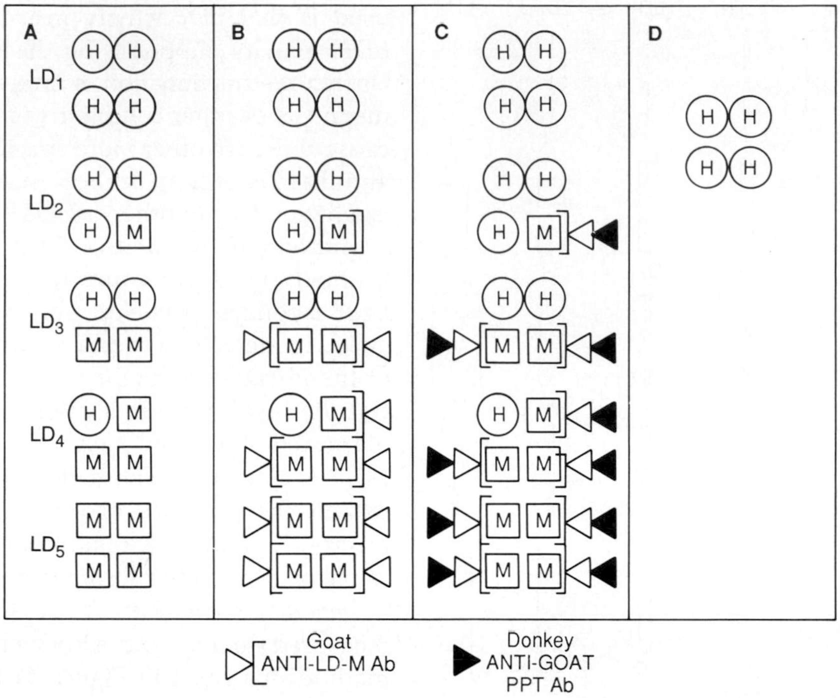

Figure 11.17. Immunoprecipitation assay for LDH isoenzymes. **A**, Major LDH isoenzymes represented as tetrameric combinations of M and H subunits. **B**, Addition of goat anti-LD-M antibody to label LD_{2-5} isoenzymes. **C**, Addition of donkey anti-goat IgG precipitating antibody to remove LD_{2-5} isoenzymes. **D**, Measurement of residual LDH activity attributed to LD_1 only. (Reproduced with permission from Wu AHB. Clinical chemistry. Bethesda, MD: Health Education Resources, 1991.)

vated in conditions such as leukemia, some tumors, gangrene, and a variety of other processes, aldolase is not as useful as creatine kinase for the elevation of muscle diseases, and is not considered useful for diagnostic purposes (12).

MYOGLOBIN

Myoglobin is a low–molecular weight protein (less than 18 kd) found in all skeletal muscle and myocardial tissues. Myoglobin is an oxygen-binding protein, serves as a reserve for oxygen, and facilitates the movement of oxygen within muscle cells. Concerning use of myoglobin for the diagnosis of AMI, myoglobin released from the heart is indistinguishable from that released from skeletal muscle tissues. Myoglobin can be measured using isotopic and nonisotopic immunoassay. Because of its small size, myoglobin appears in the serum very soon after its release from necrotic tissues, is filtered by the glomerulus, and returns to normal within 24 hours. Reference limits are below 100 ng/ml.

TROPONIN

Troponin is a regulatory protein complex located on the thin filament of striated muscles, and consists of three isotypes. Troponin-T has a molecular weight of 38 kd, and binds the troponin complex to tropomyosin. Troponin-I has a molecular weight of 24 kd, and functions to inhibit actomyosin ATPase. Troponin-C has a molecular weight of 18 kd, and regulates troponin-I activity by binding calcium. Troponin-T and troponin-I have the potential for being better diagnostic markers for AMI than existing enzymes such as CK-MB because cardiac isotypes are distinctly different from skeletal isotypes. Monoclonal antibodies have been developed to cardiac troponin that do not cross-react with skeletal muscle forms. Commercial immunoassays for troponin have been approved for use in Europe.

Diagnosis of Acute Myocardial Infarction

The diagnosis of acute myocardial infarction is defined by the World Health Organization, based on clinical signs and symptoms (e.g., chest pain), specific changes in electrocardiographic recordings, and the presence of elevated serum levels of enzymes such as total CK, CK-MB, LDH, and LD isoenzymes (13). New markers that are currently being studied include CK isoforms, myoglobin, and troponin.

EFFICIENCY OF AMI MARKERS WITH DIFFERENT DECISION LIMITS

The clinical sensitivity and specificity of biochemical markers for acute myocardial infarction are func-

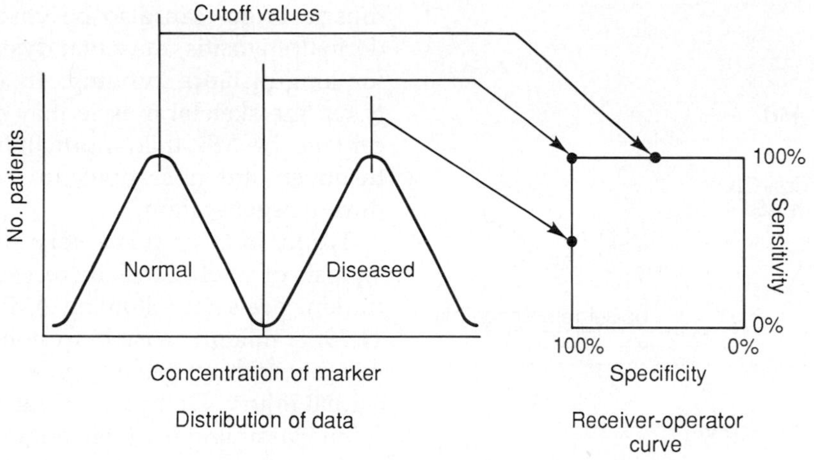

A

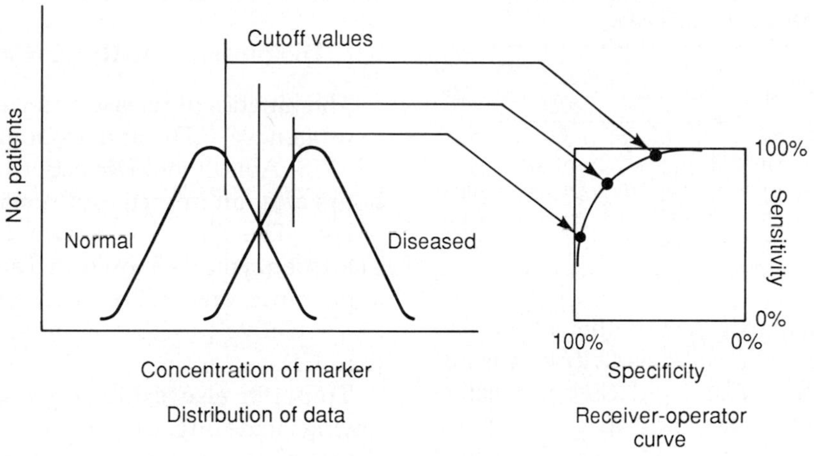

B

Figure 11.18. Use of receiver-operator characteristic (ROC) curves for determination of decision limits. **A**, ROC curve with non-overlapping distribution of test results. **B**, ROC curve with an overlapping distribution of test results. Clinical sensitivity and specificity are functions of the cutoff limit selected.

tions of the decision limits and the population studied. These are evaluated by use of receiver-operating characteristic (ROC) curves, which plot clinical sensitivity (number of true positives) versus specificity (number of true negatives) at different decision limits for a set of data. In an ideal situation, 100% sensitivity and specificity could be achieved if the data from the two populations do not overlap (Fig. 11.18*A*).

In practice, the diagnosis of AMI must be made from a population of patients with ischemic heart diseases of varying severity, congestive heart failure, and a variety of other problems. When plotting data of MI and non-MI patients, considerable overlapping will be observed. Selection of the decision limit will dictate the sensitivity and specificity for the marker in question (Fig. 11.18*B*). Low cutoff values will increase sensitivity, while high values will increase specificity.

EFFICIENCY OF AMI MARKERS WITH SAMPLING TIME

Early Diagnosis: Myoglobin and CK Isoforms

An important factor that affects the efficiency of biochemical markers for AMI diagnosis is the sampling time from the onset of chest pain. Figure 11.19 shows the activity-time curves for cardiac enzymes. As shown, myoglobin and CK-MM and MB isoforms have the earliest diagnostic windows of the markers shown. Myoglobin is increased early after AMI because of its small size. CK isoforms appear early because serum levels normally contain only trace levels of CK isoforms, and a low cutoff can be used to detect the very earliest release of tissue isoforms following myocardial necrosis. Myoglobin and CK isoforms assays are currently being studied to determine if

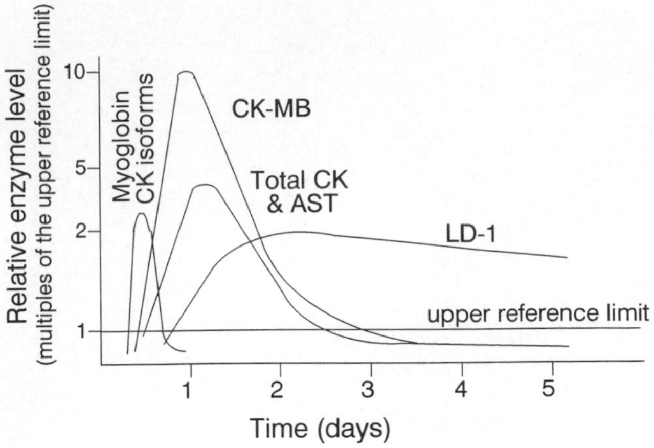

Figure 11.19. Activity versus time curves for biochemical markers of acute myocardial infarction.

Table 11.3. Estimates of Clinical Sensitivity and Specificity of Diagnostic Tests for Acute Myocardial Infarction

	Sensitivity				
Marker	2–8 hr	8–24 hr	24–72 hr	>72 hr	Specificity
Myoglobin	95	75	0	0	70
CK-MB isoforms	90	60	0	0	90
CK-MB	60	95	98	50	95
LD_1	40	85	95	90	85
Troponin	75	95	98	98	90

they can be used to diagnose AMI within 4 hours after onset. Estimates for clinical sensitivity at various time intervals after chest pain, and clinical specificity, are shown in Table 11.3. Early diagnosis is important in the management of AMI, particularly if thrombolytic therapy is to be used. Myoglobin and CK-MM isoforms are falsely elevated in patients with skeletal muscle injury or disease. Therefore, the clinical specificity of these tests is not as high as for CK-MB isoforms. Utilization of MB isoforms for routine use, however, warrants improvements in the methodology.

Definitive Diagnosis of AMI: CK-MB and Troponin

The creatine kinase MB isoenzyme is the most widely used enzyme for the diagnosis of acute myocardial infarction. Levels begin to rise 6 to 10 hours after onset, peak at 18 to 24 hours, and return to normal within 3 days (Fig. 11.19). The sensitivity of CK-MB is about 95 to 98% (see Table 11.3). The specificity of CK-MB when sampled at the optimum time after the onset of AMI ranges from 92 to 99%. CK-MB is more specific than total CK because the total can increase in a variety of nonmyocardial diseases. False-positive results do occur when myocardial tissue is damaged by other means, such as trauma to the heart or open heart surgery. CK-MB of skeletal muscle origin can also be observed in serum with dermatomyositis, muscular dystrophies, and training for long-distance running. In each of these conditions, the skeletal muscle may contain a higher percentage of MB than normal because of increased turnover and alterations in isoenzyme expression during regeneration.

Troponin (T or I) is a very efficient marker for diagnosis of AMI. Gross increases of troponin concentrations are seen following AMI, as shown in Figure 11.19. A mild increase in troponin is also observed in patients with unstable angina, reflecting minor myocardial injury. Detection of minor injury may be useful in classifying unstable angina patients who are at high risk for developing AMI (14). Because of the increasing availability of commercial troponin assays, troponin may eventually replace CK-MB as the "gold standard" for diagnosis of AMI.

Late Diagnosis of AMI: LDH and Troponin

The kinetics of release and clearance for lactate dehydrogenase, LD_1, and troponin are different from CK-MB. Abnormal LDH activity first appears 12 to 18 hours after an infarct, and remain elevated for about 7 days. The clinical sensitivity and specificity for the LD_1 isoenzyme is shown in Table 11.3. The delayed appearance and subsequent prolonged increase of LDH relative to CK is because LDH is much larger than CK.

Troponin also exhibits a prolonged increase following acute myocardial infarction. Concentrations are increased for up to 2 weeks after the onset of injury (Fig. 11.19). Unlike LD_1, the extended increase is due to ongoing destruction and clearance of the structural complex of muscle cells. Once released into the circulation, troponin has a half-life of 90 minutes.

LD_1 and troponin measurements are most useful in a patient who presents with chest pain 2 to 3 days after the initial onset. In such a patient, the activity of CK and CK-MB are often within normal limits. With electrophoresis, the diagnosis of AMI is based on detection of the "flipped pattern," i.e., $LD_1/LD_2 > 1$. If chemical or immunoinhibition assays are used, the absolute LD_1 concentration and calculation of the LD_1/total LDH ratio is used for the diagnosis of AMI. For troponin, concentrations exceeding the cutoff limits (e.g., 0.1 ng/ml for troponin-T) indicate myocardial injury. Because troponin has a much larger diagnostic window for AMI, assays for LDH isoenzymes may eventually be replaced.

The optimum use of enzyme markers for diagnosis of acute myocardial infarction requires careful selection of decision limits and correct timing of blood samples. Because false positives can occur, the best

Table 11.4. CK Levels Before and After a Marathon Race[a]

Pre-race CK	Post-race CK[b]	Post-race MB[b]	%MB/total CK
U/liter	*U/liter*	*U/liter*	
202	1293	85	6.6
322	1654	108	6.5
232	2261	138	6.1
340	1768	85	4.8
147	683	80	11.7

[a]Data from Apple FS, Rogers MA, Sherman WM Ivy Jr. Comparison of serum creatine kinase and creatine kinase MB activities post marathon race versus post myocardial infarction Clin Chim Acta 1984;138:111–118.
[b]Values taken 24 hr after the race.

information is obtained when serial collections are analyzed to construct activity versus time curves. Emergency or "stat" measurement of CK-MB is not usually necessary to establish a diagnosis but can be helpful in triaging suspected patients to an appropriate level of care.

Enzymes in Skeletal Muscle Disease

The important enzyme markers of skeletal muscle necrosis include total creatine kinase, CK-MB, and, to a lesser extent, aspartate aminotransferase and aldolase. Elevations of total CK with a normal relative index for CK-MB indicate skeletal muscle disease, necrosis, or injury. When both total CK and CK-MB are elevated, the diagnosis of skeletal muscle injury may be difficult. Patients with muscular dystrophies can have a higher than normal proportion of CK-MB in their muscle tissue because of increased muscle turnover. Also, individuals who run long distances can exhibit significant levels of noncardiac CK-MB in serum. Table 11.4 shows typical results of CK and CK-MB levels following a marathon race (15). In most cases, the clinical history is sufficient for differentiating acute skeletal muscle damage from acute myocardial injury. In cases of concomitant skeletal muscle injury and AMI, measurement of troponin will allow differentiation between skeletal muscle injury and myocardial damage.

CK in Cerebrovascular Injury

Although CK-BB is found in high concentrations in the brain, only small amounts appear in the serum following cerebral injury. Levels of mitochondrial CK and CK-MM are released in stroke victims. High levels of CK-BB have been found in the serum of some patients with breast and prostate cancer, but the incidence of this finding is low and it therefore has no clinical use.

PANCREATIC DISEASES

Enzymes of Pancreatic Origin

AMYLASE (EC 3.2.1.1)

Amylase (α-1,4-glucan,4-glucanohydrolase) catalyzes the hydrolysis of complex carbohydrates at the α-1,4 linkages of adjacent glucose residues. The amylases have a molecular weight of about 50 kd, are small enough to pass through the glomerulus, and are among the few serum enzymes that appear in urine. Amylase is found in the highest concentrations in the acinar cells of the pancreas, but other isoenzymes are found in the salivary gland, testis, and ovary. Each isoenzyme is encoded by a separate gene. Serum amylase consists primarily of the pancreatic and salivary isoenzymes. Macroamylase is a complex of immunoglobulin (usually IgG) with amylase (usually the salivary isoenzyme). Because of the high molecular weight of this complex, macroamylase is not cleared by the kidneys, and high amylase levels persist in the serum, often without any clinical disorder. Macroamylasemia is estimated to account for 2 to 5% of all patients with hyperamylasemia (16).

Analytical Measurements

Numerous methods have been developed for measuring serum amylase. Viscometric, nephelometric, and iodometric assays have been largely replaced with saccharogenic and chromogenic assays that are very precise and can be adapted to automated chemistry analyzers. Saccharogenic assays use small oligosaccharide substrates.

$$\text{maltopentaside} \xrightarrow{\alpha\text{-amylase}} \text{maltotrioside} + \text{maltose}$$

$$\text{maltotrioside} \xrightarrow{\alpha\text{-glucosidase}} \text{glucose}$$

$$\text{maltose} \xrightarrow{\alpha\text{-glucosidase}} \text{glucose}$$

The reaction can be monitored by following the production of glucose as conventionally measured, for example with glucose oxidase and an O_2-specific electrode, or hexokinase coupled with glucose 6-phosphate dehydrogenase and NAD^+. These assays must correct for the presence of variable amounts of endogenous glucose in serum.

Chromogenic assays make use of synthetic substrates containing a chromogen that is either liberated directly by amylase, or after coupling with α- or β-glucosidase. These assays eliminate the additional steps needed to measure glucose. A common chromogen is *p*-nitrophenol (PNP).

$$p\text{-nitrophenylmaltoheptaoside} \xrightarrow{\alpha\text{-amylase}} p\text{-NP-maltotetraoside} + \text{PNP-maltotrioside}$$

$$p\text{-NP-maltotrioside} + H_2O \xrightarrow{\alpha\text{-glucosidase}} p\text{-NP} + \text{glucose}$$

In this example, the reaction rate is monitored by measuring the absorbance of *p*-nitrophenol at 405 nm. The assay has an optimum pH of 7.0 and requires calcium and anions as cofactors. The reference interval for amylase is dependent on the type of assay and the substrate used. For the chromogenic assay, the reference interval is 20 to 160 U/liter at 37°C.

Renal Clearance of Amylase

Because amylase is normally excreted into the urine, the amylase clearance can be calculated by using simultaneous serum and urine amylase measurements. Corrections for differences in glomerular filtration rates are made by including serum and urine creatinine measurements:

$$\text{amylase/creatinine clearance} = \frac{[\text{amylase}]_u \times [\text{creatinine}]_s}{[\text{amylase}]_s \times [\text{creatinine}]_u}$$

where [amylase] is the activity of serum (s) and urine (u) amylase, and [creatinine] is the concentration of serum and urine creatinine. This ratio can be used to detect the presence of macroamylasemia in patients with hyperamylasemia. Normally, the ratio is in the range of 2 to 5%. In patients with pancreatitis, an increased ratio is expected because of the increased turnover of pancreatic amylase and subsequent urinary excretion. In macroamylasemia, a low ratio is expected because the macromolecular form is not filtered by the glomerulus.

Amylase Isoenzymes and Isoforms

Human serum contains two amylase isoenzymes originating from the salivary gland (S-type) and pancreas (P-type). Each isoenzyme exists as one of three isoforms. The pure gene product for the salivary and pancreatic isoforms are S_1 and P_2, respectively. These are converted to S_2 and S_3, and to P_3, respectively, by posttranslational deglycosidation, and deamidation of asparagine and glutamine residues. The P_1 isoform of amylase is a genetic isoenzyme variant. Isoenzyme measurements are used to differentiate the causes of hyperamylasemia, such as those of salivary and pancreatic origin, or the presence of macroamylase.

Amylase isoenzymes can be measured by electrophoresis, ion-exchange chromatography, isoelectric focusing, and selective inhibition and precipitation with lectins and monoclonal antibodies. Using electrophoresis, amylase isoenzyme bands can be made visible by use of a dyed-starch suspension (e.g., Phadebas Tablets, Pharmacia Diagnostics, Piscataway, NJ), which produces a color upon hydrolysis by amylase. Quantitative measurement of each band can be made scanning bands with a densitometer. In normal individuals, there are roughly equal amounts of S-type and P-type isoamylases in serum. Other methods are available to determine the total P-type amylase isoenzyme content of serum. Salivary amylase is about 90% inhibited by lectins from wheat germ. The estimation of pancreatic amylase is made by measuring the residual amylase activity after incubation with the lectin. Macroamylase of the S type is also inhibited by this technique. Monoclonal antibodies directed toward either salivary or pancreatic amylase can also be used to measure amylase isoenzymes in a variety of formats such as selective immunoinhibition, immunoprecipitation, immunoextraction, or enzyme immnoassay. Immunoassays are very specific and do not cross-react with other isoamylase forms.

LIPASE (EC 3.1.1.3)

Lipase (triacylglycerol acylhydrolase) catalyzes the hydrolysis of triglycerides sequentially into β-monoglyceride and two free fatty acids. Lipase activity depends on the substrate being present as an emulsion in contrast to related enzymes such as lipoprotein lipase and other hydrolases, which are active with short fatty acid chain substrates that are water soluble. The most commonly used assay for lipase involves measuring the clearing of a substrate emulsion by the action of lipase. Measurements can be made by either nephelometry or turbidimetry:

$$\underset{\text{(cloudy emulsion)}}{\text{triolein}} \xrightarrow{\text{lipase}} \text{glycerides} + \underset{\text{(clear solution)}}{\text{free fatty acids}}$$

The optimum pH for this reaction is 8.8. In this assay, both lipase and lipoprotein lipase are measured. However, if colipase and a bile salt such as sodium deoxycholate are included, the reaction rate and analytical sensitivity of pancreatic lipase is increased, while that for lipoprotein lipase is eliminated (17). Colipase, aided by the addition of bile salts, binds to lipase to form a complex. This association produces a conformational change in lipase, such that the latter can now more efficiently bind to the substrate. The mechanism of how colipase and bile salts interact with the enzyme in vivo is shown in Figure 11.20. The reference range for lipase depends on the substrate and whether or not colipase is used. The upper

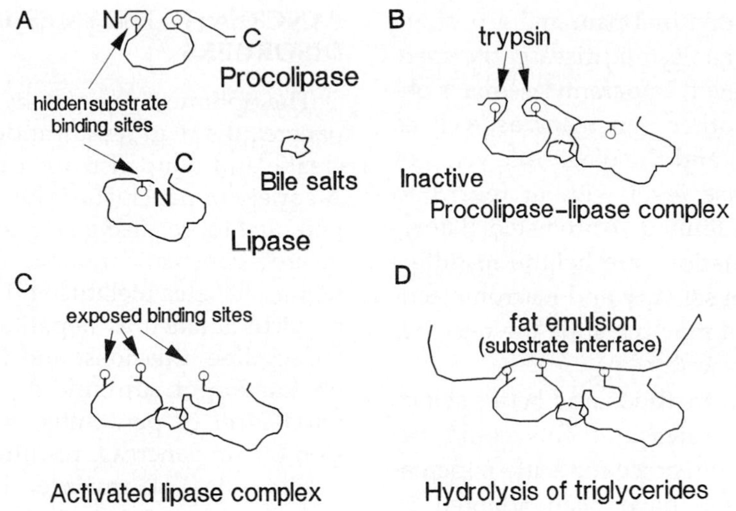

Figure 11.20. Mechanism for the hydrolysis of fat in the intestine by lipase-colipase. **A**, Lipase and procolipase are secreted as separate proteins from the pancreas. The binding sites for the triglyceride substrates are hidden for both enzymes. **B**, In the intestine, the two proteins associate to form an inactive complex. The binding is favored by the addition of mixed-chain bile salts. **C**, Trypsin converts procolipase to colipase by removal of the N- and C-terminal residues, exposing the substrate binding sites. This also produces a conformational change for lipase, thereby exposing its substrate binding site. **D**, The lipase-colipase can now attach to the fat particles, facilitating the hydrolysis of triglycerides. (Adapted from Borgstrom B. Lipase. Amsterdam: Elsevier, 1984, with permission.)

reference limit is 200 U/liter at 37°C when triolein is used as the substrate in the presence of colipase and bile salts.

Electrophoresis of lipase reveals the presence of at least two true isoforms in serum, labeled L_1 and L_2. A third form labeled L_3 also appears on electrophoresis and is thought to be pancreatic carboxyester lipase.

TRYPSIN (EC 3.4.21.4)

Trypsin is a pancreatic proteolytic enzyme that specifically cleaves peptide bonds at carboxyl groups of lysine and arginine. Trypsin originates from inactive trypsinogens produced by pancreatic acinar cells. Activation of trypsin occurs in the intestinal tract by an enterokinase. Measurement of serum trypsin is seldom performed because amylase and lipase measurements are readily available and provide much the same information. However, immunoreactive trypsin from dried blood spots is being used as a neonatal screen for cystic fibrosis (18). Because of the existence of antiproteases in the blood, trypsin must be measured immunologically by using specific antisera rather than by the use of enzymatic activity.

Clinical Uses of Pancreatic Enzymes

ACUTE PANCREATITIS

Pancreatitis results when digestive enzymes of the exopancreas find their way into the endocrine parenchyma and autodigestion of pancreatic tissue ensues. Key among these digestive enzymes is trypsin, which together with other bile components activates other proteolytic enzymes that are collectively responsible for pancreatic necrosis. The most consistent clinical symptom of acute pancreatitis is abdominal pain. Risk factors include excessive alcohol use, the presence of gallstones, and hyperlipidemias. The disease can take either of two forms: the edematous form, which is relatively mild and occurs in about 80% of all cases, and the hemorrhagic form, which is more serious and results in most of the fatalities attributed to acute pancreatitis (19).

The diagnosis of acute pancreatitis is made on the basis of clinical presentation and medical history, in addition to radiographic and laboratory studies. Laboratory findings include an elevated serum amylase, amylase clearance, and lipase. Amylase and lipase levels rise within a few hours after onset, and remain elevated for 36 to 48 hours. The extent of amylase and lipase elevations are not strongly correlated to the severity of the disease. The clinical sensitivity of serum amylase and lipase are both about 90% when blood is sampled in the first 36 hours, and highly sensitive assays are used. False negatives result when pancreatitis occurs in patients who have had recurrent attacks and have little or no functional pancreatic tissue remaining.

The clinical specificity for the diagnosis of acute pancreatitis is only 40% for amylase and 60% for lipase. The specificity for amylase is low because of the existence of nonpancreatic sources of the enzyme such as the salivary gland. The specificity of lipase is influenced by the design of the assay used. When serial amylase levels are measured in patients with a presentation of acute abdominal pain and a positive history of alcohol use or cholestatic disease, the specificity is increased. However, hyperamylasemia is observed in a variety of other pancreatic as well as nonpancreatic disorders, and the diagnostic value of a single elevated amylase level without regard to other clinical findings is limited. Automated P-amylase isoenzyme determinations are helpful in differentiating pancreatic from salivary and macromolecular hyperamylasemia and may preclude the need for a total amylase measurement.

With improvements in methods and better standardization, serum lipase measurements could become the laboratory test of choice for acute pancreatitis. Turbidimetric assays have been adapted to automated clinical chemistry analyzers for routine and stat determinations. Further improvements in diagnostic efficiencies are obtained with the measurement of amylase and lipase isoforms. Among the markers studied, the P_3 amylase and the L_2 lipase isoforms have the highest clinical specificity for the diagnosis of acute pancreatitis. Whether or not the increase in clinical efficiency justifies the use of more labor-intensive electrophoretic assays remains to be determined.

CHRONIC PANCREATITIS

Chronic inflammation of the pancreas can be caused by either recurrent episodes of acute pancreatitis, or continual subclinical pancreatic damage occurring over many months. Chronic pancreatitis often presents in patients with a history of acute pancreatitis together with diabetes in adults, and cystic fibrosis in children. Gradual degradation of exocrine function often leads to steatorrhea. Approximately 40% of chronic pancreatitis patients have vitamin B_{12} malabsorption. Examination of fecal fat and administration of the D-xylose tolerance and secretin stimulation tests are useful in determining the presence of these complications.

Serum enzyme levels in chronic pancreatitis are less useful than in the acute presentation. Amylase and lipase levels are very often within normal limits and may actually be low during the end stages of the disease, because of the small amount of functional pancreatic tissue. Patients with low-grade disease will also not be detectable by enzyme studies. The most useful procedure for diagnosis appears to be endoscopic retrograde choledochopancreatography (ERCP), which permits direct viewing of pancreatic ducts.

PANCREATIC ENZYMES IN OTHER DISORDERS

The optimum use of enzymes for the diagnosis of pancreatitis requires an understanding of other pancreatic and nonpancreatic causes of enzyme release. A variety of pancreatic injuries and diseases have the potential for releasing enzymes into the blood. These include pancreatic trauma, abdominal surgery, carcinoma, diabetes mellitus and ketoacidosis, and injury by viruses (such as hepatitis B) and drugs (such as tetracycline, thiazides, and furosemide). Injury to or obstruction of surrounding tissue, such as a perforated ulcer or peritonitis, may also cause compression of the pancreas, resulting in enzyme release.

Elevations of amylase, immunoreactive trypsin, and, to a lesser extent, lipase also occur in other nonpancreatic disorders. Since amylase and trypsin are largely cleared by glomerular filtration, high values are seen in patients with renal failure. The existence of parotid lesions and inflammation will produce salivary hyperamylasemia. Amylase isoenzyme measurements can be used to detect this form. Macroamylasemia can also cause high serum amylase values, resulting in a false-positive diagnosis for pancreatitis. Amylase isoenzyme and clearance measurements can be used to detect the presence of this form.

ENZYMES IN CANCER

Enzymes and Markers in Prostatic Carcinoma

ACID PHOSPHATASE (EC 3.1.3.2)

The acid phosphatases (ACP, orthophosphoric-monoester phosphohydrolase) are a collection of enzymes that catalyze the hydrolysis of phosphate from a variety of natural and synthetic substrates. The optimum pH is on the acid side, usually between 5 and 6. Acid phosphatase is found in the liver, red cells, platelets, bone marrow, and prostate. Several isoenzymes of acid phosphatase can be identified in serum by electrophoresis or isoelectric focusing. However, since measurement of acid phosphatase in a clinical laboratory is used primarily for monitoring patients with prostatic cancer, isoenzyme classification is generally limited to simply prostatic and nonprostatic.

ANALYTICAL MEASUREMENTS

Enzymatic Assays

Total acid phosphatase activity can be measured using a variety of substrates, including *p*-nitrophenylphosphate (*p*-NPP), phenylphosphate, thymolphthalein monophosphate, α-naphthyl phos-

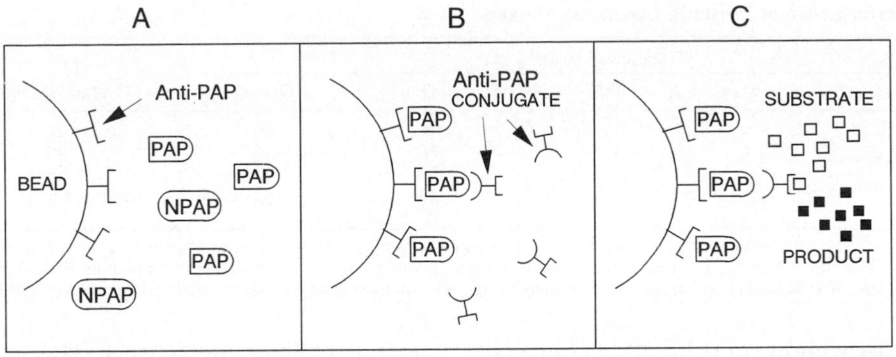

Figure 11.21. Immunoenzymometric assay for prostatic acid phosphatase. **A**, Monoclonal antibodies to prostatic acid phosphatase are immobilized onto a large bead. A serum sample containing prostatic (PAP) and nonprostatic acid phosphatase (NPAP) is added. Only PAP binds to the bead. **B**, The beads are washed to remove nonadhering proteins including NPAP, and anti-PAP antibodies conjugated to alkaline phosphatase are added. The bead is washed again to remove excess unbound conjugate. **C**, Substrate to the alkaline phosphatase conjugate is added, which reacts to produce a product that is measured at 405 nm. The activity of the conjugate is proportional to the PAP concentration of the original sample.

phate, and, most recently, 2,6-dichloro-*p*-nitrophenyl phosphate. After removal of the phosphate, these compounds absorb light in either the visible or the ultraviolet region.

The reaction of acid phosphatase with *p*-NPP is identical to that described for alkaline phosphatase (described above under Enzymes Useful In Liver Disease). *p*-NPP is a nonspecific substrate that is hydrolyzed in the presence of both prostatic and nonprostatic acid phosphatase. When separation of these two activities is desired, L-tartrate can be used to inhibit the prostatic isoenzyme. The difference between the total activity and the activity in the presence of tartrate provides an estimate of the prostatic isoenzyme. The reference intervals for total acid phosphatase using *p*-NPP at 37°C are 2.5 to 11.7 and 0.3 to 9.2 U/liter for men and women, respectively, and 0.2 to 3.5 and 0 to 0.8 U/liter, respectively, for the tartrate-inhibitable fraction.

Other substrates are more specific for the prostatic acid phosphatase isoenzyme, negating the need to perform tartrate inhibition. The reaction with thymolphthalein monophosphate is shown below:

$$\text{thymolphthalein monophosphate} \xrightarrow{\text{PAP}} \text{thymolphthalein} + \text{phosphate}$$

The reaction occurs at pH 5.6 and is stopped by the addition of alkali, which also intensifies the absorbance of thymolphthalein at 600 nm. The reference interval using this substrate at 37°C is 0.1 to 0.6 U/liter.

Immunologic Assays for Prostatic Acid Phosphatase

Measurements of prostatic acid phosphatase (PAP) can be made using specific immunoassays, which measure mass rather than enzyme activity. An example is the nonisotopic sandwich (immunoenzymometric) assay, such as the Hybritech Tandem-E and Abbott PAP-EIA assays. A schematic of one of these assays is shown in Figure 11.21. Antibodies to PAP are immobilized by linking to a bead or tube. Samples containing prostatic and nonprostatic acid phosphatase are added. After a washing step to remove all nonadhering proteins, an enzyme-linked conjugate antibody is added. After a second washing, substrate to the conjugated enzyme is added and the concentration of PAP is determined from a calibration curve. These immunologic assays are more specific for prostatic acid phosphatase than the corresponding enzyme assays, and have greater clinical sensitivity for prostatic disease. However, the increased sensitivity is not sufficient to warrant mass screening for prostatic carcinoma with PAP, even in the highest risk groups, because immunologic assays also suffer from lower clinical specificity. That is, more elevations are seen with nonmalignant disorders such as bening prostatic hypertrophy.

STAGING AND MONITORING PROSTATIC CARCINOMA

Prostatic carcinoma in men has been divided into four main clinical stages. Stage A is the earliest stage, when recognition is possible only by histologic examination of biopsied tissue. Stage B tumors can be palpated by rectal examination. Stage C is defined when the tumor has progressed to surrounding pelvic areas. Distant metastases define stage D. Extensive studies have been published concerning the diagnostic performance of both enzymatic and immunologic acid phosphatase measurements (20). In addition, prostate-specific antigen (PSA) has become an important assay for prostatic carcinoma. PSA is a glycopro-

Table 11.5. Clinical Performance of Prostatic Carcinoma Markers

Marker	Sensitivity by Stage A	B	C	D	Overall	Overall Specificity
	%	%	%	%	%	%
ACP[a]	7	13	34	76	36	95
PAP[b]	18	37	53	82	48	92
PSA[c]	57	68	81	87	80	76

[a]Data from 685 cancer patients and 591 benign prostatic hypertrophy (BPH) patients from five reports using an enzymatic acid phosphatase assay
[b]Data from 2039 cancer patients and 1734 BPH patients from 24 reports using an immunoassay for prostatic acid phosphatase (RIA, IRMA, EIA, and IEMA)
[c]Data from 1489 cancer patients and 400 BPH patients from five reports using an immunoassay for prostate-specific antigen (IRMA and IEMA).

tein with a molecular weight of 34 kd and is found in prostatic tissues. The clinical efficiency of acid phosphatase assays and PSA varies greatly with the stage of the disease. As shown in Table 11.5, none of the assays is particularly useful for early diagnosis, when surgical treatment would be most beneficial. When the assays are used for patients in stages C and D, however, the efficiencies increase considerably. PAP and PSA are much more useful for monitoring the effect of therapy for prostatic carcinoma than for making the diagnosis itself. Increases above a pre-established baseline in any of these assays suggest tumor progression or recurrence.

Other Enzymes and Isoenzyme Markers of Malignancy

Malignant tumors often produce dramatic elevations in serum enzyme levels. Among the possible causes are local tissue necrosis, obstruction caused by "space-occupying" tumors, shedding of enzymes from tumor surfaces and membranes, and, more rarely, ectopic production and secretion of enzymes by the malignant cells. Total enzyme elevations have not been successfully linked to any particular tumor and are not particularly useful in diagnosis as an isolated finding. Some isoenzymes, however, have a higher degree of specificity, and many have been examined as potential cancer markers.

ALKALINE PHOSPHATASE

One of the first isoenzymes to be linked with cancer is a placental-like isoenzyme of alkaline phosphatase that has been termed the Regan isoenzyme. This isoenzyme is identical to the placental isoenzyme in terms of heat stability, electrophoretic migration, and immunologic recognition. This isoenzyme is thought to be produced ectopically by some tumor tissue, but its presence is not linked with any specific tumor and it has such a low incidence that is not useful clinically. In contrast to the Regan isoenzyme, the α-isoenzyme, sometimes termed the fast liver fraction because of its electrophoretic migration anodic to the normal liver fraction, has more promise. This marker has been reported to have a sensitivity of 97% for detection of liver metastases. The specificity and efficiency are lower, however, because this fraction can also be found in the serum of patients with obstructive liver diseases, particularly when it is extrahepatic.

OTHER ISOENZYMES

Numerous other isoenzymes have been studied as potential markers for various malignancies. Some of these are listed in Table 11.6. Except for acid phosphatase, none of these enzymes is currently in routine use because of either low sensitivity for a particular malignancy or low specificity, or both. Those that are normally found in blood, such as lactate dehydrogenase isoenzymes, are usually not very specific. Also, some isoenzymes are detected only during the terminal stages of a malignancy, such as with macro CK type 2, and are therefore of limited use. Other markers serve specialized functions such as terminal deoxynucleotidyl transferase, which is used for the classification of leukemias.

MISCELLANEOUS ENZYMES

Cholinesterase

ANALYTICAL MEASUREMENT

The cholinesterases are enzymes that hydrolyze acetylcholine. True cholinesterase (acetylcholine acetylhydrolase, EC 3.1.1.7) is found in the red cells, lungs, spleen, and brain. In the serum, however, only pseudocholinesterase (PCHE acylcholine acylhydrolase, EC 3.1.1.8) is found. These enzymes differ in their specificity for substrates and sensitivities to inhibitors. Of particular clinical interest is the response of serum cholinesterase genetic variants to inhibition by dibucaine and fluoride.

Serum cholinesterase is measured by monitoring the hydrolysis of acetylthiocholine esters to form thiocholine:

$$\text{acetylthiocholine} + H_2O \xrightarrow{\text{PCHE}} \text{thiocholine} + \text{acetate}$$

Table 11.6. Enzymes as Tumor Markers

Enzyme	Cancer
Alkaline phosphatase	
Bone isoenzyme	Bone metastasis
Regan isoenzyme	Nonspecific
Fast liver isoenzyme	Liver metastasis
Nagao	Pancreas
Acid phosphatase	
Prostatic isoenzyme	Prostatic carcinoma
Creatine kinase	
CK-BB	Prostatic carcinoma
Macro CK type 2	Liver metastasis
5′-Nucleotidase phosphodiesterase	
V isoenzyme	Liver metastasis
Lactate dehydrogenase	
LD_1, LD_2, and LD_3	Germ cell tumors
LD_5	Colon & breast cancer
γ-Glutamyltransferase	
Albumin-migrating isoenzyme	Hepatic carcinoma
Glycosyltransferase	Colon, ovarian, & breast cancer
Terminal deoxynucleotidyl transferase	Lymphoblastic leukemia
Ribonuclease	Pancreatic carcinoma
Neuron-specific enolase	Small cell lung cancer
Ornithine decarboxylase	Colon cancer

The enzyme rate is monitored by reacting thiocholine with a disulfide agent that forms a chromogen after rearrangement, and can be measured at 340 nm:

$$\text{thiocholine} + 4,4'\text{-dithiopyridine} \rightarrow \rightarrow \text{chromogen}$$

CLINICAL SIGNIFICANCE

Serum levels of cholinesterase can be used in three different areas. Low levels of PCHE are found in patients with various forms of liver disease, including acute and chronic hepatitis, cirrhosis, and metastatic liver disease. Nonhepatic disorders, such as acute myocardial infarction, infections, and pulmonary embolism have also been shown to decrease PCHE levels. Due to the existence of more specific markers for the latter disorders, serum cholinesterase is not used for detecting or monitoring these processes.

The activity of PCHE is also important in monitoring industrial and agricultural workers who use and are exposed to organophosphate insecticides. Commonly used agents such as parathion and malathion inhibit both erythrocyte and serum cholinesterase activity, leading to neurologic and neuromuscular deficits. Levels of these enzymes are useful in determining the extent of exposure to these toxic pesticides.

The third area of clinical application of cholinesterase measurements involves the use of succinylcholine (suxamethonium) as a muscle relaxant in anesthesia. Because of a genetic variant of cholinesterase, there is a substantial difference in the rate of suxamethonium clearance by PCHE in some individuals. Patients who have the atypical cholinesterase gene can suffer prolonged apnea (due to extended relaxation of respiratory muscles) following administration of the drug. Recognition of these individuals is important and can be accomplished by measuring serum cholinesterase activity with and without inhibitors such as dibucaine or fluoride. Because atypical PCHE is more resistant to inhibitors than the normal PCHE, measurement of the percentage of inhibition (e.g., the "dibucaine number") provides a measure of the amount of the atypical enzyme that is present. Normal individuals exhibit 80 to 90% inhibition. Those who are heterozygous for one of the several possible variant genes exhibit 70 to 80% inhibition, and persons with two variant genes exhibit 10 to 30% inhibition. The individuals of the latter group are most prone to breathing complications following administration of suxamethonium.

Angiotensin-Converting Enzyme (EC 3.4.15.1)

Angiotensin-converting enzyme (ACE, peptidyl-dipeptide hydrolase) is produced by the lungs and catalyzes the conversion of the decapeptide angiotensin I to the octapeptide angiotensin II. It is a vital enzyme in the control of aldosterone secretion and regulation of blood pressure. ACE can be measured by the use of synthetic peptide substrates or by immunoassay.

Although ACE is an important step in the renin-aldosterone metabolic pathway, serum measurements of ACE are not useful for studying the etiologies of hypertension. However, it has been found that ACE is elevated in roughly 50 to 80% of cases of sarcoidosis, a multisystem granulomatous disease that most commonly involves the lungs. ACE is useful for differentiation between this disease and other granulomatous disorders, and between active and dormant sarcoidosis. Unfortunately, the specificity of ACE measurements is not high because a variety of other conditions can produce elevated activities. These include Gaucher's disease, leprosy, active histoplasmosis, pulmonary embolism, Hodgkin's disease, alcoholic cirrhosis, and chronic hepatitis.

Glucose-6-Phosphate Dehydrogenase (EC 1.1.1.49)

Glucose-6-phosphate dehydrogenase (G6PD) is an important erythrocyte enzyme in the hexose monophosphate shunt for the utilization of glucose. The in vivo reaction of G6PD is used in its laboratory analysis:

$$\text{glucose-6-phosphate} + \text{NAD}^+ \xrightarrow{\text{G-6-PD}} \text{6-phosphogluconate} + \text{NADH}$$

The reaction is monitored at 340 nm by following the production of NADH. Measurements of G6PD are clinically useful for the detection of individuals who are deficient for the X-linked G6PD gene. Glucose-6-phosphate dehydrogenase deficiency affects black males and Caucasians of Mediterranean descent. These individuals develop varying degrees of hemolytic anemias when exposed to certain drugs such as sulfa drugs, aspirin, and antimalarial medications.

Osseous Alkaline Phosphatase

As mentioned previously, the major sources of alkaline phosphatase (ALP) in the serum are liver and bone. Since osteoblasts produce alkaline phosphatase, elevations in ALP levels are seen in patients with increased osteoblastic activity, such as in rickets, osteomalacia, Paget's disease, acromegaly, osteoblastic sarcoma, bone fractures, and metastatic bone disease. Levels of ALP can exceed 10 times the upper limit of normal in severe cases. These disorders are also associated with changes in the levels of calcium, phosphorus, parathyroid hormone, and vitamin D, as discussed in Chapter 17. Patients with osteoporosis and multiple myeloma generally have normal ALP levels.

References

1. LaDue JS, Wroblewski F, Karmen A. Serum glutamic oxaloacetic transaminase activity in human acute transmural myocardial infarction. Science 1954;12:497–499.
2. Pappas NJ Jr. Theoretical aspects of enzymes in diagnosis. Clin Lab Med 1989;9(4):595–626.
3. Lehninger AL. Biochemistry. 2nd ed. New York: Worth, 1970: 183–216.
4. Nemesanszky E, Lott JA. γ-Glutamyltansferase and its isoenzymes: progress and problems. Clin Chem 1985;31:797–803.
5. Zimmerman HJ. Function and integrity of the liver. In: Henry JB, ed. Clinical diagnosis and management. 17th ed. Philadelphia: WB Saunders, 1984.
6. Cohen JA, Kaplan MM. The SGOT/SGPT ratio—an indicator of alcoholic liver disease. Dig Dis Sci 1979;24:835–838.
7. Okuno F, Ishii H, Kashiwazaki K, et al. Increase in mitochondrial GOT (m-GOT) activity after chronic alcohol consumption: clinical and experimental observations. Alcohol 1988;5: 49–53.
8. Hearse DJ. Cellular damage during myocardial ischaemia: metabolic changes leading to enzyme leakage. In: Hearse DJ. Enzymes in cardiology: diagnosis and research. New York: John Wiley, 1979.
9. Gruemer HD, Prior T. Carrier detection in Duchenne muscular dystrophy: a review of current issues and approaches. Clin Chim Acta 1987;162:1–18.
10. Lott JA, Wolf PL. Clinical enzymology. A case-oriented approach. New York: Year Book, 1986.
11. Wu AHB, Schwartz JG. Update on creatine kinase isoenzyme assays. Diagn Clin Test 1989;27(8):16–20.
12. Giesker D, Bowers GN Jr. The comparative utility of serum creatine kinase versus serum aldolase in the evaluation of muscle disorders. Conn Med 1979;43:699–704.
13. Report of the Joint International Society and Federation of Cardiology/World Health Organization Task Force on Standardization of Clinical Nomenclature: nomenclature and criteria of diagnosis of ischemic heart disease. Circulation 1979;59: 607–609.
14. Hamm CW, Ravkilde J, Gerhardt W, Jorgensen P, Peheim E, Ljungdahl L, et al. The prognostic value of serum troponin T in unstable angina. N Engl J Med 1992;327:146–150.
15. Apple FS, Rogers MA, Sherman WM, Ivy JL. Comparison of serum creatine kinase and creatine kinase MB activities post marathon race versus post myocardial infarction. Clin Chim Acta 1984;138:111–118.
16. Remaley AT, Wilding P. Macroenzymes: biological characterization, clinical significance, and laboratory detection. Clin Chem 1989;35:2261–2270.
17. Borgstrom B. Lipase. Amsterdam: Elsevier, 1984.
18. Ranieri E, Ryall RG, Morris CP, et al. Neonatal screening strategy for cystic fibrosis using immunoreactive trypsinogen and direct gene analysis. Br Med J 1991;302:1237–1240.
19. Wong WCC, Butch AW, Rosenblum JL. The clinical chemistry laboratory and acute pancreatitis. Clin Chem 1993;39:234–243.
20. van Dieisen-Visser MP, Delare KPJ, Gizen AHJ, Brombacher PJ. A comparative study on the diagnostic value of prostatic acid phosphatase (PAP) and prostatic specific antigen (PSA) in patients with carcinoma of the prostate gland. Clin Chim Acta 1988;174:131–140.

12 Lipids, Lipoproteins, and Apolipoproteins

Donald A. Wiebe and Joseph D. Artiss

Most chemicals produced by living organisms, such as peptides, enzymes, and carbohydrates, are soluble in water. Lipids, on the other hand, are soluble only in organic solvents (such as alcohol, chloroform, hexane, and diethyl ether). Lipids include a variety of compounds that have different metabolic and physiological functions but share the characteristic of limited solubility in water.

Lipid compounds are commonly referred to as fats. The term "fat" tends to generate negative connotations. However, fats (lipid compounds) are necessary for the very existence of life—e.g., lipids are an essential component of cell membranes. Some lipids function as hormones (steroid hormones), as metabolic mediators (prostagladins), and as sources of stored energy (adipose tissue).

This chapter first introduces specific lipid compounds, some of which have become routine analytes used for diagnostic purposes. Lipoproteins, including the role of lipoproteins and apolipoproteins in lipid metabolism, are also discussed. Finally, analytical methods used by clinical laboratories for lipid, lipoprotein, and apolipoprotein measurement are described.

LIPIDS

The importance of lipids in medicine was recognized long before laboratory analyses were available to measure individual classes of lipids. The total lipid content of serum was determined by extracting all of the lipids with an organic solvent(s) (such as chloroform/methanol) and reporting the weight of the extractable material versus the volume of fluid extracted. In this assay, the four major classes of lipids—sterols (cholesterol), triglycerides, phospholipids, and free fatty acids—were all reported collectively as one value. Improved laboratory methods are now available to measure the various classes of lipids separately.

Cholesterol

Cholest-5-en-3β-ol (cholesterol) belongs to a class of 3β-hydroxy sterols that share the same basic steroidal structure (Fig. 12.1). Mixtures of 3β-hydroxy sterols can be isolated from plants, fish, and other forms of life, but cholesterol is the principal sterol in the higher life forms. In humans, cholesterol is present in all body tissues, and most cells can synthesize cholesterol. Only erythrocytes (red cells) lack this ability. Typically, cholesterol can be isolated in two forms from biological specimens, either as free alcohol or esterified with a long-chain fatty acid (cholesterol esters). Serum and plasma specimens contain a higher percentage of cholesterol esters (75 to 85%) compared to free cholesterol.

The physiological role of cholesterol may be divided into two functions. Cholesterol is one of the major constituents of cellular membranes and thus serves as a structural component in all cells. The other major function of cholesterol is as a metabolic precursor molecule for other steroids. Small quantities of cholesterol are required for the synthesis of other biologically active steroids such as the female and male sex hormones (estrogens and androgens) and adrenal-corticosteroids (aldosterone and corticosterone). In addition, about 0.5 g of cholesterol is converted daily into bile acids, which serve as detergents in the gastrointestinal tract to solubilize and therefore promote digestion and absorption of dietary fats. Unlike triglycerides and phospholipids, the human body possesses no enzymes to metabolize cholesterol. Consequently, cholesterol plays no role as an energy source to human cells.

HISTORICAL PERSPECTIVE

As recently as the mid-1970s, serum cholesterol was routinely measured using methods that required

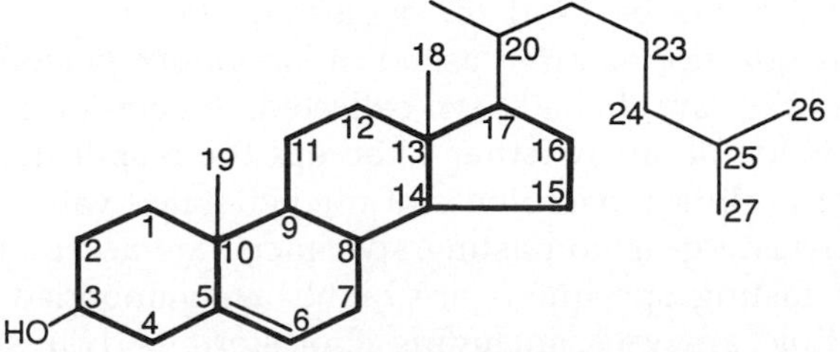

Figure 12.1. Cholesterol structure. Steroids, such as cholesterol, all share the common four-ring structure highlighted in dark lines.

Table 12.1. Comparison of Chemical and Enzymic Methods

Chemical	Enzymic
Sample pretreatment	Direct sample analysis
Large sample volume	Micro sample volume
Caustic reagents	Biological reagents
Difficult automation	Easily automated
Primary standards	Secondary calibration

Table 12.2. Sample Collection Requirements

1. Patient fasting 12–14 hours, especially no alcohol, sugar, or fat
2. Subject in a sitting position
3. Tourniquet use for less than 2 minutes
4. Properly evacuated collection device

caustic materials such as concentrated sulfuric acid, acetic anhydride, and acetic acid. Cholesterol and cholesterol esters were reacted to form ionized species that absorb between 560 and 620 nm and thus were quantitated by spectrophotometry. Automated systems were used in most clinical laboratories to measure cholesterol levels in patient specimens. The National Cholesterol Reference Method (a modified Abell, Levy, Brodie, and Kendall [Abell-Kendall] procedure) uses these same caustic materials. However, in the past 10 to 15 years, laboratories have discontinued these hazardous methods in favor of enzymic cholesterol assays. Table 12.1 compares the advantages and disadvantages of chemical versus enzymic cholesterol assays. Enzymic methods gained rapid acceptance due to ease of automation, ability to use small sample volumes, and absence of caustic reagents. The cost of performing enzymic assays is comparable to that of chemical methods.

PREANALYTICAL VARIATION/PATIENT PREPARATION

Specimen collection and patient preparation must be standardized to minimize the impact of preanalytical variation on cholesterol assays. Major preanalytical variables include fasting status and posture of the patient and use of a tourniquet during blood collection. Laboratories should standardize specimen collection processes, as shown in Table 12.2.

Should serum specimens from fasting or nonfasting patients be used for cholesterol determination? This question is often asked of laboratory personnel after the sample has been collected. A decision must be made about whether to accept the responsibility for the clinical usefulness of the generated value. Either fasting or nonfasting specimens are acceptable, but fasting specimens are highly recommended for *all* lipid analyses, including cholesterol. Advantages of fasting specimens are the standardization of specimen collection, the ability to perform other lipid tests that require fasting using the same sample, and the absence of analytical interferences caused by lipemia, which is increased in nonfasting specimens. Typically, a 12-hour fast should include avoidance of any food, sugar, cream, and alcohol prior to collection of the specimen. Coffee (without sugar or cream) will generally not significantly affect the cholesterol value. Total restriction of water and medications during the fasting period is in most cases unnecessary and may be contraindicated in some patients. The fasting status of the patient has negligible effect when screening generally healthy individuals for hypercholesterolemia.

SPECIMEN CONSIDERATIONS

The majority of cholesterol analyses are performed on venous blood. However, capillary blood (finger stick) is commonly used in physician offices or for cholesterol screening programs, and the cholesterol values from such specimens may be unrepresentative of a venous specimen. Capillary specimens have been reported to be almost 9% lower in lipids and lipoproteins than venous samples. Because lower capillary cholesterol values may result from dilution of the specimen by lymph or interstitial fluids, capillary specimens must be collected under strict protocols, and excessive "milking" must be avoided. The individual performing the test should be aware of the manner in which the instrument was calibrated, since manufacturers of physician office testing instruments may calibrate their instrument at the factory to compensate for the difference between capillary and venous blood.

Either serum or plasma specimens may be used for cholesterol analysis, but the values obtained may be different. Plasma values are generally lower than those from serum because of dilution factors that occur as anticoagulants initiate a release of intracellular fluid from blood cells into plasma (Table 12.3). Improper specimen handling may promote lipid peroxidation, lipolysis, or exchange of lipids and apoprotein between lipoproteins.

ENZYMIC CHOLESTEROL METHODS

Clinical laboratories have universally accepted enzymic cholesterol methods for routine applications,

Table 12.3. Anticoagulants

Anticoagulant	Dilution
	%
EDTA	3
Oxalate	9
Citrate	14
Fluoride	18

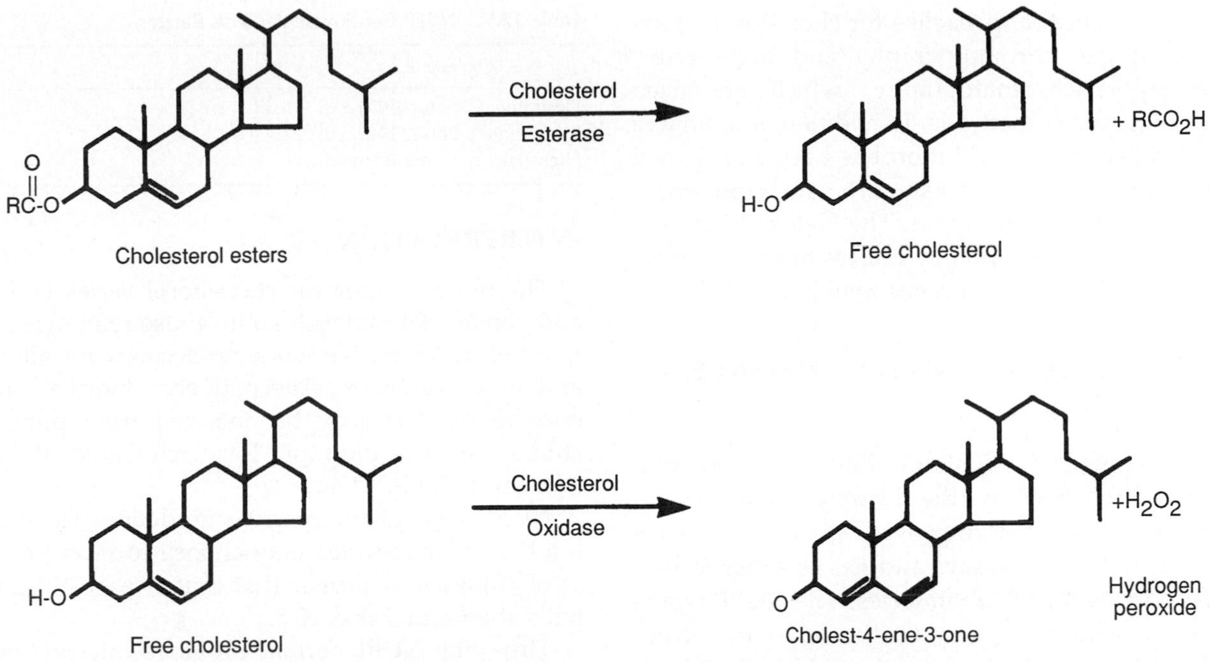

Figure 12.2. Enzymic cholesterol scheme. All enzymic assays for cholesterol utilize a cholesterol esterase to cleave the ester linkage of cholesterol esters and cholesterol oxidase to produce hydrogen peroxide from all resultant free cholesterol.

and the enzymes cholesterol esterase and cholesterol oxidase are common reagents in all commercial procedures (Fig. 12.2). Cholesterol esterase hydrolyzes esterified cholesterol to cholesterol and free fatty acids. The free cholesterol is oxidized by cholesterol oxidase in the presence of oxygen to form cholest-4-ene-3-one and hydrogen peroxide (H_2O_2).

Assays for cholesterol quantitation with enzymes have used both consumption of oxygen and formation of hydrogen peroxide as indicators. The majority of commercial procedures measure peroxide formation by coupling the enzymic reaction to a second peroxide detection system, e.g., the "Trinder" reaction. In this reaction, peroxidase catalyzes the oxidative coupling of 4-aminoantipyrene and phenol by H_2O_2 to form a quinoneimine dye and water. This quinoneimine dye absorbs maximally at 500 nm and may be quantitated spectrophotometrically.

Various derivatives of phenol and aniline have been substituted for phenol to increase the absorptivity of the quinoneimine dye and thus the sensitivity of the assay.

$$H_2O_2 + \text{4-aminoantipyrene} + \text{Phenol} \xrightarrow{\text{Peroxidase}} \text{Quinoneimine dye}$$

Enzymic methods typically use the serum or plasma directly. Consequently, hemolysis, elevated bilirubin, and lipemia may cause significant spectral interference with enzymic cholesterol methods. Because it competes with the chromogen for peroxide, bilirubin contributes additional interference to enzymic procedures. The addition of bilirubin oxidase or ferrocyanide reduces the bilirubin interference. Extremely high levels of ascorbate (vitamin C) have been reported to decrease the measured cholesterol, presumably due to competition between ascorbate and chromogen for the peroxide generated during the cholesterol oxidase reaction.

ACID AND IRON-BASED CHOLESTEROL METHODS

Acid and iron-based cholesterol methods have been largely abandoned in clinical laboratories because many of these assays required pretreatment steps to isolate cholesterol and used caustic materials, making these methods difficult to automate. However, a modified Abell-Kendall procedure remains in use and is recognized as a reference method by several professional clinical laboratory groups.

In the Abell-Kendall method, cholesterol, cholesterol esters, and other lipids are extracted from the serum with a mixture of chloroform/methanol or isopropanol. Cholesterol esters are then hydrolyzed to free cholesterol with alcoholic KOH. An aliquot of the organic extract (which contains free cholesterol) is mixed with sulfuric acid, acetic anhydride, and acetic acid to produce a chromogen with an absorption maximum at 620 nm. The method is calibrated directly against a cholesterol standard dissolved in organic solvent. A proficient technologist may process 50 to 60 samples per day, compared with automated enzymic assays that can perform several hundred tests per hour.

Other analytical approaches for cholesterol analysis include gas chromatography and high-performance liquid chromatography, which are used mainly as research methods. In addition, a definitive method called isotope dilution has been established for cholesterol that uses gas chromatography/mass spectrometry for quantitation. The National Institute of Standards and Technology utilizes this assay to assign target values for reference materials.

STANDARDIZATION AND PERFORMANCE REQUIREMENTS

The National Cholesterol Education Program (NCEP) established by the National Institutes of Health has promoted improved laboratory performance of cholesterol assays and has established performance goals for all laboratories. The NCEP works through a laboratory standardization panel composed of laboratory experts in the field of lipids and lipoproteins, including representatives from various government agencies, professional organizations, and laboratory personnel. The current goal states that cholesterol methods must be documented to have precision and bias of 3% or less.

Once a method has been demonstrated to meet the NCEP goals, a monitoring program must be implemented to ensure that performance is maintained. The quality control program must consider the source of reagents and controls, number of controls, and frequency of analysis. Obtaining either lyophilized or frozen control materials from commercial sources is most convenient. Control material should be selected to include levels through the critical decision points for cholesterol, such as 150, 200, and 240 mg/dl; performance of the method at 300 mg/dl and higher is less critical than lower concentrations.

Table 12.4. LRC Cholesterol Data (mg/dl)

	Males			Females		
Age	5%	50%	95%	5%	50%	95%
5–9	125	153	189	131	164	197
10–14	124	161	204	125	159	205
15–19	118	152	191	119	157	208
20–24	118	159	212	121	165	237
25–29	130	176	234	130	178	231
30–34	142	190	258	133	186	227
35–39	147	195	267	139	186	249
40–44	150	204	260	146	193	259
45–49	163	210	275	148	204	268
50–54	156	211	274	163	214	281
55–59	161	214	280	167	229	294
60–64	163	215	287	172	226	300
65–69	166	213	288	176	233	291
70+	144	214	265	173	226	280

Table 12.5. NCEP Cardiovascular Risk Ranges

Cholesterol	
Desirable:	0–199 mg/dl
Borderline:	200–239 mg/dl
High risk:	≥240 mg/dl

INTERPRETATION

The normal range for cholesterol varies with age and gender. To establish an in-house reference range requires an extensive study to account for all these and other variables. Alternatively, "normal" reference range data may be obtained from published studies, such as the Lipid Research Clinics Program (shown in Table 12.4).

NCEP has set interpretive guidelines for cholesterol, and laboratories may choose to report cholesterol values in a format that matches NCEP guidelines shown in Table 12.5.

Thus, the NCEP format provides interpretive information that is more useful than the traditional "normal" ranges. Clinical laboratory data may be reported in either conventional units (mg/dl) or standardized SI units (mmol/liter). To convert cholesterol data from the conventional units to SI units, multiply mg/dl by 0.026: 200 mg/dl converted to SI units equals 5.20 mmol/liter.

Triglycerides (Triacylgylcerols)

Triglycerides are composed of three long-chain fatty acids esterified to glycerol. Triglycerides are the major component of glycerides in circulating blood and tissues; small quantities of both mono- and diglycerides are also present and contain one or two fatty acids, respectively. Triglycerides are the primary form of long-term energy storage. Metabolism of 1 g of triglyceride produces 9 kcal of energy, compared with 4 kcal from 1 g of carbohydrates. Large amounts of triglycerides are stored in adipose tissue as concentrated fat droplets.

HISTORICAL PERSPECTIVE

Chemical assays for triglycerides have been used extensively in clinical laboratories. Organic solvents (such as chloroform, hexane, and isopropanol) are used to isolate triglyceride from serum proteins and interfering substances. The extraction solvent denatures serum proteins, and glycerides (mono-, di-, and triglycerides) are captured in the organic phase. Most older assays for triglycerides performed the analysis directly with this crude lipid extract, although some laboratories used thin-layer chromatography to further separate the lipid extract into the respective mono-, di-, and trigyceride fractions to permit analysis of each fraction individually. The mono- and diglycerides normally represent only a small fraction of the total glycerides found in fresh patient specimens; however, prolonged storage of specimens may result in increased concentrations of mono- and diglycerides due to lipolysis.

PREANALYTICAL VARIATION/PATIENT PREPARATION

Consumption of a number of foods will markedly increase triglyceride concentrations, so a 12-hour fast is required before triglyceride measurement to ensure that the specimen is obtained in a standardized fashion. Fluids, except water, should be avoided. However, such fasting is too difficult for some patients, and collection of the specimen should proceed with notation of any deviation from the protocol. Early morning specimen collections are usually preferable to afternoon blood draws, but the laboratory should try to make drawing time convenient for the patient. Because concentration is influenced by recent dietary habits, alcohol consumption, weight changes, and exercise patterns, triglyceride levels within an individual patient are highly variable. Triglyceride values may change by 20 to 30% within an individual because of these factors; therefore, it is necessary to perform a series of triglyceride measurements to establish a representative concentration.

SPECIMEN CONSIDERATIONS

Plasma and serum differences in triglycerides are similar to those of cholesterol. In the past, glycerol contamination of the specimen was a major problem because the stoppers of some evacuated specimen collection tubes were lubricated with glycerin, resulting in a significant positive bias for triglyceride assays. Manufacturers no longer use glycerin-based lubricants. Accordingly, this interference has been greatly reduced.

Whole blood should be processed within the first hour after collection. If a sample is to be analyzed on the same day, the temperature of storage is unimportant; however, samples should be stored under one of the following conditions if analysis is delayed: 4°C for 1 to 7 days; −20°C for 1 week to 3 months; and −70°C for up to 5 years.

TRADITIONAL METHODS FOR TRIGLYCERIDE DETERMINATION

Early methods for triglyceride determination involved measurement of liberated glycerol. The first step is extraction of the sample with organic solvents, followed by removal of the phospholipids and other interfering substances by adsorption of the extract onto an insoluble material (Lloyd's reagent,

$$\text{Triglycerides} \xrightarrow{\text{Alcoholic KOH}} \rightarrow \rightarrow \text{Glycerol} + 3 \text{ Fatty acids}$$

$$\text{Glycerol} + \text{ATP} \xrightarrow[\text{Kinase}]{\text{Glycerol}} \text{Glycerol-3-phosphate} + \text{ADP}$$

$$\text{ADP} + \text{Phosphoenolpyruvate} \xrightarrow[\text{Kinase}]{\text{Pyruvate}} \text{ATP} + \text{Pyruvate}$$

$$\text{Pyruvate} + \text{NADH} + \text{H}^+ \xrightarrow{\text{LDH}} \text{Lactate} + \text{NAD}^+$$

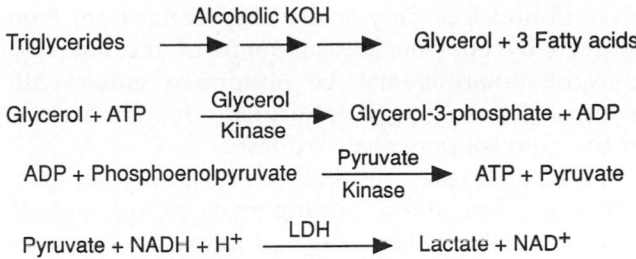

Figure 12.3. Initial enzymic triglyceride procedure. Alcoholic potassium hydroxide solution was an effective approach used to hydrolyze triglycerides prior to the availability of lipases. Glycerol kinase, pyruvate kinase, and lactate dehydrogenase enzymes to monitor production of glycerol were generally used for a number of enzymic triglyceride methods.

zeolite, diatomaceous earth, silicic acid, alumina, or Florisil). The triglycerides are then hydrolyzed to glycerol and free fatty acids by alkaline saponification, after which periodate is added to oxidize the glycerol to two molecules of formaldehyde and one of formic acid. At this point, three methods exist for glycerol determination: (*a*) reaction with phenylhydrazine and ferricyanide to produce a red-colored formazan; (*b*) condensation in a sulfuric acid medium with chromotropic acid; or (*c*) condensation with acetylacetone and ammonia to form 3,5-diacetyl-1,4-dihydrotoluidine (Hantzsch reaction). The latter method may be quantitated colorimetrically or fluorimetrically. Of these three variations, the Hantzsch reaction is the most popular. The U.S. Centers for Disease Control (CDC) uses a modified version of the chromotropic acid procedure as the reference method for triglycerides.

ENZYMIC METHODS FOR TRIGLYCERIDE DETERMINATION

Early enzymic methods for triglycerides were only "partly enzymic" in that these procedures followed the same steps as the previously noted methods up to and including alkaline hydrolysis of the lipids. An example of this approach, as well as the reaction sequence for the subsequent determination of glycerol, are shown in Figure 12.3.

The next significant advance in methods for enzymic determination of triglycerides came when lipase (from *Rhicopus delemar*) and α-chymotrypsin were incorporated into reagents to enzymatically hydrolyze fatty acid esters from the glycerol backbone. Inclusion of the protease α-chymotrypsin in the reagent improves kinetics of the ester hydrolysis by some unknown mechanism.

Currently, numerous commercial procedures are available for enzymic triglyceride assays. All start with lipolytic enzymes to hydrolyze triglyceride to glycerol and free fatty acids. Triglycerides are then assayed by enzymic measurement of the liberated glycerol. Analysis may be performed either with glycerol kinase, glycerol phosphate dehydrogenase, or the glycerol phosphate oxidase.

Glycerol kinase uses ATP to phosphorylate glycerol at the 3-position, forming glycerol-3-phosphate and ADP. Glycerol is measured indirectly by monitoring the production of ADP, as shown below in Figure 12.4. ADP is coupled with pyruvate kinase and phosphoenolpyruvate to generate ATP and pyruvate. Pyruvate, in turn, reacts with lactate dehydrogenase in the presence of NADH and a source of protons to yield lactate and NAD+. Although this method lacks sensitivity at low triglyceride concentrations, the reaction can be followed by monitoring the disappearance of NADH at 340 nm.

The glycerol-3-phosphate dehydrogenase method also uses glycerol kinase to generate a phosphorylated derivative. The dehydrogenase enzyme is coupled with glycerol-3-phosphate in the presence of NAD+ to form dihydroxyacetone phosphate and NADH (Fig. 12.5), with the increase in NADH monitored at 340 nm. This method offers greater sensitivity at lower triglyceride concentrations than the glycerol kinase assay.

The glycerol-3-phosphate oxidase method for triglycerides is based on the ability of this enzyme to oxidize glycerol in the presence of oxygen to dihydroxyacetone phosphate–generating hydrogen peroxide. The hydrogen peroxide is then measured, as in the cholesterol oxidase assays.

Advantages of enzymic assays are that these methods are easily automated and permit the direct use of serum/plasma specimens without prior extraction. Serum or plasma ordinarily contains a small amount of free glycerol, which will falsely elevate the triglyceride level. When exacting work is desired, the reaction scheme must be modified with a "blanking" approach to correct for the free glycerol by mixing the specimen with triglyceride reagent minus the lipase. Free glycerol in the specimen reacts with the reagent as if it came from triglyceride. An initial spectrophotometric reading is taken, and lipase is added to the reaction mixture, after which a second absorbance measurement is taken. The difference between the two represents the true triglyceride concentration.

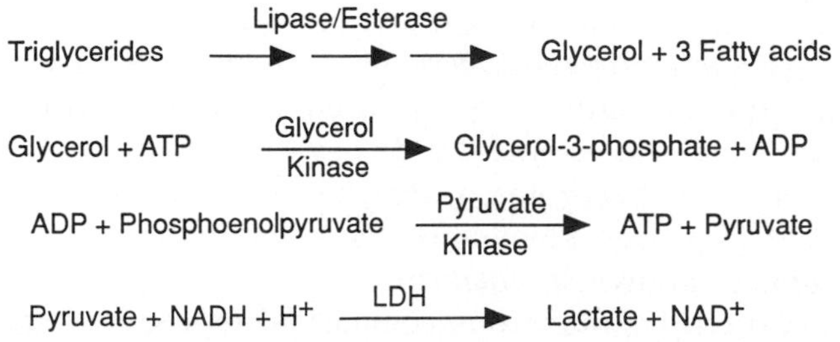

Figure 12.4. Glycerol kinase reaction scheme. Includes the lipase and esterases to generate glycerol from triglycerides.

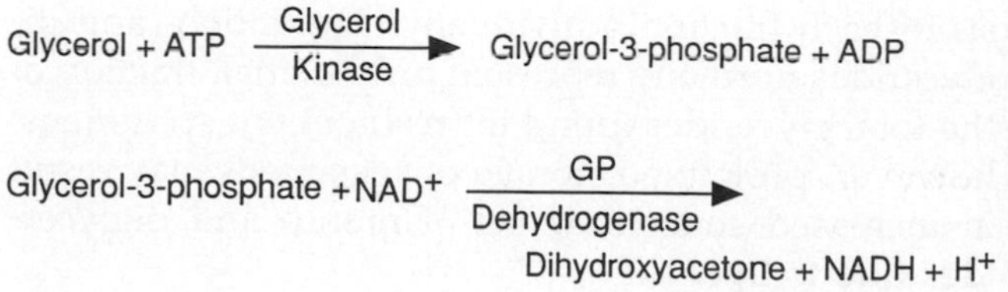

Figure 12.5. Glycerol-3-phosphate dehydrogenase scheme.

STANDARDIZATION AND PERFORMANCE REQUIREMENTS

A variety of approaches are available to calibrate triglyceride assays. Chemical methods can be calibrated with pure triglyceride standards (such as triolein) dissolved in organic solvents. Enzymic methods cannot use these primary standards because of incompatibility between organic solvents and enzymes. Activity of the enzymes is diminished or nonexistent in this environment. Although water rather than organic solvents is used, most enzymic calibrators are glycerol-based materials that can be prepared as primary standards similar to triolein. Unfortunately, glycerol per se does not function as a calibrator for the entire enzymic process. To avoid these problems, human serum-based secondary calibrators with known triglyceride values are preferred.

INTERPRETATION

Fasting triglyceride concentrations increase with age, but the gender-based difference is minimal. Laboratories can construct age-adjusted normal ranges for triglyceride based on their own studies or on published information, such as that of the Lipid Research Clinics (LRC) Program. In general, a low triglyceride value has little significance with the exception of patients being evaluated for malabsorption. Likewise, triglyceride values that exceed LRC limits on a single sample may be meaningless since the triglyceride concentration is highly variable in a given individual. Collecting a series of specimens at intervals of several weeks is more useful than an isolated value. Occasionally, a lipemic specimen with a triglyceride concentration of 500 to 10,000 mg/dl can provide important information. In this situation, without collection of a second specimen, additional lipid and lipoprotein tests are appropriate. The LRC prevalence data for triglycerides provide a range of values that are typical of the general population (Table 12.6).

As with cholesterol, triglyceride data may be expressed in either conventional units (mg/dl) or SI units (mmol/liter). To transform mg/dl to mmol/liter, multiply by 0.0113.

Nonroutine Lipid Assays

Research and reference laboratories may offer tests that are unavailable in routine clinical laboratories. Some of these specialized tests are described below.

PHOSPHOLIPIDS

Phospholipids (phosphoglycerides) have structural similarities to triglycerides in that both contain glycerol and long-chain fatty acids. However, phospholipids contain a phosphate group attached to the α-hydroxy moiety. A variety of small nitrogen-containing alcohols or carbohydrates are esterified through the phosphate group to phosphatidic acids, forming a family of phospholipids. The alcohol groups include ethanolamine, choline, serine, and inositol. Since the alcohol moiety contains a charged group, phospholipids behave as surfactants because they have both hydrophobic and hydrophilic characteristics. Therefore, phospholipids provide an ideal interface between neutral lipids and water (Fig. 12.6).

Phospholipids are among the principal components of cellular membranes. Serum or plasma phospholipids are occasionally measured in the clinical laboratory; specifically, phosphatidylcholine and sphingomyelin ratios are used to assess fetal lung maturity. Basic phospholipid measurements are performed to give a more complete analysis of individual lipoprotein structure.

Table 12.6. LRC Triglyceride Data (mg/dl)

Age	Males 5%	Males 50%	Males 95%	Females 5%	Females 50%	Females 95%
5–9	28	48	85	32	57	126
10–14	33	58	111	39	68	120
15–19	38	68	143	36	64	126
20–24	44	78	165	37	80	168
25–29	45	88	204	42	76	159
30–34	46	102	253	40	73	163
35–39	52	109	316	40	83	205
40–44	56	123	218	45	88	191
45–49	56	119	279	44	94	223
50–54	63	128	313	53	103	223
55–59	60	117	261	59	111	279
60–64	56	111	240	57	105	256
65–69	54	108	256	56	118	260
70+	63	115	239	60	110	289

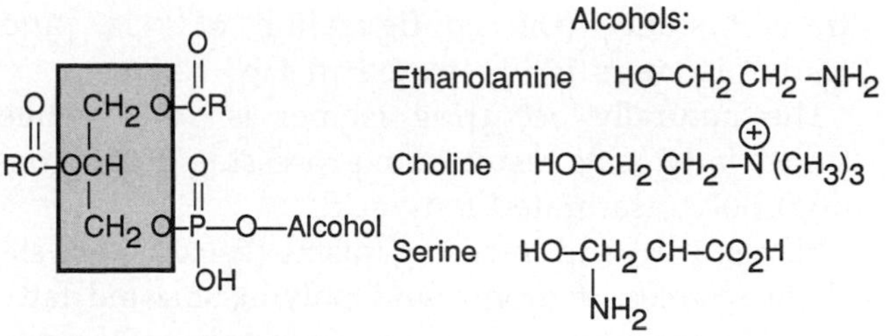

Figure 12.6. Basic phospholipid structure. The general structure of phospholipids is presented along with typical alcohols that represent a significant portion of phospholipids in serum.

Determination of serum total phospholipid is performed by various modifications of two different approaches. Enzymic procedures involve hydrolysis of choline-containing phospholipids (which constitute 91 to 97% of the total) by microbial phospholipase D to phosphatidic acid and choline. The choline is subsequently oxidized in the presence of choline oxidase to betaine aldehyde and then to the acid betaine, generating two molecules of hydrogen peroxide (H_2O_2). The H_2O_2 is utilized in a color-generating "Trinder" reaction.

Older techniques for measuring serum total phospholipids required separation of the organic from inorganic phosphorus, followed by digestion of the organic material, and subsequent phosphorus determination. These methods, which require hazardous reagents, measure total phospholipid phosphorus rather than just the choline-containing fraction.

FREE FATTY ACIDS

Nonesterified (free) fatty acids are a minor constituent in circulating plasma. The majority of free fatty acids (FFA) in circulation is bound to albumin. Naturally occurring fatty acids vary in length from 14 to 24 carbon atoms (including the carboxylic acid carbon). Only fatty acids with even numbers of carbon atoms are produced in humans, and fatty acids are further categorized by their degree of unsaturation. Saturated fatty acids lack double bonds and are the principal type of fatty acid in animal tissue. Monounsaturated fatty acids contain one double bond, whereas polyunsaturated fatty acids contain two or more double bonds. The presence of double bonds has a significant influence on the spatial configuration of the molecule. In long-chain saturated fatty acids, the carbon atoms stay within a line with free rotation. Double bonds restrict the rotation at the site of the bond and cause the carbon atoms to move offline. Double bonds can exist with either a "cis" or "trans" isomer (the configuration of "cis" and "trans" isomers is illustrated in Fig. 12.7.

The naturally occurring isomer is "cis," while "trans" fatty acids result from processing (hydrogenating) polyunsaturated fatty acids.

Plants, fish, and microorganisms (bacteria) are excellent sources of mono- and polyunsaturated fatty acids. Polyunsaturated fatty acids may be referred to as "essential" in humans who are unable to synthesize specific unsaturated fatty acids. Linoleic acid is an essential fatty acid from plants that must be part of human diets.

The primary physiological function of long-chain fatty acids is to provide energy to cells by an oxidative process referred to as β-oxidation. Considerable energy is generated by β-oxidation of fatty acids, but only half of the released energy can be used by the cells, with the remainder being released in the form of heat. Essential fatty acids are necessary precursors for prostaglandins, which function as metabolic mediators and play a vital role in regulating a wide variety of physiological functions.

Determination of FFA in serum or plasma is rarely performed in clinical medicine. Generally, FFA concentrations in healthy individuals are 0.30 to 1.10 mmol/liter, but increased amounts occur when FFA is released into blood in large quantities from adipose tissue stimulated by disorders with excessive hormones—especially ACTH, epinephrine, and norepinephrine. FFA is also increased in patients following prolonged fasting or after receiving intravenous heparin therapy.

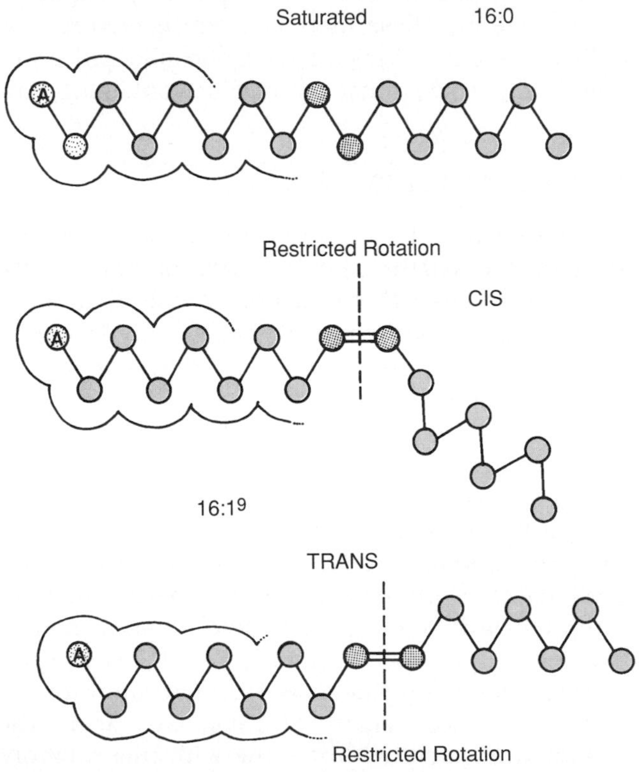

Figure 12.7. Saturated and unsaturated fatty acids. Note the restricted rotation associated with unsaturation and the impact on space dependent on the cis or trans configuration.

Table 12.7. Typical Fatty Acids in Blood

Code[a]	Generic Name	Scientific Name
12:0	Lauric	Dodecanoic
14:0	Myristic	Tetradecanoic
16:0	Palmitic	Hexadecanoic
16:1^{9}	Palmitoleic	9-Hexadecenoic
18:0	Stearic	Octadecanoic
18:1^{9}	Oleic	9-Octadecenoic
18:2^{9,12}	Linoleic	9,12-Octadecadienoic
18:3^{9,12,15}	Linolenic	9,12,15-Octadecantrienoic
20:0	Arachidic	Eicosanoic
20:4^{5,8,11,14}	Arachadonic	5,8,11,14-Eicosatetraenoic

[a]The first number refers to carbon atoms, and the second number indicates double bonds, with their position from the carboxyl end noted by superscripts.

Traditional methods for FFA determination involve either titration of the total free acid or measurement of the amount of copper reagent complexed by FFA. Both of these procedures involve organic extraction of fatty acids from the sample, either free or complexed with copper. More recently, two enzymic approaches have been introduced. Both enzymic systems involve acyl-CoA synthetase–catalyzed formation of a fatty acid–CoA complex from FFA, ATP, and CoA. One method then utilizes the AMP (a by-product of the first reaction) along with the acyl-CoA, which, in the presence of ATP and myokinase, form two molecules of ADP. ADP is subsequently measured by the decrease in absorbance at 340 nm since NADH is oxidized by phosphoenolpyruvate, pyruvate kinase-, and the lactate dehydrogenase-coupled system. The second enzymic approach requires complex formation of unreacted CoA with *N*-ethylmaleimide, followed by oxidation of the fatty acid–CoA complex with acyl-CoA oxidase to form 2,3-trans-enol-CoA and hydrogen peroxide. The amount of generated peroxide is subsequently measured by a peroxidase-coupled "Trinder" reaction. The latter method is available through commercial sources and has been favorably compared to the previously mentioned copper complexation.

LIPOPROTEINS

Lipid compounds must be capable of movement between cells and tissues to perform their various functions. Because lipids are insoluble in aqueous solution, a system is needed to transport these compounds in the body. This is accomplished by packaging lipids into structures called lipoproteins.

Lipoproteins are composites of lipid and protein that provide solubility in aqueous media. Lipoproteins are large macromolecular complexes that have a spherical shape with neutral lipid (triglycerides and cholesterol esters) at the center surrounded by free cholesterol, phospholipids, and proteins on the surface. Specific proteins (apolipoproteins) constitute the protein component of lipoproteins. Apolipoproteins have both hydrophilic and hydrophobic domains, such that part of the apolipoprotein prefers to be in an aqueous environment and the other protein portion wants to interact with lipid material at the core of the complex.

Nomenclature for lipoproteins depends on the methods used to isolate these proteins. For example, electrophoresis separates the individual lipoprotein families based on their electrophoretic mobility relative to serum proteins. Chylomicrons, triglyceride-rich lipoproteins, do not migrate on electrophoretic gels and are not classified by this method. Ultracentrifugation separates lipoproteins on the basis of their density; therefore, ultracentrifugation uses relative density of the lipoprotein for classification. Table 12.8 compares two systems of nomenclature based on ultracentrifugation and electrophoretic methods.

Lipoprotein families are designed by initials derived from their ultracentrifugation classification—VLDL, LDL, and HDL. Chylomicrons are the exception since they have a lower density than serum (less than 1.006 g/ml). The nomenclature is further complicated since each lipoprotein family represents a mixture of lipoprotein complexes. For example, HDL may be further subdivided into HDL-2 and HDL-3 fractions. The density of lipoproteins is related to both triglyceride and protein content, with lower densities associated with increasing triglyceride content and decreasing content of protein. Size is another useful characteristic that can distinguish various lipoprotein classes. The triglyceride-rich lipoproteins (chylomicrons and VLDL) are the largest particles, with approximate diameters ranging from 80 to 1000 nm and from 30 to 80 nm, respectively. LDL and HDL are much smaller particles, with diameters ranging from 20 to 25 nm and 5 to 10 nm, respectively. These size differences are shown schematically in Figure 12.8.

Table 12.8. Lipoprotein Nomenclature

Ultracentrifugation	Electrophoretic Mobility
Chylomicron	
Very low-density lipoprotein (VLDL)	Pre-β
Low-density lipoprotein (LDL)	β
High-density lipoprotein (HDL)	α

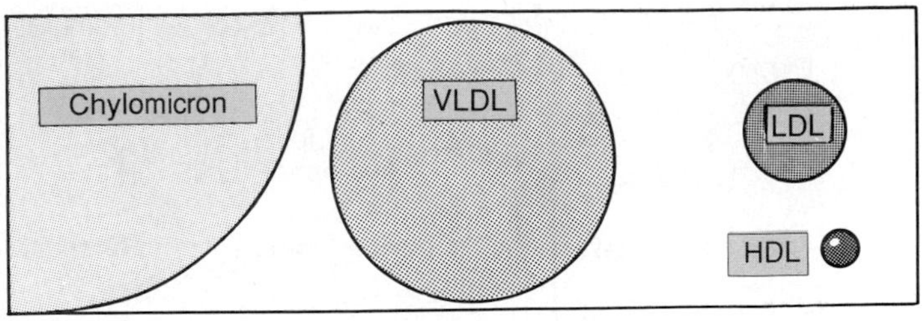

Figure 12.8. Relative lipoprotein sizes. The spheres are generally representative of typical sizes of the various lipoproteins. Considerable fluctuation and variability occur within each individual lipoprotein class.

Lipoprotein Metabolism

Lipoprotein metabolism may be divided into two separate but interrelated parts. The first part—designated exogenous metabolism—deals with lipids derived from outside sources (food). The second part concerns endogenous metabolism, which involves lipid and lipoproteins derived from the liver and other internal sources (Fig. 12.9).

EXOGENOUS METABOLISM

About 40% of the calories in a typical American diet come from fats, with protein and carbohydrate contributing the remaining 60%. As food enters the small intestine, pancreatic digestive enzymes (amylase, peptidases, and lipases) are released. These enzymes digest complex molecules from the food into metabolites that are more readily absorbed than the parent molecules. Fats (triglycerides) are hydrolyzed by lipases to free fatty acids and monoglycerides. These metabolites are readily absorbed by the intestinal mucosa and subsequently are resynthesized into triglycerides and phospholipids. These newly formed lipids are packaged into large triglyceride-rich lipoproteins called chylomicrons, which pass into the lymphatics. The chylomicron-rich lymph ultimately drains into circulating blood through the thoracic duct. Absorption of dietary triglycerides occurs rapidly following a meal, and peak serum triglyceride concentrations can be observed within 30 to 90 minutes. In the blood, triglyceride-rich chylomicrons interact with lipoprotein lipase, an enzyme bound to the capillary surface of the vascular endothelium. The function of lipoprotein lipase is to hydrolyze triglyceride to fatty acids and glycerides. These metabolites are absorbed by cells to which the enzyme is bound. Inside the cell, the hydrolyzed products are resynthesized to triglycerides for energy storage. Repeated lipolytic action by lipoprotein lipase reduces the triglyceride content of the chylomicron, ultimately forming a chylomicron rem-

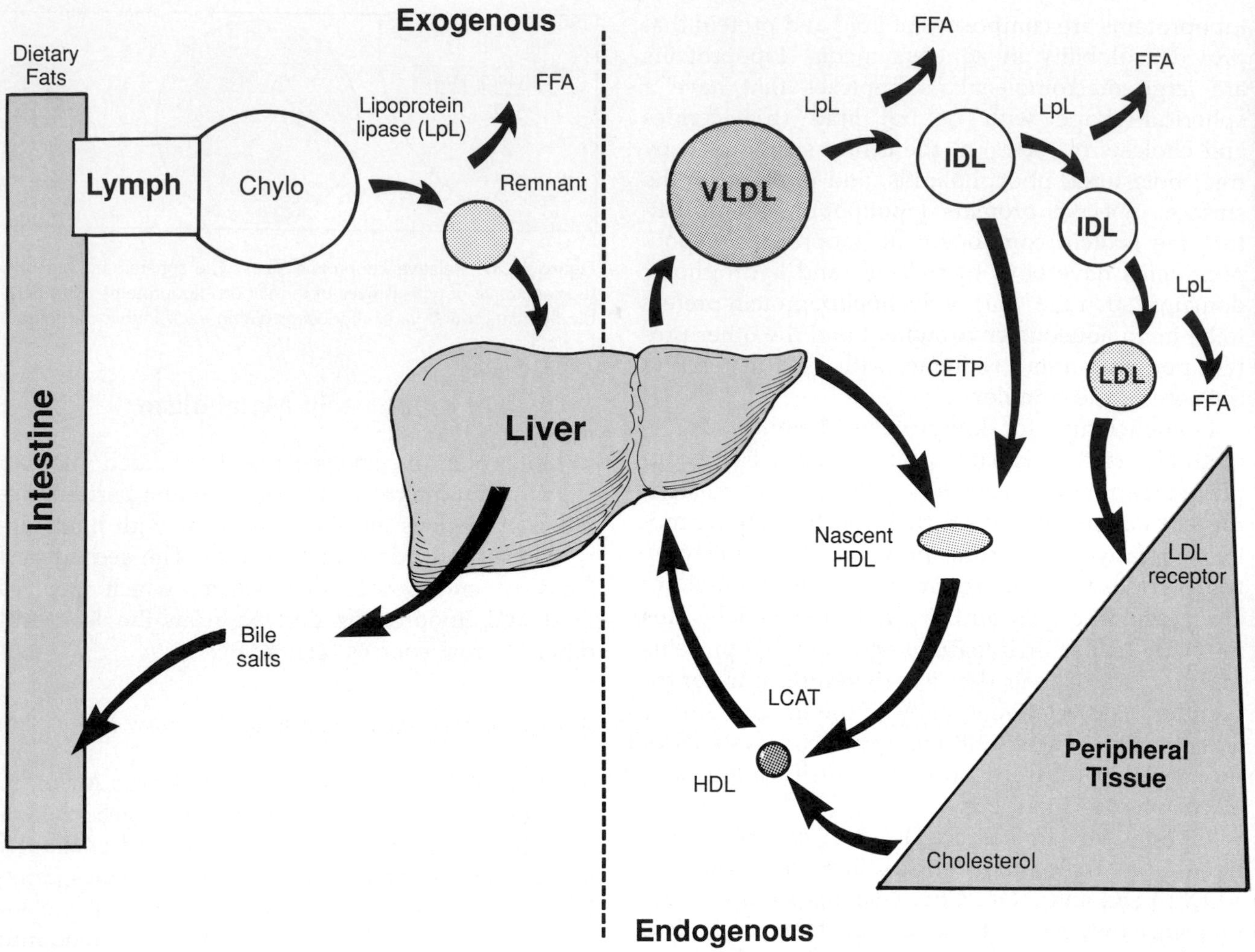

Figure 12.9. Lipid metabolism. Endogenous and exogenous lipid and lipoprotein metabolic system centered on the liver.

nant that is rapidly cleared by the liver, which has receptors for the remnant.

ENDOGENOUS METABOLISM

The liver is the principal organ for lipid metabolism and is the primary site of lipoprotein synthesis. Triglyceride and cholesterol in hepatic cells are packaged and secreted into the circulation as triglyceride-rich VLDL. Lipoprotein lipase interacts with VLDL in the same manner as with chylomicrons by hydrolyzing the triglyceride. In the case of VLDL, loss of triglyceride results in intermediate-density lipoproteins (IDL) of increasing cholesterol content. LDL is the final product from extensive lipolysis of VLDL.

LDL is the principal transport mechanism of cholesterol to peripheral tissues. LDL binds to cell surface receptors and is incorporated into the cell, so cholesterol content of the LDL complex is added to the intracellular pool and provides a mechanism to down-regulate cellular cholesterol synthesis.

HDL is derived from liver and intestine and is released into circulation in a form that does not resemble typical spherical lipoproteins. HDL acts like a sponge, absorbing lipid from other lipoproteins or cells. As lipid is absorbed by HDL, the lipoprotein assumes a spherical shape. HDL is thought to function as a reverse cholesterol transport system regulating the movement of cholesterol from peripheral tissue back to the liver. Reverse cholesterol transport is important to prevent the formation of cholesterol-rich plaques in vascular tissues. Free cholesterol from the cells is esterified within HDL catalyzed by an enzyme, lecithin-cholesterol acyl transferase (LCAT). In addition, cholesterol ester transport proteins (CETPs) present in serum interact with HDL to exchange triglyceride from VLDL and LDL with cholesterol esters. Cholesterol transported to the liver by HDL can be recirculated as VLDL or serve as a precursor for the synthesis of bile salts. Bile salts are transported to the intestine through the bile duct to promote additional lipid absorption.

Thus, VLDL, LDL, and HDL interact to maintain necessary intracellular lipid needs. Lipids are transported to peripheral tissues to provide substrate for

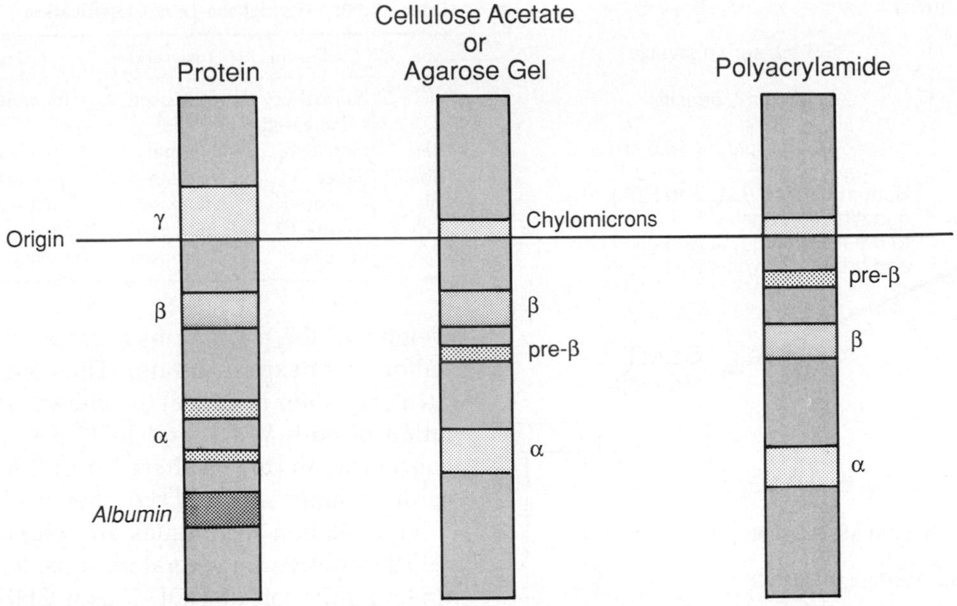

Figure 12.10. Comparison of electrophoresis systems. Lipoprotein separation patterns for cellulose acetate and agarose gel are similar. Polyacrylamide separates lipoproteins based on size and, therefore, pre-β and β lipoproteins are opposite from the cellulose acetate/agarose gels. Both systems are compared to protein electrophoresis, from which the lipoprotein fractions derive their nomenclature.

energy metabolism and synthetic functions. For example, cholesterol is transported to the adrenal cortex where it is required to synthesize corticosteroids, mineral corticoids, and adrenal androgens.

Separation/Isolation of Lipoproteins

Lipoproteins can be separated and isolated by exploiting their physicochemical characteristics, including size, buoyancy, and charge. Nondenaturing electrophoresis separates lipoproteins based on both their size and charge differences, whereas ultracentrifugation separates lipoproteins based on their hydrated densities.

LIPOPROTEIN ELECTROPHORESIS

Numerous electrophoretic techniques have been used for lipoprotein analysis, including paper, cellulose acetate, agarose gel, and polyacrylamide. For identification, lipid dyes may be used to stain the resulting bands. Common lipid stains (fat red 7B, oil red O, and Sudan black) are nonspecific for cholesterol, triglycerides, or phospholipids; thus, the ability to quantitate lipoproteins by electrophoresis is limited. One approach that has been used is to stain gels with enzymes specific for cholesterol. However, these enzyme systems are limited by sensitivity and have not been widely used.

Nomenclature for lipoproteins separated by electrophoresis is based on their mobility to other serum proteins (Fig. 12.10). Chylomicrons are too large to enter the gel, so chylomicrons remain at the origin. Agarose gel electrophoresis systems separate lipoproteins based on charge and size of the complex, and three classes of lipoproteins are resolved with the following relative mobility: β less than pre-β less than α.

ULTRACENTRIFUGATION

Lipoproteins can be separated on the basis of their hydrated densities using ultracentrifugation by adjusting the density of the plasma with high-salt solutions. Ultracentrifugation procedures have been used in clinical and research laboratories to isolate lipoprotein fractions that are quantitated by lipid analysis. Some of the disadvantages of this approach are long spin times (18 to 20 hours), large sample requirements (3 to 5 ml), and the technical skill required to prepare density gradients. The advantage of ultracentrifugation is that large volumes of serum or plasma can be processed to isolate individual lipoprotein fractions. The CDC Lipid Standardization Laboratory utilizes ultracentrifugation as part of the reference method for HDL analysis. The CDC spins the specimen at a density of 1.006 g/ml with the ultracentrifuge to remove the triglyceride-rich chylomicrons and VLDLs that may be present (illustrated in Fig. 12.11). The resultant bottom fraction is subsequently used for selective precipitation of the LDL with heparin and manganese chloride to isolate HDL. Finally, the cholesterol content of HDL is measured with the modified Abell-Kendall method.

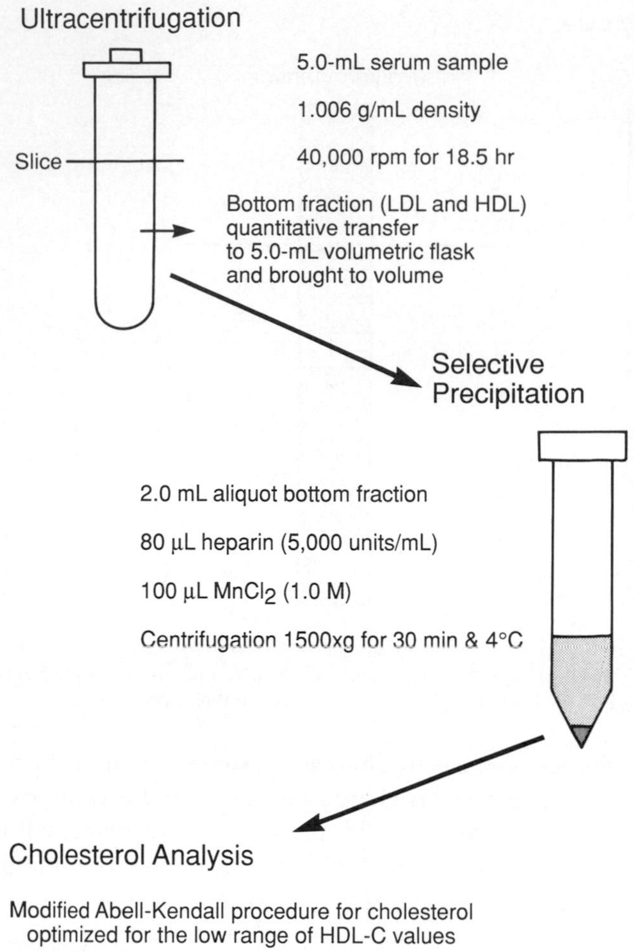

Figure 12.11. CDC HDL-C reference method. The Centers for Disease Control use a tedious three-step procedure to assign HDL-C reference values to human-based serum pools used for standardization efforts.

Table 12.9. HDL Reagents

Heparin and $MnCL_2$
Heparin and $CaCl_2$
Dextran sulfate and $MgCl_2$
Phosphotungstate and $MgCl_2$
Polyethylene glycol

SELECTIVE PRECIPITATION

Solutions of polyanionic compounds (heparin, dextran sulfate, and phosphotungstic acid) with divalent cations added to serum alters the solubility of specific lipoproteins, causing them to precipitate. Apo B-containing lipoproteins (chylomicrons, VLDL, and LDL) become insoluble as they interact with these reagents, and HDL supernatants are recovered following centrifugation. Table 12.9 lists several common reagent combinations used for selective precipitation.

Several variations of each of these methods include the use of different polymeric molecular weights of the polyanions (such as 50,000 or 500,000 daltons for dextran sulfate). The concentration of the divalent cation is critical to achieve complete precipitation of both VLDL and LDL. The apparent cation concentration can be altered if EDTA plasma is used as the sample, since EDTA chelates Mn^{2+} or Mg^{2+}.

Precipitation techniques are widely used by clinical laboratories for several reasons: (*a*) interest in routine quantitation of HDL-C as a CHD risk factor; (*b*) expensive equipment (such as the ultracentrifuge) is unnecessary; (*c*) cholesterol analysis is performed directly on the supernatant; and (*d*) the method can be partially automated for high-volume laboratories.

HDL-C is more readily and accurately quantitated by selective precipitation than with ultracentrifugation or electrophoresis. Currently, most clinical laboratories use either dextran sulfate or sodium phosphotungstate procedures for HDL-C analysis. Future approaches may include direct and selective isolation of lipoprotein fractions using immune complexes (antigen-antibody) to permit independent analysis of HDL-C, LDL-C, or even VLDL-C.

Table 12.10. Fredrickson-Levy Classification

Type	Cholesterol	Triglycerides	Abnormal Lipoproteins
I	Normal or increased	Increased	Increased chylos
IIa	Increased	Normal	Increased LDL
IIb	Increased	Increased	Increased VLDL and LDL
III	Increased	Increased	Increased IDL
IV	Normal	Increased	Increased VLDL
V	Increased	Increased	Increased chylos and VLDL

LIPOPROTEIN INTERPRETATION

Over 20 years ago, Fredrickson and Levy introduced their method of classifying hyperlipidemias, and their approach has become the standard procedure. The Fredrickson-Levy classification is a systematic scheme of assigning abnormal lipid and lipoprotein patterns to specific groups based on concentrations. Table 12.10 lists the various classifications and general lipid and lipoprotein characteristics.

Once an individual's lipid and lipoprotein patterns have been assigned to one of the aforementioned types, the physician must determine if the abnormal pattern is the result of a primary (hereditary) problem or a secondary cause. Several diseases or disorders can result in an abnormal lipoprotein pattern, and treatment for any individual should focus on the secondary problem prior to treating the abnormal lipid status. Correcting secondary disorders (Table 12.11) may normalize the lipid pattern.

A hypercholesterolemic (increased cholesterol) pattern in an individual who has no secondary cause

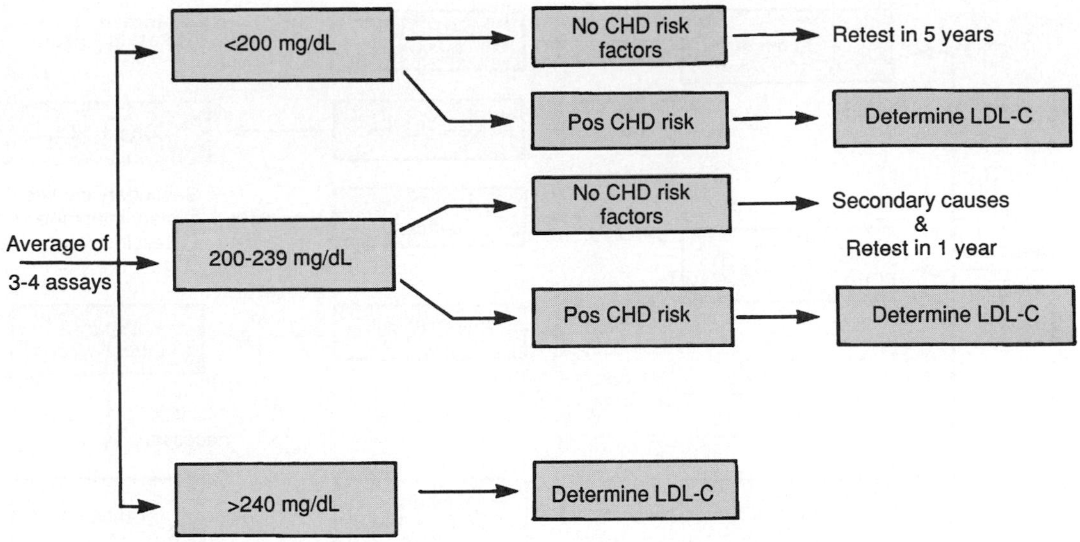

Figure 12.12. Assessment of initial cholesterol results. The National Cholesterol Education Programs recommend that individual cholesterol be assessed on the basis of concentration of cholesterol and the presence of coronary heart disease risk factors.

Table 12.11. Secondary Lipid Disorders

Increased Cholesterol	Increased Triglycerides
Cholestasis	Diabetes
Hypothyroidism	Nephrotic syndrome
Liver disease	Alcoholism
Porphyria	Pancreatitis
	Glycogen storage disease

Table 12.12. CHD Risk Assessment

Risk Factors	Definitive Disease
Male	Previous MI
Family CHD history	Angina
Hypertension	
Cigarette smoking (>10/day)	
Low HDL (<35 mg/dl)	
Diabetes mellitus	
Vascular disease	
Obesity (30% overweight)	

for high cholesterol is considered to represent increased risk for cardiovascular disease. The National Institutes of Health, through the NCEP and its Adult Treatment Panel, developed uniform guidelines for treating hypercholesterolemia. The Adult Treatment Panel recommends assessment of an individual's risk for coronary heart disease (CHD) on the basis of two or more of the risk factors listed in Table 12.12 or definitive disease.

Physicians manage patients based on specific risk factors. For example, hypertension, diabetes, cigarette smoking, and obesity are all cardiovascular disease risk factors that can be managed through proper therapy, diet, or behavior modification. Other risk factors, such as age, sex, and family history of cardiovascular disease, are beyond the control of the physician or patient. To further establish a patient's risk for CHD, cholesterol testing must be performed with possible follow-up including additional lipoprotein analyses (Fig. 12.12).

Table 12.13. LDL-Cholesterol CHD Risk Assessment

LDL-Cholesterol	CHD Risk
mg/dl	
<130	Desirable LDL
130–159	Borderline high
≥160	High LDL

Cholesterol analysis is only the first step a physician uses to assess an individual's potential hyperlipidemia. Since cholesterol measurement can be performed on nonfasting specimens, this test serves as a good screening test. Actual follow-up and treatment guidelines for adults with increased cholesterol are based on the combination of individual CHD risk factors and LDL-cholesterol value as outlined in Table 12.13 and in Figure 12.13.

APOLIPOPROTEINS

Apolipoproteins are specialized proteins that are capable of binding lipid material while simultaneously interacting with aqueous media. Portions of apolipoproteins have hydrophobic properties that associate with lipid material, while other areas of the protein exhibit hydrophilic characteristics that permit interaction with the aqueous phase of plasma. Apolipoproteins function as the interface between lipid and water and allow lipid to be transported in aqueous media. Apolipoproteins are associated with specific lipoproteins. Table 12.14 shows the amount of

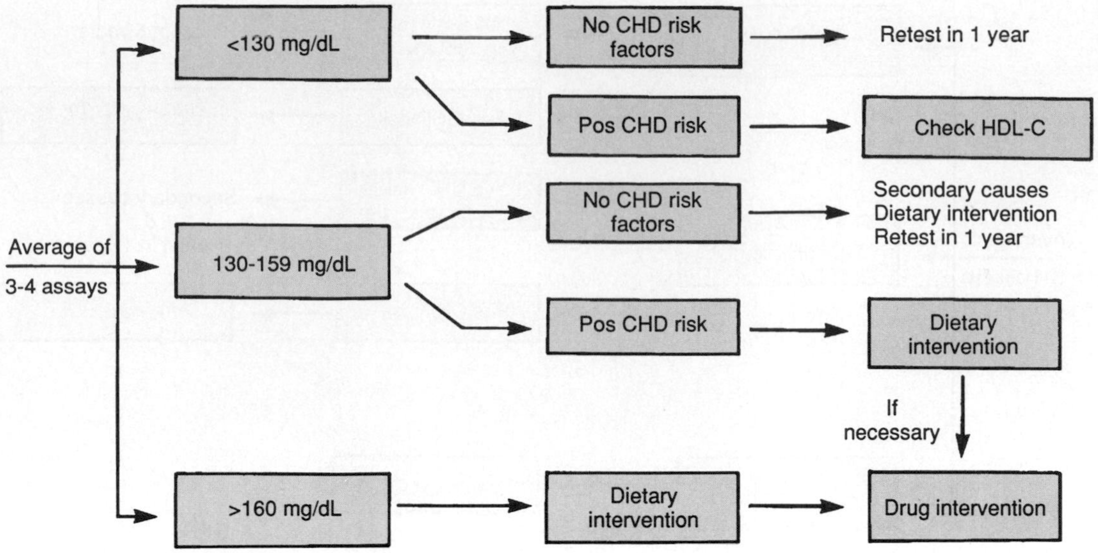

Figure 12.13. Assessment of LDL-cholesterol results. Recommendation and guidelines for the treatment of adult hypercholesterolemia are based on both LDL-cholesterol results and existing cardiovascular disease. All treatment regimens start with dietary intervention before the use of cholesterol-lowering drugs.

Table 12.14. Apolipoproteins

Abbreviation	Quantity	Lipoprotein Association
	mg/dl	
A–I	70–180	Chylos and HDL
A–II	20–50	HDL
A–IV	10–15	Chylos and HDL
(a)	0–60	Lp(a)
B–48	—	Chylos
B–100	50–160	VLDL and LDL
C–I–III	20–100	Chylos, VLDL, and HDL
E	10–60	Chylos, VLDL, and HDL

Table 12.15. General Apolipoprotein Functions

1. Transport and bind lipophilic compounds
2. Regulation of lipoprotein metabolism
3. Expression of lipoprotein immunogenicity
4. Recognition for tissue receptor
5. Backbone of lipoprotein structure

specific apolipoproteins found in plasma and lipoproteins in which they are found.

In addition to the function of lipid transport, apolipoproteins mediate several enzyme activities, such as lipoprotein lipase. Apolipoprotein molecules are recognized by receptors on the surface of cells, thus facilitating lipid uptake by cells. Table 12.15 lists some of their important functions.

In biological specimens, the ability of apolipoproteins to associate with lipids affects the choice of methods used to quantitate these proteins. Conventional techniques for protein analysis cannot be directly applied to apolipoproteins since the lipid material must first be removed by extraction techniques to isolate apolipoproteins. Measurement of the apolipoprotein content of lipoproteins by immunoassay must include a delipidation step to free the apolipoprotein from lipid. This step is necessary to expose antigenic binding sites on the apolipoprotein. A variety of delipidation procedures are available, and the apolipoprotein value is dependent on the selected method. Considerable disagreement arises regarding the different methods for apolipoprotein analysis in that the process of delipidation may alter conformation of the protein. With lipid removed, apolipoproteins change their protein structure and may aggregate when concentrated for use as calibration materials. In addition, some purified apolipoproteins have problems of limited solubility in aqueous media, especially apolipoprotein B. Collectively, these problems have limited the application of apolipoprotein methods in routine clinical work.

Apolipoprotein B

Apolipoprotein B (apo B) is the largest of the apolipoproteins (molecular weight of approximately 500,000). Apo B is difficult to study because the delipidated protein is insoluble in aqueous media. Most apo B in serum is associated with LDL, with lesser amounts in chylomicrons and VLDL. Apo B exists in two forms: apo B-100 and apo B-48. Apo B-100 is synthesized in the liver and is the primary protein of LDL and VLDL. Apo B-48 is derived from the intestine and is associated with chylomicrons. Apo B-100 is the principal transport mechanism for endogenous cholesterol, and apo B-48 serves to transport exogenous lipid. Apo B-100 binds to the LDL receptor located on cell surfaces in peripheral tissue and is

Table 12.16. Immunoassay Methods

Radioimmunoassay (RIA)
Electroimmunoassay (EIA)
Radial immunodiffusion (RID)
Enzyme-linked immunoassays (ELISA)
Nephelometric immunoassay (NIA)
Turbidometric immunoassay (TIA)

involved with cellular deposition of cholesterol. Apo B-48 does not bind to the LDL receptor and its half-life is just a few hours, whereas the half-life of B-100 is a few days. Therefore, assays for apo B using fasting specimens measure primarily the B-100 protein.

IMMUNOASSAYS FOR APO B

Several options are available to measure apolipoprotein B. Table 12.16 lists some analytical approaches that are commercially available. The precision of the method should have a coefficient of variation (CV) of less than 5%.

STANDARDIZATION AND PERFORMANCE REQUIREMENTS

Apolipoprotein assays have been developed in research laboratories, and each laboratory prepares its own source of antigen and antibodies. As a result, there is a significant lack of agreement between laboratories. Part of the reason for the disagreement lies in the variation in techniques used to delipidate apo B. For example, some apo B methods perform the assay directly on the intact lipoprotein without delipidation, while other procedures use detergents to remove lipid from apo B. A coordinated effort is needed to standardize apo B methods. In addition, standard reference materials and calibrators need to be developed to resolve the lack of consistency in results.

INTERPRETATION

Only recently have apolipoproteins been commercially available for routine use. Previously, apolipoproteins were reserved for specialized research laboratories. Because apolipoprotein assays have not been standardized, the responsibility of interpretation belongs to individual laboratories that generally must rely on manufacturers to provide interpretive information. The time and costs required to establish in-house "normal" value studies are prohibitive.

Apolipoprotein B values are generally higher in males than in females—an expected outcome because the same trend is seen with LDL, the principal source of apo B in serum or plasma. Typical apo B adult reference ranges are 45 to 120 mg/dl for females and 50 to 125 mg/dl for males. These values represent the 5 to 95% reference range. However, the use of a 5 to 95% reference range as "normal" may be misleading, since patients in the upper normal range may exhibit an increased risk for cardiovascular heart disease. It may be more appropriate to consider individuals having apo B values above the 75% limit as having increased risk toward CHD. NCEP has ignored apo B as part of its CHD risk assessment and treatment recommendation.

Apolipoprotein A-I

Apolipoprotein A-I (apo A-I) is synthesized in the liver and intestine and is released into circulation in association with nascent HDL (liver) and chylomicrons (intestine). Apo A-I is the major protein constituent of HDL, and lesser amounts are found in chylomicrons. Trace levels are also associated with VLDL. Apo A-I plays an important role in the reverse cholesterol transport system. LCAT, the enzyme that esterifies cholesterol in the reverse cholesterol transport system, requires apo A-I for activation.

IMMUNOASSAYS FOR APO A-I

Numerous techniques are available to measure apo A-I in patient specimens. All the methods listed for apo B can also be applied to apo A-I. Generally, the nephelometric and turbidimetric assays for apo A-I have been the most widely used in clinical laboratories. Radiolabeled and radial immunodiffusion assays have been used to a lesser extent because of the tendency to avoid the use of radioactive materials and imprecise methods.

STANDARDIZATION AND PERFORMANCE REQUIREMENTS

Since apo A-I is considerably smaller and exhibits greater solubility in water than apo B, many of the difficult problems associated with apo B are more readily solved. Comparative data with many of the commercially available methods show good agreement. Key considerations for selecting a method are reproducibility (precision) and available instrumentation.

INTERPRETATION

Interpretation of the apo A-I values is difficult. In general, as HDL increases, apo A-I increases. Reference ranges for apo A-I vary with the method used and the sex of the individual being tested. Since apo A-I reflects the HDL content of the serum or plasma, and HDL levels are greater in females, apo A-I values are also higher in females than males. Typical 5 to 95% reference ranges for apo A-I are 75 to 160 mg/dl for males and 80 to 175 mg/dl for females. Until methods for measuring apo A-I are standardized, quantitation of this apolipoprotein will have only limited clinical usefulness.

Electrophoretic Assays for Apolipoproteins

Immunoassays are useful for measuring specific proteins, but electrophoresis permits evaluation of the pattern of multiple proteins in the same sample. Several electrophoretic approaches for apolipoproteins include polyacrylamide gel, isofocusing, and two-dimensional electrophoresis.

Prior to electrophoresis, intact lipoproteins must be isolated using chromatographic (gel permeation, ion exchange, and affinity chromatography) or ultracentrifugation techniques. For example, VLDL can be isolated by using ultracentrifugation at density 1.006 g/ml. Delipidation of the isolated lipoproteins can then be performed with solvent mixtures, such as chloroform and methanol. Delipidated proteins are then resolubilized in buffer and subjected to electrophoresis.

POLYACRYLAMIDE GEL ELECTROPHORESIS

Polyacrylamide gel electrophoresis (PAGE) in the presence of sodium dodecyl sulfate (SDS) separates proteins based on size. A wide range of molecular weights exists among the apolipoproteins—from 500,000 (apo B) to 6,000 (C-I). Therefore, gradient or discontinuous polyacrylamide gels are used to separate apolipoproteins. Reducing agents, such as mercaptoethanol and dithiothreitol, may be added to cleave disulfide linkages between the apolipoproteins (especially with apo A-II, which exhibits significant dimerization). A comparison between the reduced and unreduced samples will assist with identification of apolipoprotein bands.

ISOELECTRIC FOCUSING

Some of the apolipoproteins, such as apo E, exist in several phenotypes (isoforms) that can be separated based on their electrophoretic mobilities in a polyacrylamide gel containing a pH gradient. The apo E isoforms are separated on the basis of their respective cysteine/arginine content. Various apo E isoforms have been designated E-2, E-3, and E-4 and are inherited traits. Individuals homozygous for apo E-2 have an apo E with a lower affinity for the apo E receptor. These individuals have a reduced ability to clear or metabolize VLDL remnants or intermediate-density lipoproteins (IDL). Type III hyperlipidemic patients have the apo E-2 phenotype, but not all individuals with apo E-2 are Type IIIs. Performing isoelectric focusing may therefore provide useful information in some patients with hyperlipidemia.

TWO-DIMENSIONAL ELECTROPHORESIS

Combining multiple electrophoretic techniques adds significantly to the resolving power of individual methods. Two-dimensional electrophoresis generates a complex electrophoretic pattern that requires interpretation by skilled personnel. Typically, isoelectric focusing is performed in one dimension and gradient polyacrylamide electrophoresis in the second. In the future, computer-assisted pattern recognition programs will assist in the interpretation of patterns generated with this technique. However, at present the method is limited to research laboratories.

Suggested Readings

Lipids and Lipoproteins

Atherosclerosis: metabolism, risk, and control. The Eleventh Annual Arnold O. Beckman Conference on Clinical Chemistry. Clin Chem 1988;34:B1–B135.

Fortmann SP, Maron DT. Disorders in lipid metabolism. In: Rubenstein E, Federman DD, eds. Scientific American medicine. New York: Scientific American, 1978–1991;9(2):1–21.

Laboratory

Albers JJ, Segrest JP, eds. Methods in enzymology: plasma lipoproteins. Part B, characterization, cell biology and metabolism. Orlando, FL: Academic Press, 1986;129.

Mills GL, Lane PA, Weech PK. Laboratory techniques in biochemistry and molecular biology: a guidebook to lipoprotein technique. Amsterdam: Elsevier, 1984.

Rafai N, Warnick GR, eds. Methods for clinical laboratory measurement of lipid and lipoprotein risk factors. Washington, DC: AACC Press, 1991.

Segrest JP, Albers JJ, eds. Methods in enzymology: plasma lipoproteins. Part A, preparation, structure and molecular biology. Orlando, FL: Academic Press, 1986;128.

13 Endocrine Function and Carbohydrates

Bruce F. Bower and Robert E. Moore

Hormones are a group of diverse biomolecules that are carried by the circulation and interact with specific cells and receptors to produce a precise cellular response. These hormones may be of low molecular weight such as steroids or thyronines or they can be more structurally complex peptides such as thyroid stimulating hormone (TSH) and growth hormone (GH). Each hormone is under the influence of stimulatory and inhibitory factors that act to provide the exquisite control of biological processes—the hallmark of endocrine systems.

Recognizing the extremes in molecular size, it is not difficult to anticipate a similar extreme in physical and chemical characteristics. Since the circulation is essentially a water-based system, the insolubility of organic compounds with extensive ring structures has been overcome by attaching these small molecules to large soluble proteins called binding or transport proteins. This serves several purposes. First, the secreting cells have few limitations in terms of distance from the target tissue. Second, this stabilizes the concentration of circulating hormone and is a reserve of inactive hormone that can be readily converted to the active form. The active hormone is usually an unbound or free form in equilibrium with the bound form. This relationship between bound and unbound hormone is under biological control. In other words, the concentration of free hormone can be rigorously controlled independent of the concentration of bound hormone.

In the case of peptides, which are generally soluble and of sufficient size to make instantaneous synthesis and secretion improbable, the existence of prohormones or hormone precursors has been demonstrated. In this instance the peptide is synthesized in a form that has little, if any, biological or pharmacological activity. The precursor hormone is stored and can subsequently undergo enzymatic alteration to be converted to the active peptide. Analogous to the bound-unbound state of small hormones, the active-inactive form of proteins and peptides gives rise to a point of control. Another type of control mechanism common to all hormones is feedback control. This can be either positive or negative. When the secretion of one hormone is stimulated by the increased concentration of a different hormone, the effect is called positive feedback. The observed increase in luteinizing hormone concentration following the administration of estrogen is an example of positive feedback. Negative feedback is what the name implies. A hormone concentration that is increasing under the influence of a stimulatory or releasing hormone will cause the secretion of that releasing hormone to diminish or stop. Pituitary TSH will stimulate the thyroid gland to secrete thyroid hormone until the concentration of active thyroid hormone reaches physiologic levels. Then the thyroid hormone will inhibit further release of TSH from the pituitary. This is accomplished in one of two ways. If the hormone acts directly on the cells secreting either the hormone itself or its releasing hormone, then the process is called a short-loop feedback system. However, if the hormone acts on the target tissue and a second hormone is released that returns through the circulation to inhibit the original hormone or its releasing hormone, the process is called long loop feedback. These feedback loops are illustrated in Figure 13.1.

A common and diagnostically useful characteristic of hormones is rhythmicity. Hormones are generally secreted on a periodic cycle that is referred to as circadian if the cycle is approximately 24 hours. Cycles shorter than this are called ultradian, and those that are longer are referred to as infradian. In addition to these cyclic secretions there are also instances of pulsatile release of hormone triggered by other events. These events may be neurological, environmental, or biochemical in character and can often be initiated by the clinician under carefully controlled conditions to elucidate the underlying pathology. Often the observation that the natural rhythm of secretion has been lost is enough to direct the diagnostic workup.

The preceding description is concerned with normal physiological events. There are instances of ectopic hormone production. Ectopic production describes a disorder in which a hormone is being produced at a site not normally associated with the production of that hormone. These tissues are generally neoplastic and can produce hormones that can either

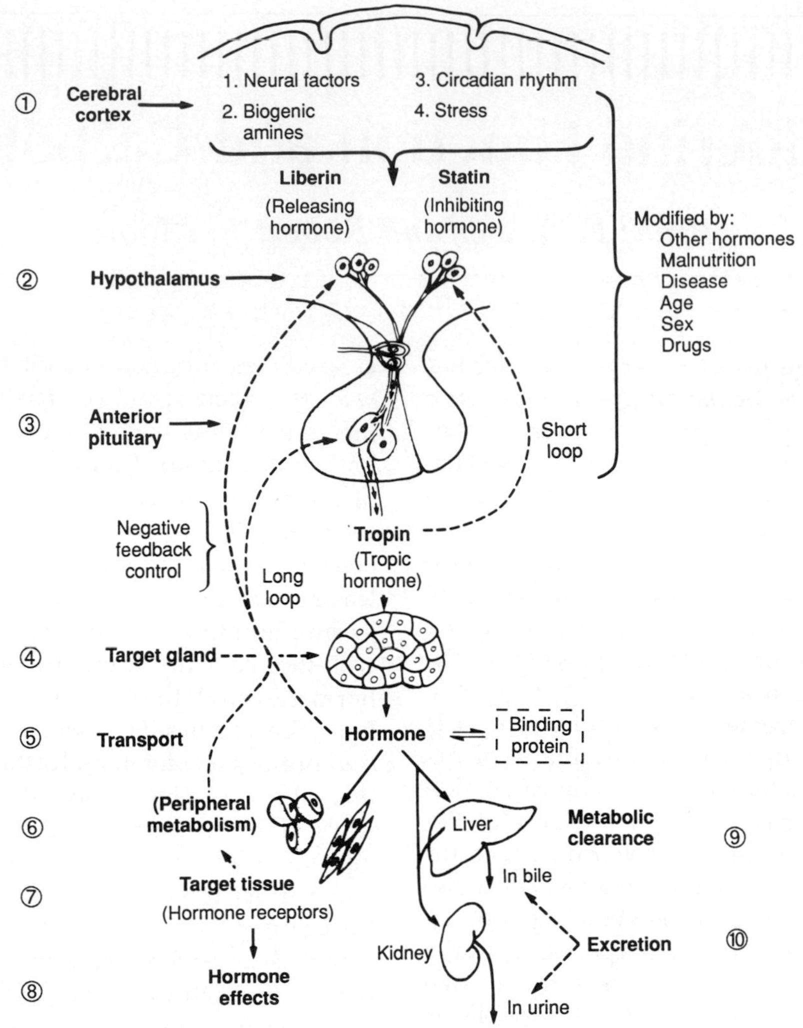

Figure 13.1. Stimulation, production, control, and metabolism of hormones. (1) Stimulation of the cerebral cortex resulting in (2) stimulation of the hypothalmus to release tropic hormones from the anterior pituitary (3). The hormone circulates to a target gland (4), where a second hormone can be produced. This hormone is bound to transport or binding proteins (5) and can undergo peripheral metabolism (6) or bind to receptors in target tissues (7), which results in the specific hormone effect (8). Hormones can then be cleared metabolically (9) or excreted from the system (10). If the tropin acts upon the hypothalmus, this is an example of the "short-loop feedback" while if the hormone or peripheral metabolic products circulate to act upon the hypothalmus, the control is termed "long-loop negative feedback." (Reproduced, with permission, from Gornall AG, Luxton AW. Endocrine disorders. In: Gornall AG, ed. Applied Biochemistry of clinical disorders. 2nd ed. Philadelphia: JB Lippincott, 1986.)

be biologically and structurally identical or variants of normal hormones.

Endocrinology addresses the various clinical disorders that arise from circulating hormone concentration excesses or deficiencies, regulatory system failures, extraneous sources of hormone production, molecular variants, and receptor abnormalities. The clinical laboratory has a crucial role in the evaluation of the patient. The laboratory must be aware of the possible approaches to measuring hormones, their metabolites, and receptor function so a clear understanding of the biological processes can be deduced by the clinician. In the following sections the biochemistry, physiology, laboratory measurement, and clinical interpretation of the more commonly encountered endocrine disorders are reviewed.

RECEPTORS

The circulating concentration of hormones is very low—in the range of 10^{-7} to 10^{-12} M—and only some of the organs and tissues they come into contact with are hormonally responsive. The mechanism of hormonal sensitivity and specificity is attributed to receptors. Receptors are cell-associated proteins that are unique in their ability to bind selected molecules, then translate that binding to initiate subsequent cellular processes. These receptors can be located in the cellular membrane where the binding sites are on the external surface of the cell, and the remainder of the protein extends through the membrane to the cytosolic surface. These receptors are referred to as plasma membrane receptors. Plasma membrane receptors move about within the confines of the cellular membrane and interact with the molecules that are unable to diffuse through the membrane.

Other receptors are intracellular and bind with the hormones that are able to diffuse through the plasma membrane. Binding to the intracellular receptor allows the hormone to be translocated to the nucleus. To regulate cell function of all the elements, hormone, receptors, and the receptor-hormone complex must become activated. Receptors are capable of binding other molecules in addition to the specific hormone. Some of these other molecules will be less effective than the primary hormone or they can be totally ineffective. Molecules that bind and have some activity are referred to as agonists, while those that bind and prevent hormone activity are referred to as antagonists. This difference in hormone-receptor activity is attributed to the fact that while receptors can bind more than one type of molecule, all hormone-receptor complexes are not equivalent in their ability to become activated and regulate cell function.

The binding process is dependent on several types of weak chemical attractive forces. These are ionic bonds, hydrogen bonds, van der Waals forces, and hydrophobic hydrophilic repulsion. Since these forces act over relatively short molecular distances, it is not surprising that there is a stereochemical requirement to maximize the binding. The better the fit between the receptor and its hormone, the greater the affinity of the hormone-receptor complex.

Experimental evidence indicates that the cell contains "spare receptors," i.e., more receptors than are required for maximal cellular response (1). Hormone-receptor binding follows the laws of mass action. Therefore, extra receptors allow the cell to be responsive to lower concentrations of hormone than if the number of receptors were limited. All of the cellular receptors are functional and equivalent. At times when hormone concentration is high these receptors bind hormone, but because the cell is already at maximum stimulation no effect is produced. At other times when hormone concentrations are low, small changes in hormone will be effective, since only a small percentage of receptors must be occupied to cause maximum stimulation. This is also a point of control. By regulating the number of receptors available, the cell can vary its sensitivity to the circulating concentration of hormone. This phenomenon of reducing receptors on the cell surface when hormone concentrations are high may explain the pulsatile secretion of some hormones. Pulsatile secretion allows target cells to maintain maximal sensitivity without being exposed to high concentrations of hormone for extended periods and consequently reducing the number of receptors on the cell surface ("down-regulation"). Additionally, the entire hormone-receptor complex can be removed from the cell membrane and degraded inside the cell with recycling of the receptor or total loss of the receptor and ligand. This internalization of hormone-receptor complexes renders them inactive and reduces the number of receptors available on the cell wall (2). All of the mechanisms of hormone-receptor deactivation have not been worked out, and there is probably more than one mechanism involved. It is thought that some of the changes in receptor number and function on cell surfaces is due to the normal turnover of receptor protein. This description of hormone-membrane receptor interactions is generic, and each of the hormone types—i.e., steroids, thyroid hormones, peptides, and catecholamines—alters cellular function in a slightly different manner.

Steroid and thyroid hormones circulate bound to much larger proteins and are in equilibrium with a very low concentration of free hormone. Because of the hydrophobic nature of these hormones, they are able to penetrate the lipid membrane of the cell by simple diffusion. Following hormone binding to a cytosolic receptor and translocation there is a conformational change that permits the activated hormone-receptor complexes to bind to a specific region on DNA, to initiate new messenger RNA and ultimately new protein synthesis (3). Figure 13.2 illustrates this process.

Large peptides and amine hormones follow a different pathway for transmembrane signaling (4). There are at least three elements on or in the cell membrane that interact to affect cellular function (3, 5). The first of these is the externally oriented receptor protein that binds to the hormone (6). This activated hormone-receptor complex is able to move about in the lipid bilayer of the cellular membrane. The activated hormone-receptor complex binds with a G protein. G proteins are composed of three subunits α, β, and γ. The α subunit binds a molecule of guanosine diphosphate (GDP) when it is in the inactive state (6). Immediately upon binding with the activated receptor complex, the G protein exchanges a guanosine triphosphate (GTP) for the GDP, and the G protein α subunit plus GTP dissociates from the $\beta\gamma$ subunit complex, activating effector proteins (5). An activated receptor is capable of activating multiple G proteins and, in turn, the activated G protein GTP or $\beta\gamma$ subunit can activate multiple effectors. This series of events is responsible for the "amplification effect" of some hormones (5). The effector protein can be an enzyme such as adenylate cyclase, which converts

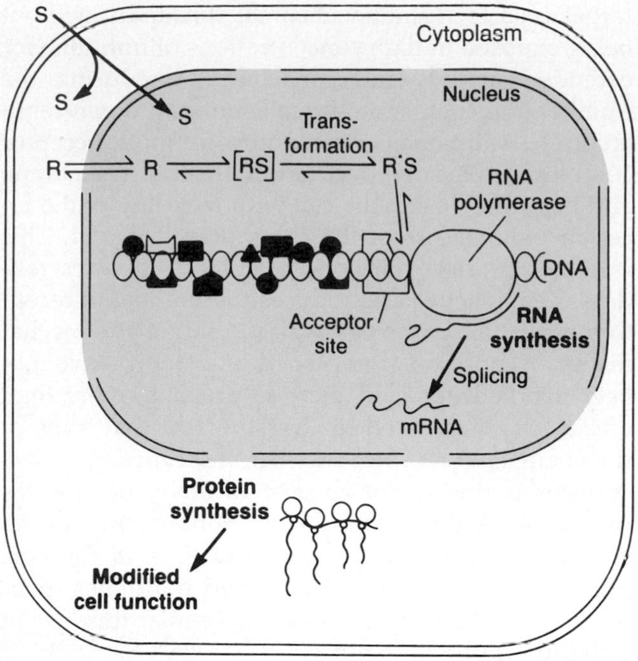

Figure 13.2. Steroid hormone initiation of protein synthesis. Steroid diffuses into the cell through diffusion or active transport mechanism, and binds with a receptor in the nucleus to form a steroid-receptor complex. This activated complex then activates DNA, which in turn activates the RNA synthesis to eventually lead to protein synthesis and cellular response. *S*, steroid; *R*, receptor; *RS*, steroid-receptor complex. (Reproduced, with permission, from Walters MR: Endocr Rev 1985;6:512.)

ATP to cyclic AMP. This process continues until the GTP on the subunit is dephosphorylated back to GDP. This terminates activation of effector proteins, and the cascade ceases. Once the generation of cyclic AMP is halted, the intracellular level of cyclic AMP is reduced by cyclic AMP phosphodiesterases and the hormone effect on the cell is terminated. Other cyclic nucleotides may be generated by analogous systems. There are other G proteins that inhibit effector proteins, giving the cell both stimulatory and inhibitory pathways activated by hormone binding to receptors (6, 7).

Cyclic AMP has been referred to as a "second messenger" since it is the intracellular agent responsible for the direct alteration of cellular function (8). There are, however, other intracellular ions and molecules that qualify as second messengers. Ionic calcium (Ca^{2+}) is an example (9). The intracellular free calcium concentration is very rigidly controlled through a series of transport processes or binding to intracellular structures (9). An important binding protein for intracellular calcium is calmodulin. The calcium-calmodulin complex represents another activated complex that can stimulate intracellular enzymes.

Calcium ion can be released in the cell through the action of a membrane-bound phosphodiesterase (phospholipase C), which generates the second messengers inositol triphosphate (IP3) and diacylglycerol (DAG) (4, 10). The inositol triphosphate can liberate calcium from bound stores within the cell. The diacylglycerol and the released calcium can activate protein kinase C, which will ultimately phosphorylate proteins. These phosphorylated proteins, generally enzymes, can either activate or inhibit further cellular processes.

Larger molecules such as insulin and epidermal growth factor (EGF) bind to the extracellular domain of a transmembrane spanning receptor, which is linked through a transmembrane sequence to an intracellular enzymatic domain often possessing tyrosine and serine kinase activity (10). Autophosphorylation of the enzymatic site leads to serine and tyrosine phosphorylation of a variety of intracellular proteins, including enzymes, which results in intracellular response.

There is an additional small group of hormones that appear to effect phosphorylation through kinases without the aid of a second messenger (8). Insulin and epidermal growth factor activate receptor-localized tyrosine kinases, which phosphorylate tyrosine residues on a variety of intracellular enzymes following hormone-receptor binding on the cell surface. This receptor complex spans the cell membrane, with the receptor binding site presented to the external environment and the tyrosine kinase on the inside of the cell.

The awareness of specific tissue receptors is clinically relevant. This is because hormone abnormalities can arise both from failures in hormone production and from failure of hormone action due to receptor abnormalities.

HYPOTHALAMIC-PITUITARY AXIS

The hypothalamic-pituitary axis can be thought of as an integrated neuroendocrine transducer in which central neural input, neuropeptide release, and both positive and negative long-loop systemic hormonal feedback regulate the production and secretion of no fewer than six anterior pituitary hormones (11). The control of anterior pituitary function by hypothalamic peptide releasing hormones is mediated via the hypophyseal portal vascular plexus, which links the hypothalamus and the hypothalamic releasing peptides with their corresponding anterior pituitary hormones. Table 13.1 lists these releasing peptides and their associated pituitary hormones. These central stimulating effects are modified by feedback loops from the peripheral endocrine glands in which a product hormone is secreted: adrenal—cortisol; thy-

Table 13.1. Releasing Peptides and Hormones[a]

Hypothalamic Releasing Peptides	Associated Hormone
Growth hormone releasing hormone (GRH)	Growth hormone
Somatostatin (SS)	Growth hormone
Thyrotropin releasing hormone (TRH)	Thyrotropin (TSH)
Gonadotropin releasing hormone (GnRH)	Follicle stimulating hormone (FSH) and luteinizing hormone (LH)
Corticotropin releasing hormone (CRH)	Adrenocorticotropic hormone (ACTH)

[a]Growth hormone releasing hormone (GRH) and somatostatin (SS) peptides regulate pituitary growth hormone secretion; thyrotropin releasing hormone (TRH) regulates pituitary thyrotropin (TSH) secretion; gonadotropin (luteinizing hormone) releasing hormone (GnRH, LRH) regulates both pituitary follicle stimulating hormone (FSH) and luteinizing hormone (LH); corticotropin releasing hormone (CRH) regulates adrenocorticotropic hormone (ACTH).

roid—thyroxine and triiodothyronine; ovary and testis—estrogen, testosterone, and the gonadal peptide inhibin; and growth hormone—somatomedin C/insulin-like growth factor 1 (SM-C/IGF-1).

A key feature of the hypothalamic-pituitary axis is episodic secretion of hypothalamic hormones with resultant episodic secretion of pituitary hormones. Pulsatile secretion is defined by frequency of pulse, amplitude, and resultant quantity of hormone secreted. Episodic secretion complicates endocrine analysis by introducing temporal variations in the serum concentration of pituitary hormone, but appears necessary to avoid down-regulation of the hormone receptors through which these peptides exert their biological influence. An additional complexity is the marked diurnal variations in pituitary peptide secretion, particularly of ACTH and GH, in which sleep-related nocturnal secretion predominates with resultant high early morning values and much lower late afternoon and evening values. Documentation of the loss of this physiologic diurnal variation may be useful clinically and requires appropriate morning and evening reference intervals for hormones such as ACTH and cortisol.

ANTERIOR PITUITARY

The pituitary gland (hypophysis) weighs about 0.5 and is located in the sella turcica, a depression of the sphenoid bone. The anterior pituitary or adenohypophysis develops from ectodermal cells of the CNS together with neuroectodermal cells from the neural crest and eventually comprises 75 to 80% of the total pituitary mass. The anterior pituitary is further subdivided into a pars tuberalis and a pars distalis, the latter containing the cells that synthesize and secrete all the anterior pituitary hormones. The major anatomical features of the pituitary are seen in Figure 13.3.

The hypothalamus is connected to the pituitary through the pituitary stalk. Blood and hormones from the hypothalamus communicate with the anterior pituitary through the portal venous plexus. The venous circulation of the brain and the pituitary is illustrated in Figure 13.4.

Growth Hormone

Growth hormone (GH), a single-chain peptide composed of 191 amino acids, is the most abundant of the anterior pituitary hormones. It is released in a pulsatile manner from the somatotropic cells, and is under the direct control of two other hormones, growth hormone releasing hormone (GHRH), which stimulates GH secretion, and somatostatin (SS), which inhibits secretion (12). Growth hormone releasing hormone and somatostatin are controlled and secreted into the hypophyseal portal circulation by the neuropeptide cells of the hypothalamus.

The association of GH with skeletal growth has been recognized for some time. However, GH is not a true growth factor since its effect is mediated through the somatomedins, a group of peptides synthesized by liver and cartilage. Somatomedin C, also referred to as insulin-like growth factor 1 (IGF-1), is one of these somatomedins and is a true cellular growth factor acting upon skeletal components to produce linear growth.

There is a general rhythmicity to the secretion of growth hormone, with the greatest secretion taking place during deep sleep. However, this circadian character has superimposed on it evoked responses to physiologic and biochemical stresses.

Growth Hormone Releasing Hormone

Growth hormone releasing hormone (GHRH) is a small peptide, present in three molecular forms having 37, 40, and 44 amino acids. All three of these molecular forms have a biologically active segment in the first 29 amino acids of the sequence. The two larger forms of GHRH are more potent than the smaller form in the human. It has been suggested that the different forms arise from a post-translational enzyme cleavage. The active GHRH reaches the pituitary by way of the portal circulation.

Somatostatin

Somatostatin was actually observed before GHRH when an extract of hypothalamus was noted to inhibit the release of growth hormone. Occurring as a 28–amino acid precursor that is enzymatically cleaved to the biologically active 14–amino acid form, somatostatin has an inhibitory effect on several hormones in addition to growth hormone, including in-

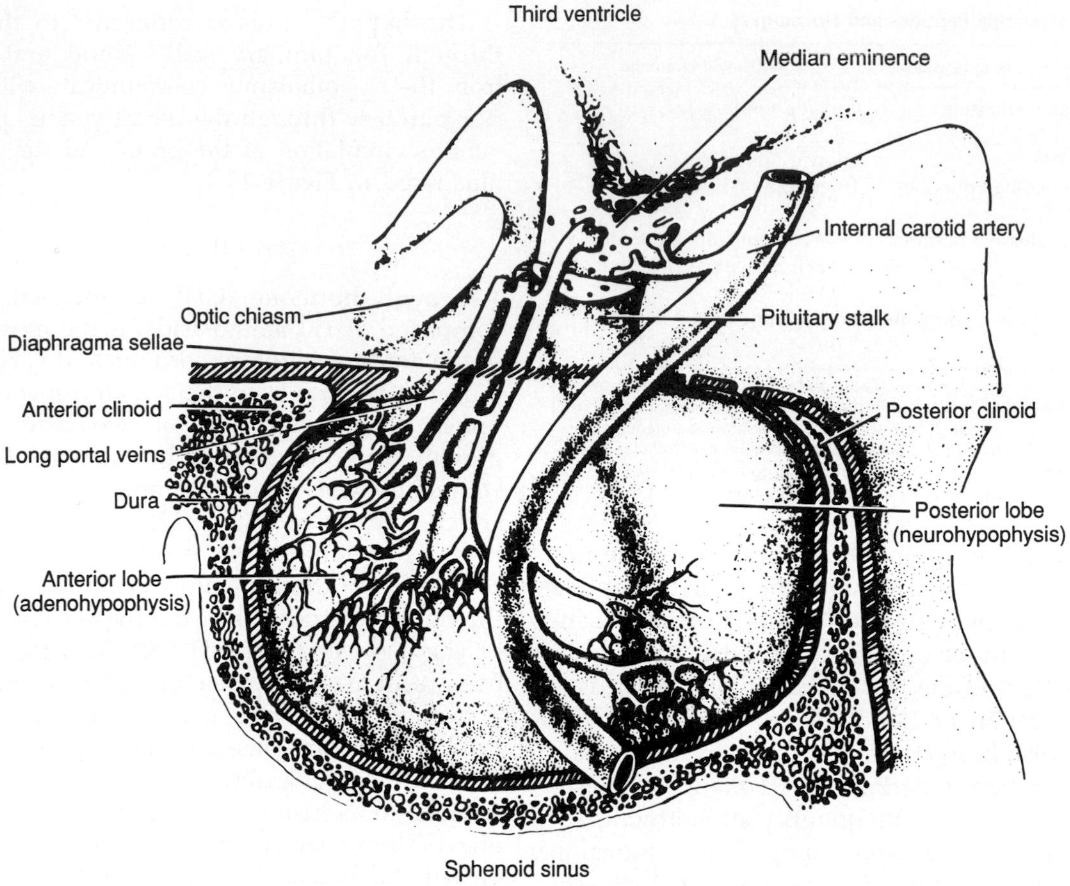

Figure 13.3. Major anatomical features of the pituitary gland. (Reproduced, with permission, from Frohman LA. Diseases of the anterior pituitary. Endocrinology and metabolism. New York: McGraw-Hill 1981:151–231.

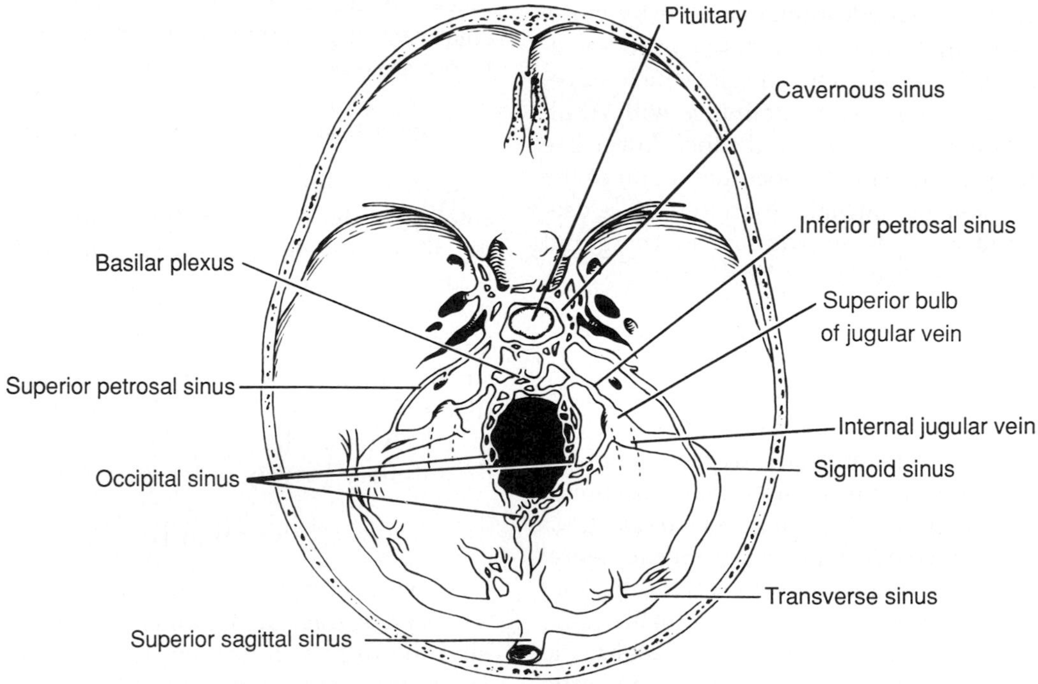

Figure 13.4. Venous system of the pituitary gland communicating with the systemic circulation. (Reproduced, with permission, from Findling JW et al. Selective venous sampling for ACTH in Cushing's syndrome: Differentiation between Cushing's disease and the ectopic ACTH syndrome. Ann Intern Med 1981;94–647.)

Table 13.2. Growth Hormone Reference Intervals

Condition	Preparation	Collection Time	Results	Increased Levels	Decreased Levels
Normal	Fasting	Early AM		Giantism Acromegaly Ectopic secretion Stress Exercise Prolonged fasting	Growth hormone deficiency Hypopituitarism Adrenal cortical hyperfunction
Child			1–10 μg/liter		
Adult					
Female			<10 μg/liter		
Male			<2 μg/liter		
L-Dopa stimulation	500 mg adult 10 mg/kg child	0, 30, 60, 90, 120, 180 min	>10 μg/liter or >5 μg/liter above baseline		No response if glucose >120 mg/dl; poor response in hypopituitarism
Arginine stimulation	Child 0.5 g/kg Adult 30 g IV 30 min	0, 30, 60 min	Fasting <5 μg/liter Peak >10 μg/liter at 30–60 min		Hypopituitarism no response
Insulin stimulation	0.1 U/kg adult 0.05 U/kg child IV	0, 15, 30, 45, 60, 90 min	>10 μg/liter or >5 μg/liter above baseline Glucose level ≤50% of baseline		Poor response in: Hypopituitarism Hypothyroidism
Exercise (vigorous)	20 min		>5 μg/liter		
Glucose suppression	75 g or 1.75 g/kg after fast	0, 30, 60, 90, 120 min	Decrease to <5 μg/liter	None to poor suppression in acromegaly, giantism, and ectopic secretion	

sulin, glucagon, and thyrotropin. Growth hormone inhibition is considered to take place at the pituitary by the binding of somatostatin to membrane receptors, which causes both a decrease in cAMP concentration and a reduction in cAMP effect. Somatostatin also inhibits hTSH at the pituitary level, as well as several other hormones throughout the body.

Growth Hormone Abnormalities

GROWTH HORMONE EXCESS

Excess growth hormone is the cause for two pathological conditions, each of which is associated with a particular age group. In children excess GH leads to giantism, while in adults it produces acromegaly. The acromegalic has a distinctive physical appearance associated with acral growth of flat bones with large, broad features such as hands, feet, and nose. Additional facial characteristics are impressive supraorbital ridges and prognathism. The skin of these individuals is thick and oily, and physical examination will reveal enlarged organs. Laboratory findings supporting the diagnosis include an elevated and nonsuppressible serum GH and an elevated serum somatomedin C/insulin-like growth factor-1 (SM-C/IGF-1). The most convenient method to demonstrate GH nonsuppressibility is glucose administration. This is usually accomplished by giving an oral glucose load of 1.75 g/kg, up to 100 g, and then measuring GH levels at 30-minute intervals for up to 2 hours. Table 13.2 lists the more common stimulation and suppression tests and their expected reference intervals.

GROWTH HORMONE DEFICIENCY

Growth hormone deficiency is primarily a problem of children before they have reached normal stature. Children with short stature with decreased growth velocity who are not malnourished or genetically predisposed to short stature and who have no underlying systemic illness should be suspected for GH deficiency. Serum somatomedin C/IGF-1 provides a useful screening technique. Insulin-induced hypoglycemia (insulin tolerance test), arginine administration arginine tolerance test) with blood samples drawn over a 60- to 90-minute period, and stimulation with α agonists such as dopamine and clonidine, will provide sufficient information to confirm the diagnosis. The GH should peak at levels greater than 10 mg/liter in normally responsive individuals.

A literature consensus of reference values for provocative testing is summarized in Table 13.2. Although normal reference intervals are listed for fasting specimens, it is generally agreed that single random specimens for GH are neither cost effective nor diagnostically informative.

Prolactin

Prolactin (hPrL) is a 198–amino acid protein with an approximate molecular weight of 22 kd. Prolactin can occur as polymers, with the dimeric form being approximately 40 to 50 kd, and a much larger form with a molecular weight in excess of 100 kd. The dimeric form is usually referred to as big prolactin, while the much larger aggregate is referred to as big big prolactin. When the polymeric forms are present in the circulation, they generally constitute less than 2% of the total prolactin. In addition to being present in low concentration, these polymeric forms are significantly less active biologically and pharmacologically and do not seem to represent serious pathologic conditions.

Monomeric prolactin is secreted from the anterior pituitary and enters the general circulation. Inhibitory control of prolactin is accomplished by the neurotransmitter dopamine. Dopamine secretion is initiated by stimulation of the neurons in the median eminence in response to high concentrations of prolactin in either the general circulation or the hypophyseal portal circulation. Although dopamine is capable of suppressing the secretion of prolactin, it does not appear that dopamine concentrations are sufficient to be the only control mechanism, and it is speculated there may be other inhibitory factors. In any event, prolactin appears to be the only anterior pituitary hormone without a long-loop feedback control.

Prolactin secretion is stimulated by thyrotropin releasing hormone (TRH) and perhaps some other prolactin releasing factor (PRF). In addition to the biochemical stimulation, prolactin secretion can be initiated by suckling, whereby stimulation of the nipple through the sucking process causes a neuroreflex of the spinal cord to the neurosecretory cells of the hypothalmus. It is felt that TRH stimulates prolactin secretion at the pituitary level while drugs such as levodopa and insulin (as well as stress) stimulate at the level of the hypothalmus. Secretion of prolactin is episodic, and concentrations are generally increased during the sleep period, with the highest concentrations of prolactin occurring just at the time of awakening.

LACTATION

Breast development through puberty requires the presence of estrogen and progesterone in conjunction with growth hormone, adrenal steroids, and prolactin. Although estrogen and progesterone are the most important steroids for development, all of these seem to be necessary but not sufficient conditions for breast development. Development is only partial until pregnancy, at which time ducts and acini mature but the process of lactation is inhibited. Through pregnancy placental lactogen, estrogen, progesterone, and prolactin increase dramatically, and the breast development is completed. The roles of prolactin and placental lactogen during this time are unclear.

After parturition estrogen and progesterone concentrations decrease and prolactin concentration remains high, stimulating the synthesis of enzymes and milk components as well as initiating milk secretion. If at this time there is no suckling, prolactin concentrations decrease and milk secretion will slowly taper off and cease. It is evident from this process that prolactin is the primary hormone of lactation. Suckling, in addition to stimulating prolactin secretion, stimulates an increase in the concentration of oxytocin. Oxytocin causes constriction of the tissue around the acini, forcing the milk into the primary collection ducts. During this feeding cycle, hPrL concentration increases, with peak levels being attained between 30 and 60 minutes. The ultimate concentration is dependent on the length and intensity of the suckling taking place. This elevated concentration of hPrL then causes the synthesis of milk components that will be available for the next feeding.

Gonadotropin releasing hormone (GnRH), inhibited by the lactation process, is responsible for depressed levels of LH and FSH, and this is probably the reason there is a contraceptive effect associated with lactation. Nonlactating females will resume normal menses with normal levels of gonadotropins two to three times sooner than women who continue to lactate after delivery.

HYPERPROLACTINEMIA

There are multiple etiologies of hyperprolactinemia, with prolactin-secreting adenomas being among the most common pituitary neoplasms (13). However, drugs such as estrogens, certain antihypertensives, phenothiazines, tricyclic antidepressants, metoclopramide, and methyldopa can all cause an increase in prolactin concentration. Hypothyroidism, renal insufficiency, and the natural states of pregnancy and lactation are also reasons for increased prolactin. In cases of prolactinoma, gonadotropin releasing hormone secretion is inhibited by the elevated prolactin, which leads to ovarian dysfunction and amenorrhea. In women, the most common prolactinoma is the microadenoma measuring less than 1 cm in diameter. Microadenomas are generally slow growing and can be monitored with periodic measurement of the prolactin level, provided the patient is willing to accept the consequences of elevated prolactin such as galactorrhea and amenor-

Table 13.3. Prolactin Reference Intervals

Condition	Patient Preparation	Specimen Collection	Results
Normal	Fasting 12 hr.	Serum early AM collection	*μg/liter*
Male			9.5–16.1
Female		Chilled	12.4–18.1
		Process in cold	
Pregnancy	Same	Same	
1st trimester			<80
2nd trimester			<160
3rd trimester			<400

rhea. In the case of macroadenoma (i.e., lesions in excess of 1 cm in diameter), the lesion is generally less common, more aggressive, associated with much higher levels of prolactin, and may produce neuroanatomical symptoms such as headache and visual impairment.

LABORATORY RESULTS

Commercial immunoassays for prolactin (hPrl) are available that employ chemiluminescent, enzymatic, fluorescent, or radioactive labels with no method having a particular advantage. Therefore, the choice of methodology should be the one that is the most familiar to the laboratory. The patient should be fasted for 12 hours and should not be on phenothiazines, estrogens, MAO inhibitors, tricyclic antidepressants, antihypertensives, or methyldopa. In addition, hypothyroidism should be ruled out and if that cannot be done with certainty by history and physical examination, then a concomitant TSH should be drawn. The specimen preferred is serum, which should be drawn into an appropriate container and placed immediately in the cold to clot. Blood specimens should be drawn before physical examination of the breast as breast manipulation can elevate serum prolactin concentrations. After clotting is complete, the specimen should be centrifuged in a refrigerated centrifuge, the serum separated from the cells, and the serum frozen if it is not to be processed immediately. If the specimen is to be analyzed within 4 to 6 hours, it is the experience of this laboratory that refrigeration until time of assay is acceptable. Storage for longer periods requires freezing. Reference intervals for normal as well as some selected clinical situations are tabulated in Table 13.3.

Follicle Stimulating Hormone and Luteinizing Hormone

GONADOTROPINS

Luteinizing hormone (LH) and follicle stimulating hormone (FSH) are synthesized and released from gonadotrophs located in the anterior pituitary in response to the stimulatory effect of gonadotropin releasing hormone (GnRH) (sometimes called luteinizing hormone releasing hormone [LHRH]). Biologically active gonadotropin releasing hormone is a decapeptide that is derived from a much larger, biologically less active propeptide of approximately 70 amino acids. The active gonadotropin releasing hormone is secreted by neurons in the median eminence, where it enters the capillaries and is carried to the anterior pituitary through the hypophysial portal system. Gonadotropin releasing hormone is secreted in a pulsatile fashion and seems to be sensitive to the circulating level of estrogen in the female and testosterone in the male. It has been demonstrated that GnRH is synthesized early in the development of the fetus and stimulates the secretion of LH and FSH until peak concentrations are reached at approximately 20 weeks of gestation. Then from the 20th week to birth LH and FSH, along with testosterone, decline in concentration to the levels normally associated with the newborn.

Luteinizing hormone and follicle stimulating hormone are glycoproteins composed of two subunits referred to as the α and β subunits. This polypeptide character is shared with two other hormones, human chorionic gonadotropin (hCG) and thyroid stimulating hormone (TSH). The α subunit of these four hormones is identical, and experiments have shown that dissociation of the α and β subunits and recombination of the α subunit of any one of the four hormones to a β subunit of another hormone, will produce the hormonal activity associated with the hormone of the original β subunit. The α subunit is a necessary component for hormone binding to receptor sites, but specificity and hormone effect are conferred by the β subunit. In addition, these four hormones show considerable homology in the structure of the β subunit. This was a serious problem in the early immunoassays, in which antibodies could not distinguish between hCG and LH and even had some cross-reactivity with FSH and TSH. Today, with the advent of monoclonal antibodies and a better knowledge of the structure of these β subunits, it is possible to construct assays that are very specific and very sensitive for the individual hormones. Table 13.4 lists one set of reference intervals for males and females. Other reference values may be found, depending on the assay and the calibrators used.

The glycoprotein character of these hormones is the result of several carbohydrate residues, of which sialic acid seems to be the most important. The sialic acid content is variable and appears to be influenced by the endocrine environment at the time of synthesis. Sialic acid residues are protective of the gonadotropin, and as the sialic acid content increases there

Table 13.4. Gonadatropin (LH/FSH) Reference Intervals

Condition	Patient Preparation	Collection Time	LH Results	FSH Results
Normal			*IU/liter*	*IU/liter*
Male	Serum (refrigerate)	Random specimen acceptable	1–8	1–7
Female				
Follicular phase	Same	Same	1–12	1–10
Ovulatory peak			15–105	6–26
Luteal phase			1–12	1–10
Postmenopausal			15–70	30–120

is an extension in the half-life and biologic activity of the particular gonadotropin.

Once luteinizing hormone and follicle stimulating hormone have been secreted from the gonadotrophs, they are carried through the general circulation to the gonads. In the female, FSH stimulates follicle development and receptors for LH binding while LH stimulates follicular production of estradiol, ovulation, and formation of the corpus luteum. In the male, FSH stimulates Sertoli cell development and LH induces testosterone secretion. It is these end product hormones from the gonads that can feed back through the long-loop system and control the gonadotropin releasing hormone and the gonadotropin secretion.

One of the first symptoms of pituitary insufficiency can be gonadal failure. The most direct approach to ruling out primary gonadal insufficiency from pituitary insufficiency is a direct measurement of the pituitary gonadotropins. If the pituitary hormones are depressed, that is highly suggestive of pituitary insufficiency. If, on the other hand, the circulating levels of luteinizing hormone and follicle stimulating hormone are high, that rules out pituitary deficiency. In Klinefelter's syndrome, a disorder of sexual differentiation, it is common to measure elevated pituitary gonadotropins and depressed testosterone. In some individuals this picture can be altered by the finding of a normal testosterone level. This problem arises because the assay measures total circulating testosterone, which includes the very large bound fraction. The biologically active fraction, or free testosterone, is low and can only be determined by an assay that measures free testosterone in the presence of bound testosterone.

LABORATORY METHODS

In the measurement of luteinizing hormone and follicle stimulating hormone, as in many other polypeptides, there is no unusual patient preparation required. That is, fasting is not an absolute requirement since most immunoassays are tolerant of mild lipemia. Fresh serum specimens are preferred because they are the least troublesome to the laboratory, but plasma is certainly an acceptable specimen. As mentioned above, current assays are able to specifically measure any of the glycoproteins, and therefore cross-reactivity and sensitivity are no longer measurement problems. In making measurements on specimens derived from female patients the most critical piece of information, with the exception of the actual level, is the menstrual status of the woman. As Figure 13.5 demonstrates, the LH and FSH concentrations vary considerably throughout the menstrual cycle. It is imperative that the physician have access to accurate menstrual information when interpreting gonadotropin results.

POSTERIOR PITUITARY

Physiology

Antidiuretic hormone (ADH, vasopressin) is secreted from hypothalamic neurons of the supraoptic nuclei and transported to the posterior pituitary by axoplasmic flow. From these storage sites it is released into the systemic circulation in response to osmotic and volume stimuli, following which it circulates to the kidney. At the renal tubule level the effect of antidiuretic hormone is accomplished by increasing water permeability of the distal tubule collecting duct, permitting water resorption and concentration of the final urine. The osmoreceptors responsible for ADH release are located in the anterior hypothalamus near the supraoptic nuclei and are responsive to small changes in extracellular tonicity.

A physiologic setpoint for ADH secretion exists at an approximate plasma osmolality of 280 mOsm/kg. Below this setpoint ADH secretion is suppressed. ADH secretion rises rapidly above this setpoint, with maximal ADH levels achieved at extracellular tonicities of approximately 300 mOsm/kg, at which point thirst and water seeking are also stimulated in an integrated fashion. The threshold and sensitivity for ADH secretion vary among individuals and are increased by hypovolemia and hypercalcemia, as well as by many drugs, including lithium and carbamazepine. The threshold is lowered by hypervolemia, glucocorticoids, alcohol, and opiates.

ADH secretion is also altered by isosmotic changes in extracellular volume. Decreases in vol-

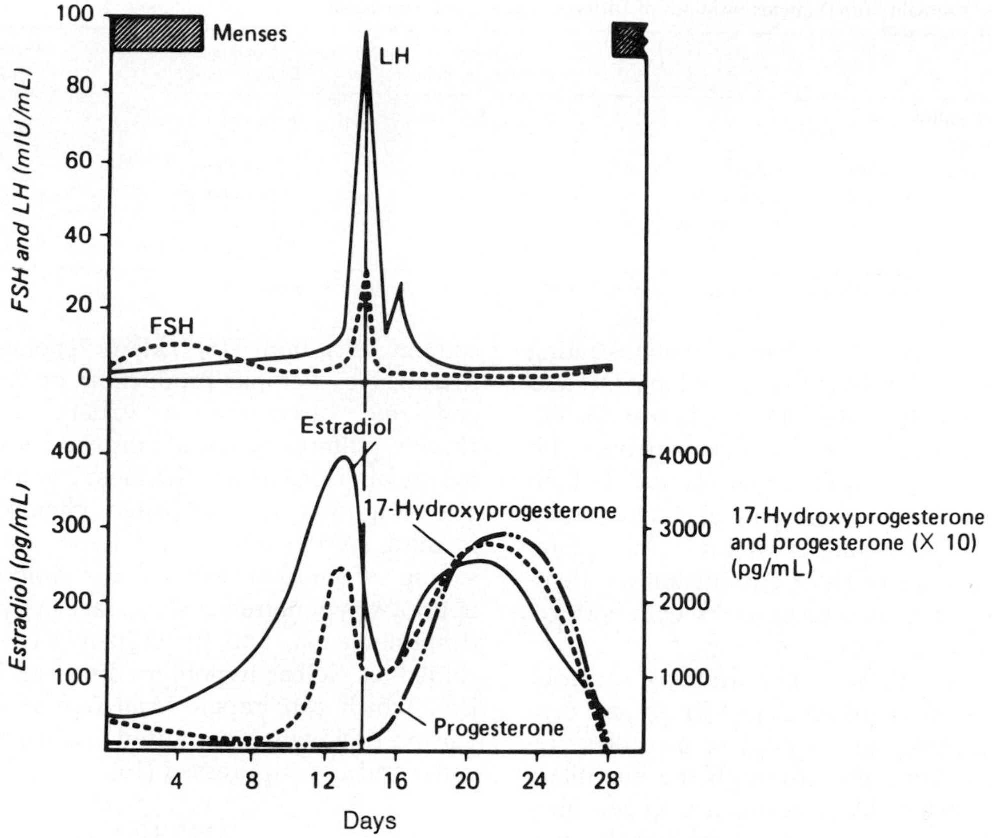

Figure 13.5. The cyclic secretion of gonadotropins and sex steroids during the normal 28-day menstrual cycle. Note that the estradiol and 17-hydroxyprogesterone peak precedes the mid-cycle surge of the gonadotropins LH and FSH. After the mid-cycle gonadotropin peak there is a second peak of 17-hydroxyprogesterone and progesterone, which decreases to baseline levels when the cycle begins again. (Reproduced, with permission, from Odell WD, Moyer DL. Physiology of reproduction. St Louis; CV Mosby, 1971.)

ume amplify the ADH release to any given osmotic stimulus, and increased volume suppresses ADH secretion in a similar manner.

Nausea, pain, and many drugs such as narcotics are also potent nonosmotic stimulators of ADH secretion.

Clinical Disorders

DIABETES INSIPIDUS

Defects in antidiuretic hormone secretion (central) or renal tubular action (nephrogenic) result in chronic polyuria, polydipsia, and thirst. In addition, functional suppression of antidiuretic hormone occurs with chronic psychogenic water drinking, producing a similar clinical picture (14). Central diabetes insipidus can result from a variety of hypothalamic etiologies, including trauma, various neoplasms, and granulomatous and infectious disorders. A heritable familial autosomal dominant central disorder is also described. In a significant percentage of patients with central diabetes insipidus no specific etiology can be determined and the patients are labeled idiopathic.

Nephrogenic diabetes insipidus can occur as a result of renal parenchymal disorders such as amyloidosis, polycystic renal disease, and sickle cell disease, as well as following relief of urinary tract obstruction. Drugs such as lithium, demeclocycline, and methoxyflurane can also produce nephrogenic diabetes insipidus. A familial X-linked recessive disorder is also recognized (15).

The diagnosis of diabetes insipidus and the differentiation between central and nephrogenic etiologies is achieved by a structured dehydration test. Fluid is withheld to achieve a decrease in body weight of approximately 3 to 5%. Weight and plasma osmolality are monitored to document the adequacy of the dehydration stimulus, and plasma ADH levels and urine osmolality are measured to monitor the clinical response. In patients with central diabetes insipidus despite an adequate dehydration stimulus there is a failure to achieve urine osmolalities greater than 300 mOsm/kg, and plasma ADH levels remain low. Confirmation is achieved by the administration of exogenous ADH in the form of parenteral or intranasal desamino-D-arginine vasopressin (DDAVP), an ADH analogue that produces urine concentration greater

Table 13.5. Urine Osmolality for Diabetes Insipidus of Different Origins and Polydipsia[a]

	Neurogenic Diabetes Insipidus	Nephrogenic Diabetes Insipidus	Psychogenic Polydipsia
Random plasma osmolality	↑	↑	↓
Random urine osmolality	↓	↓	↓
Urine osmolality during mild water deprivation	No change	No change	↑
Urine osmolality during nicotine or hypertonic saline	No change	No change	↑
Urine osmolality following vasopressin intravenously	↑	No change	↑
Plasma vasopressin	Low	Normal or high	Low

[a]Reprinted with permission from Greenspan FS. Basic endocrinology, 3rd ed., Norwalk, CT: Appleton & Lange, 1991.

than that achieved with dehydration, demonstrating the ability of the renal tubule to respond to ADH and hence confirming failure of ADH secretion as the etiology of the diabetes insipidus. In patients with nephrogenic diabetes insipidus there is usually both an easily measurable baseline and postdehydration plasma ADH concentration as well as a lack of response to exogenous, DDAVP administration, demonstrating a lack of tubular response to both endogenous and exogenous ADH.

Patients with excessive water drinking (primary polydipsia) have an acquired defect in urinary concentration attributable to washout of medullary tonicity by high volume flow through the medullary countercurrent system. As a result urine concentration during dehydration may be submaximal but will exceed 300 mOsm/kg and there is no further increment in urine osmolality following exogenous ADH or DDAVP administration. More prolonged fluid restriction or therapeutic ADH administration restores full urine concentrating ability.

PRIMARY HYPODIPSIA

In some patients with or without coexistent central diabetes insipidus, defects in thirst perception due to destruction of hypothalamic osmoreceptors are also present. These defects lead to failure of appropriate thirst response to dehydration and at times striking asymptomatic hypernatremia and hyperosmolality. Other etiologies of hypernatremia, including inadequate fluid intake secondary to coma or physical restraints preventing access to fluids need to be excluded. Plasma ADH levels are usually appropriate for the degree of osmolality unless diabetes insipidus is also present. Table 13.5 lists some common plasma and urine laboratory results for polyuria.

SYNDROME OF INAPPROPRIATE SECRETION OF ANTIDIURETIC HORMONE (SIADH)

The continued secretion of ADH despite appropriate extracellular concentration and volume and continued unrestricted water intake, results in dilutional hypoosmolality and hyponatremia, inappropriately increased urinary osmolality, and increased urinary sodium excretion (16). Many etiologies may be responsible. Ectopic production of ADH by nonendocrine carcinoma, a variety of acute and chronic pulmonary conditions, and a variety of intracranial disorders are the most common etiologies. The diagnosis is established clinically by documenting hyponatremia and hypoosmolality in the setting of normal extracellular volume integrity. Spurious hyponatremia secondary to hyperglycemia, dysproteinemia, and hyperlipemia needs to be excluded, as well as hypothyroidism and hypoadrenalism, which can impair renal free water excretion. Plasma ADH when measured is inappropriately elevated and nonsuppressed (16).

THYROID

Thyroid Physiology

Iodine is concentrated by the thyroid gland, organified into tyrosine units on thyroglobulin, and stored in colloid-containing thyroid follicles until secretion. The metabolism of iodine is shown in Figure 13.6. Synthesis and secretion of thyroxine (T_4) and triiodothyronine (T_3) is controlled by pituitary thyrotropin (TSH) secretion through classic negative feedback regulation in combination with the stimulatory effects of hypothalamic thyrotropin releasing hormone (TRH). Serum T_3 arises both from direct thyroid T_3 secretion (15%) and from peripheral monodeiodination of the outer tyrosine ring of secreted T_4 (85%). The synthesis and control of thyroid hormones is diagrammed in Figure 13.7. A biologically inactive reverse T_3 (RT_3) also arises from peripheral monodeiodination of the inner tyrosine ring of T_4.

Thyroid Transport

Circulating T_3 and T_4 are bound to a variety of thyroid transport proteins, including thyroid binding globulin (TBG), thyroid binding pre-albumin (TBPA), and albumin. Only approximately 0.03% of T_4 and 0.3% of T_3 are "free" and hence biologically active. It is the excess or deficiency of the free thyronine fractions that determine hyperthyroidism and hypothy-

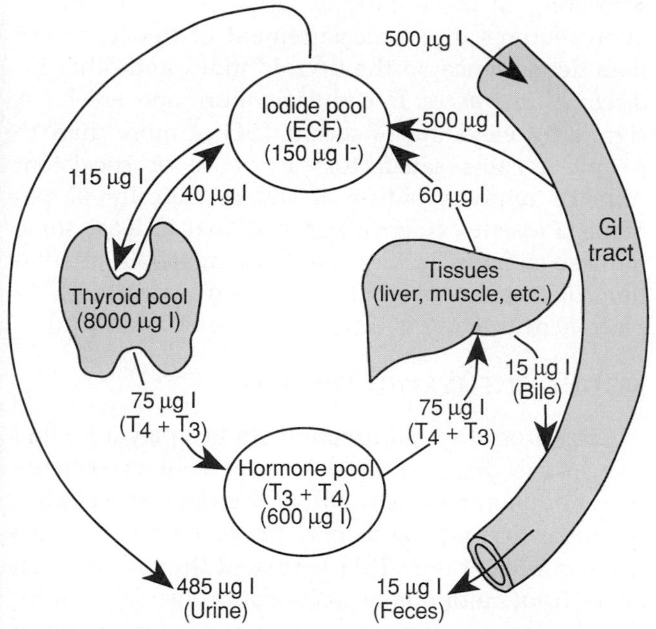

Figure 13.6. Daily iodine adsorption, synthesis and excretion in a healthy subject. (Reproduced, with permission, from Greenspan FS, Rapoport B. Thyroid gland. In: Basic and clinical endocrinology. 3rd ed. Norwalk, CT: Appleton & Lange, 1991:188–246.)

roidism. Since many drugs and disease states affect the concentrations of the thyroid transport proteins, it is critical that appropriate thyroid function studies distinguish between elevations or depressions of the bound or total, and free components of T_4 and T_3 (17).

The most common abnormalities in thyroid function evaluation are related to the widespread use of oral estrogens for contraception and postmenopausal estrogen replacement therapy. The estrogen-related increase in production of hepatic thyroid binding globulin (TBG) produces an elevation of serum total T_4, although with preservation of normal free thyroxine levels. Hereditary excess and deficiency of TBG also occurs on an X-linked familial basis in approximately one in 5000 newborns as estimated by neonatal screening programs.

Clinical Disorders

HYPERTHROIDISM

Hyperthyroidism can arise from multiple etiologies. The diagnosis of hyperthyroidism is established and documented by thyroid function studies. Determination of the etiology of hyperthyroidism requires other measures such as radioactive iodine uptake and thyroid scans. The most common etiology of hyperthyroidism is Grave's disease, or diffuse toxic goiter, in which thyroid stimulating immunoglobulins (TSIG) binding to TSH receptors stimulate the entire

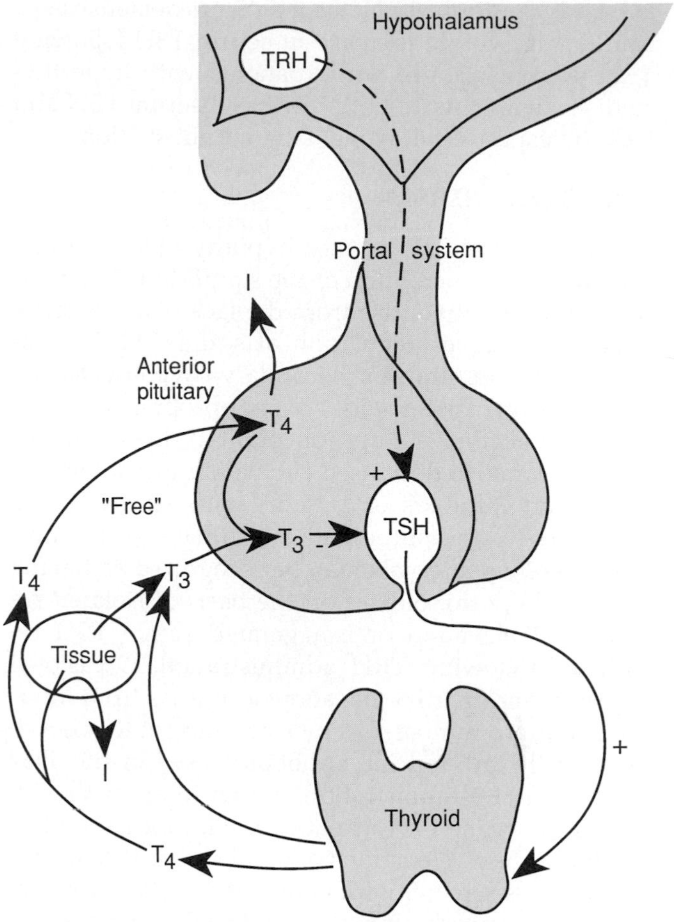

Figure 13.7. The hypothalamic-hypophyseal-thyroid axis in the production of thyroid hormones. Pathways marked with a (−) indicate inhibition, while those with a (+) indicate stimulation. I indicates deiodination of the parent T_4 molecule to produce T_3. (Reproduced, with permission, from Greenspan FS, Rapoport B. Thyroid gland. In: Greenspan FS, ed. Basic and clinical endocrinology. 3rd ed. Norwalk, CT. Appleton & Lange, 1991:188–246.)

thyroid gland to produce excess thyroid hormone secretion. Other etiologies of hyperthyroidism include toxic solitary or multinodular thyroid disorders, inflammatory disorders of the thyroid gland such as subacute thyroiditis, hyperthyroidism secondary to chorionic thyroid stimulators, excess exogenous thyroid administration, and, rarely, TSH production from a pituitary adenoma. With the exception of the latter, circulating free T_4 and free T_3 levels, as determined directly or by indexing techniques, are elevated and serum TSH levels as measured by "sensitive" immunoassay methods are suppressed. In addition an occasional patient may have only selective T_3 excess ("T_3 toxicosis"), requiring measurement of serum T_3 levels for appropriate diagnosis (17).

Confirmation of serum TSH suppression in patients with hyperthyroidism can be further achieved by TRH testing (TRH, 250 to 500 mg i.v., serum TSH at 0 and 30 minutes) . Normal patients demonstrate a significant twofold increase in serum TSH following TRH administration, while patients with hyperthyroidism demonstrate both low basal serum TSH and lack of response following TRH administration.

HYPOTHYROIDISM

The diagnosis of primary hypothyroidism is simplified by documentation of the significant elevations of serum TSH that arise from the lack of appropriate negative feedback regulation of serum TSH. In patients with central or secondary hypothyroidism (5%), serum TSH levels are inappropriately "normal," indicating failure of pituitary-hypothalamic TSH response to decreased circulating thyroid levels. Significant numbers of patients with serum T_4 and serum free T_4 measurements or estimates within normal reference intervals may be recognized as having primary hypothyroidism on the basis of isolated serum TSH elevation or exaggerated serum TSH responses following TRH administration. Occasional spurious serum TSH elevations can arise from interference in immunoassays by circulating autoantibodies to TSH anti-murine antibodies used in the TSH assays. TRH administration results in an excess increase in serum TSH in patients with indeterminate or "borderline" elevations of basal serum TSH levels.

Neonatal screening for congenital hypothyroidism has become nearly universal. Initial screening is performed using serum T_4 determinations by methods adapted to filter paper techniques. Confirmation of primary hypothyroidism is accomplished by demonstration of serum TSH elevation by similar filter paper methods. The incidence of neonatal primary hypothyroidism is approximately 1:5000. The disorder is sporadic and usually nonfamilial, requiring universal screening of newborns to permit early diagnosis and prompt institution of thyroid replacement therapy. False-positive decreases in serum T_4 may occur with heritable TBG deficiency and decreased serum TBG concentrations related to prematurity.

THE EUTHYROID SICK STATE

A unique problem arises in the thyroid laboratory evaluation of critically ill hospitalized patients. A complex series of events—including decreased serum thyroid binding protein concentration, circulating inhibitors of thyroid binding, decreased peripheral T_4 deiodination to T_3, qualitative abnormalities in serum TSH glycosylation, and quantitative abnormalities in TSH secretion—combine to produce distortions of conventional thyroid function tests in these patients. These effects are further complicated by the common use of drugs such as glucocorticoids and DOPA (which directly suppress pituitary TSH secretion), in these critically ill patients. Resolution often requires direct measurement of free T_4 rather than dependence on the thyroid index and other indirect estimates of free thyroid hormone levels. A significant elevation of serum TSH of more than 15 μU/ml remains satisfactory evidence of coexistent primary hypothyroidism in these critically ill patients. Present evidence suggests that at least some of these changes are the result of a metabolic adaptation to catabolic systemic illness and that thyroid replacement therapy is unwarranted and unhelpful.

NODULAR THYROID DISEASE

Laboratory thyroid function studies play a limited role in the diagnosis and management of patients with nodular and multinodular thyroid disease. Multinodular thyroid glands may produce hyperthyroidism if sufficient non–TSH-regulated thyroid function arises from autonomous nodules. Conversely, multinodular thyroid disease can be a secondary result of chronic TSH hypersecretion in patients with underlying hypothyroidism. In either case the functional diagnosis needs to be separated from the anatomical etiology or consequence.

Patients with carcinoma of the thyroid present with isolated thyroid nodules and are usually euthyroid. The initial diagnosis and monitoring of subsequent therapy of papillary and follicular thyroid carcinoma may be supplemented by measurement of serum thyroglobulin levels by radioimmunoassay and, in the case of medullary thyroid carcinoma, by serum calcitonin measurements. The latter may be enhanced by stimulatory tests employing pentagastrin and intravenous calcium administration.

Thyroid Therapy

Thyroid function studies are employed not only in the initial diagnosis of thyroid dysfunction but also in the subsequent monitoring of response to therapy. It is essential to understand the consequences of therapy on thyroid function and laboratory thyroid function testing. Increasingly, the third generation of serum TSH assays are becoming an integrated index of appropriateness of antithyroid therapy of hyperthyroidism, thyroid replacement therapy in primary hypothyroidism, and thyroid suppression in patients with benign and malignant thyroid disorders (18).

LABORATORY DIAGNOSIS

The basis for all laboratory methods used in a thyroid workup is immunochemical. The exquisite sensitivity and specificity of current antibodies have made thyroid testing a routine event in almost all clinical laboratories. Thyroxin (T_4), triiodothyronine

Table 13.6. Thyroid Function Studies

	Serum					
Clinical Disorder	T_4	T_3U	fT_4I	T_3	fT_3I	TSH
Elevated T_4						
Hyperthyroidism	↑	↓	↑	N/↑	↑	↓
Increased TBG						
Estrogens	↑	↓	N	↑	N	N
Pregnancy	↑	↓	N	↑	N	N
Drugs						
1-Thyroxine Rx	N/↑	N	N/↑	N	N	↓
Glucocorticoids	N/↑	N	N/↑	↓	↓	N
Propranolol	N/↑	N	N/↑	N/↓	N/↓	N
Amiodorone	↑	↑	↑	↓	↓	N
Thyroid resistance	↑	↑	↑	↑	↑	N/↑
T_3 toxicosis	N	N	N	↑	↑	↓
Depressed T_4						
Hypothyroidism						
Primary	↓	↓	↓	N	N	↑↑
Secondary	↓	↓	↓	N	N	N/↓
Decreased TBG						
Androgens	↓	↑	N	↓	N	N
Hepatic failure	↓	↑	N	↓	N/↓	N
Nephrosis	↓	↑	N	↓	N/↓	N
Drugs						
Triiodothyronine	↓	N	↓	N/↑ [a]	↓	N
Phenytoin	↓	↑	N/↓	↓	N	N
Thyroid carcinoma	N	N	N	N	N	N

↑ = increased
↓ = decreased
N = normal

[a]Time-dependent value.

(T_3), free T_4, free T_3, TSH, TBG, and even some of the by-products such as reverse T_3, can be measured accurately and precisely with only a fraction of the effort required several years ago. Because of this state of technology, laboratories are capable of choosing thyroid procedures that will fit in with the existing work flow and other techniques employed in the clinical laboratory.

Significant patient preparation is not required for biochemical thyroid studies. If possible, the patient should fast from the evening before so that an early-morning serum specimen may be obtained. However, if time or circumstance do not permit a fasting specimen, a random specimen can be used. Serum should be separated from the cells and refrigerated until the time of assay, or frozen for assays that will be performed longer than 8 hours after the collection of the specimen. There is an extensive list of drugs that interfere with thyroid physiology, and therefore the laboratory should periodically refer to one of the publications that deals with drug interferences in common laboratory tests. Some of the more commonly occurring drugs that are known to affect testing are prostaglandins, estrogen, oral contraceptives, androgens, aspirin, corticosteroids, lithium, some antibiotics, phenothiazines, dexamethasone, propranolol, and certainly many others (19).

As is the case with all laboratory procedures, each laboratory should establish their own reference intervals for their normal population. As a guide, serum thyroxine is between 4.5 and 12 mg/dl, T_3 resin uptake between 20 and 35%, serum total T_3 between 100 and 220 ng/dl, serum TSH between 0.5 and 5.0 IU/liter. Because of the diversity of these reference intervals, Table 13.6 lists thyroid function studies in terms of increase, decrease, or normal. This is a common technique used to show the relationship among the thyroid studies without having to be concerned about the specific reference intervals of a method or geographic location.

A recent addition to the routine clinical laboratory is the ability to measure free T_4. In the past, free T_4 measurements have been done by equilibrium dialysis, which was best done in research laboratories or large clinical reference laboratories. Attempts have been made to approximate the free T_4 concentration by using calculated indices, but these have generally proved to be inadequate. Attempts to estimate free T_4 using analog procedures were better than the calculated indices but they have some disadvantage in the sick euthyroid patient. If the laboratory is thoroughly familiar with the limitations of the analog procedures, they could prove useful in free T_4 assessment. Recently, however, commercial systems have become available that allow the routine clinical laboratory to perform the "gold standard" equilibrium dialysis in a cost-effective and reliable manner. It is anticipated that this approach will become widely available and could influence the way thyroid evaluation is done. There is growing enthusiasm for measuring serum TSH (by a third-generation ultrasensitive TSH assay) and free T_4 as an initial step in thyroid evaluation as opposed to the total T_4 and T_3 resin uptake that is currently done by a large number of laboratories.

THYROXINE (T_4) AND TRIIODOTHYRONINE (T_3)

Total T_3 measurements are influenced by many factors, including protein concentration. Free T_3 measurement fulfills a similar function to free T_4 since it is a direct measurement of the physiologically active hormone and is not affected by protein concentration.

T_3 UPTAKE (T_3U)

This is the historical way of measuring thyroid hormone binding to serum proteins. Although there are many approaches to this assay, all T_3U assays attempt to estimate the relative saturation of all the serum proteins capable of binding thyroxin. This result, when multiplied by the total thyroxine result, produces a value referred to as "free thyroxine index" (FTI). Before there were direct measurements for free thyroxine this approach gave a reasonable estimate of free T_4. Today there are several methods available for the quantitation of free thyroxine, so the FTI is less commonly used.

THYROTROPIN (TSH)

Many commercial immunoassays are available that are in the ultrasensitive or super-sensitive category, meaning that circulating TSH at levels of 0.01 U/liter to 0.03 U/liter can be accurately measured (20). It is this generation of TSH assay that is being considered as one of the first assays for thyroid screening.

THYROID BINDING GLOBULIN (TBG)

Immunoassays are available that are sufficiently reliable and simple so that most laboratories can perform them on a routine basis. It should be remembered that the specificity of immunoassays is such that the TBG is not a replacement for T_3 uptake. The uptake assays measure total thyroid binding sites, while the TBG measures only thyroid binding globulin.

PROVOCATIVE TESTING

Stimulation by the intravenous administration of thyrotropin releasing hormone (TRH) amplifies the information available from measurement of steady-state thyroid and TSH levels. TRH (250 to 500 mg) is administered intravenously over approximately 1 minute. Serum TSH levels are obtained at time zero and at 30 or 60 minutes. In normal subjects an increase of from 5 to 20 mIU/ml over baseline is obtained. In patients with hyperthyroidism the low serum TSH does not increase following TRH administration. In patients with primary hypothyroidism an excessive rise in serum TSH occurs at 30 and 60 minutes. In hypothyroidism secondary to pituitary or hypothalamic disease serum TSH increase is either absent, suboptimal, or delayed.

ADRENAL CORTEX

Physiology of Adrenal Biosynthesis and Regulation

The adrenal cortex is composed of three distinct anatomical layers, each associated with specific steroid hormone synthesis and secretion. The glomerulosa is the most superficial and is responsible for mineralocorticoid biosynthesis and resultant renal sodium:potassium homeostasis. The glomerulosa is controlled principally by the renin-angiotensin system.

The fasciculata is the second layer of the adrenal cortex, is the thickest and most prominent on examination, and is responsible for glucocorticoid production, including cortisol. The fasciculata is regulated by pituitary adrenocorticotropin (ACTH) by long-loop negative feedback from peripheral cortisol production in combination with central hypothalamic corticotropin releasing hormone (CRH) stimulation. ACTH is produced by anterior pituitary processing of a large precursor peptide, pro-opiomelanocorticotropin (POMC), which also contains MSH and endorphin sequences. Cortisol circulates bound to a specific transport protein, cortisol binding globulin (CBG), as well as being bound nonspecifically to serum albumin. Approximately 10% of circulating cortisol is free and therefore biologically active.

The reticularis is the innermost zone of the adrenal cortex and is responsible for androgen and estrogen production. Regulation is achieved through pituitary ACTH levels but only in response to cortisol feedback from the fasciculata, an important interrelationship in congenital adrenal hyperplasia syndromes related to adrenal enzyme defects.

Another important regulator of adrenal steroid synthesis and secretion is the renin-angiotensin axis, which selectively regulates adrenal mineralocorticoid production. This axis is also strongly influenced by adrenergic factors and by sodium and potassium concentrations.

Clinical Disorders

CUSHING'S SYNDROME

Cushing's syndrome is the clinical disorder that results from sustained glucocorticoid excess. Clinical features include central weight gain, weakness, and facial plethora as well as hirsutism and menstrual irregularity in female patients. When Cushing's syndrome is suspected, screening laboratory studies are indicated to document glucocorticoid excess followed by additional studies to define the etiology of the disorder and to plan specific therapy.

The most common etiology of Cushing's syndrome is pituitary-dependent bilateral adrenal hyperplasia (Cushing's disease). Other etiologies include primary tumors of either adrenal gland, bilateral macronodular adrenal hyperplasia, or pigmented micronodular hyperplasia. Finally, certain nonendocrine neoplasms of the lung and pancreas as well as carcinoid tumors of the bronchi and thymus can produce ectopic nonpituitary ACTH syndromes (21).

Elevated urinary excretion of cortisol and cortisol metabolites is reflected in urinary cortisol, 17-hydroxysteroid, and 17-ketosteroid determinations. Urinary creatinine should always be included to ensure adequate collections. Elevated serum cortisol and loss of normal physiologic diurnal variation of serum cortisol are complementary or alternative methods of establishing *quantitative* glucocorticoid excess. Obesity alone may increase urinary cortisol metabolite excretion and estrogens—either endogenous secondary to pregnancy, or exogenous secondary to anovulatory or estrogen replacement therapy—may increase cortisol binding globulin (CBG) and result in false-positive serum cortisol elevations.

Dexamethasone, a potent glucocorticoid derivative, may be used to document *qualitative* glucocorticoid abnormality by demonstrating lack of physiologic adrenal suppressibility. Normal patients or those with uncomplicated obesity will demonstrate a decrease of 50% or more in urinary cortisol or cortisol metabolite excretion when treated with dexamethasone 0.5 mg orally every 6 hours for 48 hours. A single dose of dexamethasone, 1 mg orally at 11 PM, will suppress serum cortisol at 8 AM the following morning. Patients with any of the Cushing's syndrome etiologies will not demonstrate physiologic serum or urinary suppression. False positives may arise from estrogen administration, which increases serum cortisol binding (cortisol binding globulin), or the administration of drugs such as phenobarbital and analeptics, which accelerate metabolic clearance of dexamethasone.

Patients with bilateral adrenal hyperplasia suppress urinary cortisol excretion with larger doses of dexamethasone, 2 mg orally every 6 hours, for a subsequent 48 hours (22). Those with autonomous primary adrenal disorders such as adrenal adenoma or carcinoma or those with autonomous ACTH secretion such as those arising from para-endocrine neoplasms will also fail to suppress with the larger dose of dexamethasone (23).

Alternatively, exogenous ACTH or endogenous ACTH stimulated through inhibition of cortisol synthesis by pharmacologic agents such as metyrapone may also provide useful supplementary information (Table 13.7).

Pituitary localization as well as lateralization can be accomplished by measurement of plasma ACTH obtained by bilateral petrosal sinus catheterization (24). This information is particularly helpful when transsphenoidal pituitary surgery for correction of ACTH-dependent Cushing's disease is anticipated.

ADRENAL INSUFFICIENCY

Adrenal insufficiency (Addison's disease) can arise from either primary adrenal cortical failure or as a result of secondary pituitary ACTH deficiency. The disorder can present as both a chronic and an acute syndrome.

The most common etiology of chronic adrenal insufficiency is autoimmune adrenalitis. Other etiologies include granulomatous disorders such as tuberculosis, sarcoidosis, adrenal leukodystrophy, and metastatic adrenal involvement. Autoimmune adrenalitis may occur as an isolated phenomenon or as a component of polyglandular autoimmune syndromes. Polyglandular autoimmune syndrome type I includes patients with adrenal insufficiency, hypoparathyroidism, and mucocutaneous moniliasis. Polyglandular autoimmune syndrome type II includes patients with adrenal insufficiency, diabetes mellitus, and thyroid dysfunction. Fatigue, weight loss, nausea, and hyperpigmentation are clinical presentations in patients with chronic adrenal insufficiency. The latter is related to the overproduction of pituitary ACTH and MSH sequences, which are derived from pituitary processing of pro-opiomelanocortin (POMC). Acute adrenal insufficiency is most often seen in the intensive care setting in stressed and anticoagulated patients. Hypotension and shock dominate the clinical picture of acute adrenal insufficiency.

Secondary adrenal insufficiency arises as a result of infiltrative or destructive disorders of the hypotha-

Table 13.7. Cushing's Syndrome

	Normal	Cushing's Syndrome			
Screening studies					
Urinary free cortisol	<80 μg/24 hr	>100 μg/24 hr			
Overnight dexamethasone suppression study[a]	<5 μg/dl	>5 μg/dl			
	Normal	**Pituitary Dependent**	**Adrenal Adenoma**	**Adrenal Carcinoma**	**Ectopic ACTH**
Definitive studies					
Baseline					
Urinary					
17-OHCS (mg/24 hr)	2–8	>100%	>100%	>100%	>>100%
17-Ketosteroid	5–15			>>100%	
Cortisol (μg/24 hr)	20–80	>100%	>100%	>100%	>100%
Serum					
Cortisol 8 AM (μg/dl)	6–26				
4–8 PM	4–14				
DHEA Sulfate (μg/dl)	40–360			>>100%	
Plasma ACTH pg/ml	20–80	>50	<20	<20	>>50
Suppression					
Dexamethasone (0.5 mg every 6 hr × 48 hr)	<50%	>50%	>50%	>50%	>50%
Dexamethasone (2.0 mg every 6 hr × 48 hr)	>90%	>90%	>50%	>50%	>50%
Stimulation					
ACTH stimulation:			often		
(0.5 mg iv/8 hr)	>50%	>100%	>50%	10%	variable
Metapyrone stimulation:					
(750 mg every 6 hr × 24 hr)	>50%	>50%	<50%	<50%	<50%
Corticotropin releasing hormone (CRH) (100 μg iv)					
Serum cortisol		>20%	<20%	<20%	<20%
Plasma ACTH		>50%	<20%	<20%	<20%

lamic-pituitary axis or from functional suppression by exogenous glucocorticoid administration.

Congenital adrenal hyperplasia syndromes are the result of heritable defects in the enzymes required for cortisol biosynthesis. The resultant disorders are characterized both by cortisol deficiency and often by androgen excess resulting from ACTH stimulation secondary to cortisol deficiency. The most common disorders involve deficiencies of the 21-hydroxylase enzyme involved in cortisol and mineralocorticoid synthesis. In the newborn, syndromes of glucocorticoid and mineralocorticoid deficiency as well as ambiguous external genitalia in females are common. In later pediatric and adolescent years disorders of hirsutism, virilization, and menstrual irregularity are seen.

ISOLATED MINERALOCORTICOID DEFICIENCY

A syndrome of isolated mineralocorticoid deficiency is seen in older patients who present with recurrent hyperkalemia but normal cortisol and ACTH secretion. This disorder is particularly common in patients with diabetes mellitus and underlying kidney diseases such as interstitial nephritis. Evaluation requires exclusion of primary adrenocortical insufficiency by serum cortisol and ACTH testing followed by documentation of defective plasma renin and serum aldosterone response to sodium restriction and upright posture.

ADRENAL VIRILIZATION AND CONGENITAL ADRENAL HYPERPLASIA

Virilization secondary to adrenal disorders occurs in patients with congenital adrenal hyperplasia syndromes and as a component of Cushing's syndrome secondary to adrenocortical androgen excess. Rarely, adrenal cortical adenoma may secrete androgens alone, producing isolated adrenal androgen excess. Elevated serum DHEA sulfate, an excellent marker of adrenal androgen excess, is the most consistent finding, as are selective elevations of urinary 17-ketosteroids when measured.

The syndromes of congenital adrenal hyperplasia are a group of inborn disorders of adrenal cortisol biosynthesis that have in common defects in cortisol biosynthesis and often androgen excess as a consequence of increased ACTH secretion. The most common enzyme defect is at the 21-hydroxylase step (25). Affected female newborns present with ambiguous genitalia as a result of intrauterine exposure to excessive adrenal androgens. Affected male newborns have normal external genitalia and share with their female counterparts variable renal sodium loss as a result of mineralocorticoid deficiency. Affected individuals not properly diagnosed at birth may present in later pediatric years with sexual precocity in males and virilization in females as a result of ongoing adrenal androgen production. The diagnosis of congenital adrenal hyperplasia is established by measurement of serum 17-hydroxyprogesterone, which is the precursor for the 21-hydroxylase enzyme. Recently, a more subtle defect in 21-hydroxylase has been recognized in girls at puberty with resultant hirsutism and menstrual irregularity. Diagnosis requires measurement of 17-hydroxyprogesterone before and 60 minutes following ACTH (Cortrosyn) administration. Other relatively common adrenal enzymatic disorders occur at the 11-hydroxylase and 3β-dehydrogenase steps. The former is associated with increased desoxycorticosterone synthesis, resulting in hypertension rather than sodium loss, and the latter by profound cortisol, mineralocorticoid, and androgen deficiency. The laboratory diagnosis is established by documentation of increased 11-desoxycortisol in the 11-hydroxylase disorder and by the ratio of pregnenolone:progesterone, 17-hydroxypregnenolone:17-hydroxyprogesterone or DHEA:androstenedione in the 3β-dehydrogenase deficiency. Finally, it should be noted that all steroid hormones exert their biologic actions through cellular receptors and that clinical disorders that mimic adrenal biosynthetic abnormalities may arise as a result of receptor abnormalities.

ADRENAL HYPERTENSION

Hypertension resulting from primary adrenal mineralocorticoid excess can be caused either from mineralocorticoid-secreting solitary adrenal adenomas (aldosterone-secreting adenomas) or from bilateral adrenal adenomatous hyperplasia. Hypokalemia and elevated urinary potassium excretion are related to increased mineralocorticoid biosynthesis, and plasma renin is suppressed by the resultant extracellular volume expansion. Failure of serum aldosterone to suppress following intravenous saline infusion and of plasma renin to increase following sodium restriction, upright posture, and diuretic administration are additional characteristics (26). The specific etiology can then be distinguished by the use of adrenal computed tomographic scanning, I-131 iodocholesterol adrenal scanning, or differential adrenal vein catheterization studies. Rarely, other mineralocorticoid-secreting adrenal adenomas may produce a similar clinical picture.

Secondary aldosterone hypersecretion as a result of increased renin secretion is associated with renal artery stenosis, accelerated hypertension of any etiology, and in some patients following oral estrogen administration, particularly anovulatory agents, as a result of estrogen-mediated hepatic angiotensinogen secretion.

THE ENDOCRINE PANCREAS AND GASTROINTESTINAL PEPTIDES

The islet cells of the pancreas and the endocrine cells of the foregut constitute an integrated endocrine system functionally related to alimentation and metabolic fuel integration. The islets of Langerhans of the pancreas contain alpha, beta and delta cells respectively secreting glucagon, insulin, and somatostatin. The close proximity of these cells permits both paracrine, (i.e., local interactions at a cell-to-cell level) and more traditional endocrine actions. The common embryologic origin of these endocrine cells from histochemically distinct APUD (amine uptake and decarboxylation) cells of the embryologic neuroectoderm results not only in the presence of cells in the adult foregut that secrete gastrin, motilin, vasoactive intestinal peptide (VIP), and somatostatin but also in peptide-secreting cells that are distributed from the hypothalamic pituitary axis, through the thyroid and bronchial epithelium, to the distal small bowel. These foregut peptides are involved in the integration of intestinal secretion and motility. All of these sites may become clinically involved in endocrine neoplastic syndromes.

Diabetes Mellitus

The most common endocrine disorder of the endocrine pancreas is type I insulin-dependent diabetes mellitus (IDDM). In this disorder there is progressive loss of pancreatic beta cell function and without treatment the ultimate development of hyperglycemia and ketoacidosis. Antibodies to islet cells are present in a high percentage of cases at the time of clinical onset and there is a relationship between IDDM and the HLA histocompatibility loci DR3 and DR4 on the sixth chromosome.

IDDM accounts for approximately 10% of patients with diabetes. Ninety percent of patients with diabetes have Type II diabetes, non–insulin-dependent diabetes (NIDDM), which is often associated with obesity and is present particularly in patients over the age of 40. In this disorder insulin resistance complicates a quantitatively less severe defect in insulin secretion. Islet cell antibodies are negative and there is no relation to HLA abnormalities.

An additional category of impaired glucose tolerance (IGT) is reserved for patients with abnormalities of glucose tolerance testing but without fasting hyperglycemia or other overt evidence of diabetes mel-

Table 13.8. Criteria for the Diagnosis of Diabetes Mellitus

	FBS	1 hr	2 hr	3 hr
Adult	*mg/dl*	*mg/dl*	*mg/dl*	*mg/dl*
Diabetes mellitus				
Fasting	>140			
Glucose tolerance test (75 g glucose or 1.75 g glucose/kg body weight)	>140	>200	>200	—
Impaired glucose tolerance (75 g glucose)	>200	140–200		
Gestational diabetes mellitus				
Screening (50 g glucose)		>140		
Definitive (100 g glucose)	>105	>190	>165	>145
Pediatric				
Diabetes mellitus				
Fasting	>140			
Glucose tolerance test (1.75 g glucose/kg body weight)	>140	>200	>200	

litus. Diabetes can also occur secondary to other endocrine disorders such as acromegaly or Cushing's disease, in which elevations of counterregulatory hormones develop. IGT may initially present during pregnancy in patients with subclinical insulin deficiency as a result of the secretion of placental hormones, which antagonize insulin action.

DIAGNOSIS OF DIABETES MELLITUS

The diagnosis of diabetes mellitus is usually straightforward when fasting hyperglycemia is present. A fasting blood sugar greater than 140 mg/dl on two occasions is diagnostic of diabetes mellitus.

Greater sensitivity but decreased specificity are achieved by the use of oral glucose tolerance testing, which is unnecessary if fasting hypoglycemia is documented (27). The patient should have eaten at least 150 g of carbohydrate for 3 days preceding the test. Glucose (75 g) is administered to nonpregnant adults at time zero (1.75 g/kg in children) and serum samples are obtained at zero, 1 and 2 hours. For screening during pregnancy 50 g of glucose is administered without respect to fasting between the 24th and 28th weeks of pregnancy. If blood sugar exceeds 140 mg/dl 60 minutes after the administration of glucose a formal glucose tolerance test is performed with 100 g of glucose and with serum samples obtained at zero, 1, 2, and 3 hours. For the evaluation of patients with suspected reactive hypoglycemia 75 to 100 g of glucose is administered and blood sugars obtained at zero, 1, 2, 3, 4, and 5 hours and additionally with spontaneous symptoms. In nonpregnant adults blood sugars greater than 200 mg/dl at either 1 or 2 hours is diagnostic of diabetes. In pregnant adults gestational diabetes is diagnosed if two of the following are achieved: fasting blood sugar greater than 105, 1-hour blood sugar 160, 2-hour blood sugar 165, or 3-hour blood sugar 145 mg/dl. A summary of the criteria for making the diagnosis of diabetes mellitus is given in Table 13.8.

MANAGEMENT OF DIABETES MELLITUS

The contemporary management of diabetes mellitus relies heavily on the use of frequent capillary blood sugars, which are monitored by patients with fingerstick samples obtained with disposable lancets and reagent strips that are read visually or by glucose meters. Urinary glucose monitoring is not sufficiently precise for optimal diabetic control, although the measurement of urinary ketones may be helpful during episodes of acute illness and potential ketoacidosis. These blood sugar results are supplemented by the measurement of one of several glycolated proteins, including glycosylated hemoglobins, hemoglobin A_{Ic}, glycosylated albumin, and fucosamine. These proteins undergo non-insulin glycation as a function of integrated blood sugar levels (28). The concentrations of these glycated proteins is a function of the degree of hyperglycemia and the half-life of the involved cells or proteins. Glycosylated hemoglobin, as an example, gives an integrated estimate of blood sugar over the aproximately 4-month life span of the erythrocyte.

Hypoglycemia

Hypoglycemia, either documented or clinically suspected, can be divided into disorders in which symptoms occur when fasting and that are often associated with decreased levels of consciousness or mentation (i.e., fasting hypoglycemia) and disorders that typically occur within several hours following eating and that are typically associated with sympathomimetic symptoms such as anxiety, palpitations, and anxiety (29).

Fasting hypoglycemia can arise from disorders of insulin secretion, from autoimmune mechanisms involving either the insulin molecule or the insulin receptor, from defects in counter-regulatory hormone secretion such as cortisol and growth hormone, and from exogenous means such as insulin or sulfonylurea administration. Measurement of blood sugar and serum insulin levels following overnight fast and during spontaneous symptoms is essential. With blood sugars below 50 mg/dl, serum insulin should be undetectable and the ratio of serum insulin (uU/ml) blood glucose (mg/dl) less than 0.3. In addition, measurement of the serum insulin C peptide or serum proinsulin may be useful in identifying endogenous versus exogenous insulin, since C-peptide and proinsulin are not present in exogenous insulin preparations. Finally, antibodies to insulin may be helpful in identifying both exogenous insulin administration and spontaneous insulin antibodies with partial agonist actions.

Patients with postprandial symptoms may have reactive hypoglycemia. The symptoms are dominated by shakiness, anxiety, fatigue, and hunger rather than loss of consciousness. Postgastrectomy patients and patients with early Type II diabetes mellitus with delayed but ultimately normal or even elevated serum insulin levels may present in this manner.

The criteria for the diagnosis of reactive hypoglycemia are problematic, and blood sugars obtained at the time of spontaneous symptoms are more appropriate and preferred when this diagnosis is being considered. The diagnosis of reactive hypoglycemia is frequently made uncritically by patients and physicians alike. Many subjective symptoms that may or may not be related to eating or are associated with food relief are attributed to "low blood sugar." This tendency is compounded by the excessive and uncritical use of the glucose tolerance test to establish this diagnosis.

The mean blood glucose nadir in normal subjects following glucose administration is 64 mg/dl, and 10% of normal subjects have blood sugars below 47 mg/dl. Failure of recognition of these variances has led to the overdiagnosis of hypoglycemia by glucose tolerance testing and has led many authorities to recommend that glucose tolerance tests *not* be employed in the evaluation of patients with suspected hypoglycemia.

Islet Cell–Foregut Peptides

Neoplasms of the cells of the pancreatic islet and the neuroectodermal cells of the foregut arise infrequently but may produce distinctive and characteristic endocrine syndromes (30). Benign and malignant tumors of the beta cells of the pancreas produce the insulinoma syndrome, characterized by fasting hypoglycemia and inappropriately elevated serum insulin levels, which is reviewed under fasting hypoglycemia.

GASTRIN

Tumors of the delta cells of the islets or of gastrin secreting cells of the foregut produce the gastrinoma syndrome (Zollinger-Ellison syndrome,) characterized by recurrent duodenal and distal small bowel peptic ulcer disease and diarrhea secondary to increased gastric acid secretion and resultant small bowel pH disruption. These tumors are often malignant and may be multifocal. The diagnosis is based on the documentation of elevated fasting serum gastrin levels by immunochemical methods (above 100 pg/ml) in the setting of increased gastric acid secretion or by the paroxysmal increase (more than 200 pg/ml) in serum gastrin following intravenous secretin administration (2 units/kg i.v.) when basal serum gastrin levels are not clearly elevated.

VASOACTIVE INTESTINAL PEPTIDE

A second syndrome associated with watery diarrhea and resultant hypokalemia as a result of increased diarrheal potassium loss is the watery diarrhea-hypochlorhydria-hypokalemia (WDHHK) syndrome or Verner-Morrison syndrome. Gastric acid secretion is not elevated in this disorder which results from the excessive secretion vasoactive intestinal peptide (VIP) from pancreatic islet cell tumors. Serum VIP levels by immunoassay are elevated (more than 50 pg/ml) in the majority of patients with this disorder.

GLUCAGON

A syndrome characterized by hyperglycemia, anemia, weight loss, and a characteristic migratory necrotizing dermatitis skin rash is related to glucagon-secreting neoplasms of the islet cells of the pancreas. These tumors are often malignant and extensive before diagnosis is established. Serum glucagon levels are elevated (above 100 pg/ml). The etiology of the rash, which is seen in approximately two-thirds of the patients, is unknown.

SOMATOSTATIN

Several patients with diabetes, diarrhea, and gallstones secondary to decreased gallbladder contractility have been described secondary to somatostatin-secreting islet cell pancreatic tumors. These actions are consistent with the known actions of somatostatin on insulin secretion and gastrointestinal and biliary tract motility. Serum somatostatin levels by radioimmunoassay (RIA) are elevated.

Table 13.9. Calcium Regulation by Hormone and Site of Action[a]

	Bone	Kidney	Intestine
Parathyroid hormone (PTH)	Increases resorption of calcium and phosphate	Increases reabsorption of calcium, decreases reabsorption of phosphate; increases conversion of 25-OHD_3 to 1,25$(OH)_2D_3$; decreases reabsorption of bicarbonate	No direct effects
Calcitonin (CT)	Decreases resorption of calcium and phosphate	Decreases reabsorption of calcium and phosphate. Questionable effect on vitamin D metabolism	No direct effects
Vitamin D	Maintains Ca^{2+} transport system	Decreases reabsorption of calcium	Increases absorption of calcium and phosphate

Reprinted with permission from Greenspan FS. Basic endocrinology. 3rd ed. Norwalk, CT: Appleton & Lange, 1991.

CARCINOID SYNDROME

The syndrome characterized by flushing, diarrhea, asthma, and right-sided endocardial valvular thickening and dysfunction is produced by carcinoid tumors of the chromaffin cells of the distal intestine and bronchial epithelium. These symptoms are related to episodic serotonin and bradykinin secretion. Diagnosis is usually confirmed by documentation of elevated urinary excretion of 5-hydroxyindoleacetic acid (5-HIAA) (a metabolite of serotonin) or by increased serum serotonin levels.

OTHER GI PEPTIDE SYNDROMES

Many other gastrointestinal peptides are known, including pancreatic polypeptide (PP), gastric inhibitory peptide (GIP, bombesin), secretin, and cholecystokinin. No recognized endocrine syndromes are associated with these peptides. Elevation of serum levels by RIA may serve as markers in other APUD endocrine syndromes. Serum β-hCG, α-fetoprotein, and chromogranin-A may also be useful as serum markers of pancreatic-gastrointestinal pancreatic syndromes.

HYPERCALCEMIA/HYPOCALCEMIA METABOLIC BONE DISEASE

Physiology

SERUM CALCIUM REGULATION

Maintenance of serum ionized calcium stability is essential to a variety of critical biological functions, including nerve transmission, muscle contractility, and exocrine secretion. Serum calcium regulation is achieved by the interactions of parathormone, vitamin D and its activated metabolites, and calcitonin. These hormones act at the skeletal, gastrointestinal, and renal levels to maintain a stable ionized serum calcium concentration in the setting of highly variable dietary calcium intake. The major hormones responsible for calcium homeostasis and their modes of action are listed in Table 13.9.

Dietary calcium intake is approximately 1000 mg daily. Eighty percent of dietary calcium is initially absorbed, although 60% is subsequently secreted into the gastrointestinal tract as calcium-containing exocrine pancreatic secretion and sulcus entericus, with a resultant net absorption of dietary calcium of approximately 20%. Calcium is also available from the skeletal system, which serves as a reservoir of calcium through the integrated process of new bone formation and resorption of existing bone, which occurs in the process of continuous bone remodeling. Approximately 10,000 mg of ionized calcium is filtered at the glomerulus of the kidney, although efficient proximal and distal tubule resorption limit urinary calcium excretion to only 100 to 300 mg daily.

A fall in serum ionized calcium results in a rise in serum parathormone as a result of the direct negative feedback regulation of parathormone by serum ionized calcium. The rise in serum parathormone simultaneously increases bone resorption of calcium, increases urinary calcium tubular resorption, and activates the 1-hydroxylation of 25-hydroxyvitamin D to its active metabolite 1,25-dihydroxyvitamin D, which in turn increases gastrointestinal calcium absorption and amplifies parathormone mediated bone resorption. These actions serve to return the serum calcium to a normal range. Spontaneous increases in serum calcium have the opposite effects with resultant decrease in serum calcium. Calcitonin appears to have little influence on steady-state serum calcium regulation but moderates the rise in serum calcium during unsteady-state serum calcium changes. Through these hormonal, dietary, and physical activity relationships both serum calcium and bone mineral remodeling are maintained.

Clinical Disorders

HYPERCALCEMIA

Clinical hypercalcemia results from the pathologic disruption of serum calcium regulation by a variety of clinical disorders (31).

Primary hyperparathyroidism is the most common etiology of hypercalcemia and is characterized by a rise in serum ionized calcium as a result of increased parathormone secretion, most commonly from a parathyroid adenoma (90%) involving one of the four parathyroid glands, although occasionally as a result of multiple adenomas or hyperplasia involving all four parathyroid glands. The resultant hypercalcemia can produce symptoms of lassitude; increased bone calcium fatigue and increased resorption can produce demineralization and fractures; and increased urinary calcium secretion can lead to renal calculi. With newer and widespread monitoring of serum calcium by biochemical profile determinations, many older patients are found to have relatively asymptomatic hypercalcemia and hyperparathyroidism In all of these instances, serum parathormone is elevated when determined by appropriate immunoassay techniques (32). This is in contradistinction to other causes of hypercalcemia in which serum parathormone levels are suppressed by non-parathyroid-dependent hypercalcemia. Hyperparathyroidism may occur alone or as a component of multiple endocrine neoplasia (MEN) syndromes type I and II, in which case parathyroid hyperplasia involving all four parathyroid glands is seen. In MEN I hyperparathyroidism is associated with pancreatic islet cell neoplasms and pituitary adenomas. In MEN II hyperparathyroidism is associated with medullary thyroid carcinoma and pheochromocytoma, often bilateral. Both disorders are inherited as autosomal dominant disorders.

Hypercalcemia is one of the most common metabolic complications of malignancy, and several unique mechanisms are recognized. Hematologic malignancies such as multiple myeloma are associated with the production of osteolytic cytokines such as interleukin-I (IL-I) and tumor necrosis factor (TNF). In addition, some lymphomas are associated with increased 1,25-dihydroxyvitamin D levels as a result of tumor-related extrarenal 1-hydroxylase enzyme systems. Certain epithelial tumors produce a parathyroid hormone related peptide (PTH-RP), or humoral hypercalcemia of malignancy (HHM) peptide, which is similar in amino acid composition to parathormone in the amino acid terminus of the molecule, although it is highly distinct in its complete structure (33). Hypercalcemia in these patients is generally severe and is associated with decreased serum parathormone levels and by both hypercalcuria and hypochloremia as a result of suppression of parathormone tubular actions on calcium and hydrogen ion resorption.

Sarcoidosis and other granulomatous disorders such as tuberculosis, coccidiomycosis and berylliosis may be associated with extrarenal 1-hydroxylase enzyme activity, which results in hypercalcemia from increased dietary calcium absorption.

Certain drugs may elevate serum calcium, including vitamins A and D, thiazide diuretics, and lithium. The mechanisms are quite distinct. Vitamin D excess leads to increased circulating vitamin D levels, thiazides decrease urinary calcium excretion, and lithium appears to alter transmembrane calcium transport.

The syndrome of familial hypocalcuric hypercalcemia (FHH) is associated with mild hypercalcemia, normal to slightly elevated serum calcium concentrations, and low urinary calcium excretion (urinary calcium clearance:urinary creatinine clearance <0.01). The disorder is an autosomal dominant abnormality in which a heritable disorder of transmembrane calcium transport is present similar to that in patients with lithium-associated hypercalcemia. Care should be exercised to avoid unnecessary parathyroid surgical exploration in these patients.

HYPOCALCEMIA

Hypocalcemia results from failure of the parathormone–vitamin D system to maintain stable ionized calcium levels. It is important to recall that approximately 50% of serum calcium is bound to serum albumin. As a result, a decrease in serum total calcium can arise from decreased serum albumin concentration without any change in biologically active ionized serum calcium. Ionized serum calcium needs to be either measured directly or estimated by adding 0.8 mg/dl of serum calcium to the observed serum total calcium for every 1.0 g/dl decrease in serum albumin concentration.

Hypoparathyroidism results from failure of appropriate parathormone secretion or action. Hypoparathyroidism may follow thyroid or parathyroid surgery in which parathyroid glands are compromised or may arise as idiopathic hypoparathyroidism as a result of immunologic parathyroid dysfunction. The latter may arise as a component of one of two multiple endocrine immunodeficiency syndromes: Type I with idiopathic hypoparathyroidism, adrenal insufficiency, and mucocutaneous moniliasis; or type II with idiopathic hypoparathyroidism, immunologic thyroid dysfunction (such as Hashimoto's thyroiditis or Graves' disease), and insulin-dependent diabetes mellitus.

Pseudohypoparathyroidism is an uncommon disorder in which parathormone secretion is normal but parathormone action is deficient as a result of blunted parathormone receptor activity. Serum parathormone levels are elevated and the patients do not respond to exogenous parathormone administration by either a rise in serum calcium or urinary cyclic AMP excretion. In some patients this defect is associated with a defective guanidine nucleotide coupling protein, which serves to integrate the external parathormone binding receptor with the internally located adenyl cyclase catalytic subunit.

Since magnesium is necessary for both parathormone secretion and action, magnesium depletion is associated with hypocalcemia and decreased serum parathormone levels. Replacement of magnesium corrects both the hypocalcemia and the impaired PTH secretion, which is not responsive to calcium replacement alone.

DEMINERALIZATION

The participation of the skeletal system in the maintenance of serum calcium homeostasis gives rise to several significant clinical syndromes in which loss of skeletal mineral content may progress to the point of demineralization and fracture.

Osteoporosis

The most common demineralization disorder is osteoporosis. Osteoporosis is responsible for over 1.5 million fractures annually in the United States, with annual costs estimated to be over 15 billion and with a substantial increase in mortalty particularly in relation to hip fractures (34). The majority of patients have primary osteoporosis related to age, sex, and menopausal status in which a gradual loss of bone mineral occurs as a result of decreased bone formation relative to bone resorption. The residual bone is qualitatively normal although quantitatively reduced in mass. Additional contributory factors include limited dietary calcium intake, excessive alcohol or tobacco use, and family history. Osteoporosis can arise secondary to hyperthyroidism, Cushing's disease (particularly related to steroid use), and malabsorptive disorders. As a result of the relatively low levels of negative calcium balance, laboratory parameters are usually quite unremarkable. Contributory secondary factors can be excluded by laboratory means.

Osteomalacia

Defective bone mineralization despite adequate bone matrix formation is seen in osteomalacia. The resultant bone is qualitatively abnormal, with wide osteoid seams of unmineralized bone collagen as a result of inadequate bone mineralization. Malabsorption and chronic acidotic disorders are common contributing abnormalities. Drugs such as phenytoin and barbiturates may be factors as a result of hepatic enzyme induction and increased clearance of vitamin D. Inborn errors of vitamin D metabolism and action, such as vitamin D–dependent rickets and vitamin D–resistance rickets, also occur. Although serum calcium levels are well maintained despite the lack of adequate calcium for mineralization, decreased serum phosphorus levels as a result of secondary hyperparathyroidism, increased alkaline phosphatase activity, and low urinary calcium excretion are commonly seen. Definitive diagnosis may require bone biopsy.

PAGET'S DISEASE

Paget's disease, a common disorder of older patients is characterized by increased osteoclastic bone resorption, chaotic new bone formation, and elevated serum alkaline phosphatase levels. The latter may lead to the initial diagnosis of Paget's disease in asymptomatic patients without fracture or other skeletal abnormality.

Azotemic osteodystrophy is the complex metabolic bone disease that is commonly seen in patients with chronic renal insufficiency. As dialysis extends life in these patients the combination of chronic acidosis, secondary hyperparathyroidism as a result of phosphate retention, vitamin D abnormalities as a result of decreased renal 1-hydroxylation of vitamin D, and skeletal aluminum accumulation all lead to a progressively disabling metabolic bone disease.

METABOLIC STONE DISEASE

Renal calculi can arise from increased solute excretion (calcium, uric acid, cysteine), from decreased urinary volume or pH (uric acid, calcium oxalate, calcium phosphate), as a result of loss of biological inhibitors of urinary crystallization (citrate, pyrophosphate, magnesium, others), or secondary to underlying obstruction and infection. Evaluation requires exclusion of hypercalcemic disorders; quantitation of urinary calcium, oxalate, and uric acid excretion; and exclusion of underlying obstruction or infection (35).

REPRODUCTIVE ENDOCRINOLOGY

Physiology

Pituitary gonadotropin secretion in both males and females is initiated by the secretion of hypothalamic gonadotropin releasing hormone (GnRH) into the hypothalamic-hypophyseal portal vasculature in pulsatile fashion at 60- to 90-minute intervals (36). The resulting stimulation of pituitary follicle stimulating hormone (FSH) and luteinizing hormone (LH) secretion is further modulated by both positive and negative feedback of gonadal steroids and peptides.

In males LH binds to receptors on the interstitial Leydig cell of the testis, where it stimulates the production of testosterone and estradiol. FSH binds to receptors on the Sertoli cell of the seminiferous tubule, leading to the production of inhibin and an androgen binding protein produces the high local concentrations of testosterone needed for spermatogenesis. Inhibin feeds back through the systemic circulation to downregulate pituitary FSH secretion, while estradiol and testosterone feed back to downregulate pituitary LH secretion.

In females similar but much more dynamic hypothalamic-pituitary-ovarian relationships are present. FSH binds to the granulosa cells of the developing follicle, where it stimulates oocyte maturation, estradiol secretion, and inhibin production. Estradiol and inhibin downregulate FSH secretion by feedback inhibition. LH stimulates estrogen and androgen secretion from the interstitial cells of the ovary. These steroid hormones feed back initially to negatively inhibit LH secretion. At a critical threshold of estradiol, however, positive feedback—probably from a different set of hypothalamic neurons—results, with a resultant estrogen-stimulated peak in LH and FSH secretion which is necessary for ovulation. Thereafter the site of ovulation undergoes luteinization and becomes morphologically the corpus luteum, the site of progesterone secretion during the second half or luteal phase of the cycle. Under the influence of estrogen the endometrial lining of the uterus undergoes proliferative changes. These proliferative changes are further modified by progesterone-dependent glycogen deposition during the luteal phase of the cycle to prepare the endometrium for implantation should fertilization occur. If fertilization does not occur the decline and withdrawal of estradiol and progesterone brings about loss of the endometrium as a menstrual cycle preliminary to initiation of the subsequent menstrual cycle.

Fetal testicular androgen secretion is necessary for intrauterine male external genital differentiation. Female external genital differentiation occurs passively in the absence of directive testosterone secretion. Pituitary gonadotropin secretion is low during pediatric development in both sexes. At puberty an increase in serum FSH and LH secretion occurs as a result of increased hypothalamic GnRH secretion, initially leading to secondary sexual maturation in both sexes and ultimately to reproductive function.

Clinical Disorders

MALE

Hypogonadism

Delayed or absent sexual maturation in males can occur as a result of lack of hypothalamic-pituitary gonadotropin secretion, failure of gonadal response to pituitary gonadotropins, or failure of androgen action at the target cell receptor or postreceptor level.

When the defect is at the pituitary-hypothalamic level, low serum FSH and LH levels will be present as well as low testosterone levels. With organic lesions such as pituitary adenomas, craniopharyngiomas, or infiltrative or granulomatous disorders, other pituitary functions such as growth hormone, TSH, and ACTH function may be defective. The association of isolated hypogonadotropic hypogonadism with anosmia is known as Kallman's syndrome.

Not all abnormalities are organic. A common clinical problem is functional delay, in which ultimately normal physiologic sexual maturation may be delayed into late adolescence or early adulthood.

When the defect is at the testicular level, testosterone levels are low and pituitary gonadotropin levels elevated as a result of lack of physiologic feedback regulation of both testosterone and inhibin. In addition to traumatic testicular injury, Klinefelter's syndrome, a relatively common chromosomal disorder associated with an additional X chromosome (i.e., 47,XXY or 47,XXY/46,XY versus 46,XY in normal males), may be present.

Sexual Dysfunction

Sexual dysfunction—including decreased libido and failure of erection and ejaculation—often prompts pituitary-testicular endocrine evaluation. Although endocrine factors, including low testosterone states, may be present, other nonendocrine etiologies, including vascular and neurogenic disorders, must be considered. Disorders resulting in serum prolactin elevation may also be present.

Gynecomastia

Gynecomastia is the presence of clinically significant subareolar breast tissue in male subjects. The disorder can arise as a result of testosterone deficiency, inhibition of testosterone action by drugs such as spironolactone or cimetidine, and from neoplastic disorders with either ectopic chorionic gonadotropin or estrogen secretion. Pubertal gynecomastia is a common disorder in male adolescents associated with the initiation of physiologic pubertal gonadotropin secretion, which is usually self-limited and not associated with sustained androgen abnormality.

FEMALE

Amenorrhea

Primary amenorrhea, the absence of menses by age 16, may result from endocrine, chromosomal, anatomical, or functional disorders. With endocrine abnormalities there is usually an associated lack of appropriate physiologic sexual maturation. Turner's syndrome, with a 45/XO karyotype including mosaic variations in which only a portion of cells express a loss of the X chromosome, is usually associated with short stature. Elevated serum FSH levels implicate primary ovarian failure. Decreased serum gonadotropins indicate either organic or functional hypothalamic-pituitary dysfunction, the latter often related to low body weight and vigorous physical activity. Normal gonadotropin levels generally indicate loss of the physiologic cycle necessary for ovulation and menses. In patients with amenorrhea, pregnancy should always be excluded by appropriate hCG determinations.

Secondary amenorrhea is the cessation of periods in a previously menstruating patient. Pregnancy must again be excluded by hCG determination. The history of previous periods documents an intact uterus and functional endometrium in the absence of gynecologic intervention. Prolactin excess, either as a result of psychotropic medications such as phenothiazines, and pituitary microprolactinomas and macroprolactinomas require exclusion by serum prolactin measurement. Premature ovarian failure is associated with elevated serum gonadotropin levels. In patients with the polycystic ovary syndrome, variable clinical and laboratory evidence of androgen excess is present.

Hirsutism and Virilization

Excessive hair growth in androgen-responsive areas is a common clinical problem (37). Many drugs such as danazol, minoxidil, phenytoin, glucocorticoids, and cyclosporine may produce hirsutism. If other signs of androgen expression in addition to hirsutism are present—such as acne, amenorrhea, temporal hair recession, and masculinization—systemic androgen excess or virilization is present. Laboratory evaluation of hirsutism should include measurement of serum testosterone to document biochemical androgen excess and serum DHEA sulfate, an adrenal androgen, to distinguish adrenal from ovarian etiology. Additional laboratory studies may include measurement of serum free testosterone to distinguish free biologically active versus bound testosterone, androstenedione, cortisol, and pituitary serum FSH and LH levels. In patients with adrenal and ovarian neoplasms the elevated serum androgen levels also qualitatively fail to suppress following dexamethasone administration.

Patients with latent-onset 21-hydroxylase congenital adrenal hyperplasia may have elevated serum 17-hydroxyprogesterone levels, although often only following Cortrosyn stimulation testing (Cortrosyn, 0.25 mg i.v.; serum 17-hydroxyprogesterone at 0 and 60 minutes). Such tests should not be performed during the luteal phase of the menstrual cycle, when 17-hydroxyprogesterone secretion by both the ovarian corpus luteum and the adrenal gland may be present. Androgen suppression with dexamethasone may also be demonstrated.

Menopause

Physiologic cessation of menses occurs in the mid to late forties in a majority of patients secondary to ovarian senescence. This change is monitored most appropriately by elevation of serum FSH levels as a result of decreased estrogen and inhibin negative feedback suppression. Premature ovarian failure may occur at any age. The disorder may occur either as an isolated defect or as a component of a polyglandular autoimmune syndrome and the diagnosis documented by premature serum FSH elevation.

Laboratory Diagnosis

Figure 13.8 illustrates a diagnostic workup to determine the various causes of amenorrhea.

ADRENAL MEDULLA

The adrenal medulla is composed of chromaffin cells, which produce and secrete the vasoactive catecholamines, epinephrine and norepinephrine. These cells share a common embryologic origin with the cells of the sympathetic nervous system and with chromaffin cells of extrasympathetic distribution ranging from the carotid bodies to the organ of Zuckerkandl at the bifurcation of the aorta. The symptoms attributable to catecholamine excess are usually related predominantly to their cardiovascular effects.

Clinical Disorders

Pheochromocytomas are tumors arising from the adrenal medulla or sympathetic ganglia that produce hypertension which may either be labile or sustained and which is often associated with episodic symptoms of anxiety, headache, tremor, and weight loss. Such tumors may present sporadically or as a component of multiple endocrine neoplasia syndrome types IIA and IIB in association with medullary carcinoma of the thyroid and hyperparathyroidism. The diagnosis is often first considered as a result of labile hypertension noted at the time of general anesthesia and surgery.

A high index of suspicion is warranted in the presence of labile hypertension, particularly in younger patients with episodic symptoms including anxiety, tremulousness, and weight loss.

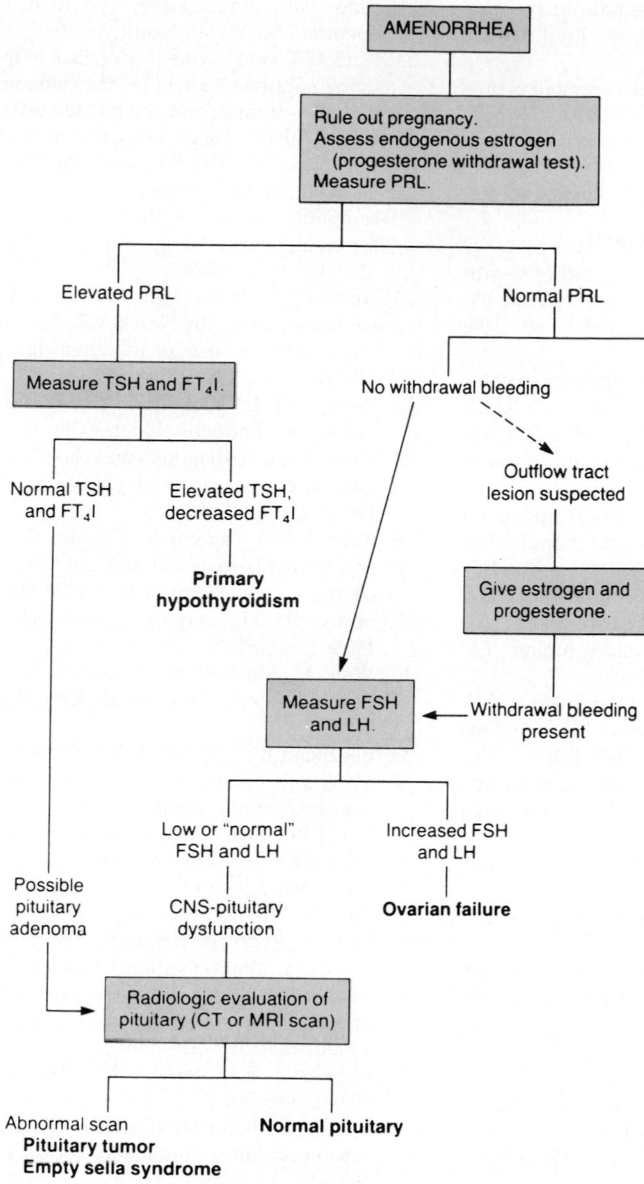

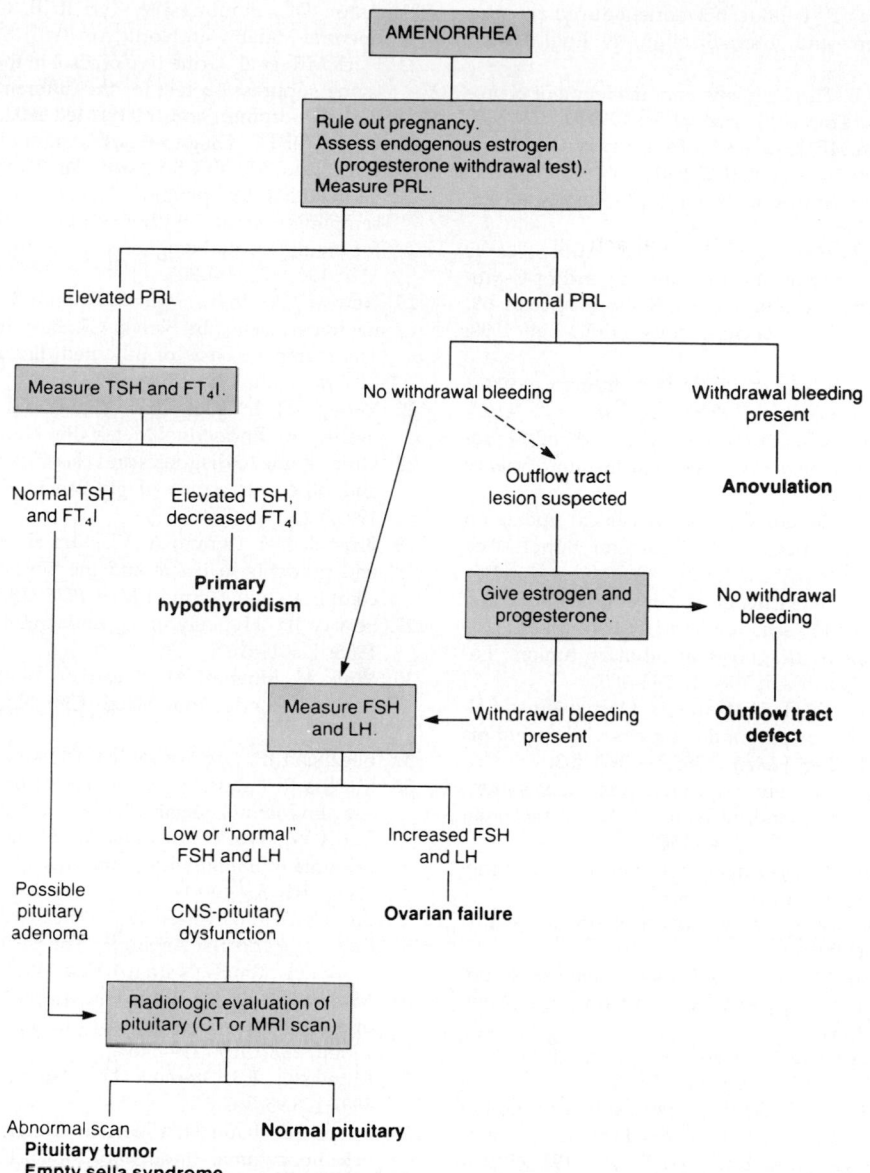

Figure 13.8. Potential decision tree for evaluation of amenorrhea. (Reproduced, with permission, from Goldfien A, Monroe SE. Ovaries. In: Greenspan FS ed. Basic and clinical endocrinology. Norwalk CT: Appleton & Lange, 1991:442–490.)

Laboratory Diagnosis

The diagnosis of pheochromocytoma is based on the demonstration of increased concentrations of the catecholamines and their metabolites supplemented by anatomical localization employing CT scanning (38). Due to the labile and variable nature of plasma catecholamines, more integrated urinary collections for measurement of urinary catecholamines and their metabolites, metanephrines and vanillylmandelic acid (VMA) are preferred. All collections should include urinary creatinine to ensure adequacy of collection and to permit expression of catecholamines and metabolites per 1000 mg of creatinine excretion. Such collections may encompass brief periods of spontaneous symptomatology or 24-hr periods with or without spontaneous symptoms. Attention must be given to the exclusion of multiple potential interfering medications. Initial anatomical localization is attempted with abdominal CT imaging. Arteriography or nuclear medicine localization by adrenal imaging with metaiodobenzylguanidine is reserved for those patients who fail to localize with CT scanning or in whom extraadrenal pheochromocytoma is suspected.

References

1. Thompson EB. Comment: single receptors, dual second messengers. 1992;6(4):551–556.
2. Williams, JA. Mechanisms of hormone secretion and action. In: Greenspan FS, (ed). Basic and clinical endocrinology. 1991.

3. King AC, Cuatrecasas P. Peptide hormone-induced receptor mobility, aggregation, and internalization. N Engl J Med 1981;305:77.
4. Findlay J, Eliopoulos E. Three dimensional modeling of G protein-linked receptors. Trends Pharmacol Sci 1990;11:492–499.
5. Simon MI, Strathman MP, Gautam N. Diversity of G proteins in signal transduction. Science 1991;252:802–808.
6. Gilman AG. G proteins: transducers of receptor-generated signals. Annu Rev Biochem 1987;56:615–649.
7. Spiegel AM, Simonds WF, Jones TL, et al. Antibodies as probes of G-protein receptor effector coupling and of G-protein membrane attachment. Biochem Soc Symp 1990;56:61–69.
8. Rink TJ. Receptor-mediated calcium entry. FEBS–Lett 1990; 268(z):381–385.
9. Dreyer M, Rudiger HW. Genetic defects of human receptor function. Trends Pharmacol Sci 1988;9(3):98–102.
10. Rarick HM, Artemyev NO, Hamm HE. A site on rod G protein alpha subunit that mediates effector activation. Science 1992;256(5059):1031–1033.
11. Page MD, Webster J, Dieguez C, et al. A clinical update on hypothalamic-pituitary control. Acta Neurochir Suppl Wien 1990;47:48–57.
12. Dieguez C, Page MD, Peters JR, et al. Growth hormone and its modulation. JR Coll Physicians Lond 1988;22(2):84–91.
13. Abboud CF, Laws ER Jr. Diagnosis of pituitary tumors. Endocrinol Metab Clin North Am 1988;17:241–280.
14. Goldman MB, Luchins DJ, Robertson GL. Mechanisms of altered water metabolism in psychotic patients with polydipia and hyponatremia. N Engl J Med. 1988;318:397–403.
15. Merendino JL, et al. Brief report: A mutation in the vasopressin V-2 receptor gene in a kindred with X-linked diabetes insipidus. N Engl J Med 1993:328;1538–1541.
16. Vokes TJ, Robertson GL. Disorders of antidiuretic hormone. Endocrinol Metab Clin North Am 1988;17:281–299.
17. Bayer MF. Effective laboratory evaluation of thyroid status. Med Clin North Am 1991;75:1–26.
18. Wartofsky L. Use of the sensitive TSH assay to determine optimal thyroid hormone therapy and avoid osteoporosis. Annu Rev Med 1991;42:341–345.
19. Wenzel KW. Pharmacologic interference with *in vitro* tests of thyroid function. Metabolism 1981;30:717–728.
20. Ross DS, Ardisson LJ, Meskell MJ. Measurement of thyrotropin in clinical and subclinical hyperthyroidism using a new chemiluminescent assay. J Clin Endocrinol Metab 1989;69:684–648.
21. Aaron DC, Findling JW, Tyrrell JB. Cushing's disease. Endocrinol Metab Clin North Am 1987;16:705–730.
22. Flack MR, et al. Urine free cortisol in the high dose dexamethasone suppression test for the differential diagnosis of Cushing's Syndrome. Ann Intern Med 1992;116:211–217.
23. Carpenter PC. Diagnostic evaluation of Cushing's syndrome. Endocrinol Metab Clin North Am 1988;17:445–473.
24. Oldfield EH, Doppman JL, Nieman, LK, et al. Petrosal venous sampling with and without corticotrophin-releasing hormone for the differential diagnosis of Cushing's syndrome. N Engl J Med 1991;325:897–905.
25. New MI, White PC, Paug S, Dupont B, Speiger PW. The adrenal hyperplasias. In: Scriver CR, Beaudet AL, Sly WS, Valle D. The metabolic basis of inherited disease. 6th ed. New York: McGraw-Hill, 1989:1881–1917.
26. Young WF Jr, Klee GG. Primary aldosteronism. Diagnostic evaluation. Endocrinol Metab Clin North Am 1988;17:367–395.
27. Office guide to diagnosis and classification of diabetes mellitus and other categories of glucose intolerance. Diabetes Care 1993;16(Suppl 2):4.
28. Brownlee M, Cerami A, Vlassara H. Advanced glycosylation end products in tissue and the biochemical basis of diabetic complications. N Engl J Med 1988;318:1315–1321.
29. Service JH. Hypoglycemia. Endocrinol Metab Clin North Am 1988;17:601–616.
30. Vinik AI, Moattari AR. Treatment of endocrine tumors of the pancreas. Endocrinol Metab Clin North Am 1989;18(2):483–518.
31. Bilezikian JP. Hypercalcemia. Dis Mon 1988;34(12):737–799.
32. Marcus R. Laboratory diagnosis of primary hyperparathyroiism. Endocrinol Metab Clin North Am 1989;18(3):647–658.
33. Burtis WJ, Wu TL, Insogna KL, Stewart AF. Humoral hypercalcemia of malignancy. Ann Intern Med 1988;108(3):454–457.
34. Riggs, RL, Melton LJ. The prevention and treatment of osteoporosis. N Engl J Med 1992;327:620–626.
35. Coe, FL, Parks JH, Asplin JR. The pathogenesis and treatment of kidney stones. N Engl J Med 1992;327:1141–1152.
36. Marshall JC, Kelch RP. Gonadotropin-releasing hormone: role of pulsatile secretion in the regulation of reproduction. N Engl J Med. 1986;315:1459–1468.
37. Rittmaster RS, Loriaux DL. Hirsutism. Ann Intern Med 1987;106:95–107.
38. Sheps SG, Jiang N, Klee GG. Diagnostic evaluation of pheochromocytoma. Endocrinol Metab Clin North Am 1988;17: 397–414.

14 Electrolytes and Acid-Base Balance

Robert W. Burnett, Elizabeth Lee-Lewandrowski, and Kent Lewandrowski

The essential concepts necessary to understanding the mechanisms underlying acid-base, fluid, and electrolyte disorders are described here. For more details, an excellent discussion of this topic by Rose is recommended (1).

SODIUM, POTASSIUM, AND CHLORIDE

Normal Physiology and Homeostasis

Measurements of electrolyte concentrations are among the most commonly performed tests in the clinical laboratory, both because there are a wide variety of disorders that may cause electrolyte abnormalities and because the administration of intravenous and parenteral fluids necessitates periodic reassessment of serum electrolytes and osmolality.

In a healthy person homeostatic mechanisms maintain the water and electrolyte composition of intracellular and extracellular fluids within relatively narrow limits. The total body water constitutes 60% of the lean body mass and is distributed as intracellular fluid (ICF) and extracellular fluid (ECF). The distribution of water in a lean 70-kg man is shown in Table 14.1. Note that by convention "extracellular" fluid includes both blood plasma and the fluid inside blood cells.

A distinction should be made between the ECF and the effective circulating volume (ECV). The ECV is the portion of the ECF that is effectively perfusing tissue cells. Ordinarily the ECF and the ECV are closely related, but in some pathologic states (such as heart failure, cirrhosis with ascites, and edema) a portion of the ECF does not perfuse the tissues and thus does not contribute to the ECV. In these situations the effective circulating volume is decreased despite an increase in the total ECF. The importance of distinguishing the ECV from the ECF is that the ECV is the component that is sensed and therefore regulated by the body's volume receptors. A fall in the ECV is interpreted as a signal to retain sodium and water even in the face of edema and ECF volume expansion.

Cell membranes are freely permeable to water. Therefore osmotic forces are the major factor determining the distribution of water in the body. The ECF and ICF are in osmotic equilibrium but the electrolyte composition of the two compartments differs. Table 14.2 shows the composition of the major electrolytes in plasma. Sodium is the predominant cation in ECF, whereas potassium ion predominates in the cells. Sodium salts are thus the major contributor to plasma osmolality. If the osmolality of one compartment is changed, water moves across cell membranes to reestablish osmotic equilibrium.

The regulation of plasma sodium concentration, osmolality, and the effective circulating volume are complex and closely interrelated. Regulation of the plasma sodium and osmolality is accomplished largely by alterations in water balance, whereas volume regulation is achieved by changes in sodium balance (2). The plasma osmolality equals the sum of all of the osmolalities of the individual solutes.

Plasma osmolality (and thus the plasma sodium) are maintained within narrow limits by changes in water intake and renal water excretion. Renal water

Table 14.1. Water Distribution in a 70-kg Person

Component	Volume
	liters
Total body water (60% of lean body mass)	42
Intracellular fluid (66% of total body water)	28
Extracellular fluid (34% of total body water)	14
Interstitial fluid	10.5
Vascular compartment (including blood cells)	3.5

Table 14.2. Electrolyte Composition of Plasma[a]

Cations	
Sodium	135–145 mmol/liter
Potassium	3.2–5.0 mmol/liter
Calcium (total)	2.3–2.6 mmol/liter
Magnesium	0.7–1.1 mmol/liter
Trace elements	ca. 1 mmol/liter
Anions	
Chloride	95–105 mmol/liter
Bicarbonate	24–32 mmol/liter
Phosphate	0.8–1.5 mmol/liter
Other (proteins, anions of organic acids, sulfate)	ca. 21 mmol/liter

[a]Adapted from Cambel J, Frisse M, eds. Manual of medical therapeutics. 24th ed. Boston: Little, Brown, 1986.

excretion is regulated by the pituitary secretion of antidiuretic hormone (ADH). Changes in plasma osmolality are sensed by osmoreceptors in the hypothalamus. An increase initiates the thirst mechanism, thus increasing water intake, and stimulates ADH secretion. ADH acts on the renal collecting tubules to promote renal water conservation, resulting in concentrated urine and restoration of normal plasma osmolality. Conversely, a fall in osmolality results in a decreased thirst stimulus, a fall in ADH, increased renal water excretion, and dilute urine. Collectively the thirst mechanism and ADH are highly effective in maintaining normal plasma osmolality and sodium concentration. Other stimuli can also promote ADH secretion, including hypotension and a decreased blood volume (3). This mechanism is mediated by aortic and carotid baroreceptors and by atrial volume receptors. Thus a decrease in the effective circulating volume also results in ADH secretion and renal water conservation.

The kidney is the major organ responsible for sodium and water homeostasis. Sodium intake must be balanced by urinary excretion. A number of factors influence renal sodium excretion, including aldosterone, atrial natriuretic peptide (ANP), the activity of the sympathetic nervous system and catecholamines, the plasma sodium itself, and the glomerular filtration rate (2).

Maintenance of the ECV is accomplished by a series of sensors and effectors. Volume receptors are present in the carotid sinuses, the aortic arch, and in the afferent juxtaglomerular arterioles. The juxtaglomerular sensors regulate the activity of the renin-angiotensin-aldosterone system, whereas the extrarenal sensors regulate release of ANP and influence the activity of the sympathetic nervous system. Aldosterone acts on the renal collecting tubules to increase sodium resorption and potassium secretion, and sodium resorption leads to an expansion of the ECF volume. ANP promotes sodium excretion. Aldosterone and ANP are the major factors responsible for the day-to-day regulation of sodium balance and therefore volume regulation. A decrease in the ECV results in vasoconstriction, an increase in cardiac output and blood pressure, a decrease in ANP, and an increase in aldosterone with increased renal sodium and water resorption. An increase in the ECV has the opposite effect. Thus the ECV is an important determinant of renal sodium excretion, and the rate of renal sodium excretion regulates the ECV.

Potassium salts are the major intracellular solutes. Only 2% of the total body potassium is extracellular. The normal plasma potassium is 3.2 to 5.0 mmol/liter, while the normal intracellular concentration is about 150 mmol/liter. Redistribution of potassium ions between cells and the ECF occurs in a number of situations. For example, if renal loss of potassium increases for some reason, the plasma level does not drop as much as might be expected because of the large reservoir of intracellular potassium that is available for redistribution. Thus a fall in the plasma concentration of 1 mmol/liter requires a loss of 100 to 200 millimoles of potassium, most of which is lost from the intracellular compartment. Likewise, a sudden infusion of a large amount of potassium produces less of a rise in the plasma concentration than might be expected, due to cellular uptake of the ion. Potassium balance is dependent on both the daily intake and the rate of renal excretion. Normally only a small percentage of the daily potassium load is excreted by the gastrointestinal tract, but this fraction may increase markedly in some hyperkalemic states. Potassium balance is also affected by exchange of the ion between the intracellular and extracellular spaces. Unlike sodium, for which the urinary excretion may be reduced to nearly zero, there are always obligatory urinary and gastrointestinal losses of potassium that total roughly 20 mmol/day.

Potassium is filtered by the glomerulus, but most of the filtered load is resorbed in the proximal tubule. Thus, potassium secretion by the distal tubule is required for potassium excretion in the urine. The rate of transport of potassium into the distal tubular epithelial cells (and thus into the urine) is largely governed by aldosterone and the plasma potassium concentration. Aldosterone enhances potassium secretion in the distal tubule. Secretion of potassium is also dependent on the rate of urine flow (increased flow enhances excretion) and by the rate of delivery of sodium to the distal tubule. In the presence of nonresorbable anions, tubular sodium resorption necessitates excretion of another cation (potassium or hydrogen ion) to maintain electroneutrality.

Laboratory Measurement

FLAME PHOTOMETRY

In this method for sodium and potassium a sample is diluted and introduced into a high-temperature air-propane flame. In the flame, electrons in sodium and potassium ions are excited and then emit light as they return to their ground state. The wavelength of emitted light is characteristic of the particular ionic species, resulting in very high specificity for this method. Flame photometry is a robust method in that the result is not generally affected by the matrix of the specimen. Thus aqueous calibration materials may be used, and flame photometry is suitable for analysis of sodium and potassium in serum, plasma, urine, or other body fluids.

Most flame photometers use an internal standard such as a cesium or lithium salt, which is added to the diluent to compensate for dilution imprecision and for signal fluctuations due to changes in the aspiration rate of the sample. Instruments for clinical use are generally dual-channel, so that sodium and potassium may be measured simultaneously. Because of the excellent accuracy and precision of flame photometry, this technique is the basis for the reference method for sodium and potassium in serum.

ION-SELECTIVE ELECTRODES

An ion-selective electrode (ISE) is a device that develops a small voltage when in contact with a solution containing a particular ion. The critical element in the electrode is a thin membrane of a material chosen for its ability to bind one ion species much more than other ions in the sample.

Sometimes these membranes are made of glass; for example, the well-known pH electrode and some sodium electrodes. More often the membrane contains a large organic molecule, called an ionophore, which has different affinities for different ions.

To measure the voltage at the ISE, a second (reference) electrode must be used to complete a circuit, and because the voltage at the reference electrode must be constant, it is isolated from the sample (or calibrator) solution by a "salt bridge" or "liquid junction." A small voltage also exists at the interface between the salt bridge and the sample solution that is dependent on the composition of both the sample and the bridge solution. This voltage is called the liquid junction potential, Ej, and is one of the largest sources of error in ISE methods.

The difference between Ej with the unknown solution and Ej with the calibration solution is called the residual liquid junction potential. This quantity must be zero in order for the total cell voltage to accurately reflect the activity of the ion of interest. In other words, the voltage at the ISE itself should be the only voltage that varies when the test solution is changed. Although this is never completely true, the contributions of the bridge solution and the test solution to the liquid junction potential are not equal, and consequently the composition of the bridge solution can be chosen to minimize the variation in Ej with different test solutions.

A saturated, or nearly saturated, solution of potassium chloride is one popular choice of bridge solution for general-purpose ISE methods. However, electrode systems designed specifically for measurements on blood or plasma may use a different bridge solution to minimize the residual liquid junction potential in the particular test solution matrix.

Another common source of error in ISE methods is imperfect selectivity of the electrode for the ion of interest. For example, some ISEs intended for chloride measurements also respond, to a lesser but measurable extent, to bicarbonate ions in the sample. The matrix of the samples to be measured determines how selective the ISE must be. For example, for measurements in plasma, which has a sodium concentration about 30 times higher than its potassium concentration, a sodium electrode that responds slightly to potassium might be acceptable, while a potassium electrode with a significant sodium response could not be tolerated. Ion-selective electrodes are available for determination of sodium, potassium, and chloride as well as several other ions in body fluids.

COULOMETRY

One of the most accurate methods for serum chloride uses the principle of coulometry. This method measures the number of coulombs (which is proportional to the number of electrons) transferred in an electrochemical reaction. An apparatus called a chloride titrator has been designed for the determination of chloride in serum. A sample is added to an acid diluent in a cell containing a silver anode and a reference electrode, and a constant current is imposed, which generates silver ions at a constant rate. Insoluble silver chloride is formed until all of the chloride ion in the sample has been used. Excess silver ions are then generated and are detected, either potentiometrically or amperometrically, using a third electrode, and the titration is stopped. Because a constant current is used for the duration of the titration, the number of silver ions generated (which equals the number of chloride ions in the sample) are directly proportional to the duration of the titration, which is usually on the order of 1 or 2 minutes.

This method is both accurate (in the absence of other halides) and precise, and is the accepted reference method for serum chloride. Possible interferences include iodide, bromide, and any other anion that will react with the silver ion. Coulometry is also a robust method with respect to the sample matrix and is thus suitable for chloride analysis in serum, plasma, urine, and other body fluids.

SPECTROPHOTOMETRY (SODIUM AND POTASSIUM)

A spectrophotometric method for sodium and potassium measurement has been developed based on the affinity of these ions for certain large synthetic, cyclic organic molecules. These molecules, called macrocyclic ionophores, include crown ethers, cryptanols, spherands, and related structures (4). Like the ionophores used in ion-selective electrodes, these molecules are designed to selectively complex ions such as sodium and potassium. The difference is that in this case the formation of the complex results in a change in color, which is measured spectrophotometrically. The color change can be accomplished either by extracting the cation of interest along with an anionic dye into a nonaqueous phase containing the ionophore, or by using an ionophore that includes a chromophore and is water soluble. In the latter case, binding of the cation by the ionophore results in a spectral shift in the chromophore. The change in absorbance is proportional to the sodium or potassium concentration in the sample.

These methods are suitable for use with very small sample volumes, and since the methods are based on spectrophotometry, they can be readily integrated into multi-test analyzers without requiring an additional instrument module for ISEs or flame photometry.

SPECTROPHOTOMETRY (CHLORIDE)

Chloride in serum and other body fluids can be measured spectrophotometrically using a reagent containing mercuric thiocyanate and ferric ion. Chloride displaces thiocyanate to form mercuric chloride, and free thiocyanate then combines with ferric ion to form a reddish complex with an absorbance maximum around 500 nm. The sensitivity of the method can be increased by adding mercuric nitrate to the reagent. The free mercuric ions combine with the first available chloride ions so that only excess chloride is responsible for the formation of the colored ferric thiocyanate, as shown below.

$$Hg(NO_3)_2 + Cl^- \rightarrow HgCl_2 + 2\ NO_3^-$$

$$Hg(SCN)_2 + Cl^-\ \text{(excess)} \rightarrow HgCl_2 + 2\ SCN^-$$

$$3\ SCN^- + Fe^{3+} \rightarrow Fe(SCN)_3\ \text{(reddish color)}$$

This method was once the most widely used method in clinical laboratories, but is being replaced by the adaptation of ISE technology to clinical laboratory instruments.

ION ACTIVITY AND ION CONCENTRATION

When a sodium ISE is brought into contact with a sample, the electrode signal reflects the activity, not the concentration, of sodium ions in the sample. The activity of an ion may be thought of as an "effective" concentration that takes into account the influence of all other ionic species present in the solution. The activity is always less than the concentration, and the two quantities are related by the equation

$$a = \gamma c$$

where a is activity, c is concentration and γ is called the activity coefficient. The activity coefficient of an ion depends primarily on the total ionic strength of the solution, which for normal plasma is about 160 mmol/liter.

It can be argued that activity measurements are desirable because biochemical reactions involving ions proceed at rates that are dependent on activity, and are only indirectly related to concentration. However, because the ionic composition of plasma is closely regulated, the activity coefficients of ions in solution stay within narrow limits, and there is nearly a constant relationship between the activity and the concentration of the ion. Thus the distinction between activity and concentration is of more theoretical than practical importance in the clinical laboratory.

PLASMA VOLUME VERSUS WATER VOLUME

The distinction between the total volume of a plasma (or serum) sample and the volume of water contained in the sample is of much more importance than that between activity and concentration, because the water fraction of plasma can vary greatly in different patient samples. Normally, plasma contains 93% water, by volume. Most of the remaining volume results from dissolved proteins. If the protein concentration is markedly abnormal, the water fraction of plasma will change correspondingly. Triglycerides, either in solution or as chylomicrons, can also significantly reduce the water space when present at high concentrations.

The important point is that homeostatic mechanisms for electrolytes respond to the activity of ions in the *water space* of plasma. A condition such as hyperproteinemia or hyperlipidemia may result in a marked decrease in the water fraction, but the activity of sodium ions in the water space will not change, and thus the osmoreceptors controlling sodium balance will not be affected. The sodium concentration as measured by an ISE in an undiluted sample will likewise be unaffected. In contrast, a flame photometer or an ISE measurement on a *diluted* sample will reflect the amount of sodium in a fixed volume of sample. The result will be lower because of the volume occupied by the increased protein or lipid, and is misleading because it implies an electrolyte imbalance where none exists. This artifact of methods that utilize sample dilutions with specimens containing abnormally high protein or lipid concentrations has been referred to as "pseudohyponatremia."

ISE methods that use undiluted samples are sometimes called "direct" methods, while those that require dilution of a sample are called "indirect." It has been recommended that methods using undiluted samples be calibrated to agree with methods using diluted samples, for specimens of normal protein and lipid composition. This avoids having two different (and overlapping) sets of reference intervals for sodium, potassium, and chloride. Unfortunately, a single method of calibration has not yet been widely adopted, resulting in some variability of results from different instruments even on samples of normal composition.

SPECIMEN AND SPECIMEN HANDLING

Although sodium, potassium, and chloride ions are inherently stable, the large difference between concentrations in plasma and in blood cells, especially for potassium, means that if plasma levels are desired care must be taken to avoid hemolysis and to promptly separate blood cells after the specimen is obtained. If visible hemolysis is present in a plasma sample for potassium analysis, either another specimen should be obtained, or a note of the presence of hemolysis should be included with the laboratory report.

Serum concentrations of potassium are normally about 0.3 mmol/liter higher than in plasma because of potassium released from platelets and leukocytes during the clotting process. This difference can be much greater if the platelet or leukocyte count is very high. Many instruments that use ISEs in undiluted samples will work with whole blood as the sample. This is advantageous in situations where short turnaround time is especially important, but has the disadvantage that hemolysis cannot be detected.

OSMOLALITY

The major contributors to plasma osmolality are sodium salts, glucose, and urea. Plasma osmolality can be measured directly by osmometry (normally 275 to 290 mosm/kg) or estimated by summing the concentrations of the major solutes (sodium, chloride, bicarbonate, urea, glucose) as shown in the formula below. Since sodium is the major cation, the sum of the anions and cations can be approximated by multiplying the sodium concentration by 2. Thus only sodium, urea, and glucose need to be measured.

$$\text{Calculated osmolality (mosm/kg)} \cong 2C_{\text{sodium}}\ \text{(mmol/liter)} + \frac{C_{\text{glucose}}\ \text{(mg/dl)}}{18} + \frac{C_{\text{urea N}}\ \text{(mg/dl)}}{2.8}$$

A more complete discussion of formulas for calculated osmolality has been given (5). The factors 18 and 2.8 are used to convert mg/dl to mmol/liter and would not be required for glucose and urea concentrations reported in SI units.

Urea is considered an ineffective osmole because, unlike sodium and glucose, urea distributes freely across cell membranes and thus does not affect the distribution of water between cells and the ECF (3). Therefore, the effective plasma osmolality can be calculated by dropping the term for urea and is more useful than the measured osmolality for evaluating disorders of fluid and electrolyte balance in patients with renal failure.

INTERPRETATION OF ELECTROLYTE DISORDERS

Hyponatremia

Hyponatremia is defined as a plasma sodium less than 135 mmol/liter. Usually hyponatremia is associated with hypoosmolality, and to restore osmotic equilibrium water moves into cells, resulting in cellular swelling. The effects of hyponatremia are most pronounced in the brain and lead to cerebral edema and metabolic encephalopathy. The severity of the consequences of hyponatremia depend on both the level of hyponatremia and the rate of decline in the sodium concentration. Acute hyponatremia less than 125 mmol/liter may result in coma and death. However, if the hyponatremia develops slowly, a plasma sodium below 110 mmol/liter may be tolerated.

In principle, hyponatremia could result from either sodium loss or a gain in body water. Loss of sodium salts occurs in a number of conditions, including losses through the skin or through the gastrointestinal or respiratory tract, but in most cases these represent an isosmotic or hyposmotic loss of both fluid and electrolytes and will not cause hyponatremia unless the losses are replaced with water. The kidney possesses a large capacity for excreting excess water. Consequently, almost all cases of hyponatremia are associated with a defect in renal water excretion. This includes effective circulating volume depletion, renal failure, diuretic administration, adrenal insufficiency, hypothyroidism, and inappropriate ADH secretion (6). An approach to the differential diagnosis of hyponatremia is shown in Figure 14.1. Three categories of hyponatremia may be distinguished based on the plasma osmolality.

HYPOOSMOLAL HYPONATREMIA

Effective circulating volume depletion stimulates the secretion of ADH (thus promoting water conservation by the kidney) and initiates the thirst mechanism (resulting in an increased water intake). Collectively these adaptations cause hypoosmolality and

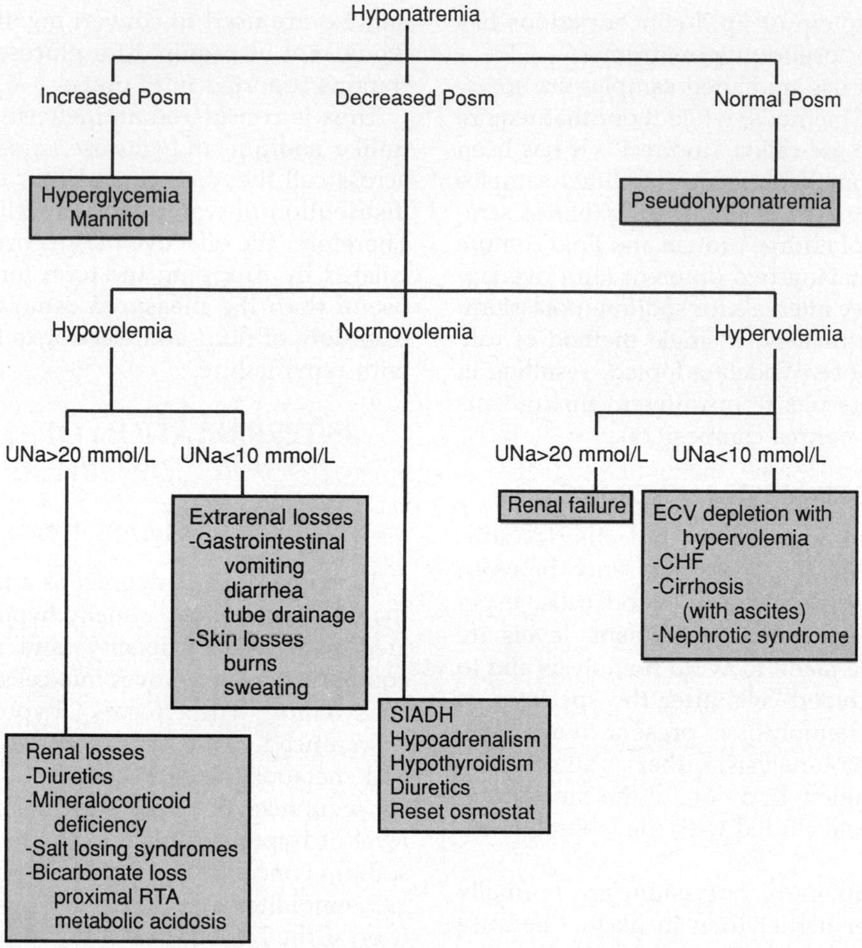

Figure 14.1. The differential diagnosis of hyponatremia. (Adapted from Kirkpatrick W, Kreisberg R. Acid-base and electrolyte disorders. In: Liu P, ed. Blue book of diagnostic tests. Philadelphia: WB Saunders, 1986:239–254.)

hyponatremia. It is important to distinguish the effective circulating volume in these patients from the extracellular volume, since some of these patients will have volume expansion (heart failure, ascites, edema) despite ECV depletion. Hyponatremia due to ECV depletion may therefore be associated with either an increased ECF (heart failure, cirrhosis, nephrotic syndrome) or a decreased ECF (vomiting, diarrhea, skin losses).

Renal disease can cause hyponatremia, but this generally occurs only with severe renal failure. Ordinarily up to 10% of the water filtered by the kidney can be excreted in the urine. However, in a severely oliguric patient, water retention with hyponatremia is common.

Diuretics induce volume depletion, inhibit solute resorption, and impair the ability of the kidney to excrete water. Water intake in excess of the ability to excrete the water will result in hyponatremia. Mineralocorticoid deficiency is associated with renal sodium losses, as are renal salt losing syndromes including medullary cystic disease, polycystic kidney disease, interstitial nephritis, analgesic nephropathy, and partial urinary tract obstruction. Hypothyroidism and hypocortisolism are both associated with a reduction in the ECV, resulting in water retention by the kidney.

The syndrome of inappropriate secretion of ADH (SIADH) is a common cause of hyponatremia. SIADH occurs in a variety of conditions, including ectopic production by tumors (e.g., bronchogenic carcinoma especially of the small cell type, thymoma, pancreatic carcinoma, and other neoplasms), pulmonary disorders (e.g., tuberculosis, pneumonia, pulmonary abscess, asthma, aspergillosis, acute respiratory failure), central nervous system (CNS) diseases (e.g., brain tumors, CNS infections, CNS trauma, cerebrovascular accidents, Guillain-Barré syndrome, acute intermittent porphyria, systemic lupus erythematosus, acute psychosis), a variety of drugs, and a variety of miscellaneous conditions (3). Some drugs produce an SIADH-like syndrome by potentiating the effects of ADH (e.g., chlorpropamide, carbamazepine, tolbutamide). Criteria for the diagnosis of SIADH include hyponatremia with hypoosmolality, a urinary osmolality above 100 mosm/kg, an inappropriately high urine sodium concentration, normal renal, adrenal, and thyroid function, normovolemia in a patient not taking diuretics, and correction of the defect with water restriction.

More rarely, hyponatremia occurs in patients with no defect in water excretion. Some patients exhibit a "reset osmostat" with a reduced threshold for ADH secretion and thirst. A condition called primary polydipsia may produce hyponatremia due to excessive water intake, but this occurs only with massive intakes beyond the capacity of the kidney to excrete the excess water. Primary polydipsia may be seen in some psychotic patients, in anxiety disorders, hypothalamic disorders, and in association with certain drugs. Miscellaneous rare causes of hyponatremia include the cerebral salt wasting syndrome and a severe decrease in salt intake.

HYPEROSMOLAR HYPONATREMIA

Causes of hyperosmolar hyponatremia include hyperglycemia and mannitol administration. Both glucose and mannitol are osmotically active and thus draw water out of cells, resulting in hyponatremia. As an approximation, each 100 mg/dl increase in glucose will lower the plasma sodium by 1.6 mmol/liter. Patients with renal failure may exhibit hyperosmolality due to urea, but this does not cause hyponatremia because urea crosses cell membranes freely and does not affect the distribution of water between cells and the ECF.

PSEUDOHYPONATREMIA

A condition called pseudohyponatremia may occur with serum or plasma samples containing large amounts of lipids (hyperlipidemia) or proteins (e.g., paraproteinemia). This condition is a laboratory artifact, which has been discussed above, and has no clinical significance other than calling attention to the underlying cause of the hyperlipidemia or hyperproteinemia. The osmolality is unaffected since osmometers measure only the solutes in the plasma water.

LABORATORY DIFFERENTIAL DIAGNOSIS

The initial laboratory evaluation of hyponatremia should include measurement of the serum or plasma osmolality, sodium, potassium, chloride, bicarbonate, glucose, and urea, and the urinary sodium concentration and urine osmolality (or specific gravity). The plasma osmolality is useful to divide hyponatremic states into three categories (Fig. 14.1), and in patients with renal failure the effective plasma osmolality should be used. The urine osmolality is useful to assess renal water excretion. Hyponatremia with a low urine osmolality (less than 100 mosm/kg or a specific gravity less than 1.004) indicates an appropriately suppressed ADH secretion as seen in primary polydipsia or a reset osmostat, whereas urine osmolality above 100 mosm/kg is indicative of impaired renal water excretion (6). Measurement of the urinary sodium concentration is useful to assess patients with impaired water excretion and hypoosmolal hyponatremia, as shown in Figure 14.1. A low urinary sodium concentration (less than 10 mmol/liter) is indicative of hypovolemia (due to extrarenal salt and water losses) or of effective circulating volume depletion. In contrast, renal diseases that produce hyponatremia are associated with a high urinary sodium concentration (above 20 mmol/liter).

Hypernatremia

Hypernatremia is defined as a serum sodium greater than 150 mmol/liter and is always associated with an increased osmolality. The symptoms of hypernatremia are mainly neurologic (metabolic encephalopathy) and depend on the degree of hyperosmolality and the rapidity of change in the serum sodium. Acute hypernatremia may produce severe symptoms with a sodium concentration below 160 mmol/liter, whereas in chronic hypernatremia sodium levels up to 180 mmol/liter may be tolerated.

Hypernatremia can result from loss of water in excess of solute, or from a gain in sodium. Ordinarily the body responds to hyperosmolality by attempting to conserve water (ADH secretion) and by stimulating the thirst mechanism. These defenses are highly effective in protecting the osmolality and preventing the development of hypernatremia. Thus, significant hypernatremia is always associated with a defect in the thirst response or else it occurs in patients who do not have access to water (coma, infants, etc.). The differential diagnosis of hypernatremia is shown in Fig. 14.2.

Fluid losses from the lungs, skin, and gastrointestinal tract are always isotonic or hypotonic, as are those associated with osmotic diuresis. The normal thirst mechanism will ordinarily correct these deficits, but a variety of hypothalamic disorders may affect the thirst response (hypodipsia) or osmoreceptor function (hyperaldosteronism, Cushing's disease) and produce hypernatremia. Examples of causes of hypodipsia due to hypothalamic disorders include brain tumors, sarcoidosis and other granulomatous disease, vascular disorders, and essential hypernatremia. Finally, hypernatremia may occasionally re-

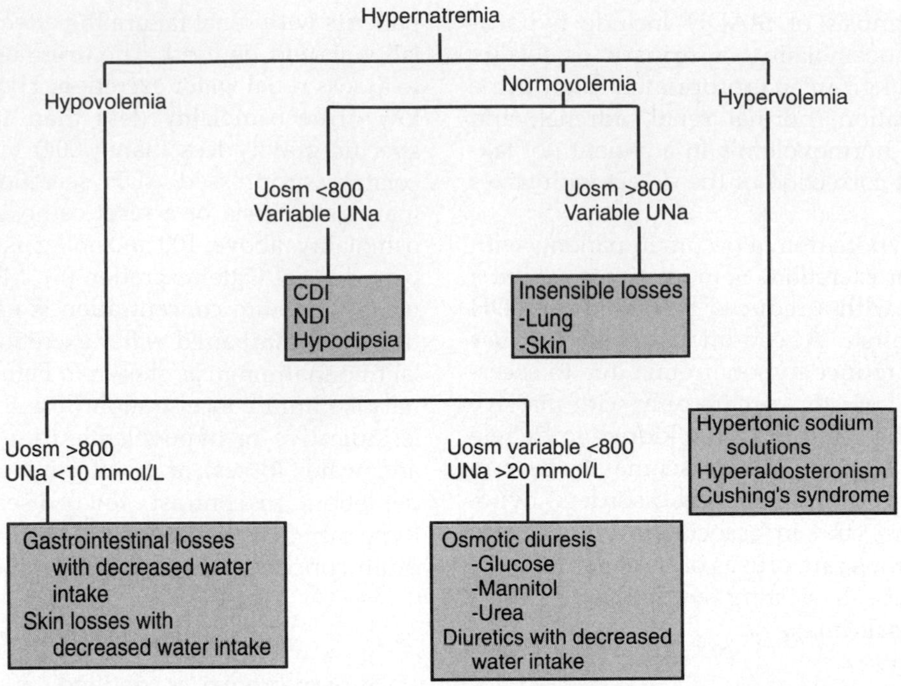

Figure 14.2. The differential diagnosis of hypernatremia. (Adapted from Kirkpatrick W, Kreisberg R. Acid-base and electrolyte disorders. In: Liu P, ed. Blue book of diagnostic tests. Philadelphia: WB Saunders, 1986:239–254.)

sult from excessive sodium intake. This can occur after the administration of hypertonic solutions of NaCl or $NaHCO_3$, or in infants given hypertonic formulas.

Strenuous exercise or seizures may be associated with a transient hypernatremia, presumably because these conditions induce a temporarily increased intracellular osmolality that draws water into the cells.

Diabetes insipidus (DI) is an important cause of hypernatremia that results either from a defect in ADH secretion (central DI) or from an impaired renal response to ADH (nephrogenic DI). In either case, the result is a defective renal concentrating ability. Unless the thirst mechanism or access to water is impaired, most of these patients maintain a nearly normal osmolality and sodium concentration (6). Patients with DI usually present with polyuria or polydipsia or both. Central DI results from a complete or partial impairment of ADH synthesis or release. The differential diagnosis includes a large number of central nervous system disorders, most commonly anoxic brain damage, head trauma, or as an idiopathic form. Other causes include primary and metastatic brain tumors, CNS infections, granulomatous diseases, and neurosurgery. Nephrogenic DI may occur in association with renal failure, hypokalemia, hypercalcemia, various drugs (diuretics, lithium, demeclocycline, methoxyflurane), pregnancy, sickle cell anemia, osmotic diuresis, and as a congenital form.

LABORATORY DIFFERENTIAL DIAGNOSIS

The majority of cases of hypernatremia occur in patients with altered mental status or in infants, both of whom cannot obtain or drink fluids in response to the normal thirst mechanism. An alert patient with hypernatremia should therefore be assumed to have a hypothalamic disorder affecting the thirst center (6). In patients with hypernatremia the urine should be maximally concentrated (more than 800 mosm/kg) with a high specific gravity (above 1.023). If this is not found, a defect in ADH secretion or response is indicated (see Fig. 14.2).

Hypokalemia

Signs and symptoms of hypokalemia generally do not occur until the plasma potassium has fallen below 3.0 mmol/liter (7) and include neuromuscular disturbances (muscle weakness, paralysis), impaired urinary concentrating ability, rhabdomyolysis, cardiac arrhythmia, and increased digitalis sensitivity. The electrocardiogram may show flat or inverted T waves, prominent U waves, and S-T segment depression (8). Hypokalemia may result from decreased potassium intake; changes in the distribution of potassium between cells and the ECF; gastrointestinal, renal, or sweat losses; and hemodialysis. The differential diagnosis is shown in Figure 14.3.

A number of conditions produce a transient hypokalemia by shifting potassium into the intracellular compartment. Respiratory or metabolic alkalosis ele-

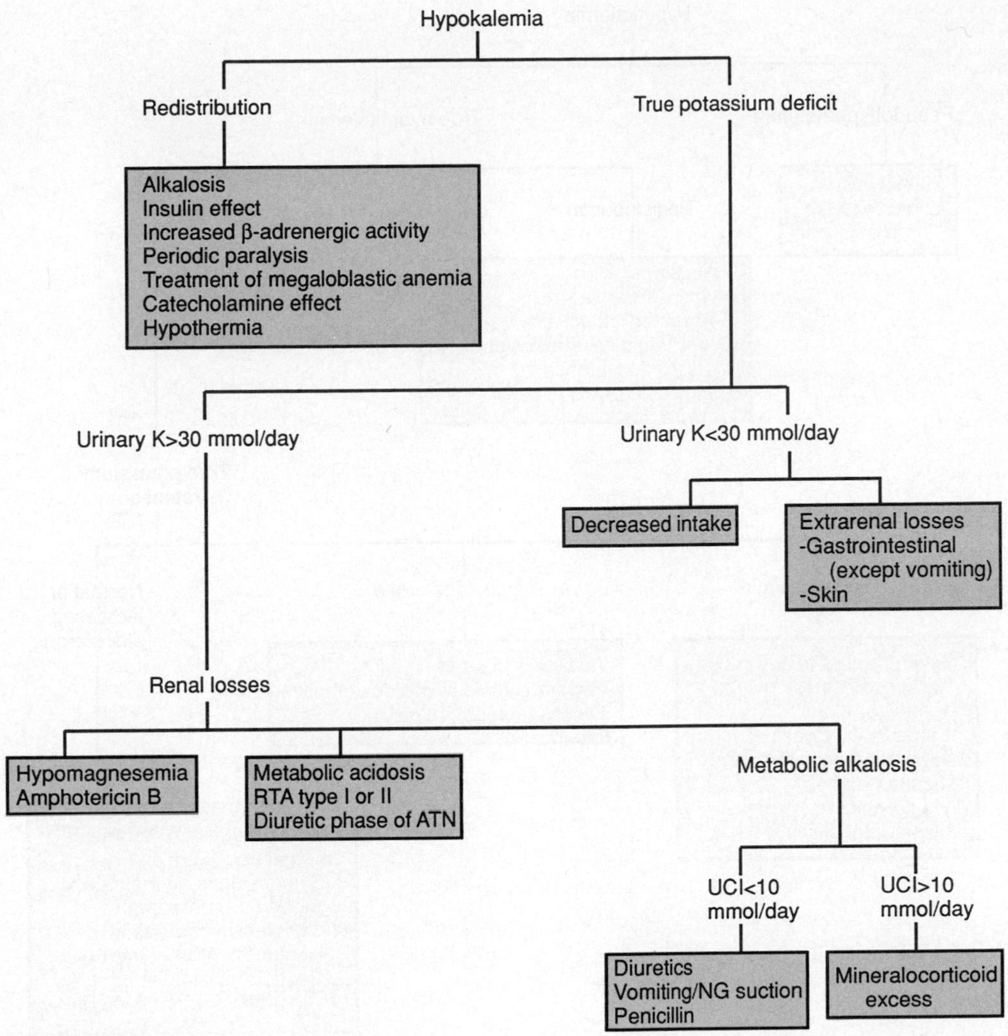

Figure 14.3. The differential diagnosis of hypokalemia. (Adapted from Kirkpatrick W, Kreisberg R. Acid-base and electrolyte disorders. In: Liu P, ed. Blue book of diagnostic tests. Philadelphia: WB Saunders, 1986:239–254.)

vates the extracellular pH, resulting in an exchange of ECF potassium for intracellular hydrogen ions. Likewise insulin, catecholamines, and increased β-adrenergic activity (as seen, for example, in severe stress or with β-agonist drugs) promote cellular uptake of potassium. Potassium uptake by newly formed cells is the mechanism for hypokalemia associated with the treatment of megaloblastic anemia. Periodic paralysis is a rare disorder that can be familial (autosomal recessive) or acquired (thyrotoxicosis) and can produce profound episodic hypokalemia with muscle weakness or paralysis often following exercise, a carbohydrate meal, or insulin administration. The mechanism causing the hypokalemia is not fully understood but involves cellular uptake of potassium ions.

Rarely, decreased potassium intake will produce hypokalemia, but only if the dietary deficiency is severe. More often hypokalemia associated with reduced intake occurs in patients who are being maintained on intravenous fluids without potassium supplementation. In these patients a 100 mmol/liter potassium deficit can occur over a 1-week period (7).

Extrarenal potassium losses produce hypokalemia when significant amounts of potassium are lost in the gastrointestinal secretions (diarrhea, villous adenoma, vomiting, laxative abuse, nasogastric suction, Zollinger-Ellison syndrome, ureterosigmoidostomy) or through the skin (e.g., sweating, burns). In these cases the hypokalemia may be exacerbated by an associated metabolic alkalosis and volume contraction, the latter resulting in increased aldosterone production with increased urinary potassium losses. A similar mechanism occurs with prolonged vomiting or nasogastric suction.

Hypokalemia resulting from increased urinary losses is commonly observed in patients taking diuretics, in those with primary or secondary hyperaldosteronism, Bartter's syndrome, the diuretic phase of acute tubular necrosis, salt wasting ne-

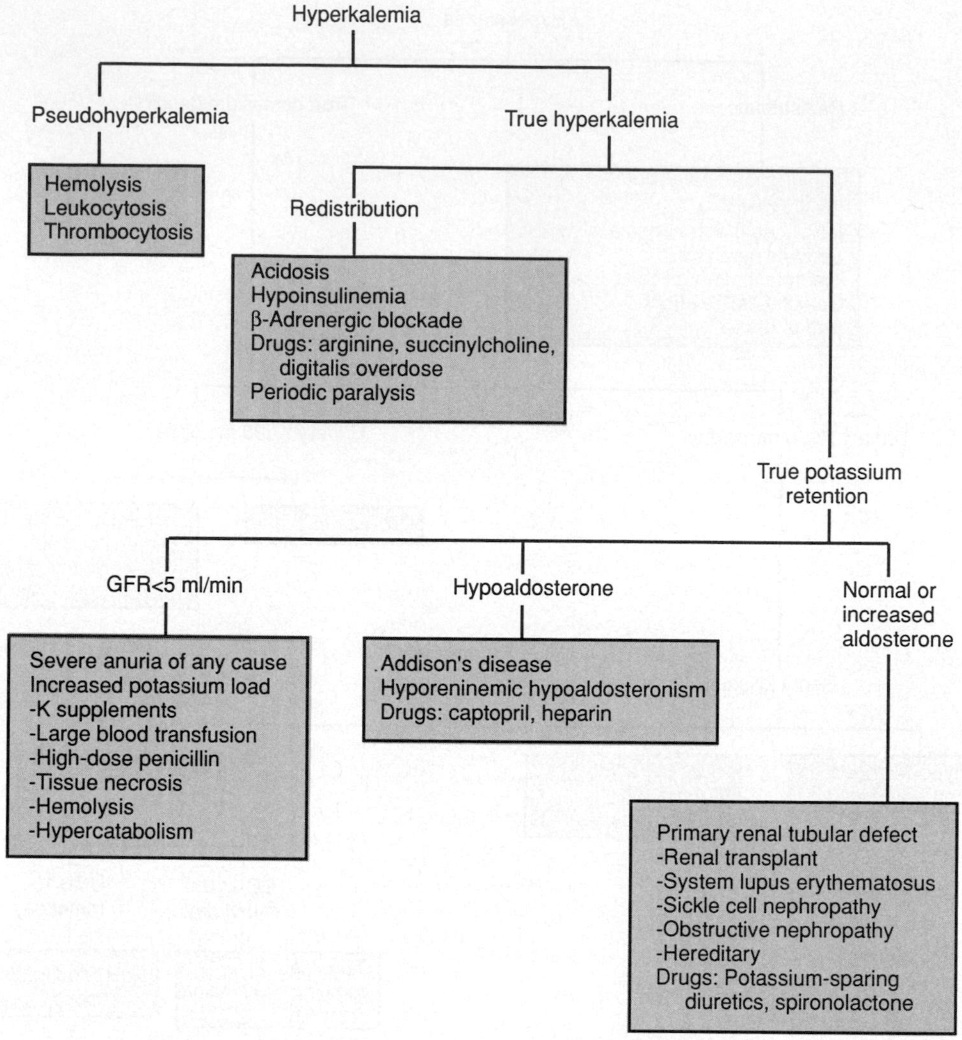

Figure 14.4. The differential diagnosis of hyperkalemia. (Adapted from Kirkpatrick W, Kreisberg R. Acid-base and electrolyte disorders. In: Liu P, ed. Blue book of diagnostic tests. Philadelphia: WB Saunders, 1986:239–254.)

phropathy, renal tubular acidosis, or hypomagnesemia, and in patients being administered amphotericin B or high-dose penicillin.

The initial evaluation of hypokalemia should include a consideration of the patient's potassium intake, potential sites of potassium losses, and of the specific conditions that may predispose to hypokalemia. Serum electrolytes, arterial blood gases, and urinary electrolytes may be useful in arriving at a correct diagnosis as shown in Figure 14.3. Further tests (e.g., aldosterone, plasma renin activity, serum magnesium) can be requested when appropriate. The urinary potassium concentration is particularly helpful, since this will differentiate renal from other causes of hypokalemia.

Hyperkalemia

The signs and symptoms of hyperkalemia include muscle weakness (impaired neuromuscular conduction) and abnormal cardiac conduction. Muscle weakness generally does not occur until the serum potassium is above 7 mmol/liter but may be potentiated by hypocalcemia. ECG changes can be seen with plasma levels above 6 mmol/liter. More severe hyperkalemia (above 8.0 mmol/liter) is associated with a sine wave pattern on the ECG with imminent ventricular fibrillation and cardiac arrest (7).

The differential diagnosis of hyperkalemia is shown in Figure 14.4. Hyperkalemia can result from increased intake, redistribution between cells and the ECF, and decreased renal potassium excretion. Since the normal kidney will efficiently excrete excess potassium, chronic hyperkalemia is always associated with impaired urinary excretion.

Hyperkalemia resulting from a sudden increase in potassium intake normally produces only a transient elevation in the serum potassium, but persistent elevations may occur in patients with impaired renal excretion.

Acidemia promotes the transcellular exchange of hydrogen ions for potassium ions and thus is a cause of hyperkalemia. The increase in the plasma potassium ranges from 0.2 to 1.7 mmol/liter for every 0.1 unit reduction in pH (7). The resulting hyperkalemia is greatest with hyperchloremic metabolic acidosis, less marked with respiratory acidosis, and negligible in high–anion gap metabolic acidosis (8).

It is important to understand that hyperkalemia may occur despite a deficit of total body potassium stores. In patients with diabetes mellitus, insulin deficiency leads to hyperkalemia, since insulin promotes cellular uptake of both glucose and potassium. β-Adrenergic blocking drugs produce hyperkalemia by inhibiting the β_2-facilitated sodium/potassium ATPase–mediated uptake of potassium by cells. Severe exercise, rhabdomyolysis, and any state of tissue breakdown (e.g., trauma, hemolysis, or tumor lysis following chemotherapy) can release large amounts of cellular potassium and cause hyperkalemia. A number of drugs promote potassium loss from cells, including cationic amino acids (arginine) and succinylcholine, whereas digitalis overdose interferes with the cellular sodium/potassium ATPase pump. Hyperkalemic periodic paralysis is a rare autosomal dominant condition characterized by recurrent intermittent episodes of paralysis associated with acute hyperkalemia.

A number of conditions may produce hyperkalemia by impairing the ability of the kidney to excrete potassium. Renal failure of any cause is a common cause of hyperkalemia, but usually significant oliguria must be present. Less severe degrees of renal failure will contribute to the development of hyperkalemia in patients with other reasons for an elevated potassium. Mineralocorticoid deficiency is another important cause of hyperkalemia resulting in an impaired renal potassium excretion. The differential diagnosis of hypoaldosteronism is extensive but includes hyporeninemic hypoaldosteronism, a number of drugs (NSAIDS, ACE inhibitors, cyclosporine), decreased aldosterone synthesis (adrenal insufficiency, congenital hyperplasia, heparin effect), and aldosterone resistance (potassium-sparing diuretics, pseudohypoaldosteronism, cyclosporine) (9).

Hyperchloremia and Hypochloremia

Chloride is quantitatively the most important extracellular anion. As such, abnormalities in the serum chloride may occur in a variety of settings as a component of acid-base, fluid, or electrolyte disorders. From a clinical perspective, the abnormality in the serum chloride itself is of little concern. Rather, attention is focused on the underlying disorder causing the hyperchloremia or hypochloremia. The differential diagnosis is shown in Table 14.3.

Table 14.3. Differential Diagnosis of Hyperchloremia and Hypochloremia[a]

Hyperchloremia
Metabolic acidosis associated with gastrointestinal bicarbonate loss
Renal tubular acidosis
Mineralocorticoid deficiency
Respiratory alkalosis
Hyponatremia with sodium losses in excess of chloride
Bromism
Administration of NH_4Cl, amino acids (hyperalimentation), saline, carbonic anhydrase inhibitors
Some cases of hyperparathyroidism
Hypochloremia
Gastrointestinal HCl losses (vomiting, nasogastric suction)
Anion-gap metabolic acidosis
Salt-losing nephropathies
Mineralocorticoid excess
Compensated respiratory acidosis
Metabolic alkalosis
Hyponatremia
Adrenocortical insufficiency

[a]Adapted from Wallach J. Interpretation of diagnostic tests: a handbook synopsis of laboratory medicine. 4th ed. Boston: Little, Brown, 1986.

Of the various conditions listed in Table 14.3, only one, bromism, merits specific discussion here. Elevations of serum bromide once occurred in patients ingesting bromide ion in the form of over-the-counter drug formulations or as an anticonvulsant. These drugs are less often used today and, as a result, the incidence of bromism has declined. Aside from its toxic properties, bromide ion causes falsely elevated chloride levels with ion-selective electrodes, coulometric, and, to a lesser degree, mercurimetric methods. Other conditions listed in Table 14.3 are discussed elsewhere in this chapter.

pH, P_{CO_2}, AND BICARBONATE

Physiology of Acid-Base Balance

An optimal pH in body fluids is required for the efficient functioning of a large number of cellular enzymes. The pH of the blood is normally maintained within narrow limits (Table 14.4) by a combination of the body's buffering systems and by renal and respiratory regulatory mechanisms. As a general rule, acidemia below pH 6.8 or alkalemia above pH 7.8 is not compatible with life. Less dramatic alterations in acid-base balance may cause significant morbidity and mortality, especially when superimposed on other serious illnesses.

It is useful in discussing acid-base balance to distinguish between abnormalities in blood pH (acidemia and alkalemia) and abnormal conditions that tend to produce acidemia and alkalemia (acidosis and alkalosis). As will be discussed, different

Table 14.4. Reference Intervals for Arterial Blood pH and Gases

pH	7.36–7.44
P_{O_2}	80–100 mm Hg
P_{CO_2}	35–45 mm Hg
Oxygen saturation	>95%
Bicarbonate	22–26 mmol/liter
Total CO_2	23–27 mmol/liter
Base excess	−2 to +2 mmol/liter

types of acidosis and alkalosis can be present simultaneously, and the resultant blood pH may be either high, low, or normal.

Acidemia is defined as an arterial pH below 7.36 and alkalemia as a pH above 7.44. Acid-base disorders affect a variety of metabolic processes, ultimately leading to impairment of essential functions, but the clinical signs and symptoms of acidosis and alkalosis are relatively nonspecific. Therefore, the diagnosis requires laboratory confirmation by measurement of blood pH and gases.

Normal metabolism generates a mixture of acids and bases that must be continuously neutralized or eliminated to achieve homeostasis. Carbon dioxide is produced by cellular respiration and is quantitatively the most important substance to challenge the acid-base balance of the body. Acid is produced by the association of CO_2 with water, forming carbonic acid, which dissociates to hydrogen ion and bicarbonate.

$$CO_2 + H_2O \leftrightharpoons H_2CO_3 \leftrightharpoons H^+ + HCO_3^-$$

Almost all of the CO_2 produced by respiration is normally eliminated in the lungs. A 70-kg person produces about 20 moles of CO_2 (volatile acid) per day. An additional acid load is imposed by the metabolism of proteins and the hydrolysis of phosphoester bonds, resulting in the production of nonvolatile acids, predominantly sulfuric and phosphoric acids. Other metabolic processes produce alkali in the form of bicarbonate, mainly by the oxidation of organic anions. The net result of normal metabolism is to produce an excess of 50 to 100 millimoles of hydrogen ions per day (10).

Pathologic or physiologic processes may increase or decrease the production of acid or impair the ability of the body to main acid-base homeostasis. Consequently, the body requires a finely regulated but flexible mechanism to cope with acid or base challenges.

The Body Buffering Systems

The immediate defenses against alterations in acid-base status are the buffering systems of the body. The Henderson-Hasselbalch equation is used to describe the relationship between pH and the acidic and basic forms of a buffer. The general relationship is

$$pH = pK' + \log\left(\frac{C_{\text{basic form of buffer}}}{C_{\text{acidic form of buffer}}}\right)$$

where C represents concentration and pK′ represents the negative logarithm of the equilibrium constant for the buffer pair.

The principal buffering system of plasma is the bicarbonate/carbonic acid system. Carbonic acid in plasma is in equilibrium with dissolved CO_2. This in turn is directly measurable as P_{CO_2}, and the two quantities are related by the solubility coefficient of CO_2 in plasma, which is 0.03 mmol·liter^{-1}·mm Hg^{-1}

$$C_{CO_2}\ (\text{dissolved}) = 0.03\ P_{CO_2}$$

For the bicarbonate/carbonic acid system the Henderson-Hasselbalch equation can thus be written as

$$pH = 6.1 + \log\left(\frac{C_{HCO_3^-}}{0.03\ P_{CO_2}}\right)$$

where $C_{HCO_3^-}$ is expressed in millimoles per liter and P_{CO_2} is expressed in millimeters of mercury.

Normally the ratio of bicarbonate to dissolved CO_2 is 20/1. Changes in either the bicarbonate concentration or the P_{CO_2} will affect the ratio and thus change the pH of the blood. Familiarity with the Henderson-Hasselbalch equation is essential to understanding the principles of acid-base balance and the calculations often performed in the blood gas laboratory. Blood gas analyzers measure pH, P_{CO_2}, and P_{O_2}, and the Henderson-Hasselbalch equation is used by the microprocessor built into the analyzer to calculate other quantities such as bicarbonate and total CO_2 concentrations.

The Henderson-Hasselbalch equation could also be written for any of the other buffer pairs in the body. Other buffers in the body include inorganic phosphate, proteins (mainly through the imidazole groups of histidine), and, in red blood cells, hemoglobin and 2,3-diphosphoglycerate. Since all buffers must be in equilibrium simultaneously, the acid-base status of the plasma is usually expressed in terms of only one, the carbonic acid/bicarbonate system.

Respiration and Acid-Base Regulation

The rate of alveolar ventilation affects acid-base status through changes in P_{CO_2}. The major factors determining the rate of respiration are the arterial P_{O_2} and pH. A change in the arterial pH is detected by chemoreceptors in the aortic arch and carotid bodies (peripheral) and in the brainstem (central). Acidemia stimulates respiration, resulting in a fall in the PCO_2 and an increase in arterial pH. Conversely, alkalemia induces hypoventilation with CO_2 retention and a decrease in pH toward normal. This forms the basis of the respiratory compensatory mechanism. Conversely, a pathologic alteration in alveolar ventilation may itself be the cause of an acid-base disorder by inducing CO_2 retention (respiratory acidosis) or excessive CO_2 elimination (respiratory alkalosis).

Renal Acid-Base Regulation

The kidney plays an important role in acid-base balance through its ability to regulate bicarbonate resorption and to excrete acid, primarily in the form of ammonium ion. Plasma bicarbonate is filtered by the glomerulus at a rate of roughly 4300 millimoles per day. Resorption of the daily filtered bicarbonate load is essential to maintain acid-base balance, since the loss of bicarbonate in the urine is equivalent to a gain in acid by the body. However, in alkalotic states, the kidney can excrete bicarbonate to compensate for an elevated pH.

Normally the body produces a net excess of acid (50 to 100 mmol/day) that must be excreted by the kidney. In humans the minimum attainable urinary pH is about 4.5 (9), and at this pH only a small number of free hydrogen ions can be excreted. Consequently the kidney requires an alternate mechanism to trap secreted hydrogen ions in the tubular lumen in order to excrete the normal daily acid load. The two most important species in this regard are phosphate (HPO_4^{2-}) and ammonia, both of which can combine with hydrogen ions secreted by renal tubular cells and are excreted in urine as $H_2PO_4^-$ and NH_4^+. The amount of phosphate available for combination with H^+ cannot be increased significantly from its normal level; however, the production of ammonia can be greatly augmented in response to increased acid production. Ammonia is generated within the renal tubular epithelium and diffuses freely through the cell membrane into the tubular lumen. In the lumen, it combines with secreted hydrogen ions to form ammonium ion, which is charged and cannot diffuse back into the cell. The hydrogen ions are thus trapped and are excreted in the urine. Ammonia formation is the main mechanism of the kidney to augment hydrogen ion excretion in states of acidosis.

Measurement of pH, PCO_2, and Bicarbonate

ANALYTICAL METHODS

Modern blood gas analyzers measure three quantities, pH, PCO_2, PO_2. All other quantities—including bicarbonate, total CO_2, dissolved CO_2, and base excess—are calculated by the microprocessor in the instrument.

pH Measurement

The method for measuring the pH of blood is essentially the same as that in any other liquid. The pH is determined by measurement of the voltage in an electrochemical cell containing a glass electrode that is selective for hydrogen ions. The principles of ion-selective electrode measurements were discussed previously, so only those factors unique to blood pH measurement are included here.

The reference electrode is usually a saturated calomel electrode and the bridge solution is usually saturated, or nearly saturated, potassium chloride, although other solutions are sometimes used. Calibration of the system is performed with two phosphate buffers that are traceable to the primary pH standards certified by the National Institute of Standards and Technology (NIST). The buffers most often used have a pH between 6.84 and 7.39 at 37°C. This narrow range is appropriate because the physiologic range of the blood pH is also quite narrow.

Blood pH, PCO_2, and PO_2 are all temperature dependent. By convention, measurements are made at 37.0°C, and the temperature is controlled to within (± 0.05°C) to ensure accurate results. This is important because the temperature coefficient of blood pH is about 10 times larger than that of the phosphate buffers used as calibrators. Therefore, if the instrument temperature drifts it will not be detected (or compensated) by a shift in the pH of the calibrators and will result in a measurement error.

The other source of significant systematic bias in blood pH measurements is residual liquid junction potential. As explained earlier, this error arises in potentiometric measurements when the potential at the liquid junction between the salt bridge and the solution is not the same for the calibrators and the test solutions. In the case of blood pH, two different sources of bias arise at the liquid junction.

The first is known as a "suspension effect" and is a result of the presence of red cells at the interface with a concentrated KCl bridge solution. A bridge of 4 mol/liter KCl causes the pH of whole blood to appear about 0.01 lower than the pH of the corresponding plasma. This effect can be eliminated by changing the bridge solution to sodium formate, but it is often simply ignored.

is no inherent reason to prefer calculation of extracellular fluid base excess to use of an equivalent diagram, or to some other approach to data interpretation.

Temperature Corrections

pH, PCO_2, and PO_2 are all temperature-dependent quantities, and by convention measurements are always made at 37.0°C. However, if the body temperature of the patient is different from 37°C, then the question arises of whether to adjust the measured values to the temperature of the patient. There has always been some controversy about the desirability of making this adjustment. On the one hand it is reasonable to do so because the adjusted values would correspond to the actual conditions in vivo. On the other hand, the reference intervals used to interpret the pH, PCO_2, and PO_2 were determined at 37°C, and the question of what values should be considered "normal" at other temperatures is unresolved. To minimize confusion it is wise to report only the values measured at 37°C, or to report *both* these and the values adjusted to body temperature. Most blood gas analyzers include software to automatically calculate adjusted values if the body temperature of the patient is known, and algorithms suggested for these adjustments have been published (16).

SPECIMENS AND SPECIMEN HANDLING

The collection and handling of specimens for blood pH and gas analysis have requirements unlike those for other clinical laboratory tests. These apply to the site and technique of collection, the specimen container, the anticoagulant, and the transport and storage of the specimen. All of these topics and several others have been recently reviewed by a subcommittee of the National Committee for Clinical Laboratory Standards (NCCLS), and a guideline document has been published covering specimen collection as well as calibration and quality control issues (17). The essence of the NCCLS recommendations on specimen collection and handling are covered in this section.

Site and Technique

In the majority of requests for blood gas testing there is a need to evaluate the degree of oxygenation of the blood in addition to the acid-base status. A specimen of arterial blood is therefore required. The technique of obtaining an arterial blood specimen is more difficult and more hazardous to the patient than venous sampling. Another NCCLS publication (18) contains detailed procedures and precautions to be observed in arterial blood sampling, and is recommended.

If it is not practical to obtain arterial blood, capillary blood may be used, but with some constraints (19). The capillaries, usually of the foot or the finger tip, must be dilated by warming the skin so that the PO_2 will be close to the arterial level. In spite of this, the correlation of capillary PO_2 to arterial PO_2 is not very good, in part due to the difficulty in obtaining a capillary sample without exposing the blood to room air. The correlation is good, however, for PCO_2 and pH.

If arterial PO_2 is not a concern, the acid-base status of the blood can be fully evaluated by analysis of venous blood for pH and PCO_2, and this should be done whenever possible to avoid the discomfort and hazard of arterial puncture.

Container and Storage

Capillary specimens are collected in preheparinized glass capillary tubes. Recommended specifications for the tubes have been published (20). The blood must be well mixed in the tube to ensure homogeneity and dissolution of the anticoagulant.

Venous specimens (for pH and PCO_2 only) may be collected in either syringes or evacuated tubes, but the latter must be completely filled. Arterial specimens should be collected in a syringe. Both glass and plastic syringes are used for blood gas specimens, and two factors influence the choice: (*a*) the expense of maintaining a system to clean, sterilize, and reuse glass syringes, and (*b*) the length of time that may elapse before the specimens are analyzed. Glass is superior to plastic, as explained below.

It now seems well established that plastic syringes can alter the PO_2 (and, to a lesser extent, the PCO_2) of a blood specimen, presumably due to room air dissolved in the plastic syringe barrel and plunger tip (21, 22). The size of the error depends on the PO_2 and the temperature of the blood, but is complicated because the buffering of PO_2 by hemoglobin changes with PO_2, as reflected by the oxygen-hemoglobin association curve. The error is increased when the specimen is cooled in ice water because oxygen solubility increases at lower temperatures.

Beginning at a PO_2 of 100 mm Hg, the oxygen level of a specimen in a plastic syringe stored in ice water may increase as much as 8 mm Hg in 30 minutes. This error is much smaller at lower PO_2 because hemoglobin is unsaturated, and is also much smaller if the specimen is kept at room temperature instead of being iced. A complication of not chilling the specimen is that metabolic processes utilizing oxygen proceed at a faster rate in the blood specimen, which constitutes yet another source of error. This error is particularly significant in blood with an elevated leukocyte or platelet count.

It is recommended that if plastic syringes are used, the blood not be chilled, but that the analysis be completed within 20 minutes to reduce the probability of error due to metabolic changes. Conversely, if glass syringes are used, the specimens should be cooled in ice water so that metabolic changes will be insignificant even with moderate elevations in leukocytes or platelets, and most specimens can then be held at least an hour before analysis, if necessary.

Room air has a PO_2 of about 150 mm Hg and a PCO_2 of less than 1 mm Hg. Obviously, contact between the blood and room air must be prevented. No air bubbles may be present in the specimen, and the needle should be replaced with an airtight cap as soon as the specimen is drawn.

Anticoagulant

Sodium or lithium heparin is the anticoagulant to be used for blood pH and gas analysis. This is available in both dry and liquid forms.

If the liquid preparation is used, care must be taken not to use more volume than necessary, because the errors caused by sample dilution can be significant. If a heparin strength of 1000 IU/ml is used, the volume in just the syringe dead space (needle and hub) is sufficient to anticoagulate a specimen in a 3-ml syringe. More concentrated heparin solutions are not recommended.

Heparin in solid form is used in some capillaries and prepacked syringes, either as a pellet or as a coating on the container wall. Dilution errors are obviously avoided but extra care must be taken to dissolve the heparin in the blood by vigorous mixing.

QUALITY CONTROL AND PROFICIENCY TESTING FOR BLOOD pH AND GAS ANALYSIS

The basic principles and issues of quality control and proficiency testing (QC/PT) that apply to all analytes in clinical chemistry apply also to blood pH and gases, but there are some additional aspects that are unique to blood gas QC/PT.

Materials and Matrix Effects

A universally accepted principle in QC/PT is that the sample used must have the same characteristics as fresh patient samples. However, this is often impractical. As a result, QC/PT materials may give results that are different from those expected on patient samples. Such differences are known as matrix effects and are of particular concern in blood gas QC/PT (23).

Commercially available controls for blood pH and gases usually are sold in the form of sealed glass ampules containing a solution in equilibrium with a gas phase above it. The solution matrix is one of three types: (*a*) aqueous; (*b*) blood-based, either stabilized whole blood or a hemolysate; or (*c*) a perfluorocarbon emulsion. In all cases the solution is buffered to stabilize the pH. The most important differences are related to the PO_2 stability in the QC material when exposed to room air. This is an important issue, because it is impossible to completely avoid contact between a QC sample for blood gas analysis and room air.

Blood gas analyzers have been carefully designed to give accurate results when whole blood is used as the sample. Matrix effects with other materials are primarily due to differences in the solubility of oxygen and carbon dioxide in these materials, and the effect is especially noticeable for PO_2. The solubility of oxygen in whole blood is much greater than in aqueous solutions because of the presence of hemoglobin. Exposure of a whole blood sample to a small amount of room air will change the PO_2, but hemoglobin will tend to buffer this change as long as it is not fully saturated with oxygen. Aqueous solutions, having no hemoglobin, will show relatively large changes in PO_2 when exposed to room air. Perfluorocarbon emulsions are used because the solubility of oxygen in perfluorocarbons is much higher than in water, and this will minimize the error caused by contamination of the sample with room air.

In PT programs in which both perfluorocarbon emulsions and aqueous materials are used, data from perfluorocarbons show significantly better precision for PO_2 than do aqueous materials (23). On the other hand, perfluorocarbons do not resemble a whole blood matrix, and this material may not be usable in analyzers containing a potassium ion–selective electrode because of interaction between perfluorocarbons and the potassium ionophore.

Blood-based controls do not necessarily behave like fresh patient samples either. Often the hemoglobin present in such controls is fully saturated with oxygen at a very low PO_2, and the sensitivity to room air contamination approaches that of aqueous solutions. However, some blood-based materials, or fresh whole blood, can be used for blood gas QC using a procedure called tonometry. Tonometry is the process of equilibrating a liquid with a gas of known composition. The apparatus used to accomplish this is called a tonometer. Tonometry makes it possible to prepare QC materials with an *accurately* known PO_2 and PCO_2, one of the rare instances in clinical chemistry when a QC material can be used as a test of accuracy as well as precision. Tonometers are readily available and the procedure and sources of error have been well described (17, 24), but the technique is underutilized because of the perception that it is too time-consuming to be performed routinely. Nevertheless, tonometry is the basis for the reference method for blood PO_2 and PCO_2.

Further details and recommendations for quality control programs in a blood gas laboratory have been published by the NCCLS (17).

Temperature and Altitude Effects

Control materials that are packaged in sealed ampules containing a gas bubble are subject to a source of preanalytical error not seen with patient samples. As the temperature of the sealed ampule rises and falls, the solubility of oxygen and carbon dioxide in the liquid changes, and the amount of gas dissolved in the liquid phase changes. Thus the measured PO_2 and PCO_2 will depend on the temperature of the ampule when it is opened, and the instructions for handling QC/PT materials must specify what this temperature should be. This effect does not occur in patient samples because care is taken to exclude bubbles from the specimen.

Another source of error in blood gas analysis that can be important in PT is the effect of ambient pressure. It has been observed that the PO_2 and, to a lesser extent, the PCO_2 measured in PT samples tend to be lower if the laboratory is at high altitude. The effect is too small to be important clinically. However, the bias can be a significant fraction of the allowable error in PT programs, and laboratories at high altitude should use a correction factor if available (25).

INTERPRETATION OF ACID-BASE DISORDERS

Acid-base disorders are classified into one of four categories: respiratory acidosis, respiratory alkalosis, metabolic acidosis, and metabolic alkalosis. Each of these categories includes a number of possible causes. The evaluation of an acid-base abnormality therefore requires the correct classification of the disorder, followed by a consideration of the differential diagnostic possibilities that may have caused it. The interpretation may be complicated by differences in acute versus chronic acid-base disorders, by the effects of renal and respiratory compensatory mechanisms, and by the presence of mixed acid-base abnormalities.

In response to a change in pH, the body initiates renal and/or respiratory compensatory mechanisms in an effort to restore the pH toward normal. The renal compensatory mechanisms include the ability of the kidney to alter bicarbonate resorption and to augment acid excretion, primarily as ammonium ion. The respiratory compensatory mechanism operates by changing the alveolar ventilation, and thus retaining CO_2 (hypoventilation) or releasing additional CO_2 (hyperventilation). The effect of compensatory mechanisms is to create a mixed acid-base disorder in which the compensatory response is superimposed on the primary acid-base abnormality. Mixed disorders may also occur in a patient with two simultaneous but unrelated primary acid-base abnormalities.

Table 14.5. Characteristics of Primary Acid-Base Disorders

Disorder	Primary Change	Compensatory Response
Metabolic acidosis	Decreased HCO_3 Decreased pH	Hyperventilation Decreased PCO_2
Metabolic alkalosis	Increased HCO_3 Increased pH	Hypoventilation Increased PCO_2
Respiratory acidosis	Increased PCO_2 Decreased pH	Increased acid excretion and HCO_3 resorption
Respiratory alkalosis	Decreased PCO_2 Increased pH	Decreased acid excretion and HCO_3 resorption

The ability of renal and respiratory compensation to normalize the arterial pH is limited, since complete correction of the pH would shut off the physiologic mechanisms driving the compensatory response. For this reason the arterial pH usually remains somewhat abnormal even in the compensated state. Also, in some cases the ability of the kidneys or respiratory system to compensate for acid-base disorders may be impaired due to intrinsic disease of the organ. For example, a patient in renal failure may not be able to modulate renal acid excretion and bicarbonate resorption and thus may fail to exhibit the expected compensatory response or show only a blunted response.

Table 14.5 shows the various types of primary acid-base disorders, the principal mechanism causing the disorder, the expected laboratory abnormalities, and the effects of compensatory responses.

There are several general approaches to the evaluation of acid-base disturbances. One system utilizes an acid-base nomogram such as the one shown in Figure 14.5. If the pH and the PCO_2 are measured, then a presumptive diagnosis may be made by locating the point corresponding to the two values on the nomogran to see which one of the seven diagnostic zones it falls into. For example, a patient with an arterial pH of 7.3 and a PCO_2 of 30 would be classified as having a metabolic acidosis. The advantages of this method are that it is simple, it requires no calculations, and it provides a reliable classification of the disorder, even with mixed acid-base abnormalities. The disadvantage of using a nomogram is that these charts are not always readily available, especially at the bedside in emergency situations. For this reason it is essential to have a simplified system for interpreting acid-base disorders that does not rely on a nomogram or the use of complex calculations.

Various textbooks describe sets of rules of thumb that permit a rapid interpretation of acid-base abnormalities (26–28). The major drawback to the use of

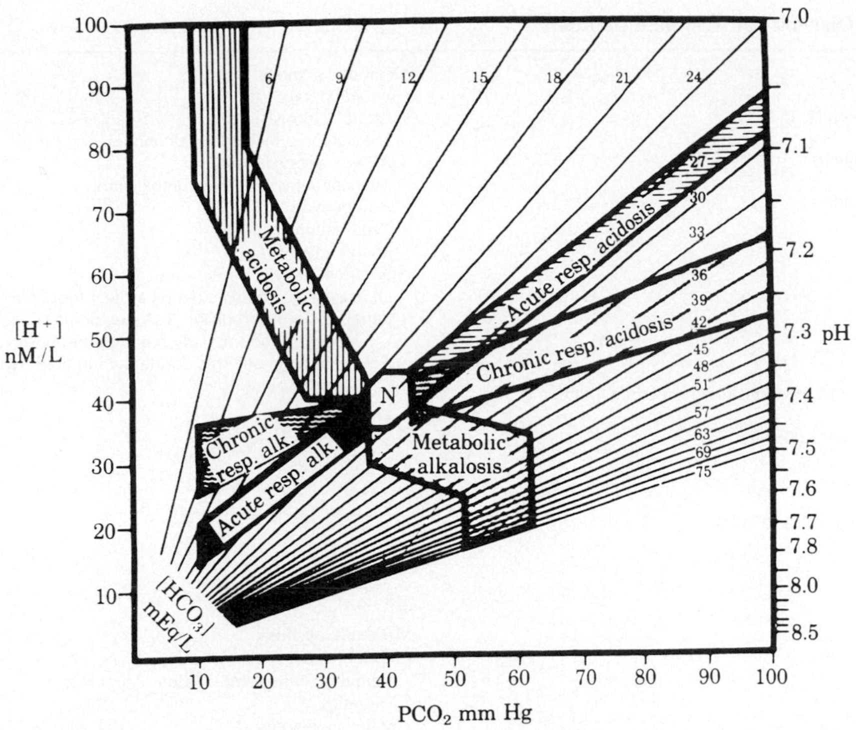

Figure 14.5. Diagram for interpretation of acid-base data. (Reprinted with permission from JAMA 1973;223:269.)

Table 14.6. Simplified Rules for the Interpretation of Acid-Base Disorders[a]

Rule 1.	A change in P_{CO_2} of 10 mm Hg will change the pH by 0.08.
Rule 2.	A change in bicarbonate of 10 mmol/liter will change the pH by 0.15.
Rule 3.	The dose of bicarbonate (millimoles) needed to correct a metabolic acidosis is given by the formula, $\frac{\text{Base deficit (mmol/liter)} \times \text{Patient weight (kg)}}{4}$

[a]Adapted from Comella L, Braen R, Olding M. Blood gases and acid-base disorders. In: Clinician's pocket reference. 4th ed. Laguna Niguel, CA: Capistrano Press, 1983:157–168.

these rules is that complex acid-base disorders are difficult to interpret. The clinical history must be considered whenever possible, rather than attempting a diagnosis based on laboratory data alone. Recognizing the need for a practical approach to the interpretation of acid-base data, the American Heart Association has recommended the use of a set of simplified rules that permit rapid interpretation of acid-base data (26, 27). These rules are shown in Table 14.6 and should be memorized and practiced, although most acid-base disorders can be interpreted by using only the first rule.

The usefulness of rule 1 is best ilustrated by example. Suppose a patient has a pH of 7.32 and a P_{CO_2} of 50 mm Hg. In this case the P_{CO_2} is elevated by 10 mm Hg. Using rule 1 this should produce a decrease in pH of 0.08, and therefore the predicted pH is 7.32 (7.40 − 0.08). Because the measured pH and the calculated pH are the same (or close), all of the change can be explained by respiratory dysfunction. The most likely diagnosis is therefore acute respiratory acidosis. Now consider a second patient with a pH of 7.35 and a P_{CO_2} of 52 mm Hg. The elevated P_{CO_2} again indicates a component of respiratory acidosis. However, rule 1 predicts a pH of approximately 7.30. The measured pH is greater (closer to normal) than predicted by 0.05, indicating that compensation has occurred. The correct diagnosis is respiratory acidosis with partial renal compensation (chronic respiratory acidosis).

Either the acid-base nomogram or these rules permit a classification of acid-base disorders into one of the categories shown in Table 14.5. The next step is to consider the differential diagnostic possibilities that comprise each category.

Respiratory Acidosis

Respiratory acidosis results from any condition that impairs CO_2 elimination by the lungs and is characterized by an increased P_{CO_2} and a decreased pH. A large number of disorders may produce respiratory acidosis, as seen in Table 14.7. These disorders may be classified as neuromuscular diseases, airway obstruction, and cardiopulmonary-thoracic disorders. Neuromuscular diseases may affect the respiratory apparatus at any level, including the central nervous system respiratory center in the brainstem, the peripheral nerves innervating the diaphragm and

Table 14.7. Differential Diagnosis of Acid-Base Disorders[a]

Respiratory acidosis *Neuromuscular* Brainstem/high spinal cord injury Sedative overdose Primary alveolar hypoventilation Sleep apnea syndrome Primary alveolar hypoventilation Sleep apnea syndrome Guillain-Barré syndrome Myasthenia gravis Poliomyelitis Botulism Diaphragmatic paralysis Myopathy of respiratory muscles *Cardiopulmonary* Airway obstruction (foreign body, tumor bronchospasm, COPD) Cardiac arrest Severe pneumonia or pulmonary edema Pulmonary embolus Mechanical underventilation Pneumothorax, plural effusion Restrictive disease of thorax (kyphoscoliosis) Flail chest *Metabolic* Myxedema	**Metabolic acidosis** *High anion gap* Lactic acidosis Ketoacidosis (diabetic or alcoholic) Aspirin overdose (late) Methanol/ethylene glycol intoxication Paraldehyde Renal failure Rhabdomyolysis *Normal anion gap* GI loss of bicarbonate (diarrhea, ileal loop, cholestyramine) Renal loss of bicarbonate (RTA, tubulointestitial diseases, hypoaldosteronism, early renal failure, posthypocapnia) Acid gain (ammonium chloride, amino acid hydrochlorides)
Respiratory alkalosis *Central nervous system* Anxiety Aspirin overdose (early) Fever Cerebrovascular accident Head trauma Brain tumor CNS infection Hypoxia *Pulmonary* Pulmonary emboli Pneumonia Interstitial lung disease ARDS Pulmonary edema (mild) High altitude Mechanical overventilation *Metabolic/other* Liver failure Pregnancy Gram-negative sepsis, endotoxemia	**Metabolic alkalosis** *Chloride responsive* Vomiting, nasogastric suction Diuretics Villous adenoma Cystic fibrosis Posthypercapnia Congenital chloridorrhea *Chloride resistant* Hyperaldosteronism Cushing's syndrome Exogenous glucocorticoids or mineralocorticoids Bartter's syndrome Excessive licorice ingestion Severe potassium depletion *Miscellaneous* Alkalinizing agents Milk alkali syndrome Hypoparathyroidism Drugs: carbenicillin, penicillin (large doses) Nonparathyroid hypercalcemia

[a]Adapted from Kirkpatrick W, Kriesberg R. Acid-base and electrolyte disorders. In: Liu P, ed. Blue book of diagnostic tests. Philadelphia: WB Saunders, 1986:239–254.

chest wall muscles, or the respiratory muscles themselves. The result is hypoventilation and retention of CO_2. A number of drugs produce respiratory acidosis by depressing the central respiratory center. Narcotic overdose is a classic example of this effect. Airway obstruction can occur at any level of the respiratory tract. If a large enough number of alveoli are affected, then the remaining nonobstructed portions of the lungs may not be able to maintain gas exchange at a sufficient level to prevent retention of CO_2 and respiratory acidosis. Cardiopulmonary-thoracic disorders also include a variety of other conditions that impair gas exchange.

In acute respiratory acidosis the bicarbonate level and total CO_2 are normal. The increase in P_{CO_2} will stimulate the central respiratory center, resulting in an attempt to increase the depth and rate of respiration. This effect occurs quite rapidly in response to an increase in the P_{CO_2}. However, if the cause of the respiratory acidosis is due to a central disorder then the respiratory response may not occur. Renal compensatory mechanisms require considerably more time to show an effective response—generally 6 to 12 hours. The effect of renal compensation is to convert CO_2 and water to hydrogen ion, which is excreted, and bicarbonate, which is reabsorbed into the plasma. When this occurs the acid-base disorder is classified as chronic respiratory acidosis, characterized by an increased P_{CO_2}, a decreased pH, and an increase in the plasma bicarbonate and total CO_2.

There are also effects on other electrolytes, notably the plasma potassium and chloride. Acidemia promotes the exchange of plasma hydrogen ions for cellular potassium ions, resulting in mild hyperkalemia, increased renal potassium excretion, and ultimately potassium depletion. Also, the increase in renal bicarbonate resorption associated with compensated respiratory acidosis is balanced by increased excretion of chloride to maintain electroneutrality. Thus, hypochloremia and chloride depletion may accompany respiratory acidosis.

The treatment of respiratory acidosis centers on improving ventilation through either mechanical or pharmacologic means. Administration of potassium and sodium chloride may be required to correct potassium and chloride depletion.

Respiratory Alkalosis

Respiratory alkalosis results from any condition that causes hyperventilation and is characterized by a decreased P_{CO_2} and an increased pH. The differential diagnosis includes primary disorders of the central respiratory center, pulmonary diseases associated with hypoxemia, and a variety of miscellaneous causes of hyperventilation (Table 14.7). Symptoms of respiratory alkalosis include lightheadedness, paresthesias, tetany, and, in severe cases, syncope. The two most common causes are hyperventilation produced by acute anxiety and hyperventilation in response to hypoxemia from various sources. A less obvious cause of respiratory alkalosis is the rapid correction of a metabolic acidosis, for example by bicarbonate infusion. Although the blood pH may return to normal the central nervous system requires some time to equilibrate with the periphery. The temporary persistence of CNS acidosis continues to stimulate the respiratory control center with the resultant hyperventilation and peripheral respiratory alkalosis.

Acute respiratory alkalosis is characterized by a low P_{CO_2}, a high pH, and a normal bicarbonate and total CO_2. Alkalemia depresses the respiratory control center, which tends to limit the hyperventilation in some cases, but the primary compensation is renal. The kidneys respond by decreasing acid excretion and bicarbonate resorption, which causes the plasma bicarbonate to fall. In chronic respiratory alkalosis, therefore, the P_{CO_2} is low, the pH high (but not as high as in the acute condition), and the plasma bicarbonate and total CO_2 are decreased.

Other electrolytes may show abnormalities as well. Persistent alkalemia promotes the movement of hydrogen ions out of cells in exchange for potassium, resulting in mild hypokalemia. Increased renal bicarbonate excretion is accompanied by chloride retention, resulting in hyperchloremia.

The treatment of respiratory alkalosis is centered on correcting the underlying disorder. Persistent hyperventilation may be treated in the short term by instructing the patient to rebreathe into a bag (thus promoting CO_2 retention) or, in the longer term, by the use of a special rebreathing apparatus. In general the alkalosis itself does not require specific therapy.

Metabolic Alkalosis

Metabolic alkalosis is characterized by increased pH, bicarbonate, and total CO_2. The causes are often divided into two categories, designated chloride-responsive and chloride-resistant types (Table 14.7). The laboratory distinction is made by measuring the urine chloride; a level below 20 mmol/liter is classified chloride-responsive, and above 20 mmol/liter is chloride-resistant.

One of the more common subcategories of chloride-responsive metabolic alkalosis is called contraction alkalosis. This condition results from a depletion of salt (NaCl) and water without a concomitant loss of bicarbonate (7). Contraction of the extracellular fluid volume without an equivalent loss of bicarbonate results in an increase in the plasma bicarbonate concentration and thus metabolic alkalosis. Ordinarily the kidney would excrete the excess bicarbonate, but in the setting of salt and water depletion, the kidney avidly conserves sodium to maintain the circulating volume and thus cannot excrete the bicarbonate. Contraction alkalosis may be a component of maintaining the metabolic alkalosis associated with vomiting or prolonged nasogastric suction. It is also seen with diuretic administration, although the major cause of the alkalosis in these cases is an enhanced renal acid excretion caused by these drugs (28).

A number of causes of chloride-responsive metabolic alkalosis are associated with the loss of hydrogen ions from the gastrointestinal tract. Gastric secretions contain large amounts of HCl and lesser amounts of KCl. Consequently, prolonged vomiting or nasogastric suctioning can produce metabolic alkalosis. The associated volume and salt depletion also contribute to the metabolic alkalosis and inhibit the ability of the kidney to excrete the excess bicarbonate, as mentioned above. The loss of KCl induces hypokalemia, further aggravating the problem since hypokalemia itself leads to alkalemia.

Villous adenomas of the intestine may cause metabolic alkalosis by secreting large amounts of sodium, chloride, and water without a proportionate loss of bicarbonate (contraction alkalosis). In cystic fibrosis, large amounts of sodium chloride may be lost in the sweat.

As discussed earlier, chronic respiratory acidosis is associated with compensatory renal bicarbonate resorption. Therefore, rapid correction of the hypercapnia with mechanical ventilation will leave only the compensatory metabolic alkalosis, which is called post-hypercapnic (28).

The treatment of chloride-responsive metabolic alkalosis is directed at the underlying disorder, but NaCl solutions are also administered to restore the extracellular fluid volume and salt deficit. This in turn enables the kidney to excrete the excess bicarbonate (22). KCl may also be given to correct hypokalemia.

The major causes of chloride-resistant metabolic alkalosis are mineralocorticoid excess (primary or secondary aldosteronism), Cushing's syndrome, Bartter's syndrome, and severe potassium depletion. Excess aldosterone promotes renal hydrogen and potassium ion excretion, and sodium resorption. The loss of hydrogen ions is partially responsible for the metabolic alkalosis, but in addition hypokalemia stimulates ammonia formation, chloride excretion, and cellular hydrogen ion/potassium ion exchange, all of which contribute to the alkalosis. Cushing's syndrome (glucocorticoid excess) may cause metabolic alkalosis because cortisol has weak mineralocorticoid activity. Bartter's syndrome, a rare disorder characterized by juxtaglomerular cell hyperplasia, produces a hypokalemic metabolic alkalosis as a result of increased renin production and resultant hyperaldosteronism. Licorice contains the steroid glycyrrhizic acid, which has weak mineralocorticoid activity (28).

The treatment of chloride-resistant metabolic alkalosis is centered on correcting the potassium deficit with KCI and treating the underlying disorder. Spironolactone, an aldosterone antagonist, may be effective in states of mineralocorticoid excess (7).

Metabolic Acidosis

Metabolic acidosis is caused by an increased production of organic acids, decreased renal hydrogen ion excretion, or loss of bicarbonate. Any of these mechanisms causes a decrease in the pH, the bicarbonate concentration, and the total CO_2. The respiratory compensatory mechanism will partially correct the acidosis by increasing the rate of respiration, thereby lowering the P_{CO_2}. The renal compensatory mechanism is to increase hydrogen ion excretion and bicarbonate resorption. Metabolic acidosis is the most complicated of the various acid-base abnormalities; a more detailed discussion is presented by Black (10).

Metabolic acidosis is usually classified on the basis of whether or not the anion gap is increased. The anion gap is a calculated quantity that reflects the difference between the measured cations and the measured anions, as discussed earlier in this chapter. The anion gap (AG) is usually defined as

$$\text{Anion gap} = (C_{Na^+}) - (C_{Cl^-}) - (C_{HCO_3^-})$$

The reference interval for the anion gap is 8 to 14 mmol/liter. Although many conditions can alter the anion gap (5), its only clinical use is in the differential diagnosis of metabolic acidosis (Table 14.7).

There are five conditions that may cause a high-AG metabolic acidosis: renal failure, lactic acidosis, ketoacidosis, rhabdomyolysis, and certain drugs and toxins.

Renal Failure

Renal failure can actually cause either a normal-AG or a high-AG metabolic acidosis. Renal disease may impair hydrogen ion excretion due to a decrease in ammonia synthesis in the cells of the renal tubule. Impaired hydrogen ion excretion necessitates a decrease in renal HCO_3^- resorption and thus the plasma HCO_3^- falls. Chloride replaces bicarbonate in the blood, resulting in a normal-AG (hyperchloremic) acidosis. On the other hand, severe renal failure (glomerular filtration rate less than 20 to 30% of normal) is associated with renal retention of phosphate and sulfates (both unmeasured anions) and thus a high-AG acidosis.

Lactic Acidosis

Lactic acidosis is a common cause of high-AG acidosis, especially in acutely ill patients. The differential diagnosis is extensive and usually involves both increased production of lactic acid and decreased metabolism. Lactic acid is produced as a product of anaerobic metabolism. Major causes of lactic acidosis include tissue hypoxia (type A lactic acidosis) (e.g., severe exercise, seizures, hypotension, cardiac failure, hypoxemia, carbon monoxide poisoning, or severe anemia); drugs and toxins (type B lactic acidosis) (e.g., phenformin, catecholamines, salicylate, isoniazid, cyanide), congenital forms of lactic acidosis (such as defects in gluconeogenic enzymes), and a variety of severe illnesses, including sepsis, liver failure, and neoplasms (10). Lactate levels in excess of 5 mmol/liter (reference interval 0.5 to 2.2 mmol/liter) are diagnostic of lactic acidosis. The increase in the AG results from the unmeasured lactate anion.

Ketoacidosis

Ketoacidosis may occur in uncontrolled diabetes mellitus, starvation, or excessive alcohol ingestion. Ketoacids (acetoacetic acid and β-hydroxybutyric acid) are overproduced by the liver, resulting in an increase in their unmeasured anions and a high-AG acidosis.

Rhabdomyolysis

Massive destruction of muscle tissue releases organic acids from damaged myocytes, leading to a high-AG metabolic acidosis.

Drugs and Toxins

The four most common substances in this group are aspirin, methanol, ethylene glycol, and paraldehyde.

1. Salicylate overdose initially causes a respiratory alkalosis because the drug has a stimulatory effect on the central respiratory center. Eventually a high-AG acidosis occurs due to the salicylate itself and to the effects of salicylate on peripheral metabolism, resulting in the production of a variety of organic acids, including lactate and ketoacids.
2. Methanol is metabolized to formaldehyde and formic acid. Accumulation of formate causes a high-AG acidosis. Methanol intoxication causes severe damage to the eye, including retinal edema, optic papillitis, and optic nerve damage that may cause blindness.
3. Ethylene glycol, a component of antifreeze, is metabolized to glycolic, oxalic, and other organic acids. The toxic effects may include respiratory failure and acute renal failure, the latter due to precipitation of calcium oxalate and hippurate crystals in the kidney. Urinalysis may therefore reveal oxalate and hippuric acid crystals.
4. Paraldehyde has sometimes been used to treat seizures. The drug is metabolized to acetic acid, although the metabolic acidosis may actually be caused by the presence of ketoacids in patients treated with this drug.

The differential diagnosis of a high-AG acidosis may be simplified by calculation of the osmolal gap. The osmolal gap is the difference between the measured serum or plasma osmolality and the calculated osmolality as defined earlier in this chapter.

The osmolal gap is normally less than 10 mosmol/kg. If the measured osmolality exceeds the calculated osmolality by more than 10, the presence of a hidden osmotically active substance should be suspected (10). A high osmolal gap with a high-AG metabolic acidosis is suggestive of methanol or ethylene glycol poisoning.

Normal–Anion Gap Metabolic Acidosis (Hyperchloremic Acidosis)

A normal-AG acidosis can occur in several situations, including bicarbonate losses in the gastrointestinal tract, infusion of acids, and the recovery phase of ketoacidosis.

The pancreatic and biliary secretions add bicarbonate to the intestine that is subsequently resorbed in exchange for chloride. Excessive gastrointestinal bicarbonate losses may occur in patients with prolonged diarrhea, pancreatic or biliary drainage or fistulas, or ureterosigmoidostomies. Oral anion-exchange resins such as cholestyramine can exchange chloride for bicarbonate and in high doses might also produce hyperchloremic acidosis.

A normal-AG acidosis can also result from a net gain in acid. This is usually due to the use of acidifying agents such as ammonium chloride, arginine hydrochloride, and lysine hydrochloride or to the administration of hyperalimentation fluids containing amino acids (10).

Renal tubular acidosis (RTA) encompasses a number of conditions (10) associated with either decreased renal hydrogen ion excretion or renal bicarbonate wasting. Type 1 RTA (distal or classic RTA) results from an inability to secrete hydrogen ions in the distal tubule. The urine pH is high (above 5.3) despite acidemia. The causes include a primary idiopathic form(s), various autoimmune disorders, nephrocalcinosis, certain drugs, a number of congenital conditions, pyelonephritis and urinary obstruction, and cirrhosis (10). Type 2 RTA (proximal RTA) results from renal bicarbonate wasting as evidenced by a rapid excretion of a bicarbonate load and fractional excretion of bicarbonate above 15%. Like type 1 RTA the differential diagnosis includes a long list of conditions (10), and many patients also exhibit Fanconi's syndrome. Type 4 RTA (there is no type 3 RTA) results from a deficiency of aldosterone or from aldosterone resistance. The causes include adrenal insufficiency, congenital adrenal hyperplasia, hyporeninemic hypoaldosteronism, and administration of angiotensin converting enzyme (ACE) inhibitors.

Finally, a transient metabolic acidosis may occur in patients with chronic compensated respiratory alkalosis when the alkalosis is rapidly corrected (posthypocapnic metabolic acidosis). In these patients the bicarbonate level is low (due to renal compensation for the alkalosis) and cannot return to normal as rapidly as the P_{CO_2}.

References

1. Rose B. Clinical physiology of acid-base and electrolyte disorders. 3rd ed. New York: McGraw-Hill, 1989.
2. Rose B. The total body water and the plasma sodium concentration. In: Clinical physiology of acid-base and electrolyte disorders. 3rd ed. New York: McGraw-Hill, 1989:211–224.
3. Black R. Disorders of serum sodium and serum potassium. In: Irwin R, Alpert J, Fink M, eds. Intensive care medicine. Boston: Little, Brown, 1985:610–224.

4. Kumar A, et al. Chromogenic ionophore-based methods for spectrophotometric assay of sodium and potassium in serum and plasma. Clin Chem 1988;34(9):1709–1712.
5. Tietz N, Siggaard-Andersen O, Pruden E. Acid-base balance and acid-base disorders. In: Teitz N, ed. Textbook of clinical chemistry. Philadelphia: WB Saunders, 1986:1221–1254.
6. Rose B. Hypo-osmolal states—hyponatremia. In: Clinical physiology of acid-base and electrolyte disorders. 3rd ed. New York: McGraw-Hill, 1989:601–638.
7. Delmez J. Fluid and electrolyte disturbances. In: Cambell W, Frisse M, eds. Manual of medical therapeutics. 24th ed. Boston: Little, Brown, 1983:23–43.
8. Tannen R. The patient with hypokalemia or hyperkalemia. In: Manual of nephrology. 2nd ed. Boston: Little, Brown, 1985: 31–48.
9. Rose B. Hyperkalemia. In: Clinical physiology of acid-base and electrolyte disorders. 3rd ed. New York: McGraw-Hill, 1989:715–756.
10. Black R. Metabolic acid-base disturbances. In: Irwin R, Albert J, Fink M, eds. Intensive care medicine. Boston: Little, Brown, 1985:596–609.
11. Burnett RW. On the use of phosphate buffers of physiological ionic strength for standardizing blood pH measurements. In: Siggaard-Andersen O, ed. Copenhagen: Private Press, 1981.
12. Stow RW, Baer RF, Randall BF. Rapid measurement of the tension of carbon dioxide in the blood. Arch Phys Med Rehabil 1957;38:646–650.
13. Severinghaus JW, Bradley AF. Electrodes for blood pO_2 and pCO_2 determination. J Appl Physiol 1958;13:515–520.
14. Dijkhuszen P, Fongers TME, Rispens P, Zijlstra WG. A new reference method for the determination of total CO_2 in biological fluids. Clin Chim Acta 1978;86:339–347.
15. Maas AHJ, Rispens P, Siggaard-Andersen O, Zijlstra WG. On the reliability of the Henderson-Hasselbalch equation in routine clinical acid-base chemistry. Ann Clin Biochem 1984;21: 26–39.
16. Ehrmeyer S et al. Definitions of quantities and conventions related to blood pH and gas analysis. 2nd ed. Document C12-T2. Villanova, PA: National Committee for Clinical Laboratory Standards, 1991.
17. Ehrmeyer S et al. Blood gas pre-analytical considerations: specimen collection, calibration and controls. Document C27-A. Villanova, PA: National Committee for Clinical Laboratory Standards, 1993.
18. Wiseman JD et al. Percutaneous collection of arterial blood for laboratory analysis. 2nd ed. Document H11-A2. Villanova, PA: National Committee for Clinical Laboratory Standards, 1992.
19. Bruck E et al. Procedures for the collection of diagnostic blood specimens by skin puncture. 3rd ed. Document H4-A3. Villanova, PA: National Committee for Clinical Laboratory Standards, 1991.
20. Wiseman JD et al. Devices for collection of skin puncture blood specimens. 2nd ed. Document H14-A2. Villanova, PA: National Committee for Clinical Laboratory Standards, 1990.
21. Mahoney JJ et al. Changes in oxygen measurements when whole blood is stored in iced plastic or glass syringes. Clin Chem 1991;37(7):1244–1248.
22. Müller-Plathe O, Heyduck S. Stability of blood gases, electrolytes, and haemoglobin in heparinized whole blood samples: influence of the type of syringe. Eur J Clin Chem Clin Biochem 1992;30:349–355.
23. Burnett RW. Matrix effects in blood gas measurement. Arch Pathol Lab Med 1993;117:365–368.
24. Burnett RW, Covington AK, Maas AHJ, Müller-Plathe O, Weisberg HF, Wimberley PD, Zijlstra WG, Siggaard-Andersen O, Durst RA. IFCC Method (1988) for tonometry of blood: reference materials for pCO_2 and pO_2. Clin Chim Acta 1989;185: S17–S24.
25. Burnett RW, Itano M. An interlaboratory study of blood gas analysis: Dependence of pO_2 and pCO_2 results on atmospheric pressure. Clin Chem 1989;35:1779–1781.
26. Sladen A. Acid-base balance. In: McIntyre K, Lewis J, eds. Textbook of advanced cardiac life support. American Heart Association, 1983:135–142.
27. Comella L, Braen R, Olding M. Blood gases and acid-base disorders. In: Clinician's pocket reference. 4th ed. Laguna Niguel, CA: Capistrano Press, 1983:157–168.
28. Rose B. Metabolic alkalosis. In: Clinical physiology of acid-base and electrolyte disorders. 3rd ed. New York: McGraw-Hill, 1989:501–555.

15 Respiration and Measurement of Oxygen and Hemoglobin

Michael Pins, Kent Lewandrowski, and Robert W. Burnett

NORMAL PHYSIOLOGY

Respiration is the exchange of oxygen and carbon dioxide between the environment and cells. In the lungs, gas exchange is accomplished by diffusion of oxygen from alveoli into the blood and of carbon dioxide from the blood into the alveoli. At the cellular level, respiration requires the transport of oxygen into the cells and the removal of carbon dioxide. A brief review of normal physiology is necessary to understand pathophysiology.

Components of Respiration

Respiration depends on the proper functioning of the following components:

1. Ventilation (moving air in and out of the lungs),
2. Gas exchange between the lungs and the blood,
3. Oxygen binding to hemoglobin, and
4. Adequate cardiac output to deliver oxygenated blood to cells.

The efficient exchange of oxygen and carbon dioxide in the lungs requires adequate alveolar ventilation and the matching of ventilation to pulmonary blood flow. When the chest muscles and diaphragm expand the chest, a negative pressure relative to the atmosphere is created in the space surrounding the lungs (a negative intrathoracic pressure). The pressure differential causes the lungs to expand and allows outside air to flow through the respiratory passages, which terminate in sac-like outpouchings called alveoli. Gas exchange is therefore dependent on the rate and the depth of ventilation. The amount of work required for inspiration is a function of the compliance (stretchability) of the lung and the airway resistance.

The airways are divided into two zones: a conducting and a respiratory zone. The conducting zone consists of the trachea, right and left mainstream bronchi, lobar bronchi, segmental bronchi, and terminal bronchioles. The respiratory zone comprises the structures in which gas exchange occurs. This includes the respiratory bronchioles, alveolar ducts, and alveoli. Passive diffusion of gases takes place primarily at the level of the alveolar-pulmonary capillary membrane. The pulmonary capillary membrane must be thin (0.3 μm) to permit efficient diffusion of gases. This membrane consists of the alveolar epithelium, the underlying basement membrane, and the pulmonary capillary endothelium.

A constant flow of blood is essential to allow proper gas exchange. Systemic (venous), deoxygenated blood carrying CO_2 is transported to the right side of the heart, and from there to the pulmonary arteries. Gas exchange then occurs in the pulmonary capillary bed, and the oxygenated blood is transported via the pulmonary veins to the left side of the heart and then to the systemic arterial circulation.

At a normal respiratory rate of 12 to 15/minute, about 0.2 liter/minute of CO_2 and 0.25 liter/minute of O_2 are exchanged. Ventilation can increase 20- to 30-fold with increased oxygen demand such as occurs with strenuous exercise. The exchange of gases across the pulmonary capillary membrane is governed by gradients in the partial pressures of individual gases. Dry inspired room air is composed of 78% nitrogen, 21% oxygen, 0.03% carbon dioxide, and 0.1% inert gases. Inspired air is rapidly warmed to 37°C in the upper respiratory passages and becomes saturated with water (P_{H_2O} = 47 mm Hg at 37°C). Normal values for the partial pressures of gases at different levels of the respiratory tract and in arterial and venous blood are shown in Table 15.1.

The respiratory system is designed such that (*a*) forces exerted by the respiratory muscles counteract the elastic recoil and airway resistance of the lungs, (*b*) a minimal pulmonary capillary membrane thickness is maintained, (*c*) right and left heart output are balanced, and (*d*) ventilation ($\dot{V}$) and perfusion ($\dot{Q}$) within the lung are matched.

Compliance is a measure of the stretchability of the lung and is inversely proportional to elasticity. Most of the energy required for expiration is derived from the elastic recoil properties of the lung. Con-

Table 15.1. Partial Pressures of Gases in the Respiratory Tract and Blood[a]

Compartment	P_{O_2}	P_{CO_2}	P_{H_2O}
	mm Hg	*mm Hg*	*mm Hg*
Inspired air	160	0.25	Variable
Upper airways	149	0.25	47
Alveolar air	102	36	47
Arterial blood	100	40	—
Venous blood	40	46	—
Expired air	115	30	47

[a]For atmospheric pressure = 760 mm Hg.

versely, inspiration requires energy expenditure from the respiratory muscles that is proportional to the pulmonary compliance. Low compliance results in difficulty with inspiration (restrictive disease), whereas a high compliance decreases the work of inspiration but impairs expiration. A similar concept applies at the level of the alveoli. Laplace's law describes the relationship between the alveolar volume (radius, R), surface tension of the alveolar fluid (T), and the pressure (P) required to maintain an inflated alveolus ($P = 2T/R$). In theory the smaller the alveolar radius, the greater the pressure required to maintain the alveolar volume, assuming that the surface tension is the same. Pressure differences between alveoli might result in collapse of smaller alveoli were it not for the type II pneumocytes that secrete pulmonary surfactant. Surfactant is a mixture of phospholipids (chiefly lecithin) that lowers alveolar surface tension and thus prevents the collapse of small airspaces. A deficiency of surfactant results in stiff, noncompliant lungs. This condition underlies the pathogenesis of respiratory distress syndrome (RDS) in premature infants. The level of surfactant produced by the fetal lung increases during fetal development, with a large increase after 35 weeks' gestation. Infants born between 32 and 36 weeks exhibit a 15 to 20% risk of developing RDS, compared to 5% born after 37 weeks.

Ventilation, Perfusion, and the Ventilation-Perfusion Ratio

VENTILATION

Ventilation ($\dot{V}$) is the exchange of gases between ambient air and the lungs. At the end of expiration a certain amount of gas remains in the conducting airways and alveoli. Thus with inspiration, fresh air mixes with retained gases in the lung. The inspired volume, termed the tidal volume, is normally 0.5 liter. Therefore, an average respiratory rate of 12 to 15 breaths per minute accounts for a minute ventilation of 6 to 7.5 liters/minute. Ventilation to nonperfused areas is termed dead space ventilation and includes anatomic dead space (conducting system) and alveolar dead space (nonperfused alveoli). Essentially no alveolar dead space exists in the normal physiologic state.

The distribution of ventilation in the lungs is dependent on two variables: airway resistance and the ability of alveoli to accommodate pressure differentials (Laplace's law). Resistance to airflow is equal throughout the pulmonary tree in the normal lung, but variances in small airway resistance are a common cause of uneven ventilation in disease states. However, the ventilation distribution is not uniform even in healthy persons because of a gradient in pleural pressure between the uppermost and lowermost regions of the lung. As a consequence, alveoli are larger at the apex than at the base of the lungs.

PERFUSION

Perfusion ($\dot{Q}$) refers to the flow of blood through the lungs, and specifically to the flow through the pulmonary capillaries that are in close proximity to alveoli. The distribution of perfusion is dependent on several variables: gravity, cardiac output, and pulmonary vascular autoregulation. The pulmonary vasculature normally operates under low pressure. Therefore, gravity has a significant impact on the distribution of perfusion. Perfusion is greater at the base of the lung (dependent area) than at the apex. As cardiac output increases, pulmonary vascular pressure increases, and nondependent areas are better perfused.

VENTILATION-PERFUSION MATCHING ($\dot{V}/\dot{Q}$ RATIO)

Although both ventilation and perfusion are unevenly distributed in the normal lung, the critical feature is that ventilated areas are perfused and that perfused areas are ventilated. Most of the total ventilation, and an even greater proportion of the pulmonary blood flow, is directed to dependent areas of the lungs. The result is a slightly higher $\dot{V}/\dot{Q}$ ratio in nondependent areas (the lung apices in a standing person) than in dependent areas (the lung bases in a standing person). Since alveolar ventilation is approximately 4 liters/minute and cardiac output averages 5 liters/minute, the overall $\dot{V}/\dot{Q}$ ratio is normally about 0.8. Pathological mismatches of $\dot{V}$ and $\dot{Q}$ ($\dot{V}/\dot{Q}$ mismatch) are the most common cause of hypoxemia in disease states.

ALVEOLAR-ARTERIAL P_{O_2} DIFFERENCE (A-a O_2 gradient)

The alveolar-arterial O_2 gradient is the difference between the partial pressure of oxygen in alveolar air

(P_{AO_2}) and the partial pressure of oxygen in the arterial blood (Pa_{O_2}). The alveolar-arterial O_2 gradient is the single best indicator of the effectiveness of gas exchange between the alveoli and pulmonary capillaries and is extremely useful in evaluating patients with hypoxemia. The Pa_{O_2} is a measured value, whereas P_{AO_2} is calculated from the alveolar gas equation:

$$P_{AO_2} = (P_{total} - P_{H_2O})\ F_{IO_2} - Pa_{CO_2}/RQ$$

where Ptotal is the barometric pressure (760 mm Hg at sea level); P_{H_2O} is the water vapor pressure (47 mm Hg at 37°C); F_{IO_2} is the mole fraction of inspired oxygen (0.21 in room air); Pa_{CO_2} is the arterial P_{CO_2} (normally 40 mm Hg); and RQ is the respiratory quotient (the ratio of CO_2 production to O_2 consumption, usually 0.8). This equation describes the effect of a change in F_{IO_2} on alveolar oxygenation. It also takes into account displacement of O_2 molecules (decreased P_{AO_2}) when arterial and alveolar CO_2 are elevated. Normally the alveolar-arterial O_2 gradient is less than 15 mm Hg in a young person breathing room air and increases approximately 3 mm Hg per decade after the age of 30. An alveolar-arterial O_2 gradient above 20 mm Hg is considered abnormal at any age.

To calculate the alveolar-arterial O_2 gradient the patient should be breathing room air. Under these conditions the inspired O_2 is 150 mm Hg, R=0.08, and the Pa_{CO_2} is measured (normally 40 mm Hg). The P_{AO_2} is then calculated as follows:

$$P_{AO_2} = 150 - (40/0.8) = 100 \text{ mm Hg}$$

If the P_{AO_2} is normally 100 mm Hg and the Pa_{O_2} is, for example, 70 mm Hg, then the alveolar-arterial gradient would be 30 mm Hg.

The value of calculating the alveolar-arterial gradient is that it differentiates hypoventilation (in which the alveolar-arterial gradient is normal) from other causes of hypoxemia such as ventilation-perfusion mismatch, in which the alveolar-arterial gradient is increased.

Regulation of Respiration

Respiration is regulated by the interaction of the medullary respiratory center in the brain, peripheral chemoreceptors, and mechanoreceptors, and by the effects of local mediators. Involuntary changes in the rate or depth of respiration are directed by the medullary respiratory center, which is influenced by peripheral and central chemoreceptors. Central chemoreceptors, located beneath the ventral surface of the medulla oblongata, respond to changes in the pH of the cerebrospinal fluid. Peripheral chemoreceptors, which include the carotid and aortic bodies, respond to both pH and P_{O_2}. A decrease in pH stimulates both the central and peripheral chemoreceptors, whereas a decrease in P_{O_2} stimulates only the peripheral chemoreceptors. Stimulation of these receptors results in an increase in ventilation with a subsequent increased gas exchange. To the extent that the P_{CO_2} affects the arterial pH, changes in the P_{CO_2} will also affect the rate and depth of respiration.

Local decreases in oxygen tension cause constriction of the pulmonary vasculature. The result is shunting of blood away from unventilated areas of the lung to ventilated areas. This phenomenon occurs in the normal physiologic state (such as in dependent areas of the lung where the $\dot{V}/\dot{Q}$ ratio is relatively low) as well as in a number of disease states. The opposite effect (vasodilation) occurs in the systemic circulation, thus facilitating delivery of oxygen to peripheral tissues.

Mechanoreceptors (J receptors) in the lung respond to the stretching forces exerted on the lung during inspiration and reflexively excite expiration.

An additional sensor of hypoxia deserves brief mention. Juxtaproximal tubular cells in the kidney sense hypoxia and respond by stimulating erythropoiesis via erythropoietin. The result is an increased red blood cell mass and an increased O_2 carrying capacity of the blood.

Hemoglobin and the Oxygen Dissociation Curve

In addition to adequate ventilation and gas exchange with blood, respiration requires transportation of oxygen to cells. The solubility of oxygen in plasma is relatively low. Hemoglobin in erythrocytes provides the means, through binding of oxygen molecules, of transporting enough oxygen to cells to satisfy the demands of normal metabolism. Hemoglobin is a protein made up of four subunits, each of which contains a heme moiety. Heme is a ferrous iron tetrapyrrole complex that can bind one oxygen molecule. One molecule of hemoglobin can therefore bind four oxygen molecules.

The binding of one oxygen molecule to hemoglobin alters the quaternary structure of the tetramer such that subsequent binding of additional O_2 molecules is facilitated. This effect results in the sigmoidal shape of the oxygen-hemoglobin equilibrium curve (also called the oxygen dissociation curve), which relates the P_{O_2} to the oxygen saturation of hemoglobin (S_{O_2}), as shown in Figure 15.1.

At the P_{O_2} normally present in arterial blood, hemoglobin is more than 95% saturated with oxygen,

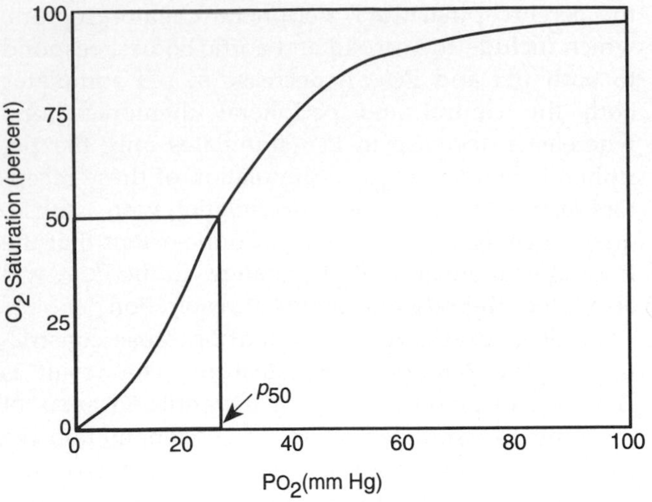

Figure 15.1. Oxygen-hemoglobin equilibrium curve.

and at a PO_2 above 100 to 120 mm Hg, is almost 100% saturated. At this point increases in inspired oxygen will increase only the dissolved oxygen content of blood and not the amount bound to hemoglobin. Thus, once hemoglobin is saturated, a higher FIO_2 will not appreciably increase the oxygen content of the blood (although the PO_2 may be markedly elevated).

The position of the oxygen dissociation curve reflects the affinity of hemoglobin for oxygen. Hemoglobin-oxygen affinity is influenced by a number of factors. Affinity is reduced by increases in temperature, decreases in pH, increases in PCO_2 (at constant pH), and increases in the erythrocyte 2,3-diphosphoglycerate (DPG) concentration. An increase in hemoglobin-oxygen affinity shifts the oxygen dissociation curve to the left, whereas a decrease in affinity shifts the curve to the right. Thus a right shift in the curve is observed with elevated DPG concentration, acidemia, and hypercapnia. The effect of these variables in normal physiology is important to the delivery of oxygen to the tissues. In the lung, where the PO_2 is high, hemoglobin takes up O_2 and releases CO_2, whereas in the tissues PO_2 is low and the reverse occurs. The comparatively high pH and PCO_2 found in the tissues further enhances oxygen release from hemoglobin. Conversely, pathologic changes in pH, PCO_2, or temperature may impair oxygen delivery. DPG is an intermediate in normal glycolysis in red blood cells. The effect of DPG is to lower the hemoglobin-oxygen affinity and thus promote O_2 delivery to tissues. DPG concentrations increase in red blood cells in response to states of anemia or alkalosis, which tends to compensate for the primary disorder. DPG concentrations tend to decrease with length of storage of blood.

MEASUREMENT OF OXYGEN AND HEMOGLOBIN SPECIES

The Oxygen Electrode

The routine measurement of PO_2 in blood became practical with the development of the oxygen electrode by Clark in 1956. In contrast to ion-selective electrode methods used for hydrogen, sodium, potassium, and other ions, which are based on potentiometry, the oxygen electrode method is amperometric; that is, the PO_2 is related to the amount of current flowing in an electrochemical cell. In this cell, oxygen is reduced at a platinum wire cathode. The other half-cell is usually a silver–silver chloride electrode. When a voltage of about −0.6 volt is applied to the cathode, oxygen is reduced according to the following reaction:

$$O_2 + 2H^+ + 4e^- \rightarrow 2OH^-$$

The current depends on the number of oxygen molecules reaching the cathode per unit time, which in turn depends on the concentration of dissolved oxygen in the sample, which is proportional to the PO_2. The area of the cathode is kept very small so that only a tiny fraction of the total dissolved oxygen is reduced, and the current then assumes a constant value proportional to the PO_2.

A diagram of the oxygen electrode is shown in Figure 15.2. The platinum cathode is in contact with a very thin layer of buffer, which is separated from the blood sample by a gas-permeable membrane. The membrane serves to keep other reducible substances in blood from reaching the cathode, which would add to the cell current and could foul the electrode surface. The membrane itself adsorbs small amounts of protein from the blood samples and needs to be replaced periodically in most electrode designs.

Calibration of the oxygen electrode is usually done with two gas mixtures whose composition is known with very high accuracy. One contains no oxygen, which allows a zero point to be established, and the other contains a known oxygen percentage, usually either 12 or 20% (±0.03%) by volume. Further details about the calibration of blood gas analyzers and the preanalytical variables that affect PO_2 measurements are discussed in Chapter 14.

Spectrophotometry of Hemoglobin Species

The measurement of total hemoglobin is a routine part of a hematology profile. The measurement of oxyhemoglobin, deoxyhemoglobin, carboxyhemoglobin, and methemoglobin by spectrophotometry is

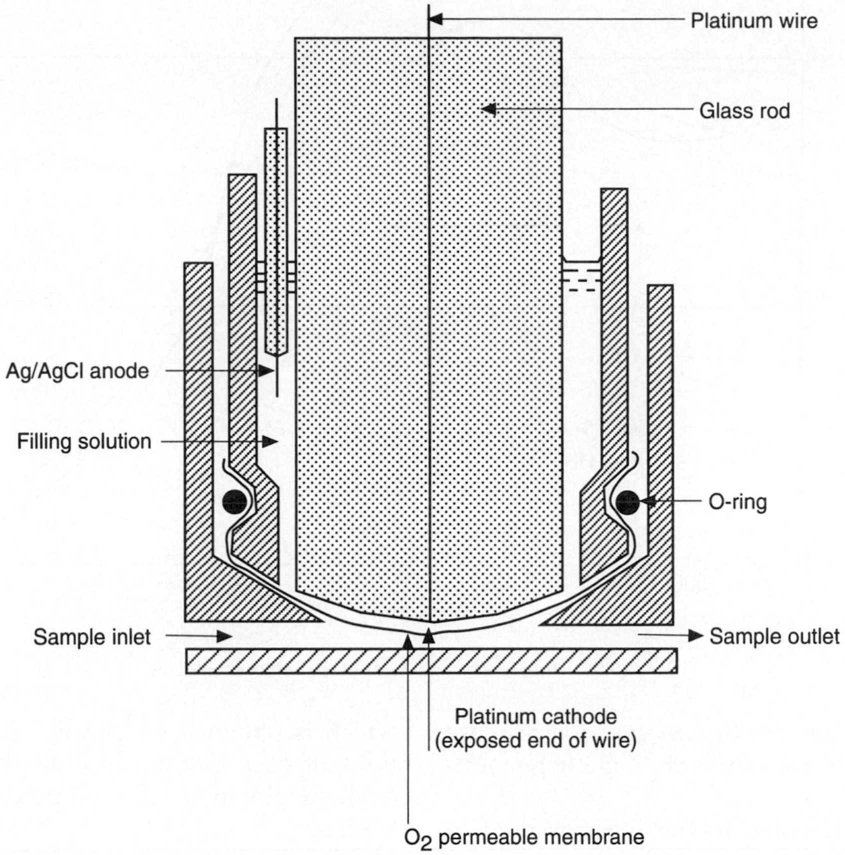

Figure 15.2. Schematic illustration of a P_{O_2} electrode. (Adapted from Siggaard-Andersen O. The acid-base status of the blood. 4th ed. Baltimore: Williams & Wilkins, 1974.)

often performed as an adjunct to blood gas measurements and is therefore discussed here.

Each of the hemoglobin species of interest has a unique absorbance spectrum in the visible region, as illustrated in Figure 15.3. Once the spectrum of each species is established with solutions of known concentration, the analysis of a mixture is carried out by simply measuring the absorbance of a hemolysate at multiple wavelengths—one wavelength for each of the species to be determined. Beer's law applies to the absorbance at each wavelength.

$$A_{\lambda 1} = E_{\lambda 1}(1)\,C(1) + E_{\lambda 1}(2)\,C(2) + \ldots + E_{\lambda 1}(n)\,C(n)$$

$$A_{\lambda 2} = E_{\lambda 2}(1)\,C(1) + E_{\lambda 2}(2)\,C(2) + \ldots + E_{\lambda 2}(n)\,C(n)$$

$$A_{\lambda n} = E_{\lambda n}(1)\,C(1) + E_{\lambda n}(2)\,C(2) + \ldots + E_{\lambda n}(n)\,C(n)$$

where $E_{\lambda 1}(1)$ is the absorptivity at wavelength $\lambda 1$ and $C(1)$ is the concentration of the first component, and so forth.

Thus, to determine the concentrations of oxyhemoglobin (O_2Hb), deoxyhemoglobin (Hb), carboxyhemoglobin (COHb) and methemoglobin (metHb) in blood, the absorbance is measured at four wavelengths, giving four equations of the form above, which can be solved simultaneously to yield the concentrations. The absorptivities are constants that are permanently stored in the instrument. The absorbance scale may be calibrated with a total hemoglobin standard, and a microprocessor in the instrument then performs the calculations necessary to give concentrations of each hemoglobin species as well as calculations for the several derived quantities commonly reported. It should be recognized that if all four of the hemoglobin species mentioned are to be measured, a minimum of four different wavelengths must be used. Some older laboratory oximeters and oximeters used in point-of-care testing use two or three wavelengths and are intended to measure only oxyhemoglobin. With such devices it is important to understand what errors will be seen if significant amounts of carboxyhemoglobin or methemoglobin are present (1, 2).

SPECIMENS AND SPECIMEN HANDLING

Often, the measurement of oxyhemoglobin and other hemoglobin species is requested in conjunction

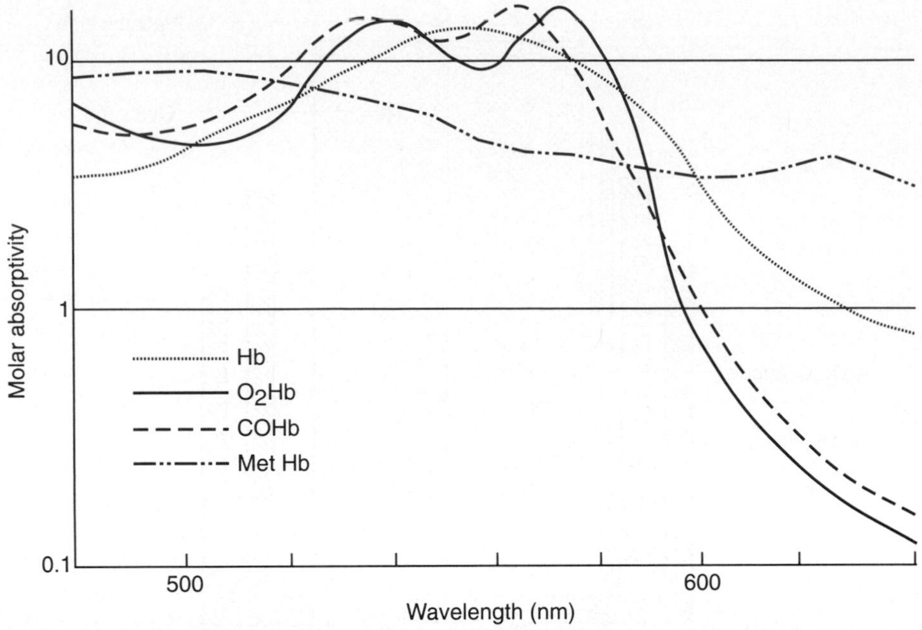

Figure 15.3. Absorbance spectrum of hemoglobin species.

with arterial blood gas measurements. In this case the same specimen is used for both, namely heparinized arterial blood.

If one is only interested in the measurement of carboxyhemoglobin or methemoglobin, then venous blood is preferred, to avoid the discomfort and difficulty of an arterial puncture. In addition, the issues of the type of container and whether or not to store the specimen on ice are not relevant. Both carboxyhemoglobin and methemoglobin are relatively stable, so a specimen anticoagulated with heparin or EDTA and transported at ambient temperature is satisfactory.

The most important aspect of specimen handling is to ensure that the blood is thoroughly mixed. Incomplete mixing of whole blood cannot be detected by eye but can produce significant errors in either direction in the total hemoglobin measurement.

Derived Quantities

There has long been confusion about definitions and conventions used in the field of blood gas analysis. This has been addressed by two different organizations, the (U.S.) National Committee for Clinical Laboratory Standards and the International Federation of Clinical Chemists, and their documents are recommended for a more complete description of the various derived quantities that are in use (3, 4).

OXYHEMOGLOBIN FRACTION AND OXYGEN SATURATION

Results are usually expressed as a fraction (or percentage) of the total hemoglobin concentration, which is obtained by simply adding the concentrations of each of the components. For example, the oxyhemoglobin fraction (in percent) would be calculated as

$$\mathrm{FO_2Hb}\ (\%) = \frac{100\ \mathrm{CO_2Hb}}{\mathrm{CO_2Hb + CHb + CCOHb + CmetHb}}$$

Fractions of carboxyhemoglobin and methemoglobin are calculated similarly.

Care must be taken not to confuse oxyhemoglobin fraction with a related quantity, oxygen saturation ($\mathrm{SO_2}$). The latter quantity, also called oxygen saturation of available hemoglobin, is defined as the concentration of oxyhemoglobin expressed as a percentage of only the hemoglobin available for oxygen binding.

$$\mathrm{SO_2}\ (\%) = \frac{100\ \mathrm{CO_2Hb}}{\mathrm{CO_2Hb + CHb}}$$

Thus, $\mathrm{SO_2}$ can also be calculated from the measured concentrations of oxyhemoglobin and deoxyhemoglobin, and many oximeters perform this calculation automatically.

Comparison of these two equations shows that the two quantities are equal if no carboxyhemoglobin or methemoglobin is present. This is partly why the two are often confused, and the term ''oxygen saturation'' is unfortunately still loosely used to refer to either oxygen saturation or oxyhemoglobin fraction. However, it is quite important for the laboratory to clearly identify which quantity is being reported so that clinicians are not confused when treating a patient with carbon monoxide poisoning or methemoglobinemia.

OXYGEN CONTENT

The concentration of total oxygen (CtO_2) in blood, also called oxygen content, is the sum of hemoglobin-bound oxygen and oxygen dissolved in blood. Oxygen content can therefore be calculated as

$$CtO_2 = CO_2Hb + \alpha O_2 \, PO_2$$

where αO_2 is the solubility coefficient of oxygen in blood plasma.

Because 98 to 99% of the total oxygen is normally bound to hemoglobin, the term for dissolved oxygen is often ignored, in which case O_2 content can be closely estimated from oximeter data alone. Oxygen content is often expressed in milliliters of oxygen (at standard temperature and pressure) per deciliter of whole blood, and the measured quantities available are oxyhemoglobin fraction and total hemoglobin. Oxygen content is then estimated as

$$CtO_2 \text{ (ml } O_2/\text{dl)} = 1.39 \; FO_2Hb \; CtHb$$

where CtHb is total hemoglobin in grams per deciliter and 1.39 is the oxygen binding capacity of hemoglobin expressed as milliliters of O_2 per gram of hemoglobin.

P_{50}

The partial pressure of oxygen corresponding to an oxygen saturation of 50% is called P_{50} and is a measure of hemoglobin oxygen affinity. In principle, if one assumes a normal shape of the oxygen dissociation curve and measures both the PO_2 and oxygen saturation, then this point on the curve can be used to calculate the PO_2 that would give 50% saturation. In practice this can be done accurately as long as the oxygen saturation is less than about 90%. To interpret the calculated P_{50} one must also measure the quantities mentioned above that affect the position of the oxygen dissociation curve. The determination of P_{50} is not commonly performed but can be useful, for example in determining in vivo oxygen affinity or in testing for hemoglobin variants with abnormal oxygen affinity. Further details and the calculation procedure are given in reference 5.

Quality Control and Proficiency Testing

Quality control (QC) of PO_2 measurements is discussed with pH and PCO_2 in Chapter 14. This brief discussion relates to QC of oximetry measurements. One of the primary difficulties with QC and proficiency testing (PT) in blood gas analysis applies also to oximetry measurements, namely the lack of a control material that closely resembles whole blood. Materials used for QC fall into three categories: (*a*) a dye mixture, (*b*) stabilized hemolysates, and (*c*) stabilized whole blood.

Dye mixtures are, in principle, adequate for QC of the spectrophotometer module of an oximeter. The principal drawbacks are that readings may not correspond to values encountered in patient samples, and also that different readings are usually obtained on various makes and models of oximeters. These problems are avoided by using a stabilized hemolysate. The main limitation of both these matrices is that they cannot check the functioning of the hemolyzer portion of the oximeter. This is important, because incomplete hemolysis of samples can result in inaccurate readings that may not be noticed; for example, the errors may appear as moderate elevations of carboxyhemoglobin or methemoglobin. Although stabilized whole blood would seem to be a logical matrix, the products commercially available may not work satisfactorily in all oximeters. For example, stabilized erythrocytes may be more resistant to lysis than normal red cells, leading to erratic results on QC materials even when the instrument is functioning well with patient samples.

A useful adjunct to any quality control program is to run occasional patient samples in duplicate on two different instruments. This is one way of using fresh whole blood for QC, and this should be done whenever two or more instruments are used. Also, the accuracy of the total hemoglobin measured by an oximeter can be checked by using fresh whole blood together with the cyanmethemoglobin reference method for total hemoglobin.

Point-of-Care Testing

Some tests, including blood gas analysis and oximetry, can now be performed at the patient's bedside. This has several advantages but also raises some concerns (6–8). Advantages include minimizing turnaround time, limiting iatrogenic blood loss and patient discomfort, and eliminating problems relating to specimen transport (9, 10). Areas of concern include cost, adequate quality control, adequate training of nonlaboratory personnel, and differences in reference ranges that may affect the interpretation of results. Several problems are particular to the acute care setting. Precision, for example, may be more important than accuracy in situations where an acute change in an analyte is more important than absolute values (11, 12).

Important parameters in the critical care setting include the PO_2, the O_2 saturation, the PCO_2, pH, elec-

Table 15.2. Methodologies Used in Point-of-Care Instrument[a]

Analytes	Electrochemical	Optical
PO_2	Amperometric Clark-type electrode	Optode based on: • Fluorescence quenching, or • Absorbance change of O_2 binding molecules
PCO_2	Potentiometric Severinghaus-type electrode	Optode based on pH sensor and gas permeable membrane
pH	Glass or polymer membrane electrodes	Optode based on fluorescence or absorbance measurement of immobilized pH indicator
Electrolytes	Ion selective electrodes (potentiometric)	Solution phase complexing reagents or colorimetric strip test
Hematocrit	Conductivity cell or ISEs (measure change in electrolytes after RBC lysis)	Microcentrifuge or cell counter
Total hemoglobin	—	Direct absorbance measurement or colorimetric measurement of pseudoperoxidase activity
Glucose	Amperometric enzyme electrodes based on immobilized glucose oxidase	Colorimetric measurement of glucose metabolite

[a]Adapted from Misiano DR, et al. Current and future directions in the technology relating to bedside testing of critically ill patients. Chest 97 (Suppl):204S–214S.

trolytes (Na^+, K^+, Ca^+), and glucose. Table 15.2 summarizes the methodologies employed by a number of bedside instruments.

Bedside testing instrumentation can be divided into four major groups: (*a*) continuous noninvasive methods, (*b*) discrete sample analyzers, (*c*) extracorporeal sensing systems, and (*d*) continuous invasive methods.

CONTINUOUS NONINVASIVE METHODS

Continuous noninvasive analyte testing is conceptually the ideal. "Real-time" continuous values are provided without the need to withdraw blood or utilize indwelling catheters. Currently, this technology is limited to the transcutaneous measurement of oxygen and carbon dioxide, and O_2 saturation by pulse oximetry. Future innovations may allow for noninvasive measurement of other analytes, including electrolytes and glucose.

Transcutaneous sensors use methods similar to conventional blood gas instruments (13, 14). Clark-style amperometric oxygen and Stow-Severinghaus–style potentiometric carbon dioxide sensors have modified electrode designs to allow attachment of the monitor to the skin. Correlation studies comparing conventional PO_2 and PCO_2 measurements to transcutaneous values demonstrate significant biases, particularly in adults. Establishing appropriate reference ranges is therefore essential. Transcutaneous measurements are most commonly used for monitoring infants and neonates, in whom the discrepancies from established methods are less pronounced. Differences between the transcutaneous PO_2 and the PaO_2 are particularly pronounced in shock and low-flow states. In some cases this discrepancy is helpful to identify patients with these disorders (15).

Pulse oximetry measures the percentage of O_2 saturation of hemoglobin by the transmission of light at 660 nm (oxyhemoglobin peak) and 940 nm (deoxyhemoglobin peak) through a finger. The relative absorbance at each wavelength is measured and a ratio of oxyhemoglobin to total hemoglobin is calculated. The measurement is conducted to coincide with the arterial pulse, thereby reflecting arterial blood (16). Advantages of pulse oximetry include simplicity, the performance of real-time measurements, and blood conservation. However, potential technical or mechanical problems may arise in patients with hypothermia, peripheral vascular disease, hyperbilirubinemia, or altered heme species, or from stray ambient lighting (1, 2, 17–19). Nevertheless, pulse oximetry is one of the most widely used continuous noninvasive methodologies, particularly in settings where early warning of sudden change is essential.

DISCRETE SAMPLE ANALYZERS

Discrete sample analyzers include single-use, disposable analyzers (e.g., glucose meters) and multitest (PO_2, PCO_2, pH, Na, K, Ca, Hct, Hgb, glucose, etc.) analyzers. All of these instruments require withdrawing blood from the patient, and therefore the test results are not true real-time values. The multitest analyzers may be placed in a central location in the critical care unit and function in a manner similar to a "stat lab." Smaller, more portable analyzers may be moved closer to the patient for easier access and more rapid results. As instruments move from the central laboratory to the bedside, issues of quality control and operator training and proficiency become more problematic (8). Establishing protocols for the use of bedside devices is mandated by the Clinical Laboratory Improvement Act (CLIA), and is often the responsibility of the clinical laboratory.

EXTRACORPOREAL SENSING SYSTEMS

Extracorporeal sensors are instruments that sample arterial blood, measure analytes, and return the blood to a vein (in-line) or pass the blood to a waste receptacle (on-line). The advantage of these systems is that they can provide "real-time" measurements of analytes by conventional methods. The disadvantages include the risk of infection, thrombotic complications, and mechanical damage to erythrocytes, all of which mandate short-term use of these devices. The use of extracorporeal monitoring systems is currently limited to dialysis and cardiac surgery settings.

CONTINUOUS INVASIVE (IN VIVO) METHODS

Continuous invasive monitoring is achieved by attaching the sensor directly to an indwelling catheter. Analytes are measured continuously and in real time at sites such as the pulmonary artery. Catheter tips with miniaturized O_2, CO_2, and pH sensors have been devised, and implantable sensors for glucose are being developed (20). Disadvantages include the complications usually associated with indwelling catheters, such as thrombosis and infection. The present technological obstacle is the development of miniaturized, durable, and biocompatible sensors that can function reliably at the end of an indwelling catheter.

Mechanical and technical variables remain the major obstacles to refining and implementing cost-effective point-of-care testing. Newer technologies—such as near infrared (NIR) spectroscopy (for the transcutaneous measurement of blood glucose) (21–23), magnetic resonance spectroscopy (24, 25), and diffuse-sink sampling (26)—as well as advances in instrumentation (27) have the potential to significantly advance point-of-care testing and improve patient care.

PATHOPHYSIOLOGY AND INTERPRETATION

Respiratory failure is a clinical condition that is best defined by abnormalities in arterial blood gas values. While in some cases the diagnosis is obvious based on the patient's signs and symptoms (e.g., dyspnea, respiratory rate, cyanosis), the diagnosis usually requires analysis of arterial blood gases (PO_2, PCO_2, and pH). The clinical signs and symptoms of hypoxemia and hypercapnia are unreliable in predicting blood gas values. Reference intervals are shown in Table 14.4 of Chapter 14. As a general guideline, respiratory failure may be defined as a PaO_2 below 50 to 60 mm Hg or a $PaCO_2$ above 50 mm Hg. In acute respiratory failure the arterial pH may be decreased due to retention of CO_2 (acute respiratory acidosis), whereas in chronic respiratory failure the pH is less affected because of renal compensation. The evaluation of blood gas results is closely related to the topic of acid-base balance (see Chapter 14). In this section the discussion is limited to the evaluation from the perspective of identifying patients with respiratory failure, and the differential diagnosis of hypoxemia (decreased PO_2) and hypercapnia (elevated PCO_2).

It is important to distinguish between the terms hypoxemia and hypoxia. Hypoxemia refers to a decreased blood PO_2, whereas hypoxia is a condition in which inadequate amounts of oxygen are available to the tissues. Hypoxemia is one cause of hypoxia, but hypoxia can exist with normal PO_2 (e.g., arterial thrombosis). Delivery of oxygen to the tissues is dependent on cardiac output, intact vasculature, and the oxygen content of the blood. Clinical assessment of these variables is an important adjunct to arterial blood gas measurements.

Abnormalities in blood gases may be viewed in terms of which compartment of the respiratory system is failing (extrapulmonary versus pulmonary), in terms of pathophysiologic mechanisms (hyperventilation, $\dot{V}/\dot{Q}$ mismatch, shunts), or from the perspective of specific disease entities (e.g., asthma, pneumonia). Each approach has its advantages and is discussed below. An excellent discussion of this topic may also be found in reference 28.

Compartment Analysis

One approach to the evaluation of abnormal arterial blood gases is to consider which component of the respiratory system is failing. For example, extrapulmonary causes of respiratory failure may arise from diseases of the respiratory center, motor neurons and neuromuscular junction, respiratory muscles, chest wall, pleura, or upper airway. All of these produce a decrease in the PaO_2 and an elevation in the $PaCO_2$ due to hypoventilation. Pulmonary causes of respiratory failure may result from diseases of the lower airways, the pulmonary circulation, the pulmonary interstitium, or the alveolar-capillary unit. Some of these produce hypoxemia alone, while others are associated with both hypoxemia and hypercapnia. Thus diseases of the pulmonary compartment can be further subdivided into hypercapnic and nonhypercapnic failure. In hypercapnic failure, the major underlying problem is inadequate ventilation, whereas in nonhypercapnic failure the major problem is with oxygenation.

Table 15.3. Pathophysiologic Classification of Respiratory Failure

Mechanism	Blood Gas Values	Alveolar-Arterial O_2 Gradient	Response to O_2
Low inspired oxygen concentration	Low P_{O_2} and a normal or low P_{CO_2}	Normal	Increased P_{O_2}
Hypoventilation	Low P_{O_2} and elevated P_{CO_2}	Normal	Increased P_{O_2}
Ventilation/perfusion ($\dot{V}/\dot{Q}$) mismatch	Low P_{O_2}, elevated P_{CO_2} when severe	Increased	Increased P_{O_2}
Right to left shunt	Low P_{O_2} and normal P_{CO_2}	Increased	No or minimal improvement
Diffusion impairment	Low P_{O_2} and elevated P_{CO_2}	Increased	No or minimal improvement

Pathophysiologic Approach

This approach divides hypoxemia or hypercapnia according to the underlying mechanism producing the abnormality in gas exchange. Once the mechanism has been identified, consideration can be given to the differential diagnostic possibilities within each category.

There are five conditions that can cause arterial hypoxemia (Table 15.3). Hypoxemia due to breathing air with a low oxygen content may be seen in subjects at high altitudes or breathing abnormal gas mixtures, but for practical purposes this mechanism does not occur in a typical patient population. A similar statement can be made regarding diffusion impairment as a cause of hypoxemia. In principle, diffusion impairment can occur whenever the alveolar-capillary membrane is thickened or infiltrated by blood, edema, fluid, fibrosis, or other substances. In practice, diffusion impairment contributes relatively little to the development of hypoxemia in most pulmonary diseases. This is because complete gas exchange across the alveolar-capillary membrane is accomplished in approximately one-third of the time that blood spends in transit in the alveolar capillary. Severe pulmonary interstitial fibrosis or edema, pulmonary amyloidosis, and some types of pneumoconioses may produce hypoxemia as a consequence of diffusion impairment, but this situation is uncommon.

Since two of the five mechanisms can usually be excluded, the vast majority of patients with hypoxemia can be classified into one of three types: hypoventilation, ventilation-perfusion mismatch, or shunting. In some cases, more than one of these mechanisms may be operating simultaneously.

HYPOVENTILATION

A decrease in minute ventilation resulting in a decrease in alveolar ventilation for a given level of CO_2 production is termed hypoventilation. This produces both an increase in arterial P_{CO_2} (CO_2 retention, or hypercapnia) and a decrease in arterial P_{O_2} (hypoxemia). The fall in the arterial P_{O_2} is due solely to a decrease in the alveolar P_{O_2}. Hypoventilation is always due to an extrapulmonary process, including diseases of the central nervous system that affect the respiratory center (narcotic overdose, stroke, hypothyroidism), neuromuscular disorders (Guillain-Barré syndrome, myasthenia gravis, tetanus, poliomyelitis), abnormalities of the chest wall or diaphragm (trauma, diaphragmatic paralysis, kyphoscoliosis), upper airway obstruction (foreign bodies, epiglottitis, laryngospasm, tumors), or pleural disease (restrictive pleuritis). Patients with hypoventilation exhibit no intrinsic pulmonary abnormality; therefore distal gas exchange is unaffected and the alveolar-arterial O_2 gradient is normal.

The treatment of patients with hypoventilation is directed at improving alveolar ventilation to correct the hypercapnia (and the resultant respiratory acidosis) and the hypoxemia. This may be accomplished by relieving obstruction, administering the appropriate pharmacologic agents (bronchodilators, naloxone, physostigmine), or applying mechanical ventilation. The response of the patient to oxygen administration has both therapeutic and diagnostic implications (Fig. 15.4). Patients with hypoxemia due to hypoventilation or ventilation-perfusion mismatch exhibit a dramatic improvement in their P_{O_2} in response to oxygen therapy, whereas hypoxemia resulting from left to right shunting shows only a minimal or no response (see below).

VENTILATION-PERFUSION MISMATCH

Ventilation-perfusion mismatch is the most common cause of hypoxemia. In healthy subjects there is always some degree of physiologic ventilation-perfusion mismatching, because the basal portions of the lungs receive a disproportionate percentage of the pulmonary arterial blood flow, while the apices of the lungs are better ventilated. There are two types of ventilation-perfusion mismatch: (*a*) Low $\dot{V}/\dot{Q}$—inadequate ventilation for a given level of perfusion, and (*b*) High $\dot{V}/\dot{Q}$—inadequate perfusion for a given level of ventilation.

Areas of low $\dot{V}/\dot{Q}$ result in a decrease in the P_{O_2} and the oxygen content of the affected pulmonary blood. This is compensated to some degree by a slight increase in oxygen content occurring in areas of high $\dot{V}/\dot{Q}$, but the compensatory effect is small due

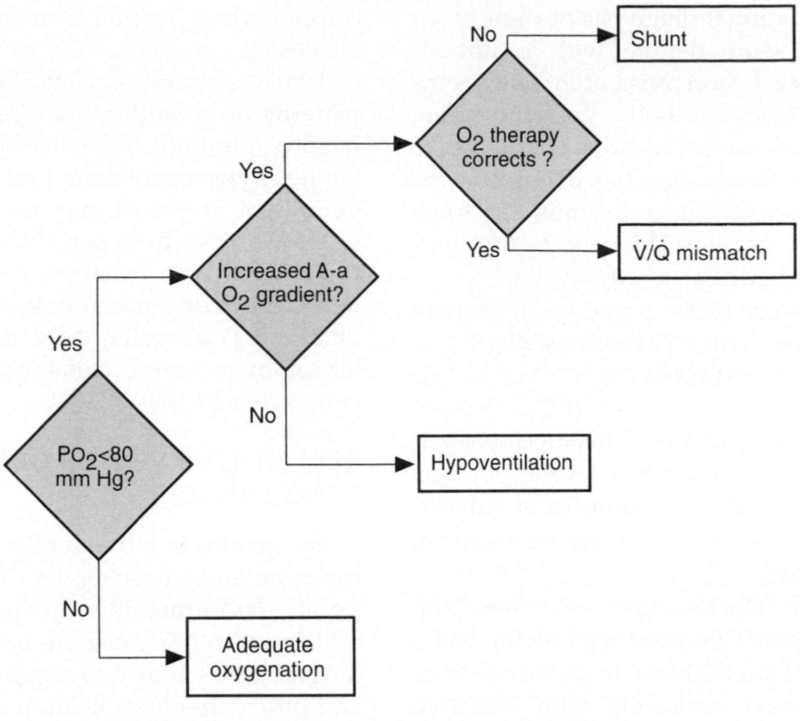

Figure 15.4. Algorithm for the evaluation of hypoxemia.

to the fact that hemoglobin in the pulmonary capillary circuit is ordinarily saturated with oxygen. As a result, areas of low $\dot{V}/\dot{Q}$ decrease the pulmonary capillary oxygen content more than the areas of high $\dot{V}/\dot{Q}$ can increase it. Mixing of the pulmonary capillary blood in the pulmonary venous system and left atrium then produces blood with a low Po_2, a low oxygen content, and an increased alveolar-arterial gradient. The Pco_2 may also be elevated, but this occurs only with severe ventilation-perfusion mismatching. Part of the explanation for this is that CO_2 transport across the alveolar-capillary membrane is more efficient than O_2 transport. Consequently, areas of high $\dot{V}/\dot{Q}$ can compensate for areas of low $\dot{V}/\dot{Q}$ much more effectively for carbon dioxide than for oxygen. The presence of CO_2 retention in a patient with ventilation-perfusion mismatch is a poor prognostic sign, since it reflects more profound respiratory failure than does hypoxemia alone.

The differential diagnosis of ventilation-perfusion mismatch is extensive and includes some of the most common pulmonary disorders encountered in clinical practice (e.g., asthma, emphysema, atelectasis, pneumonia, pulmonary embolus, adult respiratory distress syndrome, pneumothorax, cystic fibrosis, lower airway obstruction, pulmonary edema). Hypoxemia due to ventilation-perfusion mismatching may show a dramatic response to oxygen administration, because airways to poorly ventilated alveoli are not completely occluded.

SHUNTING

Arteriovenous (right to left) shunts are defined as any process that permits unoxygenated venous blood to mix with oxygenated arterial blood. The term for mixing of blood from nonventilated (or markedly underventilated) air spaces with blood from ventilated areas is called venous admixture, and can be expressed as a percentage of the cardiac output. Shunting of venous blood into the arterial circulation (including pulmonary arterial blood into the pulmonary venous system) reduces the arterial O_2 content and Po_2 and results in an increased alveolar-arterial O_2 gradient. Shunts may be normal (anatomic) or pathologic.

Normal anatomic (physiologic) shunts contribute a small amount to venous admixture. The thebesian veins, which drain the myocardium, partially empty into the pulmonary veins, and intrapulmonary anatomic arteriovenous shunts bypass ventilated areas. Collectively these normal shunts account for approximately 5% of right heart output.

Pathologic shunts may be intrapulmonary or extrapulmonary. Right to left cardiac shunts are examples of extrapulmonary shunts, as are shunts occurring in the great vessels. Most intrapulmonary shunts represent an extreme case of ventilation-perfusion mismatch and occur when blood perfuses areas of lung in which the alveoli are not ventilated (atelectasis, obstruction) or are filled with fluid or blood (e.g., pulmonary edema, pneumonia, hemorrhage). Thus the differential diagnosis of right to left shunts overlaps to some degree with conditions causing ventilation-perfusion mismatch, and some patients exhibit features of both. In pure form, shunts exhibit a poor or absent response of the PO_2 to oxygen therapy. This observation has diagnostic and therapeutic significance, since hypoxemia due to either hypoventilation or ventilation-perfusion mismatch will respond to administered oxygen.

Hypoxemia may occur in the presence or absence of arterial hypercapnia. Three pathophysiologic processes may produce hypercapnia:

1. Breathing air with a high PCO_2. This mechanism is not relevant in the usual clinical setting but may occur in some states of suffocation or in subjects rebreathing expired air (e.g., in the treatment of respiratory alkalosis).
2. Hypoventilation. In this situation ventilation is insufficient to eliminate CO_2 produced by the body. This occurs either by a decrease in minute ventilation or in conditions associated with increased CO_2 production without an effective increase in the ventilatory response (e.g., fever, sepsis, seizures).
3. Severe ventilation-perfusion mismatch. Mild to moderate degrees of low $\dot{V}/\dot{Q}$ do not cause hypercapnia, because adequate CO_2 elimination is easier to accomplish than oxygenation. Thus a patient with mild asthma will exhibit hypoxemia, but hypercapnia is observed only in severe cases. The finding of an elevated PCO_2 in a patient with ventilation-perfusion mismatch indicates more severe respiratory failure than does hypoxemia alone.

Specific Diseases

The differential diagnosis of hypoxemia and hypercapnia encompasses a large number of disease entities. A detailed discussion of this topic is beyond the scope of this chapter, but some additional comments concerning the more common disease entities are given below.

PATTERNS OF BREATHING

Various patterns of breathing may suggest specific disease states or result from compensatory mechanisms for ineffective respiration. Hyperventilation may be a pathologic primary event (resulting in respiratory alkalosis) or may result from stimulation by the chemoreceptors as an appropriate compensatory response to correct acidosis and hypoxia. Likewise, hypoventilation may be pathological, resulting in respiratory acidosis, or may occur as a compensatory response in the setting of metabolic alkalosis.

Two examples of clinically significant abnormal patterns of breathing are Cheyne-Stokes and Kussmaul respirations. Cheyne-Stokes breathing is alternating hyperventilation and hypoventilation with periods of apnea. It may result from asynchronous sensory output from peripheral and central chemoreceptors and can occur in patients with congestive heart failure or cerebral vascular accidents. Kussmaul breathing is a regular, deep, and rapid breathing pattern seen in severe metabolic acidosis (such as diabetic ketoacidosis).

RESTRICTIVE VERSUS OBSTRUCTIVE LUNG DISEASE

Spirometry is a frequently used method to assess the ventilatory function of the lungs, although it is usually performed in some location outside the clinical laboratory. The test can be used to classify certain lung diseases into two categories termed restrictive and obstructive (see below). Spirometry is useful in monitoring patients with chronic pulmonary diseases to assess the progress of disease activity.

CHRONIC OBSTRUCTIVE PULMONARY DISEASE

Chronic obstructive pulmonary disease (COPD) refers to a group of related disorders characterized by chronic, progressive airway obstruction resulting either from narrowing of the bronchial lumina as a consequence of inflammation and mucus hypersecretion (chronic bronchitis) or constriction (bronchial asthma), or loss of lung parenchyma and elastic recoil (emphysema). Proximal bronchial narrowing and mucus plugging leads to inadequate alveolar ventilation (ventilation-perfusion mismatch), hypoxemia, and, when severe, CO_2 retention. A component of pulmonary parenchymal shunting is also typically present. The major physiologic defect in COPD is an increase in resistance to airflow with limitation of expiratory airflow rates during expiration. COPD can be divided into two clinical types. Type A patients have been called "pink puffers" or "fighters" because they increase ventilation to prevent hypercapnia. Type B patients are termed "blue bloaters" or "nonfighters" because their ventilatory response is blunted. The former generally have a mildly decreased or normal PO_2 and a normal PCO_2, while the latter exhibit a low PO_2 and an elevated PCO_2. Although type A is typically associated with emphysema and type B with chronic bronchitis, most patients with COPD have features of both. Hypoxia may be the primary mechanism driving ventilation in advanced COPD. Overzealous oxygen therapy may therefore aggravate hypercapnia and respiratory acidosis by decreasing the patient's respiratory drive. For this reason oxygen is usually given judiciously to maintain a moderately low P_{O_2}.

DIFFUSE INTERSTITIAL DISEASES

In contrast to COPD, which results from airway obstruction, diffuse interstitial diseases are characterized by a restrictive process producing a reduced expansion of the lung and a decreased total lung capacity. While patients with COPD cannot expire normally, patients with restrictive diseases typically exhibit a normal rate of airflow. Thus the respiratory cycle as seen on spirometry is normal but with reduced volumes. The differential diagnosis of diffuse interstitial disease is extensive and includes disorders induced by occupational and environmental inhalants, drugs, and toxins. All are characterized by alveolitis and variable degrees of interstitial fibrosis. The primary underlying pathophysiology is inadequate ventilation, and hence interstitial diseases are characterized by ventilation-perfusion mismatch. Interstitial fibrosis results in decreased lung compliance, increased work of ventilation, and a rapid and shallow breathing pattern. A minor contributor to hypoxemia is impaired diffusion across a thickened alveolar-capillary membrane, but this occurs only in severe cases. Blood gas measurements may be normal in mild disease but demonstrate a fall in the P_{O_2} with exercise. The alveolar-arterial O_2 gradient is typically increased. Severe disease produces increasing hypoxemia and hypercapnia.

ATELECTASIS

Atelectasis is characterized by incomplete expansion of the lung (or part of the lungs) or collapse of previously inflated tissue. Atelectasis may result from many causes including airway obstruction with resorption of residual air, inadequate respiratory effort, extrinsic compression of the lung (e.g., pneumothorax), contraction of pleural or pulmonary scars, or loss of pulmonary surfactant (e.g., adult respiratory distress syndrome).

PULMONARY EDEMA

Theoretically, pulmonary edema can result from alteration of any of the components of Starling's law. Increased hydrostatic pressure occurs in left ventricular failure, mitral stenosis, and pulmonary vein occlusion. Decreased plasma oncotic pressure can be seen in hypoproteinemic states such as nephrotic syndrome, hepatic failure, and massive crystalloid infusion. The capillary membrane permeability may be altered in septic shock, pneumonia, lung trauma, oxygen toxicity, disseminated intravascular coagulation (DIC), systemic lupus erythematosus (SLE), and many other conditions. Finally, compromise of lymphatic drainage may occur in lymphangitic carcinomatosis or radiation pneumonitis. The most common cause of pulmonary edema is left ventricular failure.

Generally, the interstitial compartment is the initial site of fluid accumulation. Eventually fluid accumulates in the pulmonary alveolar spaces as well. Compromised ventilation and subsequent hypoxemia usually are not present until alveolar filling occurs. In early (interstitial) pulmonary edema the P_{O_2}, P_{CO_2}, and respiratory rate may be normal but exertion (e.g., climbing a flight of stairs) can cause dyspnea as the oxygen requirement is increased. Alveolar filling generally results in hypoxemia, an increased alveolar-arterial O_2 gradient, a normal or decreased P_{CO_2}, and dyspnea. The P_{CO_2} is increased only in very severe cases.

ADULT RESPIRATORY DISTRESS SYNDROME

Adult respiratory distress syndrome (ARDS) (also called diffuse alveolar damage or shock lung) is a condition caused by diffuse alveolar capillary damage with rapid onset of severe respiratory failure. A wide variety of insults may lead to ARDS, including sepsis, shock, lung trauma, head injury, aspiration of gastric contents, smoke inhalation, drug overdose, pancreatitis, burns, oxygen toxicity, and diffuse pneumonia (especially viral). ARDS results from a derangement of alveolar-capillary permeability, resulting in extravasation of fluid into the lung. The initial injury is to the capillary endothelium, but ultimately the epithelium is also affected (29). The mechanism responsible for the alveolar capillary damage is variable and includes aggregation of leukocytes in the pulmonary vessels, oxygen-derived free radicals, toxins, and other factors (4). The morphologic features of ARDS include congestion, edema, epithelial cell necrosis, and the formation of hyaline membranes. Clinically patients exhibit hypoxemia, decreased pulmonary compliance, diffuse pulmonary infiltrates, and cyanosis. The low P_{O_2} is typically only minimally responsive to oxygen therapy due to pulmonary vascular shunting, but the hypoxemia may respond to positive end-expiratory pressure (PEEP) induced by mechanical ventilation.

PULMONARY EMBOLISM

Pulmonary embolism is the principal cause of death in about 10% of hospitalized patients. Nonfatal emboli are even more common. Ordinarily pulmonary emboli do not cause infarction of the lung because the bronchial circulation is usually sufficient to prevent ischemic necrosis of the lung parenchyma. However, infarcts may occur in patients with preexistent cardiac or lung disease. Most emboli arise from thrombi that form in the deep veins of the legs, but some may originate from thrombi in the pelvic veins or other sites. Large pulmonary emboli are one cause of sudden death, whereas smaller emboli can produce a spectrum of symptoms from none at all to severe respiratory distress. A number of factors predispose to the development of deep venous thrombi, including congestive heart failure, immobilization, pregnancy, oral contraceptive use, venous disease of the lower extremity, and pelvic or lower-extremity surgery. Arterial blood gases show a low PO_2, often a low PCO_2 (due to hyperventilation) and an increased alveolar-arterial O_2 gradient (due to severe ventilation-perfusion mismatch).

PULMONARY INFECTIONS

A variety of organisms may infect the lungs, and the degree of respiratory compromise is also quite variable. Inflammation, edema, congestion, and hemorrhage may produce hypoxemia, an increased alveolar-arterial O_2 gradient, and either a normal, elevated, or decreased PCO_2 depending on the degree of intrapulmonary shunting and ventilation-perfusion mismatch. Initially a fall in the arterial PO_2 induces hyperventilation, which may lower the PCO_2, but as with other causes of respiratory failure, with severe disease there may be CO_2 retention.

METHEMOGLOBINEMIA

In normal hemoglobin the iron atoms are in the reduced (ferrous) state. Oxidation of the iron to the trivalent ferric state produces a brown hemoglobin called methemoglobin (metHb). Methemoglobin cannot combine with oxygen, and if the concentration of metHb is significantly elevated, cyanosis and hypoxia (not hypoxemia) occur. In normal subjects methemoglobin is produced in small quantities and is reduced back to the ferrous state by various red blood cell enzymes (methemoglobin reductases) or by reducing agents (e.g., glutathione, ascorbic acid). The normal concentration of metHb is less than 1.5% of the total hemoglobin, whereas levels above 10% produce cyanosis, levels above 35% produce symptoms, and concentrations above 60% may be fatal.

Increased levels of methemoglobin may be hereditary (due to enzyme deficiencies, most commonly an autosomal recessive methemoglobin reductase deficiency) or acquired (due to ingestion of oxidant drugs or toxins). Homozygous methemoglobin reductase deficiency produces elevated metHb levels with cyanosis. Heterozygotes exhibit normal metHb concentrations unless subjected to an oxidant stress. Rare cases of inherited methemoglobinemia are caused by one of a group of abnormal hemoglobins called hemoglobin M's, in which the iron atom cannot be reduced from the ferric state.

Acquired methemoglobinemia (and that occurring in reductase-deficient heterozygotes) results from ingestion of a variety of chemicals and drugs that oxidize hemoglobin (e.g., nitrites, nitrates, sulfones, aniline dyes, sulfonamides, phenacetin).

Effective therapy for methemoglobinemia may be accomplished by the administration of methylene blue, which accelerates the activity of the reductase system, or reducing agents such as ascorbic acid, glutathione, cysteine, and British anti-lewisite (BAL).

CARBOXYHEMOGLOBINEMIA

Carboxyhemoglobin (COHb) normally constitutes a small fraction (0.5%) of the total hemoglobin. It is formed by the reversible interaction of carbon monoxide with hemoglobin. Carbon monoxide binds hemoglobin with high affinity (210 times that of O_2), resulting in a left shift of the oxygen dissociation curve and a characteristic cherry red color of the blood. Due to the high affinity of CO for hemoglobin, carboxyhemoglobin will steadily accumulate in acute or chronic CO exposure. Inhalation of CO may occur in subjects exposed to the products of incomplete combustion of organic compounds, including fires, charcoal grills, heating appliances, internal combustion engines, and tobacco products. Smokers may exhibit carboxyhemoglobin levels of 4 to 8% of total hemoglobin.

In some patients, symptomatic CO toxicity (exertional dyspnea) can occur at levels as low as 10%, but overt symptoms usually do not occur until the blood level exceeds 30% (headache, syncope, confusion). Levels above 60% produce loss of consciousness or death. Oxygen therapy is effective treatment for CO poisoning because the CO-hemoglobin bond is reversible. The half-life of COHb in a patient breathing room air is roughly 4 to 5 hours, and this can be shortened to approximately 1 hour by breathing 100% oxygen.

References

1. Barker SJ, Tremper KK, Hyatt J. Effects of methemoglobinuria on pulse oximetry and mixed venous oximetry. Anesthesiology 1989;70:112–117.
2. Barker SJ, Tremper KK. The effect of carbon monoxide inhalation on pulse oximetry and transcutaneous PO_2. Anesthesiology 1987;66:677–679.
3. Definitions of quantities and conventions related to blood pH and gas analysis. 2nd ed. NCCLS document C-12T2. Villanova, PA: The National Committee for Clinical Laboratory Standards, 1991.
4. Burnett RW et al. Definitions of quantities and conventions related to blood gases and pH. J Int Fed Clin Chem (in press).
5. Wimberley PD, Burnett RW, Covington AK, Fogh-Andersen N, Maas AHJ, Müller-Plathe O, Siggaard-Andersen O, Zijlstra WG. Guidelines for routine measurement of blood hemoglo-

bin oxygen affinity. Scand J Clin Lab Invest 1990;50(Suppl)203: 227–234.
6. Misiano DR, Meyerhoff ME, Collison ME. Current and future directions in the technology relating to bedside testing of critically ill patients. Chest 1990;97:204s–214s.
7. Zaloga GP. Evaluation of bedside testing options for the critical care unit. Chest 1990;97:185s–190s.
8. Pemberton JO. The role of the laboratorian on the critical care team. Medical Laboratory Observer (MLO) 1991;23(9s):16–19.
9. Chernow B. The bedside laboratory. A critical step forward in ICU care. Chest 1990;97:183s–184s.
10. Rock RC. Why testing is being moved to the site of patient care. Med Lab Obs 1991;23(9s):2–5.
11. Thorson SH, Marini JJ, Pierson DJ, Hudson LD. Variability of arterial blood gas values in stable patients in the ICU. Chest 1983;84:14.
12. Zaloga GP. Monitoring versus testing technologies: present and future. Med Lab Obs 1991;23(9s):20–31.
13. Severinghaus JW. Transcutaneous blood gas analysis. Respir Care 1982;27:152–159.
14. Tremper KK, Barker SJ. Transcutaneous oxygen-studies and adult application. Int Anesthesiol Clin 1987;25:67–96.
15. Tremper KK, Waxman K, Bowman R, Shoemaker WC. Continuous transcutaneous oxygen monitoring during respiratory failure, cardiac decompensation, cardiac arrest, and CPR. Crit Care Med 1980;8:377–381.
16. Mendelson Y. Pulse oximetry: theory and applications for noninvasive monitoring. Clin Chem 1992;38:1601–1607.
17. Barrington KJ, Finer NN, Ryan CA. Evaluation of pulse oximetry as a continuous monitoring technique in the neonatal intensive care unit. Crit Care Med 1988;16:1147–1153.
18. Mansouri A. Methemoglobinemia. Am J Med Sci 1985;289: 200–209.
19. Eisenkraft JB. Pulse oximeter desaturation due to methemoglobinemia. Anesthesiology 1988;68:279–282.
20. Wilson GS, Zhang Y, Reach G, Moatti-Sirat D, Poitout V, Thevenot DR, Lemonnier F, Klein JC. Progress toward the development of an implantable sensor for glucose. Clin Chem 1992;38:1613–1617.
21. Robinson MR, Eaton RP, Haaland DM, Koepp GW, Thomas EV, Stallard BR, Robinson PL. Noninvasive glucose monitoring in diabetic patients: a preliminary evaluation. Clin Chem 1992;38:1618–1622.
22. Hall JW, Pollard A. Near-infrared spectrophotometry: a new dimension in clinical chemistry. Clin Chem 1992;38:1623–1631.
23. Rosenthal R. Research into noninvasive measurement of blood glucose by near-infrared technology [Abstract]. Clin Chem 1992;38:1645.
24. Hornung PA, Schuff N. Noninvasive imaging and spectroscopy—broad applications of magnetic resonance. Clin Chem 1992;38:1608–1612.
25. Otvos JD, Jeyarajah EJ, Bennett DW, Krauss RM. Development of a proton nuclear magnetic resonance spectroscopic method for determining plasma lipoprotein concentrations and subspecies distributions from a single, rapid measurement. Clin Chem 1992;38:1632–1638.
26. Wade SE. Less invasive measurement of tissue availability of hormones and drugs: diffuse-sink sampling. Clin Chem 1992;38:1639–1644.
27. Schembri CT, Ostoich V, Lingane PJ, Burd TL, Buhl SN. Portable simultaneous multiple analyte whole-blood analyzer for point-of-care testing. Clin Chem 1992;38:1665–1670.
28. Irwin R, Pratter M. A physiologic approach to managing respiratory failure. In: Rippe J, Irwin R, Alpert J, Fink M, eds. Intensive care medicine. 2nd ed. Boston: Little, Brown, 1991: 449–454.
29. Cotran R, Kumar V, Robbins S. The respiratory system. In: Cotran R, Kumar V, Robbins S, eds. The pathologic basis of disease. 4th ed. Philadelphia: WB Saunders, 1989:755–810.

16 Nitrogen Metabolites and Renal Function

Alfred E. Hartmann

RENAL PHYSIOLOGY

The kidneys are regulatory organs responsible for the maintenance of extracellular fluid volume and electrolyte balance, along with the excretion of toxic metabolites, drugs, and metabolic waste products. The primary kidney functions are the formation of urine by ultrafiltration in the glomerulus, selective tubular reabsorption of water and solutes, and selective tubular secretion of solutes. The kidney also has an endocrine role, it produces erythropoietin, which regulates red cell mass, produces renin, which affects sodium balance and regulates blood pressure, and metabolizes vitamin D, which influences calcium balance.

The two bean-shaped kidneys, which lie in the retroperitoneal space on either side of the aorta, are each approximately 10 to 12 cm in length and weigh approximately 150 g. Each kidney has an outer cortex averaging 40 mm thick surrounding the inner medulla. The medulla consists of a number of conical renal pyramids, which terminate in a papilla. The papillae protrude into the renal pelvis, which collects urine. Within the cortex and medulla are the functional units of the kidney, called the nephrons. Each kidney contains approximately 1.25×10^6 nephrons, which operate in parallel with each other. A nephron is composed of a glomerulus, proximal convoluted tubule, loop of Henle, distal convoluted tubule, and collecting duct.

The glomerulus is composed of a cluster of capillaries formed from an afferent arteriole and is surrounded by an epithelial saccular expansion of the proximal tubule, forming Bowman's space. The proximal convoluted tubule coils extensively in the cortex and penetrates the deeper layers of the cortex to the outer medulla. The thick descending and thin ascending loops of Henle are located in the medulla in a hairpin configuration. The distal convoluted tubule arises from the ascending thin loop of Henle and traverses through the cortex, terminating in a collecting duct near the original glomerulus. The collecting duct is formed in the outer cortex by the junction of two or more distal convoluted tubules and traverses through the cortex into the medulla, where several collecting ducts fuse to form the papillary ducts that terminate in the renal pyramid of the medulla. The total length of the nephron is 40 to 60 mm. The afferent arteriole leaves the glomerulus as the efferent arteriole and penetrates deep into the medulla, forming a network around the loop of Henle called the vasa recta. Tubular function is dependent on the anatomy of the loop of Henle and the surrounding vasa recta. The close proximity of the vasa recta to the loop of Henle is responsible for maintaining the medullary osmotic gradient, by a counter-current exchange between the renal tubule and the corresponding arteriole (Fig. 16.1).

Glomerular filtration is the initial event in the formation of urine. As blood flows through the glomerulus, ultrafiltration occurs due to hydrostatic pressure within the glomerular capillaries, forcing plasma water and smaller solutes across the capillary membrane, opposed by the oncotic pressure of plasma proteins remaining in the glomerular capillaries and the hydrostatic pressure in Bowman's space. The glomerular filtration rate is dependent on the balance of these Starling forces: the permeability of the capillary wall to water and solutes, the total surface area of the capillaries, and the rate of plasma flow through the capillaries. The glomerular filtration rate is the total glomerular filtrate formed by all the glomeruli per unit time. In the average-sized person, the glomerular filtration rate is 125 ml/minute, or 180 liters/day. The glomerular filtration rate can be determined with clearance studies using solutes that are filtered and neither subsequently reabsorbed nor secreted. The determination of the glomerular filtration rate provides an estimation of the functional renal mass and can be of considerable importance in the initial evaluation and follow-up of patients with renal disease. Certain extrarenal conditions will also cause the glomerular filtration rate to rise or fall significantly. Most important is the volume of the extracellular fluid. Expansion of the extracellular fluid volume is accompanied by an increase in the glomerular filtration rate, and an actual or perceived depletion of the extracellular fluid volume causes a marked reduction in the glomerular filtration rate.

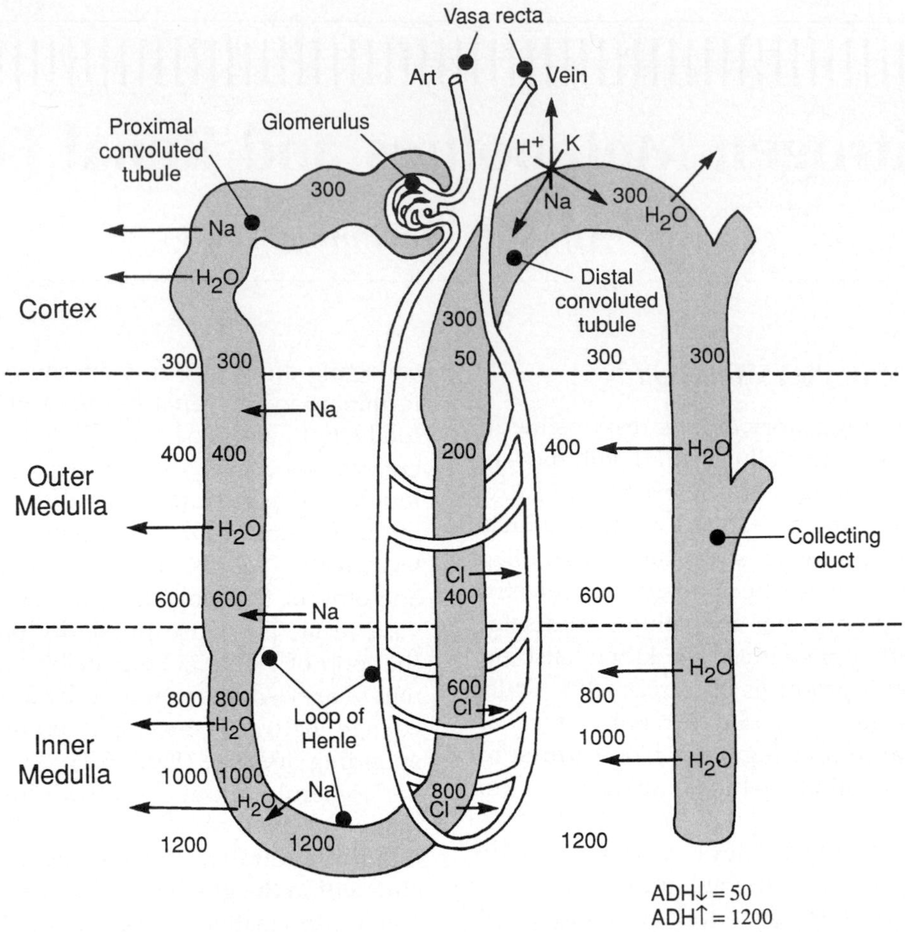

Figure 16.1. Diagram of the renal nephron. The numerals indicate the changes in osmolality (mosm/kg H_2O) in the interstitium and the tubular fluid. The tubular exchanges of water and ions during the course of the production of urine are indicated.

A large amount of ultrafiltrate (180 liters/day) containing 300 mosm/kg H_2O of solute enters the tubules, and only 1% of that filtrate with a markedly altered solute content reaches the renal pelvis as urine. In the renal tubules there is both selective reabsorption and secretion. Tubular reabsorption facilitates the conservation of substances essential for homeostasis. Examples are water, bicarbonate, glucose, amino acids, and electrolytes. The reabsorption may be passive (for example, urea and water) or active, defined as a net movement of the substance against an electrochemical potential gradient with the loss of metabolic energy (for example, sodium). Tubular secretion involves the movement of substances from the tubular cell into the tubular fluid. Tubular secretion may also be passive or active. Many of the substances are weak acids or bases, such as drugs, or metabolic end products that can be eliminated from the body in the urine.

In the proximal convoluted tubule, 70 to 80% of the filtered solute and water are reabsorbed into the renal circulation. Sodium is reabsorbed actively, while chloride follows sodium passively. Water is reabsorbed by osmosis. At the end of the proximal convoluted tubule the tubular fluid is sharply reduced in volume to approximately 20% of the original filtrate, while the osmolar concentration remains isotonic. As the tubular fluid flows through the loop of Henle, a countercurrent multiplication occurs. In the thick descending loop of Henle, water diffuses out of the tubule into the hypertonic interstitium of the medulla, while a small amount of sodium diffuses into the tubule. At the hairpin curve deep in the medulla, the tubular fluid is maximally concentrated to nearly 1200 mosm/kg H_2O. In the ascending loop of Henle, the tubule is impermeable to water, while chloride is actively reabsorbed with sodium into the interstitium. The osmolar concentration decreases in the ascending loop of Henle until the tubular fluid is hypotonic (50 to 100 mosm/kg H_2O) entering the distal convoluted tubule. The marked osmotic gradient established in the medullary interstitium is established by the passive reabsorption of urea and the active reabsorption of chloride followed by sodium in the ascending loop of Henle. The rich capillary network (vasa recta) enveloping the tubule allows a counter-

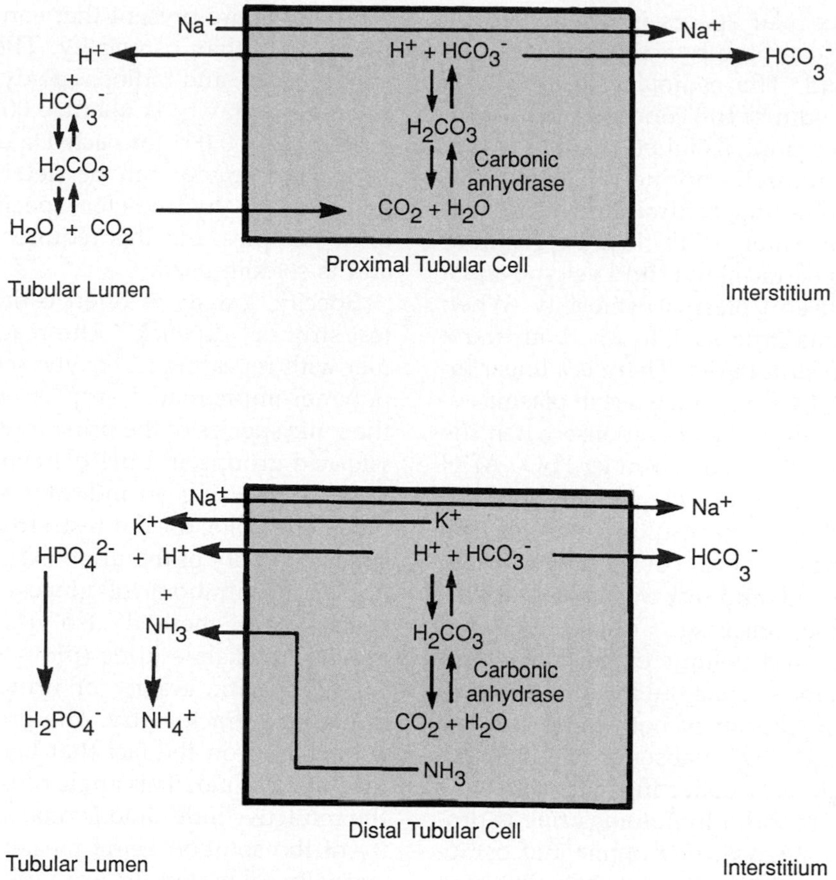

Figure 16.2. Hydrogen ion secretion in the proximal and distal renal tubular cells.

current exchange to occur between the interstitial fluid and the renal blood flow. This exchange allows the reabsorption of water and electrolytes from the medullary interstitium into the renal circulation and is responsible for maintaining the hyperosmolality of the interstitium. In the distal convoluted tubule and collecting ducts, water reabsorption is regulated by antidiuretic hormone (ADH). Under the influence of ADH, the distal convoluted tubule and collecting duct become permeable to water. Water is reabsorbed into the hyperosmolar medullary interstitium and tubular fluid becomes hypertonic. In the absence of ADH, the distal tubule is relatively impermeable to water and the tubular fluid remains hypotonic. The distal convoluted tubule also can be stimulated by aldosterone to reabsorb 5 to 10% of the original filtered sodium against a steep concentration gradient. The renal nephron is also responsible for the maintenance of acid-base balance through the elimination of hydrogen ions and the regulation of plasma bicarbonate by either conserving, regenerating, or eliminating bicarbonate.

The renal tubular cells are capable of hydrogen ion secretion along much of the length of the nephron (Fig. 16.2). In the tubular cell, carbon dioxide is used as a source of hydrogen ion and bicarbonate. The hydrogen ion is secreted into the tubular lumen in exchange for a cation, usually sodium. In the proximal convoluted tubule, the hydrogen ion that is secreted into the tubular fluid is used up almost entirely in reabsorbing filtered bicarbonate, and the pH of the tubular fluid changes very little. In the distal convoluted tubule, hydrogen ion and potassium ion are secreted into the tubular lumen in exchange for sodium. In addition to combining with bicarbonate in the distal tubular fluid, hydrogen ion can combine with other buffer ions such as hydrogen phosphate or can combine with ammonia to form ammonium ion. The secretion of hydrogen ion in the distal tubules changes the pH of the urine dramatically due to the relatively small amount of bicarbonate remaining in the tubular fluid after proximal reabsorption of bicarbonate.

WATER BALANCE, SPECIFIC GRAVITY, AND OSMOLALITY

Water accounts for 50 to 60% of total body weight. Two-thirds of total body water is intracellular, and one-third is located in the extracellular fluid space. Water is freely diffusible across cell membranes. The distribution of water beween the intracellular and extracellular spaces is determined by the concentration of osmotically active particles (osmolality) in each fluid. The osmolality of a fluid is roughly equal to the sum of the concentrations of individual solutes in the fluid. Total body water is regulated by thirst, antidiuretic hormone (ADH), and renal function, which in turn control fluid intake and renal conservation of water. With fluid deprivation, there is a decrease in extracellular fluid volume and a corresponding increase in plasma osmolality. When osmolality increases as little as 1 to 2%, both thirst and ADH release are stimulated. There is a linear increase in plasma ADH with an increase in plasma osmolality, with a maximum ADH response when the plasma osmolality reaches 290 mosm/kg H_2O. ADH increases water reabsorption in the distal tubule and collecting ducts of the kidney, resulting in water conservation and excretion of a concentrated urine. Urine volume is reduced, and urine osmolality is typically greater than 800 mosm/kg. Conversely, when there is extracellular fluid volume expansion, receptors in the hypothalamus sense the fall in plasma osmolality and cause inhibition of both thirst and the pituitary release of ADH. The absence of ADH renders the distal tubule and collecting duct relatively impermeable to water, and a hypotonic urine is produced with relatively high urine volume and osmolality typically less than 100 mosm/kg. Actually, both thirst and ADH release are also regulated directly by extracellular fluid volume in addition to osmolality. A change in extracellular fluid volume is sensed by carotid baroreceptors and stretch receptors in the left atrium of the heart, and signals are sent to the hypothalamus via the vagus nerve to modify thirst and ADH release. Extracellular fluid volume can override the regulation from plasma osmolality if there is a disparity between the two. For example, decreased extracellular fluid volume with low osmolality can actually cause stimulation of thirst and ADH release.

The concentrating and diluting function of the kidney is reflected in the solute concentration of the urine, which can be measured by specific gravity or osmolality. Specific gravity is defined as the ratio of the weight of a volume or urine to the weight of an equal volume of water. The specific gravity, like osmolality, is related to the concentration of dissolved solutes.

The specific gravity of a 24-hour urine specimen normally varies between 1.015 and 1.025, while the specific gravity of random urine samples can vary between 1.003 and 1.030, depending on fluid intake and state of hydration. After an overnight fast, a random urine specific gravity over 1.020 is considered to reflect normal renal concentrating ability.

There will be disparity between urine specific gravity and osmolality when significant amounts of compounds are present that contribute more to specific gravity than osmolality. These can include protein, glucose, and radiopaque dyes. The contribution to specific gravity is about 0.003 for each 1 g/dl of protein, and 0.004 for each 1 g/dl of glucose.

Specific gravity can be determined with a "urinometer," a hydrometer specifically designed for urine samples, but this requires a large sample size and is seldom used.

Specific gravity is often estimated using a urine test strip or "dipstick." The reagent includes a polymer with repeating carboxylic acid groups. When the polymer-impregnated strip is immersed into urine, the ionic species of the urine interact with the carboxylic acid groups and the pH change on the test strip is detected using an indicator such as bromthymol blue. The color on the test strip correlates with the specific gravity of the urine except in the presence of high concentrations of glucose or other non-ionic species. The method also underestimates specific gravity in alkaline urine (pH > 6.5).

The specific gravity of urine can also be determined by refractometry. The principle of refractometry is based on the fact that light bends as it passes through a liquid. This angle of refraction is known as the refractive index and is related to the specific gravity of the solution being measured. A refractometer specially calibrated for use with urine is available.

The urine osmolality is a better measure of renal concentrating ability than the urine specific gravity. The sum of the "active" concentrations of all species dissolved in a solution determines the osmolality.

The colligative properties of a solution are directly related to the number of particles dissolved per unit mass of solvent, and the measurement of osmolality is based on one of these colligative properties. A 1-molal "ideal" solution will lower the freezing point by 1.86°C, lower the vapor pressure by 0.3 mm Hg, raise the osmotic pressure by 22.4 atmospheres, and raise the boiling point by 0.52°C. The colligative properties most commonly used in the laboratory to measure osmolality are depression of the freezing point and depression of the vapor pressure. Real solutions usually have somewhat lesser effects on the freezing point and vapor pressure of the solvent than an ideal solution. The osmolality of a real solution is expressed as

$$\text{osmolality (mosm/kg } H_2O) = \phi\, n\, C$$

where ϕ is the osmotic coefficient, which is 1.0 for an ideal solution and somewhat less than 1 for electrolytes that are incompletely dissociated or for solutes that tend to associate because of electrostatic or other forces; n is the number of particles formed by complete dissociation of the molecular species (mosm/mmol); and C is the molality of the solute in mmol/kg H_2O.

Clinical Use of Urine Osmolality

The osmolality of urine can vary from 50 to 1200 mosm/kg H_2O, depending on the state of hydration. A random urine sample is usually in the range of 300 to 800 mosm/kg H_2O. With a water load and corresponding decreased plasma osmolality, there is an inhibition of thirst and ADH release, which leads to diuresis with low urine osmolality. With water deprivation and a corresponding high plasma osmolality, thirst and ADH release are stimulated, and renal water conservation occurs, with a resultant high urine osmolality. While the measurement of urine osmolality alone is of limited use in the diagnosis of water and electrolyte imbalance, a ratio of the urine osmolality to plasma osmolality can be extremely helpful in the differentiation of water imbalance states. In normal individuals, the urine osmolality to serum osmolality ratio is usually between 1.0 and 2.5. In chronic renal failure, the concentrating ability of the renal tubules is progressively lost. The urine to plasma osmolality ratio is less than 1.2 if there is predominantly tubular damage, but is over 1.2 if there is predominantly a decrease in glomerular filtration rate. In acute tubular necrosis, the urine osmolality can be less than or equal to the plasma osmolality. Normal renal concentrating ability should result in a urine osmolality above 800 mosm/kg H_2O after an overnight fast.

The urine to plasma osmolality ratio is also helpful in the diagnosis of polyuria. Polyuria can be caused by water diuresis induced by insufficient ADH; suppression of ADH by excessive water consumption seen in such entities as psychogenic polydipsia, organic brain disease, and iatrogenic water ingestion; or failure of the kidney to respond to ADH, as seen in congenital nephrogenic diabetes insipidus, chronic renal disease, and acquired tubular defects from drugs such as lithium, dilantin, ethanol, and amphotericin B.

Diabetes insipidus is a partial or total lack of the ability to produce ADH. Diabetes insipidus can be an inherited condition or can result from an insult to the hypothalamus or posterior pituitary gland. Nephrogenic diabetes insipidus is a different condition in which the distal nephron remains relatively impermeable to water reabsorption despite large amounts of ADH. The condition may also be inherited but is more commonly related to nephrotoxic drugs such as lithium, dilantin, ethanol, and amphotericin B.

Either a lack of ADH, suppression of ADH, or a failure of the kidney to respond to ADH will result in copious volumes of a dilute urine due to the distal convoluted tubule and collecting duct being impermeable to water. There may be 10 to 15 liters of urine a day, with osmolalities of less than 100 mosm/kg H_2O. Serious dehydration will occur unless water intake matches the urine output. Water diuresis states can be studied by concentration tests. The principle of a concentration test is that polyuria should be corrected by either fluid deprivation or ADH administration. With the patient fasting, plasma osmolality is determined every 2 hours. All urine excreted is also collected. The patient is adequately prepared when the plasma osmolality reaches 300 mosm/kg, or when the urine has a level plateau of osmolality. Baseline plasma and urine osmolality and ADH levels are then determined. The patient is then given 5 mU of ADH subcutaneously and the urine osmolality measured 1 hour later. With diabetes insipidus the result will be high plasma osmolality, low urine osmolality, absent plasma ADH level, and rise in urine osmolality after ADH injection. With suppression of ADH due to psychogenic polydipsia the results will usually be normal to low plasma osmolality with low urine osmolality, low plasma ADH level, and a rise in urine osmolality after administration of ADH. With nephrogenic diabetes insipidus the results will be high plasma osmolality, low urine osmolality, high plasma ADH level, and absent rise in urine osmolality after ADH injection (Table 16.1).

Other concentration test such as the Hickey-Hare test utilizing hypertonic saline can be used in the differential diagnosis of polyuria. In the Hickey-Hare test, samples for plasma osmolality and ADH levels are obtained at 20-minute intervals after hypertonic saline is started intravenously. In diabetes insipidus, there are undetectable ADH levels even when the plasma osmolality reaches 300 mosm/kg H_2O.

The ratio of urine to plasma osmolality (U/P osm) is also helpful in the diagnosis of the syndrome of inappropriate ADH. In this syndrome there is an excessive amount of ADH, producing the opposite biochemical effects of diabetes insipidus. The excess ADH causes increased permeability of the distal tubule to water, leading to water retention and hyponatremia. The urine osmolality will be elevated in comparison to the plasma osmolality (U/P osm > 2). The increased extracellular fluid volume leads to an increased glomerular filtration rate (GFR). Increased tubular fluid flow, and a resultant sodium washout into the urine. There can be a substantial urinary loss of sodium in this condition, with urine sodium concentrations exceeding 20 mmol/liter. The syndrome of inappropriate ADH can be seen in a variety of conditions, most commonly in pathologic lesions of the central nervous system or pulmonary system, and in malignant tumors producing ADH, such as small cell carcinoma of the lung.

Table 16.1. Laboratory Differentiation of Polyuria

Laboratory Parameter	Psychogenic Polydipsia	Diabetes Insipidus	Nephrogenic Diabetes Insipidus	Osmotic Diuresis
Posm	N, ↓	↑	↑	N, ↑
Uosm	↓	↓	↓	↑
Plasma ADH	↓	↓	↑	↑
Uosm after ADH	No increase	Increase	Nil	Slight increase

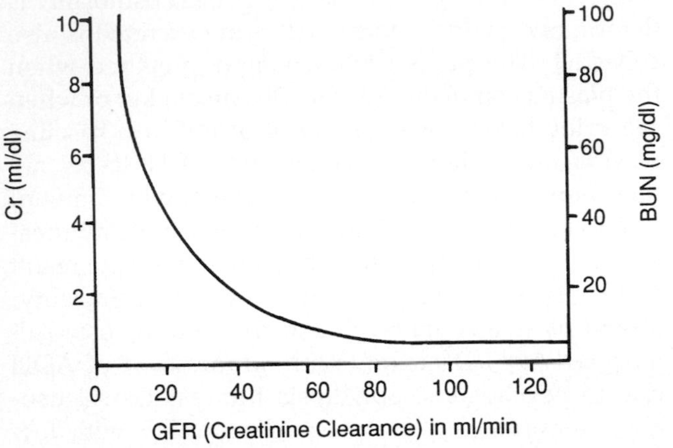

Figure 16.3. Relationship of serum creatinine or blood urea nitrogen (BUN) to the GFR as measured by the creatinine clearance.

UREA

Urea is the major nitrogen-containing metabolite from the degradation of protein. The formation of urea occurs primarily in the liver, with minor amounts of urea formation occurring in the kidney and brain. The concentration of urea in the bloodstream depends on several factors. These are the rate of urea production, the volume of body water in which the urea is distributed, and the rate of urea elimination. The rate of urea production depends on the amount of protein in the diet, protein and blood in the gastrointestinal tract, catabolic states, and liver function. Urea is freely diffusible across cell membranes and is equally distributed in the total body water. Urea excretion depends on the glomerular filtration rate and the subsequent tubular reabsorption of urea. Urea is freely filtered across the glomerular membrane, with approximately 25% of the urea reabsorbed into the extracellular fluid from the tubule. The reabsorptive process is passive and depends on the fraction of filtered water that is reabsorbed.

Plasma urea will rise as the GFR decreases in patients with renal disease. The urea level is insensitive to a minimal fall in GFR and rises sharply only after 40 to 60% of the nephrons have ceased to function. Plasma urea increases progressively with a hyperbolic relationship to the GFR as renal disease progresses, such that a 50% drop in the GFR results in an approximate doubling of plasma urea (Fig. 16.3).

Table 16.2. Etiologies of Elevated Serum Urea

Prerenal
Increased synthesis of urea
- Catabolic states: fever, stress, burns
- High-protein diet
- GI bleeding
- Hyperthyroidism
- Cushing's syndrome
- Hemolysis
- Antianabolic drugs—tetracycline

Decreased perfusion of kidney
- Congestive heart failure
- Hypotension, shock
- Renal vein thrombosis
- Dehydration
- Cirrhosis, ascites

Intrinsic renal disease
Glomerular disease
Tubular disease—acute tubular necrosis
Interstitial disease

Postrenal
Urinary tract obstruction
- Benign prostatic hyperplasia
- Prostatic carcinoma
- Carcinoma of bladder or ureters
- Retroperitoneal tumor
- Calculi

Extravasation of urine into tissues

Etiologies of elevated urea level can be categorized as prerenal, renal, and postrenal (Table 16.2). Prerenal causes are related to increased production of urea or decreased renal perfusion. Renal causes are related to a loss of functioning nephrons with a corresponding decrease in GFR. Postrenal causes are related to obstruction of the urinary tract with a decreased urine flow.

Urea may be abnormally low in several conditions in which there is a low rate or urea production, hemodilution, or increased rate of urea excretion. Decreased urea synthesis can occur with a low protein intake, administration of androgens or growth hormone, and severe liver dysfunction. Hemodilution can occur with overhydration, psychogenic polydipsia, and diabetes insipidus. Increased rates of elimination can be seen in hemodilution, pregnancy, and postdialysis states.

Analysis of Urea

1. *Urease with glutamate dehydrogenase (EC 1.4.1.3) coupled reaction.* This is the most common method for analysis of urea. The highly specific urease enzyme converts urea into ammonia. A coupled reaction utilizing glutamate dehydrogenase with NADH and α-ketoglutarate is monitored by measuring the decrease in absorbance at 340 nm as NADH is converted to NAD^+. Interferences may be seen in the assay if other enzymes that can also oxidize NADH are elevated in the specimen.
2. *Conductimetric urease.* There is an increase in conductivity of the specimen following the addition of urease (EC 3.5.1.5). The liberated bicarbonate and ammonium increase the conductivity of the solution. The rate of change of conductivity of the mixture as non-ionized urea is transformed to the ionic species and can be monitored with a conductivity cell.
3. *Diacetyl.* Diacetyl monoxime is hydrolyzed to form diacetyl and hydroxylamine. The diacetyl complexes with urea in an acid solution containing an oxidizing agent to form a yellow diazine compound (Fearon reaction), which can be measured at 550 nm, or fluorometrically at 415 nm. This method is easily automated. The disadvantage of this method is that nonspecific substances may produce chromogens and there is a low specificity compared to the enzymatic assays. The end color fades and usually a stabilizer such as thiosemicarbazide is added to enhance and stabilize the end product. An oxidizing agent may also be added to remove hydroxylamine and ensure a complete reaction.
4. *O-Phthalaldehyde.* Urea binds to O-phthalaldehyde to form a colored chromogen that can be monitored at 510 nm. The disadvantage of this method is interference by other primary amines.
5. *Urease with quinolinium dye.* The urease (EC 3.5.1.5) enzyme liberates ammonia from urea. The ammonia reacts with merocyanine dye, which can be measured at 670 nm.
6. *Berthelot reaction.* Urea is hydrolyzed with urease to carbonic acid and ammonia. Sodium phenate and hypochlorite react with ammonia in the presence of sodium nitroprusside to produce a blue indophenol complex with maximum absorbance at 630 nm. The disadvantages of this reaction are nonspecificity and long reaction times. The advantages are that protein precipitation is not required and turbidity is not a problem.

The earliest methods for urea in the clinical laboratory used whole blood as the sample, and an analytical method that measured nitrogen in urea. This led to the convention of reporting concentrations in terms of milligrams of *nitrogen* per deciliter of sample, which is still used except in areas where SI units have been adopted. The misnomer BUN (for blood urea nitrogen) is also still commonly used today, even though plasma or serum urea nitrogen is meant. The reference interval for plasma (or serum) urea nitrogen is 7 to 25 mg/dl.

CREATININE

Creatine is synthesized in the liver from arginine and glycine and is transported to muscle, which contains 98% of the total body stores of creatine. The creatine pool is related primarily to muscle mass, which is affected primarily by sex and age, and to a lesser extent by dietary intake of creatine. Approximately 1.5% of the total body creatine is degraded to creatinine each day by non-enzymatic dehydration. Creatinine is not bound to protein it is freely distributed through the total body water and is excreted from the body by glomerular filtration, with an additional 10 to 20% of creatinine secreted through the tubule. Creatinine is not reabsorbed in the tubule.

The serum creatinine level is determined by creatinine production, state of hydration, and creatinine excretion. Increased creatinine production is seen in acute muscle disease such as dermatomyositis, and decreased creatinine production is seen in muscle wasting diseases. Decreased renal perfusion, as in shock, hypotension, congestive heart failure, or cirrhosis will decrease the GFR and raise the serum creatinine. Creatinine will also be elevated whenever the GFR is low due to renal disease or postrenal obstruction. Like urea, the etiologies of elevated creatinine level can be categorized as prerenal, renal, or postrenal, and are summarized in Table 16.3.

Also like urea, creatinine has a nonlinear relationship to the GFR and does not become significantly elevated until the GFR decreases by 40 to 60% (Fig. 16.3).

Simultaneous determination of the serum creatinine and urea levels and calculating the urea nitrogen:creatinine ratio may be of benefit in separating prerenal and postrenal conditions from renal diseases as the cause of an elevated serum creatinine or urea level. The normal urea nitrogen:creatinine ratio is in the range of 10:1 to 20:1. An elevated urea nitrogen:creatinine ratio is seen in prerenal and postrenal conditions, while a normal urea nitrogen:creatinine ratio is seen in renal disease. The ratio is elevated in prerenal or postrenal conditions due to either increased tubular reabsorption of urea or increased production of urea. In renal disease, the urea nitrogen:creatinine ratio remains in the normal range due

Table 16.3. Etiologies of Elevated Serum Creatinine Level

Prerenal
Increased synthesis of creatinine
Muscle hypertrophy
Muscle necrosis
Anabolic steroid use
High-meat diet
Drug—phenacemide
Severe exercise
Decreased renal perfusion
Hypotension, shock
Congestive heart failure
Cirrhosis, ascites
Renal
Glomerular
Tubulointerstitial
Decreased tubular secretion
Drugs—cimetidine, trimethroprim, probeneoid
Postrenal
Urinary tract obstruction
Benign prostatic hyperplasia
Carcinoma of prostate, bladder, or uterus
Calculi
Retroperitoneal tumor

to both being similarly affected by the loss of functioning nephrons.

The amount of creatinine excreted in a 24-hour urine depends primarily on the muscle mass of the individual. A male excretes 14 to 26 mg of creatinine per kilogram per day, and a female excretes 11 to 20 mg/kg/day in the urine, but the amount is fairly consistent for a given individual. The urine creatinine therefore provides a rough estimate of the completeness of a timed urine collection.

Creatinine Methods

The most common methods for the analysis of creatinine are based either on the Jaffé reaction or on one of several enzymatic reactions. The Jaffé reaction, first described in 1886, is the reaction between creatinine and picrate in an alkaline medium, forming a red-orange complex that absorbs in the range of 480 to 520 nm. Optimal performance of the reaction depends on the concentrations of the various reagent components, especially the concentration of the alkali, which determines the rate of the reaction and the wavelength of maximal absorbance. Most manual methods are endpoint assays with 10 to 15 minutes allowed for the reaction. The Jaffé reaction is not specific for creatinine, as a variety of other substances can also react with the picrate. These are called noncreatinine chromogens, and the most common are protein, acetoacetone, glucose, ascorbic acid, guanidine, acetone, α-ketoacids, urea, and cephalosporin antibiotics. Many modifications have been introduced to minimize these interferences. These include pretreatment with Lloyd's reagent (aluminum silicate) to remove most of the noncreatinine chromogens, dialysis or precipitation to remove protein, the addition of buffers to complex glucose and ascorbic acid, and the introduction of a kinetic approach rather than an endpoint determination. The kinetic analysis is useful because there is a time interval (usually 25 to 60 seconds) during which the reaction rate is predominantly due to the formation of a creatinine picrate complex. There is still some positive interference due to acetoacetone, and bilirubin causes a negative interference. The Jaffé rate method is more specific, faster, and can easily be automated.

There are several enzymatic methods for the analysis of creatinine, which are usually based on one of two enzymes. Creatininase (creatinine iminohydrolase) (EC 3.5.4.21) catalyzes creatinine degradation to n-methylhydantoin and ammonium ion. This is then followed by detection of the ammonium ion. Creatinine hydrolase (creatinine amidohydrolase) (EC 3.5.2.10) catalyzes hydrolysis of creatinine to creatine. The creatine can be coupled to other enzymatic reactions that, for example, usually culminate in measuring a change in NADH absorbance at 340 nm.

3,5-Dinitrobenzoic acid—this method involves creatinine reacting with the 3,5-dinitrobenzoic acid at an alkaline pH to give a purple color. The method correlates with the alkaline picrate methods.

High-pressure liquid chromatography—Several high-pressure liquid chromatography (HPLC) methods have been described involving the separation of creatinine from interfering substances using an isocratic reverse-phase method. Although this method is not practical for routine clinical use, it is useful for validating other methods because of its high specificity. A description of a definitive method using isotope dilution gas chromatography/mass spectrometry has also been published. This method is also extremely specific, and the creatinine values of the definitive method are approximately 20% lower than values from the alkaline picrate method when serum samples are used.

CLEARANCE TESTS

The renal clearance of a substance can be thought of as the volume of plasma that can be completely cleared of that substance each minute by the kidney. The renal clearance of any substance can be calculated with the following relationship:

$$\text{Clearance (ml/min)} = \frac{\text{Urine concentration}}{\text{Plasma concentration}} \times \text{Timed urine volume (ml/min)}$$

The clearance is proportional to the renal parenchymal mass, which in turn is roughly proportional to the total body surface area. To compare clearance studies of individuals with varying body sizes, the clearance can be expressed in terms of a standard body surface area of 1.73 m^2. This is done by dividing 1.73 by the patient's body surface area and multiplying the observed clearance by this corrected surface area. Nomograms can be used to calculate body surface area from the patient's body weight and height.

The clearance of a substance that is freely filtered through the glomerulus and is not subsequently reabsorbed or secreted by the tubule is a measure of glomerular filtration rate (GFR). Inulin is such a substance. Inulin is an inert polysaccharide with a molecular weight of about 5000 that is not bound to plasma proteins. The measurement of inulin clearance necessitates a continuous intravenous infusion of inulin to maintain a plasma inulin steady state. Intravenous administration of radiolabeled substances such as ^{51}Cr-EDTA, ^{125}I-iothalamate, and ^{99m}Tc-DTPA can also be used to obtain clearances that directly measure the GFR.

Because determination of the clearance of these compounds is time consuming and impractical to perform routinely, the endogenous creatinine clearance is commonly used for the estimation of GFR. Creatinine is produced in muscle at a relatively constant rate, is not bound to plasma protein, and is freely filtered through the glomerulus. Because a small amount (less than 10%) of creatinine is also secreted by the tubules, the creatinine clearance is slightly higher than a simultaneously measured inulin clearance, and thus slightly overestimates the GFR. With increasing renal failure, the creatinine clearance overestimates the GFR even more due to increased tubular creatinine secretion.

The creatinine clearance averages 125 ml/min in adult males and 115 ml/minute in adult females. The GFR is relatively stable from the first year of life through the fourth decade. After the fourth decade, the GFR decreases approximately 1 ml/minute per year, and thus the normal range for creatinine clearance in elderly adults is lower than in younger individuals.

There are several other important factors to consider in interpreting the creatinine clearance. The coefficient of variation of creatinine clearance varies from 10 to 20% due to the imprecision of the creatinine measurement, biological variation of creatinine synthesis, variations in the urinary excretion of creatinine, and variations in the timing and collection of urine specimens.

The relationship between plasma creatinine and urea and the GFR is nonlinear (see Fig. 16.3). It is evident that with normal to moderately low values of GFR, a large change in the GFR results in only a small rise in the plasma creatinine or urea level, while with lower values of GFR, the increase in urea or plasma creatinine level becomes increasingly greater as the GFR falls. Thus urea and creatinine are relatively insensitive tests of early renal disease; the GFR must fall by approximately 50% before these tests become significantly abnormal.

An abnormal creatinine clearance is not a specific indication of renal disease because of other things that influence the GFR. With decreased renal perfusion (e.g., congestive heart failure, cirrhosis, dehydration, hemorrhage) or decreased tubular fluid flow seen in postrenal obstruction (e.g., benign prostatic hyperplasia, urinary bladder or prostatic carcinoma, calculi) the GFR will fall, with a corresponding decrease in the creatinine clearance. The GFR also increases in high renal perfusion states such as pregnancy and inappropriate ADH, leading to a corresponding increase in the creatinine clearance.

Other types of renal clearances can be used to determine parameters other than the GFR. For example, renal plasma flow can be estimated by *p*-aminohippurate (PAH) clearance, tubular function by sodium clearance, and osmolar excretion by osmotic clearance.

CREATINE

Creatine can be measured directly by (*a*) the condensation of creatine with diacetyl-1-naphthol to form a pink product, (*b*) the use of creatine kinase enzyme with a fluorometric assay, and (*c*) the use of guanidine with ninhydrin in an alkaline solution to produce a fluorescent product. Creatine is commonly measured indirectly by converting creatine to creatinine through heating the sample with acid in the presence of a heavy metal. Creatinine is measured before and after the addition of the reagent and creatine is calculated from the difference in the concentrations. Plasma creatine is increased with muscle necrosis and most muscle diseases, but the utilization of plasma creatine measurements has declined sharply in favor of the analysis of muscle enzymes such as creatine phosphokinase.

URIC ACID

Uric acid is the major end product of purine metabolism, specifically the catabolism of the purine nucleosides adenosine and guanosine. The metabolism of these nucleosides is as follows:

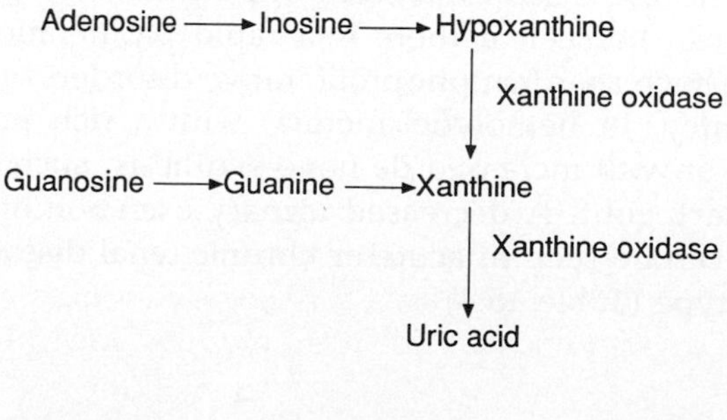

Uric acid production occurs primarily in the liver and intestinal mucosa because of the high xanthine oxidase enzyme activity in these two tissues. Daily synthesis of uric acid is approximately 700 mg, with dietary nucleoprotein contributing 300 mg to the daily total uric acid production. The body pool of uric acid is about 1.2 g, and about 60% of this pool turns over every day. Since the pKa of uric acid is 5.75, the majority of uric acid in the body exists as the urate ion.

The only effective route for excretion of uric acid from the body is through the kidney. Uric acid excretion is complex. 98 to 100% of filtered uric acid is actively reabsorbed in the proximal portion of the proximal convoluted tubule, is secreted in the distal portion of the proximal convoluted tubule, and finally is actively reabsorbed in the distal convoluted tubule. Only 6 to 12% of the original filtered uric acid is excreted in the urine, which amounts to 400 to 800 mg excreted in the urine daily.

Plasma uric acid levels show day-to-day and seasonal variations in the same patient. The uric acid level is higher in the summer than in the winter in most individuals. Plasma levels are lower during childhood, reaching adult levels by age 18. The reference range depends on the method that is used to analyze uric acid, and is in the range of 4.0 to 8.5 mg/dl for adult males and 2.7 to 7.3 mg/dl for adult females when a uricase method is used. Several factors influence the uric acid level, most of which are poorly understood. Increases in exercise, stress, and weight, along with hypertension, diabetes mellitus, and type A personalities are associated with higher values of uric acid. Drugs can affect uric acid levels by altering the rate of synthesis and/or excretion. Drugs that have been reported to elevate uric acid are ethanol, acetaminophen, androgens, low-dose aspirin, furosemide, and mercurial diuretics; the following drugs have been reported to lower uric acid: high-dose aspirin, allopurinol, chlorpromazine, cortical steroids, Coumadin, estrogens, and phenothiazines.

Hyperuricemia is seen in several pathologic conditions. These conditions can be due to either an increased production of uric acid or decreased renal excretion of uric acid. Increased production of uric acid is seen with increased nucleic acid turnover, which leads to increased catabolism of purines. This condition can be seen if there is a rapid proliferation of cells, such as in lymphoproliferative disorders or malignancy, in hemolytic anemia, with a rich purine diet, or with increased de novo synthesis, such as in primary gout. A decreased urinary excretion of uric acid can be seen in acute or chronic renal disease of any type (Table 16.4).

Table 16.4. Etiology of Hyperuricemia

Increased uric acid synthesis
Gout
Purine rich diet—organ meats
Tissue catabolism—necrosis, radiation
Myeloproliferative disorders
Lymphoproliferative disorders
Chemotherapy of malignancy
Lesh-Nyhan syndrome
Decreased renal excretion of uric acid
Renal failure
Drugs
Diuretics
Small-dose aspirin (< 2 g/day)
Metabolic acidosis
Toxemia or pregnancy
Miscellaneous etiologies
Intoxications—ethanol, methanol
Endocrine—acromegaly, hyperparathyroidism
Psychosocial, hypertension, type A personality
Psoriasis

Gout is a disorder of purine metabolism or renal excretion characterized by an increase in the total body uric acid and the precipitation of monosodium urate as deposits (tophi) in and around joints, bursae, periarticular cartilage, bone, and subcutaneous tissue. There can be recurrent attacks of arthritis and nephropathy with nephrolithiasis. The deposits of urate crystals are responsible for the clinical signs and symptoms of the disease. There is thought to be a genetic disposition, although fewer than one-third of patients have a positive family history. Males make up 90% of all cases, and gout is uncommon in females before menopause. The peak age of onset of gout is in the fifth decade. The plasma level of uric acid correlates roughly with the clinical severity of gout; however, there is extreme variability from individual to individual with the same level of uric acid producing different degrees of clinical symptoms.

Hypouricemia, defined as a uric acid level below 2.0 mg/dl, can be seen in severe liver disease with a decreased synthesis of purines, a hereditary deficiency of xanthine oxidase, administration of allopurinol (a xanthine oxidase inhibitor) or uricosuric drugs, and a defect in renal tubular reabsorption of uric acid seen in Fanconi's syndrome.

Analytical methods for uric acid fall into two categories: phosphotungstic acid and uricase methods.

Phosphotungstic acid oxidizes uric acid to allantoin. The reduction product of phosphotungstate in an alkaline medium is blue and can be quantitated by measuring absorbance at about 700 nm. Phosphotungstic acid methods differ in the reagents used to intensify the blue color. The reaction is nonspecific, and positive interferences can be seen for glucose, ascorbic acid, glutathione, cystine, and drugs such as aspirin, acetaminophen, caffeine, and theophylline. Protein must be removed to avoid turbidity and quenching of the color development. Phosphotungstic acid methods give plasma uric acid values 0.2 to 0.4 mg/dl higher than uricase methods.

Uricase methods are based on the oxidation of uric acid to allantoin and hydrogen peroxide by the enzyme uricase (urate oxidase, EC 1.7.3.3) and have the advantage of greater specificity and accuracy. There are many adaptations of this method. Uric acid is maximally absorbed between 290 and 295 nm at an alkaline pH. This absorbance disappears as uric acid is oxidized with uricase. The concentration of uric acid can therefore be calculated from the difference in absorbance before and after the action of uricase. In another approach, coupled uricase methods utilize the hydrogen peroxide produced as a substrate for a chemical indicator reaction catalyzed by peroxidase or catalase. The reference method for uric acid analysis is based on the uricase reaction, and there is also a definitive method using mass fragmentography and gas chromatography/mass spectrometry.

AMMONIA

Ammonia is a product of amino acid metabolism, primarily in the liver, where oxidative deamination of L-glutamate occurs to form α-ketoglutarate and ammonia. The major source of ammonia, however, is absorption from the gastrointestinal tract where bacteria proteases, ureases, and amine oxidases act on protein contents in the colon, and simultaneous hydrolysis of glutamine occurs in the small and large bowels to form a large amount of ammonia. Ammonia is absorbed into the portal blood system and is ultimately metabolized to urea in the liver through the urea cycle. A small amount of ammonia is converted into glutamine and stored in the liver, brain, and skeletal muscle. The ammonia concentration in the systemic circulation is low, in the range of 10 to 80 μg/dl. Elevated ammonia levels can be seen in congenital deficiencies of any of the enzymes of the urea cycle, in Reye's syndrome, and in severe liver disease. In severe hepatic failure, hepatic encephalopathy and coma are associated with high blood ammonia and glutamine but the severity of the clinical signs does not correlate well with the blood ammonia level.

The most common method for the analysis of ammonia uses the enzyme glutamate dehydrogenase (GLDH) (EC 1.4.1.3) in the following reaction:

$$NH_4^+ + \alpha\text{-ketoglutarate} + NADPH \xrightarrow{GLDH} \text{L-glutamate} + NADP^+ + H_2O$$

The ammonia level is determined by measuring the decrease in absorbance at 340 nm as NADPH is converted to $NADP^+$.

Two-stage assays are also available. In the first stage, the plasma is mixed with a cation exchange resin that binds ammonium ion. The ammonium is eluted off the resin and quantitated with Nessler's reagent or the Berthelot reaction (phenolhypochlorite).

Ammonia analysis in the clinical laboratory is particularly subject to preanalytical sources of error because of the very low concentration of ammonia that is normally present. The ammonia content of blood rises rapidly after collection due to the in vitro metabolism of nitrogenous compounds and the degradation of glutamine. These can be minimized by keeping the sample on ice and beginning the analysis within 30 minutes. Ammonia is stable for at least 2 days if plasma is frozen at −20°C.

RENAL DISORDERS

Acute Renal Failure

An abrupt decline in renal function is a common clinical problem. This is manifested clinically by the onset of oliguria (less than 500 ml of urine per day) and an acute rise in serum creatinine and urea. Approximately 70 to 75% of cases have a prerenal etiology associated with decreased renal perfusion, and 25% of cases are due to intrinsic renal disease from ischemia or toxins. Decreased renal perfusion can be the result of volume depletion from hemorrhage or gastrointestinal tract fluid loss, hypotension associated with septic shock, congestive heart failure, and cirrhosis. The most common renal disease associated with acute renal failure is acute tubular necrosis (ATN). ATN is manifested by sloughing of renal tubular cells and occlusion of the tubules by cellular debris. ATN is associated with hypoxic injury of the tubule due to renal ischemia or tubular injury due to toxins or drugs, such as aminoglycosides, radiologic contrast media, heme pigments, amphotericin B, and cisplatin. The oliguric phase of ATN lasts 7 to 21 days and is followed by a diuretic phase. Azotemia decreases 1 to 3 weeks after the onset of diuresis. The mortality rate is 40 to 60%. It is important to differentiate between decreased renal perfusion and ATN as the cause of acute renal failure, because the treatment for the two conditions is quite different. In general, the treatment for decreased renal perfusion is fluid administration to expand blood volume, while ATN requires careful management of fluid to control water and electrolyte imbalance.

In acute renal failure due to decreased renal perfusion, serum urea tends to be elevated proportionately more than creatinine due to increased reabsorp-

Table 16.5. Laboratory Differentiation of ATN and Renal Hypoperfusion

Value[a]	Hypoperfusion	ATN
UN/cr	> 20	< 15
Uosm	> 500	< 350
U/P osm	< 1.5:1	1:1
U/P cr	> 15	< 15
UNa	< 20	> 30–40
SG	> 1.015	< 1.010
FE_{Na}	< 1	> 2

[a]Abbreviations: UN/cr, urea nitrogen: creatinine ratio; FE_{Na}, fractional excretion of sodium; SG, specific gravity; UNa, urinary sodium (mEq/liter); Uosm, urinary osmolality; U/Pc, ratio of urinary to plasma creatinine; U/Posm, ratio of urinary to plasma osmolality.

tion of urea in the renal tubule. The urea to creatinine ratio is generally greater than 20. The decreased plasma volume stimulates ADH and aldosterone, resulting in production of smaller urine volume. The urine is relatively concentrated with a high osmolality, but with a low sodium concentration.

Renal tubular damage seen in ATN results in marked tubular dysfunction with a loss of concentrating ability and inability to conserve sodium. The urine osmolality is similar to plasma osmolality, and the urine sodium is over 40 mg/dl (see Table 16.5 for differentiation between ATN and decreased renal perfusion).

The fractional excretion of sodium (FE_{Na}) may also be of help in differentiating between ATN and decreased renal perfusion. The FE_{Na} is an index of the ability of the kidney to conserve sodium and represents the percentage of filtered sodium that is excreted in the urine. The FE_{Na} can be calculated by simultaneously measuring urinary and plasma sodium (U_{Na}, P_{Na}) and creatinine (U_{cr}, P_{cr}) and using the following formula:

$$FE_{Na}\ (\%) = \frac{U_{Na} \times P_{cr}}{U_{cr} \times P_{Na}} \times 100$$

In decreased renal perfusion the FE_{Na} will be less than 1%, while in ATN it will generally be greater than 2%.

Chronic Renal Disease

Patients with early renal disease are usually asymptomatic. However, there may be complaints relating to the urinary tract, such as urinary frequency, hematuria, and pain, or there may be systemic complaints such as edema, hypertension, lassitude, and weakness. The urinalysis is one of the most important tests to detect early renal disease. The kinds of abnormalities seen in the urinalysis are related to the type of renal disease present.

Renal disease can be divided into glomerular, tubular, and interstitial diseases. Glomerular diseases are usually caused by immunologic factors and are defined by specific pathologic changes seen on microscopy. Usually the first manifestation of glomerular disease is altered permeability of the glomerulus, causing proteinuria or hematuria. Additional glomerular damage leads to a decreased GFR, seen as a progressive decrease in the creatinine clearance, and finally an elevation in plasma urea and creatinine. Due to the hyperbolic relationship between plasma urea or creatinine and the GFR, as mentioned earlier, these measurements are poor indicators of early renal disease.

Tubular and interstitial damage can be secondary to multiple myeloma, ATN, nephrotoxic drugs, and pyelonephritis. Tubular dysfunction can be detected by abnormal tests of urinary concentration such as changes in specific gravity, urine and plasma osmolality ratios, inability to conserve sodium, and defects in acidification of the urine.

Progressive and irreversible deterioration of renal function will lead to the kidney's progressive inability to perform its excretory, secretory, and regulatory functions. When over 90% of the nephrons are nonfunctioning, signs and symptoms known as the uremic syndrome can develop. The uremic syndrome consists of anorexia, nausea and vomiting, lassitude, anemia, bleeding tendency, altered endocrine function, neuromuscular symptoms, and hypertension. Characteristic laboratory findings include anemia, abnormal urinalysis, elevated urea and creatinine, low creatinine clearance, elevated phosphorus, hyperkalemia, hypocalcemia, hyperuricemia, hypermagnesemia, elevated alkaline phosphatase, metabolic acidosis, and a loss of concentrating ability. Diabetes mellitus and essential hypertension are contributing factors in a sizable portion of all chronic renal disease patients. When the GFR decreases below 25 ml/min, most patients require dialysis or renal transplantation to prevent the onset of the uremic syndrome.

Renal Tubular Acidosis

Renal tubular acidosis is a term applied to a group of diverse disorders in which the kidneys are unable to acidify urine normally. The common feature is a mild hyperchloremic metabolic acidosis caused by abnormal renal acid-base handling. These disorders show little alteration in the glomerular filtration rate. There are two major types of renal tubular acidosis, involving either the proximal or the distal convoluted tubules, and a third subtype of distal disorder.

Table 16.6. Causes of Distal RTA (Type I)

Hereditary
Diseases associated with gammopathy
  Amyloidosis
  Systemic lupus erythematosus
  Sarcoidosis
  Macroglobulinemia
Tubulointerstitial disease
  Analgesic nephropathy
  Sickle cell disease
  Chronic pyelonephritis
  Obstruction of the urinary tract
Nephrocalcinosis
  Hyperparathyroidism
  Vitamin D intoxication
Drugs
  Amphotericin B
  Lithium
  Analgesics

Type I renal tubular acidosis was the first renal tubular acidosis described. It is caused by a reduced ability of the distal convoluted tubule to acidify urine. Patients with type I distal renal tubular acidosis cannot produce urine with a pH below 6.0. The exact mechanism is uncertain. The presence of a urine pH below 5.2 excludes the diagnosis of distal renal tubular acidosis. There may be an associated abnormal loss of potassium, phosphorus, and calcium in the urine, with the formation of renal calculi. Type I renal tubular acidosis may be familial, autosomal-dominant, or secondary to toxic or metabolic etiologies such as hyperparathyroidism, hypergammaglobulinemia, vitamin D deficiency, use of amphotericin B, and hydronephrosis (Table 16.6). Diagnosis can be made with an ammonium chloride challenge test, in which the urine pH remains inappropriately high in relation to the degree of induced systemic acidosis.

Type II renal tubular acidosis is caused by an inability of proximal renal tubular cells to conserve bicarbonate. In the renal tubule the majority of renal hydrogen ion secretion occurs in the proximal convoluted tubule, which is responsible for reabsorbing 85% of the filtered bicarbonate. In this disorder, the proximal reabsorption of bicarbonate is impaired, and thus bicarbonate is lost in the urine. Distal hydrogen ion secretion is normal in these patients. In some patients with type II renal tubular acidosis, the net acid secretion may be normal if the serum bicarbonate is low. When the serum bicarbonate falls, a level is reached at which the proximal tubular cells are able to recover all of the filtered bicarbonate. The distal tubule then can acidify the urine in a normal manner. A bicarbonate loading test will reveal that over 15% of the filtered bicarbonate is lost in the urine. Type II proximal renal tubular acidosis may be an isolated hereditary defect, but it is more commonly associated with other proximal defects, such as aminoaciduria, glycosuria, and phosphaturia (Fanconi's syndrome). Type II renal tubular acidosis can be secondary to multiple myeloma, cystinosis, galactosemia, heavy-metal intoxication, carbonic anhydrase inhibitors, tetracycline use, hyperparathyroidism, and amyloid infiltration (Table 16.7). The treatment is large dosages of bicarbonate.

Table 16.7. Causes of Proximal Renal Tubular Acidosis (Type II)

Idiopathic or hereditary
Vitamin D deficiency
Hyperparathyroidism
Fanconi's syndrome
Chronic renal disease
Amyloidosis
Systemic lupus erythematosus
Drugs
  Tetracycline
  Carbonic anhydrase inhibitors
  Streptozotocin
  Gentamicin
Heavy metal intoxication
Wilson's disease
Multiple myeloma
Cystinosis
Galactosemia

Table 16.8. Differentiation of Type I, II, and IV Renal Tubular Acidosis

Clinical or Laboratory Features	Type I	Type II	Type IV
Urinary pH with			
$HCO_3 > 20$	> 5.5	> 5.5	> 5.5
$HCO_3 < 15$	> 5.5	< 5.5	> 5.5
K	↓	↓	↑
Calculi	Y	N	N
NH_4Cl loading	> 5.5	< 5.5	> 5.5
Fanconi's	N	Y	N
% HCO_3 excretion	< 10	> 15	< 10
Bone disease	Y	N	N

Type IV renal tubular acidosis is a type of distal renal tubular acidosis associated with a hyporenin hypoaldosterone state. Due to a decreased response or absence of aldosterone, there is a failure of potassium and hydrogen ion secretion in the distal tubule and a failure of the distal convoluted tubular cells to produce ammonia. This type of renal tubular acidosis may also be seen in generalized renal disease.

Laboratory differentiation of the different types of renal tubular acidosis is tabulated in Table 16.8.

Suggested Readings

Renal Physiology

Harrington AR, Zimmerman SW. Renal pathophysiology. New York: John Wiley & Sons, 1982.

Kassirer JP. Clinical evaluation of kidney function—glomerular function. N Engl J Med 1971;285:365–385.

Kassirer JP. Clinical evaluation of kidney function—tubular function. N Engl J Med 1971;285:499–501.

Pitts RF. Physiology of the kidney and body fluids. 3rd ed. Chicago: Year Book Medical Publishers, 1974.

Renkin EM, Robinson RR. Glomerular filtration. N Engl J Med 1974;290:785–792.

Renal Tubular Acidosis

Battle D. Renal tubular acidosis. Med Clin North Am 1983;67:859–878.

Maher ER, Scoble JE. Renal tubular acidosis. Br J Hosp Med 1989;42:116–119.

Roth KS. Diagnosis of renal tubular transport disorders. Clin Pediatr 1988;27:463–470.

Rothstein M, Obialo C, Hruska KA. Renal tubular acidosis. Endocrinol Metab Clin North Am 1990;19:869–887.

Water Metabolism

Carroll HJ, Oh MS. Water, electrolyte and acid-base metabolism: diagnosis and management. Philadelphia: JB Lippincott, 1978.

Kleeman CR, Fichman MP. The clinical physiology of water metabolism. N Engl J Med 1967;277:1300–1306.

Valtin H. Mechanisms preserving fluid and solute balance in health. 2nd ed. Boston: Little, Brown & Co, 1983.

Zerbe RL, Robertson GL. A comparison of plasma vasopressin measurements with a standard indirect test in the differential diagnosis of polyuria. N Engl J Med 1981;305:1539–1546.

Specific Gravity

Burkhardt AE, Johnston KG, Waszak CE, et al. A reagent strip for measuring the specific gravity of urine. Clin Chem 1982;28:2068–2072.

Rubini HE, Wolfe AV. Refractometric determination of total solids and water of serum and urine. J Biol Chem 1957;225:869–874.

Wolf AV, Fuller JB, Goldman EJ, Mahoney TD. New refractiometric methods for the determination of total proteins in serum and urine. Clin Chem 1962;8:158–165.

Osmolality

Dorwart WV, Chalmers L. Comparison of methods for calculating serum osmolality from chemical concentrations and the prognostic value of such calculations. Clin Chem 1975;21:190–194.

Gennari FJ. Serum osmolality. N Engl J Med 1984;310:102–105.

Jacobson MH, Levy SE, Kaufman RM, et al. Urine osmolality: a definitive test of renal function. Arch Intern Med 1962;110:83–86.

Weisberg HF. Osmolality. Lab Med 1981;12:81–85.

Urea

Baum N, Dichoso CC, Carlton CE. Blood urea nitrogen and serum creatinine—physiology and interpretations. Urology 1975;5:583–588.

Lum G, Leal-Khouri S. Significance of low serum urea nitrogen concentrations. Clin Chem 1989;35:639–640.

Lyman JL. Blood urea nitrogen and creatinine. Emerg Med Clin North Am 1986;4:223–233.

Passey RB, Gillum RL, Fuller JB, et al. Evaluation of three methods for the measurement of urea nitrogen in serum as used on six instruments. Am J Clin Pathol 1980;73:362–368.

Ward PC. Renal dysfunction: urea and creatinine. Postgrad Med 1981;69:93–104.

Creatinine

Bjorkhem I, Blomstrand R, Ohman G. Mass fragmentography of creatinine proposed as a reference method. Clin Chem 1977;23:2114–2121.

Bowers LD, Wong ET. Kinetic serum creatinine assays. II. A critical evaluation and review. Clin Chem 1980;25:555–561.

Levey AS, Perrone RD, Madias NE. Serum creatinine and renal function. Annu Rev Med 1988;39:465–490.

Narayanan S, Appleton HD. Creatinine: a review. Clin Chem 1980;26:1119–1126.

Perakis N, Wolff CM. Kinetic approach for the enzymic determination of creatinine. Clin Chem 1984;30:1792–1796.

Rosano TG, Ambrose RT, Wu A, et al. Candidate reference method for determining creatinine in serum: method development and interlaboratory validation. Clin Chem 1990;36:1951–1955.

Weber JA, Van Zanten AP. Interferences in current methods for measurement of creatinine. Clin Chem 1991;37:695–700.

Creatinine Clearance

Apple FS, Benson P, Abraham PA, et al. Assessment of renal function by insulin clearance: comparison with creatinine clearance as determined by enzymatic methods. Clin Chem 1989;35:312–314.

Bauer JH, Brooks CS, Burch RN. Clinical appraisal of creatinine clearance as a measurement of glomerular filtration rate. Am J Kidney Dis 1982;2:337–346.

Bennett WM, Porter GA. Endogenous creatinine clearance as a clinical measure of glomerular filtration rate. Br Med J 1971;4:84–86.

Camara AA, Arnk D, Reimer A, et al. The twenty-four hour endogenous creatinine clearance as a clinical measure of the functional state of the kidneys. J Lab Clin Med 1951;37:743–763.

Cockcroft DW, Gault MH. Prediction of creatinine clearance from serum creatinine. Nephron 1976;16:31–41.

Rhodes PJ, Rhodes RS. Evaluation of eight methods for estimating creatinine clearance in man. Clin Pharm 1987;6:399–406.

Uric Acid

Bendersky G. Etiology of hyperuricemia. Ann Clin Lab Sci 1975;5:456–467.

Carroll JJ, Coburn H, Douglass R, et al. A simplified alkaline phosphotungstate assay for uric acid in serum. Clin Chem 1971;17:158–160.

Duncan PH, Gochman N, Cooper T, et al. A candidate reference method for uric acid in serum: 1. Optimization and evaluation. Clin Chem 1981;28:284–290.

Elin RJ, Johnson E, Chester R. Four methods for determining uric acid compared with a candidate reference method. Clin Chem 1982;28:2098–2100.

Paulus HE, Coutts A, Calabro JJ, et al. Clinical significance of hyperuricemia in routinely screened hospitalized men. JAMA 1970;211:277–281.

Ammonia

Flannery DB, Hsia VE, Wolf B. Current status of hyperammonemic syndromes. Hepatology 1982;2:495–506.

Forman DT. Rapid determination of plasma ammonia by an ion-exchange technic. Clin Chem 1964;10:497–499.

Gerron GG, Ansley JD, Isaacs JW, et al. Technical pitfalls in measurement of venous plasma NH_3 concentration. Clin Chem 1976;22:663–666.

Miller GE, Rice JD. Determination of the concentration of ammonia nitrogen in plasma by means of a simple ion exchange method. Am J Clin Pathol 1963;39:97–103.

Pesh-Iman M, Kumar S, Willis CE. Enzymatic determination of plasma ammonia: evaluation of Sigman and BMC kits. Clin Chem 1978;24:2044–2046.

Willems D, Steenssens W. Ammonia determined in plasma with a selective electrode. Clin Chem 1988;34:2372.

Renal Disease

Cohen EP, Lemann J Jr. The role of the laboratory in evaluation of kidney function. Clin Chem 1991;37:785–796.

Espinel C. The FE_{NA} test: use in the differential diagnosis of acute renal failure. JAMA 1976;236:579–581.

Harrington JT, Cohen JJ. Acute oliguria. N Engl J Med 1975;292: 89–91.

Bricker NS, Kirschenbaum MA. The kidney: diagnosis and management. New York: John Wiley & Sons, 1984.

Pillay VRG. Clinical testing of renal function. Med Clin North Am 1971;55:231–241.

Wolfson M. Laboratory values in renal failure. Lab Med 1985;16: 107–110.

17 Calcium, Magnesium, and Phosphate

John G. Toffaletti

The electrolytes calcium, magnesium, and phosphate are the principal inorganic constituents of bone and are vital in the function of membranes, hundreds of enzymes, genetic regulation, muscle contraction, and energy utilization. Their distribution between bone, soft tissues, and extracellular fluids is regulated by parathyroid hormone and vitamin D. As with most electrolytes, the kidneys are the most important regulators of the concentration of these ions in blood.

With the exception of parathyroid dysfunction and occult causes of hypercalcemia, the usefulness of these electrolytes in diagnostic tests was of only moderate interest through the 1970s. During the past 10 years the discovery and awareness of the importance of calcium and magnesium in cellular regulation, ischemia, and pathophysiology, especially of myocardial and smooth muscle cells, has led to a much more prominent role for these tests in monitoring during surgery, in critical care, and in the neonate. The role of intracellular calcium ions in reperfusion injury following ischemia, the potentially fatal complications from hypomagnesemia in cardiovascular disease, and the importance of adequate phosphate for regulation of oxygen delivery and energy utilization are some examples of the vital importance of these electrolytes in critically ill patients.

Although there is no doubt of the importance of these electrolytes to health and cellular survival, the measurement of their physiologically active forms remains quite difficult. While reliable measurements of ionized calcium are readily available, reliable methods for measuring ionized magnesium are still being developed. An even greater challenge arises in measuring and interpreting intracellular concentrations of magnesium and phosphate. Techniques that measure intracellular concentrations of any of these electrolytes remain relatively crude and too slow to be of value for clinical decision making in an acute care setting, but they are the subject of current research and development.

CALCIUM

Biochemistry and Physiology

In 1883, Ringer showed that calcium was essential for myocardial contraction (1). While studying the actions of bound and free forms of calcium on frog heart contraction, McLean and Hastings showed that the ionized (free) calcium concentration was proportional to the amplitude of frog heart contraction, while protein-bound and citrate-bound calcium had no effect (2). From this observation, they used isolated frog hearts to develop the first assay for ionized calcium. While the method had poor precision by today's standards, they were able to show that blood ionized calcium was both closely regulated and had a mean concentration in humans of about 1.18 mmol/liter.

Because of recent evidence that decreased ionized calcium can impair myocardial function, an important goal both during surgery and with critically ill patients is to maintain ionized calcium at a nearly normal concentration (3). The flow of calcium ions into cells in the myocardium helps control cardiac rhythm. Calcium binds to contractile proteins, which initiates the contractile process. The rate at which calcium ions flow into smooth muscle cells influences the tension of arterioles, which regulates blood pressure. A diagram showing these basic intracellular movements of calcium ions is shown in Figure 17.1.

Since the intracellular concentration of calcium ions is the critical factor responsible for muscle contraction, the regulation of calcium ion flow into and out of cells is extremely important. Two types of calcium channels on the cell membrane are known to regulate this flow: a voltage-dependent and a phosphorylation-dependent channel. These gates function as follows: the voltage-dependent gate opens when the membrane is depolarized, while the phosphorylation-dependent gate requires a cAMP-activated protein kinase. The cardiotropic drugs epinephrine and isoproterenol facilitate transport of calcium ions through these channels, while acetyl choline hinders the transport of calcium ions (4).

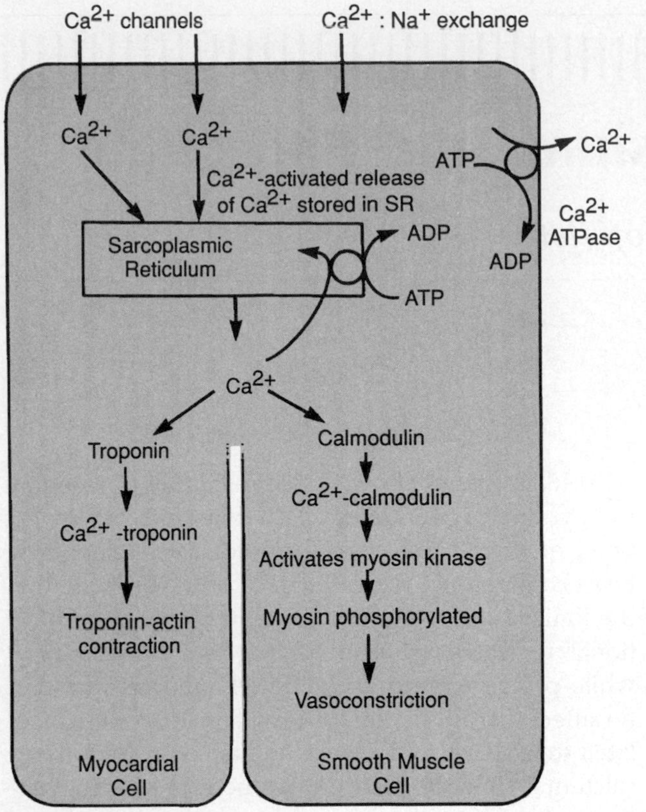

Figure 17.1. Basic intracellular movements of calcium ions that result in the contraction of myocardial or smooth muscle cells. The reactions characteristic of a myocardial cell are shown in the bottom left, while the reactions in a smooth muscle cell are shown in the bottom right of the figure.

Note that this inward flux of calcium ions does not directly trigger contraction of the myocardial cell. Rather, these ions amplify intracellular calcium by releasing calcium ions from both the sarcoplasmic reticulum and the inner cell membrane.

To remove the excess calcium ions that have accumulated inside the cell, ATPases are necessary: a membrane-bound ATPase extrudes calcium ions from the cell, while a magnesium ATPase transports calcium ions back into the sarcoplasmic reticulum for future release.

Calcium ions are also important as "second messengers" in controlling the secretion of many hormones such as insulin, aldosterone, vasopressin, and renin. Following stimulation at the cell surface by a specific molecule (first messenger) the inward flux of calcium ions (second messenger) initiates intracellular events, such as production of a hormone.

Decreased ionized calcium concentrations in blood can cause both cardiovascular disorders such as cardiac insufficiency and arrhythmias, and neuromuscular irritability, which may become clinically apparent as irregular muscle spasms, called tetany. Studies have shown that the rate of fall of ionized calcium in blood initiates tetany as much as the absolute concentration of ionized calcium (5).

Regulation of Calcium in the Blood

Three hormones are known to participate in serum calcium regulation, and have rates of secretion that depend on ionized calcium concentration. These hormones are parathyroid hormone (PTH), vitamin D, and calcitonin. Their actions are depicted in Figure 17.2. Parathyroid hormone related protein (PTHRP) has hypercalcemic actions similar to PTH. However, the role of PTHRP in normal calcium homeostasis has yet to be clearly defined.

PTH secretion into blood is stimulated by a decrease in ionized calcium (6) and, conversely, PTH secretion is stopped by an increase in ionized calcium. PTH acts on both bone and kidney to increase calcium in blood. In the bone, PTH activates osteoclasts that break down bone and subsequently release calcium into the extracellular fluid. In the kidneys, PTH conserves calcium by increasing tubular reabsorption of calcium ions. PTH also activates a specific hydroxylase enzyme in the kidney that increases renal production of active vitamin D.

Vitamin D_3, a cholecalciferol, is most often obtained either in the diet or from exposure of the skin to sunlight. Vitamin D_3 from either source is converted in the liver to 25-hydroxycholecalciferol (25-OH-D_3), an inactive form of vitamin D. In the kidney, 25-OH-D_3 is specifically hydroxylated by a 1α-hydroxylase to form 1,25-dihydroxycholecalciferol (1,25-$(OH)_2$-D_3), the most active form. This form of vitamin D increases calcium and phosphate absorption in the intestine and enhances the effect of PTH on bone resorption and calcium retention by the kidneys.

Calcitonin, which originates in the medullary cells of the thyroid gland, is secreted when the concentration of calcium in blood increases. Calcitonin inhibits osteoclast activity and apparently exerts its calcium-lowering effect by inhibiting the actions of both parathyroid hormone and vitamin D.

Distribution Of Calcium in Blood and Cells

Over 99% of the calcium in the body is part of bone. The remaining 1% is mostly in the blood and other extracellular fluid. Very little is intracellular. In fact, the concentration of ionized calcium in blood plasma is 5,000 to 10,000 times higher than in the cytosol of cardiac or smooth muscle cells. Maintenance of this large gradient is vital to allowing the rapid inward flux of calcium ions that is essential for the initiation of muscle contraction.

Calcium in blood is distributed among several forms. About 45% circulates as ionized calcium (i.e.,

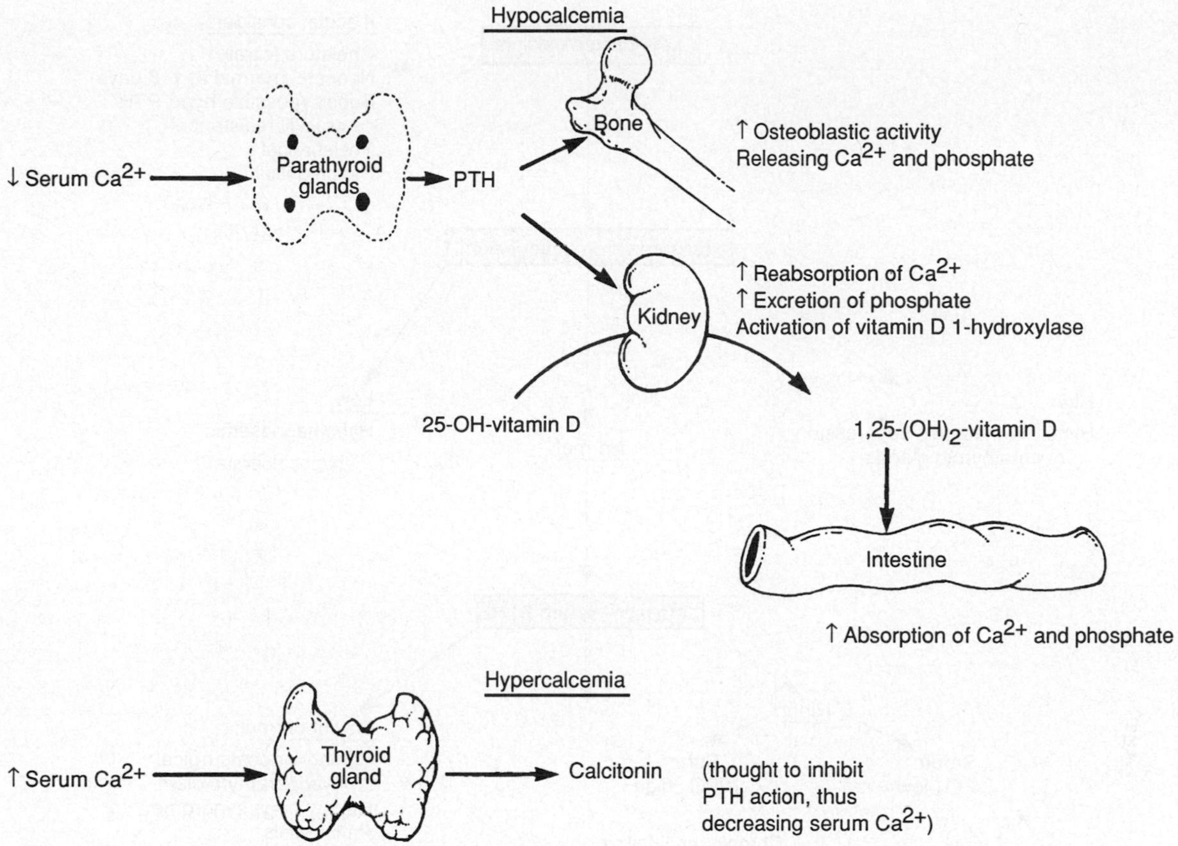

Figure 17.2. Hormonal responses to hypocalcemia and hypercalcemia.

free calcium ions), 40% is bound anionic sites on protein (mostly albumin), and 15% is bound to anions such as bicarbonate, citrate, phosphate, and lactate (7). This distribution can change in disease because concentrations of citrate, bicarbonate, lactate, phosphate, and albumin can change dramatically, especially during surgery or in critically ill patients. This is the principal reason why ionized calcium cannot be calculated from total calcium measurements. In addition, this binding is dependent on pH. As pH falls, more hydrogen ions are available to combine with anions and anionic sites on protein, thus in effect displacing calcium ions and increasing ionized calcium concentrations. As a rough guide, a lowering of pH by 0.1 pH unit will increase ionized calcium by about 0.05 mmol/liter.

Clinical Interpretation of Calcium Measurements

Most cases of abnormal serum calcium concentration are related to one of the following:

- A defect in parathyroid function,
- A defect in vitamin D metabolism,
- Malignancy,
- Renal disease,
- An iatrogenic cause (e.g., administration of citrate, calcium, or saline).

In addition, calcium measurements are useful in the monitoring of neonates, critically ill patients, and patients undergoing surgery.

The use of calcium measurements is complicated somewhat by having both total calcium and ionized calcium measurements available in many laboratories. The relative merits of each test are briefly mentioned in this section. As best emphasized by Ladenson et al. (8), ionized calcium cannot be accurately calculated from a total calcium concentration, and thus this should never be attempted. Ionized calcium concentrations can be determined only by direct measurement.

A further complication to interpreting ionized calcium measurements has been caused by the creation of the pH-adjusted ionized calcium parameter ($[Ca^{2+}]_{7.4}$). This was introduced as a convenience to allow the measurement of ionized calcium in serum collected for the performance of routine chemistry tests. These samples are usually exposed to room air, and the pH-adjusted parameter attempts to correct for loss of carbon dioxide, which increases pH. The increased pH increases calcium-ion binding by proteins, which lowers the ionized calcium concen-

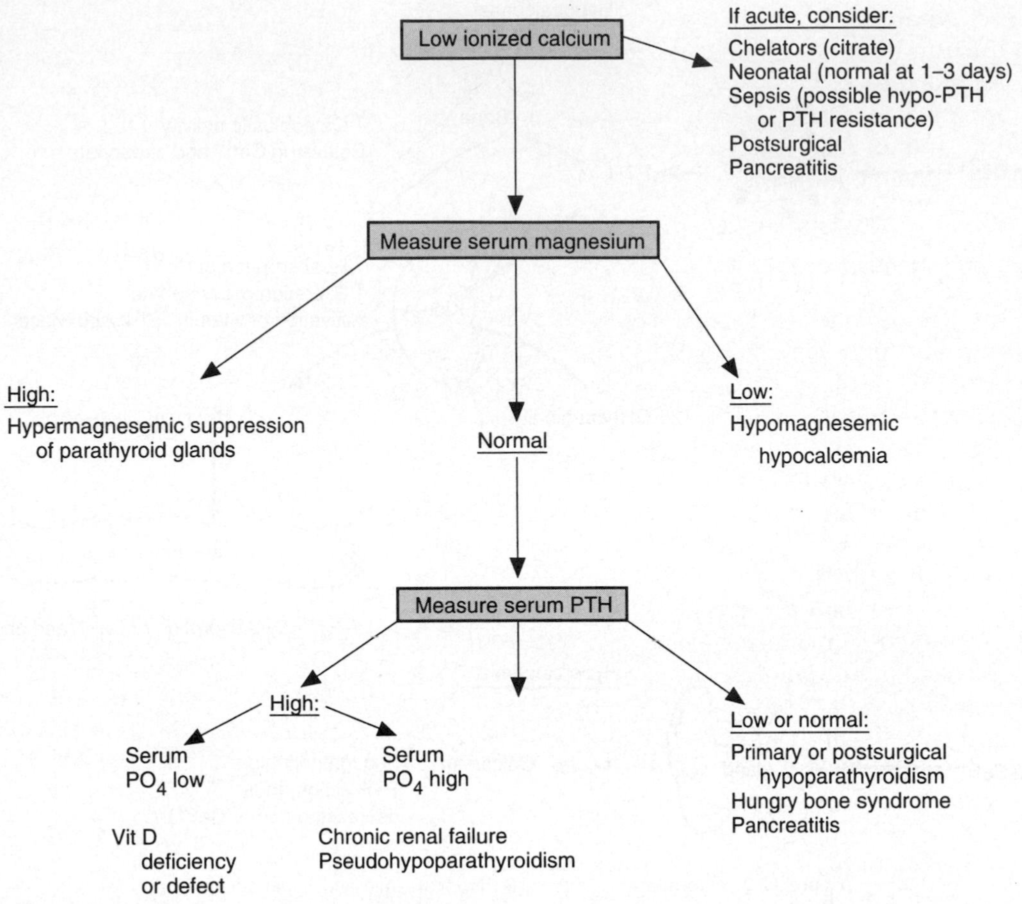

Figure 17.3. Evaluation of hypocalcemia.

tration. Since it has been reported that the pH correction is not accurate for patients undergoing surgery, patients who are critically ill, patients with renal disease, or neonates, it is recommended that actual ionized calcium measured on anaerobically collected blood should be used.

Hypocalcemic Disorders

Hypocalcemia occurs most commonly in patients receiving citrated blood products during major surgery, in patients with renal disease, in patients with parathyroid gland insufficiency following surgery, in neonates, in patients with a magnesium deficiency, and in patients with pancreatitis. A flow diagram for the evaluation of hypocalcemic disorders is shown in Figure 17.3.

HYPOPARATHYROIDISM

While hypoparathyroidism may be acquired by autoimmune or other chronic processes cases of hypocalcemia due to hypoparathyroidism result from surgical removal of tissue during parathyroid or thyroid surgery. Hypocalcemia is usually transient (lasting less than 5 days) unless surgery has removed too much parathyroid tissue or has interfered with the parathyroid blood supply. Zaloga and Chernow recommend that serum ionized calcium should be monitored every 12 hours after neck surgery until a rise in the ionized calcium concentration indicates recovery of the parathyroid gland (4).

Pseudohypoparathydroidism is a condition in which renal cells do not respond to PTH. The combined effects of PTH resistance and hyperphosphatemia may suppress renal 1α-hydroxylase activity, leading to vitamin D deficiency and hypocalcemia.

RENAL DISEASES

Patients with renal glomerular disease often have altered concentrations of calcium, phosphate, albumin, magnesium, and hydrogen ion (pH). Since these conditions tend to change ionized calcium independently of total calcium, ionized calcium is the preferred test for accurately monitoring calcium status in renal disease (9). In chronic renal disease, secondary hyperparathyroidism frequently compensates for hypocalcemia caused either by hyperphosphatemia, in which phosphate binds calcium, or by altered vitamin D metabolism. Controlling ionized calcium by monitoring its concentration can avoid problems due to hypocalcemia, such as osteodystrophy, unstable cardiac output or unstable blood pressure, and problems arising from hypercalcemia such as renal stones or other soft-tissue calcifications.

NEONATAL MONITORING

The ionized calcium concentration in the blood of neonates is typically high at birth, then declines by 10 to 20% after 1 to 3 days. After about a week, ionized calcium concentrations in the neonate stabilize at concentrations slightly higher than in adults (10), and no treatment is usually needed.

Neonatal hypocalcemia may be either of two types. The first type, which normally develops within 1 to 3 days after birth, is associated with parathyroid immaturity and usually resolves by the first week of life. This type of neonatal hypocalcemia in healthy infants may be a normal stimulus to activate parathyroid gland function. The second type of neonatal hypocalcemia is usually seen about 1 week after birth and is associated with both hyperphosphatemia from a high phosphate intake from milk and hypomagnesemia caused by decreased intestinal absorption of magnesium (4). Other factors that increase the incidence and severity of hypocalcemia during this period are prematurity, maternal diabetes mellitus, complications during delivery, and birth asphyxia (4). Hypocalcemia may even become life-threatening if it is severe, prolonged, or accompanied by seizures, hypotension, hypoglycemia, or sepsis.

Ionized calcium measurements are more useful than total calcium in monitoring calcium status in the neonate (10). Rather large changes in the concentration of ionized calcium may occur in the early neonatal period, because calcium may be lost rapidly and not readily reabsorbed. Several possible etiologies have been suggested, including abnormal PTH and vitamin D metabolism, hypercalcitoninemia, hyperphosphatemia, and hypomagnesemia (10).

MONITORING IN SURGERY AND ACUTE CARE

Largely because of the importance of both transcellular and intracellular movement of calcium ions in myocardial and vascular smooth muscle cells, the maintenance of a normal ionized calcium concentration in blood is especially important to the patient in either surgery or intensive care. Adequate calcium concentrations promote good cardiac output and maintain adequate blood pressure. Monitoring and adjusting calcium concentrations may be most critical in open heart surgery when the heart is restarted. Normalizing ionized calcium by administering calcium as a cardiotropic agent is preferred before giving drugs such as epinephrine or isoproterenol (3). Monitoring of ionized calcium is also especially important during liver transplantation, because large volumes of citrated blood are given at a time when the function of the liver (the major organ for metabolizing citrate) is compromised or absent.

Because patients in surgery may receive large amounts of citrate, bicarbonate, calcium salts, and fluids, clear discrepancies between total calcium and ionized calcium are common in these patients. In these cases ionized calcium measurements should be used wherever possible.

CRITICALLY ILL PATIENTS

In critically ill patients, including those with sepsis, thermal burns, renal failure, and/or cardiopulmonary insufficiency, hypocalcalemia occurs in as many as 70% of cases (11). These patients frequently have abnormal acid-base balance and may also be losing protein and albumin. Again there is a clear advantage to monitoring calcium status with ionized calcium measurements instead of total calcium. A direct relationship has been shown between serum ionized calcium and mean arterial pressure in a study of 112 patients admitted to a medical intensive care unit (12).

HYPOMAGNESEMIA

Chronic hypomagnesemia has become recognized as a frequent cause of hypocalcemia. There are three possible mechanisms:

- Inhibition of transport of PTH across the parathyroid gland membrane (13),
- Impairment of PTH action at its receptor site on bone (4), and
- Interference with the action of vitamin D (14).

Hypercalcemic Disorders

A flow chart for the evaluation of hypercalcemia is presented in Figure 17.4. While a total calcium results of 3 mmol/liter or above virtually always indicates hypercalcemia, a total calcium lower than 3 mmol/liter should be confirmed by measurement of ionized calcium, if available. Malignancy and primary hyperparathyroidism are the most common causes of hypercalcemia, accounting for 80 to 90% of cases. Hypercalcemia due to malignancy is more common in hospital populations, while primary hyperparathyroidism is more commonly found in the outpatient setting.

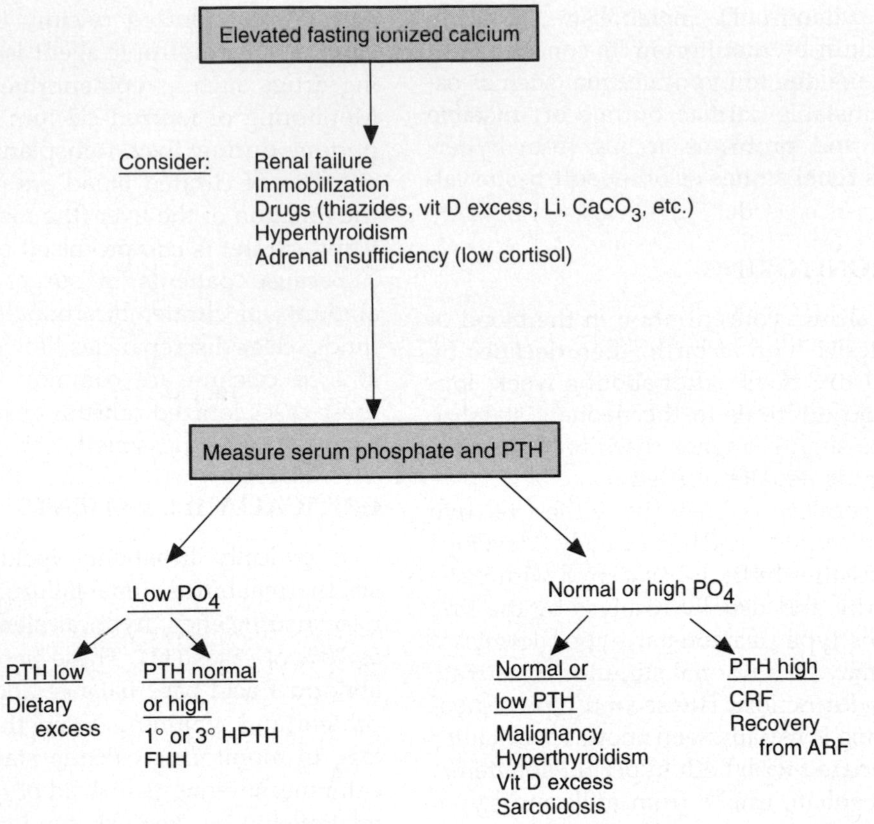

Figure 17.4. Evaluation of hypercalcemia. Abbreviations: 1° HPTH, primary hyperparathyroidism; 3° HPTH, tertiary hyperparathyroidism; FHH, familial hypocalciuric hypercalcemia; ARF, acute renal failure; CHF, chronic renal failure.

While hyperparathyroidism refers to excessive secretion of parathyroid hormone, this excess can range from slight to a very large amount. Hyperparathyroidism may therefore either show obvious clinical signs or be asymptomatic. Several studies have shown that, while both total and ionized calcium measurements are elevated in severe hyperparathyroidism, ionized calcium is more frequently elevated in subtle or asymptomatic hyperparathyroidism. Ionized calcium measurements have been reported to be elevated in 90 to 95% of cases of hyperparathyroidism, while total calcium is elevated in 80 to 85% of cases (15).

Hypercalcemia is present in up to 20% of various types of malignancy, with calcium measurements sometimes serving as biochemical markers for otherwise inapparent disease (Table 17.1). The increase may be caused by direct lysis of bone by tumor or by the secretion of substances, such as PTH isolated protein, that have PTH-like activity in both bone and kidney resorption. Although ionized calcium may have slightly higher diagnostic sensitivity, ionized and total calcium measurements have about equal utility in the detection of occult malignancy (16). Carcinoma of the bronchus, breast, urogenital tract, and head and neck area, and multiple myelomas account for 75% of hypercalcemia in malignancy.

Table 17.1. Interpretation of Laboratory Tests in Differentiating Primary Hyperparathyroidism (HPTH) from Malignancy

Test	Favors HPTH	Favors Malignancy
Total Ca (mmol/liter)	<3.13	>3.13
Serum Cl (mmol/liter)	>103	<103
Intact PTH	Elevated	Low or normal
Serum PO_4	N to low	N to high
Hematocrit	Normal	Low
Urine Ca	High	Very high
1,25-$(OH)_2$ vit D	High	Low
PTHRP	Normal (undetected)	Elevated

Proper Collection and Handling of Samples

Total calcium determinations may be performed on either serum or heparinized plasma. Because anticoagulants such as EDTA and oxalate bind calcium very tightly and interfere with its measurement, even by atomic absorption, they must not be used.

The proper collection of samples for either total or ionized calcium measurements requires both care and appreciation of the problems that can occur. Tourniquet application should be as brief as possible (less than 1 minute) before a specimen is collected:

the combined effects of hemoconcentration (causing hyperproteinemia) and localized lactic acid production can alter total calcium by up to 10% (17) and ionized calcium by about 2 to 3% (17, 18). Since loss of CO_2 will increase pH, all samples for ionized calcium measurements must be collected anaerobically. The metabolic activity of cells during storage affects pH and therefore ionized calcium. Although the effects of the lactate anion and the hydrogen cation partly offset each other (18), blood should be centrifuged within 1 hour to prevent acidosis from affecting the ionized calcium concentration (19, 20). While anticoagulated whole blood can be analyzed more rapidly, serum from sealed evacuated blood collection tubes is satisfactory for ionized calcium if clotting and centrifugation are done within 1 hour. Because of dilutional effects, no liquid heparin products should be used. Heparin also binds a small amount of calcium and tends to lower ionized calcium concentrations. However, if the heparin concentration is less than 30 IU/ml, the interference should be less than 4%. Dry heparin products are available that virtually eliminate the interference by heparin. These products are available either as heparin titrated with small amounts of calcium or zinc ions or as a small amount of heparin dispersed in an inert soluble material.

For analysis of calcium in urine, an accurately timed urine collection is preferred. The urine should be acidified with 6 mol HCl per liter, with approximately 1 ml of the acid added for each 100 ml of urine.

Methods for Measurement of Total and Ionized Calcium

While atomic absorption spectroscopy remains the reference method for total calcium, accurate measurements require care, both in maintenance and calibration of the instrument and in preparation of samples. In routine testing of serum, many automated analyzers give results that are comparable to atomic absorption. However, for analysis of total calcium in urine and other fluids, atomic absorption is still preferred.

Atomic absorption involves introducing a diluted sample into an air-acetylene flame and measuring the absorption of light at 422.7 nm.

Many automated methods for total calcium measurement are based on the complexometric reaction between calcium and the dye ortho-cresolphthalein complexone, often with 8-hydroxyquinoline added to prevent magnesium interference (21, 22). This methodology is used on the duPont aca, Beckman Astra 8 and Technicon SMAC. Some automated analyzers, including the Kodak Ektachem and Beckman CX3 use another dye, Arsenazo III.

Table 17.2. Reference Ranges for Calcium[a]

	mmol/liter	*mg/dl*
Total calcium		
Child	2.20–2.68	8.8–10.7
Adult	2.10–2.55	8.4–10.2
Ionized calcium		
At birth	1.30–1.60	5.2–6.4
Neonate	1.20–1.48	4.8–5.9
Child	1.20–1.38	4.8–5.5
Adult	1.16–1.32	4.6–5.3

[a]Urine reference ranges will vary with diet. Adults on an average diet should excrete 12 to 75 mmol/day (50 to 300 mg/day).

Ionized calcium is measured using an ion-selective electrode system. These electrodes use membranes impregnated with molecules (ionophores) that selectively, but reversibly, bind calcium ions (23). As calcium ions bind to these membranes, an electric potential develops across the membrane that is related to the ionized calcium concentration. The potential is measured with a sensitive voltmeter in the same way that pH is measured.

Reference Ranges for Calcium

Ionized calcium concentrations can change rapidly during the first 1 to 3 days of life. Following this, they stabilize at relatively high levels with a gradual decline through adolescence. For total calcium, the reference range varies slightly with age. Calcium concentrations are relatively high through adolescence when bone growth is most rapid (see Table 17.2).

MAGNESIUM

Biochemistry and Physiology

Awareness of the physiological role and the clinical importance of magnesium has developed relatively recently. The first clinical symptoms of hypomagnesemia were not reported until 1934 by Hirschfelder and Haury. In 1969, Shils reported that magnesium depletion was associated with hypomagnesemia, hypokalemia, and hypocalcemia (24). While hypomagnesemia has been frequently overlooked in the past, there is now a much greater awareness of the clinical importance of magnesium. This is the result of many recent articles describing the effects of magnesium on myocardial function and blood pressure (25), the role of magnesium as a calcium channel–blocking agent (26), the clinical consequences of hypomagnesemia (27), and the implications of magnesium depletion during open heart surgery (28) and critical care (29, 30).

The clinical importance of magnesium reflects its biochemical importance. Magnesium is an essential activator of over 300 enzymes, including those important in glycolysis, gene replication, transcellular ion transport, muscle contraction, and oxidative phosphorylation. In fact, the magnesium complex of ATP is probably the true substrate in energy production, rather than ATP alone. It can be fairly said that magnesium is equal in importance to any of the other electrolytes in the body, many of which have been much more intensively studied and are more commonly measured.

Regulation of Magnesium in the Blood

The average dietary intake of magnesium is 10 to 15 mmol/day. Rich sources are green vegetables, meat, grains, and seafood. The small intestine may absorb from 20 to 63% of the dietary magnesium, depending on the need. The overall regulation of body magnesium is controlled largely by the kidney, which can avidly reabsorb magnesium in deficiency states or can readily excrete excess magnesium in overload states. The renal threshold for magnesium is about 0.60 to 0.85 mmol/liter. Because this is close to the normal serum concentration, slight excesses of magnesium in serum are rapidly excreted by the kidneys. Since renal magnesium reabsorption competes with reabsorption of calcium in the ascending limb of the loop of Henle, the loss of calcium by diuretics, hypercalcemia, or saline infusion will also cause loss of magnesium (31).

While the regulation of magnesium appears to be related to that of calcium, it has not been as well characterized. Parathyroid hormone increases renal reabsorption of magnesium and enhances absorption of magnesium in the intestine. However, for equivalent decreases in ionized calcium and magnesium in blood, changes in ionized calcium have a far greater effect on PTH secretion (32). Paradoxically, chronic or severe acute hypomagnesemia can depress secretion of PTH, which is one mechanism by which hypomagnesemia can cause hypocalcemia. Aldosterone apparently has the opposite effect of PTH, increasing the renal excretion of magnesium. Insulin appears to increase both intestinal and renal absorption of magnesium, yet also increases intracellular concentrations of magnesium.

Distribution of Magnesium in Tissues and Blood

The human body contains about 1 mol (24 g) of magnesium, with about 50% in the skeleton and relatively high concentrations in skeletal muscle, liver, and myocardium. Magnesium is primarily an intracellular ion, with only about 1% being in the blood and extracellular fluid (33). Magnesium in serum exists as protein-bound (24%), complex-bound (10%), and ionized (66%) forms (data derived from reference 32). Of course, these proportions vary with the concentration of proteins and other anions in blood, and, as with calcium, the extent of binding is affected by blood pH.

Table 17.3. Causes of Hypomagnesemia

Diarrhea
Diuretics
Diabetes
Dietary
Drinking
Diverted to free fatty acids
Drugs, such as cyclosporin
Decompensated heart, lungs, liver
Delivery of pregnancy: toxemia or eclampsia
Denuded skin and burns

Clinical Importance of Magnesium Measurements

Spontaneous hypermagnesemia is rarely observed in clinical practice, with most cases resulting from administration of magnesium-containing antacids, enemas, or parenteral nutrition to patients with renal insufficiency (31). In contrast, hypomagnesemia can arise from a number of causes (34–36), which often begin with the letter "D" as listed in Table 17.3 (37). Magnesium should be measured during the initial examination of acutely or chronically ill patients, especially those with poor food intake, malabsorption disorders, hypokalemia, or hypocalcemia, and in those taking diuretics (34). The incidence of hypomagnesemia in hospitalized patients has been reported to be from 5 to 50%, with differences among populations studied accounting for some of this variation.

CARDIAC DISORDERS

The detection of hypomagnesemia is critical in cardiovascular disease because magnesium deficiency is associated with coronary vasospasm, arrhythmias, acute infarction, and sudden death (25, 38). These conditions may arise because hypomagnesemia both contributes to the loss of myocardial potassium and increases the ratio of calcium to magnesium, both of which alter myocardial electrophysiology (39). Magnesium plays several important roles in metabolism, and the heart, with its high metabolic activity, is particularly vulnerable to magnesium deficiency. The extracellular concentration of ionized magnesium apparently controls arterial tone and blood pressure by regulation of Mg-Ca exchange sites on the membrane

(40). A reduction of ionized Mg in the extracellular fluid produces sustained constriction of arterioles and venules, produces coronary vasospasm, and increases the potency of vasoconstrictive agents. Magnesium may also control an Na-Ca pump that maintains the normal tone of coronary and peripheral vessels. Magnesium affects vascular tone by modulating the vasoconstrictive effects of hormones such as norepinephrine and angiotensin II: a high magnesium concentration antagonizes their effects, while a low magnesium concentration enhances their activity (41).

One of the most important consequences of hypomagnesemia in cardiovascular disease may be that cellular loss of magnesium uncouples oxidative metabolism which, by depleting ATP, leads to disruption of mitochondrial function and structure. Moreover, in congestive heart failure (CHF), cardiac output is diminished and inadequate for the metabolic needs of tissues. Since deficiencies of magnesium and potassium lead to high blood pressure, causing increased vascular resistance, the problems of diminished cardiac output of CHF are further intensified (40). Again, this shows the importance of detecting deficiencies in magnesium as well as potassium.

DRUG EFFECTS ON MAGNESIUM CONCENTRATION

Several drugs—including diuretics, gentamicin and other aminoglycoside antibiotics, cisplatin, and cyclosporine—increase renal loss of magnesium and frequently result in hypomagnesemia. The loop diuretics, such as furosemide, are especially effective in increasing renal loss of magnesium. Thiazide diuretics usually require chronic use to develop hypomagnesemia (42). Gentamicin inhibits reabsorption of magnesium in the renal tubule. Hypomagnesemia intensifies the toxic side effects of gentamicin, and so should be especially avoided (43). Cisplatin is also nephrotoxic, and profound hypomagnesemia can be caused by cyclosporine, an immunosuppressant widely used following organ transplantation. Cyclosporine also severely inhibits the renal tubular reabsorption of magnesium in addition to its other side effects, which include hypertension and hepatotoxicity (44).

DIABETES MELLITUS

Hypomagnesemia has been reported in from 25 to 75% of patients with diabetes (45). Hypomagnesemia can aggravate the neuromuscular and vascular complications commonly found in this disease. Although it is not well understood, the mechanism of magnesium deficiency appears to be hormonal both because insulin increases intestinal and renal reabsorption of magnesium, and because diabetic patients often have decreased PTH and altered vitamin D metabolism and/or insulin resistance. Because of this, it is important for diabetic patients to have adequate dietary magnesium. Acute hypomagnesemia can result from intracellular shifts of magnesium following the administration of glucose or amino acids (35, 36). This effect is pronounced following starvation or insulin treatment for hyperglycemia.

ALCOHOLISM

Although hypomagnesemia is frequently observed in patients admitted for alcoholism, alcohol does not appreciably increase renal magnesium excretion. Therefore, hypomagnesemia in alcoholic patients apparently results from a combination of dietary deficiency, ketosis, vomiting, diarrhea, and hyperaldosteronism. Alcoholic patients may become hypomagnesemic after treatments such as dextrose infusion, which induces insulin secretion. This would also be the result of a shift of magnesium back into cells to correct a chronic intracellular deficiency. Frequent monitoring of magnesium is needed in such cases.

OTHER DISEASES

Because magnesium requirements increase during pregnancy, hypomagnesemia may develop if intake is not also increased. Premature labor and preeclampsia/eclampsia are clearly associated with the development of hypomagnesemia. Treatment with magnesium salts has long been an accepted practice in these conditions, although hypermagnesemia sometimes results from excessive doses. The fetus may also be affected by hypermagnesemia in such cases.

Magnesium deficiency may be an important risk factor in renal stone formation and other renal calcification (46). Magnesium ion probably inhibits calcification by pairing with anions that would otherwise form insoluble salts with calcium.

Patients with Paget's disease who also have hypomagnesemia tend to have more active disease as measured by increased serum alkaline phosphatase and urinary hydroxyproline. Since urinary magnesium is not significantly increased in Paget's disease, the low serum magnesium is apparently caused by increased uptake of magnesium into bone. For these reasons, patients with Paget's disease should increase their intake of magnesium to about 10 mmol per day (47).

Proper Collection and Handling of Samples

Because of the threefold higher concentration of magnesium in erythrocytes, serum should not remain in contact with the clot for an extended period of time. Hemolyzed samples are not acceptable. The anticoagulants citrate, oxalate, and EDTA bind magnesium tightly and must not be used.

Measurement of Magnesium

While measurement of total magnesium concentrations in serum remains the usual diagnostic test for the detection of magnesium abnormalities, serum concentrations have two limitations. First, about 25 to 30% of magnesium is protein bound. Therefore, as with total and ionized calcium, total magnesium may not reflect the physiologically active magnesium. While measurement of ultrafiltrable magnesium may be of some use (30), it would not detect citrate-induced hypomagnesemia. Second, and probably of greater significance, because magnesium is primarily an intracellular ion, serum concentration will not necessarily reflect the status of intracellular magnesium. Even when cellular magnesium is depleted by 20%, serum magnesium concentration may remain normal.

A magnesium load test may detect body depletion of magnesium in patients with a normal concentration in serum. However, a magnesium load test requires over 48 hours to complete. After collecting a baseline 24-hour urine, $MgSO_4$ is administered while another 24-hour urine is collected. Individuals with adequate body stores of magnesium will excrete 60 to 80% of the magnesium load within 24 hours, while magnesium-deficient patients excrete less than 50% (31).

Of the numerous methods developed for measurement of magnesium over the years, at least four have accuracy and precision that are acceptable for clinical laboratories (48, 49). These methods are atomic absorption spectroscopy, colorimetric methods using either calmagite or methylthymol blue, and a dry-slide colorimetric method using a formazan dye and a calcium chelator.

Calmagite is a metallochromic derivative of naphthol sulfonic acid that can be used to measure magnesium without deproteinization of the sample. The blue-colored reagent forms a pink magnesium-calmagite complex, with the absorbance measured at around 532 nm. The use of ethylene glycol tetraacetic acid (EGTA) prevents interference by calcium, and cyanide is used to bind heavy metals, preventing them from binding to the dye. The reaction is completed within 60 seconds, which allows the calmagite method to be used on automated analyzers (50).

Table 17.4. Reference Ranges for Magnesium[a]

	mmol/liter
Serum (newborns)	0.50–0.90
Serum (adults)	0.65–1.05
Erythrocytes	1.65–2.65
CSF	1.0–1.40
Urine	1–5 mmol/day

[a]Concentrations of magnesium in serum are lower at birth than in older children or adults.

Methylthymol blue is also widely used for determination of magnesium, with calcium chelators added to increase the specificity. This method is used on the duPont aca, with the absorbance measured at both 510 and 600 nm (50). The dry-slide method uses a multilayered reagent with both a calcium chelator and a magnesium-sensitive formazan dye. The magnesium-formazan complex is measured at 630 nm (49).

The reference method for magnesium measurement is atomic absorption spectroscopy. This method is capable of excellent accuracy and precision (48) in the hands of an experienced operator. Neutron activation analysis with the radioactive isotope magnesium-27 has been proposed as a definitive method (50).

Magnesium ion–selective electrodes have only recently become available, but free magnesium has been quantitated as ultrafiltrable magnesium (30, 32, 51). This may give a reasonable estimate of ionized magnesium in many cases, but ultrafiltrable measurements may seriously overestimate the concentration of both ionized magnesium and ionized calcium following administration of citrate (6). Reference ranges for magnesium are shown in Table 17.4.

PHOSPHATE

Biochemistry and Physiology

Compounds of phosphorus are in all cells and participate in many biochemical processes. The genetic materials DNA and RNA are complex phosphodiesterases. Phosphate is a component of nucleotides, phospholipids, and most coenzymes. The most important reservoirs of biochemical energy are adenosine triphosphate (ATP), creatine phosphate, and phosphoenol pyruvate. One explanation for the widespread occurrence of phosphate in biochemical systems is that phosphate has three oxygen radicals. This allows linkage with two other molecules while still leaving one basic oxygen, which can be protonated or can participate in other reactions (52). Inorganic phosphate is important for maintaining adequate cellular stores of compounds such as ATP,

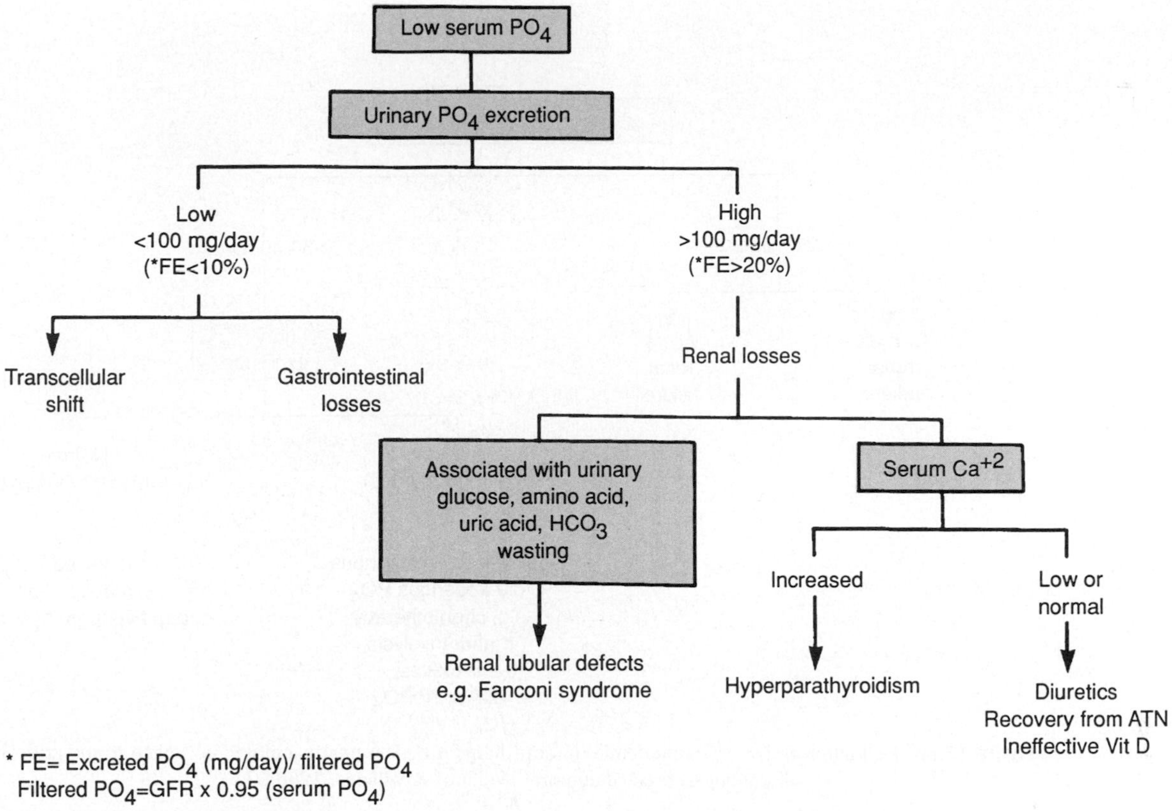

Figure 17.5. Evaluation of hypophosphatemia. (From Chernow B. The pharmacologic approach to the critically ill patient. 2nd ed. Baltimore: Williams & Wilkins, 1988:629.)

and 2,3-DPG (53). Phosphate deficiency can lead to ATP depletion, which is ultimately responsible for many of the clinical symptoms observed in hypophosphatemia.

About 80% of the 700 to 800 g of phosphate in the body is contained in bone, mostly in the form of hydroxyapatite [$Ca_{10}(PO_4)_6(OH)_2$]. Phosphate in blood is either absorbed from dietary sources or resorbed from bone. Most phosphate is found within cells, and the transport of glucose into cells is accompanied by an influx of phosphate. Intracellular phosphate is then used in the synthesis of phosphorylated compounds (54).

The kidney plays an important role in the regulation of serum phosphate concentration, and the renal reabsorption of phosphate is affected by several factors, including acid-base status, vitamin D, and parathyroid hormone (PTH). PTH inhibits the normal tubular reabsorption of phosphate, increasing loss in the urine and decreasing serum phosphate concentrations. Therefore PTH can have a dramatic effect on phosphate regulation, because the renal tubules normally reabsorb over 90% of phosphate filtered at the glomerulus.

While PTH lowers serum phosphate, vitamin D increases phosphate concentrations in the blood by promoting both phosphate absorption in the intestine and phosphate reabsorption in the kidney. Growth hormone, which helps regulate skeletal growth, can also affect circulating concentrations of phosphate. With excessive secretion or administration of growth hormone, phosphate concentrations in the blood tend to increase because of decreased renal excretion. However, growth hormone administered together with parathyroid hormone increases renal excretion of phosphate (55).

Although the total concentration of phosphate (expressed as phosphorus) in blood is about 12 mg/dl, most of this is organic phosphate; only about 3 to 4 mg/dl is inorganic phosphate. HPO_4^{2-} and $H_2PO_4^-$ are an important buffer pair; at pH 7.4 inorganic phosphate is about 75% HPO_4^{2-} and 25% $H_2PO_4^-$.

Clinical Interpretation of Phosphate Measurements

Both hyperphosphatemia and hypophosphatemia are seen frequently in clinical medicine, and both conditions are important to recognize. Flow diagrams for the elevation of hypophosphatemia and hyperphosphatemia are shown in Figures 17.5 and 17.6, respectively.

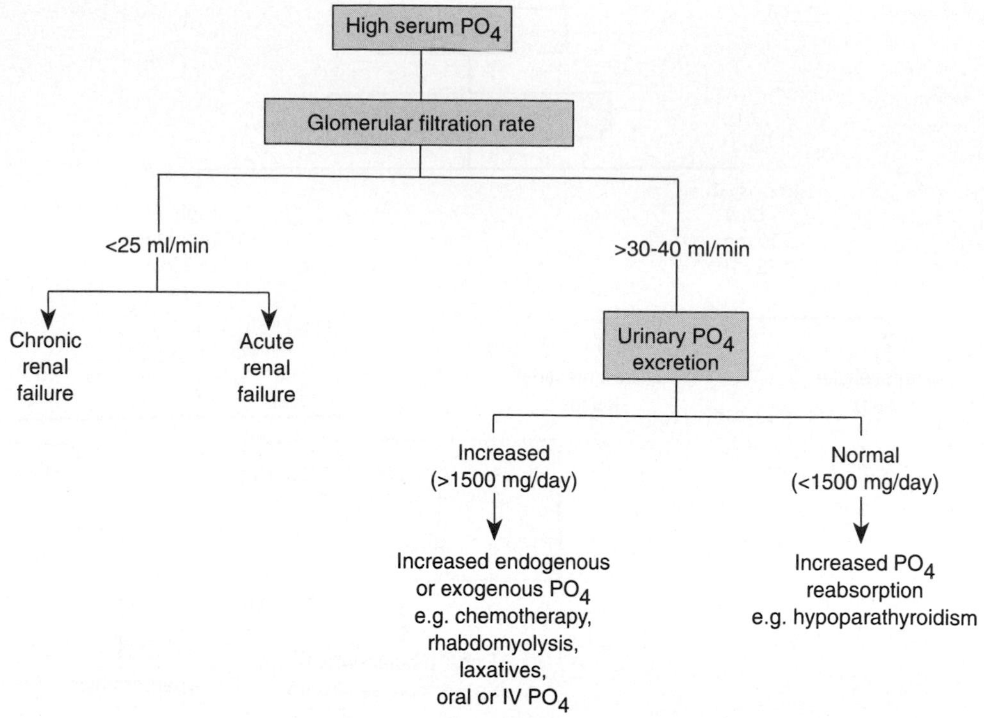

Figure 17.6. Evaluation of hyperphosphatemia. (From Chernow B. The pharmacologic approach to the critically ill patient. 2nd ed. Baltimore: Williams & Wilkins, 1988:633.)

HYPOPHOSPHATEMIA

The incidence of hypophosphatemia in hospitalized patients varies from 2 to 40%, depending on the population studied (56). Severe hypophosphatemia usually results in decreased concentrations of phosphate-containing compounds, such as ATP and membrane phospholipids. These deficiencies in turn are responsible for symptoms of hypophosphatemia, including muscle weakness, respiratory and myocardial insufficiency, and hepatocellular damage (56). Because phosphate is present in nearly all foods, a pure dietary deficiency rarely causes hypophosphatemia. More commonly, hypophosphatemia is caused by renal loss, gastrointestinal malabsorption, or transcellular shifts of phosphate. Mild hypophosphatemia is common in hospitalized patients and is usually not treated, but severe hypophosphatemia (less than 1.0 g/dl or 0.3 mmol/liter) requires monitoring and possible replacement therapy. Causes of severe hypophosphatemia in hospitalized patients are as follows:

1. *Infusion of dextrose solution*. The flow of glucose into cells is often accompanied by an influx of phosphate, with the cellular uptake of phosphorus substantially enhanced by either insulin administration or respiratory alkalosis (57). In addition, the renal tubular reabsorption of glucose and phosphate seem to be linked, with glycosuria accompanied by decreased tubular reabsorption of phosphate.
2. *Nutritional recovery syndrome*. This syndrome occurs as people who are severely malnourished are refed. Severe hypophosphatemia is often seen, probably also because of a shift into cells (54).
3. *Use of antacids that bind phosphate*. The divalent cations in antacids such as aluminum hydroxide, magnesium hydroxide, or aluminum carbonate bind phosphate and prevent its absorption in the gut. Hypophosphatemia is usually associated with chronic excessive use of antacids (54).
4. *Diabetic ketoacidosis*. The combined effects of acidosis, glycosuria, ketonuria, and insulin therapy can lead to severe depletion of phosphate, with serum concentrations decreasing to less than 1 mg/dl within 24 hours. Acidosis induces mobilization of phosphate from bone and tissues, and both glycosuria and ketonuria are accompanied by renal loss of phosphate. Insulin induces movement of phosphate, glucose, and potassium into cells (56).
5. *Thermal burns*. During recovery from burns, phosphate is shifted into cells and secreted into renal tubules, both of which cause hypophosphatemia.

HYPERPHOSPHATEMIA

The most common cause of hyperphosphatemia is decreased phosphate excretion due to renal failure. In the early stages of a chronic loss of renal function, the remaining nephrons increase excretion of phosphate. Therefore, severe hyperphosphatemia does not occur until renal disease is well advanced and when the glomerular filtration rate is less than 25 ml/min. Other causes of hyperphosphatemia include increased intake of either phosphate or vitamin D and increased breakdown of cells by severe infections, intensive exercise, or neoplastic diseases. Immature lymphoblasts have about 4 times the phosphate content of mature lymphocytes, so patients with lymphoblastic leukemia may develop hyperphosphatemia. Neonates are especially prone to hyperphosphatemia caused by increased intake because they may not have mature PTH and vitamin D metabolism.

On the other hand, in acute renal failure serum phosphate may rise even more rapidly than urea or creatinine. Consequently, serum phosphate should be monitored in acutely ill patients (55, 56).

If renal function is normal, a urinary phosphate excretion above 1500 mg/day suggests hyperphosphatemia caused by chemotherapy, rhabdomyolysis, malignant hyperthermia, or excessive administration of phosphate by enema or intravenous route. A urinary phosphate excretion less than 1500 mg/day with normal renal function suggests some form of hypoparathyroidism (56).

Proper Collection and Handling of Samples

Hemolysis will falsely elevate serum phosphate concentrations, and serum should be removed or separated from cells promptly to avoid intracellular loss of phosphate into the plasma or serum phase. Phosphate concentrations will be slightly lower after meals, so the patient should be fasting before the sample is drawn to obtain an accurate baseline level. Intravenous administration of glucose or fructose lowers serum phosphate by promoting the intracellular shift of phosphate.

Methods for Measurement of Serum Phosphate

Since the 1920s, phosphate has been measured by methods in which molybdate reacts with phosphate to form complex molecules of phosphomolybdate. Fiske and Subbarow used a reducing reagent, 1-amino-2-naphthol-4-sulfonic acid (ANS), to form molybdenum blue, a complex polymer with a high molar absorptivity at 660 nm (58). While utilization of the basic reaction of phosphate with molybdate has remained essentially the same through the years, several different reducing agents have been developed. In addition to ANS, agents used have included stannous chloride (with and without hydrazine) and ferrous ammonium sulfate (59).

Table 17.5. Reference Ranges for Phosphate[a]

	Serum Phosphate[b]	
	mgp/dl	mmol/liter
Newborn (1–2 days)	5.5–9.5	1.78–3.07
Infant	4.5–6.5	1.45–2.10
Child	4.5–5.5	1.45–1.78
Adult male	2.3–3.7	0.74–1.20
Adult female	2.8–4.1	0.90–1.32

[a]Serum phosphate concentrations are relatively high at birth, then decline by 3 to 4 days, about the time the parathyroid gland becomes functional. Adults on an average diet should excrete 0.4–1.3 g of phosphorus per day.
[b]Expressed as phosphorus.

Simonsen showed that the unreduced phosphomolybdate complex has a high absorptivity at 340 nm, and Daly and Ertingshausen optimized this method for centrifugal analysis (59). Garber and Miller proposed a selected method for phosphate in serum that utilizes protein precipitation with semidine HCl as a reducing agent (60). A dry-slide method for phosphate determination utilizes *p*-methylaminophenol sulfate as reducing agent while monitoring light reflection at 680 nm (61). Several enzymatic methods for measuring phosphate have been developed (62) but have not been widely used in clinical laboratory practice. Reference ranges for phosphate are shown in Table 17.5.

References

1. Ringer, S. A further contribution regarding the influence of different constituents of blood on contractions of the heart. J Physiol 1883;4:29–42.
2. McLean FC, Hastings AB. A biological method for the estimation of calcium ion concentration. J Biol Chem 1934;107:337–350.
3. Drop LJ. Ionized calcium, the heart, and hemodynamic function. Anesth Analg 1985;64:432–451.
4. Zaloga GP, Chernow B. Calcium metabolism. In: Geelhoed GW, Chernow B, eds. Endocrine aspects of acute illness. New York: Churchill Livingstone, 1985:169–204.
5. Gray TA, Patterson CR. The clinical value of ionized calcium assays. Ann Clin Biochem 1988;25:210–219.
6. Toffaletti J, Nissenson R, Endres D, et al. Influence of continuous infusion of citrate on responses of immunoreactive PTH, calcium and magnesium components, and other electrolytes in hormal adults during plateletapheresis. J Clin Endocrinol Metab 1985;60:874–879.
7. Toffaletti J, Gitelman HJ, Savory J. Separation and quantitation of serum constituents associated with calcium by gel filtration. Clin Chem 1976;22:1968–1972.
8. Ladenson JM, Lewis JW, Boyd JC. Failure of total calcium corrected for protein, albumin, and pH to correctly assess free calcium status. J Clin Endocrinol Metab 1978;46:986–993.

9. Burritt MF, Pierides AM, Offord KP. Comparative studies of total and ionized serum calcium values in normal subjects and patients with renal disorders. Mayo Clin Proc 1980;55:606–613.
10. Wandrup J. Critical analytical and clinical aspects of ionized calcium in neonates. Clin Chem 1989;35:2027–2033.
11. Desai TK, Geheb MA, Haupt MT, et al. Hypocalcemia in critically ill patients [Abstract]. Chest 1984;86:282.
12. Desai TK, Carlson RW, Thill-Baharozian M, Geheb MA. A direct relationship between ionized calcium and arterial pressure among patients in an intensive care unit. Crit Care Med 1988;16:578–582.
13. Anast CS, Winnacker JL, Forte LF, Burns TW. Impaired release of parathyroid hormone in magnesium deficiency. J Clin Endocrinol Metab 1976;42:707–717.
14. Medalle R, Waterhouse C, Hahn TJ. Vitamin D resistance in magnesium deficiency. Am J Clin Nutrition 1976;29:854–858.
15. Ladenson JH, Lewis JW, McDonald JM, Slatopolsky E, Boyd JC. Relationship of free and total calcium in hypercalcemic conditions. J Clin Endocrinol Metab 1979;48:393–397.
16. Boyd JC, Lewis JW, Slatopolsky E, Ladenson JH. Parathyrin measured concurrently with free or total calcium in the differential diagnosis of hypercalcemia. Clin Chem 1981;27:574–579.
17. Renoe BW, McDonald JM, Ladenson JH. The effects of stasis with and without exercise on free calcium, various cations, and related parameters. Clin Chem Acta 1980;103:91–100.
18. Toffaletti J, Abrams B. Effects of in vivo and in vitro production of lactic acid on ionized, protein-bound, and complex-bound calcium in blood. Clin Chem 1989;35:935–938.
19. Graham G, Schoen I, Johnson L. The effect of specimen choice, collection, processing, and storage on ionized calcium determinations. In: Moran RF, ed. Ionized calcium: its determination and clinical usefulness. Galveston, TX: MVI Publishing, 1986:88–92.
20. Toffaletti J, Blosser N, Kirvan K. Effects of storage temperature and time before centrifugation on ionized calcium in blood collected in plain vacutainers and SST tubes. Clin Chem 1984;30:553–556.
21. Gitelman HJ. An improved automated procedure for the determination of calcium in biological specimens. Anal Biochem 1967;18:521–531.
22. Moorehead WR, Biggs HG. 2-Amino-2-methyl-1-propanol as the alkalizing agent in an improved continuous-flow cresolphthalein complexone procedure for calcium in serum. Clin Chem 1974;20:1458–1460.
23. Toffaletti J. Ionized calcium. In: Pesce AJ, Kaplan LA, eds. Methods in clinical chemistry. St. Louis: CV Mosby, 1987: 1010–1020.
24. Gambling DR, Birmingham CL, Jenkins, LC. Magnesium and the anaesthetist. Can J Anaesth 1988;35:644–654.
25. Altura BM, Altura BT. New perspectives on the role of magnesium in the pathophysiology of the cardiovascular system. I. Clinical aspects. Magnesium 1985;4:226–244.
26. Iseri LT, French JH. Magnesium: nature's physiologic calcium blocker [Editorial]. Am Heart J 1984;108:188–193.
27. Gums JG. Clinical significance of magnesium: a review. Drug Intell Clin Pharm 1987;21:240–246.
28. Turner ET, Osborn JJ, et al. Magnesium and open-heart surgery. J Thorac Cardiovasc Surg 1972;645:695–704.
29. Chernow B, Bamberger S, et al. Hypomagnesemia in patients in postoperative intensive care. Chest 1989;95:391–397.
30. Zaloga GP, Wilkins R, Tourville J, Wood D, Klyme DM. A simplified method for determining physiologically active calcium and magnesium concentrations in critically ill patients. Crit Care Med 1987;15:813–816.
31. Zaloga GP, Chernow B. Divalent ions: calcium, magnesium, and phosphorus. In: Chernow B, ed. The pharmacoligic approach to the critically ill patient, 2nd ed. Baltimore: Williams & Wilkins, 1988:621–627.
32. Toffaletti J, Cooper D, Lobaugh B. The response of parathyroid hormone to specific changes in either ionized calcium, ionized magnesium protein-bound calcium, in humans. Metabolism 1991;8:814–818.
33. Elin RJ. Assessment of magnesium status. Clin Chem 1987;33: 1965–1970.
34. Shils ME. Magnesium in health and disease. Annu Rev Nutrition 1988;8:429–460.
35. Berkelhammer C, Bear RA. A clinical approach to common electrolyte problems: hypomagnesemia. Can Med Assoc J 1985;132:360–368.
36. Brautbar N, Massry SG. Hypomagnesemia and hypermagnesemia. In: Maxwell MH, Kleeman CR, Narins RG, eds. Clinical disorders of fluid and electrolyte metabolism. 4th ed. New York: McGraw Hill, 1987:831–849.
37. Iseri LT, Allen BJ, Brodsky MA. Mg therapy of cardiac arrythmias in critical care medicine. Magnesium 1989;8:299–306.
38. Hanline M. Hypomagnesemia causes coronary artery spasm. JAMA 1985;253:342.
39. Sheehan JP, Seelig MS. Interactions of Mg and K in the pathogenesis of cardiovascular disease. Magnesium 1984;3:301–314.
40. Altura BM, Altura BT. Biochemistry and pathophysiology of CHF: is there a role for Mg? Magnesium 1986;5:134–143.
41. Rude R, Manoogian C, Ehrlich L, et al. Mechanism of BP regulation by Mg in man. Magnesium 1989;8:266–273.
42. Ryan MP. Diuretics and potassium/magnesium depletion: directions for treatment. Ann J Med 1987;82(suppl 3A):38–47.
43. Whang R, Oei To, Watanabe A. Frequency of hypomagnesium in hospitalized patients receiving digitalis. Arch Int Med 1985;145;655–656.
44. June CH, Thompson CB, Kennedy MS. Profound hypomagnesemia and renal magnesium wasting associated with the use of cyclosporine for marrow transplantation. Transplantation 1985;39:620–624.
45. Durlach J, Collery P. Magnesium and potassium in diabetes and carbohydrate metabolism: review of the present status and recent results. Magnesium 1984;3:315–323.
46. Revusova V, Zvara U, Karlikova L, Suchane KB, et al. Prognosis of urolithiasis and nephrocalcinosis in hypomagnesemia. Czech Med 1985;8:207–213.
47. Taylor WM. Low serum magnesium concentration in Paget's disease of bone (osteitis deformans). Ann Clin Biochem 1985;22:591–595.
48. Wills MR, Sunderman FW, Savory J. Methods for estimation of serum magnesium in clinical laboratories. Magnesium 1986;5:317–327.
49. Toffaletti J, Abrams B, Bird C, Schwing M. Clinical validation of an automated thin-film reflectance method for measurement of magnesium in serum and urine. Magnesium 1988;7: 84–90.
50. Farrell EC Jr. Magnesium. In: Pesce AJ, Kaplan LA, eds. Methods in clinical chemistry. St. Louis: CV Mosby, 1987:1021–1026.
51. D'Costa M, Cheng PT. Ultrafiltrable calcium and magnesium in ultrafiltrates of serum prepared with the Amicon MPS-1 System. Clin Chem 1983;29:519–522.
52. Westheimer FM. Why nature chose phosphates. Science 1987;235:1173–1178.
53. Ditzel J. Effect of plasma inorganic phosphate on tissue oxygenation during recovery from diabetic keotacidosis. Adv Exp Med Biol 1973;37A:163–172.

54. King AL, Sica DA, Miller G, Pierpaoli S. Severe hypophosphatemia in a general hospital population. South Med J 1987;80: 831–835.
55. Slatopolsky E, Rutherford WE, Rosenbaum R, et al. Hyperphosphatemia. Clin Nephrol 1977;7:138–146.
56. Chester WL, Zaloga GP, Chernow B. Phosphate problems in the critically-ill patient. In: Geelhoed GW, Chernow B, eds. Endocrine aspects of acute illness. New York: Churchill Livingstone, 1985:205–216.
57. Knochel JP. Hypophosphatemia. Clin Nephrol 1977;7:131–137.
58. Fiske CH, Subbarrow Y. The colorimetric determination of phorphorus. J Biol Chem 1925;66:375–400.
59. Farrell EC Jr. Phosphorus. In: Pesce AJ, Kaplan LA, eds. Methods in clinical chemistry. St. Louis: CV Mosby, 1987: 1038–1042.
60. Garber CC, Miller RC. Revisions of the 1963 semidine HC1 standard method for inorganic phosphorus. Clin Chem 1983;29:184–188.
61. Toffaletti J. Automated dry-film method for phosphorus in serum evaluated. Clin Chem 1985;31:148–149.
62. Adam A, Boulanger J, Azzouzi M, Ers P. Colorimetric versus enzymatic determination of serum phosphorus. Clin Chem 1984;30:1724–1725.

18 Porphyrins, Bilirubin, and Other Bile Pigments

Thomas R. Koch

A series of compounds, collectively termed porphyrins and bile pigments, derive from metabolic pathways involved in synthesis and degradation of heme. These compounds serve as important biochemical markers of various disorders associated with these pathways.

The porphyrins are metal-free tetrapyrroles found in virtually all cells, but in greatest quantities in bone marrow. These compounds apparently have no primary biological function other than to serve as intermediates in the synthesis of heme. However, the metalloporphyrins, such as heme, carry out essential functions in both animals and plants. Porphyrins are pigmented compounds that share the common property of exhibiting fluorescence when exposed to light near 400 nm. The reduced porphyrins, termed porphyrinogens, are colorless but undergo oxidation to the corresponding porphyrins in the presence of molecular oxygen. Measurement of porphyrins and associated bile pigments is usually required in the investigation of various genetic defects affecting heme synthesis pathways.

When hemoglobin is liberated as a result of the degradation of the erythrocyte in the reticuloendothelial system, the molecule is catabolized, resulting in free iron and the waste product bilirubin. Of no value to the body, bilirubin is transported to the liver, conjugated, and excreted via the bile in the stool.

Most compounds that exist only as excretory products receive little attention in clinical medicine. Bilirubin, however, serves as an important marker of diseases involving accelerated erythrocyte destruction, liver disease, certain inherited disorders, and obstructive diseases. Because the clinical indications associated with bilirubin abnormalities are largely distinct from those involving porphyrins and other bile pigments, bilirubin is considered in a separate section from the other compounds in this chapter.

PORPHYRINS AND BILE PIGMENTS

Heme Synthesis and Metabolism

The pathway for biosynthesis of heme is shown in Figure 18.1. The first reaction in this sequence consists of condensation of succinyl CoA with glycine, mediated by the mitochondrial enzyme δ-aminolevulinic acid synthase (ALA synthase, EC 2.3.1.37). This step is rate-limiting in the synthetic sequence; ALA synthase activity is regulated by feedback inhibition of heme. Because this first step in the biosynthetic pathway is rate-limiting, the product δ-aminolevulinic acid (ALA) and subsequent intermediary products are found only in low, steady-state concentrations in normal cells, and consequently normal concentrations of these compounds in body fluids are quite low.

Synthesis of ALA occurs in the mitochondrion, but afterward ALA transfers to the cytoplasm, where two molecules of ALA are condensed with the aid of ALA dehydratase (PBG synthase, EC 4.2.1.24) to form porphobilinogen (PBG). The amino group is removed from the side chain of each of four PBG molecules which are condensed into the intermediate hydroxymethylbilane by PBG deaminase (uroporphyrinogen I synthase, EC 4.3.1.8). In the presence of uroporphyrinogen III cosynthase, hydroxymethylbilane is converted to uroporphyrinogen III. By a minor alternative pathway, hydroxymethylbilane undergoes cyclization to form the functionless uroporphyrinogen I.

Uroporphyrinogen III contains acetic acid groups at positions 1, 3, 5, and 8. In the presence of the cytosolic enzyme uroporphyrinogen III decarboxylase (EC 4.1.1.37), these acetic acid groups are converted to methyl groups forming coproporphyrinogen III, which reenters the mitochondrion. There, the propionic acid groups at positions 2 and 4 are decarboxylated by the action of the enzyme coproporphyrinogen oxidase (EC 1.3.3.3), resulting in vinyl groups at those positions in the compound protoporphyrinogen IX.

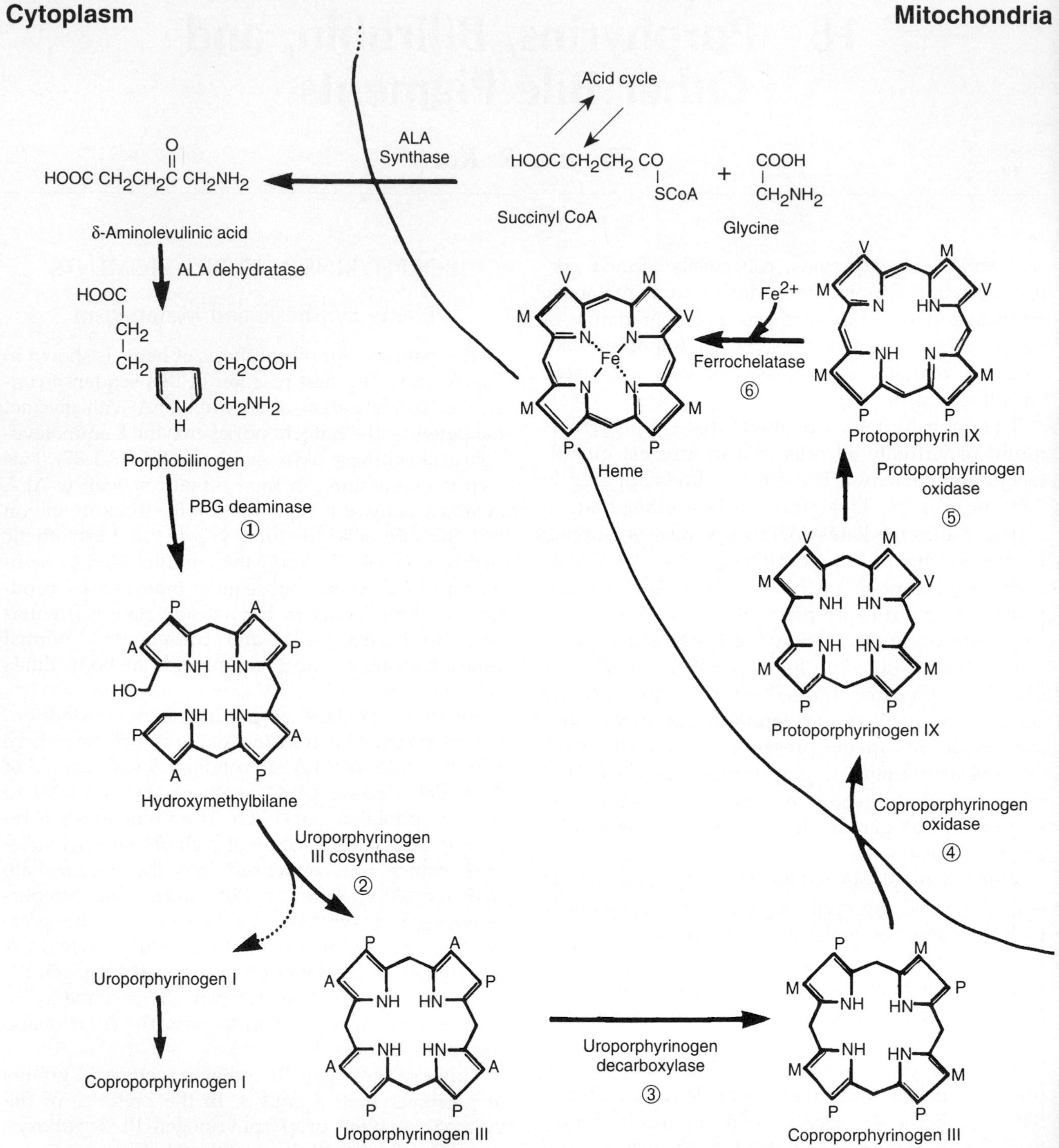

Figure 18.1. Heme biosynthetic pathway. V, vinyl ($-CH{=}CH_2$); M, methyl ($-CH_3$); A, acetyl ($-CH_2COOH$); P, propionyl ($-CH_2CH_2COOH$). Enzymes deficient in the porphyrias are as follows: **1**, Acute intermittent porphyria; **2**, Possible cause of congenital erythropoietic porphyria; **3**, Porphyria cutanea tarda; **4**, Hereditary coproporphyria; **5**, Possible cause of variegate porphyria; **6**, erythropoietic protoporphyria.

Table 18.1. The Porphyrias

Disorder	Primary Diagnostic Tests[a]	Photosensitive?	Neurologic Signs	Latent	Acute Disease Induced by	Approx. Prevalence
Acute intermittent porphyria	PBG, Quant(U)[b] ALA, Quant(U)[b] PBG, Qual(U)[c]	No	May be severe	Yes	Drugs, stress	1:100,000
Variegate porphyria	Protoporphyrin(F)[b] PBG, Quant(U)[c] ALA, Quant(U)[c]	Often	Often	Yes	Sun, drugs, trauma	1:250,000
Hereditary coproporphyria	Copro(U)[b] Copro(F)[b] PBG, Quant(U)[d] ALA, Quant(U)[d]	Occasionally	Mild	Yes	Drugs	<1:250,000
Porphyria cutanea tarda	Uropor(U)[e] Copro(U) Copro(F)	Yes	No	Yes	Liver disease, hypertrichosis	1:25,000
Congenital erythropoeitic porphyria	Uropor(U)[f] Copro(U)[f]	Extreme	No	No	Presents acutely in infancy	<1:1,000,000
Erythropoeitic protoporphyria	Protopor(RBC) Protopor(F)	Mild	No	Yes	Sun	1:200,000

[a]F, fecal; U, urinary.
[b]Consistently elevated.
[c]May be normal between acute attacks.
[d]Elevated during acute attack.
[e]Exceeds coproporphyrin elevation.
[f]Extremely elevated.

The mitochondrial enzyme protoporphyrinogen oxidase catalyzes the oxidation of protoporphyrinogen IX to protoporphyrin IX. Finally, with catalysis by ferrochelatase (EC 4.99.1.1). Fe^{2+} is complexed with protoporphyrin IX to form heme.

Heme synthesis takes place aerobically and mostly in the bone marrow and liver, although it can occur in many cells.

The Porphyrias

A variety of primary disorders of porphyrin metabolism, involving defects of enzymes in the heme synthetic pathway, are known. Each of these disorders is expressed through characteristic symptoms, and accordingly the disorders are classified by the pathologic characteristic of each disease. In addition, disorders of porphyrin metabolism may occur secondary to another primary event or process; secondary causes of porphyria are considered separately.

Primary porphyrias result in either neurological symptoms or cutaneous lesions of varying severity. Because diseases in each of these groupings have certain common characteristics, this classification approach will be followed in preference to other systems (Table 18.1).

NEUROLOGICAL PORPHYRIAS

Three disorders constitute the group of primary porphyrin diseases with significant neurological sequelae: acute intermittent porphyria, variegate porphyria, and hereditary coproporphyria. These diseases have in common the occurrence of acute attacks coincident with increased excretion of the porphyrin precursors characteristic of each disease. The onset may occur over a period of hours to days, and the episode can last for 1 day to several weeks. In all three disorders, δ-aminolevulinic acid and porphobilinogen are substantially increased in urine during the acute attack. Although usually somewhat elevated, the concentration of these compounds may occasionally be within reference ranges between acute attacks.

Neurological symptoms during acute episodes often include abdominal pain, weakness, nausea, and constipation. Other symptoms sometimes seen include excessive perspiration, hypertension, and tachycardia. In about 60% of patients, peripheral neuropathy occurs. At least 75% of acute attacks are precipitated by starvation or by ingestion of alcohol and certain drugs, including steroids (1). These disorders are more common in women than in men; acute attacks may be associated with oral contraceptive agents, the menstrual cycle, or pregnancy. Patients are managed primarily by avoiding factors that tend to precipitate acute attacks.

An additional disorder, termed porphobilinogen synthase deficiency, has recently been described (2) that causes similar symptoms.

Acute Intermittent Porphyria

The autosomal dominant disease called acute intermittent porphyria (AIP) results from four distinct mutants for PBG deaminase. In the most common genotype, patients typically have half the normal erythrocyte PBG deaminase. In the other three, rarer types, defective enzyme function results from (*a*) selective deficiency of the non–erythroid tissue form of the enzyme in the presence of normal concentrations of the erythrocyte form; (*b*) a mutant enzyme that has increased affinity for substrate or low activity toward intermediate complexes; or (*c*) another mutant form of the enzyme that has compromised ability to release the reaction product (1).

With regard to the most common genotype, decreased concentrations of PBG deaminase may be found both in patients with clinical disease and in latent carriers of this gene defect. Most patients with decreased PBG deaminase activity owing to this gene defect never develop porphyria. However, such individuals may be at risk of developing disease if exposed to stimuli associated with the disorder. PBG and ALA are usually elevated in urine, even during latent phases. Unfortunately, PBG deaminase is of limited value in the diagnosis of acute intermittent porphyria.

Abdominal pain is the hallmark symptom of this disorder, and may be accompanied by constipation, diarrhea, nausea, vomiting, and distention. Hyponatremia may be observed either as a result of vomiting or diarrhea, or due to inappropriate ADH secretion. Bladder dysfunction may also be present. Commonly, hypertension and tachycardia are present. Other signs of the peripheral neuropathy of acute intermittent porphyria include weakness, particularly of the extremities, and sometimes symptoms associated with involvement of the optic and cranial nerves. Seizures may occur during an acute attack.

Acute or chronic mental disturbances may be present; patients may be violent, disoriented, depressed, restless, etc., and may be treated for a primary mental illness if the correct diagnosis is not made.

The principal laboratory tests useful in screening for AIP are measurements of ALA and PBG in urine. Whereas tests for ALA are generally quantitative and are most often performed in reference laboratories, many laboratories have used qualitative screening test methods for PBG. The Watson-Schwartz test (3), in which urine is reacted with *p*-dimethylaminobenzaldehyde (Ehrlich's reagent), is simple but is subject to false-positive results. Specificity is improved somewhat by modifications of the Watson-Schwartz test employing extraction with chloroform and *n*-butanol to remove interferences. Specificity is also improved in a commercially available test, in which PBG is isolated with an ion-exchange column prior to the Ehrlich reaction (4). Even in the absence of interfering substances, these qualitative, subjective methods suffer from variable interpretation of the resultant color. It is essential to perform the assay on a known positive PBG control simultaneously with the unknown so that a true positive color reaction is available for comparison.

A test used for initial evaluation for a rare disorder such as AIP must have very high sensitivity for the detection of disease. Although empirical evidence suggests that the Watson-Schwartz test is suitable for detection of the majority of cases of AIP, this author knows of no systematic study of the diagnostic sensitivity of this test when applied to a typical population evaluated for AIP. In any case in which the diagnosis of AIP is seriously considered, quantitative analysis of a timed urine sample for ALA and PBG should be performed, since the sensitivity of the Watson-Schwartz test is uncertain. In questionable cases, repeated tests over a course of several weeks should provide definitive information.

On theoretical grounds, measurement of the deficient enzyme, PBG deaminase, would be expected to provide definitive information for diagnosis. However, levels of PBG deaminase vary widely among normal individuals and with red cell age. Consequently, the range of activities found in normal individuals is wide, overlapping the range found in persons with AIP. Thus, although measurement of PBG deaminase activity may add information to the evaluation of patients for AIP, a normal result does not exclude the diagnosis. Additionally, very few laboratories perform this analysis.

Variegate Porphyria

Unlike many other porphyrias, the precise biochemical defect responsible for variegate prophyria is not known. This disease is believed to be due to a deficiency of protoporphyrinogen oxidase, but it is also possible that a defect of ferrochelatase, different from that which causes erythropoietic porphyria, may be the cause.

Variegate porphyria is an autosomal dominant disorder that can present with variable symptoms: either cutaneous or neurological presentation or a mixed presentation is possible. Most often, patients exhibit symptoms of acute intermittent porphyria at the time of first discovery; chronic cutaneous symptoms are also commonly present, and resemble those in porphyria cutanea tarda. This disorder is most common among Dutch descendants in South Africa; this familial pattern is repeated in other societies as well.

Like acute intermittent porphyria, acute attacks are characterized by excretion of large amounts of δ-aminolevulenic acid and porphobilinogen, but with variegate porphyria normal urinary excretion is common between acute attacks. However, stool protoporphyrin is characteristically increased in patients with variegate porphyria, and this is the key test in laboratory diagnosis. In addition, fecal coproporphyrin and uroporphyrin may also be elevated. The discussion regarding laboratory methodology for diagnosis of acute intermittent porphyria also applies here; in fact, due to the frequent finding of normal urinary concentrations between acute attacks, the use of qualitative screening tests in suspected cases of variegate porphyria cannot be encouraged.

Hereditary Coproporphyria

A decreased tissue content of coproporphyrinogen oxidase is the cause of hereditary coproporphyria, a disorder with autosomal dominant inheritance. Symptoms of this disease resemble a mild manifestation of the more common acute intermittent porphyria, except that patients with hereditary coproporphyria may also experience photosensitivity.

Abdominal pain is the most common symptom; other symptoms of acute intermittent porphyria are present with similar frequency. Hepatic function is generally not impaired. As with AIP, many individuals apparently inherit this enzyme defect but never experience clinical disease. The onset is usually after puberty.

The characteristic laboratory finding in hereditary coproporphyria is increased excretion of coproporphyrin in urine and in stool. Stool protoporphyrin is normal or mildly elevated. Excretion in urine of δ-aminolevulinic acid and porphobilinogen is often normal in these patients, but these compounds are excreted in excess along with uroporphyrin during acute attacks.

Because erythrocytes lack mitochondria, assay of the enzyme deficient in this disorder requires preparation of enriched leukocytes from the buffy coat, or another cellular preparation for analysis. When, rarely, the enzyme assay is used in diagnosis, the activity is about half that found in normal subjects. Carriers of the enzyme defect who do not develop clinical disease exhibit similar reductions in activity.

CUTANEOUS PORPHYRIAS

Although two of the porphyrias classified as neurological diseases sometimes exhibit cutaneous symptoms (photosensitivity), three diseases have been identified for which photosensitivity is the dominant clinical observation: porphyria cutanea tarda, erythropoietic protoporphyria, and congenital erythropoietic porphyria. The degree of skin damage varies markedly between these disorders. Whereas the neurological porphyrias have in common the occurrence of acute attacks, which usually lead to initial diagnosis, the cutaneous porphyrias are chronic diseases that tend to be discovered early in life.

The occurrence of photosensitivity is related to the presence in the skin of elevated concentrations of porphyrins. Elevated blood concentrations of porphyrins are observed in the cutaneous porphyrias. Plasma screening tests for porphyrins may therefore be useful in excluding these diseases from the differential diagnosis of patients with hypersensitivity of the skin.

Porphyria Cutanea Tarda

The most common porphyria, porphyria cutanea tarda (PCT), is caused by a decrease in uroporphyrinogen decarboxylase in tissues. The disease is most common in the elderly and in men, and almost always occurs in a sporadic manner (although some causes of familial inheritance have been described). Porphyria cutanea tarda is often found in association with liver disease; a history of significant alcohol abuse is common to most cases. PCT is also found in association with other diseases: uremia, diabetes mellitus, and certain immunologic disorders. Iron overload and excessive hepatic iron stores are often present. Other factors that have been associated with development of PCT include estrogen therapy and exposure to chlorinated hydrocarbons.

Patients with porphyria cutanea tarda develop cutaneous lesions on areas of the skin exposed to the sun—the face, dorsa of the hands, forearms, and the legs and feet in women. These lesions may not develop immediately after sun exposure.

Deposition of porphyrins in the cytoplasm of hepatocytes is common, as is impaired liver function, evidenced by elevations of transaminases and γ-glutamyl transferase.

Skin lesions and other clinical findings are characteristic but not pathognomonic of porphyria cutanea tarda, so laboratory tests fulfill a confirmatory role. Measurements of porphyrin precursors are usually normal; however, these tests may be helpful in differentiating PCT from variegate porphyria, which has similar skin lesions and in which the precursors are elevated.

Measurements of urinary and stool coproporphyrin are elevated in porphyria cutanea tarda. Elevations of uroporphyrin in urine are also found, exceeding the elevation of coproporphyrin. Additionally, protoporphyrin in stool is elevated. These elevations result from increased concentrations of certain isomers of porphyrins in this disease: 7-carboxylate porphyrin (measured as uroporphyrin), 5-carboxylate porphyrin (measured as coproporphyrin), and other isomers are present, but analysis of isomeric composition is not necessary for the diagnosis.

The possible role of the analysis of uroporphyrinogen decarboxylase in the diagnosis of patients with porphyria cutanea tarda is unclear. It is generally agreed that patients with familial PCT consistently have reduced activity of the enzyme in tissues, cultured skin fibroblasts, and erythrocytes. However, most presentations of PCT are sporadic, and in these cases erythrocyte enzyme activities often appear normal. Enzyme deficiency in erythrocytes has not consistently been demonstrated in porphyria caused by chlorinated hydrocarbon exposure. Therefore porphyrin measurements in urine, stool, and plasma must be combined with clinical observation for the diagnosis of porphyria cutanea tarda.

Congenital Erythropoietic Porphyria

This very rare disease is characterized by excretion of unusual quantities of type I porphyrins rather than the usual type III isomers. This is thought to be due to a deficiency of uroporphyrinogen III cosynthase, but definitive proof is lacking.

Congenital erythropoietic porphyria (CEP) is usually discovered soon after birth because patients excrete red-pigmented urine, although some individuals have first been diagnosed as adults. Intravascular hemolysis occurs to a variable extent. Severe skin photosensitivity begins at an early age, resulting in blistering lesions that may rupture and become infected. Fine hair may cover much of the skin, which becomes scarred with age due to repeated injury. Some patients develop blindness. Patients with this disorder have decreased life expectancy due to the risk of infection and sequelae of the disease.

Because of the early and severe presentation of most patients with this rare disease, it is a diagnosis that is seldom considered in most patients evaluated for porphyrias. Urinary excretion of uroporphyrin and coproporphyrin is extremely high—sometimes over 100 times normal. The type I isomers constitute most of the porphyrins excreted, although the type III isomers may be somewhat elevated. Additionally, stool coproporphyrin I excretion is quite elevated. Urine color is typically reddish to dark red and plasma porphyrin concentration is also elevated.

Erythropoietic Protoporphyria

Erythropoietic protoporphyria is probably caused by deficiency of ferrochelatase. Symptoms of this disease vary greatly in severity. Some individuals may not experience photosensitivity, but many patients are moderately sensitive to sunlight and experience symptoms including itching, inflammation, redness, and swelling of exposed areas of the skin. Severe scarring is not seen.

Elevated levels of protoporphyrin may be detected in erythrocytes and stool. Most of the protoporphyrin is present as the free form, not as the usual zinc chelate. Urine porphyrins and porphyrin precursors are normal.

Laboratory methods that measure "free erythrocyte protoporphyrin" are suitable for use in the evaluation of patients for erythropoietic protoporphyria. However, it is not appropriate to use methods that directly measure the fluorescence of blood (hematofluorometery). This approach, intended for measuring protoporphyrin elevations in the detection of lead poisoning, predominantly measures the zinc chelate of protoporphyrin and underestimates the concentration of free protoporphyrin.

Because ferrochelatase is a mitochondrial enzyme, attempts to measure enzyme activity in blood require preparation of a buffy coat to enrich the population of leukocytes. Additionally, direct analysis of this enzyme is technically difficult. Because of the ease of performing protoporphyrin analysis and the high specificity of this test in symptomatic patients, enzyme analysis is rarely used in diagnosis of this disorder.

Secondary Disorders of Porphyrin Metabolism

LEAD POISONING

At concentrations encountered in patients with clinical effects of lead poisoning, two steps in the heme synthetic pathway are interfered with by lead: ALA dehydratase is inhibited, and the incorporation of iron by ferrochelatase is incomplete (likely due to inadequate iron transport). In consequence, the substrates of these enzymes, δ-aminolevulinic acid and protoporphyrin, are increased in lead poisoning. Additionally, coproporphyrin is often elevated in urine in lead poisoning; however, this is an insensitive diagnostic test and coproporphyrin measurements are not recommended for the detection or monitoring of lead poisoning.

Urinary measurement of ALA is a quite sensitive indicator of lead poisoning. However, the difficulty of collecting accurate 24-hour urine specimens from young children who are outpatients precludes the widespread use of this test.

Measurement of protoporphyrin in the erythrocyte (present predominantly in the form of the zinc chelate) was until recently an important test for population screening for lead poisoning, and is used by some physicians for monitoring treated patients. The U.S. Centers for Disease Control and Prevention has now established 10 μg/dl as the maximum acceptable blood lead concentration in unexposed individuals. Measurement of zinc protoporphyrin is not sufficiently sensitive to detect lead poisoning at this threshold, although the test is still useful in monitoring therapy for lead poisoning.

OTHER SECONDARY DISORDERS

Various forms of liver disease can cause increased excretion of porphyrins in the urine. Most commonly, only coproporphyrin elevations are seen, and generally no clinical signs or symptoms associated with primary porphyrias occur. This is also the case in some patients with hemolytic diseases.

In Dubin-Johnson syndrome (see Bilirubin), the presence of large amounts of δ-aminolevulinic acid results in increased biliary excretion of protoporphyrin and decreased excretion of coproporphyrin III.

Rarely, hepatic tumors elaborate excess porphyrins. Interestingly, patients with porphyria cutanea tarda are at increased risk for hepatocellular carcinoma.

Another disorder related to porphyrin metabolism is hereditary tyrosinemia; succinylacetone, a byproduct of the degradation of tyrosine, inhibits ALA dehydratase. Patients with hereditary tyrosinemia exhibit symptoms resembling those with acute intermittent porphyria, among them abdominal pain and increased urinary ALA.

Protoporphyrin may be elevated secondary to various diseases involving the heme system. These include iron deficiency, sideroblastic anemia, secondary polycythemia, and any cause of excessive erythrocyte destruction.

Laboratory Tests for Porphyrin Disorders

TESTING FOR PORPHOBILINOGEN IN URINE

Screening Tests

The classic method for screening for porphobilinogen in urine is the Watson-Schwartz test (3), in which porphobilinogen is reacted with *p*-dimethylaminobenzaldehyde (Ehrlich's reagent) to yield a magenta product. The product is extracted into chloroform and re-extracted into *n*-butanol to improve specificity. Some authors recommend performing the Hoesch test (3) in positive cases, to increase specificity. This test employs the same reagent but is not interfered with by urobilinogen.

Lamon et al. (5) reported the limit of detection of the Watson-Schwartz and Hoesch tests for PBG to be approximately 9 mg/liter. However, when Schreiber et al. (6) submitted unknowns to four laboratories using the Watson-Schwartz method, none detected porphobilinogen at concentrations below 25 mg/liter. These detection limits (compared to the usual reference interval for porphobilinogen of less than 1.0 mg/day) are sufficient only for the detection of acute intermittent porphyria during an acute episode.

Another modification uses an anion-exchange column for isolation of porphobilinogen prior to reaction (4), which probably results in improved specificity.

Schreiber et al. (6) recently described an ion-exchange method for porphobilinogen with improved sensitivity. The method was able to identify two patients with acute intermittent porphyria in the latent phase; both tested negative with the Watson-Schwartz method.

In all of these qualitative screening tests, the colored product is subjectively judged as positive or negative. Since true positive results are rare, it is essential to run a negative urine and a urine sample supplemented with porphobilinogen as negative and positive controls. The positive control should be at a concentration near the desired limit of detection for the test method. Samples with equivocal results must be retested using a quantitative method.

Quantitative Measurement

Most methods for quantitative measurement of porphobilinogen in urine employ chromatographic isolation followed by reaction with Ehrlich's reagent. For example, the method of Moore and Labbe (7) has found widespread acceptance. A method employing anion exchange for the isolation of PBG is commercially available (4).

MEASUREMENT OF PORPHYRINS IN URINE

Because porphyrins are strongly fluorescent, it is often possible to detect elevations of porphyrins in urine merely by examining the urine under an ultraviolet light. Direct spectrophotometric analysis can also be performed. However, these approaches are neither sensitive nor specific, because the presence of many other compounds can result in nonspecific fluorescence or absorption or in the quenching of fluorescence from porphyrins.

Quantitative methods generally employ solvent extraction from acidified urine or anion-exchange column separation, followed by fluorometric or spectrophotometric measurement. The method of Westerlund et al. (8) is an example of such methods.

A simple screening test is commercially available (4) that employs an anion-exchange column to exclude many possible interfering compounds. A similar method is available for quantitative measurement of porphyrins.

MEASUREMENT OF δ-AMINOLEVULINIC ACID IN URINE

Reliable measurement of δ-aminolevulinic acid in urine requires chromatographic separation of the analyte from other compounds, especially porphobilinogen. The isolated ALA is reacted with acetylacetone or a related compound to form a pyrrole, which is then reacted with Ehrlich's reagent. At least one version of this method is commercially available (4).

MEASUREMENT OF PROTOPORPHYRIN IN BLOOD

The method of Chisholm (9) or of Piomelli (10) is usually employed to test for protoporphyrin in blood. Protoporphyrin is extracted in the presence of acid, which dissociates zinc from the porphyrin molecule (thus, the measure resulting from such methods is termed "free erythrocyte protoporphyrin"). Measurement of fluorescence in the acid extract provides a measure of the protoporphyrin concentration.

Direct measurement of protoporphyrin in blood can be accomplished using a simple, direct-reading instrument called a hematofluorometer. This approach provides a simple measure of zinc protoporphyrin. It is important to appreciate that such an approach is not appropriate for use in evaluating patients for porphyrias, in which conditions excess porphyrin may be present in the free state. It should be noted that some laboratories employing the hematofluorometer express results as "free erythrocyte protoporphyrin," although only the zinc chelate is actually measured.

BILIRUBIN

Bilirubin Production and Elimination

PRODUCTION FROM HEMOGLOBIN

Of the 250 to 400 mg of bilirubin formed in the body daily, about three-fourths is derived from the degradation of hemoglobin. Other hemoproteins, including catalase, cytochrome P-450, myoglobin and others, contribute the remainder. None of these sources is known to contribute significantly to bilirubin concentrations in disease.

In the cells of the reticuloendothelial system, microsomal heme oxygenase in the presence of NADH and oxygen catalyzes the oxidation of Fe^{2+} in heme to Fe^{3+} (Fig. 18.2). The resulting compound, termed α-hydroxyhemin, is oxidized nonenzymatically by molecular oxygen. The iron atom is removed and enters the iron pool for reuse. The α-methine carbon is converted to carbon monoxide, the ring is opened, and a green pigment called biliverdin is produced. In the presence of NADH, the enzyme biliverdin reductase catalyzes the reduction of biliverdin to bilirubin.

The compound commonly referred to as "bilirubin" is the predominant of several isomers that exist in bile. The IX-α isomer, derived from protoporphyrin IX, constitutes 99.5% of the bilirubin produced. Isomers other than the IX-α are found in trace quantities, and are of no known importance. In the acid form (pK is near neutral pH) bilirubin has a very low water solubility (approximately 10^{-14} mol/liter), owing to the molecule's extensive intramolecular hydrogen bonding.

TRANSPORT TO THE LIVER

Bilirubin is transported to the liver in the form of a reversible ionic complex with albumin. Albumin has one high-affinity binding site ($K = 5.9 \times 10^7$) capable of binding one molecule of bilirubin in the di-anionic form to each molecule of albumin. Binding at this site is responsible for the transport of bilirubin to the liver. In principle bilirubin may also be bound at other sites, but these are of little practical significance since binding is weak and bilirubin is more readily displaced by other anions than at the primary binding site.

One other form of bilirubin-albumin complex has been described in which bilirubin is covalently bound to albumin. This fraction has been given several names, including "biliprotein" and the "δ" fraction of bilirubin. In the absence of a consensus regarding naming, the term "bili-albumin" will be used here. Bili-albumin is normally present at very low concentrations but can be a significant fraction of total bilirubin during and following obstructive liver disease.

Other anions can compete with bilirubin for the primary binding site on albumin, or may bind at a different location but nevertheless displace bilirubin. These include certain contrast media, sulfonamides, and salicylate and other anti-inflammatory drugs. Binding may also be disrupted by high concentrations of fatty acids.

UPTAKE BY THE LIVER AND EXCRETION

In the liver, bilirubin dissociates from albumin and enters the hepatocyte. The mechanism of removal from albumin and entry into the hepatocyte has not been completely characterized, but it is known to be saturable, is not entirely specific (in that some other

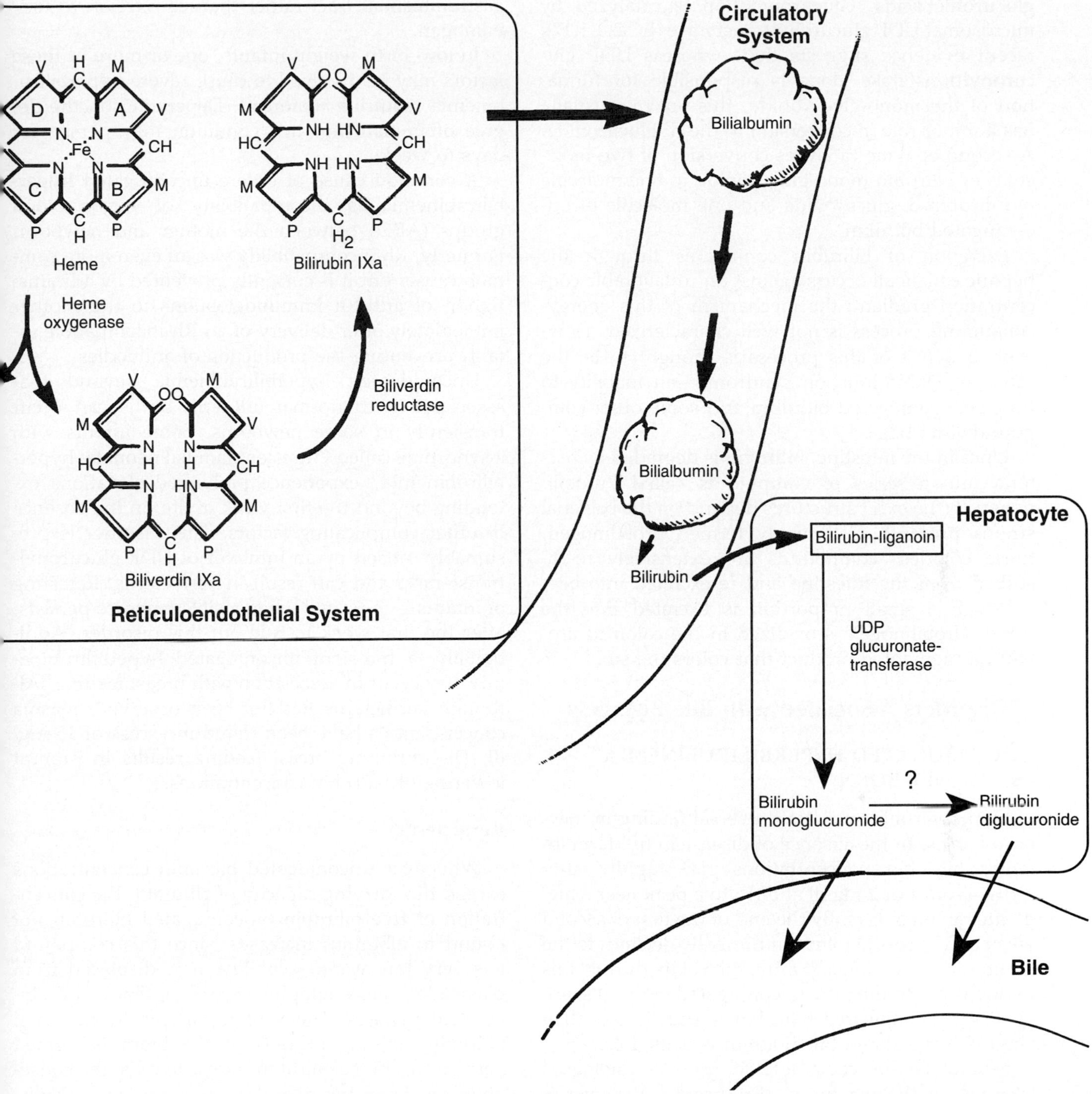

Figure 18.2. Bilirubin biosynthesis. V, vinyl (–CH=CH$_2$); M, methyl (–CH$_3$); A, acetyl (–CH$_2$COOH); P, propionyl (–CH$_2$CH$_2$COOH).

organic anions compete with bilirubin for hepatic uptake), and may be mediated by a carrier protein.

After removal from plasma, bilirubin is stored in the hepatocyte until its subsequent elimination in bile. In the cytosol of the hepatocyte, bilirubin is bound to a major cytoplasmic protein called ligandin. (Ligandin binds bilirubin more weakly than albumin; this and other evidence support the suggestion that ligandin does not have a primary role in the extraction of bilirubin from plasma).

While in the hepatocyte, bilirubin is metabolized into forms that are more polar and thus more water soluble. This conversion is essential for excretion of bilirubin. Esterification of one or both of the propionic acid functional groups with glucuronic acid results in the formation of bilirubin mono- and di-glucuronic acids. Glucuronidation is catalyzed by microsomal UDP glucuronyltransferase (EC 2.4.1.17); recent evidence suggests that, whereas UDP glucuronyltransferase alone is responsible for formation of the mono-glucuronide, this enzyme usually has a minor role in conversion to the di-glucuronide. A second enzyme catalyzes conversion of two molecules of bilirubin mono-glucuronide to one molecule of bilirubin di-glucuronide and one molecule of unconjugated bilirubin.

Excretion of bilirubin conjugates through the hepatic canaliculi occurs against an unfavorable concentration gradient; the mechanism of this energy-consuming process is not well characterized. However, a defect of this process is thought to be the cause of Dubin-Johnson syndrome—an inability to transport conjugated bilirubin and some other compounds into bile.

Once in the intestine, bilirubin is degraded by bacteria into a series of compounds called "urobilinogens" (the exact structures depend on the bacterial strains present). Collectively termed urobilinogen, these colorless compounds are extensively re-absorbed from the intestine and re-excreted into bile, although a small proportion is excreted into the urine. Urobilinogen is oxidized in the colon to urobilin, a pigmented product that colors the stool.

Disorders Associated with Bile Pigments

UNCONJUGATED HYPERBILIRUBINEMIA IN THE NEWBORN

Hyperbilirubinemia is a universal finding in newborn babies. In the absence of disease in full-term infants, bilirubin concentrations rise rapidly after birth—from 1 or 2 mg/dl at birth to a peak near 6 mg/dl after about 3 days. By the end of the first or second week of life, serum bilirubin normally declines to the adult reference range. Serum bilirubin during this period is predominantly unconjugated in the absence of disease; conjugated bilirubin is usually less than about 0.3 mg/dl and bili-albumin is negligible.

Several factors contribute to this "physiological jaundice of the newborn." Erythrocyte turnover is accelerated in the newborn, resulting in an increased bilirubin load being presented to the liver for conjugation and excretion. Uptake of bilirubin by the liver is decreased at birth. Additionally, the fetal liver is deficient in UDP glucuronyltransferase at birth, although adult levels of this enzyme are reached within a few days.

In addition to these factors, bilirubin may be elevated in the newborn due to delayed canalicular excretion, and due to the lack of intestinal bacteria, resulting in increased absorption of bilirubin from the gastrointestinal tract rather than conversion to urobilinogen.

In low–birth weight infants, one or more of these factors may be involved to cause severe hyperbilirubinemia requiring treatment. Depending on the degree of immaturity, this condition may persist for days to weeks.

A common cause of severe unconjugated hyperbilirubinemia is incompatibility of major blood groups (ABO) between the mother and newborn. Formerly, Rh incompatibility was an even more common cause, but it is currently prevented by administration of anti-Rh immunoglobulins to the mother immediately after delivery of an Rh-incompatible infant, preventing the production of antibodies.

Unconjugated hyperbilirubinemia beyond that associated with normal full-term births can occur transiently in some newborns. Some infants with a syndrome called "transient familial neonatal hyperbilirubinemia" experience prolonged elevations extending beyond the first week of life, in the absence of other complicating factors. This disorder is presumably caused by an inhibitor of UDP glucuronyltransferase, and can result in kernicterus. Retesting of infants is indicated when visible jaundice persists, after the first week to rule out this disorder. Additionally, a transient unconjugated hyperbilirubinemia may occur in association with breast feeding. Although kernicterus has not been observed, plasma concentrations have been found in excess of 15 mg/dl. Discontinuing breast feeding results in prompt lowering of bilirubin concentrations.

Kernicterus

Whenever unconjugated bilirubin concentrations exceed the carrying capacity of albumin, the concentration of free bilirubin (unconjugated bilirubin not bound to albumin) increases; since this compound has very low water solubility, it is displaced from plasma into more lipophilic matrices, that is, into intracellular spaces. This is of importance in the brain; bilirubin staining of cells of the brain is termed kernicterus. Since bilirubin is toxic to cells, the consequence is brain injury and, in extreme cases, death.

Classically plasma bilirubin concentrations above 20 mg/dl are considered to represent significant risk of kernicterus. However, it is now recognized that this limit is too high for premature infants. In the presence of lowered plasma pH, increased free fatty acids, or certain drugs that compete for binding, kernicterus can occur at concentrations as low as 12 mg/dl in low–birth weight infants.

Phototherapy (exposure of the infant to high-intensity visible light) is commonly used to lower plasma bilirubin concentrations—a procedure that takes advantage of the photosensitivity of bilirubin. The products of irradiation of bilirubin, various photoisomers of the compound, are more water soluble than bilirubin and are rapidly excreted. (Isomers resulting from irradiation of bilirubin do not interfere with commonly used methods for bilirubin measurement). In extreme cases in which phototherapy is unsuccessful in preventing the rise of bilirubin in plasma to dangerous levels, exchange transfusions can be used to rapidly remove bilirubin from the circulation.

EXCESSIVE PRODUCTION OF UNCONJUGATED BILIRUBIN

A common cause of unconjugated hyperbilirubinemia is excessive producton of bilirubin, resulting in a bilirubin burden exceeding the capacity of the liver for uptake, conjugation, and excretion. Regardless of the mechanism, hyperbilirubinemia is generally mild except in the event of liver failure.

Hemolytic conditions are frequently associated with unconjugated hyperbilirubinemia; causes include sickle cell anemia, drug reactions, and hereditary spherocytosis. Additionally, ineffective erythropoiesis in hematological disorders such as thalassemia can be associated with elevations of unconjugated bilirubin. Usual bilirubin concentrations in these conditions are in the range of 2 to 4 mg/dl, but higher concentrations can occur.

GILBERT'S SYNDROME

A relatively common disorder diagnosed in young adults, Gilbert's syndrome is typically detected as a result of mild icterus with unknown cause, icterus secondary to fasting or carbohydrate restriction or to administration of certain drugs, or as an incidental finding upon biochemical screening.

The prevalence of Gilbert's syndrome in the general population has been estimated as high as 5%. However, due to the asymptomatic nature of the disorder and the small degree of plasma bilirubin elevation, many individuals with Gilbert's syndrome go undiagnosed.

Presumably Gilbert's syndrome results from defects in hepatic uptake and/or conjugation of unconjugated bilirubin. It is likely that the syndrome consists of several distinct but similar disorders of differing etiologies. Bilirubin concentrations in the plasma of patients with Gilbert's syndrome fluctuate with time and under the influence of a variety of factors, including illness, exertion, stress, administration of drugs that induce the microsomal enzyme system, and fasting.

Gilbert's syndrome is usually diagnosed by elimination of other causes of mild jaundice in an otherwise healthy adult. Absolute confirmation of the syndrome is often not attempted, since the disorder is essentially harmless. Diagnostic protocols have been proposed involving a 48-hour fast, or administration of nicotinic acid to induce a rise in plasma bilirubin, but both are of limited value. Liver biopsy is usually not considered justified. An increased proportion of bilirubin monoglucuronide in the bile of subjects with Gilbert's syndrome has been reported, but this measurement is rarely available and requires an invasive procedure for sample collection.

CRIGLER-NAJJAR SYNDROME

Two distinct syndromes resulting from absence or partial deficiency of UDP glucuronyltransferase in the liver are termed Crigler-Najjar syndrome types I and II. Both disorders are rare.

Fewer than 100 patients have been reported with Crigler-Najjar syndrome type I. This disorder, usually fatal in infancy, is caused by the absence of UDP glucuronyltransferase. Occasional patients survive beyond infancy, but death (caused by kernicterus) occurs in childhood in virtually all cases.

Transmission is by autosomal recessive inheritance and is common in families with consanguinity. There is no association with any race.

Serum bilirubin concentrations exceed 20 mg/dl and may be as high as 50 mg/dl. All of the serum bilirubin is unconjugated. However, nonspecific methods for conjugated (or "direct") bilirubin may falsely indicate the presence of conjugated bilirubin. Bilirubin is not detected in the urine.

The lives of some patients with Crigler-Najjar syndrome type I have been extended by one or more therapeutic modalities: exchange transfusion, phototherapy, and plasmapheresis. Because of several factors, principally increased skin thickness, phototherapy is of decreasing effectiveness with older children.

Crigler-Najjar syndrome type II is a distinct disorder characterized by reduced but measurable UDP glucuronyltransferase in the liver and by a benign course. Serum bilirubin is often over 10 but usually below 20 mg/dl and again is entirely composed of unconjugated bilirubin. Urine bilirubin is negative.

Crigler-Najjar syndrome type II exhibits a pattern of occurrence within families, but a specific mode of inheritance has not been elucidated.

Patients with Crigler-Najjar syndrome type II usually do not experience neurological symptoms or adverse effects from the disease. It has been speculated that this disorder might be better classified as a more severe form of Gilbert's syndrome. The exact etiology is unknown.

DUBIN-JOHNSON SYNDROME

Dubin-Johnson syndrome, an autosomal recessive disorder of unknown etiology, is characterized by mild jaundice caused by elevated conjugated bilirubin. Total bilirubin concentrations are sometimes normal but usually mildly elevated (less than 5 mg/dl). However, greater elevations are occasionally observed, especially in conjunction with stress such as pregnancy or illness. Some medications, including oral contraceptives, may exacerbate the usual mild jaundice. The disease is usually first discovered after puberty. Patients experience few if any symptoms from this disease.

The liver of Dubin-Johnson syndrome patients is black, owing to the accumulation of an unidentified pigment in the hepatocyte. Despite the presence of this pigment, hepatocytes appear functionally normal. However, organic anion excretion follows an abnormal pattern, indicating delayed release from the hepatocyte. Additionally, coproporphyrin excretion in the urine is reduced to about half normal, and the proportion of coproporphyrin I to coproporphyrin III is greatly altered. The latter pattern can be useful in the differential diagnosis of Dubin-Johnson syndrome.

ROTOR'S SYNDROME

Once considered a form of Dubin-Johnson syndrome, Rotor's syndrome is a rare disorder characterized by conjugated hyperbilirubinemia. Unlike in Dubin-Johnson syndrome, the appearance of the liver is normal. Excretion of organic anions is prolonged. Urinary excretion of coproporphyrin is somewhat increased.

The etiology of Rotor's syndrome is unknown. Some evidence suggests the disease follows an autosomal recessive inheritance.

LIVER DISEASE

Disease processes either within the liver or causing obstruction of the common bile duct lead to elevated bilirubin in serum. Gross obstruction of the bile duct causes backup of bile in the canaliculi of the liver. As a result, bilirubin (primarily conjugated) and other components of bile are released into the blood stream. Common causes of obstructive disease include inflammation of the gallbladder, cancer or other disease of the head of the pancreas, and strictures secondary to abdominal surgery.

Similar consequences result from intrahepatic diseases that culminate in inflammation and swelling. Flow of bile through the bile canaliculi is restricted, resulting in increased conjugated bilirubin in blood. In both intrahepatic and posthepatic jaundice, bili-albumin as well as conjugated bilirubin are elevated in serum. Additionally, bilirubin is present at elevated concentrations in urine. Following removal of the cause of flow restriction, clinical jaundice persists beyond the time when urine bilirubin returns to normal. This is the result of elevated blood concentrations of bili-albumin, which has the same half-life as albumin.

Measurement of Bilirubin

In the normal adult, up to about 1 mg/dl of bilirubin is found in plasma. Most of this bilirubin consists of unconjugated bilirubin resulting from erythrocyte destruction. Only trace concentrations of conjugated bilirubin and bili-albumin are found in normal plasma. Laboratory methods need to be capable of measuring unconjugated bilirubin concentrations between 0.1 and 1 mg/dl, conjugated bilirubin concentrations near 0.1 mg/dl, and total bilirubin concentrations near the critical decision limits in neonates in the range of 10 to 20 mg/dl.

TOTAL BILIRUBIN

Direct Photometric Measurement

Bilirubin is a pigment with maximum absorption near 455 nm in aqueous solution. Although the various forms do not have identical spectra, molar absorptivities at 455 nm are similar, so that the absorbance at this wavelength can be used as a basis for total bilirubin quantitation.

Direct photometry is used, however, only for measurements in newborn infants. In children and adults, due to the consumption of solid foods, a number of other pigments are present that invalidate direct photometric measurements of total bilirubin. These pigments include carotenoids, and perhaps bilifuscin and mesobilifuscin.

Hemolysis is present in a substantial proportion of blood specimens obtained by heelstick from newborns. Oxyhemoglobin also absorbs light at 455 nm, and thus is a potential source of interference. Direct spectrophotometric methods must include a measurement at a second wavelength (typically 575 nm) to estimate the hemoglobin concentration. This is then used to correct the measured absorbance at 455 nm for the contribution due to hemoglobin.

Bilirubin measurements with this approach are quite accurate as long as the spectrophotometer used has high wavelength and absorbance accuracy.

Alternatively, dedicated instruments ("bilirubinometers") may be used for direct spectrophotometric estimation of total bilirubin in serum. Although such instruments are capable of accurate measurements, frequent recalibration, linearity checks, and regular quality control are required.

Methods Employing the Diazo Reaction

Bilirubin undergoes coupling with diazo compounds to form two isomeric pigments collectively termed "azobilirubin." In acidic solution the pigment is red (absorbing at 540 nm); in strong acid or alkaline solution azobilirubin turns blue (absorption at 600 nm). Conjugated bilirubin reacts rapidly with reagents that promote coupling, but unconjugated bilirubin requires the addition of a chemical agent termed an "accelerator" to promote its reaction.

A wide variety of diazo methods are available, differing in reagent formulation, reaction conditions, and measurement wavelength. The reference method (11) (modified from that of Jendrassik and Grof) employs diazotized sulfanilic acid; caffeine and sodium benzoate serve as accelerators, and measurement is performed at 600 nm in alkaline solution. This method is virtually free from hemoglobin interference, provides equivalent reactivity for all bilirubin fractions, and is thoroughly characterized. Some diazo methods, particularly those that perform measurement at acidic pH, are susceptible to interference from hemoglobin and are poorly documented with regard to accuracy. Some methods exhibit a bias caused by matrix differences between calibrator and quality control materials and fresh human serum.

Reagents for diazotization are usually prepared shortly before their use, since many such reagents are unstable. Various attempts have been made to stabilize diazo reagents, often by the use of compounds other than sulfanilic acid. It is important to realize that diazonium compounds may be chemically unstable and have explosive potential in the dry state.

BILIRUBIN FRACTIONS

Traditionally, analysts have exploited the relatively slow reaction of unconjugated bilirubin with diazotization reagents to attempt measurement of conjugated bilirubin. When serum is reacted in the absence of an accelerator for a fixed time between 1 and 10 minutes, the resultant concentration, termed "direct" bilirubin, is an estimate of the conjugated bilirubin and bili-albumin concentration.

The limitations of this approach have recently been clarified (12). Seventy-five percent or less of the conjugated bilirubin present is measured by this approach; additionally, some unconjugated bilirubin (usually more than 5% of the amount present) reacts under these conditions. Thus the "direct" bilirubin is a crude measure only of the conjugated bilirubin and bili-albumin concentrations in serum. Estimates are especially inaccurate in the presence of high concentrations of unconjugated bilirubin.

A recent approach employing measurement by reflectance photometry on thin-film slides permits accurate measurement of unconjugated and conjugated bilirubin concentrations (13). When these species are bound to a mordant in a film layer, they may be differentiated and quantitated spectraphotometrically.

Bili-albumin, usually measured by high-performance liquid chromatography, is seldom measured in clinical laboratories due to its limited clinical value. The bili-albumin concentration may be estimated with the thin-film approach, as the difference between a diazo-based measure of total bilirubin and the sum of conjugated and unconjugated fractions. Additionally, a method has been described based on separation of diazotized biliprotein from other fractions using anion-exchange chromatography (14).

References

1. Elder GH, Smith SG, Smyth SJ. Laboratory investigation of the porphyrias. Ann Clin Biochem 1990;27:395–412.
2. Doss M. Enzymatic deficiencies in acute hepatic porphyrias: porphobilinogen synthase deficiency. Semin Dermatol 1985;5:161.
3. Labbe RF, Lamon JM. Porphyrins and disorders of porphyrin metabolism. In: Tietz NW, ed. Textbook of clinical chemistry. Philadelphia: WB Saunders, 1986.
4. Biorad Laboratories, Hercules, CA.
5. Lamon JM, Frykholm BC, Tschudy DP. Screening tests in acute porphyria. Arch Neurol 1977;34:709–712.
6. Schreiber WE, Jamani A, Pudek MR. Screening tests for porphobilinogen are insensitive. Am J Clin Pathol 1989;92:644–649.
7. Moore DJ, Labbe RF. A quantitative assay for urinary porphobilinogen. Clin Chem 1964;10:1105–1111.
8. Westerlund J, Pudek M, Schreiber WE. A rapid and accurate spectro-fluorometric method for quantification and screening of urinary porphyrins. Clin Chem 1988;34:345–351.
9. Chisholm JJ, Brown DH. Microscale photofluorometric determination of "free erythrocyte porphyrin" (protoporphyrin IX). Clin Chem 1975;21:1669–1682.
10. Piomelli S. Free erythrocyte porphyrin in the detection of undue absorption of lead and of iron deficiency. Clin Chem 1977;23:264–269.
11. Doumas BT, Poon PKC, Perry BW, Jendrzejczak B, McComb RB, Schaffer R, Hause LL. Candidate reference method for determination of total bilirubin in serum: development and validation. Clin Chem 1985;31:1779–1789.
12. Lo DH, Wu TW. Assessment of the fundamental accuracy of the Jendrassik-Grof total and direct bilirubin assays. Clin Chem 1983;29:31–36.
13. Wu TW, Dappen GM, Spayd RW, Sundberg MW, Powers DM. The Kodak Ektachem clinical chemistry slide for simultaneous determination of unconjugated and sugar-conjugated bilirubin. Clin Chem 1984;30:1310.

14. Seligson D, Seligson H, Wu TW. An anion-exchange chromatographic method for measuring bilirubin covalently bound to albumin. Clin Chem 1985;31:1317–1321.

Suggested Readings

Porphyrins and Bile Pigments

Elder GH, Smith SG, Smyth SJ. Laboratory investigation of the porphyrias. Ann Clin Biochem 1990;27:395–412.

Hindmarsh JT. The porphyrias: recent advances. Clin Chem 1986;32:1255–1263.

Kappas A, Sassa S, Galbraith RA, Nordmann Y. The porphyrias. In: Scriver CR, et al., eds. The metabolic basis of inherited disease, 6th ed., New York: McGraw-Hill, 1989.

Labbe RF, Lamon JM. Porphyrins and disorders of porphyrin metabolism. In: Tietz NW, ed. Textbook of clinical chemistry. Philadelphia: WB Saunders, 1986.

Straka JG, Rank JM, Bloomer JR. Porphyria and porphyrin metabolism. Annu Rev Med 1990;41:457–469.

Bilirubin

Balistreri WF, Shaw LM. Liver function. In: Tietz NW, ed. Textbook of clinical chemistry. Philadelphia: WB Saunders, 1986.

Wolkoff AW, Chowdhury JR, Arias IM. Hereditary jaundice and disorders of bilirubin metabolism. In: Scriver CR, et al., eds. The metabolic basis of inherited disease, 6th ed. New York: McGraw-Hill, 1989.

19 Therapeutic Drug Monitoring

Thomas P. Moyer and George M. Lawson

Therapeutic drug monitoring is a clinical laboratory practice that crosses many of the classic boundaries of medicine. It is based in the analytical capabilities of the clinical chemistry laboratory, but also requires a thorough knowledge of pharmacology, cardiology, gastroenterology, immunology, infectious diseases, nephrology, neurology, psychiatry, vascular medicine, and other specialties.

Therapeutic drug monitoring (TDM) involves providing the patient the right dose of a drug to achieve the optimal therapeutic effect while avoiding toxic side effects. It is a practice that is usually reserved for drugs that have a narrow therapeutic index—those drugs that have proven efficacy but are also toxic if administered at too large a dose. Many drugs have a wide therapeutic index; thus, there is a large margin of safety in their use. Propranolol is an example of such a drug; it is safe when administered at therapeutic doses, and it requires a large dose to induce toxicity. There is no reason to measure propranolol levels and adjust the dose accordingly, since standard dosing guidelines are more than adequate to provide safe dosage. Indeed, the measurement of blood pressure provides an easy and rapid biological monitor of the effectiveness of the drug. Propranolol levels are almost never measured. Digoxin, on the other hand, is very effective at enhancing the force of contraction of a failing heart, yet it can be very toxic when the blood level just exceeds the safe limit. When digoxin is used, the drug level must be monitored and the dose adjusted based on the blood level to ensure safe use.

This chapter describes the fundamental principles of pharmacology that the practitioner must know and understand thoroughly to use this technique. Correct application of drug monitoring and interpretation of results require that the practitioner understand the principles of absorption, distribution, clearance rate, half-life, volume of distribution, zero- and first-order elimination kinetics, and drug-drug interactions. Following this discussion, the chapter briefly describes techniques commonly employed to measure drug levels. It is important for the practitioner to understand the potential limitations of the analytical procedures used so that incorrect interpretation based on invalid test results can be avoided. The chapter concludes with a detailed discussion of individual drugs by drug group. With this information, the practitioner can adjust the dose correctly and be aware of the known drug-drug interactions affecting the interpretation of the drug level.

Readers are referred to the sample case described in the section on digoxin. This application of TDM is a classic example of how this technique is applied in a real case situation to predict the dose needed to achieve optimal effect in the presence of compromising disease.

BASIC PRINCIPLES OF PHARMACODYNAMICS AND PHARMACOKINETICS AS USED IN TDM

Several comprehensive courses are available that discuss drug pharmacodynamics and pharmacokinetics (1–6) and with specific reference to TDM (7, 8). The purpose of the following discussion is to provide a general overview of these topics with emphasis on those aspects that are most relevant to the interpretation of plasma drug levels. Readers interested in a more detailed analysis should consult the aforementioned references.

Pharmacodynamics

The pharmacodynamics of a drug describe the repertoire of physiological effects resulting from the administration of that drug, including the desired therapeutic effects as well as the undesired side effects or toxicities. The physiological actions of many drugs are mediated through interaction with specific receptor molecules localized in target tissues. In such cases, maximum therapeutic efficacy is achieved when the drug concentration in the target tissue results in an optimal degree of receptor saturation; increases in concentration beyond this optimal level generate no additional therapeutic benefits but may increase the probability for toxicity. Other drugs interact in a more nonspecific manner with biological components, and toxicity may ensue from a direct extension of the therapeutic mechanism (e.g., generalized binding of lyophilic anesthetic agents to neuronal membranes or intercalation of antineoplastic drugs between DNA nucleotide pairs). Therapeutic efficacy (i.e., the effective dose) can be described by the parameter ED_{50}, which is defined as the drug dose required to achieve the desired therapeutic effect in 50% of test subjects. Toxicity can be described by the parameter LD_{50}, which is defined as the drug dose that is lethal in 50% of test animals. The therapeutic index, which is strictly defined as LD_{50}/ED_{50} but can be applied to any specific drug-related toxicity (not necessarily lethal), is an indicator of the safety margin associated with a given drug. In a given individual, a drug having a narrow therapeutic index may induce toxic symptoms at doses only slightly greater than those required to achieve therapeutic efficacy. Such drugs are often associated with greater frequencies of toxicity within the population and may be appropriate candidates for TDM.

Pharmacokinetics

Pharmacokinetics is the study of drug disposition within the body and is usually discussed in terms of drug absorption, distribution, metabolism, and elimination.

ABSORPTION AND DISTRIBUTION

Numerous routes are available for drug administration including oral, parenteral (intravenous, intramuscular, subcutaneous), sublingual, buccal, intranasal, and rectal. Following a discrete dose, the increase in serum drug concentration as a function of time depends upon both the extent and rate of drug absorption. For a given drug, the extent of absorption is related to the bioavailability, which is defined as the fraction of administered drug that reaches the systemic circulation, not including the hepatic portal system. A bioavailability of 1.0 is assigned to the intravenous route of administration, with other routes having bioavailabilities ranging from 0 to 1.0. For drugs taken orally, various factors can affect the overall bioavailability as well as the rate of absorption. These include the type of drug formulation; the rate of gastric emptying (since absorption of most drugs is optimal in the small intestine); the pH of the gastric and duodenal contents (because most drugs are more readily absorbed in their nonionized form); the simultaneous presence of food or coadministered drugs that may inhibit or accelerate absorption; the presence of intestinal flora that may inactivate a given drug or alternatively convert an inactive prodrug to its active form; and the extent to which the drug undergoes hepatic metabolism when delivered via the portal vein (i.e., first-pass effect). Following absorption into the systemic circulation, the drug becomes available for distribution from the vascular compartment into the peripheral tissues. The free drug fraction (i.e., the fraction not bound to protein) is available to diffuse across cell membranes and is subsequently distributed into tissues. Some drugs circulate almost exclusively in the unbound form (e.g., gentamicin), while others are extensively bound to plasma proteins (e.g., warfarin). For those drugs exhibiting significant binding to plasma proteins, it is generally true that acidic drugs bind predominantly to albumin, whereas basic drugs bind to α_1-acid glycoprotein, although, depending upon the specific drug, other plasma proteins may be involved as well.

Factors that affect the ability of a given drug to localize into extravascular tissues include the extent to which the drug is bound to plasma and tissue proteins as well as the capacity to penetrate lipid bilayer membranes. The extent of distribution is most conveniently expressed by the pharmacokinetic parameter, V_d, known as the apparent volume of distribution. When distribution from the vascular space to the extravascular tissues is complete and plasma and tissue drug concentrations are in equilibrium, V_d is defined as follows:

$$V_d = \frac{\text{Amount of drug in body}}{C_p} \quad (1)$$

where: C_p = plasma drug concentration

Under conditions of constant drug infusion at steady-state equilibrium, where infusion and elimination rates are equal and distribution is complete, the tissue and plasma concentrations of unbound drug will be equal, and V_d can be expressed as follows (6):

$$V_d = V_p + V_t \cdot \frac{f_p}{f_t} \quad (2)$$

where: V_p = plasma volume
V_t = actual tissue volume
f_p = fraction of unbound drug in plasma
f_t = fraction of unbound drug in tissue

The presence of the factor f_p/f_t in equation 2 underscores the importance of the relative degree of drug binding by plasma and tissue proteins in determining V_d. For a series of different drugs, as the binding affinity for tissue protein relative to serum protein increases, f_p/f_t increases and is reflected as an increase in V_d. The apparent volume of distribution as calculated from the total body burden of drug and the plasma concentration (equation 1) is actually a composite parameter, which is a summation of the individual V_d's of the different tissues that can bind the drug (equation 2). Without knowledge of these individual tissue components, which in practice are difficult to obtain, V_d as calculated from equation 1 provides no information on the actual drug distribution pattern within the body. Thus, two drugs having very different distribution patterns (e.g., one highly bound to a single target tissue, the other less avidly bound but showing a more general tissue distribution) can have identical V_d's. Therefore, the V_d for a given drug does not correspond to an actual physiological compartment. Rather, it represents a theoretical volume into which the drug would need to distribute uniformly so that its concentration in tissue would be equal to its concentration in plasma. Apparent volumes of distribution typically range between 0.25 and 20 liters/kg of body weight, with the larger volumes indicating a high degree of extravascular tissue binding.

METABOLISM AND ELIMINATION

The rate at which a drug is eliminated from the body is usually expressed as its clearance (Cl), which is defined as the volume of plasma that is completely cleared of drug in a given unit of time (usually expressed in units of ml/min). This definition is equivalent to the following expression:

$$\text{Rate of elimination} = \text{Cl} \cdot C_p \quad (3)$$

The major organs involved in drug elimination are the kidney and liver, although other organs may contribute to a lesser extent. Each organ has its own associated clearance that contributes to the total systemic clearance, and, depending upon the specific drug, one or the other may predominate.

Drugs cleared predominantly by the liver are usually metabolized by an enzyme or enzymes associated with the cytochrome P-450 mixed function oxidase system. Typical biotransformation reactions include oxidations, reductions, and hydrolyses (phase I reactions), often followed by conjugation to glucuronic acid, sulfate, or glycine (phase II reactions) to increase water solubility and facilitate subsequent excretion, usually by biliary or renal mechanisms. Factors that affect hepatic clearance include hepatic blood flow, intrinsic activity of the metabolizing enzyme(s), and the fraction of drug bound to plasma proteins.

A drug molecule is considered to have been cleared following hepatic biotransformation, even though the metabolite has not yet been physically eliminated from the body. Since most metabolites are either pharmacologically inactive or much less active than the parent drug, this is a reasonable assumption. If the metabolite does possess significant activity, it may have to be analyzed as a separate entity.

For drugs cleared predominantly by the kidney, clearance will depend upon renal blood flow, glomerular filtration rate, and fraction of drug bound to plasma proteins; tubular secretion and reabsorption may play roles as well. For drugs subject to reabsorption, urine pH can significantly affect clearance because acidic urine favors the reabsorption of acidic drugs (which are un-ionized at acidic pH and more readily diffuse across tubular cell plasma membranes). Conversely, more alkaline urine favors the reabsorption of basic drugs, which tend to be un-ionized at higher pH.

KINETICS OF DISTRIBUTION AND ELIMINATION

For simplification this discussion assumes that the drug is administered intravenously, but the principles discussed are essentially independent of the route of administration. Following intravenous administration of a drug, two processes begin to occur: distribution of the drug into the extravascular tissue, and elimination of the drug by clearance mechanisms. Although both processes begin to occur simultaneously, it is possible to resolve them into their separate components through appropriate pharmacokinetic modeling. A popular two-compartment model accurately describes the behavior of many drugs. The central compartment consists mainly of the intravascular space and any closely affiliated systems into which drug disperses and equilibrates very rapidly. The peripheral compartment represents the extravascular tissue. Distribution of drug occurs from the central to the peripheral compartment until an equilibrium is attained, at which time the distribution phase is complete. In the simplest version of the model, elimination occurs only from the central compartment. Elimination causes a decline in drug concentration in both compartments. These compartments continue to maintain their postdistribution equilibrium during the elimination phase.

This model predicts a biphasic decline in plasma concentration (C_p) when log C_p is plotted as a function of time following administration of an intravenous bolus, as shown in Figure 19.1. At any time following drug administration, C_p can be calculated as a sum of two exponential functions, one representing distribution from the central into the peripheral compartment, and the other representing elimination from the central compartment:

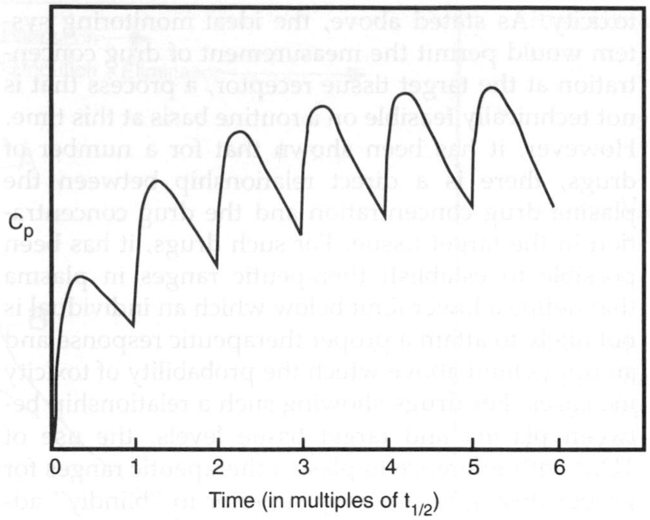

Figure 19.2. Plasma drug concentration (C_p) as a function of time following oral administration where the dosing interval is equal to the elimination half-life.

proximately 5 half-lives will also be required for the drug to clear completely or to attain a new steady state, respectively. These principles also apply to drugs administered intravenously, either as discrete bolus or continuous infusion, although in the latter case, peaks and troughs are not observed.

In the present example, the patient was administered a fixed dose at a fixed dosing interval, and 5 half-lives were required to attain steady state. In the absence of any factors that would alter clearance or bioavailability, $C_{p(ave)}$ will be maintained indefinitely, and the dose administered is referred to as a maintenance dose. In situations where it is critical to attain the desired C_p rapidly, a bolus loading dose can be administered. The loading dose is determined by V_d and is derived from equation 1:

$$\text{Dose} = \frac{C_p \cdot V_d}{f} \quad (14)$$

C_p is then maintained at the desired level by administering appropriate maintenance doses.

Inspection of equation 13 indicates that for a given drug, knowledge of the drug's clearance (Cl) and bioavailability (f) allow the calculation of the dose required to achieve a desired steady state $C_{p(ave)}$. Although these values are available, they are derived from population studies and represent the mean values of the study group. Unfortunately, for many drugs, both Cl and f can show significant interindividual variation within the population as well as intraindividual variation over time. Recommended dosage as provided by the pharmaceutical industry, although a logical place to start, is based upon mean population parameters, and any given individual may deviate significantly from the mean; in such cases, the recommended dose may result in subtherapeutic or toxic levels, situations that can be avoided by the appropriate use of TDM.

Indications for Therapeutic Drug Monitoring

Because of the large number of drugs currently in use, it is not practical to monitor all of them. In fact, on theoretical grounds alone, the need for TDM is restricted to a fairly limited number of drugs. The characteristics of those drugs that are typically monitored as well as some conditions that merit judicious use of TDM to enhance patient management are listed in the sections that follow.

DRUGS SHOWING A DEFINITE RELATIONSHIP BETWEEN PLASMA DRUG LEVEL AND CLINICAL RESPONSE

A fundamental assumption in the use of TDM is that the plasma drug concentration is proportional to the drug concentration in the target tissue. Such a relationship permits the establishment of a plasma therapeutic range that serves as a reference for assessing the appropriateness of drug dosage. A plasma level ordered for a drug showing a poor correlation between plasma concentration and clinical response serves no purpose other than to assess compliance. Plasma therapeutic ranges have been established for many drugs through clinical correlation studies. Although these ranges are valid for a large percentage of the patient population, they may not strictly apply to all individuals. For a given drug, some patients may be adequately treated with doses giving "subtherapeutic" plasma concentrations, while other patients may experience toxicity with plasma levels within the therapeutic range. As with most laboratory results, the plasma drug concentration contributes additional information to be used in patient management, but it should always be interpreted in conjunction with an assessment of the patient's clinical status.

DRUGS HAVING A NARROW THERAPEUTIC INDEX

Drugs having a narrow safety margin between the upper limit of the therapeutic range and the lower limit of the toxic range are prime candidates for TDM. Interindividual differences in pharmacokinetic parameters, particularly clearance, which are to some extent genetically determined, can result in one individual becoming toxic while another is optimally dosed. This can occur even if both are administered the same dose per unit weight. Even for patients receiving successful long-term therapy, subtle decreases in clearance can elevate the plasma level into the toxic range even though no change in dosing regimen has occurred. Physiological changes associated with the normal aging process or disease onset and coadministration of other drugs are among the most common causes.

DRUGS SUBJECT TO ZERO-ORDER ELIMINATION KINETICS

For drugs cleared by first-order kinetics, the plasma concentration (and total body burden) is proportional to the dose, and alterations in dose result in predictable changes in plasma levels. This relationship does not hold for drugs cleared by zero-order kinetics, where an increase in drug dose may yield an unpredictable and disproportionate increase in plasma concentration. Many drugs will exhibit zero-order elimination kinetics when administered in high enough doses, particularly in overdose situations. From the perspective of TDM, the drugs that require careful monitoring are those that may change from first-order to zero-order kinetics at concentrations only slightly above or possibly within the high end of the therapeutic range, such as phenytoin.

DRUGS USED TO TREAT SYMPTOMS THAT LACK A DEFINITE CLINICAL ENDPOINT

For relatively nontoxic drugs that have an easily measured clinical endpoint, the dose can be increased until the desired clinical response is achieved. If the response is not always clear-cut and may be based on a more subjective assessment, as in the treatment of depression, plasma levels can assist in verifying the adequacy of dosage. Likewise, the plasma monitoring of anticonvulsant drugs may prevent a therapeutic failure due to inadequate medication or noncompliance.

PATIENTS EXPERIENCING PHYSIOLOGICAL OR PATHOLOGICAL CHANGES

Changes in physiology associated either with the normal aging process or with the onset of disease can significantly affect drug disposition. Drug clearance in neonates is prolonged until the hepatic metabolizing enzymes have developed (9). Children generally have a more rapid rate of drug metabolism than adults, and it is maintained until the onset of adolescence. In healthy individuals, the adult rate is maintained well into middle age but gradually declines thereafter (10). Alterations in drug dose over time may be required to compensate for these changes in metabolic rate. Alterations in pharmacokinetic parameters resulting from physiological changes associated with pregnancy may also necessitate modifications in drug dosage (11).

Hepatic and renal disease can significantly affect the elimination of drugs cleared by these organs, thus necessitating lower dosage to maintain the same plasma concentration. Patients receiving digoxin who experience acute renal failure can rapidly develop digoxin toxicity if plasma levels are not carefully monitored and the dose adjusted accordingly. Gastrointestinal disease can result in decreased absorption, thereby reducing the bioavailability of orally administered drugs. Congestive heart failure can alter pharmacokinetics by causing alterations in the volume of distribution and by reducing blood flow to the liver and kidney. Monitoring plasma drug concentrations can be important under such pathological conditions, particularly for drugs that have a narrow therapeutic index or that are subject to zero-order elimination kinetics.

COADMINISTRATION OF MULTIPLE DRUGS

Administration of a new drug may affect the pharmacodynamics of pharmacokinetics of any drugs already being administered. Pharmacodynamic interactions, which can occur between drugs that interact with tissue receptors mediating similar physiological responses, are of less interest from the perspective of TDM. Of greater importance are drugs that interact pharmacokinetically. Such interactions often occur when a drug that induces or inhibits hepatic metabolizing enzyme activity is added to the therapeutic regimen. Phenobarbital and phenytoin are potent inducers of hepatic P-450 enzymes and can result in a significant increase in clearance with concomitant decrease in plasma concentration of other drugs metabolized by the same enzymes. Conversely, cimetidine, which is an inhibitor of P-450 activity, can have the opposite effect. Coadministration of cimetidine to a patient taking theophylline can cause theophylline toxicity in the absence of any change in theophylline dose. Cigarette smoking and chronic ethanol consumption also induce hepatic metabolizing enzymes. Interactions between drugs cleared predominantly by the kidney can also occur if active tubular secretion contributes significantly to renal clearance and the drugs compete for the same saturable secretion pathway.

Interaction between drugs that are strongly bound to plasma proteins can occur by competitive displacement from protein binding sites. Most analytical methods are designed to measure total (i.e., the sum of bound and unbound) plasma drug concentration. The total concentration approximates the bound concentration for drugs that are strongly bound. Addition of a second drug that competes with and displaces the first drug will initially increase the unbound fraction. Since the unbound drug is available to diffuse out of the vascular space into target tissues, an increase in pharmacologic response may ensue. However, unbound drug may also be more readily accessible to clearance mechanisms that will attenuate the initial increase in unbound concentration. Although the overall effect may be difficult to predict, the total plasma concentration of displaced drug is usually decreased because of the decrease in its bound concentration. The effect is most pronounced when two competing drugs are coadministered in doses that yield significantly different plasma concentrations, with the less concentrated drug showing the greater effect. As an example, the plasma concentrations of valproic acid normally exceed that of phenytoin by approximately fivefold; addition of valproic acid to a patient stabilized on phenytoin will cause a decrease in the total phenytoin concentration (possibly to "subtherapeutic" levels), even though the unbound concentration may remain relatively unchanged and may provide appropriate prophylaxis against seizures. In such cases, the measurement of unbound drug may be useful (12), but at this time, reliable assays for the routine measurement of unbound plasma concentrations of most drugs are not readily available.

ASSESSING COMPLIANCE

Monitoring plasma drug concentrations is the most reliable method of assessing compliance, since patient histories can be notoriously unreliable. Obviously, this indication applies to all drugs for which assays are available, not just those mentioned in the aforementioned categories.

Practical Considerations

When applied in those situations where TDM is indicated, useful results will be ensured only if the specimen is collected under appropriate conditions. The timing of collection relative to drug administration is especially important. When therapy is initiated with a new drug, approximately 5 half-lives are required before steady state is attained (Fig. 19.2). The measurement of plasma concentration prior to steady state will give low values that are not indicative of the true steady-state concentration and may lead to an inappropriate increase in drug dose. Likewise, if a dose change is instituted in a patient who is at steady state, 5 half-lives will also be required before the new steady-state level is attained, and samples should not be obtained before such time has elapsed.

Figure 19.2 illustrates that even at steady state, plasma drug concentrations will fluctuate between peak and trough values for drugs administered orally. The relative difference between peak and trough concentrations is dependent upon the drug half-life relative to the dosing interval. Ideally, to minimize toxicity and to maximize therapeutic efficacy, both peak and trough concentrations will be within the therapeutic range and, theoretically, samples collected at any time during the dosing interval will provide meaningful results. In actual practice, however, trough values on samples collected shortly before administration of the next dose are usually preferred. This is because trough samples tend to show less variability over time compared to samples collected near the peak when the rate of change is greater and the time to peak is less predictable. For some drugs, such as the aminoglycoside antibiotics (which are administered intravenously), both peak and trough concentrations may be desired to assess the efficacy and probability of toxicity from the respective values.

Another rationale for routinely obtaining trough concentrations is related to the basic assumption that plasma concentrations are proportional to target tissue concentrations. For drugs for which such proportionality has been demonstrated, the relationship is valid during the postdistributive phase when an equilibrium has been established between plasma and tissue. Plasma levels obtained on samples collected prior to the completion of distribution will be disproportionately elevated relative to the tissue concentration. For many drugs, this is not a great concern since the distributive process is usually quite rapid. However, for drugs having a prolonged distributive phase, samples collected too soon after the last dose will provide misleading values. As an example, digoxin normally requires approximately 12 hours to complete its distributive phase. In a properly dosed patient, plasma concentrations obtained on samples collected a few hours after the last dose will indicate toxicity even though the digoxin concentration in myocardial tissue is entirely appropriate. A sample correctly collected at least 12 hours after the last dose would be well within the therapeutic range.

For these reasons, the laboratory should request that information documenting the date, time, and amount of the last dose be submitted along with the specimen to be tested. This information should be included on the actual laboratory report and, in conjunction with the specimen collection time, would greatly facilitate interpretation of the plasma drug concentration. In actual practice, it is often difficult to convince the ordering service to provide this information on a regular basis.

Although the majority of drug metabolites are not pharmacologically active, this is not always the case. If an active metabolite is produced in significant quantity, it should be measured in conjunction with the parent drug and related to its own therapeutic range. Alternatively, a therapeutic range should be established for the sum total of the parent drug and its metabolite.

Finally, the reliability of the assayed drug concentration is dependent upon the analytical process used to perform the measurement. Drug assays having high levels of analytical accuracy, precision, sensitivity, and specificity have been developed in recent years. The methods enjoying most widespread use are described in the following section.

METHODOLOGY

The methods for measuring serum drug levels fall into two general categories: (*a*) immunoassays, in which detection is based upon the specific interaction between the drug and an antibody directed against that drug, and (*b*) chromatographic techniques where the drug is first separated from potentially interfering endogenous and exogenous substances and then subsequently identified based upon its physicochemical characteristics. Both methodologies have their strengths and limitations, and depending upon the specific application, one is usually preferred over the other.

Immunoassays have been utilized extensively for TDM in recent years. This can be attributed mainly to ease of performance and access to commercially available reagents. Homogeneous immunoassays that do not require separation of antibody-bound drug from unbound drug prior to measurement can be adapted to automated instruments and have become most popular. Two of the more widely used systems are the enzyme-multiplied immunoassay technique (EMIT) and fluorescence polarization immunoassay (FPIA).

The EMIT assay (Syva Company) incorporates a reagent that contains a bacterial enzyme, glucose-6-phosphate dehydrogenase (G6PD) covalently linked to the drug in question so that the drug-enzyme conjugate maintains full enzymatic activity toward its substrate, NAD. When a drug-specific antibody, contained in a second reagent, binds to the drug-enzyme conjugate, enzymatic activity is lost, presumably due to stearic hindrance or an allosterically induced conformation change that prevents the interaction of substrate with the active site. The assay is conducted by combining the two reagents and an aliquot of the patient's plasma; drug in the plasma competes with the drug-enzyme conjugate for antibody binding so that the rate of enzymatic conversion of NAD to NADH is quantitatively related to the plasma drug concentration. The assay is monitored by following the absorbance change at 340 nm (ΔA_{340}). Since human G6PD utilizes NADP as substrate, there is no interference from endogenous enzyme activity. The plasma concentration is calculated from a calibration curve relating ΔA_{340} to drug concentration constructed from known standards. Although the relationship between ΔA_{340} and drug concentration is nonlinear, an appropriate mathematical transformation can be applied to linearize the data, a function that can be performed automatically by the software packages available on many automated analyzers.

The FPIA method (Abbott Laboratories) incorporates a reagent containing a fluorescent probe (fluorescein) covalently linked to the drug in question. When the fluorescent probe is excited by absorption of polarized light under the hypothetical condition of zero molecular rotation, it subsequently emits light having the same plane of polarization as the incident light. When free in solution, the rate of rotation of the fluorescein-drug conjugate is rapid relative to the time elapsed between the absorption and subsequent emission of light (relaxation time). Consequently, if an incident beam of polarized light is absorbed by the fluorescein-drug conjugate, the plane of polarization of the emitted light will be randomized, resulting in an overall depolarization of the incident beam. However, when an antibody specific to the drug (contained in a second reagent) binds to the fluorescein-drug conjugate, the effective molecular size of the probe is increased so that the rate of rotation becomes less than the relaxation time, and the plane of polarization is maintained during the absorption-emission process. Since drug in the plasma sample competes with the drug-fluorescein conjugate for binding to the antibody, the plasma drug concentration is related to the extent of depolarization. The assay is conducted by combining the two reagents with an aliquot of the patient's serum and measuring the absorbance in two detectors oriented at 0° and 90° relative to the plane of polarization of the incident light. The plasma concentration is calculated from a calibration curve relating depolarization to drug concentration constructed from standards of known concentration.

The EMIT and FPIA methods can generate rapid, reliable results and do not require extensive technical expertise on the part of the technologist performing the tests. Because the principle of measurement is the same regardless of the specific drug in question (i.e., the differences in assays reside in the specific drug-G6PD or drug-fluorescein conjugates and the antibodies), a large number of different drugs can be measured on the same instrument. The stability and precision of many contemporary automated analyzers allow storage of calibration data for extended periods, thereby reducing operation time and reagent costs. Since the EMIT method requires only standard spectrophotometry, it permits more flexibility in that it can be adapted to most chemistry analyzers currently available. This property may be important to laboratories wishing to perform TDM on existing instrumentation. Alternatively, laboratories performing high-volume testing may select instruments based on low reagent volume requirements in order to reduce costs. Because FPIA requires a polarization detector, a dedicated instrument for this purpose is required.

In contrast to the original immunoassays that utilized polyclonal antibodies, contemporary immunoassays often use monoclonal antibodies, which result in greater specificity due to less cross-reactivity with drug metabolites or other structurally related, potentially interfering compounds.

Chromatographic methods are based upon the selective partitioning of a drug between a stationary phase, usually immobilized within a column, and a mobile phase that perfuses the column. The drug elutes from the column with a retention time that is characteristic of that drug under specified conditions. Among the chromatographic methods available, high-performance liquid chromatography (HPLC) (13) and gas-liquid chromatography (GLC) (14) have proved most versatile for TDM.

Reversed-phase HPLC methods utilizing columns containing solid nonpolar stationary phases and more polar liquid mobile phases have been developed for many drugs. Preanalytical separation of the drug from protein and potentially interfering exogenous (e.g., other drugs) or endogenous compounds using liquid-liquid or solid phase extractions with organic solvents is usually required prior to analysis. The extract is resuspended in the mobile phase and injected onto the column, which is eluted with the mobile phase under elevated pressure. For a given flow rate, the drug's retention time on the column is dependent upon its relative affinity for mobile and stationary phases. The compounds eluting from the column are most commonly detected and quantitated by measuring absorption of ultraviolet light or fluorescence. The concentration of drug in the original serum sample is proportional to the area (or height) of the peak having a retention time characteristic of that drug and is quantitated relative to standards of known concentration taken through the entire procedure. By varying the extraction conditions, stationary and mobile phases, and elution program (isocratic or gradient), the procedure can be optimized to reduce elution time to a minimum while ensuring adequate separation of the drug from any interfering substances.

Gas-liquid chromatography is analogous to HPLC except that the stationary phase is a high boiling liquid, and the mobile phase is a gas, typically helium, hydrogen, or nitrogen. Conventional GLC columns are packed with small particles of an inert support material coated with stationary phase, usually a silicone polymer. Capillary columns in which the stationary phase forms the inner lining of a thin silica tube provide greater resolution and have become increasingly popular in drug analysis laboratories in recent years. The column is encased in an oven whose temperature can be varied during the run to optimize resolution. Various detectors are available that are sensitive to all drugs (flame ionization detector) or only to drugs containing specific atoms such as nitrogen or halogens (nitrogen-phosphorus detector, electron capture detector). By coupling a mass spectrometer to the gas chromatograph, a molecular fragmentation pattern can be obtained that is virtually unique to the drug being assayed (14), however, such specificity is rarely required for TDM, and this technology is not available in most clinical laboratories. Analysis by GLC is restricted to drugs that are sufficiently volatile or can be rendered volatile by chemical derivatization. Preanalytical sample preparation is similar to that for HPLC.

Chromatographic methods require more specialized instrumentation and substantial technical expertise to operate and maintain the instruments. The preanalytical extractions are labor intensive, and throughput is slow due to the sequential nature of the analysis. Chromatographic methods are therefore usually applied to the more esoteric, less prescribed drugs for which commercial immunoassays have not been developed. However, a major advantage of chromatographic techniques is that methods can often be developed that allow simultaneous measurement of metabolites along with the parent drug, which is important for those metabolites exhibiting pharmacologic activity.

PHARMACOLOGY AND PHARMACOKINETICS OF DRUGS COMMONLY MONITORED

The following sections review the indications and contraindications for the use of drugs that are commonly monitored. The order in which the drugs are listed is typical of the order in which a physician might consider them for use. Each drug is reviewed with respect to its pertinent pharmacokinetic and pharmacodynamic properties and the known relationships of blood concentration to efficacy and toxicity. Some of the information about each drug is extracted from the *Physicians' Desk Reference* (15), *Goodman and Gilman's The Pharmacological Basis of Therapeutics* (16), *Medical Toxicology: Diagnosis and Treatment of Human Poisoning* (17), or *Textbook of Clinical Chemistry* (18), unless specifically listed otherwise. At the conclusion of the chapter are listed references for proven methodologies that are used by many laboratories.

Antiarrhythmics

This term describes the drugs used to control cardiac rhythm disturbances.

LIDOCAINE

Lidocaine is indicated in the acute management of ventricular arrhythmias following myocardial infarction or during cardiac manipulation such as surgery.

Lidocaine is administered intravenously at a dose of 0.35 to 0.7 mg/kg to achieve a therapeutic blood concentration of 2 to 6 mg/liter. At therapeutic concentrations, lidocaine is 50% bound to plasma proteins, primarily α_1-acid glycoprotein. Lidocaine undergoes more than 80% first-pass hepatic metabolism, with an average renal clearance of 9 ml/min/kg. The drug has a volume of distribution of 1 liter/kg and an elimination half-life of approximately 1.5 hours (19). Toxicity occurs when the concentration of lidocaine exceeds 6 mg/liter and is usually associated with symptoms of central nervous system excitation, lightheadedness, confusion, dizziness, tinnitus, blurred or double vision, and can be accompanied by bradycardia and hypotension, leading to cardiovascular collapse.

Because lidocaine has such a high first-pass hepatic extraction, the drug is never administered orally. Diseases that reduce hepatic and renal function (e.g., congestive heart failure) reduce clearance and prolong elimination half-life. Approximately 24 hours after a myocardial infarction, the concentration of α_1-acid glycoprotein increases, causing higher rates of protein binding and requiring larger doses of lidocaine to achieve pharmacologic efficacy. During the interval of days 2 to 5 postinfarct, patients may require blood concentrations in the range of 6 to 8 mg/liter to achieve rhythm control without exhibiting signs of toxicity. Thereafter, the α_1-acid glycoprotein concentration declines, requiring that the dose and blood concentration be reduced to avoid signs of toxicity. Because of these difficulties, Harrison has suggested that lidocaine should always be monitored whenever it is administered (20).

PROCAINAMIDE

Procainamide is indicated in the treatment of premature ventricular contractions, ventricular tachycardia, atrial fibrillation, and paroxysmal atrial tachycardia. Procainamide is contraindicated in patients with complete A-V block.

Administration of a dose of 50 mg/kg will usually yield the optimal plasma concentration in the range of 4 to 8 mg/liter (21). Patients who are undergoing aggressive antiarrhythmic therapy under intensive medical surveillance can often tolerate (and may require) plasma concentrations up to 16 mg/liter to maintain good rhythm control (22). Procainamide is metabolized to an active metabolite, *N*-acetylprocainamide (NAPA); metabolism is controlled by genetically determined enzymes. Patients who are fast metabolizers will have a PA:NAPA ratio less than 0.5 3 hours after the dose is administered. Slow acetylators (PA:NAPA greater than 2 after 3 hours) are more likely to develop a positive test for antinuclear antibodies and present with systemic lupus erythematosus–like symptoms. Patients who have prolonged exposure to procainamide more than 12 mg/liter (or the sum of procainamide plus NAPA concentration more than 30 mg/liter) are very likely to exhibit symptoms of toxicity that are characterized by hypotension, ventricular fibrillation, widened QRS complex, junctional tachycardia, oliguria, confusion, nausea, and vomiting.

Renal disease, hepatic disease, cardiac failure, and states of low cardiac output reduce the metabolism and clearance of procainamide and NAPA. Coadministration of histamine H_2 receptor antagonists such as cimetidine and ranitidine reduce renal clearance of procainamide and NAPA, resulting in higher plasma concentrations of each (23).

QUINIDINE

Quinidine is indicated in the treatment of premature atrial and ventricular contractions, paroxysmal atrial tachycardia, paroxysmal A-V junctional rhythm, and atrial flutter. Quinidine is contraindicated in A-V block and in digitalis-induced A-V conduction disorders.

Quinidine dose is highly variable to achieve optimally effective serum concentrations in the range of 2 to 5 mg/liter. Quinidine is 70% protein bound in plasma with a volume of distribution of 2.7 liter/kg. It undergoes renal clearance at a rate of 5 ml/min/kg with an elimination half-life of 6 to 8 hours. There are no significant active metabolites, and toxicity is invariably observed when concentrations are greater than 8 mg/liter (24). Symptoms of toxicity include cinchonism, tinnitus, lightheadedness, premature ventricular contractions, and atrioventricular node block. Gastrointestinal distress is a frequent side effect but becomes more severe and is associated with nausea and vomiting at higher blood concentrations.

Physiological processes that generally reduce metabolism and clearance increase the blood concentration of quinidine (25). Coadministration of drugs that activate the cytochrome oxidase enzymes enhance clearance, resulting in lower blood concentrations.

While digoxin coadministration does not affect quinidine concentration, quinidine does reduce digoxin clearance (26).

DISOPYRAMIDE

Disopyramide is indicated in the treatment of unifocal premature (ectopic) ventricular contractions and ventricular tachycardia. Disopyramide is contraindicated in cardiogenic shock, second- and third-degree A-V block, and congenital Q-T prolongation.

Disopyramide administered in a daily dose ranging from 6 to 15 mg/kg yields blood concentrations in the range of 2 to 5 mg/liter. Protein binding is concentration dependent, ranging from 70% at 0.4 mg/liter to 30% at 4 mg/liter. At steady state, the volume of distribution is 0.8 liter/kg. Disopyramide undergoes renal clearance at a rate of 1.3 ml/min/kg with a half-life of approximately 8 hours (27). Toxicity is observed when the concentration exceeds 5 mg/liter and is characterized by dry mouth, urinary hesitancy, and blurred vision. Severe toxicity occurs when the concentration exceeds 8 mg/liter and is characterized by excessive widening of the QRS complex and Q-T interval, worsening congestive heart failure, hypotension, bradycardia, and a systole in the worst cases (28).

Disopyramide is metabolized by dealkylation to nordisopyramide, a compound having approximately 25% of the antiarrhythmic activity of disopyramide. Dealkylation is accomplished by hepatic microsomal enzymes that are induced by phenobarbital and other related compounds. Coadministration of any "hepatic enzyme inducers" such as phenobarbital will increase the rate of clearance, resulting in lower blood concentrations.

TOCAINIDE

Tocainide is indicated for the treatment of life-threatening ventricular arrhythmias, but its use is restricted to patients in whom the benefit of treatment outweighs the risk of the leukopenia or agranulocytosis, side effects of the drug observed in about 0.2% of patients treated. Tocainide is contraindicated in patients with second- or third-degree A-V block.

Tocainide has electrophysiological properties similar to lidocaine. It is useful in the management of ventricular arrhythmias, where it reduces the amplitude and rate of depolarization of the action potential by decreasing the effective refractory period. Tocainide is particularly useful in the treatment of ventricular arrhythmias associated with prolonged Q-T interval (29).

Optimal therapeutic effect occurs when the blood concentration is within the range of 8 to 12 mg/liter. Dosage to achieve optimal effect is widely variable, ranging from 15 to 25 mg/kg/day. Tocainide is administered intravenously at a rate of 0.5 to 0.75 mg/kg/min for a period of 15 minutes as a loading dose followed by oral doses not to exceed 15 mg/kg/day, usually administered in the three daily doses (30). The dose of tocainide is adjusted to achieve the therapeutic concentration of 8 to 12 mg/liter. At therapeutic concentrations, tocainide is 10% protein bound, does not undergo significant first-pass metabolism, has a volume of distribution of 3 liters/kg, and undergoes renal clearance at a rate of 2.6 ml/min/kg. The elimination phase half-life of tocainide is approximately 13 hours. Toxicity due to tocainide occurs at concentrations in excess of 15 mg/liter and is characterized by gastrointestinal disturbance, central nervous system irritability culminating in convulsions, and cardiopulmonary depression culminating in cardiac arrest.

Congestive heart failure and uremia reduce renal clearance and the volume of distribution and increase the clearance half-life. Dosage reduction in association with these disease states is appropriate, and blood level monitoring is frequently used to determine optimal dose and dose interval. The drug is not highly protein bound, so tocainide does not exhibit the protein-binding phenomena described for lidocaine following myocardial infarction.

MEXILETINE

Mexiletine is a class I B antiarrhythmic with electrophysiological properties similar to lidocaine and is useful in the suppression of ventricular arrhythmias, Mexiletine reduces the effective refractory period and inhibits sodium influx, reducing the rate of rise of the action potential at phase 0. Mexiletine has no significant negative inotropic effects, nor does it affect the QRS or Q-T interval (31).

Mexiletine is administered orally at a dose of 15 mg/kg or less to achieve a therapeutic concentration of 0.7 to 2 mg/liter. The drug has a high degree of oral bioavailability, is approximately 60% protein bound, and undergoes renal clearance at a rate of 10.3 ml/min/kg. Mexiletine has a volume of distribution of 9.5 liter/kg at a half-life of 11 hours (32).

Myocardial infarction and uremia reduce the rate of clearance and increase the half-life of mexiletine, requiring dosage adjustment guided by drug monitoring. Mexiletine toxicity occurs at concentrations in excess of 2 mg/liter and is characterized by symptoms of nausea, hypotension, sinus bradycardia, paresthesia seizures, intermittent left bundle-branch block, and temporary asystole (33).

PROPAFENONE

Propafenone is a weak β-blocker and calcium antagonist that has an effect on the HIS-Purkinje cells that slows the rate of action potential and decreases action potential duration (34).

Propafenone is administered at approximately 4 mg/kg t.i.d. to achieve a therapeutic concentration in the range of 0.5 to 2.0 mg/liter. Administered orally, the drug is readily absorbed. The drug has a relatively short half-life ranging from 2 to 10 hours, with an average of 8 hours. The clinical efficacy of propafenone is maintained through the formation of active metabolites, such as 5-hydroxypropafenone, that are more pharmacologically active than the parent drug and have longer elimination half-lives (35).

AMIODARONE

Amiodarone is a class III antiarrhythmic used for the treatment of life-threatening recurrent ventricular arrhythmias that have not responded to adequate doses of other available antiarrhythmics. Amiodarone is reserved for the treatment of recurrent ventricular fibrillation and recurrent hemodynamically unstable ventricular tachycardia that is demonstrated to be nonresponsive to other antiarrhythmics because of its significant side effects.

Amiodarone is administered orally at a dose of 1.5 to 8 mg/kg to achieve a therapeutic blood concentration of 1.0 to 2.5 mg/liter. Oral bioavailability is 35 to 50%, and amiodarone is metabolized to an active metabolite, *N*-desethylamiodarone, which has equal pharmacologic activity. At equilibrium, the known pharmacokinetic properties of amiodarone and *N*-desethylamiodarone are approximately equal, as are their blood concentrations. In blood, amiodarone is 95% protein bound with a volume of distribution of 60 liters/kg (the largest volume of distribution of any drug described in this chapter). It undergoes renal clearance at a rate of 1.9 ml/min/kg. Amiodarone elimination is predicted by a multiphasic elimination pattern made up of an early elimination phase with a half-life of 2 to 3 days (not hours) followed by a slower elimination phase with a mean half-life of 53 days (36).

Because amiodarone has numerous side effects, it is reserved as a last-resort treatment. Side effects that are not concentration related include pulmonary toxicity (interstitial pneumonitis/alveolitis), liver toxicity, keratopathy, photosensitivity, and hypothyroidism. Significant heart block or sinus bracycardia have been observed in approximately 5% of all patients treated. The symptoms of pulmonary toxicity, keratopathy, hypothyroidism, and cardiac toxicity have been noted to be significantly worse in patients with blood concentrations exceeding 2.5 mg/liter (37).

Amiodarone is highly concentrated in tissue, where it maintains activity. Because of the prolonged elimination half-life, dosage adjustments are made based on the degree of pulmonary and thyroid toxicity noted. The grade of corneal keratopathy correlates directly with the concentration—grade 1 noted in patients with blood concentrations in the range of 1.0 to 1.7 mg/liter; grade 2 noted in patients with levels of 1.7 to 2.5 mg/liter; and grade 3 keratopathy observed in patients with blood levels greater than 2.5 mg/liter.

Numerous drug interactions have been observed for amiodarone (38). Amiodarone potentiates the anticoagulant effect of warfarin. It also inhibits the clearance of digoxin, and it is associated with *torsades de pointes* when coadministered with quinidine, disopyramide, mexiletine, propafenone, procainamide, or aprindine. Bradycardia may be observed with β-blockers, and sinus arrest with calcium channel blockers.

DIGOXIN

Digoxin is administered intravenously or orally to produce increased cardiac output following heart failure and to control atrial flutter or fibrillation.

Digoxin dosage is dependent upon a wide range of factors. An empirical approach to digoxin dosing is provided in the *Physicians' Desk Reference* (15), and a pharmacokinetic approach is provided in the sample problem found at the end of this section. Oral bioavailability of digoxin is approximately 70% but is highly variable between products; some digoxin products not subjected to Food and Drug Administration review (from outside the U.S.) have had bioavailability as low as 30%. Digoxin is 25% protein bound. Clearance of digoxin is directly dependent upon renal function and is predicted by the equation $Cl = 0.88\ Cr_{cl} + 0.33$, yielding a half-life of 40 to 48 hours in patients with normal renal function that is prolonged to 72 to 100 hours during compromised renal function. Volume of distribution is also dependent upon renal function (16) and is predicted by the equation $V = 3.12\ Cr_{cl} + 3.84$. The therapeutic range of digoxin is 0.8 to 2.0 μg/liter in a specimen collected more than 8 hours after the last dose (39, 40). Toxicity is characterized by severe ventricular arrhythmias, progressive bradycardia, second- or third-degree heart block not responsive to atropine, and elevation in serum potassium associated with a blood concentration in excess of 3 μg/liter in a specimen collected more than 8 hours after the last dose (41, 42).

Treatment of heart failure or atrial rhythm disturbances with digoxin is complicated because these diseases are frequently associated with reduced renal

CHLORAMPHENICOL

Chloramphenicol is used in life-threatening infections caused by *Salmonella* species, *Haemophilus influenzae* (specifically meningeal infections), *Rickettsia*, Lymphogranuloma-psittacosis group, and susceptible Gram-negative bacteria causing bacteremia and meningitis that do not respond to other antibiotics.

Chloramphenicol is administered intravenously at a dose of 50 mg/kg/day in divided doses to produce blood concentrations adequate to kill the organism as demonstrated by MIC studies but not to exceed a peak serum blood concentration of 20 mg/liter within 30 minutes of dose administration. Chloramphenicol is 50% protein bound and undergoes renal clearance at a rate of 2.4 ml/min/kg. It has a volume of distribution of 0.9 liter/kg and a normal elimination half-life of 4 hours. Chloramphenicol administered in doses resulting in blood concentrations persistently in excess of 25 mg/liter have been associated with the development of blood dyscrasias (aplastic anemia, hypoplastic anemia, thrombocytopenia, and granulocytopenia). Cardiovascular collapse ("gray syndrome") has been observed in newborns that are exposed to chloramphenicol concentrations in excess of 50 mg/liter (59).

Chloramphenicol is administered intravenously as a pro-drug, chloramphenicol succinate, which must be metabolized to chloramphenicol by serum esterases to achieve activity. The active drug circulating in the blood is chloramphenicol. Oral versions of chloramphenicol are available as either parent drug or chloramphenicol palmitate. These forms of chloramphenicol are not as toxic as the intravenous form.

SULFONAMIDES

Sulfonamides, typified by sulfamethoxazole and administered in conjunction with trimethoprim, are used for the treatment of infections due to *Chlamydia*, susceptible strains of *Enterobacter* species such as *Escherichia coli, Klebsiella* species, *Morganella morganii, Proteus mirabilis,* and *Proteus vulgaris,* and Gram-positive cocci such as *Staphylococcus pyogenes, Streptococcus pyogenes, Streptococcus pneumoniae,* and *Streptococcus viridans*.

Monitoring of sulfonamides in indicated only when prolonged (greater than 3 months) therapy is required. Minimal inhibitory concentrations of the sulfonamides are invariably less than 25 mg/liter for susceptible organisms, whereas toxicity associated with sulfonamides occurs with prolonged exposure to serum concentrations in excess of 125 mg/liter. Toxicity is expressed as renal disease characterized by formation of sulfonamide crystals in the kidney, resulting in the development of calculi. Maintenance doses of sulfonamide to achieve serum concentrations less than 100 mg/liter should avoid this phenomenon.

The common sulfonamides are absorbed readily after oral administration. Following a typical oral dose of 2 g/day administered b.i.d., the serum concentration peaks in approximately 3 hours at or near 100 mg/liter. The average elimination half-life is 6 to 10 hours. Sulfonamides undergo significant protein binding, ranging from 60 to 95% bound. The volume of distribution is 0.2 to 0.4 liters/kg; while they do not distribute at high concentrations outside the serum, sulfonamides are effective against infections located in deep tissue sites because high serum concentrations can be achieved relatively safely, resulting in organ concentrations that exceed the MIC.

Antidepressants

These drugs are used to control mental depression. Therapeutic drug monitoring of antidepressants has become an integral part of the practice of psychiatry. A task force of the American Psychiatric Association concluded that "plasma level measurements of imipramine, desmethylimipramine, and nortriptyline are unequivocally clinically useful in certain situations, (and) that these measurements are helpful in many situations" (60).

AMITRIPTYLINE

Amitriptyline is administered for the relief of symptoms of endogenous depression. Amitriptyline is administered orally in doses from 75 to 150 mg/day in divided doses. Because amitriptyline has a sedating effect, patients are usually started on the drug at lower doses administered at bedtime, adding a second morning dose 2 weeks later. The optimal dosage of amitriptyline yields trough (just before the next dose) blood levels of 75 to 200 μg/liter (61, 62).

Amitriptyline is metabolized to nortriptyline, which has similar pharmacologic activity. The relative blood levels of amitriptyline and nortriptyline are highly variable between patients; there is no normal A:N ratio. Nortriptyline pharmacokinetics are described in the next section. Amitriptyline exhibits approximately 50% bioavailability and is 95% bound to plasma proteins. The drug is cleared by hepatic metabolism and renal clearance of 12 ml/min/kg. Amitriptyline has a volume of distribution of 14 liters/kg and a half-life of 16 to 20 hours. Amitriptyline displays major cardiac toxicity when the concentration is in excess of 800 μg/liter, characterized by QRS widening in excess of 120 msec, leading to ventricular tachycardia and asystole (63).

Amitriptyline is the drug of choice in the treatment of depression when the side effect of mild sedation is desirable. Coadministration of perphenazine prolongs the elimination of amitriptyline, requiring reduced doses to maintain therapeutic levels. Amitriptyline is metabolized by the cytochrome P-450 system; all drugs that activate the P-450 system (for example, phenobarbital) will increase the rate of clearance of amitriptyline.

NORTRIPTYLINE

Nortriptyline is indicated for the relief of symptoms of endogenous depression when stimulation of the patient is desired.

Nortriptyline is administered in doses of 25 mg t.i.d to yield optimal blood levels of 50 to 150 μg/liter. Like amitriptyline, nortriptyline is approximately 50% bioavailable and 92% bound to plasma proteins. It is cleared by hepatic oxidation and renal excretion with a clearance rate of 7 ml/min/kg. Nortriptyline has a volume of distribution of 18 liters/kg and a normal excretion half-life of 25 to 35 hours. Toxicity is the same as described for amitriptyline and occurs when the blood concentration exceeds 800 μg/liter (63).

Nortriptyline is used when its stimulatory side effect is considered to be of clinical advantage. Nortriptyline is unique among the antidepressants in that its blood level exhibits the classic "therapeutic window" effect. The optimal effectiveness of the drug occurs between 50 and 150 μg/liter. When the concentration is less than 50 μg/liter, the drug shows little effectiveness, and when the drug concentration exceeds 150 μg/liter, nortriptyline will actually induce depression (64). Thus, therapeutic monitoring to ensure that the blood level is within the therapeutic window is critical to accomplish successful treatment with this drug.

IMIPRAMINE

Imipramine is used for the relief of symptoms of endogenous depression, requiring 1 to 3 weeks of treatment before therapeutic effectiveness becomes apparent.

Imipramine is administered in doses of 75 to 150 mg/day in divided doses. Optimal response to the drug usually occurs when the blood concentration is in the range of 125 to 250 μg/liter (65). Imipramine is metabolized to desipramine, which is described in the next section. Imipramine has a limited bioavailability of approximately 25% and is 95% protein bound. It undergoes hepatic metabolism and renal elimination with a clearance of 15 ml/min/kg. Volume of distribution of imipramine is 23 liters/kg, and the elimination half-life is 15 to 20 hours (66). Toxicity associated with imipramine is as described for amitriptyline.

DESIPRAMINE

Desipramine is used for the treatment of endogenous depression when the patient needs a drug with significant stimulatory side effects.

Desipramine is administered in doses of 100 to 200 mg/day to yield therapeutic levels of 50 to 200 μg/liter (65). Desipramine exhibits 38% bioavailability and is approximately 90% protein bound. As with the other antidepressants, it undergoes hepatic metabolism and renal elimination with a clearance rate of 30 ml/min/kg. The volume of distribution is 34 liters/kg, and the elimination half-life is 15 to 20 hours. Toxicity is as described for amitriptyline.

Desipramine is the antidepressant of choice in patients for whom maximal stimulation is indicated. Of the four tricyclic antidepressants described here, desipramine has the strongest stimulating effect. Desipramine exhibits clearance phenomena when coadministered with other drugs, as described for amitriptyline.

TRAZODONE

Trazodone is indicated for the treatment of depression characterized by prominent and persistent dysphoric mood that interferes with daily function.

Trazodone is administered in oral doses of 150 to 400 mg/day in divided doses to yield blood levels of 500 to 1100 μg/liter that correlate with response to the drug (67). Within the therapeutic range, trazodone is 93% protein bound. It exhibits a volume of distribution of 1.0 liter/kg and an elimination half-life of 6 hours. Oral bioavailability ranges from 60 to 90%. Priapism and hypotension are side effects that occur at therapeutic doses of the drug. There are no known major drug interactions that affect the pharmacology of trazodone.

Toxicity occurs at blood concentrations in excess of 1500 μg/liter and is characterized by respiratory arrest, seizure, and EKG changes typical of A-V conduction block. There is no specific antidote to trazodone overdose; treatment is symptomatic and supportive.

FLUOXETINE

Fluoxetine recently became the most widely prescribed antidepressant on the market. The drug is popular because it is effective as an antidepressant, lacks side effects, and has relatively mild toxicity in overdose. Fluoxetine acts by inhibiting uptake of serotonin in the central nervous system with relatively little antimuscarinic or antihistaminic activity, which is atypical of the other antidepressants.

Fluoxetine is administered in doses of 20 to 80 mg/day. Doses in excess of 20 mg/day are administered b.i.d. Blood concentrations observed after therapeutic doses range from 90 to 300 ng/ml. Fluoxetine has an active metabolite, norfluoxetine, which is usually present at concentrations in the range of 50 to 400 μg/liter. Pharmacokinetic properties of fluoxetine and norfluoxetine are similar except for their half-lives: fluoxetine has a half-life of approximately 2 days, while norfluoxetine has a half-life of 6 to 10 days. Both compounds are highly protein bound (95%) and have very large volumes of distribution (35 ± 21 liters/kg). Clearance of fluoxetine is predominantly hepatic, so liver disease will significantly prolong the action of fluoxetine.

Because of the very long half-life and the very large volume of distribution of the active metabolite norfluoxetine, there is little correlation between the blood concentration of fluoxetine and clinical response to the drug. Measurement of norfluoxetine provides a slightly better correlation; the use of blood vessels is generally limited to documenting that the patient is compliant.

Toxicity associated with drug overdose occurs when the patient has greatly exceeded typical therapeutic doses, and is typified by nausea, vomiting, agitation, and other signs of CNS excitation. Seizure activity has been observed only in animal models of overdose. No cardiac toxicity has been reported, although cardiac monitoring of overdose patients is recommended because polydrug abuse is common. Blood concentrations associated with overdose are frequently 5 times therapeutic or more. The very large volume of distribution of fluoxetine and metabolite make dialysis of limited value; the treatment of overdose is supportive and symptomatic.

LITHIUM

Lithium is used in the treatment of the manic phase of manic-depressive illness, typified by hyperactivity, feelings of grandiosity, poor judgment, aggressiveness, and reduced need for sleep.

The typical maintenance dose of lithium is approximately 900 mg/day. If the drug is administered as the quick-release form, the dose is split and given t.i.d. or q.i.d. If the slow-release form is administered, the dose is split and administered b.i.d. Blood concentrations achieved after therapeutic administration of lithium range from 0.8 to 1.2 mmol/liter. Lithium is usually 100% bioavailable and is not bound to plasma proteins. It has a typical volume of distribution of 0.7 liter/kg and an elimination half-life of 22 hours. The pharmacokinetics of lithium are significantly altered in states of diuresis; the normal physiological response in diuresis is to conserve electrolytes by enhanced reabsorption in the renal tubules. When patients are administered diuretics or develop severe diarrhea or vomiting such that they become dehydrated, lithium levels increase. Blood level monitoring is important in these cases to guide dosage adjustment.

Toxicity occurs when the blood concentration exceeds 1.5 mmol/liter, and becomes life threatening above 2.0 mmol/liter. Symptoms of early toxicity include diarrhea, vomiting, drowsiness, muscular weakness, and lack of coordination. Severe toxicity is signaled by ataxia, giddiness, tinnitus, and large output of dilute urine.

Antiepileptics

These drugs are used to control seizure disorders.

PHENOBARBITAL

Phenobarbital is a general CNS suppressant that has proven effectiveness in the control of generalized and partial seizures. It is frequently coadministered with phenytoin for control of complex seizure disorders and with valproic acid for complex partial seizures.

Phenobarbital is administered in doses of 60 to 300 mg/day in adults or 3 to 6 mg/kg day in children. Clinical response to the drug correlates strongly with blood concentration; dosage adjustments are made after 2 weeks of therapy to achieve steady-state blood levels in the range of 20 to 35 mg/liter (68, 69). Phenobarbital is slowly but completely absorbed, with bioavailability in the range of 100%. It is approximately 50% protein bound with a volume of distribution of 0.5 liters/kg. Phenobarbital has a long half-life of 96 hours, with no known active metabolites. Sedation is common at therapeutic concentrations for the first 2 to 3 weeks of therapy, but this side effect disappears with time. Patients chronically administered phenobarbital usually do not experience sedation unless the blood level exceeds 40 mg/liter. There are no known drug interactions that significantly affect the pharmacokinetics of phenobarbital; conversely, phenobarbital affects the pharmacokinetics of other drugs significantly (see below) because it induces the synthesis of enzymes associated with the hepatic cytochrome P-450 metabolic pathway (70).

Toxicity due to phenobarbital overdose is characterized by CNS sedation and reduced respiratory function. Mild symptoms characterized by ataxia, nystagmus, fatigue, and attention loss occur at blood levels in excess of 40 mg/liter. They become severe at concentrations in excess of 60 mg/liter, and life-threatening above 100 mg/liter. Death usually occurs from respiratory arrest when pulmonary support is not supplied manually.

PHENYTOIN

Phenytoin is the drug of choice to treat and prevent tonic-clonic and psychomotor seizures. If phenytoin alone will not prevent seizure activity, coadministration with phenobarbital is usually effective.

Initial therapy with phenytoin is started at doses of 100 to 300 mg/day for adults or 5 mg/kg/day for children. Because absorption is variable and the drug exhibits zero-order (nonlinear) kinetics, the dose must be adjusted within 5 days, using blood concentration to guide therapy. The dose should be adjusted to achieve steady-state blood levels between 10 and 20 mg/liter. Oral bioavailability ranges from 80 to 95% and is diet dependent. Phenytoin exhibits zero-order pharmacokinetics; the rate of clearance of the drug is dependent upon the concentration of drug present. Therefore, phenytoin does not have a classic half-life like other drugs, since it varies with blood concentration (71). At a blood level of 15 mg/liter approximately half the drug in the patient's body will be eliminated in 20 hours. But, as the blood level drops, the rate at which it is excreted increases. Phenytoin has a volume of distribution of 0.65 liters/kg and is highly protein bound (90%), mostly to albumin (72). Some drug side effects occur in the therapeutic range; these include gingival hyperplasia, hyperglycemia, and skin rash.

Phenytoin pharmacokinetics are significantly affected by a number of other drugs. Again, phenytoin and phenobarbital are frequently coadministered. Induction of the cytochrome P-450 enzyme system by phenobarbital will increase the rate at which phenytoin is metabolized and cleared. At steady state, enzyme induction will increase the rate of clearance of phenytoin such that the dose must be increased approximately 30% to maintain therapeutic levels.

Phenytoin is highly bound to protein. Under normal circumstances, 90% of the drug is bound to albumin. Ten percent of the phenytoin circulates in the free, unbound form; thus, the normal range for free phenytoin is 1 to 2 mg/liter. Valproic acid, which is an antiepileptic frequently coadministered with phenytoin, will compete for the same binding sites on albumin as phenytoin (73). Valproic acid displaces phenytoin from albumin, reducing the fraction bound and increasing the free fraction. Free phenytoin is the active form of the drug, available to cross biological membranes and bind to receptors; increased free phenytoin produces an enhanced pharmacologic effect. At the same time, the free fraction is more available to the liver to be metabolized, so it is cleared more quickly. The overall effect of coadministration of a therapeutic dose of valproic acid is that the total concentration of phenytoin decreases because of increased clearance, but the free fraction increases. The free concentration of phenytoin, which is the active form, remains virtually the same. Thus, when valproic acid is added, no dosage adjustment is needed to maintain the same pharmacologic effect, but the total concentration of phenytoin decreases.

Uremia has a similar effect on phenytoin protein binding. In uremia, byproducts of normal metabolism accumulate and bind to albumin, displacing phenytoin, which causes an increase in the free fraction. Unlike the valproic acid circumstance, however, there is not the same opportunity for the free phenytoin fraction to be cleared. The result is that both the total and free concentrations of phenytoin increase, with the free concentration increasing faster than the total. Dosage must be reduced to avoid toxicity. The free phenytoin level is the best indicator of adequate therapy.

Toxicity is a constant possibility because of the manner in which phenytoin is metabolized. Small increases in dose can lead to very large increases in blood level, resulting in early signs of toxicity such as nystagmus, ataxia, and dysarthria. Severe toxicity occurs when the blood level exceeds 30 mg/liter and is typified by tremor, hyperreflexia, and lethargy. The outcome of phenytoin toxicity is not as severe as phenobarbital toxicity because phenytoin is not a CNS sedative.

CARBAMAZEPINE

Carbamazepine is used to control partial seizures associated with both temporal lobe and psychomotor symptoms and for generalized tonic-clonic seizures. It is also used for analgesia of trigeminal neuralgia.

Initially, carbamazepine is administered as an oral dose of 200 mg/day b.i.d. for adults or 100 mg/day b.i.d. for children, with dosage increases as the patient adapts to the medication. At steady state, adults are usually given no more than 1200 mg/day, and children no more than 1000 mg/day. Dosage adjustments are usually guided by monitoring blood levels. Most patients respond well when the blood concentration is in the range of 4 to 10 mg/liter (74). Carbamazepine exhibits a volume of distribution of 1.4 liter/kg with an elimination half-life of 15 hours. Protein binding averages 75%. Carbamazepine-10,11-epoxide (CBZ10-11) is an active metabolite that represents the predominant form of the drug in children. Optimal response occurs when the CBZ10-11 level is in the range of 0.5 to 2 mg/liter. The volume of distribution of CBZ10-11 is 1.1 liters/kg, and the half-life is 8 hours. It is 50% protein bound. Aplastic anemia and agranulocytosis are rare side effects of treatment

19. Tucker GT, Mather LE. Clinical pharmacokinetics of local anesthetics. Clin Pharmacokinet 1979;4:241–278.
20. Harrison DC. Should lidocaine be administered routinely to all patients after acute myocardial infarction? Circulation 1978;58:581–584.
21. Federman J, Vlietstra RE. Clinical pharmacology: II. Antiarrhythmic drug therapy. Mayo Clin Proc 1979;54:531–542.
22. Myerburg RJ. Relationship between plasma levels of procainamide, suppression of premature ventricular complexes and prevention of recurrent ventricular tachycardia. Circulation 1981;64:280–290.
23. Somogyi A, Heinzow B. Cimetidine reduces procainamide elimination. N Engl J Med 1982;307:1080.
24. Ochs HR, Greenblatt DJ, Woo E. Clinical pharmacokinetics of quinidine. Clin Pharmacokinet 1980;5:150–168.
25. Kessler KM, Lowenthal DT, Warner H, Gibson T, Briggs W, Reidenberg MM. Quinidine elimination in patients with congestive heart failure or poor renal function. N Engl J Med 1974;290:706–709.
26. Hooymans PM, Merkus FW. Effect of quinidine on plasma concentration of digoxin. Brit Med J 1978;2:1022.
27. Nayler WG. The pharmacology of disopyramide. J Int Med Res 1976;4(suppl 1):8–12.
28. Rangno RE, Warnica W, Ogilvie RI, Keeft J, Bridger E. Correlation of disopyramide pharmacokinetics with efficacy in ventricular tachyarrhythmia. J Int Med Res 1976;4(suppl 1): 54–58.
29. Maloney JD, Nissen RD, McColgan JM. Open clinical studies at a referral center: Chronic maintenance tocainide therapy in patients with recurrent sustained ventricular tachycardia refractory to conventional antiarrhythmic agents. Am Heart J 1980;100:1023–1030.
30. Graffner C, Conradson TB, Hovendahl S. Tocainide kinetics after intravenous and oral administration in healthy subjects and in patients with acute myocardial infarction. Clin Pharmacol Ther 1980;27:64–71.
31. Horowitz JD, Anavekar SN, Morris PM, Goble AJ, Doyle AE, Louis WJ. Comparative trial of mexiletine and lignocaine in the treatment of early ventricular tachyarrhythmias after acute myocardial infarction. J Cardiovasc Pharmacol 1981;3: 409–419.
32. Campbell DPS, Kelly JG, Adgey AAJ, Shanks RG. The clinical pharmacology of mexiletine. J Clin Pharmacol 1978;6:103–108.
33. Simon JP, Holt DW. Electrophysiological properties of mexiletine assessed with respect to plasma concentration. Eur J Cardiol 1980;11:115–121.
34. Hammill SC, Sorenson PB, Wood DL, et al. Propafenone for the treatment of refractory complex ventricular ectopic activity. Mayo Clin Proc 1986;61:98–103.
35. Connolly SJ, Kates RE, Lebsack CS, Harrison DC, Winkle RA. Clinical pharmacology of propafenone. Circulation 1983;68:589–596.
36. Riva E, Gerna M, Latini R, Giani P, Volpi A, Maggioni A. Pharmacokinetics of amiodarone in man. J Cardiovasc Dis 1982;4:264–269.
37. Heger JJ, Prystowsky EN, Zipes DP. Relationships between amiodarone dosage, drug concentrations, and adverse side effects. Am Heart J 1983;106:931–935.
38. Marcus FI. Drug interactions with amiodarone. Am Heart J 1983;106:924–930.
39. Appelfeld MM, Adir J, Crouthamel WG, Roffman DS. Digoxin pharmacokinetics in congestive heart failure. Clin Pharmacol 1982;21:114–120.
40. Cusack B, Kelly J, O'Malley K, Noel J, Lavan J, Horgan J. Digoxin in the elderly: pharmacokinetic consequences of old age. Clin Pharmacol Therp 1979;25:772–776.
41. Ingelfinger JA, Goldman P. The serum digitalis concentration—does it diagnose digitalis toxicity? N Engl J Med 1976;294:867–870.
42. Muller JE, Turi ZG, Stone PH, et al. Digoxin therapy and mortality after myocardial infarction: experience in the MILIS study. N Engl J Med 1986;314:265–271.
43. Kleinbloesem CH, van Brummelen P, Hillers J, Moolenaar AJ, Breimer DD. Interaction between digoxin and nifedipine at steady state in patients with atrial fibrillation. Ther Drug Monit 1985;7:372–376.
44. Leahey EB, Reiffel JA, Drusin RE, Heissenbuttel RH, Lovejoy WP, Bigger JT. Interaction between quinidine and digoxin. JAMA 1978;240:533–534.
45. Bresnahan JF, Vlietstra RE. Clinical pharmacology: III. Digitalis glycosides. Mayo Clin Proc 1979;54:675–684.
46. Koren G, Beatie D, Soldin S, Einerson TR, McLeod S. Interpretation of elevated postmortem serum concentrations of digoxin in infants and children. Arch Pathol Lab Med 1989;113:758–761.
47. Skogen WF, Rea MR, Valdes R. Endogenous digoxin-like immunoreactive factors eliminated from serum samples by hydrophobic silica-gel extraction and enzyme immunoassay. Clin Chem 1987;33:401–404.
48. Stone JA, Soldin SJ. Improved liquid chromatographic/immunoassay of digoxin in serum. Clin Chem 1988;34:2547–2551.
49. McGoon MD, Vlietstra RE, Holmes DR, Osborn JE. The clinical use of verapamil. Mayo Clin Proc 1982;57:495–510.
50. Dominic JA, Bourne DWA, Tan TG, Kirsten EB, McAlister RG. The pharmacology of verapamil: III. Pharmacokinetics in normal subjects after intravenous administration. J Cardiovasc Pharmacol 1981;3:25–38.
51. Anderson P, Bondesson U, Sylven C, Astrom H. Plasma concentration-response relationship of verapamil in the treatment of angina pectoris. J Cardiovasc Pharmacol 1982;4:608–614.
52. Schwartz JB, Keefe D, Kates RE, Kirsten E, Harrison DC. Acute and chronic pharmacodynamics interaction of verapamil and digoxin in atrial fibrillation. Circulation 1982;65: 1163–1170.
53. Hull JH, Sarubbi FA. Gentamicin serum concentrations: pharmacokinetic predictions. Ann Intern Med 1976;85:183–189.
54. Davey PG, Geddes AM, Gonda I, Harpur ES, Scott DK. Clinical experience with a method for adjusting gentamicin dose from measured drug clearance. J Antimicrob Chemother 1983;12:613–622.
55. Smith GR, Lipsky JJ, Laskin OL, et al. Double-blind comparison of the nephrotoxicity and auditory toxicity of gentamicin and tobramycin. N Engl J Med 1980;302:1107–1109.
56. NCCLS Standard PSM-7. Standard methods for dilution antimicrobial susceptibility tests for bacteria which grow aerobically. Villanova, PA: National Committee on Clinical Laboratory Standards, 1980.
57. Schaad VB, McCracken GH, Nelson JD. Clinical pharmacology and efficacy of vancomycin in pediatric patients. J Pediatr 1980;96:119–126.
58. Cook FV, Farrar WE. Vancomycin revisited. Ann Intern Med 1978;88:813–818.
59. Meissner HC, Smith AL. The current status of chloramphenicol. Pediatrics 1979;64:348–356.
60. Task Force on the Use of Laboratory Tests in Psychiatry. Tricyclic antidepressants—blood level measurements and clinical outcome: an APA Task Force Report. Am J Psychiatry 1985;142:155–162.
61. Biggs JT. Clinical pharmacology and toxicology of antidepressants. Hosp Pract 1978;15:79–84.

62. Vandel S, Vandel B, Sandoz M, Allers G, Bechtel P, Volmat R. Clinical response and plasma concentration of amitriptyline and its metabolite nortriptyline. Eur J Clin Pharmacol 1978;14:185–190.
63. Bailey DN, Van Dyke C, Langou RA, Jatlow PI. Tricyclic antidepressants: plasma levels and clinical findings in overdose. Am J Psychiatry 1978;135:1325–1328.
64. Preskorn SH, Irwin HA. Toxicity of tricyclic antidepressants—kinetics, mechanism, intervention: a review. J Clin Psychiatry 1982;43:151–156.
65. Zeigler VE, Biggs JT, Rosen SH, Meyer DA, Preskorn SH. Imipramine and desipramine plasma levels: relationship to dosage schedule and sampling time. J Clin Psychiatry 1978;39:660–663.
66. Ereshefsky L, Tran-Johnson T, Davis CM, LeRoy A. Pharmacokinetic factors affecting antidepressant drug clearance and clinical effect: evaluation of doxepin and imipramine—new data and review. Clin Chem 1988;34:863–880.
67. Monteleone P, Gnocchi G, Delrio G. Plasma trazodone concentrations and clinical response in elderly depressed patients: a preliminary study. J Clin Psychopharmacol 1989;9:284–287.
68. Faero O, Kastrup KW, Nielson EL, Melchior JC, Thorn I. Successful prophylaxis of febrile convulsions with phenobarbital. Epilepsia 1972;13:279–285.
69. Painter MJ, Pipenger C, MacDonald H, Pitlick W. Phenobarbital and diphenylhydantoin levels in neonates with seizures. J Pediatrics 1978;92:315–319.
70. Penry JK, Newmark ME. The use of antiepileptic drugs. Ann Intern Med 1979;90:207–218.
71. Richens A. Clinical pharmacokinetics of phenytoin. Clin Pharmacol 1979;4:153–169.
72. Graves NM, Leppik IE, Termond E, Taylor JW. Phenytoin clearances in a compliant population: description and application. Ther Dug Monit 1986;8:427–433.
73. Perucca E, Hebdige S, Frigo GM, Gatti G, Lecchini S, Crema A. Interaction between phenytoin and valproic acid: plasma protein binding and metabolic effects. Clin Pharmacol Ther 1980;28:779–789.
74. Cereghino JJ, Van Meter JC, Brock JT, Penry JK, Smith LD, White BG. Preliminary observations of serum carbamazepine concentration in epileptic patients. Neurology 1973;23:357–366.
75. Bruni J, Wilder BJ, Willmore LJ, Villarreal HJ, Thomas M, Crawford LEM. Clinical efficacy of valproic acid in relation to plasma levels. Can J Neurol Sci 1978;5:385–387.
76. Cotariu D, Zaidman JL. Valproic acid and the liver. Clin Chem 1988;34:890–897.
77. Gerber N, Dickinson RG, Harland RC, et al. Reye-like syndrome associated with valproic acid therapy. J Pediatr 1979;95:142–144.
78. Riva R, Albani F, Franzoni E, Perucca E, Santucci M, Baruzzi A. Valproic acid free-fraction in epileptic children under chronic monotherapy. Ther Drug Monit 1983;5:197–200.
79. Reidenberg MM, Levy M, Warner H, et al. Relationship between diazepam dose, plasma level, age, and central nervous system depression. Clin Pharmacol Ther 1978;23:371–374.
80. Browne TR. Clonazepam: a review of a new anticonvulsant drug. Arch Neurol 1976;33:326–332.
81. Van Dellen RG. Theophylline: practical applications of new knowledge. Mayo Clin Proc 1979;54:733–745.
82. Bredon JW, Bootman JL, Jones WN, et al. Theophylline serum concentration in ambulatory patients with chronic obstructive pulmonary disease. Ther Drug Monit 1985;7:168–173.
83. Vestal RE, Thummel KE, Musser B. Climetidine inhibits theophylline clearance in patients with chronic obstructive pulmonary disease: a study using stable isotope methodology during multiple oral dose administration. Br J Clin Pharmacol 1983;15:411–418.
84. Stults B, Felice-Johnson J, Higbee MD, Hardigan K. Effect of erythromycin stearate on serum theophylline concentration in patients with chronic obstructive lung disease. South Med J 1983;76:714–718.
85. Zwillich CW, Sutton FD, Neff TA, Cohn WM, Matthay RA, Weinberger MM. Theophylline-induced seizures in adults: correlation with serum concentrations. Am Intern Med 1975;82:784-787.
86. Ou CN. Efficacy of caffeine in the treatment of neonatal apnea. Am Assoc Clin Chem TDM-LIP 1985;6:1–5.
87. Wenk M, Follath F. Temperature dependency of apparent cyclosporin A concentration in plasma. Clin Chem 1983;29:1865.
88. Agarwal RP, Threatte GA, McPherson RA. Temperature-dependent binding of cyclosporine to an erythrocyte protein. Clin Chem 1987;33:481–485.
89. Hamberger C, Urien S, Barre J, et al. Distribution of cyclosporin A between blood cells and plasma of cardia and renal transplant recipients. Ther Drug Monit 1988;10:28–33.
90. Grevel J, Kahan BD. Area under the curve monitoring of cyclosporine therapy: the early posttransplant period. Ther Drug Monit 1991;13:89–95.
91. NACB/AACC Task Force on Cyclosporine Monitoring. Critical issues in cyclosporine monitoring: report of the task force on cyclosporine monitoring. Clin Chem 1987;33:1269–1288.
92. Kahan BD, Shaw LM, Holt DM, Grevel J, Johnston A. Consensus document: Hawk's Cay meeting on therapeutic drug monitoring of cyclosporine. Clin Chem 1990;36:1510–1516.
93. Myers BD, Ross J, Newton L, Luetscher J, Perlroth M. Cyclosporine-associated chronic nephropathy. N Engl J Med 1984;311:699–705.
94. Canadian Multicentre Transplant Group. A randomized clinical trial of cyclosporine in cadaveric renal transplantation. N Engl J Med 1986;314:1219–1225.
95. Maiorca R, Cristinelli F, Scolari F, et al. Cyclosporine toxicity can be minimized by careful monitoring of blood levels. Trans Proc 1985;17(suppl 2):54–60.
96. Moyer TP, Post GR, Sterioff S, Anderson CF. Cyclosporine nephrotoxicity is minimized by adjusting dosage on the basis of drug concentration in blood. Mayo Clin Proc 1988;63:241–247.
97. de Groen PC. Cyclosporine: a review and its specific use in liver transplantation. Mayo Clin Proc 1989;64:680–689.
98. Brat DJ, Windebank AJ, Brimijoin S. Emulsifier for intravenous cyclosporin inhibits neurite outgrowth, causes deficits in rapid axonal transport, and leads to structural abnormalities in differentiating N1E.115 neuroblastoma. J Pharmacol Exp Ther 1992;261:803–810.
99. Thompson CB, Sullivan KM, June CH, Thoman ED. Association between cyclosporin neurotoxicity and hypomagnesemia. Lancet 1984;2:1116–1120.
100. Ochiai T, Nakjima K, Nagata M, Hori S, Asano T, Isono K. Studies of induction and maintenance of long-term graft acceptance by treatment with FK-506. Transplantation 1987;44:734–738.
101. Kay JE, Moore AL, Doe SE, et al. The mechanism of action of FK-506. Transplant Proc 1990;22(suppl 1):96–99.
102. Starzl TE, Fung J, Jordan M, et al. Kidney transplantation under FK-506. JAMA 1990;264:63–67.

Method References[a]

Antiarrhythmics

Lidocaine

EIA: Walberg CB. Lidocaine by enzyme immunoassay. J Anal Toxicol 1978;2:121–123.

FPIA: Bertol E, Mari F, Torracco F. Comparison of lidocaine by fluorescent polarization immunoassay, enzyme immunoassay, and high resolution gas chromatography. J Anal Toxicol 1987;11: 122–124.

HPLC: Moyer TP, Pippenger CE, Blanke RV, et al. Therapeutic drug monitoring. In: Tietz NW, ed. Textbook of clinical chemistry. Philadelphia: WB Saunders, 1986:1644–1645.

Procainamide

EIA: Griffiths WC, Dextraze P, Hayes M, et al. Assay of serum procainamide and *N*-acetylprocainamide: a comparison of EMIT and reverse phase high performance liquid chromatography. Clin Toxicol 1980;16:51–54.

FRIA: Sonsalla PK, Bridges RR, Jennison TA, Smith CM. Evaluation of the TDx fluorescence polarization immunoassay for procainamide and *N*-acetylprocainamide. J Anal Toxicol 1985;9:152–155.

HPLC: Stearns FM, Broussard LA, Early RJ, Shaw LM, Spratt B, Frings CS. Determination of procainamide and *N*-acetylprocainamide by "high performance" liquid chromatography. Clin Chem 1981;27:2064–2067.

Quinidine

HPLC: Drayer DE, Restivo K, Reidenberg MM. Specific determination of quinidine and (3S)-3-hydroxyquinidine in human serum by high-pressure liquid chromatography. J Lab Clin Med 1977;90:816–822.

EIA: Drayer DE, Lorenzo B, Reidenberg MM. Liquid chromatography and fluorescence spectroscopy compared with a homogeneous enzyme immunoassay technique for determining quinidine in serum. Clin Chem 1981;27:308–310.

FPIA: Bridges RR, Smith CM, Jennison TA. Comparison of quinidine by fluorescence polarization immunoassay and high performance liquid chromatography. J Anal Toxicol 1984;8:161–164.

Disopyramide

EIA: Raghow G, Meyer MC, Straughn AB. Determination of free disopyramide plasma concentrations using ultrafiltration and enzyme multiplied immunoassay. Ther Drug Monit 1985;7:466–471.

HPLC: Meffin PJ, Harapat SR, Harrison DC. Analysis of disopyramide and its mono-*N*-dealkylated metabolite in plasma and urine. J Chromatogr 1977;132:503–510.

GLC: Vasiliades J, Owens C, Pirkle D. Gas chromatographic determination of disopyramide in serum, with use of nitrogen-selective detector. Clin Chem 1979;25:311–313.

Tocainide

HPLC: Reece PA, Stanley PE. High performance liquid chromatographic assay for tocainide in human plasma: comparison with gas-liquid chromatographic assay. J Chromatogr 1980;183:109–114.

GLC: Venkataramanan R, Axelson JE. Electron-capture detector GLC technique for estimating tocainide in biological fluids. J Pharmaceut Sci 1978;67:201–205.

Mexiletine

HPLC: Mastropaolo W, Holmes DR, Osborn MJ, et al. Improved liquid-chromatographic determination of mexiletine, an antiarrhythmic drug, in plasma. Clin Chem 1984;30:319–322.

GLC: Smith KJ, Meffin PJ. Mexiletine analysis in blood and plasma using gas chromatography and nitrogen-selective detection. J Chromatogr 1980;181:469–472.

Propafenone

HPLC: Harapat SR, Kates RE. High-performance liquid chromatographic analysis of propafenone in human plasma samples. J Chromatogr 1982;230:448–453.

GLC: Marchesini B, Bosci S, Mantovi MB. Determination of propafenone in serum or plasma by electron-capture gas chromatography. J Chromatogr 1982;232:435–439.

Amiodarone

HPLC: Flanagan RJ, Storey GCA, Holt DW. Rapid high-performance liquid chromatographic method for the measurement of amiodarone in blood plasma or serum at the concentrations attained during therapy. J Chromatogr 1980;187:391–398.

Digoxin

RIA: Smith TW, Butler VP, Haber E. Determination of therapeutic and toxic serum digoxin concentrations by radioimmunoassay. N Engl J Med 1969;281:1212–1216.

EIA: Clark DR, Inloes RL, Kalman SM, Sussman HH. Abbott Tdx, Dade Stratus, and DuPont aca automated digoxin immunoassays compared with a reference radioimmunoassay method. Clin Chem 1986;32:381–385.

FPIA: Erickson KA, Green PJ. Intercomparison of seven radioimmunoassay kits and a fluorescence polarization immunoassay kit for digoxin. Clin Chem 1984;30:1225–1227.

Verapamil

HPLC: Harapat SR, Kates RE. High-performance liquid chromatographic analysis of verapamil. J Chromatogr 1980;181:484–489.

GLC: McAlister RG, Tan TG, Bourne DWA. GLC assay of verapamil in plasma: identification of fluorescent metabolites after oral drug administration. J Pharm Sci 1979;68:574–577.

GC/MS: Hynning P, Anderson P, Bondesson U, Boreus LO. Liquid-chromatographic quantification compared with gas-chromatographic-mass-spectrometric determination of verapamil and norverapamil in plasma. Clin Chem 1988;34:2502–2503.

Antibiotics

Aminoglycosides

HPLC: Anhalt JP. Assay of gentamicin in serum by high-pressure liquid chromatography. Antimicrob Agents Chemother 1977;11: 651–655.

EIA: O'Leary TD, Ratcliff RM, Geary TD. Evaluation of an enzyme immunoassay for serum gentamicin. Antimicrob Agents Chemother 1980;17:776–778.

FPIA: Amina-Watson RA, Landon J, Shaw EJ, Smith DS. Polarization fluoroimmunoassay of gentamicin. Clin Chim Acta 1976;73: 51–55.

Bioassay: Edberg SC, Chu A. Determination of antibiotic levels in blood. Am J Med Technol 1975;41:99–105.

Vancomycin

HPLC: Uhl JR, Anhalt JP. High performance liquid chromatographic assay of vancomycin in serum. Ther Drug Monit 1979;1: 75–83.

RIA: Kirby WMM. Vancomycin therapy in severe staphylococcal infections. Rev Infect Dis 1981;3:S236–239.

FPIA: Schwenzer KS, Wang CHJ, Anhalt JP. Automated fluorescence polarization immunoassay for monitoring vancomycin. Ther Drug Monit 1983;5:341–345.

Chloramphenicol

GC: Pickering LK, Hoecker JL, Kramer WG, Liehr JG, Caprioli RM. Assays for chloramphenicol compared: radioenzymatic, gas

[a]Abbreviations: Color, classic colorimetric technique; EIA, homogeneous enzyme immunoassay; Fluor, fluorescence-based technique; FPIA, Fluorescence polarization immunoassay; GC/MS, gas chromatography/mass spectrometry; GLC, gas-liquid chromatography; HPLC, high-performance liquid chromatography; RIA, radioimmunoassay.

chromatographic with electron capture, and gas chromatographic-mass spectrometric. Clin Chem 1979;25:300–305.

HPLC: Gerson B, Anhalt JP, eds. High pressure liquid chromatography and therapeutic drug monitoring. Chicago: ASCP Press, 1980.

EIA: Schwartz JG, Castro DT, Ayo S, Carnahan JJ, Jorgenssen JH. A commercial enzyme immunoassay method (EMIT) compared with liquid chromatography and bioassay methods for measurement of chloramphenicol. Clin Chem 1988;34:1872–1875.

Sulfonamides

Color: Weinfeld RE, Lee TL. Simultaneous automated determination of free and total sulfisoxazole and sulfamethoxazole in plasma and urine. J Pharmaceut Sci 1979;68:1387–1392.

HPLC: Gerson B, Anhalt JP, eds. High pressure Liquid chromatography and therapeutic drug monitoring. Chicago: ASCP Press, 1980.

Antidepressants

Tricyclic Antidepressant Method References

GC/MS: Biggs JT, Holland WH, Chang S, Hipps PP, Sherman WP. Electron beam ionization mass fragmentographic analysis of tricyclic antidepressants in human plasma. J Pharm Sci 1976;65: 261–268.

HPLC: Wong SHY. Measurement of antidepressants by liquid chromatography: a review of current methodology. Clin Chem 1988;34:848–855.

EIA: Pankey S, Collins C, Jaklitsch A, et al. Quantitative homogeneous enzyme immunoassays for amitriptyline, nortriptyline, imipramine, and desipramine. Clin Chem 1986;32:768–772.

Trazodone

GC/MS: Anderson WH, Archuleta MM. The capillary gas chromatographic determination of trazodone in biological specimens. J Anal Toxicol 1984;8:217–219.

HPLC: Wong SHY, Waugh SW, Draz M, Nita J. Liquid-chromatographic determination of two antidepressants, trazodone and mianserin, in plasma. Clin Chem 1984;30:230–232.

Fluoxetine

GLC: Nash JF, Bopp RJ, Carmichael RH, Fario KZ, Lemberger L. Determination of fluoxetine and norfluoxetine in plasma by gas chromatography with electron-capture detection. Clin Chem 1982;28:2100–2102.

HPLC: Orsulak PJ, Kenney JT, Debus JR, Crowley G, Wittman PD. Determination of the antidepressant fluoxetine and its metabolite norfluoxetine in serum by reversed-phase HPLC, with ultraviolet detection. Clin Chem 1988;34:1875–1878.

Lithium

Atomic Absorption: Franzier A, Secunda SK, Mendels J. A method for the determination of sodium, potassium, magnesium, and lithium concentrations in erythrocytes. Clin Chem 1972;36:499–509.

Ion Electrode: Okorodudu AO, Burnett RW, McComb RB, Bowers GN. Evaluation of three first-generation ion-selective electrode analyzers for lithium: systematic errors, frequency of random interferences, and recommendations based on comparison with flame atomic emission spectrometry. Clin Chem 1990;36:104–110.

Antiepileptics

Phenobarbital

HPLC: Reidmann M, Rambeck B, Meijer JWA. Quantitative simultaneous determination of eight common antiepileptic drugs and metabolites by liquid chromatography. Ther Drug Monit 1981;3: 397–413.

EIA: Nandedkar AKN, Kutt H, Fairclough GF. Correlation of the "EMIT" with a gas-liquid chromatographic method for determination of antiepileptic drugs in plasma. Clin Toxicol 1978;12: 483–494.

FPIA: Wang ST, Peter F. The Abbott Tdx fluorescence polarization immunoassay and liquid chromatography compared for five anticonvulsant drugs in serum. Clin Chem 1985;31:493–494.

Phenytoin

Color: Svensmark O, Kristensen P. Determination of diphenylhydantoin and phenobarbital in small amounts of serum. J Lab Clin Med 1963;61:501–507.

HPLC: See phenobarbital reference.

EIA: Nandedkar AKN, Williamson R, Kutt H, Fairclough GF. A comparison of plasma phenytoin level determinations by EMIT and gas-liquid chromatography in patients with renal insufficiency. Ther Drug Monit 1980;2:427–430.

FPIA: See phenobarbital reference.

Fluor: Gonzalez G, Cid-Amador A, Steele B, Castro A. Results of fluorescent immunoassay for phenytoin compared with those by enzyme immunoassay, liquid chromatography, and discrete analysis (DuPont aca). Clin Chem 1982;28:1494–1496.

Carbamazepine

HPLC: See phenobarbital reference.

EIA: See phenobarbital reference.

FPIA: See phenobarbital reference.

Primidone

HPLC: See phenobarbital reference.

EIA: See phenobarbital reference.

FPIA: See phenobarbital reference.

Valproic Acid

GLC: Dusci LJ, Hackett LP. Gas chromatographic determination of valproic acid in human plasma. J Chromatogr 1977;132:145–147.

EIA: Kumps AH, Kumps-Grandjean B, Mardens Y. Enzyme immunoassay and gas-liquid chromatography compared for determination of valproic acid. Clin Chem 1986;27:1788–1789.

FPIA: Haidukewych D. Fluorescence polarization immunoassay and enzyme immunoassay compared for free valproic acid in serum ultrafiltrates from epileptic patients. Clin Chem 1985;31: 156.

Ethosuximide

HPLC: See phenobarbital reference.

EIA: See phenobarbital reference.

FPIA: See phenobarbital reference.

Benzodiazepines

GLC (Diazepam): Kelly RC, Anthony RM, Krent L, Thompson WL, Sunshine I. Toxicological determination of benzodiazepines in serum: methods and concentrations associated with high-dose intravenous therapy with diazepam. Clin Toxicol 1979;14: 445–457.

GLC (Clonazepam): de Silva JA, Puglisi CV, Munno N. Determination of clonazepam and flunitrazepam in blood and urine by electron-capture GLC. J Pharmacol Sci 1974;63:520–527.

Bronchodilators

Theophylline

HPLC: Ou CN, Frawley V. Concurrent measurement of theophylline and caffeine in neonates by an interference-free liquid-chromatographic method. Clin Chem 1983;29:1934–1936.

EIA: Chang J, Gotcher S, Gushaw JB. Homogeneous enzyme immunoassay for theophylline in serum and plasma. Clin Chem 1982;28:361–367.

FRIA: Lalande RL, Bottorff MB, Straughn M. Comparison of high performance liquid chromatography and fluorescence polarization immunoassay methods in a theophylline pharmacokinetic study. Ther Drug Monit 1985;7:442–446.

Caffeine

HPLC: Ou CN, Frawley V. Concurrent measurement of theophylline and caffeine in neonates by an interference-free liquid-chromatographic method. Clin Chem 1983;29:1934–1936.

EIA: Ou CN, Frawley VL, Ellis JM. Evaluation of the EMIT reagent system for measurement of caffeine with the EMIT Lab 5000 system and a centrifugal analyzer. Clin Chem 1984;30:887–889.

GLC: Floberg S, Linstrom B, Lonnerholm G. Simultaneous determination of theophylline and caffeine after extractive alkylation in small volumes of plasma by gas chromatography-mass spectrometry. J Chromatogr 1980;221:166–169.

Immunosuppressants

Cyclosporine

Polyclonal RIA: Donatsch P, Abisch E, Homberger M, et al. A radioimmunoassay to measure Sandimmune in plasma and serum samples. J Immunoassay 1981;2:19–32.

Monoclonal RIA: Holt DW, Johnston A, Marsden JT, et al. Monoclonal antibodies for radioimmunoassay of cyclosporine: a multicenter comparison of their performance with the Sandoz polyclonal radioimmunoassay kit. Clin Chem 1988;34:1091–1096.

Monoclonal EIA: Yatscoff RW, Copeland KR, Faraci CJ. Abbott TDx monoclonal assay evaluated for measuring cyclosporine in whole blood. Clin Chem 1990;36:1969–1973.

Monoclonal EIA: Dasgupta A, Soldana S, Desai M, et al. Analytical performance of EMIT cyclosporine assay evaluated. Clin Chem 1991;37:2130–2133.

HPLC: Moyer TP, Johnson P, Faynor SM, et al. Cyclosporine: a review of drug monitoring problems and presentation of a simple, accurate liquid chromatographic procedure that solves these problems. Clin Biochem 1986;19:83–89.

FK-506

RIA: Tamura K, et al. A highly sensitive method to assay FK-506 levels in plasma. Trans Proc 1987;19(suppl 6):23–29.

20 Toxicology

Tai C. Kwong

SCOPE OF CLINICAL TOXICOLOGY

Clinical toxicology in laboratory medicine can be defined as the analysis of drugs in human biological fluids for the purpose of patient care (1). The two traditional clinical toxicology services provided by clinical laboratories are therapeutic drug monitoring and emergency toxicology. Therapeutic drug monitoring, which is the measurement of serum drug concentration to aid in optimizing drug therapy, is the topic of another chapter. Emergency toxicology is the accumulation of laboratory data to assist in the diagnosis and treatment of poisonings due to self-poisoning, accidental ingestion, or exposure.

In the last few years, the widespread abuse of illicit drugs has placed additional demands on the health care system. Consequently, clinical toxicology laboratories have moved beyond their traditional activities and are now routinely performing urine testing of drugs of abuse for the purposes of documentation and management of drug dependency. As patient enrollment in treatment for chemical dependency has increased, so has the need for the laboratory to assist in the counseling and monitoring of these patients by urine drug testing.

Some clinical toxicology laboratories have extended their expertise in analytical toxicology of drugs of abuse into the new arena of workplace drug testing. This is nonmedical testing, and is a departure from the traditional mission of clinical toxicology. The forensic nature and specific requirements of workplace drug testing are discussed at the end of this chapter.

ROLE OF THE CLINICAL TOXICOLOGY LABORATORY

The role of the clinical toxicology laboratory is to provide toxicology data to assist the clinician in the diagnosis, management, and monitoring of poisonings and substance abuse (2, 3). Because of the complexity of the diagnosis and treatment of poisoning and substance abuse, a team effort of the clinical staff and laboratory personnel is required.

In the emergency department, the clinician first makes an assessment based on history and physical examination, and the patient is treated symptomatically to support vital signs and vital functions. Toxicological data, if available at this point, can influence the diagnosis and subsequent treatment of the patient. If the patient is obtunded or comatose, a drug history may not be available. Drug history, even if available, is frequently inaccurate. Hence an emergency toxicology screen can validate drug history or identify drugs that are not previously suspected (4). In those cases where specific treatments are effective, expeditious laboratory identification of the toxic agents is invaluable for prompt institution of treatment: for example, the initiation of *N*-acetylcysteine therapy for acetaminophen overdose, hemoperfusion for massive barbiturate overdose, or administration of ethanol for methanol poisoning. A drug screen that fails to identify specific toxic agents is still an important laboratory result because it will influence the clinician to evaluate the differential diagnosis and to explore other diagnostic studies to explain the patient's clinical presentation. The determination of serum drug levels can, in some instances, help to gauge the severity of intoxication and prognosis. Ensuing determinations can be useful in monitoring and evaluating the effectiveness of the treatment procedure.

The demand for drugs of abuse testing has come not only from the emergency department, but also from other clinical services such as obstetrics for pregnant drug abusers, pediatrics for their newborns and drug dependency treatment programs. Such testing usually focuses on a small panel of the most frequently abused drugs such as cocaine, cannabinoids, and the benzodiazepines, rather than the broad spectrum screening performed in emergency toxicology.

Pregnant patients with a chemical dependency, particularly that of cocaine, are at high risk for obstetric complications (5). Urine testing for drugs of abuse provides evidence for the diagnosis of drug dependency and subsequent monitoring of drug use during the course of the pregnancy. For babies born of drug-dependent mothers, there is a higher risk of congenital malformations and neurobehavioral impairment (6). Therefore, early identification of their addiction not only allows better medical care; it will also permit prompt social evaluation and intervention. In many localities, the hospital, upon the demonstration of illicit drug in an infant's urine, may be required to report it to a governmental agency. This may trigger a sequence of events that in extreme cases may result in the removal of the infant from the mother's custody. While the mother's family and social environment are important considerations, the confirmed positive urine drug test result is frequently the overriding medical evidence in this contest of custody. In these instances, the clinical toxicology testing has taken on an additional evidentiary role. Therefore, the laboratory must be prepared to defend its data against challenges.

Urine drug testing is an objective way to identify these infants. However, because urine collection for infants is difficult and drug concentration is low, urine screening probably underestimates the number of babies at risk. Recent data suggested that testing for drugs in meconium may be a better approach (7).

The emphasis on treatment and rehabilitation of chemical dependency has led to higher numbers of patients enrolled in drug treatment programs. Many clinical toxicology laboratories now routinely perform urine testing in support of the diagnosis of these patients' chemical dependency. Urine testing also is an adjunct to the counseling and management of these patients by monitoring their progress during rehabilitation. Enrollment in drug treatment programs is not always voluntary. A drug-addicted employee may have enrolled because his employer's substance abuse policy mandates that all employees with a drug problem must be rehabilitated as a condition for continued employment. Successful rehabilitation is evidenced in part by negative urine drug test results obtained during and after the treatment program. Therefore, although the toxicology laboratory is performing testing for medical reasons, test results may ultimately be used for administrative purposes, and the potential for legal challenge by dismissed employees is real.

TOXICOLOGY SERVICE

Cost constraints and staffing problems limit the kind of toxicology service a laboratory can provide. The laboratory has to design a drug screen that is cost-effective and that can still meet the basic needs of clinicians. Furthermore, programmatic issues that need to be considered include what drugs comprise a drug screen, which assays should be qualitative or quantitative, what type of sample is required, when the specimen should be obtained, and how much time is involved in completing a drug screen (8–10).

Ideally, the laboratory will be one that can analyze for any drug the clinician might encounter, and can do so in the shortest turnaround time. In reality, this goal is difficult to achieve. Methodologies for many drugs are not suitable for a clinical toxicology laboratory, either because they require costly and sophisticated instrumentation, or the turnaround time is too long for them to be clinically useful. Even in laboratories blessed with experienced staff and advanced instrumentation, the financial and personnel requirements for performing timely comprehensive drug screening are prohibitive. Therefore, a drug screen should be one that is designed to detect a shorter list of drugs, the selection of which is based on the prevalence of these drugs in the population served by the emergency department, the clinical usefulness of their early identification, and the ability of the laboratory to perform the analyses within an acceptable turnaround time. This list should be determined jointly by the emergency department and the laboratory. A basic clinical toxicology service should include tests for ethanol, salicylate, acetaminophen, barbiturates, and the tricyclic antidepressants. Serum iron and total iron binding capacity (TIBC), carboxyhemoglobin, and methemoglobin should also be available (usually analyzed in the clinical chemistry laboratory). Any drugs that have a high prevalence in the locality should also be included. The importance of turnaround time for a drug screen is directly related to the impact the results have on patient management. Therefore, these drug tests are recommended available on an immediate (stat) basis. With additional resources and expertise, the laboratory may enlarge its service to include other drug assays: e.g., cocaine, opiates, benzodiazepines, phenothiazines, sedative-hypnotics. The laboratory should encourage clinicians to inquire about drugs that are not on this list and whether they can be identified by the laboratory or by a reference laboratory.

A drug screen is a compromise among rapid turnaround time, analytical specificity, and sensitivity, and it may be a combination of qualitative and quantitative analyses. An initial screen might be a targeted search for a small number of drugs by a series of tests, each of which is specific for a drug or group of drugs (e.g., spot tests or immunoassays). Obviously, this approach is restricted, as the availability of specific methodologies is limited. Moreover, the time required for these individual assays is cumulative, and the turnaround time rapidly deteriorates as the number of drug assays increases. If the number of drugs in a screen has to be expanded, a broad-spectrum screen utilizing a methodology such as thin-layer chromatography or gas chromatogra-

Urine Qualitative		
TLC	Broad-spectrum screen → Confirmation	
Spot test	Salicylate → Serum quantitation	
Enzyme Immunoassays	Benzodiazepines Cocaine/benzoylecgonine → Confirmation Opiates THC	
Serum Quantitative		
	Alcohols Acetaminophen* Salicylate* Hypnotic sedatives* Theophylline*	Phenytoin* Digoxin* Lithium* Iron/TIBC*

* Quantitation when indicated.

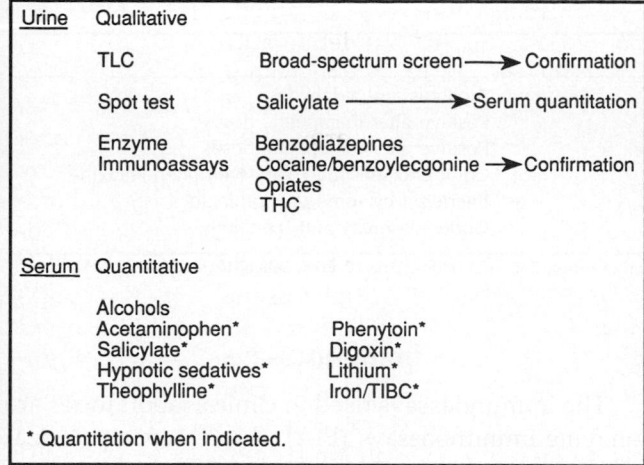

Figure 20.1. A thin-layer chromatography based comprehensive drug screen.

phy can be employed at the expense of lower sensitivity compared to immunoassays.

The specimens most frequently submitted for analysis are urine, blood, serum/plasma, and gastric fluid. Drug screens in most clinical laboratories are performed on urine. The advantage of urine is that a large volume can be obtained, allowing analysis of drugs in low concentration. Urine, however, contains metabolites, which may complicate identification. For those drugs that are extensively metabolized, the parent drug may not be present; therefore an assay should be chosen that will identify the metabolites that are present in the greatest concentrations. Urine tests are qualitative, as quantitation offers little correlation with clinical effects. Blood (and serum or plasma), although limited by sample volume, is the specimen of choice for quantitative analysis of those drugs for which therapeutic and toxic levels are known.

Quantitative tests are usually more time consuming. If knowledge of a specific level does not influence patient management, quantitation should not be performed. Some tests that provide useful quantitative information include those for acetaminophen, alcohols, salicylates, barbiturates, phenytoin, theophylline, lithium, digoxin, and iron/TIBC. Quantitative level, however, can be misleading for drugs for which tolerance can develop. For example, a supposedly lethal barbiturate level for a novice user may be well tolerated by a chronic barbiturate abuser. First gastric aspirate, vomitus, or stomach washings are appropriate specimens if they are obtained soon after ingestion and particularly if pill fragments are noted. Drug concentrations in these specimens are high, and metabolites that may interfere with some analyses are absent, but drugs that are rapidly absorbed or that are not taken orally will not be detected.

An example of a thin-layer chromatography (TLC)-based comprehensive drug screen is presented in Figure 20.1. The urine TLC screen is supplemented by a spot test for salicylate and four immunoassays. These analytes are not adequately detected by TLC due to poor extraction from urine (salicylate and benzoylecognine), or low sensitivity without prior hydrolysis of conjugates (opiates and benzodiazepines). A urine that tests positive for one of the drugs will often be processed for confirmatory testing. Quantitation in serum is always necessary for an alcohol; for some other drugs, serum levels may be informative and quantitation will be performed when indicated.

Although much emphasis has been placed on the rapidity with which a drug screen can be performed and reported, the importance of accuracy needs to be addressed (11). The analytical methods used in performing a drug screen, including colorimetric assays, immunoassays, TLC, and gas chromatography (GC), do not necessarily give unequivocal identification of a drug. Some assays are group-specific rather than analyte-specific (e.g., an immunoassay for the opiates rather than morphine). Some chromatographic methods do not separate isomers (e.g., quinine and quinidine by TLC and GC) or closely related drugs (e.g., the tricyclic antidepressants by GC). Hence there is a need for confirmation of a presumptive positive result obtained by the screening test.

Repeat analysis of the presumptive positive specimen using the same screening test method does not constitute confirmation, although it does serve to reduce random error. Confirmation requires testing a new aliquot of the original specimen using a different technique that has greater specificity and at least equal sensitivity to that of the initial test. For example, a presumptive positive result obtained by an immunoassay for opiates cannot be confirmed by a different opiate immunoassay. It can be confirmed by TLC, however, which can identify the opiate involved. While confirmation testing is mandatory in forensic toxicology, in clinical toxicology, where rapid turnaround time to support a diagnosis of a suspected drug overdose is required, it is not always possible to meet these requirements. Presumptive positives are routinely reported by the clinical laboratories, but interpretation by the clinician is done within the context of both clinical and other laboratory findings. The laboratory, however, should make every attempt to do confirmatory testing whenever possible. The laboratory report must state accurately whether the positive result is a confirmed positive or an unconfirmed (presumptive) positive so that clinicians can properly evaluate toxicologic results.

Table 20.1. Spot Tests[a]

Drug(s)	Test	Comments
Volatiles (U, S)[b]	Dichromate	Alcohols and aldehydes
Salicylates (U, S)	Trinder's	Positive after therapeutic doses
Acetaminophen (U)	Cresol-ammonia	Positive after therapeutic doses
Phenothiazines (U)	FPN	Color and sensitivity vary with phenothiazine
Imipramine/desipramine/trimipramine (U)	Forrest	Interfered by some phenothiazines
Ethchlorvynol (U, S)	Diphenylamine	Good sensitivity and specificity

[a]From Stevens HM. Colour tests. In: Moffat AC, ed. Clark's isolation and identification of drugs. 2nd ed. London: The Pharmaceutical Press, 1986:128–147.
[b]U, urine; S, serum.

METHODOLOGIES

Spot Tests

Spot tests are among the simplest, most rapid, and inexpensive screening tests. Urine or serum is added directly to the reagents either in a test tube or on a white tile or porcelain dish. The formation of a color product indicates the presence of a specific drug, but more often, a class of drugs (e.g., a positive Folin-Ciocalteu test for phenolic compounds). Interpretation of the color test should take into consideration that a range of color is possible (e.g., phenothiazines give red, orange, blue, or violet colors with the Forrest Reagent), colors may vary dependent on the conditions of the test, amount of substance present, and the presence of other drugs and extraneous material. A positive test should trigger more definitive testing. Examples of spot tests routinely performed in clinical laboratories are in Table 20.1 (12).

Ultraviolet Spectroscopy

Identification of a compound by ultraviolet (UV) spectroscopy is based on the compound's UV absorbance spectrum. Specificity is enhanced by scanning in acidic and basic pH and in solvent (e.g., methanol) to generate a family of curves with characteristic peaks and troughs. Absorptivity ratios of the peaks and the change in these ratios, and spectral shift when pH changes occur are criteria for identification. Excellent compilation of spectral data are available (13, 14). Selectivity can be enhanced by techniques such as difference and higher derivative spectrophotometry, which are available on modern computer-driven instrumentation (15).

The use of UV spectral data with other analytical techniques, e.g., HPLC, is a powerful combination for specific identification of a compound. The recent development of coupling HPLC to rapid-scanning photodiode array detector permits spectrum acquisition during elution of peaks and microcomputer technology enables identification based on library searches (16).

Immunoassays

The immunoassays used in clinical laboratories are enzyme immunoassays (EIA), fluorescence polarization immunoassays (FPIA), and radioimmunoassays (RIA). These assays have sensitivity more than adequate for drug overdose situations, and with no preliminary extraction required before analysis, they can give a fast positive or negative result. The nonisotopic assays (EIA and FPIA) have the advantage over RIA in that they are homogeneous assays. Therefore they are more rapid and easily automated. RIAs, although more sensitive, and less susceptible to signal interference, are less frequently used because the long incubation time precludes short turnaround time.

A drug screen utilizing immunoassays is a combination of individual tests. Although each individual test is fast, the time required for several accumulates. Also, the spectrum of drugs that can be detected in such a screen is limited to those for which assay kits are available. The immunoassay kits are designed specifically for use with either urine or serum/plasma. When a kit is used with a different matrix (e.g., analyzing serum with a urine assay), the laboratory needs to validate this modification.

Not all immunoassays are specific for an analyte (17). Many will detect a family of closely related compounds with different degrees of cross-reactivity. For example, the opiates assay will detect morphine, codeine, and synthetic narcotics such as hydromorphone, hydrocodone and oxycodone. Therefore, a positive result will require additional testing by confirmation assays that can differentiate among members of this family. Forensic urine drug testing has been the driving force behind the development of more specific assays. For example, new amphetamine assays are highly specific for amphetamine and methamphetamine with much lower cross-reactivity with phenylpropanolamine and other phenethylamines. While this approach was intended to reduce the number of presumptive positives needing gas chromatography-mass spectrometry confirmation, the use of such an assay of limited specificity is less useful in clinical toxicology. The users of immunoassays should be familiar with assay specificities for proper interpretation of test results.

Thin-Layer Chromatography

The simplicity, reliability, and low cost of a thin-layer chromatography (TLC) system are the reasons why this technique is widely used for drug screening and confirmation. Its selectivity of detection is enhanced through the use of various stationary and mobile phases, and color reagents. For larger laboratories, the ability to perform simultaneous analyses of several specimens is an advantage. Drug spots on the chromatogram can be scraped off and eluted for further testing (18).

The disadvantage of TLC is lower sensitivity (usually greater than 1 mg/liter) compared with GC or HPLC, although the limits of detection are adequate for a large number of commonly encountered drugs in overdose cases. TLC also has lower resolution compared with GC or HPLC, particularly when small size (10 cm) plates are used. Recent developments in high-performance TLC (HPTLC) have demonstrated improvement in both sensitivity and resolution. Despite the simplicity of TLC procedures, proper interpretation of a TLC chromatogram requires highly skilled and experienced personnel. A commercially available TLC system in kit form facilitates a broad spectrum TLC screen by providing accelerated development and a systematized color detection scheme (19).

Gas Chromatography

Gas chromatography (GC) is a powerful tool for separating a mixture of drugs (20). GC is the method of choice for volatile compounds (e.g., anesthetic gases, organic solvent, alcohols). It is less suitable for compounds of low volality or those with polar functional groups. Careful use of chemical derivatives can overcome these problems. More problematic are compounds that are thermally unstable (e.g., benzodiazepines).

Although a wide choice of stationary phases is available, only a few are commonly used in drug analysis such as the roughly equivalently nonpolar dimethyl silicone phases of SE-30, OV-1, and OV-101, and the relatively more polar phenylmethyl silicone, OV-17. A single column of SE-30 (and its equivalents) or OV-17 can elute most of the drugs of interest, and is therefore sufficient for a drug screen. More definitive identification can be based on the retention data obtained by simultaneous chromatography on two different columns linked to the injector by a splitter. Separation has further been advanced by the use of capillary columns. The higher efficency of these columns results in tall narrow peaks that improves detection limits.

Among the detectors, the flame ionization detector (FID) is probably the most widely used. It responds with good sensitivity to nearly all classes of compounds with excellent linearity over a wide range of concentrations. The nitrogen-phosphorus detector (or NPD) has enhanced response to compounds containing nitrogen and phosphorous. Since most drugs contain nitrogen atoms NPD is particularly useful for drug analysis and has sensitivity up to 100 times that of an FID. By adjusting detector operating conditions, an NPD can have virtual specificity for phosphorus compounds, making it especially useful for detection of phosphorus-containing pesticide.

The electron capture detector (ECD) has very high sensitivity for compounds with high affinity for electrons such as those containing halogen, nitro, or carbonyl groups. The selectivity of the ECD and its high sensitivity (down to 1 pg) makes it very useful for drugs such as benzodiazepines and phenothiazines, which are present in very low concentrations. The higher selectivity of this detector, however, makes it unsuitable for drug screening.

The use of a mass spectrometer (MS) as a GC detector provides sensitivity and specificity unsurpassed by other detectors. Mass spectrometry in combination with chromatographic separation is the most effective method for identification of drugs (21, 22). The mode of ionization most widely used is electron impact (EI), which is the only mode available in the low cost MS equipment. Since fragmentation can be quite extensive with EI, the molecular ion may not be detectable. Therefore, the molecular weight cannot be deduced. In chemical ionization, soft ionization results in fragmentation, which is minimal, and a prominent molecular ion or quasimolecular ion (frequently the base peak) allows molecular weight elucidation. Less fragmentation, however, means less structural information for unambiguous identification. Operation of an MS in the CI mode gives even higher sensitivity than EI, but the best performance will require more critical conditions.

Identification of unknowns by MS can be based on the computer matching of the unknown mass spectrum against those that are commercially available in libraries. Alternatively, a laboratory can build its own library of the most frequently encountered drugs.

The main disadvantages of MS are the complexity and cost of the instrumentation. Recently, low-cost bench top instruments have been designed for routine analysis, multiple-operators, easy maintenance, and good reliability. These instruments have made GC-MS affordable and technologically accessible for many clinical laboratories. Still, GC-MS analysis is costly in terms of equipment, personnel, and required time. It is not cost-effective for screening and is more suitable for confirmation testing. In forensic urine drug testing, confirmation by GC-MS analysis is the standard of practice and is mandated in federally regulated programs.

High-Performance Liquid Chromatography

High-performance liquid chromatography (HPLC) is similar to GC in its ability to separate complex mixture of drug compounds, and the availability of a variety of detectors (spectrophotometric, fluorometric, electrochemical, mass spectrometric) that can be used to attain high sensitivity (23). HPLC has the advantage over GC in that compounds which are nonvolatile and thermally labile can be analyzed. Until recently, HPLC has found its place in a toxicology laboratory mostly as an instrument for quantitative analysis of targeted groups of drugs (e.g., tricyclic antidepressants, benzodiazepines, barbiturates) rather than for broad spectrum drug screen. Structural information helpful for identification of unknown compounds eluting from HPLC can be obtained using an MS detector or photodiode array detector. Recently, an automated LC system equipped with extraction and analysis columns was reported. Identification of up to 300 basic drugs and metabolites is based on retention and scanning UV data. This approach seems promising for performing routine drug screens by HPLC (16).

CLINICAL TOXICOLOGY OF SELECTED DRUGS

Ethanol

Ethanol is the most widely used social drug, and its abuse is one of the most important causes of injury and disease. Recent attempts to combat the problems of driving while under the influence of alcohol (DUI) have placed additional responsibilities on hospitals and clinical laboratories because the results of blood alcohol analyses, although obtained for medical reasons, may be used for legal purposes.

Ethanol is usually consumed in beers (3 to 6% ethanol), wines (10 to 12%), and distilled beverages (40 to 50%). The term "proof" means two times the percent of ethanol by volume. Ethanol is rapidly absorbed, and there is significant intersubject variability in the peak blood alcohol concentration attained and the time for its achievement due to food intake and physiological variables (24). Ethanol distributes in total body water. Therefore, at equilibrium ethanol concentration in any tissue or fluid is a function of water content of that specimen. A plasma/blood ratio of 1.18 (range of 1.10 to 1.35), urine/blood ratio of 1.3, and breath/blood ratio of 2180 (range of 1837 to 2863) have been determined (25).

Ethanol is metabolized mostly by liver alcohol dehydrogenase to acetaldehyde at a rate that follows first order kinetics at low concentration (less than 20 mg/dl). At higher concentration, metabolism proceeds at zero order kinetics, which is independent of dose or initial blood alcohol concentration. The average rate of metabolism is approximately 16 mg/dl/hr for men with significant variability (10 to 25 mg/dl/hr) and may be 10 to 20% lower for women (26). Individuals with high blood ethanol concentration (greater than 3 g/liter) have a rate of metabolism that is higher and more unpredictable (27).

Ethanol is a central nervous system (CNS) depressant. In intolerant subjects, ethanol-induced CNS dysfunction ranges from limited muscular incoordination at blood concentrations less than 50 mg/dl to coma, respiratory failure, and death at 400 mg/dl or higher. It is difficult to interpret blood levels in tolerant subjects. Seemingly alert patients with ethanol levels in excess of 600 mg/dl have been reported.

The clinical signs of alcohol intoxication can be simulated by other diseases such as diabetic ketoacidosis and subdural hematoma. Blood alcohols are ordered for the investigation of those patients who present with anion gap metabolic acidosis or those who are comatose. Medically, it may be desirable, or necessary, to know the patient's blood alcohol concentration before administrating anesthetics or medications.

Clinical toxicology laboratories are increasingly involved in the collection and analysis of blood for ethanol that subsequently has forensic implications. A set of guidelines has been developed in response to the need for information that deals with various aspects of blood alcohol analysis (28).

TYPE OF SPECIMEN

Plasma or serum is usually analyzed in clinical laboratories. Most state laws on drinking and driving, however, define alcohol concentration in terms of whole blood. Alcohol concentration in whole blood is lower than in plasma or serum; the frequently used serum/whole blood ratio is 1.18. The analysis of either serum or whole blood yields results with the same clinical significance. However, the difference between serum and whole blood ethanol concentration is significant in forensic analysis particularly when a "blood" alcohol result falls in the vicinity of a statutory threshold pertaining to drinking and driving. Conversion of results of alcohol analysis performed on serum or plasma to whole blood using a population mean ratio of 1.18 is discouraged. For legal purposes it is best to analyze whole blood. Laboratories that analyze serum samples for alcohol should identify them in their reports.

Urine is not a suitable specimen because blood alcohol concentration cannot be established with sufficient reliability from alcohol concentration of a pooled bladder urine specimen and because of the great variability of the blood:urine ratio of alcohol.

Venipuncture sites should be cleansed by non–alcohol-containing disinfectant such as benzalkonium chloride or aqueous povidone-iodine. If analysis will be delayed for a few hours, sodium fluoride at 1.5 g/liter (higher for longer-term storage) is an effective perservative.

ANALYTICAL METHODS

Many methods for alcohol analysis are in use in clinical laboratories (29). They can be grouped into the following categories:

- Chemical oxidation of ethanol with acid dichromate. The reduction of dichromate is proportional to ethanol concentration. This is a nonspecific reaction; other alcohols and paraldehyde (as its metabolite acetaldehyde) will also give positive results. It is used in some breath analyzers.
- Enzymatic oxidation using alcohol dehydrogenase (ADH)

$$C_2H_5OH + NAD^+ \xrightarrow{ADH} CH_3CHO + NADH + H^+$$

The specificity of this assay depends on the source of ADH; interference by methanol and isopropanol varies substantially among kits. The alcohol assay available on the Abbott TDx is an ADH-based assay that measures the attenuation of fluorescence. Enzymatic methods are simple and the most commonly used methods in clinical laboratories. Laboratories, however, must be prepared to investigate ingestion of alcohols other than ethanol or the coingestion of ethanol and another alcohol.
- Gas chromatography. Gas chromatography is the most specific method (30, 31). It yields information on both identity of the alcohol as well as concentration. For emergency analysis, direct injection of a diluted sample is preferred because it eliminates the 15- to 30-minute equilibration period required for head space analysis. The use of an internal standard (e.g., n-propanol) will improve precision.

In emergencies where better methods are not available, the difference between the measured serum osmolality and the calculated serum osmolality can serve as an indirect approximation of ethanol concentration (32). A formula to estimate serum osmolality is:

$$\left[1.86 \times \text{Na (mmol/liter)} + \frac{\text{Glucose (mg/dl)}}{18} + \frac{\text{BUN (mg/dl)}}{2.8}\right] \div 0.93$$

The calculated osmolality is divided by 0.93 as serum is approximately 93% water. The measured osmolality must be determined by freezing point depression osmometry (not by using a vapor pressure osmometer). The expected contribution to measured osmolality of a serum ethanol concentration of 100 mg/dl is 21.7 mOsm/kg. Ethanol is the most common cause for elevation of serum osmolality. Users of this approach must be aware of its nonspecificity since other alcohols, acetone and ethylene glycol can also raise serum osmolality if present in sufficient concentration.

CONCENTRATION UNITS

Clinical laboratories most commonly report alcohol concentration as milligram alcohol per 100 ml (dl) of blood (or serum). Many state laws define blood alcohol concentration as percent by weight/volume (% w/v). A concentration of 100 mg/dl is equivalent to 0.1% w/v.

Methanol and Isopropanol

Methanol and isopropanol are important industrial chemicals that are also available as household items—methanol as a constituent of some antifreeze and windshield washer solutions; isopropanol as a disinfectant (30 to 99.9% solution) or as rubbing alcohol (70% solution). Intoxication with methanol and isopropanol can be due to accidental ingestion, industrial exposure, self-poisoning as in suicide attempts, or as substitutes for ethanol.

Both methanol and isopropanol are readily absorbed following ingestion. They are metabolized by hepatic alcohol dehydrogenase at rates one-tenth or less of that for ethanol. Methanol is oxidized to highly toxic formaldehyde and then to formic acid. Formic acid is much more toxic than methanol and accounts for the profound anion gap metabolic acidosis and its occular toxicity. Ingestion of as little as 10 ml of methanol has caused permanent blindness, and the fatal dose for adults is 100 ml. Since methanol is a CNS toxin, symptoms may include inebriation, headache, dizziness, seizure, and coma. Nausea, vomiting, stiff neck, abdominal pain, and malaise are also common complaints. There may be a latent period of up to 8 to 12 hours when there is a deceiving lack of severe toxic manifestation but during which appropriate treatment is critical.

Isopropanol is metabolized to acetone, which accounts for the CNS effects and ketonemia. There is no metabolic acidosis. Hemorrhagic tracheobronchitis and gastritis are characteristic findings. A lethal ingested dose of isopropanol has been estimated to be 250 ml for an adult.

Since the toxicity of both methanol and isopropanol are due to their toxic metabolites generated by alcohol dehydrogenase, the treatment is similar (33, 34). The alcohol dehydrogenese activity with methanol and isopropanol is inhibited with a saturating concentration (100 to 150 mg/dl) of the preferred substrate, ethanol. At the same time hemodialysis may be performed to remove these alcohols and their toxic metabolites until they reach undetectable levels.

The method of choice for the identification and measurement of methanol and isopropanol is gas chromatography. The GC methods for ethanol are generally also applicable to these two alcohols if acetone is adequately resolved from the alcohols (30, 31).

The popular enzymatic assay for ethanol is not applicable for methanol and isopropanol because of the weak enzyme activity when these alcohols are substrates. Toxic serum levels of these osmotically active substances, however, will result in a significant osmolal gap between measured osmolality and calculated serum osmolality, thus allowing the evaluation of an acute situation when specific assays for methanol and isopropanol are not available.

Ethylene Glycol

Ethylene glycol is the principal component of antifreeze products and brake fluids. It has a sweetish taste and is occasionally consumed by children. More frequently it is used in suicide attempts or by alcoholics as a substitute for ethanol-containing beverages (35). It is metabolized by oxidization to glycolic acid, glyoxylic acid and formic acid by alcohol dehydrogenese and glycolic acid oxidase (36). Ethylene glycol itself is only mildly toxic. Its metabolites, however, are highly toxic. Persistent vomiting, and gradual onset of CNS depression appear within 4 to 8 hours and are accompanied by a large anion gap metabolic acidosis. A common urinalysis finding is the presence of calcium oxalate or hippurate crystals. Acute renal tubular necrosis developing within 12 hours to 2 days is due to the precipitation of oxalate crystals or the direct toxic effect of the metabolites. An oral dose of 100 ml of ethylene glycol is believed to be fatal to most adults.

Treatment of ethylene glycol poisoning consists of correction of metabolic acidosis, inhibition of metabolism by ethanol, and hemodialysis (35). Hemodialysis rapidly clears both ethylene glycol and its toxic metabolites from the bloodstream and is recommended for patients who are symptomatic or have blood levels of ethylene glycol greater than 25 to 50 mg/dl.

The half-life of ethylene glycol is 3 to 7 hours in animals, but has not been established in humans. Therefore, diagnosis of toxicity based on serum ethylene glycol measurement must be done soon after ingestion. Later on, measurement of glycolic acid has been suggested due to its accumulation in blood following ingestion (36).

There is no easy assay for ethylene glycol, and most clinical laboratories do not provide ethylene glycol analysis (37). Serum osmolality measurement, and the calculation of the osmolal gap can provide a rough approximation of ethylene glycol concentration, but only if ethanol and other alcohols are known to be absent.

Early gas chromatographic methods, including those based on direct injection, were plagued by trailing peaks, "ghost peaks," and variable recovery (38) although columns packed with Porapack Q appear to be more reproducible than the frequently used Carbowax 20M columns. More recent GC (39) and HPLC procedures (40) based on derivatization have improved precision and accuracy, and capillary columns also improve method performance. An enzymatic method specific for ethylene glycol in small volumes of plasma or serum has been reported (40).

Acetaminophen

Acetaminophen is an effective analgesic and antipyretic drug that lacks antiinflammatory action. It is available in pure form and also in combination with other drugs such as codeine and propoxyphene. It presents less risk for producing gastrointestinal ulceration and hemorrhage than aspirin and other nonsteroidal anti-inflammatory drugs. With the reported link of Reye's syndrome to aspirin use, usage of acetaminophen as an over-the-counter medication in recent years has surpassed that of aspirin. At typical nonprescription doses of 325 to 1000 mg every 4 hours, acetaminophen is a safe drug. At higher doses acetaminophen is hepatotoxic, although toxic dosage is variable. Liver damage may occur after single doses of 7.5 g or greater in healthy adults or 150 mg/kg in children (41). Individuals on other medications that are hepatotoxic or those who have liver diseases or who are alcoholics, however, will be susceptible to acetaminophen toxic effects at lower doses (42).

Acetaminophen after a therapeutic dose is eliminated mostly as glucuronide or sulfate conjugates. Following overdosage, the conjugation pathways are saturated, and formation of a highly reactive intermediate (probably N-acetyl-benzoquinoneimine) (43) takes place via the cytochrome P-450 mixed-function oxidase system. This metabolite, normally detoxified by endogenous glutathione, reacts with and destroys hepatocytes once glutathione stores are depleted.

Acetaminophen is rapidly absorbed with peak plasma concentration reached within 30 to 120 minutes after therapeutic doses. Delayed peaks may occur with slower gastric emptying following large doses. Clinically, an acetaminophen-overdosed patient may present in four phases (41). In the initial phase, lasting 12 to 24 hours after ingestion, the patient usually exhibits GI irritability, nausea, and vomiting. Some patients may be asymptomatic. During the second phase (24 to 72 hours postingestion) the patient may feel reasonably well while liver function tests prove abnormal. If significant hepatic necrosis has occurred, the third phase (72 to 96 hours postingestion) is characterized by the sequelae of hepatic necrosis including coagulopathy, jaundice, encephalopathy, and renal failure. If the patient survives phase 3, complete resolution of hepatic dysfunction will ensue (4 days to 2 weeks).

N-Acetylcysteine is an effective antidote. In the U.S. the standard oral dosage consists of a loading dose of 140 mg/kg followed by 17 doses of 70 mg/kg every 4 hours. Treatment is most successful when started within 8 hours of ingestion, and its effectiveness appears to extend to those high-risk patients who are treated as late as 24 hours postingestion (44). In Canada and Europe intravenous administration (300 mg/kg) over a 20-hour period is recommended up to 16 hours postingestion.

A nomogram relating time since ingestion, plasma drug concentration, and risk of hepatotoxicity is used in evaluating the need for *N*-acetylcysteine treatment (Fig. 20.2) (45). Since early treatment is critical to a favorable outcome, and initial plasma drug concentration is a crucial deciding factor to initiate therapy, prompt and reliable measurement of plasma acetaminophen level is an importance emergency toxicology service. Numerous methods are available for the analysis of acetaminophen. Colorimetric tests such as the cresol-ammonia spot test or the quantitative Glynn and Kendal (40) method are fast and sensitive. The Glynn and Kendal method is interfered by salicylates, and various modifications have been proposed to minimize the inference (47). The colorimetric method based on the prior hydrolysis of acetaminophen *and* its conjugated metabolites to indophenol is not recommended because the aforementioned nomogram is based on serum concentration of unconjugated acetaminophen only (48). HPLC procedures, though simple and rapid, are not as convenient as the FPIA and EMIT methods that are available in most clinical laboratories.

Salicylates

Salicylate, as one of the least expensive and most widely used drugs, has been the cause of many drug overdose cases, particularly in the very young and the elderly. Safety measures enacted in the 1950s and 1960s have resulted in a decline in the incidence of salicylate poisoning in children. Salicylate, however, still ranks as a leading cause of childhood poisoning deaths and still is commonly used in self-poisoning by adults (49). Many derivatives of salicylic acid are commercially available; the most important is acetysalicylic acid (aspirin) which is rapidly hydrolyzed to salicylic acid, and circulates in the blood in the ionized form, salicylate. In serum, salicylate at therapeutic concentration is highly protein bound, and the extend of binding varies with total salicylate concentration. The apparent volume of distribution of salicylate increases with increasing plasma concentration, due in part to the saturable binding of salicylate to albumin.

The major metabolic pathways of salicylate conjugation with glycine and with glucuronic acid are saturable. Thus, the half-life of elimination of salicylate as well as the serum level of salicylate will increase disproportionately with increasing dosage (49).

The primary pathophysiological effects of salicylism are complex (50). They include direct stimulation of the respiratory center resulting in hyperventilation, respiratory alkalosis and compensatory excretion of base, uncoupling of oxidative phosphorylation, interference with the Krebs cycle, and accumulation of organic acids leading to metabolic acidosis. In children, respiratory alkalosis is transient and a late-stage dominant metabolic acidosis is common. In adult patients the most common acid-base disturbance is mixed respiratory alkalosis and metabolic acidosis. Associated with acid-base disturbances are fluid and electrolyte imbalance and dehydration. Other metabolic effects of salicylate toxicity are hyperthermia and impaired glucose metabolism with either hyperglycemia or hypoglycemia. In overdosed patients who are acidemic, the lower blood pH will increase the amount of nonionized salicylate (pKa = 3.0) for transfer into the central nervous system. Thus, central nervous system disturbances often accompany those intoxicated patients who are severely acidemic.

The toxic severity after acute ingestion is related to the amount of drug ingested. Ingestion of less than 0.15 g/kg is unlikely to result in toxic symptoms. Mild to moderate toxic reactions can be expected from an ingested dose of 0.15 to 0.39 g/kg, and doses in excess of 0.3 g/kg lead to severe reactions. Ingestion of greater than 0.5 g/kg is potentially lethal (49).

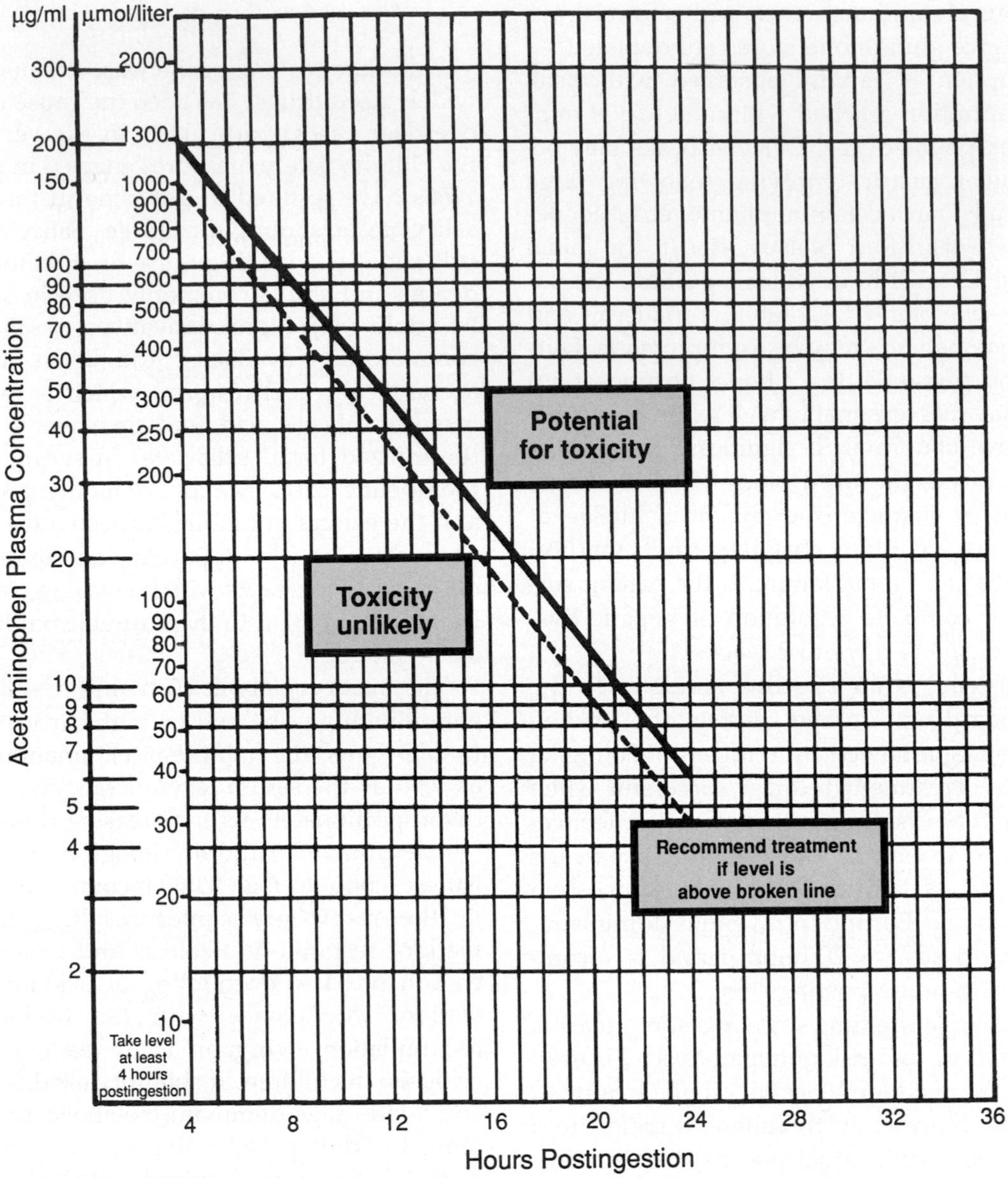

Figure 20.2. Nomogram relating acetaminophen plasma concentration, time since ingestion, and risk of toxicity. (Modified from Rumack BH, Matthew H. Acetaminophen poisoning and toxicity. Pediatrics 1975;55:871–876.)

Chronic intoxication or therapeutic overdose is a result of excessive therapeutic administration of salicylate over a period of 12 hours or longer, and zero order kinetics lead to accumulation of salicylate in serum to toxic levels (51). Chronic salicylate intoxication is a diagnostic problem particularly among elderly patients because the presenting symptoms are often ascribed to other causes. Thus, the intoxication often goes unrecognized, and as a result, appropriate therapy is delayed. These patients suffer significant morbidity and mortality (52).

Treatment for salicylate intoxication includes measures to prevent further absorption of salicylate by induction of emesis or gastric lavage and the administration of activated charcoal. Medically, the intoxicated patients should be treated aggressively to correct the metabolic imbalances such as fluid and electrolyte depletion and acid-base disturbances. Alkalinization to enhance the renal elimination of the drug should be considered in adults with serum salicylate level exceeding 0.5 g/liter and children with levels greater than 0.35 g/liter (51). If the salicylate level is greater than 1 g/liter, hemodialysis or hemoperfusion is indicated (53).

The availability of salicylate assay on an emergency basis is critical to confirm the clinical suspicion of acute salicylate intoxication. Diagnosis of chronic salicylate intoxication, particularly in the elderly, is much more difficult without a high degree of suspicion because patients may have become drowsy and

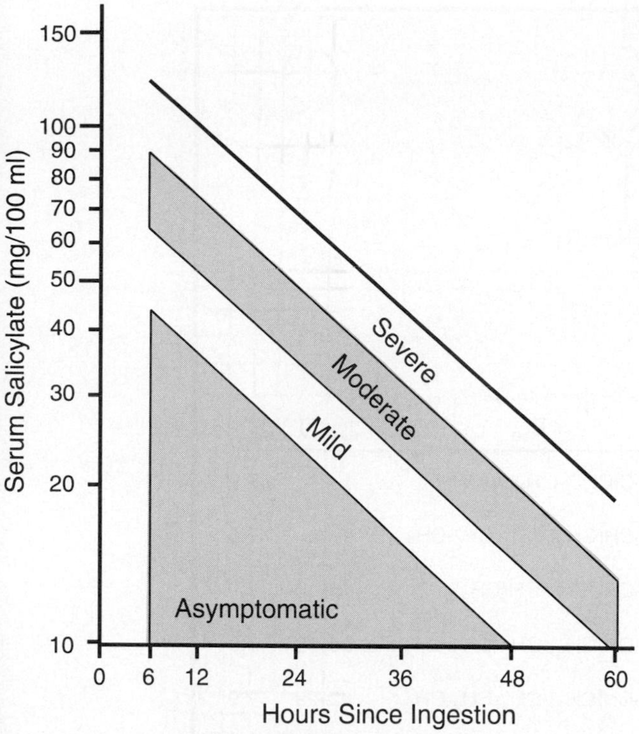

Figure 20.3. Nomogram for salicylate poisoning. (From Done AK. Salicylate intoxication. Significance of measurements of salicylate in blood in cases of acute ingestion. Pediatrics 1960;26:800–807.)

confused and are unable to offer a reliable drug history. Therefore, documentation of elevated serum salicylate levels becomes very important in the differential diagnosis (49).

A nomogram (Done nomogram) (54) has been constructed to facilitate the interpretation of salicylate levels at different intervals after ingestion in order to predict the severity of intoxication (Fig. 20.3). The greatest clinical value of the nomogram lies in early estimation of the severity of the intoxication for appropriate patient disposition and in identifying those high-risk patients requiring prompt alkalinization therapy or hemoperfusion. Done's nomogram is not useful in the prediction of the rate of salicylate elimination or future serum salicylate levels. Furthermore, this nomogram is applicable only to acute ingestion, and is not to be used for the assessment of severity of chronic salicylate intoxication.

If the ingested salicylate is of an enteric-coated or sustained-released formulation, the absorption of salicylate will be delayed. The diagnosis of salicylate intoxication based on an elevation of serum level on admission can be missed due to delayed absorption (55). If ingestion of enteric-coated or sustained-release salicylate is suspected, the patient must be observed for at least 24 hours, and serum salicylate determination should be repeated. Peak salicylate level may not be attained until 60 to 70 hours postingestion. The use of Done's nomogram in these patients is inappropriate because a different ingestion time-serum concentration relationship is involved.

Simple qualitative screening tests such as ferric chloride, Trinder's reagent and Phenistix for urine salicylate are useful for quick confirmation of salicylate overdose if quantitation of serum levels is not available immediately (49). These tests are not specific for salicylate; therefore, all positive urine results should be confirmed using quantitative assays and serum samples. Colorimetric assays based on the reaction of salicylic acid with ferric ion to give a purple color are not specific but have proven acceptable for the routine clinical use of salicylate levels in the diagnosis of salicylate intoxication. The assay based on Trinder's method is the most commonly used, although newer techniques such as FPIA, HOPLC and enzymatic assay using salicylate hydrolase are available (49).

Barbiturates

Barbiturate poisoning either by accident or more often in suicide attempts was a major health problem in the past. It has lessened in recent years because their use as anxiolytics has been replaced by the safer benzodiazepines. Today, medical use of barbiturates is primarily for treatment of insomnia and convulsive disorders, and as anesthetic and preanesthetic medications.

The barbiturates are derivatives of barbituric acid (Fig. 20.4). Pharmacologically, they can be broadly divided into ultra-short (e.g., thiopental), short- to intermediate- (e.g., secobarbital and butalbital), and long- (e.g., phenobarbital) acting groups depending on their duration of action (56). The short- to immediate-acting barbiturates are preferred by drug abusers because of the relative rapid onset of action (15 to 40 minutes), which may last up to 6 hours. Duration of drug action is dependent on lipid solubility. Thus, the short-acting barbiturates have higher lipid solubility, greater potency, and more rapid clearance from the central compartment. In contrast, the long-acting barbiturates have less lipid solubility, lower potency, and much longer half-lives of elimination.

The barbiturates are weak acids with pKa values ranging between 7.2 and 7.9. Hence, at pH 7.4 a barbiturate such as phenobarbital (pK = 7.2) will be about 40% nonionized, whereas secobarbital (pK = 7.9) is 76% nonionized and is therefore more lipid soluble and more rapidly distributed to tissues. This explains the observation that phenobarbital administration is accompanied by higher plasma concentrations (but lower tissue concentrations) than those observed after equivalent doses of secobarbital.

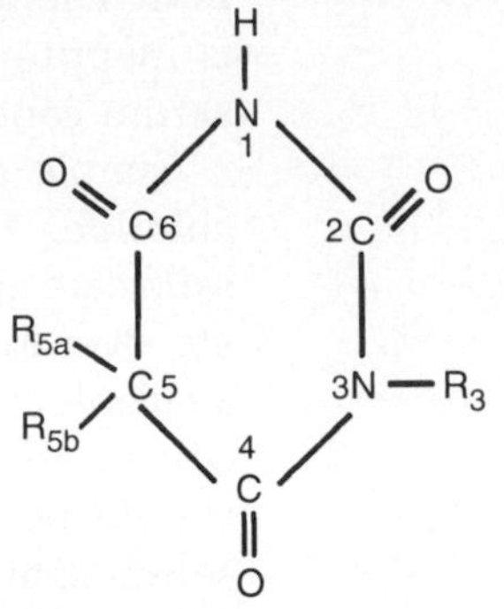

Generic (Trade) Name	R_{5a}	R_{5b}	$t_{1/2}$(h)	pKa
Methohexital (Brevital)	$-CH_2-CH=CH_2$	$-C(CH_3)-C{\equiv}CH_2-CH_3$	1–2	7.9
Thiopental (Pentothal)	$-CH_2-CH_3$	$-CH(CH_3)-CH_2-CH_2-CH_3$	4–60	7.6
Amobarbital (Amytal)	$-CH_2-CH_3$	$-CH_2-CH_2-CH(CH_3)_2$	15–40	7.9
Pentobarbital (Nembutal)	$-CH_2-CH_3$	$-CH(CH_3)-CH_2-CH_2-CH_3$	20–30	7.9
Secobarbital (Seconal)	$-CH_2-CH=CH_2$	$-CH(CH_3)-CH_2-CH_2-CH_3$	22–29	7.9
Butabarbital (Butisol)	$-CH_2-CH_3$	$-CH(CH_3)-CH_2-CH_3$	34–42	7.9
Butalbital (Fiorinal)	$-CH_2-CH=CH_2$	$-CH_2-CH(CH_3)_2$	35–88	7.6
Phenobarbital (Luminal)	$-CH_2-CH_3$	$-C_6H_5$	48–144	7.2

R_3 = H, except for methohexital, for which $R_3 = CH_3$.

Figure 20.4. Common barbiturates.

The major actions of the barbiturates are their depressant action on the CNS and cardiovascular system. Acute barbiturate intoxication is characteristically associated with coma and shock; the former must always be differentiated from other forms of coma or CNS injury. Plasma barbiturate levels may be helpful in making a diagnosis, but they are of limited value in predicting the severity of the overdose or the duration of the coma, which are related more closely to brain than plasma barbiturate concentration. Also, chronic barbiturate users are expected to have higher plasma concentration for any grade of coma due to the tolerance they have developed. Moreover, the depth of coma can be greater than might be expected from plasma concentration if other central nervous system depressants, such as alcohol, have also been ingested.

Treatment of barbiturate intoxication consists of aggressive support to combat shock and hypoxia in addition to lavage and charcoal treatment. Alkalinization of urine to pH 7.5 to 8.0 with sodium bicarbonate will increase the fraction of ionized drug and will enhance excretion in urine. It is helpful for long-acting barbiturates because their principal means of elimination is renal. Alkalization is less effective for short-acting barbiturates since they have higher pKa values, are more highly protein-bound, and they are primarily metabolized by the liver (56).

The classic method for barbiturate quantitation is UV spectrophometry at different pH values (57). Identification of the specific barbiturate(s) requires chromatographic separation. Thin-layer chromatography can effectively separate phenobarbital from other barbiturates, but the short- and intermediate-acting group—ambobarbital, butabarbital, butalbital, secobarbital and pentobarbital—have similar migration, and identification requires skill and experience (58). Gas chromatography and HPLC methods for identification of the commonly encountered barbiturates are available (59, 60). Mass spectral identification of the barbiturates must be done with care because these drugs are structurally similar and yield similar spectral data (61).

Immunoassays detect barbiturates as a group and provide rapid results. However, barbiturates other than the one used as the calibrator may have differ-

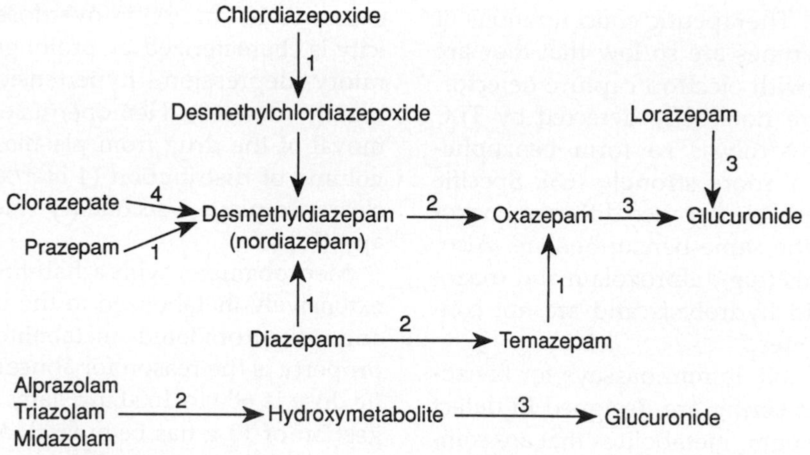

Figure 20.5. Major biotransformation pathways of common benzodiazepines. 1, dealkylation; 2, hydroxylation; 3, glucuronidation; 4, decarboxylation.

Table 20.2. Common Benzodiazepines

Generic Name	Trade Name	Half-life
Diazolobenzodiazepines		*hr*
Chlordiazepoxide	Librium	6–27
Diazepam	Valium	21–37
Oxazepam	Serax	4–11
Clorazepate	Tranxene	2
Flurazepam	Dalmane	2–3
Lorazepam	Ativan	9–16
Temazepam	Restoril	3–13
Halazepam	Paxipam	14–16
Prazepam	Centrax	1.3
Triazolobenzodiazepines		
Alprazolam	Xanax	10–12
Trialzolam	Halcion	2.6
Midazolam	Versed	1–4

ent cross-reactivities to the antibody. For example, an enzyme immunoassay that uses secobarbital as the calibrator will detect the less reactive phenobarbital only at higher concentrations.

Benzodiazepines and Sedative Hypnotics

BENZODIAZEPINES

The benzodiazepines are among the most frequently prescribed drugs. They vary in their potency in anxiolytic, hypnotic, muscle relaxant, anticonvulsant, and anesthetic effects. One useful classification of the benzodiazepines is according to their half-lives: long (greater than 24 hour), intermediate-short (5 to 24 hours) and ultrashort-acting (less than 5 hours) (Table 20.2). A long-acting benzodiazepine such as diazepam is well suited as an anxiolytic agent, whereas a short-acting benzodiazepine such as triazolam is more appropriate as a hypnotic. Benzodiazepines are also useful for treating neuromuscular diseases, sleep disorders, seizure, drug withdrawal, and as preanesthetic agents. Continuous use has led to tolerance, addiction, dependence, and abuse (62).

All the benzodiazepines are metabolized and cleared by the kidney as glucuronides or sulfates. Many of the metabolites are active, and some benzodiazepines such as clorazepate and flurazepam are considered to be prodrugs (Fig. 20.5). The major biotransformation routes are demethylation (e.g., chlordiazepoxide, temazepam) and hydroxylation (diazepam, nondiazepam).

With the popularity of these drugs, overdosage is a frequent occurrence, yet fatalities resulting from benzodiazepines alone are very rare. Patients intoxicated with benzodiazepines are minimally sedated. Side effects include respiratory depression, weakness, headache, blurred vision, nausea, and diarrhea. Serious intoxication with benzodiazepines usually results from coingestion with other CNS depressants (e.g., ethanol). Addicts have abused methodone and benzodiazepines to enhance their effect (63). Therefore, in the evaluation of a patient suspected of benzodiazepine intoxication, it is important to investigate if other drugs have also been ingested. Plasma benzodiazepine concentration does not predict the severity of intoxication or outcome. Both physostigmine and naloxone have been used to treat benzodiazepine toxicity, but a specific benzodiazepine antagonist flumazenil has been reported to effectively reverse benzodiazapine-induced central nervous system depression (64).

Benzodiazepine levels in blood and plasma can be determined by HPLC or GC. Some benzodiazepines, such as chlordiazepoxide and oxazepam, are heat-labile, and are more suitable for HPLC analysis. GC methods using electron capture detection have the best sensitivity, whereas those dependent on FID detection are adequate for drug levels in the high therapeutic or toxic ranges. Therapeutic concentrations of the newer benzodiazepines are so low that they are best analyzed by GC with electron capture detector.

Benzodiazepines are not easily detected by TLC without prior acid hydrolysis to form benzophenones, which fluoresce more strongly (65). Specific identification is not possible because different benzodiazepines can form the same benzophenone. Also, newer benzodiazepines (e.g., alprozolam and triazolam) are stable to acid hydrolysis and are not converted to benzophenones.

Commercially available immunoassays for benzodiazepines in urine or serum are designed to detect oxazepam or nordiazepam, metabolites that are common to several benzodiazepines (Fig. 20.5). Immunoassays have sufficient cross-reactivity with many of the newer benzodiazepines to detect therapeutic levels of some (e.g., alprazolam), but only higher levels for others (e.g., triazolam) (66, 67).

SEDATIVE HYPNOTICS

The sedative hypnotics include a wide range of drugs ranging from over-the-counter (OTC) sleep aids to benzodiazepines to nonbarbiturate sedative hypnotics such as ethchlorovynol and glutethimide.

The active compound in OTC sleep aids are antihistamines such as diphenhydramine, pyrilamine, and doxylamine. Although these have a wide margin of safety, acute intoxication causes sedation, anticholinergic effects (pyrilamine and doxylamine), respiratory depression, and coma (68).

The nonbarbiturate, nonbenzodiazepine sedative hypnotics share common pharmacological features (56). They are CNS depressants. The resulting coma from overdose is deep and prolonged. Drug tolerance develops with chronic use, and physiological and psychological dependence can occur if high doses are taken for a prolonged period of time. Abrupt discontinuance can precipitate acute withdrawal symptoms similar to those associated with barbiturate or alcohol withdrawal. Management of intoxication is mainly supportive. Laboratory analysis of plasma or urine for these drugs requires GC (59) or TLC (58) procedures. A spot test based on a reaction with diphenylamine is a very effective test for ethchlorvynol which in some TLC systems does not separate well from glutethimide.

Chloral hydrate, once a popular hypnotic, is now used infrequently. Trichlor ethanol, a metabolite formed by alcohol dehydrogenase is responsible for the hypnotic effect. Acute chloral hydrate intoxication resembles barbiturate poisoning.

Ethchlorvynol has a half-life of 19 to 32 hours. It localizes in adipose tissues, and the slow release from these depots account for the long half-life (in excess of 100 hours) in overdose. Ethchlorvynol toxicity is characterized by prolonged deep coma, respiratory depression, hypertension, and a pungent breath odor (69). Hemoperfusion can hasten the removal of the drug from plasma, but due to its large volume of distribution (4 liter/kg), complete plasma clearance plays a secondary role to supportive therapy (70).

Meprobamate, with a half-life of 6 to 17 hours, is extensively metabolized to the inactive hydroxylated and glucuronidated metabolites. Its euphorigenic property is the reason for abuse. The usual therapeutic dose is 600 to 1600 mg daily in divided doses. Ingestion of 12 g has been fatal, although survival has been reported after a 40 g dose. Massive overdosage has been reported to cause respiratory depression, coma, and hypertension (71). Drug clearance has been successfully enhanced by hemoperfusion.

Glutethimide is extensively metabolized to a number of compounds, some of which, especially 4-hydroxyglutethimide, are pharmacologically active. Glutethimide overdose is associated with profound and prolonged coma. An ingested dose of 10 g or more and plasma concentration exceeding 30 mg/liter have been reported to associate with deep coma (72). Patients who have also ingested barbiturates are a higher risk even if the glutethimide dose ingested or plasma concentration is low (72). Glutethimide is erratically absorbed from the GI tract, and enterohepatic circulation is significant. As a result, the CNS depression can sometimes occur cylically. Thus, although extracorporeal therapy can reduce the elimination half-life of glutethimide, its use does not significantly alter the course of intoxication.

Cyclic Antidepressants

The cyclic antidepressants are a major cause of life-threatening drug overdose, and are responsible for nearly 25% of all fatal drug exposures, more than any other drug classes (73). Drugs in this class of commonly prescribed antidepressants include the tricyclic compounds, such as imipramine, desipramine, trimipramine, amitriptyline, nortriptyline, doxepin, and loxapine, the tetracyclic compounds maprotiline and miaserin, and the bicyclic fluoxetine. Trazadone, a triazolopyridine, and amoxapine, a dibenoxapine, while structurally unrelated to the tricyclic compounds, are often classified or described with them.

These cyclic compounds are rapidly absorbed by the GI tract, but absorption may be delayed at higher blood levels due to the anticholinergic effect of delayed gastric emptying. The volumes of distribution of these drugs are large (10 to 50 liters/kg) and extent of binding to plasma protein is high (greater than 90%). There is extensive first pass metabolism, and the major hydroxylated metabolites of the tricyclic, and demethylated metabolites of the bi- and tetracyclic compounds are pharmacologically active.

The toxic effects of the tricyclic and tetracyclic antidepressants are similar and are mostly related to their anticholinergic and cardiotoxic effects. Anticholinergic effects result in agitation, seizure, coma, and hallucination. Circulatory collapse, serious cardiac arrhythmias, conduction disturbances and heart block can occur; arrhythmia is the leading cause of death in tricyclic overdoses. The toxicity of trazadone is different from that of the tricyclic and tetracyclic antidepressants in that there are no anticholinergic signs or symptoms and that the primary manifestations are CNS effects and hypertension. Fluoxetine adverse effects are anxiety, nervousness, and insomnia.

A patient presenting with convulsion or coma, anticholinergic syndrome, and cardiac arrhythmias should be strongly suspected of tricyclic or tetracyclic antidepressant poisoning. The first 24 hours of a cyclic antidepressant overdose are critical and require close monitoring in a continuous care setting. The use of physostigmine to reverse anticholinergic toxicity is diminishing (74). Hemoperfusion is ineffective due to the large volume of distribution of these drugs (73).

Although tricyclic antidepressant-intoxicated patients who had peak (not admission) serum drug levels of 100 mg/dl or greater were more frequently associated with seizures and ventricular arrhythmias (75), there was no correlation between drug levels and toxic symptoms over a wide range of tricyclic antidepressant levels (33 to 487 mg/dl) (76). Therefore, the measurement of serum tricyclic antidepressant level as an indicator of the clinical severity of acute tricyclic antidepressant poisoning is not indicated.

The tricyclic antidepressants can be detected and identified in urine by TLC. Because the toxic effects due to an overdose of these compounds are so similar, demonstration of the presence of one of these drugs without specific identification is often sufficient for management. Qualitative serum or plasma immunoassays (EMIT-st EMIT-tox, TDx) are designed primarily for detection of the major tricyclic antidepressants (imipramine, desipramine, amitriptyline, nortriplyline) but, due to the cross-reactivities of the antibody for other members of the tricyclic antidepressant family, these immunoassays are also capable of screening for the presence of other tricyclic antidepressants and metabolites (77). Although a positive result does not necessarily indicate a toxic concentration of the drug, a negative response will rule out the possibility of an overdose. Quantitative immunoassays (EMIT) for the four major tricyclic antidepressants are also available. These assays require solid-phase extraction from serum or plasma prior to analysis.

Table 20.3. Elemental Iron Equivalents in Iron Salts

Salt	% Fe	mg Fe/Tablet[a]
Sulfate	20	65
Gluconate	12	38
Fumarate	33	106
Lactate	19	—
Chloride	28	—
Ferrocholinate	13	—

[a]325-mg tablet.

Gas chromatographic and HPLC assays are available. For higher than therapeutic concentrations of tricyclic antidepressant, GC procedures using an FID detector are adequate. GC methods, however, do not separate the different tricyclic antidepressants as well as the HPLC assays.

Iron

Iron salts are readily available and acute iron poisoning is particularly common in the pediatric population, with 75% of the reported exposure occurring in children less than 6 years of age (78).

Ferrous sulfate, the cheapest and most common iron salt, is frequently involved in overdose. Other iron salts are gluconate, fumarate, succinate, lactate, chloride, ferrocholinate, and glutamate. The elemental iron dose ingested can be calculated from the percentage of elemental iron in the formulation (Table 20.3).

In acute iron poisoning, an estimation of the amount of elemental iron is important in assessing potential toxicity. An ingestion of less than 20 mg/kg has little risk of toxicity. A dose of 20 to 60 mg of elemental iron/kg can cause cause mild GI distress and poses moderate risk, whereas a dose greater than 60 mg/kg has high risk for toxicity (79).

Four clinical stages of acute iron poisoning have been described. The first stage is the initial postingestion period lasting up to 6 hours. As iron is absorbed in the duodenum and upper small intestine, GI symptoms manifested at this stage are a direct result of the corrosive action of iron. During the next stage (latent period) of up to 12 hours, the patient may appear to improve. If the dose ingested is sufficiently large, the patient's condition may progress directly to a third stage (12 to 48 hours postingestion) of systemic toxicity with cardiovascular collapse, seizure, coma, shock, renal failure, and hepatic necrosis. Patients who survive the three stages of acute intoxication are still at risk of developing late strictures and some GI tract obstruction (2 to 4 weeks) (79).

Ingestion of iron can be documented by abdominal x-ray and a qualitative color test performed on gastric fluid. Abdominal x-ray can reveal iron-containing pills prior to dissolution as much as 6 hours or longer after ingestion of adult-strength tablets. Pediatric preparations, which are chewable iron supplements, dissolve rapidly in 30 to 60 minutes and are not always seen (80). In the qualitative color test, deferoxamine is added to gastric fluid (81). An immediate color change indicates the presence of iron. If performed within 2 hours of ingestion, a negative test indicates the patient needs no further evaluation, but a negative test obtained more than 2 hours after ingestion does not rule out iron ingestion because absorption may have been completed.

A qualitative test to predict potential for toxicity is the deferoxamine challenge test. A sufficiently large deferoxamine dose is given to bind free iron in plasma and forms the reddish feroxamine complex, which is excreted in urine. The appearance of feroxamine in urine within 4 to 6 hours implies potential toxicity. This test is sometimes used when serum iron levels are not readily available, but false-negative results have been reported, and a negative challenge test should not rule out toxicity (82).

Serum iron level is usually determined along with total iron binding capacity (TIBC). Theoretically, if the serum iron value is greater than the TIBC, then the free circulating iron is potentially toxic. Following a clinically toxic dose of elemental iron, TIBC has been reported to rise. Although TIBC always remained above serum iron levels (83), symptoms of iron toxicity still occurred. Serum iron levels greater than 350 μg/dl are associated with toxicity, although a lower level does not rule out toxicity. Serum iron levels in the 350 to 500 μg/dl range may require chelation therapy if the patient is exhibiting signs of systemic toxicity. Serious toxicity and death have been reported in cases with serum levels in excess of 500 μg/dl. Sampling of blood should be 4 to 6 hours post-ingestion of adult preparations and 2 hours following ingestion of pediatric preparations.

The management of acute iron poisoning includes removal of residual iron in the GI tract by emesis or lavage and standard support therapy (84). Deferoxamine therapy is used to chelate free serum iron.

Most methods for measuring serum iron levels are based on spectrophotometric measurement of a color complex formed by the chelation of ferrous iron with bathophenanthroline, ferrozine, tripyridyltriazine (TPZ) or other dyes. Deferoxamine, as a competing chelator, interferes with dye-binding colormetric assays by giving falsely low results (85). Therefore, serum iron levels should be drawn prior to deferoxamine chelation therapy. Atomic absorption spectroscopy for serum iron levels is not usually routinely available but is a method that can be used in the presence of deferoxamine.

Cannabinoids

The term cannabinoids denotes a group of more than 60 compounds found in the plant *Cannabis sativa L.* and includes their metabolites in animals and humans. Δ^9-Tetrahydrocannabinol (THC) is the major psychoactive compound of marijuana, and its content (percentage THC by weight of plant material) in street marijuana in the U.S. has been increasing in recent years. It now averages 4%, and is four to five times greater than it was in the mid-1970s. Even more potent is the carefully cultivated sinsemilla varieties of cannabis whose THC content averages 7% and can reach as high as 14%. This is as potent as hashish (up to 10%) (86).

The effects of THC, when smoked, appear within minutes and seldom last for longer than 2 or 3 hours. Oral intake delays the onset of symptoms for 30 minutes to 2 hours but the duration of action of the drug is longer. The effects of THC are tempered by dose, route of administration, and experience of the user. There is usually a sense of euphoria, an altered perception of time, a keener sense of hearing, and more vivid visual imagery. Frequently, there is increased hunger, and dry mouth and throat are quite common. Both short-term memory and task performance are impaired. Higher doses can induce frank hallucinations, delusions, and paranoid feelings. The most consistent cardiovascular effects are an increase in pulse rate and conjunctival reddening (87).

The effects of chronic use of THC are less certain. Field studies failed to detect any major health consequences, although many objections have been raised about the adequacy of these studies (87).

THC is a lipophilic drug whose volume of distribution is estimated to be about 10 liters/kg. There is high sequestration of THC in certain organs such as liver and lung.

In man, THC is rapidly transformed first by the hepatic cytochrome P450 enzyme system to 11-hydroxy-Δ-9-THC (11-hydroxy-THC) which is then oxidized by alcohol dehydrogenase to 11-nor-Δ-9-THC-9-carboxylic acid (carboxy-THC). 11-hydroxy-THC is a psychoactive metabolite, whereas carboxy-THC is devoid of psychoactivity (88).

The primary urinary metabolite is carboxy-THC, which exists both as the free acid and glucuronide conjugate. Because of the large tissue storage of THC, continuous re-entry of THC from tissues into the central compartment followed by metabolism means that carboxy-THC is excreted into the urine long after a person has stopped using marijuana. The duration of positive urine samples is dependent on the dose, metabolism of THC, route and frequency of use, the timing of the urine collection, the quantity of liquid taken prior to specimen collection, and the assay cutoff. Generally, urine of infrequent users tested positive from 2 to 5 days after each dose when a 20-μg/liter cutoff is used. In a study of heavy users, positive EMIT results (greater than 20 μg/liter) were obtained for over 40 days since the user was last exposed to marijuana (89). There was also a significant day-to-day fluctuation in the excretion pattern near the cutoff. An individual may test positive one day and negative the next; it took the same patient 75 days to drop below the cutoff for 10 consecutive days. Thus, a positive urine result indicates only that the subject has been exposed to marijuana 1 hour to weeks prior to the collection of the urine specimen, and the result cannot be used to estimate the time of exposure.

Since marijuana is commonly smoked in social situations, it is possible that nonsmokers could inhale a sufficient amount of cannabinoids present in sidestream smoke to produce a positive urine cannabinoid test. Studies have shown that this can occur, but only after exposure to high concentrations of marijuana smoke in a small unventilated area (90). Such extreme exposure conditions are not encountered in the usual social situations, and with higher cutoffs (e.g., 100 μg/liter) used by many screening assays, the detection of a positive urine due to passive inhalation is unlikely (91).

Screening is usually done with immunoassays as they have good sensitivity and they can be automated for batch analysis of large numbers of samples. The immunoassay (EMIT, RIA, and FPIA) antibodies detect not only carboxy-THC, the major urinary metabolite, but also have cross-reactivity to many of the other metabolites of THC. These assays, therefore, measure the sum of the immunoreactive THC metabolites. In contrast, the chromatographic assays (TLC, HPLC, GC, GC-MS) separate and specifically measure carboxy-THC. The threshold concentrations of these chromatographic methods, if they are used as confirmatory assays for immunoassays, are usually set lower than those of the initial tests. For example, a confirmation threshold of 15 μg/liters might be used with an immunoassay cutoff of 100 μg/liter (92).

If a chromatographic assay is used, hydrolysis of the glucuronide metabolites is necessary. TLC has a detection limit as low as 25 μg/liter, whereas GC-MS methods, using a deuterated internal standard and selected ion monitoring, can have a limit of quantitation of 5 μg/liter.

Opioids

The opioid drugs can be divided into naturally occurring, semisynthetic, and synthetic groups. The naturally occurring opioids are morphine and codeine, which are derived from the opium poppy, *Papaver somniferum L.* Semisynthetic opioids include heroin, hydromorphone, oxycodone, and oxymorphone. Synthetic opioids are meperidine, methadone, diphenoxylate, propoxyphene, and the fentanyls. Opioids have similar pharmacological effects and potential for addiction and tolerance. They vary only in their potency for analgesia, duration of action, and extent of abuse (93).

Opioids produce analgesic respiratory depressant, euphorigenic, and emetic effects. The triad of miosis, coma, and respiratory depression are pathognomonic of opioid poisoning (94). The response to the pure opioid antagonist, naloxone, is both diagnostic and therapeutic for opioid intoxication.

Heroin and methadone are the most frequently abused opioids. In recent years concomitant use of heroin or methadone with cocaine has been reported. Methadone abusers are known to use benzodiazepines, such as diazepam and alprazolam, to enhance drug effect (63). The preferred route of heroin administration is intravenous, although smokeable heroin is now available, and concomitant use of heroin with cocaine has been reported. Heroin (diacetylmorphine) is rapidly deacetylated to 6-monoacetylmorphine (MAM), which then undergoes a second deacetylation step to form morphine (95). Morphine and MAM are equally potent in their opioid effects. Thus, heroin acts as a prodrug for providing the active metabolites, MAM and morphine. The hydrolysis of heroin to morphine is very rapid, with a half-life of 3 minutes. Consequently, only MAM and morphine are found in the urines of heroin users.

Codeine is rapidly absorbed from an oral dose, with plasma concentration peaking 1 hour postingestion. It is extensively metabolized to norcodeine, but at least 10% of the dose is transformed to morphine. Most of the dose is excreted in the urine as glucuronide conjugates of codeine, norcodeine, and morphine. Thus, morphine is a metabolite of both heroin and codeine. Consumption of baked goods containing poppy seeds can result in detectable amounts of morphine and codeine in urine (96, 97) because these opiates are contained in poppy seeds. When a urine contains both morphine and codeine, it becomes important to ascertain whether the morphine comes from codeine in prescription medications, from heroin/morphine abuse, or from poppy seed ingestion. A set of guidelines has been proposed to help in the interpretation of urine opiates results and the determination of the source of morphine and codeine in urine (97, 98). Test results that can rule out poppy seeds as the sole source for morphine and codeine are (*a*) codeine levels greater than 0.3 mg/liter with a morphine-to-codeine ratio less than 2 (indicative of codeine use); (*b*) high levels of morphine (greater than 1 mg/liter) when codeine is undetectable; (*c*) total morphine levels exceeding 5 mg/liter (indicative of abuse of heroin, morphine, or codeine); (*d*) the presence of MAM (a positive indication of heroin use) (97).

The fentanyls are analgesic-anesthetic drugs that are many times more potent then morphine. Many analogs of fentanyls (3-methyl-, α-methyl-, and parafluoro-derivatives) have appeared on the street as "China white" (100). Heroin containing fentanyl is a grave risk to heroin abusers. A standard urine drug screen will most likely fail to detect a fentanyl overdose because fentanyl concentration in urines is very low (μg/liter), and the available urine immunoassays for opiates have no reactivity for fentanyls.

Immunoassays (EMIT, RIA and FPIA) are commonly used as preliminary tests for the opiates (morphine and codeine), methadone and propoxyphene because they have adequate sensitivity, and they can be easily automated. The synthetic narcotics (dihydrocodone, hydrocodone, hydromorphone, and oxycodone) are also detected by the opiates' immunoassays, thus necessitating a confirmation test that can distinguish between morphine and the other opioids (TLC, HPLC, GC, and GC-MS). Conventional TLC has a detection limit of 1 mg/l, which makes it suitable for use in overdose cases but not for drug abuse testing.

Cocaine

Cocaine (benzoylmethylecgonine) is an alkaloid extracted from the leaves of the *Erythroxylon coca* plant and purified as the hydrochloride salt (cocaine HCl). It is a powerful central nervous system stimulant, and in recent years the illicit use of cocaine has increased rapidly.

Cocaine hydrochloride is snorted or administered intravenously. Many cocaine users used to prepare free-base crystals for smoking ("free-basing") by dissolving cocaine HCl in a solution of baking soda or ammonia, and extracting it with a solvent (ether) that is evaporated, leaving relatively pure cocaine crystals. This dangerous process to obtain smokeable cocaine has decreased in popularity in recent years due to the availability of "crack." Crack (so named because of the crackling sound made by the crystals when heated) is also a free-base form of cocaine, prepared by precipitation from an alkaline solution. Crack is relatively pure cocaine (80 to 90%), and when heated, is vaporized rather than pyrolysed. Its low cost and wide availability have worsened the cocaine epidemic.

Cocaine, a powerful CNS stimulant, produces heightened alertness, self-confidence, and an intense feeling of euphoria ("rush"). These stimulatory effects are followed by depression ("crash"). It is the positive reinforcement of the "rush" to escape the "crash" that leads to chronic cocaine abuse (101). Psychosis, repeated grand mal seizures, and coma are common following acute intoxication. Other clinical manifestations include arrhythmias, myocardial infarction, hypertensive crisis, cerebral vascular accidents, hyperthermia, and respiratory arrest. Spontaneous abortion and abruptio placentae are obstetric complications for women who use cocaine during pregnancy (5). Low birth weight and higher risk of congenital malformations, perinatal mortality, and neurobehavioral impairment are common results of a fetus exposed to cocaine in utero (6). Necrosis of the nasal septum from "snorting" cocaine, lung damage, and pulmonary edema are some of the other complications associated with cocaine use.

Bioavailability of intranasal cocaine is variable (20 to 60%) and appears to be dose dependent. Smoking free-base provides a more effective absorption of cocaine (57% bioavailability) (102), and a rapid peaking in its plasma concentration within 5 minutes. The euphoric effects of smoking cocaine usually lasts for only 20 minutes. Similar results were obtained in subjects given cocaine intravenously. In contrast, the effects of intranasal administration may last for 60 to 90 minutes with the maximum plasma concentration occurring later in 1 hour. Cocaine is lipid soluble and readily crosses cell membranes and distributes rapidly across the blood-brain barrier and the placenta.

The main routes of metabolism of cocaine are enzymatic and nonenzymatic hydrolysis of the methyl ester giving benzoylecgonine (BE) and enzymatic hydrolysis of the benzoyl group by plasma and liver esterases, yielding ecgonine methyl ester (EME) (103). Further hydrolysis of both of these compounds gives ecgonine. Norcocaine, the product of *N*-demethylation, undergoes similar hydrolysis and is believed to be pharmacologically active, but it is present in very small amounts. The two major metabolites in human urine, BE and EME, are excreted in about equal amounts (40 to 50%) (104). Cocaine itself is excreted in very small amounts, less than 1% of the dose in 3 days. Elimination half-lives for BE, EME, and cocaine have been calculated from literature data to be 7.5, 3.6, and 1.5 hours, respectively.

A pharmacologically active metabolite called cocaethylene has been identified following concurrent use of cocaine and ethanol (105).

Addition of sodium fluoride to inhibit esterase activity and low temperature will stabilize cocaine in blood specimens for long-term storage. The major urine metabolites, BE and EME, are relatively stable.

Immunoassays (RIA, EMIT, FPIA) are popular because they do not require sample pretreatment, and they are fast and easy to perform. Since these assays were designed primarily for use with urine specimens, the target analyte is the major urinary metabolite benzoylecognine (106). All three immunoassays have little cross-reactivity with norcocaine or ecognine methyl ester, and Roche RIA is the only immunoassay that has substantial cross-reactivity with cocaine. Benzoylecognine is not effectively extracted by nonpolar solvents and requires the addition of an alcohol (e.g., ethanol) or chloroform to make the extraction solvent more polar. The resulting extract can be used for various chromatography techniques (TLC, HPLC, GC, and GC-MS).

Thin-layer chromatography sensitivity is generally at 1 to 2 mg/liter, which is adequate for cocaine overdose cases. Sensitivity has been improved to 0.25 mg/liter for use in drug abuse testing. A disadvantage of the most commonly used TLC procedure is that there is limited migration of BE away from the origin.

Gas chromatography procedures require derivatization of the carboxylic side group of benzoylecognine before chromatography (for a review, see reference 22). Procedures using a flame ionization detector have sensitivity down to 0.2 mg/liter which can be further enhanced 50- to 100-fold by the use of nitrogen-phosphorus detector.

The high specificity and sensitivity of GC/MS are utilized for confirmation of cocaine and benzoylecognine in urine. Both electron impact and chemical ionization modes have been used. To detect and quantitate cocaine and benzoylecognine in the same procedure, two internal standards should be employed. The preferred internal standards are deuterated cocaine and deuterated benzoylecognine.

Ecognine methyl ester is a major urinary metabolite of cocaine. Its presence in urine is an indicator as sensitive and specific as that of benzoylecognine for cocaine use. The use of EME has the advantage that, unlike benzoylecognine, it can be easily extracted and it has good chromatographic qualities in common TLC and GC systems (107).

Urine BE levels typically decline rapidly to below the usual 0.3 mg/liter cutoff in 24 to 96 hours since last exposure, but among long-term, high-dose abusers BE was reportedly detectable after 10 to 22 days (108). Detection times, however, are assay-dependent. In a study of human subjects given 20 mg of cocaine HC1 intravenously, the mean times of detection of the last positive urine specimen (greater than or equal to 0.3 mg/liter BE) after cocaine administration varied from 16.9 to 52.9 hours depending on the commercial tests used (TLC, EIA, FPLA, RIA) (106).

FORENSIC URINE DRUG TESTING

One of the initiatives for achieving a drug-free workplace is to implement urine drug testing programs for job applicants as well as for workers in occupations that are considered critical to public safety and health, e.g., those in nuclear power plants and the transportation industry. Urinalysis programs remain a controversial approach to dealing with the substance abuse problem in the workplace. Among the issues being intensely debated are the accuracy of the tests and the reliability of the laboratories conducting them (109, 110).

It is important to appreciate that urine drug testing for the workplace differs from clinical testing in several critical respects (109). For example, workplace drug testing results may be used for administrative purposes such as disciplinary action, dismissal, or denial of employment. Moreover, such test results stand on their own and are interpreted without the usual benefit of the physician-patient relationship or the clinical context in clinical testing. Thus, workplace drug testing must produce definitive test results that are both scientifically and legally defensible, the latter requiring comprehensive documentation to show that the integrity of the specimen has been maintained (chain of custody). This forensic aspect of substance abuse testing is usually unfamiliar to clinical laboratorians.

In addition to standard good laboratory practice, stringent requirements are needed for forensic urine drug testing (FUDT) laboratories (109). A discussion of these requirements follows.

Laboratory Facility

The FUDT laboratory where specimens and records are kept and where analytical work is performed should be separate from areas of clinical activities, and the laboratory should be a limited access area to authorized personnel. The laboratory should have protocols to protect the confidentiality of all records, to ensure the security of computer files relating to FUDT, and to limit computer access to authorized users.

Initial and Confirmation Tests

FUDT is a two-stage process—initial testing followed by confirmatory analysis of the presumptive positive specimens by quantitative GC-MS. Both initial and confirmation testing must be performed at the same laboratory site.

SPECIMEN CHAIN OF CUSTODY

Specimen (blood, urine, etc.): ______________________

Specimen Identification: ______________________

Specimen sealed: Yes No

Remarks: ______________________

____

Laboratory Accession #: ______________________

Date	Released By	Received By	Purpose of Change in Custody

ALIQUOT CHAIN OF CUSTODY

Date	Released By	Received By	Purpose of Change in Custody

Figure 20.6. Specimen/aliquot chain of custody form.

Chain of Custody Documentation

In FUDT, every urine specimen is treated as evidence. Therefore, there is a need to show proof of integrity of the specimen from specimen collection to its final disposition after analysis is completed. This requires documentation of *what* was done with the specimen (or aliquot), *who* handled the specimen (or aliquot), and *when* it was handled. A sample chain of custody form is shown in Figure 20.6.

Since the chain of custody procedures are the most challenged aspect of FUDT, they should be an important part of a laboratory's quality assurance program. The chain of custody of every specimen must be checked to assure that it has been appropriately completed before certifying results for reporting.

Personnel

The qualifications of a FUDT laboratory director are stringent, requiring training, experience, and expertise in forensic analytical toxicology comparable to that of a diplomate of the American Board of Clinical Chemistry in Toxicological Chemistry or the American Board of Forensic Toxicology.

The forensic aspect of drug testing creates the need for a laboratory certifying scientist (LCS) that does not exist in clinical laboratories. The LCS performs the final review of the entire laboratory process: the chain of custody documentation, and standards, blanks and quality control data of preliminary and confirmation tests before certifying the reports for release.

Accreditation and Licensure

In some states, e.g., New York, FUDT laboratories must meet state regulatory licensure requirements. At the national level there are two certification programs: The College of American Pathologists (CAP) Forensic Urine Drug Testing program and the Department of Health and Human Services (HHS) National Laboratory Certification Program (NIDA Certification). The federal program is based on a set of guidelines issued by NIDA (National Institute on Drug Abuse) (111), and certification by this program is required for laboratories engaged in the testing of employees of the federal government or industries regulated by the Department of Transportation (112). Both programs require acceptable performance in proficiency testing programs, and laboratories must successfully pass on-site inspection for obtaining and maintaining accreditation or certification.

References

1. Jatlow PI. Analytical toxicology in the clinical laboratory. An overview. Lab Med 1975;6:10–14.
2. McCarron MM. The role of the laboratory in treatment of the poisoned patient: clinical perspective. J Anal Toxicol 1983;7: 142–145.
3. Helliwell M, Hampel G, Sinclair E, Huggett A, Flanagan RJ. Value of emergency toxicologial investigations in differential diagnosis of coma. Br Med J 1979;2:819–821.
4. McCarron MM. The use of toxicology test in emergency room medicine. J Anal Toxicol 1983;7:131–135.
5. Chasnoff IJ, Burns KA, Burns WJ. Cocaine use in pregnancy: perinatal morbidity and mortality. Neurotoxicol Teratol 1987;9:291–293.
6. Gingras JL, Weese-Mayer DE, Hume RF Jr, O'Donnell KJ. Cocaine and development: mechanisms of fetal toxicity and neonatal consequences of prenatal cocaine exposure. Early Hum Dev 1992;31:1–24.
7. Ortrea EM Jr, Brady M, Gause S, Raymundo AL, Stevens M. Drug screening of newborns by meconium analysis: a large scale prospective, epidemiologic study. Pediatrics 1992;89: 107–113.
8. Bailey DN. The role of the laboratory in the treatment of the poisoned patient: laboratory perspective. J Anal Toxicol 1983;7:136–141.
9. Walberg CB. Comprehensive approaches to emergency toxicology. J Anal Toxicol 1983;7:146–148.
10. Hepler BR, Sutheimer CA, Sunshine I. The role of the toxicology laboratory in emergency medicine. J Toxicol-Clin Toxicol 1982;19:353–365.

11. Ingelfinger JA, Isakson G, Shine D, Costello CE, Goldman P. Reliability of the toxic screen in drug overdose. Clin Pharmacol Ther 1981;29:570–575.
12. Stevens HM. Colour tests. In: Moffat AC, ed. Clark's isolation and identification of drugs. 2nd ed. London: The Pharmaceutical Press, 1986:128–147.
13. Moffat AC. Clark's isolation and identification of drugs. 2nd ed. London: The Pharmaceutical Press, 1986.
14. Jatlow P. UV spectrophotometry for sedative drugs frequently involved in overdose emergencies. In: Sunshine I, ed. Methodology for analytical toxicology. 2nd ed. Cleveland: CRC Press, 1975:414–420.
15. Fell AF. Ultraviolet, visible, and fluorescence spectrum photometry. In: Moffat AC, ed. Clark's isolation and identification of drugs. 2nd ed. London: The Pharmaceutical Press, 1986:221–236.
16. Binder S, Regalia M, Biaggi-McEachern M, Mazhar M. Automated liquid chromatographic analysis of drugs in urine by on-column sample cleanup and isocratic multi-column separation. J Chrom 1989;473:325–341.
17. Allen L, Jr., Stiles ML. Specificity of the EMIT drug abuse urine assay methods. Clin Toxicol 1981;18:1043–1065.
18. Moffat AC. Thin layer chromatography. In: Moffat AC, ed. Clark's isolation and identification of drugs. 2nd ed. London: The Pharmaceutical Press, 1986:160–177.
19. Michaud JD. Thin layer chromatography for broad spectrum drug detection. Am Lab 1980;12:104–107.
20. Poklis A. Gas chromatography. In: Kaplan LA, Pesce AJ, eds. Clinical chemistry. 2nd ed. St. Louis: CV Mosby, 1989:110–125.
21. Message GM. Practical aspects of gas chromatography: mass spectrometry. New York: John Wiley & Sons, 1984.
22. Foltz RL, Fentiman AF, Foltz RB, eds. GC/MS assays for abused drugs in body fluids, NIDA Research Monograph No 32. DHHS Pub. No. (ADM) 80-104. Washington, DC: U.S. Government Printing Office, 1980.
23. Bowers LD. Liquid chromatography. In: Kaplan LA, Pesce AJ, eds. Clinical chemistry. 2nd ed. St. Louis: CV Mosby, 1989:94–109.
24. Dubowski KM. Absorption, distribution and elimination of alcohol: highway safety aspects. J Stud Alcohol 1985;(Suppl 10):98–108.
25. Basalt RC, Cravey RH. Disposition of toxic drugs and chemicals in man. 3rd ed. Chicago: Year Book Medical Publishers, 1989:322–326.
26. Whitfield JB, Starmer GA, Martin NG. Alcohol metabolism in men and women. Alcohol Clin Exp Res 1990;14:785–786.
27. Bogusz M, Pach J, Stasko W. Comparative studies on the rate of ethanol elimination in acute poisoning and in controlled conditions. J Forensic Sci 1977;22:446–451.
28. Dubowski KM, ed. Blood alcohol testing in the clinical laboratory. Proposed guideline TDMG-P. Villanova, PA: National Committee for Clinical Laboratory Standards, 1988.
29. Dubowski KM. Recent developments in alcohol analysis. Alcohol, Drugs, and Driving 1986;2:13–46.
30. Dubowski KM. Manual for analysis of ethanol in biological liquids. Report HS 802 208. Washington, DC: Department of Transportation, National Highway Traffic Safety Administration, 1977.
31. Gadsden RH, Terry CS, Thompson BC. Alcohols in biological fluids by gas chromatography (automated head-space method). In: Frings CS, Faulkner WR, eds. Selected methods of emergency toxicology. Washington: AACC Press; 1986:40–43.
32. Geller RJ, Skyker DA, Herold DA, Bruns DE. Serum osmolal gap and ethanol concentration: a simple and accurate formula. Clin Toxicol 1986;24:77–84.
33. McCoy HG, Cipolle RJ, Ehlers SM, et al. Severe methanol poisoning. Am J Med 1979;67:804–807.
34. Lacouture PG, Wason S, Abrams A, Lovejoy FH Jr. Acute isopropyl alcohol intoxication: diagnosis and management. Am J Med 1988;76:680–686.
35. Peterson CD, Collins AJ, Himes JM, Bullock ML, Keane WF. Ethylene glycol poisoning. Pharmacokinetics during therapy with ethanol and hemodialysis. N Engl J Med 1981;304:21–23.
36. Hewlett TP, McMartin KE, Lauro AJ, Ragan FA. Ethylene glycol poisoning. The value of glycolic acid determinations for diagnosis and treatment. Clin Toxicol 1986;24:389–402.
37. Doedens DJ. Methods for the determination of ethylene glycol. Vet Hum Toxicol 1983;25:96–101.
38. Porter WH, Avansakul A. Gas chromatographic determination of ethylene glycol in serum. Clin Chem 1982;28:75–78.
39. Gupta RN, Eng F, Gupta ML. Liquid-chromatographic determination of ethylene glycol in plasma. Clin Chem 1982;28:32–33.
40. Standefer J, Blackwell W. Enzymatic method for measuring ethylene glycol with a centrifugal analyzer. Clin Chem 1991;37:1734–1736.
41. Linden CH, Rumack BH. Acetaminophen overdose. Emerg Med Clin North Am 1984;2:103–119.
42. Lauterburg BH, Velez ME. Glutathione deficiency in alcoholics: risk factor for paracetamol hepatoxicity. Gut 1988;29:1153–1157.
43. Cocoran GB, Mitchell JR, Vaishnav YN, Horning EC. Evidence that acetaminophen and N-hydroxyacetaminophen form a common arylating intermediate, N-aceyl-p-benzoquinoneimine. Mol Pharmacol 1980;18:536–542.
44. Smilkstein MJ, Knapp GL, Kulig KW, Rumack BH. Efficacy of oral N-acetylcysteine in the treatment of acetaminophen overdose. N Engl J Med 1988;319:1557–1562.
45. Rumack BH, Matthew H. Acetaminophen poisoning and toxicity. Pediatrics 1975;55:871–876.
46. Glynn JR, Kendal SR. Paracetamol measurement. Lancet 1975;i:1147–1148.
47. Longlands MG, Wiener K. Minimisation of salicylate interference in the Glynn and Kendal paracetamol procedure. Am Clin Biochem 1982;19:187–190.
48. Stewart MJ, Chambers AM, Watson ID. Letter to the editor. Clin Chem 1984;30:1885.
49. Kwong TC. Salicylate measurement: clinical usefulness and methodology. CRC Crit Rev Clin Lab Med 1987;25:137–159.
50. Goldfrank LR, Bresnitz EA, Hartnett L, Flomenbaum NE. Salicylates. In: Goldfrank LR, Flomenbaum NE, Levin NA, Weisman RS, Howland MA, eds. Goldfrank's toxicological emergencies. 4th ed. Norwalk, CT: Appleton & Lange, 1990: 261–269.
51. Proudfoot AT. Toxicity of salicylates. Am J Med 1983; 75(suppl 5A):99–103.
52. Anderson RJ, Potts DE, Gabow PA, Rumack BH, Schrier RW. Unrecognized adult salicylate intoxication. Ann Intern Med 1976;85:745–748.
53. Brenner BE, Simon RR. Management of salicylate intoxication. Drugs 1982;24:335–340.
54. Done AK. Salicylate intoxication: significance of measurements of salicylate in blood in cases of acute ingestion. Pediatrics 1960;26:800–807.
55. Kwong TC, Laczin J, Baum J. Self poisoning with enteric coated aspirin. Am J Clin Pathol 1983;80:888–890.
56. Rall TW. Hypnotics and sedatives; ethanol. In: Gilman AG, Rall TW, Nies AS, Taylor P, eds. Gooman and Gilman's the Pharmacological basis of therapeutics. 8th ed. New York: Pergamon Press 1990;345–382.
57. Bath R, Kananen G. Barbiturates: type B procedure. Methods for Analytical Toxicology Cleveland: CRC Press, 1975;34–44.

58. TOXI-LAB AB Drug Detection System, TOXI-LAB, Inc., Irvine, CA, 1989.
59. Soo VA, Bergert RJ, Deutsch DG. Screening and quantification of hypnotic sedatives in serum by capillary gas chromatography with a nitrogen-phosphorus detector, and confirmation by capillary gas chromatography-mass spectrometry. Clin Chem 1986;32:325–328.
60. Atwell SH, Green VA, Haney WG. Development and evaluation of a method for simultaneous determination of phenobarbital and diphenylhydantoin in plasma by high-pressure liquid chromatography. J Pharm Sci 1975;64:806–809.
61. Mulé SJ, Casella GA. Confirmation and quantification of barbiturates in human urine by gas chromatography/mass spectrometry. J Anal Toxicol 1989;13:13–16.
62. Woods JH, Katz JL, Winger G. Use and abuse of benzodiazepines. Issues relevant to prescribing. JAMA 1988;260:3476–3480.
63. Weddington WW, Carney AC. Alprazolam abuse during methadone maintenance therapy. JAMA 1987;257:3363.
64. Geller E, Crome P, Schaller MO, Marchant B, Ectors M. Scollo-Láuizzari G. Risks and benefits of therapy with flumazenil (Anexate) in mixed drug intoxications. European Neurology 1991;31:241–250.
65. Roets E, Hoogmartens J. Thin layer chromatography of the acid hydrolysis products of nineteen benzodiazepine derivatives. J Chrom 1980;194:262–269.
66. Fraser AD, Bryan W, Isner AF. Urinary screening for alprazolam and its major metabolites by the Abbott ADx and TDx analyzers with confirmation by GC-MS. J Anal Toxicol 1991;15:25–29.
67. Fraser AD. Urinary screening for alprazolam, triazolam, and their metabolites with EMIT d.a.u. benzodiazepine metabolite assay. J Anal Toxicol 1987;11:263–266.
68. Osborn H, Goldfrank LR, Howland MA, Bresnitz EA, Kirstein RH. Barbiturates and other sedatives—hypnotics. In: Goldfrank LR, Flomenbaum NE, Levin NA, Weisman RS, Howland MA, eds. Goldfrank's toxicological emergencies. 4th ed. Norwalk, CT: Appleton & Lang, 1990:449–463.
69. Kelner MJ, Bailey DN. Ethylchlorvynol ingestion: interpretation of blood concentrations and clinical findings. J Toxicol Clin Toxicol 1983–84;21:399–408.
70. Benowitz N, Abdin C, Tozer T, et al. Resin hemoperfusion in ethylchlorvynol overdose. Clin Pharmacol Ther 1980;21:236–242.
71. Gomolin I. Meprobamate. Clin Toxicol 1981;18:757–760.
72. Greenblatt DJ, Allen MD, Harmatz JS, Noel BJ, Shader RI. Correlates of outcome following acute glutethimide overdosage. J Foren Sci 1979;24:76–86.
73. Frommer DA, Kulig KW, Marx JA, Rumack BH. Tricyclic antidepressant overdose. A review. JAMA 1987;257:521–526.
74. Lewin NA, Goldfrank LR. Physostigmine. In: Goldfrank LR, Flomenbaum NE, Levin NA, Weisman RS, Howland MA, eds. Goldfrank's toxicological emergencies. 4th ed. Norwalk, CT: Appleton & Lange, 1990:409–410.
75. Spiker DG, Weiss AN, Chang SS, Ruwitch JF, Biggs JT. Tricyclic antidepressant overdose: clinical presentation and plasma levels. Clin Pharmacol Ther 1975;18:539–546.
76. Boehnert MT, Lovejoy FH. Value of the QRS duration versus the serum drug level in predicting seizures and ventricular arrhythmias after an acute overdose of tricyclic antidepressants. N Engl J Med 1985;313:474–479.
77. Orsulak PJ. Therapeutic monitoring of antidepressant drugs: guidelines updated. Ther Drug Monit 1989;11:497–507.
78. Litovitz TL, Schmitz BF, Matyunas N, Martin TG. 1987 annual report of the American Association of Poison Control Centers National Data Collection Center. Am J Emerg Med 1988;6:479–515.
79. Schauben JL, Augenstein WL, Cox J, Sato R. Iron poisoning: report of three cases and a review of therapeutic intervention. J Emerg Med 1990;8:309–319.
80. Everson GW, Oudjhane K, Young LW, Krenzelock EP. Effectiveness of abdominal radiographs in visualizing chewable iron supplements following overdose. Am J Emerg Med 1989;7:459–463.
81. McGuigan MA, Lovejoy FH, Marino SK, Propper RP, Goldman R. Qualitative deferoxamine color test for iron ingestion. J Pediatr 1979;94:940–942.
82. Proudfoot AT, Simpson D, Dyson EH. Management of acute iron poisoning. Med Toxicol 1986;1:83–100.
83. Burkhart KE, Kulig KW, Hammond KB, Pearson JR, Ambruso D, Rumack BH. The rise in the total iron-binding capacity after iron overdose. Am J Emerg Med 1991;20:532–535.
84. Goldfrank LR, Kulberg AG, Kirstein RH. Iron. In: Goldfrank LR, Flomenbaum NE, Nevin NA, Weisman RS, Howland MA, eds. Goldfrank's toxicological emergencies. 4th ed. Norwalk, CT: Appleton & Lang, 1990:277–287.
85. Helfer RE, Rodgerson DO. The effects of deferoxamine on determination of serum and iron binding capacity. J Pediatr 1966;68:804–806.
86. Turner CE. Marihuana and cannabis research: why the conflict? In: Harvey DJ, ed. Marihuana. Oxrord: IRL Press 1985: 31–36.
87. Hollister LE. Health aspects of cannabis. Pharmacol Rev 1986;38:1–20.
88. Wall ME, Sadler BM, Brine D, Taylor H, Perez-Reyes M. Metabolism, disposition, and kinetics of δ-9-tetrahydrocannabinoid in men and women. Clin Pharmacol Ther 1983;34:352–363.
89. Ellis GM, Maun MA, Judson BA, Schram T, Tashchian A. Excretion patterns of cannabinoid metabolites after last use in a group of chronic users. Clin Pharmacol Ther 1986;38:572–578.
90. Cone EJ, Johnson RE. Contact highs and urinary cannabinoid excretion after passive exposure to marijuana smoke. Clin Pharmacol Ther 1986;40:247–256.
91. Mulé SJ, Lomax P, Gross SJ. Active and realistic passive marijuana exposure tested by three immunoassays and GC/MS in urine. J Anal Toxicol 1988;12:113–116.
92. Schwartz RH, Hawks RL. Laboratory detection of marijuana use. JAMA 1985;254:788–792.
93. Jaffe JH, Martin WR. Opioid anagesics and antagonists. In: Gilman AG, Goodman LS, Rall TW, Murad F, eds. Goodman and Gilman's The pharmacological basis of therapeutics. 7th ed. New York: Macmillan, 1985:491–531.
94. Goldfrank LR, Bresnitz EA. Opioids. In: Goldfrank LR, Flomenbaum NE, Levin NA, Weisman RS, Howland MA, eds. Goldfrank's toxicological emergencies. 4th ed. Norwalk, CT: Appleton & Lange, 1990:433–447.
95. Inturrisi CE, Max MB, Foley KM, Schultz M, Shinn SJJ, Houde RW. The pharmacokinetics of heroin in patients with chronic pain. N Engl J Med 1984;310:1213–1217.
96. Mulé SJ, Casella GA. Rendering the "poppy-seed defense" defenseless: identification of 6-monoacetylmorphine in urine by gas chromatography/mass spectroscopy. Clin Chem 1988;34:1427–1430.
97. ElSohly HN, ElSohly M, Stanford D. Poppy seed ingestion and opiates urinalysis: a closer look. J Anal Toxicol 1990;14: 308–310.
98. ElSohly M, Jones AB. Morphine and codeine in biological fluids: approaches to source differentiation. Forensic Sci Rev 1989;1:13–22.
99. Cone EJ, Welch P, Mitchell JM, Paul BD. Forensic drug testing for opiates: 1. Detection of 6-acetylmorphine in urine as an indicator of recent heroin exposure: drug and assay considerations and detection times. J Anal Toxicol 1991;15:1–7.

100. Henderson GL. Designer drugs: past history and future prospects. J Forensic Sci 1988;33:569–575.
101. Gawin GH, Ellinwood EH Jr. Cocaine and other stimulants. N Engl J Med 1988;318:1173–1182.
102. Jeffcoat AR, Perez-Reyes M, Hill JM, Sadler BM, Cook CE. Cocaine deposition in humans after intravenous injection, nasal insufflation (snorting), or smoking. Drug Metab Dispos 1989;17:153–159.
103. Jatlow P. Drug of abuse profile: cocaine. Clin Chem 1987;33: 66B–72B.
104. Ambre J. The urinary excretion of cocaine and metabolites in humans: a kinetic analysis of published data. J Anal Toxicol 1985:241–245.
105. Landry MJ. An overview of cocaethylene, an alcohol-derived, psychoactive, cocaine metabolite. J Psychoactive Drugs 1992;24:273–276.
106. Cone EJ, Menchen SL, Paul BD, Mell LD, Mitchell J. Validity testing of commercial urine cocaine metabolite assays. 1. Assay detection times, individual excretion patterns, and kinetics after cocaine administration to humans. J Forensic Sci 1989;34:15–31.
107. Clark DR, Hajar TM. Detection and confirmation of cocaine use by chromatographic analysis for methylecgonine in urine. Clin Chem 1987;33:118–119.
108. Weiss RD, Gawin FH. Protracted elimination of cocaine metabolites in long-term, high-dose cocaine abusers. Am J Med 1988;85:879–880.
109. Critical issues in urinalysis of abused substances: report of the Substance-Abuse Testing Committee, American Association of Clinical Chemistry. Clin Chem 1988;34:605–632.
110. Schottenfeld RS. Drug and alcohol testing in the workplace—objectives, pitfalls, and guidelines. Am J Drug Alcohol Abuse 1989;15:413–427.
111. Mandatory guidelines for federal workplace drug testing programs. Federal Register 1988;53:11979–11989.
112. Procedures for transportation workplace drug testing programs; interim final rule. Federal Register 1988;53:47001–47177.

21 Nutrition, Vitamins, and Trace Elements

Michael D. D. McNeely and Gordon N. Hoag

NUTRITION AND MALNUTRITION

Nutrition is the process whereby an organism takes in the raw materials it requires for energy production, metabolism, and synthetic activities. The basic food substances required by humans are carbohydrates, fats, and proteins. These must be ingested in appropriate amounts to meet the nutritional needs of the body. In addition, there are specific requirements for micronutrients such as essential amino acids, vitamins, and trace elements.

Inappropriate nutrition is the single greatest cause of illness in the world today. The majority of the world's population is subject to some degree of malnutrition in either protein, calories, or essential micronutrients. Up to 700 million children worldwide suffer from malnutrition. In contrast, a large segment of the population in developed countries experience a state of overnutrition leading to obesity and its assorted adverse health effects. The recommended dietary allowance (RDA) represents the minimum recommended dietary amount of a specific nutrient. However, the amount of a nutrient that is actually required depends on what is to be achieved. For example, the basal requirement is the amount of a nutrient required to maintain normal functioning of the organism. On the other hand, the normative storage requirement is the amount of a nutrient required to maintain a reserve in body tissues. Thus, it is possible to have "iron deficiency with anemia" and "iron deficiency without anemia."

The laboratory assessment of nutritional status is complicated by several factors (1). For example, establishing "cut-off" values may not in all cases separate deficient from adequately nourished subjects. This occurs for several reasons. First, the ability of laboratory tests to predict nutritional status varies across the spectrum from undernutrition to overnutrition. Second, the correlation between dietary intake and laboratory measurements is at best rough, partly because of normal biological variation and also because dietary intake and laboratory test responses are rarely correlated in a linear fashion.

MALNUTRITION

Starvation is a condition in which the human body cannot obtain sufficient calories or nutrients to sustain normal bodily functions. This disorder is rarely seen in the general population of North America but is endemic in many Third World countries, and local factors may create periodic epidemics. Less organized is the prevalence of malnutrition in selected populations in the developed world (2). Patients with chronic illnesses, the uncared-for elderly, and mentally deficient persons are particularly susceptible to malnutrition. About 40% of hospital patients have some degree of nutritional deficiency, and 15% of those in acute care hospitals have clinically significant protein calorie malnutrition (PCM). Severe PCM impairs the recovery of hospital patients, increases the risk of infection, and delays wound and tissue repair. In hospitalized patients there is a 3-fold increase in morbidity and mortality with untreated malnutrition. In the surgical population, preoperative nutritional support may decrease postoperative complications 2.5-fold and mortality 5-fold.

Malnutrition in the hospitalized patient may result from a combination of factors. For example, some patients cannot eat (coma, severe gastrointestinal disease), others will not eat (nausea, anorexia, apathy), while others have high losses (diarrhea, vomiting, burns). Although many patients have deficiencies of vitamins or minerals, the most common nutritional problem affecting the hospitalized patient is PCM.

The laboratory is of limited usefulness in the evaluation of malnutrition. Sophisticated methods such as nitrogen-balance studies can be performed for research purposes but are impractical for routine clinical use. Of the common laboratory tests, albumin is often used as a test of visceral protein status, but it is insensitive and nonspecific, and is depleted only when severe protein malnutrition occurs. Other measures of visceral protein status include transferrin, prealbumin, and retinol-binding protein. The measurement of the 24-hour urinary creatinine excretion provides a good assessment of somatic protein status (lean body mass). Urinary hydroxyproline levels have been used to assess collagen catabolism and as an indicator of protein status. Other tests that may be of value in the evaluation of nutritional status include the total lymphocyte count and serum levels of vitamins A and C. See also the discussion below of nutritional assessment.

Kwashiorkor

Kwashiorkor is a syndrome caused by a severe protein deficiency despite an adequate caloric intake, usually in the form of carbohydrates. In countries where kwashiorkor is endemic, the syndrome may occur as early as the time of weaning. The syndrome is characterized by growth retardation, muscle wasting, edema, hair loss, anemia, anorexia, flaky skin with hypopigmentation, a swollen abdomen (ascites), a characteristic fretful facies, and susceptibility to infection. Unlike marasmus (see below) subcutaneous fat is present (albeit reduced) and there is increased fat in the liver (steatosis), leading to hepatomegaly. Ultimately, cardiac failure may occur. The increased susceptibility to infection in patients with kwashiorkor presumably results from a defective barrier function in the skin and mucous membranes; impaired granulocyte, humoral, and cell-mediated immune functions; and impaired complement activity. All patients with kwashiorkor will die without treatment; however, due to the severity of this disorder, up to 40% die despite medical intervention. There are no characteristic biochemical findings of this condition.

Marasmus

Marasmus is a condition in which the diet is extremely deficient in both protein and carbohydrate. These patients exhibit wasting of both muscle and fat. This is in contrast to kwashiorkor, in which body fat may be normal. There is no edema or anorexia, the liver is normal in size, and the skin does not exhibit hyperpigmentation or hypopigmentation. The subcutaneous fat is extremely depleted.

Obesity

Obesity is defined for men as having more than 20% of the body weight as fat and, for women, more than 30%. It affects approximately 15% of the North American population. The cause of obesity has in the past been attributed to psychological problems within the sufferers, but this is probably not the explanation in the majority of cases. The causes are more likely to represent a change in physical activity, alteration of body image, the availability of food, and the social connotations associated with eating it (3). There is no evidence that a biochemical abnormality leads to obesity except in rare but specific conditions such as Cushing's syndrome (4).

Most people, whether obese or lean, remain at relatively the same weight for long periods of time. This suggests an endogenous weight control mechanism.

Studies into the mechanism of obesity have revealed the following facts:

1. Food intake: Obese people eat more than nonobese persons, and in most retrospective studies of food intake, the obese person will underestimate significantly. Obese people are much more susceptible to environmental change and during such times will increase their food intake.
2. Energy expenditure: Energy expenditure is greatest in infants and declines with age. The increase in body fat with age can be partially attributed to this. It is also recognized that energy expenditure may vary up to 20% among persons with the same lean body mass. Similarities in metabolic rate can be seen in family clusters, which may explain the familial predisposition to obesity.

Obesity may exacerbate or initiate certain disorders. It is recognized that when fat deposition increases, the number of insulin receptors also increases. This exacerbates diabetes mellitus in certain individuals. In addition, the risk and severity of hypertension is exacerbated by obesity. In general, obesity beyond 15% of the ideal body weight is detrimental to overall health. There is some evidence that the distribution of body fat may also be an important factor. It has been shown that a high ratio of abdominal/gluteal circumference carries a twofold or greater risk of heart attack, stroke, hypertension, diabetes, gallbladder disease, and death.

There are various methods to assess body fat. Unfortunately, most simple methods are not accurate, and accurate methods are not widely available or are very expensive. The simple approaches include caliper measurements, abdominal/limb circumference, body density (water immersion or isotope dilution with ^{40}K), electromagnetic conductivity, bioelectric impedance, and CT scanning. The best approach is the Quetelet index. This is the weight (in kilograms) divided by the height (in centimeters) squared (W/H^2). The result can be compared to tables. There are no routine laboratory tests available to assess total body fat.

The obvious treatment for obesity is the reduction of calories. For a diet to be effective, an individual must enter negative caloric balance. In such a diet, there will be an initial diuretic phase. This is due to the fact that the reduction of calories is also associated with a reduction in protein intake, which causes a depletion of urea and this diminishes the renal tubular concentrationg power. The result is a diuresis, which causes a large, early, rapid weight loss of up to 2 kg, which often gives a false impression that the diet is doing extremely well. Those who accept such diets are then subsequently discouraged by the fact that there is no weight loss over the ensuing 2 to 3 weeks. Caution is therefore advised when choosing or evaluating a dietary regimen. In general, the best weight-loss diets are nutritionally balanced and palatable and serve as a model for the regular diet that must eventually be taken.

When obesity reaches a crisis situation, then surgical intervention may be warranted. In the past, the conventional surgical intervention was intestinal bypass. In this procedure, a rerouting of the intestinal passageway was made so that food would be delivered from the stomach into the large intestine in a relatively shortened time frame. Regrettably, this form of surgery had a 4% operative mortality, with death occurring as a result of pulmonary embolism, wound infections, gastrointestinal hemorrhage, and renal failure. Even when the surgery was successful, the recipients suffered from hyperoxaluria and calcium oxalate renal stones. They also developed toxic megacolon from bacterial overgrowth, anemia, acute cholecystitis from deranged intrahepatic circulation, diarrhea, electrolyte abnormalities, hypoproteinemia, and fatty infiltration of the liver (3).

A recent surgical approach has been surgical stapling of the stomach. This allows the physical size of the stomach to be reduced, causing early satiety. Dental splinting, in which the mouth is completely closed by wires, has also been attempted. Recipients of this treatment must ingest a liquid dict.

These are obviously very radical approaches that are only applied in extreme situations.

PARENTERAL NUTRITION

It is now possible to sustain the nutritional requirements of hospitalized patients entirely through intravenous feeding. Over the past 2 decades, significant advances have been made in refining the intravenous solutions to provide optimal nutrition (5). Initially, the problem was to provide sufficient caloric intake while avoiding the use of highly osmolar solutions. As this problem was solved, and patients were kept for longer periods of time on total parenteral nutrition, other complications due to vitamin and trace substance deficiencies began to emerge. To a large degree these have been corrected by the inclusion of trace materials in the intravenous solutions or by regimens that allow them to be added at intervals.

Currently, the major complications of total parenteral nutrition (TPN) are problems with the intravenous site (including systemic infections and clotting of the line), generalized septicemia produced through the intravenous site, overhydration or underhydration, inappropriate nutritional balance, and acid-base imbalances (6).

The major assessment of patients undergoing such therapy remains clinical. However, several laboratory parameters are extremely helpful (5).

The measurement of urine specific gravity (or more specifically, the measurement of urine osmolality) is an excellent test to monitor hydration. In addition, urinary sodium and potassium are important measures of salt balance.

The measurement of urine urea provides a rough guide to overall nitrogen balance. If an individual is in negative nitrogen balance, then almost no urine urea will be excreted. This test suffers from differences in urea handling that occur at various levels of nutritional status. A better assessment of nitrogen balance can be obtained by the measurements of urine urea, creatinine, uric acid, and total protein. Obviously, the direct measurement of total urinary nitrogen is the single best procedure, but this is technically difficult and is not justified over the measurement of the individual components.

Measuring urinary ketones and glucose is easily performed and provides useful information. Ketosis is observed when body stores of fat are being mobilized for calories. The presence of ketones in the urine indicates either an inappropriate use of the TPN solution or a starvation state. Excess glucose in the urine may indicate that spilling of the TPN fluid through the glomerulus is taking place. This will lead to calorie, fluid, and electrolyte loss and hampers the calculation of nutritional parameters. Another possibility is, of course, lack of carbohydrate control.

Blood tests are less valuable for monitoring TPN, except as outlined below for general nutritional assessment. Many TPN solutions are rich in lipids and will render the serum almost opaque. They also have high concentrations of glucose and other substances. Therefore, it is mandatory to avoid collecting blood from a patient in whom a TPN solution has recently been administered, since the components of the solution may significantly alter test results.

A suggested monitoring panel for monitoring adults on TPN is albumin, prealbumin, magnesium, inorganic phosphorus, ionized (free) calcium, copper, zinc, prothrombin time, and zinc protoporphyrin.

NUTRITIONAL ASSESSMENT

Nutritional assessment is best performed by evaluation of the patient's history, physical examination (including anthropomorphic measurements), and laboratory parameters.

Clinical examination provides a number of clues about the general nutritional status of the patient and specific deficiency states. For example, the loss of subcutaneous fat and muscle indicates general nutritional deficiencies, while various skin and mucous membrane changes can be extremely good indicators of vitamin deficiencies.

A careful nutritional history and dietary evaluation are important components in the assessment of nutritional status. However, this information is not always reliable. Even the most skilled dietitian cannot conduct an entirely accurate dietary history. Direct measurement of consumption over a fixed period of time does not assess the natural diet, nor can it be extrapolated over a long time frame.

Anthropomorphic measurements may be helpful. The simplest is the measurement of body weight. A weight less than 85% of ideal usually indicates a nutritional deficiency. Measurements of both height and weight can be compared to tables such as those developed by the Metropolitan Life Insurance Company. These tables are best suited for analysis of populations but, because of person-to-person variability, are less useful for evaluating a single subject. Fat stores can be assessed by measuring the triceps skinfold thickness of the dominant arm. Multiple measurements of other sites can be used to establish the percentage of body weight as fat. This approach gives a 20% overlap between normal and abnormal populations. By measuring the mid-arm circumference and the triceps skinfold thickness, an estimate of the mid-arm muscle circumference can be derived by the formula shown below (6).

$$\text{Mid-arm muscle circumference} = \text{Mid-arm circumference} - \pi \times \text{Triceps skinfold thickness}$$

Laboratory measurements are of limited use in nutritional assessment. Serum albumin responds slowly to nutritional change and may also be altered by liver or renal disease. The body has large extravascular pools of albumin, and the half-life is long (19 days). Consequently, the serum albumin level responds slowly to changes in nutritional status. Nevertheless, in the absence of liver and renal disease a serum albumin less than 20 g/liter indicates severe malnutrition, and values between 20 and 30 g/liter indicate moderate malnutrition. Serum transferrin has been used for the general assessment of visceral protein status, but its sensitivity is low. Transferrin has a half-life of 8 days, and therefore the serum level changes somewhat faster than albumin but the half-life is altered by a variety of diseases. Prealbumin, with a half-life of 1.9 days, provides a good short-term nutritional index, whereas retinol binding protein (RBP) provides the most sensitive index of protein status and is the quickest protein to respond to refeeding. RBP is also decreased rapidly in liver disease and is increased in kidney disease and following estrogen administration. However, assays for RBP are less widely available than those for albumin or transferrin.

The measurement of urinary creatinine is closely correlated with body nitrogen loss from the urinary tract. Values 60 to 80% of normal indicate moderate nitrogen deficiency, and values less than 60% of normal indicate severe depletion. By measuring three consecutive 24-hour urines and averaging the creatinine content, an estimate of lean body mass (LBM) can be made by the formula shown below.

$$\text{LBM (kg)} = 7.38 + 0.02909 \text{ Creatinine (mg/day)}$$

Urinary amino acid patterns change as nutritional status declines. For example, with chronic protein calorie deficiency the total amount of urinary amino acids decreases with a relative deficiency of branched chain amino acids and an increase in glycine and serine.

Muscle breakdown (somatic protein) can be evaluated by measuring the 24-hour excretion of 3-methylhistidine in the urine. 3-methylhistidine is almost exclusively found in myofibrillar protein. It is released from actin and myosin but is not reutilized. 3-Methylhistidine (4.2 μmol per 24 hours) is derived from 1 gram of mixed muscle protein. This amount will increase in muscle breakdown and fever. An amino acid analyzer is required for this measurement.

The ability to develop ketosis after a fast is good evidence of fat stores, and the rate of clearance of an IV injection of fat has been used as a measure of fat utilization.

Skin sensitivity testing using intradermal injections of antigens (e.g., PPD) has been attempted for assessment of nutritional status because the immune response is impaired by states of severe nutritional deficiency. Unfortunately, this test is nonspecific and difficult to quantitate, and is therefore unreliable.

VITAMINS

The term "vitamin" comes from the words "vital" and "amine," reflecting the long-held knowledge that such substances are essential for normal growth and development and the somewhat narrower vision that these substances were nitrogen-containing. Vitamins include a number of trace substances that are essential but that cannot be synthesized at all or in large enough amounts to provide the basic bodily requirements. Vitamins often act as coenzymes in enzymatic reactions (Table 21.1). Each vitamin-depend-

Table 21.1. Clinical Syndromes Due to Abnormal Vitamin Intake

Vitamin	Deficiency State	Toxic State
Vitamin A	Night blindness Blindness	Cerebral syndrome Skin desquamation Carotenemia
Vitamin B_6 (pyridoxine)	Isolated deficiency is rare Genetic disorders of pyridoxine resistance Drug interference with B_6 may cause polyneuritis	
Vitamin C (ascorbic acid)	Scurvy	Kidney stones
Vitamin E (tocopherols)	Edema and hemolytic anemia in infants	Interference with the absorption of other fat-soluble vitamins
Vitamin K	Bleeding disorder	
Niacin (nicotinic acid)	Pellegra Secondary pellegra Hartnup's disease Isoniazid administration	Flushing and pruritus
Vitamin B_2 (riboflavin)	Glossitis, dermatitis, neuropathy and anemia	
Vitamin B_1 (thiamin)	Beriberi	
Vitamin H (biotin)	Alopecia totalis and scaly dermatitis	

ent enzyme requires the combination of an apoenzyme (protein) and a coenzyme (vitamin or a mineral element) (7).

The mass media and fringe medical practitioners advocate the use of various vitamins in different and generally unproven ways (1, 8). In general, the overemphasis on vitamins as a source of health does little harm. However, the use of vitamins in massive doses has resulted in a number of toxic effects. For this reason, megavitamin therapy is usually inappropriate. There are some situations, such as vitamin D-resistant rickets, in which large doses of a vitamin has proved useful, but these conditions are rare. For normal subjects it is generally accepted that an adequate diet will supply all of the essential nutrients.

Vitamin A

METABOLISM

Vitamin A is made up of a group of compounds that have the biological action of retinol. Vitamin A is essential for vision, reproduction, growth, epithelial differentiation, and mucus secretion. The main vitamin A compounds are retinol (vitamin A_1) and 3-dehydroretinol (vitamin A_2).

Vitamin A is found in the livers of many animals and fish. It is stored there predominantly as fatty acid esters of vitamin A. Meat, fat, eggs, and dairy products are considered good sources of vitamin A. It is also found as plant carotenoid pigments (β-carotene) in yellow and green vegetables and fruits. These substances can be converted into retinol.

Neither vitamin A nor carotene is soluble in water, but both will dissolve in organic solvents. For this reason they cannot be directly absorbed in the gastrointestinal tract but must be coabsorbed with fats as part of the micelles that form in the intestine. Fatty acid esters are hydrolyzed by retinyl-ester hydrolase, an enzyme secreted by the pancreas, and by brush-border enzymes.

Free retinol is absorbed in the gastrointestinal tract and reesterified with fatty acids intracellularly. Carotenoids are converted into retinal and then to retinol, which is esterified in the same way. Retinol esters are packaged into chylomicrons, which pass into the lymphatics and are carried to the liver, where they are reconverted to retinol and linked to an intracellular retinol binding protein. When needed by the body, the retinol is transferred to a circulating retinol binding protein (MW 20,000) or may form a complex with prealbumin. Serum levels of retinol binding protein (RBP) vary with the amount of vitamin A that must be carried.

Vitamin A influences cell division, RNA synthesis, protein glycosylation, lysosomal-membrane stabilization, and prostaglandin biosynthesis and determines the rate of keratinization and differentiation of epithelial-cell layers.

Vitamin A has a vital role in vision. Retinal is the prosthetic group of the photosensitive pigment in the eye. Retinol has the ability to be isomerized and then dehydrogenated during dark adaption, where it can be linked to opsin to form a substance known as rhodopsin. When the eye is subjected to light, there is a reversal of this process, which creates an electron flux and triggers the optic nerve.

CLINICAL SYNDROMES

Vitamin A deficiency is endemic in the Third World and is one of the most common causes of blindness. In the Third World, vitamin A deficiency is primarily due to dietary deficiency. Deficiency may also occur as a result of fat malabsorption.

The initial symptom of vitamin A deficiency is night blindness, but with severe deficiency total blindness may occur. In addition, there is disordered maturation and keratinization of epithelial surfaces, resulting in tissue breakdown. Vitamin A deficiency is often a component of general malnutrition. Zinc deficiency may mimic certain aspects of vitamin A deficiency, since the enzyme retinol dehydrogenase is zinc dependent. This enzyme is responsible for the formation of retinolaldehyde (active vitamin A).

Toxicity with vitamin A has been primarily observed in infants in whom a cerebral syndrome with epithelial changes has been described. Symptoms of acute toxicity in adults include abdominal pain, nausea, vomiting, severe headaches, dizziness, lethargy, and irritability. The skin lesion is characterized primarily by desquamation. Chronic toxicity results in bone and joint pain, hair loss, dryness of the lips, and hepatomegaly.

An excess of carotene can result from a diet high in carotenoid-containing vegetables, such as lettuce and carrots. This imparts an orange tinge to the skin, which is not harmful but may cause cosmetic embarrassment or be misinterpreted as jaundice.

The ingestion of large amounts of vitamin A has been suggested as possible anticancer treatment (8). The theoretical basis of this strategy is to reverse the loss of cellular differentiation characteristic of malignant tumors. Other unproven uses of vitamin A include the treatment of schizophrenia, learning disabilities, and autism.

MEASUREMENT

The measurement of carotene in the serum provides an indirect assessment of vitamin A, and the assay for serum carotene is easier to perform than the measurement of vitamin A. Its primary use in the clinical laboratory is as a rough guide to fat absorption. The procedure involves denaturation of serum proteins with alcohol and extraction with petroleum ether, followed by spectrophotometric measurement of the yellow pigment.

Increased serum carotenes may occur in subjects consuming high vegetable diets and in hypothyroidism, while low serum carotene levels are seen with low vegetable diets and with fat malabsorption.

Vitamin A assays involve precipitation of serum binding proteins with alcohol extraction followed by evaporation of the ether and reextraction into chloroform. The classic reaction to quantitate vitamin A is the Carr-Price method, which uses antimony trichloride. The assay is very susceptible to water and is therefore unreliable, although it is the most popular approach. More recently, it has been shown that reaction with trifluoroacetic acid in an organic extract is more reliable, but vitamin A determinations are rarely performed in the clinical laboratory.

High-pressure liquid chromatography (HPLC) may also be used to assess vitamin A in serum.

Normally, the liver stores large amounts of vitamin A. Consequently, in vitamin A–deficient subjects the serum level of vitamin A remains in the normal range for a very long time as the liver stores are gradually depleted. Only when the liver stores are almost completely depleted does the serum level begin to fall.

High levels of vitamin A are seen in subjects taking vitamin supplements. Low values may occur in liver disease, vitamin A deficiency, and fat malabsorption. The normal vitamin A concentration of serum varies directly with the level of retinol-binding protein.

Vitamin B_6 (Pyridoxine)

METABOLISM

Vitamin B_6 is composed of three substances: pyridoxine, pyridoxal, and pyridoxamine. All of these are phosphorylated to pyridoxal phosphate, which is a cofactor for many enzymes. Its primary role is as a cofactor for amino acid transferases. It is therefore vital for protein synthesis.

Dietary sources of vitamin B_6 include meat, yeast, seeds, and bran. Vitamin B_6 compounds are sensitive to heat and may be destroyed by cooking. Vitamin B_6 compounds are separated from their esters in the intestinal lumen by alkaline phosphatase. They are then readily absorbed and are trapped within cells by phosphorylation. Hydrolysis will release the vitamin back into the cell and into the circulation.

CLINICAL SYNDROMES

An isolated deficiency of vitamin B_6 is rare, but deficiency may occur as a component of generalized vitamin deficiency or malnutrition. Vitamin B_6 deficiency is characterized by dermatitis with cheilosis and glossitis, an anemia (pyridoxine-responsive microcytic anemia), and convulsions.

The drugs isoniazid, hydralazine, penicillamine, and cycloserine all interfere with vitamin B_6 metabolism and may therefore cause polyneuritis.

A number of genetic disorders may respond to increased levels of vitamin B_6. These include (*a*) infantile convulsions (a deficiency of glutamate dehydrogenase); (*b*) pyridoxine-responsive microcytic anemia, (*c*) xanthurenic aciduria; (*d*) primary cystathioninuria; and (*e*) homocystinuria.

MEASUREMENT

Vitamin B_6 may be measured using a microbiological assay. Different bacterial species respond to various forms of vitamin B_6 and, therefore, assays can be customized for each of the components. A fluorometric method has also been described. HPLC methods have been used for research purposes. It is also possible to assess the amount of vitamin B_6 in serum by performing an aspartate aminotransferase (ASAT) assay before and after the addition of vitamin B_6. Vitamin B_6 serves as an essential cofactor for ASAT.

Deficiency of the vitamin will therefore result in a greater difference between the unsupplemented and supplemented assays.

Pyridoxine may be reduced in the bloodstream by oral contraceptives, isoniazid, methotrexate, and excess alcohol.

A good screening test for vitamin B_6 deficiency is the tryptophan loading test (9). In this procedure, 2 grams of tryptophan is administered orally. If vitamin B_6 levels are normal, then the urinary xanthurenic acid level will be greater than 50 μmol/24 hours. A failure to achieve this level implies a vitamin B_6 deficiency.

Vitamin C (Ascorbic Acid)

METABOLISM

Vitamin C is a strong reducing agent, an important property in its metabolic function.

The vitamin is found in citrus fruits, berries, melons, tomatoes, green peppers, and leafy vegetables. It is susceptible to destruction by heat and various food processing methods.

Vitamin C is water soluble and is readily absorbed in the stomach by both passive diffusion and active transport mechanisms. It is found in most tissues, with high concentrations in the retina. Its half-life in the body is 16 days. Iron absorption is enhanced by the presence of vitamin C. Vitamin C is metabolized in the body, and one of its metabolic products is oxalate, which is excreted in the urine.

The reducing properties of vitamin C are important for the hydroxylation of proline and lysine during collagen synthesis. It acts as a cofactor for protocollagen hydroxylase. It is important in tyrosine metabolism, drug metabolism, the synthesis of epinephrine, and fatty acid metabolism.

CLINICAL SYNDROMES

Vitamin C deficiency may result from a diet that is lacking in citrus fruits and leafy vegetables. The most severe form of deficiency is known as scurvy which is characterized by swollen and bleeding gums, arthralgias, fatigue, tender edematous legs, and subcutaneous hemorrhages.

Toxicity due to vitamin C has also been reported. Chronic overdosage of vitamin C may be a cause of uric acid and cystine kidney stones. In susceptible individuals, it clearly is associated with oxalate renal calculi. High levels of vitamin C in the urine will cause false-negatives with some conventional methods of dipstick chemistry (glucose, blood, bilirubin, and nitrite), and with quantitative measurements of oxalate.

MEASUREMENT

Vitamin C can be measured by colorimetric, fluorometric, and HPLC methods.

The colorimetric method is the most convenient. In this technique, serum ascorbic acid is oxidized by Cu(II) to form dehydroascorbic acid. This reacts with 2,4-dinitrophenylhydrazine to form a red hydrazone, which can be quantitated spectrophotometrically.

Another method to assess vitamin C status is to conduct a 24-hour urine ascorbic acid test on a baseline sample and after 2 days of 200 mg oral ascorbic acid. If the second 24-hour urinary collection contains less than 50 mg of ascorbic acid, then ascorbic acid deficiency can be presumed.

Serum ascorbic acid concentrations of less than 11 μmol/liter suggest vitamin C deficiency. Low values are also found in smokers, in the postoperative period, and in association with barbiturate and aspirin ingestion.

Vitamin E (Tocopherols)

METABOLISM

Vitamin E includes a group of compounds known as tocopherols (namely D-α-tocopherol). They are synthesized by plants and are found in high concentrations in vegetable oils. They are also present in egg yolk, liver, and milk. Vitamin E is insoluble in water, is soluble in fats, and is easily oxidized.

Vitamin E is coabsorbed with fats and enters the lymphatic system. There is no specific serum carrier. The vitamin is stored in most tissues, with higher concentrations in adipose tissue. The dietary requirement of tocopherols is closely related to the dietary intake of polyunsaturated fats, in which they are found in abundance.

Chemically, vitamin E is an antioxidant and is thought to protect membrane lipids from oxidation. The vitamin may decrease oxidative damage to the lungs, red blood cells, and neurons by absorbing the free radicals produced during normal metabolism. Vitamin E is required for reproduction in animals, but evidence for this role in humans has never been proved (10).

CLINICAL SYNDROMES

Deficiency of vitamin E has been described in premature infants. This syndrome is characterized by edema, hemolytic anemia, thrombocytosis, and erythematous, papular skin lesions.

Adult vitamin E deficiency is rare but may occur in severe malabsorption and fat malabsorption.

Toxicity due to vitamin E is not well described, but large amounts may compete for absorption with other fat-soluble vitamins.

There is a popular belief that vitamin E can cure a variety of ailments. It is a component of some skin creams and may be beneficial for the treatment of skin wounds and other dermatologic ailments. It has also been suggested that vitamin E will retard the aging process, presumably due to its antioxidant properties, but all such suggestions are unproven at present.

MEASUREMENT

The serum or blood level of vitamin E does not correlate with body storage of the vitamin (11).

Vitamin E assays usually employ saponification, solvent extraction, and then separation on HPLC or GLC, but the measurement is rarely performed.

Recently, various ratios of tocopherol to lipids (cholesterol and triglyceride) have been studied as a means to assess vitamin E body stores (12).

Vitamin K

METABOLISM

There are a number of different vitamin K compounds (13). Chemically, these compounds are methylnaphthoquinones. Plant vitamin K_1 and bacterial vitamin K_2 occur naturally. There is also a synthetic analogue of vitamin K that is structurally similar to the natural form of K_3.

All vitamin Ks are coabsorbed with fat and transported to the liver for storage.

Vitamin Ks are required for the production of prothrombin and clotting factors VII, IX, and X. Vitamin K can be synthesized by intestinal bacteria, and up to 50% of the vitamin K requirement is provided by the normal GI flora (14).

CLINICAL SYNDROMES

Newborns are susceptible to vitamin K deficiency because they do not have an active bacterial flora. Vitamin K deficiency is also seen in persons with fat malabsorption or biliary obstruction. The disorder is characterized by a prolonged prothrombin time and possible hemorrhagic disease and is easily corrected by administering parenteral vitamin K.

Coumarins are used as anticoagulants. They prevent the production of the reduced form of vitamin K, which is required for the synthesis of clotting factors.

MEASUREMENT AND INTERPRETATION

A variety of direct measurements are available for vitamin K, involving chromatography or spectrophotometry. However, these methods are rarely used except in research applications (15), and it is usually adequate to rely on the measurement of the prothrombin time to assess the activity of the vitamin K system.

Low vitamin K levels with an associated prolongation of the prothrombin time are seen in fat malabsorption, in patients receiving broad-spectrum antibiotics, and with coumarin administration. Conditions that predispose to vitamin K deficiency include liver disease, biliary insufficiency, prolonged salicylate administration, alterations of the intestinal flora, uremia, and ingestion of mineral oil.

Niacin (Nicotinic Acid)

METABOLISM

Niacin, or nicotinic acid, is a derivative of tryptophan. Dietary sources include yeast, legumes, lean red meat, liver, and poultry. Protein, which contains tryptophan, can be converted by pyridoxine to niacin.

Niacin is hydrolyzed in the gastrointestinal tract and is readily absorbed.

The vitamin is transported to many tissues, where it is converted into its coenzyme forms. Nicotinic acid niacin as niacinamide (nicotinic acid amide) is a component of nicotinamide adenine dinucleotide (NAD) and nicotinamide adenine dinucleotide phosphate (NADP). These are found in virtually every cell of the body. There are numerous enzymes that require NAD or NADP (mostly dehydrogenases).

CLINICAL SYNDROMES

The most dramatic niacin deficiency syndrome is pellagra, which is characterized by diarrhea, dementia, dermatitis, and death (the four "Ds"). This syndrome generally occurs as a result of dietary deficiency. Persons who eat corn as their main dietary staple are susceptible to pellagra because corn is low in tryptophan, and its niacin is complexed and therefore not readily available.

Hartnup's disease is a disorder of the kidney tubules that causes massive urinary loss of monoamino-monocarboxylic acids. One of the amino acids lost in the urine is tryptophan, and this loss can be large enough to cause niacin deficiency. The condition is diagnosed by its characteristic urinary amino acid pattern.

Isoniazid administration in the treatment of tuberculosis may cause a pellagra-like syndrome. Isoniazid is a pyridoxine antagonist, and pyridoxine is necessary for the conversion of tryptophan into niacin. Patients receiving isoniazid may require vitamin supplements.

Finally, carcinoid tumors are rare endocrine neoplasms that may produce extremely large amounts of serotonin from tryptophan. The tumor may consume much of the tryptophan in the body and thereby cause a form of pellagra.

A syndrome of niacin excess characterized by flushing, pruritus, nausea, vomiting, and diarrhea has been reported in persons taking large doses of the drug.

MEASUREMENT

Niacin status is usually evaluated by urinary measurement of the principal metabolites of the vitamin, namely N^1-methylnicotinamide and its pyridone (16). Normally, more than 12 mg per day of this metabolite is found in the urine. In pellegra, the values are less than 2 mg per day.

Vitamin B_2 (Riboflavin)

METABOLISM

Dietary sources of vitamin B_2 include liver, kidney, heart, eggs, and vegetables. Small amounts are found in cereals. The vitamin is present in raw milk but disappears with pasteurization (17).

Vitamin B_2 is hydrolized in the stomach and is linked to a binding protein. It is absorbed in the gastrointestinal tract by a specific transport system in the intestine. In the circulation the vitamin is complexed to proteins (mainly albumin).

The precursors flavin mononucleotide (FMN) and flavin adenine dinucleotide (FAD) are cofactors for electron transport, liver enzyme action, and corticosteroid production.

CLINICAL SYNDROMES

Riboflavin deficiency is characterized by glossitis, dermatitis, neuropathy, and anemia. However, these findings are nonspecific, and the syndrome is usually found in association with other B vitamin deficiencies.

MEASUREMENT AND INTERPRETATION

Blood and urine measurements of riboflavin have little clinical application. The best test for vitamin B_2 involves measurement of red cell glutathione reductase before and after the addition of FAD. An increase in activity of less than 20% is normal, whereas an increase greater than 40% indicates a deficiency state (17–19).

An isolated deficiency of B_2 is very unusual. Low values may be seen during times of increased B_2 requirement (tissue repair and testosterone therapy) and in B vitamin deficiencies.

Vitamin B_1 (Thiamin)

METABOLISM

Vitamin B_1 in its coenzyme form is thiamin pyrophosphate. The vitamin is found in most plant and animal tissues, but the best source is unrefined cereal grains, enriched flour, liver, heart, and kidney.

Thiamin can be inactivated by gastric secretions, especially in achlorhydria. It is readily absorbed in the small intestine by an active transport mechanism. The vitamin is phosphorylated in the gastrointestinal mucosa and transported to the liver. Thiamin diphosphate is the predominant form of the vitamin.

CLINICAL SYNDROMES

Thiamin is essential for the oxidative decarboxylation of α-keto acids and is therefore important in the Krebs cycle. It is also needed for the hexosemonophosphate (HMP) shunt transketolase activity. The vitamin plays an important role in myelin lipid maintenance and is therefore important for the functioning of the CNS.

Thiamin deficiency occurs in populations that depend on rice as a staple in their diet. If the rice is milled, the outer, thiamin-containing portion of the grain is lost. Thiamin deficiency occurs predominantly in children in underdeveloped nations and in adult alcoholics in the developed world (20, 21). There are various clinical presentations.

Dry beriberi is due to chronic thiamin deficiency and is characterized by a prominent neurological involvement. Wet beriberi is characterized by severe edema. Acute beriberi presents with congestive heart failure.

Combined vitamin B_1 and B_6 deficiency has a detrimental effect on the transport of calcium, cadmium, and zinc and may be associated with deficiencies of these trace materials. There are also thiamin antagonists in coffee, tea, betel, and raw fish, which may have an influence on the thiamin level in the body.

MEASUREMENT

Whole-blood thiamin levels can be measured but are very difficult to perform. The measurement of urinary thiamin is of no clinical value.

The most reliable indicator of thiamin status is the measurement of erythrocyte transketolase (20, 21). This is a thiamin-dependent enzyme of the HMP shunt. The enzyme is measured in red cells before and after the addition of thiamin monophosphate.

INTERPRETATION

Low transketolase activity may be due to thiamin deficiency (20). The deficiency may be exacerbated by increased thiamin requirements due to fever, malignancy, increased carbohydrate intake, and TPN. Diuretics may cause a urinary thiamin loss.

Vitamin H (Biotin)

METABOLISM

Biotin is found in liver, kidney, pancreas, eggs, and milk. It is readily absorbed as biotin and biocytin in the gastrointestinal tract. Biocytin is quickly converted into biotin by a biocytinase found in the plasma and red blood cells. Biotin is then taken up by cells stored in the cytosol.

There are nine biotin-dependent enzymes. These enzymes are involved in CO_2 fixation, the synthesis and oxidation of fatty acids, the deamination of some amino acids, and in cholesterol metabolism and storage.

CLINICAL SYNDROMES

Biotin deficiency is rare, but when it occurs, the syndrome is characterized by alopecia totalis and a fine scaly dermatitis.

An inborm error of generalized carboxylase deficiency that is similar has been described and is characterized by vomiting and ketoacidosis at birth and an acrodermatitis at 3 to 6 months of age.

MEASUREMENTS

Although biotin assays are rarely performed, the vitamin can be measured by microbiological techniques and by isotope dilution. Reciprocal assay techniques, ELISA, and a chemiluminescence assay have recently been described (22, 23).

Choline

METABOLISM

Although the body can synthesize choline from methionine and serine, it cannot synthesize enough for its basic needs. Choline is a source of labile methyl groups in several biological reactions in the body and is involved in the detoxification of certain toxins, the synthesis of phospholipids, lecithins, sphingomyelins, and acetylcholine. It is also involved in lipid transport from the liver.

CLINICAL SYNDROMES

Choline deficiency is rare (24). The condition is associated with fatty infiltration of the liver and is seen in alcoholics and persons with kwashiorkor.

TRACE ELEMENTS

Trace elements are elemental substances that collectively constitute less than 1% of the total body mass. Many of the trace elements are found in the transition metal series of the periodic table. They are capable of forming complex bonding arrangements with large organic molecules and are often found as a component of metallo-enzymes. Many trace elements, like vitamins, are essential nutrients.

Sampling and Analysis

Because the concentrations of many trace elements in the general laboratory environment greatly exceed those in a serum or urine specimen, extreme care is required when collecting specimens for trace element analysis. Specially designed vacutainers and syringes that have been acid-washed and specially cleaned are available for trace metal collections.

Various analytical methods are now available for the measurement of trace elements. Essential to all methods is the need for extreme cleanliness of glassware and purity of reagents. Glassware must be cleaned in dilute nitric acid and thoroughly rinsed with purified water (ACS type I). The laboratory area for trace metal analysis should be isolated from the main clinical laboratory for better control of the environment.

Atomic absorption spectrophotometry is the most popular method for the measurement of trace metals, since a number of metals can be assayed in various clinical fluids (25, 26). The use of flameless (electrothermal) techniques is required in most instances for adequate sensitivity.

Emission spectrometry, neutron activation, mass spectrometry, and x-ray fluorescence spectrometry are applicable in principle, but require expensive apparatus and expertise not usually warranted in a clinical laboratory. Colorimetry is useful in some cases, and anodic stripping voltametry has some limited applications (27, 28).

Clinical Relevance of Trace Element Measurements

Interpretation of trace element values can be difficult because these substances are stored in various parts of the body, and the serum or urine level may be a poor reflection of these stores. It is important, therefore, to select the most appropriate body fluid for measurement.

The trace substances may be divided into those that are required for nutritional well-being (essential) and those that are nonessential (28). Proving that a substance is essential is a complex problem, but it usually involves (*a*) finding a definite level in most humans, (*b*) finding a metallic protein of which it is an intrinsic part, and (*c*) finding a deficiency state that can be regularly reproduced by withholding the substance.

Trace metals can be toxic when present in excessive amounts. These situations are rare, but high levels of trace metals are occasionally observed in water and food or with industrial exposures and may result in toxicity (28).

There are numerous claims for the correlation between trace metal abnormalities and a variety of disorders. Most of these are unproven. Charlatans abound who would lead us to believe that replacement of certain metals will result in curing virtually every disorder that has plagued mankind. Such claims must always be considered with great skepticism until they have been confirmed by several independent investigators.

Hair Analysis

The analysis of metals in hair has been frequently performed. Hair analysis is appealing because the samples are easier to collect than blood (especially when surveying large populations or the deceased), are easier to transport and store, and may provide a better reflection of cellular metal burden. Some metals may concentrate selectively in hair, and, as the hair grows, the levels may change at different points along the hair shaft, reflecting changes in the metal burden over time. However, there are a number of problems with hair sampling (29).

External contamination of the hair is the most significant problem. Pollutants, industrial fumes, shampoos, sprays, bleaches, and dyes may bind permanently to the hair. Some of these contain metals that will invalidate assay results, and attempts to remove these agents can alter the true elemental content of the hair. For this reason, a standardized washing technique should be employed.

Sample selection is also a problem. The concentration of metals varies in hairs from different sites, and the level can change as the hair grows. Hair analysis is more difficult than the analysis of body fluids because it requires destruction of a solid matrix.

The interpretation of hair metal analysis is fraught with difficulty. There are no widely accepted normal values. Age, sex, and hair color differences have not been defined, and the correlation between hair metal concentrations and the levels in other organs has not been established.

In conclusion, there are insufficient data to support the use of hair samples in clinical medicine, and caution is advised in using the results of hair metal analysis.

Table 21.2. Essential Trace Metals

Metal	Clinical Syndromes
Iron	Deficiency: anemia Excess: hemosiderosis (excess iron intake), Hemochromatosis (excess absorption) Acute intoxication
Cobalt	Deficiency: not known for elemental cobalt Excess: beer drinker's cardiomyopathy
Copper	Deficiency: scorbutic joints, hematologic abnormalities, CNS damage, Menke's kinky hair syndrome Excess: Wilson's disease Acute copper toxicity
Manganese	Deficiency: one case Excess: basal ganglion disturbance
Molybdenum	Deficiency: not well recognized Excess: not well recognized
Zinc	Deficiency: juvenile dwarfism, hypogeusia, delayed wound healing, night blindness, acrodermatitis enteropathica Excess: acute pulmonary syndrome
Chromium	Deficiency: atherosclerosis, impaired glucose tolerance
Selenium	Deficiency: Keshan disease Muscular dystrophy-like disorder in animals Excess: garlic breath, teratogenic, hepatotoxic, neurotoxic, carcinogenic
Nickel	Deficiency: experimental animal evidence only Excess: carcinogenic as organometal compound
Vanadium	Deficiency: experimental only

ESSENTIAL TRACE METALS (see Table 21.2)

Iron

METABOLISM

Iron is an essential component of hemoglobin, myoglobin, and cytochromes.

Iron is absorbed in the gastrointestinal tract in the ferrous (Fe^{2+}) form. Stomach acid interacts with ligands (such as fructose, ascorbic acid, and citric acid) and gastroferrin from the stomach mucosa to form complexes that maintain the solubility of iron in the alkaline fluid of the duodenum. In a similar manner, phytates and phosphates may bind iron and impair its absorption.

Ferrous iron combines with apoferritin (MW 450,000) in the cells of the intestinal epithelium to form ferritin. If iron is needed in the body, it enters the serum through mass action from the mucosal cells. If iron is not required, it stays within the epi-

Table 21.3. Variations of Tests of Iron Metabolism in Disease

Test	Iron Deficiency	Anemia of Chronic Disease	Renal Rheumatoid Failure Disease	Acute Toxicity	Hemochromatosis
Serum iron	– –	+ +	– –	+ + +	+ + +
TIBC	+ +	N	N	N	N
% Saturation	– –	+	+	+ +	+ + +
Ferritin	– – –	–	N or +	N	+ + +

thelial cells, where it is eventually shed into the GI lumen.

The human body is in precarious iron balance. The requirement for men is 1 mg/day. In women the requirement is larger (2 mg/day) due to menstrual losses. In pregnant females 4 mg/day is required. Most iron is recycled within the body, but there is an obligate loss of 0.1 mg/day in the urine, 0.2 mg/day by skin desquamation, and 0.7 mg/day by gastrointestinal losses.

Circulating iron exists in equilibrium with iron in all body tissues. Therefore, the level of serum iron correlates with the amount of iron in body tissues.

Iron is transported in the blood loosely bound to a specific binding protein called transferrin (siderophilin). Thirty to forty percent of the sites on transferrin are normally occupied by iron. Iron is delivered to the bone marrow, where it is stored as ferritin.

The measurements of iron carried out in the clinical laboratory reflect this protein binding. Total serum iron (SI) measurements quantify the iron bound to transferrin plus the small additional amount (1%) that is present as a free ion, complexed to other ions, or bound to albumin. The total iron binding capacity (TIBC) is a measure of the total amount of iron that the serum is capable of binding. TIBC correlates with the amount of transferrin present. The product SI/TIBC × 100 is the percent saturation. It is usually computed to define the relationship between these two measures. The measurement of ferritin is now favored as providing the best correlation with iron stores (except when the iron stores are affected by inflammation or increased cell production).

CLINICAL SYNDROMES

Iron deficiency may be due to a dietary deficiency, abnormal absorption, or excessive losses (Table 21.3).

Iron excess syndromes also occur. When iron is present in excess over long time periods, cell and tissue damage may result. One form of iron overload is called hemosiderosis. This condition may result from excessive parenteral administration (by injections or transfusions), chronic or excessive oral iron administration, alcoholic cirrhosis, or cooking with iron pots.

Another cause of iron overload is known as primary hemochromatosis. This disorder is genetically inherited and is characterized by overabsorption of iron from the gastrointestinal tract, leading to widespread accumulation of iron in body tissues. The toxic effect is most pronounced in the liver, the pancreas, and the myocardium. The classic presentation of hemochromatosis includes the trial of hyperpigmentation, hepatic cirrhosis, and secondary diabetes mellitus (bronzed diabetes). The primary treatment is to recognize the situation before damage can occur. Transferrin saturation with iron usually exceeds 80%, and ferritin concentrations will be raised above 200 μg/liter. The administration of 10 mg/kg of desferrioxamine followed by the measurement of iron excretion over the next 24 hours can be used to assess total body burden of iron. Normally, less than 2 mg (35 μmol) of iron is excreted, but in hemochromatosis the amount is often 10 mg (180 μmol) or more.

Cobalt

METABOLISM

The only known role of cobalt in the body is as the metal component of vitamin B_{12}. Cobalt can also substitute for zinc in zinc metal enzymes, but the significance of this is not clear.

Cobalt is readily absorbed in the gastrointestinal tract and is excreted in the urine.

CLINICAL SYNDROMES

There is no known deficiency state of elemental cobalt.

Excess amounts of cobalt are nontoxic, since the metal is easily excreted in the urine. However, cobalt was once used as a foam stabilizer in beer production, which caused a form of cardiomyopathy known as "beer drinker's cardiomyopathy." The toxicity was determined to be due to the combination of the cobalt-organic compound and ethanol. Chronic ingestion of large amounts of cobalt have been reported to cause polycythemia, pericardial effusions, thyroid hyperplasia, and a variety of neurological abnormalities.

MEASUREMENT

Cobalt can be measured by atomic absorption spectrometry, flameless atomic absorption spectrometry, and neutron-activation analyses. These assays are difficult to perform, and there is no demonstrated clinical application for these measurements.

Copper

METABOLISM

Copper is an intrinsic part of a number of metal enzymes that catalyze oxidation-reduction reactions. Copper is readily absorbed from the small intestine by a mechanism shared with zinc. Accordingly, there is a reciprocal relationship between zinc and copper absorption. The metal is bound in the intestinal epithelium to a binding protein and is then transported to the liver by albumin. Copper is rapidly cleared from the blood. Within 2 hours, 60 to 95% of the absorbed copper is deposited in the liver. Within the hepatocyte, copper is trapped by incorporation into proteins. Some of the copper is incorporated into ceruloplasmin. The remainder is excreted into the bile (30).

Copper is found in cytochrome C oxidase, lysyl oxidase (required in collagen elastin formation), tyrosinase, superoxide dismutase, erythrocuprein, dopramine-β-hydroxylase, and uricase.

CLINICAL SYNDROMES

Dietary copper deficiency has been reported in premature infants and in persons undergoing parenteral nutrition (30). It produces a syndrome of neutropenia, scorbutic joint changes (characterized by swollen joints that result from inadequate connective tissue formation like that of scurvy), and anemia. The anemia is partially explained by the fact that copper is required to incorporate iron into heme. In severe cases, there is a central nervous system disorder characterized by spinal demyelination, low brain catecholamines, hypotonia, psychomotor retardation, and decreased visual acuity. Depigmentation of the skin may occur due to inactivation of tyrosinase.

Low serum copper is also found in two syndromes that are not associated with generalized copper deficiency (30).

In Wilson's disease (hepatolenticular degeneration), an autosomal recessive disorder, there is a defective incorporation of copper into ceruloplasmin and a failure to excrete copper into the bile. The result is an accumulation of copper in various tissues, including the cornea, brain, liver, and renal tubules.

Menke's kinky hair syndrome (trichopoliodystrophy) is a sex-linked, recessive disorder in which there is an inability to absorb copper or metabolize the copper intracellulary. The syndrome is characterized by retarded growth development, pili torti (kinky hair), arterial tortuosity, scorbutic bone changes, and cerebral degeneration. The serum copper and ceruloplasmin are both low and hepatic, and hair copper concentrations are very low. Copper therapy does not cure this disease.

Ceruloplasmin is an acute phase reactant and will be increased in a variety of conditions. In these situations the increase in ceruloplasmin will result in an apparent increase in serum copper.

Acute copper toxicity has been reported in hemodialysis patients, various industrial workers, and in persons who have ingested copper salts. The most serious consequence is an acute hemolytic anemia.

MEASUREMENT

Copper measurement can be performed using atomic absorption spectrometry of either serum or urine.

The superoxide dismutase activity in red blood cells is a promising assay to assess body copper status.

Manganese

METABOLISM

Manganese is an essential cofactor in a large number of biochemical processes. Manganese is absorbed through the small intestine and is excreted in the bile. Very little is known concerning its absorption and homeostatic control.

CLINICAL SYNDROMES

A deficiency syndrome consisting of impaired growth, skeletal abnormalities, decreased reproductive function, and ataxia has been described in one isolated report. Overdosages of manganese have been demonstrated with manganese-dust inhalation and are associated with basal ganglion impairment.

MEASUREMENT

Atomic absorption spectrometry may be used to measure manganese. Other possible techniques include colorimetry, neutron activation analysis, and emission spectrometry (31). Recently, the assay of manganese in lymphocytes has been suggested as a means of evaluating body burden (32).

Molybdenum

METABOLISM

Molybdenum is an essential element but its metabolism is not well understood (33). It is absorbed in the gastrointestinal tract and excreted in both the urine and bile.

Molybdenum is a component of three enzymes: xanthine oxidase, aldehyde oxidase and sulfite oxidase.

CLINICAL SYNDROMES

There is no well-recognized molybdenum deficiency syndrome. A combined defect due to an absent molybdenum cofactor has been reported that resulted in a deficiency of sulfite oxidase and xanthine dehydrogenase. This patient (an infant) presented with mental retardation, seizures, bilateral lens dislocation, sulfaturia, and thiosulfaturia.

Chronic molybdenum poisoning is not known. Acute molybdenum intoxication has been said to cause inhibition of ceruloplasmin, cytooxidase, glutaminase, cholinesterase, and sulfite oxidase. Molybdenum may have a protective influence on the dental enamel, but this has not been generally supported.

MEASUREMENTS

There is no generally accepted method for the measurement of molybdenum in biological fluids.

Zinc

METABOLISM

Zinc is an essential cofactor in many enzymes, including carboxypeptidases A and B, carbonic anhydrase, alkaline phosphatase, RNA and DNA polymerase, and alcohol dehydrogenase.

Zinc is obtained from protein sources. The zinc found in vegetables and cereals is not well absorbed because it is complexed to phytates. Absorption is inhibited by the presence of fiber. Zinc is absorbed in the duodenum and jejunum by an active transport mechanism specific for zinc. The metal is then transported in the blood, bound to albumin and α_2-macroglobulin. Zinc is readily eliminated in the urine and bile (34).

Low plasma zinc concentrations may occur in liver and lung disease, myocardial infarction, uremia, malnutrition, increased catabolic states, some cancers, pernicious anemia, leukemia, pregnancy, and steroid therapy.

Cadmium and mercury compete with zinc for intestinal absorption. Therefore, zinc therapy offers some protection against cadmium toxicity.

CLINICAL SYNDROMES

There are several distinct syndromes associated with zinc deficiency (35, 36).

Juvenile zinc deficiency was reported over 20 years ago, in Egypt and Iran. In this syndrome a low dietary zinc combined with chelation of zinc by dietary phytic acid and chronic gastrointestinal loss (due to intestinal parasitism) caused a serious zinc deficiency. A group of boys suffering from this condition exhibited dwarfism and delayed sexual maturation.

Zinc deficiency may also be caused by severe burns, total parenteral nutrition, and penicillamine therapy (due to chelation and excretion of zinc).

Zinc deficiency causes hypogeusia (impaired taste) and delayed wound healing (particularly of ischemic ulcers and decubitus ulcers), and may contribute to night blindness.

Another syndrome of zinc deficiency is known as acrodermatitis enteropathica or Danbolt's disease. This lethal condition may be caused by a deficiency of body zinc. It is an autosomal recessive disorder characterized by progressive bullous, pustular skin lesions.

Maternal zinc deficiency has been associated with congenital abnormalities in fetuses, but this remains controversial.

Zinc is involved in the immune system. Animal studies have demonstrated that immune deficiency can be caused by zinc deficiency and then reversed by zinc repletion. Curiously, excessive zinc (20 times dietary) can also suppress the immune system.

ZINC TOXICITY

Zinc toxicity has resulted from zinc ingestion by children chewing on toys. An acute pulmonary syndrome may occur on exposure to high zinc levels. A single-dose poisoning may cause necrosis and atrophy of the testes. Zinc salts are soluble and are not known to be toxic.

Zinc is increased in a variety of acute-phase reactions and in hypothermia; however, the most common cause of apparently elevated zinc levels in serum and urine is contamination of the specimen.

MEASUREMENT

Zinc can be measured using atomic absorption spectrometry. However, plasma or serum levels correlate only roughly to total body zinc concentrations; consequently there is no satisfactory test to evaluate body zinc status.

It is very important to avoid hemolysis when separating serum or plasma since carbonic anhydrase is concentrated in red cells, making the red cell zinc concentration very high in comparison to serum.

Chromium

METABOLISM

Chromium is important in glucose and lipid metabolism (37). It is absorbed in the upper small intestine. In the bloodstream the metal is bound to a β-globulin (possibly transferrin) and to a protein known as glucose tolerance factor (GTF).

Chromium affects glucose tolerance in type II diabetics by facilitating insulin release and promoting tissue binding. This action has been attributed to a low–molecular weight complex containing chromium (III), which is found in brewer's yeast. This "glucose tolerance factor" binds to insulin and enhances its activity.

Chromium also has a role in stimulating fatty acid and cholesterol synthesis.

CLINICAL SYNDROMES

Chromium deficiency may play a role in the pathogenesis of atherosclerosis. Chronic deficiency of chromium impairs glucose tolerance and is associated with accelerated progression of aortic atheromas. Chromium deficiency has also been linked to growth retardation.

Two cases of TPN-induced chromium deficiency have been reported. These instances were accompanied by weight loss, decreased glucose tolerance, and the onset of peripheral neuropathy.

There may be an increased requirement for chromium during times of stress.

The threshold for toxicity of trivalent chromium (Cr III) is very low. Chromium IV is even more toxic. This form is involved in occupational exposure, which is prevalent in the electroplating, photographic processing, and steel making industries. Chronic exposure may lead to GI disorders, hepatitis, lung cancer, and dermatitis. Treatment for chromium toxicity is usually supportive, but BAL (dimercaprol, a chelating agent) may be administered in some situations.

The best method for diagnosing chromium deficiency is to demonstrate improvement in glucose tolerance after chromium supplementation. A modified glucose tolerance test is used in which fasting, 30-, 60-, 90-, and 120-minute samples are measured and the area under the resulting glucose curve is calculated using the formula shown below:

$$\text{Area} = (\text{fasting}/2) + (30\ \text{min}) + (60\ \text{min}) + (90\ \text{min}) + (120\ \text{min}/2)$$

MEASUREMENT

The measurement of chromium is extremely difficult, and there are no reliable methods that reflect body chromium content. The normal range for serum chromium has been reported to be between 0.03 ng/ml and 18 ng/ml. Urinary chromium can be used as a measure of chromium overexposure.

Selenium

METABOLISM

The common source of selenium is seafood and organ meats. Cereals are also an important source. Selenium is the least abundant and potentially the most toxic of all the essential elements (38).

Selenium is absorbed from the gastrointestinal tract and readily excreted into the urine. The site and mechanism of its absorption are not well known. The metal is preferentially carried in red blood cells, but there is also nonspecific, loose binding to plasma proteins.

Selenium is part of the erythrocyte enzyme glutathione peroxidase (39). This enzyme contains four atoms of selenium per molecule. The purpose of the enzyme is to break down peroxides, thereby preventing oxidative damage in red blood cells. For example, the enzyme prevents the peroxidation of hemoglobin and red blood cell membranes. The enzyme may be nutritionally important when vitamin E is low, since the body needs this compensatory increase of another antioxidant.

In white blood cells glutathione peroxidase provides protection from peroxides generated during the oxidative destructive actions of the leukocytes.

In the liver, lipid hydroperoxides are destroyed, as are a variety of unusual toxins.

CLINICAL SYNDROMES

A deficiency of selenium in animals leads to hepatic necrosis, retarded growth, muscular degeneration, and infertility.

Keshan disease has been described in China, in which selenium deficiency leads to a form of dilated cardiomyopathy in children.

Selenium deficiency in patients undergoing long-term TPN therapy has been associated with myalgia. Decreased selenium is known to increase platelet aggregation.

Selenium deficiency causes a muscular dystrophy–like syndrome in sheep and cattle, pancreatic insufficiency in poultry, and liver necrosis in rats. For this reason selenium is added to chicken and turkey feed.

The most highly publicized consequence of selenium deficiency is its possible association with cancer and the suggestion that selenium supplementation may reduce the chance of developing a malignancy. There is currently no evidence to support this claim.

The safe dietary intake of selenium is between 50 and 200 μg/day. Many of the so-called anticancer supplementation diets exceed this amount and, ironically, may increase the risk of developing a malignancy.

Selenium toxicity syndromes are well recognized. The most characteristic clinical feature is a garlic odor of the breath due to pulmonary excretion of dimethyl selenide.

Selenium is known to be teratogenic, hepatoxic, and neurotoxic.

The metal is known to accumulate in plants, which, if eaten by animals, may cause a dramatic overdosage with a bizarre syndrome known as the blind staggers (or alkali disease in cattle).

Selenium administration in high quantities is carcinogenic in animals, but there has never been any link between selenium and malignancy in humans.

MEASUREMENT

The direct measurement of selenium may be accomplished using neutron activation analysis, spectrofluorometry, or atomic absorption spectrometry. Selenium forms covalent organic compounds and therefore can be underestimated if these compounds are not analyzed in these techniques. For this reason the best approach is atomic absorption spectrometry employing a hydride generation method.

Selenium in 24-hour urine samples gives an indication of excessive exposure. The body burden of selenium may be approximated by a combination of fluid estimations and by measurement of glutathione peroxidase activity in red cells (this is only valid at low levels).

Nickel

METABOLISM

The role of nickel is not well established. There is some evidence that it is essential. Nickel is poorly absorbed through the gastrointestinal tract. The metal is transported loosely bound to albumin and is incorporated into α_2-macroglobulin (nickeloplasmin). It is readily excreted by the kidney (40).

CLINICAL SYNDROMES

Nickel in the serum is increased following myocardial infarction, cerebral vascular accidents, and burns. It is decreased in cirrhosis and uremia. The reason for the decrease in the latter two conditions is due to a reduction in albumin binding.

Both serum and urine nickel concentrations reflect environmental exposure to the metal.

Nickel, when linked to organic compounds, is known to be carcinogenic. This is particularly true of nickel carbonyl ($Ni(CO)_4$), which is a biproduct of the Mond nickel refining technique. Acute exposure to nickel carbonyl may cause a fatal cardiopulmonary syndrome. Chronic exposure is associated with an extraordinarily high incidence of nasopharyngeal carcinoma.

Urinary nickel monitoring of exposed workers is recommended.

MEASUREMENT

The most difficult aspect of nickel measurement is sample collection. Urinary collections must be made in plastic containers which have been thoroughly acid cleaned and extensively washed with distilled, deionized water. Blood collections must be made using plastic syringes and cannulas.

The analysis of nickel in bodily fluids is performed using an atomic absorption technique developed by Sunderman (41). The normal serum level for humans is 26 to 76 nmol/liter.

Vanadium

METABOLISM

Vanadium is probably essential. It probably inhibits the sodium potassium ATPase and thereby modifies the sodium pump. It has a questionable role as an enzyme regulator. It may also play a role in cholesterol and fatty acid metabolism, calcium flux, bone development, and cardiac and renal function. It is poorly absorbed from the gastrointestinal tract.

MEASUREMENT

The measurement of vanadium currently has no clinical value. It has been assayed using neutron activation analysis and flameless atomic absorption spectrometry (42).

NONESSENTIAL TRACE METALS (see Table 21.4)

Aluminum

METABOLISM

There is no demonstrated biological role for aluminum. The average oral intake of this metal is between 10 and 100 mg/day. Only a very small percentage of this is absorbed.

CLINICAL SYNDROMES

Overdosage from aluminum is seen in patients with renal disease taking antacids containing aluminum, persons on TPN, and those undergoing renal dialysis in which aluminum has not been removed from the dialysis fluid (43).

There is a recognized syndrome known as dialysis dementia in which a combination of telangiectases,

Table 21.4. Toxic Effects of the Nonessential Trace Metals

Metal	Toxic Effect
Arsenic	Carcinogenic
	Neuropathic
	Renal cortical necrosis
Cadmium	Metal fume fever
	Acute poisoning
	Increased cardiovascular disease
	Chronic pulmonary fibrosis
	Proximal kidney tubular damage
	Itai-Itai
Fluoride	Gastric ulcerations
	Fluorosis
Gold	Bone marrow suppression
	Renal tubular damage
Lead	Anemia, neurological damage, encephalopathy, GI disturbances, porphyria
Mercury	Dementia, neurological damage
	Minamata disease in newborns

myoclonus, dementia, behavioral changes, and dysphagia are seen.

Excessive amounts of aluminum are known to cause osteomalacia, since aluminum blocks the incorporation of calcium into osteoid.

MEASUREMENT

Measurement of aluminum in bodily fluids is performed using atomic absorption spectrometry.

Arsenic

METABOLISM

Exposure to inorganic arsenicals (particularly arsenic trioxide and sulfide) may occur in the smelting of nonferrous ores (copper and gold). There is a higher incidence in this industry of lung cancer and hepatic angiosarcoma, which has been attributed to this exposure.

Fowler's solution (1% potassium arsenite) has been used as a tonic and as a treatment for psoriasis and asthma. The drug was withdrawn in the 1950s but occasionally is still used in nontraditional medications. Fowler's solution been shown to cause skin cancers in long-term users.

Long-term low-dose administration of arsenic causes palmar and plantar keratosis, squamous cell carcinoma, and neuropathy. Low-dose arsenic poisoning may present as a syndrome characterized by an insidious onset of fatigue, generalized muscle weakness, paresthesias, numbness, anorexia, and malaise. The syndrome may be caused by exposure to pesticides and herbicides, in gold refining, in poisoning, or from contaminated water (44, 45).

Acute arsenic poisoning is characterized by renal cortical necrosis and subsequent chronic renal insufficiency.

Arsenic toxicity may result from ingestion of contaminated water. Surface water (particularly when acidic and with a high iron content) promotes the formation of insoluble iron arsenic complexes that precipitate when the water is oxygenated. These precipitates sink to the bottom of deep wells. If the wells become contaminated, they may turn alkaline and thereby change the solubility of the precipitate. This allows the arsenic to be released into the water supply.

MEASUREMENT

Blood measurements of arsenic are of little use except to identify arsenic as the cause of acute toxicities (45). Arsenic is rapidly cleared from the blood, with a half-life of less than 6 hours. It is rapidly excreted into the urine as a methalate derivative. Therefore, urine arsenic levels can be used only as a measure of recent exposure. The recent ingestion of seafood will cause an increase in urinary arsenic and must be considered as a cause of a false-positive elevation. The normal urine arsenic level is less than 50 μg/day. Up to 1.68 mg/liter is seen after a seafood meal.

In the investigation of chronic arsenic poisoning, hair and fingernail analyses may be performed. Hair analysis is useful, provided external contamination of the sample can be eliminated. In forensic analysis it is important to check the concentration of arsenic in the soil around any exhumed body.

Arsenic measurements may be carried out using atomic absorption spectometry.

Gutzeit's test may be used as a screen for excess urinary arsenic. Potassium iodide and stannous chloride reduce pentavalent arsenic (As(V)) to trivalent arsenic (As (III)), which is liberated from the specimen as arsine gas. The liberated gas is trapped and reacted with one of a number of different compounds, including silver diethyldithiocarbomate in pyridine to form a red iodine-potassium iodide solution, or mercuric bromide (filter paper technique).

This latter technique is the basis of a commercial kit in which urine is mixed with zinc and HCl to produce arsine gas. The gas reacts with mercuric bromide impregnating a paper strip. The color change produced is visually compared to a scale.

Methods using GLC and HPLC have also been used.

Cadmium

CLINICAL SYNDROMES

Cadmium is an extremely toxic metal. Its fumes may cause metal fume fever, a syndrome characterized by a restrictive lung disease, which may kill the patients within hours after exposure to hot metal fumes.

Acute cadmium intoxication is characterized by nausea and vomiting, diarrhea, renal failure, and hepatic failure. Long-term exposure to cadmium may cause testicular tumors, renal damage of the proximal tubular type, hypertension, arteriosclerosis, growth retardation, premature aging, and cancer. It is well recognized that high levels of cadmium in the environment are associated with increased cardiovascular mortality in the residents of the affected area.

Chronic industrial exposure to cadmium is associated with chronic pulmonary fibrosis and renal damage (proximal kidney tubule disorders). Exposed workers should be monitored by serial pulmonary function studies, by serial measurement of β_2-microglobulin in the urine to assess proximal kidney integrity, and by cadmium determinations.

In the Jintsu River valley of Japan, the industrial contamination of a river led to soil contamination with cadmium. Women working in the fields irrigated by the river absorbed excessive amounts of cadmium, producing a syndrome of brittle bones known as Itai-Itai or "ouch-ouch" disease.

MEASUREMENT

Measurement of cadmium may be performed on serum or urine using atomic absorption spectrometry.

Fluoride

Fluoride is readily absorbed in the small intestine and excreted by the kidney. Once absorbed, it is taken up by bone and teeth, replacing hydroxyl groups in the apatite crystal of these structures.

Excessive amounts of naturally occurring fluoride in drinking water were once observed to cause mottling of the teeth. However, the persons in these areas did not have any dental cavities. Subsequently, it was determined that adding fluoride in small amounts to drinking water results in a reduction in dental cavities without mottling (41). The same theory has been applied to the treatment of osteoporosis, in which fluoride may promote increased calcification of the bone. This latter therapy is controversial because, while the bones are definitely harder, there may be no reduction in the number of bone fractures.

Massive fluoride overdose causes a syndrome characterized by serious gastric ulcerations.

MEASUREMENT

Fluoride is best measured using a fluoride-sensitive electrode. The normal range for serum is 10 to 370 ng/ml. Values of up to 450 ng/ml are seen in red blood cells. Values of 0.2 to 1.9 mg/liter are seen in urine. It is best to make collections for fluoride measurement in plastic containers, since the silicon in glassware may react with fluoride to form volatile compounds that can be lost during the analysis.

Gold

Gold sodium thiomalate and gold sodium thioglucose have both been employed as a treatment for rheumatoid arthritis. These substances inhibit lysosomal enzymes and thereby reduce inflammation in the joints. There is no correlation between serum or urine measurements of gold and the efficacy of therapy or the onset of toxicity (47). Therefore, measurement of gold is almost never performed.

Gold can cause bone marrow suppression and renal tubular damage. Patients receiving gold therapy should be monitored by measuring platelet count, urinary protein, and serum aspartate aminotransferase.

Lead

The exposure of humans to excessive amounts of lead is a major public health concern. Indeed, the Centers for Disease Control (CDC) state that lead poisoning is one of the most common and preventable pediatric health problems today (48).

Lead interferes with porphyrin syntheses at a number of sites. It inhibits the activity of red blood cell aminolevulinic acid dehydrase, preventing the normal conversion of aminolevulinic acid to porphobilinogen. This causes an increased aminolevulinic acid level in the urine.

Lead also interferes with the incorporation of iron into the tetrapyrrole ring of hemoglobin, allowing replacement of iron by zinc. This causes sideroblastic anemia. Free erythrocyte protoporphyrin levels will rise.

The effect of even low levels of lead on the nervous system, particularly the developing nervous system of children, may be significant. Poisoning by lead will cause anemia, encephalopathy, neuropathy, GI disturbances, and porphyria. Chronic exposure over a long period of time may cause mental deficiency and neurological disease.

Industrial exposure is generally due to the inhalation of automobile exhausts or exposure to lead-containing compounds such as in lead battery refining industries, battery workers, and automobile radiator repair shops (49).

Table 21.5. Centers for Disease Control Recommendations on Lead Poisoning in Children

Class	Blood Lead Concentration µg/dl	µmol/liter	Comment
I	< 10	< 0.5	Not considered to be lead poisoned.
IIA	10–14	0.5–0.7	Many children (or a large proportion of children) with blood lead levels in this range should trigger community-wide childhood lead poisoning prevention activities. Children in this range should be rescreened frequently.
IIB	15–19	0.7–0.97	Child should receive nutritional and educational interventions and more frequent screening. If the blood lead level persists in this range, environmental investigation and intervention should be done.
III	20–44	1–2.1	Child should receive environmental evaluation and remediation and a medical evaluation. Such a child may need pharmacologic treatment of lead poisoning.
IV	45–69	1.2–3.3	The child will need both medical and environmental intervention, including chelation therapy.
V	> 70	> 3.3	The child should be considered a medical emergency. Medical and environmental intervention must begin immediately.

Children are particularly susceptible to lead poisoning and classically are exposed through the ingestion of lead paint.

Whole blood lead levels are between 0 and 20 µg/dl (0 to 1 µmol/liter) in urban populations and less than 10 µg/dl (0.5 µmol/liter) in rural populations that are not exposed to lead in the environment.

Overt toxicity in adults is almost always seen at levels of 100 µg/dl (5 µmol/liter), but seizures and coma can occur in children at 50 µg/dl. Any value over 40 µg/dl (2 µmol/liter) should be considered toxic in adults.

The action level in children has been lowered over the years. By 1985, the recognized level for lead toxicity was considered to be 25 µg/dl (1.2 µmol/liter). In 1991, the CDC published a recommendation that this level be revised downward to 10 µg/dl (0.48 µmol/liter) (48). The CDC recommendations in children are listed in Table 21.5.

MEASUREMENT

Urine measurements must be carried out in a lead-free container (usually a polyethylene bottle that has been acid-washed). The volume of urine excreted is best assessed by weighing the container rather than by pouring the sample into a potentially contaminated measuring vessel.

The collection tube for blood must have a lead-free anticoagulant, and special tubes for this purpose are commercially available. Venipuncture is preferred over capillary sampling because of the potential for contamination during fingerstick sample collection. If capillary sampling is carried out, the guidelines presented in the 1991 CDC recommendations should be followed. Results from capillary samples should always be confirmed using a venipuncture. The measurement of plasma or serum lead has no clinical value. Lead standards and whole blood samples deteriorate due to adsorption onto the wall of glass tubes.

The assay can be carried out using atomic absorption spectrometry or anodic stripping voltametry. Graphite tube flameless atomic absorption methods have been well developed. Whatever method is selected, it must be capable of producing reliable results at the level of 10 µg/dl (0.5 µmol/liter).

Screening for the presence of lead poisoning has been done using erythrocyte protoporphyrin measurements using a specially designed flurometer, but this approach is not sufficiently sensitive to detect lead poisoning at levels less than 25 µg/dl (1.2 µmol/liter).

High-quality lead standards are now available in the United States through the National Institute of Science and Technology (SRM 3121). In addition, a set of whole blood reference materials (SRM 955A, Lead in Blood) may also be obtained.

Mercury

Mercury has no known biological function but is a well-recognized toxin. There are various forms of mercury poisoning (50, 51).

Inorganic mercury salts are not hazardous since the mercury is easily absorbed and excreted through the kidneys.

Liquid mercury will not cause poisoning if ingested; however, liquid mercury is highly toxic because it is easily vaporized and will contaminate the environment. Mercury vapor, if inhaled, passes through the alveoli and diffuses into tissues, notably the CNS, where it causes a form of dementia. One cause of mercury vapor poisoning is clothing contaminated with liquid mercury droplets. When the clothing is ironed, the heat causes instant vaporization and potential toxicity.

The most common cause of serious mercury toxicity is organic mercury compounds. The organic compounds easily cross cell membranes, particularly in the nervous system. Examples of these compounds are phenyl, methoxyethyl, and other alkyl mercury

36. Prasad AS. Clinical, endocrinological and biochemical effects of zinc deficiency. Clin Endocrinol Metab 1985;14:567–589.
37. Anderson RA. Chromium metabolism and its role in disease processes in man. Clin Physiol Biochem 1986;4:31–41.
38. Lockitch G. Selenium: clinical significance and analytical concepts. CRC Crit Rev Clin Lab Sci 1989;27:483–541.
39. Shamberger RJ. Selenium metabolism and function. Clin Physiol Biochem 1986;4:42–49.
40. Sunderman FW Jr, Hopfer SM, Crisostomo MC, Stoeppler M. Rapid analysis of nickel in urine by electrothermal atomic absorption spectrophotometry. Ann Clin Lab Sci 1986;16:219–230.
41. Sunderman FW Jr, Hopfer SM, Sweeney KR, Marcus AH, Most BM, Creason J. Nickel absorption and kinetics in human volunteers. Proc Soc Exp Biol Med 1989;191:5–11.
42. Ishida O, Kihira K, Tsukamoto Y, Marumo F. Improved determination of vanadium in biological fluids by electrothermal atomic absorption spectrometry. Clin Chem 1989;35:127–130.
43. McCarthy JT, Milliner DS, Kurtz SB, Johnson WJ, Moyer TP. Interpretation of serum aluminum values in dialysis patients. Am J Clin Pathol 1986;86:629–636.
44. Hindmarsh JT, McCurdy RF. Clinical and environmental aspects of arsenic toxicity. CRC Crit Rev Clin Lab Sci 1986;23:315–347.
45. Lee-Feldstein A. A comparison of several measures of exposure to arsenic. Matched case-control study of copper smelter workers. Am J Epidemiol 1983;129:112–124.
46. American Academy of Pediatrics Committee on Nutrition. Fluoride supplementation. Pediatrics 1986;77:758–761.
47. Heath MJ, Gillett GT, Swannell AJ, Williams CR, Palmer T. Patterns of gold levels in urine, serum, and saliva in patients with rheumatoid arthritis undergoing therapy. Ann Rheum Dis 1982;16:827–828.
48. Preventing lead poisoning in young children: a statement by the Centers for Disease Control. Washington, DC: US Department of Health and Human Services, October 1991.
49. Rempel D. The lead exposed worker. JAMA 1989;262:532–534.
50. Sunderman FW. Perils of mercury. Ann Clin Lab Sci 1988;18:89–101.
51. Curtis HA, Ferguson SK, Kell RL, Samuel AH. Mercury as a health hazard. Arch Dis Child 1987;62:293–295.

22 Inborn Metabolic Errors

Miriam G. Blitzer and Tina M. Cowan

An inborn error of metabolism is classically defined as a genetic defect in which reduced or absent enzyme function leads to a specific block in a metabolic (usually catabolic) pathway. Such a block can lead to abnormal accumulation of metabolites, often in turn causing disease. Inherited metabolic diseases are typically grouped according to the general type of molecule for which catabolism is altered, such as the aminoacidemias, organic acidemias, or sphingolipidoses. Clinically, most inborn errors of metabolism present with symptoms that could be compatible with more than one category of metabolic disease (e.g., inborn errors of amino acid and organic acid metabolism), or with more than one disease within a single category (e.g., the mucopolysaccharidoses Hunter's and Hurler's syndromes). A patient's presenting symptoms can also be suggestive of a nongenetic disease (e.g., sepsis, Reye's syndrome). Therefore, metabolic disorders must be considered in the differential diagnosis of a variety of conditions. The definitive diagnosis for most of the metabolic disorders comes from the laboratory, usually following either qualitative or quantitative determinations of abnormal metabolites, or, more directly, reduced or absent enzyme activity.

An understanding of the basic clinical and laboratory features of inherited metabolic disorders is essential for the rapid and accurate diagnosis and subsequent management of patients. Treatment of many of the inborn errors is feasible using a variety of approaches, such as dietary restriction of a particular compound or supplementation of a missing cofactor, provided that the specific metabolic block is known. In the absence of diagnosis and treatment, however, recurrent, life-threatening illnesses often result. Even for disorders for which treatment is not feasible, a rapid, accurate diagnosis is a prerequisite for effective genetic counseling, which includes a discussion of the expected prognosis, the recurrence risks, the availability of heterozygote testing, and prenatal diagnosis for future pregnancies.

An important concept to be emphasized in discussions of metabolic disorders is that of heterogeneity. Examples of heterogeneity can be seen at all levels, from clinical and biochemical to molecular. Thus, the same clinical entity (e.g., hepatomegaly) can have a variety of genetic and nongenetic causes; the same biochemical phenotype (e.g., hyperphenylalaninemia) can be caused by several different genetic mutations; and the same molecular phenotype (e.g., deficient activity of the lysosomal enzyme hexosaminidase A) can be caused by one of several mutations within a single gene. With emerging understanding of the contribution of molecular heterogeneity to clinical variability, combined with the powerful tools of DNA technology, the complexities of metabolic disease at the molecular level are now beginning to be unravelled. As a practical consequence, we will eventually be able to give patients and their families more accurate estimates of recurrence risk, prognosis, and optimum management and treatment approaches.

This chapter presents clinical and classic biochemical approaches for the diagnosis and management of patients with inherited metabolic diseases. It is meant not as an exhaustive review, but rather focuses on several disorders as a means of highlighting clinical and laboratory features which help to distinguish between the many metabolic disorders. Although specific laboratory tests and approaches will be discussed, detailed protocols are not given, and the reader is referred to the Suggested Readings at the end of the chapter for descriptions of these methods.

METABOLIC DISORDERS

Disorders of Amino Acid Metabolism

NORMAL AMINO ACID CHEMISTRY AND PHYSIOLOGY

Amino acids, the fundamental building blocks of proteins, are small molecules with a tetrahedral carbon covalently bound to an amino group, a carboxyl group, a variable (R) group, and a hydrogen atom. R groups are classified as either hydrophobic, neutral, acidic, or basic, and determine the unique chemical properties of the individual amino acids. There are 20 commonly occurring amino acids found in proteins, and at least 150 other nonprotein amino acids.

Normal turnover of amino acids occurs through a series of enzymatically controlled steps, the first of which is often a deamination, or removal of the primary amine group, to form the corresponding α-ketoacid. These compounds are metabolized in a step-wise fashion, ultimately entering the tricarboxylic acid (TCA) cycle, leading to the formation of ATP. Several amino acids are intermediates in the urea cycle, the main pathway of ammonia detoxification through the formation of urea. Amino acids are also found as intermediates in the transsulfuration pathway, as well as in pathways involved in the generation and utilization of single carbon units.

Free amino acids normally are found in all body fluids, including plasma, urine, cerebrospinal fluid (CSF), amniotic fluid, semen, sweat, and tears. Normal levels of amino acids depend to a great extent on the age of the individual, as well as nutritional status and overall health. Circulating plasma amino acids are the products of protein catabolism, and are filtered in the kidneys by the renal glomeruli. Specific amino acids are then reabsorbed in the proximal tubules via specialized transport systems, while others are efficiently excreted in the urine. The pattern of urinary amino acid excretion therefore depends largely on the function of transport mechanisms governing tubular reabsorption.

Abnormal concentrations of amino acids in the plasma (aminoacidemias) or urine (aminoacidurias) arise when either the normal degradation or excretion of amino acids is altered.[a] These disorders are classified as either primary or secondary, depending on the nature of the underlying defect.

PRIMARY DISORDERS OF AMINO ACIDS

A primary aminoacidemia results from a mutation in a gene governing the activity of a specific degradative enzyme. The defective enzyme cannot catabolize a particular amino acid, which in turn accumulates. These blocks can also lead to abnormal accumulations of secondary metabolites and to depletions of "downstream" intermediates. Primary aminoacidemias refer solely to metabolic blocks in the first or second step of amino acid catabolism; blocks further downstream, although in the same overall pathway, are classified as organic acidemias and often differ in both clinical presentation and laboratory approach to diagnosis (see below). The vast majority of aminoacidemias follow an autosomal recessive pattern of inheritance.

[a]The distinction between aminoacidemia and aminoaciduria is somewhat arbitrary, since for many disorders abnormal concentrations of amino acids occur in both plasma and urine. The terms are therefore often used interchangeably.

Clincial findings associated with the primary aminioacidopathies range from severe and life-threatening to benign. Examples of the most commonly encountered of these disorders are highlighted below; a summary of common aminoacidemias is presented in Table 22.1.

Hyperphenylalaninemia Syndromes

Hyperphenylalaninemia is a heterogenous group of disorders involving either a complete or partial block in the phenylalanine hydroxylase (PH) enzyme system, which converts phenylalanine to tyrosine. Classic phenylketonuria (PKU) involves a virtual absence of PH activity, while some variant forms demonstrate significantly reduced, but not absent, activity. Other variants result from a block in either the recycling or synthesis of tetrahydrobiopterin, the cofactor necessary for PH activity. Specific diagnosis is made on the basis of phenylalanine and/or cofactor levels in plasma; assay of the PH enzyme, a liver-specific protein, is usually not necessary. An elevation of phenylalanine and its metabolites and/or a deficiency of tyrosine lead to early, irreversible brain damage and impairment of mature brain function. Clinical consequences include mental retardation, microcephaly, seizures, eczema, and a characteristic musty odor. These symptoms are avoided if dietary restriction of phenylalanine is started within the first weeks to months of life and continued throughout the patient's life. Benign forms of hyperphenylalaninemia also exist for which no treatment is necessary. Finally, maternal PKU is seen in children born to women with untreated hyperphenylalaninemia; prenatal exposure to high concentrations of phenylalamine leads to congenital malformations, microcephaly, and mental retardation in patients who themselves have normal levels of phenylalanine.

Hyperphenylalaninemia occurs in approximately 1 of 12,000 live births, and all states in the U.S. offer newborn screening for this disorder to identify asymptomatic infants and to institute therapy, if needed, prior to the onset of symptoms. Accurate prenatal diagnosis of PKU and its variants is now available using DNA analysis and linkage studies in informative families, i.e., families with a sufficient degree of molecular polymorphism to allow the tracking of mutant alleles.

Homocystinuria

Excretion of homocysteine in the urine can have a variety of inherited causes. The most common of these is deficient activity of cystathionine-β-synthase, the vitamin B_6 (pyridoxine) dependent enzyme catalyzing the conversion of homocysteine to

Table 22.1. Primary Disturbances in Amino Acid Metabolism

Disorder	Clinical Findings	Laboratory Findings	Deficient Enzyme
Homocystinuria	Marfanoid features; optic lens dislocation, ± mental retardation, osteoporosis, thromboemboli. Variable responsiveness to pyroxidine (B_6).	↑ Homocyst(e)ine in plasma and urine; ↑ methionine in plasma.	Cystathione-β-synthetase.
	Lethargy, seizures, feeding difficulties, variable responsiveness to folic acid.	↑ Homocyst(e)ine and cystathione, ↓ or normal methionine and methylmalonic acid in plasma and urine.	N^5-methyltetrahydrofolate-homocysteine methyltransferase.
	Mental retardation, seizures, proximal muscle weakness. Variable responsiveness to folic acid.	↑ Homocyst(e)ine in plasma and urine.	$N^{5,10}$-methylene-tetrahydrofolate reductase.
Nonketotic hyperglycinemia	Failure to thrive, seizures (hypsarrhythmia), coma, death in early infancy or childhood.	↑ Glycine in urine, plasma, and CSF; ↑ CSF [gly]/plasma [gly] ratio.	Glycine cleavage system.
Hyperornithinemia (gyrate atrophy of the choroid and retina)	Progressive chorioretinal degeneration, mypopia, night-blindness, loss of peripheral vision in 1st decade, blindness by 3rd or 4th decade.	↑ Ornithine in plasma and urine (and CSF).	Ornithine-δ-aminotransferase.
Hyperphenylalaninemia			
Phenylketonuria	If untreated, profound mental retardation, microcephaly, seizures, musty odor. Treatable by dietary restriction of phenylalanine, supplementation of tyrosine.	↑ Plasma phenylalanine (≥20 mg%); ↓ or normal tyrosine in plasma; ↑ phenylpyruvic and 2-OH phenyl-acetic acids in urine.	Phenylalanine hydroxylase (in liver).
Persistent hyperphenylalaninemia	Normal neurological development; no dietary restriction required.	↑ Plasma phenylalanine (<17 mg%), ↓ or normal tyrosine in plasma.	Phenylalanine hydroxylase (in liver).
Transient mild hyperphenylalaninemia	Clinically benign; seen most often in premature infants.	↑ Plasma phenylalanine in early life (transient).	—
Dihydropteridine reductase deficiency	Seizures, mental retardation, choking, eczema, hypotonia. Not treatable by phenylalanine restriction. Treated with dopamine, 5-OH tryptophan and carbidopa.	↑ Phenylalanine in plasma (>20 mg%). Abnormal biopterin/neopterin ratio in urine.	Dihydropteridine reductase (fibroblasts).
Abnormal dihydrobiopterin function	Pseudobulbar palsies, athetoid movements, abnormal EEG. Treated with dopamine, carbidopa, and 5-OH tryptophan.	↑ Phenylalanine in plasma (>20 mg%); ↓ and abnormal biopterin metabolites in urine; abnormal neopterin/biopterin ratio in urine.	Unknown (dihydrobiopterin synthesis defect?).
Tyrosinemia			
Type I (hereditary or acute tyrosinemia)	Failure to thrive, fever, vomiting, bleeding manifestations, hepatomegaly, hepatic failure, cabbage-like odor. Rapidly progressive, fatal by age 12 months.	↑ Tyrosine in plasma. ↑ Urine organic acid metabolites including 4-OH-phenyllactic and 4-OH-phenylpyruvic acids.	Possible fumarylacetoacetate hydrolase or 4-OH-phenylpyruvate dioxygenase.
Subacute	Renal tubular dysfunction, vitamin D-resistant rickets, anemia, progressive cirrhosis. Onset after age 1 year, death by age 10 years. Treatment by dietary restriction of tyrosine, methionine, phenylalanine.	Same as for acute tyrosinemia.	Same as for acute tyrosinemia.
Type II (Richner-Hanhart syndrome)	Mental retardation, palmar and plantar hyperkeratosis, and keratitis. Attempted therapy with tyrosine/phenylalanine restriction.	↑ Urine organic acid metabolites including 4-OH-phenylacetic, 4-OH-phenyllactic and *N*-acetyl-tyrosine; ↑ tyrosine in plasma.	Tyrosine aminotransferase (in liver).

cystathionine. This block also leads to secondary hypermethioninemia. Some, but not all, of these patients respond to therapy with pyridoxine. Clinical features include dislocation of the optic lens, skeletal abnormalities including osteoporosis, increased tendency for thromboembolic events, and variable metal retardation. Homocystinuria with methylmalonic aciduria and hypomethioninemia is caused by defects in the remethylation of homocysteine to methionine, a reaction dependent on the vitamin B_{12} derivative, methylcobalamin (MeCbl). Remethylation defects can arise from (a) failure in the matabolic conversion of hydroxycobalamin to MeCbl; (b) nutritional or intestinal absorption deficiencies of vitamin B_{12}; or (c) failure to synthesize 5-methyltetrahydrofolate, the cosubstrate in the remethylation reaction (note that methylmalonic aciduria) is not seen in this last group). Clinical findings are highly variable, and range from severe, life-threatening illness presenting in infancy, to neuropathy and thrombocytopenia of juvenile or adult onset. Some, but not all of these patients respond to therapy with vitamin B_{12} or MeCbl.

Nonketotic Hyperglycinemia

Nonketotic hyperglycinemia (NKHG) is a primary disorder of glycine metabolism clinically characterized by neonatal seizures, neurological deterioration, and death in infancy or early childhood. Patients who survive have uncontrollable seizures and are severely mentally retarded. Diagnosis is based on abnormal elevations of glycine in all fluids, particularly cerebrospinal fluid. A ratio of CSF glycine/plasma glycine in the range of 0.2 or above is considered diagnostic (normal ratio less than or equal to 0.02). Because abnormal elevations of glycine are also seen in many of the organic acidurias, a complete workup must include urinary organic acid analysis. Ketones are characterisically absent in NKHG but are often present in the organic acidurias with secondary hyperglycinemia. There is no successful treatment for altering the outcome of NKHG, although various management strategies focusing on lowering glycine levels and controlling the seizures have been attempted. Confirmation of diagnosis by enzyme assay is not routinely performed, but there is a growing research interest in delineating the specific biochemical and molecular defects in patients. Several different prenatal dianostic approaches are currently being offered.

Urea Cycle Defects

The urea cycle is central to the excretion of nitrogen via conversion of ammonia to urea, and is also involved in the synthesis of arginine. The urea cycle defects represent disruptions in the five different enzymatically controlled steps in the pathway (Table 22.2). All are inherited as autosomal recessive disorders except orithine transcarbamylase deficiency, which is X-linked. Although considerable clinical and genetic heterogeneity exists, the typical and most severe presentation occurs at 1 to 3 days of life with progressive lethargy, hypothermia, and apnea accompanied by profound hyperammonemia (often in the range of 600 to 1200 μg/dl). Later-onset forms can include episodes of vomiting, abnormal mental status, and hyperammonemia, as well as developmental delay and poor growth. Patients in this latter group often have enzyme activity that is reduced but not entirely absent. Laboratory studies leading to the diagnosis of a urea cycle defect include plasma and urine amino acids and urine organic acids, including orotic acid. The specific pattern of metabolites that are elevated indicates the point at which the pathway is impaired (see Table 22.2). Confirmation of diagnosis can be performed by enzyme assay, and there is a growing research interest in defining the specific molecular mutations in patients.

Clinically Benign Aminoacidemias

In some cases, abnormal elevations of amino acids do not lead to any predictable pattern of clinical findings, and any symptoms present are only coincidental to, but not caused by, the metabolic disturbance. Such conditions are thought to include histidinemia, sarcosinemia, prolinemia, and hydroxprolinemia. Therefore, caution must be exercised in attributing specific clinical findings to abnormal elevations in amino acids.

SECONDARY DISORDERS OF AMINO ACIDS

Secondary changes in amino acid concentrations result from a physiological disturbance not directly involving the primary metabolic pathways. These include transport and absorption defects (Table 22.3), changes secondary to prematurity, kidney and/or liver failure, starvation, overfeeding, fever, organic acidemia, hyperammonemia, and interference from drugs and their metabolites. Some of these disorders have significant clinical consequences, such as the failure to thrive in lysinuric protein intolerance or renal stones in cystinuria. Other secondary changes in amino acid levels can be indicators of other clinical problems, including generalized aminoaciduria in renal tubular dysfunction and hypertyrosinemia in liver failure. A wide variety of medications can also lead to secondary changes in amino acid profile. Those most commonly encountered include antibiotics, antiseizure medications (e.g., valproate leading to hyperglycinuria) and contrast dyes given for diag-

Table 22.2. Urea Cycle Defects

Disorder/Enzyme Defect	Clinical	Laboratory Findings
Carbamoyl phosphate deficiency	Severe mental retardation, failure to thrive, seizures, vomiting, encephalopathy. Death in infancy.	Hyperammonemia. ↑ plasma glutamine, alanine, glycine, and lysine. Generalized aminoaciduria. Deficient enzyme activity in liver.
Ornithine carbamoyl transferase deficiency	X-linked inheritance. Clinically indistinguishable from carbamoyl phosphate synthetase deficiency. Males die in infancy. Variable expression in females.	Hyperammonemia, ↑ orotic acid in plasma and urine. ↑ plasma glutamine, glycine, and alanine. Deficiency enzyme activity in liver.
Argininosuccinate synthetase deficiency (citrullinemia)	Neonatal form: hypertonicity, vomiting, seizures, mental retardation, and coma. Subacute form: mental retardation and ataxia in older children. Exacerbations with vomiting and encephalopathy.	Hyperammonemia. ↑ citrulline in plasma and urine. ↓ plasma arginine. Deficient enzyme activity in liver, fibroblasts, lymphocytes.
Argininosuccinate lyase deficiency (argininosuccinic aciduria)	Failure to thrive, seizures, coma, mental retardation, and eventually death. In older children, ataxia, trichorrhexis nodosa, and hepatomegaly. Exacerbations with vomiting and encephalopathy.	Hyperammonemia. ↑ argininosuccinic acid in plasma, urine. ↑ plasma glutamine, glycine, alanine, and citrulline. Deficient activity of enzyme in red blood cells, fibroblasts.
Arginase deficiency (argininemia)	Only a few patients described. Mental retardation, spasticity, ataxia, seizures, vomiting, hepatomegaly. Exacerbations with vomiting and encephalopathy.	Moderate hyperammonemia. ↑ CSF, plasma, urine arginine. Orotic aciduria during exacerbations. Deficiency of arginase in red blood cells, leukocytes, and liver.

Table 22.3. Transport Defects Leading to Secondary Aminoaciduria

Disorder	Clinical Findings	Laboratory Findings	Defect
Cystinuria	Nephrolithiasis, kidney complications, mental retardation in some patients.	Marked urinary excretion of cysteine and dibasic amino acids.	Defective transport of cystine dibasic amino acids in renal tubules and intestinal mucosa.
Lysinuric protein intolerance	Failure to thrive, periods of nausea and vomiting, aversion to protein-rich foods.	Increased urinary excretion of lysine, arginine and ornithine; low levels in plasma, intermittent hyperammonemia.	Defective transport of lysine, arginine, and ornithine in intestinal epithelia and renal tubules.
Hartnup disorder	Intermittent and variable, photosensitivity, motor abnormalities, and psychotic behavior. Some patients respond to nicotinamide; others show spontaneous remission.	Characteristic aminoaciduria of the monoamino-monocarboxylic group.	Impaired transport of neutral amino acids by intestinal mucosa and renal tubules.
Lowe's syndrome (oculocerebrorenal syndrome)	Renal tubular damage, congenital cataracts, hypotonia, hyporeflexia and psychomotor retardation. Inherited as X-linked recessive.	Nonspecific aminoaciduria, proteinuria, phosphaturia, renal acidosis.	Metabolic defect unknown.

nostic imaging procedures. Because of the large number of situations that can potentially confound the interpretation of an altered amino acid profile, it is important that the laboratory be made aware of any pertinent clinical information, including relevant physical and routine laboratory findings, drug history, and diet and nutritional status.

LABORATORY INVESTIGATIONS OF AMINOACIDEMIAS

Amino acid analysis should be undertaken in any patient (*a*) who presents with life-threatening illness in the neonatal period, particularly if the illness coincides with the introductiuon of protein into the diet; (*b*) with unexplained mental retardation or developmental delay, particulary if the patient was noted to be neurologically normal early in life and/or if there is a family history of a similarly affected sibling; or (*c*) with unexplained systemic findings that could be compatible with one of the aminoacidopathies. Note that abnormalities in amino acid concentration often depend on protein intake, such that important clues may be missed if the patient was restricted from protein prior to sample collection. It is therefore imperative that specimens be collected prior to altering the diet or giving medication.

The specimens evaluated most frequently are plasma, urine, and, less often, CSF. The analysis of amino acids in newborns and young infants is best accomplished in plasma. Evaluation of newborn urine can be relatively unreliable and uninformative, because the sample is often dilute and contains interfering drug metabolites (e.g., antibiotics given because of a clincial picture resembling sepsis). Furthermore, the immature renal reabsorption systems of premature infants can lead to secondary changes in urinary amino acid profile that can mask a primary abnormality. For older children and adults, analysis of urine is a relatively reliable screening approach, although valuable information is also gained by evaluating plasma. The most appropriate specimen(s) for analysis are also dictated by the clinical presentation of the patient.

Urine Spot Tests

Simple urinary screening tests have been developed for patients suspected of having a metabolic defect. While these tests have the advantage of being rapid and relatively inexpensive to perform, they are limited in both sensitivity and specificity. However, especially when results of several tests are taken together, these "spot tests" can give useful clues that a more extensive metabolic workup may be warranted. The most commonly used spot tests for amino acid disorders include the ferric chloride test for PKU and tyrosinemia, the nitroprusside-cyanide test for cystinuria and homocystinuria, and the silver-nitroprusside test for homocystinuria.

Thin-Layer Chromatography

More precise information about amino acid composition is gained by chromatographic separation of amino acids by thin-layer chromatography (usually on cellulose or silica) in either one or two dimensions. This technique can be applied using either plasma or urine; urine amounts are usually standardized against creatinine concentration. Samples are deproteinized prior to chromatography, typically with acid precipitation, such that only free amino acids are analyzed. Amino acids are visualized with a stain such as ninhydrin, which reacts with primary amine groups of all compounds, including those of amino acids (for this reason, many drugs also give rise to seemingly abnormal bands). The resulting pattern is interpreted by comparing the position and intensity of the bands with the pattern of normal, age-matched controls. This semiquantitative approach to amino acid analysis is useful for detecting relatively large changes in amino acid concentration, such as those resulting from generalized aminoaciduria, hyperglycinuria, or phenylketonuria. Many of the more subtle changes may be missed by this method, and are assessed much more accurately by quantitiative amino acid analysis using liquid column chromatography.

Quantitative Amino Acid Analysis

The most accurate method of assessing amino acid abnormalities is quantitative amino acid analysis. Modern systems are fully automated high-pressure liquid chromatography analyzers. In a typical setup, amino acids are separated on a single ion-exchange column using a gradient of elution buffers of increasing pH and ionic strength, allowed to react with ninhydrin, and then detected spectrophotometrically. The resulting peaks are then integrated, quantitated, and compared with normal, age-matched controls. The entire analysis takes less than 3 hours per specimen, with the most sophisticated systems resolving at least 40 different amino acids. Because of the ease of operation and accuracy of results, some laboratories with automated systems routinely offer quantitative amino acid analysis in lieu of spot tests and thin-layer chromatography.

Disorders of Organic Acid Metabolism

Organic acids are carboxylic acids that contain a variety of functional groups, but do not contain the primary amine group of amino acids. This implies that organic acids will not be stained by ninhydrin, and will therefore not be detected by standard methods of amino acid analysis. Organic acids are metabolic intermediates from a variety of pathways including the metabolism of amino acids, fatty acids, carbohydrates, and steroids. Organic acids are also derived from the diet (e.g., benzoic acid, a common food preservative), a wide variety of drugs, as products of bacterial metabolism in the gut, or as contaminants from plastic urine containers, lotions, or other exogenous sources.

Primary disorders of organic acid metabolism occur as a result of an enzymatic block in a metabolic pathway, leading to the abnormal accumulation of organic acid intermediates in the blood and urine. As with the majority of inborn errors of metabolism, the block can be due to a mutation in a gene either encoding the degradative enzyme itself, or an enzyme involved in the synthesis or utilization of a cofactor required for enzyme activity. There are currently 50 to 60 known disorders of organic acid metabolism and their variants, most following an autosomal recessive mode of inheritance.

ORGANIC ACIDURIAS ARISING FROM BLOCKS IN AMINO ACID METABOLISM

The endpoint of amino acid metabolism is the generation of carbon skeletons and acetyl-CoA, which enter the TCA cycle for reutilization or energy production. Organic acidurias arising from blocks in amino acid metabolism most often involve the degrative pathways of valine, leucine, isoleucine (the branched-chain amino acids) or lysine; the specific pattern of accumulating intermediates gives important diagnostic information in determining which metabolic pathway is affected. Analysis of urinary organic acids is therefore an important step in pinpointing the specific metabolic block. For many disorders, diagnosis is confirmed by demonstrating deficient enzyme activity, most often in peripheral leukocytes or cultured skin fibroblasts. Table 22.4 outlines the more commonly encountered organic acidurias.

Clinical findings tend to be overlapping and nonspecific. The typical course involves acute, life-threatening illness in the neonatal period, with altered mental status (e.g., lethargy, hypotonia, coma), tachypnea, and vomiting. Symptoms are usally not seen until after the first protein feeding. Less severe forms include failure to thrive and vomiting beginning during the first year of life, progressive psychomotor delay, and episodes of ketoacidosis and neurological deterioration exacerbated by infection, immunization, or other metabolic stress. Finally, some patients may experience onset of symptoms only after the first year of life, with episodes of ketoacidosis and neurological deterioration following a minor infection, often accompanied by lethargy, seizures, or coma. Organic acidurias may also be accompanied by unusual odors caused by accumulation of organic compounds. Because of the nonspecific clinical findings, a definitive diagnosis can be made only through evaluation of urinary organic acid profile, most often with gas chromatography and mass spectrometry.

The accumulation of abnormal organic acid metabolites and their coenzyme A derivatives also leads to secondary laboratory findings, giving strong indications that an underlying organic aciduria is present. These include metabolic acidosis (including ketosis and lactic acidosis), hypoglycemia, hyperglycinuria, hyperammonemia, and carnitine deficiency. Abnormal metabolites are often present only during acute illness, and levels frequently return to normal between episodes.

Maple Syrup Urine Disease

Maple syrup urine disease (MSUD), or branched-chain ketoacidosis, is a heterogenous group of disorders resulting from defects in branched-chain α-ketoacid dehydrogenase. This multienzyme complex is common to the catabolic pathways of the branched-chain α-keto acids (BCKA) derived from valine, leucine, and isoleucine. The classic MSUD phenotype occurs in neonates or young infants, and includes sudden apnea, poor feeding, lethargy, profound ketoacidosis, and coma, possibly leading to death. The urine often has a sweet smell resembling maple syrup. Intermediate, intermittent and thiamine-dependent forms of branched chain ketoacidosis also exist with variable onset and outcomes; clinical heterogeneity may be a reflection of molecular heterogeneity. The abnormal accumulation of BCKA in MSUD leads to secondary elevations of branched chain amino acids, which are readily detectable in plasmas by amino acid analysis; a characteristic, abnormal pattern of urinary organic acid excretion is also seen. Alloisoleucine, a transamination product of the ketoacid of isoleucine can be identified by amino acid analysis and is essentially pathognomonic for MSUD. Treatment of classic MSUD is accomplished by dietary restriction of the branched-chain amino acids. Confirmation of diagnosis by assay of enzyme activity can be performed.

Isovaleric Acidemia

Isovaleric acidemia results from a deficiency in isovaleryl-CoA dehydrogenase, the enzyme that converts isovaleryl-CoA to 3-methylcrotonyl-CoA in the degradative pathway of leucine. Roughly half of patients have the neonatal form of this disorder, similar in presentation to neonatal MSUD, with acute episodes of severe metabolic acidosis and ketosis, vomiting, and coma often leading to death. A chronic intermittent form also exists, with acidotic episodes often involving neutropenia, thrombocytopenia, or pancytopenia. An abnormal "sweaty feet" odor is often present during acute episodes. The major abnormal urinary organic acid detected by gas chromatography is the glycine conjugate of isovaleric acid, isovalerylglycine; diagnosis is confirmed by demonstration of absent or severely reduced activity of isovaleryl-CoA dehydrogenase in cultured fibroblasts. Normal growth and development can be seen in patients treated with moderate protein restriction, and carnitine and glycine supplementation.

Other Organic Acidurias from Altered Amino Acid Metabolism

A variety of other organic acidurias are clinically indistinguishable from MSUD or isovaleric acidemia and are differentiated solely by organic acid profile. These include propionic aciduria, methylmalonic aciduria and glutaric aciduria type I (see Table 22.4).

Table 22.4. Organic Acidurias

Disorder	Clinical Findings	Laboratory Findings	Defect
Disorders of leucine metabolism			
Isovaleric acidemia	Neonatal presentation: poor feeding, vomiting, ketoacidosis, coma, "sweaty feet" odor. Chronic course: exacerbations with encephalopathy, mental retardation.	Severe acidosis, with ↑ blood lactate and pyruvate. ↑ Urine isovalerylglycine and 3-hydroxyisovaleric acid; pancytopenia.	Isovaleryl-CoA dehydrogenase.
3-Hydroxy-3-methyl-glutaric acidemia	Hepatomegaly. Exacerbations with a Reye's syndrome-like presentation.	Acidosis, profound nonketotic hypoglycemia. No ketonuria. ↑ Urine 3-hydroxy-3-methylglutaconic acid.	3-hydroxy-3-methyl-glutaryl-CoA lyase.
3-Methylcrotonyl-glycinemia	Failure to thrive, erythematous rash, alopecia, developmental delay, hypotonia. "Cat's urine" odor.	↑ Urine 3-hydroxy-isovaleric acid and 3-methylcrotonylglycine.	3-methyl-crotonyl-CoA-carboxylase.
Disorders of isoleucine and valine metabolism			
2-Methyl-3-hydroxybutyric acidemia	Failure to thrive, encephalopathy, mental retardation.	Ketoacidosis, variable hyperammonemia. ↑ Urine 2-methyl-3-hydroxybutyric acid; frequently also ↑ methylaceto-acetic acid and triglycine.	β-ketothiolase.
Propionic acidemia	Acute presentation with lethargy, vomiting, seizures. Chronic presentation with failure to thrive, mental retardation.	Ketoacidosis, hypoglycemia, hyperglycemia, hyperammonemia, neutropenia. ↑ Urine 3-hydroxypropionic and methylcitric acids.	Propionyl-COA carboxylase.
Methylmalonic acidemia	Mut group: vomiting, hypotonia, failure to thrive. Usually unresponsive to B_{12}.	All groups: acidosis, hypoglycemia, hyperammonemia; ↑ urine methylmalonic acid; frequently ↑ lactic, 3-hydroxybutyric, acetoacetic, 3-hydroxy-n-valeric, 3-keto-n-valeric acids.	Methylmalonyl-CoA mutase.
	CblC and CblD groups: severe CNS dysfunction, megaloblastic anemia.	Groups C & D: Also ↓ serum methionine and ↑ serum and urine cystathionine.	Defective synthesis of both methyl- and adenosylcobalamin
	CblA and CblB groups: vomiting, hypotonia, failure to thrive. Usually responsive to B_{12}.		Defective synthesis of adenosylcobalamin.
Multiple carboxylase deficiency	Skin rash, mental retardation, alopecia, hypotonia, abnormal urinary odor.	Acidosis: ↑ urine β-methylcrotonylglycine and 3-hydroxyisovaleric acids.	Biotinidase or holocarboxylase synthetase.
Maple syrup urine disease (branched-chain ketoaciduria)			
Type I (classic)	Mental retardation, recurrent cerebellar ataxia, feeding difficulty, CNS deterioration, seizures. Maple syrup odor.	Acidosis, hypoglycemia, ketonuria. ↑ Urine 2-oxoisosocaproic, 2-oxo-3-methylvaleric, and 2-oxoisovaleric acids. ↑ Serum and urine branched-chain amino acids.	Branched-chain α-ketoacid dehydrogenase complex.
Type II (intermediate)	Mental retardation, anemia; no obvious ketoacidotic episodes. Variable urine odor.	Acidosis; variable excretion of organic acids as type I.	
Type III (intermittent)	Acute onset of CNS symptoms, including seizures and coma. Precipitated by infection, stress, or protein load.	Acidosis. Variable excretion of organic acids as in type I.	Aminoacidemia and aminoaciduria of branched chain amino acids when symptomatic.
Type IV (thiamine-responsive)	Mental retardation; no obvious ketoacidotic episodes.	Hyperuricemia. Variable excretion of organic acids as in type I.	Aminoacidemia and aminoaciduria of branched chain amino acids.

Table 22.4—*continued*

Disorder	Clinical Findings	Laboratory Findings	Defect
Disorders of lysine and tryptophan metabolism			
2-Ketoadipic acidemia	Varying degrees of metal retardation, metabolic acidosis, and hypotonia.	Acidosis. ↑ Urine 2-ketoadipic and 2-ketoglutaric. 2-aminoadipic acidemia.	Probably deficient activity of 2-oxoadipic acid dehydrogenase.
Glutaric acidemia, type I	Normal early development. Encephalopathy, seizures, and hepatomegaly. Slow, incomplete recovery. Deteriorating course.	Acidosis, hypoglycemia. ↑ Urine glutaric acid, 3-hydroxyglutaric acid, and glutaconic acid.	Deficiency of glutaryl-CoA dehydrogenase.
Glutaric acidemia, type II (multiple acyl-CoA dehydrogenase deficiency)	Hypotonia, poor weight gain, episodic vomiting, polycystic kidneys, and smell of "sweaty feet." Death in early childhood.	Acidosis. Hypoglycemia. Hyperammonemia. ↑ Urine glutaric, 2-hydroxyglutaric, ethylmalonic, and others.	Electron transfer flavoprotein.

Therefore, urinary organic acid analysis by gas chromatography/mass spectrometry is an essential step in diagnosing the individual metabolic defects in patients presenting with symptoms compatible with one of these disorders.

ORGANIC ACIDURIAS ARISING FROM BLOCKS IN FATTY ACID METABOLISM

The endpoint of normal fatty acid β-oxidation is the formation of acetyl-CoA and ketone bodies. Fatty acid oxidation is an important source of energy in heart and skeletal muscle, and occurs in all tissues except brain. Following the entry of fatty acids into the cell, these molecules are activated to their acyl-CoA esters, and subsequently linked to carnitine via the action of carnitine palmitoyl transferase I. Fatty acylcarnitines are then translocated across the inner mitochondrial membrane, where the carnitine is removed and fatty acyl-CoA enters the β-oxidation cycle (carnitine esterification is necessary only for long-chain fatty acids to transverse the mitochondrial membrane, while medium- and short-chain fatty acids enter as free acids without the need for carnitine). Sequential rounds of fatty-acyl CoA dehydrogenation are catalyzed by long-, medium-, and short-chain acyl-CoA dehydrogenases (LCAD, MCAD, and SCAD, respectively). Genetic defects in each of these enzymes have been described, as well as simultaneous blocks in all three enzymes (leading to multiple acyl-CoA dehydrogenase deficiency or glutaric aciduria, type II). Defects in fatty acid oxidation also arise due to systemic carnitine deficiency caused by a variety of genetic factors. Patterns of abnormal fatty acid metabolites seen on urinary organic acid anaylsis give important clues about which enzyme(s) may be defective; definitive diagnosis through enzyme assay in leukocytes or cultured fibroblasts is possible in most cases. Genetic defects in fatty acid metabolism are outlined in Table 22.4.

Medium-Chain Acyl CoA Dehydrogenase Deficiency

Medium-chain acyl CoA dehydrogenase deficiency (MCAD) is an enzyme involved in the oxidation of medium-chain (C_6 to C_8) fatty acids. Its deficiency results clinically in episodes of vomiting and lethargy following a period of fasting or stress, accompanied by profound hypoglycemia and characteristically low ketones. Initial presentation typically occurs within the first 2 years of life and can include hepatomegaly and fatty infiltration of hepatocytes. Patients with MCAD deficiency have been misdiagnosed as having Reye's syndrome or, because the initial presentation may be as extreme as sudden death, sudden infant death syndrome (SIDS). Recent studies have suggested that MCAD deficiency may be a significant contributor to cases of SIDS (see Bennett et al., 1990). Accumulation of medium-chain fatty acids leads to elevated excretion of medium-chain dicarboxylic acids (adipic, suberic, and sebacic acids) in urine, which can be detected by gas chromatography. More detailed studies are also available for the efficient workup of patients. Diagnosis is confirmed by demonstrating decreased MCAD activity in cultured fibroblasts and/or the presence of the specific gene mutation by DNA analysis. Treatment involves maintaining adequate caloric intake with a low-fat, high-carbohydrate diet, and chances for favorable outcome appear to be excellent. Although the exact incidence of this disease is unknown, the frequency of heterozygotes may be as high as 1 in 100.

Systemic L-Carnitine Deficiency

Primary systemic carnitine deficiency results from inherited defects in the active transport of carnitine in the kidney and small intestine, leading to increased urinary loss of carnitine. Secondary deficiencies result from the abnormal accumulation of acyl-CoA compounds, such as those accumulating in many of the organic acidurias involving amino acid or fatty acid metabolism. Acyl-CoA derivatives readily bind to free carnitine to form acylcarnitines, which are efficiently excreted in the urine. This leads to a secondary decrease in circulating free and total carnitine, and an increase in urinary acylcarnitines. Clinical abnormalities associated with carnitine deficiency itself resemble those of Reye's syndrome, including hepatic dysfunction, encephalopathy, hypoglycemia, and hyperammonemia. There may also be signs of muscle dysfunction, including cardiomyopathy. There are no known defects in the synthesis or degradation of carnitine. Treatment of carnitine deficiency is by supplementation with L-carnitine, with the efficacy of various treatment protocols currently under investigation.

LABORATORY INVESTIGATIONS OF ORGANIC ACIDURIAS

Organic acids are effectively excreted by the kidneys and concentrated in the urine. For this reason, organic acids are most accurately measured in urine rather than blood. Patients presenting with clinical indications of an organic aciduria, especially neonates or young infants, should also be evaluated for plasma amino acids, since several of the aminoacidemias can present with similar findings. In addition, plasma and urine caritine levels should be determined. A complete metabolic workup should also include the following routine studies: blood lactate and pyruvate, complete blood count and differential, ammonia, glucose, electrolytes, ketones, and pH, and urine reducing substances and ketones. Because metabolic abnormalities are often not detectable once the patient has been stabilized, it is imperative that all studies be ordered at the time of acute illness, and not after the more likely possibilities (e.g., sepsis, poisoning, starvation) have been ruled out.

Urine Spot Tests

As for the aminoacidemias, a variety of simple spot tests have been developed that can give indications of the presence of an organic aciduria. Although the limitations in sensitivity and specificity of these tests must be recognized, results can provide important clues that a more extensive metabolic workup is warranted. The most commonly used spot tests for the organic acidurias are the dinitrophenylhydrazine (DNPH) test for ketoaciduria, Clinitest (Ames) for urine reducing substances, ferric chloride test for aromatic organic acids, and the methylmalonic acid spot test for methylmalonic aciduria.

Gas Chromatography and Mass Spectrometry

The general procedure for organic acid analysis involves the acidic extraction of urine organic acids, followed by derivitization (alteration of chemical structure such that compounds are suitable for chromatography) and separation by gas chromatography (GC). Creatinine is used as a reference for urine concentration. Extraction of organic acids is typically done using a combination of organic solvents such as ethyl acetate and ether. Oximization, or replacement of the keto groups of α-ketoacids with oxime groups, can be done prior to extraction to decrease artifacts introduced by the solvents.[b] Following extraction, the organic acids are converted to their trimethylsilyl derivatives and separated by GC. The separated organic acids are identified by comparing their retention times with those of known individual organic acids. This semiquantitative method is the one most often employed for routine screening for organic acid disorders.

Any suspected abnormalities detected by GC should be confirmed by mass spectrometry (GC/MS), which provides positive identification of organic acids. Compounds are separated by GC coupled to a mass spectrometer, giving rise to a characteristic mass/charge ratio for each ionizable species. Computer programs then compare the resulting mass spectra to libraries containing mass spectra of known compounds.

Further Studies of Organic Acidurias

Specialized methods have recently been developed for the detailed evaluation of patients suspected of having certain organic acid defects. Fast atom bombardment-mass spectrometry (FAB-MS) is a highly sensitive technique used for the identification and quantitation of urinary acylcarnitines, such as those that accumulate in patients with MCAD deficiency. Alternatively, the stable-isotope dilution measurement of urinary glycine conjugates also identifies compounds accumulating in MCAD deficiency patients, particularly n-hexanoylglycine,

[b]This type of solvent extraction, with or without oximization, favors the extraction of nonvolatile organic acids; extraction of the volatile short-chain compounds (such as pyruvic, propionic and isovaleric acids) is nonquantitative using this approach. Patients with disorders in which volatile acids accumulate also have abnormal elevations of nonvolatile derivatives (e.g., glycine conjugates such as isovalerylglycine in patients with isovaleric acidemia) that are readily detected by standard procedures of solvent extraction. Therefore, although methods for the specific determination of volatile compounds are available, they are for the most part considered unnecessary for the routine screening of organic acids.

3-phenylpropionylglycine and suberylglycine, as well as in patients with other fatty acid oxidation defects. These tests are performed by only a few specialized laboratories throughout the U.S., but are particularly useful in the efficient diagnostic workup of patients with clinical findings suggestive of MCAD deficiency or other defects in fatty acid oxidation.

Disorders of Carbohydrate Metabolism

DISORDERS OF GALACTOSE METABOLISM

Classic Galactosemia

Classic galactosemia is an autosomal recessive disorder caused by deficient activity of galactose-1-phosphate uridyltransferase (transferase), the enzyme responsible for the conversion of galactose-1-P (gal-1-P) and UDP-glucose to UDP-galactose and glucose-1-P. The resulting clinical signs and symptoms usually appear within a few days following milk ingestion, and include failure to thrive, vomiting, diarrhea, and liver dysfunction presenting as jaundice and/or heptomegaly. Cataracts resulting from punctate lesions on the lens nucleus can be present within a few days of life. Galactosuria, generalized aminoaciduria, proteinuria, and hyperchloremic acidosis are commonly present. There is an increased susceptibility to infection, particularly by *E. coli.*, and an increase frequency of death from *E. coli.* sepsis is seen in affected infants. If left untreated, irreversible mental retardation will develop.

Many of the clinical symptoms appear to be reversible and/or avoidable by early diagnosis and dietary restriction of galactose by avoidance of lactose ingestion. Liver abnormalities resolve, weight gain ensues, and the aminoaciduria, proteinuria, and galactosuria decrease. In general, the cataracts will regress, and if not extensive at the outset, do not result in impaired vision. Mental retardation is not severe, but is irreversible. Long-term studies have shown that IQ scores are often somewhat lower in treated patients than in their unaffected siblings. In addition there may be some specific learning disorders involving spatial relationships and mathematics, as well as an increased incidence of attention deficit and behavioral problems, even in patients under strict dietary control. A high incidence of ovarian failure and hypergonadotropic hypogonadism is seen in female patients, including those who have been well managed by dietary therapy; however, pregnancies have occurred in several patients. No abnormalities have been reported in male gonadal tissue.

Because galactosemia is a treatable disease that can be diagnosed prior to the onset of symptoms, many states screen for this disorder in newborn infants using dried blood specimens. Measurement of galactose and/or gal-1-P levels by microbiological assays or transferase activity (by enzyme activity or bacterial inhibition assays) are routinely employed. The suspicion of galactosemia is strengthened by the finding of nonglucose-reducing substances in urine by Clinitest. (Caution must be stressed since many hospital laboratories test only for glucose, such as with the glucose oxidase test [Clinistix], and therefore do not detect elevated galactose.) When abnormal screening results are found, diagnostic tests are performed for quanitative determinations of red cell transferase activity and gal-1-P; absence of enzyme activity accompanied by elevated levels of gal-1-P indicates the need for immediate implementation of dietary therapy.

Transferase Variants

Once screening was implemented on a large scale, numerous infants identified by abnormal screening results were found on follow-up testing to have abnormally low, rather than absent levels of transferase activity. The subsequent workup of these patients has led to the characterization of several variants of the transferase enzyme. Their classification is based on characteristic variations in the electrophoretic migration pattern of the enzyme. Duarte, the most common transferase variant, is identified by two distinct electrophoretic bands that migrate faster than the single band seen in normal individuals. Patients homozygous for the Duarte allele have roughly 50% of normal red cell transferase activity, and Duarte/normal heterozygotes have about 75% normal activity. Patients who carry both the Duarte and classic galactosemia alleles have approximately 25% normal activity, and can present with clinical symptoms resembling classic galatosemia and elevated gal-1-P levels, warranting dietary galactose restriction. Several other, rarer mutant alleles have also been described.

Other Genetic Causes of Elevated Galactose

Galactokinase and UDP-gal-4-epimerase (epimerase) deficiencies are two other inherited enzyme defects in the galactose utilization pathway that can result in elevations of galactose or gal-1-P. Galactokinase deficiency results in the inability to convert galactose to gal-1-P, in turn leading to elevations of galactose and its byproduct galactitol in blood and urine. The clnincal findings of galactokinase deficiency are cataracts and pseudotumor cerebri, both of which can occur very early in infancy. Patients can be identified by the newborn screening tests for classic galactosemia as having elevated galactose but normal transferase activity. Definitive diagnosis is based on demonstration of deficient galactokinase activity in red cells. This disorder occurs much less frequently than classic galactosemia: estimates from newborn screening suggest a frequency of about 1 in 250,000.

Patients with epimerase deficiency can be identified by newborn screening as having elevated red cell gal-1-P but normal transferase activity. Enzyme activity is deficient in red cells and leukocytes but it is thought to be normal in other tissues. This condition is typically clinically benign. Two patients with systemic, rather than isolated red cell, epimerase deficiency have presented with symptoms similar to classic galactosemia.

GLYCOGEN STORAGE DISORDERS

Glycogen, the principal storage form of carbohydrate in animals, is present in virtually all cells in varying concentrations. It is comprised of glucose molecules linked to form a polymeric, highly branched structure. Glycogen is synthesized from glucose via a series of enzymatic steps, and is degraded by a phosphorylase, causing the stepwise cleavage of glucose (yielding glucose-1-phosphate), with other enzymes cleaving the branched linkages.

The glycogen storage disorders (GSDs) are caused by defects in the enzymes involved in glycogen synthesis and degradation. Some present mainly with liver or muscle involvement, while others have a more generalized picture. The hepatic forms are most common and are characterized by growth retardation, hepatomegaly, and fasting hypoglycemia. Other forms primarily affecting muscle usually have no liver involvement, but may present with fatigue and muscle weakness. It is the combination of clinical, biochemical, and pathological findings that must be considered in the differential diagnosis of these diagnosis.

GSD Type I (von Gierke's Disease)

This disorder is caused by deficient activity of glucose-6-phosphatase, a liver enzyme that normally converts glucose-6-phosphate to glucose. This results in severe hypoglycemia and lactic acidosis (with no ketosis), that can be life-threatening. Neonates often present with large livers at birth, which continue to increase in size. There is a protruding abdomen from hepatomegaly (but no splenomegaly), short stature, and a characteristic doll-like facial appearance. There is no neurological involvement. Laboratory findings include hyperuricemia, hypertriglyceridemia, and bleeding tendencies from deficient platelet adhesiveness. Progressive renal dysfunction is a frequent complication in older patients. In the second decade, a high incidence of adenomatous nodules in the liver develop, but cirrhosis does not occur. There are several clinical variants of GSD I, probably with different genetic causes. Since definitive diagnosis by assaying enzyme activity can be done only with a liver biopsy, the diagnosis is usually inferred from functional tests. These include glucagon or epinephrine challenges, as well as glucose or galactose tolerance tests (for details, see Scriver et al., pp. 433–436; Fernandes et al., pp. 70–71). Dietary treatment focuses on preventing hypoglycemia and controlling the lactic acidemia. Management strategies involve frequent feedings along with nocturnal nasogastric infusion of high glucose-containing formula.

GSD Type II (Pompe's Disease)

GSD type II is a lysosomal storage disorder caused by deficient activity of the enzyme α-glucosidase (acid maltase). The infantile form presents during the first few months of life with muscle hypotonia, macroglossia, cardiomegaly, and hypertrophic muscles. The liver is normal in function but progressively increases in size. Hypoglycemia and ketosis are not present. Infants usually die withn the first year of life from cardiac failure. The juvenile or adult forms typically present with delay and/or difficulty in walking, and progress much more slowly than the infantile form. Muscle weakness can develop even in the third or fourth decade, appearing as chronic myopathy. GSD type II is diagnosed by measuring α-glucosidase activity in leukocytes or fibroblasts.

GSD Type III (Limit Dextrinosis or Forbes' Disease)

GSD type III is caused by deficient activity of the debranching enzyme, resulting in the accumulation of limit dextrin, a polysaccharide with short outer branches. The clinical picture is similar to, but milder than, GSD type I, with hepatomegaly as the predominant feature. The clinical and metabolic abnormalities usually decrease at puberty, while muscle and heart involvement may become more pronounced in adulthood. The disorder can be diagnosed by measuring activity of the debrancher enzyme in liver, leukocytes, or fibroblasts. Management is similar to but not as demanding as that for type I GSD.

GSD Type IV (Andersen's Disease)

GSD type IV is a rare disorder in which patients appear normal at birth, but present with hepatosplenomegaly, progressive failure to thrive, hypotonia and muscle atrophy within the first several months of life. Cirrhosis develops, and death occurs usually by the age of 3 years. GSD type IV is caused by deficient activity of the brancher enzyme resulting in the accumulation of structurally abnormal glycogen. The enzyme deficiency can be demonstrated in liver or fibroblasts.

GSD Type V (McArdle's Disease)

GSD type V is caused by complete deficiency of muscle phosphorylase. Characteristically, patients present in their third or fourth decade with muscle cramps following vigorous exercise. Myoglobinuria commonly is seen. Serum creatine kinase can be elevated at rest and increases dramatically following exercise. There is significant clinical and molecular heterogeneity between patients. Diagnosis can be confirmed by demonstrating deficient phosphorylase activity in a muscle biopsy.

GSD Type VI (Hers' Disease)

In contrast to GSD type V, this disorder is caused by a deficiency either in liver phosphorylase or phosphorylase *b* kinase. Both are characterized by significant hepatomegaly in childhood that resolves before puberty, as well as mild hypoglycemia, muscle hypotonia, motor and growth delay. Diagnosis is made by enzyme analysis in liver or leukocytes. Phosphorylase *b* kinase deficiency, unlike all the other GSDs, is inherited in an X-linked recessive manner. Treatment for this disorder is usually not necessary.

GSD Type VII (Tarui's Disease)

GSD type VII is the rarest of the GSDs and the most severe of the muscle glycogenoses. It is caused by a deficiency of muscle phosphofructokinase. Clinically, its presentation is similar to but more severe than GSD type V, with onset usually in childhood. There is an increased reticulocyte count; red cells are affected causing a hemolytic anemia. Diagnosis is made by measuring phosphofructokinase activity in leukocytes or fibroblasts.

DISORDERS OF FRUCTOSE METABOLISM

Fructose is the predominant sugar in honey, vegetables, and fruit, and is a component of the disaccharide sucrose, one of the most common sweeteners in food, medications, and infant formula. Fructose metabolism occurs mainly in the liver, kidney, and small intestine. The clinical consequences of metabolic blocks in fructose metabolism range from life-threatening to benign.

Hereditary Fructose Intolerance

Hereditary fructose intolerance (HFI) is an autosomal recessive disorder that presents with symptoms including failure to thrive, poor eating, vomiting, jaundice and hepatomegaly, hypoglycemia, generalized aminoaciduria, and proteinuria. Symptoms appear only following ingestion of fructose or sucrose and can be so severe as to be life-threatening. Since there is no fructose in breast milk, breast-fed infants with HFI do not experience symptoms until weaning or the introduction of fruits and vegetables into the diet.

HFI is caused by deficient activity of fructose-1,6-biphosphate aldolase (aldolase B), which normally catalyzes the conversion of fructose-1-phosphate to *d*-glyceraldehyde and dihydroxyacetone phosphate. Its absence leads to an abnormal accumulation of fructose-1-phosphate in liver, kidney, and small intestine, resulting in hyperuricemia, lactic acidosis, and hypoglycemia. The diagnosis of HFI is suspected in patients with clinical findings and fructosuria following fructose ingestion. Although enzymatic studies can be performed using liver tissue, the diagnosis is usually made by demonstrating hypoglycemia and hypophosphatemia following an intravenous fructose load. The complete elimination of fructose and sucrose from the diet results in normal physical growth and development. Interestingly, some affected individuals learn to selectively avoid fructose-containing foods.

Fructose-1,6-Biphosphatase Deficiency

Fructose-1,6-biphosphatase catalyzes the conversion of fructose-1,6-biphosphate to fructose-6-phosphate and inorganic phosphate. Because this enzyme plays an important role in gluconeogenesis, its deficiency leads to the accumulation of gluconeogenic precursors once liver glycogen stores are depleted. Symptoms are similar to those seen for many of the organic acidurias, with severe metabolic acidosis, hypotonia, apnea, and hypoglycemia usually appearing within the first week of life. These patients do not develop an aversion to fructose, and there is no renal tubular dysfunction or liver abnormalities, as seen in HFI. Outcome is good with appropriate dietary management.

Essential Fructosuria

This is a benign condition usually identified by elevated reducing substances following routine urinalysis. Essential fructosuria is caused by a deficiency in hepatic fructokinase activity, the enzyme that catalyzes the conversion of fructose to fructose-1-phosphate. No clinical or pathological findings have been reported.

Disorders of Lysosomal Storage

Lysosomes are single-membrane bound, acidic organelles that contain degradative hydrolases involved in the normal turnover of macromolecules.

Lysosomal storage disorders result from deficient activity of a particular lysosomal enzyme or enzymes, leading to the abnormal accumulation of macromolecular substrates and ultimately to clinical pathology. Deficient enzyme activity can be caused by a mutation in a gene encoding the degradative enzyme itself, an activator protein required for proper enzyme function, or a protein involved in the synthesis and processing of the enzyme.

The general clinical course for the lysosomal storage disorders is one of regression. Patients most often appear normal at birth and begin to experience symptoms in late infancy or early childhood (although neonatal-, juvenile- and adult-onset variants of many of these disorders are known). Symptoms can include progressive loss of developmental milestones, psychomotor retardation, and variable visceral involvement, usually leading to early death. The variation in symptoms between the different disorders is explained in part by the different tissue distributions of the various substrates. For example, many of the sphingolipids are components of brain and other nervous tissue; therefore, enzymatic defects in sphingolipid catabolism often lead to mental retardation and other neurological involvement. Significant clinical variability also is seen within the various groups of disorders, and the specific clinical phenotype is, to a large extent, determined by the molecular mutation(s) present in a given patient.

MUCOPOLYSACCHARIDOSES

The mucopolysaccharides are a heterogeneous group of macromolecules predominantly involved in the structural integrity of the extracellular matrix. They consist of unbranched polysaccharide chains containing both acidic and amino sugars and are also referred to as acidic mucopolysaccharides, glycosaminoglycans, or, when linked to protein, proteoglycans. There is varied tissue distribution for the different mucopolysaccharides: keratan sulfate is found predominantly in cartilage, cornea, and intervertebral discs; dermatan sulfate is found in heart, blood vessels and skin; and heparan sulfate is a component of lung, arteries, and cell surfaces in general.

Mucopolysaccharidoses (MPSs) are disorders resulting from defects in the stepwise degradation of mucopolysaccharides due to enzymatic blocks at various points in the catabolic pathways of keratan, heparan, or dermatan sulfate. Although clinically heterogeneous, the MPSs are generally characterized by a chronic progressive course, organomegaly (including hepatomegaly and splenomegaly), dysostosis multiplex, and coarsening of facial features. Profound mental retardation is seen in types IH, II, and III (Hurler's, Hunter's, and Sanfilippo's syndromes), but normal intelligence is retained in types IS, IV, and VI (Scheie's, Morquio's, and Maroteaux-Lamy syndromes). Morquio's syndrome is also characterized by distinctive skeletal abnormalities arising from abnormal storage of keratan sulfate. Although still considered experimental, treatment of the MPSs has been attempted by enzyme replacement with bone marrow transplant. Results are potentially encouraging, especially for those disorders lacking neurological involvement (refer to Krivit et al., 1990). There are currently 10 different known enzyme deficiencies leading to abnormal mucopolysaccharide storage, including four genetically distinct deficiencies leading to Sanfilippo's syndrome and two leading to Morquio's syndrome. All of the MPSs are inherited in an autosomal recessive manner except Hunter's syndrome, which is X-linked. A list of the MPSs and their subtypes is given in Table 22.5.

Patients characteristically excrete mucopolysaccharides in their urine; the specific pattern gives an indication of the site of the enzymatic defect. The preliminary workup of a patient suspected of having an MPS therefore includes a urinary screening test for abnormal mucopolysaccharides, including thin-layer chromatography (TLC) or electrophoresis to identify the specific macromolecular species. Such screening tests are subject to false-negatives, particularly for Sanfilippo's syndrome; if clinical findings are suggestive of an MPS, further workup is warranted even with negative screening results. Histologic changes include large, empty-appearing vacuoles, inclusions resembling zebra bodies, and metachromatic granules (seen upon staining with a cationic dye such as Alcian blue) that are lysosomes distended by stored material. Definitive diagnosis of a specific disorder is based on the demonstration of deficient enzyme activity in leukocytes or cultured fibroblasts.

Prenatal diagnosis is possible for all of the MPSs by enzyme assay on chorionic villus tissue or cultured aminocytes. Heterozygotes have roughly half of normal enzyme activity, making carrier testing for these disorders feasible. Care must be taken when interpreting results of carrier testing for Hunter's syndrome because of the influence of X chromosome inactivation on enzyme activity.

OLIGOSACCHARIDOSES

Oligosaccharides, or the carbohydrate portion of glycoproteins, consist of 10 to 20 sugar residues with a characteristic branched structure. These molecules play an integral role in determining the specificity of protein structure, function, and antigenicity, and are found throughout the body. The group of disorders known as the oligosaccharidoses arise

Table 22.5. Mucopolysaccharidoses (MPS)

Disorder	Clinical Findings	Laboratory Findings
Hurler's syndrome (MPS I H)	Onset 6–8 months. Severe mental and motor regression, coarse facial features, early corneal clouding, cardiac insufficiency, stiff joints, protuberant abdomen, deafness, dysostosis multiplex. Death usually before age 10.	Urinary excretion of dermatan and heparan sulfate. Deficient activity of α-L-iduronidase in leukocytes and fibroblasts.
Scheie's syndrome (MPS I S)	Milder variant of type IH. Late corneal clouding, stiff joints, and cardiac insufficiency. Normal intelligence. Shortened life expectancy.	Same as type IH.
Hunter's syndrome (MPS II)	Onset in infancy and childhood. Mental deterioration, dwarfing, coarse facial features, progressive deafness, stiff joints, and ivory-colored skin lesions. Mild and severe clinical forms with varying degress of neurological involvement. X-linked inheritance.	Urinary excretion of dermatan and heparan sulfate. Deficient activity of iduronate sulfatase in serum, leukocytes, and fibroblasts.
Sanfilippo's syndrome (MPS III)	Onset in first few years oflife. Progressive mental retardation, severe behavioral disturbances, hirsutism, moderate dwarfing, joint stiffness and moderate hepatosplenomegaly. Four genetically distinct forms, distinguishable by enzyme assay.	Variable urinary excretion of heparan sulfate. Deficient activity of heparan-*N*-sulfatase (type A), α-*N*-acetyl-D-glucosaminidase (type B), acetyl CoA:α-glucosaminide-*N*-acetyltransferase (type C), *N*-acetyl-α-D-glucosaminide-6-sulfatase in leukocytes and fibroblasts. Type B also diagnosed in serum.
Morquio's syndrome A (MPS I V A)	Onset 12–18 months. Severe progressive skeletal changes, cardiovascular changes (aortic regurgitation), progressive deafness, hypoplastic odontoid process, and cervical myelopathy. Usually normal intelligence.	Variable urinary excretion of keratan sulfate. Deficient activity of galactosamine-6-sulfate sulfatase in leukocytes and fibroblasts.
Morquio's syndrome B (MPS I V B)	Onset in childhood. Milder form of Morquio's A. Mild bone changes, corneal clouding, hypoplastic odontoid.	Urinary excretion of keratan sulfate. Deficient activity of acidic-β-galactosidase in leukocytes and fibroblasts. Indistinguishable from GM_1 gangliosidosis when evaluated using synthetic substrate.
Maroteaux-Lamy syndrome (MPS VI)	Onset 2–3 years. Growth retardation, coarse facial features, corneal clouding, dysostosis multiplex, and cardiac failure. Mild, moderate, and severe clinical forms.	Urinary excretion of dermatan sulfate. Deficient activity of arylsulfataste B (*N*-acetylgalactosamine-4-sulfatase) in leukocytes and fibroblasts.
MPS VII	Onset in infancy and childhood. Coarse facies ± mental retardation, hepatosplenomegaly, and dysostosis multiplex.	Urinary excretion of dermatan and heparan sulfate. Deficient activity of β-glucuronidase in leukocytes and fibroblasts.

from enzymatic defects in the stepwise degradation of N-linked oligosaccharides. This degradation normally occurs by the action of (*a*) a series of exoglycosidases acting in sequential fashion at the nonreducing termini; and (*b*) aspartylglycosaminidase, which cleaves the bond between asparagine and the adjacent sugar, *N*-acetylglucosamine. Defects in each of the degradative steps are known, and are summarized in Table 22.6. All oligosaccharide storage disorders follow an autosomal recessive pattern of inheritance.

Clinically, the oligosaccharidoses are similar to the MPSs, with a chronic progressive course, often following a period of normal growth and development. Specific findings can include mental retardation, facial coarsening, hepatosplenomegaly, cataracts or corneal opacities, and hearing loss. There are clinical subtypes for each of the oligosaccharidoses, representing a broad range of variability in both age of onset and severity of symptoms, and probably resulting from specific molecular mutations.

Abnormal urinary oligosaccharide excretion is seen in patients with oligosaccharidosis, as well as in some patients with mucolipidosis, sphingolipidosis, or glycogen storage disease. The diagnostic approach for patients suspected of having an oligosaccharidosis therefore begins with screening for abnormal urinary oligosaccharides by TLC; these results are used as a guideline for proceeding with specific diagnostic enzyme assays in leukocytes or cultured fibroblasts. Because of the clinical overlap between the MPSs and oligosaccharidoses, the MPSs should be considered in the differential diagnoses and workup of these patients. Prenatal diagnosis and carrier detection are possible for all of the oligosaccharidoses.

SPHINGOLIPIDOSES

The sphingolipids comprise a heterogeneous group of macromolecules containing the fatty alcohol sphingosine, which is covalently linked to a fatty acid side-chain to form ceramide. Sphingolipids can

Table 22.6 Oligosaccharidoses

Disorder	Clinical Findings	Laboratory Findings
Fucosidosis	Onset at 1 year. Coarse facies, growth retardation, dysostosis multiplex, and severe psychomotor regression. Variants with milder presentations, as well as angiokeratomas, have been described.	Deficient activity of α-L-fucosidase in leukocytes and fibroblasts. ↑ sweat electrolytes in most patients. Urinary excretion of fucosyl-rich oligosaccharides.
Mannosidosis	Onset during infancy. Rapid progression of psychomotor and mental retardation, facial coarsening, dysostosis multiplex, marked hepatosplenomegaly, and death beween 3–10 years. Milder clinical variants have been described.	Deficient activity of α-mannosidase in leukocytes, fibroblasts. Vacuolated lymphocytes. Urinary excretion of mannose-rich oligosaccharides.
β-Mannosidosis	Milder than α-mannosidosis. Variable mental retardation, facial dysmorphism, hepatosplenomegaly, and bone disease.	Deficient activity of β-mannosidase in leukocytes, fibroblasts and plasma. Urinary excretion of a characteristic mannose-containing disaccharide.
Aspartylglycosaminuria	Rare. Onset during the first few months of life. Recurrent infections, hernias, coarse facies, sagging skin folds, sun sensitivity, and mental deterioration. Ethnic predilection in Finns.	Deficient activity of aspartylglycosaminidase in leukocytes and fibroblasts. Aspartylglucosaminuria present.
Sialidosis (Mucolipidosis I)		
Type I	Onset in second decade. Myoclonus, ocular cherry-red spot, decreased visual acuity, gait abnormalities.	Deficient activity of neuraminidase (sialidase) in leukocytes and fibroblasts. Urinary excretion of sialyl-containing oligosaccharides.
Type II	Multiple dysmorphic findings similar to MPS IH. Hepatosplenomegaly, dysostosis multiplex, coarse facies, and dwarfism. Clinical variants with congenital or juvenile onset have been described.	As above, with or without associated β-galactosidase deficiency (galactosialidosis).

be divided into different subclasses based on chemical modifications of ceramide: glycolipids (glycosphingolipids) result from the linkage of ceramide to one or more sugar residues; cerebrosides from the linkage of ceramide to a single sugar residue; sulfatides (or sulfolipids) from a cerebroside containing a sulfate group; and sphingomyelin from ceramide linked to phosphocholine. In addition, the gangliosides are a complex group of glycolipids containing one or more negatively charged sialic acid (*N*-acetylneuraminic acid) residues. The sphingolipids are distributed throughout the body as structural components of plasma membranes, and many are particularly abundant in brain and other nervous tissue. Table 22.7 summarizes the known genetic defects of sphingolipid catabolism. All follow an autosomal recessive pattern of inheritance except Fabry's disease, which is X-linked. Diagnosis is made directly from results of enzyme assays ordered on the basis of clinical, laboratory, and histologic findings.

Although there is clinical overlap between the different disorders, it is useful to distinguish between those with a progressive neurodegenerative course and those characterized by more severe visceral involvement. The sphingolipidoses characterized by progressive psychomotor deterioration include metachromatic leukodystrophy, Krabbe's disease (globoid-cell leukodystrophy), G_{M1} gangliosidosis, and G_{M2} gangliosidosis (inclduing Tay-Sachs disease and Sandhoff's disease). These disorders are usually considered in the evaluation of patients with clinical findings suggestive of neurodegenerative disease.

The sphingolipidoses characterized by more severe visceral involvement include Gaucher's diasease and Niemann-Pick disease. Both of these diseases are characterized by hepatosplenomegaly and variable neurological involvement. Histopathological changes represent lyosomes swollen with stored material: Gaucher's disease is typified by the presence of Gaucher cells, and Neimann-Pick by foamy histiocytes. More rarely encountered disorders such as Farber's disease and acid lipase deficiency are discussed elsewhere (see Suggested Readings); Pompe's disease (glycogen storage disease type II) is discussed elsewhere in this chapter.

Tay-Sachs Disease Carrier Testing

Current treatment strategies for the sphingolipidoses are aimed at prevention rather than cure. This involves the identification of at-risk couples (i.e., both partners are carriers for the same disorder), who can then make informed decisions regarding their reproductive future. This approach is well suited for Tay-Sachs disease (TSD), which is found at a significantly increased frequency among Ashkenazi Jewish individuals, as well as a subset of French Canadians. There is roughly a 10-fold increase in heterozygote frequency among these groups compared to the general population, making it feasible to conduct screening programs aimed at identifying TSD carriers.

Table 22.7. Sphingolipidoses

Disorder	Clinical Findings	Laboratory Findings
G_{M1} Gangliosidosis		
Type I	Infantile onset. Rapid mental and motor regression. Seizures, hypotonicity to decerebrate rigidity, blindness, coarse facial features, macrocephaly, cherry-red spots, macroglossia, moderate hepatosplenomegaly, dysostosis multiples; death 1–2 years.	Deficient activity of an acidic β-galactosidase (G_{M1}-ganglioside β-galactosidase) in leukocytes and fibroblasts. Foamy histiocytes in bone marrow.
Type II	Juvenile onset. Slower progression than type I. May present with ataxia, seizures, strabismus, loss of speech; death 3–10 years.	Same as in type I
Type III	Adult onset. Progressive cerebella dysarthria with progressive spasticity and ataxia.	Same as in type I
G_{M2} Gangliosidosis		
Tay-Sachs disease	Onset 3–6 months. Exaggerated startle reaction. Seizures, mental and motor deterioration, blindness, dysphagia, doll-like facies, cherry-red spots, and macrocephaly; death by 3 years.	Deficient activity of β-hexosaminidase A in serum, leukocytes, and fibroblasts.
Sandhoff's disease	Clinically indistinguishable from Tay-Sachs	Deficient activity of hexosaminidase A and B in leukocytes and fibroblasts.
Juvenile G_{M2} gangliosidosis	Onset 2–6 years. Ataxia, progressive spasticity, seizures, late blindness; death by 5–15 years.	Same as in Tay-Sachs disease.
Adult (chronic) G_{M2} gangliosidosis	Progressive deterioration of gait and posture, muscle weakness and wasting, and ataxia. Gradual loss of motor and intellectual milestones.	Same as in Tay-Sachs disease.
Metachromatic leukodystrophy		
Late infantile form	Onset 6 months–24 months. Rapid neurological regression, gait disturbance, blindness, peripheral neuropathy, and quadriparesis.	Deficient activity of arylsulfatase A (cerebroside sulfatase) in leukocytes and fibroblasts. Elevated CSF protein, decreased nerve conduction velocity.
Juvenile form	Onset 5–10 years. Mental regression, gait disturbance, blindness, peripheral neuropathy, loss of speech, quadriparesis.	Same as above.
Adult form	Onset midteens–60 years. Dementia, symptoms similar to juvenile form.	Same as above.
Krabbe's disease (globoid cell leukodystophy)	Onset 3–6 months. Irritability progressing to severe mental and motor deterioration. From flaccidity to hypertonicity, blindness, deafness, and peripheral neuropathy; death by 12–18 months.	Deficient activity of galactocerebroside β-galactosidase.
Fabry's disease	X-linked inheritance. Pain and paresthesia in extremities, corneal opacities, angiokeratomas, cardiovascular angiectasis and renal failure.	Deficient activity of α-galactosidase A.
Gaucher's disease		
Type I (chronic nonneuropathic; adult form; visceral form)	Onset in childhood or later. Most patients are Ashkenazi Jews (incidence 1:2,500). Hepatosplenomegaly, episodic bone pain, hypersplenism, and pulmonary infiltrates.	Deficient activity of acidic β-glucosidase (glucocerebrosidase). Typical foam cells in bone marrow.
Type II (acute neuronopathic)	Onset birth–18 months. Rapid progressive neurological regression with seizures, dysphagia, spasticity, and hepatosplenomegaly; death by 24 months.	Same as above.
Type III (subacute neuronopathic)	Signs may appear early in life, but their progression is slower.	Same as above.
Niemann-Pick disease		
Type A (acute neuronopathic form)	Most common type. Onset in infancy. Rapidly progressive neurological regression, cherry-red spots, hepatosplenomegaly; death by 3 years.	Deficiency of sphingomyelinase. Foam cells in bone marrow.
Type B (chronic; visceral form)	Onset in infancy or childhood. Only the visceral findings of type A.	Same as above.
Type C (chronic neuronopathic form)	Later onset than type A; usually after 2 years. Hepatosplenomegaly, ataxia, seizures, hypertonia, loss of mental and motor skills; death before age 20 years.	Enzymatic defect unresolved. Foamy macrophages in marrow.
Type D (Nova Scotia variant)	Onset 2–4 years. Resembles type C with a protracted course and neurological abnormalities.	Enzymatic defect unkown. Foam cells in spleen and lymph nodes.
Type E (Adult form, non-neuronopathic form)	Adult onset. Hepatosplenomegaly. No neurologic difficulties.	Enzymatic defect unknown. Foam cells in marrow.

The assay for TSD carrier detection is routinely performed using serum, although certain medications (particularly oral contraceptives) and medical conditions (pregnancy, liver disease) can interfere with the serum assay. In these cases, evaluation of enzyme activity in leukocytes usually yields reliable results. Carriers of Sandhoff's disease also will be detected by this assay in either tissue.

MUCOLIPIDOSES

These disorders are so named because they share clinical features of both the MPS and sphingolipidoses. Mucolipidoses (ML) I and IV represent deficiencies in sialidase (neuraminidase) activity specific for glycoproteins and gangliosides, respectively. ML-II (I-cell disease) and ML-III (pseudo-Hurler's polydystrophy) are single gene disorders characterized biochemically by deficient intracellular activity of multiple lysosomal enzymes involved in the degradation of mucopolysaccharides, oligosaccharides, and sphingolipidoses, leading to abnormal storage of these compounds. The primary defect for both disorders is deficient activity of *N*-acetylglucosaminyl-1-phosphotransferase, the enzyme necessary for normal intracellular targeting of lysosomal enzymes. As a result, the enzymes are secreted extracellularly. The distinction between ML-II and ML-III is made on clinical grounds, with ML-II patients being much more severely affected. Biochemical diagnosis is made by demonstrating low intracellular activity of several lysosomal enzymes together with abnormally high activity outside cells (serum or culture medium). Diagnosis can be confirmed by demonstration of deficient phosphotransferase activity.

POPULATION SCREENING FOR GENETIC DISORDERS

Screening for genetic disorders falls into three categories: (*a*) neonatal screening, or the identification of infants with treatable metabolic disorders prior to the onset of clinical symptoms; (*b*) prenatal screening, or the identification prior to birth of fetuses with certain genetic disorders; and (*c*) carrier screening, or the identification of phenotypically normal individuals who are heterozygous for a particular mutation and therefore at risk of having affected offspring. There are numerous issues that must be addressed in determining which disorders are amenable to population screening. This section focuses on neonatal screening and the disorders typically included in these programs.

Newborn screening first became feasible in 1961, with the development of the Guthrie bacterial inhibition assay for measuring phenylalanine in dried blood specimens. The purpose of this test was to identify infants at risk for phenylketonuria (PKU) prior to the onset of symptoms, so that dietary management could be instituted and serious clinical sequelae avoided. PKU screening has subsequently been instituted throughout the U.S. and other countries, and has also been expanded to include other metabolic and nonmetabolic disorders.

At least three aspects of PKU render this disorder amenable to newborn screening. First, untreated PKU leads to severe clinical symptoms, including mental retardation. Secondly, dietary management prevents the mental retardation, provided the treatment is begun early. Finally, PKU can be detected in the newborn period as an elevation of blood phenylalanine in affected individuals. Newborns are now screened prior to discharge from the hospital at 1 to 3 days of age; some states retest at 2 weeks of age to assure that all infants have ingested sufficient protein for the screen to identify an affected infant. The most effective screening programs are those in which all newborns are tested.

Many general issues must also be considered in the establishment of an optimal screening test. The test must be simple and inexpensive to perform, as well as reliable, reproducible, and accurate. Ethical, legal, and economic considerations also determine the appropriateness of a given test, including the estimation of both the adverse and advantageous consequences of the proposed screening. These are determined in part by the frequency of the disorder in the population, as well as by the number of affected individuals who will be successfully identified. In addition, the practicality and cost of preventative treatment must be considered and constantly reevaluated in the context of advances being made in biomedical technology. Finally, the test sensitivity (the proportion of people with the disease whose results are positive) and specificity (the proportion without the disease whose results are negative) must be balanced for each screening test, thereby minimizing the number of false-negative results while holding false-positive cases to an acceptably low number.

Many of the newborn screening tests rely on the detection of abnormally elevated blood metabolites that accumulate as a consequence of a particular metabolic block. These include the tests for PKU, homocystinuria, and tyrosinemia. In contrast, other metabolic disorders are instead identified by the deficient activity of a specific enzyme, rather than the accumulation of substrate. These include the screening tests for biotinidase deficiency and the Beutler test for classic galactosemia. For these disorders in which enzyme activity itself is measured from the dried newborn blood spot, the accuracy of the test is independent of both dietary intake and clinical status of the infant.

An effective screening program is one in which all affected newborns are detected, leading to the expedient diagnosis and initiation of treatment. Referral centers capable of performing the confirmatory diagnostic tests by more specific analyses must be available to the physician and family. Finally, initiation of treatment must be prompt, and management, follow-up, and counseling should be continually offered to the patient and family by professionals trained in the management of metabolic disorders.

Suggested Readings

Bennet MJ, Allison, F, Pollitt RJ, Variend S. Fatty acid oxidation defects as causes of unexpected death in infancy. In: Tanaka K, Coates PM, eds. Fatty acid oxidation. Clinical biochemical and molecular aspects. New York: Alan R. Liss, Inc., 1990:349–364.

Benson PF, Fensom AH. Genetic biochemical disorders. Oxford: Oxford University Press, 1985.

Fernandes J, Saudubray JM, Tada K, eds. Inborn metabolic diseases. Diagnosis and treatment. New York: Springer-Verlag, 1990.

Hommes FA, ed. Techniques in diagnostic human biochemical genetics. A laboratory manual. New York: Wiley-Liss, 1991.

Krivit W, Whitley CB, Chang PN, et al. Lysosomal storage diseases treated by bone marrow transplantation: review of 21 patients. In: Johnson FL, Pochedly C, eds. New York: Raven Press, 1990:261–287.

Scriver CR, Beaudet AL, Sly WS, Valle D, eds. The metabolic basis of inherited disease. 6th ed. New York: McGraw-Hill, 1989.

Shapira E, Blitzer MG, MIller JB, Africk DK. Biochemical genetics. A laboratory manual. New York: Oxford University Press, 1989.

Section IV

Section Chief: *Meryl H. Haber*

Medical microscopy can be defined as the discipline of clinical laboratory medicine that deals with the examination of body fluids, other than blood, using macroscopic, physicochemical, and microscopic techniques. The term "microscopy" is therefore a misnomer, since the modern clinical laboratory performs many other important nonmicroscopic examinations on specimens. However, the old terminology has remained and serves a purpose in distinguishing analyses performed on body fluids from those performed on blood.

Urine is the most frequently examined body fluid, but other fluids such as joint, pleural, peritoneal, cerebrospinal, amniotic, seminal, and ocular also receive a fair degree of attention, especially in larger laboratories. Most often, when examination of a particular fluid includes microbiological examination with culture or requires cytologic appraisal, all or a portion of the fluid sample is sent to the appropriate laboratory for that specific analysis.

The urine reagent strip, a 20th century invention, has all but replaced complicated individual chemical analyses for the determination of the presence of various bodily products in urine. Estimations of glucose, albumin, hemoglobin, and bile levels, for example, as well as the determination of physical properties such as pH and osmolality, can all be accomplished using dipstick methodology. Advances in the analysis of urine are constantly being achieved, especially in the area of immunodiagnostic testing. Abnormal products of body metabolism may be expected to be found in the various fluids of the body, and fluids, especially urine, are more easily obtained than tissue. Medical microscopy and the physicochemical examination of body fluids will therefore continue to be an important source for obtaining information to assist in diagnosis and patient care.

MEDICAL MICROSCOPY AND URINALYSIS

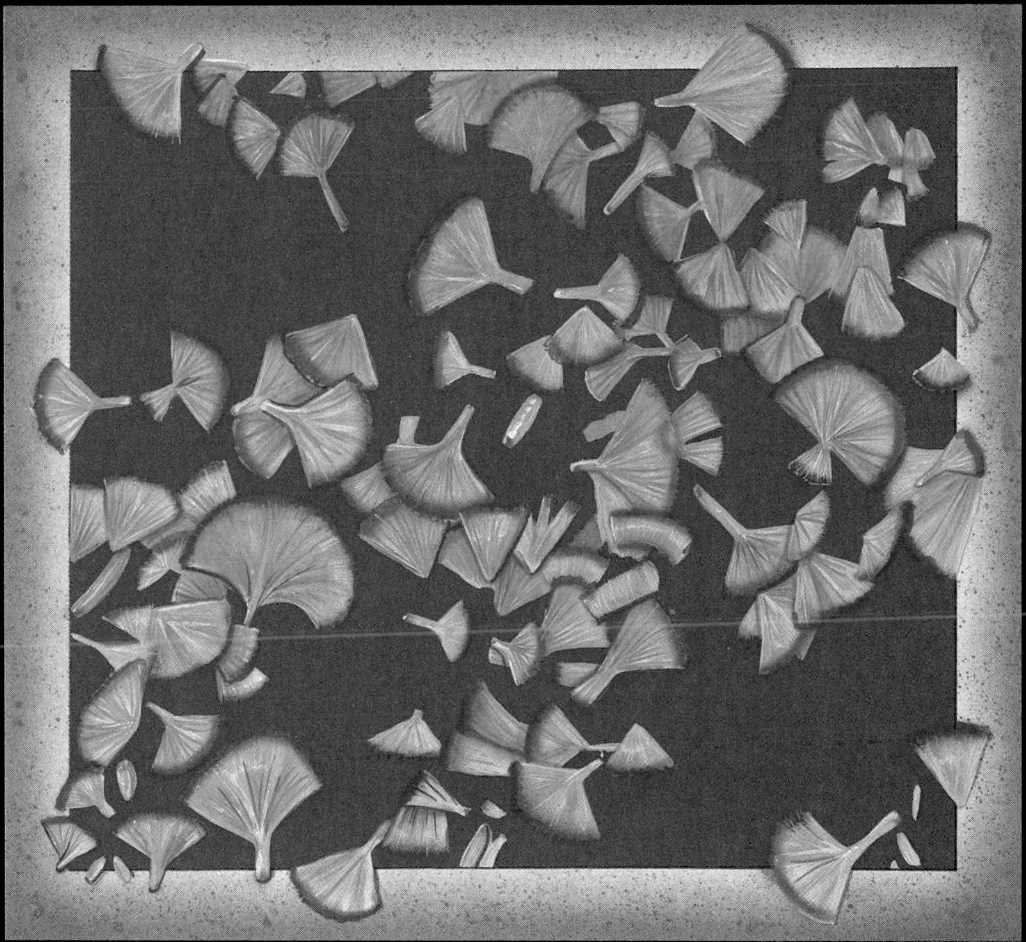

23 Urine

Meryl H. Haber

Examination of urine as an aid in diagnosis has long been an important part of medical practice. Ancient physicians recognized various discolored urines and associated these changes with prognosis (1). With the advent of the microscope, microscopy of various substances, fluids, organs, tissues, and cells became a commonly applied procedure, with great reliance being placed on it for diagnosis. Frequently performed by well-educated physicians, "uroscopy" was also performed by untrained charlatans, called "pisse-mongers" or "pisse-prophets." The unrestricted proliferation of these quacks finally led, in England in the 17th century, to the enactment of regulations and licensure laws, which protected the public from these individuals (2).

The modern microscope was first applied to the analysis of urine by Golding Bird in the mid-19th century. Bird, in his masterful textbook on urine published in 1842 (3), described certain elements in the sediment that are now commonly diagnosed; crystals and casts were correctly identified and named and were also accurately illustrated by means of engravings. Richard Bright, working at the same hospital as Bird (Guy's Hospital, London), in 1827, correctly recognized the presence of "red corpuscles" in the urine in a series of patients with severe renal disease, although apparently he did not identify them microscopically (4).

Present-day microscopy is a far cry from that used by Bird in the 19th century. Although the basic fundamentals of bright-field microscopy were in use then, the advent of the binocular microscope with better optics and the development of planar and apochromatic lenses have facilitated recognition of various elements. Analysis of urine exemplifies the use of modern microscopic techniques; here, phase-contrast microscopy, polarized microscopy, and interference-contrast microscopy have provided enhanced images that ultimately improve the accuracy of reporting. Staining the elements in a body fluid, be it urine or any other, has become an accepted procedure, often with considerable enhancement of cell identification (5).

Aside from the microscopic techniques performed in the modern clinical laboratory, body fluids may also undergo a variety of physicochemical evaluations. Medical science has come a long way from the ancient and medieval "pisse prophets" who used visual examination of the urine almost exclusively to diagnose and prognosticate. The advent of the science of chemistry introduced distillation, and it was made part of the uroscopy ritual. Various substances were added to the distillation flask or "urine vesicle," and these, in turn, often produced changes in urine color and precipitation of proteins, which caused lines or bands to form at various levels in the distillation flask. The flask was frequently molded into a human-like shape and contained an alembic "nose." If a band formed, a marking on the vesicle flask could be established, which would then represent a portion of the human form of the flask (e.g., a band across the abdominal region of the flask). The location of the band would then be interpreted by the physician as indicating the seat of the patient's disease—in this example, the umbilicus (1). This crude application of chemistry to urinalysis was the beginning of modern urine chemistry. Rapid advances in chemistry occurred during the past 300 years. Many substances were specifically identified in urine (sugar, uric acid), and these tests became available and were subsequently applied to other body fluids. Now chemical analysis is performed routinely, and the most advanced of techniques are utilized, including spectrophotometry, gas chromatography, and a variety of immunologic methods.

The urine reagent strip, a 20th century invention, has all but replaced complicated individual chemical analyses for the determination of various bodily products in urine. Estimations of glucose, albumin, hemoglobin, and bile, for example, as well as the determination of physical properties such as pH and osmolality, can all be accomplished using dipstick methodology. Advances in the analysis of urine are continually being made, especially in the area of immunodiagnostic testing. Abnormal products of body metabolism may be expected to be found in the various fluids of the body, and these (especially urine) are more easily obtained than tissue. Medical microscopy and the physicochemical examination of body fluids will therefore continue to be an important source of information to assist in diagnosis and patient care.

QUALITY ASSURANCE IN URINALYSIS

Urinalysis, although more frequently performed than any other laboratory test, often does not receive the same quality assurance (QA) attention given to other common tests. When conducting a urinalysis it is important to ensure that the results are accurate, reproducible, and precise (6). Standards of performance and QA procedures must be adopted and applied in the urinalysis laboratory; these measures may be followed with a minimal amount of inconvenience in the modern well-equipped laboratory, but they should be described and documented appropriately (7, 8). The procedure for the performance of a routine urinalysis has several parts; each is discussed separately below to delineate major issues of quality assurance. Ordinarily, the attending physician or house-staff officer writes an order for a urinalysis; a nurse, clerk, or other individual then completes a request form.

Urinalysis Request Form

The request form itself should be readily recognized and easy to complete. Color coding the form and using bold labeling are helpful. Space should be available for patient information, including name, sex, age, race, ID number (whether an outpatient or inpatient), the reason for ordering the test (i.e., chief complaint, symptoms and clinical impression, surgery), any medications, the time and date of collection, and how the specimen was obtained (i.e., midstream, catheter, aspiration, etc.). The form may also serve for reporting the results. If so, ample space should be included for this report. On the other hand, if the report form is separate, it should have a design similar to that of the request form as far as the color coding and patient information are concerned.

Equipment and Supplies

An overriding consideration when performing a urinalysis is the possibility that the specimen contains an infectious organism that may be transmitted to the technologist. Thus, the test itself, and the design of all supplies and equipment used in its performance, must ensure protection for the person performing the test; universal precautions must be adhered to in the handling of all specimens.

Equipment needed for the performance of a routine urinalysis generally consists of a microscope, a centrifuge, and a refractometer. In higher-volume laboratories, some of the physicochemical procedures (e.g., dipstick) may be automated or semi-automated, and appropriate instruments necessary for this automation must be available. High-quality work necessitates the use of modern equipment with known performance characteristics.

The microscope should be modern and binocular and should have an adjustable condenser with a built-in light source (8). The lenses should be of high quality and should consist of at least three magnifications: low and high power and oil immersion. A lower-power "scanning" lens can be added and often is of value in assessing the general characteristics of the urine sample and in determining whether or not the field being examined is representative of the entire specimen. The microscope should be kept clean and properly aligned at all times.

The microscopic technique most frequently utilized for examination of urine sediment is bright-field (BF) microscopy. Tungsten-filament light is transmitted through an adjustable condenser to produce parallel rays of light, so-called Köhler illumination. It is important to be able to reduce the level of light to enhance contrast, since many sediment elements have a low refractive index and are difficult to see. High contrast is provided by stopping down the iris diaphragm and lowering the condenser to the level at which the elements are best seen. Light is transmitted through the sediment, and whatever elements are present are observed through the eyepiece lenses (usually 10×). For the most accurate and reproducible results of a sediment examination, it is important that the same microscope be used daily; significant variations in element counts may occur if different microscopes are used. For example, if one observer uses a microscope with wide-field 10× eyepieces and another with ordinary 10× eyepieces, there will be a discrepancy in counts, since the field of view is significantly greater with wide-field eyepieces.

The best microscopic lenses are plano to provide a "flat" field of view. Lenses without chromatic aberration are called apochromatic lenses. Some manufacturers produce a lens that gives both a flat field and essentially no chromatic abnormalities, the plan-apo lens; these are usually more expensive and are not essential for ordinary everyday work.

Polarized microscopy is a simple and inexpensive addition to the bright-field microscope. All specimens that demonstrate abnormalities, whether macroscopically, chemically, or microscopically, should be examined using two polarizing lenses, a polarizer and an analyzer. The polarizer is inserted between the condenser and the microscopic slide, and the analyzer between the slide and the eyepiece. Certain substances, such as crystals and some lipids, have a peculiar property of being *birefringent* or *anisotropic* (also called being doubly refractile). Through polarized microscopy, objects that have this property are easily observed; objects that do not show birefrigence are totally obscured from the field of view. Cholesterol esters, present in the nephrotic syndrome when there is lipiduria, demonstrate a "Maltese Cross" pattern in in the urine; these same lipids may be entirely missed, or misdiagnosed, if polarization is not applied to the sediment. Enhancement of ordinary polarization with the use of retardation plates may be helpful in crystal identification. These plates are inserted into the light path to change the path of light vibration. Most commonly used in a first-order red plate, which is useful in distinguishing urate from calcium pyrophosphate crystals, especially in joint fluids. Plates made of mica may be similarly employed.

Phase-contrast (PC) microscopy is a technique that has proved to be very useful in examination of the urinary sediment. Phase-contrast microscopy utilizes a special microscope condenser that produces parallel and in-phase light rays, causing the peaks and troughs of the light to be in synchrony. As these waves pass through an object, the wave becomes asynchronous and out of phase. Elements viewed in this manner appear to have a white "halo" around them, greatly enhancing observation and facilitating diagnosis. Phase-contrast microscopy equipment is available from nearly every optical product manufacturer at relatively modest cost and should be standard equipment in the urinalysis laboratory.

Interference-contrast microscopy (ICM) is a valuale microscopic technique that provides a "three-dimensional" or "shadow-cast" image of the element under study (9). This is accomplished by inserting a pair of beam-splitting prisms in the light path (Nomarski interference), one to actually divide the light and reorient it into phased and perpendicular waves of light (a reference beam and an object beam), and the second to recombine the light *after* it has passed through the element. As the object beam courses through the specimem, both its amplitude and its phase are altered; the reference wave, on the other hand, does not pass through the element and thus no change occurs in its amplitude or phase. When these two light waves are recombined by passing through the second Nomarski prism, the image of the object appears to be three-dimensional when viewed through the eyepieces of the microscope. ICM is of particular value in teaching because of the ease in demonstrating fine points of structure. The cost of ICM equipment is somewhat high, and therefore it is difficult to justify in most routine laboratories where the urinalysis microscope is used exclusively for patient care.

The centrifuge, necessary for sediment concentration for microscopic evaluation, must be calibrated to provide a constant relative centrifugal force (RCF) of 400 (8). Spinning the urine for 5 minutes will provide a sediment in which there are no artifacts. Neither the exact time of centrifugation nor the RCF are "set in stone"; each laboratory must determine for itself what settings to use—and be certain to check the exact same time and RCF are applied to each urine every time. Regular periodic maintenance and calibration checks of the centrifuge are essential to ensure a standardized procedure that will eliminate variations in results.

Refractometers measure the total solids (TS) in a solution by comparing the refractive index of the specimen to water: solids dissolved in urine change the refractive index in proportion to their concentration (10). These instruments are operated with ease and provide a quantitative estimate of the specific gravity using a single drop of urine. Most commercially available refractometers are temperature corrected, and these have replaced the older (and far less accurate) urinometers (or hydrometers) for the measurement of specific gravity. Reference solutions with known quantities of dissolved substances, such as salt, are prepared to check the calibration of refractometers. Water is used as a standard and is given a value of 1.00. Calibration should be done frequently and at least daily in high-volume laboratories (8).

Osmolality, although not usually tested in the urinalysis laboratory when a routine urinalysis is requested, is a measurement of the number of particles in a solution. Instruments employed to measure osmolality are based on the principle that when a solution is frozen, or vaporized, the point at which this occurs is proportional to the number of particles present. This relationship may not always be a direct one, since larger molecules, such as protein, affect the proportionality more than simple molecules, such as sodium chloride. The measurement of urine osmolality is a valuable test when estimating the kidney's concentrating ability, as in the case of possible tubular disease or in the calculation of free water clearance (11). Reference solutions, both high and low, should be utilized at frequent intervals in the testing procedure for instrument calibration to ensure precision and accuracy. Instruments that measure osmolality are complex and need to be treated with the utmost care, always making certain that the manufacturer's instructions are followed exactly.

The supplies used in routine urinalysis should be disposable (7, 8). These include a specimen collection system consisting of a collection container, a cover for it, a graduated centrifuge tube with a leakproof cap, labels, and disposable microscopic slides containing a constant-volume chamber for sediment quantitation. Reagent strips are available from a number of different suppliers and can be obtained with several configurations of tests. Most, however, include the following physicochemical tests: pH, hemoglobin, glucose, protein, bilirubin, urobilinogen, ketone bodies, and nitrites. Other commonly available pads test for leukocyte esterase and measure specific gravity (10). Each of these tests is discussed separately in a later section of this chapter.

It is important to conclude this section with a brief comment about reporting. No matter how accurate and precise a procedure may be, or how relevant the results, if one is not consistent in the method of reporting misinterpretations may result (8). It is therefore incumbent on the laboratory to standardize reporting and to be certain that whoever is performing the test uses the same terminology and utilizes identical criteria for the identification of elements. A procedures manual should contain diagnostic criteria and specific definitions; all personnel performing the test should use these criteria. A definition of what constitutes "normal" urine should be included. Separate mention should be given to abnormal values, and those that should prompt a phone call to the attending physician—the so-called "panic values"—should be defined.

MACROSCOPIC, PHYSICOCHEMICAL URINALYSIS

The Physical Examination of Urine

An adult human produces 1 to 2 liters of urine every 24 hours. The urine is formed in the kidney and contains predominantly water in which are admixed mostly urea and salts, especially sodium chloride (11). The amount of solute is directly related to the amount and kind of ingested foods and fluids. Urea is predominantly a byproduct of protein metabolites. Numerous other dissolved constituents are also found in urine, including sugars, bile, other electrolytes such as potassium, products of protein metabolism such as nucleic acids, hormones and their metabolites, vitamins, and certain trace metals.

The routine macroscopic, physical and chemical examination of urine includes appearance, "dipstick" testing, and measurement of specific gravity (8, 10). Normally, urine is pale yellow and has an ammoniacal odor. This odor increases significantly when the urine has been allowed to stand for any length of time and is primarily due to the release of nitrogenous compounds from bacterial action. The urine is more deeply pigmented as its concentration increases.

PHYSICAL URINALYSIS

Appearance

When freshly voided, normal urine should be clear and pale yellow to amber in color. Many ingested foods, dyes, or pharmaceuticals may produce a color change. The normal yellow color is due to the presence of urochrome pigment, a product of hemoglobin metabolism. Color intensity may vary and depends on the concentration of the urine; in highly concentrated urine such as in the early morning, the colors may be more vivid.

Abnormal color of urine occurs in the normal state and also in certain diseases. Various foods, such as carrots and beets, produce abnormally colored orange to red urine. Although color by itself is not a particularly sensitive indicator of abnormality, any variation from the normal should be investigated and the specific cause determined. Some conditions may be associated with abnormally colored urine: hemoglobinuria—red; melanin—black; bile pigments—green; chyluria—white; porphyria—red-purple, to mention a few. Also, certain dyes and pharmaceuticals and some food colorings are notorious for discoloring urine. Specific examples are phenolphthalein—red; methylene blue—blue; pyridium—yellow-orange (11).

Normal urine is not always clear, especially after refrigeration. Urate and phosphate crystals often form a cloudy precipitate when urine is subjected to low temperatures. Simply rewarming the urine to room temperature will frequently cause the crystals to dissolve and the urine to become clear once again. Urine contaminated with seminal fluid or vaginal secretions and mucous may be cloudy. A clear urine that has been permitted to stand at room temperature for any length of time may become cloudy due to bacterial growth. Turbid urine is commonly associated with abnormal conditions, especially hematuria, leukocyturia, and bactiuria. Chyluria, or the appearance of lymph in the urine causing cloudiness, is an extremely rare complication of blockage of the lymph passages with the production of a fistula and flow of the lymph into the urinary outflow tract.

Odor

Normal urine has a distinct and easily recognized odor, albeit ill defined. Upon standing, the same urine acquires a pungent ammoniacal odor due to the action of bacteria and the release of ammonia. Food, such as asparagus, gives the urine a distinct odor promptly after eating. The odor of urine is given little importance in clinical diagnosis, but if an unusual odor is recognized during analysis, it too should be reported. Foul-smelling odors may be associated with urinary tract infections and "fruity" odors with diabetes mellitus when ketones are present.

Collection of Urine

An early-morning, freshly voided specimen is preferred. This should be a clean-catch midstream voided urine (8). The patient is instructed to cleanse the area surrounding his or her urethra using a mild soap and water solution and then to urinate into a clean (not necessarily sterile) collection container that is properly labeled, free of interfering chemicals, can be capped, and is leakproof.

The specimen should be transported to the urinalysis laboratory promptly, and examined within 2 hours after voiding. Although refrigeration of the specimen is not necessary due to frequent precipatation of urate or phosphate crystals, in certain instances it is preferable to allow the urine to stand at room temperature. The addition of antibacterial agents such as formaldehyde or thymol crystals to the urine to prevent bacterial growth is not advised, since these substances interfere with the chemical evaluation.

Once received in the laboratory, the urine is decanted into a graduated centrifuge tube and centrifuged to obtain sediment for evaluation. Transfer pipettes and microscopic slides, preferably with graduated, consistent-volume chambers, are desirable for use. None of the materials mentioned above should be reused.

A major and most important concept in the analysis of urine must be that of quality assurance that ensures consistency and accuracy of results (6–8). Basically, this concept is one of careful control and consistency in every step of the urinalysis procedure to ensure that each and every urine sample is treated and examined in exactly the same manner, and the results obtained are compared with nonsamples to ensure that when and if a discrepancy occurs, corrective action will be taken.

Equipment such as microscopes, centrifuges, reagent strip readers, and refractometer all need to be clean, calibrated, and frequently checked to provide consistency and accuracy in evaluations. The reader is referred to NCCLS Document GP16-P for guidelines with regard to routine urinalysis (8).

Chemical Urinalysis

The performance of a "routine" physicochemical urinalysis has evolved into a sophisticated, but easily performed procedure mainly due to the advent of urine dipsticks (10). These are plastic strips on which are attached a series of chemically impregnated absorbent pads. Each pad contains certain chemicals that react with a substance in the urine, producing a color change in the pad. This color change is then compared with a series of known standards so that any reaction seen in the patient's urine may be evaluated and quantified. This methodology is simple and easily taught, is rapid, and provides a means of analysis that, although not without some drawbacks, offers an inexpensive and highly useful assessment of several urinary constituents. Most of the available dipsticks contain pads for determination of pH, hemoglobin, glucose, protein, urinary ketones, bilirubin, urobilinogen, and nitrites (12). Other available pad tests, depending on the manufacturer, measure specific gravity and leukocyte esterase (13).

Along with the bottle containing the dipsticks, each manufacturer provides an insert that describes in detail the proper use of the product. Care must be taken to follow these directions exactly. Before using the sticks, one must be certain that they are not outdated and that they have been stored in their original container at the recommended temperature. The bottle should remain unopened until the dipsticks are required for use. The strips should be removed from the container only a few at a time and, once opened, the container should be closed tightly for storage of the remaining dipsticks until further need (8).

In use, the dipstick is immersed into the urine by a rapid, deliberate motion and is then removed. During removal, the edge of the stick is guided over the lip of the urine container, usually a centrifuge tube, to allow excess urine to run off the stick and flow back into the container. Each manufacturer provides a time sequence for the interpretation of each test pad; it is important to follow these instructions, since the color reactions on the pads change with prolonged exposure. As pad colors are compared with a colored comparison chart provided by the manufacturer, test results are recorded by the observer. For accurate interpretations, lighting conditions should be good and should simulate daylight. Visual reading of the pads is subject to variation from observer to observer; automated strip readers have improved this variability.

QA procedures need to be employed during the chemical analysis of urine (6). This is performed by utilizing solutions with known concentrations of the analytes being tested for on the dipstick. When spurious or unexpected results are obtained in any given patient, or if a trend toward abnormal results occurs, the source of potential error must be searched for and corrected. Confirmatory testing is performed on the urine sample on occasion. In such instances, it may be desirable to obtain results that exceed those provided by the semiquantiative methodology of the dipstick (8). Confirmatory tests are available for essentially all urine dipstick pads.

Certain substances may produce interference with the reaction on the dipstick pad. Many of these are well known and consist of pharmaceutical products, various foodstuffs, and dyes (10, 11). In addition, certain physicochemical changes in the urine may interfere with the pad's color reaction and can result in inaccurate false-positive or false-negative readings. As an example, bilirubin, when exposed to light, breaks down and a false-negative reaction on the dipstick pad occurs if the urine has been exposed to direct light for long time periods. An excellent example of an interfering substance is ascorbic acid (vitamin C), which is frequently taken in high concentrations in the belief that it affords better overall health and prevents the common cold from occurring. This substance is excreted by the kidneys, and when present in the urine may obscure the dipstick pad for hemoglobin, giving a false-negative reaction. It is of primary importance to provide the laboratory with a good clinical history prior to the performance of a urinalysis to ensure useful clinical correlations and consistent and accurate interpretations.

Glucose

Glucose is one of a variety of reducing substances that may be present in the urine, but from a clinical standpoint it is the most important one. Small amounts of glucose may normally be present in the urine, especially after ingesting foods or beverages that have a high concentration (11). Glucose is freely filtered by the glomerulus and almost entirely reabsorbed by the renal tubules, so under normal circumstances little is found in the urine. *Glycosuria* is defined as the presence of detectable glucose in the urine. This generally occurs when blood levels of glucose exceed 180 mg/dl. At these levels, with similar concentrations occurring in the glomerular filtrate, the *renal threshold* for glucose is exceeded, and any glucose that exceeds this concentration cannot be reabsorbed by the renal tubules and is excreted in the urine. The renal threshold is not an absolute number, and varies somewhat from individual to individual, in the range of 160 to 200 mg/dl.

Diabetes mellitus, a common clinical condition in which serum concentrations of glucose may reach very high levels, is frequently diagnosed and monitored by the detection of glucose in the urine. Elevated blood levels of glucose lead to similarly elevated levels in the glomerular filtrate, which then exceed the renal threshold for glucose, and glycosuria results. Glucose may be found in the urine in conditions other than diabetes; these affect the central nervous system (stroke, neoplasms), kidneys (uremia), endocrine system (overproduction of adrenocorticotropic hormone), and liver (glycogen storage disease), or may be related to general metabolic problems, such as starvation and obesity (10, 11, 14). Certain pharmaceutical agents, such as diuretics and birth control pills, may also cause glycosuria.

Although glucose may be measured in various ways, the method employed on dipsticks utilizes an enzymatic methodology (10). This method takes advantage of the specific reaction of the enzyme glucose oxidase, which catalyzes the conversion of glucose to gluconic acid and hydrogen peroxide. A second enzyme, peroxidase, promotes the reaction of the H_2O_2 generated with a chromogen (iodine complex) to form a brown oxidized compound. The chromogen varies with the manufacturer, as does the sensitivity (10, 12).

$$\text{Glucose} + O_2 \xrightarrow{\text{glucose oxidase}} \text{Gluconic acid} + H_2O_2$$

$$H_2O_2 + \text{Chromogen} \xrightarrow{\text{peroxidase}} \text{Oxidized colored chromagen} + H_2O$$

Color charts are provided with the dipsticks to enable semi-quantitative determination of the amount of glucose present in the specimen. Reporting is commonly given in a 1+ to 4+ format, which may then be equated to concentrations ranging from approximately 100 to 2000 mg/dl. Sensitivity of the various dipsticks varies with the manufacturer, but is usually in the range of 50 to 100 mg/dl. Reagent strip testing for glucose has its problems, since at the higher concentrations (i.e., 1 to 2 g/dl) color differences in the pads are more difficult to interpret.

Reducing substances, especially other sugars, do not give a positive dipstick test because the method, which utilizes glucose oxidase, is specific for glucose. However, false-positive reactions may occur if the urine container used is not disposable and strong oxidizing detergents remain from prior washings (11, 14). False-negative results may be encountered when any part of the chemical reaction is interfered with, such as when high doses of aspirin or ascorbic acid are present in the urine and these compounds, both reducing agents, prevent the formation of the chromogen by preventing its oxidation by H_2O_2. One other relatively frequent cause of false-negative results is glucose being metabolized by bacteria when the urine sample has been allowed to stand for any length of time after voiding.

A second method for the measurement of reducing sugars, including glucose, in urine is by means of the copper reduction test (Benedict's reaction) (Table 23.1). This test is performed by adding urine to a tablet composed of copper sulfate, sodium citrate, sodium carbonate, and sodium hydroxide, (Clinitest, Ames Division, Miles Laboratories) (10). The cupric ion ($CuSO_4$), in the presence of a base (NaOH), re-

Table 23.1. A Comparison of the Reactions of Glucose Oxidase and Copper Sulfate Tests for Urine Sugars

Substance	Glucose Oxidase Dipstick	Copper Sulfate Tablet
Glucose	Positive	Positive
Other reducing sugars	Negative	Positive
Pharmaceutical agents	Negative	Some false-positives
Detergent contaminants (peroxide or strong oxidants)	False-positive	Negative

acts with reducing substances in the urine to produce cuprous ions plus heat. Depending on the amount of sugar present, a color change occurs, which can then be compared with reference charts to quantitate the reaction. This test is performed by simply adding urine and water to a test tube containing a Clinitest tablet, waiting a brief period of time for the chemical reaction to occur (the solution boils with heat liberation and color development; the bottom of the test tube should not be touched), and then quantitating the amount of sugar present by comparing the color of the reactants with a color chart. The manufacturer's directions should be followed in their entirety; accuracy is related to adding the correct amounts of urine and water as well as to the timing of the reaction and the development of color.

Reducing sugars other than glucose are infrequently seen in urine, but are sometimes discovered in a pediatric population. They may be overlooked unless careful attention is paid to the possibility of their existence. This is accomplished by means of testing each pediatric patient's urine with Clinitest or by using another similiar nonenzyme specific methodology. This copper sulfate method will detect the presence of all reducing sugars, some of which may not be glucose. To verify the presence of a nonglucose reducing sugar, comparisons should be made with dipstick results from the same patient; if the sugar is not glucose the dipstick test is negative. Thin-layer chromatography may be utilized in the specific identification of nonglucose reducing sugars when inherited inborn metabolic diseases of sugar metabolism are considered.

Galactosemia, an inborn error of metabolism, must be screened for using the copper sulfate methodology. The use of a dipstick will not discern galactose. Lactase deficiency in the infant results in lactosuria; early diagnosis is of importance since failure to thrive and intestinal damage may result if ordinary milk, which contains lactose, is not removed from the diet. Sucrase deficiency, less common than lactase deficiency, also results in mellituria (sucrosuria), which can be diagnosed by means of Clinitest table use. Symptoms are similar to those seen in lactosuria. Other sugars that may be present in the urine are fructose and pentose. Fructosuria and pentosuria are infrequent causes of nonglucose mellituria.

Protein

Relatively small quantities of protein are normally excreted in the urine, usually no more than 100 to 150 mg/day (15, 16). Normal urine volume is between 1,000 and 1,500 ml/day, thus the expected protein concentration in a normal sample is somewhere in the range of 8 to 10 mg/dl (10, 14). The predominant protein present in the urine is albumin, which is filtered by the glomerulus and is not reabsorbed by the tubules; albumin accounts for approximatley one-third of normal urine protein. The other main source of urinary protein are the renal tubules, especially the distal tubules. These tubules account for the other two-thirds of urine protein excretion, and of this portion approximately half is Tamm-Horsfall mucoprotein (THP), which is secreted by the distal tubular epithelium and collecting ducts and is of importance in the formation of urinary casts. Small quantities of other urinary proteins come from filtered low-molecular weight proteins of the blood plasma that are not reabsorbed by the tubules, microglobulins from renal tubular epithelial cells, and prostatic and vaginal secretions (15).

Proteinuria, defined as increased protein in the urine, is a frequent finding in intrinsic diseases of the kidney and urinary tract. Proteinuria, often associated with urine sediment abnormalities, frequently serves as a basis for the diagnosis of intrinsic renal disease (15). Albumin is most often the predominant protein excreted in excess in urine in disease states and may account for as much as 80 to 90% of the total protein present. In multiple myeloma, a neoplastic condition affecting plasma cells, large quantities of a low–molecular weight globulin (Bence Jones protein) may be present in the urine, replacing albumin as the predominant protein. Proteinuria may accompany generalized non–urinary tract conditions such as hemorrhage, systemic infections, heart failure, dehydration, and starvation.

Normal persons may excrete abnormal quantities of protein, mainly albumin, in some situations; among these are strenuous physical exercise (17), pregnancy, exposure to extreme cold, and psychological stress.

Orthostatic proteinuria is a condition, mainly found in adolescents and young adults, in which increased quantities of protein are found in the urine when the patient is in a vertical position; the proteinuria disappears when the patient is resting horizontally (14). Pressure on the renal veins when standing is thought to be the cause of this condition, and it frequently disappears with increasing age. Testing the first urine specimen of the morning for protein and comparing the result with that obtained from a specimen collected later in the day after physical activity will usually provide the correct diagnosis and may eliminate the need for a more elaborate workup.

Dipstick screening for protein is designed to differentiate between what is considered a random normal amount (i.e., less than 10 mg/dl) in a given urine sample, preferably an early morning one, and quantities that exceed these norms. One reason for the early-morning collection of urine is that samples of urine obtained after eating or drinking may produce false-negative dipstick tests for protein because of the dilutional effects of food and water. Whenever unsuspected proteinuria is found, confirmatory tests for protein are essential, since a diagnosis of proteinuria carries with it considerable clinical importance (8). Any diagnosis of proteinuria should be verified and substantiated. Clinically, proteinuria is considered mild (less than 0.5 g/day), moderate (0.5 to 4 g/day), or severe (more than 4 g/day) (10). Most patients with intrinsic renal disease such as acute glomerulonephritis or pyelonephritis present with moderate proteinuria, but patients with the nephrotic syndrome commonly excrete over 4 grams of protein a day in the urine.

Testing urine for the presence of protein has been performed for centuries. It was well known in ancient times that when heat was applied to urine containing large amounts of protein, a white coagulum formed (similar to boiling an egg and seeing the mucoid albumin become a white gelatinous precipitate) (1). It was realized, over time, that other substances interfered with this simple test; acetic acid was added to clear some of these compounds, as was sodium chloride. The addition of these chemicals to proteinaceous urine ensure that protein precipitation occurs even when there are small amounts of protein present. Today, the heat and acetic acid method has been replaced with a turbidimetric test utilizing sulfosalicylic acid (11). This test is performed without heat.

Quantitative protein concentrations can be determined by setting up standards containing measured amounts of protein and comparing the precipitation obtained on an unknown urine sample with these standards using a nephelometer or spectrophotometer. Immunoassays have recently been employed for the accurate determination of urinary protein content (15). In practice, a qualitative estimation of protein is initially made by comparing the degree of precipitation (i.e., turbidity) with a set of standard tubes containing known concentrations of protein. This reaction may be classified as 1 to 4+ or may be quantified as milligrams per deciliter. A trace reaction is one in which is there is perceptible, but minimal, turbidity (≈ 20 mg/dl); a 1+ reaction (≈ 50 mg/dl) shows definite turbidity, but no white precipitation granules; in a 2+ reaction (≈ 250 mg/dl) reaction, granules and turbidity are seen; a 3+ reaction (≈ 500 mg/dl) demonstrates granules and flocculation; and in a 4+ reaction (more than 1 g/dl) large clumps of white precipitate are seen.

Present-day dipsticks for the determination of urine protein use a colorimetric methodology based on the concept of "the protein error of indicators." This method utilizes a physicochemical property of protein that causes certain indicators (e.g., Tetrabromphenol Blue) to change color in the presence of varying concentrations of protein when the pH is kept constant (the dipstick pad is impregnated with buffers kept at a pH of about 3). This method provides a rapid means of testing for protein, but one that is somewhat difficult to interpret when low concentrations of protein are encountered, generally in the "trace" to 1+ range. This difficulty is due to subtle color changes that occur in the indicators in this range (i.e., yellowish tan). As protein levels increase, the colors become more intense and easier to interpret (i.e., green and blue). Results are read as trace and 1+ to 4+. A dipstick trace reaction corresponds to approximately 15 to 30 mg/dl of protein, whereas a 4 + reaction corresponds to more than 2 g/dl. Dipstick urine testing is best for albumin. Other proteins, such as Bence Jones (BJ) protein, which is a globulin, give negative or less than optimal results, therefore making confirmatory testing using other methods a necessity.

Bence Jones protein is found in the urine in approximately half of patients with multiple myeloma; it may also be present in malignant lymphoma and macroglobulinemia (14, 18). Reagent strip testing for Bence Jones protein often is not reflective of the type or amount of protein present in the urine since they are globulins, and the protein pad may even show a completely negative result (10). Urine electrophoresis or immunoelectrophoresis are the procedures of choice for recognizing this protein (15), but other tests may also prove helpful, especially as screening tests, because of the peculiar solubility properties of BJ protein.

When gradual heat in a water bath is applied to a test tube of urine containing BJ protein, precipitation occurs between 40° and 60°C. However, if the heat is continued by putting the tube in boiling water, precipitated BJ protein will redissolve at approximately 100°C after a few minutes. Cooling the tube reverses the process, so a precipitate will reform at 40° to 60°C and will redissolve when the temperature falls below 40°C (12). Severe proteinuria in myeloma, if left untreated, often produces renal tubule injury (myeloma kidney), which may lead to clinical manifestations of the nephrotic syndrome and to renal failure. If large amounts of protein other than BJ protein are present in urine, they may interfere with the heat test. Filtering the urine after boiling it and heating it to 100°C and then cooling it to room temperature will remove these interfering substances.

Clinically, it is often valuable to know the total amount of protein excreted in the urine in 24 hours (15). A single urine sample is not sufficient to provide this information, therefore a 24-hour sample must be collected. Chemicals that cause no interference with the tests for protein are added to the urine collection bag to preserve the specimen. At the end of the timed collection period, the urine is analyzed for its protein content using a precipitation test (i.e., sulfosalicylic acid turbidity). The results are reported as milligrams of protein per deciliter and, depending on the total volume of urine voided, the amount of protein excreted by the kidneys in a given day can easily be calculated.

Blood

Hematuria, defined as increased numbers of red blood cells (RBCs) in the urine, is an important indicator of diseases involving the genitourinary tract. Normal urine may contain up to 5 RBCs/μl. Increased numbers of erythrocytes may come from a variety of sources, including the kidneys, ureters, bladder, urethra, prostate gland, and uterus and vagina. Erythrocytes may be found intact, or they may lyse and release their contained hemoglobin into the urine, resulting in *hemoglobinuria.* Frank bleeding into the urine causes a reddish discoloration, but lesser numbers of RBCs or hemoglobin in the urine (i.e., occult bleeding) has been described by some patients as a "smoky" urine. Normally, there are small numbers of RBCs in the urine sediment, but these are not detectable using dipstick methodology.

The causes of hematuria are many (18). Among the more common are bladder and kidney tumors, trauma to the kidneys, glomerulonephritis, pyelonephritis, renal calculi, and bleeding disorders related to anticoagulant use. Hemoglobinuria, on the other hand, is far less common. It may be associated with trauma or transfusion reactions and is seen in severe burns or poisonings. *Myoglobinuria,* the presence of myoglobin in the urine, is found, on occasion, after severe physical exercise or in trauma where muscle fiber necrosis has occurred. Myoglobin gives a positive dipstick reaction for hemoglobin, and therefore the distinction between myoglobinuria, which indicated rhabdomyolysis, and hemoglobinuria must be made using other tests (14). Myoglobinuria should be considered when the dipstick pad is positive for hemoglobin, but microscopic analysis of the sediment does not show RBCs.

Dipstick testing for hemoglobin is based on the property of hemoglobin to catalyze the oxidation of a chromogen because of the release of the RBC enzyme hemoglobin peroxidase (10). Various manufacturers use different chromogens that, when catalyzed by hemoglobin peroxide in the presence of an organic peroxide buffer, form a green to dark blue chromogen.

$$H_2O_2 + \text{chromogen} \xrightarrow{\text{hemoglobin peroxidase}} \text{colored chromogen} + H_2O$$

Reagent strip pads for hemoglobin are impregnated with the benzidine chromogen and buffered organic peroxide. If hemoglobin is present in the urine, the hemoglobin peroxidase catalyzes the reaction shown above so that a color develops on the pad. This colored pad can then be compared with color charts for a semiquantitative determination of the amount of hemoglobin present. The readings are 1+ to 3+ and indicate trace, small, moderate, and large amounts of blood. Intact red blood cells are lysed when they come in contact with the pad, resulting in a speckled pattern. In most urine containing blood, intact RBCs, as well as free hemoglobin from lysed RBCs, combine to provide the positive reaction on the strip.

Hemoglobin dipstick testing, especially for microscopic hematuria, has been very effective (19). However, there are well-known interfering substances that must be considered whenever the clinical history or the sediment examination does not substantiate the results of the dipstick test. Interference by ascorbic acid (vitamin C) is a prime example of this. False-negative reaction errors can be avoided if a careful clinical history is taken and a check is made for the presence of vitamin C in the urine (12). Other methods used to detect hemoglobin when interfering substances are present include direct chemical analysis using a spectrophotometer or by use of another dipstick with a hemoglobin pad that does not produce false-negative results for hemoglobin in the presence of ascorbic acid.

pH

The kidneys, along with the lungs, are prime regulators of acid-base balance. Depending on the foods ingested, the state of health or disease, lung and renal function, medications being used, and a host of other issues, urine pH may vary from 4.5 to 8. pH is a measure of the hydrogen ion content of the urine. Acid urine, by definition, has a pH less then 7, whereas the pH of alkaline urine is greater than 7.

The usual finding in freshly voided samples from normal patients is acidic urine with pH between 5 and 6. If fresh urine is allowed to stand at room temperature before analysis, the pH will change from acid to alkaline due to the growth of bacteria and the breakdown of urea in the urine with the liberation of ammonia. The kidneys constantly regulate acid-base balance and tend to conserve various ions, especially sodium. This process is accomplished primarily by sodium reabsorption in the renal tubules with concomitant excretion of ammonium and hydrogenic ions (20). In metabolic acidosis such as occurs in diabetes, for example, the urine is acidic; in metabolic alkalosis, the urine is alkaline. Control of the urine pH becomes important in the treatment of certain diseases, such as renal stone formation and bacterial infections of the urinary tract. Maintaining alkaline urine provides a more effective environment for certian antibiotic agents, and drugs that keep the urine alkaline therefore assist in the use of these agents. Renal calculi may form from soluble inorganic ions, and by controlling pH, the formation may be slowed or prevented (i.e., uric acid stones tend to develop in acid urine, and calcium carbonate stones in alkaline urine).

Measurement of urine pH is facilitated by dipstick methodology and comparison with a color chart (21). Confirmatory testing may be performed with a pH meter, but this is usually not necessary. The pH pad is impregnated with two indicators, methyl red and bromthymol blue, which change color when immersed in urine. Two indicators are usually used to provide a broad range of color change, orange-green-blue. QA checks of pH dipsticks should be made regularly with known solutions (7, 8).

Ketone Bodies

Ketonuria, or the presence of ketone bodies in the urine, occurs in conditions in which there is incomplete metabolism of fat. In normal metabolism, the body completely metabolizes fat to carbon dioxide and water. However, in disease conditions such as diabetes, especially when poorly controlled, the supply of carbohydrate is ineffectually utilized, more energy from fat is required, and fat is frequently broken down as an energy source, with the products of fat metabolism appearing in the blood (ketosis) and urine (ketonuria). These intermediary products, which are formed in the liver, are called ketone bodies; they are acetoacetic acid, acetone, and betahyroxybutyric acid (14). The latter two are derivatives of acetoacetic acid. Nearly 80% of the ketone bodies found in the urine are betahydroxybutyric acid, with acetone accounting for only 2% and acetoacetic acid making up the remainder (10). Ketones are excreted in the urine along with basic ions, depleting the body of its anions and producing acidosis.

Diabetes is the most common disease in which ketosis and ketoacidosis are found, but there are many other conditions in which ketosis also occurs. Among the most important on a worldwide basis is starvation, but in the United States ketosis is also produced in acute dieting. Under this condition the body begins to break down its own fat surplus, which results in the production of ketone bodies. Other conditions in which ketones are found in the urine are anorexia nervosa, prolonged vomiting, and in several gastrointestinal diseases.

Dipstick testing for ketone bodies is based on the principle that both acetone and acetoacetic acid react with sodium nitroprusside in an alkaline buffer medium to produce a purple complex (Legal's test). β-Hydroxybutyric acid does not react. When the color is fully developed, it is compared with a color chart to determine the amount present; the test is interpreted as trace (5 mg/dl) to 4+ (more than 100 mg/dl) (purple color) (10). Acetoacetic acid is the most sensitive reactant, and since the proportions of the three ketone bodies are similar in ketotic states, it is not clinically important that β-hydroxybutyric acid is not measured.

Certain dyes, such as phthaleins, may produce a red color on the test pad. However, this color is different from the violet-purple of acetoacetic acid and should not be confused with it. Similarly, phenylketones may give an orange-red color that may be misinterpreted as a positive dipstick reaction. If the urine stands too long before analysis, there is a potential for ketones to be broken down by bacterial action and give a false-negative reaction. Specific chemical tests are available to measure individual ketone bodies, but these are rarely used today, since they have little clinical importance.

Reagent tablet tests exist for the determination of urinary ketones and can also be used on serum samples (10). These tablets are sometimes used to follow the course of strict dieting or when the concentration of acetoacetic acid is so high that dilution is required for accurate estimation. In the use of this product, Acetest, lactose is added to the other reactants on the test strip to provide enhanced color differentiation.

Bilirubin

Bilirubinuria, the presence of bilirubin in the urine, is an important early indicator of liver dysfunction and of intrinsic or extrinsic biliary obstruction. Bilirubinuria may be diagnosed before clinical jaundice appears. Bilirubin is formed from the breakdown of RBC hemoglobin. It attaches to albumin (indirect or unconjugated bilirubin) and is carried to the liver to be processed by the hepatocyte into a water-soluble form (direct or conjugated bilirubin). Unconjugated bilirubin is water insoluble and cannot be excreted by the kidneys because of its albumin binding and the fact that albumin is not generally filtered by the glomerulus. Conjugated bilirubin, on the other hand, is excreted in the urine because of its water solubility and ease of transport across the glomerular basement membrane (GBM). In normal circumstances, conjugated bilirubin never reaches the kidneys; it is entirely secreted into the bile after conjugation as bilirubin diglucuronide and then into the intestines, where it is broken down by bacteria into urobilinogen. In pathologic conditions, however, such as bile duct obstruction or hepatitis, conjugated bilirubin enters the bloodstream due to very high concentrations of processed bilirubin, and is then found in the urine because of its water solubility and ease of passage across the GBM (14).

Small quantities of conjugated bilirubin are normally present in urine ($\approx$ 0.02 mg/dl), but concentrations this low are not detectable using ordinary dipstick methodolgy. Unconjugated bilirubin is not normally found in the urine. A crude but rapid method for the determination of bilirubin in urine is often performed by house-staff officers when they want a quick answer to the question of whether a patient is jaundiced. Since conjugated bilirubin is water soluble, vigorous shaking of the test tube containing the suspect urine will produce a yellow foam if increased quantities of bilirubin are present, whereas if the urine contains normal amounts of bilirubin, the foam will be white.

Methodology for the semiquantitative determination of conjugated bilirubin in the urine depends on the color produced by the reaction of a diazotized aniline dye and bilirubin; a purplish azobilirubin compound develops. Reagent tablets (Ictotest), utilizing similar diazotized dyes, are available for use to confirm dipstick results and are more sensitive than the dipstick pads and less affected by interfering substances (10). The exact aniline dye used in dipsticks varies with the manufacturer. Results are interpreted as negative to 1+ (small amounts of bilirubin) to 3+ (large amounts of bilirubin).

It is of considerable importance that the urine be tested for bilirubin immediately after voiding, since bilirubin is unstable and breaks down rapidly, especially after exposure to light; prolonged exposure to room air will also cause the dipstick pad reaction to become negative due to oxidation of the bilirubin to biliverdin, a substance that is nonreactive to the diazo dyes. False-negative results are obtained on the bilirubin pad when the tested urine contains large quantities of ascorbic acid (vitamin C) or nitrites (released because of bacterial growth).

Urobilinogen

Urobilinogen is also a product of hemoglobin metabolism and is formed with the degradation of bilirubin in bacteria in the intestine. About half of the urobilinogen is excreted in the feces and the other half is reabsorbed into the circulation from the intestines. This reabsorbed urobilinogen is then filtered by the kidneys and appears in the urine if increased in amount. In normal persons, only small amounts of urobilinogen are excreted in the urine daily, usually less than 4 mg; a random urine sample contains 0.1 to 1 mg/dl. Serum and urine urobilinogen levels increase when there is increased bilirubin production: this may occur in severe liver disease such as cirrhosis or hepatitis (the liver cannot remove reabsorbed urobilinogen from the blood) and in hemolytic disorders (excess urobilinogen is produced in the intestines due to excessive bilirubin production and the liver cannot handle it all). Blockage of the biliary system, such as occurs in ampullary carcinoma or with gallstones in the common bile duct, does not lead to an increase in urine urobilinogen levels since bilirubin never reaches the intestinal tract where it can be broken down into urobilinogen.

The dipstick method for the detection of urobilinogen (Urobilstix and Multistix makes use of the Ehrlich reaction; when urobilinogen is mixed with diethylaminobenzaldehyde in an acid buffer, a tan to orange colored compound is formed (10). Using the Ehrlich reactants, some compounds other than urobilinogen (i.e., porphobilinogen, sulfonamides and aminosalicylic acid) also produce a colored reaction and, if present, cause false-positive results. A relatively new and more specific method for the detection of urobilinogen utilizes a stable diazonium salt (4-methoxybenzenediazonium fluoborate) in an acid buffer. With the Chemstrip dipstick, a red azo dye color is produced when urobilinogen is present in urine in excess (22). After the dipstick is immersed in urine, the color produced is compared with a color chart to interpret the urobilinogen concentration. No color development on the pad suggests that a normal amount of urobilinogen is present in the specimen (i.e., less than 1 mg/dl); development of significant color implies an abnormal concentration of urobilinogen in the urine. Compounds other than urobilinogen do not produce color on the pad.

False-negative results for urobilinogen can be obtained whenever the urine is allowed to remain in daylight for extended time periods after voiding, as the urobilinogen breaks down. If formaldehyde is used as a urine preservative, it will inhibit the reaction and produce a false-negative result. Pharmaceuticals that contain azo dyes may mask the colors of the urobilinogen pad and lead to erroneous interpretations. Finally, the Ehrlich reaction may be inhibited by high concentrations of nitrites, a product of bacterial metabolism (11, 23).

Determination of the presence of excess urobilinogen in urine in a jaundiced patient may be of primary importance in differentiating between obstruction of the biliary tract or upper intestines and hepatic or hemolytic disease. If the upper bowel or common bile duct is obstructed, bilirubin does not reach the intestines and urobilinogen is not produced and therefore is not found in the urine. On the other hand, in the same conditions, bilirubin is greatly elevated in both serum and urine, and the bilirubin test pad will show a positive result.

Nitrite

This test provides an effective and rapid method for screening urine for the presence of a bacterial infection (24). The test is based on the principle that most bacteria found in urine have the ability to reduce urine nitrate, a plentiful constituent of urine, to nitrite. These organisms include *Escherichia coli, Klebsiella, Proteus, Staphylococcus,* and *Pseudomonas*, to mention a few that are frequent causes of urinary tract infections. The determination of clinical *bacteriuria*, is of major significance when culture shows the presence of more than 10^5 colonies per milliliter. Bacterial infections of the urinary tract are usually accompanied by the presence of large numbers of white blood cells in the urine, most often neutrophils. Occasionally, urinary tract infection may give rise to no clinical symptoms; in these asymptomatic individuals the urine examination is of prime importance in diagnosis and in the prevention of long-term complications, especially in the kidneys. Urine nitrite determinations are not designed to replace culture as a means of identification of specific organisms or to replace sediment examination to determine whether or not the bacterium is a contaminant. However, the nitrite test does serve as a valuable screening tool, along with the leukocyte esterase dipstick test, in defining whether a urinary tract infection is present (25). Concomitant negative dipstick results from both tests provide a predictive value of over 95% that culture for urinary tract infection will be negative (10).

The chemical basis of the nitrite reaction is that in an acid environment, nitrite reacts with an aromatic amine (sulfanilamide or *p*-arsanilic acid) to form a colored diazonium salt that in turn reacts with a hydroxy-benzoquinoline to provide a pink color (Griess reaction). A positive reaction occurs when the bacterial content is greater than 10^5/ml. It is imperative that fresh urine samples are used when this test is interpreted to eliminate the possibility that the nitrate has been produced by bacterial contamination. First-voided morning specimens are best for detecting bactiuria. If bacterial infection is present in the urinary tract, a single dipstick test will be positive in 80 to 90% of patients when the first morning specimen is promptly examined (10). The nitrite test is qualitative, and any shade of pink produced is considered a positive result and indicative of bacterial infection of the urinary tract.

Negative test results for nitrite are found when the particular species of bacteria does not reduce nitrate in the urine. Therefore, a negative dipstick result when the patient is suspected of having an infection of the urinary tract should always be verified by urine culture and/or microscopy of the sediment. Fortunately, most bacteria that cause infections of the urinary tract are Gram negative and are nitrite forming. However, yeasts and a significant number of non–nitrite producing, Gram-positive cocci may cause infections of the urinary tract and produce a negative nitrite dipstick reaction. Other causes of false-negative results are the presence of high levels of ascorbic acid and urobilinogen in the urine (22). Adequacy of diet, especially in vegetables, to allow for sufficient nitrates to be formed is essential to the proper interpretation of this test. A diet deficient in vegetables may lead to erroneously false-negative dipstick reactions in urinary tract infections. Antibiotic agents may inhibit the growth of bacteria, even if present, and a false-negative test result is reported. False-positive results are obtained when various dyes, such as pyridium, discolor the strip test pad pink or red.

Leukocyte Esterase

Leukocyturia, or *pyuria*, is a valuable indicator of the presence of urinary tract inflammation (26, 27). The relatively recent advent of an enzymatic test for the presence of leukocyte esterase has provided a simple means for the detection of increased numbers of white blood cells in the urine (22). Neutrophils are nearly always present in infections and inflammations of the kidneys and lower urinary tract. They are nearly always associated with bacterial infections and are thus found in the urine in these conditions in elevated numbers. WBCs are normally present in a centrifuged urinary sediment in relatively small numbers, usually fewer than 5/hpf. Counts of WBCs of more than 10/hpf may be considered abnormal and should be investigated further (20). Pyelonephritis, cystitis, urethritis, renal calculi, interstitial nephritis, and glomerulonephritis all give rise to leukocyturia. On close examination, the WBCs are predominantly polymorphonuclear neutrophils (PMNs), although a scattering of other WBC types may be seen. Until the initiation of the leukocyte esterase test, the presence of leukocyturia was verified by microscopic analysis of the sediment (28).

The leukocyte esterase test is based on the release from neutrophils of the enzyme leukocyte esterase, and on the ability of this enzyme to split an ester and form a pyrrole. Depending on the test, the pyrrole either reacts with a diazo compound to form a colored azo dye (Multistix) or becomes oxidized to form an indigo dye that then reacts with a diazo salt to form a colored reaction within 2 minutes (Chemstrip) (10, 22). The color produced is dependent on the number of PMNs present in the urine. The sensitivity of the dipstick test has been adjusted to provide a negative reaction when fewer than 5 WBCs/hpf are present and a trace when there are from 5 to 15 WBCs/hpf. False-positive results are usually not seen, except when oxidizing agents have been mistakenly added to the urine container. Cells other than leukocytes that may be present in the urine, such as RBCs, epithelial cells, and bacteria, do not contain the leukocyte esterase enzyme in their cytoplasm and cannot produce a positive strip reaction. However, large numbers of eosinophils or a heavy infestation of the vaginal parasite *Trichomonas vaginalis* may provide sufficient esterase to give a false-positive result (10). False-negative results are found when there are high levels of vitamin C, oxidizing agents, formalin, or albumin in the urine (22). Mention should be made of the fact that the leukocyte esterase test may occasionally be positive even when neutrophils cannot be demonstrated in the urinary sediment. This may be due to lysis of neutrophils in the urine prior to microscopic examination and release of their cytoplasmic contents. If such a circumstance occurs, a repeat of the urinalysis using a freshly voided specimen will usually reveal many intact WBCs in the sediment.

Specific Gravity

Waste product excretion and reabsorption of vital chemicals are two of the most important functions of the kidneys (20). A measure of their reabsorptive capacity provides a valuable test of renal function, and estimation of urine specific gravity provides just such a measurement. The specific gravity of a liquid provides an estimation of the density of the solid substances dissolved in it. As a measure of density, specific gravity varies according to the size and number of the particles present in the liquid. The specific gravity of urine is a useful indicator of the ability of the renal tubules to concentrate or dilute the urine. Normally functioning kidneys are able to alter the specific gravity of urine in a range of 1.003 to 1.035; early-morning urine specimens are usually more concentrated than random samples taken at various times during the day and tend to have specific gravity readings above 1.020, while urine voided at other times during the day, especially after ingestion of water and food, are lower. A specific gravity over 1.025 in a random urine sample serves as reasonably good evidence that the concentrating ability is preserved. Specific gravity may be at the upper end of the normal scale (i.e., above 1.025) in patients with congestive heart failure, severe liver disease, dehydration and vomiting, and diarrhea who have experienced severe water loss. Kidneys lose their concentrating abilities in severe end-stage renal disease; in these cases the urine may have a "fixed" specific gravity near 1.010. Low values are also obtained in diabetes insipidus, in which antidiuretic hormone excretion is compromised.

In the past, an instrument called a urinometer was employed for the estimation of specific gravity. The principle of its use is simple: a weighted float displaces a volume of urine proportional to the amount of dissolved substances present in the urine in which it is immersed (10). The more dissolved substances that are present, the more the float is pushed out of the urine or the less it sinks (with distilled water being calibrated at 1.000). This testing method is no longer advised for use in clinical laboratories due to the considerable error that is encountered because the urinometer is standardized for a certain temperature (20°C) and it is difficult to obtain constant temperatures for urine and the environment. Also, because the instrument cannot touch the sides of the urine container during reading, use of the urinometer requires a large container and therefore a large volume of urine.

The refractometer, which is temperature corrected, is the most accurate and widely used instrument for the estimation of urine specific gravity (6–8). It measures the amount of dissolved substances in a liquid by measuring the refractive index of the liquid. This task is performed by comparing the velocity of light in air with the velocity of light in the urine. Increases in the concentration of dissolved substances in a solution change the velocity of light penetrating the solution and therefore the angle of the light as it enters a prism. This angle is then converted to specific gravity by the use of standard scales. The most important advantages of the refractometer over the urinometer is that it can provide an accurate measurement of specific gravity with only a few drops of urine, and that the instruments in current use are temperature corrected, facilitating standardization. When large amounts of protein or glucose are present in the urine, certain corrections are necessary to ensure accuracy because of the significantly increased density of the solution, but these corrections are less significant than with the urinometer. Maintaining the refractometer requires little more than cleaning the glass prism and cover after each use (quality control procedures are considered elsewhere in this chapter).

Specific gravity can be estimated with a dipstick available from one manufacturer (Multistix, the Ames Company, Elkhart, Indiana) (10). This colorimetric method provides a fast and convenient way of estimating the specific gravity of urine without the use of a refractometer (29). Specific gravity estimation by dipstick is an indirect method based on the principle that a change in ionic concentration of a solution initiates a change in the dissociation constant (pK) of pretreated polyelectrolytes (polymethylvinyl ether/maleic acid) embedded in the dipstick pad. This change is then detectable by the use of a pH indicator dye (bromthymol blue). The polyelectrolyte is sensitive to the electrolyte ions in solution in the urine; when these ions increase in number, the pK of the dipstick pad is decreased, thus reducing the pH. This pH change is reflected by a change in the color of the indicator on the dipstick pad; i.e., the indicator, bromthymol blue, changes from blue to yellowish-green (more acidic), and this transformation is directly related to specific gravity.

Another method to assess specific gravity is by the use of the "falling drop" procedure. This method is useful for equipment that automates the reading of dipsticks (e.g., Yellow IRIS, Clintek Auto 2000); it is a more specific measure of specific gravity than the one provided by refractometry. A water-immiscible silicon oil that has a predetermined constant specific gravity is utilized (10). As the urine drops in a carefully designed column filled with this oil, the time it takes for a urine drop to fall a given distance is determined; the falling time is accurately measured by electronic means and is then directly converted to specific gravity units.

Ascorbic Acid

Vitamin C is a frequently administered pharmaceutical that often interferes with several of the usual dipstick reactions (e.g., glucose, bilirubin, leukocyte esterase, hemoglobin, nitrite). For this reason, it became important to develop a convenient means of testing for its presence in the urine so that if interferences were suspected, alternate testing for specific substances could be initiated. Erroneous results should be suspected when a microscopic sediment evaluation shows RBCs, but the dipstick is negative for hemoglobin. The various dipstick reactions are based on the powerful reducing property of vitamin C and the change in indicator dye color when this reduction occurs (10).

Phenylpyruvic Acid

It is clinically important to determine whether phenylpyruvic acid is present in the urine of very young infants, since its presence is diagnostic of phenylketonuria (PKU) (14). PKU is an inherited metabolic disease in which there is absence of an enzyme, phenylalanine hydroxylase, that is necessary for the conversion of phenylalanine, present in milk, to tyrosine. In the absence of this enzyme, metabolites of phenylalanine, such as phenylpyruvic acid, accumulate and cause brain damage. Treatment is dietary with removal of foods and milk containing phenylalanine. If undiagnosed and untreated, PKU results in permanent brain damage and mental insufficiency, thus early diagnosis by screening urine for phenylpyruvic acid is an important preventive measure. Strip testing is available for the detection of phenylpyruvic acid (Phenstix) and when present, phenylpyruvic acid reacts with a buffered ferric ion solution on the strip to form a bluish-green reaction; the color develops in 30 seconds and it is compared with a color chart for an estimate of the concentration of phenylpyruvic acid (10).

Miscellaneous Tests

Several other tests may be performed on urine samples using various technologies (10, 11, 14). Melanin may be present in the urine in metastatic malignant melanoma, and several different methods for its detection are available. Serotonin, a metabolite of tryptophan, is found in the urine of some patients with tumors of argentaffin cells (carcinoid tumors). Testing urine for its metabolite, 5-hydroxy-indoleacetic acid, is a valuable means of diagnosing this condition. In porphyria, a group of inherited enzyme-deficient diseases of hemoglobin metabolism, intermediary metabolic products may appear in the urine. Specific methods for the detection of these products (i.e., porphobilinogen, uroporphyrin, and coproporphyrin) are available and should be utilized when a clinical diagnosis of one of the porphyrias is suspected because of the presence of such symptoms as skin lesions, photosensitivity, recurrent acute abdominal pain, neurologic symptoms, or urine that changes color in light.

MICROSCOPIC URINALYSIS

A microscopic evaluation of the urinary sediment often produces valuable information that provides the clinician with a more specific diagnosis or an assessment of therapy that could not otherwise be obtained if only a physicochemical examination of the urine were performed (30). Recent controversy concerning the cost efficiency of the microscopic part of the urinalysis procedure has centered around the relatively low rate of positive results from sediments in which the chemical examination was negative (28, 31, 32). Without debating this issue, it should be the responsibility of each laboratory to establish its own guidelines for urine analysis that include when to perform a microscopic evaluation; these guidelines should be based on sound scientific evidence (8). As a general "well population" screening procedure, urine microscopics are not particularly cost effective; on the other hand, in a hospitalized population, especially in patients on urology or general medical wards, this part of the examination has been shown to be very valuable.

The procedure for the performance of microscopic urinalysis is quite simple and requires little additional equipment other than what is ordinarily found in any well-equipped laboratory; i.e., a calibrated centrifuge, a modern, clean binocular microscope, and a means of ensuring that strict quality assurance procedures are followed (7). There is no substitute for experience and training on the part of the technologist or physicial for accurate sediment evaluation (30). Constituents in the sediment can be varied, and accurate interpretation often depends on prior experience. Although some have advocated not centrifuging the urine when doing a microscopic examination (this is a common practice in England), this author is not one of those. Centrifugation of 10 or 12 ml of urine at a constant time of 5 minutes and a relative centrifugal force (RCF) of 400 to 500 is the usual standard of practice in the United States (11, 20). The sediment is produced at the bottom of the centrifuge tube. There are a number of commercial products that offer a "system" for the processing of urine to obtain a sediment; these all yield a constant volume of sediment admixed with urine so that an aliquot may be decanted and then viewed with a microscope (20). As an example, if the initial volume of urine is 12 ml and the volume of the sediment remaining after decanting the supernatant urine is 1 ml, the resulting concentration of the sediment is 12:1. If a "system" is utilized—and the use of one is highly recommended—the concentrated sediment is pipetted into a constant-volume chamber on a microscopic slide. In such instances, this procedure ensures that the volume of the concentrated urine observed in the chamber will be constant from patient to patient and from day to day—an important consideration in quality assurance (6). Since constant volumes of urine are utilized, when sediment elements are recognized, these can be quantitated on a volume basis (i.e., numbers per milliliter), rather than as numbers per microscopic field. Prior to the advent of constant-volume slide chambers, the usual procedure for microscopic examination of the urine was to place a drop of the concentrated centrifuged urine sediment on a glass microscopic slide and observe it with a microscope. Great discrepancies could be found in the quantitation of the elements because of the variability of the size of the urine drop and the weight of the coverslip. The use of a standardized system for this examination permits much greater consistency in the reporting of results.

Table 23.2. Constituents of Normal Urine Sediment

Cells	Crystals	Casts	Other
Blood cells	Acid urine	Hyaline	Mucus
RBC	Amorphous	Granular	Sperm
WBC	Uric acid		Microorganisms
Epithelial cells	Neutral urine		Bacteria
Squamous	Calcium oxalate		Fungi
Urothelial	Hippuric acid		Contaminants
Renal tubular	Alkaline urine		Fibers
	Triple phosphate		Pollen
	Ammonium biurate		
	Calcium carbonate		

Centrifugation at an RCF of 400 to 500 for 5 minutes produces a concentrated sediment in which all elements present may be easily found and are not artifacturally distorted by compacting during centrifugation (8). Since most modern centrifuges can be adjusted for rpm but not for RCF, the following formula is used, which takes into consideration the radius of the centrifuge head.

$$\text{RCF} = 1.118 \times 10^{-5} \times \text{radius of centrifuge head in cm} \times \text{rpm}^2$$

Normal Urinary Sediment

Recognition of sediment elements depends on a "good eye," knowing what should be present in normal urine and being able to accurately define and contrast the normal with the potentially abnormal. Certain particles or elements may appear in the urine in normal persons. These are blood cells, cells lining the urinary tract, mucus secretions of glands, cylindrical proteinaceous particles that have formed in the nephron (casts), crystals that have formed in the urine, and foreign cells (e.g., spermatozoa in a female), microorganisms, or contaminants (Table 23.2) (12, 20, 30). Each of these constituents is discussed separately.

BLOOD CELLS

Erythrocytes (RBCs) and leukocytes (WBCs) may be found in small numbers in the normal sediment. Both of these cells may pass through the glomerulus and enter the urinary flow. Quantitation of these cells over a given time period, such as 12 hours, is uncommonly performed today due to the great varia-

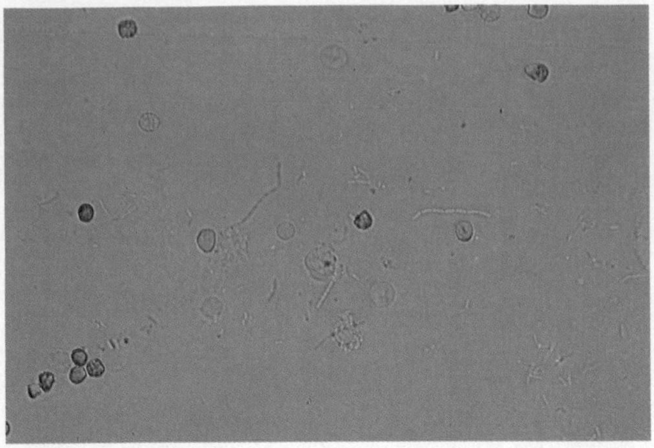

Figure 23.1. Red blood cells and bacteria in urine sediment. This field contains a scattering of RBCs and bacillary forms. This is slightly more than the usual number of RBCs one would expect to find in a high-power field and would generally warrant further investigation. Two leukocytes are also present in the center of the field. (Bright field microscopy [BF], ×160.)

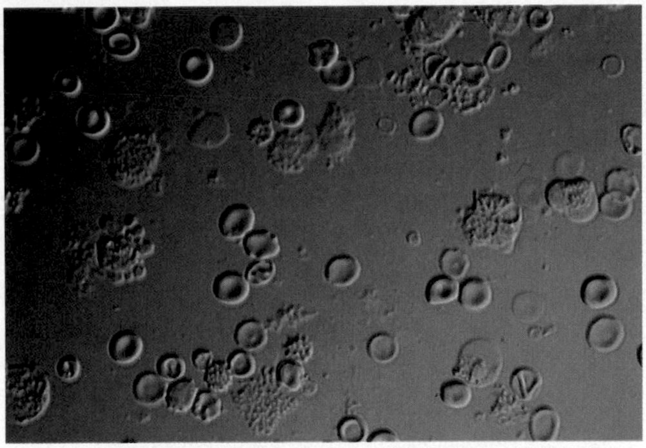

Figure 23.2. PMNs and RBCs in urine. This unstained photomicrograph vividly demonstrates the biconcavity of RBCs and also the multilobed nuclei and granular cytoplasm of the neutrophils. A few RBCs are crenated. (Interference contrast microscopy [ICM], ×200.)

tion in cellular excretion from person to person and the difficulties associated with the collection of the urine and the counting technique (Addis count; a hemocytometer counting chamber is utilized) (33). A normal person may eliminate up to 750,000 RBCs and 1,750,000 WBCs in 12 hours.

RBCs

In any given urine sediment obtained from a normal person, small quantities of erythrocytes may be present (Fig. 23.1); these vary in number from none per high-power microscopic field (hpf) to as many as 5/hpf (30). The usual normal sediment will contain an occasional RBC per every other field; counts greater than 5/hpf should be thoroughly investigated and an explanation for the hematuria sought. Microscopically, the RBCs appear similar to those found in the peripheral blood, i.e. biconcave discs that have a pale faint orange color confirming their hemoglobin content (Fig. 23.2). In hypertonic urine, RBCs may be crenated and in hypotonic urine they may swell, become spherical, and burst in due course, leaving only the cell membrane or "ghost" visible. Small globules of oil may simulate the appearance of RBCs. The oil is frequently from the skin of the microscopist. Oil droplets may be differentiated from RBCs on the basis of variable size, absence of hemoglobin, and a spherical rather than biconcave disc shape.

WBCs

Leukocytes are frequently found in the normal urine sediment, but their numbers are small and should not exceed 5/hpf (12, 20). Although all the WBC types that appear in the peripheral blood may also be found in urine (i.e., lymphocyte, monocyte, eosinophil), the most common cell present is the polymorphonuclear neutrophil (PMN). In fact, it is unusual to find any leukocyte other than a PMN in a normal person's sediment. PMNs have a phagocytic function, are actively motile, and move by means of ameboid action with the extension of pseudopods. Leukocytes measure 10 to 20 μm in diameter, with lymphocytes being on the smaller end of that range and PMNs at the upper. PMNs are readily recognized in urine due to their multisegmented nuclei and their granular cytoplasm in which brownian movement is often noted.

Staining the sediment enables the observer to diagnose PMNs more readily since the multilobed nucleus is clearly apparent and confusion with nonleukocytic cells, such as renal tubular epithelial cells, is less likely. Differential staining with Wright's or Giemsa stain provides an accurate means of identifying the various other leukocytes, such as lymphocytes and eosinophils (30). This becomes important when WBCs are increased in number, but is unnecessary in the normal sediment evaluation.

EPITHELIAL CELLS

Normal urine contains three main varieties of epithelial cells: renal tubular, urothelial or transitional, and squamous (30). These cells provide the lining for the urinary tract and compose the tubules of the nephron. Table 23.3 lists some differentiating features of each of these epithelial cell types.

Renal Tubular Epithelial Cells

Renal tubular epithelial cells (RTEs) are infrequently present in the urine sediment in the normal person (0 to 1 per 5 hpf). When observed, they are usually single, but may also be seen in pairs. If a

Table 23.3. Epithelial Cells of Urine

	Renal Tubular	Urothelial	Squamous
Origin	Nephron	Renal pelvis, ureter, bladder, proximal urethra	Terminal urethra, vagina
Size	15–25 μm	20–30	30–50
Shape	Polyhedral	Polyhedral, "tadpole," spherical	Flattened
Other	Microvilli if from proximal tubule		

microvillus border is present, their origin can be presumed to be the proximal tubule. Specific immunohistochemical identification may be made, when warranted, by means of acid phosphatase staining, since the RTEs have a high intracellular content of this enzyme (30). Their shape is most often polyhedral, but they may also be somewhat flattened (indicating that they originate from the loop of Henle). Their nucleus is usually eccentric but may be central; it is spherical, with nucleoli readily apparent if there are no autolytic changes. In certain disease states, primarily those that affect the tubular portions of the nephron, the number of RTEs in the sediment may be significantly increased.

RTEs are normally found in the urine because of the constant process of tubular cell renewal and regeneration. In a renal biopsy, tubular lining cells show frequent mitotic activity; the older cells are sloughed into the urine flow and may then be seen in the sediment after having been replaced by the newly fashioned cell. This type of cell regeneration occurs in the most proximal nephron, rather than the distal.

Transitional Epithelial Cells

These cells (also called urothelial cells) constitute the lining epithelium for a large portion of the urinary tract and are frequently present in the sediment (0 to 1/hpf) due to their high turnover rate. Transitional epithelium is stratified and is ordinarily several cell layers thick. Only the most superficial cells are found in the urine and these take three main shapes: spherical (Fig. 23.3), polyhedral, and "tadpole." Urothelial cells have the peculiar characteristic of being able to absorb water and thus swell to as much as 2 times their original size, when they acquire a spherical contour (20). Polyhedrally shaped transitional cells may present difficulties in differentiation from RTEs if they have no microvillus surface and have a central rather than an eccentric nucleus. The cytoplasm of transitional cells does not contain large quantities of acid phosphatases. Tadpole-shaped urothelial cells are frequently observed in urine.

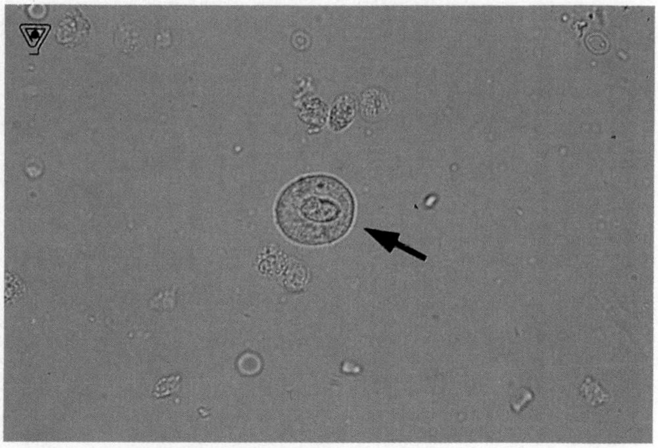

Figure 23.3. Urothelial cell *(arrow)* and occasional red and white cells in urine. Note the spherical shape and central nucleus of this cell. (BF, ×160.) (Reproduced by permission from the College of American Pathologists.)

They probably derive from the mid-stratification layers of the transitional epithelium (12). Tadpole transitional cells appear in groups or pairs, as well as singly. Their nucleus is usually central, and they have a fusiform-shaped cytoplasm. Transitional cells increase in number in the urine in certain inflammatory conditions affecting the urinary tract.

Squamous Epithelial Cells

Squames are the easiest of all the epithelial cells to recognize in the urine because they are large, flat, and frequent (Fig. 23.4). In a well-collected midstream "clean catch" specimen, their numbers should be small (i.e., less than 1/hpf). The finding of numerous squamous cells in urine from a female patient usually indicates vaginal contamination. Squamous epithelium normally lines the terminal third of the urethra in both men and women, and it is also the epithelium that lines the vagina. A "clean catch" urine collection is a more difficult achievement in women than in men, and contamination with vaginal fluid and cells is common, especially when the patient has not been instructed beforehand on how to collect the specimen properly (8).

CRYSTALS

Finding crystalline forms in urine sediment is common if the urine has been allowed to stand after voiding, but this finding is infrequent in fresh urine. The formation of crystals is related to the concentration of various salts in the urine and this in turn is related to the patient's metabolic state, diet, and fluid intake as well as to the effects of the changes that occur in the urine after voiding (i.e., changes in pH and temperature, which change the solubility of salts in the urine and promote crystal formation). Since

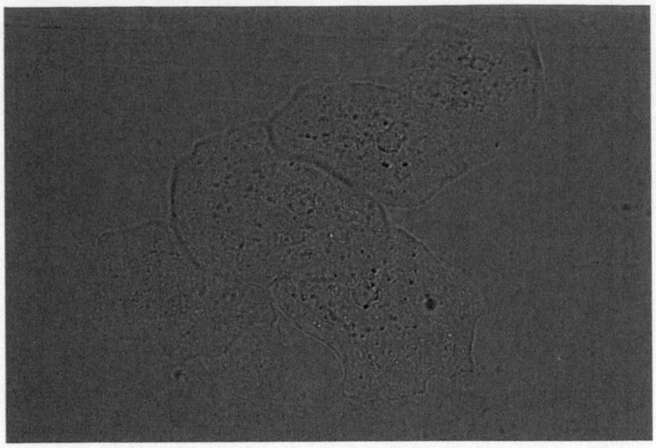

Figure 23.4. A group of squamous epithelial cells in urine. The cells are large and flat and have some granules in their cytoplasm. The central nucleus is approximately the size of a large lymphocyte. (BF, ×160.)

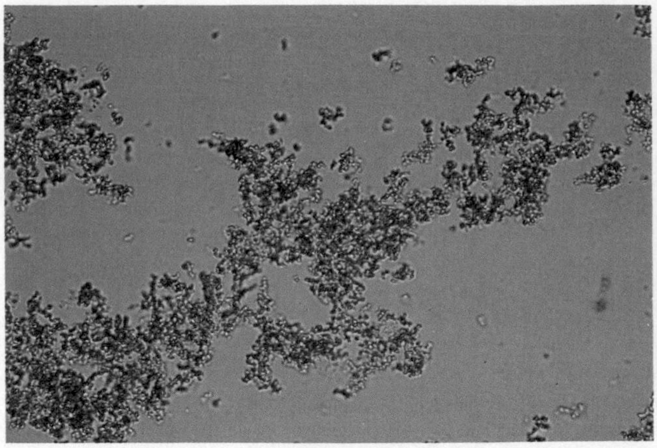

Figure 23.5. Amorphous urate crystals in urine. (BF, ×160.) (Reproduced by permission from the College of American Pathologists.)

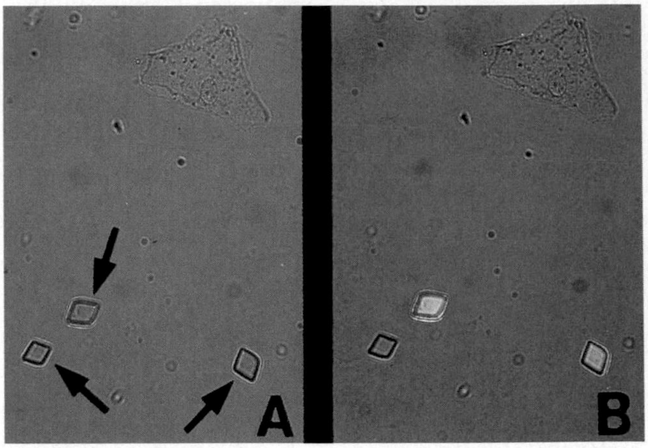

Figure 23.6. Uric acid crystals *(arrows)* and squamous cell. In this view, the urate crystals are rhomboid (**A**) and display anisotropism under polarized light (**B**). (BF and polarized [POL], ×80.) (Reproduced by permission from the College of American Pathologists.)

the kidneys play a major role in metabolite excretion and the maintenance of homeostasis, the end products of metabolism are found in high concentrations in the urine, and these tend to precipitate and form crystals (10). The pH of normal urine varies from acid to alkaline, and certain crystals are associated with an acid pH, whereas others may be more commonly found in alkaline urine (20). There are relatively few crystals associated with a normal state, and the student is well advised to become aware of their various morphological forms and characteristics. Most normally occurring crystals have little if any pathologic significance. The more common varieties are described here. In a later section of this chapter, several "abnormal" crystals are considered.

Uric Acid Crystals

Uric acid, a metabolic product of protein breakdown, is present in the urine in high concentrations and commonly produces a wide assortment of crystalline structures. Amorphous urates may be described as granular, birefringent, colorless to pale yellow crystals without a particular microscopic structure; they appear as fine granules when observed with the 10× or 40× microscopic objectives (Fig. 23.5). These crystals frequently develop when urine has been refrigerated, and they may be so plentiful that they obscure any other sediment elements present. When urine is prepared for microscopic examination, these crystals are noted as the compacted "pink button" of sediment at the bottom of the centrifuge tube. Most amorphous urates dissolve when alkali is added to the sediment or when the urine is warmed (to at least room temperature) after refrigeration.

Uric acid crystals are among the most pleomorphic of all urine crystals; they assume a wide variety of forms, including rods, cubes (Fig. 23.6), rosettes, six-sided plates, rhombi, and a whetstone shape. They are strongly birefringent and vary greatly in size. Uric acid crystals are soluble in alkaline solutions and insoluble in acid (14). They are colorless to pale yellow to pinkish-brown. Uric acid crystals have been associated with renal stones, but their presence in the urine in the normal person is so common that this association has little if any clinical significance.

Other urate salts may form crystals in the urine; i.e., sodium and potassium urates. These can be seen as colorless, needle-shaped crystals and brownish spherules, respectively.

Calcium Oxalate

Aside from uric acid crystals, calcium oxalate is the most frequently observed crystal in both acid and

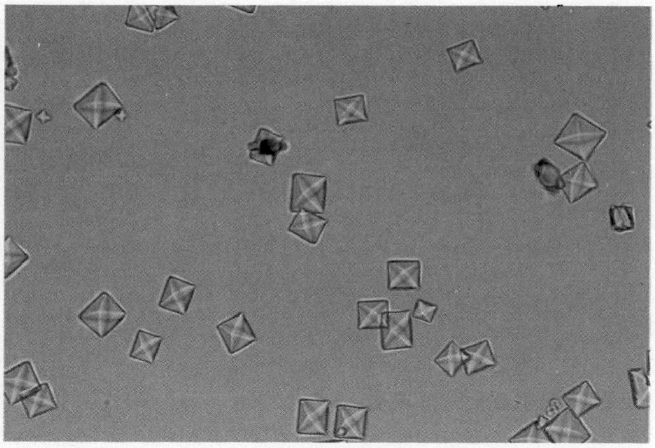

Figure 23.7. Calcium oxalate crystals. Their square shape and "starred," envelope-like appearance are characteristic. (BF, ×160.)

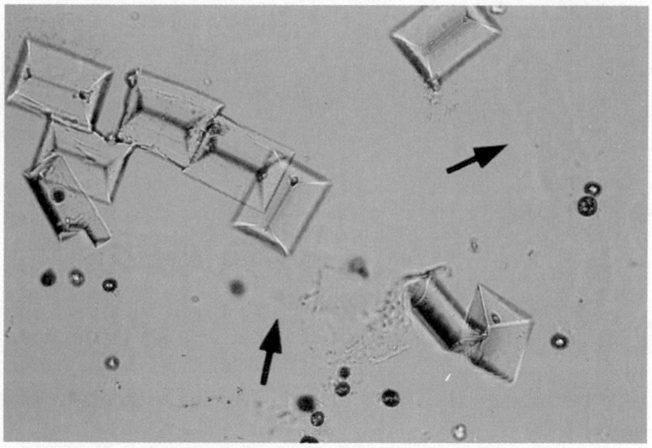

Figure 23.8. Triple phosphate crystals in urine. Hyaline casts *(arrows)* are seen in the background. (BF, ×160.) (Reproduced by permission from the College of American Pathologists.)

neutral urine (Fig. 23.7). This colorless, birefringent crystal is identified by its characteristic octahedral shape, for which it is called the "envelope" crystal (30). These crystals are found in abundance in normal persons, especially if they have ingested ascorbic acid in high doses or have eaten foods rich in oxalic acid (tomatoes, asparagus). Oxalic acid crystals may also take other forms in urine such as dumbbell and elliptical shapes.

Hippuric Acid Crystals

While they are not often diagnosed in urine, hippuric acid crystals are also associated with a neutral pH. These crystals are usually seen as colorless, elongate prisms with pyramidal ends; they may also be thin and needle-like. They are birefringent and are associated with diets high in fruits and vegetables containing large quantities of benzoic acid (10, 11).

Amorphous Phosphate Crystals

Crystals derived from phosphates are the most frequently observed crystals associated with alkaline urine. The most common of these is the amorphous phosphate crystal. Microscopically, these cannot be distinguished from amorphous urate crystals present in acid urine. They are fine, granular, birefringent crystals that produce a white precipitate in the bottom of the centrifuge tube. They may also obscure other sediment elements, since they are often formed in large quantities.

Triple Phosphate Crystals

Triple phosphate (ammonium-magnesium phosphate) crystals are birefringent crystals that assume a "coffin-lid" appearance (Fig. 23.8). They are usually colorless and birefringent, and they vary greatly in size, they may also be found in neutral urine. These crystals are soluble in acetic acid.

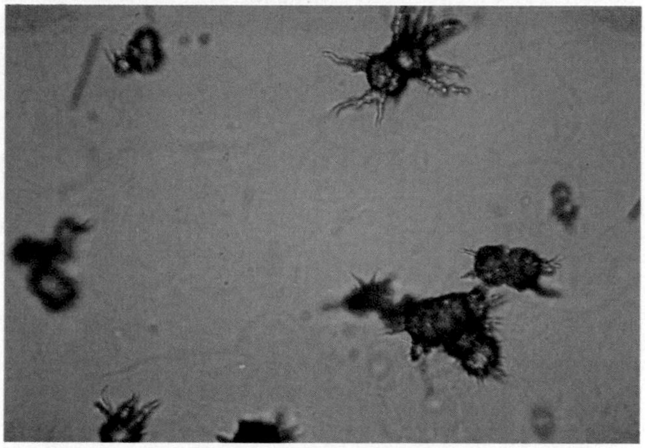

Figure 23.9. Ammonium biurate crystals in urine. These "crab-shaped," spiculated crystals are characteristic and are associated with alkaline urine. (BF, ×400.) (Reproduced by permission from the College of American Pathologists.)

Ammonium Biurate Crystals

Ammonium biurate crystals have a peculiar "crab-like" or "thorn-apple" shape (Fig. 23.9). They are yellowish-brown and often demonstrate radial or concentric striations in a central sphere with "arms" or spicules radiating from it. They are uncommonly present in normal urine and are soluble in sodium hydroxide.

Calcium Carbonate Crystals

Calcium carbonate crystals are small spherules of dumbbell-shaped birefringent crystals found in alkaline urine. Because of their small size they are often mistaken for bacteria. A ready means of differentiation is by the use of polarization, since bacteria are

Table 23.4. Classification of Urinary Casts

Acellular Casts	Cellular Casts
Normal	Normal
Hyaline	None
Granular	None
Abnormal	Abnormal
Hyaline	RBC
Granular	WBC
Waxy	Epithelial (RTE)
Pigment	Fatty/oval fat bodies
Fatty	Bacterial/fungal

not birefringent. These crystals dissolve in acetic acid and, in the process, effervesce.

CASTS

Urine casts are defined as cylindrical microscopic structures that form in the distal nephron and occur in the urine in both health and disease (34). These "cylinders" are composed primarily of a kidney-specific protein that is produced only in the distal tubule and collecting duct of the nephron (Tamm-Horsfall mucoprotein, THM) (35, 36). As THM is excreted by lining cells of the distal tubules and collecting ducts, certain events occur in the glomerular filtrate in the lumen of the nephron that induce this soluble protein to become insoluble and to form thin, proteinaceous bands that may then coalesce or be molded into a cast. The cast thus formed represents an exact model of the shape of the lumen of the renal tubule in which it originated, much as a mold of gelatin assumes the exact shape of the container the liquid gelatin is placed in. In experimental studies, changes in certain physical factors are necessary to induce soluble THM to become fibrillar. These include changes in urine flow, ionic strength, concentration, salinity, and pH of the glomerular filtrate. It is likely that in both normal and disease states similar changes occur in human urine, especially in physiologic stress, which induces previously soluble THM to become insoluble and to form fibrils, which then coalesce into casts.

The classification of renal casts is simple and is based on morphologic appearances (Table 23.4) (34). In the normal state, only two varieties of casts appear in the urinary sediment: hyaline casts and granular casts (17). Any additional cast forms must be considered "abnormal" and are most often associated with generalized metabolic or intrinsic renal diseases. Each cast type is discussed separately in detail below. Casts, in contrast to cells, are quantitated in the sediment as number per low-power microscopic field (lpf).

In the normal person, the presence of small numbers of hyaline or granular casts in the urine is a frequent occurrence and does not ordinarily present diagnostic difficulty or imply renal disease. The microscopist usually scans the sediment using the 10× objective, and occasionally casts are found, somewhere in the order of one or two per 10 lpf. These two forms of casts have a low refractive index and are therefore somewhat difficult to see with the ordinary light microscope unless the contrast is enhanced. Stopping down the iris diaphragm on the condenser while lowering it and keeping the light intensity the same will produce the optimal contrast for this observation. A quick scan of the entire microscopic slide will reveal if any casts are present and their numbers; and subsequent specific identification can be made using the 10× or 40× lens.

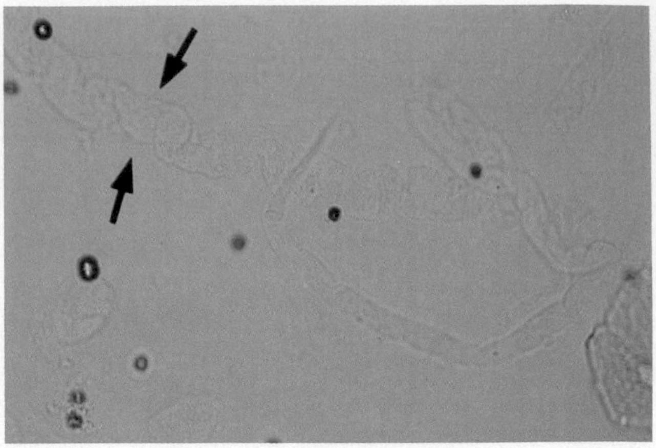

Figure 23.10. Hyaline casts. These translucent, colorless proteinaceous structures *(arrows)* are frequently found in normal urine sediment. Their low refractive index makes them difficult to discern using ordinary BF microscopy. (BF, ×100.) (Reproduced by permission from the College of American Pathologists.)

Hyaline Cast

This is the most frequently observed cast in the urine. It is typically translucent and somewhat difficult to see because of its low refractive index. Careful inspection shows a smooth outer perimeter and a matrix that is most often smooth but may be wavy (Fig. 23.10) (37). Occasional granular inclusions may be present in the matrix, and sometimes a cell or two may also be seen. The cast may have one end that, instead of being curved, is drawn out into a "tail" or point. In the past, these casts with tails were called "cylindroids"; this term is considered antiquated and is not commonly used today (Fig. 23.11).

Staining the sediment, or using phase microscopy (38), is very helpful in the identification and quantitation of all casts, but is especially useful for hyaline casts in particular; with ordinary bright-field microscopy and an unstained sediment sample, hyaline casts are somewhat difficult to find.

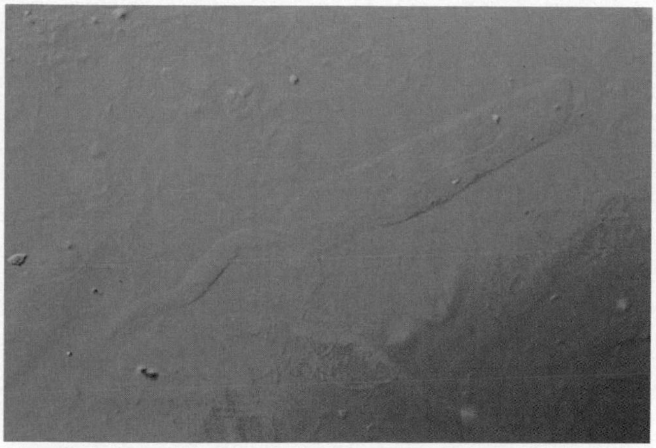

Figure 23.11. Urine cylindroid—a hyaline cast with a tail. The term "cylindroid" is antiquated. (ICM, ×160.)

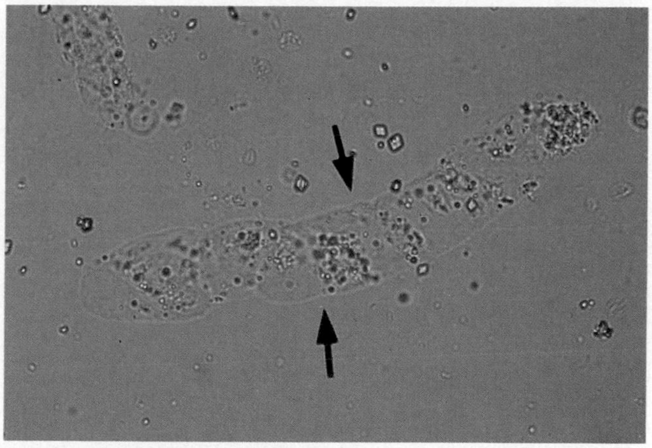

Figure 23.12. Granular cast. This type of cast is fundamentally a hyaline cast to which granules have attached along its surface. In the example shown here *(arrows)*, the granules do not cover the entire surface of the cast but are relatively evenly dispersed. (BF, ×160.) (Reproduced by permission from the College of American Pathologists.)

The effects of stress and strenuous physical exercise on the production and appearance of hyaline casts (also granular casts) in the urine have been well documented (17). Running a mile race or participating in a vigorous physical sport may induce the production of a large number of these casts (39). Stressful emotional situations, such as having to take an examination, can invoke the same phenomenon. *Cylindruria*, or the finding of increased numbers of casts in the urine, when the patient has undergone physical or emotional stress within the past 24 hours, should not be considered a pathologic condition. In such instances, the urine reverts to a normal state within 24 to 48 hours if the stressful situation or the physical exercise has stopped (17).

Granular Cast

These casts may also be observed in increased numbers in the urine if the patient has been involved in an emotionally stressful situation or has undergone recent strenuous physical exercise (17, 30). Compared to hyaline casts, granular casts are found in a ratio of approximately four hyaline for each granular. Once again, on removal of the stress or ending the exercise, the number of granular casts in the urine diminishes to normal within 24 to 48 hours. The reasons for the increased production of these casts in stress or exercise is unknown.

Granular casts have a higher index of refraction than do hyaline casts and are therefore easier to find. They are also cylindrical, although some may have "tails," and have a smooth, well-defined perimeter. Generally, in the normal person, granules covering the cast surface are small and regular (Fig. 23.12). The origin of these granules in the normal person appears to be at least in part from intracellular lysosomal particles that are expelled into the urine as metabolic products of the renal tubular epithelium (37, 40). Once in the urinary flow, the lysosomal granules are incorporated into a preformed hyaline cast matrix and thereby transform a previously smooth-surfaced hyaline cast into a granular cast.

MUCUS

It is thought that various glands that line the GU tract, such as those present in the prostatic urethra and urinary bladder, secrete this mucopolysaccharide into the urine. In addition, recent immunological studies have shown that at least some of the mucus present in the urine is in fact Tamm-Horsfall protein—a specific immunoprotein secreted exclusively in the nephron by the distal tubule and collecting duct lining cells (36). The clinical significance of THM in the urine is unknown. When large quantities of mucus are present in the sediment, vaginal secretions may be contaminating the specimen.

Mucus is a low-density substance that is often difficult to see unless sufficient contrast has been obtained with the microscope. It appears as thin, fibrillar, wavy, fiber-like bands or lines across the field that have no particular form or shape (Fig. 23.13). The inexperienced observer may sometimes confuse mucus with a hyaline cast due to coalescence of the individual ribbons into what may at first glance appear as a cylindrical object. Mucus has a low refractive index and is not birefringent. Sometimes, cells or microorganisms may get caught up in it.

MICROORGANISMS

Bacteria (Fig. 23.1), and occasionally yeast (Fig. 23.14), are often found in what is considered "normal" urine (41). Theoretically, at least, microorgan-

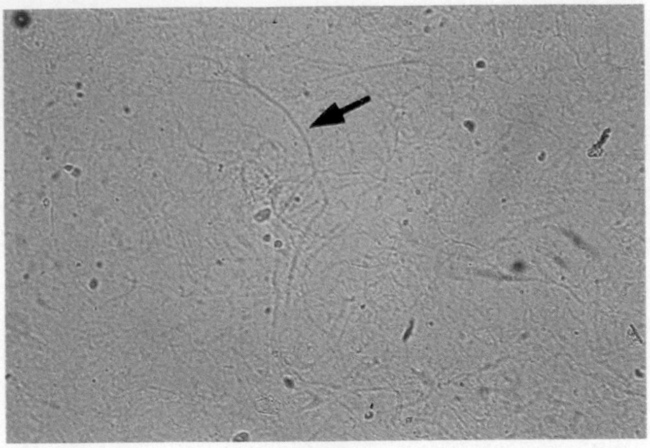

Figure 23.13. Mucus threads in urine. Thin, fibrillar mucus is a common feature of urine sediment and should not be confused with cast structures, as these threads do not acquire a cylindrical form. (BF, ×112.) (Reproduced by permission from the College of American Pathologists.)

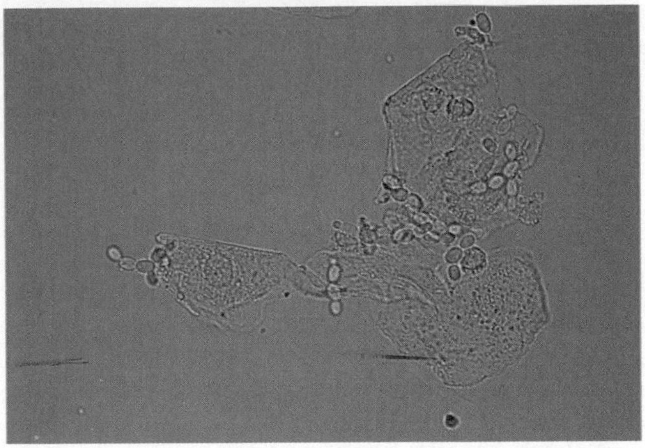

Figure 23.14. Budding yeast forms and squames in urine. When not accompanied by leukocytes, yeast forms are most likely growing contaminants, rather than pathogenic. They appear as spherical to elliptical transparent microorganisms about the same size as an RBC, with which they may be confused. (BF, ×160.)

isms should not be a part of the normal sediment. However, they are commonly found in normal urine because collection of the sample is performed without the use of adequate or effective precautionary techniques that would insure that no (or few) organisms contaminate the specimen. Additionally, collection systems frequently used to collect and transport the urine for examination are not sterile and may also serve as a source of microbiological contamination.

Urine is an excellent culture medium in which microorganisms grow with great rapidity. Therefore, when bacteria or yeast forms are present in the sediment and are *unaccompanied by PMNs*, they are most likely the result of contamination of the specimen. The bacteria may be either cocci or bacilli; yeasts often show budding, but no hyphae.

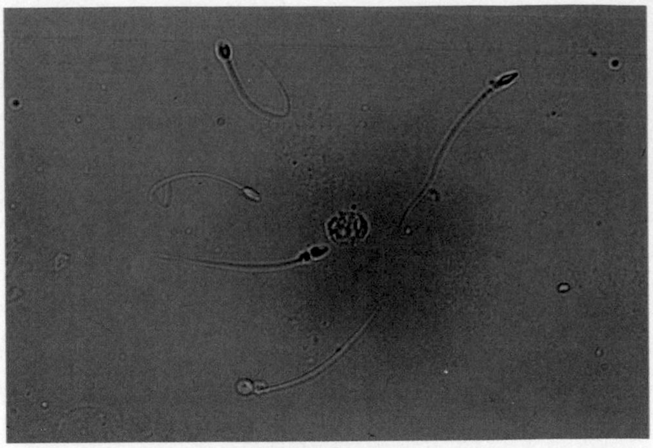

Figure 23.15. Spermatozoa. Several sperm are present around the neutrophil in the center of the field. Sperm may normally be found in urine from both men and women. (BF, ×200.)

Now, having said that normal urine should ordinarily be sterile, one qualifying statement may be made: bacteria normally inhabit the distal urethra. Therefore, should a sample consist of the first part of the voided specimen, rather than a midstream collection, one might expect to find a few bacterial forms in the sediment. This occurrence is more common in women than men, since a urine sample obtained from a female patient is more likely to be contaminated than one received from a male.

SPERMATOZOA

Spermatozoa are frequently found in male urine, but may also be present in female urine (Fig. 23.15). Since urine is naturally spermicidal, the sperm are usually nonmotile when found, except when ejaculation and/or intercourse has been very recent. The presence or absence of spermatozoa in the urine of a female has been used as evidence in rape cases but is not a reliable determinator of the actual time of the rape.

CONTAMINANTS AND ARTIFACTS

Contaminants, especially fibers, appear in abundance in urine sediments. The importance of the correct recognition of these substances—be they fibers (Fig. 23.16), pollen grains, plant cells, starch granules (Fig. 23.17), or other substances—is that they must not be mistaken for actual constituents of the sediment and result in an incorrect diagnosis. To avoid these errors, it is important to keep in mind the following: (*a*) most fibers and other contaminants have a high refractive index and are easily seen, whereas most actual constituents of the sediment are much more difficult to detect; (*b*) many artifacts and contaminants are far larger than any sediment element and can be differentiated by size alone; and (*c*) plant

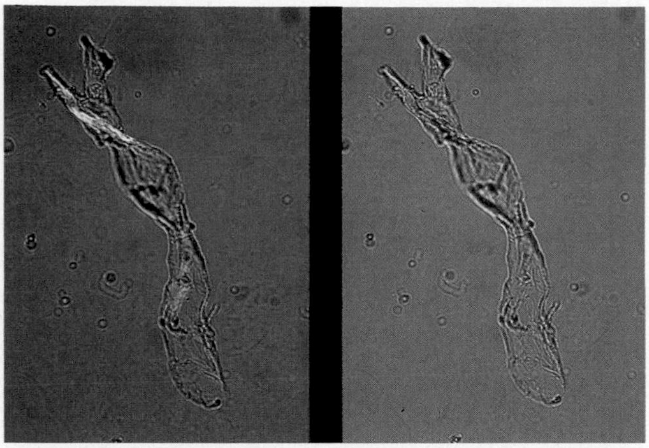

Figure 23.16. Fiber in urine. Fiber artifacts are frequently present in urine sediment and should not be confused with "real" elements that may be pathological. Polarization will usually reveal their true characteristic as they display anisotropism. (BF and POL, ×80.) (Reproduced by permission from the College of American Pathologists.)

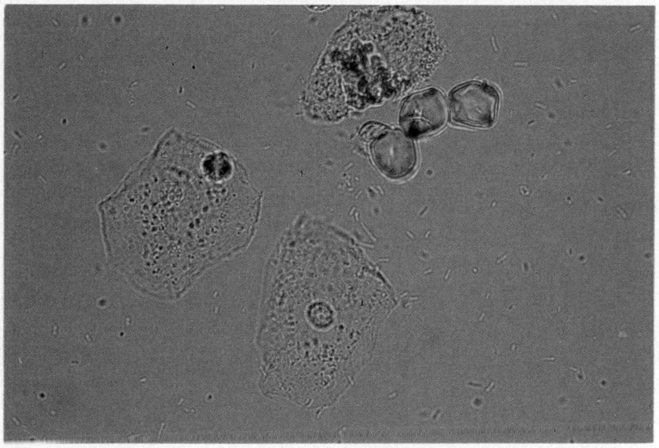

Figure 23.17. Starch granules in urine. These highly refractile, irregularly shaped, dense granules are easily identified in urine and are commonly found, since starch is the material used to powder latex gloves and to dry the skin (i.e., baby powder). They are birefringent. In this field, three squamous cells and bacteria are also present. (BF, ×160.)

and synthetic fibers nearly always show birefringence with polarized light (Fig. 23.16), whereas urine casts do not (except fatty casts, which do not look like fibers). In general, the best and most effective means of avoiding a misdiagnosis due to a contaminant is to be certain about the appearance of and the ways to identify normal sediment elements. If what is seen does not fit the normal pattern, the structure is either abnormal or a contaminant.

Abnormal Urinary Sediment

Once the normal contents of urinary sediment can be recognized, it is not particularly difficult to identify deviation from normal and make a diagnosis of abnormal. Most frequently, abnormal sediment is defined by an *increase* in the number of cells or casts present, not by an alteration in the type of cell or cast. However, different sediment elements are found in the urine in various disease states, and each of these is discussed in this section (Table 23.5). It should be pointed out once again that often there are subtle differences between normal and abnormal, and when these differences depend on quantitative or semiquantitative measurements, as in cell and cast counting, the examiner must be exceptionally aware of producing results that are consistent, accurate, and reproducible.

Table 23.5. Constituents of Abnormal Urine Sediment

Cells	Crystals	Casts	Other
Blood cells	Acid urine	Acellular	Parasites
RBCs	Bilirubin	Hyaline	
WBCs	Cholesterol	Granular	
Epithelial cells	Cystine	Waxy	
Renal tubular	Leucine	Fatty	
Oval fat bodies	Tyrosine	Cellular	
	Hemoglobin	RBC	
	Drug-related	WBC	
		Bacterial	
		Epithelial	
		Crystal	

BLOOD CELLS

Erythrocytes and leukocytes are increased in number in urine in a wide variety of diseases. The patient may complain of having a "smoky" urine if hematuria is present, or of having a foul-smelling "white" urine if pyuria is the cause. In each instance, a careful examination of the sediment is needed with a quantitation of the number and type of blood cells present. RBCs or WBCs in quantities greater than 5/hpf should be considered abnormal (30).

RBCs

Hematuria accompanies a wide variety of clinical conditions (Fig. 23.18). However, the most frequent cause is not pathological, but represents contamination of the urine with menstrual blood. One of the first questions to ask when hematuria is encountered in an adult premenopausal female is whether she is having her period. A subsequent urinalysis, when the urine has been collected after appropriate patient instruction and preparation, will produce a normal number of red blood cells in the sediment if menstrual contamination is the cause of the hematuria.

Another common cause of hematuria is related to exercise. Contact sports such as football, boxing, wrestling, and ice hockey may cause trauma to the kidney or bladder and induce hematuria. This is usually self limited and disappears after a day or two.

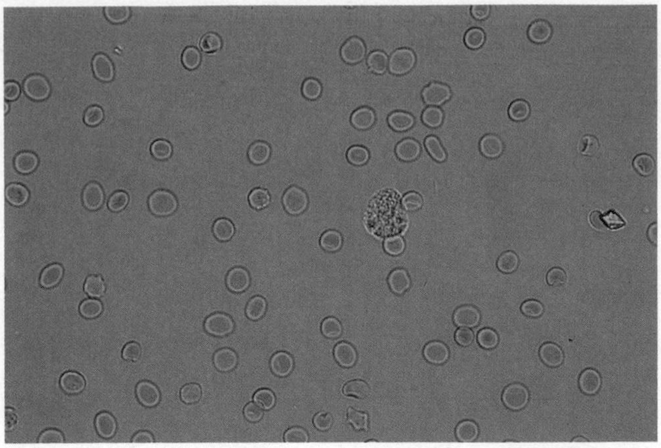

Figure 23.18. Hematuria. This field shows a large number of RBCs, accompanied by a single PMN, in the sediment. Note that the RBCs appear to be regularly shaped biconcave disks. (BF, ×160.)

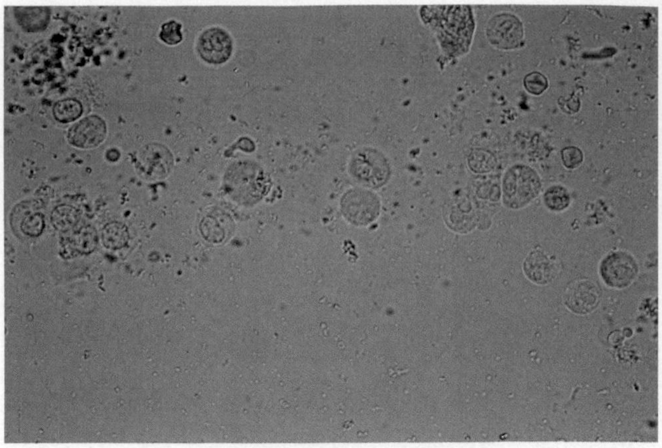

Figure 23.19. Leukocytes (PMNs) in urine. Across the center of the photomicrograph are a large number of white blood cells; most are PMNs, but there are occasional mononuclear forms as well. Bacteria and a few erythrocytes are present in the background. (BF, ×160.)

The terms "pseudoathletic nephritis" and "sports anemia," coined in the 1950s, have been used to describe the findings in patients with hematuria, and sometimes hemoglobinuria, after strenuous physical exercise (42, 43). Before it was recognized that this was an unusual, but not pathologic, response to exercise, many dollars were spent on medical workups of patients presenting with these symptoms. It has been shown that the hematuria in these patients is induced by the stress of the exercise and/or the trauma associated with the constant pounding of bladder urine against the bladder wall, irritating and traumatizing the lining to the point that bleeding into the urine occurs. In addition, continual pounding of the feet of runners against the pavement causes the RBCs in the foot capillaries to be crushed and rupture, thus releasing their hemoglobin into the circulation where it is then cleared by the kidneys and found in the urine. Abatement of the exercise in these cases produces a normal urine within 48 hours.

Medical causes of hematuria include glomerulonephritis, pyelonephritis, cystitis, and neoplasms of the kidney and urinary tract, to mention a few. The hematuria may be microscopic, usually less than 20 RBCs/hpf to gross or macroscopic, more than 50 RBCs/hpf. In bladder or renal cell carcinoma, microscopic hematuria is often an early and important finding that is manifested during a routine laboratory workup in an asymptomatic patient.

Dysmorphic erythrocytes have been described when the hematuria originates in the kidneys (44). These deformed RBCs become an important indicator of intraglomerular hemorrhage and are often overlooked by the inexperienced observer. When dysmorphic RBCs are seen, they are easily recognized. Dysmorphic RBCs have been bent out of shape and into peculiar angles, but are not disrupted (see Fig. 23.24). The peculiar contortions of the red cells are thought to be caused by squeezing through a damaged glomerular basement membrane.

WBCs

Leukocytes in the sediment in numbers greater than 5/hpf are considered pathologic. This number is not absolute and may vary from laboratory to laboratory, depending on the established "normal values." Norms for WBCs in urine may be slightly higher for females. WBCs appear in increased numbers in the urine primarily when an inflammatory process affects the urinary tract. Pyuria is a common finding in cystitis, urethritis, and pyelonephritis. The white cells are predominantly PMNs, but careful study has shown that lymphocytes, monocytes and eosinophils may also be present (Fig. 23.19). PMNs are actively motile. They enter the urine in the kidney or in the remainder of the urinary tract by actively migrating to the site of the inflammatory process moving through the glomerular or tubular basement membranes in the kidney, or across the lining epithelium of the renal pelvis, ureter, bladder, or urethra (30).

Phase microscopy greatly facilitates the recognition of PMNs because their characteristic spherical shape, granular cytoplasm in which Brownian motion is often evident, and multilobed nuclei are readily seen (Fig. 23.20) (38). PMNs are actively phagocytic and serve the body well in protective functions as destroyers of microorganisms and as scavengers and destroyers of microorganisms (Fig. 23.21). "Glitter cells" are PMNs in which the intracytoplasmic vacuoles are large and in motion and appear to be twinkling when observed in the fresh state. Supravital staining of urine (e.g., Sternheimer-Malbin) provides a ready means of specific identification

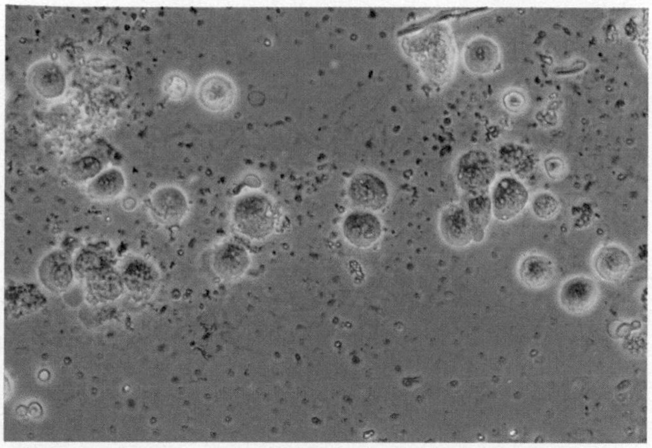

Figure 23.20. Phase microscopy of leukocytes in urine. This photomicrograph represents the same field as seen in Figure 23.19. Here, the cytoplasmic granules in the PMNs and the multilobed nuclei are prominent. (PH, ×160.)

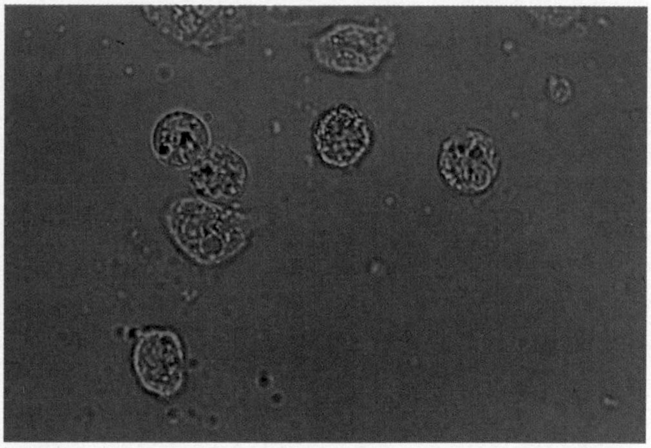

Figure 23.21. Glitter cells. These PMNs display amoeboid motion. PMNs may show active motility, as is seen in the large cell near the center of the field. They do this by extending pseudopods from their cytoplasm. (BF, ×250.)

of PMNs since their granules and individual nuclear lobes are prominently displayed (5).

In interstitial nephritis, an infrequent condition associated with allergic reactions to therapeutic agents, eosinophils are often present in the sediment in greatly increased numbers (45, 46). Eosinophils may not be readily identified without the use of special stains, such as Wright's or Giemsa's stain, or a specific stain for eosinophils, Hansel's stain. Eosinophiluria has recently been reported to be associated with atheroembolic renal disease, a condition in which renal emboli occur in patients with severe atherosclerosis of the aorta (47).

EPITHELIAL CELLS

Epithelial cells may occur in the urine sediment in increased numbers in pathologic conditions. For practical purposes, only the presence of increased numbers of RTEs is of clinical significance. However, it is important to recognize that large numbers of squamous cells are generally a sign of contamination of the specimen by vaginal fluid, whereas an increased number of transitional cells, if not accompanied by PMNs, most often indicates that some type of medical manipulative procedure involving the urethra and/or bladder has been recently performed, such as catheterization.

Renal Tubular Epithelial Cells

RTEs are increased in the urine when there has been damage to the renal tubules and these cells are sloughed. This increased sloughing is most often accompanied by cylindruria, especially the presence of RTE casts in the urine. The specific etiologies for increased numbers of RTEs in the urine are varied and multiple; renal tubular necrosis (48) heavy metal poisoning, cytomegaloviral, renal transplantation (49), aminoglycoside nephrotoxicity (50), and renal vein thrombosis are among the more common causes. Tubular lining cells are 15 to 25 μm in diameter and are usually polyhedral and contain an eccentric single nucleus that is about the size of a mature lymphocyte; they must be differentiated from similar-appearing transitional cells, which can be a difficult task.

Generalized viral diseases, such as viral hepatitis and cytomegaloviral disease, tend to affect the RTEs and cause their sloughing (30, 51). Common diseases, such as the common cold and measles, produce similar damage to the RTEs, resulting in large numbers being sloughed into the urine. Tubular lining cells are active metabolically and may show bile staining, since bilirubin is actively excreted by the kidney when the patient is jaundiced and has severe liver disease. Heavy metals such as lead, bismuth, antimony, and mercury, when ingested in toxic amounts, produce tubular cell death with the result being the presence of increased numbers of these cells in the sediment. Lead toxicity induces an acid-fast inclusion body to form in some RTEs, which, if recognized in the sediment, is of great diagnostic assistance in the identification of the clinical problem. Viruses may also induce the formation of inclusion bodies in RTEs, best demonstrated in herpes, cytomegaloviral disease, and measles.

Oval Fat Bodies

Oval fat bodies (OFBs) (Fig. 23.22) are renal tubule epithelial cells in which globules of lipid have become visible (30). These deformed cells are frequently associated with a nephrotic syndrome but may be seen in various diseases that affect the tubule

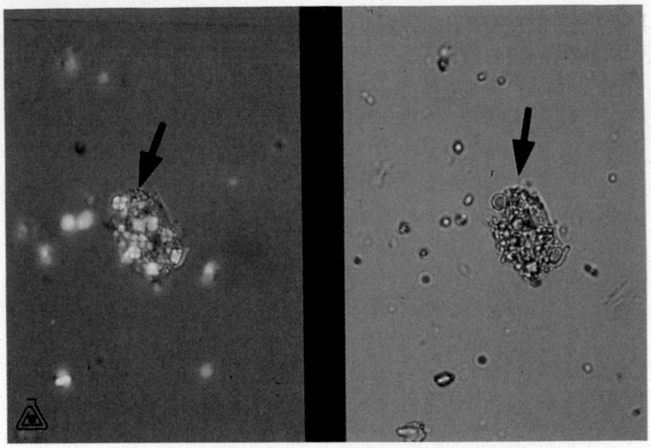

Figure 23.22. Oval fat bodies in urine. This renal tubule epithelial cell contains spherical globules of lipid *(arrow)* which, when polarized *(left)*, show a Maltese Cross pattern. (BF and POL, ×160.) (Reproduced by permission from the College of American Pathologists.)

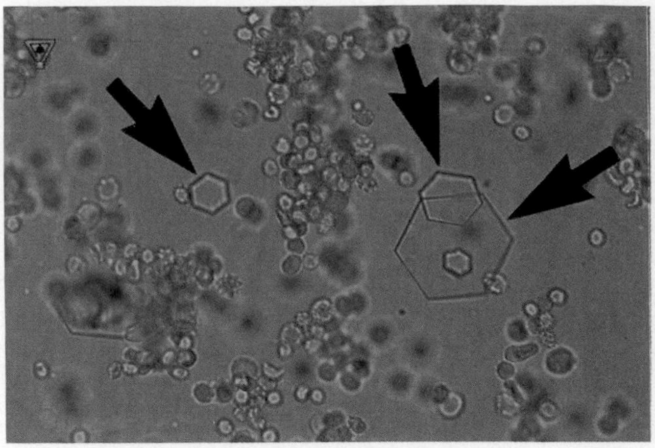

Figure 23.23. Cystine crystals in urine *(arrows)*. These are flat, colorless, hexagonal crystals. Numerous red blood cells are present in the background. (Wright's stain, BF, ×400.) (Reproduced by permission from the College of American Pathologists.)

portion of the nephron. The lipid globules are of varying size, are usually spherical, and because cholesterol is a major component (rather than neutral fat) demonstrate anisotropic properties (Fig. 23.22) by showing a Maltese Cross pattern (52). OFBs may occur singly or in pairs or groups.

Transitional Epithelial Cells

These cells are rarely of pathologic significance unless there are large numbers present; even then, the usual etiology is that the patient has undergone a recent urinary tract procedure, such as a cystoscopy. In these circumstances, the cells may be observed in groups due to traumatic removal of the epithelium during the procedure. Inflammatory conditions of the bladder and urethra, especially, may give rise to increased numbers of urothelial cells in the sediment. However, they are usually accompanied by large numbers of PMNs since inflammation causes a degeneration and sloughing of transitional lining cells of the bladder or urethra. The morphology of these cells is as previously described, and most assume either spherical or caudate shapes. On occasion, irregular forms of transitional cells are observed in the sediment. Some of these cells may be larger than normal and irregularly shaped and have huge and irregular nuclei. Since bladder cancer is a relatively common entity, and a suspicion of it may be considered, an additional sediment sample should be obtained for submission to the cytology laboratory for analysis (53, 54).

Squamous Epithelial Cells

The presence of large numbers of squamous cells in the urine usually represents contamination from vaginal contents. If these cells are accompanied by many bacteria this is especially true. In patients with rectovesical or rectovaginal fistulas, many squamous cells may be seen in conjunction with fecal matter and bacteria. One form of squamous cell that has recently been identified is the "clue cell." It has been shown that this cell, a squamous cell with bacillary forms adhering to its surface, is a frequent finding in *bacterial vaginosis*, an inflammatory condition of the vagina caused by the bacillus *Gardnerella vaginalis* (20). Clue cells should be diagnosed and reported when present.

ABNORMAL CRYSTALS

Of primary importance in the recognition of abnormal crystals is the fact that they are found only in urine of acid or neutral pH. For definitive crystal diagnosis, chemical analysis is performed. A few of the more frequently seen varieties are discussed in detail.

Cystine

These crystals are usually flat, six-sided plates that are clear and colorless (Fig. 23.23) (30). The sides of the hexagon may not be equal in length. Polarization demonstrates a negative birefringent pattern (55). Sometimes, in very fresh urine, the hexagonal shapes are incomplete, and aberrations of these forms may be observed. The crystals may be layered or joined. They are soluble in ammonia water and can be distinguished from six-sided uric acid crystals, also soluble in ammonia water, when they dissolve in dilute hydrochloric acid.

Cystine crystals appear in the urine in an inherited disorder that prevents the reabsorption of the amino acid cystine by the epithelial cells of the nephron and causes *cystinuria*. This disease is one of the more

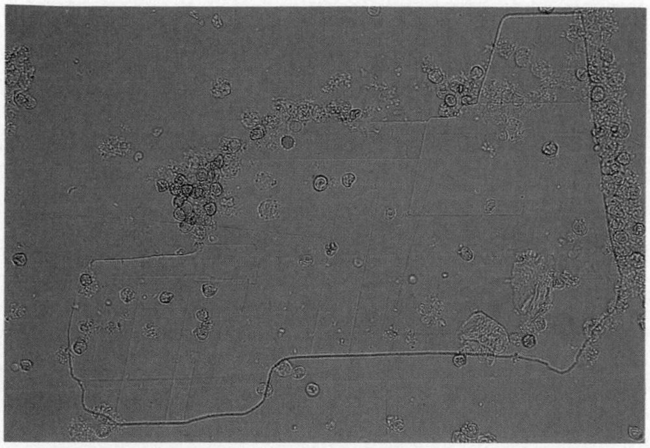

Figure 23.24. Cholesterol crystals in urine. These colorless, flat plates are characteristic because of their rectangular shape and "staircase" patterns. In the background are many red blood cells and an occasional leukocyte. Some of the red cells demonstrate dysmorphic shapes. (BF, ×160.)

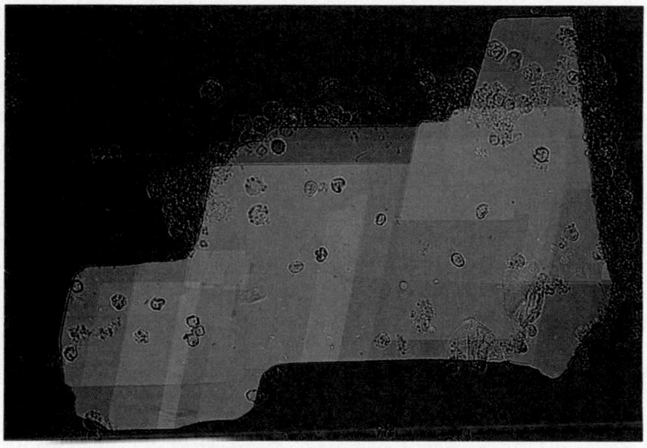

Figure 23.25. Cholesterol crystals, polarized (same as Fig. 23.24). These crystals are anisotropic and often overlap. (POL, ×160.)

common inherited diseases and is expressed equally in each sex as an autosomal-recessive trait. Cystinuria also occurs in diseases affecting the liver (Wilson's disease) and in other diseases of the renal tubules.

Cholesterol

These crystals are most frequently found after refrigeration of the urine; lipid appears in globular form in urine at body temperature but crystallizes on refrigeration. Cholesterol crystals are large, flat, colorless thin plates that assume rectangular shapes of various diameters (Fig. 23.24) (30). One peculiar feature is that the crystals often show a "staircase" pattern or contain an indentation of one or more of the corners of the rectangular plate. They are birefringent and often overlap or appear together (Fig. 23.25).

Cholesterol crystals are occasionally found in the urine sediment of patients with lipoid nephrosis, membranous glomerulonephritis, or polycystic renal disease and in patients with the nephrotic syndrome (edema, lipiduria, lipidemia, and hypercholesterolemia). In lymphatic obstruction due to neoplasms or parasitic disease (filariasis), chyluria may be a consequence if the dilated lymphatics rupture into the kidney or urinary tract.

Leucine

Leucine crystals are rarely found in the urine sediment. They appear as spheroids with a central nidus surrounded by concentric bands with apparent radiations originating from the center and crossing the bands (30). They are brownish-yellow, are highly refractile, and show birefringence. Patients with severe liver disease, such as fulminant hepatitis and advanced cirrhosis, as well as patients with congenital metabolic conditions, such as maple sugar urine disease, excrete these crystals in their urine. They may occur in association with tyrosine crystals. Microscopically, they should not be confused with prostatic concretions or pollen grains and, if there is doubt, chemical testing of the urine for leucine is warranted.

Tyrosine

This crystal is one of the most difficult to see due to its relatively low refractive index; it is birefringent. Tyrosine crystals occur as fine, delicate, colorless or pale yellow elongate needles that may be single or may appear together in clusters or sheaves (Fig. 23.26). Microscopically, the sheaves look as if they have a black central focus, which is a useful point in diagnosis. Tyrosine crystals in the urine are uncommon, even in severe liver disease.

Bilirubin

This brownish-red crystal appears in the sediment as amorphous granular material or as short needles. It may be difficult to distinguish from amorphous urates or phosphates without confirmatory chemical testing. For these crystals to form, high levels of direct-reacting bilirubin need to be reached in the blood and urine, usually as a result of obstructive jaundice.

Hemoglobin

Granules of hemoglobin and hemosiderin may be found in the urine sediment on occasion. When concentrations of hemoglobin in the urine are excessive, as in massive hematuria with RBC lysis, or in severe hemolytic anemia and crush syndrome after trauma,

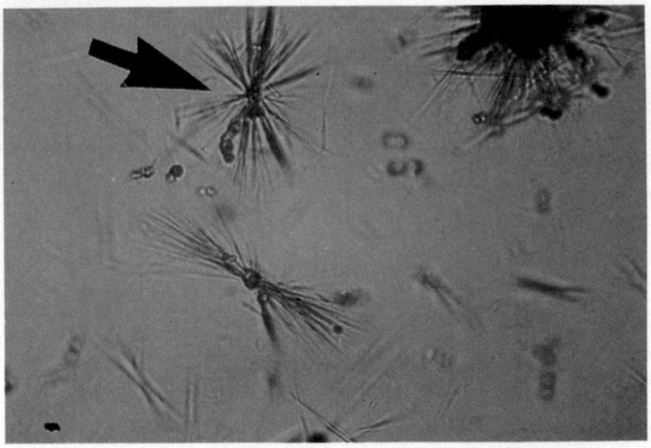

Figure 23.26. Tyrosine crystals in urine. These fine needle-like crystals commonly occur in clusters or sheaves. The black central focus depicted in the photomicrograph *(arrow)* is a useful characteristic for diagnosis. (BF, ×320.) (Reproduced by permission from the College of American Pathologists.)

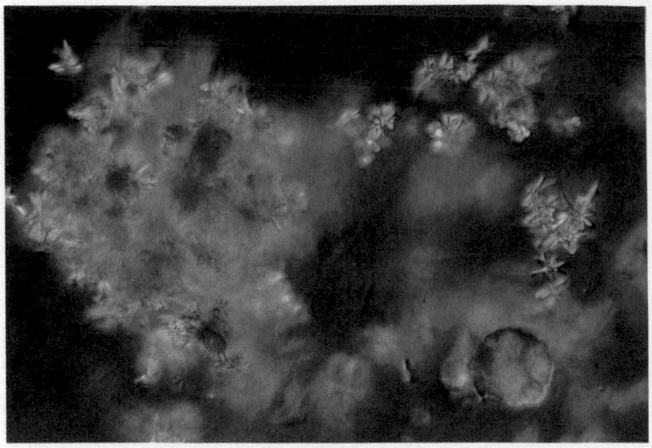

Figure 23.27. Sulfadiazine crystals. Sulfa drugs under manufacture today are water soluble, and finding sulfa crystals in urine is unusual. (ICM, ×250.)

hemoglobin crystals form and appear as tiny, refractile, reddish-brown, amorphous granules. These may be difficult to distinguish microscopically from other granular crystals, and chemical testing along with staining for hemoglobin (e.g., Prussian blue) may be required.

Pharmaceutical Agents

A whole host of pharmaceutical products may, on occasion, produce urinary crystals. Perhaps the most common of these are the dyes associated with radiologic visualization of the urinary tract (i.e., meglumine diatrizoate, Hypaque, and Renografin). These crystals produced by these dyes are colorless crystals, highly refractile, and assume needle-like or elongate rectangular shapes with indented or notched ends. The urine specific gravity is frequently over 1.040 in patients with these crystals (10). A careful history will reveal the true origin of the crystal.

Ampicillin

The crystal produced in the urine by this drug is an elongate, needle-like, colorless crystal that is found in acid urine. It may be difficult to distinguish from radiographic dye crystals, and a history helps in making a correct diagnosis.

Sulfa Drugs

Now that most sulfanilamide drugs are manufactured with water solubility in mind, finding their crystalline products in the urine is uncommon, but does occur infrequently. Sulfadiazine is the most commonly found. The urine is acid, with the pH usually less than 6. The sulfa crystals each assume various needle-like shapes, are birefringent, and are most often seen as bundles of brownish-yellow "sheaves of wheat" with eccentric binding (Fig. 23.27). A lignin test confirms their presence.

ABNORMAL CASTS

Both hyaline and granular casts are commonly found in the urine sediment of patients with renal disease. Each of these cast forms has been discussed previously and is associated with the "normal" state, but there are some morphologic variations that are worthy of comment. All other casts are abnormal, for all practical purposes, and each is discussed in detail.

Casts originate in the distal tubules and collecting ducts of the kidney and are molds of the tubular lumen; therefore, a damaged nephron may have an abnormal tubular lining epithelium that may be atrophic, degenerating, necrotic, or absent, which results in a dilated lumen (34). In such instances of nephron damage, casts form that represent this pathologic dilatation by being wider than normal, i.e., *broad cast* (Fig. 23.28). Although the evaluation is subjective, the uroscopist is quickly able to recognize broad casts, as they may be as much as 5 or 6 times wider than ordinary casts. A large number of broad casts present in a sediment is representative of considerable tubular alteration and nephron injury and, for this reason, they have also been called "renal failure casts."

Damage to either the glomerular or tubular portions of the nephron may give rise to products in the sediment not normally found there, some of which may then become incorporated into casts (30). These products may be present in the glomerular filgrate (e.g., fat, hemoglobin, myoglobin, RBCs, WBCs) or may be directly related to tubular damage or destruction (e.g., epithelial cells or cell products). Casts, on

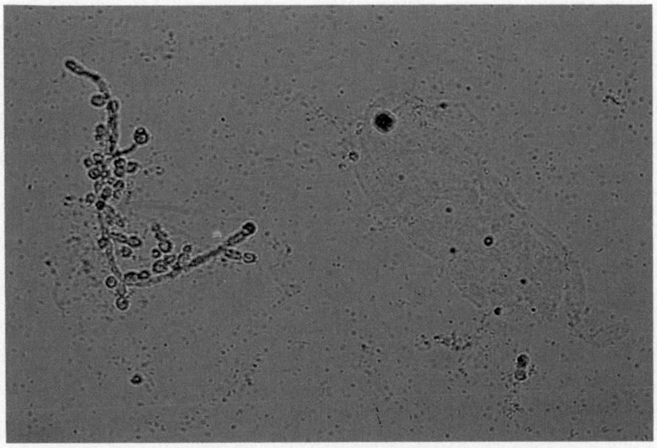

Figure 23.28. Broad hyaline cast. When looking at this cast, it is easy to determine that it has a greater breadth than any cast associated with a "normal" state (cf. Figs. 23.10 and 23.11). The cast depicted here shows some disruption at one end. The background contains budding yeast and hyphae, as well as a bacterium. (BF, ×100.)

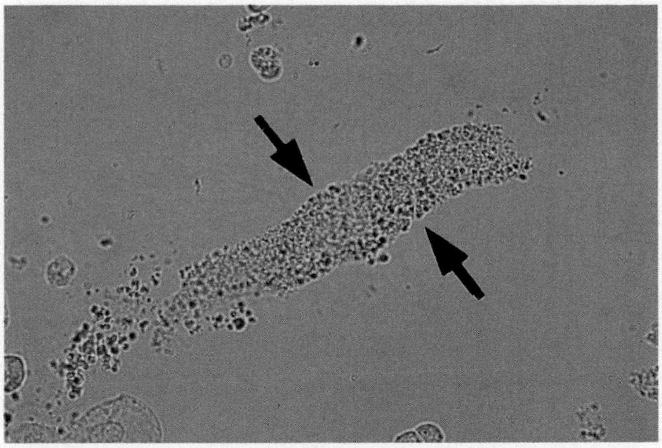

Figure 23.29. Granular cast. This cast *(arrows)* is composed of a diffuse scattering of fine granules over its entire surface. (BF, ×160.) (Reproduced by permission from the College of American Pathologists.)

the other hand, are produced only when the environment in the renal tubule is appropriate for their formation. Although it is a little-understood phenomenon, it is known that alterations in urine flow, pH, and ionic strength of the glomerular filtrate and a sufficient concentration of Tamm-Horsfall protein are all necessary for the production of these casts (20).

Hyaline Casts

In disease states, hyaline casts may increase significantly in number in the sediment, but their morphologic appearances are not different than what is associated with the normal, except where broad forms are noted (Fig. 23.28). Broad hyaline cast forms are usually an indication of some serious intrinsic renal abnormality and require further clinical and laboratory investigation. Generally, in disease states, increased numbers of hyaline casts are found in conjunction with other sediment or chemical abnormalities, such as the presence of additional cast types and/or proteinuria. It is uncommon to find only large numbers of hyaline casts in the urine in disease.

Granular Casts

Large numbers of granular casts are rarely seen in the sediment in health, but this not an infrequent finding in various diseases. These casts may be small or large or broad. The granules may be diffusely scattered over the entire cast surface (Fig. 23.29) or may be concentrated in one or more sections of the cast. Granule size has long been a topic of discussion. In the normal person, the granules are most often small and regular, and the casts are considered to be finely granular (37). Finely granular casts are also found in diseased urine. On the other hand, in diseases in which there has been considerable cellular damage and death (e.g., acute tubular necrosis), the granules may be large and vary greatly in shape and size, and the resulting casts are called coarsely granular (Fig. 23.30). The difference between fine and coarse granules is somewhat subjective, and there is little reason to make this distinction in reports. Cellular destruction leads to the formation of granules that vary in size; when these granules are incorporated into a cast, the resulting granular cast is readily recognized. In some granular casts, cell wall remnants are observed. Due to this fact, the concept arose that some preexistent cellular casts degenerate during their transit through the nephron and evolve into granular casts. In turn, some granular casts continue this evolution and become waxy casts.

Waxy Casts

Morphologically, waxy casts are the most easily recognized of all urinary casts. This is due to their high refractility, characteristic shape, and peculiar "tallow-wax" surface appearance. Classically, waxy casts appear as cylinders with ends that appear to have been sharply cut or broken off (not rounded), and whose sides are notched (Fig. 23.31) (11, 30). Their surface is smooth, for the most part, but may contain a few granules or an occasional cell or cell membrane.

The origin of waxy casts is not clear, and scanning electron microscopy provides little in the way of solution (37). On electron microscopic study, the surface of a waxy cast is composed of what probably is a boilerplate-like protein material (most likely derived from cells) that coats the cast. Waxy casts often appear as broad casts; finding large numbers of waxy

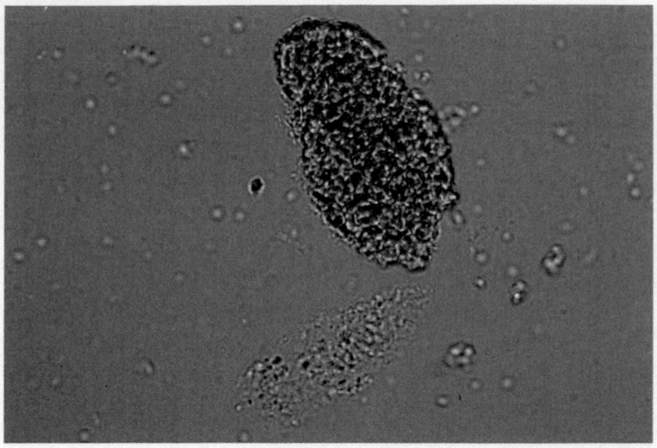

Figure 23.30. Broad coarsely granular cast. In this cast, from a jaundiced patient, the cast has adsorbed the bile pigment in the urine. The granules composing it are irregularly shaped and far larger than those seen in the cast in Figure 23.29. A second, less obvious granular cast is also present in this photomicrograph—just below the broad granular cast initially described. (BF, ×100.)

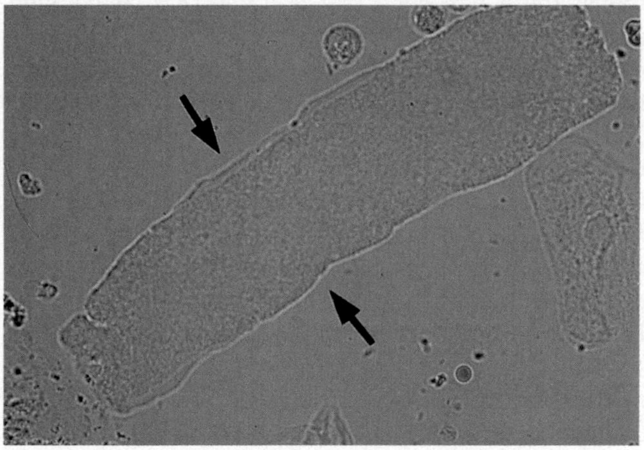

Figure 23.31. Waxy cast *(arrows)*. This cast presents the typical appearance of a waxy cast in the urine. It has sharp, angular, squared-off ends and an irregularly notched margin. Its surface is relatively smooth and looks like it has a "tallow-wax" consistency. (BF, × 160.) (Reproduced by permission from the College of American Pathologists.)

casts in the sediment portends a poor prognosis and is often associated with severe nephron destruction, oliguria, and renal failure.

Pigment Casts

Mention should be made of a variety of cast that contains one of the pigments or abnormal products excreted in the urine. These pigments are most commonly bilirubin, hemoglobin, or myoglobin. Melanin pigment casts also occur but are rarely present in melanuria, a complication of malignant melanoma that has metastasized. Pigment casts usually appear hyaline or waxy but appear as if stained when in fact no sediment stain has been applied (Fig. 23.32).

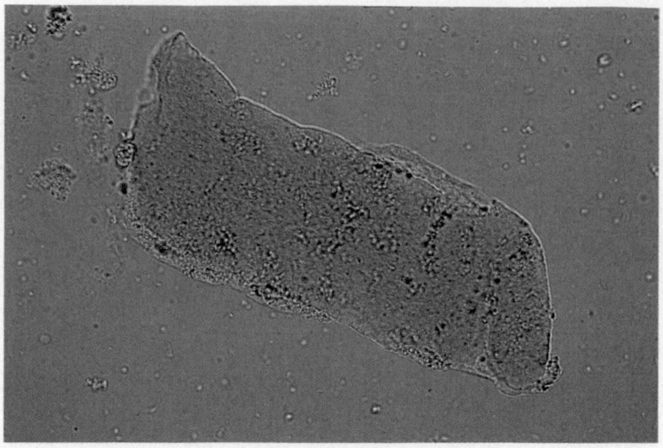

Figure 23.32. Waxy cast, bile stained (pigment cast). This broad cast has a relatively smooth-appearing surface with blunt ends and notched sides. Bile has been absorbed by its matrix to give it a brown surface appearance. (BF, ×160.)

Some pigments can be differentially stained (i.e., hemoglobin). In multiple myeloma, a neoplastic disease of plasma cells, Bence Jones protein may be excreted by the kidneys in large quantities (see Chemical Urinalysis, Protein, earlier in this chapter), and casts composed of this low–molecular weight protein may form and be found in the urine.

Fatty Casts

Lipid may be present in a cast in two forms: either as free globules or within cells. Cholesterol and cholesterol esters demonstrate anisotropism and can be seen with the use of a polarizing microscope (Fig. 23.33). It is observed as having a "Maltese Cross" pattern (30, 52). Neutral fats and triglycerides, on the other hand, do not have this anisotropic property but can be stained with Sudan III or oil red O dye.

Whether the fat is contained within cells (oval fat bodies) or is present as free lipid spherules on the cast surface, accurate recognition is essential. Fatty casts are associated with renal diseases that affect both tubules and glomeruli. These casts are most commonly associated with the nephrotic syndrome but are also present in diseases in which there is severe tubular damage, such as heavy metal poisoning. Fatty casts may form as a result of glomerular injury, which causes a leakage of serum lipids into the glomerular filtrate. The newly formed fatty globules are either absorbed by the tubular epithelium with the formation of OFBs or become a component of the cast by adhering to its surface.

Fatty casts are easily confused with RBC casts because of the globular nature of the free lipid. Careful observation assists in distinguishing them since the lipid globules are of varying size, spherical, and have a rather pale golden-brown color. Simple polariza-

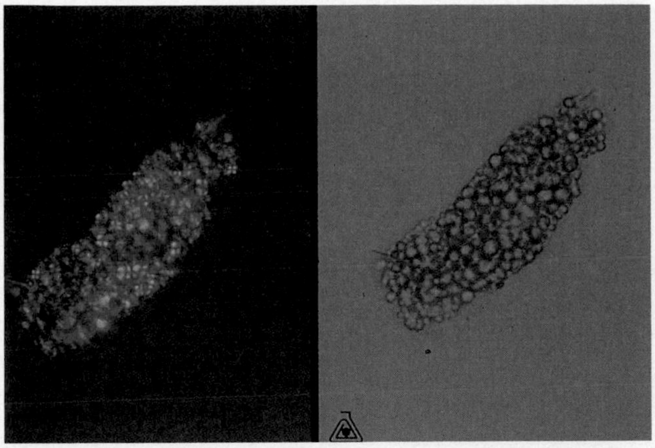

Figure 23.33. Fatty cast. This cast contains multiple different-sized lipid globules which, when subjected to polarized light, are anisotropic and display a Maltese Cross pattern *(left)*. (BF and POL, ×160.) (Reproduced by permission from the College of American Pathologists.)

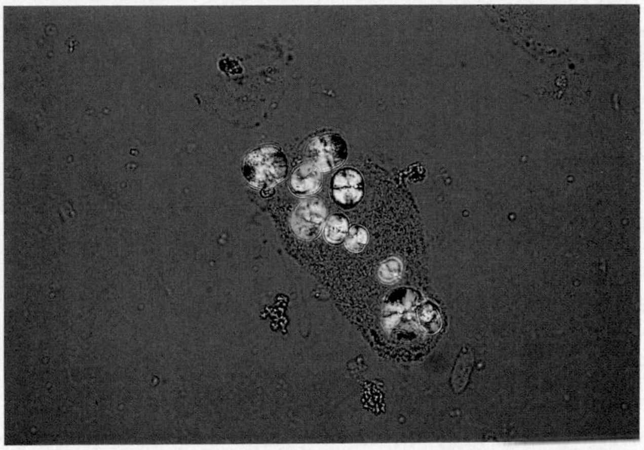

Figure 23.34. Crystal casts in urine. Note that the crystals are irregularly scattered over the hyaline cast matrix, which shows fine granularity. This urine sediment sample was from a liver transplant patient who was severely jaundiced. (BF, ×100.)

tion reveals a "Maltese Cross" pattern of the globules. RBC casts, on the other hand, are not anisotropic, contain reddish-brown RBCs of uniform size and in the typical nonspherical, biconcave disc shape.

Crystal Casts

These casts are infrequently present in the urine sediment and may be a helpful indicator of renal obstruction. In obstruction when casts form, precipitation of various crystals occurs in the nephron, and these crystals become incorporated into the cast matrix (Fig. 23.34). The basic crystal cast has a hyaline matrix. Crystal casts might contain uric acid, calcium oxalate, and rarely, sulfadiazine. Since all of these crystals are anisotropic, simple polarization of the cast should demonstrate their true nature if there is

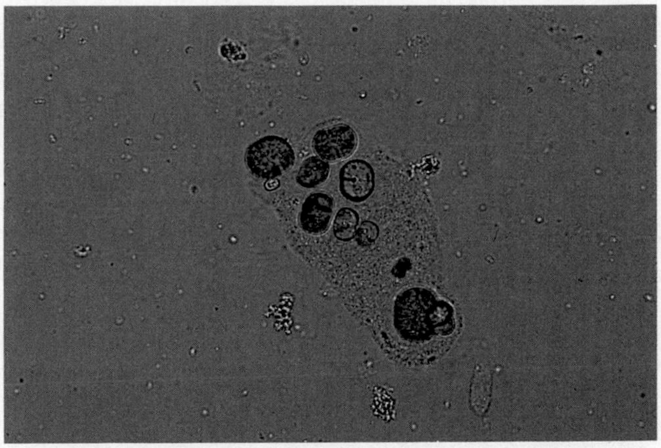

Figure 23.35. Crystal cast, polarized. The same cast shown in Fig. 23.34 is depicted under polarized light. The crystals in the cast show anisotropic properties that enable them to be distinguished. These casts may be associated with renal obstruction. (Polarized, ×100.)

any doubt about their diagnosis (Fig. 23.35). It is important to distinguish crystal casts from crystalline pseudocasts (compacted amorphous urate or phosphate crystals assuming a cylindrical cast-like shape), since crystal casts may be associated with pathological conditions while pseudocasts have no clinical significance.

Red Blood Cell Casts

Red blood cell casts are among the most diagnostically important of all elements in the urine sediment; their presence usually indicates glomerular injury (i.e., acute glomerulonephritis, IgA nephropathy, lupus erythematosus nephropathy) (56, 57). RBC casts can also be found, but far less frequently, in disease states that do not primarily involve glomeruli (i.e., pyelonephritis and renal infarction). RBCs enter the urinary flow via two major mechanisms: they either pass through the glomerular basement membrane (GBM)—a transglomerular route—or they cross the tubular basement membrane (TBM)—a transtubular route (34). Both mechanisms are of importance in the formation of RBC casts. When serious glomerular injury occurs, as in acute poststreptococcal glomerulonephritis, the GBM is damaged and increased numbers of RBCs transgress it; some of these RBCs become incorporated into a preexistent cast matrix and form an RBC cast. A similar mechanism occurs in instances of transtubular bleeding. Here, the TBM is damaged, as in renal infarction or pyelonephritis, and RBCs leak across it and into the urine flow, there to become incorporated into the cast (Fig. 23.36).

An RBC cast is basically a hyaline cast to which RBCs adhere. Scanning electron micrographs of this cast type demonstrate that the RBCs are attached to the matrix by means of thin fibrils, presumably in

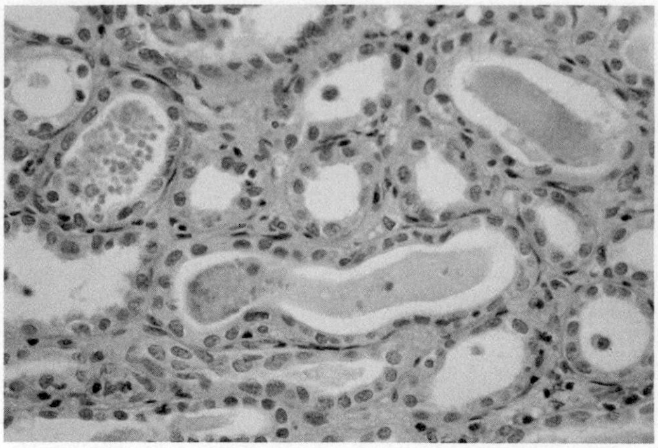

Figure 23.36. Red blood cell casts forming in the distal nephron. This histologic section shows three casts in the lumens of the tubules. Two of the casts contain red blood cells, while the third is purely hyaline. (Hematoxylin and eosin, ×100.)

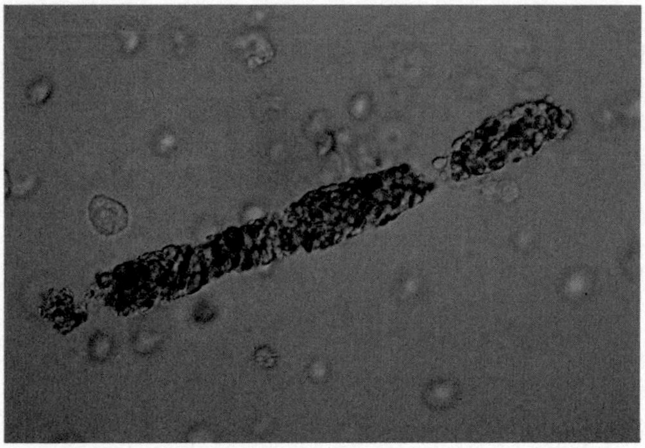

Figure 23.37. Red blood cell cast. In this cast, the RBCs are easily identified and closely compacted and have the typical color of hemoglobin. Many RBCs are also present in the background. (BF, ×200.)

part Tamm-Horsfall mucoprotein, which serve as a kind of glue to attach the cells to the cast surface. The RBCs apparently attach *after* the cast has been formed in the distal tubule or collecting duct.

Recognition of RBC casts requires careful microscopic observation since they may be confused with other cast forms such as fatty casts (Fig. 23.37). The RBCs in the cast may be sparse, with only a few present in any one area, or they may be closely packed so that the underlying cast matrix can hardly be seen. The RBCs themselves may be intact, thereby facilitating a diagnosis, but they frequently show degeneration and disruption. If the disruption is severe enough, one may be left with only RBC membranes and brownish-red hemoglobin pigment in the cast; these are named blood or hemoglobin casts. To diagnose an RBC cast, the cast surface should contain sufficient numbers of RBCs, or their disrupted membranes, so that no doubt exists regarding the specific diagnosis. Often, RBCs within the cast will show dysmorphism, and appear in twisted and irregular shapes (44). In most patients with RBC casts, proteinuria and hematuria are seen concurrently in the chemical evaluation and the urine sediment surrounding the casts contains free-floating RBCs.

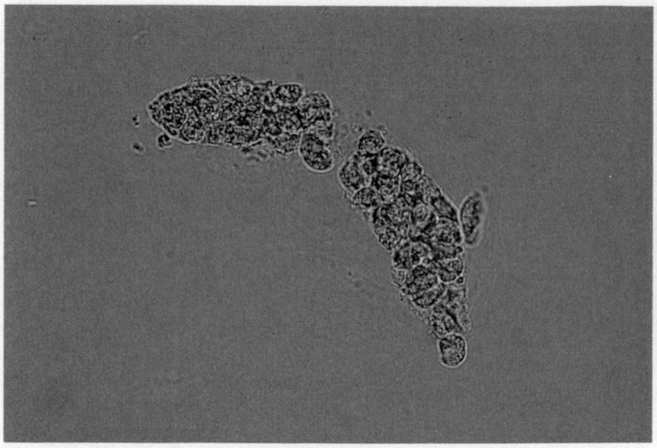

Figure 23.38. White blood cell cast. The cast depicted in the photomicrograph is basically a hyaline cast to which PMNs have adhered. The leukocytes on the cast surface show a granular cytoplasm and multilobed nuclei. (BF, ×160.)

White Blood Cell Casts

Leukocyte casts in the urine usually indicate that an inflammatory process is occurring in the kidney, most frequently involving the interstitium in pyelonephritis and interstitial nephritis. WBCs migrate to the affected region of the kidney and then across the TBM, where they enter the urine flow and become incorporated into the cast matrix. These WBCs are secured to the hyaline matrix by means of fibrillar protein bands, similar to those found in RBC casts (37). Glomerular damage that induces an immune response, and the subsequent chemotactic attraction of leukocytes to the site of injury, also causes WBC casts to form (i.e., lupus nephritis).

Leukocyte casts may be difficult to recognize accurately because of the possibility of confusion with renal tubular epithelial cell (RTE) casts. The white cells occupying the cast surface are most often neutrophils (PMNs) (Fig. 23.38). These cells measure approximately 20 μm across and can be identified by their multilobed nuclei and granular cytoplasm. However, neutrophils in these casts are frequently disrupted, fragmented, or undergoing degeneration, and the individual nuclear lobes may be difficult to distinguish. Phase-contrast or interference-contrast microscopy or differential staining may assist in making the distinction between leukocytes and tubular epithelial cells.

Lymphocytes and eosinophils may occasionally be found in WBC casts. Lymphocytes, being much

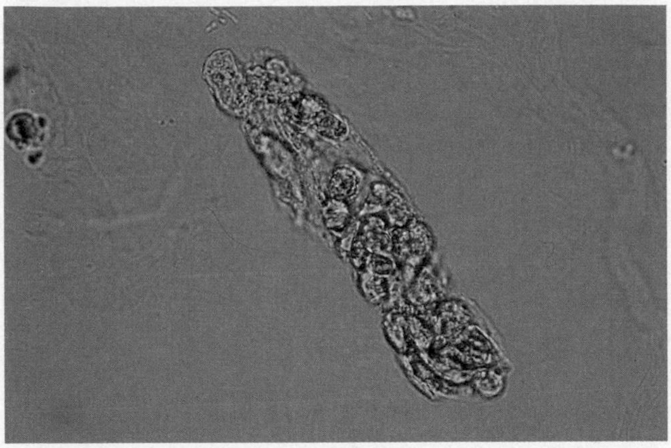

Figure 23.39. Renal tubule epithelial cell cast. The basic matrix of this cast is hyaline and RTE cells coat its surface. The cells are large (approximately 20 μm) and have a large central nucleus. Their cytoplasm contains far fewer granules than do PMNs and the single nucleus distinguishes their character. They may present difficulty in differentiation from WBC casts. Mucus strands are present in the background. (BF, ×160.)

smaller cells than neutrophils (12 μm), and having a large central nucleus, are easily recognized. Eosinophils, on the other hand, may present diagnostic difficulties unless Giemsa's or Hansel's stains are applied. The author has never observed a pure eosinophil cast in interstitial nephritis, but has noted occasional eosinophils in WBC casts in this disease.

Renal Tubular Epithelial Cell Casts

RTE casts are cellular casts composed of renal tubular epithelium that has been sloughed off. Tubular lining cells are easily affected by various poisons, especially the heavy metals, such as lead and mercury, ethylene glycol (antifreeze), and viruses (cytomegalovirus and hepatitis) and are also sensitive to alterations in blood flow in instances of prolonged shock and also in renal transplantation. In these examples, the RTE cells are caused to exfoliate. If hyaline casts are forming in the distal portions of the nephron, the cells become attached to the cast matrix and form an RTE cast (37).

RTE casts are sometimes difficult to distinguish from WBC casts since the two cell types are of approximately the same size (20 μm). One means of accurate identification is to look for a single large central nucleus in the cell (Fig. 23.39). In contrast, neutrophils have a smaller nucleus with multiple lobes. Both cell types have intracytoplasmic granules, although those in RTE cells are usually less prominent than those in neutrophils. When the RTEs begin to degenerate, their cell and nuclear membranes become permeable and the cytoplasmic granules may leak into the surrounding cast matrix, giving a granular appearance. The tendency for microscopists to incorrectly diagnose RTE casts as WBC casts is pervasive, since WBC casts are far more common than RTE casts. This mistake should and can be avoided by careful observation of the cells that make up the cast.

Oval Fat Body Casts

In diseases that cause severe degeneration and necrosis of renal tubular epithelial cells, such as heavy metal poisoning or acute tubular necrosis, the intracellular lipids become visible and the resulting sloughed OFBs are incorporated into a cast. These are truly RTE casts but have been designated OFB casts because of the peculiar appearance of the damaged epithelial cells and their visible and anisotropic intracytoplasmic lipid droplets. The lipid may be cholesterol or cholesterol esters, in which case it demonstrates anisotropism in a typical "Maltese Cross" pattern, or it may consist of neutral fats and triglycerides, which can be differentially stained with Sudan III or oil red O dye. The fat globules within the RTE cells are of varying size and are usually spherical, but may be somewhat irregular. If the RTE cell has a disrupted membrane, the fat droplets may leak out into the surrounding cast matrix.

Bacterial/Fungal Casts

The recognition that microorganisms could be included within the cast matrix is an observation that has often been overlooked in routine urinalysis (58). Bacterial forms, being as small as they are, are frequently not diagnosed within a cast since they appear as granules, and a granular cast is diagnosed when ordinary bright-field microscopy is used in analysis. In studies of women with acute pyelonephritis, WBC casts were often present in the urine and it became apparent that some of the granules within these WBC casts were in fact bacteria. Studies using scanning electron microscopy verified this conclusion (Fig. 23.40). It is therefore of prime importance to carefully analyze all abnormal sediments that contain granular or WBC casts and to look for bacterial and/or fungal forms in these casts. This analysis is significantly aided by using a phase-contrast or interference-contrast microscope or by staining with Sternheimer-Malbin sedistain; in either instance bacilli will be readily identifiable.

The importance of recognizing bacterial and fungal casts is the fact that their presence is pathognomonic for acute infections of the kidney (58). Bacterial forms are generally scattered throughout the entire cast matrix and are bound to its surface by bands of fibrillar protein, probably Tamm-Horsfall protein. WBCs are often admixed with the bacteria or fungi. Pure bacterial casts are uncommon. Fungal

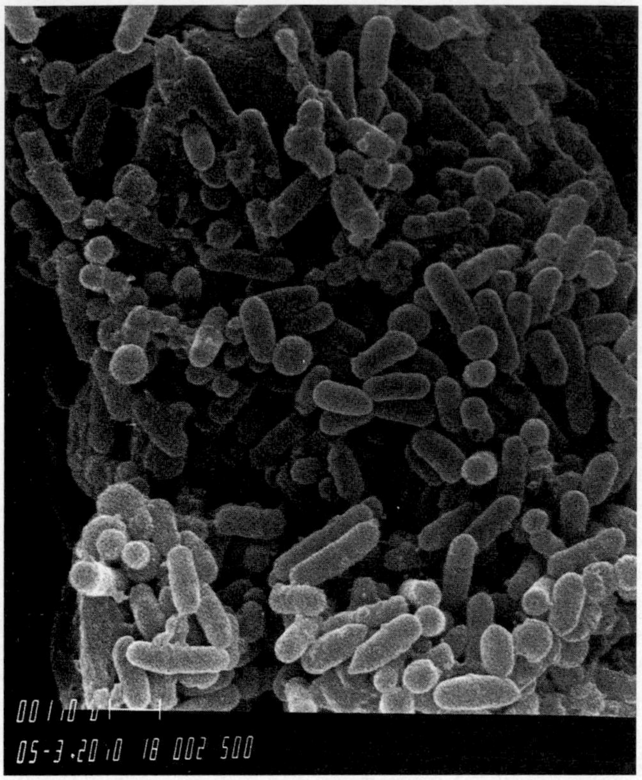

Figure 23.40. Bacterial cast. Numerous bacillary forms completely occupy the cast surface. (Scanning electron microscopy, ×5000.)

casts are being diagnosed more frequently today than before because of the recent increase in transplantation surgery and the extensive use of chemotherapeutic and immunosuppressive agents in these patients and in the many patients with malignant neoplasms. Patients with a decreased immune response are more susceptible to various infectious diseases, especially bacterial and fungal (e.g., AIDS). Fungal forms are somewhat easier to recognize in casts than are bacteria due to their larger size. Yeasts are often budding and, on occasion, even hyphae may be found in the cast.

PARASITES

Parasitic organisms are rarely present in the urinary sediment (30). In the United States, the eggs of *Enterobius vermicularis* (pinworm) are occasionally found, especially in children, and are the result of fecal contamination. The female worm lays her eggs in the perirectal region and during urine collection they may be carelessly carried into the urine collection bottle, especially if the collection is not performed under supervised and controlled conditions and the genital area has been inadequately cleaned. Other parasites, such as pubic lice and fleas, may be present in the sediment as contaminants when proper collection procedures have not been followed.

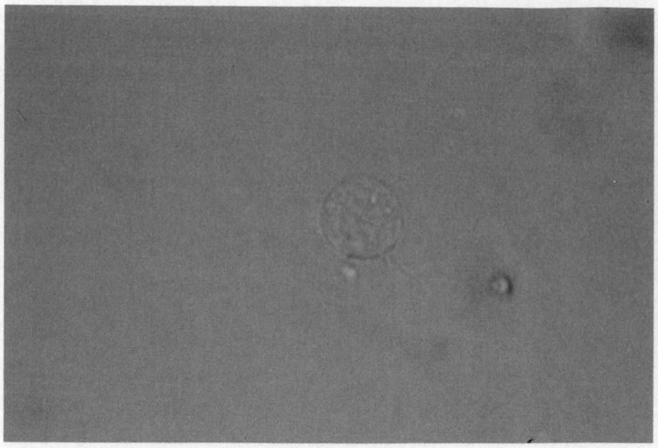

Figure 23.41. *Trichomonas vaginalis* in urine. Note the flagella and the spherical character of this parasite. These organisms are easily misdiagnosed as white blood cells. (BF, ×400.)

The single parasite that inhabits the urinary tract (bladder) as part of its life cycle is *Schistosoma hematobium*. The egg of this parasite is difficult to see with ordinary microscopic techniques, as it is clear and colorless. It has a characteristic terminal spine or spike and a elliptical shape. Schistosoma eggs measure approximately 150 μm in length and 60 μm in diameter. A particular species of snail is necessary for the maturation of this organism, which, fortunately, is not present in the United States. In other parts of the world, especially Africa and Egypt, however, schistosomiasis or genitourinary bilharziasis is a significant public health problem, and the finding of these parasitic eggs in urine is not unusual.

Trichomonas vaginalis is the most frequently encountered parasite in urine sediment in the United States and is usually a contaminant from the vagina. This organism typically inhabits the distal urethra of men and women, the vagina, and, rarely, the prostate gland. These flagellated protozoans are actively motile in freshly voided urine, and have a characteristic appearance. The body measures 10 to 30 μm in length and typically has an undulating membrane running about half its length; there are four anterior flagella (Fig. 23.41). The inexperienced observer may easily misdiagnose these organisms as neutrophils, since they usually occur in the company of PMNs and are about the same size. Careful scrutiny must be given to the sediment to detect their motility, elliptical shape, and flagella.

ARTIFACTS

As previously discussed, the ability to distinguish between actual urinary constituents and artifactual or contaminant material that may appear in the sediment is of primary importance in sediment analysis. The experienced observer will have little difficulty in

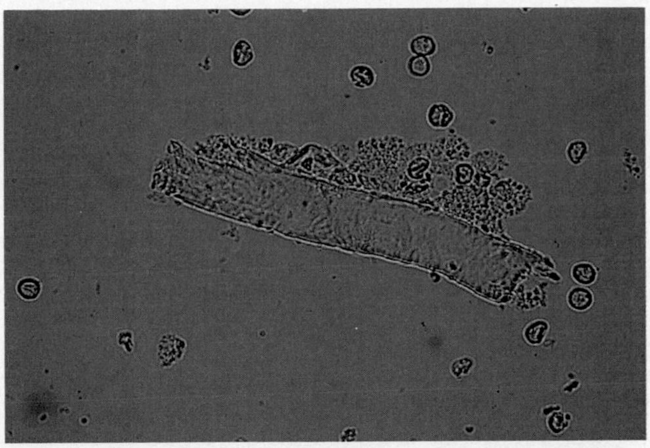

Figure 23.42. Fiber artifact in urine. This fiber from a disposable diaper may be easily confused with a waxy cast as it has some of the same morphologic features. A clear distinction may be made using polarized microscopy (cf. Fig. 23.43). RBCs and occasional WBCs are present in the background. (BF, ×160.)

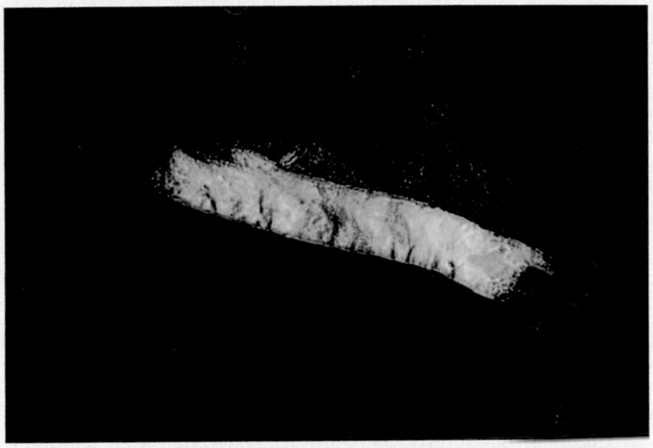

Figure 23.43. Fiber artifact in urine, polarized. Note the birefringence of the fiber. Waxy casts do not display anisotropism, and therefore any misdiagnosis of this fiber as a waxy cast should be prevented. (Polarized, ×160.)

making this distinction and will use the microscopic "tools" of polarization, phase contrast, and staining to this end. Fibers, precipitated stains, oil droplets, and scratches will frequently be observed and should not be confused with, or misdiagnosed as, abnormal elements (Figs. 23.42, and 23.43).

Summary

Microscopic evaluation of urine sediment is often a valuable diagnostic part of "routine" urinalysis. It provides a means of evaluating the urine or of confirming an abnormal physicochemical finding, which is clinically useful. For this part of the urine examination to be most effective, however, a regularly employed standardized approach must be followed. Whether a laboratory purchases one of the many "systems" commercially available or develops one of its own, the results of performing the microscopic examination by doing the same thing to each and every urine sample every time a urinalysis is ordered will undoubtedly pay dividends in the long run by producing more accurate and reliable results. Table 23.6 presents an approach to the performance of urine microscopic examination once the urine has been prepared for sediment evaluation.

Table 23.6. Methodology in Performing a Urine Microscopic Examination

View concentrated sediment with low-power objective (100×)
Observe sediment for cells, casts, and crystals
Count casts as number per low-power field
Search for any other type of abnormality, i.e., yeast, parasites
Polarize sediment to look for lipid (i.e., cholesterol)
If any part of physicochemical examination is abnormal, or
If urine is cloudy, or
If increased numbers of cells or casts are present, THEN
View sediment under high power (400×)
Identify *all types* of cells present
Count blood cells as numbers per high-power field
Count renal tubular epithelial cells as number/hpf
Identify all types of casts present, specify type
If casts are increased in number then:
Normal vs. abnormal
If abnormal, acellular vs. cellular
Identify crystals present; determine if
Normal, or
Abnormal (only in acid or neutral urine)
Identify any microorganisms, bacteria, fungi, or parasites
Produce report and sign

References

1. Haber MH. Pisse prophecy: A brief history of urinalysis. In: Haber, MH, Corwin HL, eds. Clinics in laboratory medicine. Philadelphia: WB Saunders, 1988:415–430.
2. Brian T. The Pisse-prophet or, certaine pisse-pot lectures. London, 1637.
3. Bird G. Urinary deposits. London: John Churchill, 1844.
4. Bright R. Reports of medical cases selected with a view of illustrating the symptoms and cure of diseases by a reference to morbid anatomy. London: Longman, 1827:1.
5. Sternheimer R. A supravital cytodiagnostic stain for urinary sediments. JAMA 1975;231(8):826–832.
6. Haber MH. Quality assurance in urinalysis. In: Haber MH, Corwin HL, eds. Clinics in laboratory medicine. Philadelphia: WB Saunders, 1988:431–448.
7. Fisher A. Quality assurance program for urinalysis. In: Haber MH, ed. A primer of microscopic urinalysis. Garden Grove, CA: Hycor Biomedical, 1991:12–18.
8. Free HM, Baker J, Haber MH, et al., eds. Routine urinalysis. Proposed guidelines. NCCLS Document GP 16-P. Villanova, PA: National Committee for Clinical Laboratory Standards, 1991.
9. Haber MH. Interference contrast microscopy for identification of urinary sediments. Am J Clin Pathol 1972;57:316–319.
10. Free HM. Modern urine chemistry. Elkhart, IN: Miles Laboratories, 1987.
11. Schumann GB, Schweitzer SC. Examination of urine. In: Henry JB, ed. Clinical diagnosis and management by labora-

tory methods. 18th ed. Philadelphia: WB Saunders, 1991:387–444.

12. Strasinger SK: Urinalysis and body fluids. A self-instructional text. 2nd ed. Philadelphia: FA Davis, 1991.
13. Gillenwater JY. Detection of urinary leukocytes by Chemstrip-L. J Urol 1981;125:383–384.
14. Freeman JA, Haber MH. Urinalysis. In: Freeman JA, Beeler MF, eds. Laboratory medicine/urinalysis and medical microscopy. 2nd ed. Philadelphia: Lea & Febiger, 1983:1–260.
15. Kim MS. Proteinuria. In: Haber MH, Corwin HL, eds. Clinics in laboratory medicine. Philadelphia: WB Saunders, 1988:527–540.
16. Hindmarsh JT. Microalbuminuria. In: Haber MH, Corwin HL, eds. Clinics in laboratory medicine. Philadelphia: WB Saunders, 1988:611–616.
17. Haber MH, Lindner LE, Ciofalo LN. Urinary casts after stress. Lab Med 1979;10:351–355.
18. Schoolwerth AC. Hematuria and proteinuria: their causes and consequences. Hosp Pract 1987;22:45–62.
19. Corwin HL, Silverstein MD. Microscopic hematuria. In: Haber MH, Corwin HL, eds. Clinics in laboratory medicine. Philadelphia: WB Saunders, 1988:601–610.
20. Haber MH. A primer of microscopic urinalysis. 2nd ed. Garden Grove, CA: Hycor Biomedical, 1991.
21. James GP, Bee DE, Fuller JB. Accuracy and precision of urinary pH determinations using two commercially available dipsticks. Am J Clin Pathol 1978;70(3):368–374.
22. Anonymous. Urinalysis today. Indianapolis: Boehringer Mannheim Diagnostics, 1987.
23. Binder L, Smith S, Kupka T, et al. Failure of prediction of liver function test abnormalities with the urine urobilinogen and urine bilirubin assays. Arch Pathol Lab Med 1989;113:73–76.
24. Monte-Verde D, Nosanchuk JS. The sensitivity and specificity of nitrite testing for bacteriuria. Lab Med 1981;12(12):755–757.
25. With T. Bile pigments. New York: Academic Press, 1968.
26. Kusumo RK, Grover PJ, Kunin CM. Rapid detection of pyuria by leukocyte esterase activity. JAMA 1981;245(16):1653–1655.
27. Sadof MD, et al. Dipstick leukocyte esterase activity in first-catch urine specimens. JAMA 1987;258(14):1932–1934.
28. Morrison MC, Lum G. Dipstick testing of urine—can it replace urine microscopy? Am J Clin Pathol 1986;85:590–594.
29. Hensey OJ, Cooke RWI. Estimation of urine specific gravity and osmolarity using a simple reagent strip. Br Med J 1983;286(6358):53.
30. Haber MH. Urinary sediment: a textbook atlas. Chicago: American Society of Clinical Pathologists, 1981.
31. Koepke JA. Hematology and urinalysis testing in the physician's office. Pathologist 1986;40:17–20.
32. Schumann GB, Greenberg NF. Usefulness of macroscopic urinalysis as a screening procedure. A preliminary report. Am J Clin Pathol 1979;71:452–456.
33. Addis T. Glomerular nephritis. New York: Macmillan, 1948.
34. Haber MH. Urine casts, their microscopy and clinical significance. Chicago: American Society of Clinical Pathologists, 1975.
35. Tamm I, Horsfall FL Jr. A mucoprotein derived from human urine which reacts with influenza, mumps, and Newcastle disease viruses. J Exp Med 1952;95:71–97.
36. McKenzie JK, McQueen EG. Immunofluorescent localization of Tamm-Horsfall mucoprotein in human kidney. J Clin Pathol 1969;22:334–339.
37. Haber MH, Lindner LE. The surface ultrastructure of urinary casts. Am J Clin Pathol 1977;68:547–552.
38. Brody L, Webster MD, Kark RM. Identification of elements of urinary sediment with phase-contrast microscopy. JAMA 1979;206:1977–1981.
39. Behrman RA. Urinary findings before and after a marathon race. N Engl J Med 1939;225:801–802.
40. Lindner LE, Vacca D, Haber MH. Identification and composition of types of granular urinary casts. Am J Clin Pathol 1983:353–358.
41. Jenkins RD, Fenn JP, Matsen JM. Review of urine microscopy for bacteriuria. JAMA 1986;255:3397–3403.
42. Roberts AM. Some effects of exercise on the urinary sediment. J Clin Invest 1935;14:31–33.
43. Dressendorfer RH, Wade CE, Amsterdam EA. Development of pseudoanemia in marathon runners during a 20-day road race. JAMA 1981;246:1215–1218.
44. Fairley FK, Birch DF. Hematuria: a simple method for identifying glomerular bleeding. Kidney Int 1982;21:105–108.
45. Corwin HL, Korbet SM, Schwartz MM. Clinical correlates of eosinophiluria. Arch Intern Med 1985;145:1097–1099.
46. Corwin HL, Bray RA, Haber MH. The detection and interpretation of urinary eosinophils. Arch Pathol Lab Med 1989;113:1256–1258.
47. Wilson DM, Salazer TL, Farkouh ME. Eosinophiluria in atheroembolic renal disease. Am J Med 1991;91:186–189.
48. Dunnil MS. A review of the pathology and pathogenesis of acute renal failure due to acute tubular necrosis. J Clin Pathol 1974;27:2–13.
49. Schumann GB, Palmieri LJ, Jones DB. Differentiation of renal tubular epithelium in renal transplantation cytology. Am J Clin Pathol 1977;67:580–584.
50. Mandal AK. Analysis of urinary sediment by transmission electron microscopy. An innovative approach to diagnosis and prognosis in renal disease. In: Haber MH, Corwin HL, eds. Clinics in laboratory medicine. Philadelphia: WB Saunders, 1988:463–481.
51. Bolande RP. Inclusion bearing cells in the urine in certain viral infections. Pediatrics 1959;24:7–12.
52. Hudson JB, Dennis AJ, Gerhardt RE. Urinary lipid and the Maltese cross. N Engl J Med 1978;299:586.
53. Papanicolaou GN. Cytology of urine sediment in neoplasms of the urinary tract. J Urol 1947;57:375–379.
54. Holmquist N. Detection of cancer with urinary sediment. J Urol 1980;123:188–201.
55. Bradley M. Urine crystals: identification and significance. Lab Med 1982;13:348–353.
56. Heptinstall RH. Pathology of the kidney. 4th ed. Boston: Little, Brown, 1991.
57. Schreiner GE. The identification and clinical significance of casts. Arch Intern Med 1957;99:356–369.
58. Lindner LE, Jones RN, Haber MH. A specific urinary cast in pyelonephritis. Am J Clin Pathol 1980;73:809–811.

24 Body Fluid Analysis

Karl S. Theil

SYNOVIAL FLUID

Synovial fluid analysis can reveal critical diagnostic information in the evaluation of patients with joint disease. The classic signs of inflammation—redness, pain, swelling, and warmth—are typical presenting complaints of arthritis that have various causes. Distinction of infectious from crystal-induced arthritis can readily be made by examination of synovial fluid. Inflammatory and noninflammatory or traumic conditions can frequently be separated, allowing a differential diagnosis to be narrowed and early treatment instituted. Like other body fluids, changes in the macroscopic, microscopic, and chemical characteristics of synovial fluid permit recognition of pathological conditions.

Synovial fluid analysis usually includes evaluation of fluid volume, color, clarity, and viscosity; microscopic examination noting total white blood cell count (WBC), total red blood cell count (RBC), and differential WBC, evaluation of a wet preparation to search for crystals or other abnormalities by compensated polarized microscopy, and microbiological studies including culture and Gram stain. The value of additional studies, such as glucose, protein, and lactate dehydrogenase, is less certain (1).

Anatomy and Physiology

The synovium, the lining tissue that covers the surface of the joint space except the contact surfaces of articular cartilage and menisci, is composed of a fibrillar interstitial matrix of collagen and glycosaminoglycans containing loosely interdigitating synovial cells (2). Unlike usual epithelial cells, synovial cells do not have desmosomal junctions, and there is no basement membrane between the synovial lining and subsynovial tissue. Nerves, lymphatics, and capillaries with fenestrated endothelial cells are also located in synovial tissue (Fig. 24.1).

Synovial fluid is a colorless to light yellow, highly viscous fluid that functions both as a lubricant and as a source of nutrients for articular cartilage in diarthrodial joints. The fluid, formed from the synovium, consists of an ultrafiltrate of plasma, trace nonplasma proteins, trace amounts of lipids, and hyaluronic acid. While essentially all plasma proteins are represented in synovial fluid, high–molecular weight proteins such as fibrinogen, α_2-macroglobulin, β_2-macroglobulin, and β_1-lipoprotein are present only in trace amounts. Thus, normal synovial fluid does not clot. The paucity of high–molecular weight proteins in the ultrafiltrate may be related to endothelial permeability in synovial capillaries, charge interactions in the synovial matrix, and metabolism of proteins by synovial cells (3). Lubricin, a protein produced by synovial cells, appears to aid in lubricating cartilage-cartilage interactions (4). Studies of knee aspirates from normal male volunteers established a normal synovial protein concentration of 1.3 mg/dl (5) with an albumin/globulin ratio of 1.88 (3). Whether there are variations in normal synovial fluid protein concentration due to sex, age, or joint location is currently unknown. Hyaluronic acid, a high–molecular weight glycosaminoglycan, is secreted by synovial cells and tends to increase the viscosity of synovial fluid.

The small amount of synovial fluid normally present within a joint provides a medium for the transport of oxygen, glucose, and other nutrients from the blood in the synovial capillaries to the avascular articular cartilage. Similarly, metabolic wastes from the

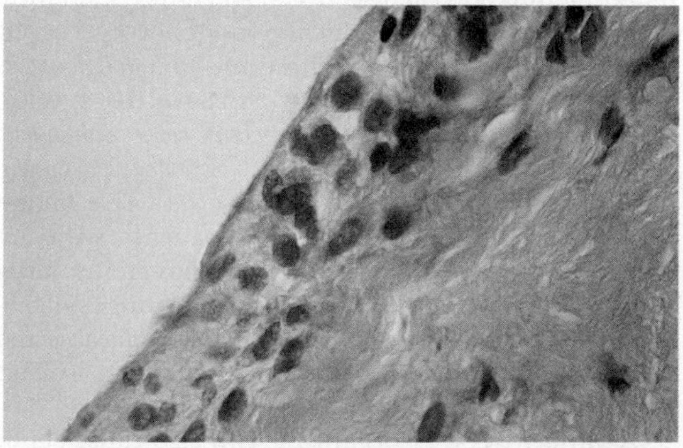

Figure 24.1. Synovial membrane from a normal knee joint shows joint space, synovial membrane composed of synovial cells embedded in a loose connective tissue stroma overlying dense collagen (hematoxylin & eosin).

cartilage cells are carried back to the bloodstream. Proteins are removed from synovial fluid by lymphatic clearance.

Disease States

TRAUMA

Acute trauma to a joint may result from a variety of causes. Hemorrhage is the most frequent consequence of trauma. Acute hemorrhage is characterized by frank blood. Evidence of previous bleeding may be inferred by finding hemosiderin-laden macrophages or erythrophagocytosis.

SEPTIC ARTHRITIS

Bacterial infections are the most common cause of septic arthritis. Early diagnosis of septic arthritis is important to prevent rapid destruction of the joint by proteolytic enzymes released from neutrophils. Bacteria most frequently reach the joint space by hematogenous spread across the synovial membrane. The synovial membrane is quite vascular and lacks a basement membrane and intercellular bridges; these features facilitate the spread of bacteria into the joint. Direct inoculation through trauma, contiguous wound extension, arthroscopy, or surgery is a less frequent mechanism for septic arthritis. All bacteremic patients are at risk to develop septic arthritis; however, most patients with bacteremia do not develop septic arthritis. Host interactions with the infecting organism modify the likelihood of developing a septic joint: immunologic defects, impaired defense mechanisms, trauma, and joint damage from surgery or chronic inflammation all increase the risk (6).

Neisseria gonorrhoeae is the most common cause of septic arthritis in young adults, especially in women. Gonococcal arthritis may be mimicked by disseminated meningococcal infections, so culture identification of the organism is critical. Nongonococcal septic arthritis in adults is most often due to *Staphylococcus aureus*, followed by group A *Streptococcus* species, Gram-negative bacilli (*Escherichia coli, Salmonella* species, *Pseudomonas aeruginosa*), *Streptococcus pneumoniae*, and *Staphylococcus epidermidis*. The Gram-negative bacilli tend to occur in patients with impaired resistance to infection, intravenous drug abuse, or underlying infections of the urinary, biliary, or intestinal tracts (7). *Haemophilus influenzae* and *Streptococcus pyogenes* are the most frequent isolates in neonates and children, respectively (7).

A variety of other organisms can also cause septic arthritis and may not be detected unless special cultures are initiated (8). Tuberculous arthritis may be the result of underlying osteomyelitis. The most common organism is *Mycobacterium tuberculosis*. Culture of a synovial biopsy specimen may be necessary to establish a diagnosis. *Fungal arthritis* may be due to any of the deep tissue invasive fungi, including histoplasmosis, *Candida* species, coccidiodomycosis, blastomycosis, aspergillosis, and sporotrichosis. Actinomycosis and nocardiosis are also causes of septic arthritis. *Mycoplasma pneumoniae* has been isolated from the synovial fluid of patients with atypical pneumonia on rare occasions (9).

Viral arthritis can develop as a primary manifestation of the virus itself or as a complication related to immune complex deposition. Viral causes of arthritis include coxsackieviruses, hepatitis B virus, lymphocytic choriomeningitis virus, mumps, parvovirus (10), rubella, and varicella (7). Diagnosis is established through serology rather than culture of synovial fluid. Although there is no evidence that human immunodeficiency virus (HIV) causes an arthritic process directly, HIV has been isolated from synovial fluid (11, 12). HIV antigen p24 has been demonstrated in synovial fluid when peripheral blood was negative for the antigen (13).

CRYSTAL-INDUCED ARTHRITIS

Monosodium urate (MSU) and calcium pyrophosphate dihydrate (CPPD) are the two most common crystals encountered in synovial fluid, and are associated with disorders termed gout and CPPD deposition disease, respectively. While joint manifestations of both disorders may be clinically indistinguishable, treatment is different. Other crystals, including calcium hydroxyapatite and calcium oxalate, are usually associated with osteoarthritis.

Gout is a multisystem disorder characterized by hyperuricemia (14). The clinical spectrum of hyperuricemia varies from asymptomatic to full-blown gout with arthritis; crystalline deposits of MSU (tophi) in and around joints, soft tissues, and renal interstitium; and nephrolithiasis. Gout is primarily a male disease, with the highest incidence in the fifth decade. Gouty arthritis is usually monoarticular at first, exquisitely painful, and characterized by granulomas containing MSU crystals within neutrophils or macrophages. Joints of the lower extremity (instep, ankle, heel, knee) are most commonly involved; wrists, fingers, and elbows may also be affected. The diagnosis of gouty arthritis is established by demonstrating MSU crystals in synovial fluid by compensated polarized microscopy. Over 95% of patients with acute gout have demonstrable crystals. Treatment is directed toward relieving the acute attack with anti-inflammatory agents in the short term and decreasing serum uric acid in the long term. MSU crystals can persist in synovial fluid for months in patients following treatment, even when the WBC is only slightly elevated (15).

CPPD deposition disease is most common in the elderly. The cause of crystal deposition is unknown but may be associated with age-related changes in cartilage, because many patients have preexisting joint damage. Clinical presentations vary from asymptomatic to subacute, acute, or chronic arthritis. The most common joint affected is the knee; the wrist, shoulder, elbow, ankle, and hand may also be involved. Acute attacks (pseudogout) may be precipitated by trauma, infection, joint surgery, or even walking (16). The definitive diagnosis of pseudogout is based on identification of characteristic CPPD crystals by compensated polarizing microscopy of synovial fluid. Nonsteroidal anti-inflammatory drugs are the mainstay of treatment.

RHEUMATOID ARTHRITIS

Rheumatoid arthritis (RA) is a multisystem disorder of unknown cause characterized by chronic synovial inflammation (17). Although the disease has a varied course from patient to patient, the potential for joint destruction and deformity is a major cause of morbidity. RA affects approximately 1% of the population, and women are 3 times more frequently affected than men. Most patients develop the disease between the ages of 35 and 50. Joints typically are affected in a symmetrical fashion, with the hands (especially proximal interphalangeal and metacarpophalangeal joints), wrists, knees, and feet most commonly involved. Signs and symptoms include joint pain aggravated by movement, and generalized stiffness greatest after periods of inactivity ("morning stiffness").

Pathological examination of rheumatoid joints shows hypertrophy and hyperplasia of synovial lining cells, edema, vascular proliferation, and infiltration of synovium by macrophages and T lymphocytes. The release of immune mediators and chemotaxins in the synovium causes an acute inflammatory response in the synovial fluid. Proliferation of the inflammatory synovium gradually results in destruction of articular cartilage and limitation of movement due to pain. Clinical diagnostic criteria are well established (18).

REACTIVE ARTHRITIS

Reactive arthritis describes an acute nonpurulent arthritis that complicates an infection elsewhere in the body. Reiter's syndrome (arthritis, nongonococcal urethritis, and conjunctivitis) is a classic example of reactive arthritis. Frequent mucocutaneous lesions, linkage with HLA-B27 antigen in 75% of patients, an association with enteric bacteria (*Shigella, Salmonella, Yersinia, Campylobacter* species), and genital infection with *Chlamydia trachomatis* as precipitating agents make it clear that there are a variety of causes of reactive arthritis. The role of HLA-B27 antigen in the pathogenesis of the arthritis is unclear.

Clinical manifestations vary from involvement of one joint to a multisystem disease. A history of recent infection may be obtained, but is not invariable. The joints most commonly involved include the knee, ankle, and foot; however, the wrist and hand may also be affected. Relapses of the acute symptoms may occur as late sequelae (19).

OSTEOARTHRITIS

Osteoarthritis (OA) is the most common joint disease in humans, especially in the elderly (20). OA, or degenerative joint disease, increases in prevalence with increasing age. The pattern of joint involvement appears to be related to joint usage, with the hip in men, and the fingers in women being the most common sites. OA typically involves one or a few joints, with pain aggravaged by use and relieved by rest. OA can be classified into primary, when the cause is unknown, or secondary types related to an underlying disorder.

A defect in articular cartilage integrity at sites of wear is common to both types of OA. Articular cartilage is weakened, fibrillated, and thinned. Thinning of the articular cartilage surface exposes bone. Further distortion of the joint occurs with the formation of osteophytes at the joint margins, cystic changes beneath the articular surface, fibrosis of the joint capsule, proliferation of synovium, and replacement of articular cartilage by fibrocartilage. Synovial effusions, if present, are small; however, crystals of calcium pyrophosphate or calcium hydroxyapatite may be found.

OTHER DISORDERS

Ankylosing spondylitis (AS) is an inflammatory disorder that primarily involves the axial skeleton. AS is more prevalent in men than in women, and most patients are HLA-B27 positive. The inflammatory process causes articular cartilage erosion, followed by fibrocartilage regeneration and, ultimately, ossification of the joint. Peripheral joints show synovial hyperplasia, lymphocytic infiltration, and pannus formation (19). Inflammatory arthritis is also associated with psoriasis (21) and inflammatory bowel disease (22).

Table 24.1. Laboratory Examination of Synovial Fluid

Macroscopic examination
Volume
Viscosity
Clarity
Color
Cell counting
Leukocyte count
Erythrocyte count
Microscopic examination
Wet preparation
Stained preparation
Polarized microscopy for crystals
Microbiological examination
Gram stain
Culture
Special studies
Chemical examination
Immunologic examination

Methodologies

SPECIMEN COLLECTION

The techniques for physical examination and needle aspiration of joint fluid are outlined in textbooks of rheumatology and orthopaedics (23–25). The sample should be collected in a sterile, plastic disposable syringe using aseptic technique. Care should be taken to ensure that a sterile joint is not iatrogenically contaminated with bacteria from a local infection in adjacent soft tissue or from bacteremia (25). The syringe may be moistened with sodium heparin (26) (25 U/ml synovial fluid). Lithium heparin, oxalate, and powdered ethylenediaminetetraacetic acid (EDTA) should be avoided because artifacts that confound crystal analysis may result (26–28).

The specimen is dispensed into three sterile tubes: 5 to 10 ml in a heparinized tube for microbiological studies, 5 ml in a tube containing heparin or liquid EDTA for microscopic examination, and the remainder in a nonanticoagulated tube for other studies. If lesser amounts are obtained, fluid may still be examined. Only several drops are necessary for a wet mount, leukocyte count and differential, and bacteriologic studies (29). When selecting studies on limited amounts of fluid, examinations for crystals and for microorganisms (Gram stain and culture) should receive top priority (Table 24.1).

GROSS EXAMINATION

Gross examination of joint fluid is the first step in establishing a differential diagnosis of arthritis. While a precise diagnosis is rarely made from gross examination alone, a careful look at the fluid can provide valuable clues to underlying pathology.

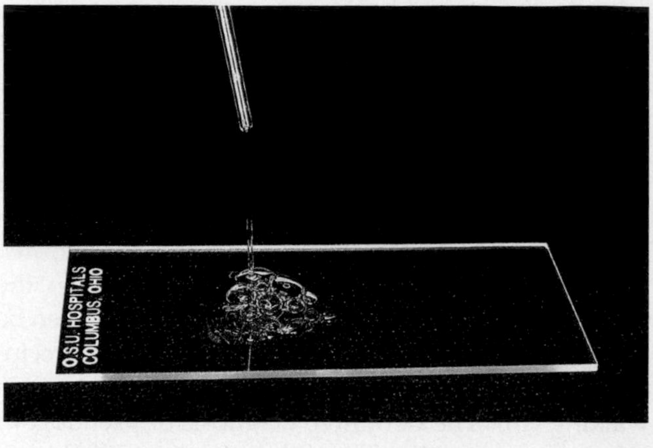

Figure 24.2. The viscosity of synovial fluid is demonstrated by the "string test"—the normally viscous synovial fluid forms a thin strand between the pipette tip and the surface of the slide.

Volume

Normal joints contain very small amounts of fluid; the normal knee joint—the largest synovial joint—contains from a few drops to as much as 4 ml. There is sufficient fluid to coat synovial surfaces and little more, thus making it difficult to sample fluid from a normal joint. Increased amounts of fluid can be seen in conditions causing edema such as myxedema, congestive heart failure, or anasarca. High-dose corticosteroid therapy may be associated with transient, asymptomatic, noninflammatory effusions (30). Difficulty in obtaining fluid from an obvious effusion may occur because of rice bodies, thick fibrin exudates, or loculations that prevent aspiration.

Viscosity

Normal joint fluid is viscous because of a high concentration of hyaluronate. An estimate of viscosity can be made by watching the fluid "string" as it is expressed from a syringe, or by suspending a drop between a glass slide and the tip of a glass rod. Normal fluid will stretch to a string of 1 to 2 inches in length, having a viscosity like egg white (Fig. 24.2). A watery consistency indicates low viscosity, and is usually associated with inflammation. Enzymes released by inflammatory cells, primarily neutrophils, degrade hyaluronate and visibly reduce the joint fluid viscosity. Low viscosity is often caused by inflammation; however, edema or a sudden effusion after trauma can decrease viscosity by dilution in the absence of inflammation. Very viscous fluids can be seen in hypothyroidism and in fluid aspirated from ganglia. More precise quantification of viscosity is generally not necessary.

The mucin clot test is a qualitative test used to estimate the degree of polymerization of hyaluronic

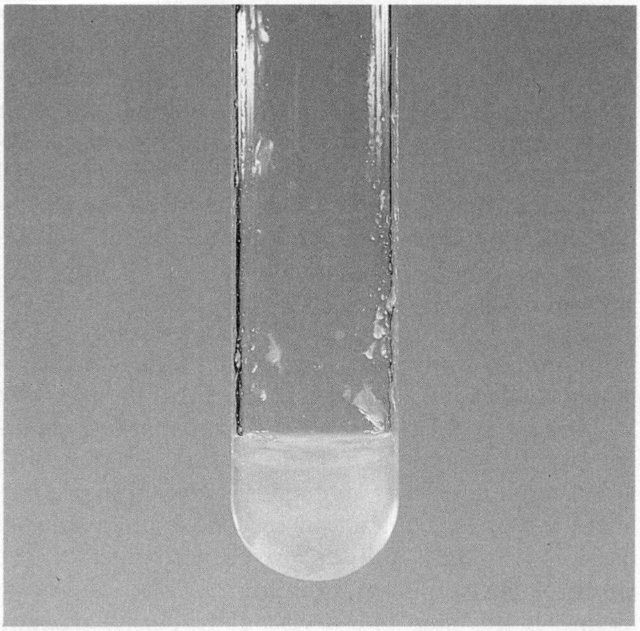

Figure 24.3. Poor mucin clot formation is marked by friable, poorly formed shreds.

acid. Both protein and hyaluronate are required for a mucin clot to form (31). The supernatant from a centrifuged specimen is transferred to a clean glass tube. A few drops of glacial acetic acid are gently layered on the surface of the fluid. As the acid settles to the bottom of the tube, a dense white precipitate (clot) of protein hyaluronate forms. The quality of the clot is graded as "good," "fair," or "poor." A "good" clot will remain intact even when the tube is shaken; a "poor" clot resembles a few formed shreds in a turbid solution (Fig. 24.3). An alternate method is to prepare a 1:4 solution of joint fluid and 2% acetic acid. The solution is mixed and examined for the presence of a mucin clot. The quality of the clot is graded as just described. The cause of poor mucin clot formation is uncertain. The quality of the mucin clot is not solely related to the fluid leukocyte count and the percentage of neutrophils; abnormal synovial cell metabolism resulting in production of altered forms of hyaluronate may also be a factor (32).

Synovial fluid is metachromatic if stained with 0.2% aqueous toluidine blue. This feature can help identify synovial fluid if there is doubt whether the joint or soft tissue has been aspirated (dry tap). To perform the *metachromatic stain test*, spot a filter paper with a drop of fluid. Use a drop of normal saline as a control. After drying, add a few drops of toluidine blue. A positive reaction is marked by a color change to purple when the control spot remains blue (Fig. 24.4). This procedure may be misleading if the fluid has come in contact with heparin, since heparin is also metachromatic with toluidine blue (28).

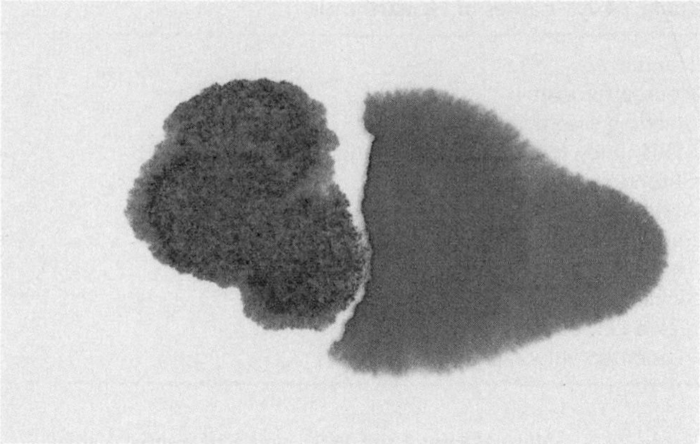

Figure 24.4. Metachromatic stain test illustrates metachromasia of normal synovial fluid. Toluidine blue stained synovial fluid (left) is purple. Compare with toluidine blue alone (right).

Clot Formation

Normal joint fluid does not clot because it lacks high–molecular weight coagulation proteins, including fibrinogen, prothrombin, factors V and VII, antithrombin, and tissue thromboplastin (33). The absence of a clot can help distinguish a truly bloody effusion from a traumatic aspiration or inflammatory effusion.

Clarity

Normal joint fluid is transparent. Since erythrocytes and leukocytes may settle out in the collection tube after aspiration, it is important to ensure that the fluid is well mixed before assessing clarity. If newsprint cannot be read easily through it, the fluid is designated cloudy or opaque. Cloudy fluids may reflect an increase in cellular or protein components, and are usually due to inflammation. Rice bodies, products of degenerating, fibrin-infiltrated synovial membrane, may appear as flecks resembling polished white rice. Flecks of dark particles resembling ground pepper may be a clue to ochronosis (34). Black or gray pigmented debris due to metal or plastic fragments after prosthetic surgery has been described (35). Cholesterol crystals can lend an oily quality to the fluid.

Color

Normal synovial fluid is colorless to light yellow. Grossly bloody fluid can be seen in a variety of conditions listed in Table 24.2. Streaks of blood, or the appearance of blood at the beginning of aspiration that decreases as aspiration continues, suggests a traumatic tap. Examination of the supernatant of centrifuged fluid may help distinguish true hemorrhage from a traumatic tap: if the supernatant is

Table 24.2. Causes of Hemarthrosis

Trauma
Neuroarthropathy
Bleeding disorders
Malignancy (primary vs. metastatic)
Chrondrocalcinosis
Anticoagulant therapy
Joint prostheses
Thrombocytosis
Sickle cell trait
Sickle cell disease
Pigmented villonodular tenosynovitis

Table 24.3. Normal Joint Fluid WBC and Differential Values[a]

Item	Mean	Range
WBC (× 10^9/liter)	0.063	0.013–0.180
Differential count (%)		
Neutrophils	7	0–25
Lymphocytes	24	0–78
Monocytes	48	0–71
Histiocytes	10	0–26
Synovial lining cells	4	0–12

[a]From McCarty DJ. Synovial fluid. In: McCarty DJ, ed. Arthritis and allied conditions: a textbook of rheumatology. 11th ed. Philadelphia: Lea & Febiger, 1989: 70.

xanthochromic, blood has probably been present for some time. Comparison of the hematocrit of the fluid with the venous hematocrit can help resolve the question of whether venous blood (acute bleed) or a hemorrhagic effusion is present. Noninflammatory fluids are generally yellow or straw-colored. Massive numbers of crystals can make the fluid appear opalescent. Cream-colored to off-white fluids usually contain pus with or without crystals. Fluid may be discolored by various bacterial pigments in septic arthritides. Milky white or chylous effusions are typically related to chronic arthritis or lymphatic obstruction secondary to filariasis, but can be seen following trauma and pancreatitis (36, 37). The presence of free-floating fat droplets suggests trauma with or without fracture. Golden cloudy fluids may contain cholesterol crystals. A gray fluid has been attributed to a retained bullet fragment (38).

CELL COUNTING

In addition to the macroscopic examination, the leukocyte count is critically important in classifying joint fluids as noninflammatory, inflammatory, or septic. The total leukocyte count and percentage of neutrophils are good discriminators between inflammatory and noninflammatory disease (1). Normal synovial fluids are paucicellular; most studies indicate that a WBC of less than 0.1×10^9/liter (100/mm^3) is normal (39), with an upper limit of less than 0.2×10^9/liter (200/mm^3) being generally accepted (Table 24.3) (28). Red cell counts (RBCs) are valuable in distinguishing frank blood from a hemorrhagic effusion.

The total cell count is obtained using a hemacytometer chamber viewed with a standard light or phase-contrast microscope. The count should be performed promptly to minimize the effects of cell clumping and cell death, which can decrease the total leukocyte and neutrophil counts within several hours (40). The presence of clots should be noted as a sign of spuriously low cell counts. The fluid should be well mixed to avoid cell sedimentation before counting. In contrast to other body fluids, normal saline (0.9 N) rather than acetic acid must be used as a diluent to avoid clogging of the pipette and consequent cell entrapment by a protein clot. Staining with 0.1% methylene blue dye aids in identifying leukocytes if a phase-contrast microscope is not available. Hypotonic saline (0.3 N) can be employed to lyse erythrocytes when performing a total leukocyte count. If the fluid is too viscous to permit dilution and cell counting, 0.05% hyaluronidase in phosphate buffer may be added as a diluent (28); however, leukocyte counts are said to be slightly higher in hyaluronidase-treated fluids (41).

In the absence of a hemacytometer chamber, a rough estimate of the leukocyte count in undiluted fluid can be made by counting leukocytes per high-power (400×) microscopic field (HPF). When a WBC of less than 2/HPF is noted, the chamber count frequently shows less than 1000 cells/mm^3. In cases where the WBC is higher than 2/HPF, chamber counts should be done to ensure accuracy (42). Electronic counters have been used as a substitute for manual counts, but they are subject to counting errors if debris, lipid droplets, or proteinaceous material are mistaken for leukocytes (43).

MICROSCOPIC EXAMINATION

The microscopic examination includes analysis of a wet preparation, leukocyte differential count, cytologic evaluation using stained slides, and crystal examination using compensated polarized microscopy.

Wet Preparation

A wet preparation is made for immediate examination by placing a drop of fresh, well-mixed fluid onto the center of a clean glass slide. The drop of fluid is covered with a coverslip, the edges of which may be sealed with nail polish to prevent drying. Examine the center of the coverslipped area for white blood cells, red blood cells, crystals, and other materials. Be careful to avoid artifacts introduced during slide preparation, such as paper fibrils or drying artifacts near the nail polish seal. The wet preparation may reveal crystals that cannot otherwise be seen af-

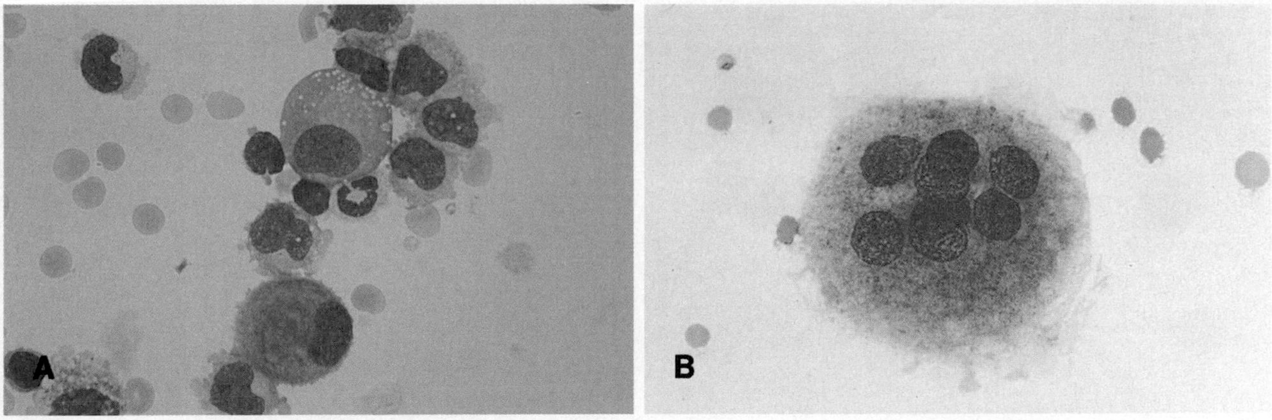

Figure 24.5. **A**, Normal cellular elements found in synovial fluid include neutrophils, lymphocytes, monocytes, histiocytes, and synovial lining cells. A few red blood cells are almost always present in joint effusions (Wright-Giemsa). **B**, Synovial lining cells may be multinucleate (Wright-Giemsa).

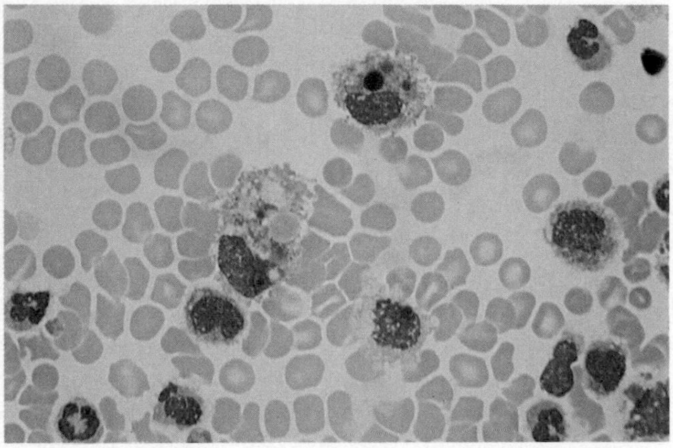

Figure 24.6. Indicators of previous hemorrhage in synovial fluid include erythrophagocytosis by a macrophage *(center)* and breakdown products of hemoglobin, including hemosiderin pigment *(brown)* and hematoidin crystal *(yellow)* in macrophage *(top)* (Wright-Giemsa).

ter routine fixation with alcohol and staining with Wright's stain. Examination of the sediment following centrifugation can help concentrate cellular material and crystals, especially in the clear fluids. Addition of a drop of synovial fluid to special slides coated with dry methylene blue and cresyl violet offers promise as a rapid supravital stain (44).

Light Microscopy

Air-dried Wright-stained cytocentrifuge preparations are used for cellular differential counts. In the absence of a cytocentrifuge, smears of the centrifuged sediment are acceptable, provided there is no delay in processing the sample and the smears are as thin as possible. Thick smears may have a bluish background from heparin or mucopolysaccharides in the fluid, which can prevent cytoplasmic spreading and make examination difficult (28).

Normal cellular elements found in synovial fluid (Table 24.3) include monocytes, lymphocytes, histiocytes, neutrophils, and synovial lining cells or synoviocytes (Fig. 24.5). The appearance of blood cells in Wright-stained preparations is identical to that of peripheral blood. The predominant cell type is a monocyte. Phagocytic vacuoles help identify histiocytes, but the distinction from monocytes is not always clear-cut. Occasional lymphocytes may show reactive changes, including larger nuclear size, nuclear indentations, and a small nucleolus, but the majority are small with round nuclei similar to those in peripheral blood. Synovial lining cells resemble mesothelial cells and do not have diagnostic significance. A few red blood cells are almost always present in joint effusions.

Abnormal cellular elements can suggest a specific diagnosis in some cases. *Erythrophagocytosis* by macrophages indicates previous hemorrhage. *Hemosiderin* pigment and *hematoidin crystals* are breakdown products of hemoglobin, and are seen after hemorrhage. Hematoidin crystals are golden yellow, refractile, rhomboidal crystals that may be seen intracellularly or extracellularly (Fig. 24.6). *Cartilage cells*, or their fragments, are not normally present in synovial fluid and are recognized as individual cells with deep purple cytoplasm and a small nucleus surrounded by a halo (Fig. 24.7). Cartilage may be seen following trauma or in osteoarthritis. Iron-laden chondrocytes can point to a diagnosis of hemochromatosis. Yellow chondrocytes are described in ochronosis (45). *Ragocytes* or *RA cells* are neutrophils containing refractile round cytoplasmic inclusions and are best seen in wet preparations using phase-contrast microscopy. These cells are frequently found in inflammatory effusions and are not diagnostic of a specific disorder. The inclusions represent phagocytosed immunoglobulin, immune complexes, DNA particles, rheumatoid

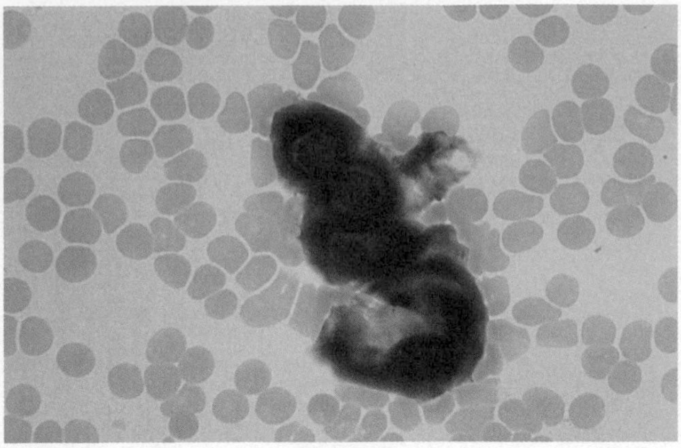

Figure 24.7. Cartilage is recognized by its deep purple cytoplasm and nucleus in a lacuna. Chrondrocytes may also be seen as single cells rather than the cluster shown here (Wright-Giemsa).

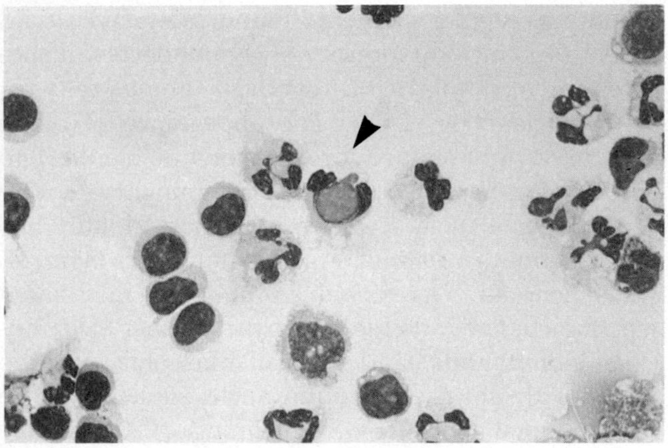

Figure 24.8. LE cell *(arrow)* is a neutrophil containing a phagocytized homogeneous nucleus (Wright-Giemsa).

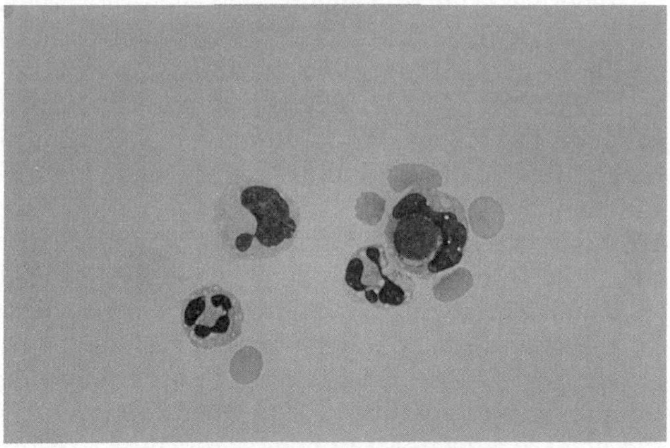

Figure 24.9. Tart cell is a macrophage containing a phagocytized nucleus that retains some nuclear detail (Wright-Giemsa).

factor, fibrin, and antinuclear factors (29). *Lupus erythematosus (LE) cells* are neutrophils that contain a phagocytized homogenized nucleus (Fig. 24.8). While LE cells may be present in the synovial fluid of patients with systemic lupus erythematosus (SLE),

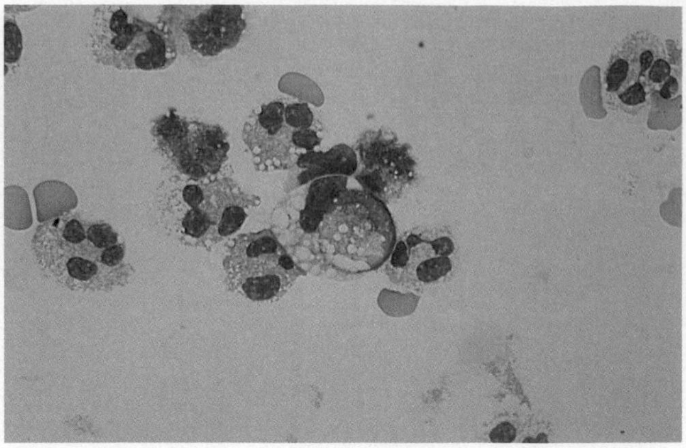

Figure 24.10. Rieter's cell *(center)* is a macrophage that has phagocytosed one or more neutrophils. This finding is not specific for Reiter's syndrome.

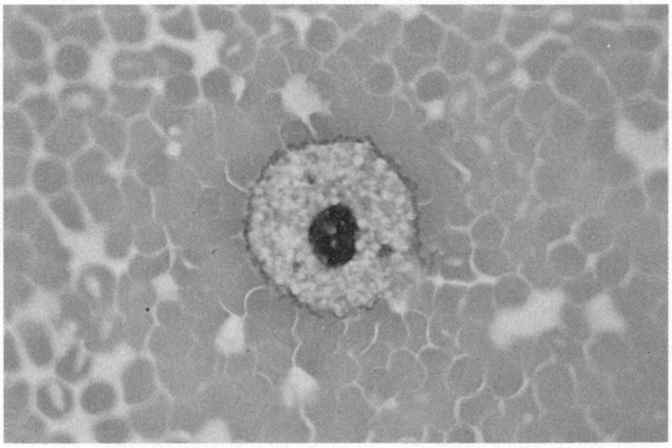

Figure 24.11. Lipid-laden macrophage in synovial fluid (Wright-Giemsa).

even when peripheral blood LE preparations are negative (28), they are not diagnostic. LE cells have also been described in rheumatoid arthritis (46), and their absence does not exclude a diagnosis of SLE. LE cells should be distinguished from *tart cells,* which are neutrophils or macrophages containing a phagocytized nucleus that retains some chromatin detail (Fig. 24.9). Tart cells are a nonspecific finding without diagnostic significance. So-called *Reiter's cells* are macrophages containing one or more phagocytized neutrophils (Fig. 24.10). They are not diagnostic of Reiter's syndrome, and can be found in a variety of inflammatory effusions.

Lipid-laden macrophages (Fig. 24.11) may be seen in traumatic arthritis as a late finding (47), in chronic arthritis with chylous effusion, and in pancreatitis (37). The lipid in chronic arthritis probably originates from a breakdown of cells damaged by inflammation. Lipid may appear as extracellular or intracellular isotropic fat globules or as anisotropic lipid droplets that show "Maltese cross" birefringence under polarized

Table 24.4. Causes of Synovial Fluid Eosinophilia

Rheumatic diseases
Hypereosinophilic syndromes
Bacterial infections
Allergic disease
Parasitic arthritides
Metastatic adenocarcinoma
Arthrography
Air
Dye
Therapeutic x irradiation
Urticaria
Acute
Chronic
Idiopathy

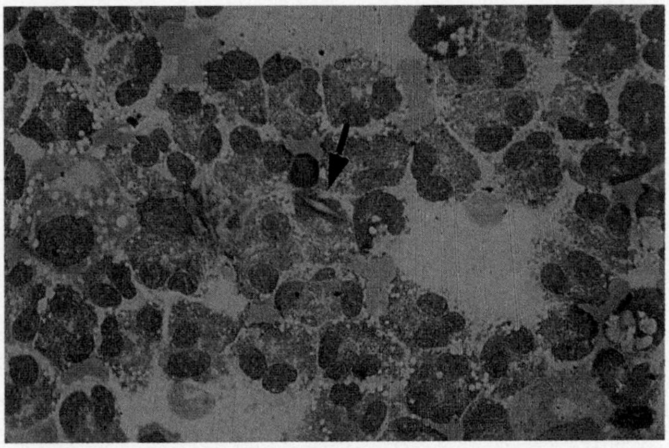

Figure 24.12. Diamond-shaped Charcot-Leyden crystal *(arrow)* within an eosinophil in eosinophilic effusion (Wright-Giemsa).

light. Oil red O or Sudan black B fat stains may be used to identify lipid material. Prominent intracellular and extracellular *lipid microspherules* or *lipid liquid crystals* may be observed under polarized microscopy as small Maltese crosses (48, 49). They are of uncertain origin and have been seen in pigmented villonodular synovitis (50) and chronic arthritis (51). The role of the microspherules in the pathogenesis of the arthritis remains to be determined.

Eosinophils are not found in normal synovial fluid, and are uncommon in pathological fluids. Increased eosinophils (more than 2% of the leukocytes) are noted in a variety of disorders listed in Table 24.4 (52). *Charcot-Leyden crystals* are elongated diamond-shaped crystals of lysolecithinase from eosinophils that stain pink or purple with Wright stain (Fig. 24.12). They have been noted in conditions associated with chronic eosinophilia, but their appearance in joint fluid is very rare. Charcot-Leyden crystals have been described in a patient with an allergic reaction following intra-articular injection of steroids (53) and also in a patient with chronic myelogenous leukemia (54). *Mast cells* (Fig. 24.13) have been identified in small numbers in synovial fluid, with variable

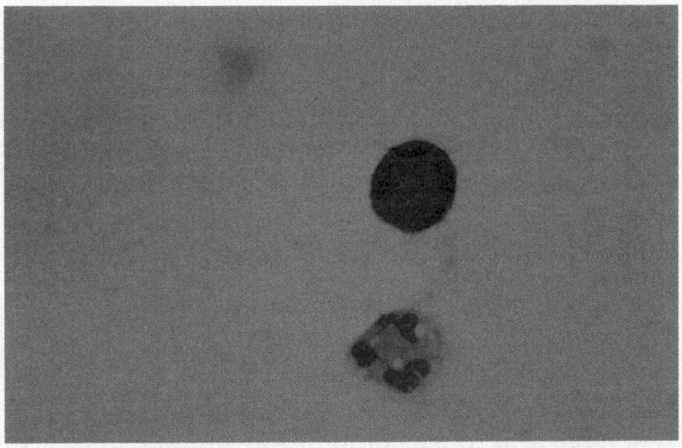

Figure 24.13. Mast cell in synovial fluid (Wright-Giemsa).

quantities observed in patients with diverse disorders, including ankylosing spondylitis, Reiter's disease, psoriatic arthritis, and enteropathic arthritis (55). Mast cells have been observed in greatly increased numbers in patients with systemic mastocytosis (56).

Sickled erythrocytes may provide a clue to an underlying sickle disease, trait, or combination SC or S-thalassemia (57, 58). The presence of sickled cells does not necessarily indicate that the hemoglobinopathy is responsible for the joint pathology. *Platelets* may be found in synovial fluid of patients with osteoarthritis and rheumatoid arthritis (59, 60). *Marrow spicules* are a clue to fracture with involvement of joint (61).

Although they are rare, primary and metastatic malignancies can involve the joint space, and the malignant cells can be recognized on microscopic examination. *Non-Hodgkin's lymphoma* (62), *Hodgkin's lymphoma* (63), *blast transformation of chronic myeloid leukemia* (64, 65), *acute lymphocytic leukemia* (66–68), adult T-cell leukemia (66), *acute myelomonocytic leukemia* (69), *chronic lymphocytic leukemia* (70, 71), and *metastatic squamous carcinoma* (72, 73), and *adenocarcinoma* (74, 75) are described.

Collagen can be seen to advantage by lowering the microscope condenser. Under polarized light, collagen is weakly birefringent. *Amyloid* appears as amorphous deposits that are green and weakly birefringent when stained with Congo red and viewed under polarized light. Identification of amyloid in synovial fluid correlates well with synovial biopsy findings, so biopsy may be avoided in patients with positive fluid findings (76, 77). Rarely, fragments from metal or polymer prostheses can be seen (35, 78).

Some medications and radiographic contrast media can affect the leukocyte differential count. One study found significantly lower numbers of lymphocytes in patients with rheumatoid arthritis treated with nonsteroidal anti-inflammatory drugs (NSAIDs) plus methotrexate, gold, or hydroxychloroquine than in those receiving NSAIDs alone (79). Injection of ionic contrast media with epinephrine was associated with a leukocytosis, whereas no inflammatory changes were noted after injection of nonionic contrast media (80).

Polarized Microscopy: Examination for Crystals

A polarizing light microscope is equipped with two polarizing filters: one over the light source, called the polarizer, and one between the stage and the observer's eye, called the analyzer. Polarizing filters have a fixed axis of light transmission. For crystal analysis, a first-order red compensator is placed between the polarizer and the analyzer to allow compensated polarized microscopy. In some microscopes, the analyzer is located in the barrel between the objective and the analyzer. In others, the analyzer fits over the polarizer. A convenient feature of some microscopes is a rotating stage. This facilitates the alignment of crystals with the orientation of the compensator. Phase-contrast optics may be added to improve the visibility of cytoplasmic granularity.

When viewing crystals in a wet preparation or stained smear, it is helpful to first scan the slide at low power using polarized light without the compensator. Objects of interest are then viewed with high-power objectives (40× or 100×). The polarizing filters should be "crossed," i.e., with their axes of transmission oriented perpendicular to one another, so that light transmitted by the polarizer will not be transmitted by the analyzer. The background of the field is its darkest black when the polarizer and analyzer are oriented at 90°. If a birefringent crystal is placed between the polarizer and analyzer, polarized light entering the crystal is refracted into two rays (both oriented perpendicular to one another), neither of which is parallel to the plane of the entering light. The fraction of refracted light that is shifted to the plane of the analyzer passes, and the crystal appears as a white object on a dark background. Only birefringent materials behave this way in polarized light.

Birefringence is a property of materials that have two optical axes; not all crystals are birefringent, and not all birefringent objects are crystals. The optical axis of an object is the path through which light passes unrefracted. Plane polarized light entering a birefringent object out of alignment with the optical axis is refracted into two rays: the one that deviates greatest from the optical axis travels a greater distance and is designated the slow ray; the one deviating least is the fast ray (Fig. 24.14). The exiting rays, by virtue of traveling at different velocities through the object, are out of phase with each other. The difference in the degree of refraction between the fast and slow ray, along with the thickness of the object, determines the strength of birefringence.

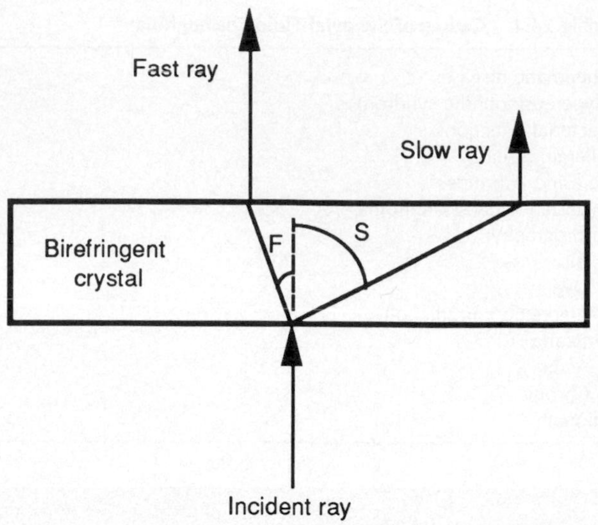

Figure 24.14. Light entering a birefringent crystal is refracted into fast and slow rays that are mutually perpendicular. The fast ray has the lesser degree of deviation from the optical axis of the crystal. (Modified from Gatter RA. Use of the compensated polarizing microscope. Clin Rheum Dis 1977;3:91–103; used with permission.)

A first-order red compensator is itself a birefringent crystal, usually quartz, that, based on its birefringence and thickness, selectively retards the transmission of green light (540 to 575 nm). When the compensator is oriented at 45° to the polarizer, transmitted light from the compensator that passes through the analyzer appears red or rose-colored. Compensators are named based on the color of light transmitted; hence the red designation. The orientation of the slow ray (axis) of the compensator is marked on it to permit proper alignment; most are fixed in the 45° position with respect to the polarizer and analyzer. Improvised compensators have been created using cellophane tape (81). These do not work as well as professional equipment, and the kind of tape used is critical.

Crystals are further classified optically as positively or negatively birefringent. For crystals with two optical axes (biaxial), this designation is based on the orientation of the fast and slow refractive rays to the optical axes of the crystal. The optical axes are roughly in line with the physical long dimension of the crystal, and cross obliquely in the center of the crystal. By definition, when the fast ray of the crystal bisects the acute angle of the optical axes, the crystal is termed negatively birefringent (Fig. 24.15). When the slow ray of the crystal bisects the acute angle of the optical axes, the crystal is termed positively birefringent.

How is the orientation of the slow and fast rays within a crystal determined? The rays of light passing through a crystal cannot be seen, but the color

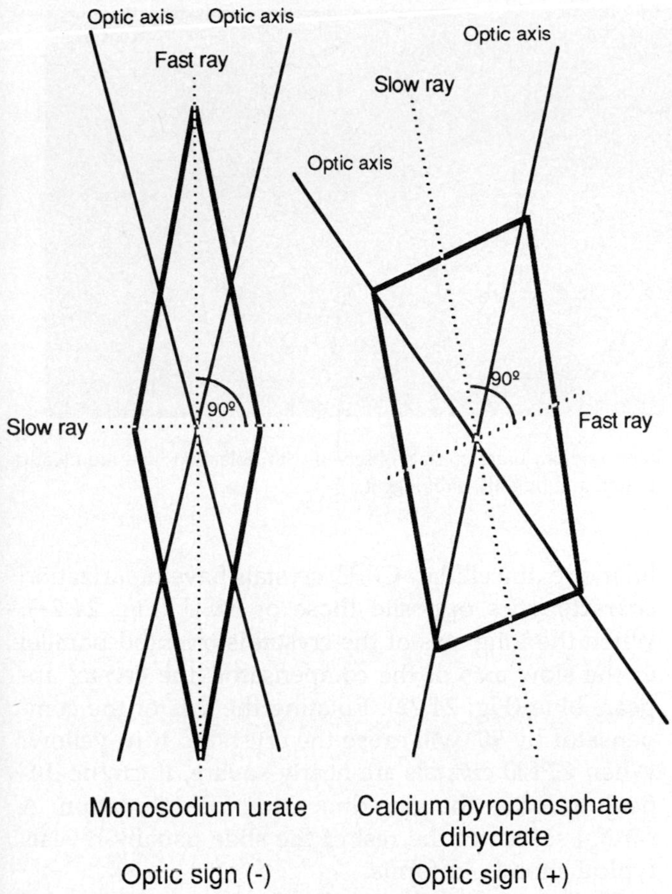

Figure 24.15. The optical sign of biaxial crystals is determined by the relationship of the fast and slow axes to the optical axis of the crystal. If the fast axis of the crystal bisects the acute angle of the optical axis, the crystal is optically negative. If the slow axis of the crystal bisects the acute angle of the optical axis, the crystal is optically positive. (Modified from Gatter RA. Use of the compensated polarizing microscope. Clin Rheum Dis 1977;3:91–103; used with permission.)

and physical orientation of a crystal can be compared with a known crystal, such as the red compensator. A birefringent crystal produces interference colors by adding to or subtractng from the incident ray when that ray is oriented parallel to the slow ray (axis) of the compensator. The wavelength of emitted light is shifted higher, to blue, if the *slow* ray of the crystal is parallel to the slow axis of the compensator, and is shifted lower, to yellow, if the *fast* ray of the crystal is parallel to the slow axis of the compensator. The colors are described with respect to the wavelength of the red compensator and represent the sum of the wavelengths produced by the compensator and crystal when both are placed between two polarizing filters. As seen in Figure 24.16, blue and yellow are spectrally equidistant from the red of the red compensator and reflect the additive or subtractive effect of the crystal on the red wavelength. Thus, the color of the crystal when its long dimension is parallel to the slow axis of the compensator defines the direc-

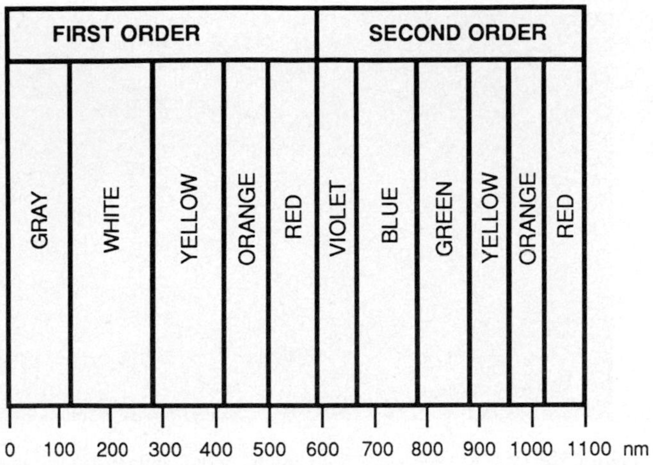

Figure 24.16. Orders and colors resulting from the use of compensators in a polarized light system theoretically from 0 to 1100 nm. Yellow and blue are spectrally equidistant from the red of a red compensator. (From Gatter RA. Use of the compensated polarizing microscope. Clin Rheum Dis 1977;3:91–103; used with permission.)

tion of the crystal's slow axis: a crystal that appears blue when its long dimension is parallel to the slow axis of the compensator has its slow ray oriented parallel to the long dimension of the crystal, and is also positively birefringent. A crystal that appears yellow when its long dimension is parallel to the slow axis of the compensator has its slow ray oriented perpendicular to the long dimension of the crystal (the fast ray bisects the acute angle of optical axes) and is negatively birefringent. Several reviews provide detailed discussions of polarized microscopy (25, 81–83).

Any crystals seen under low power should be examined under high power. Weakly birefringent crystals may be difficult to see if the light is not properly adjusted; too bright a background can "overexpose" the crystals; too little light makes the already weak birefringence too weak to see. The slide should be screened under high power even if no crystals are noted under low power, with the knowledge that light microscopy alone cannot definitively exclude the presence of crystals (29, 84). Estimate the number of crystals as few, moderate, or many, and note their location as intracellular, extracellular, or both. Next, with a crystal in view, insert the red compensator. Align the long dimension of the crystal with the slow axis of the compensator, using a rotating stage or by rotating the slide, and note the color and shape of the crystal. Remember that more than one type of crystal may be present (85). Unidentifiable crystals may be subjected to x-ray diffraction, electron microscopy, or other esoteric tests when the crystals are suspected to be responsible for the joint complaints (25).

Monosodium urate (MSU) crystals are needle-shaped, 5 to 20 µm long, strongly negatively birefrin-

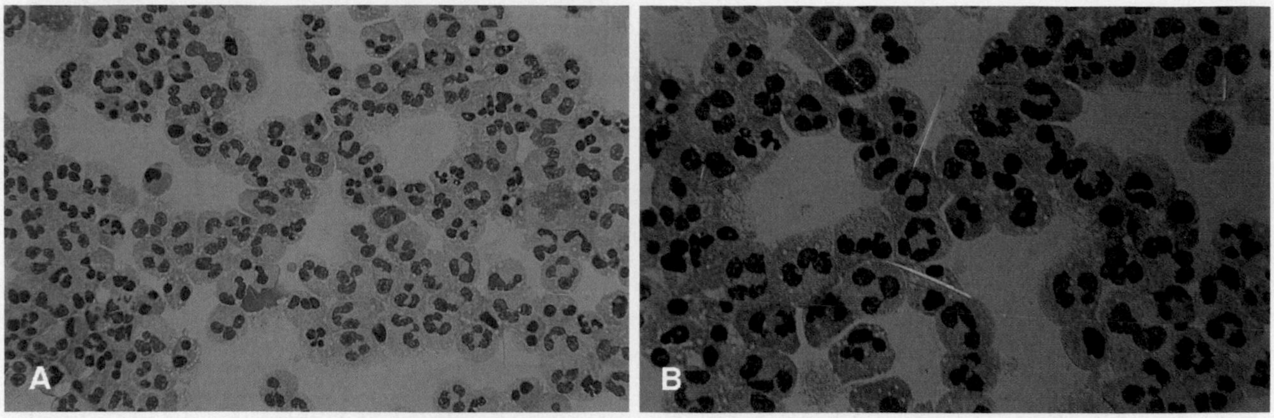

Figure 24.17. A, Synovial fluid with acute inflammation and monosodium urate crystals. The needle-shaped crystals are more difficult to recognize without polarized microscopy (Wright-Giemsa). B, Monosodium urate crystals observed with polarized light are clearly visible and brightly birefringent.

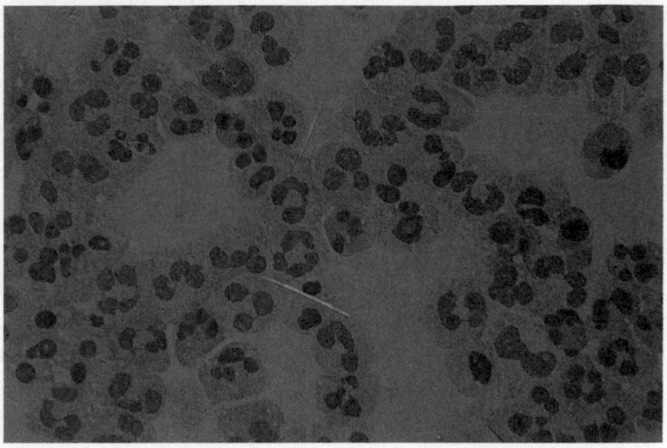

Figure 24.18. Monosodium urate crystals observed with compensated polarized light. The slow axis of the compensator is oriented parallel to the long axis of the yellow crystal.

gent crystals (Fig. 24.17) that may be located intracellularly or extracellularly (29). When the long axis of the crystal is oriented parallel to the slow axis of the red compensator, the crystal is bright yellow (Figs. 24.18 and 24.19). Rotating the axis of the compensator by 90° causes the crystal to change to blue. These crystals are usually easy to see under low power with polarized light; occasionally, microcrystals 1 to 2 μm in length may be the only ones found, and require high-power examination for detection (86). MSU crystals can be provisionally recognized by their size and color in Wright-stained preparations in the absence of a polarizing microscope (Figs. 24.17) (87). Rarely, spherules of MSU are present, which may be difficult to recognize as urate (88).

Calcium pyrophosphate dihydrate (CPPD) crystals are rod- to rhomboidal-shaped, 1 to 20 μm in length, and up to 4 μm in width, weakly positive birefringent crystals (Fig. 24.20) that are often more difficult to see than MSU crystals. CPPD crystals can be intracellular or extracellular. CPPD crystals have polarization characteristics opposite those of MSU (Fig. 24.21). When the long axis of the crystal is oriented parallel to the slow axis of the compensator, the crystal appears blue (Fig. 24.22). Rotating the axis of the compensator by 90° will cause the crystal to turn yellow. When CPPD crystals are nearly square, it can be difficult to locate the long dimension for orientation. A careful search of the rest of the slide usually reveals typical rhomboid forms.

Cholesterol crystals usually appear as large, flat rhomboidal plates and have notched corners. They are strongly positively birefringent, especially when stacked on top of one another. Cholesterol crystals are associated with chronic and chylous effusions in inflammatory and degenerative arthritis (89). Negatively birefringent, needle-shaped forms have been described that can resemble MSU (90). Cholesterol crystals are never phagocytosed (29), and have no known etiologic role in the pathogenesis of arthritis. Both rhomboidal and needle-shaped forms can be seen in the same specimen.

Basic calcium phosphate (BCP) crystals, including hydroxyapatite and calcium phosphates, are ultramicroscopic in size and can be diagnosed as individual crystals only with transmission electron microscopy. Under the light microscope, these crystals appear as spheroidal clumps that vary from 1 to 50 μm in diameter (29). BCP crystals are usually not birefringent unless they are oriented along a common axis. Alizarin red S, a stain for calcium salts, has been used to identify clumps of crystals within cells, though its value as a screening test for these crystals has been questioned (84).

Calcium oxalate (CO) crystals are bipyramidal, 1 to 2 μm in size, and positively birefringent. They are associated with primary oxalosis as a manifestation of extensive tissue oxalate deposition, and chronic

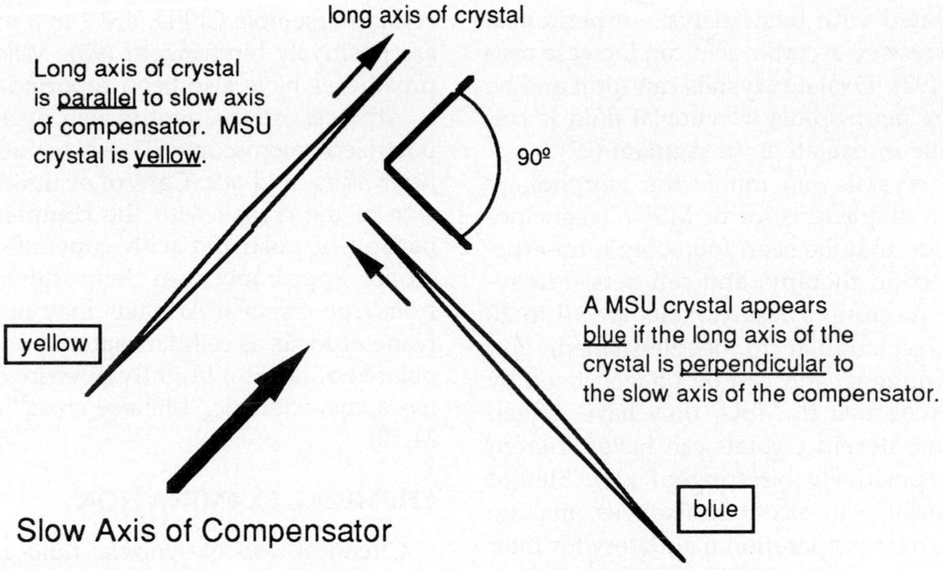

Figure 24.19. Polarization characteristics of monosodium urate crystals.

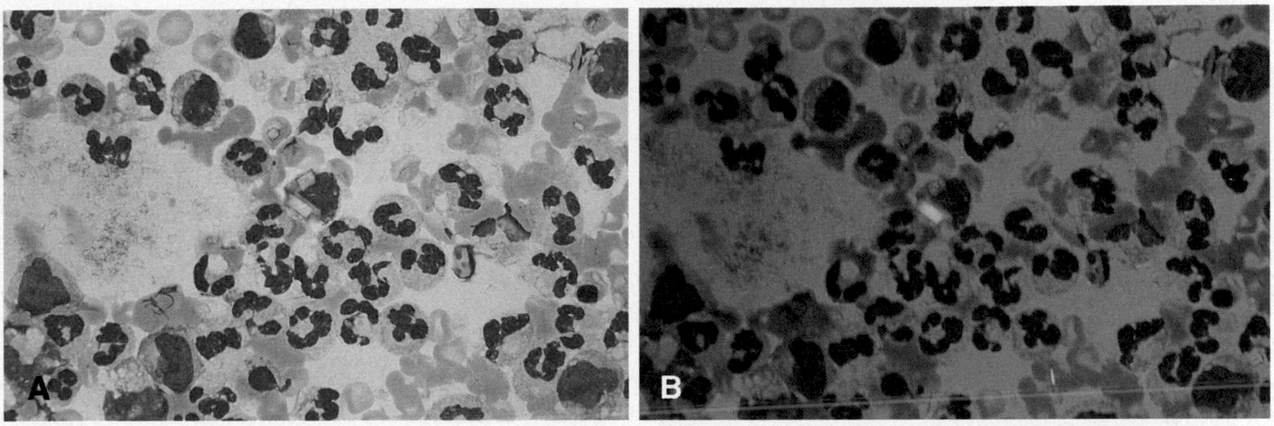

Figure 24.20. **A**, Synovial fluid with acute inflammation and calcium pyrophosphate dihydrate crystals. The rhomboidal intracellular crystals *(center)* are characteristic (Wright-Giemsa). **B**, Calcium pyrophosphate dihydrate crystals observed with polarized light show weak birefringence.

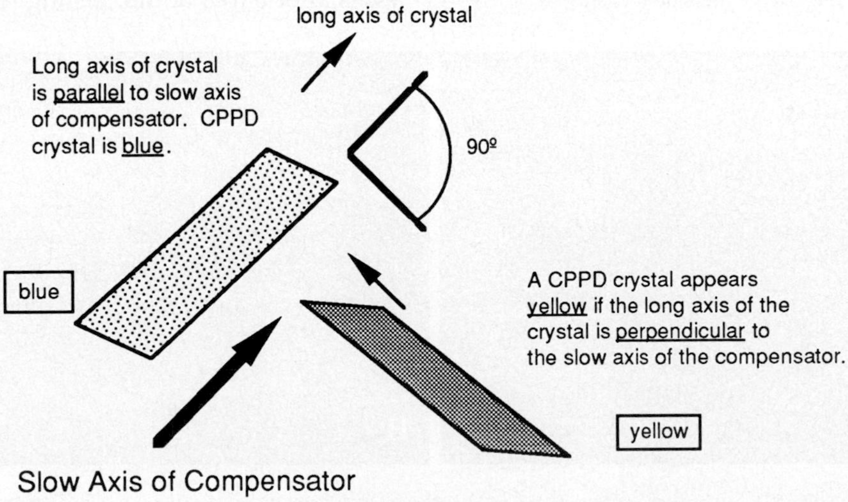

Figure 24.21. Polarization characteristics of calcium pyrophosphate dihydrate crystals.

renal failure treated with hemodialysis or peritoneal dialysis (91). Excessive ascorbic acid can increase oxalate deposition (92). Oxalate crystals can form and be phagocytized by neutrophils if synovial fluid is collected by mistake in oxalate anticoagulant (27).

Corticosteroid crystals can mimic the morphology and polarization characteristics of MSU. Triamcinolone hexacetonide may be seen following intra-articular steroid injection therapy, and can persist in synovial fluid for months. These crystals are 10 to 20 μm in length, rectangular to needle-shaped, and negatively birefringent, and can be phagocytized by neutrophils. In contrast to MSU, they have ragged edges (29). Other steroid crystals can have different shapes and be positively birefringent (25). Steroid crystals may dissolve in alcoholic fixatives, making examination of a wet preparation mandatory for their identification.

Other crystalline objects that have been described in synovial fluid include *cryoprotein and immunoglobulin* (93), and *aluminum phosphate* (94). *Lithium heparin* crystals resemble CPPD, are 2 to 5 μm in length, and are positively birefringent (95). *Metal fragments* from prostheses have also been reported (35).

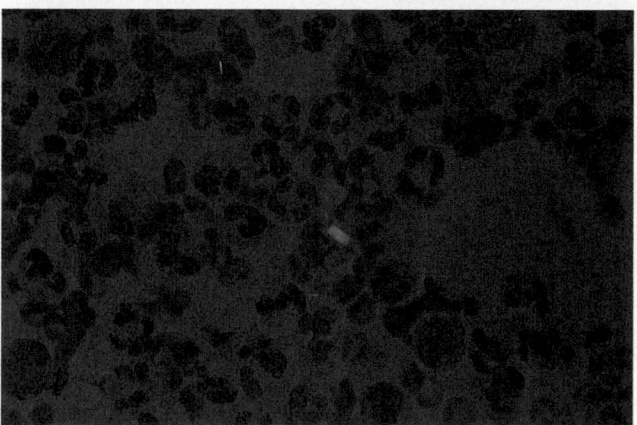

Figure 24.22. Calcium pyrophosphate dihydrate crystals observed with compensated polarized light. The slow axis of the compensator is oriented parallel to the long axis of the blue crystal.

Artifacts are frequently seen during compensated polarized microscopy. These include *dust* and *dirt*, *paper fibers*, and *talc*. Careful evaluation of the optical sign of the crystal with the compensator, and comparison of polarized with conventional light microscopic appearance can help differentiate artifacts from true crystals. Artifacts may not be in the same plane of focus as cellular material on the slide. When polarized, talc is a brightly birefringent spherule and has a characteristic "Maltese cross" appearance (Fig. 24.23).

CHEMICAL EXAMINATION

Chemical tests of synovial fluid generally contribute little to establishing a clinical diagnosis. Normal values for synovial fluid are shown in Table 24.5. Of the analytes, joint fluid protein, glucose, and uric acid may be requested in the usual clinical laboratory setting. Other tests, including lipids (96), enzymes, lactate, hyaluronidase, and ferritin, are more often performed in research studies. These are reviewed in several texts (25, 28, 29). If viscosity presents a problem in clinical analyzers, the fluid can be sonicated or pretreated with hyaluronidase. Analyzers built to analyze serum may not perform as well with synovial fluid (97).

Glucose

Historically, low synovial fluid glucose has been used to differentiate infection from inflammatory effusions. Synovial fluid and plasma specimens should be collected at the same time in tubes containing fluoride to minimize cellular metabolism of glucose in vitro. Joint fluid glucose equilibrates with serum levels after 6 to 8 hours; fasting levels are most relia-

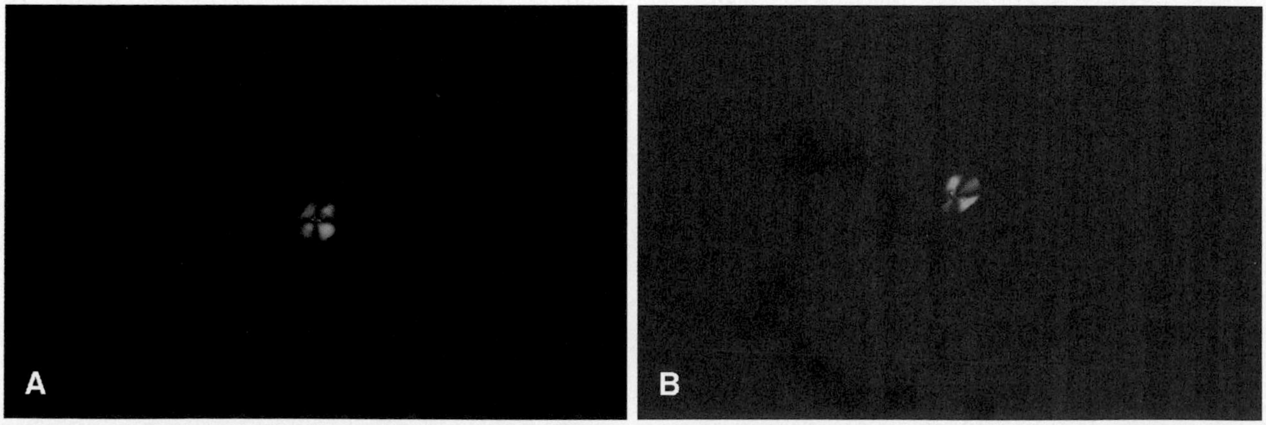

Figure 24.23. **A**, Talc observed under polarized light shows typical "Maltese cross" appearance. **B**, Talc viewed under polarized light with red compensator.

Table 24.5. Normal Joint Fluid Chemical Values[a]

Item	Range	Mean
pH	7.3–7.43	7.38
Total protein (g/dl)	1.2–3.0	1.8
Albumin (%)	56–63	60
Globulin (%)	37–44	40
Hyaluronate (g/dl)		0.3

[a]From McCarty DJ. Synovial fluid. In: McCarty DJ, ed. Arthritis and allied conditions: a textbook of rheumatology. 11th ed. Philadelphia: Lea & Febiger, 1989: 70.

ble. In noninflammatory effusions, there is a glucose difference of less than 10 mg/dl between serum and joint fluid. With increasing inflammation, glucose levels in joint fluid fall. Infections should be considered when fluid glucose is less than 20 mg/dl (98). The large variation in glucose concentration in inflammatory and infectious disorders minimizes the usefulness of this test. Low glucose levels have been noted with CPPD in the absence of infection (99).

Protein

Measurement of synovial fluid protein does not distinguish transudates from exudates as in serous effusions. Increases in protein concentration above 2.5 g/dl are not normal, and concentrations above 4.5 g/dl are often associated with inflammation (31). Unfortunately, the protein concentration does not provide a specific diagnosis and is not of practical clinical value.

Urate

Urate is not concentrated within joints, and joint levels mirror serum levels (100). Therefore, there is little need to measure synovial fluid uric acid.

IMMUNOLOGIC EXAMINATION

There are few immunologic tests performed on synovial fluid that are helpful in establishing a clinical diagnosis. Many studies pertain to rheumatoid arthritis. Normal synovial fluid *immunoglobulin* concentrations are about 10% of those serum. Synovial fluid immunoglobulins in rheumatoid arthritis are typically increased and are derived both from peripheral blood and also local synthesis by plasma cells in the synovium. IgG, IgA, and IgM are all produced as part of the inflammatory response, and at least a portion of the IgM and IgG has *rheumatoid factor* activity. In most cases, the synovial rheumatoid factor titer is similar to the serum titer, but cases have been reported in which serum is negative in the presence of a positive synovial titer. Rheumatoid factors are unique to rheumatoid arthritis (29).

Measurements of total hemolytic complement activity (CH_{50}) in synovial fluid need to be correlated with serum levels. The CH_{50} level is low in normal joints, and parallels serum CH_{50} in diseased joints with altered protein permeability. In the absence of local consumption, the CH_{50} is 33 to 50% of the serum value (29). A significant decrease in synovial fluid complement compared with peripheral blood levels correlates with activation by local immune complexes, and is a usual finding in RA. However, similar patterns may be seen in septic arthritis and gout (101). Decreases in both serum and synovial complement may be found in systemic lupus erythematosus. In general, because the levels do not permit separation of similar entities, complement levels are not of diagnostic assistance (102). Analysis of B and T cell subsets in RA demonstrates that the percentage of B cells is similar to peripheral blood, while T cell fractions are increased. Analysis of synovial B and T cell subsets in inflammatory disorders is largely a research tool.

MICROBIOLOGICAL EXAMINATION

Microbiological examination includes Gram stain of fluid smears and culture for microorganisms. While the Gram stain provides an immediate diagnosis when bacteria are visualized, its sensitivity is inadequate to detect all bacterial infections. Negative smears are not uncommon in gonococcal arthritis and in patients who have been treated with antibiotics before arthrocentesis (7). Thus, cultures should be initiated whenever a joint infection is a possibility. Clinical history, physical findings, and radiographic examinations narrow the differential diagnosis, and guide which organisms should be considered for culture.

Samples for culture should be collected in a sterile container and transported to the laboratory as soon as possible. Special handling and media are necessary for *Neiserria gonorrhoeae*, anaerobic bacteria, mycobacteria, and fungal cultures. Viral cultures are rarely indicated.

Rapid analysis of fungal or bacterial antigens by latex agglutination or counterimmunoelectrophoresis, examination of metabolites by gas chromatography, and *Limulus* lysate assay for bacterial endotoxin are all applicable to synovial fluid samples.

INTERPRETATION

Based on the gross examination, WBC, and differential, most fluids can be classified into one of several categories (Table 24.6) to narrow the diagnosis. Examples of disorders representative of each category are shown in Table 24.7. Synovial fluid findings are often nonspecific, and clinical information and results of other laboratory tests are necessary to establish a specific diagnosis. From the laboratory per-

Table 24.6. Classification of Synovial Effusions[a]

Gross Examination	Normal	Noninflammatory (Group I)	Inflammatory (Group II)	Septic (Group III)	Crystal (Group IV)	Hemorrhagic (Group V)
Volume (ml) (knee)	<3.5	Often >3.5	Often >3.5	Often >3.5	Often >3.5	Often >3.5
Viscosity	High	High	Low	Variable	Variable	Variable
Color	Colorless to straw	Straw to yellow	Yellow Cloudy	Yellow-white Cloudy	Yellow Cloudy	Red Xanthochromic
Routine laboratory examination						
WBC (mm³)	<200	200–2,000	2,000–75,000	Often >100,000	2,000 to 75,000	50-10,000
PMN leukocytes (%)	<25	<25	>50 often	>75[b]	>50 often	<50
Crystals present	No	No	No	No	Yes	No
Culture	Negative	Negative	Negative	Often positive	Negative	Negative
Mucin clot	Firm	Firm	Friable	Friable	Friable	
Glucose (AM fasting)	Nearly equal to blood	Nearly equal to blood	<50 mg% lower than blood	>50 mg% lower than blood	>50 mg% lower than blood	Nearly equal to blood

[a]Adapted from Schumacher HR. Synovial fluid analysis and synovial biopsy. In: Kelley WN, Harris ED, Ruddy S, Sledge CB, eds. Textbook of rheumatology. 3rd ed. Philadelphia: WB Saunders, 1989:638, and Kjeldsberg CR, Knight JA. Body fluids: laboratory examination of amniotic, cerebrospinal, seminal serous, and synovial fluids. 2nd ed. Chicago: ASCP Press, 1986:134.
[b]WBC and %PMN leukocytes will be less if organism is less virulent or partially treated.

Table 24.7. Differential Diagnosis by Joint Fluid Groups[a]

Group I Noninflammatory	Group II Inflammatory	Group III Septic	Group IV Crystal-induced	Group V Hemorrhagic
Osteoarthrosis	Rheumatoid arthritis	Bacterial	Gout	Traumatic arthritis
Traumatic arthritis	Lupus erythematosus	Mycobacterial	CPPD crystal deposition disease	Hemophiliac arthropathy
Osteochondritis dissecans	Reiter's syndrome	Fungal	Apatite-associated arthropathy	Anticoagulation
Osteochondromatosis	Ankylosing spondylitis			Pigmented villonodular tenosynovitis
Neuropathic osteoarthropathy	Regional eneritis			Neuropathic osteoarthropathy
Pigmented villonodular tenosynovitis	Ulcerative colitis			Synovial hemangioma
	Psoriasis			

[a]From Kjeldsberg CR, Knight JA. Body fluids: laboratory examination of amniotic, cerebrospinal, seminal, serous, and synovial fluids. 2nd ed. Chicago: ASCP Press, 1986:133.

spective, fluid analysis may be approached with the following questions in mind: Is this septic or inflammatory arthritis? Is this crystal-related or septic arthritis? If crystals are present, is this gout or pseudogout? Is this a bloody effusion or a traumatic tap? The answers to the questions are not mutually exclusive, because two processes (e.g., bacteria with rheumatoid arthritis [103]) may be occurring simultaneously in the same joint.

The highest WBC and neutrophil counts are encountered in septic arthritis. WBCs are typically in the 50,000/mm^3 range, but vary from 150 to greater than 100,000 (31, 104). Neutrophils generally account for more than 90% of the differential count. Previous treatment or diagnostic procedures may modify the WBC and percentage of neutrophis. Finding more than 80% neutrophils in a joint fluid should prompt a search for bacteria no matter what the WBC. Definitive diagnosis is established when an organism is cultured from the fluid or synovium. When organisms are identified on Gram stain, a presumptive diagnosis can be made. However, a negative Gram stain does not exclude infection. Gram-stained smears are positive in 75% of patients with staphylococcal infections and in 50% of those with Gram-negative bacilli, but in less than 25% of patients with gonococcal arthritis (6).

Cell counts and percentage of neutrophils in joint fluid in septic arthritis overlap with those of crystal-induced arthritis. WBCs in crystal-related arthritis range from less than 100/mm^3 to greater than 100,000, with approximately 80% neutrophils (range: 2 to 100) (31). Identification of the characteristic crystal will establish a diagnosis. Both CPPD and MSU can occur in the same joint.

Inflammatory noncrystal, nonseptic arthritis is characterized by more than 50% neutrophils and WBCs ranging from 2,000 to greater than 100,000/mm^3. This group is largely diagnosed by the exclusion of crystals and organisms. A specific diagnosis is not always possible from joint fluid analysis alone.

A WBC of less than 2,000/mm^3 distinguishes noninflammatory from inflammatory disorders. This number is clearly not absolute, since there is much overlap between diagnostic categories. Most noninflammatory fluids will have variable numbers of neutrophils, lymphocytes, monocytes, and synovial cells. Fluid analysis alone will not usually provide a specific diagnosis.

Macroscopic examination of the fluid may help distinguish traumatic aspiration from hemarthrosis. A xanthochromic or dark red-brown supernatant after centrifugation of a bloody fluid favors hemarthrosis. Comparison of WBC/RBC ratios in fluid and peripheral blood may also be helpful.

Interpretation of synovial fluid findings must be done in the appropriate clinical context. Algorithms for evaluation of synovial fluid microscopy have been proposed and evaluated (105). Careful evaluation by an educated observer gives the best chance for an accurate diagnosis (106, 107).

References

1. Shmerling RH, Delbanco TL, Tosteson ANA, Trentham DE. Synovial fluid tests: what should be ordered? JAMA 1990;264: 1009–1014.
2. Simkin PA. Physiology of normal and abnormal synovium. Semin Arthritis Rheum 1991;21:179–183.
3. Weinberger A, Simkin PA. Plasma proteins in synovial fluids of normal human joints. Semin Arthritis Rheum 1989;19:66–76.
4. Swann DA. Structure and function of lubricin, the glycoprotein responsible for the boundary lubrication of articular cartilage. In: Franchimont P, ed. Articular synovium: anatomy, physiology, pathology, pharmacology, and therapy. Basel: Karger, 1982:45–58.
5. Balazs EA, Watson D, Duff ID, et al. Hyaluronic acid in synovial fluid. I. Molecular parameters of hyaluronic acid in normal and arthritic human fluids. Arthritis Rheum 1967;10:357–376.
6. Goldenberg DL, Reed JI. Bacterial arthritis. N Engl J Med 1985;312:764–771.
7. Ayers LW, Fritsche TR, Lancz G, Pindur A, Specter S. Skin, wound, and tissue specimens. In: Howanitz JH, Howanitz PJ, eds. Laboratory medicine: test selection and interpretation. New York: Churchill Livingstone, 1991:765–719.
8. Freeman R, Jones MR. Microbiology. Clin Rheum Dis 1983;9: 3–26.
9. David CP, Cochran S, Lisse J, et al. Isolation of *Mycoplasma pneumoniae* from synovial fluid samples in a patient with pneumonia and polyarthritis. Arch Intern Med 1988;148:969–970.
10. Dijkmans BAC, Van Elsacker-Niele AMW, Salimans MMM, Van Albada-Kuipers GA, DeVries E, Weiland HT. Human parovirus B19 DNA in synovial fluid. Arthritis Rheum 1988;31:279–281.
11. Withrington RH, Cornes P, Harris JRW, et al. Isolation of human immunodeficiency virus from synovial fluid of patients with reactive arthritis. Br Med J 1987;294:484.
12. Forster SM, Seifert HJ, Keat AC, et al. Inflammatory joint disease and human immunodeficiency virus infection. Br Med J 1988;296:1625–1627.
13. Madariaga L, Aramburu JM, Suarez MD, et al. Presence of HIV antigen p24 in the synovial fluid of a patient without antigenemia suffering from staphylococcal arthritis. AIDS 1991;5:337–348.
14. Kelley WN, Palella TD. Gout and other disorders of purine metabolism. In: Wilson JD, Braunwald E, Isselbacher KJ, et al., eds. Principles of internal medicine. 12th ed. New York: McGraw-Hill, 1991:1834–1843.
15. Pascual E. Persistence of monosodium urate crystals and low-grade inflammation in the synovial fluid of patients with untreated gout. Arthritis Rheum 1991;34:141–145.
16. Hoffman GS. Arthritis due to deposition of calcium crystals. In: Wilson JD, Braunwald E, Isselbacher KJ, Petersdorf RG, et al., eds. Principles of internal medicine. 12th ed. New York: McGraw-Hill, 1991:1479–1482.
17. Lipsky PE. Rheumatoid arthritis. In: Wilson JD, Braunwald E, Isslebacher KJ, et al., eds. Principles of internal medicine. 12th ed. New York: McGraw-Hill, 1991:1437–1443.
18. Arnett FC, Edworthy SM, Bloch DA, et al. The American Rheumatism Association 1987 revised criteria for the classification of rheumatoid arthritis. Arthritis Rheum 1988;31:315–324.
19. Taurog JD, Lipsky PE. Ankylosing spondylitis and reactive arthritis. In: Wilson JD, Braunwald E, Isselbacher KJ, eds. Principles of internal medicine. 12th ed. New York: McGraw-Hill, 1991:1451–1455.
20. Brandt KD, Kovalov-St. John K. Osteoarthritis. In: Wilson JD, Braunwald E, Isselbacher KJ, et al., eds. Principles of internal medicine. 12th ed. New York: McGraw-Hill, 1991: 1475–1479.
21. Laurent MR. Psoriatic arthritis. Clin Rheum Dis 1985;11:61–85.
22. Gravallese EM, Kantrowitz FG. Arthritis manifestations of inflammatory bowel disease. Am J Gastroenterol 1988;83:703–709.
23. Owen DS. Aspiration and injection of joints and soft tissues. In: Kelley WN, Harris ED, Ruddy S, Sledge CB, eds. Textbook of rheumatology. 3rd ed. Philadelphia: WB Saunders, 1989:621–636.
24. Samuelson CO, Cannon GW, Ward JR. Arthrocentesis. J Fam Pract 1985;20:179–184.
25. Gatter RA, Schumacher HR. A practical handbook of joint fluid analysis. 2nd ed. Philadelphia: Lea & Febiger, 1991:1–122.
26. Naib AM. Cytology of synovial fluids. Acta Cytol 1973;17: 299–309.
27. Schumacher HR. Intracellular crystals in synovial fluid anticoagulated with oxalate. N Engl J Med 1966;274:1372–1373.
28. Kjeldsberg CR, Knight JA. Body fluids: laboratory examination of amniotic, cerebrospinal, seminal, serous, and synovial fluids. 2nd ed. Chicago: ASCP Press, 1986:129–165.
29. McCarty DJ. Synovial fluid. In: McCarty DJ, ed. Arthritis and allied conditions: a textbook of rheumatology. Philadelphia: Lea & Febiger, 1989:69–90.
30. Lally EV. High-dose corticosteroid therapy: association with noninflammatory synovial effusions. Arthritis Rheum 1983;26:1283–1287.
31. Cohen AS, Goldenberg D. Synovial fluid. In: Cohen AS, ed. Laboratory diagnostic procedures in the rheumatic diseases. 3rd ed. New York: Grune & Stratton, 1985:1–54.
32. Hogan DB, Pritzker KPH. Synovial fluid analysis—another look at the mucin clot test. J Rheumatol 1985;12:242–244.
33. Cho NH, Neuhaus OW. Absence of blood clotting substances from synovial fluid. Thromb Diath Haemorrh 1960;5: 108–111.
34. Hunter T, Gordon DA, Ogryzlo MA. The ground pepper sign of synovial fluid: a new diagnostic feature of ochronosis. J Rheum 1974;1:45–53.
35. Kitridou R, Schumacher HR, Sbabaro JL, Hollander JL. Recurrent hemarthrosis after prosthetic knee arthroplasty: iden-

tification of metal particles in the synovial fluid. Arthritis Rheum 1969;12:520–528.

36. Reginato AJ, Feldman E, Rabinowitz JL. Traumatic chylous knee effusion. Ann Rheum Dis 1985;44:793–797.
37. Simkin PA, Brunzell JD, Wisner D, Fiechtner JJ, Carlin JS, Willkens RF. Free fatty acids in the pancreatic arthritis syndrome. Arthritis Rheum 1983;26:127–132.
38. Roberts RD, Wong SW, Thiel GB. An unusual case of lead nephropathy. Arthritis Rheum 1983;26:1048–1051.
39. Coggeshall HC, Warren CF, Bauer W. The cytology of normal human synovial fluid. Anat Rec 1940;77:129–144.
40. Kerolus G, Clayburne GH, Schumacher HR. Is it mandatory to examine synovial fluid promptly after arthrocentesis? Arthritis Rheum 1989;32:271–278.
41. Palmer DG. Total leukocyte enumeration in pathologic synovial fluids. Am J Clin Pathol 1968;49:812–814.
42. Clayburne G, Baker DG, Schumacher HR. Estimated synovial fluid leukocyte numbers on wet drop preparations as a potential substitute for actual leukocyte counts. J Rheumatol 1992;19:60–62.
43. Vincent J, Korn JH, Podewell C, Tully E. Synovial fluid pseudoleukocytosis. Arthritis Rheum 1980;23:1399–1400.
44. Reginato AJ, Maldonado I, Reginato AM, Falasca GF, O'Connor CR. Supravital staining of synovial fluid with Test-simplets. Diagn Cytopathol 1992;8:147–152.
45. Schumacher HR, Holdsworth DE. Ochronotic arthropathy. I. Clinicopathologic studies. Semin Arthritis Rheum 1977;6: 207–246.
46. Krieg AF, Kjeldsberg CR: Cerebrospinal fluid and other body fluids. In: Henry JB, ed. Clinical diagnosis and management by laboratory methods. 18th ed. Philadelphia: WB Saunders, 1991:459.
47. Baer AN, Wright EP. Lipid laden macrophages in synovial fluid: a late finding in traumatic arthritis. J Rheumatol 1987;14:848–851.
48. Reginato AJ, Schumacher HR, Allan DA, Rabinowitz JL. Acute monoarthritis associated with lipid liquid crystals. Ann Rheum Dis 1985;44:537–543.
49. Gardner GC, Terkeltaub RA. Acute monoarthritis associated with intracellular positively birefringent Maltese cross appearing spherules. J Rheumatol 1989;16:394–396.
50. Ugai K, Kurosaka M, Hirohata K. Lipid microspherules in synovial fluid of patients with pigmented villonodular synovitis. Arthritis Rheum 1988;31:1442–1446.
51. Astorga GP, Carvajal PR. Lipid spherule associated arthritis. J Rheumatol 1990;17:1720.
52. Kay J, Eichenfeld AH, Athreya BH, Doughty RA, Schumacher HR. Synovial fluid eosinophilia in Lyme disease. Arthritis Rheum 1988;31:1384–1389.
53. Ménard HA, de Médicis R, Lussier A, Brown J. Charcot-Leyden crystals in synovial fluid. Arthritis Rheum 1981;24:1591–1593.
54. Del Blanco J, Valverde J, Mateo L, Juanola X, Pons M, Ferrer J. Charcot Leyden crystals in synovial fluid. J Rheumatol 1991;18:1944.
55. Freemont AJ, Denton J. Disease distribution of synovial fluid mast cells and cytophagic mononuclear cells in inflammatory arthritis. Ann Rheum Dis 1985;44:312–315.
56. Malone DG. Mast cell numbers and histamine levels in synovial fluid from patients with diverse arthritides. Arthritis Rheum 1986;29:953–963.
57. Hasselbacher P. Sickled erythrocytes in synovial fluid. Arthritis Rheum 1980;23:127–128.
58. Glickstein SL, Melton JW, Katz P. Sickled cells in synovial fluid: clue to unsuspected hemoglobinopathy. South Med J 1989:769–771.
59. Yaron M, Djaldetti M. Platelets in synovial fluid. Arthritis Rheum 1978;21:607–608.
60. Endresen GKM. Investigation of blood platelets in synovial fluid from patients with rheumatoid arthritis. Scand J Rheumatol 1981;10:204–208.
61. Lawrence C, Seife B. Bone marrow in joint fluid: a clue to fracture. Ann Intern Med 1971;74:740–742.
62. Dorfman HD, Siegel HL, Perry MC, Oxenhandler R. Non-Hodgkin's lymphoma of the synovium simulating rheumatoid arthritis. Arthritis Rheum 1987;30:155–161.
63. Barton A, Hickling P. Synovial involvement in Hodgkin's disease. Br J Rheumatol 1986;25:391–392.
64. Li CY, Yam LT. Blast transformation in chronic myeloid leukemia with synovial involvement. Acta Cytol 1991;35:543–545.
65. Fam AG, Voorneveld C, Robinson JB, Sheridan BL. Synovial fluid immunocytology in the diagnosis of leukemic synovitis. J Rheumatol 1991;18:293–296.
66. Harden EA, Moore JO, Haynes BF. Leukemia-associated arthritis: identification of leukemic cells in synovial fluid using monoclonal and polyclonal antibodies. Arthritis Rheum 1984;27:1306–1308.
67. Gramatzki M, Burmester GR, König KJ, Henschke F, Kalden JR. Synovial fluid involvement in null cell acute lymphoblastic leukemia diagnosed with monoclonal antibodies. J Rheumatol 1988;15:500–504.
68. Holdrinet RSG, Corstens F, VanHorn JR, Bogman JJT. Leukemic synovitis. Am J Med 1989;86:123–126.
69. Marsh WL, Bylund DJ, Heath VC, Anderson MJ. Osteoarticular and pulmonary manifestations of acute leukemia. Cancer 1986;57:385–390.
70. Gagnerie F, Taillan B, Euller-Ziegler L, Kermarec J, Commandre F, Ziegler G. Arthritis of the knees in B cell chronic lymphocytic leukemia: a patient with immunologic evidence of B lymphocytic synovial inflammation. Arthritis Rheum 1988;31: 815–816.
71. Fort JG, Fernandez C, Jacobs SR. Abruzzo JL. B cell surface marker analysis of synovial fluid cells in a patient with monoarthritis and chronic lymphocytic leukemia. J Rheumatol 1992;19:481–484.
72. Flint A, Remick DG. Metastatic squamous-cell carcinoma: diagnosis by synovial fluid aspiration. Acta Cytol 1984;28:776–777.
73. Villanueva T, Schumacher HR. Cytologic examination of synovial fluid. Diagn Cytopathol 1987;3:141–147.
74. Goldenberg DL, Kelley W, Gibbons RB. Metastatic adenocarcinoma of synovium presenting as an acute arthritis. Arthritis Rheum 1975;18:107–110.
75. Fam AG, Kolin A, Lewis AJ. Metastatic carcinomatous arthritis and carcinoma of the lung. J Rheumatol 1980;7:98–104.
76. Muñoz-Gómez J, Gómez-Pérez R, Solé-Arques M, Llopart-Buisán E. Synovial fluid examination for the diagnosis of synovial amyloidosis in patients with chronic renal failure undergoing haemodialysis. Ann Rheum Dis 1987;46:324–326.
77. Lakhanpal S, Li CY, Gertz MA, Kyle RA, Hunder GG. Synovial fluid analysis for diagnosis of amyloid arthropathy. Arthritis Rheum 1987;30:419–423.
78. Crugnola A, Schiller A, Radin E. Polymeric debris in synovium after total hip replacement: histological identification. J Bone Joint Surg 1977;59:860–862.
79. Bahremand M, Schumacher HR. Effect of medication on synovial fluid leukocyte differentials in patients with rheumatoid arthritis. Arthritis Rheum 1991;34:1173–1176.
80. Corbetti F, Malatesta V, Camposampiero A, et al. Knee arthrography: effects of various contrast media and epinephrine on synovial fluid. Radiology 1986;161:195–198.

81. Fagan TJ, Lidsky MD. Compensated polarized light microscopy using cellophane adhesive tape. Arthritis Rheum 1974:256–262.
82. Gatter RA. The compensated polarized light microscope in clinical rheumatology. Arthritis Rheum 1974:253–255.
83. Gatter RA. Use of the compensated polarizing microscope. Clin Rheum Dis 1977;3:91–103.
84. Gordon C. Swan A, Dieppe P. Detection of crystals in synovial fluids by light microscopy: sensitivity and reliability. J Rheum Dis 1989;48:737–742.
85. Halverson PB, Ryan LM. Triple crystal disease: monosodium urate monohydrate, calcium pyrophosphate dihydrate, and basic calcium phosphate in a single joint. Ann Rheum Dis 1988;47:864–865.
86. McCarty DJ. Crystal identification in human synovial fluids: methods and interpretation. Rheum Dis Clin North Am 1988:253–267.
87. Pascual E. The ordinary light microscope: an appropriate tool for provisional detection and identification of crystals in synovial fluid. Ann Rheum Dis 1989;48:983–985.
88. Fiechtner JJ, Simkin PA. Urate spherulites in gouty synovia. JAMA 1981;245:1533–1536.
89. Riordan JW. Dieppe PA. Cholesterol crystals in shoulder synovial fluid. Br J Rheumatol 1987;26:430–432.
90. Ettlinger RE, Hunder GC. Synovial effusions containing cholesterol crystals. Mayo Clin Proc 1979;54:366–374.
91. Hoffman GS, Schumacher HR, Paul H, et al. Calcium oxalate microcystalline-associated arthritis in end stage renal disease. Ann Intern Med 1982;97:36–42.
92. Schumacher HR, Reginato AJ, Pullman S. Synovial fluid oxalate deposition complicating rheumatoid arthritis with amyloidosis and renal failure. Demonstration of intracellular oxalate crystals. J Rheumatol 1987;14:361–366.
93. Langlands DR, Dawkins RL, Matz LR, et al. Arthritis associated with crystallizing cryoprecipitable IgG paraprotein. Am J Med 1980;68:461–465.
94. Netter P, Delongeas JL, Faure G, et al. Inflammatory effect of aluminum phosphate. Ann Rheum Dis 1983;42[suppl]:114.
95. Tanphaichitr K, Spilberg I, Hahn B. Lithium heparin crystals simulating calcium pryophosphate dihydrate crystals in synovial fluid. Arthritis Rheum 1976;19:966–968.
96. Wise CM, White RE, Agudelo CA. Synovial fluid lipid abnormalities in various disease states: review and classification. Semin Arthritis Rheum 1987;16:222–230.
97. Georgewill DA, Graham GA, Schoen I. Applicability of the Ektachem 400 analyzer for assaying analytes in miscellaneous body fluids. Clin Chem 1988;34:2534–2539.
98. Owen DS. Synovial fluid glucose. JAMA 1978;239:193.
99. Wheeler AR, Graham BS. Case report: pseudogout presenting with low synovial fluid glucose: identification of crystals by Gram stain. Am J Med Sci 1985;289:68–69.
100. Seegmiller JE. Serum uric acid. In: Cohen AS, ed. Laboratory diagnostic procedures in the rheumatic diseases. Boston: Little, Brown, 1975.
101. Schumacher HR. Synovial fluid analysis and synovial biopsy. In: Kelley WN, Harris ED, Ruddy S, Sledge CB, eds. Textbook of rheumatology. 3rd ed. Philadelphia: WB Saunders, 1989:637–649.
102. Kim HJ, McCarty DJ, Kozin F, Koethe S. Clinical significance of synovial fluid total hemolytic complement activity. J Rheumatol 1980;7:143–152.
103. Goldenberg DL. Infectious arthritis complicating rheumatoid arthritis and other chronic rheumatic disease. Arthritis Rheum 1989;32:496–502.
104. McCutchan HJ, Fisher RC. Synovial leukocytosis in infectious arthritis. Clin Orthop Rel Res 1990;257:226–230.
105. Freemont AJ, Denton J, Chuck A, Holt PJL, Davies M. Diagnostic value of synovial fluid microscopy: a reassessment and rationalisation. Ann Rheum Dis 1991;50:101–107.
106. Schumacher HR, Sieck MS, Rothfuss S, et al. Reproducibility of synovial fluid analyses: a study among four laboratories. Arthritis Rheum 1986;29:770–774.
107. Hasselbacher P. Variation in synovial fluid analysis by hospital laboratories. Arthritis Rheum 1987;30:637–642.

Section V

Section Chief: *Daniel L. Van Dyke*

Clinical cytogenetics was born in 1959 with the description of trisomy 21 in Down's syndrome, monosomy X in Turner's syndrome, and XXY in Klinefelter's syndrome. The field came of age in 1970 with the introduction of chromosome banding techniques. Cytogenetics is maturing further today because of the rapid development of fluorescence-labeled DNA probes that can mark whole chromosomes, centromere regions, or specific genes of interest. Thus, chromosome analysis has become a major independent discipline in clinical pathology, and an ever-increasing number of medical centers and reference laboratories have a cytogenetics laboratory. Most clinical cytogenetics laboratories have experienced dramatic growth throughout the 1980s, and that growth continues into the 1990s. The importance of cytogenetics will continue to expand with the wider application of new technologies such as maternal serum screening in pregnancy, cytogenetic analysis of solid cancers, in situ hybridization of DNA probes, and chromosome painting.

Throughout this section the authors offer critical technical information related to the preparation of specimens for karyotype analysis, such as the fine points of cell culture for analysis of hematologic malignancy, and the problem of confined chorionic mosaicism in the interpretation of prenatal diagnostic results. Newer concepts and insights into understanding the molecular genetic effects of cytogenetic abnormalities are detailed, such as genomic imprinting in Prader-Willi and Angelman's syndromes; amplification of short "nonsense repeats" in fragile X syndrome; the molecular genetic defects associated with the inherited chromosome instability syndromes; and alterations involving oncogenes and tumor-suppressor genes in cancer and leukemia.

CYTOGENETICS

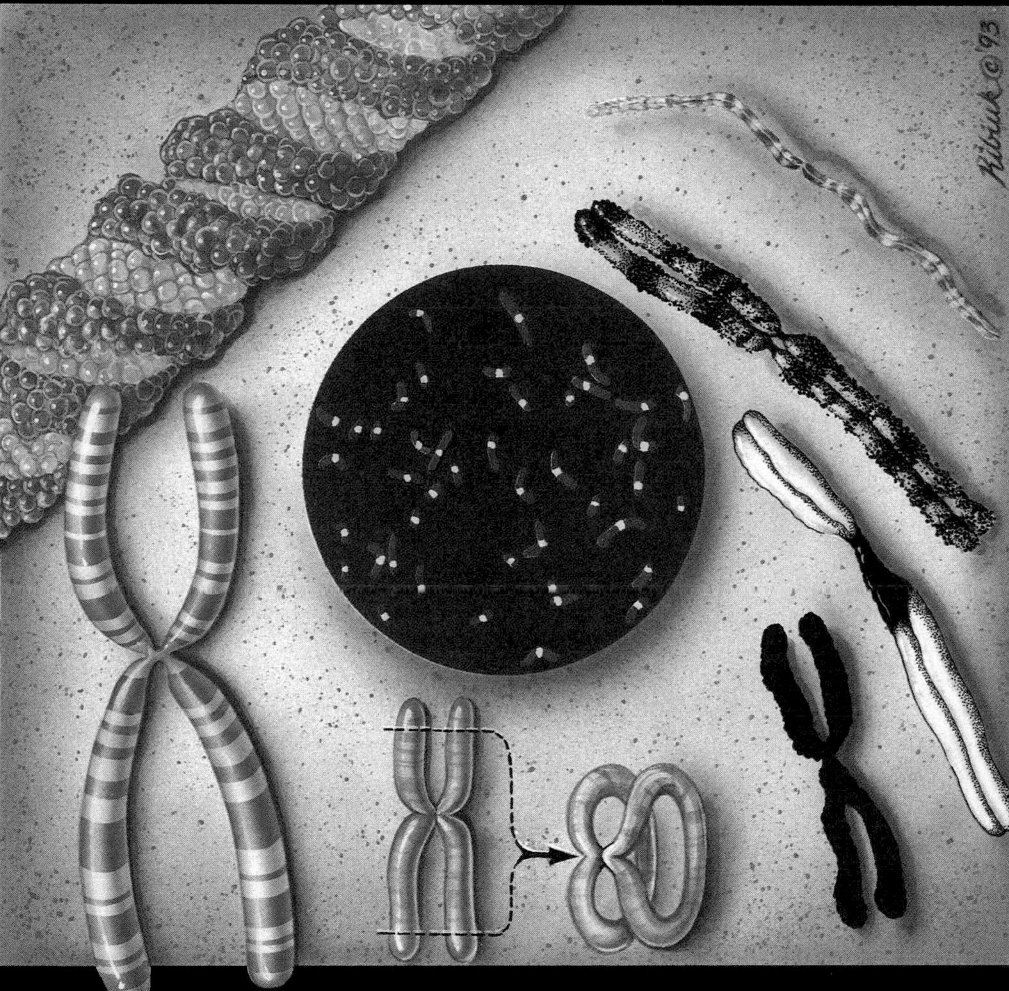

25 Basic Cytogenetics

Catherine G. Palmer

HISTORY OF HUMAN CYTOGENETICS

The initial discoveries leading to the discipline of human cytogenetics occurred in the early 1950s, but their advent was based on a period of technical development extending back to the turn of the century. The understanding of human chromosome behavior is based on chromosome methodology and an understanding of aberrations gained from plant and insect cytogenetics, supplemented by methods developed in studying animal tumors and tissue cultures.

The early studies of human chromosomes beginning in the 1890s to the l920s used testicular tissue to observe the meiotic divisions occurring in gametogenesis. The tissue, obtained from recently executed criminals, was fixed immediately postmortem and usually was sectioned. The chromosome counts varied widely, but the work of Winiwarter in 1912 established chromosome counts of 47 in spermatogonia and 48 in oogonia and an XX/XO sex-determining mechanism. T.S. Painter confirmed Winiwarter's work in 1923 and established the human chromosome number to be 48, but disagreed with the sex-determining mechanism, considering it to be XX/XY.

Further progress required tissue culture technology and methodology for handling mitotic cells, not the least of which was the discovery by T.C. Hsu in 1952 of the usefulness of hypotonic pretreatment of tissue culture cells prior to fixation to disperse the metaphase chromosomes.

Among the methods derived from plant cytogenetics was the use of agents that interfered with the organization of tubulin into the mitotic apparatus. Blakeslee and Avery used the alkaloid colchicine for this purpose and prepared plant chromosomes by a technique involving squashing the cells under a coverglass with gentle pressure. Another plant cytogeneticist, Albert Levan, in John Biesle's tissue culture laboratory, was the first to combine the colchicine and hypotonic pretreatments to obtain chromosome preparations of metaphases from tissue cultures. In 1956, he and Tjio used the same methodology on tissue cultures of human embryonic cells and found the chromosome number of these mitotic cells to be 46 rather than the previously accepted 48. The work was shortly thereafter confirmed by Ford and Hamerton, who observed 23 sets of paired chromosomes or bivalents in squash preparations of human male meiosis.

Once the correct normal chromosome number was established, the identification of chromosome abnormalities soon followed. Jerome Lejeune in 1959 described trisomy of a small chromosome in Down's syndrome, and in rapid succession sex chromosome abnormalities, occurring in already described syndromes were identified: 45,X in Turner's syndrome by Ford and coworkers in 1959, 47,XXY in Klinefelter's syndrome, and 47,XXX by Jacobs and associates in the same year. The next year saw the other two viable trisomic syndromes described, trisomy 13 by Patau and trisomy 18 by Edwards.

Some of these investigators used tissue cultures of skin biopsies, others bone marrow preparations; but the squash methodology was in use until Rothfels and Simonivitch discovered that rapid air drying on slides of drops of fixed cells resulted in spreading of the metaphases. The culmination of this series of technical advances occurred when Peter Nowell in 1960 discovered that cultures of leukocytes that had been separated from red blood cells using phytohemagglutinin, an extract of the broad bean, were stimulated to divide in culture. This technique, still used today, provided a readily available source of dividing cells and led to the identification of many chromosomal abnormalities.

The rapid progress of cytogenetics during these few years required that a common system of nomenclature for the chromosomes be developed, and a series of conferences involving the major investigators in cytogenetics was convened. The first conference, in Denver in 1960, resulted in a system to group the chromosomes based on relative length, arm ratio, and centromeric index and proposed a standard system of nomenclature of the groups using a numerical designation, i.e., chromosomes 1–3,4–5,6–12, etc. (Figs. 25.1 and 25.2). The London Conference in 1963 further described the system and added letters to the groups, A to G plus the sex chromosomes. The meeting in Chicago in 1966 adopted a shorthand system for describing human chromosome abnormalities.

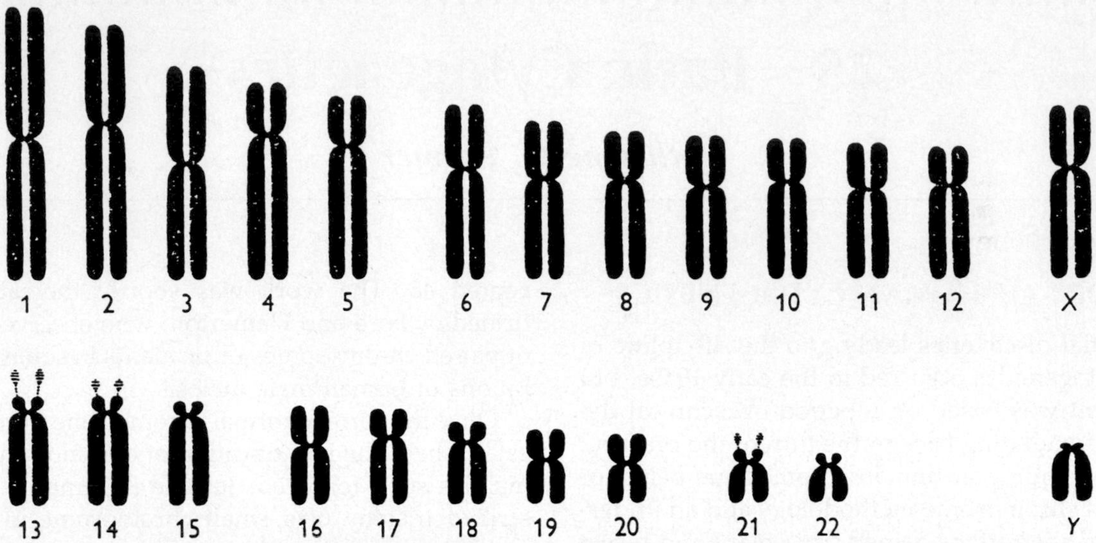

Figure 25.1. Idiogram drawn from standard measurements of human chromosomes from the 1960 Denver conference. (Reprinted from Editorial Comments, Ann Hum Genet 1960;24:319.)

Chromo-some No.	Relative length A	B	C	D	Centromere index A	B	C	D
1	9.08	9.08 ± 0.611	9.11 ± 0.53	8.44 ± 0.433	48.0	49.4 ± 3.04	48.6 ± 2.6	48.36 ± 1.166
2	8.45	8.17 ± 0.250	8.61 ± 0.41	8.02 ± 0.397	38.1	39.4 ± 2.05	38.9 ± 2.6	39.23 ± 1.824
3	7.06	6.96 ± 0.352	6.97 ± 0.36	6.83 ± 0.315	45.9	47.6 ± 2.10	47.3 ± 2.1	46.95 ± 1.557
4	6.55	6.62 ± 0.403	6.49 ± 0.32	6.30 ± 0.284	27.6	29.2 ± 2.97	27.8 ± 3.3	29.07 ± 1.867
5	6.13	6.34 ± 0.366	6.21 ± 0.50	6.08 ± 0.305	27.4	29.2 ± 3.03	26.8 ± 2.6	29.25 ± 1.739
6	5.84	6.19 ± 0.516	6.07 ± 0.44	5.90 ± 0.264	37.7	39.1 ± 2.63	37.9 ± 2.5	39.05 ± 1.665
7	5.28	5.60 ± 0.435	5.43 ± 0.47	5.36 ± 0.271	37.3	35.3 ± 2.90	37.0 ± 4.2	39.05 ± 1.771
X	5.80	5.45 ± 0.377	5.16 ± 0.24	5.12 ± 0.261	36.9	41.4 ± 6.16	37.5 ± 2.7	40.12 ± 2.117
8	4.96	5.13 ± 0.307	4.94 ± 0.28	4.93 ± 0.261	35.9	32.7 ± 2.80	32.8 ± 2.8	34.08 ± 1.975
9	4.83	4.81 ± 0.194	4.78 ± 0.39	4.80 ± 0.244	33.3	37.0 ± 3.04	32.7 ± 4.1	35.43 ± 2.559
10	4.68	4.66 ± 0.512	4.80 ± 0.58	4.59 ± 0.221	31.2	35.4 ± 3.81	32.3 ± 2.9	33.95 ± 2.243
11	4.63	4.70 ± 0.289	4.82 ± 0.30	4.61 ± 0.227	35.6	40.7 ± 3.07	40.5 ± 3.3	40.14 ± 2.328
12	4.46	4.66 ± 0.410	4.50 ± 0.26	4.66 ± 0.212	30.9	30.5 ± 3.64	27.4 ± 4.0	30.16 ± 2.339
13	3.64	3.22 ± 0.310	3.87 ± 0.26	3.74 ± 0.236	14.8	-	16.6 ± 3.6	17.08 ± 3.227
14	3.55	3.09 ± 0.212	3.74 ± 0.23	3.56 ± 0.229	15.5	-	18.4 ± 3.9	18.74 ± 3.596
15	3.36	2.83 ± 0.262	3.30 ± 0.25	3.46 ± 0.214	14.9	-	17.6 ± 4.6	20.30 ± 3.702
16	3.23	3.46 ± 0.353	3.14 ± 0.55	3.36 ± 0.183	40.6	42.2 ± 3.57	42.5 ± 5.6	41.33 ± 2.74
17	3.15	3.06 ± 0.377	2.97 ± 0.30	3.25 ± 0.189	31.4	36.6 ± 5.86	31.9 ± 3.3	33.86 ± 2.771
18	2.76	2.98 ± 0.316	2.78 ± 0.18	2.93 ± 0.164	26.1	31.5 ± 4.15	26.6 ± 4.2	30.93 ± 3.044
19	2.52	2.55 ± 0.269	2.46 ± 0.31	2.67 ± 0.174	42.9	48.1 ± 2.48	44.9 ± 4.0	46.54 ± 2.299
20	2.33	2.61 ± 0.144	2.25 ± 0.24	2.56 ± 0.165	44.6	46.5 ± 3.59	45.6 ± 2.5	45.45 ± 2.526
21	1.83	1.34 ± 0.189	1.70 ± 0.32	1.90 ± 0.170	25.7	-	28.6 ± 5.0	30.89 ± 5.002
22	1.68	1.53 ± 0.178	1.80 ± 0.26	2.04 ± 0.182	25.0	-	28.2 ± 6.5	30.48 ± 4.932
Y	1.96	1.82 ± 0.353	2.21 ± 0.30	2.15 ± 0.137	16.3	-	23.1 ± 5.1	27.17 ± 3.182

Figure 25.2. Relative length and arm ratios of human chromosomes. A, B, C, and D represent different data sets. Sets B, C, and D were identified by Q-banding and stained with orcein or Giemsa 9. Set A is the Denver-London data not preidentified by Q-banding. The relative length of each chromosome is the length of the chromosome compared to the length of the haploid (1N) set of chromosomes. There are two ways of designating the centromere position: the arm ratio, which is the length of the longer arm relative to the shorter one, and the centromere index, the ratio of the length of the shorter arm to the total length of the chromosome. (Reprinted from Harnden DG, Klinger HP, eds. An international system for human cytogenetic nomenclature. Basel, Switzerland: S Karger, 1985:114.)

Although many chromosome abnormalities were described by 1966, the abnormalities were relatively easily visualized—gains or losses of whole chromosomes or easily observed deletions or rearrangements. Some chromosomes could not be readily differentiated from each other; a few were separable by autoradiographic methods based on differences in the completion of replication of similarly appearing chromosomes. Caspersson in 1970 used a fluorescing dye, quinacrine mustard, to stain human chromosomes and was able to demonstrate a different pattern of fluorescence for each of the 22 pairs of autosomes and the X and Y chromosomes. Each chromosome could now be defined by a specific pattern of light and dark bands, and the banding pattern was shown to be reproduced by other staining techniques using Giemsa stain or other fluorescent dyes. This technique permitted identification of further rearrangements, deletions, duplications, and inversions not previously recognized. The Paris Conference of 1971 addressed the identification of individual chromosomes, regions, and bands and detailed a method of describing structural changes using the banding nomenclature. All of the nomenclature was consolidated in the International System for Human Cytogenetic Nomenclature (ISCN) in 1978 (see Chapter 26, Table 26.1).

The major change in the subsequent years was the use of prophase and prometaphase chromosomes to obtain a greater number of recognizable bands, which permitted recognition of even more subtle abnormalities. This was achieved by Yunis, who synchronized the dividing cells to obtain the early stages of division in sufficient quantity to make them useful.

The description of the prophase chromosomes—the size, width, and number of bands at different levels of band resolution—was incorporated into the ISCN in 1981 in *An International System for Human Cytogenetic Nomenclature—High Resolution Banding 1981;* some further revisions were made in 1985 (Fig. 25.3).

In 1991, recognizing the complexity of describing acquired abnormalities with the current nomenclature, the Study Committee on Human Cytogenetic Nomenclature established new guidelines specific for describing abnormalities encountered in cancer cytogenetics (ISCN 1991).

The most recent advance in cytogenetics has been the advent of molecular cytogenetics, in which techniques of molecular biology are applied to cytogenetic preparations. These procedures include in situ hybridization for localizing DNA probes to specific chromosomes and bands. While radioactive probes labeled with tritiated thymidine were initially used, recently developed procedures utilize immunologic reactions coupled with staining of the product with a fluorescent dye (immunofluoresence). These techniques have not only been useful for gene localization but also have been directed to the identification of fragments or rearrangements in dividing and nondividing cells.

Competitive in situ supression (CISS) hybridization uses complex probes derived from sorted human chromosomes labeled with biotin and visualized by fluorochrome staining and fluorescence microscopy. This method permits staining of individual chromosomes and allows identification of specific chromosome rearrangements in either metaphase or interphase cells.

Cytogenetics has now become an integral part of the gene mapping attempts and has a wide application to medical questions regarding the relationships between such chromosome abnormalities as infertility, miscarriage, birth defects, mental retardation, and cancer.

CHROMOSOME STRUCTURE

Studies of chromosomes of a wide variety of organisms have led to the conclusion that the chromosome is composed of a single continuous DNA fiber in each chromatid (i.e., one of the two daughter strands of a replicated chromosome). The basic subunit is a 10-nm fiber that has been described following digestion by micrococcal nuclease as the "nucleosome"—the familiar beads-on-a-string structure, the core particle of which contains 145 base pairs of DNA helix coiled about an octomer of histones H2a, H2b, H3, and H4 (Fig. 25.4). Adjacent nucleosomes are separated by DNA linkers of varying length associated with H1 histone, which stabilizes the structure (Fig. 25.5). This fibril is in turn compacted into a 30-nm thick fibril, which undergoes further condensation to form the metaphase chromosome (Fig. 25.6). Observations of higher chromosome structure derived from whole-mount or histone-depletion electron microscopy give different perspectives of chromosome architecture and have resulted in several models of chromosome structure.

When chromosomes are digested to remove most of the histones, leaving only protein and DNA and observed by electron microscopy after spreading, a loose fibrillar protein structure extending through the chromatids and surrounded by a halo of loops of DNA is revealed. These observations have suggested a chromosome structure in which radial loops of DNA are supported by a cytoskeleton or scaffold of fibrillar protein (Fig. 25.7).

Another model derived from whole-mount electron microscopy and light microscopy observations of coiled chromatids suggests that the chromosome is based on a successive series of helical coils of the

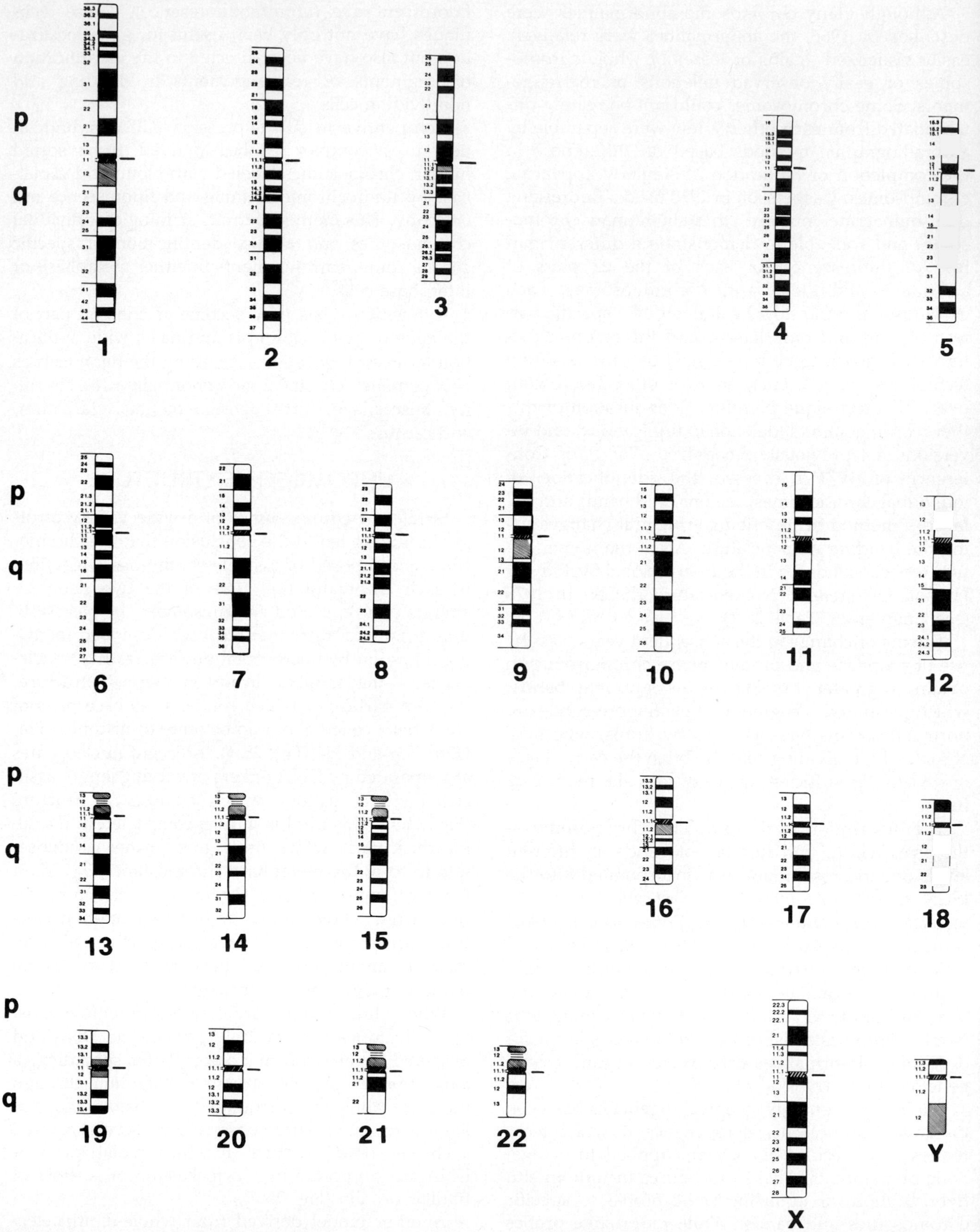

Figure 25.3. Diagram showing G-banding pattern of normal human chromosomes at 400 band level. (Adapted from Harden DG, Klinger HP, eds. An international system for human cytogenetic nomenclature. Basil, Switzerland: S Karger, 1985:114.)

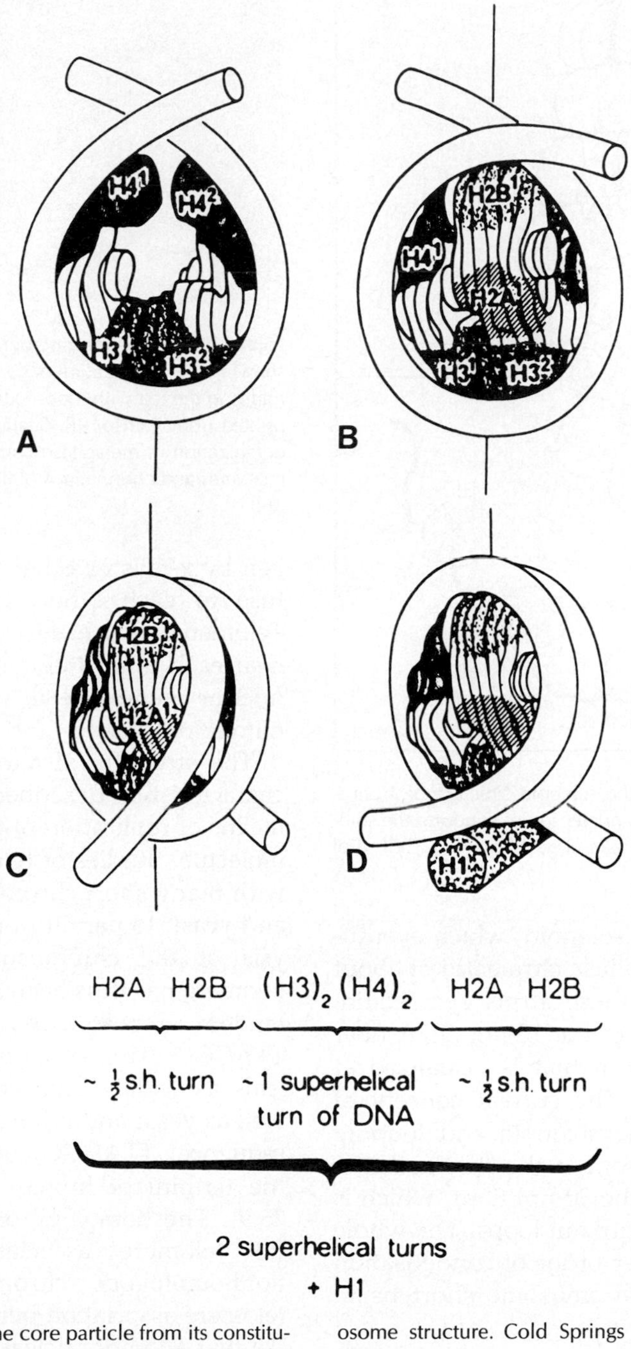

Figure 25.4. Assembly of nucleosome core particle from its constituents. (Reprinted from Richmond TJ, Finch JT, Klug A. Studies of nucleosome structure. Cold Springs Harbor Symposium 1982; 47:493–501.)

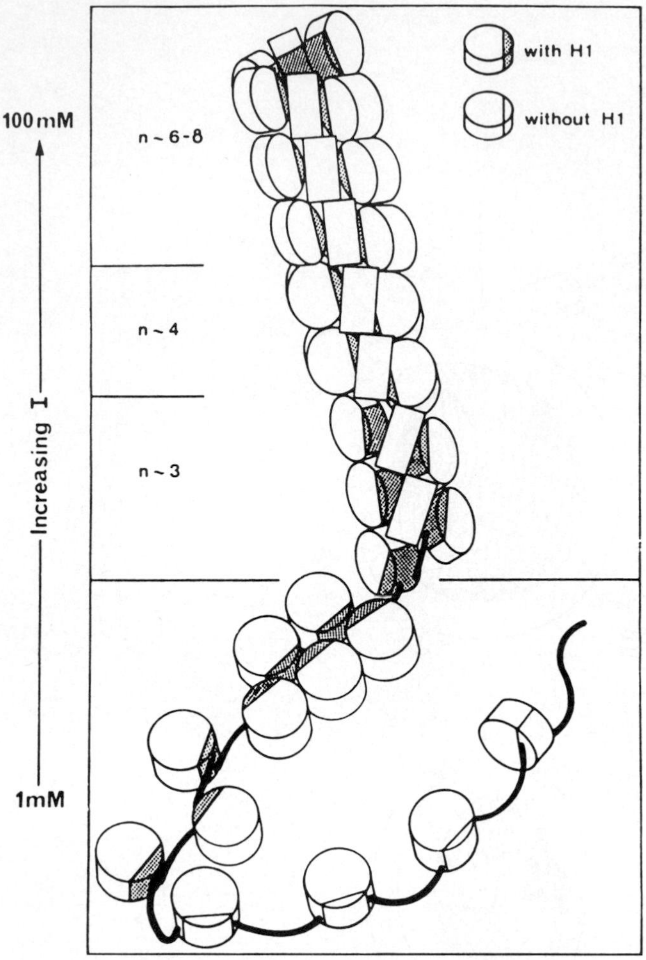

Figure 25.5. Idealized drawing of the solenoid structure of a chromosome showing the open zig-zag of nucleosomes that form the solenoid. (Reprinted from Thoma F, Koller TH, Klieg A. J Cell Biol 1979;83:403–427.)

30-nm fiber to form a super solenoid, which eventually results in a coiled metaphase chromatid of about 1000 nm in width. All of these structures require some degree of compaction of the 10-nm DNA fiber into the condensed chromatin that is visualized at mitotic or meiotic division. The current concept of the chromosome is that the solenoid and looping conformations are both present in the chromosome. The solenoidal structure is the 30-nm fibril, which is attached to a scaffold-like matrix in loops. The whole structure undergoes a higher order of condensation by further coiling as the chromosome shortens in progress toward metaphase.

Specialized Regions of Chromosomes

The ends of the chromosomes, the telomeres (Fig. 25.8), are required for the maintenance of stability and necessary for the completion of replication of the chromosome. The concept of the telomere is based on the observation that when chromosomes are broken by x-rays or other means, the broken ends will fuse to each other, but not to unbroken ends. Telomeres also have the tendency to be positioned near each other (telomere association) and with the nuclear membrane in meiosis and, on occasion, in mitotic prophase.

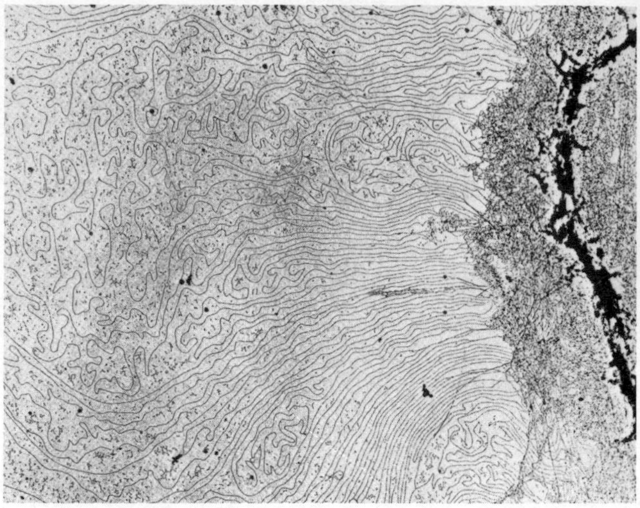

Figure 25.6. Electron micrograph of histone-depleted chromosomes showing the organization of the DNA in loops. The chromosome scaffold is to the left with loops extending outward from the scaffold. (Reprinted from Paulson JR. Scaffolding and radial loops, the structural organization of metaphase chromasomes. In: Adolph KW, ed. Chromosomes and chromatin, Vol III. Baco Raton, FL: CRC Press, 1988:3–36.)

The structure of telomeres must account for the characteristics described above as well as for the means of replication of the terminus of a linear DNA molecule. Studies of telomeres have used organisms with many short chromosomes, such as *Tetrahymena* and yeast, to permit purification and molecular analysis of the chromosome ends. The *Tetrahymena* telomere has thus been found to contain 1500 to 6000 tandem repeats of the nucleotide sequence, TTAGGG. This structure has been found in organisms as widely separated as birds and reptiles, as well as yeast and other microorganisms. A repeating sequence, TTAGGG, or similar sequences occur at the termini of human chromosomes as well (Fig. 25.9). The homology of base sequence can account for telomere association of homologous and nonhomologous chromosomes. In cases where telomere association persists to metaphase it is possible that an endonuclease involved in replication has failed to function.

Although the mechanism for replication of the telomeres of eukaryotes is not yet completely resolved, there has been rapid progress during the past 5 years. There are special problems in replicating the ends of the DNA strand—namely the requirement of a DNA polymerase to have both a template to copy

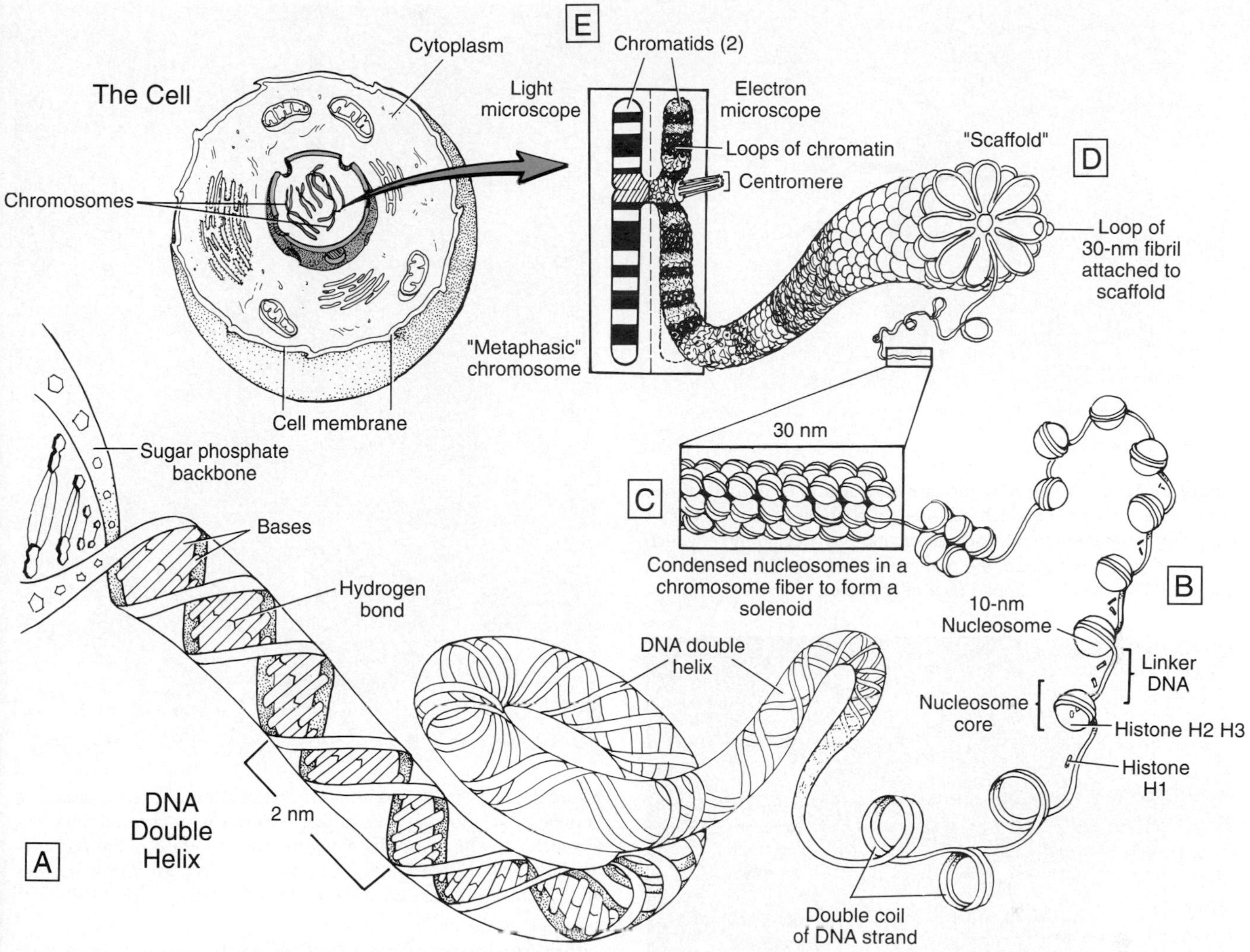

Figure 25.7. Model of chromosome structure showing the hierarchy of coiling and looping in the DNA helix (**A**), nucleosomal 10-nm fiber (**B**), 30-nm solenoidal fiber (**C**), the looping of the 30-nm fibers and their attachment to the chromosome scaffold (**D**), and the chromosome as seen on electron microscopy (**E**).

and a primer to extend, since polynucleotide synthesis can proceed in only one direction (from 5′ to 3′). The 3′ ends of the strands cannot be replicated because there is no more DNA left on which to synthesize the RNA primer. How then does the telomere replicate?

An unusual telomerase that functions as a special reverse transcriptase has been found in *Tetrahymena*. The RNA of the telomerase provides its own template for the synthesis of the telomeric repeats that are added on during replication of the ends of the chromosome. A similar telomerase has been identified in human HeLa cells, suggesting that the *Tetrahymena* system may be present in all cells.

The centromere, the region of the chromosome also referred to as the primary constriction, divides the chromosome into arms (Fig. 25.8). The centromere may be in the middle of the chromosome, resulting in a metacentric chromosome; or may be asymmetrically placed on the chromosome, to give a submetacentric and/or acrocentric chromosome; or may be at the end of a chromosome in a telocentric chromosome. The centromere is composed of the kinetochore and associated constitutive heterochromatin (see below).

The kinetochore, a locus at the centromere, functions as the region of attachment of the subunits of the spindle apparatus, the microtubules, to the DNA of the chromosome during division. The kinetochore of a mammalian chromosome is a multilayered disk that stains with heavy metals; when visualized by electron microscopy it appears to have a trilaminar structure composed of an outer plate of condensed fibrillar or granular material 40 nm thick that contains DNA (Fig. 25.10). The kinetochore microtubules appear to terminate in this outer plate. Beneath this is a middle and more electron translucent 30-nm thick layer that appears to be loosely aggregated and fibril-

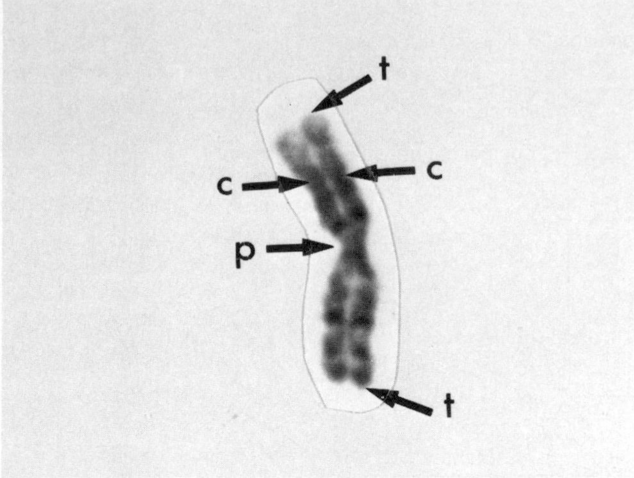

Figure 25.8. Each chromosome at metaphase is composed of two chromatids (c), each of which has a single continuous strand of DNA extending from end to end. Each chromatid has a centromere, which is located in a constriction, the primary constriction (p), and at each end each chromatid is capped by a telomere (t).

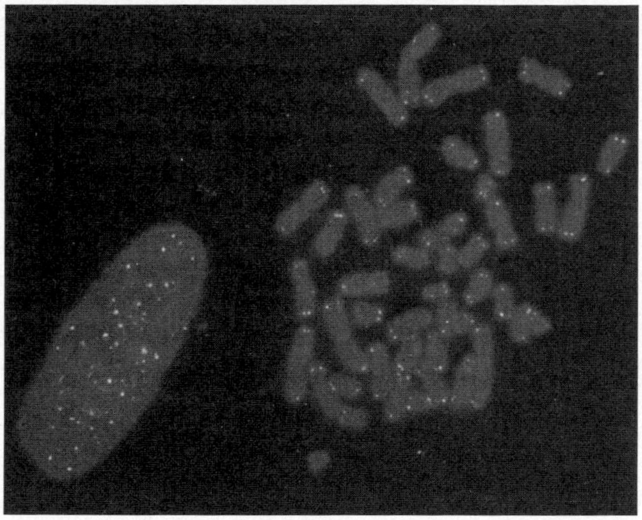

Figure 25.9. Telomeres of chromosomes shown after in situ hybridization with biotin-labeled repetitive telomeric sequences to metaphase chromosomes. (Reprinted from Moyzes RK, Buckingham JM, Scott Cram L, et al. A highly conserved repetitive DNA sequence (TTAGGG), present at the telomeres of human chromosomes. Prac Natl Acad Sci USA 1988;85:6622–6626.)

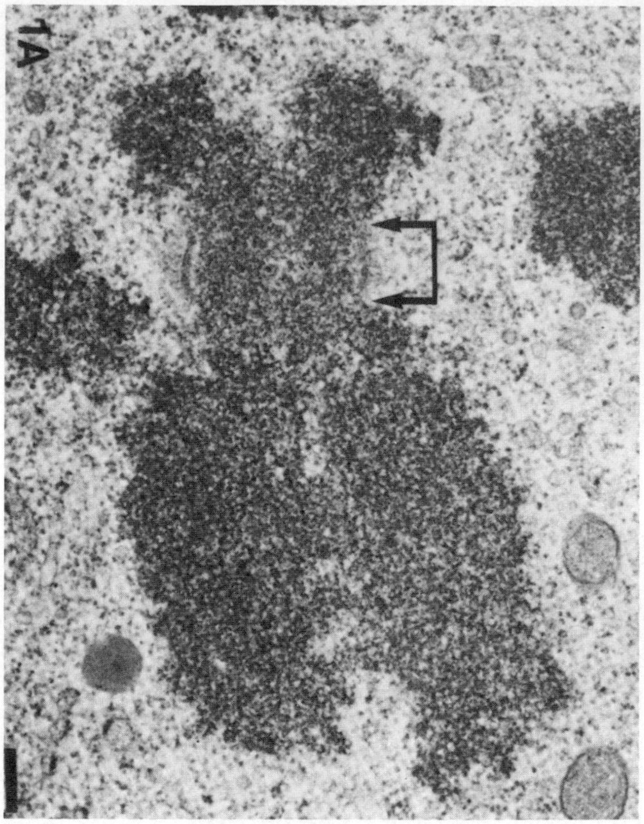

Figure 25.10. An electron micrograph of a thin section of a mouse chromosome showing the primary constriction (*arrows*) and the kinetochore, which appears along the lateral surface of the constriction. (Reprinted from Rattner JB. In: Adolph KW, ed. Chromosomes and chromatin. Vol II. Boca Raton, FL: CRC Press, 1988:29–49.)

lar in nature. The inner layer, also composed of DNA, is similar in thickness to the outer layer and approximates the underlying chromatin. In addition to DNA and RNA which are contained in the kinetochore, there are specific proteins associated with the outer and inner kinetochore plates. These may be demonstrated using anticentromere antibodies derived from patients with the CREST variant of scleroderma. These autoantibodies are of practical value in identifying active centromeres. Reduced or absent reaction with anticentromere antibodies provides evidence of an inactive centromere (for example, one of the centromeres of a dicentric chromosome resulting from a chromosome rearrangement).

Heterochromatin

A major component of the centromeric region is constitutive heterochromatin. First described by Heitz in 1928, heterochromatin is chromatin that remains condensed telophase and remains visible during interphase. This out-of-phase or allocyclic behavior of heterochromatin is also reflected in its DNA synthesis, which occurs late in the replication of the chromosome. Two types of heterochromatin may be differentiated. One, the constitutive heterochromatin, contains genes that are not transcribable and is located mainly at centromeric and telomeric sites, although in some organisms its location is not limited to these regions. In human chromosomes constitutive or c-heterochromatin is centromeric in all the chromosomes, with additional paracentromeric areas in chromosomes 1, 9, and 16. It makes up much of the long arm of the Y chromosome and may be readily demonstrated by C-banding (described later in this chapter).

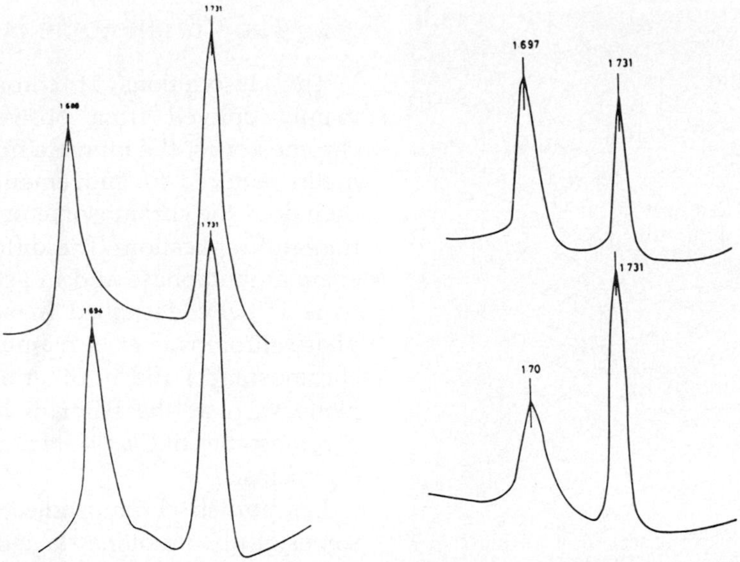

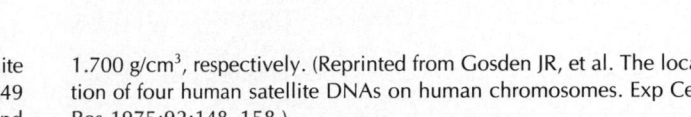

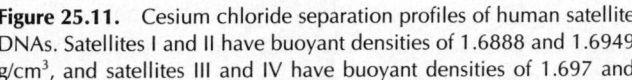

Figure 25.11. Cesium chloride separation profiles of human satellite DNAs. Satellites I and II have buoyant densities of 1.6888 and 1.6949 g/cm^3, and satellites III and IV have buoyant densities of 1.697 and 1.700 g/cm^3, respectively. (Reprinted from Gosden JR, et al. The location of four human satellite DNAs on human chromosomes. Exp Cell Res 1975;92:148–158.)

The second kind of heterochromatin, facultative heterochromatin, is composed of transcribable DNA that has been inactivated and that has assumed the other characteristics of heterochromatin, including allocyclic condensation and late replication.

Constitutive heterochromatin is composed largely of a type of DNA—satellite DNA—that differs in base composition and physical characteristics from the remainder of the DNA. When DNA is fragmented and ultracentrifuged, the lightest and heaviest fragments settle at a different rate than the remainder of the DNA, appearing as separate "satellite" bands (Fig. 25.11). Satellite DNA is composed of multiple tandem repeats of simple-sequence DNA, 2 to 12 base pairs in length, resulting from amplification of these simple sequences. Divergence due to mutation produces related but distinct satellites within an organism. In addition to the satellite DNAs, other repeated sequences are found in the human genome. These include short interspersed repeated sequences (SINES), which are about 300 bp in length, Alu elements (which are repeated DNA sequences cleaved by the restriction indonuclease Alu I), and long interspersed repeated sequences, or LINES. Eight different satellites identified by gradient centrifugation have been defined in human DNA and have been localized in the centromeric and telomeric regions of the chromosomes by in situ hybridization. Analysis of human genomic DNA using restriction endonucleases (enzymes that cleave DNA molecules at specific recognition sites) has revealed additional satellite DNA composed of tandem repeats that also hybridize to centromeric regions. One of these, alpha satellite DNA, is composed of a number of subfamilies that differ with respect to the sequence and location of sites of cleaving by restriction endonucleases. Alpha satellite sequences are located at the centromeres of human chromosomes. The alpha satellite regions of most human chromosomes differ from each other.

Heterochromatin may affect the expression of genes located in adjacent euchromatic segments. Chromosome rearrangements in which euchromatic segments are positioned next to heterochromatin result in variation in condensation of the euchromatin at the cellular level. The expression of the euchromatic gene is repressed in the condensed segments, and a mosaic or variegated expression pattern results. This is known as position effect. In humans, the best example of the effect of heterochromatin on the expression of genes in euchromatin is in X-autosome translocations in which the autosomal genes are inactivated by the spreading of inactivation from the facultative heterochromatin of the X chromosome to the autosomal genes (see X Inactivation, below).

A number of effects of heterochromatin occur at meiosis, suggesting a role for heterochromatin during the meiotic divisions. Homologous heterochromatic segments fail to form chiasma, the microscopic manifestation of crossing over, and regions approximating heterochromatic segments may also show decreased chiasma formation. Thus, heterochromatin may affect chiasma formation and distribution. In plants and in *Drosophila*, in which the amount of heterochromatin may be manipulated experimentally, extra segments of heterochromatin have been re-

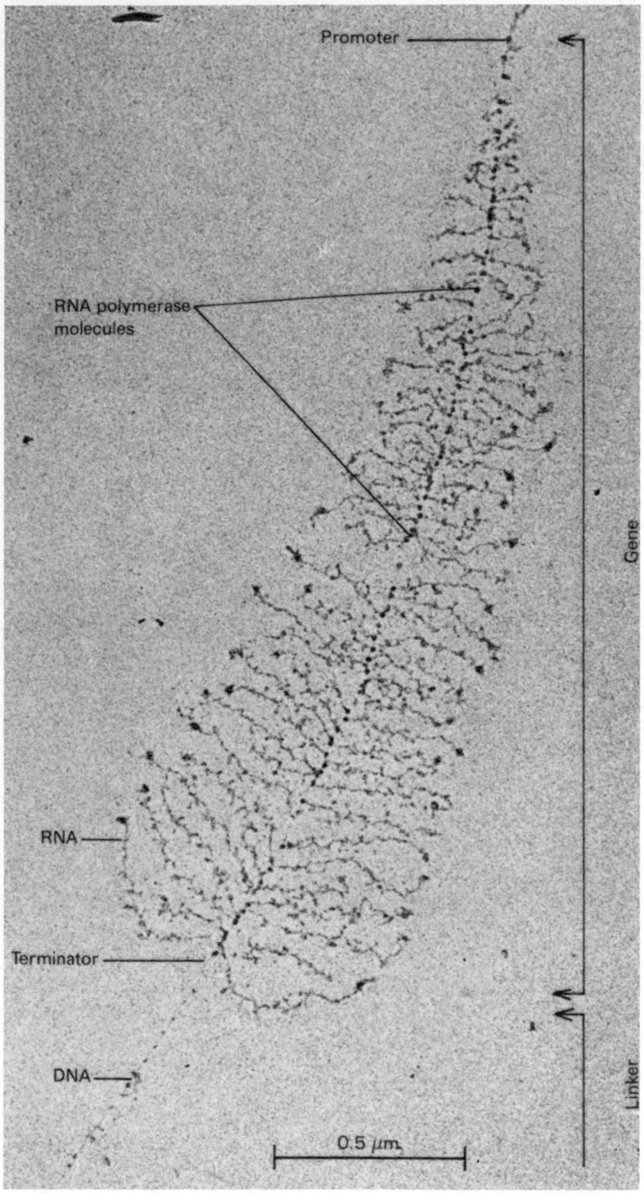

Figure 25.12. Chromatin in transcription. The central DNA stalk with "knobs" of RNA polymerase, in the process of transcribing a gene. The lateral fibers are growing RNA transcripts. The bare part of the stalk is the untranscribed linker between genes. (Reprinted from deDuve C. A guided tour of the living cell. New York: The Rockefeller University Press, 1984:295–296, by copyright permission of the American Society for Clinical Investigation.)

ported to reduce chiasma frequency, and in corn the presence of extra heterochromatic "knobs" induces directed segregation (in lieu of random segregation found in meiosis) of other heterochromatin-bearing chromosomes to one pole. Although these effects of heterochromatin have been described, no specific function for constitutive heterochromatin, either at mitosis or at meiosis, has been defined. This is also true of dispersed repetitive DNA families, which continue to remain without known function.

The Chromosome in Transcription

The descriptions of chromosome structure are mainly derived from observations of metaphase chromosomes, the ultimate in the packaging of chromatin required for movement on the spindle. How then does the chromosome unfold to allow transcription and replication? The differences in the chromosome at metaphase and in actively transcribing cells were initially described in studies of meiotic prophase chromosomes of mammalian eggs (lampbrush chromosomes) and in other actively transcribing regions such as the Balbiani rings of salivary gland chromosomes of *Chironomus*, and spermatocytes during meiosis.

Lampbrush chromosomes are extended chromosomes of the diplotene stage of meiosis (see Meiosis, below) held together by chiasma and closely in apposition at the centromere by c-heterochromatin. These large chromosomes, which may be visualized with a dissecting microscope, are composed of an axial strand of the paired chromatids, interrupted at intervals by chromomeres—compact refractile granules, to which one or more pairs of loops covered with ribonucleoproteins are attached. Each loop in turn has a single axis of DNA with RNA polymerase molecules attached to it and the RNA transcript attached to the polymerase. Each loop shows a thick to thin progression as transcription proceeds from an initiation site and moves around the loop axis transcribing RNA. In other organisms there is a similar arrangement of DNA polymerase and ribonucleoprotein, giving a typical Christmas tree or fern-like structure to the chromatin (Fig. 25.12).

In the multistranded, polytene chromosomes of the salivary glands of larvae of dipterans darkly and lightly stained bands, or Balbiani rings, change as gene activity increases. The bands swell and there are local extensions of the DNA of the bands, forming puffs at the locations of active RNA synthesis. These changes in the chromosome occur at a particular developmental stage and then regress as differentiation continues.

Changes also occur at the level of the nucleosome during transcription. The chromatin becomes extended with a decreased frequency or absence of the nucleosomes, and, as the chromatin is extended, there is an increase in nuclease (DNase I) sensitivity. The level of DNase I sensitivity corresponds to the extension of the chromatin as it proceeds through the mitotic cycle and is accompanied by other changes in chromatin structure, including acetylation of core nucleosomes, hypomethylation of DNA, and an open configuration of nucleosomes coincident with association of nonhistone proteins.

MITOSIS

DNA packaging changes during the cell cycle. From great extension during transcription there is an increasing formation of loops as metaphase approaches, concurrent changes in the methylation of chromatin, and the presence of a variety of associated histone and nonhistone proteins as the chromosome is again compacted.

The culmination of contraction of the interphase chromosome is the mitotic division. Mitosis, which is necessary to distribute the chromosomes equally at cell division, is only a transient phase occupying about 1 hour of a cell cycle, which comprises some 18 to 24 hours (Fig. 25.13). At the initiation of the cell cycle, cells may be activated from a resting state, G-0, and enter the cell cycle. During the G-1 stage of the cell cycle, events occur that are necessary for the subsequent S (synthesis) phase in which the chromosomes are replicated. DNA replication is followed by G-2, a period in which further changes occur in preparation for formation of the spindle, in nuclear membrane breakdown, and in further shortening of the chromosomes composed now of two chromatids. At the beginning of metaphase, the chromosomes align themselves on the metaphase plate so that each short thick chromatid is oriented toward one pole of the mitotic spindle. As anaphase occurs, the two chromatids of each chromosome separate beginning at the kinetochores and move to opposite poles of the spindle. By telophase, the chromosomes are grouped at the poles. A nuclear membrane is reformed and the chromosomes uncoil, forming the interphase nuclei of the daughter cells (Fig. 25.14).

MEIOSIS

While mitotic divisions result in two identical daughter cells, the essence of meiosis is pairing, recombination, and a reduction in chromosome number to the haploid, 1N, number. DNA replication during premeiotic S is 3 to 6 times longer than the S phase of mitotic cells. The DNA is almost completely replicated, a small portion remaining unreplicated until replication is finally completed at zygotene. Meiosis results in a reduction to the haploid chromosome number because two cell divisions occur with only one replication of DNA. The synaptonemal complex, a unique structure not found in mitotic divisions, holds the paired homologous chromosomes together during meiosis I and facilitates the exchange of chromatin that results in crossing over.

Meiosis is characterized by a series of stages that are microscopically distinct, with significant changes in chromosome behavior seen as well at the electron microscope level (Fig. 25.15).

The chromosomes are at their greatest length at leptotene. They are still unpaired but, since DNA replication has occurred, two chromatids may be observed. At this stage, the telomeres are attached to the nuclear membrane and synapsis of the chromosomes begins from these ends. The homologous chromosomes are brought together by the protein chromosome cores to which the loops of chromatin are attached. Synapsis is complete at zygotene, the core proteins from the homologous chromosomes forming the synaptonemal complex (SC). This structure, specific to meiosis, is essential for maintaining the alignment of the homologous chromosomes, which are now closely paired (Fig. 25.16).

At the pachytene stage of meiosis, the paired homologous chromosomes (or bivalents), each composed of four chromatids (tetrads), are held in register by the SC as crossing over occurs. The SC, a ladderlike structure composed of two lateral elements on either side of the chromosomes and a central fibrillar region, is complete. Recombination nodules, units that mediate the molecular process of exchange, appear on the SC and chiasmata are visible. The latter are evidence that crossing over has occurred. The recombination nodules correspond in number and position with chiasmata.

At diplotene, the SC begins to disappear, but the chromosomes are held together by chiasmata. If no chiasmata are present, the bivalent falls apart and the homologous chromosomes will segregate independently. Thus, the chiasmata have an additional important function in holding the paired homologous chromosomes together.

At diakinesis, the chromosomes shorten and, as they shorten, the chiasmata appear to move to the ends of the chromosomes (terminalize), and there is a reduction in the total number of chiasmata. The bivalents move to the periphery of the nucleus. The nuclear membrane disappears and chromosomes align on the spindle. At metaphase as the paired homologs align, the kinetochores are widely separated facing opposite poles of the spindle. Orientation of centromeres of nonhomologous chromosomes in the metaphase spindle is random, resulting in independent assortment of the several pairs of chromosomes.

When the homologs separate, the telophase groups of chromosomes at the poles contain half the number of chromosomes of the original cell. However, each chromosome still has two chromatids, and each is referred to as a dyad.

The subsequent interphase is short and without a period of DNA replication, and the dyads separate at the second meiotic division. Each of the products of meiosis now has half the number of chromosomes and half the amount of DNA of the original germinal cells.

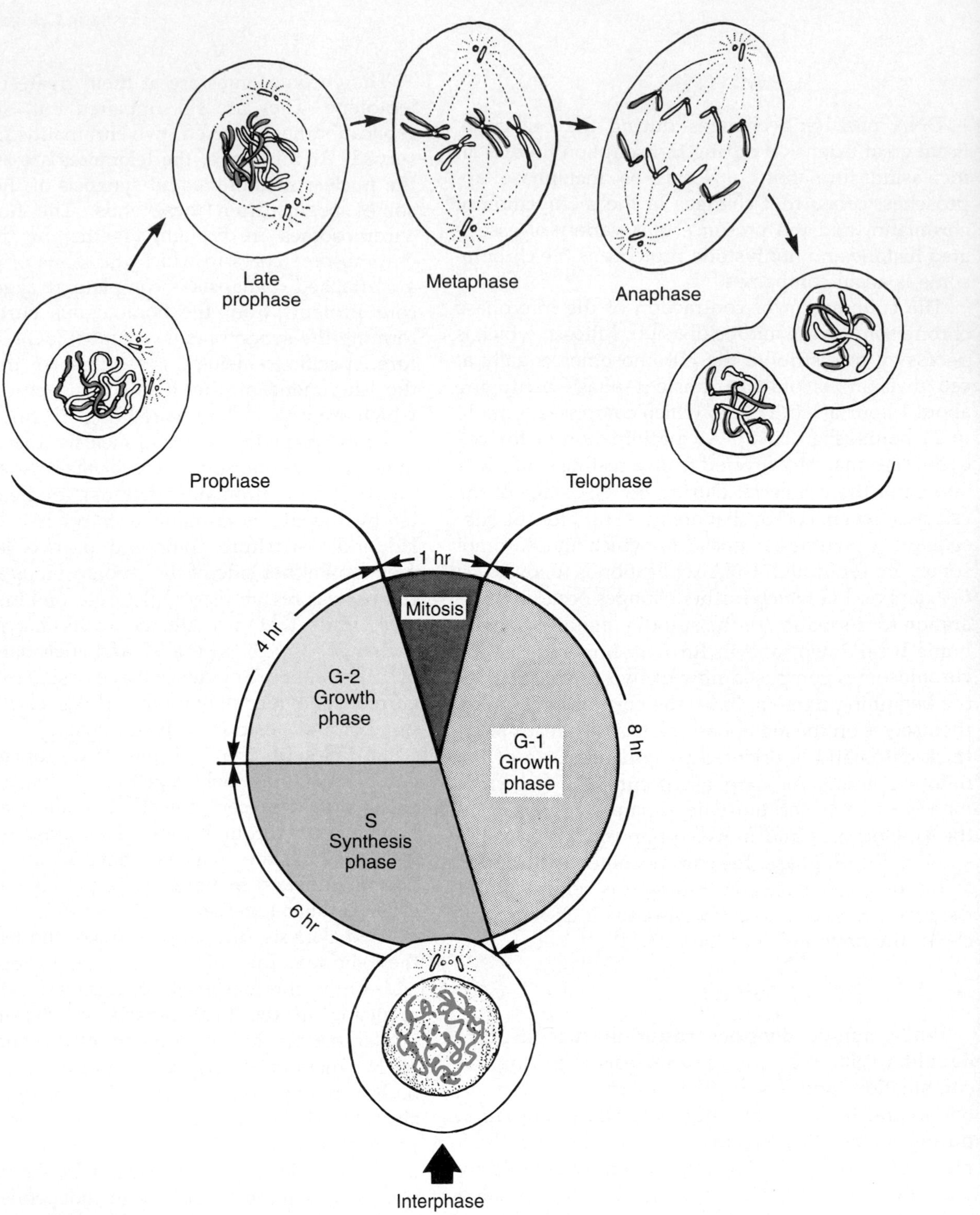

Figure 25.13. The mitotic cycle. The mitotic division comprises only a small segment (0.75 to 1.0 hour) of the cycle, which is characterized by an S or synthesis phase and two growth phases, all occurring during interphase.

Figure 25.14. Components of the mitotic apparatus after staining with specific antibodies and fluorescent stains. Cells are from a mammalian cell line (PtK). **A,** The microtubules are stained green with antitubulin antibodies and fluorescein-labeled secondary antibodies. **B,** The kinetochores are stained red with anticentromere antibodies from a patient with scleroderma plus rhodamine-labeled secondary antibodies. **C,** The chromatin of an early prophase cell. The chromosomes are stained blue with DAPI stain. Centrosome activity is revealed in the two asters of the cytoplasmic microtubules (green), but the nuclear envelope blocks interaction with kinetochores. **D–F,** Prometaphase through anaphase. The chromosomes are stained blue with DAPI and the spindle green with antitubulin antibodies and fluorescein-labeled secondary antibodies. **G–I,** Prometaphase through anaphase stained to show kinetochores (with anticentromere antibodies and rhodamine-labeled secondary antibodies). **J** and **K,** A pair of cells in late telophase-interphase, when nuclei are essentially reestablished, but the two cells are connected by a cytoplasmic bridge. **J,** Stained to show chromatin and spindle as above. **K,** Same cell stained to show kinetochores. (Reprinted from McIntosh J, Koonce MP. Mitosis. Science 1989;246:622–628, copyright 1989 by the American Association for the Advancement of Science.)

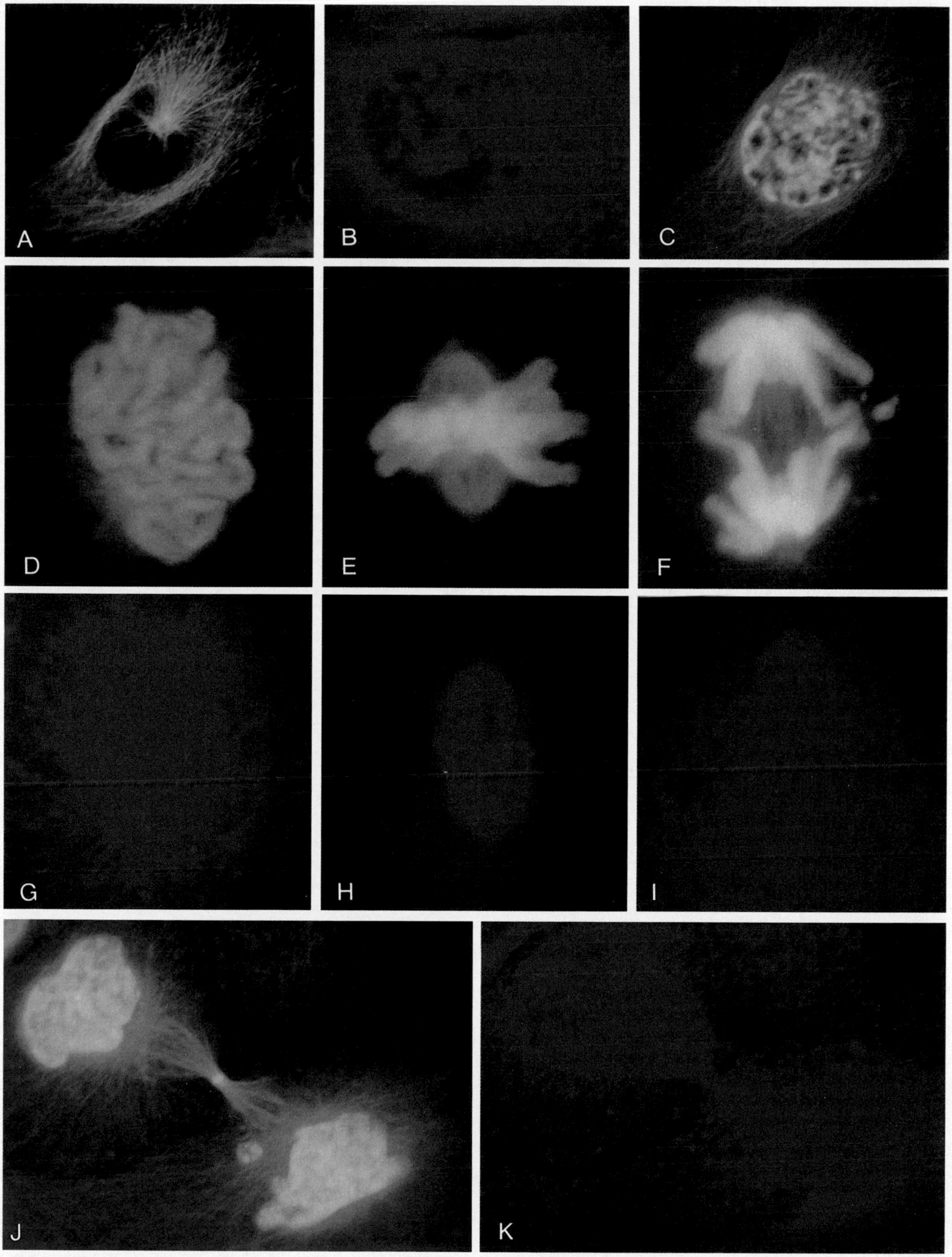

A
B
C
D
E
F
G
H
I
J
K

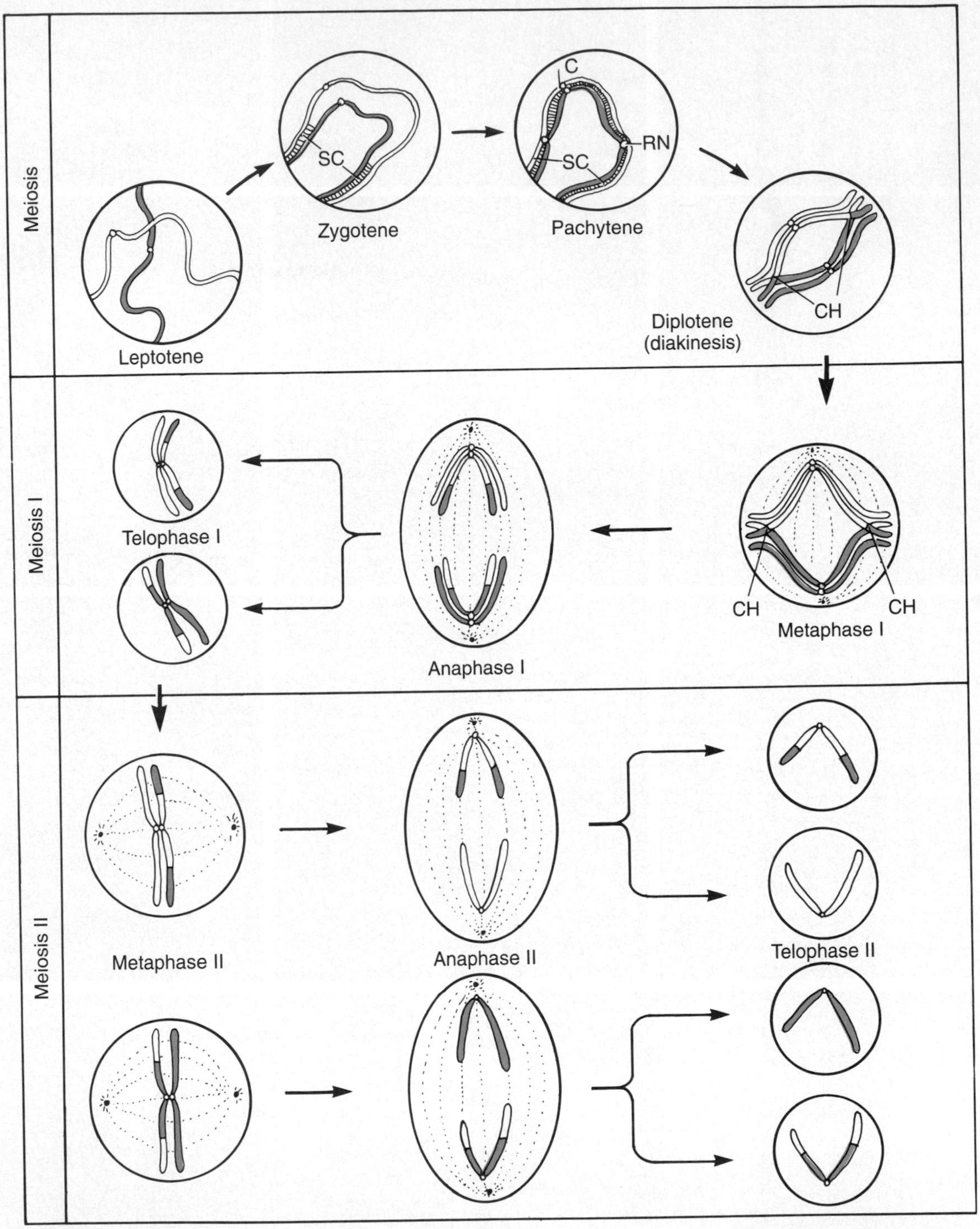

Figure 25.15. The meiotic division. Note the extended chromatin of leptotene; the beginning of the formation of the synaptonemal complex (SC) at zygotene; the completed synaptonemal complex showing recombination nodules (RN) at pachytene; the four strands showing crossing over at diplotene to diakenesis, with the centromeres (C) widely separated and the chromosomes held together by chiasmata (CH); and the alignment of homologs at metaphase I and separation at anaphase I (only one daughter cell shown). Prophase II is short and is not shown. At metaphase II the sister chromatids separate, and at telophase II the haploid number results.

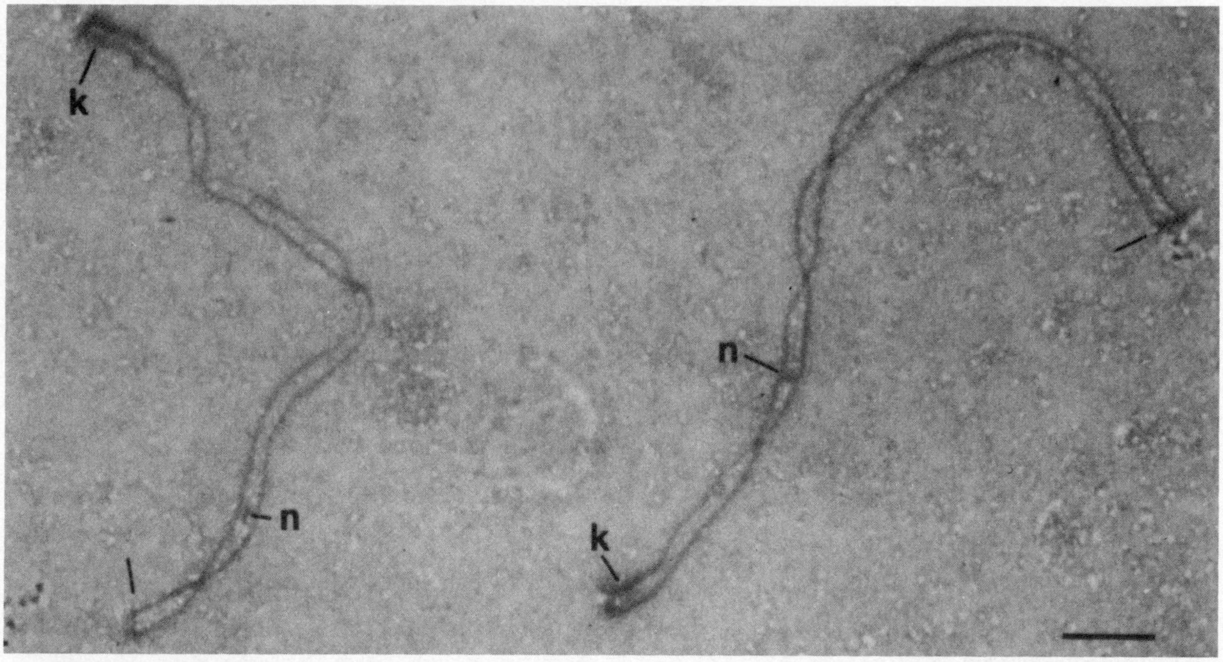

Figure 25.16. Electron micrograph of mouse synaptonemal complex showing attachment plaques (—) to nuclear envelope; kinetochore (k); and recombination nodules (n). The kinetochores are terminal in mouse chromosomes. The synaptonemal complex holds the chromosomes in register. The recombination nodules correspond in position and number to chiasmata. (Reprinted from De La Chapelle A, Sorsa M. Microspreading and the synaptonemal complex in cytogenetic studies. In: Chromosomes today. Vol 6. Amsterdam: Elsevier Science Publishers, 1977:71–82.)

In males, meiosis occurs in germ cells, which begin to divide meiotically at puberty. Meiotic divisions are of much longer duration than mitosis, requiring 15 to 32 hours to complete the division. The transition from spermatogonia to mature sperm requires 8 to 9 weeks.

In females, the first meiotic division is initiated prenatally at about 3 to 6 weeks of gestation and is completed as each egg matures and is released from the follicle. This may occur at any time from puberty to menopause. The second meiotic division occurs in the fallopian tube after fertilization; each division produces a polar body so that at maturation, the egg and two polar bodies result (Fig. 25.17).

CHROMOSOME IDENTIFICATION

Human chromosome morphology is usually based on the appearance of mitotic metaphase chromosomes. Metaphase chromosomes are composed of two identical chromatids resulting from the prior replication of DNA during the S phase. Chromosomes may differ in length and in position of the centromeres. The chromosomes appear constricted at the centromere or primary constriction, and this constriction usually divides each chromosome into two arms. The arms are designated p (the short arm) and q (the long arm) (Fig. 25.18). These arms may be equal, in which case the chromosome is referred to as metacentric; if the arms are unequal, the chromosome is called submetacentric. The centromere may be near one end of the chromosome (acrocentric chromosome) or terminal (telocentric chromosome).

The morphology of the human chromosome was initially defined by the relative length of the chromosome compared to the total length of a normal X-containing haploid set and by two parameters relative to the position of the centromere: the arm ratio and the centromeric index (see Fig. 25.2).

Another defining feature of the chromosome is the occurrence of secondary constrictions, a thinning or indentation of the chromosomes, which may be visible in only a portion of the cells. These constrictions occur in areas of heterochromatin and at the tip of the acrocentrics, where they separate a small segment, the satellite, from the chromosome. The secondary constrictions are variable in size; in human acrocentric chromosomes, the region of the constriction between the main part of the chromosome and the satellite contains the nucleolar organizing region.

Chromosome Staining Patterns

Chromosome bands in human chromosomes were first demonstrated by Caspersson in 1970. A band is defined as an area of the chromosome that is darker or lighter than its adjacent segments. The chromosome consists of a continuous series of dark and light

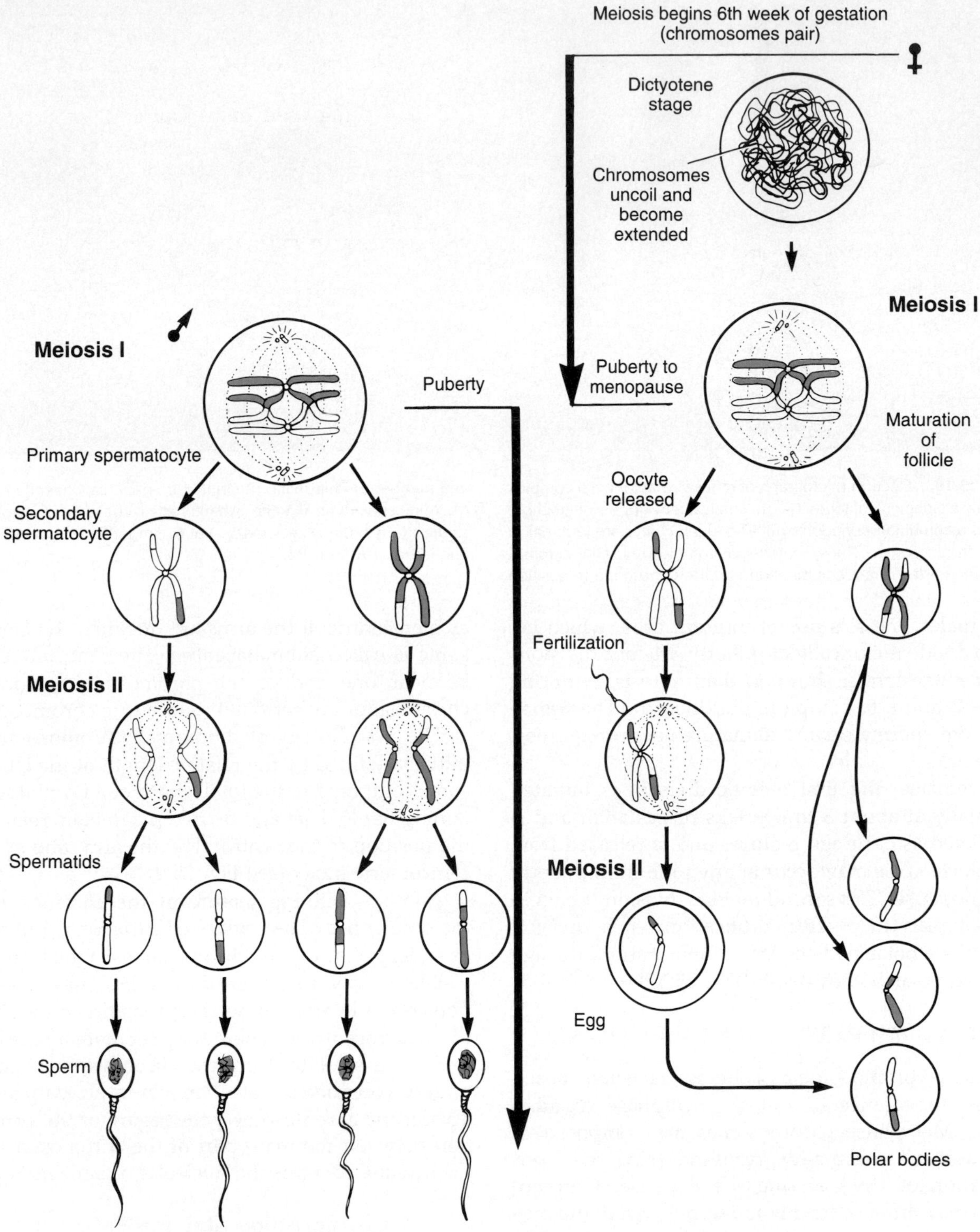

Figure 25.17. Comparison of meiosis in male and female gametogenesis.

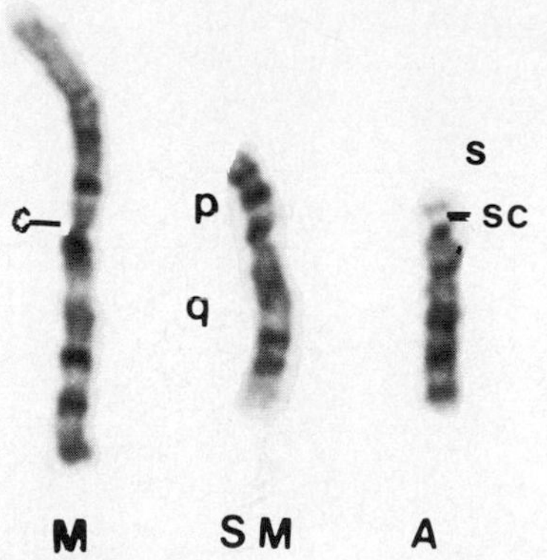

Figure 25.18. Morphological characteristics used to group human chromosomes. M, metacentric; SM, submetacentric; A, acrocentric; c, centromere, p, short arm; q, long arm, s, satellites; sc, secondary constriction.

bands. A variety of staining procedures have been developed, and bands that appear dark with one procedure may be light with another. Chromosome banding patterns are a means of identifying individual chromosomes.

Q and G Bands

Caspersson used quinacrine mustard, a fluorescent dye, to demonstrate areas of bright and dull fluorescence on the arms of the chromosomes. The bands produced are referred to as Q bands. Q-banding permits identification of each chromosome in the human karyotype. In particular, the Y chromosome is readily differentiated from the remaining acrocentric chromosomes by the brilliant fluorescence of the distal half of Yq, which is also visible in the interphase nucleus as a brilliant Y body. With Q-banding, centromeric regions and satellites demonstrate variations in staining intensity and size that are inherited (Fig. 25.19).

The staining reaction of Q-banding is based on interaction with specific bases, adenine and thymidine. Other adenine-thymidine (AT)-specific fluorochromes such as Hoechst 33258 and DAPI produce a similar banding pattern.

G bands are produced by pretreatment with mild salt or proteolytic enzymes, followed by staining with one of the Romanowski dyes (Giemsa, Wright's or Leischmann's stain) (Fig. 25.20). The patterns of G and Q bands are similar and correspond to the pattern of chromomeres seen in the chromosomes of meiotic pachytene. The G/Q bands condense early in mitosis and meiosis, and replication studies with tritiated thymidine (^{3}HT) or bromodeoxyuridine (BrdU) show that these regions replicate late in the cell cycle.

Although darkly staining G bands generally correspond to bright Q bands, there are some differences in staining, particularly in some paracentromeric regions that stain negatively by Q-banding but stain darkly with G-banding. Similarly, the segment of the Y chromosome that stains brilliantly with Q-banding stains with G-banding uniformly with the remainder of the chromosome. Thus, although there are similarities in banding patterns, the two banding methods have different uses in cytogenetic studies, G-banding being used more routinely for cytogenetic studies, and Q-banding reserved for special purposes requiring visualization of polymorphisms on the Y chromosome.

METHOD FOR G-BANDING WITH TRYPSIN

To obtain sharply defined bands with trypsin banding, slides must be aged. Freshly prepared slides are placed in a drying oven at 65°C overnight or longer, depending on humidity, and then trypsinized.

Materials: 0.1 g Difco powdered trypsin (1:250) in 100-ml isotonic buffered saline (Isoton)
Isotonic buffered saline
Phosphate buffer pH 6.8
Giemsa working solution: 1 ml Giemsa and 49 ml phosphate buffer at pH 6.8

Slides are treated in trypsin solution for 3 to 7 seconds, rinsed in Isoton and fetal calf serum and then in Isoton alone. The slides are then stained for approximately 2 to 4 minutes in Giemsa solution, rinsed in phosphate buffer (pH 6.8) and then in distilled water, and allowed to dry.

METHOD FOR QM STAINING

Materials: 5 mg of quinacrine mustard dihydrochloride in 80 ml of KH_2PO_4 buffer (store in light-tight container).
Buffer 18.16 g of KH_2PO_4 in 2 liters of distilled H_2O.

Slides do not need to be aged. Stain slides 1 to 2 minutes and rinse in distilled water. Place slides in KH_2PO_4 buffer for 1 to 2 minutes. Place 2 or 3 drops of KH_2PO_4 buffer on slide, coverslip, blot excess buffer and seal edges of coverslip. Store in the dark. Observe with fluorescent microscope using a wavelength of 450 to 500 nm.

R Bands

R-banding is produced by treatments that selectively denature AT-rich DNA; for example, heat denaturation of chromosomes at 85°C followed by staining with Giemsa (RHG—R-banding with heat and Giemsa stain) or with acridine orange (RFA—

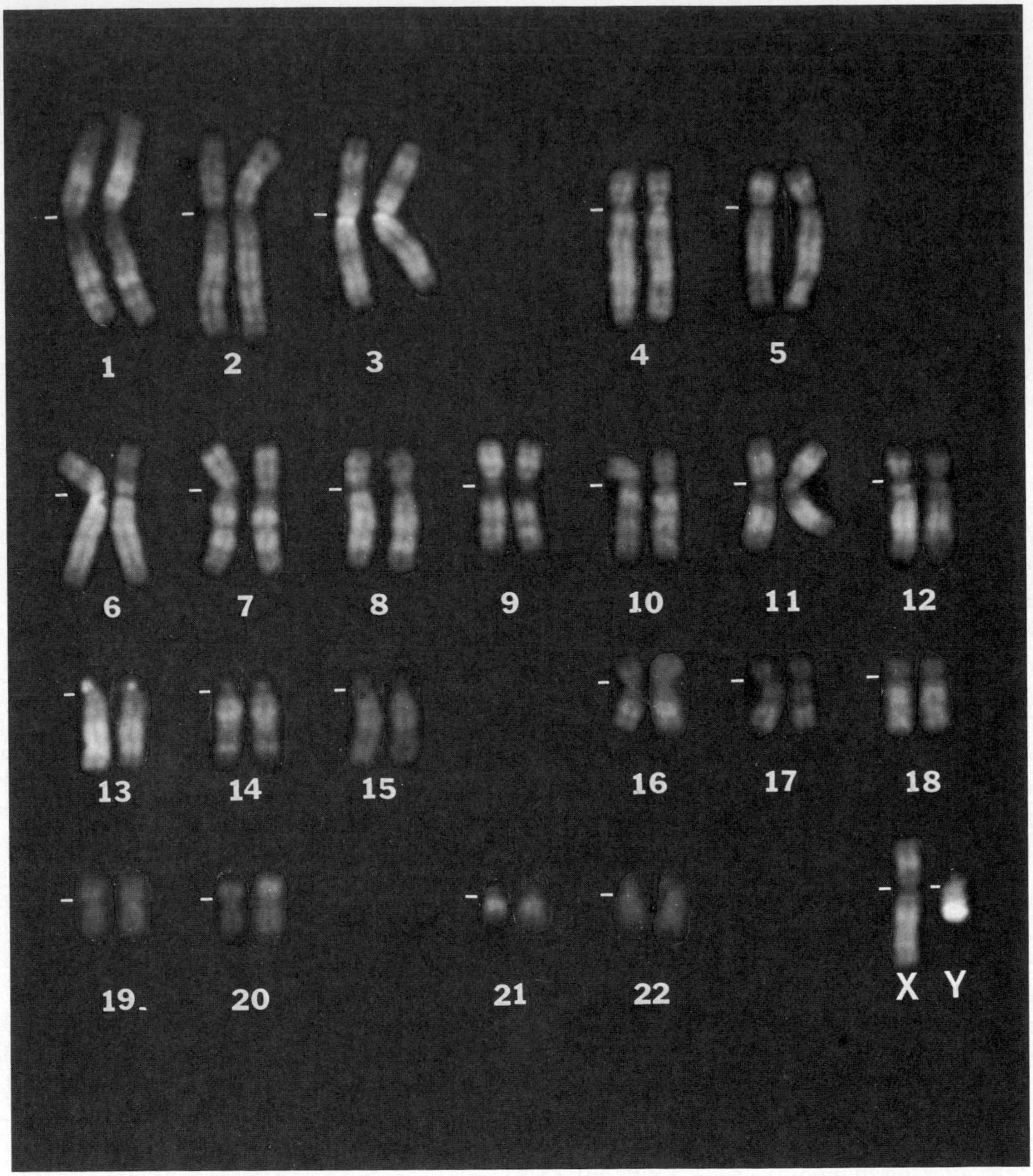

Figure 25.19. Q-band karyotype. (Reproduced with permission from C. C. Lin.)

R-banding with acridine orange). Fluorochromes with an affinity to GC base pairs such as chromomycin A3 or olivomycin will also produce a fluorescence pattern similar to that of R bands. R-banding may also be produced by BrdU incorporation, a replication banding technique (RBG) that takes advantage of the late replication of R bands (discussed under Replication Banding).

R-banding is the reverse of G/Q banding. Regions that appear light with G-banding are darkly stained with R-banding (Fig. 25.21). After R-banding, the ends of the chromosomes appear darkly stained. Thus, it is useful to utilize R-banding when an abnormality involving the chromosome ends, such as a terminal deletion, is suspected. The extent of deletions may be more precisely determined from the darkly staining R bands than with G-banding, in which the same band is lightly staining.

R bands are relatively guanine-cytosine (GC) rich, replicate in the first half of the S phase, and condense late in prophase. In situ hybridization of DNA complementary to mRNA sequences indicates that the coding DNA is localized in R bands. Among genes and genetic diseases localized to specific bands on the chromosome, the greatest proportion (74%) are located in G-negative bands.

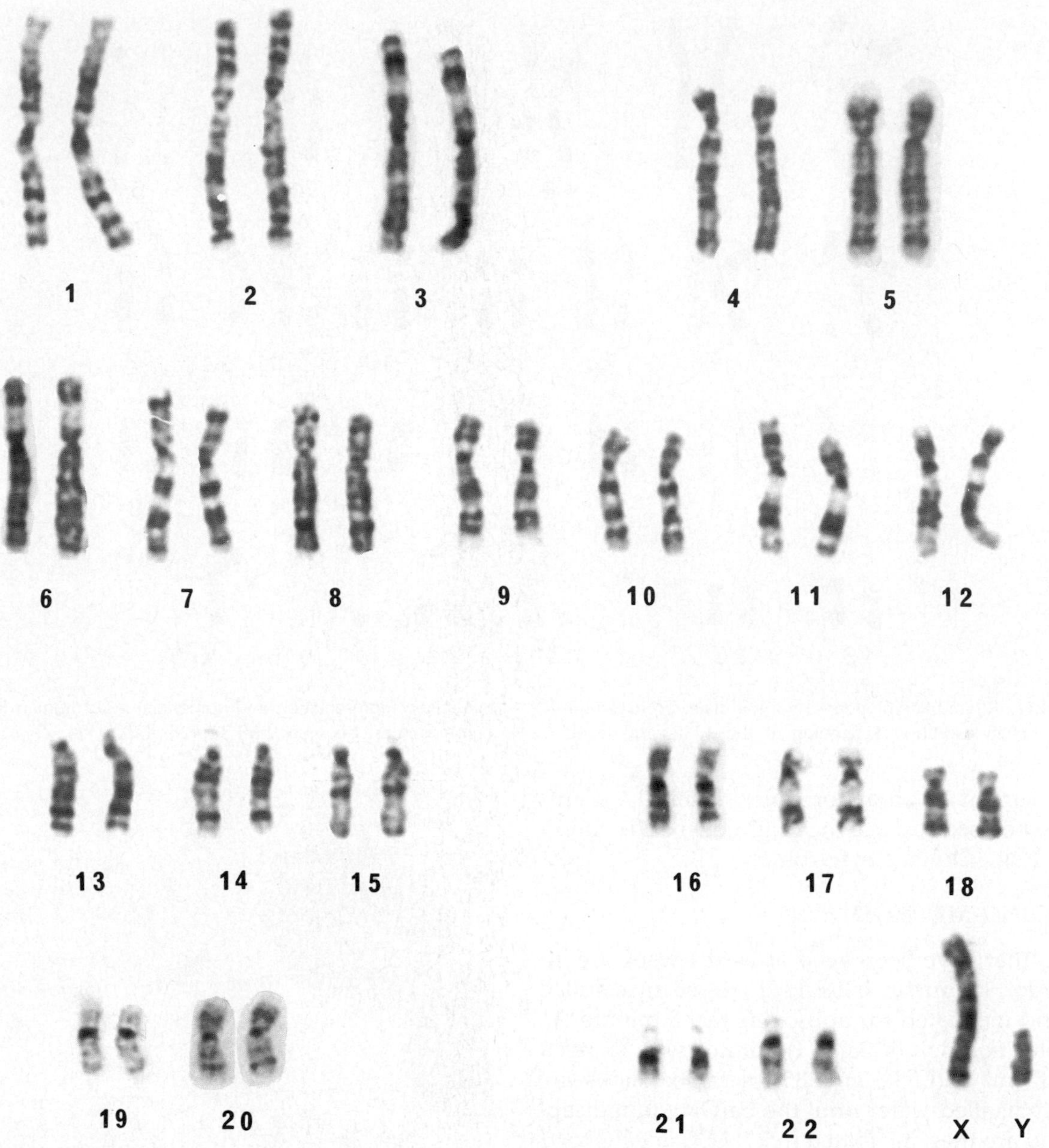

Figure 25.20. G-band karyotype of a normal male.

R-BANDING METHOD

Aged slides are incubated in Sorensen's buffer pH 6.5 at 85°C for approximately 8 minutes, rinsed in the same buffer at room temperature, stained in Giemsa 5 to 10 minutes, rinsed in distilled water, and allowed to dry.

C Bands

C-banding is derived from the methodology used by Pardue and Gall for in situ hybridization of mouse satellite DNA to mouse centromeric heterochromatin. Arrighi and Hsu found that this method produced darkly staining centromeric heterochromatin without the hybridization step by staining with Giemsa after denaturation with sodium hydroxide (barium hydroxide may be substituted) and subsequent incubation in a salt solution. The bands at the centromeres are readily observed (Fig. 25.22). These heritable regions are variable in size, may differ in homologs, and may vary in position in the long or short arm pericentromeric region. C-banding may also be obtained after treating fixed cells on slides with the restriction endonucleases AluI, DdeI, HaIII, MboI or RoaI, or HinfI.

C-banding is used to identify the heterochromatic segments (for example, in suspected dicentric chromosomes) and to identify chromosome variants when there is question of whether an unusual find-

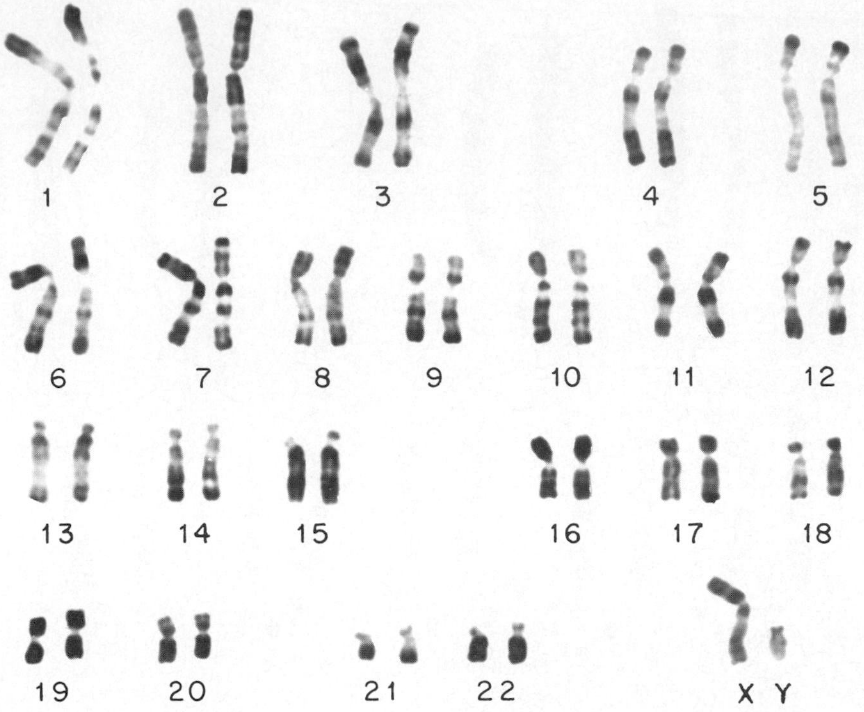

Figure 25.21. R-band karyotype of a normal male. (From Drouin R, Richer CL. High-resolution R-banding at the 1250-band level. II. Schematic representation and nomenclature of human RBG-banded chromosomes. Genome 1989;32:428, 429.)

ing is a variant or an abnormality. Familial variants may also be used to trace the origin of specific abnormalities (e.g., Down's syndrome).

C-BANDING METHOD

Slides that have been aged at least 1 week are incubated for 1 hour in 0.2N HCl, rinsed in distilled water and incubated for approximately 3 minutes in a saturated solution of $Ba(OH)_2$ diluted with distilled water (15 ml $Ba(OH)_2$ and 35 ml H_2O). Slides are rinsed in distilled water until the $Ba(OH)_2$ film disappears and are then incubated in 2× SSC at 60°C for 1 hour. They are rinsed and stained in Giemsa for 10 minutes, rinsed again, and dried.

The Significance of Banding and Chromosome Structure

A number of lines of evidence have suggested that G bands are more AT rich than R bands. Evidence from base-specific fluorochromes such as Hoechst 33258 supports this observation. Autoradiographic studies using tritiated thymidine or tritiated guanidine and buoyant density data suggest that G and R band DNA differ in base ratio. The differences in R and G bands may be related to the distribution of families of interspersed repeated sequences. The short interspersed repeated sequences (SINES), of which the Alu DNA sequence family is predominant, occur mainly in R bands. Alu is 56% guanine plus cytosine. In G bands, the long interspersed repeated sequences (LINES), or L_1 family, occur more fre-

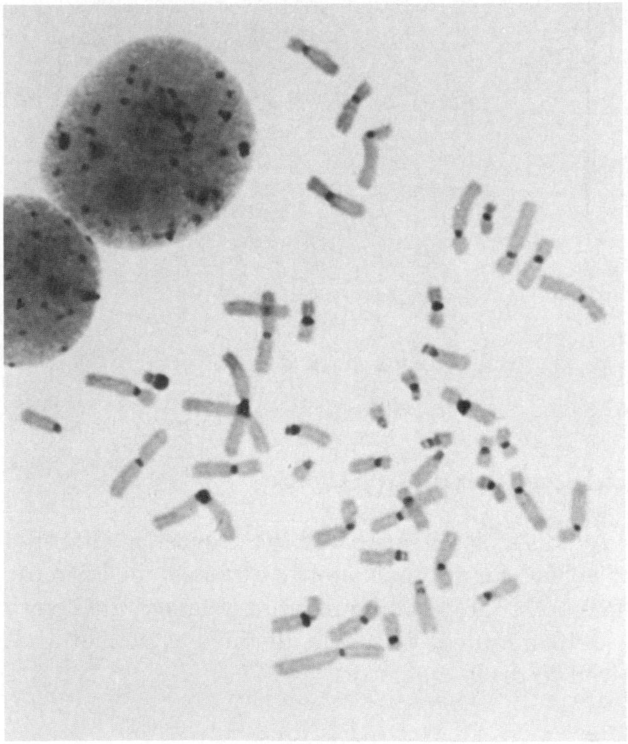

Figure 25.22. C-banded metaphase: centromeric and paracentromeric regions of chromosomes 1, 9, 16, and Yq stain. (Courtesy of J. Zunich.)

Table 25.1. Functional and Biochemical Attributes of Chromosome Bands

Bands	G/Q	R	C
Base composition of DNA	AT rich	GC rich	Mainly AT rich
Timing of DNA replication	Last half of S	First half of S	Late S
Time of condensation	Early mitosis	Late mitosis	Remains condensed in interphase
Concentration of expressed genes	Low	High	None
Enriched repeated DNA sequences	Lines (Li)	Sines (Alu)	Satellite

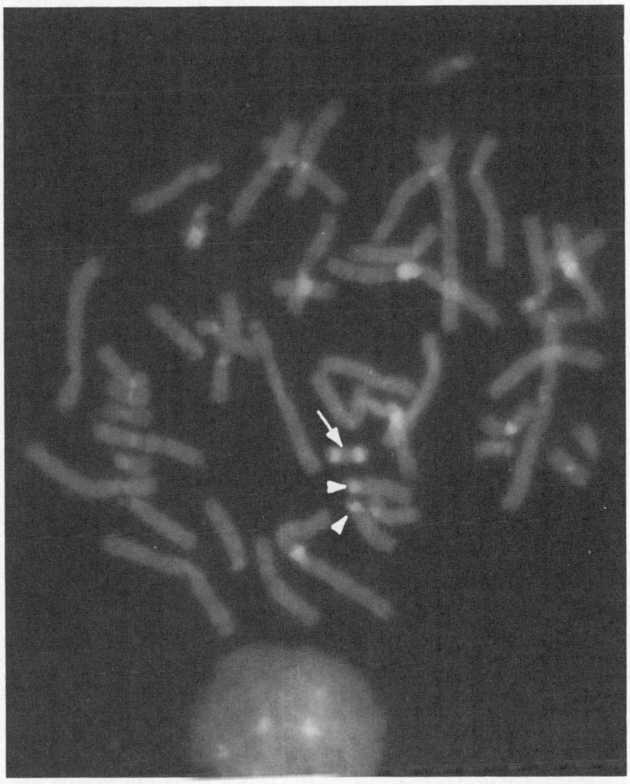

Figure 25.23. Cell with an i(15p) marker after DA/DAPI staining. The paracentric heterochromatin of chromosomes 1, 9, 16, Yq, and 15p (*arrowheads*) stain brightly. An extra marker chromosome (*arrow*) derived from 15p is also shown to fluoresce after DA/DAPI staining.

quently. L_1 is composed of 58% adenine plus thymidine. Thus, the difference in distribution of these repeated sequences may account for the banding with fluorescent dyes and the reaction with base-specific antibodies. The basis for banding with proteolytic enzymes and Giemsa staining may be related to differences in the distribution of interacting proteins.

C bands are areas of the chromosome that are composed of condensed and highly repetitive, nontranscribed satellite DNA, which is highly methylated (see Heterochromatin). C-banding procedures result from the differential extraction of DNA in which more DNA remains in the C band region. This may be related to a difference in protein-DNA interaction interfering with DNA extraction. Alpha satellite DNA has been found by restriction analysis and in situ hybridization to be located in the C heterochromatin of all human chromosomes. Subsets of alpha satellite sequences have been localized to specific centromeric regions (although some are present in more than one chromosome). The alphoid sequences are hypermethylated and may be related to the inactivity of C heterochromatin. Thus, the studies of the basis for staining procedures used for the identification of human chromosomes have led to a further understanding of the structure of chromosomes. Some of the functional and biochemical characteristics of chromosomes are summarized in Table 25.1.

Distamycin/DAPI

DAPI (4′6-diamidino-2-phenylindole) is a fluorochrome that, when combined with a nonfluorescent counterstain, distamycin A (DA), shows bright fluorescence at secondary constrictions of chromosomes 1, 9, 16, the proximal 15 (15p11), and distal Yq (Fig. 25.23). It is particularly useful in identifying marker chromosomes that have originated from 15p, which fluoresce brightly after DA/DAPI staining. Both DAPI and DA bind preferentially to AT-rich DNA.

DA/DAPI METHOD

Slides are flooded with DA (Distamycin A-HC 0.2 mg/ml of McIlvaine's citric acid—Na_2HPO_4 buffer at pH 7.0), covered with a coverslip and incubated at room temperature for 15 minutes. The coverslip is removed and the slide rinsed with buffer at pH 7.0.

The DAPI solution (0.2 to 0.4 μg/ml) is added to the slide, the slide is coverslipped and incubated in the dark at room temperature for 15 minutes, rinsed, mounted in buffer, and sealed. The slides are observed with a fluorescence microscope using a 360-nm excitation filter and a 460-nm emission filter.

NOR Bands

The specific chromosome region in the satellite stalk that organizes the nucleolus, the nucleolar organizing region (NOR) may be observed in metaphase chromosomes by a silver impregnation method (Ag-NOR banding) (Figure 25.24). This technique stains nonhistone residual proteins that appear to be located specifically at functional NORs and localizes the areas coding for the 18s and 28s ribosomal RNA. Each of the acrocentric chromosomes may bear

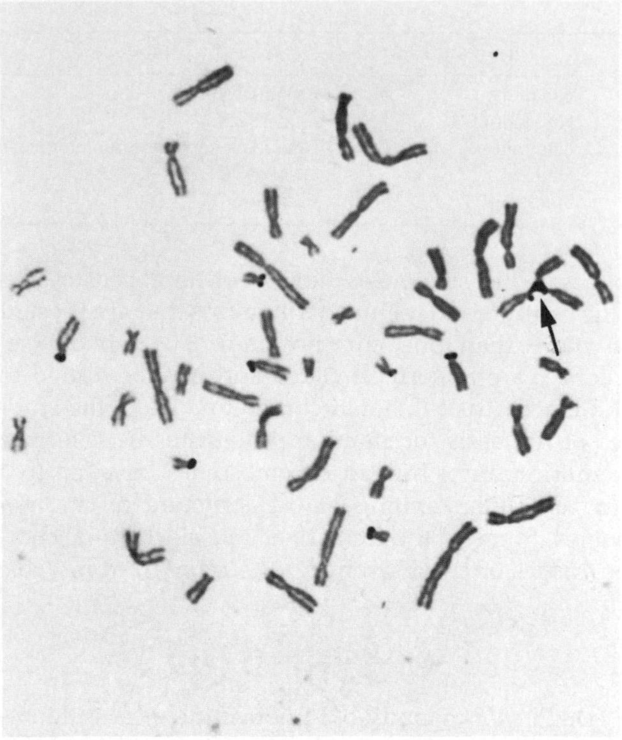

Figure 25.24. Ag-NOR staining. The active "NOR" regions are seen as darkly staining areas at the ends of each of the ten acrocentric chromosomes. *Arrow* indicates three acrocentric chromosomes in association and the NOR regions of the three fused.

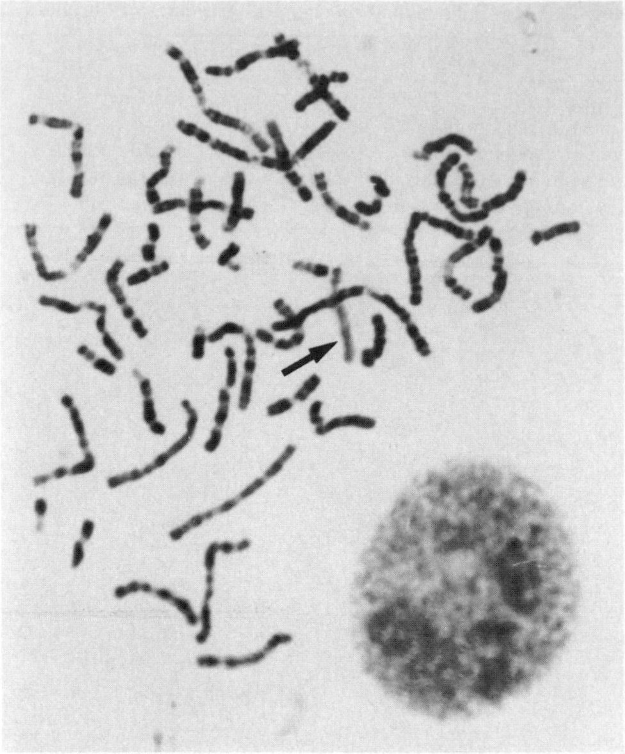

Figure 25.25. Replication banding (RBG). Banding after treatment of the cell for the last 5 hours with BrdU. This technique is frequently used to demonstrate the late-replicating X (*arrow*). The chromosomes show an R-banding pattern.

an active NOR. Usually not all ten of the acrocentric NOR regions are active in any one cell. NORs may vary in size, and in some cases double NORs may be present in a chromosome. These variations are consistent and heritable from parent to child.

Replication Banding

Early cytogenetic studies using ^{3}H thymidine and autoradiography demonstrated that different chromosomes and regions of chromosomes completed their replication at different times during the S phase. More recently, it has been possible to demonstrate these replication differences and the differences in replication time of G (late) and R (early) bands by use of BrdU, an analog of thymidine. When BrdU is added to the culture, it is incorporated into DNA during the cell cycle. If the cells are treated with Hoechst 33258 and subjected to photolysis and differential staining with acridine orange (RFA technique) or with Giemsa (FPG technique), R bands are produced. BrdU also interferes with chromosome condensation. This banding technique is often used to produce R bands in previously synchronized cultures. Since R bands have completed their replication early in S phase, the regions incorporating BrdU during the last half of S will be G bands. Thus, the R bands will be dark and the G bands light after FPG staining. Alternatively, the same staining procedure may be used to show G bands if the cells are grown initially in 2 BrdU and thymidine is added late in replication (Fig. 25.25).

The BrdU/FPG method is most useful in demonstrating the differences in the two X chromosomes, since the late-replicating X chromosome stains light and the early-replicating one dark with this method.

FPG METHOD

Lymphocytes are grown for 48 to 54 hours in RPMI 1640 and are synchronized with excess thymidine (Concentration 1.24×10^{-3} M) for 17 hours. The block is released after rinsing by resuspending in TC199 plus BrdU (10^{-3} M) for 4.5 hours, and cells are harvested without colcemid exposure.

Slides are stained with Hoechst 33258 (2.5 g/ml) for 15 minutes. The slides are exposed to ultraviolet light for 120 to 150 minutes and stained with Giemsa (1%) for 5 minutes.

High-Resolution Banding

Although most laboratories use metaphase chromosomes for routine chromosome analysis, the need for procedures that demonstrate subtle gains or losses of single bands has led to the development of methodology for high-resolution imaging of chromosomes. Identification of small deletions involved in Prader-Willi, Miller-Dieker, and other deletion syndromes requires the use of methods that will provide chromosomes with identifiable bands in the order of 800 to 1000 bands. High-resolution chromosomes may be obtained by the use of compounds such as ethidium bromide or actinomycin D that interfere with the condensation of the chromosomes and produce longer chromosomes with subdivided bands. Alternatively, Yunis' method of synchronization of cells (which uses antimetabolites to arrest cells in S phase) may be used, followed by release with thymidine for specific periods to accumulate cells in particular stages of prophase or prometaphase. While standard metaphase chromosomes demonstrate 400 to 500 bands, high-resolution methods may resolve 800 to 1200 bands in prometaphase or prophase chromosomes. (The latter technique may also be used in conjunction with replication banding with BrdU to give high-resolution R banding.) The chromosomal procedures may also be altered by increasing hypotonic treatment and reducing colcemide time to permit maximum length and greatest spreading of the more extended chromosomes.

High-resolution chromosomes are not only extended compared to metaphase chromosomes, but also have a greater number of bands. Both light and dark bands seen at the 400-band level may be resolved at the earlier stages of division into multiple light and dark bands (Fig. 25.26).

METHOD OF SYNCHRONIZATION FOR HIGH-RESOLUTION CHROMOSOMES

After incubation of leukocyte cultures grown in RPMI 1640 for 72 hours, methotrexate (final concentration 10^{-7} M) is added to the cultures. Seventeen hours later the incubated cells are released from the block by rinsing in RPMI 1640 and are grown for an additional 5 to 5½ hours, treated with colcemid (0.05 μg/ml at room temperature) for 10 minutes, and harvested. Alternatively, the block may be released with 0.1 ml thymidine (1×10^{-3} M) added to each 10-ml culture.

ETHIDIUM BROMIDE METHOD FOR PROMETAPHASE CHROMOSOMES

Leukocyte cultures grown for 72 hours are harvested by addition of 0.05 ml of 6 mg/ml of colcemide and 0.1 ml of a 1 mg/ml solution of ethidium bromide for 2 hours. The cells are fixed and processed in a standard manner.

Chromosome Heteromorphisms

Constitutive heterochromatin in human chromosomes may vary in size or position in the chromosome. This variation in amount of highly repetitive DNA results in chromosome variants or heteromorphism. Homologous chromosomes may vary in the amount or position of C bands and in the intensity of fluorescence or size of Q bands. Individual variation in C heterochromatin is inherited and the heteromorphisms segregate in a mendelian fashion (Fig. 25.27).

The quinacrine heteromorphisms are seen mainly as variations in the intensity of fluorescence of short arms and satellites of chromosomes 13, 14, 15, 21, and 22 and the length of the distal portion of the Y chromosome. Additional QFQ variation in the intensity of staining at the centromeric regions of chromosomes 3 and 4 and pericentric inversions of the centromeric heterochromatin of chromosome 3 are frequently recognized (Fig. 25.28). The nonuniformity of fluorescence may be compared in individuals by the use of internal standards to indicate the approximate intensity of fluorescence. These standards were defined at the Paris Conference of 1971.

Negative	No or almost no fluorescence
Pale	As in distal 1p
Medium	As the two broad bands in 9q
Intense	As the distal half of 13q
Brilliant	As a distal Yq

Pericentric inversion of Q fluorescent regions may also occur. The variably fluorescent region of chromosome 3 in the European population may appear proximally in the p arm rather than the usual proximal q location.

C band heteromorphisms include variation in the size and position of the centromeric heterochromatin of all chromosomes and of the paracentromeric heterochromatin of chromosomes 1, 9, and 16 and the distal long arm of Y. Variation in the size of short arms or satellites may also be documented by C banding. The variation in size is continuous and may be classified by length into very small, small, intermediate, large, and very large. In some cases, large C bands may appear to be composed of two segments. The position of C bands may be in the long or short arm, or part may be in the long arm and part in the short arm.

Variations in the C bands, in particular of chromosomes 1 and 9, are clearly defined after G-11 staining. Variation in size and number of active NORs may be observed after silver staining (Ag-NOR) and are seen as silver deposits at the site of activity. Rarely, variation in the position of the NOR may be

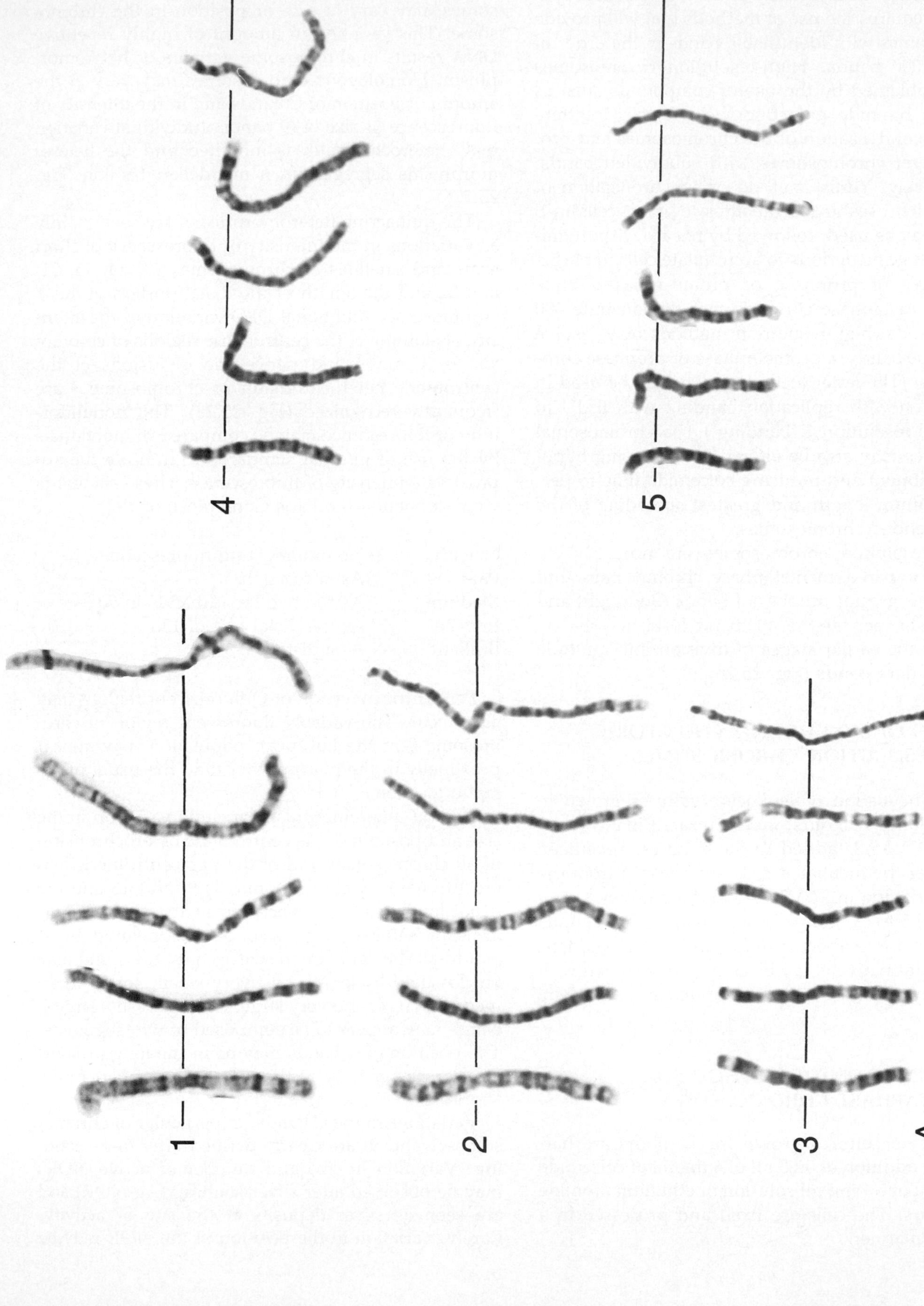

Figure 25.26. A-D, High-resolution banding of human chromosomes. The first chromosome of each series is shown at about the 475-band level, with increasing length and band resolution as the chromosomes become more extended in prometaphase.

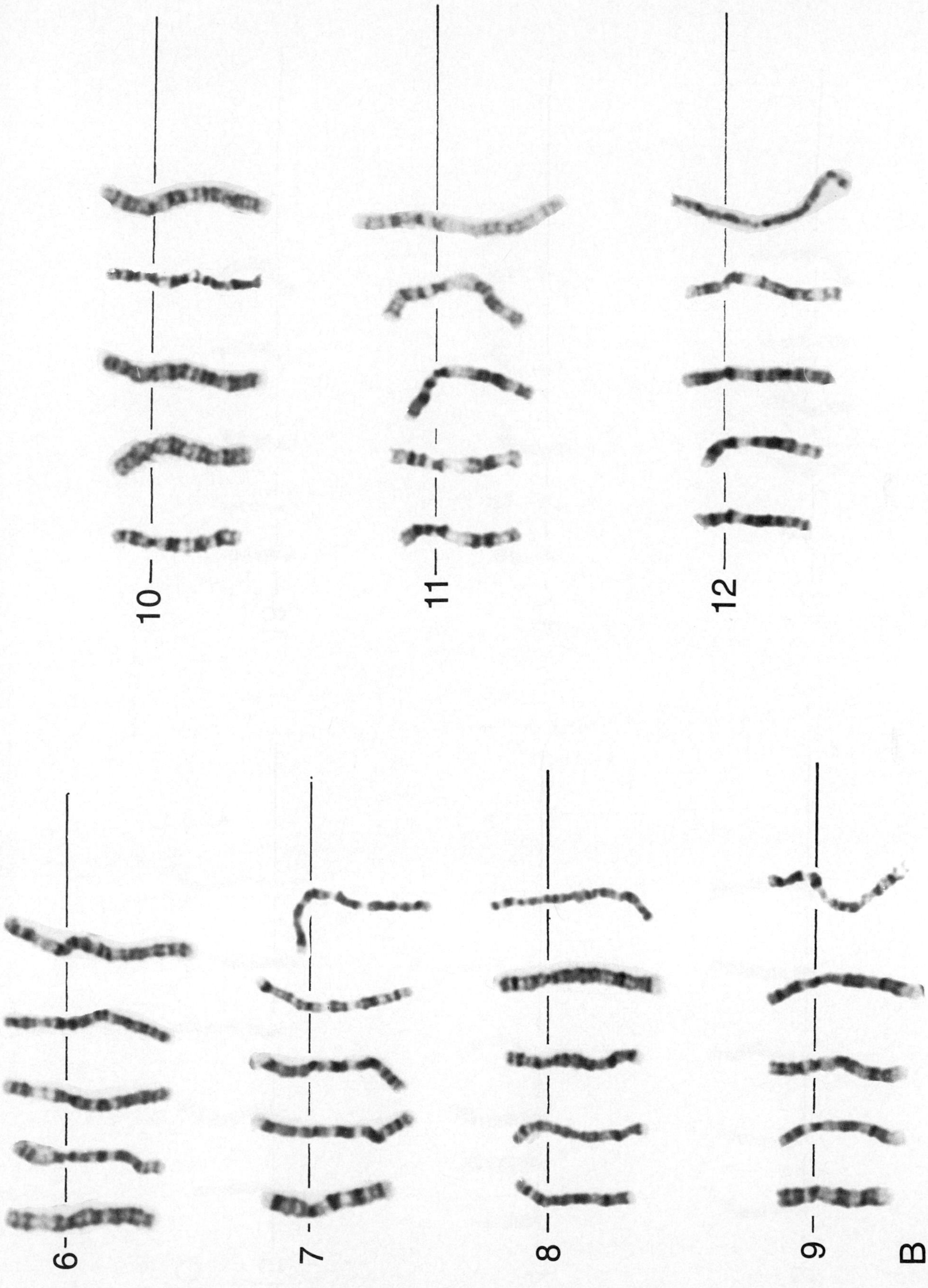

Figure 25.26. B.

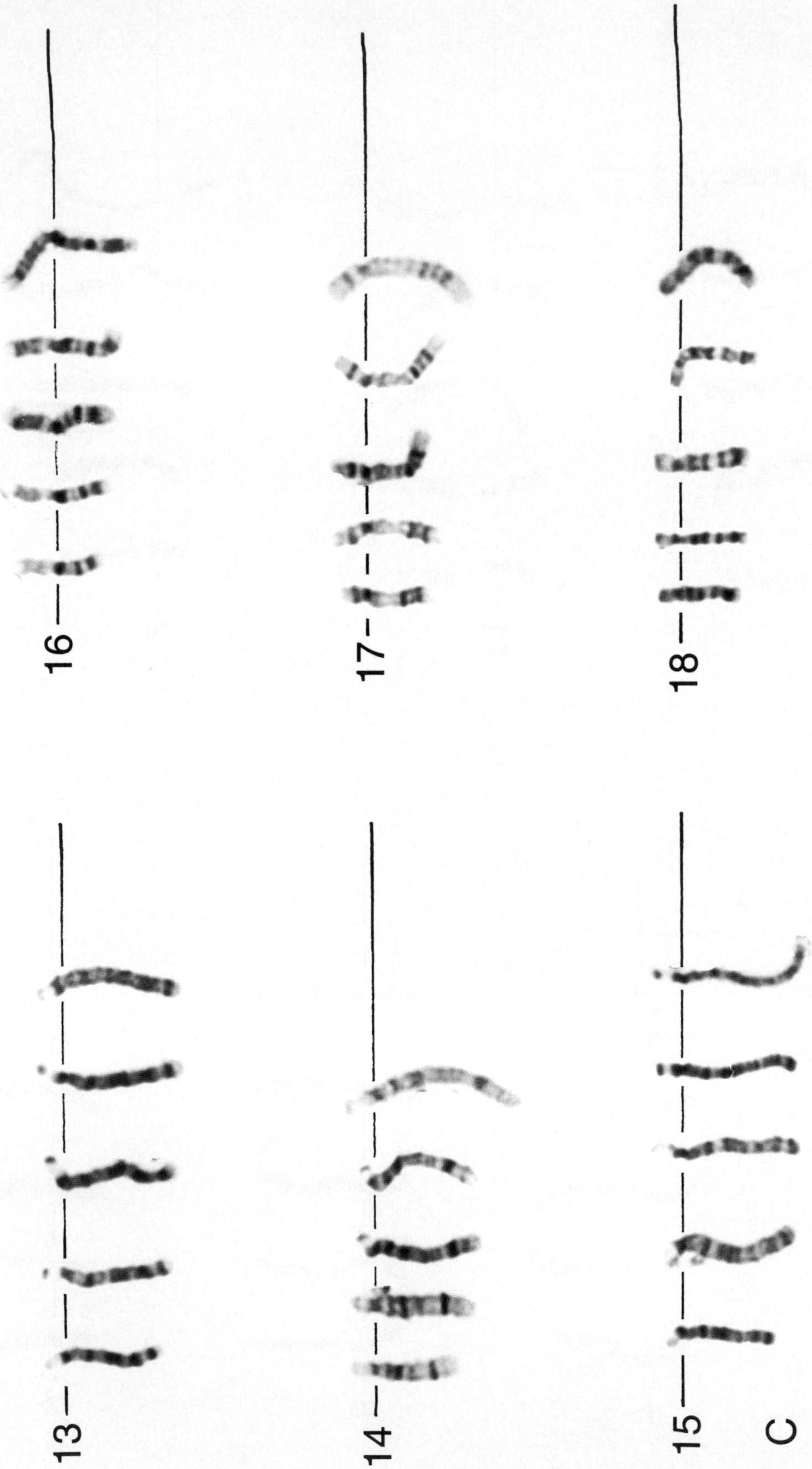

Figure 25.26. C.

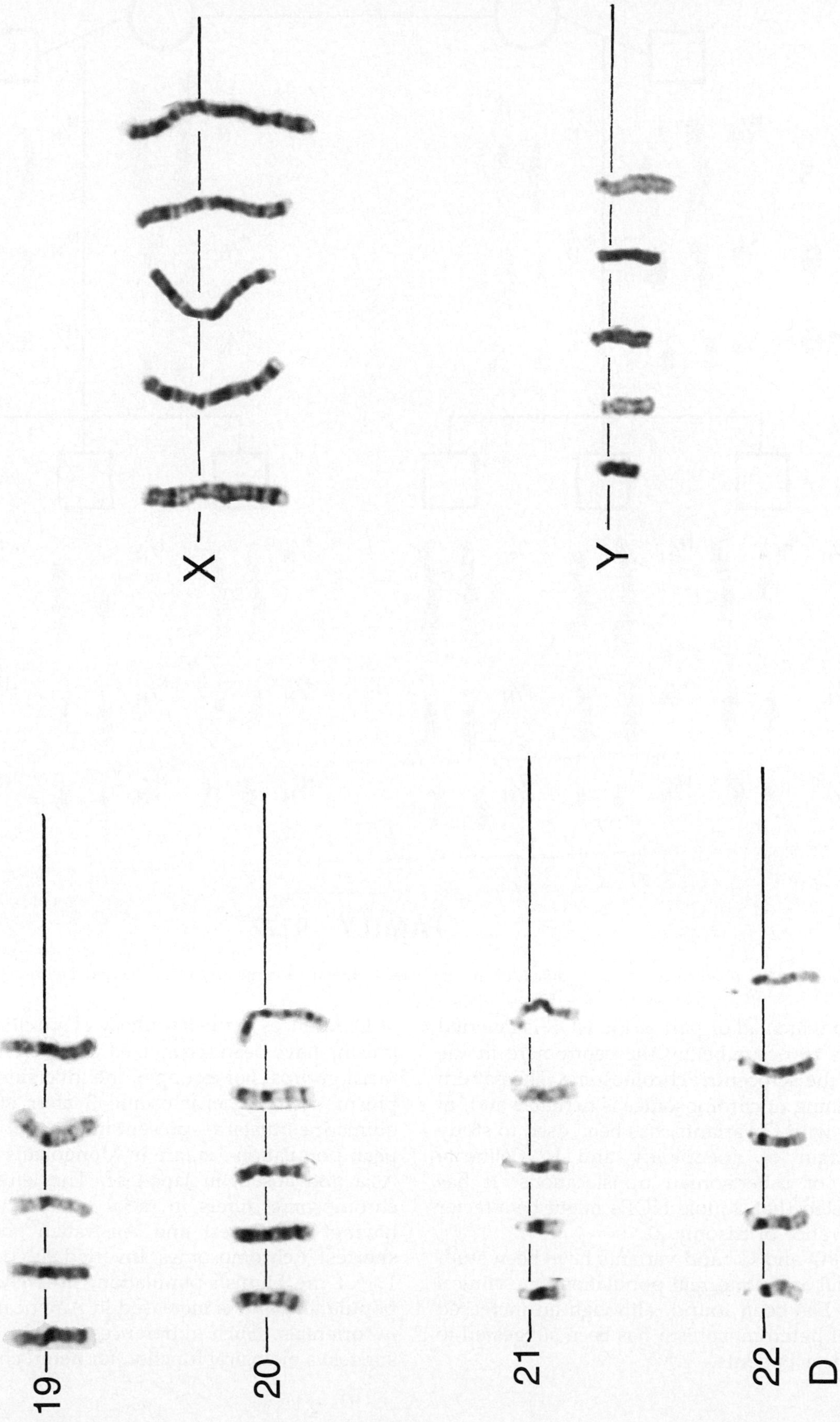

Figure 25.26. D.

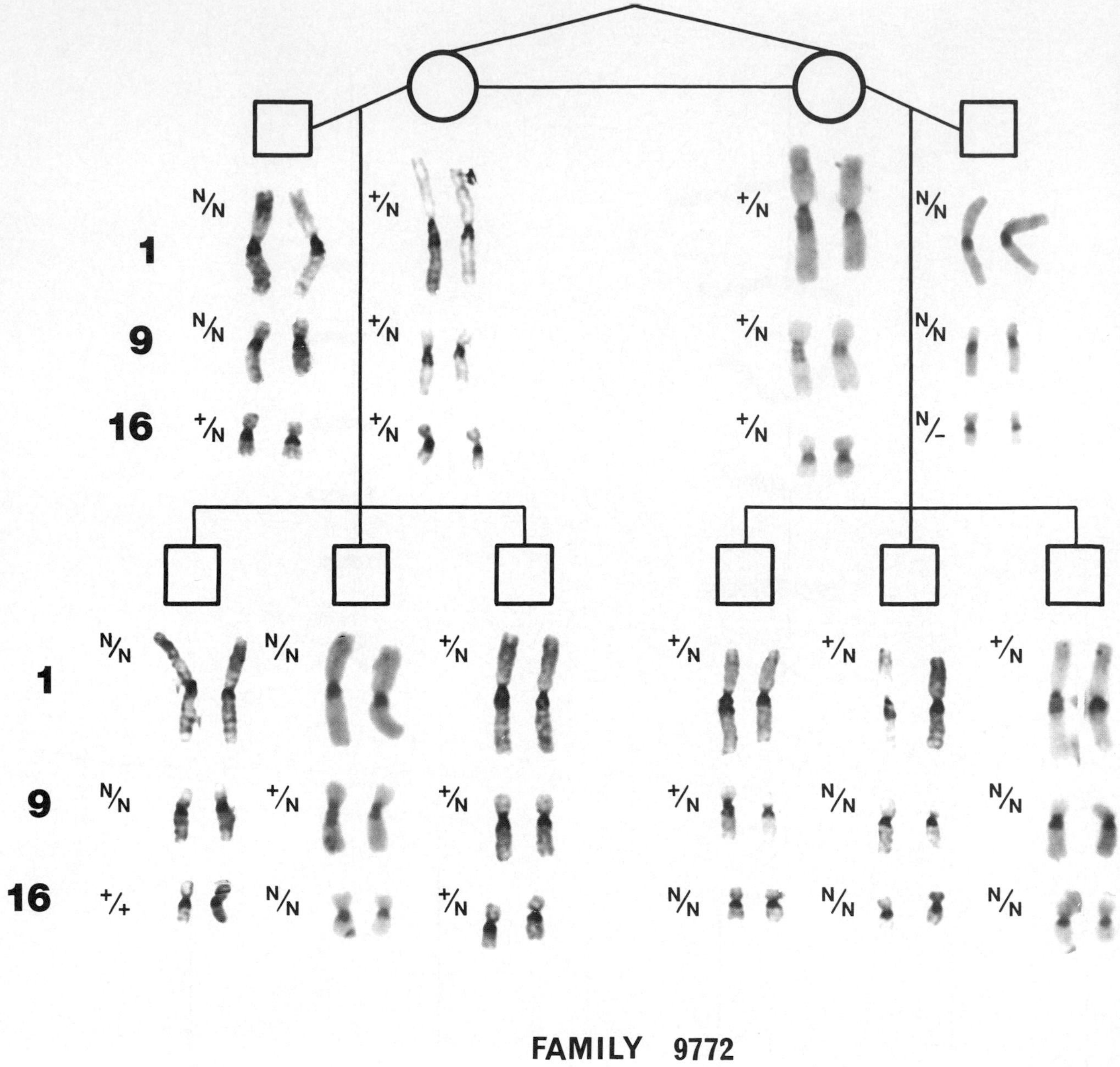

Figure 25.27. Inheritance of C band variants of chromosomes 1, 9, and 16 in monozygotic twins and their offspring.

observed, in which all or part of the NOR is inverted and appears to occur below the centromere in the long arm of the acrocentric chromosome. The pattern of NOR staining of chromosomes is heritable and, in conjunction with Q variants, has been used to study parental origin of aneuploidy and to delineate breakpoints of robertsonian translocations. It has been suggested that double NORs might be a factor in the recurrence of trisomy 21.

Although Q and C band variants have been studied in normal and abnormal populations, no clinical significance has been found, although an increased frequency of heteromorphism has been suggested to occur in cancer patients.

Differences in the frequency of specific heteromorphisms have been recognized in different ethnic and racial groups. For example, the inversion heteromorphism seen in chromosome 3 after staining with quinicrine mustard—present in 6 to 11% of the European population—is rare in Mongolians in northeast Asia and absent in Japanese. The length of the Y chromosome differs in racial groups, the Japanese having the longest and Australian aborigines the shortest Y chromosomes. Inverted 9qh occurs in only 1% of the Finnish population, in 4% of the Greek population, and is increased in American blacks and in orientals. Such differences among populations suggest a biological function for heterochromatin and

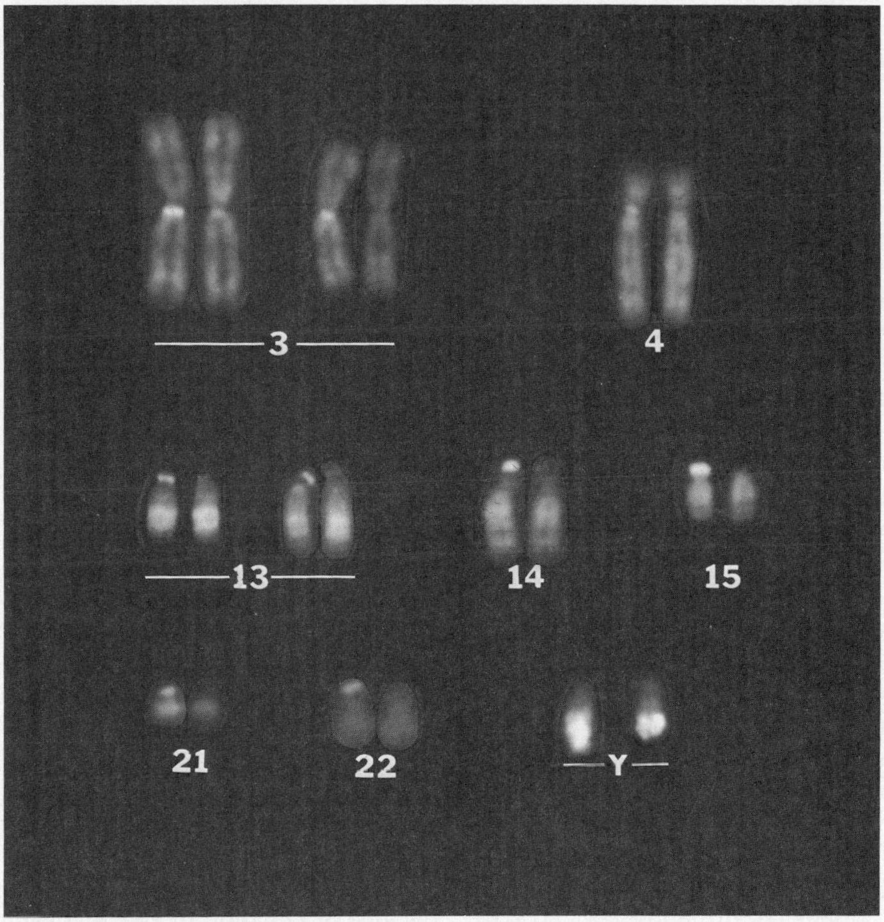

Figure 25.28. Q-banding polymorphisms. Variations in size and fluorescent intensity are shown in the pericentric regions of homologous chromosomes 3 and 4 and in the short arm and satellite regions of group D (13–15), and G (21–22) chromosomes. The brightly fluorescent region in the distal long arm of the Y chromosomes also show polymorphism. (Courtesy of C. C. Lin.)

have been used to demonstrate the evolutionary origins of populations.

C heteromorphisms were used in early linkage studies. The "uncoiler" locus, a large heteromorphism of chromosome 1, was useful in localizing the Duffy blood group to that chromosome. Other uses of heteromorphisms have included zygosity determination of twins and the origin (donor or recipient) of repopulating cells in bone marrow transplants.

THE SEX CHROMOSOMES

In humans, females have two X chromosomes and males an X and a Y chromosome. The fact that this difference in the number of Xs did not result in differences in expression of X-linked genes between males and females led H. J. Muller in 1931 to propose the concept of dosage compensation. In humans and most mammals, dosage compensation is achieved by inactivation of excess copies of the X chromosome, and equal amounts of gene product result from transcription of the single active X in both males and females.

The X Chromatin Body

In 1948, Murray Barr and his graduate student E. C. Bertram identified a nucleolar satellite that was present in histologic preparations of neurons of female cats but not of male cats. After further verification on human preparations, they called the sex-specific chromatin mass "sex chromatin." (Sex chromatins are now also called Barr bodies.) Subsequently, Barr observed that individuals with ovarian dysgenesis (Turner's syndrome) had male type nuclei—lacking a sex chromatin body—and that biopsies from males with Klinefelter's syndrome were similar to normal females in that a sex chromatin body was present. When the chromosome defects in these syndromes were observed, the correspondence of the number of Barr bodies to the number of inactive X chromosomes became evident.

Further contribution to an understanding of X chromatin came with the demonstration of asynchronous replication of the sex chromosomes, one of the two X chromosomes replicating later in the S phase, and of the mosaicism in the expression of X-linked genes.

In humans, females heterozygous for glucose-6-phosphate dehydrogenase (G6PD) deficiency demonstrated two types of erythrocytes, and in the mouse, coat color variegation resulting from X-linked coat color mutants or autosomal genes translocated to the X chromosomes occurred in female mice but not in male mice.

These observations led Lyon in 1961 to propose the single active X hypothesis that one of the two X chromosomes in each cell of a female is inactive, that inactivation occurs early in embryogenesis at which time random inactivation of maternally and paternally derived X chromosomes occurs, and that inactivation in the lineage of an X is stable and is transmitted to all descendants.

This hypothesis received confirmation from a variety of experiments demonstrating mosaicism in the expression of X-linked genes in mice, humans, and other mammals. Single cells cloned from tissue cultures derived from females heterozygous for glucose-6-phosphate dehydrogenase demonstrated either A or B electrophoretic variants of G6PD, but never both. Similar behavior of other X-linked enzymes and the presence of two cell populations in heterozygous females who carry the gene for disorders such as ocular albinism and hypohydrotic ectodermal dysplasia provided additional confirmation and acceptance of the Lyon hypothesis.

The Timing of Inactivation

The onset of inactivation may be demonstrated by the appearance of the sex chromatin body, the change to asynchronous replication of one of the X chromosomes, or the appearance of differences in X-linked enzyme activity. These may be shown directly at different stages of embryogenesis or indirectly by the use of chimeric mice. By transplanting single cells from an embryo heterozygous for pigment mutants at different stages of embryogenesis into blastocysts carrying a different mutant it has been possible to demonstrate (*a*) lack of inactivation by the appearance of three different colors in patches, or (*b*) if inactivation has occurred, by the occurrence of only two of the pigment mutants.

Using the tools described above, it has been shown that inactivation does not occur in all tissues simultaneously, but occurs at different times in cell lineages as differentiation occurs. Thus, in the blastocyst that occurs at 3 days in the mouse, X inactivation is limited to the trophectoderm. Inactivation occurs between 6 and 13 days in the inner cell mass and at the differentiation of the primitive ectoderm. Inactivation in the germ cell progenitors appears to occur by day 12, but, since both Xs are active in the mature oocyte, reactivation of the X chromosomes must occur prior to meiotic prophase.

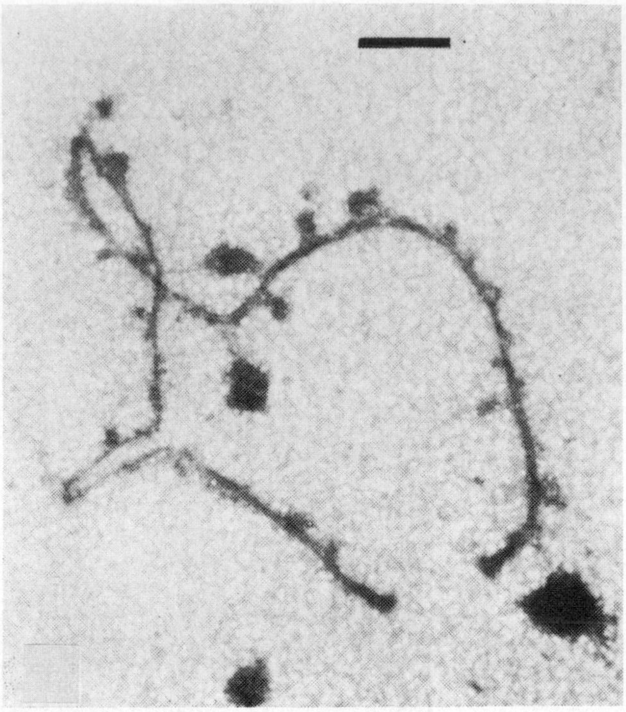

Figure 25.29. Human synaptonemal complex showing pairing of X and Y chromosomes in human meiosis. (Reprinted from Solari AJ. Synaptonemal complexes and associated structures in microspread human spermatocytes. Chromosoma 1980;81:315–337.)

There is evidence that the inactivated X chromosome is not completely inactive. The pseudoautosomal region, the distal portion of the Xp—a segment of the X that undergoes recombination with the Y chromosome (Fig. 25.29)—escapes inactivation in man and in mice. In this region is MIC2, a cell surface antigen that is located at the proximal end of the pseudoautosomal region in humans. A number of DNA probes have been localized to the human pseudoautosomal region with DXYS14 at the telomeric end. Steroid sulfatase (STS), a gene resulting in X-linked ichthyosis, and the Xga blood group map close to the pseudoautosomal region and escape inactivation in humans.

Nonrandom Inactivation

Exceptions to random inactivation of maternally and paternally derived X chromosomes occur in apparent nonrandom inactivation of X chromosome abnormalities, in nonrandom inactivation of paternal X chromosomes in trophoblastic tissues, and in nonrandom inactivation of X chromosomes bearing certain X-linked genes.

Apparent preferential inactivation of X chromosome abnormalities such as isochromosome X, ring

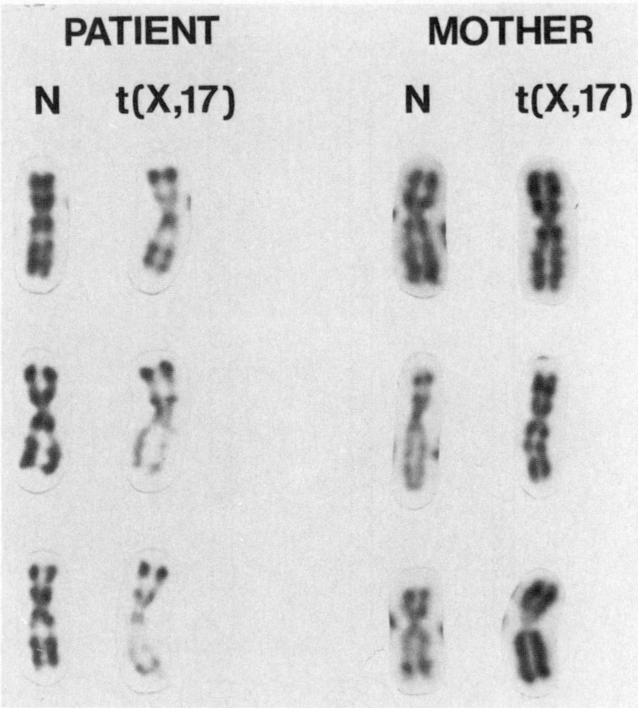

Figure 25.30. Nonrandom inactivation of X-autosome translocation in patient and mother. The cells were stained after replication banding (RBG). The late-replicating, inactive X is lightly stained; the early-replicating X is darkly stained. The mother carries a balanced translocation between the X and chromosome 17, but the daughter carries an unbalanced form of the translocation. The normal X chromosome is preferentially inactivated in the mother, but in the daughter, the structurally abnormal X is inactivated. In each case, selection favored the greatest degree of genetic balance.

X, and deleted Xs occur regularly in humans. In each case, random inactivation of the normal X would result in cells nullisomic for a portion of the X chromosome and inviability or lessened viability. In balanced X-autosomal translocations, random inactivation appears to be followed by selection, presumably as a result of the spreading of inactivation into autosomal segments. Cells with such autosomal segments inactivated will have reduced viability and, as a result, cells with the translocation active and the normal X inactivated usually predominate.

On the other hand, in unbalanced X-autosome translocations, the abnormal X appears to be preferentially inactivated as a result of selection of cells with a balanced karyotype (Fig. 25.30). In these instances, spreading of inactivation to the autosomal segment may be incomplete, and phenotypic expression of the extra segment may occur.

Preferential expression of the maternally derived X chromosome has been shown to occur in tissues of marsupials and in the extraembryonic membranes of rodents and of humans. Unlike X rearrangements, the preferential inactivation of paternal alleles does not result from selection, but appears to be initial nonrandom inactivation due to differences in parental origin—"imprinting."

Inactivation Center

Studies of X-autosome translocations in mice and humans suggest that inactivation proceeds from a region controlling inactivation, the inactivation center, and spreads to the rest of the chromosome. Thus, in reciprocal translocations between an X and an autosome, only one of the two segments will show inactivation. The X controlling element, the X_{ce} locus, is considered to be the major controlling center for X inactivation in mice. Evidence from allelic variants of X_{ce} suggests that this locus controls the probability of inactivation of the X chromosome and can also control the preferential inactivation of paternal X chromosomes in extraembryonal membranes.

In humans, Therman proposed the presence of an inactivating center between Xq11.2 and Xq21.1 on the basis of failure of inactivation in the absence of this segment in various deletions and rearrangements and on the evidence of the occurrence of bipartite sex chromatin when this region of the X is duplicated (Fig. 25.31).

The XIST (X inactive specific transcripts) gene, which is close to and may represent the inactivating center, has now been identified by Hunt Willard to be at Xq13.

Once inactivation has been initiated, it spreads outward on the inactive X. Evidence from X-autosome translocations in humans and mice suggests that autosomal regions close to the point of translocation are more likely to be inactivated, although studies of similar translocation in human chromosomes suggest that inactivation may skip some regions and inactivate others farther from the translocation point.

To attribute X inactivation to any mechanism, it is necessary to explain both the initiation and the maintenance of X inactivation and to consider whether the same method pertains to both random and preferential paternal inactivation. DNA methylation has been proposed as this mechanism. This concept is supported by evidence for differences in methylation of specific gene sequences in active and inactive Xs. Although the stability of the inactive state has been shown in somatic cells, in cell hybrids, and by the failure of selection in culture to identify revertants of hypoxanthine-guanine phosphoribosyl transferase (HPRT) cells, it has been possible by treatment with 5-azacytidine, an antagonist of methylation, to reactivate localized regions of the inactive X chromosome in cell hybrids.

The inability of DNA from the inactive X of these hybrid cells to function in DNA-mediated cell trans-

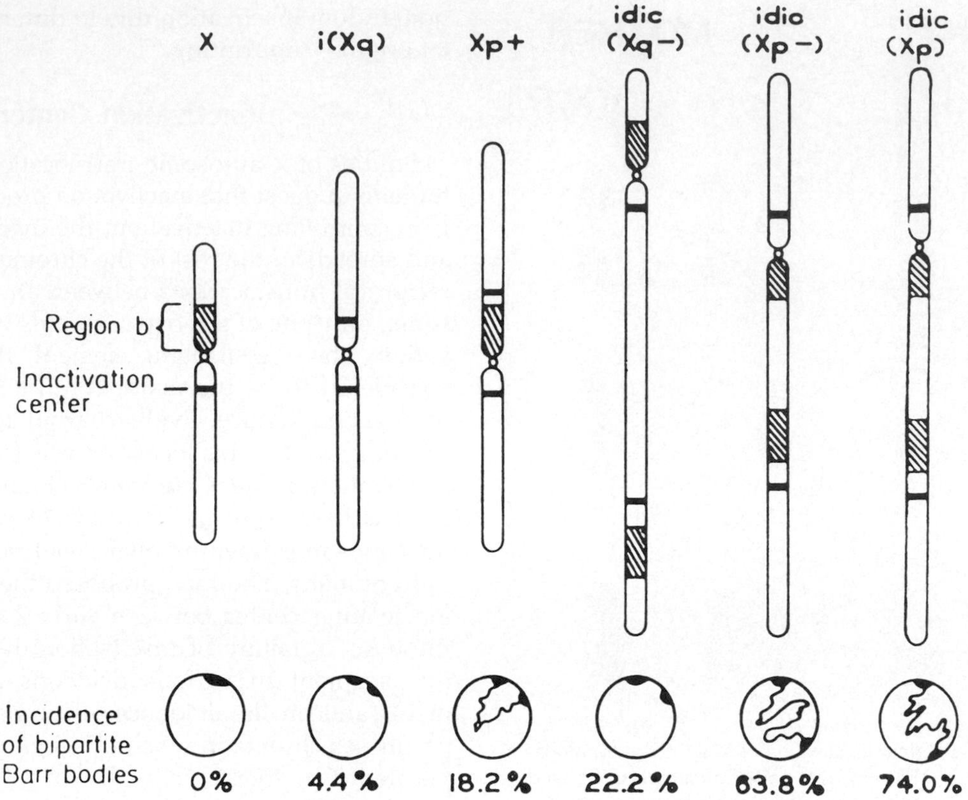

Figure 25.31. The location of the X inactivation center of Xq and the presumably active (b) region on Xp in six structurally different X chromosomes, plus the incidence and hypothetical structure of bipartate Barr bodies formed by them. (Reprinted from Therman E, Sarto GE. Inactivation center on the human X chromosome. In: Sandberg AA, ed. Cytogenetics of the mammalian X chromosome. Part A. New York: Alan R. Liss, 1983:315–325.)

formation, but the ability of DNA isolated from 5-azacytidine–reactivated X chromosomes to so function suggests that methylation of the DNA is involved. Methylation may also be involved in imprinting DNA in preferential paternal inactivation.

As a corollary to inactivation by methylation, maintenance of inactivation by a maintenance methylase has been suggested. Recently, demonstration of age-related reactivation of randomly inactivated X-linked genes and autosomal coat color loci in X-autosome translocations in mice suggest that there may be a waning of X inactivation with age. Examples of instability of imprinted Xs are not merely the result of aging. Fusion of chorionic villus cells with adult somatic cells in culture will cause complete reactivation of the inactive X of the chorionic villus cells. Partial activity of paternal alleles in the preferentially inactivated paternal X of marsupials and the ability to demonstrate activity of both alleles of G6PD in cultured chorionic villus cells suggest a difference in the maintenance of inactivation in imprinted Xs. These examples suggest that an understanding of X inactivation continues to evolve and with it an understanding of the X chromosome.

Sex Determination and Mapping of X and Y Chromosomes

The search for the sex-determining genes has been closely related to the mapping of the X and Y chromosomes. Such a gene or genes would be responsible for inducing differentiation of the neutral gonad to become a testis. There have been several candidates for the sex-determining gene or genes. One, the HY antigen, a male-specific antigen, was for many years considered to be the testis-determining factor (TDF). More recently, ZFY, a zinc finger gene on the Y chromosome, was enthusiastically received as the possible TDF. Both are now considered to be related to sperm maturation rather than to the initial differentiation of the testes.

The HY antigen was initially demonstrated when skin transplanted from male isogenic mice was rejected by females of the same strain. The antigen has also been demonstrated by serological tests using antisera produced after inoculation of females with male cells or by cytotoxicity assays with T cells. When interspecific comparisons demonstrated conservation of the soluble antigen in evolution, it was hypothesized that the HY antigen and TDF were one

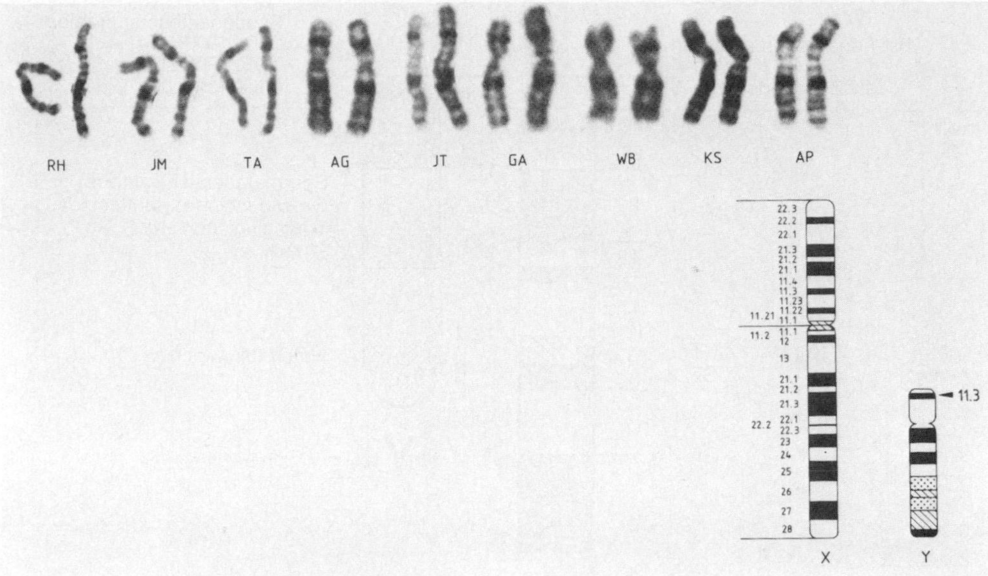

Figure 25.32. Examples of X chromosomes from XX males. The X chromosome on the right in each case can be distinguished from its homolog by a G-positive band at distal Xp. This is believed to be Yp11.3 to pter, which has been interchanged. (Reprinted from Ferguson-Smith MA. Genotype-phenotype correlations in XX males and their bearing on current theories of sex determination. Hum Genet 1990;84:198–202.)

and the same. More recent evidence indicates that the serologic and transplantation antigens are coded by two different genes and further evidence indicates that neither are the TDF. A gene with properties similar to the serologically detected antigen has been localized to chromosome 6 and its presence in females as well as X chromosome abnormalities removes it from contention as TDF. The T cell toxicity antigen has been localized to the long arm of the Y while evidence from XX males indicates that TDF is on the short arm of the Y chromosome.

The identification of XX males in whom the distal portion of the Yp chromosome has been transferred to the X (Fig. 25.32) and t(Y;15) females with a corresponding deletion of the Y chromosome led to the cloning of a 140-kb segment of the Y chromosome that coded for a regulatory protein, a zinc finger protein (the human gene is designated ZFY). Although it was suggested that the H-Y antigen may be the biochemical expression of the TDF (since both have at least one locus in or close to the pseudoautosomal region), evidence has now accumulated to indicate that ZFY is not the sex-determining gene. In mice, where the H-Y antigen has been mapped to the X chromosome, the testis-determining factor (Tfy in mice) can be separated genetically from this locus.

Recently the association of ZFY and testes determination has been questioned based on evidence from mice where fetal testes lacking germ cells do not express ZFY, and the occurrence in humans of XX males who do not demonstrate ZFY sequences. In addition, genes closely homologous to ZFY were found to be present on the X chromosome and on the autosomes of mice and marsupials. Most recently, another gene, SRY, has been identified in sex-reversed individuals, i.e., a female with X and a t(Y;22) in which there are two regions deleted from the Y, one ZFY, and another that includes sequences present in all XX males. The gene cloned from the latter region, SRY, is present in all XX males and absent in all XY females. Its counterpart in mice, Sry, appears to be testis specific and expressed during testis differentiation prior to the appearance of mature sperm. Figure 25.33 is an abbreviated map of the X and Y chromosomes including the location of the pseudoautosomal region, the inactivating center, and the critical area—a segment that must be intact in both X chromosomes to permit normal ovarian development in females.

The usefulness of chromosome abnormalities of X and Y and of cytogenetic analyses of unusual XX males and XY females in resolving the question of the location of the sex-determining gene cannot be discounted. The usefulness of chromosome abnormalities to mapping of the human genome is discussed further in the following section.

CYTOGENETICS AND GENE MAPPING

The development of chromosome banding methods and a system of nomenclature to identify individual chromosome arms and bands was an important step needed to allow the assignment of human genes and DNA probes to individual chromosomes, regions, and bands (gene mapping). As banding pro-

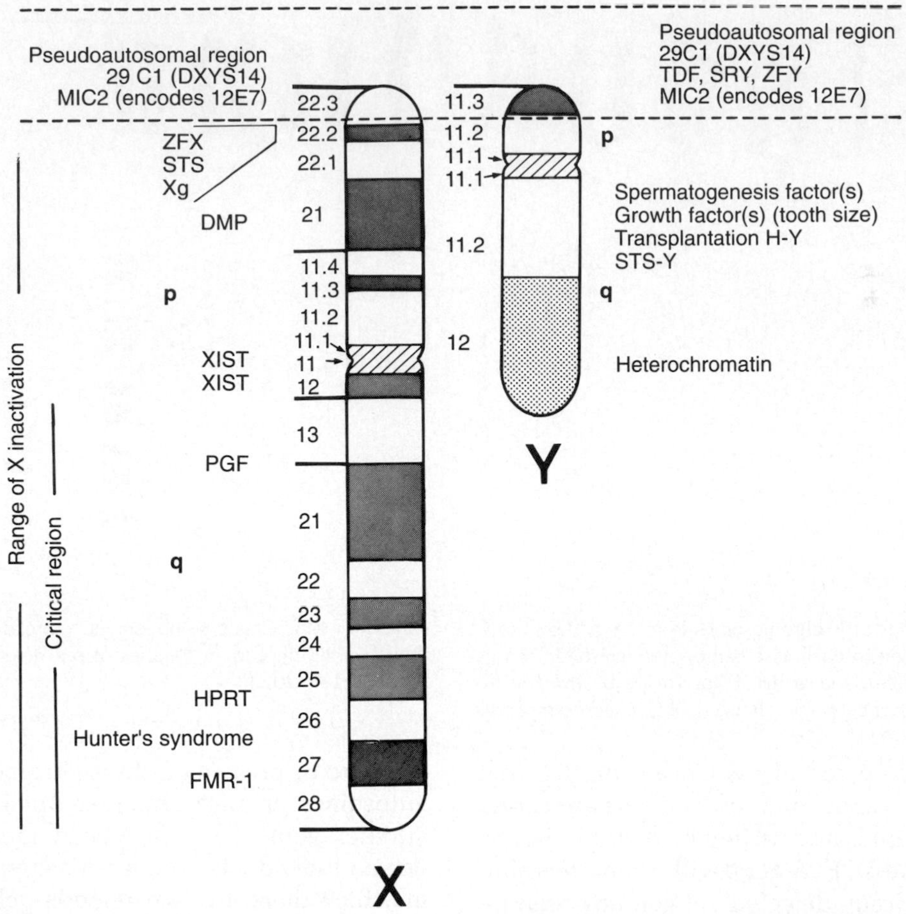

Figure 25.33. An abbreviated map of the X and Y chromosomes showing loci and areas related to sexual differentiation. ZFX and ZFY, Loci for zinc finger protein on X and Y chromosomes. DXYS14, Pseudoautosomal locus defined by probe 29C1, the most distal of a group of probes localized to this region. MIC2, pDP1002 encoding cell surface antigen 12E7. Pseudoautosomal region, Region of pairing of X and Y chromosomes. This region is not inactivated. STS and Xg, Steroid sulfatase and Xga blood group. Both are located close to the pseudoautosomal region, and both escape inactivation. SRY, Sex determining region of the Y chromosome. HY, Locus encoding transplantation histocompatibility HY. MIC2, Locus encoding histocompatibility cell surface antigen 12E7. Gonadal development, Regions of Xp and Xq which, when deleted, result in gonadal dysgenesis. Critical region, Region whose integrity is important in gonadal development of balanced X/autosomal translocation carriers. Inactivation center, Region controlling X inactivation.

cedures and identification of chromosome variants and chromosome abnormalities became available, techniques of gene mapping were simultaneously developed.

Cytogenetics has made important contributions to gene mapping by a number of different approaches, including the use of classic mapping techniques with chromosome variants and abnormalities used as markers, deletion mapping with and without concurrent dosage studies, cell hybridization, and in situ hybridization.

Although assignment of genes to the X chromosome based on sex linkage was possible prior to cytogenetic studies, the assignment of genes to specific autosomes was possible only after chromosome variants were observed. The first gene assignment, the Duffy blood group, used the segregation of a familial chromosome 1 variant, an extended paracentric heterochromatic band of chromosome referred to then as "uncoiler," and the concurrent segregation of the Duffy blood group.

The presence of chromosome variants in a family made it possible to establish how often the variant was inherited with specific markers. The degree of linkage of genes on a chromosome is related to their closeness in position on a particular chromosome. Those farther apart are more likely to undergo crossing over and separation at meiosis. Recombination, when genes are close together, may be close to zero; if far apart or on different chromosomes, it will approach 50%. This is the recombination frequency. Gene mapping is based on the degree of recombination, the frequency serving as a measure of genetic distance and the relative distance apart of variant and gene on a genetic map.

Thus, investigators used C-band variants to localize and order a number of genes on chromosome 1. Similarly, segregation in families of translocations or other cytogenetically marked chromosomes have been used to localize genes to chromosomes. For example, it was possible to use a fragile site on chromosome 16 (at 16q21–22), segregating as an autosomal dominant trait, to demonstrate linkage with α-haptoglobin by following segregation and recombination of the two in a large family and thus to localize the α-haptoglobin gene close to this fragile site.

A second approach to gene mapping, somatic cell hybridization, involves the fusion of human cells, fibroblasts, or lymphoblastoid cell lines with rodent cells. If both parental lines are drug sensitive, the use of selective media will allow growth of the cell hybrids, but not the parental cell lines. Fusion is facilitated by use of Sendai virus, or polyethylene glycol. Although the hybrid cells initially contain chromosomes of both parent lines, human chromosomes are gradually lost from unstable hybrid cells. Eventually only one or a few human chromosomes are retained in a stable cell line. Cytogenetic recognition of the individual human chromosomes or, alternatively, recognition of a protein associated with a specific chromosome permits identification of a number of unique cell lines. A collection of such cell lines, each with a different chromosome or chromosomes—a cell panel—allows the presence of a particular chromosome to be correlated with a unique gene product. Thus, a specific gene is localized to a chromosome.

More recently, linkage studies using cell hybridization have employed lymphoblastoid cell lines derived from individuals with different chromosomal abnormalities to develop panels with multiple overlapping rearrangements of the same chromosome. These facilitate localization of a particular gene to a specific region or band.

The first use of deletions to map chromosomes was in *Drosophila*. A series of chromosome deletions seen in the salivary gland chromosomes were compared to the expression of specific genes, and the position of the gene on the *Drosophila* chromosomes established. In human chromosomes, deletion mapping has taken several forms. One relates reduced enzyme levels, loss of an allele, and occurrence of a deletion to localize a gene. For example, Ferguson-Smith used a series of abnormalities of chromosome 2 to localize red cell phosphatase (ACP_1) to the region 2p23. Trisomies and duplications have also been used to localize genes by gene dosage studies or by the presence of three different alleles. For example, individuals trisomic for 6p21–6pter with three different histocompatibility haplotypes facilitated the localization of the histocompability locus to 6p21 to 6pter.

A panel of abnormalities of chromosome 9, including duplications and deletions, has been used in dosage studies of human red cell adenylate kinase (AK-1). Demonstration of an increase of AK-1 activity by 43% in one duplication permitted the assignment of AK_1 to 9q33–qter. In this case, the chromosome involved had been previously identified by cell hybridization, and dosage studies with the panel of cell lines permitted further localization to a region.

The most direct cytogenetic method of gene localization has been in situ hybridization, which permits direct visualization of the location of a probe on a chromosome. This method originated in attempts to localize satellite DNA by hybridizing DNA labeled with tritiated nucleotides to chromosomes that had been previously denatured. After a period of incubation, slides that had been dipped in photographic emulsion subsequent to hybridization were observed. The appearance of silver grains on the slides showed the location of the decaying isotope and hence of the hybridizing DNA.

Although this method was initially used for localizing satellite DNAs and other repetitive DNAs and RNA to chromosomes, Harper and Saunders subsequently adapted the methodology to permit its use with single-copy probes. Their adaptations included the use of dextran sulfate in the hybridization reaction and probes contained in a vector that had been nick translated to label the DNA with tritiated nucleotides. These adaptations resulted in networking of vectors and accumulation of the label at specific sites on the chromosome. The labeled chromosomes may be photographed for grain location and then banded and rephotographed or the grain developed and the chromosomes banded, usually with a fluorescent dye, and observed simultaneously (Fig. 25.34).

A further development of in situ hybridization was the use of chromosomally abnormal cells, such as those bearing a translocation, for regional mapping. In such cases, the mapping of the probe to the translocated segment can identify the specific region or band to which the grain is confined (Fig. 25.35).

Most recently, hybridization with radioactive probes has been replaced by the use of immunofluorescence. With this method, the nick-translated probe is commonly a biotin-labeled probe; random primer, also conjugated with avidin, can be used to label and can be subsequently visualized by use of anti-avidin antibodies and immunofluorescence with fluorescein on counterstained chromosomes. This method has the advantage that, by use of two separate fluorescent dyes, it is possible to visualize the chromosomes at two different wavelengths, one producing banding and the other demonstrating the localization of the probe. The process is faster and the hybridized probe is more specifically localized (Fig. 25.36). One of the problems with the use of radioactive probes was the occurrence of grain on other chromosomes of the cell as a result of scatter of radio-

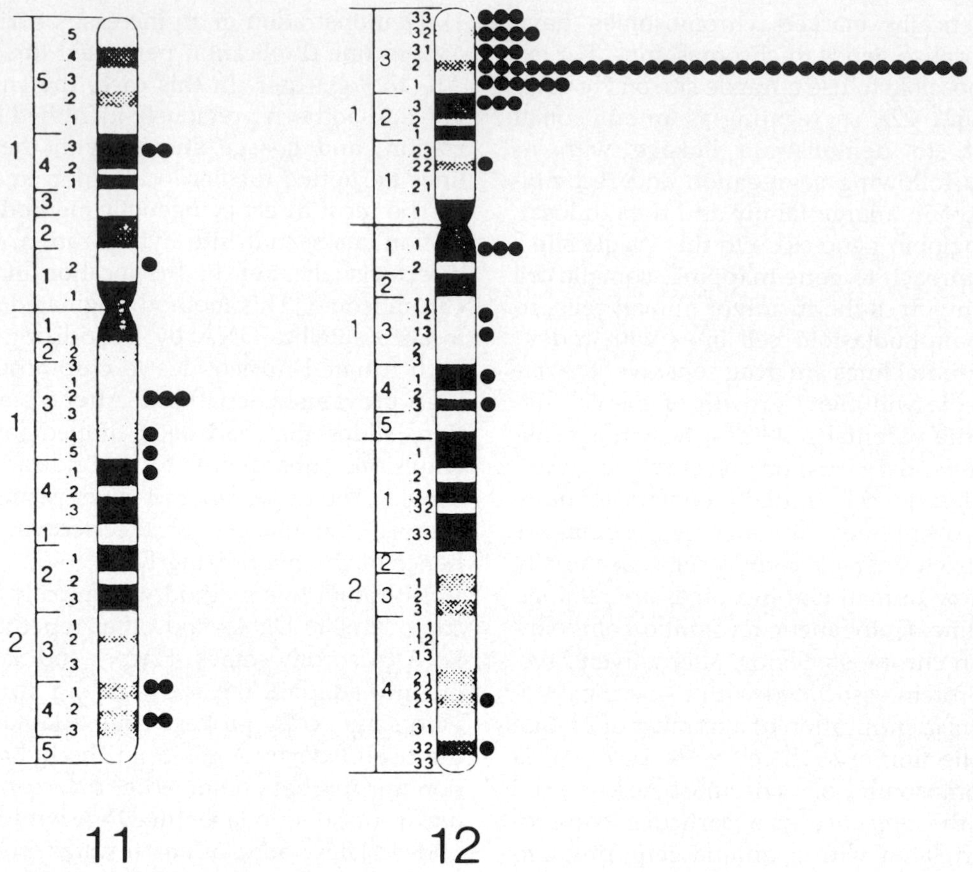

Figure 25.34. Labeled sites after in situ hybridization with a probe PRP-1, a genomic clone with human salivary proline–rich protein gene sequences. The illustration shows the distribution of grain on the labeled metaphases localized to the chromosomes. (Reprinted from Mamula PW, Heerema NA, Palmer CG, et al. Localization of the human salivary protein complex (SPC) to chromosome band 12p13.2. Cytogenet Cell Genet 1985;39:279–284.)

active emissions, which necessitated grain counting and statistical evaluation of the results. The immunofluorescent approach is more specific and is useful for both repetitive and single-copy probes. Its usefulness has been demonstrated by its ability to delimit the position of linked genes on a chromosome by using interphase cytogenetics and labeling with several fluorescent dyes emitting in different wavelengths.

Gene mapping studies have included combinations of the above techniques with molecular methods. While chromosome variants were initially useful, the variation in DNA by the use of restriction endonuclease digestion has been so much greater that chromosome variants are now rarely used for conventional linkage studies. In these studies, DNA is cut with restriction endonucleases and separated by size using agarose gel electrophoresis. This procedure takes advantage of natural variations in DNA sequence occurring in genes. When radioactively labeled DNA probes, fragments of genes, or randomly isolated DNA are hybridized with the separated fragments followed by autoradiography of the gel, polymorphisms are seen as variations in the banding pattern of the gel. The cosegregation and recombination frequency of these markers in families can be used for genetic linkage studies. It is this approach that has led to the identification of probes diagnostic for genetic disorders and ultimately to their chromosomal localization, either by linkage to previously located genes or by in situ hybridization.

Since 1973, International Human Gene Mapping Workshops have met regularly to summarize the assignment of genes to chromosomes. From 25 genes mapped in humans in 1973, the conference of 1989, the Tenth International Workshop, reports 1808 genes identified and localized. The data generated at these conferences have been summarized in published reports and include information on the genetic constitution of each of the chromosomes, assignment of mendelian disorders and clinical disorders, and catalogs of cloned genes and DNA fragments. The reader is referred to the current edition of the human gene map in the most recent workshop report, which was Human Gene Mapping 10 as of this writing (see Suggested Readings). An example of the extent of

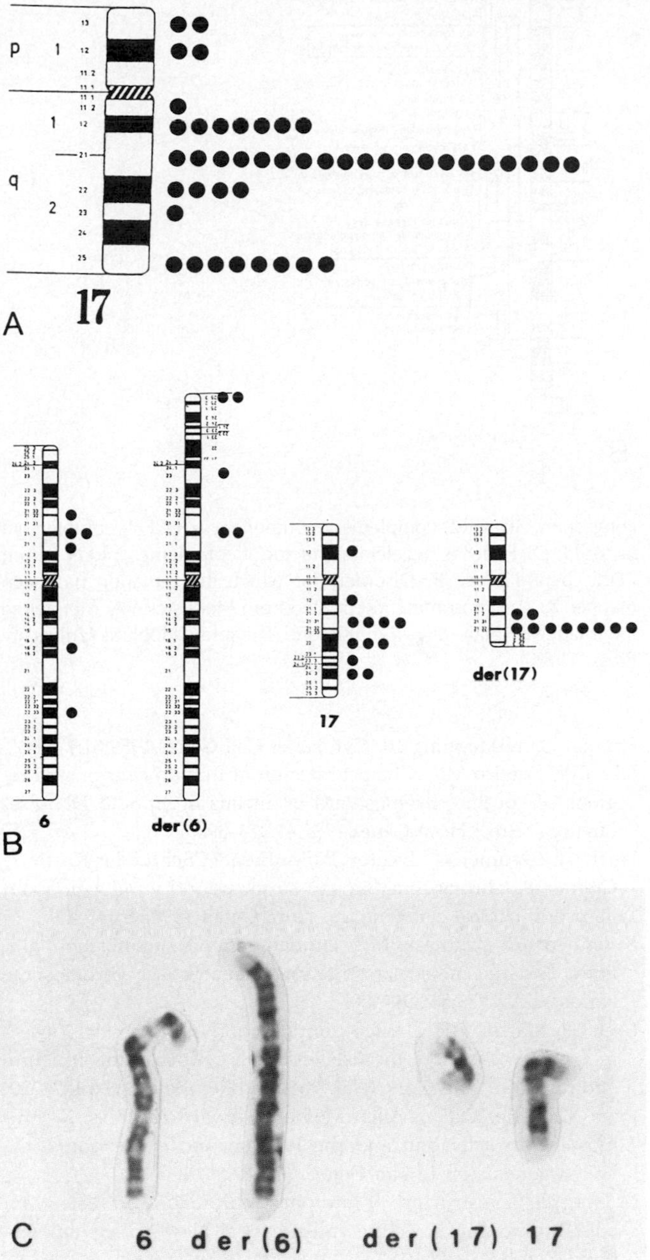

Figure 25.35. Localization of probes by in situ hybridization using chromosome abnormalities. **A**, Ideogram of chromosome 17 showing localization of acetyl-CoA carboxylase cDNA probe to normal 17. **B** and **C**, Grain distribution on a rearranged chromosome 17. In this case, the distal portion of chromosome 17q has been translocated to 6p, but the breakpoint in chromosome 17 at 17q21.33 is distal to the location of the probe, thus localizing the probe to 17q21.33. (Reprinted from Milatovich A, Plattner R, Heerema NA, et al. Localization of the gene for acetyl CoA carboxylase to human chromosome 17. Cytogenet Cell Genet 1988;48:190–192.)

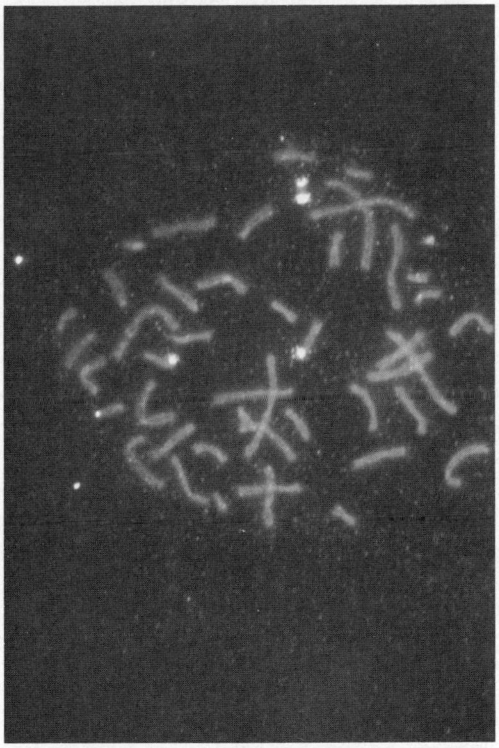

Figure 25.36. Localization of alpha satellite probe from chromosome 15 to both chromosome 15s and to a marker chromosome derived from chromosome 15, i(15p).

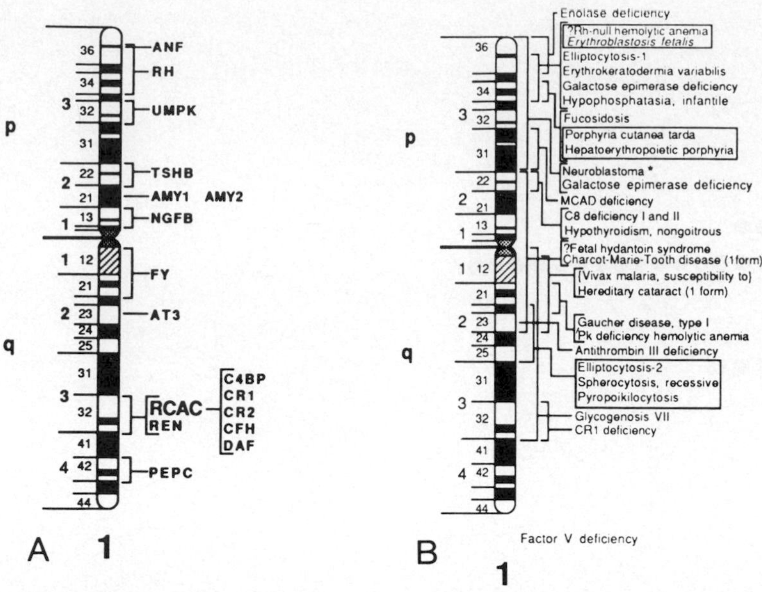

Figure 25.37. Gene localization on chromosome 1. **A**, Selected anchor loci: ANF, natriuretic factor; RH, rhesus blood group; UMPK, uridine monophoshate kinase; TSHB, thyroid-stimulating hormone—β subunit; AMY1, amylase (salivary); AMY2, amylase (pancreatic); NGFB, nerve growth factor β; FY, Duffy blood group; AT3, antithrombin III; RCAC, regulator of complement activation center; C4BP, complement component 4 binding protein; CR1, complement component 3b; CR2, complement component 3d; CFH, complement factor H; DAF, decay accelerating factor of complement; REN, renin; PEPC, peptidase C. **B**, Disorders for which the mutation has been mapped to chromosome 1. (Reprinted from McKusick VA. Mendelian inheritance in man. 8th ed. Baltimore: The Johns Hopkins University Press, 1988.)

mapping is shown in Figure 25.37, where selected "anchor" loci are indicated for chromosome 1, and a human disease phenotype for that chromosome is also shown. The progress of mapping the human genome is rapidly increasing, with international cooperation in this effort and with molecular biology, computer science, and technology making contributions to progress in this field.

Suggested Readings

Adolph KW. Chromosomes and chromatin. Vols. I, II, and III. Boca Raton, FL: CRC Press, 1988.

Bergsma D, ed. Chicago Conference: Standardization in human cytogenetics. Birth defects. New York: Alan R. Liss, Original Articles Series, Vol. II, No.2, 1966.

Bickmore WA, Sumner AT. Mammalian chromosome banding—an expression of genome organization. Trends Genet 1989;5:144–148.

Blackburn EH. Telomeres: do the ends justify the means? Cell 1984;37:7–8.

Craig I. Sex determination: zinc fingers point in the wrong direction. Trends Genet 1989;6:135–137.

Ellis N, Goodfellow PN. The mammalian pseudoautosomal region. Trends Genet 1989;5:389–429.

Gartler SM. Mammalian X chromosome inactivation. Annu Rev Genet 1983;17:155–190.

Harnden DG, Klinger HP, eds. An international system for human cytogenetic nomenclature. Basel, Switzerland: S Karger, 1985.

Holmquist G, Gray M, Porter T, Jordan J. Characterization of Giemsa dark- and light-band DNA. Cell 1982;31:121–129.

Hsu TC. Human and mammalian cytogenetics: an historical perspective. New York: Springer-Verlag, 1979.

Human Gene Mapping 10. Cytogenet Cell Genet 1989;51:1–1147.

Jabs EW, Persico MG. Characterization of human centromeric regions of specific chromosomes by means of alphoid DNA sequences. Am J Hum Genet 1987;41:374–390.

Jauch A, Daumer C, Lichter P, Murken J, Schroeder-Kurth T, Cremer T. Chromosomal in situ suppression hybridization and its use in clinical cytogenetics. Hum Genet 1990;85:145–150.

Korenberg JR, Rykowski MC. Human genome organization: alu, lines, and the molecular structure of metaphase chromosome bands. Cell 1988;53:391–400.

Lock LF, Martin, GR. Dosage compensation in mammals: X chromosome inactivation. In: Risley MS, ed. Chromosome structure and function. New York: Van Nostrand Reinhold, 1986:187–220.

Lyon MF. The William Allen Memorial Award Address: X chromosome in activation and the location and expression of X-linked genes. Am J Hum Genet 1988;42:8–16.

McGhee D. The structure of interphase chromatin. In: Risley MS, ed. Chromosome structure and function. New York: Van Nostrand Reinhold, 1986:1–37.

McKusick VA. Mendelian inheritance in man. 8th ed. Baltimore: The Johns Hopkins University Press, 1988.

Magenis RE. Application of structural rearrangements and DNA probes to gene mapping. In: Daniel A, ed. The cytogenetics of mammalian autosomal rearrangements. New York: Alan R. Liss, 1988:855–893.

Marsden MPF, Laemmli U. Metaphase chromosome structure: evidence for a radial loop model. Cell 1989;849–858.

Moyzis RK, Buckingham JM, Scott-Cram L, et al. A highly conserved repetitive DNA sequence, (TTAGGG), present at the telomeres of human chromosomes. Proc Natl Acad Sci USA 1988;85:6622–6626.

Page DC, Fisher MC, McGillivray B, Brown LG. Additional deletion in sex determining region of human Y chromosome resolves paradox of X, t(Y;22) female. Nature 1990;346:279–281.

Pluta AF, Zakian VA. Recombination occurs during telomere formation in yeast. Nature 1989;337:429–433.

Risley MS. The organization of meiotic chromosomes and synaptonemal complexes. In: Risley MS, ed. Chromasome structure and function. New York: Van Nostrand Reinhold, 1986:126–151.

Sandberg AA, ed. Cytogenetics of the mammalian X chromosome. Part A. Basic mechanisms of X chromosome BEH. Progress and Topics in Cytogentics Series, Vol. 3A. New York: Alan R. Liss, 1983.

Sandberg AA, ed. The Y Chromosome. Part A. Basic characteristics of the Y chromosome. Progress and Topics in Cytogenetics Series, Vol 6A. New York: Alan R. Liss, 1985.

Szostak JW. Telomerase: the beginning of the ends. Nature 1989;3378:303–304.

Sumner AT. The nature and mechanisms of chromosome banding. Cancer Genet Cytogenet 1982;6:59–87.

Verma RS, Babu A. Human chromosomes: manual of basic techniques. Elmsford, NY: Pergaman Press, 1989.

26 Clinical Cytogenetics

Daniel L. Van Dyke and Anne Wiktor

In Chapter 25, normal chromosome structure and the normal karyotype were described. This chapter addresses cytogenetic pathology associated with birth defects, mental retardation, infertility, and pregnancy loss. About 0.5% of newborns have a chromosome abnormality, constituting a major cause of lethal or debilitating birth defects and mental retardation. Among couples who experience two or more miscarriages, 5% have a balanced chromosome rearrangement. Most of these are familial and some also confer an increased risk of having a liveborn child with an abnormal karyotype. About 50% of first-trimester miscarriages have a chromosome abnormality, making this by far the most common cause of pregnancy loss, and perhaps 100% of leukemias and cancers acquire an abnormal karyotype. We begin with a discussion of the variety of numerical and structural chromosome abnormalities and continue with examples and descriptions of cytogenetic changes associated with birth defects, mental retardation, and male and female infertility. The main indications for chromosomal study are summarized, followed by techniques for chromosome preparation and guidelines for analysis. The recommendations of the International System for Human Cytogenetic Nomenclature (ISCN 1985) are used to describe karyotypes throughout this section (1) (Table 26.1).

CHANGES IN CHROMOSOME NUMBER AND STRUCTURE

Changes in Chromosome Sets (Ploidy)

The normal karyotype contains two copies of every autosome plus two sex chromosomes. This is diploid, or 2n. A sperm or ovum is haploid, or 1n, and normally contains one copy of each autosome plus an X or a Y chromosome.

Triploidy (three haploid sets, or 3n) results when two sperm fertilize one ovum (Figure 26.1). About 7% of first-trimester miscarriages are triploid. Rare triploid stillbirths and livebirths have occurred. The karyotypes 69,XXY and 69,XXX are most common, whereas 69,XYY is far less common, and 69,YYY is never seen. Triploidy can also occur from fertilization of a diploid ovum, but recent evidence suggests that most of these conceptions are unable to survive long enough to be observed among miscarriage specimens. This implies that two maternal contributions are more detrimental than are two paternal contributions. Triploidy appears to occur sporadically among miscarriages, and the risk of recurrence in subsequent pregnancies is not increased. In the in vitro fertilization laboratory, a higher concentration of sperm in the fertilization culture can increase the rate of formation of triploids.

Tetraploidy (4n) usually results from failure of cell division after a round of mitosis, and the karyotype is typically 92,XXXX or 92,XXYY (Fig. 26.1). There is evidence from tumor studies that tetraploidy can also arise from fusion of two diploid cells. About 2.5% of first-trimester miscarriages are tetraploid. A few patients with birth defects have been reported as having a mixture of diploid and tetraploid cells. However, since tetraploidy can also arise as a technical artifact, this is a difficult diagnosis to confirm, and the significance of such cells must be questioned. Tetraploidy appears to arise sporadically, and there is no increased risk of recurrence in subsequent pregnancies.

Changes in Chromosome Number in a Diploid Background

In the haploid, diploid, triploid, and tetraploid karyotypes there are one, two, three, or four copies of each chromosome, respectively. The normal karyotype is euploid (Latin, true number). When an individual chromosome is gained or lost the karyotype is aneuploid (Latin, not true number). The loss or gain of a single chromosome from a diploid background is monosomy or trisomy, respectively.

Down's syndrome (trisomy 21), identified by Lejeune in 1959, was the first clinical condition in which a gain of a single chromosome was reported (Fig. 26.1). Trisomy 18 and 13 (Edward's and Patau's syndromes, respectively, after the men who described their chromosomal etiologies in 1960) are also classic trisomy syndromes associated with major birth defects, mental retardation, and a high risk of

Table 26.1. Standard Cytogenetic Nomenclature[a]

International System for Human Cytogenetic Nomenclature (ISCN) Abbreviations

cen	centromere	mar	marker
del	deletion	mat	maternal origin
der	derived chromosome	p	p arm, the short arm
dic	dicentric	pat	paternal origin
dup	duplication	pter	p terminal, the end of the short arm
dir dup	direct duplication	q	q arm, the long arm
inv dup	inverted duplication	qter	q terminal, the end of the long arm
fra	fragile site	r	ring chromosome
i	isochromosome	rec	recombinant chromosome
inv	inversion	t	translocation
ins	insertion		

Nomenclature Examples

Chromosome count
Sex chromosomes

Normal karyotype	46,XX	Female, diploid
	46,XY	Male, diploid
Gamete karyotype	23,X	Haploid with X
	23,Y	Haploid with Y
Triploid	69,XXX	Three haploid sets
Tetraploid	92,XXYY	Four haploid sets

Other numerical changes follow a comma

Monosomy	45,XY,−7	One copy of chromosome 7
	45,X	Monosomy X
Trisomy	47,XX,+21	Three copies of chromosome 21 (primary trisomy)
	47,XXX	Trisomy X
Double trisomy	48,XX,+8,+21	Trisomy 8 and 21
Tetrasomy	48,XX,+8,+8	Four copies of chromosome 8
	48,XXXX	Tetrasomy X
Pentasomy	49,XXXXX	Pentasomy X

Multiple cell lines are separated by a solidus, in numerical order irrespective of the proportion of cells with each karyotype

Mosaic	46,XY/47,XY,+21	Mosaic with some normal and some trisomy 21 cells

Abbreviation for structural change
Chromosome
Breakpoint or breakpoints; proximal breakpoint first

Deletion	46,XX,del(13)(q12q14)	Interstitial deletion with breaks at 13q12 and 13q14
	46,XY,del(18)(p11)	Terminal deletion from 18p11 to pter
	46,XY,18p−	Older nomenclature, still used to denote a deletion with breakpoints not specified
Ring	46,XX,r(1)(p36q44)	Breakage and fusion of 1p36 and 1q44 to form a ring
Duplication	46,XY,dup(1)(q11.2q22)	Duplication of 1q11.2–1q22 (direction uncertain)
	46,XY,dir dup(8)(p21p23)	Direct duplication of 8p21–p23
	46,XY,inv dup(8)(p23p21)	Inverted duplication of 8p21–p23; note order of breakpoints

For monocentric isochromosomes the chromosome and arm are within the same parentheses

Isochromosome (monoisodisomy)	46,X,i(Xq)	One copy of the X chromosome contains two long arms and no short arm
	46,XX,i(17q)	One copy of 17 contains two long arms and no short arm
Isochromosome (secondary trisomy)	47,XX,+i(18p)	There are two normal copies of 18 plus an isochromosome of 18p
Dicentric isochromosome	46,X,dic(X)(p11)	Very similar to i(Xq), except the breakpoint is at Xp11 and the isochromosome consists of Xqter-p11-qter
	47,XY,+dic(15)(q13)	There are two normal copies of 15 plus a dicentric isochromosome consisting of 15pter-q13-pter

Table 26.1—*continued*

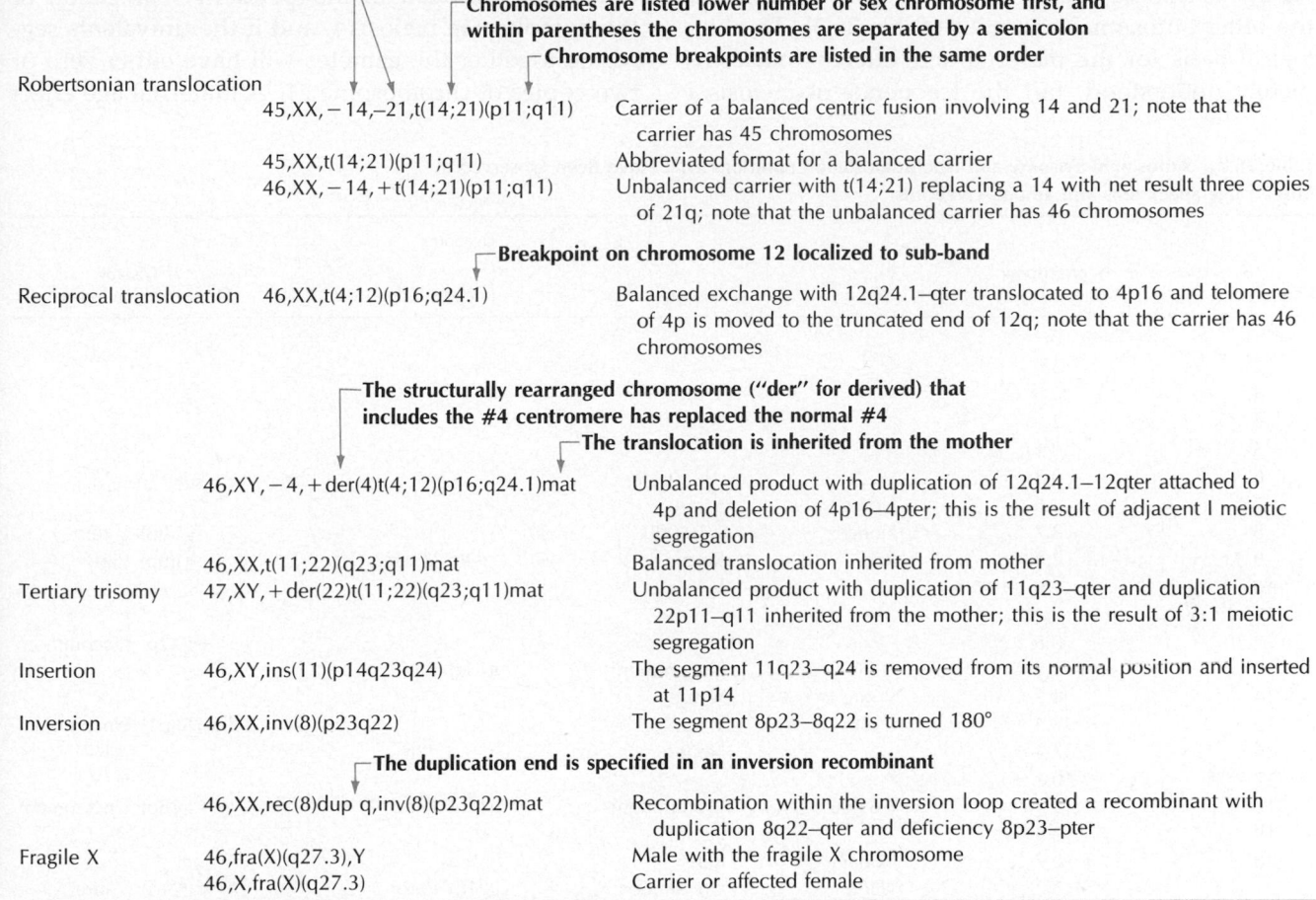

	Numerical changes are listed before structural changes; Chromosomes are listed lower number or sex chromosome first, and within parentheses the chromosomes are separated by a semicolon; Chromosome breakpoints are listed in the same order	
Robertsonian translocation	45,XX,−14,−21,t(14;21)(p11;q11)	Carrier of a balanced centric fusion involving 14 and 21; note that the carrier has 45 chromosomes
	45,XX,t(14;21)(p11;q11)	Abbreviated format for a balanced carrier
	46,XX,−14,+t(14;21)(p11;q11)	Unbalanced carrier with t(14;21) replacing a 14 with net result three copies of 21q; note that the unbalanced carrier has 46 chromosomes
	Breakpoint on chromosome 12 localized to sub-band	
Reciprocal translocation	46,XX,t(4;12)(p16;q24.1)	Balanced exchange with 12q24.1–qter translocated to 4p16 and telomere of 4p is moved to the truncated end of 12q; note that the carrier has 46 chromosomes
	The structurally rearranged chromosome ("der" for derived) that includes the #4 centromere has replaced the normal #4; The translocation is inherited from the mother	
	46,XY,−4,+der(4)t(4;12)(p16;q24.1)mat	Unbalanced product with duplication of 12q24.1–12qter attached to 4p and deletion of 4p16–4pter; this is the result of adjacent I meiotic segregation
	46,XX,t(11;22)(q23;q11)mat	Balanced translocation inherited from mother
Tertiary trisomy	47,XY,+der(22)t(11;22)(q23;q11)mat	Unbalanced product with duplication of 11q23–qter and duplication 22p11–q11 inherited from the mother; this is the result of 3:1 meiotic segregation
Insertion	46,XY,ins(11)(p14q23q24)	The segment 11q23–q24 is removed from its normal position and inserted at 11p14
Inversion	46,XX,inv(8)(p23q22)	The segment 8p23–8q22 is turned 180°
	The duplication end is specified in an inversion recombinant	
	46,XX,rec(8)dup q,inv(8)(p23q22)mat	Recombination within the inversion loop created a recombinant with duplication 8q22–qter and deficiency 8p23–pter
Fragile X	46,fra(X)(q27.3),Y	Male with the fragile X chromosome
	46,X,fra(X)(q27.3)	Carrier or affected female

[a]Many of the abnormalities described here are shown in figures throughout the section. The "short form" ISCN nomenclature is shown here. For the long form, refer to ISCN (1985). A clinical cytogenetics laboratory can hardly function without a copy of the ISCN (1985) report (see reference 1).

perinatal death. Trisomy X is mild by comparison. Most of the other autosomal trisomies are associated with fetal demise and are not commonly found among livebirths (Table 26.2). Trisomy 8 is a common abnormality in leukemia and trisomy 7 is common in many solid cancers.

During meiosis I (see Chapter 25) the chromosome homologs segregate to opposite sides of the meiotic cell. During meiosis II or mitosis, sister chromatids segregate to opposite sides of the cell. This is normal disjunction. If sister chromatids fail to segregate normally (nondisjunction), the daughter cells become aneuploid (Fig. 26.2). Most individuals with penta-X syndrome (49,XXXXX) or 49,XXXXY probably arise as a result of maternal nondisjunctional events during both meiosis I and meiosis II, with a normal paternal contribution of an X- or Y-bearing sperm.

The parents of trisomic individuals typically have normal chromosomes. From a genetic counseling point of view, it is not common practice to study the karyotypes of the parents of a baby with known trisomy 13, 18, or 21. However, an individual who is trisomic, such as a female with trisomy X or 21, has an increased risk for having offspring with the same trisomy. The formation of a 24,X,+21 or 24,XX ovum in a trisomy 21 or trisomy X female, respectively, is called secondary nondisjunction. One would expect 50% of the conceptions of a 47,XXX mother to be either 47,XXX or 47,XXY and 50% of the conceptions of a 47,XX,+21 mother to have trisomy 21, as products of secondary nondisjunction.

Because trisomy 21 (Down's syndrome) is the most common single identified cause of mental retardation, the biological basis of nondisjunction is of great interest. The parental origin and meiotic stage of the nondisjunctional error can often be identified from studies of chromosome 21 short arm variants and restriction fragment length polymorphism (RFLP) using DNA probes from 21q in Down's syndrome patients and their parents. From such studies it has been established that 94% of the nondisjunctional events occur during maternal meiosis and 6% during paternal meiosis. Most of these errors occur during meiosis I. The average maternal age for trisomy 21 children is about 30 years compared to the population average maternal age of about 25 years. Maternal age is also advanced for 47,XXX and 47,XXY and the other autosomal trisomies (Table 26.3). The biological basis for the maternal age effect is not completely understood, but the frequency of meiosis I univalents (Fig. 26.2**B**) is known to increase with maternal age. The presence of chromosome 21 univalents can lead to independent segregation of the homologs in meiosis I, and if the univalents segregate together the gametes will have either zero or two copies of chromosome 21. A maternal age effect

Table 26.2. Autosomal Trisomy and Isochromosome Conditions That Have Been Observed in Miscarriage Specimens and among Liveborns

		Liveborns[b]			
Chromosome	% of Trisomic Miscarriages[a]	Trisomy[b]	Trisomy Mosaic	Isochromosome	2° Trisomy (47,+isochromosome)
1	0				
2	5.6				
3	0.8		V rare		
4	2.5		V rare		
5	0.1				
6	0.3				
7	4.5	None?	V rare		
8	3.7	None?	1/10,000		+i(8p) V rare
9	2.8	Rare	Rare	i(9q) V rare	+i(9p) Rare[c]
10	1.9		V rare		
11	0.2				
12	0.8		V rare		+i(12p) Uncommon[c]
13	5.7	1/5,000[c]	Uncommon[c]	i(13q) Rare	
14	4.2	V rare	V rare		
15	7.3	V rare	V rare		+dic(15)(q1) Uncommon[c]
16	32.4		None?		
17	0.7				
18	5.1	1/6,000[c]	Uncommon[c]	i(18q) Rare	+i(18p) Uncommon[c]
19	0.3		None?		
20	2.7	None?	Rare[c]		
21	8.3	1/800[c]	Uncommon[c]	i(21q) Rare[c]	+i(21q) V rare
22	10.1	V rare	V rare	i(22q) V rare	+dic(22)(q11) Rare[c]

[a]Autosomal trisomy is identified in 25 to 30% of miscarriage specimens. The percentage of each chromosome among autosomal trisomies is shown. Data from Bond DJ, Chandley AC. Aneuploidy. Oxford: Oxford University Press, 1983:13.
[b]More than 50 reported cases but less than 1 per 10,000 livebirths is considered uncommon, 10 to 50 reported cases is considered rare, and fewer than 10 reported cases is considered very rare. The designation "none?" means that this has been reported but the finding is controversial. A blank space indicates that the condition has not been observed.
[c]Syndrome is described in the text.

Table 26.3. Chromosome Abnormality Rates per Thousand in Livebirths by 5-Year Maternal Age Intervals[a]

Maternal Age	Down's Syndrome[b]	Edwards' Syndrome	Patau's Syndrome	47,XXY	47,XXX
15–19	0.6	0.06	0.03	0.4	0.4
20–24	0.7	0.07	0.04	0.4	0.4
25–29	0.9	0.09	0.05	0.4	0.4
30–34	1.4	0.14	0.07	0.6	0.4
35–39	4.2	0.42	0.21	1.1	0.7
40–44	14.2	1.42	~0.60	2.6	1.9
45–49	~50	? 1.42	? 0.6	6.6	3.5

[a]The statistics are from Hook EB. Cytogenetics: incidence, risks, and recurrence of chromosome abnormalities. In: Brock DJH, Rodeck C, Ferguson-Smith MA, eds. Prenatal diagnosis and screening. London: Churchill Livingstone, 1992:351–392.
[b]Average of studies of rates in New York and Sweden.

Figure 26.1. Numerical changes. An abnormal number of haploid sets (n) is found in triploidy (3n) (**A**) and tetraploidy (4n) (**B**). Monosomy X (**C**, *arrow*) is the most common monosomy (loss of a single chromosome, 2n − 1), and trisomy 21 (**D**, *arrows*) is the most common trisomy among liveborns (gain of a single chromosome, 2n + 1).

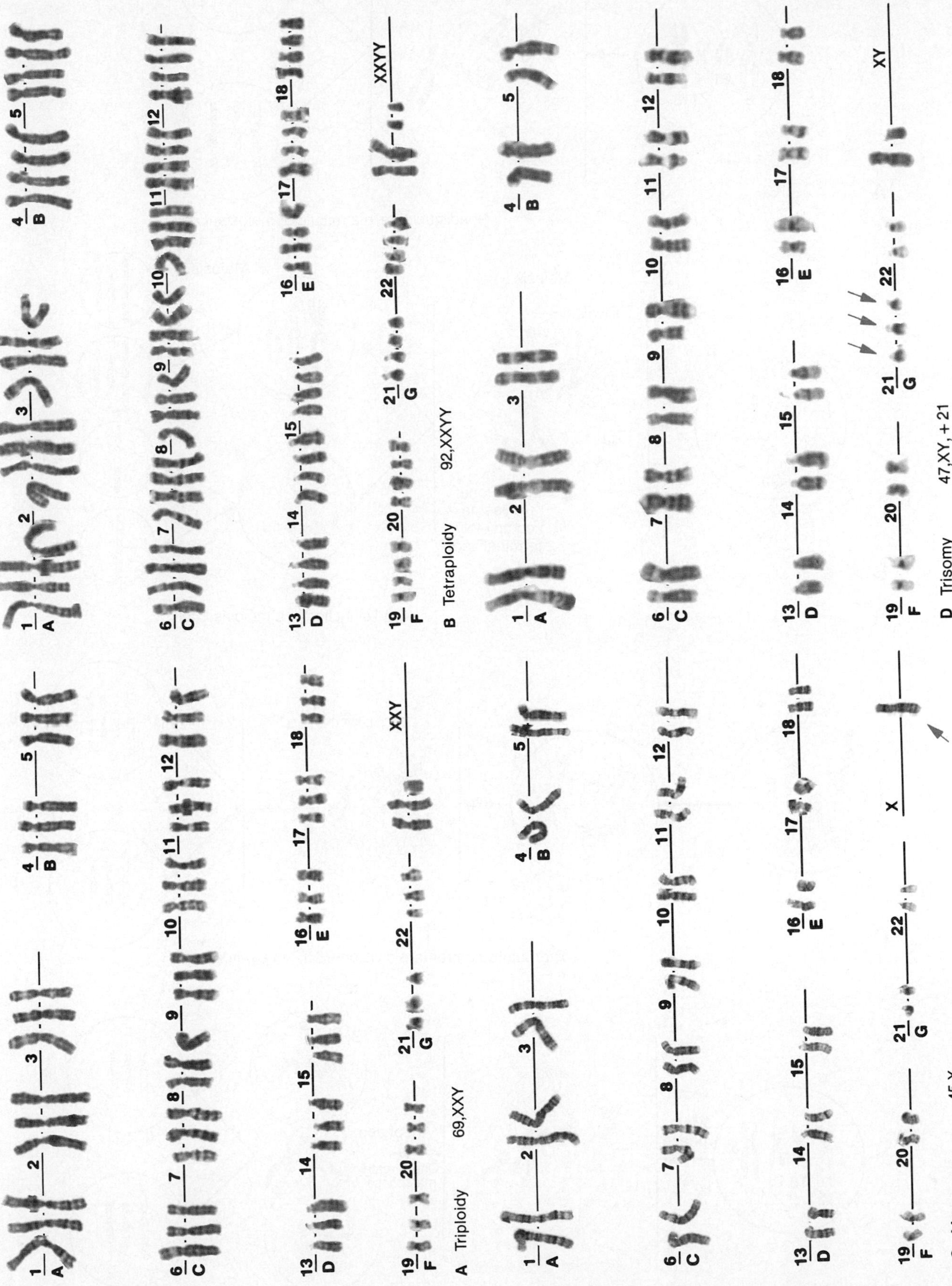
A Triploidy 69,XXY
B Tetraploidy 92,XXYY
C Monosomy 45,X
D Trisomy 47,XY,+21

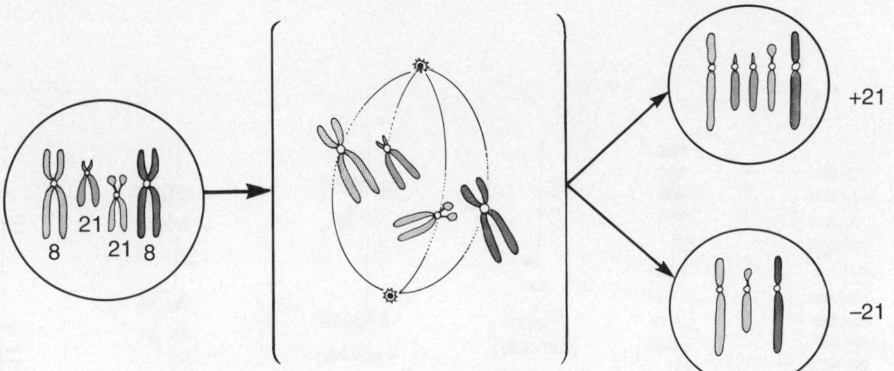

A

Nondisjunction in a mitotic or meiosis II cell

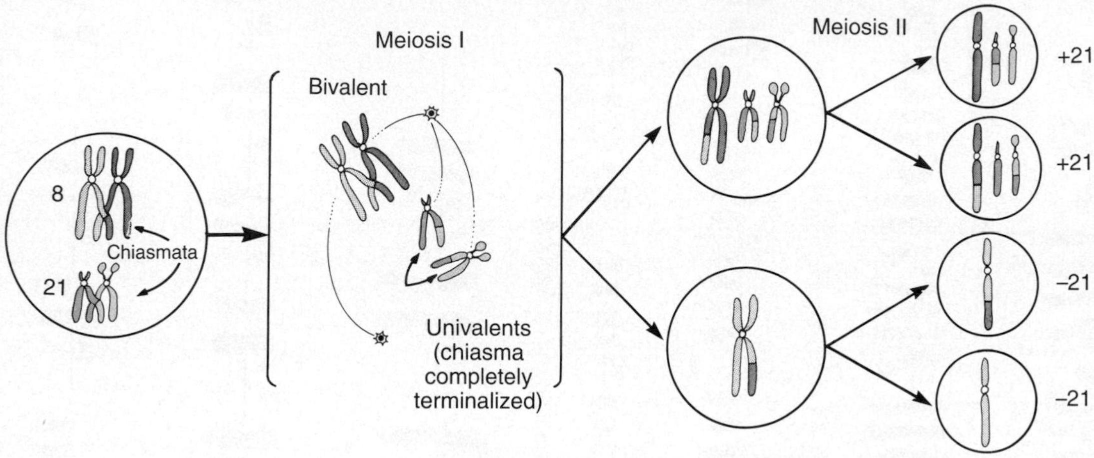

B

Nondisjunction in a meiosis I cell

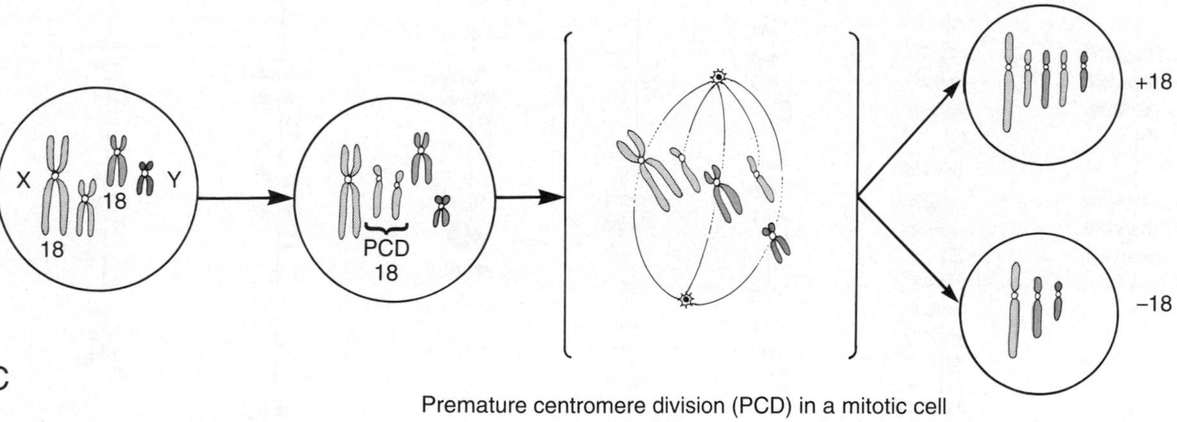

C

Premature centromere division (PCD) in a mitotic cell

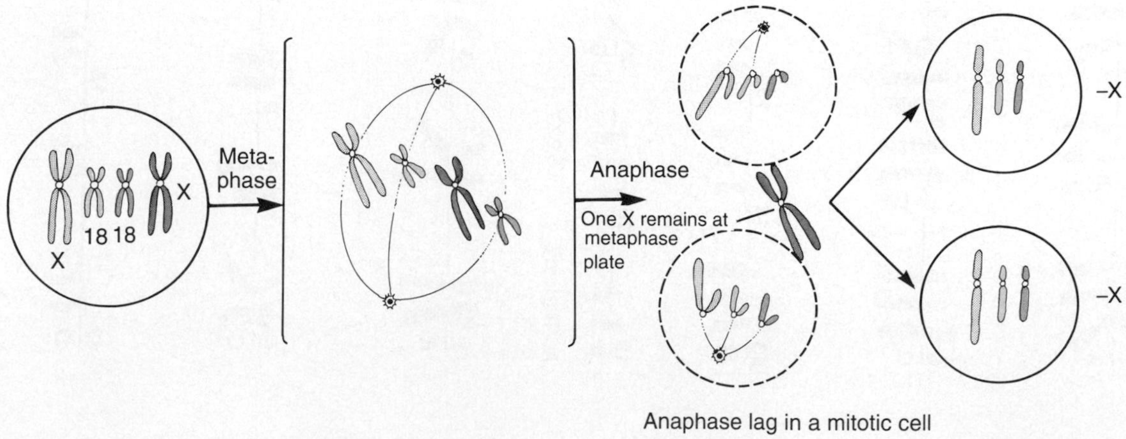

D

Anaphase lag in a mitotic cell

for maternal meiosis II errors may be associated with delayed fertilization because couples have decreasing sexual activity with advancing age.

Many other risk factors for nondisjunction have been postulated, but none have been clearly demonstrated as important, including paternal age, ionizing radiation, maternal thyroid dysfunction, inbred population groups, chromosome 21 short arm variants, and rearrangements involving other chromosomes.

The only nonmosaic monosomy observed in liveborns or miscarriages is 45,X. This is important in Ullrich-Turner syndrome (Fig. 26.1) and is observed in about 12% of miscarriages. Monosomy 21 and 22 are rarely identified in miscarriages. Conceptions with autosomal monosomy appear unable to survive long enough to be recognized, and are probably lost before the time of implantation. On the other hand, monosomy 7 is a common change in acute nonlymphocytic leukemia, and our laboratory has reported that monosomy 9 is important in bladder carcinoma (see also Chapters 29 and 30). Although maternal age is a major risk factor in trisomy, it is not advanced in monosomy X.

MOSAICISM

Nondisjunction or anaphase lag in mitotic cell division creates mosaicism, a mixture of cells with different karyotypes. Mosaics for trisomies 13, 18, and 21 and monosomy X are all well known and in general have a similar but less severe phenotype than the nonmosaics. Several other mosaic trisomies have been observed in liveborns (Table 26.2). Patients with trisomy 8 are probably all mosaic with a normal and a trisomic cell line. It has been suggested that cultured fibroblast cells from trisomy 8 mosaics typically have a higher proportion of +8 cells than do lymphocytes. Different cell types probably tolerate certain chromosome abnormalities differently. A variety of tissue-limited or tissue-dependent mosaic chromosome abnormalities have been identified in patients who have mental retardation, asymmetric skeletal or other malformations, and a variegated, swirled, or linear streak pattern of skin pigmentation. Many of these subjects were studied years ago and had a normal blood karyotype, but recent studies of cultured fibroblasts were found to be abnormal. Although the true frequency of clinically important mosaicism is uncertain, trisomy 8 and diploid/triploid mosaicism are among the most important distinct mosaicism syndromes.

Mosaic autosomal monosomy is very rare (other than in cancer cells), and we are aware of only a very few cases of −21 or −22 mosaicism in liveborns, prenatal diagnostic specimens, or miscarriages. We have seen one amniotic fluid specimen with −21/diploid mosaicism. The parents elected to interrupt the pregnancy, so it is uncertain whether the fetus would have been viable. The source of mosaic monosomy/diploidy could be mitotic nondisjunction, premature centromere division, or anaphase lag (Fig. 26.2). Since lymphocyte chromosome preparations in most laboratories have about 5% of cells with 45 chromosomes, it is difficult to detect a low-frequency mosaic monosomy against this background level of aneuploidy. Cell cultures from some subjects with autosomal rings or dicentrics (see below) have a low frequency of monosomy due to loss of the mitotically unstable chromosome, but the in vivo viability of such cells is unclear. Mosaic monosomy X, with either 46,XX or 46,XY or altered sex chromosome structure, is common among patients with Ullrich-Turner syndrome, gonadal dysgenesis, and ambiguous genitalia. About one in 2500 prenatal studies is 45,X/46,XY, usually resulting in a phenotypically normal male infant. The frequency of cells 45,X,−Y in males and 45,X,−X and 47,XXX in females increases with advancing age. In females, this age effect becomes evident by age 30.

Changes in Chromosome Structure

Changes in chromosome structure fall into three broad categories: deletion, duplication, and rearrangement. A structural change can involve a single base pair or millions of bases of DNA. The lower limit of visibility through the microscope—thus the limit for classic cytogenetic techniques—is about 2,500,000 base pairs (2500 kb). The average chromosome contains about 100,000 kb, much of it nontranscribed, and the average gene is about 40 kb in length. The average 2500-kb segment is thought to contain about 60 genes.

DELETION

A deleted chromosome has lost part or all of one of its arms (Fig. 26.3). A chromosome with a deletion of its centromere region (acentric) is usually lost

Figure 26.2. Origins of aneuploidy. Nondisjunction (**A**), an important source of trisomy and monosomy, occurs during mitosis or meiosis II when sister chromatids (or when homologs in meiosis I, as shown in **B**) move together to the same daughter nucleus. A second source of aneuploidy (**C**) is premature division of the centromere, which permits the site chromatids to drift apart and segregate independently during anaphase to daughter nuclei. Monosomy can also arise through anaphase lag (**D**), in which one chromatid is excluded from either daughter nucleus.

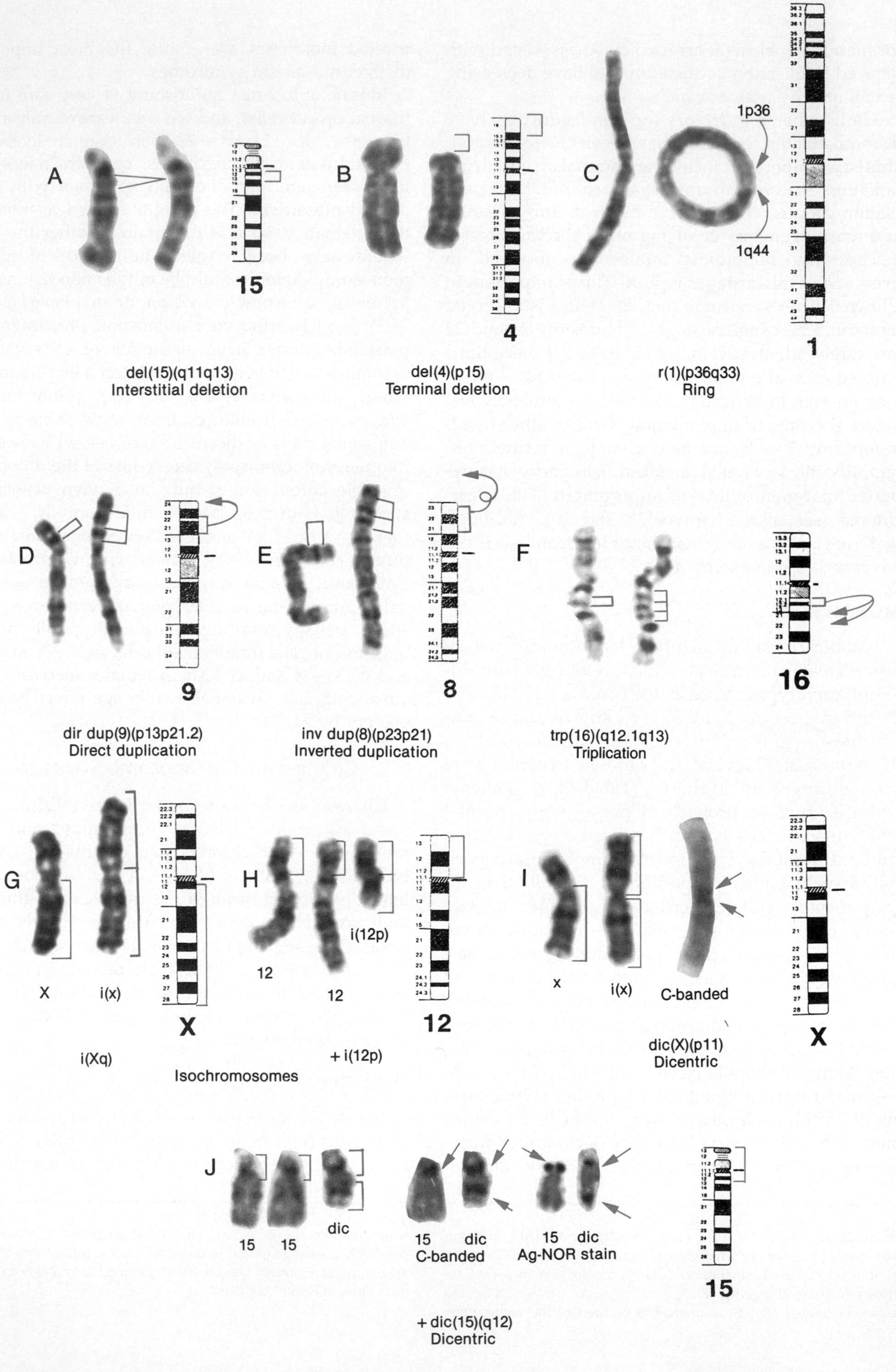
A
15
del(15)(q11q13)
Interstitial deletion
B
4
del(4)(p15)
Terminal deletion
C
1p36
1q44
1
r(1)(p36q33)
Ring
D
9
dir dup(9)(p13p21.2)
Direct duplication
E
8
inv dup(8)(p23p21)
Inverted duplication
F
16
trp(16)(q12.1q13)
Triplication
G
X
i(x)
X
i(Xq)
H
12
12
i(12p)
12
+ i(12p)
Isochromosomes
I
x
i(x)
C-banded
X
dic(X)(p11)
Dicentric
J
15
15
dic
15
dic
C-banded
15
dic
Ag-NOR stain
15
+ dic(15)(q12)
Dicentric

within a few cell divisions. Most chromosome deletions appear through the microscope to be terminal. That is, the telomere (chromosome end) appears to have been lost. However, it is doubtful whether a chromosome with a terminal deletion is stable, since the telomere appears to be an essential structure (discussed in more detail in Chapter 25). For example, deletions induced by ionizing radiation have "sticky ends" and frequently form unstable chromosome rearrangements, whereas deletions associated with birth defects are highly stable. Some R-banding studies have suggested that the terminal R band is not lost from deletions that appear by G-banding to be terminal. Nevertheless, the ISCN (1985) (1) provides for interpretation of a deletion as terminal if it appears to be so through the microscope.

Deletions have been observed for many but not all regions of the karyotype. Several deletion syndromes (a syndrome is a constellation of features typical of patients with the defect) were characterized prior to the advent of chromosome banding because the structural change was obvious even on uniformly stained chromosome preparations. These include 4p– and 5p– (Wolf-Hirschhorn and cri-du-chat syndromes, respectively), 18p– and 18q– syndromes, and X chromosome deletions associated with gonadal dysgenesis. Some patients with the "classic" deletion syndromes have been identified only by using high-resolution cytogenetics, since the deletion can be quite small (the 4p– in Figure 26.3 was not seen in metaphase spreads with shorter chromosomes). For genetic counseling, the parents of patients with deletions need to be karyotyped, since 10 to 15% are derived from parental chromosome rearrangements. If the parents' karyotypes are normal, the risk of recurrence is very low. Deletions are also important in carcinogenesis, in permitting the loss of expression of tumor suppressor genes (see Chapter 30).

RING

Breakage in both arms of a chromosome and repair by fusion at the two breakpoints results in a circular chromosome, or ring (Fig. 26.3). A ring can arise in any cell, and many patients with rings are mosaic with a normal cell line. Complicated structures that arise during replication can produce daughter cells with rings that have zero, two, or even more centromeres. This instability often generates cell lines with rings of different sizes and with monosomy for the chromosome involved. Rings of every chromosome have been observed, and a few have been sufficiently common to delineate syndromes. However, differences among patients in breakpoints of the rings and the frequent mitotic rearrangement of rings lead to wide variation in the phenotypes of patients who appear to have the same ring.

Although the risk of recurrence in future pregnancies is considered very low, chromosome studies of parents are necessary because some familial rings have been found. If the deletion at both ends of the chromosome is minimal, the phenotypic effects can be minimal as well. Some individuals with rings have had a normal or nearly normal phenotype and have reproduced, but their offspring are at an increased risk for birth defects. In our department, we identified a four-generation family with a ring chromosome 21. One mildly mentally retarded child had a ring 21 with more material lost than the ring in her mother's cells. An individual who is mosaic with normal diploid cells probably had a mutation early in embryogenesis and the parents would be expected to have normal chromosomes, although reversion from a ring to a stable rod chromosome has been reported.

DUPLICATION

A cytogenetically visible duplication is almost invariably incompatible with normal embryogenesis and results in a miscarriage or a liveborn with birth defects and mental retardation. The exceptions primarily involve duplications of heterochromatic (C band–positive) segments and acrocentric short arm variants. Gene duplication has been important in evolution, allowing species to "experiment" with nonessential duplicate genes. The hemoglobin and immunoglobulin gene families are classic examples of evolution after gene duplication.

A segment can be duplicated on the same chromosome or on a nonhomologous chromosome (intrachromosomal or interchromosomal duplication, respectively). An intrachromosomal duplication can be immediately adjacent to the normal segment (tandem or contiguous, ABCD*E*EFG) or, less frequently, separated by nonduplicated material (noncontiguous, ABCDEF*E*G). When the duplicated segment has a normal orientation with respect to the centromere, it is a direct duplication (ABCcenD*EF*EFG), otherwise

Figure 26.3. Structural changes. A chromosome deletion can be interstitial (**A**), terminal (**B**), or involving both chromosome ends to form a ring (**C**). A tandem duplication can be inverted (**E**) or direct (**D**) with respect to the centromere. A tandem triplication is shown in **F** (courtesy of The Children's Hospital, Denver). A monocentric or dicentric isochromosome can replace a normal homolog (**G** and **I**) or represent an extra element in the karyotype (**H** and **J**).

it is an inverted duplication (ABCcenD*EFFE*G) (Fig. 26.3). In practice it is not always possible to determine the orientation of a duplicated segment or whether the duplication is contiguous or not. The source of a small duplicated segment is often somewhat speculative, and biochemical, molecular, or molecular cytogenetic studies have sometimes been useful to confirm a cytogenetic impression.

A direct tandem duplication is the most common intrachromosomal duplication, probably because it can arise from a simple unequal exchange between sister chromatids in a mitotic or meiotic cell, whereas an inverted tandem duplication requires three chromosome breaks (Fig. 26.4**A** and **B**). The mean parental age is significantly advanced in patients with inverted duplications, suggesting a meiotic origin, but it is normal in patients with direct duplications. The majority of tandem duplications are new mutations with a low risk of recurrence. Chromosome studies of the parents are necessary in all duplication cases, to look for a familial chromosome rearrangement and to provide accurate genetic counseling. For an intrachromosomal duplication, the odds that a parent carries a balanced translocation are greater than the 10 to 15% for a deletion. Duplications and deletions associated with familial chromosome rearrangements are discussed further below.

ISOCHROMOSOME

In an isochromosome, the arms are mirror images (Figs. 26.3 and 26.4 **C** to **F**). The isochromosome can replace a normal chromosome (monoisodisomy) or be an extra chromosome in an otherwise normal karyotype (secondary trisomy). It can be monocentric with two long or two short arms of the chromosome, or dicentric with the material between the centromeres continuing the mirror image: ABCDcenDCBA or ABCDcenEF::FEcenDCBA, respectively. Isochromosome Xq is associated with gonadal dysgenesis and features of Ullrich-Turner syndrome. Isochromosome Yp and Yq are associated with male infertility and disorders of sex differentiation, and several autosomal isochromosomes cause birth defects (Table 26.2). Even though the origin of secondary trisomies is often a meiotic error, mosaicism is frequent because the cell genotype reverts to normal in cells that lose the isochromosome, and dicentric chromosomes are typically unstable in mitotic division. Parental karyotypes are usually normal but should be studied since some rearrangements, mainly paracentric inversions (see below), can give rise to an apparent isochromosome. Parental mosaics have also been described. Isochromosomes are also important in the cytogenetic evolution of leukemias and solid cancers.

REARRANGEMENT

The three main categories of balanced chromosome rearrangements are robertsonian translocations, reciprocal translocations, and inversions. One in 200 to 300 phenotypically normal subjects carries a balanced rearrangement (Table 26.4). The identification of balanced rearrangements is important because carriers have increased risks for having miscarriages and malformed liveborns, and some male carriers have reduced fertility. A rearrangement can be carried by many family members, conferring risk to many relatives. Furthermore, new mutation carriers of apparently balanced reciprocal translocations and inversions (but not centric fusions) are overrepresented among the mentally retarded. There are several possible explanations for this, including loss of gene function because of breakpoints within genes, undetected deletion at one or both chromosomal breakpoints, or position effects (changes in gene expression because of different location in the genome, such as movement away from or adjacent to controlling elements or heterochromatin).

ROBERTSONIAN TRANSLOCATION

A centric fusion or robertsonian translocation arises from the fusion of two acrocentric chromosomes (chromosomes 13, 14, 15, 21, and 22) (Fig. 26.5). During the resting phase of the cell cycle multiple nucleoli form, each involving the nucleolar organizing region (NOR) of one acrocentric chromosome. With time, the number of nucleoli becomes fewer and their size larger as they coalesce. In a metaphase chromosome preparation, remnants of nucleolar activity are evidenced by frequent acrocentric associations and by strands of silver stain running between acrocentric chromosomes when the Ag-NOR staining technique is applied (Fig. 26.5**B**). Acrocentric association no doubt plays a role in the formation of centric fusions. For reasons that are not understood, the frequency of different robertsonian translocations is nonrandom (Table 26.5).

Individuals who carry a de novo balanced robertsonian translocation have no increased risk for having malformations or mental retardation; these are not seen in increased frequency among patients with mental retardation or birth defects. However, rare patients with a de novo "centric fusion" involving chromosome 15 have been described as having Prader-Willi or Angelman's syndrome (described later).

Some patients with trisomy 21 (Down's syndrome) and trisomy 13 (Patau's syndrome) have un-

Table 26.4. Frequency of Balanced Rearrangements (per Thousand) in the General Population[a]

	Newborn (Unbanded)[a]	Prenatal + Newborn (banded, to 1982)	Prenatal (1982–1990)
Sample size	56,952	12,923	11,500
Translocations			
Robertsonian	0.9	0.9	1.4
Reciprocal	0.9	1.5	1.8
Inversions			
Pericentric	0.1	0.7	1.7
Paracentric	0	0.3	0.9
Total	1.9	3.4	5.8

[a]Estimates from newborn surveys using routine stained (unbanded) chromosome preparations were accurate for robertsonian translocations because the chromosome count is 45. Reciprocal translocations and pericentric inversions were identified only if centromere positions changed. No paracentric inversions were found. Estimates based on prenatal genetic studies using banded chromosomes vary somewhat, the differences being at least partly due to improvements in the quality of banding over time. The statistics are from various sources summarized in Hook EB, Hamerton JL. The frequency of chromosome abnormalities detected in consecutive newborn studies—differences between studies—results by sex and by severity of phenotypic involvement. In: Hook EB, Porter TH, eds. Population cytogenetics studies in humans. New York: Academic Press, 1977:63–79; Van Dyke et al. The frequency and mutation rate of balanced autosomal rearrangements in man estimated from prenatal genetic studies for advanced maternal age. Am J Hum Genet 1983;35:301–308; Bourrillou G, Colombies P, Dastugue N. Chromosome studies in 2136 couples with spontaneous abortions. Hum Genet 1986;74:399–401; and Van Dyke et al., unpublished data.

Table 26.5. Distribution of Each Type of Robertsonian Translocation in Three Population Samples[a]

Translocation	Unbiased Surveys	Multiple Miscarriages	Unbalanced Translocations
	%	%	%
13;13	2.3	3.6	3.3
13;14	71.0	59.6	12.8
13;21	0.9	0.4	2.6
14;21	9.3	8.0	40.7
15;21	0.9	1.2	3.8
21;21	2.3	0.4	28.4
21;22	0.5	0.8	2.8
All others[b]	12.6	26.0	5.5

[a]The statistics summarize the distribution of robertsonian translocations among subjects karyotyped in newborn surveys and routine screening programs such as prenatal diagnostic studies; couples who experienced multiple miscarriages or reduced fertility; and probands with malformations and an unbalanced robertsonian translocation (about two-thirds of whom had Down's syndrome). The unbiased surveys show that t(13;14) is by far the most common robertsonian translocation. The pattern for the multiple miscarriage and infertility group is similar to that of the unbiased surveys. The t(14;21) and t(21;21) are relatively more important clinically than their frequencies in the general population would suggest. Together they comprise only 12% of robertsonian translocations, but because of their association with Down's syndrome, they account for two-thirds of those with unbalanced translocations. Statistics are adapted from Therman et al. The non-random participation of human acrocentric chromosomes in Robertsonian translocations. Ann Hum Genet 1989;53:49–65, pooled with data from our laboratory.
[b]All other robertsonian translocations include t(14;14), t(15;15), t(22;22), t(13;15), t(13;22), t(14;15), t(14;22), and t(15;22).

balanced forms of robertsonian translocations (Fig. 26.5). This is the primary reason for studying the karyotype of a Down's syndrome patient, since the diagnosis can usually be made clinically. The risk that a carrier of a balanced translocation will have chromosomally unbalanced offspring depends on the translocation involved, the sex of the parent, and the likelihood of survival of the abnormal conceptus. The expected 1:1 ratio of normal to balanced karyotypes among offspring is not found, as more than half of the normal offspring are translocation carriers. This observation is not yet understood.

Robertsonian translocations are more common among couples with multiple miscarriages, and males with infertility. In studies of consecutive newborns or prenatal diagnosis specimens, the sex ratio of centric fusion carriers is about equal, whereas among the parents of carriers or unbalanced progeny, many more mothers are carriers. The difference is probably related to the observed reduced fertility in some male carriers of centric fusions.

RECIPROCAL TRANSLOCATION

A reciprocal translocation involves the exchange of chromosome segments, usually involving breakpoints on each of two nonhomologous chromosomes. One in 500 to 700 livebirths carries a balanced reciprocal translocation. Unbalanced translocations and complex rearrangements involving more than two breakpoints are less common. One translocation, t(11;22)(q23;q11), is seen in roughly 1 in 5000 normal subjects. Other than recurring translocations in cancer and leukemia, this is the only important exception to the practically random distribution of chromosomal breakpoints among reciprocal translocations. Why bands 11q23 and 22q11 constitute "hot spots" for reciprocal translocation is the subject of current research.

A major factor in the reproductive risks to a translocation carrier is the viability of the possible unbalanced meiotic products (Fig. 26.6). [Several chapters in A. Daniel's book (2) are devoted to this issue.] In general, risks of having a child with an unbalanced

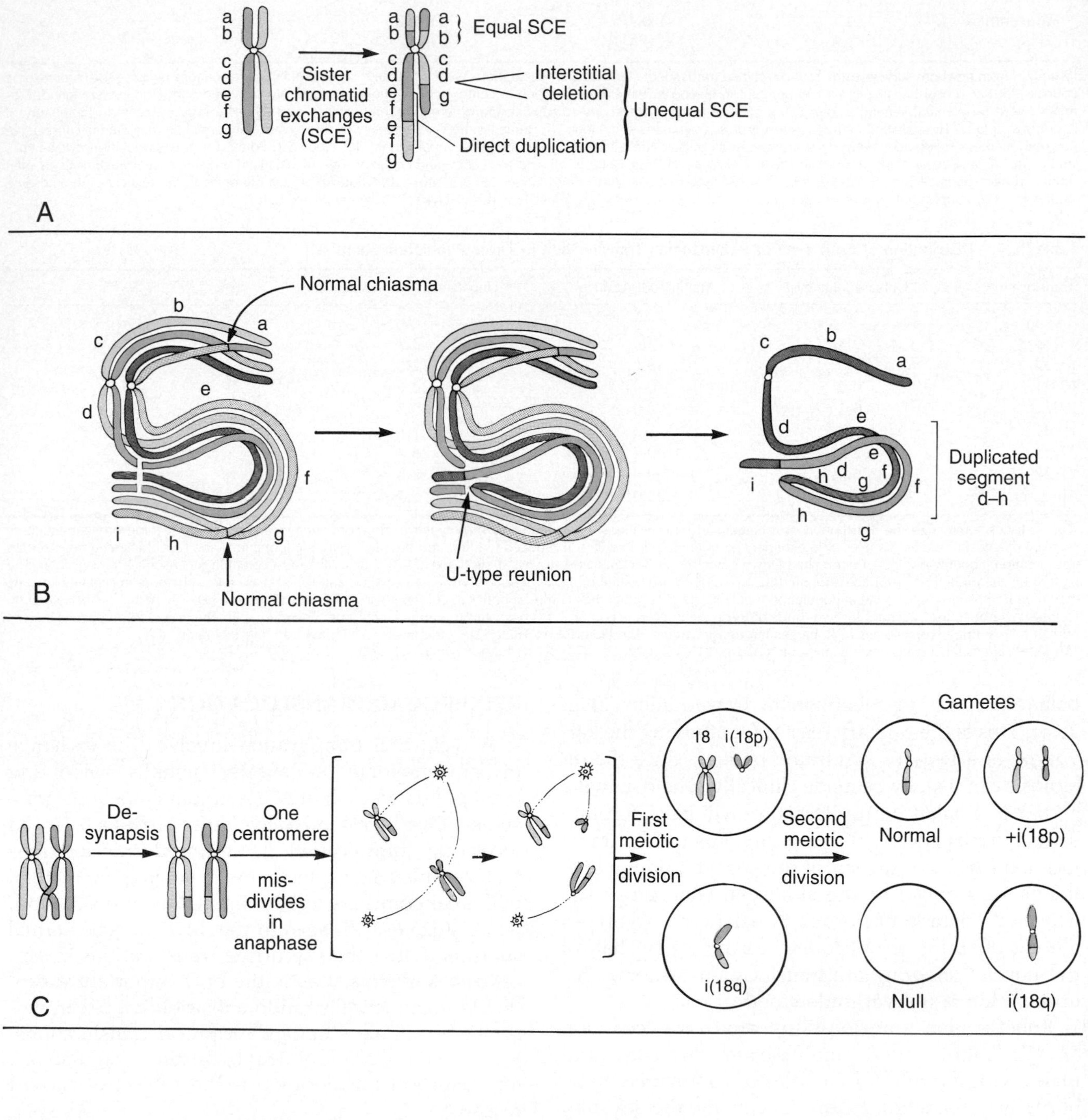

a
b
c
d
e
f
g
Sister
chromatid
exchanges
(SCE)
Equal SCE
Interstitial
deletion
Unequal SCE
Direct duplication
A
Normal chiasma
U-type reunion
Normal chiasma
Duplicated
segment
d–h
B
De-
synapsis
One
centromere
mis-
divides
in
anaphase
First
meiotic
division
Second
meiotic
division
18
i(18p)
i(18q)
Gametes
Normal
+i(18p)
Null
i(18q)
C

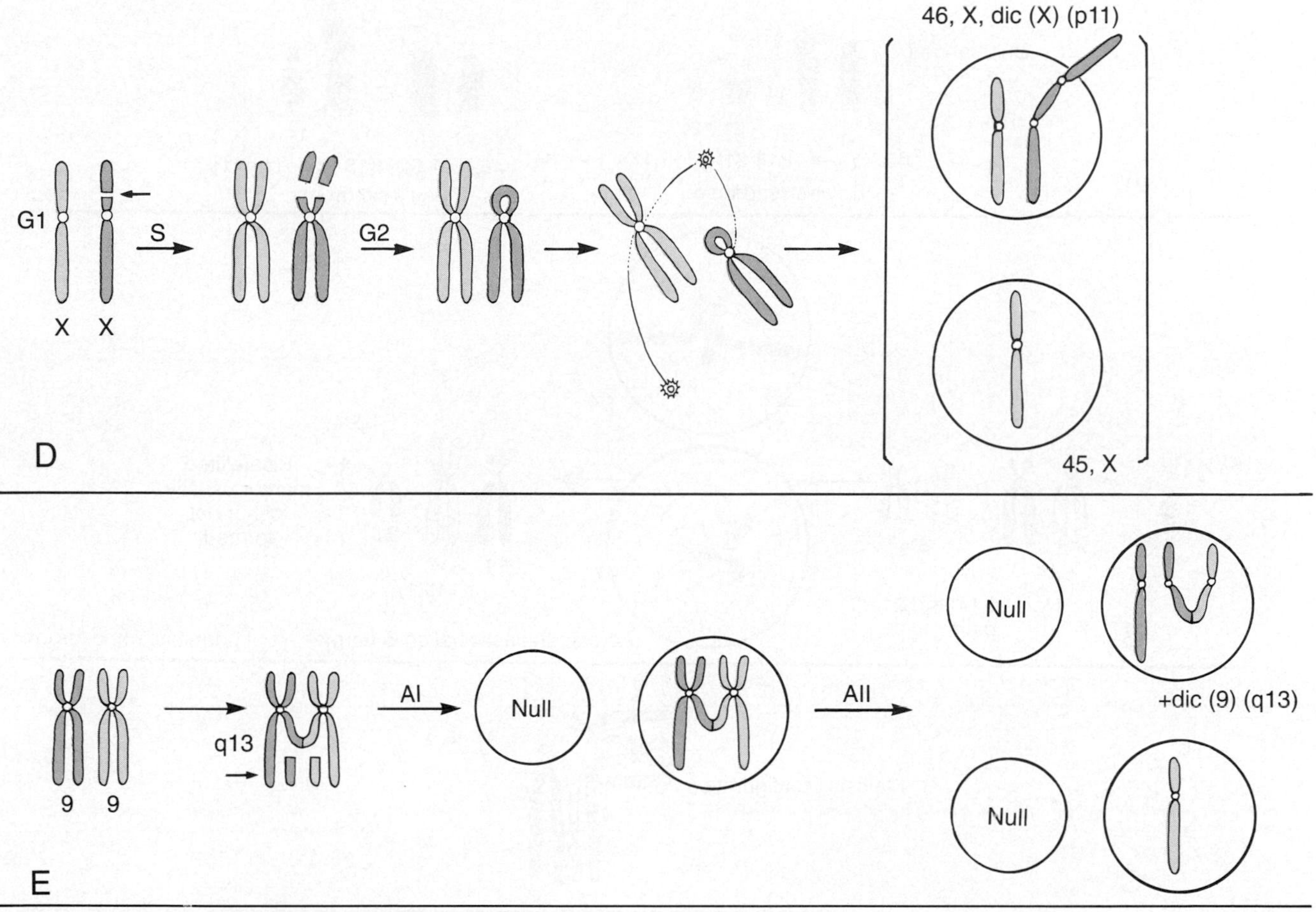

Figure 26.4. Origins of duplications and isochromosomes. A direct duplication (**A**) can arise in a mitotic or meiotic cell by unequal sister chromatid exchange or recombination. The reciprocal product is a deletion. An inverted duplication (**B**) probably results from a three-break rearrangement between homologous or sister chromatids during meiosis I. The repair of the three-breaks would include a U-type reunion. Here it is shown arising in meiosis I, with one break in the proximal long arm and two breaks in the distal long arm. The repair process results in duplication of the intervening segment. Several mechanisms of isochromosome formation have been proposed. The models for the origins of isochromosomes are speculative, but the application of RFLP analysis to patients and their families is expected to provide new information. In meiosis I, desynapsis of the two chromosome 18s can lead to misdivision of a centromere in anaphase I to form monocentric isochromosomes of each chromosome arm (**C**), and gametes could have either an i(18q) replacing a normal 18, or a supernumerary i(18p). As shown in this example, both 46,−18,+i(18q) and 47,+i(18p) have been observed. Formation of a dicentric isochromosome X can result from repair of a chromosome break with a U-type reunion. In a mitotic cell (as shown in **D**) this would produce an individual with 45,X/46,X,dic(X) mosaicism and in some cases a 46,XX line as well. The acentric short arm remnants would be lost. In contrast to the mitotic origin of the dicentric that replaces a normal homolog (as in **D**), during meiosis a supernumerary dicentric isochromosome is more likely to arise. In **E**, a chromatid break in both chromosome 9s and U-type reunion is shown. In anaphase I, the homologous chromosomes are attached by the rearrangement and travel together to the same daughter cell. One might expect an anaphase bridge to occur because the two centromeres typically are drawn to opposite poles, but "centromere cooperation" can occur in a dicentric chromosome. The final result is one gamete with a normal chromosome 9 plus the dicentric, one normal gamete, and two null gametes. The acentric fragments are lost.

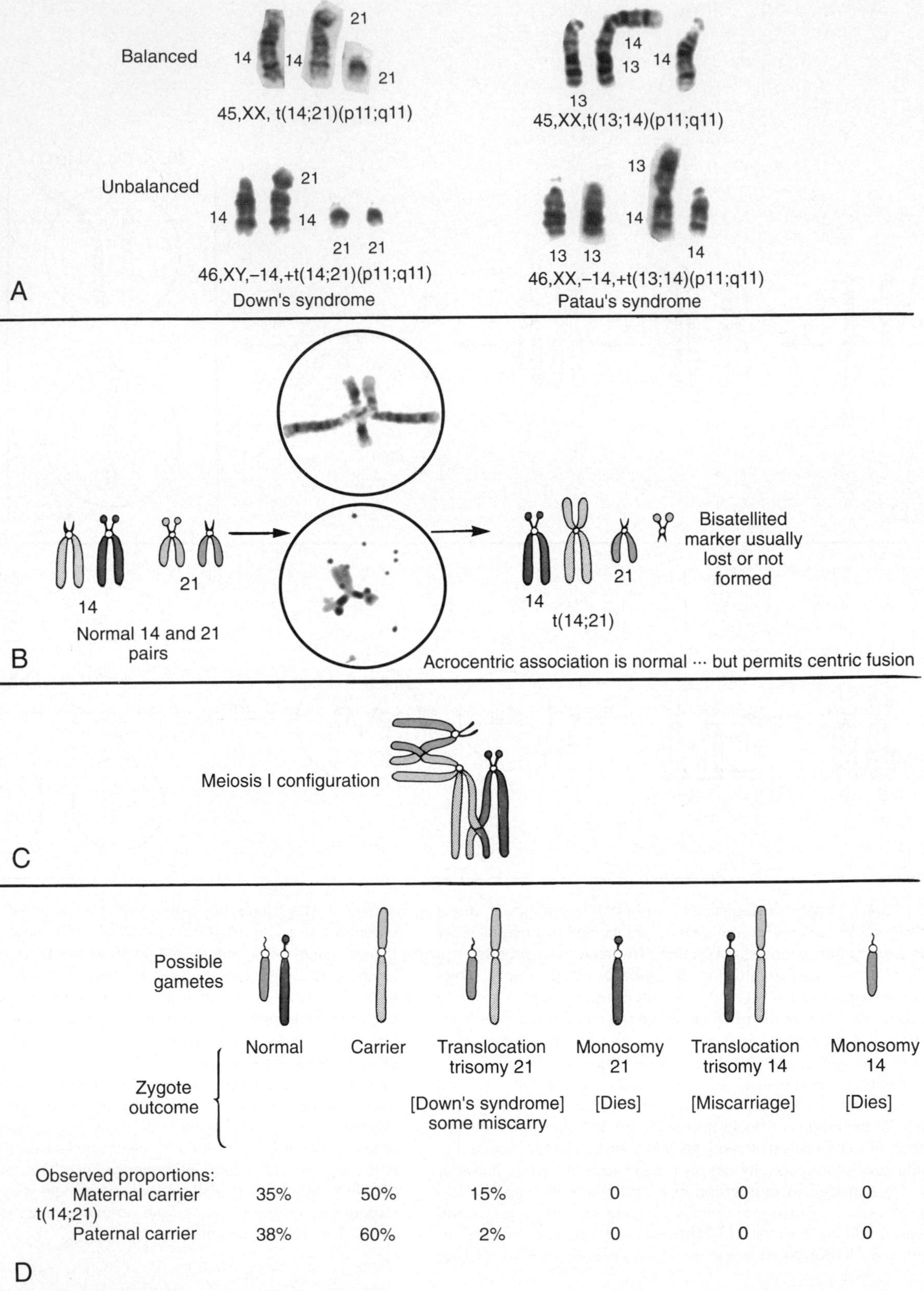

Figure 26.5. Robertsonian translocation (centric fusion). The most important robertsonian translocations are t(14;21) and t(13;14). Partial karyotypes of a balanced and an unbalanced set are shown in **A**. Satellite association (in **B**) is normal chromosome behavior. It is a remnant of nucleolar activity, as shown by the common stream of silver staining (Ag-NOR staining). This close association probably accounts for the relatively high frequency of centric fusions compared to other balanced rearrangements. The reciprocal product of a centric fusion, a bisatellited marker chromosome, is usually not found. A meiosis I configuration (**C**) formed in a carrier of a t(14;21) is shown, along with the six possible gametic products (**D**), of which only three are ever observed. Frequency statistics are based on prenatal diagnosis results in carriers. (Boue A, Gallano P. A collaborative study of the segregation of inherited chromosome structural rearrangements in 1356 prenatal diagnoses. Prenatal diagnosis 1984;4(special issue):45–68).

form of a reciprocal translocation range from nearly zero to 25 to 30%; the risk of miscarriage averages about 25%; and some males have reduced fertility. Unbalanced products with small duplications or deletions are more likely to be viable, and a gain of 1% or loss of 0.5% of the haploid complement is usually viable, whereas a gain of 4% or loss of 2.5% is likely to be lethal. The short arms of chromosomes 17 and 20 each constitute about 1% of the haploid complement, so either arm is a handy device for predicting the viability of a rearrangement. However, viability is determined more by the genes that reside on a chromosomal segment than by its length, so there is wide variation in viability, with some larger chromosomal segments viable as duplication or deletion and a few smaller segments never observed in a chromosomal imbalance.

Of the unbalanced meiotic segregants, adjacent I segregants are the most commonly observed (Fig. 26.7). Adjacent II segregants usually have great imbalances and are rarely seen. If one of the translocation products is small, then a 3:1 segregation product may result in a viable tertiary trisomy. For the t(11;22) mentioned above, the risk is about 5% for the viable tertiary trisomy, and a maternal age effect may be superimposed upon this risk, analogous to the maternal age effect in primary trisomy.

INSERTION AND SHIFT

An insertion is a three-break translocation resulting from removal of a chromosomal segment (two breakpoints) to another site in the karyotype (third breakpoint). A shift is an insertion within the same chromosome (Fig. 26.8). Although insertions are uncommon, they are important because the risk of a chromosomally unbalanced conception in a carrier can be 50%. As with a reciprocal translocation, the risk to have a viable liveborn with a deletion or duplication depends greatly on the size of the inserted segment.

INVERSION

An inversion is a two-break rearrangement in which a chromosome segment is turned 180° (3) (Fig. 26.9). A paracentric inversion involves only one arm. A pericentric inversion includes the centromere and material from both arms. Balanced pericentric and paracentric inversions are more difficult to identify than translocations, so estimates of their frequency in the general population have continued to increase as the quality of chromosome preparations has improved (Table 26.4). Inversions have been called "crossover suppressors" because the meiosis crossover products are often inviable recombinants. Meiotic pairing is expected to create an inversion loop, but an inverted or noninverted segment that is small may remain unpaired during meiosis. Recombination within the inversion loops creates unbalanced products with duplication of material from one end of the chromosome and loss of material from the other end; the inverted segment is neither duplicated nor deleted. For a paracentric inversion one recombinant product is dicentric and one acentric.

Among pericentric inversions, the risk for producing a malformed liveborn or a recognized miscarriage with a recombinant chromosome varies greatly. In general, a small inversion has a lower likelihood of meiotic exchange between the inverted region and the normal homolog, and therefore a smaller proportion of gametes carry an unbalanced recombinant. Moreover, the recombinants have a greater imbalance and the consequence is lower viability. Conversely, a larger inversion has a greater chance of recombination within the inversion loop, and the recombinants have a smaller imbalance, increasing the chance of producing a miscarriage or malformed liveborn. One can apply some of the same empirical risk data from translocations to pericentric inversions: that viability is dramatically reduced if the imbalance is greater than 0.5% deletion or 1% duplication.

The frequency of balanced pericentric inversions in the general population is roughly one in 600. Pericentric inversions are found more frequently among couples with multiple miscarriages, and probands with unbalanced recombinants are found among patients with birth defects and occasionally in miscarriage specimens. A pericentric inv(3) (p25q21) is responsible for at least 30 patients with a recombinant chromosome having duplication of 3q21–qter and deficiency 3p25–pter (Fig. 26.9*A*). This inv(3) may have originated in France and been carried by descendants to Canada and the United States, including Detroit, where we identified a branch of the family that came from Newfoundland to Ontario and southeast Michigan. Several other pericentric inversions are considered normal variants because they are not known to create unbalanced recombinants or interfere with fertility. These include small pericentric inversions of chromosome 2 and a metacentric Y chromosome inv(Y) (p11q11). An inv(2) (p12q14) appears to be more frequent among descendants of Sephardic Jewish people from North Africa and Spain. A common normal variant, inv(9) (p11q12), has a C band–positive block in the short arm in addition to the long arm but may not be a true inversion. It may instead have originated by amplification of a small segment of repetitive DNA in the proximal short arm.

The frequency of balanced paracentric inversions in the general population is almost one in 1000, based on our experience from prenatal genetic stud-

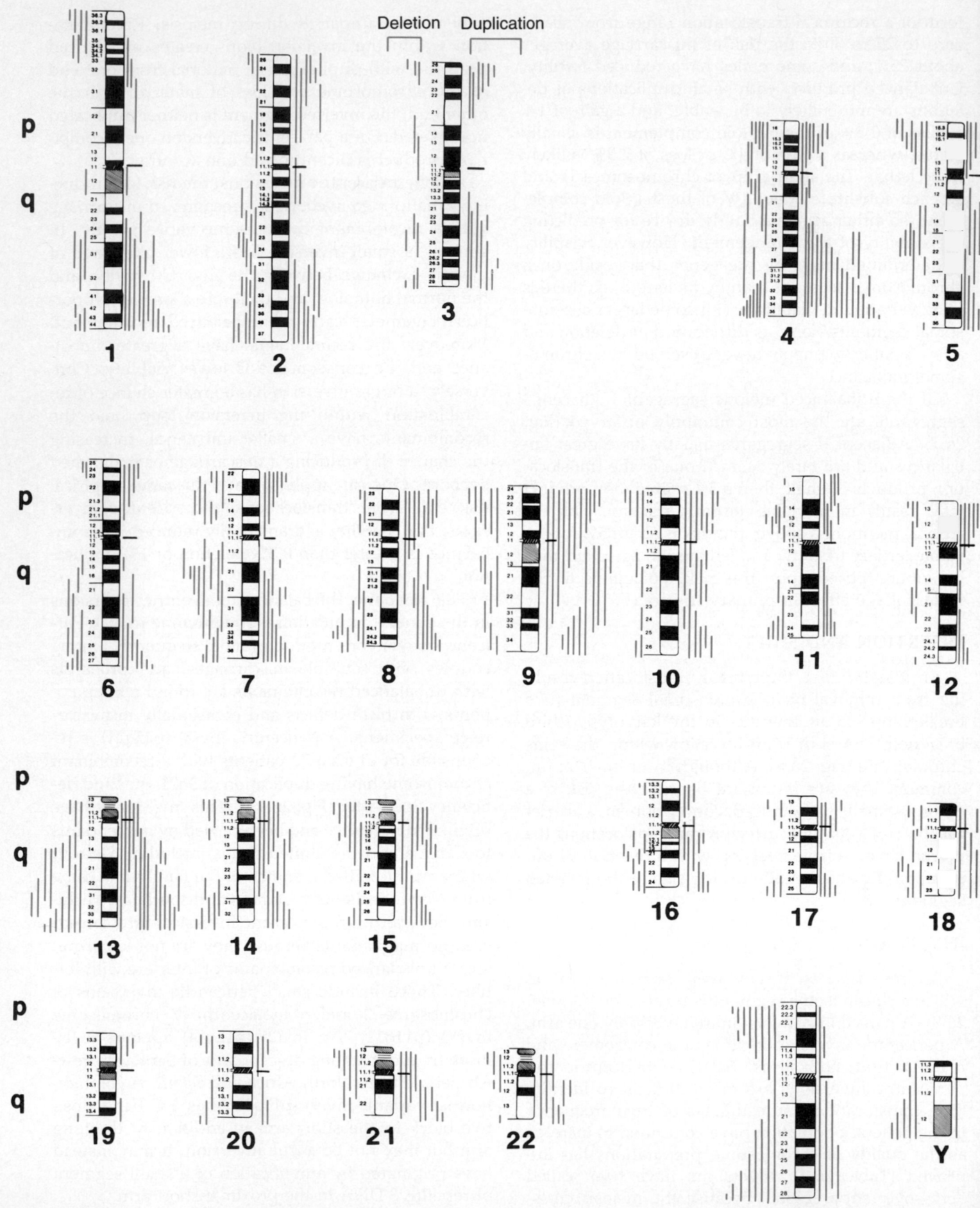
Deletion
Duplication
p
q
1
2
3
4
5
6
7
8
9
10
11
12
13
14
15
16
17
18
19
20
21
22
X
Y

ies. Many paracentric inversions are not detected in routine studies because the altered pattern of chromosome banding can be quite subtle. Most have been identified by chance (mainly prenatal genetic studies) and only a very few from unbalanced recombinant offspring or de novo mutations in patients with birth defects or mental retardation. For a paracentric inversion carrier, the risk of producing a viable conception carrying a recombinant is low because, in general, the acentric and dicentric recombinant products are lost. Nevertheless, our laboratory has identified a girl with a stable dicentric recombinant chromosome whose mother carries a paracentric inv(9) (q22.1q34.3), and a girl with an unusual monocentric recombinant whose mother carries an inv(8) (p21p23) (Fig. 26.9). Since only one other dicentric and five other monocentric recombinants from paracentric inversions have been reported in the literature, it is clear that viable recombinants of paracentric inversions are rare. On the other hand, there may be significant underreporting, since in our single laboratory we have identified two cases. Although the risks for having offspring with unbalanced recombinant chromosomes are probably extremely low for most carriers of paracentric inversions, one must recognize that stable dicentric and monocentric chromosome imbalances can occur.

AUTOSOMAL CHROMOSOME SYNDROMES

The diversity of autosomal chromosome imbalances is immense, so it follows that the variety of phenotypes associated with autosomal imbalance is great. Only a minority of chromosome syndromes can be identified by physical examination alone. Rather than compare and contrast all chromosome syndromes in detail, it is appropriate to examine the features common to many conditions. The two features found in almost all chromosome imbalances are growth retardation and mental retardation. Congenital heart disease, microcephaly, dysmorphic facial features (including hypo- or hypertelorism, broad nasal bridge, micrognathia, and low-set ears) and, in males, cryptorchidism are also common and reflect the complexity of embryogenesis of the brain, face, urogenital tract, and heart and the sensitivity of these processes to perturbations of genetic balance. In general, any individual with mental retardation and more than two minor or major congenital anomalies is a candidate for chromosome studies unless a clearly defined nonchromosomal cause is evident.

As stated earlier, gain of a chromosome segment is tolerated better by the developing organism than is loss of the same segment. In addition to trisomy 13, 18, and 21, several other autosomal trisomies have been reported in liveborns (Table 26.2). Likewise, duplication of whole arms in isochromosomes has been observed, as well as triplication through secondary trisomy. The map of reported duplications and deletions in liveborns (Fig. 26.6) shows visually that the amount of autosomal duplication tolerated is usually greater than that of deletion. It also shows the variety of potential chromosomal imbalance—virtually any segment can be duplicated or deleted.

Many chromosomal syndromes have been described in the *Clinical Atlas of Human Chromosomes* (4), the *Catalog of Unbalanced Chromosome Aberrations in Man* (5), and *Smith's Recognizable Patterns of Human Malformation* (6). In this section, we present brief descriptions of selected classic chromosomal syndromes and two main categories of new syndromes: those associated with a small deletion or duplication involving loss or gain of a small number of genes, called contiguous gene syndromes (7), and those associated with tissue-limited mosaicism. Each syndrome has a constellation of associated birth defects. Few patients exhibit the entire constellation, but each defect is more common in that condition, and in well-defined syndromes, most of the patients will have some of the features.

The contiguous gene syndromes (Table 26.6) have several features in common. They result from duplications or deletions of small segments of chromosome material, containing only a few genes that are functionally unrelated, but by chance are closely linked on the chromosome. The phenotype tends to be variable because of different chromosomal breakpoints, making delineation of a clear syndrome difficult. The occurrence of a contiguous gene syndrome is usually sporadic, but clusters within families are known. The familial clusters are due to balanced chromosome rearrangements that carry a risk for producing unbalanced offspring with the syndrome. Before their chromosomal basis was identified, many of these syndromes were thought to represent autosomal recessive conditions or new dominant mutations.

Figure 26.6. Chromosome deletions and duplications. The idiogram depicts the deletions (at left of each chromosome) and duplications (at right) that have been observed among liveborns. Mosaic cases with a normal cell line are excluded. The length of each line represents the chromosome segment that was lost or duplicated. Variation in the relative frequency of each chromosomal imbalance is not represented here. In general, smaller amounts of imbalance are more common, but there are many exceptions. For example, gain and loss of chromosome 13 and chromosome 18 segments are among the most common, whereas even the smallest changes to chromosome 19 are very rare.

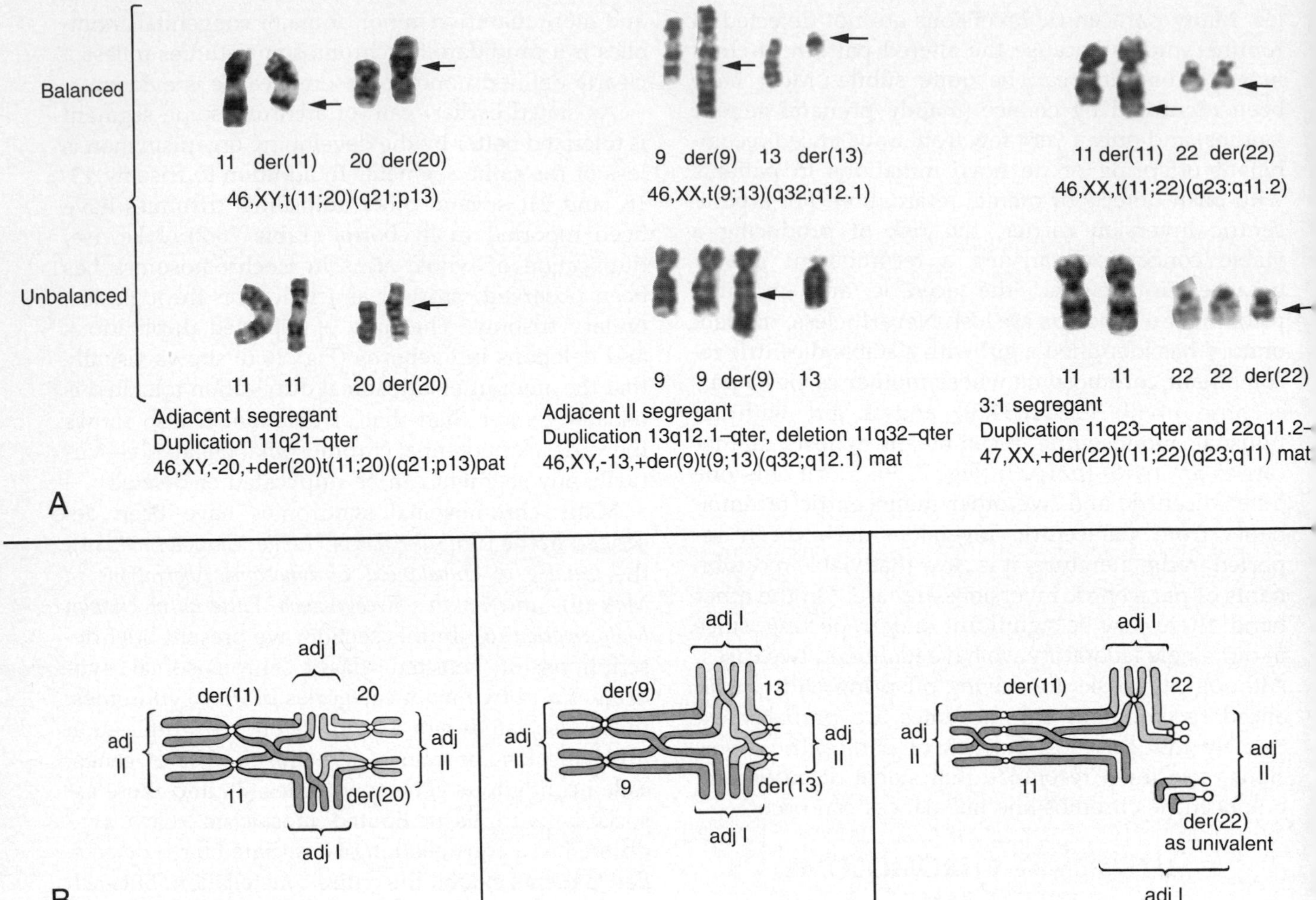

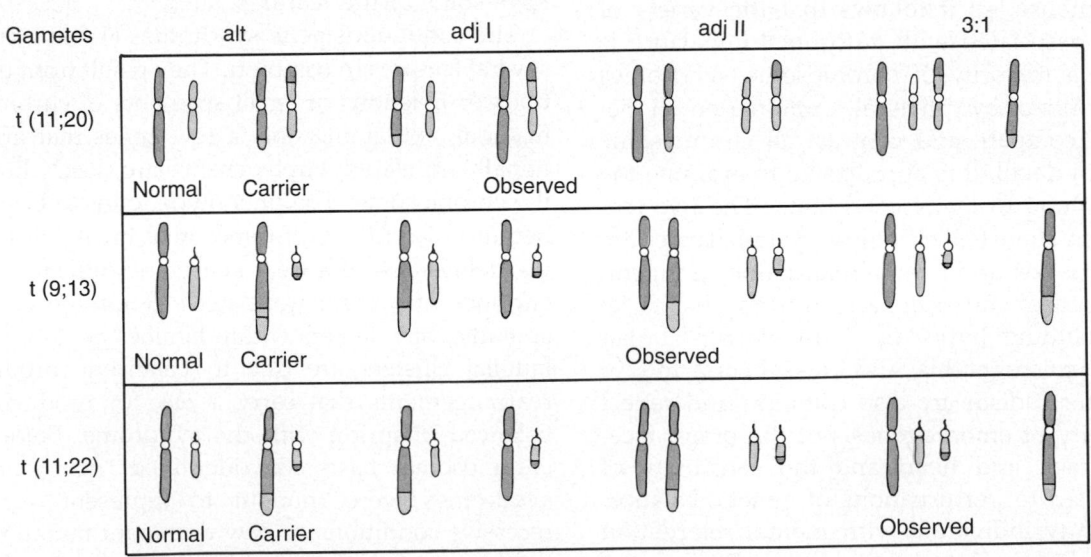

Figure 26.7. Segregation in reciprocal translocations. In **A**, three different translocations are shown in their balanced form and in an unbalanced form. In **B**, a meiosis I prophase quadrivalent is depicted for each translocation. The theoretically possible meiosis I segregants include alternate (alternate chromosomes segregate together), adjacent I (non-homologous centromeres segregate together), adjacent II (homologous centromeres segregate together), and 3:1 segregation (more common when one element is small). Only alternate segregation leads to chromosomally balanced gametes. The meiotic products are shown in **C**, and for the specific translocation used as an example in **A** and **B**, the viable gametes that have been observed are noted.

Table 26.6. Contiguous Gene Syndromes[a]

Autosomal		X Chromosomal	
Vander Woude syndrome, MR[b]	1q32–q41	Ichthyosis, chondrodysplasia punctata, and Kallmann's syndrome, MR	Xp22.3
Piebald trait, MR	2q34–q36	Microphthalmia, iridoschisis, goiter, labium synechia, and craniotabes	Xp22
Rieger's syndrome, MR	4q25–q27	Choroideremia, deafness, MR	Xp21.1–21.3
Schizophrenia	dup 5q11.2–q13.3	Duchenne's/Becker's dystrophy, MR	Xp21
Adenomatous polyposis, MR	5q21	DMD, CDG, McLeod phenotype, retinitis, and MR	Xp21
Craniosynostosis, MR	7p21.2–p21.3	DMD, glycerol kinase deficiency, Aland's eye disease, and MR	Xp21
Greig's cephalopolysyndactyly, MR	7p13	Glycerol kinase deficiency, adrenal hypoplasia, hypogonadotropic hypogonadism, and MR	Xp11.2–p21
Zellweger's syndrome	7q11.23		
Spherocytosis I, MR	8p11.2–p21.1		
* Langer-Giedeon syndrome	8q24.11–24.13		
Tricho-rhino-phalangeal, type I	8q24.12		
DiGeorge sequence	10p13		
* Wilms' tumor—aniridia (WAGR)	11p13		
* Beckwith-Wiedemann syndrome	dup 11p15.5		
* Retinoblastoma, MR	13q14		
* Prader-Willi syndrome	15q11–q12 pat		
Angelman's syndrome	15q11–q12 mat		
Smith-Magenis syndrome	17p11		
* Miller-Dieker syndrome	17p13.3		
Alagille's syndrome (arteriohepatic dysplasia), MR	20p11.23–p12.1		
DiGeorge sequence, MR	22q11		

[a]Asterisks indicate "classic" contiguous gene syndromes. All of the contiguous gene syndromes are deletions except Beckwith-Wiedemann syndrome. (Adapted from Harper et al., Cytogenet Cell Genet 1989;51:563–611.)
[b]MR, mental retardation.

For the study of contiguous gene syndromes, high-resolution cytogenetic techniques are essential. The mid- to early metaphase analysis that is the accepted standard in most cytogenetics laboratories is not sufficient for reliable identification of these syndromes. The smallest karyotype changes can appear normal, even when using high-resolution banding methods, because the imbalance is below the resolution of the light microscope. With advances in molecular cytogenetic technology, DNA probes for several contiguous gene syndromes are commercially available, including Wolf-Hirschhorn, cri-du-chat, Miller-Dieker, Angelman's and Prader-Willi syndromes, and others are being developed. For some syndromes, DNA probe technology (discussed later) is likely to become the standard of care as an adjunct to high-resolution cytogenetic analysis, because it provides sensitive and specific assays for the smallest chromosomal deletions and duplications.

Triploidy and Diploid/Triploid Mosaicism

Triploidy is identified in 7% of miscarriages and is found rarely in stillborns, with 60% being 69,XXY, 35% 69,XXX, and only 5% 69,XYY. Triploids with 69,XYY are less common and tend to be found in earlier miscarriages, suggesting less viability compared to XXY or XXX triploids. The liveborn incidence may be as great as one in 2500 births, but most escape detection because of neonatal death. The mean parental age is not advanced. Probably all liveborns with triploidy have a mixture of diploid and triploid cells. The diagnosis of diploid/triploid mosaicism is typically made by karyotyping cultured skin fibroblast cells. This syndrome is surely underdiagnosed, since the lymphocyte population is primarily diploid. It is possible that triploid lymphocytes are inviable or do not respond to the mitogen.

Several plausible origins have been proposed for diploid/triploid mosaicism. A relatively common origin of this mosaicism may be fertilization of both the egg and a first or second polar body, one with a single sperm and the other with two sperm. Subsequently, the two zygotes develop as a single organism. This sequence of events actually results in chimerism, not mosaicism. (A chimera is an organism that results from fusion of more than one zygote.) An alternative origin is fertilization of separate ova, with postzygotic fusion during the earliest stages of embryogenesis.

PHENOTYPE

Triploid miscarriages are often associated with cystic villi or a hydatidiform mole. The embryos often have retarded limb development and generalized growth retardation, facial malformations, open spine defects, syndactyly, and subectodermal hemorrhage. We have identified several triploids in amniotic fluid cell cultures studied because of an elevated maternal serum AFP level or anatomic malformations observed on ultrasound. Key physical features of stillborns and liveborns include low birth weight, syndactyly, asymmetry of the body or face, and

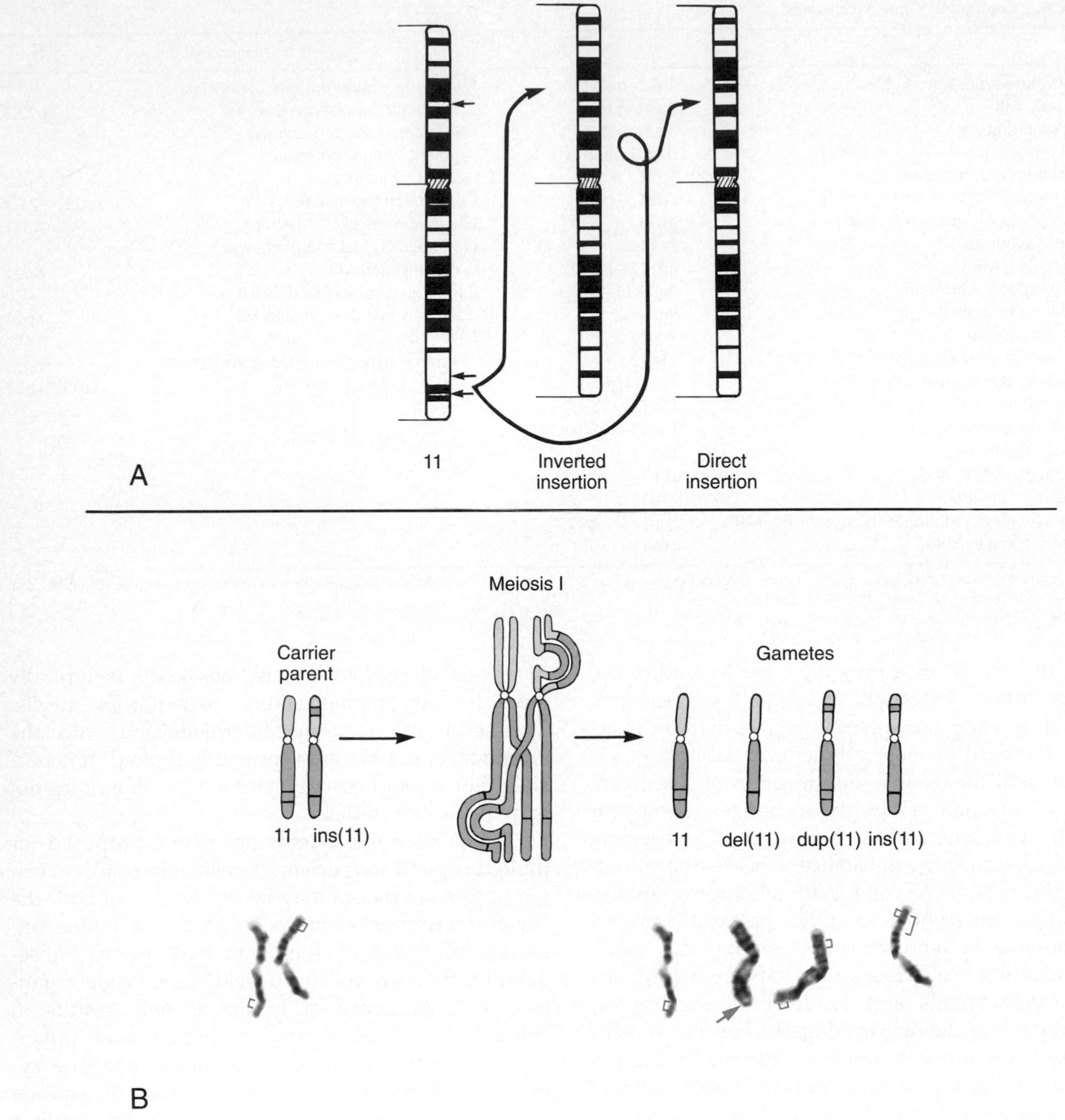

Figure 26.8. Recombination in insertion (shift). An intrachromosomal shift requires three breakpoints, as shown in **A** for a chromosome 11 shift. The insertion can be inverted with respect to the original centromeric orientation, or direct. In **B**, the chromosome 11s of the carrier parent are shown diagrammatically and as a partial karyotype. Since the inserted segment is small, it is appropriate to show the meiosis I prophase configuration without synapsis of the insertion segment. Nonrecombinant gametes perpetuate the parental karyotypes, whereas recombination will produce deletion and duplication gametes. Both were observed in siblings with mental retardation and mild malformations. (From Forsythe et al. Duplication and deletion 11q23–q24 recombinants in two offspring of an intrachromosomal insertion ("shift") carrier. Henry Ford Hosp Med J 1988;36:183–186.)

Figure 26.9. Recombination in inversion. Three examples are provided to show the results of recombination in pericentric and paracentric inversions. A partial karyotype of the carrier parent and affected offspring is provided at top and bottom, respectively, with an illustration of the meiosis I prophase configuration and recombinant and nonrecombinant products. A pericentric inversion 3 (in **A**) and a paracentric inversion 9 (in **B**) are shown. A two-break exchange within the paracentric inversion loop (in **C**) during meiosis I in a paracentric inversion 8 carrier mother resulted in a child with an inverted duplication of 8p. (The inv(9) family was reported by MJ Worsham et al. A dicentric recombinant 9 derived from a paracentric inversion: phenotype, cytogenetics, and molecular analysis of centromeres. Am J Hum Genet 1989;44:115–123, the inv(8) family by GL Feldman et al. Inverted duplication of 8p: Ten new patients and review of the literature. Am J Med Genet, in press, 1993.)

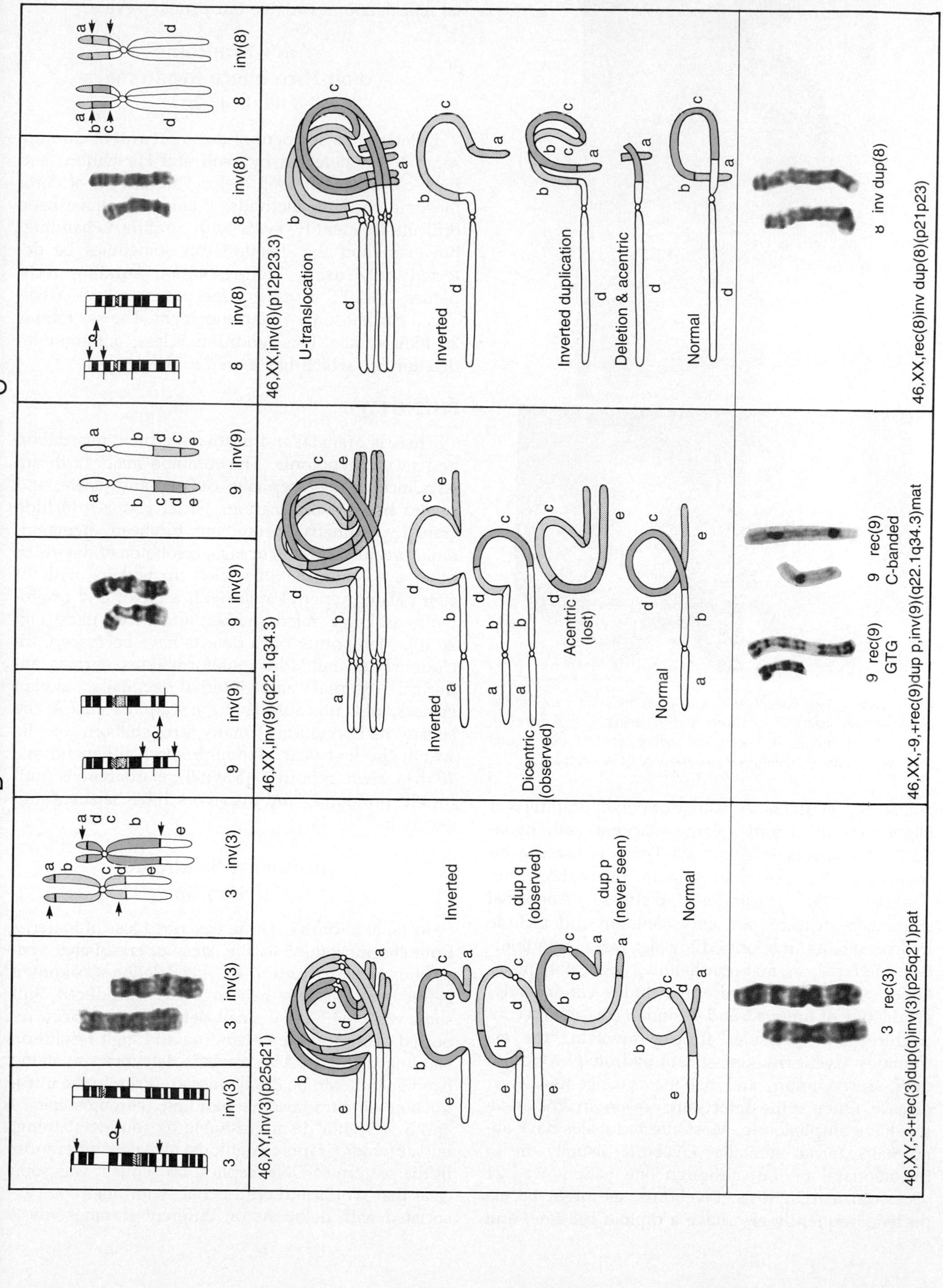

3 inv(3)
3 inv(3)
3 inv(3)
46,XY,inv(3)(p25q21)
Inverted
dup q (observed)
dup p (never seen)
Normal
3 rec(3)
46,XY,-3+rec(3)dup(q)inv(3)(p25q21)pat
9 inv(9)
9 inv(9)
9 inv(9)
46,XX,inv(9)(q22.1q34.3)
Inverted
Dicentric (observed)
Acentric (lost)
Normal
9 rec(9) GTG
9 rec(9) C-banded
46,XX,-9,+rec(9)dup p,inv(9)(q22.1q34.3)mat
C
8 inv(8)
8 inv(8)
8 inv(8)
46,XX,inv(8)(p12p23.3)
U-translocation
Inverted
Inverted duplication
Deletion & acentric
Normal
8 inv dup(8)
46,XX,rec(8)inv dup(8)(p21p23)

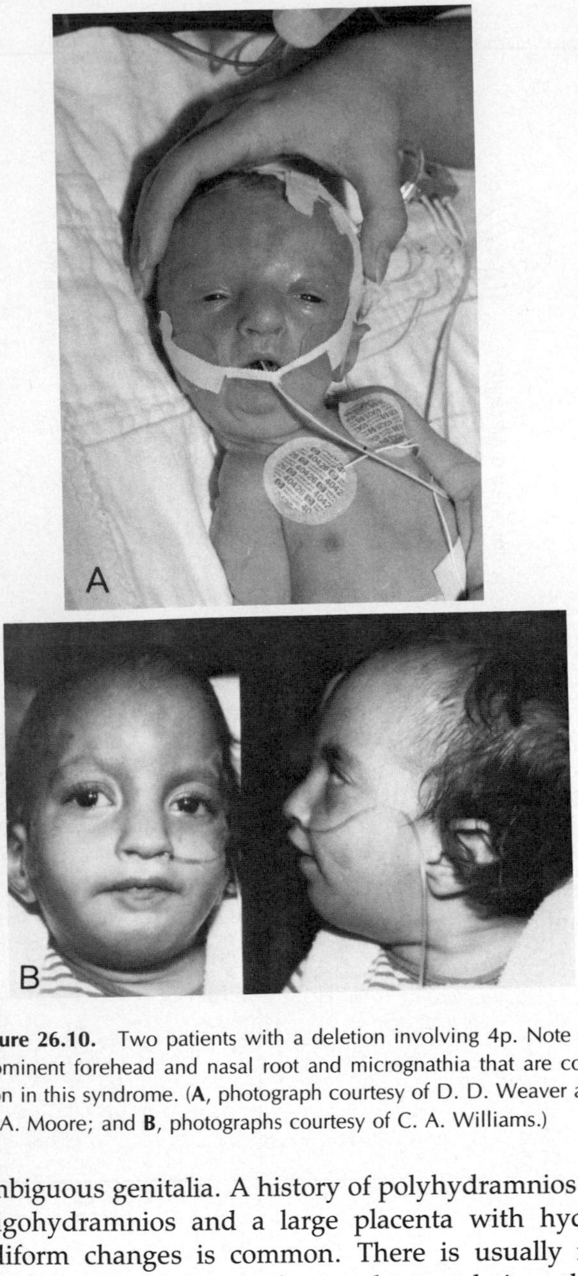

Figure 26.10. Two patients with a deletion involving 4p. Note the prominent forehead and nasal root and micrognathia that are common in this syndrome. (**A**, photograph courtesy of D. D. Weaver and C. A. Moore; and **B**, photographs courtesy of C. A. Williams.)

ambiguous genitalia. A history of polyhydramnios or oligohydramnios and a large placenta with hydatidiform changes is common. There is usually intrauterine and postnatal growth retardation, hypotonia, and respiratory distress. Abnormal craniofacial features are very common and include hydrocephalus, malformed low-set ears, hypertelorism, cleft palate, microphthalmia, and colobomata. Other abnormal features include clinodactyly, syndactyly of fingers 3 and 4, simian crease, and contractures and muscular atrophy involving the extremities. Cystic, hypoplastic, or hydronephrotic kidneys are common, and half have congenital heart disease. Open spine defects are present in 25% and a few have omphalocele. Most affected males have abnormal external genitalia. Liveborns usually die in the neonatal period, although one patient was 21 years old at diagnosis. Liveborns, as might be expected, frequently also have a diploid cell line, and can present with bodily and facial asymmetry. Mental retardation is variable but usually severe.

Wolf's Syndrome (Wolf-Hirschhorn Syndrome) Deletion 4p

Deletion of a segment of the short arm of chromosome 4 was detected by Wolf and Hirschhorn and their coworkers in 1965, before the advent of chromosome banding methods. Some cases have been difficult to identify even with routine G-banding, however, and the deletion can sometimes be detected only using high-resolution banding techniques. In 10% of cases, one parent carries a balanced chromosome 4 rearrangement. The sex ratio is 2:1 female:male. This syndrome is less common than deletion 5p, which has a milder phenotype.

PHENOTYPE

There is prenatal and postnatal growth retardation and severe hypotonia. The common major birth defects include microcephaly, cleft lip and palate, and severe heart malformation. Facial features include cranial asymmetry, prominent forehead, hemangioma, preauricular pits or tags, coloboma of the iris or other eye malformations, cleft lip with or without cleft palate, hypertelorism with a broad and prominent nasal root, micrognathia, and a long neck (Fig. 26.10). Many other birth defects have been seen, including brain and kidney malformations, hernias, abnormal external and internal genitalia, simian creases, and cutis aplasia of the scalp. Because of the severe malformations, many are stillborn or die within the first year, although survival beyond age 20 has been reported. Mental retardation is uniformly profound, and survivors have seizures and severe hypotonia.

Cri-du-chat Syndrome Deletion 5p

In 1963, Jerome Lejeune described loss of material from chromosome 5 as the cause of cri-du-chat syndrome. As with deletion 4p, this deletion was known before chromosome banding was introduced, but some cases with very small deletions have been reported using routine G-banding and high-resolution banding methods. The smallest deletions, involving band 5p15.1, can be easily missed. (Prior to the introduction of chromosome banding, chromosomes 4 and 5 were not distinguishable by routine staining, but autoradiographic methods revealed differences in the pattern of DNA replication. Thus it was soon clear that Wolf's and cri-du-chat syndromes were associated with deletions on different chromosomes.)

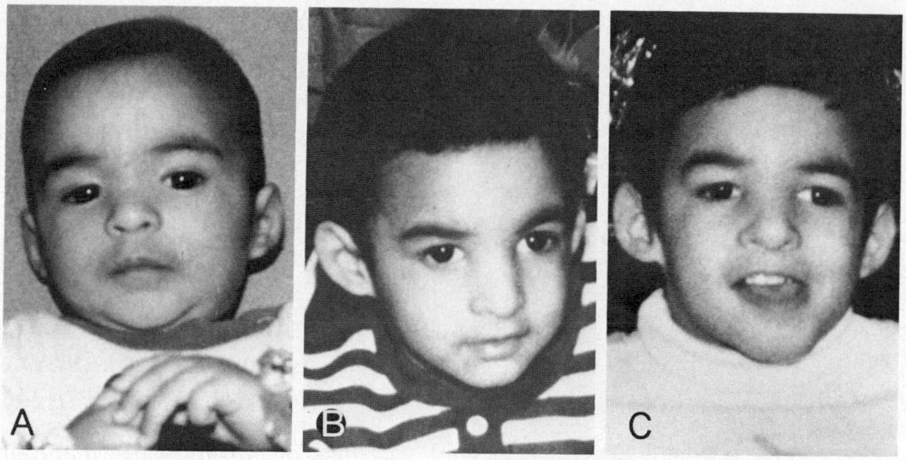

Figure 26.11. Three photographs of a patient with cri-du-chat syndrome depict the characteristic facial appearance at ages 5 (**A**), 24 (**B**), and 36 (**C**) months.

The incidence of cri-du-chat syndrome is about one in 45,000 newborns, and 12% result from familial rearrangements involving chromosome 5. The mean parental age is normal. Among de novo deletions, about 80% represent a mutation in the chromosome 5 inherited from the father. Slightly more females than males are affected (8).

PHENOTYPE

Cri-du-chat syndrome can be suspected in infants with a plaintive, meowing cry, low birth weight, and failure to thrive. Some mothers have described weak fetal movements. Life-threatening birth defects are uncommon, but because of neonatal complications about 10% do not survive beyond the first few months. The newborn frequently has low birth weight and small head circumference. The weak kitten-like cry that gives the syndrome its name is at least partly due to an anatomic abnormality of the larynx, is very common among affected infants, and is very distinct to the parents and medical personnel. Although the cry changes with age, it does not become normal. Facial features include microcephaly, a round face, low-set ears, strabismus, broad nasal bridge and epicanthus which give the impression of hypertelorism, micrognathia, and occasionally facial asymmetry (Fig. 26.11). The hands and feet appear small, and hands often have a simian crease, fifth digit clinodactyly, and single flexion crease. With age, premature gray hair, dental malocclusion, inguinal hernia, diastasis recti, and scoliosis are common. Infants have hypotonia, but older individuals can have normal tone or hypertonia. The IQ varies mostly between 20 and 50 but can range up to mildly retarded, with skills approaching those of 5- or 6-year-olds.

Trisomy 8 Mosaicism (Warkany's Syndrome)

Most and perhaps all cases are mosaic with a normal cell line. One commonly finds dramatic differences in the proportion of abnormal cells between tissues. The proportion of trisomy 8 cells appears to decrease with age, especially in the lymphocyte population. The incidence of this condition is estimated to be one in 10,000 newborns, but it is certainly underdiagnosed. The mean parental age is advanced and the sex ratio is 3:1 male:female.

PHENOTYPE

A normal birth weight with postnatal growth retardation is typical. The face is only mildly dysmorphic with a prominent forehead, malformed ears, bulbous nose with upturned nares, everted lower lip, protruding lower helix of ear, downslanting palpebral fissures, and mild micrognathia (Fig. 26.12). Multiple skeletal abnormalities are common, including additional vertebrae or hemivertebrae, spina bifida occulta, broad dorsal ribs, hypoplastic iliac wings, and hypoplastic patellae. Other features include a long and slender body habitus, simian creases, deep plantar and palmar furrows (which may disappear in late childhood) and a similar deep furrow on the lower lip, mild joint contractures, mild congenital heart defects, and absent corpus callosum. Males often have hypospadias, cryptorchidism or inguinal hernia. Life threatening birth defects are unusual. Mental retardation is usually moderate but widely variable.

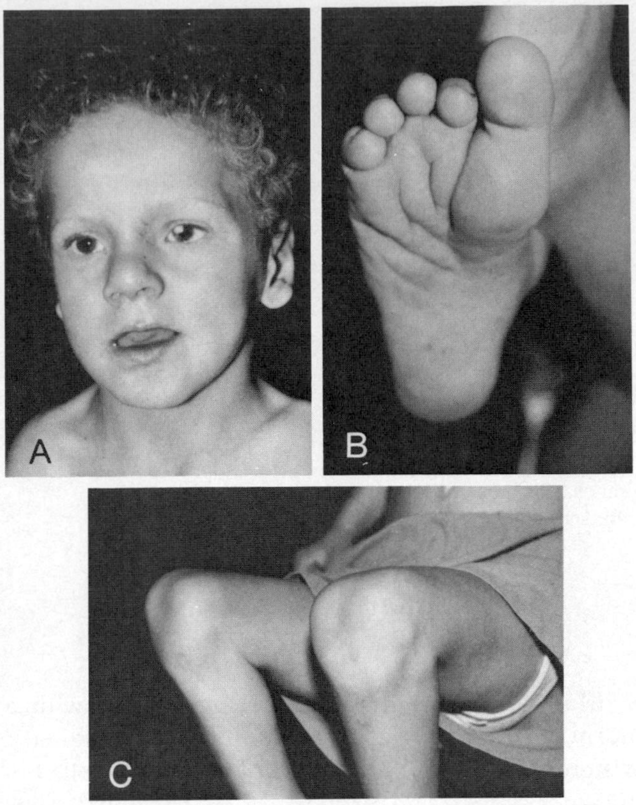

Figure 26.12. Trisomy 8 mosaic syndrome includes (**A**) malformed ears with protruding lower helix, bulbous nose, and downward-slanting palpebral fissures. Deep creases are common in the palms and soles (**B**), and absent or hypoplastic patellae (**C**) are characteristic. (Photographs courtesy of C. A. Williams.)

Secondary Trisomy 8p
47,+i(8p)

This recently recognized chromosome abnormality, associated with mental retardation and dysmorphic features, is probably rare, but its apparent tissue-limited mosaicism (fewer abnormal cells in fibroblasts than in lymphocytes) makes it interesting. Only three cases have been reported so far. One patient had the extra i(8p) in 13 of 50 blood cells, the only tissue studied. A second patient had the isochromosome in 7% of lymphocytes and 3% of fibroblasts. A third patient had the isochromosome in 27% of lymphocytes and 15% of fibroblasts, but the isochromosome was not seen in any of 50 cultured amniocytes. A prenatal study had been done because of advanced maternal age and, apparently, the extra isochromosome was not identified because of tissue-limited mosaicism. It is likely that more cases will be missed by prenatal testing in the future, particularly if secondary trisomy 8p has the advanced parental age effect and mosaicism that is typical of other secondary trisomies.

PHENOTYPE

The phenotype appears to include normal birthweight, short stature, rib and vertebral anomalies, heart defect (ventricular septal defect in one patient), absent corpus callosum, and enlarged cerebral ventricles. One patient was ventilator dependent until death at age 8 months, and surviving patients have IQs in the range of 50 to 70.

Trichorhinophalangeal Syndrome Type II (Langer-Giedion Syndrome)
del(8)(q24.11q24.13)

A loss of chromosome material, including del(8)(q24.11q24.13) can be demonstrated in at least half of cases. About 50 cases have been published thus far, and most of those with a chromosome deletion appear to be new mutations. DNA markers within the deleted region showed maternal origin of the deletion in the only case studied so far.

PHENOTYPE

The physical findings include loose skin during infancy and multiple exostoses (benign osteoid tumors). Facial features include microcephaly, sparse hair, large protruding ears, bulbous nose with tented alae, long and prominent philtrum, thin upper lip, and micrognathia. Radiographs characteristically show cone-shaped epiphyses by age 3 or 4. Mild to severe mental retardation is typical in those with a visible deletion. Patients with dominantly inherited Type I trichorhinophalangeal syndrome have many of the features of Langer-Giedion syndrome but normal intelligence, normal head circumference, no exostoses, and a normal karyotype. The recent observation of deletion of band 8q24.12 only, in association with severe mental retardation and other features of Langer-Giedion syndrome, but without exostoses, has led to the hypothesis that the two conditions are overlapping contiguous gene syndromes with the phenotype depending on the extent of the deletion.

Secondary Trisomy 9p
47,+dic(9p) or 47,+i(9p)

An extra isochromosome 9p has been identified in 13 patients, and we have identified it once in a prenatal genetic study. The karyotypic interpretation can be confirmed by the observation of elevated GALT enzyme activity. The GALT gene, galactose-1-phosphate uridylyltransferase, resides within band 9p13. In at least half of cases the isochromosome is dicentric. There is tissue-limited mosaicism in which most lymphocyte metaphases carry the isochromosome, whereas cultured fibroblasts show wide variability. This reduced expression in fibroblasts may carry over to amniocytes and chorionic villus cells and make prenatal diagnosis more difficult. The average maternal age (31 years) is advanced.

PHENOTYPE

Birth defects have included congenital heart disease, cleft lip and palate, joint dislocations, hemivertebrae, scoliosis and kyphosis, hypoplastic clavicles, kidney malformations, cryptorchidism in males, and simian creases. Facial features include hypertelorism and micrognathia. About half have died within a year. The severity of mental retardation has been variable, and one affected man has been described as semi-independent with an IQ of 63.

Beckwith-Weidemann Syndrome Duplication of Band 11p15

The overall incidence of Beckwith Wiedemann syndrome (or EMG syndrome—*e*xomphalos, *m*acroglossia, and *g*igantism) has been estimated as one in 14,000 live births, and a duplication involving band 11p15 is present in about 10% of cases. Most patients apparently represent new mutations, although a familial chromosome rearrangement is involved in some instances. Paternal origin of the de novo duplication was identified in all of the patients evaluated so far. The autosomal dominantly inherited form of Beckwith-Wiedemann syndrome has been localized to 11p15.5.

PHENOTYPE

Patients with the visible chromosome change have mental retardation and usually congenital heart disease; some have been stillborn. Other features of the syndrome include gigantism and generalized organomegaly, a large tongue, and omphalocele (Fig. 26.13). Neonatal hypoglycemia is identified in 35 to 50% of subjects. Craniofacial features include microcephaly, linear creases on ear lobes, indentations on the posterior edge of the helix, and nevus flammeus. Cleft lip is an occasional finding. Among the dominantly inherited cases there is about a 6% risk of cancer: Wilms' tumor (60% of tumors), adrenocortical carcinoma (15%), and other tumors, including gonadoblastoma, hepatoblastoma, and rhabdomyosarcoma. Presumably the cases with a visible duplication have a similar risk. Genes that reside in this region include insulin and insulin-like growth factor. If they are duplicated, they may account for some of the phenotypic features, such as macrosomia and neonatal hypoglycemia. In tumor cells, loss of heterozygosity is observed for 11p genes, including the HRAS1 locus (see Chapter 30). Mental retardation can be secondary to the associated hypoglycemia or the chromosome abnormality, but is not a constant feature of the autosomal dominantly inherited syndrome.

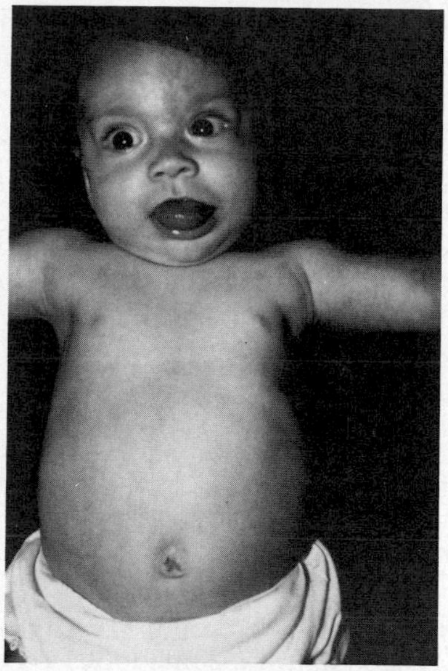

Figure 26.13. Patient with Beckwith-Wiedemann syndrome. (Photograph courtesy of C. A. Williams.)

WAGR Syndrome Deletion of Band 11p13

This contiguous gene syndrome is associated with the loss of band 11p13, and occasionally with a familial chromosome rearrangement. The incidence of WAGR (*W*ilms' tumor, *a*niridia, *g*enitourinary malformations, and mental *r*etardation) syndrome is about one in 50,000 live births, and the association between aniridia and Wilms' tumor was known many years before the chromosomal basis was identified. Either aniridia or Wilms' tumor alone can be inherited as a discrete autosomal dominant trait with normal intelligence and no visible deletion. Two loci for aniridia have been identified, AR1 and AR2, on chromosomes 2 and 11, respectively, and the Wilms' tumor locus (WT1) appears to reside at the same site as the deletion in WAGR syndrome. About one in 70 Wilms' tumor patients has aniridia. The closely linked catalase gene locus is often deleted, and reduced catalase activity can be detected in about 95% of cases. The sex ratio is 2:1 male:female.

PHENOTYPE

The four major features of WAGR syndrome are Wilms' tumor, aniridia, genitourinary malformations, and mental retardation. Wilms' tumor (nephroblastoma) is identified in 35 to 50% of patients with the deletion, and males have an increased risk of gonadoblastoma. Genitourinary malformations are present in 90%, including ambiguous genitalia in most males. Aniridia is present in 97% of patients who have the other three major features. Craniofacial features include microcephaly in 50%, prominent lips, micrognathia, and malformed ears. Moderate to severe mental retardation is present in 90% of cases.

Secondary Trisomy 12p (Killian's or Pallister-Killian Syndrome, or Mosaic Tetrasomy 12p) 47,+i(12p)

This syndrome results from an extra isochromosome 12p. The isochromosome looks very much like an i(21q), and many cases have been misidentified as such and called "tetrasomy 21." The phenotype is not at all similar to Down's syndrome, however, and increased expression of the LDHB enzyme (lactate dehydrogenase B, located within band 12p12) has confirmed the abnormality to be a +i(12p). More than 40 cases have been reported, and we have seen at least three cases in our laboratory since 1985. Early perinatal death and dramatic tissue-limited mosaicism have probably resulted in most diagnoses being missed, and therefore the true clinical significance of this syndrome has been underestimated. Over 99% of lymphocytes have a normal karyotype, whereas at least 10% of fibroblasts typically have the extra i(12p). Cells with the isochromosome are probably present in the blood prenatally, but disappear very soon after birth. Alternatively, patients who are identified in the newborn period may be more severely affected because of the involvement of other tissues, including peripheral blood. A high proportion of abnormal cells has been reported in bone marrow preparations from subjects who had very few cells in PHA-stimulated blood cultures, suggesting poor PHA response by or in vitro selection against lymphocytes that carry the isochromosome. Parental age is more advanced than in trisomy 21, with mean maternal age 31 years and mean paternal age 34 years.

PHENOTYPE

The birth weight is usually normal. Massive diaphragmatic hernia is a key feature and a common cause of perinatal death. Associated features include short limbs, imperforate anus, talipes; craniofacial features include a high forehead, sparse hair, small dysplastic ears, hypertelorism, irregularly shaped bushy eyebrows, flat nasal bridge with short nose and anteverted nares, and thin upper lip. Other findings include supernumerary nipples, sacral dimple, short fingers, broad hands and feet, vetebral and joint deformities, and disordered or dysplastic skin pigmentation, dental eruption and hair distribution. The pigmentary dysplasia can suggest hypomelanosis of Ito or incontinentia pigmenti with swirls of hypopigmentation or can be expressed as sparse hypopigmented macules that are clearly seen only with a Wood's lamp. Those who live beyond the neonatal period usually have seizures and severe mental retardation. The first described cases were bedridden patients who had mental retardation, seizures, and joint contractures.

Trisomy 13 (Patau's Syndrome)

Trisomy 13 is present in one in 5000 newborns. Primary trisomy 13 is present in 75% of cases, 4% are mosaics, 10% have an unbalanced t(13;13), and 10% have an unbalanced t(13;14). Other robertsonian translocations associated with trisomy 13 are rare. At least half of the t(13;14), but fewer than 10% of the t(13;13) cases are familial. The t(13;14) is the most common balanced rearrangement in humans, with a frequency of about one in 5000 in the general population. The reproductive risk to a t(13;13) carrier parent is 100%, and for a t(13;14) carrier parent the reproductive risk is estimated to be 1% for a carrier female and under 1% for a carrier male. The majority of t(13;14) carrier parents of unbalanced progeny are female, and as far as we know all of the t(13;13) carrier parents of unbalanced progeny have been female. The average maternal age of trisomy cases is advanced, as with other autosomel trisomies.

PHENOTYPE

Many trisomy 13 conceptions result in miscarriage or stillbirth. In the liveborn, the common and key physical features are microcephaly, localized areas of cutis aplasia on the scalp, microphthalmia, bilateral cleft lip, and polydactyly with hyperconvex and narrow fingernails (Fig. 26.14). Midline facial defects are commonly associated with holoprosencephaly, and can be as severe as cyclopia. Multiple ocular malformations have been reported, with microphthalmia or anophthalmia most common. Other features include malformed low-set ears, micrognathia, short neck with extra skin folds at the nape of the neck, broad flat nose, and hemangiomata. Other malformations include heart defects (ventricular or atrial septal defect or patent ductus arteriosus), kidney malformations, single umbilical artery, crytorchidism in males, and a single palmar crease. Polymorphonuclear cells have characteristic nuclear projections, and persistent embryonic hemoglobin has been reported. Men-

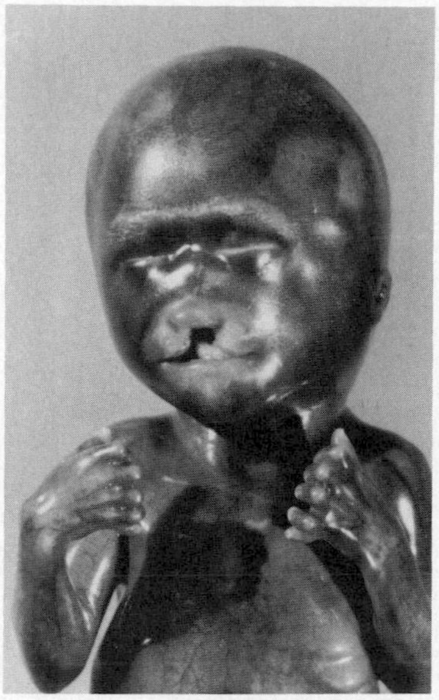

Figure 26.14. Fetus with trisomy 13, with bilateral clefts and postaxial polydactyly. (Photograph courtesy of J. R. Roberson and L. Weiss.)

tal retardation is profound and seizures are common. Half of trisomy 13 liveborns die within the first month and 90% die within the first year. Survival beyond age 5 years is unusual.

Retinoblastoma Deletion of Band 13q14

A contiguous gene syndrome of retinoblastoma and birth defects is associated with an interstitial deletion of a small segment of chromosome 13 including band 13q14. The deletion usually arises as a new mutation of paternal origin. The dominantly inherited retinoblastoma gene (RB1) resides within band 13q14. The incidence of retinoblastoma is about one in 23,000 liveborns. Among patients with retinoblastoma, the tumors are bilateral in about 20%, and 5% of the bilateral cases have a visible chromosome 13 deletion. Retinoblastoma patients without birth defects (sporadic or dominantly inherited type) have normal 13s, although some of their tumors have visible del(13) or loss of heterozygosity at 13q14. This is discussed in greater detail, along with the two-mutation model for carcinogenesis, in Chapter 30. The esterase D gene is closely linked to the RB1 locus and is deleted in about 95% of deletion cases.

PHENOTYPE

The craniofacial features are variable but include macrocephaly (or, with larger deletions, microcephaly), prominent eyebrows, nasal bridge with a bulbous nasal tip, and a wide mouth with a thin vermilion border. There is a high risk of retinoblastoma and osteosarcoma, and most patients have been ascertained because of the association of retinoblastoma and birth defects. In about half of the cases with retinoblastoma, the tumor is unilateral. A few patients who have a deletion in this region, including loss of the esterase D gene, do not have retinoblastoma. Even so, these patients may remain at risk for other neoplasias. Molecular genetic studies to detect submicroscopic mutations within the retinoblastoma gene may be useful in such patients. Mental deficiency can be severe, but some patients who have a visible deletion reportedly have normal intelligence. Familial deletions and balanced chromosome 13 rearrangements have been reported, as well as duplication of band 13q14 associated with a normal phenotype in a few relatives.

Prader-Willi Syndrome (Prader-Labhart-Willi Syndrome) del(15)(q11.2q12)

The majority of patients (65%) have an interstitial deletion of 15q11.2–q12 or q13 that always includes the loss of sub-band 15q11.2. Another 5% have other changes involving chromosome 15, 10% have a submicroscopic deletion detectable by molecular or molecular cytogenetic methods, and 20% have a normal 15 pair even using probes for DNA fragments that are known to be lost in the deletion patients. The incidence of this contiguous gene syndrome is at least one in 25,000 and the recurrence risk is under 1%, with very few familial cases reported. Numerous DNA probes have located RFLPs within and around the Prader-Willi locus, and the genetics of this region is under intense investigation. The deletion is of paternal origin in at least 90% of cases.

PHENOTYPE

Birth weight and head circumference are generally normal. Prematurity, decreased prenatal movement, and breech presentation are common. As infants, these patients have hypogonadism (cryptorchidism and micropenis in males and hypoplastic labia in females), mild ocular and cutaneous hypopigmentation, strabismus, extreme hypotonia, and failure to thrive; many need to be gavage fed because of a weak suck. Some parents have commented about the child having cold hands and feet and skin mottling. Craniofacial features include narrow bitemporal diameter, high forehead, almond-shaped eyes, epicanthus, malar hypoplasia, and small mouth with downturned corners. By age 3, hyperphagia leading to marked obesity, and small hands and feet are characteristic features (Fig. 26.15). The patients with normal 15s usually do not have hypopigmentation. Mental retardation is usually moderate (average IQ is

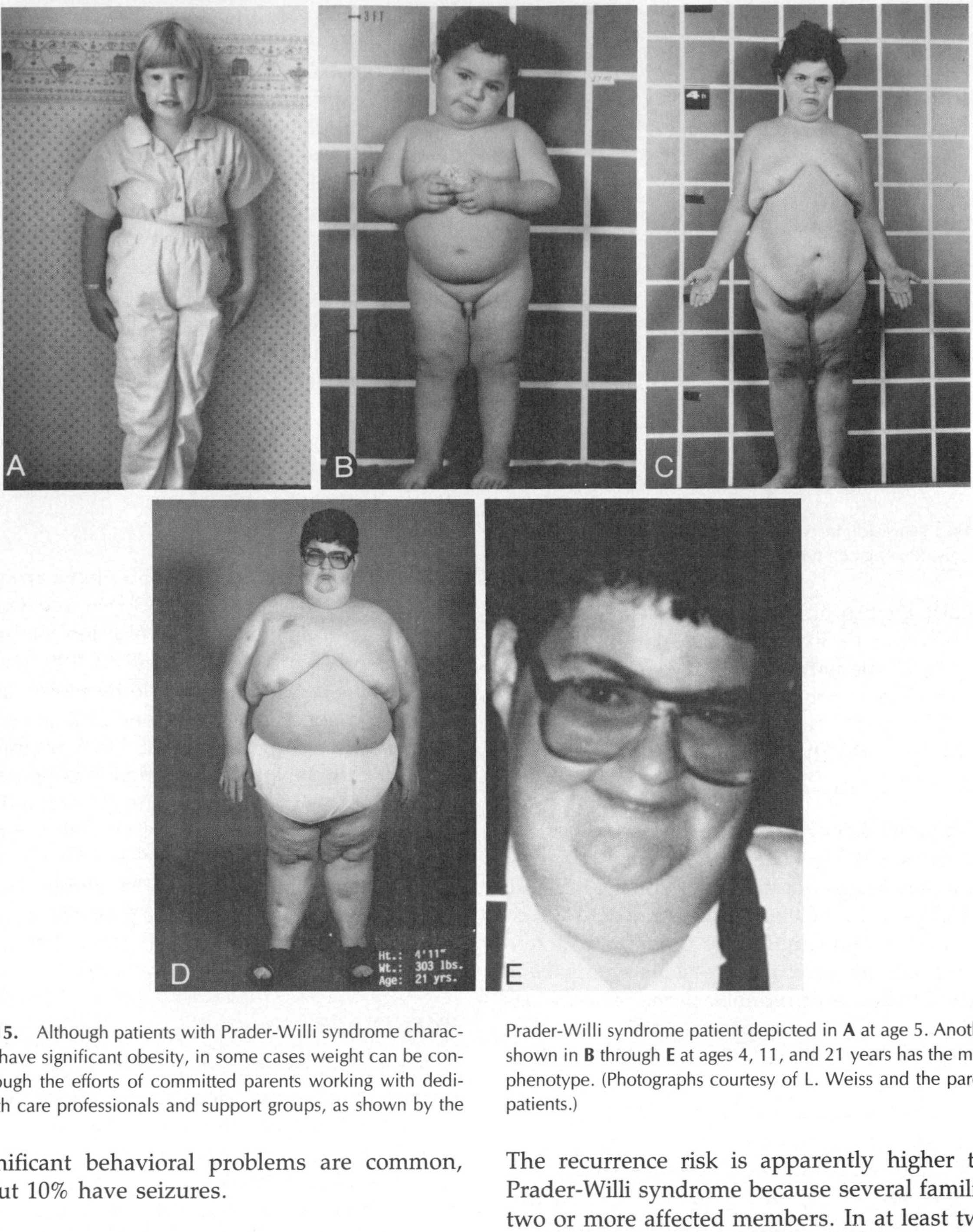

Figure 26.15. Although patients with Prader-Willi syndrome characteristically have significant obesity, in some cases weight can be controlled through the efforts of committed parents working with dedicated health care professionals and support groups, as shown by the Prader-Willi syndrome patient depicted in **A** at age 5. Another patient shown in **B** through **E** at ages 4, 11, and 21 years has the more typical phenotype. (Photographs courtesy of L. Weiss and the parents of the patients.)

65), significant behavioral problems are common, and about 10% have seizures.

Angelman's Syndrome (Happy Puppet Syndrome) del(15)(q11.2q12)

The incidence is about one in 25,000 births, perhaps somewhat lower, with most cases diagnosed after 2 years of age. This is a contiguous gene syndrome in which about 50% of patients have a de novo 15q11.2–q13 deletion or less common other rearrangement, and up to 85% have a deletion detectable by cytogenetic or molecular cytogenetic methods. The recurrence risk is apparently higher than for Prader-Willi syndrome because several families have two or more affected members. In at least two families the chromosome 15 pair appears normal in the affected siblings. Some families appear to show autosomal recessive inheritance of a defective gene at this or some other locus, and others have a chromosome 15 rearrangement that is unbalanced in the affected family members. The sex ratio is 1:1. Parental ages are not advanced.

PHENOTYPE

In Angelman's syndrome, there is microcephaly of postnatal onset, developmental delay, hypotonia

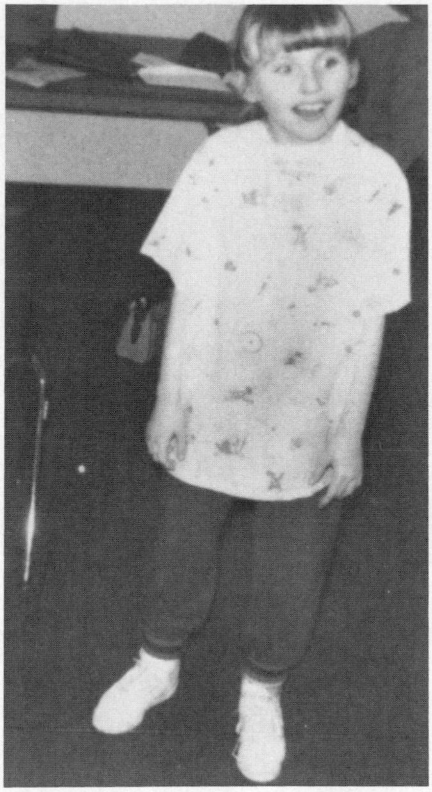

Figure 26.16. Patient with Angelman's syndrome. (Photograph courtesy of L. Weiss.)

with brisk reflexes, blue eyes and fair skin compared to other family members, and choroid and iris pigment hypoplasia (25% have oculocutaneous albinism). Seizures and an abnormal EEG are typical with onset by age 10 months. The diagnosis is usually not suspected until at least age 2, after the appearance of the characteristic hyperkinetic behavior with a stiff, ataxic gait. The facial expression is alert with frequent and inappropriate smiling and laughter. The ataxia, posture, and facial features led to the original designation of the condition as the "happy puppet syndrome" (Fig. 26.16). Mental retardation is severe.

UNIPARENTAL DISOMY IN PRADER-WILLI AND ANGELMAN'S SYNDROMES

The deletion in Angelman's syndrome tends to be larger than that in Prader-Willi syndrome, but the deleted segment cannot be distinguished from that in Prader-Willi syndrome using available DNA probes. However, whereas the deleted 15 is of paternal origin in Prader-Willi patients, its origin is maternal in all of the patients with Angelman's syndrome studied so far. Therefore, parental origin of the deletion appears to be a critical factor in the development of the phenotype in Prader-Willi and Angelman's syndromes. The reason for this can only be speculated at present. In experimental situations, the level of expression of some autosomal genes depends on the parental origin of the chromosome carrying the gene; this has been termed genomic imprinting. For Prader-Willi and Angelman's syndromes, imprinting of chromosome 15s by one parent has been proposed, with both an imprinted and an unimprinted copy of chromosome 15 being essential for normal development. The concept of genomic imprinting is consistent with the finding of two maternal copies and no paternal copies (termed maternal disomy) of chromosome 15 in the chromosomally normal Prader-Willi patients who have been studied so far. Another Prader-Willi patient with an apparently balanced robertsonian t(13;15) inherited from his mother also inherited his structurally normal 15 from his mother (termed maternal heterodisomy). Conversely, several chromosomally normal Angelman's syndrome patients have inherited two paternal and no maternal copies of chromosome 15. It is probable that in most patients with Prader-Willi or Angelman's syndrome who have structurally normal 15s the syndrome is due to maternal and paternal disomy, respectively, in which the gamete from one parent had disomy 15 and the other gamete had nullisomy 15, with fertilization providing a balanced chromosome 15 set except for the unusual parentage. Uniparental disomy cannot be very frequent because it depends on independent nondisjunctional events in both gametes, but it nevertheless appears to be a significant factor in these two syndromes and probably others yet to be identified. For Prader-Willi and Angelman's syndromes, molecular cytogenetic evaluation for deletion, and RFLP analysis for uniparental disomy appear to be reliable diagnostic tools.

Genomic imprinting has also been invoked as a model to explain the phenotypic differences described for triploids with two maternal versus two paternal contributions, and some of the peculiar features of expression of the fragile X chromosome (described below).

Secondary Trisomy 15q1-pter 47,+dic(15)(q1)

A dic(15)(q1) present as a 47th chromosome has been described in numerous patients with mental retardation, and we have identified at least four subjects since 1975. The phenotype depends to some degree on the amount of material duplicated, although a clear syndrome is not well defined as yet. In the smallest dicentrics, with a karyotype of 47,+dic(15)(q11.1), the two centromeres are very close together with little 15q material duplicated; such "bisatellited markers" are often familial and consistent with an entirely normal phenotype. Slightly larger dic(15)(q11.2) chromosomes are usually new mutations and

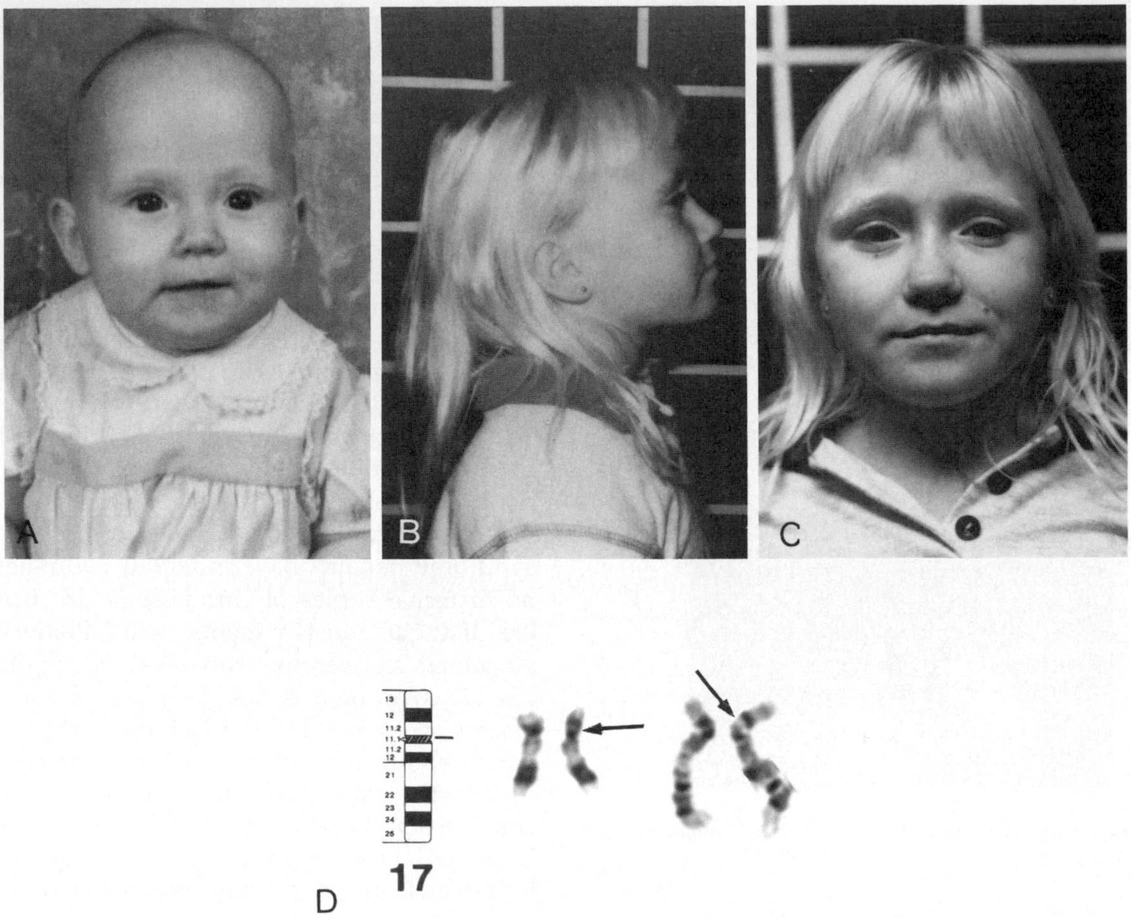

Figure 26.17. Patient with Smith-Magenis syndrome at age 9 months (**A**) and 8 years (**B** and **C**). She has an IQ of about 70 and suffers from a significant sleep disturbance. She has a de novo interstitial deletion involving band 17p11 only (**D**). Two chromosome 17 pairs are shown, with *arrows* pointing to band 17p11 in the normal homolog. The deletion homolog is at the left in each pair. (**A–C**, photographs courtesy of J. R. Roberson and L. Weiss.)

have been associated with mental retardation, including a few cases of Prader-Willi syndrome. In two patients with Prader-Willi syndrome the dicentric was of maternal origin. Still larger dic(15)(q12–q15) chromosomes that have an acrocentric appearance on G-banding are associated with mental retardation and mild dysmorphic features. They are typically new mutations, most often maternal in origin, and the average maternal age is advanced (mean 35 years).

Smith-Magenis Syndrome Deletion of Band 17p11

This uncommon contiguous gene syndrome is associated with an interstitial deletion involving band 17p11 only. Only about 50 cases have been identified in the United States. In all but one case the deletion represented a new mutation (the mother in one case appears to be mosaic), and the deletion apparently involves the paternal chromosome 17 in most cases. One mildly affected patient has a de novo translocation with a breakpoint within band 17p11.

PHENOTYPE

Failure to thrive is common. The phenotype is variable but includes brachycephaly, prominent forehead, microcephaly, flat and broad midface, broad nasal bridge, malformed ears, high or cleft palate, prognathism, short and broad hands and feet, scoliosis, and cryptorchidism (Fig. 26.17). The voice is hoarse and there may be hearing loss. Mental retardation is variable but usually severe with seizures, and hyperactivity. Unusual features of the syndrome include decreased reflexes, decreased sensation, and other features of peripheral neuropathy; specific self-destructive behavior, including insertion of foreign bodies into bodily orifices and pulling out finger and toe nails; and disturbed REM sleep that is most troublesome to the family because the patient sleeps very little, effectively requiring nearly 24-hour supervision.

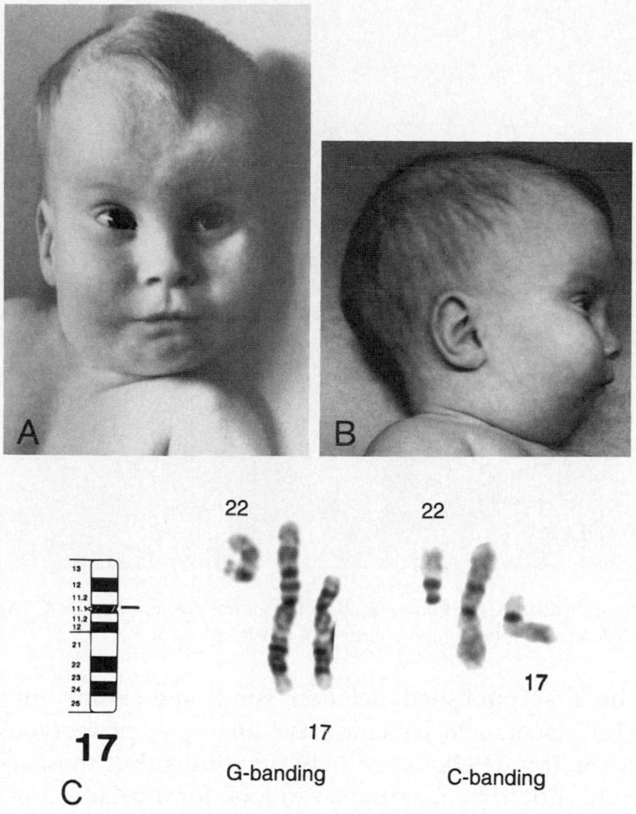

Figure 26.18. The sole Miller-Dieker syndrome patient identified by our laboratory had a de novo dicentric translocation between chromosomes 17 and 22. At age 12 months (**A** and **B**) she was beginning to smile socially but still had very poor head control. There may be as few as two genes deleted to create this syndrome, one probably more distal that is responsible for the lissencephaly and one more proximal that is responsible for the heart and kidney defects. Karyotype studies showed this patient had one normal copy of chromosomes 17 and 22. The other 17 and 22 were represented by a dicentric chromosome that contained most of 22p and appeared to have lost at least part of band 17p13. Two partial karyotypes are shown (**C**). Molecular genetic studies confirmed the deletion of this region and demonstrated the paternal origin of the chromosome rearrangement (unpublished results from David Ledbetter, Houston, TX). (**A, B,** photographs are courtesy of L. Weiss.)

Miller-Dieker Syndrome Deletion of Sub-band 17p13.3

This rare contiguous gene syndrome has been associated with the loss of sub-band 17p13.3, due to either a simple deletion or an unbalanced chromosome rearrangement. Several different rearrangements were identified by David Ledbetter and coworkers in the original families. This discovery excluded the originally proposed autosomal recessive mode of inheritance in most if not all cases. In de novo deletion cases, parental origin of the mutation can be either maternal or paternal. Nearly half of the patients have normal-appearing chromosomes even under high-resolution analysis, but studies using polymorphic DNA probes to 17p13.3 reveal a submicroscopic deletion of perhaps one million base pairs in 90%. In some patients with isolated lissencephaly, a submicroscopic deletion of the proximal segment of band 17p13.3 has been identified.

PHENOTYPE

A key feature is microcephaly and a prominent forehead with vertical skin furrowing and bitemporal narrowing (Fig. 26.18). The phenotype includes type I lissencephaly (cerebral agyria or smooth brain with a four-layered cortex), profound EEG abnormality, seizures, profound hypotonia, severe to profound mental retardation, and prenatal and postnatal growth retardation. Other facial features are ptosis, upturned nares, long philtrum with thin upper lip, mild micrognathia, and malformed ears. Heart and kidney defects are common. Most die in infancy. Isolated lissencephaly without the dysmorphic facial features is not Miller-Dieker syndrome and is not associated with a visible or submicroscopic deletion, although it may result from a point mutation within the postulated lissencephaly gene at the same locus.

Trisomy 18 (Edwards Syndrome)

Primary trisomy 18 is identified in one per 6000 to 8000 liveborns but is much more common among stillborns and represents about 6% of second-trimester miscarriages with an autosomal trisomy. Translocations are very uncommon. There is a maternal age effect, and the nondisjunctional event occurs during maternal meiosis in about 95% of cases. The sex ratio is about 4:1 female:male.

PHENOTYPE

Prenatal movement is weak, and polyhydramnios and a single umbilical artery are common. There is significant prenatal and postnatal growth retardation (Fig. 26.19). Newborns are hypotonic but later become hypertonic. The head is microcephalic with a prominent occiput, narrow midface, and micrognathia. Ears have a simple helix, the nose is small with upturned nares, and the mouth is small with a high-arched palate. Heart, kidney, and genitourinary tract malformations are common. The hands are typically clenched with the second finger overlapping the third finger, and fifth overlapping the fourth. Among the many other features of trisomy 18 syndrome are single palmar crease, multiple fingertips having a simple arch dermatoglyphic pattern, loose skin at the nape of the neck, hypoplastic nipples, dislocated hips, rocker-bottom feet, and diaphragmatic hernia. Mental retardation is profound. Half of liveborns die within 2 months and fewer than

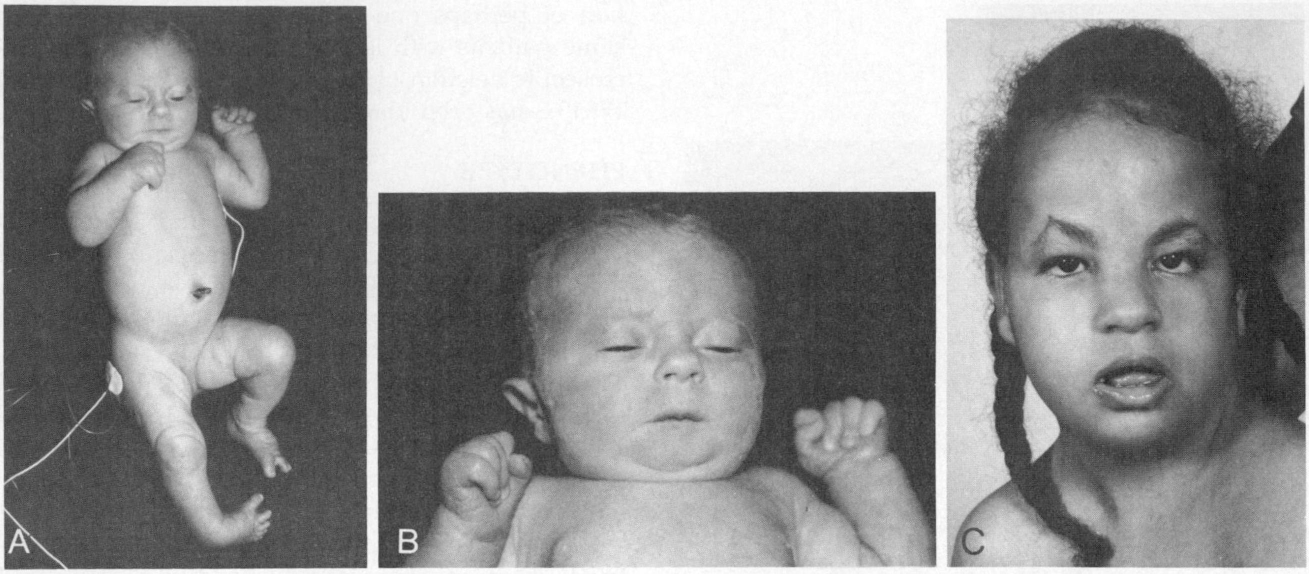

Figure 26.19. Infant (**A, B**) with trisomy 18. **C**, This 25 year-old female with nonmosaic trisomy 18 is one of the longest surviving patients with this syndrome. (**A, B**, photographs are courtesy of C. A. Williams. **C**, photograph courtesy of L. Weiss.)

10%, mostly girls, survive 1 year. Survival beyond age 5 is exceptional. Chromosomal mosaics with a normal cell line constitute about 10% of liveborns, and the phenotype can be somewhat moderated in these patients.

Secondary Trisomy 18p 47,+i(18p)

Patients with an extra isochromosome 18p are uncommon but have been seen by most large laboratories. Unlike most extra isochromosomes, mosaicism with a diploid line is unusual. Most are new mutations, but in one case the mother had a deleted 18p plus the isochromosome. The cytogenetic impression can be confirmed using a chromosome 18–specific DNA probe. The average maternal age (31 years) is advanced.

PHENOTYPE

Birth weight is normal or low. Craniofacial features include microcephaly, low-set and malformed ears, small nose with upturned nares, high-arched palate, and micrognathia. Facial asymmetry is common after infancy. Hands have campyodactyly, syndactyly, overlapping fingers, and contractures, and about half of patients have renal malformations. Infants are hypertonic and irritable and children have spasticity, an abnormal gait, moderate to severe mental retardation, and behavior problems.

Deletion 18p

Deletion of part of this small arm was identified before the use of banding techniques and in fact was the first published deletion syndrome. Some ring chromosome 18 patients have an 18p− phenotype. Most 18p deletions are new mutations, but the parents should be karyotyped to look for a balanced rearrangement. The average parental age is advanced, which is atypical for chromosome deletions and is unexplained. Slightly more females than males are affected. This has been said to be the most common deletion syndrome in humans.

PHENOTYPE

About 10 to 15% of patients have gross craniofacial malformations including holoprosencephaly, but in the patients without major brain malformations there are usually no life-threatening birth defects. The physical features include growth retardation and facial features of mild microcephaly, low-set, soft and malformed ears, strabismus, ptosis, epicanthus, flat nasal bridge, upturned nares, Cupid's bow of upper lip, and micrognathia. Dentition is poor and severe caries are very common. A short neck, broad chest, and mild edema of hands and feet can be reminiscent of Ullrich-Turner or Noonan's syndrome. Other features include hernias and IgA deficiency. Mental retardation is typical but severity varies.

Trisomy 20

This unusual trisomy is found in miscarriage specimens, and mosaic trisomy 20 is found in about 1 per 2500 amniotic fluid chromosome studies (9). There is no syndrome of birth defects associated with trisomy 20 mosaicism, and the majority of newborns have been phenotypically normal. The mosaicism has

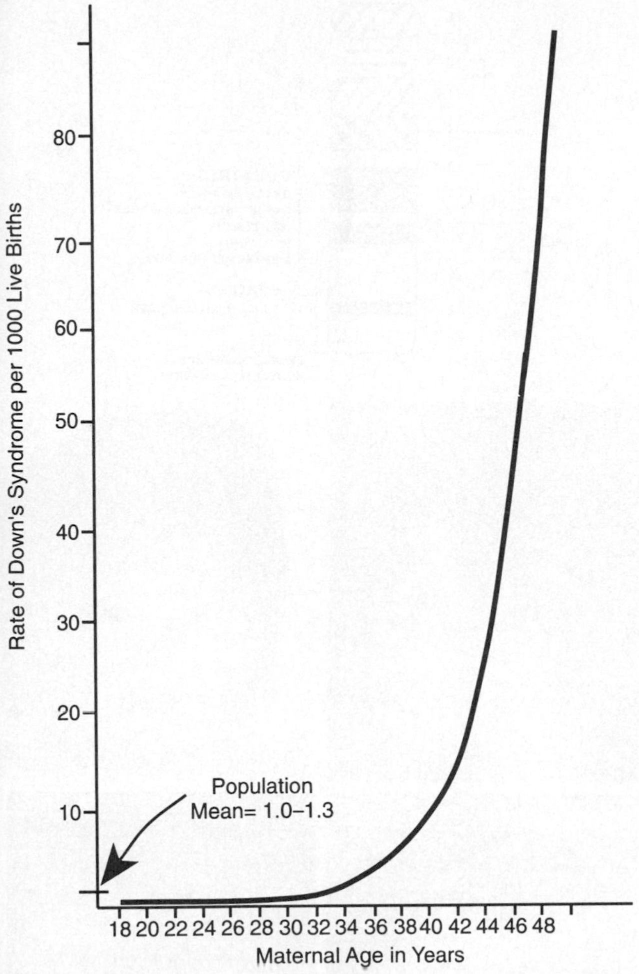

Figure 26.20. Frequency of Down's syndrome among livebirths, by maternal age. (Statistics from Hook EB. Cytogenetics: incidence, risks, and recurrence of chromosome abnormalities. In: Brock DJH, Rodeck C, Ferguson-Smith MA, eds. Prenatal diagnosis and screening. London: Churchill Livingstone, 1992:351–392.

been confirmed in foreskin fibroblasts and other tissues but never in peripheral blood cells. The risk of malformation or mental retardation seems low for cases identified prenatally, but this tissue-limited mosaicism is still poorly understood.

Trisomy 21 (Down's Syndrome)

One infant in 800 to 1000 has Down's syndrome (10–12). Primary trisomy 21 accounts for about 93% of all cases. Another 2 to 3% are mosaics, 3.5 to 5% have a robertsonian translocation, and fewer than 1% have other rearrangements. The sex ratio among Down's syndrome liveborns is about three males to two females. In 1960, 11% of births were to women over age 35, whereas this frequency is only about 5% today, and in the United States nearly half of pregnant women over age 35 obtain prenatal diagnosis. This has resulted in a small decrease in Down's syndrome births overall but a relative increase of Down's syndrome babies born to younger women. Screening the pregnant population for low maternal serum AFP, a risk factor for Down's syndrome, is decreasing the incidence of Down's syndrome further.

The maternal age effect in trisomy 21 is illustrated in Figure 26.20, and rates of Down's syndrome and other trisomies are provided in Table 26.3. There is also a maternal age effect in mosaic trisomy 21; this finding and other studies suggest that most mosaics begin as trisomic conceptions and anaphase lag gives rise to the diploid cell line. The normal cell line may have a selective growth advantage that results in an increase in the proportion of normal cells with age, especially in lymphocytes.

In a few trisomy cases (3% in one study, 0.3% in another study), one parent appears to be a trisomy 21 mosaic, and presumably the trisomy 21 offspring resulted from secondary nondisjunction. The incidence of parental mosaicism is probably greater among parents with more than one child with the same trisomy, and may be lower in older parents. The mosaic parents in general have normal intelligence and no obvious Down's syndrome stigmata. It has not become standard practice to study the chromosomes of parents of trisomy 21 patients, partly because it is impossible to disprove that a parent is a low-level mosaic, and partly because even if one or two +21 cells are observed among 100 cells, the chance remains that this is a technical artifact rather than a clear demonstration of +21 mosaicism. Instead, it seems reasonable based on the available data to advise the parents of a risk of recurrence of at most 1% over the maternal age-associated risk. Experience shows about a 0.5% recurrence risk for trisomy 21 plus 0.5% for other chromosome abnormalities (the latter risk does not appear to be significantly greater than the general population risk). It has also been proposed that a woman who has a trisomy 21 miscarriage has an increased risk of having a trisomy 21 liveborn, but the evidence for this, independent of maternal age effects, is weak. In general, other relatives of a trisomy 21 individual (e.g., siblings) do not have an increased risk of having a trisomy 21 child beyond their maternal age-associated risk.

The majority of translocations associated with Down's syndrome are t(14;21) or t(21;21). About half of t(14;21) cases are inherited but only 5% of t(21;21) cases are inherited (Table 26.7). This low frequency of inherited t(21;21) cases, together with recently presented molecular genetic studies, is consistent with the hypothesis that these are often isochromosomes rather than robertsonian translocations, but another factor in their high mutation rate is that a t(21;21) cannot be inherited through multiple generations. In most inherited cases the mother is the carrier, which is consistent with the observation of reduced fertility

Table 26.7. Robertsonian Translocations in Down's Syndrome[a]

	% of Cases[a]	% Inherited[b]	Risk to Carrier[c] Female	Male
			%	%
t(14;21)	51.7	50	14	4
t(13;21)	2.9	—[d]	—	—
t(15;21)	4.6	—	—	—
t(21;21)	37.2	5	100	100
t(21;22)	3.5	—	7	≤ 3

[a]Based on data in Therman E et al. The nonrandom participation of human acrocentric chromosomes in robertsonian translocations. Ann Hum Genet 1989;53:49–65, plus cases from our laboratory.
[b]Based on a sample of 4760 cases of Down's syndrome from Giraud F, Mattei JF. Aspects epidemiologiques de la trisomie 21. J Genet Hum 1975;23:1–30.
[c]Risk of bearing an offspring with Down's syndrome due to an unbalanced form of the translocation. Statistics for t(14;21) are from Daniel A, Hook EB, Wulf G. Risks of unbalanced progeny at amniocentesis to carriers of chromosome rearrangements: Data from United States and Canadian laboratories. Am J Med Genet 1989;33:14–53. Statistics for t(21;22) are from Chapman CJ, Gardner RJM, Veale AMO. Segregation analysis of a large t(21q22q) family. J Med Genet 1973;10:362–366.
[d]"—" indicates that the data are insufficient to make an estimate. The proportion of inherited t(13;21), t(15;21) and t(21;22) may be similar to that of t(14;21). The estimate for t(21;21) also includes our experience of 10 de novo and zero inherited cases. Still, the 5% seems to be an overestimate. When the translocation is inherited, it is much more often inherited from the mother than from the father.

in some carrier males and lower empirical risk of Down's syndrome in the offspring of carrier males. Recurrence has been reported in several instances of apparently de novo t(21;21) or other robertsonian translocation Down's syndrome cases, suggesting germ line mosaicism in a parent, and as with trisomy 21, it is reasonable to advise parents of de novo translocation cases that the risk of recurrence is roughly 1% over the maternal age-associated risk.

The increase in trisomy with advancing maternal age is reflected in a relative decrease in translocation cases with advancing maternal age. This is helpful in genetic counseling situations when the karyotype of the affected person and the parents is unknown and they are unavailable for evaluation. If the mother's age was under 30 when the affected person was born, the chance of a familial translocation is about 1.5%, whereas that chance is 0.4% if maternal age was 35 years, and 0.04% if maternal age was 40 years.

Rare patients with duplication of small segments of chromosome 21 have been instructive in the development of a "phenotype map" of chromosome 21 in which duplication of band 21q22.3 is essential for the expression of the Down's syndrome phenotype (Fig. 26.21**A**). Although a very large number of unrelated genes are duplicated in trisomy 21, investigators such as Charles Epstein (San Francisco) and Julie Korenberg (Los Angeles) are making progress in understanding the relationship between specific genes on chromosome 21 and the Down's syndrome phenotype. One line of investigation is to use a mouse model: mouse chromosome 16 contains many of the same genes as human chromosome 21, and trisomy 16 in the mouse has many comparable birth defects.

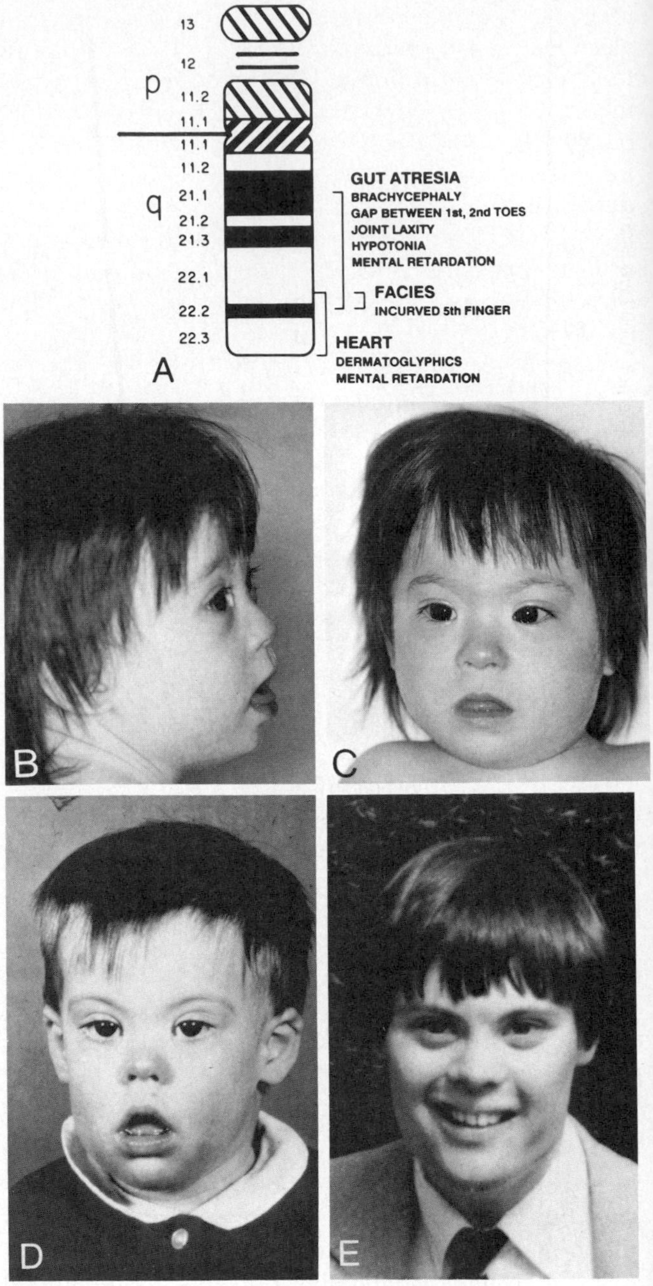

Figure 26.21. The phenotype of Down's syndrome. In **A**, individual stigmata of the Down's syndrome phenotype have been mapped by molecular analysis of small duplications involving chromosome 21. In **B, C,** and **D**, the childhood phenotype is illustrated, showing many of the features detailed in the text. The male shown in **D** is shown in **E** at age 18 years. (**B** and **C**, photographs courtesy of D. D. Weaver and C. A. Moore; **D** and **E**, photographs courtesy of L. Weiss and J. R. Roberson.)

PHENOTYPE

As many as 75% of trisomy 21 conceptions result in miscarriage (cf. Table 26.2), and 1% of stillborns have trisomy 21. Among trisomy 21 pregnancies identified by mid-trimester amniocentesis and not electively interrupted, about one-fourth abort spontaneously or are stillborn. There is significant prenatal and postnatal growth retardation with reduced birth weight. Heart defects, mainly endocardial cushion defects (atrial or ventricular septal defect, patent ductus arteriosus, or tetralogy of Fallot) are present in 40% of subjects. The facial features in Down's syndrome commonly include a round and flat face, ear malformations such as a folded upper helix, epicanthus, upward-slanting palpebral fissures, Brushfield spots, flat nasal bridge, and open mouth with a protruding tongue (Fig. 28.21B–D). The hands frequently have a transverse palmar crease, short fifth finger with a single flexion crease, and clinodacytly. There is often a gap between toes 1 and 2. Many have an umbilical hernia. Radiologically, there is a small pelvis with hypoplastic iliac wings and small acetabular angle. A multitude of less-common birth defects in Down's syndrome include strabismus, cataracts, duodenal atresia, imperforate anus, and an increased risk of leukemia.

Newborns are hypotonic, especially if a heart defect is present, and have poor reflexes. Many have loose skin on the back of the neck that is a remnant of prenatal lymphatic edema. They do not have a significant adolescent growth spurt. Adolescents and adults have short stature (standard growth charts for Down's syndrome are available in Cronk et al.) (13). A tendency to be overweight is typical. Hypothyroidism is common (and treatable) among infants and children with Down's syndrome. There is also an increased risk of diabetes mellitus, depression, premature aging of the skin, and dementia.

Only one male is known to have reproduced (one chromosomally normal offspring). Females have reproduced and about 40% of their offspring have had Down's syndrome due to secondary nondisjunction. (The expected 50% risk is not met, perhaps because of reduced viability of the +21 embryos.) Congenital heart disease and heart failure, respiratory tract infection, intestinal obstruction, and leukemia are major factors in mortality. Of patients without heart defects, 90% survive 1 year and 80% survive to age 30. Those who have heart disease are smaller on average, with 75% surviving 1 year and 50% to age 30. Only 45% of Down's syndrome patients are expected to survive to age 60, compared to 86% of the general population.

Developmental delay is not always evident until after age 1, since the infants tend to be content and only modestly delayed in milestones that are normally attained by 12 to 18 months. Mental retardation is usually mild to moderate, and children are often placed in education programs for the trainably or educably mentally impaired. In institutionalized populations, there is an excess of males among the Down's syndrome patients, probably because affected males present more severe behavior problems. Whereas most were institutionalized years ago, today adults with Down's syndrome live with family or in a group home, and many work in sheltered situations. As marketplace demands increase for unskilled labor, an increasing number of adults with Down's syndrome are finding employment in cafeterias, hotels, laundries, and similar industries.

Many patients with Down's syndrome become afflicted with an Alzheimer-like disease at a relatively early age, and an autosomal dominantly inherited form of Alzheimer's disease is apparently caused by a defective β-amyloid precursor protein gene localized to chromosome 21q11–q22. The nature of the mutation is unclear, but recent findings seem to exclude a simple duplication in the familial form of Alzheimer's disease.

As is true of other mosaics, the phenotype of trisomy 21 mosaics is not as severe as with full trisomy 21, with fewer major malformations. As stated earlier, a few individuals with low level +21 mosaicism have been identified after having a Down's syndrome child. Nevertheless, infants who are karyotyped because they have Down's syndrome clinically and then are shown to be mosaics do in general remain clinically indistinguishable from their nonmosaic counterparts.

Cat's Eye Syndrome Secondary Trisomy 22q11-pter

Patients with this phenotype often have a de novo extra bisatellited chromosome derived from chromosome 22 (an example of a bisatellited chromosome 15 is provided in Fig. 26.3). In situ hybridization using a chromosome 22q11 DNA probe has shown that this band is consistently duplicated. Although the defect usually arises de novo, in two cases of cat's eye syndrome the parent carried the extra isochromosome but had normal intelligence and a diagnosis of Duane's syndrome (radial ray abnormalities and deafness). Maternal origin of the de novo extra chromosome was shown in at least two cases. Tissue-dependent mosaicism is probable—one patient had 3% normal cells in lymphocytes, but 70% of cultured fibroblasts had normal chromosomes.

PHENOTYPE

The common facial features are coloboma of the iris, down-slanting palpebral fissures, preauricular tag or pit, and imperforate anus. None of these features are seen in every instance, however. Mental retardation is usually mild to moderate, but congenital heart disease or severe kidney defects can cause death in infancy.

DiGeorge Syndrome
Deletion of Band 22q11

A chromosome abnormality is identified in 20% of patients with this contiguous gene syndrome. Half of these have a deletion involving band 22q11, and the remainder have a deletion of 10p13 or other deletion or duplication. The deletion frequently results from an unbalanced form of a familial translocation. Thus far, all chromosome 22 deletions have involved the maternally inherited copy.

PHENOTYPE

Many of the malformations result from a sequence of flawed embryonic development due to a defect involving the third and fourth branchial arches. Patients have thymic and parathyroid hypoplasia with associated hypocalcemia, seizures and cellular immune deficiency, and aortic arch and conotruncal heart defects. Affected individuals often have a "pixie face" with low-set ears and hypertelorism, and cleft lip and palate are common. Most patients die in infancy because of the heart defects or severe infections. Survivors who have a visible chromosome defect have mild to moderate mental retardation. Patients with other birth defects, such as diaphragmatic hernia, or severe mental retardation may have deletion of a larger segment from chromosome 22.

Tertiary Trisomy from t(11;22)(q23;q11.2)

A European collaborative study has identified over 100 families with this particular translocation. Our laboratory has identified five unrelated families, three through prenatal genetic studies and two through studies of couples with multiple miscarriages. Many families have been identified through an abnormal proband who carries an extra small chromosome (Fig. 26.7), and the risk of 3:1 meiotic segregation is 5%, with the vast majority of the affected individuals having 47 chromosomes with two normal 11s and 22s plus the small derived 22 from the translocation. The net result is duplication of proximal 22q and distal 11q. Many patients have diploid/trisomy mosaicism, and extra care must be exercised in prenatal studies of these families to identify affected mosaics. The carrier parent is the mother in about 90% of cases, and many males have reduced fertility. A peculiar pattern of segregation has also been observed in female carriers: nearly 70% of the normal offspring of carriers are themselves carriers, and more than half of the carrier progeny are females. This deviation from randomness is not yet understood. The pattern of segregation to offspring of male carriers appears to be normal.

PHENOTYPE

The phenotype includes hypotonia, microcephaly, malformed ears with preauricular pits and tags, cleft or high-arched palate, micrognathia, dislocated hips, anal atresia or anal stenosis, and cryptorchidism. Two-thirds have congenital heart defects (atrial or ventricular septal defect or patent ductus arteriosus). Mental retardation is moderate to severe.

SEX CHROMOSOME SYNDROMES

As reviewed in Chapter 25, our understanding of the sex chromosomes has improved greatly over the past few years. Males have an X and a Y chromosome and females have two X chromosomes, one of which is inactivated to compensate for the single-X dosage in males. Most of the genes on the X and the Y are unique to each, but some are shared. Many of the genes that are shared by the X and the Y are not inactivated on the "inactive" X in females, and are confined to the pseudoautosomal region on distal Xp and Yp. Other recently described genes that reside in proximal Xp and Xq are expressed on both the active and the inactive X, and these also appear to have counterparts on the Y, thus maintaining the equivalence of gene expression between the sexes. A small number of expressed genes on the Y, including SRY (sex determining region of Y), appear to be responsible for male sexual differentiation. As our understanding of these various groups of X- and Y-linked genes improves, so will our understanding of their effects in the sex chromosome syndromes (14).

Monosomy X and Structural Abnormalities of the X Chromosome

The incidence of monosomy X is about one in 3000 newborns. An apparently nonmosaic 45,X chromosomal constitution is identified in 50% of girls with Ullrich-Turner syndrome, 15% have some 46,XX cells (45,X/46,XX mosaicism), 20% have an isochromosome Xq, 10% have mosaicism with a Y chromosome (45,X/46,XY), and most of the remainder have X or Y rearrangements (e.g., deletions, rings, isochromosomes). Among 45,X cases, the nondisjunctional event results from loss of the paternal X in the majority (70 to 80%). This is a striking difference from the more frequent maternal meiotic error associated with autosomal trisomy.

X chromosome deletions, rings, translocations, and other rearrangements are seen in some women with primary or secondary amenorrhea who do not have other features of Ullrich-Turner syndrome. Al-

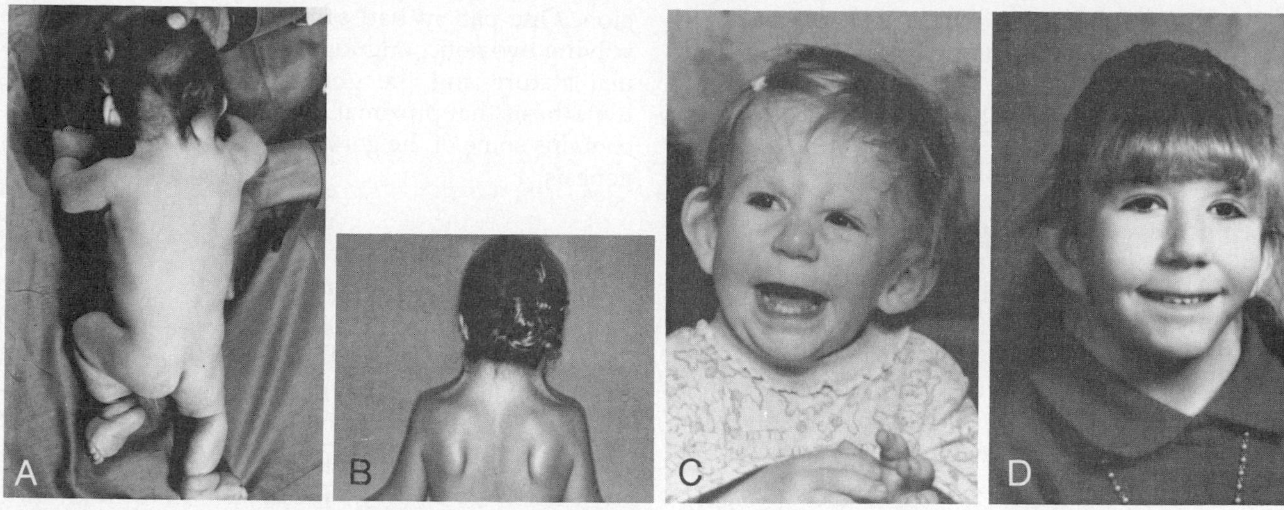

Figure 26.22. **A**, Ullrich-Turner syndrome in infancy is sometimes suspected on the basis of lymphedema involving the hands and feet and loose skin at the back of the neck. **B**, Neck webbing is shown in an older patient. The girl depicted in **C** and **D** at ages 16 months and 11 years is a well-adapted middle school student. (Photographs are courtesy of L. Weiss.)

though structural X abnormalities represent less than 10% of all Ullrich-Turner syndrome patients, if women with primary or secondary amenorrhea without the Ullrich-Turner phenotype are included, about 25% of all females with an X abnormality are of these variant types.

PHENOTYPE

The phenotype of Ullrich-Turner syndrome patients is variable, and depends in large measure on the karyotype (Fig. 26.22). The nearly universal features are decreased birth weight and short stature (in the range of the fifth percentile on a growth curve), and gonadal dysgenesis. Common features (25 to 75% of cases) include high-arched palate; visual defects (usually strabismus); webbed or short, broad neck; low posterior hairline; shield chest; pigmented nevi; cubitus valgus; short fourth metacarpal; and thyroid disease. Lymphedema is common and is severe in abortuses and stillborns. One-third of patients have bicuspid aortic valves, and 12% have other severe heart defects such as a ventricular septal defect or coarctation of the aorta. Over half have kidney malformations (including double collecting system, malrotation, or malformation), making recurrent urinary tract infections common, although life-threatening renal malfunction is uncommon.

In a population survey of consecutive newborns, 13 subjects with a 45,X chromosomal constitution were identified. Three of the 13 died neonatally and one died at age 11. All four of these had serious congenital heart disease. Of the nine survivors, five had multiple stigmata of Ullrich-Turner syndrome, two had pedal edema only, and two had high-arched palate only.

The majority of Ullrich-Turner syndrome patients have streak gonads at birth; their ovaries appear normal at 12 weeks of gestation, but the ovarian follicles degenerate after that time. One-fifth of Ullrich-Turner syndrome patients have spontaneous menstruations, and most of these are 45,X/46,XX mosaics. The available data on their pregnancy outcomes suggest a high risk for miscarriage and 45,X liveborns, and possibly an increased risk of trisomy 21.

Mosaic individuals have a better prognosis, including lower risk of Ullrich-Turner syndrome stigmata and lower risk for gonadal dysgenesis, whereas 45,X without obvious mosaicism is more often associated with Ullrich-Turner syndrome. Ring X and isochromosome X patients usually have features of Ullrich-Turner syndrome, but these patients typically have a 45,X cell line as well. Many females with Xq deletions are less severely affected. A few patients with Xq deletion have been fertile, and the chance of fertility may depend on the breakpoint or perhaps to a greater extent on whether a 45,X or 46,XX cell line mosaicism is present. Those with Xp deletions often have features of Ullrich-Turner syndrome, including short stature and primary or secondary amenorrhea, although a few have been fertile.

The incidence of mental retardation among patients with Ullrich-Turner syndrome is not dramatically increased, and the majority have normal intelligence. They are more likely to have problems with spatial relations and numerical identification. There is often a deficiency in perceptual motor organization or in fine motor execution. Therefore the nonverbal IQ is lower than the verbal IQ. Personality traits commonly include inertia to emotional arousal, a high capacity to deal with stress, and strong traditional femininity. An increased risk of mental retardation is, however, associated with ring X mosaicism if the ring is very small, and some females with X/autosome translocations have mental retardation.

45,X/46,XY Mosaicism

The phenotype of 45,X/46,XY mosaics is extremely varied, ranging from typical Ullrich-Turner syndrome to ambiguous genitalia to normal male. Females with a 45,X/46,XY karyotype or ring (Y) cell line have a 15 to 25% risk of gonadoblastoma. The gonads of XY mosaics should be removed before school age because of this risk. Molecular studies are in progress to determine the frequency of low-level Y-positive mosaicism in Ullrich-Turner syndrome subjects who have cytogenetically nonmosaic 45,X. Further studies will be required to determine whether these low-level 46,XY mosaics have an increased risk of gonadoblastoma. A large number of phenotypically normal males with 45,X/46,XY mosaicism have been identified in prenatal studies, but their fertility has not been evaluated, as they have not yet reached reproductive age. However, this mosaicism does not appear to be overrepresented in studies of male infertility, nor is there an increased risk of gonadoblastoma in phenotypically normal males who have 45,X/46,XY mosaicism.

46,XY Females

Females with nonmosaic 46,XY typically have gonadal dysgenesis and little secondary sexual development but few other features of Ullrich-Turner syndrome, and a high risk of developing gonadoblastoma. The majority of 46,XY females have a structurally normal X and Y chromosome, and have a mendelian inherited disorder of sexual differentiation, such as testicular feminization syndrome (X-linked recessive) or 5α-reductase deficiency (autosomal recessive). As mendelian traits, such disorders carry a significant risk of recurrence.

A few 46,XY females have been identified with del(Y) (p11) who are probably affected because their Y chromosome has lost the sex-determining region of the Y chromosome. Females with a Y chromosome deletion are more likely to exhibit some of the features of Ullrich-Turner syndrome, although most appear to have normal stature. As with the nondeletion cases, there is a high risk of gonadoblastoma. In distinction to the nondeletion cases, the Y deletions are not known to have an increased risk of recurrence in a family. Molecular genetic studies by Christine Disteche and coworkers showed that Yp-specific DNA probes did not hybridize with the deleted Y chromosome. The deletion breakpoints differed slightly, but the deletions overlapped in the sex-determining region. One patient had a more complex deletion involving two noncontiguous DNA segments. The normal stature and the gonadoblastoma support the hypothesis that proximal Yp or the long arm of the Y contains some of the genes for stature and spermatogenesis.

Triple X Syndrome 47,XXX

The incidence of 47,XXX is about one in 1000 liveborn females. There is a maternal age effect, with maternal meiosis I errors in 50% of cases; paternal errors account for fewer than 10% of cases. Triple X women do not appear to have an increased risk for having XXX or XXY offspring. The phenotype typically is within normal limits, with development of secondary sexual characteristics and normal fertility. Many but not all triple X females are developmentally normal, although the exact risk of mild or more severe mental retardation is uncertain. Among females with mild mental retardation, the frequency of triple X is increased to about one in 200. Ten 47,XXX females who were identified in unselected newborn surveys have been followed to age 20 to 22 (15). As children, they had less motor coordination and more speech and language problems than their peers, but standard speech therapy seems to have been sufficient for most of them. One was in a school program for the educationally mentally impaired, three were mainstreamed with some remedial education, and six were in regular classes. Four of the 10 have an IQ of 60 to 80, so in this small, unselected sample 40% had mild mental retardation. At age 20 to 22 years, nine of the 10 appear to cope well in society, and hold a job or have a family.

Klinefelter's Syndrome 47,XXY

The incidence of 47,XXY is about one in 700 male newborns. Because of the maternal age effect in 47,XXX and 47,XXY, these karyotypes are seen more frequently in prenatal genetic studies. For 47,XXY, maternal and paternal meiotic errors are responsible in about equal proportions.

PHENOTYPE

The phenotype of Klinefelter's syndrome includes tall stature, small testicles and prostate, and infertility. Half have a eunuchoid habitus and half have gynecomastia. A few have a varicocele, undescended testes, or a small penis.

The diagnosis of Klinefelter's syndrome is usually made during adolescence or adulthood because of small testicles, gynecomastia, or infertility. Mosaics, mostly 46,XY/47,XXY, constitute about 10% of Klinefelter patients, and as a group have milder symptoms. Most have azoospermia and most of those who have oligospermia are chromosomal mosaics. As children, many have mild speech and language deficits, which respond to standard speech therapy. They also tend to have a poor attention span and memory, and low self-esteem. Early educational intervention appears to be effective in overcoming these potential liabilities. Nielsen and Sorensen in Denmark (16) have recommended mass newborn screening to identify infants with X chromosome aneuploidy and institute early topical testosterone therapy for XXY infants who have a small penis. Twelve men with Klinefelter's syndrome who were identified in unselected newborn surveys have been followed to age 20 to 22. Eight had a normal IQ and have coped well in society. Four had IQs of 80 to 90, and had learning problems in school. Two of these men were said to cope well as adults and have found employment. The other two had psychiatric problems as well as learning difficulties and were said not to cope well. Nevertheless, the XXY men as a group were said to be not as severely affected as the XXX women.

More severely affected variants of XXY include 48,XXYY; 49,XXXYY; 49,XXXXY, and other karyotypes. Their cumulative incidence is probably about one in 2500 males. Hypogonadism is present, and cryptorchidism is more common. Adult height is over 6 feet (180 cm) in 80% of variants, and skeletal abnormalities are not uncommon. Mental retardation is more likely than in 47,XXY, and is more severe.

46,XX Males

The incidence of 46,XX males is about one in 20,000 liveborn males. These are phenotypic males who have normal or slightly shorter stature and normal external genitalia, but who have reduced testosterone levels, reduced facial and body hair, dysgenetic testes, and azoospermia, and may have gynecomastia. There is strong cytogenetic and molecular genetic evidence favoring an aberrant paternal meiotic exchange between the X and Y chromosomes, such as unequal meiotic exchange, resulting in an X;Y rearrangement. Some of these are cytogenetically visible (see Fig. 25.32). Many other XX males have molecular evidence of a rearrangement between the X and Y that results in the sex-determining region of the Y being moved to one X chromosome, i.e., Yp-specific DNA is present. A minority of XX males (10%) do not have evidence of Yp-specific DNA, and their phenotype includes gynecomastia and hypospadias or a small penis.

47,XYY Males

The frequency of XYY is about one in 800 males, with no maternal age effect since the nondisjunctional event occurs during male meiosis or as a postzygotic error. Stature is taller than average; one in 200 males over 6 feet (180 cm) have an XYY constitution. Fertility appears to be normal in most but not all cases, since about 1% of men with oligospermia have XYY. The personality is described as impulsive in nature but variable in how that is expressed. Some XYY males are overtly aggressive and others are timid and have autistic features. For reasons that are not entirely clear, about one in 200 prisoners have 47,XYY. As children, XYY boys tend to have a high activity level, poor emotional control, and a weak self-concept, and tend to be clumsy and easily frustrated. There may be a higher frequency of XYY boys with severe behavior disorders, and on average, the IQ appears to be slightly lower. However, most XYY males have intelligence and personality traits within normal limits. The frequency of tall stature, lower IQ, and criminal records is similar in XYY and XXY males, so the phenotype cannot be attributed directly to the extra Y chromosome. Early intervention education programs may be useful in 47,XYY as well as in 47,XXX and 47,XXY.

FRAGILE X SYNDROME

FRA-X, Martin-Bell Syndrome, X-Linked Mental Retardation with Fragile X Chromosome

This is not a classic cytogenetic syndrome, caused by gain or loss of a chromosomal segment (17). Rather, under certain conditions of tissue culture (see Methods section), fragile X patients express a chromosome break at sub-band Xq27.3 in 4 to 50% of leukocyte metaphases (Fig. 26.23). Estimates vary, but the fragile X syndrome (FRA-X) appears to be expressed in 1 per 1200 to 1500 males and 1 per 2000 females. Many more females carry the fragile X chromosome but are not affected with the syndrome. The fragile X syndrome accounts for about 5% of mental retardation among males, and 40 to 50% of all X-linked mental retardation. The total frequency of fragile X syndrome in the population is often compared with that of Down's syndrome.

The pattern of inheritance of the fragile X syndrome is X-linked. Although 80% of males with the gene are retarded, the penetrance of the gene (odds of retardation in one who inherits the fragile X) is further complicated because expression of the phenotype depends partly on which parent transmits the gene (Table 26.8). The risk of retardation in new

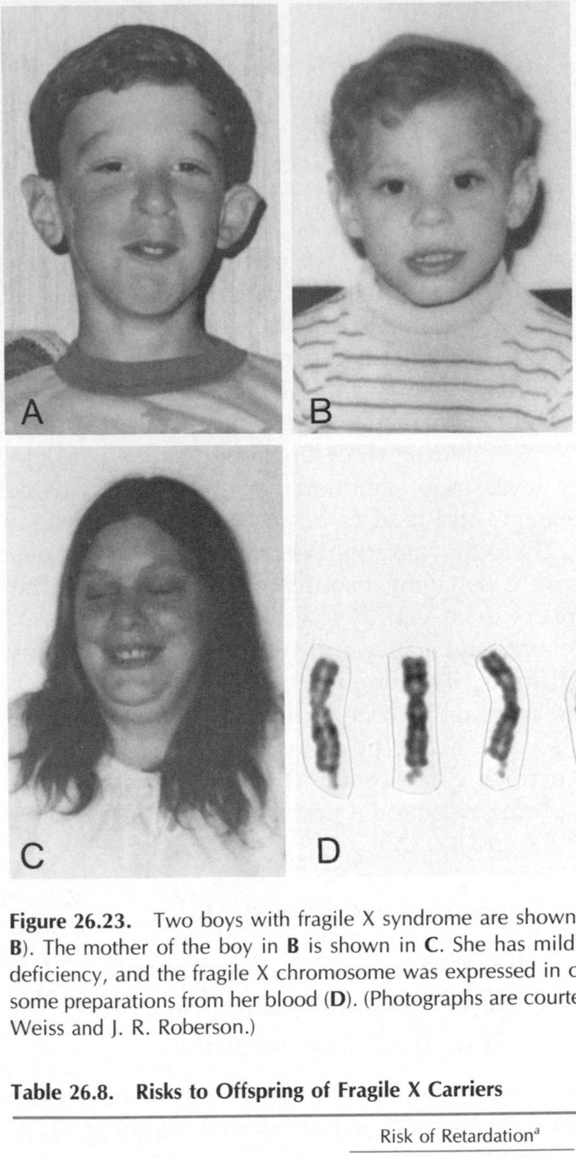

Figure 26.23. Two boys with fragile X syndrome are shown (**A** and **B**). The mother of the boy in **B** is shown in **C**. She has mild mental deficiency, and the fragile X chromosome was expressed in chromosome preparations from her blood (**D**). (Photographs are courtesy of L. Weiss and J. R. Roberson.)

Table 26.8. Risks to Offspring of Fragile X Carriers

	Risk of Retardation[a]	
Carrier Parent	Son	Daughter
	%	%
Father is a transmitting male	—	<4
Mother is a normal carrier	38	16
Mother is a retarded carrier	50	27

[a]The carrier mother has a 50% risk of transmitting the gene to each offspring. The transmitting male transmits the fragile X chromosome to all of his daughters but none of his sons. Estimates are based on Weaver DD, Sherman SL. A counseling guide to the Martin-Bell syndrome. Am J Med Genet 1987;26:39–44, Sherman SL, et al. Further segregation analysis of the fragile X syndrome with special reference to transmitting males. Hum Genet 1985;69:289–299.

mutants appears to be exceedingly low. There are many pedigrees with unaffected males who have transmitted the gene to their daughters. Most of these "transmitting males" have 0 to 5% fragile X cells in culture, and their obligate carrier daughters are normal and have 0 to 5% fragile X cells in culture. Many of these obligate carrier daughters have affected offspring. Most carrier females inherit the fragile X from their mothers, and although estimates vary, 25% of carrier females express the fragile X and have mental retardation, 25% express the fragile X but have borderline to normal intelligence, and 50% have normal intelligence and do not express the fragile X. Thus, about two-thirds of the carriers who have normal intelligence do not express the fragile X.

The gene (familial mental retardation 1, FMR1) that is associated with fragile X syndrome was identified in 1991. The common mutation in FMR1 involves instability in a repeating DNA sequence, $(CGG)_n$, the length of which is increased in fragile X syndrome. Most normal individuals have 2 to 50 repeats of the sequence. Phenotypically normal carrier females and transmitting males have 50 to 200 copies. This increase is termed a premutation, because it precedes the development of the full mutation in future generations. In fragile X syndrome, more than 200 more copies of the CGG repeat are found. Although cytosines within the mutated gene are highly methylated in affected individuals and unmethylated in premutation carriers, the clinical significance of methylation is unclear. Likewise, the association between phenotype and preferential X chromosome inactivation in females with the full mutation is unclear. The FMR1 mutation continues to be the focus of active research. Molecular assays have been developed that can identify the number of repeats within the FMR1 gene (18), and thereby differentiate between normal individuals and carriers of the premutation and full mutation. These assays are likely to replace the cytogenetic assays for fragile X syndrome. Related research findings suggest that other disorders that exhibit a "maternal effect"—such as myotonic dystrophy, Kennedy's disease, Huntington's disease and spinocerebellar ataxia—have a similar class of mutation (19, 20).

Prenatal testing for fragile X is available (21). The relatively high frequency of fragile X syndrome among the mentally retarded, the familial nature of the syndrome, and the availability of family screening and prenatal diagnosis combine to present a compelling case in support of screening programs for fragile X syndrome by state and regional health departments. In a survey of a developmental center in Saint Clair County, Michigan, we identified fragile X syndrome in 6% of the mentally retarded subjects (4% of the families) who were screened. Population studies in New South Wales, Australia, have identified 79 probable carrier women who did not know they were at risk, and who may now make informed decisions about childbearing.

PHENOTYPE

The phenotype is variable and can be subtle. There are no major birth defects, but perinatal complications (e.g., premature birth, asphyxia, or seizures) are rather common and there is evidence of a high rate of sudden infant death syndrome. Intrauterine or postnatal growth deficiency is not characteristic, although adult males average 3 to 5 cm shorter than their normal brothers. Head circumference is often large at birth, leading to occasional confusion with Sotos' syndrome (cerebral gigantism).

Over half of the affected males and females, and even some normal-IQ female carriers and transmitting males, have features consistent with a connective tissue defect, including hyperextensible joints and skin, velvety soft skin texture, a high palate, pectus excavatum, large ears, and flat feet. After puberty, a long and narrow face, a prominent jaw and nasal bridge, and mitral valve prolapse become more evident. Macroorchidism is also common, especially after puberty. Mean testicular volume in fragile X males is 40 ml (most of the sample were Caucasian) compared to a mean of 15 ml, 20 ml, and 30 ml in normal oriental, Caucasian, and black males. Carrier females have been reported to have large ovaries.

The personality is variable, with hyperactive, extremely anxious and tremulous behavior common. Perhaps 10 to 20% of males who are characterized as autistic have fragile X syndrome. Although most fragile X males do not have classic autism, some do exhibit autistic features such as poor eye contact, characteristic speech patterns, and anxiety.

The IQ in affected males is highly variable with a mean of 50. Verbal IQ is 15 points lower than performance IQ. Those with seizures (10 to 15%) have a lower mean IQ. The average IQ is higher in affected females. As a partial explanation for the IQ variability in carrier females, there is limited evidence of a correlation between intelligence and the proportion of cells that have the FRA-X chromosome genetically inactivated.

INDICATIONS FOR CHROMOSOME STUDIES (SUBPOPULATIONS)

Miscarriages, Stillbirths, and Livebirths

Miscarriage occurs in roughly 15% of all recognized pregnancies, with stillbirth representing another 1%. A chromosome abnormality is observed in 11% of stillbirths and 5% of perinatal deaths, compared with less than 1% of liveborns. Although the frequency of chromosome abnormalities is highest in macerated or malformed fetuses, many anatomic defects are not obvious, particularly those associated with trisomy 18, which constitutes about 25% of chromosome defects in stillborns. Therefore, it is appropriate to karyotype all stillbirths as part of a formal protocol that should also include family and obstetrical history, photographs of the face and any malformations, a whole body x-ray, bacterial cultures, and autopsy. When malformation or a chromosome abnormality is identified, genetic counseling is warranted. The resources are unavailable to karyotype all miscarriage specimens, but for couples with two or more pregnancy losses it is appropriate to carry out chromosome studies of the abortus as well as peripheral blood karyotype studies of the couple.

Table 26.9. Incidence of Chromosome Abnormalities in Miscarriages and Stillborns Compared to Newborns[a]

	Miscarriages[b]	Stillborns	Newborns
	%	%	%
Normal karyotype	50	95	99.
Abnormal karyotype	50	5	0.
Tetraploid	2.5	≪1%	—
Triploid	7	0.2	—
Trisomy (autosomal)	30	3.0	0.14
+22	2.8	—	—
+21	2.6	0.8	0.
+18	1.8	1.4	0.01
+16	9.9	—	—
+15	2.3	—	—
+13	1.5	0.5	0.
all other	9.1	0.3	0.
Monosomy X	8.6	0.05	0.01
XXX, XXY, XYY, variants	0.6	0.5	0.2
Other	3	1.4	0.4

[a]Statistics compiled from Angell RR et al. Chromosome variation in perinatal mortality: a survey of 500 cases. J Med Genet 1984;21:39–44; Simpson and Bombard in Bennett MJ, Edmonds DK, eds. Spontaneous and recurrent abortion. Oxford: Blackwell Scientific Publications, 1987; and Hook EB, Hamerton JL. The frequency of chromosome abnormalities detected in consecutive newborn studies—differences between studies—results by sex and severity of phenotypic involvement. In: Hook EB, Porter IH, eds. Population cytogenetics studies in humans. New York: Academic Press, 1977:63–79.
[b]Mostly first-trimester miscarriages.

About 50% of first-trimester, 25% of second-trimester, and 11% of third-trimester miscarriages have a chromosome abnormality (Table 26.9). For the earliest recognized miscarriages (under 8 weeks from last menstrual period), however, there is some evidence that the frequency of chromosome abnormalities may be only about 10%, although this may be an underestimate, since 20% of normal-appearing in vitro fertilization embryos have a chromosome abnormality. Ectopic pregnancies do not have a substantially increased frequency of chromosome abnormalities.

Polyploidy is observed in 10% of abortus specimens, with 3% being tetraploid and 7% being triploid. These are often associated with an empty sac or a severely disorganized embryo, but mosaics are often less severely affected and some liveborns are known with polyploidy mosaicism.

Hydatidiform degeneration of the placenta is frequent in triploid conceptions, and although some hydatidiform moles are triploid, the majority of com-

Table 26.10. Frequency of Recurrent Trisomic and Chromosomally Normal Miscarriages, among 125 Pairs of Abortuses[a]

Karyotype of first loss	Karyotype of Second Loss		
	Normal	Trisomic	Other
Normal	55	6	7
Trisomic	8	24	2
Other	9	8	6

[a]Adapted from Hassold TJ. A cytogenetic study of repeated spontaneous abortion. Am J Hum Genet 1980;32:723–730.

plete moles (which carry a risk of malignant degeneration) are diploid with two paternal and no maternal contribution to the zygote. Diploid moles appear to arise from fertilization of an empty (degenerating) egg by a haploid sperm with subsequent duplication of the paternal chromosomes, or by dispermy (fertilization by two sperm). The absence of embryonic development in diploid moles is consistent with the hypothesis that a paternal chromosome set is required to form the placenta and a maternal set required to form the embryo.

Trisomy for the autosomes (chromosomes 1 to 22) as a group comprises about 30% of all miscarriages (Table 26.2). By far the most common is trisomy 16, which accounts for about a third of cases. Trisomy 16 is frequently associated with an empty sac and hydatidiform degeneration of the placenta. Trisomy 1 has not yet been seen in a miscarriage specimen. As with liveborn trisomy, there is a maternal age effect, and most trisomic miscarriages result from nondisjunction during maternal meiosis I.

In general, women who have one or more miscarriages have an increased risk of miscarriage in future pregnancies compared to women who have no history of miscarriage (25% versus 12%). However, this information is based on unkaryotyped miscarriages, so it is unclear whether there is a maternal age–independent increased risk of pregnancy loss subsequent to a trisomic miscarriage.

After a couple experiences a trisomic miscarriage, there is an increased likelihood that any subsequent miscarriage will also be trisomic, although not necessarily for the same chromosome (Table 26.10). Some centers recommend prenatal diagnosis in future pregnancies for women who have had a trisomic miscarriage, but there is only weak evidence that such women have a maternal age–independent increased risk for having a liveborn trisomic.

Monosomy for an autosome is extremely rare, and most monosomies have never been observed. One plausible reason is that loss of a chromosome or chromosome segment has a much more severe effect on phenotype than does gain of the same chromosome or chromosome segment. In contrast, monosomy X accounts for about 10% of miscarriages. Although 45,X is compatible with full-term development, the great majority do not survive to term. In one study only 1 to 6% of 45,X miscarriages had cytogenetic or molecular evidence of mosaicism, whereas at least 50% of liveborns are mosaics.

Other chromosome abnormalities seen in miscarriages and stillborns include unbalanced rearrangements, and the balanced translocation or inversion is sometimes identified in a parent.

The reasons for miscarriage or stillbirth in chromosomally normal conceptions are legion, but there are major categories that can be explored in women who have more than one chromosomally normal miscarriage. Smoking, alcohol, cocaine, and infections are major environmental factors in chromosomally normal miscarriages. On the other hand, the identification of a chromosome abnormality in an abortus is generally sufficient to exclude a teratogenic or other nonchromosomal cause. This can be useful to some couples who are concerned about teratogenic exposures or other factors as a cause for their miscarriage. If one of two miscarriages is aneuploid and the other euploid, it is also safe to conclude that the multiple miscarriages are not causally related.

Multiple Miscarriages

Since 15% of recognized pregnancies end in miscarriage or stillbirth, simple probability dictates that 2% of couples with two pregnancies will have two miscarriages, and 6% of couples with three pregnancies will have two miscarriages. Nonetheless, in 4% of couples (2% of subjects) who experience multiple pregnancy losses (more than one miscarriage or stillbirth), one member of the couple carries a balanced chromosome rearrangement. By comparison, the incidence of balanced chromosome rearrangements in the general population is only 0.6% (Table 26.4). This increased frequency of rearrangements justifies a chromosome study in all couples who experience more than one pregnancy loss.

The rearrangements found in couples with multiple miscarriages include reciprocal translocations (50%), robertsonian translocations (35%, mostly t(13;14), inversions (13%, mostly pericentric), and 2% others (e.g., X deletion or normal/ring mosaic). The majority (75%) of the identified carriers are female. The nature of the chromosome rearrangement in a specific family influences the risk of miscarriage or malformed liveborn, but it is reasonable to suggest family studies and offer prenatal diagnosis to the carriers. Couples with three or more *consecutive* miscarriages may have a lower frequency of rearrangements as obstetric, immunologic, and endocrinologic risk factors become more likely.

Table 26.11. Chromosomes in Azoospermia and Oligospermia[a]

Azoospermia: 15% abnormal (73 of 489 men)	
56	47,XXY
5	47,XYY mosaics
1	47,XYY mosaic
5	46,XX males
1	45,X/46,XY mosaic (30:70 ratio)
5	balanced rearrangements
Oligospermia (under 10 million/ml sperm count): 6% abnormal (58 of 959 men)	
7	47,XXY
4	47,XXY mosaics
7	47,XYY
1	47,XYY mosaic
32	balanced rearrangements
1	46,X,del(Y) (q12) new mutation
6	46,XY/47,XY,+marker

[a]Data from Retief AE, et al. Chromosome studies in 496 infertile males with a sperm count below 10 million/ml. Hum Genet 1984;66:162–164, and Bourrouillou G, et al. Chromosome studies in 952 infertile males with a sperm count below 10 million/ml. Hum Genet 1985;71:366–367.

Many women who have multiple miscarriages have a small proportion of 45,X or 47,XXX cells in their peripheral blood chromosome preparations. This finding is age-related and does not indicate an increased risk for subsequent miscarriages or conceptions with an abnormal karyotype beyond the patient's age-related risk. The frequencies of 47,XXX and 47,XYY constitutions are probably no greater in multiple miscarriage subjects than in the general population. There have been suggestions of an association between miscarriages and chromosome variants, especially 9qh and Yqh, but the evidence favoring this association is weak.

Male Infertility

A chromosome abnormality is detected in 15% of men with azoospermia and in 6% with sperm counts above zero but below 10 million (Table 26.11). Among men with sperm counts ranging from 10 to 20 million, about 2% have a chromosome abnormality. Men with a 47,XXY karyotype are in the majority in the azoospermic group, but balanced rearrangements are more important among the oligospermic men. 47,XYY is not overrepresented among azoospermic men but is more frequent in oligospermia.

A 45,X/46,XY mosaicism does not appear to be a significant risk factor for infertility. Most prenatally diagnosed cases have normal-appearing male external genitalia at birth, but long-term follow-up will be of interest to determine prospectively their level of fertility.

Female Infertility

A chromosome abnormality is detected in 25% of primary amenorrhea and gonadal dysgenesis patients, with about 10% numerical and 10% structural changes of the X, and 5% 46,XY or structural changes involving the Y chromosome. In one study, 33% of patients with secondary amenorrhea had an X abnormality, and in our experience 10% of women karyotyped because of premature menopause have an isochromosome Xq or other structural abnormality of the X chromosome. There are many nonchromosomal, genetic causes of female infertility, and there is no significant increase in chromosome abnormalities among women with reduced fertility who have normal menstrual histories.

Ambiguous Genitalia

An important point for the reader to understand is that ambiguous genitalia in a newborn becomes a social emergency for the family, whether it appears as an isolated birth defect or as part of a syndrome. Abnormalities of the external genitalia can be associated findings in several sex chromosome abnormalities. For an infant with hypotonia as well as hypogonadism, Down's syndrome and Prader-Willi syndrome should be considered, and high-resolution cytogenetic studies should be done. The biochemistry of abnormal sexual differentiation in chromosomally normal 46,XX and 46,XY newborns—and the many nonchromosomal causes of ambiguous genitalia—are beyond the scope of this text (22–25).

The karyotype is essential and should be done as a stat specimen. It is standard practice to order also serum 17-hydroxyprogesterone and testosterone measurements, either at the same time or depending on the cytogenetic result. Since many hospitals send these tests to reference laboratories, the urgency of the karyotype result is accentuated. Until the question of gender is answered, anxiety is tremendous. The physicians and other medical staff generally prefer to avoid mention of gender, and use the ambiguous term "gonads" rather than "testes" or "ovaries."

Mental Retardation and Multiple Congenital Anomalies

Estimates of the frequency of chromosome abnormalities among the mentally retarded vary widely, but we find the following estimates have been workable. Among the moderately to severely retarded, Down's syndrome is present in 10 to 15%, and 3 to 5% have other chromosome abnormalities, including other trisomies, and balanced and unbalanced structural changes. The fragile X syndrome can be identified in 3 to 6% of males and in 3 to 4% of females whose IQ is between 55 and 75. The frequencies of de novo balanced reciprocal translocations and inversions are increased, but inherited balanced rearrangements and de novo robertsonian translocations are not more frequent among the mentally retarded. The likelihood of finding a chromosome abnormality is greater if multiple minor or major malformations are present. Of patients with congenital heart disease, 13% have a chromosome defect, mainly Down's syndrome, and to a lesser extent trisomy 8, 13, 18, monosomy X, and unbalanced chromosome rearrangements.

Fibroblast tissue–limited mosaicism is present in 3 to 10% of subjects with multiple malformations, mental retardation, a normal blood karyotype, and no clear nonchromosomal syndrome.

PIGMENTARY DYSPLASIA

A number of recent studies have drawn attention to an association between swirls and lines of hyperpigmentation or hypopigmentation of the skin and chromosomal mosaicism (26). In some patients the pigmentary changes can be seen better using an ultraviolet lamp. The terms hypomelanosis of Ito and incontinentia pigmenti achromiens have been used to describe these pigmentary abnormalities, which traverse the trunk in a generally horizontal pattern and linearly along the arms and legs. The lines may reflect migration of melanocytes from the neural crest region during early embryogenesis. The associated chromosome abnormalities include XX/XY chimerism, diploid/triploid mosaicism, secondary trisomy 12p, and a variety of rings with normal/ring mosaicism, including patients who have some features of Ullrich-Turner syndrome, seizures, mental retardation, and a small ring X. Several X; autosome translocation cases are represented in this group and the X breakpoint is often near the locus of a hypothesized gene for incontinentia pigmenti, although the patients do not have classic incontinentia pigmenti.

In patients with pigmentary dysplasia and mental retardation, seizures, or other birth defects, chromosome studies should be extended to cultured fibroblasts if the blood karyotype is normal, and biopsies should be taken from skin with each pigmentary expression or from the borders between areas of different pigment.

ARTHROGRYPOSIS (CONGENITAL CONTRACTURES)

Of patients with arthrogryposis and delayed development or mental retardation, about 15% have a karyotype abnormality, and half of these are mosaics (27). Trisomy 8 mosaicism is perhaps most common, but contractures have been associated with a variety of other chromosome abnormalities.

A blood karyotype should be obtained if multiple joint contractures are associated with developmental delay, and especially if other birth defects are present. If the blood karyotype is normal, a cultured skin fibroblast chromosome study should be done.

Paternity and Forensics

Chromosome studies have been used for paternity and other medicolegal studies but are not as useful as other available methods (e.g., DNA fingerprinting), mainly because the scoring of chromosome variants is too subjective. Complaints of birth trauma and teratogenic exposures are common subjects of litigation. Each case needs to be evaluated by a pediatric geneticist, since some individuals with malformations have a chromosome abnormality or other known syndrome with an etiology independent of the complaint.

METHODS

Chromosome preparations for cytogenetic analysis can be obtained from many tissue sources. Peripheral blood is the most frequently used specimen for routine chromosome analysis, as it is the easiest tissue to obtain. Blood karyotypes are usually ordered because of the presence of birth defects, mental retardation, infertility, or multiple miscarriages. Lymphocytes are incubated under appropriate conditions, during which blast transformation is induced by one of several lectins, such as phytohemagglutinin (PHA). Cell harvest begins with the addition of an agent (e.g., Colcemid or vinblastine) to arrest cell division at the metaphase stage. Other treatments may be employed to inhibit chromosome condensation or prepare the cells for specialized banding patterns such as RBG-staining (Chapter 25). The cultures are then treated with a hypotonic solution to swell the cells and allow dispersion of the chromosomes within the cell membrane. Fixative is used as a wash solution to lyse the remaining red cells and remove some chromosomal proteins. Microscope slides are prepared and treated with one of several staining or banding methods. Chromosome preparations are then analyzed through the microscope for numerical and structural abberations, and findings are documented with photographs or computer-generated images.

Chromosome analysis in newborns requires special consideration since a smaller volume of specimen is usually received and decisions regarding life support systems or surgical intervention require rapid or "stat" analysis and interpretation. Direct preparations can be obtained from bone marrow cells harvested from specimens immediately after being received in the laboratory, although the quality is inconsistent. Whole blood specimens or bone marrow aspirates can be cultured as briefly as overnight.

Thus analysis of numerical and major structural changes can be performed within 6 hours, but normal results from marginal preparations must be confirmed with better material. This technique or a 48-hour method can be employed for prenatal percutaneous umbilical blood samples (PUBS).

Fibroblast monolayer cultures can be established from miscarriage material to help identify the cause of the loss, and from skin biopsies to look for sex chromosome mosaicism or tissue-limited mosaicism. Cultures are established using small tissue pieces (explants) or dissociated cell suspensions obtained by treatment of tissue pieces with enzymes that break collagen fibers in tissues. Harvest techniques follow the basic principles used in harvesting lymphocytes.

The use of other tissues for chromosome analysis has been described in the literature but is not routinely done. Culture of urine sediment cells from newborns has been employed to confirm a prenatally detected trisomy mosaicism. Sperm chromosome analysis (28) is being used by a few laboratories to detect germ cell mosaicism.

Many methods for tissue culture, banding techniques, and differing protocols for cell analysis have been published. Each institution must modify procedures to suit their laboratory conditions and needs. The methods described on the following pages are those currently used in our laboratory and meet the requirements of accrediting agencies.

Cytogenetic Procedure for Peripheral Blood

REAGENTS

Blood culture media: 100 ml RPMI 1640 (GIBCO) with 20 ml fetal bovine serum, 0.13 ml penicillin-streptomycin, 1.4 ml L-glutamine, and 4 ml phytohemagglutinin. Dispense 10-ml aliquots into sterile T-25 flasks and store at 4°C for up to 2 weeks.

Fetal bovine serum (Flow Laboratories).

Penn-Strep (GIBCO): 10,000 IU/ml penicillin and 10,000 μg/ml streptomycin.

L-Glutamine (GIBCO): 200 mM.

Phytohemagglutinin (GIBCO).

Ethidium bromide (BioRad): 1 mg/ml. Warning: Mutagenic.

Colcemid (GIBCO): 10 μg/ml

Fixative: 3 parts anhydrous methanol: 1 part glacial acetic acid. Prepare fresh for each use.

Hypotonic: 0.075M KCl (5.59 g/liter).

Microscope slides can be washed in a sonicator using methanol. Sonicate for 10 to 15 min, rinse in distilled water, and store at 4°C in distilled water.

All centrifugation steps are performed under the same conditions: 10 min at about 165 × G (e.g., 900 rpm using a 175-mm radius head).

CULTURE

This method is used to obtain routine mid to early metaphase preparations. To obtain prometaphase chromosomes for high-resolution analysis, a modification of the method is provided in Chapter 25.

1. Obtain 10 ml of heparinized blood (usually drawn in a Vacutainer) and allow the blood to settle at room temperature. For small volumes of blood, cultures can be established using whole blood.
2. With a sterile pipette, collect the buffy coat layer between the plasma and red blood cells and transfer to a sterile tube. Obtain 1.5 ml plasma and white cells and mix well in the tube.
3. Using sterile technique, establish two cultures per patient by inoculating blood culture medium with 0.75 ml of buffy coat suspension or 0.5 ml whole blood.
4. Incubate flasks in 5% CO_2 at 37°C.

HARVEST

5. On the third day, after 65 to 68 hours of incubation, add 0.1 ml ethidium bromide and 0.1 ml Colcemid to each flask. Return flasks to the incubator for 2 hours. *Variation:* Rush or stat cultures can be harvested after 48 hours' incubation.
6. Gently swirl the culture to loosen cells that have adhered to the flask and transfer culture to a conical centrifuge tube.
7. Centrifuge and aspirate the supernatant.
8. Add 10 ml of prewarmed (37°C) hypotonic solution and mix gently with a pipette to a smooth suspension. Incubate in 37°C water bath for 20 minutes, remixing cells at 5-minute intervals.
9. Add 2 ml of freshly prepared cold (4°C) fixative and mix well with pipette.
10. Centrifuge and aspirate the supernatant.
11. Resuspend cell pellet in residual supernatant (about 0.5 ml) using a pipette. Add 10 ml fresh cold fixative, mix well, and allow to stand for 20 minutes.
12. Centrifuge and aspirate the supernatant.
13. Continue the wash procedure with fresh fixative until the cell pellet is clean and white. After the final wash, resuspend the cells in fresh fixative to form a cloudy suspension. The cells are now ready to be dropped onto slides. If the cells are to be stored, add fresh fixative but do not resuspend the pellet. Store in a tightly capped tube at 4°C.

cultures. For flask cultures, use the following protocol. Sterile technique is not required unless the culture is to be carried for additional harvests. Cultures are examined using an inverted microscope. Cultures are ready for harvest when they are approximately 60% confluent. Slower-growing cultures may give a better yield of mitotic cells if harvested at 80% confluency.

1. Add Colcemid, 0.01 ml per milliliter of medium in flask.
2. Return the culture to the incubator for 2 hours or until rounded-up (mitotic) cells are evident.
3. Pour medium from the flask into a 15-ml centrifuge tube.
4. Add 3 ml of 1× HBSS to the flask, swirl gently, and decant into tube containing the medium.
5. Add 2 ml 1× trypsin-EDTA solution to the flask. Incubate at 37°C for 5 minutes.
6. When most of the cells are free floating, gently tap the base of the flask against a large rubber stopper to loosen any cells still adhered to the flask.
7. Add 2 ml of F-10 medium to each flask to inactivate the trypsin.
8. Gently swirl and immediately decant into the tube. If the culture is to be maintained, add 3 ml of fresh media and return the flask to the incubator.
9. Centrifuge and aspirate the supernatant.
10. Add approximately 8 ml of prewarmed hypotonic solution and mix well. Incubate in 37°C water bath for 15 minutes.
11. Add 4 ml of freshly prepared cold (4°C) fixative and mix well with a pipette.
12.. Centrifuge and aspirate the supernatant.
13. Resuspend the cell button by flicking the bottom of the tube with a finger. Add 4 to 6 ml of fresh cold fixative and mix well with a pipette.
14. Centrifuge and aspirate the supernatant.
15. After the final wash, the cells are ready to be dropped onto slides, or the pellets can be stored as a cell-fixative suspension in a tightly capped tube at 4°C.

SLIDE PREPARATION

Slides are prepared in much the same way as lymphocyte metaphase slides, but because of the small pellet extra care is taken to conserve material.

Technical Variations

FRAGILE X TESTING

Fragile sites in chromosomes, whether expressed in response to culture conditions or chemically induced, have not been associated with any clinical condition with one significant exception. A fragile site in the long arm of the X chromosome (Xq27.3) is expressed in patients with the fragile X syndrome. Patients, as well as suspected carriers with this syndrome, can be screened for the fragile X. Fragile X analysis ought not to be used without serious consideration of a full G-banding analysis except in special circumstances (e.g., for an otherwise normal female member of a known fragile X family).

Blood samples to be analyzed must be cultured in a manner that will induce expression of the fragile X. Lymphocytes are cultured in folate-deficient media or chromosome breakage is induced with chemical agents (e.g., methotrexate, FUdR, or thymidine). Analysis of chromosome breakage is highly subjective, and guidelines must be established within the laboratory to ensure that chromosome breakage is induced in each case, and to ensure consistent criteria for scoring breakage. It is suggested to use two different induction methods to verify results.

Reagents

5-Fluorodeoxyuridine (FUdR): 4×10^{-7} M. Warning: Mutagenic

Thymidine: 1.3 mg/10 ml. Store at 0°C.

Procedure

1. Establish lymphocyte cultures as previously described. For comparative breakage studies between FUdR and thymidine, three flasks are established.
2. At approximately 41 hours of culture (morning of the second day), add 0.1 ml FUdR to two flasks and 0.1 ml thymidine solution to one flask, and continue incubation.
3. Harvest cultures and prepare G-banded microscope slides following previously described protocol.

FLUORESCENCE IN SITU HYBRIDIZATION

The mapping of the human genome has made it possible to extend the applications of molecular biology to cytogenetics. Fluorescence in situ hybridization (FISH) techniques allow for the highly sensitive detection of specific nucleic acid sequences in specimens on fixed microscope slides.

Several types of DNA probes have been developed and each has unique applications. A repetitive sequence probe (usually centromere-specific alphoid sequence probes) has unique DNA sequence repeats in hundreds to thousands of copies, and is useful in determining ploidy and in identifying small marker chromosomes (Fig. 26.24*A*). Chromosome paints consist of a cocktail of different repeat and unique se-

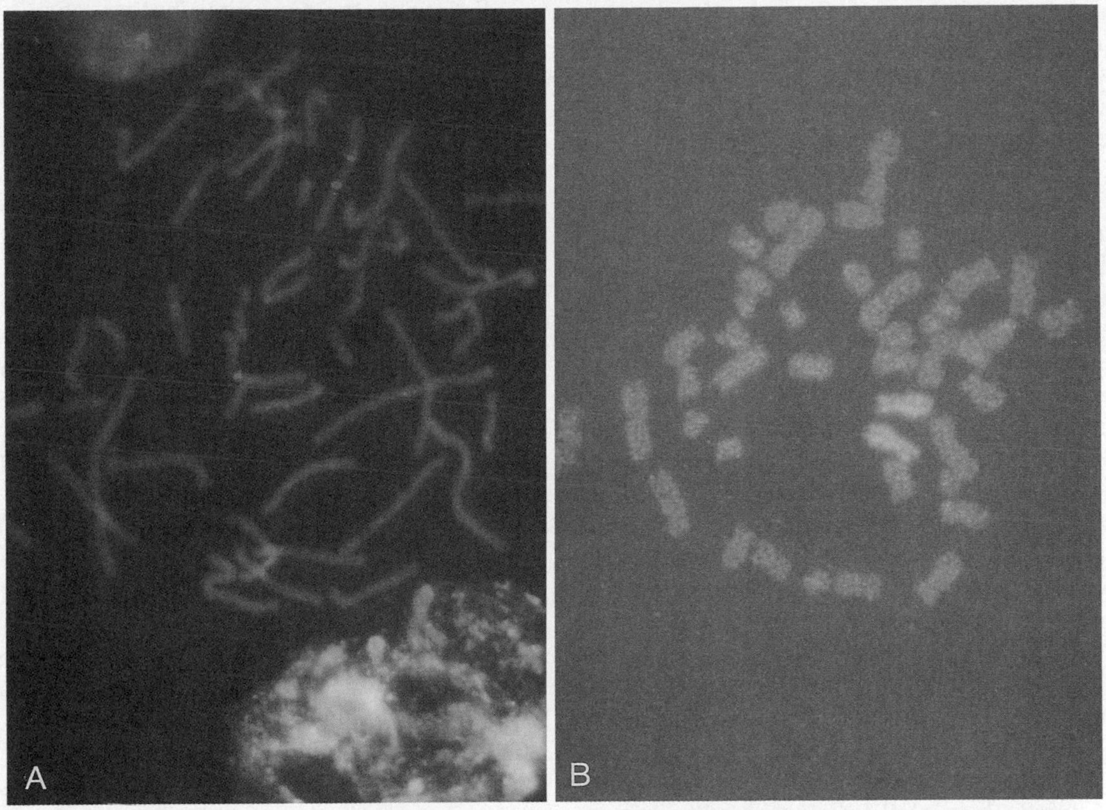

Figure 26.24. Fluorescence In situ hybridization (FISH) in **A** employed an X chromosome–specific probe for centromeric alphoid sequences (Oncor, Inc., Gaithersburg, MD) on a cell from a patient with Ullrich-Turner syndrome who has a large isodicentric X. Her karyotype is 45,X/46,X,dic(X) (p21). A single biotin-avidin hybridization signal is present over the centromere of the normal X, and two signals over the abnormal X chromosome. In **B**, a whole chromosome probe cocktail specific for chromosome 6 (Imagenetics, Inc., Framingham, MA) was applied to cells from a normal subject. The chromosome 6 pair exhibits a uniform yellow fluorescence, the biotin-avidin hybridization signal, against a background of propidium idodide fluorescent dye staining the other chromosomes.

quence probes, all located on the same chromosome. The unique sequences are homologous to DNA sequences along the entire length of the chromosome (Fig. 26.24**B**). Chromosome painting is useful in identifying translocation segments and in studies using somatic cell hybrids. Single-gene probes are isolated for the identification of a specific gene or unique DNA sequence. For example, a unique sequence probe from the short arm of chromosome 5 can be employed to look for a deletion associated with cri-du-chat syndrome.

For most FISH protocols, slides are prepared from cultures using the standard protocols. Slides are pretreated to eliminate cross-hybridization with RNA and to decrease nonspecific staining. After the chromosomal DNA and labeled probes are denatured, the probe is applied to the slide in a solution that promotes the formation of DNA-DNA hybrids between the target and probe. Many probes are commercially available prelabeled, with a detector molecule so that a hybridization signal can be visualized through the microscope. Hybridization conditions vary depending on the probe and target size. After hybridization, excess probe must be removed from the slides through a series of stringent washing steps.

Our laboratory uses a modification of a technique, originally described by Pinkel (29), that incorporates biotin-labeled or digoxigenin-labeled probes in a nonradioactive system based on the strong binding capacity of avidin to biotin, or anti-digoxigenin to digoxigenin. Depending on the label of the probe, a fluorescent stain conjugated to avidin or anti-digoxigenin is applied to the slide and binds to the hybridized probe/target DNA sequences. The slides are counterstained and the hybridization signal is analyzed using a fluorescence-equipped microscope. With the increasing availability of commercially produced probes, FISH is becoming a valuable tool for cytogenetic analysis.

Analysis of Chromosome Preparatioı

Cells in mid or early metaphase are usually suitable for analysis. Shorter chromosomes with fewer bands are easier to analyze but may mask subtle deletions or inversions. Selection of cells should be appropriate for each specimen type, and each laboratory should establish criteria for its own standards. A chromosome band resolution similar to that depicted in Figure 26.6 is reasonable for most applications other than high-resolution analysis for the contiguous gene syndromes. We specifically look for bands 17p13, 17p11.2, and 17q23 as markers of adequate resolution for routine analysis.

Preparations are analyzed using a light microscope. There are several fine manufacturers; we use a Zeiss Axioscope equipped with a 12-V, 100-W halogen lamp, mechanical, stage with verniers, 10×, 20× phase 2, and 100×/1.30 oil planneofluar objectives, and a basic top-mounted 35 mm camera. A complete system cost about $19,000 in 1993. Suitable metaphase cells have a sharp banding pattern and a small number of overlapping chromosomes, with the chromosome spread having a roughly circular shape. Excessively spread, teardrop-shaped metaphase cells are frequently broken, with one or more chromosomes lost. The location of each analyzed cell is recorded. The number of chromosomes in each spread is counted. The counts are pooled to determine the modal number (the count representative of most cells).

After the chromosomes are counted, each chromosome is carefully inspected and compared to its homolog. Band-to-band comparison studies are done on each pair and any structural differences are noted. Any abnormality should be confirmed in other cells, since morphologic changes can occur within any cell as an artifact. Since banding intensity and condensation of chromosomal material varies between cells, thorough analysis of an adequate number of cells is essential for the proper interpretation of results. A structural or numerical abnormality found in one cell should be sought when scoring other cells. It is reasonable to assume the presence of a second clone if, among 30 cells scored, at least two cells have the same extra chromosome or the same chromosome rearrangement, or at least three cells have the same chromosome loss. In an abnormal karyotypic background, the presence of one normal cell usually indicates that a normal cell line is present.

The number of cells to be analyzed depends on the specimen type and the indication for the study (30). If there is any question of chromosomal mosaicism we analyze at least 30 cells (e.g., abnormal sex differentiation, suspected sex chromosome syndrome, or infertility). For situations where mosaicism is occasional but is not a strong consideration, we analyze at least 20 cells (e.g., multiple congenital anomalies, mental retardation, possible Down syndrome, or stillborns). When mosaicism is rarely a consideration, we analyze at least 10 cells (e.g., translocation family member or couple with multiple miscarriages).

Following the analysis, photographs are taken of metaphase cells representative of the analyzed cells (31, 32). Photographs serve as a permanent record of what was observed, and we do not recommend their use as an alternative to routine analysis through the microscope. Black-and-white enlargements are made and individual chromosomes are cut to arrange a karyotype. The final report includes at least two full karyotypes.

Guidelines and recommendations for culture and analysis for all specimen types have been established by the College of American Pathologists and the Association of Cytogenetic Technologists (33), and are pending from the American College of Medical Genetics. Chromosome nomenclature should conform to standards established by the Standing Committee of Human Cytogenetic Nomenclature (ISCN 1985) (1).

Automated systems for cytogenetic analysis have been developed by several companies. Basic systems allow the technologist to scan for metaphases on a slide and store cell locations in the computer memory. Metaphases, which in some systems are quality ranked by the computer, can be displayed and analyzed using a video display terminal. Sophisticated systems are able to automatically locate metaphase cells on slides, count the chromosomes, and produce a karyotype of the cell, using the technologist to isolate and identify some or all of the chromosomes in an interactive process. The karyotype image can be printed in hard copy format and can be archived on a disk or other memory system.

FRAGILE X ANALYSIS

The autosomal fragile sites that are expressed universally serve as an internal control to determine whether the fragile site at Xq27.3, if present in the patient, would be expressed. If at least 4% of the cells have a break at the fragile sites 1p31, 3p14, and 16q23, then the medium is inducing sufficient breakage to induce the fragile Xq27.3 site. If fewer than 4% of cells have a break at these three fragile sites, but at least 12% of cells have at least one break at other bands, then the medium is inducing sufficient breakage. The autosomal breakage rate is highly variable, but if there is an insufficient number of autosomal breaks, then confidence is low in a negative result of the fragile X analysis and a second specimen is requested.

In a female, 100 cells should be scored for the fragile X, whereas 50 cells are sufficient for analysis on a male. Examples of positive fragile X chromosome are provided in Figure 26.23*D*.

If the fragile X is present in 4% of the cells, the patient is considered to be positive. The fragile X is probably not present if an adequate number of autosomal breaks are observed but no cells have a break at Xq27. If autosomal breaks are adequate but only 2 to 4% of the cells have a break at Xq27, the interpretation of the results becomes more difficult. Generally, repeat testing is advised along with the evaluation of other family members or possible carriers in the family and formal evaluation by a clinical geneticist if that was not done prior to the chromosome study.

SEX CHROMATIN STUDIES (BARR BODIES)

The Barr body, formed during interphase from the inactivated X chromosome, can be observed in cells from normal females and males with Klinefelter's syndrome, but not in normal males or females with 45,X or 46,XY constitutions. Females with more than two X chromosomes have some cells with multiple Barr bodies, and some structurally abnormal X chromosomes show smaller or larger Barr bodies. Scoring Barr bodies in buccal mucosal cells is less costly than karyotype analysis, but the technical limitations of the test are considerable, and presence of the Y chromosome is not addressed without application of a second stain for the Y-body (the quinacrine-brilliant segment of Yq). Because of the obvious benefit of a full cytogenetic study, sex chromatin studies have fallen out of favor.

References

1. Harnden DG, Klinger HP, eds. An international system for human cytogenetic nomenclature (1985). Basel: S Karger, 1985.
2. Daniel A, ed. The cytogenetics of mammalian autosomal rearrangements. New York: Alan R Liss, 1988.
3. deGrochy J, ed. Special issue on pericentric and paracentric inversions in man. Ann Genet 1986;29:126–214.
4. deGrouchy J, Turleau C. Clinical atlas of human chromosomes. 2nd ed. New York: John Wiley & Sons, 1984.
5. Schinzel A. Catalog of unbalanced chromosome aberrations in man. Berlin: Walter de Gruyter, 1984.
6. Jones KL. Smith's recognizable patterns of human malformation. 4th ed. Philadelphia: WB Saunders, 1988.
7. Schmickel RD. Contiguous gene syndromes: a component of recognizable syndromes. J Pediatr 1986;109:231–241.
8. Niebuhr E. The cri du chat syndrome. Epidemiology, cytogenetics, and clinical features. Hum Genet 1978;44:227–275.
9. Van Dyke DL, Roberson JR, Babu VR, Weiss L. Trisomy 20 mosaicism identified prenatally and confirmed in foreskin fibroblasts. Prenat Diagn 1989;9:601–602.
10. Epstein CJ. Down syndrome (trisomy 21). In: Scriver CR, Beaudet AL, Sly WS, Valle D, eds. The metabolic basis of inherited disease. 6th ed. New York: McGraw-Hill, 1989:291–326.
11. Hook EB. Down syndrome frequency in human populations and factors pertinent to variation in rates. In: de la Cruz FF, Gerald PS, eds. Trisomy 21 (Down syndrome) research perspectives. Baltimore: University Park Press, 1981:3–67.
12. Pueschel SM, Tingey C, Rynders JE, Crocker AC, Crutcher DM, eds. New perspectives on Down syndrome. Baltimore: Paul H Brookes, 1987.
13. Cronk C, Crocker AC, Pueschel SM, Shea AM, Zackai E, Pickens G, Reed RB. Growth charts for children with Down syndrome: 1 month to 18 years of age. Pediatrics 1988;81:102–110.
14. Ratcliffe SG, Paul N, eds. Prospective studies on children with sex chromosome aneuploidy. New York: Alan R Liss, 1986.
15. Stewart DA, ed. Children with sex chromosome aneuploidy: follow-up studies. March of Dimes Birth Defects: Original Article Series 18 (4). New York: A R Liss, 1982.
16. Bandmann HJ, Breit R, eds. Klinefelter's syndrome. Berlin: Springer-Verlag, 1984.
17. Davies KE. The fragile X syndrome. Oxford: Oxford University Press, 1989.
18. Rousseau F, Heitz D, Biancalana V, Blumenfeld S, Kretz C, Boue J, et al. Direct diagnosis by DNA analysis of the fragile X syndrome of mental retardation. N Engl J Med 1991;325:1673–1681.
19. Caskey CT, Pizzuti A, Fu YH, Fenwick RG Jr, Nelson DL. Triplet repeat mutations in human disease. Science 1992;256:784–789.
20. Richards RI, Sutherland GR. Heritable unstable DNA sequences. Nature Genet 1992;1:7–9.
21. Jenkins EC, Krawczun MS, Brooks SE, Sklower Brooks SL, Sherman SL, Brown WT. Laboratory aspects of prenatal Fra(X) detection. In: Proceedings of the Birth Defects Symposium XX: Fragile X/Cancer Genetics. New York: Wiley/Liss, 1991.
22. Blethen SL, Weldon VV. Disorders of external genital differentiation. In: Kelley VC, ed. Practice of pediatrics. rev. ed. Philadelphia: Harper and Row, 1987;7:1–23.
23. Lanes RL. Ambiguous genitalia, micropenis, and cryptorchidism. In: Lifshitz F, ed. Pediatric endocrinology: a clinical guide, 2nd ed. New York: Marcel Dekker, 1990.
24. Moore DC. Disorders of gonadal differentiation. In: Kelley VC, ed. Practice of pediatrics, rev. ed. Philadelphia: Harper & Row, 1987;7:1–30.
25. Styne DM. The testes: disorders of sexual differentiation and puberty. In: Kaplan SA, ed. Clinical pediatric endocrinology. Philadelphia: WB Saunders, 1990:367–425.
26. Flannery DB. Pigmentary dysplasia, hypomelanosis of Ito, and genetic mosaicism. Am J Med Genet 1990;35:18–21.
27. Reed SD, Hall JG, Riccardi VM, Aylsworth A, Timmons C. Chromosomal abnormalities associated with congenital contractures (arthrogryposis). Clin Genet 1985;27:353–372.
28. Martin RH. A detailed method for obtaining preparations of human sperm chromosomes. Cytogenet Cell Genet 1983;35:252–256.
29. Pinkel D, Straume T, Gray JW. Cytogenetic analysis using quantitative, high-sensitivity fluorescence hybridization. Proc Natl Acad Sci USA 1986;83:2934–2938.
30. Knutsen T, Bixenman H, Lawce H, Martin P. Chromosome analysis guidelines preliminary report. Karyogram 1989;15:131–135.
31. Bradbury S. An introduction to the optical microscope. Oxford: Oxford University Press, 1984.
32. Delly JG. Photography through the microscope. Rochester, NY: Eastman Kodak Company, 1988.
33. Barch MJ, ed. The Association of Cytogenetics Technologists cytogenetics laboratory manual. 2nd ed. New York: Raven Press, 1991.

27 Prenatal Cytogenetic Diagnosis

Daniel L. Van Dyke, Jacquelyn R. Roberson, and Anne Wiktor

With advancing maternal age, there is an increased risk of having a child with Down's syndrome. This finding has led to the development and wide acceptance of prenatal diagnosis of Down's syndrome and many other chromosomal and nonchromosomal birth defects and inherited conditions. The methods used to obtain fetal cells for prenatal diagnosis include amniocentesis, chorionic villus sampling (CVS), and blood sampling from the umbilical cord (percutaneous umbilical blood sampling—PUBS). Methods to obtain fetal cells from the maternal blood circulation are being developed. Including all accepted reasons (Table 27.1), prenatal diagnosis is indicated in 5 to 8% of all pregnancies. Other than screening for neural tube and abdominal wall defects, nonchromosomal prenatal diagnostic studies are beyond the scope of this chapter. For a detailed discussion of these topics the reader is referred to the books edited by Milunsky and Weaver (1, 2).

Amniocentesis for prenatal genetic diagnosis is typically performed at 14 to 20 weeks. The procedure has been performed as early as 9 weeks, and some groups advocate early amniocentesis, although its practicality seems limited prior to 12 gestational weeks. Genetic amniocentesis has become widely available since it was introduced in the late 1960s, is regarded as safe to the mother and fetus, and has a culture success rate of 99.5% or better.

Although CVS for prenatal diagnosis got off to a rocky start, with several patients experiencing severe intrauterine infections, the technical problems associated with obtaining the specimen have been resolved. The risks of the procedure to the mother and the embryo are now considered acceptable after 10 gestational weeks, with over 96% of procedures providing a satisfactory cytogenetic result (3–6). CVS for first-trimester prenatal diagnosis is routinely done between gestational age of 10 and 12 weeks using an ultrasound-guided biopsy catheter or needle passed through the cervix (transcervical CVS, or TC-CVS) or abdominal wall (transabdominal CVS, or TA-CVS). TA-CVS is gaining popularity among obstetricians because it is easier and faster to learn and has fewer contraindications. TA-CVS is also preferred by many women for reasons of modesty and its similarity to amniocentesis. Transabdominal CVS can also be performed during the second and third trimesters and is sometimes useful to evaluate the karyotype when oligohydramnios or fetal defects are found on ultrasound examination.

For CVS, two general chromosome preparation methods have been developed. Short-term tissue culture of fibroblasts, mainly originating from the mesenchymal core of the chorionic villus, has the disadvantage of a longer reporting time. However, this is offset by the advantages of better-quality preparations, the opportunity to use clonal analysis, no greater frequency of false-positive results (0.5 to 1% of specimens), and a much lower frequency of false-negative results. (With a false-positive analysis, the karyotype interpretation is abnormal but the fetal karyotype is actually normal. With a false-negative, the karyotype interpretation is normal but the fetal karyotype is actually abnormal.) Placental villi, rich in blood vessels and buds, grow well in vitro. The buds are newly growing villi full of actively dividing cells. Extraplacental villi (chorion lavae) appear edematous and with few blood vessels or buds, but appear to grow equally well in vitro. Early technical problems with maternal cell contamination due to adherence of decidual fragments to the villi have been resolved by most laboratories.

The alternative CVS method is a direct preparation of uncultured, rapidly dividing cytotrophoblast cells that comprise the outer sheath of the villus, after 24 to 48 hours of incubation of these cells. This has the advantage of more rapid reporting time but the disadvantages of a higher false-negative rate and poorer-quality preparations. The false-negative rate of 0.03 to 0.1%, missing roughly 1% of the true fetal

Table 27.1. Indications for Prenatal Cytogenetic or AFP Diagnosis

Advanced maternal age
One parent carries a chromosome rearrangement
Previous offspring with a chromosome abnormality
Previous offspring with a neural tube defect or hydrocephalus
High maternal serum AFP
Low maternal serum AFP (or similar screening result)
Fetal abnormality detected by ultrasound exmination
Fetus at risk for X-linked or prenatally diagnosable inherited disease

Table 27.2. Rate per Thousand of Chromosome Abnormalities at CVS and Amniocentesis, and in Live Births, By Maternal Age.[a]

	Trisomy 21			All Abnormalities		
Maternal Age	CVS	Amnio	Livebirth	CVS	Amnio	Livebirth
35	4.2	4.0	2.6	8.8	8.0	5.2
36	5.7	5.2	3.4	11.5	9.9	6.4
37	7.5	6.7	4.4	15.1	12.2	7.9
38	10.0	8.7	5.7	19.8	15.2	9.8
39	13.4	11.2	7.3	26.0	19.0	12.1
40	17.9	14.5	9.4	34.1	23.8	15.2
41	23.8	18.7	12.2	44.7	29.9	19.0
42	31.7	24.1	15.7	58.6	37.6	23.9
43	42.3	31.1	20.2	76.8	47.2	30.2
44	56.4	40.1	26.1	100.8	57.8	37.3
45	75.1	51.8	33.7	132.1	71.3	46.6
46	~100	66.8	43.4	~170	88.6	58.4
47	~130	86.2	56.0	~230	110.9	73.6
48	~180	111.2	72.3	~300	139.9	90.4

[a]The statistics are from Hook EB. Cytogenetics: incidence, risks, and recurrence of chromosome abnormalities. In: Brock DJH, Rodeck C, Ferguson-Smith MA, eds. Prenatal diagnosis and screening. London: Churchill Livingstone, 1992:351–392.

chromosome abnormalities, has been a major factor leading to broader acceptance of CVS culture techniques. For second- and third-trimester CVS, the direct method, or percutaneous umbilical blood sampling (PUBS), may be preferable to culture of amniocytes or CVS cells if a very rapid result is the first consideration, although false-negative CVS direct preparation results have been reported for all three trimesters. Thus, cultures should be employed for any CVS chromosome studies. The false-negative rate is unknown for second- and third-trimester CVS studies.

PUBS has also been used to obtain fetal cells for chromosome analysis, although it is not widely used for this purpose, being more applicable to studies of fetomaternal infections and Rh incompatibility.

INDICATIONS FOR PRENATAL CHROMOSOME ANALYSIS

Maternal Age

Two-thirds of genetic amniocenteses and 80 to 90% of CVS procedures are performed because the mother will be age 35 years or over when the baby is born. The risks of trisomy 13, 18, 21, X, and 47,XXY all increase with maternal age, dramatically so after age 35 (7) (Table 27.2). There is an increased risk of some other chromosome defects with maternal age as well, including deletion 18p, extra isochromosomes, and other small accessory marker chromosomes. In our experience, such nontrisomic chromosome imbalances that are or may be associated with maternal age constitute 10% of prenatally diagnosed chromosome abnormalities. In the United States, a maternal age of 35 years at the expected date of confinement (EDC) is the usually accepted age at which physicians routinely offer prenatal diagnosis; age 34.5 at midgestation is another accepted cutoff date. Some centers have suggested lowering the age criterion to age 32 at EDC. In fact, any criterion is to some extent arbitrary. Some women would like to have prenatal diagnosis no matter what their risk; others think it wholly unnecessary.

A chromosome abnormality is identified in 5 to 8% of CVSs from women age 35 or over, compared to 1.5 to 3% of amniotic fluid samples from the same age group. The abnormality rate is higher in earlier gestational weeks. However, if detailed ultrasound examination is employed to exclude deceased embryos, the rate for CVS is about the same as for amniocentesis. Most centers do not attempt CVS if the embryo is dead, but perhaps it is worth considering, since nearly all of this subset have an abnormal karyotype.

Positive Family History

About 3% of prenatal chromosome studies are performed because one parent carries a balanced chromosome rearrangement or the couple has had a child or stillborn with a chromosome abnormality. The risk of a liveborn with an unbalanced chromosome rearrangement varies with the specific rearrangement. In general, the risk is higher if the carrier is female. The risk of recurrence for a de novo abnormality averages 1.4% but varies with the specific defect, and for some abnormalities varies with parental age.

If there is a family history of a neural tube defect or hydrocephalus, a genetics consultation may be useful. In addition, depending on the specific defect and relationship to the present pregnancy, prenatal studies may be appropriate, including amniotic fluid α-fetoprotein (AFP) and ACHE, and a detailed ultrasound examination.

Prenatal Screening

Prenatal screening of maternal serum α-fetoprotein (MSAFP) or related tests (described below) has become part of routine obstetric care. Abnormal serum AFP or triple screen results account for 25% of amniocentesis procedures at our institution. The proportion of women tested and the proportion of tests for these indications vary somewhat among centers. Most centers study the karyotype for both high and low MSAFP as an indication, even though a high MSAFP is not generally considered a risk factor for a chromosome abnormality. In our experience, a clinically significant karyotype abnormality is identified in 0.6 to 1% of amniotic fluid chromosome studies done because of either a high or a low MSAFP.

Ultrasound-Identified Abnormalities

About 2% of prenatal genetic studies are done because an anatomic defect, obstructive uropathy, intrauterine growth retardation (IUGR), nonimmune hydrops, or oligohydramnios or polyhydramnios is identified by ultrasound examination. Of these, 10 to 20% have a chromosome defect. Fetal nuchal skin thickening observed between gestational weeks 15 and 20 is used in some centers as a risk factor for trisomy 21. Cystic hygroma identified at ultrasound examination is associated with 45,X in 50 to 75%. There is usually more generalized fetal lymphedema or fetal hydrops, and if so, spontaneous fetal death is very likely. Cystic hygroma is less commonly associated with trisomy 21 and other chromosome abnormalities, although nonimmune hydrops without cystic hygroma has about a 25% rate of chromosome abnormalities with about half of these trisomy 21, one-fourth 45,X, and one-fourth other abnormalities. If amniotic fluid is inaccessible, it is possible to obtain cells for both PHA-stimulated culture and for standard monolayer culture from a sample of cystic hygroma fluid, or to obtain a CVS.

Fragile X Syndrome

Fragile X syndrome can be diagnosed prenatally, but the cytogenetic procedures are still complicated, requiring multiple tissue culture protocols, and should be considered experimental. (Molecular genetic assays are available and are likely to become the preferred methods within a few years.) The test should be done in collaboration with a laboratory well experienced in the prenatal diagnosis of this condition. This necessitates early booking of the patient, and extra effort to confirm the diagnosis cytogenetically and to obtain specimens from other family members for cytogenetic and molecular studies. The parents should be advised of the experimental nature, that a low breakage rate at Xq27.3 may be difficult to interpret, and that several false-negative results have been reported in the literature. Great caution should be exercised in performing this test in a family with no clear family history or fragile X syndrome (e.g., a woman whose brother is mentally retarded but was never karyotyped.) Although few families can benefit from molecular genetic techniques for prenatal diagnosis of fragile X syndrome, this is an area of active research, and the expectation of success is high for developing widely applicable techniques (8).

Chromosome Instability Syndromes

Prenatal diagnosis of the mendelian chromosome instability syndromes are described in Chapter 28.

X-Linked Mendelian Disorders

A large number of X-linked conditions such as Duchenne's and Becker's muscular dystrophy, hemophilia A and B, and Hunter's syndrome can be prenatally diagnosed with confidence. Others cannot as yet be diagnosed (2). In either situation, it may be useful to determine the fetal sex. This can be done by chromosome analysis, but when information is needed more quickly, FISH analysis of X and Y chromosome–specific DNA sequences may be preferable.

GENETIC COUNSELING

Prior to any prenatal diagnostic procedure, it is important to obtain a family history including, at a minimum, all first-degree relatives of both parents for birth defects, mental retardation, heritable diseases; and to look for other risk factors (e.g., maternal diabetes or seizures, exposure to alcohol, cocaine, or other teratogenic agents) that can be addressed in a constructive way. If the indication is a positive family history of a specific birth defect, a known syndrome, or an inborn error of metabolism, it is imperative that the specific diagnosis be confirmed. Failure to do so can cause a prenatal diagnostic error. For routine obstetric use, several brief questionnaires have been devised to assist in identifying genetic and teratogenic risk factors.

Informed consent for a prenatal diagnostic procedure should include the estimated risk to the mother and the fetus and accuracy of the tests being done on the sample. If the patient is trying to choose between CVS and amniocentesis, a discussion of the advantages and limitations of each technique should be provided (Table 27.3). For amniocentesis, there is about a 1/500 risk of miscarriage or infection. Infection is a potentially serious risk to the mother and her future fertility. For CVS, the risk of miscarriage is estimated at 1/125 to 1/300. Although the risk of severe maternal infection after transcervical CVS has been estimated at roughly 1/500, as experience with the procedure has increased this risk seems to have decreased very dramatically. Because of the potential of a vascular disruption sequence (e.g., limb reduction or hypoglossia-hypodactyly sequence), CVS is no longer recommended prior to 10 gestational weeks. It is uncertain whether the relatively small increased risks of miscarriage due to CVS or amniocentesis procedures are statistically different from each other. It is important to state that the tests are specific and do not identify structural birth defects or mental retardation, and that some results are difficult to interpret or need further studies before interpretation is possible.

A follow-up study, usually involving amniocentesis, is necessary in 1 to 2% of CVS cases because of an inadequate sample or an indeterminate cytogenetic result (usually mosaicism). In addition, about 1% of women who have CVS also need an amniocentesis because of an elevated MSAFP result.

Table 27.3. Comparative Advantages of Prenatal Cytogenetic Diagnosis Using the CVS and Amniocentesis Techniques

Chorionic villus sampling
- Earlier gestational age provides more personal privacy
- Pregnancy termination at an earlier gestational age is quicker and safer
- Preferred by many women, assuming similar risks to fetus and mother
- Anxieties relieved sooner, although amniocentesis follow-up, necessary in 1 to 3%, is a source of new anxiety

Amniocentesis
- Usually less expensive
- Risks to fetus and mother are probably slightly lower
- Wide availability
- Available after MSAFP screening
- Ability to assay amniotic fluid AFP and AChE
- Better experience with false-positive and false-negative results

An unexpected result is obtained in about 3% of all prenatal studies (Table 27.4). Half of these are autosomal or sex chromosomal trisomies. Many of the rest require follow-up studies and can be difficult to interpret.

Some pregnancies are already nonviable when they are ultrasound-scanned in preparation for CVS, or miscarriage occurs between the date the appointment is set and the day of the scheduled CVS procedure. At the CVS scan about 10 to 13% fetal nonviability or an abnormal gestational sac is discovered (this is the frequency in the CVS population, not the entire pregnant population). About 6% of women age 35 to 39, and about 20% of women age 40 or over miscarry between weeks 7 and 11. Among women age 35 or over who schedule amniocentesis, about 4% miscarry prior to their appointment date. When fetal demise is discovered at ultrasound, the prenatal clinic staff must be prepared to help the family deal with their grief.

Parents do not need to commit themselves to interrupt their pregnancy should a chromosome abnormality be identified. One cannot be expected to make such decisions in the abstract. These are complicated, personal decisions in which the genetics counseling team can and should play a supporting role. The burdens of a developmentally disabled child can be tremendous on a family, and may lead to high divorce rates and other less obvious outcomes, including annual costs of care well over $100,000. The decision whether to continue the pregnancy depends to some extent on the perceived burden of the defect

Table 27.4. Chromosome Abnormality in Prenatal Studies, and Parental Decisions Regarding Continuation of the Pregnancy, in Our Program

	Proportion of All Results[a]	Proportion of All Abnormals	Proportion Who Continued
47,+21	0.7%	31%	8%
47,+13	0.1	5	0
47,+18	0.1	5	0
46/47,+20	0.05	2	75
45,X[b]	0.1	4	(None have survived)
47,XXX	0.1	4	25
47,XXY	0.1	5	66
47,XYY	0.07	3	0
45,X/46,XX or XY[b]	0.1	4	100
Inherited balanced rea	0.6[c]	26	100
De novo balanced rea	0.1	5	100
Inherited extra marker	0.07	3	100
De novo extra marker	0.05	2	50
Other abnormalities	0.02	1	—

[a]About 2 to 3% of prenatal studies have an abnormal cytogenetic result, and 0.3% are true mosaics (or roughly 10% of the abnormal results).
[b]The nonmosaic 45,X cases were associated with ultrasound-diagnosed abnormalities. The 45,X mosaics all appeared normal on ultrasound and had a normal outcome at birth.
[c]Between 75 and 85% are inherited from the mother.

(Table 27.4), but some parents will continue the pregnancy whatever the diagnosis: others will terminate the pregnancy in relatively low-risk situations. When a trisomic pregnancy is continued, the remaining chance of spontaneous miscarriage is about 30% for trisomy 21, 40% for trisomy 13, and 70% for trisomy 18. For monosomy X, the chance of a miscarriage approaches 100%.

For laboratory and clinic quality assurance, we strongly urge postcard or telephone follow-up of every continued pregnancy with a normal karyotype result. One cannot assume that a discrepant result will be automatically reported. We urge long-term follow-up of continued pregnancy after an abnormal or unclear cytogenetic result.

SCREENING FOR NEURAL TUBE DEFECTS

Prenatal diagnosis for spina bifida defects is the second most common reason for amniocentesis. Open neural tube defects, including anencephaly, meningocele, and meningomyelocele, occur in approximately one to two newborns per thousand in the United States. The rate should fall worldwide with the institution of dietary folic acid supplementation for women of childbearing age.

Anencephaly is a lethal condition, and most affected fetuses are stillborn. The prognosis for meningocele and meningomyelocele can be quite variable, depending on the anatomic site of the defect, the extent of spinal cord damage, and the presence or absence of associated hydrocephalus.

The familial nature of spina bifida has been well documented, although many genes influence the risk (multifactorial inheritance). For a couple who have one child with spina bifida, the empirical risk for recurrence is in the range of 2 to 5%. However, 95% of infants with spina bifida are born to couples with no family history.

Some cases of spina bifida are associated with other anomalies as part of a genetic syndrome such as Meckel's syndrome or Roberts' syndrome, both autosomal recessive conditions with a 25% risk of recurrence. Some can be associated with other risk factors such as maternal diabetes or prenatal medication exposure (i.e., isotretinoin or valproic acid).

Prior to the availability of maternal serum α-fetoprotein (MSAFP) screening, only patients with a positive family history of spina bifida were offered prenatal diagnosis. Although ultrasound examination can identify between 50 and 75% of spina bifida defects in the second trimester of pregnancy (9), its high cost has prevented its adoption as a screening test.

α-Fetoprotein (AFP) is the major protein in fetal plasma in early pregnancy. Peak levels of AFP are attained in fetal plasma at 12 to 14 weeks' gestation. The concentration falls rapidly thereafter. AFP levels in amniotic fluid (AFAFP) parallel fetal serum levels at 1/100th concentration. In maternal serum, however, AFP levels rise throughout the first and second trimesters, and peak at 28 to 30 weeks' gestation (Fig. 27.1). In 1972, Brock and Sutcliffe were the first to diagnose spina bifida defects prenatally by elevated AFAFP levels (10).

In 1973, Brock and coworkers first reported on the use of MSAFP assays to identify pregnancies at increased risk for spina bifida, introducing the concept of mass screening for open neural tube defects. Patients with elevated MSAFP values could then be offered diagnostic testing such as amniocentesis and ultrasound evaluation.

Antenatal Screening for Spina Bifida

Although neonatal screening for certain genetic disorders such as phenylketonuria was commonplace by the early 1960s, the idea of prenatal screening evoked considerable anxiety. The anxiety was partly related to the fact that an elevated MSAFP level was not always associated with a birth defect in the fetus. Furthermore, an elevated MSAFP did not identify all of the fetuses that had a neural tube defect. However, the element of false-positive and false-negative test results is inherent in the concept of screening tests. A valid screening test identifies a subgroup of patients who have a sufficient likelihood of an abnormality to warrant further diagnostic investigation. Over time, MSAFP screening gained broad acceptance, and during 1990, about half of all pregnancies in the United States were screened.

The United Kingdom was the first to apply population-based screening for spina bifida defects. Maternal serum samples obtained between 15 and 20 weeks' gestation were found to have the best predictive value. Approximately 85% of affected fetuses were identified with MSAFP cutoffs of 2.5 multiples of the median (MoM). Approximately 5% of all pregnant women would have values above this level, but only one woman in 50 in this high-risk group would actually carry a fetus with anencephaly or spina bifida. Half of the women with initially elevated MSAFP values had an inaccurate estimate of gestational age, fetal demise, or twin gestation as the cause of the elevation. Since an elevated MSAFP result is not diagnostic of a fetal abnormality, MSAFP screening can be effective only within a well-integrated program offering genetic counseling, ultrasound evaluation, and amniocentesis (11). The

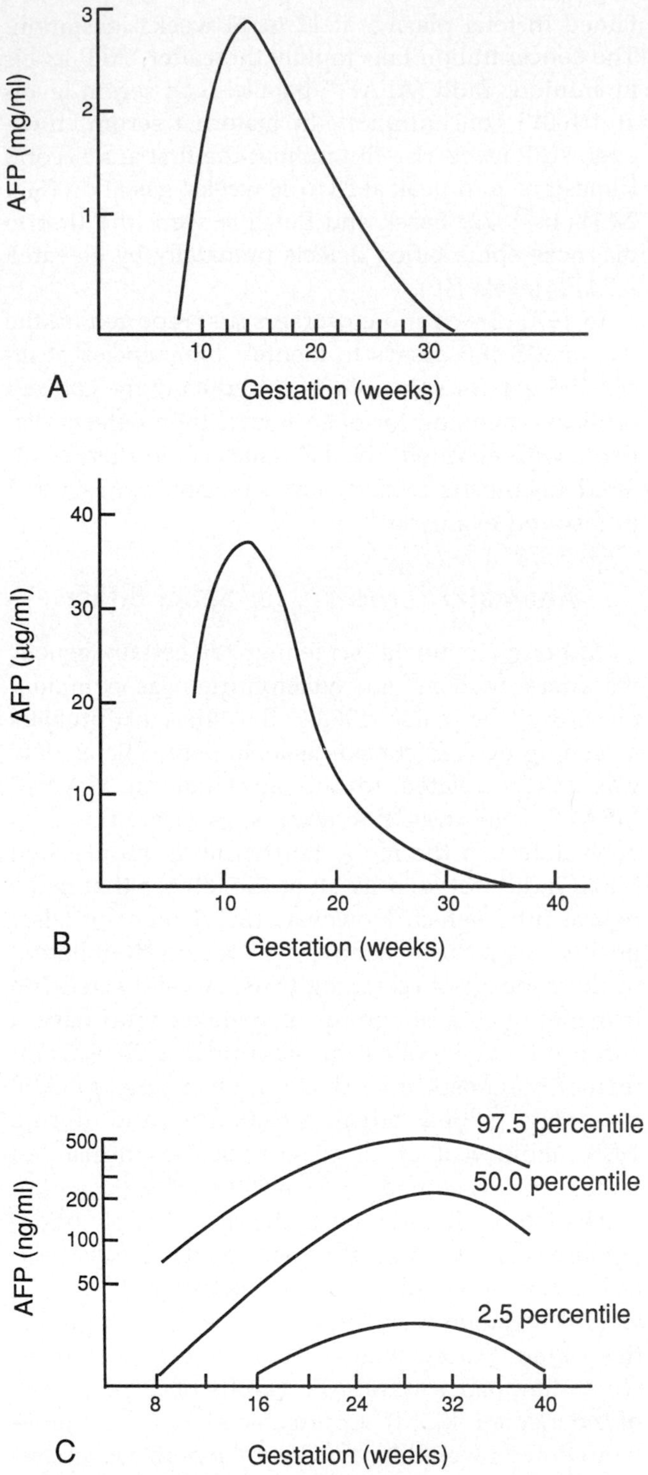

Figure 27.1. Approximate relationship between AFP values in (**A**) fetal serum, (**B**) amniotic fluid, and (**C**) maternal serum. Different units of measurement are used for each graph. (From Habib A. Maternal serum alpha-fetoprotein: its value in antenatal diagnosis of genetic disease and in obstetrical-gynecological care. Acta Obstet Gynecol Scand (suppl) 1977;61:1–72. Used with permission.)

United Kingdom's nationalized health care system offered an ideal setting for such a coordinated program (Table 27.5). After encouraging data were presented concerning MSAFP screening programs in the United Kingdom, and after extensive confirmatory studies, MSAFP test kits were released in the United States in 1983.

Table 27.5. Requirements for a Worthwhile Screening Program[a]

Aspect	Requirement
Disorder	Well defined
Prevalence	Known
Natural history	Medically important disorder for which an effective remedy is available
Finance	Cost-effective
Facilities	Available or easily installed
Ethics	Procedures following a positive result are generally agreed upon and acceptable to screening authorities and patients
Assay	Simple and safe
Test performance	Distributions of test values in affected and unaffected individuals are known. The extent of overlap is small. A suitable cutoff level is defined.

[a]From Cuckle HS, Wald, NJ. Principles of screening. In: Wald, NJ, ed. Antenatal and neonatal screening. London: Oxford University Press, 1984:1–22.

MSAFP Methods

Maternal serum AFP determinations are usually made by radioimmunoassay techniques. Values may be expressed in either ng/ml or IU/ml. Commercial MSAFP kits have been tested in clinical trials and "kit" normal ranges are published for each gestational week, but there is considerable variability among laboratories. Therefore, "kit normal values" are not recommended in establishing upper (or lower) limits of normal. Each laboratory must establish its own median for each gestational week between 15 and 20 weeks of gestation. To facilitate interlaboratory communication, AFP values are expressed as multiples of the median (MoM). For example, if laboratory A has a median value of 30 IU/ml at 16 weeks and laboratory B's median is 39 IU/ml, both values would be called 1.0 MoM at 16 weeks' gestation.

Determination of the appropriate cutoff for AFP depends on several criteria (Table 27.6). Most laboratories set a cutoff in the range of 2.0 to 2.5 MoM. MSAFP cutoffs in this range usually result in an 85 to 90% detection rate for open spina bifidas, with a false-positive rate of 3 to 5%.

ISSUES IN THE INTERPRETATION OF MSAFP SCREENING RESULTS

By midtrimester, the primary source of AFP in amniotic fluid is fetal urine. If a fetus has an open body wall defect, additional AFP leaks into the amniotic fluid as a transudate from the fetal serum.

Table 27.6. Prevalence, Detection Rate, and Specificity in Screening for Spina Bifida.

The *birth prevalence* of spina bifida varies in a specific geographic region. In the United States the prevalence is greater in the Northeast than in the Southwest. The prevalence in the United States also varies by ethnic group: about 1/700 in whites compared with 1/1500 in blacks. The overall incidence in the United States is 1/1,000 live births.

The *detection rate* (sensitivity): The proportion of affected individuals with a positive test result.

The *false-positive rate:* The proportion of unaffected individuals with a positive test result.

Steps in determining an AFP screening policy:
1. What is the local birth prevalence of open spina bifida?
2. What risk of open spina bifida is acceptable after screening?
3. The likelihood ratio (LR) is determined by considering the factors in 1 and 2.
4. $\text{LR} = \dfrac{\text{Detection rate (DR)}}{\text{False-positive rate (FPR)}}$
5. There is only one AFP cutoff that corresonds to a given LR.

[a]From Wald NJ, ed. Principles of screening. Antenatal and neonatal screening. London, Oxford University Press, 1984:1–22.

Gestational Age

MSAFP normally increases by approximately 15% per week from 15 to 21 weeks' gestation. Prior to 15 weeks' gestation, fetal urine is not the primary source of amniotic fluid. After 22 weeks' gestation, the fetal liver gradually switches from production of AFP to production of other serum proteins such as albumin. Therefore, outside of this gestational range, AFP is an unpredictable marker for spina bifida. In addition, discrepancies in gestational dating can have a significant impact on AFP interpretation. The first step in interpretation of abnormal AFP results is usually an ultrasound examination to check gestational dates (Fig. 27.2). Ultrasound gestational dating in the second trimester by biparietal diameter (BPD) is usually considered accurate within 7 days. Gestational weeks are calculated through the last completed week (e.g., 16.1 to 16.9 weeks' gestation are within the 16th week). MSAFP interpretations are usually revised if the ultrasound examination findings change the gestational dating by at least 10 days.

Race

MSAFP values tend to be 12 to 15% higher in patients of African American descent compared with Caucasians, and blacks have a lower prevalance of spina bifida defects. Because of these differences, application of a uniform cutoff without regard to race would label a larger proportion of black patients as "elevated," leading to a higher amniocentesis rate in blacks. For screening programs with a significant black patient population, racially pooled samples would also raise the medians for the entire population, and this in turn could lead to a lower detection rate in nonblacks. This problem can be addressed in one of two ways. Some laboratories establish separate medians for black and nonblack patients. Others calculate medians for nonblacks and use a correction factor to provide race-adjusted medians for black patients.

Diabetes

Pregnant women with insulin-dependent diabetes mellitus have an increased risk for birth defects, including open and closed central nervous system defects and congenital heart defects. Some studies suggest a 15 to 20% rate of birth defects compared with the general population incidence of 3 to 5%. For this reason, some programs use a lower cutoff MoM in diabetic patients. Many geneticists recommend more thorough diagnostic evaluation in pregnancies of insulin-dependent diabetic women, including amniotic fluid AFP, acetylcholinesterase, and detailed fetal ultrasound examination. In addition, diabetic mothers have 70 to 80% lower MSAFP levels at each week of gestation. To compensate for this, many laboratories use a correction factor to adjust the MoM.

Twins

MSAFP cutoffs for singleton pregnancies (2.0 to 2.5 MoM) label 56% of twin gestations as "elevated" (Fig. 27.3). This is not surprising, since each normal fetus contributes approximately 1.0 MoM of AFP to the maternal circulation. Therefore, many laboratories set the upper limit of normal for twin gestations at double the singleton cutoff (4.0 to 5.0 MoM). However, since twins are not usually concordant for spina bifida, a more important screening concern is the expected MSAFP results for discordant twins; i.e., when one twin is affected and one is not. In singleton pregnancies, the median MSAFP value for a fetus with open spina bifida is 3.7 MoM, so screening programs that set their twin cutoff below 4.7 MoM (1.0 MoM + 3.7 MoM) can expect at least a 50% detection rate for discordant twins.

Procedure-related Elevations of MSAFP

Both amniocentesis and CVS are associated with fetomaternal bleeding, which causes a transient elevation in MSAFP of 2 to 4 weeks' duration. Genetics programs that obtain blood samples for MSAFP on amniocentesis patients must obtain samples prior to performing the procedure.

First-trimester CVS or early amniocentesis (11 to 14 weeks' gestation) offers the advantage of earlier fetal chromosomal or biochemical diagnosis, but spina bifida prenatal diagnosis by assay of AFAFP is not yet available at that gestational age. Therefore, all

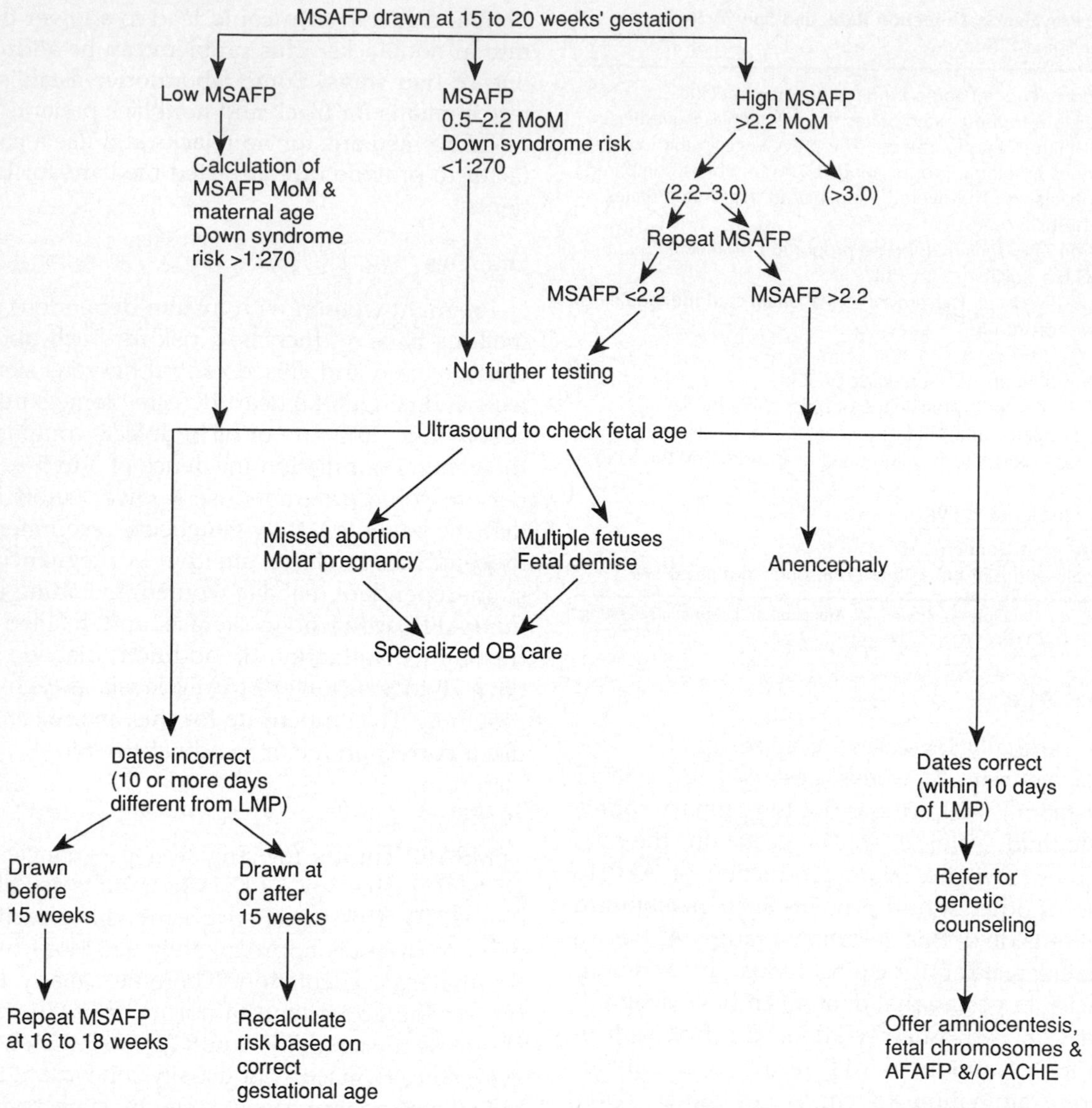

Figure 27.2. Protocol used at Henry Ford Hospital for the management of patients with abnormal MSAFP levels.

such patients should be offered the option of MSAFP screening at 16 weeks' gestation. Approximately 1% of CVS patients have an elevated MSAFP at 16 weeks and require amniocentesis and detailed ultrasound evaluation.

AFP elevations are not specific for neural tube defects. Other open body wall defects, such as gastroschisis and omphalocele, also allow excess AFP transudation. Many other fetal anomalies may also be associated with elevated MSAFP (Table 27.7). Since many of these can be identified prenatally, complete diagnostic evaluation is recommended, including amniocentesis for AFAFP, acetylcholinesterase, fetal karyotype, and ultrasound examination.

LOW MSAFP

An association between low MSAFP values and chromosome abnormalities was first reported in 1984(12). The MSAFP median for Down's syndrome fetuses is approximately 0.7 MoM for normal singleton pregnancies (Fig. 27.4). Some reports have suggested that trisomy 18, triploidy, and sex-chromosome abnormalities also have lower median MSAFP values. The etiology of low MSAFP in chromosomal syndromes is unclear, although placental immaturity has been suggested (13).

Prior to MSAFP screening, maternal age was shown to be the strongest indicator of risk for Down's syndrome and other trisomies. However, only 20% of Down's syndrome fetuses were born to women age 35 or older. Screening for low MSAFP provides an independent indicator of increased risk for Down's syndrome. Studies showed that approximately 20% of Down's syndrome fetuses had MSAFP values below 0.4 MoM, whereas only 5% of all MSAFP values fall below this level (14).

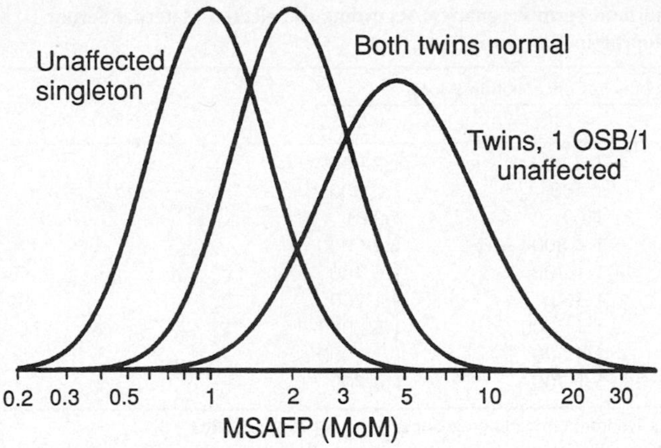

Figure 27.3. Distribution of MSAFP values for singleton and twin pregnancies. Median MoM for normal singletons is 1.0 MoM. Median MoM for normal twins is 2.0 MoM. Median MoM for twins—one twin normal and with open spina bifida (OSB) is 4.8 MoM. (Reprinted with permission of Palomaki G, Foundation of Blood Research, Scarborough, Maine.)

Table 27.7. Other Causes of Elevated MSAFP Values

Oligohydramnios
Renal anomalies
Bilateral renal agenesis
Congenital nephrosis
Urinary tract obstruction
Infantile polycystic kidney disease
Sacrococcygeal teratoma
Chorioangioma of the placenta
Fetal demise
Chromosome abnormality (e g , triploidy or autosomal trisomy)

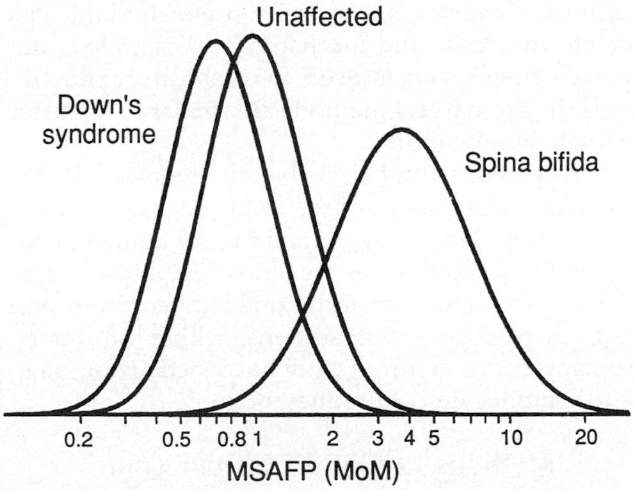

Figure 27.4. Distribution of MSAFP values in controls and a series of patients with Down's syndrome. (Reprinted with permission of Palomaki G, Foundation of Blood Research, Scarborough, Maine.)

Most laboratories now employ age-adjusted MSAFP cutoffs that assign a likelihood for Down's syndrome and detect an additional 20 to 25% of Down's syndrome cases. Newer triple-screen assays detect 60% of all Down's syndrome cases. In our program, women whose risk for Down's syndrome is at least one in 270 (the midtrimester risk for Down's syndrome in a 34-year-old woman) are offered further diagnostic evaluation including an ultrasound examination to confirm gestational dates and amniocentesis. Irrespective of a normal range MSAFP or triple-screen result, it remains the standard of obstetrical care to offer amniocentesis to all women over age 35 at the estimated date of confinement.

Maternal Weight

Shortly after the introduction of low-MSAFP screening, genetics centers noted a disproportionately high number of obese patients in the "low-MSAFP" group. This association was due to dilution of fetal AFP in the greater serum volume in heavier women. Most laboratories now use a weight correction factor to lessen this bias.

As for elevated MSAFP, a low MSAFP interpretation is also dependent on accurate gestational dating. Very low values are often associated with gestational age less than 14 weeks, molar pregnancy, or missed abortion. MSAFP values are reinterpreted if an ultrasound examination demonstrates a change in dates of at least 10 days (Fig. 27.2).

Since 1987, investigators have identified two additional fetoplacental chemicals in maternal serum, estriol and human chorionic gonadotropin (HCG), which have predictive association with Down's syndrome. Bogart and coworkers (15) reported a 56% detection rate for chromosomally abnormal fetuses using a simple cutoff of 2.5 MoM for maternal serum HCG. Canick and coworkers (13, 16) found that the median value of maternal serum estriol in 22 Down's syndrome fetuses was approximately 0.79 MoM. Using multivariate analysis of these three biochemical markers plus maternal age, Down's syndrome detection rates of 60% can be achieved (Table 27.8). Many screening programs are implementing these multiple assays for Down's syndrome and trisomy 18 screening; our program employs the three markers AFP, estriol, and human chorionic gonadotropin.

Amniotic Fluid AFP

Prenatal diagnosis of open spine defects by amniotic fluid AFP analysis has been routinely available since the early 1970s. More than 98% of cases of anencephaly and open spine defects have AFAFP levels above 2.5 MoM, compared to less than 1% of normal fetuses that have values above 2.5 MoM.

Other anomalies associated with defects in the fetal skin, such as omphalocele and gastroschisis, also result in elevated AFAFP.

False-positive AFAFP values may be associated with fetal blood admixture in the amniotic fluid sam-

Table 27.8. Probability of a 35-Year-Old Woman Having a Down's Syndrome Term Pregnancy According to Selected Maternal Serum Human Chorionic Gonadotropin (HCG), Unconjugated Estriol, and α-Fetoprotein Concentrations.[b]

		α-Fetoprotein Concentration (MoM)		
Unconjugated Estriol (MoM)	HCG (MoM)	0.4	1.0	2.5
0.4	0.5	1:370	1:2,800	1:22,000
	1.0	1:84	1:480	1:2,800
	2.0	1:16	1:69	1:310
1.0	0.5	1:820	1:4,800	1:28,000
	1.0	1:330	1:1,400	1:6,400
	2.0	1:110	1:360	1:1,200
1.4	0.5	1:2,200	1:11,000	1:52,000
	1.0	1:1,300	1:4,600	1:17,000
	2.0	1:630	1:1,700	1:4,700

[a]From Wald NJ, Cuckle HC, Densem JD, et al. Maternal serum screening for Down's syndrome in early pregnancy. Br Med J 1988;297:883–887.
[b]MoM, multiple of median value for unaffected pregnancies of same gestational age.

ple. A Kleihauer-Betke test on the sample can confirm the presence of fetal red cells.

Amniotic fluid acetylcholinesterase (AChE) is a second biochemical marker that is positive in 95% of fetuses with an open neural tube defect (17). The likelihood of an open spine defect is greater than 99.5% when AFAFP and AChE are both positive. Some fetuses with ventral wall defects may also have positive AChE results. Nicholas Wald and coworkers (18) found that the ratio of pseudocholinesterase to acetylcholinesterase was a useful tool to differentiate open spina bifida from ventral wall defects.

Some patients may present with the diagnostic dilemma of elevated amniotic fluid AFP and negative AChE assay. This biochemical pattern may be seen in one-third of fetuses with ventral wall defects, which can usually be identified by an ultrasound examination. The most common reason for positive amniotic fluid AFP and negative AChE is fetal hemorrhage into the amniotic fluid, and this pattern is observed in 90% of fetal blood contamination cases because the concentration of AChE is lower in fetal blood than in fetal cerebrospinal fluid. In the remaining 10%, the hemorrhage is so extensive that AChE is also elevated. Positive amniotic fluid AFP associated with negative AChE has also been reported in congenital nephrosis. Most pregnancies with a positive AFP and negative AChE pattern end in the delivery of a normal full-term infant.

Detailed ultrasound evaluation in the midtrimester is useful to identify the level of the spinal defect and to detect early changes of fetal hydrocephalus in most cases (Fig. 27.5).

SPECIMEN COLLECTION, CELL CULTURE, AND SLIDE PREPARATION

So far, amniocentesis has been the most commonly used procedure to obtain fetal cells at 14 to 20 weeks of gestation. Many laboratories prefer to culture amniocyte monolayers on coverslips in small Petri dishes and harvest the mitotic cells in situ for analysis of chromosomes from cells of distinctly different colonies. Harvesting of amniocyte culture follows the same principles used in harvesting lymphocytes or tissues. Colcemid is added to arrest cell division at metaphase, and treatment with a hypotonic solution disperses chromosomes within the cell membrane. The cells are then fixed in situ, chromosome preparations are stained usually using GTG-banding, and metaphase spreaders are analyzed microscopically.

Chorionic villus sampling is generally performed during the first trimester. The villi can be used to obtain chromosome preparations by direct harvest or monolayer culture methods. By using a direct harvest method, metaphase spreads can be prepared within a few hours after sampling. For monolayer cultures, which we prefer, cells in the chorionic villi are enzymatically and mechanically dissociated, and the cell suspension is used to establish in situ cultures. In situ harvest methods are similar to those for amniotic fluid cultures.

Percutaneous umbilical blood samples (PUBS) provide a fetal tissue source from pregnancies at 20 weeks' gestation or beyond, and up to term depending on the indication for the study. Fetal blood samples drawn directly from the umbilical cord can provide chromosome preparations within 48 hours. Specimens are cultured and harvested using standard lymphocyte culture methods.

Methods to Obtain Chromosome Preparations for Prenatal Testing

REAGENTS

Chang complete media: 100 ml (Irvine Scientific) with 10 ml supplement C, 0.25 ml penicillin-streptomycin and 2.0 ml L-glutamine. Store at 4°C for up to 5 days.

Transport media for villi: 100 ml RPMI 1640 with 1.5 ml glutamine, 1.0 ml heparin, 5.25 ml fetal bovine

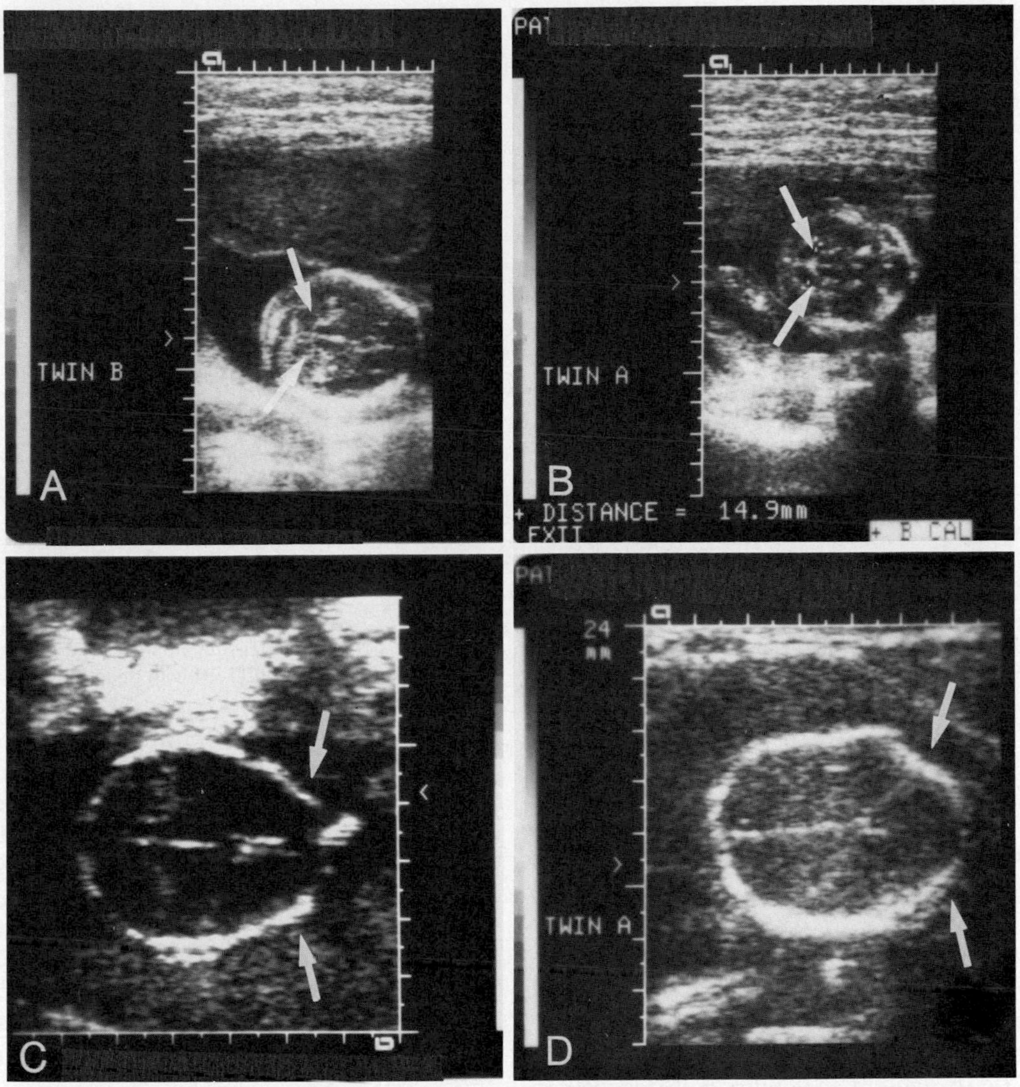

Figure 27.5. Comparison of midtrimester cranial ultrasound findings in fetuses with and without open spina bifida. **A**, Normal transverse scan of cranium at the level of the cerebellum (*arrows*). **B**, Scan at the same level of a fetus with open spina bifida, demonstrating a positive "banana sign," compression of the cerebellum due to Arnold-Chiari malformation. **C**, Transverse scan of a normal fetus at the level of the lateral ventricles. **D**, Scan at the same level of a fetus with open spina bifida, demonstrating the positive "lemon sign," reflecting a narrowing of the frontal calvarium.

serum, and 0.25 ml gentamicin. Store at 4°C for up to 7 days.

Gentamicin (GIBCO): 10 mg/ml.

L-Glutamine (GIBCO): 200 mM.

Penicillin-streptomycin (GIBCO): 10,000 IU/ml penicillin and 10,000 IU/ml streptomycin.

Colcemid (GIBCO): 10 μg/ml.

Fetal bovine serum (Flow Laboratories).

Hand's buffered salt solution (HBSS) (GIBCO) 1X: 100-ml bottle with 0.25 ml gentamicin.

Hypotonic: 0.8% sodium citrate.

Fixative: 3:1 anhydrous methanol:glacial acetic acid or 5 parts anhydrous methanol:2 parts glacial acetic acid. Prepare fresh before each use.

Trypsin solution (GIBCO): 0.05% 1× with EDTA.

Ethidium bromide (BioRad): 0.3 mg/ml. Warning: mutagenic.

Sterilized 22-mm^2 coverslips are prearranged in sterile 35-mm culture dishes.

All centrifugation steps are performed under the same conditions: 10 min at 140 × G (e.g., 800 rpm using a 185-mm radius centrifuge head.)

All tissue culture work is performed in a laminar flow hood using sterile technique. All cultures are incubated in 5% O_2/5% CO_2/90% N_2 incubators. The cultures grow more quickly in a low-oxygen atmosphere, but traditional incubators with 5% CO_2 can be used.

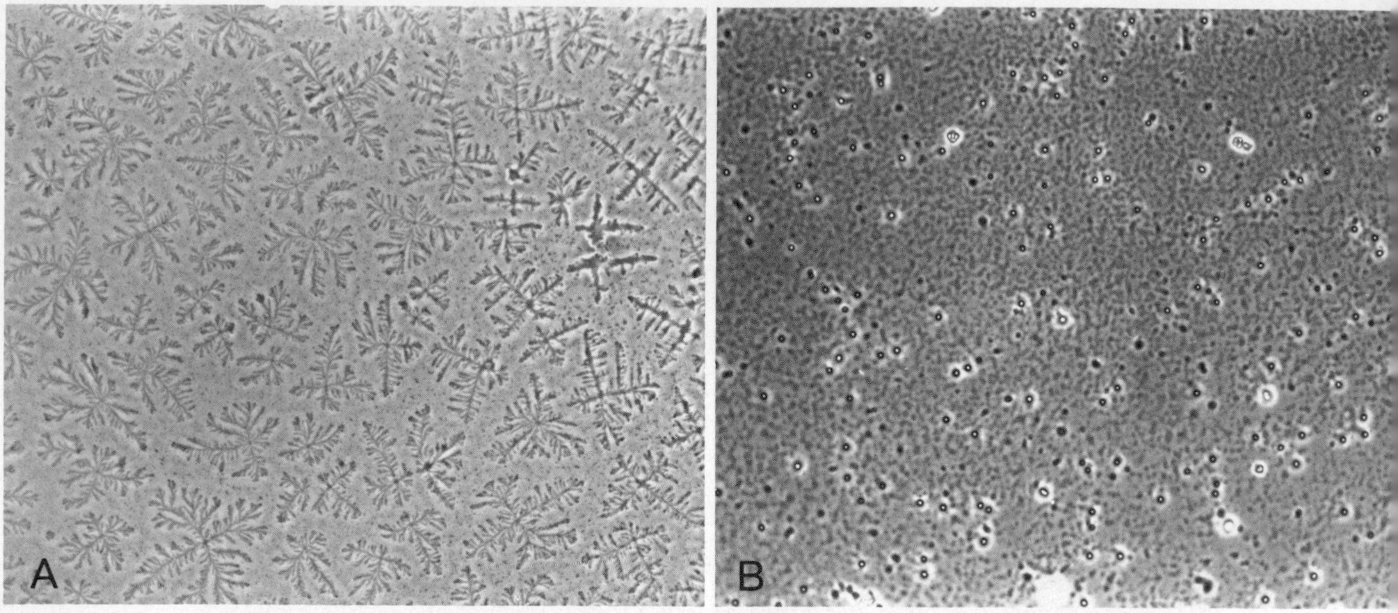

Figure 27.6. Urine and amniotic fluid can be distinguished by microscopic examination of a droplet of the fluid spread, dried on a microscope slide. The proteins in amniotic fluid give the appearance of ferning (**A**) that is not observed with urine (**B**).

Culture of Amniotic Fluid Cells

1. Two tubes of amniotic fluid (Fig. 27.6), with 20 ml total, are generally sent to the laboratory. If AFP and/or AChE assays are requested, aliquot 1 to 2 ml per test into a sterile tube. Centrifuge both tubes.
2. Remove all but 0.5 ml of supernatant from each tube. Add 1 to 2 ml media to each of the original tubes and resuspend the cells.
3. Distribute the cell suspension from each tube among a total of eight coverslip cultures. When specimens are grossly bloody or when a large number of cells is required for special testing protocols, establish cultures in T-25 flasks. Add another 3 ml of media to each flask culture. *NOTE*: Extreme care must be taken in labeling specimens for prenatal testing. A name and/or ID number should appear on each culture as well as identifying which amniotic fluid tube was used to establish the culture. Analysis should be performed on cells cultured from each tube.
4. Incubate cultures at 37°C.
5. After 12 to 24 hours' incubation, gently add 1 to 1.5 ml prewarmed media to each coverslip, taking care not to dislodge cells that have adhered to the coverslip.
6. On days 3 to 5 of culture, aspirate the media from the culture dish and flask and replenish with 1.5-ml prewarmed media (4-ml media for flask cultures). Flask cultures should be maintained by replenishing the media every third day with 4 ml prewarmed media. Coverslip cultures should be fed every third day until they are ready to harvest.
7. Cultures are examined on the 5th to 6th day of culture and every day thereafter until all cultures are harvested. An inverted microscope is used to evaluate cell growth. A coverslip is ready to harvest when there are 2 or more feathery colonies (separate areas of growth) with 100 to 200 cells per colony.

Culture of Chorionic Villus Cells

1. A 5- to 15-mg sample of chorionic villi (Fig. 27.7), or more, is transported to the laboratory in transport media. A sample of less than 5 mg of villi is only marginally satisfactory.
2. Transfer the specimen to a large culture dish, and using two TB syringes, dissect away any blood clots and tissue that do not appear to be villus in origin.
3. Select villi with buds and visible capillaries and rinse several times in HBSS.
4. Transfer villus pieces into a 60-mm culture dish containing 5 ml of trypsin-EDTA solution. Swirl the dish gently and incubate at 37°C for at least 2 hours.
5. With sterile forceps, pick each piece and shake vigorously in the trypsin solution. Place the pieces in a 60-mm culture dish containing 5 ml Chang media and 2 mg/ml collagenase V. Using two sterile tuberculin syringes or two scalpels, mince the tissue into small pieces, about 1 to 2 mm in diameter. Incubate the collagenase-cell suspension for 2 hours.

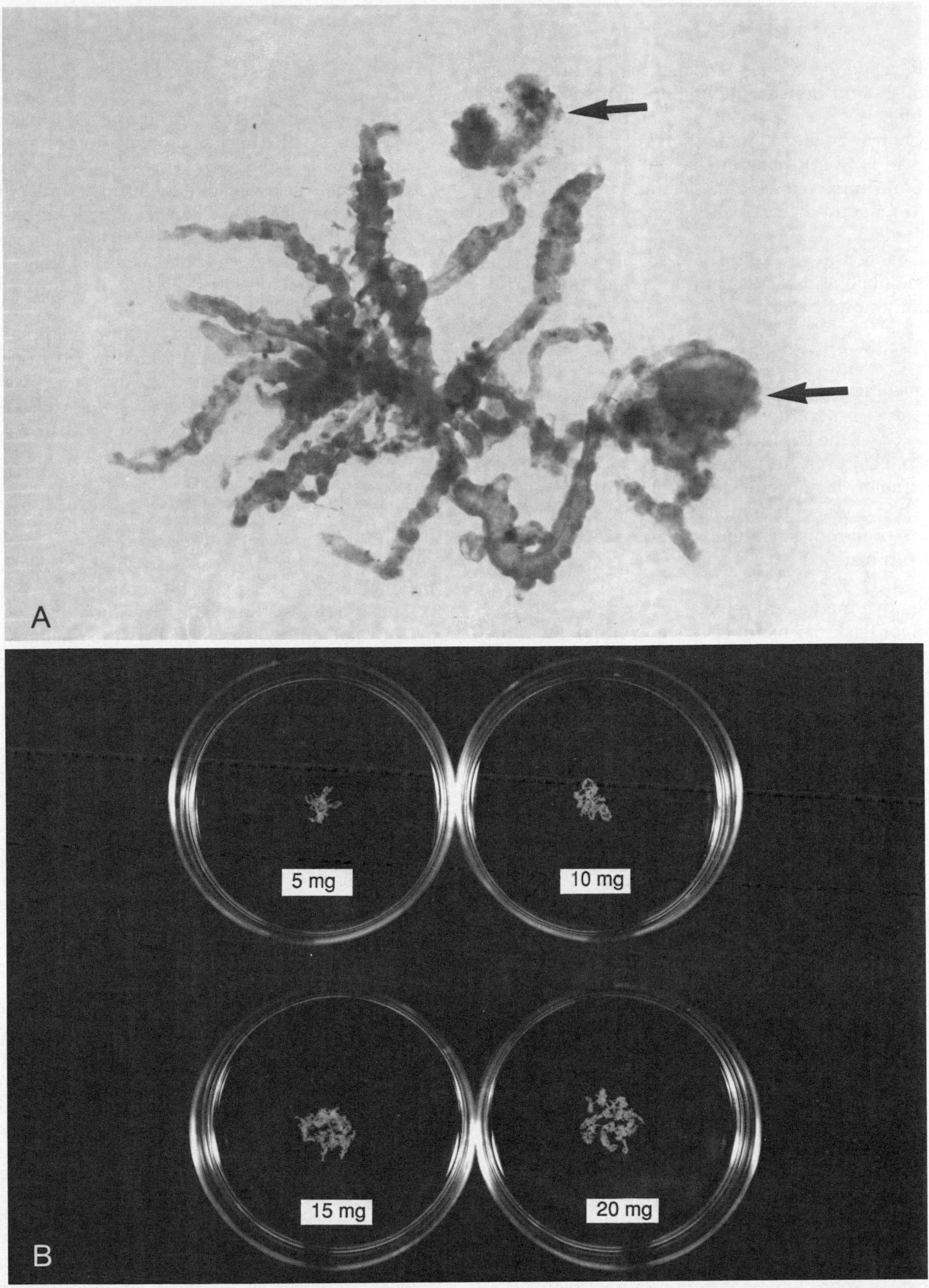

Figure 27.7. Chorionic villi (**A**) have a characteristic appearance of fronds of coral, whereas decidua (*arrows*) appear spongiform. **B** shows the appearance of 5, 10, 15, and 20 mg of villi in 60-mm small Petri dishes.

6. Resuspend the villus/collagenase mixture vigorously and transfer the mixture to a sterile 15-ml tube.
7. Centrifuge and aspirate the supernatant.
8. Add 5 ml of Chang media and mix well.
9. Centrifuge and aspirate the supernatant.
10. Resuspend the cell pellet in 2 ml of fresh Chang media.
11. Establish in situ cultures as for amniocytes, and maintain and harvest cultures following protocol for amniotic fluid.

Subculture of Flasks and Coverslips

Subculture of a flask or coverslip culture may be necessary if a culture is needed for noncytogenetic studies or if the culture becomes confluent. Harvests from subcultures are usually better quality if carried out either 1 day after feeding or 2 days after subculture. For flask cultures, follow the protocol for subculture of fibroblast cultures (Chapter 26). For coverslip cultures:

1. Remove media and replace with Hank's BSS (3.0 ml for flask, 1.5 ml for coverslip culture). Swirl the culture to rinse and remove the Hank's BSS.
2. Add trypsin EDTA (2 ml for flask, 1 ml for coverslip culture).
3. Incubate at 37°C for 5 minutes.
4. Lightly tap the culture vessel to dislodge some of the cells.
5. Add complete media to inactivate the trypsin and split the culture into one or more vessels.
6. Feed with media on the following day.

Harvest

Sterile technique is not required. For harvest of tissue culture flasks, follow the protocol described in Chapter 26 for fibroblast cultures. For coverslip cultures:

1. Add 4 drops (about 20 μl) of ethidium bromide to each coverslip culture using a tuberculin syringe, and return it to the incubator for 45 minutes. Add 1 drop (about 5 μl) colcemid from a tuberculin syringe and return the culture to the incubator for an additional 10 minutes.
2. Using a Pasteur pipette held against the side of the dish, aspirate all of the media, taking care not to touch the coverslip.
3. Gently add 2 ml of hypotonic solution and incubate at room temperature for 25 minutes.
4. Gently add 2 ml of fixative to the dish and incubate at room temperature for 3 minutes.
5. Aspirate most of the liquid from the dish but do not allow the coverslip to dry out.
6. Add 3 ml of fresh fixative and let stand for 20 minutes.
7. Aspirate fixative and repeat fixative "washes" two times with incubation times of 20 and 10 minutes.
8. After final wash, aspirate the fixative until a thin layer remains on the coverslip and the edges around the coverslip begin to dry.
9. Immediately invert the culture dish over an alcohol lamp flame until the cell side of the coverslip is nearly dry. The intensity of heat required for good spreading varies with room humidity.
10. Write the coverslip identification number on the back of the coverslip and place in drying oven at 65°C overnight or at 90°C for 1 hour.
11. Chromosomes are G-banded using trypsin as described in Chapter 25.

Robotic Harvesting of Cultures

In situ cultures can be processed using a robotic harvesting system (e.g., Tecan by Tecan U.S., Chapel Hill, NC, or Ser-Gen by Sermeter Co., Niles, IL). This is a time-saving, consistent tool for harvesting and can improve the quality and quantity of metaphases. After incubation in colcemid, all cultures for harvest are placed on the base of the instrument. The aspiration and dispensing of media, hypotonic, and fixative are all done automatically through a computer-programmed process. The rate of aspiration, amount of solution dispensed, and incubation time between each step can be individually programmed to adapt to each laboratory's individual procedure. After the harvesting procedure is completed, cultures can be placed under an air-flow hood to control evaporation of fixative and spreading of the chromosomes.

Culture of PUBS

Lymphocyte cultures are established following the protocol for peripheral blood (Chapter 26). The amount of blood sent is usually 1 ml or less, and whole blood (rather than a buffy coat suspension) is used to inoculate the cultures. Two cultures are established, one to be harvested after 48 hours of incubation, and one generally incubated for a standard 66- to 72-hour harvest.

Fluorescent In Situ Hybridization Using Multiple Probes

Since chromosomes 13, 18, 21, X, and Y are responsible for most of the numerical chromosome abnormalities identified prenatally, a single rapid screening assay that could detect these trisomies might be desirable. Fluorescent in situ hybridization

(FISH) using DNA probes, either singly or in a cocktail with each probe labeled with a different fluorochrome, could be used to screen for aneuploidy by scoring the hybridization signals in interphase cells. Methods are currently being developed for the application of this technology to amniotic fluid cells, chorionic villus cells, or fetal cells isolated from the maternal blood circulation. Molecular cytogenetic techniques in prenatal screening may become more popular, but it is doubtful whether prenatal screening programs will ever supplant complete karyotype analysis.

CHROMOSOME ANALYSIS FOR PRENATAL DIAGNOSIS

The analysis of prenatal specimens is done in much the same way as for blood or tissue samples, as described in Chapter 26. The major difference with this specimen type is that cells for analysis can be selected from multiple distinct colonies. A laboratory ideally should be able to provide a reporting time of 3 to 6 days for PUBS, 6 to 12 days for CVS cultures, and 7 to 14 days for amniotic fluid cell cultures.

For in situ harvests we suggest analysis of at least 12 metaphase cells taken from 12 different colonies, and representing at least two independent cultures. For laboratories using a suspension harvest method, a minimal study should include analysis of 15 cells representing at least two culture vessels. In general, one cell per colony is analyzed, but other cells in the colony should be analyzed if an abnormal cell is found. In actual practice, we routinely analyze cells from three, four, or more cultures. We try to sample the greatest variety of cells to increase the likelihood of finding mosaicism and to reduce the risk of maternal cell contamination. We also recognize that these recommendations may be somewhat controversial, since the CAP inspection checklist has the general analysis requirement of 20 cells, or 15 in situ colonies. We would argue that for this specimen type the lower numbers are more than adequate since chromosomal mosaicism is not a screening target for prenatal diagnosis. Moreover, based on our long experience with analysis of 20 to 30 cells, the majority of mosaics can be identified with a 12-cell analysis.

For CVS, some laboratories attempt both direct and culture harvests, but this nearly doubles the cost of the analysis, with marginal benefit over the culture technique alone. We do not recommend reliance on direct chromosome preparations alone; cultured cells or pooled analysis from direct preparations and cultures is preferable. If both methods are employed, at least 15 cells should be analyzed, with at least 10 cells coming from the culture harvests.

We discourage the use of preliminary reports based on an unfinished analysis. The parents are usually but not always given the correct answer, and a false sense of security can be engendered in the parents, the physicians, and worst of all the laboratory personnel. The urgent need for a result does not justify the risk of an incorrect preliminary result.

We encourage the practice of confirming abnormal prenatal diagnosis results. This is a laboratory test that, on the basis of a single result, determines whether a desired pregnancy will be continued. The parents very often benefit from certain knowledge of a correct result, and the practice serves as a powerful quality control device for the cytogenetics laboratory. For a urea termination, fetal tissues are usually inviable in tissue culture, but an amniotic fluid sample can be obtained prior to instillation of the urea, and chorionic villi obtained after delivery are also usually viable.

CYTOGENETIC RESULTS

Growth Failure

For amniotic fluid samples, growth failure is rare in an experienced laboratory. Aside from technical catastrophe, sources of growth failure include maternal urine or hygroma fluid submitted as amniotic fluid, or heat or cold damage during transport of the specimen to the laboratory. A bloody amniotic fluid sample may grow more slowly, but a result can usually be expected. First-trimester CVS growth failure should be well under 1% for specimens that contain 5 mg or more of chorionic villi and have visible blood vessels (19, 20). The amniotic fluid cell culture failure rate should be 0.1% or less.

Maternal Cell Contamination

Maternal cell contamination (MCC) has been observed in about 0.3% to 0.5% of amniotic fluid cultures. We request at least two aliquots of fluid and find that maternal cell contamination is usually confined to cultures established from the first tube collected during amniocentesis. Some laboratories prefer to discard the first 2 ml of amniotic fluid. MCC is usually not an interpretive problem, since in almost every recognized case the majority of colonies in the culture are not maternal, and diagnostic errors (wrong sex or missed chromosome abnormality) are rare. Clusters of maternal cell contamination can be caused by an inexperienced person performing the amniocentesis procedure.

In CVS direct preparations, the very low rate (below 0.1%) of MCC is due to the relative absence of

Table 27.9. Estimate of the Increased Risk of Mental Retardation (with or without Birth Defects) Associated with Chromosome Rearrangements[a]

Type of Rearrangement	Risk Estimate
Unbalanced rearrangement	Nearly 100%
Balanced rearrangement	
Familial	0
De novo	
Robertsonian translocation	0–1
t(15;15)(p11;q11)	May be increased
Reciprocal translocation	3–15
Inversion	6–20
Extra marker, familial	Near 0
Extra marker, de novo:	
Not satellited	15–25%
Monosatellited	10–20%
Bisatellited	
Monocentric	Probably <5
Dicentric, 1 G-light band	Probably <10
Dicentric, > 1 bands	High risk

[a]The background risk is estimated to be 3%, so total risk is the sum of the two risk estimates. The total frequencies of each class of abnormality are summarized in Table 27.4. Statistics are from many sources, including Hsu LYF. Prenatal diagnosis of chromosome abnormalities. In: Milunksy A, ed. Genetic disorders and the fetus. 2nd ed. New York:Plenum Press, 1986;115–183; Hsu LYF, Perlis T. United States survey on chromosome mosaicism and pseudomosaicism in prenatal diagnosis. Prenat Diagn 4 1984:97–130; Warburton D. Outcome of cases of de novo structural rearrangements diagnosed at amniocentesis. Prenat Diagn 1984;4:69–80; Steinbach P, Djalali M, Hansmann I, et al. The genetic significance of accessory bisatellited marker chromosomes. Hum Genet 1983;65:155–164, and Van Dyke, unpublished data.

mitotic activity in the decidual fragments. The experience varies among laboratories, but MCC is identified as a 46,XX/46,XY admixture in 1 to 2% of CVS cultures. Undoubtedly, there is an equal frequency of unrecognized admixtures of maternal and 46,XX fetal cells. The maternal cells are usually in the minority and have caused few cytogenetic errors in experienced laboratories, although their presence can be problematic for biochemical or DNA studies.

The theoretical concern is that a mixture of 46,XX and 46,XY may represent a true chimera. The incidence of chimeras has been estimated at one in 60,000 newborns. Weighing this incidence against the rate of 46,XX/46,XY cell admixture in prenatal genetic cell cultures, the likelihood of maternal cell contamination in any individual case seems very high, even if 46,XX cells are seen in multiple culture vessels. When the 46,XX cells are confined to one or a minority of the cultures, they almost certainly represent maternal cell contamination. When an XX/XY admixture is identified, some laboratories raise the question of chimerism and some do not. Exceedingly few true chimeras identified in prenatal genetic studies have been described in the literature, and it is likely that a chimera presenting at prenatal diagnosis will not be identified as such. Other possible sources of XX/XY admixture include cross-contamination of samples, twins, or a resorbed twin.

Chromosome Rearrangement

If a chromosome rearrangement is identified, the risk to the fetus depends on whether or not the rearrangement is balanced and on whether or not it is familial (21, 22) (Tables 27.4 and 27.9). A balanced familial translocation or inversion does not confer a significantly increased risk for birth defects or mental retardation, nor does a familial extra marker chromosome (also termed extra small accessory chromosome or ESAC). A duplication or deletion involving euchromatin generally results in mental retardation with or without birth defects.

Extra Marker Chromosomes

For an extra marker chromosome (22, 23), whether mosaic or not, the karyotypes of both parents need to be studied with specific attention to the presence of a similar marker in a small proportion of their blood cells, and for the relatively common t(11;22) translocation associated with cat's eye syndrome (Tables 27.4 and 27.9). If the marker appears to be a new mutuation, C-banding should be done to determine whether it is dicentric. Ag-NOR staining or scoring satellite associations should be done to determine whether the marker is monosatellited or bisatellited. If the marker is bisatellited and either monocentric or dicentric with only a tiny amount of light-staining material between the centromeres, there is little to suggest an increased risk to the fetus for having birth defects or mental retardation. DA-DAPI staining can help to evaluate whether the marker is a dic(15) (q11–q13), but this knowledge does not improve the prediction of the risk to the fetus, at the present. FISH is also being used experimentally to identify the chromosomal origin of small markers.

Polyploidy

A diagnosis of tetraploidy or mosaic tetraploidy should be confirmed by an independent specimen and follow-up detailed ultrasound examination, unless defects were observed by ultrasound. Tetraploidy is a common artifact of harvest procedures in monolayer cultures. Triploidy is an occasional finding in prenatal studies, and, when seen in an amniocentesis culture, unambiguous abnormalities are usually evident on ultrasound examination.

Autosomal Monosomy Mosaicism

Rare cases of true mosaicism for monosomy 21 and monosomy 22 have been reported. A diagnosis of monosomy mosaicism should be considered if multiple cultures have colonies with the same monosomy. The diagnosis is sufficiently uncommon that detailed ultrasound and a confirmatory study (amniocentesis or PUBS) can be considered.

Trisomy 20 Mosaicism

About one in 2500 amniotic fluid cell cultures reveals true trisomy 20 mosaicism, which in many cases has been confirmed in fibroblast cultures from various tissue sources from the fetus or newborn, including urine sediment cells (originating from the bladder and kidney) and extrafetal membranes, although never from peripheral blood cultures. The clinical significance of this finding is still poorly understood, but a trisomy 20 syndrome has never been described. Also, the majority of newborns with this prenatal diagnosis have had a normal phenotype at birth and throughout the few follow-up studies extending into early childhood. Long-term investigation of such subjects is needed to provide better information to parents.

Sex Chromosome Aneuploidy

The phenotypes of the nonmosaic sex chromosome abnormalities 45,X; 47,XXX; 47,XXY; and 47,XYY are described in Chapter 26. The incidences of 47,XXY and 47,XXX increase with advancing maternal age, and together they constitute nearly 10% of the chromosome abnormalities we have detected prenatally.

45,X/46,XY Mosaicism

In our experience, this cytogenetic diagnosis constitutes about 2% of all abnormalities found prenatally. In the majority of the first such cases identified, the pregnancies were terminated because of the known association with Ullrich-Turner syndrome, mixed gonadal dysgenesis, and ambiguous genitalia. However, since most of the fetuses had normal-appearing male external genitalia, the parents of most more recent cases have continued the pregnancies. Although further research is required, the risk of abnormal sexual differentiation in prenatally diagnosed 45,X/46,XY is 5%. Detailed ultrasound examination of the external genitalia can be useful. The mosaicism is occasionally confirmed in fetal or extrafetal tissues. Confirmatory cytogenetic studies and long-term clinical follow-up are encouraged (24).

45,X/46,XX Mosaicism

This prenatal diagnosis requires further study, but in the absence of ultrasound evidence of a cystic hygroma or nonimmune hydrops, there may be little risk of fetal death or an Ullrich-Turner syndrome phenotype. As with 45,X/46,XY, this result appears to be consistent with a normal phenotype in most instances. The risk of isolated gonadal dysgenesis without an Ullrich-Turner phenotype is uncertain in this group. Many have normal puberty and fertility, although there is a suggestion of an increased risk of miscarriage or early menopause, so the 45,X/46,XX mosaic would want to take this into consideration in her own family planning. As with other prenatally diagnosed mosaics, cytogenetic confirmation and long-term follow-up are encouraged.

Prenatal Diagnosis of Mosaicism

The diagnosis of chromosomal mosaicism is one of the most difficult problems in clinical cytogenetics, and has been particularly troublesome in prenatal cytogenetic studies (25–27). When an abnormality is found in some but not all cells, the clinical significance is not always clear, and several possibilities need to be considered, including maternal cell contamination (discussed earlier), true fetal mosaicism, mosaicism confined to placental villi, and tissue culture artifact (false-positive, or pseudomosaicism).

About 0.2% of prenatal genetic studies reveal fetal mosaicism that can be confirmed by cytogenetic studies of fetal tissues. Another 1 to 5% have some degree of mosaicism (more than one cell with the same abnormality among the 10 to 20 cells scored) that is probably limited to the chorionic villi or to the tissue culture and has no clinical significance. A large proportion of studies have single cells with a missing or extra chromosome or a structural rearrangement. The challenge is to identify the clinically significant mosaicism.

Confined Placental Mosaicism

Among pregnancies in which mosaicism is detected in chorionic tissue by CVS but not confirmed at amniocentesis or in the fetus, the rate of pregnancy loss or growth retardation may be increased. These possibilities require further study but are supported by other observations of mosaicism limited to the placenta in 5 to 7% of pregnancies with spontaneous abortion or intrauterine growth retardation. Moreover, in trisomy 13 and 18 liveborns, confined placental mosaicism with a normal cell line has been reported, and it is plausible that the karyotypically normal placenta may play a role in the survival of these two nearly lethal trisomies. Other studies of placental cells have demonstrated confined placental mosaicism in pregnancies in which mosaicism was identified by CVS but not confirmed by amniocentesis. This is a source of false-positive results in direct CVS preparations.

Confined placental mosaicism has also been documented in amniocentesis mosaics, in which a mosaic trisomy identified in amniotic fluid cultures could not be confirmed in any of multiple fetal tissues but was found in cells from cultured chorion and chorionic villi. In these cases, the placental cells were apparently drawn into the amniocentesis needle as it traversed the extraembryonic tissue. Confined placental mosaicism has typically involved trisomies that are not associated with fetal viability.

Pure or mosaic "nonviable" trisomies (e.g., 2 and 16) have been observed in several direct preparations and cultures from CVS. These have not thus far been confirmed at amniocentesis or PUBS, and several normal infants have been delivered, although growth retardation was a complication in some, and one died in utero at gestational age 37 weeks. Many mosaic trisomies identified with CVS probably arise as trisomic conceptions. Fetal viability is salvaged by a compensating mitotic nondisjunction that produces a karyotypically normal cell population. Academic interest in this phenomenon is high, partly because of the possibility that the compensating nondisjunction can produce a normal appearing karyotype with isodisomy (both homologs from the same parent; see Chapter 26.)

Protocol for Mosaicism

Several protocols have been proposed to distinguish the true mosaicism from pseudomosaicism. Since we employ an in situ harvest method for both amniotic fluid and chorionic villus cell cultures, our protocol for dealing with possible mosaicism is similar for both cell types. Stated briefly, true fetal mosaicism is likely only when abnormal colonies are detected in independent preparations.

MIXED COLONY

If one colony has a mixture of abnormal and normal cells, and no other colony shows that abnormality, the abnormal cells are usually considered an in vitro artifact.

Many colonies represent single clones, but some do not. A colony can arise from several cells attached together in the original inoculum; cells can be dislodged during handling; and the cells do have limited mobility, so they can infiltrate nearby colonies or establish new, apparently independent colonies. Furthermore, independent clones can form a single colony as they enlarge. We have observed mosaicism limited to one side of a colony, with normal cells on the other side. This might be interpreted as a mixed colony, but examination of the clonal growth patterns under lower magnification can sometimes reveal that there were originally two separate colonies, each cytogenetically pure.

PURE COLONY

If we identify one colony that is abnormal, we usually attempt to score 10 or 20 additional colonies for that abnormality, particularly colonies in other cultures. In most cases, the additional cells scored do not have the same abnormality, and the abnormal colony is interpreted as a probable artifact of no clinical significance (pseudomosaic).

It is understood that classic cytogenetic techniques cannot identify 100% of all mosaics. The available data suggest that apparent pseudomosaicism in amniotic fluid cell cultures actually does reflect true fetal mosaicism in about 1% of cases. For CVS, the rate of true mosaicism interpreted only as pseudomosaicism is not known. Some laboratories use different protocols depending on whether the possible mosaicism is or is not consistent with viability, but since many unusual autosomal aneuploidies have been reported as mosaics in liveborns, we treat almost all cases of possible mosaicism in much the same way, as just described.

SINGLE ABNORMAL CELL

If a colony has only one metaphase spread, it is abnormal, and the abnormality is not consistent with a viable mosaicism (see Table 26.2), it is reasonable to interpret it as an artifact (pseudomosaic) (28). A single hypodiploid cell (even 45,X) almost always represents an artifact of culture or slide preparation. However, if the defect is consistent with a viable numerical or structural mosaicism, we follow the same protocol as for a pure abnormal colony, and score 10 to 20 additional colonies for that abnormality.

MULTIPLE PURE COLONIES IN ONE CULTURE

If multiple colonies have the same chromosome abnormality, all from the same culture vessel, we attempt to score 20 or more additional colonies from other culture vessels. In actual practice, the technologists often score all colonies from all available cultures. It seems highly unlikely that a mutation in tissue culture could produce more than two or three abnormal colonies. In an amniotic fluid cell culture, as well as in a CVS culture, multiple abnormal colonies may reflect confined placental mosaicism with fragments of cytogenetically abnormal chorionic villi having been introduced into just one culture vessel. If the mosaicism is not seen in any of at least 20 colonies from other cultures, the finding is usually interpreted as an artifact (pseudomosaic) or confined placental mosaicism.

Although follow-up at birth is strongly encouraged, aggressive prenatal follow-up studies, such as repeat amniocentesis, or amniocentesis after

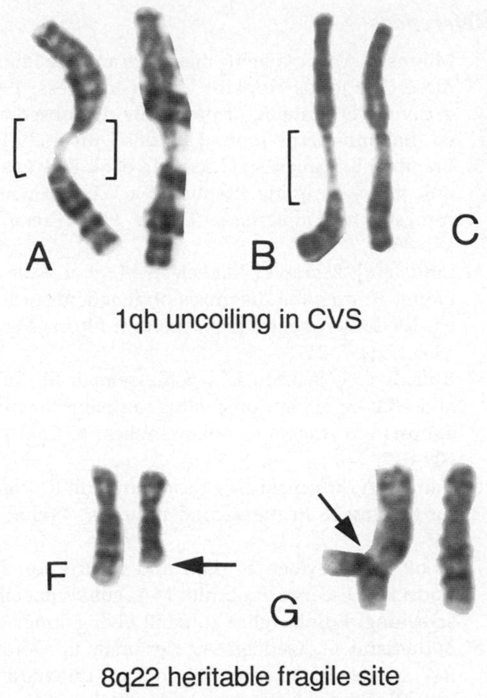

Figure 27.8. The fragile site at 8q22 and the uncoiler locus. Chromosome 1 uncoiling (**A** through **D**), usually not seen in chromosome preparations from other cell types, is a common artifact in CVS preparations. Both homologs (as in **A**) are frequently involved, and in occasional cells (**E**), an entire arm is lost. A chromosomal fragile site can give the appearance of chromosomal mosaicism by producing multiple colonies with the same abnormality, yet have no clinical significance. The case depicted here had three colonies with one or two cells (**F**) having a del(8)(q22); the remaining cells in each colony had a normal karyotype. One cell (**G**) had a triradial configuration at 8q22. Many other cells had a chromatid break or chromosome break (**H**) at the same site. This finding was interpreted as a heritable fragile site with a high rate of chromosome breakage located at the common fragile site, 8q22.

CVS for analysis of another tissue, are generally not done if the mosaicism is limited to a single culture vessel, since these would increase the risks to the fetus without ensuring an accurate cytogenetic diagnosis. If *all* of the colonies in one culture have the same abnormal karyotype, but no colonies from other cultures have it, one must consider the possibility of mixed-up samples.

MULTIPLE MIXED COLONIES IN MULTIPLE CULTURES

This situation is very unusual but may raise questions of an unstable chromosome such as a ring or dicentric, or of a chromosomal instability syndrome, which would need further investigation. Tetraploid and diploid cells appearing together within multiple colonies probably reflect a tissue culture artifact.

Chromosomal fragile sites other than the fragile site at Xq27.3 are considered to be of no clinical significance but can present themselves in this way (Fig. 27.8). Region 1q11–q12 is a C band–positive variable region, also known as 1qh or, in the older literature, the "uncoiler locus." In CVS preparations 1qh is true to its original moniker, because in some individuals it uncoils dramatically (Fig. 27.8). This behavior is not observed to the same extent in routine preparations of other cell types, and is of no known clinical significance when observed in a CVS preparation.

MULTIPLE CULTURE VESSELS

If an abnormality is observed in multiple colonies grown in more than one culture vessel, true mosaicism is likely. From U.S., Canadian, European, and other large surveys of mosaicism in amniocentesis, mosaicism was confirmed in 60 to 70% of cases, but this is considered a minimal figure of the proportion of true mosaics in this group. True mosaicism is also likely if observed in both direct and cultured CVS cells. In our experience, more than half of true mosaics have involved the sex chromosomes, often 45,X/46,XX or XY, and pregnancies usually were continued with a normal outcome.

FOLLOW-UP STUDIES FOR MOSAICISM

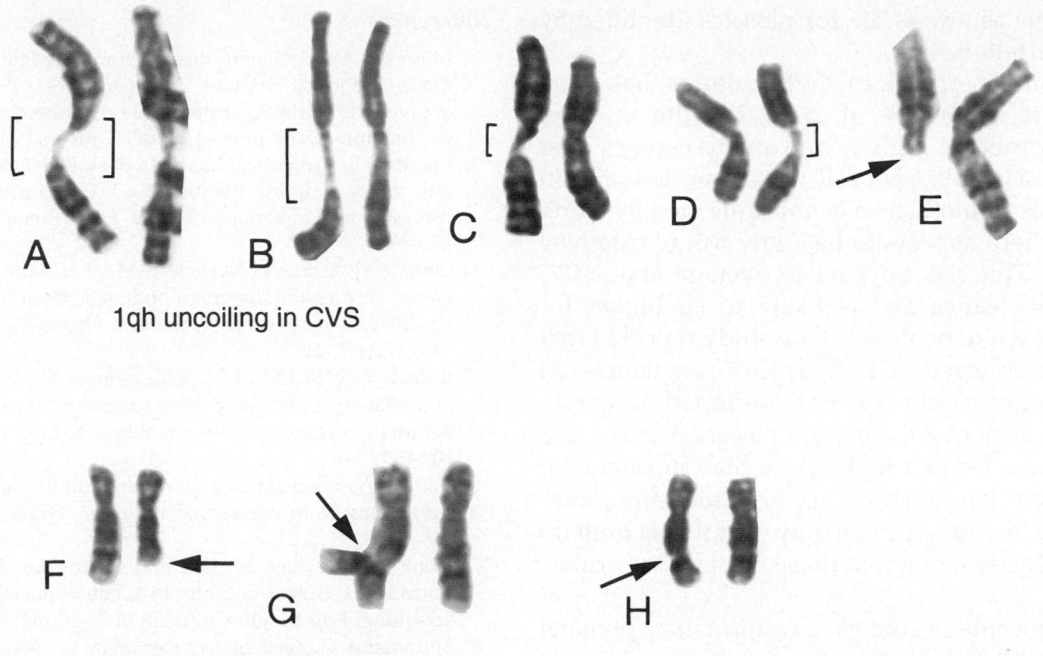

If mosaicism is detected in a direct CVS preparation but not in the cultures, there is a low chance of true fetal mosaicism, especially if the mosaicism involves a "lethal trisomy." Mosaicism found on a direct CVS is usually not confirmed in amniotic fluid or fetal blood cells, and direct CVS is especially weak at detecting true fetal mosaicism. The rate of true mosaicism may be as low as 5% for mosaics identified by direct preparation.

Mosaicism identified in CVS cultures has been confirmed in 40 to 70% of cases, but the true frequency is probably higher, and many centers offer amniocentesis confirmation if mosaicism is found in CVS cultures. If mosaicism is not confirmed by amniocentesis, there appears to be a low risk of true fetal mosaicism. This risk appears to average about 1%, but probably varies and is likely to be higher for mosaics known to be viable. One study reported that miscarriage occurred in 13 to 17% of pregnancies in which CVS mosaicism was not confirmed at amniocentesis. In such cases, confined placental mosaicism may be detectable at a higher rate than normal (29). The relatively long wait for confirmatory amniocentesis results is a source of anxiety, but this is preferable to simply assuming that these mosaics are artifactual.

For amniocentesis studies, a confirmatory prenatal study is usually not undertaken when mosaicism is confined to a single culture vessel. A follow-up study and a detailed ultrasound examination of the fetus may be appropriate when (*a*) the physicians and family agree to confirm mosaicism (or other abnormal result) when the decision would be to interrupt the pregnancy only if the abnormality is confirmed; (*b*) only a single culture is available or an uncertain result is obtained from a very small sample of amniotic fluid or villi; (*c*) the quality of the cytogenetic preparation is below usual standards and has led to an uncertain result; and (*d*) a 46,XX and 46,XY admixture in multiple cultures is observed. In some circumstances, tissue-limited mosaicism is possible (e.g., trisomy 20 or extra marker chromosome), so a PUBS is not always an appropriate sample for confirming mosaicism. The staff and the family must recognize that a normal result on confirmatory studies cannot rule out mosaicism nor ensure a normal outcome of the pregnancy, and that even when mosaicism is confirmed by amniocentesis or CVS, the clinical interpretation is subject to uncertainties as to risk to the fetus and the likelihood of the mosaicism in the fetus.

There are many unknowns in the clinical interpretation of mosaicism, de novo balanced rearrangements, and extra marker chromosomes. For this reason we strongly urge all groups involved in prenatal diagnosis to participate in cytogenetic and clinical follow-up studies, including long-term clinical follow-up when pregnancies are continued, and cytogenetic studies of placenta, amnion, circumcision skin, and other tissues when possible.

References

1. Milunsky A, ed. Genetic disorders and the fetus. 3rd ed. Baltimore: The Johns Hopkins University Press, 1992.
2. Weaver DD. Catalog of prenatally diagnosed conditions. 2nd ed. Baltimore: The Johns Hopkins University Press, 1992.
3. Brambati B, Kuliev A, Jackson L, et al. Risk evalution in chorionic villus sampling. Report of a WHO consultation on first trimester fetal diagnosis, 1 June 1985. Prenat Diagn 1986;6: 451–456.
4. Lindsten J, Marsk L, Mikkelson M, et al. Role of chorion villi biopsy in prenatal diagnosis of genetic disorders. In: Berg K, ed. Medical genetics: past, present, future. Prog Clin Biol Res 1985;177:195–212.
5. Rhoads GG, Jackson LG, Schlesselman SE, et al. The safety and efficacy of chorionic villus sampling for early prenatal diagnosis of cytogenetic abnormalities. N Engl J Med 1989;320: 609–617.
6. Canick JA, Palomaki GE, Osanthanondh R. Prenatal screening for trisomy 18 in the second trimester. Prenat Diagn 1990;10: 546–548.
7. Hook EB. Prevalence, risks and recurrence. In: Brock DJH, Rodeck CH, Ferguson-Smith MA, eds. Prenatal diagnosis and screening. Edinburgh: Churchill Livingstone, 1992:351–392.
8. Sutherland G, Gedeon A, Kornman L, Donnelly A, Byard RW, Mulley JC, Kremer E, Lynch M, Pritchard M, Yu S, Richards RI. Prenatal diagnosis of fragile X syndrome by direct detection of the unstable DNA sequence. N Engl J Med 1991;325: 1720–1722.
9. Nyberg DA, Mack LA, Hirsch J, et al: Abnormalities of fetal cranial contour in sonographic detection of spina bifida: evaluation of the "lemon" sign. Radiology 1988;167:387–392.
10. Brock DJH, Sutcliffe RG. Alpha-fetoprotein in the antenatal diagnosis of anencephaly and spina bifida. Lancet 1972;2:197.
11. Cuckle HS, Wald NJ. Principles of screening. In: Wald NJ, ed. Antenatal and neonatal screening. London: Oxford University Press, 1984:1–22.
12. Merkatz IR, Nitowsky HM, Macri JN, Johnson WE. An association between low maternal serum alpha-fetoprotein and fetal chromosome abnormalities. Am J Obstet Gynecol 1984;148: 886–892.
13. Canick JA. Screening for Down syndrome using maternal serum alpha-fetoprotein, unconjugated estriol, and HCG. J Clin Immuno 1990;13:30–33.
14. Palomaki GE, Haddow JE. Maternal serum alpha fetoprotein, age, and Down syndrome risk. Am J Obstet Gynecol 1987;156: 460–463.
15. Bogart MH, Pandian MR, Jones OW. Abnormal maternal serum chorionic gonadotropin levels in pregnancies with fetal chromosome abnormalities. Prenat Diagn 1987;7:623–630.
16. Canick JA, Knight GJ, Palomaki GE, Haddow JE, Cuckle HS, Wald NJ. Low second trimester maternal serum unconjugated oestriol in pregnancies with Down's syndrome. Br J Obstet Gynaecol 1988;95:330-333.
17. Burton BK. Positive amniotic fluid acetylcholinesterase: distinguishing between open defects of the neural tube and ventral wall defects. Am J Obstet Gynecol 1986;155:984–986.
18. Wald NJ, Barlow RD, Cuckle HS, et al. Ratio of amniotic fluid acetylcholinesterase as an antenatal diagnostic test for exomphalos and gastroschisis. Br J Obstet Gynaecol 1984;91:882.
19. Ledbetter DH, Martin AO, Verlinsky Y, et al. Cytogenetic results of chorionic villus sampling: high success rate and diagnostic accuracy in the United States collaborative study. Am J Obstet Gynecol 1990;162:495–501.

20. Ledbetter DH, Zachary JM, Simpson JL, et al. Cytogenetic results from the U.S. collaborative study on CVS: high diagnostic accuracy in over 11,000 cases. Prenat Diagn 1992;12:317–345.
21. Warburton D. Outcome of cases of de novo structural rearrangements diagnosed at amniocentesis. Prenat Diagn 1984;4:69–80.
22. Warburton D. De novo balanced chromosome rearrangements and extra marker chromosomes identified at prenatal diagnosis: clinical significance and distribution of breakpoints. Am J Hum Genet 1991;49:995–1013.
23. Steinbach P, Djalali M, Hansmann I, et al. The genetic significance of accessory bisatellited marker chromosomes. Hum Genet 1983;65:155–164.
24. Hsu LYF. Prenatal diagnosis of 45,X/46,XY mosaicism—a review and update. Prenat Diagn 1989;9:31–48.
25. Hsu LYF, Perlis TE. United States survey on chromosome mosaicism and pseudomosaicism in prenatal diagnosis. Prenat Diagn 1984;4:97–130.
26. Vejerslev LO, Mikkelsen M. The European collaborative study on mosaicism in chorionic villus sampling: data from 1986 to 1987. Prenat Diagn 1989;9:575–588.
27. Worton RG, Stern R. A Canadian collaborative study of mosaicism in amniotic fluid cell cultures. Prenat Diagn 1984;4:131–144.
28. Bui TH, Iselius L, Lindsten J. European collaborative study on prenatal diagnosis: mosaicism, pseudomosaicism and single abnormal cells in amniotic fluid cell cultures. Prenat Diagn 1984;4:145–162.
29. Jackson A, Wapner RJ, Davis GH, Jackson LG. Mosaicism in chorionic villus sampling: an association with poor perinatal outcome. Obstet Gynecol 1990;75:573–577.

28 Chromosome Breakage Syndromes

Maimon M. Cohen

The clinical entities that constitute the chromosome instability syndromes are a group of inherited disorders that share some common characteristics. In affected individuals, findings include elevated rates of spontaneous chromosome damage, cellular hypersensitivity to exogenous physical and chemical agents, and a predisposition to the development of cancer. These characteristics can be found in most of the syndromes, but each manifests its own constellation of features. Significant clinical heterogeneity exists, and variant forms have been described. Although 11 chromosome instability syndromes are listed in Table 28.1, the four conditions investigated in detail and always considered in this group are ataxia-telangiectasia (A-T), Bloom's syndrome (BS), Fanconi's anemia (FA), and xeroderma pigmentosum (XP). The other entities included in this list are less thoroughly studied.

As indicated in Table 28.1, almost all of these conditions clearly demonstrate a recognized inheritance pattern. Most are transmitted in an autosomal recessive pattern of inheritance, which by necessity defines the parents of an affected individual as phenotypically normal heterozygotes with no outward manifestations of disease. One of every four children born to such a pair of carrier parents will be affected (Fig. 28.1A). Therefore, the risk for subsequent affected siblings in each pregnancy is 25%. In sex-linked recessive inheritance (Fig. 28.1B), the female parent is usually the carrier of the mutant gene, which is masked by its normal allele on the second X chromosome. Because she is heterozygous at this locus, she usually manifests no phenotypic effects of the abnormal gene. However, because the affected male inherits the mutation and is hemizygous at this locus (only the abnormal copy is present), he is affected. Therefore, half of all male offspring born to carrier mothers will be affected, but none of the female offspring will be affected (although half of her daughters will be carriers). These two modes of inheritance account for the genetic control of the clearly heritable chromosome breakage syndromes, and such mendelian segregation accounts for the "clustering" or familial aggregation of the disease in certain families. Most frequently, this is seen as pairs of affected siblings or first cousins.

CHROMOSOME INSTABILITY

Various cellular processes exist for the repair of DNA damage occurring through both endogenous and exogenous factors. Such events may occur during either normal meiosis or mitosis, leading to the rearrangement of genetic material within a single chromatid or between sister chromatids of the same pairs of chromosomes, or between nonhomologous chromosomes in various types of chromosomal aberrations (See Fig. 28.2). DNA damage may also result from exposure to exogenous physical, chemical, and biological agents (e.g., radiation, drugs, viruses). Such induced chromosome damage has provided the investigational tool for the elucidation of the "DNA repair processes." It is beyond the scope of this chapter to detail the specifics of these sometimes very complicated systems, but they exist nonetheless, and they maintain the viability of the cells exposed to such intrinsic DNA damage.

Observed cytogenetic damage usually results from chromosome breakage, and in some cases, the broken chromosomes are rearranged, yielding new morphologic elements. Such events are best observed at metaphase in cells prepared for microscopic exami-

Table 28.1. Chromosome Instability Syndromes

Name	Mode of Inheritance
Ataxia telangiectasia	Autosomal recessive
Fanconi's anemia	Autosomal recessive
Bloom's syndrome	Autosomal recessive
Xeroderma pigmentosum	Autosomal recessive
Nijmegen breakage syndrome	Autosomal recessive
Werner syndrome	Autosomal recessive
Multibranched chromosome syndrome	?Autosomal recessive
Roberts syndrome	Autosomal recessive
Systemic sclerosis (scleroderma)	Unknown
Dyskeratosis congenita	X-linked recessive; autosomal recessive
"N" syndrome	X-linked recessive

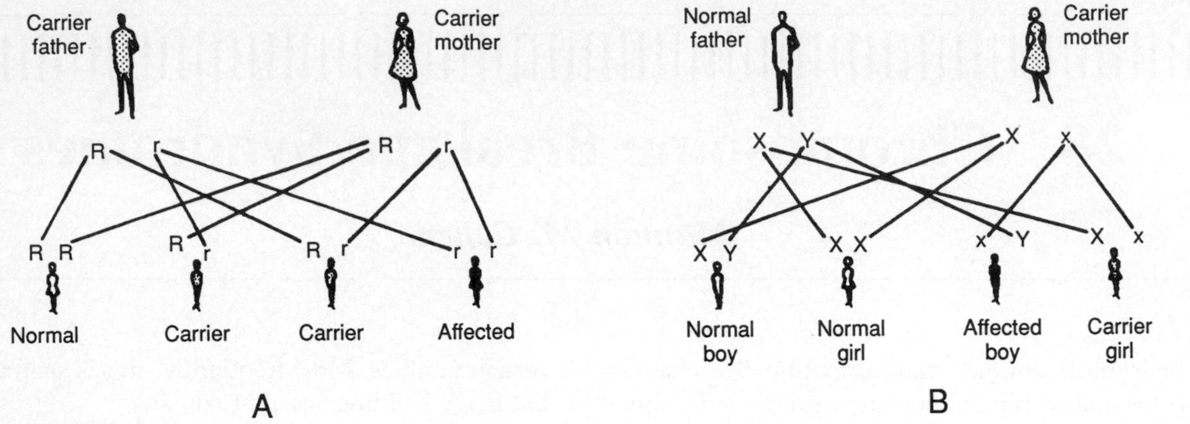

Figure 28.1. Patterns of inheritance. **A**, Autosomal recessive—both parents are phenotypically normal carriers of the mutant gene. There is a 25% risk of an affected offspring in each pregnancy. Both sexes are affected equally. **B**, Sex-linked recessive—both parents are phenotypically normal. The mother is a heterozygote for a mutant gene on one of her X chromosomes. Half of her sons will be affected; all daughters will be normal, but 50% will be carriers, like the mother.

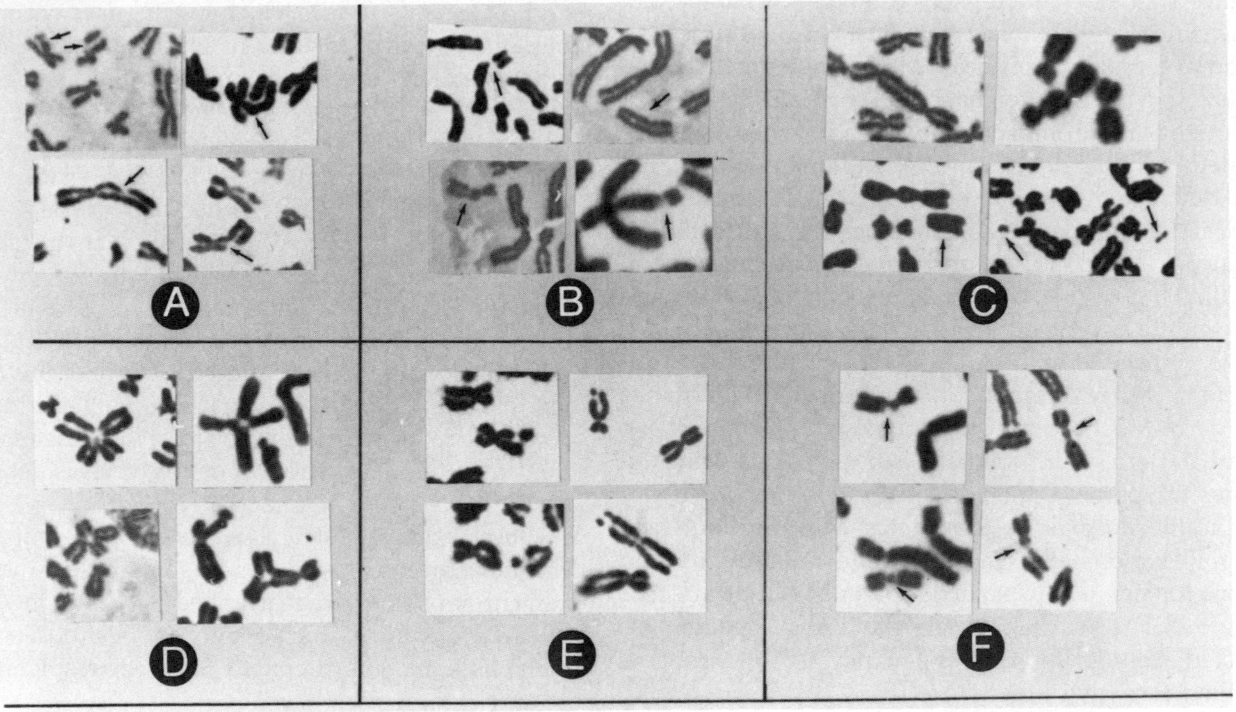

Figure 28.2. Examples of chromosome breakage. **A**, *Arrows* indicate chromatid breaks; note the displacement of distal fragments from the axis of chromatid orientation. **B**, *Arrows* indicate isochromatid breaks. **C**, Dicentric chromosomes; note the "double" acentric fragments (*arrows* in lower row). **D**, Multiradial configurations; both asymmetrical quadriradials and asymmetrical triradial (lower right). **E**, Single chromatid terminal fragments (chromatid breaks). **F**, *Arrows* indicate attenuation and breakage at heterochromatic secondary constrictions.

nation by methods identical to those used for diagnostic cytogenetics.

The microscopic evaluation to quantify these types of chromosome damage most frequently utilizes peripheral lymphocytes, although cultured skin fibroblasts are less commonly used. In fact, any cell that can be arrested in mitosis can be used for cytogenetic scoring. In most cases, chromosomal breakage experiments use lymphocytes following either a 48- or a 72-hour culture period. To minimize the possible loss of induced aberrations in subsequent division cycles, first-metaphase cells after putative clastogen exposure should be evaluated. However, cells may also be exposed for the last 24 hours of a 72-hour culture, allowing the accumulation of more metaphases to provide the larger population of dividing cells necessary for statistical analyses. For establishment of spontaneous damage (i.e., controls), chromosome preparations following routine culturing techniques are used. Either banded or unbanded metaphases

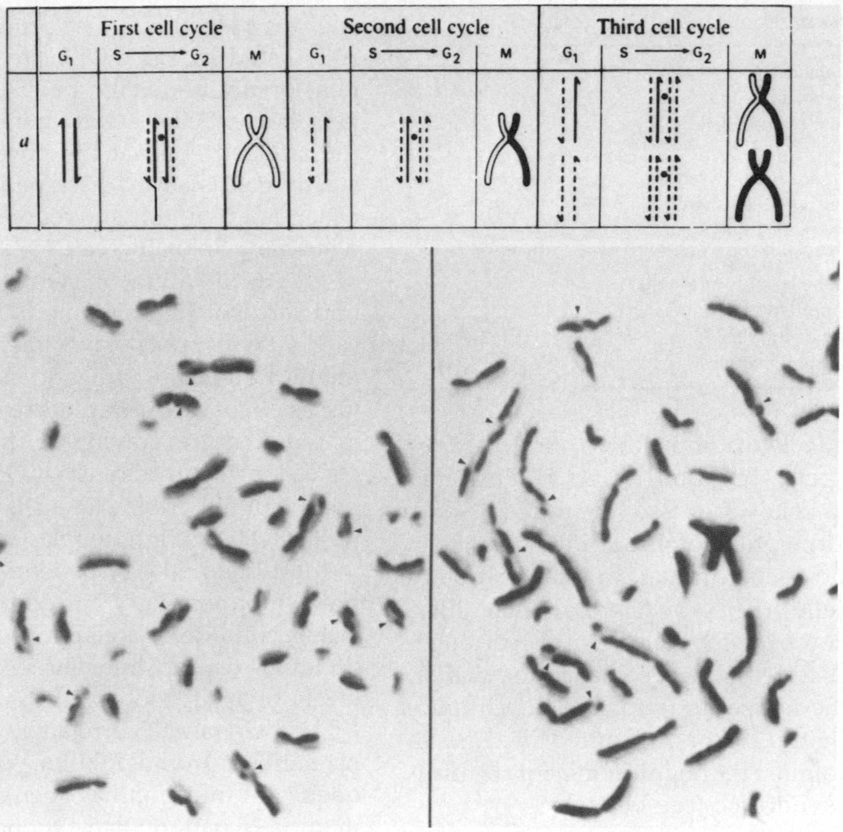

Figure 28.3. Sister chromatid exchange (SCE). *Top*, Incorporation of 5-bromodeoxyuridine in during several cell cycles, leading to differential staining of the chromatids. The *solid lines* represent DNA containing thymidine, while the *dotted lines* are DNA with incorporated BrdU. *Bottom*, *Arrowheads* indicate the occurrence of sister chromatid exchanges in normal metaphases. Note the "switch" of staining intensity between chromatids at the point of SCE.

can be utilized for the evaluation of clastogenic damage, with unbanded preparations used most frequently if only quantitation of cytogenetic damage is desired. However, if the localization of damage to specific areas of given chromosomes is a goal of the investigation, then G-banded preparations would obviously serve to study possible specificity of the distribution of breaks.

Cytogenetic damage (Fig. 28.2) is usually scored as a break only if clear discontinuity and displacement of the chromatid from the longitudinal axis, by at least its width, are visible. Breaks are classified as *chromatid* if only one chromatid is affected, and as *isochromatid* if both sister chromatids are broken at the same location. Both of these abnormalities are scored as single breaks. Single fragments are included with chromatid breaks, and double fragments are scored as isochromatid breaks. Gaps, or visual discontinuities of the chromatid material without displacement of the distal portion of the arm, are noted. Chromosome rearrangements resulting from breaks in two or more chromosomes, with subsequent reunions, lead to exchange figures (chromosome translocations) or dicentric and ring chromosome. Each of these chromosome rearrangements is counted as two breaks.

In the chromosome instability syndromes, all of the types of abnormalities described above are observed spontaneously, with greater or lesser frequencies, in routine cytogenetic preparations derived from circulating lymphocytes of affected individuals. A notable exception is xeroderma pigmentosum, in which the cytogenetic phenotype is discernible only after exposure of the cells to ultraviolet radiation or UV-mimetic drugs. However, each syndrome demonstrates a hypersensitivity to either chemical or physical (radiation) agents and elevated rates of chromosome damage are manifested when affected persons are exposed to the appropriate clastogen. Details of these such hypersensitivities and disease specificity are presented below in the discussions of the individual diseases.

SISTER CHROMATID EXCHANGE

A specific type of chromosome damage, possibly representative of DNA repair, is sister chromatid exchange (SCE) (Fig. 28.3). This phenomenon is observed under special conditions utilizing the incorpo-

Table 28.2. Clinical Features of Ataxia-Telangiectasia

Progressive cerebellar ataxia
Oculocutaneous telangiectasia
Recurrent pulmonary infections (50%)
Growth retardation
Nystagmus, strabismus, drooling, dysarthria
Hypogonadism, ovarian dysgenesis (?)
Humoral immunodeficiency (↓ IgA, IgE)
Absent or hypoplastic thymus
Deficient cellular immune response (T cells)
Increased serum α-fetoprotein
Radiosensitivity (in vivo or in vitro)
Propensity to lymphoid malignancies

ration of bromodeoxyuridine (BrdU) in place of thymidine during DNA replication. As is illustrated in Figure 28.3*A*, following two rounds of DNA sythesis and incorporation of BrdU into the newly synthesized strand, one chromatid of each chromosome is differentially stained by Giemsa. Such differential staining allows for the detection of rearrangements between sister chromatids (hence the name), as indicated by the harlequin nature of the chromosomes seen in Figure 28.3*B*. A marked increase in SCE frequency is almost pathognomonic for the diagnosis of Bloom's syndrome (see below).

CLINICAL CONSIDERATIONS IN THE CHROMOSOME INSTABILITY SYNDROMES

Comprehensive reviews of the clinical symptoms of these syndromes have been published periodically. Although each condition represents a distinct and recognizable entity, they all manifest dermatological abnormalities, immune dysfunction, neurological abnormalities, and a predisposition to cancer. Of the syndromes presented in Table 28.1, only four are discussed in detail because the most information is available on these entities: ataxia-telangiectasia (A-T), Fanconi's anemia (FA), xeroderma pigmentosum (XP), and Bloom's syndrome (BS). These four chromosome instability syndromes all result from homozygosity for rare recessive genes whose true gene frequencies are difficult to determine due to incomplete ascertainment and possible population differences. Calculation of actual gene frequencies and prevalance figures for these diseases is further complicated variability and the apparent existence of multiple mutations that yield several subgroups with the same phenotype (genetic heterogeneity) in each of the disorders.

Ataxia-Telangiectasia

Ataxia-telangiectasia is estimated to affect one in 40,000 individuals, although an incidence as high as one in 20,000 can be calculated via various pedigree analysis procedures. The principal clinical findings in A-T, listed in Table 28.2, involve almost every system, organ, and cell type. The first symptom to appear is cerebellar ataxia, which is clearly evident in the affected child at the onset of walking. The unsteady gait is easily discerned (in most cases) by the observant mother, who reports this finding to the pediatrician. Soon thereafter, telangietasia, principally of the sclera and the malar region constitutes the second cardinal finding. In addition, in some patients, café au lait spots have been reported along with manifestations of progeric skin changes, including losses of cutaneous fat, decreased elasticity, atrophy, and premature graying of the hair. A-T is a lethal condition; death almost always occurs by the third decade of life. Most patients succumb to either recurrent infections or a neoplastic disease (see below).

More than 50% of patients with A-T suffer recurrent sinopulmonary infections. Both humoral and cellular immunity are abnormal. Up to 80% of the individuals demonstrate absence or severely decreased levels of IgA, and almost as many are deficient in IgE. Obviously, a correlation between the low levels of these immunoglubulin subclasses and the frequency of infection has been suggested. In addition, many A-T patients have a poorly developed or completely absent thymus, which may also be responsible for abnormal cell-mediated immunity and delayed hypersensitivity responses. Thymic hypoplasia may also be related to the humoral abnormalities, since defects have been demonstrated not only in the function of the antibody-producing B cells but also in helper T cells. Peripheral blood lymphocytes from A-T patients showed decreased in vitro proliferative response to mitogenic stimulation.

Neurologic abnormalities in A-T are quite significant. As indicated above, the cerebellar ataxia, noted shortly after walking begins, is invariably progressive, and the patient becomes wheelchair dependent or bedridden in the second decade of life. All patients also suffer dysarthria, and most manifest choreoathetosis, hypotonia with poor or absent deep tendon reflexes, apraxic eye movements and nystagmus, and one-third characteristic facies and postural attitudes. Mental retardation has been reported in as many as one-third of cases, but it is difficult to evaluate because of the dysarthria. Their mental capacity has been referred to as "arrested cognitive development."

There is a striking, persistent elevation of α-fetoprotein levels throughout life in A-T patients. Normally, the level of this fetal protein decreases rapidly after birth, but in A-T, it may remain elevated throughout life. Hypogonadism, especially ovarian dysgenesis in affected females is a frequent finding. Growth retardation is also common.

Table 28.3. Clinical Features of Fanconi's Anemia

Shortness of stature
Pancytopenia
Skeletal anomalies
Absent or rudimentary thumbs
Hypoplastic radius
Abnormal skin pigmentation
Café au lait spots
Renal anomalies
Aplasia
Horseshoe kidney
Genital hypoplasia (50%)
Increased propensity to neoplasia

An increased propensity for the development of neoplasia is a consistent feature of all of the chromosome instability syndromes; however, the type of malignancy observed is variable. The most common cancer observed in A-T are lymphoproliferative non-Hodgkin's lymphoma and lymphoid leukemias. Other tumors include gastric, basal cell, and hepatic carcinomas and ovarian dysgerminoma. Lymphomas and leukemias in A-T patients usually appear before age 16, whereas epithelial carcinomas occur in patients who survive beyond this age. Estimates of the lifetime risk that any A-T patient will develop cancer range from 10 to 20%.

The treatment of malignancies in A-T patients led to the discovery of a clinical hypersensitivity to the effects of ionizing radiation. Following standard doses of radiation for malignant lymphomas, several patients died from a severe radiation reaction. This repeated observation, along with the in vitro demonstration in fibroblasts derived from A-T patients, confirmed the clinical observations and identified a dose-related hypersensitivity to the effect of ionizing radiation on A-T cells. This observation has had a significant impact on the investigations into the basic defect in ataxia-telangiectasia.

An increased risk of cancer among the relatives of A-T patients has also been reported. The most common malignancy among A-T heterozygote is breast cancer; others include lymphoma and leukemia as well as ovarian, gastric, and biliary carcinomas. It has been estimated that as many as 5% of all cancer deaths before the age of 45 and 8.8% of breast cancer deaths occur in A-T heterozygotes.

Fanconi's Anemia

Compared to A-T, Fanconi's anemia is a less common disease with a homozygote frequency of approximately 1 in 360,000. Dermatological changes include both hyper- and hypopigmentation but are most commonly seen as café au lait spots. Immunologically, FA patients manifest pancytopenia, although they apparently suffer no increased infection and demonstrate no immunological defects. The most prevalent clinical characteristics of Fanconi's anemia are listed in Table 28.3. Unique clinical findings of FA include congenital skeletal anomalies (specifically hypoplasia or absence of the thumb and/or radius), gradual onset of progressive pancytopenia leading to eventual bone marrow failure, and, in some cases, congenital renal anomalies and hypogenitalism. Although FA was initially described in 1927, reports of the associated malignacies did not appear until the mid-1960s. It has since become recognized that FA patients demonstrate a more marked increase in neoplasia, especially acute leukemias and hepatic tumors. Possible reasons for the delayed recognition of this relationship (approximately 40 years after the syndrome was described) have been the subject of much dispute. Of significance is the fact that preferred treatment for aplastic anemia (androgen therapy) was instituted in 1959, a few years prior to the first reports of cancer in FA patients, and has been associated with hepatic neoplasia. However, leukemia and/or hepatocellular carcinoma have also been reported in FA patients receiving no androgen therapy. Alternative explanations suggest that androgen therapy somehow enhances a predisposition to cancer in FA patients, or that current treatment modalities have extended patient survival in spite of bone marrow failure, allowing expression of malignancy. Whether the increased incidence of neoplasia results from a basic genetic disposition or is induced by treatment, FA patients develop cancer more frequently than the general population. It has been estimated that 5 to 10% of all FA patients will die from leukemia.

As in A-T, there is an increased risk of cancer in the family members of persons with FA (i.e., heterozygotes). However, no statistically significant excess of any specific cancer type is recognized among the relatives of FA patients.

Bloom's Syndrome

No frequency estimate of Bloom's syndrome has been published. Although Bloom's syndome was intitially reported to be much more common among Ashkenazi Jews, subsequent studies, including more widespread reporting, have not confirmed this observation. A clinical description of Bloom's syndrome can be found in Table 28.4. Persons affected by BS are easily recognized by a marked short stature at birth and severe growth retardation. They also have a very characteristic narrow face with a beaked nose, hypoplastic malar region, and small mandible. BS patients also manifest telangiectasia and pronounced sun sensitivity, with an onset of an associated erythema in the malar area during the first or second

Table 28.4. Clinical Features of Bloom's Syndrome

Growth retardation (proportional)
Characteristic facies
Narrow face
Beaked nose
Hypoplastic malar area
Retarded mandible
Telangiectatic facial erythema
Sun sensitivity
Immunologic impairment
Increased propensity to neoplasia

Table 28.5. Clinical Features of Xeroderma Pigmentosum

Sun sensitivity of exposed areas
Dermatological anomalies
Numerous freckles
Cutaneous atrophy
Hyperpigmentation
Hypopigmentation
Ocular abnormalities
Photophobia
Tearing
Atrophy of eyelid
Conjunctival drying
Corneal ulceration
Microcephaly
Neurologic involvement—De Sanctis-Cacchione type mental retardation
Cutaneous neoplasia

summer of life. The telangiectatic erythema in BS patients tends to resolve during the second decade. These patients also suffer extensive scarring and atrophy of the skin.

Immunologically, BS patients suffer chronic infections of the respiratory and gastrointestinal tracts. Immunodeficiency, particularly decreased IgM, is a common finding; some patients also manifest a delayed-type hypersensitivity response and a decreased in vitro proliferative response to mitogens. No consistent neurologic abnormalities have been reported in Bloom's syndrome.

Information concerning neoplasia in BS derives mainly from analysis of the International Bloom's Syndrome Registry. Approximately one in four BS patients develops cancer. Leukemias, especially the acute lymphocytic variety, occur more frequently than in the general population; other tumors, including lymphomas and gastrointestinal carcinomas, are no more frequent but appear at significantly earlier ages than in the general population. The onset of leukemia in BS is usually before age 30, whereas solid tumors have a mean onset age of 36. Patients with Bloom's syndrome demonstrate hypersensitivity to many antileukemic drugs and manifest bone marrow failure when treated with these agents. There is a suggestion of increased cancer incidence in Bloom's syndrome heterozygotes, but analytical data are scarce.

Xeroderma Pigmentosum

The worldwide frequency of XP has been estimated at 1 in 250,000, but it may reach as high as 1 in 40,000 in Japan. Predominant clinical manifestations are listed in Table 28.5. The most striking clinical characteristic of XP patients is the extreme sensitivity to ultraviolet radiation, manifested not only in cutaneous abnormalities but also in photophobia and other ocular symptoms such as corneal ulceration, dryness of the cornea and conjunctiva, and atrophy of the eyelids. Telangiectasia may also appear in some XP patients, although the main dermatological finding in this syndrome is an erythematous rash, often with freckling, that results from sensitivity to sunlight and appears around 3 years of age. Pigmentary changes, including both hyperpigmentation and hypopigmentation, occur. These patients also have dry, scaly skin and atrophy and develop actinic keratoses, which eventually give rise to multiple skin cancers.

XP patients have normal serum immunoglobulin levels but with reduced numbers of T_4 (primarily helper) T cells, a decreased mitogenic response to phytohemagglutinin (PHA), and an impaired delayed-type hypersensitivity reaction. Decreased ability to mount a skin contact allergic reaction to sensitizing agents has also been reported; the degree of deficiency may correlate with the severity of sun-induced cutaneous disease. Approximately 18% of XP patients develop CNS symptoms, including progressive neurologic deterioration, mental retardation, or areflexia, dysarthria, deafness, ataxia, and an abnormal electroencephalogram. De Sanctis-Cacchione syndrome is a clinical subtype of XP in which the patients have severe neurologic involvement. However, most XP patients with neurologic abnormalities manifest only a few of these symptoms.

In XP, tumors occur most frequently in exposed areas of the skin, the tongue, and the eye. This is consistent with the known hypersensitivity of these patients (and their cells) to the effects of ultraviolet radiation. Basal cell and squamous cell carcinomas represent the most common cancer types. These tumors are locally invasive, but they do not usually metastasize and can be treated surgically. The squamous cell carcinomas typically develop from actinic keratoses, which are the end stage of the characteristic skin changes occurring in XP. The mean onset of these tumors in XP is 8 years of age, some 50 years younger than in the general U.S. population. Malignant melanoma is also a common neoplasm in XP; this aggressively metastatic cancer is often the cause of death. Cancers other than those mentioned above

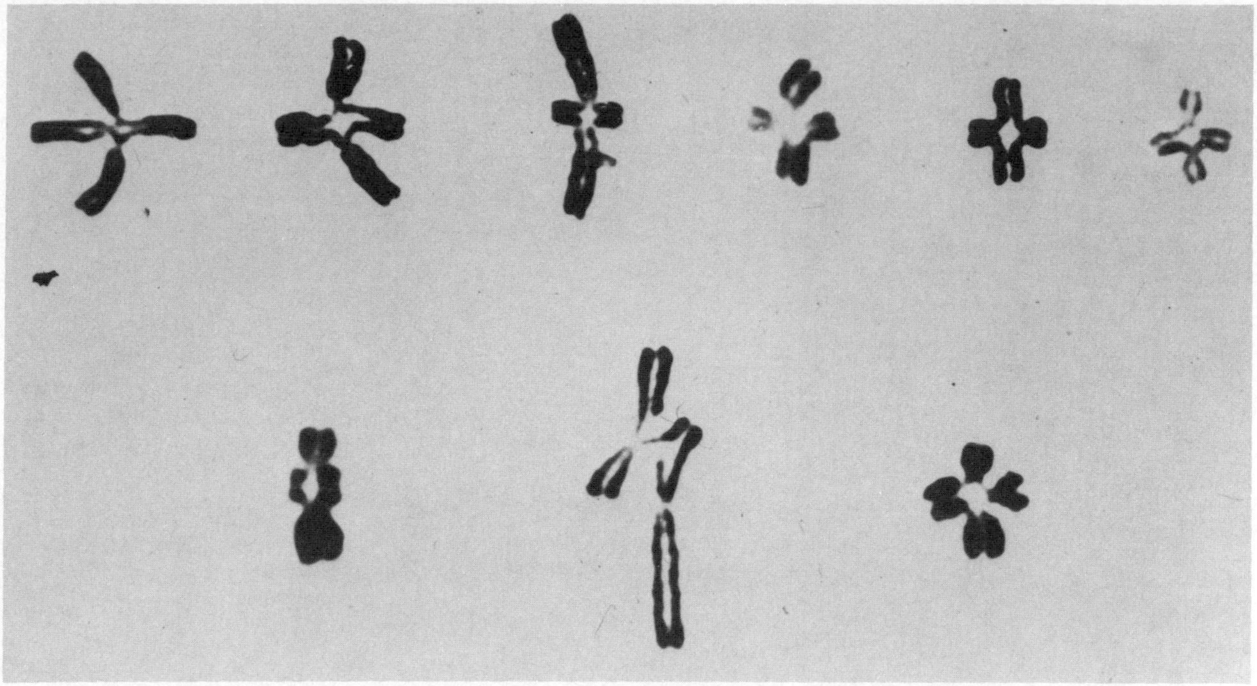

Figure 28.4. Quadriradial configurations that are the cytogenetic hallmark of Bloom's syndrome cells. Both symmetrical (*top row*) and asymmetrical (*second row*) figures can be observed.

are rare in XP patients, although the risk of developing internal neoplasis (mostly sarcomas) is increased by 12.5% over the general population. It is unclear at this time whether heterozygote carriers of XP genes are at increased risk for developing malignant neoplasias.

The epidemiological consequences of the heterozygote condition for at least two of these diseases (AT and FA) are clearly evident. For BS and XP, the data are not as convincing. However, this group of carriers, who possess only a single dose of the genes responsible for the chromosome instability syndromes, constitutes a population at significant risk for the development of neoplasia.

CYTOGENETIC CONSIDERATIONS

Spontaneous Chromosome Breakage

Each of the syndromes manifests as a unique spectrum of spontaneous chromosome damage.

ATAXIA-TELANGIECTASIA

Increased frequencies of both chromatid and isochromatid breaks have been observed; however a few patients do not demonstrate this finding. Although spontaneous chromosome damage is an integral component of A-T, it may not be observed in a single sample derived from any given patient, which suggests the need for repeated studies over a period of time. Nonetheless, cases in which chromosome damage is not observed may represent one of the variant A-T syndromes described below. A more striking cytogenetic feature of A-T is the increased frequency of structural rearrangements (particularly translocations and multiradial configurations) that occur both sporadically and as particular marker chromosomes in clonally derived subpopulations of cells. Multiradial configurations that occur are often of the nonhomologous, asymmetrical type (Fig. 28.4). The frequency of spontaneous sister chromatid exchange in A-T patients is normal.

An increased frequency of chromosome damage and rearrangement has been observed in both PHA-stimulated lymphocytes and cultured dermal fibroblasts of A-T patients. Although A-T fibroblasts demonstrate significantly more chromosome damage than lymphocytes, the fibroblasts show only slightly more damage than is seen in normal fibroblasts. Interestingly, long-term lymphoblastoid cell lines (LCLs) established from A-T patients fail to demonstrate increased spontaneous chromosome breakage despite the increased rates observed in lymphocytes and fibroblasts of the same patients. The in vivo situation has been investigated through examination of bone marrow cells, and, with only one exception, neither increased breaks, rearrangements, nor clones bearing marker chromosomes have been found. However, recent evaluation of micronuclei in exfoliated cells demonstrates substantial increases in the frequency of chromosome aberrations of A-T patients, and this suggests that chromosome instability

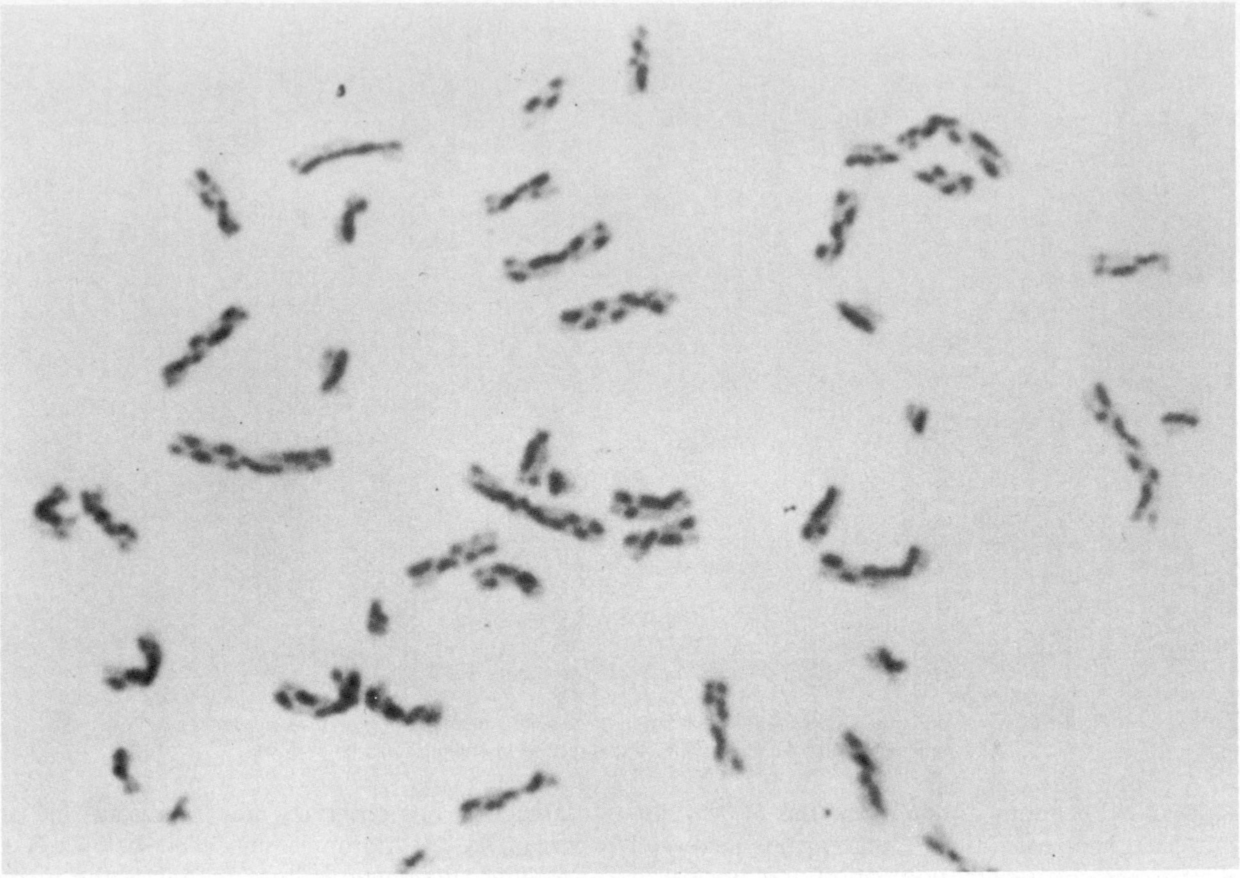

Figure 28.5. Sister chromatid exchanges in Bloom's syndrome cells. Note the marked increase in frequency and "harlequin" appearance of the chromosomes. For comparison, see normal cells in Fig. 28.3**B**.

does occur in vivo despite the negative bone marrow findings.

Studies investigating the preferential involvement of certain chromosome bands in the cytogenetic damage of A-T cells have been quite informative. There seems to be a marked specificity for the involvement of chromosome 7 and 14. Both single cells and clones bearing rearrangements involving these two chromosomes have been reported in A-T lymphocytes. The most common breakpoints were 7p13, 7q35, 14q11–q12 and 14q32. Rearrangements involving these loci have been reported both in inversions such as inv(7)(p13q35) and inv(14)(q12q32), and in translocations, the most frequent being a tandem translocation, t(14;14)(q12;q32). Clones bearing these abnormal rearrangements increase in frequency with the age of the patient. An association of clonal rearrangements of chromosome 14 with T-cell lymphocytic leukemia in A-T patients has been demonstrated supporting the theory that the selective advantage conferred by these rearrangements may be associated with the development of lymphoid malignancies. However, clones carrying similar rearrangements of chromosomes 7 and 14 also exist in A-T patients who fail to develop a malignancy. Therefore, the presence of the rearrangement itself does not appear to be sufficient for carcinogenesis. It must be remembered that these same breakpoints are the most common sites of chromosome rearrangements in normal individuals in the general population, although they are approximately 40 times more frequent in A-T patients.

BLOOM'S SYNDROME

Increased chromosome breakage manifested as isochromatid breaks and acentric fragments, as well as some nonhomologous asymmetric multiradial configurations, are an integral component of BS. However, the hallmark of spontaneous cytogenetic instability in BS is the presence of homologous symmetrical rearrangements (quadriradials) in as many as 10% of the patients' lymphocytes (Fig. 28.4).

Spontaneous SCEs are about 15 times more frequent in BS than in normal cells. This observation is pathognomonic for BS, and it has not been associated with any of the other chromosome instability syndromes (Fig. 28.5).

Fibroblasts from BS patients also manifest chromosome damage. The question of in vivo versus in vitro effects has been addressed in BS, with results very similar to those in A-T. Evaluation of the bone marrow in a small number of patients does not give clear-cut evidence of chromosome damage. However, increased frequencies of micronuclei have been observed in cells of both urinary tract and oral mucosa, suggesting that chromosome instability occurs in vivo as well.

Study of LCLs derived from BS patients demonstrates that some, but not all, retain the cytogenetic characteristics of lymphocytes. Of significant interest is the fact that multiple LCLs established from several BS patients demonstrate either normal or increased frequencies of SCEs.

Nonrandom involvement of particular chromosomes has been reported in BS. Specifically, chromosomes 1, 17, and 18 and some members of groups C, D, and F are preferentially involved in quadriradial formation, and most exchanges tend to cluster around the centromeric and Q-dark regions of these chromosomes.

FANCONI'S ANEMIA

In contrast to the specific types of cytogenetic damage found in BS (homologous exchanges and increased SCEs), the chromosomal instability in FA patients is primarily characterized by single chromatid breaks and gaps as well as multiradials of the nonhomologous type. Increased spontaneous cytogenetic damage is a consistent finding in nearly all FA patients and in some cases is manifested prior to the onset of pancytopenia. The total frequency of breakage in these individuals is nearly twice that observed in A-T or BS patients. In addition to chromosome breaks and gaps, the cytogenetic abnormalities include a high rate of endoreduplication, and then there are occasional reports of isochromatid breaks and acentric fragments. Clonal populations of cells bearing unique marker chromosomes have been reported, but this by no means as frequent a finding as in A-T.

The chromosomal instability of FA lymphocytes is also observed in cultured fibroblasts. In most cases, bone marrow preparations also reveal chromatid breaks as well as mitotic and interphase disturbances (such as bridges, aberrant fragments, and micronuclei) suggestive of chromosome instability. However, the bone marrow findings are not uniform in all cases. Analysis of FA bone marrow cells has also shown the existence of clones bearing rearranged chromosomes, even though clonal abnormalities are not characteristic of this disorder. Although bone marrow aberrations are not a consistently reported phenomenon, there seems to be little doubt that chromosome instability does occur in vivo. FA LCLs also exhibit increased spontaneous breakage, although not to the degree observed in PHA-stimulated lymphocytes. Nonrandom chromosomal anomalies also occur in FA. However, rather than involving specific chromosomes, the breakpoints appear to occur preferentially at the junctions between light and dark G bands and the sites of SCE in FA lymphocytes.

XERODERMA PIGMENTOSUM

Chromosome instability is apparent in XP patients only after UV exposure, although a single patient with a low level of spontaneous chromosome rearrangements and subclones of dermal fibroblasts has been reported. An increased spontaneous frequency of dicentrics and breaks has been reported in cultured fibroblasts from some XP patients, but these are observed only in later passages, shortly before senescence of the cell strains. These cells had normal karyotypes at earlier passages, but they may have derived from sun-exposed areas of the skin, thereby manifesting chromosomal instability following UV exposure.

Induced Chromosomal Aberrations

In addition to spontaneous chromosome damage, the cells of patients with the instability syndromes demonstrate hypersensitivity to various clastogens (chromosome breaking agents), mutagens, and carcinogens following in vitro treatment.

IRRADIATION

Following exposure to ionizing radiation, extensive breakage has been reported in skin fibroblasts, PHA-stimulated lymphocytes, and LCLs derived from A-T patients.

In FA cells, exposure to short-wave (254 nm), but not long-wave, radiation causes an increase in chromatid breaks. Ionizing radiation yields conflicting results, with increased chromosome breakage in some patients but no effect in others. In FA fibroblasts, normal chromosomal sensitivity to ionizing radiation is observed; however, an inconsistent elevation of chromatid breaks can also be observed in lymphocytes from the same patient. This phenomenon varies both among patients and in repeated studies of the same patients.

The response of BS cells to physical agents is variable, with UV-induced chromosome breakage and SCEs observed in some fibroblast strains but not in others. Thus, BS cells are heterogeneous in their cytogenetic response following exposure to both UV and ionizing radiation.

Patients with XP demonstrate a hypersensitivity to UV radiation. At the cellular level, this is expressed as increased chromosome breakage.

CHEMICAL AGENTS

In addition to ionizing radiation, A-T cells are cytogenetically hypersensitive to chemicals whose mode of action mimics radiation (radiomimetic). The most thoroughly studied agent is bleomycin, a chemotherapeutic antibiotic whose clastogenic effects have been demonstrated in lymphocytes, fibroblasts, and LCLs of A-T patients. Certain chemicals, when used in conjunction with exposure to ionizing radiation, also increase the clastogenic response of these cells (e.g., caffeine, as well as a combination of cytosine arabinoside and UV radiation). Although ionizing radiation and radiomimetic chemicals induce oxidizing free radicals, A-T cells are not cytogenetically hypersensitive to either paraquat (a free radical-generating drug) or increased oxygen tension with or without x-ray irradiation.

The chromosomal hypersensitivity of BS cells is not restricted to a particular class of drugs. However, certain agents increase the frequency of breaks and SCEs. Chief among these is mitomycin C, although hypersensitivity to specific agents is not especially apparent.

The chromosomal hypersensitivity of FA cells is specific for bifunctional DNA cross-linking agents, including nitrogen mustard, mitomycin C, UV-activated 8-methoxypsoralen, and diepoxybutane. However, FA cells demonstrate no cytogenetic hypersensitivity to monofunctional alkylators. FA lymphocytes manifest fewer SCEs than normal lymphocytes. However, many of the mitomycin C–induced chromatid breaks in these cells occur at the site of sister chromatid exchange. Although cytogenetic hypersensitivity to cross-linking agents appears to be uniform in FA, a significant discrepancy exists between the clinical classification of several patients and the diagnosis suggested by clastogenic response to chemical agents. This indicates that definitive diagnosis cannot be reliably based solely on in vitro cytogenetic findings.

In XP cells, increased chromosome breakage occurs after treatment with chemical agents that are UV-mimetic drugs (e.g., 4-nitroquinoline-1-oxide). SCEs in XP cells are also induced by both 4-nitroquinoline-1-oxide and nitrogen mustard.

BIOLOGICAL FACTORS

Biological factors inducing a clastogenic effect ("active" factors) have been reported in a number of the chromosome instability syndromes. "Corrective" factors, which are capable of reducing levels of chromosome damage, have also been inferred. Such factors have been observed in A-T, FA, XP, and BS. However, controversy exists over the exact identification of these factors. Although preliminary investigations indicate that these are small, low–molecular weight peptides, their detailed biochemical identification and molecular characterization are currently unknown.

FAMILIAL CONSIDERATIONS

Various types of physical and chemical "stress" tests have demonstrated specific hypersensitivities following exposure to different clastogens. These results suggest possible heterozygote screening methods for the various genes that control the chromosome instability syndromes to identify unaffected carriers of these syndromes. These persons may constitute more than 1% of the general population and, as indicated above, may be at increased risk for the development of neoplasia. Therefore, the ability to detect such individuals presymptomatically may be important from the standpoint of preventive medicine. Additionally, reliable heterozygote screening tests would also contribute significantly to the genetic counseling of individual families.

Techniques that attempt to identify heterozygotes have been developed for A-T, FA, and XP, but not BS. However, these procedures do not absolutely distinguish between normal individuals and carriers. In addition, many of the suggested assays are labor intensive and require extensive use of fibroblast strains. These difficulties preclude their implementation in large screening programs for heterozygote detection.

Prenatal Diagnosis

Based on the cellular phenotypes that demonstrate hypersensitivity to chemical clastogens, experimental approaches to the prenatal diagnosis of several of the chromosome instability syndromes have been devised. Such attempts must be considered preliminary, and extreme caution is advised due to the paucity of cases examined. The complicated nature of these studies demands specific expertise, and they are currently being performed in only a very few laboratories. Utilizing diepoxybutane induced chromosome breakage in cultured amniocytes and chorionic villus samples, fetuses at risk for FA can be identified. However, it must be stated that such attempts are limited to families in which an affected proband has already been born, and that the condition of the proband must be clearly identified and characterized before prenatal diagnosis can be attempted on subsequent pregnancies.

Exclusion of the presence of A-T in fetuses has been accomplished based on the normal frequencies of spontaneous and x-ray induced chromosome breakage in amniocytes. Several fetuses affected with A-T have been identified by detecting an increased frequency of spontaneous and induced chromosome breakage in cultured amniocytes as well as by demonstrating the clastogenic potential of the amniotic fluid from a pregnant woman suspected of having A-T, presumably because of the presence of an active biological clastogenic factor. Currently, the use of periumbilical blood sampling or chordocentesis provides a ready source of fetal lymphocytes for the direct assessment of chromosome breakage rates.

The prenatal exclusion of BS has been accomplished after the finding of normal chromosomal integrity in the amniocytes of several at-risk fetuses. To date, there has been no positive prenatal diagnosis of BS.

The feasibility of the prenatal detection of XP was suggested by the presence of reduced levels of DNA repair in cultured fibroblasts following UV exposure; amniocytes from at-risk fetuses can be investigated by similar approaches. However, for all of these techniques it is important to confirm and thoroughly characterize the abnormal phenotype in cells from an affected sibling, if possible, before attempting the prenatal diagnosis of a chromosome instability syndrome in later pregnancies

HETEROGENEITY AND COMPLEMENTATION

Variability and heterogeneity of both clinical and cellular phenotypes of the chromosome instability syndromes is common. For example, in De Sanctis-Cacchione syndrome, a unique clinical subtype of XP, patients demonstrate neurological findings, although the majority of XP patients do not. Before the development of complementation analysis, XP was divided into three clinical subtypes based on clinical findings: classic XP with severe symptomatology, classic XP with mild to moderate manifestations, and the De Sanctis-Cacchione type. Clinical differences in the recurrence rate of immunopulmonary infections, as well as the extent of neurological development and the frequency of chromosomal abnormalities, also indicated genetic heterogeneity among patients with A-T. Based on the cellular phenotype, complementation studies have suggested that such variability exists at the molecular level as well. The principle behind such an approach relies on the correction of the in vitro defect by cocultivation or hybridization of cells from two patients with the same disease. Correction of the defect is evidence that the mutations involve two different genes and that these patients belong to different complementation groups (Fig. 28.6). Utilizing tests based on the specific cellular responses to various treatments of the individual conditions, a series of complementation groups has been demonstrated for many of the syndromes.

More definitive proof of complementation groups came through a variety of in vitro approaches that demonstrated differences between certain groups of patients. XP can be divided into nine DNA excision repair deficiency complementation groups. The clinical variability described above does not correlate strictly with the established genetic heterogeneity. Each complementation group has a characteristic residual excision repair capability, but intragroup heterogeneity also exists. Thus, at least nine genes, and possibly more, may be involved in the maintenance of normal cellular incision repair capacity. Moreover, there are probably several mutant alleles (different mutations of the same gene) for some of these genes, as suggested by the intragroup heterogeneity.

In A-T, complementation studies have shown the existence of at least five (and possibly nine) complementation groups. These differences are based on the results of the various laboratory assays evaluating the response to ionizing radiation and other approaches used to evaluate different groups of patients. Variations of classic A-T have also been described in patients who show minimal chromosome instability but have a high incidence of neoplasia, and in patients who have normal radiosensitive DNA synthesis and bleomycin-induced increase in the frequency of chromosome breakage. Some patients are without ataxia, others without telangiectasia. Thus, A-T is also a broadly heterogeneous disorder. The defined complementation groups have been established using fewer than 20 cell strains, suggesting that genetic heterogeneity in A-T may be even greater than is currently appreciated.

A unique clinical subtype of Fanconi's anemia, the Estren-Dameshek subtype (FA-ED), describes patients who manifest hypoplastic anemia and chromosome instability but none of the characteristic congenital anomalies normally associated with the syndrome. Some of the patients have developed leukemia and other types of neoplasia. Increased spontaneous, as well as mitomycin-induced, chromosome breakage has been observed in these patients. Using classic complementation analysis, two and possibly three different groups of FA patients have been described.

Evidence for genetic heterogeneity in BS is sparse. Although the heterogeneity demonstrated by the high- and low-SCE lymphoblastoid cell lines discussed above may be indicative of different cell types within individuals, absolute demonstration of genetic heterogeneity (i.e., multiple complementation

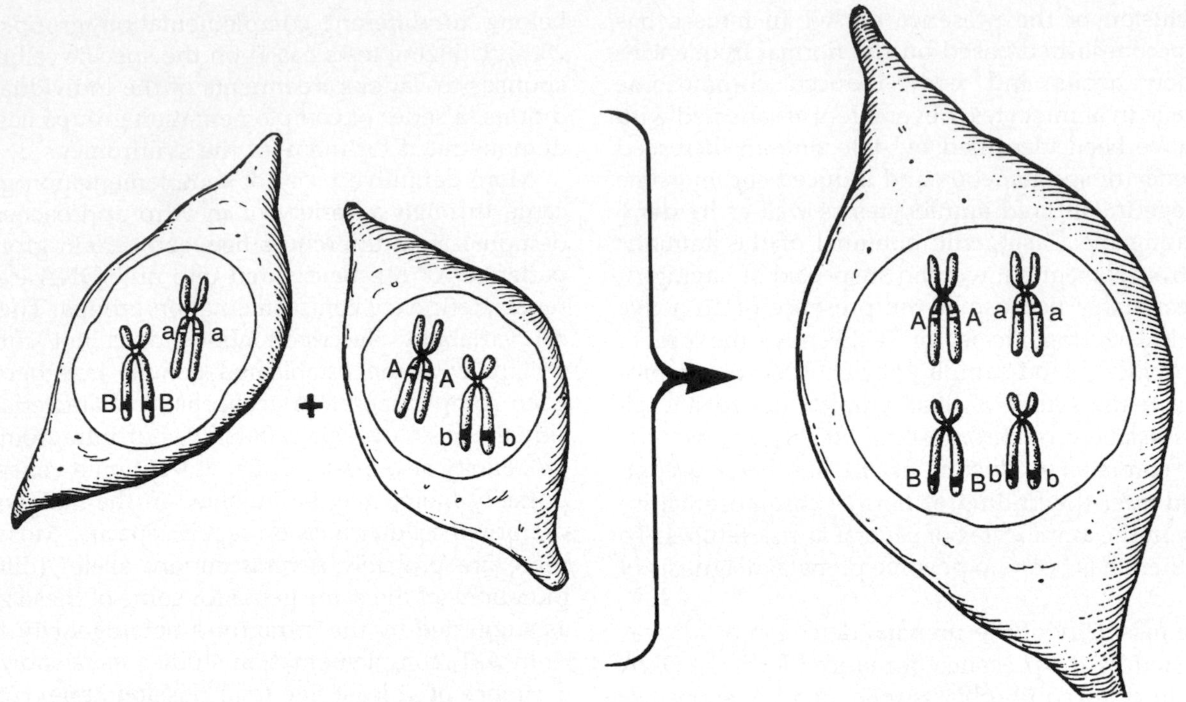

Figure 28.6. Complementation analysis to identify multiple mutations within a single syndrome. If different mutations exist in the cells to be tested, they should be corrected in the heterokaryon of the fused cells. The absence of complementation indicates identical mutations in both cells; i.e., the patients from whom the cells were derived belong to the same complementation group.

groups) has yet to be accomplished in Bloom's syndrome.

MOLECULAR CONSIDERATIONS

Xeroderma Pigmentosum

Although the molecular defect in XP—failure to repair UV-induced DNA lesions—was initially reported in 1968, detailed understanding of the exact lesion is still lacking. In most complementation groups, a defect in one of the initial steps of incising the DNA to remove the thymine dimers formed by UV radiation is believed to be present. However, in one complementation group, DNA repair assays are perfectly proficient and this suggests a defect of a different type. These latter patients, nonetheless, demonstrate the classic clinical findings of XP. Therefore, at least two distinct mutations must exist. Voluminous literature that details the biochemical and/or molecular basis of XP exists. Current efforts to identify the gene(s) responsible for XP are directed toward isolating DNA sequences or chromosome segments capable of correcting various mutant XP phenotypes in vitro. Most of these studies utilize somatic cell hybrids and the transfer of genetic material capable of complementing XP phenotypes. This approach has been successful with respect to XP complementation group A, whose phenotype has been corrected in vitro.

In ataxia-telangiectasia, the underlying defect is not as clearly defined as in XP. A large variety of studies have examined both the proficiency of DNA repair following exposure to x-rays or radiomimetic chemicals and the control and regulation of DNA synthesis. The A-T cellular phenotype demonstrates hypersensitivity to ionizing radiation and radiomimetic agents, disturbances of the cell cycle, radioresistant DNA synthesis, cytogenetic instability, and abnormalities in the levels or activities of several proteins and enzymes. The primary defect is probably not a failure in excision repair of radiation-induced DNA damage, but may instead involve a defect in the recognition of, or response to, the DNA strand breakage that is induced by exposure to ionizing free radicals.

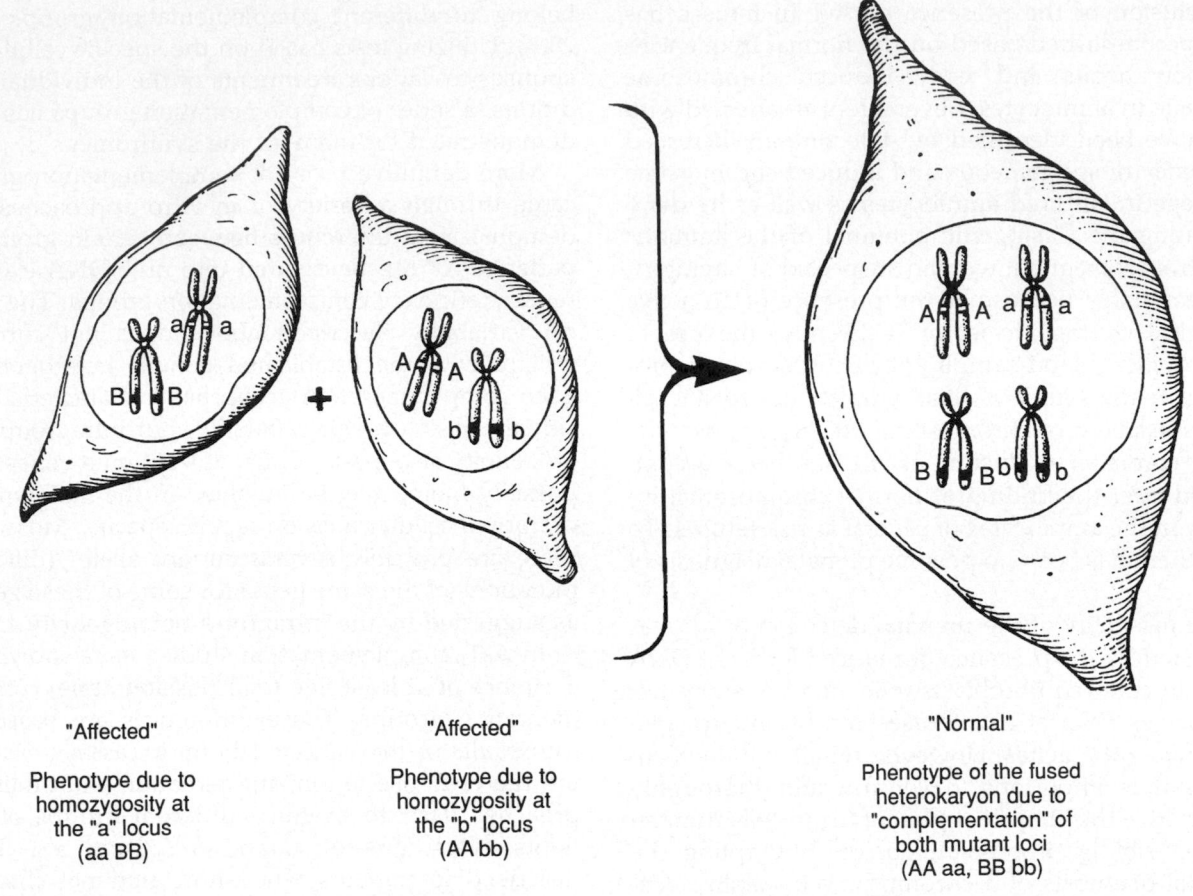

In contrast to XP and A-T, there is little evidence for a DNA repair defect in Bloom's syndrome. Although they are neither conclusive nor definitive, some studies have shown a deficiency in DNA ligase I activity in several cell strains derived from patients with Bloom's syndrome. This is currently the working hypothesis for the basic defect in this particular syndrome.

A potentially unifying theory capable of explaining the diverse clinical cellular and molecular manifestations of Fanconi's anemia has yet to emerge. The cytogenetic hypersensitivity to bifunctional alkylating agents is suggestive of a defect in the repair of DNA interstrand crosslinks. A variety of enzymatic studies indicate a large array of deficiencies in isolated patient cell strains, but no single abnormality has been found in a large number of patients. Therefore, the basic defect in this syndrome remains unknown.

PRACTICAL DIAGNOSTIC CONSIDERATIONS

Unfortunately, our knowledge of the chromosome instability syndromes is insufficient to develop presymptomatic population screening tests for affected individuals. Because none of the basic defects is well understood, it is necessary to detect an affected individual before recognizing that an entire family is at risk. Nonetheless, for autosomal-recessive syndromes, each birth or pregnancy following the birth of the proband will carry a 25% risk of a similar outcome. Additionally, it is virtually impossible, based on currently available tests and techniques, to identify phenotypically normal individuals who carry the gene for any of these syndromes in a heterozygous condition. Therefore, diagnostic capability is possible only for homozygous recessive individuals who are phenotypically abnormal. Nonetheless, it is still important to make the diagnosis because diagnosis based on clinical manifestations alone can be misleading, particularly with regard to the prognosis and possible outcome of the condition. In other words, absolute clinical and cytological diagnoses are both necessary because some of these conditions overlap clinically, and a mistaken diagnosis can lead to significantly different outcomes.

The diagnostic capability to identify affected individuals is based on a combination of unique clinical phenotypes with cytogenetic evaluation of the pattern of chromosome instability. Obviously, the presence of an abnormal phenotype is the primary indication of a chromosome instability syndrome. The laboratory component of making the diagnosis is the cytogenetic evaluation of levels of chromosome breakage using both untreated (spontaneous levels) and clastogen-treated cells. Because they are easily obtained, peripheral lymphocytes are most frequently used, but cultured fibroblasts and (with utmost caution) amniotic fluid cells or chorionic villus samples can also be used for diagnosis. In other words, cell types amenable to cytogenetic evaluation may be used for diagnostic purposes. The typical experiment for such a diagnosis involves the use of treated and untreated cells from the patients which are usually compared with cells from their parents (if available) as obligate heterozygotes for the condition. Cells of unrelated normal individuals are included as controls. Usually, peripheral blood lymphocyte cultures are established and exposed to the clastogen to which the particular hypersensitivity associated with the syndrome has been demonstrated (stress test). For example, XP cells are subjected to ultraviolet radiation, A-T cells to x-rays or bleomycin, and FA cells to diepoxybutane or mitomycin C. BS cells are examined for increased frequency of spontaneous sister chromatid exchanges. The cultures are established, and the experiment is completely coded both at the stage of establishing cultures and on examining the microscope slides. Because of the subjective nature of scoring procedures for the evaluation of chromosome breakage, it is extremely important that the observer be totally unaware of the source of the slides being examined. A statistically sufficient scored sample of cells is counted (usually a minimum of 100 to 200 cells per treatment) and 2 or 3 replicates are established for each data point. The cells are then scored for the types of chromosome damage described above (Fig. 28.2), and the results are totaled.

Various types of statistical comparison are necessary for appropriate data analysis. At the spontaneous breakage level, comparisons between the affected and unaffected individuals or with induced breakage will usually be the first indication of a positive diagnosis. That is, at least a three-fold to four-fold increase in spontaneous breakage rates will be suggestive of an affected individual. Similarly, comparisons between the spontaneous breakage levels and the "clastogen stress level" within an affected individual or between clastogen-stressed normal cells and the putative affected cells can be made (see Table 28.6). Again, statistically significant differences, based on the sizes of the individual samples, should be obtained to confirm the diagnosis.

Statistical analyses usually employed in such comparisons are varied, and there is no definitive protocol for the interpretation of such data. Depending on the complexity of the design of the particular experiment and the number of variables involved, these techniques range from relatively simple chi-square approaches to highly complex analyses of variance, correlation, regression, etc. The type of analysis used depends on how the experiment is constructed. However, the investigator is cautioned to consult

Table 28.6. Comparisons of Spontaneous and Induced Cytogenetic Damage in Various Cell Types in the Chromosome Breakage Syndromes[a]

Spontaneous Breakage Frequencies—Peripheral Lymphocytes			
Individuals	No. of Individuals	No. of Cells	Breaks/Cell
Probands:			
Ataxia-telangiectasia	7	785	0.47
Bloom's syndrome	3	200	0.34
Fanconi's anemia	6	600	0.28
A-T heterozygotes	7	632	0.19
A-T siblings (phenotypically normal)	10	1250	0.20
FA heterozygotes	10	1000	0.03
Controls:			
Newborns	580	8700	0.014
Cytogenetic patients (Non–chromosome instability syndromes)	50	1300	0.016
Total controls		10,000	0.015[b]

Clinical "Stress Tests" in Ataxia-Telangiectasia and Fanconi's Anemia Demonstrating Cytogenetic Hypersensitivity			
Cell Type	No. of Individuals	No. of Cells	Breaks/Cell
	Lymphoblastoid lines treated with 2.0 μg/ml bleomycin for final 24 hours of culture		
Ataxia-telangiectasia	5	750	0.52
Xeroderma pigmentosum	3	450	0.13
Normal	4	600	0.09
	Lymphocytes treated with 0.10 μg/ml of diepoxybutane for final 24 hours of culture		
Fanconi's anemia	5	650	1.62
Controls	25	10,500	0.09

[a]Adapted from: Cohen *et al*, Cytogenet. Cell Genet. 15:338-356, 1975. Cohen *et al*, Am. J. Hum. Genet. 34:794-810, 1982. Cohen *et al*, Cancer Res 41:1817-1823, 1981.
[b]Average of controls.

with a biostatistician to ascertain the best experimental design and method of data analysis prior to embarking on a diagnostic trial.

These cytogenetic diagnoses are subject to several types of difficulties and pitfalls, and caution is therefore advised. From a technical point of view, consideration must be given to the dosage levels of the clastogen used to ensure viability of the cells treated and to avoid cytotoxic levels because results at those levels will be highly questionable. Moreover, the lymphocyte assay itself contains inherent variability that must be considered. Most importantly, emphasis must be placed on the "blind coding" of slides and sufficiently large samples to be representative of the actual results. With regard to diagnosis, the differences between rates of spontaneous and induced chromosome damage for affected and normal individuals are usually sufficiently large to be apparent without intricate statistical testing. However, it must be remembered that the initial suspicion of an instability syndrome is generally a clinical impression, and this impression must always be considered in interpreting the cytogenetic data. These two approaches—clinical phenodeviation and cytogenetic results—are both necessary components of the diagnostic decision.

The prenatal diagnosis of affected individuals is a much more tenuous situation. As indicated above, the procedures used to arrive at such diagnoses are often complex and highly specialized. Therefore, only laboratories with considerable experience will undertake such analyses. The number of patients prenatally diagnosed to date is extremely limited, and experience has been concentrated in only a few laboratories around the world. If such a situation does arise, the reader is directed to contact one of these laboratories.

OTHER SYNDROMES

In addition to the four syndromes described in detail, other entities have been included among the chromosome instability syndromes. These have not been as thoroughly studied, and the basis of their cellular phenotypes is not well understood. Nonetheless, they do show some common characteristics with the major instability syndromes.

Nijmegen Breakage Syndrome

In addition to the clinical heterogeneity mentioned above, patients have been reported with manifestations suggestive of, but not entirely consistent with, the diagnosis of A-T. The best described of these has become known as the Nijmegen breakage syndrome (NBS). These patients manifest microcephaly, short statute, mental retardation, café au lait spots, and an immunodeficiency characteristic of A-T. However, they have neither ataxia nor telangiectasia. They do demonstrate increased spontaneous, radiation-induced, and bleomycin-induced chromosome breakage, as well as x-ray hypersensitivity and the molecular hallmark of A-T: radioresistant DNA synthesis. Normal levels of α-fetoprotein are observed in these patients. Even within NBS, two complementation groups have been defined.

Werner's Syndrome

A rare autosomal recessive disorder characterized by progeria-like premature aging, early onset of cataracts, generalized osteoporosis, diabetes, atherosclerosis, hypokeratosis, leg ulcers, and a high frequency of cancer. These cancers are predominantly mesenchymal in origin and are a principal cause of death.

The cytogenetic instability in Werner's syndrome has been termed "variegated translocation mosaicism" and has been described in both fibroblasts and lymphoblasts of these patients. The observed chromosomal abnormalities consist primarily of stable structural chromosome rearrangements ranging from partial deletions to multiple translocations. However, to date, no specific hypersensitivity to any physical or chemical clastogen has been found that is capable of identifying persons with Werner's syndrome or their cells. No molecular abnormalities that could explain the basic defect in Werner's syndrome have been suggested.

Multibranched Chromosome Syndrome

Multibranched chromosome syndrome is a relatively new entity that, to date, has been observed in only seven patients. Clinical findings include immunodeficiency and facial abnormalities, most commonly hypertelorism, a flat nasal bridge, epicanthal folds, protrusion of the tongue, and micrognathia. In addition to these common findings, the following are reported in fewer patients: cerebral atrophy, cardiac murmur, cleft palate, hydrocephalus, and chorioretinitis. Mental retardation can range from severe to borderline; speech development is usually impaired. Growth retardation is variable and is usually below the third percentile. The cytogenetic observations include a peculiar branching of the chromosome from the centromere. Chromosomes 1 and 9 and, less frequently, 16 are involved in this syndrome and show large secondary constrictions (Fig. 28.7). Other chromosomes are rarely involved, but chromosomes 2 and 10 and the acrocentrics have been implicated. Although a clear mode of inheritance is not apparent, the occurrence of affected siblings suggests an autosomal-recessive pattern. No known hypersensitivity to clastogens has been reported, and an underlying defect has not been suggested.

Roberts Syndrome

Roberts Syndrome (RS) is another autosomal recessive condition that shares many of the features of the chromosome instability syndromes. Patients with RS are affected with a broad spectrum of physical abnormalities, including tetraphocomelia, bilateral cleft lip and palate, ectrodactyly and syndactyly, ocular hypertelorism and exophthalmos, growth retardation, and failure to thrive. Approximately 70 cases have been reported to date. Most commonly, the chromosome abnormality observed in Roberts syndrome consists of centromere "splaying" or "popping" (Fig. 28.8). These abnormalities are observed spontaneously in both lymphocytes and fibroblasts derived from RS patients. Hypersensitivity to a series of clastogens, including UV radiation, methylnitrosurea, mitomycin C, and cisplatin, has been observed. These data suggest that RS cells, like FA cells, are sensitive to cross-linking agents.

Systemic Sclerosis (Scleroderma)

Scleroderma is a multisystem disease of unknown etiology characterized by immune dysfunction, excess accumulation of collagen and ground substance leading to fibrosis of the skin and viscera, and spontaneous chromosome breakage. Two clinical subsets of generalized scleroderma have been described: (a) diffuse scleroderma, characterized by extensive skin involvement, including the trunk, hands, and face, and widespread, progressive visceral involvement; (b) CREST syndrome (*c*alcinosis, *R*aynaud's phenomenon, *e*sophageal hypomotility, *s*clerodactyly, *t*elangiectasia), in which the organ involvement is similar to the diffuse type, but the progression is slower. Throughout the course of the disease, patients have malaise, weight loss, and depression, as well as more specific symptoms related to systemic involvement of the connective tissue in the skin, gastrointestinal tract, lungs, heart, and kidneys. In rare instances, familial segregation has been tested, but no clear inheritance pattern has been demonstrated. None of the familial cases has been associated with any specific environmental exposure. Although the reports have not all been consistent, approximately 95% of patients with scleroderma demonstrate increased frequencies of spontaneous chromosome damage.

Dyskeratosis Congenita

Dyskeratosis congenita is a rare multisystem disorder that shows both X-linked and autosomal reces-

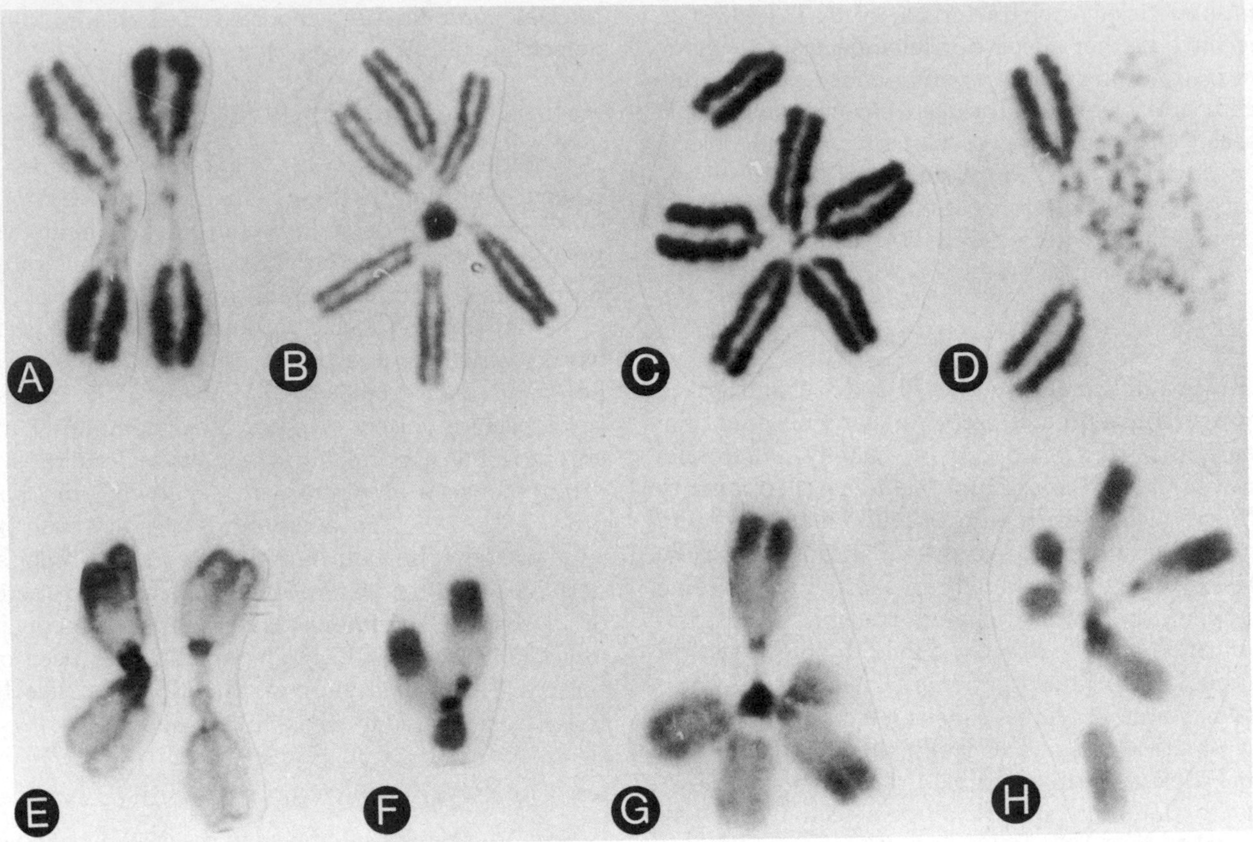

Figure 28.7. Examples of chromosome 1 pairs and branched configurations (BCs). *Upper row*, standard Giemsa staining. **A**, Elongated secondary constriction; **B**, BC with heterochromatin block; **C**, BC with heterochromatin block; **D**, Pulverization. *Lower row*, C-banding; **E**, Elongated secondary constriction; **F**, BC involving chromosomes 1 and 16; **G**, **H**, BC with and without chromatin block. Note that in all instances the centromere is conserved. (Reprinted with permission from Turleau C, Cabanis MO, Girault D. Multibranched chromosomes in the ICF syndrome: immunodeficiency, centromeric instability, and facial anomolies. Am J Med Genet 1989;32:420–424.)

sive inheritance patterns. The characteristic clinical features include nail dystrophy, cutaneous and mucosal pigmentation changes, and chronic bone marrow failure. The dermatological abnormalities usually develop during childhood but may be described at birth. An increased susceptibility to infection and a predisposition to malignancy are the most serious features of this disease. Increased cytogenetic instability is not a constant feature of this syndrome, but elevated rates of chromosome breakage and sister chromatid exchanges have been observed in many of the patients. Specific chromosomal anomalies noted include premature centromeric disjunction (similar to Roberts syndrome) and fibroblast hypersensitivity to G_2 chromosome damage (similar to A-T, FA, XP groups C and E, and BS fibroblasts).

"N" Syndrome

This multiple congenital anomaly/mental retardation syndrome was described in two brothers, leading to the suggestion of X-linked recessive inheritance. Both brothers died of an acute malignancy resembling T-cell leukemia. Lymphocytes and fibroblasts of the probands and lymphocytes of their unaffected mother showed a greatly elevated rate of chromosome damage. Preliminary experimental evidence suggests that the basic defect in this syndrome may be associated with a mutation affecting the gene controlling DNA polymerase alpha, an enzyme essential for DNA synthesis and repair.

CONCLUSIONS

With recent advances in molecular DNA technology, the successful cloning and characterization of the genes responsible for the chromosome instability syndromes is in the offing. Although such an accomplishment may represent the successful conclusion of one chapter of research into these conditions, it will simultaneously begin several additional lines of investigation. The careful analysis of the molecular pathophysiology of these syndromes will be facilitated, thereby helping to elucidate the multifaceted cellular characteristics and diverse, yet specific, individual cellular sensitivity observed. Of even greater interest is the understanding of the tissue and organ abnormalities re-

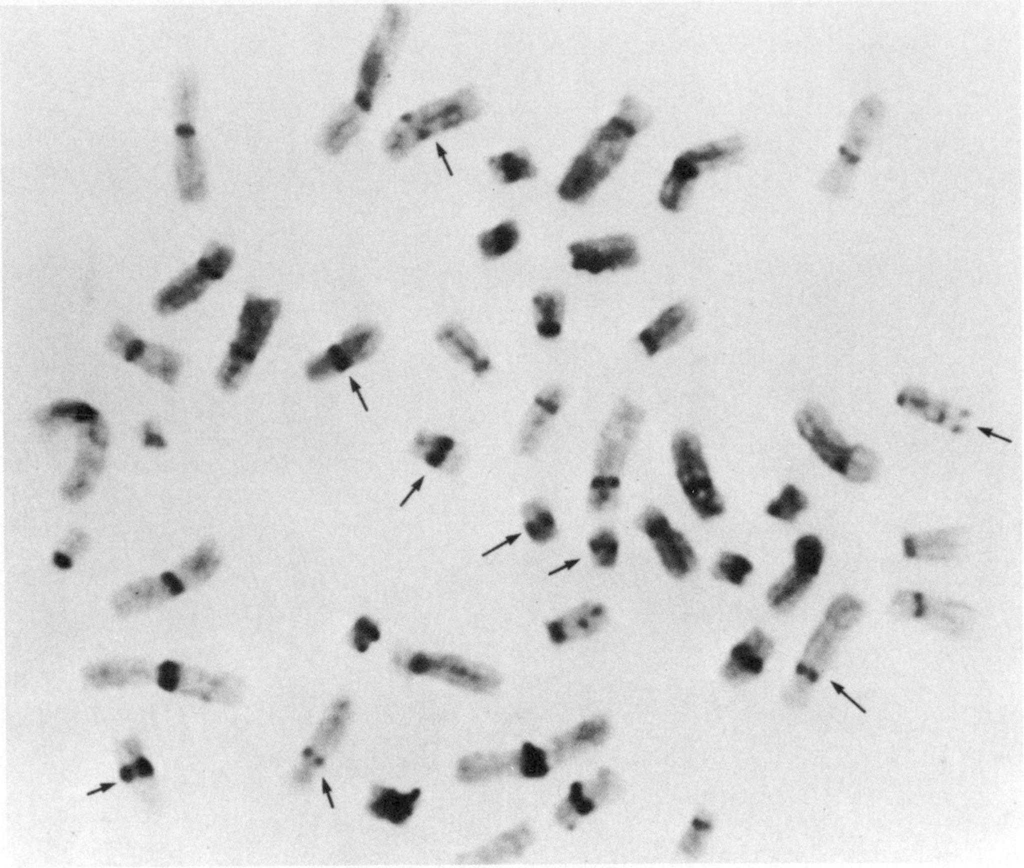

Figure 28.8. Metaphase from a patient with Roberts syndrome. *Arrows* indicate premature centromere separation, or "centromere splaying." (From Parry DM, Mulvihil JJ, Tsai S, Kaiser Kupfer MI, Cowan JM, SC phocomelia syndrome, premature centromere separation, and congenital cranial nerve paralysis in two sisters, one with malignant melanoma. Am J Med Genet 1986;24:653–672.)

sponsible for the disparate manifestations unique to each syndrome. New and more powerful techniques may facilitate both the prenatal and early, presymptomatic diagnosis of affected individuals and the detection of heterozygotes. Model therapeutic regimens may be designed based on knowledge of the particular genetic defect, and morbidity and mortality in both carriers and affected patients may be reduced or at least delayed. Research into the chromosome instability syndromes is beginning a new era, and the questions that lie ahead should prove both challenging and exciting.

Suggested Readings

Bridges BA, Harnden DG, eds. Ataxia-telangiectasia: a cellular and molecular link between cancer, neuropathy and immune deficiency. New York: John Wiley & Sons, 1982.

Cohen MM, Levy HL. Chromosome instability syndromes. In: Harris H, Hirschhorn K, eds. Advances in human genetics. New York: Plenum Publishing, 1989;18:43–149.

Gatti RA, Swift M, eds. Ataxia-telangiectasia: genetics, neuropathy, and immunology of a degenerative disease of childhood. Kroc Series, vol. 19. New York: Alan R Liss, 1985.

German J. Patterns of neoplasia associated with chromosome breakage syndromes. In: German J, ed. Chromosome mutation and neoplasia. New York: Alan R Liss, 1983:97–134.

Jaspers NGJ, Gatti RA, Baan C, Linssen PCML, Bootsma D. Genetic complementation analysis of ataxia telangiectasia and Nijmegen breakage syndrome: a survey of 50 patients. Cytogenet Cell Genet 1988;49:259–263.

Kraemer KH, Lee MM, Scotto J. Xeroderma pigmentosum. Cutaneous, ocular, and neurologic abnormalities in 830 published cases. Arch Dermatol 1987;123:241–250.

Parry DM, Mulvihill JJ, Tsai S, Kaiser-Kupfer MI, Cowan JM. SC phocomelia syndrome, premature centromere separation, and congenital cranial nerve paralysis in two sisters, one with malignant melanoma. Am J Med Genet 1986;24:653–672.

Schroeder-Kurth TM, Auerbach AD, Obe G, eds. Fanconi anemia: clinical cytogenetic and experimental aspects. New York: Springer-Verlag, 1989.

Turleau C, Cabanis MO, Girault D, et al. Multibranched chromosomes in the ICF syndrome: immunodeficiency, centromeric instability, and facial anomalies. Am J Med Genet 1989;32:420–424.

29 Chromosome Studies in Neoplastic Hematologic Disorders

Gordon W. Dewald, Mary Ann Morris, and Virginia C. Lilla

A recent survey by the Association of Cytogenetic Technologists indicates that approximately 39,800 chromosome studies were done in 1988 on patients with neoplastic hematologic disorders (1). These studies were done by 192 cytogenetic laboratories located throughout the United States. This figure is conservative because not all cytogenetic laboratories in the United States participated in the survey. The survey also indicates that more cytogenetic laboratories perform chromosome studies on specimens for hematologic disorders (192 laboratories) than on amniotic fluids (180 laboratories), chorionic villi (77 laboratories), or fibroblasts (26 laboratories). The only type of specimen studied by more laboratories was peripheral blood for congenital disorders (234 laboratories). This survey demonstrates the wide use of cytogenetic studies in the United States for patients with neoplastic hematologic disorders.

Today, chromosome studies are used to diagnose clonal neoplastic processes. Because specific chromosome abnormalities are associated with certain hematologic disorders, cytogenetic studies can help classify diseases. The observation of cytogenetic subclones can provide clues to disease progression. Classification and disease progression are important criteria for making decisions related to treatment. Cytogenetic studies can be used to monitor remission and to distinguish between donor and recipient cells in bone marrow transplants. The mechanisms that produce disease progression in malignant disorders are not understood, but the study of chromosome evolution could provide important clues. For these reasons and others, cytogenetic studies have become important in the repertoire of new tests used by hematologists.

This chapter presents some applications of cytogenetic studies in hematologic disorders. A model is proposed for the role of chromosome abnormalities in the origin and progression of malignant hematologic disorders. The kinds of chromosome abnormalities that occur and their association with the classification schemes for hematologic disorders are presented. How chromosome studies can be used in the workup of patients suspected of having hematologic disorders is emphasized. Information is provided about the types of specimens to collect, the procedures for transporting specimens to cytogenetic laboratories, and the interpretation of the results of chromosome analysis. Finally, some new techniques that may facilitate the use of chromosome studies in hematologic disorders are discussed. The reader can find more information in the list of references at the end of the chapter.

CHROMOSOMAL BASIS OF MALIGNANCY

Kinds of Chromosome Abnormalities

Chromosome abnormalities are generally classified as either numerical or structural (Fig. 29.1). The numerical abnormalities are subclassified into polyploid and aneuploid. The term *polyploid* refers to chromosome complements that are multiples of the haploid number of chromosomes; for example, triploidy refers to 69 chromosomes, and tetraploidy refers to 92 chromosomes. Polyploid clones are sometimes found, especially in advanced tumors. In neoplastic disorders, most polyploid clones are derived from the fusion of cells.

Aneuploid refers to chromosome complements that involve irregular multiples of the haploid number; for example, a cell that has trisomy 8 is characterized by 47 chromosomes, including three number 8 chromosomes. A cell that is monosomy 7 contains 45 chromosomes and is lacking a chromosome 7. The aneuploid abnormalities usually occur as a consequence of some malfunction in cell division, such as nondisjunction.

Structural abnormalities are usually classified as translocations, deletions, inversions, duplications, or isochromosomes. Most structural abnormalities originate during the replication or repair of DNA; this is a time when the DNA is particularly vulnerable to breakage and fusion. Thus, structural abnormalities of chromosomes usually form in interphase, during a time when the chromosomes are uncoiled and the

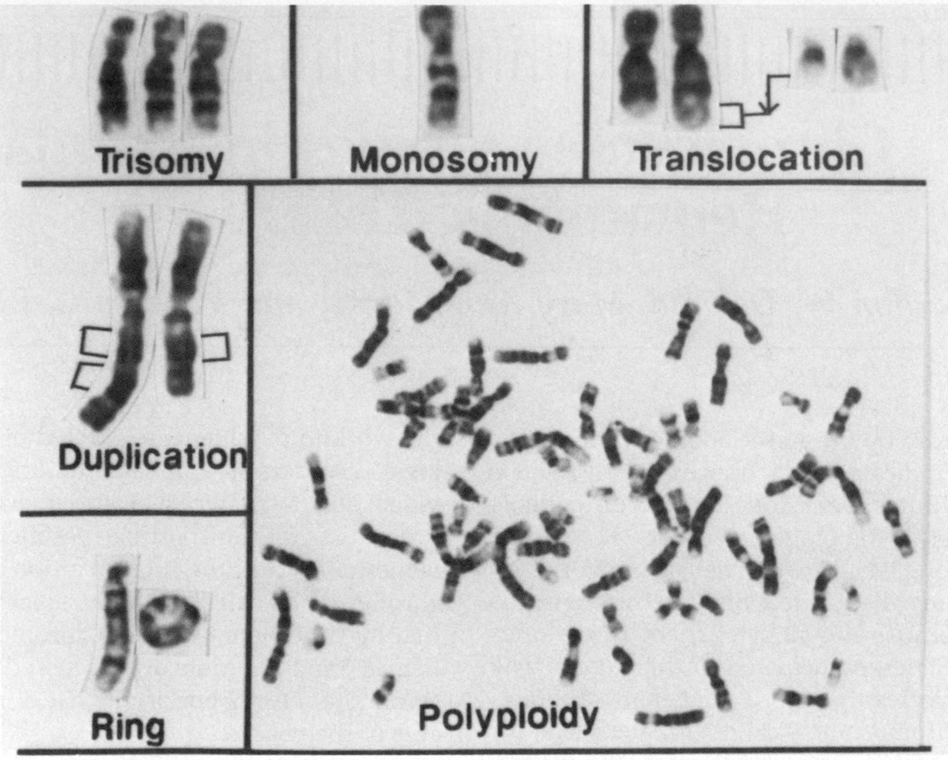

Figure 29.1. Some examples of common chromosome abnormalities. Trisomy is the presence of three copies of any chromosome. Monosomy denotes the presence of a single copy of any chromosome. Translocations involve the exchange of chromatin between any two nonhomologous chromosomes. Duplications produce structural abnormalities with multiple portions of genes present in duplicate. Deletions result in the loss of a portion of a chromosome; a ring chromosome is an example of a deletion. Polyploid cells involve 69 or 92 chromosomes or some exact multiple of the haploid chromosome number.

DNA of different chromosomes is overlapped or in association with each other. Because cytogenetic studies are usually performed on cells in mitosis, most investigators are accustomed to the morphology of chromosomes in metaphase, when chromosomes are considerably more condensed than in interphase.

Although several types of translocations exist, reciprocal translocations are the most common in hematologic disorders. Reciprocal translocations involve the interchange of parts of different chromosomes. Deletions involve the loss of part of a chromosome and may be either terminal or interstitial (i.e., occurring at a nonterminal site). Inversions produce a reversal in the direction of an interstitial part of a chromosome. Inversions may be either pericentric or paracentric. They are considered pericentric if both arms are involved and paracentric if only one arm is involved. Duplications produce two or more copies of a particular segment of a chromosome on the same chromosome. Isochromosomes have a mirror-image band pattern with respect to the center of the chromosome. Isochromosomes arise from a break and fusion of sister chromatids. Although isochromosomes are usually dicentric, some may appear to be monocentric.

Origin of Chromosome Abnormalities

Chromosome abnormalities are formed in sporadic cells of every person on a regular basis. In the authors' cytogenetic practice, structural chromosome abnormalities are seen in about six of 1000 metaphases. Isolated cells with chromosome abnormalities can even be seen in patients who do not have malignant disorders. Sporadic cells with chromosome abnormalities occur in amniotic fluid, tissue biopsy specimens, fibroblasts, peripheral blood, bone marrow, and other tissues. These chromosome abnormalities probably represent new mutations rather than clinically significant clones because it is rare that more than one cell with the same abnormality is observed. If more than one metaphase in 30 has structural abnormalities, most cytogeneticists become concerned that the patient has a breakage syndrome or was exposed to toxic substances such as chemotherapy or dangerous agents at home or at work. Another possibility is a problem with the laboratory procedure.

People who are exposed to agents that cause structural damage to chromosomes or to the mitotic apparatus may have a higher than usual incidence of sporadic cells with chromosome abnormalities. Several genetic mechanisms to repair DNA damage exist

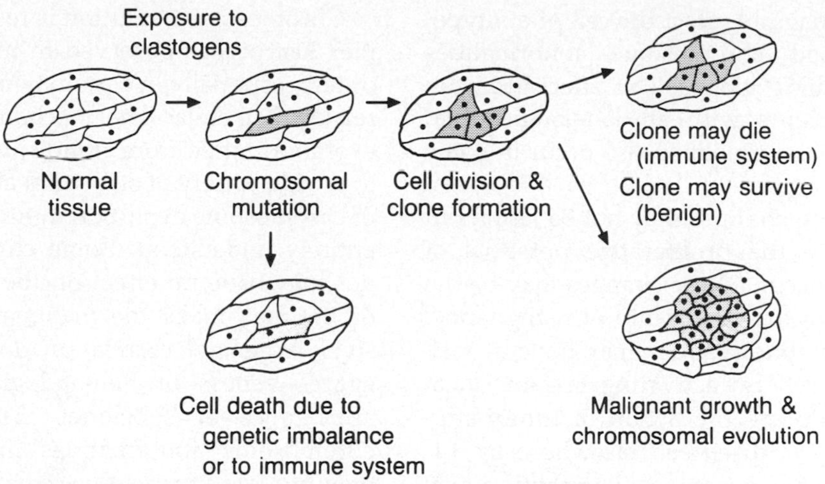

Figure 29.2. Formation of a clone. In the early stages, chromosomally abnormal clones may die as a consequence of genetic imbalance or may be destroyed by the immune system. If not, the clone may proliferate and form a malignant tumor, and subclones may form due to chromosome evolution. (From Dewald GW. Possible role of chromosome abnormalities in the origin and progression of lymphoma. In: Muller SA, ed. Parapsoriasis: Proceedings of the First International Parapsoriasis Symposium, September 7 and 8, 1989. Rochester, MN: Mayo Foundation, 1990:43–51. By permission of Mayo Foundation.)

in every human. One repair mechanism corrects for thymidine dimer formations. Others repair damage due to alkylating agents or radiation. Repair mechanisms for other special forms of DNA damage are also known. The damaged DNA can usually be repaired without producing chromosome abnormalities. Any mutation in the genes that control the repair processes can significantly affect the proportion of cells with chromosome abnormalities. This explains the considerable incidence of cells with structurally abnormal chromosomes in patients with chromosome breakage syndromes.

The most common chromosome breakage syndromes include ataxia-telangiectasia, Bloom's syndrome, xeroderma pigmentosum, and Fanconi's anemia (see Chapter 28). The incidence of malignant disorders is higher among people with these genetic disorders than among people with normal DNA repair mechanisms. The chromosomes of patients with different breakage syndromes are sensitive to particular DNA agents. This sensitivity is evidence that each of these disorders is due to a different gene mutation for DNA repair. The chromosomes of patients with Fanconi's anemia are particularly sensitive to bifunctional alkylating agents such as mitomycin C. The chromosomes of patients with ataxia-telangiectasia are hypersensitive to ionizing radiation and radiomimetic chemicals such as bleomycin. Patients with xeroderma pigmentosum are particularly sensitive to ultraviolet light.

Formation of Clones

Most investigators now believe that nearly all malignant disorders are clonal. The clonal pattern of malignancies has been demonstrated with cytogenetic studies, X-linked enzyme markers, molecular genetic methods, immunocytochemical techniques, and many other procedures. Cytogenetic studies done for research purposes suggest that nearly all malignant disorders are associated with chromosomally abnormal clones. Hundreds of cytogenetic reports have been published in recent years recording the presence of chromosomally abnormal clones in a wide variety of hematologic disorders and solid tumors. However, in clinical practice, many patients do not appear to have a chromosomally abnormal clone. The reasons for the discrepancies between research and clinical practice are discussed elsewhere in this chapter.

The formation of each chromosomally abnormal clone probably begins with the origin of a chromosome abnormality in a single cell. The formation and consequences of an abnormal clone are shown in Figure 29.2. The observation of identical chromosome abnormalities in different cells of the same tumor is accepted evidence of clonality.

The formation of structural abnormalities of chromosomes may be relatively random with respect to the site of breakpoints. Thus, a break theoretically could affect any site on any chromosome. Considering that the human diploid genome has approximately 6 billion base pairs distributed among 46 chromosomes, about 36×10^{18} different chromosome rearrangements are theoretically possible. Certain chromosome abnormalities may produce biologically significant genetic imbalances that affect important cellular pathways. Cells with these abnormalities may die without having the chance to proliferate. Other chromosome abnormalities may be balanced and may or may not affect the cell phenotype. Cells with balanced chromosome abnormalities might produce "benign" clones. This effect has been noted in some patients with ataxia-telangiectasia. Balanced structural abnormalities also occur in some congenital disorders.

Some chromosome changes may not be lethal but rather may enhance the proliferative potential of cells in which they occur. These changes may be the most important from the standpoint of malignancy. These chromosome abnormalities may have a positive effect on the cell by activating certain oncogenes or by interrupting the action of tumor-suppressor genes. This is discussed elsewhere in this chapter. Different chromosome abnormalities may influence different genetic and cellular pathways. This might partially explain why various malignant neoplastic disorders are associated with different prognoses. It may also partially explain why certain chromosome abnormalities are associated with specific neoplastic disorders.

It is possible that the breakage of chromosomes is not entirely random. The likelihood of developing a chromosome abnormality with oncogenic significance may be affected by the presence of fragile sites on various chromosomes, the association of specific portions of chromosomes during interphase, and specific modes of action by the mutagens. In fact, since the number of possible chromosome arrangements is 36×10^{18}, the likelihood of developing one of the common hematologic abnormalities by accident seems so remote that chance alone would not explain the relatively high frequency of hematologic disorders.

Chromosome Evolution and Tumor Progression

In most tumors, as the abnormal cells proliferate, additional chromosome abnormalities appear in sporadic malignant cells by "chromosome evolution." Some of these chromosome abnormalities produce subclones, each containing the initial or primary chromosome abnormality as well as one or more so-called secondary chromosome abnormalities. For example, if a t(9;22)(q34;q11) is observed in all the cells analyzed, this abnormality can be considered the primary chromosome anomaly of the clone. If some cells also have trisomy 8, this is evidence of chromosome evolution and is consistent with the appearance of a subclone. All cells in this subclone would contain both a t(9;22)(q34;q11) and trisomy 8. It is not uncommon to observe more than one subclone in hematologic disorders.

Chromosome evolution is responsible for the complex karyotypes observed in many hematologic disorders, especially in certain lymphomas and therapy-related leukemia. The mechanisms of chromosome evolution range from nondisjunction and cell fusion to a wide variety of structural abnormalities. The role of chromosome evolution in tumor progression is not entirely understood. Some chromosome abnormalities may have no effect on the tumor cells, whereas others may make the malignant cells more aggressive. A general correlation does exist between the aggressiveness of hematologic disorders and the appearance of subclones. Thus, the number of chromosome abnormalities in an abnormal clone may provide a crude measurement of tumor progression. Indeed, many high-grade lymphomas have very complex karyotypes, and low-grade lymphomas often have only one or two chromosome abnormalities.

The correlation between karyotype complexity and the extent of tumor progression is not perfect. With only a few exceptions, karyotype complexity has not been reliably used in clinical practice to estimate prognosis or to decide forms of treatment. Two exceptions are chronic granulocytic leukemia and the 5q− syndrome, in which the more aggressive stages often exhibit chromosome evolution.

Chromosome evolution may affect how tumors respond to therapy. It would be difficult to imagine the development of a specific therapy for any tumor that involves multiple subclones. Treating a tumor with multiple subclones may be akin to dealing with a patient who has several malignant neoplastic disorders at the same time. For these patients, it may be necessary to develop more than one form of treatment to combat the genotype of each subclone.

Role of the Immune System

The immune system may prevent the progression of at least some malignant clones. The immune system may be most effective early in the formation of a clone, when the number of abnormal cells is small. Not everyone has a perfect immune system. Some people may have better immune systems for warding off malignant processes than others. This difference may not be surprising if one considers that the immune system itself is under genetic control. Exposure to immune-suppressing substances, such as chemotherapy and radiotherapy, can also affect the chances of developing malignancies. These treatments may increase the frequency of chromosome damage and impair the ability of the immune system to destroy malignant clones.

CHROMOSOME ABNORMALITIES AND THEIR FREQUENCY OF OCCURRENCE

Frequency of Abnormal Clones

Nearly all patients with malignancies probably have one or more clones of neoplastic cells that contain abnormal chromosomes. However, in clinical practice the frequency with which chromosomally abnormal clones are found in patients with hematologic disorders varies considerably among laboratories. One major factor that contributes to this interlaboratory variation is the mixture of patients with different hematologic disorders seen by the physicians who refer specimens. In the authors' cytogenetic and clinical practice, abnormal clones are found in about 58% of patients with acute nonlymphocytic leukemia, 69% with acute lymphocytic leukemia, 100% with chronic granulocytic leukemia, 39% with myelodysplastic syndromes, 39% with polycythemia vera, and 79% with non-Hodgkin's lymphoma. Except for polycythemia vera, the specimens used to estimate the frequency of detection of abnormal clones in routine practice are all collected at the time of initial diagnosis. Considerably higher frequencies of chromosomally abnormal clones are observed among patients in the more advanced stages of each of these hematologic disorders.

Why All Patients Do Not Appear to Have Chromosomally Abnormal Clones

The referral patterns of physicians differ with regard to the type of disease, treatment, and stage of illness of patients, and these factors can all contribute to the variation among laboratories with respect to the frequency of detecting chromosomally abnormal clones. The technical experience of the laboratory staff, the processing time for specimens, and the cost of testing can also affect the chances of finding chromosomally abnormal clones. In practice, many cytogenetic studies are done as part of the initial examination of a patient, when a diagnosis has not yet been established. This step often occurs relatively early in the disease, when normal cells predominate. The typical cytogenetic study is usually done on a single bone marrow specimen. Frequently, the most cellular part of the specimen is used for other laboratory tests, such as standard hematologic studies. In such cases, the cytogenetic study is relegated to the "bloody" part of the specimen, which contains few mitotic cells. In routine practice, usually no more than 4 or 5 hours can be allotted to the analysis of metaphases for each case. The cytogenetic results are often needed within a few days so that the physician can use the results to manage the patient. In addition, investing excessive hours to each test would significantly affect the cost of cytogenetic studies. The introduction of new and more efficient preparation procedures may someday result in a higher yield of chromosomally abnormal clones.

Frequency of Specific Chromosome Abnormalities

Prior to 1985, approximately 43 chromosome abnormalities that were either common or discussed frequently in the literature were encountered in routine practice (2). These abnormalities are included in the list of structural anomalies in Table 29.1 and in all of the numerical abnormalities in Table 29.2. In 1985, the authors attempted to estimate the frequency of occurrence for each of these abnormalities in our practice by reviewing the cytogenetic findings of 748 consecutive patients with an abnormal clone who were studied between 1975 and 1984. Patients were excluded who had only normal metaphases or in whom the minimal criteria for an abnormal clone were not met. These persons were excluded because there was uncertainty about whether they actually had malignant disease or whether, for some technical reason, an abnormal clone was not seen.

Table 29.1. Status I and II Chromosome Aberrations in Hematologic Disorders[a]

Abnormality[b]	Example	Associated Disorders[c]	Status	Frequency in 748[d] patients: Total Patients	Patients with Only One Abnormality	Patients with Other Abnormalities
Translocations						
t(X;18)(p11;q11)		SS	I			
t(1;1)(p36;p11-12)		ML	II			
t(1;3)(p36;q21)		MDS, ANLL	I			
t(1;6)(q23-25;p21-25)	Fig. 29.4*w*	MPD	II			
t(1;7)(p11;p11)	Fig. 29.4*a*	MPD, MDS, ANLL	I	13	7	6
t(1;11)(p32;q23)	Fig. 29.4*b*	ALL	I			
t(1;11)(q21;q23)		ANLL	I			
t(1;14)(p32-34;q11)	Fig. 29.4*x*	T-ALL	II			
t(1;14)(q21-q25;q32)		ML	I			
t(1;14)(q42;q32)		B-ML	II			

Table 29.1—*continued*

Abnormality[b]	Example	Associated Disorders[c]	Status	Frequency in 748[d] patients: Total Patients	Patients with Only One Abnormality	Patients with Other Abnormalities
t(1;17)(p11 or q11;p11 or q11)		CGL, MPD, ANLL, ML	I			
t(1;17)(p36;q21)		ANLL-M3	II			
t(1;19)(q23;p13)	Fig. 29.4*y*	pre-B cell ALL	I	1	1	0
t(2;3)(p13-p22;q26-q29)	Fig. 29.4*z*	ANLL	I			
t(2;3)(q21-q23;q27)		ML	II			
t(2;5)(p23;q35)	Fig. 29.4*aa*	MH, T-ML	I			
t(2;8)(p12;q24)	Fig. 29.4*bb*	BL, ALL-L3	I			
t(2;11)(p21;q23)	Fig. 29.4*c*	MDS, ANLL	I			
t(2;14)(p13;q32)	Fig. 29.4*d*	B-CLL	II			
t(3;3)(q21;q26)	Fig. 29.4*cc*	ANLL, MDS, MPD	I			
ins(3;3)(q26;q21q26)	Fig. 29.4*e*	ANLL, MDS, MPD	I	2	1	1
t(3;5)(q21;q31)	Fig. 29.4*f*	ANLL	I			
t(3;5)(q24-25;q32-34)		ANLL	I			
t(3;14)(p21;q32)	Fig. 29.4*dd*	ML	II			
t(3;21)(q26;q22)	Fig. 29.4*g*	CGL, MDS	I			
t(4;11)(q21;q23)	Fig. 29.4*h*	ALL, ANLL	I	5	3	2
t(6;9)(p23;q34)	Fig. 29.4*i*	ANLL	I	1	1	0
t(6;11)(q27;q23)	Fig. 29.4*j*	ANLL-M5	I			
t(6;14)(p21;q32)		ML	II			
dic(7;9)(p11-13;p11)		ALL	I			
t(7;11)(p15;p15)	Fig. 29.4*ee*	ANLL, MPD	I			
t(7;11)(q35;p13-14)		T-ALL	II			
t(8;9)(p11;q34)		MPD	II			
t(8;14)(q22;q32)		ML	II			
t(8;14)(q24;q11)	Fig. 29.4*k*	T-ALL	I			
t(8;14)(q24;q32)	Fig. 29.4*l*	BL, ALL-L3, ML	I	8	4	4
t(8;16)(p11;p13)	Fig. 29.4*ff*	ANLL-M5, ANLL	I			
t(8;21)(q22;q22)	Fig. 29.4*m*	ANLL-M2	I	15	6	9
t(8;22)(q24;q11)	Fig. 29.4*gg*	BL, ALL-L3	I			
t(9;11)(p21-p22;q23)	Fig. 29.4*n*	ANLL-M4, ANLL-M5	I	6	3	3
t(9;12)(p11-12;p12)		ALL	I			
dic(9;12)(p11-p13;p11-p12)		ALL	I			
t(9;22)(q34;q11)	Fig. 29.4*o*	CGL, ALL, ANLL, T-ML	I	378	292	86
t(10;11)(p11-p15;q23)	Fig. 29.4*p*	ANLL-M5	I			
ins(10;11)(p11;q23q24)		ANLL-M5	I			
t(10;11)(p14;q13-q14)		ANLL-M4, ANLL-M5	II			
t(10;14)(p11;q32)		ML	II			
t(10;14)(q24;q11)		T-ALL	I			
t(11;14)(p13;q11-q13)	Fig. 29.4*q*	T-ALL	I	3	1	2
t(11;14)(q13;q32)	Fig. 29.4*r*	ML, B-CLL, MM/PCL, B-PLL	I	5	0	5
t(11;14)(q21;q32)		ML	II			
t(11;14)(q23;q32)		ML	II			
t(11;17)(q23;q25)		ANLL-M4, ANLL-M5	I			
t(11;19)(q23;p13)	Fig. 29.4*hh*	ANLL	I			
t(11;20)(p15;q11)		ANLL	II			
t(12;17)(p13-12;q11)		ALL	I			
t(14;17)(q32;q23)		B-CLL	I			
t(14;18)(q32;q21)	Fig. 29.4*s*	ML	I	5	0	5
t(14;19)(q32;q13)	Fig. 29.4*t*	CLL	I			
t(14;22)(q32;q11)	Fig. 29.4*u*	ALL	I			
t(15;17)(q22;q11-q12)	Fig. 29.4*v*	ANLL-M3	I	1	1	0
t(16;16)(p13;q22)		ANLL-M4Eo	I			
Isochromosomes						
idic(X)(q13)	Fig. 29.5*s*	MDS, ANLL	I	5	3	2
i(1q)	Fig. 29.5*b*	ML	I			
i(6p)	Fig. 29.5*g*	ML, ALL	I	2	1	1
i(7q)	Fig. 29.5*ii*	ML, ALL, MDS, ANLL	I			
i(8q)	Fig. 29.5*m*	T-CLL, T-PLL	I			

Table 29.1—*continued*

Abnormality[b]	Example	Associated Disorders[c]	Status	Frequency in 748[d] patients: Total Patients	Patients with Only One Abnormality	Patients with Other Abnormalities
i(9q)	Fig. 29.5*jj*	ALL	I			
i(17q)	Fig. 29.5*w*	CGL, MDS, ANLL, ML, ALL, CLL	I	33	1	32
i(18q)		ML	I			
i(21q)	Fig. 29.5*z*	ANLL, MDS	I			
Inversions						
inv(3)(q21q26)	Fig. 29.5*d*	ANLL, MDS, MPD	I	3	3	0
inv(14)(q11q32)	Fig. 29.5*u*	ATL, T-CLL, T-PLL	I			
inv(16)(p13q22)	Fig. 29.5*v*	ANLL-M4Eo	I	3	0	3
Duplications						
dup(1)(q12q31)	Fig. 29.5*cc*	BL, ALL-L3, ML	I			
dup(1)(q21q32)	Fig. 29.5*c*	MPD	I	12	5	7
dup(11)(q13q23)		ML	II			
dup(11)(q13q25)	Fig. 29.5*ll*	ML	II			
dup(12)(q13q21-q22)	Fig. 29.5*mm*	ML	I			
Deletions						
del(1)(p13)	Fig. 29.5*a*	ML	I			
del(1)(q21)	Fig. 29.5*dd*	ML	II			
del(1)(q32)		ML	I			
del(1)(q42)	Fig. 29.5*ee*	ML	I			
del(1)(p32-p36)	Fig. 29.5*bb*	ML	I			
del(2)(p21)		ML	II			
del(2)(q31)	Fig. 29.5*ff*	CLL, ANLL	I			
del(2)(q32)		ML	II			
del(3)(p21)	Fig. 29.5*gg*	ML	I			
del(4)(p13-p14)	Fig. 29.5*e*	ML	II			
del(5)(q11-q35)	Fig. 29.5*f*	MDS, ANLL	I	101	32	69
del(5)(p13)	Fig. 29.5*hh*	ML	II			
del(6)(q14-q27)	Fig. 29.5*i*	ML, ALL, ATL,HCL, PLL	I	21	1	20
del(6)(p21-p23)	Fig. 29.5*h*	T-ML	I			
del(7)(p13-p14)	Fig. 29.5*j*	ML	II			
del(7)(q22-q36)	Fig. 29.5*k*	ANLL, MDS	I	29	5	24
del(7)(q32)	Fig. 29.5*l*	ML	II			
del(9)(p13)	Fig. 29.5*n*	ML	II			
del(9)(p21)	Fig. 29.5*o*	ALL	I			
del(9)(q11-q32)	Fig. 29.5*p*	ANLL	I	10	2	8
del(10)(q22-23)	Fig. 29.5*kk*	ML	II			
del(11)(q14)		MDS	I			
del(11)(q23)	Fig. 29.5*q*	ML	I	19	8	11
del(12)(p11-p13)	Fig. 29.5*r*	ANLL, ALL, CMML	I			
del(12)(p11-p12)		ML	II			
del(12)(q22)	Fig. 29.5*nn*	ML	II			
del(13)(q12-q22)	Fig. 29.5*t*	MPD, MDS	I	20	9	11
del(13)(q22)		ML	II			
del(14)(q22-q24)	Fig. 29.5*oo*	B-CLL	I			
del(14)(q22 or q24)		ML	I			
del(16)(q22)	Fig. 29.5*pp*	ANLL-M4Eo	I	3	2	1
del(20)(q11)	Fig. 29.5*x*	PV, MDS, ANLL	I			
del(20)(q11q13)	Fig. 29.5*y*	PV, MDS, ANLL	I	65	31	34
del(22)(q11-q12)	Fig. 29.5*aa*	ML	II			

[a]Data from Trent JM, Kaneko Y, Mitelman F. Report of the committee on structural chromosome changes in neoplasia. Cytogenet Cell Genet 1988; 49:236–253.
[b]The terminology is from the International System for Human Cytogenetic Nomenclature. The following standard notations are used for chromosome anomalies: del, deletion; der, derived; dup, duplication; i, isochromosome; idic, isodicentric; ins, insertion translocation; inv, inversion; p, short arm; q, long arm; t, translocation. The numbers within the first set of parentheses adjacent to the type of anomaly identify the chromosome or chromosomes involved. The numbers within the second set of parentheses identify the breakpoints. Thus, the expression t(9;22)(q34;q11) indicates a reciprocal translocation between parts of chromosomes 9 and 22 with breakpoints at 9q34 and 22q11.
[c]ALL, acute lymphocytic leukemia (subtype L3 where indicated); ANLL, acute nonlymphocytic leukemia (subtype M1-M5 where indicated); ATL, acute T-cell lymphoma; B-CLL, B-cell chronic lymphocytic leukemia; BL, Burkitt's lymphoma; B-ML, B-cell malignant lymphoma; B-PLL, B-cell peripheral lymphocytic leukemia; CGL, chronic granulocytic leukemia; CLL, chronic lymphocytic leukemia; CMML, chronic myelomonocytic leukemia; HCL, hairy cell leukemia; MDS, myelodysplastic syndrome; MH, malignant histiocytosis; ML, malignant lymphoma; MM, multiple myeloma; MPD, myeloproliferative disorder; PCL, plasma cell leukemia; PLL, peripheral lymphocytic lymphoma; PV, polycythemia vera; SS, Sézary's syndrome; T-ALL, T-cell acute lymphocytic leukemia; T-CLL, T-cell chronic lymphocytic leukemia; T-ML, T-cell malignant lymphoma; T-PLL, T-cell peripheral lymphocytic lymphoma.
[d]Frequency of each chromosome abnormality seen among 748 patients with an abnormal clone seen at Mayo Clinic. Data from Dewald GW, Noel P, Dahl RJ, Spurbeck JL. Chromosome abnormalities in malignant hematologic disorders. Mayo Clin Proc 1985;60:675–689.

Table 29.2. Common Aneuploid Abnormalities Associated with Malignant Neoplastic Hematologic Disorders[a]

	No. of Specimens			
Type of Anomaly	Total	Only Abnormality	With Other Abnormalities	Reported Associated Disorders[b]
Near haploid	1	1	0	ALL
Monosomy				
−5	25	0	25	MDS
				ANLL
				Therapy-related ANLL
−7	97	21	76	CGL in blast crisis
				MDS
				ANLL
				Therapy-related ANLL
−Y	118	66	52	Age-associated disorder and CGL
				MDS
				ANLL
−X	20	4	16	ANLL
Trisomy				
+3	5	0	5	ATL
+7	10	1	9	ATL
				ML
+8	161	55	106	CGL in blast crisis
				MDS
				ANLL
				Therapy-related ANLL
+9	20	4	16	MM
				Therapy-related ANLL
				Various disorders
+11	20	2	18	MM
+12	5	0	5	CLL
				HCL
				ML
+15	9	3	6	MM
+18	8	0	8	ML
+19	31	4	27	CGL in blast crisis
				ANLL
+21	53	8	45	CGL in blast crisis
				MDS
				ANLL

[a]From Dewald GW, Noel P, Dahl RJ, Spurbeck JL. Chromosome abnormalities in malignant hematologic disorders. Mayo Clin Proc 1985;60:675–689. Reproduced by permission of the Mayo Foundation.
[b]For explanation of abbreviations, see footnote c in Table 29.1

Collectively, these 748 patients had 1352 chromosome abnormalities. Many patients had more than one chromosome abnormality. About 61% of these specimens had one or more of the selected chromosome abnormalities. The remaining 39% of specimens had other chromosome abnormalities that either were not yet associated with any hematologic disorder or occurred infrequently in routine practice.

Since 1985, many other chromosome abnormalities associated with hematologic disorders have been reported (3). Because these newly discovered chromosome abnormalities are relatively rare, it is doubtful whether their frequency would be much different if this survey were done today. Nevertheless, it may be only a matter of time before the clinical disorders associated with nearly all chromosome abnormalities will be characterized. For the time being, physicians and cytogeneticists who have to interpret the finding of chromosome abnormalities that have not been described will need to limit their interpretation of cytogenetic results to evidence for a neoplastic process.

The relative frequencies for the chromosome anomalies investigated by the authors are shown in Table 29.1 and 29.2. The frequencies for each of the more common abnormalities are summarized in Figure 29.3. In this series of patients, translocations were the most common chromosome abnormalities, followed by trisomies, deletions, and monosomies. The most common specific chromosome abnormality was the Ph chromosome, followed by +8, −Y, 5q−, −7, 20q−, and +21. The most common trisomy was trisomy 8, followed by trisomy of chromosomes 21, 19, 9, 11, and 7. Loss of the Y chromosome was the most common monosomy, followed by monosomy of chromosomes 7, 5, and X. The most common dele-

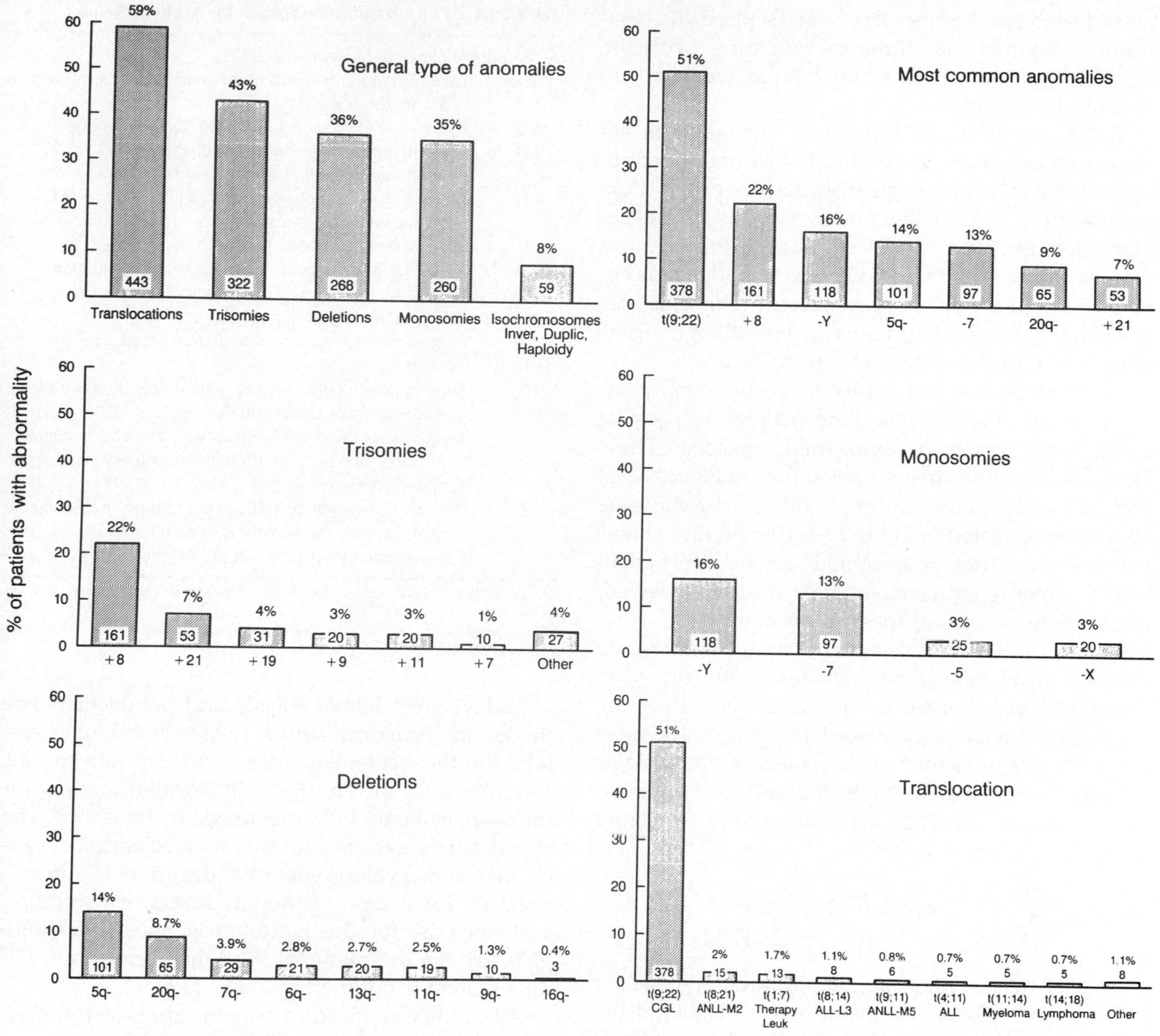

Figure 29.3. Frequency of different kinds of chromosome abnormalities in hematologic disorders. Inver, inversions; Duplic, duplications; ALL, acute lymphocytic leukemia (L3, subtype of ALL); ANLL, acute nonlymphocytic leukemia (M2 and MS, subtypes); CGL, chronic granulocytic leukemia; Therapy Leuk, therapy-related leukemia.

tion was 5q−, followed by 20q−, 7q−, 6q−, 13q−, 11q−, 9q−, and 16q−. The most common translocation was t(9;22), followed by t(8;21), t(1;7), t(8;14), t(9;11), t(4;11), and t(14;18). Isochromosomes, inversions, duplications, haploidy, and polyploidy were infrequent in this series of patients.

Specific Abnormalities in Hematologic Disorders

In recent years, hundreds of reports have been published describing chromosome abnormalities in a wide variety of hematologic disorders and solid tumors (3). It is beyond the scope of this chapter to discuss all of these chromosome abnormalities. The reader may want to refer to the publications listed at the end of the chapter for more information.

Recently, a Committee on Structural Chromosome Changes in Neoplasia was formed as part of the gene mapping organization (4). The purpose of this committee is to monitor the cytogenetic literature and to establish a grading system to correlate chromosome abnormalities with neoplastic disorders. The committee has established rules of "correlation rating," classifying each chromosome abnormality as I or II. Status I classification requires that at least five cases involving the same chromosome abnormality be reported from two or more laboratories. Status II classification requires that three or four cases with the same chromosome abnormality be reported from two or more laboratories.

The Committee on Structural Changes has assigned a correlation status for 113 chromosome abnormalities in hematologic disorders. A list of these chromosome abnormalities and their associated hematologic disorders is shown in Table 29.1. Because this committee meets periodically to update the information, the list of chromosome abnormalities achieving a correlation status in hematologic disorders can be expected to grow in the future.

We attempted to provide examples of as many status I and II chromosome abnormalities as possible using cases from our cytogenetic practice. These chromosome abnormalities are shown in Figures 29.4 and 29.5 and are cross-indexed with the chromosome abnormalities listed in Table 29.1. Certain rare abnormalities were not represented among more than 30,000 patients with hematologic disease reviewed; therefore, examples of these are not given.

So far, the Committee on Structural Chromosome Changes in Neoplasia has not dealt with numerical changes. Nevertheless, numerical abnormalities are common in hematologic disorders. Some of the most common trisomies and monosomies in hematologic disorders are listed in Table 29.2 and their frequencies in routine practice are summarized in Figure 29.3.

CLASSIFICATION OF HEMATOLOGIC DISORDERS

A brief overview of the classification systems for hematologic disorders is given here to highlight the relationship between cytogenetics and hematologic disorders.

Neoplastic hematologic disorders are classified according to the primary site of involvement and predominant cell type. The leukemias usually develop and evolve in the bone marrow and may be either myelocytic or lymphocytic. Leukemias are considered acute when more than 30% of the cells in the bone marrow are blasts. If less than 30% of the cells are blasts, the hematologic disorder is either myelodysplastic or myeloproliferative. The rare myeloid neoplasms that metastasize into lymph nodes are termed *chloromas*.

Lymphomas involve lymphocytes and usually develop and evolve in lymph nodes, although lymphomas may involve the bone marrow, spleen, and other tissues. A system of staging for lymphomas has been developed that is based on the tissues and organs involved.

Table 29.3. FAB Classification System for Acute Leukemias

Acute nonlymphocytic leukemia[a]	
M1	Lack of maturation beyond the blast stage, with less than 3% maturation.)
M2	Maturation to the progranulocyte stage or beyond
M3	Abnormal (hypogranular or hypergranular) progranulocytes that display bundles of Auer rods
M4	Blasts with both monocytic and granulocytic characteristics. Monocytes exceed 20% of the nucleated cell population
M5a	Monoblastic cells > 50% monocytic differentiation
M5b	Monocytic cells > 50% monocytic differentiation
M6	Erythrocytic cells predominantly erythroid
M7	Megakaryocytic cells predominantly megakaryocytes
Acute lymphocytic leukemia[b]	
L1	Small blasts, regular nuclear outline, few or no visible nucleoli, scant cytoplasm
L2	Larger blasts (X2 small lymphocyte), irregular or clefted nucleoli, one or more prominent nucleoli, variable to abundant cytoplasm
L3	"Burkitt's" type, large cells, dense chromatin, round or oval nucleus, moderately abundant cytoplasm, deeply basophilic cytoplasm with prominent vacuoles

[a]Acute nonlymphocytic leukemia is classified into seven categories on the basis of cell type.
[b]Acute lymphocytic leukemia is classified into three categories on the basis of cell morphology.

Today, most hematologists and pathologists use the French-American-British (FAB) classification system for the acute leukemias and myelodysplastic syndromes (5, 6). The FAB classification system for the acute leukemias is summarized in Table 29.3. The classification system for the myelodysplastic syndromes and myeloproliferative disorders is summarized in Table 29.4. Although several classification systems exist for the lymphomas, most hematologists use the International Working Formulation (7). This system is outlined in Table 29.5.

All of the classification systems are based primarily on the predominant cell type as defined by morphologic criteria. The classification of any specimen is based on the hematologic picture at the time a specimen is collected. Thus, these classification systems do not provide much historical or prognostic information about the disease. In practice, these classification schemes are very useful, but they are subjective, and different hematologists and pathologists often disagree about the classification of specimens.

Because the determination of cell morphology is often difficult, many physicians use supplemental methods such as cytogenetics, cytochemistry, immunologic markers, biochemical markers, B-cell and T-cell rearrangement studies, electron microscopy, and cell culture methods to help classify hematologic disorders. The application of these procedures has produced some significant changes in the various classification schemes in hematology. They have also

Table 29.4. FAB Classification System for Myelodysplastic Syndromes and for Myeloproliferative Disorders

Myelodysplastic Disorders		
Subtype	Peripheral Blood	Bone Marrow
Refractory anemia	<1% blasts	Erythroid hyperplasia Dyserythropoiesis <5% blasts No or few ringed sideroblasts
Refractory anemia with ringed sideroblasts	<1% blasts Occasional dysplastic neutrophils and platelets Dimorphic erythrocytes	Dyserythropoiesis Dysmegakaryocytopoiesis Dysgranulocytopoiesis >15% ringed sideroblasts
Refractory anemia with excess blasts	Cytopenias Dysgranulopoiesis Dysthrombopoiesis <5% blasts	Dyshematopoiesis 5 to 20% blasts
Refractory anemia with excess blasts in transition	Cytopenias Dysgranulopoiesis Dysthrombopoiesis >5% blasts	Dyshematopoiesis 20 to 30% blasts
Chronic myelomonocytic syndrome	>1 × 10^9/liter monocytes Left shift granulocytes Dysthrombopoiesis <5% blasts	20% blasts Increase in monocytes and precursors

Myeloproliferative disorders	
Predominant Abnormal Cell Line	Myeloproliferative Disorder
Erythroid	Polycythemia vera
Granulocytic	Chronic granulocytic leukemia
Megakaryocytic	Primary thrombocythemia
Fibroblast	Myelofibrosis with myeloid-metaplasia

Table 29.5. International Working Formulation for non-Hodgkin's Lymphomas

Low grade
Small lymphocytic
Follicular, predominantly small cleaved
Follicular, small cleaved and large cell
Intermediate grade
Follicular, predominantly large cell
Diffuse, small cleaved cell
Diffuse, mixed, small and large cell
Diffuse, large cell
High grade
Diffuse, large cell, immunoblastic
Lymphoblastic
Small, noncleaved cell

produced new subtypes and have refined the definition of other subtypes.

Much effort has been expended by cytogeneticists, hematologists, and pathologists attempting to correlate the findings of cytogenetic studies with the hematologic classification systems. Since 1978, six International Workshops on Chromosomes in Leukemia and Lymphoma have been convened for this purpose (8–15). These workshops have contributed significantly to the establishment of relationships between specific chromosome abnormalities and the hematologic classification systems. Their results have demonstrated a strong correlation between some specific chromosome abnormalities and certain classification categories. These findings have helped document the biological validity of the classification schemes. The participants in these workshops have also recorded many other chromosome abnormalities that do not correlate well with any classification category. These findings suggest that the existing classification systems are not perfect and could still be improved.

At this time, the evidence indicates that cytogenetic studies are an important supplement to standard hematology in the classification of hematologic disorders. When considered together with the clinical picture and the results of standard hematology and other laboratory tests, cytogenetic studies can help with the classification of hematologic disorders in many ways. As discussed in more detail below, cytogenetic studies can sometimes (*a*) distinguish between benign and malignant disorders, lymphoid and myeloid processes, de novo and therapy-related diseases, and active and indolent disease; (*b*) help accurately classify some problematic cases; and (*c*) identify the presence of multiple and independent clones, the appearance of subclones, the emergence of new disorders, and many other important clinical problems.

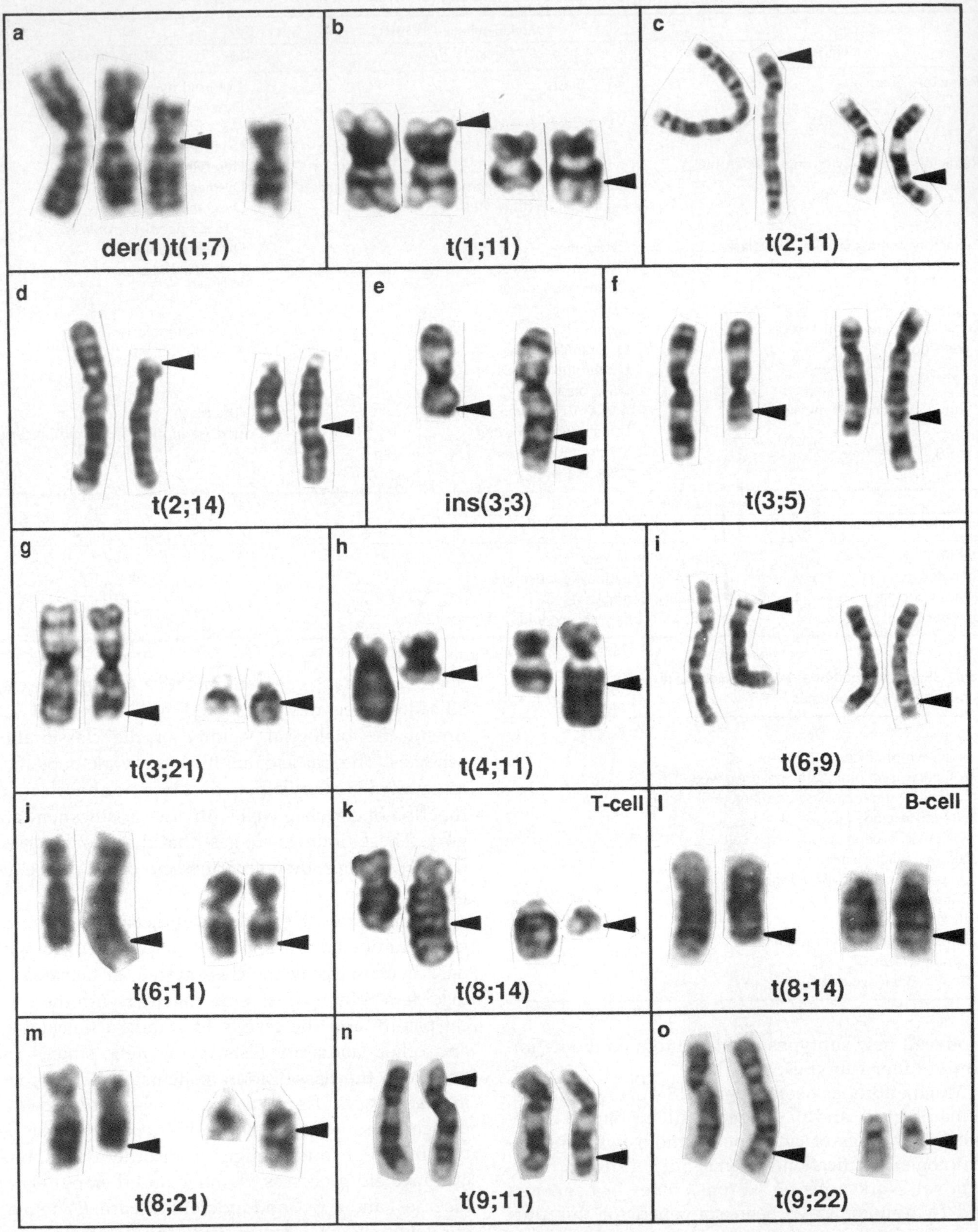

Figure 29.4. Examples of status I and II chromosome translocations in hematologic disorders according to the Committee on Structural Changes in Neoplastic Disorders. See Table 29.1 for more information about the breakpoints, associated hematologic disorders, and correlation status.

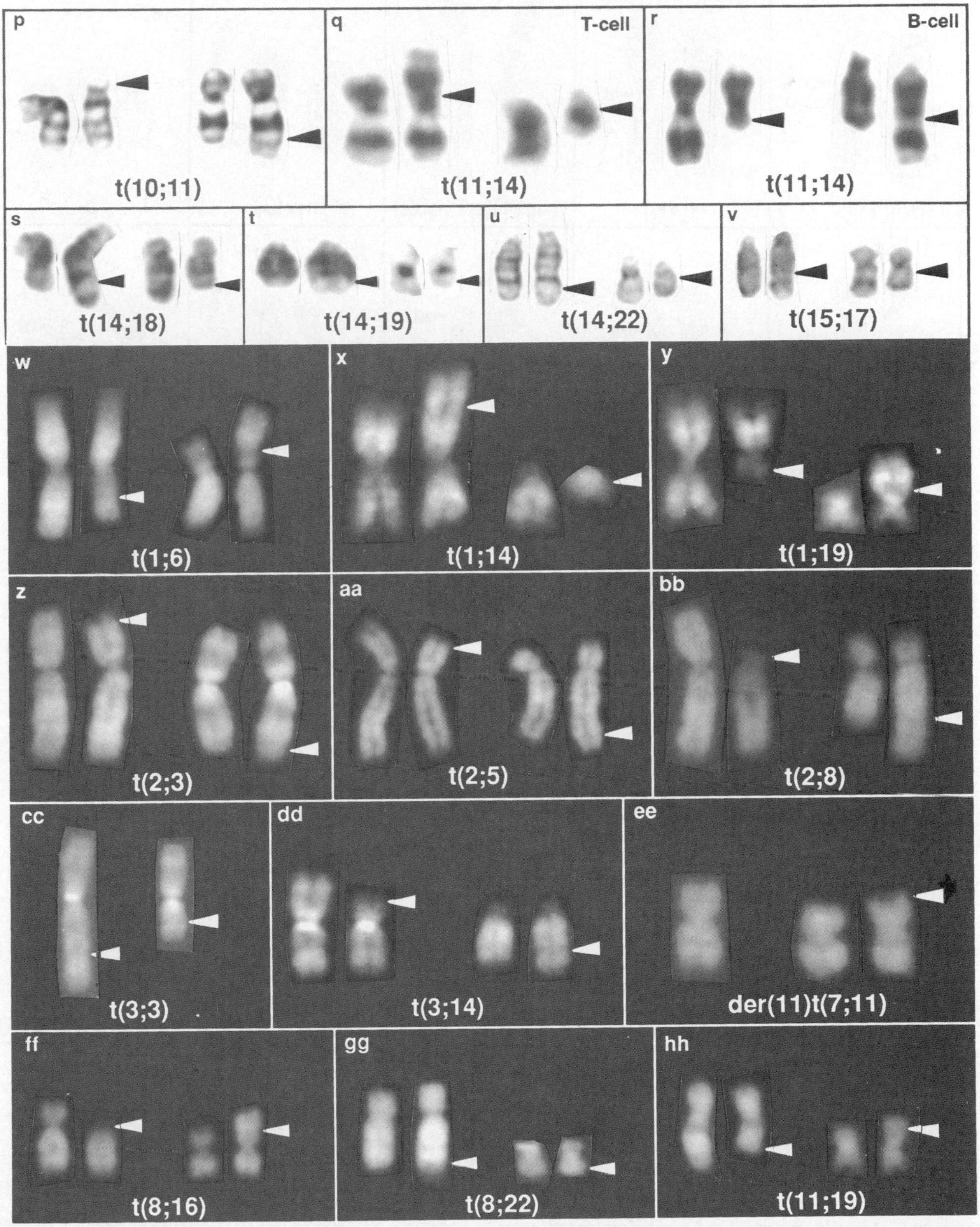

Figure 29.4. p–hh.

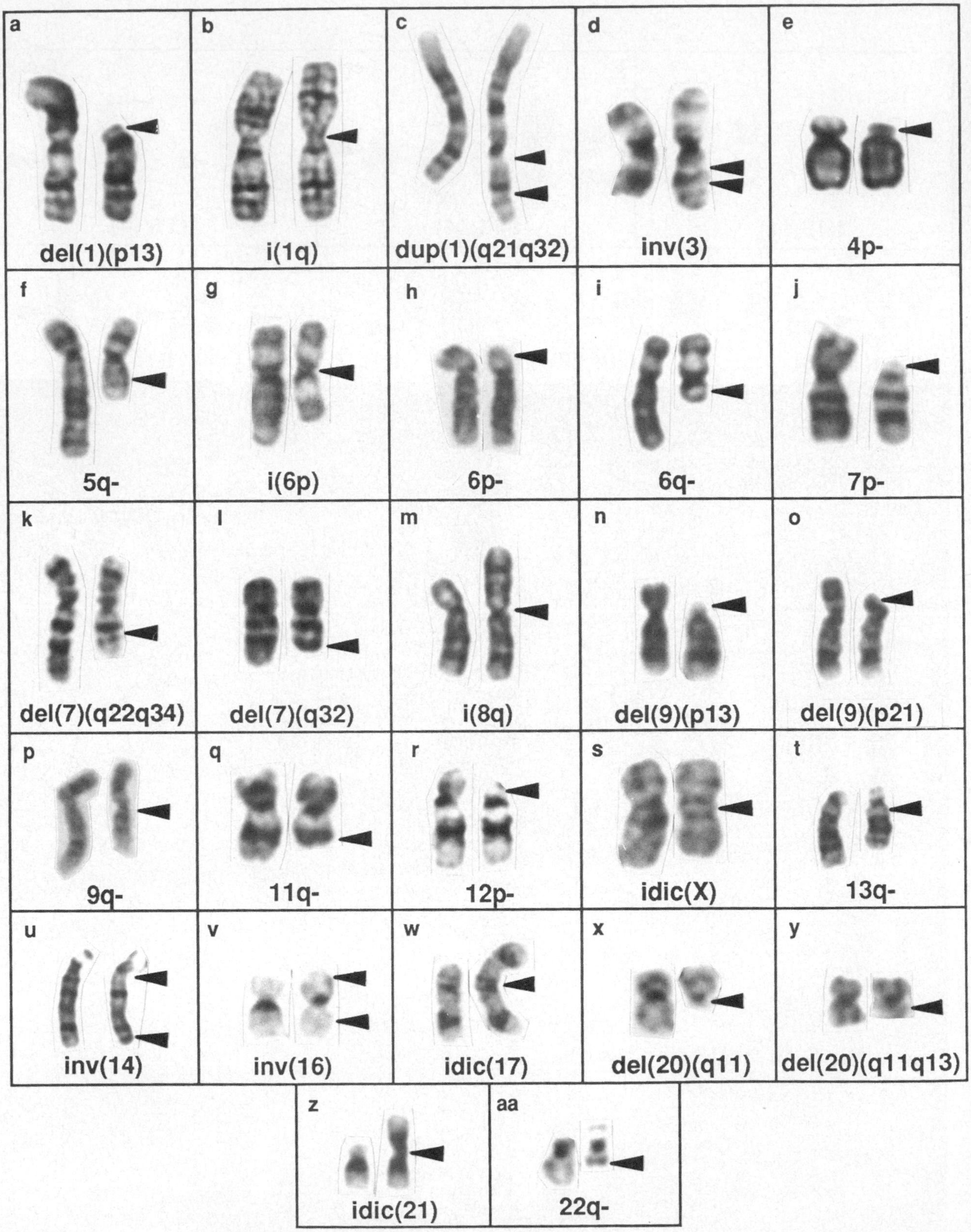

Figure 29.5. Examples of status I and II chromosome isochromosomes, deletions, inversions, and duplications in hematologic disorders according to the Committee on Structural Changes in Neoplastic Disorders. See Table 29.1 for more information about the breakpoints, associated hematologic disorders, and correlation status.

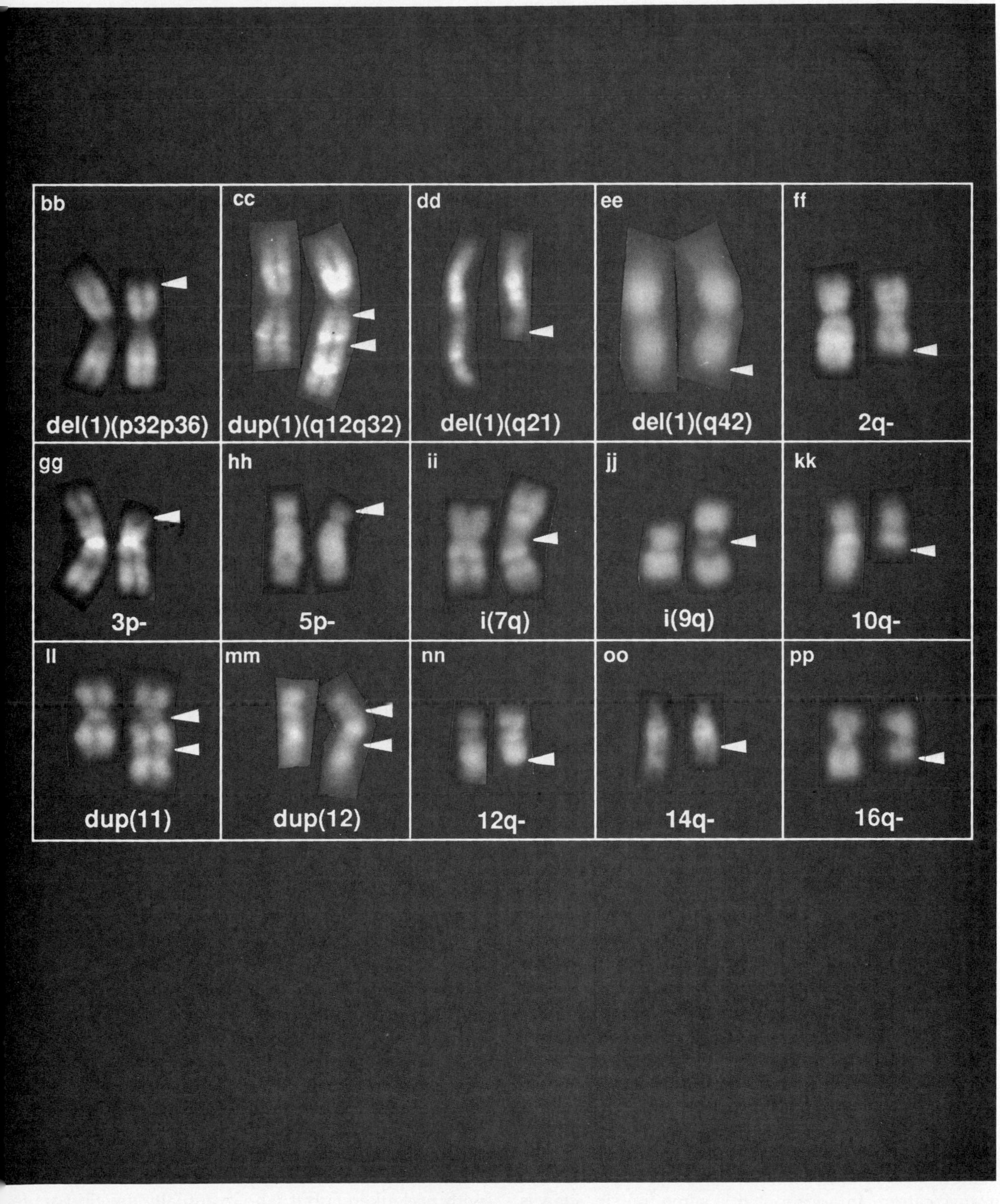

Figure 29.5. bb–pp.

ACUTE LEUKEMIA

The leukemias are a group of disorders involving the neoplastic proliferation of a bone marrow cell line with the accumulation of immature malignant hematopoietic precursors. Diagnosis is made by examination of the peripheral blood and bone marrow. In the past, the classification of leukemias was partly based on the duration of illness. Acute leukemia was characterized by survival of less than 6 months, whereas chronic leukemia involved survival of more than 1 year. Survival of 6 to 12 months was considered subacute or intermediate.

Among adults who develop leukemia each year, approximately 50% have acute leukemia, 20 to 30% have chronic granulocytic leukemia, and 20 to 30% have chronic lymphocytic leukemia. By definition, blast forms, either lymphocytic or myelocytic, constitute 30% or more of the bone marrow cells in acute leukemia. If the blasts are lymphocytic, the disorder is called acute lymphocytic leukemia; if the cells are myeloid, the disorder is called acute nonlymphocytic leukemia. The FAB classification system for the acute leukemias is summarized in Table 29.3.

Role of Cytogenetics in Classification

Cytogenetic studies have helped establish the overall biological accuracy of the FAB classification system for the acute leukemias by demonstrating that certain chromosome abnormalities are associated with FAB subtypes. Some of the chromosome abnormalities linked with FAB subtypes are listed in Tables 29.1 and 29.2. Examples for many of these chromosome abnormalities are shown in Figures 29.4 and 29.5. Cytogenetic studies have helped refine certain FAB subtypes. For example, certain 15;17 translocations have been strongly associated with acute nonlymphocytic leukemia (ANLL)-M3 and with no other FAB subtypes. Recently, a variant of ANLL-M3 was discovered with very small cytoplasmic granules and fewer Auer rods than is ordinarily associated with ANLL-M3. Because affected patients have a 15;17 translocation, it is appropriate for this variant to be added to the M3 subtype.

The results of cytogenetic studies correlate better with some FAB subtypes of acute leukemia than with others. This suggests that some FAB subtypes may be more heterogeneous or the criteria less reliable than for other subtypes. ANLL-M2 is an example of a FAB subtype that may be heterogeneous. Approximately 10% of patients with ANLL-M2 have an 8;21 translocation. In addition, this same translocation is occasionally seen in patients with other FAB subtypes, especially ANLL-M4. ANL-M3 and Burkitt's leukemia are two examples of nearly perfect correlation between cytogenetic abnormalities and FAB subtype. Many cytogeneticists believe that nearly all patients with ANLL-M3 have a 15;17 translocation. Burkitt's leukemia and Burkitt's lymphoma are also strongly associated with certain 8;14 translocations.

The occurrence of different chromosome abnormalities among patients with the same FAB subtype suggests that chromosome studies may help further subclassify the acute leukemias. This conclusion is supported by evidence indicating that ANLL patients with certain chromosome abnormalities respond better to therapy and survive longer than do other patients with acute nonlymphocytic leukemia. The 8;21 translocation associated with ANLL-M2 is an example of a chromosome abnormality that is associated with a better prognosis than that for most patients with acute nonlymphocytic leukemia. The 4;11 translocation is an example of a chromosome abnormality associated with a hematologic disorder and a poor prognosis.

Cytogenetics in Acute Leukemia versus Preleukemia

Some hematologists and pathologists regard the acute leukemias and the preleukemias as different disorders. Others believe that preleukemia is, as the name implies, a stage in disease progression before acute leukemia. The diagnosis of acute leukemia requires the presence of more than 30% blasts in the bone marrow. Any neoplastic hematologic disorder involving less than 30% blasts may be preleukemia. The empirical data suggest that, whenever 30% of bone marrow cells are blasts, the condition is usually so serious that the use of chemotherapy and other aggressive forms of treatment is reasonable. This criterion takes into account the likelihood of the patient surviving without treatment as well as the dangers and discomfort associated with aggressive therapy.

The evidence from cytogenetic studies and other modern methods of laboratory testing strongly suggests that neoplastic hematologic disorders originate from a single cell. This abnormal cell then forms an abnormal clone by cell division. At some point in the progression of the disease, enough abnormal cells accumulate to affect the phenotype of the patient. Thus, the patient's disorder is classified according to the hematologic picture at that time. Thus, it seems reasonable to think of preleukemia as a prelude to acute leukemia rather than as a separate disorder.

Hematologists see many patients who present with overt acute leukemia and others who present with preleukemia but who eventually develop acute leukemia. Certain chromosome abnormalities have been strongly associated with overt acute leukemia and others with preleukemia. This suggests that somehow these chromosome abnormalities play an important role in the origin and progression of these disorders. Two examples of chromosome abnormalities associated specifically with acute leukemia are t(8;21)(q22;q22) and t(15;17)(q22;q11). These and other chromosome abnormalities in acute leukemia are discussed in more detail below.

Patients with chromosome abnormalities that are specifically associated with acute leukemia may actually experience a short preleukemic phase, but they usually present with overt acute leukemia. We have studied hundreds of patients with these abnormalities and have seen only one patient for whom the hematologists classified the hematologic disorder as preleukemia. This patient had an 8;21 translocation, and his hematologic disease was classified as refractory anemia with excess blasts in transition. Within 3 weeks after the specimen for chromosome study was collected, the hematologic disorder met the criteria for ANLL-M2, with more than 30% blasts in the bone marrow.

t(8;21)(q22;q22) and ANLL-M2

Approximately 10% of patients with ANLL-M2 and 7% with ANLL-M4 have a t(8;21)(q22;q22). An example of this anomaly is shown in Figure 29.4*m*. Because this abnormality occurs in both adults and children with acute nonlymphocytic leukemia, a cytogenetic similarity for this neoplastic disorder in different age groups is suggested. This chromosome abnormality is often associated with loss of a sex chromosome. Perhaps up to 70% of males with a t(8;21)(q22;q22) also lack a Y chromosome. Some females with this abnormality also lack an X chromosome, but the incidence is not nearly as great as that of loss of the Y chromosome in males.

Patients with a t(8;21)(q22;q22) are thought to have a better prognosis than other patients with acute nonlymphocytic leukemia. The remission rate with this abnormality is higher than with other forms of acute nonlymphocytic leukemia. The median duration of survival with treatment is about 15 months. This is also better than the overall survival for acute nonlymphocytic leukemia. Patients with a t(8;21)(q22;q22) are usually young; the average age is about 25 years.

The participants of the early International Workshops on Chromosomes in Leukemia had the impression that the prognosis may be better for patients with a t(8;21)(q22;q22) who were lacking a sex chromosome. More recent studies involving many more cases suggest that survival is not affected by the loss of a sex chromosome.

t(15;17)(q22;q11) and ANLL-M3

A t(15;17)(q22;q11) is thought to occur in nearly all patients with ANLL-M3. An example of this anomaly is shown in Figure 29.4*v*. This chromosome abnormality has not been reported in patients with other hematologic disorders. It is relatively easy to miss in routine practice. Many patients with this abnormality have mixtures of normal and abnormal metaphases. The proportion of normal cells is often far greater than that of abnormal cells. In addition, the morphology and banding pattern of the t(15;17)(q22;q11) can be deceptive because they resemble some normal chromosomes. To complicate things, variants of this translocation are also known.

Some investigators believe that t(15;17)(q22;q11) may be more readily detected in bone marrow when culture techniques rather than direct techniques are used. Several laboratories have reported observing this abnormality in cells of short-term, unstimulated cultures and not in cells of direct preparations. The study of patients with t(15;17)(q22;q11) demonstrates the importance of using the appropriate laboratory procedures for specific disorders.

inv(16)(p13q22) and Abnormal Eosinophils

Patients with an inv(16)(p13q22) often have ANLL-M4 with abnormal eosinophils and, frequently, eosinophilia. An example of this chromosome anomaly is shown in Figure 29.5*v*. The eosinophils appear abnormal by morphology, by cytochemical reactions, and by ultrastructure. A new FAB subtype for this hematologic disorder has been established and named ANLL-M4Eo to denote the importance of eosinophils in this classification.

Nearly 50% of patients with an inv(16)(p13q22) or a variant of this abnormality have ANLL-M4Eo. One variant of this inversion involves a reciprocal translocation between the two chromosome 16 homologs in a cell to form an abnormality described as t(16;16)(p13;q22). This variant resembles inv(16)(p13q22) because bands 16p13 and 16q22 are involved in both cases. A few patients with apparent deletions of the long arm of one chromosome 16 have also been described. The breakpoints on the deletions appear to involve only 16q22. Some investigators believe that the hematologic disorder associated with the del(16)(q22) abnormality may be somewhat different from ANLL-M4Eo. An example of this chromosome abnormality is shown in Figure 29.5*pp*.

Abnormalities of 11q and ANLL-M5

Perhaps as many as 35% of patients with ANLL-M5 may have an abnormality of the long arm of chromosome 11. This cytogenetic-hematologic correlation approaches 50% for patients with poorly differentiated types of ANLL-M5, known as ANLL-M5a. Abnormalities of the long arm of chromosome 11 are also common in childhood ANLL-M5. Abnormalities of 11q have been observed in patients with ANLL-M4 and occasionally in other FAB subtypes. Similar abnormalities have even been observed in patients with acute lymphocytic leukemia. The occurrence of abnormalities of chromosome 11 in both lymphoid and myeloid disorders has not been explained, but some investigators have suggested that these chromosome abnormalities may occur in multipotential stem cells.

The abnormalities of chromosome 11 involve a wide variety of interstitial deletions and translocations. The most specific abnormality is a t(9;11)(p22;q23). An example of this anomaly is shown in Figure 29.4*n*.

inv(3)(q21q26), Variants, and Abnormal Thrombocytosis

Certain abnormalities of chromosome 3 have been associated with thrombocytosis. These abnormalities usually involve bands 3q21 and 3q26. The most common abnormalities are inv(3)(q21q26), t(3;3)(q21;q26), and certain insertion translocations such as ins(5;3)(q14;q21q26). An example of a t(3;3)(q21;q26) is shown in Figure 29.4*cc*, and an inv(3)(q21q26) is shown in Figure 29.5*d*. Patients with any of these chromosome abnormalities may have elevated platelet counts and an increased number of megakaryocytes. The megakaryocytes are often smaller than usual. The prognosis of patients with this chromosome abnormality may be poor.

t(6;9)(p23;q34) and Basophilia

The t(6;9)(p23;q34) abnormality is relatively rare. An example of this anomaly is shown in Figure 29.4*i*. Perhaps only about 2% of patients with acute nonlymphocytic leukemia have a t(6;9)(p23;q34). This abnormality is often associated with an increased number of basophils in the bone marrow, but it does not correlate well with any specific FAB subtype. It has been observed in ANLL-M1, ANLL-M2, and ANLL-M4.

In the t(6;9)(p23;q34) abnormality, the breakpoint on chromosome 9 is at 9q34. This is the same band that is involved in the Ph chromosome. Because basophilia is common in chronic granulocytic leukemia, it has been suggested that the breakpoint on chromosome 9 in both the t(6;9)(p23;q34) and t(9;22)(q34;q11) may affect a gene for basophil proliferation. However, the breakpoints in the t(6;9)(p23;q34) have not yet been characterized at the molecular level.

t(8;14)(q24;q32) and Burkitt's Leukemia

The observation of a t(8;14)(q24;q32) is strongly associated with Burkitt's leukemia and Burkitt's lymphoma. An example of this anomaly is shown in Figure 29.4*l*. This abnormality occurs in both African and non-African Burkitt's disease. The occurrence of a t(8;14)(q24;q32) in both leukemia and lymphoma of the Burkitt type suggests that these disorders may be biologically similar. The formal FAB classification for Burkitt's leukemia is acute lymphocytic leukemia (ALL)-L3.

In a t(8;14)(q24;q32), the breakpoint on chromosome 14 is at 14q32, which is the site of the gene for the heavy-chain locus of immunoglobulin. This is most likely no coincidence because ALL-L3 and Burkitt's lymphoma are B-cell disorders. The relationship between this 8;14 translocation, the heavy-chain immunoglobulin locus, and the *myc* oncogene is discussed in more detail later in this chapter.

Two variants of the 8;14 translocation are also associated with ALL-L3 and Burkitt's lymphoma. These chromosome abnormalities are t(2;8)(p12;q24) and t(8;22)(q24;q11). Examples of these are shown in Figures 29.4*bb* and 29.4*gg*, respectively. Chromosome 2p12 is the site of the κ light chain of immunoglobulin, and chromosome 22q11 is the site of the λ light chain of immunoglobulin.

t(4;11)(q21;q23) and Lymphocytic and Undifferentiated Leukemia

A t(4;11)(q21;q23) occurs in about 8% of patients with acute lymphocytic leukemia and in many patients with acute undifferentiated leukemia. An example of this anomaly is shown in Figure 29.4*h*. Many patients with t(4;11)(q21;q23) have a mixed leukemia involving both myeloid and lymphoid cells. The cells often have features of monocytes and clonal rearrangements of both immunoglobulin heavy- and light-chain genes. The t(4;11)(q21;q23) abnormality has been associated with a particularly poor prognosis. The median duration of survival appears to be about 7 months.

t(1;19)(q23;p13) and Pre-B Cell Acute Lymphocytic Leukemia

A t(1;19)(q23;p13) translocation occurs in about 30% of patients with pre-B cell acute lymphocytic leukemia. An example of this chromosome anomaly is shown in Figure 29.4*y*. The prognosis for patients with this 1;19 translocation is thought to be poor. Pre-B cell acute lymphocytic leukemia can be distinguished from other acute leukemias by virtue of rearrangements in the immunoglobulin heavy-chain genes and expression of immunoglobulin μ chain in the cytoplasm. Children with pre-B cell acute lymphocytic leukemia and a t(1;19)(q23;p13) also frequently have low leukocyte counts and a poor prognosis.

Hyperdiploidy and Acute Lymphocytic Leukemia

Many patients with acute lymphocytic leukemia have neoplastic clones with 50 to 60 chromosomes but few, if any, apparent structural abnormalities. This karyotype has been associated with the type of childhood acute lymphocytic leukemia that often responds well to standard therapy for this disease. Approximately 86% of these patients achieve a remission, and the median duration of survival is about 34 months. These patients usually have acute lymphocytic leukemia that can be non-T, non-B ALL-L1 or ALL-L2.

Near Haploidy and Acute Lymphocytic Leukemia

Near haploidy is a rare karyotype in somatic cells, but it has been associated with acute lymphocytic leukemia. In this disorder, the number of chromosomes is not exactly haploid but is usually in the range of 26 to 36 chromosomes. The prognosis associated with this karyotype is poor, and the duration of survival is about 9 months. In routine practice, cytogenetic technologists often exclude metaphases with so few chromosomes from study because they believe these metaphases are broken and have lost chromosomes for technical reasons. Care should be taken to avoid missing near haploidy in chromosome analysis by examining at least some metaphases with few chromosomes. Nearly haploid cells can be recognized because they usually have at least one member of each chromosome homolog and more than one metaphase with a nearly haploid karyotype. Broken metaphases usually show random loss of different chromosomes among the cells.

THERAPY-RELATED LEUKEMIA

Certain chromosome abnormalities are associated with therapy-related hematologic disorders. The therapy-related disorders are said to be secondary disorders because they probably result from treatment for solid tumors, lymphoma, monoclonal gammopathies, acute leukemia, and other neoplastic disorders. The therapy-related disorders are commonly associated with the more aggressive forms of treatment, such as chemotherapy and radiotherapy. Similar chromosome abnormalities occur among patients with hematologic disorders due to exposure to chemicals, pesticides, and other environmental carcinogens. Apparently, therapy-related leukemia and some environmental carcinogen-related leukemias are similar. The secondary leukemias may resemble acute leukemia or myelodysplastic syndromes, but the FAB classification scheme does not provide any specific subtype for them.

Hypodiploidy and Abnormalities of Chromosomes 5 and 7

In therapy-related leukemia, the number of chromosomes is often less than 46 (hypodiploid), and the karyotype frequently involves either structural abnormalities or loss of chromosome 5 or 7 (or both). Examples of typical structural abnormalities of chromosomes 5 and 7 are shown in Figures 29.5*f* and *k*. Unlike many hematologic disorders, it is relatively easy to detect chromosomally abnormal clones in patients with therapy-related leukemia. Chromosomally abnormal clones can be observed in nearly 90% of these patients even with routine cytogenetic techniques. This high rate could be due to both the high proportion of neoplastic cells in the bone marrow of affected patients and the fact that the chromosome abnormalities are so gross that they can be readily detected by routine chromosome studies.

Unbalanced 1;7 Translocations and Therapy-Related Myelodysplasia

Approximately 70% of patients with an unbalanced 1;7 translocation have a therapy-related hematologic disorder. The remaining patients appear to have de novo disorders without a history of treatment or exposure to environmental carcinogens. This abnormality is formally written +der(1)t(1;7)(p11;p11). An example of this anomaly is shown in Figure 29.4*a*. The unbalanced 1;7 translocation is the third most common translocation in our practice.

In our series of 12 patients with this abnormality, nine had either a myeloproliferative disorder or a myelodysplastic syndrome, one had acute leukemia, and two had been treated for multiple myeloma but had no morphologic evidence of evolving myeloproliferative disease. These patients usually do not develop acute leukemia; rather, they persist with a chronic myeloproliferative disorder or myelodysplastic syndrome, although some patients do progress to acute leukemia.

Seven patients in our series had a history of exposure to chemotherapy or radiotherapy for another malignant disorder. In one other patient, we were unable to establish whether prior therapy had been given. Only four patients had no evidence of prior therapy. The frequency of de novo myelodysplastic syndromes is considerably greater than the incidence

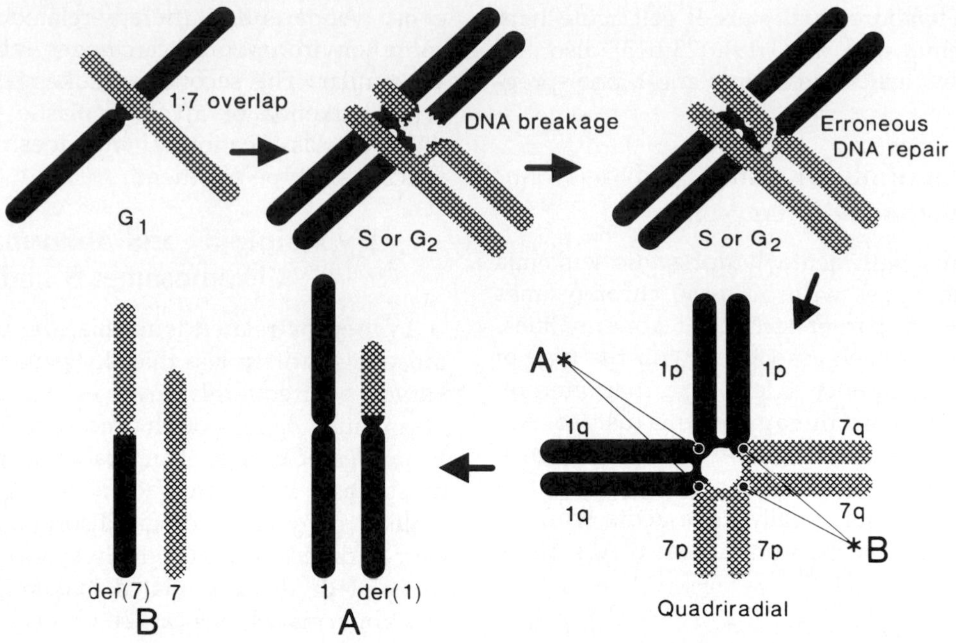

Figure 29.6. Hypothetical origin of an unbalanced 1;7 translocation. DNA breakage occurs in chromatid of both chromosomes 1 and 7 in S or G_2. Reciprocal translocation of chromatids occurs from erroneous DNA repair. This leads to quadriradial formation at metaphase. Adjacent II segregation would produce the types of chromosomes shown in daughter cells A and B. (From Morrison-DeLap SJ, Kuffel DG, Dewald GW, Letendre L. Unbalanced 1;7 translocation and therapy-induced hematologic disorders: a possible relationship. Am J Hematol 1986;21:39–47. Copyright © 1986 by Wiley-Liss. Reprinted by permission.)

of therapy-related myelodysplastic syndromes. Thus, the occurrence of an unbalanced 1;7 translocation in so many patients with a history of therapy suggests an association between this chromosome abnormality and therapy.

As illustrated in Figure 29.6, this unbalanced 1;7 translocation probably develops during DNA replication or in the G_2 stage of the cell cycle. The carcinogen causes a translocation between a chromatid of a chromosome 1 and a chromatid of a chromosome 7. This translocation leads to the formation of a quadriradial configuration involving these two chromosomes at metaphase. When the chromatids separate in anaphase, one of the daughter cells receives two copies of a normal chromosome 1, a copy of the 1;7 translocation chromosome, and one normal chromosome 7. Thus, the karyotype is unbalanced because there are three copies of the long arm of chromosome 1 and only one copy of the long arm of chromosome 7.

The *erb* B gene has been mapped to a site on the short arm of chromosome 7 at band 7p11, and this is the same band associated with this 1;7 translocation. Thus, this translocation may exert its neoplastic influence by activating the *erb* B oncogene.

MYELODYSPLASTIC SYNDROMES

Myelodysplastic disorders involve pluripotential stem cells. They may present as neoplastic disorders that are either primary or secondary to chemotherapy, radiation, or environmental mutagens. The FAB classification system for myelodysplastic disorders is summarized in Table 29.4. Some hematologists would include the 5q− syndrome with the myelodysplastic disorders, but this has not yet been officially recognized by the FAB group.

Cytogenetic studies may be particularly useful in the workup of patients with myelodysplastic disorders. Some patients have myelodysplastic bone marrow due to exposure to chemicals, vitamin deficiencies, and other nonneoplastic problems. Cytogenetic studies can sometimes help distinguish neoplastic from nonneoplastic disorders. The observation of a chromosomally abnormal clone is evidence that the disorder is neoplastic.

Some myelodysplastic syndromes are difficult to distinguish from other hematologic disorders. For example, numerous publications have described patients with so-called Ph-negative chronic granulocytic leukemia. Several groups have now demonstrated that most of these patients do not have chronic granulocytic leukemia; rather, they have chronic myelomonocytic leukemia. These two disorders can be readily distinguished from each other by either cytogenetic or cytochemistry techniques. Chronic granulocytic leukemia is associated with a Ph chromosome, and chronic myelomonocytic leukemia is not. Often, patients with chronic myelomonocytic leukemia have abnormalities of the long arm of chromosome 11.

In routine practice, approximately 40% of patients with myelodysplastic syndromes have a demonstrable clone with chromosome abnormalities. In their bone marrow, patients with these disorders often have many normal metaphases mixed with neoplastic metaphases. Thus, it is easy to miss the detection of an abnormal clone because of sampling error. Most likely, nearly all patients with myelodysplastic syndromes have a chromosomally abnormal clone. When many more cells than usual are examined or multiple chromosome studies are done on patients in whom no abnormality was apparent by routine chromosome studies, it is usually possible to identify a chromosomally abnormal clone.

The incidence of chromosomally abnormal clones among patients with myelodysplastic syndromes is about 40%. This figure is fairly similar among the different FAB subtypes for myelodysplastic syndromes. In a series of 166 patients with myelodysplastic syndromes, we found chromosomally abnormal clones in 31% of patients with refractory anemia, 29% with refractory anemia with ringed sideroblasts, 46% with refractory anemia with excess blasts, 50% with refractory anemia with excess blasts in transition, 45% with chronic myelomonocytic leukemia, and 100% with the 5q− syndrome.

Except for certain abnormalities of the X chromosome and 5q− abnormalities, no specific chromosome abnormality correlates with any FAB subtype of the myelodysplastic syndromes. This lack of association may suggest that the myelodysplastic disorders either are heterogeneous or readily evolve from one FAB subtype to another. Many patients with myelodysplastic syndromes progress to acute leukemia before they succumb to their disease. Thus, in some patients with acute leukemia, it is not unusual to see chromosome abnormalities that are similar to those seen in myelodysplastic syndromes.

5q− Chromosomes and the 5q− Syndrome

The 5q− chromosome is associated with the 5q− syndrome. The 5q− syndrome, among other things, involves macrocytic and oval macrocytes with marked anisopoikilocytosis, erythroid hypoplasia, and dyserythropoiesis. The definition of the 5q− syndrome requires the presence of a 5q− chromosome. Thus, the apparent perfect association between 5q− abnormalities and the 5q− syndrome is artificial.

The expression "5q−" actually refers to an interstitial deletion of part of the long arm of chromosome 5 and is formally written del(5)(q13q31). Thus, in the 5q− chromosome, the entire long arm is not missing, as might be inferred from the expression 5q−. (Deletion of the entire long arm of chromosome 5 would be expressed as −5q.) We distinguish at least four different types of 5q− chromosomes. In our series of 50 patients with a 5q− chromosome, 39 had a del(5)(q13q33), nine had del(5)(q31q35), one had del(5)(q22q33), and one had del(5)(q13q35). An example of a 5q− chromosome is shown in Figure 29.5*f*. The portion of chromosome 5 that is lacking may not be as important as the genes at the site of the breakpoints. The 5q− chromosome may alter the expression of certain genes at the breakpoints. Although the underlying molecular basis of the 5q− syndrome has not been resolved, this problem is under extensive investigation by several laboratories.

The 5q− chromosome is the most common deletion we encounter in routine practice. About 50% of the patients have other chromosome abnormalities associated with a 5q− chromosome. Patients with chromosome abnormalities in addition to a 5q− chromosome have a significantly worse prognosis and are much more likely to have a history of chemotherapy or exposure to radiation.

Many patients with a 5q− chromosome do not have the 5q− syndrome. In a series of 50 patients that we studied, six had the 5q− syndrome, 12 had refractory anemia, 16 had refractory anemia with excess blasts, 13 had acute nonlymphocytic leukemia, and three had an unclassifiable myeloproliferative disorder (16). This suggests that the natural history of the 5q− chromosome anomaly may evolve from an indolent disorder resembling the 5q− syndrome to a myelodysplastic disorder to acute leukemia.

idic(X)(q13) and Pathological Ringed Sideroblasts

Structural abnormalities of X chromosomes involving breakpoints at Xq13 are strongly associated with pathological ringed sideroblasts. We studied a series of 26 patients with X chromosome abnormalities and hematologic disorders (17). Among 13 patients with abnormalities of the X chromosome involving Xql3, we found pathological ringed sideroblasts in 12. Among 13 patients with abnormalities involving chromosome bands other than Xq13, none had pathological ringed sideroblasts.

The most common abnormality of the X chromosome involving Xq13 has been isodicentric X chromosomes. An example of this anomaly is shown in Figure 29.5*s*. Translocations involving Xql3 may produce a similar hematologic disorder. So far, the patients with Xq13 abnormalities have all been females. Most of these patients have been older than 60 years, but we have seen at least two patients in their 30s. The evidence now suggests that (*a*) Xq13 is the most common breakpoint involved in structural abnormalities of the X chromosome in hematologic disorders; (*b*) Xq13 may be associated with refractory anemia; (*c*) Xq13 may contain a gene for the formation of pathological ringed sideroblasts; and (*d*) Xq13 may contain a gene associated with myelodysplasia or leukemia.

20q− Abnormality and Myelodysplasia

The 20q− chromosome has been associated with polycythemia vera, but it also occurs in many patients with myelodysplastic syndromes. These diseases may evolve to acute nonlymphocytic leukemia in many cases. In our series of 20 patients with a 20q− chromosome, three had polycythemia vera, one had pancytopenia, one had chronic myelomonocytic leukemia, one had agnogenic myeloid metaplasia, eight had an unclassifiable preleukemia, and six had acute leukemia (18). In our experience, this anomaly is found in about 6% of patients with polycythemia vera, 3% with acute nonlymphocytic leukemia, and 1% with myelodysplastic syndromes.

The 20q− chromosome is the second most common deletion among patients with hematologic disorders. The expression 20q− might imply that the entire long arm is lacking. However, the 20q− abnormality is actually an interstitial deletion with breakpoints usually in band 20q11.2 and 20q13.3. (Deletion of the entire long arm of chromosome 20 would be expressed as −20q.) Occasional patients may have a breakpoint at 20q13 rather than 20q11.2. Examples of 2q− chromosomes are shown in Figures 29.5*x* and *y*.

Trisomy 8

Trisomy 8 frequently occurs among patients with different myelodysplastic syndromes. Trisomy 8 is the second most frequently seen chromosome abnormality in our practice and the most common trisomy in hematologic disorders. Trisomy 8 may occur alone or with other chromosome abnormalities as a consequence of chromosome evolution. When Trisomy 8 occurs secondary to another condition, it is usually associated with the more aggressive stages of hematologic disorders, such as acute leukemia or blast crisis of chronic granulocytic leukemia. This association suggests that trisomy 8 has neoplastic potential as either a primary or a secondary chromosome abnormality.

In our series of 69 patients with myelodysplastic syndromes, seven (10%) had trisomy 8. Among these patients, two had refractory anemia, three had refractory anemia with ringed sideroblasts, one had refractory anemia with excess blasts, and one had chronic myelomonocytic leukemia. The occurrence of trisomy 8 in various myelodysplastic syndromes, myeloproliferative disorders, and acute leukemia suggests that the natural history of trisomy 8 may involve hematologic disorders with a preleukemic phase of considerable duration with frequent evolution to acute leukemia (19).

Monosomy 7

Monosomy 7 is a common chromosome finding in myelodysplastic syndromes. It is the fifth most common chromosome abnormality and the second most frequent monosomy in hematologic disorders. In our series of 25 patients with monosomy 7, two had an unclassifiable myelodysplastic syndrome, two had refractory anemia, one had refractory anemia with ringed sideroblasts, four had refractory anemia with excess blasts, one had refractory anemia with excess blasts in transition, four had a therapy-related myelodysplastic syndrome, and 11 had acute leukemia. Some evidence suggests that isolated monosomy 7 has a significantly better survival rate than monosomy 7 in combination with other chromosome abnormalities.

MYELOPROLIFERATIVE DISORDERS

The myeloproliferative disorders are a group of diseases that result from an autonomous proliferation of one or more cellular elements. These disorders are characterized by panhypercellular marrows and expression of abnormal hematopoiesis in peripheral blood. Myeloproliferative disorders are classified by the predominant cell type (Table 29.4). Myeloproliferative disorders are considered chronic diseases and include polycythemia vera, agnogenic myeloid metaplasia, idiopathic thrombocythemia, and undifferentiated myeloproliferative disorders.

t(9;22)(q34;q11), Ph Chromosome, and Chronic Granulocytic Leukemia

Chronic granulocytic leukemia is also known as chronic myelogenous leukemia. This disorder has been studied extensively with cytogenetic techniques and often serves as a model for chromosome abnormalities in hematologic disorders. The initial or chronic phase of this disorder usually lasts about 30 to 36 months. After this time, the condition may accelerate into a blastic phase that may last 3 to 6 months.

Chronic granulocytic leukemia is associated with the Philadelphia (Ph) chromosome, which is usually the result of a translocation between chromosomes 9 and 22 with breakpoints at 9q34 and 22q11. This anomaly is written formally as t(9;22)(q34;q11). An example of this anomaly is shown in Figure 29.4*o*.

Most likely, all patients with chronic granulocytic leukemia have this 9;22 translocation or a variant of it. In our experience, a 9;22 translocation occurs in about 90% of patients with true chronic granulocytic leukemia. The remaining patients with this disorder have a variant of the 9;22 translocation.

The variant translocations of t(9;22)(q34;q11) are classified into two categories: simple and complex. The complex variant Ph chromosomes clearly involve three or more chromosome abnormalities. Two of the chromosomes are always 9 and 22, and the breakpoints invariably involve 9q34 and 22q11. The other abnormalities present in complex translocations may involve any chromosome and any breakpoint. An example of a complex variant Ph chromosome is t(4;9;22)(q31;q34;q11).

Simple variant translocations of the Ph chromosome appear to involve chromosome 22 and another chromosome other than chromosome 9. However, this anomaly is deceptive because the portion of chromosome 9 involved in the usual t(9;22)(q34;q11) is so small that it can be overlooked in simple variant translocations. With the use of high-resolution chromosome techniques and molecular genetic methods, it has been demonstrated that simple variant Ph chromosomes actually do involve chromosome 9 with breakpoints at 9q34. Thus, both simple and complex variant Ph chromosomes are the molecular equivalent of the typical t(9;22)(q34;q11). The sites at 9q34 and 22q11 on the chromosome contain the *abl* oncogene and *bcr* region, respectively. The mRNA and protein hybrid produced is composed of both *abl* and *bcr* information and may be responsible for the proliferative potential of the t(9;22)(q34;q11).

In the chronic phase, usually only a Ph chromosome is observed. In blast crisis, it is not uncommon to observe other chromosome abnormalities in addition to a Ph chromosome. It has been suggested that these "additional" chromosome abnormalities are the result of chromosome evolution and are associated with disease progression. Thus, the observation of chromosome abnormalities besides the Ph chromosome can be a clue that the disease is in the accelerated phase and suggests the onset or occurrence of blast crisis.

In most patients with chronic granulocytic leukemia, all the metaphases examined will be chromosomally abnormal. Only about 10% of patients will show a mixture of normal and Ph-positive cells. Many patients with a mixture of normal metaphases and Ph-positive metaphases develop a lymphoid form of blast crisis. This criterion by itself is not sufficiently consistent to reliably predict a lymphoid blast crisis. In our experience, about 50% of patients with a mixture of normal and abnormal metaphases develop a lymphoid blast crisis. By comparison, nearly 90% of patients with myeloid blast crisis appear to have a pure population of Ph-positive cells.

Some evidence now suggests that the observation of certain chromosome abnormalities may be useful to predict whether the blast crisis is myeloid or lymphoid. Trisomy 8 and i(17q) (Fig. 29.5*w*) are usually associated with myeloid blast crisis. A second Ph chromosome is also frequently associated with myeloid blast crisis, but we have seen at least two patients with two Ph chromosomes who have developed a lymphoid blast crisis. Chromosome abnormalities other than trisomy 8, i(17q), and multiple Ph chromosomes are frequently associated with lymphoid blast crisis, especially if structural abnormalities of chromosomes 7 and 14 are involved. Chromosome 7 is known to contain two genes for T-cell receptor sites, and chromosome 14 contains genes for heavy-chain immunoglobulin and a T-cell receptor site. This evidence is preliminary, and these associations should not be used as diagnostic criteria alone until more data are accumulated.

One question that arises in cytogenetic practice relates to the observation of the Ph chromosome in some patients with acute lymphocytic leukemia and a few with acute nonlymphocytic leukemia. The fact that some patients with chronic granulocytic leukemia develop a lymphoid blast crisis and others develop a myeloid blast crisis suggests that these disorders may not be so different. The child who develops acute lymphocytic leukemia with a Ph chromosome may simply be experiencing a disease that is similar to chronic granulocytic leukemia in lymphoid blast crisis. Some molecular evidence suggests that the breakpoint on chromosome 22 may be slightly different in these two disorders. Most likely, the patients in lymphoid blast crisis will be shown to have the same molecular breakpoints as patients with acute lymphocytic leukemia.

Patients with chronic granulocytic leukemia who undergo standard treatments for this disease may achieve a remission, but the mitotic cells of the bone marrow continue to be predominantly Ph chromosome-positive. If very aggressive treatment is used or if bone marrow transplantations are performed, Ph-positive cells are not usually evident in routine chromosome studies. If the disease relapses, the cells of the bone marrow are again predominantly Ph-positive. In this respect, chronic granulocytic leukemia is different from other hematologic disorders. In most other hematologic disorders, cells with chromosome abnormalities are not usually evident in remission.

Polycythemia Vera, +8, +9, and 20q−

Polycythemia vera is a chronic myeloproliferative disorder that, in the early stages, can be confused with chronic granulocytic leukemia. Cytogenetic studies can be useful to distinguish between the two diseases because chronic granulocytic leukemia is associated with the Ph chromosome and polycythemia vera is not.

Approximately 30% of patients with polycythemia vera have a chromosome abnormality; however, the incidence varies according to the stage of disease. The incidence of chromosome abnormalities is about 15% among patients at the time of diagnosis, 19% in the chronic phase, 40% when extensive myelofibrosis occurs, 78% in the spent phase, and nearly 100% when acute leukemia develops. Many patients with polycythemia vera are treated with alkylating agents and other forms of treatment that may cause therapy-related leukemia. Thus, polycythemia vera appears to be a myeloproliferative disorder with an unpredictable course. Some patients may remain in the chronic phase all their lives; others may develop a fibrotic phase or spent phase, and others may develop de novo myelodysplastic disorders or acute leukemia.

The results of cytogenetic studies in polycythemia vera are consistent with the clinical variation in this hematologic disorder (20). Polycythemia vera may originate as a submicroscopic gene or physiologic abnormality. Patients who develop chromosomally abnormal clones may do so as a consequence of excessive DNA replication due to the mitotic activity of the disease or to DNA repair related to treatment.

Trisomy 8, trisomy 9, and a 20q− anomaly are common in polycythemia vera, but they do not seem to affect the duration or survival of patients with this disease. These abnormalities occur in some patients at the time of diagnosis and in others who have been treated with only phlebotomy. These abnormalities probably suggest the onset of a de novo myelodysplastic disease or another undifferentiated myeloproliferative disorder whose natural history is not too different from that of polycythemia vera. Some patients with myelofibrosis and polycythemia vera have 13q− abnormalities. Interestingly, 13q− abnormalities have been associated with agnogenic myeloid metaplasia, as discussed below. Abnormalities such as 5q− and unbalanced 1;7 translocations occur in some patients with polycythemia vera, but these patients usually have a history of aggressive treatment and probably have therapy-related leukemia. Cytogenetic studies may not be helpful in the diagnosis of polycythemia vera, but they may provide important clues to the appearance of leukemia or alteration in the course of the disease.

13q− Abnormalities and Myelofibrosis

Evidence has emerged to suggest that structural abnormalities of chromosome 13 may be associated with myelofibrosis. Patients with this chromosome abnormality often have hematologic disorders that are classified as agnogenic myeloid metaplasia or myelofibrosis. In our series of 13 patients with a 13q− chromosome abnormality, five had agnogenic myeloid metaplasia (21). Although the association between myeloid metaplasia and 13q− abnormalities may not be perfect, it is strong and may be a clue to the presence of a gene or genes on chromosome 13 that are linked with myelofibrosis.

The 13q− chromosome does not lack the whole long arm, as the name may imply. This abnormality is actually an interstitial deletion with breakpoints commonly at 13q12 and 13q22. An example of this anomaly is shown in Figure 29.5*t*. The 13q− chromosomes have also been observed in chronic granulocytic leukemia and polycythemia vera as secondary chromosome abnormalities. Patients with secondary 13q− chromosome abnormalities often have myelofibrosis. This suggests that the 13q− chromosome may have neoplastic potential as either a primary or a secondary chromosome abnormality.

LYMPHOMAS AND LYMPHOPROLIFERATIVE DISORDERS

Lymphoproliferative disorders occur in the bone marrow, peripheral blood, lymph nodes, spleen, or other organ systems. When neoplastic cells are found primarily in the blood or bone marrow, the term *lymphocytic leukemia* is used. If the neoplastic cells occur predominantly in the lymphoreticular system, the term *lymphoma* is used. Many of the chromosome abnormalities associated with lymphomas also occur in the lymphocytic leukemias. This strongly suggests a similarity in the pathogenesis of lymphomas and lymphocytic leukemias. For this reason, we have chosen to deal with these two hematologic disorders in the same section.

T-Cell versus B-Cell Lymphoproliferative Disorders

A strong correlation exists between certain chromosome abnormalities and the immunotype in lymphoproliferative disorders. Chromosome abnormalities with breakpoints at any of the T-cell receptor sites on chromosomes 7 and 14 are usually associated with T-cell disorders (Fig. 29.7). An example of a chromosome abnormality involving a T-cell receptor site is shown in Figure 29-4*q*. Abnormalities with

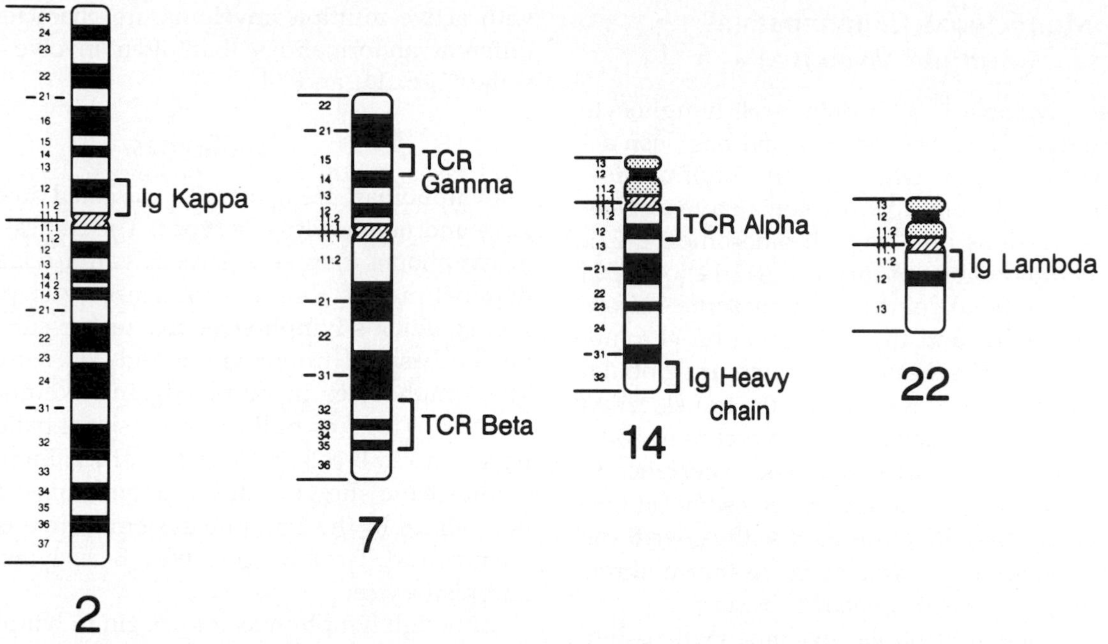

Figure 29.7. The immunoglobulin loci on chromosomes 2, 14, and 22; chromosome abnormalities involving any of these sites are usually B-cell disorders. The T-cell receptor (TCR) loci on chromosomes 7 and 14; chromosome abnormalities involving these sites are usually T-cell disorders. (From Dewald GW, Jenkins RB. Cytogenetic and molecular genetic studies of patients with monoclonal gammopathies. In: Wiernik PH, Canellos GP, Kyle RA, Schiffer CA, eds. Neoplastic diseases of blood. 2nd ed. New York: Churchill Livingstone, 1991:427–438. By permission of the publisher.)

breakpoints involving one or more of the light-chain immunoglobulin loci on chromosomes 2 and 22, or the heavy-chain immunoglobulin locus on chromosome 14, are usually associated with B-cell disorders. An example of a chromosome abnormality involving the heavy-chain immunoglobulin locus is shown in Figure 29.4*r*. These observations suggest that certain normal genes functioning in any particular cell type may play an important role in the origin of the chromosome abnormalities that have neoplastic potential.

Chronic Lymphocytic Leukemia

Chronic lymphocytic leukemia is a progressive clonal proliferation and accumulation of mature or nearly mature lymphocytes leading to replacement of the bone marrow, absolute peripheral blood lymphocytosis, and replacement of lymphoid tissues. This produces bone marrow failure and disruption of normal immunologic functions. This disease rarely occurs in patients younger than 40 years. The symptoms are often mild, and the diagnosis is usually made incidentally during a routine physical examination. The disease is characterized by an increased leukocyte count (10 to 150 × 10^9/liter) and monotonous lymphocytosis. The bone marrow may contain foci of lymphocytes or diffuse lymphocytes with the same morphology as in the peripheral blood.

More than 90% of patients have B-cell chronic lymphocytic leukemia. Several chromosome abnormalities have been associated with B-cell chronic lymphocytic leukemia. Two examples of structural abnormalities are t(11;14)(q13;q32) and del(6)(q14 – q27). These two abnormalities are discussed in more detail below. The most common numerical abnormality is trisomy 12.

About 10% of patients with chronic lymphocytic leukemia have T-cell disorders as demonstrated by immunologic, immunocytochemical, and T-cell gene rearrangement studies. T-cell chronic lymphocytic leukemia may be divided into helper and suppressor subtypes. T-cell suppressor disorders are characterized by an indolent course, whereas T-cell helper disorders are aggressive, with a median survival of 15 months.

The neoplastic cells in the chronic lymphocytic leukemias divide infrequently. Thus, it is not uncommon to observe only normal metaphases in patients with chronic lymphocytic leukemia. Attempts have been made to use various T-cell and B-cell mitogens, but in practice, the most consistent procedure for identifying abnormal clones is a short-term unstimulated culture without any mitogens. If abnormal metaphases are detected using this method, they suggest that the disease is actively proliferating. The use of mitogens in the procedure may interfere with this application of cytogenetic studies.

Monoclonal Gammopathies (Multiple Myeloma)

Multiple myeloma is a chronic B-cell lymphocyte disorder that involves plasma cells and has been associated with various chromosome abnormalities. Many patients with multiple myeloma have translocations or inversions involving chromosome 14 (22). The most common abnormality is a t(11;14)(q13;q32) (Fig. 29.4*r*). The breakpoint on chromosome 11 contains a gene for *bcl*, and the breakpoint on chromosome 14 contains the heavy-chain immunoglobulin locus. A t(8;14)(q24;q32) resembling the translocation linked with Burkitt's lymphoma also occurs in some patients with multiple myeloma. The occurrence in multiple myeloma of different chromosome abnormalities that are usually associated with other B-cell lymphoproliferative disorders suggests that multiple myeloma may be a heterogeneous disease.

In some patients, multiple myeloma evolves into or may present as plasma cell leukemia. The karyotype of plasma cell leukemia is often complex, but it involves chromosome abnormalities similar to those in multiple myeloma. This may be evidence that multiple myeloma evolves directly into plasma cell leukemia.

Chromosome studies can be useful in the workup of newly diagnosed patients with multiple myeloma and other monoclonal gammopathies because they can sometimes distinguish patients who have a poor prognosis. We studied a series of five patients with multiple myeloma and a chromosomally abnormal clone who at the time of diagnosis did not appear to have aggressive myeloma on the basis of routine hematologic studies. Follow-up studies on these patients showed that three actually did have an aggressive myeloma and died within 12 months. The other two patients were alive at the time of the study. One had a possible benign chromosome abnormality (−Y) and was still alive after 4 months. The other patient was alive after 13 months but was developing resistant multiple myeloma at the time the study ended.

An increasingly important application for chromosome studies in monoclonal gammopathies is to distinguish patients with an active plasma cell proliferation process from those with cytopenia due to an evolving preleukemia. This information can be helpful in the clinical management of such patients, especially in cases of monoclonal gammopathies in which the source of cytopenia is unknown. The results of several investigations now indicate that patients with evolving therapy-related leukemia are often characterized by either loss of or alteration in the structure of chromosome 5 or 7 (or both). In contrast, patients with active multiple myeloma are characterized by different abnormalities that often involve chromosomes 1, 6, 11, and 14.

Lymphomas

Lymphomas are generally classified into Hodgkin's and non-Hodgkin's types. The clinical findings in lymphoma involve enlarged lymph nodes or abdominal masses that are not sensitive to pain. The non-Hodgkin's lymphomas are further subclassified on the basis of tumor grade and cell morphology. The lymphocytes in non-Hodgkin's lymphoma can be B cell, T cell, or null cell. Occasional patients may have a mixed B-cell and T-cell disorder. Immunologic studies have shown that lymphoma arises from abnormalities in the immune system. Three cell types are involved: T-cell lymphocytes, B-cell lymphocytes, and histiocytes.

Although lymphomas may begin in lymph nodes, evidence of disease in other sites such as liver, bone marrow, and spleen is common. Occasionally, lymphomas metastasize to the bone marrow. Staging is an important criterion for prognosis. Some laboratories use cytogenetic studies to help stage lymphomas because chromosomally abnormal clones can be found in bone marrow, spleen, or peripheral blood if metastasis has occurred.

Many chromosome abnormalities have been associated with non-Hodgkin's lymphoma. Because the cytogenetic investigation of lymphomas is relatively recent, many new chromosome abnormalities are still being described. Among those already discovered, four stand out as the most common: t(14;18)(q32;q21), t(8;14)(q24;q32), t(11;14)(q13;q32), and del(6)(q14q23). Each of these abnormalities is discussed in more detail below.

t(14;18)(q32;q21) and Follicular Center Cell Lymphomas

A t(14;18)(q32;q21) translocation occurs in up to 80% of lymphomas with follicular center cell morphology and in up to one-third of diffuse large cell lymphomas. An example of this chromosome anomaly is shown in Figure 29.4*s*. A t(14;18)(q32;q21) can be found in both lymphomas with follicular center cell morphology and diffuse cell lymphomas. This may be evidence that some follicular lymphomas evolve into diffuse lymphomas. Because it is unusual to see this chromosome abnormality in bone marrow specimens, it may be related more to lymphoma than to lymphocytic leukemia. Thus, the observation of this chromosome abnormality in a bone marrow specimen may suggest metastatic lymphoma of the B-cell follicular center cell variety.

t(8;14)(q24;q32) and Burkitt's Lymphoma

Nearly 100% of cases of Burkitt's lymphoma and Burkitt's leukemia may have a t(8;14)(q24;q32). An example of this chromosome anomaly is shown in Figure 29.4*l*. Two variants of this 8;14 translocation are also recognized: t(2;8)(p12;q24) and t(8;22)(q24;q11). Examples of these anomalies are shown in Figure 29.4*bb* and *gg*, respectively. The association of these translocations with the *myc* oncogene and immunoglobulin loci is discussed in another section of this chapter.

The t(8;14)(q24;q32) abnormalities occur in ALL-L3 or Burkitt's leukemia as well as Burkitt's lymphoma. This association suggests that these two disorders may have a similar pathogenesis. This hypothesis is further supported by a similar cell morphology in both ALL-L3 and Burkitt's lymphoma. The t(8;14)(q24;q32) abnormalities occur in African and non-African Burkitt's lymphoma. Thus, the origins of Burkitt's lymphoma and ALL-L3 are probably more related to the t(8;14)(q24;q32). The Epstein-Barr virus has been implicated in Burkitt's lymphoma and is known to be a B-cell mitogen. Perhaps Epstein-Barr virus plays a role in the origin of t(8;14)(q24;q32) abnormalities simply by increasing the number of B cells undergoing DNA replication. This could increase the chances of developing a chromosome abnormality with neoplastic potential.

t(11;14)(q13;q32) and Small Cell Diffuse Lymphoma

An example of t(11;14)(q13;q32) is shown in Figure 29.4*c*. Although most patients with t(11;14)(q13;q32) who have lymphoma have small cell diffuse lymphoma, this translocation has also been observed in B-cell chronic lymphocytic leukemia and multiple myeloma. This suggests that these disorders may have a similar pathogenesis. The association of this translocation with the *bcl* oncogene and the heavy-chain immunoglobulin locus is discussed in more detail elsewhere in this chapter.

del(6)(q14q23) and Large Cell Lymphoma

Approximately 80% of patients with a del(6)(q14q23) have large cell lymphoma, but this abnormality is also common among the lymphocytic leukemias, including some of the cutaneous T-cell lymphomas such as the Sézary syndrome. An example of such an interstitial deletion from the long arm of chromosome 6 is shown in Figure 29.5*i*. The observation of some of the abnormalities in both lymphomas and the lymphocytic leukemias strongly suggests a similarity in the pathogenesis of these disorders.

Numerical Abnormalities

Several trisomies are common in lymphomas. Trisomy 12 occurs in about 50% of patients with lymphocytic lymphoma. Trisomy 3 has been linked with adult T-cell lymphoma. Trisomy 7 is common in follicular lymphomas and diffuse large cell tumors.

Cutaneous T-Cell Lymphomas

Results of chromosome studies have been reported for about 169 patients with cutaneous T-cell lymphomas, and about 55% of these patients had a chromosomally abnormal clone. The publications include three large series of patients with cutaneous T-cell lymphoma and one with unselected patients with the Sézary syndrome. The combined results of these series suggest that a chromosomally abnormal clone can be found in about 40% of patients with cutaneous T-cell lymphomas. The rest of the studies were case reports, and each patient was chromosomally abnormal.

The largest series of unselected patients with Sézary syndrome was reported from the Mayo Clinic. The results of this series probably reflect what might be expected in routine clinical practice for patients with cutaneous T-cell lymphomas. Use of 72-hour cultures with phytohemagglutinin and peripheral blood showed a chromosomally abnormal clone in 5 of 17 patients. In six other patients, more than 20% of the metaphases showed random aneuploidy and sporadic structural anomalies but no apparent abnormal clone. In four patients, only normal metaphases were observed, and in two patients no metaphases were found. Four of the five patients with a chromosomally abnormal clone died by the time of the report. The median duration of survival of these patients from the time of chromosome analysis was 6 months. The six patients with random chromosome anomalies had long survivals. Perhaps chromosome analysis can help physicians estimate prognosis for patients with cutaneous T-cell lymphomas.

The results of chromosome analysis in cutaneous T-cell lymphoma have demonstrated many different chromosome abnormalities among patients with this disorder. Thus, cutaneous T-cell lymphoma may be either a group of different disorders or a single heterogeneous disorder. The cytogenetic results favor the first hypothesis. The most common abnormality in the Sézary syndrome and other cutaneous T-cell lymphomas appears to be del(6)(q14–q27). Abnormalities of chromosome 14 with breakpoints involving 14q11–14q12 have been reported in two patients. This finding is consistent with other T-cell disorders because 14q11–q12 is the locus of the α chain T-cell receptor. Other chromosome abnormalities that may be associated with cutaneous T-cell lymphomas are abnormalities of the long arm of chromosome 1, 14q32, i(17q), and abnormalities of chromosome 9.

CHROMOSOME ABNORMALITIES AND ONCOGENES

Cell division is initiated and regulated by numerous genes. Under normal circumstances, the genes that govern cell division serve important functions during embryogenesis, growth, and cell repair to ensure the production of new cells. In mature cells in which mitosis is no longer necessary, these genes are inactive. Unfortunately, through genetic mutation, one or more of the genes that control cell division may become activated. When this happens, the DNA sequences of these genes become unregulated and continuously transcribe certain genes that cause cancer. These genes have become known as oncogenes.

Recent evidence indicates that one or more oncogenes are located near the sites of chromosome breakage for several of the specific chromosome abnormalities associated with malignant neoplastic disorders (23). This might suggest a molecular pathway to explain the pathogenesis of chromosome abnormalities in neoplastic disorders.

Some cytogeneticists believe that structural changes in chromosomes may be more significant than numerical abnormalities in the activation of oncogenes. Trisomy of any given chromosome may amplify the copy number of an oncogene. Monosomy for any given chromosome may decrease the copy number of an oncogene. Nevertheless, numerical imbalances of chromosomes may still be regulated by the usual cellular processes, and the degree of genetic imbalance is seldom more than one gene copy. In contrast, structural changes can alter gene expression by position effect or gene mutation at the site of chromosome breakage. This could lead to continual transcription of an oncogene.

Although at least 57 oncogenes are now known in humans, only 4 have been directly linked to chromosome changes: *bcl*-2 with t(14;18)(q32;q21); *myc* with t(8;14)(q24;q32), t(2;8)(p12;q24), and t(8;22)(q24;q11); *abl* with t(9;22)(q34;q11); and *erb-b* with der(1)t(1;7)(p11;p11). The lack of more cytogenetic and oncogene correlations could suggest that not all oncogenes lead to malignancy through the formation of chromosome abnormalities. To illustrate how chromosome abnormalities may exert their influence in neoplastic processes by activating oncogenes, two examples are provided: t(8;14)(q24;q32) and t(14;18)(q32;q21).

t(8;14)(q24;q32) and *myc* Oncogene

The activation of the *myc* oncogene by the t(8;14)(q24;q32) translocation in Burkitt's lymphoma is an example of how a chromosome abnormality may deregulate cell division. In this translocation, the breakpoints on chromosome 14 are at 14q32, the site of the heavy-chain immunoglobulin gene. The breakpoint on chromosome 8 in this translocation is at 8q24, the site of the *myc* oncogene. As a consequence of the 8;14 translocation, the *myc* oncogene is moved adjacent to part of the heavy-chain immunoglobulin locus on chromosome 14. The transcription of the *myc* gene is then controlled by the heavy-chain immunoglobulin gene.

Two other translocations associated with Burkitt's lymphoma provide further evidence for the activation of *myc* in lymphoproliferative disorders. Some patients with Burkitt's lymphoma have a t(8;22)(q24;q11); this variant translocation brings the gene for the λ light chain of immunoglobulin into juxtaposition with the *myc* oncogene on chromosome 8. Other patients with Burkitt's lymphomas have a t(2;8)(pl2;q24); this translocation brings the κ light-chain gene into juxtaposition with the *myc* oncogene. Each of these translocations is known to activate transcription of the *myc* oncogene.

t(14;18)(q32;q21) and *bcl*-2 Oncogene

The t(14;18)(q32;q21) translocation provides further clues to the importance of structural changes in neoplasms. The breakpoint of this translocation involves the immunoglobulin gene on chromosome 14. The breakpoint on chromosome 18 is at 18q21.3, the site of the *bcl*-2 oncogene. Up to 60% of the t(14;18)(q32;q21) breakpoints on chromosome 18 occur within about 500 DNA base pairs; this DNA section has become known as the major breakpoint cluster region. The 14;18 translocation produces a hybrid *bcl*-2/immunoglobulin heavy-chain transcript. How this protein is related to the pathogenesis of follicular lymphoma is not yet known.

WHY CYTOGENETICS CORRELATES WITH SPECIFIC MALIGNANCIES

Molecular studies suggest that chromosome abnormalities move certain oncogenes into juxtaposition with functional normal genes. The transcription of the normal gene overlaps with the oncogene, producing a hybrid mRNA and protein that is derived partly from the oncogene and partly from the normal gene. How the hybrid protein causes the cell to become malignant is unknown. Nevertheless, this scenario offers an explanation as to why specific chromosome abnormalities may be associated with

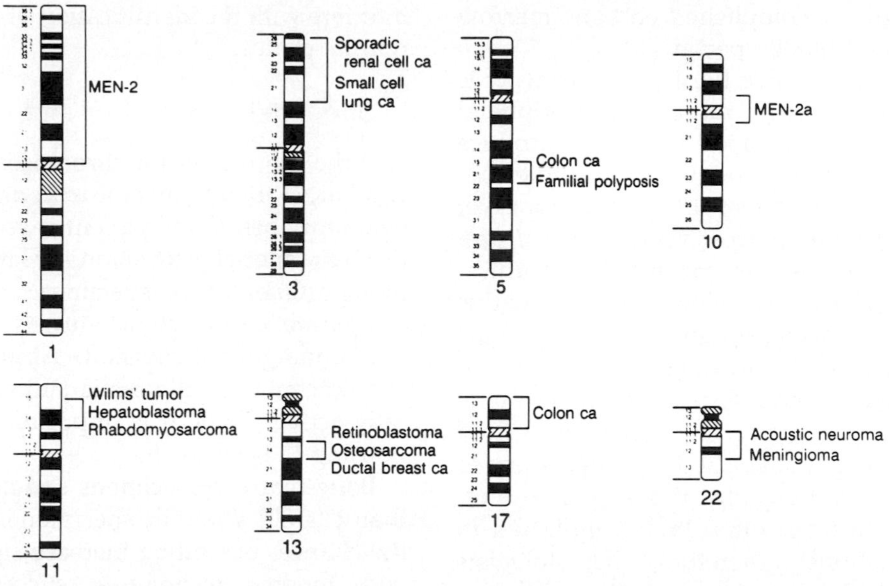

Figure 29.8. Chromosome sites associated with loss of heterozygosity in solid tumors that provide evidence for tumor-suppressor genes. Abbreviations: ca, carcinoma; MEN, multiple endocrine neoplasia. (From Dewald GW. Possible role of chromosome abnormalities in the origin and progression of lymphoma. In: Muller SA, ed. Parapsoriasis: Proceedings of the First International Parapsoriasis Symposium, September 7 and 8, 1989. Rochester, MN: Mayo Foundation, 1990: 43–51. By permission of Mayo Foundation.)

particular neoplastic disorders. For example, a malignancy involving a t(8;14)(q24;q32) may effectively induce translocation in B cells because the heavy-chain immunoglobulin locus is involved. This same translocation may not have neoplastic potential in cells in which the heavy-chain immunoglobulin locus is not normally transcribed.

CHROMOSOME ABNORMALITIES AND TUMOR-SUPPRESSOR GENES

Recent evidence suggests that tumor-suppressor genes may provide a mechanism for tumorigenesis (24). In normal cells, tumor-suppressor genes may be important in preventing excessive cell growth. Individuals who are heterozygous for mutant recessive tumor-suppressor genes may be predisposed to developing malignancies. The malignant process is probably initiated by a mutation or loss of the normal dominant gene, allowing the recessive gene to be expressed. Loss of heterozygosity can happen by loss of a chromosome through nondisjunction or by structural rearrangements such as deletions and unbalanced translocations.

The inactivation of tumor-suppressor genes through loss of heterozygosity has not been associated with any specific hematologic disorder. However, there are many possibilities to investigate because loss of all or part of any chromosome is a potential tumor-suppressor problem. For example, monosomy 7, del(5)(q13q33), del(6)(q14q32), and other losses of chromosomes would be candidates for this mechanism. The best candidates for investigation may be abnormalities in which no specific oncogene has yet been identified because this may implicate another process.

The importance of loss of heterozygosity and expression of tumor suppressor genes has been demonstrated in many solid tumors. One example is the development of retinoblastoma and osteosarcoma associated with the loss of heterozygosity of a gene located at 13q14. Possibly, the same process relates to the 13q− chromosomes associated with agnogenic myeloid metaplasia and other hematologic disorders. A more complete list of tumor-suppressor genes and their apparent association with neoplastic disorders is summarized in Figure 29.8.

CHROMOSOME ANALYSIS

Choice of Tissue

Physicians who use chromosome studies in their hematology practice need to provide appropriate specimens for chromosome analysis. The tissue of choice should include malignant cells. For lymphomas, involved lymph node biopsy specimens are most suitable. Bone marrow specimens are best for analyzing specimens from patients with myeloproliferative and myelodysplastic syndromes, chronic lymphocytic leukemias, and acute leukemias. In certain instances, it can be useful to collect a peripheral blood specimen. This can be done for chronic lymphocytic leukemia and some cutaneous T-cell lymphomas. For dry bone marrow taps, chromosome studies can often be accomplished on bone marrow biopsy or peripheral blood specimens.

For disorders that involve the bone marrow, it is better to use bone marrow rather than peripheral blood. Only about 60% of blood specimens produce adequate metaphases, and bone marrow studies are diagnostically more sensitive. In general practice, more than 95% of bone marrow specimens can provide suitable specimens for chromosome studies. Chromosome analysis on blood is informative mainly in advanced disorders and is used as a last resort if bone marrow is not available.

In special instances, other types of specimens may need to be collected. If metastasis to the spinal fluid or to some other site is suspected, it is necessary to collect the specimen from the tissue in question. Chromosome studies can often be accomplished in unexpected situations; therefore, hematologists should not exclude the use of cytogenetics because of small fluid samples or lack of apparent cells. We have successfully done chromosome studies on the vitreous fluid of the eye to demonstrate the relapse of chronic granulocytic leukemia in this location. Chromosome studies can identify malignant hematologic disorders that cause pleural effusions. In pleural fluids, lymphomas are often more readily diagnosed by cytogenetic techniques than by standard cytologic examination.

It is helpful to provide some clinical information with the specimen. The cytogenetic laboratory benefits from knowing what hematologic disorder is suspected and the reason why the specimen has been referred. This information can help the laboratory select the most appropriate cytogenetic procedure. Some laboratories want to know certain information, such as the leukocyte count. This information may be used to set up cultures to avoid adding too many cells to the media. Some laboratories believe that a high leukocyte count is more likely to yield metaphases than a low count. This theory has not worked well in our experience. A blood specimen may have a high leukocyte count, but the number of mitotic cells may be too low for a suitable chromosome study.

Most therapeutic agents may interfere with attempts to recover metaphases from specimens. The function of most therapeutic agents in neoplastic diseases is to prevent cells from undergoing division. Some of these agents are alkylating agents; others intercalate into DNA, interfere with the spindle fiber apparatus, or act through different mechanisms. It is usually possible to do successful chromosome studies 2 to 3 weeks after treatment. This happens to be the approximate time before treatment can significantly affect any malignant clone. Although the agents used to treat malignancies may induce sporadic abnormalities in chromosomes, they should not interfere with the identification of chromosomally abnormal clones.

Specimen Collection and Transportation

If the procedures for chromosome analysis are unfamiliar, it may be useful to contact the cytogenetic laboratory before the patient is seen. Many laboratories have special instructions or kits for collection and transportation of the specimen.

Routine chromosome studies are done on cells that undergo cell division. Appropriate specimens should contain living malignant cells that are mitotically active. Thus, it is important to avoid fixing or freezing the cells.

Bone marrow specimens should involve no more than 1.0 ml. When the specimen is more than 1.0 ml, the chances of clotting increase significantly. In fact, with modern techniques, successful chromosome studies can be accomplished routinely on 0.25 to 0.50 ml of bone marrow. The specimen should be collected with heparin sodium using sterile technique. It is useful to collect a fresh specimen for chromosome analysis. This can be done without interfering with the collection of fresh specimens for standard hematologic examination by redirecting the needle at the time the bone marrow is collected.

If it is necessary to transport the bone marrow specimen to a cytogenetic laboratory located some distance away, then particular attention should be paid to transportation methods. Some laboratories transport the specimens in media, but others prefer to have the specimen partially processed before mailing. We use a special kit for processing bone marrow specimens that includes a 50-ml centrifuge tube with a Colcemid solution, hypotonic solution, and a set of instructions (25). It is usually best for the referring laboratory to prepare fresh fixative. Although fixative is not readily provided in kits, it consists of methanol and glacial acetic acid, which are common commodities in many clinical laboratories.

In our experience, this kit has been used successfully on about 92% of specimens. It permits the use of a direct technique to analyze bone marrow specimens. Once the cells are fixed, transportation time is not a problem. At our institution, we use both a direct technique and a short-term unstimulated culture method for local specimens. This combination method results in a 96% success rate.

If peripheral blood is the specimen for chromosome study, most laboratories request 7.0 to 10.0 ml collected in a sterile syringe containing heparin sodium. The specimen should be immediately transferred to a vial with heparin sodium. The blood should not be hemolyzed or clotted. Some anticoagulants are harmful to the viability of the cells. Heparin sodium is highly recommended as the anticoagulant of choice.

Chromosome studies can be done on lymph node biopsy specimens of 1.0 to 3.0 ml. The specimen should be transported in a screw-capped, sterile container with sterile tissue medium or in sterile Hank's balanced salt solution. The specimen can be refrigerated or sent to the cytogenetic laboratory at ambient temperature.

For unusual specimens, it is best to contact the cytogenetic laboratory for instructions. Successful analysis has been performed on 10 ml of pleural effusion, 5 ml of spinal fluids, and many other specimens.

Processing Specimens for Chromosome Analysis

Various methods exist to process specimens for chromosome analysis. Specimens can be processed immediately after collection with a direct technique. The cells are first treated with Colcemid for 1 hour. Then they are treated with warm hypotonic solution (0.075 M KCl) for about 15 minutes and fixed with 3:1 methanol–glacial acetic acid. This method is favored by many laboratories for bone marrow specimens and has a success rate of more than 92%. With this technique, a report can be issued within 24 hours. Some laboratories find the direct technique especially valuable in the study of acute lymphocytic leukemia. Others think this method is not as good for certain hematologic disorders, such as for acute progranulocytic leukemia (ANLL-M3).

Short-term cultures of 24 to 48 hours are used by many laboratories. These cultures use standard media such as RPMI 1640, fetal bovine serum, and antibiotics. No T-cell or B-cell mitogens are used in this procedure. The cells are incubated at 37°C for 24 to 48 hours. It is desirable to use a low-oxygen environment (5% oxygen, 5% carbon dioxide, and 90% nitrogen) with these cultures. The cells are harvested for chromosome analysis using the standard procedures with Colcemid, hypotonic solution, and fixative. In our experience, this method can be successfully used for more than 90% of bone marrow specimens. Some laboratories believe this method is particularly good for certain disorders, such as ANLL-M3.

In most laboratories, short-term cultures of bone marrow are done in 25-ml T-flasks, but in situ techniques can be used. Most laboratories set up from one to three cultures in T-flasks for each case. The harvest procedures then involve transferring the specimen to centrifuge tubes. Several washes using a pipette to bubble the cells are required. Finally, the cells are drawn into a pipette and dropped onto slides. This procedure results in the loss of many cells and therefore limits the harvest procedure to manual methods.

The in situ method involves culturing the cells in chamber slides. We usually set up eight chamber slides for each bone marrow specimen. The cells are then cultured in low oxygen using RPMI 1640. The cells are harvested in the chamber slides, thus avoiding the loss of cells associated with the flask technique. One advantage of the in situ method is the ability to process the cultures with a robotic harvesting machine (Tecan, Inc.). This technique also allows different cultures to be processed easily with different methods (e.g., with or without mitogens). The in situ method conserves cells and can be used with small specimens.

For chromosome studies of blood or bone marrow specimens from patients with chronic lymphocytic leukemia, it can be helpful to use certain mitogens to stimulate the neoplastic cells to divide. Mitogens such as phytohemagglutinin, 12-*O*-tetradecanoylphorbol-13-acetate (TPA), pokeweed, and inactivated Epstein-Barr virus have been used successfully. Some laboratories have successfully used combinations of these and other mitogens. However, mitogens may also stimulate the normal B cells and T cells to divide. Furthermore, not all the cells in specimens taken from patients with neoplastic lymphocytic disorders are capable of responding to such mitogens, even though they may actually be derived from B cells or T cells.

What is the best way to process specimens from patients with hematologic disorders for chromosome analysis? The answer to this question varies among laboratories and according to the hematologic disorder being studied. In an attempt to answer this question for routine practice, we compared the direct technique with 24-hour unstimulated cultures and with methotrexate synchronization methods in a blind study of 100 unselected bone marrow specimens (26). No consistent differences were noted among any of these methods in terms of chromosome morphology, mitotic index, or the chance of detecting a chromosomally abnormal clone. Nevertheless, one method was often more successful than another. Thus, we recommend routinely using at least two methods with each case, one of which should be a direct technique.

Staining

Numerous techniques are available to stain the chromosomes for analysis. The most common staining methods are G-banding and Q-banding. Many methods produce G bands. We use a brief treatment with trypsin, followed by staining with Leishman's stain. This technique produces permanent preparations with sharp-contrast bands that are easily viewed and photographed with light microscopy, permitting the identification of each chromosome and the detection of subtle structural abnormalities. This staining method is somewhat inconsistent and is best used when numerous metaphases are available.

Q-banding involves staining the chromosomes with quinacrine mustard for 1 or 2 minutes and viewing the chromosomes with a fluorescence microscope system. This stain usually fades in a few minutes, but the rate of fluorescence loss can be reduced using *n*-propyl gallate. This method permits the identification of all chromosomes and subtle structural abnormalities. The Q-banding patterns may not be as apparent as G-banding, but Q-banding is more consistent than G-banding. Q-banding is the staining technique of choice when there are only a few metaphases or when chromosome morphology is poor.

Analysis of Metaphases

Most laboratories analyze at least 20 metaphases. It has been suggested that the analysis of 20 metaphases could exclude a clone that accounts for more than 14% of the cells with 95% confidence. The analysis of 30 cells would exclude a clone that accounts for more than 10% of the cells with 95% confidence. This assumes that the metaphases are selected randomly for analysis and does not attempt to meet the minimal criteria for identifying clones as described below. In actual practice, many technologists do not randomly select metaphases, and they usually examine far more metaphases than they actually report. This is because not all metaphases provide equal information. To completely analyze any metaphase, a technologist needs to establish the number of chromosomes, identify the number of each type of chromosome, and examine the band pattern of each chromosome, looking for any structural abnormalities. The level of resolution should be at least the 400-band stage. This would permit the identification of 400 or more separate bands on a haploid set of chromosomes in the best metaphases. Usually, it is not possible to accomplish all this in each metaphase because of overlapping chromosomes, inconsistent staining, lack of metaphases, and many other reasons.

In the face of all these obstacles, technologists can only do their best. Nevertheless, it is important that the technologist not select only "beautiful" metaphases. Frequently, the poorest metaphases represent the neoplastic clone. Nor should the technologists select only bad metaphases. We have had cases in which the metaphases from the neoplastic clone stained better than the normal cells. It is best to select all kinds of metaphases regardless of staining pattern. The goal of a laboratory that does neoplastic studies should not be to analyze the 550 band metaphases in all cases if this has to be done at the expense of poor turnaround time and success rate.

Experience is the most valuable tool of the cytogenetic technologist. A technologist who is familiar with the classic chromosome abnormalities in hematologic disorders is most likely to find them. Furthermore, the task will be accomplished efficiently and economically. The technologist should establish as much information about each metaphase as possible and record the identity of extra or missing chromosomes as well as any structural abnormalities.

Karyotype Preparations

Each metaphase that is analyzed should be photographed. Film is inexpensive, and the photographic negative makes an excellent permanent record of the study. For each case, several formal karyotypes should be prepared from representative metaphases. This permits a more objective comparison of band patterns between homologous chromosomes and the detection of subtle abnormalities. It also helps identify the chromosome abnormalities in a more objective manner than is possible from microscopic analysis alone. Each of the laboratory-certifying agencies requires the preparation of at least two karyotypes from the primary clone. Some certifying agencies suggest the preparation of at least one karyotype from each subclone. This is not always feasible, because in some cases all the metaphases analyzed may have some differences due to considerable chromosome evolution and technical artifacts.

Definition of a Clone

The hallmark of malignant hematologic disorders is the presence of a neoplastic clone. The standard cytogenetic definition of a clone requires the observation of at least two metaphases with the same extra chromosome or the same structural abnormality. This definition also requires the presence of three or more metaphases that are missing the same chromosome. The stricter definition for chromosome loss helps to exclude overinterpretation of errors due to technical artifacts. Loss of chromosomes during processing of the specimen is more likely than the introduction of multiple cells with the same extra chromosome or the same structural abnormality.

Because chromosome abnormalities are a part of normal events, the definition of a clone should include a maximal number of metaphases to be analyzed. We prefer to analyze no more than 30 metaphases in each study because this limit keeps the study economical and uses the overall time of the laboratory most efficiently. Nevertheless, the observation of even one cell with a classic chromosome abnormality should be reported. The report should explain that this discovery does not meet the minimal criteria for a clone but that it could be diagnostically important.

Reporting Results

The report should include a complete and formal cytogenetic description using standard cytogenetic nomenclature. A brief description of the findings for nongeneticists should be provided. We discourage overanalysis of the data. For example, it may not be appropriate to say that trisomy 8 is evidence of acute leukemia, because this diagnosis is based on the percentage of blasts in the bone marrow rather than on the cytogenetic findings. It would be appropriate to say that a clone of cells with trisomy 8 is consistent with the observation of a neoplastic clone.

Some laboratories report results as NN, AN, or AA. This is an unofficial abbreviated report indicating that all the metaphases are normal (NN), all are abnormal (AA), or some metaphases are abnormal and some normal (AN). Not long ago, it was thought that this information might have some prognostic value, but as techniques for chromosome analysis have improved and the experience of laboratories has increased, more and more patients with neoplastic clones are proving to be AN or AA. Thus, the prognostic significance of this classification system is now in question. We still provide this information in our reports because it is widely recognized by hematologists.

Some laboratories provide a representative karyotype preparation with the report. Most hematologists do not readily appreciate this information, but we think it is still useful. This picture can be useful to any hematologists who review their cases with individuals who might be familiar with chromosome banding patterns. Pointing out the structural and numerical abnormalities on the picture can be helpful to hematologists.

PATIENT MANAGEMENT AND CYTOGENETICS

Evidence of a Neoplastic Clone

The observation of a chromosomally abnormal clone usually provides objective evidence that a patient has a neoplastic process, regardless of the nature of the chromosome abnormality. Thus, chromosome studies can help distinguish between acquired clonal neoplasms and most other normal cellular reactions. If only normal metaphases are observed, it should not be concluded that the patient does not have a neoplastic clone. It may be that cells from the abnormal clone were overlooked in the chromosome study. However, normal cytogenetic information, taken together with the results of all other laboratory tests and clinical impressions, may indicate the absence of a clonal disorder.

Multiple Clones

The occurrence of multiple clones is not synonymous with chromosome evolution. When two or more clones each exhibit completely different karyotypes, the patient probably has more than one neoplasm. Chromosome evolution produces one or more subclones derived from an original abnormal clone, thereby indicating that a single neoplasm is progressing, usually to a higher grade of malignancy. For example, we studied a patient with multiple myeloma who had three different chromosomally abnormal clones in his bone marrow. One clone had the 11;14 translocation observed in multiple myeloma. Another had an unbalanced 1;7 translocation like those associated with therapy-related leukemia. The patient had, in fact, been treated. The karyotype of the third clone was trisomy 8. These three separate clones may indicate three different hematologic neoplasms, one of which may have been therapy related, one associated with active multiple myeloma, and one related to some other de novo hematologic disorder. Multiple clones do not necessarily imply a poor prognosis, but those that evince chromosome evolution are usually associated with refractory disease and short survival.

Myeloid or Lymphoid Process

Chromosome studies can help classify disorders as either myeloid or lymphoid. This distinction is important because these hematologic disorders are often treated differently. For example, a t(8;14)(q24;q32) abnormality in the bone marrow is evidence that the patient has a B-cell disorder. Because this chromosome abnormality is specifically associated with ALL-L3 or Burkitt's lymphoma, this finding also helps to classify the disorder. Other abnormalities are specifically associated with myeloid disorders. For example, the presence of a clone of cells with trisomy 8 is evidence that the neoplastic process is most likely myeloid.

Subclassification of Hematologic Disorders

Chromosome studies can help subclassify disorders. For example, by morphologic and immunocytochemical determinations, a disorder may be classified as ANLL-M2. Patients with ANLL-M2 can sometimes be further subclassified by cytogenetic studies into important chromosomal categories that are associated with different prognoses and responses to therapy. For example, patients with ANLL-M2 who have a t(8;21)(q22;q22) are thought to have a better prognosis than other patients with ANLL-M2.

Distinguishing between Similar Disorders

Certain hematologic disorders may be confused with one another by using only morphologic and immunocytochemical determinations. For example, essential thrombocythemia can sometimes be difficult to distinguish from the early stages of chronic granulocytic leukemia. This distinction is readily apparent on routine chromosome studies because chronic granulocytic leukemia is associated with a Ph chromosome, whereas essential thrombocythemia is not. It is not unusual in routine practice to encounter patients in whom the referring physician suspects one hematologic disorder but instead finds another after performing chromosome analysis and other tests.

Monitoring Remission

Most patients who have an apparent chromosomally abnormal clone before therapy will not have one when remission is achieved. Thus, cytogenetic studies can be used to help establish when remission is achieved and to monitor the patient in subsequent follow-up visits. The reappearance of metaphases with the same chromosome abnormalities is evidence of disease relapse. Abnormal metaphases are probably still present during remission, but the number of malignant cells is probably too small to detect by routine chromosome studies. Thus, the reappearance of abnormal metaphases with the same karyotype as observed before therapy indicates a reemergence of the original disease and not a second de novo disorder that by coincidence happens to have the same chromosome abnormality.

Unlike most other disorders, chronic granulocytic leukemia does not demonstrate the usual disappearance of chromosomally abnormal metaphases in remission. Unless very aggressive treatment or bone marrow transplants are given to patients with chronic granulocytic leukemia, most metaphases will remain Ph-positive, even in apparent remission.

Identifying Patients with Aggressive Disease

In multiple myeloma, considerable evidence has accumulated to suggest that chromosome studies can help identify patients who have an aggressive disease and a poor prognosis, even at the time of diagnosis. The observation of a chromosomally abnormal clone at the time of diagnosis should be considered evidence of aggressive disease. These patients have a median survival of about 6 months and need treatment for their disorder. Alternatively, when a chromosomally abnormal clone is not observed, the median survival is considerably greater and the patient may not need immediate treatment.

Establishing the Emergence of Therapy-Related Disease

For patients who have had chemotherapy for one disease and then develop cytopenia, chromosome analysis can sometimes help decide whether the cytopenia is a response to the treatment, a resurgence of the original hematologic disorder, or an evolving therapy-induced leukemia. For example, consider a patient with multiple myeloma who has received chemotherapy and then develops cytopenia. If a multiple myeloma–like karyotype is found, the physician should be concerned about aggressive myeloma and treat the patient accordingly. If the karyotype is typical of therapy-related leukemia, the physician should be concerned about an evolving leukemia that is separate from the myeloma and treat it accordingly.

Bone Marrow Transplant Programs

Chromosome analyses can be particularly useful to physicians in bone marrow transplant programs. Chromosome studies can be used before transplantation to help decide the precise hematologic classification and karyotype of the neoplastic process. This information is useful in subsequent chromosome studies on these patients because it provides important cytogenetic markers of the original hematologic disorder. Chromosome studies help physicians in their attempts to achieve remission in patients before bone marrow transplantation. The persistence of cells with the original leukemic karyotype is evidence that a complete remission has not been achieved. This information is especially helpful if a physician is considering autologous bone marrow transplantation.

Cytogenetic studies can also characterize the chromosomal polymorphisms in the karyotype of the patient as well as in the donor. These polymorphisms are not clinically important variations in chromosome structure, but they can provide useful chromosome markers that can help identify the origin of cells. These polymorphisms are particularly helpful for distinguishing between normal donor and recipient cells after bone marrow transplantation. Some examples of normal polymorphisms include variations in the size and staining pattern of chromosome satellites and C-bands. In opposite-sex transplants, the Y chromosome is an especially good marker because it is readily distinguishable from other chromosomes by Q-banding.

In the event of a relapse after bone marrow transplantation, chromosome studies can help determine whether the leukemic cells have the karyotype of the original clone. In most cases, it is possible to distinguish between a new kind of leukemia that has emerged and the relapse of the original disorder because the cells have a different karyotype than the original leukemic cells. Inspection of the chromosomal polymorphisms can sometimes help determine whether the new leukemia involves the donor's cells or the recipient's cells.

Constitutional Chromosome Abnormalities

With routine cytogenetic techniques, it is not possible to accurately establish the cell lineage of any given metaphase. This information is usually suggested by the tissue being studied and the culture technique used. For example, if a T-cell mitogen such as phytohemagglutinin is used in the culture, most metaphases will be T cells. Certain chromosome abnormalities are present at birth and are not directly associated with neoplastic disorders. In routine practice, it is important to distinguish between acquired chromosome abnormalities associated with neoplastic processes and abnormalities that are congenital.

Congenital chromosome abnormalities are part of the constitutional karyotype and, except in cases of mosaicism, occur in all tissues of the patient. These abnormalities may be either balanced or unbalanced. A reciprocal translocation is an example of a balanced abnormality because it involves the exchange of chromatin between the two chromosomes and results in neither extra chromatin nor loss of chromatin. Trisomy 21 is an example of an unbalanced abnormality because the patient has three copies of chromosome 21. Approximately one in 500 adults carries a balanced chromosome abnormality. Carriers of balanced chromosome abnormalities are usually phenotypically normal, but they may be at risk for having children with birth defects. About one in 100 newborns has unbalanced chromosome abnormalities. Some of these abnormalities are associated with classic syndromes such as Down's and Klinefelter's syndromes.

Constitutional structural abnormalities of chromosomes are usually different from the abnormalities associated with hematologic disorders. When a balanced structural abnormality is observed in a patient with a neoplastic process that has not been associated with hematologic disease, it can be difficult to determine whether the abnormality is constitutional or acquired. If both normal and abnormal metaphases are observed, this can be an important clue that the abnormality is acquired. Likewise, if the cells contain more than one chromosome abnormality, a congenital cause is less likely. It is rare for more than one chromosome abnormality to occur in the constitutional karyotype. For classic congenital chromosome disorders, such as trisomy 21, the diagnosis is often readily evident on physical examination. A structural abnormality that is frequently associated with certain hematologic disorders in a patient with a hematologic disorder can usually be assumed to be acquired.

Occasional cases are encountered in which there are no clinical or cytogenetic clues as to whether a chromosome abnormality in the bone marrow is constitutional or acquired. In these difficult cases, more extensive cytogenetic studies may be needed. Usually, constitutional chromosome abnormalities occur in cells of every tissue, whereas acquired abnormalities are present only in cells of the neoplastic tissue. Chromosome analysis on peripheral blood cultured in medium containing phytohemagglutinin to stimulate T-cell mitosis may be helpful in these cases. This permits a comparison of the karyotype of T cells with those of neoplastic hematopoietic cells. This procedure may not be useful if the patient has a T-cell disorder. In these cases, it may be necessary to do chromosome studies on fibroblast cells using a skin biopsy to initiate the culture.

The incidence of hematologic disorders may be higher among patients with constitutional chromosome abnormalities than among normal individuals. The predisposition for patients with Down's syndrome to develop hematologic disease is well known. Also, trisomy 21 is common in hematologic disorders. Thus, in cases of trisomy 21, distinguishing between an abnormal clone that is associated with neoplastic disease and a constitutional abnormality that reflects Down's syndrome can be difficult. Fortunately, in hematologic disorders, trisomy 21 is usually associated with many other chromosome abnormalities. In these cases, the chromosomally abnormal cells are unbalanced and are associated with neoplastic disease.

We have seen at least 13 patients without Down's syndrome who had neoplastic disorders associated with only trisomy 21 (27). We have also studied patients with neoplastic clones containing other classic karyotypes, including 45,X (Turner's syndrome), 47,XXY (Klinefelter's syndrome), and 47,XXX (triple X syndrome). Thus, when a classic congenital karyotype is encountered in the study of patients with hematologic disorders, the possibility that the karyotype is part of an acquired neoplastic disease should not be discounted.

RECENT ADVANCES IN CYTOGENETIC METHODOLOGY

In recent years, many advances in methodology have greatly enhanced the power of cytogenetics. It may soon be possible to produce slide preparations containing hundreds of metaphases. Then, chromosome studies should become more informative, less expensive, less time-consuming, and hence even more useful in the diagnosis of neoplastic disorders.

High-Resolution Techniques with DNA Intercalating Agents

New techniques to produce metaphases with high-resolution banding have been introduced. One method is to treat cells in culture using substances, such as methotrexate, to block DNA synthesis. Then the culture medium is changed. This frees the cells from this block, so that cell division is synchronized. By processing the cells from several cultures that are harvested at slightly different times, it is possible to produce slides with cells in different stages of mitosis. These slides will show chromosomes in different degrees of contraction. One may then examine a few slides from each culture to find the preparations that show the morphology of the chromosomes most clearly. Longer chromosomes can be produced by adding DNA intercalaters such as actinomycin D or ethidium bromide to the culture media. Further refinement can be achieved with low concentrations of Colcemid for periods of only 10 to 15 minutes.

We find the synchronization technique excessively time-consuming for a busy diagnostic laboratory. Instead, we simply add 10 μl/ml ethidium bromide to the culture 1 hour before harvesting, and this significantly improves the band resolution of the chromosomes. This procedure also avoids the reduction of the mitotic index that occurs with synchronization techniques. Ethidium bromide can also be used in direct preparations by adding it at about the same time as the Colcemid.

Media with Growth Factors and Special Mitogens

Some culture media are enriched with lymphokines, growth hormones, and other growth-promoting substances that increase the number of metaphases after short-term cultures. An example is Chang's medium. There has also been some work with culture media that contain substances that stimulate colony stem cells. The main drawback of such media is the fact that the mitogens often stimulate the division of normal cells rather than malignant cells.

In lymphoproliferative disorders, it is sometimes useful to use certain mitogens such as phytohemagglutinin, interleukin-2, pokeweed antigen, Epstein-Barr virus, and 12-*O*-tetradecanoylphorbol-13-acetate (TPA) or a combination of these mitogens to stimulate cells to undergo mitosis.

One mitogen combination often used in chronic lymphoproliferative disorders is interleukin-2 and tetradecanoylphorbol-acetate. This combination of mitogens may stimulate both T cells and B cells.

Use of Low-Oxygen Gas Mixtures to Increase the Number of Metaphases

Culture systems can be improved by using special gas mixtures to stimulate cell growth. Many laboratories now culture cells in an atmosphere of 5% carbon dioxide, 5% oxygen, and 90% nitrogen. This gas mixture provides culture media with conditions that are not unlike those of venous blood and bone marrow. This gas mixture simulates in vivo conditions and reduces the detrimental effects of higher oxygen concentrations on cells in culture.

Use of Flame Drying to Produce Better Metaphase Spreads

The use of flame drying can improve the quality of metaphase spreads. This method was popular before the banding techniques were introduced, but it then fell into disfavor because it was thought to denature the chromosomes and interfere with the banding procedures. This may be true, but this method is still effective for improving the spreading of chromosomes. The interference with banding can be reduced by using a "cool flame" technique. This is done by using slides moistened with water to reduce the concentration of methanol, the flammable component of the fixative.

Flow Cytometry and DNA Aneuploidy

Flow cytometry is sometimes used to identify "aneuploid clones" in hematologic disorders. This technique does not provide information about the number of chromosomes in any cell; rather, it gives an estimate of the amount of DNA in individual cells. Briefly, the technique involves staining the cells with a DNA-specific stain such as ethidium bromide and then passing the cells through a laser beam in a flow cytometer. By comparing the estimates of DNA in cells from any patient with the DNA content in cells from normal individuals, it is possible to determine whether there are cells with more or less than the normal amount of DNA. This ratio is usually referred to as the DNA index. A DNA index of 1 is equivalent to diploid, less than 1 to hypodiploid, and greater than 1 to hyperdiploid. Because an actual count of the chromosomes is not determined, it is recommended that the results be expressed in units of DNA ploidy rather than chromosome ploidy.

Flow cytometry is considerably faster than routine cytogenetic studies and permits the analysis of thousands of cells. However, the DNA index does not permit the detection of balanced chromosome abnormalities or subtle structural abnormalities. Unfortunately, these are very common in all neoplastic disorders, especially in patients with early disease. Furthermore, the DNA index does not permit the detailed characterization of the karyotype. This is a serious limitation because important clinical information can be gleaned from a complete karyotype characterization. Nevertheless, flow cytometry may someday complement traditional chromosome analysis. Perhaps flow cytometry will help isolate certain cell types for further cytogenetic analysis.

Automated Karyotyping and Metaphase Finding

Automated karyotyping machines are now commercially available. Although these systems are expensive to purchase and to operate, they may be helpful in many laboratories, especially if a good photographic darkroom is not readily available. Some commercial companies are developing automated metaphase finders. The perfection of these machines may be particularly useful for chromosome studies in hematologic disorders because the number of metaphases is often small. This makes locating metaphases the most time-consuming part of chromosome analysis in hematologic disorders.

Simultaneous Cytogenetic and Immunocytochemical Metaphase Analysis

A recently developed method permits the staining of metaphases by both cytogenetic and immunocytochemical techniques. This permits the simultaneous characterization of the karyotype, morphology, and immunotype of metaphases. Unlike conventional cytogenetic methods, this procedure uses a milder hypotonic solution and a different fixative. With this procedure, the metaphase cell remains intact and the cytoplasmic structure is maintained. Any of the cytogenetic staining methods can be used to study the chromosomes. The cell morphology and immunology can be established with any routine hematologic stains and immunofluorescence techniques using various anitsera.

This combined cytogenetic-immunocytochemical procedure is not recommended for routine cytogenetic studies because the chromosomes are not adequately fixed and satisfactory examples of morphology are not consistently produced. Nevertheless, these studies have been useful to show that chromosome abnormalities exist in the predominant cell type of patients with certain kinds of leukemia. In some cases, studies with this method have suggested that more cell types may be involved in the neoplastic process than are apparent from routine studies of cell morphology. For example, in some patients with chronic granulocytic leukemia, the Ph chromosome occurs in all types of hematopoietic cells, not only in the granulocytes.

Chromosome-Specific Probes to Study Interphase Nuclei

New staining methods are under investigation that will permit chromosome analysis on interphase cells. These methods would permit the analysis of hundreds of interphase nuclei with little effort. Probes unique to each chromosome have been identified and can be labeled with fluorescent molecules to permit the identification of numerical abnormalities in interphase nuclei (28). This method may even be developed to the point where it is suitable to detect certain structural abnormalities of chromosomes (29). If this procedure proves useful and reliable, it may provide a simple and consistent technique that can be used to supplement routine chromosome studies.

References

1. Association of Cytogenetic Technologists. International cytogenetic laboratory directory. Pasadena, CA: The Association of Cytogenetic Technologists, 1989.
2. Dewald GW, Noel P, Dahl RJ, Spurbeck JL. Chromosome abnormalities in malignant hematologic disorders. Mayo Clin Proc 1985;60:675–689.
3. Mitelman F. Catalog of chromosome aberrations in cancer. 3rd ed. New York: Alan R Liss, 1988.
4. Trent JM, Kaneko Y, Mitelman F. Report of the Committee on Structural Chromosome Changes in Neoplasia. Cytogenet Cell Genet 1988;49:236–253.
5. Bennett JM, Catovsky D, Daniel MT, et al. Proposed revised criteria for the classification of acute myeloid leukemia: a report of the French-American-British Cooperative Group. Ann Intern Med 1985;103:620–625.
6. Bennett JM, Catovsky D, Daniel MT, et al. Proposals for the classification of the myelodysplastic syndromes. Br J Haematol 1982;51:189–199.
7. The Non-Hodgkin's Lymphoma Pathologic Classification Project. National Cancer Institute sponsored study of classifications of non-Hodgkin's lymphomas: summary and description of a working formulation for clinical usage. Cancer 1982;49: 2112–2135.
8. First International Workshop on Chromosomes in Leukaemia. Chromosomes in Ph^1-positive chronic granulocytic leukaemia. Br J Haematol 1978;39:305–309.
9. Second International Workshop on Chromosomes in Leukemia, 1979. Morphological analysis of acute promyelocytic leukemia (M3) and t(8;21); cytogenetic, morphologic, and clinical

correlations in acute nonlymphocytic leukemia with t(8q−;21q+); chromosomes in acute promyelocytic leukemia; chromosomes in preleukemia. Cancer Genet Cytogenet 1980;2:89–113.
10. Third International Workshop on Chromosomes in Leukemia, 1980. Chromosomal abnormalities in acute lymphoblastic leukemia: structural and numerical changes in 234 cases; clinical significance of chromosomal abnormalities in acute lymphoblastic leukemia; report on essential thrombocythemia. Cancer Genet Cytogenet 1981;4:95–142.
11. Fourth International Workshop on Chromosomes in Leukemia, 1982. A prospective study of acute nonlymphocytic leukemia. Cancer Genet Cytogenet 1984; 11: 249–360.
12. Fifth International Workshop on Chromosomes in Leukemia-Lymphoma. Correlation of chromosome abnormalities with histologic and immunologic characteristics in non-Hodgkin's lymphoma and adult T cell leukemia-lymphoma. Blood 1987;70:1554–1564.
13. Pierre RV, Catovsky D, Mufti GJ, et al. Clinical-cytogenetic correlations in myelodysplasia (preleukemia). (Sixth International Workshop on Chromosomes on Leukemia, 1987.) Cancer Genet Cytogenet 1989;40:149–161.
14. Garson OM, Hagemeijer A, Sakurai M, et al. Cytogenetic studies of 103 patients with acute myelogenous leukemia in relapse. (Sixth International Workshop on Chromosomes in Leukemia, 1987.) Cancer Genet Cytogenet 1989;40:187–202.
15. Arthur DC, Berger R, Golomb HM, et al. The clinical significance of karyotype in acute myelogenous leukemia. (Sixth International Workshop on Chromosomes in Leukemia, 1987.) Cancer Genet Cytogenet 1989;40:203–216.
16. Dewald GW, Davis MP, Pierre RV, O'Fallon JR, Hoagland HC. Clinical characteristics and prognosis of 50 patients with a myeloproliferative syndrome and deletion of part of the long arm of chromosome 5. Blood 1985;66:189–197.
17. Dewald GW, Brecher M, Travis LB, Stupca PJ. Twenty-six patients with hematologic disorders and X chromosome abnormalities: frequent idic(X)(q13) chromosomes and Xq13 anomalies associated with pathologic ringed sideroblasts. Cancer Genet Cytogenet 1989;42:173–185.
18. Davis MP, Dewald GW, Pierre RV, Hoagland HC. Hematologic manifestations associated with deletions of the long arm of chromosome 20. Cancer Genet Cytogenet 1984;12:63–71.
19. Knapp RH, Dewald GW, Pierre RV. Cytogenetic studies in 174 consecutive patients with preleukemic or myelodysplastic syndromes. Mayo Clin Proc 1985;60:507–516.
20. Swolin B, Weinfeld A, Westin J. A prospective long-term cytogenetic study in polycythemia vera in relation to treatment and clinical course. Blood 1988;72:386–395.
21. Johnson DD, Dewald GW, Pierre RV, Letendre L, Silverstein MN. Deletions of chromosome 13 in malignant hematologic disorders. Cancer Genet Cytogenet 1985;18:235–241.
22. Dewald GW, Jenkins RB. Cytogenetic and molecular genetic studies of patients with monoclonal gammopathies. In: Wiernik PH, Canellos GP, Kyle RA, Schiffer CA, eds. Neoplastic diseases of the blood. 2nd ed. New York: Churchill Livingstone, 1991:427–438.
23. Seemayer TA, Cavenee WK. Molecular mechanisms of oncogenesis. Lab Invest 1989;60:585–599.
24. Friend SH, Dryja TP, Weinberg RA. Oncogenes and tumor-suppressing genes. N Engl J Med 1988;318:618–622.
25. Dewald G, Allen JE, Strutzenberg DK, Pierre RV. A cytogenetic method for mailed-in bone marrow specimens for the study of hematologic disorders. Lab Med 1982;13:225–229.
26. Dewald GW, Broderick DJ, Tom WW, Hagstrom JE, Pierre RV. The efficacy of direct, 24-hour culture, and mitotic synchronization methods for cytogenetic analysis of bone marrow in neoplastic hematologic disorders. Cancer Genet Cytogenet 1985;18:1–10.
27. Dewald GW, Diez-Martin JL, Steffen SL, Jenkins RB, Stupca PJ, Burgert EO Jr. Hematologic disorders in 13 patients with acquired trisomy 21 and 13 individuals with Down syndrome. Am J Med Genet Suppl 1990;7:247–250.
28. Jenkins RB, LeBeau MM, Kraker WJ, et. al. Fluorescence in situ hybridization; a sensitive method for trisomy 8 detection in bone marrow specimens. Blood 1992;79:3307–3315.
29. LeBeau MM. Detecting genetic changes in human tumor cells: have scientists "gone fishing?" Blood 1993;81:1979–1983.

30 Solid Tumor Cytogenetics

V. Ramesh Babu and Thomas E. Carey

INTRODUCTION

Historical Perspective

The discovery of a consistent, specific chromosome abnormality in chronic myelogenous leukemia (CML) in 1960 by Nowell and Hungerford gave birth to the field of cancer cytogenetics. The visibly altered copy of chromosome 22 that they described became known as the Philadelphia chromosome (Ph). This marker, which is the result of a reciprocal translocation between chromosomes 9 and 22, is present in more than 95% of CML cases and is so commonly known that, even among noncytogeneticists and nonhematologists, the Philadelphia chromosome is regarded as pathognomonic for CML.

In the years following the description of the Philadelphia translocation in CML, multiple specific chromosome changes have been identified in various hematologic neoplasms. Some chromosome abnormalities are highly specific for a restricted set of malignant diseases; e.g., t(15;17)(q22;q11) is found in nearly all acute nonlymphocytic leukemias of the French-American-British (FAB) M3 type, but it has not been reported in other hematologic diseases (see Chapter 29). Other rearrangements—such as t(8;14), t(2;8), and t(8;22) involving the loci for *MYC* (c-myc) on chromosome 8 and the immunoglobulin genes on chromosomes 14, 2, and 22 originally observed in Burkitt's lymphoma—are common to several types of B-cell neoplasms.

Thus, as described in Chapter 29, specific chromosome changes can be used to distinguish tumors of a specific type (e.g., B-cell leukemias can be distinguished from T-cell leukemias by rearrangements affecting the immunoglobulin genes and the T-cell receptor genes, respectively). Specific chromosome rearrangements in some cases have also been shown to be independent prognostic indicators. For example, t(8;21)(q22;q22) is associated with a relatively good prognosis in acute nonlymphocytic leukemia, whereas t(4;11)(q21;q23) is associated with a poor prognostic outlook in acute lymphocytic leukemia and acute undifferentiated leukemia.

Applications of Tumor Cytogenetics

As indicated above, specific chromosome alterations are useful in classifying hematologic tumors according to type. They may also have prognostic significance and, perhaps most importantly, can provide essential clues to the location of genes associated with tumor development and progression. This chapter discusses specific chromosome rearrangements that have been identified in a variety of solid human tumors. By the end of the chapter, we hope to have conveyed to the reader how knowledge of the consistent chromosome abnormalities in solid tumors will serve as a map to the genes that are altered during the neoplastic process. We will illustrate how some cancer-associated chromosome abnormalities have already led to the isolation of genes and the identification of gene products that are not only important in the cancer process but are essential for normal cell growth and development. The elucidation of how gene expression is altered by chromosome rearrangement will provide the basis for predicting the clinical behavior of individual tumors and should lead to the development of novel strategies for cancer treatment and prevention.

METHODOLOGICAL CONSIDERATIONS

Although the role of chromosome changes in hematologic cancers is well established, until recently only a small proportion (6 to 13%) of cancer cytogenetic studies concerned solid tumors. Of these, the majority dealt with benign tumors and pediatric tumors which generally contain relatively few chromosome abnormalities. Therefore, by 1989 only 1% of the published cytogenetic reports about cancer dealt with common epithelial tumors or carcinomas, which represent 80% of all human cancers. Thus, cytogenetic analysis of the common malignant tumors is still in its early stages of development, but rapid progress is being made. Several factors impeded progress in the cytogenetic analysis of solid tumors. How these problems have been overcome is dealt with in the next section.

Complicating Factors in the Cytogenetic Analysis of Solid Tumors

To analyze chromosomal integrity with standard techniques, it is necessary to examine the cells during mitosis. However, in a significant proportion of solid tumors, the mitotic index is low, making it difficult to obtain sufficient mitotic cells for cytogenetic characterization. This is further complicated by the fact that epithelial tumors are surrounded by stromal components that limit access to the mitotic cancer cell populations. This difficulty in gaining access to the tumor cells often results in chromosome preparations that are fuzzy, incomplete, and less than optimal for complete characterization. Compounding these problems, solid tumors usually show multiple chromosome changes, many of which are complex and some of which have been unidentifiable. Solid tumors also frequently have high ploidy with near triploid or tetraploid counts or more, especially in more advanced tumors. Furthermore, carcinomas, which arise from epithelial surfaces such as the upper areodigestive tract, the gastrointestinal tract, the lower urogenital tract, and the skin, may be contaminated with microorganisms that can destroy even short-term cultures. Additionally, for a thorough cytogenetic examination, analysis of a minimum number of metaphases is necessary, and without adequate recovery of viable tumor cells, it is difficult to accurately determine the consensus karyotype. For many solid tumors, these problems have now been overcome with the development of more effective culture techniques. As a result, the field of solid cancer cytogenetics is expanding rapidly.

Advances in Culture Techniques for Cytogenetic Analysis of Solid Tumors

Advances in culture methodology include the careful selection by the surgeon of viable, uninfected tissue for culture; the adequate washing of tumor specimens with antibiotics, including antifungal agents, to prevent microbial outgrowth; improvements in disaggregation techniques; better media formulations for epithelial cells; use of feeder layers; a better understanding and application of growth factors and hormones; the use of decreased serum supplements for certain tumor types and increased serum supplements for others; and the development of methods for removing stromal cell contamination. For disaggregation of solid tumors, probably the most important advance has been in the commercial development of highly purified enzymes, such as collagenase, to break down tumor stroma without damaging the tumor cells. Early preparations contained other proteolytic enzymes that had detrimental effects on tumor cell viability. Currently available purified enzymes effectively digest stromal components and release viable tumor cells in large numbers for direct study and for in vitro cultivation. Other improvements have included modifications of culture media, such as supplementation with hormones, particularly hydrocortisone, insulin, and transferrin; the addition of trace elements such as selenium; and the appropriate use of growth factors in the culture media. The elimination of stromal cell contamination by selective trypsinization or by growing tumor cells in soft agar is important, as is the use of irradiated fibroblast feeder layers or the use of extracellular matrix materials such as collagen, fibronectin, or bovine endothelial matrix for better tumor cell attachment.

In addition to these improvements in culturing, techniques for better chromosome resolution, such as cell synchronization to increase the mitotic fraction, reducing the time of exposure to Colcemid to improve chromosome morphology, and the use of ethidium bromide to maximize chromosome length, have also played a role in obtaining better results in dealing with solid tumors.

In attempting the in vitro cultivation of solid tumors, it is important to recognize that methods that have worked for one histologic type are not necessarily effective on other tumor types. For example, standard culture media were ineffective for small cell carcinoma of the lung (SCLC), but great progress was made in the in vitro cultivation of this tumor type when a novel medium formulation was used. Use of the HITES medium—containing hydrocortisone, insulin, transferrin, estradiol, and selenium, with low (2.5%) or no serum—resulted in a 72% success rate for SCLC, which had previously been resistant to culture. For other tumor types such as squamous cell carcinoma (SCC), misunderstandings regarding their properties may have led to the widely held belief that these tumors were difficult if not impossible to grow in vitro. In fact, when appropriate techniques were employed, success rates exceeding 30% were routinely obtained in several laboratories. Explant techniques either on plastic or on irradiated feeder cell layers were most effective for this tumor. Squamous cells are nearly always substrate dependent, probably because they require attachment molecules for mobility and mitotic activity. Because the attachment to substrate is critical to success with SCC, the simple expedient of using only a small volume of media to cover primary explant cultures prevents the tumor fragments from floating away from the substrate and increases the opportunity for squamous cell outgrowth. Another important factor for cultivating SCC is the application of a satisfactory method for removing fibroblasts. Fibroblasts tend to outgrow the tumor cells in early mixed cultures, surrounding and sometimes undermining the epithelial islands. Removing fibroblasts with brief exposures to trypsin-EDTA while monitoring the culture under the microscope to ensure that tumor cells are not detaching eliminates this problem and increases the culture success rate. In some cases, we have also discovered tumor cell islands completely buried under sheets of fibroblasts. The tumor cells were not apparent when the culture was viewed under the microscope; if the fibroblasts had not been removed these tumor cultures might have been discarded.

Advantages Derived from Cultured Tumor Cells

Improved culture methods have increased not only the yield and quality of solid tumor karyotypes but also the accuracy of the characterization of the breakpoints and rearrangements. This is because, in many cases, the tumor cells persist in culture, making additional harvests possible. As a result, it is possible to accurately determine whether a chromosome is missing due to a random loss from a cell or because monosomy was one of the events in the genesis of the tumor. Similarly, persistent cell cultures can be harvested repeatedly to obtain early-metaphase chromosomes, which are more informative because they are longer and more bands can be clearly discerned.

Cells in culture provide excellent material for special chromosome staining techniques such as C-banding, Q-banding, and silver staining. These techniques are valuable for identifying rearranged chromosomes, for helping the cytogeneticist to determine breakpoints more accurately, for identifying centromeres, and for detecting dicentric chromosomes. Sometimes C-banding can even help to identify which chromosome of a pair is present in case of monosomy or to determine if both copies might be the same homologue as a result of loss that has been compensated for by duplication and nondisjunction of the remaining chromosome. Silver staining to detect the nucleolus organizing regions (NORs) of acrocentric chromosomes is valuable for determining if acrocentrics are involved in rearrangements and for distinguishing NORs from homogeneously staining regions (HSRs). This distinction is important because the latter are considered to be indicative of amplified genes. Examples of special staining techniques to identify rearranged chromosomes are provided in Chapter 25.

In vitro cultures also provide pure populations of tumor cells for studies to further investigate the mechanisms at work at the level of the DNA and RNA molecules in tumor cells with rearranged or deleted chromosomes. Just a few examples of such studies include (*a*) Southern analysis to detect and study amplified, mutated, or deleted genes, (*b*) restriction fragment length polymorphism (RFLP) analysis to investigate loss of alleles, (*c*) Northern analysis to detect abberant gene expression or inactivation of alleles, and (*d*) gene isolation and sequencing to determine the nature of mutations that alter genes or affect gene expression (see Chapters 26 through 29). Finally, cultured cells provide a test system for examining the cell biology associated with altered gene expression.

Controversy Over the Use of Cell Cultures

In spite of the many advantages gained through the use of cultured cells for studies of the genetic changes in cancer, there is controversy over the validity of the karyotypic changes that are defined using cultured cells. Some investigators suggest that culture conditions are not physiologic and may introduce selective pressures that result in clones of cells that are not representative of the in vivo tumor population. It has also been suggested that cells grown in culture are unstable and undergo frequent changes or continuous karyotypic evolution in vitro.

Addressing the Cell Culture Controversy

To analyze these objections, several points should be considered. As a starting point, it should be noted that following amniocentesis, short-term culture is employed for expanding mitotic cells to detect chromosome abnormalities in utero (see Chapter 27), yet accurate results are obtained consistently, suggesting that short-term culture does not routinely introduce karyotypic artifacts. With solid tumors, it is difficult to entirely eliminate some time in culture from the process of karyotyping tumors since it is necessary to harvest mitotic cells to observe the chromosomes in their condensed state. Nevertheless, in some cases it is possible to make "direct preparations" in which karyotypes are prepared from cells released directly from tumor tissue. Direct preparations can serve as controls for evaluating the effects of culture on the tumor populations by comparing results obtained by this method to those obtained after culture. To minimize the possible selective effects of in vitro culture, we have also used an "in situ" technique, in which metaphase spreads are prepared from relatively few mitotic cells in short-term cultures by directly treating primary cultures on coverslips with hypotonic solution. In addition, conventional harvests from very early cultures can also minimize selective or evolutionary effects of in vitro culture. If random chromosome aberrations arise as a result of in vitro culture, then in vitro events should accumulate with time in culture. To evaluate this, early preparations can be compared to early passages and to long-term cultures from the same tumors to document whether in vitro changes are significantly skewing the results. In our laboratories, we have observed only one example of an in vitro change or in vitro evolution during long-term culture. In a cell line that was studied repeatedly over a period that spanned more than 60 in vitro passages, a normal 7 was replaced by an i(7p). Results from direct preparations, in situ preparations on early cultures, and long-term culture have shown that the karyotypes obtained immediately or after days, weeks, and months of in vitro culture are remarkably consistent. Thus, in our experience, tumor cultures examined after different periods of time in culture nearly always contain the same chromosome rearrangements and the same numerical changes and, in most cases, even maintain similar fractions of near-diploid and near-tetraploid populations. Incidentally, we have also noted that when there are near-diploid and near-tetraploid populations within the same tumor, each population contains the same rearrangements, and they differ from one another only in copy number.

If in vitro culture selects for nonrepresentative cell populations with certain rearrangements, then there should be frequent discrepancies between in vitro and in vivo findings. In earlier studies of leukemias and lymphomas, when the chromosome abnormalities obtained from leukemia cell lines in long-term culture were compared to those found in marrow or blood samples from patients, the same consistent changes and rearrangements for each leukemic type were noted. For example, the original studies of Burkitt's lymphoma (BL) showed the same t(8;14) translocation in both fresh specimens and BL cell llnes.

If tumor cells grown in culture are not representative of the cells that persist in the patient, then we would expect that separate tumor samples from the same patient would represent different clones. When we examine karyotypes from cell cultures taken from primary tumors and metastatic or recurrent tumors from the same donors, the same clonal abnormalites are present in both primary and metastatic or recurrent cultures. (For examples of this type of analysis, see the discussion of chromosome changes in squamous carcinomas of the head and neck below). Taken together, these observations support the concept that in vitro cultures are a reasonable model of the in vivo tumor.

Molecular Allelotyping

It should become possible to determine the validity of karyotypic analyses on cultured cells by using new techniques such as molecular allelotyping and interphase cytogenetics by chromosome painting to confirm that the tumor cells in culture and in the tumor specimen have the same chromosome changes. In molecular allelotyping, DNA is harvested from tumor cells and normal cells and assessed for loss of restriction fragment length polymorphisms (RFLP). Multiple probes are used for each arm of the chromosome to detect loss of heterozygosity (LOH) that corresponds to chromosome deletion. This method has been used to great advantage by Bert Vogelstein and his colleagues to define chromosomal loci important in the genesis of colon carcinomas. Essential to this kind of analysis is good separation of normal and tumor tissue. If normal cells are included in the tumor DNA extractions, there will be significant loss of resolution.

Interphase Cytogenetics

Interphase cytogenetics or chromosome painting, which employs fluorescent, chromosome-specific probes, can be used on cells in interphase to identify individual chromosomes either in tissue sections or in cultures. As discussed above, it is not unusual to obtain only a few metaphase cells in some solid tumors, although there may be abundant interphase cells. In situ hybridization of chromosome-specific probes to the nuclei of nonmitotic cells makes it possible to examine the interphase cells for specific genetic changes. For numerical changes, repetitive satellite DNA probes that are specific for the centromere of a given chromosome can be used. This method is already effective for characterizing ploidy changes, trisomies, and monosomies, and it may become useful for identifying specific rearrangements as well. To detect specific translocations, a mixture of DNA probes for different arms of the chromosomes can be used. With such approaches, it will be possible to confirm that the findings that are identified and characterized on in vitro cultures preexisted the culture.

Premature Chromosome Condensation

Some authors have proposed another novel method of examining the chromosomes of tumor cells during interphase by using premature chromosome condensation. This method employs hybridization of cell suspensions from fresh tumor with a population of cultured mitotic cells that induce the interphase cells in the fresh tumor to undergo premature condensation of their chromatin. This method is still in the early stages of application, and it is not yet clear how effective it will be. Regardless of methodology, the final proof of the chromosome loci important in solid tumors will come from the summed results of multiple laboratories employing varieties of tests. In fact, the consistent and most important changes are already emerging in numerous solid tumor types.

CYTOGENETIC CHANGES IN SOLID TUMORS

Types of Cytogenetic Changes in Solid Tumors

In general, solid tumors have more numerous and more complicated chromosome changes than hematologic tumors. This may be because, by the time the initial diagnosis is made for solid tumors, the tumor has already advanced to a higher grade and stage than a comparable hematologic neoplasm. Alternatively, solid tumors may require more genetic changes to overcome the conditions that usually drive epithelial differentiation and restrict the growth of epithelial cells. Nevertheless, in a small number of solid tumors, there will be only one chromosome change at the time of diagnosis. To find the tumors with a sole abnormality, it is necessary to study a large series of tumors of a specific type. When such a single chromosome abnormality is encountered, it is regarded as a "primary" change. A chromosome change is also considered primary if it occurs with an appreciable frequency in a given tumor type. In the solid tumors, most primary changes are determined by the frequency of occurrence. All other changes are regarded as "secondary." Primary and secondary changes are implicated in tumor initiation and progression, respectively.

In contrast to hematologic neoplasms, in which the primary abnormalities are usually balanced translocations, the most common chromosome changes in solid tumors result either in the loss of genetic material (i.e., chromosome deletions or allelic losses) or in the gain of genetic material (i.e., trisomies of various chromosomes, duplication/amplification of chromosome segments, or amplification of activated oncogenes). The frequency and extent of ploidy change is often much greater in solid tumors than in hematologic tumors. In general, higher grade tumors tend to have polyploid karyotypes, which sometimes contain 100 or more chromosomes. It appears that all polyploid solid tumors have structural rearrangements. This is in contrast to the hyperdiploid karyotypes that have been observed in cases of acute lymphocytic leukemia in which there are more than 50 chromosomes without any visible structural changes.

Classification of Solid Tumors

Solid tumors can be classified in a variety of ways. They may be grouped by the cell of origin or tissue type (e.g., adenocarcinomas arise from glandular cells, transitional cell carcinomas from the transitional epithelium that lines the ureters and bladder, squamous cell carcinomas from stratified squamous epithelium of the skin and mucous membranes, and malignant melanomas from melanocytes). Alternatively, they may be classified by the site of origin (e.g., adenocarcinoma from breast and colon, transitional cell carcinoma from the bladder, and squamous cell carcinomas from a variety of sites such as lung, skin, mouth and throat, uterine cervix, vulva, and vagina). Finally, they may be organized by histopathology, i.e. by the degree of differentiation, pattern of infiltration, or appearance (e.g., clear cell carcinoma). However, tumors classified by site are not always histologically similar; for example, the major categories of malignant lung tumors include small cell carcinomas, squamous cell carcinomas, and adenocarcinomas. For the purposes of this chapter, we will classify the solid tumors as benign or malignant and then by histologic type and site. No attempt will be made to be exhaustive; rather, we will concentrate on tumors that have been relatively well characterized, and we will attempt to identify the genetic changes that are most consistent or characteristic for a given tumor type.

Chromosome Alterations in Benign Tumors

After the long history of cytogenetic evaluation in leukemias, in which normal karyotypes frequently prevailed even in known leukemic states, a surprising observation in the cytogenetics of benign tumors was that chromosome abnormalities could be identified in a high proportion of cases. More importantly, specific chromosome changes could be described for several benign tumors. Perhaps even more surprising in the study of malignant neoplasms is the fact that several types of benign tumors were studied effectively before significant progress was made with malignant tumors. This is surprising because benign tumors are more generally more difficult to cultivate than malignant tumors. The more rapid progress made with benign tumors is thus most likely due to the greater complexity and number of chromosomal abnormalities usually encountered in the common malignant solid tumors. Although the solid tumor types presented a daunting challenge only a few years ago, excellent progress is now being made, and consistent chromosome changes are now being identified in the common carcinomas as well as in the benign tumor types (Table 30.1).

Meningiomas

Of the benign tumors, meningiomas are one of the types most extensively studied by cytogenetic analysis. The majority of meningiomas have a simple

Table 30.1. Characteristic Chromosome Changes in Human Solid Tumors[a]

Tumor Type	Chromosome Rearrangement	Incidence
		%
Rhabdomyosarcoma	t(2;13)(q37;q14)	?
Bladder carcinoma	Structural changes of 1	30
	i(5p)	20
	Trisomy 7	22
	Monosomy 9 or deletion 9q	37
	11p deletion	42
	6q deletion	20
Breast carcinoma	Structural changes of 1	80
	t/deletion (16q)	20
Ewing's sarcoma/Askin's tumor/neuroepithelioma	t(11;22)(q24;q12)	>90
Glioma	dmin (EGF receptor)	50
	9p rearrangements	
Kidney carcinoma	t/deletion (3)(p11–p21)	80
	t(5;14)(q13;q22)	?
Large bowel carcinoma	Structural changes of 1	20
	Trisomy 7	30
	Trisomy 12	10
	Structural changes of 17	?
Lipoma (benign)	t(1,3,21;12)(p33,q28,q12;q13–q14)	50
Liposarcoma (malignant, myxoid type)	t(12;16)(q13–q14;q11)	?
Malignant melanoma	t/deletion (1)(p12–p22)	60
	t(1;19)(q12;p13)	?
	t/deletion (6q)/i(6p)	80
	Trisomy 7	50
Meningioma	Monosomy 22, del(22q), t(14;22)	>90
Neuroblastoma	deletion (1)(p31–p32)	70
	HSR/dmin (n-myc)	70
Ovarian carcinoma	Structural changes of 1	80
	t(6;14)(q21;q24)/deletion 6q	?
Pleomorphic adenoma	t(3;8)(p21q12)	50
	t/deletion (8)(q12)	50
	t/deletion (12)(q13–q15)	20
Prostatic adenocarcinoma	deletion (7)(q22)	?
	deletion (10)(q24)	?
	Trisomy 7	?
Retinoblastoma	Structural changes of 1	50
	i(6p)	30
	deletion (13)(q14)/−13	20
Small cell lung cancer	deletion (3)(p14p23)	>90
Squamous cell carcinoma (head and neck)	loss 3p, 4p, 8p21–p22, 18q22–qter	≥70
	loss 1c-p22,9p,10p,13q12–q14	50–70
Squamous cell carcinoma (vulva)	loss 3c-p14, 8p, 22q13, inactXp	80
Synovial sarcoma	i(X;18)(p11;q11)	?
Testicular teratoma/seminoma	i(12p)	90
Uterine carcinoma	Structural and numerical changes of 1	80
Uterine leiomyoma	t(12;14)(q14-15;q22-q24)	?
Wilms' tumor	Structural changes of 1	50
	t/deletion (11)(p13)	30

[a]Adapted from Heim S, Mitelman F, eds. Cancer cytogenetics. New York: Alan R Liss, 1987:229. Copyright © 1987, Wiley-Liss.

monosomy 22 or deletion of the long arm of 22. However, other nonrandom changes include loss of chromosomes 8, 14, 17, and Y. In addition, translocation involving chromosomes 22 and 14 has been reported. It appears that most meningiomas start out with a normal karyotype, then the change arises in chromosome 22 and subsequently the tumors acquire additional changes. These later changes are observed mostly in recurrent tumors of advanced grade and poorly organized histology.

Acoustic Neuromas

Acoustic neuromas have also been linked to a locus on chromosome 22. This tumor type occurs in both a sporadic form in which tumors are unilateral and a familial form characterized by bilateral tumors. The familial form is also referred to as bilateral acoustic neurofibromatosis or neurofibromatosis type 2 (NF-2). Initially, NF-2 was thought to be a variant of von Recklinghausen's disease, which is also called neurofibromatosis type 1 (NF-1). However, studies of families with NF-2 have shown that acoustic neuromas are genetically more closely linked to meningiomas than to NF-1. There are two sets of evidence for this distinction. First, some members of the NF-2 pedigrees also develop meningioma, but individuals with NF-1 do not develop acoustic neuromas. Second, consistent loss of alleles from the region of chromosome 22 affected in the meningioma tumors has also been documented in tumor DNA from patients with bilateral acoustic neuroma, even though cytogenetic evidence linking chromosome 22 to acoustic neuromas is sparse.

Neurofibromatosis Type 1 (von Recklinghausen's Disease)

Consistent chromosome changes have not been observed in tumors from patients with von Recklinghausen's neurofibromatosis (NF-1). However, using constitutional chromosome 17 translocations in two unrelated individuals with NF-1 as a guide, the gene locus for NF-1 has been mapped to chromosome 17q11.2 through molecular genetic and linkage analysis.

Benign Salivary Gland Tumors

Cytogenetic changes in pleomorphic adenoma of the salivary gland are frequently observed and are relatively well characterized. A specific rearrangement t(3;8)(p21;q12) is the most common change in these myxoid salivary gland tumors, and chromosome 8 band q12 is the most common site of change. However, at least three subsets of characteristic rearrangements seem to exist. These include rearrangements (deletions, translocations, and other changes) involving the regions 3p21, 8q21, and 12q13–q15.

Lipomas

Of the benign tumors that have been well studied, lipomas exhibit the greatest heterogeneity. At least three and possibly four different groups of tumors have been identified: tumors with normal karyotypes, tumors with no rearrangements but numerical changes (usually chromosome losses), tumors with abnormalities of 12q involving a translocation of 12 and another chromosome; and tumors with other clonal changes. Recent studies of a large cohort of tumors revealed that clonal changes are present in about 50% of tumors. Translocations involving region q13–q15 of chromosome 12 and a variety of other chromosomes have been identified most frequently. Translocations t(1;12)(p33;q14),t(3;12)(q28;q14), and t(12;21)(q13;q12) were all observed in three to five tumors each, with t(3;12) being the most common. Complex rearrangements involving region 12(q13–q15) and several other chromosomes have also been observed. Other clonal abnormalities not involving chromosome 12 included rearrangements of 13q, most commonly del(13)(q12–q22), translocations affecting 11q13, and rearrangements of 6p21–p23.

Adenomas of the Colon

The vast majority of adenomas of the colon and rectum have diploid karyotypes, in contrast to the higher ploidy often found in adenocarcinomas of the colon. Even in nondiploid benign tumors of the colon, no specific changes have been identified in cytogenetic studies. This is most likely due to the poor quality of most preparations and the complex rearrangements present. Recurrent numerical changes have been noted, including trisomies of 7, 8, 13, and 14. More recent studies, guided by an interstitial deletion of 5q in a patient with familial adenomatous polyposis (FAP, also called familial polyposis coli or FPC), led to the discovery of a polymorphism for an anonymous DNA probe (c11p11) linked to affected family members in six informative FAP families. These studies localized the FAP/FPC gene to 5q21–q22. Subsequent studies of colon carcinomas showed that 20% of malignant tumors also had loss of alleles on chromosome 5q. Because FAP is a predisposing condition for colon carcinoma, these findings support the concept that 5q is a locus for a predisposing cancer gene. Molecular genetic studies of individual adenomas and polyps of the nonfamilial type and colon carcinomas have helped to clarify additional chromosomal loci that are important in colon cancer. These studies, pioneered by Bert Vogelstein and his collegues, have also helped to define the changes that occur during the progression from adenomas and polyps to invasive cancer.

Leiomyomas

Few studies exist for uterine leiomyomas. Although the majority of these neoplasms have normal karyotypes, a specific translocation, t(12;14)(q14–q15;q22–q24), has been identified. Other changes affecting chromosomes 12 and 14 are also common.

At the present, there is little information available to clarify the basis for these consistent changes in benign tumors. However, the combination of cytogenetic studies and molecular genetic studies is rapidly closing these gaps in our knowledge.

Chromosome Alterations in Embryonal and Pediatric Malignant Tumors

Several tumors, including Wilms' tumor (or embryonal nephroblastoma), retinoblastoma, Ewing's sarcoma, neuroblastoma, and rhabdomyosarcoma, make up this group. Unlike many tumors of adult life, these tumors are not the result of long-term accumulation of genetic damage from carcinogens; therefore, they have been heavily studied to detect the primary changes associated with tumor induction. This study has paid off reasonably well and in fact has provided important insight into the molecular mechanisms responsible for cancer.

RETINOBLASTOMA, THE KNUDSON HYPOTHESIS, AND TUMOR SUPPRESSOR GENES

Important progress toward understanding what appears to be a central genetic mechanism in the genesis of malignant solid tumors began with the study of retinoblastoma, a common pediatric tumor. The primary driving force for genetic studies in this tumor came from what has been termed the Knudson hypothesis, first articulated by Alfred Knudson in the early 1970s and based on observations of patients with retinoblastoma. In this section, we provide the basic cytogenetic data on retinoblastoma; the combination of cytogenetic data, familial inheritance patterns, distributions of affected individuals that led Knudson to formulate his hypothesis that two hits are necessary for tumor induction; and the molecular genetic analysis that proved Knudson to be right. This model is central to our current understanding of one of the most important mechanisms in cell transformation, loss of tumor suppressor function.

Retinoblastoma

The important locus in retinoblastoma was first identified because constitutional deletions of the long arm of chromosome 13 were detected in certain unrelated individuals with mental retardation, multiple congenital anomalies, and bilateral retinoblastoma. Although the deletions were of different sizes, band 13q14 was common among the deleted regions, suggesting that this was the locus of the gene that predisposes retinoblastoma. Cytogenetic analysis of retinoblastoma tumor cells, including about 20% of nonsyndromic sporadic cases, also revealed chromosomal deletions involving 13q14. Other common changes in retinoblastoma are isochromosome 6p and abnormalities of chromosome 1. However, the primary chromosomal change in retinoblastoma is loss of band 13q14.

The Knudson Hypothesis

In addition to the syndromic and sporadic cases, retinoblastoma also occurs in a hereditary form. Because enucleation of the affected eye has been an effective treatment for retinoblastoma for many years, it has been possible to examine the offspring of affected individuals. The hereditary pattern in retinoblastoma is autosomal dominant with a high penetrance. The tumors tend to occur earlier in life in hereditary cases than in sporadic cases, and the hereditary tumors tend to be bilateral or multifocal, whereas the sporadic types are unifocal. Based on these observations, Knudson proposed that there must be two events that lead to the development of these cancers. In the hereditary form, the first event or predisposing mutation is transmitted from one of the parents and is carried in all somatic cells of the affected offspring. Therefore, since not all cells of the body become tumorigenic, the second mutation must be a rare event even in hereditary and bilateral cases. Knudson reasoned that the second mutation must occur at the same genetic locus and similarly affect the remaining wild-type allele in the target somatic cell. In the sporadic cases, he postulated, a single somatic cell must undergo both rare events, which would explain why such tumors develop late and are unifocal. Subsequent studies have proved this hypothesis to be correct and have identified the genetic locus that is affected by these two events. Further studies have extended this hypothesis to other tumors and to other genetic loci as well.

Molecular Genetic Events in Retinoblastoma

In a tour de force of molecular genetic analysis carried out during the mid-1980s, Webster Cavenee and his collaborators demonstrated that the molecular events in retinoblastoma begin with a mutation or deletion that inactivates the *RB1* gene located in chromosome band 13q14. This is followed by mutation or loss of the wild-type allele from the other chromosome 13 as predicted. In a few cases, the first event is a deletion like that represented by the deleted chromosome 13 observed in children born with the syndromic effects and predisposition to retinoblastoma. In most cases, however, the first event is an invisible change, often a point mutation, and the second event is inactivation or loss of the remaining normal allele from the other chromosome. As a result, the chromosomal abnormality that we see in the 20% of tumors with chromosome 13q deletions is the evidence of the second event, namely the deletion of the chromosome carrying the normal allele. Ironically, the remaining apparently normal copy of chromosome 13 is the one with the mutated gene. The chromosomal mechanisms that have been demonstrated to be involved in retinoblastoma by the loss of heterozygosity for alleles adjacent to 13q14 are illustrated in Figure 30.1.

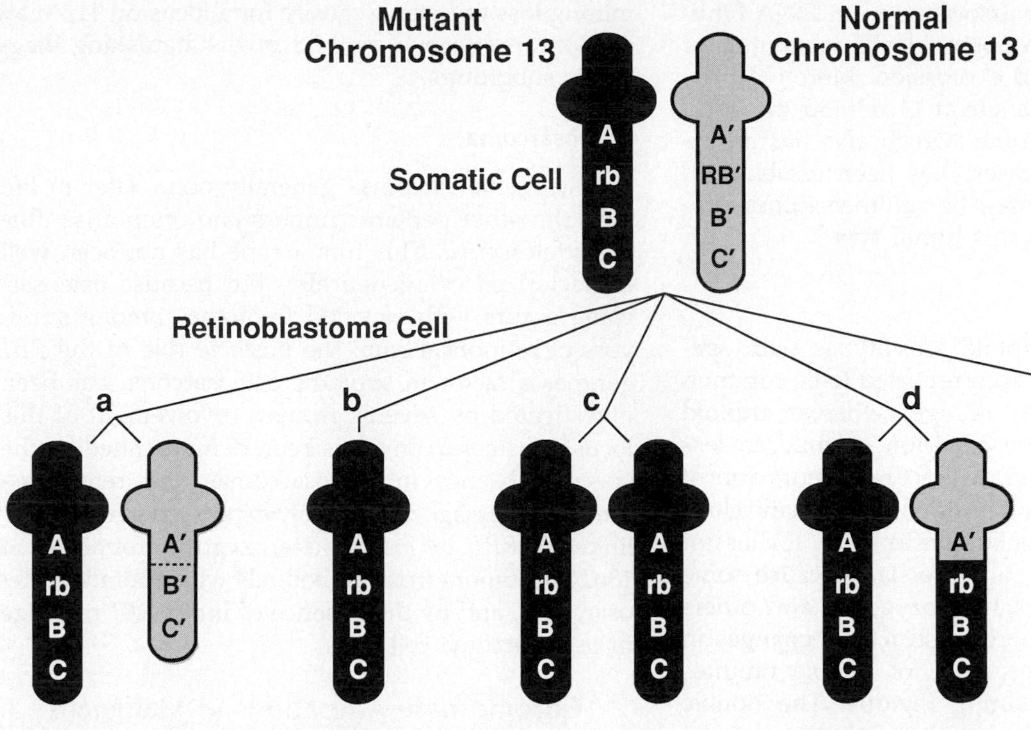

Figure 30.1. Chromosomal mechanisms leading to loss of the *RB* gene in retinoblastoma. The first event is a recessive inactivating mutation of the retinoblastoma gene shown as rb. The second event is the loss of the normal allele, shown as RB′, from the other chromosome. The chromosomal mechanisms include (a) loss of part of the normal chromosome 13 (deletion); (*b*) all of the normal chromosome 13 (monosomy); (c) loss of normal 13 and duplication of the abnormal 13 (appears as disomy); (*d*) mitotic recombination resulting in homozygosity for the distal portion of chromosome 13, including the abnormal rb allele (appears as disomy); and (e) point mutation or gene conversion at the corresponding (13q14) locus (appears as disomy). Each of these events has been demonstrated in retinoblastoma families by analysis of restriction fragment polymorphisms for multiple loci on 13q. Of these mechanisms, cytogenetic studies can detect only the first two (chromosome deletion or loss), which explains why only a relatively small proportion of tumors have visible chromosome 13 abnormalities. (Adapted from Cavenee WK, Dryja TP, Phillips RA, et al. Expression of recessive alleles by chromosomal mechanisms in retinoblastoma. Nature 1983;305:779–784. Reprinted with permission.)

RB1—The Prototype Tumor-Suppressor Gene

Tumor genes that, like the retinoblastoma gene, have a mutated gene that is recessive to the normal allele have been termed tumor-suppressor genes. Generally, when there are consistently deleted regions in tumors, it raises the possibility that a tumor-suppressor gene may be included within the deleted region. The molecular mechanisms by which tumor suppressor genes are involved in neoplasia have now been partially elucidated. These mechanisms and the importance of replacing the defective gene in tumor cells will be discussed further in the significance section.

Wilms' tumor

Wilms' tumor, or nephroblastoma, is similar to retinoblastoma in that there are two forms, a sporadic form and a form associated with congenital syndromes, in which constitutional deletion of 11p has been described. In tumor cells, deletion of 11p, structural changes of chromosomes 1 and 16, and duplication of chromosomes 9 and 12 are found. As in the case of retinoblastoma, chromosome abnormalities associated with the congenital syndromes have been important in identifying a specific chromosomal site, chromosome 11p, as the site of tumor-specific deletions and of a possible tumor-suppressor gene or genes.

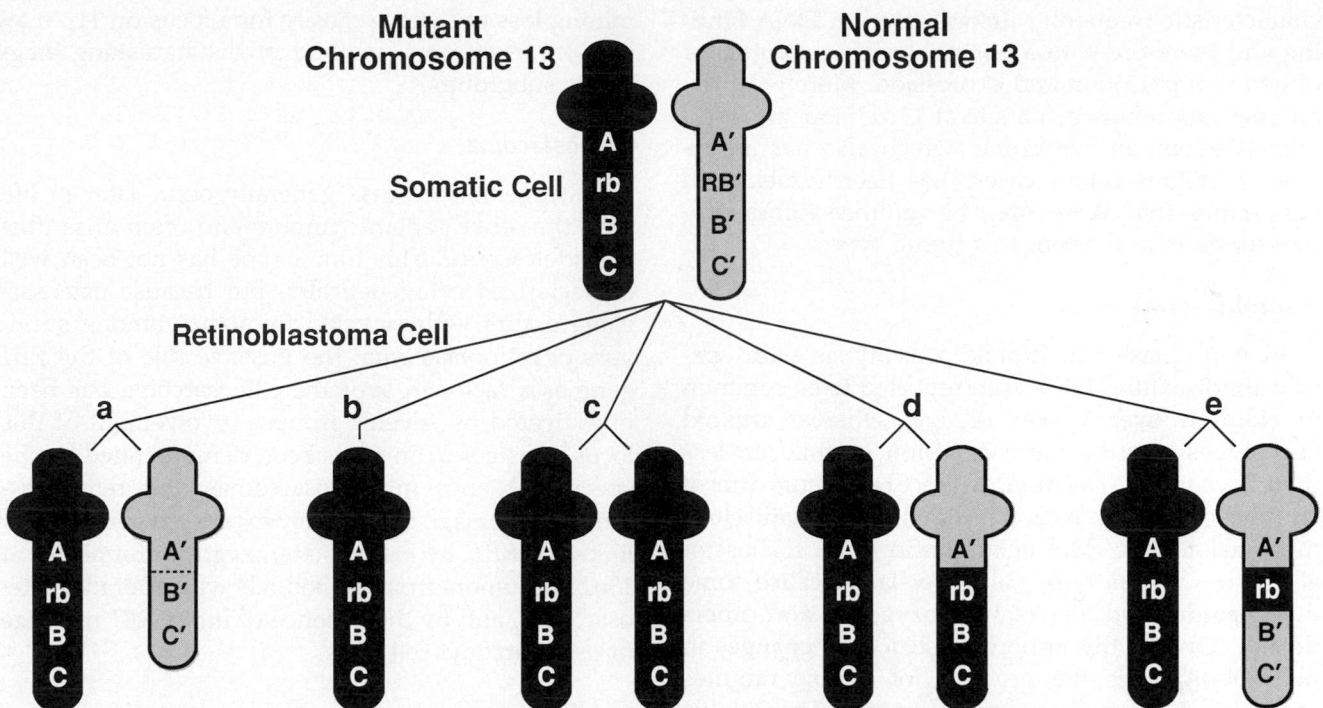

Wilms' tumor occurs with greatly increased frequency in children born with either of two congenital syndromes. The first syndrome, which includes Wilms' tumor, aniridia, genitourinary anomalies, and mental retardation (WAGR), provided the evidence for 11p13 as the likely site of a deleted gene in Wilms' tumor. Affected individuals with WAGR often have a deletion of 11p with the smallest region of overlap corresponding to band 11p13. Analysis of normal and tumor DNA using restriction fragment length polymorphisms has demonstrated consistent loss of heterozygosity for alleles mapped to 11p13, and now a candidate tumor-suppressor gene, *WT1*, has been isolated. This *WT1* gene, which is expressed in normal kidney but is homozygously deleted from a number of Wilms' tumors, has sequences that encode zinc finger regions. This is a characteristic frequently associated with DNA binding and therefore with a potential role as a regulator of gene transcription and expression. More recently, an association between a site at 11p15 and the Beckwith-Wiedemann syndrome, which also has an excess of Wilms' tumor cases, has been established, suggesting that there may be another tumor-suppressor gene at work in this tumor type.

Neuroblastoma

In neuroblastoma, diploid karyotypes with specific abnormalities have been reported to be common in children over 1 year of age, whereas triploid karyotypes may be more common in children less than 1 year old. Deletion of the distal short arm of chromosome 1 has been identified as a specific chromosomal change. Molecular confirmation for loss of alleles on 1p has been controversial, because some investigators find loss of heterozygosity and others do not. One of the important structural changes in neuroblastoma is the presence of double minutes and homogeneously staining regions. The double minutes are associated with amplification of the protooncogene *MYCN* (N-myc). More recently, autonomously replicating submicroscopic episomes have also been identified that carry amplified copies of this oncogene. There is a correlation of amplification of *MYCN* with the chromosome 1 deletion. This is surprising because this oncogene is mapped to chromosome 2, and no consistent change has been specifically defined there. *MYCN* amplification and 1p deletion are associated with a poor prognosis.

Ewing's Sarcoma, Rhabdomyosarcoma, and Neuroendocrine Tumors

Duplication of the long arm of chromosome 1 is a frequent change in each of these embryonal tumors. In Ewing's sarcoma, a specific translocation, t(11;22)(q23–q24;q11–q12), has been described in more than 90% of tumors. An indistinguishable translocation has been identified in two other neuroendocrine tumors: Askin's tumor and neuroepithelioma. An unbalanced translocation, t(1;16), may be a secondary change in some Ewing's sarcomas.

In rhabdomyosarcoma, t(2;13)(q37;q14) was originally described as a specific change for the alveolar subtype. Because tumors of the alveolar and embryonal types have different clinical behavior, an objective marker would be an important diagnostic indicator in tumors with indeterminant histologic features. In one study, however, the same translocation has been observed in advanced tumors of both alveolar and embryonal subtypes. Rearrangements affecting the 3p14 region are also common in rhabdomyosarcomas. Molecular analysis suggests that determining loss of heterozygosity for a locus on 11p may be a more effective method of distinguishing diagnostic subgroups.

Osteosarcoma

Osteogenic sarcomas generally occur later in life than the other pediatric tumors and often arise during adolescence. This tumor type has not been well characterized cytogenetically, but because osteosarcoma occurs with elevated frequency among survivors of retinoblastoma, the possible role of the *RB1* gene as a factor in sporadic osteosarcoma has been investigated by several groups. Involvement of this locus in osteosarcoma has been demonstrated by the specific absence in osteosarcomas and retinoblastomas of message for a widely expressed gene closely linked to *RB1*, by loss of heterozygosity for alleles at 13q14 in tumors from individuals with sporadic osteosarcoma, and by the absence of intact *RB1* message in osteosarcoma cell lines.

Chromosome Alterations in Malignant Tumors of Adults

Testicular Tumors

Testicular tumors for which there are cytogenetic data include teratomas and seminomas. Isochromosome 12p has been observed in more than 90% of these tumors, and this characteristic change is usually present in one extra copy, although several tumors have been described with multiple copies of i(12p).

Bladder Cancer

Transitional cell carcinomas of the bladder are a heterogeneous group of tumors. Reflecting the heterogeneity of tumor grade (1 to 4) and stage (noninvasive to invasive), several nonrandom chromosome changes have been identified in bladder cancer. Isochromosome 5p or deletion 5q, monosomy 9 or deletion 9q, trisomy 7, and deletion of the short arm of 11 are the more common changes (Fig. 30.2). Other changes such as trisomy 20, 13, or 15; deletion of the long arm of 6, 10, and 21; or duplication of 1q and 3p have been reported. In general, low-grade, noninvasive tumors have near-diploid karyotypes and high-grade, invasive tumors have polyploid karyotypes with multiple marker chromosomes. Bladder cancer is one of the best-studied human cancers in terms of clinical heterogeneity, and histopathologically similar tumors have divergent karyotypes with different tumor behavior (prognosis). RFLP analysis has confirmed that LOH is most commonly found, affecting 9q, 17p, and, to a lesser extent, 11p.

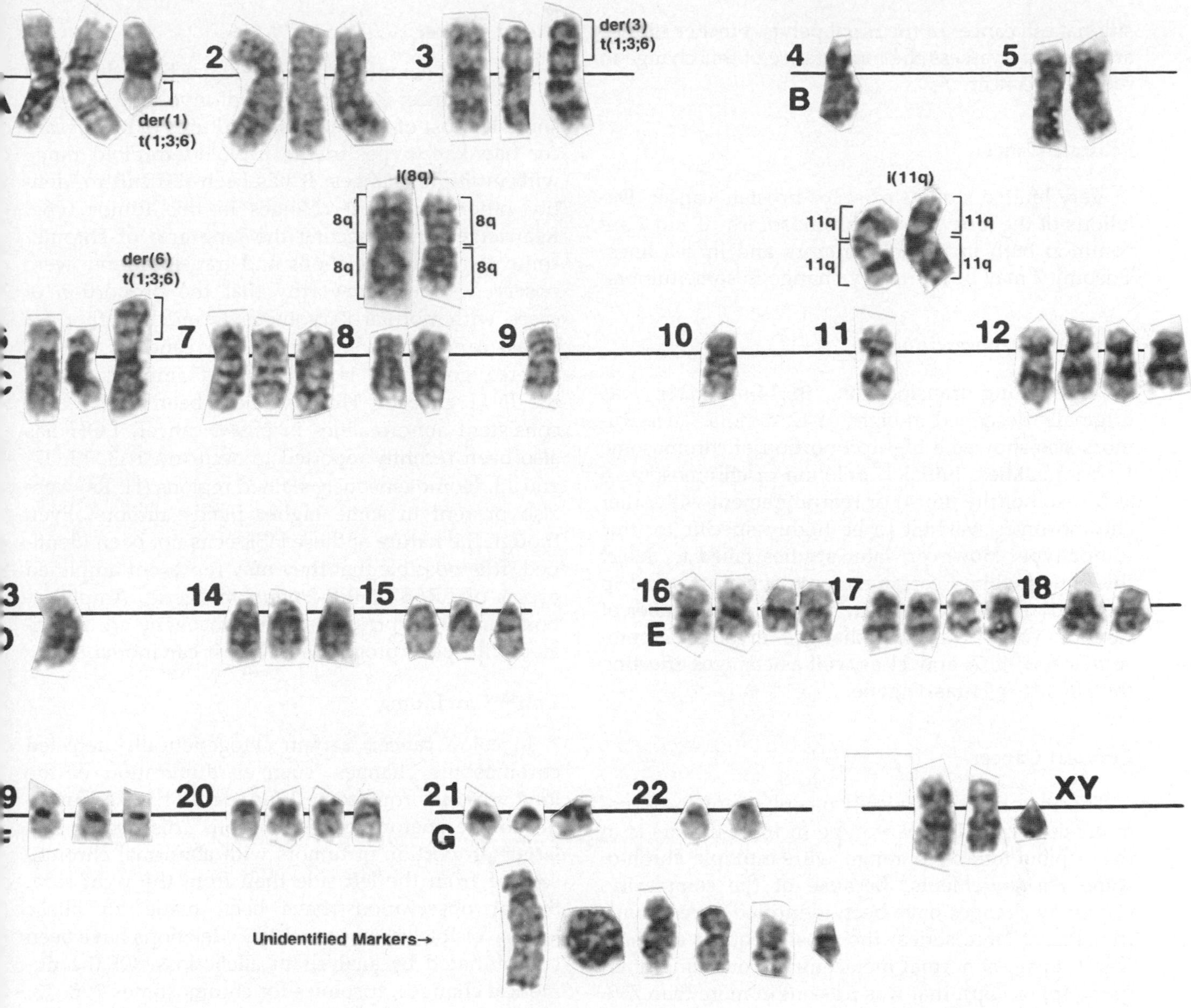

Figure 30.2. Near tetraploid karyotype of an invasive grade 3 bladder carcinoma showing representative hanges associated with this tumor type. Structural abnormalities include a t(1;3;6)(q21;p14;p23), two i(8q)s, and two i(11q)s. This cell also contains six unidentified markers. In other cells from this tumor, the der(1) and der(3) chromosomes are lost and, in additon to the der(6), there are three or four normal 3s and two or three normal 6s. Note also that there is only one identifiable copy of 4, 9, 10, 11p, and 13, as well as only two copies of 5, 18, and 22 against a tetraploid background. These changes suggest that loss of genetic material may had occurred at these sites, which are commonly involved in other solid tumors. (Reprinted with permission from Babu VR, Lutz MD, Miles DJ, Farah RN, Weiss L, Van Dyke DL. Tumor behavior in transitional cell carcinoma of the bladder in relation to chromosomal markers and histology. Cancer Res 1987;47:6800–6805.)

Renal Cell Carcinoma

In one family, a specific constitutional rearrangement, t(3;8)(p21;q24), was strongly associated with the development of renal cell carcinoma. In these cases, the *MYC* oncogene located on chromosome 8 was translocated to chromosome 3. This suggested the involvement of chromosome 3 as a primary site of chromosome change in renal cell cancer. Subsequent cytogenetic analysis of tumor cells from other patients revealed deletions and translocations involving the region 3p11–21, confirming the role of 3p genes in the genesis of this tumor type. The common region of overlap for the deletions was 3p13 to 3pter. The finding of 3p deletions as sole abnormalities in a few tumors and loss of 3p alleles by molecular genetic studies adds further evidence for the role of 3p genes, perhaps by loss of one or more tumor suppressor genes in the etiology of this cancer.

A nonreciprocal translocation t(5;14)(q13;q22) that results in the deletion of 14q has been observed in two different renal tumors: renal cell cancer and transitional cell cancer of the renal pelvis. Further studies are needed to assess the importance of this change in renal cell cancer.

Prostate Cancer

Very limited studies exist for prostate cancer. Deletions of the long arm of chromosomes 10 and 7 are common both in primary tumors and in cell lines. Trisomy 7 may be a primary change in some tumors.

Ovarian Adenocarcinoma

A recurring translocation, t(6;14)(q21;q24), was originally described in eight of 12 tumors. These tumors also showed a high proportion of chromosome 1 abnormalities. Initially, deletion of chromosome 6 as a result of the t(6;14) or rearrangement with other chromosomes was felt to be highly specific for this tumor type. However, later studies failed to detect this abnormality. Rearrangements of chromosome 3p have now been observed in a significant number of tumors. Other common changes involve chromosomes X, 1, 3, 7, and 11 as well as changes affecting the *HRAS1* (c-H-ras-1) gene.

Cervical Cancer

The majority of cervical cancers are of the squamous cell type. The karyotype in most tumors is in the triploid/tetraploid range with multiple chromosome rearrangements. Because of the complexity, not many changes have been identified as recurrent. In a recent large series, the most frequent anomaly was a small, abnormal metacentric, consisting of either i(4p) or i(5p), that was present in more than 75% of tumors. Loss of 1p or i(1q) was present in two-thirds of cases, and translocations of 1q to the short arms of chromosomes 17 and 11 were also observed.

Endometrial Carcinoma

As in many of the solid tumors, the initial changes in these tumors were thought to involve mostly chromosome 1. Subsequent studies in a small number of tumors have identified several chromosomal locations that appear to be quite consistent. These include deletions of distal 18q, rearrangements with breakpoints involving the short arm of chromosome 22, and breakpoints involving 12q. Loss of chromosome 4, deletion 9q and 13q, and a breakpoint on 8p may be associated with aggressive tumors. An example of a karyotype from an endometrial carcinoma containing the common changes is shown in Figure 30.3.

Breast Cancer

The most common change that has been described in breast cancer is rearrangement involving chromosome 1. Most of the successful cultures of breast cancer had karytoypes in the triploid/tetraploid range with multiple changes. It has been difficult to identity other consistent changes in this tumor type. Rearrangements affecting the long arm of chromosome 16, mostly deletions and translocations, were observed. It is noteworthy that the proportion of cases with normal karyotypes is much higher for breast cancer than for most other cancers. Loss of heterozygosity for 11p alleles and amplification of the *INT2* gene on 11q have both been reported as consistent abnormalities in breast cancer. LOH has also been recently reported to occur on 1, 3, 13, 17, and 18. Homogeneously stained regions (HSRs) were also present in some higher ploidy tumors. Even though the nature of these HSRs has not been identified, it is possible that they may represent amplified copies of *ERB*B2 (HER-2/neu) oncogene. Amplification and overexpression of this oncogene are associated with poor prognosis in breast carcinoma.

Colon Carcinoma

In colon cancer, certain cytogenetically detected chromosome changes, such as duplication of the long arm of chromosome 1, appear to have a disproportionate anatomical distribution. This results in a larger proportion of tumors with abnormal chromosome 1 from the left side than from the right side. Similar observations have been made for allelic losses. Visible chromosome 1p35 deletions have been substantiated by analysis of allelic loss. Of the numerical changes, trisomies for chromosomes 7, 8, 13, 19, 20, and 21 and monosomy 17 and 18 are very common, as are relative deficiencies of 17 and 18. Of the structural changes, deletion of the short arm of chromosome 17 is common, followed by 20q+ and 1p−. Deletions and loss of heterozygosity (LOH) for alleles on 5q in the region thought to contain the locus for familial polyposis coli is also observed in a lower proportion of tumors. Point mutations of the *RAS* oncogene have been identified as early changes in colon cancer. Recently, Bert Vogelstein and his colleagues have performed molecular alleleotyping using multiple syntenic probes for each chromosome and carefully microdissected tissue sections from polyps, adenomas, and colon cancers to identify a series of genetic changes that corroborate the cytogenetic findings from multiple studies. In particular, LOH of 17p and 18q affecting the loci for the *p53* and *DDC* (deleted in colon cancer) genes, respectively, are very common abnormalities.

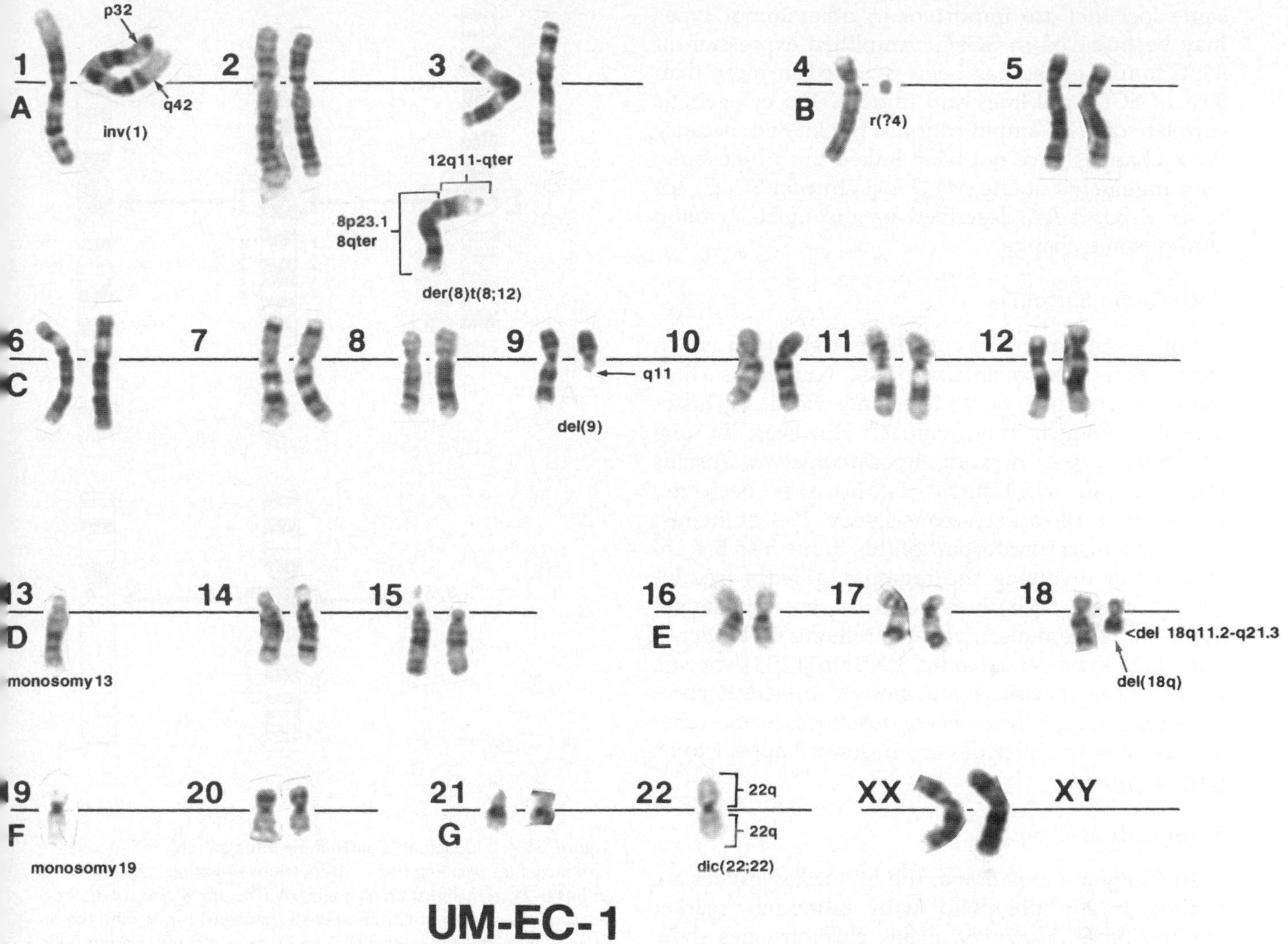

Figure 30.3. Karyotype from a hypodiploid endometrial carcinoma demonstrating several consistent changes found in this tumor type. Note that there is monosomy 4, 13, and 19. In addition, there is a pericentric inversion of chromosome 1, deletion of 9q, deletion of 18q, and isochromosome or Robertsonian fusion 22q. There is also a der(8)t(8;12)(p23.1;q22). The small ring chromosome found in about half the cells is most likely derived from chromosome 4. (Reprinted with permission from Grenman SE, Van Dyke DL, Worsham MJ, et al. UM-EC-1, a new hypodiploid human cell line derived from a poorly differentiated endometrial cancer. Cancer Res 1988;48:1864–1887.)

Gastric Cancer

Relatively few studies have been done with gastric cancer. Structural and numerical changes of chromosomes 8 and 9 are common. In a few cases, trisomy 12 was observed as the sole abnormality. Structural changes of 1p, 3p, and 19p are also frequent.

Lung Cancers

The most extensive cytogenetic studies in lung cancer have been carried out on oat cell or small cell lung carcinomas (SCLC), which is one of three major histologic types at this site. In addition to SCLC, which accounts for 35 to 60% of lung cancers, squamous cell carcinoma and adenocarcinoma are also prevalent tumor types. SCLC is the best studied cytogenetically because cell culture methods developed by Adi Gazdar, John Minna and their co-workers made tumor cells from many patients available for study. Using these cultures, Jacqueline Whang-Peng identified a deletion of the short arm of chromosome 3 as a highly consistent change in SCLC cell lines. This change has been shown by molecular genetic studies to be present in primary tumors as well. Later studies have demonstrated that chromosome 3 deletions are not specific for SCLC, but are also found in non–small cell lung cancers and are also consistent abnormalities in squamous cancers at other sites. Some other nonrandom changes, such as abnormalities of chromosomes 1, 6, and 11, have also been described as being common in SCLC. Loss of heterozygosity for chromosome 13q and 17p alleles have also been documented, suggesting that the same loci that are important in other tumor types may be involved in SCLC. Amplified expression of *MYC* family genes has been reported in more than 80% of SCLC cell lines and tumors. The cytogenetic correlate of *MYC* amplification is not known, because these changes have not been linked to chromosome, rearrangements at the *MYC* loci. In non-SCLC, trisomy 7 has been described as the most common chromosome change.

Soft Tissue Sarcomas

Soft tissue sarcomas constitute a group in which tremendous heterogeneity exists. Numerous chromosome changes have been described in histologically distinct liposarcomas. However, in one particular type, myxoid liposarcoma, a specific translocation, t(12;16)(q13–q14;q11), has been described with remarkable consistency. It is of interest that the benign counterpart of this tumor also has abnormalities involving the region 12q13–q14 (see Lipomas, above). Whether or not the breakpoints are identical at the molecular level remains to be determined. In synovial sarcoma, t(X;18)p11;q11) appears to be highly specific. Even though numerous chromosome changes have been described in mesotheliomas, abnormalities of chromosome 3 appear to be more frequent.

Malignant Melanomas

In malignant melanoma, the tumor karyotypes are usually highly polyploid with numerous marker chromosomes. However, a few chromosomes show preferential involvement in both numerical and structural changes. These include chromosomes 1, 6, 7, 11, and 9. The simple abnormalities include trisomy 7 and duplication of the long arm of 1. Trisomy 7 has been reported to be more common among males and younger patients. In a few patients, an identical unbalanced translocation, t(1;19)(q12;p13), has been described. This translocation is associated with one of the most consistent abnormalities in melanoma, deletion of 6q. Consistent translocations were found to be indicators of specific gene loci involved in the development and progression of lymphoid neoplasms, but consistent translocations have been relatively uncommon as indicators in solid tumors. Jeffrey Trent and his coworkers noted a consistent t(1;6)(p22,q12–q21;q11–q13) in several melanomas and after review of the literature observed that band region 6q11–q13 was consistently the recipient of nonreciprocal translocations from several other chromosomes as well. These included (in order of frequency) two regions of chromosome 1 (p22,q12–q21), chromosomes 5, 3, 4, and 17. An ideogram provided by Dr. Trent illustrating the translocation breakpoints and the region of 6q affected by chromosome deletion, either as a result of translocation or loss by deletion alone, is presented in Figure 30.4. The 6q region is now the site of an intensive search for a tumor-suppressor gene.

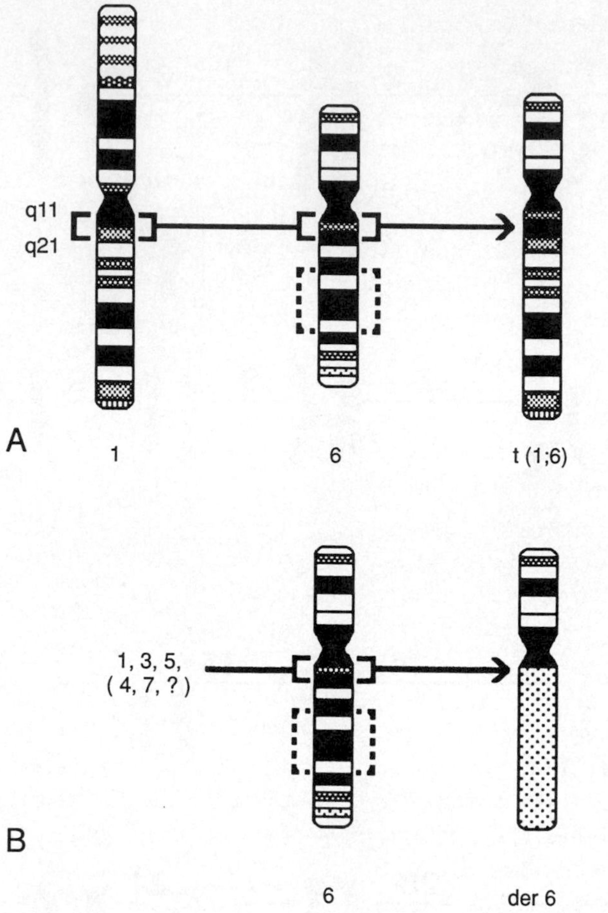

Figure 30.4. Ideogram diagramming breakpoints and derivative chromosomes resulting from translocations of various chromosomes to 6q11–21 in malignant melanomas. **A**, The *arrow* and *solid brackets* show the region of chromosome 1 (bands q11–q21) and the region of proximal 6q involved in the breakpoints and, on the right, the resultant derivative t(1;6), consisting of the short arm and centromere of 6 and most of the long arm of 1. The *dashed bracket* shows the region of 6 most frequently involved in simple deletions. **B**, This illustrates the other chromosome regions frequently translocated to the same region of 6, including 1p, 3, 5, 4, 7, and unknown chromosome regions to yield the other derivative chromosome 6s found in malignant melanomas. (Figure generously provided by Dr. Jeffrey Trent. Reprinted with permission from Trent JM, Thomspon FH, Meyskens FJ Jr. Identification of a recurring translocation site involving chromosome 6 in human malignant melanoma. Cancer Res 1989;49:420–423.)

There is a familial predisposition to melanoma in kindreds with the dysplastic nevus syndrome. In most studies of nevi and dysplastic nevi, the karyotypes have been normal. When abnormalities were detected, they were specific and did not include chromosomes 1, 6, 7, or 11, which have been implicated in the malignant tumors.

Astrocytoma and Glioblastoma Multiforme

These malignant neurogenic tumors have been well studied. Several specific chromosome changes have been described. The most frequent changes are trisomy 7 and double minutes. The double minutes have been shown to correlate with gene amplification for the epidermal growth factor receptor, which resides on chromosome 7. Other common changes include monosomy or deletion of the long arm of chromosome 10, monosomy 22, rearrangements involving the short arm of 9, and loss of the Y chromosome. Except for double minutes, most of these changes have been identified in both high- and low-grade tumors. However, LOH for alleles on 10q and 17p are found almost exclusively in the two most malignant variants of the astrocytic tumors, anaplastic astrocytoma and glioblastoma multiforme.

Squamous Cell Carcinoma of the Vulva

Vulvar carcinomas are relatively rare tumors, with an incidence of 1 or 2 tumors per 100,000 women. As a result, there are relatively few studies of this tumor type. The etiologic factors for these tumors are not well understood and may differ from squamous cancers that arise at other sites after prolonged exposure to carcinogens. We studied a consecutive series of six patients and found each tumor to have a unique and complex karyotype. However, there was a surprising degree of similarity in the rearrangements. Five of the six tumors had losses of 3p14–cen, 8pter–p11, 22q13.1–q13.2, and the short arm of the inactive X; the same proportion of tumors had gains of 3q25–qter, band 11q21, and rearrangement breakpoints in 5cen–q12. In this same series, two regions of relative chromosome loss involving 10q and 18q were observed in all four tumors in patients who died from progression of their tumors, whereas the two patients whose tumors did not have these losses were alive and well several years later. In some cases, the loss affected the whole chromosome, but in others there were specific deletions in which the smallest region of loss corresponded to del(10)(q23q25) and del(18)(q22q23). These regions provide targets for additional study as possible sites of genes important in prognosis. An example of a hypotetraploid karyotype from a vulvar carcinoma is presented in Figure 30.5. Note that many of the regions already mentioned as important in other tumors are also affected in this squamous cancer. For example, i(5p) and loss of 5q as well as loss of 18q are changes in this tumor that are also associated with colon cancer.

Squamous Cell Carcinoma of the Head and Neck

Like other squamous carcinomas, head and neck tumors usually have complex karyotypes. In spite of the complexity of most squamous cancers, by carefully evaluating all changes it has been possible to sort out the consistent changes. An example of two relatively simple karyotypes from this tumor type are shown in Figure 30.6. One of these is a hyperdiploid laryngeal cancer from a female patient, and the other is a squamous cancer of the head and neck from a male patient with xeroderma pigmentosum. In the first case, 13 chromosomes are rearranged. In the latter case, the only visible changes are loss of 4, loss of 21, i(9p) and i(9q), and a rearrangement of chromosomes 10 and 11. This is the least complicated karyotype we have observed in a squamous cancer, yet the breakpoints and changes that are present in this tumor correspond to some of the most frequently observed changes in other squamous cancers. The most common consistent changes in head and neck tumors, present in more than 70% of tumors, include loss of 3p13–p14, loss of chromosome 4, loss of 8p21–p22, and loss of 18q22–qter. Between 50 and 70% of the tumors had loss of 1q13–p22, loss of 9q13–p13, loss of 10p11.2–pter, loss of 13q14–q12, loss of 21p, and breakpoints in 11p14–p15. The most commonly duplicated regions, observed in one-third to one-fifth of tumors, included 3q, 5p, 7p, and 1qter–q25.

Although the information obtained by cancer cytogenetics can serve as a roadmap to the sites of genes involved in neoplasia, not all chromosome changes are detectable by karyotype. This was illustrated in retinoblastoma, in which tumors with homozygous loss or inactivation of the *RB1* allele had visible chromosome 13 changes in only 20 to 30% of cases. In some cases tumor progression may be accompanied by chromosomal gains that can obscure the loss of whole chromosomes. Figure 30.7 presents a set of karyotypes from cultures of a primary tumor and a metastatic tumor in the same patient. UM-SCC-21A is derived from a squamous carcinoma of the skin that was placed in culture several years before a metastasis became palpable in the soft tissues of the neck. UM-SCC-21B was derived from that metastatic tumor. The karyotypes show that both tumors are derived from the same clone. Note the presence in both tumors of i(1q), i(5p), t(5;6), i(7p), and t(13;del(13)). However, several changes from the primary tumor have been lost, and others have developed in the metastatic tumor. Of particular interest are monosomy 6, 18, and 19 in the primary tumor, all of which are represented by two copies in the metastasis. This finding suggests that the single homologue in the primary tumor was duplicated in the metastasis and replaced through nondisjunction. If

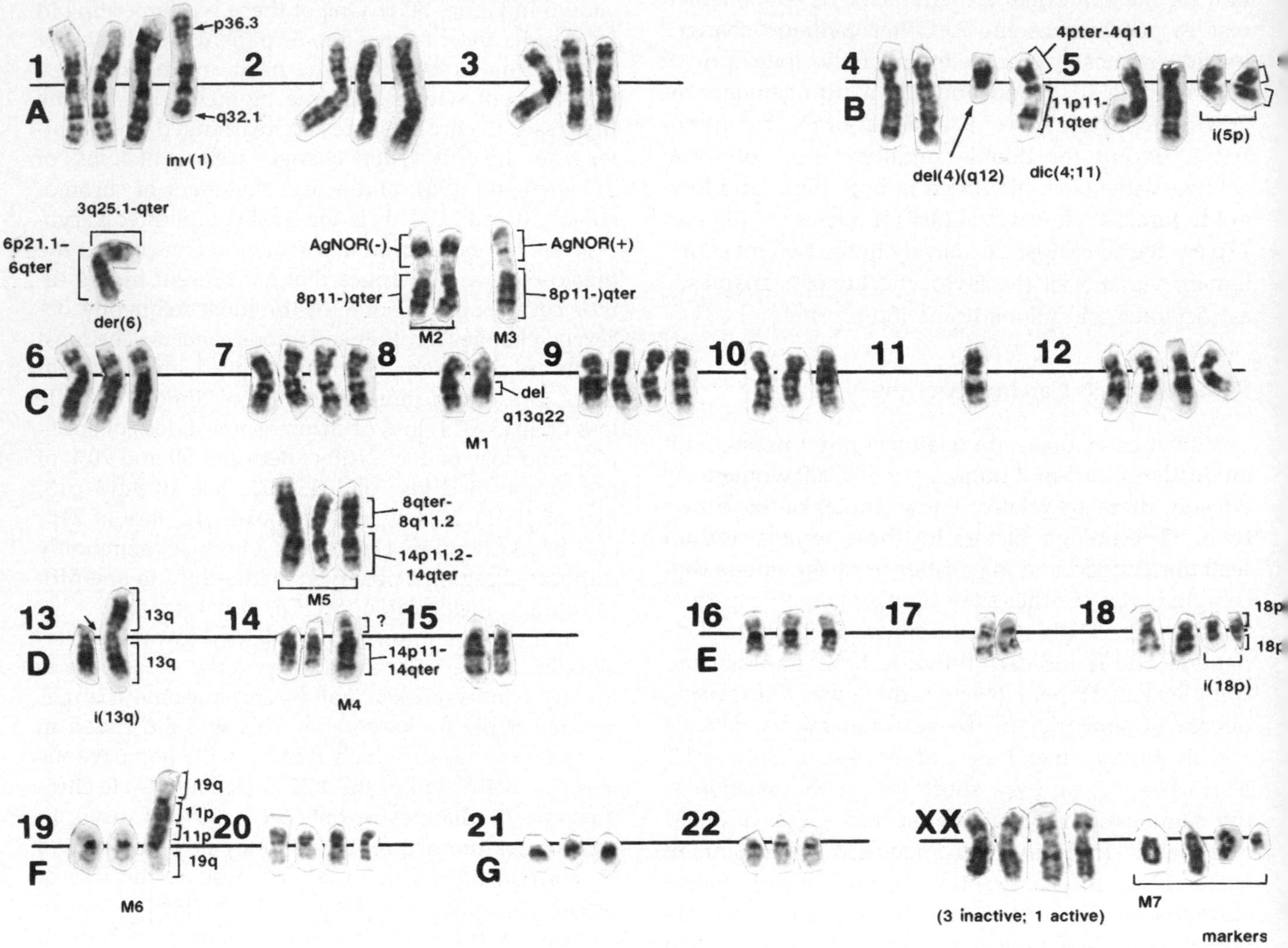

UM-SCV-1

Figure 30.5. Representative karyotype from a hypotetraploid squamous carcinoma of the vulva. In this figure, the rearranged chromosomes are identified. Prominent abnormalities against the tetraploid background are the loss of 4q, 5q, 8p, 11 (there is only one intact 11, a total of three copies of 11p, and two copies of 11q), 15, 17, and 18q, as well as the gain of 5p, 8q, 14q, and 18p. (Reprinted from Grenman SE, Van Dyke DL, Worsham MJ, et al. Phenotypic characterization, karyotype analysis and in vitro tamoxifen sensitivity of new ER-negative vulvar carcinoma cell lines, UM-SCV-1A and UM-SCV-1B. Int J Cancer 1990;45:920–927.)

this is true, then apparently normal pairs of chromosomes may mask loss of heterozygosity in some tumors. RFLP analysis will help to determine if this is the case in UM-SCC-21A and 21B.

Clonality in Squamous Carcinoma

The majority of studies of solid tumors and hematologic neoplasms find that tumors are clonal and can usually be tracked to a single precursor cell. In the examples given above, we have illustrated some examples in which related clones can be found in the same tumor, and we take these to be evidence of progression. In some cases, however, studies of primary tumors have revealed as many as 12 unrelated clones in a single tumor. These studies by Felix Mitelman and his coworkers raise the possibility that there may be multiple independent malignant clones in some tumor types, and this may substantiate the theory of "field cancerization," which was proposed some years ago to account for the high frequency of multiple primary cancers in the upper aerodigestive tract. Alternatively, the culture methods employed for these studies may allow the outgrowth and proliferation of karyotypically abnormal but not malignant cells that might be present in the tissues surrounding the primary tumor. The growth of the malignant clone itself might be suppressed by the epidermal growth factor in the medium, whereas other cells could proliferate in the same formulation. Further work is necessary to determine if only a single clone predominates in vivo in such patients and to determine the origin of the multiple clones in these cases.

SIGNIFICANCE OF CHROMOSOME REARRANGEMENTS

Translocations, Point Mutations, and Amplification of Protooncogenes

Activation of Protooncogenes

Protooncogenes are normal cellular genes involved in the process of cell replication. When the protooncogenes go awry by any of several mechanisms, the involved cell acquires the ability for autonomous replication, which results in uncontrolled proliferation. As discussed in Chapter 29, in hematologic neoplasms protooncogene activation commonly occurs by chromosome translocations.

Translocations

The classic example of oncogene activation by this type of mechanism is the translocation of the *MYC* oncogene from chromosome 8 to the immunoglobulin heavy–chain (*IGH*) locus on chromosome 14. As a result of the juxtaposition of *MYC* to the active *IGH* gene, there is increased expression of MYC and deregulation of cell growth, driven by the promoter and enhancer elements of the *IGH* gene.

As discussed in Chapter 38, the translocation of chromosomes 9 and 22 in CML provides another example. This translocation juxtaposes the *ABL* protooncogene locus on 9 and a gene locus called breakpoint cluster region (*BCR*) on 22. This translocation results in the active production of both message and a protein called $P210^{bcr/abl}$ that is similar to the oncogene product of the Abelson murine leukemia virus designated $P160^{gag/v\text{-}abl}$. Both of these rearranged genes encode fusion proteins with deregulated tyrosine-kinase activity. Expression of the $P160^{gag/v\text{-}abl}$ fusion protein induces acute leukemia in mice, and recent studies from David Baltimore's laboratory have shown that mice given murine bone marrow cells transfected with the human $P210^{bcr/abl}$ hybrid construct also develop hematologic tumors and myeloproliferative disorder that closely resembles CML humans. This demonstrates most conclusively the significance of the translocation that gives rise to the Philadelphia chromosome.

The consistent translocations in T-cell tumors are not yet as well characterized as the *IGH/MYC* or *ABL/BCR* rearrangements. Nevertheless, early rearrangements in T-cell leukemias have been shown by Carlo Croce and others to often involve the T-cell receptor gene loci and a breakpoint region containing a gene or genes whose function is not yet well defined. By analogy to the B-cell neoplasms, we can predict that this type of rearrangement involves an active gene, the T-cell receptor, whose promoters and enhancing elements can presumably affect the expression of a gene related to growth regulation on the recipient chromosome.

Based on these observations, several authors have concluded that consistent chromosome rearrangements in cancers are very likely to occur at the sites of protooncogenes. Several authors have collected consistent breakpoint data from the literature and compared these sites to known oncogene loci. These comparisons show a strong concordance, which adds further support to the concept that chromosome rearrangements in cancer are functionally related to the cancerous behavior of the tumor cells.

Oncogene Activation

In solid tumors, a major mechanism of oncogene activation appears to be activation by point mutations and gene amplification, rather than activation by translocation. The point mutations that have been best studied and most strongly implicated in the genesis of solid tumors belong to the *RAS* gene family, which consists of three members: *HRAS*, *NRAS*, and

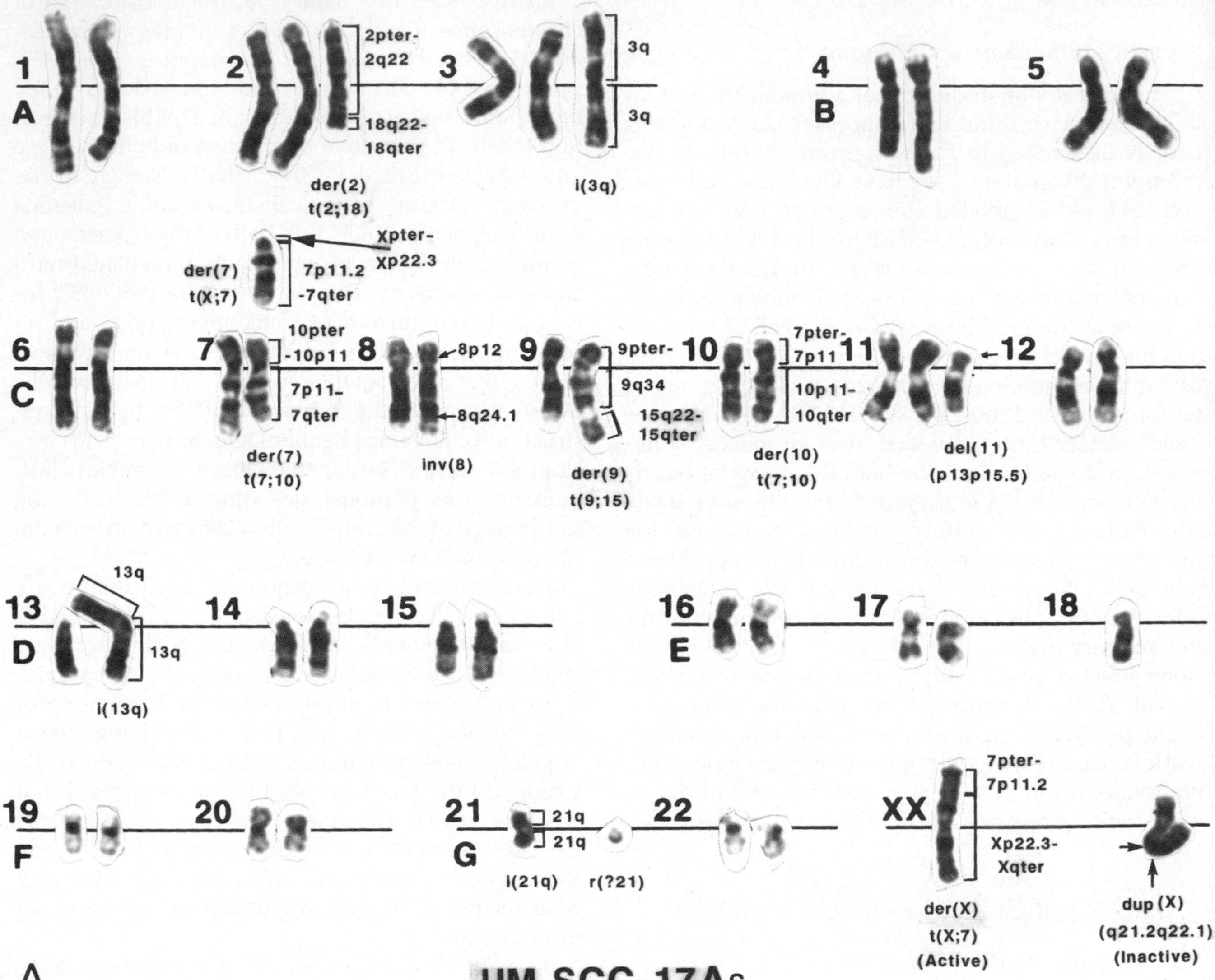

Figure 30.6. Examples of relatively simple tumor karyotypes from patients with squamous carcinomas arising in the head and neck region. **A**, Karyotype from a laryngeal carcinoma cell line UM-SCC-17As. This cell line is one of three tumor lines derived from the same female patient. Two lines, UM-SCC-17A and UM-SCC-17As, represent clones derived from the primary tumor. UM-SCC-17B was derived from a metastatic extension into the soft tissues of the neck. The prominent changes in this tumor are a t(2;18), i(3q), reciprocal translocations of 7, 10, and X [der(7)t(X;7), der(7)t(7;10), der(10)t(7;10), and der(X)t(X;7)], inv(8), t(9;15), del(11p), i(13q), loss of 18, i(21q), r(21?), and dup(X). Several chromosomes that are rearranged or lost in other, more aggressive cancers are apparently not affected in this tumor, and this may correlate with the long-term survival of the patient. **B**, Karyotype from a squamous carcinoma arising in a male patient with xeroderma pigmentosum. This figure illustrates one of three closely related clones that all contained the monosomy 4 and the i(9p), i(9q), which must represent the initial changes in this tumor. The change in clone 1 associated with progression was t(5;7)(q11.2;p22). Clones 2 (shown here) and 3 shared the loss of chromosome 21 and differed by the der(11)t(10;11)(q21;p14) present in this cell and a t(13;14)(q14;q32) present in clone 3. In spite of the simplicity of the changes in this tumor, it was an aggressive neoplasm that recurred and spread rapidly, eventually causing the death of the patient. The involvement of genes on chromosomes 4 and 9 must be considered important in tumor initiation and perhaps also important in tumor progression, since loss of chromosome 4 has been associated with aggressive behavior in other tumors.

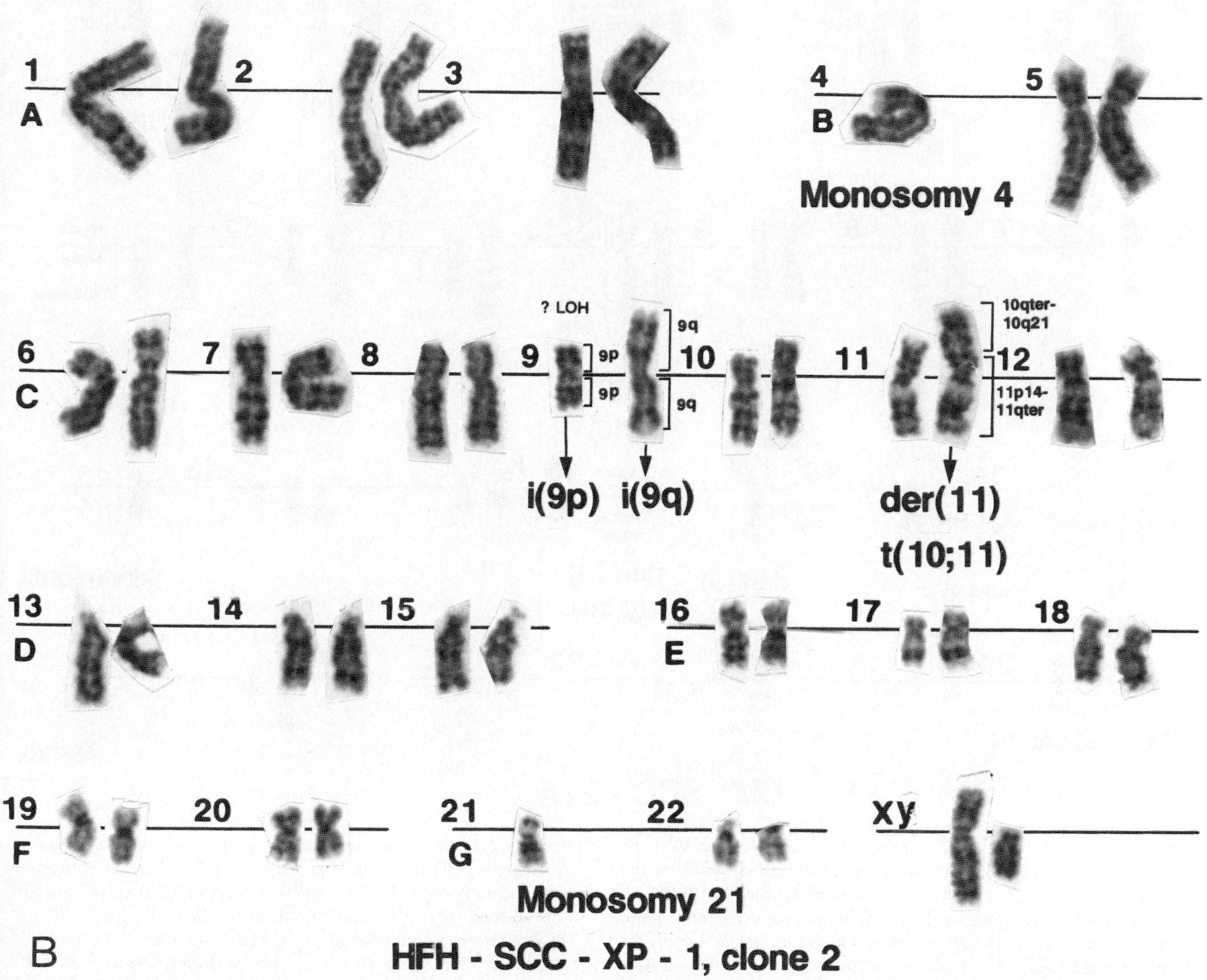
1
A
2
3
4
B
5
Monosomy 4
6
C
7
8
9
? LOH
9p
9p
9q
9q
10
11
10qter-
10q21
12
11p14-
11qter
i(9p)
i(9q)
der(11)
t(10;11)
13
D
14
15
16
E
17
18
19
F
20
21
G
22
XY
Monosomy 21
B
HFH - SCC - XP - 1, clone 2

Figure 30.6. B.

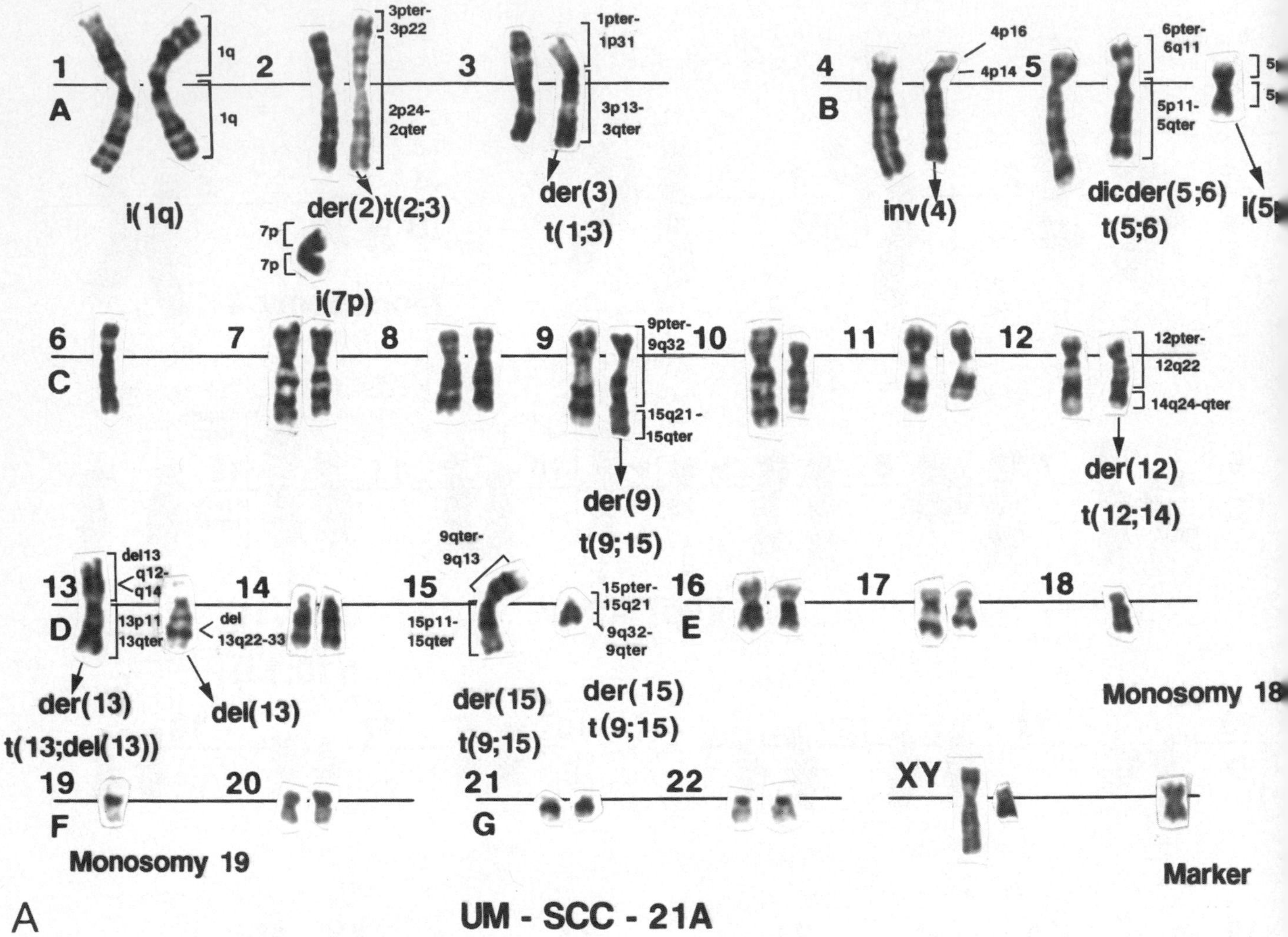

Figure 30.7. Karyotypes from a primary squamous carcinoma of the facial skin (UM-SCC-21A) (**A**) and a metastatic tumor that was detected a year later in the neck of same patient (UM-SCC-21B) (**B**). Although there has been independent evolution of some rearrangements and accumulation of additional changes in the metastatic tumor, the similar clonal origin of both tumors is attested to by the shared rearrangements i(1q), i(5p), t(5;6), i(7p), and der(13)t(13;del(13)(q12q14)) that are evident in both karyotypes. The differences between UM-SCC-21A and 21B are as follows: A der(2) in 21A is replaced by two apparently normal copies of chromosome 2 in 21B; the der(3)t(1;3) in 21A is replaced by a different der(3) and a normal chromosome 3 in 21B; the inv(4) is replaced by two normal chromosome 4s; the normal chromosome 5 is replaced by an i(5q); monosomy 6 is replaced by disomy 6; i(7p) is duplicated; two normal chromosome 8s are replaced by i(8p) and der(8)t(8;21); der(9)t(9;15) is lost and replaced by a normal chromosome 9; a new i(11q) is present in 21B; the der(12)t(12;14) is lost and replaced by a normal chromosome 12 and an i(12p); a del(13)(q22–q23) is lost and replaced by an apparently normal chromosome 13; two different der(15)t(9;15) copies are lost and replaced by two normal chromosome 15s and a der(15)t(8;15). There is an extra chromosome 16 in 21B, monosomy 18 is replaced by disomy, monosomy 19 is replaced by disomy, there is an extra chromosome 20, both normal sex chromosomes and a small marker are lost and replaced by a der(X)t(X;X). Two changes, loss of chromosomes 13 and 15, must have occurred in 21A after the separation of the two populations in vivo, otherwise there would be no normal copies of these chromosomes in the metastatic line. This example gives some idea of the magnitude of the evolution that can occur in tumors and in particular suggests that chromosome loss may be compensated by duplication and nondisjunction. This pair of cell lines provides an example in which to determine if loss of heterozygosity has occurred for multiple chromosomes.

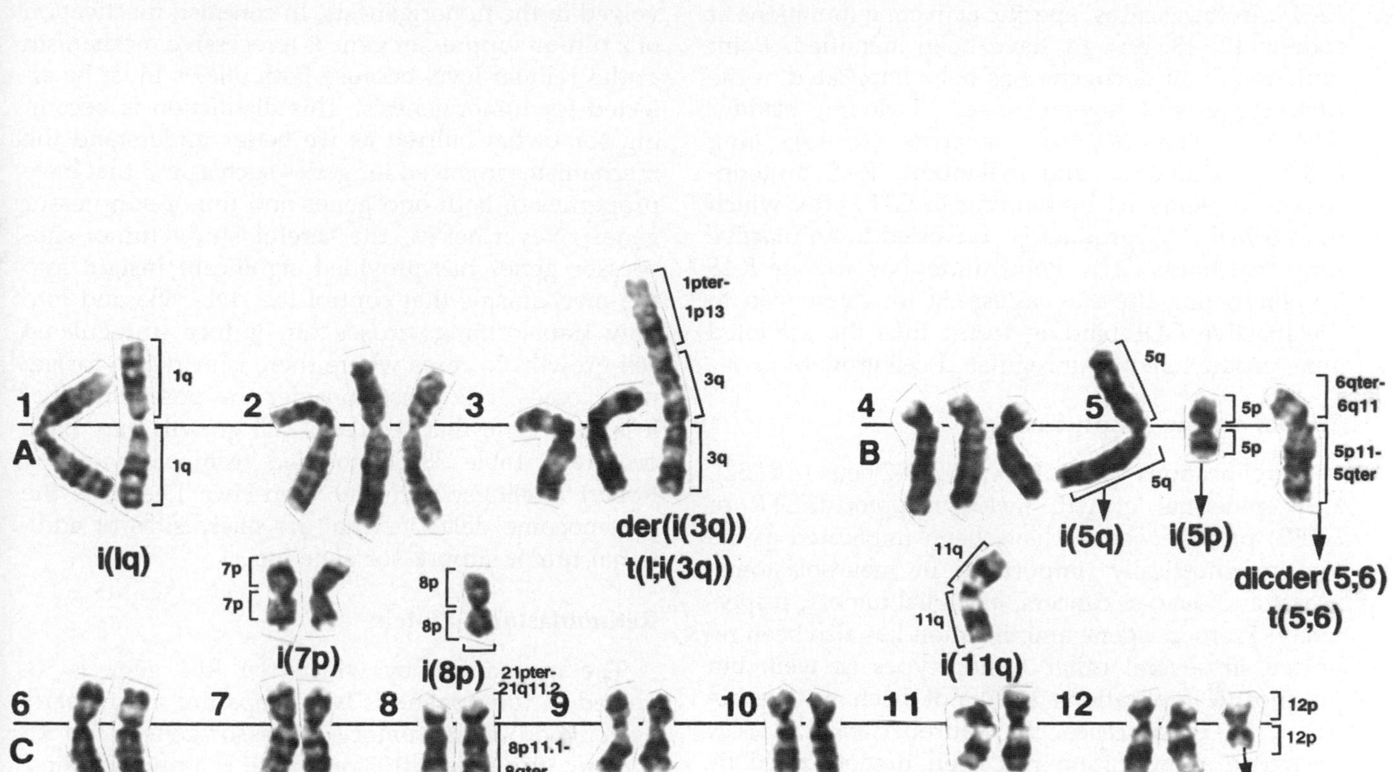
1
A
1q
1q
i(lq)
2
3
1pter-
1p13
3q
3q
der(i(3q))
t(l;i(3q))
7p
7p
i(7p)
8p
8p
i(8p)
4
B
5
5q
5q
i(5q)
5p
5p
i(5p)
6qter-
6q11
5p11-
5qter
dicder(5;6)
t(5;6)
11q
11q
i(11q)
6
C
7
8
21pter-
21q11.2
8p11.1-
8qter
der(8)
t(8;21)
9
10
11
12
12p
12p
i(12p)
13
D
del13
<q12-q14
13p11-
13qter
der(13)
t(13;del(13))
14
15
8qter -
8q11.2
15p11-
15qter
der(15)
t(8;15)
16
E
17
18
19
F
20
21
G
22
XY
Xqter-Xq13
Xp23-Xqter
der(X)
t(X;X)
B
UM - SCC - 21B

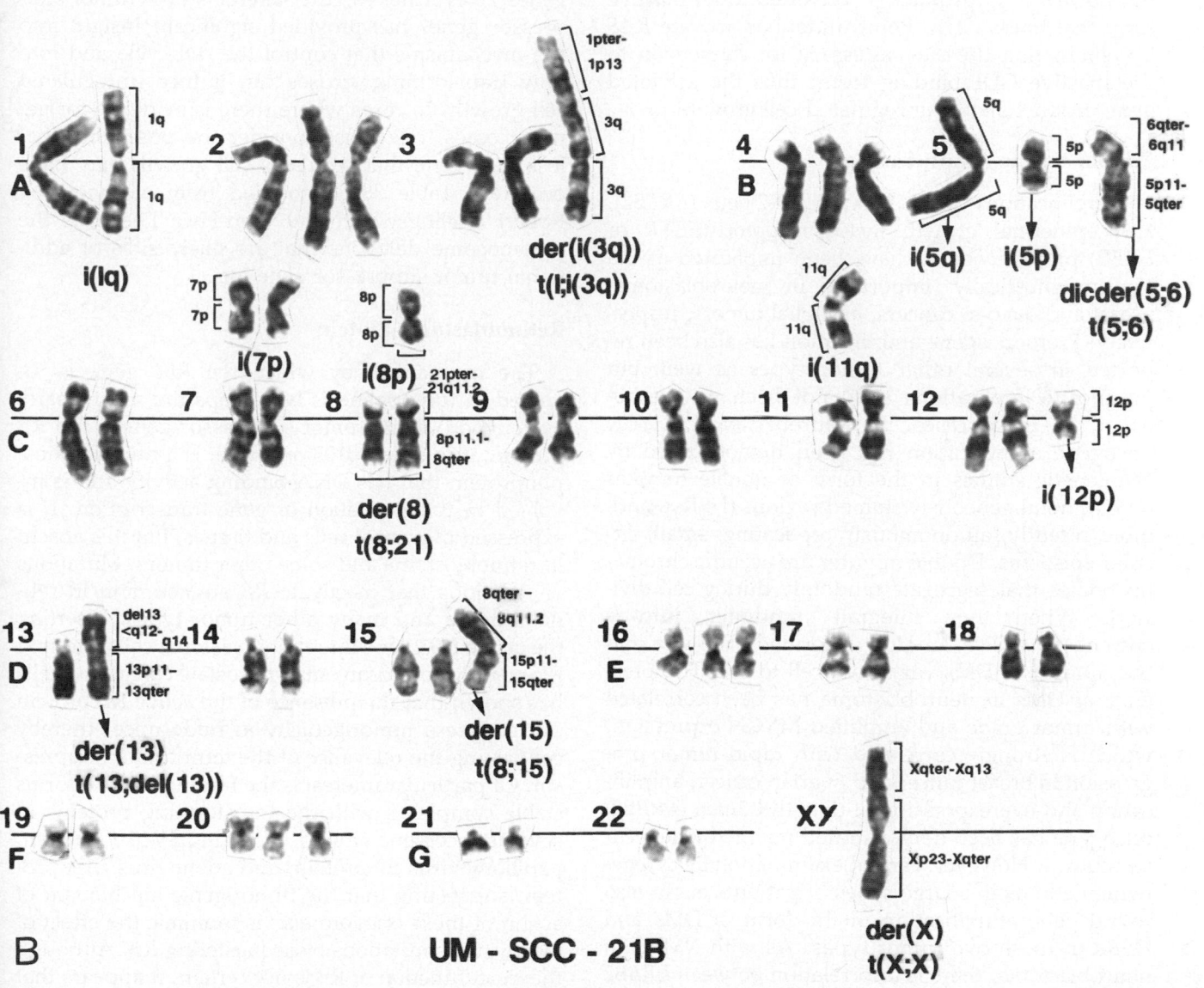

Figure 30.7. B.

KRAS. In these cases, specific activating mutations at codons 12, 13, and 61 have been identified. Point mutation of an oncogene has been implicated in the tumorigenesis of several cancers, including bladder (*HRAS*), colon (*KRAS*), pancreas (*KRAS*), lung (*KRAS*), seminoma, and melanoma. RAS protooncogene proteins act by binding to GTP, after which the normal RAS product is converted to an inactive form that binds GDP. Point mutations activate *RAS* by eliminating the site necessary for conversion to the inactive GDP-binding form, thus the activated gene product allows unregulated cell growth.

Protooncogene Amplification

Amplifications of *MYCN*, HER-2/neu (*ERB*B2), and epidermal growth factor receptor (*EGFR* or *ERB*B) protooncogenes have been implicated as being prognostically important in neuroblastoma, breast and ovarian cancers, and glial tumors, respectively. Protooncogene amplification has also been reported in several other tumor types as well, but prognostic implications have not been well established in these cases. In neuroblastoma, *MYCN* oncogene amplification has been demonstrated by cylogenetic studies in the form of double minutes (DMs), homogeneously stained regions (HSRs), and, more recently, autonomously replicating, small, circular episomes. Double minutes are acentric chromatin bodies that segregate randomly during cell division. When they integrate randomly into a chromosomal site, an HSR is formed. The size and the number of DMs vary from cell to cell. The presence of DMs in neuroblastoma has been correlated with tumor grade and amplified MYCN expression, which is strongly correlated with rapid tumor progression in breast cancer and ovarian cancer, amplification and overexpression of the HER-2/neu (*ERB*B2) oncogene has been demonstrated mainly by molecular studies. However, careful examination by cytogenetic methods in a large series of patients might also reveal gene amplification in the form of DMs and HSRs in these two tumor types. As with *NMYC* in neuroblastoma, there is a correlation between *ERB*B2 amplification and elevated *ERB*B2 expression and highly malignant behavior in breast cancer and ovarian cancer. In glial tumors, amplification of *EGFR* (*ERB*B) has been observed in the form of DMs and HSRs, and this is associated with an advanced grade and a poor prognosis.

Chromosome Deletion and Inactivation of Tumor-Suppressor Genes

Activation of an oncogene by translocation, point mutation, or amplification is a dominant phenomenon because malfunction of only one allele is involved in the tumorigenesis. In contrast, inactivation of a tumor-suppressor gene is a recessive mechanism at the cellular level because both alleles must be affected for tumorigenesis. This distinction is becoming somewhat blurred as we better understand the mechanisms involved for genes such as *p53* that have properties of both oncogenes and tumor-suppressor genes. Nevertheless, the careful study tumor-suppressor genes has provided significant insight into the mechanisms that control the cell cycle and into how transforming viruses can induce unregulated cell growth. In cases where there is evidence for genetic losses, one must consider the possibility that loss of a gene that regulates cell growth may have occurred. Table 30.2, modified from a review by Robert Hollingsworth and Wen-Hwa Lee, lists the chromosome deletions that are likely sites of additional tumor-suppressor gene loci.

Retinoblastoma Protein

The mechanism by which the *RB1* gene is involved in tumorigenesis is perhaps the most clearly understood of the tumor-suppressor genes, The RB protein, also called p105 or pp110, is a nuclear phosphoprotein that has DNA binding activity and is involved in the regulation of gene transcription. It is expressed in normal cells and tissues, but it is absent in retinoblastoma and some other tumors. Mutations or deletions that inactivate *RB* are common in retinoblastoma and many other tumor types. Inserting the active *RB1* gene into retinoblastoma cells and into RB-negative osteosarcoma or prostate carcinoma cells has shown that the presence of the active RB protein can suppress tumorigenicity in nude mice, thereby confirming the relevance of the term tumor suppressor. Of particular interest is the finding that RB forms stable complexes with the transforming proteins of several oncogenic viruses, including SV40 T antigen, papillomavirus E7 protein, and adenovirus E1A protein, suggesting that the tumorigenic mechanism of action of these oncoproteins is to mimic the effect of inactivating mutations by sequestering RB. Although the exact function of RB is not certain, it appears that one of its actions in suppressing cell growth is to bind to control elements for *FOS* and repress its expression, thereby blocking the assembly of the AP-1 transcriptional regulator that inhibits cells from leaving G_0 and entering G_1.

p53 Protein

The *p53* gene was at first thought of as an oncogene because it was found to be overexpressed in many tumor cells compared to normal cells and because transfection of the *p53* gene isolated from tumor cells into rodent cells conferred immortalization.

Table 30.2 Chromosome Deletions Associated with Cancer[a]

Chromosome Deletion	Associated Tumor-Suppressor Gene	Type of Cancer
1p		Melanoma, neuroblastoma, medullary thyroid carcinoma, pheochromocytoma, MEN-2, ductal breast carcinoma
1q		Breast carcinoma
3p		Small-cell lung carcinoma; renal cell carcinoma; squamous carcinoma of the cervix, vulva, head, and neck; bladder carcinoma; von Hippel-Lindau disease
4		Squamous carcinoma, endometrial carcinoma
5q		Familial adenomatous polyposis, sporadic colorectal carcinoma, bladder carcinoma
6q		Melanoma
10q		Glioblastoma multiforme, squamous carcinoma
11p	*WT1*	Wilms' tumor, breast carcinoma, rhabdomyosarcoma, hepatoblastoma, transitional cell bladder carcinoma
13q	*RB1*	Retinoblastoma, osteosarcoma, small-cell lung carcinoma, ductal breast carcinoma, squamous carcinoma
17p	*p53*	Small cell lung carcinoma, colorectal carcinoma, breast carcinoma, osteosarcoma
17q	*NF1*	Neurofibroma
18q	*DCC*	Colorectal carcinoma, squamous carcinoma
22		Meningioma, acoustic neuroma, pheochromocytoma

[a]Modified from Hollingsworth RE, Lee WH. Tumor suppressor genes: new prospects for cancer research. JNCI 1991;83:91–96. Reprinted with the permission of the Journal of the National Cancer Institute.

This made it difficult to resolve the finding that the *p53* gene was frequently deleted from the short arm of chromosome 17 in colon carcinoma. However, when *p53* alleles from normal cells and tumor cells were compared, mutations were found at a variety of sites within the gene, suggesting that perhaps these were inactivating mutations. Subsequent studies showed that when the mutant protein is over-expressed it can act in a dominant fashion by forming stable but inactive complexes with the normal protein. Thus, its mechanism may be to inactivate the function of the active *p53* protein. Nevertheless, when the normal wild-type allele is introduced into tumor cells that lack the *p53* gene, tumorigenicity is suppressed. Additionally, as in the case of the RB protein, viral transforming proteins, including SV40 T antigen, papillomavirus E6 protein, and adenovirus E1B, can bind to p53 protein. Of particular interest is the fact that the T antigen binding sites for *RB* and *p53* are distinct and that the papilloma and adenovirus oncoproteins are different than those that inactivate *RB*. Furthermore, papillomavirus E6 and E7 alone are ineffective as transforming agents, but together these proteins have high transforming activity. This suggests that inactivation of both RB and p53 proteins is important for transformation to occur.

CLINICAL APPLICATIONS OF CHROMOSOME CHANGES

The importance of chromosome changes in the diagnosis and prognosis of hematologic cancers has been well established and is discussed in Chapter 29. In solid tumors, a few clinical correlations have been established as well. Some of these deal with differential diagnosis, and the others relate to prognosis.

Differential Diagnosis

Small cell and round cell tumors in children pose a considerable diagnostic dilemma because it is often impossible to make a diagnosis based on histology alone. The presence of a specific translocation, t(11;22), will make a definite diagnosis of Ewing's sarcoma, whereas the presence of a 1p deletion will establish the diagnosis of neuroblastoma. Similarly, neuroblastoma can be distinguished from Askin's tumor and neuroepithelioma by the presence of t(11;22) in the latter tumors. For a long time, neuroepithelioma and Askin's tumor were considered to be atypical neuroblastomas and were treated accordingly. However, because, like Ewing's sarcoma, they contain t(11;22), they have since been reclassified as primitive neuroectodermal tumors, and they now receive the more favorable therapy used for Ewing's sarcoma.

The presence of a specific change, t(12;16), can be used to make the diagnosis of a subset of liposarcomas, i.e., myxoid liposarcoma. Even though the distinction between benign and malignant tumors is clear in most soft tissue tumors, the t(12;16) can also be utilized to make this distinction because the benign tumors never show the chromosome 16 involvement in this translocation. Abnormalities in chromosomes 2, 13, and 3 can be used to distinguish rhabdomyosarcoma from other neuroepithelial tumors. A specific translocation, t(2;13), might even distinguish the alveolar subtype.

Cytogenetics has been clearly underutilized in the area of diagnosis of malignant disease in body fluids such as pleural and peritoneal effusions. Several studies have provided evidence for the correlation between the presence of a clonal abnormality and the presence of neoplastic cells. Thus, cytogenetic analysis can be a useful adjunct to standard cytology in the differential diagnosis of neoplasia versus inflammation or other causes.

Prognostic Implications

In bladder cancer, chromosome abnormalities were recognized as predictors of clinical outcome even before the banding era. Banding techniques have refined the accuracy of identifying chromosome changes in this tumor type, and some specific changes, such as the deletion of 11p, have been shown to be associated with tumor progression. In general, low-grade, noninvasive bladder tumors have diploid karyotypes with few markers, and the higher-grade, invasive tumors have polyploid karyotypes with multiple marker chromosomes. The presence of marker chromosomes is also correlated with recurrence and mortality. Patients whose tumors did not have marker chromosomes had only a 5% rate of recurrence and achieved a 5-year survival rate of 90%, whereas patients whose tumors had markers had a 50% recurrence rate and a 5-year survival rate of only 75%. Thus, the karyotype can be a prognostic indicator in bladder cancer.

In neuroblastoma, the presence and the copy number of double minutes (*MYCN* amplification) has clinical implications. Patients with low-grade tumors and low copy numbers of double minutes have a much better likelihood of survival compared to patients with high-grade tumors and higher numbers of double minutes. Even among patients with high-grade tumors, those with low numbers of double minutes do well compared to those with high numbers. In general, patients with high numbers of double minutes also have chromosome 1 deletions, and this group of patients has the poorest prognosis.

Another prognostic indicator already mentioned above is the amplification of HER-2/neu (*ERB*B2) oncogene at the DNA, mRNA, and protein level which has been correlated with a shortened disease-free interval and decreased overall survival in breast and ovarian cancers.

In colon cancer, tumors from the left side often have more genetic changes, including chromosomal as well as allelic losses, than tumors from the right side. These genetic changes are correlated with disease-free interval and ultimate survival.

Tumor-Specific Reciprocal Chromosome Translocations and Other Changes

Certain rearrangements of chromosomes are specific for particular tumor types. For example, rearrangements involving the immunoglobulin loci are specific for neoplasms of the antibody-producing cell lineage, and rearrangements involving the T-cell receptor loci are specific for neoplasms of the T lymphocyte lineage. These chromosome rearrangements are specific for certain tumor types because they involve genes that are specifically expressed in these cell lineages. It may also be important that, in the process of differentiation, these cell types rearrange the DNA of the chromosome loci for the immunoglobulin genes and the T-cell receptor genes. The reason for tumor type specificity for other rearrangements is less clear.

During the early stages of the analysis of the chromosome changes in solid tumors, several tumors types were found to have characteristic chromosome abnormalities. Initially, it appeared that these changes, such as the chromosome 13 deletion associated with inactivation of the retinoblastoma gene in retinoblastoma and the loss of alleles on chromosome 11 in Wilms' tumor, were specific for those tumor types. However, as more solid tumor types were adequately studied, it was shown that changes in chromosomes 11p, 13q, 17p, and 18q were common to multiple types of tumors. The basis for the commonalities among different tumor types is now known for the retinoblastoma gene because this regulator of cell growth is expressed in many cell types. The same appears to hold true for the *p53* gene on 17p. In the case of *WT1*, the Wilms' tumor suppressor gene, it is uncertain whether the changes in the 11p chromosome observed in other tumor types involve altered expression of this gene, because so far its expression has been detected only in kidney tissues and in CEM, a cultured T-cell leukemia line. Likewise, too little is known about the *DCC* gene on chromosome 18q to determine if this gene is active in the tissues from which 18q-deficient tumors arise. At this point it seems likely that chromosome rearrangements associated with the loss or mutation of tumor-suppressor genes will have relatively wide distribution among tumors. Based on what we know about the leukemias and lymphomas, it is likely that genetic changes in solid tumors that are tissue specific may involve genes that undergo natural rearrangement during the process of differentiation. Such genes are probably more susceptible to abnormal translocation because of the natural chromosome rearrangement events used to select specific gene segments for expression. Possible candidates for such tissue-specific expression in solid tumors are keratin genes, extracellular matrix components, matrix receptors, and glycosyltransferases. Much more work will be required before we have a clear sense for such tissue-specific changes in solid neoplasms.

Summary

Remarkable progress has been made with regard to the nature of the genetic changes in the hematologic tumors and their clinical implications. Similar progress has been lacking for solid tumors mainly because of problems in the technical, analytical, and interpretive areas. The technical difficulties include the lack of sufficient mitotic cells, poor morphology of the chromosomes, and normal stromal cell contamination. The analytical difficulties include the highly complex karyotypes with multiple rearangements, which occasionally make the identification of the individual marker chromosomes impossible. Finally, the identification and differentiation of primary changes from secondary changes as well as elucidation of the genetic changes of prognostic significance have all been very challenging.

Recent improvements in tissue culture methodology have allowed the identification of a few consistent chromosoma, and genetic changes. These improvements include the use of low-serum media, cell synchronization techniques, the use of feeder layers, and the enzymatic disaggregation of tumor tissue. The field of "interphase cytogenetics" is in its infancy, and the applications of fluorescent in situ hybridization will increase in the near future. This will result in better characterization of genetic changes in solid tumors.

Currently, the more consistent chromosome changes include t(3;8)(p12;q12) in pleomorphic adenoma of the salivary gland; deletion of the short arm of chromsome 3 in renal cell carcinoma and small cell carcinoma of the lung; trisomy 7, monosomy 9, isochromosome or deletion 5q, and 11p deletion in bladder cancer; i(12p) in germ cell tumors; translocations involving 12q13–q14 in lipoma and t(12;16)(q13–q14;q11) in liposarcoma; t(X;18) in synovial sarcoma; monosomy 22 in meningioma; t(11:22)(q24;q12) in Ewing's sarcoma and other neuroendocrine tumors; deletion 13q14 in retinoblastoma; and deletion 11p13 in Wilms' tumor.

Some of the genetic changes have proved to be of diagnostic value; for example, t(X;18) for synovial sarcoma, t(12;16) for myxoid liposarcoma, t(2;13) for rhabdomyosarcoma, t(11;22) for neuroendorcine tumors, and i(12p) for germ cell tumors. As more studies are done, there is no doubt that additional specific rearrangements will be uncovered. With respect to prognosis, karyotype has been shown to be an independent prognostic indicator in bladder cancer; gene amplification has been shown to be a predictor of clinical outcome in neuroblastoma and in breast and ovarian cancers; and the loss of genetic information (i.e., chromosome deletions and allelic losses) is a predictor of clinical outcome in colorectal cancers. As more prospective studies are done, the results for solid tumors will prove to be akin to those for hematologic cancers.

Acknowledgments

The authors wish to acknowledge the expert assistance of Tim Drumheller, Maria Worsham, and Margaret Conlon. We are also indebted to our friend and colleague Dr. Daniel Van Dyke for his helpful suggestions.

Suggested Readings

Baker SJ, Fearon ER, Nigro JM, et al. Chromosome 17 deletions and p53 gene mutations in colorectal carcinomas. Science 1989;244:217–221.

Bodmer WF, Bailey CJ, Bodmer J, et al. Localization of the gene for familial adenomatous polyposis on chromosome 5. Nature 1987;328:614–616.

Brodeur GM, Green AA, Hayes FA, Williams KJ, Williams DL, Tsiatis AA. Cytogenetic features of human neuroblastomas and cell lines. Cancer Res 1981;41:4678–4686.

Call KM, Glaser T, Ito CY, et al. Isolation and characterization of a zinc finger polypeptide gene at the human chromosome 11 Wilms' tumor locus. Cell 1990;60:509–520.

Cavenee WK, Dryja TP, Phillips RA, et al. Expression of recessive alleles by chromosomal mechanisms in retinoblastoma. Nature 1983;305:779–784.

Daley GQ, Van Etten RA, Baltimore D. Induction of chronic myelogenous leukemia in mice by the P210$^{bcr/abl}$ gene of the Philadelphia chromosome. Science 1990;247:824–830.

Dryja TP, Cavenee W, White R, et al. Homozygosity of chromosome 13 in retinoblastoma. N Engl J Med 1984;310:550–553.

Fearon ER, Vogelstein B, Feinberg AP. Somatic deletion and duplication of genes on chromosome 11 in Wilms' tumours. Nature 1984;309:176–178.

Fearon ER, Feinberg AP, Hamilton SH, Vogelstein B. Loss of genes on the short arm of chromosome 11 in bladder cancer. Nature 1985;318:377–380.

Francke U, Holmes LB, Atkins L, Riccardi VM. Aniridia-Wilms' tumor association: evidence for specific deletion of 11p13. Cytogenet Cell Genet 1979;24:185–192.

Friend SH, Dryja TP, Weinberg RA. Oncogenes and tumor-suppressing genes. N Engl J Med 1988;318:618–623.

Gessler M, Poustka A, Cavenee W, Neve RL, Orkin SH, Bruns GAP. Homozygous deletion in Wilms' tumours of a zinc-finger gene identified by chromosome jumping. Nature 1980;343:774–778.

Haluska FG, Tsujimoto Y, Croce, CM. Oncogene activation by chromosome translocation in human malignancy. Annu Rev Genet 1987;21:321–345.

Hollingsworth RE, Lee WH. Tumor suppressor genes: new prospects for cancer research. J Natl Cancer Inst 1991;83:91–96.

Huang HJS, Yee JK, Shew JY, et al. Suppression of the neoplastic phenotype by replacement of the RB gene in human cancer cells. Science 1988;244:1563–1566.

Knudson AG, Mutation and cancer: statistical study of retinoblastoma Proc Natl Acad Sci USA 1971;68:820–823.

Milburn MV, Tong L, deVos A, et al. Molecular switch for signal transduction: structural differences between active and inactive forms of protooncogenic *ras* proteins. Science 1990;247:939–945.

Robbins PD, Horowitz JM, Mulligan RC. Negative regulation of human c-*fos* expression by the retinoblastoma gene product. Nature 1990;346:668–671.

Seeger RC, Brodeur GM, Sather H, et al. Association of multiple copies of the N-*myc* oncogene with rapid progression of neuroblastomas. N Engl J Med 1985;313:1111–1116.

Slamon DJ, Clark GM, Wong SG, Levin WJ, Ullrich A, McGuire WL. Human breast cancer: correlation of relapse and survival with amplification of the HER2/*neu* oncogene. Science 1987;235: 177–182.

Solomon E, Voss R, Bodmer WF, et al. Chromosome 5 allele loss in human colon carcinomas. Nature 1987;328:616–619.

Sreekantaiah C, Leong SG, Karakousis CP, et al. Cytogenetic profile of 109 lipomas. Cancer Res 1991;51:422–433.

Vogelstein B, Fearon ER, Hamilton SR, et al. Genetic alterations during colorectal tumor development. N Engl J Med 1988;319: 525–532.

Whang-Peng J, Kao-Shan CS, Lee EC, et al. Specific chromosome defect associated with small-cell lung cancer; deletion 3p(14–23). Science 1982;215:181–182.

Section VI

Section Chief: *Emanuel Hackel*

In an area of rapidly evolving technology, with its resultant expansion of understanding, great care must be exercised in preparing a textbook on methodology. Including the "hot" topics such as HLA is done only at great peril. Nonetheless, the chapters on HLA methods and applications are herewith presented with the full knowledge that changes are afoot. Current practices and procedures are widely used and lead to useful interpretations with effective results in clinical medicine as well as in research. The certainty that these procedures will change in the near future does not detract at all from their importance as clinical tools and their fruitfulness in research.

HLA testing has evolved over the years through a variety of different methods. Some of these have persisted, with minor variations, for a long time. Given the diverse nature of the demonstrated structural differences between the class I, II, and III HLA antigens, it is not surprising that a number of diverse typing methods should be required to identify them. These methods are subject to constant review and are revised when it is appropriate. The methods presented here are those in use at the time of writing, but it should come as no surprise that variations of these may soon become standard.

The use of DNA probes for typing class II HLA antigens has become widespread. It is emerging as the standard method. Many of the newer specificities are identified only by polymerase chain reaction–sequence specific oligonucleotide probe (PCR-SSOP) techniques. But for the class I antigens, and others of the class II group, lymphocytotoxicity still remains the method of choice. However, the caveat is clear: as we hone our understanding of the major histocompatibility complex ever more sharply, so will our need for more precise typing methods be the driving force behind the development of these methods.

HLA TYPING

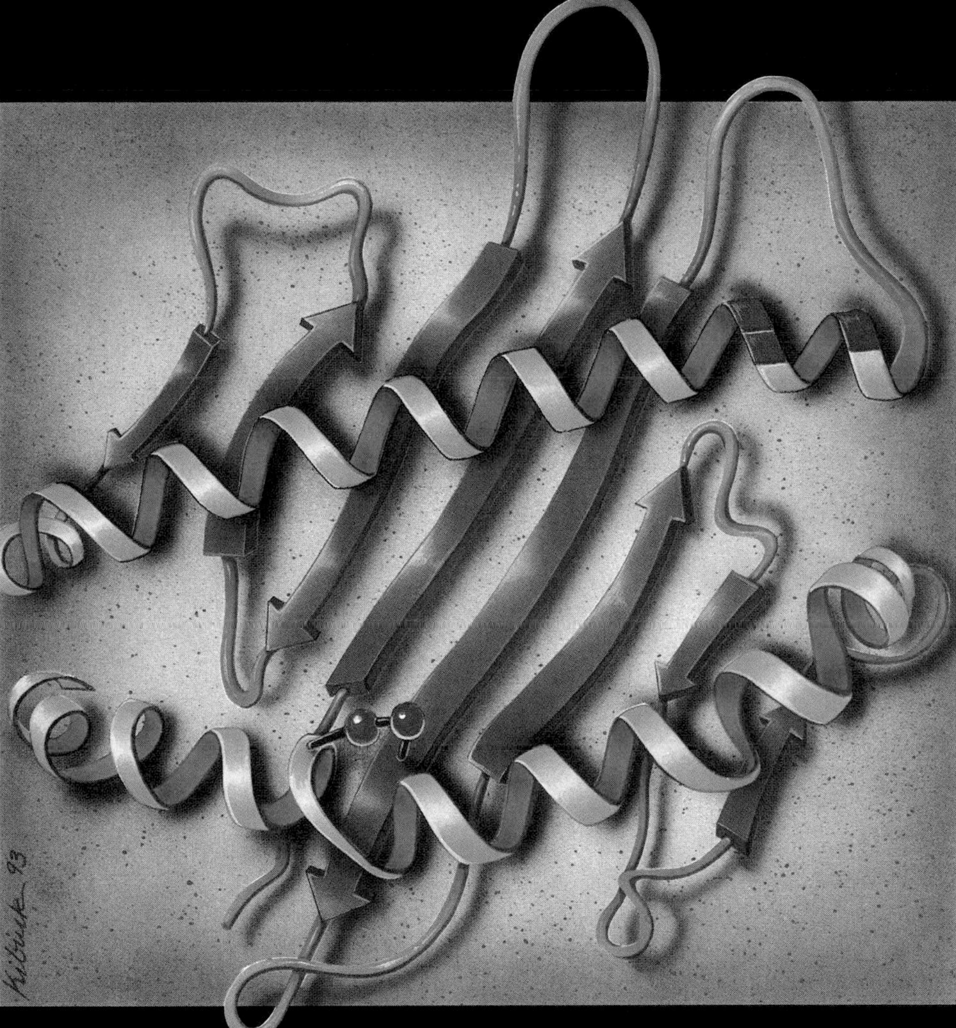

31 HLA: The Major Histocompatibility Complex—Methodologies

Chester M. Zmijewski

Organ transplantation has long held fascination for scientists of many persuasions. Workers in diverse specialties have been attracted to this area for many reasons and it has burgeoned into activity requiring multidisciplinary input. Attempts to transplant tissues and organs for the purpose of studying oncogenesis or aging were thwarted by the failure of the engrafted tissues or organs to thrive in the body of the host. Characteristically, grafts of skin exchanged between animals belonging to the same species begin to heal shortly after surgery. Blood vessels from the host extend into the grafted tissue and circulation is thereby established. After 10 to 12 days, the vessels become occluded, circulation ceases, and necrosis begins. This culminates in the formation of an eschar and rejection of the graft at about day 14.

When skin grafts were exchanged between animals of the same inbred strain, which are akin to identical twins, healing occurred without incident and survived for the life of the animal. However, grafts exchanged between animals of different strains were rejected, as expected. Finally, the F1 offspring from the mating of two different inbred strains would accept grafts from animals of either parental strain. On the other hand, either parent rejected grafts from an F1 donor. This offered experimental evidence indicating that graft rejection was under genetic control.

As early as 1944, Medawar clearly demonstrated that the homograft reaction had an immunologic basis (1). He showed that, although the rejection of skin did occur in 14 days, a second graft from the same donor was rejected much more rapidly. Such a secondary response implied immunologic memory. Furthermore, subsequent grafts were rejected even more rapidly until finally a situation took place in which vascularization failed to occur, giving rise to a so-called "white graft."

Microscopic examination of biopsies taken from the site of these grafts revealed the presence of a large number of small lymphocytes clustered around capillary venules, inflammatory cells, and, in the case of white grafts, massive thrombi with relatively little lymphocytic involvement.

Based on these observations and other experiments involving the generation of tolerance, Medawar postulated that there existed a set of alloantigens under genetic control that are present on donor tissues and recognized by the host. The host mounts an immune response to these antigens that is not unlike a delayed hypersensitivity response consisting of immune lymphocytes as effectors. Upon continued exposure to antigen or after repeated challenges, antibodies directed against these antigens are formed. Indeed, it was eventually demonstrated that the features of the white graft were caused primarily by circulating antibodies that had been formed in response to previous grafts. This was the origin of the idea of histocompatibility antigens, which were first described by Gorer, elucidated through the use of inbred strains by Snell, and extended to humans by Dausset, Payne, Van Rood, and others (2, 3).

Histocompatibility antigens were conceived as being a set of alloantigens that were significant only as targets for the allograft reaction. However, shortly after their definition, it became clear that these antigens, which are controlled by a genetic complex referred to collectively as the major histocompatibility complex (MHC), are involved in immunologic self-recognition and therefore have a much deeper biological function. It is now clear that histocompatibility antigens serve as self-recognition molecules. In this capacity they help to trigger the T cell–dependent immune response and actively participate in the immune elimination of cells infested with foreign substances.

The antigens of the HLA system comprise the histocompatibility antigens in man. The genetic complex controlling the production of these antigens is located on the distal third of the short arm of chromosome 6. Counterparts of this system exhibiting the same general characteristics have been found in all mammalian species studied to date and are similarly genetically controlled. For example, the mouse equivalent, called H-2, is found on mouse chromo-

Table 31.1. The HLA Specificities 1991

D				B			C	A
DPw1	DQ1	DR1	Dw1	B5	B40	B59	Cw1	A1
DPw2	DQ2	DR103	Dw2	B7	B4005	B60(40)	Cw2	A2
DPw3	DQ3	DR2	Dw3	B703	B41	B61(40)	Cw3	A203
DPw4	DQ4	DR3	Dw4	B8	B42	B62(15)	Cw4	A210
DPw5	DQ5(1)	DR4	Dw5	B12	B44(12)	B63(15)	Cw5	A3
DPw6	DQ6(1)	DR5	Dw6	B13	B45(12)	B64(14)	Cw6	A9
	DQ7(3)	DR6	Dw7	B14	B46	B65(14)	Cw7	A10
	DQ8(3)	DR7	Dw8	B15	B47	B67	Cw8	A19
	DQ9(3)	DR8	Dw9	B16	B48	B70	Cw9(3)	A23(9)
		DR9	Dw10	B17	B49(21)	B71(70)	Cw10(3)	A24(9)
		DR10	Dw11(7)	B18	B50(21)	B72(70)		A2403
		DR11(5)	Dw12	B21	B51(5)	B73		A25(10)
		DR12(5)	Dw13	B22	B5102	B75(15)		A26(10)
		DR13(6)	Dw14	B27	B5103	B76(15)		A28
		DR14(6)	Dw15	B35	B52(5)	B77(15)		A29(19)
		DR15(2)	Dw16	B37	B53	B7801		A30(19)
		DR16(2)	Dw17(7)	B38(16)	B54(22)			A31(19)
		DR17(3)	Dw18(6)	B39(16)	B55(22)			A32(19)
		DR18(3)	Dw19(6)	B3901	B56(22)	Bw4		A33(19)
			Dw20	B3902	B57(17)	Bw6		A34(10)
		DR51	Dw21		B58(17)			A36
		DR52	Dw22					A43
		DR53	Dw23					A66(10)
			Dw24					A68(28)
			Dw25					A69(28)
			Dw26					A74(19)

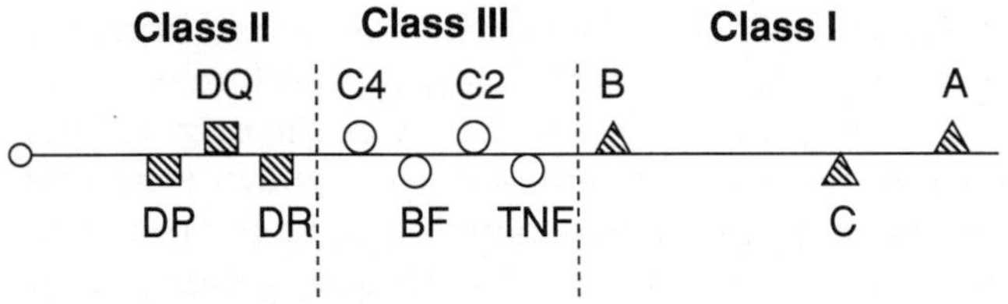

Figure 31.1. A diagrammatic representation of the distal third of the short arm of human chromosome 6 carrying the major loci of HLA. The region is divided into three areas which control the production of the class I, class II, and class III molecules.

some 17. This system has been studied extensively and continues to serve as a model for the investigation of basic questions in immunology centered on immune responsiveness and tolerance. Among the other species in which the MHC systems have been studied are horses (ELA), cows (BLA), cats (FLA), dogs (DLA), rats (RtLA) and rhesus monkeys (RhLA).

GENETICS AND SPECIAL FEATURES OF HLA

The HLA region on chromosome 6 is composed of a set of very closely linked loci. The general arrangement of these loci is shown in Figure 31.1 (4). The genetic complex can be divided into three major regions, each of which controls the production of molecules that have distinct biological functions. These are called class I, which encompasses the HLA-A, B, and C loci; class II, which includes the HLA-D region loci HLA-DR, DQ, and DP; and class III, which are loci whose gene products are molecules that belong to the complement system and include C2, C4, and Bf as well as the cytokines referred to as tumor necrosis factors (TNFs).

The HLA system is highly polymorphic. Indeed, it is the most polymorphic genetic system in man. Associated with each of the loci is a set of alleles each of which gives rise to the production of a unique antigenic specificity, which is expressed on the cell surface and can be detected by specific antibodies. The recognizable antigens of the HLA system are shown in Table 31.1 (5, 34). The nomenclature for the alleles of the HLA system has been established and is controlled by a select committee of the World Health Organization (WHO). The antigen name is composed of a letter designating the locus, (e.g., A, B, C, DR, DP, DQ) and a number.

Originally, before it was known that multiple loci controlled HLA, the numbers were assigned in the order of their discovery. Therefore, some inconsistencies occur, such as 1, 2, and 3 assigned to the A locus; 5, 7, and 8 assigned to B; and 9, 10, and 11 reverting to A. The more recently described antigens now follow in logical sequence. Another noticeable peculiarity is the absence of antigens 4 and 6 from the original list. These numerical assignments were reserved for some very special antigens that did not seem to follow the accepted patterns of inheritance

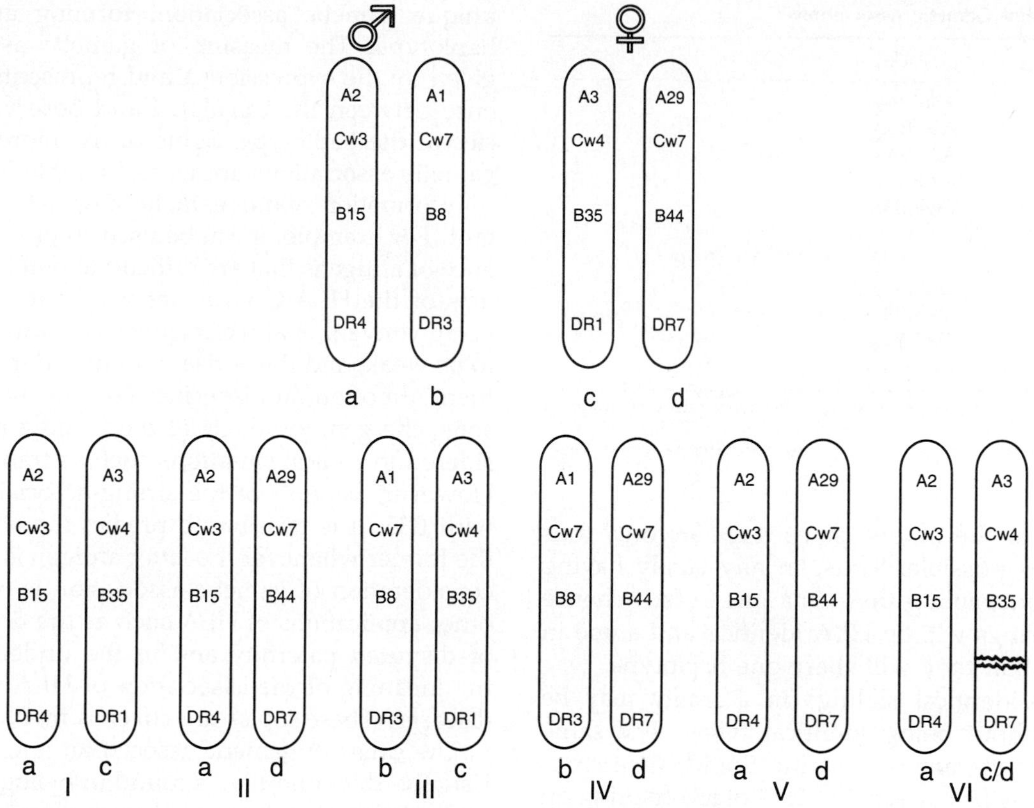

Figure 31.2. A pedigree of a family consisting of two parents and six siblings. The HLA haplotypes of paternal origin are labeled a and b. The maternal haplotypes are labeled c and d. Siblings I through IV represent the different combinations. Sibling V is HLA-identical to sibling II. Sibling VI carries a maternal haplotype that is a recombinant in which the A, C, and B loci come from chromosome c and the DR locus comes from chromosome d.

or serology. Since then they have been shown to be "supertypic" or public antigens. These are the products of specific epitopes found on the HLA-B molecule and are described in a subsequent section. They are now called Bw4 and Bw6.

Some of the antigens in Table 31.1 carry a "w" designation. In previous versions of the HLA nomenclature, this prefix indicated a provisional designation pending confirmation based on extensive serologic testing. This was often involved and the results clouded by the fact that the antisera used for the testing were frequently multispecific, and being products of biological immune responses, they carried the expected variations normally associated with such responses.

Current practice calls for serologic specificities to be named based on correlation with an identified DNA sequence. Therefore, there is no need for a provisional designation since the antigens will have a primary definition. The "w" prefix, however, will be retained in the case of the Bw4 and Bw6 epitopes to distinguish them from alleles; the C locus specificities to distinguish them from the complement components; and in the case of the bioassay determined specificities Dw and DP.

The new system of nomenclature also allows for the differentiation between the currently accepted classic serologic splits and what might be termed allelic variants. Thus, for example, B51 and B52 are splits of the B5 specificity, distinguishable serologically, while B5101 and B5102 are allelic variants of B51, discernible by biochemical techniques. In the future, however, new serologically defined splits that may be due to epitopes corresponding to combinations of alleles will not be given official names.

The individual loci of the HLA complex are tightly linked; thus, genetic recombination or crossing over is a rare event occurring for the most part no more than 1% of the time between A and B and between B and DR and 0.6% between A and C and 0.2% between B and C (6). Accordingly, the alleles of the HLA system for the most part are inherited en bloc from each parent as a unit called a haplotype.

Figure 31.2 shows the typical inheritance pattern of the HLA antigens in a hypothetical family with six siblings. Each of the first four siblings is different with respect to the HLA antigens he or she has inherited; however, the group can be divided into pairs that share either identical maternal or identical paternal chromosomes. But the fifth sibling must be iden-

Table 31.2. Major Gametic Associations[a]

Whites	Blacks
A1,B8	A36,B44
A30,B13	A30,B42
A25,B18	A29,B44
A3,B7	A2,B45
Cw4,B35	Cw4,B35
Cw2,B27	
Cw5,B44	
DR2,B7	DR2,B7
DR3,B8	DR3,B8
DR7,B13	DR7,B13
	DR11,B18

[a]From Baur MP, Neugebauer M, Albert ED. Reference tables of two-locus haplotype frequencies for all MHC marker loci. In: Albert ED, Baur MP, Mayr WR, eds. Histocompatability testing 1984. New York: Springer-Verlag, 1984: 677–755.

tical to one of the others, since there are only four combinations possible. Thus, in any family having more than one sibling there is a one in four chance that two siblings will be HLA identical and a one in two chance that they will share one haplotype.

The HLA-identical siblings in a family may be identical without being identical twins. The same combinations of gametes bearing the MHC of chromosome 6 may be expected in 25% of all offspring on the basis of chance combination alone. Nevertheless, the extremely low frequency of recombination within the HLA region due to tight linkage is the phenomenon that permits transplantation between ordinary siblings.

Although recombination in the HLA system is an infrequent event, it does occur, and usually between the B and the DR loci. An example of this type of recombination is given by sibling 6 in Figure 31.2. In this case offspring number 6 is identical to siblings numbered 4 and 5 with respect to class I antigens but differs with respect to class II antigens. Such recombination can have important clinical implications for transplantation. Highly polymorphic multilocus systems such as HLA are usually found in the population at large in a state of genetic equilibrium. This equilibrium is such that the frequency with which two or three alleles from the linked loci occur together in a single haplotype is equal to the product of the individual gene frequencies in the population being observed. Although this holds true to a certain extent in the HLA system, there are some notable exceptions. The phenomenon of genetic disequilibrium, or more properly, gametic association, is one of the hallmarks of the HLA system.

Gametic associations are regularly found between certain alleles of A and B, C and B, B and DR, and DR and DQ. In addition, there are instances in which certain haplotypes containing even the sequences controlling the class III antigens are found in a unique gametic association, forming an extended haplotype. The measure of gametic association is given by the expression Δ and represents the difference between the calculated and observed frequencies of the haplotype. Some of the more prominent gametic associations are listed in Table 31.2 (7).

Information about gametic association is important. For example, it can be used to predict the presence of antigens that are difficult to detect. The products of the HLA-C locus are very difficult to detect using conventional techniques. The antigens appear to be weak, and the antisera produced in response to them are often multispecific. For this and other reasons, the gene products of the C locus are not considered in clinical situations such as transplantation. However, because of the strong association of Cw4 with B35, it is possible to predict the occurrence of the former whenever the latter antigen is detected. A consideration of gametic association is important in other applications of HLA such as the determination of disputed paternity and in the understanding of the meaning of the association of HLA with certain diseases. These topics are covered in Chapter 32.

The cause of gametic association is unknown (9). Usually, this condition is found in biological systems with alleles that have undergone recent mutation and that have not yet had an opportunity to reach equilibrium. This does not appear to be the case with the HLA system. The gametic associations observed extend throughout widely divergent populations, suggesting simultaneous and identical mutations. This is a highly unlikely event.

In the mouse system there is a set of genes at the telomeric end of the MHC region that preferentially inhibit recombination in haplotypes that carry them, thereby favoring gametic association (10). A search for a similar set of genes in man has been under way, but thus far has been without reward. Genes have been found telomeric to HLA-A that give rise to putative MHC molecules. However, their function does not appear to be equivalent to that found in rodents.

Another theory often proposed to explain such a finding is selective advantage. With respect to HLA this is difficult to rationalize since many of the haplotypes in gametic association are also associated with certain diseases. The common haplotypes HLA-A3,B7 and HLA-A1,B8 are strongly associated with multiple sclerosis and myesthenia gravis, as described later in this chapter. Although this is far from a convincing argument for advantage, some proponents of the idea point out that there may be other very beneficial genes associated with these haplotypes, which by far outweigh the occasional detrimental effects.

As with many of the other alloantigens such as the blood groups of the human red cells, the alleles of

Table 31.3. HLA Gene Frequencies in Various Populations[a]

HLA	White	Black	Oriental
A1	**.149**	.033	.005
A2	**.269**	**.147**	**.246**
A23	.025	**.108**	.005
A24	.066	.029	**.356**
A11	**.059**	.006	**.090**
A34	.006	**.065**	.001
B7	**.098**	**.089**	**.059**
B8	**.090**	.029	.001
B38	**.032**	.000	.002
B42	.003	**.077**	.006
B53	.009	**.065**	.001
B54	.000	.000	**.073**
DR3	**.118**	**.173**	.016
DR4	**.148**	.049	**.235**
DR5	**.103**	**.133**	.022
DR9	.011	.027	**.122**

[a]From Baur MP, Danilovs JA. Population analysis of HLA-A, B, C, DR and other genetic markers. In: Terasaki PI, ed. Histocompatability testing 1980. Los Angeles: UCLA Tissue Typing Laboratory, 1980:955–993.

the HLA system have gene frequencies that vary from one population to the next. The variability exists not only among the different races but also among various ethnic groups. Some of the more prominent differences in gene frequencies are shown in Table 31.3 (8). Key frequencies of antigens common to all three racial groups or peculiar to a given group are listed in bold type. Thus, some antigens may be present in high frequency in caucasians but altogether absent in orientals. Other antigens may be present in blacks in fairly high frequency and virtually absent from caucasians. Although not shown, such distinctions may be present among various ethnic populations within the same race. Thus, there may be certain antigens that are characteristic of eastern Europeans such as the Poles and Russians which are rarely found among the English. Similar analogies in antigen distribution may be found among the various black tribes of Africa and among various oriental peoples such as the Japanese, Chinese, and Koreans.

Although the majority of the HLA alleles present in caucasians have been discovered as evidenced by gene frequencies that total almost 100%, the same may not be true of the other races. In considering the HLA-A and B loci one would expect that an individual should have at least four antigens: two HLA-A antigens, one from each parent, along with two HLA-B antigens inherited in the same fashion. In testing black families, for example, it is not uncommon to find individuals who appear to lack one or more HLA antigens. It is usually clear from the familial pattern of inheritance that the individuals in question are not homozygous for a given allele and therefore phenotypically express it only once but rather they have inherited what appears to be an undetectable characteristic, a so-called "blank." The obvious explanation for such a finding is that the individual has a gene that causes the expression of an antigen that cannot be detected with the currently available battery of anti-HLA antisera. Indeed, studies of such individuals among blacks have revealed the existence of unique black antigens. Similar race-specific antigens have been reported in the Japanese.

These antigens become an important consideration in transplant programs associated with large metropolitan hospitals. The random organ donor population available to such institutions as well as their patient populations will be composed of different racial groups. Therefore, the knowledge of these special antigens and the ability to detect them are essential. In addition, a knowledge of the variation in the gene frequency of HLA is important because it can have an effect on the ability to find an HLA-matched random cadaveric donor from the general population in a given geographic area. It might be very difficult to locate a suitable donor for a black patient with one or more unique antigens in some midwestern city populated primarily with whites of Scandinavian ancestry. Numerous other examples could be cited for other regions of the U.S. where there are widely divergent racial and ethnic backgrounds. For this reason, a national system of organ sharing, though currently impractical, might be considered in the future to give patients the maximum potential for obtaining a well-matched graft.

The majority of antigens in the HLA system are detected by means of serologic methods employing specific antibodies. One of the characteristic phenomena that has been observed when using anti-HLA alloantibodies is the frequent appearance of serologic cross-reactivity. This is a condition in which an antiserum previously shown to react with one particular HLA specificity, upon further testing is shown to react either wholly or partially with another specificity. An example of this is shown in Table 31.4.

The occurrence of serologic cross-reactivity is most easily attributed to the presence of a mixture of antibodies having specificities directed against several but perhaps related antigens. However, this does not appear to be the cause of cross-reactivity in the HLA system (11). Usually, the repeated absorption of the HLA antiserum in question with cells bearing one of the specificities totally removes all reactivity for the other specificity. Such a finding indicates that the antiserum is truly monospecific and establishes that the cross-reactivity may be attributable to factors at the level of the antigenic determinant. This outcome is supported by the results of experiences with in vivo immunization. In some cases an antigenic challenge with a given primary antigen may result in the development of antibodies that react with another antigen

Table 31.4. Cross-Reactivity due to Shared Epitopes

HLA Specificity	Epitopes	Possible Antibodies	Observed Specificity	Reaction with: B5	B35	B18
B5	1,2,3	Anti-1 Anti-2 Anti-3	Anti-B5	+++	+	+
B35	1,4,5	Anti-1 Anti-4 Anti-5	Anti-B35	+	+++	+
B18	3,6,5	Anti-3 Anti-6 Anti-5	Anti-B18	+	+	+++

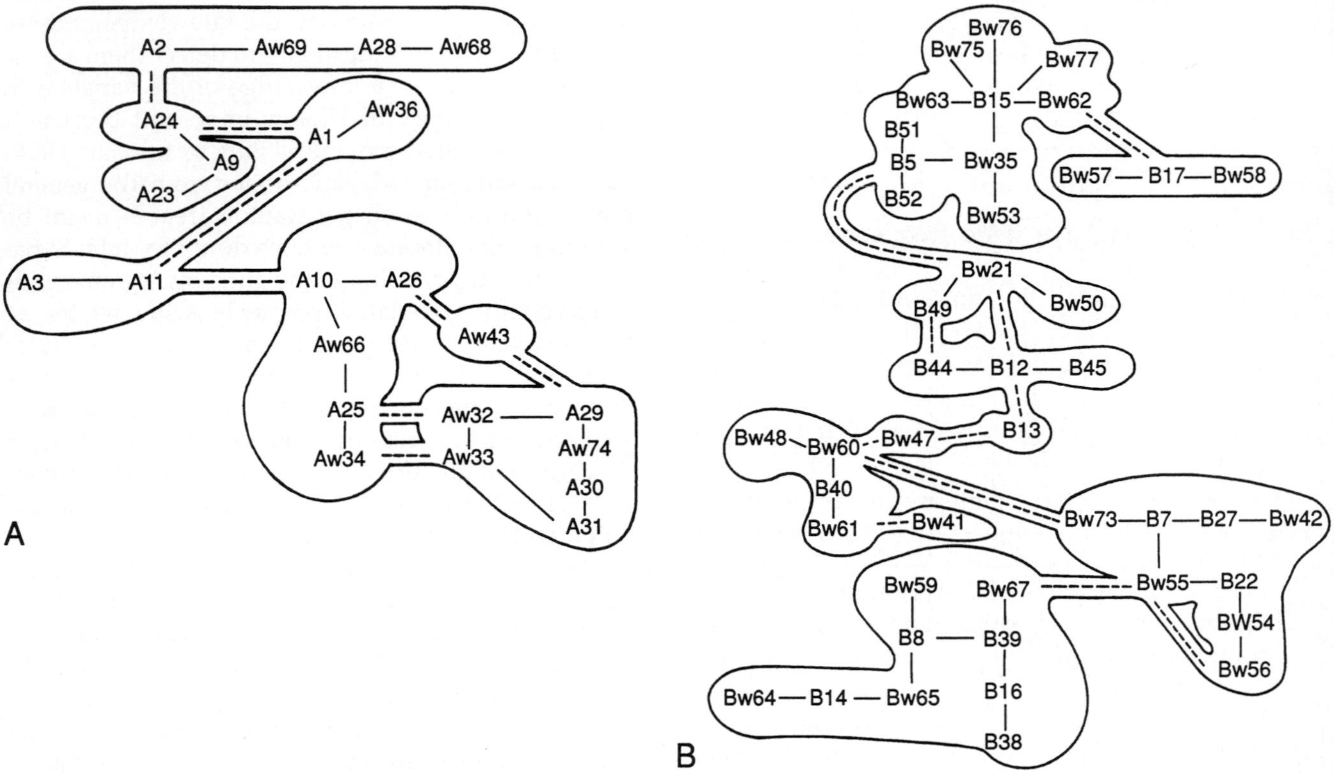

Figure 31.3. The prominent cross-reactive groups (CREGs) of the HLA antigens. The CREGs of the HLA-A antigens are shown in **A** and those of the HLA-B antigens in **B**. The antigens form tightly bound clusters that are strongly cross-reactive. In addition, some weaker cross-reactivity shown by the dotted lines exists between the clusters.

not present in the immunizing dose. Furthermore, an attempt to immunize an individual with an antigen that he or she is lacking but which is cross-reactive with one of his or her own antigens may not result in an immune response.

The phenomenon of antigenic cross-reactivity is due to the sharing of specific epitopes on the antigenic molecule. It is a regular feature of the HLA system whose antigens may be arranged in "cross-reactive groups" or CREGs. The most prominent CREGs of the HLA-A and HLA-B loci are shown in Figure 31.3.

CREGs are important in that they allow for greater latitude in donor-recipient HLA matching and at the same time may be used to predict potential problems with graft outcome. So, for example, transplantation or platelet transfusion within a CREG can often be performed without eliciting any great uncontrollable immune response. By the same token, if a patient is shown to have an antibody of a particular specificity, it is possible that under the proper circumstances his or her serum will react as well with tissues bearing other antigens within the same CREG.

The so-called Public and Private specificities of the HLA system are a special type of CREG and constitute a prominent feature of the antigens in the HLA system. Public antigens are specific epitopes that are found to be associated with each of the different specificities of an entire family of HLA molecules. Two such public specifications are the HLA-Bw4 and Bw6 mentioned previously. As the HLA system unfolded, it became clear that many of the antisera belonging to a number of investigators in the field and supposedly detecting a variety of different antigens were in fact detecting a common antigen that could be given an HLA designation. However, the supposedly allelic antigens 4a and 4b originally described by van Rood did not appear to fit the scheme. Further investigation revealed that 4a and 4b were not products of antithetical allelic genes but rather were found associated with all antigens of the HLA-B locus. Since these specificities cross the boundaries of all of the other specificities of this locus, they were envisioned as public specificities.

In contrast to public specificities, which tend to group antigens into large categories, private specificities tend to divide the groups. For example, the specificity HLA-A9 has two private specificities—HLA-A23 and A24. Cells expressing either of these antigens will react not only with anti-HLA-A23 or A24 antisera but also with anti-HLA-A9. Thus, the private specificities are true specificities in their own right. In addition, HLA-A23 and A24 each have a different gene frequency in whites and in blacks, indicating that they probably arose from a common ancestral gene after the divergence of the races.

Although the idea of public and private HLA specificities has been somewhat diminished by the introduction of an allele-based nomenclature, it still carries practicality from a clinical standpoint. The antigenic structure is defined by DNA sequence, but the extent of an individual's humoral immune response is strongly influenced by the collection of epitopes expressed on the antigenic molecule. Evidence for this is given by the diversity of antibody specificities directed toward the HLA specificities, which were used to define them in the first place. Therefore, in those clinical situations that could be adversely affected by HLA antibodies, an appreciation for the epitopic relationships of the antigens such as that given by the public and private designations can be most useful.

BIOLOGY AND BIOCHEMISTRY OF HLA

In the previous section the HLA chromosomal region was divided into sections that controlled the production of three different types of molecules that were called class I, class II, and class III. Each of these is unique in terms of its tissue distribution, biochemical structure, and biological function.

Class I molecules are expressed constitutively on the surface of all nucleated cells in the body with the possible exception of the cells of the central nervous system. They can be demonstrated readily on mature lymphocytes, granulocytes, monocytes, platelets, epithelial cells, endothelial cells, and fibroblasts grown in culture. However, they are not found as normal components of the surface of mature human erythrocytes.

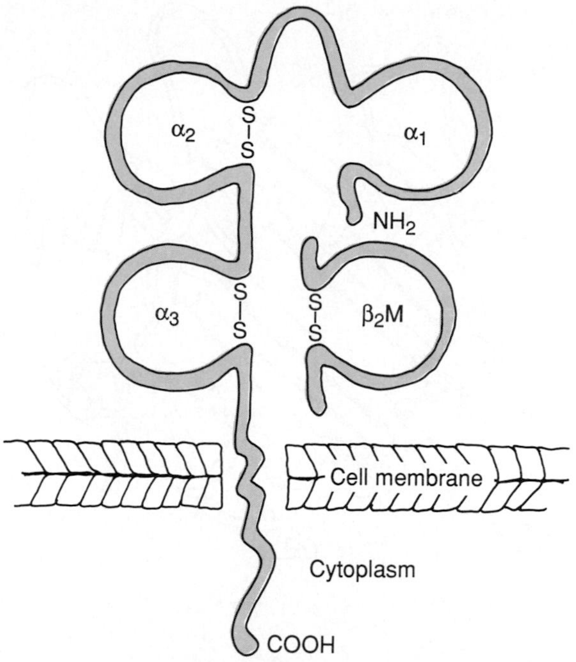

Figure 31.4. A diagrammatic representation of the HLA class I molecule. The α chain carries the specificity. It is always found in association with β_2-microglobulin.

There have been numerous reports that class I antigens may be found on red blood cells in humans just like their murine counterparts, the H-2 antigens. These observations are best explained by the finding that free HLA antigens may be present as soluble substances in the plasma. Most likely they are shed from the surface of nucleated cells and maybe even from maturing erythroblasts. Occasionally, these soluble class I HLA antigens may become attached to the surface of mature red cells as they float freely in the plasma (12). It is highly unlikely that the antigens can be synthesized by anuclear mature red cells.

The class I MHC molecules, Figure 31.4, consist of heterodimers composed of two noncovalently linked polypeptide chains. The larger of the two, the α chain, is glycosylated and has a molecular weight of approximately 45 kd. It is produced as a direct result of genetic information within the MHC and bears amino acid sequences that are part of the allospecific epitopes. The α chain is anchored in the lipid bilayer of the cell membrane. This form of attachment allows the molecule to move freely on the surface of the cell and is loose enough to permit shedding.

The smaller, β_2-microglobulin chain does not penetrate the cell surface. It has a molecular weight of

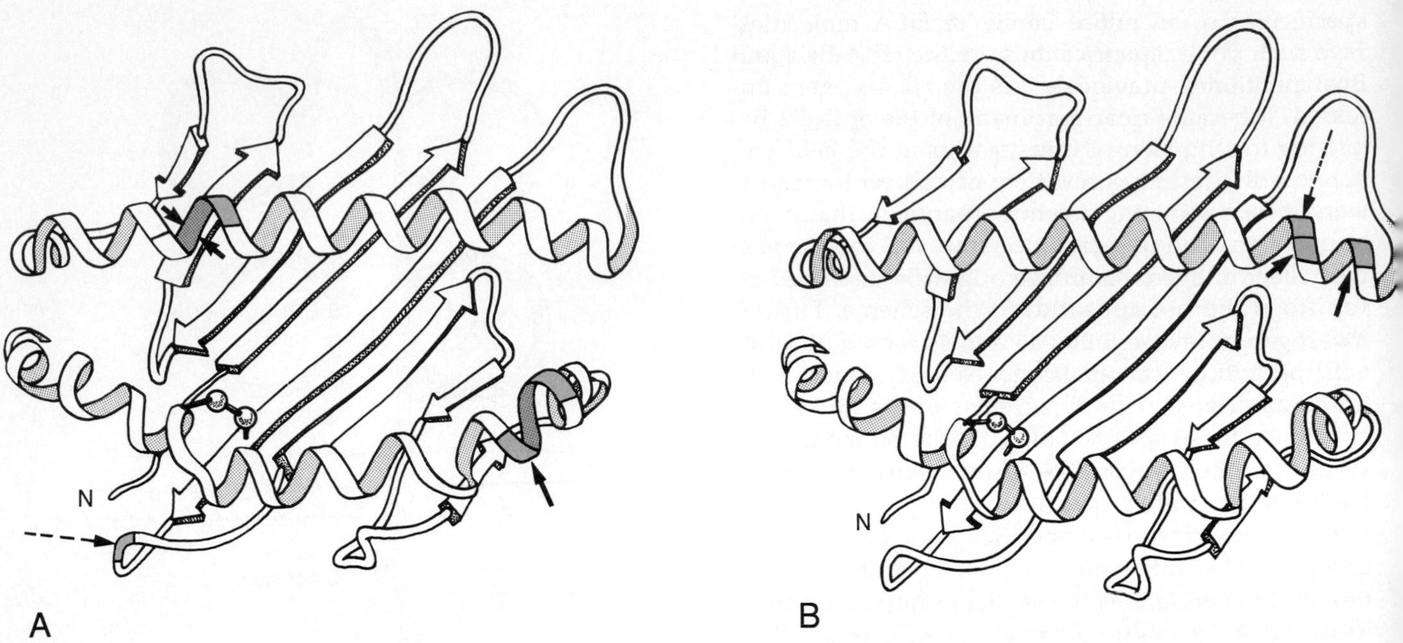

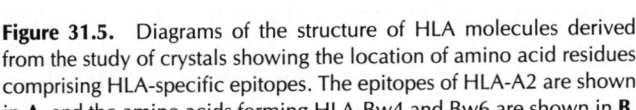

A2, w69	107	←----
A2, B17	62–65	→ ←
A2, A28	142–145	←

	79	80	83
Bw4	Arg	Ile Leu/Thr	Arg
Bw6	Arg	Asp	Gly
Not Bw4/Bw6	Gly	Thr/Lys	Gly
	↑	↑	↑

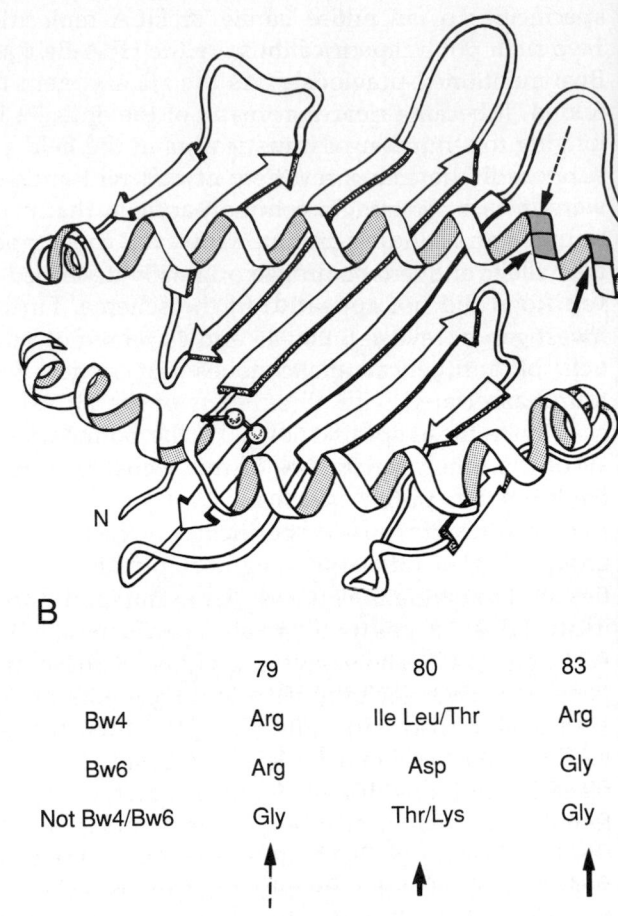

Figure 31.5. Diagrams of the structure of HLA molecules derived from the study of crystals showing the location of amino acid residues comprising HLA-specific epitopes. The epitopes of HLA-A2 are shown in **A,** and the amino acids forming HLA-Bw4 and Bw6 are shown in **B.** (Reprinted with permission from Parham P, Lawlor DA, Slater RD, Lomen CE, Bjorkman PJ, Ennis PD. HLA-A, B, C: patterns of polymorphism in peptide binding proteins. In: Dupont B, ed. Immunobiology of HLA, II. New York: Springer-Verlag, 1989:17.)

12 kd. Its production in man is controlled by nonpolymorphic genes found on chromosome 15. Thus, the two polypeptides that form class I HLA antigen are produced independently and associate posttranslationally to produce the final molecule.

The presence of β_2-microglobulin is required to maintain the stability of the class I molecule, and it has been found to be an integral part of such molecules from all species studied.

An analysis of the amino acid sequence of the α chain has shown that it is divided into five domains consisting of three extracellular regions—α_1, α_2, and α_3—a transmembrane domain and a cytoplasmic domain. The α_2 and α_3 domains each have intrachain loops held by disulfide bonds having strong sequence homology to immunoglobulin domains. The α_1 domain is not held in a loop and contains a glycosylation site at position 86. The amino acid sequencing of α chains from MHC antigens of different specificities and even from diffrent species shows a remarkable degree of conservation in some of the domains (13). Most of the variability occurs in the α_1 domain, which is the region expressing allospecificity. The transmembrane domain consists primarily of hydrophobic amino acids with some highly charged residues that may help to anchor the molecule. The cytoplasmic domain contains serine residues that may be phosphorylated and could be involved in intracytoplasmic signaling.

The associated β_2-microglobulin consists of a single domain formed by one disulfide loop. It is associated with the heavy chain through interaction with the α_3 domain.

Recently, the class I molecule has been crystallized and its structure deduced by x-ray diffraction and computer-assisted analysis (14). The resultant image, shown diagrammatically in Figure 31.5, is a globular structure containing an immunoglobulin-like groove that acts as a peptide-binding site. The α_1 and α_2 domains combine to form a structure composed of two α helices that form the walls of the groove and a β-pleated sheet that forms the floor.

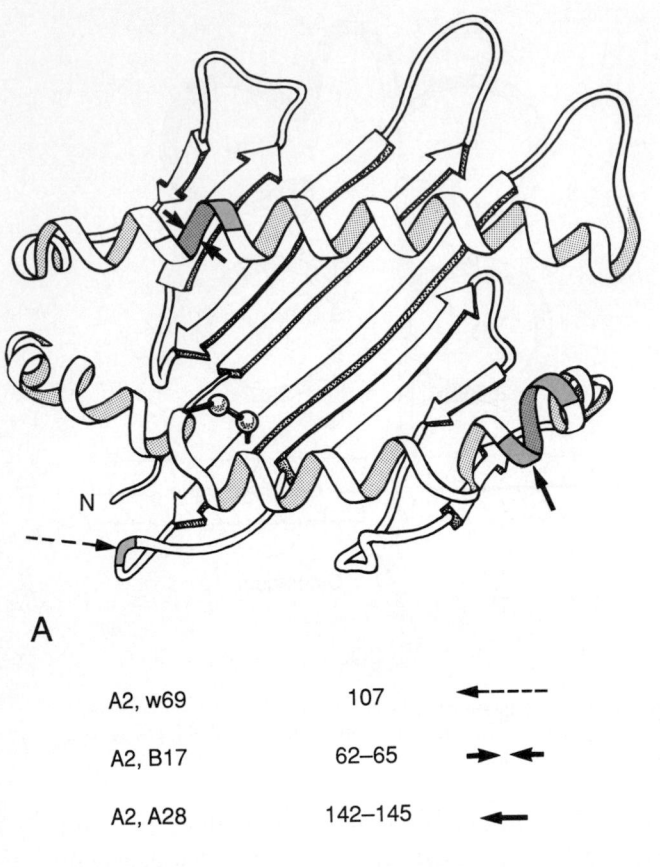

Amino acid sequence analysis of the α chains of class I molecules of different HLA specificities has revealed the presence of at least 20 residues of high variability (13). Eighteen of these residues are situated in a region of the molecule that can potentially interact with bound peptide or the T-cell receptor. Some of these, found along the inner walls of the α helices and within the area of the β-pleated sheets have their side chains pointing into the groove. These are involved in peptide binding, the high degree of variability allowing the binding of a wide range of peptides. Other residues found along the top surfaces of the α helices have their side chains pointing outward. These contribute to interaction with the T-cell receptor.

Linear sequences identifying residues critical to the expression of allospecificities are found in the helices of the α_1 and α_2 domains as well as external portions of the β structure.

These findings explain certain phenomena that confounded serologists working in the HLA system. The public specificities Bw4 and Bw6 are the result of amino acid substitutions in residues 79 to 83 of the α_1 domain. Asparagine at position 80 is essential for the expression of the Bw6 epitope, while arginine at position 83 is responsible for the Bw4 specificity. These amino acid positions are different from those that confer the private specificities. Therefore, the so-called inclusion of private specificities within public ones can be explained because the HLA molecule has several epitopes in different locations.

The finding that within the HLA-A2, A28, A69 CREG a combination of three epitopes is required for the expression of HLA-A2 could be the basis for cross-reactivity. While all three epitopes are required for the expression of A2, the expression of A28 depends only on residues at positions 142 to 145 and Aw69 at position 107. HLA-B17, a loose member of this CREG, is defined by residues at positions 62 to 65.

In contrast to class I antigens, the class II antigens, which include the products of the HLA-DR, DQ and DP loci are limited in their distribution. In general, these antigens do not appear to be constitutive products of nucleated cells. Rather, they are produced in conjunction with an immune response by means of lymphokines such as IL-2 and γ-interferon.

Most regularly, the class II antigens are found on B lymphocytes, monocytes, macrophages, endothelial cells, Langerhans cells and activated T cells. However, they may also be induced in other types of cells such as renal epithelial cells and pancreatic β cells by means of lymphokines. The latter finding has led to the formation of a hypothesis regarding a possible mechanism for autoimmunization with subsequent tissue damage and disease.

Class II antigens (Figure 31.6) are heterodimers consisting of two noncovalently linked polypeptide

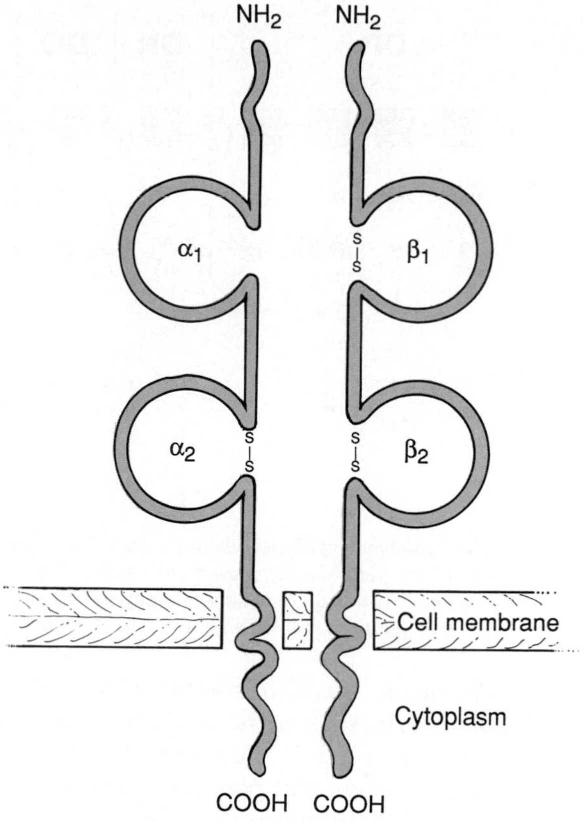

Figure 31.6. A diagrammatic representation of the HLA class II molecule. The carboxy-terminal ends of both the α and the β chains are embedded in the lipid bilayer of the cell membrane.

chains, each of which is a product of genes in the HLA region. The chains each have two external domains, a transmembrane portion anchored in the lipid bilayer of the cell wall, and a cytoplasmic domain. One of the chains, the α chain, has a molecular weight of 34 kd and only its α_2 domain is arranged as a disulfide loop. It bears structural homology to the constant region of immunoglobulin. The α chains of DR molecules are not polymorphic. All of the DR specificities thus share identical α chains. However, the α chains of DQ molecules have some degree of limited polymorphism.

The second polypeptide or β chain has a molecular weight of 29 kd. It is highly polymorphic in all class II molecules and carries sequences appropriate to the allospecificity in three hypervariable regions of its β_1 domain situated between residues 9 to 13, 26 to 33 and 67 to 74. In contrast to the α chain, both the β_1 and β_2 domains contain disulfide loops. Glycosylation sites are found in the α_1, α_2, and β_1 domains which are not involved in the allospecificity of the intact molecule (15).

The class II molecule has not yet been crystallized, so its conformational structure is not known. However, given its function, most investigators believe that it has a structure not too different from that of

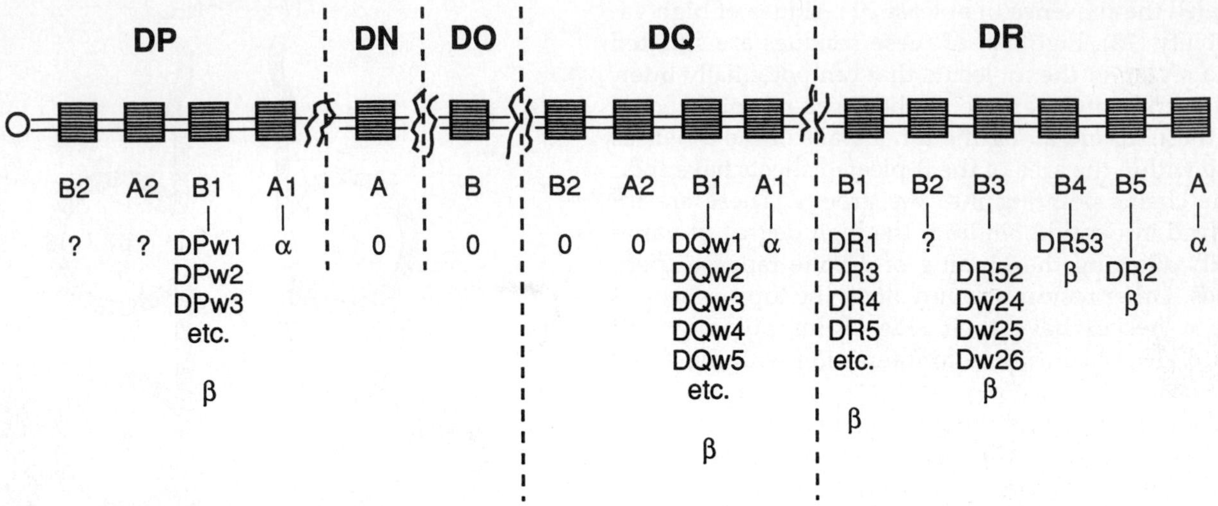

Figure 31.7. The arrangement of loci within the HLA class II region. The specificities of the gene products are listed below the loci that control the specificity. The loci containing pseudogenes are marked with a "?." The gene products marked with a "0" have not been detected. (Adapted from Carroll MC, Katzmann P, Alicot EM, et al. Linkage map of the human major histocompatibility complex including the tumor necrosis factor gene. Proc Nat Acad Sci USA 1987;84: 8535–8539.)

the class I molecule. Thus, it is assumed to contain a pair of α helices that form the walls of an antigen-binding groove and a β-pleated sheet that form the floor. Key amino acids that play a role in conveying specificity would be found in the α helices of such a model.

The genetic region of the class II segment of the HLA locus is quite complex, as illustrated in Figure 31.7. There are a number of separate loci, each coding for the individual α and β chains of the DR, DQ, and DP molecules (16). In addition, there are a number of pseudogenes in the DR, DQ, DO, DN, and DP regions with no apparent products discernible using current techniques. As with the class I antigens, the α and β chains are synthesized independently and then associate posttranslationally to form the individual molecules.

Within the DR region, the β chain locus B1 has polymorphic alleles that give rise to the private DR specificities, DR1, DR3, DR4, etc., while B3 carries the gene that codes for DR52 and B4 the gene that codes for DR53. Originally these two specificities were thought to be supertypic or public antigens similar to the class I antigens Bw4 and Bw6 because they were always found along with one of the other DR specificities. DR3, DR5, DR6, and DR8 are associated with B52 and DR4, DR7, and DR9 with DRw53. The elucidation of this region at the level of the gene has shown that this is not the case. Rather, the observed phenotypic association occurs because of the tight linkage and almost absolute gametic association between the two β chain loci involved.

The DR2 expressing haplotype is a special case. The DR2 specificity of this antigen is imparted as the result of polymorphic alleles at the B1 locus that result in the serologically defined splits, DR15 and DR16. These genes are in gametic association with a nonpolymorphic gene at the B5 locus in lieu of a gene at either the B3 locus or the B4 locus. Thus, the DR2 haplotype expresses neither DR52 or DR53 (5). The nonpolymorphic specificity has been named DR51.

The DQ antigens were likewise thought to be public specificities of DR since DR1, 2, and 6 are associated with DQ1; DR3 and 7 with DQ2, and DR4 and 5 with DQ3. However, this too is the result of gametic association. The posttranslational bonding of the α and β chains in the formation of the DQ heterodimers offers some interesting possibilities. In the heterozygous individual there are two α chain genes for DQ, one from each parent. These may be different because the responsible genes exhibit at least limited polymorphism. In addition, there are two different DQ β chain genes. It is possible for the products of genes in the *trans* position to associate posttranslationally, as shown diagramatically in Figure 31.8. Therefore, a paternal DQ α chain could associate with a maternal DQ β chain, giving rise to a hybrid molecule. Such a molecule would display the maternal DQ allospecificity, since this is controlled by the β chain. However, the specificity of this molecule arising from the complementarity of the two chains could be entirely unique to antigen recognition cells and contribute to further polymorphism.

The early studies of the HLA system additionally defined a set of antigens that could be detected only in biological assays. These behaved as polymorphic class II antigens from a functional standpoint and were called HLA-D. A whole list of these specificities was identified, and many are still found in the table

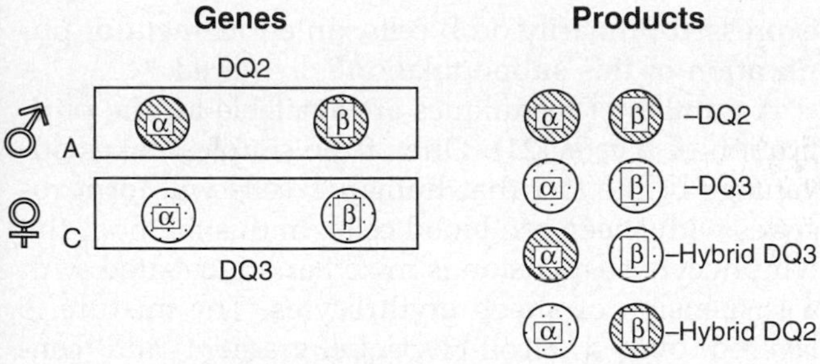

Figure 31.8. A scheme showing how the posttranslational combination of DQ α and β chains in a DQ-heterozygous individual can result in four different molecules.

of current alleles. It is now recognized that the HLA-D specificities are controlled by the DR molecules. However, they may be different from those recognized serologically.

It is clear that immune cells are more robust than antibodies in their ability to detect very small molecular differences. Thus, two DR β chains coming from two different individuals and having identical DR epitopes, but differing by only a single amino acid substitution in another part of the molecule, could not be distinguished by anti-DR antibodies. The cells expressing these chains, however, could be recognized by other cells. Such differences and their impact on class II antigen detection will be reconsidered in the section dealing with biochemical techniques and the mixed lymphocyte culture (MLC).

The biological function of the molecules of the MHC has been the subject of a great deal of basic research. In studying the biology of the immune response to rodent systems, it became clear that the response to certain well-defined antigens was under genetic control (17). Furthermore, it could be demonstrated that the genes responsible for this function could be mapped to the MHC region of the chromosome.

In vitro experiments designed to study the immune response at the cellular level showed that both antigen presentation and antigen destruction by immunologically transformed cytotoxic cells was restricted by the MHC antigens (18). For example, cytotoxic lymphocytes induced in response to challenge with influenzavirus can kill only other cells infected with such a virus if two conditions are met. First, the virus has to be antigenically identical with the one used for induction. Second, the MHC of the infected cell to be destroyed has to be identical to the MHC of the cell that harbored the immunizing virus. The primary biological role of the class I antigens that make up the HLA-A, B, and C repertoire described in this section is to function in such a capacity. Their behavior as alloantigens in transplantation by serving as the targets of the allograft response is a secondary activity of iatrogenic origin.

Class II molecules function biologically in antigen presentation. In vivo, pathogens and other foreign substances are processed by antigen and delivered to specific T-cell receptors on immunologically competent lymphocytes in the context of class II antigen. The T-cell receptor must recognize both the foreign antigen and the self-class II molecule in order to transmit a signal. Therefore, class II antigens play a very important role in the initiation of the immune response. Furthermore, in this context they can act in the capacity of controlling the response.

Although the genetic control of the immune response in man has never been established due to the lack of an appropriate experimental model, it is believed to exist. Rodent model systems clearly demonstrate that the ability of an animal to respond to certain antigens is under genetic control. In the mouse this activity can be mapped to the MHC region of the chromosome and a set of antigens called IA. Biochemical studies indicate that the human counterparts of IA appear to be the DQ antigens, which show sequence homology with the mouse molecules.

Class III MHC antigens are molecules that participate in the complement cascade; these are discussed further elsewhere in the book.

CLASSIC TECHNIQUES FOR DETECTING HLA ANTIGENS

The most widely used technique for the detection of HLA antigens of class I are based on the microlymphocytotoxicity method originally developed by Terasaki and McClelland (19, 20). This is a complement-mediated serologic assay in which peripheral blood lymphocytes are first mixed with an antiserum containing specific anti-HLA antibodies. After a period of incubation, complement is added and the mixture is further incubated. If the lymphocytes carry the HLA antigen against which the antibodies in the antiserum are directed, an antigen-antibody reaction that activates the complement will occur. The ensuing enzymatic cascade culminates in membrane damage that ultimately kills the lymphocytes. A positive reaction is ascertained by examining the cell suspension for cell death. This can be accomplished in a number of ways, including phase-contrast microscopy coupled with the use of supravital stains.

The test has been reduced in size to the point where only microliter volumes of cells and serum are used. This is done to conserve not only the very valuable antisera, but also the amount of blood required to obtain an adequate cell suspension. As noted later in this chapter, several examples of each antiserum

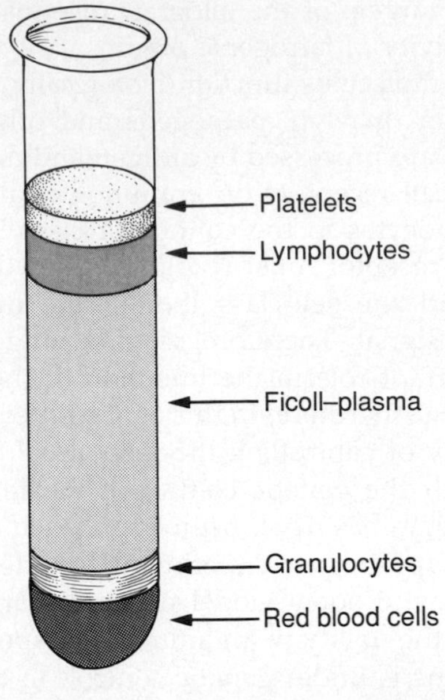

Figure 31.9. The gradient formed after the centifugation of whole blood layered on a mixture of Ficoll-Hypaque. (From White TJ, Arnheim N, Erlich HA. The polymerase chain reaction: the basic technique. Trends Genet 1989;5:6.)

must be used for the optimum definition of each specificity. With the number of specificities in the HLA system, a large quantity of cell suspension would be required in conventionally scaled assays.

Variations of this general method have been developed to increase its sensitivity and to distinguish live cells from dead ones. These will be described later.

The target cells of choice for HLA typing are the small lymphocytes of the peripheral blood. These cells fully express all of the class I antigens. They can be isolated and purified and easily remain stable during in vitro manipulation.

The most widely used separation method is based on the density of small lymphocytes, which ranges from 1.077 to 1.080. Diluted whole blood that has been collected in preservative-free heparin or ACD is carefully layered over a solution of Ficoll-Hypaque that has a corresponding specific gravity. The resultant gradient is centrifuged, allowing the mononuclear cells consisting primarily of lymphocytes to settle at the Ficoll-blood interface. Because they are denser, the erythrocytes and granulocytes settle to the bottom of the tube while most of the platelets remain floating in the uppermost layer (Figure 31.9).

Small lymphocytes isolated in this manner consist of a mixture of T cells and B cells. Such a suspension is perfectly adequate for the detection of class I HLA-A, B, and C antigens since these are well represented on all subsets of lymphocytes. However, in order to identify class II HLA-DR and DQ antigens that are expressed primarily on B cells, an enrichment or purification of this subpopulation is required.

A number of techniques are available for the purification of B cells (21). One of the simplest takes advantage of the fact that human T cells will form rosettes with sheep red blood cells. In this method, the lymphocyte suspension is mixed and incubated with a suspension of sheep erythrocytes. The mixture is layered over a Ficoll-Hypaque gradient and centrifuged. The B cells will come to rest at the blood-Ficoll interface because of their relative density. The T cells, however, are heavier because of the red cells rosetted around them. Therefore, they will be forced through the gradient to the bottom of the tube. Almost pure B cells can be aspirated from the interface, the gradient poured off, and T cells harvested from the bottom. The red cells adhering to the T cells can be lysed away with a hypertonic solution of ammonium chloride.

Another method for isolating B cells takes advantage of their adhesive properties. In this case the lymphocyte suspension is poured onto a small flexible column conveniently made from a plastic drinking straw, filled with washed nylon wool, and moistened with Hank's balanced salt solution. The column is incubated at 37°C to allow the B cells to attach themselves to the fibers of nylon. Following the incubation, the column is allowed to drain, and the nonadherent T cells flow off. This is followed by a gentle wash to eliminate all residual T cells. Finally, the column is gently kneaded and, with a little more washing, the adherent B cells are forced out. This is a good technique, which in skilled hands can result in pure and viable quantities of both T cells and B cells.

Cell suspensions can be enriched for B cells by selectively removing T cells using specific antibody and complement. T cells carry on their surface a number of differentiation antigens that are not found on B cells. Complement-fixing monoclonal antibodies that react specifically with these determinants are available. In practice, a cell suspension is mixed with such an antibody and incubated. When complement is added, the T cells coated with the monoclonal antibody are lysed, leaving behind a suspension of B cells.

In one of the most novel methods currently available, the lymphocyte suspension is mixed with specially prepared magnetic beads that are coated with IgM antibody. The B cells express Fc receptors that couple with the Fc portions of the antibody molecules attached to the beads. This results in a suspension containing B cells attached to magnetic beads. By placing the test tube of cells in a strong magnetic field, the bead-coated B cells are attracted to the magnet and immobilized against one wall of the tube while the T cells remain in suspension and can easily be poured off. The B cells come through this procedure unscathed except for having a coating of beads that precludes the use of routine microlymphocytotoxic detection methods. Therefore, the user is limited to more sophisticated procedures using fluorescent dyes that can differentiate between lymphocytes and beads. Nevertheless, the procedure is quite efficient and useful in cases having a relatively low number of B cells in the peripheral blood.

The antisera used for HLA typing are available from a number of commercial sources both as bulk reagents and on prepared typing trays. The prepared trays are the most economical since they contain a wide range of antisera capable of detecting the majority of clinically relevant antigens. In addition, much of the initial quality control on the finished product has been performed by the manufacturer. Bulk sera, on the other hand, need to be selected according to some predetermined criteria based on their specificity and then dispensed into the typing trays. Finally, extensive primary quality control procedures must be carried out to ensure that the reagents are working and that the assortment of sera selected can accurately delineate an individual's HLA phenotype.

In addition to commercial reagents, typing sera may be prepared in the individual laboratory or obtained from individuals or organizations engaged in basic research on HLA. In some cases this may be the only source of some particularly rare specificity or one newly defined in a recent workshop. However, these sources are not recommended except for those laboratories having a great deal of experience in the use of such materials. Often such reagents require the use of specialized modifications in technique, and the results obtained may be ambiguous, requiring considerable expertise for their interpretation.

The majority of typing sera used for the detection of class I and class II HLA antigens are derived from the sera of multiparous women. HLA antibodies are frequently produced as a result of alloimmunization during pregnancy (22, 23). Approximately 25% of para 3 or greater have them in their serum. This event does not result in any harm to the fetus even though these antibodies are almost exclusively IgG and capable of crossing the placenta. Most likely, the protection is afforded by the placenta, which carries the fetal tissue antigens and acts like a sponge to absorb the antibodies. In fact, placentae are a rich source of HLA antibodies. One of the benefits of antisera produced in this manner is their relatively limited specificity. The fetal antigens that act as the immune stimulus in these cases are those of paternal origin. Therefore, in most instances the antigenic challenge associated with multiple pregnancies involving the same father is restricted by the limited number of different paternal antigens.

Anti-HLA antibodies may be produced as the result of other forms of exposure to antigenic stimuli including transplantation and blood transfusion. Sera from transplanted patients who have rejected their grafts are not a good source of reagent antibody. Such antisera are often of poor quality as reagents since they are low titer and broadly reactive. Furthermore, the patients, having recently undergone the trauma of organ rejection, are poor candidates for serum donation.

The sera from multitransfused patients are the least desirable for use as typing reagents. The immunizing antigens in these cases come mostly from platelets and sometimes from the relatively few nucleated cells found in a unit of transfused blood. Thus, the antigenic dose is small, administered intravenously—a poor route of immunization—over a short period of time. Since this antigenic challenge is inefficient, a large number of transfusions must be given before patients develop antibodies of sufficient titer to work as typing sera. However, exposure to many units of blood from different random donors results in the development of multispecific antisera that are not useful as typing reagents.

The method developed for the production of monoclonal antibodies has been employed to make some anti-HLA reagents (24). This procedure, which was thought to have the potential for revolutionizing HLA typing, had yielded results that were somewhat disappointing at first. Although a number of good reagents useful for HLA typing had been developed, most of the antibodies produced in this manner recognized either very private specificities or, by contrast, very public ones. Reagents such as these were excellent for basic research on the HLA molecule but had limited usefulness in the clinical arena.

Currently, this area has been revisited with somewhat more promising results. The clinically significant allospecific epitopes on the antigen molecules have been better defined, and the procedure for monoclonal antibody production, including antigen preparation and clonal selection, has become more sophisticated. As a result, some of the newer reagents appear to be quite specific in their ability to distinguish clinically significant HLA types; yet they offer all the advantages of a monoclonal reagent. For example, they are specific for either class I or class II antigens. Thus, B-cell separation is not required to type for HLA-DR. In addition, they are free of many interfering substances found in human sera containing alloantibody, thereby allowing for the development of novel and perhaps more rapid techniques for HLA typing.

Regardless of their source, the antisera used for HLA typing are quite different from the alloantisera used for typing in other systems such as the red cell

	A9	210	108	306	53	A23	A24
67	–	–	–	–	–	–	–
1	–	–	–	–	–	–	–
98	–	–	–	–	–	–	–
85	–	–	–	–	–	–	–
59	–	–	–	–	–	–	–
4	–	–	–	■	–	–	–
90	–	–	–	–	–	–	–
6	–	–	–	–	–	–	–
7	–	–	–	–	–	–	–
35	–	–	–	–	–	–	–
59	–	–	–	–	–	–	–
91	–	–	■	–	–	–	–
68	–	–	–	–	–	–	–
57	–	–	■	–	–	–	–
75	–	■	–	–	–	–	–
61	■	■	■	■	–	■	–
94	■	■	■	■	–	■	–
3	■	■	■	■	–	■	–
76	■	■	■	–	■	■	–
5	■	■	■	■	■	■	–
63	■	■	■	■	■	■	–
99	■	■	■	■	–	■	–
10	■	■	■	■	■	■	–
52	■	■	■	■	■	■	–
18	■	■	■	■	■	■	–
16	■	■	■	■	■	■	–
9	■	■	■	■	■	■	–
28	■	■	■	■	■	■	■
84	■	■	■	■	■	■	■
25	■	■	■	■	■	■	■
90	■	■	■	■	■	–	■
50	■	■	■	■	■	–	■
32	■	■	■	■	■	–	■
29	■	■	■	■	■	–	■
77	■	■	■	■	■	–	■
75	■	■	–	■	■	–	■
40	■	■	■	■	■	–	■
80	■	■	■	■	■	–	■
22	■	■	■	■	■	–	■
30	■	■	■	■	–	–	■

– Negative
■ Positive

Figure 31.10. A serogram showing the reaction patterns of four sera reacting with cells positive for HLA-A9. The occurrence of the A23 and A24 antigens among the cells of the panel is shown in the last two columns. Serum 108 is "long" and serum 53 is "short" compared to the index specificity, HLA-A9.

blood groups. Over the years, for example, very few sera directed apparently against the same specificity have been shown to be identical when tested on a cell panel from a large number of donors. In other words, each serum is bound to give both false-negative and false-positive reactions with the lymphocytes of various individuals.

Over the years various descriptive terms have been coined to describe these phenomena. Some of them are derived from the habit of most investigators to represent the reactivity of a serum by means of a histogram or serograph, as shown in Figure 31.10. The test cells are listed along the side, the sera across the top, and each block represents the reaction of a single serum with a single cell. The positive reactions are represented by a solid block, while the negatives are assigned a dash. The cells are arranged so that those expressing the key antigen, graphed on the left side of the diagram, are at the bottom of the chart. In this type of an illustration a serum giving false-positive reactions will cause its serum bar to be longer than the occurrence of the antigen. Therefore such sera were often referred to as "long." On the other hand, sera that tend to give false-negative reactions result in reaction bars that are shorter than the occurrence of the antigen. These sera were called "short."

Absorption studies performed using the cells giving the false-negative reactions with short sera often showed that they were able to fully absorb the specific antibody from such sera. Still, they failed to give a positive cytotoxicity reaction. A finding of this type has been called cytotoxicity negative absorption-positive (CYNAP). This phenomenon may be due to a number of factors including poor antigen expression on the cell at the time of the test, low antibody affinity, or the presence of anticomplementary factors in the cell preparation or the antiserum containing the antibodies.

Figure 31.10 also shows the reaction patterns of the public specificity HLA-A9 along with the private specificities HLA-A23 and A24. The pattern is such that the private specificities are "included" in the public one. The practice of resolving the reaction patterns of anti-HLA sera into serograms has resulted in a wealth of information regarding the relationships of the various specificities to each other. It formed the basis from which many of the features of the system could be defined and served as a template for further studies employing molecular biology and biochemistry.

The complement source used in the microlymphocytotoxicity test is normal rabbit serum. The sera from a large number of different animal species have been tested for their usefulness in cytotoxicity, and the rabbit was found to be the best. This is in contrast to most complement-dependent serologic reactions in which guinea pig serum is used. Guinea pig complement is excellent in those situations requiring a good cytolytic endpoint. However, cell lysis is not desirable in the cytotoxicity procedure in which the endpoint is measured by ascertaining the percentage of dead cells. Furthermore, guinea pig serum is innately toxic for human lymphocytes.

Normal rabbits naturally produce a small amount of anti-human antibody in response to environmental stimuli. This is why rabbit serum is an efficient source of complement. These antibodies act in synergy with anti-HLA antibodies to promote rapid complement activation. This synergism may be explained as follows. First, the majority of anti-HLA antibodies are almost exclusively IgG immunoglobulins; therefore, two adjacent molecules of such antibodies are required for complement activation. Second, the HLA antigens are floating on the cell surface anchored through the lipid bilayer of the cell wall. Two molecules of antigen may therefore not be oriented on the cell surface in a configuration favoring the attachment of adjacent IgG molecules. The presence of anti-human antibody obviates this problem because a single human IgG anti-HLA molecule may be complemented by an adjacent rabbit anti-human molecule to achieve the appropriate configuration for complement activation.

The amount of anti-human antibody present in normal rabbit serum varies from one animal to another. Its concentration is critical to the success of the test system. If the concentration of these antibodies is too low, the desired synergy will not take place, and false-negative results will be obtained. On the other hand, if the concentration of this component is too high, the anti-human antibodies may activate complement in the absence of anti-HLA antibodies and lead to false-positive results. For this reason, the sera of individual rabbits must be prescreened for their effectiveness in the cytotoxic reaction. In addition, stringent quality control procedures must be observed with each lot, and adequate positive and negative controls must be employed with each test.

In some cases, the presence of even small amounts of anti-human antibody in the rabbit serum used as a complement source can interfere with the test procedure. This can occur at times when either B cells from lymphoblastoid lines or fibroblasts are used as the target cells for antibody. These cell types are highly susceptible to killing by even very small amounts of anti-human antibody and complement. In such instances it is preferable to sacrifice some sensitivity for the sake of specificity by using sera from baby rabbits that lack such antibodies. Alternatively, the rabbit serum may be preabsorbed with cultured human cells or even platelets to reduce nonspecific cytotoxic effects.

Currently, a number of commercial sources supply excellent rabbit complement. Indeed, some suppliers of reagent anti-HLA sera provide complement specifically tailored for use with their reagents. Nevertheless, it is considered good laboratory practice to

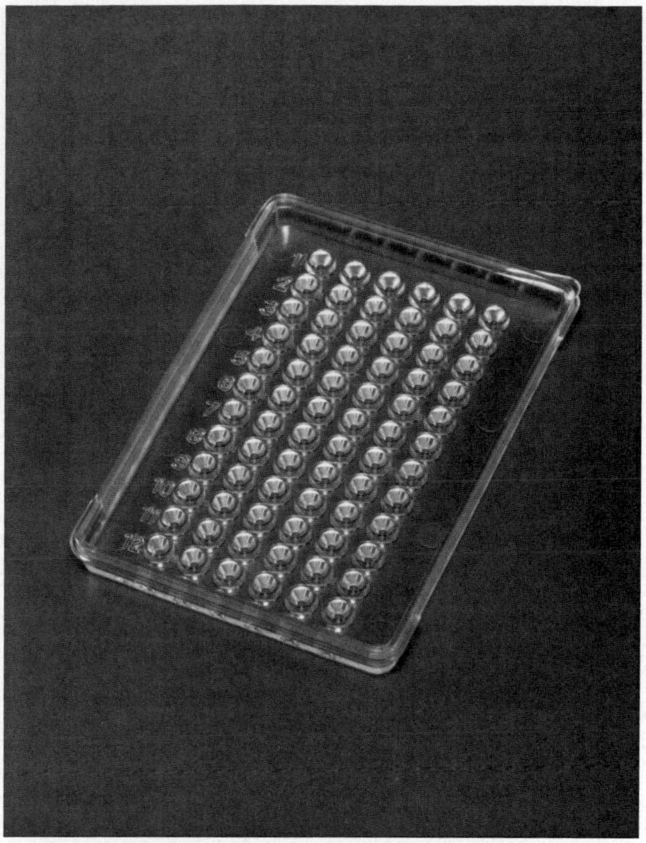

Figure 31.11. A standard 55 × 80 mm tray used for HLA typing. The reactions are carried out in the individual wells, whose contents can be observed from below by means of an inverted microscope. (Courtesy of Robbins Scientific Corporation, Sunnyvale, CA.)

ensure the quality of each new lot of complement. In this way, consistency of testing and typing results can be assured.

The standard microlymphocytotoxicity test is performed in specially designed plastic trays containing wells with optically flat bottoms (Fig. 31.11). In practice, the wells are first filled with biologically inert mineral oil that is used to retard the evaporation of the minute volumes of reactants. One microliter of antiserum containing antibodies is added to the bottom of the well followed by 1 μl of cell suspension containing approximately 2000 cells.

This mixture is incubated at room temperature for 30 minutes to allow the antibodies in the serum to react with antigens on the cell surface. At the conclusion of the incubation, 5 μl of rabbit complement are added, and the reaction is further incubated for 60 minutes at room temperature. During this period, complement is activated by the antigen-antibody complexes at the cell surface, resulting in cell death. At this point, a 5% solution of Eosin-Y dye is added to stain the cells and to make the test easier to read. Finally, a solution of neutralized formalin is added to

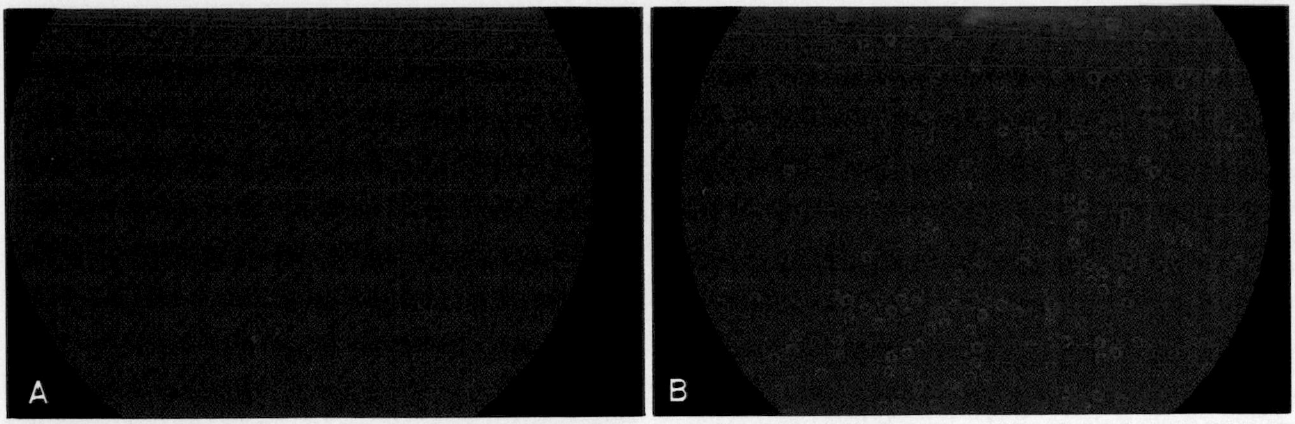

Figure 31.12. Microscopic appearance of the lymphocytotoxicity reaction. **A,** A positive reaction. The cells have taken up the eosin Y dye. They are swollen and have prominent nuclear detail. **B,** A negative reaction. Most of the cells appear clear, glistening, and refractile.

Table 31.5. Cytotoxicity Scoring

Score	% Cell Death	Interpretation
1	0–10	Negative
2	10–25	Possibly negative
4	25–50	Possibly positive
6	50–80	Positive
8	80–100	Strong positive

stop the reaction and to preserve the architecture of the cells.

The reaction is read using an inverted microscope equipped with phase-contrast illumination. Under these conditions, live lymphocytes appear as clear glistening small round cells not too different from red cells. For this reason it is imperative to remove as many red cells from the final cell suspension as possible. The red dye used for staining penetrates the cells but can be excreted by live ones, giving them a golden tone on a light red background. The dead cells cannot excrete the dye, thus staining with an intense maroon color. They appear as dark, opaque, swollen cells with prominent nuclear detail (Fig. 31.12).

The reaction is scored by determining the percentage of cell death in each well. This can be done by actually counting the number of live cells versus the number of dead ones. In practice, however, skilled workers estimate the percentage of cell death by trained optical pattern analysis. The results are expressed according to the grading scheme shown in Table 31.5. A score of 8 is maximum, but the reaction is considered positive with a score of 6. A negative is defined by a score of 1.

In the performance and the reading of this type of test, which depends so heavily on a biological endpoint, there is always the possibility of some doubtful reactions. These are indicated by the scores of 4 and 2. A score of 4 is usually interpreted to mean, "I don't know, but I think it's positive." A score of 2 means, "I don't know, but I think it's negative." Although this may seem subjective, it does have some precision. Skilled workers are remarkably consistent in coding these reactions, and very little variation is observed between duplicate readings performed by the same or different individuals.

There are a number of variations to this basic test that were introduced in attempts to make it more sensitive (25). The first of these, which is known as the Amos Mod technique, calls for the cells to be washed with tissue culture fluid after their initial incubation with antiserum. This modification is based on the fact that the source of antiserum is frequently a patient whose serum may contain factors that bind complement nonspecifically. These could be aggregated γ-globulins, antigen-antibody complexes, or even the products of bacterial contaminants in stored sera. Any of these materials could deplete the system of complement and lead to false-negative reactions. Therefore, their elimination prior to the addition of complement effectively increases sensitivity.

Another modification that increases the sensitivity of the standard microlymphocytotoxicity test is based on the use of an anti-human globulin reagent (26). The reagent of choice in this case is directed against the light chain of human IgG. An anti-κ-containing serum is the most popular. The underlying principle of this modification is different from that of classic anti-human globulin or Coombs tests used in red cell serology in which anti-heavy chain reagents are used. In this case the antiglobulin serum serves as a source of additional Fc fragments to interact with those on bound anti-HLA to help activate complement rather than as an antibody bridge to promote agglutination. Using this approach, it is possible to achieve complement activation even with a relatively small number of anti-HLA antibody molecules bound per cell, thereby giving extreme sensitivity.

This method must be carefully controlled since its high degree of sensitivity can result in false-positive reactions.

These procedures are most useful in those cases in which patients' sera are used as a source of potential anti-HLA antibody, such as in cross-matching (see Chapter 32). However, this and other modifications should be avoided when using commercial typing sera that have been standardized according to routine methods. The instructions found on the direction circulars accompanying such products should be followed exactly.

A totally different approach to the microlymphocytotoxicity test is given by a technique called cytofluorochromasia (27). The basis for this modification is that living lymphocytes possess esterases in their cytoplasm. One of these enzymes is capable of converting the colorless compound fluorescein diacetate into fluorescein, which glows with a green fluorescence under ultraviolet light. In the test procedure, the lymphocyte suspension is pretreated with fluoresceine diacetate before any exposure to antibody. Then the cells are incubated, first with antibody and then with complement in the usual fashion. The reaction is read with an inverted microscope equipped with an ultraviolet light source and the appropriate excitation filters. Under these conditions only the live cells can be seen glowing with an apple-green fluorescence. The fluorescent compound leaks from the dead cells and leaves them colorless. Therefore, the degree of fluorescence is proportional to the number of remaining live cells. A totally dark well indicates 100% cell death and a positive test. A negative reaction is given by a well filled with glowing cells. To improve the accuracy of the reading and subsequent interpretation, the dead cells can be counterstained with ethidium bromide, a red fluorescing compound that can penetrate the damaged membranes of dead cells and stain their nuclei.

An interesting variation of this technique was developed by van Rood and his colleagues. This method can be used to test for class II HLA antigens without preparing suspensions of pure B cells (28). It can work because B cells express immunoglobulins on their surface.

A cell suspension prepared from peripheral blood containing both B cells and T cells is treated with a predetermined dose of a reagent containing goat anti-human immunoglobulin antibodies that have been conjugated with fluorescein diisothiocyanate. This reagent reacts with the immunoglobulins expressed on the B cells, effectively coating them with a fluorescent compound. In addition, the reagent cross-links the immunoglobulins expressed on the cell surface, causing them to form a cap that migrates to one pole of the cell.

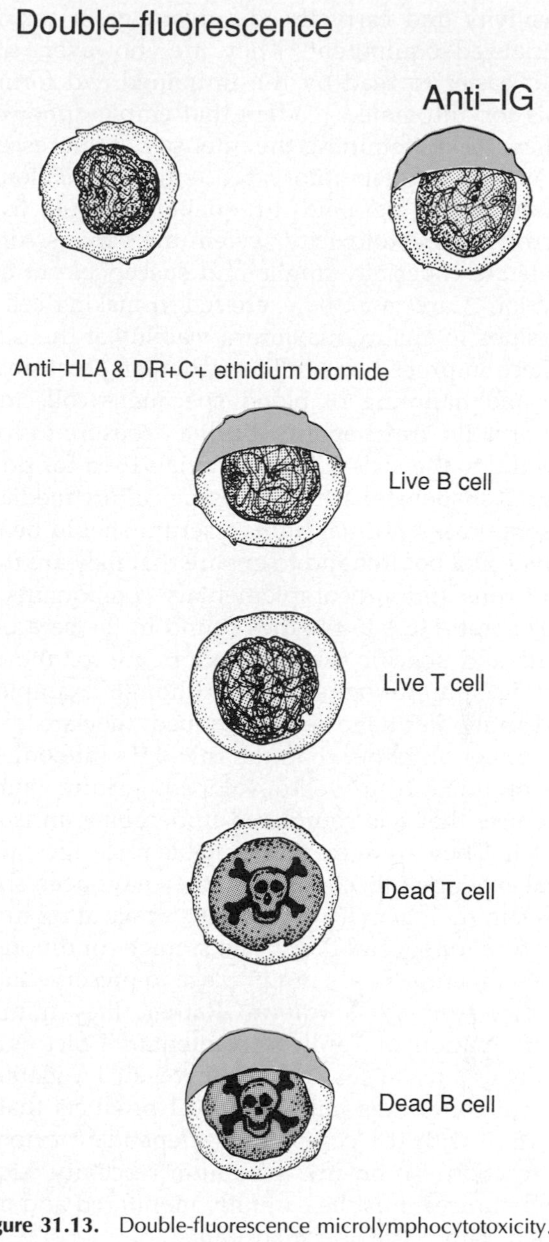

Figure 31.13. Double-fluorescence microlymphocytotoxicity.

The microlymphocytotoxicity test is performed in the usual way with the exception that ethidium bromide is added as the final stain instead of eosin. This dye will penetrate the damaged walls of dead cells and will stain their nuclei. Live cells having intact membranes exclude this material, leaving their nuclei unstained.

The reaction is read using an ultraviolet microscope equipped with filters capable of exciting both green and red fluorescence. Under these conditions, dead B cells will fluoresce red with green caps, live B cells will have only green caps, dead T cells will be red but with no caps, and live T cells will be colorless (Fig. 31.13).

The fluorescent methods offer no advantage over the standard cytotoxicity procedures with respect to sensitivity and carry the disadvantage of requiring specialized equipment. They are, however, somewhat easier to read by the untrained and form the basis for automated readers that employ photomultipliers for determining the intensity of fluorescence.

As with any laboratory procedure, meticulous attention must be paid to quality control. In the microlymphocytotoxicity system the various components are especially fragile and susceptible to denaturation. Care must be exercised in making cell suspensions to ensure maximum viability at the outset. Collection procedures call for room temperature storage and handling of blood specimens collected in preservative-free heparin. Undue exposure to cold is harmful to the cells. Other materials used for preparing cell suspensions such as tissue culture media and in some cases normal human serum should be carefully tested beforehand to ensure that they are free of cytotoxins and anticomplementary components.

The anti-HLA antibodies found in the sera of patients and specific reagent donors are for the most part IgG immunoglobulins. Although examples of IgM antibodies have been described, they are usually the exception rather than the rule. IgG antibodies are the products of a well-developed, mature immune response that has completed undergoing an isotype switch. They are remarkably stable molecules; under ideal experimental conditions, they have been shown to retain their activity even after storage at room temperature for several days. The storage conditions imposed on antisera are not in place to preserve the antibodies from denaturation. Rather, they minimize the formation of "anticomplementary" factors consisting of substances such as aggregated γ-globulins, protein complexes, and microbial products that can interfere with the complement-dependent cytotoxicity reaction. To ensure maximum reactivity, storage temperatures must be carefully monitored and maintained within the specified limits.

Controls should be used with each test to ensure a minimum viability of 10% at the start, and maximum viability with a negative control serum. A positive control must be included to ensure that the complement is working and that the cell suspension being used is susceptible to its action.

Complement must be carefully controlled. Each new lot of complement should be compared with a previous lot to determine its optimum working titer. This assay should be performed using several antisera having different specificities and antibody titers to demonstrate that the new source of complement works with equal facility with strong as well as weak sera. In addition, since complement has a natural denaturation time that is related to temperature, storage temperature for this reagent must be carefully monitored.

The anti-κ antiserum used in the antiglobulin modification of the standard procedure needs to be controlled in much the same manner as complement. Each new lot should be tested along with a previously used working lot to determine its optimum working dilution. It should be aliquoted into small volumes to avoid repeated freezing and thawing.

Finally, in performing quality control on the cytotoxicity procedure, the proficiency of the operator performing the test cannot be overlooked. This test is highly dependent on individual skills, especially those required for reading the test. These skills must be carefully monitored by the periodic performance of blind repeats of HLA typings and the duplicate reading of tests by more than one individual. Readings should differ by no more than a single score value.

When populations of lymphocytes from two different individuals are mixed in culture, the cells from one individual are able to recognize foreign antigens on the cells of the other and to respond to these antigens by undergoing blastogenic transformation (29). This forms the basis of the mixed lymphocyte culture (MLC), a method used to investigate class II HLA antigens. This reaction is dependent only on the cellular components of the immune system, and some investigators have likened it to an in vitro model of the delayed hypersensitivity reaction.

The antigens recognized in this reaction are class II HLA antigens. Originally they were called HLA-D and were believed to be recognizable only by lymphocytes. When the HLA-DR antigens were detected serologically on the surface of B lymphocytes, it became clear that they were the targets of MLC reactivity. However, the serologically defined specificities alone cannot fully explain cellular reactivity. Therefore, the HLA-D designations have been retained.

In order for the MLC reaction to occur, there must be a difference between the HLA-DR antigens of the two cell populations. Discrepancies in the HLA-A and/or HLA-B antigens alone will not result in stimulation. However, cytotoxic T lymphocytes (CTL), which are directed against class I antigens, are generated as a by-product of this reaction. This will be discussed further in the description of the primed lymphocyte typing test (PLT).

One of the applications of the test is to compare the identity of two individuals with respect to their class II antigens. In the test, lymphocytes from the two individuals being compared are prepared in the usual fashion. Care must be taken that the cells remain viable and that the suspension contains both T cells and B cells.

If these suspensions were mixed without further treatment, it would be impossible to determine if the resulting blastogenesis was due to the response of

Table 31.6. MLC Test Protocol[a]

	Patient cells Irradiated	Donor Cells Irradiated	Control Cell Irradiated
Patient cells	P + Px	P + Dx*	P + Cx
Donor cells	D + Px*	D + Dx	D + Cx
Control cells	C + Px	C + Dx	C + Cx

[a]Cell combinations indicated with an asterisk are test combinations; all others are controls.

cells from individual A to the antigens of individual B or vice versa. Consequently, one of the populations must be rendered immunologically inactive. Cells treated in this way can stimulate but not respond. Normally the test is set up in a manner that allows the cells from each individual to act in turn as stimulators and as responders. Immunologic inactivation can be accomplished by treating the stimulating population with mitomycin-C, a drug that will inhibit mitosis; or by exposing the cells to a low dose of γ irradiation (1500 to 3000 R) under controlled conditions. The use of irradiation is the method of choice.

The lymphocyte suspensions are mixed in appropriate combinations in multiwelled tissue culture trays according to a set protocol. A typical pattern of mixtures is shown in Table 31.6. It can be seen that two-thirds of the test consists of controls. The mixtures are incubated at 37°C with 5% CO_2 for 5 days. At the conclusion of the incubation the cells are pulsed with tritiated thymidine, ^{3}HTdr. This material is a DNA precursor that will be incorporated into the nuclei of dividing cells. Eighteen hours later, the cell suspensions are washed to remove excess radioactivity, a scintillation cocktail is added, and the amount of radioactivity present in the cells is counted in a β-scintillation counter. The amount of incorporated radioactivity is proportional to the degree of blastogenic transformation, which in turn is somewhat proportional to the degree of antigenic disparity between the two cell types.

The degree of antigenic disparity may be expressed in one of two ways. The most common is the relative response (RR). This describes the degree of reactivity obtained with the test cell compared with maximum reactivity to an indifferent control cell tested at the same time.

$$\text{RR} = \frac{(\text{cpm test combination}) - (\text{cpm autologous control})}{(\text{cpm unrelated stimulator}) - (\text{cpm autologous control})} \times 100$$

The second expression is called the stimulation index (SI). This value represents the number of times the test counts per minute exceed the autologous counts per minute. Some workers feel that this is a much better measure of reactivity than the RR. However, in most cases involving HLA typing by the MLC (discussed in the next section), the RR remains the value of choice.

$$\text{SI} = \frac{(\text{cpm test combination})}{(\text{cpm autologous control})}$$

A number of controls are required in this test. The responding cell suspension of each individual must be mixed with an autologous stimulating cell suspension. Any population of lymphocytes maintained under culture conditions undergoes a certain degree of spontaneous blastogenesis due to normal growth. The autologous cell combination is used to measure the cpm attributable to spontaneous transformation. This must then be subtracted from the cpm obtained in the test. A control consisting of a stimulator cell suspension derived from a widely disparate random donor is used to establish that a given responder population is able to respond. The response obtained using this combination not only establishes that the responder can respond but also serves as a measure of the maximum response possible. Finally, a mixture in which the stimulator cell population is tested against an unrelated random donor responder cell population must be included to establish that the stimulator population can indeed stimulate. Often cell populations may be derived from patients who, because of disease or therapy, may lack functional B cells. These would fail to stimulate a responder population and lead to the false conclusion that stimulator and responder are identical with respect to class II antigens.

All of the media used in the MLC must be carefully controlled using the criteria similar to those employed by any good microbiology lab. Each lot should be tested for sterility and its ability to support the growth of cells. In addition, the media should not contain contaminants that could induce blastogenesis. The normal human group AB serum that is used as a supplement must be tested for cytotoxicity as well as for the presence of anti-HLA antibodies that could inhibit the MLC reaction.

The results of a typical MLC performed on a family consisting of a father, mother, and three siblings is shown in Table 31.7. In this table, the responder cells are listed along the side. The stimulators are listed across the top and are designated by an "X" to indicate that they have been irradiated. Each of the individuals exhibits very little incorporation of the radioactive label when challenged with an autologous stimulator. The RRs are 0, by definition, and the SIs are 1.0.

The indifferent stimulators in this example consist of a pool of several cells designed to elicit the maximum response from each of the test subjects, indicating that each is capable of responding. The control

Table 31.7. A Typical MLC Result

Responders		Stimulators Father X	Mother X	Patient X	Sib 1 X	Sib 2 X	Indifferent Control Pool X
Father	CPM[a]	0.2	67.6	52.7	48.2	12.4	192.4
A28, B53, DR2/	SI	**1.0**	338.0	263.5	241.0	62.0	962.0
A , B14, DR7	RR	**0.0**	35.1	27.3	25.0	6.3	100.0
Mother	CPM	47.5	0.3	46.3	60.3	17.5	235.8
A1, B7, DR11/	SI	158.3	**1.0**	154.3	201.0	58.3	786.0
A29, B63, DR6	RR	20.0	**0.0**	19.5	25.5	7.3	100.0
Patient	CPM	39.8	46.7	0.3	0.4	32.5	201.4
A28, B53, DR2/	SI	129.7	155.7	**1.0**	**1.3**	108.3	671.3
A29, B63, DR6	RR	19.2	23.1	**0.0**	**0.0**	16.0	100.0
Sib 1	CPM	38.9	46.7	0.3	0.4	32.5	201.4
A28, B53, DR2/	SI	127.5	171.7	**1.0**	**1.0**	88.8	521.5
A29, B63, DR6	RR	24.3	32.7	**0.0**	**0.0**	16.9	100.0
Sib 2	CPM	44.1	54.1	60.2	59.9	0.3	205.2
A28, B53, DR2/	SI	147.0	180.3	200.7	199.7	**1.0**	684.0
A1, B7, DR11	RR	21.4	26.3	29.2	29.1	**0.0**	100.0
Control cell	CPM	64.0	172.4	89.1	138.1	44.9	287.2
	SI	53.3	143.7	74.3	115.1	37.4	239.3
	RR	22.0	59.9	30.7	47.9	15.3	100.0

[a]Counts per minute (in 1000s).

responding cells are stimulated by each of the test subjects, indicating that the system is working.

The parents in this family stimulate and respond to each other as expected. The patient is serologically identical to sibling 1. This is confirmed by the results of the MLC in which they fail to stimulate or respond to each other, yielding RRs of 0.0 and SIs of 1.3 and 1.0. Sibling 2 shares one paternal haplotype with the other two siblings and differs by one maternal haplotype. Both the RRs and the SIs obtained in combination with each of the other two siblings are high, indicating nonidentity. In addition, they are of the same order of magnitude as those obtained in the mixtures between the mother and the father. This result was obtained in spite of the fact that this individual shares one haplotype with his siblings and the parents share none with each other. Findings such as these are common and indicate that the degree of blastogenesis may not always be quantitatively proportional to the extent of the HLA mismatch.

In addition to serving as a method for assessing class II identity between two individuals, the MLC reaction can be used as a tool to type for the HLA-D series of antigens (30). This is accomplished by using cell suspensions from individuals who are known homozygotes as stimulators for the HLA-D alleles. Such cells, called homozygous typing cells (HTC), express only one HLA-D antigen. Therefore, when they are used as stimulators, if they fail to induce a response in the cells of another individual under the conditions of the MLC, it can be assumed that the individual shares at least one HLA-D antigen with the HTC. Thus, if the HTC expressed HLA-Dw1 and fails to stimulate the cells of an individual, the individual must be HLA-Dw1 as well. Naturally, a person could have a second HLA-D antigen of a different specificity in addition to HLA-Dw1. However, the presence of a single copy of the antigen is adequate to prevent a response.

Individuals who are homozygous for alleles of the MHC usually occur as the offspring of first-cousin matings (Fig. 31.14). These individuals are not only homozygous in that they have two identical copies of an allele, but in this special case they have duplicate copies of the same allele that was inherited from each of the parents, who were first cousins. Homozygous individuals have also been found in the general population; however, in this case the two alleles may be the same but they are not exact duplicates of the same gene.

The results obtained in HLA-D typing using HTCs in the MLC reaction may not give a definitive answer as to the presence or absence of a given HLA-D type. Depending on the particular HTC used and the responding cell being tested, a lack of response does not always result in a low RR (10% or less). In practice, when more than one HTC of the same specificity is used to test cells (as dictated by proper procedure), a range of reactivities and resultant RR values is obtained. Furthermore, a single HTC tested on the

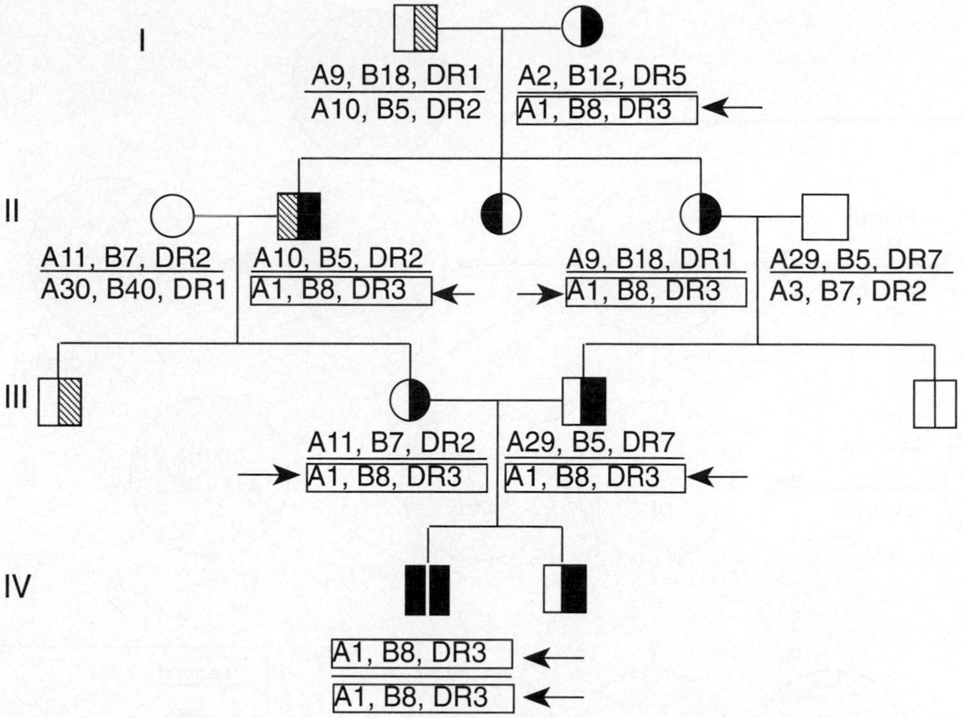

Figure 31.14. The pedigree of a family showing a mating of first cousins. The critical haplotype is boxed. The offspring in generation IV shown with an arrow is homozygous for the haplotype of maternal origin in generation I.

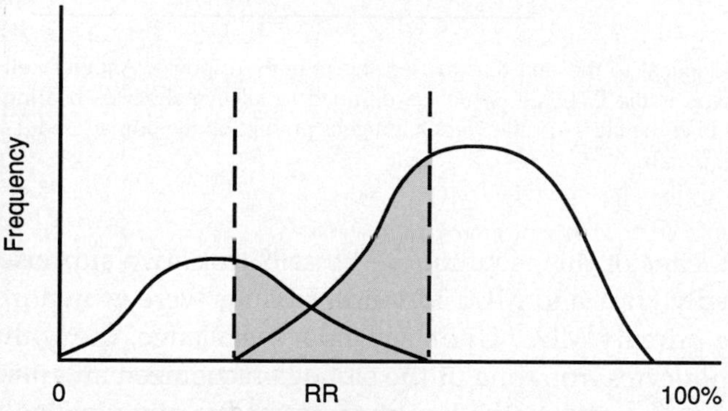

Figure 31.15. The bimodal frequency distribution of relative responses (RR) obtained in the population using a single HTC. Cells falling within the area of the left-hand curve give a low or negative response; therefore, they are assumed to have the antigen expressed by the HTC. Those within the right-hand curve give a high or positive response, indicating that they lack the antigen expressed on the HTC. It is impossible to interpret the meaning of the values in the region where the two curves overlap. This has been referred to as the "gray zone."

cells from a population of individuals will give a range of RR values whose frequency distribution is bimodal (Fig. 31.15). The bimodality results from the summation of two normal distributions. The distribution, having a mean at a low RR, represents the normal distribution of the antigen-positive nonresponders. The other, with a mean in the range of high RR, is the normal distribution of the antigen-negative responders. These curves are often skewed and result in a bimodality containing a significant overlap. It is impossible to make accurate antigen assignments to cells giving RRs that fall in this region. Therefore, the assignment to a given HLA-D type depends on statistical manipulation in which a series of responses is normalized with respect to the stimulation potential of the HTCs and the responding potential of the cells being tested. Given these values, a range of RR values can be generated that correspond to a negative response and indicate the presence of the antigen. Even so, the system carries with it some degree of uncertainty.

Because of these shortcomings, HLA-D typing by this procedure has been avoided except in certain highly specialized laboratories. As a result, the true clinical significance of the cosmic HLA-D types has been difficult to assess. Currently it is possible to type for these antigens using serologic methods for DR and DQ coupled with molecular techniques. Though more sophisticated to perform, these techniques offer some readily quantifiable and unambiguous data that are easier to interpret and are far more reliable.

In the normal MLC, 5 days of culture are required for the cells from a given individual to respond to the antigens of another individual and to undergo blastogenesis. However, if this reaction is allowed to continue until all of the stimulating cells are expended, the multiplying responding cells return to a mature steady state. A rechallenge with fresh stimu-

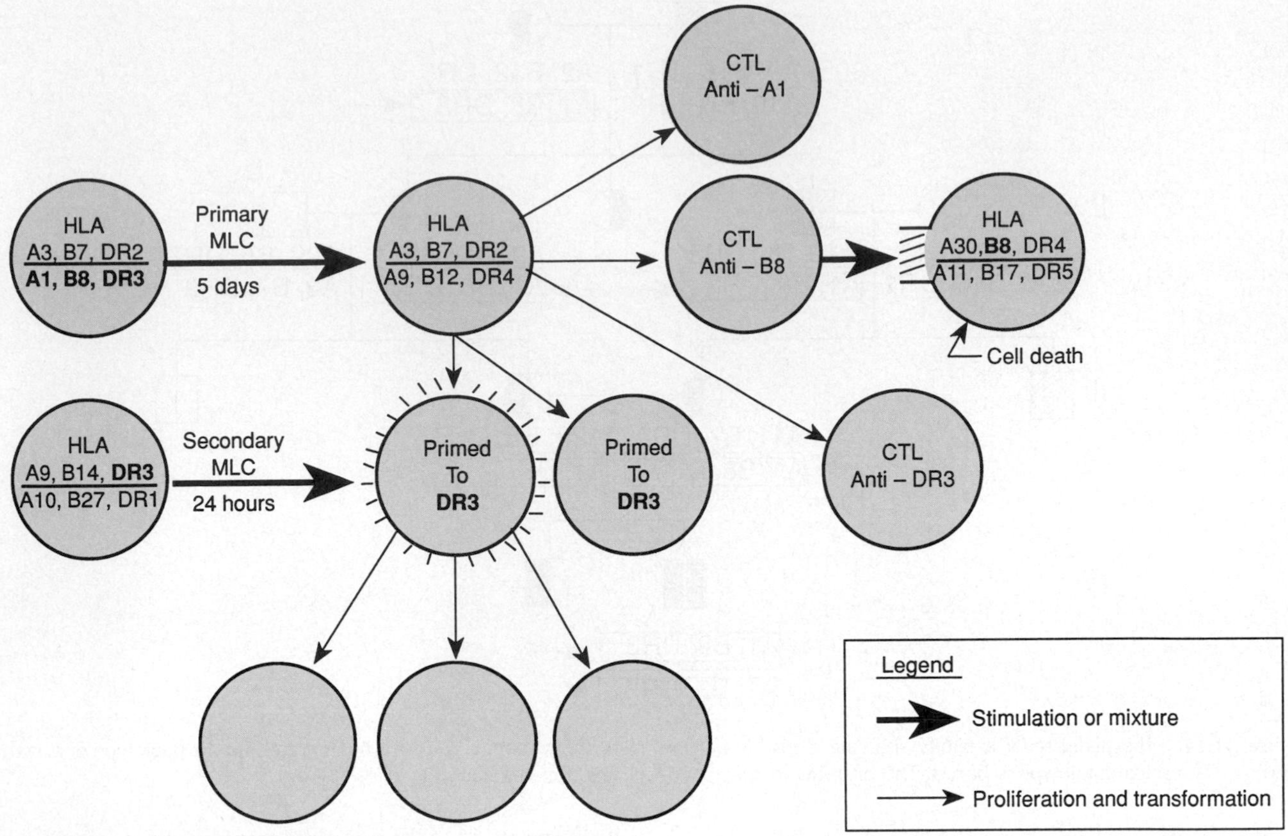

Figure 31.16. A schematic representation of the events following the mixture of lymphocytes from two different individuals. The "primary MLC" results in the proliferation of at least two different cell types. One of these (the PLT cell) is primed to undergo an immediate response to secondary challenge with cells bearing a class II antigen identical to the one that caused the primary response. Another cell type is the CTL cell, which is destined to kill lymphocytes bearing either the class I or the class II antigens present on the primary inducing cells.

lating cells from the original donor will result in a brisk blastogenic response within the first 24 hours. This is a secondary response and takes place because the responding cells have been primed to recognize the stimulating antigen (Fig. 31.16). This phenomenon forms the basis of the primed lymphocyte test (PLT) (31).

The PLT has been used for a number of different assays, but the most interesting is for the identification of cellularly defined HLA antigens. An HTC can be used to generate a specific PLT cell that will instantly recognize and respond to a specific HLA-D antigen. The test cell to be typed is used to challenge a set of PLT cells that have been primed to recognize the array of HLA-D specificities. The specific PLT cell responding to this challenge effectively labels the HLA-D antigen expressed by the stimulating cell population.

This reaction is highly specific, and the responsible cells are remarkably efficient in detecting minute epitopic differences in antigenic molecules not ordinarily detected by antibodies. As an example, the antigens of the DP locus were originally detected by means of this technique. The cells from two supposedly HLA and MLC identical siblings were grown in a primary MLC. Upon secondary challenge, the lymphocytes from one of the siblings recognized an antigen present on the lymphocytes of the other sibling. Further genetic analysis and family studies revealed that the antigen being recognized was not HLA-D but the product of a new locus in the class II region.

The lymphocytes that are generated in a primary MLC are composed of one population educated to recognize the antigens that elicited the response (PLT cells) and another population consisting of cytotoxic lymphocytes (CTL) that can destroy a cell carrying the specific HLA antigen against which the CTL cell is directed (32) (Fig. 31.16). Thus, these cells can be thought of as cellular counterparts of antibody molecules produced in response to antigen. The initial stimulation is brought about by the class II antigens on the cell. However, the cytotoxic cells produced are capable of recognizing not only class II antigens that were expressed on the inducing cells but the class I antigens as well.

CTL cells generated in the MLC directed against class I antigens have been used to subtype some of the better-known specificities such as HLA-A2, B27, and B44 in a method referred to as cell-mediated lympholysis (CML). In this method CTL cells are mixed in short-term culture with the target lymphocytes of the test subject. The targets are prelabelled with ^{51}Cr. After incubation the suspensions are washed and the radioactivity in the supernatants is measured to indicate the degree of target cell lysis.

Cytotoxic lymphocytes are capable of detecting private epitopes and subtypes that are unrecognizable with alloantibodies but have been shown by biochemical methods to be unique variants. In this regard CTLs constitute a powerful set of highly specialized reagents that have many applications, particularly in the research laboratory.

Once generated, CTL cells and PLT cells can be cryopreserved and later thawed and expanded in culture when needed. However, the techniques for their use are not without problems, and successful results can be achieved only with experience. The PLT and the CML are methods that depend on biological activity and are subject to the variabilities inherent in all biological systems. Fortunately, most of the unique epitopes recognized in these systems can also be detected quite reliably using biochemical approaches or in some cases serological procedures with monoclonal antibodies.

TECHNIQUES OF MOLECULAR BIOLOGY APPLIED TO HLA TYPING

Many new techniques originally developed for use in molecular biology have recently been applied to the study of the HLA system. Some of these techniques have resulted in data that contribute significantly to a better understanding of the system. Others are in the process of being used for special applications in the diagnostic and forensic laboratory.

One biochemical method shown to be very useful is two-dimensional gel electrophoresis, a technique that has been applied extensively to the investigation of the β chains of DR molecules. Individuals whose cells express HLA-DR4 have been found to belong to one of several HLA-D types, including Dw4, Dw10, Dw13, and Dw14. These studies have shown that cells from individuals belonging to HLA-DR4 can be sorted by this method into groups corresponding to their particular HLA-D specificity. In this method, lymphocytes are cultured in the presence of ^{35}S methionine, which biosynthetically labels the HLA gene products. The harvested cells are lysed and their HLA molecules immunoprecipitated with monoclonal antibody directed against epitopes present on the constant region of the DR β chain.

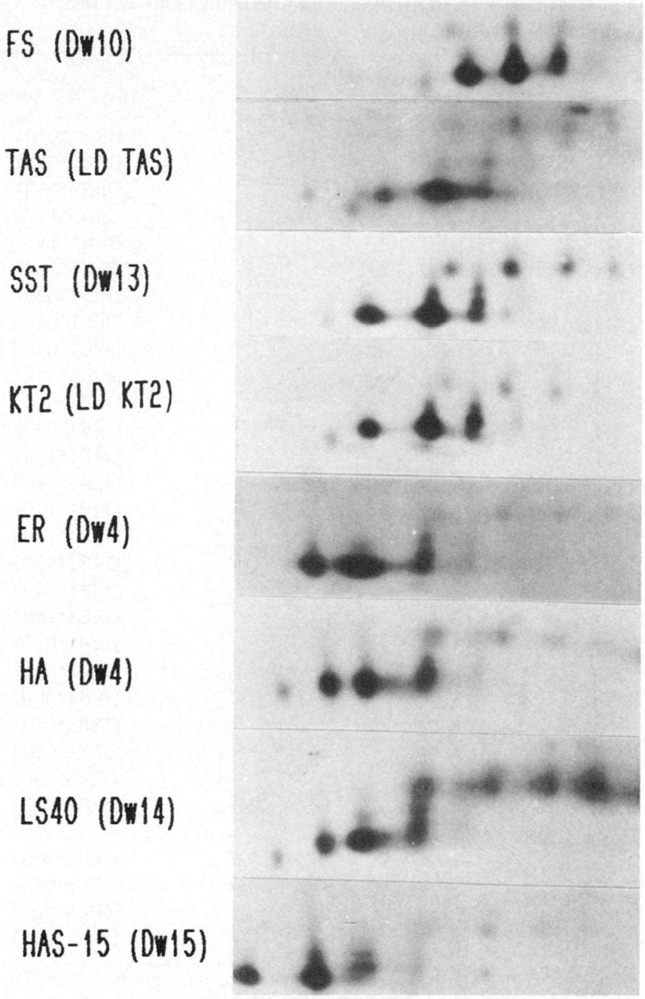

Figure 31.17. Two-dimensional gel electrophoresis of immunoprecipitated DR4 molecules. The β chains appear as three separate spots due to differences in glycosylation. The chains migrate in different areas depending on their individual amino acid composition. Even though these examples all behave serologically as DR4, they have different HLA-D specificities. (Reprinted by permission of Elsevier Science Publishing Co., Inc. from Monos DS, Mickelson E, Hansen JA, Baker L, Zmijewski CM, Kamoun M. Analysis of DR and DQ gene products of the DR4 haplotype in patients with IDDM: possible involvement of more than one locus. Hum Immunol 1988;23;289–299. Copyright 1988 by the American Society for Histocompatibility and Immunogenetics.)

The immunoprecipitated molecules are first separated on a gel containing a pH gradient according to their isoelectric point. The focusing gel is then transferred to an electrophoretic gel. Further separation according to size and electrical charge takes place in a second dimension, which is 90° to the first. The resulting radioactive spots are developed by exposure to photographic film. A typical result is shown in Figure 31.17 (33). Each DR molecule separates into several spots. The invariant α chain forms a single

Table 31.8. Some HLA-DR and HLA-D Equivalents and the Responsible Alleles[a]

HLA-DR Specificity	HLA-D Specificity	HLA-DR B Allele
DR1	Dw1	DRB1*0101
DR1	Dw20	DRB1*0102
DR15(2)	Dw2	DRB1*1501
DR15(2)	Dw12	DRB1*1502
DR16(2)	Dw21	DRB1*1601
DR16(2)	Dw22	DRB1*1602
DR17(3)	Dw3	DRB1*0301
DR4	Dw4	DRB1*0401
DR4	Dw10	DRB1*0402
DR4	Dw13	DRB1*0403
DR4	Dw14	DRB1*0404
DR4	Dw15	DRB1*0405
DR11(5)	DW5	DRB1*1101
DR11(5)	Dw"FS"	DRB1*1104
DR12(5)	Dw"DB6"	DRB1*1201
DR13(6)	Dw18	DRB1*1301
DR13(6)	Dw19	DRB1*1302
DR14(6)	Dw9	DRB1*1401
DR14(6)	Dw16	DRB1*1402
DR7	Dw17	DRB1*0701
DR8	Dw8.1	DRB1*0801
DR9	Dw23	DRB1*0901
DR52	Dw24	DRB3*0101
DR52	Dw25	DRB3*0201
DR52	Dw26	DRB3*0301
DR53	Dw4, Dw10, Dw14, Dw15, Dw17, Dw23	DRB4*0101
DR51	Dw2	DRB5*0101
DR51	Dw12	DRB5*0101
DR51	Dw21	DRB5*0201
DR51	Dw22	DRB5*0202

[a]From Bodmer JG, Marsh SGE, Albert ED, et al. Nomenclature for factors of the HLA system, 1991. Tissue Antigens 1992;39:161–173.

Table 31.9. Isoelectric Focusing Variants of HLA-A and HLA-B[a]

HLA Specificity	10th W IEF[b] Variants
A2	A2.1
A2	A2.2
A2	A2.3
A2	A2.4
B7	B7.1
B7	B7.2
B27	B27.1
B27	B27.2
B27	B27.3
B27	B27.4
B27	B27.5
B27	B27.6

[a]From Bodmer JG, Marsh SGE, Albert ED, et al. Nomenclature for factors of the HLA system, 1991. Tissue Antigens 1992;39:161–173.
[b]IEF = Isoelectric focusing.

large spot. The β chains, however, usually separate into three spots that reflect different levels of the glycosylation of individual metabolically labeled molecules. This technique, coupled with the DNA methods described below, has been applied to the study of DR β chains from other DR specificities. The relationship between HLA-DR detected serologically and HLA-D detected by means of lymphocyte interactions is now becoming clearer. The various HLA-D types are due to specific DRB1 alleles, some of which are shown in Table 31.8. Several of these alleles may result in the production of β chains with identical epitopes recognizable by anti-DR antibody, and distinctly different epitopes recognizable by lymphocytes.

Isoelectric focusing alone has been used to study the HLA-A and HLA-B molecules. For the most part this technique has been able to detect all of the common class I variants currently detected serologically. These are listed in Table 31.9 (34).

HLA typing can also be accomplished at the DNA level. Restriction enzymes produced by certain bacteria can cut the DNA strands at specific palindromic sequences known as restriction sites. There are a number of different restriction sites in the vicinity of the HLA genome that can be used advantageously.

When single-stranded DNA is digested with one of these enzymes, it is cut into fragments of varying lengths and molecular weights corresponding to the distance between similar restriction sites. The distance between restriction sites differs from one individual to another because of so-called variable number tandem repeats (VNTRs), i.e., randomly repetitive sequences within the region of the introns. Additionally, mutations in the exons encoding for structural proteins that affect adjacent restriction sites also result in differing lengths of DNA fragments. Therefore, it is possible to associate a specific series of fragments of a certain size with a gene that is responsible for the production of a given antigen. Differences in fragment length produced in this fashion are collectively referred to as restriction fragment length polymorphisms (RFLPs).

In performing RFLP analysis, the DNA of an individual to be tested is prepared from some convenient source such as peripheral blood. The isolated DNA is denatured to separate the strands, followed by digestion with the appropriate enzyme. The digested DNA fragments are then separated by electrophoresis in a gel matrix. Under these conditions, the fragments migrate according to their charge and size. The heavier fragments will migrate slowly and therefore localize near the origin. The smaller fragments will move through the gel more readily and become localized at points farther from the origin at a distance proportional to their size.

The electrophoretic separation is followed by performing a Southern blot during which the separated DNA fragments are transferred to a nitrocellulose membrane. The membrane is flooded with a radiolabeled single-stranded DNA probe complementary to the genes being identified. Under ap-

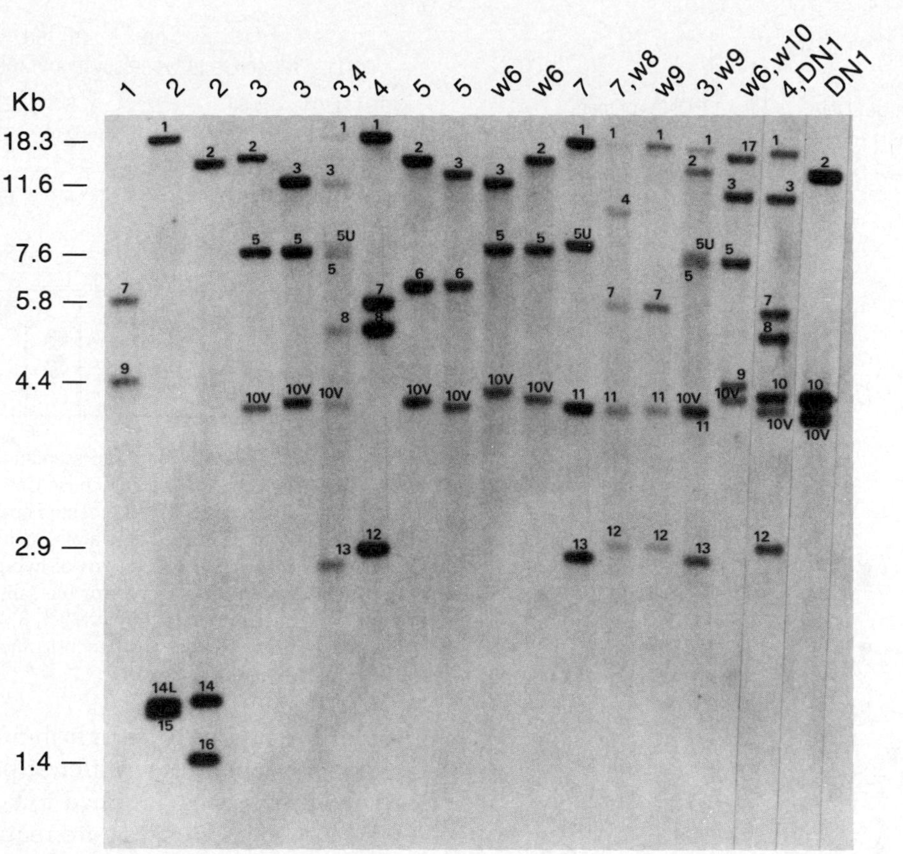

Figure 31.18. The RFLP patterns of the different DR specificities. The bands are numbered to indicate the pattern found within each DR antigen. The DNA was cut using the restriction enzyme TaqI, and the patterns were developed using a DR β probe. (Reprinted with permission of The University of Chicago Press and The American Society of Human Genetics. From Cox NJ, Mela PA, Zmijewski CM, Spielman RS. HLA-DR typing "at the DNA level": RFLP, and subtypes detected with a DRB cDNA probe. Am J Hum Genet 1988;43:956.)

propriate conditions, the labeled cDNA will anneal to the single-stranded genomic DNA fixed to the membrane at sites corresponding to the sizes of the restriction lengths. Thus, the genes toward which the probe is directed can be observed by exposing the membrane to photographic film. A typical radiograph showing a series of bands corresponding to a number of different DR β genes is shown in Figure 31.18 (35).

Some even more powerful techniques have emerged as a direct result of the biochemical characterization of the HLA antigens. The amino acid sequence of a given HLA specificity provides the information needed to ascertain the exact nucleic acid sequence of its gene and vice versa. To date the nucleotide sequences of the majority of the HLA class I and class II alleles have been ascertained and are published (36, 37). This has made it possible to construct highly specific nucleic acid oligomers complementary to the individual genes. These site-specific oligomers (SSOs) may be labeled with radioisotopes and handled similarly to the cDNAs used in RFLP testing. However, newer methods currently in use in most laboratories avoid the use of isotopes. Typically the SSOs are coupled to the enzyme terminal deoxynucleotidyl transferase (TdT), which binds to the 3′ ends of DNA. After hybridization, the membranes are exposed to the substrate digoxigenin-11dUTP, which will undergo a color change subsequent to digestion by the enzyme coupled to the annealed SSO and permit direct observation.

This procedure can be further enhanced and extended to the typing of extremely small amounts of DNA containing the critical gene by means of the polymerase chain reaction (PCR). This is a procedure of enzymatic gene amplification and involves repeated cycles consisting of the denaturation of the DNA followed by the annealing of primers (38, 39). These primers are custom-made oligonucleotides homologous to sequences flanking the region of interest. The annealing process is coupled with primer extension by DNA polymerase, causing the doubling of discrete DNA. The product is a strand having termini corresponding to the 5′ ends of the oligonucleotide primers employed and containing the sequence of interest. The repeated cycling of the process results in the production of a large amount of DNA. This process is shown in Figure 31.19.

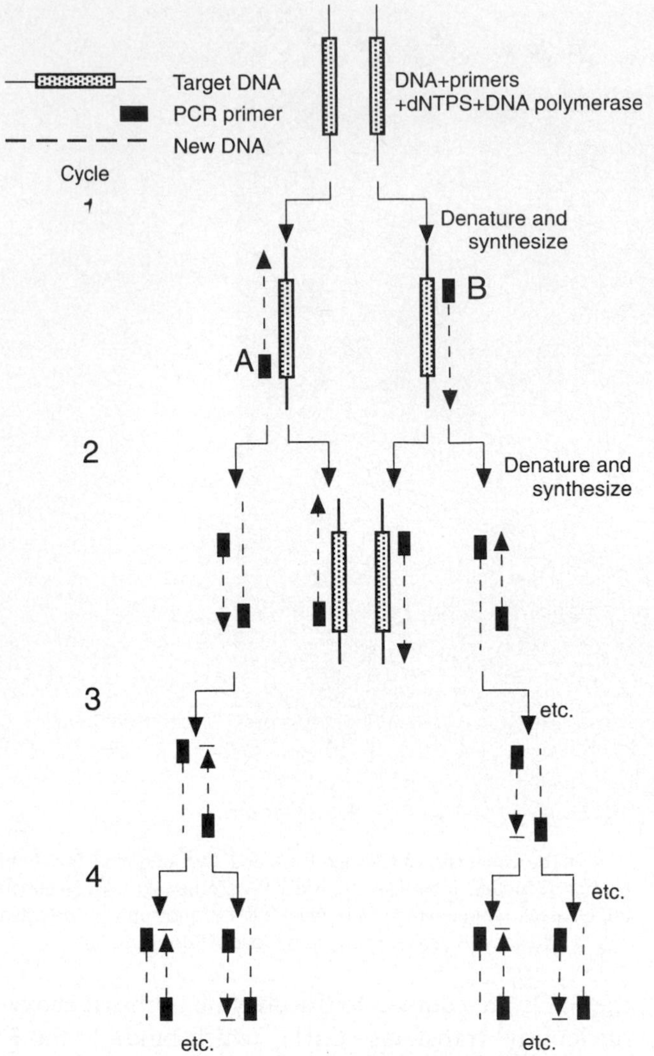

Figure 31.19. The polymerase chain reaction. The DNA is denatured at 95°C; oligonucleotide primers A and B, which define the limits of the targeted sequence, are annealed and extension of a complementary DNA strand occurs in the presence of a thermostabile Taq polymerase and the four deoxyribonuclease triphosphates. Subsequent cycles result in the amplification of the target DNA. (From White TJ, Arnheim N, Erlich HA. The polymerase chain reaction. Trends Genet 1989;5:185–189.)

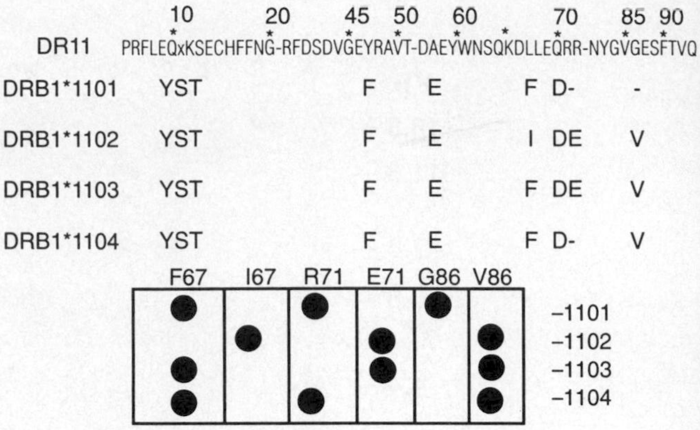

Figure 31.20. Diagrammatic representation of oligonucleotide typing for HLA-DR11 variants. The consensus sequence of amino acids 1–95 is given according to the accepted code. Differences among the DR11 alleles can be noted in the amino acids at positions 67, 71, and 86. Characteristic dot blot patterns of hybridization to the sequence specific oligonucleotide probes for the salient regions are shown for each of the alleles. (Adapted from Mach B, Tiercy JM. Genotypic typing of HLA class II: from the bench to the bedside. Hum Immunol 1991;30:278–284.)

The availability of such products has simplified the procedure considerably, making it much more specific. These oligonucleotide probes will anneal only to their specific genes. Therefore, it is unnecessary either to cut the DNA with restriction enzymes or to separate the resultant fragments. Intact DNA can be denatured, spotted on a membrane, and probed with the specific probe. The appearance of a radioactive or otherwise colored spot is indicative of the presence of the gene. A typical oligonucleotide typing for four of the variants of HLA-DR11 is shown diagramatically in Figure 31.20 (40).

The consensus sequence for the first 95 amino acids of the B1 chain of HLA-DR11 is listed across the top of the figure. Although the four variants are remarkably similar, they differ at positions 67, 71, and 86. Specific probes designed to be complementary to the DNA sequences that are required to code for the amino acids at each of these key positions have been applied to the individual membranes on which the DNA to be typed has been spotted. After the development of the colored spots and the alignment of the membranes, the pattern of spots corresponding to the individual allelic variants can be identified.

In practice, this technique is somewhat complicated because individual DR and DQ alleles share large portions of sequence and may differ from each other by only a few base pairs. This is especially true of the alleles within a given specificity such as DR4. This situation can result in the nonspecific annealing of certain probes, leading to difficulties in interpretation. In addition, certain heterozygous combinations of alleles can mimic an entirely different single specificity or combination of specificities. Although this problem can be controlled to some extent by carefully defining the annealing conditions in terms of stringency, time, and temperature, it is often difficult to predict in any given test sample.

This problem has resulted in the development of a number of strategies for DNA typing along with a series of technical variations, similar to the evolution of HLA typing by serology. Some of these methods include sequence-specific amplification in which primers bearing a sequence complementary to a particular allele are used in the PCR (41). DNA amplification alone indicates the presence of the allele, and an annealing to an oligo probe is not required. Other methods such as PCR/RFLP combine amplification of allele-specific regions of DNA with the subsequent analysis of restriction fragment polymorphisms (42). Still other methods include PCR/heteroduplex formation (43), PCR/single-strand conformation polymorphism (SSCP) (44) analysis, and DNA sequence analysis (45). Heteroduplex analysis is based on the fact that single-stranded DNA can form double strands that are derived from two or more different alleles. Such heteroduplexes are different in physical size from homoduplexes derived from two identical alleles and can therefore be separated and identified by electrophoresis. SSCP analysis is based on the unique conformation in the secondary structure of HLA alleles in single-stranded DNA. These may result in characteristic migration patterns in nondenaturing gels.

The entire field of HLA typing by DNA techniques is changing rapidly, with newer methods and variations of older methods emerging. An ideal technique applicable to all situations does not yet exist. However, in spite of the vagaries that are encountered, the DNA methods as they exist have a practical application. They are particularly useful, for example, in the clinical setting for the HLA class II typing of patients whose B cells are present in low numbers or are difficult to isolate for other reasons. Such situations may be encountered in very young children, in patients with hematologic disorders such as aplastic anemia or various forms of leukemia, and in patients undergoing chemotherapy or immunosuppressive therapy. Frequently, patients such as these are being considered for bone marrow transplantation in which class II identity is essential. Prior to the development of this approach, repeated serologic and MLC tests had to be performed, which more often than not yielded poor results.

The newer methods have contributed a great deal to a better understanding of the HLA system. In particular, they have helped to explain some of the inconsistencies that were experienced by earlier workers. For example, the original discovery of antibodies reactive with HLA antigens on B cells heralded a serologic solution to the lengthy and troublesome MLC. With the greatest confidence, the new HLA-DR antigens were assigned numbers corresponding to the then-defined HLA-D types since they were considered equivalent. Unfortunately, it became apparent that quite often lymphocytes from unrelated individuals who had identical HLA-DR types stimulated and responded to each other in the MLC. Information obtained using two-dimensional gel electrophoresis and RFLP analysis (Fig. 31.17 and Table 31.8) has revealed that the β chains conferring a given DR specificity may differ slightly in other areas along their length. Lymphocytes can detect these differences, resulting in MLC reactivity among cells with the same DR type but differing in their DR β molecules.

The isolation, crystalization, and amino acid sequencing of the class I molecules can explain how the HLA-Bw4 and Bw6 antigens are related to the rest of the HLA-B series. These studies have shown that the amino acid sequences responsible for the Bw4 and Bw6 specificities are located at positions 79 and 83, whereas the private specificities are controlled by amino acids at positions 107 and 142 to 145 (see Fig. 31.5).

Studies at the genomic level have explained the relationship of the supposed public antigens DR52 and DR53 and their relationship to the other DR antigens. There are at least two loci in the DR region that result in the formation of DR-specific β chains (see Fig. 31.7). One of these, the B1 locus, is responsible for the formation of the β chains that carry the DR specificities DR1 and DR3 through DR18, while genes at the B3 and B4 loci result in the production of DR52 and DR53, respectively. The DR2 specificity appears to be the product of the B1 locus, which gives rise to DR15 and DR16 and the B5 locus, which gives rise to DR51 (34, 46). Thus, every cell has two DR specificities—a private and a public—but unlike Bw4 and Bw6, these are found on two separate molecules. The relationship among the specificities is due to gametic association between the genes at the adjacent β chain loci.

These newer techniques, though vastly more robust than the routine serologic and culture techniques, may not replace them altogether in the clinical arena. Most certainly, they do have their place. In addition, oligonucleotide probes have proven to be extremely useful in determining accurate DR types in patients lacking adequate B cells and for the selection of unrelated bone marrow donors and in certain forensic applications.

However, these methods may be too sensitive for routine use in solid organ transplantation. For example, unrelated donor selection is complicated by the high degree of polymorphism in the HLA system as defined by existing methodologies. Evidence clearly indicates that the newer methods are able to distinguish even more polymorphisms, further complicating the picture. In addition, little is known about the true clinical significance of these minor antigenic differences. Until this significance can be established and a system is established for dealing with the extreme degree of polymorphism, many of these newer methods will have limited clinical application and will remain within the scope of reference and research laboratories.

References

1. Medawar PB. Behavior and fate of skin autografts and homografts in rabbits. J Anat 1944;78:176–200.
2. Snell GD, Smith P, Babrielson F. Analysis of the histocompatibility-2 locus in the mouse. J Natl Cancer Inst 1953;14:457–480.
3. Bach FH, van Rood JJ. The major histocompatibility complex Part 1. N Engl J Med 1976;295:806–813.
4. Albert E, Amos DB, Bodmer WF, et al. Nomenclature for factors of the HLA system. Tissue Antigens 1977;11:81–86.
5. Bodmer WF, Albert E, Bodmer JG, et al. Nomenclature for factors of the HLA system 1987. In: Dupont B, ed. Immunobiology of HLA I. New York: Springer-Verlag, 1989;72–79.
6. Koller BH, Geraghty D, Orr HT, Shimizu Y, DeMars R. Organization of the human class I major histocompatibility complex genes. Immunol Res 1987;6:1–10.
7. Baur MP, Neugebauer M, Albert ED. Reference tables of two-locus haplotype frequencies for all MHC marker loci. In: Albert ED, Baur MP, Mayr WR, eds. Histocompatibility testing 1984. New York: Springer-Verlag, 1984;677–755.
8. Baur MP, Danilovs JA. Population analysis of HLA-A, B, C, DR and other genetic markers. In: Terasaki PI, ed. Histocompatibility testing 1980, Los Angeles: UCLA Tissue Typing Laboratory, 1980:955–993.
9. Thomson G. The effect of a selected locus on linked neutral loci. Genetics 1987;85:753–788.
10. Hammerberg C, Klein J. Linkage disquilibrium between H-2 and t complexes in chromosome 17 of the mouse. Nature 1975;258:296–299.
11. Schwartz BD, Luehrman LK, Lee J, Rodey GE. A public antigenic determinant in the HLA-B5 cross-reacting group—a basis for cross-reactivity and a possible link with Behçet's disease. Hum Immunol 1980;1:37–54.
12. Krangel MS. Two forms of HLA class I molecules in human plasma. Hum Immunol 1987;20:155–165.
13. Parham P, Lawlor DA, Salter RD, Lomen CE, Bjorkman PJ, Ennis PD. HLA-A, B, C: Patterns of polymorphism in peptide binding proteins. In: Dupont B, ed. Immunobiology of HLA. II. New York: Springer-Verlag, 1989;10–33.
14. Bjorkman PJ, Saper MA, Samraoui B, Bennett WS, Strominger JL, Wiley DC. Structure of human class I histocompatibility antigen, HLA-A2. Nature 1987;329:506–512.
15. Kaufman JE, Auffray C, Korman AJ, Shackelford DA, Strominger J. The class II molecules of the human and murine major histocompatibility complex. Cell 1984;36:1.
16. Carroll MC, Katzman P, Alicot EM, et al. Linkage map of the human major histocompatibility complex including the tumor necrosis factor gene. Proc Natl Acad Sci USA 1987;84:8535–8539.
17. Benacerraf B. Role of major histocompatibility complex in genetic regulation of immunologic responsiveness. Transplant Proc 1977;9:825–831.
18. McMichael AJ, Ting A, Sweerink HJ, Askonos BA. HLA restriction of cell-mediated lysis of influenza virus-infected human cells. Nature 1977;270:524.
19. Terasaki PI, McClelland JD. Microdroplet assay of human serum cytotoxins. Nature 1964;204:998–1000.
20. Hopkins KA. Basic microlymphoytotoxicity test. In: Zachary AA, Teresi GA, eds. ASHI laboratory manual. 2nd ed. Lenexa, KS: American Society for Histocompatibility and Immunogenetics, 1990:195–201.
21. Falk JA, Goeken NE, eds. Cell Isolation. In: ASHI laboratory manual. 2nd edition. Lenexa, KS: American Society for Histocompatibility and Immunogenetics, 1990:49–80.
22. Payne R, Rolfs MR. Fetomaternal leukocyte incompatibility. J Clin Invest 1958;37:1756–1763.
23. Zmijewski CM, Zmijewski HE, Honeycutt HC. The relationship of the frequencies of white cell antibodies and red cell antibodies in the sera of multiparous women. Int Arch Allergy 1967;32:574–582.
24. Brodsky FM, Parham P, Barnstable CJ, Crumpton MJ, Bodmer WF. Monoclonal antibodies for analysis of the HLA system. Immunol Rev 1979;47:3–61.
25. Amos DB, Baskin H, Boyle W, MacQueen M, Tiilikaineen A. A simple microytotoxicity test. Transplantation 1969;7:220–222.
26. Johnson AH, Rossen RD, Butler WT. Detection of allo-antibodies using a sensitive antiglobulin microcytotoxicity test: identification of low levels of preformed antibodies in accelerated allograft rejection. Tissue Antigens 1972;2:215–255.
27. Bodmer WF, Tripp M, Bodmer JG. Application of a fluorochromatic cytotoxicity assay to human leukocyte typing. In: Curtoni ES, Mattiuz PL, Tosi RM, eds. Histocompatibility Testing 1967. Copenhagen: Munksgaard, 1967;341–350.
28. van Rood JJ, van Leeuwen A, Ploem JS. Simultaneous detection of two cell populations by two color fluoresence and application to the recognition of B cell determinants. Nature 1986;262:795–797.
29. Hirschhorn K, Bach F, Kolodny RL, et al. Immune response and mitosis in human peripheral blood lymphocytes *in vitro*. Science 1963;142:1185–1187.
30. Mempel W, Grosse-Wilde H, Baumann P, et al. Population genetics of the MLC response: typing for MLC determinants using homozygous and heterozygous reference cells. Transplant Proc 1973;5:1529–1534.
31. Sheehy MJ, Sondel PM, Bach ML, et al. HL-A LD (lymphocyte defined) typing a rapid assay with primed lymphocytes. Science 1975;188:1308–1310.
32. Mickelson EM, Nepom GT, Nisperos B, Hansen JA. DQw3 variants defined by cloned alloreactive T cells. Hum Immunol 1988;21:63–73.
33. Monos DS, Mickelson E, Hansen JA, Baker L, Zmijewski CM, Kamoun M. Analysis of DR and DQ gene products of the DR4 haplotype in patients with IDDM: possible involvement of more than one locus. Hum Immunol 1988;23:289–299.
34. Bodmer JG, Marsh SGE, Albert ED, et al. Nomenclature for factors of the HLA system, 1991. Tissue Antigens 1992;39:161–173.
35. Cox NJ, Mela PA, Zmijewski CM, Spielman RS. HLA-DR typing "at the DNA level": RFLPs and subtypes detected with a DRβ cDNA probe. Am J Hum Genet 1988;43:954–963.
36. Zemmour J, Parham P. HLA class I nucleotide sequences, 1991. Hum Immunol 1991;31:195–206.
37. Marsh SGE, Bodmer JG. HLA class II nucleotide sequences, 1991. Hum Immunol 1991;31:207–227.
38. Mullis KB, Faloona F. Specific synthesis of DNA in vitro via a polymerase-catalyzed chain reaction. Methods Enzymol 1987;155:335–350.
39. White TJ, Arnheim N, Erlich HA. The polymerase chain reaction. Trends Genet 1989;5:185–189.
40. Mach B, Tiercy JM. Genotypic typing of HLA class II: from the bench to the bedside. Hum Immunol 1991;30:278–284.
41. Gao X, Fernandez-Vina M, Shumway W, Stastny P. DNA typing for class II HLA antigens with allele-specific or group specific amplification. I. Typing for subsets of HLA-DR4. Hum Immunol 1990;27:40–50.
42. Inoko H. PCR-RFLP method holds great promise of complete HLA class II genotyping. Tissue Antigens 1990;36:88–92.
43. Sorrentino R, Cascino I, Tosi, R. Subgrouping of DR4 alleles by DNA heteroduplex analysis. Hum Immunol 1992;33:18–23.

44. Orita M, Iwakana H, Kanazawa H, et al. Detection of polymorphism of human DNA by gel electrophoresis as single-strand conformation polymorphisms. Proc Natl Acad Sci USA 1989;86:2766–2770.
45. Bugawan TL, Horn GT, Long CM, et al. Analysis of HLA-DP allelic sequence polymorphism using the in vitro enzymatic amplification of DPα and DPβ loci. J Immunol 1988;141:4020.
46. Tiercy JM, Jeannet M, Mach B. Oligonucleotide typing analysis for the linkage disequilibrium between the polymorphic DRB1 and DRB5 loci in DR2 haplotypes. Tissue Antigens 1991;37:161–164.

32 HLA: The Major Histocompatibility Complex—Applications

Chester M. Zmijewski

TRANSPLANTATION—SOLID ORGANS

The critical need for allogeneic renal transplantation as a therepeutic modality in end-stage renal disease served as the impetus for the investigations that led to the rapid discovery and understanding of the HLA system.

The concept of donor-recipient matching for histocompatibility antigens prior to transplantation is founded on the same principles underlying those used for the selection of blood for transfusions. An allograft is rejected as a result of an immune response directed against alloantigens expressed on the graft that are absent from the host. Matching for the most prominent antigens should result in some abrogation of the antigenic stimulus, resulting in a response that is more amenable to control by immunosuppressive drugs. It is recognized that exact matching for all possible antigens may be a practical impossibility. However, closer matches for major antigens will result in lesser degrees of antigenic challenge and will therefore require lower levels of immunosuppressive drugs, resulting in better overall outcomes.

Renal transplantation is carried out successfully using two groups of donors as sources for allografts. The first of these are living donors, usually relatives of the patient, who have two functioning kidneys, are in good health, and consent to donate. The second source is from cadaveric donors who were in reasonable health before death and whose kidneys were not affected by the fatal disease or circumstances of death. The most suitable donors in this category are victims of head trauma or other situations that result in irreversible brain damage. There are advantages and disadvantages to the use of each of these types of donors, and each presents a different set of problems with respect to matching.

Although the HLA system automatically comes to mind in the consideration of donor-recipient matching for transplantation, its importance is not exclusive. The strongest and probably more signficant transplantation antigens in humans are the antigens of the ABO blood group system (1). These antigens, in addition to being present on erythrocytes, are fully expressed in all tissues of the human body with the exception of those of the central nervous system. In addition, all people possess antibodies against the antigens (of the ABO system) they lack, developed as a result of natural environmental stimuli. These antibodies have the potential of reacting with antigens expressed on the vascular endothelium of the donor organ and can result in a hyperacute rejection similar to the white graft reaction described in the previous section. Therefore, matching for ABO within the same general guidelines used for blood donor selection is an essential prerequisite for organ transplantation.

The HLA matching of living related donors is performed with respect to the sharing of haplotypes containing the HLA-A, HLA-B, and HLA-DR antigens. Data excerpted from the UCLA transplant registry are shown in Table 32.1 (2). The overall 1-year survival among 1282 Caucasians with grafts matched for both haplotypes was 93% and the survival at 3 years was 89%. Among 2320 patients with grafts matched for only one haplotype the 1-year survival was slightly lower (87%) and the 3-year survival was only 76%. The overall survival among blacks was significantly lower—86% at 1 year and 76% at 3 years with two haplotype matches, and 79% and 57% with one haplotype match. From these data it is clear that HLA typing has a significant influence on the survival of kidneys from living, related donors.

Table 32.1. Living Related Kidney Graft Survival According to Haplotype Matches[a]

	Caucasians		Blacks	
Years After Graft	2 Matches n=1282	1 Match n=2320	2 Matches n=197	1 Match n=312
1	93%	87%	86%	79%
2	90%	82%	80%	66%
3	89%	76%	76%	57%

[a]Data from Cicciarelli J. Living donor kidney transplants. In: Terasaki PI, ed. Clinical transplants 1988. Los Angeles: UCLA Tissue Typing Laboratory, 1988: 293–299.

The striking difference in the overall outcome of transplantation between whites and blacks is noteworthy. These differences, which have been observed not only with living, related donors but with cadaveric donors as well, cannot be readily explained. The inability to type for certain antigens prevalent only in blacks plays no part in the cases of living, related donors since they are matched for haplotypes derived from family studies. However, so-called center effects, physiology, and lack of patient compliance have been cited as possible contributory causes.

The center effect must be considered whenever analyzing data of this type, which has been collected in a central registry from a large number of individual transplant centers. The effect originates from a collection of events that may exert a significant influence on outcome but that are not attributable to the condition being measured: for example, HLA matching. These influences would include such factors as surgical technique, standards for organ harvesting, immunosuppressive protocols, clinical condition of the patient prior to transplantation, nursing care, socioeconomic status of the patient, patient compliance, postgraft monitoring, and assessment of clinical condition. Interestingly enough, this collection of factors, which contribute to the center effect and therefore may obfuscate the interpretation of collated data to some extent, may have a marked effect on the results from a single center. Thus, any single center might appear to show either a very high or a very low correlation of graft survival with typing. Therefore, the analysis of pooled data from a large number of patients gives the best picture since the center effect is minimized.

HLA matching appears to have an effect on long-term graft survival. In one analysis of long-term survivors of kidney transplantation from cadaveric donors the average half-life of grafts was 10.1 years for those with no HLA-A or B mismatches and 6 years for those with no HLA antigens in common. When both HLA-A,B and HLA-DR matching are considered the results are clearly superior, with patients receiving organs with zero mismatches for the entire constellation of HLA antigens and achieving a graft survival half-life of 11.3 years compared to a half-life of 6.3 years for grafts that were completely mismatched for HLA-A,B and DR (3).

HLA matching is especially beneficial in second transplants and in patients with preformed antibodies (4). Patients matched with their donors for both DR antigens (disregarding any HLA-A,B matching) have a 1-year survival of 83% versus 76% for those with one match and 74% for those with no matches. At 5 years 64% of the fully matched grafts are still functioning while only 55% of those with one or no matches survive. Matching for the HLA-A and B antigens in addition to HLA-DR has an enhancing effect. In the study cited, the patients matched for both HLA-DR antigens achieve a 1-year graft survival of 87% if they are also matched for a single HLA-A antigen and a single HLA-B antigen versus 74% for those with no HLA-A or B match. Additional analyses have confirmed these findings and have shown that HLA-A, B matching has a significant effect on long-term graft survival (5). Interestingly, the same study revealed that HLA-DR matching alone does not improve long-term graft survival even though it appears to have an effect during the early period after transplantation.

There has been some controversy regarding the benefit of HLA matching in the era of newer modalities of immunosuppression. One of these is cyclosporine, a remarkable immunosuppressive drug that made liver transplantation a reality. Studies have shown that it can improve graft survival by 10 to 15%. However, even in these cases graft survival can be improved even more by donor selection based on HLA matching.

Figure 32.1 shows some long-term extrapolation of graft survival with respect to the degree of mismatching (6). The solid line represents the average survival of all grafts prior to the use of CsA. In the post-cyclosporine era, matching significantly improves kidney graft survival in the long term.

A new donor-recipient matching scheme has been proposed that is based on the matching for the relevant immunogenicity of shared epitopes in AB and DR (7). The examination of the antibodies from 50,000 pregnancies revealed that most of the specificities were directed against public and private specificities defined by molecules with shared epitopes (8). Furthermore, this analysis allowed the calculation of an immunogenicity score for each specificity, based on the chance of immunization. This immunogenicity score varied by more than 10 times between different specificities. In addition, the shared epitopes based on the cross-reactivity between different DR types could be defined. This approach to matching is receiving a great deal of attention and is being supported by the ever-increasing understanding of the HLA antigens at the amino acid level (9). Hopefully this should lead to a better definition of allowable mismatches like those that are routinely applied to the choice of blood for transfusion.

Still another sophisticated procedure for donor recipient matching is being explored at the peptide level. Using a computer-generated table of peptides unique to each HLA specificity, Takemoto and Terasaki (10) used this system for matching. They claim that this approach was more effective in identifying patients with extremely poor outcomes than conven-

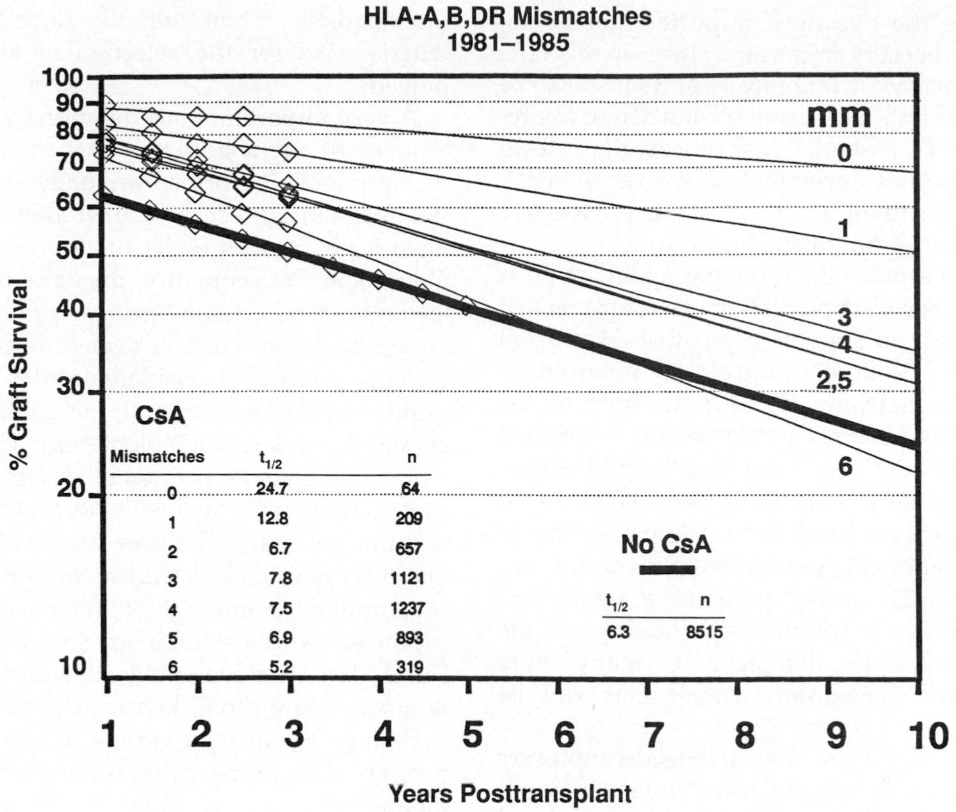

Figure 32.1. The projected survival of the first patients to receive cadaver-donor renal transplants performed in conjunction with cyclosporine (CsA) treatment. The data are plotted according to linear regression transformed to a log scale. The *heavy line* represents the survival of grafts prior to the use of cyclosporine. Even with the use of this drug, only the 0- and 1-antigen mismatches (MM) show a 10-year survival of 50% or more. (Reprinted with permission from Cook D. HLA-A, B, DR. Mismatches 1981-85. In: Terasaki PI, ed. Visuals of the Histocompatibility Workshop—Palm Springs Invitational 1988. Los Angeles: One Lambda, Inc., 1988:14.)

Table 32.2. UNOS Point System for Organ Sharing

Degree of HLA Matching	Points
0 A,B,DR mismatch	10
0 B,DR mismatch	7
0 A,B mismatch	6
1 B,DR mismatch	3
2 B,DR mismatch	2
3 B,DR mismatch	1
High PRA-negative cross-match	4
Waiting time	up to 1 + 0.5/year

tional techniques. Although such a tool is far from practical in its present state of development, it may offer new insights to the problem.

Under ideal circumstances it would be most desirable to obtain donors who are perfectly matched with respect to all six HLA antigens of the recipient. In spite of the polymorphism of the HLA system, some haplotypes are more prevalent in the population than others. Therefore, in certain cases it is possible to find exact matches, even among random donors. Unfortunately, this can take time, and for many patients with end-stage renal disease the time needed to find an exact match may not be available. For this reason, each case must be evaluated individually, and compromises based on both scientific and clinical judgment must be made.

The analysis of data such as those presented earlier has led to the development of a hierarchy of matching: A,B,DR >B,DR >A,DR >DR >B >A. A convenient way to select a recipient for any given random donor is based on the awarding of points. The points assigned by the United Network for Organ Sharing (UNOS) for the various degrees of matching are give in Table 32.2. In addition to HLA matching, this scheme also allows for the awarding of points for other factors related to the quantity of preformed anti-HLA antibody in the recipient serum and the length of time on the waiting list.

In contrast to the kidney, donors of nonpaired organs such as the heart and liver must be of cadaveric origin, although single hepatic lobes from living donors have been used. Furthermore, in these cases clinical considerations play a very prominent role because, unlike the kidney patient who can be supported on dialysis, end-stage coronary and liver diseases are not amenable to long-term maintenance therapy. In the case of these organs ABO compatibility and size are the two most important considerations. Size is especially important since these grafts must fit when placed orthotopically and must also be capable of handling the physiologic burden of the recipient. Speed is essential, as preservation techniques either are not developed or are very critical. For these reasons there is little time for prospective donor-recipient matching based on HLA.

Retrospective studies on the significance of HLA matching in cardiac transplantation are controversial. Some data appear to support a positive effect from DR matching, while others indicate no apparent effects from such matching (11, 12). In spite of the fairly large number of cardiac transplants performed to date, the data base is still too small and heterogeneous to permit any significant conclusion to be reached. Experience gained from the evaluation of renal transplantation suggests that the myriad of factors associated with cardiac patients is even more complicated. This contributes significantly to the center effect, requiring the study of many more cases before any meaningful conclusions can be reached.

In liver transplantation, clinical considerations are even more important than in heart transplantation; as a result, a careful prospective study has never been attempted. However, data from retrospective studies performed at the largest liver transplant center in the United States are showing some interesting, although somewhat ironic, results. They seem to suggest that HLA matching for DR has a reverse effect; that is, patients with grafts poorly matched for class II antigens appear to do better than those with well-matched grafts (13).

This finding seems to parallel results from rodent models of endocrine organ transplantation. In these systems, it has been suggested that the graft failure stems from the ability of the cells in the matched tissue to act as antigen-presenting cells to the host immune system. Class II antigen expression by the nonlymphoid cells being transplanted may be induced by IL-2 and interferon gamma released during the normal inflammatory stages of the transplant procedure. Class II identity with the host allows these cells to act as antigen-presenting cells. The antigens being presented are thought to be minor histocompatibility antigens expressed on the donor cells that are absent from the host. If this is indeed the cause of the failure of DR-matched livers in humans it could lead to a better understanding of human minor histocompatibility antigens (14).

Pancreas is transplanted both as a solid organ and as dissociated islet cells. Both of these tissues are exceptionally susceptible to the action of HLA antibodies. The greatest success is obtained when pancreas and kidney from the same donor are transplanted simultaneously. Therefore, the same HLA matching criteria used for the selection of kidneys are employed.

A very important consideration in the selection of a donor of any solid organ is the antibody status of the recipient. Preformed antibodies in the serum of the recipient directed against donor antigens can have a deleterious effect on the outcome of transplantation. Consequently, presence of such antibodies must be ascertained prior to donor selection.

Antibodies to HLA antigens are produced by recipients awaiting transplantation in response to a number of different stimuli, including blood transfusion and previous transplantation. The dose of challenging antigen is presented differently in each of these situations. This results in a variety of different immune reponses that may vary with respect to the quantity, biochemical affinity, and in some cases the predominant immunoglobulin class of the antibodies produced as well as their specificity and persistence. In addition to developing alloantibodies, some patients awaiting renal, heart, or pancreas transplants may have produced a variety of autoantibodies as a result of their primary disease or pregraft therapeutic modalities.

In marked contrast to the well-developed and sharply defined response obtained in alloimmunization of pregnancy, the immunologic response to a clinical allograft is somewhat immature. Under these circumstances the antibody producer is an unhealthy individual whose immune system has been compromised as a result of disease; this unhealthy immune system has been further compromised deliberately by immunosuppressive drugs. This doubly impaired immune system is then presented with an antigenic challenge as a single bolus containing a large variety of antigenic specificities. The result is a broad polyclonal response directed against a host of cross-reactive antigens, some of which may not even be represented on the graft.

The quality of the antibody response to blood transfusion may be classified as falling somewhere between that of pregnancy and that of transplantation. In this case the subject is an unhealthy individual whose immune system may be somewhat depressed as a result of uremia, but the patient has not been pharmacologically immunosuppressed. The antigen is introduced intravenously in small and overlapping doses. The antigens constituting the challenge are relatively weak; therefore, a substantial quantity is required to achieve a response. On the other hand, the number of antigen-bearing cells, leukocytes, and platelets in a unit of blood is relatively small and decreases even further with time after the unit is drawn. As a result, multiple transfusions of units of blood are required to constitute an adequate antigenic dose. These units come from different blood donors whose cells display a variety of private specificities. The antigens that are most readily recognized by the immune system, therefore, are those directed against public specificities shared by the donors and those directed against private specificities that occur with relatively high frequencies in the general population. Patients undergoing transfusion routinely produce a spectrum of antibodies, including anti-HLA-A, B, C, and DR.

The antibodies produced as a result of either of these challenges are IgG and IgM, though the IgG antibodies are frequently of low affinity. They are directed against a variety of HLA antigens and tend to react with the public specificities of the HLA cross-reactive groups. In addition, IgM antibodies with very broad specificities may be produced as well. Current data seem to indicate that, with some exceptions, these antibodies tend to disappear with time, and, in the case of transfusion-induced antibodies, fail to reappear upon secondary challenge (15).

Antibodies to class I HLA antigens can be directed specifically against private specificities or public specificities. Antibodies with private specificities are clinically relevant and are directed against epitopes formed by a unique amino acid sequence that forms a single specificity. Antibodies to public specificities, on the other hand, define various cross-reactive groups. They have been the subject of a great deal of study to establish their importance in clinical transplantation.

Antibodies to the class II HLA antigens DR and DQ appear to be clinically significant with respect to adversely affecting graft survival. On the other hand, other antibodies that preferentially react with B cells but that have no apparent specificity for class II MHC antigens may have little or no clinical significance. Many of these antibodies are composed of IgM immunoglobulin and react preferentially at 20°C or below. They are not very stable and can be inactivated by treatment with dithiothreitol (DTT) or other similar reducing agents (16).

Autoantibodies may occasionally be found in the sera of pretransplant patients who are suffering from diseases with a heightened immune response such as lupus nephritis. They tend to react with a patient's own cells in in vitro serologic tests and may sometimes have HLA specificity (17). In addition, autoantibody-like substances may be produced in response to certain drugs such as hydralazine or procainamide. These may not be true antibodies at all; they may be aggregated γ-globulins or other macromolecules that become attached to cell surfaces nonspecifically and cause complement activation.

Autoantibodies appear to play no role in transplantation rejection, but they serve as an indicator of a patient's abnormal immune status and frequently interfere with the interpretation of serologic tests for alloantibody detection. Most often these antibodies are IgM and react preferentially at room temperature or below. However, their thermal amplitude is occasionally higher and they will react at 37°C. For the most part, such antibodies can be inactivated with DTT or removed by absorption with the patient's own cells.

Screening procedures used in the pretransplant patient for antibody detection and identification must be designed to take all of the aforementioned characteristics into consideration. The approach is designed to uncover the total antibody content of a patient's serum and its characteristic reaction patterns. This information is then used to render a judgment regarding the interpretation of the pretransplant test between the serum of the patient and the cells of the donor with respect to the suitability of a given donor-patient combination. Therefore, it is essential to fully ascertain all of the properties of any antibodies involved. Are they public, private, or auto? Are they class I or class II? Do they react by the standard testing method, or do they require enhanced antiglobulin procedures? Finally, what is their expected frequency of positive reactions with the general population?

From these data, much important information may be derived, including an estimate of the likelihood of finding a cross-match compatible donor among the random cadaver population in a given region. This, in turn, serves as the basis for a prediction of the waiting time for a given patient on the list. Additionally, from these data it is possible to predict the HLA types of donors who are likely to cause a positive cross-match and thus avoid unnecessary testing. Finally, the data derived above permit the selection of optimal serologic cross-matching methods to ensure maximum sensitivity for antibody detection as well as the interpretation of any unexpected positive or equivocal results.

The patient's serum to be screened is tested serologically against a panel of cells whose antigenic composition has been predetermined according to rigorous standard typing criteria. The distribution of positive reactions is compared with the distribution of each of the known HLA antigens in the cell panel. The specificity of the antibody in the serum is equivalent to the antigenic specificity in the panel that most closely matches the distribution of positive reactions. The match will hardly ever be exact, since most frequently the sera contain a mixture of antibodies. In addition, the sera may contain a heterogeneous population of antibody molecules that have a spectrum of affinities for antigen. As a result, although the observed pattern may be similar to that for a particular antigen distribution, discrepancies will occur and a certain degree of uncertainty will be experienced.

To interpret the results, the reaction patterns are normally analyzed using statistical methods that allow for a measure of this uncertainty. If the level of uncertainty is small, being due to chance alone, the similarity observed between the reactions of the serum and the distribution of an antigen in the cell panel is probably real. On the other hand, if the level of uncertainty is large, then the differences may be real and the plausibility of similarity diminishes. The most frequently used statistic for this purpose is the 2 × 2 contingency chi-square test.

The following is an example of a 2 × 2 analysis showing the comparison of the reactions of serum S.J. with the distribution of HLA-B7 in the test cell panel.

		HLA–B7 +	HLA–B7 -	
Serum S.J.	+	43	2	45
	-	3	27	30
		46	29	75

$$\chi^2 = \frac{[(43 \cdot 27) - (3 \cdot 2)]^2\, 75}{(45 \cdot 30 \cdot 46 \cdot 29)} = 55.5$$

The theoretical distribution of chi-square against which the computed value will be compared is a continuous distribution. The data, on the other hand, lead to a discontinuous distribution of computed chi-square values. In practice it is customary to correct for continuity by employing the Yates correction factor (18). For the example given above, the corrected chi-square is computed as follows:

$$\chi^2 \text{ CORRECTED } = \frac{(|(43 \cdot 27) - (3 \cdot 2)| - [0.5 \cdot 75])^2\, 75}{(45 \cdot 30 \cdot 46 \cdot 29)} = 52.01$$

If the two events—namely the occurrence of the antigen and the positive reactions of the serum—are independent, then the chi-square value will be low. On the other hand, if the occurrence of a positive reaction depends on the presence of the antigen in a given cell (or, stated another way, the antibody defines the specific antigen in the panel), then the chi-square value will be high and will approach *n*, the number of cells tested, but will never quite reach it. In addition, the customary use of the Yates correction factor to correct for discontinuity further lessens this chance. The hypothesis that the serum is detecting the given antigen in the panel is accepted or rejected depending on the probability corresponding to the calculated chi-square value obtained from a table of the chi-square distribution for 1 df (degree of freedom). When the chi-square is low the probability of independence between reaction patterns and specificity is high. When the chi-square is high, the probability is low. A probability in the range of 0.01 to 0.001 or less indicates that the serum reaction patterns most likely correspond to the antigen distribution pattern.

In the example given above, the probability is less than 0.001. Therefore, the hypothesis that the serum S.J. most likely contains antibodies with HLA-B7 specificity may be accepted.

In practice, these calculations are performed with the aid of computer programs. The chi-square values are then ranked. Frequently sera will give high values with more than one antigen because they are multispecific. A crude approximation of the range of specificities that is adequate for clinical work can be obtained by performing a careful examination of the antigen distribution among the cells in the panel and the resultant chi-square values that are significant. Extensive screening against highly selected cell panels to confirm the specificities implied by the initial studies is usually not performed for diagnostic purposes in pretransplant patients. A careful consideration of the preliminary screening data along with the HLA type of the patient and the typing data of the previous grafts, if any, will usually give a good indication of the HLA antigens to be avoided in future grafts.

The knowledge of the specificity of antibodies in patients' sera is essential to making a sound decision regarding the suitability of a given donor for a particular patient. In addition, it serves as the basis for computing a predictive measure of the possibility of finding a suitable donor among the cadaveric organs available from the general population. The predictive value is given by the percent or panel reactive antibody (PRA). It is computed from the frequency in the local population of the antigens defined by the patient's serum when it was tested and gives a reasonable reflection of how the sera might be expected to react in cross-matches with donors from the random population. Over the years this value has become a standard parameter for judging a patient's transplantability and is used as one of the criteria that govern a patient's clinical management.

The serologic methods used in screening patient sera should be the most sensitive available. One of the purposes is to learn as much as possible about the reactivity of a given patient's serum during a time of relative leisure and to predict how it will behave in the cross-match procedure performed under more stressful conditions and time constraints.

Ordinarily, the screening is performed using panels of purified T cells for the detection of class I antigens and purified B cells for the detection of class II antigens, as well as the patient's own cells to detect autoantibodies.

The practice of treating all sera prior to screening and cross-matching with dithiothreitol (DTT) to eliminate bothersome and clinically insignificant reactions due to IgM antibodies has been advocated. Although this practice saves some time, it masks the presence of IgM antibodies and occasionally may dilute weak IgG antibodies, thus inhibiting their activity beyond their threshold of detectability. It is preferable to recognize that the serum of a particular patient may contain an IgM antibody so that it can be dealt with accordingly and the serum's reactivity interpreted intelligently.

In summary, antibody screening can be defined as the systematic examination, under controlled conditions, of a serum for its content of antibodies directed against surface antigens of nucleated cells, and the analysis of the resultant data. The information sought from these data determines the methods and extent of the systematic examination and the resultant data analysis.

The useful information required for patient antibody screening includes an exhaustive characterization of the antibody reactivity under a variety of very sensitive serologic methods, a general feeling for the scope and range of its reactivity with an array of different specificities, and a measure of the frequency of its reactivity with cells from the random population (PRA). Therefore, the major emphasis is on serologic conditions with a cell panel that is broadly inclusive.

Donor-specific HLA antibodies in the serum of a recipient prior to transplant are especially significant. Such antibodies can readily combine with antigens on the grafted organ immediately after a blood supply is established and result in hyperacute or accelerated graft rejection. This can be avoided by performing a pretransplant cross-match in which a serum sample from the recipient is tested against lymphocytes obtained from the intended donor. A negative cross-match is an essential prerequisite for the performance of a transplant.

The serum sample from the patient must be one that best represents a sampling of the patient's anti-HLA antibody repertoire at the time the transplant will be performed. Ideally this should be one collected just prior to surgery. Quite frequently, however, this may not be possible due to practical considerations. For example, the test itself is time consuming: if the intended recipient is not readily available to provide a serum sample, donor organ ischemia time might be prolonged to the point where irreversible damage could occur. Similarly, the recipient is usually one of several candidates; therefore the identity of the actual recipient might not be known. For these reasons, serum samples are collected from potential recipients of cadaveric organs at monthly or more frequent intervals, especially those coinciding with the peak of an immunizing event such as a blood transfusion. These samples are carefully preserved in the frozen condition to be used for cross-matching with a potential donor.

Standard immunologic dogma dictates that once a patient formed an HLA antibody it would be of significance even after it had disappeared from the serum. Such antibodies might remain at undetectable levels or could be rapidly produced in a secondary response upon reexposure to antigen. Consequently, historical serum samples containing the maximum levels of antibody reactivity should be used routinely in cross-matches along with current samples. A positive historic cross-match would be considered to be a contraindication to transplantation with that particular donor. Recent evidence indicates that this does not hold true in cases in which HLA antibodies disappear prior to a first transplant (15). In such cases, the antibodies developed before the graft are most likely the result of exposure to HLA antigens present in blood transfusions. Apparently the response produced to such an immunization does not result in long-term immunologic memory. Therefore, positive cross-matches with historical sera are frequently disregarded in such cases. On the other hand, in cases involving a second or third transplant, the reactions of historically positive sera with the potential donor are most important (16). It seems that patients immunized or in conjunction with a previous graft develop strong immunologic memory and can produce a brisk secondary response when rechallenged with the offending antigen.

Traditionally, the cross-match is performed using a sensitive modification of the microlymphocytotoxicity test. Many centers employ the antiglobulin technique; others opt for an extended incubation of the antibody-lymphocyte mixture; still others favor some modification incorporating one or more wash steps prior to the addition of complement. However, any method selected should be capable of detecting the varieties of antibody found in the patient's serum during the pretransplant antibody screening. Thus the importance of pretransplant screening cannot be overemphasized. This procedure allows a detailed and accurate assessment of the antibody repertoire carried by the patient in a relatively leisurely manner rather than under the stresses associated with a cadaveric donor organ harvest and the overzealous anticipation of a possible transplant.

When using a cadaveric donor the lymphocytes of choice are prepared from excised lymph nodes or a section of spleen obtained in conjunction with organ harvesting. The nodes should be kept moist after their removal and during delivery to the laboratory. Some workers advocate the use of peripheral blood from the potential donor in order to save time. This is a debatable point. The peripheral blood cells of patients who have been kept on life support systems may be unsuitable for use in the cytotoxicity test for a number of reasons, including the effects of antemortem steroids administered to reduce cerebral edema. Consequently, uninterpretable results may often be obtained, requiring the tests to be repeated. Thus, little time is saved and the expense of duplicate work is incurred.

It is best to perform the cross-match using pure T cells as targets (20). This is good practice, since anti-HLA class I antibodies are the most frequently encountered and the most clinically significant. In addition, many types of patients such as those with lupus erythematosus, certain diabetics, and others often demonstrate nonspecific autoreactivity. This is most frequently directed against B cells and seems to have no clinical significance. If mixtures of T and B cells are used in the cross-match with the sera of such patients, they would give a positive result. Therefore a transplant would be denied because of a false-positive reaction.

In contrast to nonspecific B-cell antibodies, those directed against class II HLA antigens are of definite clinical relevance. Pretransplant antibody screens should be designed for their detection and identification. In addition, cross-matches with the serum of patients containing such antibodies should be performed using suspensions of B cells.

Flow cytometry is currently being investigated as a sensitive adjunct for performing cross-matches (21). In addition to being extremely sensitive, this method has the advantage of being able to dissect the reaction between the serum of the recipient and the cells of the donor with respect to the cell types involved (T or B), the immunoglobulin class (IgM or IgG), and the quantity of antibody being bound. Such information allows for a more sophisticated judgment to be made as to the suitability of a particular donor for a given recipient. Furthermore, the technique has the advantage of being complement independent. Therefore it is capable of detecting noncomplement binding antibodies as well as avoiding some of the pitfalls associated with complement binding reactions. However, it is not entirely free of disadvantages. It is time consuming, requires expensive equipment, and demands highly skilled operators and expertise in interpretation.

TRANSPLANTATION—BONE MARROW

In patients who have never been previously immunized to HLA antigens, the single most important consideration in the grafting of bone marrow is the prevention of a reaction of the engrafted cells against the recipient. Immunologically competent donor cells reacting with recipient tissues can lead to a serious disorder known as graft versus host disease (GVH). Most patients who require a bone marrow transplant have a nonfunctioning immune system because of their underlying disease or therapy. If this is not the case, deliberate immunologic incompetence is induced by cytoreductive chemotherapy and/or irradiation prior to transplantation. Under these conditions, the recipient cannot respond easily to foreign antigens in the donor and therefore the problem of graft rejection is not as important as in other forms of transplantation. However, since the donor cells have full immunologic potential, they can recognize the recipient antigens and react against them. Total identity for all antigens of the major histocompatibility complex appears to be an important factor in keeping the GVH reaction to a minimum. For this reason, the assessment of nonreactivity between donor and host as defined by the mixed leukocyte culture (MLC) is a paramount consideration prior to transplantation. The early attempts at marrow grafting were carried out using HLA-identical siblings as donors. Further clinical trials indicated that sibling donors who differed from the recipient by only one or two HLA antigens could be used successfully. Sibling donors who demonstrated class II identity and class I mismatch in part of a haplotype due to recombination could be used as donors. Current data indicate that unrelated donors may be used with some degree of success if they are well matched for HLA. The degree of permissible mismatch among unrelated donor-recipient combinations is being investigated (22).

Large numbers of HLA-typed potential donors of bone marrow are being developed in England, the United States, and elsewhere to satisfy the needs of patients lacking appropriate siblings. The selection of an unrelated donor is made through a comparison of the total HLA type. The cells of the potential donor identified from a donor file by such a comparison are

Table 32.3. Selective Match Grades for Platelet Transfusion[a]

Match Grade	Extent of HLA Matching	Example
A	Four HLA-A,B antigen match	A2,30,B12,7 → A2,30,B12,7
B1U	One HLA antigen is unknown	A2,?,B12,7 → A2,30,B12,7
B2U	Two HLA antigens are unknown	A2,?,B12,? → A2,30,B12,7
B1X	One antigen is cross-reactive	A2,30,B12,**27** → A2,30,B12,7
B2X	Two antigens are cross-reactive	A2,**33**,B12,**27** → A2,30,B12,7
BUX	One antigen unknown, one cross-reactive	A2,?,B12,**27** → A2,30,B12,7
C	One major antigen mismatch	A2,30,B12,**5** → A2,30,B12,7
D	Two or more major mismatches	A2,**10**,B12,**5** → A2,30,B12,7

[a]Adapted from Dahlke MB, Weiss KL. Platelet transfusion from donors mismatched for crossreactive HLA antigens. Transfusion 1984;24:299–302.

sent to the patient's institution for confirmation of class II identity by means of an MLC. If this is found to be nonreactive, the donor marrow is collected and shipped for infusion into the recipient.

One of the problems associated with this procedure centers on the reliability of the MLC when using stored or shipped cells from an unrelated donor. Another problem confounding the MLC, regardless of the donor source, is that quite frequently, patients awaiting transplant have very few or inseparable B cells in their peripheral blood. Therefore they are poor stimulators and as such provide little usable information. The perfection of some of the newer molecular methods will offer a solution to both of these difficulties. For example, patient class II antigens can be defined by DNA regardless of which cell types can be harvested. Similarly, isolated DNA or even dried cells can easily be transported, allowing for an accurate comparison of the potential donor with the potential recipient. As an example, we were recently able to HLA type a very young infant who had been transfused by using DNA prepared from scrapings of the buccal mucosa.

Although minimal, the reactivity of the host against donor marrow can not be totally neglected. This can be manifested as either a failure of the transplanted marrow to engraft or as a true rejection. In most cases this can occur as the result of preformed antibody reacting against the donor cells. The antibody may be anti-HLA produced in response to blood products administered as supportive therapy prior to transplantation. In ABO-incompatible grafts, which are performed quite frequently, it can be due to the anti-A and/or anti-B antibodies that were not completely removed or neutralized prior to grafting. To avoid the problem of graft rejection, crossmatches performed between the cells of the donor and the serum of the recipient are advisable.

PLATELET TRANSFUSION

Patients receiving repeated infusions of platelet concentrate over long periods of time frequently become refractory. They fail to achieve an incremental increase in their platelet count proportional to the number of platelets transfused. It has been shown that this condition results from the development of antibodies frequently produced in response to class I HLA antigens expressed on the surface of platelets. HLA class II antigens play no role in this phenomenon.

The use of HLA-matched platelets is beneficial in many of these cases for achieving normal platelet survival in the immunized patients and the prevention of immunization in the immunologically virgin patient (23).

However, exact HLA matching for platelet transfusion may not be possible for practical reasons. Fortunately, not all HLA antigens are expressed on platelets with equal strength. Furthermore, it has been shown that matching for some of the antigens as outlined in Table 32.3, together with matching for cross-reactive groups (CREGs) is adequate to achieve successful clinical results (24). The selection of the type of matched product—whether it is matched for private antigens or matched for CREGs—depends entirely on the patient. Platelet recipients can be divided into three groups. The first consists of patients who are nonresponsive and never become refractory. The second group are those who become refractory to random donor platelets but tolerate HLA-matched products. These may be further subdivided into those who require HLA-identical products from siblings and those in whom platelets matched according to the schemes outlined above result in adequate increments and provide adequate hemostatic function. The third group are those who become refractory very quickly after a minimal number of random units and cannot tolerate even very well-matched platelets.

DISEASE ASSOCIATION

The association of HLA types with various diseases has been the subject of intense investigation (25). Originally discovered as a chance observation and later enforced by the finding of a strong association between ankylosing spondylitis and the presence of the infrequent antigen HLA-B27, this line of investigation has led to a clearer understanding of some of the disease processes themselves. For example, diabetes mellitus has been reclassified into two distinct types. Juvenile-onset, insulin-dependent diabetes, or type I diabetes mellitus, is strongly associated with HLA; whereas type II or maturity-onset diabetes shows no apparent association. As a result of these findings it is now recognized that each of these types is a clinically distinct disease entity with its own pathogenesis.

In discussing the concept of HLA and disease, it is important to recognize the distinction between association and linkage. It is tempting to speculate that the reason for the observed relationships between the occurrence of a given disease and the presence of a particular HLA antigen is linkage. However, linkage implies a formal genetic analysis of family inheritance patterns and indicates that two loci are situated closely enough on the chromosome to allow crossing over to occur less than 50% of the time. With the exception of diseases that exhibit familial tendencies, most of the studies carried out with respect to HLA and disease have been population studies that do not permit formal genetic analysis.

Indeed, such analyses have shown that genes responsible for hemochromatosis, for deficiencies in 21-hydroxylase (resulting in congenital adrenal hyperplasia), and for C2 are linked to HLA. Further studies resulting from these observations have revealed that the loci for 21-OH and C2 are not only linked to the MHC but are within the MHC itself.

However, the majority of diseases studied in this manner exhibit association rather than linkage. Association of a particular HLA antigen with a certain disease is a statistical event established by comparing the frequency of the antigen in the disease population with its frequency in the normal population. The normal population in this case should consist of random individuals matched for racial composition with the disease population. A comparison is made using the chi-square statistic in a 2 × 2 contigency table and corrected for the number of antigens tested. The strength of the association can be obtained by calculating the relative risk (RR) or the statistical chance that a patient with a certain disease will have the given HLA antigen. This may be computed either by the method of Woolf (26) or that of Haldane (27). Both of these are shown in the example given below. This example demonstrates the steps in the analysis of data obtained in a hypothetical study of the incidence of the antigen HLA-B27 among 40 patients suffering from ankylosing spondylitis and 904 normal control subjects.

HLA–B27

	+	-	
Disease	[a] 35	[b] 5	[a+b] 40
Control	[c] 67	[d] 837	[c+d] 904
	[a+c] 102	[b+d] 842	[n] 944

$$\chi^2 = \frac{(ad - bc)^2 n}{(a+b)(c+d)(a+c)(b+d)} =$$

$$\frac{[(35)(827) - (5)(67)]^2(944)}{(40)(904)(102)(842)} = 254.9$$

$$RR = \chi = \frac{ad}{bc} = \frac{(35)(837)}{(67)(5)} = 87.4$$

according to the method of Woolf; and

$$RR = \chi = \frac{[2(a+1)][2(d+1)]}{(2c+1)(2b+1)} =$$

$$\frac{(2)(35+1)(2)(837+1)}{(2)(67+1)(2)(5+1)} = 73.9$$

according to the method of Haldane. The chi-square value of 254.9 is highly significant and indicates that the higher incidence of HLA-B27 among the patient population is not due to chance. In this example, both populations were tested only for the presence or absence of HLA-B27; consequently no corrections are required. However, when studying a disease for the first time, it is customary to test for a battery of HLA antigens. Since one would expect that some deviation from the normal distribution of antigen frequencies could occur due to chance, the chi-square is corrected by dividing it by the number of antigens that were tested.

The RR of 87.4 given by the method of Woolf agrees with that published. The method of Haldane is designed to correct for small sample sizes and gives a value of 73.9. This is slightly less than the published value but is nevertheless quite significant in terms of its order of magnitude.

Associations have been shown to be of two types. Those in which the disease is associated with class I antigens are shown in Table 32.4. Those having strong associations with class II antigens are given in Table 32.5. Interestingly, the diseases have a strong immunologic flavor, being either diseases of the immune system itself or having autoimmunity as their underlying theme.

Table 32.4. Some Prominent Associations of Diseases with Class I Antigens[a]

Disease	HLA	RR
Idiopathic hemochromatosis	A3	6.77
Vitiligo (Yemenites)	B35	13.9
Acute anterior uveitis	B27	10.4
Ankylosing spondylitis	B27	87.4
Reiter's disease	B27	37.0
Duodenal ulcer	B35	2.7
Subacute thyroiditis (de Quervain)	B35	13.7
Psoriasis vulgaris	Cw6	13.3

[a]From Zmijewski CM. HLA and disease. CRC Crit Rev Clin Lab Sci 1984;20: 285–370.

Table 32.5. Some Prominent Associations of Diseases with Class II Antigens[a]

Disease	HLA	RR
Allergy (Ra 5 response)	DR2	19.0
Multiple sclerosis	DR2	4.1
Narcolepsy	DR2	129.7
Celiac disease	DR3	10.8
Goodpasture's disease	DR3	15.0
Insulin dependent diabetes	DR3	4.6
Systemic lupus erythematosus	DR3	2.6
Rheumatoid arthritis	DR4	4.2
Insulin dependent diabetes	DR4	15.4
Pemphigus vulgaris	DR4	14.4
Juvenile rheumatoid arthritis	DR5	5.2
Pernicious anemia	DR5	5.4
Nephrotic syndrome (steroid responsive)	DR7	5.9

[a]From Zmijewski CM. HLA and disease. CRC Crit Rev Clin Lab Sci 1984; 20: 285–370.

Of particular note are rheumatoid arthritis (RA) and insulin-dependent diabetes mellitus (IDDM). These diseases have been studied extensively at the molecular level and have yielded a great deal of innovative information. Studies of RA indicate that the DR4 molecules associated with this disease carry a β chain that is characteristic of the cellularly defined antigen Dw4. In addition, the DQ7 of DQ3 is the predominant DQ molecule found in disequelibrium with that particular DR4 (28).

IDDM is also found to be strongly associated with DR4. However, in this disease the DQ8 variant of DQ3 appears to be most prevalent (29). This is an interesting contrast to the findings in RA and might lead to a speculation regarding possible mechanisms. Nevertheless, at least one study indicates that susceptibility to IDDM may be due to interactive effects of both DR and DQ loci, since no clear-cut difference was found between patients and controls with respect to either of these gene products alone.

Another study delved even deeper into the molecular level (30, 31). There has been a good indication that residue #57 of the first domain sequence of DQB allelic products is involved in the susceptibility and resistance to IDDM. The DQB gene products of IDDM patients generally lack aspartic acid at residue #57. However, among haplotypes showing a negative association with IDDM, aspartic acid is usually found at position #57 of the first domain sequence of DQβ. Unfortunately, a notable exception to this otherwise straightforward association is reported in the Japanese population. Here DR9 is associated with IDDM, but the DQB products accompanying it do not show the expected universal absence of aspartate at position #57. The matter requires further investigation.

The biological mechanisms underlying the associations between HLA antigens and various diseases is not understood. A number of possibilities have been suggested, including antigenic mimicry, faulty immune response, or other susceptibility genes in gametic association with HLA. Each of these can be supported with a good deal of positive evidence. However, in each case there is an equally impressive body of contradictory evidence. Surely some of the newer approaches at the molecular level should lead to a satisfactory explanation of this most intriguing mystery.

PARENTAGE TESTING

The extensive polymorphism of the HLA system makes it a powerful tool in the resolution of litigation resulting from disputed parentage (32). The method is based on the logical genetic premise that cell membrane antigens or any other readily discernible phenotypic markers cannot appear in an offspring unless they are present in either or both of the parents. Applying this premise to the resolution of paternity, it can be concluded that if the putative father lacks an antigen expressed by the child that could not have been inherited from the mother (the obligatory gene), he is excluded from consideration as the biological father of that child. This is referred to as a first-order exclusion and is positive evidence that the accused man is not the father.

If the accused man expresses the obligatory characteristic he cannot be excluded. However, this finding does not offer proof that he is indeed the true father; it merely offers evidence against an exclusion. Nevertheless, based on the findings, a probability of the likelihood of his being the true father can be calculated. It is in this arena that the HLA system demonstrates its great potential.

The calculations used to compute the probability of true paternity are based on the frequency of the obligatory gene or combination of genes in a population of random individuals of the same race as the accused. Since the HLA system is so polymorphic, the frequency of each combination is usually very low. Thus, if an accused does indeed have the obligatory gene or combination of genes, it is a simple probability calculation to show how likely he is to be the biological father.

In practice the HLA system is used in conjunction with a number of red cell blood group systems, incuding ABO, Rh, MNSs, Kell, Duffy, and Kidd. The cumulative probability is computed and used to assess the likelihood of paternity. Using all of these systems results in a greater than 95% exclusion of falsely accused males.

The HLA system has many applications in transplantation, in platelet transfusion, in the study of the immunogenetics of disease and in forensic matters such as parentage testing. Nevertheless, its most important biological function is probably in the orchestration of the immune response through self-recognition. As such it is the only polymorphic alloantigenic system in humans whose function is known.

References

1. Starzl T, Marchioro TL, Holmes JH, et al. Renal homografts in patients with major donor - recipient blood group incompatibilities. Surgery 1964;55:195–200.
2. Cicciarelli J. Living donor kidney transplants. In: Terasaki PI, ed. Clinical transplants 1988. Los Angeles: UCLA Tissue Typing Laboratory, 1989:293–299.
3. Cho YW, Terasaki PI. Long-term survival. In: Terasaki PI, ed. Clinical transplants 1988. Los Angeles: UCLA Tissue Typing Laboratory, 1989:277–282.
4. Busson M, Raffoux C, Bouteiller AM, et al. Influence of HLA-A, B and DR matching on the outcome of kidney transplant survival in preimmunized patients. Transplantation 1984;38: 227–230.
5. Mickey R, Cho Y, Carnahan E. Long term graft survival. In: Terasaki PI, ed. Clinical transplants 1990. Los Angeles: UCLA Tissue Typing Laboratory, 1991:385–395.
6. Cook D. HLA-A, B, DR. Mismatches 1981–85. In: Terasaki PI ed. Visuals of the clinical histocompatibility workshop—Palm Springs Invitational 1988. Los Angeles: One Lambda, Inc., 1988:14.
7. Cicciarelli J, Corcoran S. An update on HLA matching, including HLA "epitope" matching: a new approach. In: Terasaki PI, ed. Clinical transplants 1988. Los Angeles: UCLA Tissue Typing Laboratory, 1989:329–337.
8. Konoeda Y, Terasaki PI, Wakisaka A, Park MS, Mickey MR. Public determinants of HLA indicated by pregnancy antibodies. Transplantation 1986;41:253–259.
9. Park MS, Barbett AA, Geer LI, Clark BD, Terasaki P, Aoki J. HLA epitopes detected by serology. In: Terasaki PI, ed. Clinical Transplants 1990. Los Angeles: UCLA Tissue Typing Laboratory, 1991:515–531.
10. Takemoto S, Terasaki P. HLA peptide matching. In: Terasaki PI, ed. Clinical transplants 1990. Los Angeles: UCLA Tissue Typing Laboratory, 1991:497–513.
11. Yacoub M, Festenstein H, Doyle P, et al. The influence of HLA matching in cardiac allograft recipients receiving cyclosporine and azathioprine. Transplant Proc 1987;19:2487–2489.
12. Opelz G. Effect of HLA matching in heart transplantation. Transplant Proc 1989;21:794–796.
13. Markus BM, Duquesnoy RJ, Gordon RD, et al. Histocompatibility and live transplant outcome: does HLA exert a dualistic effect? Transplantation 1988;46:372–377.
14. Halloran PF, Wadgymar A, Autenreid P. The regulation of expression of major histocompatibility complex products. Transplantation 1986;41:413–420.
15. Sanfilippo F, Vaughn WK, Spees EK, Bollinger PR. Cadaver renal transplantation ignoring peak-reactive sera in patients with markedly decreased pretransplant sensitization. Transplantation 1984;38:119–124.
16. Okuno T, Kondelis N. Evaluation of dithiothreitol (DTT) for inactivation of IgM antibodies. J Clin Pathol 1978;31:1152–1155.
17. Tan EM. Drug induced autoimmune disease. Fed Proc 1974;33:1984–1987.
18. Elandt-Johnson RC. Test for association and the sample correlation coefficient for a 2×2 contingency table. In: Probability model and statistical methods in genetics. New York: John Wiley & Sons, 1971:362–365.
19. Goeken NE. Outcome of renal transplantation following a positive crossmatch with historic sera: the second analysis of the ASHI survey. Transplant Proc 1985;17:2443–2450.
20. Noreen HJ. Crossmatch tests. In: Zachary AA, Teresi GA, eds. ASHI laboratory manual. 2nd ed. Lenexa, KS: American Society for Histocompatibility and Immunogenetics, 1990:307–320.
21. Thistlewaite JR, Buckingham MM, Stuart JK, et al. T cell immunofluorescence flow cytometry crossmatch results in cadaver donor renal transplantation. Transplant Proc 1987;19: 722–724.
22. Beatty PG, Cleft RA, Mickelson EM, et al. Marrow transplantation from related donors other than HLA-identical siblings. N Engl J Med 1985;313:765–771.
23. Yankee RA, Grumet FC, Rogentine GN. Platelet transfusion therapy. The selection of compatible platelet donors for refractory patients by lymphoyte HLA typing. N Engl J Med 1969;281:1208–1212.
24. Dahlke MB, Weiss KL. Platelet transfusion from donors mismatched for crossreactive HLA antigens. Transfusion 1984;24: 299–302.
25. Zmijewski CM. HLA and disease. CRC Crit Rev Clin Lab Sci 1984;20:285–370.
26. Woolf B. On estimating the relation between blood group and disease. Ann Hum Genet 1955;19:251–253.
27. Haldane JBS. The estimation and significance of the logarithm of a ratio of frequencies. Ann Hum Genet 1956:20:309–311.
28. Nepom GT, Seyfried C, Holbeck S, et al. HLA-DR4-associated disease: oligonucleotide probes identify specific class II susceptibility genes in type I diabetes and rheumatoid arthritis. In: Dupont B, ed. Immunobiology of HLA. New York: Springer-Verlag, 1990;II:404–406.
29. Monos DS, Mickelson E, Hansen JA, Baker L, Zmijewski CM, Kamoun M. Analysis of DR and DQ gene products of the DR4 haplotype in patients with IDDM: possible involvement of more than one locus. Hum Immunol 1988;23:289–299.
30. Todd JA, Bell JI, McDevitt HO. HLA DQβ gene contributes to susceptibility and resistance to insulin dependent diabetes mellitus. Nature 1987;329:599–604.
31. Morel PA, Dorman JS, Todd JA, McDevitt H, Trucco M. Aspartic acid at position 57 of the HLA DQB chain protects against type 1 diabetes: a final study. Proc Natl Acad Sci USA 1988;85:8111–8115.
32. Bias WB, Zachary AA. Genetic and statistical principles of paternity determination. In: Rose NR, DeMarcario EC, Rosner G, Fahey JL. Friedman H, Penn GH, eds. Manual of clinical laboratory immunology. 4th ed. Washington, DC: American Society for Microbiology, 1986:901–912.

Section VII

Section Chief: *Curtis A. Hanson*

The field of hematology remains as exciting as ever. As a discipline of clinical pathology, hematopathology requires expertise in a variety of areas, including instrumentation, clinical laboratory analysis, and traditional microscopic skills. These skills actually place hematopathology in the unique position of bridging the clinical laboratory sciences and anatomical pathology. Although the basic foundation of hematopathology remains unchanged, the technological advances that have characterized the field of medicine over the past decade have certainly not spared the discipline of hematopathology. Indeed, the hematopathologist is now challenged with mastering both the traditional skills of laboratory medicine and morphology, as well as newer diagnostic modalities and instrumentation. Hematopathology thus continues to be at the forefront of adapting advances in basic science research to clinical application.

The key to the future of hematopathology will be how to incorporate these newer diagnostic modalities into routine laboratory practice and balance them with traditional morphologic skills and instrumentation analysis. The reality of the current medicoeconomic environment also mandates that, now more than ever before, the laboratory must weigh the ability to provide increasingly sophisticated laboratory findings with the reality of containing the escalating cost of medical care. The major advances on the hematopathology horizon include (*a*) increasingly automated hematology instruments with more robotic function; (*b*) the evolution of laboratory information systems that contribute to laboratory and clinical decision making, such as determining the appropriate utilization for CBC/differential testing; and (*c*) simplification and automation of newer immunologic and molecular assays. Laboratorians will have to maintain their flexibility while developing, evaluating, and implementing these new advances.

HEMATOLOGY

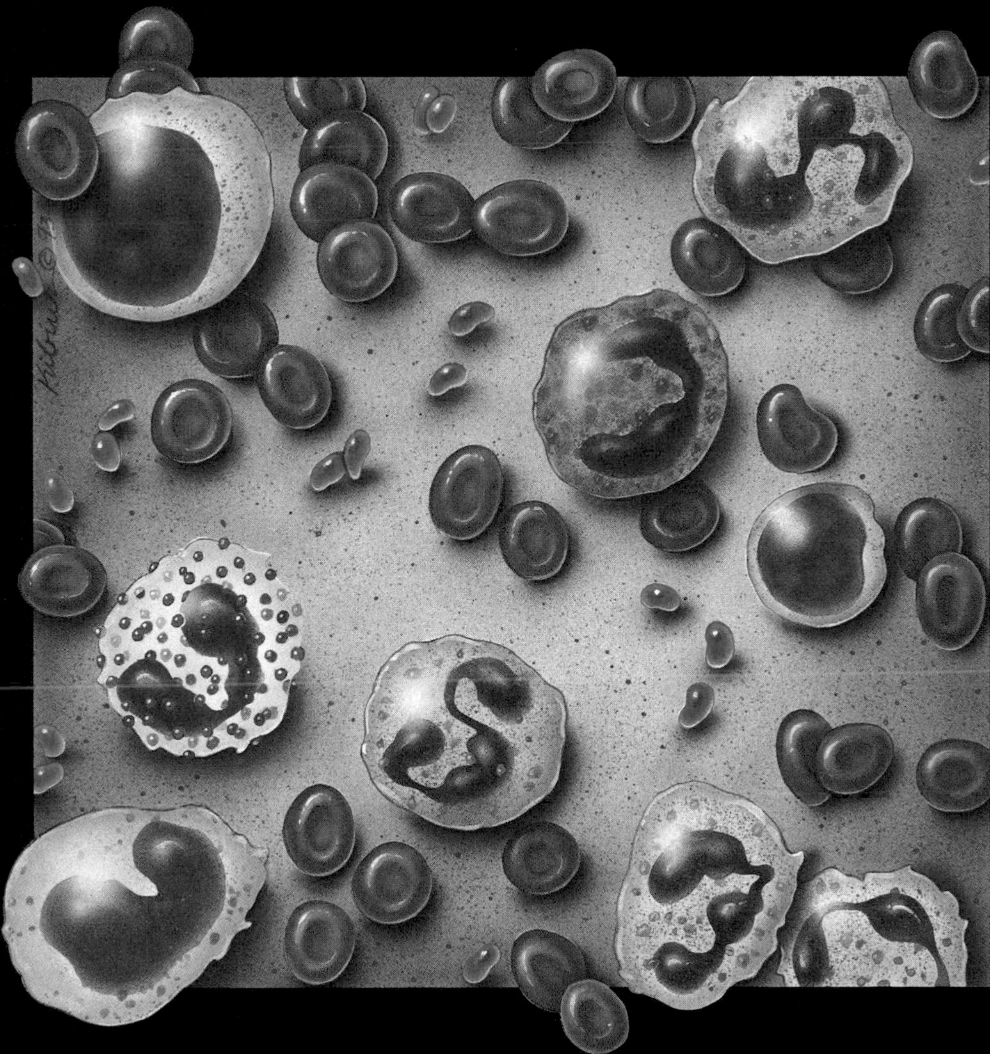

33 Hematopoiesis and the Hematopoietic Growth Factors

Stephen G. Emerson and John P. Farnen

INTRODUCTION

All of the cells observed in the adult peripheral blood derive from the bone marrow, arising through an extraordinary process termed hematopoiesis. This process results in the maintenance of the wide variety of distinct blood cells, despite the fact that each blood cell variety has its own distinct lifespan in the circulation. Our current understanding of this process is embodied in a theory called the stem cell model of hematopoiesis. This model forms the foundation for truly all of our present thinking about normal hematopoiesis, pathologic hematologic disease states, and hematologic therapies.

Stem Cell Theory

Unlike other tissues of mesodermal origin, which as a rule have little turnover in their constituent cell populations, the cellular components of the blood are constantly undergoing cell death and replacement by new cells. While red blood cells last approximately 4 months in the circulation, platelets last only about 1 week and granulocytes less than 10 hours. It is estimated that every day 1×10^{11} blood cells are lost to wear and tear and are replaced with an equal number of new blood cells. To fulfill the continual need for replacement blood cells, hematopoiesis occurs actively throughout our lifetimes. As a result, the blood-forming tissues are among the most mitotically active, along with the gastrointestinal epithelium and epidermis. The recognition of this high turnover rate for blood cells has led to the development of the stem cell theory of blood cell development and maintenance, or hematopoiesis (1). This chapter discusses this theory in detail, as well as its implications for clinical practice.

Hematopoietic Growth Factors

One of the most exciting advances in the study of hematopoiesis in the last decade has been the study of the role of hematopoietic hormones in the control of the process of blood cell differentiation. These hematopoietic hormones, also known as hematopoietic growth factors, appear to control every step in the process of the development of new blood cells. At the present time, we know principally a group of such hematopoietic growth factors that are stimulatory to hematopoietic stem cells and their progeny. However, some inhibitory factors have been discovered and appear to play an equally important role in the negative control of this process. Other hormones that are felt to have primarily nonhematopoietic functions are also known to affect the process of the production of new blood cells. This chapter concisely describes the role of both stimulatory and inhibitory hematopoietic growth factors.

Hematopoietic Microenvironment

The term hematopoietic microenvironment refers to the "stromal" elements of the organs in which hematopoiesis occurs, that is, the cellular and noncellular elements that do not directly give rise to the blood cells but rather provide a solid three-dimensional structural matrix in which the hematopoietic stem cells and their progeny proliferate and differentiate until they migrate into the blood stream. The role of the hematopoietic microenvironment in the control of the development of blood cells is believed to be of paramount importance in the process of hematopoiesis. Both the stromal cells and their secreted matrix proteins appear to influence the process of hematopoiesis as profoundly as the soluble, secreted hematopoietic growth factors, and a summary of current understanding of the contribution of the hematopoietic microenvironment is included in this chapter.

HISTORICAL CONSIDERATIONS

Early Studies

The scientific study of hematopoiesis is a recent phenomenon. Although the cellular nature of blood was discerned by van Leeuwenhoek and reported in 1674, it was not until the middle of the 19th century that interest was aroused in the origin of the cellular components of blood. The earliest observations on hematopoiesis were the studies of Weber and Kolliker, who determined in 1846 that, in the fetus, the liver is the principal site of hematopoiesis. In 1868, two scientists working independently, Ernst Neumann and Giulio Bizzozero, discovered that in the adult, erythropoiesis, the process of the differentiation of red blood cells, occurs within the bone marrow, with subsequent release of newly formed erythrocytes into the bloodstream. Bizzozero also recognized that white cells were formed in the bone marrow, and he coined the term 'platelet' for thrombocytes. The origin of the blood platelets from megakaryocytes in the bone marrow was not uncovered until 1906, however, when James Homer Wright, the inventor of the stain used most frequently for blood and hematopoietic tissues, noted the shedding of platelets from the cytoplasm of megakaryocytes.

The identification of the bone marrow as the principal hematopoietic organ in the adult was followed, at the close of the 19th century and the first half of the 20th century, by a proliferation of various theories of the cellular origin of blood cells. While it was universally understood during that time that the various blood cells must derive from some sort of ancestral cell or cells, the nature of the precursor cell(s) remained highly controversial.

Two basic theories were advanced, each with highly opinionated proponents, and each with a myriad of variations. The first theory, the monophyletic theory, postulated that all different forms of blood cells were derived from a common ancestral cell, the *totipotent* hematopoietic stem cell. The term totipotent indicated its capability of differentiating into any and all of the various forms of blood cells. The monophyletic theory was first proposed by Artur Pappenheim at the turn of the century (2) and was supported vigorously by some of the most prominent medical scientists of this century, including the Russian anatomists/embryologists Vera Dantschakoff and Alexander Maximow, Maximow's pupil William Bloom, and Hal Downey, a hematologist and the editor of an important work called the *Handbook of Hematology*.

In opposition to the monophyleticists, a second group arose, the polyphyleticists, who posited the existence of independent lines of hematopoietic cell development for various types of blood cells. For example, Paul Ehrlich, the first to apply histologic staining techniques to the study of blood tissues, proposed the 'dualist' theory, viz., that granulocytes derived from a primitive "myelocyte," whereas the lymphocytes had a completely separate origin (3). Others who were considered polyphyleticists included the Swiss hematologist Otto Naegeli, Robert Schilling of the University of Wisconsin, and Florence Sabin. Each described various modifications of the polyphyletic theory, all of which, however, basically revolved around the notion that the different morphologically recognizable lineages of blood cells derived from different populations of precursor cells that did not have the capability of giving rise to several different types of blood cells.

Experimental evidence to settle this vexing issue did not come until the middle of the 20th century, when evidence of the multilineage capability of hematopoietic stem cells was convincingly demonstrated in transplantation experiments in lethally irradiated mice (4, 5). The monophyletic viewpoint has now largely been vindicated, and at the present, most experts in hematopoiesis agree on the existence of a totipotent hematopoietic stem cell that has the capability, as a single cell, of giving rise to cells of all the different lineages of blood cells, including lymphoid, myeloid (granulocytes and monocytes/macrophages), erythroid (red blood cells), and megakaryocytic lineages (6).

HEMATOPOIESIS IN THE EMBRYO AND FETUS

Role of the Yolk Sac

The fertilized egg first develops the beginnings of blood tissue while still in the embryonic stage (7). The first step toward the development of blood tissue is thought to occur in the yolk sac, where undifferentiated cells called mesoblasts are found and are believed to migrate there from the primitive streak of the embryo. The mesoblasts are highly mitotically active, and will subsequently differentiate into cells that are clearly related to the mature blood cells of the adult, called "primitive erythroblasts," as well as into cells called primitive endothelial cells, which give rise to vascular channels in the yolk sac. Within hours after migration, the yolk sac mesoblasts have generated, by a process of cell division and differentiation, primitive erythrocytes, primarily nucleated but including a minority that are nonnucleated, all of which acquire hemoglobin and thus lend a reddish color to the clumps of yolk sac cells where blood cell formation is occurring. The clumps of hemoglobinized cells are visible to the naked eye, hence the name "blood islands" to describe these localized areas of embryonic hematopoiesis in the yolk sac. Megakaryocytes are also found in the blood islands and are presumably derived from the mesoblasts. Other mesoblasts appear to differentiate into a type of cell called the "hemocytoblast."

A second stage of hematopoiesis in the yolk sac occurs in the embryos of some mammals. In human embryos, this second stage is present but is not as vigorous as in rabbits, the mammal in which the embryogenesis of blood cells has been most extensively studied. In the second stage of yolk sac hematopoiesis, hemocytoblasts differentiate into "definitive" erythroblasts, which subsequently acquire hemoglobin and are called "definitive" or "secondary" normoblasts. These may lose their nuclei by a process of extrusion and become "definitive" erythrocytes. Vascular channels form in the blood islands, and eventually connect to form a network of blood vessels. This network of primitive blood vessels early on contains the primitive erythroblasts and hemocytoblasts, and later definitive erythroblasts and erythrocytes. By the end of the third week of embryonic development in the rabbit, all the hematopoietic activity of the blood islands has subsided and the process of hematopoiesis has gradually shifted to the liver.

The Embryonic Body Mesenchyme

A minor role in early embryonic hematopoiesis is played by primitive mesenchymal cells in the body cavity itself, particularly in the head mesenchyme. Small numbers of mesenchymal cells of the body cavity develop into erythroblasts, megakaryocytes, granulocytes, and phagocytic cells analogous to their counterparts in the adult. Quantitatively, the number of cells produced is small, and large accretions of blood cells similar to the blood islands of the yolk sac do not form in the body cavity mesenchyme. The small clusters of blood cells that do form quickly degenerate and no further blood formation occurs here to any significant degree after the third week. However, the formation of blood cells in the mesenchyme is illustrative of the fact that mesenchymal cells have potential for differentiation into hematopoietic cells, and this potential may in theory reside with mesenchymally derived cells throughout life.

Emergence of the Liver As the Principal Site of Hematopoiesis in the Embryo

Beginning at around the 12-mm stage of the human embryo, blood formation is seen to occur in the embryonic liver. The liver soon becomes the dominant site of hematopoiesis and remains active in hematopoiesis until birth. As the endodermal cords of the liver primordium grow into the septum transversum, they encounter wandering mesenchymal cells with the appearance of lymphocytes. These lymphocytoid wandering cells are subsequently trapped between the primordial liver endodermal cords and the endothelial cells of ingrowing capillaries. They give rise to hemocytoblasts similar to those of the yolk sac. These hemocytoblasts soon form foci of hematopoiesis similar to the blood islands of the yolk sac, wherein secondary erythroblasts are formed in large numbers, which subsequently divide and differentiate into definitive erythrocytes through the progressive acquisition of hemoglobin and loss of the cell nucleus. Although definitive erythrocytes may be seen in the liver at the 12-mm stage, they do not emerge into the circulation in any great numbers until much later. Thus, by the 70-mm stage, the majority of circulating erythrocytes in the embryo are secondary (definitive) erythrocytes.

Megakaryocytes also appear to form from the hemocytoblasts in the embryonic and fetal liver. Granulocytic cells are found in the embryonic liver, but they appear to develop not from the hemocytoblasts but perhaps directly from the lymphocytoid wandering cells themselves. The embryonic liver is not long the dominant site of hematopoiesis, being replaced in importance by the embryonic bone marrow beginning around the 25- to 30-mm stage in the human.

The Embryonic Bone Marrow and Myelopoiesis

Bone formation in the embryo occurs at varying times for different bones. The earliest bones to form are the long bones of the appendicular skeleton. Initially, a cartilaginous model of each bone is formed. The central core of the diaphysis of each long bone subsequently becomes ossified, and soon an area of bone resorption develops followed by the ingrowth of mesenchymal cells from the periosteum. These mesenchymal cells are accompanied by the ingrowth of capillaries. The mesenchymal cells continue to increase in number by continued influx of other mesenchymal cells as well as by division of those already within the newly forming marrow cavity. They also elaborate a noncellular ground substance, or "stroma," which fills the developing marrow cavity. Cells identical to the hemocytoblasts of the liver and yolk sac develop from these early marrow mesenchymal cells. As in the yolk sac and liver, these give rise to megakaryocytes and erythroid cells. However, there is a second population of cells, called the "lymphoid wandering cells," which appear nearly identical to lymphocytes. These cells predominate in the population of cells in the very early marrow cavity, and are thought to give rise to myeloid cells, including neutrophils, basophils, and eosinophils. The embryonic marrow differs markedly from the earlier centers of hematopoiesis in that the generation of these myeloid cells is especially vigorous and dominates the embryonic marrow hematopoietic activity. The process of formation of the early myeloid cells, or "myelopoiesis," occurs first in the central portion of the marrow cavity and spreads outward from there to eventually include the entire marrow cavity. Erythropoiesis occurs slightly later in the embryonic marrow and is generally admixed with the process of myelopoiesis. Small foci of erythropoiesis can thus be seen among the many maturing cells of myeloid lineage. After birth, hematopoiesis ceases in the liver, and the bone marrow continues to be the principal site of hematopoiesis for the remainder of life.

Hematopoiesis in the Spleen of the Embryo and Fetus

The last major site of hematopoiesis to form in embryonic life is the spleen. Although the spleen itself forms much earlier, wandering mesenchymal cells do not begin to invade the spleen until around the 70-mm stage in humans. These then differentiate into typical hemocytoblasts, which give rise to cells of primarily erythroid lineage. The spleen is thus a center of erythropoiesis until the time of birth, when erythropoiesis gradually ceases. Although some myelopoiesis occurs in the embryonic and fetal spleen, it is relatively insignificant in comparison. Much later, during the fifth month of gestation, the white pulp of the spleen forms by the differentiation of mesenchymal cells that have grouped around the splenic arterioles. The formation of the splenic lymphocytes appears to occur as a process completely separate from the origin of erythropoiesis in this organ.

Other Sites of Hematopoiesis in the Embryo and Fetus

The embryonic thymus develops as an outgrowth of the third branchial pouch. The thymic epithelium is invaded by wandering mesenchymal cells, which begin multiplying rapidly and differentiating into lymphocytes. During this process, small numbers of erythroid and myeloid cells are formed in the thymus, but the primary process is that of lymphopoiesis. The lymphocytes formed in this organ will constitute a distinct class of lymphocytes with a special function: that of cell-mediated immunity.

The lymph nodes develop as outpouchings from the primitive lymphatic vessels, which become surrounded by accretions of mesenchymal cells. Subsequently, these seem to round up and become similar in appearance to the lymphocytes of the adult. A few of the mesenchymal cells give rise to cells of other lineages, such as erythrocytes, granulocytes, and megakaryocytes, but this is a transitory phenomenon, and, as in the thymus, the principal process is that of lymphopoiesis.

Summary of Embryonic and Fetal Hematopoiesis

In all the hematopoietic organs of the embryo and fetus, a similar process takes place. Wandering mesenchymal cells are attracted to a particular site, by processes still not clearly understood, and become transformed into cells recognizable as hematopoietic precursors. These embryonic hematopoietic precursors appear to be capable of multilineage differentiation, but at any one site the process of hematopoiesis may be dominated by the formation of a particular lineage, presumably under the influence of the local environment. The various sites of embryonic hematopoiesis seem to be active only at specific times during development and follow a pattern of programmed involution, except for the bone marrow, which continues as the principal location of hematopoiesis in the adult, and the lymph nodes, spleen, thymus, and other lymphatic tissues, which continue to be active in lymphopoiesis.

HEMATOPOIESIS IN THE ADULT

After birth, the major site of hematopoietic activity shifts gradually from the liver and spleen to the bone marrow cavities of nearly all bones of the axial and appendicular skeleton. The marrow acquires a reddish color like that of blood once hematopoietic activity begins, reflecting the vigorous production of erythrocytes that contain hemoglobin. The bone marrow cavity serves primarily as a site for the production of nonlymphoid blood cells, whereas lymphopoiesis in the adult occurs primarily in the spleen, lymph nodes, thymus, and the gut-associated lymphoid tissue, including the tonsils, adenoids, and Peyer's patches. Thus, when examined with the light microscope, the adult marrow will be seen to be composed primarily of erythroid and myeloid precursor cells, together with scattered megakaryocytes and a population of cells known as "stromal cells," which are crucial for the maturation of the precursor cells and release of the fully differentiated cell types into the circulation.

As each individual ages, the marrow of bones of the appendicular skeleton gradually loses its red appearance and is transformed into yellow marrow, a reflection of the progressive replacement of hematopoietic tissue by adipose tissue. Thus, by early adulthood, the long bones no longer bear red marrow but are completely replaced by nonhematopoietic yellow marrow, and the primary sites of red marrow are confined to the sternum, ribs, vertebrae, and pelvis. Although the stimulus for this progressive transformation of red to yellow marrow is unknown, in pathologic conditions associated with vigorous hematopoietic activity, the transformation may fail to take place and the red marrow may actually expand into bones not normally associated with hematopoietic activity, such as the diploic cavities of the cranial bones. The liver, spleen, and lymph nodes may also be locations of "extramedullary hematopoiesis" in such situations. An extreme example occurs in individuals with thalassemia major, a disease in which erythropoiesis is unusually brisk throughout life, resulting in a characteristic expansion of the marrow spaces of all the cranial bones and long bones and enlargement of the liver and spleen. This is so pronounced that the diploe of the calvarium has a characteristic "hair-on-end" appearance in x-rays of the skull due to expansion of the marrow space, and maxillary hyperplasia results in a characteristic facies with prominent cheekbones and malocclusion of the teeth because the maxilla is disproportionately larger than the mandible.

THE STEM CELL MODEL OF HEMATOPOIESIS

The cell that gives rise to all other types of blood cells, the stem cell, is so rare that it has never been clearly morphologically identified. Rather, the existence of stem cells is inferred by functional assays that demonstrate the ability of single cells to generate multiple hematopoietic lineages. Thus, stem cells are currently defined not by their appearance but by their function (8). Stem cells are known to be extremely rare cells, although quantifying them is somewhat imprecise due to different degrees of rigor applied to the definition of what constitutes a stem cell. The most generous estimate is that stem cells occur in human bone marrow with a frequency of 1 per 1,000,000 nucleated bone marrow cells, while more conservative estimates place this figure at 1 per 10,000,000.

The tremendous production rate of hematopoietic cells requires that the bone marrow produce as many cells as it contains roughly every other day. To maintain this rate throughout life, the bone marrow must contain cells that have the ability to generate vast numbers of mature cells continuously, that is, without losing the ability to do so. This *self-renewal* ability is critical to the concept of the stem cell. At present there are two theories as to how this might occur. According to the first theory, every stem cell division is asymmetric, producing one undifferentiated stem cell and one more differentiated cell that is committed to producing mature blood cells (9). In the second theory, each stem cell division produces either two additional stem cells or two more mature cells. The stem cell pool is thus maintained not by precise asymmetric divisions within each stem cell, but rather by a balance between the number of stem cell divisions yielding more stem cells and divisions yielding more mature cells.

At the point the stem cell leaves the self-renewing pool to populate the differentiating pool, it is still an unrecognizable blast cell with the capacity to produce cells of all lineages. With each subsequent division, the daughter *progenitor cells* become more and more restricted in their commitment to the production of specific blood cell lineages. That is, if one isolates progenitor cells and permits them to propagate and differentiate, they will generate collections of cells that are of only one or a few lineages. The more differentiated the progenitor cell, the fewer lineages are produced and the smaller the number of cells produced (10). These concepts, which have been supported by several decades of in vivo and in vitro experiments, have now defined the hierarchical stem cell model of hematopoiesis (Fig. 33.1).

The Hematopoietic Microenvironment

If maintained in a simply nutritive environment, stem cells will die without differentiating or dividing. To support the process of hematopoietic self-renewal and differentiation, stem cells and their progeny must be maintained in the close proximity of nonhematopoietic mesenchymal cells, called *stromal cells*. These cells, which are composed of a heterogeneous group of fibroblasts, endothelial cells, and adipocytes, line the endosteal surfaces in the bone marrow cavity. These cells appear to supply two closely related requirements for the hematopoietic cells, soluble hematopoietic growth factors and membrane-bound attachment molecules (11).

The *hematopoietic growth factors (HGF), or colony-stimulating factors (CSFs)* are a class of glycoprotein hormones that obligately regulate the division and differentiation of hematopoietic cells. These hormones are required for survival, proliferation, differentiation, and function of all the hematopoietic cells. Although initially discovered as spontaneously secreted products of T cell tumors, it is clear that these hormones are normally the products of bone marrow stromal cells as well as T lymphocytes and monocytes.

CSFs are produced in a two-tiered process. First, small amounts of certain CSFs—interleukin 6 (IL-6), granulocyte-macrophage colony-stimulating factor (GM-CSF), and stem cell factor (SCF)—are produced constitutively by bone marrow stomal cells, probably in response to stimulation by plasma proteins. The production of these CSFs is responsible for basal hematopoiesis, maintaining blood counts in the normal ranges (12).

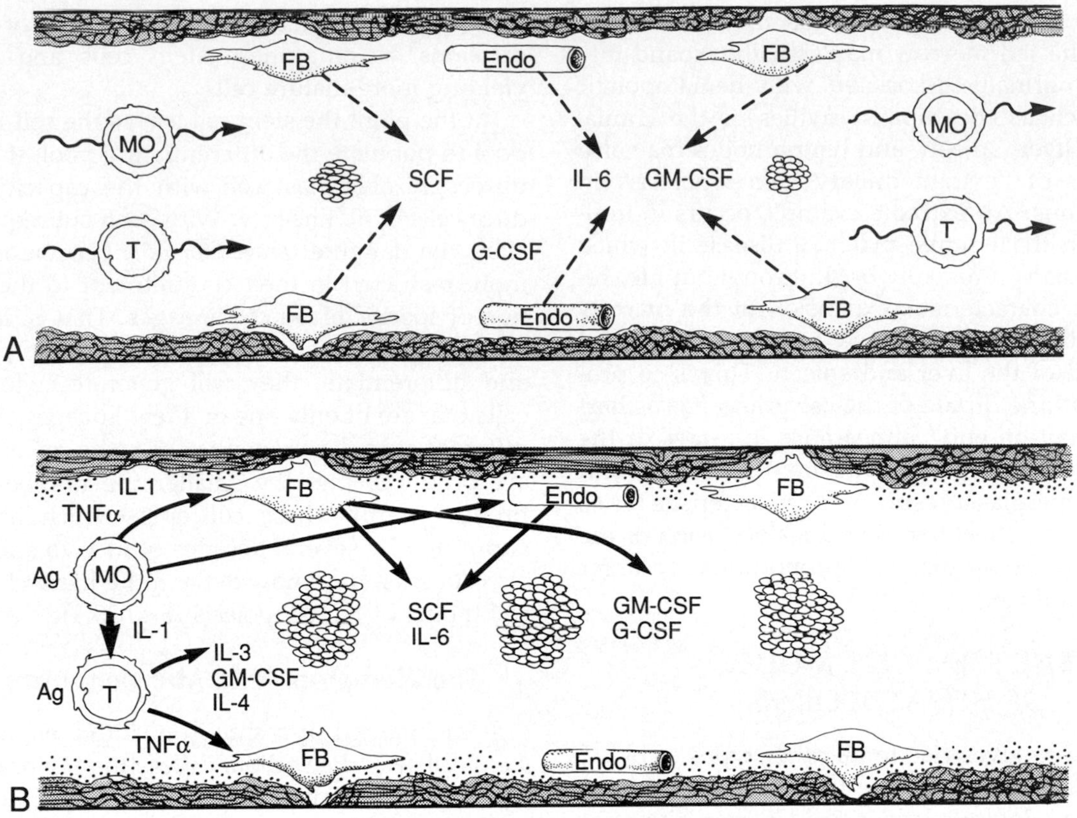

Figure 33.1. **A**, Basal hematopoiesis. **B**, Antigen-amplified hematopoiesis.

CSF secretion is greatly increased above the basal levels in response to infection. Bacterial and viral products activate monocytes, which then secrete interleukin 1 (IL-1), tumor necrosis factor α (TNFα), and granulocyte colony stimulating factor (G-CSF, as well as their own macrophage colony stimulating factor (M-CSF). These products in turn stimulate additional CSF secretion. IL-1, together with antigenic stimulation of specific receptors, activates T cells to secrete GM-CSF and interleukin 3 (IL-3) (13). IL-1 and TNFα each stimulates fibroblasts and endothelial cells in the bone marrow stromal microenvironment to increase their secretion of IL-6 and GM-CSF, and also to secrete large quantities of G-CSF (Fig. 33.2) (14). These cytokines thereby directly increase the numbers of circulating neutrophils, monocytes, and plasma cells as well as activating these same mature cells. The generation of each specific lineage of mature blood cells is in this manner regulated by a specific set of hematopoietic growth factors. Although the sets of hematopoietic growth factors that induce specific mature blood cell subsets overlap, each is characteristically distinct.

Erythropoiesis

The final stages of erythroid differentiation are regulated largely by *erythropoietin*, a glycoprotein produced in response to tissue hypoxia in the fetal liver and adult kidney. Of the 18 or so cell divisions that take place during the time that a stem cell generates a mature red blood cell, the final 8 to 10 divisions are strongly induced by erythropoietin. The transcription of the erythropoietin gene in renal peritubular endothelial cells and hepatoblasts is regulated by oxygen-sensitive transcription factors that upregulate gene expression with declining O_2 delivery. Overproduction of erythropoietin, observed in some cases of renal cell carcinoma and hepatoma, leads directly to erythroid polycythemia.

The preceding cell divisions, which give rise to erythropoietin-sensitive erythroid progenitor cells, are largely erythropoietin-independent. These proliferation and maturation events are instead induced by *granulocyte-macrophage colony-stimulating factor (GM-CSF)* and *stem cell factor (SCF)*, both of which are produced locally within the marrow microenvironment by bone marrow stromal cells. In addition, these steps can be specifically amplified by the secretion of *interleukin 3 (IL-3)* by activated T lymphocytes (15).

Granulopoiesis

Much like erythroid differentiation, the final stages in neutropoiesis and monopoiesis are induced

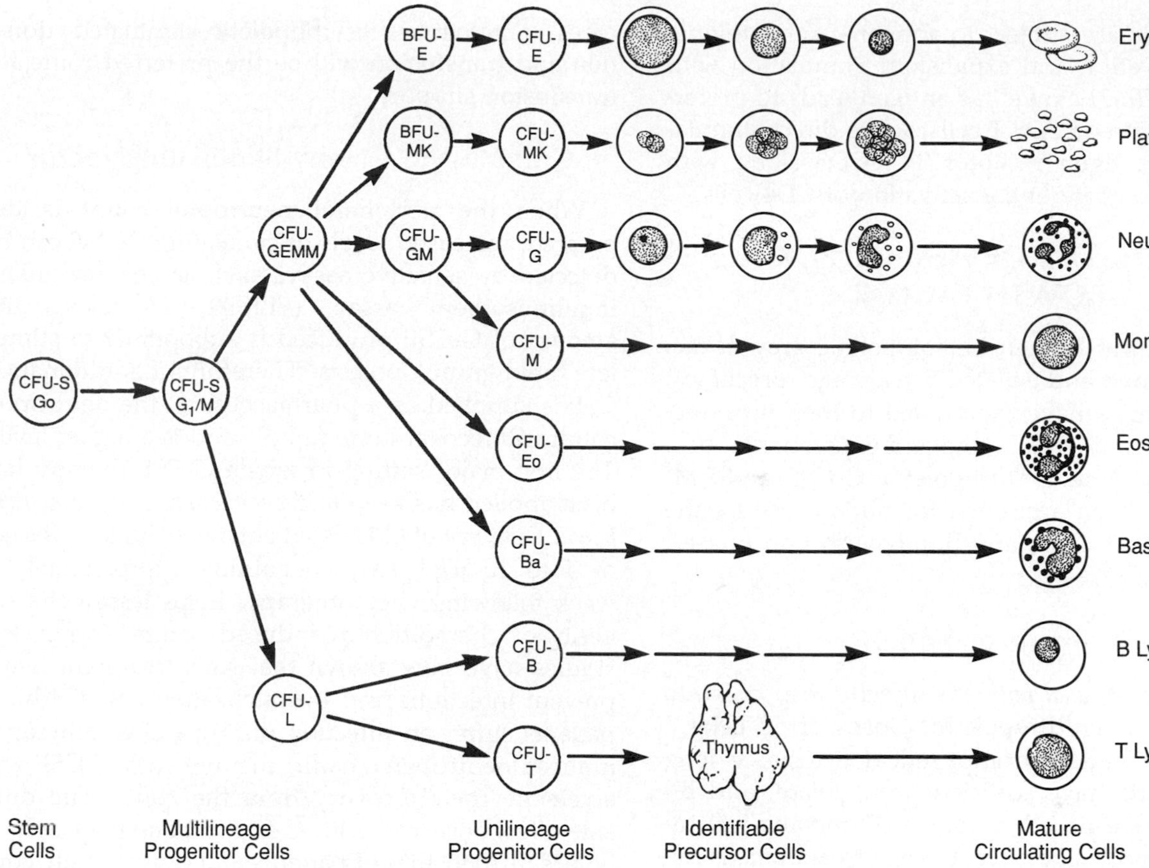

Figure 33.2.

by *granulocyte colony-stimulating factor (G-CSF)* and *macrophage colony-stimulating factor (M-CSF)*, respectively. The early divisions, which direct multipotential progenitors to become committed to individual lineages, are regulated by the synergistic interactions of GM-CSF, SCF, and IL-3. As described above, while there is a constant level of basal secretion of CSF by the bone marrow stromal fibroblasts that line the marrow endosteal surfaces, the secretion of GM-CSF and G-CSF is dramatically upregulated in the presence of inflammation in response to the secretion of IL-1 and TNFα by monocytes.

For the production of eosinophils, *interleukin 5 (IL-5)* and, to a lesser extent IL-3 and GM-CSF, play major inductive roles. Basophils and mast cells are directly stimulated by SCF and IL-3. In both of these instances, the initial afferent signals that trigger the release of these cytokines is not yet well understood.

Megakaryopoiesis

The earliest stages in the development of megakaryocytic progenitor cells also appear to be induced by IL-3 and GM-CSF, in conjunction with SCF. What induces the later stages of megakaryopoiesis is not yet certain, but recent evidence suggests that *interleukin 6 (IL-6)* plays an important role (16). IL-6 may even play a role in the terminal budding events that lead to increased platelet counts, but it would appear that the major cytokines that play this thrombopoietic role have yet to be isolated.

B Lymphopoiesis

As with the myeloid lineages, the development of B cells begins by the differentiation of pluripotent stem cells into undifferentiated but committed B cell progenitors. The initial stages in the proliferation and differentiation of these B cell progenitors are induced by *interleukin 7 (IL-7)* and SCF. Once recognizable pre-B cells and B cells are generated, further differentiation and divisions are induced by stimulation through the immunoglobulin antigen receptor, through the $F_c g$ receptor, and through stimulation by soluble *interleukin 4 (IL-4)* and interleukin 6. Once antibody-producing plasma cells are generated, additional proliferation as well as antibody secretion is stimulated by IL-6 and GM-CSF.

T Lymphopoiesis

Once pre-T cells undergo the complex processes of negative and positive selection in the thymus that generate self/nonself discrimination, the resulting mature T cells are subject to antigen- and cytokine-induced activation and expansion. Stimulation with *interleukin 2 (IL-2)* as well as antigen leads to preferential expansion of CD8 T cells, while direct stimulation of the antigen receptor TCR/CD3 along with CD28 leads to preferential activation of CD4 cells.

CLINICAL USE OF HEMATOPOIETIC GROWTH FACTORS

Since the first human hematopoietic growth factors were cloned and isolated 8 years ago, preclinical and clinical trials have rapidly led to their introduction into the clinic for routine and experimental use. At the present time, erythropoietin, G-CSF, and GM-CSF have all been approved for human use by the FDA, while IL-3, SCF, and IL-6 have begun phase I and II trials.

Erythropoietin

The *anemia of renal failure* is directly responsive to treatment with erythropoietin. Doses of 50 U/kg 3 times weekly lead to prompt reticulocytosis, as long as the patients have sufficient iron, folate, and B_{12} stores and have no other source of ongoing inflammation. The only side effect of such treatments is hypertension, if the hemoglobin level rises too high. The introduction of erythropoietin therapy in this manner has made thousands of renal dialysis patients non–transfusion dependent and has greatly improved the quality of their lives (17).

Other anemias, such as in the setting of chronic diseases such as cancer, AIDS, and rheumatologic diseases, can also respond to erythropoietin. However, the doses required are higher (150 U/kg or more 3 times weekly), and even at high doses the responses are variable. In general, the higher the baseline erythropoietin level circulating in the patient's plasma, the less the chance of response to erythropoietin therapy.

A third, growing area of application of erythropoietin therapy is to *autologous donation* of red blood cells prior to elective surgery. By administering erythropoietin under a controlled setting, hematologists can stimulate a mild erythrocytosis, which then allows safe phlebotomy and storage. In this way, it is possible to stimulate and store several units of red blood cells prior to any elective surgery, thus eliminating the need for and risk of allogeneic red cell transfusion. The only limitations on this therapy are the organizational abilities of hematologists and blood banks. Given the large fraction of blood products that go for urgent and emergent surgeries, allogeneic donation and blood transfusion will still be essential. However, for an increasing fraction of cases, autologous, erythopoietin-stimulated donation and transfusion will be the preferred route for transfusion support.

Granulocyte Colony-Stimulating Factor

When the peripheral neutrophil count is depressed, increased levels of circulating G-CSF can be detected by sensitive assays such as enzyme-linked immunosorbent assay (ELISA). However, the amount of G-CSF produced is suboptimal to stimulate rapid granulopoiesis. Therefore, if additional G-CSF is supplied as a pharmaceutical, the neutrophil count will recover more rapidly and to a higher level. The first major setting in which G-CSF therapy has been applied has been in *chemotherapy-induced neutropenia*. Delivery of G-CSF subcutaneously, in a dosage of 4 to 10 μg/kg/day, beginning approximately 1 week following chemotherapy, helps lessen the severity of chemotherapy-induced nadirs. Controlled studies have now shown that such treatment helps prevent infections and hospitalizations. Similarly, if patients suffer an infection during a chemotherapy-induced neutropenic nadir, therapy with G-CSF will accelerate their recovery from the nadir. The only side effect observed with G-CSF is bone pain, which occurs in 10 to 15% of patients and can be easily controlled with analgesics.

Pharmacologic doses of G-CSF are also effective in raising the neutrophil count in several cases of chronic neutropenia, such as congenital neutropenia (Kostmann's disease), idiopathic neutropenia, and immune-mediated neutropenias, such as thyroglobulin lymphoproliferative disease (18). In these cases, however, the doses of G-CSF required can be substantially higher, and the responses are not as uniform.

Granulocyte-Macrophage Colony-Stimulating Factor

Like G-CSF, GM-CSF increases the neutrophil count in vivo. However, it has a substantially broader range of activity and also increases the monocyte count and eosinophil count as well. Increases in reticulocytes and platelets have also been reported, but these are less reliable. Given its broad spectrum of activity, GM-CSF has been approved by the FDA for *acceleration of recovery of hematopoietic function following bone marrow transplantation*. In this setting GM-CSF clearly shortens the time to recovery, resulting in notably decreased morbidity of the transplantation procedure (19).

In addition, GM-CSF almost certainly has the same salutory effect as G-CSF in preventing and treating chemotherapy-induced nadirs. Although it is possible that its spectrum of side effects (chills, fevers, third-spacing of plasma) might make its use in this setting more problematic than G-CSF, at this time there has been no side-by-side comparison of GM-CSF and G-CSF in any setting.

One recent application of GM-CSF and G-CSF that deserves particular notice is that of *progenitor cell mobilization*. In the first trials of GM-CSF, it was found that while the density of bone marrow progenitor cells rose slightly, the density of circulating progenitor cells rose dramatically, often 50- to 100-fold over baseline. Later, very similar data were obtained for G-CSF (and the same is probably true for IL-3 and SCF as well) (20). Based on these data, several bone marrow transplant centers have used decreasing numbers of peripheral blood leukapheresis collections (from a baseline of 8 to 10 down to 2 to 4) to successfully support reengraftment following autologous peripheral blood transplantation. Although there are many questions remaining regarding the cause and the meaning of this effect, as well as the role of progenitor cell mobilization in transplantation, the application of hematopoietic growth factors to "hemotherapy" in transplantation medicine will be an exciting venue in the decade ahead.

References

1. Emerson SG. The stem cell model of hematopoiesis. In: Hoffman R, Benz E, Shattil S, Furie B, Cohen H, eds. Hematology, basic principles and practice. Baltimore: Williams & Wilkins, 1991:72–81.
2. Pappenheim A. Abstammung und Entstehung der roten Blutzelle [Abstract]. Virchows Arch 1898;151:89.
3. Ehrlich P. Uber die specifischen Granulationed des Blutes. Arch Anat Physiol Abt 1879;2:571.
4. Ford CE, Hamerton JL, Barnes DWH, Loutit JF. Cytological identification of radiation chimeras. Nature 1961;177:452.
5. Till JE, McCulloch EA. Direct measurement of the radiation sensitivity of normal mouse bone marrow cells. Radiat Res 1961;14:213.
6. Lemischka IF, Raulet CH, Mulligan RC. Developmental potential and dynamic behavior of hematopoietic stem cells. Cell 1986;45:917.
7. Lipton JM, Nathan DG. The anatomy and physiology of hematopoiesis. In: Nathan DG, Oski FA, eds. Hematology of infancy and childhood. Philadelphia: WB Saunders, 1987:128–158.
8. Metcalf D, Moore MAS. Haematopoietic cells. In: Neugberger A, Tatum EL, eds. Frontiers of biology. Amsterdam: North-Holland, 1971;25.
9. Holzer H, Biehl J, Antin P, et al. Quantal and proliferative cell cycles: how lineages generate cell diversity and maintain fidelity. Prog Clin Biol Res 1983;134:213.
10. Emerson SG, Sieff CA, Wang EA, et al. Purification of fetal hematopoietic progenitors and demonstration of recombinant multipotential colony stimulating activity. J Clin Invest 1985;76:1286.
11. Tsai S, Sieff CA, Nathan DG. Stromal cell associated erythropoiesis. Blood 1986;67:1418.
12. Guba SC, Sartor CI, Gottschalk LR, et al. Bone marrow stromal fibroblasts secrete IL-6 and GM-CSF in the absence of inflammatory stimulation. Blood 1992;80:1190.
13. Guba SC, Stella G, Turka LA, et al. Regulation of IL-3 gene induction in normal human T cells. J Clin Invest 1989;84:1701.
14. Fibbe WE, van Damme J, Billiau A, et al. IL-1 induces human marrow stromal cells in long-term culture to produce G-CSF and GM-CSF. Blood 1988;71:430.
15. Emerson SG, Thomas S, Ferra JL, Greenstein JL. Developmental regulation of erythropoiesis by hematopoietic growth factors: analysis on populations of BFU-E from bone marrow, peripheral blood, and fetal liver. Blood 1989;74:49.
16. Long MW, Hutchinson RJ, Gragowski LL, et al. Synergistic regulation of human megakaryocyte development. J Clin Invest 1988;82:1779.
17. Eschbach JW, Egrie JC, Downing MR, et al. Correction of the anemia of end stage renal disease with recombinant human erythropoietin. N Engl J Med 1987;316:73.
18. Bonilla MA, Gillio AP, Ruggiero M, et al. Effects of recombinant humans G-CSF on neutropenia in patients with congenital agranulocytosis. N Engl J Med 1989;320:1574.
19. Nemunaitis J, Singer JW, Buckner CD, et al. Long-term follow-up of patients who received recombinant human granulocyte–macrophage colony stimulating factor after autologous bone marrow transplantation for lymphoid malignancy. Bone Marrow Transplant 1991;7:49.
20. Kessinger A, Armitage JO. The evolving role of autologous peripheral stem cell transplantation following high-dose therapy for malignancies [editorial]. Blood 1991;77:211.

34 Peripheral Blood and Bone Marrow: Morphology, Counts and Differentials, and Reactive Disorders

Curtis A. Hanson

This chapter covers a variety of topics, all included under the broad category of laboratory hematology. This area is really the substantive, day-to-day component of any routine clinical hematology laboratory. Such a laboratory must have a solid foundation in (*a*) basic morphologic identification of peripheral blood and bone marrow cells; (*b*) the complete blood count (CBC) and its components; (*c*) the differential leukocyte count; (*d*) basic hematology instrumentation and automation, as related to the CBC and differential count; and (*e*) a variety of miscellaneous, hematology-associated assays, such as reticulocyte count and erythrocyte sedimentation rate.

Besides these morphologic and technological considerations, the laboratorian must have an understanding of the clinical disorders, both benign and malignant, associated with abnormalities of the CBC and differential leukocyte count. Conversely, the interpretation of hematologic data by the clinician must be based on an awareness of how the data were generated and how to avoid the production of spurious results. Thus, to gain the greatest clinical benefit from hematologic studies, a mutual understanding of both the laboratory and clinical components is required.

This chapter is divided into three broad areas: (*a*) peripheral blood and bone marrow morphology, as this is the basis for understanding normal hematopoiesis as well as clinical hematologic disease; (*b*) blood cell counting, including the CBC and its components, as well as the differential leukocyte count, reticulocyte count, and the erythrocyte sedimentation rate; and (*c*) nonmalignant disorders of white blood cells, including quantitative increases or decreases in any white blood cell count (WBC) component, benign morphologic disorders, and functional disorders of leukocytes.

PERIPHERAL BLOOD AND BONE MARROW MORPHOLOGY

The morphologic evaluation of the peripheral blood and bone marrow involves the evaluation of all components of each sample. Examination of the peripheral blood must therefore consist of evaluating the erythrocytes (red blood cells), leukocytes (white blood cells), and platelets (thrombocytes). The leukocyte component consists of five basic cell types: neutrophils, lymphocytes, monocytes, eosinophils, and basophils. Neutrophils, eosinophils, and basophils can also be referred to as granulocytes or polymorphonuclear leukocytes. Among neutrophils there are both segmented and band neutrophil types. Each of these different cell components has a particular morphologic appearance, as well as having unique and essential cellular functions.

Peripheral Blood

Neutrophil (Segmented). The segmented neutrophil is an intermediate-sized cell (10 to 15 μm) with three to five nuclear segments. Each of the segments is connected by a thin filament. The nuclear chromatin of the neutrophil is coarsely clumped, with no visible nucleoli. The cytoplasm of the neutrophil contains abundant small, azurophilic (secondary) granules that vary in size (Fig. 34.1).

Neutrophil (Band). The band neutrophil is slightly larger than the segmented neutrophil and has a U-shaped nucleus with coarsely clumped chromatin. Instead of a thin filament separating the lobes, as seen in the segmented neutrophils, a band neutrophil has a much thicker band connecting the nuclear segments. This defining criterion is somewhat vague and has led to significant variability and a lack of reproducibility between technologists in determining band counts (see the subsection on neutrophilia in this chapter). Cytoplasmic granulation is identical to that found in the segmented neutrophil.

Lymphocyte. The lymphocyte is a round or oval-shaped cell that varies from small (7 to 10 μm) to intermediate (10 to 20 μm) in size. The nucleus is usually round to slightly indented or folded, having smooth, mature chromatin; parachromatin is not typ-

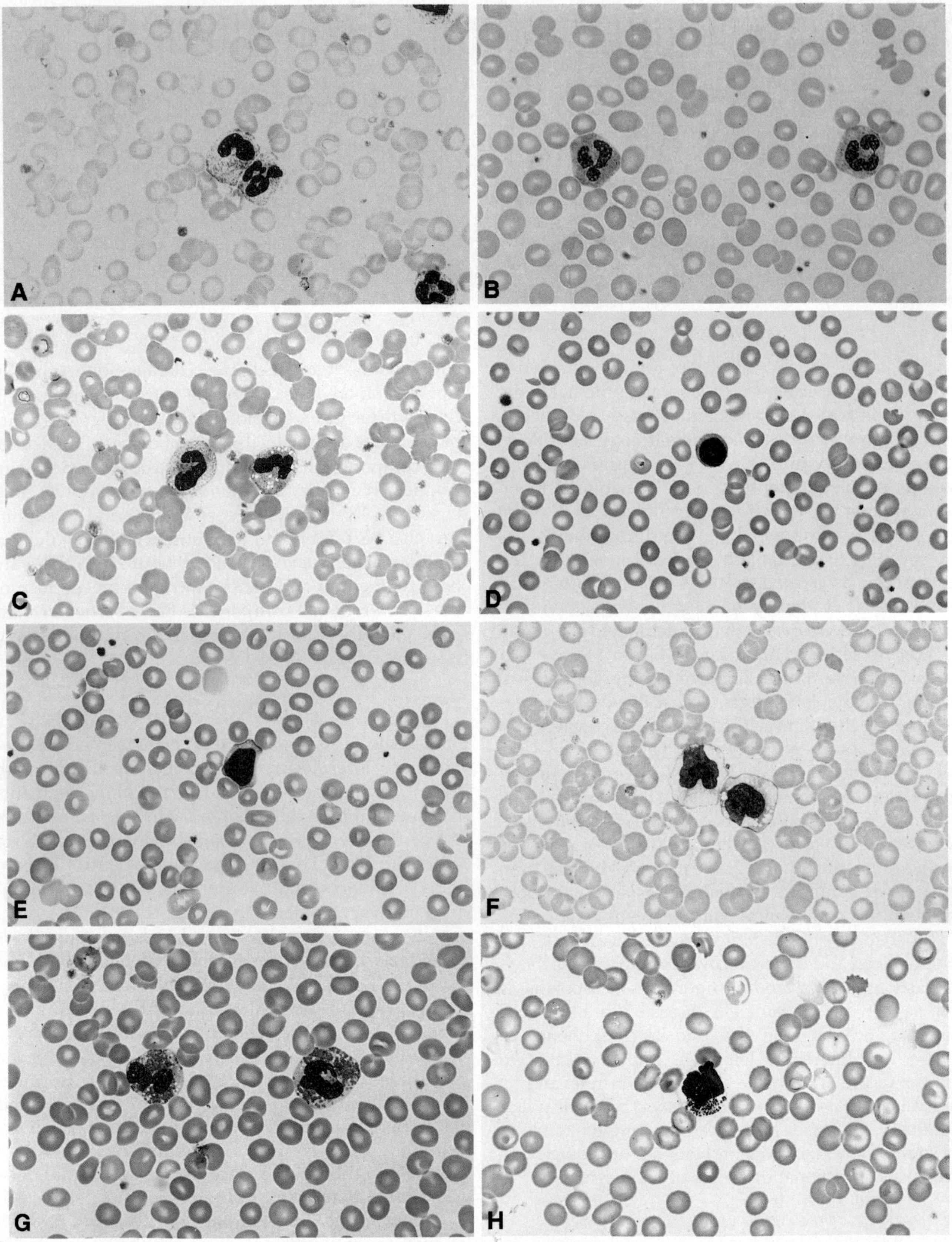

Figure 34.1. Peripheral blood smear from a normal individual. **A**, Segmented neutrophil. **B**, Segmented neutrophil. **C**, Band neutrophil. **D**, Lymphocyte. **E**, Lymphocyte. **F**, Monocyte. **G**, Eosinophil. **H**, Basophil.

ically visible. Nucleoli are faint. Cytoplasm will vary from scant to abundant and pale blue to basophilic in color. Occasional azurophilic granules may be identified. These granulated lymphocytes are thought to represent either natural killer cells or lymphocytes with cellular cytotoxic function.

Monocyte. The monocyte is an intermediate to large cell (15 to 20 μm) with an indented and irregularly folded nucleus. The nucleus consists of what has been described as "raked" chromatin. Nucleoli are typically not seen. The cytoplasm of a monocyte is "dirty," being grayish blue and occasionally having fine to very small azurophilic granules. Occasional vacuoles may also be identified.

Eosinophil. The eosinophil is an intermediate-sized (10 to 15 μm) cell characterized by large, refractile, reddish-orange granules. These eosinophilic granules are much larger than those found in neutrophils and are quite distinct in appearance. The nucleus is typically segmented into two or occasionally three lobes. The nuclear chromatin is coarsely clumped with no visible nucleoli.

Basophil. The basophil is similar in size to the neutrophil and eosinophil and contains characteristically large, round, blue-purple granules spread over the nucleus and cytoplasm. This granulation frequently obscures the nuclear features of the cell. The nucleus may contain from one to three lobes and typically has no visible nucleolus. The chromatin of the basophil is slightly different from the chromatin of an eosinophil or neutrophil and is not as coarsely clumped as those two cells. Rather, the basophil nuclear chromatin is smooth, having little visible parachromatin.

Bone Marrow: Granulopoiesis

The normal cellular maturation of the erythrocytic, granulocytic, and monocytic sequence is illustrated in Figure 34.2. The maturation of the granulocytic series is characterized by sequential steps of reductions in nuclear and cytoplasmic volume, progressive clumping of nuclear chromatin, nuclear lobulation and segmentation, and the sequential loss and gain of primary and secondary granules, respectively (Fig. 34.3). The cells in the first half of the morphologic differentiation scheme (myeloblasts, promyelocytes, and myelocytes), are capable of replication and of undergoing mitosis. The cells in the latter half of myeloid differentiation (metamyelocyte, band neutrophil, segmented neutrophil, eosinophil, and basophil) cannot divide and undergo mitosis.

Myeloblast. The myeloblast is the youngest identifiable cell in the granulocytic series. Myeloblasts are medium-sized cells (12 to 16 μm), having high nuclear:cytoplasmic ratios, finely reticular chromatin, and prominent nucleoli. The scant cytoplasm is deep blue and will show rare to few primary, azurophilic granules.

Promyelocyte. The promyelocyte is the largest cell of the granulocytic series, measuring 15 to 22 μm. The prominent azurophilic primary granules are the characteristic feature of this cell. Its nucleus remains round to oval, having fine to perhaps slightly condensed chromatin and typically one to two nucleoli. The amount of cytoplasm in the promyelocyte is slightly more than is found in the myeloblast and is basophilic to pale blue in color. No secondary granules are identified. The primary granules typically overlie both the cytoplasm and the nucleus. At the junction between promyelocyte and myelocyte development, the secondary granules appear in the cytoplasm as a pale, yellowish blush, typically in the Golgi area. It may be difficult to appreciate the specific secondary granules; rather, the early secondary granules give a "patchy," light blue appearance to the cytoplasm.

Myelocyte. The myelocyte is slightly smaller than the promyelocyte with a central to eccentrically located, round to oval nucleus. The chromatin of the nucleus has begun to clump, but no definite indentation in the nucleus has occurred. Nucleoli are absent or inconspicuous. A moderate amount of cytoplasm is present. The cytoplasm of the myelocyte contains both primary and secondary granules. The secondary granules will appear pink to light blue or purple on a Wright-Giemsa stain. The Golgi hof may be quite prominent in these cells. The amount of cytoplasm relative to the nucleus is increased as compared to the promyelocyte stage.

Metamyelocyte. The metamyelocyte is the first stage beyond the mitotically active stages of granulopoiesis. The metamyelocyte is only slightly larger than the mature neutrophil (10 to 18 μm) and shows a slightly indented or kidney bean-shaped nucleus. Chromatin is quite dense with no nucleolus evident. Obviously, secondary granules at this point are quite prominent and far outnumber the larger, darker, primary granules.

Neutrophil/Eosinophil/Basophil. The band and segmented neutrophils, eosinophils, and basophils have been previously discussed.

Bone Marrow: Monocytopoiesis

Monocytes and macrophages constitute the so-called mononuclear phagocyte system (Fig. 34.2). These cells arise from committed stem cells capable of generating either monocytic or granulocytic precursors. After differentiation into mature monocytes, circulating monocytes may eventually migrate to target tissues, where they become macrophages. These

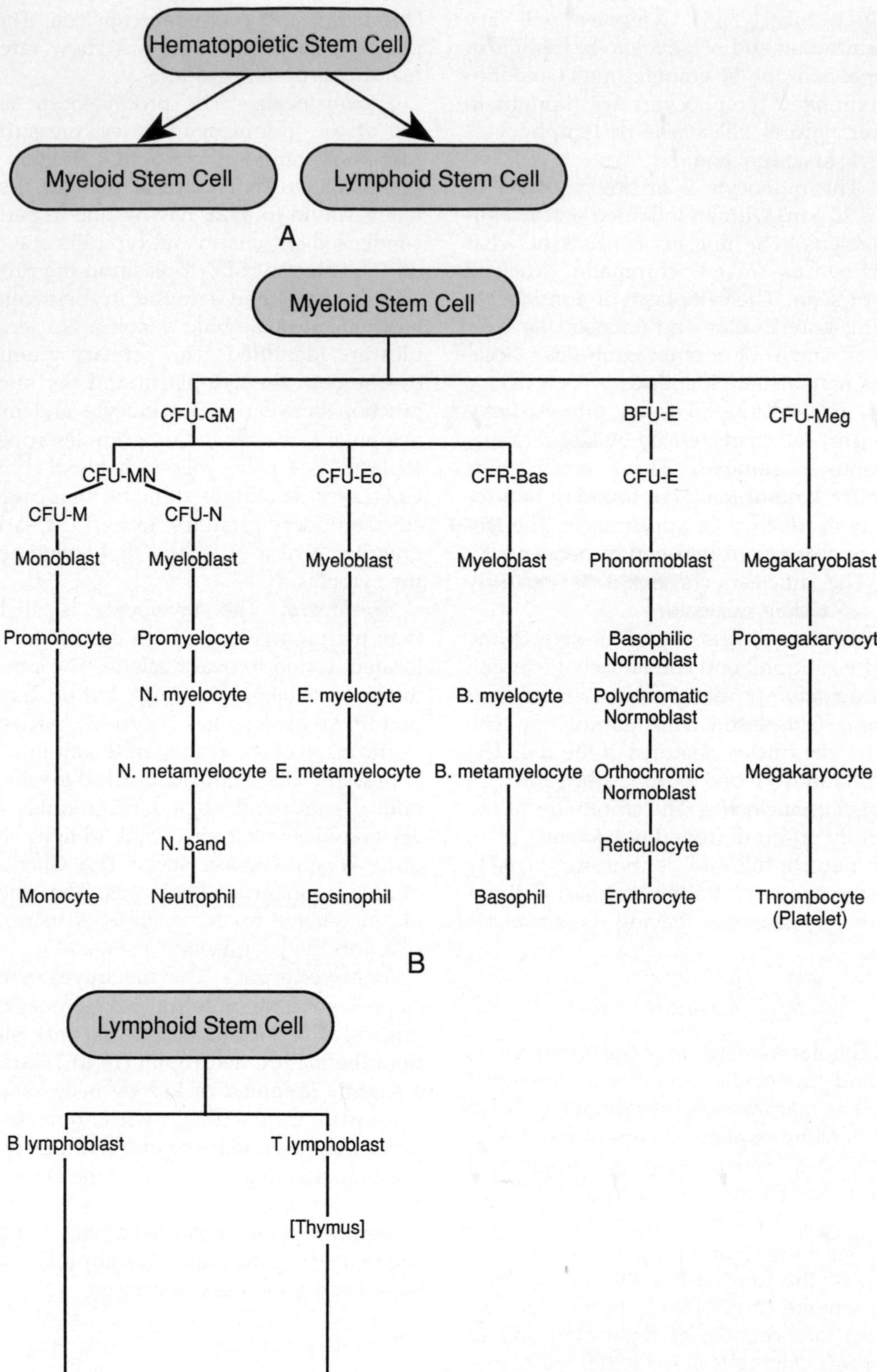

Figure 34.2. Schematic line drawing of the normal. **A**, Hematopoietic; **B**, Myeloid. **C**, Lymphoid maturation sequence. CFU, colony-forming unit; BFU, burst-forming unit; GM, granulocyte/monocyte; M, monocyte; N, neutrophil; Eo, eosinophil; Bas, basophil; E, erythroid; Meg, megakaryocyte.

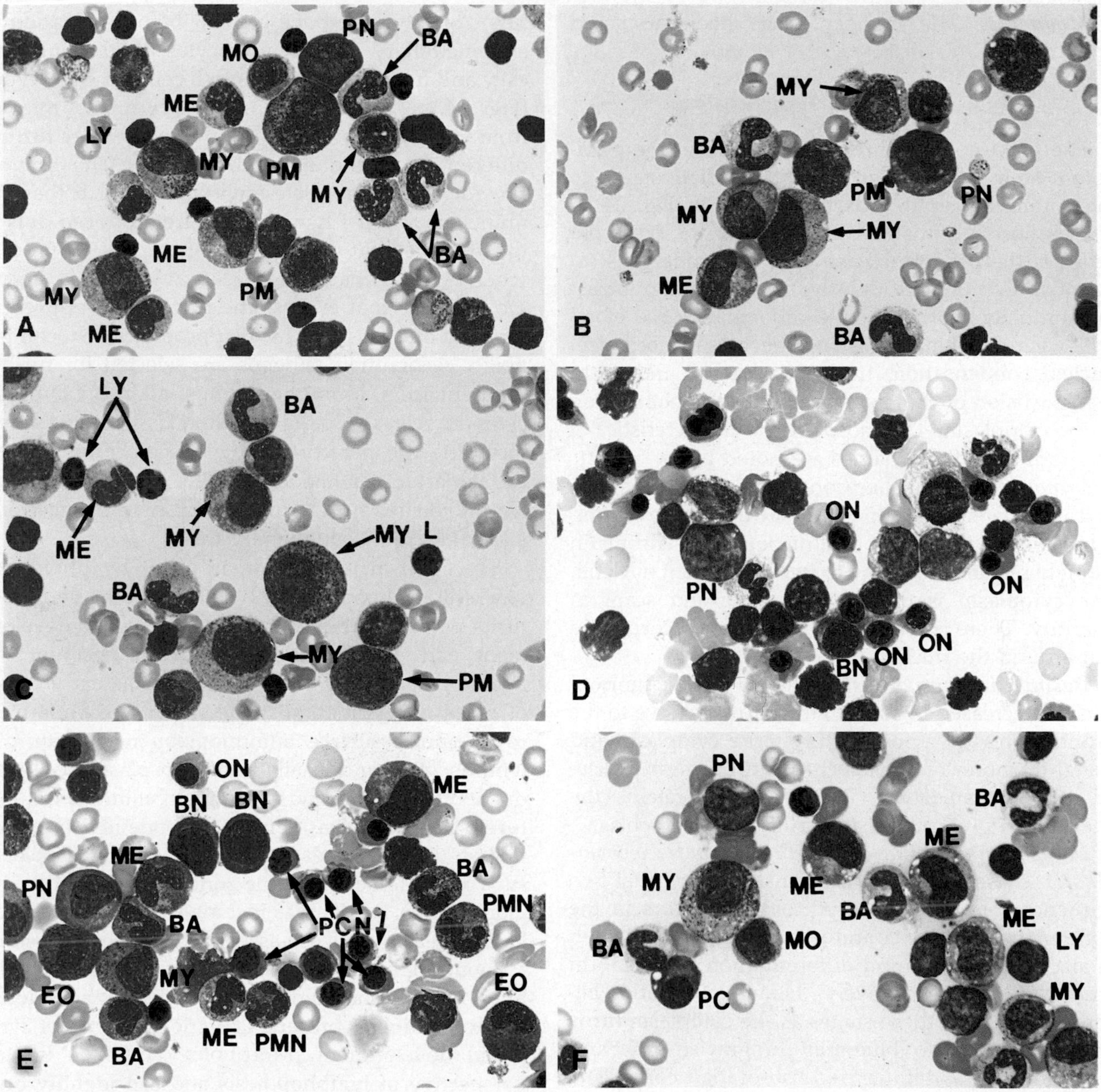

Figure 34.3. **A–F**, Photomicrographs of bone marrow aspirate smears showing erthothyroid erythroid and granulocytic maturation: MB, myeloblast; PM, promyelocyte; MY, myelocyte; ME, metamyelocyte; MO, monocyte; PN, pronormoblast; BN, basophilic normoblast; PCN, polychromatophilic normoblast; ON, orthochromatic normoblast; PC, plasma cell.

macrophages may be present in multiple tissue sites, including the spleen, liver, and lungs.

Monoblast. The monoblast is a large cell (14 to 22 μm) with a round, eccentrically placed nucleus. The nucleus has fine chromatin and prominent nucleoli. There is relatively abundant cytoplasm for such a large, "blastic"-appearing cell, with certainly more cytoplasm than a typical myeloblast. The cytoplasm is pale blue and may rarely contain some faint azurophilic granules.

Promonocyte. The promonocyte is a poorly defined cell, intermediate between a monoblast and a mature monocyte. Like the monoblast, the promonocyte is a large cell with an indented to slightly irregular nucleus. Nuclear folding does not reach the degree of indentation seen in the mature monocyte, and thus is intermediate between a monoblast and a monocyte. The nucleus typically shows one to two faint nucleoli. The nuclear chromatin has begun to show slight condensation and a coarseness beyond that of the typical monoblast. The cytoplasm retains the gray-blue color of a monocyte and typically shows some fine azurophilic granules and occasional vacuoles.

Monocyte. The monocyte has been discussed previously.

Bone Marrow: Erythropoiesis

The process of erythropoiesis begins at the pluripotent stem cell through the intermediate stages to the committed erythroid stem cell unit (Fig. 34.1). The earliest identifiable component of the erythroid series is the pronormoblast. This cell undergoes sequential divisions through the basophilic normoblast to eventually the reticulocyte and a mature red blood cell. Each division results in a decrease in cell size, nuclear condensation, nuclear pyknosis, and eventual extrusion of the nucleus and hemoglobinization of the cytoplasm. The morphologic characteristics of the normal erythroid series are noted below.

Pronormoblast. The pronormoblast is the largest erythroid precursor (15 to 22 μm), having a uniformly round to slightly oval nucleus. The chromatin is finely reticular with one to two prominent nucleoli. The cytoplasm is deeply basophilic and scant in quantity. There is typically a well-defined chromatin rim around the nucleus.

Basophilic Normoblast. The basophilic normoblast is decreased in size (10 to 16 μm) relative to the pronormoblast, having slightly more cytoplasm and a slightly more condensed chromatin pattern. Nucleoli are inconspicuous. The cytoplasm retains the deeply basophilic color seen in the pronormoblast.

Polychromatophilic and Orthochromatic Normoblast. These two cell types constitute the final two sequences of nucleated erythroid precursors in the bone marrow. They continue to show the reduction in size seen in erythroid differentiation (10 to 15 μm and 8 to 12 μm, respectively). Hemoglobinization becomes evident at these stages as the cytoplasm turns from basophilic to blue-gray to grayish-pink and eventually to a definite reddish-orange color. The nucleus shows further chromatin condensation and becomes quite pyknotic in appearance in the orthochromatic stage.

Reticulocyte. The reticulocyte is the first stage of erythroid development that lacks a nucleus. The cytoplasm has a slight grayish blue tinge to the prominent orange-staining color. Vital staining (e.g., with new methylene blue) will show fine basophilic reticulum in the red blood cell, which is the defining feature of a reticulocyte. This represents residual RNA, remaining from previous precursor stages.

Bone Marrow: Lymphopoiesis

Lymphocytes play a key role in antigen recognition and the subsequent immune response. The earliest lymphocyte precursors undergo the initial maturation steps in the bone marrow before migration to extramedullary sites; lymphocytes can be antigenically and functionally split into B cell and T cell types (Fig. 34.1). The T lymphocyte precursors migrate from the bone marrow to the thymus, where further differentiation and maturation occur. The thymus provides an appropriate environment such that immunocompetent T lymphocytes are produced. It is in the thymus that T-cell selection occurs, a process whereby cells that would react with "self" are removed; cells that express the preferred T-cell receptors and antigens and have appropriate histocompatibility recognition antigens are selected for further differentiation. From the thymus, mature T lymphocytes are released to the peripheral lymphoid tissues, including the paracortical regions of lymph nodes, the periarteriolar regions of spleen, and other nonlymphoid sites such as in the mucosa of the gastrointestinal tract and pulmonary tree.

The other major component of the lymphoid system is the B lymphocyte. B cells differentiate to maturity within the bone marrow. The normal development and differentiation of B cells begin at the hematopoietic stem cell, go through the early stages of B-cell differentiation while still in the bone marrow, acquire surface immunoglobulin as mature B lymphocytes, and finally end with plasma cell production of cytoplasmic immunoglobulin. As the mature B cells are released from the bone marrow, they migrate to B-cell areas of lymph nodes and spleen, such as the follicles, mantle zones, and medullary regions. Other B-cell areas include the follicles and follicular areas of mucosa-associated lymphoid tissue.

Lymphopoiesis can be accurately and precisely defined by immunophenotyping studies, which detect surface antigens present at various stages of lymphoid development. Morphology offers a limited perspective of lymphopoiesis and can identify only the lymphoblast, lymphocyte, and plasma cell components.

Lymphoblast. The lymphoblast is a small to intermediate-sized cell (8 to 15 μm) with a round nucleus and scant cytoplasm. The chromatin is fine, but slightly coarser than that found in myeloblasts. It has inconspicuous to prominent nucleoli, and no observable cytoplasmic granules.

Lymphocyte. The morphology of the lymphocyte has been discussed previously.

Plasma Cell. The plasma cell is a small cell (7 to 10 μm) with an eccentrically placed nucleus. The nucleus has coarsely clumped chromatin that has been described as resembling a clock face. The cytoplasm is a basophilic, cornflower-blue color and has a prominent, perinuclear hof.

Bone Marrow: Megakaryopoiesis

Megakaryopoiesis involves a much different morphologic sequence of differentiation than the other myeloid cell lines (Fig. 34.1). The megakaryoblast is closely related to the early erythroid precursor and morphologically has some resemblance to a primitive pronormoblast. Erythropoietin, which stimulates bone marrow erythroid production, also stimulates megakaryopoiesis and the production of platelets. The megakaryoblast undergoes endomitosis, which involves chromosomal division without cytoplasmic and cellular division. As endomitosis and nuclear segmentation occur, recognizable megakaryocytic precursors can be identified. Endomitosis continues until the megakaryocyte contains 8, 16, or 32 nuclear lobes. This process is accompanied by an increase in cell size and cytoplasm. Eventually the cytoplasm becomes more granular, and small platelets, which are membrane-bound portions of granular cytoplasm, break off and eventually enter the circulation.

Megakaryoblast. The megakaryoblast is a poorly defined cell that may not be easily recognizable as a distinct entity within a normal bone marrow. It may either be a small blast (8 to 15 μm) or much larger in size (18 to 30 μm). The megakaryoblast has a round to oval nucleus, prominent nucleoli, and variable amounts of blue to deeply basophilic cytoplasm. The chromatin may be finely reticular in larger cells or dark and dense in smaller cells.

Megakaryocyte. The megakaryocyte is the largest nucleated cell within the bone marrow and ranges in size from 35 to 100 μm. The megakaryocyte typically has a multilobated nucleus with 8, 16, or 32 nuclear lobes. No nucleoli are evident. The cytoplasm appears light blue and contains finely dispersed granules.

BLOOD CELL COUNTING

The complete hematologic evaluation of a peripheral blood sample can provide important clinical and diagnostic information about the three major components of the peripheral blood: (*a*) the erythrocytes or red blood cells; (*b*) the leukocytes or white blood cells; and (*c*) the platelets. These studies are useful in screening patients for potential hematologic disorders as well as providing diagnostic information for specific diseases as described in this and other chapters of this section.

The process of performing a basic hematologic analysis of peripheral blood involves four primary steps: (*a*) collection and processing of the peripheral blood sample; (*b*) determination of the CBC, including cell concentrations and red blood cell indices; (*c*) determination of the white blood cell differential count (either automated or manual); and (*d*) blood film examination for potential morphologic changes/abnormalities. Although these steps are discussed in some detail here, it may not be appropriate or necessary to perform all four steps on all samples. Rather, there must be an appropriate utilization of laboratory resources according to the presenting clinical indications.

Specimen Collection and Processing

The handling and processing of blood samples can be a forgotten component in providing quality results for the hematology laboratory. Table 34.1 lists some of the "preanalytic" and "analytic" errors that can affect hematologic results. Understanding these potential sources of errors is essential knowledge for both laboratorians and clinicians. These include, in part, specimen collection, choice of anticoagulant, specimen clotting, storage temperature, time between acquisition and analysis, hemolysis, adequate specimen mixing, hyperlipemia, and other metabolic/biochemical abnormalities. Recognition of these factors by laboratory personnel is essential in providing accurate clinical hematologic data for their clinical colleagues.

Venipuncture/Anticoagulants. Peripheral blood for hematologic tests is typically obtained from a venipuncture specimen. Blood may also be drawn from a "stick" of the fingertip, the heel, great toe, or earlobe. The blood should be collected into a tube containing an anticoagulant and thoroughly mixed. The choice of anticoagulants for hematologic studies include ethylenediaminetetraacetic acid (EDTA) (sodium or potassium salts), trisodium citrate, and heparin, with EDTA being the standard anticoagulant of choice for hematologic studies. Citrate and EDTA are, in effect, calcium chelators and thus remove calcium, which is an essential ingredient for the coagulation process. Heparin inhibits thrombin formation by complexing with antithrombin III.

EDTA specimens may produce significant morphologic artifacts on blood films if allowed to stand for more than 2 to 3 hours, although instrument analysis is stable for up to 8 hours at room temperature. If analysis cannot be performed within 8 hours, clinical specimens can be refrigerated for up to 24 hours at 4°C with little degradation of instrument results. Specimens with EDTA kept at room temperature for more than 8 hours may show an artifactual increase in the mean corpuscular volume (MCV) and a decrease in both the mean corpuscular hemoglobin concentration (MCHC) and erythrocyte sedimentation rate (ESR).

Table 34.1. The Complete Blood Count: Sources of Spurious Results[a]

CBC Component	Causes of Spurious Increase	Causes of Spurious Decrease
WBC	Cryoglobulin Heparin Monoclonal proteins Nucleated red cells Platelet clumping Unlysed red cells	Clotting Smudge cells
RBC	Cryoglobulin Giant platelets High WBC (>50,000/μl)	Autoagglutination Clotting Hemolysis (in vitro) Microcytic red cells
Hemoglobin	Carboxyhemoglobin (>10%) Cryoglobulin Hemolysis (in vivo) Heparin Hyperbilirubinemia Lipemia Monoclonal proteins	Clotting
Hematocrit (automated)	Cryoglobulin Giant platelets High WBC (>50,000/μl) Hyperglycemia (>600 mg/dl)	Autoagglutination Clotting Hemolysis (in vitro) Microcytic red cells
Hematocrit (microhematocrit)	Hyponatremia Plasma trapping	Excess EDTA Hemolysis (in vitro) Hypernatremia
MCV	Autoagglutination High WBC (>50,000/μl) Hyperglycemia	Cryoglobulin Giant platelets Hemolysis (in vitro) Microcytic red cells Swollen RBC
MCH	High WBC (>50,000/μl) Spuriously high Hgb Spuriously high RBC	Spuriously low Hgb Spuriously high RBC
MCHC	Autoagglutination Clotting Hemolysis (in vitro) Hemolysis (in vivo) Spuriously high Hgb Spuriously low Hct	High WBC (>50,000/μl) Spuriously low Hgb Spuriously high Hct
Platelets	Cryoglobulin Hemolysis (in vitro and in vivo) Microcytic red cells Red cell inclusions White cell fragments	Clotting Giant platelets Heparin Platelet clumping Platelet satellitosis

[a]Modified from Cornbleet J. Spurious results from automated hematology cell analyzers. Lab Med 1983;14:509.

Citrate is most commonly used for coagulation and special platelet studies, but may be useful for routine hematologic studies if EDTA-dependent platelet agglutination is present; blood counts should be increased by a factor of 1.1 if citrate is used to account for the sample dilution that occurs with the use of sodium citrate. Heparin is a sufficient anticoagulant for RBC analysis, but may cause clumping of platelets or leukocytes. These limitations of available anticoagulants have basically mandated that most hospital-based hematology work be performed on-site and that referral hematologic specimens be acquired within a relatively short time of analysis to minimize laboratory and morphologic artifact.

Complete Blood Count

The complete blood count (CBC) is the backbone of any hematologic evaluation. The CBC includes a determination of (*a*) red blood cell data, such as total red blood cell count (RBC); hemoglobin/hematocrit; red blood cell indices, including MCV, MCHC, and mean corpuscular hemoglobin (MCH); and the red cell distribution width (RDW); (*b*) white blood cell data; and, usually, (*c*) platelet count and, sometimes, mean platelet volume (MPV). A white blood cell differential count may also be part of a routine CBC in some laboratories, although a more judicial use of the differential count is probably warranted.

Table 34.2. Indications for Ordering the Complete Blood Count

Ambulatory population	
General population (screening)	Not useful
Specific subgroups (pregnant women, elderly, immigrants, etc.)	Possibly useful
Hospital population	
No abnormality suspected	Rarely useful
Hematologic abnormality suspected	Useful
Repetitive testing	Useful in some patients at appropriate intervals

The CBC in the broadest sense can provide important baseline information about the functional state of the bone marrow. Recognition of a "-penia," or deficiency of a blood component, is indication of either a marrow production problem or a peripheral destruction activity. Likewise, a "-cytosis," or elevation of a blood component, could indicate either a normal marrow response to a peripheral stimulation or the peripheral manifestation of an uncontrolled malignant proliferation. Thus, in general, the CBC is useful in broadly screening for hematologic disease (Table 34.2). The hemoglobin (Hb) and/or hematocrit (Hct) quantify the degree of anemia or polycythemia and the MCV/MCHC/RDW can be useful in further subclassifying the type of anemia (e.g., normocytic, microcytic, macrocytic). The white blood cell count (WBC) can provide diagnostic or follow-up information regarding either a benign response or malignant process (see later in this chapter). Obtaining a platelet count is the first step in the evaluation of the hemostatic process. Any of the CBC components can be useful in monitoring patient responses to therapy (iron, vitamin B_{12}/folate, marrow toxicity due to drugs, chemotherapy, among other things).

The appropriate ordering of the CBC is not something that has been seriously debated in the medical literature. Indeed, the role of the CBC has been considered a virtual icon in the evaluation of hospitalized as well as ambulatory patients. The challenge to the medical community will be to develop practice parameters for CBC utility in various patient settings. The CBC as a screening device in the ambulatory setting has limited utility in the general population due to the low prevalence of asymptomatic disease that would be detected by a routine CBC. Indeed, even the detection of mild asymptomatic abnormalities with the CBC, such as mild anemia, may not offer any real clinical benefit to the patient. Screening of particular subgroups, such as pregnant women, institutionalized geriatric persons, and possibly immigrants from third world countries, may be useful as the prevalence of hematologic disease is higher in those groups than in the general population. However, no studies have been done in these groups to justify the benefit of CBC screening for disease.

It is in hospitalized patients that the routine CBC has been most abused both as an admission screen as well as as a repetitive follow-up test. If no hematologic abnormality is suspected clinically, the CBC is rarely useful on patients admitted to a hospital. Those clinical situations in which a routine CBC would be of questionable value would include elective surgeries in which only minor blood loss is anticipated, for patients undergoing minor diagnostic procedures, and for patients who have no clinical indication of a hematologic abnormality. If, however, a hematologic abnormality is suspected clinically, the CBC is obviously indicated and may be useful in confirming either a primary or reactive hematologic disorder that may have an impact on disease diagnosis and management.

It is also difficult to document the effectiveness of repetitive CBC testing. Unfortunately, it has become common practice to order repetitive CBCs (e.g., daily) in patients in whom no benefit may be gleaned. If a patient clinically responds to treatment for a hematologic disease, then ordering a repetitive CBC would not be beneficial unless there is indication that such treatment has not been effective. This aspect of defining appropriate testing intervals for the CBC has not been studied extensively and remains a major challenge.

Table 34.2 provides a summary of the utility and indications for obtaining a CBC. Although laboratories have generally not sought to control the flow of CBC samples, it seems inevitable that some limitation of its use will evolve as health care cost containment grows in importance. The biggest challenge to laboratorians will be devising practice standards that will outline more effectively the indications for routine and follow-up CBCs for both hospitalized and ambulatory patients.

Hematology Analyzers/Instrumentation

Clinical hematology laboratories have undergone significant changes in the arena of automation as technological advances have continually evolved. The era of manual CBC determinations has thankfully passed, with automated blood analysis now a routine part of virtually all hematology laboratories. Automated red blood cell and white blood cell counters emerged in the clinical laboratories in the 1960s. The addition of platelet counters, seven-parameter CBC analyzers, and three-parameter differential leukocyte counters appeared in the 1970s. The 1980s were characterized by single, stand-alone instruments capable of performing 10-parameter CBCs. The greatest change in the hematology laboratory came in the latter part of the 1980s and the early 1990s with the development of more sophisticated and accurate leukocyte differential counters. Changes that have emerged over the last few years include bar code readers, closed-tube sampling, automated sampling systems, and "walk-away" analysis stations. Bar code readers have allowed for efficient and high throughput of specimens and provide more accurate patient and specimen identification. Closed-tube sampling has been a tremendous benefit in this era of universal precautions and the recognition of high-risk blood samples. The "walk-away" features of many instruments has been made possible due to the built-in mixing systems as well as simple robotics for specimen aspiration and handling.

It is improbable that more clinically relevant parameters will be extrapolated from the CBC. So one would predict that the next decade or two will show advances and changes related to two areas: increasing automation and "walk-away" capabilities of the instrument with the eventual use of robotics to handle and process specimens; and increasing use of computer analytic capabilities to control utilization of hematologic testing as well as providing more innovative ways of displaying and interpreting laboratory data.

One can envision the evolution of robotic techniques that would allow specimens to be transported from a central receiving area to the hematology instrument based on appropriate specimen bar coding. Technologist interaction would be needed at the point of trouble-shooting or manual slide making (another potential automated area). The power of today's computers to store and interrogate large clinical databases will also permit the evolution of autoverification of patient results. In addition, by interrogating the patient database, computer capabilities may allow the laboratorian better control over the utilization of the CBCs and leukocyte differential counts; in particular, controlling the frequency of repetitive CBCs and differential counts. Lastly, more sophisticated laboratory information systems will hopefully allow the laboratories to present their data in a more meaningful clinical fashion. For example, the capability to present data graphically or in combination with results from other laboratories (for example, hemoglobin values with Coomb's test, transfusion record, and bilirubin) could be a major enhancement in how laboratory data are interpreted clinically.

Total Red Blood Cell Count

For most medical technologists, the hemacytometer is but a fond reminder of how technology has improved their lives. It is safe to write that virtually all modern laboratories use some form of automated counting to determine the total red blood cell count (RBC). Nearly all modern instruments use either electrical impedance methods or laser light-scatter characteristics to determine the RBC. Although frequently ignored in the evaluation of a CBC, the RBC is the basis for calculating the hematocrit, MCH, and MCHC. In addition, the RBC may have value in and of itself when attempting to distinguish iron deficiency anemia from thalassemia in patients with an unknown microcytic anemia. In iron deficiency, the RBC diminishes in proportion with the hemoglobin concentration. This is in contrast with thalassemia, where the RBC may be normal to increased relative to the degree of anemia as shown by the hemoglobin value. Several mathematical formulas have been derived in an attempt to distinguish these disorders more accurately; none has proved perfect, and most have been too complex to remember. A simple formula published by Cornbleet takes the MCV divided by the RBC (1); a value greater than 13 favors iron deficiency and a value less than 13 favors thalassemia.

Automated counting methods for red blood cells have been based primarily on electrical impedance or light-scattering techniques. These methods allow for both the counting of total cells as well as determining the cell size (i.e., the MCV) of the red blood cells. Analyzers from the Coulter Corporation and TOA use the electrical impedance method, while light-scattering techniques have been pioneered with the Technicon analyzers. The electrical impedance method requires that cells pass an aperture through which a current is passing. As the cells cross the electrical current, the change in the electrical resistance that can be detected is proportional to the cell size. In light-scattering techniques, photomultiplier tubes detect changes in light scatter as the cells pass through a flow cell. Various cell types can be distinguished from these light-scatter characteristics based on cell size and granularity.

Very few clinical situations will result in false elevations or decreases in the total RBC. Red blood cell autoagglutination and extreme red blood cell microcytosis may lead to spurious decreases in the reported total RBC. In the latter case, the small red blood cells may be counted as large platelets and not be included in the red blood cell histograms, while autoagglutination can result in the red blood cell "clump" being counted as a single cell. Conversely, very high leukocyte counts as well as cryoglobinemia may both lead to false elevations in total RBC. High leukocyte counts, typically if greater than 100.0×10^9 cells/liter, can significantly add to the total RBC, while normal WBCs have little impact on the total RBC.

Hemoglobin

The primary function of the red blood cell is transporting oxygen and carbon dioxide. Hemoglobin within the cell takes up oxygen within the lungs and releases it in tissues in exchange for carbon dioxide. This regulated delivery and control of oxygen and carbon dioxide exchange is obviously an extremely vital component of the mammalian system. The role of oxygen delivery is dependent on the binding of hemoglobin to oxygen. The equilibrium between oxygen and hemoglobin varies according to oxygen tension (PO_2). This dissociation curve (the so-called oxygen dissociation curve) demonstrates the saturation process of hemoglobin relative to the conditions found in both lung (binding of oxygen) and peripheral tissue capillaries (release of oxygen).

Hemoglobin constitutes over 90% of the red blood cell and is composed of two pairs of globin chains ($\alpha_2\beta_2$) and four "heme" groups containing ferrous iron. A decrease in hemoglobin concentration is referred to as an anemia, while an increase in hemoglobin concentration is called polycythemia. Some clinical conditions can lead to the formation of oxidized hemoglobin (for example, Heinz body anemias); this oxidized hemoglobin is called methemoglobin, which has a reduced capacity for carrying carbon dioxide. Sulfhemoglobin is an uncommon form of hemoglobin that results from the addition of sulfur into the hemoglobin molecule during the process of oxidation. Sulfhemoglobin cannot carry oxygen and typically accounts for less than 1% of all hemoglobins. Clinically, sulfhemoglobin has been reported in some patients receiving sulfa-based drugs, as well as in some patients with clostridium bacteremia. Carboxyhemoglobin normally accounts for less than 1% of the overall hemoglobin concentration and is produced during the process of heme metabolism to bilirubin.

The interaction of carbon monoxide and hemoglobin deserves specific mention. The affinity of carbon monoxide to hemoglobin is much greater than with oxygen (more than 200 times greater). Thus, even small concentrations of carbon monoxide in the air will preferentially bind to hemoglobin and thus prevent oxygen exchange and transportation. Acute carbon monoxide poisoning is the most dramatic cause of elevated carboxyhemoglobin levels. Long-term carbon monoxide exposure as a result of smoking, or smoke exposure, may also lead to elevation of carboxyhemoglobin and a "left shift" in the oxygen dissociation curve. The differentiation of these various hemoglobin derivatives is classically based on spectrophotometric determination. The various hemoglobins have particular absorption spectra, shown in Table 34.3.

Table 34.3. Hemoglobin Derivatives: Absorption Maximas[a]

Hemoglobin	Abbreviation/Terms	Maxima
		nm
Hemoglobin	Hb	431,555
Oxyhemoglobin	HbO_2	415,542
Carboxyhemoglobin	HbCO	420,539
Sulfhemoglobin	SHb	—
Carboxysulfhemoglobin	SHbCO	—
Hemiglobin	Hi/methemoglobin	406,500
Hemiglobincyanide	HiCN/cyanmethemoglobin	421,540

[a]Modified from van Assendelft OW. Spectrophotometry of haemoglobin derivatives. Assen, The Netherlands: Royal Van Gorcum Ltd., 1970.

Hemoglobin is most commonly determined by spectrophotometry in modern instrumentation using a cyanomethemoglobin procedure; this is the standard method by which virtually all hematology instruments measure hemoglobin. This procedure involves oxidizing all hemoglobin to methemoglobin by using excess ferric iron (potassium ferricyanide). Excess cyanide ions (potassium cyanide) subsequently leads to the formation of cyanated methemoglobin (which maximally absorbs light at 540 nm). Other forms of hemoglobin besides cyanomethemoglobin, including hemoglobin, oxyhemoglobin, carboxyhemoglobin, and methemoglobin, will also absorb light at 540 nm (Table 34.3). Falsely elevated (real or apparent) hemoglobin absorbances can occur due to hyperlipemia, fat droplets (associated with hyperalimentation), hypergammaglobulinemia, cryoglobulemia, or a leukocytosis (more than 50.0×10^9 cells/liter). Improperly collected blood specimens (venipuncture or fingerstick) can also cause falsely elevated (hemoconcentrate) or falsely decreased (hemodilute) levels. Other laboratory methods for the determination of hemoglobin have been based on detecting oxyhemoglobin or by detecting the iron content of whole blood. Neither method is widely performed because of the lack of standardization or the inherent complexity of the process.

The automated determination of hemoglobin has bypassed many of the inherent errors of manual hemoglobin detection. However, variation in results can still occur from a variety of situations. As discussed earlier, sample collection problems or specimen abnormalities (hyperlipemia, etc.) can give falsely elevated or decreased hemoglobin levels. Hemoglobin concentrations are reported in grams per deciliter or grams per liter and vary according to age, sex, and ethnic background (Table 34.4). Cord blood or newborn capillary blood can be more concentrated (up to 2 g/dl) than venous blood; premature infants have lower hemoglobin values than term infants. The average hemoglobin concentration drops dramatically during the first month of life and does not significantly increase until after puberty. Adult fe-

Table 34.4A. Complete Blood Count: Normal Values[a]

Age	Hb[b]	Hct	RBC (× 10^{12}/liter)	MCV	MCH	MCHC	RDW
	(g/dl)	(%)		(fl)	(pg)	(g/dl)	(%)
At birth	13.5–19.5	42–60	3.9–5.4	98–118	31–37	30–36	—
1 day	14.5–22.5	45–67	4.0–6.6	95–121	31–37	29–37	—
1 week	13.5–21.5	42–66	3.9–6.3	88–126	28–40	28–38	—
1 month	10.0–18.0	31–55	3.0–5.4	85–123	28–40	29–37	—
6 months	9.5–13.5	29–41	3.1–4.5	74–108	25–35	30–36	—
1 year	10.5–13.5	33–39	3.7–5.4	70–86	23–31	30–36	—
6 years	11.5–13.5	34–40	3.9–5.3	75–87	24–30	31–37	—
12 years	11.5–13.5	35–45	4.0–5.2	77–95	25–34	31–37	—
Adult female	11.7–15.7	34.9–46.9	3.8–5.2	80.8–100	26.5–34.0	31.4–35.8	<15
Adult male	13.5–17.5	39.8–52.2	4.4–5.9	80.5–99.7	26.6–33.8	31.5–36.3	<15

[a]Data from Baker J, Cornbleet PJ. Erythrocyte disorders. In: Howanitz JH, Howanitz PJ, eds. Laboratory medicine—test selection and interpretation. New York: Churchill Livingstone, 1991:447–498.
[b]Mean Hb level in blacks of both sexes and all ages may be 0.5–1.0 below the mean for whites.

Table 34.4B. White Blood Cell and Leukocyte Differential Counts: Normal Values[a]

Age	WBC (× 10^9/liter)	Neutrophils (× 10^9/liter) Total	Band	Segmented	Lymphocytes	Monocytes	Eosinophils	Basophils
At birth	18.1 (9.0–30.0)	11.0 (6.0–26.0)	1.61	9.4	5.5 (2.0–11.0)	1.05 (0.40–3.1)	0.40 (0.02–0.85)	0.10 (0–0.64)
		61%	9.1%	52%	31%	5.8%	2.2%	0.6%
24 hours	18.9 (9.4–34.0)	11.5 (5.0–21.0)	1.75	9.8	5.8 (2.0–11.5)	1.10 (0.20–3.1)	0.45 (0.05–1.00)	0.10 (0–0.30)
		61%	9.2%	52%	31%	5.8%	2.4%	.05%
1 week	12.2 (5.0–21.0)	5.5 (1.5–10.0)	0.83	4.7	5.0 (2.0–17.0)	1.10 (0.30–2.7)	0.50 (0.07–1.10)	0.05 (0–0.25)
		45%	6.8%	39%	41%	9.1%	4.1%	.04%
1 month	10.8 (5.0–19.5)	3.8 (1.0–9.0)	0.49	3.3	6.0 (2.5–16.5)	0.70 (0.15–2.0)	0.30 (0.07–0.90)	0.05 (0–0.20)
		35%	4.5%	30%	56%	6.5%	2.8%	0.5%
6 months	11.9 (6.0–17.5)	3.8 (1.0–8.5)	0.45	3.3	7.3 (4.0–13.5)	0.48 (0.10–1.3)	0.30 (0.07–0.75)	0.05 (0–0.20)
		32%	3.8%	28%	61%	4.8%	2.5%	.04%
1 year	11.4 (6.0–17.5)	3.5 (1.5–8.5)	0.35	3.2	7.0 (4.0–10.5)	0.55 (0.05–1.1)	0.30 (0.05–0.70)	0.05 (0–0.20)
		31%	3.1%	28%	61%	4.8%	2.6%	0.4%
6 years	8.5 (5.0–14.5)	4.3 (1.5–8.0)	0.25 (0–1.0)	4.0 (1.5–7.0)	3.5 (1.5–7.0)	0.40 (0–0.8)	0.23 (0–0.65)	0.05 (0–0.20)
		51%	3.0%	48%	42%	4.7%	2.7%	0.6%
12 years	8.0 (4.5–13.5)	4.4 (1.8–8.0)	0.25 (0–1.0)	4.2 (1.8–7.0)	3.0 (1.2–6.0)	0.35 (0–0.8)	0.20 (0–0.55)	0.04 (0–0.20)
		55%	3.0%	52%	38%	4.4%	2.5%	0.5%
Adult	7.4 (4.5–11.0)	4.4 (1.8–7.7)	0.22 (0–0.7)	4.2 (1.8–7.0)	2.5 (1.0–4.8)	0.30 (0–0.8)	0.20 (0–0.45)	0.04 (0–0.20)
		59%	3.0%	56%	34%	4.0%	2.7%	0.5%

[a]Modified from Cornbleet J, Astanita R, Wolf PL. White blood cell and platelet disorders. In: Howanitz JH, Howanitz PJ, eds. Laboratory medicine—test selection and interpretation. New York: Churchill Livingstone, 1991:553–618.
[b]Data presented as mean (±2 S.D.)

males have hemoglobin values of 1.0 to 2.0 g/dl lower than adult males. It also has been recognized that blacks of both sexes have slightly lower mean hemoglobin levels than Caucasians. All this normal variation mandates that different normal ranges be utilized for reporting hematologic results and that the clinical interpretation of CBC findings be done in conjunction with all appropriate clinical findings.

Hematocrit

The hematocrit is simply the ratio of the volume of the red blood cells to the volume of the whole blood. Although hematocrits can be determined directly by centrifugation ("spun" hematocrits), most hematocrits are now calculated directly from the RBC and MCV: hematocrit = RBC (cells/liter) × MCV (liter/cell) (Table 34.5). Thus, any factor leading to spurious errors in RBC or MCV determination will also lead to spurious hematocrit results. Because the hematocrit is thus derived from two separate factors and all their sources of error, it should be clear that the hematocrit is a less accurate measure of anemia than the direct determination of hemoglobin concentration.

Manual or "spun" methods for determining hematocrits are still used in some circumstances and are based on centrifuging capillary blood tubes at 10,000 to 15,000 g to separate the fluid and cell components of the blood. Spun hematocrits may give spuriously high results if a significant concentration of plasma becomes "trapped" in the red cell layer. This phenomenon can be found in samples with polycythemia, macrocytosis, spherocytosis, hypochromic anemias, and RBC fragment disorders (such

Table 34.5. Components of the Complete Blood Count

CBC	Traditional Units	International Units
Hemoglobin	g/dl	g/liter
Hematocrit	dl/dl (%)	L/L (%)
Red blood cells	10^6 cells/μl	10^{12} cells/liter
White blood cells	10^3 cells/μl	10^9 cells/liter
Platelet count	10^3 plt/μl	10^9 platelets/liter
Mean corpuscular volume	fl/cell	fl (10^{-15} liter/cell
Mean corpuscular hemoglobin	pg/cell	pg (10^{-12}g)/cell
Mean corpuscular hemoglobin concentration	g/dl	g/liter

Derived CBC Values

Hematocrit (L/L;%) = [MCV (in liters per cell)] × [RBC (in cells/liter)]

MCH (pg/cell) $= \frac{\text{[HB (in g/liter)]}}{\text{[RBC (in cells/liter)]}}$

MCHC (g/dl) $= \frac{\text{[Hb (in g/dl)]}}{\text{[Hct (in L/L)]}}$

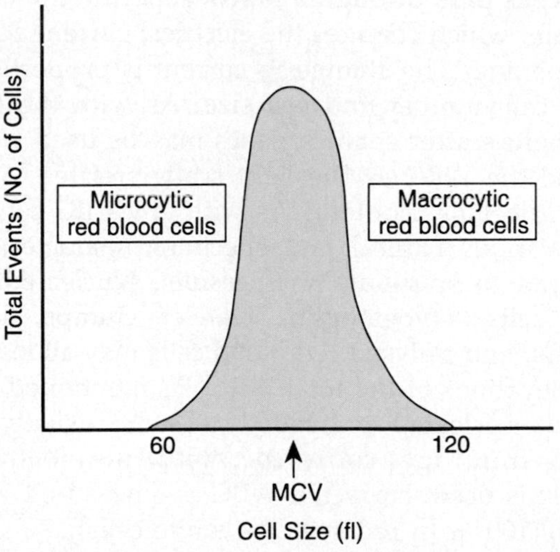

Figure 34.4. Red cell distribution histogram from an automated blood analyzer. The number of events counted (*y* axis) is plotted versus the cell size or volume (*x* axis). The median value of the histogram distribution is the mean corpuscular volume (MCV) of the sample. The coefficient of variation (or in some cases, the standard deviation) is equivalent to the red cell distribution width (RDW). Microcytic red blood cells, large platelets, and debris fall to the left portion of the curve, while macrocytic red blood cells, and small leukocytes fall to the right portion of the curve.

as sickle cell anemia or burn patients). Improper mixing and excessive dilution with anticoagulant can also lead to inaccurate "spun" hematocrit levels.

Red Blood Cell Indices

The red blood cell indices are a key component of the CBC. These include the MCV, MCH, and MCHC, which are used to determine the size, cellular hemoglobin, and hemoglobin concentration of the red blood cells, respectively. The MCV is the most useful of the red blood cell indices and is especially important in classifying anemias as either normocytic (normal MCV), microcytic (decreased MCV), or macrocytic (increased MCV) (see Chapter 35 for more details). The MCV is determined by the distribution of the red blood cell histogram (Fig. 34.4). The mean of the red blood cell distribution histogram, based on electrical impedance, is the MCV and the coefficient of variation (or sometimes, the standard deviation) is the RDW (discussed later).

The MCH is the hemoglobin concentration per cell and is calculated from the hemoglobin and RBC (Table 34.5). It is of little use clinically and typically follows the "movement" of the MCV value. The MCHC is the average hemoglobin concentration per total red blood cell volume (Table 34.5), and is of minimal diagnostic use. A decrease in MCHC provides little clinical information and may not be noted until, for example, late in the course of an iron-deficiency anemia. An increased MCHC is indicative of instrumentation or specimen problems and is a useful tool in the quality control process. When MCHCs (Hb/Hct) were determined manually (before automated instruments were widely used), a low MCHC was more commonly encountered in iron deficiency. This erroneous finding was the result of spuriously elevated "spun" hematocrits with the plasma trapping seen in microcytic anemias. Thus, the MCV is the only one of its red blood cell indices that provides consistently useful clinical information, with the MCH and MCHC useful primarily for quality control purposes.

Red Cell Distribution Width

The red cell distribution width (RDW) provides some insight and quantification into the variation in red cell size, or anisocytosis. It is derived from the red blood cell histogram and represents the coefficient of variation (or, in some cases, the standard deviation) of the red cell histogram distribution curve (Fig. 34.4). Bessman has proposed a system of classifying anemias based on RDW and has suggested that it may be a more sensitive indicator of a change in cell size than purely the MCV (Table 34.6) (2). In general, an elevated RDW has been associated with anemias from various deficiencies such as iron, B_{12}, or folate. This is to be contrasted with the normal RDW that classically characterizes the microcytic anemias seen in thalassemia. However, as in most laboratory tests, this single red blood cell parameter has been shown to have more than its share of false positives and false negatives relative to this classification scheme. Indeed, some cases of thalassemia may have an elevated RDW, and cases with anemia of chronic disease that have slightly lower MCVs appear to have slightly elevated RDWs; myelodysplastic syndromes and some malignancies may also be associated with elevated RDWs. Thus, the RDW must be

Table 34.6. Utility of RDW and MCV in Classification of Anemia[a]

	RDW Normal	RDW High
MCV—Low	Thalassemia trait Transfusion Chemotherapy Malignancy Hemorrhage Hereditary spherocytosis Posttraumatic splenectomy	Iron deficiency S-β-thalassemia Hgb H RBC fragmentations
MCV—Normal	Normal Chronic disease	Transfusion Early iron, B_{12}, or folate deficiency Homozygous hemoglobinopathy Myelofibrosis Sideroblastic anemia
MCV—High	Aplastic anemia Liver disease	Folate deficiency B_{12} deficiency Cold agglutinin Hemolytic anemia Chemotherapy

[a]Modified from Bessman, JD, Gilmer PR Jr, Gardner FH. Improved classification of anemias by MCV and RDW. Am J Clin Pathol 1983;80:322–326.

interpreted in conjunction with other CBC data in interpreting the abnormal hemogram.

White Blood Cell Count—Total

The total white blood cell count (WBC), or leukocyte count, consists of the polymorphonuclear neutrophils (PMNs) (segmented and band forms), lymphocytes, monocytes, eosinophils, basophils, and potentially any other circulating hematopoietic cells. Historically, nucleated red blood cells have been granted an exception to this rule and are typically subtracted out of the total leukocyte count. WBCs are performed on EDTA-anticoagulated blood. With automated hematology counters, the total WBC, like the total RBC, is determined by either electrical impedance methods or light-scatter techniques. Hemacytometers are thankfully not used routinely in hematology laboratories for the WBC, but may be called into action if the automated counters fail to provide accurate results, such as in leukopenic or leukemic patients. In either method, the red blood cells are lysed prior to the determination of the WBC.

The WBC can provide important diagnostic and monitoring information in patients with primary hematologic disease or acute/chronic infectious processes. The WBC also provides appropriate therapeutic data following administration of chemotherapy, radiation therapy, or antimicrobial agents. Since the WBC is composed predominantly of PMNs, any change in the total WBC typically reflects a change in the total PMN count. However, the WBC by itself is neither highly sensitive nor specific for an acute or chronic infectious process. In other words, an elevated WBC should not be inferred as evidence of an infectious process unless there is clinical evidence of such and, conversely, a low WBC does not rule out an infectious process when clinical findings favor an infectious process. Other causes of elevated WBC include trauma, postsurgery (24 to 48 hours), hemorrhage, postdelivery, tissue necrosis, corticosteroids, and numerous other medications.

Heparinized blood should not be used for determining the WBC because of its interference with lysing reagents and also its association with platelet agglutination in some specimens. As mentioned previously, citrate anticoagulant may be useful in cases with EDTA-dependent platelet agglutination; a correction factor of 1.1 is needed to account for the extra volume of anticoagulant used.

With the electrical impedance method, the red blood cells are first lysed and the remaining white blood cells pass through a narrow aperture, one cell at a time, which changes the electrical current across that opening. The change in current is proportional to the cell number and cell size. As with the total RBC, light-scatter characteristics may be used to determine the WBC as the light scatter relates to cell size and cellular content. As with any CBC component, various clinical and specimen characteristics may lead to spurious WBC results. Nucleated red blood cells, cryoglobulin, platelet clumps, large platelets, and unlysed red blood cells may all lead to false elevations of the total WBC. As mentioned previously, nucleated red blood cells are usually excluded from the corrected WBC; the following formula is used: corrected WBC = (measured WBC × 100)/(100 + [n red cells/100 white cells]).

White Blood Cell Count—Differential

The differential leukocyte count, or the white blood cell differential, remains one of the most frequently performed tests in the clinical hematology laboratory. Up until the early 1970s, the only accepted method for performing a differential count was microscopic examination of a Romanowsky-stained peripheral blood smear. Traditionally, the differential leukocyte count has included the counting and categorization of typically 100 white blood cells based on morphologic criteria, with the results being expressed as a percentage of each cell type identified. Absolute concentrations of the various cell types are calculated by multiplying the percentage by the total WBC. In addition to the differential count, morphologic evaluation of the smear provides the opportunity to morphologically evaluate all components of the peripheral blood, including red blood cells, white blood cells, and platelets. This is a key advantage of the manual differential and allows for

Table 34.7. Confidence Limits (95%) for Percentages of Cells Reported in a Manual Differential Count[a]

% Reported	n = 100	n = 1,000	n = 10,000
0	0.0–3.6	0.0–0.4	0.0–0.1
1	0.0–5.4	0.5–1.8	0.8–1.3
2	0.2–7.0	1.2–3.1	1.7–2.3
3	0.6–8.5	2.0–4.3	2.6–3.4
4	1.1–9.9	2.9–5.4	3.6–4.5
5	1.6–11.3	3.7–6.5	4.5–5.5
6	2.2–12.6	4.6–7.7	5.5–6.5
7	2.9–13.9	5.5–8.8	6.5–7.6
8	3.5–15.2	6.4–9.9	7.4–8.6
9	4.2–16.4	7.3–10.9	8.4–9.6
10	4.9–17.6	8.2–12.0	9.4–10.7
15	8.6–23.5	12.8–17.4	14.3–15.8
20	12.7–29.2	17.6–22.6	19.2–20.8
25	16.9–34.7	22.3–27.8	24.1–25.9
30	21.2–40.0	27.2–32.9	29.1–31.0
35	25.7–45.2	32.0–38.0	34.0–36.0
40	30.3–50.3	36.9–43.1	39.0–41.0
45	35.0–55.3	41.9–48.1	44.0–46.0
50	39.8–60.2	46.9–53.1	49.0–51.0
55	44.7–65.0	51.9–58.1	54.0–56.0
60	49.7–69.7	56.9–63.1	59.0–61.0
65	54.8–74.3	62.0–68.0	64.0–66.0
70	60.0–78.8	67.1–72.8	69.0–70.9
75	65.3–83.1	72.2–77.7	74.1–75.9
80	70.8–87.3	77.4–82.4	79.2–80.8
85	76.5–91.4	82.6–87.2	84.2–85.7
90	82.4–95.1	88.0–91.8	89.3–90.6
95	88.7–98.4	93.5–96.3	94.5–95.5
100	98.2–100.0	99.6–100.0	99.9–100.0

[a]Modified from Rümke CL, Bezemer PD, Kuik OJ. Normal values and least significant differences for differential leukocyte counts. J Chron Dis 1975;28:661–668.
[b]n = total cells counted.

the detection of a variety of disorders that might otherwise be lost in a totally automated system.

The manual performance of a differential count, i.e., the manual differential, is a time-consuming, labor-intensive, and relatively expensive procedure in this era of technological advances and automation. In addition to these technical and administrative disadvantages, the traditional manual differential count has other medical and scientific limitations, including poor sensitivity, specificity, and predictive value; it suffers from imprecision due to sampling error and statistical probabilities; and it is prone to subjective judgmental errors. Nonetheless, for better or worse, the manual differential count has historically remained the gold standard of differential leukocyte counts.

To accurately interpret the morphologic features of a peripheral blood film, several technical steps are required. First, the film must be well made with a good "feathered" edge and preferably with space around all slide edges. There should be a uniform distribution of cells and uniformly distributed Wright's or Wright-Giemsa stain. Though these basic requirements seem rather obvious, they can be easily forgotten in the laboratory, which can lead to inaccurate differential counts.

The area behind the feather edge of the blood film is the site of accurate counting. In this area, the red cells should show typical central pallor without being clumped. The smear is examined in a logical pattern, moving from one edge to another. Typically, 100 consecutive white blood cells are identified and classified by the morphologic reviewer. Other morphologic abnormalities are also noted during this process.

It is important to realize the statistical impact that a 100-cell count has on overall differential accuracy. The greater the number of cells counted, the greater the statistical precision of a differential count. Table 34.7 illustrates the 95% confidence interval limits for various blood cell percentages as determined by the total cell count obtained. Basically, the fewer cells that are counted, the less precise the blood cell percentage is. This is especially true with the cells that account for relatively lower percentages, as would be seen with neutrophil bands, monocytes, eosinophils, and basophils. For example, a band count of 5% obtained at one time would not represent a statistically significant change in the percentage of bands compared to a 10% count the following day if a 100-cell differential count is performed. This can be contrasted to obtaining either a 500- or 1000-cell differential count in which a change from 5% to 10% would be considered statistically significant. In addition to this statistical variation dependent on total cell counts obtained, one cannot forget the large number of errors that can result from inadequately collected or processed blood samples, poor-quality blood films, inconsistent staining, or judgmental errors by the technologist or physician performing the differential count. All of these components emphasize the deficiencies of the manual differential count. Thus, the historical reliance of the manual differential count as the gold standard of the hematology laboratory must be viewed skeptically, considering the major sources of error that can potentially contribute to the determination of the differential leukocyte count.

Because of the significant limitations of the differential leukocyte count, the clinical hematology laboratory has incorporated the use of numerous instruments with the capability to perform differential leukocyte counts. Two basic methodologies have been used as automated differential counters in the clinical laboratory. These include digital image analysis systems based on cell recognition from a stained blood smear and the determination of different leukocyte cellular characteristics that permit separation into subtypes by using various flow-cell related techniques. This latter methodology has become the standard in automated differential counts and is

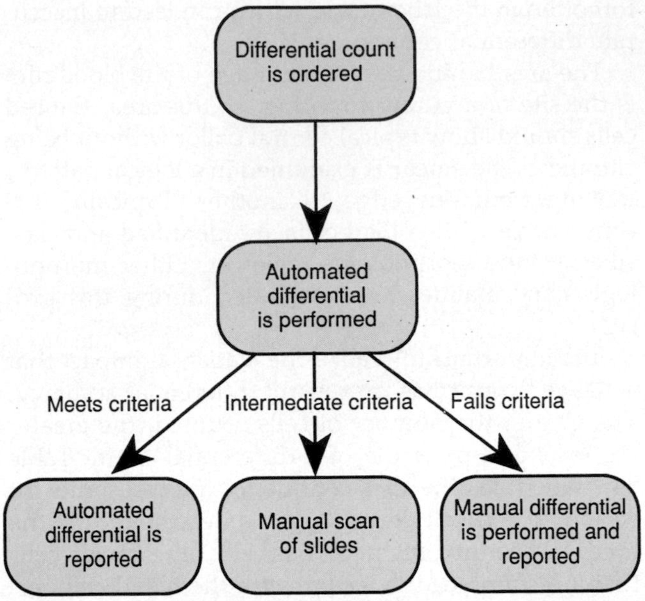

Figure 34.5. Schematic drawing showing the laboratory logistics of incorporating automated leukocyte differential counts, manual differential counts, and slide scanning.

based on the use of either electrical impedance or light-scattering techniques.

Automated differential leukocyte counts as performed by modern hematology analyzers are more accurate, more precise, more economical, faster, and safer than traditional manual differential counts. Although the goal of any automated differential leukocyte counting system is to replace the manual differential count, this has not been fully accomplished in the clinical laboratory. The automated differential leukocyte count is superior to the manual differential count in many aspects, but in some cases it fails to provide important morphologic detail that only the manual differential/review can provide. For example, red cell morphologic findings, categorization of immature granulocytes, and recognition of intracellular or extracellular organisms (for example, malaria) can be accurately identified only on a manual smear. Thus, all modern clinical hematology laboratories have to deal with the question of how an automated differential leukocyte count can be incorporated into the routine practice of that particular laboratory.

Most laboratorians would agree that the initial differential count on every patient, whether hospitalized or ambulatory, should be performed by automated methods. The key to successful implementation is based on the ability of the instrument to recognize both quantitative and qualitative abnormalities and to "flag" particular cases for further review. These flagged results may then lead to either a manual differential count or at least a manual review of the stained blood smear. Figure 34.5 demonstrates an approach to incorporating automated differential counts with manual reviews to best meet the patient's needs while still maintaining appropriate utilization of laboratory resources. It is the ability to recognize these qualitative abnormalities that determines the success of an automated differential count in a particular laboratory. The laboratorian must expect a false-negative rate that approaches "0%," while enduring a false:positive rate that is not too high. Obviously, the kinds of patients evaluated by a clinical hematology laboratory and the overall percentage of "abnormal differential counts" will also influence the degree of success of the automated differential. Thus, the type of instrument, the flagging criteria chosen, and the patient population served by the laboratory will determine the role of automated differential counts.

A wide variety of hematology analyzers are available for the clinical laboratory. Each one approaches the issue of automated differentials in slightly different ways, but all use a single-cell "flow" apparatus that allows for interrogation of each individual cell for a variety of potential characteristics. These characteristics permit separation of the various cell types. Technicon's H6000, H1, and H2 analyzers are basically flow cytometers that use myeloperoxidase cytochemistry coupled with light-scattering characteristics. Others, including Coulter's STKS, and TOA's Sysmex NE8000, use a combination of electrical impedance, low-frequency conductivity, and light-scattering characteristics to categorize white cells. Other newer analyzers, including the Cobas Argos 5 Diff by Roche, uses electrical impedance, cytochemistry, and optical absorbance, and the Cel-Dyn 3000 from Abbott uses a complex multiangle light-scattering technology to categorize white cells. As mentioned previously, image analysis–based systems have not survived their initial introduction and are no longer being actively marketed to the clinical laboratories.

The blood cell histograms as produced by the modern automated hematology analyzers provide a wealth of information about the CBC and differential count. However, these scattergrams and histograms have not gained popularity among clinicians for various reasons. It is neither important nor necessary for clinicians to routinely review these histograms, but laboratorians may find the histograms invaluable for quality control purposes as well as for evaluating difficult diagnostic cases and recognizing problem cases that need further review. Figure 34.6 provides examples of histograms from the Coulter STKS automated analyzer and depicts the typical distribution of the various peripheral blood components.

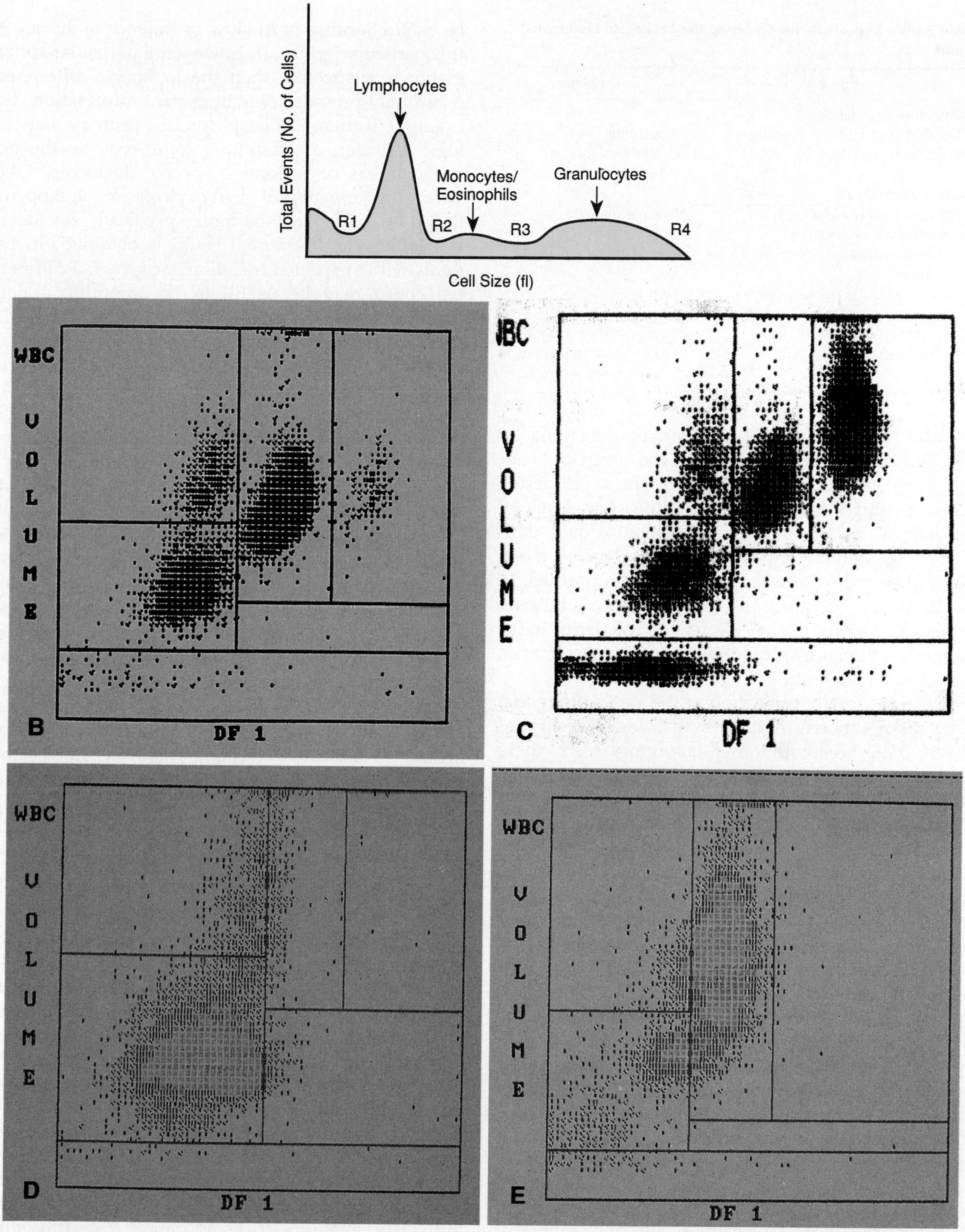

Figure 34.6. Blood cell histograms (Coulter STKS). **A**, Example of a WBC differential histogram based on volumetric studies. The various components of the WBC are shown on the graph. R_1 to R_4 correspond to flags generated by the instrument representing distribution abnormalities warranting manual observation. R_1, nucleated RBC, platelet clumps, large platelets, cryoglobulin, small lymphocytes, unlysed RBC; R_2, reactive lymphocytes, lymphoblasts, basophils, clotted sample; R_3, eosinophilia, monocytosis, blasts, clotted sample; R_4, granulocytosis. **B**, STKS—normal differential; **C**, STKS histogram—eosinophil (52%); **D**, STKS histogram—chronic lymphocytic leukemia; **E**, STKS histogram—acute myelogenous leukemia.

Table 34.8. Indications for Ordering the Leukocyte Differential Count

Indication	Usefulness
Ambulatory Population	
General population (screening)	Not useful
Specific subgroups	Possibly useful (see below)
Hospital Population	
No abnormality suspected	Not useful
Abnormality suspected	
Newly suspected infection or new fever	Useful in some patients
Suspicion of a primary hematologic disorder	Useful
Leukocytosis or leukopenia	Useful in some patients
Repeat tests	Useful in some patients at appropriate intervals

Additional parameters that can be generated by the Technicon analyzers include the mean peroxidase index, which is a measure of the myeloperoxidase staining intensity of neutrophils. Low levels of peroxidase index indicate a myeloperoxidase deficiency; the clinical importance of an elevated mean peroxidase index, however, has not been clarified. In addition, the Technicon also determines a lobularity index for neutrophils. A decreased lobularity index suggests less neutrophil lobulation and, therefore, a granulocytic "left shift."

The appropriate utilization of the WBC differential is a serious concern for most hematology laboratories (Table 34.8). As with other laboratory tests, there should be different criteria for ordering differential leukocyte counts for ambulatory patients as opposed to hospitalized patients. There is sufficient evidence to indicate that the leukocyte differential count is not useful in the routine screening of ambulatory patients. Since the prevalence of hematologically manifested disease is low in this group of patients, significant clinical disease is typically not identified from the differential count unless it has also been suspected on other clinical grounds. Even when differential counts outside the "normal range" are identified in the ambulatory population, only rarely is a specific disease process diagnosed. Therefore, in the outpatient group, a differential leukocyte count should be performed only in patients in whom the information may provide important diagnostic, prognostic, or therapeutic decisions.

In hospitalized patients, there are many clinical situations in which an abnormal differential count will correlate with a particular clinically important disease. Subsequent sections of this chapter outline the clinical situations associated with either cytopenias or cytoses of particular leukocyte components. As in the outpatient group, if no abnormality is suspected, a leukocyte differential count will not be useful because of the low prevalence of disease in this particular group. If, however, a particular abnormality is suspected, then the leukocyte differential count may provide some important information. For example, if there is a suspicion of a primary hematologic disorder, a differential count may be the primary means of making a specific diagnosis. Likewise, an unexpected leukocytosis or leukopenia found on a CBC may be more specifically elucidated if a leukocyte differential count is obtained. In patients with suspected infections or fevers, a differential count may be useful in documenting a neutrophilia if other data are inconclusive. It typically does not contribute diagnostic information if a leukocytosis has already been identified on a CBC, thus indicating a reactive process. Conversely, the differential count is seldom abnormal if the total leukocyte count is normal, even if there is an ongoing infectious process. Thus, it should be recognized that a normal WBC and differential count does not exclude the possibility of an infectious process.

A larger question that remains is the frequency at which to repeat a differential leukocyte count in hospitalized patients. A repetitive test may have diagnostic value if an infection has not shown improvement or if new symptoms evolve that are suspicious of either an infectious or hematologic disorder. Certainly, if management decisions are based on differential counts, for example, in a leukopenic or hematologic patient, then appropriate repetitive testing would be indicated. Overall, there has not been a consensus as to the appropriate testing interval for the differential count, but it would appear unlikely that daily differential counts in nonleukopenic patients would be indicated.

Platelet Count

A platelet count provides the starting point in the functional evaluation of the hemostatic system. An abnormality in the platelet count can lead to significant bleeding complications in a patient and may be indicative of a variety of underlying malignant or nonmalignant conditions. A diminished platelet count may be the result of either a marrow production problem or a peripheral destructive process. In cases in which megakaryopoiesis is decreased and platelet production diminished, evaluation of the bone marrow may reveal an infiltrative malignant process, whether metastatic or hematologic in nature. Also, various drugs and some viral infections may lead to a reduction in platelet production. In patients receiving chemotherapeutic regimens, platelets are commonly diminished to very low levels. Peripheral destructive processes of platelets are common and are frequently entertained as part of a differen-

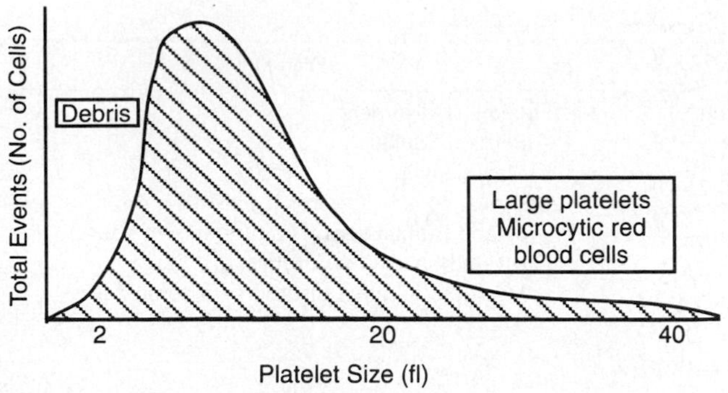

Figure 34.7. Platelet distribution histogram from 2 to 40 fl. The left portion of the curve may be contaminated with debris; the right portion of the curve may be contaminated with large platelets and microcytic red blood cells.

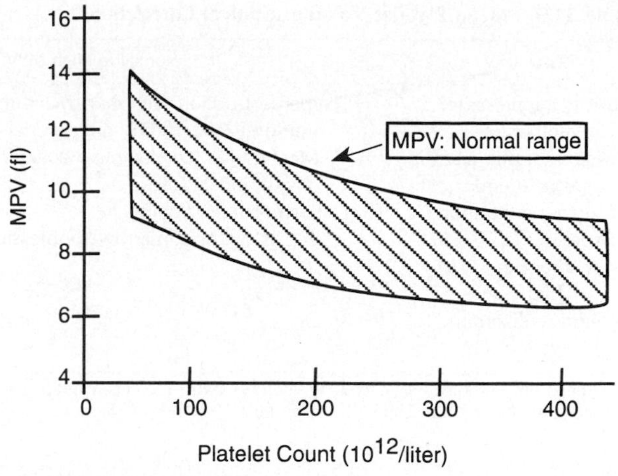

Figure 34.8. Mean platelet volume (MPV). The MPV varies inversely with total platelet count. Those samples having MPV values above the normal range for their total platelet count represent cases with adequate marrow production and, therefore, thrombocytopenia due to peripheral destructive processes. Those samples with MPV values below the normal range for their total platelet count represent cases with probable marrow suppression and diminished platelet production.

tial diagnosis. These are primarily immune-based thrombocytopenias, but may occasionally involve splenic sequestration of platelets. Further discussion of the role of platelets in hemostasis is included in Section VIII of this book, Coagulation. This chapter does not deal with the variety of platelet assays that are used to evaluate the bleeding patient. Rather, the laboratory's analysis of the total platelet count as obtained from hematology analyzers is described here.

EDTA is the preferred anticoagulant for platelet analysis and must be mixed thoroughly with the blood to avoid clotting and platelet clumping. If clotting does occur, a spuriously decreased platelet count may result. As discussed previously, in individuals with EDTA-dependent platelet agglutinin, citrate is the preferred alternative anticoagulant.

Today's automated hematology analyzers routinely obtain platelet counts over a wide range of values. However, manual hemacytometer counts are still essential in cases that have low platelet counts; for example, those cases with less than 50.0×10^9 platelets. Various red and white blood cells, platelet, and instrument artifacts may interfere with platelet counting. Newer instrumentation enhancements such as hydrodynamic focusing and pulse editing have helped to eliminate some of the crossover abnormalities seen between red cells and platelets. Some instruments, such as those manufactured by Coulter, count platelets within a particular size range—for example, 2 to 20 fl—to eliminate any possible interference by red blood cells (Fig. 34.7). The instrument's computer then fits the results to a log-normal curve and extrapolates the curve to cover the normal range of platelet size of 0 to 70 fl.

Artifacts that can specifically interfere with platelet counting include red or white blood cell fragments/debris or electronic noise that can be found at the low end of platelet distribution. Interfering microcytic red blood cells or giant platelets may skew the distribution curve to the right. Platelet clumping is the most common cause of mistaken thrombocytopenia in the automated laboratory. Clumps of platelets will look to the instrument like large, single platelets or even white blood cells and will usually be excluded from the platelet distribution curve. In such cases, phase microscopy is necessary to obtain an accurate platelet count.

Some instruments will also calculate mean platelet volumes (MPVs). The MPVs represent the mean volume (size) of platelets as determined by the platelet distribution histogram. Some studies have indicated that the presence of large platelets, i.e., those with a high MPV, is suggestive of younger platelets that are found in peripheral destructive processes such as immune thrombocytopenias. The MPV may falsely increase or decrease with EDTA anticoagulation and therefore must be interpreted with caution. This inconsistency has limited its routine use. As discussed in the previous platelet section, the MPV will be unreliable if cytoplasmic fragments, electronic noise, giant platelets, or microcytic red blood cells artifactually interfere with platelet determination. Figure 34.8 demonstrates that the typical reference range of the MPV is inversely related to the platelet count. In other words, as the platelet count decreases, the MPV typically increases. The MPV is found to be high in patients with thrombocytopenia due to ITP and other peripheral destructive processes, while patients with thrombocytopenia due to marrow suppression typically have decreased MPV values (Table 34.9). In spite of these possible uses, the clinical value of the MPV has not been clearly elucidated and must not be looked upon as a gold standard in the evaluation of the thrombocytopenic patient.

Table 34.9. Mean Platelet Volume: Clinical Correlations[a]

Low MPV	Normal to High MPV	High MPV
Marrow suppression Chemotherapy Megaloblastic anemia Aplastic anemia Marrow infiltration Sepsis Hypersplenism (variable) Hereditary disorders Wiscott-Aldrich	Hyperdestruction with marrow compensation Immune-related (ITP, drug-induced) Mechanical (consumptive coagulopathies, vasculitis) Hemorrhage (major) Sepsis (without marrow suppression)	Hereditary disorders Bernard-Soulier May-Hegglin Miscellaneous α- and β-thalassemia trait (unknown cause) Myelodysplastic syndrome Myeloproliferative disorders (in some cases)

[a]Modified from Cornbleet PJ, Astanita R, Wolf PL. White blood cell and platelet disorders. In: Howanitz JH, Howanitz PJ, eds. Laboratory medicine—test selection and interpretation. New York: Churchill Livingstone, 1991:553–618.

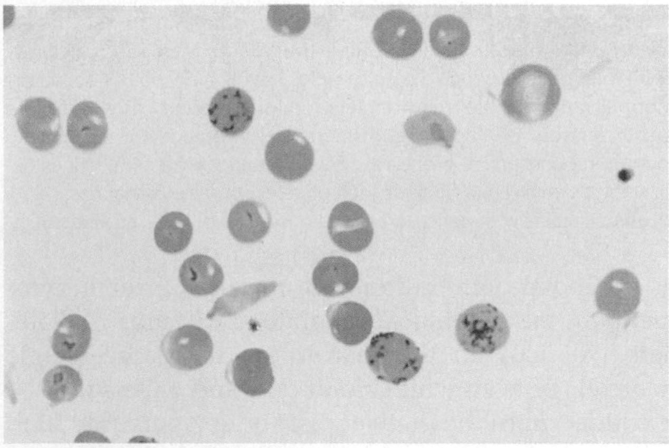

Figure 34.9. Peripheral blood smear with reticulocytes; staining is with new methylene blue dye. The blue granules represent precipitated, residual RNA.

Reticulocyte Count

A reticulocyte can be broadly defined as an erythrocyte that still contains residual ribosomes and organelles, but has ejected its nucleus from the previous orthochromatic erythroblast stage. Reticulocytes may take on a variety of morphologic appearances depending on the amount of residual ribosomes and organelles, or "reticulum" (hence, the term reticulocyte). The definition of a reticulocyte from a technologist's perspective has classically been described as an erythrocyte containing a few (two or three) scattered "dots." Although this may describe the majority of circulating reticulocytes, it may rarely appear as diffusely granular cells. The life span of a reticulocyte has been estimated to be 3 to 4 days, but probably only 24 hours of it is spent in the peripheral circulation. Clinically, the reticulocyte percentage can be used as an indicator of erythropoiesis and is often utilized for evaluating patients with anemia. Although reticulocyte counts do not absolutely correlate with bone marrow erythroid activity, the ease of obtaining and performing such a count has led to its common usage as a marker of red cell production. A normal or decreased reticulocyte count in the face of a moderate to marked anemia is strong evidence that the bone marrow is not responding in an appropriate fashion, as would be seen in iron, folate, or vitamin B_{12} deficiency, or as a result of a bone marrow infiltrative process. In contrast, an increased reticulocyte count generally reflects a rapid erythroid turnover, as would be seen in acute blood loss or acute or chronic hemolysis. In other words, the reticulocyte level can be used as a general indicator of bone marrow erythropoiesis and release.

Most current laboratory microscopic methods make the reticulocyte visible by precipitating the residual ribosomal RNA material with a dye such as new methylene blue or brilliant creosol blue; the precipitated RNA (or reticulum) will form small clumps that will stain with the dye and be visible as blue cytoplasmic dots or filaments (Fig. 34.9). Usually, a 1000-erythrocyte count is performed manually through the microscope and the percentage of stained red blood cells derived. This manual determination of reticulocyte counts is a very imprecise method and is open to subjective interpretation by the technologist. The imprecision and inaccuracy of reticulocyte counts have been well documented in several studies, with coefficients of variation ranging from 25% to over 50%. These inaccuracies are probably related to (*a*) sampling error; (*b*) interobserver bias; (*c*) supervital staining of other cytoplasmic elements, such as nuclear debris, sidersomes, Heinz bodies, etc.; and (*d*) variation in the quality of the smear and stain.

Automated reticulocyte counting methods, such as image analysis and flow cytometry, have gained respectability and use in the clinical laboratories. Both these procedures remove much of the subjective interpretation involved in manual reticulocyte counting, allow for evaluating large numbers of red blood cells to avoid sampling error, and provide for a standard and uniform analysis. Flow cytometric procedures depend on the binding of a suitable fluorescent dye to residual erythrocyte RNA. Although numerous dyes have been developed that accomplish RNA binding, not all have been successful in meeting the laboratory requirements for reticulocyte counting. To date, auramine O and thiazole orange are probably the two preferred fluorescent dyes for reticulocyte counting. Studies with both of these fluorescent dyes have shown good to excellent correlation with results obtained from manual counts of cells and have consistently shown a tight reproducibility with duplicate samples. Flow cytometric detection methods offer many advantages over manual counting methods and will undoubtedly become the method of choice for reticulocyte analysis. Improved fluorescent dyes and increasing automation will continue to promote this transition.

Erythrocyte Sedimentation Rate

The erythrocyte sedimentation rate (ESR) is one of the time-honored traditional tests in the hematology laboratory that has perhaps garnered too much importance in the clinical laboratory. In the laboratory, the ESR measures the distance a red blood cell falls in a vertical tube over a given period of time. The principle behind this process is the increased negative charge that the various inflammatory proteins (fibrinogen, α-, β-, and γ-globins) exact on the surrounding red blood cells. This promotes red blood cell separation and thus a more rapid fall of the red blood cell in the analysis tube. The resulting higher "stack" of measured red blood cells is interpreted as an elevated ESR.

Specimen collection and the anticoagulant used are crucial in the determination of the ESR. The Westergren method (3) has become the standard procedure for determining the ESR. In this procedure, the blood specimen is anticoagulated with sodium citrate and placed in a 30-cm glass tube with a 2.5-mm internal diameter. The modified Westergren procedure uses EDTA as the anticoagulant and may be the easiest method to use in the hematology laboratory because such samples can be used routinely for other hematologic parameters. The EDTA tube must be full and used within 2 hours if kept at room temperature; refrigerated samples may keep for up to 12 hours if warmed before analysis.

The Wintrobe method (4) has also historically been a popular method for ESR determination. The Wintrobe method also uses EDTA blood, but requires only 1 ml (as opposed to 2 ml of blood with the Westergren procedure), uses a shorter but wider diameter tube than with the Westergren procedure, and may be preferred in the pediatric population due to the decreased amount of blood that is required.

Various factors, both clinical well as laboratory-based, are known to disrupt the ESR. A slightly tilted ESR tube, high room temperature, or the use of heparin as an anticoagulant are all known to increase the ESR level. Conversely, a clotted blood sample, low room temperature, too short an ESR tube, or prolonged delay (longer than 2 hours if at room temperature) in analysis may all lead to a false decrease in ESR values. Clinical factors may also complicate the interpretation of the ESR. Anemia, hypercholesterolemia, chronic renal failure, as well as inflammatory disease may all produce an elevated ESR. Conversely, fragmented red blood cells (e.g., sickle cell anemia, burn patients), spherocytes, microcytic red blood cells, steroids, hypofibrinogenemia, and other miscellaneous entities may all lead to a decrease in the ESR value.

Clinically, an elevated ESR has been used as evidence for an inflammatory process. However, false-positive and false-negative results abound, and a wasteful hunt for a nonexistent underlying condition could result if only the ESR is relied on. The only consistent diagnostic use for the ESR, albeit begrudgingly, is in the diagnosis and monitoring of temporal arteritis and polymyalgia rheumatica. What then would constitute a valid indication for requesting an ESR? As with most laboratory tests, the ESR should not be used as a screening device in the healthy, asymptomatic population. No study has shown a significant contribution of an elevated ESR in detecting unsuspected disease in the asymptomatic patient. In the symptomatic patient, interpretation of ESR is complicated by the numerous factors that can lead to falsely elevated or falsely decreased values. Physicians often obtain an ESR in patients whose history and physical findings do not suggest any specific cause for their illness. Several studies have shown that ESR is not useful in those patients, such as in those for whom a diagnosis of a specific disease is not confirmed by other clinical data. In general, the ESR must be markedly elevated in such patients to be diagnostically useful, which is an exceedingly rare event in patients with no clear evidence of serious disease. A subsequent ESR in several months is the first step in evaluating an initial ESR elevation, rather than the physician instituting an extensive hunt for occult disease.

As previously indicated, the ESR is almost always increased in patients with temporal arteritis and polymyalgia rheumatica, and a normal ESR virtually excludes the diagnosis of temporal arteritis. The ESR may be useful in distinguishing inflammatory arthritic processes from other causes of joint symptoms, such as osteoarthritis. However, it is neither absolutely specific nor sensitive for rheumatoid arthritis and must be interpreted with great caution and obviously in conjunction with other clinical and laboratory findings. Some studies have also suggested the role of ESR as an indicator of Hodgkin's disease, and studies suggest a possible role as a marker for relapse of disease. Patients with a markedly elevated ESR above 100 mm/hr almost always have underlying malignancy, acute infection, or some type of connective tissue disease. However, unexplained elevations in ESR less than this level probably do not warrant evaluation and most do not have any associated disease process.

In summary, the ESR is a laboratory test that has remained essentially unchanged over its 75-year laboratory history. As such, its role in clinical diagnosis should be tempered with the reality that it is associated with numerous false-positive and false-negative results. A more judicial use of this "screening" test is definitely warranted.

BONE MARROW EXAMINATION

Components

Examination of the bone marrow ideally consists of evaluating three major components (Table 34.10): (*a*) the peripheral blood; (*b*) the bone marrow aspirate smear; and (*c*) a bone marrow tissue section (trephine biopsy and/or aspirate clot). Not all three components may contribute to a diagnosis in a given case, but each may potentially provide important diagnostic information and must be a part of the total examination process. Examination of the peripheral blood includes reviewing the CBC, differential count, reticulocyte percentage, and blood smear morphology. The bone marrow aspirate provides useful information for various studies, including (*a*) morphology and cytochemical stains; (*b*) flow cytometric immunophenotyping; (*c*) cytogenetic analysis; (*d*) molecular biological studies; and (*e*) microbiological studies, if needed. Bone marrow tissue sections provide important information regarding the overall cellular distribution and marrow architecture and may consist of either a decalcified trephine biopsy or a clotted aspirate specimen (Fig. 34.10). Miscellaneous laboratory studies are also essential in interpreting a bone marrow study. These may include studies to evaluate red cell problems such as iron studies, B_{12}/folate levels, hemoglobin electrophoresis, and Coomb's test; LDH, serum/urine immunoelectrophoresis, microbiological or virologic culture results, and other pertinent laboratory tests that may also provide important laboratory data needed to properly evaluate a bone marrow study.

Table 34.10. Bone Marrow Examination

Peripheral Blood
CBC
Differential count
Reticulocyte count
Blood smear morphology
Bone Marrow Aspirate
Morphology
Cytochemical stains
Flow cytometric immunophenotyping
Cytogenetic analysis
Molecular biological studies
Bone Marrow Tissue Section
Trephine biopsy
Clot section
Laboratory Studies—Miscellaneous
Iron studies
B_{12}/folate
Hemoglobin electrophoresis
Immunoelectrophoresis
LDH
Coomb's test
Microbiology culture/serology results
Miscellaneous

Indications for Bone Marrow Evaluation

Indications for examining a bone marrow are outlined in Table 34.11. The most common reason is for the evaluation of a known or suspected malignancy. A bone marrow study is definitely mandated if a hematologic malignancy is suspected. This suspicion may arise from either clinical or physical examination findings (e.g., splenomegaly or lymphadenopathy) or if abnormal or immature circulating cells are found in the peripheral blood smear. The bone marrow may also be involved in metastatic malignancies of nonhematopoietic origin. Evaluation of patients with either non-Hodgkin's lymphomas or Hodgkin's disease usually indicates that a bone marrow study be performed to adequately stage the patient for the presence of lymphoma. Bone marrow studies are also essential in monitoring the effect of therapy for patients with hematologic malignancies, as well as monitoring the effectiveness of bone marrow transplantation.

In nonspecialized institutions and practices, bone marrow studies are frequently required to evaluate patients with unexplained cytopenias. Patients who have unexplained thrombocytopenias or neutropenias can benefit by having a bone marrow aspirate and biopsy performed to fully evaluate whether the cytopenia is a reflection of decreased marrow production or, by inference, increased peripheral destruction. Bone marrow studies for the evaluation of an anemia are not indicated as a primary procedure unless other clinical, peripheral blood morphology, and biochemical studies have failed to reveal the etiology of the anemia. Other indications for a bone marrow biopsy include obtaining tissue for culture in patients with fever of unknown origin.

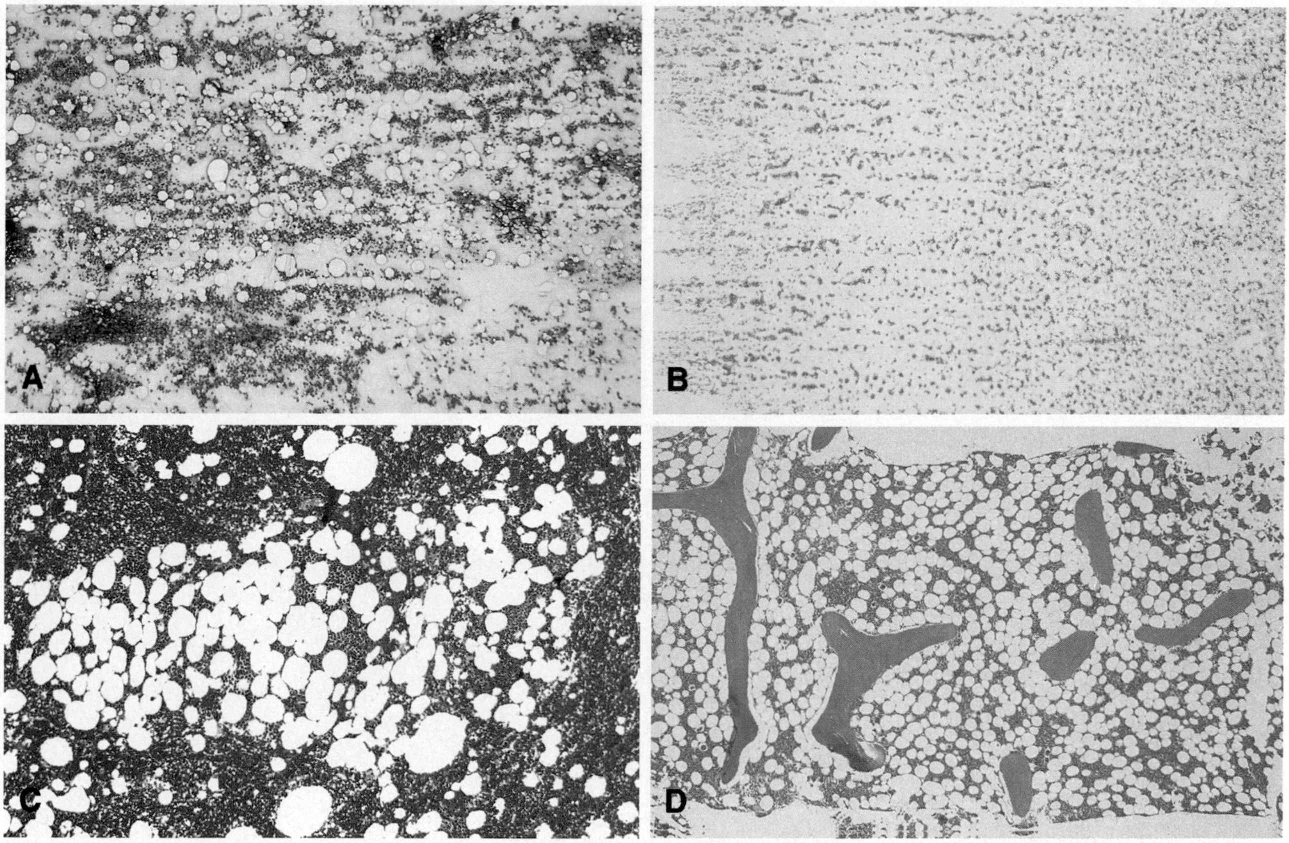

Figure 34.10. Examples of bone marrow preparation samples. **A**, Bone marrow aspirate spicule; **B**, Bone marrow aspirate buffy coat smear; **C**, Bone marrow aspirate clot section, fixed in formalin; **D**, Bone marrow biopsy section, fixed in B5-fixative.

Table 34.11. Indication for Bone Marrow Evaluation

Evaluation for Malignancy
Primary hematologic disorder
Staging for Hodgkin's disease
Staging for non-Hodgkin's lymphoma
Metastatic tumor (nonhematopoietic)
Monitoring Therapy
Postchemotherapy
Postbone marrow transplantation
Evaluation of Cytopenias
Marrow production problem
Peripheral destruction
Inadequate/ineffective marrow release
Miscellaneous
Culture (fever of unknown origin)

Interpretation of Bone Marrow Studies

Bone marrow cellularity is best determined on the bone marrow tissue sections but can be estimated from the bone marrow aspirate smear. Marrow cellularity varies with age and is expressed as an estimate of the percentage of the bone marrow area occupied by cells to the total area of cells plus background elements and fat. The normal cellularity decreases with age and for a newborn is approximately 75 to 100%, 50 to 90% in the adolescent, 30 to 80% in the adult, and 20 to 50% in the elderly (over age 65) (Fig. 34.11). Determination of cellularity is useful when evaluating patients with unexplained cytopenias; for example, increased cellularity in a patient with a cytopenia would suggest ineffective hematopoiesis (i.e., decreased cellular release) or increased peripheral destruction (Fig. 34.12). In contrast, decreased cellularity in an individual with a particular cytopenia would suggest a marrow production problem (Fig. 34.12).

The next step in evaluating a bone marrow is determining the distribution of cells within the marrow. The adequacy of megakaryocyte production is easily estimated by evaluating either the marrow biopsy, aspirate clot sections, or an aspirate spicule. Typically, one to two megakaryocytes can be seen on a 40× or 50× objective field. The determination of increased or decreased numbers of megakaryocytes relative to the overall platelet count can suggest that a production or destruction problem may exist.

The next step in the evaluation of a marrow is assessing myeloid and erythroid development both quantitatively and qualitatively. There should be a normal distribution of all cell types within each of the granulocytic and erythroid lines, indicating a normal maturational process. A 500-cell differential count of the bone marrow aspirate is useful in quantifying the

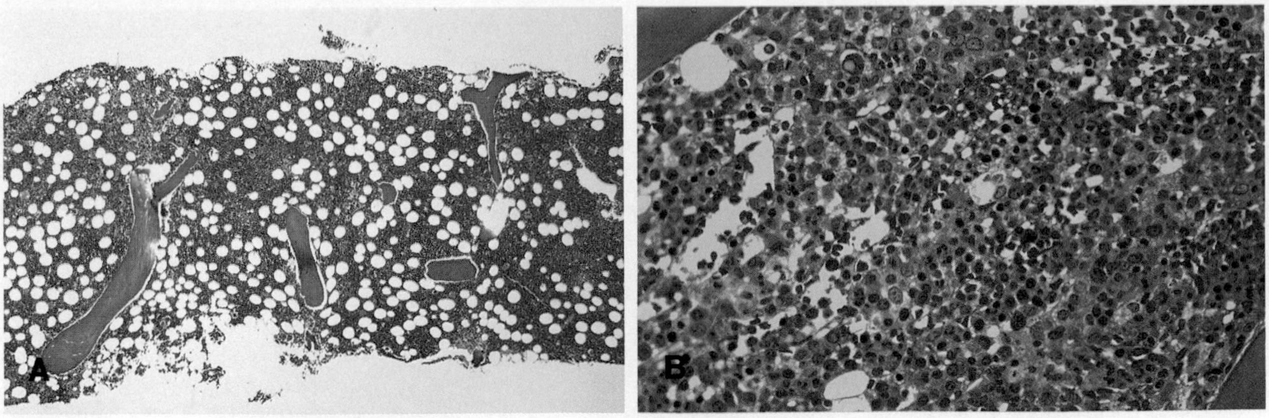

Figure 34.11. Bone marrow biopsy sections demonstrating normal cellularity. **A**, Approximately 40 to 50% cellularity in an otherwise healthy 60-year-old male; **B**, Virtually 100% cellular marrow from a newborn boy.

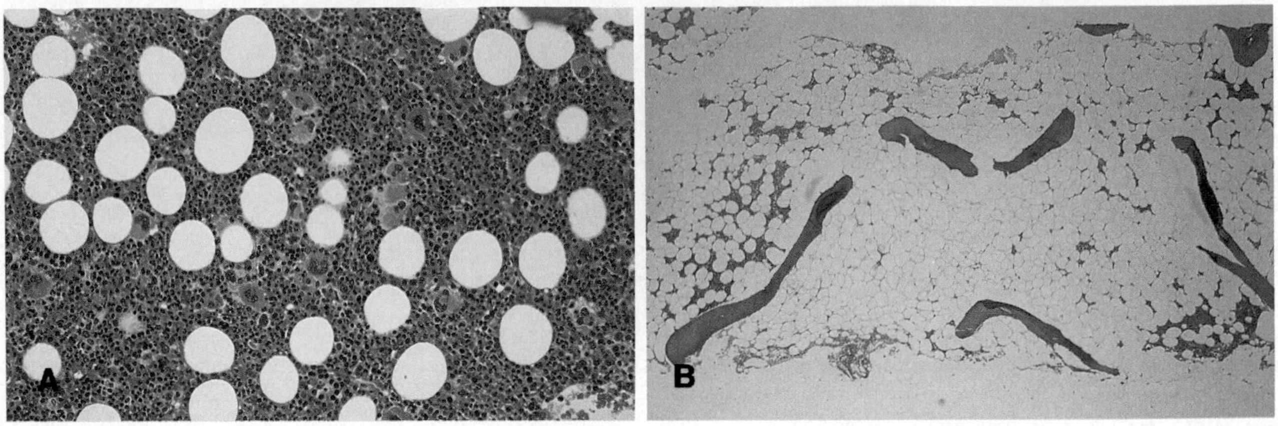

Figure 34.12. Bone marrow biopsy sections. **A**, Megakaryocytic hypercellularity from an individual with immune thromobocytopenia purpura; bone marrow from an individual with granulocytic hyperplasia due to Kostman's syndrome; **B**, Markedly hypocellular bone marrow following chemotherapy in an individual with acute lymphoblastic leukemia.

amount of granulocytic and erythroid precursors within the marrow (Table 34.12). This myeloid-to-erythroid (M:E) ratio ranges from 2:1 to 4:1 in the adult and is useful in determining whether there are relative hyper- or hypoplasias. Again, this may provide useful information in evaluating a patient with a neutropenia or anemia. In addition to quantitative abnormalities, qualitative abnormalities of myeloid development must also be assessed. Dysplastic changes in erythroid or granulocytic cells is not an uncommon finding and must be looked for when evaluating a bone marrow aspirate.

Other cell types and lesions may be identified within the bone marrow and must be assessed including the presence or absence of granuloma, necrosis, lymphoma, metastatic neoplasia, bone marrow fibrosis, lipid storage disease, benign lymphoid aggregates, and bone abnormalities such as osteosclerosis and osteoporosis. Also, a Prussian blue iron stain of the bone marrow aspirate and/or tissue section can provide useful information concerning a patient's iron stores (Fig. 34.13). Iron stains of a bone marrow trephine biopsy must be interpreted with caution. A decalcification may cause a false-negative interpretation; evaluation of the clot section for iron stores is probably superior to the trephine biopsy. In addition to iron stores, iron stains of the bone marrow aspirate smear need to be evaluated for the presence or absence of sideroblasts and, in particular, ringed sideroblasts (Fig. 34.13); detection of sideroblastic iron cannot be reliably assessed on tissue section stains.

REACTIVE DISORDERS

Disorders of white blood cells include both malignant and nonmalignant diseases. The nonmalignant disorders of white blood cells may consist of quantitative abnormalities leading to an increase or decrease of a particular WBC component, benign morphologic changes that have little if any effect on cellular function, and true functional disorders of a

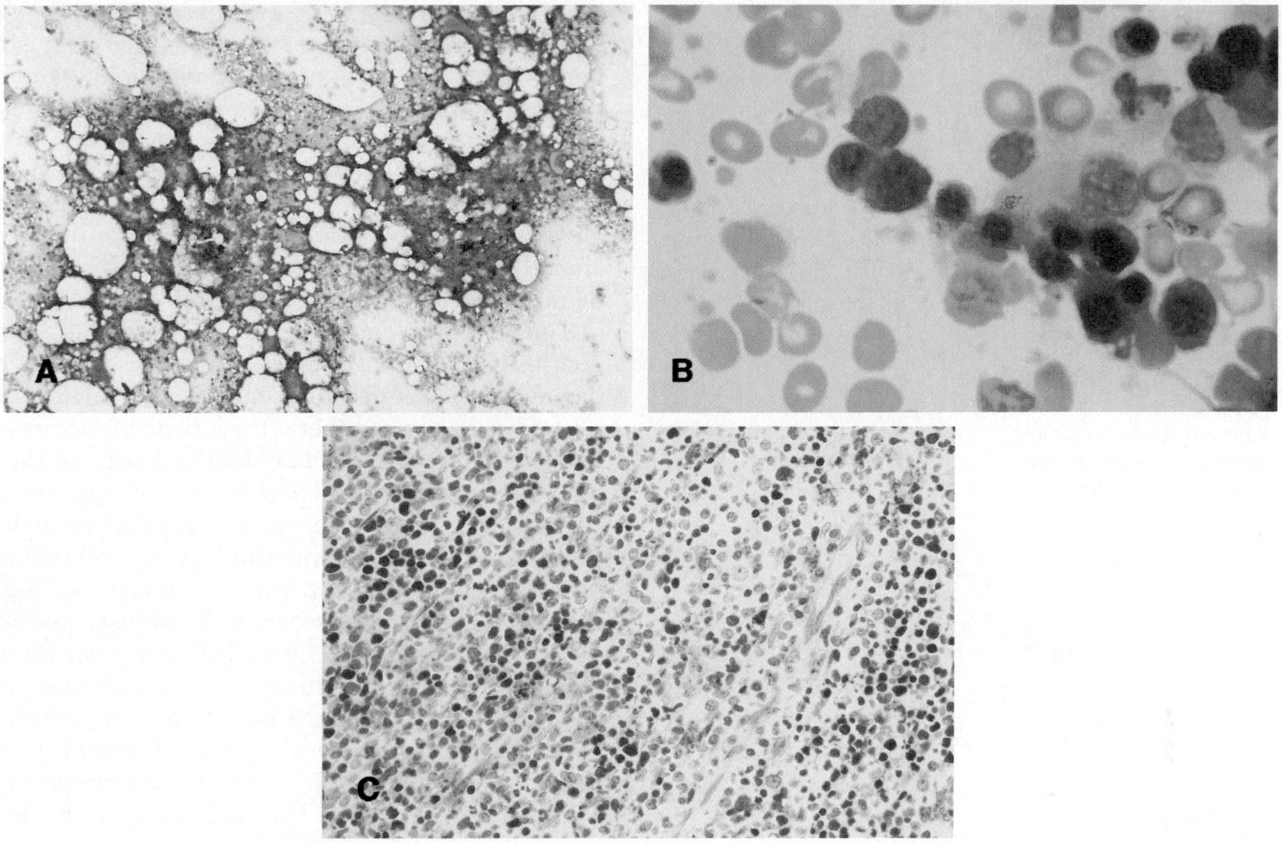

Figure 34.13. Iron stains of bone marrow. **A**, Bone marrow aspirate spicule showing iron stores; **B**, Bone marrow aspirate smear showing sideroblastic iron. Note the small green granules present in the cytoplasm; **C**, Bone marrow aspirate clot section showing iron stores.

Table 34.12. Bone Marrow Differential Cell Counts: Normal Values[a]

Bone Marrow Cells	Childhood	Adult
	(%)	(%)
Normoblasts (total)	23.1	21.5 (14.2–30.4)
Pronormoblasts	0.5 (0.0–1.5)	0.6 (0.2–1.4)
Basophilic	1.7 (0.2–4.8)	2.0 (0.7–3.7)
Polychromatophilic	18.2 (4.8–34.0)	12.4 (12.2–24.2)
Orthochromatic	2.7 (0.0–7.8)	6.5 (2.0–22.7)
Granulocytes (total)	57.1	56.0 (45.1–66.5)
Myeloblasts	1.2 (0.0–3.2)	1.0 (0.5–1.8)
Promyelocytes	1.4 (0.0–4.0)	3.4 (2.6–4.6)
Myelocytes	18.3 (8.5–29.7)	11.9 (8.1–16.9)
Metamyelocytes	23.3 (14.0–34.2)	18.0 (9.8–25.3)
Bands	?	11.0 (8.5–20.8)
Segmented	12.9 (4.5–29.0)	10.7 (8.0–16.0)
Lymphocytes	16.0 (4.8–35.8)	15.8 (10.8–22.7)
Monocytes		1.8 (0.2–2.8)
Eosinophils	3.6 (1.0–9.0)	3.2 (1.2–6.2)
Basophils	0.06 (0.0–0.8)	<0.1 (0.0–0.2)
Plasma cells	0.4 (0.2–0.6)	1.8 (0.2–2.2)
M:E ratio	2.9 (1.2–5.2)	2.5 (1.2–5.0)

[a]Data are from Mauer AM. Pediatric hematology. New York: McGraw-Hill, 1969; and Jandl JH. Blood—textbook of hematology. Boston: Little, Brown & Co., 1987.

white blood cell type that may lead to significant patient morbidity and mortality. Although the peripheral blood is obviously the easiest vehicle by which to evaluate these nonmalignant abnormalities, the effects of these changes are truly reflected in the tissues in which they circulate, for example, lymph nodes, spleen, or any other organ.

Neutrophilia

Neutrophils play an important role in the inflammatory response and are the primary cells involved in phagocytosis of foreign organisms. The number of circulating neutrophils is determined by multiple factors, including the rate of bone marrow production, the speed at which cells leave the marrow and enter the peripheral circulation, and changes in vascular margination. Clinical findings associated with neutrophilia are listed in Table 34.13. The most commonly encountered reason for neutrophilia is an acute bacterial infection. Other frequent causes include an inflammatory response to necrotic tissue (e.g., tumor necrosis), drugs (such as corticosteroids), and acute hemorrhagic episodes.

Morphologic changes in neutrophils associated with acute infection include a shift toward the release of immature granulocytes (i.e., shift to the left), toxic granulation, Döhle bodies, and cytoplasmic vacuolation (Fig. 34.14). The left shift seen in patients with

Table 34.13. Disorders Associated with Neutrophilia

Physiological Neutrophilia
Neonates
Third-trimester pregnancy
Labor and delivery
Emotional stress
Exercise
Extreme cold or heat
Nausea and vomiting
Seizures
Infection
Bacterial
Fungal
Rickettsia
Parasite (rare)
Virus (rare/first 1 to 2 days)
Inflammation/Tissue Necrosis
Myocardial infarction
Tumor necrosis
Trauma
Surgery
Tissue infarction
Burns
Collagen vascular disorders
Dermatitis
Drugs/Chemicals
Corticosteroids
Epinephrine
Digitalis
Etiocholanolone
Heparin
Lithium
Histamine
Endotoxin
Metabolic Changes
Diabetic acidosis
Gout
Hyperthyroidism
Uremia
Eclampsia
Hematologic Disorders
Acute hemorrhage
Hemolysis
Myeloproliferative disorders (see Chapter 39)
Cyclic neutrophilia
Hereditary/miscellaneous
Idiopathic neutrophilia

an acute infection consists of primarily neutrophil bands and metamyelocytes and occasionally more immature granulocytic precursors, such as myelocytes and promyelocytes; blast forms are only rarely seen. The quantitative assessment of neutrophil bands is a time-honored test within the hematology laboratory as an indicator of an acute infection. However, there are many problems in accurately determining neutrophil band counts, which mandates that some caution is necessary when interpreting band counts in isolation. Clinicians frequently use elevated band counts as evidence of acute infection and frequently may look at sequential changes in band counts as evidence of response or nonresponse to anti-infection therapy. However, this is fraught with inaccuracies for several reasons. The first is the poorly defined normal range of neutrophil bands in the peripheral blood. As gleaned from several reference laboratories and textbooks, the upper limit of normal for band counts in peripheral blood can range from 0.5×10^9/liter to 1.8×10^9/liter. This variation between laboratories is much greater than with any other peripheral blood component, such as total neutrophils, lymphocytes, and eosinophils.

The next problem is the inability to define a band accurately. Some have defined a band as any cell not having a well-defined filament between lobes, while others have required that a thick filament be present before a neutrophil band is identified (Fig. 34.15). In other words, there is a spectrum of cell appearances between the metamyelocyte and segmented neutrophil, preventing the band from being well defined. This inability to define a band accurately has led to extreme variability between technologists performing differential counts. Every laboratory has known "high banders," "intermediate banders," and "low banders." National comparison studies of neutrophil band identification have shown coefficients of variations of greater than 100% between laboratories performing band counts. This lack of reproducibility also emphasizes the inaccuracy of differential counts performed by counting only 100 or 200 cells. The classic 95% competence limit table by Rumke (5) (Table 34.7) demonstrates that at least 1000 cells must be classified to get a reasonably accurate differential count. Thus, the actual range of what the "true" count may be of a low-percentage cell such as a neutrophil band, is quite wide and leads to significant inaccuracy (Table 34.7). Any sequential use of band counts to evaluate therapeutic response is therefore inaccurate and wrought with clinical witchcraft.

There is also a significant amount of biological variability that will affect band counts. For example, it is well known that neutrophil counts may increase by several thousand, decrease by several thousand, remain the same, or be quite variable from morning to evening among individuals. Again, this variability limits the accuracy of using sequential band counts in a meaningful fashion. Conflicting reports have been published in the literature as to the utility of band counts in predicting acute infection. Some studies have shown that a "bandemia" is significantly associated with proven infection, while others have shown no correlation of band count to fever, infection, or tissue inflammation. In general, total leukocyte count and total neutrophil count provide more meaningful and consistent information in predicting an acute infection than the presence or absence of neutrophil bands. It is likely that a band count, which is carefully enumerated using clearly defined

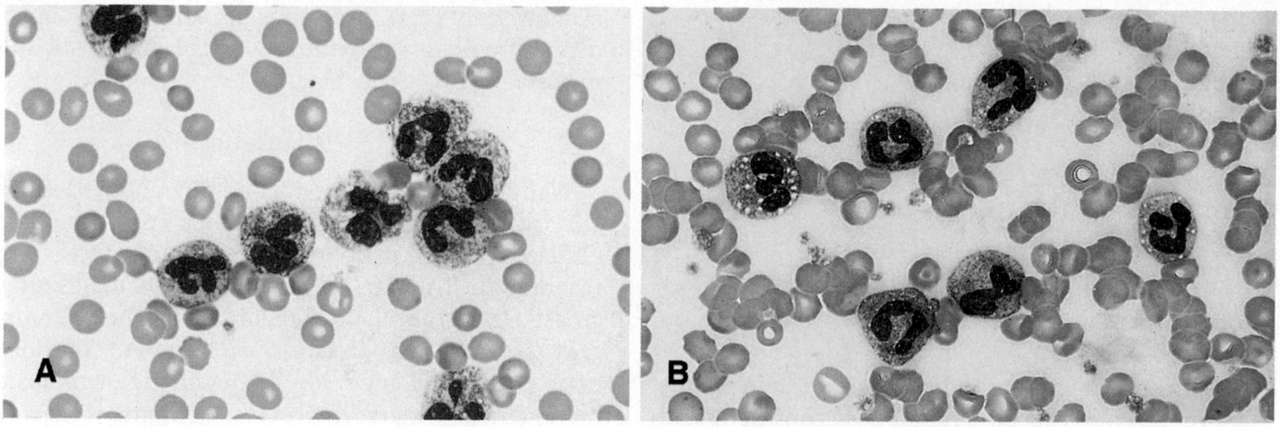

Figure 34.14. A, Toxic neutrophils with prominent azurophilic granules and cytoplasmic vacuolation. **B**, Toxic neutrophils with cytoplasmic vacuolation.

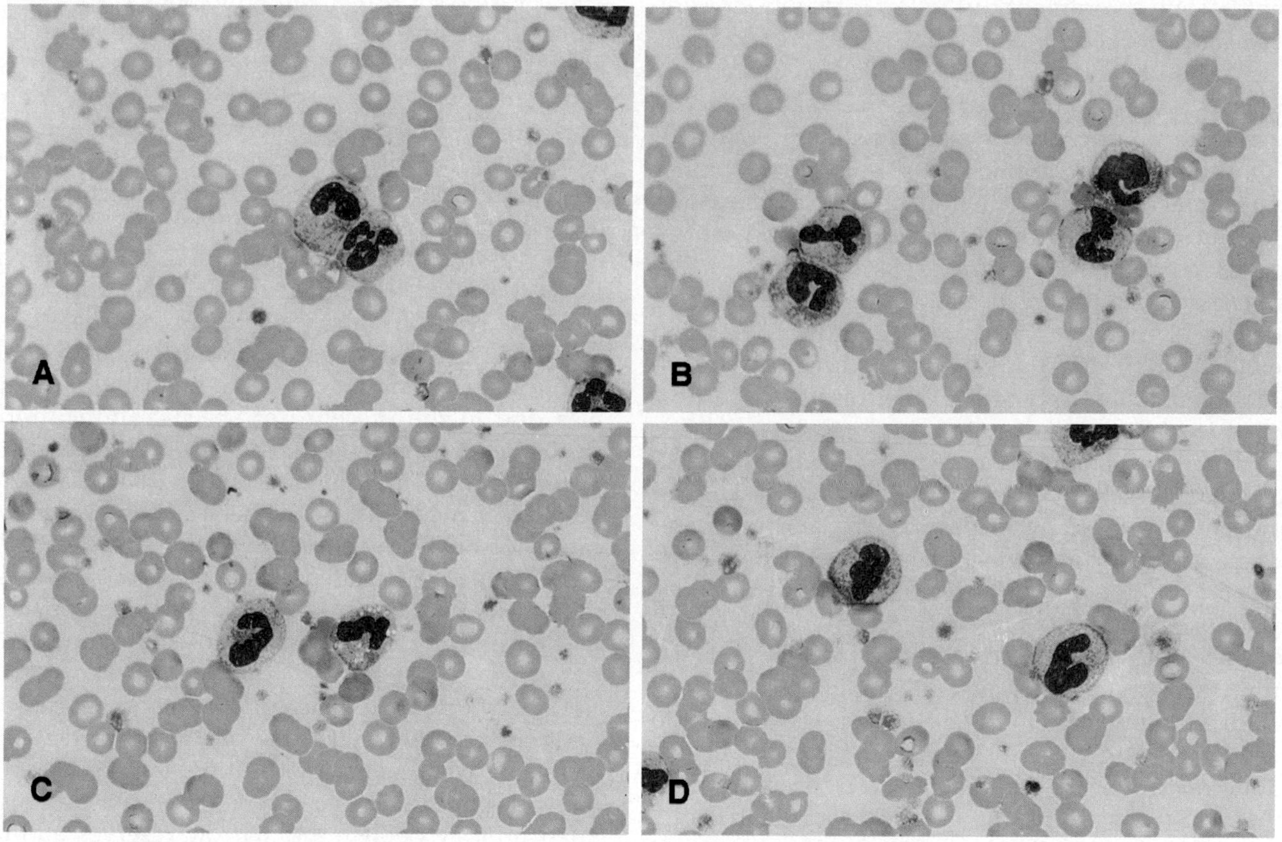

Figure 34.15. **A–D**, Examples of band neutrophils. Note the variation in nuclear appearance, complicating the exact definition of this cell type.

uniform criteria, is a useful indicator of acute inflammation. However, routine band counts performed by a clinical laboratory with multiple technologists during a 7-day work week have little value in the evaluation of acute infection and should not be considered a reliable test.

Toxic granulation is another classic sign of an infectious neutrophilia (Fig. 34.14). This is characterized by coarse cytoplasmic granules that represent prominent primary granules still present from a "rush" through the normal maturation sequences. Toxic granulation may be difficult to identify with certainty unless appropriate peripheral blood smear staining is performed. A weak or faint Wright's stain may not accentuate toxic granulation; on the other extreme, laboratories not familiar with a Wright-Geimsa stain may have the tendency to overcall toxic granulation due to the prominence of the granules

Table 34.14. Differential Diagnosis: Leukemoid Reaction Versus Chronic Myelogenous Leukemia (CML)

	Leukemoid Reaction	CML
WBC[a]	10.0–100.0 × 10^9/liter	30.0–500.0 × 10^9/liter
Eosinophilia/ Basophilia	None	Present
M:E ratio	5–10:1	>20:1
LAP	>100	<10
Organomegaly	Absent	Present

[a]WBC = white blood count; M:E = myeloid:erythroid; LAP = leukocyte alkaline phosphatase.

seen with the Giemsa portion of the stain. Thus, laboratorians need to be familiar and confident with the stain that they are observing before diagnosing toxic granulation. Döhle bodies are a faint, pale blue cytoplasmic area near the periphery of a neutrophil that become prominent during an infectious episode (Fig. 34.14). These small bodies represent endoplasmic reticulum and are a very reliable sign of an infectious process. Again, Döhle bodies may be easily overlooked if appropriate staining is not performed. Cytoplasmic vacuolation is a less common feature of acute infection and is thought to represent cellular areas in which lysosomal ingredients have been released to engulf and destroy bacteria (Fig. 34.14). Cytoplasmic vacuolation due to EDTA artifact can also occur and must be distinguished from vacuolation resulting from infectious process. The EDTA-associated vacuolation appears to be a result of the time spent in anticoagulant.

In most situations, the degree of neutrophilia in an acute infection seldom exceeds 50.0 × 10^9/liter and is more typically in the 15.0 to 30.0 × 10^9/liter range. In cases in which the neutrophilia exceeds 50.0 × 10^9/liter, the term "leukemoid reaction" has been used. The obvious differential problem that arises in cases of leukemoid reaction is differentiation from chronic myelogenous leukemia (CML). Several features that will aid in the distinction of a leukemoid reaction from CML are listed in Table 34.14. Leukemoid reactions are typically characterized by morphologic signs of infections, such as a "left shift," toxic granulation, Döhle bodies, and cytoplasmic vacuolation. The left shift in a leukemoid reaction is a gradation with greater prominence of segmented neutrophils, band forms, and metamyelocytes, whereas CML shows a prominence of both mature neutrophils and myelocytes. Leukemoid reactions lack dysplastic changes and basophilia, and should only show rare blast forms at best. Laboratory tests that may be useful in this distinction include leukocyte alkaline phosphatase (LAP) and cytogenetic karyotyping. The LAP will be increased, and no Philadelphia chromosome will be found in a leukemoid reaction. Obviously, the clinical history and physical examination (e.g., presence or absence of splenomegaly) will also provide important diagnostic information.

Neutropenia

Neutropenia is defined as having counts less than 1.5 to 2.0 × 10^9/liter. Neutropenia may result from either decreased marrow production or increased peripheral destruction of neutrophils. Causes of decreased neutrophil production in the bone marrow are vast and may include replacement of normal bone marrow elements by hematologic or metastatic malignancies, marrow fibrosis, or marrow necrosis. Chemotherapeutic or other toxic agents may also suppress normal marrow activity, including granulopoiesis; this group of "toxins" also includes alcohol and a variety of drugs and antibiotics (Table 34.15). Aplastic anemia, bone marrow irradiation, megaloblastic anemia (folate/B_{12} deficiency), myelodysplastic syndromes, and congenital abnormalities of granulopoiesis may all be associated with neutropenia. The latter inherited disorders would include Fanconi's anemia and familial benign and cyclic neutropenias (also known as Kostman's syndrome).

Increased destruction or utilization of neutrophils in the peripheral blood or tissue is not uncommon and may result from hypersplenism associated with a variety of collagen vascular disorders, liver abnormalities, among others. Immune-mediated neutropenias due to the presence of specific antineutrophil antibodies may also occur. Many viral infections, including human immunodeficiency virus (HIV), have been associated with neutropenias. Other particular causes of neutropenia are listed in Table 34.15. The neutropenias associated with viral disorders are thought to be the result of direct marrow "damage" by the infecting virus, which causes a disruption in normal myelopoiesis.

Usually in acute bacterial infection, significant neutrophilia will result. However, if the particular infection is overwhelming or if it occurs in an individual with borderline marrow reserves, the prolonged infection may deplete the marrow reserves and create more demand than what the marrow can respond to. This occurs primarily in the elderly, newborns, or in any patient with an underlying myelosuppressive process. The resulting neutropenia will prevent an adequate response to the tissue infection and may lead to an overwhelming infection with subsequent death.

Monocytosis

Monocytosis is defined as an increase in peripheral blood monocytes greater than 0.8 × 10^9/liter and is associated primarily with inflammatory and im-

Table 34.15. Neutropenia

Decreased marrow production
Agents that lead to bone marrow suppression
- Chemotherapeutic agents
- Radiation
- Benzene
- Chloroform
- Alcohol
- Arsenic

Drugs (Nonchemotherapeutic)
- Chloroamphenicol
- Semisynthetic penicillins
- Sulfonamides
- Nitrofurantoin
- Tricyclic antidepressants
- Antithyroid drugs
- Diuretics (thiozides)
- Hypoglycemic agents
- Quinidine, procanimide, alapurinol, and antihistamines

Bone Marrow Replacement
- Hematologic malignancies
- Metastatic malignancies
- Myelofibrosis
- Bone marrow necrosis
- Storage disorders

Hematologic Disorders with Suppressed Marrow Production
- Aplastic anemia
- Paroxysmal nocturnal hemoglobinuria
- Vitamin B_{12}/folate deficiency
- Myelodysplastic syndromes
- Chédiak-Higashi syndrome

Hereditary Disorders
- Fanconi's anemia
- Familial cyclic neutropenias
- Kostman's syndrome

Increased peripheral destruction/utilization
Hypersplenism
- Collagen vascular diseases
- Felty's syndrome
- Cirrhosis

Immune-mediated
- Antineutrophil antibody
- Drug-associated antibody
- Miscellaneous

Overwhelming infection (may also cause decreased production)
- Especially in elderly, newborns, or in patients with limited marrow reserve
- Some viral infections

Miscellaneous
- Pump-oxygenator in open heart surgery
- Hemodialysis

mune disorders. It is difficult to correlate monocytosis directly with specific disease states, as opposed to neutrophilia (Table 34.16). One of the classic associations of monocytosis is with tuberculosis infections. However, other infections such as subacute bacterial endocarditis, salmonella, listeria, syphilis, leprosy, and brucellosis can also be associated with a monocytosis. Monocytosis often appears during the recovery phase of an acute infection or following bone marrow suppression. This relative or absolute monocytosis heralds the marrow recovery

Table 34.16. Disorders Associated with Monocytosis

Normal newborn infections
- Tuberculosis
- Syphilis
- Leprosy
- Salmonella
- Brucellosis
- Rikettsia
- Subacute bacterial endocarditis
- Parasites (some)

Marrow recovery phase
- Acute infections
- Neutrophil suppression

Hematologic disorders
- Chronic myeloproliferative disorders
- Myelodysplastic syndromes
- Acute leukemias with monocytic component
- Hodgkin's disease
- Agranulocytosis

Collagen vascular diseases

Gastrointestinal
- Ulcerative colitis
- Regional anuritis

Miscellaneous
- Corticosteroids
- Lipid storage disorders

and usually precedes the return of granulocytes. Monocytoses may also be associated with hematologic malignancies, such as myelodysplastic syndromes and some types of acute and chronic leukemia. Interestingly, up to 25% of patients with Hodgkin's disease have been reported to have a peripheral blood monocytosis. Monocytosis may also accompany many nonhematopoietic malignancies as well as some of the collagen vascular disorders. Thus, the finding of a patient with monocytosis is relatively nonspecific and can be associated with a variety of benign and malignant hematologic and nonhematologic disorders.

The mononuclear phagocyte system is also the primary cell affected in a variety of storage disorders. These storage disorders are generally hereditary abnormalities or deficiencies of enzymes that are necessary for lipid storage and processing. The macrophages become the most obvious morphologic abnormality in these disorders as they become packed full of lipid material that cannot be further digested. Hematologic abnormalities, such as cytopenias, may result from bone marrows that are replaced with accumulated macrophages. Splenomegaly and hypersplenism may also result. Table 34.17 lists some of the hereditary disorders associated with storage diseases and the accompanying blood and bone marrow findings.

Gaucher's disease is a hereditary deficiency of glucocerebrocidase that results in an intracellular accumulation of the syphingoglycolipid glucocerebrocide. Gaucher cells appear as enlarged macrophages

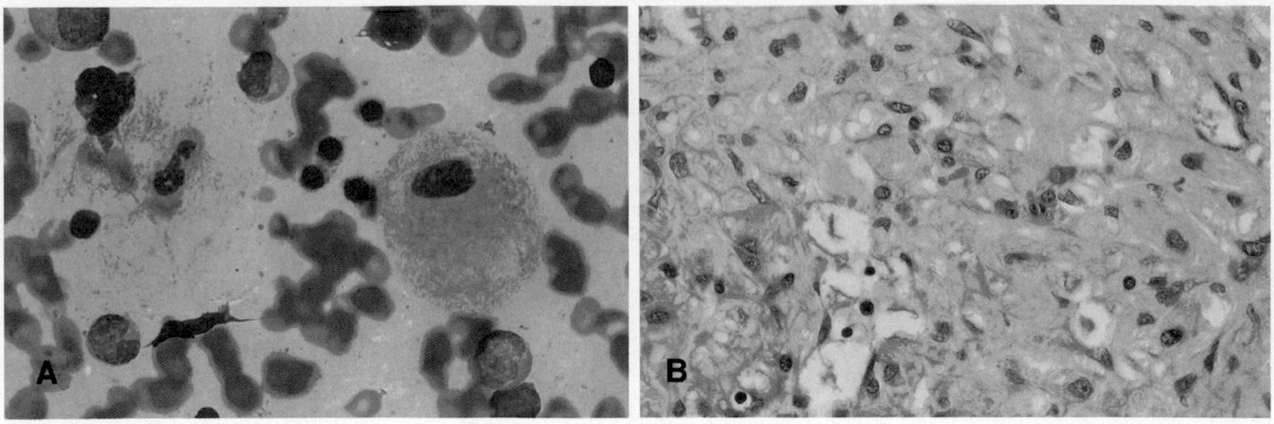

Figure 34.16. Gaucher's disease. **A**, Bone marrow aspirate showing macrophage with prominent blue cytoplasmic fibrils; **B**, Bone marrow biopsy section showing classic accumulation of Gaucher cells having a fibular cytoplasm ("tissue paper" appearance).

Table 34.17. Storage Disorders/Blood and Bone Marrow Findings

Blood	Bone Marrow	Storage Disorders
—	"Gaucher cell"	Gaucher's disease
Vacuolated lymphocyte		Tay-Sachs Batten-Spielmeuer-Vogt Glycogen storage diseases
Vacuolated lymphocyte	Foam cells	Niemann-Pick disease
Metachromatic inclusion	Metachromatic inclusion	Mucopolysaccharidosis Alder-Reilly anomaly

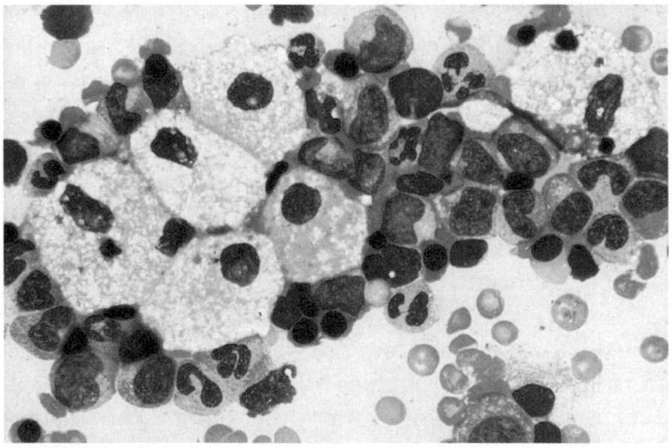

Figure 34.17. Niemann-Pick disease. Bone marrow aspirate smear showing large, foamy macrophages. These macrophages are not specific for Niemann-Pick disease and can be found in other diseases.

within the bone marrow and are engorged with distinctive cytoplasmic fibrioles that are meshed in an irregular pattern (Fig. 34.16). In bone marrow sections, Gaucher cells have been described as having a cytoplasmic appearance of "wrinkled tissue paper." Pseudo-Gaucher cells have been commonly observed in patients with chronic myelogeneous leukemia, representing increased glucocerebrocide turnover from the massive leukocyte population in CML. Pseudo-Gaucher cells have also been observed in patients with thalassemia and multiple myeloma. The pseudo-Gaucher cells of CML are thus different from true Gaucher cells in that they represent normally functioning macrophages overloaded with lipid byproducts, although they are morphologically very similar.

Neimann-Pick disease is a rare autosomal recessive disorder caused by deficiency of syphingomyelinase and results in accumulation of syphingomyelin in the mononuclear phagocytes. Numerous large, foamy macrophages are identified in the bone marrow of patients with Neimann-Pick disease (Fig. 34.17). These foamy cells are not specific for Neimann-Pick disease because such cells can be identified in other lipid disorders and various hematologic diseases.

Eosinophilia

Eosinophils are primarily associated with anaphylactic responses and hypersensitivity reactions. Bacterial killing is not a major function of eosinophils, but eosinophils probably play a minimal role in antigen recognition. The cause of an eosinophilia in a patient can be quite difficult to determine. Benign eosinophilia is associated with a variety of drugs, parasitic infections, allergic reactions, and some collagen vascular diseases (Table 34.18). These must be differentiated from malignant disorders of eosinophils, such as hypereosinophilic syndrome.

Hypereosinophilic syndrome is, in reality, a chronic myeloproliferative disorder characterized by a proliferation of mature eosinophils. The eosinophils frequently appear agranular and atypical. This disorder is characterized by splenomegaly, leukostatic problems and complications caused by the release of eosinophilic products in susceptible tissues (such as heart and brain).

Table 34.18. Disorders Associated with Eosinophilia

Drug reactions
Parasitic infestations
Trichinosis
Toxocara
Filariasis
Echinococcus
Pneumocystis carinii
Aspergillosis
Coccidiomycosis
Strongyloides
Ascaris
Schistosomiasis
Allergic reactions
Asthma
Dermatitis
Rhinitis
Graft rejection
Graft versus host disease
Pemphigus/pemphigoid
Farmer's lung
Collagen vascular diseases
Rheumatoid arthritis
Periarteritis nodosa
Hematologic disorders
Hodgkin's disease
Systemic mastocytosis
Chronic myelogenous leukemia
Pulmonary disease
Löffler's syndrome
Idiopathic/hypereosinophilic syndrome
Hypereosinophilic syndrome

Basophilia

Basophils are the least common of the peripheral blood cell components and typically number less than 0.1 × 10^9/liter. Chronic myelogenous leukemia (CML) is the most common and significant cause of basophilia. Benign basophilia may be associated with hypersensitivity reactions, renal disease, myxedema, and some inflammatory responses. Other causes of basophilia are listed in Table 34.19.

Monocytopenia/Eosinopenia/Basopenia

The determination of monocytopenia, eosinopenia, and basopenia can be made only if large numbers of cells are directly counted (Table 34.20); manual counts of 100 or 200 total cells are inaccurate for these low numbers. Eosinopenia and basopenia have both been reported to occur in situations of acute stress or acute infection, with corticosteroids of exogenous source, or with Cushing's syndrome. Monocytopenia has also been reported to occur following treatment with corticosteroids. Monocytopenia is also a well-described phenomenon in hairy cell leukemia.

Table 34.19. Disorders Associated with Basophilia

Hematologic malignancies
Chronic myeloproliferative diseases
Myelodysplastic syndromes
Mastocytosis
Acute basophilic leukemia (rare)
Hypersensitivity reactions
Hypothyroidism/myxedema
Ulcerative colitis
Radiation
Infections
Varicella
Smallpox
Miscellaneous
Renal disease (rare)

Table 34.20. Disorders Associated with Monocytopenia/Eosinopenia/Basopenia

Monocytopenia
Corticosteroids
Hairy cell leukemia
Eosinopenia
Acute stress
Acute infection
Corticosteroids
Cushing's syndrome
Basopenia
Acute stress
Acute infection
Corticosteroids
Cushing's syndrome

Reactive Lymphocytosis

Reactive lymphocytoses are polyclonal expansions of T and/or B lymphocytes. Table 34.21 lists some of the common causes associated with peripheral blood lymphocytoses. An acute viral infection is the classic disease associated with a lymphocytosis. These can include infectious mononucleosis (Epstein-Barr virus), cytomegalovirus, and a variety of other viral agents. It must be emphasized that an absolute lymphocyte count must be determined in the evaluation of a lymphocytosis, so that an "absolute" lymphocytosis can be distinguished from a "relative" lymphocytosis due to an absolute neutropenia. It must also be remembered that the normal range age of lymphocyte counts varies with age. Children under the age of 4 have a much higher absolute lymphocyte count than older children and adults (Table 34.4).

The morphologic hallmark of an acute viral infection is the so-called atypical or reactive lymphocyte (Fig. 34.18). This refers to lymphocytes that are "transformed" and are larger than the small lymphocyte with scant cytoplasm. These transformed lymphocytes have a slightly finer chromatin than a small lymphocyte and usually have a distinct nucleus and abundant cytoplasm. The cytoplasm may have a blue

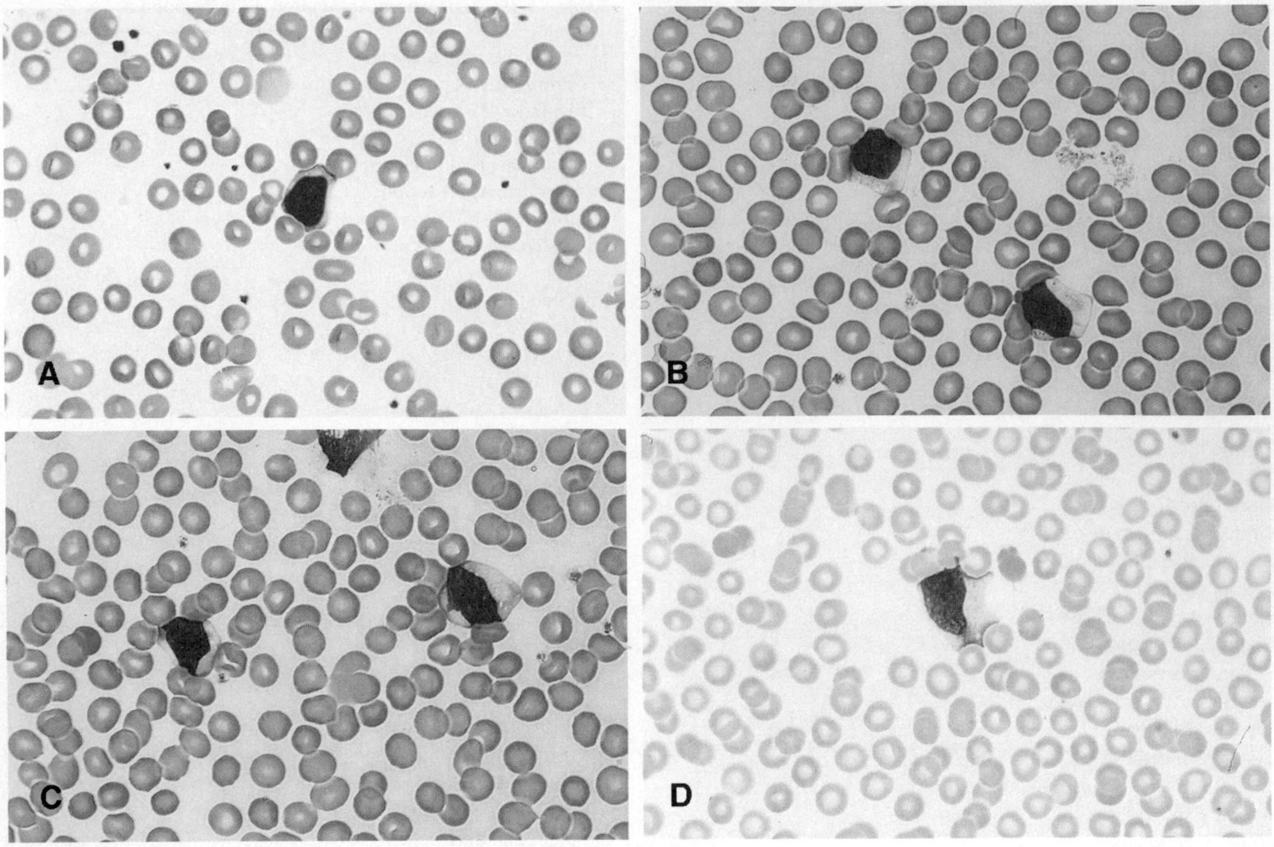

Figure 34.18. A–D, Various types of reactive, or atypical, lymphocytes.

Table 34.21. Disorders Associated with Lymphocytosis

Physiological (first week to 4 years)
Infectious
Infectious mononucleosis (Epstein-Barr virus)
Infectious lymphocytosis
Cytomegalovirus
Infectious hepatitis
Pertussis
Brucellosis
Toxoplasmosis
Mycoplasma
Chronic infections
Syphilis
Drug sensitivity
Dilantin
Para-aminosalicylic acid
Miscellaneous
Autoimmune disorders
Hyperthyroid toxicosis
Addison's disease
Graft rejection
Hematologic malignancies
Acute lymphoblastic leukemia
Chronic lymphocytic leukemia
Peripheralized lymphomas
Chronic lymphoproliferative diseases

to plasmacytoid appearance. Occasional azurophilic granules (large granular lymphocytes) may also be identified. These reactive lymphocytes have also been called Downey cells. The atypical lymphocytes often comprise more than 20% of the total lymphocyte count. Some diseases, such as cytomegalovirus infection, hepatitis, and toxoplasmosis, are more commonly associated with a lymphocytosis than with an increase in plasmacytoid-appearing lymphocytes and plasma cells. The lymphocytosis associated with *Bordetella* pertussis may appear as deeply clefted cells that can mimic the clefted cells of a peripheralized, small cleaved cell lymphoma (Fig. 34.18). Obviously, a clinical history of lymphoma or lymphadenopathy and the patient's age will aid in this differential diagnosis. The lymphocytes in the so-called infectious lymphocytosis disorder are usually small, with scant cytoplasm. This vague disorder can be associated with WBCs greater than 100.0×10^9/liter and is not associated with any known etiology.

Lymphopenia

Lymphopenia is defined as an absolute decrease in the lymphocyte count to less than 1.5×10^9/liter in adults and less than 3.0×10^9/liter in children. This decrease in lymphocytes may be the result of decreased production or increased destruction or loss

Table 34.22. Disorders Associated with Lymphopenia

Immunodeficiency syndromes: inherited
DiGeorge syndrome
Bruton-type agammaglobulinemia
Severe combined immunodeficiency (Swiss-type)
Common variable hypogammaglobulinemia
Wiskott-Aldrich syndrome
Ataxia telangectasia
Immunodeficiency syndromes: acquired
Acquired immunodeficiency syndrome (HIV)
Increased destruction
Corticosteroids
Cushing's syndrome
Radiation
Chemotherapy
Intestinal lymphocyte loss
Lymphangiectectasia
Whipple's disease
Malabsorption syndromes
Malignancies
Hodgkin's disease
Terminal carcinoma
Miscellaneous
Bone marrow aplasia
Collagen vascular diseases
Renal failure
Sarcoidosis
Tuberculosis

Table 34.23. Morphologic and Functional Leukocyte Disorders

May-Hegglin anomaly
Pelger-Huët anomaly
Hereditary hypersegmentation in neutrophils
Alder-Reilly anomaly
Chédiak-Higashi syndrome
Chronic granulomatous disease
Myeloperoxidase deficiency
Miscellaneous
CD11/CD18 (CR3) deficiency
Specific neutrophil granule deficiency
Lazy leukocyte syndrome
Various immunoglobulin deficiencies
Autoimmune diseases
Chronic renal failure
Diabetes
Malnutrition
Burns
Various malignancies

of peripheral lymphocytes. The decreased production of lymphocytes may be associated with a variety of inherited or acquired immunologic deficiencies. Rare disorders associated with abnormalities of the lymphatic system have also been associated with lymphopenias. Acquired immunodeficiency syndrome (AIDS) that is associated with human immunodeficiency virus (HIV) has become a frequent cause of lymphopenia because of the lymphocytotoxic effect of the HIV virus. Other abnormalities associated with lymphocytopenias include Hodgkin's disease, irradiation, chemotherapy, corticosteroids, Cushing's disease, and a variety of other miscellaneous diseases (Table 34.22).

Morphologic and Functional Leukocyte Disorders

A variety of qualitative disorders of neutrophils may be manifested as either morphologic or functional disorders (Table 34.23). Some of these abnormalities are little more than laboratory curiosities with little clinical impact on the patient, whereas other disorders are clinically quite significant and can lead to potentially life-threatening complications.

May-Hegglin Anomaly. The May-Hegglin anomaly is an uncommon autosomal dominant disorder characterized by large, abnormal Döhle bodies in neutrophils and monocytes, giant platelets, and a variable degree of thrombocytopenia (Fig. 34.19). Although the majority of patients with May-Hegglin anomaly are asymptomatic, some of these patients may have problems with abnormal bleeding from an unknown abnormality. Although it would be easy to surmise that a platelet defect is responsible for this abnormality, platelet function studies in the laboratory have not shown any abnormality. The Döhle bodies in May-Hegglin anomaly are quite prominent and are typically larger and bolder than the Döhle bodies associated with an acute infection. As with acute infections, the Döhle bodies in May-Hegglin anomaly consist of rough endoplasmic reticulum. The giant platelets measure anywhere from 4 to 8 μm in diameter and, when present with Döhle bodies, are quite diagnostic of the May-Hegglin anomaly.

Pelger-Huët Anomaly. The Pelger-Huët anomaly is a benign autosomal dominant disorder, characterized by the inability of the neutrophils to undergo proper segmentation. This results in a neutrophil that has a bilobed or dumbbell-shaped nucleus with coarsely clumped chromatin (Fig. 34.20). Over 75% of the neutrophils will show this bilobed segmentation. Patients who are homozygous for the Pelger-Huët anomaly are incredibly rare and have been reported to have neutrophils with a single, round nucleus without segmentation and with coarsely condensed chromatin. Both the homozygote and heterozygote state are associated with normal granulocytic function and are not thought to be associated with any clinical problems. Pseudo-Pelger-Huët neutrophils found in the myelodysplastic syndromes are morphologically identical to this hereditary type and are a characteristic finding in granulocytic dysplasia.

Hereditary Hypersegmentation in Neutrophils. This rare autosomal dominant disorder results in giant neutrophils having five or more segments. Neutrophil precursor cells, such as the promyelocyte and myelocyte, also show nuclear indentation and seg-

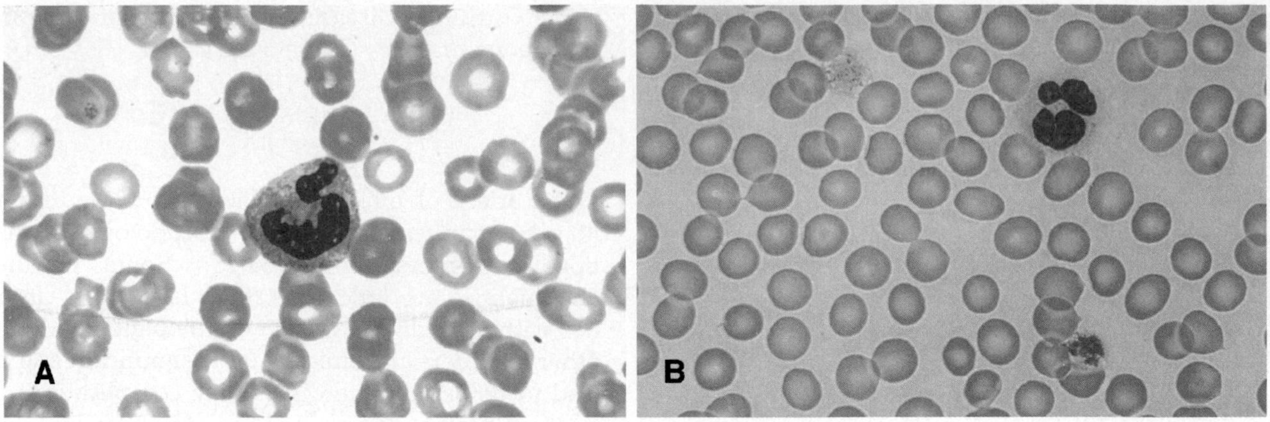

Figure 34.19. **A** and **B**, May-Hegglin anomaly, showing large platelets and prominent Döhle bodies in the cytoplasm.

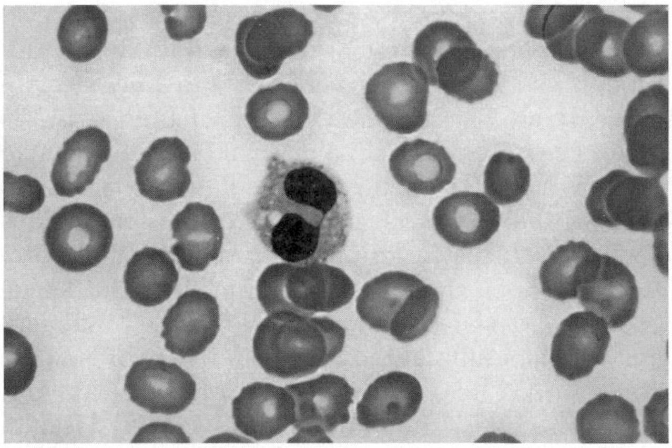

Figure 34.20. Pelger-Huet anomaly showing abnormal, bilobed segmentation of mature neutrophils.

mentation. No oval macrocytes or other megaloblastic changes are seen. These neutrophils are reported to possess normal function.

Alder-Reilly Anomaly. This anomaly relates to the dense, large, azurophilic granules that can be found in neutrophils, eosinophils, basophils, and occasionally lymphocytes and monocytes from patients with a variety of metabolic disorders, including many of the mucopolysaccharidoses, such as Hurler's, Hunter's, or Maroteaux-Lamy syndromes (Fig. 34.21). This heavy granulation is easily confused with toxic granulation, but is not associated with any infectious process and is a "permanent" feature of the circulating cells. In these syndromes, the neutrophils become constipated with granular mucopolysaccharide deposits, which stain metachromatically with tolidine blue stains. This morphologic characteristic has also been reported to be found occasionally in otherwise healthy individuals.

Inclusions within the lymphocytes are less numerous than in the neutrophils or monocytes in patients with the Alder-Reilly anomaly. These basophilic inclusions are surrounded by a clear halo and also stain metachromatically. The evaluation of the bone marrow will reveal these same inclusions in the mononuclear phagocytes, lymphocytes, and granulocytic cells.

Chédiak-Higashi Syndrome. The Chédiak-Higashi syndrome is a rare autosomal recessive disorder characterized by giant, cytoplasmic lysosomal inclusions, in all types of circulating leukocytes (Fig. 34.22). The primary granules within neutrophils fuse into large cytoplasmic structures that are deficient in the enzymes required for normal neutrophil phagocytosis and chemotaxis. The granules found in Chédiak-Higashi syndrome are myeloperoxidase positive. Patients with Chédiak-Higashi syndrome also exhibit oculocutaneous albinism, recurrent infections, and an increased bleeding tendency. These patients are functionally immunodeficient, and the majority, if they survive the infectious episodes, eventually develop high-grade lymphoproliferative processes.

Chronic Granulomatous Disease. Chronic granulomatous disease (CGD) is an X-linked (two-thirds of cases) or autosomal recessive (one-third of cases) disorder associated with a deficient functional ability of neutrophils to undergo an oxidative respiratory burst. This defect leads to an inability to succeed in the killing of bacterial organisms. These patients with CGD have recurrent and severe infections beginning early in life, typically with catalase-positive bacteria or fungi. The defect in at least the X-linked form is related to a deficiency in cytochrome b_{558}. There is also some association of CGD with the Macleod phenotype as well as Duchenne's muscular dystrophy in some patients. This relates to the close proximal location of the genes involved in these three disorders. The neutrophils and monocytes are morphologically unremarkable. Tests of phagocytic and chemotatic function are abnormal in patients with CGD. Specific tests that evaluate the oxidative

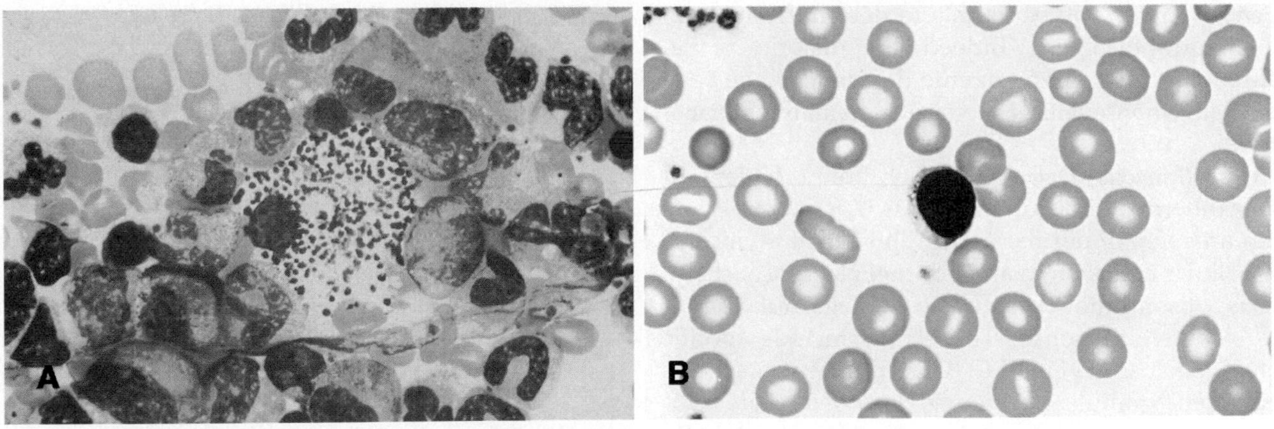

Figure 34.21. Alder-Reilly anomaly showing prominent cytoplasmic inclusions surrounded by a clear halo. **A**, Macrophage. **B**. Lymphocyte.

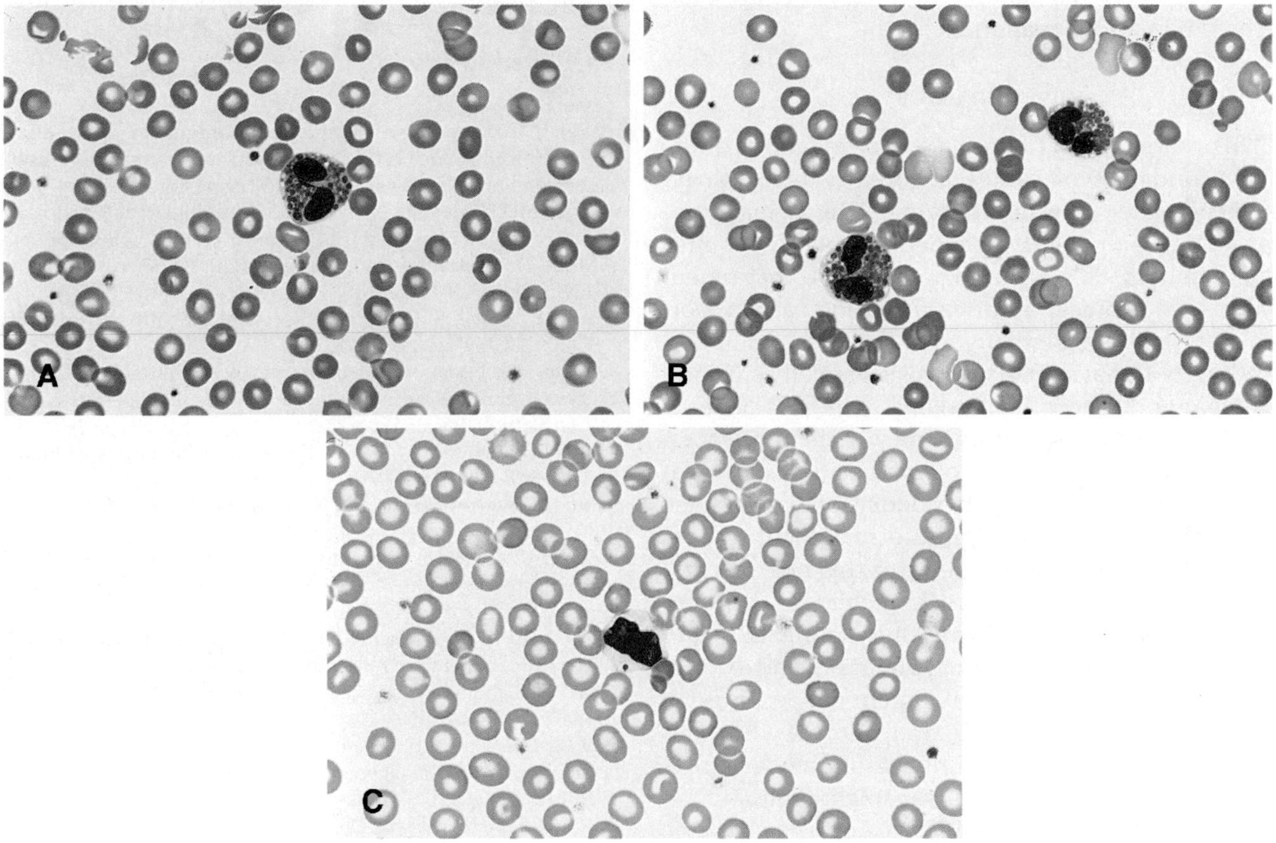

Figure 34.22. Chédiak-Higashi syndrome showing neutrophil (**A**), eosinophil (**B**), and lymphocyte (**C**), with numerous large, fused granules within the cytoplasm.

metabolic pathway, such as the nitroblue tetrazolium dye test or oxidative burst analysis by flow cytometry are used to evaluate the ability of the patient's neutrophils to undergo an intact oxidative burst and are used to confirm the diagnosis of CGD.

Myeloperoxidase Deficiency. Myeloperoxidase deficiency is a benign autosomal recessive trait associated with the absence of myeloperoxidase in neutrophils and monocytes. Paradoxically, eosinophilic myeloperoxidase is normal. Although neutrophils lack this enzyme that mediates the oxidative burst, neutrophil function remains intact and is not associated with any significant clinical problems. Morphologically, the neutrophils and monocytes appear unremarkable. However, the myeloperoxidase cytochemical stain will be negative in these patients. Likewise, hematologic blood counters that rely on peroxidase cytochemical staining for determining differential counts will be unable to determine an accurate neutrophil count. Indeed, the majority of patients with this benign enzyme deficiency have been detected when evaluated on such hematologic analyzers.

Miscellaneous Defects. There are a variety of other inherited or acquired defects that may interfere with any step of normal neutrophil function, including cellular adhesion to an endothelial surface, chemotaxis, opsonization, phagocytosis, degranulation, or the oxidative response. These may include specific defects such as CD11/CD18 (CR3) deficiency, specific neutrophil granule deficiency, lazy leukocyte syndrome, or various complement or immunoglobulin deficiencies. A variety of systemic diseases may also affect neutrophil function such as autoimmune diseases, chronic renal failure, diabetes, malnutrition, burns, and various malignancies.

SUMMARY

This chapter has attempted to outline much of the basic foundation of clinical laboratory hematology. As in no other clinical laboratory, the hematologic evaluation of a patient specimen frequently requires a combination of morphologic features, instrument analysis, and clinical findings. A strong base in morphologic skills is essential and is the basis for understanding both basic hematopoiesis as well as clinical hematology. Modern hematology analyzers have allowed for increasing automation within the laboratory and provide a wealth of information in a relatively rapid fashion. The frequency of hematologic abnormalities in both benign and malignant disease has underscored the importance of this field in clinical laboratory medicine. Important changes in the future will likely include increasing automation and robotics, computer-aided interpretation and control of specimen utilization, development of specific practice parameters related to the utilization of CBCs and differential counts, and the impact that modern therapeutic approaches, such as transplantation and cytokine/growth factors, will have on hematologic studies. The hematology laboratory is steeped in tradition, yet remains at the forefront of modern laboratory and clinical medicine.

References

1. Baker J, Cornbleet PJ. Erythrocyte disorders. In: Howanitz JH, Howanitz PJ, eds. Laboratory medicine—test selection and interpretation. New York: Churchill Livingstone, 1991:461.
2. Bessman JD, Gilmer PR Jr, Gardner FH. Improved classification of anemias by MCV and RDW. Am J Clin Pathol 1983;80: 322–326.
3. Nelson DA, Davey FR. Hematopoiesis. In: Henry JB, ed. Clinical diagnosis and management by laboratory methods. 18th ed. Philadelphia: WB Saunders, 1991:599–601.
4. Wintrobe MM, Landsberg JW. A standardized technique for the blood sedimentation test. Am J Med Sci 1935;189:102–107.
5. Rümke CL, Bezemer PD, Kuik OJ. Normal values and least significant differences for differential leukocyte counts. J Chron Dis 1975;28:661–668.
6. Cornbleet J. Spurious results from automated hematology cell counters. Lab Med 1983;14:509–514.
7. van Assendelft OW. Spectrophotometry of haemoglobin derivatives. Assen, The Netherlands: Royal Van Gorcum, Ltd., 1970.
8. Baker J, Cornbleet PJ. Erythrocyte disorders. In: Howanitz JH, Howanitz PJ, eds. Laboratory medicine—test selection and interpretation. New York: Churchill Livingstone, 1991:447–498.
9. Cornbleet PJ, Astanita R, Wolf PL. White blood cell and platelet disorders. In: Howanitz JH, Howanitz PJ, eds. Laboratory medicine—test selection and interpretation. New York: Churchill Livingstone, 1991:553–618.
10. Mauer AM. Pediatric hematology. New York: McGraw-Hill, 1969.
11. Jandl JH. Blood—Textbook of hematology. Boston: Little, Brown & Co., 1987.

Suggested Readings

General

Baker J, Cornbleet PJ. Erythrocyte disorders. In: Howanitz JH, Howanitz PJ, eds. Laboratory medicine—test selection and interpretation. New York: Churchill Livingstone, 1991:447–498.

Cornbleet PJ, Astanita R, Wolf PL. White blood cell and platelet disorders. In: Howanitz JH, Howanitz PJ, eds. Laboratory medicine—test selection and interpretation. New York: Churchill Livingstone, 1991:553–618.

Dacie JV, Lewis SM. Practical haematology. 5th ed. Edinburgh: Churchill Livingstone, 1975.

Douglas AS, Dacie JV. The incidence and significance of iron-containing granules in human erythrocytes and their precursors. J Clin Pathol 1953;26:770–772.

Hyun BH, Ashton JK, Dolan K. Practical hematology. Philadelphia: WB Saunders, 1975.

Jandl JH. Blood—Textbook of hematology. Boston: Little, Brown & Co., 1987.

Koepke JA. Practical laboratory hematology. New York: Churchill Livingstone, 1991.

Lewis SM. The constituents of normal blood and bone marrow. In: Hardisty RM, Weatherall DJ, eds. Blood and its disorders. 2nd ed. Oxford: Blackwell Scientific, 1982:3–56.

Miale JB. Laboratory medicine—hematology. 6th ed. St Louis: CV Mosby, 1982.

Nelson DA, Davey FR. Hematopoiesis. In: Henry JB, ed. Clinical diagnosis and management by laboratory methods. 18th ed. Philadelphia: WB Saunders, 1991:553–716.

Schumacher HR, Garvin DF, Triplett DA. Introduction to laboratory hematology. New York: Alan R Liss, 1984.

Sun NCJ. Hematology—an atlas and diagnostic guide. Philadelphia: WB Saunders, 1983.

Wintrobe MM, Lee GR, Boggs DR, et al. Clinical hematology. Philadelphia: Lea & Febiger, 1981.

Blood Cell Counting/Differential

Bentley SA. Alternatives to the neutrophil band count. Arch Pathol Lab Med 1988;112:883–884.

Bessman D. Microcytosis caused by RBC fragmentation. JAMA 1978;239:2475–2476.

Bessman JD. Heterogeneity of red cell volume: quantitation, clinical correlations, and possible mechanisms. Johns Hopkins Med J 1980;146:226–230.

Bessman JD. Automated blood counts and differentials. Baltimore: Johns Hopkins University Press, 1986.

Bessman JD, Banks D. Spurious macrocytosis, a common clue to erythrocyte cold agglutinins. Am J Clin Pathol 1980;74:797–800.
Bessman JD, Feinstein DI. Quantitative anisocytosis as a discriminant between iron deficiency and thalassemia minor. Blood 1979;53:288–293.
Bessman JD, Williams LJ, Gilmer PR. Mean platelet volume. Am J Clin Pathol 1981;76:289–293.
Bollinger PB, Drewinko B, Brailas CD, et al. The Technicon H*1™—an automated hematology analyzer for today and tomorrow. Am J Clin Pathol 1987;87:71–78.
Chien S, Dellenback J, Usami S, Gregerson MI. Plasma trapping in hematocrit determination. Difference among animal species. Proc Soc Exp Biol Med 1965;119:1155–1158.
Coulter WH. High speed automatic blood cell counter and cell size analyzer. Proc Natl Elect Conf 1956;12:1034–1040.
Cox CJ, Habermann TM, Payne BA, et al. Evaluation of the Coulter Counter Model S-Plus IV. Am J Clin Pathol 1985;84: 297–306.
Coyne R. The white blood cell differential count, a comparison of manual spread films and semi-automated spun films. Can J Med Technol 1976;38:18–24.
England JM, Walford DM, Waters DAW. Re-assessment of the reliability of the haematocrit. Br J Haematol 1972:247–256.
England JM, Ward SM, Down MC. Microcytosis, anisocytosis and the red cell indices in iron deficiency. Br J Haematol 1976;35:589–597.
England JM. Prospects for automated differential leucocyte counting in the routine laboratory. Clin Lab Haematol 1979;1:263–273.
Fisher SL, Fischer SP. Mean corpuscular volume. Arch Intern Med 1983;143:282–283.
Fossat C, David M, Harle JR, et al. New parameters in erythrocyte counting. Value of histograms. Arch Pathol Lab Med 1987;111: 1150–1154.
Fulwyler MJ. Electronic separation of biologic cells by volume. Science 1965;150:910–911.
Giles C. The platelet count and mean platelet volume. Br J Haematol 1981;48:31–37.
Goldner FM, Mann WN. Statistical error of differential white counts. Guys Hosp Rep 1938;88:54–56.
Griswold DJ, Champagne VD. Evaluation of the Coulter S-PLUS IV. Three-part differential in an acute care hospital. Am J Clin Pathol 1985;84:49–57.
Hillman RS, Finch CA. Red cell manual. 5th ed. Philadelphia: FA Davis, 1985.
Hughes-Jones NC, Norley I, Young JMS, England JM. Differential white cell counts by frequency distribution analysis of cell volumes. J Clin Pathol 1974;27:623–625.
Klee GG. Performance goals for internal quality control of multichannel hematology analyzers. Clin Lab Haematol 1990;12:65–74.
Koepke JA. Differential leukocyte counting. Skokie, IL: College of American Pathologists, 1978.
Koepke JA, Dotson NA, Shifman MA. A critical evaluation of the manual/visual differential leukocyte counting method. Blood Cells 1985;11:173–186.
Krause JR. Automated differentials in the hematology laboratory. Am J Clin Pathol 1990;93(suppl 1):S11–S16.
Mansberg HP, Saunders AM, Groner W. The Hemalog D white cell differential system. J Histochem Cytochem 1974;22:711–724.
O'Sullivan MB. Quality control of multichannel haematology analyzers: critique of current methods and the need for performance goals. Clin Lab Haematol 1990;12:3–12.
Pierre RV, Payne BA, Lee WK, et al. Comparison of four leukocyte differential methods with the National Committee for Clinical Laboratory Standards (NCCLS) reference method. Am J Clin Pathol 1987;87:201–209.
Rümke CL. The statistically expected variability in differential leukocyte counting. In: Koepke JA, ed. Differential leukocyte counting. Skokie, IL: College of American Pathologists, 1978:39.
Saunders AM. Development of automation of differential leukocyte counts by the use of cytochemistry. Clin Chem 1972;18:783–788.
Shapiro MF, Greenfield S. The complete blood count and leukocyte differential count. An approach to their rational application. Ann Intern Med 1987;106:65–74.
Stiene-Martin EA. Causes for poor leukocyte distribution in manual spreader-slide blood films. Am J Med Technol 1980;46:624–632.
van Assendelft OW. Reference values for the total and differential leukocyte count. Blood Cells 1985;11:77–96.
Weick JK, Hagedorn AB, Linman JW. Leukoerythroblastosis: diagnosis and prognostic significance. Mayo Clin Proc 1974;49:110–113.
Wintrobe MM. Erythrocyte in man. Medicine (Baltimore) 1930;9: 195–217.

Miscellaneous Tests

Cline MJ, Berlin NI. The reticulocyte count as an indicator of the rate of erythropoiesis. Am J Clin Pathol 1963;39:121–128.
Sox HC, Liang MH. Erythrocytes and the sedimentation rate. Guidelines for rational use. Ann Intern Med 1986:104:515–523.

Bone Marrow

Gulati GL, Ashton JK, Hyun BH. Structure and function of the bone marrow and hematopoiesis. Hematol Oncol Clin North Am 1988;2:495–511.

Reactive Disorders

Cline MJ, Lahrer RI, Territo M, et al. Monocytes and macrophages: functions and diseases. Ann Intern Med 1978;88:78–88.
Hyun BH, Gulati GL. Lymphocytosis and lymphocytopenia. Lab Med 1984;15:319–324.
Maladonado JE, Hanlon DG. Monocytosis: a current appraisal. Mayo Clin Proc 1965;40:246–251.
Wood TA, Frankel EP. The atypical lymphocyte. Am J Med 1967;42:923–936.

35 Red Blood Cell Disorders

Brian D. Kueck

ANEMIA

It is helpful to consider the circulating red blood cell and its progenitors as a single functional unit, the erythron. Many of the diseases afflicting the erythron may then be seen to result from the same basic processes that affect other organ systems: genetic disorders, disorders of immunity, neoplasia, infectious diseases, nutritional disease, and environmental disorders. The result of the majority of these disease processes is anemia.

Anemia is defined as a reduction in total red cell mass. As total red cell mass is not easily measured, anemia is considered to be present if the hemoglobin concentration or the hematocrit is below the normal range. The range of normal values is subject to variables imposed by lifestyles, geographic altitude, age, and sex.

Clinical Manifestations of Anemia

Anemia itself is not a disease, but merely an objective sign of an underlying process. Hence, the clinical manifestations of anemia are often quite similar regardless of the etiology, resulting from the diminished delivery of oxygen to the tissues. The signs and symptoms of anemia are influenced by the rate of onset, the degree of reduction in red cell and plasma volume, and the adequacy of circulatory and respiratory compensation.

Physiologic adjustments of the cardiovascular system in response to anemia include increases in cardiac output, heart rate, and stroke volume. This compensatory high-output state may result in palpitations, tinnitus, dizziness, or syncopy. High-output cardiac failure may ensue with prolonged anemia, advanced age, or underlying heart disease.

As the red cell mass decreases, blood flow is redistributed to maintain adequate visceral and cerebral oxygenation. Shunting of blood flow away from the skin results in the characteristic pallor of anemia, best observed by inspection of the oral mucosa, conjunctivae, or nail beds, since skin coloration is affected by multiple variables. To further facilitate oxygen delivery to critical tissues, the concentration of red cell 2,3-diphosphoglycerate increases shortly after the onset of anemic hypoxia.

At rest, few changes in respiration are noticeable. Most patients, however, exhibit signs of dyspnea on exertion. Respiratory failure is typically a sign of cardiac decompensation and is usually accompanied by pulmonary edema. Transfusion, in an attempt to improve the oxygen-carrying capacity of the blood, is tempting in such cases, but must be approached with extreme caution, as the risk of precipitating volume overload and further cardiovascular compromise is imminent.

A Morphologic Approach to Anemia

Although anemia may first be suspected from a patient's presenting symptoms, many times the diagnosis is based on laboratory findings. The laboratory data provided by an automated hematology analyzer provides a framework upon which further investigation can be built. Utilizing red cell indices, a morphologic classification to anemia can be structured (Table 35.1). A measure of anisocytosis, or variation in red cell size, is often offered as part of an automated hematology profile and is referred to as the red cell distribution width (RDW) or the red cell morphology index (RCMI). Adding this information may help further stratify the morphologic classification of anemias. It must be kept in mind that the red cell indices are a description of the average red cell. Important clues may be missed if evaluation does not include examination of the peripheral blood smear. A balanced population of microcytic and macrocytic red cells may otherwise go unnoticed in a normal mean corpuscular volume. Shape changes in the erythrocytes (poikilocytes) often offer clues to a number of specific disease states. Rouleaux, agglutination, or evidence of increased erythrocyte regeneration are also important in findings that may direct further investigation.

A Pathophysiologic Approach to Anemia

In addition to the information provided by the automated hematology analyzer, the history and physical examination may also provide clues directing fur-

Table 35.1. Morphologic Classification of Anemia

Microcytic hypochromic anemias
Iron deficiency anemia
Anemia of chronic disease
Thalassemias
Sideroblastic anemia
Normocytic normochromic anemias
Anemia of chronic disease
Aplastic anemia
Myelophthisic processes
Some hemolytic anemias
Some hemoglobinopathies
Macrocytic anemias
Vitamin B_{12} deficiency
Folic acid deficiency
Aplastic anemia
Liver disease
Myelodysplastic syndromes
Some hemolytic anemias

ther study. The history and review of the prior medical and laboratory data should help to establish the onset and duration of the anemia. Attention to cardiovascular complaints will also provide similar information. Blood loss may be documented by a history of menorrhagia or melena. Dietary inadequacies, current medicinal use, or history of toxin exposure may be elicited in questioning. A family history may provide evidence of an inherited red cell abnormality. Systemic symptoms such as fever or weight loss might point toward neoplasia or infection.

The physical examination should document the signs of anemia. Signs of hyperbilirubinemia, which may suggest increased red cell destruction, should be sought. Lymphadenopathy or hepatosplenomegaly, if present, may provide clues to an underlying infection, lymphoproliferative disorder, or myeloproliferative state. Changes detected in the neurologic examination may reflect nonspecific signs of global cerebral hypoxia, but might also provide clues indicative of megaloblastic anemia or hypothyroidism.

The information obtained through the history and physical examination is helpful in understanding the physiologic mechanisms underlying a decreased red cell mass. A pathophysiologic approach to the anemias can be utilized as an alternative to the morphologic classification scheme provided by the initial laboratory data (Table 35.2). Subsequent discussion of the red cell disorders will follow such a pathophysiologic approach. It is important, however, to understand both classification schemes and how they relate, as evaluation of the anemic patient requires a thorough and careful history, physical examination, laboratory investigation, and examination of the peripheral blood smear.

Table 35.2. A Pathophysiologic Approach to Anemia

1. Blood loss
2. Impaired red cell production
   a. Disorders of heme synthesis
   b. Disorders of DNA synthesis
   c. Inadequate erythroid precursors
3. Accelerated red cell destruction
   a. Intrinsic/inherited red cell abnormalities
   b. Extrinsic/acquired red cell abnormalities
   c. Paroxysmal nocturnal hemoglobinuria

POST-HEMORRHAGIC ANEMIA

Acute Blood Loss

The clinical manifestations of acute blood loss are largely related to the loss of blood volume. Healthy individuals may tolerate a loss of up to 20% of blood volume without clinical manifestations. The loss of larger quantities of blood results in cardiovascular distress; losses exceeding 50% of total blood volume typically result in death. The following discussion presumes a single episode of acute blood loss unattended by therapeutic intervention, an infrequent clinical scenario.

Immediately following acute blood loss, the hemoglobin and hematocrit remain normal as a proportional decline of plasma volume and red cell mass occurs. In an attempt to maintain an adequate blood volume, albumin and fluid are shifted from the extravascular space to the vascular compartment. As this is a slow process, the maximum fall in hematocrit is reached approximately 3 days following blood loss when plasma volume is restored; prior to this time the extent of blood loss is underestimated by the hematocrit. The resulting anemia is initially normochromic and normocytic.

A compensatory increase in red cell production is stimulated by the release of erythropoietin. A lag phase of 3 to 5 days occurs as the erythrocytes mature in the marrow. Subsequently, evidence of increased erythrocyte regeneration is seen in the peripheral blood reflected by increased numbers of polychromatophilic macrocytes or by an increased reticulocyte count. Maximal reticulocytosis is evident approximately 10 days after blood loss; at this time an increased mean corpuscular volume may be noted.

The platelet count and leukocyte count are also affected by acute blood loss. An early transient thrombocytopenia is typically followed within hours by a thrombocytosis that may reach 1000×10^9/liter. The leukocyte count may rise as high as 35×10^9/liter, in part responding to an epinephrine-induced shift of the marginating granulocyte pool to the circulating granulocytic pool. Leukocytosis, which may be accompanied by a mild left shift in granulocytic maturation, occurs within several hours of blood loss and typically resolves within 2 to 4 days.

Such changes in the peripheral blood are readily recognizable as secondary to acute blood loss when hemorrhage is external. Acute blood loss into a body space or cavity, however, may go clinically undetected. In such instances, anemia coupled with evidence of increased erythrocyte regeneration might suggest a hemolytic anemia. Hyperbilirubinemia, typical of hemolytic anemias, may also be evident as internal blood loss leads to erythrocyte breakdown and heme metabolism. Other laboratory findings often seen in conjunction with hemolytic anemia, such as erythrocyte shape abnormalities, decreased serum haptoglobin, hemoglobinemia, hemoglobinuria, and hemosiderinuria are, however, absent.

Chronic Blood Loss

The previously described changes of acute blood loss are lacking if the loss of blood occurs slowly over an extended period of time. Chronic blood loss results in anemia only when the rate of blood loss exceeds the regenerative capacity of the bone marrow or when the body's iron stores are depleted. In the latter circumstance, the resultant blood picture is one of iron deficiency.

IMPAIRED ERYTHROCYTE PRODUCTION

The anemias discussed in this section each result from the bone marrow's inability to produce adequate numbers of functional erythrocytes. This may arise from an inadequate number of erythroid precursors or from an insufficient quantity of substances essential for nuclear or cytoplasmic maturation. A deficiency of such factors vital to cell maturation often affects nonhematopoietic tissue as well; the ensuing discussion, however, focuses only on the consequences to the hematopoietic system.

Disorders of Heme Synthesis

Cytoplasmic maturation is a reflection of hemoglobin synthesis. The normal biosynthesis of hemoglobin requires that iron, protoporyphrin, and globin are present in optimal amounts within the developing erythrocyte. It follows, therefore, that abnormalities in synthesis or integration of any of these three constituents results in an anemia characterized by deficient hemoglobin synthesis, morphologically manifest as hypochromic erythrocytes. Since mitosis is terminated when a critical intracellular concentration of hemoglobin is reached, erythrocytes deficient in hemoglobin typically undergo an additional cell division, resulting in the production of small or microcytic red blood cells. As abnormalities of globin synthesis are discussed in Chapter 36, the following discussion is limited to abnormalities of heme synthesis (Fig. 35.1).

Under the influence of δ-aminolevulinic acid (ALA) synthetase and pyridoxal 5′-phosphate as a cofactor, succinyl CoA and glycine combine to form ALA. This initial step is the major rate-limiting step in heme synthesis, largely controlled as an inverse function of the intracellular concentration of heme. Two molecules of ALA then combine to form porphobilinogen, with subsequent condensation of four porphobilinogen molecules to form the tetrapyrrole ring structure of uroporphyrinogen. Uroporphyrinogen undergoes a number of changes, each under the influence of specific enzymes, eventually resulting in an oxidized molecule of protoporphyrin IX. The final step in heme synthesis occurs in the mitochondria as ferrous iron is incorporated into protoporphyrin IX.

Diminished heme synthesis will result from abnormalities at any point in this multistep pathway. Examples include a deficiency of pyridoxine, or the diminished conversion of pyridoxine to pyridoxal 5′-phosphate seen in alcoholics; the toxic effects of lead, which inhibit ALA dehydrase and inhibit iron delivery to protoporphyrin IX; and deficiencies of enzymes integral to the tetrapyrrole conversions of uroporphyrinogen that result in the rare, typically inherited group of disorders known as the porphyrias.

Normally, protoporphyrin IX is produced in slight relative excess to the amount of iron available for heme synthesis and can be measured clinically as free erythrocyte protoporphyrin (FEP). If incorporation of iron is reduced, due to either an enzymatic block or a deficiency of available iron, an excess of protoporphyrin IX results (increased FEP). In actuality, FEP is zinc protoporphyrin, a naturally fluorescent moiety. Since the action of heme synthetase is not specific for iron, and zinc is the second most plentiful transitional metal within the erythrocyte, it is not surprising that zinc is readily incorporated into protoporphyrin IX when iron is unavailable. Using the hematofluorometer, one can determine the ratio of zinc protoporphyrin to heme (or hemoglobin) absorption. This ratio is perhaps the most sensitive indicator available for iron-deficient erythropoiesis.

IRON-DEFICIENCY ANEMIA

If one excludes the clinically silent thalassemia syndromes, iron deficiency is the primary cause of anemia worldwide. To understand the multiple causes of iron deficiency and the consequent bio-

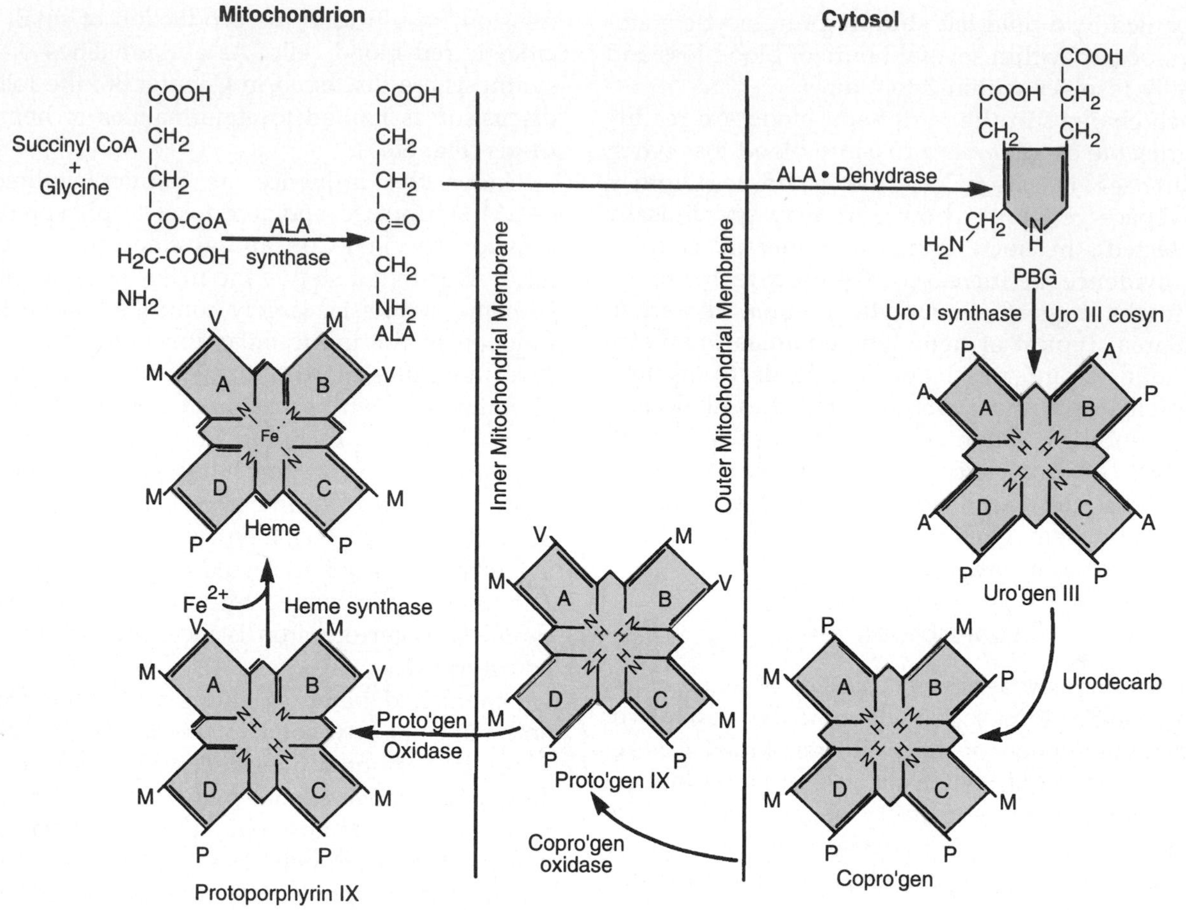

Figure 35.1. Heme biosynthesis. M, methyl (—CH_3); P, propionate (—CH_2 —CH_2 —COOH); V, vinyl (—CH=CH_2); ALA, δ-aminolevulinic acid; PBG, porphobilinogen; Uro I synthase, uroporphyrinogen I synthase; Uro III cosyn, uroporphyrinogen III cosynthase; Urodecarb, uroporphyrinogen decarboxylase. Uro'gen, uroporphyrinogen; Copro'gen, coproporphyrinogen; Proto'gen, protoporphyrinogen. (From Wintrobe MM et al. Erythropoiesis. In: Clinical hematology. 8th ed. Philadelphia: Lea & Febiger, 1981.)

chemical changes that are used clinically as aids in establishing a diagnosis of iron-deficiency anemia, one must first understand iron metabolism.

Iron Metabolism

Iron is supplied exogenously through the diet in two forms: heme iron and nonheme iron. Heme iron is derived from hemoglobin, myoglobin, or other heme proteins in foods of animal origin. Nonheme iron must be converted to or maintained in the ferrous state to facilitate absorption, a process enhanced by the acid environment of the stomach. Iron is absorbed in the duodenum or upper jejunum by means of specific mucosal receptors. It is at the level of the mucosal cell that the absorption of iron is regulated and hence, the tight balance of iron controlled (Fig. 35.2). Under normal circumstances, 5 to 10% of ingested iron is absorbed; in states of iron deficiency, absorption may increase several fold. Exactly how this process occurs and how it is controlled remain unclear.

Once absorbed, iron may be sequestered within the mucosal epithelial cell to be subsequently excreted with cell death, or it may pass through the cell to enter the circulation, where it is quickly complexed with the plasma carrier protein transferrin. The synthesis of transferrin, occurring principally in the liver, is regulated by feedback inhibition in inverse relation to the body's iron stores. Under normal circumstances, approximately one-third of the binding sites of transferrin are saturated with iron.

Transferrin provides for purposeful transport of iron by directing the transferrin-iron complex to transferrin receptors located on the surface of all cells requiring iron. The critical role of transferrin in iron transport is evident by the rare congenital disorder atransferrinemia. The absence of transferrin in this disease results in severe transfusion-dependent anemia as well as hemosiderosis due to random iron deposition throughout the body.

Once bound to the surface of the developing red cell, the transferrin-iron complex is internalized by a process of pinocytosis. Iron is then liberated from transferrin with subsequent return of the intact transferrin molecule to the plasma, where it resumes its transport function.

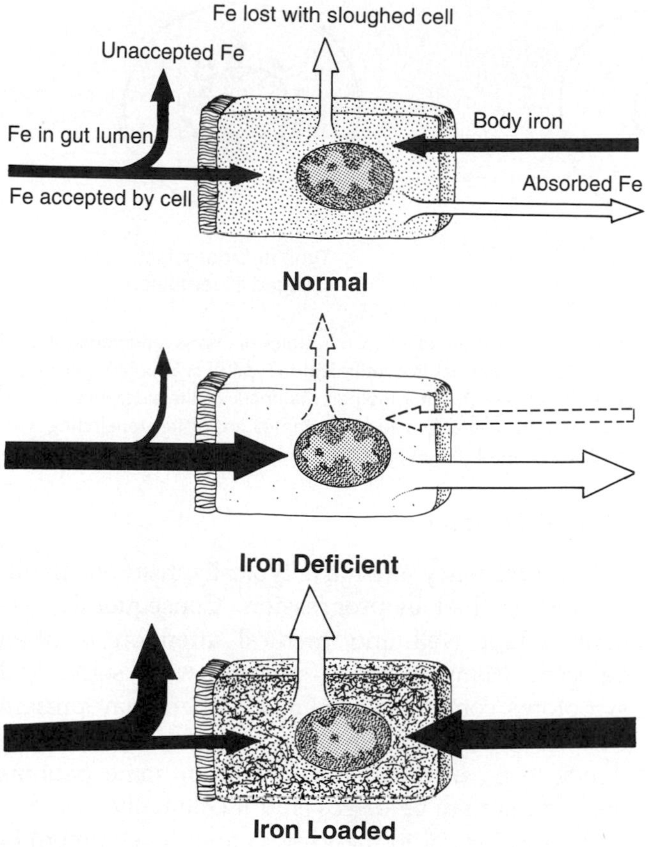

Figure 35.2. The concentration of iron within the intestinal mucosal cell likely parallels body iron stores and serves to regulate the amount of iron absorbed. Iron accepted into the mucosal cell may pass through the cell and enter the circulation, a fate which is promoted by decreased intracellular iron concentration. Alternatively, iron may be retained within the mucosal cell and subsequently lost from the body as the cell is sloughed with normal epithelial turnover. Increased Intracellular iron promotes retention of iron as well as diminishing acceptance of iron into the cell. (Modified from Crosby WH. The control of iron balance by the intestinal mucosa. Blood 1963;22:441.)

The majority of the iron delivered to the developing erythrocyte is incorporated into heme. A small amount of residual nonheme iron is accounted for as ferritin. These small ferritin granules can be visualized with a Prussian blue stain of a bone marrow aspirate. Normally, one to five small randomly distributed Prussian blue–positive granules are seen in the cytoplasm of 20 to 60% of normoblasts; these nonheme iron–containing erythroblasts are referred to as sideroblasts (Fig. 35.3). The number of sideroblasts present reflects both the availability of iron and the incorporation of iron into heme. A good correlation exists between the number of sideroblasts and the percent saturation of transferrin, defined as serum iron/total iron binding capacity × 100 or serum iron/transferrin × 100. These normal cytoplasmic ferritin deposits are removed by solubilization and extrusion of ferritin into the surrounding media, a process that requires active cellular oxidative metabolism.

Iron incorporated into heme remains in the erythrocyte throughout its life span. Erythroid senescence results in removal of the red cell from circulation, primarily by the splenic macrophages. Within the macrophage, hemoglobin is catabolized with ultimate liberation of iron, protoporphyrin, and globin. Iron is then stored in the reticuloendothelial system of the spleen, bone marrow, and liver. From these storage sites, iron is liberated to transferrin to be directed to a newly developing erythrocyte and to begin the iron cycle once again.

Iron is stored in two forms: hemosiderin and ferritin. Ferritin is well characterized and is the major physiologic storage form of iron. Hemosiderin, considered to represent an agglomerate of degraded ferritin and debris from lysozomal vacuoles, is distinguished from ferritin by its insolubility in water and its intense stainability with Prussian blue. The latter characteristic is employed in assessing iron stores in tissue sections or bone marrow aspirate smears.

Iron stores may also be assessed by quantitation of serum ferritin. Although ferritin is typically sequestered within the reticuloendothelial system, a trace amount normally leaks into the circulation. Serum quantitation by radioimmunoassay generally correlates with the body's iron stores. A low serum ferritin is usually a valid indication of decreased iron stores. An elevated serum ferritin, however, does not necessarily indicate adequate or excess body iron stores, as ferritin shows an acute phase response, which may persist for several days to weeks. Consequently, serum ferritin may not be a valid indication of iron stores when measured in the face of underlying inflammatory processes, neoplasia, or liver disease. Interestingly, immunohistochemical assessment of ferritin in bone marrow biopsy specimens has been reported to be a very sensitive tool in the evaluation of body iron stores.

Etiology

From the foregoing discussion it is evident that iron is highly conserved by the body. How then does iron-deficiency anemia develop? In general, iron deficiency arises either from an inadequate intake of iron or from a depletion of the body's iron stores. Dietary inadequacy is typically not a problem in the United States, except during periods of increased metabolic need. Rapid periods of growth, as found during the first year of life and early in adolescence, require additional dietary intake. Consequently, infants between the ages of 6 and 20 months are vulnerable, particularly those maintained solely on an unsupplemented milk diet. Increased demands for iron are also noted during pregnancy and lactation.

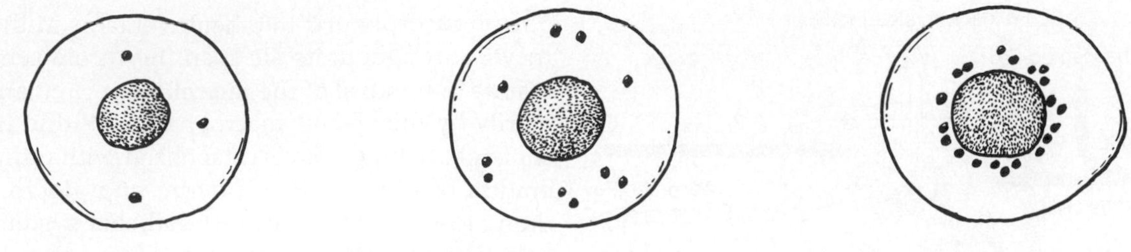

Figure 35.3. Small particles of nonheme iron may be seen in the cytoplasm of developing erythroblasts utilizing iron stains such as Prussian blue. Type I sideroblasts contain one to five small, randomly distributed iron particles and account for 20 to 60% of erythrocytes. Type II sideroblasts contain five or more coarse, randomly distributed iron granules and are often seen in states of excess reticuloendothelial iron and/or abnormal iron utilization. Type III sideroblasts, or ringed sideroblasts, are the morphologic hallmark of the sideroblastic anemias and are characterized by a ring or arc of iron encircling two-thirds or more of the erythroblast nucleus.

Table 35.3. Common Causes of Gastrointestinal Blood Loss

Esophagus
Varices
Stomach
Ulcer
Gastritis
Small intestine
Ulcer
Crohn's disease
Colon
Ulcerative colitis
Diverticulitis
Carcinoma
Rectum
Hemorrhoids

A decreased intake of iron may rise in the face of an adequate diet if the body is incapable of absorbing iron. Malabsorption of iron may be seen with achlorhydria, following partial or total gastrectomy, or as a complication of diffuse enteritis (e.g., celiac disease). Pica, the ingestion of unusual substances, may be seen both as a cause and as a manifestation of iron deficiency. When habitually ingested, substances such as clay or starch can either interfere with iron absorption or serve as an iron-poor caloric substitute.

In the adult population of the United States, depletion of the body's iron stores through chronic blood loss is a much more common cause of iron-deficiency anemia than is an insufficient intake of iron. If an average diet is consumed, a steady loss of as little as 3 to 4 ml of blood per day can result in negative iron balance. Gastrointestinal bleeding is the most frequent cause of iron deficiency in men and postmenopausal women; menstrual blood loss must be considered first in premenopausal women. Common gastrointestinal disorders resulting in blood loss are presented in Table 35.3. Unusual causes of chronic blood loss include hemoglobinuria and pulmonary hemosiderosis.

Clinical Symptoms

Iron-deficiency anemia is typically insidious in onset and gradual in progression. Consequently, patients adapt well and medical attention is often delayed. Many patients present with signs and symptoms common to anemia. Others may present with symptoms related to the cause of the iron deficiency (e.g., ulcer disease), while in some patients the anemia may be discovered incidentally.

As iron is vital to the growth and development of all cells, it is not surprising that a deficiency of iron leads to manifestations beyond the hematopoietic system. The clinical changes appear as the body becomes incapable of replacing cells at a rate equivalent to cell loss or exfoliation. Abnormalities of the nails, tongue, and upper gastrointestinal tract are common. Brittle, breakable, ridged, or spoon nails may be seen. Absence or flattening of the papillae of the tongue may be accompanied by soreness or burning (glossitis). Fissures or ulcers at the corners of the mouth (angular stomatitis) may also be noted. Upper esophageal webs or strictures may develop; the combination of dysphasia, stomatitis, and hypochromic anemia is referred to as Paterson-Kelly or Plummer-Vinson syndrome.

Laboratory Findings

Serum Chemistry. The appearance of a microcytic hypochromic anemia is actually a finding late in the course of iron deficiency. A number of laboratory changes reflective of the body's declining iron stores are observed prior to the appearance of microcytic hypochromic red cells. Decreased iron stores, reflected by a decreased serum ferritin, are found early in the course of iron deficiency, as stored iron is liberated to transferrin to maintain an adequate delivery of iron to the developing erythroblast. As iron stores are depleted, serum iron falls and a compensa-

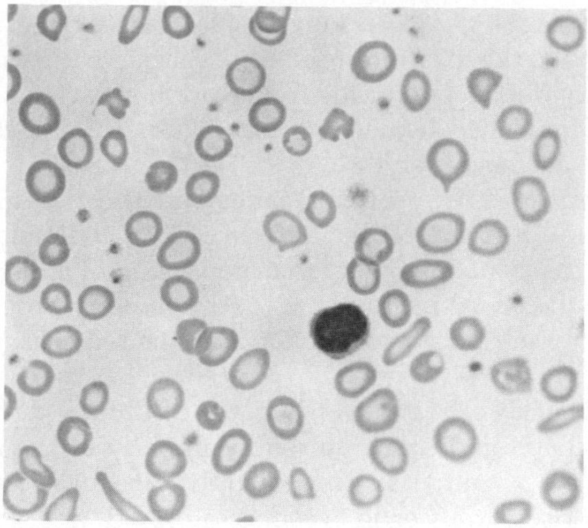

Figure 35.4. The peripheral blood smear in fully developed iron-deficiency anemia exhibits erythrocytes rich in central pallor. Although virtually all erythrocytes are microcytic, note the prominent variation in both size and shape, typical of iron-deficiency anemia.

tory increase in transferrin synthesis is begun. These two events result in a decreased transferrin saturation; by definition, iron-deficient erythropoiesis is present when the transferrin saturation falls below 16%. As insufficient iron is available for heme synthesis, an elevation of FEP becomes evident.

Blood. Early in the course of iron deficiency, the anemia appears normocytic and normochromic. As heme synthesis is impaired, hypochromic erythrocytes become evident. Microcytosis usually develops in tandem. As a result, the mean corpuscular volume (MCV), mean corpuscular hemoglobin (MCH), and mean corpuscular hemoglobin concentration (MCHC) are typically proportionally reduced.

Examination of the peripheral blood smear reveals an erythroid population, heterogeneous in both size and shape, which becomes quite striking in severe cases (Fig. 35.4). As iron deficiency becomes pronounced, many erythrocytes exhibit only a thin peripheral rim of hemoglobin. Poikilocytes often seen include ovalocytes, pencil cells, teardrop forms, fragments, and target cells.

The leukocyte count is typically normal, although slight granulocytopenia may be seen. Hypersegmented neutrophils may be present. The platelet count is often elevated, commonly up to twice normal. Values reaching 1000×10^9/liter may be seen, mimicking essential thrombocythemia.

Bone Marrow. The bone marrow often demonstrates mild erythroid hyperplasia. The developing erythroblasts appear small with scanty cytoplasm, and exhibit frayed or ragged cell borders (Fig. 35.5). Nuclear budding or fragmentation may be noted. PAS-positive erythroblasts indicative of abnormal cytoplasmic maturation may also be seen. Many of these small abnormal erythroblasts die within the marrow, resulting in ineffective erythropoiesis. A Prussian blue stain demonstrates an absence of stainable iron. Sideroblasts are decreased, often to the point of being absent.

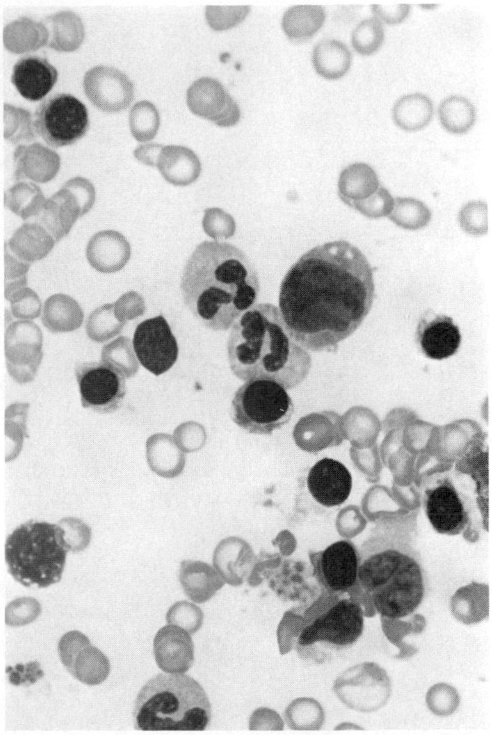

Figure 35.5. The developing erythroblasts in iron deficiency are small with scanty cytoplasm, often having a frayed, ragged, or moth-eaten appearance.

Therapy

It cannot be overemphasized that iron-deficiency anemia is not a disease but merely a sign of disease. Consequently, it is imperative that patients presenting with iron-deficiency anemia be thoroughly evaluated to establish the cause of the deficiency. Once the cause has been identified and appropriate therapy instituted, iron stores must be replenished. This is best accomplished by oral administration of ferrous sulfate. Parenteral administration of iron should be utilized only in the unusual circumstance of malabsorption.

Signs of iron deficiency usually begin to abate within days of iron therapy. Hematologic response can be monitored with the reticulocyte count, which should reach a maximum 7 to 10 days following the institution of therapy. The reticulocyte count seldom exceeds 10% and slowly falls as the hemoglobin level rises. Normalization of the hemoglobin should be complete within 8 weeks.

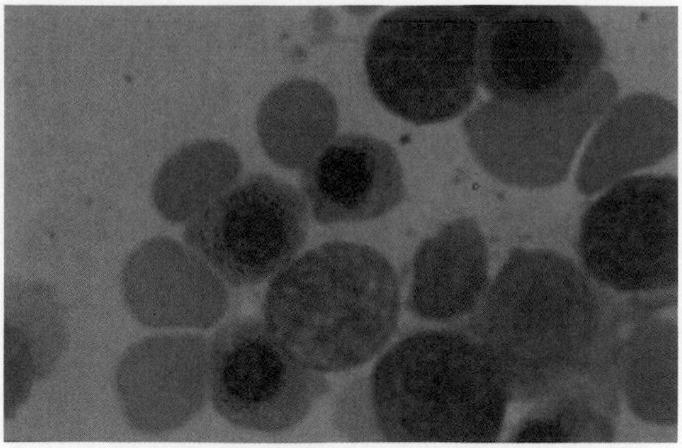

Figure 35.6. Ringed sideroblasts (Prussian blue stain). Numerous erythroblasts demonstrate deposition of granular iron nearly encircling the nucleus.

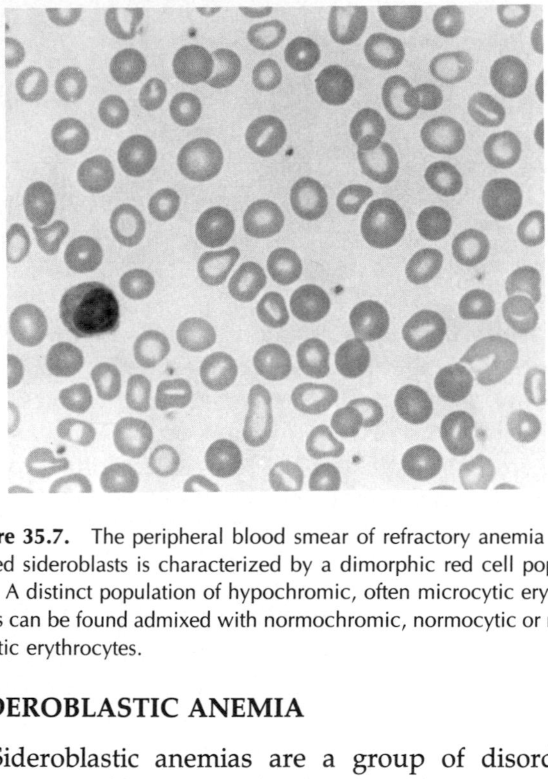

Figure 35.7. The peripheral blood smear of refractory anemia with ringed sideroblasts is characterized by a dimorphic red cell population. A distinct population of hypochromic, often microcytic erythrocytes can be found admixed with normochromic, normocytic or macrocytic erythrocytes.

SIDEROBLASTIC ANEMIA

Sideroblastic anemias are a group of disorders characterized by impaired utilization of iron resulting in diminished heme synthesis. The uptake of iron by the developing erythrocyte is partly controlled by the concentration of intracellular heme, which acts as a feedback inhibitor. The diminished heme synthesis resulting from impaired utilization of iron therefore results in a continued stimulus for iron absorption despite an adequate or increased level of intracellular iron. Excess iron is deposited in the mitochondria of the erythrocytes, the site of incorporation into protoporphyrin IX. The excessive deposition of iron is seen as rings or arcs around the nucleus of the erythroblast with a Prussian blue stain; these ringed sideroblasts are the morphologic hallmark of this group of disorders (Fig. 35.6). Ringed sideroblasts often succumb to the toxic effects of iron, leading to intramedullary destruction or ineffective erythropoiesis.

Diminished heme synthesis results in hypochromic microcytic erythrocytes. The degree of microcytosis and hypochromia varies between the different forms of sideroblastic anemia. Often a dimorphic red cell population is present consisting of a distinct population of microcytic hypochromic erythrocytes among normocytic or even macrocytic red cells (Fig. 35.7).

Iron absorption by the body continues despite the inability of the erythron to properly utilize iron in heme synthesis. Consequently, plasma (serum) iron rises, transferrin becomes saturated, and transferrin synthesis is suppressed. With time, the reticuloendothelial stores become overloaded and iron is deposited in the parenchymal cells of various tissues. Excessive iron deposition in the heart, pancreas, or liver can result in organ dysfunction and sequelae analogous to the genetic disorder hemochromatosis.

These three features—ringed sideroblasts, a population of microcytic hypochromic erythrocytes, and hyperferremia—characterize the sideroblastic anemias. As a group, these disorders may be divided into hereditary and acquired forms.

Hereditary Sideroblastic Anemia

Hereditary forms of sideroblastic anemia are distinctly less common than acquired sideroblastic anemia. The majority of the hereditary forms have been traced to an X-linked pattern of inheritance. Typically, it is only the male hemizygote who exhibits manifestations of the disease; rarely, female carriers may be moderately anemic. The severity of the anemia is variable. Often a severe microcytic hypochromic anemia is detected in infancy or early childhood. Mild forms of the disease may go undetected until early adulthood. The red cell population often exhibits marked anisopoikilocytosis, obscuring the classic dimorphic picture ascribed to sideroblastic anemia. Coarse basophilic stippling is present, and when found in microcytic hypochromic cells is a clue to the diagnosis. Ringed sideroblasts constitute 10 to 40% of erythroblasts and are typically seen only in late stages of erythroid development. Serum iron is high, and transferrin and reticuloendothelial stores are saturated. Over the course of years, parenchymal deposition may lead to cirrhosis, cardiomyopathy, and/or diabetes. Consequently, the removal of excess iron should be initiated. This may not only delay or prevent the damage of parenchymal iron deposition, but it may improve the hematologic status of the patient

Table 35.4. Drugs Implicated in Secondary Sideroblastic Anemia

Antituberculous agents
Isonicotinic acid hydrazine (INH)
Pyrazinamide
Cycloserine
Ethionamide
Chlorampheniol
Chemotherapeutic agents
Alkylating agents
Antimetabolites
Lead
Alcohol

by diminishing the toxic effects of excess iron on the erythron.

Variable defects of ALA synthetase have been implicated as the cause of X-linked sideroblastic anemia. Some forms respond to pharmacologic doses of pyridoxine; although not truly pyridoxine deficient, these patients possess ALA synthetase variants that either have an increased Michaelis constant (K_m) for pyridoxal 5′-phosphate or are unstable and abnormally sensitive to mitochondrial proteases. Clinical responses to pyridoxine are variable. Subtotal correction of the hemoglobin is common with persistence of microcytic hypochromic erythrocytes.

A few cases of hereditary sideroblastic anemias have been described that, although clinically indistinguishable from the X-linked variants, are indeterminant in their pattern of genetic transmission. An autosomal recessive pattern of inheritance has been suggested.

Acquired Sideroblastic Anemia

Acquired sideroblastic anemia is typically a disorder of adulthood. It may be idiopathic or it may occur as a secondary reversible phenomenon during administration of certain medicinal agents or after exposure to various myelotoxic chemicals (Table 35.4).

The antituberculous drugs and alcohol interfere with pyridoxine metabolism or the conversion of pyridoxine to the active pyridoxine 5′-phosphate, respectively. Ringed sideroblasts may be transiently associated with the administration of chemotherapeutic drugs or may appear years after therapy as part of a secondary or therapy-related myelodysplastic syndrome or leukemia. Lead is toxic to the erythron in a number of ways, including inhibitory effects at multiple sites in the heme biosynthetic pathway. Regardless of the etiology, the number of ringed sideroblasts and the degree of anemia and microcytosis tend to be less prominent than in either the inherited or idiopathic forms of sideroblastic anemia.

Ringed sideroblasts have also been described in association with a variety of other hematologic and nonhematologic conditions, including myeloproliferative disorders, multiple myeloma, lymphomas, megaloblastic anemia, collagen vascular disorders and myxedema. In some circumstances, this finding may be secondary to the administration of therapeutic agents, as previously described.

It is imperative that known causes of sideroblastic anemia be excluded prior to rendering the diagnosis of idiopathic sideroblastic anemia, also known as refractory anemia with ringed sideroblasts (RARS). The idiopathic form of sideroblastic anemia is grouped among the myelodysplastic syndromes, and shares with them a predilection for individuals over the age of 50, an association with various nonrandom chromosomal abnormalities, and progression to acute nonlymphocytic leukemia, estimated to occur in up to 20% of cases.

Ringed sideroblasts are typically more prevalent in RARS, constituting 40 to 95% of the erythroid population. Most patients present with anemia, reticulocytopenia, and erythroid hyperplasia, indicating ineffective erythropoiesis. Leukocytes and platelets are typically unaffected. Ringed sideroblasts must account for more than 15% of the erythroblast population and myeloblasts less than 5% of all nucleated cells to establish the diagnosis.

The anemia is unresponsive to hematinic agents, including pyridoxine. Most patients have a relatively indolent and prolonged course managed with transfusional support. Periodic bone marrow evaluation is advised, as a small number of patients progress to acute leukemia or evolve into a more aggressive myelodysplastic syndrome. Although hyperferremia is also characteristic of the idiopathic form of sideroblastic anemia, the long-term side effects of iron toxicity are unusual due to the advanced age of individuals affected by this disorder.

IRON OVERLOAD

Iron is highly conserved by the body; under normal circumstances, the 1 to 2 mg of iron lost daily through turnover of the upper gastrointestinal epithelium is balanced by absorption of ingested iron. Prolonged administration of iron or enhanced absorption of iron cannot be matched by increased iron excretion. A gradual progressive buildup of iron eventually leads to accumulation outside the reticuloendothelial system, causing injury to parenchymal cells. It is postulated that the toxic effects of iron may be related to the formation of free radicals, causing lipid peroxidation, or to the liberation of lysosomal enzymes. The clinical manifestations of parenchymal damage are referred to as hemochromatosis. Organs principally involved include the liver (cirrhosis), the heart (cardiomyopathy or arrhythmias), and the pancreas (glucose intolerance). Additionally, patients often exhibit bronze pigmentation of the skin, resulting from a combination of iron deposition and increased melanin. Arthritis, resembling rheumatoid arthritis, and manifestations of hypogonadism may also be present.

Primary Inherited Hemochromatosis

Hemochromatosis has been divided into primary inherited (idiopathic) and secondary forms. Inherited hemochromatosis results from an inborn error of metabolism that leads to increased iron absorption. Although the precise mechanism is unknown, investigation has implicated a defect in the handling of iron at the level of the duodenal or jejunal mucosal cell. The amount of iron absorbed from the diet in afflicted individuals exceeds normal by only 2 to 3 mg/day. Over the course of time, however, the body accumulates iron stores up to 10 times normal. The toxic effects of iron are related not only to the sheer bulk of total body iron but also to the preferential deposition in parenchymal cells seen in this disorder, particularly the liver. Indeed, biopsies of reticuloendothelial sites such as bone marrow may exhibit normal iron stores in the face of massive iron deposits in other tissues.

Idiopathic hemochromatosis is inherited as an autosomal recessive disorder with full expression in homozygotes and partial expression in some heterozygotes. Males are predominantly affected, likely reflecting the protective effect of iron loss occurring naturally in women during menstruation and pregnancy. The genetic locus of the disorder has been linked to chromosome 6 near the locus of the major histocompatibility complex; the tight linkage to several HLA loci is useful as an aid in tracing the pattern of inheritance of the affected allele in families once an index case has been identified. The gene frequency in the United States and Europe is such that approximately three in every 1000 persons have the potential to develop hemochromatosis, and one in 10 is a carrier.

Organ injury is a time-quantity function of iron accumulation. Treatment is therefore aimed at early identification of the disorder and repeated phlebotomy or the introduction of iron chelators as a means of removing excess iron. Unfortunately, the untoward effects are often silent until significant organ damage is initiated. Clinical manifestations of the disorder are frequently not apparent until the fifth or sixth decade. Criteria useful for detecting parenchymal iron overload are transferrin saturation exceeding 80% and serum ferritin levels above 500 μg/liter. Tissue confirmation of the disorder is established by liver biopsy.

Table 35.5. Conditions Associated with the Anemia of Chronic Disease

Chronic infections
Tuberculosis
Chronic fungal infections
Subacute bacterial endocarditis
Osteomyelitis
Pyelonephritis
Pelvic inflammatory disease
Chronic inflammatory disorders
Rheumatoid arthritis
Systemic lupus erythematosus
Sarcoidosis
Rheumatic fever
Neoplasms
Carcinoma
Malignant lymphoma

Secondary Hemochromatosis

Secondary causes of iron overload principally result in deposition of iron within the reticuloendothelial system (also referred to as hemosiderosis). Damage to parenchymal tissues indistinguishable from inherited hemochromatosis, however, occurs with time as iron becomes deposited outside the saturated reticuloendothelial stores.

Increased intake of dietary iron may rarely result in iron overloading; more frequently iron overloading is a complication of the anemias characterized by lifelong ineffective erythropoiesis. Examples include thalassemia major, inherited sideroblastic anemia, and certain forms of congenital dyserythropoietic anemia. All display hyperabsorption of iron in response to an increased rate of erythropoiesis. A program of maintenance transfusion therapy may be necessary in these disorders, further complicating the picture of iron overload through the associated parenteral administration of iron in blood products.

ANEMIA OF CHRONIC DISEASE

Anemia of chronic disease is the term used to describe the anemic state that is often seen in conjunction with a number of chronic nonhematologic disorders (Table 35.5). Considering the array of conditions with which anemia of chronic disease has been associated, it is not surprising to find that it follows closely behind iron deficiency as a cause of anemia.

Beyond the descriptive association with chronic disease, anemia of chronic disease may also be characterized as an anemia of impaired iron utilization. As such, it is defined by a reduction in both serum iron and serum transferrin. Hypoferremia typically outpaces the hypotransferrinemia, resulting in a decreased transferrin saturation. These changes occur in the face of adequate or increased iron stores, indicating a sequestration of iron in the reticuloendothelial system.

Iron trapping is but one factor in the pathogenesis of anemia of chronic disease. Additionally, there is a diminished erythrocyte survival time, which is further compounded by the inability of the bone marrow to compensate by increasing the rate of erythropoiesis. Each of these factors, in part, appears to be related to the sustained release of interleukin-1 (IL-1) found during chronic inflammation and neoplasia.

IL-1 triggers the release of lactoferrin, a glycoprotein found in the secondary granules of neutrophils, which competes with transferrin or the binding of iron. Unlike iron bound to transferrin, which is transported to tissues in need, lactoferrin-bound iron is delivered to the macrophage, where it is internalized and effectively trapped, preventing delivery to the developing erythron.

Decreased erythrocyte survival may, in part, be related to fever induced by IL-1 or to enhanced ingestion of erythrocytes by macrophages activated by IL-1. IL-1 activation of macrophages and T-lymphocytes may also alter the microenvironment of the bone marrow, creating conditions unfavorable for a compensatory erythroid hyperplasia.

Clinical and Laboratory Features

Anemia of chronic disease typically develops within 1 to 2 months following the onset of a chronic illness and remains stable throughout the disease course. It is typically mild to moderate in severity, with the hematocrit ranging from 0.30 to 0.40. As such, the signs and symptoms of the underlying disease tend to overshadow the effects of the anemia.

The anemia is frequently normocytic and normochromic; however, a microcytic hypochromic anemia may occasionally be encountered. Anisopoikilocytosis is usually minimal, in contrast to the findings in iron-deficiency and sideroblastic anemias. The reticulocyte count, when corrected for the degree of anemia, is normal or low. The bone marrow shows essentially normal numbers of erythroid precursors with no significant morphologic abnormalities. Iron stores appear adequate or increased in the marrow; however, the number of sideroblasts is decreased (less than 20%); this combination of findings is virtually diagnostic of anemia of chronic disease.

Anemia of chronic disease and iron-deficiency anemia have in common a diminished delivery of iron to the erythron, hence both are characterized by decreased serum iron. The two disorders may be distinguished by quantitation of serum transferrin and ferritin. Transferrin is normal or decreased in anemia of chronic disease, in contrast to the elevated values found in iron deficiency. Transferrin saturation is typically decreased in both disorders; however, values are often below 10% in iron deficiency, a level seldom reached in anemia of chronic disease. Ferritin is normal or increased in anemia of chronic disease, reflecting adequate iron stores, whereas ferritin is decreased in iron deficiency. Caution must be exercised, however, in interpreting serum ferritin in the face of inflammation or neoplasia, as it is an acute phase reactant.

SUMMARY: A LABORATORY APPROACH TO THE DISORDERS OF HEME SYNTHESIS

Together with the thalassemias, iron-deficiency anemia, sideroblastic anemia, and anemia of chronic disease must each be considered in the differential diagnosis of a microcytic hypochromic anemia. From the preceding discussion, however, it can be seen that the morphologic classification of anemia is not perfect; this is evident in the frequent presentation of anemia of chronic disease as a normocytic anemia and sideroblastic anemia as a normocytic or macrocytic anemia. Iron-deficiency anemia, sideroblastic anemia, and anemia of chronic disease are related beyond a common morphologic presentation; they share a defect in heme synthesis related to the deficiency, utilization, or transport of iron. Taking advantage of the altered handling of iron exhibited by these disorders, differentiation can often be achieved by simple quantitation of serum iron, transferrin, and ferritin (Fig. 35.8). As the defect in thalassemias is unrelated to iron metabolism, normal iron studies in the face of a microcytic hypochromic anemia are indicative of thalassemia. A notable exception may be encountered with the thalassemia major syndromes, in which iron overload occurs as a late complication. This latter group of disorders, however, is infrequently encountered in the U.S. population.

Disorders of DNA Synthesis: Megaloblastic Anemia

The megaloblastic anemias are a group of disorders characterized by a reduced rate of DNA synthesis. RNA synthesis, its processing and ultimately protein synthesis are, however, unaffected. The resultant dyssynchrony in nuclear (DNA) and cytoplasmic (RNA) development is the morphologic hallmark of the megaloblastic anemias. Deficiencies of vitamin B_{12} or folic acid are far and away the most frequent etiologic factors.

VITAMIN B_{12}

Metabolism

Vitamin B_{12}, or cobalamin, is composed of a corrin ring linked to a ribonucleotide through one of the ni-

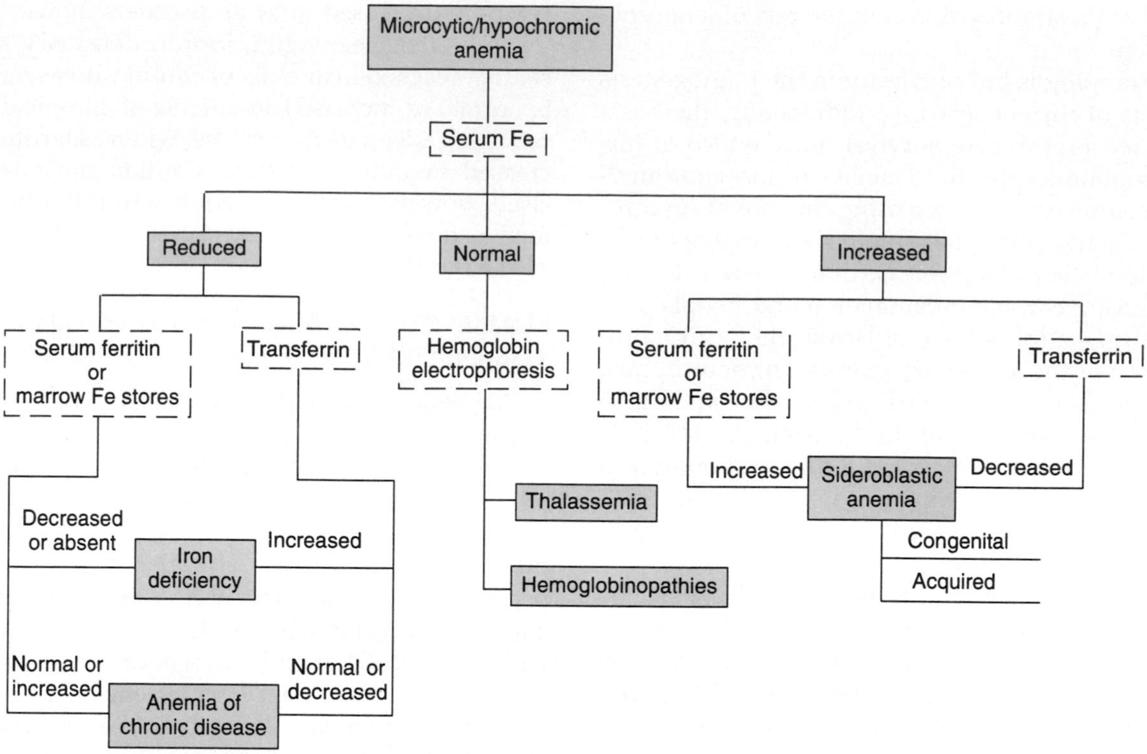

Figure 35.8. A laboratory approach to the disorders of heme synthesis.

trogens of its base. The corrin ring bears resemblance to the tetrapyrrole ring structure of heme; cobalt occupies the central position of the corrin ring analogous to the position occupied by iron in heme. The unsatisfied valence of the cobalt ion is filled in humans largely by CN^- (cyanocobalamin) or OH^- (hydroxycobalamin). These cobalamin species each have nutritional properties of B_{12} yet have no biochemical activity. Rapid tissue conversion to the active coenzymes methylcobalamin and adenosylcobalamin occurs through the action of coenzyme synthetases.

Methylcobalamin and adenosylcobalamin are vital cofactors for two independent metabolic reactions in humans. Methylcobalamin is a coenzyme needed for converting N^5-methyltetrahydrofolate to tetrahydrofolate (FH_4) (Fig. 35.9). FH_4 is a key element in a number of biochemical reactions; most important is its role as an intramediary coenzyme in DNA synthesis. Conversion of FH_4 to the folate coenzyme $N^{5,10}$-methylene FH_4 is essential for the conversion of deoxyuridine monophosphate (dUMP) to deoxythymidine monophosphate (dTMP), ultimately allowing for integration of thymidine (as deoxythymidine triphosphate (dTTP)) into DNA. Therefore, in large part, the impairment of DNA synthesis seen with vitamin B_{12} deficiency is related to abnormalities in folate metabolism. This explains the shared manifestations of vitamin B_{12} and folic acid deficiency.

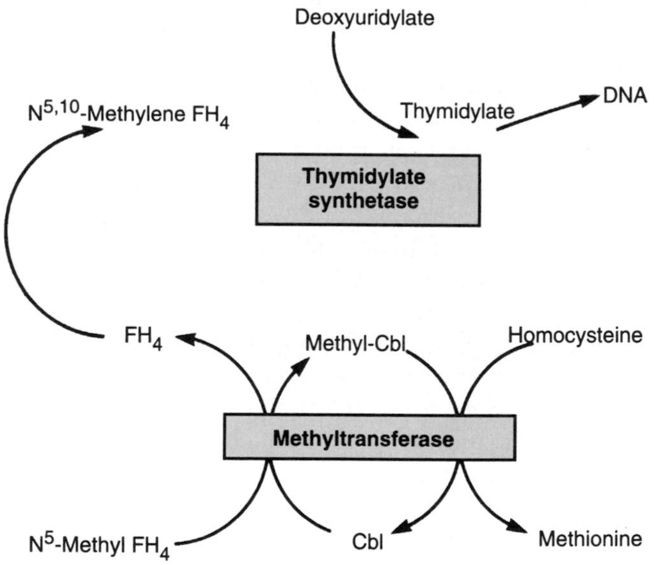

Figure 35.9. The role of methylcobalamin in methionine synthesis and its integral relationship to folate metabolism and DNA synthesis. FH_4, tetrahydrofolate; —Cbl, cobalamin. (From Williams W et al. Hematology. 3rd ed. New York: McGraw Hill, 1983:314.)

The inability to convert dUMP to dTMP, seen with both vitamin B_{12} and folic acid deficiency, alternatively results in the conversion of dUMP to deoxyuridine triphosphate (dUTP). The excess dUTP ultimately becomes incorporated into DNA in place of dTTP, since DNA polymerase is unable to distinguish between these two nucleotides. The substitu-

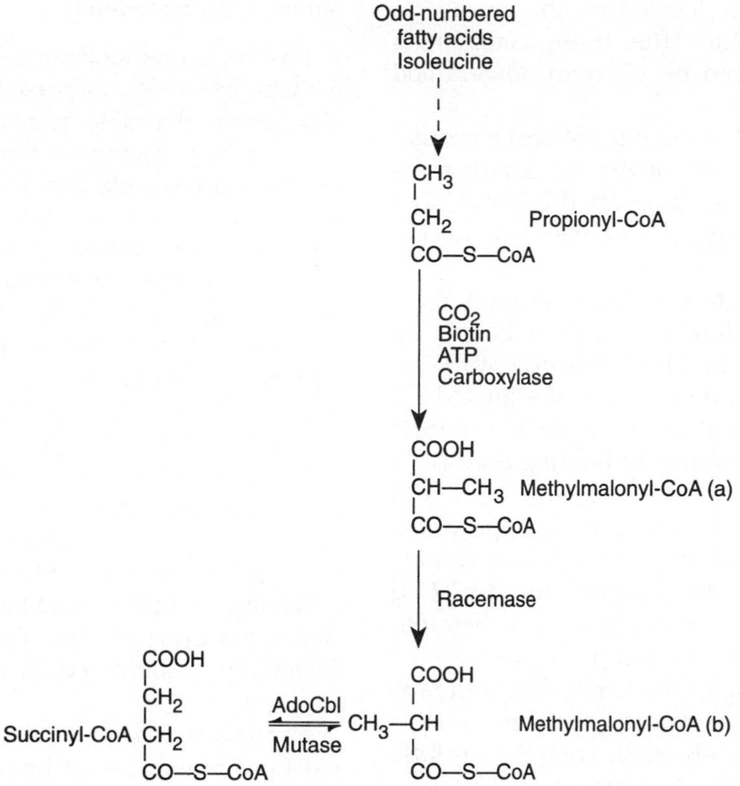

Figure 35.10. Adenosylcobalamin as a cofactor in the conversion of methylmalonyl-CoA to succinyl-CoA. AdoCbl, adenosylcobalamin. (From Williams W et al. Hematology. 3rd ed. New York: McGraw-Hill, 1983;315.)

tion of dUTP for dTTP results in errors in strand copying followed by attempts to edit the wrongfully inserted uridylate residue. Subsequent efforts to correctly synthesize DNA obviously fall short, as the requisite thymidylate is in short supply. Repeated cycles of fragmentation and attempted repair slow the synthesis of DNA and result in the characteristic nuclear chromatin pattern of megaloblastic anemia.

The other metabolically active form of cobalamin, adenosylcobalamin, is a coenzyme in humans essential to the conversion of methylmalonyl-CoA to succinyl-CoA, the basic fuel of the Krebs cycle (Fig. 35.10). While adenosylcobalamin cannot be linked to DNA synthesis, it has been postulated, but not well established, that interruption of this reaction may play a role in the development of the neurologic changes seen in vitamin B_{12} deficiency. Inhibition of the conversion of methylmalonyl-CoA to succinyl-CoA results in an accumulation of the methylmalonyl-CoA precursor propionyl. In high concentration, propionyl-CoA may replace acetyl-CoA as the usual primer for synthesis of even-chain fatty acids. Consequent errant production and insertion of odd-chained fatty acids into lipid membranes may result in lipid membrane abnormalities such as demyelination and subsequent neurologic impairment. An alternate hypothesis suggests that the impaired conversion of methionine due to the deficiency of methylcobalamin results in a deficiency of *S*-adenosylmethionine (SAM). SAM is important for certain transmethylation reactions, including some that may be important in the maintenance of myelin.

Vitamin B_{12} Absorption

Synthesized by many bacteria and certain molds, vitamin B_{12} is found only in foods of animal origin such as meat, eggs, cheese, and milk. It has been estimated that the minimal daily requirement of vitamin B_{12} is 0.6 to 1.2 μg/day, an amount easily achieved in Western diets, which commonly contain 5 to 30 μg of vitamin B_{12}.

Vitamin B_{12} is released from food sources by the digestion of animal proteins. Free B_{12} is then competitively bound either to intrinsic factor (IF), a high-affinity glycoprotein produced by the parietal cells of the stomach, or to R-proteins, a class of B_{12}-binding proteins so designated because of their rapid electrophoretic mobility. R-proteins are found in a variety of sites, including gastric juice and saliva, and serve to bind the majority of newly ingested B_{12}. Under normal circumstances, however, the R-protein–B_{12} complex is short-lived; degradation of R-protein by pancreatic proteases occurs in the proximal small intestine, liberating B_{12}, which then avidly binds to IF. IF greatly facilitates the absorption of B_{12}, providing direct and safe transport through the gastrointestinal tract to specific receptors located on the mucosa of the terminal ileum. Once the IF-B_{12} complex is bound, B_{12} is internalized by a poorly understood process.

Not to be overlooked is the enterohepatic circulation of B_{12}. More than 50% of the B_{12} entering the intestine each day arrives through this route. The majority is reabsorbed through IF-dependent mechanisms.

Following absorption in the ileum, vitamin B_{12} is released to the circulation, where it is bound by transcobalamin (TC), the B_{12} transport protein. Transcobalamin exists in three forms, designated TC I, TC II, and TC III, TC II is the major physiologic carrier of B_{12}. Although normally binding only 10 to 25% of the plasma concentration of B_{12}. TC II has great capacity for rapid B_{12} transport to appropriate receptors at sites of need (dividing cells) or storage (liver). Once bound by the receptor, the B_{12}–TC II complex is internalized by endocytosis, B_{12} liberated, and TC II degraded by lysosomal proteases.

TC I and TC III belong to the family of T-proteins. Although most of the plasma B_{12} concentration is bound to TC I, this relatively stable complex has little capacity for transfer of B_{12} to tissue sites. TC III is largely synthesized in granulocytes and, although capable of binding B_{12} in vitro, is not engaged in the transport of endogenous B_{12} to tissue cells. Under normal circumstances, TC I is approximately 50% saturated with B_{12}, whereas less than 5% of TC II is saturated. The sum of the unsaturated TC I and TC II is referred to as the unsaturated B_{12} binding capacity.

Quantitative Assays

Serum levels of vitamin B_{12} are largely determined using isotope dilution techniques, although cobalamin-dependent microbial assay systems may still be used. Universal use of intrinsic factor as a binding protein in radioisotope assays eliminates binding of cobalamin analogs and yields values that compare favorably to those obtained with a microbiological system. Normal serum levels of B_{12} typically are in the range of 200 to 900 pg/ml. The serum B_{12} concentration is but a minute fraction of the total body stores of B_{12}, estimated at 1 to 5 mg, the liver being the primary site of storage.

Abnormalities of B_{12} binding proteins have been reported in a variety of disease states. Quantitation of both serum B_{12} and (unsaturated) B_{12} binding capacity are often cited as a tool in the evaluation of the chronic myeloproliferative disorders. Increases in one or both parameters largely reflect elevations of TC I and TC III liberated from the breakdown of increased numbers of granulocytes in these disease states.

Vitamin B_{12} Deficiency

Five basic mechanisms may lead to B_{12} deficiency: inadequate intake, increased requirement, defective absorption, defective transport, and defective enzyme activity. Defective transport due to an abnormality of a transcobalamin carrier protein is rare, as are abnormalities of the coenzyme synthetases needed for conversion of B_{12} to the active forms of methylcobalamin or adenosylcobalamin. Also uncommon, given the body's reserves of B_{12}, are deficiencies occurring during transient periods of increased B_{12} requirement, e.g., during growth and development, pregnancy, or lactation. Similarly, an inadequate dietary intake of B_{12} is largely limited to strict vegetarians who abstain from all animal proteins, including milk and eggs. Assuming a previously healthy diet, strict avoidance of foods replete with B_{12} for a period of 3 to 5 years is required before achieving complete exhaustion of the body's B_{12} stores. For these reasons, deficiencies of B_{12} are most frequently encountered as a result of defective absorption.

Pernicious Anemia. Pernicious anemia is the most common cause of impaired B_{12} absorption and is the result of an acquired failure to secrete intrinsic factor (IF) by the gastric parietal cells. The markedly diminished or absent secretion of intrinsic factor is typically associated with achlorhydria; both findings are related to the universal presence of gastric atrophy. Pernicious anemia is most commonly found in individuals of northern European ancestry, although no racial or ethnic group is immune. Typically, the disorder presents after the age of 40. The etiology of the disorder remains speculative. Circumstantial evidence suggests a hereditary basis for the disorder, although neither a mode of inheritance nor a link to any genetic marker is currently known.

An autoimmune basis for pernicious anemia has also been proposed based on the frequent finding of autoantibodies in patients with pernicious anemia and the histologic findings of a lymphoplasmacytic infiltrate in the gastric biopsies of patients with pernicious anemia. Two types of autoantibodies are found in patients with pernicious anemia. Approximately 90% of patients have antibodies to parietal cell cytoplasm in their serum. The exact role, if any, of these antibodies in the pathogenesis of pernicious anemias is uncertain. Anti–parietal cell antibodies have also been found in individuals with atrophic gastritis unassociated with pernicious anemia, in persons with Hashiomoto's thyroiditis, and in a small number of normal individuals. Serum antibodies to intrinsic factor have been detected in 55% of patients, whereas assays of gastric juice allow detection of anti–intrinsic factor antibodies in 75% of patients with pernicious anemia. Anti-IF antibodies are of two types: blocking antibodies, which block the attachment of B_{12} to IF, and binding antibodies, which prevent the absorption of B_{12} in the ileum. Although these antibodies have shown functional impairment of IF activity in vivo, their temporal sequence appears to postdate the onset of disease, thereby negating their role as a primary etiologic agent in this disease process.

Variant Forms of Pernicious Anemia. Two rare variant forms of pernicious anemia (PA) are found. Juvenile PA is distinguished from classic PA solely by its clinical appearance in adolescence or early adulthood. A rare congenital form of PA has also been described. Patients with congenital PA suffer either from absence of IF or from a functionally aberrant form of IF. In contrast to other forms of PA, the defect in IF is selective; the appearance and function of the gastric mucosa in all other aspects is normal. The congenital form of PA is inherited as an autosomal recessive defect with hematologic manifestations appearing in infancy. Like classic PA, both juvenile and congenital PA respond to the administration of IF.

Gastrectomy. B_{12} deficiency typically develops 3 to 5 years following total gastrectomy as B_{12} absorption ceases and the body's B_{12} stores are gradually depleted. B_{12} deficiency is less predictable following subtotal gastrectomy; often appearing 1 to 2 decades following surgery, it may be related to the slow development of postoperative gastritis and gastric atrophy.

Pancreatic Insufficiency. Loss of the exocrine function of the pancreas, regardless of cause, may result in B_{12} deficiency. Pancreatic proteases are integral to the digestion of gastric R-proteins, which compete with IF for B_{12}. Intact R-proteins inhibit formation of the B_{12}-IF complex, thereby diminishing absorption in the terminal ileum.

Intestinal Malabsorption. A number of small intestinal abnormalities may result in diminished B_{12} absorption. Surgical resection or diseases of the terminal ileum, such as Crohn's disease, effectively remove the site of B_{12} absorption. Malformations of the intestinal tract may predispose to the development of localized pockets of bacterial overgrowth. These proliferative microorganisms may effectively deprive the host of B_{12}. Similarly, competition for B_{12} may be encountered with intestinal infestation by the fish tapeworm, *Diphyllobothrium latum*.

Laboratory Evaluation of B_{12} Deficiency. A number of tests may be employed in the laboratory investigation of megaloblastic anemia. Serum or plasma quantitation of B_{12} is the usual method of detecting a vitamin B_{12}–deficient state. Less direct and less specific measures of a B_{12} deficiency state, such as urinary excretion of methylmalonic acid or the deoxyuridine suppression test, are seldom needed.

Once B_{12} deficiency is established, the etiology must be determined. The most frequent test employed to determine if the patient lacks IF is the Schilling test. Shortly following oral administration of 0.5 to 2.0 μg of radiolabeled B_{12}, a large intramuscular flushing dose of nonlabeled B_{12} is administered, which will saturate B_{12} binding sites. Once saturated, the orally ingested radiolabeled B_{12} absorbed by the ileum will be excreted in the urine. A 24-hour urine collection normally reveals greater than 7% absorption of a 1-μg dose. If excretion is found to be diminished, the test is repeated 1 week later. The subsequent test, however, provides purified intrinsic factor with the orally administered B_{12}. Improved absorption following administration of IF implies a deficiency of IF, whereas continued poor absorption signifies intestinal malfunction. Unfortunately, the Schilling test suffers from two common pitfalls: inadequate urine collections and underlying renal dysfunction.

Anti–parietal cell and anti–intrinsic factor antibodies have been previously described and may be used as additional tests to help substantiate the diagnosis of pernicious anemia.

FOLIC ACID

Metabolism

Folic acid, or pteroylglutamic acid, consists of three parts: pteridine, *p*-aminobenzoic acid, and glutamic acid. It serves as the parent for a large family of compounds having similar nutritional value to which the generic term folate is applied. Folates are widely distributed in a variety of foods, being synthesized by higher plants and microorganisms. Green leafy vegetables, fruits, and dairy products provide the greatest sources of folate in the usual Western diet. Unfortunately, folates are thermolabile, so a large portion of dietary folates may be lost in food preparation, particularly in boiling. A normal balanced diet, however, has no difficulty in meeting the recommended daily allowance for adults of 200 to 400 μg. In sharp contrast to vitamin B_{12}, the body's stores of folate are limited. Following cessation of dietary intake, a decline in blood folate levels can be detected within a few weeks, and megaloblastic anemia may ensue in 3 to 5 months.

Most food folates are in the form of reduced methyl or formyl derivatives; about 90% are polyglutamates. Absorption occurs predominantly in the upper small intestine. When ingested in the monoglutamate form, folate is readily absorbed. The more prevalent polyglutamates, however, must first be converted to the monoglutamate form through the action of deconjugating enzymes found in the brush borders of intestinal epithelial cells as well as within intracellular lysosomes.

Following assimilation by the intestinal epithelial cell, folate is converted to N^5-methyl TH_4, in part through the action of dihydrofolate reductase; it is in this form that folate is found in circulation. Cellular incorporation occurs as N^5-methyl TH_4 relinquishes its methyl group to homocysteine, forming methionine and TH_4, a reaction requiring methylcobalamin as a coenzyme (Fig. 35.9). Intracellular TH_4 may then proceed as a precursor to DNA synthesis or may be converted to an intracellular polyglutamated storage form through the action of an ATP-dependent synthetase. The storage form may undergo later deconjugation ultimately to yield TH_4 at critical times in DNA synthesis. This interconversion of the mono- and polyglutamated forms appears to play a role in the regulation of DNA synthesis.

Table 35.6. Drug-Induced Suppression of DNA Synthesis

Folate antagonists
Methotrexate
Aminopterin
Trimethoprin
Pyrimethamine
Triamterene
Antimetabolites
5-Fluorouracil
Hydroxyurea
Cytosine arabinoside
Alkylating agents
Cyclophosphamide
Nitrogen mustard
Chlorambucil
Busulfan
Melphalan
Nitrous oxide

Folate Deficiency

Folate deficiency may arise from inadequate intake, impaired absorption, increased requirements, or defective folate metabolism. The most frequent cause of folate deficiency is a folate-poor diet. With limited folate reserves, the effects of an unbalanced diet are soon felt by chronic alcoholics, the impoverished, and the "tea and toast" elderly. Diets associated with the development of folate deficiency are characterized by a predominance of starches and grains with relatively little animal protein or fresh green vegetables. Megaloblastic anemia arising from folate deficiency in the setting of general malnutrition may also be complicated by diminished reserves of other hematinic agents.

Intestinal malabsorption is also a common cause of folate deficiency. Although folate absorption occurs principally in the proximal small intestine, receptor sites are found throughout the small bowel. Consequently, for megaloblastic anemia to occur secondary to impaired folate absorption, diffuse small intestinal disease is generally required. Tropical sprue and adult celiac disease (nontropical sprue or gluten-sensitive enteropathy) both bring about such a state of generalized malabsorption, resulting in a deficiency of a variety of nutrients, including folate. Widespread involvement of the small bowel by Crohn's disease may also result in folate deficiency.

Increased folate requirements are seen in a variety of physiologic and pathologic conditions exhibiting an overall increase in cell proliferation and DNA synthesis. Folate deficiency typically occurs during the last trimester of pregnancy, when folate requirements increase approximately fivefold. Following delivery, lactation brings further demands for additional folate. Infancy is marked by the greatest rate of growth, and hence increased folate intake is required. Pathologic hyperproliferative states also require additional folates and include a variety of chronic hemolytic anemias: sickle cell anemia, hereditary spherocytosis, thalassemia, and chronic autoimmune hemolytic anemias. This is not surprising if one considers that normal hematopoiesis is responsible for approximately half of total DNA synthesis. Rapidly dividing tumors such as leukemias, high-grade lymphomas, and small cell carcinoma may also usurp the body's folate supply.

Impaired folate metabolism is the desired effect of certain drugs. Chemotherapeutic agents such as methotrexate and aminopterin interfere with the conversion of folate to tetrahydrofolate. Consequently, administration of these agents causes megaloblastic changes in the marrow. More commonly prescribed, but much less frequently the cause of severe megaloblastic changes, are such antifolates as trimethoprim and triamterene. The induction of megaloblastic changes as a side effect of drug therapy is, however, not limited to the antifolates. A number of other chemotherapeutic agents that interfere with DNA synthesis (antimetabolites, alkylating agents) are also known to induce similar changes (Table 35.6).

Aside from these drug-induced defects in folate utilization, inborn errors of folate metabolism have been reported. These include dihydrofolate reductase deficiency and formiminotransferase deficiency, as well as congenital defects of folate absorption.

Laboratory Evaluation of Folic Acid Deficiency

Both microbiological and radioisotopic assays are available for the quantitation of serum folate. Serum levels of folate are, however, quite labile and sensitive to short-term variation in vitamin intake. Quantitation of red cell folate provides a better long-term measure of true tissue folate levels, since folate metabolism ceases in the developing red cell following nuclear extrusion. Thereafter, folate levels remain stable throughout the life span of the erythrocyte. Changes in red cell folate come about over time as red cells are released from a marrow environment of differing folate concentrations. Megaloblastic anemia caused by folate deficiency typically exhibits serum folate concentrations less than 3 ng/ml and red cell folate concentrations less than 100 ng/ml.

The following cautions must be exercised in interpreting the results of serum or red cell folate concentrations. Since serum folates are greatly influenced by short-term dietary variation, quantitation should be obtained prior to ingestion of a balanced hospital diet replete with folate. Similarly, red cell folate may be affected by the administration of transfusions, and assays should therefore be performed on samples obtained prior to the administration of red cell products. Finally, because B_{12} is a requisite cofactor for the uptake and utilization of folate by the cell, in its absence, folate is trapped in the serum. Therefore, in Vitamin B_{12} deficiency, serum folate may be elevated and red cell folate decreased.

CLINICAL FEATURES OF MEGALOBLASTIC ANEMIA

Vitamin B_{12} deficiency is most frequently insidious in onset, likely reflecting the prolonged period of time required to deplete the body's B_{12} stores. Given our capacity to compensate over time, it is not surprising that patients often present with few signs or symptoms despite a frequently marked degree of anemia. Classically, patients with pernicious anemia have been described as pale, but not wasted, with lemon-yellow skin reflecting a combination of anemia and mild hyperbilirubinemia. Blue eyes, a broad face and chest, and blond or prematurely gray hair complete the stereotype. Some of these features may reflect the Northern European ancestry of many patients with pernicious anemia. It is important to remember, however, that no race or sex is immune from this disorder; consequently, many of these features may not be present.

A diagnostic triad of weakness, sore tongue, and paresthesias is cited as the classic symptom complex of vitamin B_{12} deficiency. Indeed, weakness reflects anemia. Glossitis, present in approximately half of patients, is the most visible indicator of generalized epithelial atropy. Particularly vulnerable is the gastrointestinal tract, where rapid turnover of epithelial cells is a normal event. Gastric atrophy, occurring either as the sine qua non of pernicious anemia or as a secondary complication of other forms of B_{12} deficiency, coupled with villous atrophy of the small bowel, may lead to complaints of heartburn, bloating, loss of appetite, or diarrhea. Paresthesias are among many neurologic manifestations complicating B_{12} deficiency. Neurologic changes chiefly affect the white matter of the posterior and lateral columns of the spinal cord, leading to symmetrical numbness and tingling of the hands and feet, diminished vibratory or position sense, progressive weakness, and an unsteady or ataxic gait. The terms "subacute combined degeneration" or "combined system disease" are employed to encompass these abnormalities of multinerve pathways. The severity and rate of progression of the neurologic changes do not always correlate with the degree of anemia or other findings of B_{12} deficiency. Consequently, familiarity with this complication of vitamin B_{12} deficiency is mandatory if it is to be recognized and arrested before serious irreversible neurologic changes occur.

The manifestations of folic acid deficiency are often tainted by the myriad of health problems associated with chronic alcoholism and poverty. In fact, associated health problems may be the initiating reasons for seeking medical attention. Hematologic manifestations are similar to those found in megaloblastic anemia attributable to vitamin B_{12} deficiency. The neurologic changes typical of B_{12} deficiency, however, are absent.

PERIPHERAL BLOOD AND BONE MARROW FINDINGS

The peripheral blood and bone marrow findings in folic acid and vitamin B_{12} deficiency are indistinguishable. Recognizing that DNA synthesis is critical to all developing cell lines, it follows that patients with full-blown megaloblastic anemia typically present with pancytopenia. Red cell indices classically reveal macrocytosis; an MCV above 120 fl is common. The MCH is elevated, whereas the MCHC is normal. The reticulocyte count is normal or decreased, reflecting the inability of the bone marrow to produce red cells. Unfortunately, however, not all patients present with pancytopenia and macrocytosis. Although anemia is a fairly universal finding, the presence and degree of leukopenia and thrombocytopenia are variable. Superimposed infection may lead to an elevated white blood count at presentation. Likewise, the MCV may appear normal with coexisting iron deficiency or a silent thalassemia trait.

Examination of the peripheral blood smear reveals a number of important clues to the diagnosis (Fig. 35.11). Macroovalocytes and hypersegmented neutrophils are invariably present. Anisopoikilocytosis of moderate to marked degree is present including

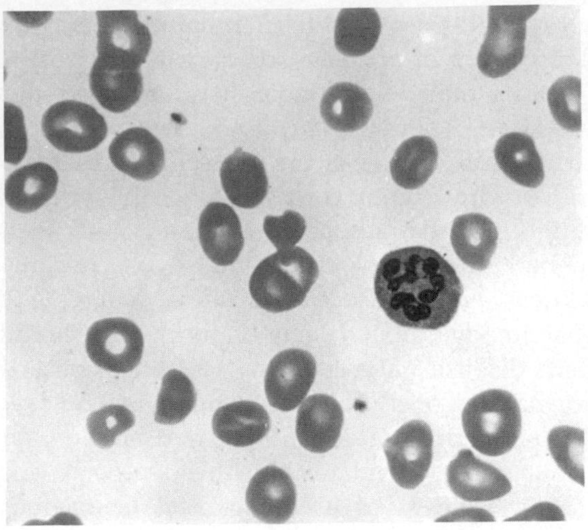

Figure 35.11. Megaloblastic anemia is characterized by hypersegmented neutrophils and the presence of well-hemoglobinized macrocytes and macroovalocytes.

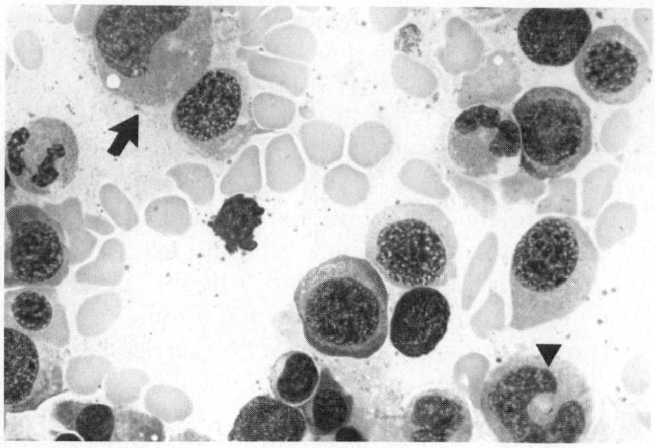

Figure 35.12. Bone marrow aspirate smear in megaloblastic anemia demonstrates numerous large erythroblasts having a fenestrated nuclear chromatin. The nuclear appearance has been likened to that of a piece of salami. Nuclear changes are also evident in the developing neutrophils: giant metamyelocytes *(arrow)* and giant bands *(arrowhead)*.

ovalocytes, teardrop forms, schistocytes, and spherocytes. Basophilic stippling and Howell-Jolly bodies may be seen; two or more Howell-Jolly bodies may be found per cell, unlike in postsplenectomy states. With severe anemia, nucleated red blood cells may be present that exhibit characteristic megaloblastic nuclear changes.

Bone marrow aspirate smears reveal an intensely cellular marrow with increased numbers of erythroblasts (Fig. 35.12). Nuclear cytoplasmic dyssynchrony may be found in all myeloid cell lines. The changes in the red cell series, however, often appear most striking. Changes are most evident in the later stages of erythroid maturation, when cellular enlargement and open fenestrated or sieve-like nuclear chromatin contrasts sharply with the smaller size and shrunken, condensed nucleus of the late polychromatophilic and orthochromatic normoblasts. Intramedullary destruction is morphologically manifested as nuclear karyorrhexis or fragmentation. Bizarre nuclear budding or lobulation may also be seen. Although megaloblastic changes in developing neutrophils tend to be overshadowed by those of the erythroid series, they offer important clues to both early and partially treated megaloblastic anemia. Giant bands and metamyelocytes are frequent; as the name implies, these cells are large and often exhibit an increased nuclear:cytoplasmic ratio. Nuclear chromatin appears less mature than anticipated for the stage of maturation indicated by nuclear shape. Premature nuclear segmentation is also common as these giant "bands" exhibit nuclear folding and twisting as if to form segments of a mature neutrophil. Such changes appear prior to those of the erythroid series and persist even after normoblastic erythroid maturation returns following therapeutic intervention. Abnormalities may also be seen in the megakaryocytes. These include complex hypersegmentation and a similar open or fenestrated nuclear chromatin pattern.

Perhaps no other disorder better exemplifies the hazards of interpreting bone marrow trephine biopsies without the benefit of aspirate smears than does megaloblastic anemia. The trephine biopsy is virtually always hypercellular, in many cases approaching 100%. The lag in nuclear maturation results in an accumulation of erythroblasts in the early to middle stages of maturation. This, coupled with the immature appearance of the nuclear chromatin, imparts the picture of a marrow overrun with primitive hematopoietic cells. The temptation to regard this picture as one of acute leukemia can be overcome by careful examination, which demonstrates the presence of all three cell lines, evidence of cellular maturation, and characteristic giant bands.

Abnormal maturation leads to intramedullary destruction of all cell lines, resulting in the paradox of ineffective hematopoiesis: pancytopenia in the face of a hypercellular bone marrow. Intramedullary red cell destruction results in a mild hyperbilirubinemia, an increased LDH, and an increase in serum iron. Red cells are rich in LD_1 and LD_2; LD_1 predominates in immature red cells, which may result in a "flip" of the normal LD_1:LD_2 ratio. Iron is liberated during the catabolism of red cells at a rate greater than it can be utilized. Consequently, serum iron increases, transferrin saturation increases while synthesis decreases, and iron stores become replete. Marrow sideroblasts may increase in number, and type II as well as type III (ringed) sideroblasts may be found.

DIFFERENTIAL DIAGNOSIS

The combined findings of pancytopenia, macrocytosis, and hypersegmented neutrophils are virtually diagnostic of megaloblastic anemia. Individually, however, these findings are not specific, each being associated with a host of disorders largely unrelated to B_{12} or folic acid metabolism. Pancytopenia generally implies diminished marrow precursors, ineffective hematopoiesis, or hypersplenism. Macrocytosis may occur in chronic liver disease, hypothyroidism, pregnancy, normal neonates, marrow failure, chronic hemolytic states with elevated reticulocyte counts, myelodysplastic syndromes, and following administration of a variety of cytotoxic drugs. Hypersegmented neutrophils, although uncommon outside of megaloblastic anemia, may be seen as a congenital anomaly and in iron deficiency, sepsis, renal disease, and chronic myeloproliferative disorders.

Megaloblastic changes in one or more cell lines of the bone marrow are frequently seen following the administration of a variety of chemotherapeutic agents. Most often these changes affect the developing neutrophils to the greatest degree and pose no diagnostic dilemma given the patient's history. Megaloblasts may be seen as one of many changes in the myelodysplastic syndromes or in erythroleukemia. The clinical history, the absence of B_{12} or folic acid deficiency, and the presence of dysgranulopoiesis, dysmegakaryopoiesis, and/or increased numbers of myeloblasts will all help separate these neoplastic conditions from megaloblastic anemia. A variety of inborn errors may also lead to megaloblastic changes or frank megaloblastic anemia, including congenital dyserythropoietic anemia, hereditary orotic aciduria, and Lesch-Nyhan syndrome.

MANAGEMENT

Therapy for megaloblastic anemia is aimed both at replenishing the body's stores of vitamin B_{12} or folic acid and at documenting and correcting the underlying cause. Parenteral administration of B_{12}, typically on a monthly basis, is required therapy for pernicious anemia and malabsorption states, which are not amenable to medical intervention. Folic acid deficiency, since most often dietary in nature, is amenable to oral administration of folic acid. Folic acid preparations for parenteral administration are available if required.

Improvement in the patient's hematologic status is initially evident within 3 to 5 days by a rise in the reticulocyte count, which typically reaches a maximum at 10 days. A prompt decrease in serum iron is noted as effective red cell production begins. Amelioration of megaloblastic changes in the red cell series is largely complete within 24 to 48 hours, whereas changes in the neutrophil line persist in the peripheral blood and bone marrow for up to 10 days. Within 1 to 2 months all peripheral blood parameters should return to normal.

Neurologic deficits are arrested following the institution of appropriate therapy. Regression is, however, not always complete. Mild deficits of short duration are more apt to resolve than are chronic or severe impairments. It is important to diagnose the cause accurately and to administer the correct hematinic agents appropriately in patients with megaloblastic anemia. This is underscored by the progression of neurologic changes that occurs in B_{12} deficiency inappropriately treated with folic acid in spite of partial hematologic correction.

Bone Marrow Failure: Inadequate Erythroid Precursors

Included in this section are the anemias that result from an inadequate number of erythroid precursors occurring either as a selective phenomenon or, more frequently, as part of the trilineage suppression that results from a reduction in pluripotent hematopoietic stem cells.

APLASTIC ANEMIA

Aplastic or hypoplastic anemia is typically an acquired defect in pluripotent stem cells, although defects in growth factors, immunoregulatory signals, or the marrow microenvironment have also been proposed as possible mechanisms. Regardless of the etiology, the net effect is a reduction in erythroid, granulocytic/monocytic, and megakaryocytic cell lines in the bone marrow and their progeny in the peripheral blood. The incidence of aplastic anemia varies worldwide; in the Western nations 5 to 10 new cases per million general population are estimated to occur annually. Cases are roughly equally divided into idiopathic and secondary forms, the latter composed largely of chemical or drug injury, radiation exposure, or infection-associated aplasia.

Etiology

Prior to labeling aplastic anemia as idiopathic, careful exclusion of known etiologic factors must be undertaken. This is particularly true in cases occurring in childhood, adolescence, or early adulthood, when a putative cause is found more frequently than in adulthood.

Drug-Related Injury. Chemical- or drug-related injury to the marrow may arise either as a dose-dependent or an idiosyncratic phenomenon. Marrow ablation is the desired dose-dependent effect of many chemotherapeutic agents. Similar dose-dependent marrow aplasia is encountered as an untoward side effect of exposure to chemicals such as benzene, its derivative trinitrotoluene, arsenic, or alcohol. Hematopoietic suppression associated with heavy alcohol intake is typically self-limited and reversible following cessation of drinking, unlike that found with benzene, trinitrotoluene, and arsenic, which often progress to fatal aplasia. Chronic benzene and arsenic exposure are both associated with the development of dysplasia, largely marked by bizarre megaloblastic changes of the erythroid series. In the case of benzene exposure, such dysplastic changes may progress and evolve to acute myelogenous leukemia (AML); not unexpectedly, the frequency of erythroleukemia is increased compared to that found in de novo AML.

Chloramphenicol is perhaps the most widely publicized example of an idiosyncratic drug reaction leading to marrow aplasia. This adverse side effect cannot be related to drug dosage or route of administration. Likewise, its occurrence and the rapidity of onset cannot be predicted. This largely fatal complication has no relation to the mild, reversible, dose-dependent erythroid suppression known to occur in approximately half of individuals exposed to large doses of chloramphenicol. Similar idiosyncratic reactions are encountered with quinacrine, phenylbutazone, carbonic anhydrase inhibitors, gold, and a variety of anticonvulsants, including phenytoin, mephenytoin, trimethadione, methsuximide, and carbamazepine. The effect of these agents upon the three hematopoietic cell lines is not always uniform, and in some cases selectively results in red cell aplasia, agranulocytosis, or thrombocytopenic purpura.

Ionizing Radiation. The hematopoietic system, like all body cells, is susceptible to damage by ionizing radiation. The untoward effects of radiation are dependent on the nature and quantity of radiant energy, the duration of exposure, and the mitotic rate of the exposed cell population. It is the high mitotic activity of the bone marrow that makes it one of the most vulnerable organ systems to the toxic effect of radiation. Aplastic anemia may ensue following a single exposure to large but sublethal doses of radiation, as well as repeated or long-term exposure to moderate doses.

Infection. A number of viruses have been associated with myelosuppression. Most notable is the rare, unexplained, and often fatal aplasia that occurs in association with hepatitis. This unpredictable sequela is most frequently associated with non-A, non-B hepatitis and exhibits no relationship to the severity of liver disease. The time to onset is variable, with most cases becoming manifest approximately 6 weeks following clinically evident hepatic disease.

Human parvovirus (serotype B19) is now recognized as a cause of aplastic anemia. This virus, as well as several others, is responsible for myelosuppression, most frequently manifesting in individuals with an underlying chronic hemolytic anemia. Although granulocytes and platelets may be reduced, a profound exacerbation of the chronic anemia is the major cause of morbidity in these cases. Due to the shortened erythrocyte survival inherent to the underlying hemolytic state, affected individuals are exquisitely sensitive to the abrupt cessation of erythropoiesis caused by the selective cytotoxic invasion of erythroblasts by the parvovirus. Such temporary erythroblastopenia is typically preceded by or associated with an upper respiratory or flu-like illness. Although short-term transfusional support may be necessary, these aplastic crises are generally self-limited.

Idiopathic. Aside from the direct toxic effect of various drugs, chemicals, and radiant energy, the pathogenesis of aplastic anemia is not fully understood. Evidence supporting an immunologic mechanism has emerged from a number of observations linking aplasia with disorders of immunoregulation. Support for this concept has been found in vitro through alterations in marrow lymphoid populations and in vivo by the success in certain individuals of anti-lymphocyte or anti-thymocyte globulin as a therapeutic modality.

Clinical Features

The onset of aplastic anemia is variable, in part dependent on etiologic factors. Signs and symptoms of generalized bone marrow failure are evident: pallor, weakness, fatigue, and dyspnea on exertion are associated with anemia; infections and fever are associated with granulocytopenia; and petechiae, ecchymoses, or overt hemorrhage may be associated with thrombocytopenia.

Peripheral Blood and Bone Marrow Findings

Pancytopenia is the rule in the peripheral blood; however, the decline in erythrocytes, leukocytes, and platelets is often not proportional. In part, this may be related to the susceptibility of the marrow cell lines to the injurious agent. Erythrocytes are usually normochromic and normocytic with little variation in size and shape, although mild macrocytosis may be evident in some cases. Neutrophils are significantly decreased, and lymphocytes predominate on examination of the peripheral smear. Dysplastic features are not common in any cell line unless there has been exposure to toxins such as benzene or arsenic.

The bone marrow trephine biopsy shows a marked reduction in cellularity, largely replaced by fat. Foci of increased cellularity may be found scattered throughout the marrow, most often dominated by erythroblasts. Such hot spots of hematopoiesis may be misleading when aspirated or when only a small core of tissue is available for examination. This underscores the need for a generous sample of tissue in cases of suspected marrow aplasia.

Aspirate smears typically reflect the marked diminution in hematopoietic elements. Lymphocytes and plasma cells predominate; increased numbers of mast cells and histiocytes, the latter often laden with iron or particulate debris, are also frequently seen. Mild cytoatypia may be seen when foci of hematopoiesis are aspirated; however, this is never a striking feature unless exposure to toxins has occurred.

Treatment

The clinical course of patients with aplastic anemia depends on the etiology, the severity of the pancytopenia, the age of the patient, and the response to therapy. In some instances, marrow recovery may ensue following discontinuation of drugs known to act as marrow suppressants. Similarly, removal from the source of a known environmental toxin may initiate marrow recovery. Transient episodes of myelosuppression are amenable to short-term transfusional support. All too often, however, marrow aplasia is severe and irreversible, requiring long-term medical intervention.

Therapy with a number of drugs has met with variable success. Corticosteroids, androgens, lithium carbonate, anti-thymocyte globulin and cyclophosphamide have been utilized as marrow stimulants or as immunosuppressive agents aimed at reversing putative immune-mediated aplasia. Repeated transfusions can obviously provide needed red cells and platelets, but do little to offset granulocytopenia. Multiple transfusions are, however, complicated by the associated morbidity of iron overload and the risk of posttransfusional infectious complications. Additionally, in young patients with HLA-matched bone marrow donors, repeated transfusions have an adverse effect on bone marrow transplantation, the treatment of choice for this group of patients.

PURE RED CELL APLASIA

As the name implies, pure red cell aplasia is characterized by anemia secondary to a marked reduction in the number of red cell precursors in the marrow. Granulocytes and megakaryocytes are unaffected. To some degree, the aplastic crises known to complicate various chronic hemolytic states can be viewed as an acute form of pure red cell aplasia. Similarly, young children may experience a transient arrest of erythropoiesis following a viral illness (transient erythroblastopenia of childhood). Idiosyncratic drug reactions may also selectively involve the red cell series.

Many cases of pure red cell aplasia are associated with a thymoma; in conjunction, some patients also exhibit myasthenia gravis. Thymectomy will restore normal hematopoiesis in a subset of these patients. Similar to aplastic anemia, an immunologic mechanism has been proposed as a pathogenetic factor in pure red cell aplasia. Accordingly, therapy has included immunosuppressive agents as well as transfusional support.

CONSTITUTIONAL AND HEREDITARY DISORDERS ASSOCIATED WITH APLASTIC ANEMIA

Several hereditary or constitutional syndromes are associated with aplastic anemia or the variant pure red cell aplasia. Manifestations are apparent in childhood and consist not only of hematologic abnormalities but of a variety of other anomalies, including skeletal malformations, pigmentary changes of the skin, retarded mental and sexual development, and renal abnormalities.

Fanconi's anemia is inherited as an autosomal recessive disorder. Patients exhibit progressive pancytopenia and marrow aplasia during the first decade of life. Associated findings include increased levels of fetal hemoglobin and expression of i antigen, reflecting reversion to fetal hematopoiesis. Like ataxia-telangiectasia and xeroderma pigmentosum, Fanconi's anemia is a disorder of defective DNA repair. Cytogenetic analysis reveals evidence of chromosome instability including chromosomal breaks and sister chromatid exchange. Not surprising, therefore, is termination in acute myelogenous leukemia in approximately 10% of cases of Fanconi's anemia.

Diamond-Blackfan anemia predominantly affects the red cell line and may therefore be viewed as a constitutional form of pure red cell aplasia. Anemia is often present at birth and invariably develops within the first 2 years of life. Macrocytosis is common. The marrow shows features common to pure red cell aplasia. Like Fanconi's anemia, fetal hemoglobin and i antigen expression are increased. Transfusional support is the mainstay of therapy, and a significant number of patients demonstrate improvement in their hematologic status with glucocorticoid therapy. Spontaneous remission has been reported in up to 20% of cases.

CONGENITAL DYSERYTHROPOIETIC ANEMIAS

Congenital dyserythropoietic anemia (CDA) amply describes this rare inherited group of anemias characterized morphologically by dyserythropoiesis. The morphologic abnormalities are also associated with premature intramedullary destruction of developing erythroblasts, i.e., ineffective erythropoiesis, resulting in a diminished reticulocyte count and signs and symptoms related to continued low grade hemolysis. The anemia is usually mild to moderate. Treatment is typically limited to periodic transfusional support. Because of the life-long intramedullary destruction, the risk of iron overload must not be overlooked. Granulocytic and megakaryocytic cell lines are unaffected. Based largely on the morphologic findings in the marrow, the CDAs are separated into three subtypes. In some cases, however, the morphologic features are overlapping and subcategorization is not easily achieved.

CDA I

This autosomal recessive disorder is characterized by the presence of 1 to 2% binucleated or multinucleated erythroblasts in conjunction with the finding of thin chromatin bridges between developing erythroblasts. Megaloblastic changes are frequently present with prominent karyorrhexis. The resulting anemia is typically mild and macrocytic with variable anisocytosis and poikilocytosis.

CDA II (HEMPAS)

This is the most frequently encountered type of CDA and is characterized by striking multinuclearity of late-stage marrow erythroblasts and the serologic finding that these defective erythroblasts lyse in acidified serum. These findings have led to the acronym HEMPAS: hereditary erythrocyte multinuclearity with positive acidified serum tests. Lysis in the Ham's (acidified serum) test occurs only with heterologous sera. This contrasts with the pattern of lysis seen in paroxysmal nocturnal hemoglobinuria that develops in either autologous or heterologous serum, as well as following complement activation by shifts in ionic strength (i.e., sucrose hemolysis tests).

Additional abnormalities associated with type II CDA include an abnormally high density of i antigen, defects in glycosylation, and a surplus of endoplasmic reticulum in late-stage erythroblasts that leads to the ultrastructural appearance of a double membrane. It is postulated that the latter finding may functionally interfere with cell division.

CDA III

This autosomal dominant disorder is characterized by prominent multinuclearity with occasional giant erythroblasts containing up to 12 nuclei.

MYELOPHTHISIC ANEMIAS

Encompassed under the term myelophthisic anemia are the peripheral cytopenias that arise as the result of bone marrow replacement by a wide variety of disorders. Although most frequently encountered in conjunction with malignant neoplasms metastasizing to or arising within the bone marrow cavity, nonneoplastic disorders may similarly result in marrow replacement. Examples of the former include metastatic carcinoma, leukemia, Hodgkin's and non-Hodgkin's lymphomas, and multiple myeloma. Marrow replacement occurring in the setting of nonneoplastic disease is typically the result of histiocytic proliferation seen either with disseminated granulomatous inflammation such as tuberculosis or in association with a variety of storage disorders.

Marrow infiltration results in variable degrees of anemia, leukopenia, and thrombocytopenia, which may occur singly or in combination. In addition, immature neutrophils and erythroblasts are often present in the circulation, a finding referred to as a leukoerythroblastic reaction. It is easy to conceptualize the reduction in peripheral counts as a crowding-out phenomenon, i.e., normal hematopoietic tissue being replaced by foreign elements. In a similar fashion, immature white and red cells may be squeezed out of the marrow by advancing tumor. It is likely, however, that other mechanisms also come into play, such as an altered and inhospitable marrow microenvironment leading to impaired development, destruction, or premature release of immature hematopoietic elements.

Other changes may also be encountered in the peripheral blood. Reticulocytes are often increased disproportionally to the degree of anemia. This finding may reflect premature release from the marrow. Teardrop-shaped erythrocytes may also be found. Although this shape change has been linked to the aforementioned infiltrative marrow disorders, it is typically a more striking finding in idiopathic myelofibrosis.

Both the diagnosis and etiology of a myelophthisic process rely on bone marrow examination. In many circumstances, the disease process does not diffusely involve the bone marrow. Changes of detection, therefore, are increased by bilateral bone marrow biopsies. Biopsies directed at sites of clinical or radiographically evident disease may also provide an increased yield. Often the aspirate smears may be unrewarding, as many focal lesions are associated with reticulin deposition and are therefore poorly aspirable. Necrosis, when encountered in the aspirate or trephine biopsy, is suggestive of marrow infiltration requiring further investigation.

ACCELERATED ERYTHROCYTE DESTRUCTION

Normal Erythroid Senescence

It is well established that the average natural life span of the human erythrocyte is 120 days. The exact mechanism or terminal events that allow these senescent cells to be recognized and removed from circulation is, however, not well understood. Erythrocytes undergo a number of age-related changes, including diminished intracellular concentrations of glycolytic enzymes, water, and solutes; altered membrane composition; and reduced surface area and volume. These factors undoubtedly have detrimental effects on deformability and functions vital to cellular integrity. Yet where and how red blood cells are actually removed from circulation is elusive, as observations to date have elucidated neither the progressive morphologic signs of aging nor the sites where active red cells are lost from circulation each second.

HEMOGLOBIN CATABOLISM

Senescent red cells liberate hemoglobin, the vast majority of which is catabolized within the reticuloendothelial system of the liver, spleen, and bone marrow. A small amount of hemoglobin is, however, released to circulation where, following dissociation to α-β dimer form, it is bound by haptoglobin, an α_2-glycoprotein synthesized by the liver. The haptoglobin-hemoglobin complex is rapidly cleared by the liver, where catabolism of both hemoglobin and haptoglobin occurs.

Human nature is to conserve, and red cell catabolism is no exception. Within the reticuloendothelial system, hemoglobin is dissociated into its three main building blocks: globin, iron, and protoporphyrin. Globin chains are rapidly degraded with return of their constituent amino acids to the plasma for future protein synthesis; iron is conserved to begin its role once again in hemoglobin synthesis; and protoporphyrin is degraded.

The protoporphyrin ring is initially cleaved by heme oxygenase, yielding biliverdin and carbon monoxide. This reaction provides the only source of endogenous carbon monoxide in the body. Biliverdin is reduced to bilirubin and bilirubin is then transported to the liver following solubilization by albumin, where the bilirubin-albumin complex (indirect bilirubin) is rapidly cleared by the liver (Fig. 35.13). Within the hepatocyte, bilirubin is conjugated and excreted in the bile mainly as bilirubin diglucuronide (direct bilirubin). Subsequent hydrolysis by bacterial enzymes present in the ileum and colon frees bilirubin, which is then reduced by anaerobic flora to a family of compounds collectively referred to as urobilinogens. Urobilinogens are largely excreted in the stool. Approximately 10 to 20% of urobilinogen is absorbed from the terminal ileum and redirected to the liver, where it is returned to the bile for excretion. A small amount of urobilinogen escapes this enterohepatic circulation and is excreted by the kidneys.

The hemolytic anemias are anemias resulting primarily from increased red cell destruction. By definition, many anemias secondarily associated with a slight reduction in red cell life span are excluded. By convention are also excluded disorders associated with defective erythropoiesis leading to marked intramedullary red cell destruction. The hemolytic anemias are therefore the disorders in which premature extramedullary red cell destruction is the primary cause of the anemia.

Often the terms intravascular and extravascular are used to denote sites of red cell destruction. The term extravascular, however, is somewhat misleading, because in fact the distinction is between lysis within the systemic circulation and destruction within the sinusoids of the reticuloendothelial system.

LABORATORY FINDINGS

Regardless of the mechanism or site of hemolysis, the hemolytic anemias share manifestations of increased red cell catabolism. Although increases in endogenous carbon monoxide production and fecal urobilinogen are measures of hemolysis, the most clinically useful laboratory parameter of increased red cell destruction is serum bilirubin. Elevated bilirubin levels, however, are nonspecific and may be found as a sign of hepatocellular or biliary disease. Elevated levels of indirect bilirubin are viewed as a better measure of hemolysis, provided that disorders of bilirubin conjugation are excluded.

Decreased levels of serum haptoglobin are also found in hemolysis. Although often suggested as an indicator of intravascular red cell destruction, diminished levels of haptoglobin are also found with extravascular or reticuloendothelial-mediated red cell destruction. It is important to note that haptoglobin is an acute phase reactant; normal values may therefore be encountered in hemolytic disorders complicated by infectious or inflammatory states.

Once haptoglobin is depleted through hepatic degradation of the haptoglobin-hemoglobin complex, free hemoglobin emerges in the circulation (Fig.

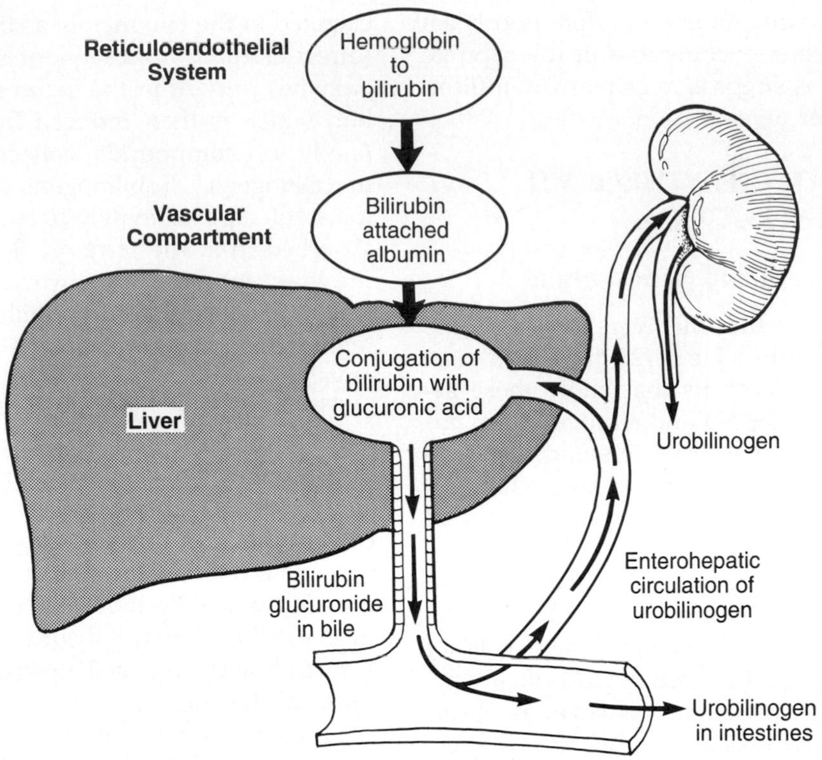

Figure 35.13. Hemoglobin liberated from senescent erythrocytes is catabolized in the reticuloendothelial system, and the protoporphyrin ring is converted to bilirubin, which is transported to the liver loosely bound to albumin. In the liver, bilirubin is conjugated and excreted in the bile as bilirubin diglucuronide. Enzymatic hydrolysis occurs in the intestine, with subsequent reduction to a family of compounds, the urobilinogens. 10 to 20% of the urobilinogen is reabsorbed and largely returned to the bile; a small amount of urobilinogen escapes the enterohepatic circulation and is excreted in the urine. Elevated levels of unconjugated hemoglobin and urinary urobilinogen are present in the hemolytic anemias. (From Petz LD, Garratty G. The diagnosis of hemolytic anemia. In: Acquired immune hemolytic anemias. New York: Churchill Livingstone, 1980:4.)

35.14). Quantitation of plasma (or serum) free hemoglobin is possible, but is fraught with the difficulty of obtaining a blood sample unbiased by the effects of a traumatic venipuncture. In circulation, the free dimeric form of hemoglobin is readily filtered by the glomerulus and absorbed by the proximal convoluted tubules of the kidney. Here hemoglobin may undergo further degradation. Liberated iron is stored in the proximal tubular epithelial cells as ferritin and hemosiderin. When sloughed in the urine, ferritin containing tubular epithelial cells can be detected by using a Prussian blue stain. This measure of increased red cell destruction is most useful in chronic hemolytic states, due to the lag phase that occurs between the onset of hemolysis and the detection of hemosiderinuria. The absorptive capacity of the proximal tubular cells for hemoglobin can be overcome, allowing free hemoglobin to pass into the urine. Hemoglobinuria, however, is not detectable until the absorptive capacity of both haptoglobin and the tubular epithelial cells is surpassed.

Plasma hemoglobin not bound to haptoglobin nor removed by the kidney is oxidized to methemoglobin. Subsequently, the oxidized heme moiety undergoes rapid dissociation and is then bound by hemopexin. This complex is cleared by the liver in a manner similar to the haptoglobin-mediated clearance of hemoglobin. Following depletion of hemopexin, oxidized heme binds to albumin, forming methemalbumin. Both the depletion of hemopexin and the presence of methemalbumin are two additional measures of hemolysis, though they offer little practical clinical utility.

Another intracellular constituent of erythrocytes that is readily measurable in the laboratory is lactic dehydrogenase (LDH). Since LDH is not restricted to erythrocytes, serum elevations may be encountered in a variety of disorders. Isoenzyme fractionation is somewhat more specific, as fractions LD_1 and LD_2 predominate in erythrocytes.

In the vast majority of uncomplicated hemolytic anemias, increased red cell destruction provides a stimulus for erythropoiesis. Invariably then, evaluation of suspected hemolytic states should include not only measures of increased red cell destruction but also parameters of accelerated erythropoiesis. These changes are readily apparent in a peripheral blood smear as an increased number of polychromatophilic erythrocytes. A more objective measure is obtained with a reticulocyte count. Brisk reticulocytosis may

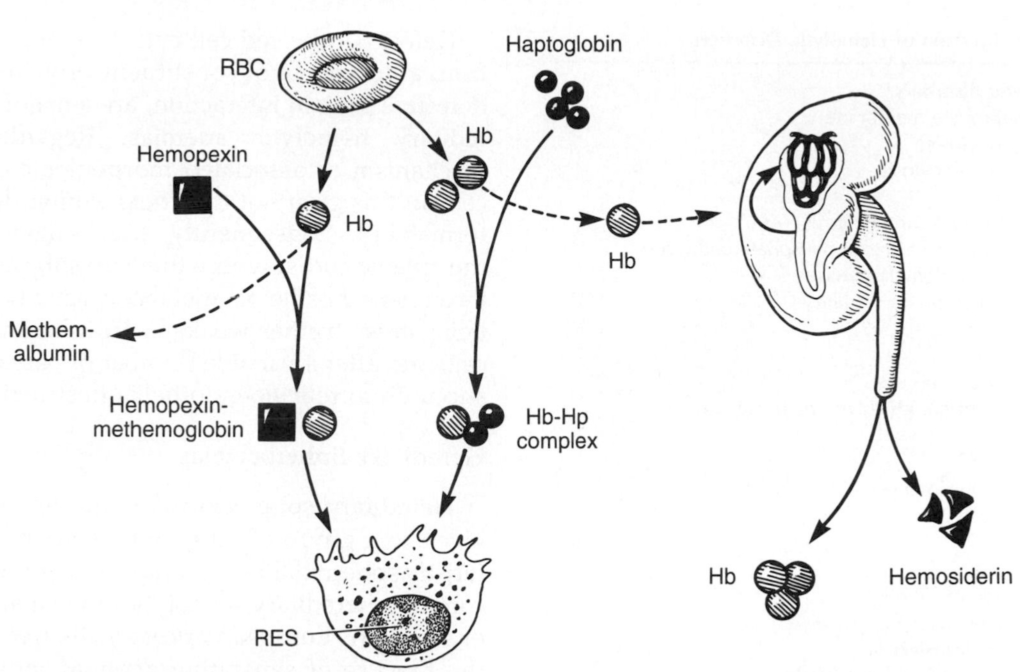

Figure 35.14. Intravascular destruction of erythrocytes liberates hemoglobin, which is bound in circulation by haptoglobin. The hemoglobin-haptoglobin complex is cleared by the liver; in the process haptoglobin is consumed. Depletion of haptoglobin results in free dimeric hemoglobin, which is readily filtered and partially excreted by the kidney. Partial reabsorption of hemoglobin occurs in the tubular epithelial cells. In chronic hemolysis, hemosiderin may be detected in the urine with turnover and sloughing of tubular epithelium. Free hemoglobin in the circulation is also oxidized to methemoglobin, which is bound by hemopexin and cleared by the liver analogous to the hemoglobin-haptoglobin complex. With depletion of hemopexin, methemoglobin is bound by albumin to form a methemalbumin. Intravascular hemolysis classically results in decreased haptoglobin; hemoglobinuria; decreased hemopexin; methemalbuminemia, and hemosiderinuria. (From Petz LD, Garratty G. The diagnosis of hemolytic anemia. In: Acquired immune hemolytic anemias. New York: Churchill Livingstone, 1980:3.)

elevate the mean corpuscular volume. Circulating erythroblasts may also be seen. Bone marrow examination typically reveals an erythroid hyperplasia, which in some cases may be quite striking, as the bone marrow is capable of increasing erythropoiesis 6 to 8 fold.

PATHOPHYSIOLOGIC CLASSIFICATION

A pathophysiologic classification of disorders resulting in shortened red cell survival is presented in Table 35.7. Broad separation is based on the nature of the abnormality: is the defect *intrinsic* to the red cell, or do *extrinsic* forces result in hemolysis? With one exception, intrinsic disorders are inherited defects, whereas extrinsic disorders are acquired. Paroxysmal nocturnal hemoglobinuria, the exception to this rule, is an acquired intrinsic abnormality.

Intrinsic and Inherited Red Cell Abnormalities

Intrinsic erythrocyte abnormalities are commonly grouped as membrane, metabolic, or hemoglobin defects. In keeping with convention, therefore, a discussion of the hemoglobinopathies is not undertaken here, but may be found in Chapter 36.

As inherited defects, these disorders may present a number of clinical features not typically seen with acquired red cell abnormalities. In large part, this reflects the chronic nature of these disorders as well as their capacity to afflict newborns in severe cases. Persistent hyperbilirubinemia often leads to cholelithiasis, in turn complicated by cholecystitis. Hyperbilirubinemia in neonates may lead to the debilitating neurologic disorder kernicterus.

Chronic hemolytic disorders may be complicated by periods or "crises" of profound anemia. As previously described, individuals may suffer an aplastic crisis. Somewhat of a misnomer, the term aplastic crisis refers to a transient, self-limited exacerbation of the underlying anemia resulting from a cessation of erythropoiesis often seen in association with a recent viral illness. A hemolytic crisis may arise as a complication of a disorder causing splenic enlargement. A sudden increase in spleen size will exacerbate the underlying anemia, since the spleen is often the site of red cell sequestration and destruction. A megaloblastic crisis may complicate chronic hemolysis as folate stores are depleted through the increased requirements of compensatory erythroid hyperplasia. Both aplastic and megaloblastic crises are characterized by reticulocytopenia. The abrupt onset and marked erythroid hypoplasia of an aplastic crisis, however, con-

Table 35.7. Classification of Hemolytic Disorders

Inherited hemolytic disorders
Defects in the erythrocyte membrane
Hereditary elliptocytosis
Hereditary pyropoikilocytosis
Stomatocytosis
Abetalipoproteinemia (acanthocytosis)
Enzyme deficiencies of the pentose phosphate pathway
Glucose-6-phosphate dehydrogenase
Defects in globin structure and synthesis
Hemoglobinopathies
Thalassemias
Unstable hemoglobin disease
Enzyme deficiencies of the glycolytic pathway
Pyruvate kinase
Hexokinase
Glucose-phosphate isomerase
Phosphofructokinase
Aldolase
Other
Defects in nucleotide metabolism
Pyrimidine 5′ nucleotidase
Acquired hemolytic disorders
Immune-mediated erythrocyte destruction
Transfusion of incompatible blood
Hemolytic disease of the newborn
Autoimmune
Infectious agents
Protozoans
Bacteria
Paroxysmal nocturnal hemoglobinuria
Traumatic erythrocyte destruction
Macrovascular
Microvascular
Chemicals/drugs/venoms
Physical agents

trasts with the slow development and megaloblastic appearance of folate deficiency.

STRUCTURAL MEMBRANE DEFECTS

The shape and reversible deformability of the normal erythrocyte are properties determined by the membrane skeleton. Lying directly beneath the external lipid bilayer membrane is a complex network of proteins that provide structural support (Fig. 35.15). Spectrin is the major component of the red cell cytoskeleton, and consists of two intercoiled, nonidentical filamentous subunits, which form heterodimers. The chain heads of each dimer pair bind with opposite subunit heads of another dimer pair to form tetramers. The tails of spectrin tetramers bind with a protein cluster of short actin protofilaments. This interaction is markedly enhanced by protein 4.1. The spectrin-actin-protein 4.1 assembly forms a two-dimensional web that is secured to the overlying lipid bilayer through ankyrin, which anchors spectrin to the cytoplasmic domain of the anion transporter. Additional linkage occurs through the binding of protein 4.1 to glycophorin.

Defects in the red cell cytoskeleton, arising either from a deficiency of constituent proteins or through defective protein interaction, are a major cause of hereditary hemolytic anemias. Regardless of the mechanism or associated morphologic changes, red cells in this group of disorders exhibit decreased deformability. Consequently, they sluggishly traverse the splenic cords, where they are subjected to an environment hostile to metabolic activity. The metabolic stress further weakens an inherently defective cell, and after a variable number of passages the cells succumb to reticuloendothelial destruction.

Hereditary Spherocytosis

Hereditary spherocytosis is the descriptive name given to a group of inherited disorders with characteristic spheroidal red cell morphology. It is the most common hereditary hemolytic anemia among people of Northern European ancestry. Its frequency led to the practice of separating anemias into spherocytic and nonspherocytic varieties, nomenclature that, in part, is still utilized today.

At least two distinct forms of spherocytosis are recognized. Approximately 75% of individuals exhibit an autosomal dominant mode of inheritance and cytoskeletal defects, which have been linked either to defective interaction of spectrin with protein 4.1 or to defects in ankyrin. In 25% of cases, an affected parent cannot be identified, negating an autosomal dominant inheritance pattern. This subset of individuals may be heterogeneous, including cases of spontaneous mutation as well as cases of autosomal recessive inheritance. A quantitative deficiency of spectrin has been identified in this group of patients, the magnitude of which directly correlates with clinical severity.

Clinical Features. The severity of the anemia varies, not only between patients, but also within a given patient over the course of time. Approximately 20% of patients have a mild form of the disease. In these individuals, hemolysis is compensated for by accelerated erythropoiesis, resulting in subclinical disease. The majority of patients with hereditary spherocytosis have a moderate life-long anemia associated with cholelithiasis, intermittent jaundice, and splenomegaly. The hemoglobin level fluctuates, reflecting the precarious balance between the hyperplastic erythron and splenic activity. In about 10% of cases, anemia is severe. Transfusional support is often required in infancy and childhood until splenectomy is logistically feasible.

Hematologic Findings. The morphologic hallmark of hereditary spherocytosis is the spherocyte, a generally smaller, spheroidal red cell lacking central pallor and consequently appearing densely hemoglo-

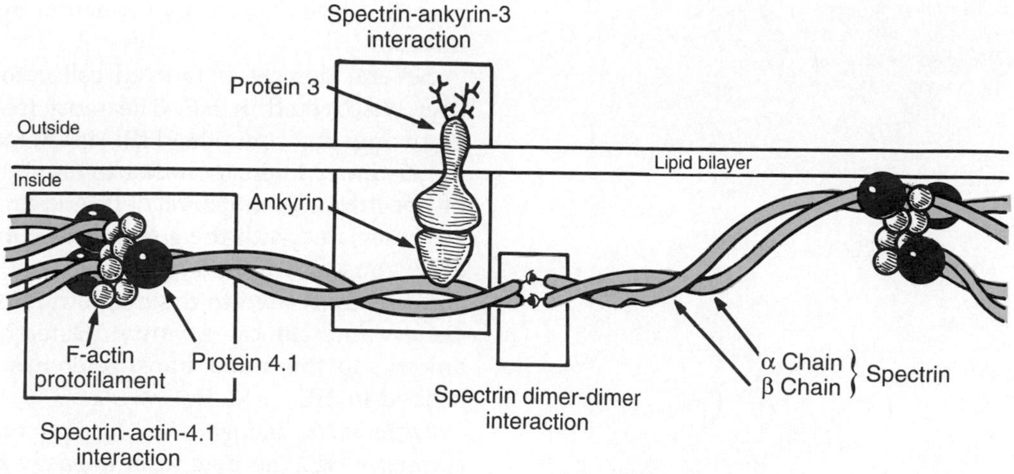

Figure 35.15. Schematic illustration of the erythrocyte cytoskeleton. (From Palek J, Lux SE. The red cell membrane skeletal defects in hereditary and acquired hematolytic anemias. Semin Hematol 1983;20(3):189.)

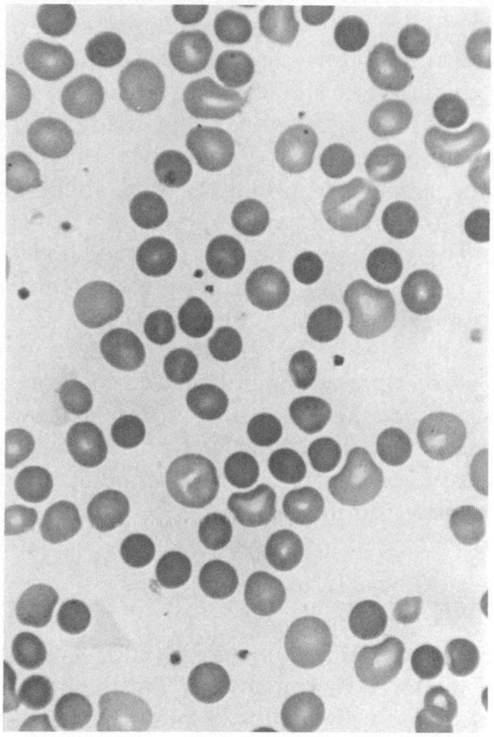

Figure 35.16. The peripheral blood smear in hereditary spherocytosis demonstrates a population of small, densely hemoglobinized, spheroidal erythrocytes that sharply contrast with the large polychromatophilic reticulocytes indicative of increased erythropoiesis.

binized (Fig. 35.16). The spherocytes contrast sharply with the increased number of large polychromatophilic reticulocytes indicative of compensatory erythroid hyperplasia. The interplay between spherocyte and reticulocyte numbers results in a widely variable MCV. Whereas the MCH is normal, the MCHC is increased, a combination of findings generally unique to hereditary spherocytosis.

The number of spherocytes present in the peripheral blood is variable, but in most cases quite striking. In the absence of other significant poikilocytosis, the presence of spherocytes is strongly suggestive of either hereditary spherocytosis or a warm autoimmune hemolytic anemia. These two conditions may be distinguished by a direct antiglobulin test.

In cases in which the diagnosis is suspected but the peripheral blood findings are inconclusive, an osmotic fragility test may be helpful. This procedure measures the red cell's capacity to withstand hypotonic stress. Since spherocytes exhibit a decreased surface area to volume ratio, their capacity to imbibe water in hypotonic salt solutions is impaired. Fifty percent lysis occurs at sodium concentrations above 0.5 g/liter. Exacerbation of this phenomenon may be induced by incubation for 24 hours, during which time the red cells additionally become metabolically stressed.

Treatment. In symptomatic patients, splenectomy is beneficial in removing the site of red cell destruction. After splenectomy, patients still exhibit spherocytes as well as the morphologic changes of a postsplenectomy state. Failure to improve following splenectomy suggests an alternative diagnosis; later relapses suggest hyperplasia of accessory splenic tissue.

Hereditary Elliptocytosis

Hereditary elliptocytosis (HE) is a clinically, genetically, and morphologically heterogeneous group of disorders that are linked through the morphologic finding of more than 20% elliptocytes in the peripheral blood (Fig. 35.17). Based on clinical findings and red cell morphology, three major categories of HE have emerged: the common form, the spherocytic form, and the stomatocytic form.

Clinical Findings. In the common form of HE, the majority of individuals exhibit numerous

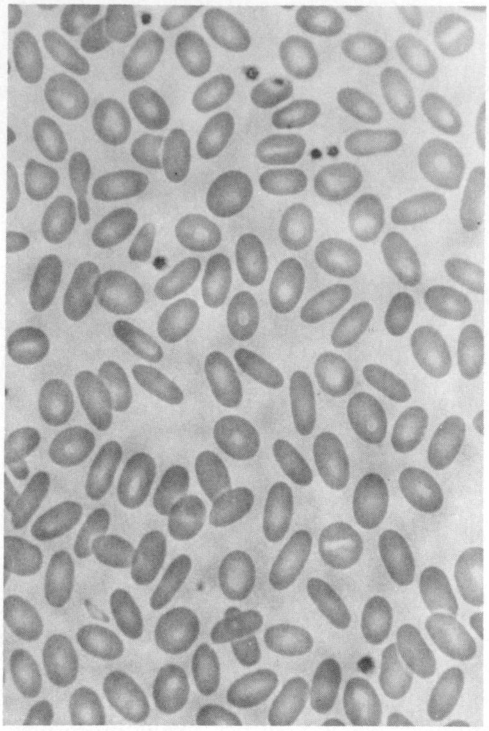

Figure 35.17. Numerous elliptocytes characterize the common form of hereditary elliptocytosis.

elliptical red cells with little or no evidence of hemolysis. Several exceptions may occur, leading to clinically symptomatic hemolysis. Moderate to severe hemolysis may occur during the first year of life in some black children, coinciding with morphologic findings in the peripheral blood similar to hereditary pyropoikilocytosis. The hematologic and clinical picture changes to one typical of common HE over the first 12 months. Unexplainedly, a small subset of individuals with common HE will exhibit significant and chronic hemolytic anemia with clinical manifestations similar to hereditary spherocytosis. Additionally, the rare homozygous form of common HE results in severe transfusion-dependent hemolytic anemia. Red cell morphology in this unusual condition found in the offspring of related HE parents resembles that of hereditary pyropoikilocytosis.

Spherocytic HE represents the dual inheritance of two nonallelic genes: one for mild HE and one for mild hereditary spherocytosis. As might be expected, the peripheral blood shows variable numbers of spherocytes and elliptocytes, either of which may predominate. Clinically mild to moderate hemolytic anemia results.

Stomatocytic HE is an unusual variant limited to Melanesia and surrounding islands. It is associated with changes in red cell antigen expression that appear to serve a protective function against malarial infection.

Several defects in the red cell cytoskeleton have been discovered in HE. The most frequent variant, occurring in common HE, is defective spectrin dimer-dimer interaction due to an abnormal α chain of spectrin. Quantitative deficiencies of protein 4.1 are associated with the spherocytic form of HE. Heterozygous and homozygous patterns of inheritance are directly related to the magnitude of protein deficiency and clinical severity. Defective binding of ankyrin to the anion transporter has also been described in HE.

Differential Diagnosis. In the typical form of common HE, the diagnosis is easily established by the finding of numerous fairly uniform elliptocytes in the peripheral blood. Other poikilocytes are few. The reticulocyte count is usually normal or mildly elevated, reflecting the asymptomatic or well-compensated nature of this disorder. The distinction between this form of HE and other disorders in which elliptocytes may be found is easily made on the basis of two observations: the frequency of elliptocytes and the presence of other size and shape changes that may give a clue to an unrelated hematologic condition. The peripheral smears of other forms of HE are not pathognomonic and may show features suggestive of hereditary spherocytosis or hereditary pyropoikilocytosis. The diagnosis in these cases requires study of family members and may necessitate analysis of cytoskeletal protein composition.

Therapy. In the common form of HE, patients are asymptomatic or very well compensated and require no specific therapy. Splenectomy is the treatment of choice in more symptomatic HE variants.

Hereditary Pyropoikilocytosis

Hereditary pyropoikilocytosis (HPP) is a rare congenital hemolytic anemia occurring most commonly in blacks. Red cells in this disorder demonstrate increased susceptibility to thermal injury. In contrast to normal erythrocytes, which can withstand temperature to 49°C, red cells in HPP begin to fragment and disintegrate at 45 to 46°C.

The mode of inheritance and the exact cytoskeletal defect(s) are not completely understood. Similar to HE, a defect in spectrin dimer-dimer association has been described that is partly due to an abnormality of the α chain of spectrin. The similarity of this structural defect to that seen in HE may explain the partial overlapping in morphologic findings seen early in the course of some cases of common HE.

The peripheral blood findings in HPP are striking and nearly pathognomonic (Fig. 35.18). Poikilocytosis is unmatched by any other disorder. Erythro-

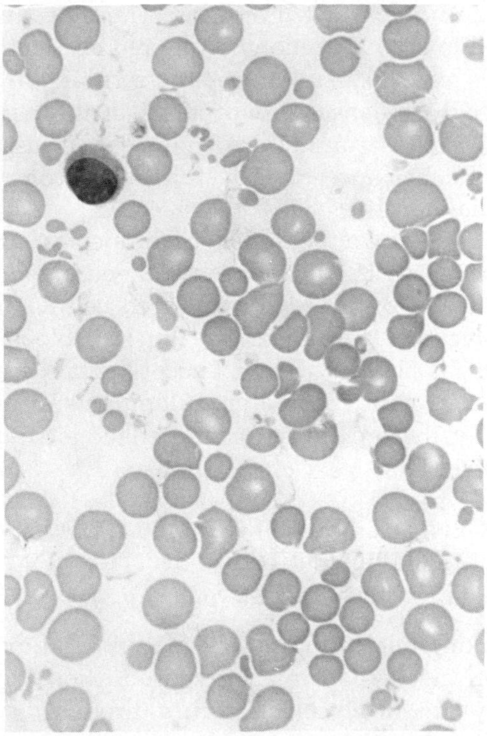

Figure 35.18. Striking poikilocytosis characterizes hereditary pyropoikilocytosis. Minute spheroidal erythrocytes result in a marked reduction in mean corpuscular volume. Note the irregular fragments of red cell membrane dusting the background of the peripheral smear.

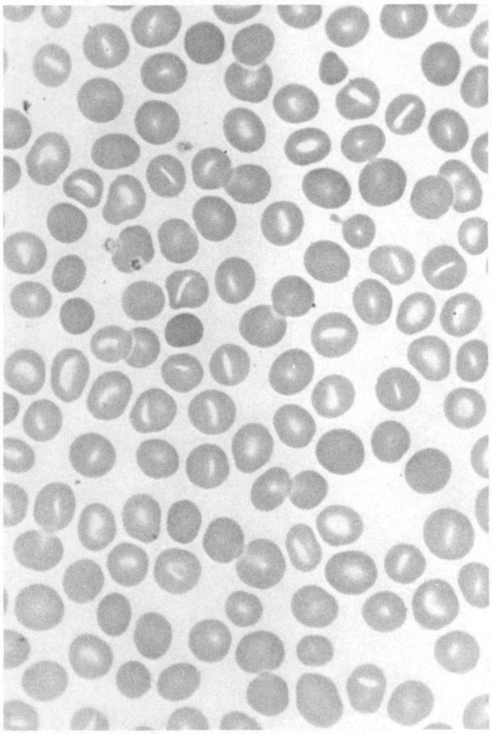

Figure 35.19. Hereditary stomatocytosis is characterized by numerous erythrocytes having slit-like central pallor.

cytes appear as if they are disintegrating, with fragments, numerous microspherocytes, and wisps of red cell membrane. These changes all lead to a markedly reduced MCV. A similar peripheral blood picture may be found in cases of third-degree burns due to thermal injury of normal red cells and in clostridial sepsis secondary to the action of a lecithinase on red cell membranes. As previously noted, infants with common HE may also exhibit similar changes in the peripheral blood, which gradually revert to a picture typical of common HE by 1 year of age.

HPP results in moderate to severe hemolytic anemia, necessitating splenectomy, which serves to diminish or abate hemolysis.

Hereditary Stomatocytosis

Although the precise structural defect is unknown, increased permeability to both sodium and potassium ions is a consistent feature of this rare disorder. Active Na^+-K^+ ATP'ase pumps are incapable of counterbalancing the flow of cations across the cell membrane. The net influx of sodium brings with it water, resulting in a swollen cell that is susceptible to osmotic and mechanical lysis.

Clinically, hereditary stomatocytosis varies in its expression. Most individuals are asymptomatic or exhibit only mild anemia because of brisk compensatory erythroid hyperplasia.

The morphologic hallmark of hereditary stomatocytosis is the stomatocyte, a cell with a slit-like or fish mouth area of central pallor (Fig. 35.19). In suspension, these cells appear uniconcave or bowl-shaped. A small number of similar-appearing cells may appear normally in air-dried smears or may be found in slightly increased numbers in association with a variety of disorders, making it difficult to conclusively establish the presence of hereditary stomatocytosis in its mild form. Evidence of hemolysis, more than 35% stomatocytes, and the absence of other poikilocytes, however, provides convincing evidence for this rare autosomal disorder. The MCV in these patients may be strikingly elevated, reflecting the reticulocytosis and the swollen nature of the stomatocytes.

Symptomatic patients may benefit from splenectomy, provided that splenic sequestration is documented.

Rh_{null} Disease

Rh_{null} disease is a rare hereditary disorder characterized by deletion of all Rh determinants, including the Landsteiner-Wiener antigen. The Rh locus, unlike many other blood group antigens, is restricted to red cells. It appears to be located in part within the red cell membrane; therefore it is not surprising the deletion results in membrane malfunction.

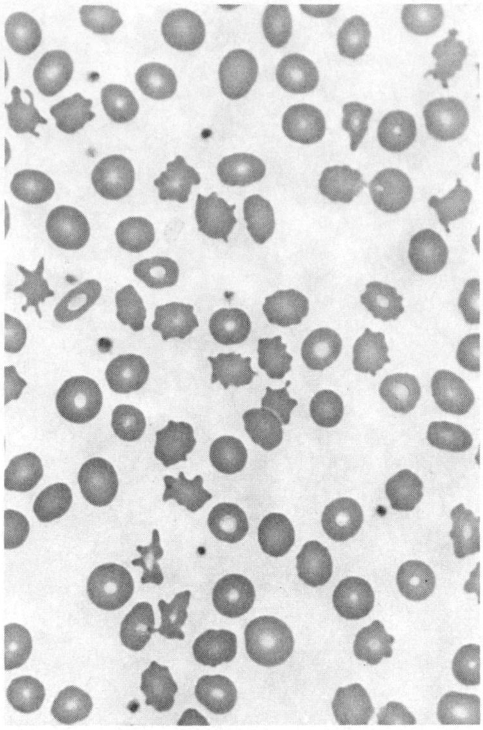

Figure 35.20. Acanthocytes are erythrocytes with irregularly placed, broad, blunted projections. They are typically found in significant numbers in abetalipoproteinemia and in end-stage liver disease. In both conditions, plasma lipid abnormalities result in alterations in the composition of the red cell membrane.

Morphologically, this disorder is associated with stomatocytes and spherocytes. Clinically, a mild compensated hemolytic anemia is found, which requires no therapy.

Abetalipoproteinemia (Acanthocytosis)

Abetalipoproteinemia is a rare disorder of lipid metabolism. The absence of apolipoprotein B results in the inability to transport triglycerides in the blood. Clinically, the syndrome presents in infancy with steatorrhea; progressive development of acanthocytosis, ataxic neuropathy, and an atypical form of retinitis pigmentosa ensues.

The acanthocytes found in the peripheral blood are dense, contracted erythrocytes with multiple irregularly spaced, broad, spiny projections (Fig. 35.20). This is presumably related to an increase in the relative sphingomyelin content of the red cell membrane, resulting in a rigid cell. The mild shortening of red cell survival is clearly overshadowed by the nonhematologic complications of this disorder.

Acanthocytes may also be found as a complication of severe hepatocellular disease. Unlike abetalipoproteinemia, acanthocytosis in this setting is associated with a severe hemolytic anemia and heralds a poor and often fatal prognosis. The defect is again related to lipid alterations of the red cell membrane, in this case excess cholesterol resulting from increased high-density lipoproteins in the peripheral blood. Similar acanthocytosis may be seen associated with the hepatocellular dysfunction accompanying neonatal hepatitis.

For unknown reasons, acanthocytes are also found in association with the McLeod blood group, an X-linked disorder in which red cell K_x antigen, the precursor substance for the Kell blood group system, is absent. The McLeod phenotype may be associated with chronic granulomatous disease because of the proximity of the genetic loci for these two disorders.

CONGENITAL NON-SPHEROCYTIC ANEMIAS: ENZYME DEFICIENCIES RESULTING IN SHORTENED RED CELL SURVIVAL

Lacking mitochondria, the mature erythrocyte relies on glycolysis for energy production. Approximately 90% of glycolysis occurs through the anaerobic Embden-Meyerhof (EM) pathway as glucose is converted to lactic acid (Fig. 35.21). The metabolically crucial byproducts of this multistep pathway are ATP and NADH. ATP, the main energy compound of the erythrocyte, is required for active cation transport across the red cell membrane. NADH is an essential cofactor for reduction of the small amount of methemoglobin normally produced each day in the red cell.

Integrally related to the EM pathway is the Rapoport-Luebering shunt, which results in the production of 2,3-diphosphoglycerate (2,3-DPG). Activity of this shunt is related to the erythrocyte's ATP and 2,3-DPG requirements. 2,3-DPG plays an essential role as a regulator of oxygen delivery to the tissues by altering the affinity of hemoglobin for oxygen.

Approximately 10% of glycolysis occurs aerobically through the hexose monophosphate (HMP) shunt, a pathway that generates the NADPH required for reduction of glutathione. Reduced glutathione is critical for the protection of hemoglobin from oxidant damage. Unlike the EM pathway, the HMP shunt can increase activity approximately 30-fold in times of oxidative stress.

Given the complexity and vital role of these pathways, it is not surprising that defects in any number of the intermediary enzymes can serve to uncouple the reaction, resulting in red cell injury. For the most part, red cell injury resulting from deficiencies of the HMP or EM pathways are not associated with significant morphologic changes and are broadly categorized as congenital or hereditary nonspherocytic hemolytic anemias.

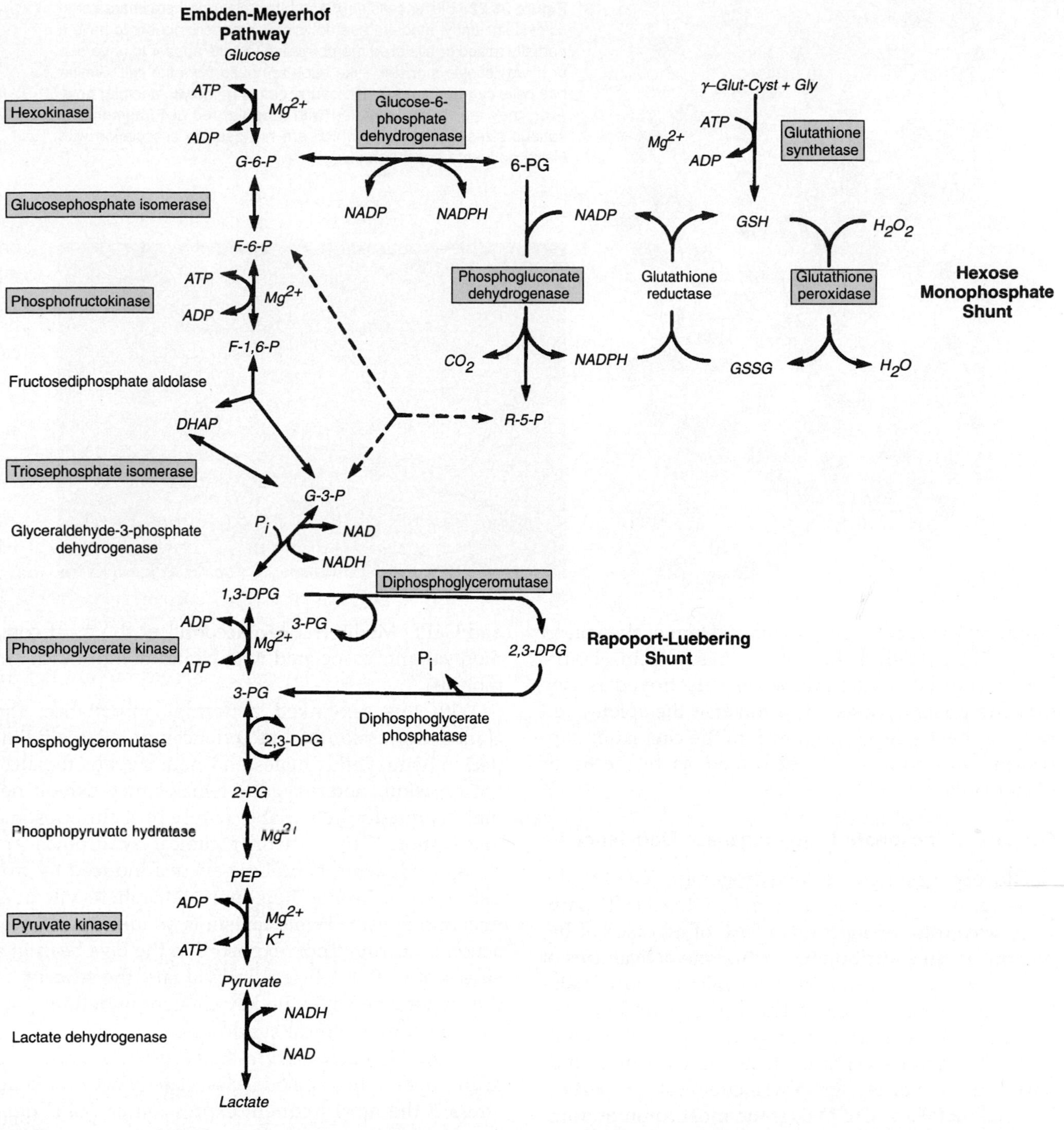

Figure 35.21. Glycolytic pathway with related hexose monophosphate shunt (glutathione metabolism) and Rapoport-Luebering shunt (2,3-diphosphoglycerate [2,3-DPG], metabolism).

ENZYME DEFICIENCIES OF THE HEXOSE MONOPHOSPHATE PATHWAY

NADPH generated by the HMP shunt is a necessary cofactor for maintaining glutathione in a reduced state. Reduced glutathione protects the red cell from naturally occurring and drug-induced oxidants that may potentially damage hemoglobin, membrane proteins, or other intracellular enzymes.

Oxidative damage to red cells is frequently manifested as Heinz bodies, small spheroidal inclusions of denatured hemoglobin visible by supravital staining. Heinz bodies exert their deleterious effects by attaching to the inner membrane of the red cell and causing deformation, alteration of cell membrane permeability, and reduction in red cell deformability. Attempted removal of these harmful inclusions occurs both through exocytosis and through active ex-

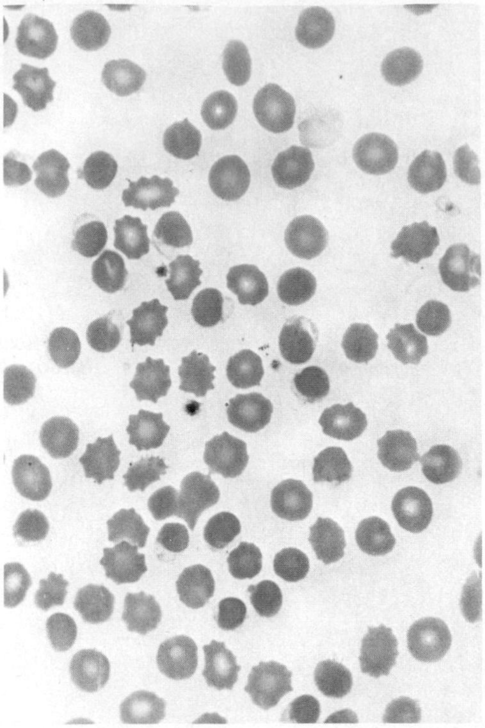

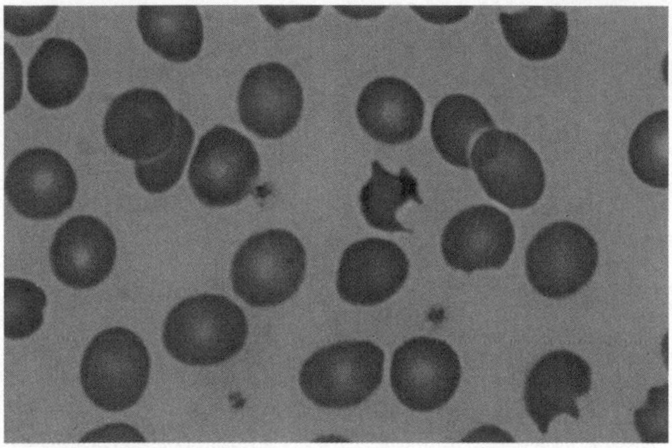

Figure 35.22. Blister cells *(left)* and bite cells *(right)* are characteristic of Heinz body–mediated hemolysis. Blister cells appear to have a partially raised or blistered membrane; bite cells appear to have one or more "cookie monster"–like bites removed from the cell. Similar bite cells can be found in microangiopathic hemolytic anemia; however, they are then associated with irregular red cell fragments of various sizes and shapes, which are not seen in association with Heinz body–mediated hemolysis.

cision by the reticuloendothelial system of the spleen (Fig. 35.22). Within the spleen, many Heinz body–laden erythrocytes are trapped and destroyed as they lose the pliability needed to traverse the splenic red pulp. Others escape and return to the circulation, appearing morphologically deformed as bite cells or blister cells.

Glucose-6-Phosphate Dehydrogenase Deficiency

Glucose-6-phosphate dehydrogenase (G6PD), the initial and rate-limiting enzyme of the HMP pathway, accounts for more than 99% of all cases of hemolytic anemia attributable to enzyme deficiencies of this pathway. It is the most prevalent inborn metabolic disorder of red cells. The structure and synthesis of G6PD are controlled by genes on the X chromosome. Numerous variants of the enzyme are found, based on a variety of physiochemical properties. Normal G6PD, or G6PD B, is the most common form of the enzyme found in all population groups. G6PD A, separated on the basis of electrophoretic mobility, exhibits normal enzyme activity and is found in approximately 20% of American black males. An unstable variant of G6PD A, designated G6PD A−, results in enzyme deficiency in aging red cells. G6PD A− is found in approximately 11% of American black males. Another variant, G6PD Mediterranean, found frequently in Sicilians, Greeks, Sephardic Jews, and Arabs, exhibits even greater instability, with a half-life measured in terms of hours as compared to 60 days for the normal G6PD B. Together, G6PD A− and G6PD Mediterranean account for the most common variants associated with clinically significant hemolysis.

With this sex-linked pattern of inheritance, the clinical expression of G6PD deficiency is largely limited to hemizygous males and homozygous females. On occasion, heterozygous females may exhibit hemolysis due to the variable nature of X chromosome inactivation. Three distinct clinical syndromes are recognized: acute hemolytic anemia induced by oxidant stress; chromic hereditary nonspherocytic anemia; and favism. While favism is an idiosyncratic reaction occurring upon exposure to the fava bean in a subset of G6PD-deficient individuals, the severity of the enzyme defect is the key element in defining the two remaining clinical syndromes.

Oxidant-Induced Acute Hemolytic Anemia. An acute hemolytic episode associated with oxidant stress is the most frequent expression of G6PD deficiency. It is seen both with G6PD A− and G6PD Mediterranean variants. Administration of a variety of drugs has been associated with acute hemolytic episodes in these individuals (Table 35.8). Additionally, infection is a common precipitating factor. Salmonellae, coliforms, β-hemolytic streptococci, rickettsiae, influenza, and viral hepatitis have each been associated with hemolysis in G6PD A− individuals through poorly elucidated mechanisms.

Laboratory and clinical evidence of acute hemolysis is usually apparent within days of onset of infection or drug administration. Signs and symptoms are

Table 35.8. Drugs or Chemicals Producing Hemolytic Anemia in Individuals Deficient in Erythrocyte Glucose-6-Phosphate Dehydrogenase

Antimalarials
Chloroquine[a]
Primaquine
Quinacrine
Quinine[a]
Antipyretics and analgesics
Acetaminophen[a]
Acetanilide[a]
Acetylsalicylic acid[a]
Aminopyrine[a]
Antipyrine[a]
Phenacetin acetophenetidin[a]
Sulfonamides
Azulfidine
Sulfacetamide
Sulfadiazine[a]
Sulfamethoxazole
Sulfamethoxypyridazine[a]
Sulfanilamide
Sulfapyridine
Sulfisoxazole[a]
Nitrofurans
Furazolidone
Nitrofurantoin
Nitrofurazone
Sulfones
Dapsone
Sulfoxone
Thiazolesulfone
Other Drugs
Acetylphenylhydrazine
Ascorbic acid[a]
p-Aminosalicylic acid[a]
Chloramphenicol
L-Dopa[a]
Methylene blue
Nalidixic acid
Naphthalene
Niridazole
Phenylhydrazine
Probenecid[a]
Quinidine[a]
Toluidine blue
Trinitrotoluene
Vitamin K (water-soluble analogues)[a]

[a]These agents can probably be safely administered in normal therapeutic doses to G6PD-deficient individuals who do not suffer from chronic nonspherocytic hemolytic anemia.

often more severe with G6PD Mediterranean, as the enzyme is much less stable. The finding of bite cells or the demonstration of Heinz bodies in this clinical setting are strong evidence for G6PD deficiency. If exposure to the inciting agent is brief, the episode of hemolysis is generally self-limited. Symptoms may also abate as compensatory release of reticulocytes into the circulation occurs. These young red cells demonstrate normal G6PD activity.

Confirmation of the diagnosis requires quantitative G6PD assays. Caution must be exercised in interpreting G6PD levels during periods of brisk reticulocytosis, as enzyme levels during these periods may not reflect steady-state conditions.

Hereditary Nonspherocytic Hemolytic Anemia. G6PD variants that lead to severe enzyme deficiency result in chronic hemolysis. On occasion, this subset of individuals may present in the neonatal period with hemolytic disease of the newborn. Moderate, partially compensated hemolytic anemia is the rule. Splenectomy is generally unsuccessful in diminishing the rate of hemolysis in these individuals.

Favism. Acute, potentially fatal intravascular hemolysis may occur as an idiosyncratic reaction upon exposure to fava beans in a subset of G6PD-deficient individuals. G6PD Mediterranean is the most commonly afflicted subtype. Signs and symptoms of brisk intravascular hemolysis occur within hours of ingestion. Maintenance of intravascular volume and renal function together with prompt transfusional support are required.

Miscellaneous Enzyme Deficiencies of the HMP Shunt

Deficiencies of the following HMP pathway enzymes have also been described: γ-glutamyl cysteine synthetase, glutathione synthetase, glutathione reductase, and glutathione peroxidase. Clinical manifestations of these enzymes are widely variable, spanning the recognized clinical syndromes of G6PD deficiency.

ENZYME DEFICIENCIES OF THE EM PATHWAY

A syndrome of hemolytic anemia has been described for deficiencies of nearly all enzymes in the EM pathway. Hemolysis occurs in these disorders as the late-developing erythroblasts lose their mitochondrial machinery and begin to rely on glycolysis for energy production.

Pyruvate Kinase Deficiency

Pyruvate kinase (PK) deficiency is the most common enzyme deficiency of the EM pathway. Numerous dysfunctional variants of the PK enzyme are known to exist, affecting, for example, enzyme activity, stability, or kinetic rate. A single copy of a defective gene usually causes no significant alteration of enzyme activity. Hemolytic anemia typically occurs in the double heterozygote, an individual inheriting two mutant genes. The clinical variability of PK deficiency likely reflects the wide range of combinational possibilities.

Hemolytic anemia presenting in infancy or childhood is usually severe, requiring maintenance transfusions and splenectomy, whereas disorders presenting in adulthood are largely compensated and result in anemia of mild to moderate severity. Paradoxically, adaptation to anemic hypoxia is facilitated by the PK deficiency itself, which results in a buildup of pathway intermediates proximal to the site of PK activity, including 2,3-DPG. Elevated levels of 2,3-DPH also lead to a peculiar laboratory finding in PK-deficient red cells. By inhibiting enzymes of the HMP pathway, red cells exhibit increased Heinz body formation upon exposure to oxidant stress.

Red cell morphology is often unremarkable. In more severe cases, echinocytes may be present, which become even more plentiful following splenectomy. Diagnosis of PK deficiency is based on enzymatic assays demonstrating quantitative or qualitative abnormalities. Hemolysates should be free of contaminating white blood cells, which normally contain high levels of PK.

An acquired form of PK deficiency may occur in conjunction with the myelodysplastic syndromes, myeloproliferative disorders, or acute myelogenous leukemia.

Miscellaneous Enzyme Deficiencies of the EM Pathway

Deficiencies of hexokinase, glucosephosphate isomerase, phosphofructokinase, aldolase, triosephosphate isomerase and phosphoglycerate kinase have all been reported to result in congenital nonspherocytic hemolytic anemia. With the exception of hexokinase, these enzyme defects have also resulted in impairment of other organ systems, most commonly involving the neuromuscular system.

DISORDERS OF NUCLEOTIDE METABOLISM

Three uncommon disorders of purine and pyrimidine metabolism in red cells are responsible for hemolytic anemia, the most frequent of which is pyrimidine-5′-nucleotidase deficiency. This enzyme is responsible for degradation of ribosomal RNA during reticulocyte maturation. A deficiency of pyrimidine-5′-nucleotidase results in aggregation of residual ribosomes, which are manifested in peripheral blood smears by coarse basophilic stippling. It is an acquired pyrimidine-5′-nucleotidase deficiency seen in lead poisoning that leads to this heralded morphologic clue to the diagnosis.

Congenital enzyme deficiencies usually result in moderate anemia. Diagnosis is established through an assay of nucleotidase activity.

A deficiency of adenylate kinase has also been described as a rare cause of congenital nonspherocytic hemolytic anemia, as has hyperactivity of the enzyme adenosine deaminase.

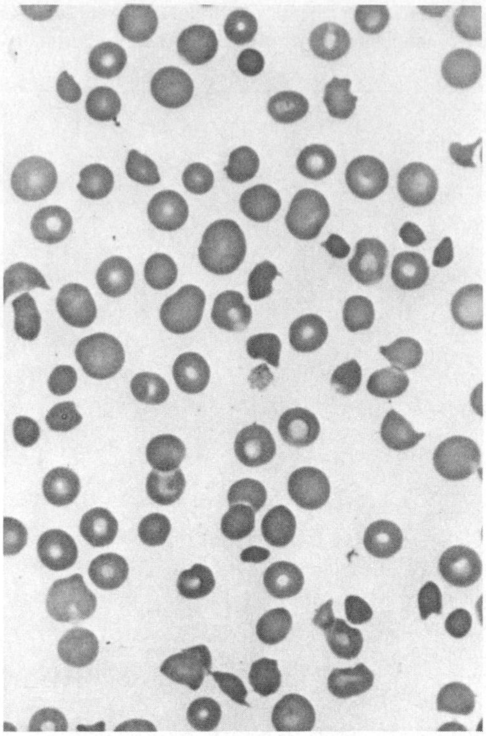

Figure 35.23. Variably sized, irregularly shaped erythrocyte fragments characterize the macroangiopathic and microangiopathic hemolytic anemias. Spherocytes may also be found. When seen in conjunction with red cell fragments, the presence of spherocytes should not raise confusion with hereditary spherocytosis or warm autoimmune hemolytic anemia.

Acquired and Extrinsic Red Cell Abnormalities

TRAUMATIC RED CELL INJURY

Excessive physical trauma to the erythrocyte on its circulatory journey may lead to intravascular lysis or cell injury predisposing to premature red cell destruction (Fig. 35.23). Red cell fragments, or schistocytes, serve as the morphologic hallmark of this type of hemolysis. These beaten and battered red cells are of various sizes and shapes. Having withstood the initial injury, these resealed erythrocyte remnants eventually succumb to splenic destruction. Traditionally, the red cell fragmentation syndromes have been separated on the basis of injury sustained in the heart or great vessels (macrovascular) versus that sustained in the prearteriolar or capillary bed (microvascular).

Macrovascular Hemolysis

Although capable of tolerating tremendous shear forces, erythrocytes become increasingly susceptible to injury with alterations in blood flow. Such changes in the macrovasculature occur with outflow

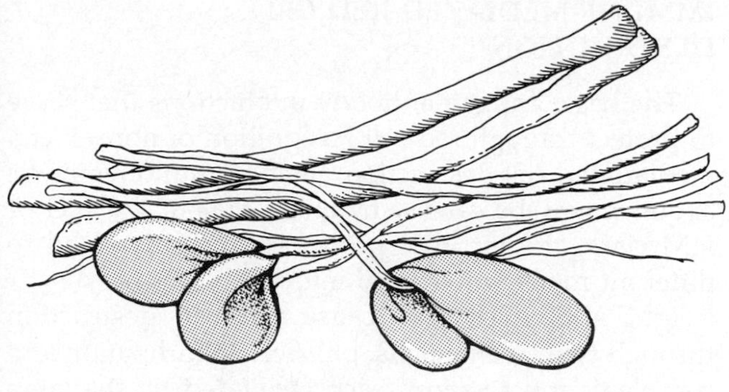

Figure 35.24. Fibrin strands in the microvasculature form a sharp mesh, causing fragmentation of circulating erythrocytes.

disease such as aortic stenosis. A calcified valve is a double-edged sword, as turbulent jet flow is created past a roughened valvular surface. Similarly, prosthetic cardiac devices employed in the surgical repair of valvular or parenchymal defects may present bare or nonendothelialized surfaces injurious to red cells. The mechanical design of early prosthetic valves, which predisposed to physical trauma and red cell fragmentation, represent another cause of macrovascular injury; this complication has now largely been resolved.

Hemolysis secondary to macrovascular injury is usually mild and well compensated. Prolonged periods of red cell injury may lead to depletion of iron stores through urinary iron loss accompanying intravascular hemolysis. Exacerbations of hemolysis may be encountered with sudden valvular incompetence, and may be a sign of a failing prosthetic implant.

Microangiopathic Hemolytic Anemia

Microangiopathic hemolytic anemia is the result of red cell fragmentation in the prearteriolar or capillary bed. Erythrocyte damage occurs as the force of the blood flow carries red cells through the narrowed or damaged microvasculature. Lysis or sublethal assault occurs through two mechanisms: deposition of a fibrin meshwork that acts as a sieve through which red cells are pushed (Fig. 35.24), or diffuse endothelial damage, which exposes flowing red cells to a rough and hostile surface. The interplay of these two mechanisms can be seen with endothelial damage, as the denuded endothelial surfaces cause fibrin deposition.

The causes of microangiopathic hemolytic anemia are numerous (Table 35.9). Disseminated intravascular coagulation, occurring as a complication of infections, disseminated carcinoma, or obstetric catastrophes; thrombotic thrombocytopenic purpura and the related hemolytic uremic syndrome; and malignant hypertension are the most frequent underlying disorders leading to red cell fragmentation and anemia.

Table 35.9. Causes of Microangiopathic Hemolytic Anemia

Thrombocytic thrombocytopenic purpura
Hemolytic uremic syndrome
Disseminated intravascular coagulation
Infections: Gram-negative septicemia
Snake bites
Hemolytic transfusion reactions
Obstetric complications: abruptio placentae, amniotic fluid embolism, retained dead fetus, eclampsia
Malignant hypertension
Immunologic disorders: vasculitis
Acute glomerulonephritis
Polyarteritis nodosa
Wegener's granulomatosis
Systemic lupus erythematosus
Scleroderma
Renal and hepatic allograft rejection
Disseminated carcinoma: gastrointestinal, breast, and pulmonary adenocarcinoma
Congenital vascular malformations
Cavernous hemangioma
Hepatic hemangioendothelioma

The peripheral blood findings are similar to those seen with macrovascular red cell injury. Additionally, thrombocytopenia is a frequent finding; this reflects the utilization of platelets and formation of platelet thrombi in thrombotic thrombocytopenic purpura and hemolytic uremic syndrome or the consumption of platelets occurring with activation of the clotting cascade in disseminated intravascular coagulation.

Multisystem support may be necessary in treatment of the complications of anemia and coagulopathy. Nonetheless, therapy of the primary underlying disease must not be neglected.

March Hemoglobinuria

Repetitive forceful contact of body parts with hard surfaces can lead to erythrocyte lysis within the local microvasculature. This phenomenon was originally described in soldiers subjected to prolonged periods of marching. Indeed, long-distance walking or running is the most frequent cause. As not all individuals are plagued by this complication, individual factors must come into play that govern the destructive forces affecting the erythrocyte.

Clinically, patients suffer self-limited bouts of hemoglobinuria following such episodes of forceful contact. Red cell morphology is generally unremarkable, suggesting immediate lysis of erythrocytes within the local microvasculature. Differentiation from myoglobinuria can be established chemically, whereas other causes of hemoglobinuria must be distinguished on the basis of clinical and laboratory features.

DRUGS, CHEMICALS, AND VENOMS

Drugs

Administration of a number of drugs may lead to red cell damage and lysis through oxidative injury to hemoglobin, red cell membranes, or intracellular enzymes. Particularly vulnerable are individuals deficient in G6PD. In rare circumstances the oxidant stress associated with administration of some drugs is sufficient to cause hemolysis in apparently normal erythrocytes.

Chemicals

Copper, arsenic, mercury, and lead are the most common heavy metals known to result in intravascular hemolysis following ingestion or inhalation. These chemicals are highly reactive with membrane thiols and interfere with red cell volume control.

Devastating intravascular hemolysis occurs within 2 to 12 hours of exposure to arsine fumes, produced by the action of water on metallic arsenide. The deficiency of ceruloplasmin found in Wilson's disease leads to the accumulation of copper in tissue, which may result in complications of hemolytic anemia. The introduction of significant amounts of water into the circulation has also been associated with hemolysis. This phenomenon has been reported as a complication of tissue irrigation accompanying prostate surgery or as a complication of near drowning in fresh water.

Venoms

The action of phospholipases released by clostridium perfringens or contained within the venoms of some snakes or spiders can lead to hemolysis through dissolution of the red cell membrane. The most devastating example is the frequently fatal hemolysis of clostridial sepsis. Rapid hemolysis in this disorder is attributable to the phospholipase activity of the α toxin and is grossly visible as deep cherry-red plasma. Microscopically, a kaleidoscope of red cell changes are visible, mimicking hereditary pyropoikilocytosis.

The bite of the brown recluse spider results in necrotic arachnidism, an intense local area of tissue necrosis and ulceration, which may be complicated within days by hemolytic anemia resulting from the sphingomyelinase activity of the spider venom. Similar enzyme activity may be found in the venom of various snakes, particularly pit vipers. The intensity of hemolysis depends on the amount of venom absorbed.

IMMUNE-MEDIATED RED CELL DESTRUCTION

The basic antigen-antibody interactions that serve to protect through red cell recognition of nonself can mediate red cell destruction. Such immunohemolytic anemias may be caused by antibodies of the IgG or IgM class, the intrinsic properties of which lead to different modes of red cell injury.

IgM antibodies may cause red cell destruction through two mechanisms: physical agglutination and complement activation, each facilitated by the large pentameric structure of the IgM molecule, which allows it to easily bridge multiple antigenic sites. The capacity of an IgM antibody to mediate red cell destruction is directly linked to its thermal amplitude, the temperature range over which it most avidly binds to an antigen. IgM antibodies are frequently referred to as cold-reacting antibodies, since they exhibit increasing binding avidity as temperatures approach 4°C. In contrast, complement activity occurs only near body temperature. Consequently, only IgM antibodies, which exhibit avid binding properties near body temperature where complement is active, cause hemolysis.

Once complement is activated, immediate red cell lysis may proceed through completion of the complement cascade. Complement activation may, however, be stalled through a series of protective checks and balances following the liberation of C3b from C3. Red cells coated with C3b may be cleared by phagocytic cells bearing C3b receptors; particularly rich in C3b receptors are the hepatic reticuloendothelial cells (Kupffer cells). Alternatively, C3b may be inactivated to C3d by a plasma inactivator. Importantly, C3d-coated red cells serve as a marker of IgM-mediated hemolysis, a property that is clinically utilized in the Coombs' or direct antiglobulin test (DAT).

In contrast to IgM, antibodies of the IgG class exhibit their greatest binding activity at body temperature. The much smaller size of the IgG molecule makes it less capable of bridging the gap between two or more red cell antigens, a prerequisite to physical agglutination or complement activation. Consequently, IgG-induced hemolysis is not mediated through complement-dependent lysis, but rather through reticuloendothelial clearance.

Once bound to the red cell surface, the Fc portion of the IgG molecule is exposed, becoming a target for the mononuclear cells of the reticuloendothelial system that bear Fc receptors. Particularly rich in Fc receptors are the splenic macrophages, making the spleen a major site of destruction of IgG-coated red cells. Unlike the rapid demise of IgM-coated red cells, red cells coated with IgG are readily found in circulation. The circulating IgG-coated erythrocytes may be detected by the DAT. The longevity of IgG-coated red cells is determined by the number of antigenic sites per red cell, the serum concentration of the IgG antibody, and the functional capacity of the reticuloendothelial system. Once bound through Fc receptor attachment the erythrocytes undergo a shape change, becoming spherical due to a loss of red cell membrane. The diminished surface area to volume ratio makes these spheroidal red cells increasingly susceptible to hypotonic (or osmotic) stress. These morphologic and physical properties are indistinguishable from the findings of hereditary spherocytosis. Destruction occurs through internalization or piecemeal destruction by macrophages, as they surround portions of the red cell membrane with fingerlike extensions.

Isoantibodies

Immunohemolytic anemias may be caused by isoantibodies (alloantibodies), i.e., antibodies to blood group antigens. For purposes of this discussion, isoantibodies are antibodies to the major and minor blood group antigens. Isoantibodies may be naturally occurring or may arise upon exposure to foreign blood group antigens through blood transfusion or during pregnancy as small amounts of fetal blood leak across the placental barrier to gain access to the maternal circulation.

Transfusion of Incompatible Blood

Antibodies to the ABO blood group antigens are of the IgM class and exhibit a broad range of thermoreactivity. Transfusion of ABO-incompatible blood results in immediate and severe symptoms related to brisk complement-mediated hemolysis. Flushing, hyperventilation, tachycardia, urticaria, and shock occur secondary to the release of vasoactive substances encountered with complement activation; severe pain results from vasoocclusion secondary to red cell agglutination. Disseminated intravascular coagulation and renal failure may also ensue.

Non–ABO-related hemolytic transfusion reactions are IgG mediated. The majority are secondary to antibodies within the Rh system, notably anti-D. Antibodies to c, E, and to the Kell, Kidd, and Duffy systems round out the most frequent causes of non–ABO-related transfusion reactions. These IgG-coated erythrocytes are predominantly cleared by the spleen. A chill/fever reaction typically occurs after approximately 1 hour, the severity of which is related to the antibody titer and the number of antigenic sites. Hemoglobinemia reflects a backwash of hemoglobin into the circulation from the splenic macrophages and consequently never reaches the magnitude seen with intravascular hemolysis of ABO transfusion reactions. Hemolysis is nonetheless thorough, as evidenced by the rise in serum bilirubin.

Very low titers of antibody may lead to a delayed transfusion reaction. In such circumstances, re-exposure to a foreign antigen through transfusion will cause an anamnestic rise in antibody titer. Clinically, hemolysis becomes evident 3 to 7 days posttransfusion as the patient exhibits jaundice and signs and symptoms of anemia.

Hemolytic Disease of the Newborn

During pregnancy, tiny amounts of fetal erythrocytes enter the maternal circulation. If these red cells bear foreign (paternally restricted) antigens, they will serve as an immune stimulus. Maternal IgG antibodies have the capacity to cross the placenta and coat fetal erythrocytes, leading to splenic sequestration and destruction. The magnitude of this hemolytic disease of the newborn is related to the titer of the maternal antibody; in severe cases, in utero exchange transfusion may be necessary to prevent fetal demise. Historically, anti-D has accounted for the majority of severe cases. With the prophylactic administration of Rh immune globulin, severe cases are now more frequently encountered with antibodies to c, E, or other minor blood group antigens.

Although ABO antibodies are largely naturally occurring and incapable of placental transfer due to their pentameric structure, small amounts of IgG type anti-A and anti-B may also be found, typically in type O individuals. These IgG antibodies are capable of placental transfer and, similar to anti-D, may cause hemolytic anemia. ABO hemolytic disease of the newborn, although much more frequent than that due to anti-D, is typically less severe.

Anemia and evidence of accelerated erythropoiesis, the hallmarks of hemolytic anemias, are present in hemolytic disease of the newborn. Nucleated red blood cells are frequent and may be striking. Hyperbilirubinemia is largely of the unconjugated type due to hepatic immaturity. Spherocytes are frequent in ABO-related hemolysis, whereas they are a minor feature of Rh incompatibility. In contrast, a strong DAT is more frequent in hemolytic disease of the newborn due to anti-D; antibodies in the ABO system are loosely bound to the erythrocyte surface, resulting in a weakly positive DAT, and may be detected in the circulation with an indirect antiglobulin test.

Autoimmune Hemolytic Anemias

Autoimmune hemolytic anemias are caused by autoantibodies, self-induced antibodies directed at one's own red cells. The autoimmune hemolytic anemias are divided into two broad categories based on the class and the corresponding thermal activity of the responsible antibody: warm (IgG) and cold (IgM) autoimmune hemolytic anemias. Both warm and cold autoimmune hemolytic anemias may be further stratified into idiopathic and secondary forms.

Warm Autoimmune Hemolytic Anemias

The warm autoimmune hemolytic anemias are predominantly mediated through the binding of IgG antibodies to the erythrocyte's surface, resulting in splenic sequestration and destruction. Consequently, the morphologic hallmarks of this group of anemias is the spherocyte. The severity of the anemia and the number of spherocytes, however, is quite variable. In severe cases, the frequency of spherocytes rivals that seen in hereditary spherocytes. In such cases, the true identity of a warm autoimmune hemolytic anemia is revealed with a positive direct antiglobulin test. Red cells are typically coated with IgG occurring alone or in combination with variable amounts of intact C3. Rarely, the red cells exhibit only C3 on their surface. The responsible antibody may be serologically nonspecific; however, in many cases preferential reactivity with the Rh locus is apparent. Seldom, however, is the antibody directed at specific Rh determinants.

Idiopathic Warm Autoimmune Hemolytic Anemia. In up to half of the cases, the warm autoimmune hemolytic anemia is not associated with an underlying disease process and is termed "idiopathic." The remaining cases are associated with or secondary to an underlying disease.

Secondary Warm Autoimmune Hemolytic Anemias. Secondary warm autoimmune hemolytic anemias most frequently arise in association with an underlying lymphoproliferative disorder or systemic autoimmune disorder. Chronic lymphocytic leukemia is the most frequently associated lymphoproliferative disease; warm autoimmune hemolytic anemia may be seen in 10 to 30% of cases sometime during the course of the disease. Other lymphoproliferative disorders are less frequently complicated by warm autoimmune hemolytic anemias, but may also give rise to cold autoimmune hemolytic anemia. The onset of the anemia may precede the diagnosis of lymphoma/leukemia by months or years. Hence, thorough systemic evaluation is necessary before labeling an individual with an idiopathic autoimmune hemolytic anemia.

Systemic lupus erythematosus is the prototype of the systemic autoimmune disorders associated with warm autoimmune hemolytic anemias. Rheumatoid arthritis, lupoid hepatitis, and ulcerative colitis may also exhibit red cell autoantibodies. Clinically significant hemolysis is less frequent than the finding of a positive DAT among these disorders. As in other forms of secondary autoimmune hemolytic anemia, treatment is directed at the underlying disease processes.

Cold Autoimmune Anemias: Cold Agglutinin Disease

As previously discussed, cold-reacting IgM antibodies may cause hemolysis through physical agglutination or complement activation. The thermal range of most IgM antibodies is sufficiently low that dissociation occurs prior to reaching temperatures compatible with complement activation. Consequently, hemolysis is frequently mild unless a broad range of thermal activity is present or ambient temperature sufficiently cool. Approximately 95% of cold-reacting antibodies show anti-I specificity, the remainder demonstrating activity with the i antigen normally found on fetal erythrocytes.

Primary Cold Agglutinin Disease. Primary cold agglutinin disease is marked by episodic painful acrocyanosis induced by agglutination of red cells in the peripheral circulation upon exposure to cold. It is typically a disease seen in the elderly and is managed largely by avoidance of cold environments. Exclusion of an underlying chronic lymphoproliferative disorder is mandatory. The diagnosis is suspected by the clinical history and the finding of red cell agglutination as blood is drawn or from blood smears prepared at room temperature. Cold agglutinin titers are established by serially diluting the patient's serum and incubating it with a suspension of group O erythrocytes. Normal individuals exhibit low concentrations of cold active anti-I, resulting in physiologic titers of less than 1:16. Pathologic titers are typically greater than 1:256 and may exceed 1:100,000 in idiopathic cold agglutinin disease. The DAT typically reveals the presence of C3.

Secondary Cold Agglutinin Disease. Secondary cold agglutinin disease is associated with a variety of infections, the prototype being mycoplasma pneumonia and infectious mononucleosis. Cold agglutinin titers are often used as a supportive test in establishing a presumptive diagnosis of mycoplasma pneumonia. Titers rise within 1 to 3 weeks following the onset of symptoms. Titers typically reach 1:640, although on occasion they may reach values exceeding 1:1000 and may be associated with symptomatic anemia. In contrast to the anti-I antibodies of mycoplasma pneumonia, cold agglutinin arising in association with infectious mononucleosis are directed against the i antigen and require fetal cells for detection.

Cold agglutinin disease may occur secondarily in association with a variety of lymphoproliferative disorders. In these cases, the monoclonal IgM antibody expressed by the malignant B-cell clone is the responsible hemolytic agent. As previously stressed, discovery of either a warm or cold autoimmune hemolytic anemia necessitates a thorough investigation to rule out an underlying occult lymphoproliferative disorder.

Paroxysmal Cold Hemoglobinuria. Paroxysmal cold hemoglobinuria (PCH) is a rare acquired hemolytic anemia that may be seen as a complication of syphilis or a recent viral illness, particularly measles, mumps, or infectious mononucleosis. It is the result of an anti-P autoantibody occurring in individuals expressing the nearly universal P_1 and P_2 red blood cell antigens. This 7S IgG antibody, termed the Donath-Landsteiner antibody, binds to the erythrocyte at temperatures below 20°C. This IgG antibody is unique not only in its binding avidity at cold temperatures, but also in its capacity to cause complement binding. Subsequent activation of complement occurs with warming; at the same time, the Donath-Landsteiner antibody dissociates from the red cell membrane. This biphasic property is utilized clinically to establish the diagnosis. Hemolysis occurs only after the blood has been chilled and then warmed to 37°C. Bound IgG can be detected in the DAT only when performed at temperatures less than 24°C; at body temperature, only C3 is detected.

Clinical hemolysis is precipitated by exposure to cold and results in symptoms similar to those seen in acute intravascular hemolysis associated with ABO incompatibility. The disorder is usually a self-limited, postviral complication. Treatment for syphilis is required for luetic PCH.

Drug-Induced Autoimmune Hemolytic Anemia

The administration of a number of pharmaceutical agents has been complicated by the development of antibody-mediated hemolysis. Although, strictly speaking, many cases are not examples of true autoantibody-mediated hemolysis, these disorders are best considered as a group. Four basic hemolytic mechanisms have been described.

Hapten Mechanism. When given intramuscularly in large doses (greater than 10 million units), penicillin is absorbed to the red cell membrane. The combination of drugs and hapten (red blood cell membrane) serves as an antigen to which formed antibody binds. The antibody is usually of the IgG type and results in hemolysis through reticuloendothelial destruction. Discontinuation of the drug results in abrupt cessation of hemolysis, although the positive DAT usually persists for several months. Penicillin analogues such as cephalothin are also known to cause similar hemolytic complications.

Immune Complex or Innocent Bystander Mechanism. A number of drugs, including quinidine, quinine, p-aminosalicylate, phenacetin, ethacrynic acid, and the nonsteroidal anti-inflammatory agents, may result in hemolysis through the formation of immune complexes that nonspecifically coat red cells. These drugs bind to plasma proteins, which act as haptens. Antibodies then bind to the circulating drug-protein complex, and the resulting immune complex is deposited on a variety of innocent bystanders such as erythrocytes, platelets, and glomerular endothelium. The antibodies are often IgM, resulting in complement deposition. The picture is usually one of acute intravascular hemolysis and does not require large amounts of drug. Renal failure becomes a problem in 50% of patients.

True Autoimmune Hemolytic Anemia—The Aldomet Model. The prototype for this type of drug-related hemolysis is Aldomet. The frequency of antibody formation with Aldomet therapy is directly linked to the dose of drug administered. Overall, approximately 15% of patients treated with Aldomet will develop a positive DAT after 3 months of treatment. The antibody is similar to the true autoantibodies encountered in idiopathic warm autoimmune hemolytic anemia, an IgG antibody exhibiting specificity toward the Rh locus. The exact mechanism of antibody formation is unknown, although it is postulated that a state of unregulated B-cell activity is created by the inhibitory effects of the drug on T-suppressor cells.

A positive DAT does not equate to hemolysis, as clinical hemolysis develops in only approximately 1% of patients. Interestingly, it is a more frequent complication with lower-dose schedules. To prevent hemolytic complications, the drug is discontinued following discovery of a positive DAT. Hemolysis seldom occurs following cessation of the drug, although a positive DAT may persist for months to years. L-Dopa, melenamic acid, flufenamic acid, chlordiazepoxide hydrochloride, cimetidine, and cefazolin have also been associated with similar induction of autoantibodies.

Nonimmunologic Absorption of Proteins. Although proven hemolysis is rare, a weakly positive DAT may develop in association with the administration of cephalothin or cephaloridine. These agents cause nonspecific absorption of a wide variety of proteins, including IgG, IgM, and complement to the red cell surface.

Paroxysmal Nocturnal Hemoglobinuria

Paroxysmal nocturnal hemoglobinuria (PNH) is a distinctly uncommon cause of hemolysis that stands apart from the myriad of hemolytic disorders previously discussed. Although an acquired disorder, hemolysis results from an intrinsic erythrocyte abnormality manifesting as a population of erythrocytes hypersusceptible to the lytic action of complement. Likely serving as the causative mechanism is a reduction in the membrane-associated regulatory protein decay accelerating factor, which serves to expedite degradation of C3 convertase on the red cell surface. Not only is this defect seen in erythrocytes, but it is shared by the granulocytes and platelets of affected individuals, implying that PNH is a disorder arising at the level of the multipotential stem cell.

The name implies that PNH is characterized by episodes of hemolysis occurring at night. This classic presentation is all too uncommon. More often, PNH manifests as pancytopenia secondary to marrow hypoplasia or aplasia and should not be forgotten in the evaluation of pancytopenia. Unexplained iron deficiency resulting from persistent hemosiderinuria or unexplained recurrent venous thromboses should also spark investigation to rule out PNH.

The peripheral blood findings are quite variable, as is the clinical presentation. Clues to the cause of the anemia are generally not present in the peripheral blood smear. Reticulocytosis may be absent in cases of marrow hypoplasia. Neutropenia and/or thrombocytopenia may be present. Similarly, the bone marrow findings are inconsistent. The marrow may be hypercellular secondary to erythroid hyperplasia or may appear hypoplastic.

That this disorder is clonal in nature is evidenced by the presence of two populations of red cells: one that is normal and another that is hypersusceptible to complement. The relative numbers of complement-sensitive erythrocytes vary from patient to patient and correlate well with the degree of hemolysis. The diagnosis rests upon demonstration of increased lysis on activation of complement. The sucrose hemolysis test is often used as a screening test. Complement is activated by the low ionic strength of the sucrose solution. Cases of PNH will show more than 5% lysis. The acid hemolysis test is used as a confirmatory test. The principle of hypersusceptibility to complement is identical, although in this test complement is activated by acidifying the serum. Although the acid hemolysis is considered diagnostic, erythrocytes in congenital dyserythropoietic anemia type II also show a positive acid hemolysis test. Other ancillary findings that may be helpful in lending support to the diagnosis are hemosiderinuria and a decreased leukocyte alkaline phosphatase.

The natural course of the disease is often prolonged but marred by episodic bouts of hemolysis and a number of often fatal complications. Marrow aplasia is accompanied by all of the complications of neutropenia and thrombocytopenia. Infection may also arise secondary to functional neutrophil defects. Anemia may be exacerbated by the development of iron deficiency with prolonged intravascular hemolysis, or folate deficiency that may accompany brisk hemolysis and reticulocytosis. Venous thromboses involving the hepatic vein may develop in up to 30% of patients. Visceral thromboses may lead to repeated bouts of abdominal pain. Cerebral and venous sinuses may also be involved. A small number of patients may develop acute myelogenous leukemia; this plus the clonal trilineage nature of the disease suggest that perhaps PNH is in reality a myelodysplastic disorder.

Hypersplenism

Anemia may arise from primary splenic sequestration or destruction through a variety of mechanisms: hyperactivity of the splenic reticuloendothelial function; impediment of transit through the splenic cords; or increased transit time due to splenic pooling. Prominent splenomegaly is common and results from a variety of conditions, including portal hypertension, extramedullary hematopoiesis, metabolic storage disorders, lymphoreticular neoplasia, and infection.

Anemia may be accompanied by thrombocytopenia and/or neutropenia mediated through the same mechanisms. The term "hypersplenism" has been used to describe such otherwise unexplained cytopenias. To properly invoke hypersplenism, one must demonstrate paradoxical peripheral cytopenia and marrow hyperplasia, both of which normalize following removal of the spleen or effective therapy of the underlying cause for splenic enlargement.

POLYCYTHEMIA

A discussion of erythrocyte disorders would not be complete without consideration of polycythemia. Polycythemia, or erythrocytosis, is defined as an increased red cell volume. As with the functional definition of anemia, red cell volume is approached in the more practical quantitative terms of hemoglobin or hematocrit. Erythrocytosis therefore equates to an increased hemoglobin level or hematocrit.

Relative erythrocytosis, or stress erythrocytosis, is secondary to diminished plasma volume and must be distinguished from an absolute erythrocytosis, a true increase in red cell volume. Absolute erythrocytosis may occur as a primary autonomous expansion of red cell mass: polycythemia vera (PV).

Table 35.10. Classification of Erythrocytosis

Relative: Diminished plasma volume
Absolute
Primary: Polycythemia vera
Secondary:
Physiologically appropriate
High altitude
Pulmonary disease
Pickwickian syndrome
Cardiovascular disease with right-to-left shunt
High–oxygen-affinity hemoglobinopathies
Congenitally decreased erythrocyte 2,3-DPG
Physiologically inappropriate
Neoplasms
Renal cell carcinoma
Cerebellar hemangioblastoma
Hepatocellular carcinoma
Uterine leiomyoma
Adrenal adenoma
Ovarian carcinoma
Nonneoplastic renal disease
Renal cysts
Hydronephrosis

PV must be differentiated from the many causes of erythrocytosis that occur secondary to the effects of excess erythropoietin. Elevated erythropoietin levels may be physiologically appropriate in response to a state of tissue hypoxia, which may arise through habitation at high altitudes, pulmonary disease, congenital heart disease with right-to-left shunts, hypoventilatory states, and high–oxygen-affinity hemoglobinopathies. If the tissue hypoxia is reversed in these conditions, erythropoietin levels fall to normal, accompanied by a return of blood hemoglobin levels to normal.

Inappropriately elevated levels of erythropoietin may be encountered in the absence of tissue hypoxia. A variety of neoplastic and nonneoplastic disorders are associated with the production or release of erythropoietin or erythropoietin-like substances (Table 35.10). A small number of endocrine disorders have also been associated with inappropriate erythrocytosis secondary to the effects of androgens on erythropoiesis. Androgens act by stimulating erythropoietin production and by directly promoting erythroid stem cells.

The approach to the patient depends on identifying the primary or secondary nature of the erythrocytosis. The peripheral blood and bone marrow findings are largely limited to the elevated red cell mass except in the case of PV, in which characteristic increases in all three cell lines are encountered. Splenomegaly, basophilia, elevated leukocyte alkaline phosphatase levels, and increased levels of vitamin B_{12} or B_{12} binding proteins are additional associated findings of PV. The underlying cause of the decreased plasma volume leading to a relative erythrocytosis is usually evident. Similarly, symptoms of hypoxemia are often readily recognizable. Geographic altitude and the extreme obesity of the Pickwickian syndrome are difficult to disguise. Hemoglobin electrophoresis, radiographic evaluation, and quantitative erythropoietin levels are useful following exhaustion of the more common causes of erythrocytosis.

Ideally, one would like to maintain the hematocrit below 52% through periodic phlebotomy. As the hematocrit rises above this level, so does blood viscosity, placing the patient at risk for thrombosis, particularly in areas of low flow rates. Additionally, as viscosity increases, the oxygen-carrying capacity of blood decreases; in cases of hypoxia-related secondary erythrocytosis, this will serve to further stimulate erythropoietin production.

36 The Thalassemia and Hemoglobinopathy Syndromes

George C. Hoffman

Much of our knowledge concerning the structure and function of proteins and the genes that control their production has its origin in studies of the hemoglobin molecule.

The history of these studies is peppered with landmark discoveries. The first observation that more than one form of hemoglobin existed, unrelated to its state of oxygenation, was that of Körber (1) who, in 1866, reported his finding of two distinct hemoglobins in the newborn based on their resistance to denaturation by acid and alkali. In 1910, Herrick (2) coined the term *sickle cell* to describe the shape of red cells seen in the blood of a student from the Caribbean who had chronic anemia. In 1925, Cooley and Lee (3) suggested that the chronic anemia, splenomegaly, and bone changes seen in a series of five children represented a distinct type of anemia. The link between Cooley's anemia and the hemolytic anemia described in the Italian literature, known as the Rietti-Greppi-Micheli type (4–6) and later as Mediterranean anemia, had to await the work of Wintrobe and his colleagues (7). The term *thalassemia*, a euphonious attempt to convert various previous titles into one word, was first suggested by Whipple and Bradford (8). In fact, the word suggests sea (thalassa) in the blood (-emia) and shows a degree of Western chauvinism since there probably are more people with thalassemia in Asia than there are people in the Mediterranean basin.

Pauling and his colleagues (9) are usually given credit for first demonstrating a chemical abnormality in an inherited hemoglobin disorder when in 1949 they observed an electrophoretic difference between adult hemoglobin (Hb A) and sickle hemoglobin (Hb S). However, 1 year earlier, Hörlein and Weber (10) suggested that an abnormal hemoglobin might explain their findings in a patient with hereditary methemoglobinemia (later shown to be Hb M Saskatoon [11]). The search for the specific defect in an abnormal hemoglobin culminated in 1956 when Ingram (12) pinpointed the amino acid substitution in Hb S. A torrent of discoveries followed this observation. Now, over 400 structurally abnormal hemoglobins (13) have been defined. Establishing the structural and functional relationships of the various molecular lesions became possible largely through the detailed x-ray crystallographic analysis of the hemoglobin molecule conducted by Perutz and his colleagues (14, 15) begun in the 1960s and still continuing.

The genetic basis for many of these disorders became evident to several investigators, and the relationship of the more common forms to malaria was suggested by Haldane (16) in 1949. The exact details of the number of globin genes and the precise definition of the lesions that underlie the various disorders had to await the explosion of knowledge resulting from the development of DNA and RNA technologies. The abilities of the cytogeneticist to look at the finer details of the chromosome have now converged with those of the "gene-prober" to produce a very complete picture of the globin genes.

The purpose of this chapter is to relate this knowledge to a discussion of the hemoglobinopathies, emphasizing the laboratory aspects of this varied group of disorders.

STRUCTURE AND FUNCTION OF NORMAL HEMOGLOBIN MOLECULES

The normal human hemoglobin molecules consist of two pairs of polypeptide (globin) chains, each of which carries a heme portion. The tetramer is roughly spherical in shape (64 × 55 × 40 Å) with a molecular weight (MW) of 64,400 daltons; the globin portion makes up approximately 96% of the molecule. The hemoglobins that are produced at various stages of embryonic, fetal, and adult life are listed in Table 36.1. Each of these hemoglobins consists of a pair of α- or α-like (ζ) globin chains and a pair of β- or β-like globin chains. There is considerable homology within each of these two groups. The structure of the various globin chains is known precisely (17) and can be considered under four headings. The primary structure consists of 141 amino acids in the α-globin chain and 147 amino acids in the β- and β-like globin chains. The secondary structure involves the α-heli-

Table 36.1. The Normal Human Hemoglobins

Hemoglobin	Globin Chains	Major Source	Embryo	Neonate	Adult
			%	%	%
Gower 1	ζ_2/ϵ_2	Yolk sac	50	0	0
Gower 2	α_2/ϵ_2	Yolk sac	25	0	0
Portland	ζ_2/γ_2	Yolk sac	25	0	0
Hb F	$\alpha_2/^G\gamma_2$[a] $\alpha_2/^A\gamma_2$	Liver, spleen	0	75	<1
Hb A	α_2/β_2	Bone marrow	0	25	97
Hb A_2	α_2/δ_2	Bone marrow	0	<1	3

[a]Two structurally and genetically distinct γ-globin chains are normally produced, one with glycine (^{G}) and the other with alanine (^{A}) as the 136th amino acid residue.

cal arrangement of amino acids present in 75% of each globin chain. The tertiary structure is represented by the larger folds superimposed on the α-helical arrangement and occurring at the junction of α-helical with nonhelical segments. Finally, the quaternary structure involves the interrelation between the four globin chains.

The heme portion (MW 614 daltons) is slung between two histidine residues in each globin chain. Thus, there are four hemes in each hemoglobin molecule, allowing it to bind up to four molecules of oxygen. The iron atom in the heme portion is covalently linked to the "proximal" histidine (F8) and is stabilized by a large number of other interatomic links within the heme pocket. A complex series of steric changes facilitate the movement of oxygen into and out of the molecule (heme-heme interaction). These differences between oxyhemoglobin and deoxyhemoglobin involve numerous amino acids in or near the heme pocket and near the points of contact between the globin chains. Therefore, amino acid substitutions in these positions can significantly alter heme function, its stability within the heme pocket, and the stability of the molecule as a whole.

The hemoglobin molecule is beautifully suited to its main function—the delivery of oxygen. It has the ability to pick up oxygen at the relatively high oxygen tension in the lungs and deliver it at the lower oxygen tension of the tissues, remaining soluble throughout, undamaged by the oxygen it carries and utilizing none of it.

Several factors facilitate the delivery of oxygen. Unrelated to the hemoglobin molecule itself are the large surface area and pliability of red cells, the blood flow that is systemically and locally controlled, and the rate of diffusion of oxygen into and through the cells adjacent to capillaries. In addition, the oxygen affinity of some cells, particularly those containing myoglobin, attracts oxygen into those cells. Factors directly related to the hemoglobin molecule and therefore of importance when considering the hemoglobinopathies include the amount of hemoglobin circulating and its ability to deliver oxygen. The latter is represented by the difference between the oxygen content of arterial and venous blood, and is dependent on the oxygen dissociation curve, which indicates the amount of oxygen delivered or released for a unit decrease in oxygen tension (PO_2).

The oxygen dissociation curve (Fig. 36.1) can be depicted as the relationship between the amount of the hemoglobin that is in the form of oxyhemoglobin (percent saturation) and the partial pressure of oxygen (oxygen tension) in the surrounding medium. The oxygen affinity of hemoglobin is often reported as the P_{50}, which is that partial pressure of oxygen at which the hemoglobin is half-oxygenated; P_{50} is inversely related to oxygen affinity. Oxygen dissociation curves of clinical import are those obtained from whole blood under standard physiological conditions—a temperature of 37°C, a PCO_2 of 40 mm Hg, and a pH of 7.4 The P_{50} for normal men is close to 27 mm Hg; it is slightly higher in women. Under normal circumstance, hemoglobin is 97% saturated in the lungs and approximately 75% saturated at the normal mixed venous oxygen tension of 40 mm Hg.

There are three main factors, other than the structure of the hemoglobin molecule itself, that affect the shape and position of the oxygen dissociation curve (Fig. 36.1): pH, temperature, and 2,3-diphosphoglycerate (2,3-DPG). Bohr and his colleagues (18, 19) were the first to show that oxygen affinity was reduced by carbon dioxide. The reciprocal relationship between oxygen affinity and carbon dioxide affinity (an obvious advantage in a system where oxygen is adsorbed in the lungs and delivered to the tissue, while the reverse is occurring for carbon dioxide) was later shown to be effected by change in pH. As carbon dioxide is expelled through the lungs, pH increases and oxygen affinity increases; there is a "shift to the left" in the oxygen dissociation curve. The lowering of pH that occurs in the tissues has the opposite effect, decreasing the oxygen affinity. Thus, at either end of the system, the Bohr effect of a change in pH is beneficial to the uptake or delivery of oxygen.

Temperature change also alters oxygen affinity (20) in an apparently appropriate fashion. Increase in temperature, with its increased metabolic demands, reduces oxygen affinity and thus increases delivery

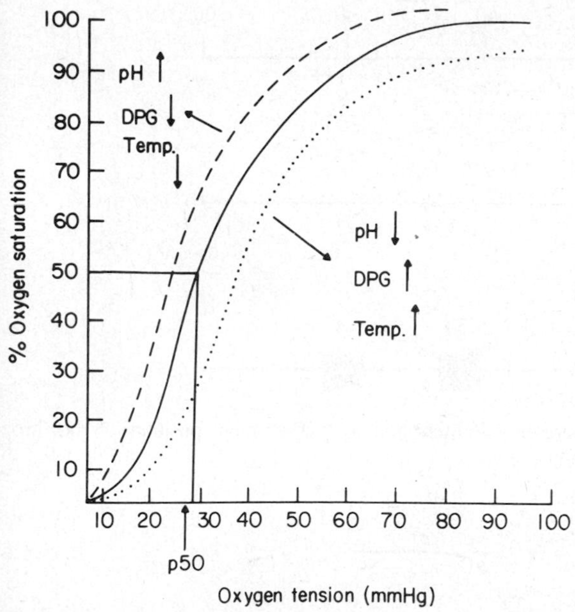

Figure 36.1. The oxygen dissociation curve of human adult hemoglobin (Hb A). Alteration in the position of the curve resulting from changes (↑ increase, ↓ decrease) in pH, 2,3-diphosphoglycerate (DPG) and temperature (temp) are indicated by the dashed and dotted lines. (Reprinted with permission from Weatherall DJ, Clegg JB. The thalassemia syndromes. 3rd ed. Oxford: Blackwell Scientific Publications, 1981.)

of oxygen. Conversely, reduction in temperature increases oxygen affinity and reduces delivery of oxygen.

2,3-DPG, the most abundant organic phosphate in the red cell at approximately 5 mM/liter of packed red cells, has a marked effect on the oxygen affinity of hemoglobin (21). 2,3-DPG lowers oxygen affinity in two ways: by binding preferentially to the β-chain of deoxyhemoglobin and thus tending to stabilize it; and by reducing intracellular pH. The concentration of 2,3-DPG within the red cell does not remain constant; it varies inversely with the hemoglobin concentration both in anemic and in normal individuals. Thus, as the hemoglobin falls, the amount of 2,3-DPG increases, oxygen affinity decreases, and more oxygen is unloaded from the hemoglobin.

In summary, hemoglobin, aided and abetted by several mechanisms active in the red cell, is a very efficient respiratory pigment. Hemoglobin within the red cell meets the four requirements suggested by Barcroft in 1928 for such a pigment, namely the ability (*a*) to carry large quantities of oxygen, (*b*) to take up and release the oxygen at appropriate pressures, (*c*) to remain soluble, and (*d*) to act as a buffer (22).

GENETIC CONTROL

Each globin chain is under separate genetic control. The α-gene cluster lies at the extreme end of the short arm of chromosome 16 (16p13.3–pter) (23) and consists of three genes and four pseudogenes[a] (Fig. 36.2) (24). There are two functional α-genes on each chromosome 16—α1 and α2; they have minor structural differences but transcribe into mRNAs that encode identical α-globin products in unequal quantities; α1 is responsible for about one-third of the α-chains and α2 for about two-thirds (25).

The β-globin gene cluster lies on the short arm of chromosome 11 distal to band p14 and between the genes for parathyroid hormone and insulin (26). It consists of six genes and two pseudogenes (Fig. 36.2). The two γ-genes encode for γ-chains that differ structurally, $^{A}\gamma$ having alanine and $^{G}\gamma$ having glycine as the 136th amino acid residue.

Each globin gene has a similar organization, consisting of three exons and two introns or intervening sequences. All five regions are transcribed into nuclear or pre-mRNA, but the RNA from the introns is spliced out in the formation of cytoplasmic mRNA, which therefore contains only information transcribed from the exons. Regions close to the gene (usually upstream at the N-terminal or 5′-end) are involved in initiating and controlling gene function. Hence, mutations occurring near a gene as well as those within a gene may significantly affect the amount or the structure of its ultimate product.

Under normal circumstances, the product of an α- or α-like gene combines with the product of a β- or β-like gene to form a hemoglobin tetramer (Table 36.1). As maturation occurs in utero and postpartum, the activity of the genes changes (Fig. 36.3). This change has a downstream direction with the embryonic genes, active in yolk sac erythropoiesis, ceasing to function at about the 10th week to be superseded by α- and γ-chain production (hepatic and splenic erythropoiesis); γ-chain production is gradually replaced by β-chain production starting at about the sixth week of fetal life and proceeding until the sixth to 12th month of extrauterine life. By that time, γ-chain production is less than 1% that of the β-chain. Production of the δ-chain is approximately 0.5% of total globin chain production at birth and rises to adult levels by 1 year. (In the vocabulary of the hemoglobin chains, adulthood is reached by about 1 year.)

Clinically, the most significant of these changes is the γ- to β-switch, which explains why at birth a normal neonate possesses approximately 75% Hb F ($\alpha_2\gamma_2$) and 25% Hb A ($\alpha_2\beta_2$), whereas by about 12

[a]Pseudogenes are segments of DNA that show significant homology to nearby genes but are not expressed, usually because of nonsense codes within them. They probably represent genes that arose as duplicates of an existing gene and lost their function as a result of mutation within them.

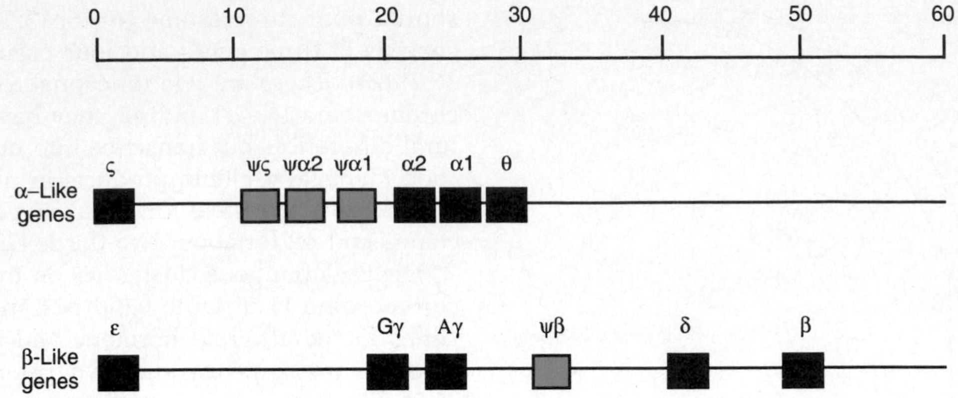

Figure 36.2. Diagrams of the relative positions of genes and pseudogenes of the α-like (chromosome 16) and β-like (chromosome 11) series. The scale represents kilobases; the sequences from left to right represent 5′ (N-terminal) to 3′ (C-terminal) positions on the chromosome.

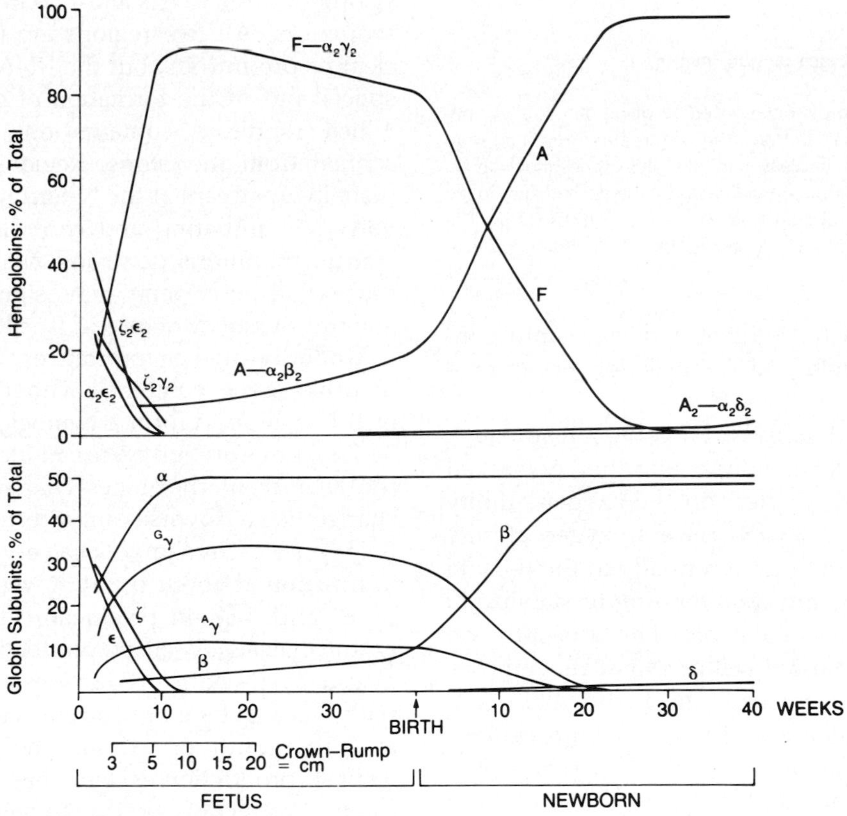

Figure 36.3. Changes in globin chain and hemoglobin production during human development. (Reprinted with permission from Bunn HF, Forget BG. Hemoglobin: molecular, genetic and clinical aspects. Philadelphia: WB Saunders, 1986.)

months the infant possesses less than 1% Hb F, approximately 96% Hb A, and approximately 3% Hb A_2 ($\alpha_2\delta_2$).

CLASSIFICATION AND NOMENCLATURE

The vast majority of hemoglobinopathies are inherited abnormalities. A few result from de novo mutation (27), and there is a small but fascinating group of acquired defects mimicking α-thalassemia and persistence of fetal hemoglobin (28, 29).

The inherited group of disorders can be divided into three broad categories (Table 36.2):

- *Structural, or qualitative abnormalities,* in which the amino acid sequence of one or more of the globin chains is altered (by substitution, addition, deletion, or fusion) as a result of an incorrect DNA code. Sickle hemoglobin (Hb S) is a common example.
- *Quantitative abnormalities,* in which the production of one or more of the globin chains is reduced or

Table 36.2. A Classification of the More Common Hemoglobinopathies

Structural defects
Involving Hb S
Without in vivo sickling:
Hb AS (sickle cell trait)
Hb AS-$G_{Philadelphia}$
Hb AS α-thalassemia
Hb S HPFH
With in vivo sickling:
Hb SS (sickle cell anemia)
Hb SC
Hb $SD_{Los\ Angeles}$
Hb SO_{Arab}
Hb Sβ-thalassemia
HB C disorders
Hb D disorders
Hb $G_{Philadelphia}$ disorders
Unstable hemoglobins
Hemoglobins with high or low O_2 affinity
Hb M (methemoglobinemia)
Globin chain imbalance (thalassemia)
α-Thalassemia
Silent (one-gene defect)
Thalassemia minor (two-gene defect)
Hb H disease (three-gene defect)
Hb Barts hydrops fetalis (four-gene defect)
Result of a structural defect
Hb Constant Spring
β-Thalassemia
β^{o}-Thalassemia
β^{+}-Thalassemia
Result of a structural defect
Hb Lepore
Hb E
Unstable hemoglobins (some)
δβ Thalassemia
Hereditary persistence of fetal hemoglobin (HPFH)
Black type
Swiss type
Greek type
Associated with structural defect:
Hb Kenya

absent (due to inadequate amounts of mRNA, to unstable mRNA, or to mRNA that contains an untranslatable "nonsense" message) resulting in an imbalance in globin chain production. These form the various thalassemia syndromes that are classified according to the globin chain whose production is deficient.

- *Hereditary persistence of fetal hemoglobin (HPFH)*, in which there is complete or partial failure of the γ- to β-switch. As noted later, there is an overlap between HPFH and the β-thalassemia, resulting in a spectrum with HPFH at one end, β-thalassemia at the other, and δβ-thalassemia as an intermediate.

Since many of these disorders are common, combinations occur as a result of compound heterozygosity for abnormal genes (Fig. 36.4). Further-

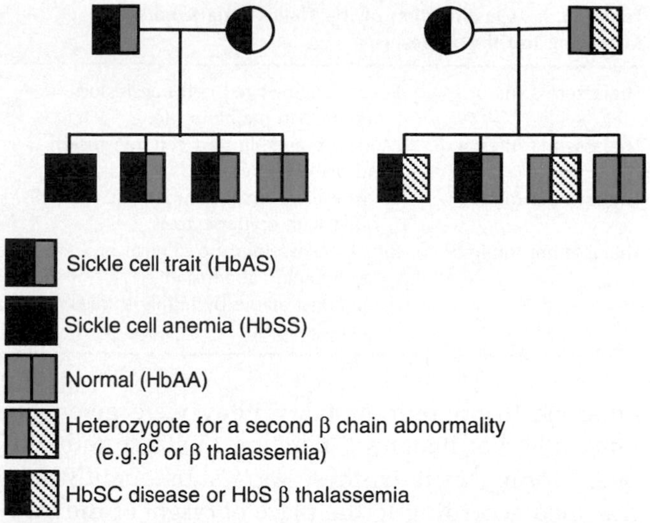

Figure 36.4. The inheritance pattern of hemoglobinopathies. β-Globin chain defects are used in these examples. α-Globin chain defects have a more complicated inheritance pattern because two α-globin genes are inherited from each parent. (Reprinted with permission from Hoffman GC. The sickling disorders. Lab Med 1990;21:797–807.)

more, structural defects, such as Hb Lepore, may cause an imbalance in globin chain production and hence a thalassemia syndrome. In general, the various genetic abnormalities are inherited in a codominant fashion.

Nomenclature commonly used for the hemoglobinopathies is somewhat confusing, because as knowledge has been accumulated, it has not always been translated into more accurate designations. The structural hemoglobin variants can be specifically named according to their structural abnormality. Thus, sickle hemoglobin is $\alpha_2\beta_2^{6glu\rightarrow val}$ or $\alpha_2\beta_2^{6(A3)glu\rightarrow val}$, indicating that the sixth amino acid residue (or the third amino acid in the first α-helical segment) of the β-globin chain, which is normally glutamic acid, is replaced by valine. However, this is difficult to verbalize, if not to write; hence, it is generally referred to as Hb S. Three hemoglobins are referred to by their initials: Hb A (adult hemoglobin), Hb F (fetal hemoglobin), and Hb S (sickle hemoglobin). Letters were given to hemoglobins as they were discovered, but it was soon realized that the alphabet would not be large enough, so various eponyms were then used in a somewhat disorganized fashion. The list of hemoglobin variants, now over 400, includes names of countries (Hb Nigeria), regions or states (Hb Ohio), cities or towns (Hb Seattle), urban areas (Hb Queens), rivers (Hb Volga), hospitals (Hb Barts), and even historic figures (Hb Abraham Lincoln). Confusion arises for two reasons. In many instances, the variant was discovered because of its electrophoretic pattern. Since several different structural defects can give rise to hemoglobins with the

Table 36.3. Classification of the Thalassemia Syndromes According to Clinical Severity

Thalassemia major	Severe anemia; red cell transfusion required to maintain life.
Thalassemia intermedia	Moderate anemia; red cell transfusion occasionally required.
Thalassemia minor	Slight if any anemia, microcytic red cells, often with erythrocytosis.
Thalassemia minima	Silent thalassemia; no clinical or hematologic abnormality. Demonstratable by family studies or gene analysis.

same electrophoretic mobility, they were given the same title. For instance, there are 13 structurally different forms of Hb D; these were subsequently subclassified according to the place of origin of the individual carrying the abnormality (Hb $D_{Los\ Angeles}$, Hb D_{Ibidan}, etc.). A second confusion arises when hemoglobins given different designations are subsequently found to be identical; the hemoglobin $\alpha_2{}^{47(CE5)Asp-Gly}\beta_2$ has had nine different names attached to it.

In the laboratory, the specific designation of the structural abnormality would seem to be the most logical nomenclature to use. However, at least for the common varieties, the exact structure is seldom verified, so the eponym is usually applied.

When referring to heterozygotes, a shorthand is used listing the hemoglobin present in greatest quantity first. Hb AS, for example, refers to a sickle cell trait in which there is approximately 55% Hb A and 45% Hb S. The same system can be applied to double heterozygotes; for instance, Hb SC indicates an individual who has inherited a β^S gene from one parent and a β^C gene from the other. Hb S β-thalassemia indicates an individual who has inherited a β^S gene from one parent and a β-thalassemia gene from the other (Fig. 36.4).

The nomenclature commonly used for the thalassemia syndromes is relatively simple but somewhat less accurate; the Greek letter of the globin chain that is reduced in quantity is used. Thus, β-thalassemia indicates reduction of β-chain production, α-thalassemia reduction of α-chain production, and so on. However, there are over 40 different lesions in or near the β-gene that can cause β-thalassemia. Attempts to name the various subsets of the thalassemias are discussed later.

The term *trait* is used for heterozygotes (sickle cell trait, Hb C trait) and *disease* for the homozygote (sickle cell disease, Hb C disease); however, not all authors would agree that *sickle cell anemia* is synonymous with *sickle cell disease*. This system becomes unwieldy when four genes are involved, as in α-chain abnormalities such as Hb G Philadelphia. The adjectives *minor* and *major*, used in describing the thalassemias, were originally used in both a clinical and a genetic (heterozygote and homozygote) sense. As the large number of different thalassemia genes with varying clinical expressions became known, the terms have reverted to a strictly clinical interpretation (Table 36.3).

INCIDENCE, DISTRIBUTION, AND THE MALARIA HYPOTHESIS

The majority of the more than 400 hemoglobinopathies are rare and known to occur in a handful of families at the most; the affected individuals are almost exclusively heterozygotes, with homozygotes occurring mainly in consanguinous families. The common abnormalities, particularly those that have reached polymorphic levels in some populations, such as Hb S, Hb C, Hb E, and the α-and β-thalassemias achieved their popularity through natural selection.

Inherited abnormalities in the three major components of the red cell—membrane, hemoglobin, and a rudimentary glycolytic pathway—represent some of the best examples of Darwinism in action among human populations. All are related to malaria (30). The remarkably high incidence of stomatocytic elliptocytosis in Melanesia is an example of a membrane abnormality that is beneficial in areas of endemic *Plasmodium falciparum* malaria (31). The parasite has difficulty entering these abnormal red cells. The Duffy blood group provides another striking example (32); *Plasmodium vivax* is unable to enter Duffy-negative red cells. In Africa, Duffy-negative individuals, Fy(a − b −), are found mainly in western regions where *P. vivax* malaria is not found. In this situation, it appears that the blood group distribution preceded and prevented the spread of *P.vivax* from the east (33).

This Duffy relationship is completely different from that with Hb S, whose incidence is greatest where malaria (in this case *P. falciparum*) is most prevalent. There are areas in central Africa in which the incidence of sickle cell trait reaches 40%. This high incidence is maintained (despite the loss of sickle genes from the gene pool with the neonatal death of most Hb SS individuals) because falciparum malaria is much milder and seldom lethal in Hb AS individuals than in normal (Hb AA) individuals. This is an example of balanced polymorphism in which the heterozygote has an advantage over both the normal and abnormal homozygote (34). The high incidence of Hb E in southeast Asia can also be explained by the malaria hypothesis (35).

The distribution of α- and β-thalassemia also matches the distribution of malaria. The classic studies of Siniscalco and his colleagues (36) in Sardinia and Flint et al. (37) in Melanesia are two among many population studies demonstrating this relationship. In Sardinia, the incidence of β-thalassemia minor (and G6PD deficiency) is directly related to the incidence of malaria, which in turn is related to the altitude at which the populations live (mosquitoes being limited to valleys by temperature and water requirements). In Melanesia, malaria and α-thalassemia were shown to be directly related, the diagnosis of α-thalassemia being proved by gene analysis. One exception to the relationship between malaria and β-thalassemia is the relatively low prevalence of the latter in central and western Africa, where Hb S is the major hemoglobinopathy. A likely explanation is that two mutations, both beneficial, are unlikely to coexist if both homozygotes are lethal. Hb S seems to have won—perhaps as the more "beneficial" trait with respect to *P. falciparum* infection.

Glucose-6-phosphate dehydrogenase (G6PD) deficiency is another "guard" against malaria, and, like sickle cell trait, has a high incidence in Africa (38).

The incidence of Hb S (present in approximately 8% of African Americans), G6PD deficiency (with a similar incidence), α-thalassemia minor (approximately 30% of African Americans have single-gene deletion type), and β-thalassemia minor (3 to 5% among African Americans and individuals of Mediterranean extraction) can be explained by their origin from areas of high malarial endemicity.

LABORATORY APPROACH

The diagnosis of all hemoglobinopathies eventually lies in the laboratory. The number and degree of sophistication of the tests needed will depend on the clinical needs of the patient population and the interests of the investigator. At one extreme, a simple solubility test to rule out the presence of Hb S may suffice, while at the other, precise amino acid sequencing or gene analysis may be required.

There are three main reasons that a laboratory may be asked to investigate the possible existence of a hemoglobinopathy. There may be a hint in the patient's history or physical examination; the blood count may indicate the possibility; or the investigation may be required as part of a screening program either of a population such as neonates or of individuals as a preoperative or other requirement. Hemoglobinopathies of real or potential clinical significance will usually present with some abnormality in the blood count. However, many of the rarer examples detected in screening programs are noticed because of an abnormal electrophoretic pattern; many of these will be of little or no clinical significance but nevertheless need to be labeled. Whatever the entry point, hemoglobin electrophoresis and a blood count, if not already performed, will almost certainly be required.

In this section, the application and value of the more commonly used tests are discussed. Some more esoteric tests, including those involving molecular and gene studies, are mentioned in later sections dealing with specific diseases.

Blood Count and Red Cell Morphology

Three types of abnormal blood counts are associated with clinically significant hemoglobinopathies: (*a*) microcytic hypochromic red cells often without significant anemia (as in thalassemia minor); (*b*) a hemolytic anemia (as in sickle cell anemia and Hb C disease); (*c*) a combination of the two (as in thalassemia intermedia and major). In addition to these common findings, a physiologically appropriate erythrocytosis is associated with high–oxygen affinity hemoglobins, and the appropriate "anemia" is associated with low–oxygen affinity hemoglobins.

Red cell morphology may provide a general or specific indication of a hemoglobinopathy. The latter include sickle cells, Hb C crystals, and the bizarre-shaped red cells seen in Hb SC disease. Less specific and often requiring additional staining techniques are Heinz bodies associated with many unstable hemoglobins and the Hb H inclusions of Hb H disease and some forms of α-thalassemia minor. Target cells are particularly common when Hb C or Hb D is present.

Heinz bodies, which consist of aggregates of denatured hemoglobin within the red cell, are seen in two main situations—oxidative hemolysis and instability of the hemoglobin. They are not visible in red cells stained with Wright's or other trichrome stains; vital or supravital stains such as those used to demonstrate reticulocytes are required. Crystal violet or methyl violet have an advantage over stains such as new methylene blue and brilliant cresyl blue because the latter redox stains are themselves able to cause Heinz body formation. However, this latter property may be advantageous in situations where few Heinz bodies are present. This concept can be carried further by the use of phenylhydrazine, a drug that in correct concentration in vitro will cause the formation of many more Heinz bodies in red cells containing an unstable hemoglobin (or with other abnormalities such as G6PD deficiency that predispose to Heinz body formation) than in normal red cells (39). Whatever staining method is use, normal controls must be incorporated in the procedure.

Hb H (β_4) is an unstable tetramer and forms a distinct type of Heinz body when exposed to a redox dye such as brilliant cresyl blue or new methylene blue (40). A suspension of red cells containing Hb H when incubated at 37°C for 1 hour with a few drops of 1% citrate-saline solution of brilliant cresyl blue will contain many round, small-blue-stained inclusions of precipitated Hb H, giving the cell a golf ball appearance. These inclusions can be distinguished from the precipitated RNA of reticulocytes and the larger Heinz bodies associated with other unstable hemoglobins under similar test conditions.

Solubility Test

The relative insolubility of deoxygenated Hb S compared with other hemoglobins is the basis of a simple test for its presence (41).

Several acceptable commercial kits are available that consist of a mixture of a lysing agent and a reducing agent in a high-phosphate buffer. When red cells containing Hb S are added, an opaque dispersed precipitate forms that is readily distinguished from the clear pink solution obtained with other hemoglobins.

False-positive results are rare and may be due to incomplete lysis of red cells because of erythrocytosis or to the presence of large amounts of protein in the patient's plasma, lending an opacity to the solution. False-negative results, on the other hand, are not uncommon and depend mainly on the amount of the Hb S present. When less than 20 to 25% Hb S is present (as may occur in a transfused or exchange-transfused patient with sickle cell anemia, in an individual with both sickle cell trait [Hb AS] and two-deletion α-thalassemia [$-\alpha/-\alpha$], in a severely anemic patient, and most importantly in a neonate with sickle cell anemia or trait), the result is often negative. Doubling the quantity of blood tested may get around this problem.

A positive solubility test indicates the presence of Hb S or any hemoglobin containing the Hb S mutation such as Hb C_{Harlem}, but does not provide a quantitative measure and does not therefore distinguish sickle cell trait, sickle cell anemia, or any combination of Hb S and another hemoglobinopathy.

Electrophoresis

Electrophoresis in or on various media is usually the first step in demonstrating and specifying a hemoglobin variant. Four commonly used techniques will be outlined here: isoelectric focusing (42), electrophoresis on cellulose acetate at alkaline pH (43), in agar at acid pH (44), and electrophoresis of separated globin chains (45).

Isoelectric focusing (IEF) is probably the method of choice for laboratories that handle a large number of specimens or for laboratories that are about to launch into the hemoglobin sea. This technique depends on the property of hemoglobins and other proteins to act as zwitterions. When placed in a pH gradient through which a direct current is flowing, hemoglobin molecules migrate to the position in the pH gradient at which they are electrically neutral (the isoelectric point or pI). The pI is virtually unique and highly reproducible for each hemoglobin. Therefore, IEF offers a one-step approach the specification of abnormal hemoglobins (Fig. 36.5). Minute quantitites of blood are needed; many laboratories involved in cord blood screening use the "filter paper" specimens submitted for detection of other genetic abnormalities. The cost of the equipment and material needed for IEF is greater than that of cellulose acetate and agar electrophoresis, but when large numbers of specimens are to be tested, the advantages of IEF make it cost-effective.

Cellulose acetate is a popular supporting medium and allows rapid separation of normal and many variant hemoglobins. In alkaline solution (tris-EDTA-borate buffer at pH 8.6), all hemoglobin molecules have a net negative charge and migrate toward the anode; the amino acid substitution in many hemoglobin variants alters their net charge and thus their electrophoretic mobility. The characteristic migration pattern of some of the more common variants is shown in Figure 36.6. Because either substitution of different amino acids or substitution of the same amino acid at different points in a globin chain may result in identical alterations in net charge, electrophoresis on cellulose acetate at alkaline pH seldom provides a specific diagnosis. However, the hemoglobins that migrate together on cellulose acetate at alkaline pH can often be separated by electrophoresis in agar using a citrate-citric acid buffer at pH 6.0. Migration under the latter conditions depends not only on electric charge but also on the counter-current of ions moving in the opposite direction that slows or reverses the migration of the hemoglobin molecules (electroendosmosis), an effect that varies with the hemoglobin under investigation (Fig. 36.6).

Using these two latter techniques, most of the common variants can be diagnosed with sufficient certainty to meet clinical demands. For instance, on cellulose acetate, Hb E and Hb O migrate with Hb C; but in citrate agar, Hb E migrates with Hb A, and Hb O remains near the point of application, forming a characteristic sharply defined band (Fig. 36.7). Hb $D_{Los\ Angeles}$ and Hb $G_{Philadelphia}$ migrate with Hb S on cellulose acetate but with Hb A in acid agar. These two hemoglobins can be separated from each other easily because Hb $D_{Los\ Angeles}$ has a β-chain defect ($\alpha_2\beta_2{}^{121Glu\rightarrow Gln}$), whereas Hb $G_{Philadelphia}$ has an α-chain defect ($\alpha_2{}^{68Asn\rightarrow Lys}\beta_2$). Since α-chains are present in all normal hemoglobins, an α-chain defect will give rise to abnormal forms of Hb A, Hb F, and Hb A_2. In the

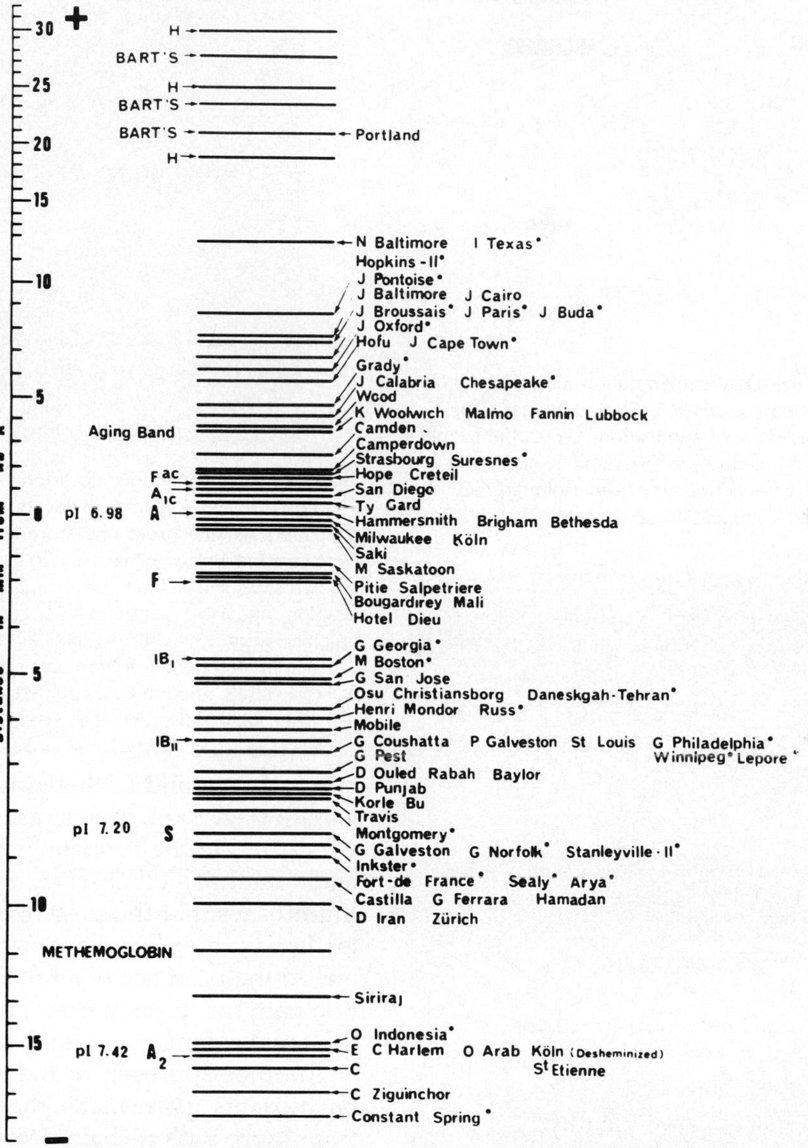

Figure 36.5. Isoelectric focusing of hemoglobin variants on polyacrylamide gels. Asterisks (*) indicate α-globin chain variants. 1BI and 1BII are the ferrous-ferric hybrids of Hb A. (Reprinted with permission from Basset P, Braconnier F, Rosa J. An update on electrophoretic and chromatographic methods in the diagnosis of hemoglobinopathies. J Chromatogr Biomed Appl 1982;227:267–304.)

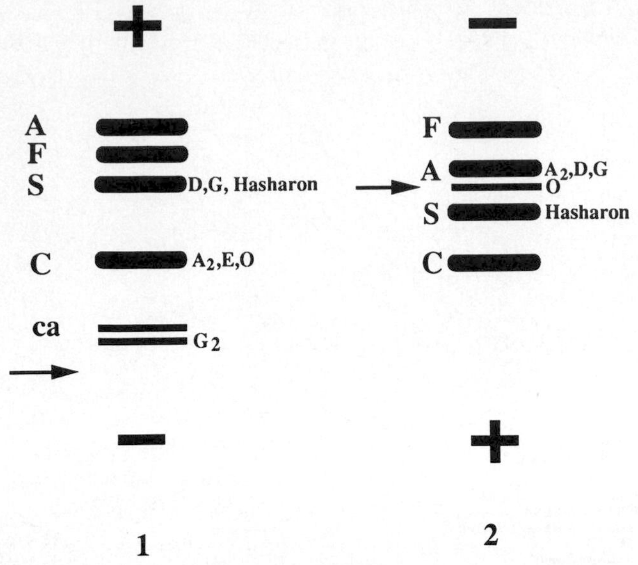

Figure 36.6. Diagram of the relative migration of some common hemoglobins on cellulose acetate at pH 8.6 (**1**), and in agar at pH 6.2 (**2**). The *arrows* indicate the point of application; CA, carbonic anhydrase; G_2, the abnormal form of Hb A_2 ($\alpha_2^G\delta_2$) found in the presence of Hb $G_{Philadelphia}$. (Reprinted with permission from Hoffman GC. The sickling disorders. Lab Med 1990;21:797–807.)

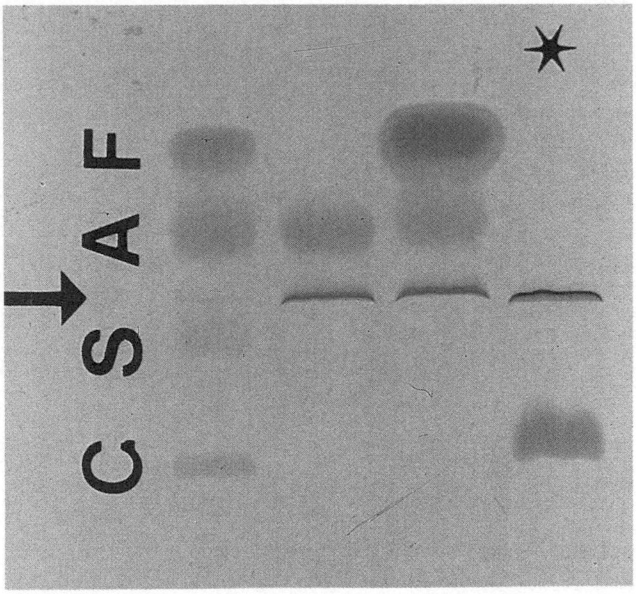

Figure 36.7. Hemoglobin electrophoresis in agar using a citrate–citric acid buffer at pH 6.0. *Arrow* indicates point of application. Left lane: Control mixture of Hb C, Hb S, Hb A, Hb F. Second lane: Adult with Hb O_{Arab} trait showing Hb A and the typically sharply defined band of the Hb O_{Arab}. Third lane: Cord blood from the daughter of patient in second lane, showing Hb F, Hb A, and Hb O_{Arab}. Fourth lane: Adult, compound heterozygote for Hb O_{Arab} and Hb C. (Reprinted with permission from Fishleder AJ, Hoffman GC. A practical approach to the detection of hemoglobinopathies: Part III. Nonsickling disorders and cord blood screening. Lab Med 1987;18:513–518.)

adult this can be recognized by the presence of an abnormal Hb A_2 band that migrates on cellulose acetate as far behind (cathodal to) normal Hb A_2 as the variant (Fig. 36.6), in this case Hb G, migrates behind Hb A, and in the neonate by the presence of normal and abnormal Hb F (Fig. 36.8). A useful rule of thumb says that the presence of more than two major bands in an electrophoretic pattern should alert one to the presence of an α-chain defect. The migration patterns of some hemoglobin variants, including the most common, are diagrammed in Figure 36.9.

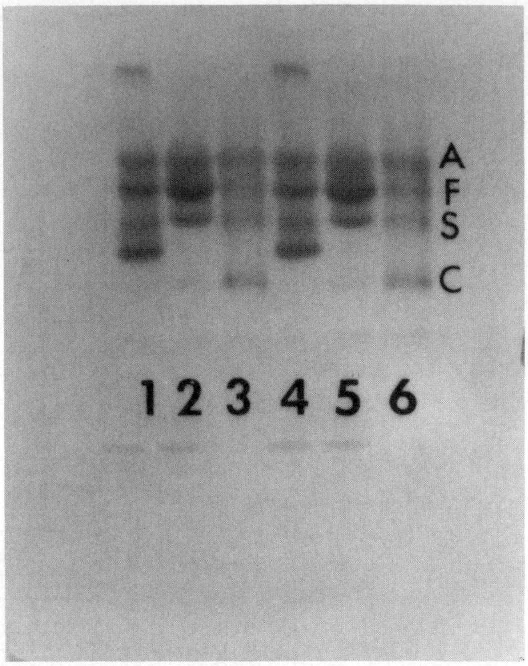

Figure 36.8. Hemoglobin electrophoresis on cellulose acetate at pH 7.4. Points of application are below the numerals. Lanes 1 and 4 show the pattern obtained from a newborn with Hb $G_{Philadelphia}$ trait and two-gene deletion type of α-thalassemia; the bands from top to bottom are Hb Bart's (γ_4), Hb A, Hb F, Hb $G_{Philadelphia}$ ($\alpha_2^G\beta_2$) migrating in the Hb S position, and Hb F variant ($\alpha_2^G\gamma_2$). Lanes 2 and 5 show the pattern obtained from a newborn with sickle cell trait (Hb A, Hb F, Hb S). Lanes 3 and 6 show the pattern obtained with a control mixture of Hb A, Hb F, Hb S, and Hb C. (Reprinted with permission from Hoffman GC. The sickling disorders. Lab Med 1990;21:797–807.)

Another approach to the separation of hemoglobin variants, particularly those with β-chain defects from those with α-chain defects, is the electrophoresis of separated globin chains (45). Globin chain separation is a simple process involving the treatment of the hemoglobin with a urea-mercaptoethanol mixture followed by electrophoresis in acid or alkaline buffer (Figs. 36.9, 36.10).

Although the references cited here and the instructions provided by manufacturers enable one to produce clear electrophoretic patterns, there are a few practical points that require emphasis. The clarity of separation will depend to a significant degree on the specimen used and its handling. Blood collected in NaEDTA as an anticoagulant is adequate for most purposes and may be stored for at least 24 hours at room temperature. This permits overnight mailing without special handling. Unstable hemoglobins are an exception because, if very unstable and therefore present in small amounts, they may disappear during such storage.

Given an adequate blood sample, there are several approaches to preparing it for electrophoresis. Since most plasma proteins such as albumin that are present in a significant quantity have an electrophoretic mobility much greater (faster) than any hemoglobin, the washing of red cells prior to preparing a lysate need not be tremendously thorough. In fact, if only a small quantity of blood is available, as in a capillary tube sample, rinsing can be omitted for screening purposes. Nevertheless, washing the red cells prior to preparing a lysate provides the best specimen.

Generally, application is best made with one of the several commercially available applicator wells, thus ensuring uniform and reproducible amounts. The quantity of lysate applied can be doubled when the amount of an abnormal hemoglobin under investigation is known to be small—in cord blood specimens, for example, where the amount of Hb A and its variants are low compared with Hb F, or when attempting to demonstrate an abnormal Hb A_2 when an α-chain defect is suspected. The concentration and the amount of lysate required for IEF is less than for the other techniques.

It is helpful to keep the concentration constant because quantitative comparisons of the electrophoretic bands are often of value. In this context, the density of the carbonic anhydrase band is often useful, since its concentration in the mature red cell is constant and therefore is usually proportional to the amount of lysate applied.

Quantitation

The quantitation of normal and variant hemoglobins is often of diagnostic importance. With a well-prepared electrophoretic pattern, "eyeballing" the plate is often as useful as more specific quantitation. Estimating the relative proportions of Hb S and Hb A can often be done in this manner (Fig. 36.11). In those circumstances in which a more precise estimate is required, densitometry can be used on cellulose acetate plates. However, this method has disadvantages, particularly when comparing large with small quantities, as when measuring Hb A_2 as a percentage of a relatively large amount of Hb A; the smaller quantity is usually overestimated. Elution of the hemoglobin bands from the electrophoretic plates and direct measurement of their hemoglobin content provides even greater accuracy, but the method is time consuming and seldom justified.

For some hemoglobins, specific methods of quantitation are readily available and simple to perform. Hb F can be quantitated on the basis of its resistance to alkali (46); toluene may be used in place of carbon tetrachloride called for in this method. Hb A_2 can be measured by elution from an anion-exchange column (47), Hb Barts and Hb H by elution from a cation-exchange column (48).

Globin Chain Synthesis

All the methods described so far provide a static view of the hemoglobin content of red cells. Under some circumstances, particularly in the thalassemia syndromes, the relative rates of production of the various globin chains provide useful information. These globin chain synthesis studies (49) require the separation and quantification of globin chains that have been generated in a reticulocyte-enriched preparation in the presence of an adequate supply of all necessary amino acids, one of which (usually leucine) is radiolabeled. The latter is then used as an indicator of the quantity of various globin chains produced. The individual globin chains are separated by high-pressure liquid chromatography. In many situations, such as in the diagnosis of the α-thalassemia syndromes, this methodology has been replaced by specific gene identification.

THALASSEMIA SYNDROMES

The thalassemia syndromes result from an imbalance in globin chain production that is almost always due to underproduction of one or two types of globin chains; rare examples in which overproduction of a globin chain causes the imbalance have been reported (50).

The thalassemia syndromes are classified according to the deficient globin chain or chains and according to their clinical severity (Table 36.3). The two largest groups are the α-thalassemias and the β-thalassemias; δ-thalassemia and γ-thalassemia are much less common and of little clinical significance. Therefore, they will be dealt with here only briefly.

δ-Thalassemia

δ-Thalassemia has been reported in the heterozygous and homozygous states (51). Hb A_2 ($\alpha_2\delta_2$) is reduced in the heterozygote and is usually absent in the homozygote because the genetic lesion results in failure to produce any δ-globin chains (δ^0); δ^+-thalassemia, in which there is a reduced production of δ-chains, has also been reported (52). Neither the heterozygote nor the homozygote exhibits any clinical or hematologic abnormality. Co-inheritance of δ-thalassemia and β-thalassemia results in a form of

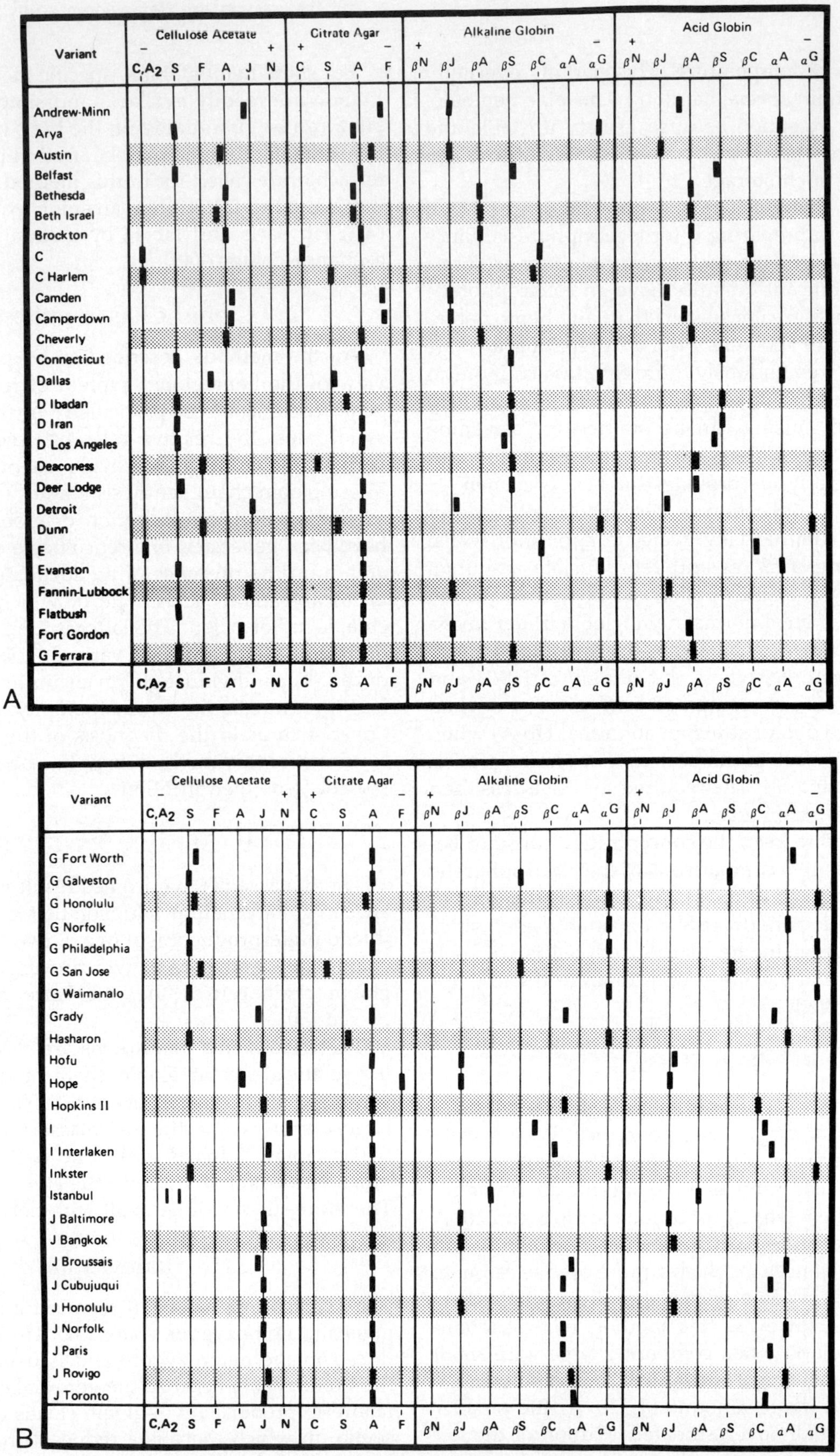

Figure 36.9. Hemoglobin electrophoresis; the relative migration of some hemoglobin variants on cellulose acetate at alkaline pH and in citrate agar at acid pH; and the relative migration of separated globin chains in alkaline and in acid buffers. (Reprinted with permission from Bunn HF, Forget BG. Hemoglobin: molecular, genetic and clinical aspects. Philadelphia: WB Saunders, 1986.)

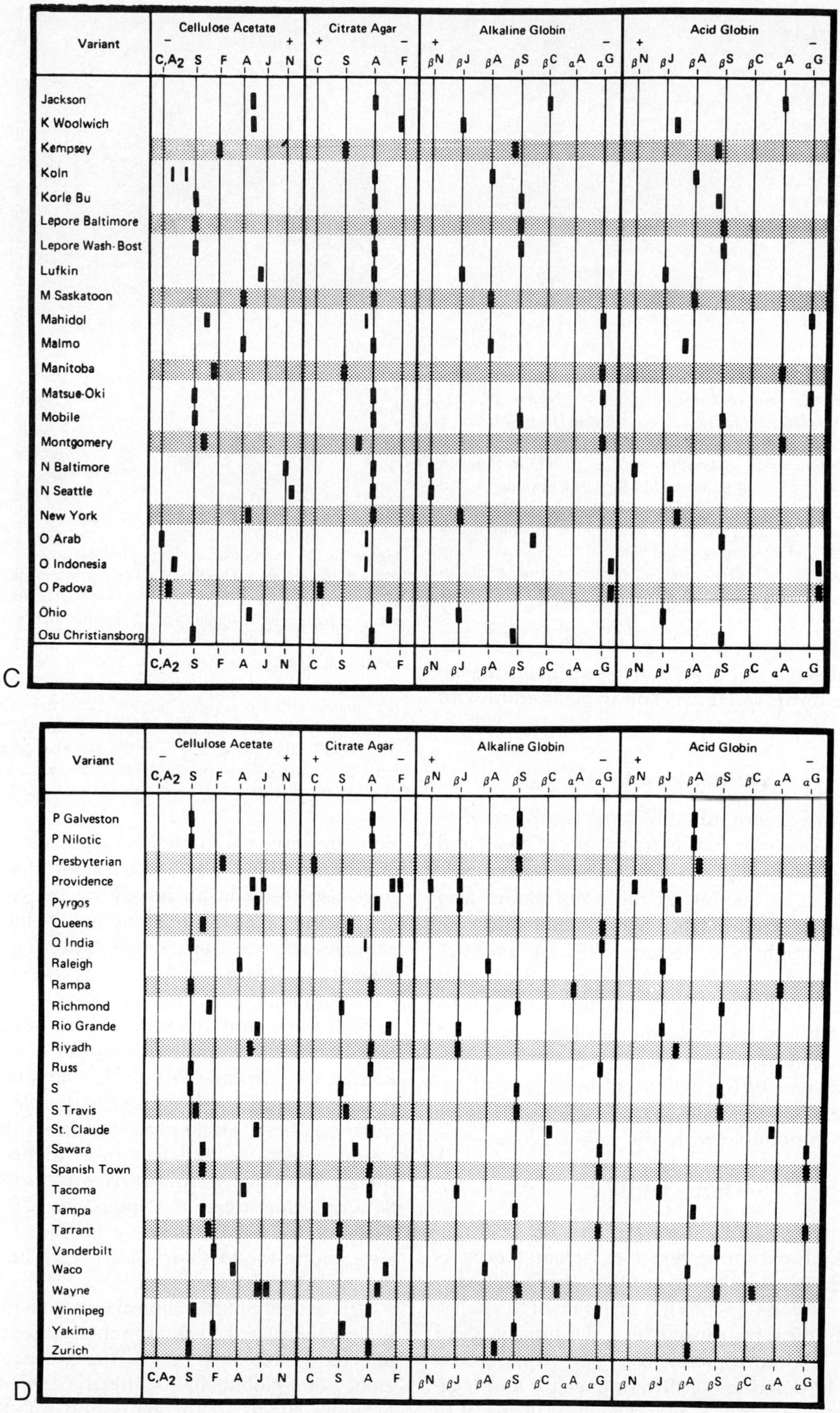

Figure 36.9. C and D.

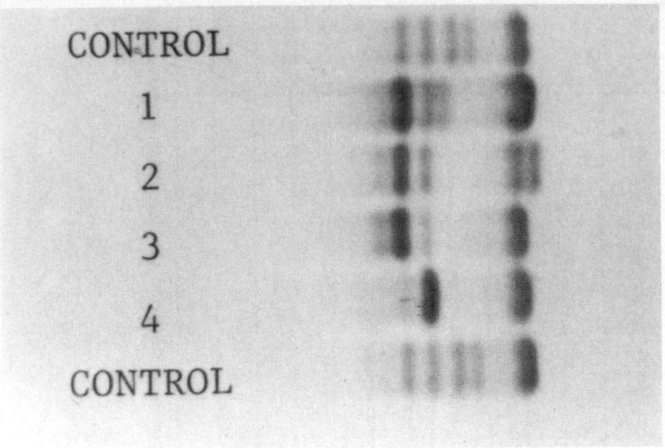

Figure 36.10. Electrophoresis of separated globin chains on cellulose acetate at pH 6.2. Controls consist from left to right of γ-, β^A-, β^S-, β^C-, and α^A-globin chains. Lane 1: Neonate with Hb D trait showing a heavy γ-chain band, β^A, β^D (note slight separation from β^S at this pH), and α^A. In electrophoresis of whole hemoglobins, Hb D migrates to the Hb S position in alkaline buffer and to the Hb A position in acid buffer. Lane 2: Neonate with Hb $G_{Philadelphia}$ trait showing a heavy γ-chain band, β^A, α^A, and α^G. Lane 3: Normal neonate showing heavy γ-chain band, β^A, and α^A. Lane 4: Adult with 5% Hb F showing faint γ-chain band, β^A, and γ^A. (Reprinted with permission from Hoffman GC. The sickling disorders. Lab Med 1990;21:797–807.)

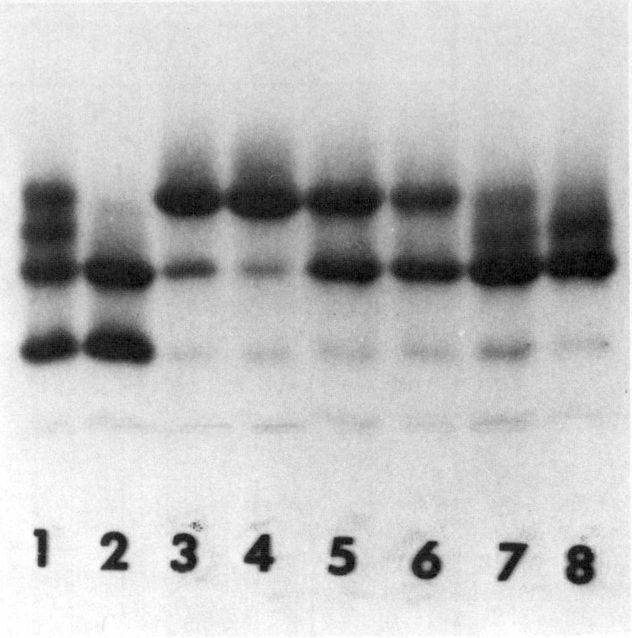

Figure 36.11. Hemoglobin electrophoresis on cellulose acetate, tris-EDTA-borate buffer, pH 8.6. Lane 1: Control mixture of Hb C, Hb S, Hb F, and Hb A. Lane 2: Hb SC disease (equal quantities of Hb S and Hb C). Lane 3: Hb S-α-thalassemia 2 (approximately 25% Hb S). Lane 4: Hb Lepore trait (approximately 10% Hb Lepore). Lane 5: Hb AS, sickle cell trait (approximately 40% Hb S). Lane 6: Hb S-β^+-thalassemia (approximately 60% Hb S). Lane 7: Hb S-β^+-thalassemia (approximately 80% Hb S, 10% Hb F, and 10% Hb A with increased Hb A_2 in the Hb C position). Lane 8: Hb SS, sickle cell anemia (approximately 90% Hb S, 10% Hb F, and 0% Hb A), a pattern also seen in Hb S-β^0-thalassemia. (Reprinted with permission from Hoffman GC. The sickling disorders. Lab Med 1990;21:797–807.)

β-thalassemia with a normal level of Hb A_2 (51). Reduction or absence of Hb A_2 is also seen in δβ-thalassemia, some forms of HPFH, and in association with Hb Lepore.

γ-Thalassemia

Since a normal individual inherits two pairs of γ-globin genes, one pair coding for $^G\gamma$-globin chain and the other for $^A\gamma$-globin chains, which differ in possessing glycine or alanine as the 136th amino acid residue, several different forms and combinations of γ-thalassemia might be expected. $^G\gamma$-Thalassemia appears to be the most common, but even in the homozygote results only in slight reduction in the total quantity of Hb F in the fetus and newborn and in no clinical or hematologic abnormality in the adult (53). Homozygous loss of the activity of both $^G\gamma$- and $^A\gamma$-globin genes has not been reported and probably would be incompatible with life.

α-Thalassemia

α-Thalassemia results from a deficiency of α-globin chains and, except in very rare circumstances, is an inherited disorder. There are three main underlying genetic lesions (54). The majority of α-thalassemia syndromes are caused by a deletion of all or part of one or both α-globin genes on chromosome 16; at least 12 deletions of differing length and location have been described. Nondeletional forms of α-thalassemia include those with single base substitutions or very small deletions in or near the α-genes and number at least 14. Unstable α-globin chains may also result in an imbalance between α and β-chains and cause a syndrome with some of the characteristics of an α-thalassemia. Since the normal complement of α-globin genes is four, there are five possible combinations of deletion (Table 36.4). Deletion of both genes from the same chromosome is called α-thalassemia 1, whereas deletion of only one gene is known as α-thalassemia 2; this apparently illogical nomenclature arose because the double deletion was described first. Single-gene deletion α-thalassemia is found worldwide and has an incidence of approximately 30% among African Americans (55) and up to 80% in some areas of Papua-New Guinea (37). α-Thalassemia 1 is particularly prevalent in southeast Asia and in the Mediterranean basin but is very rare among African Americans.

The severity of the clinical and hematologic effects is directly related to the number of genes deleted or affected (Table 36.4). As a consequence of the deficiency of α-globin chains, there is a relative excess of α-globin chains in the fetus and infant, and of β-chains in the adult; these excess chains can them-

Table 36.4. The α-Thalassemias Resulting from Gene Deletion: Nomenclature, Clinical Effect, and Percentages of Hb Barts (γ_4) and Hb H (β_4).

α-Genes	Subtype	Disorder	Hb Barts (Neonate)	Hb H (Adult)
			%	%
□-□[b] □-□	Normal	Normal	<1	0
■-□ □-□	α-Thal 2 heterozygote	"Silent" α-thalassemia	1–3	0
■-□ ■-□	α-Thal 2 homozygote	Thalassemia minor	4–10	0
■-■ □-□	α-Thal 1 heterozygote	Thalassemia minor	4–10	Trace
■-■ ■-□	α-Thal 1/α-Thal 2 compound heterozygote	Hb H disease	10–25	10–25
■-■ ■-■	α-Thal 1 homozygote	Hb Barts hydrops fetalis	75	—

[a]The 25% of hemoglobin unaccounted for in the α-thalassemia 1 homozygote consists mainly of the embryonic Hb Portland.
[b]Key: ■ Deleted α-globin gene
□ Normal α-globin gene

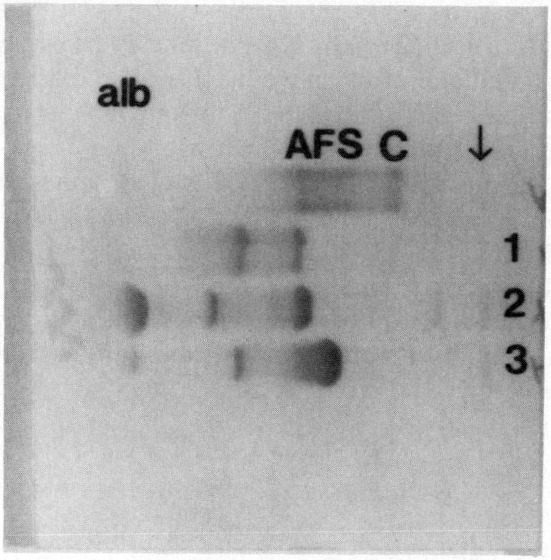

Figure 36.12. Hemoglobin electrophoresis on cellulose acetate at alkaline pH. Lane 1: Hb J trait in an adult, showing Hb A and fast-migrating Hb J. Lane 2: Hb H disease in an adult showing Hb A and fast-migrating Hb H; an albumin band is also present as an indicator that no fast-moving hemoglobin has migrated off the plate. Lane 3: Hb H disease in a neonate showing Hb F, a faint Hb A band, a fast-migrating Hb Barts band, and an albumin band. Note that the distance between Hb H (β_4) and Hb Barts (γ_4) is the same as that between Hb A ($\alpha_2\beta_2$) and Hb F ($\alpha_2\gamma_2$).

selves form tetramers: γ_4 (Hb Barts) and β_4 (Hb H). These two hemoglobins are of little physiological value because of their exceedingly high oxygen affinity. They are both unstable, a characteristic that underlies the hemolytic component of Hb H disease. On hemoglobin electrophoresis they are fast migraters (Fig. 36.12) and can be quantitated by separation on cation-exchange columns (48). Various reticulocyte stains such as brilliant cresyl MA blue and new methylene blue cause Hb H to precipitate within the red cells, giving them a typical golf ball appearance (40).

Heterozygous α-Thalassemia

This form of α-thalassemia is very common, but since it is associated with minimal imbalance between α- and γ- or β-chain production there is no clinical effect and the blood count, including the mean cell volume (MCV), is normal (56). In the adult the diagnosis may be inferred from family studies or proven by gene studies; in the neonate there is a slight increase (1 to 3%) in Hb Barts (56).

Heterozygous α-Thalassemia 1; Homozygous α-Thalassemia 2

These genetic disorders result in α-thalassemia minor (56) with the blood count typical of all forms of thalassemia minor (low MCV, minimal if any anemia). Because α-globin chains are present in all three normal hemoglobins, they are equally affected by a slight deficiency and there is no change in the relative percentages of Hb A, Hb A_2, and Hb F. It might be expected that the imbalance between α- and β-globin chain production would result in the presence of a small amount of Hb H (β_4) in the adult. This is not the case in the α-thalassemia 2 homozygote. However, in the α-thalassemia 1 heterozygote Hb H can be precipitated in a rare red cell but it is not present in sufficient quantity to be detected by routine electrophoretic methods. Because α-thalassemia 1 is exceedingly rare in African Americans but is quite common in southeast Asians the cost-effectiveness of performing Hb H stains in individuals with thalassemia minor and normal levels of Hb A_2 and Hb F will depend on the ethnic origin of the population under study.

In the neonate with either form of α-thalassemia minor an increase in Hb Barts (γ_4) in the range of 4 to 10% is usually found (56). This is a useful side benefit of neonatal screening programs for hemoglobinopathies because it provides positive evidence for a diagnosis using simple techniques, and can be helpful information when an African American child presents later in life with a microcytic hypochromic blood picture associated with normal levels of Hb A_2 and Hb F.

Hb H Disease

Hb H disease (clinically classified as a form of thalassemia intermedia) is a moderate to severe hemolytic disease (54). The Hb H tetramer (β_4) is unstable and forms Heinz bodies (denatured hemoglobin) within the red cell. These inclusions are recognized by the reticuloendothelial system, and a portion of the red cell or the complete red cell may be removed from the circulation. The morphology of the red cells is often bizarre.

The clinical severity of Hb H disease is related to the amount of Hb H in the red cells, which in turn depends on the underlying genetic lesion. The most common type is the double heterozygote for α-thalassemia 1 and α-thalassemia 2 in which three α-globin genes are deleted (since α-thalassemia 1 is rare among African Americans so also is Hb H disease). In southeast Asians, another frequent cause of Hb H disease is the combination of two deleted α-globin genes, a gene for the elongated α-globin chain of Hb Constant Spring and one normal α-globin gene ($--/\alpha^{cs}\alpha$) (57). The mutant α-globin chain of Hb Constant Spring is produced in small quantities (1 to 2%), and the α-globin chain deficiency therefore is nearly equivalent to that resulting from a deleted α-gene.

Hb Constant Spring consists of two normal β-globin chains and two abnormal α-globin chains containing 172 amino acids instead of the normal 141 (58). There is a substitution of the normal termination codon (UAA) at 142 by a codon for glutamine (CAA) in the abnormal α-globin mRNA. Downstream there is a series of 31 amino acid codons before another termination codon is reached (Fig. 36.13). Three other substitutions in the α-globin termination codon all result in elongated α-globin chains that differ from that of Hb Constant Spring only in the amino acid codon substituted for the terminator in the mRNA (AAA, lysine in Hb Icaria [59]; GAA, glutamic acid in Hb Seal Rock [60]; UCA, serine in Hb Koya Dora [61]). The heterozygotes for each of these four variants are clinically and hematologically normal, similar to heterozygotes for α-thalassemia 2. The homozygote for Hb Constant Spring has a mild normocytic hemolytic anemia with splenomegaly (62), not the typical thalassemia minor picture that might be expected. Hb Constant Spring migrates between carbonic anhydrase and Hb C on cellulose acetate at alkaline pH. The quantity is small and may be overlooked unless specifically sought (Fig. 36.14); application of twice the usual amount of hemolysate may be required. Since nondeletional forms of α-thalassemia exist, various combinations of deletional and nondeletional α-thalassemia genes and Hb Constant Spring may give rise to Hb H disease.

Homozygous α-Thalassemia 1 (Hb Barts Hydrops Fetalis)

Deletion of all four α-globin genes results in absence of α-globin chain production and is incompatible with life. Affected fetuses are hydropic, die in utero or soon after premature birth, and possess Hb Barts (γ_4) 10 to 30% Hb Portland ($\zeta_2\gamma_2$), and a small amount of Hb H (63). Hb Portland is probably the main deliverer of oxygen since it has an oxygen dissociation curve not far from the physiological one, compared to Hb Barts, which has a very high oxygen affinity (54). Hb Portland is electrophoretically similar to Hb A. The blood smear shows large hypochromic red cells with many reticulocytes, nucleated red cells, target cells, and red cell fragments. Hb Barts hydrops fetalis is rarely seen in populations outside southeast Asia and southern China, where it is the most common cause of hydrops fetalis.

β-Thalassemia Syndromes

Any imbalance in globin-chain production involving a reduction or absence of β-globin chains results in β-thalassemia. The simple concept of heterozygotes (β-thalassemia minor) and homozygotes (β-thalassemia major), although broadly applicable to these syndromes, is complicated by more than 70 different possible genetic lesions (64). In contrast with α-thalassemia, the mutations resulting in β-thalassemia are almost exclusively point mutations (65). These mutations occur in or near the β-gene and may interfere with the initiation, transcription, termination, or splicing of mRNA; mutations within the gene may produce nonsense codes that stop transcription or splicing of mRNA, or produce sense codes that result in a β-globin chain so unstable that it is found only in red cell precursors (e.g., $\beta^{\text{Indianapolis}}$) (66). The large number and variety of genetic causes are reflected in a spectrum of clinical syndromes in heterozygotes, homozygotes, and compound heterozygotes that range from "silent" β-thalassemia through thalassemia minor and intermedia to thalassemia major. For most practical purposes, it is possible to di-

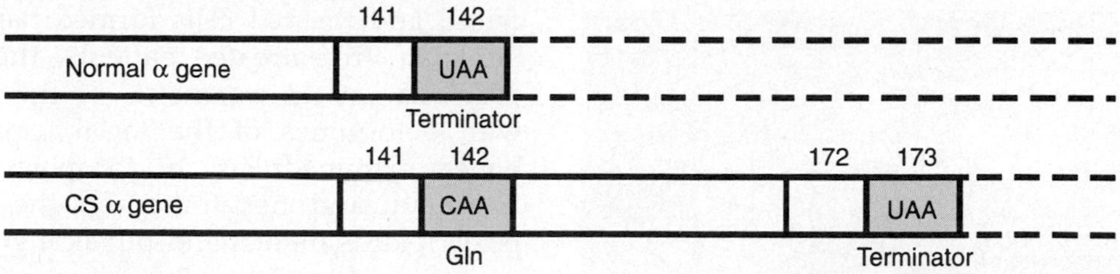

Figure 36.13. Diagram of the substitution in mRNA of the abnormal α-globin chain of Hb Constant Spring (CS). The normal terminator message at 142 position has mutated to the message for glutamine; another terminator is not reached until the 173rd message, resulting in the production of an mRNA that translates into a globin chain consisting of 172 amino acid residues.

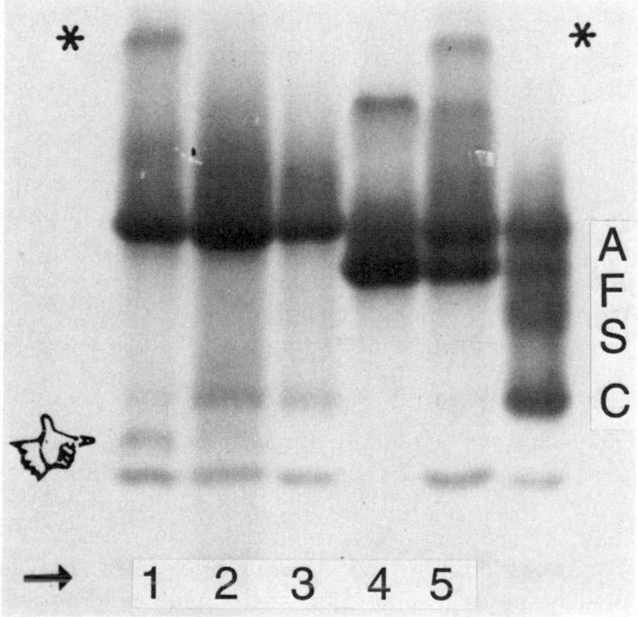

Figure 36.14. Hemoglobin electrophoresis on cellulose acetate at pH 8.6. Double quantities of hemolysate applied in each lane to emphasize minor fractions (bands identified from top to bottom). Lane 1: Hb H/Constant Spring—in adult (– –/$\alpha^{CS}\alpha$); Hb H (asterisk), Hb A, Hb A_2, Hb Constant Spring (indicator), carbonic anhydrase. Lane 2: mother of Lane 1, Hb Constant Spring trait ($\alpha\alpha$ / α^{CS}); Hb A, Hb A_2, Hb Constant Spring, carbonic anhydrase. Lane 3: father of Lane 1, α-thalassemia 1 heterozygote (– – / αα); Hb A, Hb A_2, carbonic anhydrase. Lane 4: neonate, α-thalassemia 2 homozygote (α–/α–), Hb Barts (8%), Hb A, Hb F. Lane 5: 5-month-old child, Hb H disease (– – / α–); Hb H (asterisk), Hb Barts, Hb A, Hb F. Control containing Hb A, Hb F, Hb S, Hb C, and carbonic anhydrase. (Reprinted with permission from Fishleder AJ, Hoffman GC. A practical approach to the detection of hemoglobinopathies: Part I. The introduction and thalassemia syndromes. Lab Med 1987;18:368–372.)

vide the genetic lesions into those resulting in the absence of β-globin chain production (β^0) and those resulting in reduction of β-chain production (β^+). The latter can be further divided into a "mild" β^+-gene, seen mainly in African Americans, and a "severe" β^+-gene. Many of the β-thalassemia alleles are clustered in certain populations so that, for instance, six alleles account for 92% of genes for β-thalassemia found in the Mediterranean area (65). This makes specific prenatal screening with gene probes less complicated than might be expected from the large total number of known alleles. These genetic lesions, affecting only the production of β-globin chains, underlie the "pure" β-thalassemias.

Another group of lesions, mostly relatively large deletions, in addition to the β-gene, involve other regions of the β-like gene cluster, including the γ and δ-genes. These result in the δβ- and γδβ-thalassemias and hereditary persistence of fetal hemoglobin (HPFH).

β-Thalassemia Minor

β-Thalassemia minor is seldom symptomatic and requires no therapy (65). The uniformly microcytic red cells, typical of all types of thalassemia minor, are usually the first indication of its presence. Anemia, if present, is mild, and slight erythrocytosis is common. It is not possible to distinguish between β^0-thalassemia minor and β^+-thalassemia minor (or other forms of thalassemia minor) on a hematologic basis. However, as a group, individuals, usually black, with β^+ (mild) thalassemia minor have less anemia and a higher MCV than those with β^0 or β^+ (severe) thalassemia minor (67). The three types are most easily distinguished when a sickle gene also segregates within the family; the S/β^0-thalassemia compound heterozygote will have no Hb A, the S/β^+-thalassemia compound heterozygote will have Hb A levels falling between 5 and 30% (Fig. 36.11).

An approximate doubling of the level of Hb A_2 ($\alpha_2\delta_2$) is the hallmark of β^0 and β^+-thalassemia minor (Fig. 36.15). Hb F may be normal, and when increased is seldom greater than 5%.

Normal levels of Hb A_2 and Hb F are found occasionally in phenotypic examples of β-thalassemia minor. Several families have been reported in which one parent of an offspring with typical β-thalassemia major had phenotypic β-thalassemia minor with a normal Hb A_2 level. The presence of a separate gene for β-thalassemia, either in *cis* or in *trans*, is an explanation in at least some of these families (51). Hb A_2 may be reduced in iron deficiency states (68); hence,

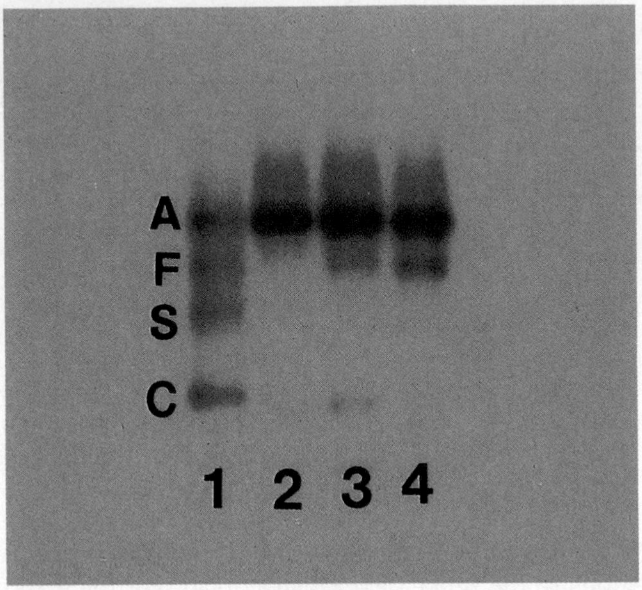

Figure 36.15. Hemoglobin electrophoresis on cellulose acetate at alkaline pH. Lane 1: α-Thalassemia (normal adult distribution of Hb A, Hb F, and Hb A_2). Lane 2: β-Thalassemia minor (visibly increased levels of Hb A_2 and Hb F). Lane 3: δβ-Thalassemia minor (approximately 10% Hb F).

Hb A_2 may fall within the reference range when iron deficiency and β-thalassemia minor coexist.

β-Thalassemia Major

Almost all β^0-thalassemia homozygotes, many β^+-homozygotes, and compound heterozygotes present as thalassemia major. The deficiency of β-globin chains is masked at birth by the production of γ-globin chains (Hb F), but as the switch from γ-globin chain production to β-globin chain production proceeds, the severity of the clinical and hematologic expression increases. Diagnosis of the majority of cases that have not been anticipated by prenatal study of the parents or antenatal study of the fetus (65) is usually made during the second month of life. Where appropriate medical facilities are available, transfusion therapy aimed at maintaining a hemoglobin level above 100 or 120 g/liter should be instituted at the time of diagnosis, to be followed by chelation therapy to reduce iron overload (69).

If no therapy or inadequate therapy is given, a series of clinical and hematologic events ensue mainly as a result of hypoxia due to the severe anemia (69). Anemia develops for two main reasons—dyserythropoiesis and hemolysis. The excess α-globin chains in the erythron do not form a soluble tetramer, α_4, comparable to the Hb Barts (γ_4) and Hb H (β_4) found in the α-thalassemias. However, the excess α-globin chains damage the red cell precursors and mature red cells so that, despite the vast erythroid hyperplasia, red cell production is reduced and the red cells formed have a shortened life span. In untreated patients, the erythroid hyperplasia causes expansion of the marrow cavity with deformities of the facial, cranial, and long bones; extramedullary erythropoiesis causes splenomegaly and hepatomegaly; the persistent hypoxia retards mental and physical growth. In many countries, this picture has been relegated to textbooks by optimal transfusion therapy.

In an untreated patient, the small amount of hemoglobin produced consists almost entirely of Hb F (90%) with little (β^+-thalassemia major) or no Hb A (β^0-thalassemia major). The distribution of Hb F among the red cells is not uniform, and those with the most Hb F have the longest life span, thus accentuating the percentage of Hb F in the circulation.

The bone marrow in untreated β-thalassemia major shows vast erythroid hyperplasia, megaloblastic, dysplastic, and bizarre precursors with many degenerate forms that reflect the intramedullary destruction of the α-globin chain-laden precursors. Although the formation of a relatively soluble tetramer α_4 comparable to Hb Barts (γ_4) and Hb H (β_4) found in α-thalassemia does not occur, aggregates of β-globin chains can be demonstrated in red cell precursors and in mature red cells (particularly after splenectomy) by supravital staining (70). The morphology may suggest erythroleukemia (FAB M6) even to the extent of exhibiting PAS-positive inclusions. Iron is present in large amounts, and ringed sideroblasts may be present in moderate numbers. Anemia is severe, MCV and MCH are low, but the MCHC may be only slightly reduced despite the apparent pallor of the red cells in a peripheral blood smear. There is marked variation in red cell size and shape. Reticulocytosis and polychromasia are present, but, because of the ineffective erythropoiesis, not in the quantity expected for the degree of anemia; erythroid precursors at various stages of maturation are also found in the peripheral blood.

There is biochemical evidence of hemolysis, including increased unconjugated bilirubin levels. Serum iron and transferrin are increased even in the untransfused individual. The urine may appear brown due to the presence of dipyrroles.

The pattern of hemoglobin electrophoresis depends on the type of β-thalassemia major. Hb A will be absent in untransfused homozygous β^0-thalassemia; a variable amount will be seen in homozygous β^+-thalassemia. Homozygous β^+-thalassemia with relatively large amounts of Hb A, clinically classified as thalassemia intermedia, is a particularly common type among Africans and African Americans. In β^0-thalassemia major Hb F represents approximately 90% of the hemoglobin present; however, this is 90%

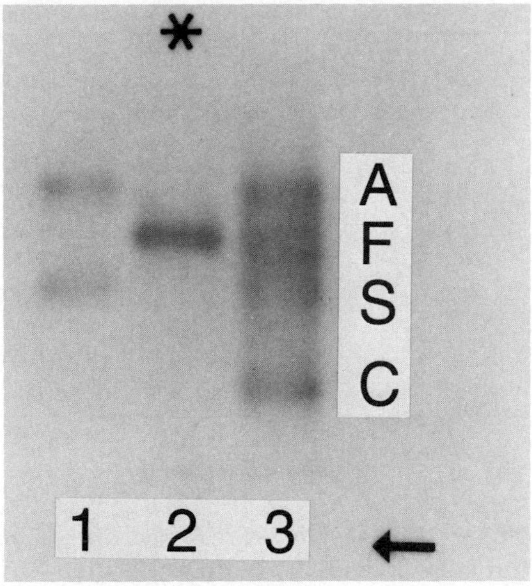

Figure 36.16. Hemoglobin electrophoresis on cellulose acetate at alkaline pH of homozygous δβ-thalassemia showing 100% Hb F(Lane 2). A similar pattern would be seen in homozygous HPFH of the common Black type. *Arrow* indicates point of application. Lane 3: Control mixture. Lane 1: Sickle cell trait, Hb AS.

of very little. Hb A_2 may be low, normal, or, less often, increased in percentage, but is always proportionally high in comparison to Hb A. Unexpectedly low levels of Hb A_2 may be accounted for by the selective survival of red cells with the greatest amount of Hb F, which also contain the lowest amounts of Hb A_2 (71).

δβ-Thalassemia

The absent or reduced production of δ- and β-globin chains that occurs in the δβ-type of thalassemia is usually the result of deletion of all or part of both the δ- and β-globin genes (72). Since two chains are underproduced, it might be assumed that the resulting thalassemias would be more severe than their β-thalassemia counterparts. This is not the case, because the deletion is associated with a significant persistent production of the γ-chains of Hb F, thus diminishing the α:non-α chain imbalance. The δβ-thalassemias form part of the spectrum that lies between β-thalassemia and HPFH.

Heterozygous δβ-thalassemia is often hematologically indistinguishable from other types of thalassemia minor, although the red cell indices may be closer to normal. In a few instances, the indices may be normal. These types can be classified as a "silent" form of thalassemia. δβ-Thalassemia minor is readily distinguished from other forms of thalassemia minor by the presence of 5 to 20% Hb F (Fig. 36.15), which is heterogeneously distributed among the red cells, and a normal or reduced level of Hb A_2.

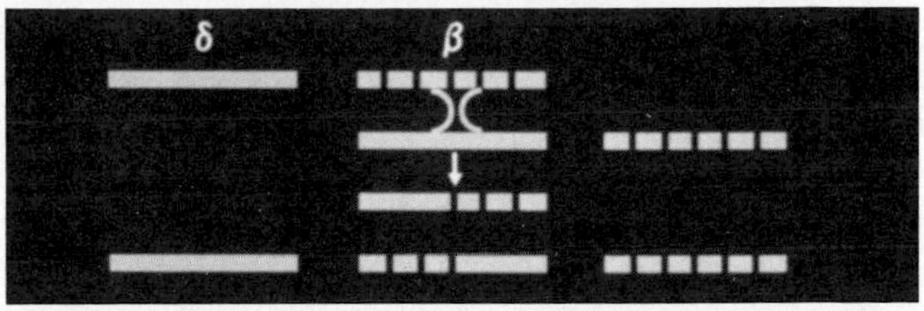

Figure 36.17. Diagram of the unequal crossover in chromosome 11 between the δ- and β-genes, resulting in the production of the δβ-fusion gene of the non-α-globin chain of Hb Lepore with no normal δ- and β-globin genes in *cis* and the βδ-fusion gene of Hb anti-Lepore with normal δ- and β-globin genes in *cis*.

Homozygous δβ-thalassemia is a mild disorder, clinically classifiable as a thalassemia intermedia or even minor (73). Anemia is mild (80 to 120 g/liter) with microcytic hypochromic red cells and evidence of reticulocytosis. Hemoglobin electrophoresis shows 100% Hb F with no Hb A or Hb A_2 (Fig. 36.16).

Hemoglobin Lepore

Hb Lepore in the heterozygote is associated with a typical thalassemia minor blood count and in the homozygote with thalassemia intermedia or even major (74). This unusual hemoglobin is composed of a pair of normal α-globin chains and a pair of non-α-globin chains that consist of the beginning (N-terminal end) of a δ-globin chain and the end (C-terminal) of a β-globin chain. This globin chain is the product of a fusion gene that has arisen from unequal chromosomal crossover (Fig. 36.17). The exact point of crossover and therefore the proportion of δ- and β-gene present in the Lepore gene varies. Three different hemoglobins have been reported: Hb $Lepore_{Hollandia}$, Hb $Lepore_{Baltimore}$, and Hb $Lepore_{Boston}$, the last being the most common (74). As a result of the crossover, the δ- and β-genes are represented only by the fusion gene that in the adult heterozygote would be expected to produce approximately 50% of the non-α-globin chains; however, Hb Lepore makes up only about 10% of the circulating hemoglobin (Fig. 36.11). This deficient production results in an imbalance between α- and non-α-globin chain production, causing thalassemia minor in the heterozygote with its typical hematologic picture. Homozygous Hb Lepore (75) presents as thalassemia major or thalassemia intermedia. The circulating hemoglobin consists of approximately 75% Hb F and 25% Hb Lepore with no Hb A or Hb A_2.

Hb Lepore migrates with Hb S on cellulose acetate in alkaline buffer (Fig. 36.11) and with Hb A in acid citrate agar. The finding of approximately 10% of a hemoglobin migrating like Hb S on cellulose acetate in an untransfused patient is virtually diagnostic of Hb Lepore.

Table 36.5. Blood Counts of 10 Patients with β-Thalassemia Minor[a]

Patient	Hb	RBC	MCV	RDW	HbA_2
Reference Range	(g/liter) 120–160	(10^{12}/liter) 4.5–5.5	(fl) 80–100	<15	% 1.5–3.5
1	124	5.7	64	13.3	6.2
2	132	7.2	65	12.5	5.2
3	127	6.2	65	12.7	6.5
4	125	6.0	64	14.4	6.3
5	140	7.2	58	14.2	6.8
6	113	6.1	58	13.6	7.3
7	120	6.0	63	14.7	6.2
8	140	6.0	61	12.8	6.5
9	126	6.0	69	15.2	6.3
10	125	5.5	71	14.4	6.6

[a]The counts, with minimal or no anemia, increased red cell count, low mean cell volume (MCV), and normal red cell distribution width (RDW) might be found in any type of thalassemia minor. The approximate doubling of the Hb A_2 percentage confirms the specific diagnosis of β-thalassemia minor.

The converse of Hb Lepore is Hb anti-Lepore (Fig. 36.17) (74). In this situation δ- and β-genes in *cis* are intact with the addition of an anti-Lepore gene that is responsible for the production of a small amount of a non-α-chain made up of the beginning of a β- and the end of a δ-globin chain. The amount of Hb anti-Lepore produced is small, and the imbalance of globin chain production is minimal. The blood count and all red cell indices are normal. Three different anti-Lepore hemoglobins have been reported; as in the case of Hb Lepore, they differ in the point at which chromosomal crossover has occurred.

Differential Diagnosis of Thalassemia Minor

Thalassemia minor is a benign syndrome with few if any symptoms but with an abnormal hematologic picture that is often described as a microcytic hypochromic anemia (Table 36.5). The anemia is slight or nonexistent in Africans but usually present in Asians, and the hypochromasia, as measured by the MCHC, is seldom more than slight. The striking features of the blood count are the low MCV, the high red cell count, and the lack of anisocytosis as measured by the red cell distribution widths (RDW). Iron-deficiency anemia and iron-deficient erythrocytosis are the main differential diagnoses. Morphologically, the red cells of thalassemia minor differ little from those of mild iron deficiency; the presence of target cells is not a useful discriminator; however, basophilic stippling occurs in thalassemia minor but is seldom seen in iron deficiency. Various regression formulas have been proposed to distinguish the blood counts of iron deficiency and thalassemia minor, indicating whether the patient's iron status or hemoglobin should be studied first. England and Fraser (76) suggested that thalassemia is the probable diagnosis if the result of the formula MCV − RBC − (5 × Hb) − 3.4 is negative. Green and King (77) suggested the formula (MCV^2 × RDW) ÷ (Hb × 100), with a result less than 73 indicating thalassemia minor.

Whatever pragmatic approach is adopted, three factors need to be kept in mind. First, since iron deficiency and thalassemia minor are common disorders, coincidence of the two is not uncommon. Second, the Hb A_2 level is reduced in iron deficiency, and ocassionally the Hb A_2 level in an individual with β-thalassemia minor and iron deficiency may fall within the normal range (68). Third, since thalassemia minor may be caused by a structurally abnormal hemoglobin (e.g., Hb Lepore) or may coexist with an abnormal hemoglobin (e.g., Hb S α-thalassemia), the complete study of a patient with the blood picture of thalassemia minor should include hemoglobin electrophoresis. In addition to indicating the presence of a hemoglobin variant, hemoglobin electrophoresis may provide other useful diagnostic information. It can be argued that with increased Hb A_2, indicated by the presence of an Hb A_2 band significantly denser than the carbonic anhydrase band, with or without an increased Hb F band in a patient with a thalassemic blood picture, is strong enough evidence for the diagnosis of β-thalassemia minor (Fig. 36.15) without specific quantification of Hb A_2. Similarly, the combination of an electrophoretic band suggesting 5 to 10% Hb F and a thalassemic blood count strongly suggests δβ-thalassemia minor (Fig. 36.15). α-Thalassemia minor is often a diagnosis of exclusion; a thalassemic blood count with normal levels of Hb A_2 and Hb F and normal iron studies is consistent with such a diagnosis. Specific evidence for the presence of one or more defective (thalassemic) α-globin genes may come from the presence of increased quantities of Hb Barts at birth (Table 36.4), the presence of rare Hb H inclusions in the αα/ − − type (heterozygous α-thalassemia 1) but not in the $\alpha-/\alpha-$ (homozygous α-thalassemia 2), and by the use of α-gene probes.

STRUCTURAL HEMOGLOBIN VARIANTS

Over 400 structural hemoglobin variants have been reported, of which the majority are rare and of no clinical or hematologic significance. An updated compendium of all reported examples is published regularly (78). A few generalizations can be made. Except in the case of two of the most common variants, Hb S and Hb C, structural alterations affecting the surface of the hemoglobin molecule seldom have any deleterious effect. On the other hand, almost all variants in which the structural defect lies near the heme pocket, lies at points of contact between globin chains, or affects their helical structure are associated with alterations in the stability or function of the molecule.

The various types of genetic lesions that underlie the structurally abnormal hemoglobins include:

- Single base substitutions within a DNA triplet codon that result in an amino acid substitution (e.g., Hb S, $\alpha_2\beta_2{}^{6\ Glu\rightarrow Val}$, A→T in GAG to GTG);
- Two separate base substitutions probably arising from chromosoml crossover involving two abnormal genes (e.g., Hb C_{Harlem}, $\alpha_2\beta_2{}^{6\ Glu\rightarrow Val,\ 73\ Asp\rightarrow Asn}$, a combination of the substitutions found singly in Hb S and Hb Korle Bu) (79);
- Deletion of one or more amino acid residues (e.g., Hb Leiden, $\alpha_2\beta_2{}^{6\ or\ 7\ Glu\rightarrow 0}$) (80);
- Shortening of globin chain by premature termination (e.g., Hb McKees Rocks) (81);
- Elongation of globin chain by insertion (e.g., Hb Grady, $\alpha_2{}^{116\text{–}118\ duplicated}\beta_2$ (82);
- Elongation by mutation in chain terminator (e.g., Hb Constant Spring $\alpha_2{}^{171}\beta_2$ (58);
- Elongation by frame-shift mutation (e.g., Hb Wayne) (83); and
- Fusion of globin chains (e.g., Hb Lepore $\alpha_2\delta\beta_2$ (74).

The Sickling Disorders

Hb S ($\alpha_2\beta_2{}^{6\ Glu\rightarrow Val}$) is present as sickle cell trait (Hb AS) in approximately 8% of African Americans, and as sickle cell anemia (Hb SS) in approximately 0.25% or one in 400. The normal DNA code for glutamic acid, GAG, is replaced by the code, GTG, for valine as the sixth amino acid code in the β-gene. This genetic abnormality is identical in all affected populations, which include those on the Mediterranean littoral, Saudi Arabians, and a small group of Indians in addition to African, American, and West Indian blacks. However, there is good evidence from studies of DNA segments near the β-globin gene locus (using restriction length polymorphisms) that the mutation probably occurred in several different population groups and then reached polymorphic levels through its beneficial effect in areas of endemic malaria (34). There are slight differences between these groups in the severity of sickle cell anemia.

The pathophysiological basis of the various sickling disorders is the tendency for molecules of Hb S to precipitate within the red cell in the form of liquid crystals or tactoids under conditions of reduced oxygen tension (Fig. 36.18). The characteristic sickle cell is the result. This tendency to precipitate is dependent on the concentration of Hb S within the red cell, on the nature of any other hemoglobin present, as well as on the oxygen tension. Thus, at the normal Po_2 of postcapillary venules, sickle cells will form in a homozygote (Hb SS, sickle cell anemia) whose red cells contain about 90% Hb S, whereas they will not form in a heterozygote (Hb AS, sickle cell trait) whose red cells contain approximately 55% Hb A and only 45% Hb S. The severity of a sickling disorder is directly related to the tendency of red cells to sickle (Table 36.6).

In Hb SS, a continuous cycle (Fig. 36.19) of peripheral deoxygenation and sickling and central oxygenation and desickling occurs as red cells pass from periphery through the lungs. Two events may alter this cycle. Repeated deformation of the red cell membranes eventually leads to the formation of irreversibly sickled red cells. Sickled red cells, unsuited to passage through small blood vessels, may block some of those vessels, causing local stasis, further deoxygenation of the red cells, and further sickling; the temporary or permanent loss of blood flow to a distal tissue segment causes the pain typical of the vaso-occlusive sickle cell crisis.

Sickle Cell Trait

Sickle cell trait (Hb AS) is an essentially benign disorder because, under normal physiological conditions, sickle cells are not formed. There is, however, some evidence that in rare hypoxic situations sickle cells may form in vivo; sudden death among individuals involved in strenuous exercise at high altitudes is more common among African Americans than among Caucasians and may be associated with in vivo sickling (84). Localized hypoxia in renal papillae is the probable explanation for the instances of painless hematuria—usually from the left kidney—which may occur rarely in sickle cell trait, but more commonly in sickle cell anemia and Hb SC disease. Isosthenuria may also occur.

The blood count is normal; hemoglobin electrophoresis shows approximately 45% Hb S, 55% Hb A, with a normal amount of Hb A_2 (Fig. 36.11); and the solubility test gives a positive result.

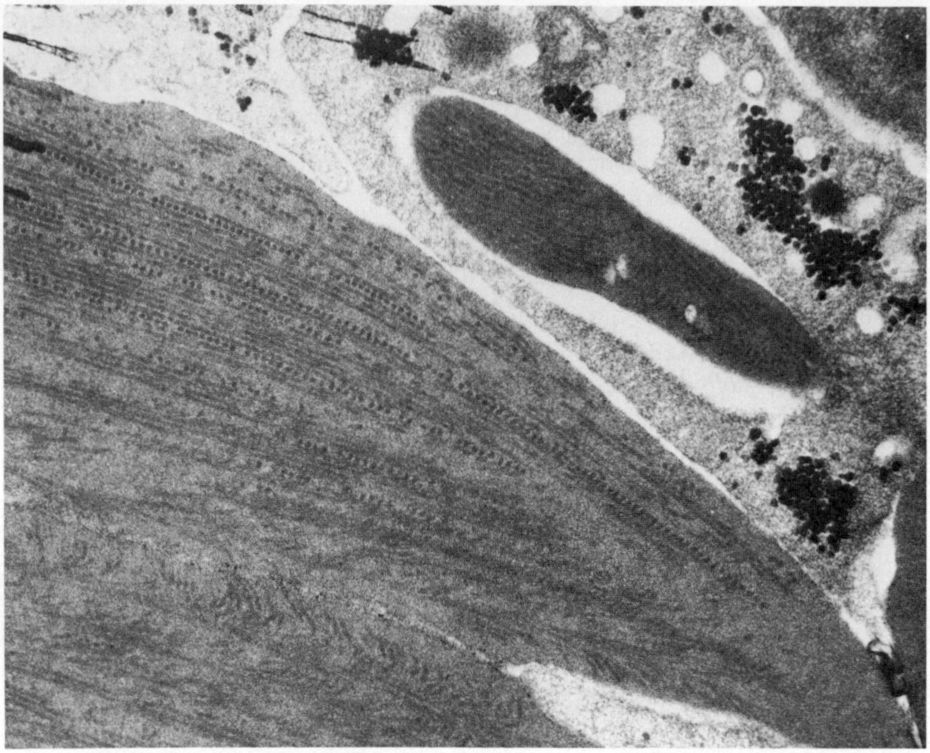

Figure 36.18. Electron micrograph of a portion of a sickled red cell in a renal biopsy. The tactoids of Hb S molecules are seen arranged in tubular fashion cut horizontally, vertically, and tangentially. (Reprinted with permission from Hoffman GC. The sickling disorders. Lab Med 1990;21:797–807.)

Table 36.6. Some Combinations of Hb S and α-Thalassemia, β-Thalassemia, or Globin Chain Structural Abnormalities

Hemoglobinopathy	Percentage in Adults[a]					Sickle Cells[b]	Clinical Severity[c]
	Hb A	Hb S	Hb X	Hb A_2	Hb F		
Sickle cell trait (Hb AS)	55–60	40–45	0	N	N	0	1
Sickle cell anemia (Hb SS)	0	90–95	0	N	5–10	+	3
Hb S α-thalassemia 1	75	25	0	N	N	0	1
Hb S β^0 thalassemia	0	90–95	0	↑	5–10	+	3
Hb S β^+ thalassemia	5–30	60–90	0	↑	5–10	+	2
Hb S HPFH	0	70–80	0	N	20–30	0	1
Hb SC	0	50	50	N	N	±	2
Hb $SD_{\text{Los Angeles}}$	0	50	50	N	N	±	2
Hb SN	0	50	50	N	N	0	1
Hb SO	0	50	50	N	N	+	3
Hb AS-$G_{\text{Philadelphia}}$	25	25	50[d]	N	N	0	1

[a]N indicates normal; Hb X, abnormal hemoglobin other than Hb S.
[b]Zero indicates sickle cells absent; plus sign, present; and plus-minus sign, possible.
[c]1, benign; 2, moderately severe; 3, similar to sickle cell anemia.
[d]Approximately 25% Hb G (migrating with Hb S) and 25% of the hybrid $\alpha_2^G \beta_2^S$ (migrating as Hb C).

Sickle Cell Anemia

The relative insolubility of deoxygenated Hb S, its tendency to gel, and the lack of deformability of sickled red cells underlie the hemolytic anemia and vaso-occlusive episodes that are the major clinical expressions of sickle cell anemia. The severity of the disease, as reflected by the degree of anemia and frequency of the painful crises, varies widely from individual to individual and between ethnic groups. The disease is usually mild among Saudi Arabians; there is little variation among the genetically distinct types of sickle cell anemia found in Africa (85). These variations depend in part on the level of Hb F, which tends to inhibit gelation, and on the number of α-genes; the coexistence of one or two α-gene deletions reduces the MCHC and the tendency for Hb S to gel. A third major factor in the morbidity and mortality of sickle cell anemia is infection, usually bacterial, that is at least in part a reflection of the functional

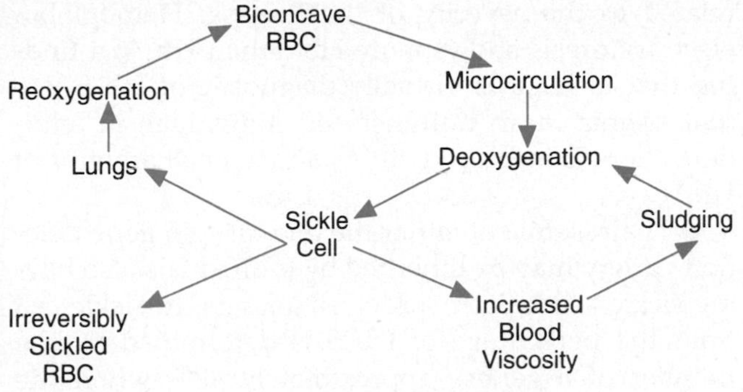

Figure 36.19. The sickling cycle that occurs in patients with sickle cell anemia. Vaso-occlusive (painful) crises may develop if "sludging" leads to blockage of blood vessels. (Reprinted with permission from Fishleder AJ, Hoffman GC. A practical approach to the detection of hemoglobinopathies: Part II. The sickle cell disorders. Lab Med 1987;18:441–443.)

asplenia of infancy and childhood and splenic infarction in the adult.

During fetal and early neonatal life, the presence of Hb F reduces the sickling tendency. Accordingly, signs or symptoms of the disease do not develop until the third or fourth month of life; in milder forms of the disease, they may not appear for several years. Rare asymptomatic cases occur.

Infancy and early childhood are particularly dangerous times for patients with sickle cell anemia, partly because of their inability to describe symptoms, but mainly because of potentially lethal complications that may occur in addition to vaso-occlusive episodes. Overwhelming infection, particularly pneumococcal, may prove lethal in a matter of hours, and acute splenic sequestration of red cells that may be equivalent to loss of one-third of the blood volume is a medical emergency. The importance of prenatal or neonatal diagnosis cannot be overstated; it allows the parent and pediatrician to take prompt action when indicated and to provide prophylaxis against infection. Vaso-occlusive episodes or painful crises may occur at any age. They occur sporadically and vary widely in frequency from patient to patient (86). A precipitating event is often not obvious; however, infection, bacterial or viral, precedes approximately one-third of crises, probably as result of pyrexia (87). Any organ may be affected. The spleen, enlarged during the first years of life, is seldom palpable after the age of 7 years due to repeated infarctions.

The degree of anemia varies widely (average hematocrit 24.6 ± 3.8) (88); the hemoglobin level may fall precipitously during the temporary "aplastic" crises that are associated with parvovirus infection (89) as well as during sequestration crises; hyperhemolytic episodes are seldom if ever the cause. The chronic hemolytic process is often associated with gallstone formation. Several long-term approaches to therapy of sickle cell anemia, in addition to supportive measures during crises, have been suggested. The roles of red cell transfusion, exchange transfusion, and hypertransfusion protocols such as those used in the treatment of β-thalassemia major remain a matter of controversy, even when considered during times of particular risk such as major surgery and pregnancy (90, 91). Some drugs, such as 5-azacytidine (92) and hydroxyurea (93) increase the production of Hb F and thus reduce the tendency for the Hb S to form tactoids. Attempts to prevent or reverse the sickling process with agents that directly interfere with the linkage of Hb S molecules have obvious advantage; however, although many such agents have been tried, few have stood the test of time, and the side effects of many often outweigh their benefits (94). Replacing the red cell factory either in toto by bone marrow transplantation (95) or in part by specific gene replacement are possible future alternatives.

The main laboratory features of sickle cell anemia include variable but usually moderate to severe normocytic anemia, primarily hemolytic, in types associated with sickle cells and reticulocytosis; the presence of Howell-Jolly bodies and target cells, indicating hyposplenism or splenic infarction; 90 to 95% Hb S with 5 to 10% Hb F and no Hb A on hemoglobin electrophoresis (Fig. 36.11); and a positive solubility test.

Sickling Disorders Involving a Second Hemoglobinopathy

The more common combinations of Hb S with other hemoglobinopathies are listed in Table 36.6. Inheritance of a β^S-gene from one parent and a second β-gene variant from the other results in a compound heterozygote such as Hb SC disease or Hb S β^0-thalassemia. An α-gene variant can be inherited by an individual who has either sickle cell trait or sickle cell anemia—for instance, Hb AS/$G_{Philadelphia}$ or Hb SS/$G_{Philadelphia}$.

Hb SC disease is a mild to moderate sickling disorder characterized by a hemolytic anemia and, in some cases, vaso-occlusive episodes. Typical sickle cells are rare or absent, but well-hemoglobinized target cells and occasional distorted angular red cells with hemoglobin condensed at one end are commonly found in the blood film. Hemoglobin electrophoresis on cellulose acetate at alkaline pH shows approximately equal amounts of Hb S and Hb C (Hb A_2 is contained within the latter) (Fig. 36.11). Acid agar electrophoresis can distinguish Hb SC from Hb SO and Hb SE, which give identical patterns on cellulose acetate. Hb SO disease is clinically and

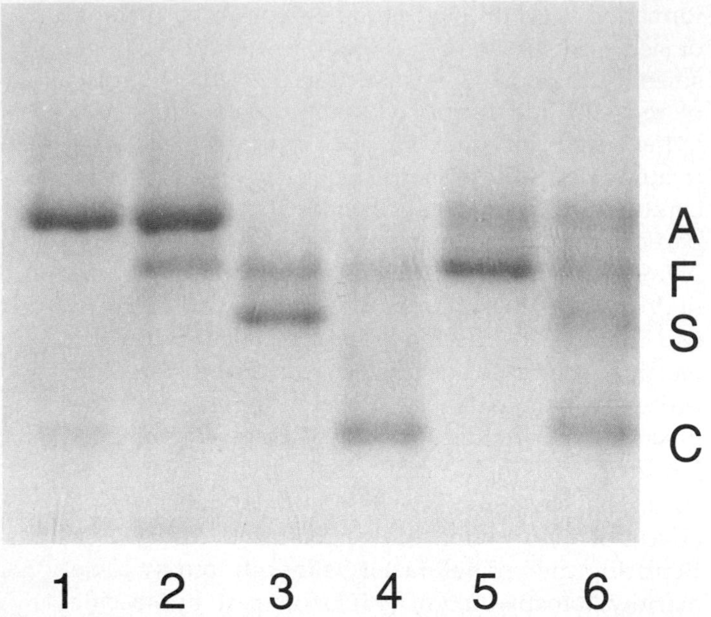

Figure 36.20. Hereditary persistence of fetal hemoglobin (HPFH). Hemoglobin electrophoresis on cellulose acetate at alkaline pH. Lane 1: Normal adult. Lane 2: HPFH trait (approximately 80% Hb A, 20% Hb F). Lane 3: Hb S HPFH (approximately 60% Hb S, 40% Hb F). Lane 4: Hb C HPFH (approximately 70% Hb C, 30% Hb F). Lane 5: Normal neonate (approximately 70% Hb F, 30% HB A). Lane 6: Control mixture.

hematologically similar to sickle cell anemia (96). Hb SE disease is similar to sickle cell trait (97).

Hb $SD_{Los\ Angeles}$ disease is a moderately severe sickling disorder, clinically similar to SC disease, with hemolytic anemia and occasional vaso-occlusive and sequestration episodes (98). On cellulose acetate, the electrophoretic pattern of Hb SD is identical to that of Hb SS. However, the two syndromes can be distinguished by citrate agar electrophoresis in which Hb D migrates with Hb A, not Hb S. Hb S HPFH is a benign disorder. Hemoglobin electrophoresis in this compound heterozygote (Fig. 36.20) usually shows approximately 60% Hb S and 40% Hb F with no Hb A (99).

Sickling Disorders Involving a Thalassemic Gene

Hb S β^0-thalassemia may be indistinguishable clinically from sickle cell anemia, although splenomegaly usually persists in the adult; hematologically, the low MCV and MCH of Hb S β^0-thalassemia help to distinguish the two (100). Hb S β^+-thalassemia is usually a less severe sickling disorder than either sickle cell anemia or Hb S β^0-thalassemia and may present as a thalassemia intermedia (101). The β^+-thalassemia gene is responsible for the production of some Hb A, ranging from 5 to 30% of the circulating hemoglobin (Fig. 36.12). The amount of Hb A is inversely related to the severity of the disease. Hemoglobin electrophoresis shows more Hb S than Hb A, a finding that in itself is virtually diagnostic of Hb S β^+-thalassemia in an untransfused individual; in addition, there is increased Hb A_2 and a small amount of Hb F.

α-Thalassemia of either the one- or two-gene deletion variety may be inherited by individuals also having sickle cell trait or sickle cell anemia. In sickle cell trait, the percentage of Hb S is determined by the number of α-genes—approximately 40% when the normal four α-genes are functioning, 35% when three α-genes are functioning (this combination of Hb AS with single-gene deletion α-thalassemia is found in approximately 30% of individuals with sickle cell trait), and 25% when only two α-genes are functioning (found in approximately 3% of individuals with sickle cell trait) (102). Iron deficiency also lowers the percentage of Hb S in sickle cell trait (68). Inheritance of α-thalassemia in individuals with Hb C trait (Hb AC) has a similar effect on the proportion of Hb C. This effect occurs because the β^S and β^C-globin chains have a positive charge relative to β^A and therefore are less likely to combine with the limited number of α-globin chains, which are also positively charged. The reverse occurs when an abnormal β-globin chain (e.g., many examples of Hb J has a relatively negative charge, and the percentage of the abnormal hemoglobin increases when combined with α-thalassemia (103).

Hb C Diseases

Hb C ($\alpha_2\beta_2{}^{6\ Glu \rightarrow Lys}$) occurs in 2.4% of African Americans; 0.02% are homozygotes (Hb CC) (104). The mutation for Hb C apparently occurred in the Ghana–Upper Volta region of western Africa, where as many as 25% of the population in some areas are heterozygotes. Hb C is found almost exclusively in blacks.

Hb C trait (Hb AC) is an entirely benign disorder. The blood count is normal, but the blood smear shows many normochromic target cells. Hemoglobin electrophoresis shows approximately 45% Hb C and 55% Hb A. Iron deficiency or the deletion of one or two α-globin genes results in a lower percentage of Hb C. Hb A_2 migrates with Hb C on cellulose acetate, and they are eluted together from ion-exchange columns; therefore, it is necessary to use chromatographic methods for the quantitation of Hb A_2 in the presence of Hb C.

Hb C disease (Hb CC) is associated with a mild to moderate chronic hemolytic anemia and splenomegaly (105). Apart from the aplastic crises and cholelithiasis, patients homozygous for Hb C have few complications and do not suffer from the vaso-occlusive crises, sequestration crises, or infections prevalent among patients with sickle cell anemia. The red cells show the unusual combination of reduced MCV but increased MCHC (106). The blood smear shows even more target cells than Hb C trait; it also contains occasional spherocytes, a reflection of the increased MCHC. Intracellular or extracellular Hb C crystals, block-like structures 1 to 3 μm in length, may be seen in the blood smear and are pathognomonic of Hb C. In Hb C disease, there is at least 90% Hb C on cellulose acetate electrophoresis at pH 8.4, with a slight increase in Hb F and no Hb A. In acid agar, pH 6.0, the normal or slightly increased amount of Hb A_2 may be visible, migrating as Hb A. This apparent combination of Hb C with a small amount of Hb A must not be confused with Hb C β^+-thalassemia; the absence of Hb A on cellulose acetate is helpful in this distinction. Hb E and Hb O migrate with Hb C on cellulose acetate but can be distinguished by acid agar eletrophoresis (Fig. 36.7).

Compound heterozygotes for Hb S and Hb C are discussed in the section on the sickling disorders. Hb C β^0-thalassemia and Hb C β^+-thalassemia are moderate and mild hemolytic anemias, respectively. The electrophoretic pattern of Hb C β^0-thalassemia is indistinguishable from that of Hb C disease (Hb CC), but the MCV is somewhat lower (50 to 70 fl) than in Hb CC (mean 72 fl) (107). In Hb C β^+-thalassemia, the quantity of Hb C exceeds that of Hb A, and in Hb C α-thalassemia, the reverse is found in a manner analogous to the proportions of Hb S and Hb A in the Hb S β^+- and Hb S α-thalassemia.

Hemoglobin E

Hb E ($\alpha_2\beta_2^{26\ Glu\rightarrow Lys}$) is the second most common hemoglobin variant after Hb S. It occurs mainly in southeast Asian populations and is particularly common in Thailand.

Hb E trait (Hb AE) is a benign disorder associated with microcytic red cells (average MCV 72 fl) but no anemia, not unlike thalassemia minor (108). The proportion of Hb E is 30 to 35% (a useful differential point from Hb C trait, in which the abnormal hemoglobin usually makes up 40 to 50%). This proportion may be even lower when there is concomitant iron deficiency or α-thalassemia.

Hb E disease (Hb EE) is also a benign disorder, but there may be a mild anemia, and the red cells are more microcytic than in Hb E trait, mimicking β-thalassemia minor (109). Red cells contain over 90% Hb E and a slightly increased quantity of Hb F, but no Hb A.

In contrast to the mild nature of Hb E disease, the combination of Hb E β^0-thalassemia may present as a thalassemia intermedia or even thalassemia major (110). The electrophoretic pattern may be similar to that of a homozygote for Hb E, but usually shows more Hb F and an increase in Hb A_2 (assayed by chromatography to separate it from Hb E).

Hb E migrates with Hb C, Hb O, and Hb A_2 on cellulose acetate at pH 8.4 but can be distinguished by electrophoresis in acid citrate agar, where it migrates with Hb A. Furthermore, Hb E is mildly unstable and may be precipitated by heat (50° to 60°C or 17% isopropanol; however, there is no evidence of hemolysis even in the homozygote. The thalassemic nature of this variant can be explained by the amino acid substitution at β^{26} which creates a new splicing sequence and interferes with mRNA processing; the α:β-synthesis ratio is increased to as much as 2:1 (111).

HEMOGLOBIN VARIANTS AFFECTING STABILITY OR FUNCTION

Amino acid substitutions, deletions, or additions that affect the heme pocket, the points of contact or interaction between globin chains, their secondary helical structure, or the hydrophobic interior of the subunit almost invariably alter the stability or function of the hemoglobin molecule. These variants may be divided into the unstable hemoglobins, hemoglobins with high or low oxygen affinity, and the hereditary methemoglobins (Hb Ms). This separation is not absolute; for instance, an unstable hemoglobin may also have an altered oxygen affinity and result in slight methemoglobinemia.

Unstable Hemoglobins

Hemolysis associated with the precipitation of denatured hemoglobin (Heinz bodies) within the red cell results from two main aberrations; oxidative hemolysis affecting either normal red cells or red cells deficient in one of the enzymes in the glycolytic pathway, and the presence of an unstable hemoglobin. Over 100 unstable hemoglobin variants have been identified (78). The majority are β-globin chain defects, which on the whole are more severe than α-globin chain defects because the latter affect only one of four α-genes as opposed to one of two β-genes. Table 36.7 contains examples chosen to demonstrate the differences in severity (which are unrelated to the quantity of unstable hemoglobin in the circulation), in the proportion of abnormal hemoglobin, and in associated functional defects.

The denatured hemoglobin in the form of single or multiple Heinz bodies becomes linked to the inner side of the red cell membrane, decreasing the pliability of the red cell and its ability to traverse the microcirculation, particularly in the spleen. The

Table 36.7. Unstable Hemoglobins—Approximately 100 Variants

Hemoglobin	Affected Globin Chain	Percent Abnormal Hb	O_2 Affinity	Clinical Severity
Koln	β	10	Increased	Mild
Gun Hill	β	30	Increased	Mild
Zurich	β	25	Increased	Mild
Hammersmith	β	30	Decreased	Severe
Cranston	β	30	Increased	Mild
Hasharon	α	15	Normal	Mild
Kansas	β	45	Decreased	Mild
Indianapolis	β	0	—	Moderate

[a]These hemoglobins are all heterozygotes and indicate the globin chain affected, the percentage of abnormal hemoglobin found in the circulation, their oxygen affinity, and clinical severity. In cases (e.g., Hb Indianapolis and Hb Hasharon) in which the percentage of abnormal hemoglobin is significantly less than 50% (β-globin abnormalities) or 25% (α-globin abnormalities), the imbalance also results in a thalassemia syndrome.

Heinz bodies may be removed from the red cell together with a portion of the red cell membrane, leaving a "bite" cell, or the whole red cell may be removed from the circulation. Not surprisingly, splenectomy results in an increased number of circulating red cells containing Heinz bodies, while at the same time lengthening the red cell life span.

In addition to the anemia, reticulocytosis, and bilirubinemia common to most hemolytic anemias, there are laboratory tests that may indicate the presence of an unstable hemoglobin. Two simple screening tests for an unstable hemoglobin involve applying a physical or ionic stress to the hemoglobin molecule. Heating a buffered lysate at 60°C for half an hour or 50°C for 1 hour will cause flocculation of any unstable hemoglobin present (112). The addition of 17% isopropanol to an equal volume of buffered lysate (the Carrell test) will also cause flocculation, within 10 minutes, of unstable hemoglobin (113). In either test, the flocculum may be small if the quantity of unstable hemoglobin is small. The flocculum is white if heme has been lost, but retains the red color of hemoglobin if heme remains attached to the precipitated hemoglobin. Hemoglobin electrophoresis may demonstrate an abnormal fraction, but a number of unstable hemoglobins migrate with Hb A.

It is always worthwhile to perform all available tests, and even repeat them on a fresh sample of blood, because the amount of unstable hemoglobin present may be small and its instability not marked.

Hemoglobins with Altered Oxygen Affinity

The presence of hemoglobins with increased or decreased oxygen affinity results in a resetting of the homeostatic mechanism that controls the amount of circulating hemoglobin. Thus, a hemoglobin with increased oxygen affinity will accept at least normal amounts of oxygen in the lungs but will unload less oxygen to the tissues. This relative hypoxia will turn on the production of erythropoietin and increase the number of circulating red cells (and hemoglobin) so that more oxygen can be delivered to the tissues. A physiological equilibrium will be reached at a hemoglobin level above or at the upper limit of a reference range based on individuals with functionally normal hemoglobin. The reverse occurs when a hemoglobin of low oxygen affinity is present, and the physiological level of hemoglobin may be below the reference range. In rare instances, the oxygen affinity of the hemoglobin (e.g., Hb Kansas ($\alpha_2\beta_2^{102\ Asn\rightarrow Thr}$) may be so low that the uptake of oxygen in the lungs is impaired. Despite the ease with which oxygen is delivered to the tissue, the level of hemoglobin lies within the normal reference range (114).

Over 40 hemoglobin variants with an oxygen affinity high enough to cause erythrocytosis have been identified (115). Affected individuals are asymptomatic except for those rare examples in which the red cell mass is large enough to cause hyperviscosity. Therapy is seldom indicated, and pregnancy involves no risk despite the high maternal oxygen affinity relative to that of the fetus.

The presence of a high-oxygen affinity hemoglobin may be first suspected from the blood count. Other laboratory findings include an abnormal electrophoretic pattern in about 70% of examples. Measurement of the P_{50} (the oxygen tension at which 50% of the hemoglobin is saturated) will confirm the diagnosis. Oxygen affinity is inversely proportional to the P_{50}, and in general the hemoglobin level or degree of erythrocytosis is directly related to the P_{50}.

Many unstable hemoglobins also have an increased oxygen affinity that may explain the high hemoglobin level found in individuals whose hemoglobin has this combination of defects. Over 15 examples of unstable hemoglobins with reduced oxygen affinity have been reported (78).

The M Hemoglobins

Seven structurally abnormal hemoglobins exist only as methemoglobin because the heme iron is stabilized in the oxidized Fe^{3+} or ferriheme form (116–118). In four, the amino acid substitution involves one of the histidines between which the heme is slung: (Hb M_{Boston} $\alpha_2^{58\ His\rightarrow Tyr}\beta_2$; Hb M_{Iwate} $\alpha_2^{87\ His\rightarrow Tyr}$ Hb $M_{Saskatoon}$ $\alpha_2\beta_2^{63\ His\rightarrow Tyr}$; Hb $M_{Hyde\ Park}$ $\alpha_2\beta_2^{92\ His\rightarrow Tyr}$). In Hb $M_{Milwaukee}$ ($\alpha_2\beta_2^{67\ Val\rightarrow Glu}$), the substituted glutamate in the heme pocket forms a similar bond, fixing the ferriheme. There are two examples of fetal M hemoglobins (Hb FM_{Osaka}($\alpha_2\gamma_2^{63\ His\rightarrow Tyr}$, Hb $FM_{Fort\ Ripley}$ $\alpha_2\gamma_2^{92\ His\rightarrow Tyr}$), which cause cyanosis at birth and disappear as γ-globin chain production switches to β-globin chain production. The substitutions in the γ-chains are analogous to those in the β-chains of Hb $M_{Saskatoon}$ and Hb $M_{Hyde\ Park}$.

The "cyanosis" seen in individuals with Hb M is only in part due to hypoxia; methemoglobin imparts a brownish color to whole blood, which appears blue when seen through the skin. The majority of patients are asymptomatic; however, Hb $M_{Saskatoon}$ and Hb $M_{Hyde\ Park}$ have been associated with compensated hemolysis and oxidant drug-induced hemolysis.

Diagnosis is often suggested by the appearance of the patient and a family history of cyanosis. In the laboratory, the absorption spectra of the hemoglobin from affected individuals when it has been fully oxidized with ferricyanide differ from methemoglobin A, but only slightly one from another, with absorption peaks in the 580- to 600-nm range (119). Electrophoresis on cellulose acetate at pH 8.6 or citrate agar at pH 6.0 does not separate hemoglobins M from A; however, isoelectric focusing, particularly if the specimen is oxidized with ferricyanide, allows wide separation of Hb Ms from Hb A (Fig. 36.6).

HEREDITARY PERSISTENCE OF FETAL HEMOGLOBIN

Hereditary persistence of fetal hemoglobin (HPFH) comprises a group of disorders, clinically benign and usually hematologically normal, in which Hb F production persists throughout life. Several distinct genetic lesions underlie the various types of HPFH (120). In four, there is a large deletion involving both the δ- and β-genes which in at least one instance may bring an enhancer at the 3′-end of the deletion into close apposition with the α-genes, probably accounting for their continued expression. A very similar deletion results in δβ-thalassemia; however, the DNA enhancer sequence is included in the deletion, perhaps accounting for the lower level of γ-globin chain (and Hb F) production and the imbalance in α:non-α-globin chain production typical of the disorder. The other types of HPFH are associated with single-base substitutions that occur in or near the γδβ-gene complex. There is even evidence that some types may be due to genetic lesions unconnected with the γδβ-gene complex (120).

The amount of Hb F varies from one type of HPFH to another (Table 36.8) as does its distribution among the red cells. HPFH may be subdivided into those in which all red cells contain Hb F (pancellular types) and those in which only a portion of the red cells contain Hb F (heterocellular types). The distinction is made based on the acid elution technique of Kleihauer and Betke (121) (Hb F is acid resistant as well as alkali resistant) or by the use of anti-Hb F antibodies (122). The latter is more sensitive; however, it may be difficult with either technique to be sure of the distribution of Hb F, particularly when at a low level. The discovery of several types of HPFH with a heterocellular distribution of Hb F reduces the value of demonstrating the type of distribution of Hb F among red cells, since a heterocellular distribution is also found in all other forms of increased Hb F in adults (29).

The heterozygote for the common type of deletional HPFH that occurs exclusively in blacks is associated with approximately 30% Hb F that is pancellular in distribution. The blood count, red cell indices and morphology, and the α:non-α-globin chain synthesis ratio are essentially normal. The hemoglobin of the homozygote consists exclusively of Hb F because the δ- and β-genes are deleted from both chromosomes 11. The blood count and morphology are similar to those seen in thalassemia minor, and the α:non-α-globin chain synthesis ratio is about 2:1; so strictly speaking, this disorder might be classified under the thalassemias. Homozygous δβ-thalassemia also has 100% Hb F (Fig. 36.16), but the deficit in δ- and β-globin chain production is greater and results in a thalassemia intermedia.

The diagnosis of HPFH is usually made from hemoglobin electrophoresis performed as part of a screen for Hb S or other hemoglobin variant. The solitary finding of increased Hb F in a healthy individual with a normal blood count is probably sufficient to make a diagnosis of HPFH. There are circumstances in which an acquired increase in Hb F may occur; however, in only a few, such as pregnancy, is the individual otherwise clinically or hematologically normal.

Compound heterozygotes for HPFH and Hb S or Hb C are not uncommon. The percentage of the abnormal hemoglobin is approximately 60% with 40% Hb F and a small amount of Hb A_2 (Fig. 36.20). Despite the high percentage of Hb S in the Hb S-HPFH compound heterozygote, the combination is benign, clinically similar to Hb S trait, with a normal blood count. The presence of Hb F in all red cells and the reduced tendency for Hb SF to sickle as compared to

Table 36.8. Hereditary Persistence of Fetal Hemoglobin. Percentage of Hb F, Ratio of γ-Globin Chains, and Distribution among Red Cells in Four Types of HPFH

Type	Hb F % Heterozygote	Hb F % Homozygote	$^{G}\gamma:^{A}\gamma$	Distribution among Red Cells
Black	17–36	100	0.4	Pancellular
Greek	10–30	—	0.1	Pancellular
British	4–12	19–21	0.08	Heterocellular
Swiss	1–5	—	Variable	Heterocellular

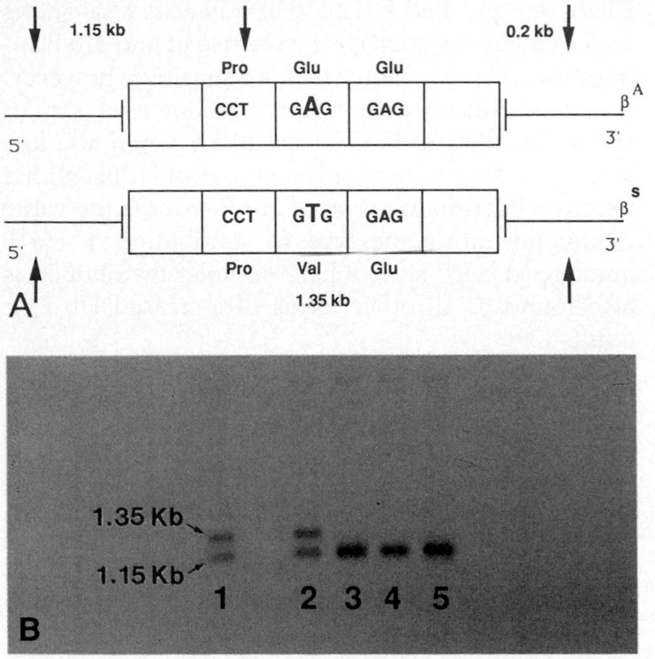

Figure 36.21. **A**, Diagram of β-globin gene with Mst II restriction sites indicated by *arrows*. The nucleotide triplets coding for the 5th, 6th, and 7th amino acids are enlarged to illustrate the mutation causing loss of a restriction site in the β^S-globin gene. (Adapted from Law et al. Gene 1984;28:153–158.) **B**, Autoradiograph of Mst II digestions using β-globin gene probe: β^A 1.15 kb, β^S 1.35 kb. Lanes 1 and 2: Sickle cell trait. Lanes 3, 4, and 5: Normal adult.

Hb SA account for the lack of sickling under normal physiological conditions.

HEMOGLOBINOPATHIES IN THE FETUS AND NEWBORN

The earlier the diagnosis of the severe hemoglobinopathies such as sickle cell anemia and β-thalassemia major can be made, the sooner appropriate therapy and prophylaxis can be instituted. Prenatal diagnosis (122, 123) is seldom available outside major hemoglobinopathy centers because it usually involves the study of DNA from chorionic villus cells, amniocytes, or a fetal blood sample. Obtaining these samples exposes the fetus to some danger; therefore, only in fetuses proven to be at risk (by study of both parents) and in situations where the parents would consider termination are such studies usually undertaken. The earliest diagnosis can be made from DNA of chorionic villus cells. DNA has the added advantage that it can survive transport across vast distanced allowing remote areas to take advantage of the gene analysis. Amplification of segments of the DNA by polymerase chain reaction (PCR) techniques increases the material available for study.

The gene for Hb S can be specifically detected (Fig. 36.21), but the situation is different for β-thalassemia major because of the many different lesions, inside and outside the β-gene that may cause it. Such techniques as restriction endonuclease mapping and linkage analysis of restriction fragment length polymorphisms and oligonucleotide probes may be required. The vast amount of genetic data (65) has shown that within any one population there are usually only a handful of lesions that need to be considered.

The ample availability of cord blood at delivery allows application of many of the methods used in studying adults (124–126). The ready availability also permits screening of all populations at risk, and in many states it is mandated that all newborns be tested for hemoglobinopathies. However, there are significant limitations and pitfalls.

In the case of sickle cell anemia, hemoglobin electrophoresis on cellulose acetate at alkaline pH will show approximately 75% Hb F and 25% Hb S with no Hb A. It is the latter that is important, and it may be difficult to confirm that no Hb A is present. Because Hb A and its variants, particularly in heterozygotes, are present in small quantities, it is advisable to double the amount of hemolysate applied. Electrophoresis in citrate agar will help to confirm the identity of Hb S and make the presence or absence of Hb A more clear-cut (Fig. 36.22). It must be remembered that Hb F and Hb S without Hb A is a pattern also present in Hb S β^0-thalassemia and Hb S HPFH; study of the parents will usually clarify the diagnosis.

The presence of maternal Hb A-may result in a diagnosis of sickle cell trait when in fact the infant has sickle cell anemia. This trap may be avoided by noticing the presence of an Hb A_2 band, which should not be present in cord blood, and therefore must be of maternal origin.

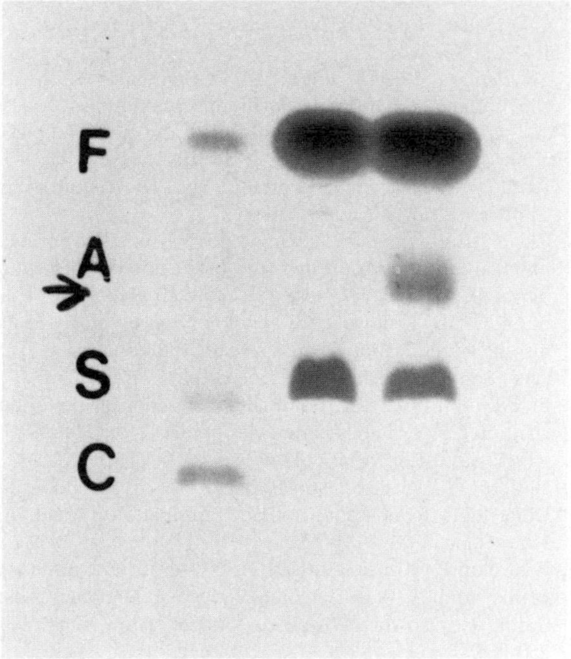

Figure 36.22. Hemoglobin electrophoresis in agar using a citric acid–citrate buffer at pH 6.2. Left lane: A control mixture of Hb C, Hb S, and Hb F. Middle lane: Cord blood from a neonate with sickle cell anemia showing Hb S and Hb F, but no Hb A (a similar pattern would be seen in Hb S-β^0-thalassemia and Hb S-HPFH). Right lane: Cord blood from a neonate with sickle cell trait showing Hb S, Hb F, and Hb A.

In β-thalassemia major, cord blood electrophoresis will show 100% Hb F. β^+-Thalassemia, on the other hand, will show a small amount of Hb A, and the pattern will be difficult to distinguish from normal.

References

1. Körber E. Inaugural dissertation: Uber differenzen blutfarbstoffes. Dorpat 1866 cited by Bischoff H. Z Gesamte Exp Med 1926;48:472–489.
2. Savitt TL, Goldberg MF. Herrick's 1910 case report of sickle cell anemia. JAMA 1989;261:266–271.
3. Cooley TB, Lee P. A series of cases of splenomegaly in children with anemia and peculiar bone changes. Trans Am Pediatr Soc 1925;37:29–30.
4. Rietti F. Ittero emolitica primitivo. Atti Acad Sci Med Nat Ferrara 1925;2:14–22.
5. Greppi E. Ittero emolitica familiare con aumento della resistanza deli globuli. Minerva Med 1928;8:1–11.
6. Micheli F, Penati F, Momigliano LG. Ulteriori richerche sulla anemia ipocromica splenomegalica con poichilocitosi. Atti Soc Ital Ematol, Hematologica 1933;16(suppl):10–20.
7. Wintrobe MM, Matthews E, Pollack R, Dobyns BM. Familial hematopoietic disorder in Italian adolescents and adults resembling Mediterranean disease (thalassemia). JAMA 1940;14:1530–1538.
8. Whipple GH, Bradford WL. Mediterranean disease—thalassemia (erythroblastic anemia of Cooley); associated pigment abnormalities simulating hemochromatosis. J Pediatr 1936;9: 279–311.
9. Pauling L, Itano HA, Singer SJ, Wells IG. Sickle-cell anemia, molecular disease. Science 1949;110:543–548.
10. Hörlein H, Weber G. Uber chronische familiare Methamaglobinamie und eine neue Modifikation des Methamaglobins. Deutsche Med Wochenschr 1948;73:746–748.
11. Staven P, Strome J, Lorkin PA, Lehmann H. Haemoglobin M Saskatoon with slight contrast haemolysis, markedly increased by sulphonamides. Scand J Haematol 1972;9:566–571.
12. Ingram VM. A specific chemical difference between the globins of normal human and sickle-cell anaemia haemoglobin. Nature 1956;178:792–794.
13. Anonymous. International Hemoglobin Information Center. IHIC variants list. Hemoglobin 1988;12:209–310.
14. Perutz MF. Molecular anatomy, physiology and pathology of hemoglobin. In: Stamatoyannopoulos G, Neinhuis AW, Leder P, Majerus PW, eds. Molecular basis of blood diseases. Philadelphia: WB Saunders, 1987:127–178.
15. Fermi G, Perutz MF, Shannon B, Fourme B. The crystal structure of human deoxyhaemoglobin at 1.7 Å resolution. J Mol Biol 1984;175:159–174.
16. Haldane JBS. The rate of mutation of human genes. Proc VIII International Congress on Genetics and Heredity. Hereditas 1948(suppl):267–273.
17. Bunn HG, Forget BG. Hemoglobin: molecular, genetic and clinical aspects. 2nd ed. Philadelphia: WB Saunders, 1986;13–35.
18. Bohr C, Hasselbach K, Krogh A. Ueber einen in biologischer Beziehung Wichtigen Einfluss den die Kohlensaurespann ung des Blutes aut dessen Sauerstoff bindung ubt. Skand Arch Physiol 1904;16:402–412.
19. Perutz MF, Muirhead H, Mazzarella L, Crowther RA, Greer J, Kilmartin JV. Identification of residues responsible for the alkaline Bohr effect in haemoglobin. Nature (London) 1969;222:1240–1243.
20. Reeves RB. The effect of temperature on the oxygen equilibrium curve of human blood. Respir Physiol 1980;42:317–328.
21. Oski FA, Gottlieb AJ. The interrelationships between red blood cell metabolites, hemoglobin, and the oxygen dissociation curve. Prog Hematol 1971;7:33–67.
22. Barcroft J. The respiratory function of the blood. Part II. Haemoglobin. London: Cambridge University Press, 1928.
23. Buckle VJ, Higgs DR, Wilkie AOM, Super M, Weatherall DJ. Localisation of human α globin to 16p13.3 pter. J Med Genet 1988;25:847–859.
24. Little PFR. Globin pseudogenes. Cell 1982;28:683–684.
25. Higgs DR, Vickers MA, Wilkie AOM, Pretorius IM, Farman AP, Weatherall DJ. A review of the molecular genetics of the human α-globin gene cluster. Blood 1989;73:1081–1104.
26. Sanders-Haigh L, Anderson WF, Francke U. The β-globin gene is on the short arm of chromosome 11. Nature 1980;283: 683–686.
27. Nute PE, Stamatoyannopoulos G. Cases of abnormal human hemoglobin produced by de novo mutation. Hemoglobin 1988;12:429–439.
28. Higgs DR, Wood WG, Barton C, Weatherall DJ. Clinical features and molecular analysis of acquired Hb H disease. Am J Med 1983;75:181–191.
29. Weatherall DJ, Pembrey ME, Pritchard J. Fetal haemoglobin. Clin Haematol 1974;3:467–508.
30. Weatherall DJ. Common genetic disorders of the red cell and the "malaria hypothesis." Ann Trop Med Parasitol 1987;81: 539–548.
31. Anonymous. Ovalocytosis and malaria [Editorial]. Lancet 1988;2:608–610.
32. Mitchell GH, Bannister LH. Malaria parasite invasion: interactions with the red cell membrane. CRC Crit Rev Oncol Hematol 1988;8:255–310.

33. Livingstone FB. The Duffy blood groups, vivax malaria and malaria selection in human populations: a review. Hum Biol 1984;56:413–425.
34. Fleming AF, Storey J, Molineaux L, Iroko EA, Attai EDE. Abnormal haemoglobins in the Sudan savanna of Nigeria. I. Prevalance of haemoglobins and relationships between sickle cell trait, malaria and survival. Ann Trop Med Parasitol 1979;73:161–172.
35. Nagel RL, Roth EF Jr. Malaria and red cell genetics. Blood 1989;74:1213–1221.
36. Siniscalco M, Bernini L, Filippi I, et al. Population genetics of human haemoglobin variants, thalassemia and glucose-6-phosphate dehydrogenase deficiency, with particular reference to the malaria hypothesis. Bull WHO 1966;34:379–393.
37. Flint J, Hill AV, Bowden DK, et al. High frequencies of α-thalassemia are the result of natural selection by malaria. Nature 1986;321:744–750.
38. Bienzle U, Guggenmoos-Holzman I, Luzzatto L. Malaria and erythrocyte glucose-6-phosphate dehydrogenase variants in West Africa. Am J Trop Med Hyg 1979;28:619–621.
39. Beutler E, Dern RJ, Alving AS. The hemolytic effect of primaquine: V1. An in vitro test for sensitivity of erythrocytes to primaquine. J Lab Clin Med 1955;45:40–50.
40. Kim HC, Schwartz E. Unstable hemoglobins. In: Williams WJ, Beutler E, Erslev AJ, Lichtman MA, eds. Hematology. 4th ed. New York: McGraw-Hill, 1990;1707–1708.
41. Schmidt RM, Wilson SM. Standardization in detection of abnormal hemoglobins. Solubility tests for hemoglobin S. JAMA 1973;225:1225–1230.
42. Basset P, Braconnier F, Rosa J. An update on electrophoretic and chromatographic methods in the diagnosis of hemoglobinopathies. J Chromatogr Biomed Appl 1982;227:267–304.
43. Anonymous. Cellulose acetate electrophoresis. In: Laboratory methods for detecting hemoglobinopathies. Atlanta: Centers for Disease Control, 1984:45–49.
44. Anonymous. Citrate agar electrophoresis. In: Laboratory methods for detecting hemoglobinopathies. Atlanta: Centers for Disease Control, 1984:53–58.
45. Anonymous. Acid globin chain electrophoresis. In: Laboratory methods for detecting hemoglobinopathies. Atlanta: Centers for Disease Control, 1984:67–69.
46. Pembrey ME, McWade P, Weatherall DJ. Reliable routine estimation of small amounts of foetal haemoglobin by alkali denaturation. J Clin Pathol 1972;25:738–740.
47. Efremov CD, Huisman THJ, Bowman K, Wrightstone RN, Shroeder WA. Microchromatography of hemoglobins. II. A rapid method for the determination of hemoglobin A_2. J Lab Clin Med 1974;83:657–664.
48. Henson J, Carver J, Wilson JB, Huisman THJ. Carboxymethyl-cellulose microchromatography for the quantitation of hemoglobin Bart's (γ_4) and its use in the detection of α-thalassemia conditions. J Chromatogr 1980;198:443–448.
49. Weatherall DJ, Clegg JB, Naughton MA. Globin synthesis in thalassemia: an in vitro study. Nature 1965;208:1061–1065.
50. Thein SL, Al-Hakim I, Hoffbrand AV. Thalassaemia intermedia: a new molecular basis. Br J Haematol 1984;56:333–337.
51. Moi P, Paglietti E, Sanna A, et al. Delineation of the molecular basis of δ- and normal HbA_2 β-thalassemia. Blood 1988;72: 530–533.
52. Pirastu M, Galanello R, Melis MA, et al. δ^+-Thalassemia in Sardinia. Blood 1983;62:341–345.
53. Heisman THJ, Reese AL, Gardiner MB, et al. The occurrence of different levels of $^G\gamma$ chain and of the $^A\gamma^T$ variant of fetal hemoglobin in newborn babies from various countries. Am J Hematol 1983;14:133–148.
54. Liebhaber SA. α Thalassemia. Hemoglobin 1989;13:685–731.
55. Pierce HL, Kurachi S, Sofroniadore K, Stamatoyannopoulos G. Frequencies of thalassemia in American blacks. Blood 1977;49:981–986.
56. Bowden DK, Hill AV, Higgs DR, Oppenheimer SJ, Weatherall DJ, Clegg JB. Different hematologic phenotypes are associated with the leftward (-alpha 4.2) and rightward (-alpha 3.7) $alpha^+$-thalassemia deletions. J Clin Invest 1987;79:39–43.
57. Wasi P, Na-Nakorn S, Pootrakul SN. The α-thalassemias. Clin Haematol 1974;3:383–410.
58. Clegg JB, Weatherall DJ. Hemoglobin Constant Spring, an unusual α-chain variant involved in the etiology of hemoglobin H disease. Ann NY Acad Sci 1974;232:168–178.
59. Efremov GD, Josifovska O, Nikolov N, et al. HbH-Hb Icaria disease: identification of the Hb Icaria mutation through analysis of amplified DNA. Br J Haematol 1990;75:250–253.
60. Bradley TB, Wohl RC, Smith EJ. Elongation of the α-globin chain in a black family: interaction with G-Philadelphia [Abstract]. Clin Res 1975;23:131A.
61. De Jong WW, Meera Kahn P, Bernini LF. Hemoglobin Koya Dora: high frequency of a chain termination mutant. Am J Hum Genet 1975;27:81–90.
62. Pootrakul P, Winichagoon P, Fucharoen S, Pravatmuang P, Piankijagum A, Wasi P. Homozygous haemoglobin Constant Spring: a need for revision of concept. Hum Genet 198;59: 250–255.
63. Weatherall DJ, Clegg JB, Boon WH. The haemoglobin constitution of infants with the haemoglobin Bart's hydrops foetalis syndrome. Br J Haematol 1970;18:357–367.
64. Kutlar A. β-Thalassemia repository. Hemoglobin 1989;13: 775–787.
65. Kazazian HH, Boehm CD. Molecular basis and prenatal diagnosis of β-thalassemia. Blood 1988;62:1107–1116.
66. Adams III JG, Boxer LA, Baehner RL, Forget BG, Isistrakis GA, Steinberg MH. Hemoglobin Indianapolis (B_{12}[G14] argenine): an unstable β-globin variant producing the phenotype of severe β-thalassemia. J Clin Invest 1979;63:931–938.
67. Millard DP, Mason K, Serjeant BE, Serjeant GR. Comparison of haematological features of the β°- and β^+-thalassaemia traits in Jamaican Negroes. Br J Haematol 1977;36:161–170.
68. Kuczynski A. The relationship between the serum iron concentration and erythrocytic hemoglobin A_2 level. J Med 1971;2:136–142.
69. Steinberg MH. Review: thalassemia: molecular pathology and management. Am J Med Sci 1988;31:308–321.
70. Yataganas X, Fessas P. The pattern of hemoglobin precipitation in thalassemia and its significance. Ann NY Acad Sci 1969;165:270–287.
71. Weatherall DJ, Clegg JB. The thalassaemia syndromes. 3rd ed. Oxford: Blackwell Scientific Publications, 1981:199–202.
72. Weatherall DJ, Clegg JB, Higgs DR, Wood WG. The hemoglobinopathies. In: Scriver CR, Beaudet AL, Sey WS, and Valle D, eds. The metabolic basis of inherited disease. 6th ed. New York: McGraw-Hill, 1989:2267–2339.
73. Weatherall DJ, Clegg JB. The thalassaemia syndromes. 3rd ed. Oxford: Blackwell Scientific Publications, 1981:428–431.
74. Baglioni C. The fusion of two peptide chains in hemoglobin Lepore and its interpretation as a genetic deletion. Proc Natl Acad Sci USA 1962;48:1880–1886.
75. Efremov GD. Hemoglobins Lepore and anti-Lepore. Hemoglobin 1978;2:197–233.
76. England JM, Fraser PM. Differentiation of iron deficiency from thalassaemia trait by routine blood-count. Lancet 1973;1:449–450.
77. Green R, King R. A new red cell discriminant incorporating volume dispersion for differentiating iron deficiency anemia from thalassemia minor. Blood Cells 1989;15:481–495.

78. Anonymous. International Hemoglobin Information Center. IHIC variants list. Hemoglobin 1989;13:221–323.
79. Konetey-Ahulu FID, Gallo E, Lehmann H, Ringelhann B. Haemoglobin Korle-Bu (β73 Aspartic acid replaced by asparagine) showing one of the two amino acid substitutions of haemoglobin C Harlem. J Med Genet 1968;5:107–111.
80. DeJong WWW, Went LN, Bernini LF. Haemoglobin Leiden: deletion of β6 or 7 glutamic acid. Nature 1968;220:778–790.
81. Winslow RM, Swenberg ML, Gross E, Chervenick PA, Buchman RR, Anderson WF. Hemoglobin McKees Rocks ($\alpha_2\beta_2$145 Tyr→Term): a human "nonsense" mutation leading to a shortened β-chain. J Clin Invest 1976;57:772–781.
82. Garel MC, Goossens G, Oudart JL, Blouquit Y, Thillet J, Rosa J. Hemoglobin Dakar = Hemoglobin Grady: demonstration by a new approach to the analysis of the tryptic core region of the α chain and oxygen equilibrium properties. Biochem Biophys Acta 1976;453:459–471.
83. Seid-Akhaven M, Winter WP, Abramson RK, Rucknagel DL. Hemoglobin Wayne: a frame shift mutation detected in human hemoglobin alpha chains. Proc Natl Acad Sci USA 1976;73:882–886.
84. Kark JA, Posey DM, Schumacher HR, Ruehle CJ. Sickle-cell trait as a risk factor for sudden death in physical training. N Engl J Med 1987;317:781–787.
85. Reider RF, Safaya S, Gillette P, et al. Effect of β-globin gene cluster haplotype on the hematologic and clinical features of sickle cell anemia. Am J Hematol 1991;36:184–189.
86. Powars DR. The natural history of sickle cell disease—the first ten years. Semin Hematol 1975;12:276–285.
87. Francis RB Jr, Johnson CS. Vascular occlusion in sickle cell disease: current concepts and unanswered questions. Blood 1991;77:1405–1414.
88. Serjeant GR, Grandison Y, Lowrie Y, et al. The development of haematological changes in homozygous sickle cell disease: a cohort study from birth to 6 years. Br J Haematol 1981;48: 533–543.
89. Davis LR. Aplastic crisis in haemolytic anaemias: the role of a parvovirus-like agent. Br J Haematol 1983;55:391–393.
90. Davies SC, Brozovic M. The presentation, management and prophylaxis of sickle cell disease. Blood Rev 1989;3:29–44.
91. Koshy M, Burd L, Wallace D, Moawad A, Baron J. Prophylactic red-cell transfusions in pregnant patients with sickle cell disease. A randomized cooperative study. N Engl J Med 1988;319:1447–1452.
92. Dover GJ, Charache S, Boyer SH, Vogelsang G, Moyer M. 5-Azacytidine increases HbF production and reduces anemia in sickle cell disease: dose-response analysis of subcutaneous and oral dose regimens. Blood 1985;66:527–532.
93. Kaufman RE. Hydroxyurea: specific therapy for sickle cell anaemia [Editorial]. Blood 1992;79:2503–2506.
94. Bunn HF, Forget BG. Hemoglobin: molecular genetic and clinical aspects. Philadelphia: WB Saunders, 1986:545–548.
95. Vermylen C, Fernandez Robles E, Ninane J, Cornu G. Bone marrow transplantation in five children with sickle cell anaemia. Lancet 1988;1:1427–1428.
96. Milner PF, Miller C, Grey R, Seakins M, DeJong WW, Went LN. Hemoglobin O Arab in four Negro families and its interaction with hemoglobin S and hemoglobin C. N Engl J Med 1970;283:1417–1425.
97. Altay C, Niazi GA, Huisman THJ. The combination of Hb S and Hb E in a black female. Hemoglobin 1976;1:100–102.
98. Kelleher JF, Park JOK, Kim HC, Schroeder WA. Life-threatening SD-Los Angeles disease. Hemoglobin 1984;8:203–213.
99. Murray N, Serjeant BE, Serjeant GR. Sickle cell-hereditary persistence of fetal hemoglobin and its differentiation from other sickle cell syndromes. Br J Haematol 1988;69:89–92.
100. Serjeant GR, Sommereux A, Stevenson M, Mason K, Serjeant BE. Comparison of sickle cell-β° thalassaemia with homozygous sickle cell disease. Br J Haematol 1979;41:83–93.
101. Gonzalez-Redondo JM, Kutlar F, Kutlar A, et al. HbS(C)-β^+-thalassemia: different mutations are associated with different levels of normal Hb A. Br J Haematol 1988;70:85–89.
102. Steinberg MH, Embury SH. α-Thalassemia in blacks: interactions with the sickle hemoglobin gene. Birth Defects 1988;23: 43–48.
103. Huisman THJ. Percentages of abnormal hemoglobins in adults with a heterozygosity for an α-chain and/or a β-chain variant. Am J Hematol 1983;14:393–404.
104. Schneider RG, Hightower B, Hosty TS, et al. Abnormal hemoglobins in a quarter million people. Blood 1976;48:629–637.
105. Redetzki JE, Bickers JN, Samuels MS. Homozygous hemoglobin C disease: clinical review of 15 patients. South Med J 1968;61:238–242.
106. Murphy JR. Hemoglobin CC erythrocytes: decreased intracellular pH and decreased O_2 affinity—anemia. Semin Hematol 1976;13:177–180.
107. Bunn HF, Forget BG. Hemoglobin: molecular genetic and clinical aspects. Philadelphia: WB Saunders, 1986:422.
108. Fairbanks VF, Gilchrist GS, Brimhall B, Jereb JA, Goldston EC. Hemoglobin E trait reexamined: a cause of microcytosis and erythrocytosis. Blood 1979;53:109–115.
109. Lachant NA. Hemoglobin E: an emerging hemoglobinopathy in the United States. Am J Hematol 1987;25:449–462.
110. Mehta BC, Agarwal MB, Verandan DJ, Joshi RH, Bhargava AB. Hemoglobin E thalassemia—a study of 16 cases. Acta Hematol 1980;64:201–204.
111. Orkin SH, Kazazian HH, Antonarakis SE, Ostrer H, Goff SC, Sexton JP. Abnormal RNA processing due to the exon mutation of β^E globin gene. Nature 1982;300:768–769.
112. Dacie JV, Grimes AJ, Meisler A, et al. Hereditary Heinz-body anaemia. A report of studies on five patients with mild anaemia. Br J Haematol 1964;10:388–402.
113. Carrell RW, Kay R. A simple method for the detection of unstable haemoglobins. Br J Haematol 1972;23:615–619.
114. Bonaventura J, Riggs A. Hemoglobin Kansas, a human hemoglobin with a neutral amino acid substitution and abnormal oxygen equilibrium. J Biol Chem 1968;243:980–991.
115. Erslev AJ. Hemoglobinopathies producing erythrocytosis. In: Williams WJ, Beutler E, Erslev AJ, Lichtman MA, eds. Hematology. 4th ed. New York: McGraw-Hill, 1990:717–721.
116. Gerald PS, Efron ML. Chemical studies of several varieties of Hb M. Proc Natl Acad Sci USA 1961;47:1758–1767.
117. Beutler E. Hemoglobinopathies producing cyanosis. In: Williams WJ, Beutler E, Erslev AJ, Lichtman MA, eds. Hematology. 4th ed. New York: McGraw-Hill, 1990:746–751.
118. Priest JR, Watterson J, Jones RT, Faassen AE, Hedlund BE. Mutant fetal hemoglobin causing cyanosis in a newborn. Pediatrics 1988;83:734–736.
119. Gerald PS, George P. A second spectrospically abnormal methemoglobin associated with hereditary cyanosis. Science 1959;129:393–394.
120. Boyer SH. The emerging complexity of genetic control of persistent fetal hemoglobin biosynthesis in adults. Ann NY Acad Sci 1989;565:23–36.
121. Anonymous. Acid elution slide test for hemoglobin F. In: Laboratory methods for detecting hemoglobinopathies. Atlanta: Centers for Disease Control. 1984:101–103.
122. Rosatelli C, Pirastu M, Cao A. The prenatal diagnosis of thalassemia [Annotation]. Br J Haematol 1986;63:215–220.

123. Driscoll CM, Lerner N, Anyane-Yeboa K, et al. Prenatal diagnosis of sickle hemoglobinopathies: the experience of the Columbia University Comprehensive Center for Sickle Cell Disease. Am J Hum Genet 1987;40:548–558.
124. Consensus conference. Newborn screening for sickle cell disease and other hemoglobinopathies. JAMA 1987;258:1205–1209.
125. Galacteros F, Kleman K, Caburi-Martin J, Beuzard Y, Rosa J, Lubin B. Cord blood screening for hemoglobin abnormalities by thin layer isoelectric focusing. Blood 1980;56:1068–1071.
126. Jacobs S, Peterson L, Thompson L, et al. Newborn screening for hemoglobin abnormalities. A comparison of methods. Am J Clin Pathol 1986;85:713–715.

37 Acute Leukemias and Myelodysplastic Syndromes

Curtis A. Hanson

ACUTE LEUKEMIA

Pathogenesis

Acute and chronic leukemias are malignancies that arise from uncontrolled clonal proliferations of hematopoietic cells. The normal cellular control mechanisms are thought to be inoperative in leukemia due to changes in the genetic code that are responsible for regulation of cell growth and differentiation. It is often mistakenly believed that acute leukemias are hyperproliferative disorders that result in the production of new cells at a rapid pace. However, it is almost paradoxically true that leukemia cells may actually have cycling times that are several times slower than normal bone marrow cells. These leukemic cells mature slowly and incompletely and survive longer than their normal marrow counterparts because of the failure to achieve normal and final maturation. It is believed, for example, that acute myelogenous leukemia cells may actually have doubling times of approximately 30 days and require 50 to 75 doubling times before there is a significant accumulation of malignant cells. This final accumulation may occur over a period of 1 to 10 years and thus make it difficult to truly access the "initiation of disease."

Leukemias undoubtedly arise as a result of multiple transformation steps, or "hits." Significant evidence has been gathered that strongly implicates cellular oncogenes as key players in this leukemic transformation process. Oncogenes typically play an important role in normal cellular control and regulation and only display their oncogenic potential when their genetic structure or control elements are mutated, rearranged, amplified, or activated. Amplification and promotion of oncogenic activity may occur when the normal transcriptional promoter and control regions of these genes are disrupted. Various retroviruses have also been implicated as a "cause" or initiator of leukemia. We also know that leukemias may secondarily arise as a result of exposures to a variety of environmental and iatrogenic therapies. Immunosuppression, for example, is known to increase the risk of leukemia and lymphoma in organ transplant patients receiving such therapy. Ionizing radiation as well as alkylating agents may also contribute to the problem of secondary leukemias.

Leukemias, in general, are defined as malignant neoplasms of the hematopoietic system arising in the bone marrow. As the bone marrow is replaced with the malignant cells, the excess malignant cells escape into the peripheral blood—hence the derivation of the name leukemia: "white" (leuk-)/"blood" (-emia). In a simplistic fashion, it is easiest to classify leukemias on the basis of (*a*) the natural course of disease, i.e., acute versus chronic, and (*b*) the basic cell type involved (lymphoid versus myeloid). Acute leukemias are the result of a block in normal hematopoietic differentiation, leading to an accumulation of immature lymphoid or myeloid cells. This accumulation of leukemic blasts, as described above, is the result of a block in maturation and differentiation rather than an increased rapidity of differentiation. Acute leukemias are characterized by a rapidly fatal course of days to weeks, if untreated. This is in contrast to the chronic leukemias, which are typically associated with an indolent, albeit progressive, course of disease. Chronic leukemias are characterized by a proliferation of differentiated cells, as opposed to the immature blasts seen in the acute leukemias. Table 37.1 outlines the various acute and chronic leukemias; Figure 37.1 is a schematic diagram of their relationship to normal hematopoiesis. The relative incidence of the four major subgroups of leukemias are as follows: acute lymphoblastic leukemia (ALL), 10%; B-chronic lymphocytic leukemia (CLL), 30%; acute myelogenous leukemia (AML), 45%; and chronic myelogenous leukemia (CML), 15%.

Clinical Manifestations

The clinical manifestations of acute leukemia are related to three major effects: (*a*) the replacement of normal bone marrow elements, leading to complications resulting from anemia, thrombocytopenia, and

Table 37.1. Classification of Leukemia

Acute leukemia
Acute lymphoblastic leukemia (ALL)
FAB: L1, L2, L3
IPh:[a] B-precursor ALL
T-cell ALL
B-ALL (Burkitt's leukemia/lymphoma)
Acute myelogenous leukemia (AML)
FAB: M0–M7
Acute biphenotypic leukemia
Myelodysplastic syndromes (pre-leukemias)
Refractory anemia (RA)
Idiopathic refractory sideroblastic anemia (IRSA)
Refractory anemia with excess blasts (RAEB)
Refractory anemia with excess blasts in transformation (RAEB-t)
Chronic myelomonocytic leukemia (CMML)
Myelodysplastic syndromes, NOS[a]
Chronic leukemia
Chronic lymphoproliferative disorders (CLPD)
B-CLPD
B-Chronic lymphocytic leukemia (CLL)
Prolymphocytic leukemia (PLL or Galton's)
Hairy cell leukemia
Variants of CLL
Waldenström's macroglobulinemia
Multiple myeloma
T-CLPD
T-Chronic lymphocytic leukemia (T-CLL)
Tγ-Lymphoproliferative disorder (TγLPD)
Adult T-cell leukemia/lymphoma (ATCL)
Sézary's syndrome
Chronic myeloproliferative disorders (CMPD)
Chronic myelogenous leukemia (CML)
Polycythemia vera (PV)
Essential thrombocythemia (ET)
Idiopathic myelofibrosis
CMPD, NOS[a]

[a]IPh, immunophenotype; NOS, not otherwise specified.

leukopenia; (*b*) the complications of either tissue infiltration or leukostasis due to a marked increase in peripheral cell counts; and (*c*) the release of physiological factors that may lead to significant complications, for example, disseminated intravascular coagulation. It is likely that the pancytopenia and suppression of normal elements seen in acute leukemia are the result of a physical displacement of normal bone marrow elements; it is also quite likely that unrecognized "suppression" factors are involved that actively suppress normal hematopoiesis. The normal bone marrow is more than a simple factory assembly line and involves complex interactions between hematopoietic stem cells and stromal cells, endothelial cells, and other "environmental" factors that lead to cellular differentiation. It is likely then, that any disturbance in this normal marrow equilibrium, such as leukemia, would be associated with marrow suppression; thus, the goal of any therapy should be to decrease and eliminate the leukemic population to allow recovery of the normal bone marrow elements.

Diagnostic Modalities

The diagnosis of acute leukemia may be a multistep process involving multiple laboratory diagnostic modalities (Table 37.2). Morphology remains the most important and significant diagnostic modality in spite of the impressive array of technology that is available in the clinical laboratories. The morphologic examination of the peripheral blood, bone marrow aspirate, and bone marrow biopsy specimen is an important ingredient in the morphologic evaluation and diagnosis of acute leukemia.

Cytochemical enzymatic stains have been available since the early part of this century and have provided investigators with a wealth of knowledge over the years concerning the various subtypes of acute leukemia. This old fashioned laboratory test remains quite effective in confirming the diagnosis and classification of acute leukemia, as various enzymatic products are more likely associated with particular myeloid or lymphoid cells. The particulars of the various cytochemical stains are described in subsequent sections.

Newer diagnostic modalities have arisen that provide important biological, diagnostic, and prognostic information in the acute leukemias. Immunophenotyping with monoclonal antibodies has provided a consistent method of subclassifying the acute leukemias into either myeloid or lymphoid origin, as well as delineating various subsets within each of these two broad leukemic subgroups. This is detailed in the subsequent sections. Cytogenetic analysis has also provided a wealth of knowledge concerning the biology of leukemia as well as important diagnostic and prognostic information. Cytogenetic studies have allowed us to recognize the importance of reciprocal translocations, deletions, and other chromosomal abnormalities, which have significantly contributed to our biological knowledge of leukemia. Specific cytogenetic abnormalities are associated with particular subtypes of acute leukemia and have been shown over the last decade to have significant, independent prognostic information. Another diagnostic modality available for the evaluation of acute leukemia is molecular diagnostics. These techniques allow for evaluation of the immunoglobulin and T-cell receptor genes, as well as analyses of various oncogenes involved with particular chromosomal translocations.

ACUTE LYMPHOBLASTIC LEUKEMIA

Pathogenesis and Clinical Manifestations

Acute lymphoblastic leukemia (ALL) is a clonal malignancy of lymphopoietic precursor cells, arising

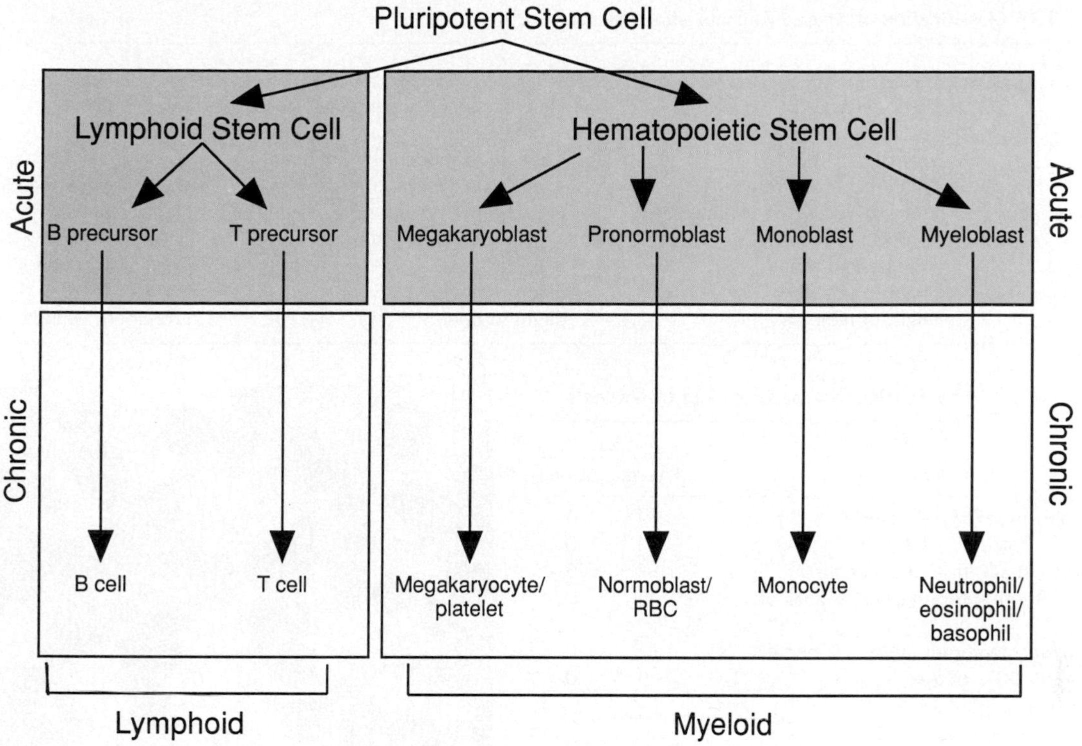

Figure 37.1. This schematic diagram outlines the relationship of the acute and chronic myeloid and lymphoid leukemias to normal hematopoietic and lymphoid development. The acute leukemias represent clonal expansions of immature precursor cells, while chronic leukemias represent proliferations of differentiated and mature lymphoid and hematopoietic elements.

Table 37.2. Diagnosis of Acute Leukemia

Routine morphology
Peripheral blood
Bone marrow aspirate
Bone marrow biopsy
Cytochemical stains
Immunophenotyping
Flow cytometry
Immunocytochemistry
Paraffin section immunoperoxidase
Cytogenetics
Karyotyping
In situ hybridization
Molecular diagnostics
Gene rearrangement studies
Oncogenes/translocations

primarily within the bone marrow. The etiology behind the development of ALL is unknown, but is not thought to be associated with radiation or exposure to toxic agents. The onset of symptoms in patients with ALL is usually acute and rapidly progressive. The clinical manifestations of ALL relate primarily to the suppression of normal bone marrow elements: weakness, fatigue, and malaise due to anemia; fever, infection, and unresponsiveness to antibiotics due to leukopenia; and bleeding due to thrombocytopenia. Skeletal pain as a result of marrow expansion is also not an uncommon finding, while lymphadenopathy and hepatosplenomegaly are common, but are usually not prominent findings. Virtually any organ may be infiltrated by the leukemic cells; involvement of the leptomeninges may result in various CNS symptoms, while the testes are a frequent source of residual disease in young boys with ALL.

Incidence

Acute lymphoblastic leukemia is the most common cancer in children under the age of 15 years and is the second or third leading cause of death in this age group. Approximately 80% of ALL cases occur in childhood and approximately 80% of childhood acute leukemia is of lymphocytic origin. Thus, ALL is typically considered a pediatric neoplasm and will be encountered much more frequently in institutions having a sizable pediatric population. Childhood ALL has a peak incidence at approximately 4 years of age, is slightly more common in boys than in girls, and is slightly more common in Caucasians than in non-Caucasians. ALL can also occur in adulthood, but has a peak incidence range between the ages of 2 and 10 years.

Laboratory Findings

Although we typically equate leukemia with disorders having markedly elevated white blood counts

Table 37.3. FAB Classification of Acute Lymphoblastic Leukemia

Cytologic Feature	L1	L2	L3
Size	Predominant small cells	Heterogeneous, intermediate to large cells	Large cells
Cytoplasm	Scant	Variable to moderately abundant	Moderately abundant
Nucleoli	Small/inconspicuous	≥ 1; prominent to large	≥ 1; prominent and large
Nuclear chromatin	Homogeneous and intermediate reticular	Heterogeneous with some having finely reticular chromatin	Finely reticular
Nuclear shape	Regular and round	Irregular	Regular to round
Basophilic cytoplasm	Slight to none	Slight to none	Intense
Vacuolation	Slight to none	Slight to none	Prominent; sharply punched out

Table 37.4. Revised FAB Scoring System for L1 and L2 Variants

Criteria	Score Present	Score Absent
High N/C[a] ratio in >75% of cells	+1	0
Low N/C[a] ratio in >25% of cells	−1	0
Nucleoli: 0–1 (small) in >75% of cells	+1	0
Nucleoli: 1 or more (prominent) in >25% of cells	−1	0
Irregular nuclear membrane in >25% of cells	−1	0
Large cells are >50% of total	−1	0
FAB-L1	0 to +2	
FAB-L2	−1 to −4	

[a]N/C, nuclear:cytoplasmic.

(WBCs), the absence of leukocytosis does not eliminate the possible diagnosis of acute leukemia. ALL is a good example of the variation in presenting WBC. Approximately 40% of ALL cases will have a presenting WBC of less than 10.0 × 10^9/liter; approximately 40% of patients will have a WBC between 10.0 × 10^9/liter and 50.0 × 10^9/liter. Only 20% of cases will have a significant leukocytosis exceeding 50.0 × 10^9/liter and only one-half of those patients will have a marked leukocytosis greater than 100.0 × 10^9/liter. The differential count of the WBC in patients with ALL shows predominantly lymphoblasts along with an expected neutropenia. Differentiation to mature lymphocytes is not seen. Other laboratory abnormalities that are commonly found in patients with ALL include elevated serum lactic acid dehydrogenase (LDH) and serum uric acid.

Morphology and FAB Classification

Acute lymphoblastic leukemia can be classified either morphologically or immunologically. The French-American-British (FAB) morphologic classification of acute leukemia has designated subtypes FAB-L1, -L2, and -L3 (Table 37.3). The revised FAB classification of ALL is based on weighing various criteria: nuclear-to-cytoplasmic ratio, the number of nucleoli, nuclear membrane irregularity, and cell size (Table 37.4).

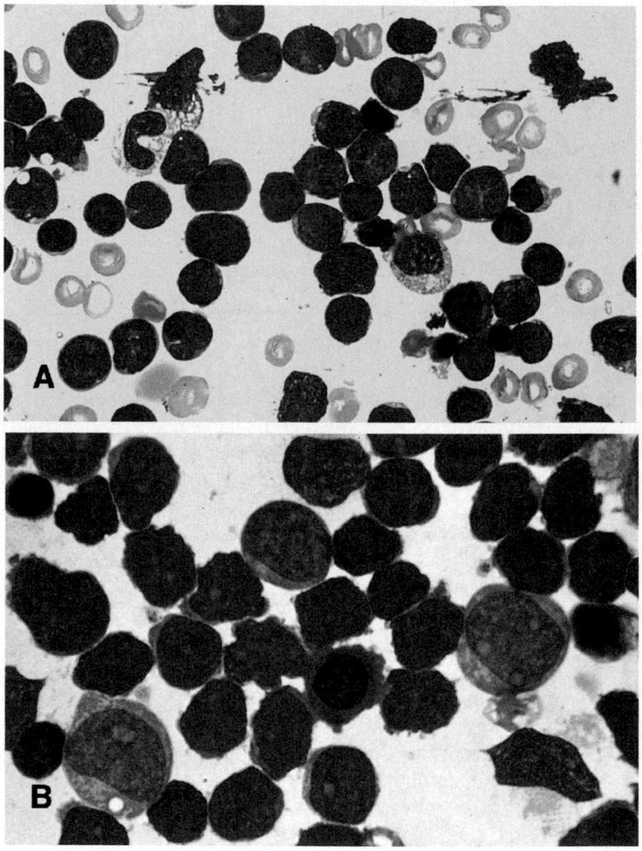

Figure 37.2. ALL-L1. **A**, Bone marrow with L1 blasts; **B**, Bone marrow with primarily L1 blasts and occasional L2 blasts.

The distribution of FAB-L1 and -L2 differs in children and adults. Approximately 80 to 85% of cases of ALL in children are FAB-L1, compared to 35 to 40% in adult ALL. The great majority of the remaining cases of ALL are classified as FAB-L2. Only 1 to 3% of ALL cases in adults and children are of the FAB-L3 subtype. This latter type of leukemia is a leukemic manifestation of Burkitt's lymphoma and is discussed in a subsequent section.

In FAB-L1 ALL, the majority of the leukemic cells are small with little to scant cytoplasm and absent, to inconspicuous at best, nucleoli. The chromatin pattern is clearly homogeneous and is not as finely reticular as those found in other types of leukemia. Nu-

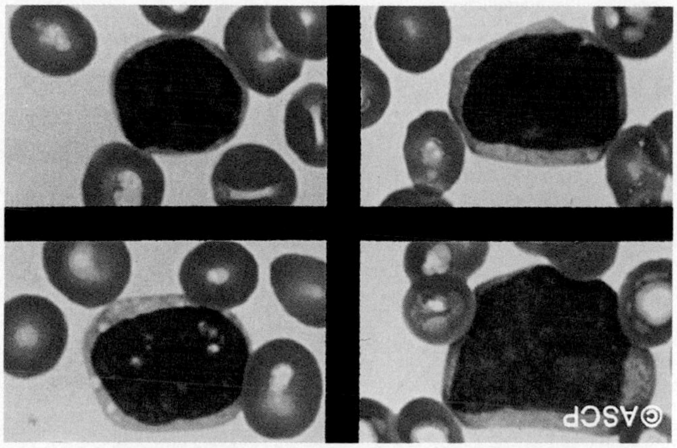

Figure 37.3. ALL bone marrow—examples of L2 blasts.

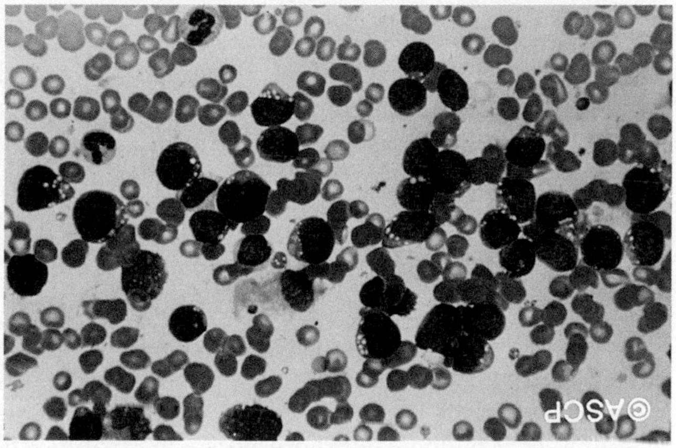

Figure 37.4. ALL-L3—Burkitt's leukemia/lymphoma.

clear irregularity is minimal (Fig. 37.2). In the FAB-L2 ALL, the most significant difference from FAB-L1 is that the leukemic cells are larger and more heterogeneous. FAB-L2 cells typically have variable to moderately abundant amounts of cytoplasm and importantly have one or more prominent nucleoli and a finer chromatin pattern compared to FAB-L1. Irregular nuclear shapes are commonly seen (Fig. 37.3). FAB-L3 ALL is characterized by a proliferation of large, homogeneous cells having deeply basophilic cytoplasm and sharply punched-out cytoplasmic vacuoles (Fig. 37.4). The nuclear chromatin is uniform and typically coarser than is found in FAB-L1 and FAB-L2. This type of ALL is in actuality the peripheralized version of Burkitt's lymphoma and thus should be considered as an acute leukemia more from a historical perceptive than a biological perspective. The WBC may be normal to slightly elevated with only a low percentage of circulating leukemic "blasts." The bone marrow typically shows only partial replacement with the leukemic cells. Because of its association with Burkitt's lymphoma, FAB-L3 ALL is typically associated with ileocecal tumor masses in the Western countries.

Morphologic Variants

Uncommon morphologic variants of ALL have been recognized. A "hand mirror" cell variant of ALL has been described in which the cytoplasm looses its spherical shape and appears to have a "handle." The elongated cytoplasmic handle has been described as being a result of cellular motility or locomotion, and has been regarded by some as a bad prognostic sign in ALL. This has not been widely accepted and is likely to be more of a laboratory artifact rather than having true biological significance.

Granular ALLs have also been described, characterized by the presence of azure granules within the cytoplasm of the leukemic lymphoblasts. These granules are reported to be negative with myeloid cytochemical stains and similar to the azurophilic structures seen in natural killer cells. This subset of ALL is not considered to have significant clinical or prognostic importance. However, recognition of this variant is important in avoiding diagnostic problems that might arise in differentiating ALL from acute myelogenous leukemia (AML).

Shen and colleagues have described a group of childhood ALL that presented with significant residual myeloid activity. These cases were referred to as "ALL with left shift." Clinically, these patients had a longer duration of complete remission that appeared to be the result of either a smaller tumor load or a lesser endogenous suppression of normal hematopoiesis. Diagnostically this may create a problem, since the marrow is only partially replaced by the leukemic blasts and may be easily confused with AML unless appropriate diagnostic tests are performed.

It has been recognized for approximately 20 years that some cases of ALL may present with significant hypereosinophilia. These patients may have their ALL present simultaneously with the hypereosinophilia, present initially as hypereosinophilia to be followed subsequently with a diagnosis of ALL, or present as ALL and relapse with a concurrent ALL and hypereosinophilic picture. The eosinophils may occasionally be slightly dysplastic in appearance, but no other evidence of myeloid differentiation is typically identified. Complications related to hypereosinophilia have been described in some patients, including endocarditis and respiratory complications. It has been postulated that the eosinophilia is secondary to release of eosinophilic growth factors from the leukemic cells. A t(5;14)(q31;q32) translocation has been identified in some cases of ALL with hypereosinophilia.

Cytochemistry

The role of cytochemical staining in the diagnosis of ALL is more relevant to exclude the diagnosis of

Table 37.5. Cytochemical Staining in Acute Lymphoblastic Leukemia

Stain[a]	L1	L2	L3
MPO	−	−	−
SBB	−	−	−
CAE	−	−	−
NSE	−[b]	−[b]	−
PAS	+(70%)	+(70%)	−
ACP	−/+[c]	−/+[c]	−
MGP	−	−	+
ORO	−	−	+
TdT	+	+	−

[a]MPO, myeloperoxidase; SBB, Sudan black B; CAE, chloroacetate esterase; NSE, nonspecific esterase; PAS, periodic acid–Schiff; ACP, acid phosphatase; MGP, methyl green pyronine; ORO, oil red O; TdT, terminal deoxynucleotidyl-transferase.
[b]Faint positivity may be seen.
[c]Most T-ALL and some B-precursor ALL will be positive.

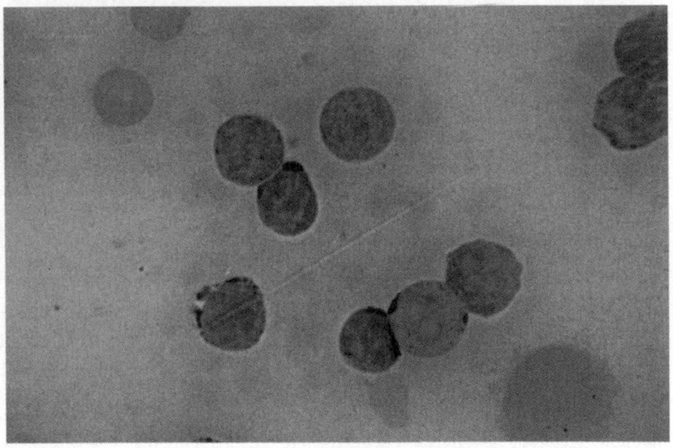

Figure 37.5. PAS stain of an ALL-L1.

AML rather than to find supportive evidence for the diagnosis of ALL (Table 37.5). Historically, the periodic acid–Schiff (PAS) reaction has classically been considered a diagnostic stain for ALL. However, only 40 to 60% of ALL cases show positivity with PAS, and PAS positivity can occasionally be found in AML. Thus, PAS lacks both sensitivity and specificity for ALL. Nonetheless, PAS positivity in ALL is characterized by large chunks or blocks of PAS-staining cytoplasmic material (Fig. 37.5). This can be distinguished from the diffuse PAS reaction seen in granulocytic cells. This enzyme is staining primarily the glycogen present within the cytoplasm of leukemic blasts. Thus, PAS positivity in an acute leukemia should be looked at as suggestive, but certainly not diagnostic, of an ALL. Acid phosphatase has been evaluated as a possible marker for T-cell ALL. T lymphocytes and most T lymphoblasts show focal, punctate, perinuclear positivity with acid phosphatase. However, not all T-cell ALLs show this pattern of staining, and a significant number of B-precursor ALL show positivity with acid phosphatase, thus limiting its utility as a differentiating stain between

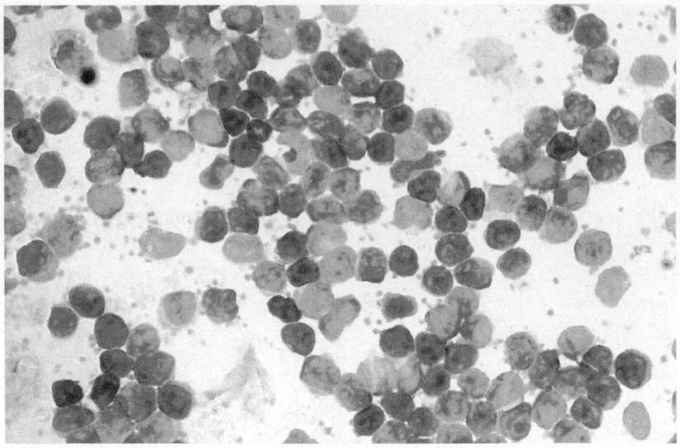

Figure 37.6. Terminal deoxynucleotidaltransferase (TdT) immunoperoxidase stain of a B-precursor ALL.

T-cell and non–T-cell ALL. Myeloblasts may also show a focal staining with acid phosphatase. Oil red O, which stains lipid material, is an excellent marker for ALL-L3 or Burkitt's leukemia/lymphoma. The oil red O stain distinctly stains the vacuoles that are seen in this subtype of leukemia/lymphoma.

Terminal deoxynucleotidyltransferase (TdT) is a DNA polymerase that contributes to the recombination heterogeneity seen in immunoglobulin and T-cell receptor gene rearrangements. This enzyme is active during lymphoblast development and is expressed in 95 to 99% of ALL cases. ALL-L3 lacks this enzyme, as it biologically represents a maturing lymphocyte rather than a true leukemic blast. Unfortunately, 5 to 10% of acute myelogenous leukemias also express this nuclear antigen, thus limiting the absolute lineage specificity of the TdT assay. TdT may be detected by either immunofluorescence, immunoperoxidase, or enzyme immunoassay methods (Fig. 37.6). TdT can be identified in ALLs of either T- or B-precursor immunophenotypes.

Immunophenotype

The most consistent and effective means of classifying ALL is based on immunophenotyping data (Table 37.6). Approximately 80 to 85% of ALLs can be classified as malignant counterparts of bone marrow B-precursor cells. 10 to 15% of ALL will be identified as T-cell ALL, thus having immunologic characteristics of immature T cells or thymocytes. The remaining 1 to 3% of ALLs will immunologically represent mature B cells having surface immunoglobulin and correspond to the FAB-L3 subgroup or Burkitt's leukemia/lymphoma.

HISTORICAL TERMINOLOGY

The terminology used in subclassifying ALLs has at best been confusing for those involved with diag-

Table 37.6. The Role of Immunophenotyping in Acute Leukemia

Distinction between ALL and AML
Identification of B-precursor ALL, T-cell ALL, and B-cell ALL subgroups
Diagnosis of acute megakaryoblastic leukemia (FAB-M7)
Recognition of acute biphenotypic leukemia

Table 37.7. Terminology Used for Acute Lymphoblastic Leukemia

B-Precursor ALL[a]
T-Cell ALL[a]
B-Cell ALL[a]
Non–T, non–B-cell ALL
Non–T-cell ALL
Common ALL
CALLA-positive ALL
Pre-B-cell ALL
Pre-pre-B-cell ALL
Pro-B-cell ALL

[a]Currently preferred terminology.

nostic hematology (Table 37.7). This growth in confusion has paralleled our increased sophistication in immunophenotyping and represents an evolution of knowledge concerning these leukemias. Rudimentary immunophenotyping initially allowed for the distinction of B-cell ALL (surface immunoglobulin positive) and T-cell ALL (E-rosette positive) from all other types of ALL. This large latter group was lumped together and sometimes referred to as non–T-, non–B-cell ALL. Others referred to this large group as "null-cell" ALL, reflecting the lack of any evidence toward a specific line of cell development. The T-cell and B-cell ALLs thus identified composed 10 to 15% and 1 to 3% of all ALL cases, respectively.

CALLA

The next breakthrough in subclassifying ALLs came with the development by Greaves and colleagues (1) of a polyclonal heteroantiserum against a case of non–T-, non–B-cell ALL; this antibody was called anti-common acute lymphoblastic leukemia antigen, or anti-CALLA. Patients with CALLA-positive ALL were found to have a much better prognosis than those with either B- or T-cell ALL. This development was considered a major breakthrough for the role of immunophenotyping in evaluating acute leukemias. These CALLA-positive ALLs made up the majority, but not all, of the non–T-, non–B-cell ALLs. Because of their reactivity with the CALLA antiserum (and subsequently with a monoclonal antibody against CALLA), these cases were called "common" acute lymphoblastic leukemias. Following this development, several B lymphocyte–associated differentiation antigens were recognized by a variety of

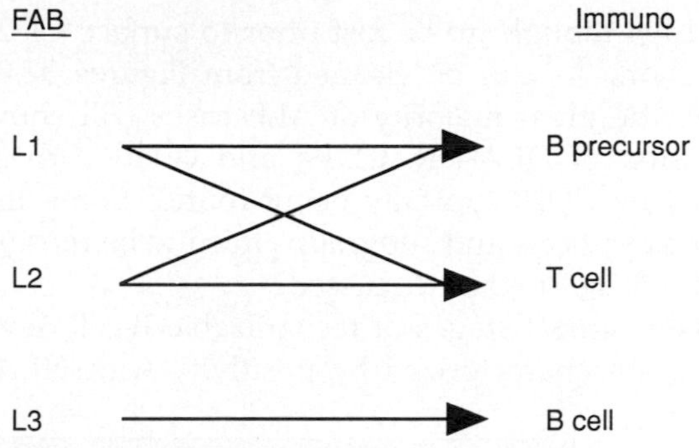

Figure 37.7. Correlation of FAB and immunophenotype in ALL.

monoclonal antibodies. This monoclonal antibody explosion led to a rapidly increasing knowledge of lymphoid development and the realization that virtually all the CALLA-positive, non–T-, non–B-cell ALLs were indeed of early B-cell lineage. Although other terminologies have been and are used to describe immunologic subgroups of ALL, we will refer to those leukemias reactive with B cell–associated antibodies as "B-precursor" ALL. Further subclassification of the B-precursor ALLs, into pro-B-cell ALL, pre-pre-B-cell ALL, etc., will not be used, as such distinctions do not currently have either therapeutic or prognostic relevance.

B-PRECURSOR ALL

A tremendous diversity of immunophenotypes can be identified in B-precursor ALL. Practical experience with immunophenotyping finds that the diagnosis of ALL is actually quite simple, to the relief of the diagnostician. However, it should also be recognized that there is only limited correlation between the FAB subtypes and immunologic results (Fig. 37.7).

The complexity of the various immunologic subgroups recognized within the B-precursor ALLs, however, has increased as the number of monoclonal antibodies to immature B-cells has grown. It has been postulated that the different stages of leukemic expression are representative of stages of normal pre–B-cell development and that, by inference, leukemias arise by clonal proliferation of cells arrested at a particular stage of normal maturation.

The CD19 antigen is recognized as an early pan–B-cell marker and is present in over 95% of ALL cases. Intracytoplasmic localization of the CD22 antigen has also been found at an early stage of normal B-cell differentiation; surface CD22 does not appear until later in immature B-cell development. The expression of CALLA or CD10 antigen occurs at the next level of development, followed by CD24. The fluorescence intensity of CD10 diminishes as the B-cell precursor undergoes maturation and CD20 expression begins.

CD10 is thought to be lost prior to surface CD22 expression. As can be gleaned from Figures 37.8 and 37.9, the great majority of ALL cases will show expression of HLA-DR, CD19, and CD10 with either CD34 or CD20 typically being found. Some important exceptions and subgroups need to be recognized and will be further discussed.

The earliest stages of recognizable B-cell development are characterized by positivity with HLA-DR, TdT, CD34, and CD19. This early B-lymphoid immunophenotype (with or without CD7) has been commonly associated with leukemias having translocations involving 11q23, in particular the t(4;11) translocation (Fig. 37.9). These t(4;11) leukemias commonly present in infancy, have a marked leukocytosis, and have an extremely short survival without response to chemotherapy. In addition, many of these leukemias will have a monocytic component at the time of diagnosis or relapse and are frequently associated with biphenotypic features. All these findings suggest that 11q23 leukemias arise very early in B-lymphocyte differentiation. Although earlier immunologic stages of B-cell differentiation are theoretically possible, characterized by HLA-DR, TdT, CD34, and CD7 expression and perhaps cytoplasmic expression of B-lineage antigens, only rare leukemias have been definitively identified with these findings.

In the latter stages of B-cell development, CD34 expression is absent, CD10 has diminished in intensity, and CD20 and/or CD22 can be identified for the first time. Cytoplasmic μ heavy chain is detectable at this latter stage and typifies the so-called pre–B-cell ALL (Figs. 37.8 and 37.9). No intact surface immunoglobulin can be identified. The terminology pre–B cell is used as an indication that these cells have evidence of B-cell commitment, i.e., cytoplasmic immunoglobulin heavy chain, but without an intact immunoglobulin molecule being identified. This subgroup

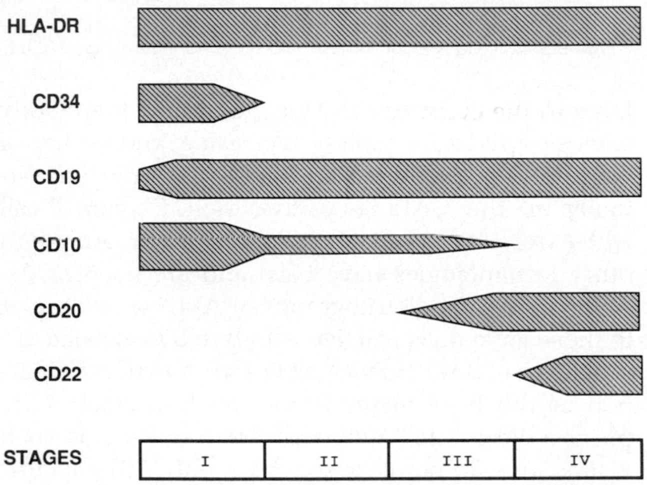

Figure 37.8. Proposed immunophenotypic stages of B-precursor lymphoid development. The narrower bars indicated decreased fluorescent intensity expression of that particular antigen (for example, CD10).

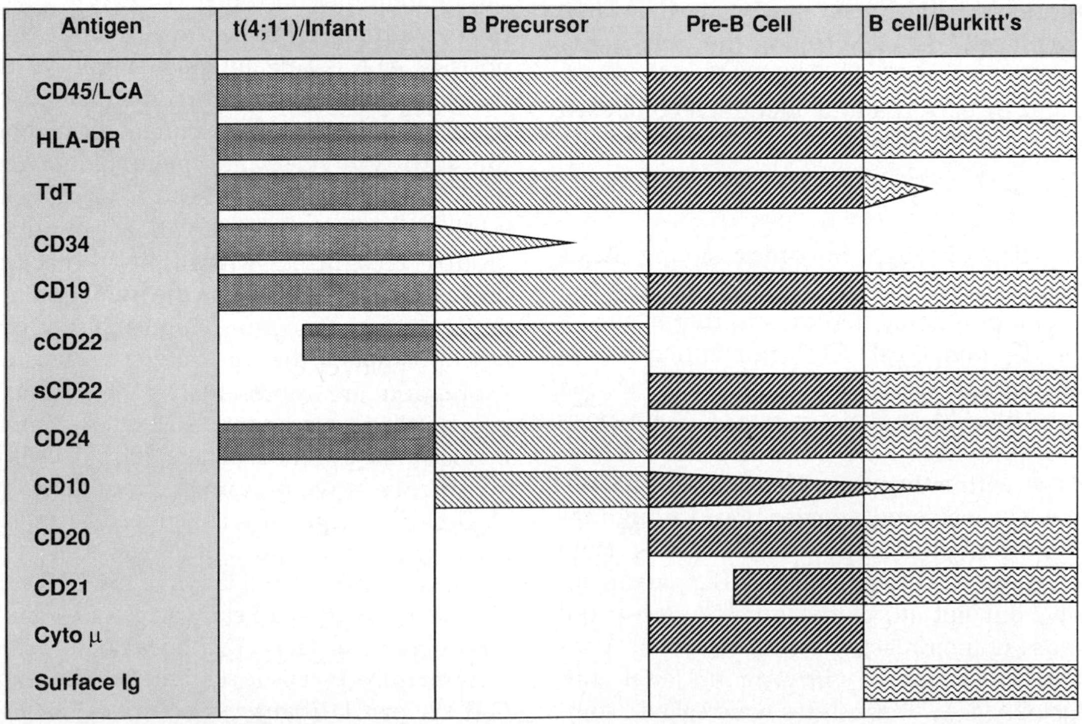

Figure 37.9. Immunophenotypes of B-precursor and B-cell ALL. The various antigens are listed in the left column. Four types of B-precursor and B-cell ALL are listed in the respective columns. cCD22 and sCD22 refer to the cytoplasmic and surface expression, respectively. Cyto μ corresponds to cytoplasmic expression of the immunoglobulin μ heavy chain.

constitutes 10 to 15% of the B-precursor ALL group and is commonly associated with a t(1;19) translocation.

The CD34 antigen also needs to be discussed in relation to the B-precursor ALL group. As mentioned earlier, CD34 is a hematopoietic progenitor cell antigen present very early in B-cell development. As the mature B cell goes through maturation and undergoes immunoglobulin heavy chain rearrangement, CD34 expression is lost. Most reports have described CD34 positivity in 50 to 60% of cases of B-precursor ALL. CD34 expression may also provide important prognostic information in ALL. A multi-institution study has shown that CD34-positive ALL has a better prognosis than CD34-negative ALL (2).

B-CELL ALL: BURKITT'S LEUKEMIA

The final and most differentiated type of ALL has detectable surface immunoglobulin. This corresponds to the original B-cell ALL group and morphologically represents ALL, FAB-L3, or what has been called "Burkitt's leukemia/lymphoma"; TdT reactivity is usually absent in such neoplasms. B-cell ALL will show positivity with CD21 in addition to the previously described B cell–associated monoclonal antibodies: HLA-DR, CD19, CD20, CD22, and CD24 (Fig. 37.9). CD10 expression is found in one-third to one half of B-cell ALL cases and is of much weaker intensity than that found in the typical B-precursor ALL.

T-CELL ACUTE LYMPHOBLASTIC LEUKEMIA

T-cell acute lymphoblastic leukemia (T-ALL) accounts for 10 to 15% of all ALL cases. It is usually associated with a marked leukocytosis; a mediastinal mass is found in over 50% of cases; male patients are favored; and median age is approximately 14 years. These patients have a high incidence of CNS relapse and a poorer survival than patients with B-precursor ALL. This survival difference has led some to conclude that immunophenotype may provide prognostic information. However, multivariate analysis has not shown that a T-cell phenotype is independent of WBC and age, both of which typically represent high risk factors in T-ALL.

The morphologic features of T-ALL are not uniquely specific for this subtype, but some findings need to be noted. The T-ALL cases are more likely to have a FAB-L1 appearance, having scant cytoplasm and relatively dense chromatin. A high mitotic rate is typically found and nuclear convolution may be evident. This latter finding, however, is neither a sensitive nor a specific feature of T-ALL and cannot be reliably used to differentiate this immunophenotypic subgroup from B-precursor ALL.

The anti-CD7, CD5, and CD2 monoclonal antibodies are the most sensitive markers that react with the leukemic blasts of T-ALL. In general, these three antigens are expressed in virtually all cases of genuine T-ALL (Fig. 37.10). Reactivity with other T-cell monoclonal antibodies in T-ALL in general correspond to intrathymic patterns of expression. The CD3 antigen has generally been reported in less than one-third of cases of T-ALL and T-lymphoblastic lymphoma, as evaluated by flow cytometric techniques. In contrast, several studies have observed CD3 expression in 95% of T-ALL/lymphoblastic lymphoma cases utilizing cryostat sections. This difference in results is related to the cytoplasmic detection of CD3 in cryostat sections. Several studies have now shown that cytoplasmic CD3 is present much earlier in thymic differentiation before the surface expression of CD3 and prior to the expression and rearrangement of the T-cell receptor gene. These data confirm that CD3 positivity is not relegated to the final stages of thymocyte development and can be a useful marker of early T-cell differentiation if a cytoplasmic method of detection is utilized. Cytoplasmic CD3 must therefore be considered as an essential antigen to be looked for if other markers of T-cell differentiation are equivocal.

Although CD7 has been promulgated as being the earliest marker of T-cell differentiation, one must use great caution in using this marker in isolation as evidence of T-cell differentiation. As will be discussed later, 5 to 10% of AMLs show expression with this marker. Likewise, the sole expression of CD2 without any other T cell–associated marker, should lead one to exercise caution before assigning the case as a definite T-ALL, since this marker can be identified in up to 5% of AML. Thus, if one identifies only one of the pan–T-cell markers listed above in a case of acute leukemia, it is essential that a wide battery of both T-cell markers, especially cytoplasmic CD3, and myeloid markers, including megakaryoblast-associated glycoproteins, be used to confidently distinguish between a T-cell and a myeloid process. Obviously, morphologic, cytochemical, and clinical findings are essential in confirming this distinction. Although CD1, surface CD3, CD4, and CD8 provide interesting information regarding the corresponding stage of thymic development of T-ALL, not much is gained from a diagnostic viewpoint, as these antigens are almost always expressed in conjunction with CD2, CD5, and CD7.

Other antigens not typically associated with T cells can be identified in T-ALL. Virtually all cases express the common leukocyte antigen CD45. CD10 (anti-CALLA) positivity is usually found in about 10 to 20% of cases of T-ALL. HLA-DR expression has also been found in 10 to 40% of T-ALL. Leukemic blasts in this disorder are also strongly positive for

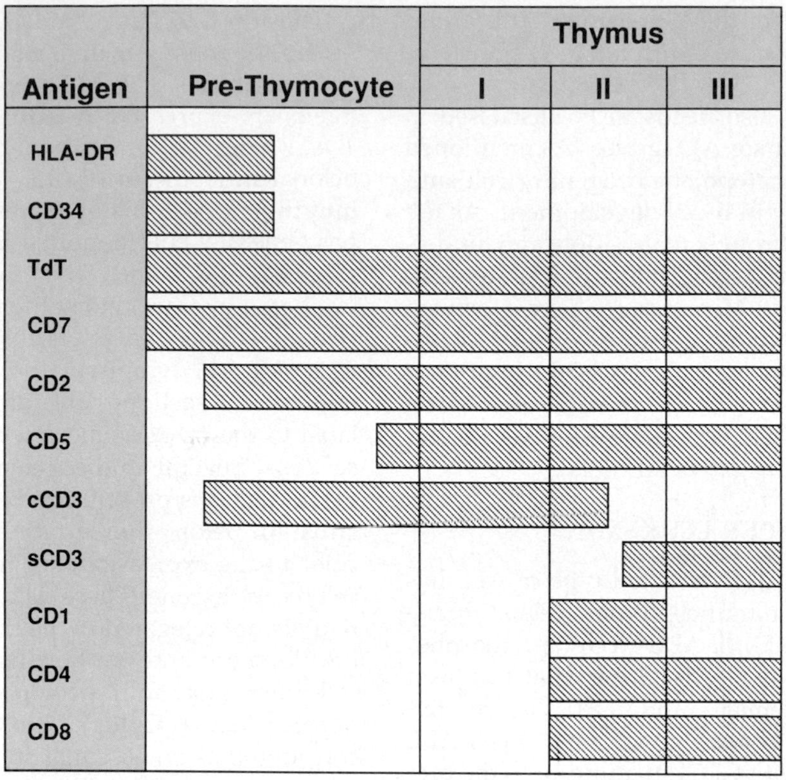

Figure 37.10. Correlation of immunophenotype and thymic stage of development in T-cell ALL. The respective antigens are listed in the left column and the various stages of thymic development in the rest of the table. cCD3 and sCD3 represent cytoplasmic and surface expression of the CD3 molecule, respectively.

TdT. CD34, a hematopoietic progenitor cell antigen, can be found in 10 to 20% of all T-ALL. This is in sharp contrast to 50 to 60% positivity found in B-precursor ALL. CD11b, CD11c, and CD15 are all antigens that are more typically associated with myeloid processes, but can also be found in 20 to 60% of T-ALL. Thus, one cannot use these antigens as strict evidence of a myeloid component.

Another interesting finding (but currently of uncertain clinical significance) is the recognition of different subtypes of T-ALL based on the type of T-cell antigen receptor present on the leukemic blasts. Over 95% of peripheral T-cell lymphocytes express the α/β heterodimer T-cell receptor, with the remainder expressing the γ/δ T-cell receptor. A higher percentage of T cells within epithelial locations express the γ/δ receptor than the α/β receptors. Within the thymus, γ/δ rearrangement is thought to occur prior to the α/β rearrangement process. Several investigators have now reported T-ALLs that express the γ/δ receptor. These have been identified primarily on the basis of expression of surface CD3 without CD4 or CD8. Although the status of the antigen receptor T-ALL has provided us with important biological information, no clinical or prognostic difference has been found between T-ALL with α/β receptor and T-ALL with γ/δ receptor. It is uncertain whether the identification of this subgroup has any clinical or prognostic importance.

Lymphoblastic Lymphoma

Malignant lymphoma, lymphoblastic type, is a high-grade lymphoma that occurs predominantly in older children and young adults; males are more frequently affected, and a mediastinal mass is often found. This neoplasm is often morphologically characterized by convoluted nuclei with fine chromatin and a high mitotic rate. Lymphoblastic lymphoma and T-ALL are closely related clinically and immunologically. The distinction between these disorders is usually based on the presentation of disease: tissue presentation generally indicates lymphoma, whereas marrow or blood presentation indicates leukemia. The proliferating cells in lymphoblastic lymphoma form E-rosettes and are reactive with multiple T cell–associated antibodies. Early studies of lymphoblastic lymphoma suggested that this type of lymphoma had a more "mature" immunophenotype than T-ALL, but this conclusion was probably falsely based on finding cytoplasmic CD3 and is not a significant finding. This lymphoma can be distinguished from other types of lymphoma on the basis of TdT positivity. Cells rarely express the pattern of reactivity seen

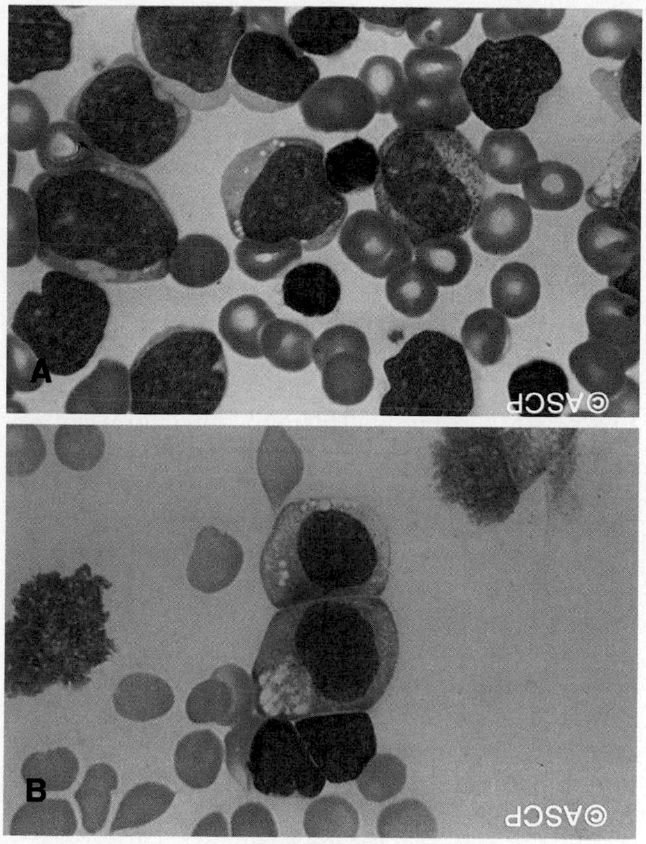

Figure 37.11. An acute leukemia with a t(4;11) translocation demonstrating both (**A**) lymphoid (L2) and (**B**) monocytic features.

in immature thymocytes; coexpression of CD4, CD8, and CD1 reactivity is also not as frequent a finding as in T-ALL.

Cytogenetics

Cytogenetic analysis may provide the most important prognostic information in childhood ALL. Several studies have now shown that by using high-resolution banding techniques over 90% of ALL patients had demonstrable clonal chromosomal abnormalities. Large international studies have shown that children and adults with ALL can be prognostically stratified according to the type of chromosomal abnormalities. Hyperdiploidy (more than 50 chromosomes) has been consistently shown to be a favorable prognostic feature and is an independent prognostic predictor of therapeutic response. In contrast, three particular translocations in ALL have been associated with very poor prognoses, short survivals, and poor responses to induction chemotherapy. These include the Philadelphia chromosome or t(9;22), t(4;11), and t(8;14). The Philadelphia chromosome occurs in approximately 5% of childhood ALL and up to 20 to 25% of adult ALL. Some of these may represent the blast crisis phase of chronic myelogenous leukemia, although molecular studies clearly indicate that many of these are de novo presentations of acute leukemia. ALL patients with the t(9;22) translocation typically are older, have marked leukocytosis, and have a B-precursor immunophenotype.

The t(4;11) translocation or any ALL involving 11q23 has been reported in up to 5% of cases of ALL. These cases typically have a FAB-L2 morphology, may frequently be associated with biphenotypia, and may occasionally show lineage switch to a monoblastic component (Fig. 37.11). The t(4;11) leukemias are most commonly identified in infant ALL (less than 2 years of age), usually present with a marked leukocytosis, and have a median survival of less than 1 year. Splenomegaly is commonly identified. The immunophenotype of this subgroup of ALL shows HLA-DR, CD34, and CD19 positivity; CD10 and CD20 are typically negative.

The t(8;14) translocation and its variants, t(2;8) and t(8;22), are always found in the B-ALL (surface immunoglobulin–positive) and FAB-L3 morphology subtype, i.e., the Burkitt's leukemias/lymphomas. These patients have short survivals and are characterized by surface immunoglobulin expression.

Survival and Prognosis

Several studies initially showed the relevance of the FAB classification in relationship to relapse rate and patient survival. The more FAB-L2 cells that were present within a bone marrow specimen, the more likely a nonresponse to chemotherapy was considered to be. Later, larger-scale comparisons failed to confirm these earlier findings of clinical differences between FAB-L1 and FAB-L2 subtypes. The main problem with using the FAB classification in ALL is the lack of reproducibility between various institutions and investigators. By using the newly defined criteria (Table 37.4), the FAB group has attempted to increase the reproducibility of classifying the ALLs.

Several clinical, hematologic, and laboratory criteria have been used to determine prognosis in patients with ALL (Table 37.8). Clinical and hematologic data have remained the stalwart of predicting therapeutic outcomes of patients with ALL, although cytogenetic data have certainly contributed positively. Major determinants for the prognosis of ALL include the initial white blood count, the degree of mediastinal involvement, and age. Children from 2 to 8 years of age do better than those younger or older, and infants less than 1 have a particularly bad prognosis. In children between the ages of 2 and 8 having white counts below 10.0×10^9/liter, a 90% cure rate can be achieved. Patients of any age presenting with WBCs above 50.0×10^9/liter have the

Table 37.8. Prognostic Groups of Childhood Acute Lymphoblastic Leukemia

Good prognosis (20%)	WBC <10.0 × 10^9/liter 2–8 Years of age
Average prognosis (60%)	WBC <10.0 × 10^9/liter <2 or >8 Years of age or WBC 10.0–50.0 × 10^9/liter Any age
Poor prognosis (20%)	WBC >50.0 × 10^9/liter

shortest survivals, and those with intermediate WBCs show intermediate survivals. The previously discussed cytogenetic factors have also been shown to be prognostically independent of age and white blood count and clearly add to the overall prognostic database. Other laboratory features that have at one time or another been used to assess prognosis include FAB-L2 morphology and T-cell immunophenotype. Both of these findings have not consistently been shown to be independent of age, WBC, and cytogenetic findings.

ACUTE MYELOGENOUS LEUKEMIA

Pathogenesis

The acute myelogenous leukemias are a heterogeneous group of malignancies originating in the hematopoietic, or myeloid, stem cell. The neoplastic proliferation seen in AML consists of myeloblasts or partially differentiated myeloid cells. This failure to show complete maturation by the neoplastic clone results in an accumulation of immature precursor cells and gradual replacement of normal bone marrow elements. To restate an earlier contention, AML is not a disorder of rapidly proliferating cells, but rather an accumulation of incompetent, long-surviving cells. The various subgroups or variants of AML basically reflect maturation arrest at various points in hematopoietic/myeloid differentiation. Thus, referring to Figure 37.1, one can rationalize the existence of the various morphologic subtypes of AML based on whether the granulocytic, monocytic, erythroid, or megakaryocytic arm of myeloid differentiation is involved.

The exact cause of this leukemia is obviously unknown. However, various risk factors for the development of AML are known, including chemical exposures, such as from benzene; alkylating agent chemotherapy; ionizing radiation; preceding myelodysplastic syndromes; aplastic anemia; paroxysmal nocturnal hemoglobinuria; syndromes with chromosome instability, such as Fanconi's anemia, ataxia-telangiectasia, and Bloom's syndrome; Down's syndrome; and rare forms of familial inheritance.

Clinical Manifestations

The most common clinical findings of AML at presentation are very similar to those described in patients with ALL. Symptoms are primarily related to increasing suppression of normal bone marrow elements leading to anemia, thrombocytopenia, and neutropenia. Splenomegaly is mild to moderate. Lymphadenopathy can be found in up to one-third of AML patients, but is not as uniform or pronounced as in ALL. Thymic involvement is exceedingly uncommon in AML. Cutaneous infiltration, however, is relatively common, occurring in up to 10% of AML patients. This and other forms of extramedullary involvement, such as the gingival tissue, are most commonly associated with those leukemias having a monocytic component. The terms chloroma, granulocytic sarcoma, and myeloblastoma all refer to the collection of leukemic cells in an extramedullary fashion. These extramedullary tumors may occur in soft tissues, the orbital region, ovaries, testes, gastrointestinal tract, breast, skin, and other sites. CNS involvement with AML is not as common as in ALL, but must still be considered as a possible complication of disease.

Incidence

AML is primarily a disease of adults. It constitutes approximately 45% of all leukemias but over 80% of all adult acute leukemias and less than 20% of childhood acute leukemia.

Laboratory Findings

In AML, the WBC is elevated in over half of patients at the time of diagnosis. Pancytopenia is a constant feature of this leukemia. The number of blasts in the peripheral blood varies according to the subtype of AML and depends on the degree of maturation and differentiation that characterizes that particular leukemic subtype. Up to 10% of patients will have WBC counts that are greater than 100.0 × 10^9/liter, with some patients approaching 500.0 × 10^9/liter. Patients with WBCs greater than 50.0 to 100.0 × 10^9/liter are at risk of developing complications due to hyperleukocytosis. Leukophoresis is mandated in these patients and is an essential part of the therapeutic process. Serum uric acid level is typically elevated in about two-thirds of patients with AML. Serum lactate dehydrogenase (LDH) level is typically not higher than in ALL.

Morphology and FAB Classification

The French-American-British (FAB) group on acute leukemia has morphologically subclassified the

Table 37.9. FAB Classification of Acute Myelogenous Leukemia

M0	Acute leukemia, undifferentiated; myeloid immunophenotype
M1	AML without maturation
M2	AML with maturation
M3	Acute promyelocytic leukemia (APL)
M3v	Hypogranular variant of APL
M4	Acute myelomonocytic leukemia (AMMoL)
M4e	M4 with eosinophilia
M5a	Acute monoblastic leukemia (AMoL)
M5b	Acute monocytic leukemia (AMoL)
M6	Acute erythroleukemia
M7	Acute megakaryoblastic leukemia

Table 37.10. Incidence of AML According to FAB Subtype

FAB Subtype	Incidence
	%
M0	?
M1	18
M2	28
M3	8
M4	27
M5	10
M6	4
M7	5

acute myelogenous leukemias into seven major subtypes: FAB-M1 to FAB-M7. The FAB classification of AML basically relies on the degree of granulocytic, monocytic, erythroid, and megakaryocytic differentiation. This is based on the morphologic appearance of cells, the number of leukemic blasts, and cytochemical findings with myeloid-associated enzymatic stains. Important variants of these seven subtypes also exist. The National Cancer Institute has proposed revised standards for the classification of AML, including another subtype based on immunophenotyping (FAB-M0). The various subtypes of AML are listed in Table 37.9. The incidences of the AML subgroups are listed in Table 37.10.

The importance of the FAB classification of AML lies not in its ability to provide important prognostic information to the patient, but rather its ability to provide precise and consistent classification of AML subtypes. The ability to reproduce the various FAB subgroups morphologically and cytochemically is well proven and allows for knowledge interaction and consistency between institutions and physicians.

The basic definition of an AML is a leukemia that has more than 30% myeloblasts in the bone marrow. Myeloblasts may be grouped into three different subtypes: type I, type II, and type III. Type I myeloblasts are undifferentiated blasts that have no evidence of granulocytic differentiation, i.e., they contain no cytoplasmic granulation or Auer rods (Fig. 37.12). Auer rods are absolutely specific for a leukemic myelogenous process and consist of abnormally fused pri-

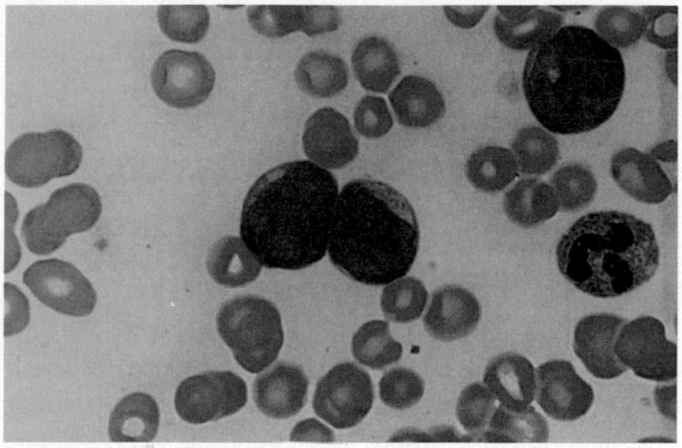

Figure 37.12. Type I (left cell) and II (right cell) myeloblasts.

mary granules. Auer rods are needle- to fusiform-like eosinophilic rods that are found in the cytoplasm of leukemic myeloid cells and stain red to purple with Wright-Giesma stain.

Type II blasts are leukemic blasts that have relatively few cytoplasmic granules (Fig. 37.12). It is too rigid to specify the exact number of these granules; however, most morphologists would define type II blasts as having fewer than 8 to 12 granules per cell. The newly defined type III blasts are cells intermediate between type II blasts and promyelocytes. Obviously, this distinction may be quite difficult to make at times, but it is generally relegated to cells that have the nuclear characteristics of blasts (fine chromatin and prominent nucleoli) but with more granules than in the type II blasts. The cytoplasm retains its basophilic appearance.

The National Cancer Institute's expanded definition of blasts is listed in Table 37.11 and includes the type I, type II, and type III blasts discussed previously. Also included in their basic definition of blasts are the abnormal promyelocytes seen in FAB-M3, the monoblasts and promonocytes of FAB-M4 and FAB-M5, and the megakaryoblasts of FAB-M7. Erythroblasts, including early pronormoblasts, are not included in the definition of a leukemic blast.

FAB-M0: ACUTE MYELOGENOUS LEUKEMIA WITHOUT MATURATION

The FAB-M0 group of AML is a recently recognized subgroup that is based on immunophenotyping analysis. These AMLs consist of small to intermediate size leukemic blasts without any evidence of granulocytic differentiation (Fig. 37.13). Cytochemical staining with myeloperoxidase, Sudan black B, and nonspecific esterase is negative. Thus, from a strict morphologic and cytochemical analysis, these cases would be classified as ALL. However, by flow cytometric immunophenotyping, these cases will show reactivity with one or more myeloid-associated markers, such as CD13, CD33, or CD15, while lacking any expression of lymphoid-associated markers.

FAB-M1: ACUTE MYELOGENOUS LEUKEMIA WITHOUT MATURATION

In these AMLs without maturation, there is minimal evidence of cytoplasmic granulation and minimal numbers of Auer rods. The blasts are intermediate in size with finely recitular chromatin, small amounts of grayish-blue cytoplasm, and typically one or more prominent nucleoli (Fig. 37.14). Basic FAB criteria for AML-M1 include the following: (*a*) the sum of total blasts is greater than 90% of the bone marrow cells; (*b*) less than 10% of bone marrow cells show evidence of granulocytic differentiation at or beyond the promyelocyte stage; and (*c*) at least 3% of the leukemic blasts demonstrate myeloperoxidase and/or Sudan black B positivity. The differential diagnosis in this disorder would include ALL-L2, AML-M5a, and AML-M7. Immunophenotyping and cytochemical staining is usually necessary to make the distinction between these subtypes of leukemias.

FAB-M2: ACUTE MYELOGENOUS LEUKEMIA WITH MATURATION

The AMLs with maturation are the most common subtype of AML. These leukemias show clear evidence of differentiation at or beyond the promyelocyte stage, and Auer rods are commonly identified (Fig. 37.15). These cells usually have more cytoplasm than is found in FAB-M1 leukemic cells, and fewer undifferentiated blasts are seen. From a diagnostic viewpoint, this subtype of AML is easy to diagnose and creates little diagnostic consternation. The basic FAB criteria for FAB-M2 include the following: (*a*) the sum of blasts is greater than 30%, but less than 90%

Table 37.11. Expanded Blast Definition: National Cancer Institute

Type I blast: no granules
Type II blast: "few" granules
Type III blast: "multiple" granules; central nucleolus; fine chromatin
Abnormal promyelocytes of M3
Monoblasts/promonocytes of M5
Megakaryoblasts of M7
Erythroblasts should *not* be included

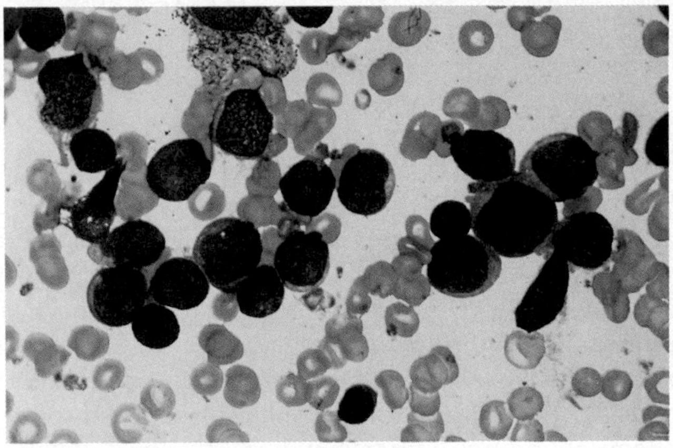

Figure 37.13. AML-M0.

Table 37.12. FAB Classification of Acute Myelogenous Leukemia

FAB Subtype	Diagnostic Criteria
M0	No morphologic evidence of differentiation Negative cytochemical staining with MPO/SBB/NSE Positivity with myeloid markers (CD13, CD33, etc.) and negative lymphoid markers
M1	≥90% blasts in bone marrow <10% of marrow showing granulocytic differentiation >3% of blasts with MPO or SBB positivity
M2	≥30% blasts and <90% blasts in marrow ≥10% of marrow showing granulocytic differentiation ≤20% monocytic cells
M3	≥30% of marrow or abnormal promyelocytes
M3v	Same as M3 except composed of hypogranular variants
M4	≥30% blasts ≤80% myeloblasts and granulocytic precursors in marrow >20% monocytic cells in marrow (morphology/NSE stain/serum lysozyme)
M4e	Same as M4 with increased number of atypical/immature marrow eosinophils
M5a	≥80% monoblasts
M5b	≥80% of monoblasts/promonocytes/monocytes <80% monoblasts in marrow
M6	≥50% nucleated RBC Prominent dyserythropoiesis ≥30% myeloblasts in nonerythroid cells
M7	≥30% blasts Identification of megakaryoblasts by ultrastructural cytochemistry or by immunophenotyping

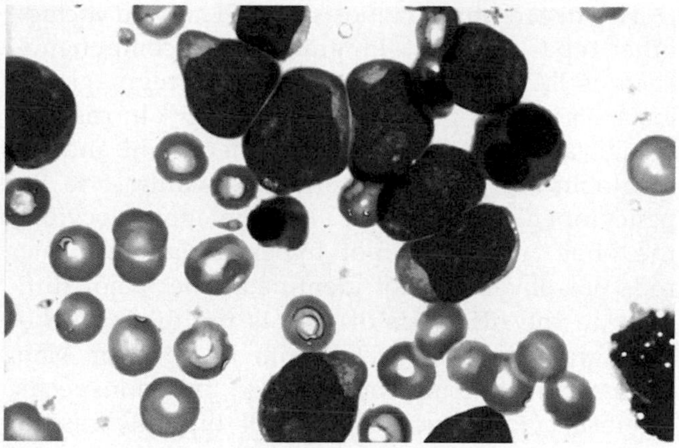

Figure 37.14. AML-M1.

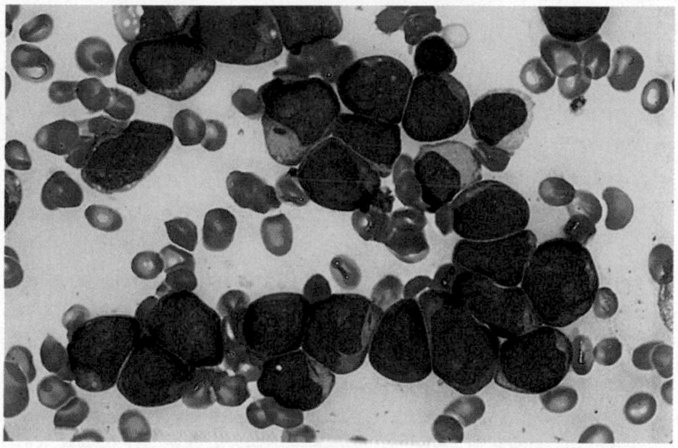

Figure 37.15. AML-M2 with numerous single Auer rods.

of the bone marrow cells; (*b*) more than 10% of the bone marrow cells show evidence of granulocytic differentiation; and (*c*) monocytic cells constitute fewer than 20% of the bone marrow cells. It should also be noted that dysplastic features may be identified in the granulocytic, erythroid, and/or megakaryocytic series. Frank panmyelosis is uncommon but can be seen in some cases. Although most bone marrow specimens are hypercellular and show frank replacement of all bone marrow elements, some patients, mainly the elderly, may have bone marrows that are moderately hypocellular.

The differential diagnosis of FAB-M2 would include a leukemoid reaction, a myelodysplastic syndrome that does not meet the criteria of AML, and possibly other types of AML having a granulocytic component such as FAB-M3, FAB-M4, or possibly FAB-M6.

A specific bone marrow chromosome abnormality, t(8;21), has been observed in some cases of FAB-M2. The percentage of patients with the t(8;21) translocation has varied from 30% to less than 5% of FAB-M2s in various literature reports. Patients having AML-M2 with a t(8;21) are believed to have a good prognosis.

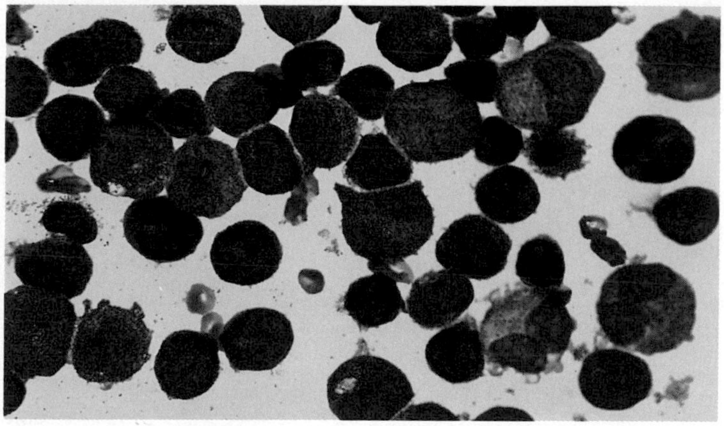

Figure 37.16. AML-M3 (APL).

The morphologic features of FAB-M2 with a t(8;21) include larger myeloblasts, easily identified and numerous Auer rods, and a distinctive dysmyelopoiesis in the developing granulocytic cells. This dysmyelopoiesis has been described as a "crushed" orange granularity in the cytoplasm of the granulocytic cells.

FAB-M3: ACUTE PROMYELOCYTIC LEUKEMIA

Acute promyelocytic leukemia (APL) can be diagnosed when more than 30% of the bone marrow cells are abnormal promyelocytes. These promyelocytes have abnormally dense and heavy granulation. One of the characteristic features of APL are the so-called faggot cells, which are cells that contain multiple Auer rods that may be bundled, intertwined, or fused together (Figs. 37.16 and 37.17). The granules of the promyelocyte are larger and darker staining than normal and at times may be so numerous as to obscure nuclear borders. Intensely basophilic cytoplasm may be present in some cells. The nuclear features, which are frequently ignored or even obscured by the granulation, typically have a "monocytoid," bilobed, or kidney-bean shape. It is uncommon for this type of AML to have a significant percentage of blasts. In a large series of APLs, the median blast count was only 12%. These patients are typically leukopenic at presentation and are clinically characterized by disseminated intravascular coagulation (DIC) and bleeding.

Approximately 20% of APLs are a variant form of FAB-M3 and are designated as microgranular or hypogranular APL (M3v). The leukemic cells in this FAB-M3 variant are characterized by sparse and/or fine granulation and a strikingly irregular nuclear shape (Fig. 37.18). Their identity as abnormal promyelocytes may be obscured by the scarcity of granulation and the nuclear shape. Cells containing multiple Auer rods are usually present, but they may be extremely difficult to identify since they are certainly

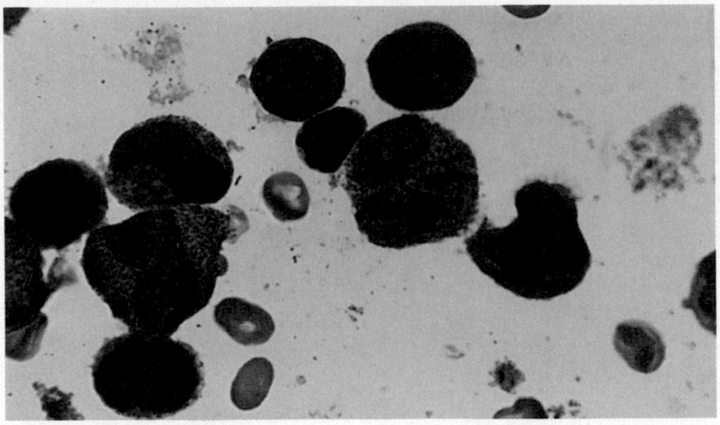

Figure 37.17. AML-M3 (APL-Faggot cell).

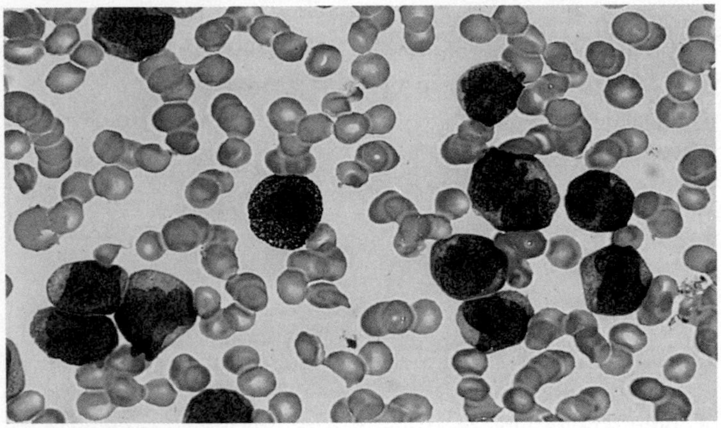

Figure 37.18. AML-M3 variant (hypogranular APL).

less abundant than in the typical hypergranular FAB-M3. The variant form of APL has the same incidence of DIC described previously, but will more likely present with leukocytosis at the time of diagnosis. The obvious differential diagnostic problem relates to the confusion with acute myelomonocytic (M4) or acute monocytic (M5b) leukemia.

APL may occur at any age but is most common in young adults, with a median age of diagnosis of 35 to 40 years. The most outstanding clinical feature associated with APL is the high frequency of DIC. This is due to the release of procoagulant factors from the cytoplasmic granules, which leads to activation of the coagulation cascade. In many patients there is severe DIC and hemorrhage prior to or during induction of therapy, when the malignant cell contents are lysed and released. Hemorrhage is the cause of death in many patients. Thus, it is essential that this subgroup of AML be accurately diagnosed rapidly so that appropriate chemotherapy and supportive care can be initiated. If the DIC and hemorrhage are adequately controlled and treated, patients with this subgroup of AML probably have the best prognostic outcome of any AML group.

The differential diagnosis of APL would include other types of AML with granulocytic components, such as FAB-M2, FAB-M4/M5, and benign agranulocytosis with a promyelocyte "arrest." In cases of benign agranulocytosis, the platelet count and hemoglobin are generally normal, in contrast to the pancytopenia seen in APL. Also, in agranulocytosis the bone marrow is not hypercellular and Auer rods are obviously not identified. The major difficulty in the diagnosis of APL is the distinction of microgranular APL (M3v) from FAB-M4 or M5b. Evaluation with myeloperoxidase and nonspecific esterase cytochemical stains will typically resolve this tissue.

FAB-M4: ACUTE MYELOMONOCYTIC LEUKEMIA

Acute myelomonocytic leukemia and FAB-M2 are the most common AMLs, together accounting for approximately two-thirds of all AML cases. The FAB-M4 subgroup of AML is probably the most difficult subgroup of AML in which to perform a reliable differential count, as this is a very heterogeneous-appearing leukemia. Both granulocytic and monocytic differentiation are present in varying proportions in the bone marrow (Fig. 37.19). It may be difficult to clearly identify the granulocytic and monocytic component, as hybrid cells clearly exist in this type of leukemia. The criteria for the diagnosis of FAB-M4 includes the following elements: (*a*) the sum of all blasts is greater than 30%; (*b*) the sum of myeloblasts and granulocytic precursor cells account for less than 80% of the bone marrow cells; (*c*) more than 20% of the bone marrow cells are of the monocytic lineage as demonstrated by morphology, nonspecific esterase cytochemical stain, or elevated serum lysozyme level (3 times normal). Thus, granulocytic and monocytic precursors coexist in proportions varying reciprocally from 20 to 80%. Auer rods may also be identified in approximately half of the cases. Because of the difficulty in the morphologic identification of both promonocytes and hybrid granulocytic/monocytic cells in bone marrow, additional diagnostic criteria utilizing nonspecific esterase and elevated serum lysozyme levels have been used. Organomegaly, lymphadenopathy, and other sites of tissue infiltration may commonly be encountered.

A variant of FAB-M4 exists, which has been called FAB-M4 with eosinophilia (M4e). Criteria for diagnosis include the usual diagnostic criteria for FAB-M4 and an increased number of atypical, immature bone marrow eosinophils (Fig. 37.20). There is not a peripheral blood esoinophilia identified in this variant. The immature and atypical eosinophils contain an abundance of large basophilic-staining granules in

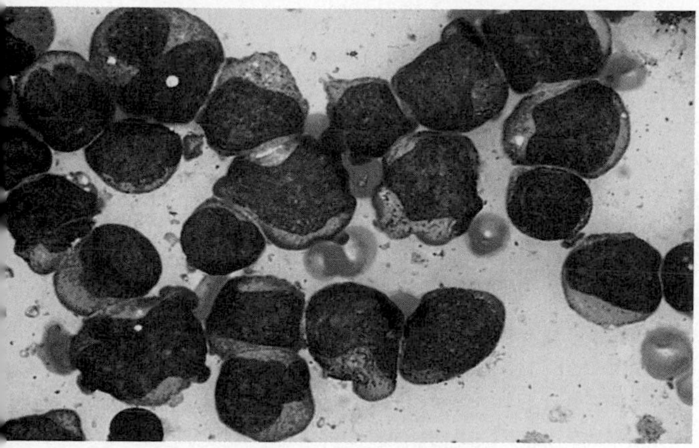

Figure 37.19. AML-M4.

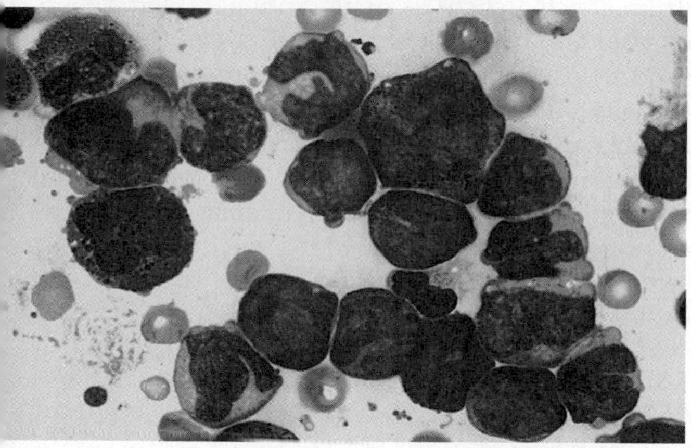

Figure 37.20. AML-M4 with eosinophilia.

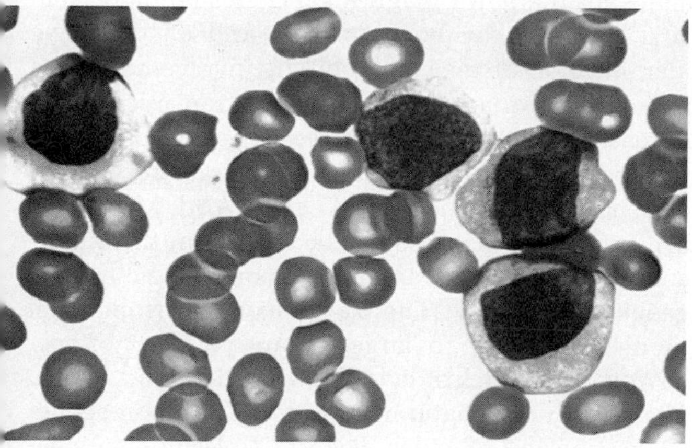

Figure 37.21. AML-M5a.

addition to the large, red eosinophilic granules that characterize a mature eosinophil. Abnormalities of chromosome 16, including inversion of 16(p13;q22) or deletion of 16q22, are consistently identified in this variant. This type of leukemia has a high rate of remission following the initial induction of therapy compared to other types of AMLs, and diagnosis of this variant is considered a good prognostic sign. Morbidity, however, due to an increased incidence of central nervous system relapse with leptomeningeal infiltration and pulmonary involvement, may occur in this subtype of AML.

FAB-M5A: ACUTE MONOBLASTIC LEUKEMIA (M5A) AND FAB-M5B: ACUTE MONOCYTIC LEUKEMIA (M5B)

FAB-M5a is characterized by a predominance of monoblasts that are large and have relatively abundant cytoplasm. Some azurophilic granules may be identified in the cytoplasm that are myeloperoxidase negative. The nucleus is typically round to oval with finely reticular chromatin and prominent nucleoli. Typically, the nucleus is displaced to one side with an ample amount of cytoplasm wrapping around the nucleus (Fig. 37.21). The sole criterion for diagnosis of FAB-M5a is the existence of more than 80% monoblasts in the bone marrow. This differs slightly from the criteria for FAB-M5b, in which more than 80% of the marrow cells are monoblasts, promonocytes, or monocytes but less than 80% of the marrow cells are monoblasts. In other words, FAB-M5b shows more differentiation than FAB-M5a. Nuclear folding and irregularity is common in FAB-M5b, and more azurophilic granulation is identified than in FAB-M5a (Fig. 37.22). Both FAB-M5a and FAB-M5b are associated with a high incidence of extramedullary infiltration; DIC may also develop in patients with FAB-M5, second in incidence only to FAB-M3 among classes of AML. Nonspecific esterase cytochemical stains are positive in the FAB-M5 leukemias. Auer rods may be seen in a small percentage of monoblasts, but are certainly much less frequent than in the granulocytic types of AML. AML-M5a is more commonly diagnosed in the pediatric age group.

FAB-M6: ACUTE ERYTHROLEUKEMIA (DI GUGLIELMO'S SYNDROME)

Acute erythroleukemia is a relatively uncommon variant of AML and may have multiple presenting appearances. One form, which has previously been called erythemic myelosis, is characterized by bizarre and markedly atypical megablastoid changes accompanied by extreme erythroid hyperplasia within the bone marrow (Fig. 37.23). Few, if any, myeloblasts can be identified. Normal granulocytic and megakaryocytic precursors are not identified and are replaced by giant, multinucleated, and markedly dysplastic erythroblasts. In other cases of FAB-M6, the marrow contains more differentiated, albeit dysplastic, erythroblasts at the time of presentation along with a definite population of granulocytic cells, in-

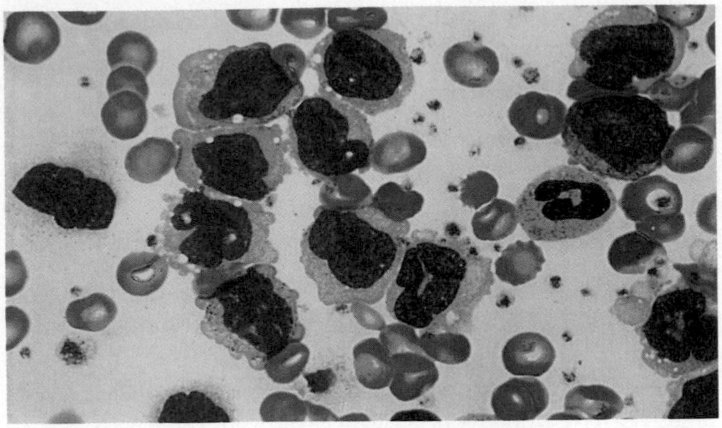

Figure 37.22. AML-M5b.

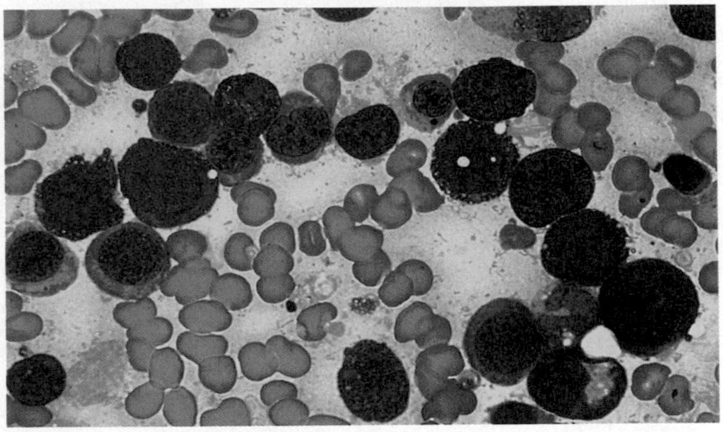

Figure 37.23. AML-M6 (erythemic myelosis).

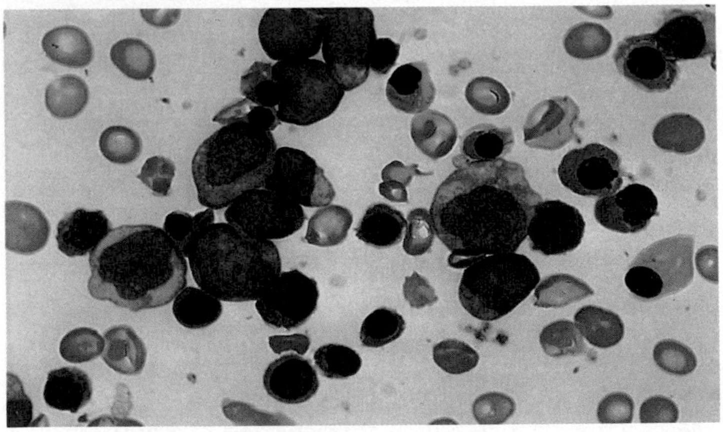

Figure 37.24. AML-M6.

cluding myeloblasts (Fig. 37.24). In 1985, the following criteria were established by the FAB group for the diagnosis of erythroleukemia in determining blast percentage: (*a*) 50% or more of all nucleated bone marrow cells must be erythroblasts; (*b*) dyserythropoiesis is prominent; (*c*) 30% or more of the nonerythroid cells in the bone marrow are myeloblasts.

Erythroleukemia will frequently evolve into other types of AML such as FAB-M1, M2, or M4. Auer rods may be identified in the myeloblasts in these cases. The leukemic erythroblasts frequently contain a "frothy" or "foamy" vacuolation in the cytoplasm. Progression of the disease is frequently marked by an increase in myeloblasts and a decrease in erythroblasts. A striking erythroblastemia may be identified in the peripheral blood. It is quite common for erythroleukemia to evolve from myelodysplastic syndromes or as a secondary leukemia in patients who have received prior radiation and/or alkylating agent chemotherapy. The differential diagnosis for erythroleukemia includes B_{12}/folate deficiency, heavy metal intoxication (such as arsenic), drug effects (such as with antineoplastic agents or chloramphenicol), congenital dyserythropoietic syndromes, myelodysplastic syndromes, and potentially other types of AML. The dysplastic erythroblasts are typically PAS positive, which reflects a cytoplasmic maturation defect. This cytochemical finding is not restricted to leukemia and can be identified in benign disorders, such as β-thalassemia, iron deficiency, sideroblastic anemia, and heavy metal intoxication.

FAB-M7: ACUTE MEGAKARYOBLASTIC LEUKEMIA

Acute megakaryoblastic leukemia has only recently been added to the FAB classification. The diagnostic criteria for diagnosis includes (*a*) more than 30% blasts in the bone marrow and (*b*) definitive identification of megakaryoblastic involvement by a platelet peroxidase reaction by electron microscopy or reactivity with megakaryocyte-specific monoclonal antibodies. The differential diagnosis of megakaryoblastic leukemia includes ALL-L2, AML-M0, AML-M1, and AML-M5a. As can be seen from this differential diagnostic list, there is a morphologic heterogeneity to FAB-M7. The blasts may vary from small to medium-sized to large, bizarre blasts typically having high, nuclear:cytoplasmic ratios (Fig. 37.25). The nuclear chromatin may be dense and homogeneous or fine and reticular. There is typically scanty basophilic cytoplasm, which may or may not be vacuolated. Indeed, the degree of basophilia may be comparable to that found in erythroleukemia, reflecting the close developmental relationship between erythroid and megakaryoblastic precursors. An irregular cytoplasmic border may be noted in some of the megakaryoblasts resembling pseudopods. Very fine granulation can be identified in the cytoplasm of some blasts. Intermediate forms between undifferentiated blasts and definitive micromegakaryocytes

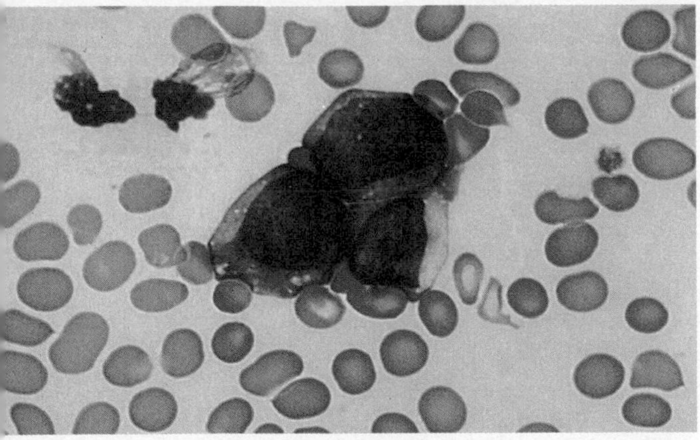

Figure 37.25. AML-M7.

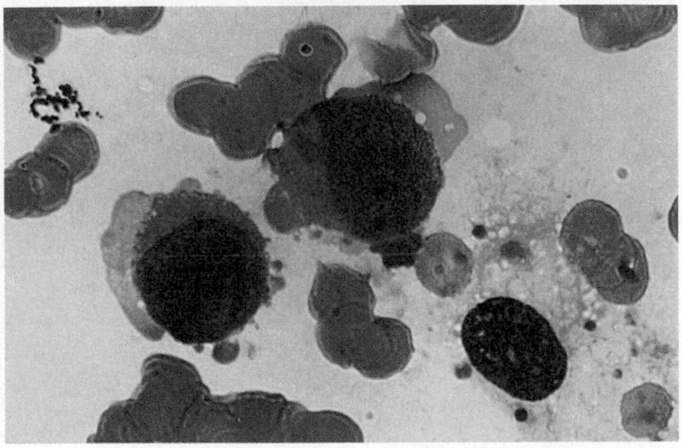

Figure 37.26. AML-M7.

Table 37.13. Diagnosis of Acute Megakaryoblastic Leukemia

Aspirate morphology
Trephine section histology
Routine cytochemistry
Immunophenotyping
Ultrastructure

may also be seen (Fig. 37.26). Some cases may show little if any differentiation and resemble the lymphoblasts of FAB-L2.

The diagnosis of FAB-M7 relies on multiple criteria including peripheral blood and bone marrow aspirate smear morphology, bone marrow trephine section histology, routine cytochemical stains, immunophenotyping, and ultrastructural studies (Table 37.13). In some cases, the peripheral blood and bone marrow aspirate morphology may be sufficient to make the diagnosis, while in other cases, more sophisticated diagnostic modalities may be needed to confirm the diagnosis of FAB-M7. Some cases of FAB-M7 have morphologic features suggestive of a megakaryoblastic process, including the presence of circulating micromegakaryocytes, atypical platelets, or the presence of myelofibrosis and atypical megakaryocytes in the bone marrow sections (Fig. 37.27).

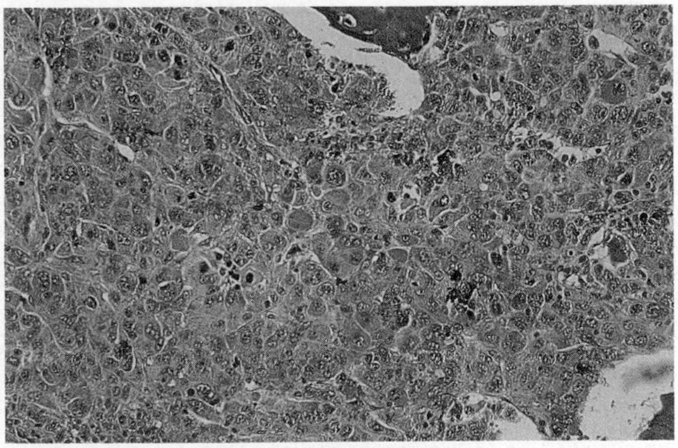

Figure 37.27. AML-M7 (bone marrow biopsy).

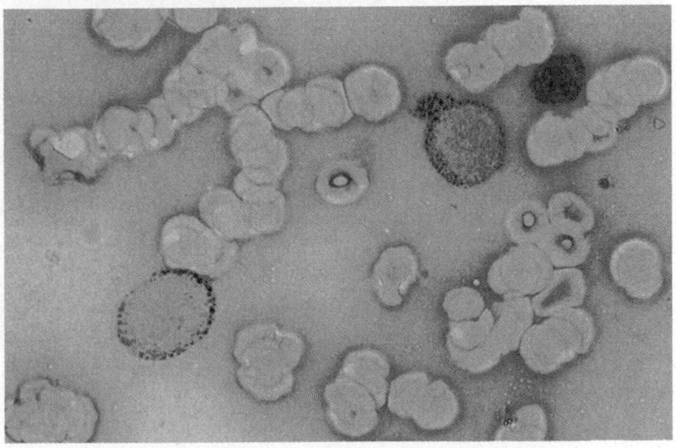

Figure 37.28. AML-M7: PAS cytochemical stain.

Cytochemically, megakaryoblasts show no reactivity with myeloperoxidase or Sudan black B. A diffuse, coarse granular positivity is typically seen with PAS, not to be confused with the chunky staining seen in ALL (Fig. 37.28). Megakaryoblasts show no reactivity with α-naphthyl butyrate esterase, but can manifest strong reactivity with the acetate substrate of nonspecific esterase (NSE) (Fig. 37.29). This latter discrepancy between the butyrate and acetate substrates of NSE can be a very useful diagnostic feature of FAB-M7. Immunophenotyping with monoclonal antibodies reactive with platelet glycoprotein (Gp) IIb/IIIa or Gp IIIa has provided for a more sensitive and reproducible method of detecting megakaryoblasts. These antibodies are discussed in more detail in the subsequent section on immunophenotyping.

The ultimate gold standard for the diagnosis of FAB-M7 is the identification of platelet peroxidase by ultracytochemistry with electron microscopy. Ultrastructural peroxidase activity is found in the nuclear

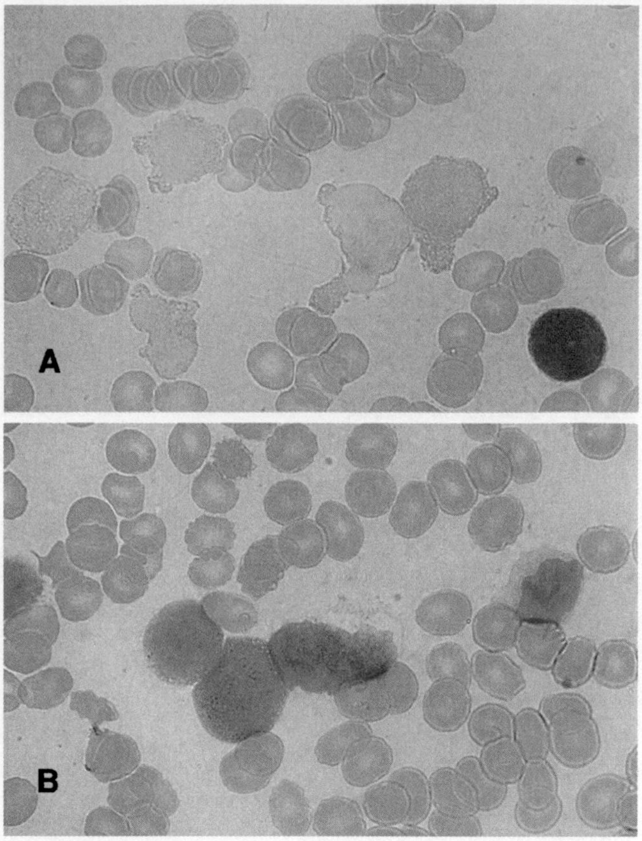

Figure 37.29. AML-M7 nonspecific esterase stain: (**A**) butyrate; and (**B**) acetate substrates.

Table 37.14. Cytochemical Staining in Acute Myelogenous Leukemia

Stain[a]	M1	M2	M3	M4	M5	M6	M7
MPO	+	+	+	+	−	+/−	−
SBB	+	+	+	+	−	+/−	−
CAE	+/−	+	+	+	+/−	+/−	−
NSE-b	−	−	−	+	+	−	−
NSE-a	−	−	−	+	+	−	+
ACP	−	−	−	+	+	−	+
PAS	−/+	−/+	−	−	+/−	+	+
TdT[b]	−	−	−	−	−	−	−

[a]MPO, myeloperoxidase; SBB, Sudan black B; CAE, chloroacetate esterase; NSE-b, nonspecific esterase butyrate; NSE-a, nonspecific esterase acetate; ACP, acid phosphatase; PAS, periodic acid–Schiff; TdT, terminal deoxynucleotidyl transferase.
[b]Between 10 and 20% of AML will be TdT positive.

envelope and endoplasmic reticulum, but is absent from the granules and golgi of the leukemic megakaryoblasts. This pattern is distinctly opposite that found in myeloblasts by ultracytochemistry.

Acute megakaryoblastic leukemia is commonly associated with patients that have Down's syndrome, therapy-related acute leukemias, and blast crises of chronic myeloproliferative disorders. Clinical features of FAB-M7 are variable and can occur in both children and adults. A marked leukocytosis is relatively uncommon in M7 and typically is not associated with extramedullary involvement, lymphadenopathy, or hepatosplenomegaly.

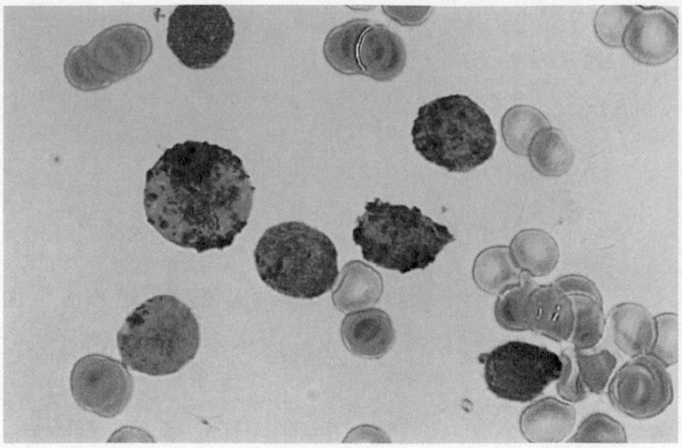

Figure 37.30. Myeloperoxidase stain of AML-M2.

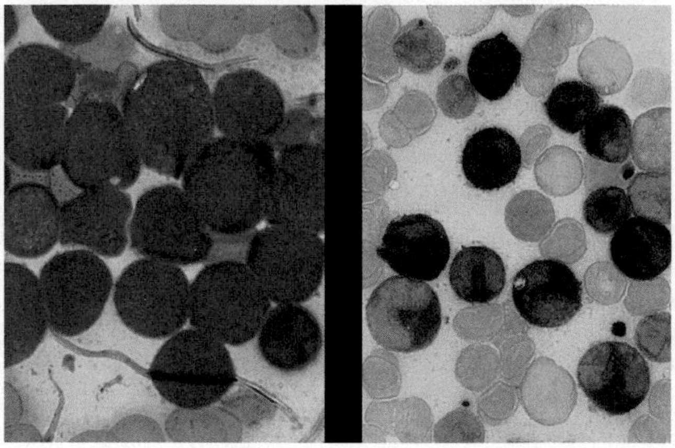

Figure 37.31. Sudan black B *(left)* and NSE (butyrate) *(right)* stain of AML-M4.

Cytochemistry

Table 37.14 shows the distribution of cytochemical staining in AML. In general, it can be noted that the AMLs with a granulocytic component will stain with myeloperoxidase (MPO), Sudan black B (SBB), and chloroacetate esterase (CAE) (Figs. 37.30 and 37.31), and those with a monocytic component will react with nonspecific esterase (NSE) and acid phosphatase (ACP) (Figs. 37.31 and 37.32). Megakaryoblastic staining has been previously discussed.

MPO is an enzyme present within the primary granules of the granulocytic series, including granulocytes, eosinophils, and some basophils. Monocytes also contain peroxidase granules but are present in very small numbers and never pose a serious problem when interpreting such a stain. Lymphoid and erythroid cells do not stain with MPO. We have found MPO to be the most sensitive marker for granulocytic differentiation; however, MPO stains will

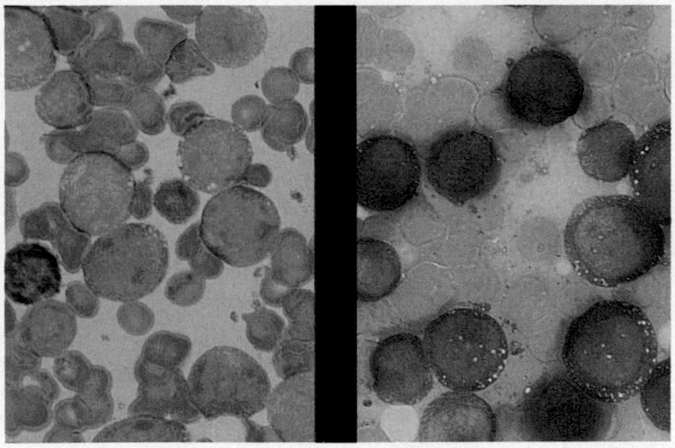

Figure 37.32. NSE (butyrate) stain of AML-M5a.

fade with time; for this reason SBB is also commonly used and is a good alternative to MPO. SBB stains intracellular lipids that are within the primary granules of the granulocyte series. This is easily detected within myeloblasts and the rest of the granulocyte series. Lymphoblasts, however, may also show an occasional rare, small positive granule. Thus, one must interpret SBB with some caution. CAE, or specific esterase/Leder stain, is confined to the primary granules of differentiated granulocytes. Myeloblasts are typically lacking in this enzyme. Monocytes, lymphocytes, and erythroid cells are negative with this enzyme stain. CAE is not as sensitive as MPO or SBB.

Nonspecific esterase (NSE) is a particularly useful stain for the monocyte series. Little, if any, staining of the granulocytic series will be found. T lymphocytes and T lymphoblasts typically show a distinct punctate, perinuclear positivity that is easily distinguished from monocyte staining. The butyrate esterase gives a clearer and more definitive stain compared to the acetate substrate of NSE and is the preferred monocyte-associated enzyme stain. It gives a deep, brick-red stain that is easy to interpret and distinguish from background staining, as opposed to the faint positivity seen with the acetate substrate of NSE. The acetate NSE activity can also be found in megakaryocytes, platelets, and some basophils and plasma cells. Fluoride sensitivity is used by some laboratories to help differentiate between different NSE-positive cells. The NSE reactivity found in monocytes is blocked by fluoride and is partially blocked in megakaryocytes. NSE staining found in lymphocytes and lymphoblasts, however, is not sensitive to fluoride treatment. Occasional cases of B-precursor ALL also show a faint blush in the golgi area of such lymphoblasts; this is also fluoride resistant.

As mentioned in the ALL section, PAS may stain some cases of AML, thus limiting its diagnostic use as a specific ALL marker. TdT reactivity can also be found in up to 20% of AML cases, although it is usually dimmer and positive in a lower percentage of cells than in typical ALL.

Immunophenotype of AML

The diagnosis of acute myelogenous leukemia is usually a straightforward diagnosis made on the basis of morphology and cytochemical staining. Immunophenotyping of potential cases of AML should be done for the following reasons (Table 37.6): (*a*) to distinguish AML from ALL (the most practical reason to analyze a potential AML), and (*b*) to provide correlation with the FAB morphologic subtype of AML. This has limited value and cannot replace the role of morphology and cytochemical stains.

The two situations that commonly pose the most difficult problem for diagnosing an AML are leukemias with no or minimal evidence of differentiation (FAB-M0 and FAB-M1) and those of megakaryoblastic differentiation (FAB-M7). Two pan-myeloid monoclonal antibodies, CD13 and CD33, have been universally used to distinguish AML from ALL on an immunologic basis. Overall, 90 to 98% of AMLs will react with CD33 and/or CD13. Moreover, these reagents have appeared to be highly specific for myeloid cells and are expressed in all FAB morphologic subtypes of AML. Some FAB-M0 and FAB-M1 AMLs tend to express CD33 only, suggesting that those leukemias are of earlier myeloid development than other AML. Also, acute megakaryoblastic leukemias (FAB-M7) may not express either CD13 or CD33 or tend to express CD13 and/or CD33 in a lower percentage of blasts with weaker intensity than in more classic AML.

The use of a panel of myeloid-associated monoclonal antibodies is necessary to access any possible correlations between an immunophenotype and the FAB morphologic classification (Fig. 37.33). Reports in the literature have demonstrated that myeloid monoclonal antibody reactivity may correspond to broad categories of morphologic differentiation: myeloblastic (FAB-M1 and M2), promyelocytic (FAB-M3), monocytic (FAB-M4 and M5), erythroid (FAB-M6), and megakaryocytic (FAB-M7). FAB-M1 and M2 acute myeloid leukemias react with the pan-myeloid markers CD13 and CD33; CD15 also reacts with a majority of cases of FAB-M1 and M2. Monocytic-associated monoclonal antibodies (CD11b, CD14, and CD36) are usually nonreactive in cases of AML-M1 and M2; CD14, however, has been detected in up to 15% of such AML cases. Monoclonal antibodies more restricted to the mature stages of granulocytic differentiation, such as CD10, CD16, CD24, and My8, do not react with the myeloblasts in these leukemias.

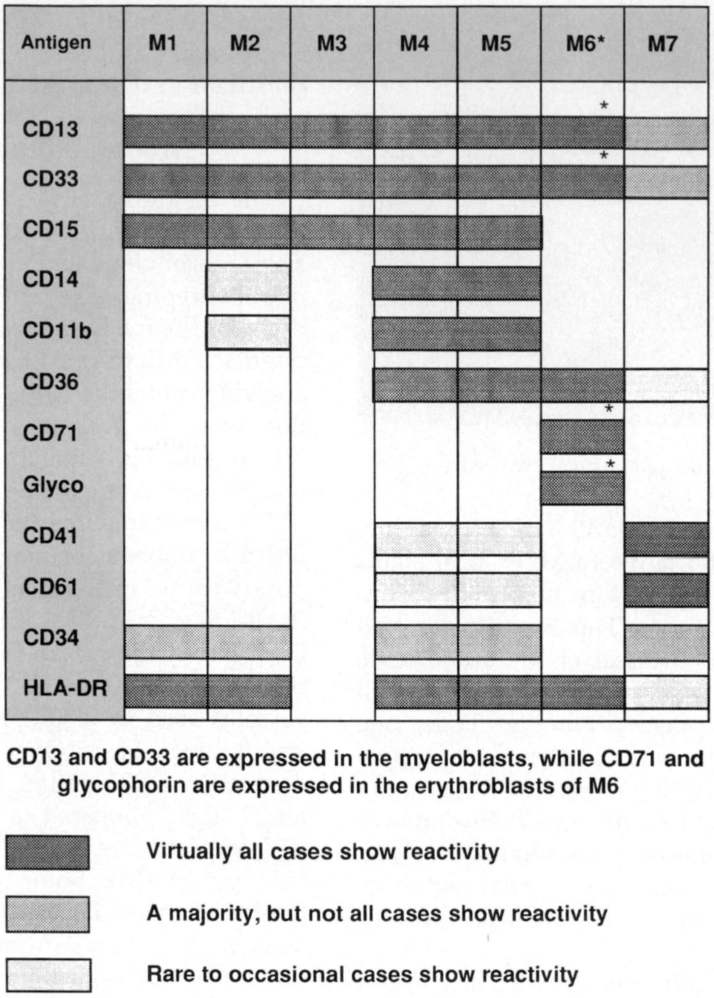

Figure 37.33. Correlation of FAB subtype of AML with immunophenotype.

HLA-DR expression is a common finding in AML. This reflects the normal distribution of HLA-DR or myeloid precursor cells up to, but not including, the promyelocyte stage. The lack of reactivity of HLA-DR antibodies in the majority of cases of APL is consistent with these observations that the normal promyelocyte is HLA-DR negative. However, occasional genuine cases of APL may be HLA-DR antigen positive. The hypogranular variant of APL has a pattern of reactivity similar to that of the typical granular form. HLA-DR negativity is not exclusive to APL, as up to 10% of AMLs (FAB-M1 and M2) may not express the HLA-DR antigen. Hence, although HLA-DR negativity is common in APL, it does not appear to be a 100% sensitive and specific diagnostic feature of this unique subtype of AML.

The monocytic leukemias (FAB-M4 and M5) are also reactive with the pan-myeloid monoclonal antibodies, CD13, CD15, and CD33, and uniformly express the HLA-DR antigen. CD11b, CD11c, CD14, and CD36 antigens are also displayed by the great majority of acute myelomonocytic and monocytic leukemias. CD14 expression is thought to be acquired at some point after the development of the monoblast and before maturation to the monocyte stage. This suggests that CD14 reactivity would be expected to be most prominent in the FAB-M4 and FAB-M5b leukemias. However, CD14 is commonly found in almost all cases of monoblastic leukemias (FAB-M5a). Interestingly, CD14 has recently been identified in a significant number of B-cell, non-Hodgkin's lymphomas, confirming that this antigen is not myeloid restricted.

No specific and sensitive marker of early erythroid development is currently available for the diagnosis of erythroleukemia (FAB-M6). The transferrin receptor CD71 is reactive with some myeloblasts in addition to all erythroblasts in the erythroleukemias. However, labeling of blasts with CD71 can also be observed in other types of AML and may be detected in some cases of ALL as well. Antiglycophorin antibodies appear to react only with cells that are morphologically obvious as erythroblasts, beginning at the basophilic normoblast stage, and thus will not label the early pronormoblasts. This finding is consistent with studies showing that these glycophorin antibodies label only the post-CFU-E stages of erythrocyte development.

The diagnosis of acute megakaryoblastic leukemia by immunophenotyping with monoclonal antibodies directed against megakaryoblast-associated antibodies has allowed for a rapid and easier method of diagnosing this poorly recognized subtype of acute leukemia. Several reports have shown that monoclonal antibodies against platelet glycoprotein IIb/IIIa or IIIa have diagnostic utility in the diagnosis of acute megakaryoblastic leukemia (FAB-M7). Although factor VIII-related antigen activity may be observed in rare cases of megakaryoblastic leukemia, the reactivity of megakaryoblasts with platelet glycoprotein IIb/IIIa or IIIa is more sensitive than labeling for factor VIII-related antigen. Preliminary data suggest that monoclonal antibodies to other glycoprotein determinants such as Ib do not react with the earliest megakaryoblasts.

Although immunophenotyping is generally accepted as the standard for diagnosing acute megakaryoblastic leukemia, it must be realized that some false positivity can be seen with these antibodies. This is most generally seen in myeloid leukemias that have a monocytic component. Whether the increased reactivity of these megakaryoblast-associated glycoproteins is due to nonspecific background labeling, reaction with platelet membrane components adhering to monocytic cells, or actual expression of the glycoprotein antigens on monocytes remains to be seen. In general, it has been our experience that the expression of these megakaryocyte-associated glycoproteins in the monocytic leukemias has been of much weaker intensity and fails to give a distinct uniform population on the fluorescence histograms, but rather a "smearing" of intensities. Our policy has been to interpret a CD61-positive immunophenotype with some caution and to correlate the findings closely with morphologic and cytochemical findings. Immunocytochemical detection of these glycoproteins on glass slide smears may also be of value in determining whether the positivity seen is truly on the leukemic cell or merely due to nonspecific adherence.

Other antigens not typically associated with myeloid cells can also be identified in acute myelogenous leukemia. CD34 can be found in 30 to 40% of all AML and has been associated with a poorer prognosis than CD34-negative AML. The CD34 antigen can be useful in evaluating a specimen containing a mixture of myeloblasts and differentiated myeloid or lymphoid cells. CD38 has classically been used as an early thymocyte marker, but is now recognized to be present on activated T cells as well as being an excellent plasma cell marker. Not surprisingly, it can also be identified in AML. CD4 is the receptor for HLA class II antigen that characterizes the "T helper" subset of T lymphocytes. This antigen is not restricted to T cells and can be identified in monocytes, monocyte precursors, and monocytic leukemias. As previously discussed, CD7 is a pan–T-cell antigen that can be found in 5 to 10% of all AMLs; CD7 can be found in all subtypes of AML. Although some have suggested that the presence of CD7 reflects an early bone marrow precursor, other data do not support this concept. CD45, the common leukocyte antigen, is found in virtually all cases of AML.

In summary, immunophenotyping with monoclonal antibodies in acute myelogenous leukemia is at its best when trying to distinguish between ALL and AML. One must use great caution in using the immunophenotype to aid in the FAB subclassification in these leukemias. Although the immunophenotype may suggest a relationship to a particular FAB subgroup, one must still rely on morphology and cytochemistry to make the final FAB morphologic distinction. The lack of DR expression suggests the possibility of an APL, expression of CD14 and CD11b are associated with monocytic leukemias, and CD71 and glycophorin antibodies certainly react with erythroid cells. The final area in which immunophenotyping has been of great diagnostic utility is the identification of megakaryoblast-associated antigens for the diagnosis of acute megakaryoblastic leukemia.

ACUTE BIPHENOTYPIC LEUKEMIA

Considerable interest has developed over the past decade in the acute leukemias that have immunophenotypes that do not fit into the accepted sequence of normal lymphoid or myeloid cell development. Perhaps the most controversial and confusing of these immunologically aberrant cases have been the so-called acute biphenotypic leukemias. A plethora of terminologies (hybrid, mixed-lineage, bilineal, biclonal, biphenotypic) has added to the confusion in this area. Such phenotypes imply that either malignant transformation leads to aberrant gene expression ("lineage infidelity") or that coexpression of "lineage-specific" markers occurs normally in the differentiation of hematopoietic cells ("lineage promiscuity"). The clinical significance of biphenotypia in acute leukemia has not been uniformly determined or accepted. Such studies have uniformly suffered from the lack of consistent guidelines for classification. Some studies have suggested that the biphenotypic leukemias have a worse clinical prognosis than nonbiphenotypic acute lymphoblastic leukemia or acute myelogenous leukemia, while other reports

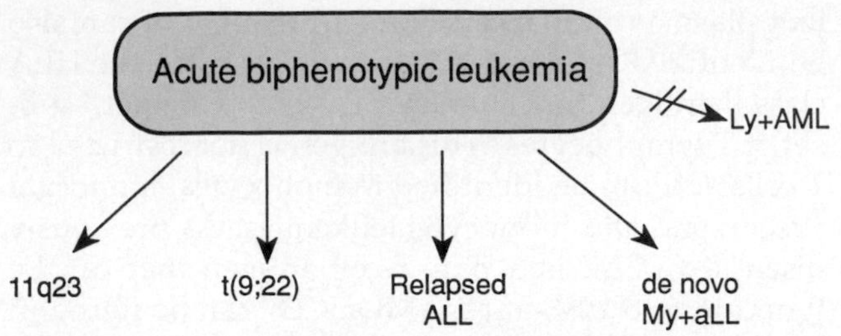

Figure 37.34. Proposed schema of subtypes of acute biphenotypic leukemia. Biphenotypic leukemias are broadly represented by cases having an 11q23 translocation, a t(9;22) translocation, relapsed ALL, and de novo myeloid antigen–positive ALL (My + ALL). Cases having lymphoid antigen–positive AML (Ly + AML) probably do not represent "true" acute biphenotypic leukemia.

have not confirmed that a clinical significance exists. The difficulty in evaluating biphenotypic leukemias may be demonstrated by looking at the reported frequency of biphenotypic leukemia in the literature. This frequency has varied from less than 1% of acute leukemia cases in some studies to almost 50% of acute leukemia cases in others. This widely variable incidence range cannot be rationally explained solely on the basis of clinical variability between different population groups. Indeed, this variability, along with the lack of consensus as to the clinical or biological significance of biphenotypia in acute leukemia is undoubtedly due to several contributing factors: the use of inconsistent and variable diagnostic criteria, the inevitable subjectiveness of immunophenotypic interpretation, and the lack of a standard and uniform panel of monoclonal antibodies utilized in immunophenotypic analyses.

Figure 37.34 is a schematic drawing outlining the diverse groups that compose what we have called biphenotypic leukemia. Leukemias with the Philadelphia chromosome or 11q23 translocations have clearly been associated with biphenotypic processes. Identification of other immunologic and cytogenetic subgroups will be essential in further characterizing and understanding these intriguing leukemias and the cellular counterparts from which they arise.

MYELODYSPLASTIC SYNDROMES

The myelodysplastic syndromes (MDSs) are a heterogeneous group of bone marrow disorders generally characterized by cytopenias and morphologic abnormalities of the erythroid, granulocytic, and megakaryocytic cell lines within a hypercellular bone marrow. Bone marrow myeloblasts may be increased but do not reach the 30% blast level necessary for a diagnosis of AML. Although MDS does not meet the morphologic criteria for the diagnosis of AML, distinction from AML may be difficult and a proportion of cases will ultimately evolve to overt AML. Patients that do not evolve into AML frequently will suffer from complications related to chronic transfusion or bone marrow failure.

MDS usually occurs in individuals over the age of 50, although genuine cases of MDS may rarely be seen in the pediatric age group. In general, however, the diagnosis of MDS in children should be made very cautiously. Patients with MDS typically present with symptoms of variable duration related to the degree of the underlying cytopenias.

Historical terms that have been used to describe MDS include preleukemia, early leukemia, smoldering leukemia, subacute leukemia, atypical leukemia, and hematopoietic dysplasia. The MDSs do not include disorders that are known to predispose an individual to the development of acute leukemia, such as chromosomal breakage syndromes. Although the MDSs are classified as distinctly different from the chronic myeloproliferative disorders, there are certainly individual cases that have features of both MDS and chronic myeloproliferative diseases. Such cases may present with neutrophilia and granulocytic hyperproliferation together with striking dysplastic features or thrombocytosis and dysplastic neutrophils and megakaryocytes.

Diagnosis

A diagnosis of MDS should be considered in a setting of unexplained cytopenias and ineffective hematopoiesis in an adult patient. Most MDSs will show quantitative and qualitative evidence of dyserythropoiesis, dysgranulopoiesis, and dysmegakaryopoiesis. An iron stain for ringed sideroblasts and the percentage of blood and bone marrow myeloblasts are essential in accurately classifying the MDS. These and other features are listed in Table 37.15 and are described below.

DYSERYTHROPOIESIS

Dyserythropoiesis may include megaloblastoid changes, irregular nuclear shapes and forms, multinucleation, internuclear bridging, abnormal chromatin, ringed sideroblasts, or nuclear karyorrhexis. Dyssynchrony between nuclear and cytoplasmic development is probably the most reliable and significant evidence of dyserythropoiesis (Fig. 37.35). For example, a red cell precursor showing evidence of hemoglobinization in the cytoplasm, while still maintaining an earlier or open chromatin pattern, would be described as "dyssynchronous." The peripheral blood smear may show significant anisopoikilocytosis and occasional nucleated red blood cells. The term "ringed" sideroblasts has been used to describe erythroblasts that contain cytoplasmic iron that

Table 37.15. Morphologic Features of Myelodysplasia

Dyserythropoiesis
Megaloblastoid changes
Multinucleation
Nuclear/cytoplasmic asynchrony
Nuclear karyorrhexis
Ringed sideroblasts
Dysgranulopoiesis
Pseudo–Pelger-Huet changes
Hypogranulation
Abnormal granules
Basophilia
Decreased or absent myeloperoxidase
Decreased leukocyte alkaline phosphatase (LAP)
Dysmegakaryopoiesis
Large, bizarre platelets
Hypogranular platelets
Bizarre megakaryocytes
Uninuclear megakaryocytes

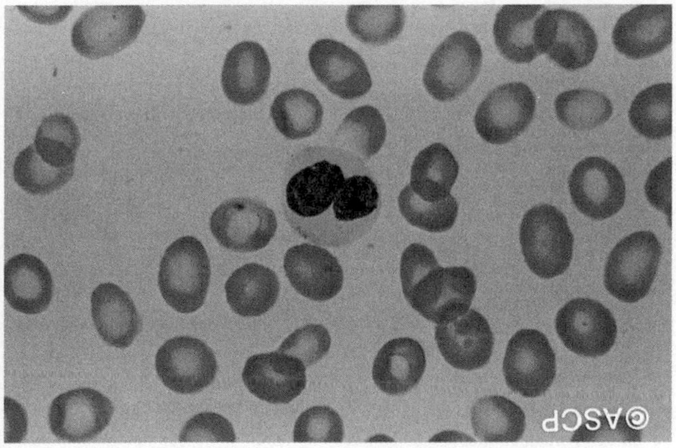

Figure 37.35. Dyserythropoiesis.

wraps around at least one-third of the nucleus. This iron is located in the mitochondria and results in ineffective erythropoiesis and subsequent marrow destruction of red cells and precursors. Ringed sideroblasts are not found in normal marrow and are easily distinguished from normal sideroblasts, which have scattered cytoplasmic iron granules.

DYSGRANULOPOIESIS

Dysgranulopoiesis can be effectively summarized as morphologic evidence of hypolobulation or hyposegmentation of the nucleus and/or hypogranulation of the cytoplasm (Fig. 37.36). The hyposegmentation of the nucleus, i.e., the presence of only two nuclear lobes, has been called "pseudo–Pelger-Huét change." The determination of this hyposegmentation must be made on a well-prepared blood or bone marrow smear, and care must be taken to distinguish that two lobes are not overlapping each other. Likewise, hypogranulation is best identified on a Wright-Giemsa stain smear. Smears stained

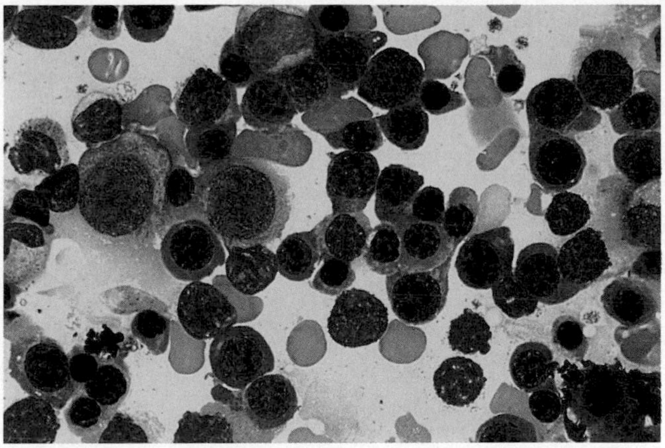

Figure 37.36. Dysgranulopoiesis (pseudo–Pelger-Huét change).

with only Wright stain may sometimes appear faint, leading to a mistaken diagnosis of hypogranulation. In addition, granulocyte enzymatic stains, such as myeloperoxidase, Sudan black B, and leukocyte alkaline phosphatase, may be negative if this dysplastic hypogranulation is marked. Occasionally, one may see abnormally dense chromatin or ringed nuclei, both of which represent uncommon forms of dysgranulopoiesis. Abnormal granulation and basophilia are other manifestations of dysgranulopoiesis.

DYSMEGAKARYOPOIESIS

Abnormalities of peripheral blood platelets and bone marrow megakaryocytes are common in the MDSs. Dysplastic platelets on the peripheral blood smear may appear as either hypogranular platelets or as large, bizarre platelet forms. Examination of the bone marrow aspirate smear and/or bone marrow biopsy specimen may show megakaryocytes with separated nuclear lobes instead of a lobulated nucleus, large bizarre nuclei with dysplastic features, open nuclear chromatin, high nuclear:cytoplasmic ratios, and large accumulations, or sheets, of megakaryocytes in the bone marrow biopsy (Fig. 37.37). Abnormally small megakaryocytes with single, round nuclei have been described in the MDSs having a chromosomal deletion of the long arm of chromosome 5 (5q− syndrome).

FAB Classification

The FAB classification scheme for MDS is listed in Table 37.16. This classification scheme uses the percentage of blasts in the bone marrow as the single most important factor. Approximately 10% of cases will not fit into one of these prescribed groups. It should also be noted that secondary or therapy-related MDS is a distinct clinical-pathologic entity occurring in patients after exposure to radiation and/or

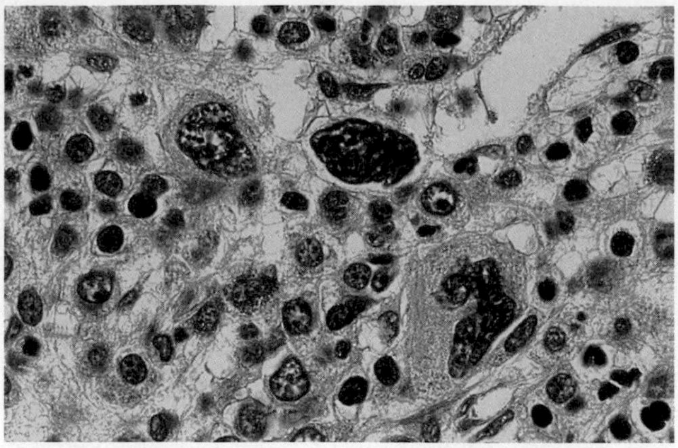

Figure 37.37. Dysmegakaryopoiesis.

Table 37.16. FAB Classification of Myelodysplastic Syndromes

Refractory anemia (RA)
Idiopathic refractory sideroblastic anemia (IRSB)
Refractory anemia with excess blasts (RAEB)
RAEB in transformation (RAEB-t)
Chronic myelomonocytic leukemia (CMML)
Myelodysplastic syndrome, unclassified (MDS, NOS)
Therapy-related myelodysplasia

alkylating agent chemotherapy for primary neoplastic or nonneoplastic disorders. Although primarily an adult disorder, two pediatric disorders that can be classified as MDS include juvenile chronic myelogenous leukemia and the monosomy 7 syndrome. These disorders are associated with organomegaly, leukocytosis, cytopenias, and increased number of bone marrow blasts without meeting the criteria for AML and are associated with the subsequent development of AML.

REFRACTORY ANEMIA

This subtype of MDS is basically a chronic, unexplained anemia occurring in adult patients over the age of 50 years. It may also be referred to as "refractory cytopenia," as it is not purely restricted to anemia (Table 37.17). Classically, patients with refractory anemia (RA) show erythroid hyperplasia in the bone marrow accompanied by a low reticulocyte count in the peripheral blood. This combination is referred to as ineffective erythropoiesis and is a characteristic hallmark of this type of MDS. Ringed sideroblasts are not increased (less than 15%) in these cases, and it is important to note that minimal to no dysplastic changes are identified in any cell line; no increase in myeloblasts are seen. This subgroup of MDS basically consists of patients who have unexplained anemias in spite of erythroid hyperplasia. Obviously, other causes of chronic anemia must be ruled out, including vitamin B12/folate deficiency,

Table 37.17. FAB Classification in Myelodysplastic Syndromes

Refractory anemia (RA)
Chronic unexplained anemia/"refractory cytopenia"
Reticulocytopenia
No blasts in peripheral blood
Bone marrow normocellular or hypercellular
Erythroid hyperplasia/mild dyserythropoiesis
Minimal to no dysplastic changes
Fewer than 5% myeloblasts
Ringed sideroblasts are not increased
Idiopathic refractory sideroblastic anemia (IRSA)
Findings similar to those described for RA
Fewer than 5% myeloblasts
Dysplastic features are uncommon
Erythroid hyperplasia; hypercellular bone marrow
Dyserythropoiesis
15% or more ringed sideroblasts
Chronic anemia; transfusion dependent
Dimorphic peripheral blood (hypochromic and normochromic)
Ineffective erythropoiesis
10% evolve to AML
Refractory anemia with excess blasts (RAEB)
Chronic clinical course
Pancytopenia
All three cell lines are dyspoietic
Bone marrow failure is common
Hypercellular bone marrow
Fewer than 5% myeloblasts in blood
5 to 20% myeloblasts in bone marrow
No Auer rods
Ringed sideroblasts may be present
30 to 40% evolve to AML
Refractory anemia with excess blasts in transformation (RAEB-t)
20 to 30% myeloblasts in bone marrow
Or "0" to 30% myeloblasts with Auer rods
Or more than 5% myeloblasts in blood
Same clinical features as RAEB
60 to 80% evolve to AML
Chronic myelomonocytic leukemia (CMML)
Males more than females
Hepatomegaly/splenomegaly in 30 to 50%
Anemia, thrombocytopenia
Leukocyte count is variable
Monocytes more than 2×10^9/liter
Hypercellular marrow
Significant myelodysplastic changes may not be found
Increased serum/urine lysozyme
Easily confused with AML-M4 or M5b

drug or toxin exposure, congenital dyserythropoietic anemias, aplastic anemia, or other uncommon causes of anemia.

IDIOPATHIC REFRACTORY SIDEROBLASTIC ANEMIA

The morphologic features of idiopathic refractory sideroblastic anemia (IRSA) are similar to those described for RA except for the additional presence of 15% or more ringed sideroblasts. The criteria for IRSA are listed in Table 37.17. The pathologic ringed sideroblasts have iron granules located in a perinuclear location, reflecting mitochondrial iron depo-

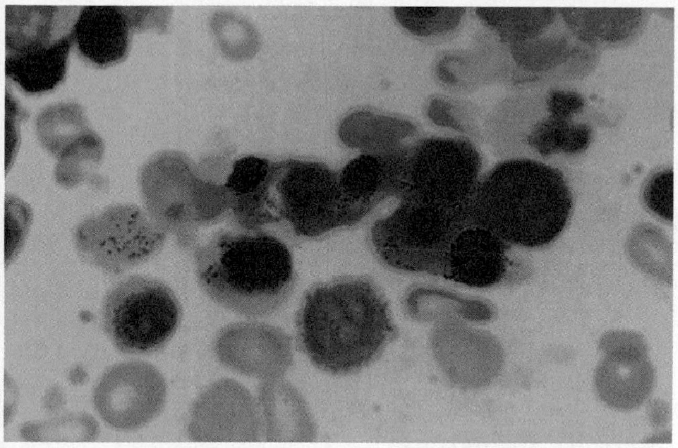

Figure 37.38. Idiopathic refractory sideroblastic anemia (IRSA) with ringed sideroblasts.

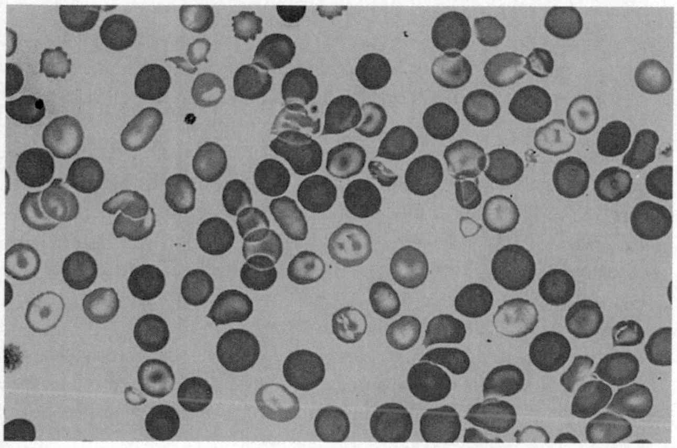

Figure 37.39. Dimorphic peripheral blood smear in IRSA.

sition (Fig. 37.38). It is important to rule out hereditary and secondary causes of sideroblastic anemia, including hereditary sideroblastic anemia, exposure to drugs (antituberculosis agents, chloramphenicol, etc.), alcohol-induced sideroblastic anemia, chronic lead poisoning, and various other diseases, including some autoimmune disorders. These patients have a significant erythroid hyperplasia, but do not have increased numbers of myeloblasts. Dysplastic features are uncommon in granulocytic and megakaryocytic precursors, and when present may portend a more aggressive clinical course. Most patients become transfusion dependent and only 10 to 15% of cases of IRSA progress to an AML. The peripheral blood smear classically shows a dimorphic blood picture with both normochromic, normocytic red blood cells and hypochromic, microcytic red blood cells (Fig. 37.39). This dimorphism reflects the heterogeneity of erythroid differentiation in the bone marrow. This dimorphic blood picture is quite distinct and should always raise the possibility of IRSA when encountered.

REFRACTORY ANEMIA WITH EXCESS OF BLASTS

Refractory anemia with an excess of blasts (RAEB) is typically associated with pancytopenia and significant dysplastic features in the granulocytic series. Erythroid and megakaryocytic dysplasia may also be found. The basic diagnostic criterion for RAEB is a hypercellular bone marrow containing between 5 and 20% myeloblasts. The peripheral blood has less than 5% circulating blasts, and no Auer rods are identified. The criteria for the diagnosis of RAEB are listed in Table 37.17. It is important to note that 30 to 40% of patients in this subgroup of MDS will eventually evolve into an overt AML. Ringed sideroblasts may be identified; however, the increased myeloblasts allow for distinction from IRSA.

REFRACTORY ANEMIA WITH EXCESS OF BLASTS IN TRANSFORMATION

RAEB in transformation (RAEB-t) has the same morphologic features as RAEB, but with differences in the percentages of myeloblasts. The criteria for diagnosis of RAEB-t are based on three possible scenarios: (*a*) more than 5% blasts in the peripheral blood; (*b*) 20 to 30% blasts in bone marrow; or (*c*) "0" to 30% myeloblasts with Auer rods. This subgroup of MDS represents an intermediate form between RAEB and overt AML. RAEB-t fails to meet the prerequisite requirement of 30% blasts, but has many features very similar to AML. Between 60 and 80% of cases progress to AML. The diagnostic criteria for RAEB-t are listed in Table 37.17.

CHRONIC MYELOMONOCYTIC LEUKEMIA

There is a current controversy over the definition of chronic myelomonocytic leukemia (CMML) and its inclusion as an MDS. It is a hematologic disorder with features common to the myeloproliferative syndromes and the MDSs. Morphologic features emphasize the presence of a blood and bone marrow monocytosis. In particular, monocytosis should exceed 2.0 $\times$ 10^9/liter. However, significant myelodysplastic changes may or may not be found. The criteria for a diagnosis of CMML are listed in Table 37.17. Some cases classified as CMML may actually represent early AML-M4 or AML-M5b. Others may represent uncommon forms of chronic myeloproliferative disorders. It obviously is also important to rule out reactive and inflammatory causes of monocytosis before making a diagnosis of CMML.

SECONDARY/THERAPY-RELATED MDS

Therapy-related MDS is a form of MDS occurring in patients previously treated with chemotherapy

Table 37.18. Prognostic Factors in Myelodysplastic Syndromes

Low-risk	
	Refractory anemia with normal platelets, WBC
	Numerous ringed sideroblasts
	Normal CFU[a] capacity
	Absence of chromosomal abnormalities
High-risk	
	Severe pancytopenia
	RAEB-t
	Low CFU capacity
	Chromosomal abnormalities

[a]CFU, colony-forming unit.

and/or radiation for neoplastic or nonneoplastic disease. The incidence of a secondary MDS or AML has been variously estimated at 2 to 10% of patients treated as such and may be related to the amount, duration, and repetition of exposure to the therapeutic agent and the age of the individual involved. Long-term alkylating agent therapy, in particular, appears to have a high leukemogenic potential. The median onset of secondary MDS is approximately within 5 years of therapy, with a range of approximately 2 to 15 years. Approximately one-third of these patients will present with an MDS prior to the evolution to a frank AML. Typically, these patients present with unexplained cytopenias and observed dysplastic abnormalities in the blood and bone marrow. Panmyelosis with dysplastic features in all myeloid lines are typically found. The prognosis of patients with therapy-related MDS is abysmal, with a median survival of less than 6 months.

Cytogenetics in MDS

Several recurring chromosome defects are found in patients with de novo MDS, including complete or partial loss of chromosome 5 or 7, loss of the long arm of chromosome 5 or 7, trisomy 8, or multiple, miscellaneous complex chromosome defects.

Prognosis

There are varying reports of the frequency that MDS evolves to overt AML. Data in the literature regarding the evolution to AML varies according to the subtypes of MDS. Table 37.18 summarizes some of these data. Generally, refractory anemia and IRSA show the lowest incidence of transformation to AML, while RAEB and RAEB-t show a much higher incidence of leukemic progression.

The survival of patients with MDS varies, with some patients surviving many years, while others only a few months. Death may be due to bone marrow failure if progression to AML does not occur. The age of patients, the degree of cytopenia, the percentage of blasts, the degree of abnormal chromosome abnormalities, and in vitro culture changes have all been used to predict the survival of patients with MDS.

References

1. Greaves MF, Hariri G, Newman RA, et al. Selective expression of the common acute lymphoblastic leukemia (gp 100) antigen on immature lymphoid cells and their malignant counterparts. Blood 1983;61:628–639.
2. Borowitz MJ, Shuster JJ, Civin CI, et al. Prognostic significance of CD34 expression in childhood B-precursor acute lymphocytic leukemia: a pediatric-oncology group study. J Clin Oncol 8:1389–1398.

Suggested Readings

Acute Lymphoblastic Leukemia

Arthur D, Bloomfield CD, Lindquist LL, et al. Translocation 4;11 in acute lymphoblastic leukemia: clinical characteristics and prognostic significance. Blood 1982;59:96–99.

Bennett JM, Catovsky D, Daniel MT, et al. The morphological classification of acute lymphoblastic leukemia: concordance among observers and clinical correlations. Br J Haematol 1981;47:553–561.

Bloomfield CD, Peterson LC, Yunis JJ, Brunning RD. The Philadelphia chromosome (Ph^1) in adults presenting with acute leukemia: a comparison of Ph^1+ and Ph^1- patients. Br J Haematol 1977;36:347–358.

Bloomfield CD, Goldman A, Alimena G, et al. Chromosomal abnormalities identify high risk and low risk patients with acute lymphoblastic leukemia. Blood 1986;67:415–420.

Brearley RL, Johnson SA, Lister TA. Acute lymphoblastic leukemia in adults: clinico-pathological correlation with the French-American-British (FAB) Cooperative Group classification. Eur J Cancer 1979;15:909–914.

Brunning RD. Philadelphia chromosome positive leukemia. Hum Pathol 1980;11:307–309.

Brunning RD, McKenna RW. Immunologic markers for acute leukemia: a morphologist's perspective. In: Berard C, Dorfman R, eds. Malignant lymphoma (IAP monograph). Baltimore: Williams & Wilkins, 1986;124–160.

Champlin R, Gale P. Acute lymphoblastic leukemia: recent advances in biology and therapy. Blood 1989;73:2051–2066.

Cossman J, Chused TM, Fischer RI, et al. Diversity of immunologic phenotypes of lymphoblastic lymphoma. Cancer Res 1983;43:4486–4490.

Crist W, Pullen J, Boyett J, et al. Clinical and biologic features predict a poor prognosis in acute lymphoid leukemias in infants. Blood 1986;67:135–140.

Crist W, Shuster J, Falletta J, et al. Clinical features and outcome in childhood T cell leukemia-lymphoma according to stage of thymic differentiation. Blood 1988;72:1891–1897.

DeKlein A, Itagemeijer A, Bartram CR, et al. bcr rearrangement and translocations of the c-abl oncogene in Ph^1 positive ALL. Blood 1986;68:1369–1376.

Flug F, Dodson L, Wolff J, et al. B-lymphocyte associated differentiation antigen expression by non-B non-T acute lymphoblastic leukemia. Leuk Res 1985;9:1051–1058.

Greaves MF, Janossy G, Peto J, et al. Immunologically defined subclasses of acute lymphoblastic leukemia in children: their relationship to presentation features and prognosis. Br J Haematol 1981;48:179–197.

Greisser H, Tkachuk D, Reis M, Mak T. Gene rearrangements and translocations in lymphoproliferative diseases. Blood 1989;73:1402–1415.

Kaneko Y, Maseki N, Takasaki N, et al. Clinical and hematologic characteristics in acute leukemia with 11q23 translocations. Blood 1986;67:484–491.

Kaplan S, Penchansky L, Stolc V, et al. Immunophenotyping in the classifications of acute leukemia in adults. Cancer 1989;63:1520–1527.

Katz F, Malcome S, Gibbons B, et al. Cellular and molecular studies on infant null acute lymphoblastic leukemia. Blood 1988;71:1438–1447.

Longacre T, Foucar K, Crago S, et al. Hematogones: a multiparameter analysis of bone marrow precursor cells. Blood 1989;73:543–552.

McKenna RW, Brynes R, Nesbit M, et al. Cytochemical profiles in acute lymphoblastic leukemia. Am J Pediatr Hematol Oncol 1979;1:263–275.

McKenna RW, Parkin J, Brunning RD. Morphologic and ultrastructural characteristics of T-cell acute lymphoblastic leukemia. Cancer 1979;44:1290–1297.

Mertelsmann R, Tzvi T, Lo T, et al. Morphological classification, response to therapy and survival in 263 adult patients with acute nonlymphoblastic leukemia. Blood 1980;56:773–781.

Mirro J, Kitchingman G, Williams D, et al. Clinical and laboratory characteristics of acute leukemia with the t(4;11). Blood 1986;67:689–697.

Nagasaka M, Maeda S, Maeda H, et al. Four cases of t(4;11) acute leukema and its myelomonocytic nature in infants. Blood 1983;61:1174–1181.

Parkin J, Arthur D, Abramson C, et al. Acute leukemia associated with the t(4;11) chromosome rearrangement: ultrastructural and immunologic characteristics. Blood 1982;60:1321–1331.

Pui CH, Williams D, Kalwinsky DK, et al. Cytogenetic features and serum LDH level predict a poor treatment outcome for children with pre B-cell leukemia. Blood 1986;67:1688–1692.

Roper M, Crist WM, Metzgar R, et al. Monoclonal antibody characterization of surface antigens in childhood T cell lymphoid malignancies. Blood 1984;63:1023–1027.

Savage RA. Utility of acid phosphatase staining of lymphoblasts. Am J Clin Pathol 1988;89:451–453.

Sobol RE, Rogaston I, LeBein TW, et al. Adult acute lymphoblastic leukemia phenotypes defined by monoclonal antibodies. Blood 1985;65:730–735.

Sobol R, Mick R, Royston I, et al. Clinical importance of myeloid antigen expression in adult acute lymphoblastic leukemia. N Engl J Med 1987;316:1111–1117.

The Third International Workshop on Chromosomes in Leukemia, Lund, Sweden, July 21-25, 1980. Cancer Genet Cytogenet 1981;4:96–98.

Turhan AG, Eaves CH, Kalousek DK, et al. Molecular analysis of clonality and bcr rearrangements in Philadelphia chromosome-positive acute lymphoblastic leukemia. Blood 1988;71:1495–1498.

van Eys J, Pullen J, Head D, et al. The FAB classification of leukemia: the pediatric oncology group experience with lymphoblastic leukemia. Cancer 1986;57:1046–1051.

Weiss LM, Bindl J, Picozzi J, Link M, Warnke R. Lymphoblastic lymphoma: an immunophenotype study of 26 cases with comparison to T cell acute lymphoblastic leukemia. Blood 1986;67:474–478.

Acute Myelogenous Leukemia

Arthur D, Bloomfield CD. Partial deletion of the long arm of chromosome 16 and bone marrow eosinophilia in acute nonlymphocytic leukemia: a new association. Blood 1983;61:994–998.

Bain B, Catovsky D, O'Brien M, et al. Megakaryoblastic leukemia presenting as acute myelofibrosis: study of four cases with platelet peroxidase reaction. Blood 1981;58:206–213.

Bennett JM, Reed CE. Acute leukemia cytochemical profile: diagnostic and clinical implications. Blood Cells 1975;1:101–113.

Bennett JM, Catovsky D, Daniel MT, et al. Proposals for classification of acute leukemias French-American-British (FAB) Cooperative Group. Br J Haematol 1976;33:451–458.

Bennett JM, Catovsky D, Daniel MR, et al. A variant form of hypergranular promyelocytic leukemia (M3). Br J Haematol 1980;44:169–170.

Bennett JM, Catovsky D, Daniel MT, et al. Proposed revised criteria for the classification of acute myeloid leukemia. Ann Intern Med 1985;103:626–629.

Bennett JM, Catovsky D, Marit-Therese D, et al. Criteria for the diagnosis of acute leukemia of megakaryocyte lineage (M7). Ann Intern Med 1985;103:460–462.

Berger R, Bernheim A, Daniel MT, et al. Cytologic characterization and significance of normal karyotypes in t(8;21) AML. Blood 1982;59:171–178.

Berger R, Bernheim A, Sigany F, et al. Acute monocytic leukemia chromosome studies. Leuk Res 1982;6:17–26.

Bitter MA, LeBeau MM, Larson RA, et al. A morphologic and cytochemical study of acute myelomonocytic leukemia with abnormal marrow eosinophils associated with inv(16)(p13q22). Am J Clin Pathol 1984;81:733–741.

Bitter MA, LeBeau MM, Rowley JD, et al. Associations between morphology, karyotype, and clinical features in myeloid leukemias. Hum Pathol 1987;18:211–225.

Bloomfield CD, Brunning RD. FAB-M7: acute megakaryoblastic leukemia—beyond morphology. Ann Intern Med 1985;103:450–452.

Breton-Gorius J, Reyes F, Duhamel G, et al. Megakaryoblastic acute leukemia: identification of the ultrastructural demonstration of platelet peroxidase. Blood 1978;51:45–60.

Cainey AE, McKenna R, Arthur DC, et al. Acute megakaryoblastic leukaemia in children. Br J Haematol 1986;63:541–554.

Catovsky D, DeSalvo Cardullo L, et al. Cytochemical markers of differentiation in acute leukemia. Cancer Res 1981;11:4824–4832.

Eber WN, Breton-Gorius J, Velleval JL, et al. Detection of cells of megakaryocytic lineage in haematological malignancies by immunoalkaline phosphatase labelling cell smears with a panel of monoclonal antibodies. Br J Haematol 1987;65:87–94.

Fan YS, Jani Sait SN, Raza A, et al. Translocation t(6;9)(p23;q34) in ANLL: two new patients without increased bone marrow basophils. Cancer Genet Cytogenet 1988;32:153–155.

Golomb HM, Rowley JD, Vardiman JW, et al. Microgranular acute promyelocytic leukemia: a distinct clinical, ultrastructural, and cytogenetic entity. Blood 1980;55:253–259.

Griffin JD, Mayer RJ, Weinstein HJ, et al. Surface marker analysis of AML: identification of differentiation-associated phenotypes. Blood 1983;62:557–563.

Griffin JD, Lowenberg B. Clonogenic cells in acute myeloblastic leukemia. Blood 1986;68:1185–1195.

Griffin JD, Davis R, Nelson DA, et al. Use of surface marker analysis to predict outcome of adult acute myeloblastic leukemia. Blood 1986;68:1232–1241.

Groupe Francais de Morphologie Hematologique: French Registry of acute leukemia and myelodysplastic syndromes. Age distribution and hemogram analysis of the 4496 cases recorded during 1982-1983 and classified according to FAB criteria. Cancer 1987;60:1385–1394.

Hanson CA, Gajl-Peczalskak J, Parkin J, Brunning RD. Immunophenotyping of acute myeloid leukemia using monoclonal antibodies and the APAAP technique. Blood 1987;70:83–89.

Holmes R, Keating M, Cork A, et al. A unique pattern of central nervous system leukemia in acute myelomonocytic leukemias associated with inv(16)(p13q22). Blood 1985;65:1071–1078.

Howe RB, Bloomfield CD, McKenna RW. Hypocellular acute leukemia. Am J Med 1982;72:391–395.

Kaneko Y, Sakura M. 15/17 translocation in acute promyelocytic leukemia. Lancet 1977;1:961.

Kaplow LS. Simplified myeloperoxidase staining using benzidine dihydrochloride. Blood 1965;26:215–219.

Koike T, Aoki S, Maruyama S, et al. Cell surface phenotyping of megakaryoblasts. Blood 1987;69:957–960.

Larson RA, Williams SF, LeBeau MM, et al. Acute myelomonocytic leukemia with abnormal eosinophils and inv(16) or t(16;16) has a favorable prognosis. Blood 1986;68:1242–1249.

Lewis DS, Thompson M, Hudson E, et al. Down's syndrome and acute megakaryoblastic leukemia. Acta Haematol (Basel) 1983;70:236–242.

McKenna RW, Bloomfield CD, Dick F, et al. Acute monoblastic leukemia: diagnosis and treatment of 10 cases. Blood 1978;45: 481–494.

McKenna RW, Parkin J, Bloomfield C, Sundberg RD, Brunning RD. Acute promyelocytic leukemia. Study of 39 cases with identification of a hyperbasophilic microgranular APL variant. Br J Haematol 1982;50:201–214.

Neame PB, Soamboonsrup B, Browman GP, et al. Classifying acute leukemia by immunophenotyping: a combined FAB-immunologic classification of AML. Blood 1986;68:1355–1362.

Ross FM, Hamilton M, Cook MK, Irving JB. A myelodysplastic syndrome with eosinophilia associated with a break in the short arm of chromosome 16. Leukemia 1987;1:680–681.

Second MIC Cooperative Study Group. Morphologic, immunologic and cytogenetic (MIC) working classification of AML. Cancer Genet Cytogenet 1988;30:1–15.

Second International Workshop on Chromosomes in Leukemia (1979): Cytogenetic, morphologic and clinical correlations in acute nonlymphocytic leukemia with t(8q-;21q+). Cancer Genet Cytogenet 1980;2:99–102.

Second International Workshop on Chromosomes in Leukemia (1979): Morphologic analysis of acute promyelocytic leukemia (M3) and t(8;21) cases. Cancer Genet Cytogenet 1980;2:97–98.

Simon JH, Tebbi CK, Freeman AI, et al. Acute megakaryoblastic leukemia associated with mosaic Down's syndrome. Cancer 1987;60:2515–2520.

Stanley M, McKenna RW, Ellinger G, Brunning RD. Classification of 358 cases of acute myeloid leukemia by FAB criteria: analysis of clinical and morphologic features. In: Bloomfield CD, ed. Chronic and acute leukemia in adults. Boston: Martinus Nijhoff, 1985:147–174.

Sultan C, Deregnaucourt J, Ko YW, et al. Distribution of 250 cases of acute myeloid leukemia (AML) according to the FAB classification and response to therapy. Br J Haematol 1981;47:545–551.

Yam LT, Li C-Y, Crosby WH. Cytochemical identification of monocytes and granulocytes. Am J Clin Pathol 1971;55:283–290.

Yunis JJ, Brunning RD. Prognostic significance of chromosomal abnormalities in acute leukemias and myelodysplastic syndromes. Clin Haematol 1986;15:597–620.

Myelodysplastic Syndromes

Alessandrino EP, Orlandi E, Brusamolino E, et al. Chronic myelomonocytic leukemia: clinical features, cytogenetics, and prognosis in 30 consecutive cases. Hematol Oncol 1985;3:147–155.

Appelbaum FR, Storb R, Ramberg RE, et al. Treatment of preleukemia syndromes with marrow transplantation. Blood 1987;69:92–96.

Belanger R, Gyger M, Perreault C, Bonny Y, St-Louis J. Bone marrow transplantation for myelodysplastic syndromes. Br J Haematol 1988;69:29–33.

Bennett JM, Catovsky D, Daniel MT, et al. Proposals for the classification of the myelodysplastic syndromes. Br J Haematol 1982;51:189–199.

Brusamolino E, Pagnucco G, Bernasconi C. Acute leukemia occurring in a primary neoplasia (secondary leukemia). A review on biological, epidemiological and clinical aspects. Haematologica 1986;71:60–83.

Cazzola M, Barosi G, Gobbi PG, Invernizzi R, Riccardi A, Ascari E. Natural history of idiopathic refractory sideroblastic anemia. Blood 1988;71:305–312.

Clark R, Peters S, Hoy T, Smith S, Whittaker K, Jacobs A. Prognostic importance of hypodiploid hematopoietic precursors in myelodysplastic syndromes. N Engl J Med 1986;314:1472–1475.

Coiffier B, Adeleine P, Viola JJ, et al. Dysmyelopoietic syndromes. A search for prognostic factors in 193 patients. Cancer 1983;52: 83–90.

Coiffier B, Adeleine P, Gentilhomme O, Felman P, Treille-Ritouet D, Byron PA. Myelodysplastic syndromes: a multiparametric study of prognostic factors in 336 patients. Cancer 1987;60:3029–3032.

d'Onofrio G, Mancini S, Tamburrini E, Mango G, Ortona L. Giant neutrophils with increased peroxidase activity: another evidence of dysgranulopoiesis in AIDS. Am J Clin Pathol 1987;87:584–591.

Delacretaz F, Schmidt P, Piguet D, Bachmann F, Costa J. Histopathology of myelodysplastic syndromes. The FAB classification (proposals) applied to bone marrow biopsy. Am J Clin Pathol 1987;87:180–186.

Dormer P, Hershko C, Wilmanns W. Mechanisms and prognostic value of cell kinetics in the myelodysplastic syndromes. Br J Haematol 1987;67:147–152.

Fenaux P, Jouet JP, Zandecki M, Lai J, Simon M, Pollet JP. Chronic and subacute myelomonocytic leukemia in the adult: a report of 60 cases with special reference to prognostic factors. Br J Haematol 1987;65:101–106.

Foucar K, McKenna RW, Bloomfield CD, Bowers TK, Brunning RD. Therapy-related leukemia: a panmyelosis. Cancer 1979;43: 1285–1296.

Foucar K, Langdon RM, Armitage JO, Olson DB, Carroll TJ. Myelodysplastic syndromes. A clinical and pathologic analysis of 109 cases. Cancer 1985;56:553–561.

Ganser A, Volkers B, Greher J, et al. Recombinant human granulocyte-macrophage colony-stimulating factor in patients with myelodysplastic syndromes—A phase I/II trial. Blood 1989;73:31–37.

Greenberg PL. The smoldering myeloid leukemic states: clinical and biologic features. Blood 1983;61:1035–1044.

Griffin JD, ed. Myelodysplastic syndromes. Clin Haematol 1986;15:909–923.

Jacobs RH, Cornbleet MA, Vardiman JW, Larson RA, LeBeau MM, Rowley JD. Prognostic implications of morphology and karyotype in primary myelodysplastic syndromes. Blood 1986;67:1765–1772.

Jacobs A. Myelodysplastic syndromes: pathogenesis, functional abnormalities, and clinical implications. J Clin Pathol 1985;38: 1201–1217.

Janssen JWG, Buschle M, Layton M, et al. Clonal analysis of myelodysplastic syndromes: evidence of multipotent stem cell origin. Blood 1989;73:248–254.

Juneja SK, Imbert M, Sigaux F, et al. Prevalence and distribution of ringed sideroblasts in primary myelodysplastic syndromes. J Clin Pathol 1983;36:566–569.

Juneja SK, Imbert M, Jouault H, Scoazec J, Sigaux F, Sultan C. Haematological features of primary myelodysplastic syndromes (PMDS) at initial presentation: a study of 118 cases. J Clin Pathol 1983;36:1129–1135.

Kaffe S, Hsu LYF, Hoffman R, Hirschhorn K. Association of 5q- and refractory anemia. Am J Hematol 1978;4:269–272.

Kantarjian HM, Keating MJ, Walters RS, et al. Therapy-related leukemia and myelodysplastic syndrome: clinical, cytogenetic, and prognostic features. J Clin Oncol 1986;4:1748–1757.

Kerkhofs H, Hermans J, Haak HL, Leeksma CHW. Utility of the FAB classification for myelodysplastic syndromes: investigation of prognostic factors in 237 cases. Br J Haematol 1987;65:73–81.

Knapp RH, Dewald GW, Pierre RV. Cytogenetic studies in 174 consecutive patients with preleukemia or myelodysplastic syndromes. Mayo Clin Proc 1985;60:507–516.

Koeffler HP. Myelodysplastic syndromes (preleukemia). Semin Hematol 1986;23;284–299.

Lyons J, Janssen JWG, Bartram C, Layton M, Mufti GJ. Mutation of Ki-ras and N-ras oncogenes in myelodysplastic syndromes. Blood 1988;71:1707–1712.

Michels SD, McKenna RW, Arthur DC, Brunning RD. Therapy-related acute myeloid leukemia and myelodysplastic syndrome: a clinical and morphologic study of 65 cases. Blood 1985;65: 1364–1372.

Mufti GJ, Stevens JR, Oscier DG, Hamblin TJ, Machin D. Myelodysplastic syndromes: a scoring system with prognostic significance. Br J Haematol 1985;59:425–433.

Napoli VM, Stein S, Spira TJ, Raskin D. Myelodysplasia progressing to acute myeloblastic leukemia in an HTLV-III virus-positive homosexual man with AIDS-related complex. Am J Clin Pathol 1986;86:788–791.

Oguma S, Yoshida Y, Uchino H, Maekaw T. Factors influencing leukemic transformation in refractory anemia with excess blasts, with ringed sideroblasts and without ringed sideroblasts. Cancer Res 1986;46:3698–3700.

Oguma S, Yoshida Y, Uchino H, Maekaw T. Factors influencing non-leukemic death in RA, RAS, and RAEB. Cancer Res 1987;47:3599–3602.

Pederson-Bjergaard J, Philip P. Cytogenetic characteristics of therapy-related acute nonlymphocytic leukaemia, preleukaemia and acute myeloproliferative syndrome: correlation with clinical data for 61 consecutive cases. Br J Haematol 1987;66:199–207.

Ribera J, Cervantes F, Rozman C. A multivariate analysis of prognostic factors in chronic myelomonocytic leukemia according to the FAB criteria. Br J Haematol 1987;65:307–311.

Schneider DR, Picker LJ. Myelodysplasia in the acquired immune deficiency syndrome. Am J Clin Pathol 1985;84:144–152.

Scoazec J, Imbert M, Crafts M, et al. Myelodysplastic syndrome or acute leukemia? A study of 28 cases presenting with borderline features. Cancer 1985;55:2390–2394.

Solal-Celigny P, Desaint B, Herrara A, et al. Chronic myelomonocytic leukemia according to the FAB classification: analysis of 35 cases. Blood 1984;63:634–638.

Teerenhovi L, Lintula R. Natural course of myelodysplastic syndromes—Helsinki experience. Scand J Haematol 1986;36:102–106.

Third MIC Cooperative Study Group. Recommendations for a morphologic, immunologic, and cytogenetic (MIC) working classification of the primary and therapy related myelodysplastic disorders. Cancer Genet Cytogenet 1988;32:1–10.

Tricot G, De Wolf-Peeters C, Hendrickx B, Verwilghen RL. Bone marrow histology in myelodysplastic syndromes. I. Histological findings in myelodysplastic syndromes and comparison with bone marrow smears. Br J Haematol 1984;57:423–430.

Tricot G, De Wolf-Peeters C, Vlietinck R, Verwilghen RL. Bone marrow histology in myelodysplastic syndromes. II. Prognostic value of abnormal localization of immature precursors in MDS. Br J Haematol 1984;58:217–225.

Tricot G, Boogaerts MA, De Wolf-Peeters C, Van Den Berghe H, Verwilghen RL. The myelodysplastic syndromes: different evolution patterns based on sequential morphological and cytogenetic investigations. Br J Haematol 1985;59:659–670.

Tricot G, Vlietinck R, Boogaerts MA, et al. Prognostic factors in the myelodysplastic syndromes: importance of initial data on peripheral blood counts, bone marrow cytology, trephine biopsy and chromosomal analysis. Br J Haematol 1985;60:19–32.

Tricot G, Boogaerts MA. The role of aggressive chemotherapy in the treatment of the myelodysplastic syndromes. Br J Haematol 1986;63:477–483.

Tricot G, Mecucci C, Van Den Berghe H. Evolution of the myelodysplastic syndromes. Br J Haematol 1986;63:609–614 (Annotation).

Vadhan-Raj S, Keating M, LeMaistre A, et al. Effects of recombinant human granulocyte-macrophage colony-stimulating factor in patients with myelodysplastic syndromes. N Engl J Med 1987;317:1545–1552.

Vallespi T, Torrabadella M, Julia A, et al. Myelodysplastic syndromes: a study of 101 cases according to the FAB classification. Br J Haematol 1985;61:83–92.

Varela BL, Chuang C, Woll JE, Bennett JM. Modifications in the classification of primary myelodysplastic syndromes: the addition of the scoring system. Hematol Oncol 1985;3:55–63.

Weisdorf DJ, Oken MM, Johnson GJ, Rydell RE. Auer rod positive dysmyelopoietic syndrome. Am J Hematol 1981;11:397–402.

Weisdorf DJ, Oken MM, Johnson GJ, Rydell RE. Chronic myelodysplastic syndrome: short survival with or without evolution to acute leukemia. Br J Haematol 1983;55:691–700.

Whang-Peng J, Young RC, Lee EC, Longo DL, Schechter GP, DeVita VT. Cytogenetic studies in patients with secondary leukemia/dysmyelopoietic syndrome after different treatment modalities. Blood 1988;71:403–414.

Worsley A, Oscier DG, Stevens J, et al. Prognostic features of chronic myelomonocytic leukaemia: a modified Bournemouth score gives the best prediction of survival. Br J Haematol 1988;68:17–21.

Yunis JJ, Rydell RE, Oken MM, Arnesen MA, Mayer MG, Labell M. Refined chromosome analysis as an independent prognostic indicator in de novo myelodysplastic syndromes. Blood 1986;61: 1721–1730.

Yunis JJ, Lobell M, Arnesen MA, et al. Refined chromosome study helps define prognostic subgroups in most patients with primary myelodysplastic syndrome and acute myelogenous leukaemia. Br J Haematol 1988;68:189–194.

Zon LI, Arkin C, Groopman JE. Haematologic manifestations of the human immune deficiency virus (HIV). Br J Haematol 1987;66:251–256.

38 Chronic Lymphoproliferative Disorders, Immunoproliferative Disorders, and Malignant Lymphoma

Fred R. Dick

The lymphoproliferative disorders represent a spectrum of diseases with a broad morphologic, functional, and clinical diversity. The classification in Table 38.1 is based on the following facts. Chronic lymphoproliferative disorders are predominantly blood- and bone marrow-based disorders with varying degrees of tissue involvement. Immunoproliferative disorders are predominantly bone marrow-based diseases. They are neoplasms of B cells at or near the terminal stage of functional development, and thus are also characterized by production of a monoclonal immunoprotein. Malignant lymphomas are predominantly tissue-based disorders that may also have a significant degree of blood and marrow involvement. Lymphoblastic leukemia is a disease of precursor B cells and T cells, and although it fits in the general category of lymphoproliferative disorders, it is discussed in the chapter on acute leukemias (Chapter 37).

CHRONIC LYMPHOPROLIFERATIVE DISORDERS

Morphologically, the chronic lymphoproliferative disorders show a "mature" appearance with condensation of nuclear chromatin and small nuclear size; however, some element of morphologic "immaturity" may be present. These disorders vary widely in their clinical course, ranging from 1 to 3 years for several of the more aggressive disorders to 7 years or more for the more clinically indolent processes.

Chronic lymphoproliferative disorders include neoplastic proliferations of the lymphocyte at the mid-stage of functional differentiation for B cells and the terminal stage of functional differentiation of T cells. Based on marker analysis, these disorders can be divided into the more common, predominantly B-cell disorders, and the much less common T-cell disorders. Although the immunophenotype cannot always be predicted by clinical and morphologic features, the presence of nuclear contour irregularity, cytoplasmic granules, or skin involvement should suggest a T-cell disorder.

Chronic Lymphocytic Leukemia

Chronic lymphocytic leukemia (CLL) is a frequently diagnosed neoplastic disease characterized by proliferation of a small, morphologically mature lymphocytes (1). CLL involves the blood and bone marrow, and also frequently the lymph nodes, spleen, and liver. It is a disease with a male predominance and a median age of approximately 65, being rarely seen in individuals less than 40 years of age (2). It usually follows an indolent course (7 years median survival), and many patients are diagnosed by finding an elevated lymphocyte count during evaluation incidental to another disease. Most cases of CLL are of B-cell type (97%), and the following discussion applies primarily to B-cell CLL. T-cell CLL is dis-

Table 38.1. Classification of Lymphoproliferative Disorders

CHRONIC LYMPHOPROLIFERATIVE DISORDERS
Chronic lymphocytic leukemia
Prolymphocytic leukemia
Hairy cell leukemia
T-Cell disorders
T-cell chronic lymphocytic leukemia
T-cell prolymphocytic leukemia
Adult T-cell leukemia/lymphoma
T-γ lymphoproliferative disease (large granular lymphocytosis)
Sézary's syndrome
IMMUNOPROLIFERATIVE DISORDERS
Plasma cell myeloma
Plasmacytoma
Waldenström's macroglobulinemia
Heavy chain disease
Benign monoclonal gammopathy
Amyloidosis
MALIGNANT LYMPHOMAS
Non-Hodgkin's lymphoma
Hodgkin's disease
Posttransplant lymphoproliferative disorders
ACUTE LYMPHOCYTIC LEUKEMIA
(Discussed in Chapter 37)

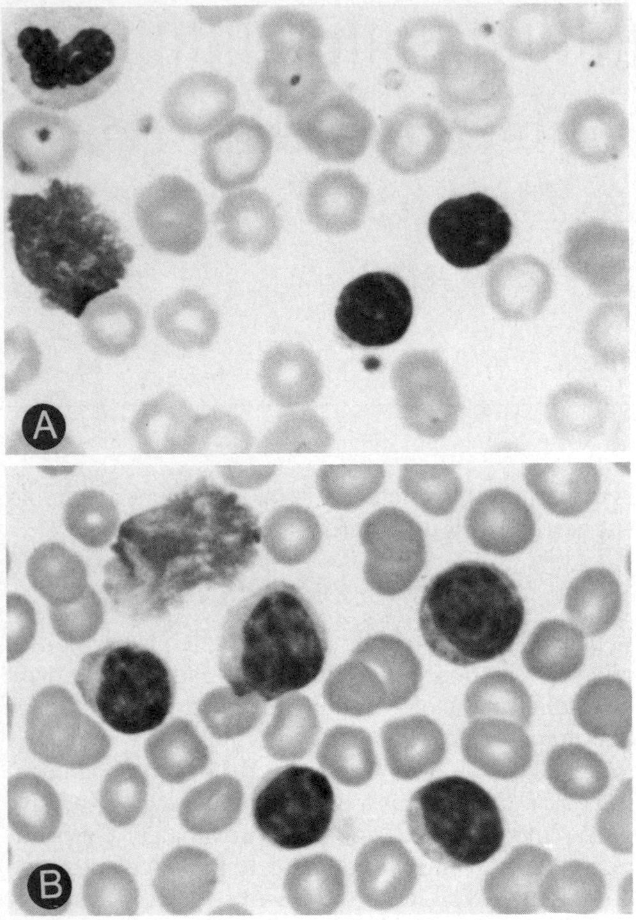

Figure 38.1. CLL lymphocytes on blood smear. Lymphocytes almost as small as erythrocytes (**A**) are rarely seen in CLL. Lymphocytes in CLL are more typically medium-sized, like those shown in **B**. Note the exaggerated chromatin clumping in some of the lymphocytes. (Wright's stain × 1200.) (From Dick FR. Chronic lymphocytic leukemia, prolymphocytic leukemia and leukemic non-Hodgkin's leukemia. In: Koepke JA, ed. Laboratory hematology. New York: Churchill Livingstone, 1984;1:325–357.)

tinctly different from B-cell CLL and is discussed in a subsequent section.

DIAGNOSTIC FEATURES

Unlike most other lymphoproliferative diseases, there is no cytologic feature of the cell in chronic lymphocytic leukemia that is diagnostic. Thus, the diagnosis rests on finding increased numbers of nearly morphologically normal-appearing lymphocytes.

To diagnose chronic lymphocytic leukemia, there should be a peripheral blood lymphocytosis greater than 5000/mm^3 and a marrow lymphocytosis greater than 30% (3). A lower limit of 4000/mm^3 has also been used as a criterion for diagnosis of CLL (4). At diagnosis, most patients have a white blood cell count (WBC) of greater than 15,000/mm^3 with a median count of about 30,000 to 40,000/mm^3. Some cases may have a WBC well over 100,000/mm^3. Because CLL is a clonal process, there is frequently a monotonous look-alike appearance to the lymphocytes on smears (Fig. 38.1). Cytoplasm is usually small to moderate in amount, pale blue, and agranular; the nuclear chromatin frequently shows exaggerated chromatin clumping compared with a normal lymphocyte.

The bone marrow in chronic lymphocytic leukemia usually aspirates freely, and marrow sections may range from normocellular to hypercellular (Fig. 38.2). When the marrow is less extensively infiltrated, the lymphocytes in the marrow may be present in focal aggregates (Fig. 38.2*A*) or may be diffusely intermixed with residual normal marrow elements (Fig. 38.2*B*). This latter pattern is called an interstitial infiltrative pattern. Frequently, a mixed focal and interstitial pattern may be seen. As the marrow becomes more extensively infiltrated, these patterns (focal or interstitial) are gradually lost, and the infiltrate diffusely obliterates the marrow space (Fig. 38.2*C*). As illustrated in Figure 38.2*D*, individual lymphocytes in CLL on sections are indistinguishable from normal mature lymphocytes.

When the blood and marrow counts are near the lower limits described above, and the diagnosis is in question, immunologic cell surface marker studies may be helpful in establishing the diagnosis and in ruling out postsplenectomy lymphocytosis or a chronic reactive lymphocytosis (5). Clonality, as evidenced by a weakly reacting surface immunoglobulin with a restricted light chain, and CD5(T1) positivity are characteristic of CLL (Table 38.2) (6). In cases with a low WBC in the range of 4,000 to 25,000/mm^3 it may be easier to make the diagnosis using peripheral blood immunology than with bone marrow examination, since the bone marrow in these cases may also show a low percentage of lymphocytes, and characteristic spreading focal aggregates may be absent. If immunulogic marker studies are available, immunologic evaluation of the peripheral blood is the method of choice to confirm the diagnosis, especially if therapy is not contemplated.

MORPHOLOGIC VARIABILITY AND DIFFERENTIAL DIAGNOSIS

Although most cases of chronic lymphocytic leukemia will fit the description above, there are some features that may lead to an altered appearance. These are listed in Table 38.3 and illustrated in Figure 38.3.

About 15 to 20% of cases of CLL will have numerous cells with a morphologic appearance similar to Downey II reactive (atypical) lymphocytes (Fig. 38.3*A*) (7). These cells are more readily identified in

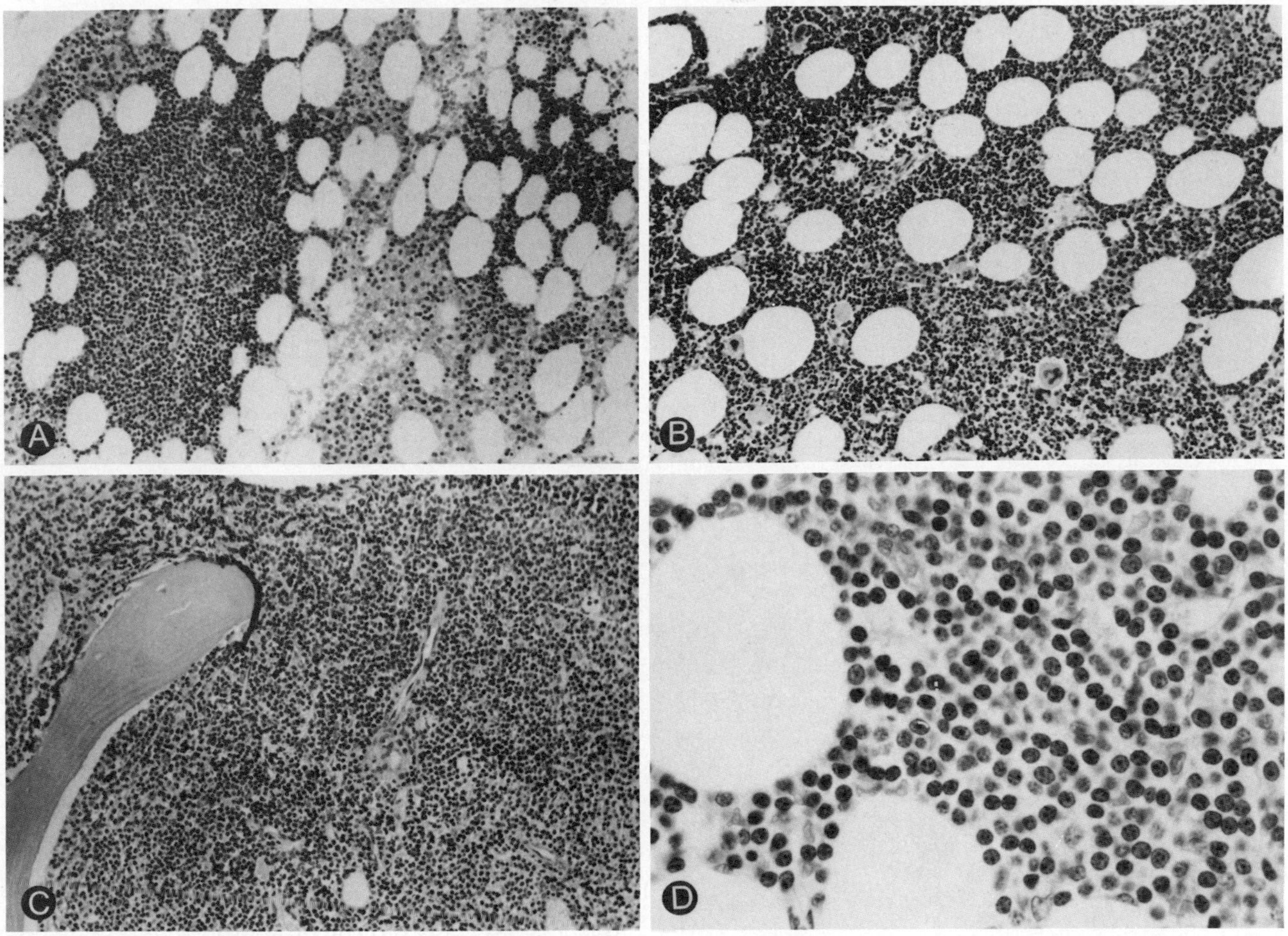

Figure 38.2. CLL bone marrow sections. The focal pattern shown in **A** is characterized by aggregates that have spreading of lymphocytes into and surrounding fat cells at the periphery. This spreading characteristic is especially evident in the aggregate in the upper right field of **A**. An interstitial pattern shown in **B** is characterized by diffuse infiltration of lymphocytes throughout the marrow space with many residual fat cells and admixed normal marrow elements. Extensive diffuse replacement of the marrow is shown in **C**. On high-power examination in **D**, note the minimal nuclear contour irregularity, clumped chromatin, uniformity, and absence of mitotic activity. (Hematoxylin and eosin, ×120 [**A, B,** and **C**], ×600 [**D**].) (*A*, From Dick FR. Chronic lymphocytic leukemia, prolymphocytic leukemia and leukemic non-Hodgkin's leukemia. In: Koepke JA, ed. Laboratory hematology. New York: Churchill Livingstone, 1984;1:325–357.)

Table 38.2. Special Studies in the Diagnosis and Differential Diagnosis of the B-Cell Lymphocytic Leukemias

	SIg[a] Intensity	SIg Subtype	CD5 (T1)	CD24 (BA-1)	CD20 (B-1)	CD25 (TAC)	TRAP
CLL	Weak	M,D>G	Most	Strong	Weak	±	Neg to weak
CLL-tr	Variable	M,D>G	Most	Strong	Weak	±	Neg to weak
PLL	Strong	M>>G,A	Some	Strong	Strong	±	Variable
HCL	Mod strong	M,D>G,A	None	Neg	Strong	+	Weak to strong
B cell lymphoma	Strong/neg	M>G,A	Rare	Weak	Strong	±	Occasional

[a]SIg, surface immunoglobulin; TRAP, tartrate-resistant acid phosphatase; CLL-tr, CLL with prolymphocytic transformation; PLL, prolymphocytic leukemia; HCL, hairy cell leukemia.

the blood than on marrow smears. In CLL, these Downey II–like lymphocytes usually have neither cytoplasmic granules nor the marked morphologic variability seen in reactive processes. A Downey II appearance in CLL tends to be associated with an earlier stage of disease but may be present throughout the course of the disease. The importance of the finding of Downey II–like lymphocytes in CLL is to recognize it as a variant and not report the cells as "atypical/reactive" lymphocytes. Since CLL is a disease of individuals more than 30 to 40 years of age, CLL should be considered in any reactive-appearing lymphocytosis in older patients.

Many cases of CLL will have rare cells with the appearance of prolymphocytes, and occasional cases may have numerous prolymphocytes at presentation

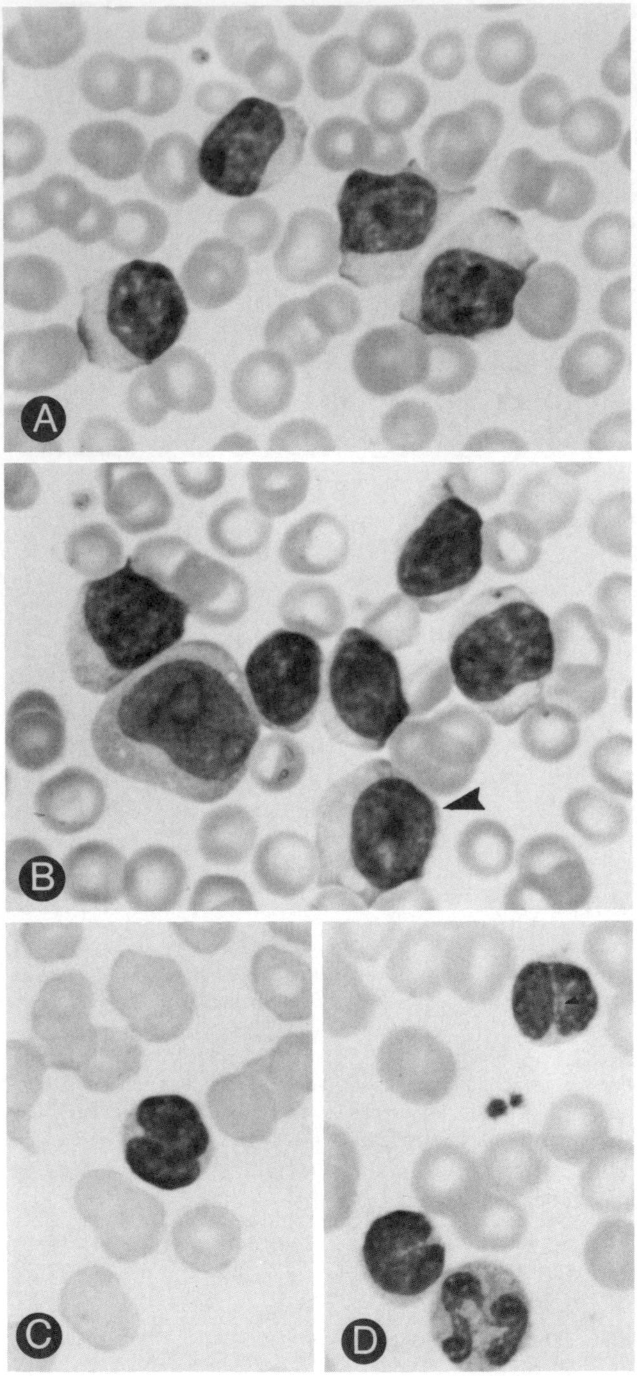

Figure 38.3. Morphologic variability in the peripheral blood of CLL. **A**, Downey II–like lymphocytes are large lymphocytes with abundant cytoplasm and peripheral basophilia. **B**, Prolymphocytes in CLL. Note the size gradation in this field from small lymphocytes to medium-sized lymphocytes to a typical prolymphocyte (*arrow*) to a large blast-like prolymphocyte. **C** and **D**, Nuclear contour irregularity in lymphocytes in CLL. Note the folded nucleus in **C** and the clefted nuclei in **D**. Clefted cells in CLL have more cytoplasm than the cells of small cleaved cell lymphoma. (Wright's stain ×1200.) (**A** and **D**, From Dick FR. Chronic lymphocytic leukemia, prolymphocytic leukemia and leukemic non-Hodgkin's leukemia. In: Koepke JA, ed. Laboratory hematology. New York: Churchill Livingstone, 1984;1:325–357.)

Table 38.3. Morphologic Variability in Chronic Lymphocytic Leukemia

Smears
Downey II appearance
Prolymphocytes
Nuclear contour irregularity (folds, clefts)
Cytoplasmic granules
Hairy cytoplasm
Sections
Prolymphocytes and growth centers
Clefted cells
Reticulin fibrosis

Table 38.4. Percentage of Prolymphocytes on Initial Diagnostic Films of CLL[a]

Percentage of Prolymphocytes	Number of Cases	Percentage of Cases
<5	198	74
6–10	40	15
11–20	24	9
>20	4	2
Total CLL cases	266	100

[a]Data from 266 cases of CLL with peripheral blood lymphocytes >15,000/mm^3 seen at the University of Iowa Hospitals and Clinics from 1960 to 1975. Differentials were done on initial diagnostic bone marrow and/or peripheral blood smears, and the percentage of prolymphocytes is per 100 lymphoid cells. Marker studies were performed on only a small percentage of the cases, and some T-cell CLLs may be included. (From Dick FR. Chronic lymphocytic leukemia, prolymphocytic leukemia and leukemic non-Hodgkin's leukemia. In: Koepke JA, ed. Laboratory hematology. New York: Churchill Livingstone, 1984;1:325–357.)

(Fig. 43.3*B*). The typical prolymphocyte in CLL has partly dispersed, partly clumped chromatin, increased cytoplasmic basophilia, and a prominent single nucleolus with perinucleolar chromatin clumping. More rarely, large blast-like prolymphocytes—also called reticular lymphoblasts (7) or paraimmunoblasts (8)—can be seen. Prolymphocytes in CLL are morphologically similar to the prolymphocytes of prolymphocytic leukemia (see later, Fig. 38.7). As shown in Table 38.4, more than 25% of cases of CLL at diagnosis will have more than 5% prolymphocytes on smears (9). When the percentage of prolymphocytes exceeds 10%, the case is said to represent an aytpical CLL with prolymphocytes (CLL/PL), and when the percentage of prolymphocytes at diagnosis exceeds 55%, an alternate diagnosis of a more aggressive disease, prolymphocytic leukemia, should be considered (10–12).

A few cells with nuclear contour irregularity can be seen in the blood and marrow smears of chronic lymphocytic leukemia (Fig. 38.3C and *D*). This nuclear contour irregularity can range from subtle nuclear folds to sharp nuclear clefts. Nuclear contour irregularity can also be seen on sections in CLL and may be confused with intermediate or small cleaved lymphoma. As illustrated in Table 38.5, 85% of cases of chronic lymphocytic leukemia have less than 5%

Table 38.5. Percentage of Lymphocytes with Irregular Nuclear Contour on Initial Diagnostic Films of CLL[a]

Percentage with Irregular Nuclear Contour	Number of Cases	Percentage of Cases
<5	225	85
6–10	30	11
11–20	11	4
Total CLL cases	266	100

[a]Data from 266 cases of CLL with peripheral blood lymphocytes > 15,000/mm^3 seen at the University of Iowa Hospitals and Clinics from 1960 to 1975. Differentials done on initial diagnostic bone marrow and/or peripheral blood smears. The percentage with irregular nuclear contour is per 100 lymphoid cells. (From Dick FR. Chronic lymphocytic leukemia, prolymphocytic leukemia and leukemic non-Hodgkin's leukemia. In: Koepke JA, ed. Laboratory hematology, New York: Churchill Livingstone, 1984;1:325–357.)

Table 38.6. Percentage of Prolymphocytes and Cells with Irregular Nuclear Contour on Initial Diagnostic Films of CLL[a]

Percentage of Prolymphocytes	Number of Cases		
21–30	3	1	0
11–20	16	4	4
6–10	30	6	4
<5	176	19	3
Percentage of cells with irregular nuclear contour	≤5	6–10	11–20

[a]Data from 266 cases of CLL with peripheral blood lymphocytes > 1,000/mm^3 diagnosed at the University of Iowa Hospitals between 1960 and 1975. Forty-five atypical CLL cases had more than 10% prolymphocytes and/or more than 10% cells with irregular nuclear contour. (From Dick FR. Chronic lymphocytic leukemia, prolymphocytic leukemia and leukemic non-Hodgkin's leukemia. In: Koepke JA, ed., Laboratory hematology. New York: Churchill Livingstone, 1984;1:325–357.)

of such cells at diagnosis (9). In one study, the presence of more than 5% lymphocytes with nuclear contour irregularity did not appear to alter the prognosis of an otherwise typical CLL (13). When the number of cells with nuclear contour irregularity is significantly greater than 5%, an alternative diagnosis of a leukemic phase of a non-Hodgkin's lymphoma such as intermediate lymphocytic lymphoma, small cleaved cell lymphoma, Sézary syndrome, or T-cell leukemia should be considered. The distinction between an atypical CLL with increased nuclear contour irregularity and a leukemic phase of intermediate lymphocytic lymphoma may be very difficult, even with marker studies (14).

Some cases of CLL will show a mixture of atypical features (Downey II–like cells, prolymphocytes, and cells with nuclear contour irregularity), giving a very heterogeneous appearance to a disease that is said to be characterized by monotony of cell type. Table 38.6 shows a combination of the data from Tables 38.4 and 38.5 (9). The data in this table indicate that 45 of 266 cases (17%) had greater than 10% prolymphocytes and/or cells with nuclear contour irregularity. The diagnosis of an atypical variant of CLL in these cases is still tenable, although it may be necessary to use immunologic marker studies or lymph node biopsy to exclude other diagnoses. In our laboratory,

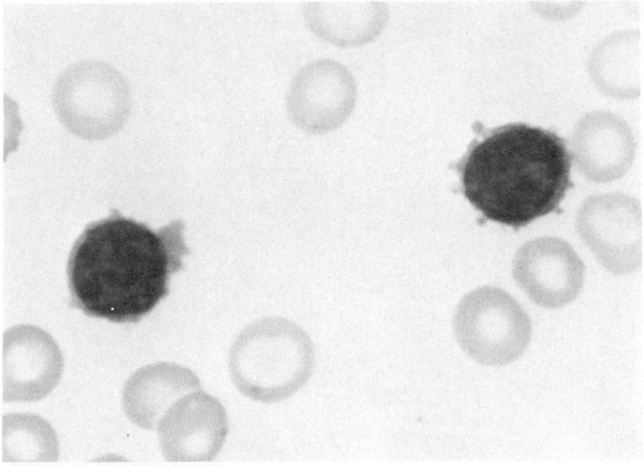

Figure 38.4. Artifactual hairy cytoplasmic projections in peripheral blood cells from CLL. The cell at the right also has a prolymphocytic appearance. (Wright's stain, ×1200.)

we enumerate the number of prolymphocytes and cells with nuclear contour irregularity in patients with chronic lymphoproliferative disorders, since greater than 10% of these cell types may have diagnostic or prognostic significance.

Cytoplasmic granulation is very uncommon in B-cell CLL, and if granules are present, a diagnosis of T-cell CLL or large granular lymphocytosis, or a reactive process should be considered. Immunologic marker studies may assist in the differential diagnosis.

Occasionally, the cells in cases of CLL (as well as prolymphocytic leukemia or low-grade lymphomas) will show artifactual hairy cytoplasmic projections (Fig. 38.4). A repeat smear or bone marrow biopsy may help solve the problem; however a tartrate-resistant acid phosphatase (TRAP) stain or immunologic marker analysis may also be helpful to distinguish CLL from hairy cell leukemia.

Growth centers (illustrated in Fig. 38.5) are frequently present in the lymph nodes of patients with chronic lymphocytic leukemia (15, 16) and less often on bone marrow sections. Growth centers are thought to be the sites of proliferation of cells in CLL since many of the cells in growth centers are large and have basophilic cytoplasm, dispersed chromatin, nucleoli, and increased mitotic activity. These cells on sections are prolymphocytes that correspond to the prolymphocytes seen on blood and marrow smears. Prolymphocytes can also be diffusely distributed throughout the marrow or be admixed with small mature cells with clefted nuclei. This may lead to confusion with lymphoma on section material.

Rare cases of CLL will aspirate poorly and show increased marrow reticulin. This finding should not cause confusion with hairy cell leukemia, which characteristically shows increased reticulin. A TRAP

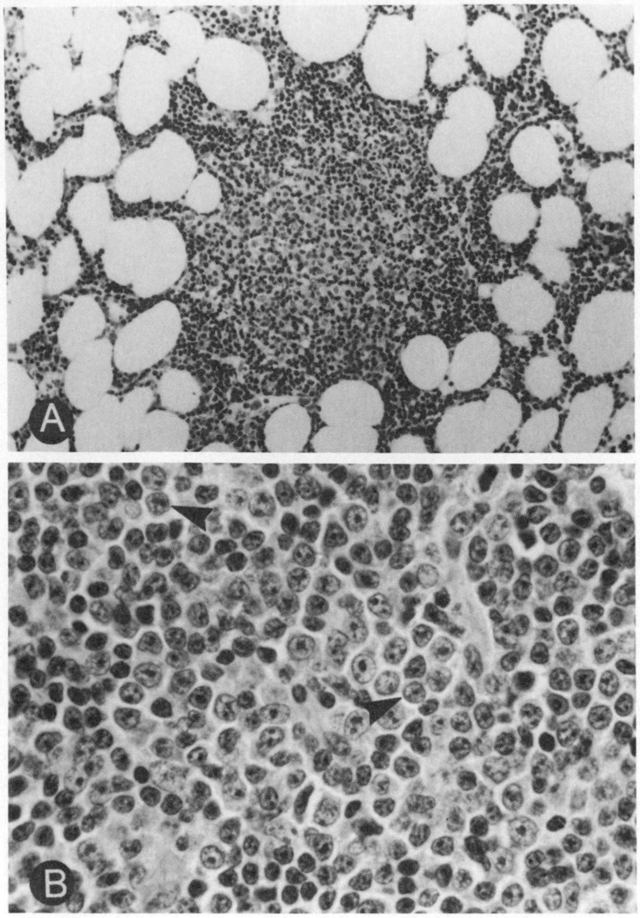

Figure 38.5. **A**, Growth center in the bone marrow of CLL. Note the central pallor of the aggregate due to focal increase in prolymphocytes. **B**, Increased concentration of prolymphocytes from a growth center. Note the gradation in size from mature lymphocytes to prolymphocytes with partly dispersed chromatin (*arrowheads*), to large blast-like prolymphocytes with dispersed chromatin, corresponding to the cells on smears illustrated in Figure 38.3**B**. (Hematoxylin and eosin, ×120 [**A**], ×600 [**B**].) (**A**, From Dick FR. Chronic lymphocytic leukemia, prolymphocytic leukemia and leukemic non-Hodgkin's leukemia. In: Koepke JA, ed. Laboratory hematology. New York: Churchill Livingstone, 1984;1:325–357.)

stain and immunophenotyping may assist in the diagnosis if cytology and histology are not characteristic of either diagnosis.

IMMUNOLOGIC AND OTHER SPECIAL STUDIES

Immunologic marker analysis is a useful adjunct to the diagnosis of CLL (Table 38.2), especially in cases with low WBC or in the differential diagnosis for other lymphoproliferative disorders. The most characteristic pattern in CLL is weakly reacting SIg coupled with CD5(T1) and CD-24(BA-1) positivity (6).

High-resolution agarose gel electrophoresis and immunofixation have shown that about 42% of patients with CLL will have a small monoclonal serum immunoglobulin, usually IgM or free light chain type (17). An additional 14% will have only free light chains in the urine. In 5% or fewer cases of CLL, the amount of monoclonal protein is large enough to be identified on conventional serum protein electrophoresis (1). A monoclonal protein on serum protein electrophoresis in chronic lymphocytic leukemia may be associated with a worsened prognosis, and its presence should stimulate a morphologic reevaluation of the case for plasmacytoid differentiation to rule out Waldenström's macroglobulinemia (4).

Table 38.7. Transformation and Secondary Tumors in CLL

Prolymphocytic transformation
Cleaved cell transformation
Large cell lymphoma (Richter's syndrome)
Plasma cell myeloma
Acute lymphocytic leukemia
Hodgkin's disease
Acute nonlymphocytic leukemia

Of special interest is the development of a warm autoimmune hemolytic anemia in about 15% of patients with CLL (1). In addition, depression of normal immunoglobulins is seen in CLL, leading to immune deficiency (1).

Over half of patients with CLL will have a clonal chromosomal abnormality after culture with B-cell mitogens; the most common finding is trisomy 12. Survival is adversely affected in patients with a clonal chromosomal abnormality (18). DNA content studies are nearly normal in a majority of cases (19, 20), and antigen-receptor gene rearrangement studies show clonal rearrangement, as would be expected of a B-cell neoplasm (21). Rarely, the additional finding of a T-cell antigen receptor rearrangement may be seen in B-cell CLL (22).

CHANGE WITH PROGRESSION AND TRANSFORMATION

Although chronic lymphocytic leukemia is a disease of the mature lymphocyte, it does not always remain morphologically mature or remain functional at the early B-cell stage. The various transformations and secondary tumors that can arise in CLL are shown in Table 38.7.

Prolymphocytic transformation of CLL is characterized by a progressive increase in prolymphocytes of more than 10 to 15%, and is similar in appearance to de novo CLL/PL, as described in Figure 43.3*B* (11, 23, 24). When there is a sustained progressive increase in the percentage of prolymphocytes, patient survival and response to therapy are adversely affected.

Increasing numbers of clefted cells may accompany an increase in prolymphocytes. However,

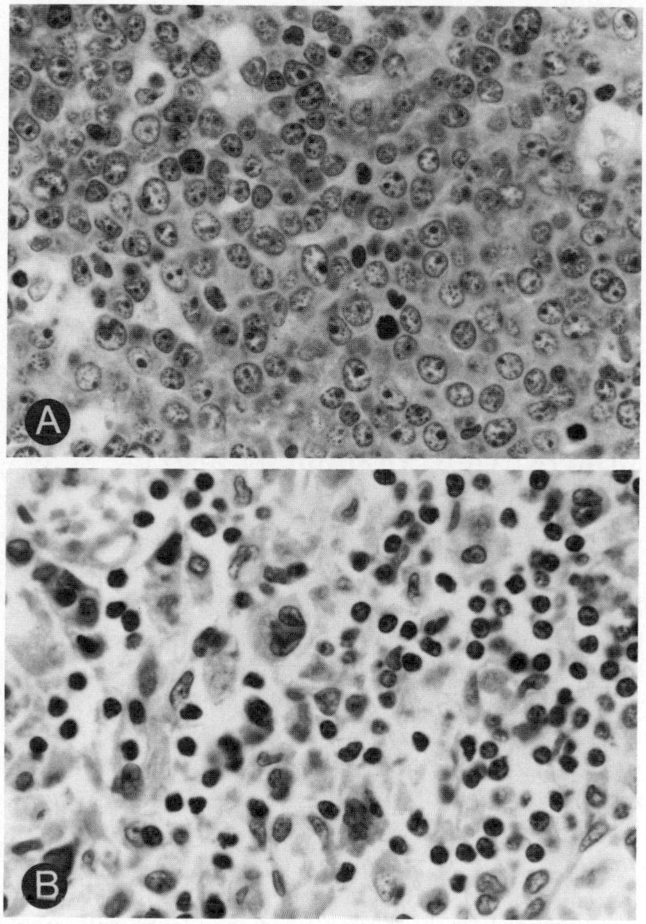

Figure 38.6. Large cell lymphomas (Richter's syndrome) arising in CLL. **A**, Cells in this lymphoma from a lymph node biopsy are the size of, or larger than, blast-like prolymphocytes. Note the marked uniformity of this tumor compared with the tumor in **B**. **B**, This lymphoma from a patient with CLL shows marked pleomorphism of the large cells (with admixed residual CLL lymphocytes). This form of Richter's syndrome can be mistaken for Hodgkin's disease. (Hematoxylin and eosin, ×600.) (**B**, From Dick FR. Chronic lymphocytic leukemia, prolymphocytic leukemia and leukemic non-Hodgkin's leukemia. In: Koepke JA, ed. Laboratory hematology. New York: Churchill Livingstone, 1984;1:325–357.)

rarely, increased nuclear clefting may be the predominant feature.

The cell of chronic lymphocytic leukemia has the ability to undergo a dramatic morphologic transformation to a cell that is much larger than a prolymphocyte, and is morphologically typical of large-cell lymphoma (24, 25). There can be marked variability in this transformation from one case to the next, as illustrated in Figure 38.6. The term "Richter's syndrome" has been applied to this transformation. Large-cell lymphoma arising in CLL frequently occurs at an extra marrow site; however, the bone marrow and occasionally the blood may be involved.

CLL may rarely present with concomitant plasma cell myeloma or may subsequently undergo apparent transformation to plasma cell myeloma, with production and secretion of immunoglobulin (26, 27).

Table 38.8. Clinical Staging in CLL[a]

Stage	Criteria	Percentage of Total	Survival
			yr
A	Fewer than three sites of involvement[b]	55	—[c]
B	Three or more sites of involvement	30	7
C	Anemia (< 10 g/dl) or thrombocytopenia (< 100 × 10 g/liter)	15	2

[a]From Dick FR. Chronic lymphocytic leukemia, prolymphocytic leukemia and leukemic non-Hodgkin's leukemia. In: Koepke JA, ed. Laboratory hematology. New York: Churchill Livingstone, 1984;1:325–357.
[b]Sites of involvement include spleen, liver, cervical nodes, axillary nodes, inguinal nodes.
[c]Survival for stage A is not significantly different from the age-matched general population.

Transformation to an entity typical of acute lymphocytic leukemia is rare (28).

When another morphologic type of lymphoproliferative disorder arises in chronic lymphocytic leukemia, it does not automatically imply that that tumor has arisen from the same clone; it may be a new tumor. This is most likely the case for Hodgkin's disease (29) and myeloproliferative disorders arising in chronic lymphocytic leukemia (24). Special studies such as chromosome analysis or gene probe analysis showing the exact pattern in both tumors will confirm that they are derived from the same clone. The appearance of a new pattern observed by these techniques suggests that either a new tumor has developed or clonal evolution of the original tumor has occurred (25, 27).

STAGING, THERAPY, AND PROGNOSTIC FEATURES

In 1981, the International Workshop on Chronic Lymphocytic Leukemia developed a simplified scheme for the staging of chronic lymphocytic leukemia (Table 38.8). A more complicated staging scheme had been developed by Rai in 1975. Either of these schemes may be used, or they may be used in combination (30).

Morphologic features have also been shown to determine prognosis in chronic lymphocytic leukemia. As stated in the previous section, increasing numbers of prolymphocytes on smears alters prognosis. Patients with CLL/PL showing more than 15,000 prolymphocytes per cubic millimeter at presentation do significantly worse than those with 15,000 or fewer prolymphocytes per cubic millimeter (12). The infiltrative pattern of marrow involvement in CLL has been correlated with survival. Patients with a focal or interstitial infiltrate (i.e., less extensive involvement) have been shown to have a better prognosis and a lower stage of disease than patients with diffuse extensive marrow involvement (31). Also, as mentioned in the previous section, clonal chromosomal abnormalities are associated with a poorer prognosis (18). The size of lymphocytes, exclusive of prolymphocytes, in chronic lymphocytic leukemia has not been conclusively shown to have prognostic significance.

Chronic lymphocytic leukemia is essentially a noncurable disease; thus, therapy is directed at treatment of symptoms and palliation. Patients with early-stage disease and low white blood cell count may be observed without therapy. If therapy is necessary due to massive adenopathy, splenomegaly, anemia, decreased platelet count, or significantly elevated white cell count, single-agent chemotherapy (chlorambucil) is used. As the disease becomes nonresponsive, multiagent therapy is instituted (30).

Prolymphocytic Leukemia

Prolymphocytic leukemia is an uncommon form of leukemia that is closely related to chronic lymphocytic leukemia (10–12, 32–34). Similar to chronic lymphocytic leukemia, it predominantly affects males and has a median age of onset in the sixth to the seventh decade. It differs from chronic lymphocytic leukemia, however, in that there is a predominance of prolymphocytes. Prolymphocytic leukemia frequently presents with a very high white blood cell count, anemia, thrombocytopenia, and splenomegaly; it differs from CLL in that adenopathy is less conspicuous in prolymphocytic leukemia. Clinically, prolymphocytic leukemia is more aggressive than chronic lymphocytic leukemia, with a median survival of approximately 2 to 3 years. A majority of cases of prolymphocytic leukemia are of B-cell type; approximately 20% of T-cell type. The discussion in this section applies primarily to B-cell prolymphocytic leukemia.

DIAGNOSTIC FEATURES

The morphology of the cell in the peripheral blood of prolymphocytic leukemia is quite characteristic. Prolymphocytes are large lymphoid cells with abundant, moderately blue cytoplasm (Fig. 38.7). The nuclear chromatin is partly condensed and partly open with a reticular pattern. A single prominent nucleolus is present and is frequently accentuated by perinucleolar chromatin clumping. The exact percentage of prolymphocytes in the blood needed to confirm a diagnosis of prolymphocytic leukemia is not well defined; however, more than 55%, with the remainder being more mature lymphocytes, is a proposed minimum (10). The bone marrow is frequently extensively infiltrated. When the marrow is not extensively involved, the distribution may be focal and/or interstitial, similar to CLL (33, 35). On high-power magnification (Fig. 38.7C), the lymphoid cells have the appearance of prolymphocytes in CLL; however, more uniformity is usually seen than in CLL with increased prolymphocytes. Cases of prolymphocytic leukemia that do not have markedly elevated WBCs have been reported (36). These may be cases of prolymphocytic leukemia that are diagnosed early in the course of the disease. When the diagnosis is in question, immunologic marker studies may be of help. B-cell prolymphocytic leukemia shows strongly reacting SIg with a restricted light chain compared with the weak-reacting SIg of CLL (see Table 38.2) (6).

MORPHOLOGIC VARIABILITY AND DIFFERENTIAL DIAGNOSIS

In some cases of prolymphocytic leukemia, the peripheral blood prolymphocytes may show considerable numbers of smaller lymphoid cells with more condensed chromatin and prominent nucleoli. This variant needs to be distinguished from CLL, which may also occasionally show evident but not large nucleoli. Blast-like prolymphocytes with completely dispersed chromatin may also be a prominent feature in some cases of prolymphocytic leukemia, suggesting a diagnosis of acute leukemia. Granules or vacuoles may be present in some cases. Very large blast-like prolymphocytes may cause confusion with peripheral blood involvement by large-cell lymphoma or monoblastic leukemia. Some cases of prolymphocytic leukemia will show a greater spectrum of cells, ranging from mature lymphocytes with marked clumping of chromatin to more blast-like cells. These cases with variability in cell type suggest the possibility that the process has evolved from a chronic lymphocytic leukemia through prolymphocytic transformation. Cases of prolymphocytic leukemia with a moderate amount of nuclear contour irregularity will suggest the possibility of a leukemic transformation of a lymphoma. Rare cases of prolymphocytic leukemia (as well as CLL and intermediate lymphoma) will have cytoplasmic projections, suggesting the possibility of a variant of hairy cell leukemia. Immunologic marker analysis may be of some assistance in resolving the differential diagnosis raised by these variant morphologies.

IMMUNOLOGIC AND OTHER SPECIAL STUDIES

As pointed out in the previous section, the majority of cases of prolymphocytic leukemia are mature B-cell phenotype with strongly reacting surface immunoglobulin (Table 38.2). Unlike chronic lymphocytic leukemia, only about half of cases of prolymphocytic leukemia express CD5(T1). FMC7 is also

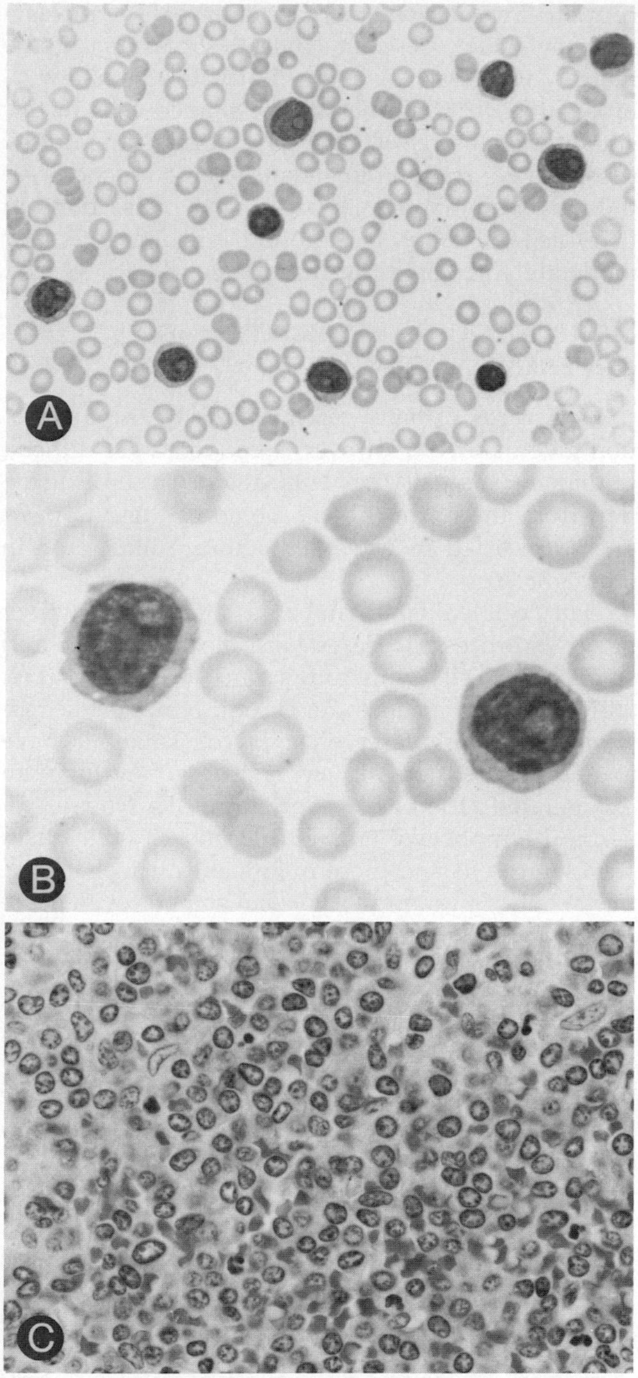

Figure 38.7. **A** and **B**, Typical prolymphocytes in the blood of prolymphocytic leukemia. **C**, Prolymphocytes on sections in prolymphocytic leukemia may have the uniform appearance illustrated here, or may show more variability in cell size with admixed mature lymphocytes and blast-like prolymphocytes. (**A**, and **B**, Wright's stain, ×1200.) **C**, Hematoxylin and eosin, ×600.) (**A** and **B**, From Dick FR. Chronic lymphocytic leukemia, prolymphocytic leukemia and leukemic non-Hodgkin's leukemia. In: Koepke JA, ed. Laboratory hematology. New York: Churchill Livingstone, 1984;1:325–357.)

more strongly expressed in prolymphocytic leukemia than in CLL (6). The intensity of surface immunoglobulin may be a useful feature to distinguish prolymphocytic leukemia from CLL with prolymphocytes (CLL/PL) and prolymphocytic transformation of CLL; however, some cases of CLL/PL and prolymphocytic transformation of CLL express strong surface immunoglobulin after the transformation (11, 23). Tartrate-resistant acid phosphatase (TRAP) stain may be positive in prolymphocytic leukemia and thus should not be used alone to distinguish prolymphocytic leukemia from hairy cell leukemia.

Serum protein studies performed on prolymphocytic leukemia have shown occasional cases with monoclonal gammopathy (34). Clonal chromosomal abnormalities are frequently seen in prolymphocytic leukemia cells using B-cell mitogens. A 14q+ was the most frequently observed abnormality in B-cell prolymphocytic leukemia in one study (37). Despite the partially transformed appearance of the cells in prolymphocytic leukemia and the chromosomal abnormalities, the cellular DNA content is normal in most cases, and there is a low percentage of cases in S-phase (38).

CHANGE WITH PROGRESSION AND TRANSFORMATION

Since prolymphocytic leukemia is uncommon and is also a tumor of relatively transformed lymphoid cells, reports of further transformation to a large-cell process are rare (24, 39).

STAGING, THERAPY, AND PROGNOSTIC FEATURES

No staging system similar to CLL exists for prolymphocytic leukemia; however, there are occasional cases of prolymphocytic leukemia with a low WBC that appear to be early-stage disease (36). Patients with prolymphocytic leukemia do not respond very well to conventional chronic lymphocytic leukemia management. Combination chemotherapy will induce remission in many patients; however, remission is usually short-lived. Some response to interferon alpha therapy has recently been reported (32).

Hairy Cell Leukemia

Hairy cell leukemia is an uncommon disease characterized by a proliferation of medium-sized lymphoid cells with hairy cytoplasmic projections (40). The disease predominantly involves the bone marrow and spleen, and the patient may or may not have a "leukemic" blood picture. There is a male predominance with a median age of onset in the sixth decade. The patient frequently presents with nonspecific constitutional symptoms, pancytopenia, and splenomegaly, and the disease usually follows a very indolent course. Virtually all cases are of B-cell origin.

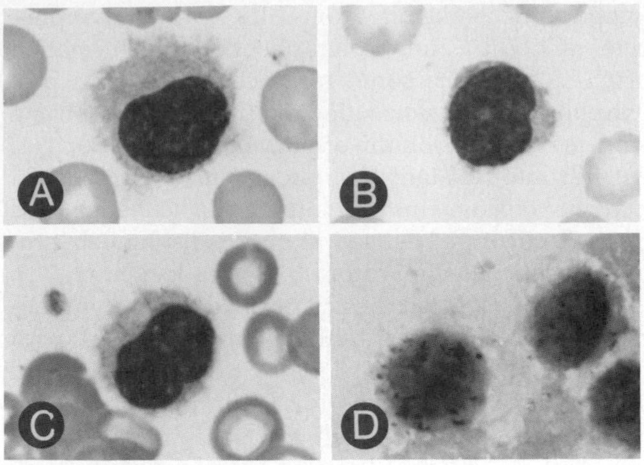

Figure 38.8. **A**, **B**, **C**, Typical hairy cells from the blood or marrow. **D**, TRAP stain. Note the dispersion of positive granules throughout the cytoplasm. (**A**, **B**, **C**, Wright's stain, ×1200. **D**, TRAP stain, ×1200.)

DIAGNOSTIC FEATURES

The most characteristic diagnostic feature of hairy cell leukemia is the appearance of hairy cells on blood and marrow smears (Fig. 38.8). Hairy cells range in size from that of a medium-sized lymphocyte to a monocyte. The cytoplasmic border has a frayed or shaggy appearance, and the cytoplasm is blue-gray with a variegated dark and light consistency. Cytoplasmic granules are uncommon. The nucleus is generally round to oval or slightly indented with a partly clumped, partly open or reticular chromatin, and a single indistinct nucleolus. The WBC is usually decreased, but hairy cells are easily found in the blood in most cases. In rare cases, it may be impossible to identify hairy cells, whereas other cases may have a markedly elevated white blood cell count with numerous hairy cells. A monocytopenia is characteristically seen in the peripheral blood and is a good differential diagnostic features. The bone marrow in hairy cell leukemia usually does not aspirate freely, and there may be a "dry tap." Thus, in some cases with a dry tap and very few hairy cells in the peripheral blood, cells showing the characteristic hairy cell morphology may be very difficult to find. Unfortunately, characteristic hairy cell morphology is not as readily identified on touch preparations of bone marrow as on aspirates. In these cases, the diagnosis must rest more heavily on the appearance of cells on the sections and a TRAP stain.

On bone marrow sections, the marrow is usually moderately to extensively replaced by hairy cells (Fig. 38.9). When the marrow is less extensively replaced, there is an interstitial pattern with varying numbers of normal marrow elements admixed. Characteristic hairy cells on sections have a bland-appearing lymphoid nucleus with mild to moderate nuclear contour irregularity and abundant pale cytoplasm between widely separated nuclei. Occasionally, the marrow will show some crush artifact resembling fibrosis (Fig. 38.9*D*). The spindle-shaped cells in this situation are hairy cells that have been strung out by the encasing reticulin fibers after being crushed. Although overt fibrosis is rarely seen on sections in hairy cell leukemia, background reticulin is usually moderately increased on reticulin stain (Fig. 38.9*E*).

MORPHOLOGIC VARIABILITY AND DIFFERENTIAL DIAGNOSIS

Most cases of hairy cell leukemia fit the description given above. However, some cases are difficult to diagnose as hairy cell leukemia because of deviation from the norm (41–47). Some of these appearances are listed in Table 38.9 and are illustrated in Figure 38.10.

Hairy cell leukemia can be mistaken for a number of other processes. Cases with elevated WBC and small hairy cells with round nuclear contour (Fig. 38.10*A*) can be mistaken for chronic lymphocytic leukemia (41). Rare cases of hairy cell leukemia have abundant clear nonhairy cytoplasm, giving them an exaggerated "fried egg" appearance of a Downey II/atypical lymphocyte (Fig. 38.10*B* and *C*) (42). Cases with large cells and more prominent nucleoli can be mistaken for prolymphocytic leukemia or even acute lymphocytic leukemia (Fig. 38.10*D*) (41, 43). Cases with a monocytoid appearance can be mistaken for monocytic leukemia (Fig. 38.10*E*) (41). Cases with multilobulated nuclei can be mistaken for lymphoma (Fig. 38.10*F*) (44, 45), and cases with minimal marrow involvement and hairy cells in the 5 to 20% range and no obvious infiltrate in sections may be mistaken for normal.

Patients with splenomegaly, pseudofibrosis on sections, and minimal numbers of hairy cells on blood and marrow smears can be misdiagnosed as having agnogenic myeloid metaplasia (51). Patients with hypoplastic marrow and minimal splenomegaly can be misdiagnosed as having aplastic anemia (46). A focal or paratrabecular infiltrative pattern can be misinterpreted as evidence of lymphoma.

Of special note is the existence of a small percentage of cases that are midway morphologically and immunologically between prolymphocytic leukemia and hairy cell leukemia and do not respond to conventional therapy for hairy cell leukemia (43). There is also a set of cases with some morphologic and immunologic overlap between CLL and hairy cell leukemia (47).

Cases of prolymphocytic leukemia and non-Hodgkin's lymphoma with hairy cytoplasm and TRAP positivity (especially splenic lymphomas of interme-

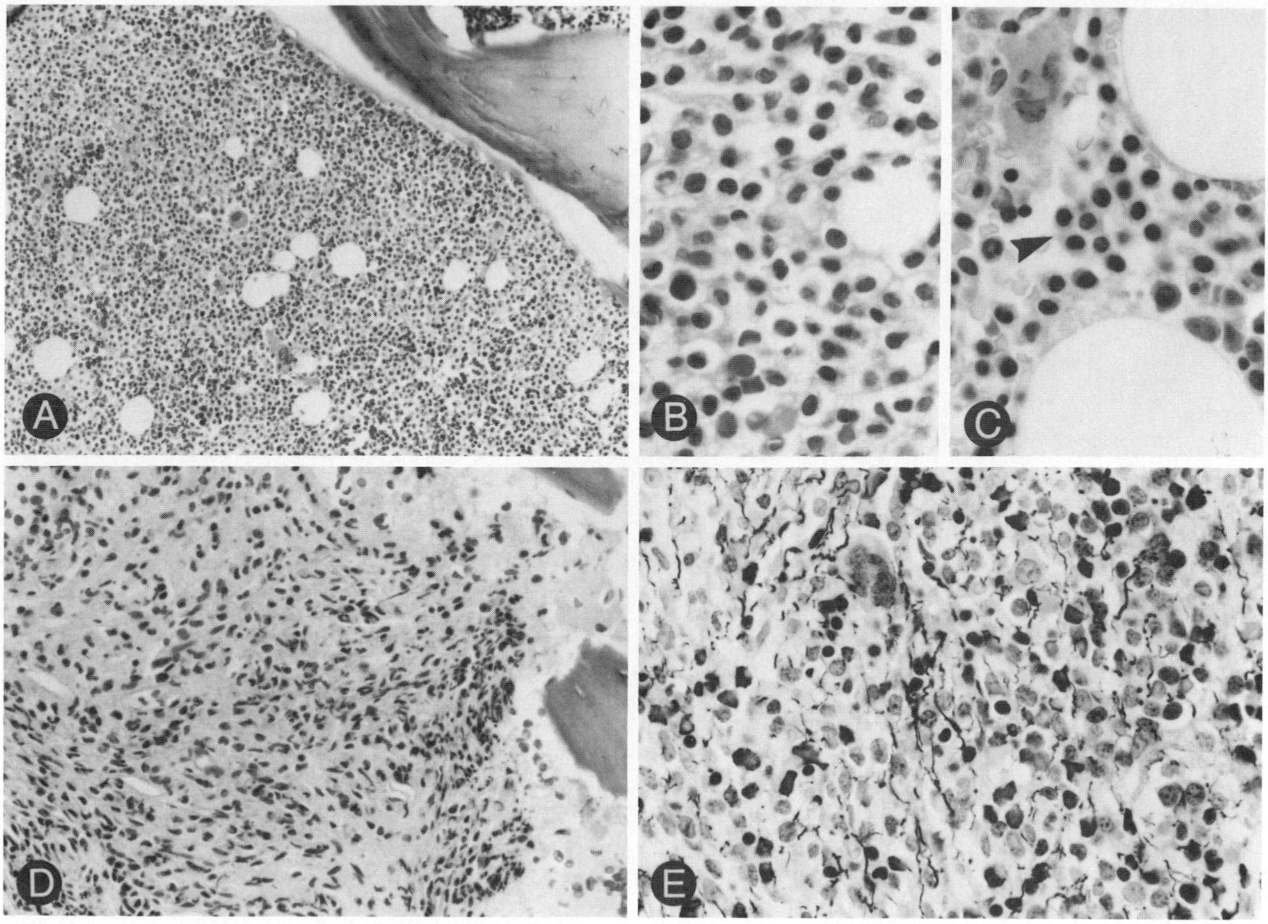

Figure 38.9. Trephine biopsy sections in hairy cell leukemia. **A**, Note the diffuse infiltrate of hairy cells with scattered normal marrow elements. **B**, Note the mild to moderate nuclear contour irregularity. The halo around the hairy cells is due to artifactual retraction in formaldehyde. **C**, Note the small collection of hairy cells in the center of the field (*arrow*) from marrow with minimal infiltration. These cells, which were fixed in B-5 fixative, do not show as much retraction artifact as those fixed in formaldehyde. **D**, Crush artifact, a frequent occurrence in hairy cell leukemia, may resemble marrow fibrosis. **E**, Reticulin frequently is extensively increased even though overt fibrosis is not seen. (Hematoxylin and eosin, ×120 [**A**], ×600 [**B, C**], ×240 [**D**].) **E**, Reticulin stain, ×600.

Table 38.9. Morphologic Variability in Hairy Cell Leukemia

Smears
Lymphoid appearance
Nonhairy cytoplasm
Downey II appearance
Prolymphocytic appearance
Monocytoid appearance
Multilobular variant
Minimal involvement
Sections
Pseudofibrosis (crush artifact)
Hypoplastic bone marrow
Focal or paratrabecular infiltrate
No obvious infiltrate

diate differentiation) should be distinguished from hairy cell leukemia (48, 49, 51). A helpful differential diagnostic feature is that most other lymphoproliferative disorders do not have the abundant pale cytoplasm in combination with the bland appearance of the nucleus seen in hairy cell leukemia on sections.

In addition, the infiltrate in hairy cell leukemia is localized in the red pulp of the spleen, and is sometimes in a more focal or white pulp distribution in other lymphoproliferative disorders.

IMMUNOLOGIC AND OTHER SPECIAL STUDIES

Hairy cells are characterized by TRAP (tartrate-resistant acid phosphatase) positivity (Fig. 38.8*D*) (50, 51). Many normal hematopoietic cells (including lymphoid cells) are acid phosphatase positive; however, the reaction in most normal and neoplastic cells is inhibited by tartaric acid. Thus, a positive TRAP stain has become a cytochemical marker for hairy cell leukemia. Unfortunately, a positive TRAP stain is not diagnostic, since a number of other processes may be TRAP positive (Table 38.2). Also, the cells of some cases of hairy cell leukemia react only weakly, or only rare strongly positive cells may be found. How-

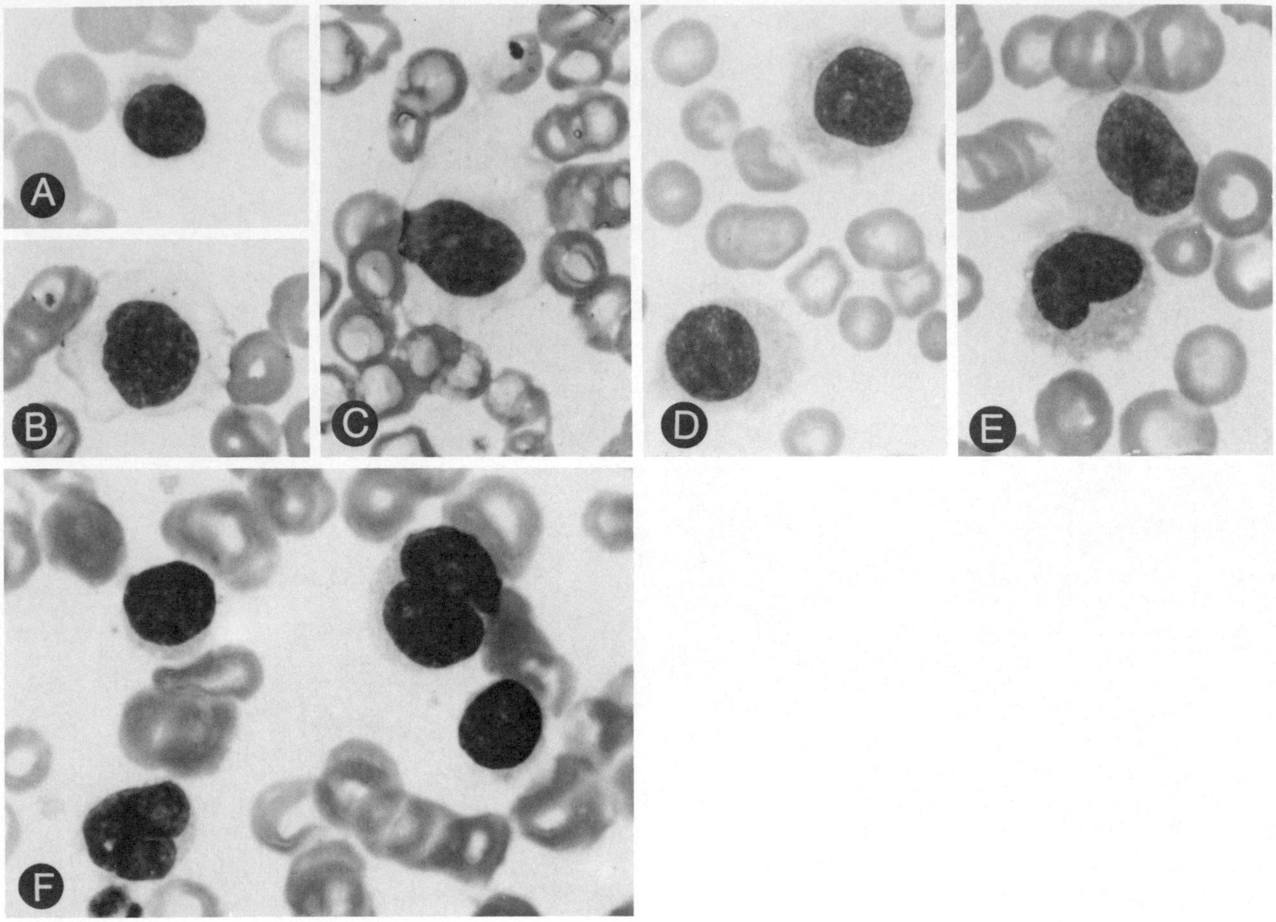

Figure 38.10. Hairy cell morphologic variants. **A**, Lymphoid appearance. **B, C**, Hairy cells with nonhairy/Downey II–like cytoplasm. **D**, Prolymphocytic appearance. Note the prominent nucleolus in the cell in the upper right of field. **E**, Moncytoid appearance. Note nuclear folds. **F**, Multilobular variant. Note the multilobular cell in the upper right of field and a deeply clefted cell in the lower left of field. (Wright's stain, ×1200.)

ever, the TRAP stain is a good screening test when the diagnosis of hairy cell leukemia is in question.

Immunologic marker studies are also of some help in the differential diagnosis of hairy cell leukemia (Table 38.6) (6). Hairy cells have moderately strong surface immunoglobulin with a restricted light chain. There are frequently strong Fc-receptors that may interfere with adequate testing. Hairy cells are also almost always positive for CD25(TAC), CD11C, and FMC7, although these markers can be positive in other lymphoproliferative diseases (6, 49, 52, 53). CD5(T1) is almost always negative in hairy cell leukemia. Immunophenotyping of paraffin sections may also be helpful when smears or frozen tissue is not available (54).

Patients with hairy cell leukemia usually have a polyclonal gammopathy; however, rare cases of monoclonal gammopathy occur. This finding, in addition to the association of PCA-1 with hairy cell leukemia, suggest to some investigators that hairy cell leukemia may be more closely related to the plasma cell than other chronic lymphoproliferative disorders (55).

Many other sophisticated studies have been performed on hairy cell leukemia, including cytogenetics (56), DNA content (19), (57, 58) and gene rearrangement (21); however, the studies of greatest diagnostic importance are the TRAP stain and immunologic markers.

CHANGE WITH PROGRESSION AND TRANSFORMATION

Transformation and secondary hematologic malignancies in hairy cell leukemia are rare (59, 60). Rarely, skeletal lesions, including osteosclerosis and lytic bone lesions, may develop (61, 62). Other extrahematopoietic complications are uncommon.

STAGING, THERAPY, AND PROGNOSTIC FEATURES

Hairy cell leukemia is an indolent disease and, if diagnosed in an asymptomatic patient, can be fol-

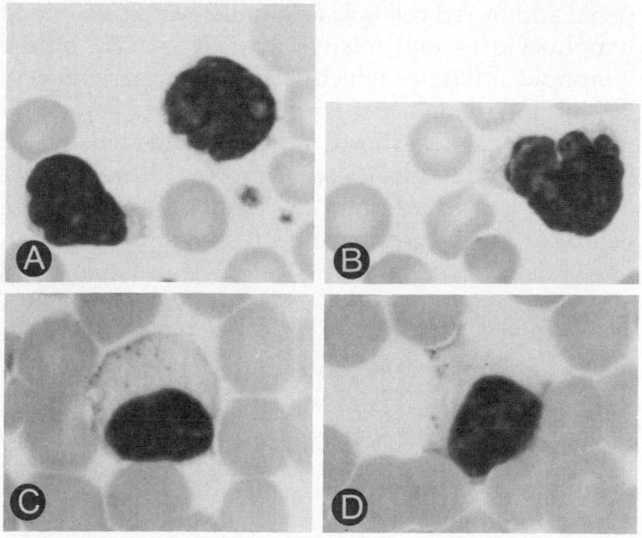

Figure 38.11. **A** and **B**, Cells of a chronic T-cell leukemia. Note the complex nuclear contour in the cells illustrated. **C** and **D**, Large granular lymphocytes. Note the abundant cytoplasm and multiple cytoplasmic granules. (Wright's stain, ×1200.) (From Dick FR. Chronic lymphocytic leukemia, prolymphocytic leukemia and leukemic non-Hodgkin's leukemia. In: Koepke JA, ed. Laboratory hematology. New York: Churchill Livingstone, 1984;1:325–357.)

lowed for many years without therapy. The therapeutic modalities available to treat symptomatic hairy cell leukemia are splenectomy and administration of interferon alpha or pentostatin, all of which are capable of inducing long-term remission of the symptoms of disease (63). Administration of interferon alpha or pentostatin can return the bone marrow to a nearly normal appearance. Treatment of hairy cell leukemia by chemotherapeutic agents used in other B-cell malignancies can result in a very poor outcome; thus, it is important to avoid erroneously diagnosing hairy cell leukemia as some other B-cell process.

T-Cell Disorders

The chronic T-cell processes listed in Table 38.1 are a heterogeneous group of rare disorders with varied clinical presentation and prognosis (64, 65). Unless these processes are thought of and studied with markers to determine their T-cell nature (66), they may not be readily diagnosed. Features that should lead to the suspicion that a patient with lymphocytosis in the blood or marrow has a T-cell lymphoproliferative disorder rather than a more common form of chronic B-cell leukemia include skin lesions, cytoplasmic granules, cytopenia, or lymphocytosis out of proportion to the extent of marrow involvement, or nuclear contour irregularity. When present in the T-cell processes listed in Table 38.1 nuclear contour irregularity generally shows more complexity (convoluted or cerebriform) (Figs. 38.11 and 38.12) than the simple clefting or folding of the nucleus seen in the B-cell processes that have nuclear contour irregularity.

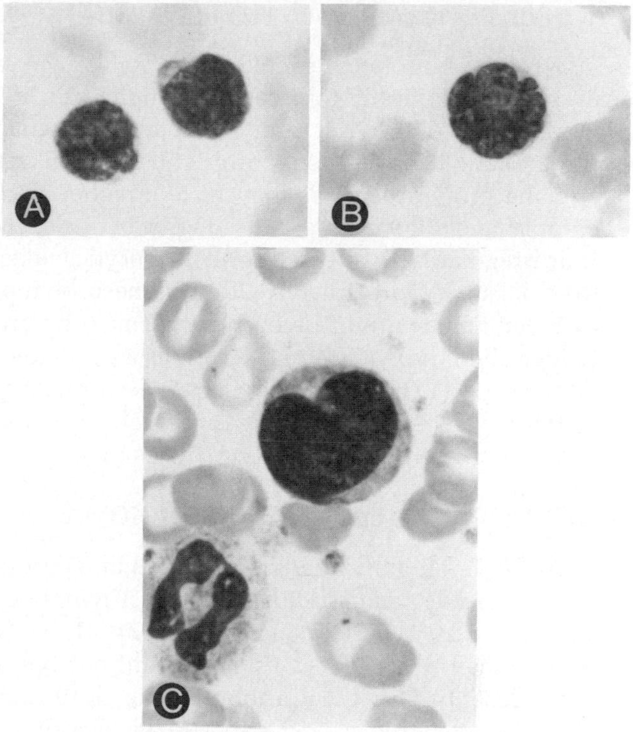

Figure 38.12. Cutaneous T-cell lymphoma cells in the peripheral blood. **A** and **B**, and Sézary cells. Note the complex internal nuclear convolutions. **C**, A large convoluted cell in the blood from a patient with disseminated mycosis fungoides. (Wright's stain, ×1200.)

T-CELL CHRONIC LYMPHOCYTIC LEUKEMIA

T-cell CLL is a very rare disease. It is seen in older individuals and is frequently associated with splenomegaly and skin involvement. Cases of T-cell CLL may have lymphocytes morphologically indistinguishable from typical B-cell CLL; however, cells with nuclear contour irregularity similar to the cells in Figure 38.11*A* and *B* may also be present. Most cases are of helper T-cell phenotype (CD4); however, rare cases of cytotoxic/suppressor (CD8) CLL have been described (67). A clonal marker such as the restricted light chain seen in chronic lymphocytic leukemia is not available to confirm clonality in T-cell lymphoproliferative disorders. Thus, in the differential between T-cell CLL (or other T-cell lymphoproliferative disorders) and a reactive T-cell lymphocytosis, a study for clonality using a probe for the T-cell CTβ receptor may be helpful (66). Some cases of T-cell CLL are less responsive than B-cell CLL to therapy (65).

T-CELL PROLYMPHOCYTIC LEUKEMIA

T-cell prolymphocytic leukemia is similar clinically and morphologically to B-cell prolymphocytic leukemia, except that T-cell prolymphocytic leukemia is more likely to have adenopathy and skin infiltrates, and the prolymphocytes may have a higher nuclear cytoplasmic ratio and a greater degree of nuclear contour irregularity than B-cell prolymphocytic leukemia (64–66, 68). Approximately 20% of the prolymphocytic leukemias are of T-cell type. A majority are of helper phenotype (CD4); however, cases of cytotoxic/suppressor (CD8) phenotype are also reported. A clonal chromosomal abnormality involving chromosome 14 is seen in a majority of cases (69).

ADULT T-CELL LEUKEMIA/LYMPHOMA

Adult T-cell leukemia/lymphoma is an aggressive T-cell disorder caused by human T-lymphocytotrophic virus 1 (HTLV-1) (64, 70, 71). It is seen predominantly in southwestern Japan, but has also been described in the Caribbean, the southeastern United States, and elsewhere. Morphologically, it is characterized by a proliferation of small- to medium-sized lymphoid cells with nuclear convolution similar to the cells illustrated in Figure 38.11*A* and *B*. These cells infiltrate lymph nodes, bone marrow, blood, and skin. There may be relative marrow sparing compared with the involvement in the peripheral blood. While a majority of patients demonstrate a "leukemic pattern," a subset of patients present with more of a "lymphoma-type" disease (71). Lytic bone lesions and hypercalcemia are common. The T cells in adult T-cell leukemia/lymphoma are of helper (CD4) phenotype (66, 71). The diagnosis is usually made by a combination of clinical, morphologic, and immunologic studies and is confirmed by antiviral antibodies or identification of the virus. This disorder usually has a very rapidly progressive course and responds poorly to aggressive combination chemotherapy, with a median survival of 1 year or less. Thus, its clinical behavior is out of proportion to the mature or chronic morphologic appearance of the process.

T-γ LYMPHOPROLIFERATIVE DISEASE

T-γ Lymphoproliferative disease (also called large granular lymphocytosis) is a fairly indolent disease characterized by a proliferation of mature-appearing lymphocytes with abundant cytoplasm and cytoplasmic granules (Fig. 38.11*C* and *D*) (64–66, 72, 73). The lymphocytes originate from natural killer cells and usually express CD16 and CD56(NKH-1) as well as CD8 (66). In a small proportion of patients with this disorder, natural killer cells are seen without CD8 positivity. The usual case presents with neutropenia and/or red cell aplasia, a mild peripheral blood lymphocytosis, and relative marrow sparing by the lymphoid infiltrate, which is focal, nonparatrabecular, or interstitial. Occasional cases are associated with rheumatoid arthritis or a positive rheumatoid factor. Although this disorder may not have a markedly elevated white blood cell count or an infiltrative character, most cases have been shown to be clonal, "neoplastic" processes by T-cell CTβ probe analysis (66). Cytogenetic studies have shown evidence of clonality in some cases; however, overall evaluation has been hampered because of the poor response of granular lymphocytes to mitogenic stimulation (74).

Granular lymphocytes may also be the cell of origin for rare cases of acute leukemia and lymphoma (74–76).

SÉZARY SYNDROME

Sézary syndrome and mycosis fungoides are closely related, uncommon disorders of older individuals, and together they constitute the category called cutaneous T-cell lymphomas (64, 70). Sézary syndrome is primarily a disorder of the skin with secondary blood involvement. It is characterized by diffuse erythroderma due to infiltration of mature-appearing helper T cells with markedly convoluted nuclear contours. The disease shows varying degrees of lymphocytosis in the peripheral blood with Sézary cells, as illustrated in Figure 38.12*A* and *B*. The bone marrow is relatively spared (77, 78). The diagnosis usually rests on a combination of clinical and morphologic features. A skin biopsy will show a band-like infiltrate of small, convoluted lymphoid cells immediately beneath the epidermis. When the skin biopsy is not diagnostic, the identification of convoluted lymphocytes (Sézary cells) in the blood may be used to help substantiate the diagnosis. A small percentage of convoluted cells indistinguishable from the neoplastic Sézary cells (similar to those shown in Figure 38.12*A*) can be seen in benign skin disorders; however, the presence of more than 15 to 20% of these cells or the presence of larger convoluted lymphoid cells similar to those shown in Figure 38.12*C* and *D* are supportive of the diagnosis of Sézary syndrome (79, 80).

Mycosis fungoides characteristically lacks blood involvement and shows multifocal skin lesions rather than the diffuse involvement of Sézary syndrome. However, late in the course of mycosis fungoides with dissemination, large, atypical, convoluted lymphoid cells similar to those shown in Figure 38.12 may be seen in the blood.

Sézary syndrome may be treated with extracorporeal photochemotherapy with variably good results.

IMMUNOPROLIFERATIVE DISORDERS

Immunoproliferative disorders are neoplastic proliferations of plasma cells and B lymphocytes at the terminal stage of functional differentiation, and are characterized by the production and secretion of a monoclonal immunoprotein called a monoclonal gammopathy. "Disease" in immunoproliferative disorders may be caused by proliferation of the neoplastic cell and by secretion of an abnormal protein that has a pathologic effect. These disorders may be indolent or more rapidly progressive.

Plasma Cell Myeloma

Plasma cell myeloma is a relatively common hematologic disease characterized by proliferation of clusters and sheets of neoplastic plasma cells primarily in the bone marrow, resulting in focal bone lesions, diffuse osteoporosis, bone pain, fractures, and cytopenia (81). The neoplastic proliferation usually produces a monoclonal gammopathy, which may result in hyperviscosity syndrome, coagulation abnormalities, immune deficiency, renal failure, or development of amyloidosis. Plasma cell myeloma is seen primarily in older individuals (in the sixth to seventh decade) with a male predominance. It is generally a progressive malignant disorder; however, its course is variable, and prognosis is based to a large degree on the tumor burden present at diagnosis.

DIAGNOSTIC FEATURES

The diagnosis of plasma cell myeloma is dependent on a combination of clinical and laboratory features (82). From a laboratory standpoint, the diagnosis of plasma cell myeloma should be suspected whenever there is a monoclonal gammopathy, and the bone marrow contains increased atypical plasma cells with a prominent single nucleolus and partially dispersed chromatin, sometimes referred to as "myeloma cells" (Figs. 38.13 and 38.14). The following morphologic changes are consistent with a diagnosis of plasma cell myeloma:

1. The presence on marrow smears of 10% or more atypical plasma cells (Figs. 38.13*A* and 38.14*A*). These cells may infiltrate in an interstitial pattern, in multiple small clusters, or in sheets. The median percentage of atypical plasma cells on smears in patients with plasma cell myeloma is about 30%. *Note*: It is important to do an actual differential (100 or more cells on three different slides) since plasma cells can easily be overestimated. Also, binucleation of plasma cells should not be considered an atypical feature; reactive plasma cells are also frequently binucleated.
2. Less than 10% atypical plasma cells on marrow smears in association with large sheets of atypical plasma cells on crush preparation or sections, with plasma cells representing nearly 100% of the cell population in the sheets (Fig. 38.13*B*) (83).

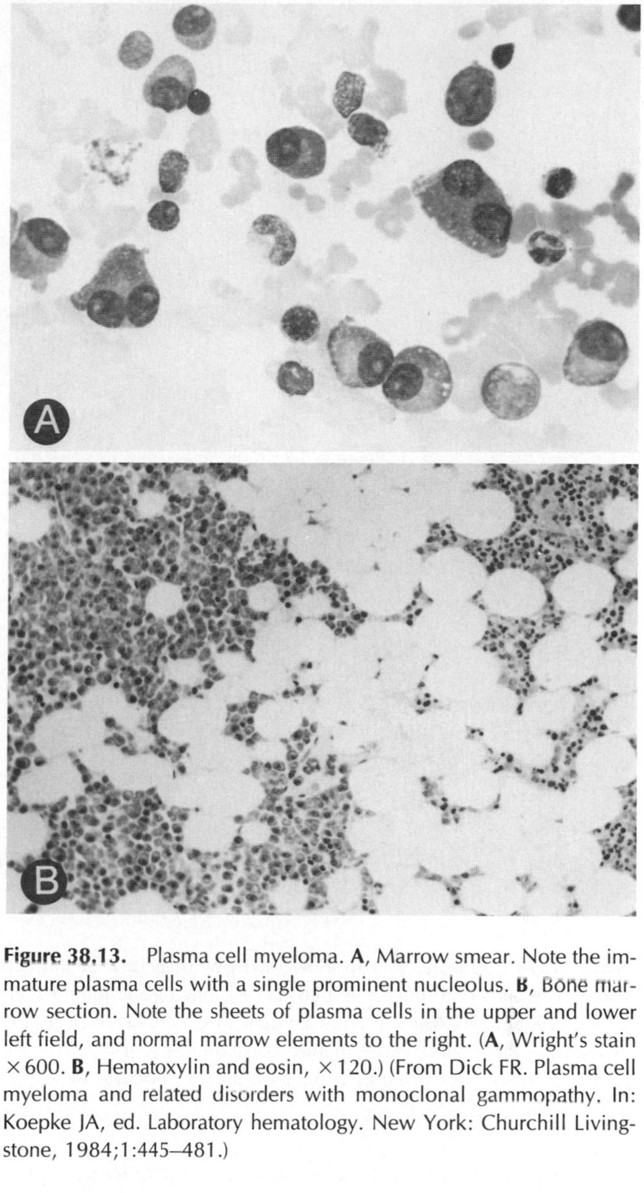

Figure 38.13. Plasma cell myeloma. **A**, Marrow smear. Note the immature plasma cells with a single prominent nucleolus. **B**, Bone marrow section. Note the sheets of plasma cells in the upper and lower left field, and normal marrow elements to the right. (**A**, Wright's stain ×600. **B**, Hematoxylin and eosin, ×120.) (From Dick FR. Plasma cell myeloma and related disorders with monoclonal gammopathy. In: Koepke JA, ed. Laboratory hematology. New York: Churchill Livingstone, 1984;1:445–481.)

Although these morphologic features are consistent with a diagnosis of plasma cell myeloma, additional clinical and laboratory evidence of disease may also be necessary to make a definitive diagnosis. Additional evidence may be a monoclonal gammopathy in serum or urine, characteristic bone lesions, or, rarely, suppression of other immunoglobulins in the absence of a monoclonal gammopathy.

Caution should be taken in making an unequivocal diagnosis of plasma cell myeloma in a patient

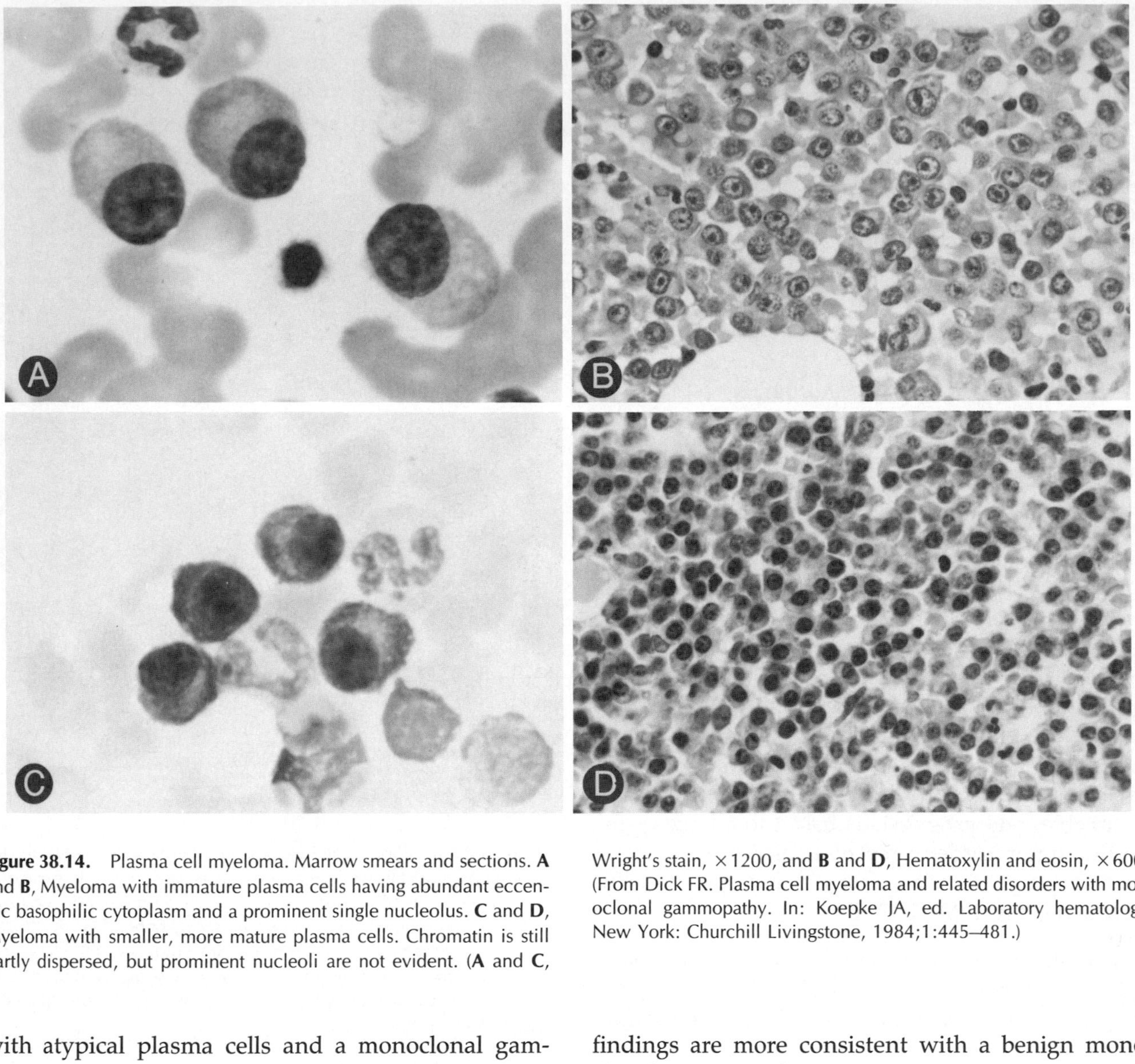

Figure 38.14. Plasma cell myeloma. Marrow smears and sections. **A** and **B**, Myeloma with immature plasma cells having abundant eccentric basophilic cytoplasm and a prominent single nucleolus. **C** and **D**, Myeloma with smaller, more mature plasma cells. Chromatin is still partly dispersed, but prominent nucleoli are not evident. (**A** and **C**, Wright's stain, ×1200, and **B** and **D**, Hematoxylin and eosin, ×600.) (From Dick FR. Plasma cell myeloma and related disorders with monoclonal gammopathy. In: Koepke JA, ed. Laboratory hematology. New York: Churchill Livingstone, 1984;1:445–481.)

with atypical plasma cells and a monoclonal gammopathy in the absence of any other evidence of disease. A small subset of patients who have 10 to 20% atypical plasma cells on marrow smears and a monoclonal gammopathy, but who are asymptomatic, may not pursue an aggressive course. These cases have been diagnosed as smoldering myeloma (84, 85).

A significant number of patients have up to 10% atypical plasma cells in the marrow with a monoclonal gammopathy and do not have disease manifestations of plasma cell myeloma. These cases usually pursue a benign course and are called benign monoclonal gammopathy, or alternatively, monoclonal gammopathy of undetermined significance (MGUS). Benign monoclonal gammopathy is discussed in greater detail later in this chapter.

Less than 10% atypical plasma cells or more than 10% normal-appearing plasma cells can be seen in patients with progressive myeloma; however, these findings are more consistent with a benign monoclonal gammopathy or a reactive process, respectively. When these morphologies are present, the diagnosis of plasma cell myeloma should rest even more heavily on clinical criteria.

Since patients can have progressive plasma cell myeloma with fewer initial morphologic changes than those described earlier, or more rarely, since progressive disease may not develop when the morphologic features described above are found, several groups have developed a set of clinical pathologic criteria (Table 38.10) that serve to ensure that patients entered on protocols are uniformly diagnosed (86, 87). Such criteria are also useful for routine diagnosis outside of protocol studies, since they emphasize the importance of radiologic, clinical, and laboratory features in arriving at the diagnosis of plasma cell myeloma. These clinical-pathological features are helpful in distinguishing plasma cell myeloma from

Table 38.10. Clinical Pathologic Criteria for Inclusion in Studies of Plasma Cell Myeloma[a]

Adapted from the Chronic Leukemia-Myeloma Task Force (78)	Adapted from SWOG[b] Criteria (86)
CRITERIA FOR DIAGNOSIS	
I Osteolytic lesions	I Plasmacytomas by biopsy
II Palpable tumors	II > 30% marrow plasmacytosis
III Monoclonal gammopathy in serum or urine	III Monoclonal gammopathy
A.1. ≥ 20% Marrow plasma cells from two sites	> 3.5 g/dl of γG
2. Tissue biopsies with plasmacytomas	> 2.0 g/dl of γA or > 1 g/day κ or λ chains in urine without other significant proteinuria
B.1. > 5% Marrow plasmacytosis	A. 10–30% Marrow plasmacytosis
2. Tissue biopsy with a plasmacytoma	B. Monoclonal gammopathy with values less than in III
3. > 500/mm Plasma cells in the blood	C. Lytic bone lesions
4. Osteolytic lesions unexplained by other reasons	D. Suppressed normal immunoglobulins < 50 mg/dl γ M, < 100 mg/dl γ A or < 600 mg/dl γ G
DIAGNOSIS CONFIRMED WITH	
I plus A.1 or 2	Symptomatic patient and
II plus A.1 or 2	I plus B, C, or D
III plus B.1, 2, 3, or 4	II plus B, C, or D
	III A, B, and C
	A, B, and D

[a]From Dick FR. Plasma cell myeloma and related disorders with monoclonal gammopathy. In: Koepke JA, ed. Laboratory hematology. New York: Churchill Livingstone, 1984;1:445–481.
[b]SWOG, Southwest Oncology Group.

potentially smoldering myeloma, and from solitary plasmacytoma and benign monoclonal gammopathy. Although these criteria may be very useful in some patients, sound judgment should be used when making the diagnosis of plasma cell myeloma based only on these criteria. The criteria of the Myeloma Task Force may not be rigid enough, and some patients with potentially smoldering myeloma, benign monoclonal gammopathy, or solitary plasmacytoma may be included as having plasma cell myeloma. On the other hand, the criteria of the Southwest Oncology Group (SWOG) may be too rigid, and some patients with progressive plasma cell myeloma may be excluded.

Note: Occasional cases of reactive plasmacytosis with polyclonal gammopathy will show a significant infiltrate in the marrow with plasma cells, sometimes in sheets (83). The author has observed two cases in which there were over 50% reactive plasma cells with atypical plasma cells in a cellular bone marrow (Fig. 38.15). This emphasizes the need to identify criteria other than plasmacytosis greater than 10% or "sheets" of plasma cells in the bone marrow to establish the diagnosis of plasma cell myeloma.

MORPHOLOGIC VARIABILITY AND DIFFERENTIAL DIAGNOSIS

The marrow in a classic case of plasma cell myeloma shows a predominance of myeloma cells, as illustrated in Figures 38.13 and 38.14*A* and *B*. Less commonly, smaller plasma cells with more mature nuclear features predominate (Fig. 38.14*C* and *D*). Other cases may show a spectrum of plasma cells ranging from nearly normal plasma cells to more classic myeloma cells (88).

Cytologic variability from the pattern described above occasionally occurs and should be recognized as part of the spectrum of plasma cell myeloma (Table 38.11).

Flame cells, thesaurocytes, and inclusions can occasionally be seen in benign plasmacytosis; however, when they are present in plasma cell myeloma, they usually represent a major percentage of the plasma cells (Fig. 38.16). Flame cells and thesaurocytes (Fig. 38.16*A* and *B*) are frequently but not exclusively associated with an IgA monoclonal gammopathy (88). A wide variety of cytoplasmic and nuclear inclusions may be seen in the cells of plasma cell myeloma, some of which are illustrated in Figure 38.16*C* and *D* (82, 89–92).

Proliferation of normal-appearing plasma cells, with only rare atypical cells, is seen in a small percentage of cases of plasma cell myeloma. In these cases, the diagnosis should be evident from other features of plasma cell myeloma.

Occasional cases may show pleomorphic, plasmablastic, or anaplastic (immunoblastic) morphology, as illustrated in Figure 38.17. Pleomorphic morphology shows marked variability in cell size with large multinucleated and bizarre forms (88). Anaplastic (immunoblastic) and plasmablastic morphology overlap (93, 94). Cases with anaplastic morphology show poor differentiation toward plasma cells, with

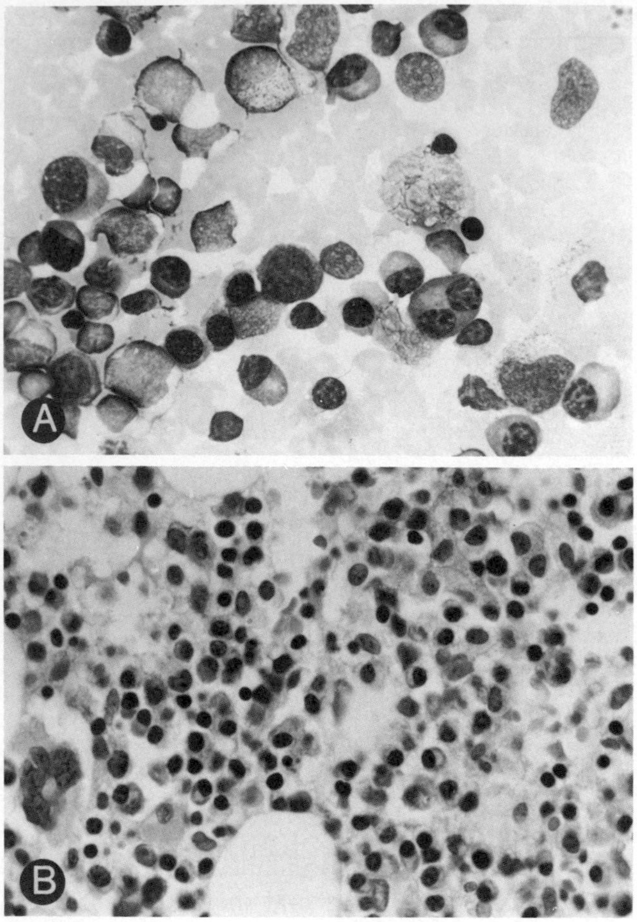

Figure 38.15. Bone marrow aspirate (**A**) and biopsy (**B**) showing a reactive plasmacytosis of greater than 50%. Note the large and binucleated plasma cells. Single prominent nucleoli are not a prominent feature, however. (**A**, Wright's stain, ×600. **B**, Hematoxylin and eosin, ×600.) (From Dick FR. Plasma cell myeloma and related disorders with monoclonal gammopathy. In: Koepke JA, ed. Laboratory hematology. New York: Churchill Livingstone, 1984;1:445–481.)

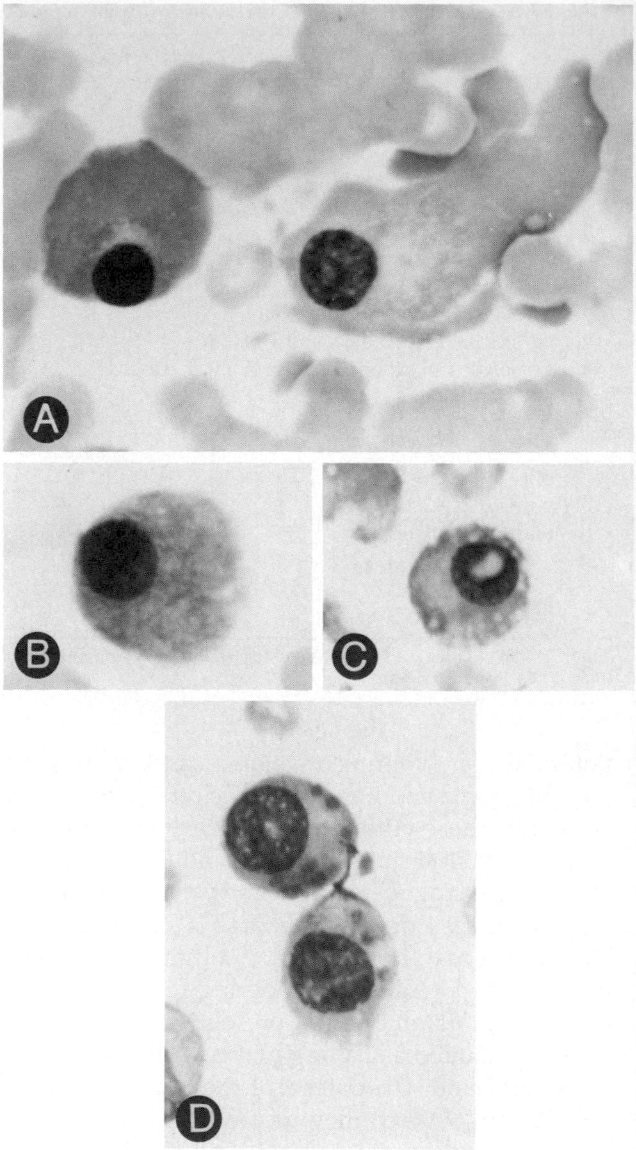

Figure 38.16. Variants of myeloma cells, bone marrow aspirate. **A**, Flame cells. The dark, flowing cytoplasmic borders on these plasma cells are red or "flaming" on Wright's stain. **B**, Thesaurocytes are plasma cells with abundant pale blue foamy or reticulated cytoplasm. **C**, Dutcher bodies on smears are pale intranuclear inclusions. **D**, Russell bodies are reddish globular cytoplasmic inclusions. (Wright's stain, ×1200.) (From Dick FR. Plasma cell myeloma and related disorders with monoclonal gammopathy. In: Koepke JA, ed. Laboratory hematology. New York: Churchill Livingstone, 1984;1:445–481.)

Table 38.11. Morphologic Variability in Plasma Cell Myeloma

Smears
Flame cells
Thesaurocytes
Inclusions
Normal-appearing plasma cells
Pleomorphic cells
Immunoblastic cells
Lymphoid cells
Monocytoid or multilobated cells
Phagocytosis
Sections
Reticulin
Fibrosis
Osteosclerosis
Amyloid
Plasma cell leukemia

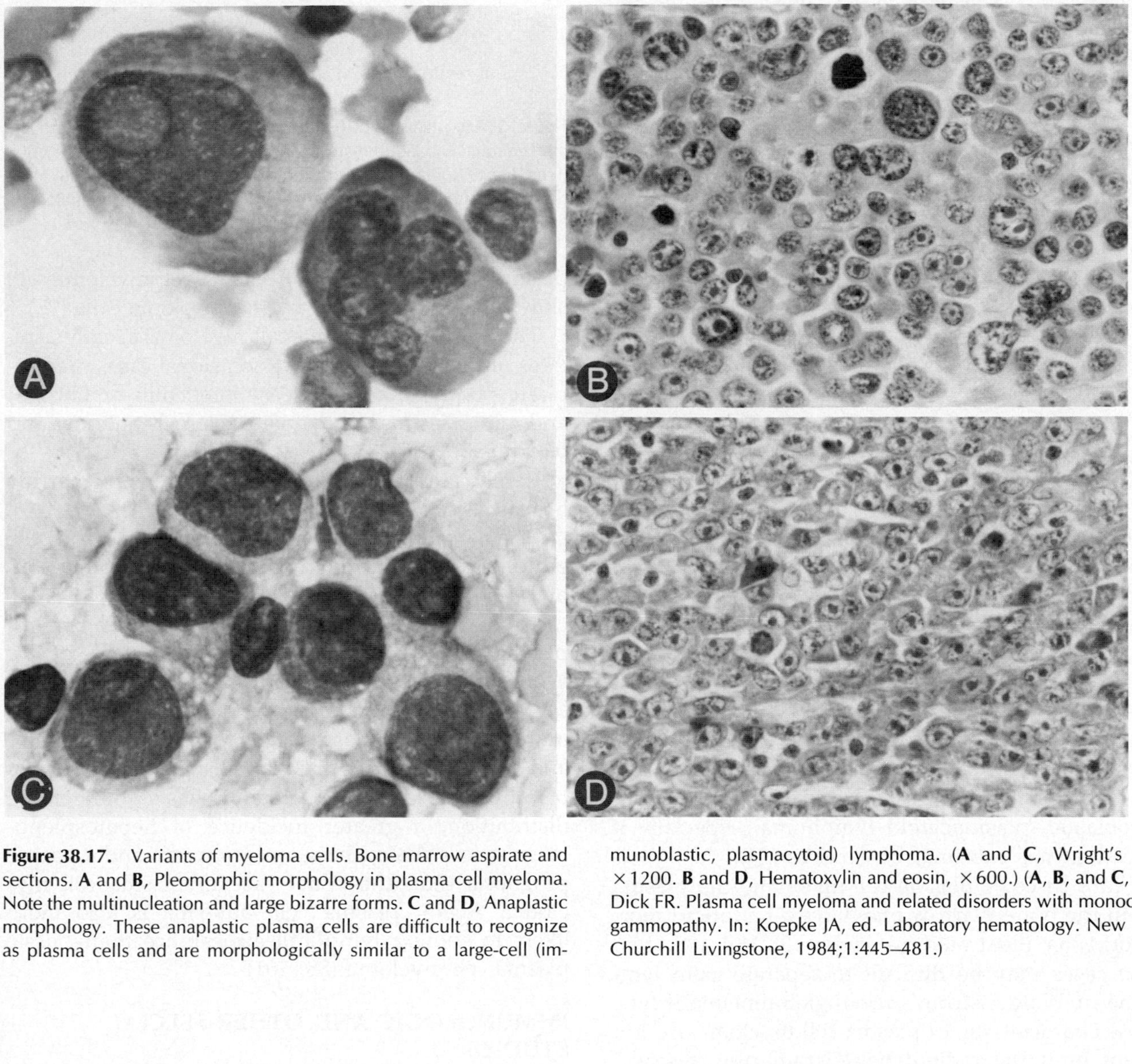

Figure 38.17. Variants of myeloma cells. Bone marrow aspirate and sections. **A** and **B**, Pleomorphic morphology in plasma cell myeloma. Note the multinucleation and large bizarre forms. **C** and **D**, Anaplastic morphology. These anaplastic plasma cells are difficult to recognize as plasma cells and are morphologically similar to a large-cell (immunoblastic, plasmacytoid) lymphoma. (**A** and **C**, Wright's stain, ×1200. **B** and **D**, Hematoxylin and eosin, ×600.) (**A**, **B**, and **C**, From Dick FR. Plasma cell myeloma and related disorders with monoclonal gammopathy. In: Koepke JA, ed. Laboratory hematology. New York: Churchill Livingstone, 1984;1:445–481.)

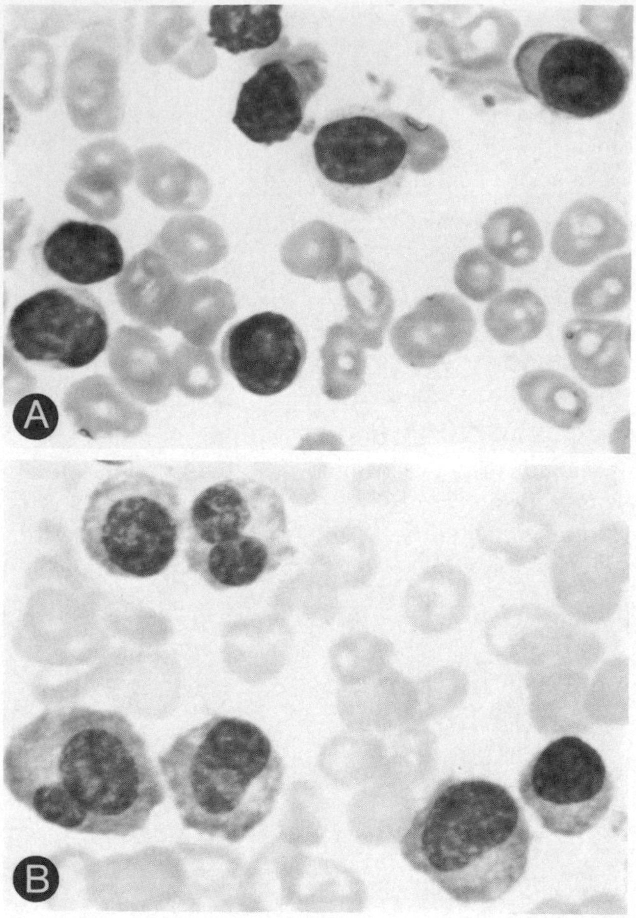

Figure 38.18. Variants of myeloma cells. **A**, Lymphoid morphology. **B**, Monocytoid or multilobated morphology. The marrow aspirates in both of these illustrations are from individuals with lytic bone lesions and IgG monoclonal gammopathy. (Wright's stain, ×1200.) (From Dick FR. Plasma cell myeloma and related disorders with monoclonal gammopathy. In: Koepke JA, ed. Laboratory hematology. New York: Churchill Livingstone, 1984;1:445–481.)

less abundant cytoplasm and absence of paranuclear pallor (hof). They are morphologically similar to, and may be difficult to distinguish from, a large-cell, immunoblastic, plasmacytoid lymphoma, especially if the patient has extramarrow masses (94).

In rare cases of plasma cell myeloma, the plasma cells in the bone marrow may have a lymphoid morphology, as illustrated in Figure 38.18*A* (88, 95). These cases may be difficult to separate from lymphoma or Waldenström's macroglobulinemia if lytic lesions characteristic of plasma cell myeloma are not present or if the patient has extramarrow disease. Plasma cells, when present in the blood in plasma cell myeloma, frequently have a more lymphoid appearance than in the marrow of the same patient.

Rare cases of myeloma will show considerable nuclear irregularity (multilobated or monocytoid), as illustrated in Figure 38.18*B* (96). On sections as well as on smears, these cells may be difficult to recognize as

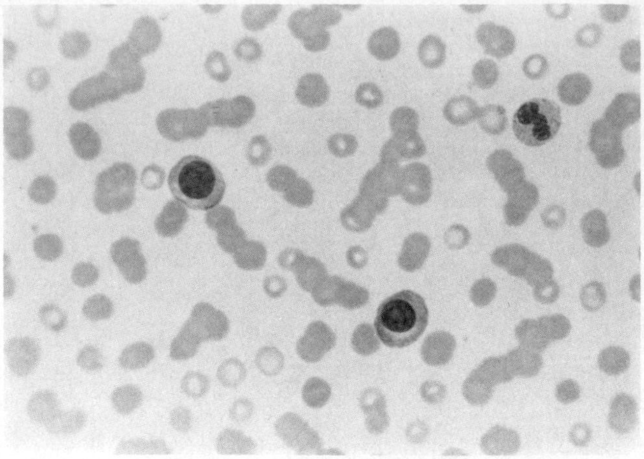

Figure 38.19. Plasma cell leukemia (peripheral blood). Note the marked rouleaux and immature plasma cells. (Wright's stain, ×600.) (From Dick FR. Plasma cell myeloma and related disorders with monoclonal gammopathy. In: Koepke JA, ed. Laboratory hematology. New York: Churchill Livingstone, 1984;1:445–481.)

plasma cells. Rare cases of plasma cell myeloma will slow phagocytic activity by the myeloma cells (97).

The marrow in plasma cell myeloma usually aspirates quite freely; however, occasional cases may aspirate poorly due to increased reticulin or fibrosis, and rare cases may show osteosclerosis on x-ray and biopsy (98, 99).

Rarely, amyloidosis is present in the bone marrow in plasma cell myeloma (100).

Plasma cells in small numbers can be seen in the peripheral blood at diagnosis in approximately 15% of cases of plasma cell myeloma (101). In about 2% of cases of plasma cell myeloma, large numbers of plasma cells will be present in the blood (Fig. 38.19). When this occurs, the patient is said to have plasma cell leukemia, which has been defined as having more than 2,000 plasma cells per cubic millimeter and more than 30% plasma cells in the peripheral blood (101). Plasma cell leukemia has a younger age distribution, a greater incidence of hepatosplenomegaly, less clinical bone involvement, and a poorer prognosis than the usual case of plasma cell myeloma. Again, plasma cell leukemia is also more likely to show a lymphoid appearance than classic plasma cell myeloma (88, 101).

IMMUNOLOGIC AND OTHER SPECIAL STUDIES

A search for a monoclonal gammopathy is the single most important test that can be done in a patient suspected of having plasma cell myeloma (Tables 38.12 and 38.13) (102). The best procedure is to perform immunofixation electrophoresis on serum and urine as a screening test. If no monoclonal gammopathy is detected by these procedures, it is highly

Table 38.12. Frequency of Type of Monoclonal Gammopathy in Plasma Cell Myeloma[a]

Monoclonal Gammopathy	Approximate Frequency of Occurrence
	%
IgG	57
IgA	20
κ or λ only	20
IgD	1
Nonsecretory	1
Biclonal	1
IgE	Rare
IgM	Rare
	100

[a]From Dick FR. Plasma cell myeloma and related disorders with monoclonal gammopathy. In: Koepke JA, ed. Laboratory hematology. New York: Churchill Livingstone, 1984;1:445–481.

Table 38.13. Other Protein Findings in Plasma Cell Myeloma[a] (82, 102)

Finding	Approximate Frequency of Occurrence in Plasma Cell Myeloma
Size of monoclonal peak	%
$<$ 2 g/dl	17
$>$ 5 g/dl	20
No obvious monoclonal peak on serum protein electrophoresis	20
Free light chains in urine	80
Hypoglobulinemia and no M-peak on serum electrophoresis	9
"Normal" serum protein electrophoresis	10–15
Location of monoclonal peak	
γ	70
β	30
α 2	Rare
Cryoglobulin	5
Pyroglobulin	1

[a]From Dick FR. Plasma cell myeloma and related disorders with monoclonal gammopathy. In: Koepke JA, ed. Laboratory hematology. New York: Churchill Livingstone, 1984;1:445–481.

unlikely that the patient has myeloma, since 1% or fewer cases of plasma cell myeloma fail to produce at least a small monoclonal protein. Serum protein electrophoresis alone is not a good screening test for a monoclonal gammopathy since it is not as sensitive as immunofixation electrophoresis. Also, in 20% of patients with myeloma, the monoclonal gammopathy will be detected by urinalysis and not by serum protein electrophoresis. A serum protein electrophoresis or quantitative immunoglobulins will, however, help detect those rare patients with myeloma who have hypogammaglobulinemia and no monoclonal gammopathy on serum immunofixation electrophoresis. As pointed out in the previous section, many patients with a monoclonal gammopathy (especially a small monoclonal gammopathy) will not have progressive plasma cell myeloma. Thus, other features in addition to a monoclonal gammopathy

Table 38.14. Transformation and Secondary Tumors in Plasma Cell Myeloma

Plasma cell leukemia
Pleomorphic/anaplastic myeloma
Immunoblastic sarcoma
Chronic lymphocytic leukemia
Extraosseous lesions
Myelodysplastic syndrome
Acute nonlymphocytic leukemia

are necessary to make the diagnosis of plasma cell myeloma.

Immunologic evaluation of the cells in myeloma is rarely needed. The morphology of the cells in myeloma is usually typical, and clonality is supported by the finding of a monoclonal gammopathy in the serum or urine. When studied, plasma cells in plasma cell myeloma will show a cytoplasmic immunoglobulin of a clonally restricted light chain in addition to a heavy chain, if present (103–105). The plasma cells in plasma cell myeloma are generally negative for SIg and B cell–associated antigens but do demonstrate plasma cell–associated antigens (6).

Immunostaining of plasma cells in the bone marrow may be useful in distinguishing benign plasma cells from nonsecretory myeloma, but may not clearly distinguish benign monoclonal gammopathy and amyloidosis with increased plasma cells from early myeloma. This is because plasma cells in the marrow of patients with benign monoclonal gammopathy and amyloidosis may also show a restricted light chain (103–106). However, in benign monoclonal gammopathy, the κ:λ ratio is usually less altered from normal than in plasma cell myeloma (103).

Numerous other special studies have been performed in plasma cell myeloma, including serum β_2-microglobulin (107, 108), plasma cell labeling indices (109, 110), CALLA (CD10) immunotyping of peripheral blood and bone marrow cells (111, 112), chromosome analysis (113), ploidy analysis (114), and growth fraction with Ki-67 (115). Some of these may have potential prognostic importance.

CHANGE WITH PROGRESSION AND TRANSFORMATION

A small percentage of patients with plasma cell myeloma may show some morphologic change with time. These changes are listed in Table 38.14.

About one-third of patients who qualify for the diagnosis of plasma cell leukemia have transformed from a more typical presentation of plasma cell myeloma (101). The remainder are de novo, as described earlier. Transformation to plasma cell leukemia

Table 38.15. Clinical Staging of Plasma Cell Myeloma[a] (82, 119)

Stage I	All of the following:
	Hg > 10 g/dl
	Calcium ≤ 12 mg/dl
	Normal bone on x-ray or solitary lesion only
	Monoclonal protein
	IgG < 5 g/dl
	IgA < 3 g/dl
	Urine light chains < 4 g/24 hr
Stage II	Fitting neither Stage I nor III
Stage III	One or more of the following:
	Hg < 8.5 g/dl
	Calcium > 12 mg/dl
	Advanced lytic bone lesions
	Monoclonal protein
	IgG > 7 g/dl
	IgA > 5 g/dl
	Urine light chains > 12 g/24 hr
Renal Status A = creatinine < 2 mg/dl	
Renal Status B = creatinine > 2 mg/dl	

[a]From Dick FR. Plasma cell myeloma and related disorders with monoclonal gammopathy. In: Koepke JA, ed. Laboratory hematology. New York: Churchill Livingstone, 1984;1:445–481.

shows many clinical features in common with de novo plasma cell leukemia.

Pleomorphic and anaplastic (immunoblastic) morphologies of myeloma can be seen at diagnosis; however, they may also develop in association with aggressive disease progression and extraosseous spread (24). A variety of other terms have been applied to this aggressive transformation, including dysplastic myeloma and immunoblastic sarcoma. These forms of transformation are probably derived from the same clone as the original tumor.

CLL associated with plasma cell myeloma is usually diagnosed simultaneously; however, rare cases of CLL developing after a diagnosis of plasma cell myeloma have been reported (116).

The increased incidence of myelodysplastic syndrome and acute nonlymphocytic leukemia in myeloma is usually attributed to prior alkalating agent therapy; however, there are isolated reports of nonlymphocytic leukemia developing in association with plasma cell myeloma without prior therapy (117, 118). Therapy-related myelodysplastic syndrome and acute nonlymphocytic leukemia have much poorer prognoses than de novo disease.

STAGING, THERAPY, AND PROGNOSTIC FEATURES

Prognosis in plasma cell myeloma is based primarily on the clinical staging scheme outlined in Table 38.15 (119). The features listed in the table, which determine the stage of the patient, in general correlate with the tumor burden present. About 15% of patients present as stage I disease, and most of these have a creatinine level of 2 mg/dl or less (status A). Stage II comprises 30% of patients, and only 5 to 10% of these have renal status B. More than half of the patients present with stage III disease, and half of these have a creatinine level above 2 mg/dl (status B).

In addition to the staging system, the following features of plasma cell myeloma have been shown to be associated with a higher stage and worsened prognosis: elevated β_2-microglobulin (107, 108) and labeling indices (108), abnormal karyotype or DNA content (113, 114), CALLA positivity (111), plasma cell morphology (93, 120), and pattern of marrow infiltration (121). β_2-microglobulin appears to be of the most use clinically.

Plasma cell myeloma is a progressive disease that, similar to CLL, is difficult to cure. Melphalan plus prednisone is usually the initial therapeutic approach for controlling disease progression; however, a variety of new therapies are under investigation (122, 123). The median survival of patients with stage I disease is 6 years; with stage II, 4 years; and with stage III, 1 year. Patients with renal status A live a median of 3 years, while those with renal status B live less than 6 months (119).

Plasmacytoma

Plasmacytoma is a rare disorder characterized by a mass lesion of neoplastic plasma cells (124, 125). Although plasmacytomas are usually seen in the surgical pathology laboratory rather than the hematology laboratory, bone marrow examination and serum and urine protein studies are frequently done subsequent to the diagnosis of plasmacytoma to rule out spread to the bone marrow. Also, as mentioned in the previous section, plasma cell myeloma may develop extramedullary plasmacytomas late in the course of disease. Plasmacytomas can be solitary or multiple and may present in the bone (spine, pelvis, femur, etc.) or as an extramedullary lesion (upper respiratory tract, lymph nodes, spleen, skin, GI tract, etc.). As with plasma cell myeloma, plasmacytomas are seen predominantly in older individuals, with a male predominance.

IMMUNOLOGIC STUDIES

When plasmacytomas are localized at presentation (solitary plasmacytoma), the presence of an associated monoclonal gammopathy is uncommon and, if present, should disappear as the solitary plasmacytoma is treated. With dissemination, the incidence of a monoclonal gammopathy increases, with IgG and κ being the predominant monoclonal gammopathies seen.

THERAPY AND CHANGE WITH PROGRESSION

Eventual dissemination of plasmacytomas is seen in about one-third to one-half of patients with solitary plasmacytoma of bone. Eventual dissemination usually results in the classic picture of plasma cell myeloma. Some cases may take up to 15 years before dissemination occurs. Extramedullary plasmacytomas have a lower incidence of eventual dissemination, and dissemination of extramedullary plasmacytoma is to lymph nodes, other extramedullary sites, and bone. Treatment for solitary plasmacytoma is radiation therapy. β_2-Microglobulin may be useful in predicting the likelihood that a patient with solitary plasmacytoma will develop disseminated plasma cell myeloma (126).

Waldenström's Macroglobulinemia

Waldenström's macroglobulinemia is an uncommon disease characterized by an IgM monoclonal gammopathy and proliferation of lymphocytes in the bone marrow, which show varying degrees of differentiation into plasmacytoid lymphocytes and plasma cells (127). Waldenström's macroglobulinemia is derived from a cell that is functionally intermediate between the lymphocyte of CLL and the plasma cell of plasma cell myeloma. The disease primarily affects the bone marrow, with frequent involvement of lymph nodes, spleen, and liver. Unlike in plasma cell myeloma, lytic bone lesions are rare. The morphology of the proliferation in Waldenström's macroglobulinemia is consistent with the diagnosis of small lymphocytic lymphoma-plasmacytoid in the Working Formulation classification of non-Hodgkin's lymphoma (discussed later). Thus, Waldenström's macroglobulinemia can be considered the bone marrow counterpart of malignant lymphoma. In Waldenström's macroglobulinemia, as in plasma cell myeloma, disease may be caused by the infiltrative nature of the neoplastic cells or by a protein abnormality. Similar to chronic lymphocytic leukemia and plasma cell myeloma, Waldenström's macroglobulinemia is a disease of older individuals and has a male predominance. Its prognosis is intermediate between CLL and plasma cell myeloma.

DIAGNOSTIC FEATURES

As stated above, the diagnosis of Waldenström's macroglobulinemia is made from a combination of bone marrow findings and the presence of an IgM monoclonal gammopathy. The bone marrow frequently aspirates poorly due to increased reticulin in the marrow infiltrate. On smears, there is a mild to marked lymphocytosis composed of mature lymphocytes with varying numbers of plasma cells, as illustrated in Figure 38.20. Plasmacytoid lymphocytes, which are morphologically intermediate between plasma cells and lymphocytes, may or may not be present to form a morphologic bridge between the lymphocytes and plasma cells. Tissue mast cells are frequently increased, and occasional Dutcher bodies may be observed. The peripheral blood in Waldenström's macroglobulinemia usually does not show lymphocytosis; however, there may occasionally be an elevated white blood cell count of up to 15,000/mm^3, with cells similar to those seen in the bone marrow aspirate.

On bone marrow sections, there are usually focal paratrabecular and nonparatrabecular infiltrates of mature lymphocytes with associated smaller numbers of plasma cells and plasmacytoid lymphocytes (Fig. 38.20*B* and *C*) (128). The degree of involvement may range from small focal aggregates to extensive diffuse replacement, or, more rarely, there may be a diffuse interstitial infiltrate. In early marrow involvement, the marrow smears may show no increase in lymphocytes and plasma cells, and the marrow sections may show only small aggregates, which are difficult to distinguish from benign aggregates.

MORPHOLOGIC VARIABILITY AND DIFFERENTIAL DIAGNOSIS

Cases of Waldenström's macroglobulinemia may show more or less plasmacytic differentiation. This is the basis for the distinction "lymphoplasmacytoid" and "lymphoplasmacytic" Waldenström's macroglobulinemia (128). Scattered transformed cells similar to prolymphocytes of CLL, or cells with increased nuclear irregularity may also be seen in Waldenström's macroglobulinemia. Cases with increased large transformed cells (immunoblasts) have been termed "polymorphous" (128).

IgM monoclonal gammopathy can be seen in a variety of processes other than classic Waldenström's macroglobulinemia (127, 129, 130). Table 38.16 summarizes the variety of morphologies associated with monoclonal IgM. Technically, only patients with a morphology of small lymphocytic lymphoma-plasmacytoid in the bone marrow have classic Waldenström's macroglobulinemia. Patients with an IgM monoclonal gammopathy and small lymphocytic lymphoma or CLL who have no plasmacytoid differentiation should not be diagnosed as having Waldenström's macroglobulinemia. The 10% diffuse lymphomas with IgM monoclonal gammopathy shown in Table 38.16 are lymphomas with more poorly differentiated morphologies such as mixed or large-cell lymphomas with immunoblastic, plasmacytoid differentiation. These cases also should not be diagnosed as Waldenström's macroglobulinemia. It is of

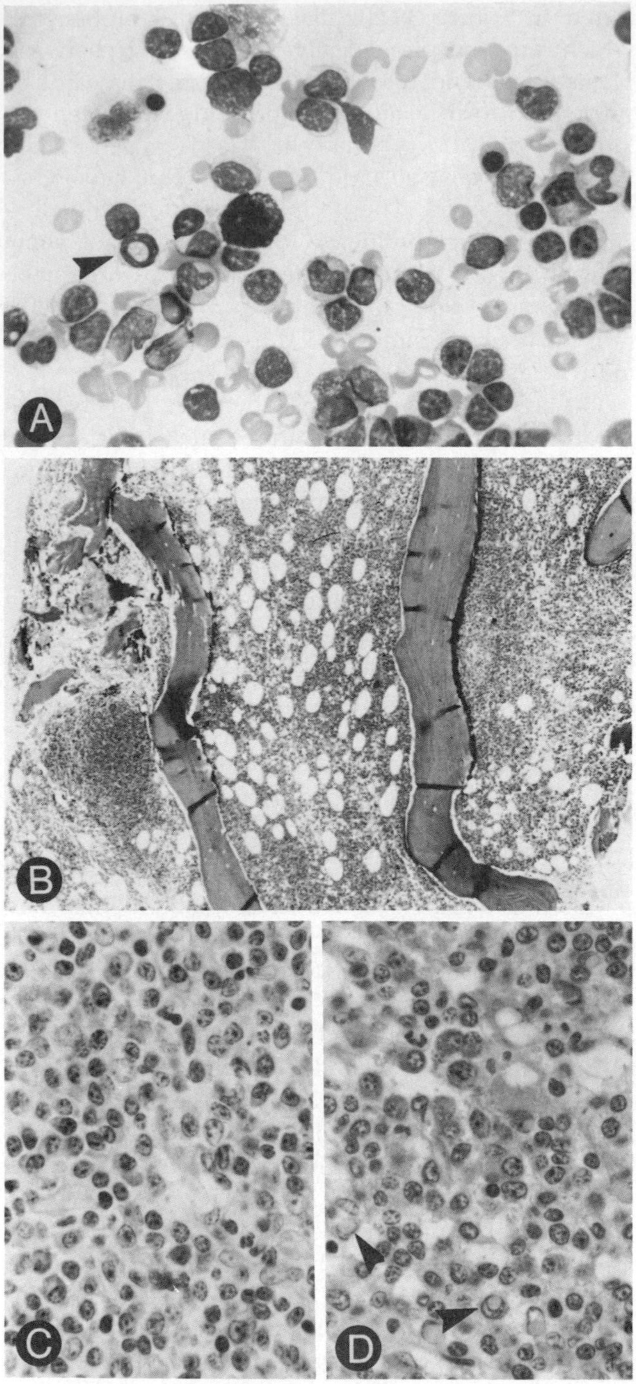

Figure 38.20. Waldenström's macroglobulinemia (small lymphocytic lymphoma, plasmacytoid). **A**, Marrow smear. Note the numerous lymphocytes, several plasma cells, a Dutcher body (*arrowhead*), and a tissue mast cell. **B**, Trephine biopsy. In the left field, the infiltrate is focal. In the center between the two long trabeculae, it is primarily interstitial, and in the right field, it is paratrabecular. **C** and **D**, Note the numerous lymphocytes and occasional plasma cells. In **D**, Dutcher bodies (pale, intranuclear inclusions) are indicated by *arrowheads*. (Hematoxylin and eosin, ×600 [**A**, **C**, **D**], ×50 [**B**].) (From Dick FR. Plasma cell myeloma and related disorders with monoclonal gammopathy. In: Koepke JA, ed. Laboratory hematology. New York: Churchill Livingstone, 1984;1:445–481.)

Table 38.16. Morphologic Entities Associated with Macroglobulinemia[a]

Morphology	Approximate Frequency in Patients with Macroglobulinemia
	%
Small lymphocytic lymphoma-plasmacytoid	50
Small lymphocytic lymphoma or CLL	10
Other lymphomas	
Diffuse	10
Follicular	Rare
Other leukemias	Rare
Plasma cell myeloma	Rare
Lymphoid aggregates in bone marrow	15
No morphologic lesion	15
	100

[a]From Dick FR. Plasma cell myeloma and related disorders with monoclonal gammopathy. In: Koepke JA, ed. Laboratory hematology. New York: Churchill Livingstone, 1984;1:445–481.

interest that lymphomas can also rarely have IgG monoclonal gammopathies (130).

Thirty percent of patients with a monoclonal IgM have no identifiable accompanying neoplastic lesion, but instead have benign-appearing lymphoid aggregates or no morphologic lesion. Such cases may be referred to as essential macroglobulinemia. These patients may have symptoms related to the protein abnormality (high serum viscosity, peripheral neuropathy cold agglutinin disease, coagulation disorders, etc.), or they may have no symptoms at all, the protein abnormality being identified incidentally on serum protein electrophoresis. This latter asymptomatic set of patients, who usually have less than 3 g/dl IgM, would fit into the category of benign monoclonal gammopathy (discussed in a later section).

IMMUNOLOGIC AND OTHER STUDIES

As for plasma cell myeloma, serum and urine immunofixation electrophoresis is of major diagnostic usefulness in patients suspected of having Waldenström's macroglobulinemia. Interestingly, a small percentage of patients with the classic clinical and morphologic features of Waldenström's macroglobulinemia have, instead of an IgM monoclonal gammopathy, an IgG or an IgA monoclonal gammopathy (131). Whether these patients should be included in the diagnostic category of Waldenström's macroglobulinemia is debatable.

Immunologic study of the cells on sections or smears in Waldenström's macroglobulinemia is usually not necessary since the monoclonal gammopathy serves as a clonal marker for the disease. When studied, the cells in Waldenström's macroglobulinemia will show cytoplasmic immunoglobulin of a clonally restricted light chain as well as B-cell surface markers and T9 (6, 132). Evaluation of bone marrow cells using flow cytometry, immunofluorescence, and immunohistochemistry has demonstrated a light-chain restricted clone of cells in a majority of patients with IgM monoclonal gammopathy but morphologically nondiagnostic bone marrow (132). That study concludes that patients with more than 20% "clonal" mononuclear cells in a morphologically nondiagnostic marrow without symptoms should be diagnosed as having small lymphocytic lymphoma-plasmacytoid (Waldenström's macroglobulinemia) rather than essential macroglobulinemia. Further investigation is necessary to confirm this conclusion.

CHANGES WITH PROGRESSION AND TRANSFORMATION

Occasional cases of Waldenström's macroglobulinemia (small lymphocytic lymphoma-plasmacytoid) show transformation to a more aggressive cell type, such as large-cell immunoblastic lymphoma (24). Like plasma cell myeloma, rare cases may also develop acute nonlymphocytic leukemia after long-term therapy with alkylating agents (24).

About 20% of patients who present initially with an apparently benign IgM monoclonal gammopathy and no definitive evidence of a lymphoid malignancy will develop a morphologically diagnosable hematologic malignancy. The median time for this to occur is slightly more than 4 years after the initial diagnosis (127).

STAGING, THERAPY, AND PROGNOSTIC FEATURES

Like chronic lymphocytic leukemia and plasma cell myeloma, Waldenström's macroglobulinemia is a progressive, noncurable disease. It has a prognosis intermediate between CLL and plasma cell myeloma, and the therapeutic approach is fairly similar to that for chronic lymphocytic leukemia. The bone marrow pattern and the degree of infiltration may have some prognostic significance, with a focal nodular pattern having a better prognosis than an extensive diffuse infiltrate (128, 133). Of the three morphologic variants described earlier, the lymphoplasmacytoid type has the best prognosis and the polymorphous type has the poorest (128).

Heavy Chain Disease

These rare disorders are characterized by a cellular proliferation of plasma cells and/or lymphoid cells and production of a monoclonal gammopathy composed of an incomplete heavy chain without an associated light chain (134). Thus, on immunofixation electrophoresis, the clonal protein reacts with antisera to heavy chains but not to light chains. Heavy chain disease involving γ, μ, and α chains have been described (135–137). The age range for heavy chain disease is wider than that of the immunoproliferative disorders described in the preceding sections. Of the three disorders, α chain disease has the youngest age distribution, being seen primarily in the second and third decades. The organ distribution of the cellular proliferation depends on the heavy chain involved.

γ HEAVY CHAIN DISEASE

Clinical findings at presentation for this disorder, in addition to organomegaly and cytopenias, include autoimmune disease, swelling of the uvula, and neuropathy (134, 135). Approximately 70% of patients with a finding of γ heavy chain disease have a neoplastic lesion, which may involve bone marrow, Waldeyer's ring, lymph nodes, spleen, and liver. The morphology of the lesion is characteristically a mixture of plasma cells, lymphocytes, and immunoblasts; however, more rarely, the lesion in γ heavy chain disease may be identical to that of chronic lymphocytic leukemia, small lymphocytic lymphoma-plasmacytoid, or large-cell immunoblastic lymphoma. The 30% of patients without a morphologic lesion associated with γ heavy chain disease will have either atypical infiltrates in the aforementioned sites or no morphologically recognizable abnormal proliferation.

μ HEAVY CHAIN DISEASE

Chronic lymphocytic leukemia and small lymphocytic lymphoma are the most common morphologic entities associated with production of μ heavy chains (134, 136). Rare cases of large-cell lymphoma may also be seen. Plasma cells in the bone marrow in this process characteristically have cytoplasmic vacuoles (138). Most patients also have free light chains in the urine. This is the rarest of the heavy chain diseases.

α CHAIN DISEASE

Patients with this disorder usually present with gastrointestinal symptoms (134, 137). This is the most common form of heavy chain disease and is characteristically seen in the Mediterranean area. A morphologic lesion in α chain disease is most commonly observed in the gastrointestinal tract and abdominal lymph nodes. The cellular proliferation in the lesion can range from a dense infiltrate of plasma cells in the lamina propria of the bowel and lymph nodes to a large-cell immunoblastic lymphoma. The bone marrow may rarely be involved (139).

"Benign" Monoclonal Gammopathy

Occasionally, a monoclonal gammopathy will be identified by serum protein electrophoresis during routine screening or workup of an elderly patient for diseases other than immunoproliferative disorders (140). A patient who has a small monoclonal gammopathy with no symptoms referable to the protein abnormality and no B-cell malignancy or amyloidosis is considered to have a benign monoclonal gammopathy, also called monoclonal gammopathy of undetermined significance (MGUS). The vast majority (80 to 90%) of these patients will follow a benign course, without developing plasma cell myeloma, lymphoproliferative disorder, or complications from protein production.

Some patients with benign monoclonal gammopathy appear to have a true benign neoplastic disorder. Evidence for this includes persistence of the monoclonal gammopathy over time in an asymptomatic patient, and the presence of a mild (less than 10%) increase in atypical clonal plasma cells. Other patients appear to have a premalignant disorder. Evidence for this is the eventual development of plasma cell myeloma or a related malignant immunoproliferative or lymphoproliferative disorder in up to 10 to 20% of cases. Currently, it is difficult to determine which patients with benign monoclonal gammopathy will experience progression to a malignant disorder. In other patients, the benign monoclonal gammopathy may represent a restricted response to some unidentified antigen. This is based on these findings: rare monoclonal gammopathies have known specificity; some benign monoclonal gammopathies are transient; and in a hospitalized setting, about 25% of benign monoclonal gammopathies are related to inflammatory, connective tissue, or neoplastic disease (140). The term essential monoclonal gammopathy has been applied to the first two sets of patients, and secondary monoclonal gammopathy to the set of patients in whom the monoclonal gammopathy may represent a restricted response (141). Although this distinction is conceptually attractive, it is not always possible to distinguish between an essential and a secondary disorder in a given patient.

DIAGNOSTIC FEATURES

Bone marrow examination, if performed in benign monoclonal gammopathy, usually shows less than 5% nearly normal-appearing plasma cells. However, up to 10% or more atypical plasma cells may also be consistent with a benign course. The term smoldering myeloma, as discussed previously, has been used to describe the asymptomatic patient who has more than 10% atypical plasma cells, has a monoclonal gammopathy above 3 g/dl, and follows a benign course (84, 85). Atypical plasma cells similar to those illustrated in Figure 38.14 can be seen in patients with benign monoclonal gammopathy. However, markedly atypical cells should raise the possibility that the patient has significant disease at another site and will have progressive disease.

Table 38.17. Classes of Serum Immunoglobulin in Benign Monoclonal Gammopathy[a] (82, 140)

Ig Class	Frequency
	%
IgG	75
IgA	15
IgM	10

[a]From Dick FR. Plasma cell myeloma and related disorders with monoclonal gammopathy. In: Koepke JA, ed. Laboratory hematology. New York: Churchill Livingstone, 1984;1:445–481.

Table 38.18. Size of M-Component in Benign Monoclonal Gammopathy[a] (82, 140)

Size	Approximate Percentage of Patients
g/dl	
≤ 1.5	30
1.6–2.5	65
> 2.5	5

[a]From Dick FR. Plasma cell myeloma and related disorders with monoclonal gammopathy. In: Koepke JA, ed. Laboratory hematology. New York: Churchill Livingstone, 1984;1:445–481.

The incidence of benign monoclonal gammopathy increases with age. Screening of healthy populations by using serum protein electrophoresis has shown that 1% of patients more than 25 years of age and 3% of patients more than 70 years of age will have a benign monoclonal gammopathy (142). Another study using more sensitive serum protein electrophoresis showed a 5% incidence in a healthy population less than 65 years old (143). The incidence may be even higher when using immunofixation electrophoresis.

IMMUNOLOGIC AND OTHER STUDIES

The class of serum immunoglobulin seen in benign monoclonal gammopathy is shown in Table 38.17, and the size of the monoclonal gammopathy is shown in Table 38.18 (144). Approximately 15% of patients with benign monoclonal gammopathy will show some decrease in other immunoglobulins, and at least 10% of patients with a serum benign monoclonal gammopathy will have free light chains (usually less than 1 g per 24 hours) in the urine (140, 144). Patients with benign monoclonal gammopathy composed of free urinary light chains and no monoclonal serum protein have also been observed (140).

Immunohistochemical studies on the bone marrow in cases of benign monoclonal gammopathy have demonstrated an excess of plasma cells with a clonally restricted light chain in a majority of patients (103–105). Thus, identification of a clonal population in this setting does not imply a malignant diagnosis.

Evaluation of β_2-microglobulinemia (140), labeling index of bone marrow plasma cells and peripheral blood lymphocytes (109, 110), cytoplasmic 5′ nucleotidase (145), and short-term bone marrow culture have been reported in benign monoclonal gammopathy (146, 147).

THERAPY AND PROGNOSIS

Approximately 10 to 20% of patients with benign monoclonal gammopathy will eventually develop plasma cell myeloma, Waldenström's macroglobulinemia, lymphoma, or amyloidosis (140). Although a progressive increase in the monoclonal protein level is a good indicator of the eventual development of progressive disease, a small percentage of patients who show an increase of 1 to 2 g in the monoclonal gammopathy are found not to have developed symptomatic neoplastic disease on long-term follow-up (140). A bone marrow examination at the time of the discovery of benign monoclonal gammopathy may or may not be indicated, depending on other clinical and laboratory findings. There is some evidence to suggest that cases of benign monoclonal gammopathy that will progress to plasma cell myeloma can be identified using peripheral blood labeling indices (110) or short-term marrow culture (146). β_2-Microglobulin has little usefulness in this regard (140). Benign monoclonal gammopathies should not be overinterpreted as evidence for plasma cell myeloma; they can be seen in patients with diseases masquerading as plasma cell myeloma, such as osteoporosis and metastatic carcinoma.

Amyloidosis

Amyloidosis may eventually develop in about 15% of patients with plasma cell myeloma, with an especially high propensity in patients with λ light chain monoclonal gammopathy (100). Amyloidosis observed on bone marrow sections usually involves vessels; however, an interstitial infiltrative pattern may also be seen, as illustrated in Figure 38.21. The presence of amyloidosis can be confirmed on marrow sections with thioflavin-T and Congo red stains.

Amyloidosis can be detected in the bone marrow in only one-fourth of patients with primary systemic amyloidosis; however, in keeping with the concept that primary amyloidosis is an immunoproliferative disorder, it has been demonstrated that, as in benign monoclonal gammopathy, there is an excess of plasma cells of restricted light chain type in almost three-fourths of the bone marrows in primary amyloidosis (106). A mild atypical plasmacytosis, as seen in benign monoclonal gammopathies or smoldering myeloma, is also seen in primary amyloidosis, sometimes with plasma cells embedded in interstitial amyloid deposits. When a patient with primary amyloidosis has more than 10% atypical plasma cells, it becomes problematic as to whether the patient should also be diagnosed as having plasma cell myeloma.

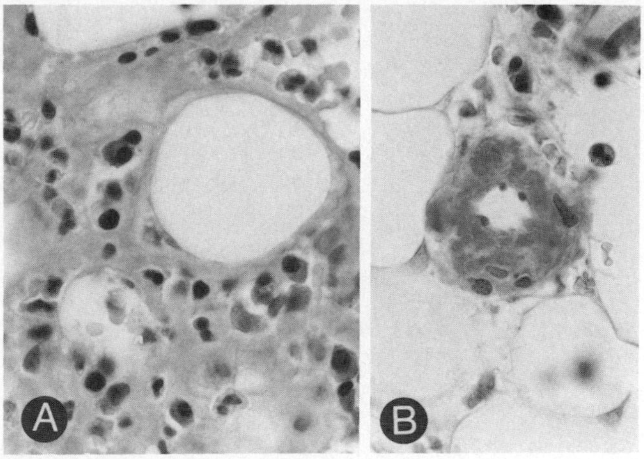

Figure 38.21. Primary amyloidosis, bone marrow section. **A**, The homogeneous interstitial deposits are amyloid. Note the scattered plasma cells embedded in the amyloid. **B**, Deposition of amyloid in a vessel wall. (Hematoxylin and eosin, ×600.)

MALIGNANT LYMPHOMA

Malignant lymphomas include a diverse group of disorders ranging from morphologically mature processes with an indolent course to highly aggressive processes with morphologic immaturity. Although these processes are diagnosed primarily by tissue biopsy, they frequently have manifestations in the blood and bone marrow. Blood and bone marrow manifestations are emphasized in this chapter; more specific details of morphologic diagnosis in extramarrow sites can be found in textbooks and articles devoted to lymph node morphology (148, 149).

Malignant lymphomas are of two major types: Hodgkin's disease and non-Hodgkin's lymphoma. There is a major difference between these two types of lymphomas: in Hodgkin's disease, the infiltrate has a minority population of a large, pleomorphic neoplastic cell (the Reed-Sternberg cell) and a major population of reactive cells including predominantly lymphocytes, with variable numbers of admixed his-

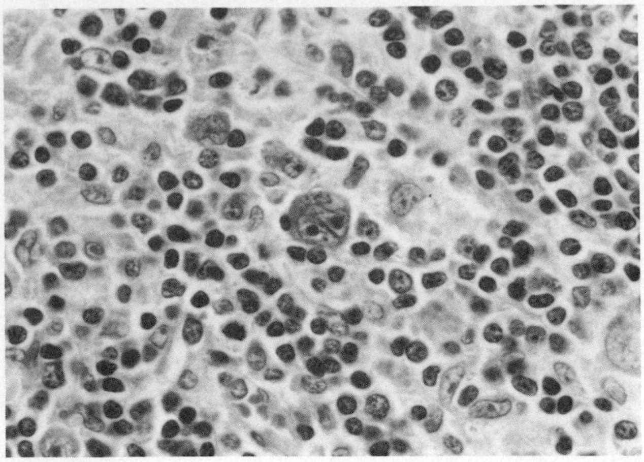

Figure 38.22. Hodgkin's disease in a lymph node with a typical large, binucleated Reed-Sternberg cell. Nucleoli in this cell are about half the diameter of a lymphocyte and are surrounded by a clear halo. Note the numerous fairly normal-appearing lymphocytes and scattered histiocytes. (Hematoxylin and eosin, ×600.)

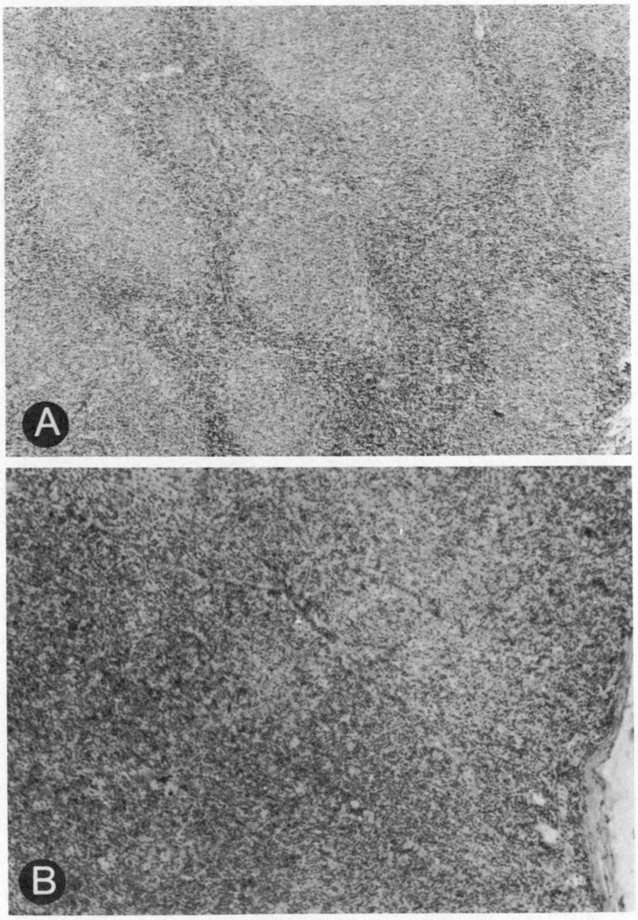

Figure 38.23. Non-Hodgkin's lymphomas. **A**, Follicular pattern. The neoplastic follicules resemble normal germinal (follicular) centers. **B**, Diffuse pattern. Note the absence of any pattern. (Hematoxylin and eosin, ×25.) (**B**, From Dick FR. Chronic lymphocytic leukemia, prolymphocytic leukemia and leukemic non-Hodgkin's leukemia. In: Koepke JA, ed. Laboratory hematology. New York: Churchill Livingstone, 1984;1:325–357.)

Table 38.19. Non-Hodgkin's Malignant Lymphomas: Classification and Incidence of Bone Marrow Involvement

Working Formulation Diagnoses	Relative Frequency	Incidence of Bone Marrow Involvement
	%	%
Low grade		
Small lymphocytic	4	70
Intermediate lymphocytic[a]	—	—
Follicular, small cleaved	23	50
Follicular, mixed small cleaved and large cell	8	30
Intermediate grade		
Follicular, large cell	4	35
Diffuse, small cleaved	7	30
Diffuse, mixed small and large cell	7	15
Diffuse, large cell	20	10
High grade		
Large cell immunoblastic	8	10
Lymphoblastic	4	50
Small noncleaved	5	15
Miscellaneous, including unclassified	10	—
	100	—

[a]Intermediate lymphocytic lymphoma was not part of the classification when it was developed in 1982. Whether it should be considered a low-grade or an intermediate-grade lymphoma is debatable.

Table 38.20. Hodgkin's Disease: Classification and Incidence of Bone Marrow Involvement

Rye Classification	Relative Frequency	Incidence of Bone Marrow Involvement
	%	%
Lymphocytic predominance	14	0
Nodular sclerosis	41	2–10
Mixed cellularity	31	5–20
Lymphocyte depleted	14	45–70

tiocytes, eosinophils, and plasma cells (Fig. 38.22). In non-Hodgkin's lymphomas, the infiltrate is composed predominantly of the neoplastic lymphoid cell.

Non-Hodgkin's lymphomas are further subclassified on the basis of infiltrative pattern into follicular and diffuse processes (Fig. 38.23) and on the basis of the cell type (discussed in detail in the next section). Hodgkin's disease is further subclassified on the basis of whether or not a nodular sclerosing pattern is present and on the basis of cellular composition (lymphocyte predominance or depletion and number of Reed-Sternberg cells).

Malignant lymphomas have variable involvement of the bone marrow and peripheral blood. The subclassification and relative frequency of lymphomas and their incidence in the bone marrow are shown in Tables 38.19 and 38.20 (148, 150).

Prognosis in lymphomas is highly dependent on the subtype of lymphoma and the extent of disease (stage). Depending on the lymphoma type, the tumor can be seen in younger or older individuals.

Low-grade and follicular non-Hodgkin's lymphomas are seen almost exclusively in older individuals, whereas lymphoblastic lymphomas are seen predominantly in younger persons.

Non-Hodgkin's Lymphoma

DIAGNOSTIC FEATURES

Non-Hodgkin's lymphomas usually are initially diagnosed by examination of lymph node or extramarrow tissue biopsy specimens rather than bone marrow sections. Diagnosis is based on the effacement of architecture by a neoplastic lymphoid infiltrate distributed in a follicular or diffuse pattern (Fig. 38.23). Once a diagnosis of a neoplastic disorder and its pattern is confirmed, the cytologic subtype is assessed. The classification currently in use for non-Hodgkin's malignant lymphomas is the Working Formulation, Table 38.19, which is essentially an amalgamation of the previously popular Rappaport classification and the Lukes-Collins classification (148). Note in this classification that small cleaved cell, mixed small- and large-cell, and large-cell subtypes may show a follicular or diffuse pattern. All the others are always diffuse (except for intermediate, which may have a mantle zone pattern).

In assessing the cell type in non-Hodgkin's lymphoma, it is useful to compare the size of the nucleus of the lymphoma cells with the nucleus of a normal histiocyte on sections (or the nucleus of a myeloblast on smears). Small lymphocytic lymphoma, small cleaved cell lymphoma, and lymphoblastic lymphoma have a nucleus that is definitely smaller than that of a histiocyte. Small noncleaved cell lymphoma has a nucleus slightly smaller than or almost the size of a histiocyte nucleus, and the nuclei in large-cell lymphomas are the size of and larger than a histiocyte nucleus. The morphologic features of the various cell types in non-Hodgkin's lymphomas are outlined in the legends to Figures 38.24 to 38.27. Small lymphocytic lymphoma is not illustrated here since it is morphologically indistinguishable from CLL or Waldenström's macroglobulinemia (see Figs. 38.1, 38.2, 38.5, and 38.20). The fine points of distinction between large-cell lymphoma of the more common type (diffuse large cell) and large-cell immunoblastic lymphoma are also not illustrated. This distinction may be morphologically quite difficult. Briefly, immunoblastic morphology is frequently associated with a T-cell phenotype, plasmacytoid differentiation, or a pleomorphic/polymorphous appearance. A true histiocytic "lymphoma" is also illustrated in Figure 38.28 for comparison with large cell lymphomas (151).

It should be stressed that, in general, the immunophenotype of a lymphoma cannot be predicted with certainty by cytologic examination of the cells, although an educated guess can sometimes be made based on the relative frequency of B-cell or T-cell phenotype for each cell type (see later, Table 38.24). Lymphomas with a follicular pattern should all be B-cell lymphomas because they are derived from the follicle, which is a B-cell domain. Immunophenotyping, rather than morphology, is the method of choice to determine the B-cell or T-cell nature of a lymphoma.

Although many lymphomas are initially diagnosed on tissue biopsy and the marrow, if involved, is diagnosed secondarily, there are situations in which a primary diagnosis can be made by examination of bone marrow sections. General principles that apply to the primary or secondary diagnosis of non-Hodgkin's lymphoma in the bone marrow are addressed below. Following this, additional features for each of the subtypes in the classification are described.

General features of non-Hodgkin's lymphoma in the marrow are as follows:

1. Bone marrow involvement can take a variety of patterns. In the early stages of involvement, the bone marrow is usually focally involved by aggregates of lymphoma cells. These aggregates may be either nonparatrabecular or paratrabecular (152). A lymphoma with a paratrabecular pattern is illustrated in Figure 38.29. Multiple paratrabecular aggregates may be diagnosed as lymphoma solely on the basis of their pattern, whereas nonparatrabecular aggregates must be diagnosed using other features. As involvement increases, the marrow becomes more diffusely infiltrated and the focal pattern is obscured. Malignant lymphomas may also have minimal involvement in an interstitial pattern; however, this is uncommon. When this occurs, it may be difficult to make a diagnosis from the examination of marrow sections, and the diagnosis may rest more heavily on identifying neoplastic lymphoid cells in aspirates or touch preparations, or on the use of immunologic markers (see later, Fig. 38.32).
2. Making the distinction between a follicular and a diffuse pattern of non-Hodgkin's lymphoma is rarely possible on bone marrow examination (152). Focal aggregates of lymphoma can be seen in diffuse and follicular lymphoma. A focal pattern in the marrow is not equivalent to follicular lymphoma.

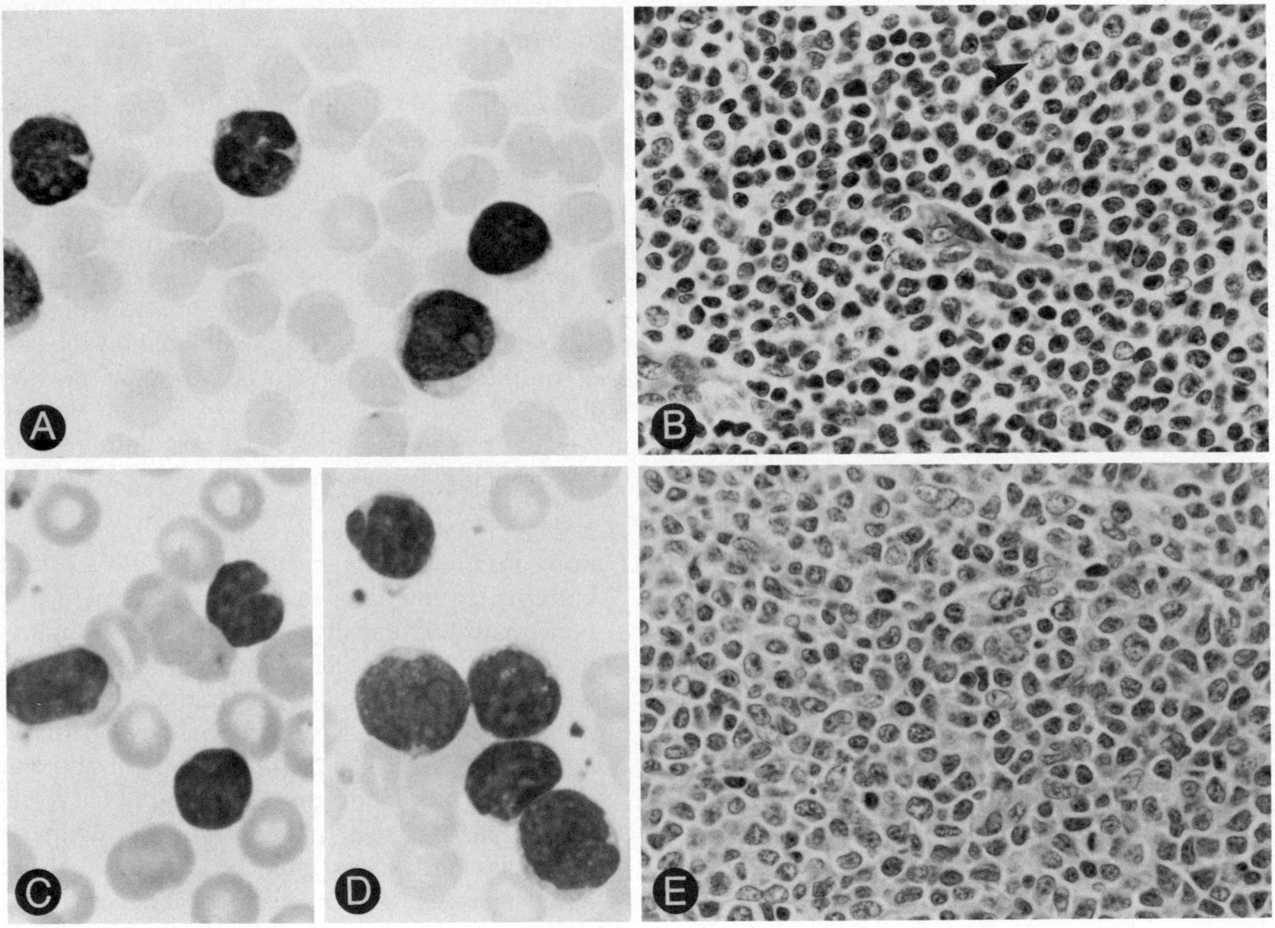

Figure 38.24. Lymphomas with a majority of cells the size of lymphocytes. **A** and **B**, Intermediate lymphocytic lymphoma. Many nearly normal-appearing lymphocytes are present; however, some cells are slightly larger, and there is moderate nuclear contour irregularity compared with small lymphocytic lymphoma. **C, D,** and **E**, Small cleaved cell lymphoma. On smears and sections, note the size range from small to large abnormal lymphocytes with scant cytoplasm and many sharply clefted nuclei. On smears, note that some of the larger, clefted lymphoid cells resemble lymphoblasts. In **E**, scattered large cells the size of large-cell lymphoma cells are also seen. A normal histiocyte nucleus is present in the upper right center field of **B** (*arrowhead*) for size comparison. (**A, C,** and **D**, Wright's stain, ×1200. **B** and **E**, Hematoxylin and eosin, ×600.) (**A, C,** and **D**, From Dick FR. Chronic lymphocytic leukemia, prolymphocytic leukemia and leukemic non-Hodgkin's leukemia. In: Koepke JA, ed. Laboratory hematology. New York: Churchill Livingstone, 1984;1:325–357.)

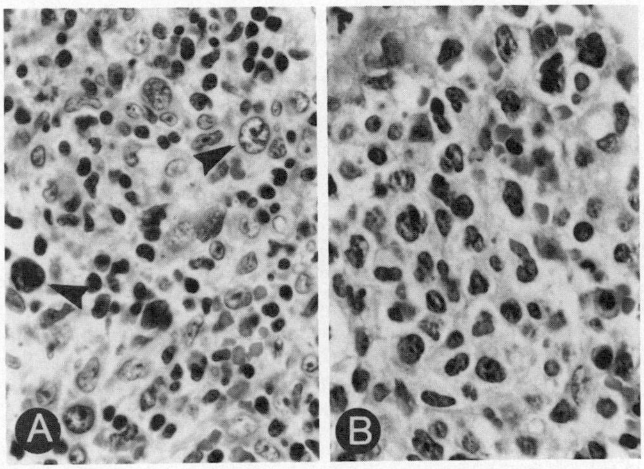

Figure 38.25. Mixed small- and large-cell lymphomas. Many cells the size of lymphocytes are present; however, atypical large cells are also numerous. Note in **A** the hyperchromatic and convoluted large cells (*arrowheads*) and in **B** the numerous small and large clefted cells. The lymphoma in **A** was immunophenotyped as a T-cell lymphoma and the lymphoma in **B** as a B-cell lymphoma. (Hematoxylin and eosin, ×600.)

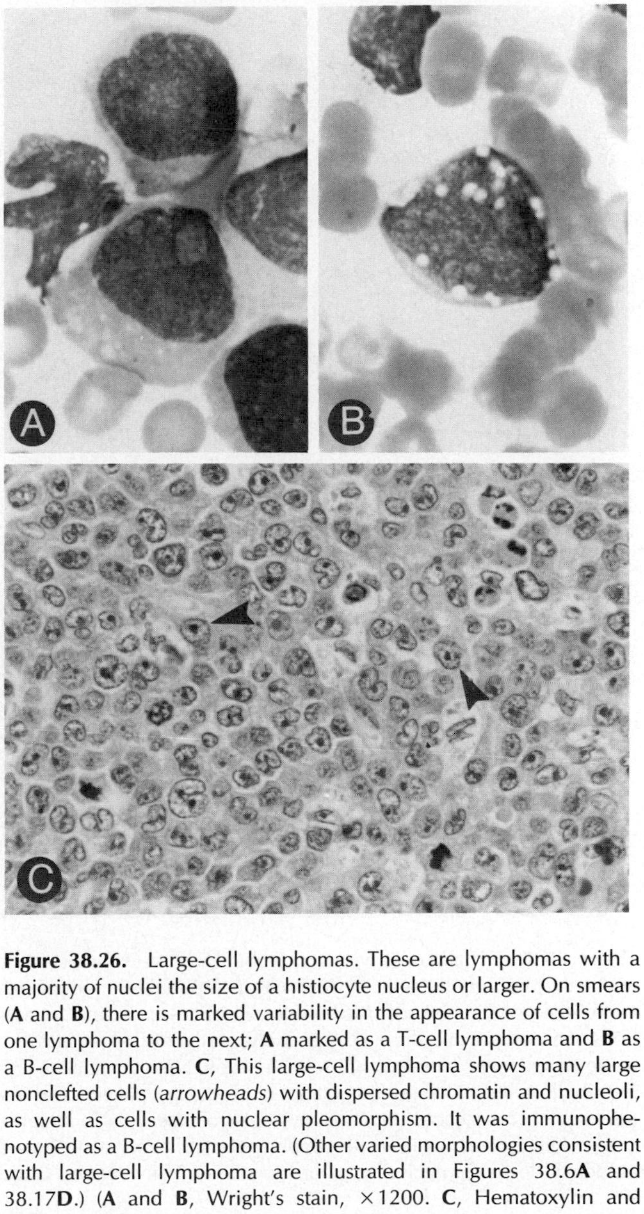

Figure 38.26. Large-cell lymphomas. These are lymphomas with a majority of nuclei the size of a histiocyte nucleus or larger. On smears (**A** and **B**), there is marked variability in the appearance of cells from one lymphoma to the next; **A** marked as a T-cell lymphoma and **B** as a B-cell lymphoma. **C**, This large-cell lymphoma shows many large noncleſted cells (*arrowheads*) with dispersed chromatin and nucleoli, as well as cells with nuclear pleomorphism. It was immunophenotyped as a B-cell lymphoma. (Other varied morphologies consistent with large-cell lymphoma are illustrated in Figures 38.6**A** and 38.17**D**.) (**A** and **B**, Wright's stain, ×1200. **C**, Hematoxylin and eosin, ×600.)

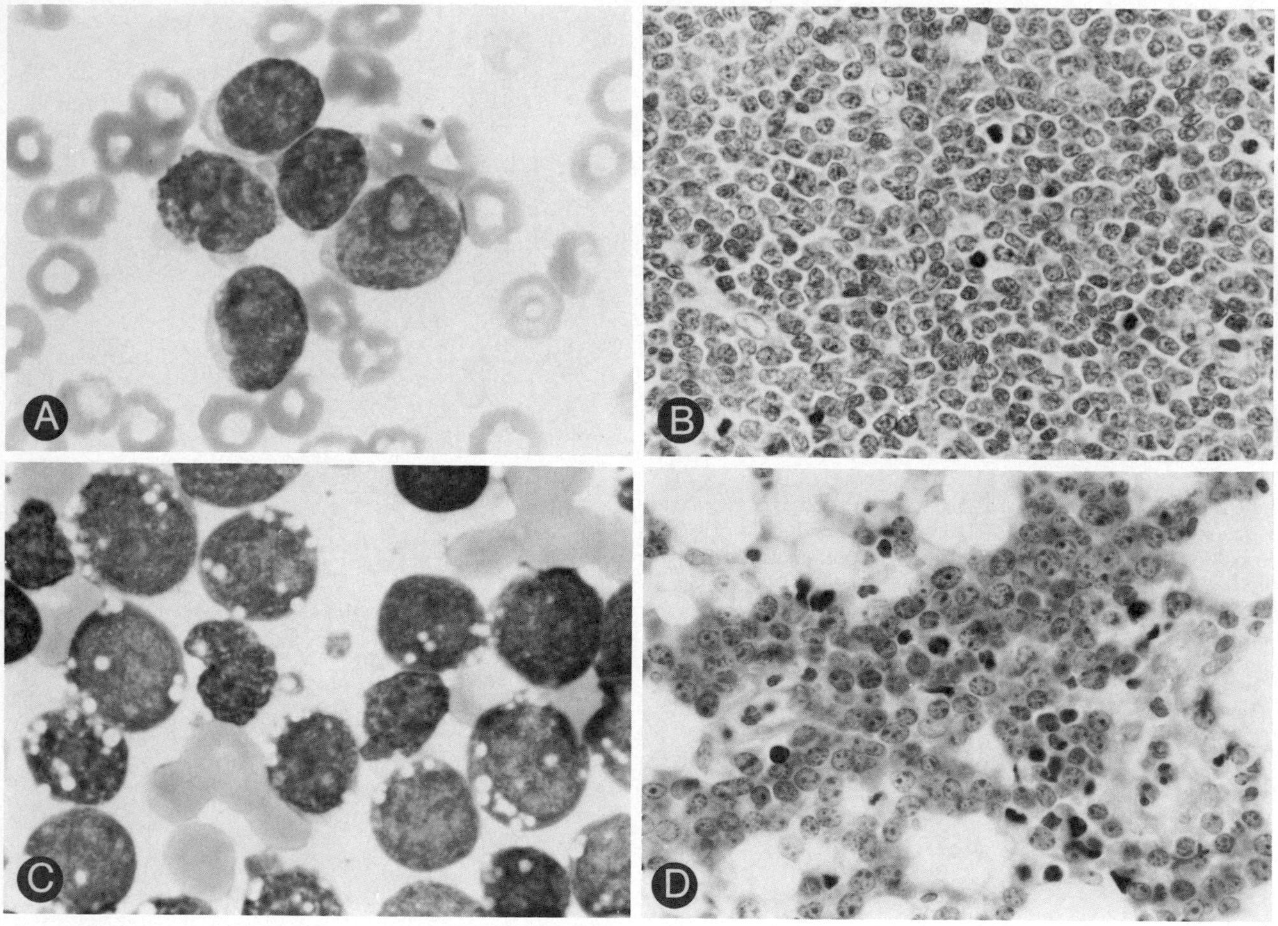

Figure 38.27. High-grade lymphomas with a blast-like appearance and very high mitotic activity. **A** and **B**, Lymphoblastic lymphoma. Lymphoma cell nuclei are smaller than a histiocyte nucleus on sections, and on smears they are morphologically similar to blasts of acute lymphocytic leukemia of L1 and L2 type. Note the relative uniformity of cellular composition, stippled chromatin pattern, and mitotic activity on sections (**B**). Cells on smears and sections in lymphoblastic lymphomas (as in acute lymphocytic leukemia) may show a moderate degree of nuclear contour irregularity (convolution). **C** and **D**, Small noncleaved lymphoma (Burkitt type). Note the marked uniformity of cellular composition, hyperbasophilic cytoplasm, and crisp cytoplasmic and nuclear vacuoles. Nuclear size is slightly smaller than or about the size of a histiocyte nucleus on sections, and on smears the cells are morphologically similar to acute lymphocytic leukemia, L3 type. Note that some large-cell lymphoma cells (illustrated in Figures 38.6**A** and 38.26**B**) may have, except for their size, some of the characteristics of small noncleaved lymphoma cells. (**A** and **C**, Wright's stain, ×1200. **B** and **D**, Hematoxylin and eosin, ×600.)

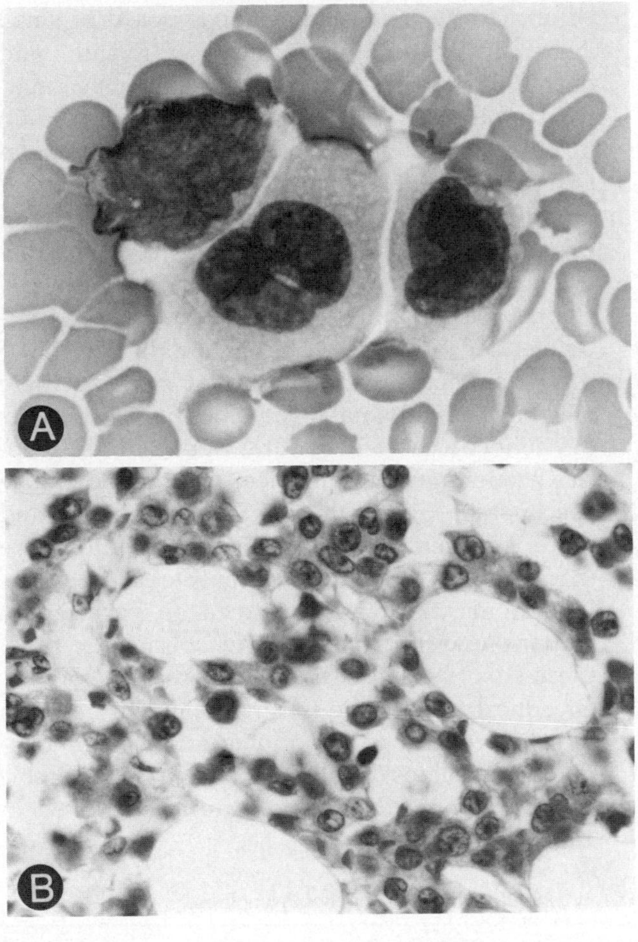

Figure 38.28. True histiocytic lymphoma/malignant histiocytosis, peripheral blood (**A**), and bone marrow section (**B**). Although this tumor resembles a large-cell lymphoma on sections, it is a malignancy of histiocytes. Note the resemblance of the cells on smears to large, highly pleomorphic monoblasts. The histiomonocytic nature of this process can be confirmed with a nonspecific esterase stain on smears or immunologic markers on sections or cell suspension. (**A**, Wright's stain, ×1200. **B**, Hematoxylin and eosin, ×600.)

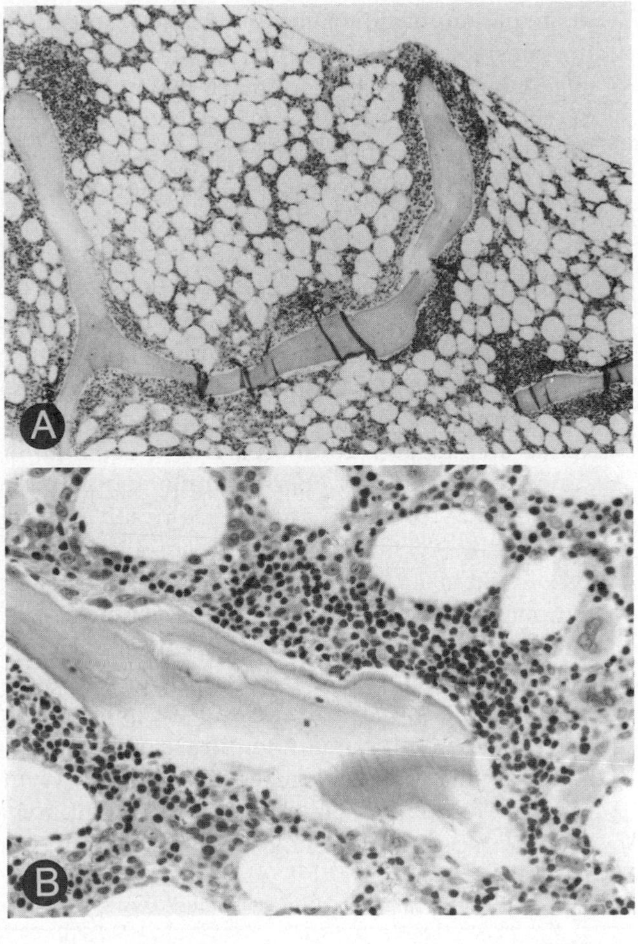

Figure 38.29. Paratrabecular pattern in non-Hodgkin's lymphoma. Note the "plastered on" or "piled up" appearance of most of the aggregates. The aggregate in the upper left field of **A** is not truly paratrabecular since its center appears to be away from the bone, and it could be touching bone by virtue of growth toward it. Note in **B** how the paratrabecular aggregate appears to be growing on the bone. Also note in **B** that the lymphocytes in this lymphoma are small and show only mild nuclear clefting, even though the lymph node biopsy showed considerable nuclear clefting. (Hematoxylin and eosin, ×50 [**A**], ×240 [**B**].)

3. The bone marrow may show a lower-grade subtype of lymphoma than an initial tissue biopsy (152–154). For example, when a lymphoma of mixed or large-cell type is initially diagnosed in an extramarrow site, the marrow may show a predominantly mixed, small cleaved, or, rarely, a small lymphocytic cell type. Thus, non-Hodgkin's lymphoma should not be definitively subtyped for purposes of therapy when a mixed, small cleaved or small lymphocytic lymphoma is seen initially in tha marrow, unless the marrow is the only site available for biopsy. A primary diagnosis of any of the other subtypes of non-Hodgkin's lymphoma (large-cell, lymphoblastic, or small noncleaved) in the marrow can be used for classification for therapy.
4. Malignant lymphomas primarily represent tissue infiltration of neoplastic lymphoid cells, whereas leukemias are bone marrow and peripheral blood manifestations of neoplastic lymphoid cells. As shown in Table 38.21, for some specific cell types, the "lymphomatous" (tissue phase) and its "leukemic or marrow" counterpart have separate diagnostic terminology. For example, a neoplastic proliferation of the mature CD4-positive B cell with weak SIg is diagnosed as chronic lymphocytic leukemia when there is a peripheral blood lymphocytosis. When it involves tissues with minimal blood and marrow involvement, it is called small lymphocytic lymphoma. Neoplastic proliferations of cells that comprise intermediate lymphocytic lymphoma; the diffuse and follicular forms of small cleaved, mixed, and large-cell lymphomas; and large-cell immunoblastic lymphoma have no specific terminology for their leukemic phase, and thus these are simply diagnosed as the leukemic phase of malignant lymphoma. In the past, some of these entities were diagnosed as "lymphosarcoma cell leukemia" (155, 156). However, because of the nonspecificity of this term, it has been dropped from our vocabulary.
5. In general, a trephine biopsy is superior to aspirate and particle sections in diagnosing malignant lymphoma in the marrow. This is because early bone marrow involvement is composed of small aggregates that may have increased reticulin and do not aspirate well. In addition, extensive marrow involvement may be partly fibrotic and result in a dry tap. In this latter situation, touch preparations are helpful in seeing cytologic detail.
6. Since bone marrow involvement is frequently focal and may be minimal, bilateral bone marrow trephine biopsies of the posterior crests with five-stepped sections on each side are generally recommended (157, 158). The volume of bone marrow examined is also important because there may be focal, minimal involvement; thus, it is recommended that between the right and left biopsies a minimum total of 3 cm of trephine biopsy specimen in aggregate length be acquired, and more is preferable (159). This may require more than one pass of the trephine needle on each side. Lymphoma may rarely be seen on particle clot sections and not on trephine specimens; thus, these should also be carefully examined (157).
7. Of critical importance is the distinction between focal aggregates of lymphoma and benign lymphoid aggregates (Fig. 38.30*A* and *B*) (160). Important differential diagnostic features are listed in Table 38.22.

Table 38.21. Terminology for "Lymphomatous" versus "Leukemic or Marrow" Manifestations of Lymphoid Neoplasms

"Lymphomatous" Counterpart	"Leukemic or Marrow" Counterpart
WORKING FORMULATION SUBTYPES	
Small lymphocytic lymphoma	CLL
with plasmacytoid features	Waldenström's macroglobulinemia
Intermediate lymphocytic	—
Follicular lymphomas	—
Diffuse small cleaved lymphoma	—
Diffuse mixed and large-cell lymphoma	—
Lymphoblastic lymphoma	ALL—L1 & L2
Small noncleaved cell lymphoma	ALL—L3
OTHER SPECIAL SUBTYPES	
—	Prolymphocytic leukemia
—	Hairy cell leukemia
Mycosis fungoides	Sézary syndrome
Adult T-cell leukemia/lymphoma	Adult T-cell leukemia/lymphoma
Small lymphocytic lymphoma (atypical)	T-cell CLL
—	T-cell prolymphocytic leukemia
—	T-γ lymphoproliferative disease
Hodgkin's disease	—
Plasmacytoma	Plasma cell myeloma

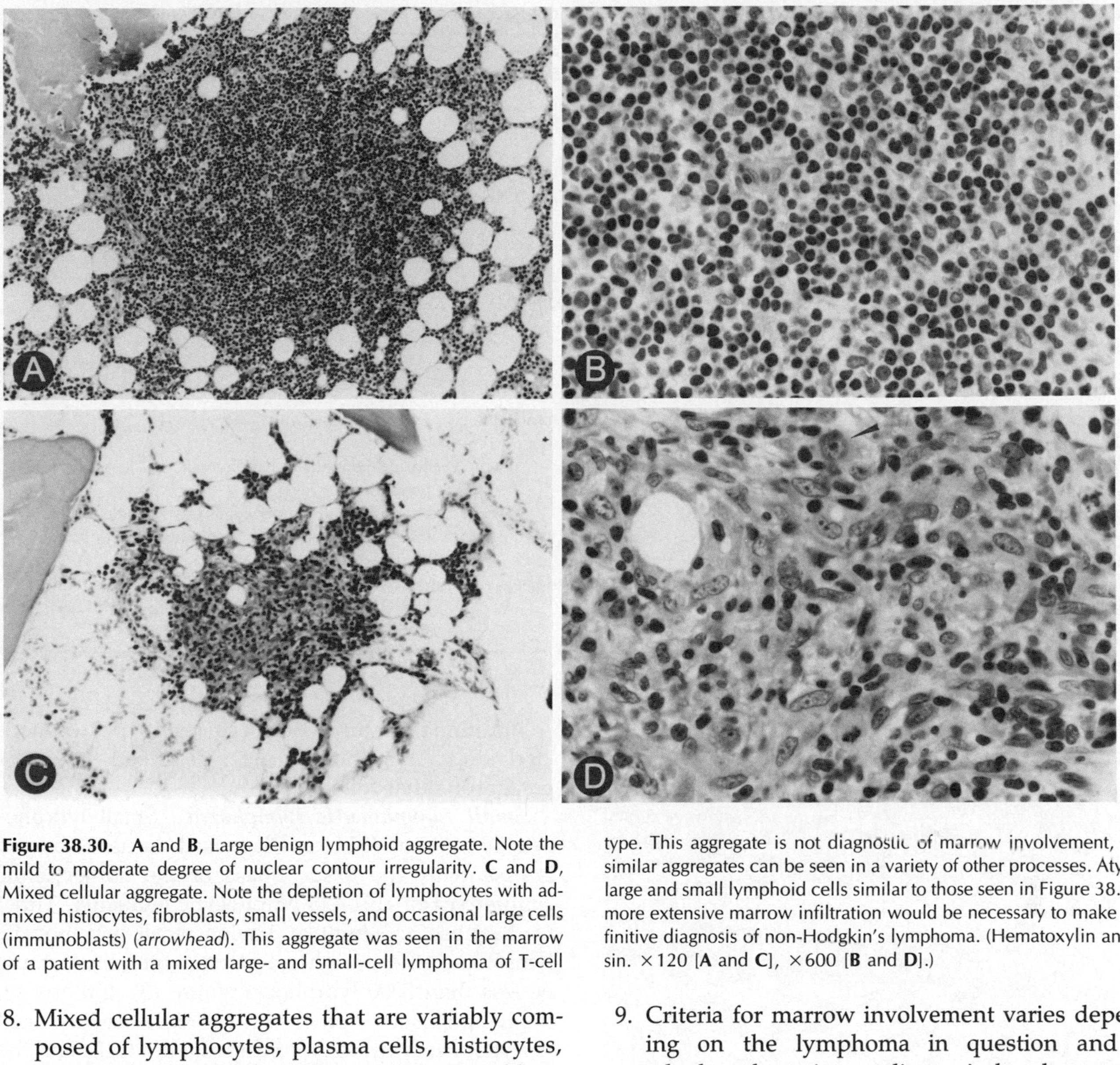

Figure 38.30. **A** and **B**, Large benign lymphoid aggregate. Note the mild to moderate degree of nuclear contour irregularity. **C** and **D**, Mixed cellular aggregate. Note the depletion of lymphocytes with admixed histiocytes, fibroblasts, small vessels, and occasional large cells (immunoblasts) (*arrowhead*). This aggregate was seen in the marrow of a patient with a mixed large- and small-cell lymphoma of T-cell type. This aggregate is not diagnostic of marrow involvement, since similar aggregates can be seen in a variety of other processes. Atypical large and small lymphoid cells similar to those seen in Figure 38.25 or more extensive marrow infiltration would be necessary to make a definitive diagnosis of non-Hodgkin's lymphoma. (Hematoxylin and eosin. ×120 [**A** and **C**], ×600 [**B** and **D**].)

8. Mixed cellular aggregates that are variably composed of lymphocytes, plasma cells, histiocytes, fibroblasts, endothelial cells, and immunoblasts may be seen in marrow involvement by lymphoma, especially peripheral T-cell lymphomas, Hodgkin's disease, and plasmacytoid lymphomas (Fig. 38.30*C* and *D*). Since these mixed cellular aggregates can also be seen in infections and in AIDS or angio-immunoblastic lymphadenopathy with dysproteinemia (AILD), which may be associated with or transform to lymphoma, the presence of mixed cellular aggregates in the marrow may result in very difficult differential diagnostic problems (161–163). Mixed cellular aggregates should not be diagnosed as lymphoma unless they contain Reed-Sternberg cells consistent with a diagnosis of Hodgkin's disease, or neoplastic lymphoid cells consistent with one of the subtypes of non-Hodgkin's lymphoma.
9. Criteria for marrow involvement varies depending on the lymphoma in question and on whether the primary diagnosis has been made elsewhere. In general, less strict evidence is needed to secondarily diagnose marrow involvement than to make a primary diagnosis of lymphoma in the bone marrow. However, the presence of aggregates without neoplastic features should not be considered definitive evidence for secondary marrow involvement, even if the aggregates are numerous.
10. Lower-grade non-Hodgkin's lymphoma may undergo transformation to a higher-grade process, especially large-cell lymphoma. In this situation, the bone marrow may be the first site biopsied, resulting in a higher-grade marrow morphology than that seen in the original biopsy specimen (153).
11. Reed-Sternberg–like cells can be seen in the marrow as well as in the lymph node in non-Hodg-

Table 38.22. Differential Diagnostic Features between Benign Lymphoid Aggregates and Focal Aggregates of Lymphoma

Feature of Aggregates	Benign	Lymphoma	Comment
Low-power features			
Paratrabecular	Rare	Yes	
Nonparatrabecular	Usually	Yes	
Uniform rounded contour	Yes	Yes	
Irregular contour	Unusual	Yes	
Benign 2° follicle	Uncommon	Rare	Neoplastic follicles are also uncommon in bone marrow
Poorly circumscribed spreading border	No	Yes	Especially in small lymphocytic lymphoma
Circumscribed border	Yes	Yes	
Associated lipoid granulomas	Yes	Uncommon	
Large size	Uncommon	Yes	
Numerous	Yes	Yes	
Rare	Yes	Yes	
Small size	Yes	Yes	
Blood vessels	Yes	Uncommon	
Cytologic features			
Minimal to mild nuclear irregularity	Yes	Yes	Seen in intermediate lymphocytic and follicular lymphoma
Distinctly atypical cell type	No	Yes	Except for small lymphocytic, intermediate, and follicular lymphoma, which may show only mild nuclear irregularity
Admixture of other elements (plasma cells, histiocytes, immunoblasts)	Yes	Sometimes	Small lymphocytic-plasmacytoid, Hodgkin's, and other non-Hodgkin's lymphomas of peripheral T cells, may show a mixed cell population

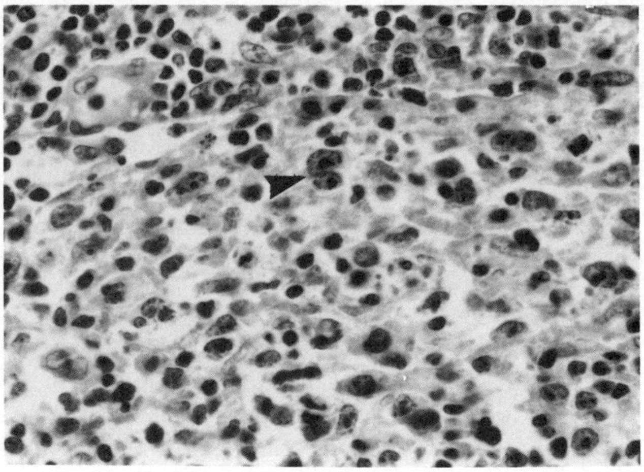

Figure 38.31. Mixed small- and large-cell lymphoma with a Reed-Sternberg–like cell (*arrowhead*). (Hematoxylin and eosin, ×600.)

kin's lymphoma, especially in peripheral T-cell lymphoma, or in other lymphomas late in the course of the disease or with transformation (Fig. 38.31 (163, 164). The best way to distinguish non-Hodgkin's lymphoma from Hodgkin's disease is to identify an atypical lymphoid population in the infiltrate characteristic of a subtype of non-Hodgkin's lymphoma, in addition to the Reed-Sternberg–like cell. It is also helpful (but not always necessary) to have a tissue biopsy diagnosis of non-Hodgkin's lymphoma.

Additional features of specific subtypes of non-Hodgkin's lymphoma are described in the paragraphs that follow.

Small Lymphocytic Lymphoma. Small lymphocytic lymphoma (SLL) as diagnosed on tissue biopsy is essentially the tissue phase or the nonleukemic counterpart of chronic lymphocytic leukemia. Thus, to diagnose a patient as having small lymphocytic lymphoma, the peripheral blood white count must be less than 5000 lymphocytes/mm^3 (3). Otherwise, the lymph node or other tissue is diagnosed as small lymphocytic lymphoma consistent with CLL, and the patient is diagnosed as having chronic lymphocytic leukemia. The pattern of marrow involvement in small lymphocytic lymphoma is similar to that of chronic lymphocytic leukemia, as illustrated in Figures 38.1 and 38.2. However, a focal pattern is seen more commonly than interstitial or diffuse extensive involvement (152). As in chronic lymphocytic leukemia, individual cell morphology is not helpful in the diagnosis of small lymphocytic lymphoma, since the tumor is made up of predominantly mature lymphocytes.

As emphasized earlier, small lymphocytic lymphoma with plasmacytoid differentiation is the characteristic marrow morphology of Waldenström's macroglobulinemia. Some studies have shown that small lymphocytic lymphoma that is extranodal and/or has plasmacytoid differentiation is less likely to show marrow involvement and is also less likely to express CD5 (6, 165).

Intermediate Lymphocytic Lymphoma. Intermediate lymphocytic lymphoma (not to be confused with intermediate-grade lymphoma) is a subtype of lymphoma that was not included in the Working Formulation, primarily because it was not recognized as a clinical pathologic entity until after the Working Formulation was devised. Since that time, it has become well established as a diagnostic entity (14, 166, 167).

It is characterized by a proliferation of small lymphocytes with a mild to moderate degree of nuclear irregularity (intermediate between small lymphocytic and small cleaved) (Fig. 38.24*A* and *B*) that in a lymph node may have a diffuse or a mantle-zone pattern. A mantle-zone pattern suggests that the lymphoma was derived from the cells of the mantle of the germinal center because of the presence of a benign-appearing germinal center in the nodules of lymphoma cells. This lymphoma commonly has marrow involvement. The distribution in early bone marrow involvement is usually focal and nonparatrabecular; however, there may also be some element of a paratrabecular pattern. With extensive involvement, the pattern becomes more diffuse. On smears, many of the cells are fairly normal-appearing lymphocytes; however, a moderate number (10 to 20%) of cells with nuclear contour irregularity are seen (Fig. 38.24*A*). When the WBC is elevated, the process has the appearance of an atypical chronic lymphocytic leukemia (14). Some cases of non-Hodgkin's lymphoma, especially those with the morphology of intermediate lymphocytic lymphoma, may have hairy cytoplasmic borders and TRAP positivity and primarily involve the spleen (168). Distinction from hairy cell leukemia may be very difficult, even with marker studies. Since the infiltrative pattern in the spleen is different in non-Hodgkin's lymphoma (white pulp) than in hairy cell leukemia (red pulp), splenectomy may be useful in the differential diagnosis.

Follicular Lymphomas. Follicular lymphomas are malignant lymphomas derived from the B cell of the germinal center, also called follicular center cells. Cells of follicular lymphomas, as described by Lukes and Collins, are small and large cleaved cells and large noncleaved (transformed) cells (169). The large cells have a nucleus about the size of a histiocyte or larger. As indicated in Table 38.19, follicular lymphomas can be composed of small clefted cells, a mixture of small clefted and large cells, or predominantly large cells.

On bone marrow sections, the early infiltrate of follicular lymphomas is characteristically focal with paratrabecular and occasional nonparatrabecular aggregates (152, 170). With more extensive involvement, the pattern becomes diffuse. To make a diagnosis of marrow involvement by follicular lymphoma when a diagnosis of lymphoma has previously been made on a nonmarrow biopsy, one should see several distinctly paratrabecular lymphoid aggregates or focal infiltrates with definitely atypical cleaved lymphoid cells. The cytology on sections of follicular lymphoma involving the marrow may range from lymphoid cells with only mild nuclear contour irregularities (similar to intermediate lymphocytic lymphoma), to markedly clefted cells, to a mixture of large cells and small clefted cells, as illustrated in Figures 38.24 and 38.25*B*. When the cytology of the cells is fairly bland and aggregates are small, the diagnosis of marrow involvement may have to be made on the basis of paratrabecular distribution of aggregates rather than on atypicality of the lymphoid cells. In follicular lymphomas, the cytologic atypicality and number of large cells in the bone marrow are frequently less than in the lymph node biopsy (152, 153).

Caution should be taken in using only nuclear contour irregularity in making a diagnosis of marrow involvement by lymphoma since lymphocytes in benign aggregates may also show mild to moderate degrees of nuclear contour irregularity. Tumors derived from follicular center cells usually attempt to mimic follicles (germinal centers) in their growth pattern when in lymph nodes; however, a follicular as opposed to a focal growth pattern, as stated previously, is rare in the bone marrow (152).

With minimal marrow involvement, malignant lymphoma cells may be difficult to recognize on bone marrow aspirates; however, when the marrow is more extensively replaced, small clefted cells similar to those shown in Figure 38.24*C* and *D* are seen on the aspirate. These cells are morphologically similar in appearance to the hematogones seen in the bone marrow of pediatric patients (152, 170, 171).

The peripheral blood may also be involved in follicular lymphomas, and when the WBC is considerably increased, the peripheral blood also contains numerous small clefted cells. If the small clefted cells are not readily identified, and a lymph node biopsy has not been done, the case may be mistakenly diagnosed as chronic lymphocytic leukemia (171).

Diffuse Small Cleaved Cell Lymphoma. Diffuse small cleaved cell lymphoma is an uncommon lymphoma. Most cases of diffuse small cleaved cell lymphoma are probably the diffuse counterpart of follicular small cleaved cell lymphoma. When the bone marrow is involved by this lymphoma, the pattern is variable and a paratrabecular pattern may be observed. Cytology is frequently similar to that seen in follicular small cleaved cell lymphoma; however, more cytologic variability may be evident from case to case (152). As stated earlier, a primary diagnosis of diffuse small cleaved cell lymphoma should not be made on the basis of bone marrow biopsy alone since a tissue biopsy may show a follicular pattern or a higher-grade cell type.

Diffuse, Mixed Small and Large Cell, and Large-Cell Lymphomas. These morphologic subtypes includes a heterogeneous group of lymphomas. Many cases represent the diffuse counterpart of follicular lymphomas; however, others represent lymphomas derived from peripheral T cells or nonfollicular B cells with plasmacytoid differentiation (148). Large-cell lymphomas included in the Working Formulation as large-cell, immunoblastic lymphoma presumably are derived from plasmacytoid immunoblasts, other nonfollicular B cells, and peripheral T cells, whereas cases included as diffuse large-cell lymphomas presumably arise from follicular derived B cells (169).

Occasionally, small lymphocytic lymphomas may have numerous prolymphocytes and blast-like cells on lymph node biopsy similar to Figure 38.5*B*, and mimic a diffuse mixed lymphoma (15, 16, 172). When the bone marrow is examined in these cases, the marrow may show an infiltrate similar to small lymphocytic lymphoma or chronic lymphocytic leukemia. This finding in the marrow should help the pathologist recognize the lymph node as a small lymphocytic lymphoma with transformation as opposed to a more aggressive diffuse mixed lymphoma (172). The lymph node in prolymphocytic transformation of chronic lymphocytic leukemia or prolymphocytic leukemia may also show a morphology suggesting a diffuse mixed lymphoma (23).

Lymphoblastic Lymphoma and Small Noncleaved Cell Lymphoma. As discussed previously, lymphoblastic lymphoma and acute lymphocytic leukemia (ALL) of types L1 and L2 are morphologically similar, and small noncleaved lymphoma and acute lymphocytic leukemia L3 are morphologically similar. When a patient has a tissue mass diagnosed as lymphoblastic lymphoma or small noncleaved cell lymphoma, and the marrow shows only a small percentage of lymphoblasts with considerable marrow sparing, it is reasonable to diagnose the patient as having lymphoma. However, if the marrow is more extensively involved, then it becomes debatable whether the patient's condition should be called a malignant lymphoma with extensive marrow involvement or a leukemia with extramarrow mass(es) (see Table 38.21). In this situation, it may be advisable to diagnose the patient as having "leukemia/lymphoma" rather than struggle with deciding which came first. On the other hand, a patient presenting with a mass and blasts in the peripheral blood will usually have a bone marrow biopsy done before a biopsy of the mass is done. At that point, a decision must be made whether to biopsy the mass, which will probably show morphology similar to the marrow. It will also be difficult to determine whether to call the process leukemia or lymphoma.

Table 28.23. Morphologic Variability in Non-Hodgkin's Lymphoma and Hodgkin's Disease in the Bone Marrow That May Lead to Diagnostic Difficulty

Non-Hodgkin's lymphoma
Morphologic discordance with tissue biopsy
Interstitial infiltrative pattern
Leukemic presentation
Reed-Sternberg cells
Fibrosis
Epithelioid histiocytes
Necrosis
Posttherapy changes
Hodgkin's disease
Fibrosis
Lack of Reed-Sternberg cells
Epithelioid histiocytes
Sheets of Reed-Sternberg cells
Posttherapy changes

Specific criteria for distinguishing leukemia from lymphoma for these cell types have been proposed; however, the criteria vary depending on the study group involved. Therapy for lymphoblastic lymphoma is frequently similar to aggressive therapy for acute lymphocytic leukemia; thus, a firm commitment to a distinction between leukemia and lymphoma in this situation may not be necessary.

Marker analysis of cells in these situations to distinguish leukemia from lymphoma is of little help. Marker analysis for ALL L3 and small noncleaved cell lymphoma is similar. Lymphoblastic lymphoma is more often a precursor T-cell type (especially late thymocyte stage) than a precursor B-cell type; however, acute lymphocytic leukemia can also be of precursor T-cell type. The morphologic features of the cells in ALL L1 and L2 and ALL L3 subtypes are also described in Chapter 37.

MORPHOLOGIC VARIABILITY AND DIFFERENTIAL DIAGNOSIS

As discussed in the preceding section, a characteristic of non-Hodgkin's lymphoma in the bone marrow is morphologic variability, in terms of both distribution and cytologic appearance. Some of the variability that may lead to confusion and difficulties in differential diagnosis are listed in Table 38.23. The first four of these have already been discussed in the previous section.

Fibrosis is an uncommon occurrence in the bone marrow in non-Hodgkin's lymphoma. When it does

Table 38.24 Immunologic Findings in Non-Hodgkin's Lymphomas

Working Formulation Diagnosis	Phenotype	Comment
Small lymphocytic	B cell >>> T cell	Clonal SIg (weak), CD5(T1), CD24(BA-1), CD20(B1)
Intermediate lymphocytic	B cell	Intermediate between small lymphocytic and diffuse or follicular small cleaved
Follicular, small cleaved	B cell	Clonal SIg, CD20(B1)
Follicular, mixed	B cell	Clonal SIg, CD20(B1), may be SIg negative
Follicular, large cell	B cell	Similar to follicular, small cleaved
Diffuse, small cleaved	B cell	Similar to follicular, small cleaved
Diffuse, mixed	B cell > T cell	B cell as above; peripheral T cells (of mature phenotype) with CD2(T11), CD5(T1), CD4, or CD8
Diffuse, large cell	B cell >> T cell	Similar to diffuse, mixed
Large cell, immunoblastic	B cell > T cell	Similar to diffuse, mixed
Lymphoblastic	T cell > B cell	Precursor B cells without SIg or CD20(B1) but with CD10(CALLA), CD19(B4) and TDT. Precursor T cells with early T cell markers and TDT.
Small noncleaved	B cell	Clonal SIg, CD20(B1)

occur, however, diagnosis may be difficult unless abnormal lymphoid cells are identified in the fibrosis.

Epithelioid histiocytes, epithelioid cell clusters, and granulomas may be admixed with non-Hodgkin's lymphoma in the bone marrow, but they may also be seen as an epiphenomenon without marrow involvement by lymphoma (173). Again, the most critical observation is to find abnormal lymphoma cells admixed with the histiocytes. Unless the histiocytes are a characteristic of the lymphoma at the previous site and lymphoma cells are admixed with histiocytes in the marrow, special stains for organisms should be performed.

Necrosis is uncommon but is very bothersome if present. This is because marrow necrosis in a patient with lymphoma is most likely due to marrow involvement with lymphoma. However, a definite diagnosis cannot be made without viable tissue evident. Taking a biopsy at another site may be helpful if it is crucial to know if the marrow is involved.

Following therapy for malignant lymphoma, the marrow may become altered by fibrosis or necrosis, making determination of residual disease difficult. In addition, aggregates in low-grade lymphoma may be reduced in size, so they are difficult to distinguish from benign lymphoid aggregates. When this occurs, it is best to not diagnose the lesion as lymphoma unless definite evidence of lymphoma is present. Instead, a comment should be made that lymphoma cannot be excluded.

IMMUNOLOGIC AND OTHER SPECIAL STUDIES

A detailed description of the immunologic findings in non-Hodgkin's lymphoma is beyond the scope of this chapter. Detailed discussions of the evaluation of non-Hodgkin's lymphoma by marker studies can be found elsewhere in the literature (6, 174, 175). A brief outline of the immunologic findings in non-Hodgkin's lymphoma is shown in Table 38.24. Except for lymphoblastic lymphomas, all of the non-Hodgkin's lymphomas show phenotypes similar to functionally mature/peripheral B or T cells. Some of the large-cell immunoblastic plasmacytoid lymphomas or small lymphocytic lymphoma with plasmacytoid differentiation may also show cytoplasmic immunoglobulin.

Usually, marker analysis is not necessary to evaluate malignant lymphoma in the bone marrow because the diagnosis has been made on another site that may already have been immunophenotyped. In addition, phenotyping is frequently predictable from the morphologic subtype, especially the first five lymphomas in the list in Tables 38.19 and 38.21. It should be emphasized that accurate immunophenotyping is best carried out on fresh unfixed tissues or aspirates. Many of the marker analyses for diagnosis and suclassification of non-Hodgkin's lymphoma cannot be readily carried out on paraffin sections. Thus, it is suggested that a fresh aspirate for flow cytometry be saved on any patient with a suspected lymphoproliferative disorder in the bone marrow until the need for immunotyping is decided. However, immunophenotyping can be done successfully on paraffin sections in some cases with monoclonal antibodies such as CD20(L26) and CD45RO(UCHL-1) and others, as illustrated in Figure 38.32 (176–178). These markers may be very useful if the diagnosis can be made by identifying the cells as lymphocytes of B-cell or T-cell phenotype; however, determining clonality based on finding a restricted light-chain SIg requires fresh cells or tissue (179).

Specific situations in which immunophenotyping is useful in the evaluation of non-Hodgkin's lymphoma in the bone marrow or blood are described below.

1. The differential diagnosis is between two morphologically similar processes that have different im-

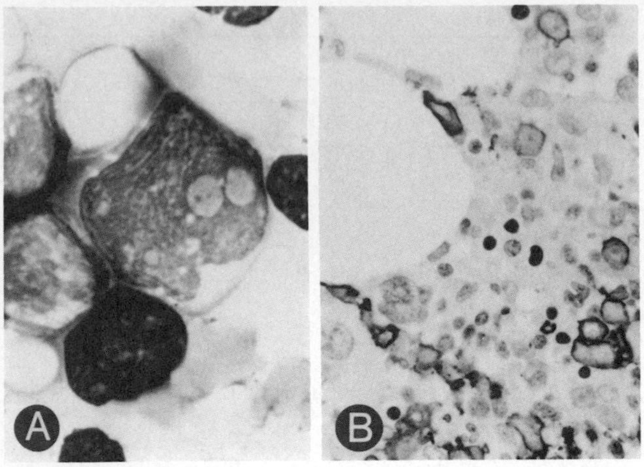

Figure 38.32. Large-cell lymphoma in bone marrow, diagnosed with the assistance of CD20 (L26) monoclonal antibody on paraffin section. **A**, On marrow smears in this case only, rare cells suspicious for large-cell lymphoma were seen. Sections (not shown) showed small clusters of large cells that could not be distinguished with certainty from reactive marrow elements. **B**, Immunoperoxidase staining with CD20 (L26) demonstrated small clusters and isolated positive cells (note dark staining of cytoplasmic outline), which were interpreted as B-cell large-cell lymphoma. (**A**, Wright's stain, ×1200. **B**, Immunoperoxidase, ×600.)

munophenotypes; for example, small noncleaved cell lymphoma can be differentiated from a large-cell lymphoma that is SIg negative or T-cell type; small lymphocytic lymphoma can be distinguished from a small cleaved cell lymphoma; lymphoma can be distinguished from reactive or neoplastic myeloid elements.

2. The morphology in the marrow has changed or is different from that of the tissue biopsy, and the question is whether a new tumor has developed or a transformation from the original tumor has occurred.
3. The differential diagnosis is a reactive lymphocytosis versus involvement with lymphoma. In this situation, identification of a clonally restricted light chain in B-cell process is particularly useful in confirming a lymphoid process as neoplastic. Marker studies are not particularly helpful in distinguishing immature B-cell lymphoblastic lymphoma or leukemia from reactive lymphocytes in children, since normal bone marrow lymphocytes in children express an immature B-cell phenotype (180). In this situation, immunoglobulin gene rearrangement studies may be helpful (175). Some neoplastic T-cell processes may be identified if an abnormal T-cell phenotype characteristic of the disease in question is identified. T-cell gene rearrangement studies may also be helpful (66, 175).
4. Benign aggregates need to be distinguished from lymphoma. The usefulness of immunohistochemistry in distinguishing benign from neoplastic aggregates of low-grade lymphoma on paraffin sections is debatable (177, 178). There are, however, cases of small lymphocytic lymphoma with plasmacytoid differentiation in which immunoperoxidase on sections may identify clonally restructed cytoplasmic immunoglobulin (132). Frozen-section material is necessary to identify a surface restricted light chain, which is the most useful criterion for distinguishing benign from neoplastic B cells (179).
5. Identification of minimal disease. Current therapy is based on morphologic interpretation of involvement in the blood and bone marrow. New techniques, such as immunophenotypic or immunogenotypic analysis, have demonstrated that lymphoma cells may be present even when they are not seen morphologically (181), especially in low-grade lymphomas. The importance of recognizing a minimal amount of marrow involvement is not yet clear. However, with the advent of autologous bone marrow transplantation techniques, identification of residual disease in transplanted marrow or stem cell harvest may become of greater importance.

A variety of other special studies have been performed on non-Hodgkin's malignant lymphomas, including chromosomal analysis (182), DNA content (19, 20), nuclear proliferation antigen Ki-67 (183, 184), and antigen receptor gene rearrangement (175). Some of these may have applicability to lymphoma in the bone marrow and blood (185, 186).

CHANGES WITH PROGRESSION AND TRANSFORMATION

Small lymphocytic lymphoma and small cleaved cell lymphoma occasionally undergo transformation to a higher-grade lymphoma with the morphologic appearance of a large-cell or mixed cell lymphoma (Table 38.25) (24). This transformation may involve the bone marrow as well as other tissue sites; therefore, when a transformation is suspected, a bone marrow examination may be performed before a tissue biopsy. Follicular small cleaved cell lymphoma can also undergo a transformation that has a morphologic appearance of acute lymphocytic leukemia in the bone marrow or blood with very blast-like cells (Table 38.25) (187). This can be distinguished from acute lymphocytic leukemia with marker studies, since the blasts in transformation still retain the phenotype of the mature B-cell lymphoma. Leukemic transformation of small lymphocytic lymphoma to chronic lymphocytic leukemia is reported by one study as occurring in at least 15% of cases (4). Likewise, lymphoblastic lymphoma and small non-

Table 38.25. Transformation and Secondary Tumors in Lymphomas

Non-Hodgkin's lymphoma
Small lymphocytic lymphoma to large-cell lymphoma
Follicular lymphoma to large-cell lymphoma
Follicular lymphoma to "lymphoblastic morphology"
Lymphoma to leukemia (see Table 38.21)
Acute myelogenous leukemia
Myelodysplastic syndrome
Hodgkin's disease
Progression toward lymphocyte-depleted
Non-Hodgkin' s lymphoma
Acute lymphoid leukemia
Acute myelogenous leukemia
Myelodysplastic syndrome

cleaved cell lymphoma may develop bone marrow and blood involvement late in the course of the disease and become morphologically indistinguishable from acute leukemia L1, L2, or L3 subtypes. Although the marrow may become extensively involved late in the course of large-cell lymphoma, a leukemic blood picture with elevated white blood count is uncommon. Development of therapy-related myeloid leukemia similar to that seen in plasma cell myeloma has been reported in non-Hodgkin's lymphoma (Table 38.25) (24).

STAGING, THERAPY, AND PROGNOSTIC FEATURES

Therapy for non-Hodgkin's lymphoma is very dependent on the stage and grade of the lymphoma. Bone marrow involvement automatically defines the patient as having widespread or stage IV disease.

A few generalizations about therapy of non-Hodgkin's lymphomas follow:

1. Low-grade lymphomas in the Working Formulation are generally widespread and not curable; thus, therapy is directed at palliation as for chronic lymphocytic leukemia. Some studies, however, have suggested that long-term disease-free survival can be achieved with aggressive therapy for follicular mixed lymphoma. A second exception is that rare, early-stage (stage I), low-grade lymphoma may be "cured" with local irradiation.
2. In intermediate and high-grade lymphomas in the Working Formulation (frequently lumped together by clinicians as "high-grade" lymphoma), even if disseminated, long-term disease-free survival may be achieved with intensive combination chemotherapy. Localized or bulky disease may also be treated with irradiation. Small noncleaved cell lymphoma has the poorest prognosis of all tumors on the list.
3. At present, autologous bone marrow transplantation is a viable option for younger patients with a higher-grade lymphoma, widespread disease, and no marrow involvement. Autologous transplantation with purging or autologous peripheral stem cell harvesting may have wider application in the future.

Hodgkin's Disease

DIAGNOSTIC FEATURES

Hodgkin's disease is usually diagnosed on the basis of lymph node or other extramarrow tissue biopsy (149, 188). On tissue biopsy, there is effacement of architecture by an infiltrate that has as its basic component numerous mature lymphocytes and less frequent Reed-Sternberg cells (Fig. 38.22). In addition, there may be varying numbers of benign histiocytes, eosinophils, and plasma cells. The subclassification of Hodgkin's disease is shown in Table 38.20. The distinction between nodular sclerosing Hodgkin's disease and the other three subtypes is made based on the presence or absence of large nodules of lymphoma surrounded by sclerotic bands of connective tissue. The cellular composition of the lymphomatous nodules in nodular sclerosing Hodgkin's disease can range in appearance from lymphocyte predominant, to mixed, to lymphocyte depleted, as described below. The three subtypes of Hodgkin's disease other than nodular sclerosing are diagnosed on the basis of the cellular composition of the lymphomatous infiltrate. Lymphocyte-predominant Hodgkin's disease has a predominance of lymphocytes with or without numerous histiocytes, and very rare Reed-Sternberg cells. Mixed-cellularity Hodgkin's disease has abundant lymphocytes but also more abundant Reed-Sternberg cells than in lymphocyte-predominant Hodgkin's disease. Lymphocyte-depleted Hodgkin's disease has a decrease in lymphoid cells, may or may not have abundant Reed-Sternberg cells, and may also have a diffuse increase in sclerosis.

When the bone marrow is involved by Hodgkin's disease, it is diagnosed by trephine biopsy and is almost never identified on clot sections, on smears, or in the peripheral blood (189–192). The marrow sections usually show focal infiltrates that are paratrabecular or nonparatrabecular. The infiltrates may be as small as lymphoid aggregates or may focally obliterate the marrow space, as in Figure 38.33. The cellular infiltrates usually have a partly cellular and partly fibrotic appearance and are somewhat lymphocyte depleted, containing varying numbers of histiocytes and eosinophils and varying degrees of fibrosis. Reed-Sternberg cells are usually difficult to find, and numerous step sections may be necessary

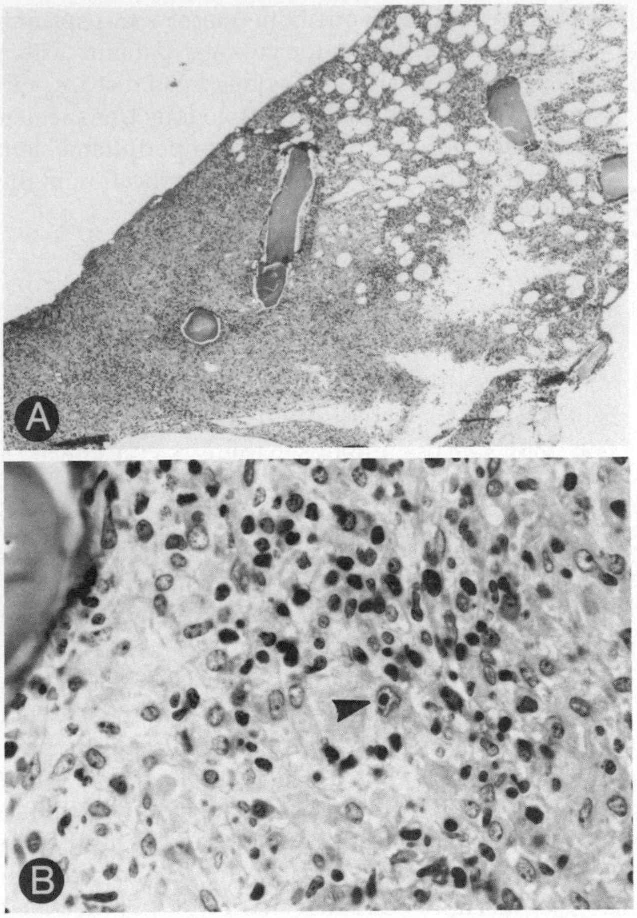

Figure 38.33. Hodgkin's disease, bone marrow. Note the extensive focal infiltrate in **A** with uninvolved normal marrow in the upper right field. Higher power (**B**) shows a mixed cellular infiltrate that is relatively lymphocyte depleted. A mononuclear Reed-Sternberg variant (half of a typical Reed-Sternberg cell) is indicated with an *arrowhead*. (Hematoxylin and eosin, ×25 [**A**], ×600 [**B**].)

to identify them. With more extensive involvement, the marrow space can become completely obliterated by the infiltrate. The lymphocyte-depleted appearance of the bone marrow in Hodgkin's disease is usually present whether the lymph node shows a nodular sclerosing, mixed, or lymphocyte-depleted morphology. Thus, a subtype diagnosis of Hodgkin's disease should not be made on the basis of the bone marrow.

Criteria for the diagnosis of Hodgkin's disease in the bone marrow are different depending on whether primary or secondary involvement is being diagnosed. When a diagnosis of Hodgkin's disease has been substantiated at another site, the requirement in the bone marrow is to see a cellular infiltrate consistent with Hodgkins' disease and at least one mononuclear variant of a Reed-Sternberg cell (Fig. 38.33*B*) (189). To diagnose Hodgkin's disease primarily in the bone marrow, which may be necessary if the only other site of disease is in the retroperitoneum, several excellent typical Reed-Sternberg cells in addition to the typical infiltrate of Hodgkin's disease must be seen. Even then, one should be cautious, since non-Hodgkin's lymphoma can have Reed-Sternberg–like cells (163, 164). Lymphocyte-depleted Hodgkin's disease may present with marrow and retroperitoneal involvement and no easily accessible peripheral nodes on which a biopsy could be performed (193).

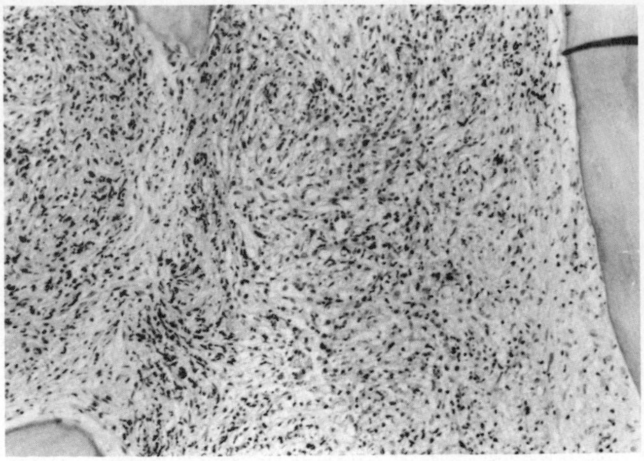

Figure 38.34. Hodgkin's disease showing extensive diffuse replacement of the marrow space by fibrosis. Lymphocytes admixed with the fibrosis suggested that this was Hodgkin's disease rather than agnogenic myeloid metaplasia, and Reed-Sternberg cells were identified after a careful search on multiple step sections. (Hematoxylin and eosin, ×120.)

MORPHOLOGIC VARIABILITY AND DIFFERENTIAL DIAGNOSIS

The morphologic variability that can be seen in Hodgkin's disease is listed in Table 38.23. In some cases of Hodgkin's disease, the marrow may be extensively fibrotic and mimic agnogenic myeloid metaplasia (Fig. 38.34) (194). Scattered lymphocytes within the fibrosis should alert one to the possibility of Hodgkin's disease. When a fibrotic bone marrow infiltrate is seen in a patient with known Hodgkin's disease at another site, and an exhaustive search reveals no Reed-Sternberg cells or variants, the marrow should be considered suspicious for Hodgkin's disease. If the lesion contains an extensive, mixed cellular infiltrate that is otherwise typical of Hodgkin's disease, but no Reed-Sternberg variants, then (after the clinician has been consulted) the marrow may be considered consistent with involvement for purposes of staging.

Because of the mixed cellular infiltrate and the frequent presence of epithelioid histiocytes, the differential diagnosis of Hodgkin's disease in the bone marrow includes infectious disease, AIDS, and AILD. In some cases of Hodgkin's disease, granulomas may accompany Hodgkin's disease in the bone marrow; however, in other cases, nonspecific granulomas may be present in the bone marrow without marrow involvement by Hodgkin's disease (173).

Peripheral T-cell lymphomas are particularly prone to mimic Hodgkin's disease in the bone marrow, especially when minimal tissue is acquired, as in a bone marrow biopsy (163). The critical feature to distinguish Hodgkin's disease from non-Hodgkin's lymphoma in the bone marrow, when the primary diagnosis is being made on the marrow, is the appearance of the background lymphocytes. In Hodgkin's disease, as opposed to non-Hodgkin's lymphoma, these lymphocytes are nearly normal in appearance and do not show transitional forms to Reed-Sternberg cells. Some variants of Hodgkin's disease may have numerous Reed-Sternberg cells and mimic large-cell lymphoma. This is usually more of a differential diagnostic problem with tissue biopsy than with bone marrow biopsy.

IMMUNOLOGIC AND OTHER SPECIAL STUDIES

In cases of Hodgkin's disease, when there is a problem in distinguishing Hodgkin's disease from a non-Hodgkin's lymphoma, immunologic studies may be of some assistance (176, 177). On paraffin sections, Reed-Sternberg cells are leukocyte common antigen negative and LeuM1 or Ki-1 positive, and the background lymphocytes are T cells. Large cells associated with anaplastic large-cell non-Hodgkin's lymphomas that might mimic Reed-Sternberg cells are leukocyte common antigen positive and should be T-cell or B-cell positive. They may also, however, be LeuM1 and Ki-1 positive, suggesting overlap between Hodgkin's disease and some anaplastic large cell lymphomas (195).

CHANGES WITH PROGRESSION AND TRANSFORMATION

In general, the natural progression of Hodgkin's disease is toward the lymphocyte-depleted variant (Table 38.25).

It is well documented that Hodgkin's disease is often associated with or develops non-Hodgkin's lymphoma (Table 38.25) (24). Cases of Hodgkin's disease that transform to large-cell lymphoma should be carefully studied to rule out the possibility of initial misdiagnosis of Hodgkin's disease or transformation of Hodgkin's disease to a syncytial or lymphocyte-depleted form of Hodgkin's disease with sheets of Reed-Sternberg cells (196, 197). Rare cases of development of "acute" lymphoid leukemias have also been reported (Table 38.25) (24). Similar to other B-cell processes, myeloid leukemia can develop subsequent to therapy in Hodgkin's disease (Table 38.25) (24).

STAGING, THERAPY, AND PROGNOSTIC FEATURES

Survival in Hodgkin's disease is dependent on the stage of disease. Furthermore, morphologic subtypes of Hodgkin's disease correlate well with stage. Lymphocyte-predominant and nodular sclerosing forms generally correlate with a low incidence of marrow involvement, early stage of disease, and good survival, whereas mixed cellularity and lymphocyte-depleted Hodgkin's disease are correlated with a higher incidence of marrow involvement, a higher stage, and poorer survival. In general, therapy for early disease is local radiation; for more advanced disease, therapy is combination chemotherapy with or without radiation. Autologous transplantation is also used for younger patients with refractory disease and negative bone marrow examination.

Posttransplant Lymphoproliferative Disorders

Posttransplant lymphoproliferative disorders usually develop months to years after transplantation and can be seen following solid organ transplantation or bone marrow transplantation (198, 199). The tumors presumably arise secondary to severe immunocompromise, are usually of B-cell phenotype, and have been very highly associated with Epstein-Barr virus. They have many features in common with non-Hodgkin's lymphoma arising in severely immunocompromised hosts in general. They are particularly likely to develop in mismatched and T cell–depleted bone marrow transplant recipients.

Clinically, these disorders can develop as isolated extranodal disease or widespread nodal disease, or they may present with peripheral blood, bone marrow, or CSF involvement (198). Morphologically, they may show a spectrum from monomorphic large-cell lymphoma to a process with a polymorphic appearance containing a mixture of large cells (immunoblasts), immature plasma cells, mature plasma cells, and lymphocytes (Fig. 38.35*A*). When the former occurs, it is usually seen on a tissue biopsy, and the diagnosis of malignant lymphoma is undisputed. However, when a polymorphous morphology is seen, distinction from a reactive process may be more difficult.

When involved by a posttransplant lymphoproliferative disorder, the peripheral blood, bone marrow, or body fluid contains large immature plasmacytoid cells that are distinctly different in appearance from reactive Downey cells (Fig. 38.35*B* to *E*). This distinction is important because Downey cells may be asso-

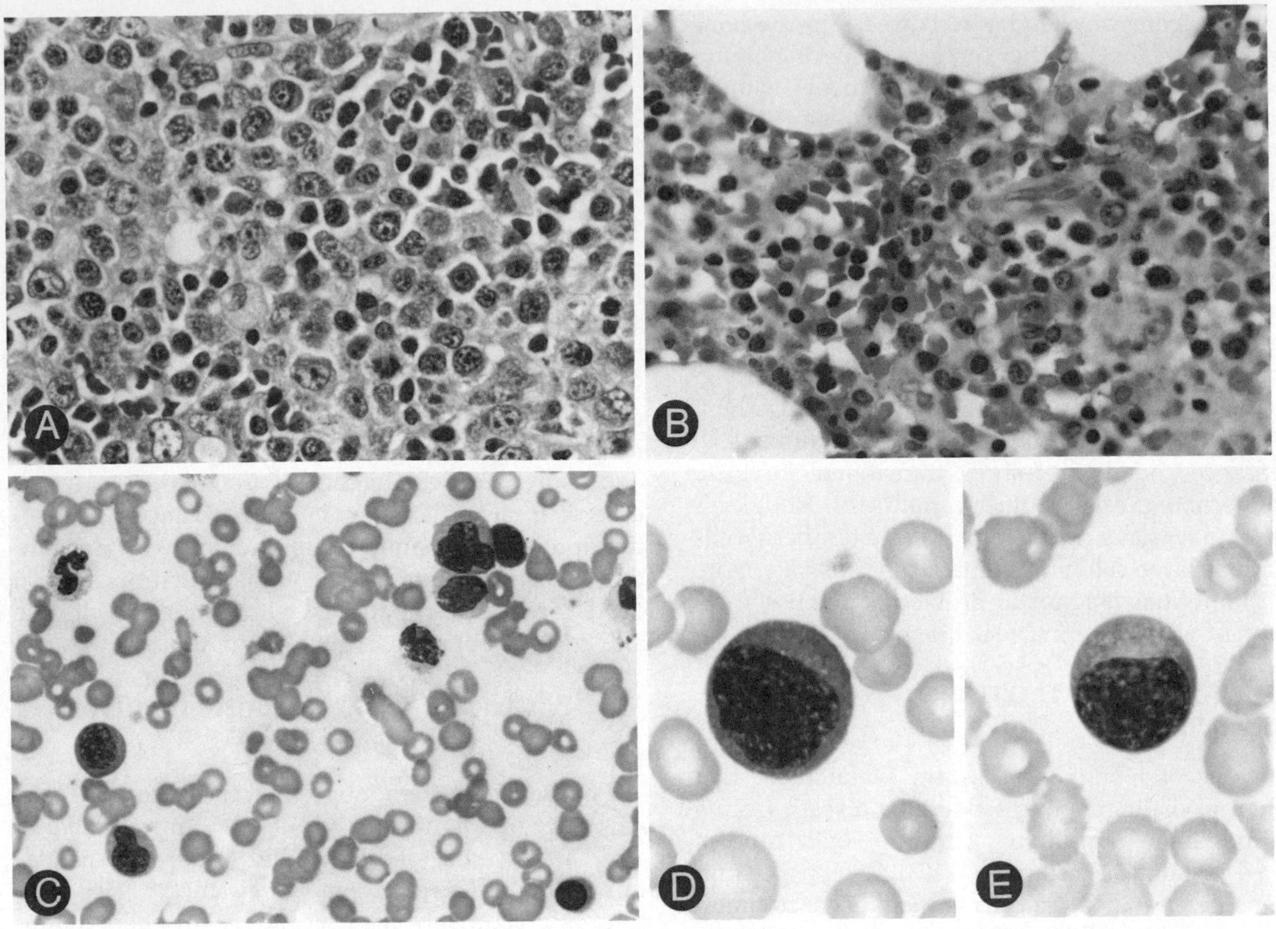

Figure 38.35. Posttransplant lymphoproliferative disorders. **A**, This polymorphous infiltrate is from a lymph node of a renal transplant patient. Note the spectrum of cells, including lymphocytes, plasma cells, immature plasma cells, and large cells (immunoblasts). **B, C, D,** and **E** are from a patient with a mismatched, T cell–depleted bone marrow transplant. Note the variety of large atypical plasmacytoid cells with deeply basophilic cytoplasm and dark, condensed nuclear chromatin. (**A** and **B**, hematoxylin and eosin, ×600. Wright's stain, ×600 [**C**], ×1200 [**D** and **E**].)

ciated with reactive processes in the posttransplant population. Immunophenotyping may be of some assistance since Downey cells are T cells, whereas the plasmacytoid cells of posttransplant lymphoproliferative disorders are usually B cells, presumably transformed by Epstein-Barr virus (EBV). Rare cases of T-cell posttransplant lymphoproliferative disorders have been described (200).

The development of posttransplant lymphoproliferative disorders is thought to be a multistep process that starts in the immunocompromised host with EBV infection of B cells, followed by a polyclonal expansion of infected B cells (199). Out of this polyclonal expansion, oligoclonal B-cell proliferation can develop, presumably due to lack of immune regulation. Subsequent to this, there may be eventual development of a monomorphic or dominant B-cell clone, which then behaves in a malignant fashion. If posttransplant lymphoproliferative disorders are studied for surface and cytoplasmic immunoglobulin at the polyclonal or oligoclonal stage, they are likely to express both κ and λ light chains, whereas the tumor at the monomorphic stage may show a clonally restricted light chain. An oligoclonal proliferation may be identified at an earlier stage by evaluating for clonal immunoglobulin gene rearrangement, clonal EBV incorporation, or clonal C-myc translocation.

Therapeutic intervention in posttransplant lymphoproliferative disorders consists of removal of immunosuppression and treatment with acyclovir and interferon alpha. For more aggressive monomorphic disease combinations, chemotherapy may be used. Prognosis for posttransplant lymphoproliferative disease is very poor; however, patients with less evidence of clonal transformation are more likely to respond to antiviral therapy and removal of immunosuppression than those with monomorphic and monoclonal proliferations (199).

Acknowledgment

The author would like to thank Barbara Ashbacher for her assistance in the preparation of this manuscript.

References

1. Gale RP, Foon KA. Biology of chronic lymphocytic leukemia. Semin Hematol 1987;24:209–229.
2. Spier CM, Kjeldsberg CR, Head DR, et al. Chronic lymphocytic leukemia in young adults. Am J Clin Pathol 1985;84:675–678.
3. Cheson BD, Bennet JM, Rai KR, et al. Guidelines for clinical protocols for chronic lymphocytic leukemia. Recommendations of the NCI-Sponsored Working Group. Am J Hematol 1988;29:152–163.
4. Pangalis GA, Nathwani BN, Rappaport H. Malignant lymphoma, well differentiated lymphocytic: its relationship with chronic lymphocytic leukemia and macroglobulinemia of Waldenström. Cancer 1977;39:999–1010.
5. Perreault C, Boileau J, Gyger M, et al. Chronic B-cell lymphocytosis. Eur J Haematol 1989;42:361–367.
6. Deegan MJ. Membrane antigen analysis in the diagnosis of lymphoid leukemias and lymphomas. Arch Pathol Lab Med 1989;113:606–618.
7. Peterson LC, Bloomfield CD, Brunning RD. Relationship of clinical staging and lymphocyte morphology to survival in chronic lymphocytic leukaemia. Br J Haematol 1980;45:563–567.
8. Pugh WC, Manning JT, Butler JJ. Paraimmunoblastic variant of small lymphocytic lymphoma. Am J Surg Pathol 1988;12:907–917.
9. Dick FR. Chronic lymphocytic leukemia, prolymphocytic leukemia and leukemic non-Hodgkin's lymphoma. In: Koepke JA, ed. Laboratory hematology. New York: Churchill Livingstone, 1984;1:325–357.
10. Melo JV, Catovsky D, Galton DAG. The relationship between chronic lymphocytic leukaemia and prolymphocytic leukaemia: I. Clinical and laboratory features of 300 patients and characterization of an intermediate group. Br J Haematol 1986;63:377–387.
11. Melo JV, Catovsky D, Galton DAG. The relationship between chronic lymphocytic leukaemia and prolymphocytic leukaemia: II. Patterns of evolution of "prolymphocytoid" transformation. Br J Haematol 1986;64:77–86.
12. Melo JV, Catovsky D, Gregory WM, et al. The relationship between chronic lymphocytic leukaemia and prolymphocytic leukaemia: IV. Analysis of survival and prognostic features. Br J Haematol 1987;65:23–29.
13. Ghani AM, Krause JR. Investigation of cell size and nuclear clefts as prognostic parameters in chronic lymphocytic leukemia. Cancer 1986;58:2233–2238.
14. Pombo De Oliveira MS, Jaffe ES, et al. Leukaemic phase of mantle zone (intermediate) lymphoma: its characterisation in 11 cases. J Clin Pathol 1989;42:962–972.
15. Dick FR, Maca R. The lymph node in chronic lymphocytic leukemia. Cancer 1978;41:283–292.
16. Ben-Ezra J, Burke JS, Swartz WG, et al. Small lymphocytic lymphoma: a clinicopathologic analysis of 268 cases. Blood 1989;73:579–587.
17. Deegan MJ, Abraham JP, Sawdyk M, et al. High incidence of monoclonal proteins in the serum and urine of chronic lymphocytic leukemia patients. Blood 1984;64:1207–1211.
18. Juliusson G, Oscier DG, Fitchett M, et al. Prognostic subgroups in B-cell chronic lymphocytic leukemia defined by specific chromosomal abnormalities. N Engl J Med 1990;323:720–724.
19. Braylan RC, Fowlkes BJ, Jaffe ES, et al. Cell volumes and DNA distributions of normal and neoplastic human lymphoid cells. Cancer 1978;41:201–209.
20. Diamond LW, Nathwani BN, Rappaport H. Flow cytometry in the diagnosis and classification of malignant lymphoma and leukemia. Cancer 1982;50:1122–1135.
21. Foroni L, Catovsky D, Luzzatto L. Immunoglobulin gene rearrangements in hairy cell leukemia and other chronic B cell lymphoproliferative disorders. Leukemia 1987;4:389–392.
22. Norton JD, Pattinson J, Hoffbrand AV, et al. Rearrangement and expression of T cell antigen receptor genes in B cell chronic lymphocytic leukemia. Blood 1988;71:178–185.
23. Kjeldsberg CR, Marty J. Prolymphocytic transformation of chronic lymphocytic leukemia. Cancer 1981;48:2447–2457.
24. York JC, Glick AD, Cousar JB, et al. Changes in the appearance of hematopoietic and lymphoid neoplasms: Clinical, pathologic, and biologic implications. Hum Pathol 1984;15:11–38.
25. Sun T, Susin M, Desner M, et al. The clonal origin of two cell populations in Richter's syndrome. Hum Pathol 1990;21:722–728.
26. Brouet JC, Fermand JP, Laurent G, et al. The association of chronic lymphocytic leukaemia and multiple myeloma: A study of eleven patients. Br J Haematol 1985;59:55–66.
27. Saltman DL, Ross JA, Banks RE, et al. Molecular evidence for a single clonal origin in biphenotypic concomitant chronic lymphocytic leukemia and multiple myeloma. Blood 1989;74:2062–2065.
28. Torelli UL, Torelli GM, Emilia G, et al. Simultaneously increased expression of the c-myc and μ-chain genes in the acute blastic transformation of a chronic lymphocytic leukaemia. Br J Haematol 1987;65:165–170.
29. Brecher M, Banks PM. Hodgkin's disease variant of Richter's syndrome. Am J Clin Pathol 1990;93:333–339.
30. Foon KA, Gale RP. Staging and therapy of chronic lymphocytic leukemia. Semin Hematol 1987;24:264–274.
31. Geisler C, Ralfkiaer E, Hansen MM, et al. The bone marrow histological pattern has independent prognostic value in early stage chronic lymphocytic leukaemia. Br J Haematol 1986;62:47–54.
32. Stone, RM. Prolymphocytic leukemia. Hematol Oncol Clin North Am 1990;4:457–471.
33. Bearman RM, Pangalis GA, Rappaport H. Prolymphocytic leukemia: clinical, histopathological, and cytochemical observations. Cancer 1978;42:2360–2372.
34. Galton DAG, Goldman JM, Wiltshaw E, et al. Prolymphocytic leukaemia. Br J Haemato 1974;27:7–23.
35. Nieto LH, Lampert IA, Catovsky D. Bone marrow histological patterns in B-cell and T-cell prolymphocytic leukemia. Hematol Pathol 1989;3:79–84.
36. Lahuerta-Palacios JJ, Valdes MD, Navas-Palacios JN, et al. Six new cases of prolymphocytic leukemia with heterogeneous prognosis: clinical and immunologic features, light microscopy, and ultrastructural findings. Cancer 1985;55:2550–2557.
37. Brito-Babapulle V, Pittman S, Melo JV, et al. Cytogenetic studies on prolymphocytic leukemia: 1. B-cell prolymphocytic leukemia. Hematol Pathol 1987;1:27–33.
38. Diamond LW, Bearman RM, Berry PK, et al. Prolymphocytic leukemia: flow microfluorometric, immunologic, and cytogenetic observations. Am J Hematol 1980;9:319–330.
39. Forman SJ, Nathwani BN, Woda BA, et al. Clonal evolution of T-cell prolymphocytic leukemia to a T-large-cell lymphoma: a morphologic and immunologic study. Arch Pathol Lab Med 1985;109:1081–1084.
40. Special Issue: The 2nd International Workshop on Hairy Cell Leukemia. Catovsky D, Golomb HM, Golde DW, guest eds. Leukemia 1987;1:284–408.
41. Yam LT, Phyliky RL, Li CY. Benign and neoplastic disorders simulating hairy cell leukemia. Semin Oncol 1984;11:353–361.

42. Woessner S, Lafuente R Sans-Sabrafen J. Unusual cytological appearance of hairy cell leukemia. Lancet 1976;2:812.
43. Sainati L, Matutes E, Mulligan S, et al. A variant form of hairy cell leukemia resistant to α-interferon: clinical and phenotypic characteristics of 17 patients. Blood 1990;76:157–162.
44. Bartl R, Frisch B, Hill W, et al. Bone marrow histology in hairy cell leukemia: identification of subtypes and their prognostic significance. Am J Clin Pathol 1983;79:531–545.
45. Hanson CA, Ward PCJ, Schnitzer B. A multilobular variant of hairy cell leukemia with morphologic similarities to T-cell lymphoma. Am J Surg Pathol 1989;13:671–679.
46. Lee WM, Beckstead JH. Hairy cell leukemia with bone marrow hypoplasia. Cancer 1982;50:2207–2210.
47. Hanson CA, Gribbin TE, Schnitzer B, et al. CD11c (Leu-M5) expression characterizes a B-cell chronic lymphoproliferative disorder with features of both chronic lymphocytic leukemia and hairy cell leukemia. Blood 1990;76:2360–2367.
48. Agnarsson BA, Kadin ME. An unusual B-cell lymphoma simulating hairy cell leukemia. Am J Clin Pathol 1987;88:752–759.
49. Melo JV, Robinson DSF, Gregory C, et al. Splenic B cell lymphoma with "villous" lymphocytes in the peripheral blood: a disorder distinct from hairy cell leukemia. Leukemia 1987;1: 294–299.
50. Katayama I, Yang JPS. Reassessment of a cytochemical test for differential diagnosis of leukemic reticuloendotheliosis. Am J Clin Pathol 1977;68:268–272.
51. Yam LT, Janckila AJ, Li CY, et al. Cytochemistry of tartrate resistant acid phosphatase: 15 years' experience. Leukemia 1987;1:285–288.
52. Vardiman JW, Gilewski TA, Ratain MJ, et al. Evaluation of Leu-M5 (CD11c) in hairy cell leukemia by the alkaline phosphatase anti-alkaline phosphatase technique. Am J Clin Pathol 1988;90:250–256.
53. Catovsky D, Cherchi M, Brooks D, et al. Heterogeneity of cell leukemias demonstrated by the monoclonal antibody FMC7. Blood 1981;58:406–408.
54. Strickler JG, Schmidt CM, Wick MR. Immunophenotype of hairy cell leukemia in paraffin sections. Mod Pathol 1990;3: 518–523.
55. Anderson KC, Boyd AW, Fisher DC, et al. Hairy cell leukemia: a tumor of pre-plasma cells. Blood 1985;65:620–629.
56. Brito-Babapulle V, Pittman S, Melo JV, et al. The 14q+ marker in hairy cell 1eukaemia: A cytogenetic study of 15 cases. Leuk Res 1986;10:131–138.
57. Katayama I, Li CY, Yam LT. Ultrastructural characteristics of the "hairy cells" of leukemic reticuloendotheliosis. Am J Pathol 1972;67:361–370.
58. Golomb HM, Braylan R, Polliack A. ("Hairy" cell leukaemia (leukaemic reticuloendotheliosis): a scanning electron microscopic study of eight cases. Br J Haematol 1975;29:455–460.
59. Jacobs RH, Vokes EE, Golomb HM. Second malignancies in hairy cell leukemia. Cancer 1985;56:1462–1467.
60. Davis KM, Spindel E, Franzine DA, et al. Anaplastic neoplasm in a patient with hairy cell leukemia. Cancer 1985;56: 2470–2475.
61. VanderMolen IA, Urba WJ, Longo DL, et al. Diffuse osteosclerosis in hairy cell leukemia. Blood 1989;74:2066–2069.
62. Demanes DJ, Lane N, Beckstead JH. Bone involvement in hairy-cell leukemia. Cancer 1982;49:1697–1701.
63. Golomb HM. The treatment of hairy cell leukemia. Blood 1987;69:979–989.
64. Knowles DM II. The human T-cell leukemias: clinical, cytomorphologic, immunophenotypic, and genotypic characteristics. Hum Pathol 1986;17:14–33.
65. Berliner N. T gamma lymphocytosis and T cell chronic leukemias. Hematol Oncol Clin North Am 1990;4:473–487.
66. Knowles DM. Immunophenotypic and antigen receptor gene rearrangement analysis in T cell neoplasia. Am J Pathol 1989;134:761–785.
67. Hui PK, Feller AC, Pileri S, et al. New aggressive variant of suppressor/cytotoxic T-CLL. Am J Clin Pathol 1987;87:55–59.
68. Matutes E, Talavera G, O'Brien M, et al. The morphological spectrum of T-prolymphocytic leukaemia. Br J Haematol 1986;64:111–124.
69. Brito-Babapulle V, Pomfret M, Matutes E. Cytogenetic studies on prolymphocytic leukemia: II. T cell prolymphocytic leukemia. Blood 1987;70:926–931.
70. Nagatani T, Matsuzaki T, Iemoto G, et al. Comparative study of cutaneous T-cell lymphoma and adult T-cell leukemia/lymphoma: clinical, histopathologic, and immunohistochemical analyses. Cancer 1990;66:2380–2386.
71. Shimamoto Y, Suga K, Nishimura J, et al. Major prognostic factors of Japanese patients with lymphoma-type adult T-cell leukemia. Am J Hematol 1990;35:232–237.
72. Pandolfi F, Loughran TP, Starkebaum G, et al. Clinical course and prognosis of the lymphoproliferative disease of granular lymphocytes: a multicenter study. Cancer 1990;65: 341–348.
73. Agnarsson BA, Loughran TP, Starkebaum G, et al. The pathology of large granular lymphocyte leukemia. Hum Pathol 1989;20:643–651.
74. Ohno Y, Amakawa R, Fukuhara S, et al. Acute transformation of chronic large granular lymphocyte leukemia associated with additional chromosome abnormality. Cancer 1989;64:62–67.
75. Imamura N, Kusunoki Y, Kawa-Ha K, et al. Aggressive natural killer cell leukaemia/lymphoma: sport of four cases and review of the literature: possible existence of a new clinical entity originating from the third lineage of lymphoid cells. Br J Haematol 1990;75:49–59.
76. Longacre TA, Listrom MB, Spigel JH, et al. Aggressive jejunal lymphoma of large granular lymphocytes: immunohistochemical, ultrastructural, molecular, and DNA content analysis. Am J Clin Pathol 1990;93:124–132.
77. Salhany KE, Greer JP, Cousar JB, et al. Marrow involvement in cutaneous T-cell lymphoma. Am J Clin Pathol 1989;92:747–754.
78. Pinto A, Zagonts el V, Carbone A. Bone marrow involvement in cutaneous T-cell lymphoma. Am J Clin Pathol 1990;94:119–120.
79. Willemze R, Van Vloten WA, Hermans J, et al. Diagnostic criteria in Sezary's syndrome: a multiparameter study of peripheral blood lymphocytes in 32 patients with erythroderma. J Invest Dermatol 1983;81:392–397.
80. Vonderheid EC, Sobel EL, Nowell PC, et al. Diagnostic and prognostic significance of Sezary cells in peripheral blood smears from patients with cutaneous T cell 1ymphoma. Blood 1985;66:358–366.
81. Proceedings of the International Conference on Multiple Myeloma—Biology, Pathophysiology, Prognosis and Treatment, June 19–22, 1989, Bologna (Italy). Eur J Haematol 1989;43(Suppl 51):11–195.
82. Dick FR. Plasma cell myeloma and related disorders with monoclonal gammopathy. In: Koepke JA, ed. Laboratory hematology. 1. New York: Churchill Livingstone; 1:1984;445–481.
83. Buss DH, Prichard RW, Hartz JW, et al. Initial bone marrow findngs in multiple myeloma: significance of plasma cell nodules. Arch Pathol Lab Med 1986;110:30–33.
84. Kyle RA, Greipp PR. Smoldering multiple myeloma. N Engl Med 1980;302:1347–1349.
85. Crowley JP. Smoldering multiple myeloma. N Engl Med 1980;303:941.

86. Durie BGM, Salmon SE. Multiple myeloma, macroglobulinemia and monoclonal gammopathies. In: Hoffbrand AV, Brain MC, Hirsh J, eds. Recent advances in hematology. New York: Churchill Livingstone, 1977.
87. Chronic Leukemia - Myeloma Task Force, National Cancer Institute. Proposed guidelines for protocol studies. Cancer Chemother Reports 1973;4:145–148.
88. Reed M, McKenna RW, Bridges R, et al. Morphologic manifestations of monoclonal gammopathies. Am J Clin Pathol 1981;76:8–23.
89. Brunning RD, Parkin J. Intranuclear inclusions in plasma cells and lymphocytes from patients with monoclonal gammopathies. Am J Clin Pathol 1976;66:10–21.
90. Hsu SU, Hsu PL, McMillan PN, et al. Russell bodies: a light and electron microscopic immunoperoxidase study. Am J Clin Pathol 1982;77:26–31.
91. Gabriel L, Escribano L, Perales J, et al. Multiple myeloma with crystalline inclusions in most hemopoietic cells. Am J Hematol 1985;18:405–411.
92. Maldonado JE, Brown AL, Bayrd ED, et al. Cytoplasmic and intranuclear electron-dense bodies in the myeloma cell. Arch Pathol 1966;81:484–499.
93. Greipp PR, Raymond NM, Kyle RA, et al. Multiple myeloma: significance of plasmablastic subtype in morphological classification. Blood 1985;65:305–310.
94. Strand, WR, Banks PM, Kyle RA. Anaplastic plasma cell myeloma and immunoblastic lymphoma: clinical, pathologic, and immunologic comparison. Am J Med 1984;76:861–867.
95. Sun NCJ, Fishkin BG, Nies KM, et al. Lymphoplasmacytic myeloma: an immunological, immunohistochemical and electron microscopic study. Cancer 1979;43:2268–2278.
96. Zukerberg I-R, Ferry JA, Conlon M, et al. Plasma cell myeloma with cleaved, multilobated, and monocytoid nuclei. Am J Clin Pathol 1990;93:657–661.
97. Kanoh T, Fujii H. Phagocytic myeloma cells: report of a case and review of the literature. Am J Clin Pathol 1985;84:121–124.
98. Krzyzaniak RL, Buss DH, Cooper R, et al. Marrow fibrosis and multiple myeloma. Am J Clin Pathol 1988;89:63–68.
99. Raman S, Frame B, Saeed SM, et al. Diffuse nonsecretory osteosclerotic myeloma with extensive erythrophagocytosis. Am J Clin Pathol 1983;80:84–88.
100. Stone, MJ. Amyloidosis: a final common pathway for protein deposition in tissues. Blood 1990;75:531–545.
101. Kyle RA, Maldonado JE, Bayrd ED. Plasma cell leukemia: report on 17 cases. Arch Intern Med 1974;133:813–818.
102. Kyle RA, Bayrd ED. The monoclonal gammopathies: multiple myeloma and related plasma cell disorders. Springfield, IL: Charles C Thomas, 1979.
103. Peterson LC, Brown BA, Crosson JT, et al. Application of the immunoperoxidase technic to bone marrow trephine biopsies in the classification of patients with monoclonal gammopathies. Am J Clin Pathol 1986;85:688–693.
104. Wolf BC, Brady K, O'Murchadha MT, et al. An evaluation of immunohistologic stains for immunoglobulin light chains in bone marrow biopsies in benign and malignant plasma cell proliferations. Am J Clin Pathol 1990;94:742–746.
105. Hitzman JL, Li CY, Kyle RA. Immunoperoxidase staining of bone marrow sections. Cancer 1981;48:2438–2446.
106. Wolf BC, Kumar A, Vera JC, et al. Bone marrow morphology and immunology in systemic amyloidosis. Am J Clin Pathol 1986;86:84–88.
107. Durie BGM, Stock-Novack D, Salmon SE, et al. Prognostic value of pretreatment serum β_2-microglobulin in myeloma: a southwest oncology group study. Blood 1990;75:823–830.
108. Greipp PR, Katzmann JA, O'Fallon WM, et al. Value of β_2-microglobulin level and plasma cell labeling indices as prognostic factors in patients with newly diagnosed myeloma. Blood 1988;72:219–223.
109. Greipp PR, Witzig TE, Gonchoroff NJ, et al. Immunofluorescence labeling indices in myeloma and related monoclonal gammopathies. Mayo Clin Proc 1987;62:969–977.
110. Witzig TE, Gonchoroff NJ, Katzmann JA, et al. Peripheral blood B cell labeling indices are a measure of disease activity in patients with monoclonal gammopathies. J Clin Oncol 1988;6:1041–1046.
111. Durie BGM, Grogan TM. CALIA-positive myeloma: an aggressive subtype with poor survival. Blood 1985;66:229–232.
112. Wearne AJ, Joshua DE, Brown RD, et al. Multiple myeloma: the relationship between CALLA (CD10) positive lymphocytes in the peripheral blood and light chain isotype suppression. Br J Haematol 1987;67:39–44.
113. Gould J, Alexanian R, Goodacre A, et al. Plasma cell karyotype in multiple myeloma. Blood 1988;71:453–456.
114. Barlogie B, Alexanian R, Dixon D, et al. Prognostic implications of tumor cell DNA and RNA content in multiple myeloma. Blood 1985;66:338–341.
115. Lokhorst HM, Boom SE, Terpstra W, et al. Determination of the growth fraction in monoclonal gammopathy with the monoclonal antibody Ki-67. Br J Haematol 1988;69:477–481.
116. Zalcberg JR, Cornell FN, Ireton JC, et al. Chronic lymphatic leukemia developing in a patient with multiple myeloma: immunologic demonstration of a clonally distinct second malignancy. Cancer 1982;50:594–597.
117. Foucar K, McKenna RW, Bloomfield CD, et al. Therapy related leukemia: a panmyelosis. Cancer 1979;43:1285–1296.
118. Mufti GJ, Hamblin TJ, Clein GP, et al. Coexistent myelodysplasia and plasma cell neoplasia. Br J Haematol 1983;54:91–96.
119. Durie BGM, Salmon SE. A clinical staging system for multiple myeloma. Cancer 1975;36:842–854.
120. Pasqualetti P, Casale R, Collacciani A, et al. Multiple myeloma: relationship between survival and cellular morphology. Am J Hematol 1990;33:145–147.
121. Carbone A, Volpe R, Manconi R, et al. Bone marrow pattern and clinical staging in multiple myeloma (Letter). Br J Haematol 1987;65:502–503.
122. Kyle RA. Newer approaches to the therapy of multiple myeloma. Blood 1990;76:1678–1679.
123. Alexanian R, Barlogie B. New treatment strategies for multiple myeloma. Am J Hematol 1990;35:194–198.
124. Knowling MA, Harwood AR, Bergsagel DE. Comparison of extramedullary plasmacytomas with solitary and multiple plasma cell tumors of bone. J Clin Oncol 1983;1:255–262.
125. Meis JM, Butler JJ, Osborne BM, et al. Solitary plasmacytomas of bone and extramedullary plasmacytomas: a clinicopathologic and immunohistochemical study. Cancer 1987;59:1475–1485.
126. Aviles A, Huerta J, Zepeda G, et al. Serum β_2-microglobulin in solitary plasmacytomata (Letter). Blood 1990;76:1663.
127. Kyle RA, Garton JP. The spectrum of IgM monoclonal gammopathy in 430 cases. Mayo Clin Proc 1987;62:719–731.
128. Bartl R, Frisch B, Mahl G, et al. Bone marrow histology in Waldenström's macroglobulinaemia: clinical relevance of subtype recognition. Scand J Haematol 1983;31:359–375.
129. Rywlin AM, Civantos F, Ortega RS, et al. Bone marrow histology in monoclonal macroglobulinemia. Am J Clin Pathol 1975;63:769–778.
130. Moore DF, Migliore PJ, Shullenberger CC, et al. Monoclonal macroglobulinemia in malignant lymphoma. Ann Intern Med 1970;72:43–47.
131. Tursz T, Brouet JC, Flandrin G, et al. Clinical and pathologic features of Waldenström's macroglobulinemia in seven pa-

tients with serum monoclonal IgG or IgA. Am J Med 1977;63: 499–502.
132. Feiner HD, Rizk CC, Finfer MD, et al. IgM monoclonal gammopathy/Waldenström's macroglobulinemia: a morphological and immunophenotypic study of the bone marrow. Mod Pathol 1990;3:348–356.
133. Chelazzi G, Bettini R, Pinotti G. Bone-marrow-patterns and survival in Waldenström's macroglobulinaemia. Lancet 1979;2:965–966.
134. Seligmann M, Mihaesco E, Preud'Homme JL, et al. Heavy chain diseases: current findings and concepts. Immunol Rev 1979;48:145–167.
135. Kyle RA, Greipp PR, Banks PM. The diverse picture of gamma heavy-chain disease: report of seven cases and review of literature. Mayo Clin Proc 1981;56:439–451.
136. Brouet JC, Seligmann M, Danon F, et al. μ-Chain disease: report of two new cases. Arch Intern Med 1979;139:672–674.
137. Galian A, Lecestre MJ, Scotto J, et al. Pathological study of alpha-chain disease, with special emphasis on evolution. Cancer 1977;39:2081–2101.
138. Ohno YI, Koya M, Yasuda N, et al. Ultrastructure of vacuolated plasma cells in macroglobulinemia associated with production of mu-chain fragment. Cancer 1982;49:2489–2492.
139. Reyes F, Piquet J, Gourdin MF, et al. Immunoblastic lymphoma involving the bone marrow in a patient with alpha chain disease: clinical and immunoelectron microscopic study. Cancer 1985;55:1007–1014.
140. Kyle RA, Lust JA. Monoclonal gammopathies of undetermined significance. Semin Hematol 1989;26:176–200.
141. Lichtman MA. Essential and secondary monoclonol gammopathies. In: Williams WJ, Bently E, Erslev AJ, et al. eds. Hematology. 4th ed. New York: McGraw-Hill, 1990:1109–1114.
142. Axelsson U, Bachmann R, Hallen J. Frequency of pathological proteins (M-components) in 6,995 sera from an adult population. Acta Med Scand 1966;179:235–247.
143. Papadopoulos NM, Elin RJ, Wilson DM. Incidence of γ-globulin banding in a healthy population by high-resolution electrophoresis. Clin Chem 1982;28:707–708.
144. Kyle RA. Monoclonal gammopathy of undetermined significance: natural history in 241 cases. Am J Med 1978;64:814–826.
145. Majumdar G, Heard SE, Singh AK. Use of cytoplasmic 5′ nucleotidase for differentiating malignant from benign monoclonal gammopathies. J Clin Pathol 1990;43:891–892.
146. Bezwoda WR, Gordon V, Bagg A, et al. Light chain restriction analysis of bone marrow plasma cells in patients with MGUS or "solitary" plasmacytoma: diagnostic value and correlation with clinical course. Br J Haematol 1990;74:420–423.
147. Majumdar G, Singh AK. Excess of monoclonal plasma cells in MGUS and diagnosis of early myeloma (Letter). Br J Haematol 1990;74:441–442.
148. The non-Hodgkin's lymphoma pathologic classification project writing committee: National Cancer Institute sponsored study of classification of non-Hodgkin's lymphomas: summary and description of a working formulation for clinical usage. Cancer 1982;49:2112–2135.
149. Jaffe ES, ed. Surgical pathology of the lymph nodes and related organs. 2nd ed. Philadelphia: WB Saunders, 1991.
150. Foucar K, Dick FR. Histopathology of non-Hodgkin's lymphoma and Hodgkin's disease. In: Keopke JA, ed. Laboratory hematology. New York: Churchill-Livingstone, 1984: 359–415.
151. Levine EG, Hanson CA, Frizzera G, et al. True histiocytic lymphoma: a review of clinical and pathologic findings. Semin Oncol 1991;18:39–49.
152. Dick F, Bloomfield CD, Brunning RD. Incidence, cytology, and histopathology of non-Hodgkin's lymphomas in the bone marrow. Cancer 1974;33:1382–1398.
153. Kluin PM, Van Krieken JH, Kleiverda K, et al. Discordant morphologic characteristics of B-cell lymphomas in bone marrow and lymph node biopsies. Am J Clin Pathol 1990;94: 59–66.
154. Fisher DE, Jacobson JO, Ault KA, et al. Diffuse large cell lymphoma with discordant bone marrow histology: clinical features and biological implications. Cancer 1989;64:1879–1887.
155. Schwartz DL, Pierre RV, Scheerer PP, et al. Lymphosarcoma cell leukemia. Am J Med 1965;38:778–786.
156. Zacharski LR, Linman JW. Chronic lymphocytic leukemia versus chronic lymphosarcoma cell leukemia. Am J Med 1969;47:75–81.
157. Brynes RK, McKenna RW, Sundberg RD. Bone marrow aspiration and trephine biopsy: an approach to a thorough study. Am J Clin Pathol 1978;70:753–759.
158. Ebie N, Lowe JM, Gregory SA. Bilateral trephine bone marrow biopsy for staging non-Hodgkin's lymphoma—second look. Hematol Pathol 1989;3:29–33.
159. Jacobs, P. Core length in bone-marrow biopsy. Lancet 1979;1: 1405–1406.
160. Maeda K, Hyun BH, Rebuck JW. Lymphoid follicles in bone marrow aspirates. Am J Clin Pathol 1977;67:41–48.
161. Pangalis GA, Moran EM, Rappaport H. Blood and bone marrow findings in angioimmunoblastic lymphadenopathy. Blood 1978;51:71–83.
162. Sun NCJ, Shapshak P, Lachant NA, et al. Bone marrow examination in patients with AIDS and AIDS-related complex (ARC). Am J Clin Pathol 1989;92:589–594.
163. Hanson CA, Brunning RD, Gajl-Peczalska KJ, et al. Bone marrow manifestations of peripheral T-cell lymphoma. Am J Clin Pathol 1986;86:449–460.
164. McKenna RW, Brunning RD. Reed-Sternberg-like cells in nodular lymphoma involving the bone marrow. Am J Clin Pathol 1975;63:779–785.
165. Evans HL. Extranodal small lymphocytic proliferations: a clinicopathologic and immunocytochemical study. Cancer 1982;49:84–96.
166. Lardelli P, Bookman MA, Sundeen J, et al. Lymphocytic lymphoma of intermediate differentiation: morphologic and immunophenotypic spectrum and clinical correlations. Am J Surg Pathol 1990;14:752–763.
167. Perry, DA, Bast MA, Armitage JO, et al. Diffuse intermediate lymphocytic lymphoma: a clinicopathologic study and comparison with small lymphocytic lymphoma and diffuse small cleaved cell lymphoma. Cancer 1990;66:1995–2000.
168. Neiman RS, Sullivan AL, Jaffe R. Malignant lymphoma simulating leukemic reticuloendotheliosis: A clinicopathologic study of ten cases. Cancer 1979;43:329–342.
169. Lukes RJ, Collins RD. Immunological characterization of human malignant lymphomas. Cancer 1974;34:1488–1503.
170. McKenna RW, Bloomfield CD, Brunning RD. Nodular lymphoma: bone marrow and blood manifestations. Cancer 1975;36:428–440.
171. Spiro S, Galton D, Wiltshaw E, et al. Follicular lymphoma: a survey of 75 cases with special reference to the syndrome resembling chronic lymphocytic leukemia. Br J Cancer 1975;31: 60–72.
172. Foucar K, Armitage JO, Dick FR. Malignant lymphoma mixed small and large cell: a clinicopathologic study of 47 cases. Cancer 1983;51:2090–2099.
173. Bhargava V, Farhi DC. Bone marrow granulomas: clinicopathologic findings in 72 cases and review of the literature. Hematol Pathol 1988;2:43–50.

174. Jaffe, ES. The role of immunophenotypic markers in the classification of non-Hodgkin's lymphomas. Semin Oncol 1990;17:11–19.
175. Kamat D, Laszewski MJ, Kemp JD, et al. The diagnostic utility of immunophenotyping and immunogenotyping in the pathologic evaluation of lymphoid proliferations. Mod Pathol 1990;3:105–112.
176. Davey FR, Elghetany MT, Kurec AS. Immunophenotyping of hematologic neoplasms in paraffin-embedded tissue sections. Am J Clin Pathol 1990;93(Suppl 1):S17–S26.
177. Kubic VL, Brunning RD. Immunohistochemical evaluation of neoplasms in bone marrow biopsies using monoclonal antibodies reactive in paraffin-embedded tissue. Mod Pathol 1989;2:618–629.
178. Horny HP, Engst U, Walz RS, et al. In situ immunophenotyping of lymphocytes in human bone marrow: an immunohistochemical study. Br J Haematol 1989;71:313–321.
179. Wood GS, Warnke RA. The immunologic phenotyping of bone marrow biopsies and aspirates: frozen section techniques. Blood 1982;59:913–922.
180. Longacre TA, Foucar K, Crago S, et al. Hematogones: a multiparameter analysis of bone marrow precursor cells. Blood 1989;73:543–552.
181. Horning SJ, Galili N, Cleary M, et al. Detection of non-Hodgkin's lymphoma in the peripheral blood by analysis of antigen receptor gene rearrangements: results of a prospective study. Blood 1990;75:1139–1145.
182. Rowley JD. Recurring chromosome abnormalities in leukemia and lymphoma. Semin Hematol 1990;27:122–136.
183. Grogan TM, Lippman SM, Spier CM, et al. Independent prognostic significance of a nuclear proliferation antigen in diffuse large cell lymphomas as determined by the monoclonal antibody Ki-67. Blood 1988;71:1157–1160.
184. Weiss LM, Strickler JG, Medeiros LJ, et al. Proliferative rates of non-Hodgkin's lymphomas as assessed by Ki-67 antibody. Hum Pathol 1987;18:1155–1159.
185. Ellison DJ, Hu E, Zovich D, et al. Immunogenetic analysis of bone marrow aspirates in patients with non-Hodgkin lymphomas. Am J Hematol 1990;33:160–166.
186. Sandhaus LM, Voelkerding KV, Dougherty J, et al. Combined utility of gene rearrangement analysis and flow cytometry in the diagnosis of lymphoproliferative disease in the bone marrow. Hematol Pathol 1990;4:135–148.
187. Come SE, Jaffe ES, Andersen JC, et al. Non-Hodgkin's lymphomas in leukemic phase: clinicopathologic correlations. Am J Med 1980;69:667–674.
188. Anastasi J, Bitter MA, Vardiman JW. The histopathologic diagnosis and subclassification of Hodgkin's disease. Hematol Oncol Clin North Am 1989;3:187–204.
189. Lukes RJ. Criteria for involvement of lymph node, bone marrow, spleen, and liver in Hodgkin's disease. Cancer Res 1971;31:1755–1767.
190. Weiss RB, Brunning RD, Kennedy BJ. Hodgkin's disease in the bone marrow. Cancer 1975;36:2077–2083.
191. Myers CE, Chabner BA, De Vita VT, et al. Bone marrow involvement in Hodgkin's disease: pathology and response to MOPP chemotherapy. Blood 1974;44:197–204.
192. Bartl R, Frisch B, Burkhards R, et al. Assessment of bone marrow histology in Hodgkin's disease: correlation with clinical factors. Br J Haematol 1982;51:345–360.
193. Kinney MC, Greer JP, Stein RS, et al. Lymphocyte-depletion Hodgkin's disease: histopathologic diagnosis of marrow involvement. Am J Surg Pathol 1986;10:219–226.
194. Meadows LM, Rosse WR, Moore JO, et al. Hodgkin's disease presenting as myelofibrosis. Cancer 1989;64:1720–1726.
195. Leoncini L, Del Vecchio MT, Kraft R, et al. Hodgkin's disease and CD30-positive anaplastic large cell lymphomas—a continuous spectrum of malignant disorders: a quantitative morphometric and immunohistologic study. Am J Pathol 1990;137:1047–1057.
196. Casey TT, Cousar JB, Mangum M, et al. Monomorphic lymphomas arising in patients with Hodgkin's disease: correlation of morphologic, immunophenotypic, and molecular genetic findings in 12 cases. Am J Pathol 1990;136:81–94.
197. Hansmann ML, Stein H, Fellbaum C, et al. Nodular paragranuloma can transform into high-grade malignant lymphoma of B type. Hum Pathol 1989;20:1169–1175.
198. Davey DD, Kamat D, Laszewski M, et al. Epstein-Barr virus-related lymphoproliferative disorders following bone marrow transplantation: an immunologic and genotypic analysis Mod Pathol 1989;2:27–34.
199. Locker J, Nalesnik M. Molecular genetic analysis of lymphoid tumors arising after organ transplantation. Am J Pathol 1989;135:977–987.
200. Zutter MM, Durnam DM, Hackman RC, et al. Secondary T-cell lymphoproliferation after marrow transplantation. Am J Clin Pathol 1990;94:714–721.

39 Chronic Myeloproliferative Disorders

Powers Peterson

The chronic myeloproliferative disorders (MPDs) represent a group of syndromes or diseases with enough in common to justify placing them in the same category of illness. These diseases are: polycythemia vera (PV), chronic myelogenous leukemia (CML), essential or primary thrombocythemia (ET), and idiopathic myelofibrosis (IMF) (or agnogenic myeloid metaplasia [AMM]). Chronic myelomonocytic leukemia (CMMoL) and the hypereosinophilic syndrome (HES) can be conceptually included within this group. The common feature is a disease process that involves a pluripotent cell capable of generating erythroid, granulocytic-monocytic, and megakaryocyte progeny (1–7). Despite the evidence that all three lines are involved, there is usually little trouble in distinguishing between patients who present with classic manifestations of these disorders. In some settings, however, the absence of classic features precludes easy assignment to one or the other of the disease categories. These patients are often referred to as having an "overlap" syndrome.

Moreover, although we have compelling evidence that CML is quite homogeneous at the molecular genetics level (8–12), there is as yet no such evidence with respect to the other diseases in the group. Chromosomal abnormalities in PV, ET, and CMMoL are of various types, and current methodologies fail to demonstrate cytogenetic abnormalities in the bone marrow of most patients at diagnosis (13, 14). The appearance of fibrosis in the marrow may be the end result of diverse disease processes (15–25).

POLYCYTHEMIA VERA

This curious hematologic disorder is neither as regal as porphyria or hemophilia, nor quite as confusing as the classification of non-Hodgkin's lymphomas (NHL). Polycythemia Vera (PV) was initially described in 1892 by Vaquez as an erythrocytosis (26). Some years later Osler characterized the clinical picture as "very distinctive," the symptoms as "somewhat indefinite," and the pathology as "quite obscure" (27). In 1938 Rosenthal and Bassen (28) recognized the generalized nature of the myeloproliferation, the chronicity, and the disorder's unusual variations over time. They divided the disease into the asymptomatic phase; the polycythemic or symptomatic phase; and the highly variable final phase, termed the anemic or spent phase. Thirty years after Vaquez's description, Minot and Buckman (29) recognized the "intimate" relation between PV and CML as "varying degrees of primary pathological activity of the myeloid tissue." Their conceptual advance was that of a shared origin in disordered growth of the pluripotent hematopoietic precursor cell. Still later, Rosenthal expanded this concept to include thrombocytosis and some leukemias (30). It was Demeshek (31), however, who stated (and took credit for) a unified theory, classifying PV as one of a group of related disorders, the chronic MPDs.

Clinical Presentation and Natural History

The plethoric patient with a palpable spleen, an elevated hematocrit, and an increased leukocyte and/or platelet count is very likely to have PV. The characteristic plethora results from engorgement of many cutaneous vessels ordinarily not perfused by the hyperviscous blood. This expansion and distention of the vasculature accounts for many of the signs and symptoms. The spleen is enlarged in most patients with PV. If not detectable on physical examination, it is often enlarged on radioisotopic scanning.

Presenting complaints vary. Many are related to the circulatory system and result from hyperviscosity and hypervolemia. They range in severity from headache and fatigue to peptic ulcer, stroke, and erythromelalgia. Sludging phenomena with resultant tissue hypoxia and thrombosis occur in at least 30% of patients. A small proportion of patients have hepatic vein thrombosis, the Budd-Chiari syndrome. On the other hand, asymptomatic patients are frequently diagnosed with PV following detection of an elevated hemoglobin and hematocrit. Figure 39.1 is an algorithm for the evaluation of the patient with an elevated hematocrit. Another frequent complaint is pruritus, which is often exacerbated after bathing or showering. Elevated blood histamine levels, an in-

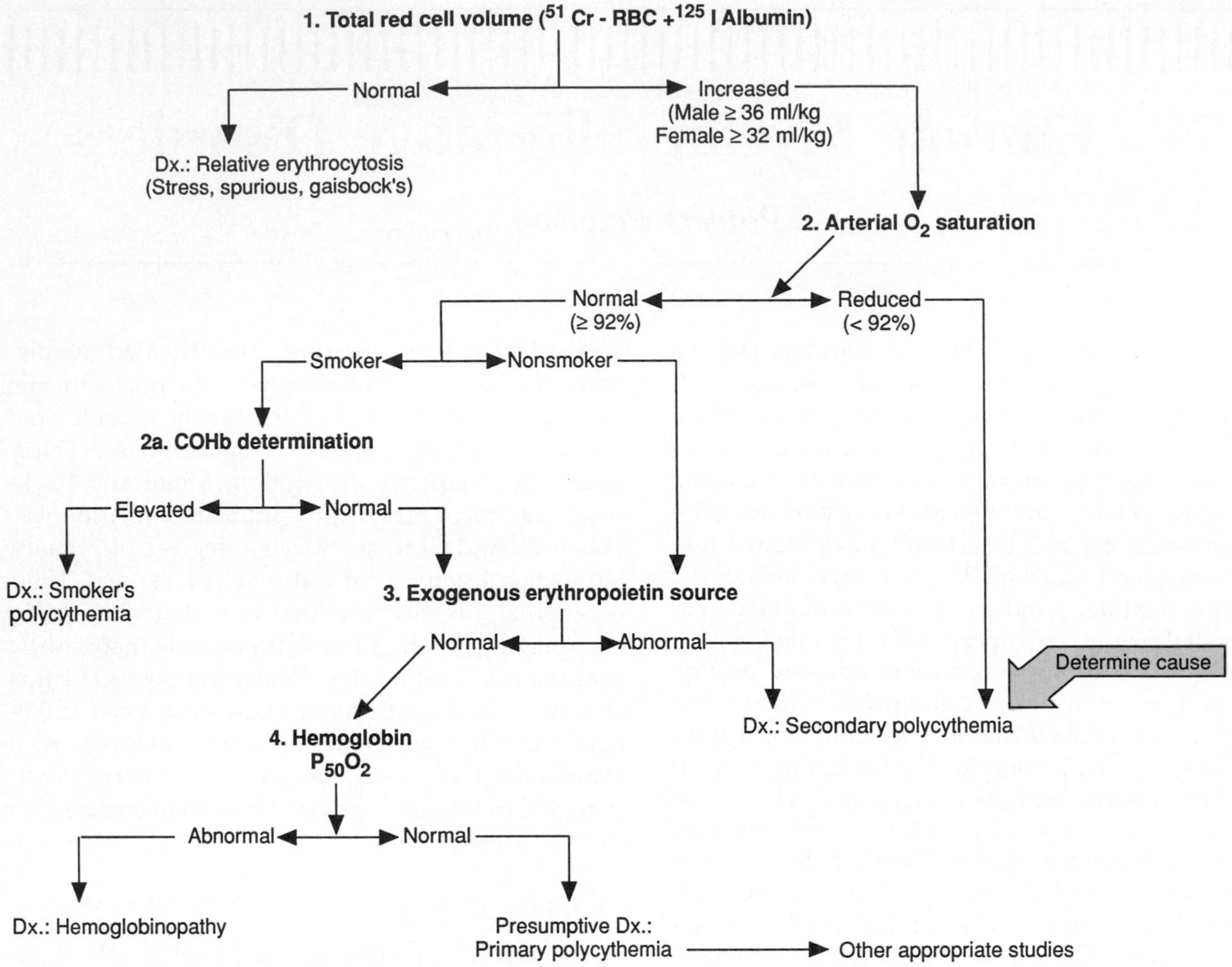

Figure 39.1. Algorithm for evaluation of an elevated hematocrit. (Adapted from Berk PH, Goldberg JD, Donovan PB, et al. Therapeutic recommendations in polycythemia vera based on polycythemia Vera Study Group protocols. Semin Hematol 1986;23:134. Reprinted with permission of Grune & Stratton.)

creased number of circulating leukocytes in the engorged peripheral blood vessels, and increased numbers of tissue mast cells may be responsible for the severe pruritus. Because of increased cell turnover, still other patients present with gout.

The natural history is complex and may be protracted. Presenting most commonly in patients over 50, PV has been reported in patients as young as 25 (32, 33). As the disease insidiously evolves from its initially asymptomatic phase through its hyperproliferative and hypoproliferative phases, the complications, symptoms, and pathological and laboratory changes all vary. If not treated, a patient's life expectancy is approximately 18 months (34). If the disease is not controlled, large numbers of patients die of thrombotic events (35, 36). Other causes of death include: acute leukemia (AL) (37–40) or blastic transformation; complications of MF (15, 41–43); solid tumors, especially gastrointestinal carcinomas (34) and non-Hodgkin's lymphomas (NHL) in patients treated with alkylating agents (15, 44, 45).

LABORATORY STUDIES

The diagnostic criteria (46) set forth by the Polycythemia Vera Study Group (PVSG) are now generally accepted (Table 39.1). Regardless of the specific diagnosis eventually made in a patient, certain basic studies are applicable to all the MPDs (Table 39.2).

Panmyelosis is a hallmark of this disease. PV is a clonal (1) disorder in which a pluripotent stem cell gives rise to the granulocytic, megakaryocytic, and erythroid lines. The increase in the red cell mass represents but one component of the proliferative process. Granulocytes and platelets are nearly always increased. Lack of a leukocytosis and thrombocytosis should initiate consideration of a different cause for the erythrocytosis.

Table 39.1. PVSG Criteria for the Diagnosis of Polycythemia Vera[a]

1. No previous treatment except phlebotomy
2. Disease diagnosed no longer than 4 years ago
3. Fulfillment of the following diagnostic criteria:

Category A	Category B
1. Total red cell volume Male ≥ 36 ml/kg Female ≥ 32 ml/kg	1. Thrombocytosis platelet count ≥ 400,000/μl (400 × 10^9/liter)
2. Arterial O_2 saturation ≥ 92%	2. Leukocytosis ≥ 12,000/μl (12.0 × 10^9/liter) (No fever or infection)
3. Splenomegaly	3. Elevated leukocyte alkaline phosphatase score ≥ 100 (No fever or infection)
	4. Serum B_{12} level ≥ 900 pg/ml or $UB_{12}BC$ ≥ 2200 pg/ml

Patient eligible if the following combinations are present: (A1 + A2 + A3) or (A1 + A2 + Any two from category B)

[a]Adapted from Berlin NI. Diagnosis and classification of the polycythemias. Semin Hematol 1975;12:342. Reprinted with permission of Grune & Stratton.

Table 39.2. Initial Evaluation of Myeloproliferative Disorders[a]

1. Clinical history.
2. Physical examination. Note: ruddiness, bone pain, splenomegaly.
3. Laboratory studies
   a. CBC with platelet and differential counts.
   b. Serum chemistries: uric acid, BUN, creatinine, alkaline phosphatase.
4. Bone marrow aspiration and biospy
   a. Cytogenetic studies: Philadelphia chromosome (Ph[1]) or a *bcr* rearrangement, other clonal abnormalities.
   b. Iron stores.

[a]From Peterson P, McIntyre OR. Myeloproliferative disorders. Chicago: American Society of Clinical Pathologists. Syllabus #5649, 1989:5. Reprinted with permission of the American Society of Clinical Pathologists.

Nearly all patients with PV have normal Po_2 levels and normal oxygen saturation. In those patients with all of the other characteristics of the disease but with low Po_2 and oxygen unsaturation, arterial blood gas studies after two or three phlebotomies should be repeated because arterial oxygen content may improve after partial relief of the polycythemia.

The elevated leukocyte alkaline phosphatase (LAP) probably results from increased granulocyte production. An elevation is characteristic of other situations in which granulocyte production is increased. Likewise, the elevated serum B_{12} levels in PV result from the increased amounts of transcobalamin I elaborated by developing granulocytes.

Elevated blood and urine histamine levels are found in two-thirds of patients. Chronically elevated histamine levels may be responsible for the frequent occurrence of peptic ulcer disease. Serum uric acid is often elevated, a consequence of increased cell turnover.

Erythropoietin levels only rarely help discriminate between a secondary polycythemia and PV. This determination is usually neither necessary nor cost-effective.

Cytogenetic studies are essential to obtain (Fig. 39.2; Table 39.2) to rule out the presence of the Philadelphia (Ph[1]) chromosome or a *bcr* rearrangement. A cytogenetically abnormal clone is detected in fewer than 10% of previously untreated patients with PV (13, 14).

Morphology

PRETREATMENT

The peripheral blood smear (PBS) in untreated early stage PV is very often normal (15, 47). It may occasionally show nucleated red blood cells, immature granulocytic elements, and increased numbers of platelets.

The marrow aspirate smear and biopsy are generally moderately to markedly hypercellular with trilineage hyperplasia being the norm. The aspirate may be misleading if it consists primarily of peripheral blood or masses of platelets and megakaryocytes. With the exception of the megakaryocyte line, overt morphologic abnormalities are generally not present in either the aspirate or biopsy in untreated early-stage PV. Megakaryocyte abnormalities include (*a*) increases in size of the nucleus and the cytoplasm; (*b*) irregular nuclear lobation; (*c*) abnormal mitoses; and (*d*) clustering (in tissue sections) (45, 47).

Marked hypercellularity is not always present: 13% of pretreatment biopsies will be normocellular (cellularity less than or equal to 60%). The aspirate is essential to assess iron stores. PV commonly presents with iron deficiency, which may mask the erythrocytosis. Only 6% of untreated PV patients can be expected to have detectable iron (smears or biopsy sections) (15, 47).

The marrow cord stromal (reticular) cells blacken with silver impregnation and form an incomplete network of reticulin fibers that is continuous with the fibers in blood vessels and sinusoidal walls. Approximately 85 to 90% of pretreatment biopsies demonstrate a normal or very slight increase in reticulin fiber content. In untreated patients, an increased reticulin fiber content correlates positively with cellularity.

DURING THERAPY—ACTIVE STAGE OF POLYCYTHEMIA VERA

With myelosuppression, whether by cytotoxic drugs or radioactive phosphorus (^{32}P), marrow cellularity generally decreases. The hypercellular marrows of patients treated by phlebotomy alone usually

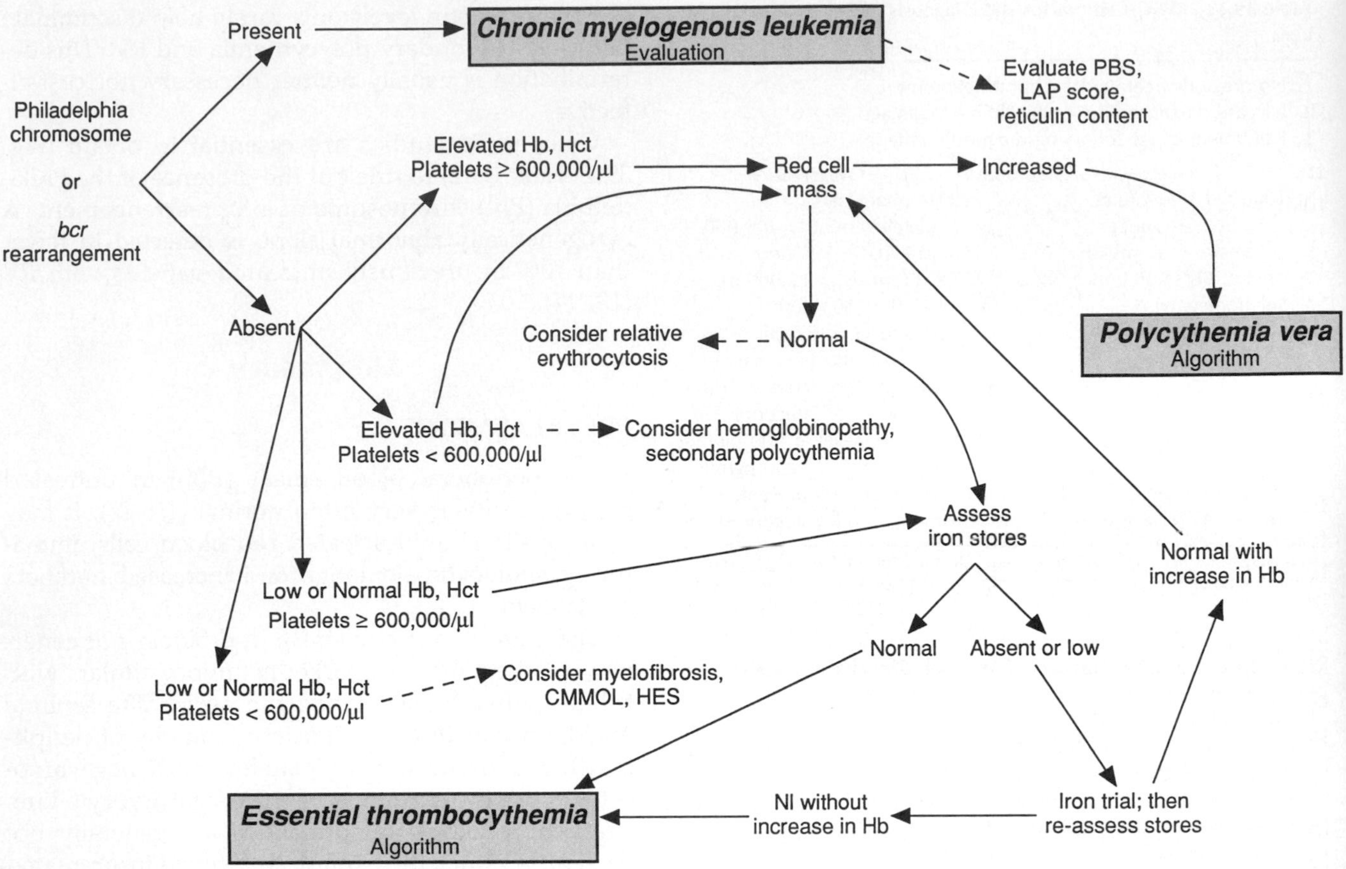

Figure 39.2. Algorithm for the diagnosis of myeloproliferative disorders. (From Peterson P, McIntyre DR. Myeloproliferative disorders. Chicago: American Society of Clinical Pathologists Syllabus 1989;6. Reprinted with permission.)

show some diminution in cellularity, but not to the same degree as those treated with myelosuppressive agents (15, 45, 47). The clustering of megakaryocytes persists, regardless of the therapy.

Following therapy, a moderate to marked increase in reticulin fiber content develops in 10% of patients. The pattern is a progressive increase over time and can occur in as short as 2 years, with 5 to 10 years probably being the norm.

Collagen determined by a trichrome stain may be present when there is a moderate increase in the reticulin fiber content and is almost invariably present when the reticulin fibrosis is marked. Characteristically, the remaining hematopoietic elements are enmeshed and distorted by the collagenous tissue.

SPENT PHASE OF POLYCYTHEMIA VERA—POLYCYTHEMIC MYELOID METAPLASIA

Nine to 10% of PV patients progress to the spent phase, also known as postpolycythemic myeloid metaplasia (PPMM). The blood and marrow changes are profound. The peripheral blood film demonstrates a typical leukoerythroblastic (LEB) picture with marked aniso- and poikilocytosis, nucleated and teardrop red cells, and reticulocytosis (15, 48). Immature cells of the granulocytic series are present, ranging from occasional myeloblasts to myelocytes. Platelet clumps and fragments of megakaryocytes may be present.

Attempts to aspirate marrow usually yield a '"dry tap" because of the fibrosis. The biopsy cellularity, however, is variable. Over time there is a progressive loss of hematopoietic tissue. As the dense connective tissue encroaches the narrow spaces, the enmeshed hematopoietic elements become distorted. Megakaryocytes may appear exceptionally bizarre.

Biopsies of patients in the spent phase show moderate (3+) to marked (4+) reticulin fibrosis with some collagen fibrosis. The fibrosis may be patchy but tends to become progressively confluent. Long-standing MF leads to the bony changes of osteosclerosis.

The spleen and liver show extramedullary hematopoiesis (EMH) in an attempt to augment the failing marrow (49). Lymph nodes and other organs may also show EMH. In addition, histologic studies of liver may show obliteration of both large and small portal veins, a consequence of thrombosis (50). The hepatic venous system may show similar changes.

Although earlier studies suggested an increased incidence of MF in PV treated with radiation (radioactive phosphorus [^{32}P]) (17, 43, 51–54), this is not the case. The development of the spent phase is independent of the type of therapy, whether phlebotomy alone, alkylating agent chemotherapy, or ^{32}P (15, 45). It is not known if this is also true in patients treated with myelosuppressive drugs with different mechanisms of action (such as hydroxyurea, a pyrimidine antagonist). More ominous than the development of the spent phase in PV, however, is the increased risk of AL the spent phase engenders (37, 42). This will be discussed in the section that follows.

ACUTE LEUKEMIA IN POLYCYTHEMIA VERA

The most frequent secondary hematologic malignancy in PV is acute leukemia (AL), or blastic transformation. There is a very low incidence of blastic transformation in PV treated by phlebotomy alone, 2 to 3% (37, 39, 41, 42, 55). This represents the natural incidence of AL in PV unmodified by therapeutic agents. Both alkylating agents and radiation are known to be leukemogenic and are associated with other neoplasias in various organs (56–64). Not surprisingly, the incidence of AL in PV is much greater following radiation therapy or alkylating agent chemotherapy than is the incidence in patients treated with phlebotomy alone (37, 39, 42). This higher incidence translates to a substantially increased risk of AL—on the magnitude of a 10 to 15 times greater risk (37, 43).

The AL in PV is usually myelogenous (nonlymphocytic) and may manifest either de novo or following the spent phase (42). The risk of developing de novo AL is approximately equal, whether treatment is an alkylating agent or ^{32}P. The major difference is the lag time, with ^{32}P-associated leukemias developing several years later than the chemotherapy-associated leukemias (37, 39, 42). In addition to the increased risk of AL associated with myelosuppressive therapy, progression to the spent phase is also a risk factor for the development of AL. A large, prospective, randomized study documented the striking and significant differences in the incidence of AL between patients with and without the spent phase of PV (37, 42). The study also demonstrated that the risk increases with time (17, 42, 45).

DIFFERENTIAL DIAGNOSIS

Because the presenting symptoms are highly variable and because other disorders may mimic PV, the diagnosis must be carefully sought and well documented. More common reasons for an absolute erythrocytosis include smoking and high oxygen-affinity hemoglobins (46, 65, 66). Much less common reasons are uterine leiomyomas, renal and hepatic carcinomas, and cerebellar hemangioblastomas (Table 39.3). Secondary polycythemia occurs in the setting of altered arterial oxygen saturation of hemoglobin, increased carboxy- or methemoglobin levels, and decreased red cell enzyme levels.

Table 39.3. Differential Diagnosis of Polycythemia[a]

- I. Nonneoplastic
  - A. Increased erythropoietin production, appropriate response
    - 1. High altitude
    - 2. Chronic obstructive lung disease
    - 3. Left-to-right cardiovascular shunt
    - 4. High-oxygen affinity hemoglobinopathy
    - 5. Congenital deficiency of red cell DPG
  - B. Increased erythropoietin production, inappropriate response
    - 1. Tumor
      - a. Uterine leiomyoma
      - b. Cerebellar hemangioblastoma
      - c. Renal cell carcinoma
    - 2. Renal disease
    - 3. Cobalt
  - C. Relative polycythemia (stress polycythemia, Gaisbock's syndrome)
  - D. Recessive familial polycythemia
- II. Neoplastic: Polycythemia vera

[a]Modified from Berlin NI. Diagnosis and classification of the polycythemias. Semin Hematol 1975;12:340. Reprinted with permission.

CHRONIC MYELOGENOUS LEUKEMIA

The demonstration of the association of CML with the Philadelphia (Ph[1]) chromosome was a major scientific advance for diagnostic and conceptual reasons. The clonal origin of CML has been confirmed by the same two techniques used to demonstrate the clonality of PV (2). In CML the Ph[1] marker is found in cells of the granulocyte-monocyte-macrophage, the erythroid, and the megakaryocytic lineages. The neoplastic stem cell in CML also has capabilities for differentiation along B-lymphoid lines (67, 68).

Clinical Presentation and Natural History

CML is a disorder of middle age but may occur at any age, including childhood (69). This is the most common of the MPDs, accounting for 20% of cases of leukemia. Similar to PV, patients usually present with palpable splenomegaly; they may complain of abdominal fullness. Asymptomatic patients may be detected because of a neutrophilic leukocytosis on a CBC. The duration of the stable or chronic phase is highly variable but averages 3 to 5 years. In 80% of patients this phase is followed by transformation to an overt AL. In some patients this transformation is preceded by the aggressive or accelerated phase.

The Ph[1] chromosome occurs in 85 to 95% of patients with CML. It results from a reciprocal translocation between chromosomes 9 and 22, designated t(9;22)(q34.1;q11.21) (3, 11, 70). In addition to the typical Ph[1] abnormality, a number of variant forms

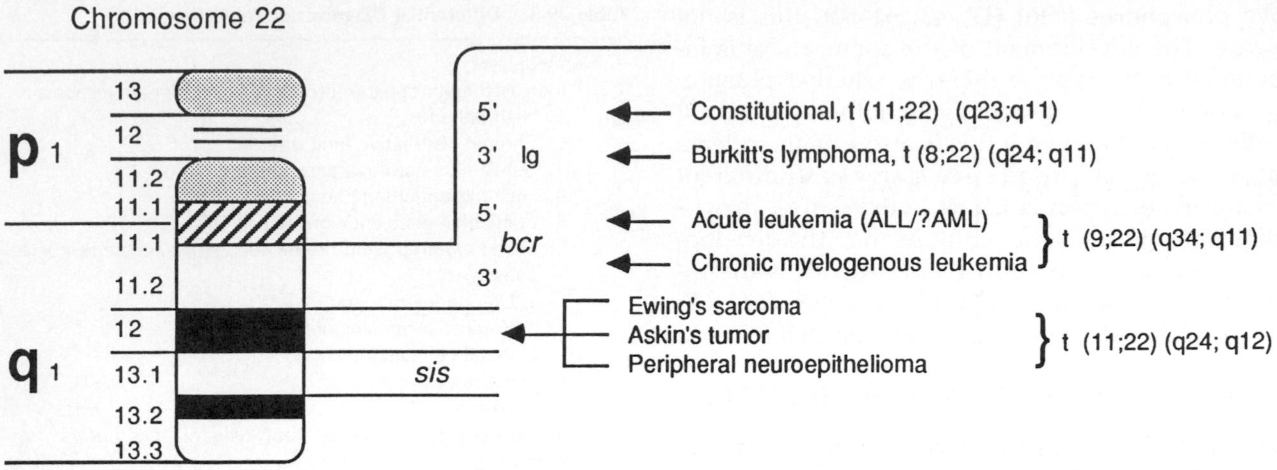

Figure 39.3. Breakpoints on chromosome 22 in band q11 and nearby regions, in various neoplasms. (From Kurzrock R, Gutterman JU, Talpaz M. The molecular genetics of Philadelphia chromosome-positive leukemias. N Engl J Med 1988;319:996. Reprinted with permission of the Massachusetts Medical Society.)

Table 39.4. Molecular Consequences of the t(9;22)(q34;q11) (Ph[1] Chromosome)[a]

Chromosome	Transcription Product	Translation Product
Normal 9	6- & 7-kb c-*abl* mRNA	145-kd c-*abl* protein ($p145^{c\text{-}abl}$)
Normal 22	4.5- & 6.7-kb *bcr* mRNA	160-kd *bcr* protein ($p160^{bcr}$)
9q+	No message found	No message found
22q−	CML: 8.5-kb *bcr-abl* mRNA	$p210^{bcr\text{-}abl}$
ALL:	7.0-kb *bcr-abl* mRNA	$p190^{c\text{-}abl}$
	or	or
	8.5-kb *bcr-abl* mRNA	$p210^{bcr\text{-}abl}$
	AML: not yet reported	$p190^{c\text{-}abl}$

[a]From Kurzrock R, Gutterman JU, Talpaz M., The molecular genetics of Philadelphia chromosome-positive leukemias. N Engl J Med 1988;319:992. Reprinted with permission of the Massachusetts Medical Society.

have been described. In almost every instance, however, chromosome 22 has been involved (71–73) (Fig. 39.3). Most patients diagnosed as having CML but lacking the Ph[1] chromosome—so-called Ph[1]-negative CML—have clinical features that set them apart from those with more typical, Ph[1]-positive disease (74, 75). Most importantly, lack of the Ph[1] chromosome generally signifies more rapid progression of the disease (10, 11, 75–77).

The cellular or protooncogenes *c-abl* anc *c-sis* map to chromosomes 9 and 22, respectively. In the typical Ph[1] abnormality these genes are reciprocally translocated. The entire *c-abl* gene is usually translocated to chromosome 22 without rearrangement. The breakpoint of chromosome 9 is variable, but that on 22 is restricted to a 5.8 kilobase protein (kbp) region, the breakpoint cluster region (*bcr*). The fusion gene *bcr-abl* encodes for a 210-Kd protein, P210; this protein has tyrosine kinase activity and is a specific marker of the translocation. Patients lacking the typical Ph[1] chromosome may still display a *bcr* rearrangement (9, 77, 78). Table 39.4 shows the molecular consequences of the *c-abl* products in normal cells or in cells with the translocation. Figure 39.4 is a schematic representation of the *bcr* and *abl* genes and the chimeric *bcr-abl* gene of the Ph[1] chromosome.

The Ph[1] chromosome is also found in up to 5% of patients with acute myelogenous leukemia (AML), in 20 to 30% of adults with acute lymphocytic leukemia (ALL) (10, 79), and in 5% of children with ALL (80). In these patients the Ph[1] encodes for a distinct 190-Kd protein, P190. When present in these conditions, it indicates a dismal prognosis. Such cases may or may not represent CML presenting in blastic transformation (80, 81).

The course of the disease may be divided into phases, proceeding from the chronic phase, to an accelerated or resistant phase, to blast crisis. These transitions may be quite gradual with indistinct boundaries, but in some patients may be abrupt and unexpected. Since CML may result from a multistep pathogenesis (82), variations are to be expected. The course of the disease is not influenced by standard chemotherapy. After a variable period during which the white count, anemia, and splenomegaly are easily controlled, all treatments fail. Following a period in which supportive measures may alleviate symptoms, a further evolution to the blast phase, as defined later, usually occurs.

Treatment with chemotherapy seldom results in clearing of the Ph[1] chromosome from the marrow, although treatment with interferon (INF) may reduce the frequency of the chromosome to a level where detection by conventional means is not possible (83–85). Bone marrow transplantation may be curative, however. Marrow transplantation is far more successful in those patients who undergo the procedure

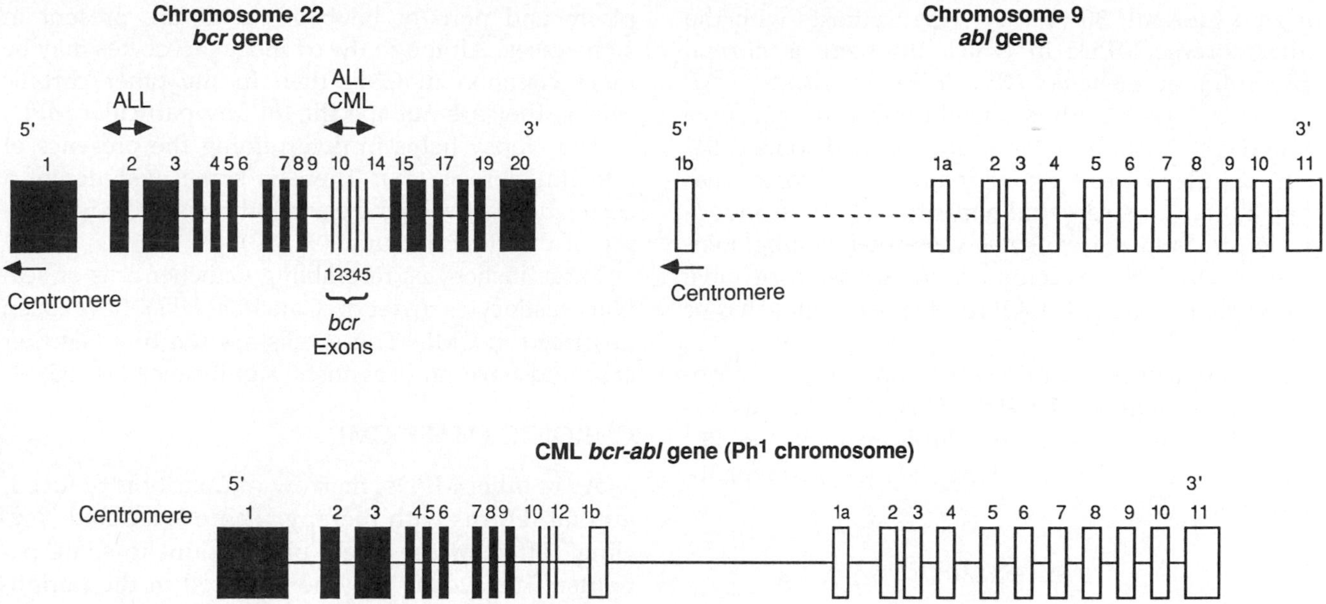

Figure 39.4. Normal c-abl and bcr genes on chromosomes 9 and 22, respectively, and the chimeric bcr-abl gene associated with CML. (From Kurzrock R, Gutterman JU, Talpoz M. The molecular genetics of Philadelphia chromosome-positive leukemias. N Engl J Med 1988;319:994. Reprinted with permission of the Massachusetts Medical Society.)

Table 39.5. Median Survival in CML after the Development of Presumed Accelerated-Phase Characteristics[a]

Characteristic	No. of Patients Developing Characteristics	Median Survival (Months)
Peripheral blasts ≥ 15%	85	8.6
Marrow blasts ≥ 15%	34	10.9
Peripheral blasts + promyelocytes ≥ 30%	32	4.7
Marrow blasts + promyelocytes ≥ 30%	38	17.4
Peripheral basophils ≥ 20%	74	16.0
Marrow basophils ≥ 20%	25	11.6
Platelets < 100,000/μl (100 × 10^9/liter)	105	14.9
Platelets ≥ 200,000/μl (200 × 10^9/liter)	76	27.2
Hemoglobin < 7g/dl (1.09)	92	16.0
Nucleated red cells ≥ 15%	60	23.5
Cytogenetic clonal evolution	54	7.0
Extramedullary disease	25	10.0

[a]Adapted from Kantarjian HM, Talpaz M. Definition of the accelerated phase of chronic myelogenous leukemia. J Clin Oncol 1988;6:181. Reprinted with permission of Grune & Stratton.

Table 39.6. Criteria for the Diagnosis of Chronic Myelogenous Leukemia

1. White blood cell count of 30,000/μl (30 × 10^9/liter) on two occasions 24–96 hours apart.
2. Absence of a reasonable cause for a leukemoid reaction.
3. Granulocytic series in peripheral blood ≥ 80% of the differential count.
4. 10% or fewer myeloblasts and/or promyelocytes in peripheral blood.
5. Hypercellular marrow.
6. Splenomegaly.
7. In the absence of splenomegaly, a leukocyte alkaline phosphatase (LAP) score of <10 or a serum B_{12} level of > 2,000 pg/ml; with splenomegaly, LAP score ≤ 25.
9. Presence of the Philadelphia chromosome (Ph^1) or a *bcr* rearrangement.

during the chronic rather than during the accelerated phase (86–88). Because of the morbidity and mortality associated with allogeneic transplantation, attempts have been made to predict the onset of the accelerated phase. This has proved difficult. Table 34.5 presents data concerning survival following the appearance of characteristics typical of the accelerated or resistant phase.

Laboratory Studies

A profound leukocytosis, frequently greater than 100,000/μl (100 × 10^9/liter), is the sine qua non of CML. The range is 50 to 250,000/μl (50 to 250 × 10^9/liter). Patients with early disease may display only a mild elevation of the granulocyte count with little or no alteration of platelet and hemoglobin levels. Because there is no evidence that early treatment benefits these patients, some patients are followed without a specific diagnosis until evidence of morbidity occurs. It is usually easy to establish the diagnosis in a patient with advanced CML. Criteria that have been set for patient eligibility for some studies are listed in Table 39.6. Quite unlike PV, anemia is frequent in CML; it is usually normochromic and normocytic. The platelet count may be normal (one-third to one-half of patients), elevated (one-half of patients), or decreased (up to one-fifth of patients).

Critical in diagnosing CML is the leukocyte (neutrophil) alkaline phosphatase (LAP) score. Performed on peripheral blood, the score is classically very low or zero (normal, 30 to 130). This contrasts with the other chronic MPDs in which the score is normal (ET, IMF) or elevated (PV, IMF). Decreased LAP levels may occur in idiopathic thrombocytopenic purpura (ITP), AML, pernicious anemia, and some collagen vascular disorders; very low LAP scores (less than 20) can occur in viral hepatitis, infectious mononucleosis, and paroxysmal nocturnal hemoglobinuria. When CML patients are in remission or have been splenectomized, LAP levels may be elevated or normal.

As the disease progresses, additional chromosomal abnormalities appear. This is known as cytogenetic clonal evolution. Duplication of the Ph^1 chromosome and trisomy 8 are the most frequent abnormalities (89).

Morphology

PRETREATMENT

A neutrophilic leukocytosis is the hallmark of CML. The peripheral blood film shows all stages of granulocytic maturation from myeloblasts to PMNs. The total of myeloblasts and promyelocytes usually does not exceed 5%. There is an excess of myelocytes, with myelocytes and metamyelocytes constituting 30–40% of the granulocytic cells. Basophils are almost always increased in number. Pseudo-Pelger-Huët cells are present in only a few patients at presentation. Red cell morphology is usually normal despite the mild anemia. Nucleated red blood cells (NRBC) are present in the great majority of patients at diagnosis, but this finding need not indicate fibrosis of the marrow. Thrombocytosis results in megakaryocyte nuclei and giant platelets.

The marrow aspirate smear is hypercellular with marked granulocytic hyperplasia. The granulocytic: erythroid ratio is altered from the normal range of 3 to 5:1 to ranges from 10:1 to 40 to 50:1. If thrombocytosis is extreme (greater than 600,000/μl [600×10^9/liter]), the megakaryocytic hyperplasia and the platelet clumping may be misleading, obscuring the changes in the granulocytic line (90).

The marrow biopsy is also hypercellular. Similar to the changes in PV, fat may be absent. As in the aspirate, granulocytic hyperplasia predominates, and the hyperplasia is found in all stages of the series. Eosinophils may appear strikingly increased. Basophils, though increased in number, are not detected unless the biopsy is plastic-embedded (91). Varying degrees of erythroid hyperplasia may also be present; erythroid maturation is usually normal. Megakaryocytic hyperplasia can be extreme (90). Micromegakaryocytes or '''dwarf'' megakaryocytes (small megakaryocytes with abundant eosinophilic cytoplasm and non- or bilobed nuclei) are present in some cases. Although dwarf megakaryocytes may be more common in CML than in the other chronic MPDs, they are not specific for any particular MPD.

The biopsy helps in determining the presence of reticulin fibrosis (18). There is some evidence of a correlation between increasing fibrosis and a worsening of the clinical course (92, 93).

Large histiocytes resembling Gaucher cells or sea-blue histiocytes (pseudo-Gaucher cells) have been described in CML. These cells are not true Gaucher cells and have no prognostic significance (94, 95).

CHRONIC PHASE CML

As in other MPDs, marrow cellularity is reduced, and fat returns with therapy. There is a noted '''cycling'' effect of the white blood count in some patients. This cycling may be reflected in the peripheral smear, especially with basophils, eosinophils, monocytes, and NRBCs, but not with lymphocytes (96).

ACCELERATED PHASE CML

The accelerated phase (89) includes the development of features associated with progressive maturation arrest and disease transformation. Morphologically, these changes are manifest by significant increases in both peripheral blood and marrow blasts and/or basophils (Table 39.5). NRBCs are 15% or more of the peripheral differential count. Extramedullary disease may also develop (97).

BLAST CRISIS (BLASTIC TRANSFORMATION)

The peripheral blood film invariably contains blasts, although their percentage may be less than the percentage of blasts in the aspirate smear (98–102). Myeloblasts plus promyelocytes, greater than 30% (either in the periphery or the aspirate), constitutes blast crisis. In addition, there is increasing immaturity of the entire neutrophilic series. The blasts are indistinguishable from those of de novo ALL or AML.

It is mandatory to perform immunologic, enzymatic, and cytochemical studies to assess the presence of terminal deoxyribonucleotidyl transferase (TdT) as well as other lymphoid and myeloid markers (80, 98, 101). The marrow may not be aspirable (''dry tap'') because of fibrosis. If aspirable, it is hypercellular, and blast cells usually constitute at least 10 to 15% of the leukocytic elements. Megakaryocytes may be either present, decreased, or absent.

The core biopsy is hypercellular in three-fourths of cases; patients with marked fibrosis tend to have bi-

Table 39.7. Differential Diagnosis of Neutrophilia

I. Nonneoplastic
  A. Infectious
    1. Bacterial, including mycobacterial
    2. Fungal
    3. Parasitic
    4. Viral (uncommon)
  B. Tissue necrosis
    1. Myocardial infarct
    2. Vasculitis
    3. Massive hemorrhage
  C. Drug-induced
    1. Steroids
    2. Epinephrine
    3. Lithium
  D. Miscellaneous
    1. Stress, physiological and nonphysiological
      a. Pregnancy and labor
      b. Electric shock
    2. Transient leukemoid reaction (TLR) in Down syndrome
    3. Hypereosinophilic syndrome (HES)
II. Neoplastic
  A. Metastatic carcinoma
  B. Hematologic
    1. MPDs
    2. Other
      a. HD and NHL
      b. AML, M4
      c. Myeloma
      d. ALL

opsies with lesser cellularity. The pattern of blastic involvement is most often diffuse, especially if the transformation is lymphoblastic. Erythroid elements are markedly reduced or absent.

Differential Diagnosis

The differential diagnosis of CML is usually that of a leukocytosis and, more specifically, that of a neutrophilia (74, 75, 90, 95). (Table 39.7) A leukemoid reaction is often a consideration. The combination of an elevated WBC count and a bimodal distribution may be helpful to distinguish CML from a leukemoid reaction: CML tends to have a '"peak" of myelocytes and metamyelocytes, whereas leukemoid reactions tend to have a PMN and bands '"peak." Changes in the PBS that may signify infection or an inflammatory state include the presence of toxic granulations and Döhle bodies. Also, the LAP score may be helpful. CMMoL may readily mimic CML; this is important because the long-term prognoses differ radically for most patients.

ESSENTIAL THROMBOCYTHEMIA

Essential thrombocythemia (ET), also known as primary thrombocythemia, is the rarest of the chronic MPDs (103–106). Patients with ET display a striking thrombocytosis in the absence of the increased red cell mass seen in PV, the leukocytosis and Ph[1] chromosome or *bcr* rearrangement of CML, and the marrow fibrosis of IMF. They also lack an underlying hemorrhagic, inflammatory, or neoplastic condition. The term "thrombocytosis" designates an elevated platelet count without regard to etiology; "thrombocythemia" should be restricted to very high platelet counts (greater than 600,000/μl [6 × 10^9/liter]) in the setting of the MPDs or an MDS. Isoenzyme studies of G6PD in female heterozygotes with ET have shown the disorder to be clonal and to involve granulocytes, erythrocytes, and platelets (4) (Fig. 39.5).

Table 39.8. Diagnostic Criteria—Essential Thrombocythemia[a]

1. Platelet count > 600,000/μl (600 × 10^9/liter).
2. Hemoglobin ≤ 13g/dl (2.02) or normal red cell mass. (males < 36 ml/kg; females < 32 ml/kg).
3. Stainable iron in marrow or failure of iron trial. (<1 g/dl [0.16] rise in Hb after 1 month of iron therapy).
4. No Philadelphia chromosome or *bcr* rearrangement.
5. Collagen fibrosis of marrow either absent or less than 1/3 biopsy area without both splenomegaly and leukoerythroblastic reaction.
6. No known cause for reactive thrombocytosis.

[a]Adapted from Murphy S, Iland HJ, Rosenthal D, Laszlo J. Essential thrombocythemia: an interim report for the polycythemia Vera Study Group. Semin Hematol 1986;23:178. Reprinted with permission of Grune & Stratton.

Clinical Presentation and Natural History

Originally known as hemorrhagic thrombocythemia (103), less is known about ET than about the other chronic MPDs. In spite of platelet numbers two, three, or more times normal, these patients bleed inappropriately, usually from the GI tract. But there is simultaneously the tendency to thrombosis, which may be venous or arterial. Transient ischemic attacks secondary to microcirculatory occlusion of the cerebral and retinal vessels are common. Erythromelalgia (digital ischemia with pain) is also frequent; it is easily treated with aspirin. Compared with the other chronic MPDs, there is a higher incidence of neurological manifestations in ET, probably also due to microvascular occlusion (107).

Established criteria for the diagnosis of ET are listed in Table 39.8. Many hematologists accept platelet counts over 600,000/μl (600 × 10^9/liter) and do not require counts in excess of one million/μl. Figure 39.6 is an algorithm for the evaluation of thrombocytosis.

The natural history of ET is more similar to that of PV than to CML or IMF/AMM (108, 109). Although more common in middle-aged patients, this disorder has been documented in both children and younger adults (110–112). Whethr ET has a more benign course in younger patients remains to be seen. Appropriate medical treatment appears to allow a nor-

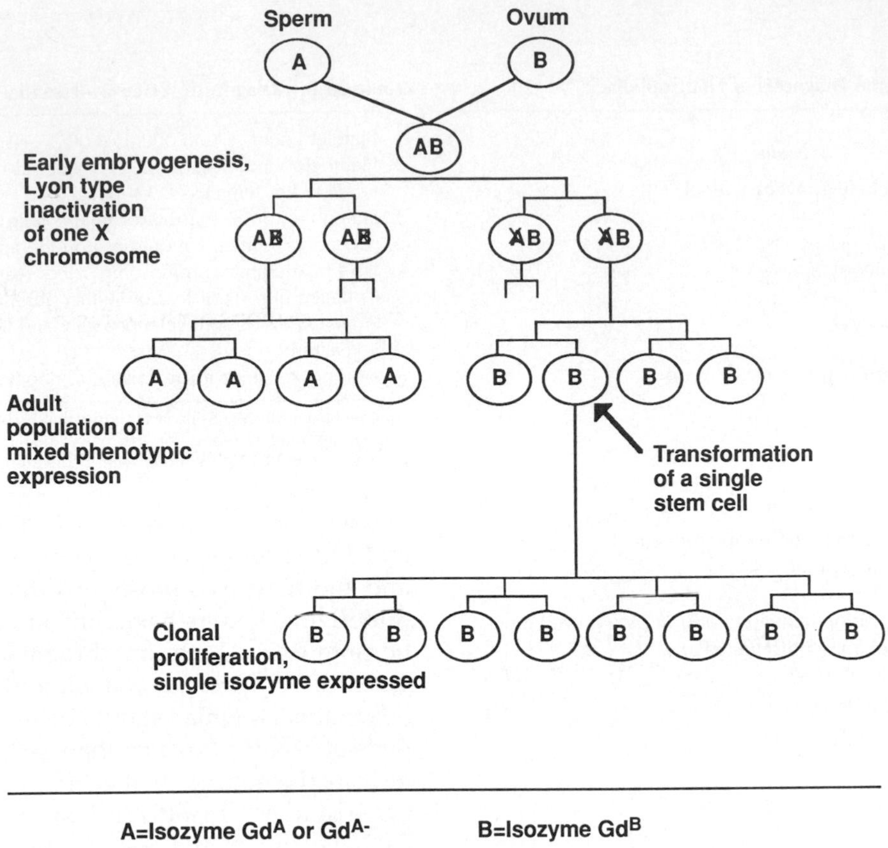

Figure 39.5. G6PD analysis in determining clonal origin of neoplasms.

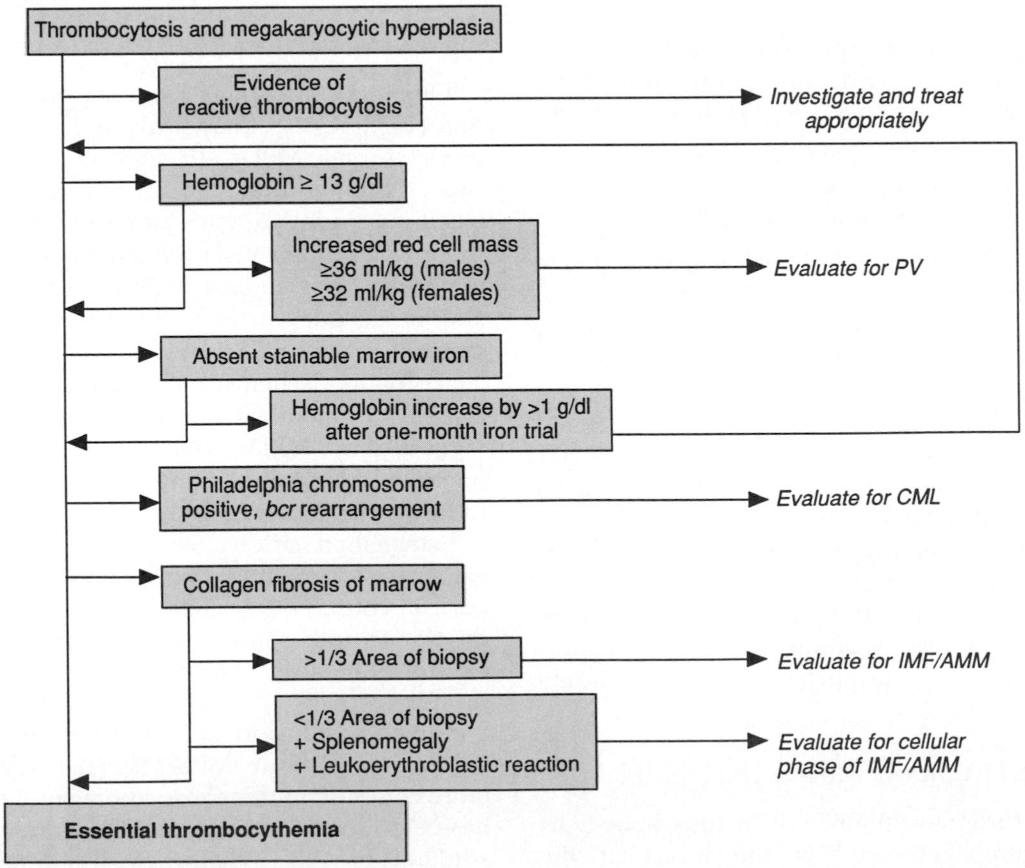

Figure 39.6. Algorithm for the evaluation of thrombocytosis. (Adapted from Iland HJ, Laszlo J, Peterson P, et al. Essential thrombocythemia: clinical and laboratory characteristics at presentation. Trans Assoc Am Phys 1983;96:167. Reprinted with permission.)

Table 39.9. Laboratory Characteristics of Patients with Essential Thrombocythemia[a]

Parameter	Median	Range
Hemoglobin (g/dl)	13.8 (2.14)	10.0–18.8 (1.55–2.91)
Red cell mass (ml/kg)	25	15–34
White cell count (/μl)	11,500 (11.5 × 10⁹/liter)	6,000–41,000 (6–41 × 10⁹/liter)
LAP score	79	0–171

[a]Adapted from Iland HJ, Laszlo J, Peterson P, et al. Essential thrombocythemia: clinical and laboratory characteristics at presentation. Trans Assoc Am Physicians 1983;96:167. Reprinted with permission of the Association of American Physicians.

mal life span (113, 114). Also, as with PV and CML, myelofibrotic and acute leukemic transformations occur, although the exact incidence is unknown (111, 114–118).

Splenomegaly is a less frequent physical finding than in PV, CML, or IMF. It occurs in fewer than 40% of patients and is of a lesser degree (less than 5 cm below the left costal margin).

Laboratory Studies

Some of the results of studies in patients who met strict criteria for ET (108) are shown in Table 39.9. Cytogenetic studies performed on patients meeting these criteria have failed to reveal a consistent cytogenetic abnormality (113, 119).

Abnormalities of platelet number are accompanied by abnormalities of platelet function (114, 120–122). A hallmark of ET (and of the other chronic MPDs) is abnormalities in platelet aggregation, most commonly a decreased responsiveness to epinephrine. One-third of patients will also exhibit aggregation defects in response to epinephrine and ADP (120).

In order to distinguish between patients with ET and thrombocytotic PV, a red cell mass determination must be performed when the tissue iron stores are documented. Otherwise, there is no single factor that separates ET patients from patients with PV (15, 109, 123).

Morphology of ET

PRETREATMENT

The peripheral blood film is most remarkable in terms of the increased numbers of platelets, often clumped, and their bizarre morphology (108, 124, 125). The qualitative abnormalities include giant platelets (megathrombocytes), atypical shapes, and irregular granulation. Fragments of megakaryocytes can be seen. NRBCs are present in 25% of patients, and there are minor degrees of anisocytosis and poikilocytosis. The leukocytes are generally unremarkable. Up to one-third of patients may display basophilia (greater than 100/μl [greater than 0.1×10^9/liter]).

The marrow cellularity ranges from normal to markedly increased; most marrows have a moderate increase in cellularity. The most striking finding is the megakaryocytic hyperplasia. In both the aspirate smear and biopsy, clumping or clustering is present, and platelet pools or lakes are common. The megakaryocytes are often bizarre and hyperlobated with abnormal mitoses. Erythroid and granulocytic hyperplasia may accompany the megakaryocytic hyperplasia, though not usually to the degree seen in PV. Iron stores are normal in this disorder, in contrast to PV. This is an important differential point (15, 47). If iron is absent in the aspirate smear, an iron trial is indicated since patients with PV may be iron deficient. Repletion of the iron stores should unmask the polycythemia.

DURING THERAPY

At present, there are very few studies of the changes that accompany therapy. At least in the short term, cellularity decreases, similar to changes seen in treated PV patients. This is reflected in normalization of the platelet count with diminished cellularity in both the aspirate smear and biopsy. Patients treated with recombinant α-INF have shown both decreased platelet counts and decreased megakaryocyte density in biopsies (126, 127).

TRANSFORMATION TO FIBROTIC STAGE AND/OR ACUTE LEUKEMIA

As in PV and CML, MF occurs in ET (114, 125). The percentage of patients who exhibit this change is not known. Those patients who do progress to MF show morphologic changes resembling those of the spent phase of PV.

Blastic or acute leukemic transformation occurs in ET, although the literature contains only sporadic case reports (114–118).

Differential Diagnosis

The differential diagnosis of an extremely elevated platelet count is long (Table 39.10). Inflammatory states and metastatic carcinomas are common causes; and iron-deficiency and postsplenectomy states may be associated with a thrombocytosis. Any other MPD may present with thrombocytosis (67, 106, 107) (90, 128, 129). A patient with an MDS, however, will more likely have thrombocytopenia; of the MDSs, the 5q- syndrome and refractory anemia with ring sideroblasts (RARS) are the two to consider.

Table 39.10. Differential Diagnosis of Thrombocytosis

I. Nonneoplastic
  A. Postsplenectomy state
  B. Iron-deficiency anemia
  C. Infections
  D. Vasculitides
II. Neoplastic
  A. Hematologic
    1. Polycythemia vera (PV)
    2. Chronic myelogenous leukemia (CML)
    3. Myelodysplastic syndromes (MDS)
      a. 5q- syndrome
      b. Refractory anemia with ring sideroblasts (RARS)
  B. Metastatic carcinoma

IDIOPATHIC MYELOFIBROSIS—AGNOGENIC MYELOID METAPLASIA

Patients are often allocated to the diagnostic category of idiopathic myelofibrosis (IMF) on the basis of splenic enlargement, a leukoerythroblastic (LEB) peripheral blood picture, and fibrosis of the marrow on biopsy. Since these findings may develop in patients with other chronic MPDs (130, 131) and with other disorders, additional tests must often be performed before assigning a patient this diagnosis.

Unlike PV, CML, and ET, G6PD isoenzyme studies show that this disorder is not clonal and does not involve a precursor to the erythroid, granulocytic-monocytic, and megakaryocytic lines (5, 6, 131–134).

Clinical Presentation and Natural History

Marrow failure results in pancytopenia. The patient's presenting complaint reflects complications of the anemia, thrombocytopenia, or granulocytopenia, or some combination thereof (19, 21–23, 135–138).

Hepatosplenomegaly is an almost invariable finding and is probably due in part to EMH; whether vascular thromboses account for some of the enlargement (as they probably do in PV) is not known.

IMF has a variable clinical course. Many patients die soon after diagnosis; others live 3 to 5 years; and still others have prolonged courses (19, 21–23, 135–138). Transformations to AL are well documented, especially in the older literature (19, 21–23, 39).

Laboratory Studies

The anemia in patients with IMF is usually normochromic and normocytic. This may be accompanied by a leukocytosis up to 30,000 to 40,000/μl (30 to 40 $\times$ 10^9/liter), although normal and decreased total white cell counts are common. The LAP score is normal or elevated.

The platelet count can vary widely. One-third of patients will have normal counts; another third will have marked thrombocytosis with counts greater than 1 million/μl (100 $\times$ 10^9/liter); the remaining third will have moderate elevations of the count. Thrombocytopenia accompanies later stages of the disease.

Consistent cytogenetic abnormalities have not been reported in several series (135, 136, 140). Indeed, cytogenetic studies may be impossible to obtain because of the impacted marrow.

Morphology of Idiopathic Myelofibrosis and Agnogenic Myeloid Metaplasia

The peripheral blood film is indistinguishable from that of patients with spent-phase PV or those with CML or ET with fibrotic marrows (22, 23). Most patients show an LEB peripheral blood picture: nucleated red blood cells and immature granulocytes. In some patients, peripheral blood examination fails to reveal the characteristic teardrop erythrocyte deformity. Attempts to aspirate marrow often result in dry taps.

The cellularity of the marrow biopsy is variable but tends to be hypocellular. There is usually both reticulin and collagen fibrosis with marked depletion of hematopoietic elements. Osteosclerosis—osteoblastic proliferation with disorganized new bone formation—frequently accompanies long-standing fibrosis (130, 136).

Any organ or tissue may show EMH. It most commonly occurs in spleen (23, 141), liver, and lymph nodes and is probably always present with a myelophthisic marrow.

The question of reversal of marrow fibrosis in idiopathic myelofibrosis (IMF) remains unanswered. Although AL "cures" MF, this is not a first-line therapeutic choice. Some studies indicate that the process is progressive and irreversible (23, 130, 135, 136). Other reports have documented regression of fibrosis, usually after intensive chemotherapy (119, 142, 143).

Differential Diagnosis

The differential diagnosis is extensive. (Table 39.11; Fig. 39.7). MF may be caused by infections: miliary tuberculosis is a well-documented cause and may be more common now than in the past 30 to 40 years. Other causes include carcinomas metastatic to marrow (breast, prostate, etc.), therapeutic and nontherapeutic radiation, and toxins (130, 137, 138). Marrow fibrosis appears to be integral to acute megakaryoblastic leukemia (AML, M7) (144). MF can also be present in other malignant hematologic disorders: Hodgkin's disease (HD), NHL, hairy cell leukemia, myeloma (121, 145, 146), and ALL (147).

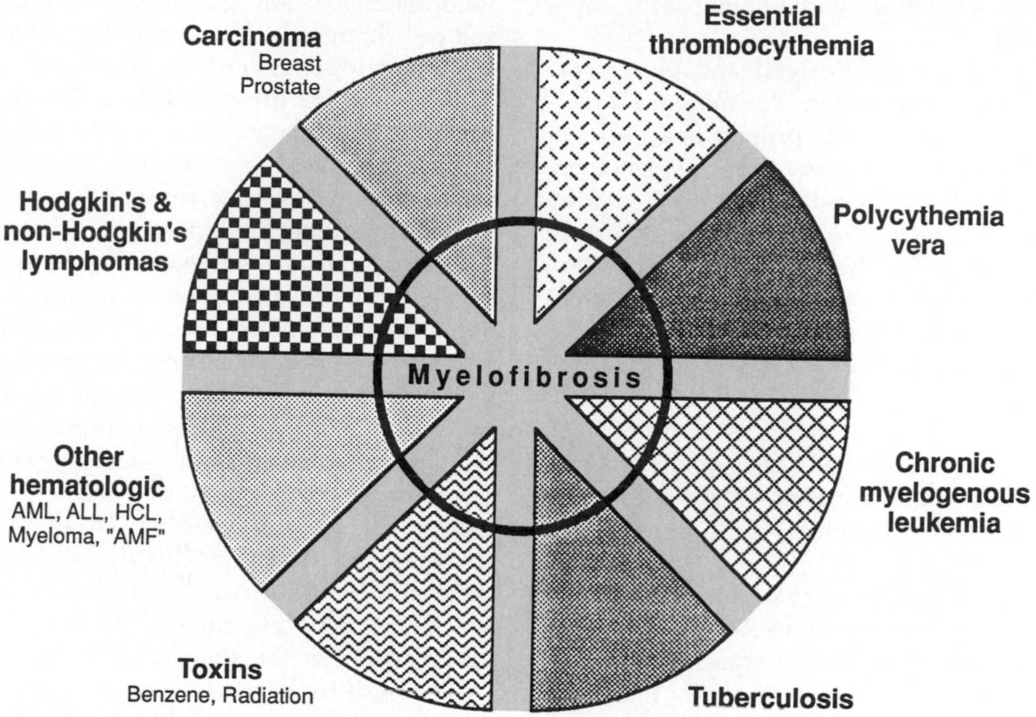

Figure 39.7. Conditions associated with myelofibrosis. (From Peterson P, McIntyre DR. Myeloproliferative disorders. Chicago: American Society of Clinical Pathologists Syllabus 1989;37. Reprinted with permission.)

Table 39.11. Differential Diagnosis of Marrow Fibrosis

- I. Nonneoplastic
  - A. Infections
    1. Miliary tuberculosis
    2. Congenital syphilis
  - B. Radiation
    1. Nontherapeutic (Hiroshima, Chernobyl)
    2. Therapeutic
  - C. Toxins
    1. Benzene
  - D. Associated with renal/endocrine disease
    1. Chronic renal failure
    2. Hyperparathyroidism
- II. Response to neoplastic process in marrow
  - A. Metastatic carcinoma
    1. Breast
    2. Prostate
    3. Other primary
  - B. Hematologic neoplasms
    1. Hodgkin's disease (HD)
    2. Myeloma
    3. Chronic MPD
       - a. PV
       - b. CML
       - c. ET
       - d. CMMoL
       - e. HES

CHRONIC MYELOMONOCYTIC LEUKEMIA

The defining feature of chronic myelomonocytic leukemia (CMMoL) is the presence of an absolute monocytosis (over 1000/µl [1.0×10^9/liter]) with at least 20% monocytes in the marrow (148). There is also an associated increase in mature granulocytes, with or without evidence of dysgranulopoiesis. The percentage of myeloblasts in the peripheral blood is less than 5% and in the marrow, 5 to 20%. Almost all patients have concomitant refractory anemia. Clinically, this disorder is characterized by special features related to the proliferation of monocytes—elevated serum lysozyme levels, leukemia cutis, and serous effusions. Splenomegaly is more common in this disorder than in the other MDSs and occurs in one-third to two-fifths of patients.

The first descriptions of CMMoL (149, 150) were followed by numerous reports (151–154) of syndromes bearing similar names. The 1982 French-American-British (FAB) classification (148) of myelodysplastic syndromes (MDS) utilized a morphologic base to define these disorders, of which CMMoL was then one. It seems more appropriate, however, to consider CMMoL as an MPD.

Clinical Course and Natural History

The clinical course of CMMoL is quite variable. Some patients behave more like true preleukemia victims, with termination in as short a period (less than 1 year) as AL; others have a relatively benign course with long (greater than 5-year) survivals (7, 153, 155–158). This disorder is more likely than any of the MDSs to be confused with another MPD, especially with CML.

CMMoL occurs in middle-aged and elderly patients, with no sex predilection. Anemia and thrombocytopenia are common. Poor prognostic features at diagnosis include high monocyte counts, splenomegaly, greater than 5% blasts in the periphery, and the biopsy finding of abnormal localization of immature precursors (ALIP) (158). The monocytic proliferation serves as the diagnostic marker and is an important feature in the assessment of prognosis, as is an increasing number of blast cells in blood and marrow (159).

Median survival in most series is 12 months (7, 152, 155–157, 159, 160), but all series document prolonged survival in some patients. Death occurs secondary to infections or bleeding, if AL does not supervene.

In the setting of peripheral cytopenias, myelodysplasia, and a hypercellular marrow, chromosomal studies are warranted. Although some CMMoL patients display chromosomal abnormalities, many will initially have a normal karyotype (161, 162). The most common karyotypic abnormalities are: 5q-, 20q-, trisomy 8, monosomy 5, monosomy 7, and loss of the Y chromosome (160, 163). No specific chromosomal abnormalities have been consistently associated with CMMoL. Not surprisingly, patients with a normal karyotype and those with '"stable" karyotypes over time are less likely to evolve into AML (7, 152, 155, 157, 159). The percentage of patients with CMMoL who progress to AL ranges from 10 to 25%. It would appear, then, that CMMoL is a clonal myeloproliferative disorder more of a qualitative than a quantitative nature.

Laboratory Studies

Because of the monocytic proliferation, serum and urine muramidase (lysozyme) levels are often elevated. The serum level has occasionally been used to predict CNS involvement. The LAP level is usually high.

Morphology of CMMoL

PRETREATMENT

A monocytosis greater than 1000/μl (1.0×10^9/liter) is the defining feature of CMMoL, and the extreme elevations in the white cell count are reflected in the peripheral blood film (164–168). The great majority of the leukocytes are monocytes. They may appear normal or may have abnormally large, variably staining granules. Granulocytes may also show hypogranulation, abnormal granulation, and nuclear abnormalities. Total myeloblasts do not exceed 5%. Red cell changes include macrocytes, ovalocytes, basophilic stippling, and a dimorphic population. NRBCs may be present. Either thrombocytosis or thrombocytopenia may be present, and platelets may be hypogranular.

The marrow aspirate smear is hypercellular with marked granulocytic hyperplasia. The granulocytic: erythroid ratio is increased. The changes observed in the PBS are also present in the aspirate: hypogranulation and/or abnormal granulation of the monocytic-neutrophilic series, hyposegmentation of nuclei, and increased numbers of myeloblasts (between 5 and 15%). There is abnormal staining of the primary granules in promyelocytes and myelocytes. The cytoplasm may show peripheral basophilia. Auer rods are not present. Dyserythropoiesis is characterized by multinuclearity, nuclear fragmentation and budding, and nuclear-cytoplasmic dyssynchrony. The cytoplasmic abnormalities include irregularities in the density of staining. Dysmegakaryopoiesis is characterized by megakaryoblasts, micromegakaryocytes (similar to CML), and mono- and bilobated forms.

The marrow biopsy (165, 166, 168) is also hypercellular. Iron is usually present. As in the aspirate, the granulocytic/monocytic series predominates and shows a shift to less mature precursors. The erythroid series shows islands of erythroblasts in the same stage of differentiation. Megakaryocytes abnormalities include: micromegakaryocytes, mono- or bilobated megakaryocytes, and size variation. An increase in reticulin fiber content and sometimes overt MF occur (169). The biopsy may show ALIP (158), a phenomenon in which blasts and promyelocytes cluster in the central marrow spaces.

TRANSFORMATION TO AL

The AL occurring in CMMoL is nonlymphocytic (170). As expected, the PBS invariably shows blasts. In addition, there is increasing immaturity of the entire monocytic/neutrophilic series. The blasts are indistinguishable from those of de novo AML. The FAB subtypes (144, 171–174) may vary, and Auer rods may or may not be present. As in CML in transformation, pseudo-Pelger-Huet cells may be seen.

Differential Diagnosis

The differential diagnosis of CMMoL includes: CML, vitamin B12 and folate deficiencies, metabolic abnormalities (renal, hepatic, endocrine), and toxic or drug-induced disorders (175, 176) (Tables 39.10 and 39.11).

IDIOPATHIC HYPEREOSINOPHILIC SYNDROME

Idiopathic hypereosinophilic syndrome (HES) is a systemic disorder with peripheral blood and marrow eosinophilia and variable organ system dysfunction with eosinophilic infiltration (177, 178). Since eosinophilia is usually associated with distinctive disease processes—parasitic infections, allergic and immunodeficient states, cutaneous disorders and tumors (bronchogenic carcinomas, HD, and T-cell leukemias and lymphomas) (179–181)—patients with a persistent eosinophilia in whom these diseases have been excluded are considered to have HES. Whether a single disease or a group of disorders, HES is rare. It occurs worldwide, affects men more than women (5 to 10:1), and is usually diagnosed between ages 20 and 50. Presenting complaints vary, ranging from weakness and fatigue to myalgias, cough, fevers, dyspnea (178, 182–184). Until the advent of immunosuppressive therapy, the prognosis in HES was poor; death occurs in less than a year (178, 182, 185). Of the nonhematologic organ systems involved, the most frequent are the cardiac and central nervous systems (CNS). One-third to three-fifths of patients will manifest cardiac symptoms sometime during their illness (158, 182–184, 186).

Thromboembolic disease involving the medium to larger blood vessels is an integral part of HES. Mural thrombi involving the mitral and tricuspid valves, subsequent embolization, and endomyocardial and endocardial fibrosis is the expected pattern of cardiac disease. The initial insult, an acute eosinophilic myocarditis (187), is thought secondary to eosinophil-induced injury to the endothelial cells of the endocardium and the microvasculature. A similar pattern of injury is postulated to explain the CNS dysfunctions. CNS dysfunction manifests as diffuse disturbances, neuropathies, or ataxia (180, 182).

The defining feature of HES is persistent eosinophilia (greater than 1500/μl [greater than 1.5×10^9/liter]) with signs and symptoms of organ involvement and without a discernible etiology (178). Anemia is present in over half of patients, and thrombocytopenia is more common than thrombocytosis (188).

MYELOPROLIFERATIVE DISORDERS IN DOWN SYNDROME

Down syndrome (DS) is the most common disorder associated with a chromosomal abnormality worldwide (189). Physiological abnormalities common in individuals with DS include cardiac anomalies, infections, mental retardation, and increased risk of malignancies. This increased risk of malignancy is almost always manifested as AL, whether ALL or ANLL. DS individuals have a 10 to 20% greater risk of developing AL before the age of 10. This risk extends into adulthood, resulting in a DS infant having a one in 95 chance of developing AL in its lifetime (190). There are bimodal peaks in the DS leukemic population: the first occurs in the newborn period and the other between 3 and 6 years. The peak occurring in the neonatal age group includes cases of congenital leukemia (CL) and the MPD, known as transient leukemoid reaction (TLR). TLR is much more common than true CL.

CL in infants with DS is usually a myelogenous leukemia. Diagnosis is often delayed because the clinical and hematologic manifestations are common in other neonatal disorders, and the distinction from TLR is difficult. Physical findings include fever and hepatosplenomegaly without lymphadenopathy. Cutaneous lesions include petechiae, purpura, and blue-gray leukemic skin nodules. Workup usually reveals an LEB reaction. Classically, the complete blood count (CNC) reveals an elevated white blood count (WBC) and thrombocytopenia. The peripheral smear and differential white cell count show numerous immature forms and nucleated RBCs. The marrow studies show markedly decreased numbers of erythroid precursors, megakaryocytes, and mature granulocytes (191). Without chemotherapeutic treatment, these children have a high mortality.

TLR is a phenomenon seen exclusively in newborns with DS and non-DS constitutional trisomy 21 mosaicism. It is characterized by circulating blasts in the peripheral blood with a spontaneous regression. Physical findings resemble those of CL; however, there may be an associated lymphadenopathy. A CBC often reveals a marked leukocytosis and thrombocytopenia. The PBS may show a myeloblastosis with megakaryoblastic proliferation and megathrombocytes with abnormal platelets (192).

The major distinction between TLR and CL appears to be in progenitor cell potential (193). Infants with CL have markedly decreased or immature CFU-GM colony growth, whereas those with TLR have normal colony growth and proliferation. The significance of these findings resides in the recognition that left untreated, TLR will spontaneously remit within a few weeks, whereas CL is fatal. A marrow aspiration and biopsy may be helpful in distinguishing between the two disorders. Despite the rather benign course of TLR, 25% of DS infants with this disease will develop acute megakaryocytic leukemia (AML, M-7) within 3 years (194).

Acknowledgments

I thank John T. Ellis, M.D., Robert V. Pierre, M.D., and O. Ross McIntyre, M.D., for their interest and support. I am grateful to Ms. R. Y. Bethea and Mrs. Barbara Whyte for their technical and secretarial help.

References

1. Adamson JW, Fialkow PJ, Murphy S, Prchal JF, Steinman L. Polycythemia vera: stem cell and probable clonal origin of the disease. N Engl J Med 1976;295:913–916.
2. Fialkow PJ, Jacobson RJ, Papayannopoulou T. Chronic myelocytic leukemia: clonal origin in a stem cell common to the granulocyte, erythrocyte, platelet and monocyte/macrophage. Am J Med 977;63:125–130.
3. Rowley JD. A new consistent chromosomal abnormality in chronic myelogenous leukaemia identified by guinicrine, fluorescence and giemsa staining. Nature 1973;243:290–293.
4. Fialkow PJ, Faguet GB, Jacobson RJ, et al. Evidence that essential thrombocythemia is a clonal disorder with origin in a multipotent stem cell. Blood 1981;58:916–919.
5. Buschle M, Jannsen JW, Drexler H, Lyons J, Anger B, Bartram CR. Evidence for pluripotent stem cell origin of idiopathic myelofibrosis: clonal analysis of a case characterized by N-ras gene mutation. Leukemia 1988;2:658–660.
6. Jacobson RJ, Salo A, Fialkow PJ. Agnogenic myeloid metaplasia: a clonal proliferation of hematopoietic stem cells with secondary myelofibrosis. Blood 1978;51:189–194.
7. Gyger M, Infante-Rivard C, D'Angelo G, et al. Prognostic value of clonal chromosomal abnormalities in patients with primary myelodysplastic syndromes. Am J Hematol 1988;28: 13–200.
8. Heisterkamp N, Stephenson JR, Groffen J, et al. Localization of the *c-abl* oncogene adjacent to a translocation breakpoint in chronic myelocytic leukaemia. Nature 1983;306:239–242.
9. Kaye FJ, Najfeld V, Singer J, Cuttner J, Fialkow RJ. Confirming evidence for the clonal development and stem-cell origin of Philadelphia-chromosome negative chronic myelogenous leukemia. Am J Hematol 1984;17:93–100.
10. Kurzrock R, Gutterman JU, Talpaz M. The molecular genetics of Philadelphia chromosome-positive leukemias. N Engl J Med 1988;319:990–998.
11. Epner DE, Koeffler HP. Molecular genetic advances in chronic myelogenous leukemia. Ann Intern Med 1990;113:3–6.
12. Hirosawa S, Aoki N, Matsushime H, Shibuya M. Undetectable *bcr-abl* rearrangements in some CML patients are due to a deletion mutation in the *bcr* gene. Am J Hematol 1988;28: 33–36.
13. Westin J, Wahlström J, Swolin B. Chromosome studies in untreated polycythaemia vera. Scand J Haematol 1976;17:183–196.
14. Wurster-Hill D, Whang-Peng J, McIntyre OR, et al. Cytogenetic studies in polycythemia vera. Semin Hematol 1976;13: 13–32.
15. Ellis JT, Peterson P, Geller SA, Rappaport H. Studies of the bone marrow in polycythemia vera and the evolution of myelofibrosis and second hematologic malignancies. Semin Hematol 1986;23:144–155.
16. Nelson B, Kniseley RM. Marrow fibrosis in myeloproliferative disorders. In: Clarke WJ, Howard EB, Hackett PL, eds. Myeloproliferative disorders of animals and man. Washington, DC: U.S. Atomic Energy Commission Symposium Series 19, 1970:533–555.
17. Peterson P, Wasserman LR. The natural history of polycythemia vera. In: Wasserman LR, Berlin NI, Berk PD, eds. Polycythemia vera and the myeloproliferative disorders. Philadelphia: WB Saunders, 1994.
18. Clough V, Geary CG, Hashmi K, et al. Myelofibrosis in chronic granulocytic leukaemia. Br J Haematol 1979;42:515–526.
19. Bouroncle BA, Doan CA. Myelofibrosis: Cinical, hematologic and pathologic study of 110 patients. Am J Med Sci 1962;243: 697–715.
20. Burston J, Pinniger JL. The reticulum content of bone marrow in haematological disorders. Br J Haematol 1963;9:172–184.
21. Pitcock JA, Reinhard EH, Justus BW, Mendelsohn RS. A clinical and pathological study of seventy cases of myelofibrosis. Ann Intern Med 1962;57:73–84.
22. Thiele J, Zankovich R, Steinberg T, Fischer R, Diehl V. Agnogenic myeloid metaplasia (AMM)—correlation of bone marrow lesions with laboratory data: a longitudinal study on 114 patients. Hematol Oncol 1989;7:327–343.
23. Ward HP, Block MH. The natural history of agnogenic myeloid metaplasia (AMM) and a critical evaluation of its relationship with the myeloproliferative syndrome. Medicine 1971;50:357–420.
24. Pagliuca A, Layton DM, Manoharan A, Gordon SM, Green PJ, Mufti GJ. Myelofibrosis in primary myelodysplastic syndromes: a clinicopathologic study of 10 cases. Br J Haematol 1989;71:499–504.
25. Maschek H, Georgii A, Kaloutsi V, et al. Myelofibrosis in primary myelodysplastic syndromes: a retrospective study of 352 patients. Eur J Haemotol 1992;48:208–214.
26. Vaquez HM. Sur une forme speciale de cyanose accompagnant d'hyperglobulie excessive et persistante. C R Soc Biol (Paris) 1892;44:384–388.
27. Osler W. Chronic cyanosis with polycythemia and enlarged spleen: a new clinical entity. Am J Med Sci 1903;126:187–201.
28. Rosenthal N, Bassen FA. Course of polycythemia. Arch Intern Med 1938;62:903–917.
29. Minot GR, Buckman TE. Erythremia (Polycythemia rubra vera). The development of anemia; the relation to leukemia; consideration of the basal metabolism, blood formation and destruction and fragility of the red cells. Am J Med Sci 1923;166:469–489.
30. Rosenthal MC. Extramedullary hematopoiesis. Myeloid metaplasia. Bull N Engl Med Cntr 1950;12:154–160.
31. Dameshek W. Some speculations on the myeloproliferative syndromes. Blood 1951;6:372–375.
32. Najean Y, Mugnier P, Dresch C, Rain J-D. Polycythaemia vera in young people: an analysis of 58 cases diagnosed before 40 years. Br J Haematol 1987;67:285–291.
33. Berglund S, Zettervall O. Incidence of polycythemia vera in a defined population. Eur J Haematol 1992;48:20–26.
34. Chievitz E, Thiede T. Complications and causes of death in polycythaemia vera. Acta Med Scand 1962;172:513–523.
35. Berk PD, Goldberg JD, Donovan PB, et al. Therapeutic recommendations in polycythemia vera study group protocols. Semin Hematol 1986;23:132–143.
36. Wasserman LR, Balcrzak SP, Berk PD, et al. Influence of therapy on causes of death in polycythemia vera. Trans Assoc Am Physicians 1981;94:30–38.
37. Berk PD, Goldberg JD, Silverstein MN, et al. Increased incidence of acute leukemia in polycythemia vera associated with chlorambucil therapy. N Engl J Med 1981;304:441–447.
38. Nand S, Messmore H, Fisher SG, Bird ML, Schulz W, Fisher RI. Leukemic transformation in polycythemia vera: analysis of risk factors. Am J Hematol 1990;34:32–36.
39. Landaw SA. Acute leukemia in polycythemia vera. Semin Hematol 1986;23:156–165.
40. Fruchtman SM, Kaplan ME, Peterson P, et al. Hydroxyurea (HU) in the management of polycythemia vera (PV): analysis

of long-term leukemogenic potential. [Abstract] Clin Res 1992;40:281.

41. Wasserman LR. Polycythemia vera—its course and treatment: relation to myeloid metaplasia and leukemia. Bull NY Acad Med 1954;3:343–375.
42. Peterson P, Ellis JT, Geller SA, Rappaport H. Increased incidence of acute leukemia in spent polycythemia following myelosuppresive therapy [Abstract]. Lab Invest 1986;54:48a.
43. Lawrence JH, Winchell HS, Donald WG. Leukemia in polycythemia vera: relationships to splenic myeloid metaplasia and therapeutic radiation dose. Ann Intern Med 1969;70:763–771.
44. Peterson P, Ellis JT, Block MH, Geller SA, Rappaport H. The occurrence of non-Hodgkin's lymphoma in polycythemia vera [Abstract]. Lab Invest 1985;52:51a.
45. Ellis JT, Peterson P. The bone marrow in polycythemia vera. In: Berlin NI, Berk PD, Wasserman LR, eds. Polycythemia and the myeloproliferative disorders. Philadelphia: WB Saunders, 1994:(in press).
46. Berlin NI. Diagnosis and classification of the polycythemias. Semin Hematol 1975;12:339–351.
47. Ellis JT, Peterson P. The bone marrow in polycythemia vera. Pathol Annul 1979;13:383–403.
48. Silverstein MN. Post-polycythemia myeloid metaplasia. Arch Intern Med 1974;134:113–120.
49. Wolf BC, Banks PM, Mann RB, Neiman RS. Splenic hematopoiesis in polycthemia vera. A morphologic and immunohistologic study. Am J Clin Pathol 1988;89:69–75.
50. Wanless IR, Peterson P, Das A, Boitnott JK, Moore GW, Bernier V. Portal hypertension in agnogenic myeloid metaplasia (AMM) and polycythemia vera (PV): a clinico-pathological study. Hepatology 1990;12:1166–1174.
51. Modan B. Lilienfeld AM. Polycythemia vera and leukemia—the role of radiation treatment: a study of 1222 patients. Medicine 1965;44:305–344.
52. Szur L, Lewis SM. The haematological complications of polycythaemia vera and treatment with radioactive phosphorus. Br J Radiol 1966;39:122–130.
53. Tubiana M, Flamant R, Attie E, et al. A study of hematological complications occurring in patients with polycythemia vera treated with ^{32}P. Blood 1968;32:536–548.
54. Silverstein MN. Myeloproliferative diseases. Postgrad Med 1977;61:206–210.
55. Berk PD, Goldberg JD, Ellis JT, et al. Malignant complications of longterm myelosuppression with ^{32}P or chlorambucil in polycythemia vera. [Abstract] Blood 1985;66:194.
56. Cronkite EP, Moloney W, Bond VP. Radiation leukemogenesis: an analysis of the problem. Am J Med 1960;28:673–701.
57. Bonnadonna G, DeLena M, Banfi A, et al. Secondary neoplasms in malignant lymphomas after intensive therapy. N Engl J Med 1973;288:1242–1243.
58. Reimer RR, Hoover R, Fraumeni JF, et al. Acute leukemia after alkylating-agent therapy of ovarian cancer. N Engl J Med 1977;297:177–181.
59. Casciato DA, Scott JL. Acute leukemia following prolonged cytotoxic agent therapy. Medicine 1979;58:32–47.
60. Fogelfeld L, Wiviott MBT, Shore-Freedman E, et al. Recurrence of thyroid nodules after surgical removal in patients irradiated in childhood for benign conditions. N Engl J Med 1989;320:835–840.
61. Pui C-H, Behm FG, Raimondi SC, et al. Secondary acute myeloid leukemia in children treated for acute lymphoid leukemia. N Engl J Med 1989;321:136–142.
62. Kaldor JM, Day NE, Pettersson F, et al. Leukemia following chemotherapy for ovarian cancer. N Engl J Med 1990;322:1–6.
63. Kaldor JM, Day NE, Clarke A, et al. Leukemia following Hodgkin's disease. N Engl J Med 1990;322:7–13.
64. Coltman CA Jr, Dahlberg S. Treatment-related leukemia. N Engl J Med 1990;322:52–53.
65. Weinreb NJ, Shih CF. Spurious polycythemia. Semin Hematol 1975;13:397–407.
66. Smith JR, Landaw SA. Smokers' polycythemia. N Engl J Med 1978;298:6–10.
67. Bakhshi A, Minowada J, Arnold A, et al. Lymphoid blast crisis of chronic myelogenous leukemia represents stages in the development of B-cell precursors. N Engl J Med 1983;309:826–831.
68. Martin RJ, Najfeld V, Hansen JA, Penfold GK, Jacobson RJ, Fialkow PJ. Involvement of the B-lymphoid system in chronic myelogenous leukemia. Nature 1980;287:49–50.
69. Chessells JM, Janossy G, Lawler SD, Secker Walker LM. The Ph[1] chromosome in childhood leukaemia. Br J Haematol 1979;41:25–41.
70. Nowell PC, Hungerford DA. A minute chromosome in human chronic granulocytic leukemia. Science 1960;132:1497.
71. Bartram CR, de Klein A, Hagemeijer A, et al. Translocation of *c-abl* oncogene correlates with the presence of a Philadelphia chromosome in chronic myelocytic leukaemia. Nature 1983;306:277–280.
72. Ishihara T, Minamihisamatsu M, Tosuji-H. Chromosome 9 in variant Ph-translocations. Cancer Genet Cytogenet 1985;14:183–184.
73. Kadam PR, Nanjangid GJ, Advani SH. The occurrence of variant Ph translocations in chronic myeloid leukemia (CML): a report of six cases. Hematol Oncol 1990;8:303–312.
74. Crisan D, Mattson JC, Al-Saadi A. Chronic granulocytic leukemia: reassessment of morphologic and cytogenetic characteristics in Ph[1]-positive and Ph[1]-negative cases. Eur J Haematol 1991;46:77–84.
75. Martiat P, Michaux JL, Rodhain J, et al. Philadelphia-negative (Ph−) chronic myeloid leukemia (CML): comparison with Ph+ CML and chronic myelomonocytic leukemia. Blood 1991; 78:205–211.
76. Kantarjian HM, Keating MJ, Walters RS, et al. Clinical and prognostic features of Philadelphia chromosome-negative chronic myelogenous leukemia. Cancer 1986;58:2023–2030.
77. Kurzrock R, Blick MB, Talpaz M, et al. Rearrangement in the breakpoint cluster region and the clinical course in Philadelphia negative chronic myelogenous leukemia. Ann Intern Med 1986;105:673–679.
78. Mills KI, Benn P, Birnie GD. Does the breakpoint within the major breakpoint cluster region (M-bcr) influence the duration of the chronic phase in chronic myeloid leukemia? An analytical comparison of current literature. Blood 1991;78:1155–1161.
79. Catovsky D. Annotation. Ph[1]-positive acute leukaemia and chronic granulocytic leukaemia: One or two diseases? Br J Haematol 1979;42:493–498.
80. Priest JR, Robinson LL, McKenna RW, et al. Philadelphia chromosome positive childhood acute lymphoblastic leukemia. Blood 1980;56:15–22.
81. Clark SS, McLaughlin J, Crist WM, Champlin R, Witte ON. Unique forms of the *abl* tyrosine kinase distinguish Ph[1]-positive CML from Ph[1]-positive ALL. Science 1987;237:85–86.
82. Fialkow PJ, Martin PJ, Najfeld V, Penfold GK, Jacobson RJ, Hansen JA. Evidence of a multistep pathogenesis of chronic myelogenous leukemia. Blood 1981;58:158–163.
83. Dowding C, Guo A-P, Osterholz J, Siczkowski M, Goldman J, Gordon M. Interferon-alpha overrides the deficient adhesion of chronic myeloid leukemia primitive progenitor cells to bone marrow stromal cells. Blood 1991;78:499–505.
84. Talpaz M, Kantarjian H, Kurzrock R, Trujillo JM, Gutterman JU. Interferon-alpha produces sustained cytogenetic responses in chronic myelogenous leukemia. Philadelphia

chromosome-positive patients. Ann Intern Med 1991;114: 532–538.

85. Talpaz M, Kantarjian HM, McCredie K, Trujillo JM, Keating MJ, Gutterman JU. Hematologic remission and cytogenetic improvement induced by recombinant human interferon alpha, in chronic myelogenous leukemia. N Engl J Med 1986;314:1065–1069.
86. Speck B, Bortin M, Champlin R, et al. Allogeneic bone marrow transplantation for chronic myelogenous leukaemia. Lancet 1984;1:665–668.
87. McGlave PB, Beatty P, Ash R, Hows JM. Therapy for chronic myelogenous leukemia with unrelated donor bone marrow transplantation: results in 102 cases. Blood 1990;75:1728–1732.
88. Thomas ED, Clift RA. Indications for marrow transplantation in chronic myelogenous leukemia. Blood 1989;73:861–864.
89. Kantarjian HM, Dixon D, Keating MJ, et al. Characteristics of accelerated disease in chronic myelogenous leukemia. Cancer 1988;61:1441–1446.
90. Stoll DB, Peterson P, Exten R, et al. Clinical presentation and natural history of patients with essential thrombocythemia and the Philadelphia chromosome. Am J Hematol 1988;27: 77–83.
91. Larson J, Kjeldsberg CR. May-Grünwald giemsa stain for plastic-embedded bone marrow specimens. Lab Med 1984;15: 412–413.
92. Dekmezian R, Kantarjian HM, Keating MJ, et al. The relevance of reticulin stain-measured fibrosis at diagnosis in chronic myelogenous leukemia. Cancer 1987;59:1739–1743.
93. Buhr T, Choritz H, Georgii A. The inpact of megakayocyte proliferation for the evolution of myelofibrosis. Histological follow-up study in 186 patients with chronic myeloid leukaemia. Virchows Archio Pathol Anat 1992;420:473–478.
94. Lee RE, Ellis LD. The storage cells of chronic myelogenous leukemia. Lab Invest 1971;24:261–264.
95. Savage RA. Specific and not-so-specific histiocytes in bone marrow. Lab Med 1984;15:467–471.
96. Vodopick H, Rupp EM, Edwards CI, Goswitz FA, Beauchamp JJ. Spontaneous cyclic leukocytosis and thrombocytosis in chronic myelogenous leukemia. N Engl J Med 1972;286:284–289.
97. Terjanian T, Kantarjian HM, Keating M, et al. Clinical and prognostic factors of patients with Philadelphia chromosome-positive chronic myelogenous leukemia and extramedullary disease. Cancer 1987;59:297–300.
98. Polli N, O'Brien M, Tavares de Castro J, Matutes E, San Migual JF, Catovsky D. Characterization of blast cells in chronic granulocytic leukaemia in transformation, acute myelofibrosis and undifferentiated leukaemia. I. Ultrastructural morphology and cytochemistry. Br J Haematol 1985;59:277–296.
99. Rosenthal S, Canellos GP, DeVita VT, Jr, Gralnick HR. Characteristics of blast crisis in chronic granulocytic leukemia. Blood 1977;49:705–714.
100. Karansas A, Silver RT. Characteristics of the terminal phase of chronic granulocytic leukemia. Blood 1968;32:445–459.
101. San Miguel JF, Tavares de Castro J, Matutes E, et al. Characterization of blast cells in chronic granulocytic leukaemia in transformation, acute myelofibrosis and undifferentiated leukaemia. II. Studies with monoclonal antibodies and terminal transferase. Br J Haematol 1985;59:297–307.
102. Kantarjian HM, Keating MJ, Talpaz M, et al. Chronic myelogenous leukemia in blast crisis: an analysis of 242 patients. Am J Med 1987;83:445–454.
103. Hardisty RM, Wolff HH. Hemorrhagic thrombocythaemia: a clinical and laboratory study. Br J Haematol 1955;1:390–405.
104. Gunz FW. Hemorrhagic thrombocythaemia: a critical review. Blood 1960;15:706–723.
105. Ozer FL, Truax WE, Miesch DC, Levin WC. Primary hemorrhagic thrombocythemia. Am J Med 1960;28:807–808.
106. Silverstein MN. Primary or hemorrhagic thrombocythemia. Arch Intern Med 1968;122:18–22.
107. Jabaily J, Iland H, Laszlo J, et al. Neurologic manifestations of essential thrombocythemia. Ann Intern Med 1983;99:513–518.
108. Iland HJ, Laszlo J, Peterson P, et al. Essential thrombocythemia: clinical and laboratory characteristics at presentation. Trans Assoc Am Physicians 1983;96:165–174.
109. Iland HJ, Laszlo J, Case DC, et al. Differentiation between essential thrombocythemia and polycythemia vera with marked thrombocytosis. Am J Hematol 1987;25:191–201.
110. McIntyre KJ, Hoagland HC, Silverstein MN, Petitt RM. Essential thrombocythemia in young adults. Mayo Clin Proc 1991;66:149–154.
111. Mitus AJ, Barbuli T, Shulman LN, et al. Hemostatic complications in young patients with essential thrombocythemia. Am J Med 1990;88:371–375.
112. Randi ML, Fabris F, Girolami A. Thrombocytosis in young people: evaluation of 57 cases diagnosed before the age of 40. Blut 1990;60;233–237.
113. Murphy S, Iland H, Rosenthal D, Laszlo J. Essential thrombocythemia: an interim report for the Polycythemia Vera Study Group. Semin Hematol 1986;23:177–182.
114. Hehlmann R, Jahn M, Baumann B, Köpcke W. Essential thrombocythemia: clinical characteristics and course of 61 cases. Cancer 1988;61:2487–2496.
115. Honma K, Nemoto K, Ohnishi Y, Kimura K. Blastic transformation of essential thrombocythemia. A case report. Acta Pathol Jpn 1989;39:670–676.
116. Sedlacek SM, Curtis JL, Weintraub J, Levin J. Essential thrombocythemia and leukemic transformation. Medicine 1986;65:353–364.
117. Kimura A, Fujimoto T, Inada T, et al. Blastic transformation in essential thrombocythemia. Cancer 1990;65:1538–1544.
118. Murphy S, Peterson P, Iland HJ, Fruchtman S, Hydroxyurea and other myelosuppressive agents in the treatment of essential thrombocythemia: analysis of leukemogenic potential. [Abstract] Thromb Haemost 1993:69.
119. Nakamura H, Hayashibara T, Kawachi T, et al. Chromosome 11 rearrangement at band 11q21 in a patient with essential thrombocythemia. Cancer Gen Cytogen 1992;58:105–107.
120. Kaywin P, McDonough M, Insel PA, Shattil SJ. Platelet function in essential thrombocythemia. N Engl J Med 1978;299: 505–509.
121. Holme S, Murphy S. Platelet abnormalities in myeloproliferative disorders. Clin Lab Med 1990;10:873–888.
122. Sehayek E, Ben-Yosef N, Modan M, Chetrit A, Meytes D. Platelet parameters and aggregation in essential and reactive thrombocytosis. Am J Clin Pathol 1988;90:431–436.
123. Buss DH, O'Connor ML, Woodruff RD, Richards F, Brockschmidt JK. Bone marrow and peripheral blood findings in patients with extreme thrombocytosis: a report of 63 cases. Arch Pathol Lab Med 1991;115:475–480.
124. Thiele J, Schneider G, Hoeppner B, Weinhold S, Zankovich R, Fischer R. Histomorphometry of bone marrow biopsies in chronic myeloproliferative disorders with associated thrombocytosis—features of significance for the diagnosis of primary (essential) thrombocythemia. Virchows Arch Pathol Anat 1988;413:407–417.
125. Burkhardt R. Bone marrow in megakaryocytic disorders. Hematol Oncol Clin North Am 1988;2:695–733.
126. Gugliotta L, Bagnara GP, Catani L, et al. In vivo and in vitro inhibitory effect of α-interferon on megakaryocyte colony

growth in essential thrombocythemia. Br J Haematol 1989;71: 177–181.
127. Chott A, Gisslinger H, Thiele J, et al. Interferon-alpha-induced morphological changes of megakaryocytes: a histomorphometrical study on bone marrow biopsies in chronic myeloproliferative disorders with excessive thrombocytosis. Br J Haematol 1990;74:10–16.
128. Murphy S. Thrombocytosis and thrombocythaemia. Clin Haematol 1983;12:89–106.
129. Frenkel EP. Southwestern internal medicine conference: the clinical spectrum of thrombocytosis and thrombocythemia. Am J Med Sci 1991;301:69–80.
130. Ellis JT, Peterson P. Myelofibrosis in the myeloproliferative disorders. In: Berk PD, Castro-Malaspina H, Wasserman LR, eds. Myelofibrosis and the biology of connective tissue. New York: Alan R Liss 1984:19–42.
131. Wang JC, Lang H-D, Lichter S, et al. Cytogenetic studies of bone marrow fibroblasts cultured from patients with myelofibrosis and myeloid metaplasia. Br J Haematol 1992;80: 184–188.
132. de la Chapelle A, Vuopio P, Börgström GH. The origin of some bone marrow fibroblasts. Blood 1973;41:783–787.
133. Hentel J, Hirschhorn K. the origin of bone marrow fibroblasts. Blood 1971;38:81–86.
134. Van Slyck EJ, Weiss M, Dully M. Chromosomal evidence for the secondary role of fibroblastic proliferation in acute myelofibrosis. Blood 1970;36:729–735.
135. Varki A, Lottenberg R, Griffith R, Reinhard E. The syndrome of idiopathic myelofibrosis: a clinico-pathologic review with emphasis on the prognostic variables predicting survival. Medicine 1983;62:353–371.
136. Visani G, Finelli C, Castelli U, et al. Myelofibrosis with myeloid metaplasia: clinical and haematological parameters predicting survival in a series of 133 patients. Br J Haematol 1990;75:4–9.
137. Pegrum GD, Risdon RA. The haematological and histological findings in 18 patients with clinical features resembling those of myelofibrosis. Br J Haematol 1970;18:475–486.
138. Hasselbalch H. Idiopathic myelofibrosis: a clinical study of 80 patients. Am J Hematol 1990;34:291–300.
139. Cervantes F, Tassies D, Salgado C, et al. Acute transformation in nonleukemic chronic myeloproliferative disorders: actuarial probability and main characteristics in a series of 218 patients. Acta Haematol 1991;85:124–127.
140. Demory JL, Dupriez B, Fenaux P, et al. Cytogenetic studies and their prognostic significance in agnogenic myeloid metaplasia: a report on 47 cases. Blood 1988;72:855–859.
141. Wolf BC, Neiman RS. Hypothesis: splenic filtration and the pathogenesis of extramedullary hematopoiesis in agnogenic myeloid metaplasia. Hematol Pathol 1987;1:77–80.
142. Talarico L, Wolf BC, Kumar A, Weintraub LR. Reversal of bone marrow fibrosis and subsequent development of polycythemia in patients with myeloproliferative disorders. Am J Hematol 1989;30:248–253.
143. Hasselbalch H, Lisse I. A sequential histological study of bone marrow fibrosis in idiopathic myelofibrosis. Eur J Haematol 1991;46:285–289.
144. Bennett JM, Catovsky D, Daniel M-T, et al. Criteria for the diagnosis of acute leukemia of megakaryocyte lineage (M7). Ann Intern Med 1985;103:460–462.
145. Krzyaniak RL, Buss DH, Cooper MR, Wells HB. Marrow fibrosis and multiple myeloma. Am J Clin Pathol 1988;89:63–68.
146. Duhrsen U, Uppenkamp M, Meusers P, Konig E, Brittinger G. Frequent association of idiopathic myelofibrosis with plasma cell dyscrasias. Blut 1988;56:97–102.
147. Wallis JP, Reid MM. Bone marrow fibrosis in childhood acute lymphoblastic leukaemia. J Clin Pathol 1989;42:1253–1254.
148. Bennett JM, Catovsky D, Daniel MT, et al. Proposals for the classification of the myelodysplastic syndromes. Br J Haematol 1982;51:189–199.
149. Block MA, Jacobson LO, Bethard WF. Preleukemic acute human leukemia. JAMA 1953;152:1018–1028.
150. Broun GO. Chronic erythromonocytic leukemia. Am J Med 1969;47:785–796.
151. Cohen JR, Creger WP, Greenberg PL, Schrier SL. Subacute myeloid leukemia: a clinical review. Am J Med 1979;66:959–966.
152. Fenaux P, Jouet JP, Zandecki M, et al. Chronic and subacute myelomonocytic leukaemia in the adult: a report of 60 cases with special reference to prognostic factors. Br J Haematol 1987;65:101–106.
153. Greenberg PL. The smoldering myeloid leukemic states: clinical and biological features. Blood 1983;61:1035–1044.
154. Zittown R. Subacute and chronic myelomonocytic leukemia: a distinct haematological entity. Br J Haematol 1976;32:1–7.
155. Ribera J-M, Cervantes F, Rozman C. A multivariate analysis of prognostic factors in chronic myelomonocytic leukaemia according to FAB criteria. Br J Haematol 1987;65:307–311.
156. Todd WM, Pierre RV. Preleukaemia: a long-term prospective study of 326 patients. Scand J Haematol 1986;36(suppl 45): 114–120.
157. Tricot G, Vlietinck R, Verwilghen RL. Prognostic factors in the myelodysplastic syndromes: a review. Scand J Haematol 1986;36(suppl 45):107–113.
158. Tricot G, DeWolf-Peeters C, Vlietinck R, Verwilghen RI. Bone marrow histology in myelodysplastic syndromes. II. Prognostic value of abnormal localization of immature precursors in MDS. Br J Haematol 1984;58:217–225.
159. Kerkhofs H, Hermans J, Haak HL, Leeksma CHW. Utility of the FAB classification for myelodysplastic syndromes: investigation of prognostic factors in 237 cases. Br J Haematol 1987;65:73–81.
160. Dewald GW, Davis MP, Pierre RV, O'Fallon JR, Hoagland HC. Clinical characteristics and prognosis of 50 patients with amyeloproliferative syndrome and deletion of part of the long arm of chromosome 5. Blood 1985;66:189–197.
161. Knapp RH, Dewald GW, Pierre RV. Cytogenetic studies in 174 consecutive patients with preleukemic or myelodysplastic syndrome. Mayo Clin Proc 1985;60:507–516.
162. Streuli RA, Testa JR, Vardiman JW, Mintz U, Golomb HM, Rowley JD. Dysmyelopoietic syndrome: sequential clinical and cytogenetic studies. Blood 1980;55:636–644.
163. Kerkhofs H, Hagemeijer A, Leeksma CHW, et al. The 5q- chromosome abnormality in haematological disorders: a collaborative study of 34 cases from the Netherlands. Br J Haematol 1982;52:365–381.
164. Juneja SK, Imbert M, Jouault H, et al. Haematological features of primary myelodysplastic syndromes (PMDS) at initial presentation: a study of 118 cases. J Clin Pathol 1983;36: 1129–1135.
165. Tricot G, DeWolf-Peeters C, Hendrickx B, Verwilghen RL. Bone marrow histology in myelodysplastic syndromes. I. Histological findings in myelodysplastic syndromes and comparison with bone marrow smears. Br J Haematol 1984;57: 423–430.
166. Delacretaz F, Schmidt P-M, Piguet D, et al. Histopathology of myelodysplastic syndromes: the FAB classification (proposals) applied to bone marrow biopsy. Am J Clin Pathol 1987;87:180–186.
167. Tricot G, Boogaerts C, DeWolf-Peeters C, Van den Berghe H, Verwilghen RL. The myelodysplastic syndromes: different

evolution patterns based on sequential morphological and cytogenetic investigations. Br J Haematol 1985;59:659–670.
168. Ríos A, Cañizo MC, Sanz MA, et al. Bone marrow biopsy in myelodysplastic syndromes: morphological characteristics and contribution to the study of prognostic factors. Br J Haematol 1990;75:26–33.
169. Ohyashiki K, Sasao I, Ohyashiki JH, et al. Clinical and cytogenetic characteristics of myelodysplastic syndromes developing myelofibrosis. Cancer 1991;68:178–183.
170. San Miguel JF, Hernández JM, González-Sarmiento R, González M, Sánchez I, et al. Acute leukemia after a primary myelodysplastic syndrome: immunophenotypic, genotypic, and clinical characteristics. Blood 1991;78:768–774.
171. Bennett JM, Catovsky D, Daniel MT, et al. Proposals for the classification of the acute leukaemias. Br J Haematol 1976;33: 451–458.
172. Bennett JM, Catovsky D, Daniel M-T, et al. Proposed revised criteria for the classification of the acute myeloid leukemia. A report of the French-American-British Cooperative Group. Ann Intern Med 1985;103:626–629.
173. Catovsky D, Matutes E, Buccheri V, et al. A classification of acute leukaemia for the 1990s. Ann Hematol 1991;62:16–21.
174. Dick FR. Evolution of the French-American-British proposals. Am J Clin Pathol 1991;96:153–155.
175. Hamblin TJ, Oscier DG. The myelodysplastic syndrome—a practical guide. Haematol Oncol 1987;5:19–34.
176. Pugh WC, Pearson M, Vardiman JW, Rowley JD. Philadelphia chromosome-negative chronic myelogenous leukemia: a morphological reassessment. Br J Haematol 1985;60:457–467.
177. Hardy WR, Anderson R. The hypereosinophilic syndromes. Ann Intern Med 1968;68:1220–1229.
178. Chusid MJ, Dale DC, West BC, Wolff SM. The hypereosinophilic syndrome. Medicine (Baltimore) 1975;54:1–27.
179. Schooley RT, Parillo JE, Wolff SM, Fauci AS. Management of the idiopathic hypereosinophilic syndrome. In: Mahmoud AF, Austin KF, eds. The eosinophil in health and disease. New York: Grune & Stratton, 1980:323–343.
180. Shurin SB. Pathologic states associated with activation of eosinophils and with eosinophilia. Hematol Oncol Clin North Am 1988;2:171–179.
181. Weller PF. The immunobiology of eosinophils. N Engl J Med 1991;324:1110–1118.
182. Fauci AS, Harley JB, Roberts WC, Ferrans VJ, Gralnick HR, Bjornson BH. The idiopathic hypereosinophilic syndrome. Clinical, pathophysiologic, and therapeutic considerations. Ann Intern Med 1982;97:78–92.
183. Parillo JE, Borer JS, Henry WL, Wolff SM, Fauci AS. The cardiovascular manifestations of the hypereosinophilic syndrome: prospective study of 26 patients, with review of the literature. Am J Med 1979;67:572–582.
184. Schooley RT, Flaum MA, Gralnick HR, Fauci AS. A clinicopathologic correlation of the idiopathic hypereosinophilic syndrome. II. Clinical manifestations. Blood 1981;58:1021–1026.
185. Parillo JE, Fauci AS, Wolff SM. Therapy of the hypereosinophilic syndrome. Ann Intern Med 1978;89:167–172.
186. Anonymous. The hypereosinophilic syndrome [Editorial]. Lancet 1983;1:1417–1418.
187. Parillo JE. Heart disease and the eosinophil. N Engl J Med 1990;323:1560–1561.
188. Flaum MA, Schooley RT, Fauci AS, Gralnick HR. A clinicopathologic correlation of the idiopathic hypereosinophilic syndrome. I. Hematologic manifestations. Blood 1981;58: 1012–1020.
189. Powers LW, Register MK. Down syndrome and acute leukemia: epidemiological and genetic relationships. Lab Med 1991;22:630–636.
190. Barber R, Spiers P. Oxford survey of childhood cancer: progress report II. Monthly Bulletin of Minnesota Health 1964;23: 46–52.
191. Weinstein HJ. Congenital leukemia and the neonatal myeloproliferative disorders associated with Down's syndrome. Clin Haematol 1978;7:147–154.
192. Cantu-Rajnoldi A, Cattoretti G, Caccamo ML, et al. Leukaemoid reaction with megakaryocytic features in newborns with Down's syndrome. Eur J Haematol 1988;40:403–409.
193. de Alacron PA, Ptil S, Goldberg J, et al. Infants with Down's syndrome: use of cytogenetic studies and *in vitro* colony assay for granulocyte progenitor to distinguish acute ANLL from TMPD. Cancer 1987;60:987–993.
194. Zipursky A. Leukemia in Down syndrome. Unpublished communication.

Suggested Readings

Hartsock RJ, Smith EB, Petty CS. Normal variations with aging of the amount of hematopoietic tissue in bone marrow from the anterior iliac crest: a study made from 177 cases of sudden death examined by necropsy. Am J Clin Pathol 1965;43:326–331.
Hyun BH, Gulati GL, Ashton JK. Myeloproliferative disorders. Classification and diagnostic features with special emphasis on chronic myelogenous leukemia and agnogenic myeloid metaplasia. Clin Lab Med 1990;10:825–838.
Richter GW. The iron-loaded cell—the cytopathology of iron storage. Am J Pathol 1978;91:361–404.

Section VIII

Section Chief: *Douglas A. Triplett*

Our understanding of the hemostatic process has increased greatly over the past decade. With the introduction of sophisticated biochemical and molecular biology techniques, the components of this process have been characterized in great detail. This section is designed to provide an overview of the hemostatic process and of disorders resulting from abnormalities of this system. In Chapter 40, the normal mechanisms of hemostasis are reviewed, including primary hemostasis (platelet plug formation), secondary hemostasis (fibrin clot formation), and regulation of hemostasis. Included in this chapter is an introduction to the approach to patients with hemostatic problems.

Disorders of primary hemostasis are discussed in Chapter 41. Congenital and acquired disorders of platelet function, including heparin-induced thrombocytopenia and thrombotic thrombocytopenic purpura, are discussed in this chapter. The characteristic laboratory findings in these disorders are reviewed. Quantitative platelet disorders are also briefly reviewed.

Disorders of fibrin clot formation are discussed in Chapter 42. These include the common congenital disorders hemophilia A and B as well as acquired abnormalities such as factor inhibitors and lupus anticoagulants. Laboratory techniques for the diagnosis of these various disorders are reviewed in detail.

Chapter 43 is devoted to problems associated with an increased risk of thrombosis. Emphasis is placed on congenital disorders associated with thrombosis (thrombophilia) and the role of the laboratory in the diagnosis of these conditions. The potential for utilizing markers of activation hemostasis is addressed in this chapter as well.

COAGULATION

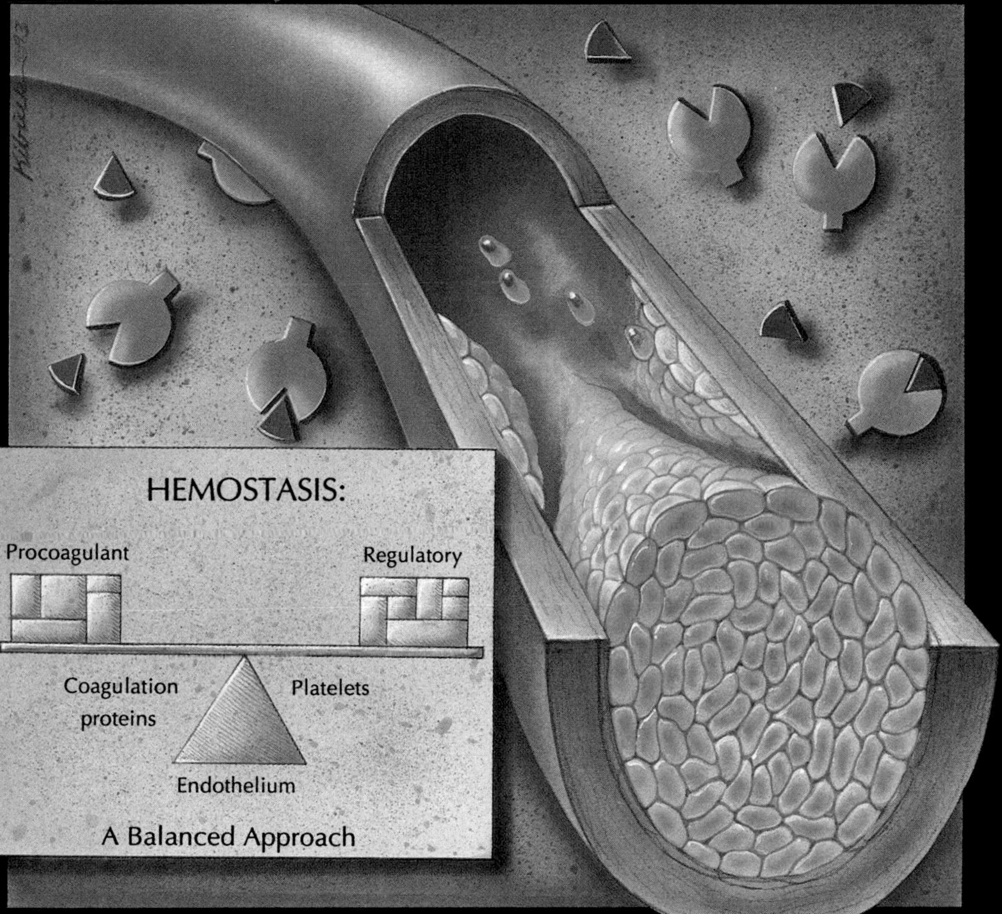

40 Overview of Hemostasis

John T. Brandt

Hemostasis may be defined as the process that maintains flowing blood in a fluid state and prevents loss of blood from sites of vascular disruption. This definition implies two major components: first, a potent procoagulant mechanism that is capable of forming hemostatic plugs at sites of vascular disruption; and second, regulatory systems that confine normal hemostatic plug formation to sites of vascular disruption. Active components in this system include circulating platelets, procoagulant and regulatory plasma proteins, and endothelial cells lining the vascular wall. Normal hemostasis is maintained by a delicate balance between the procoagulant and regulatory sides of hemostasis; disruption of this balance can lead to either excessive bleeding or clot formation.

The procoagulant mechanism is normally initiated by vascular damage or disruption. This leads to deposition of platelets at the damaged site; the platelet plug is then reinforced by a meshwork of fibrin strands. This process is normally halted as it extends out into areas of the vessel lined by intact endothelial cells (Fig. 40.1). The formation of the platelet plug is often referred to as primary hemostasis, while the formation of the fibrin meshwork is referred to as secondary hemostasis. The mechanisms involved in turning off the process are called the regulatory systems. As the limitation of clot formation to sites of vascular disruption would suggest, the process of regulation is very dependent on intact endothelial cells.

This chapter reviews the major mechanisms involved in primary hemostasis, secondary hemostasis, and regulation of hemostasis. It also outlines an approach to the evaluation of patients with hemostatic disorders. Specific disorders affecting hemostasis are discussed in subsequent chapters.

PRIMARY HEMOSTASIS

Platelet Morphology and Production

Platelets—central components of hemostasis—are anucleate cytoplasmic fragments derived from bone marrow megakaryocytes that are themselves derived from the pluripotent hematopoietic stem cell (1). At least two stages of megakaryocyte progenitors have been demonstrated by in vitro culture techniques, the burst-forming unit-megakaryocyte and the colony-forming unit-megakaryocyte. Each of these stages appears to be sensitive to a different set of cytokines. Maturation of the colony-forming unit-megakaryocyte leads to the formation of recognizable megakaryocytes. Megakaryocytes are large cells with multilobated nuclei derived from a process of endomitosis. Normal megakaryocytes are usually 8N-32N, but the ploidy number can vary depending on the rate of platelet production and consumption.

Platelets are formed and released from megakaryocytes by a process of cytoplasmic fragmentation along lines of demarcation formed by infolding of the cytoplasmic membrane. Platelet size thus depends on the size of the zone of demarcation. When platelet production is increased, the zones of demarcation are typically larger. This results in the increased mean platelet volume (MPV) characteristic of thrombocytopenia secondary to increased consumption. The peripheral platelet count appears to be regulated by the total platelet mass rather than the platelet count. This is reflected in disorders such as Bernard-Soulier syndrome and May-Hegglin anomaly, which are characterized by thrombocytopenia and an increase in MPV.

The resting platelet normally has a discoid shape that is maintained by a circumferential band of microtubules (Fig. 40.2). The platelet membrane is physically and biochemically complex. There are numerous infoldings of the plasma membrane to form the surface-connected open canalicular system. The membrane contains a variety of receptors, some of which are linked to membrane-associated enzyme systems such as phospholipase A_2, phospholipase C, and adenylate cyclase (2). Beneath the cytoplasmic membrane there is a sol-gel zone that is rich in actin and myosin. These proteins are involved in the shape change and contraction characteristic of platelet activation.

Juxtaposed to the surface-connected open canalicular system is a series of membrane-bound tubules referred to as the dense tubular system. The dense tubular system corresponds to the endoplasmic retic-

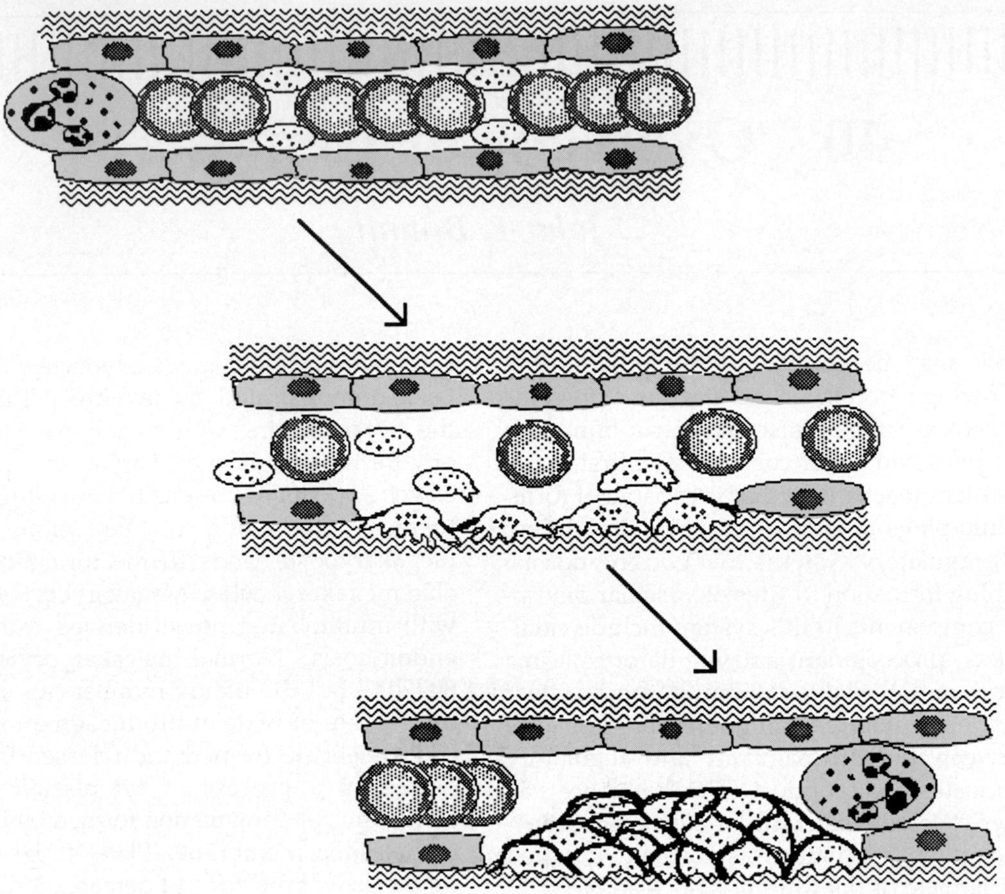

Figure 40.1. The formation of a hemostatic plug usually begins when the vessel wall is damaged, exposing the thrombogenic subendothelial tissues to blood. The initial response is platelet adhesion, with the responding platelets forming a monolayer over the exposed subendothelial tissue (**B**). During this response the platelets are activated and additional platelets are recruited to form the platelet plug. This phase of platelet-platelet interaction is known as platelet aggregation. Fibrin formation begins as the responding platelets are activated, resulting in deposition of a fibrin meshwork, which envelops the platelet plug (**C**). Hemostatic plug formation is normally limited to sites of vascular disruption by an active regulatory mechanism that is dependent upon intact endothelial cells.

ulum of smooth muscle cells and functions as a storage site for calcium.

Within the cytoplasm of the platelet are several organelles, including mitochondria, peroxisomes, α granules, and dense granules; storage pools of glycogen are also frequently present in resting platelets. α Granules contain a variety of proteins, many of which are homologues of plasma proteins (Table 40.1). A long-standing question has been whether or not such proteins are derived from passive adsorption by the platelets or active synthesis by the megakaryocyte. Evidence to date suggests that both mechanisms are important. Platelet IgG, albumin, and fibrinogen concentrations are directly proportional to the plasma concentration of these proteins. Other proteins, including platelet factor 4, β-thromboglobulin, and von Willebrand factor (vWF), are synthesized by the megakaryocyte. Some α-granule proteins are specific for the platelet; thus platelet factor 4 and β-thromboglobulin can serve as markers of platelet release. Thrombospondin, a major constituent of α granules, has a limited tissue distribution and has been used as a marker of platelet activation.

The platelet dense granules contain a variety of small organic compounds, including ADP, ATP, calcium, and serotonin. Perhaps the most important component of the dense granules is ADP, an essential platelet agonist. As circulating platelets are anucleate, their ability to synthesize new proteins is relatively limited. Thus, once a platelet has undergone release of its granule contents or inactivation of one or more of its enzymes (e.g., aspirin effect), it remains functionally impaired until it is removed from the circulation.

Platelet Response to Vascular Injury

The typical platelet response to vascular injury can be divided into three major steps (3). These are *platelet adhesion*, the interaction of platelets with nonplatelet surfaces; *platelet activation*, during which platelets undergo shape change and secrete ADP and

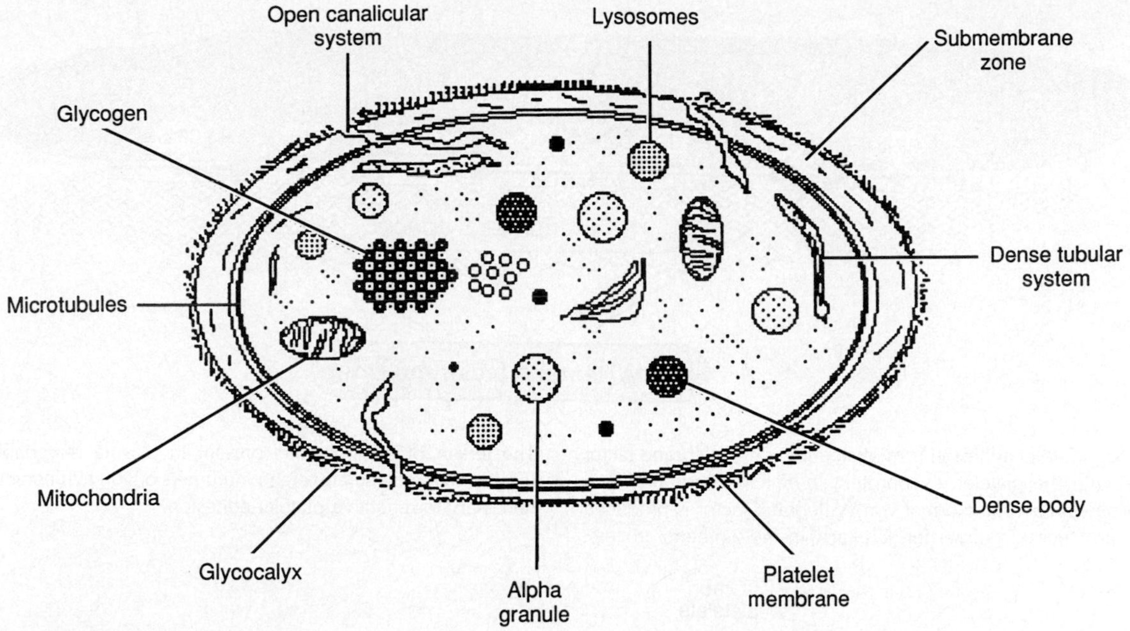

Figure 40.2. Structural features of normal resting platelets are depicted. The open canalicular system is formed by invaginations of the plasma membrane. This system becomes dilated upon platelet activation and serves as a route for platelet secretion. Closely juxtaposed to the open canalicular system is the dense tubular system, which serves as a storage site for calcium. Platelet α granules contain a variety of proteins, while the major functional constituents of the dense granules are small organic compounds such as ADP, ATP, and serotonin. The discoid shape of the resting platelet is maintained by a circumferential band of microtubules.

Table 40.1. Platelet α-Granule Proteins

Homologues of Plasma Proteins	Platelet-Specific Proteins	Platelet-Associated Proteins
Fibrinogen	Platelet factor 4	Thrombospondin
Factor V	β-Thromboglobulin	
Von Willebrand factor		
High–molecular weight kininogen		
Protein S		
Plasminogen		
Fibronectin		
Albumin		
Factor D		
β-1H-globulin		
IgG		

other granule constituents; and *platelet aggregation*, the interaction of platelets with each other.

The adhesion of platelets to exposed subendothelial structures is mediated primarily by von Willebrand factor (vWF), a large adhesive protein (Fig. 40.3). Von Willebrand factor is synthesized by endothelial cells and megakaryocytes; plasma vWF is primarily a product of endothelial cell synthesis and release, whereas platelet α-granule vWF is primarily a product of megakaryocyte synthesis. In addition, endothelial cells secrete vWF into the subendothelial cell space so that vWF is present in the subendothelial cell matrix itself. All three sources of vWF are probably necessary for normal platelet adhesion.

Current evidence suggests that when vWF interacts with subendothelial components such as collagen, it undergoes a conformational change, exposing binding sites for its platelet receptors. The primary platelet receptor for vWF is glycoprotein Ib (GP Ib). Under conditions of high shear stress, vWF can also bind to the glycoprotein IIb/IIIa (GP IIb/IIIa) complex. Von Willebrand factor is normally synthesized as a polymer consisting of a variable number of dimeric subunits. The longer polymers (high–molecular weight multimers) are capable of mediating platelet adhesion to subendothelial structures, perhaps because the larger forms maximize surface contact between the platelet and vessel wall.

Activation of the platelet membrane by adhesion or other platelet agonists leads to dynamic metabolic and morphologic changes in the responding platelet. A number of metabolic pathways are involved in this platelet response; among these, the phospholipase C–phosphatidylinositol pathway appears to be critical in initiating the platelet response (Fig. 40.4). Activation of phospholipase C by any one of a number of membrane signals leads to cleavage of phosphatidylinositol-bisphosphate (PIP_2), resulting in the release of two critical intracytoplasmic mediators, diacylglycerol (DG) and inositol trisphosphate (IP_3). Inositol trisphosphate causes rapid release of calcium from its storage sites into the platelet cytoplasm. The increase in cytoplasmic calcium activates calmodulin-dependent phosphokinases and leads directly to phosphory-

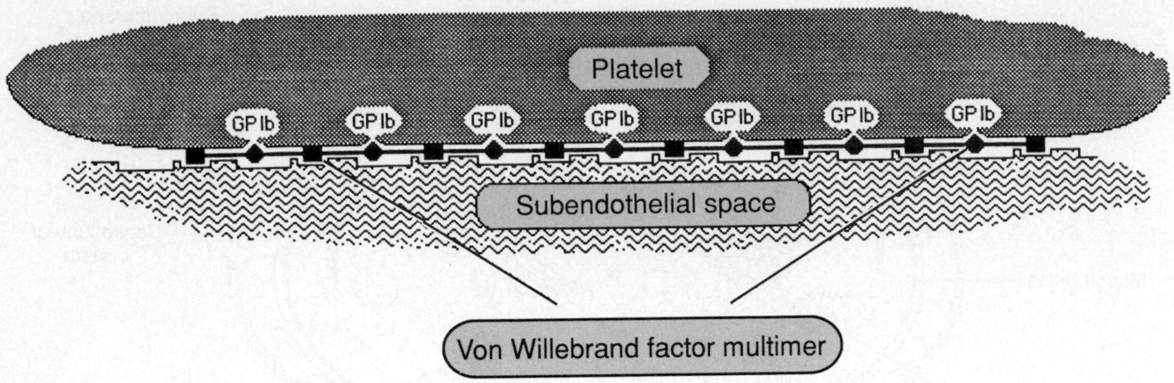

Figure 40.3. Platelet adhesion is mediated by von Willebrand factor interaction with the platelet glycoprotein Ib/IX (GPIb) complex and the subendothelial matrix. Normal von Willebrand factor is produced as a linear polymer of a dimer formed early in the synthetic process. The length of the polymers present in plasma is variable, but the longer (high molecular weight) multimers of von Willebrand factor are necessary for effective platelet adhesion.

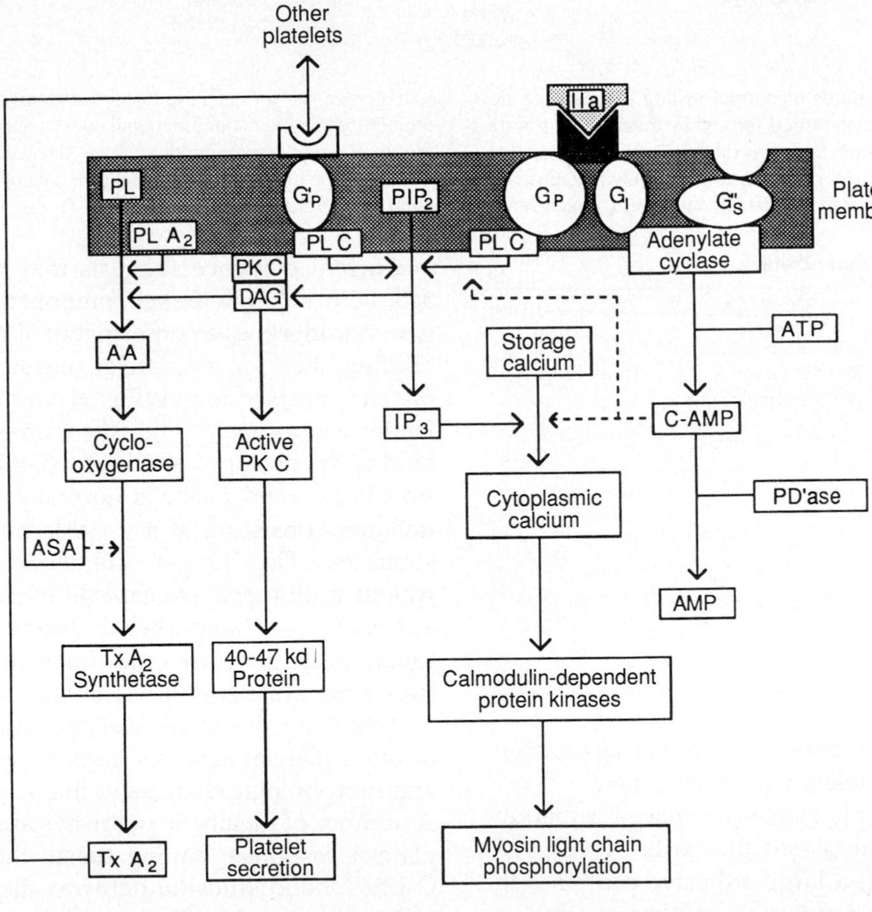

Figure 40.4. Platelet activation involves a number of biosynthetic pathways in the platelet. The phospholipase C (PLC) pathway is responsible for production of diacylglycerol (DG) and inositol trisphosphate (IP_3) from phosphatidyl inositol bisphosphate (PIP_2). DG activates protein kinase C (PK C), leading to phospholytation of a 40- to 47-kd protein necessary for platelet secretion. IP_3 releases calcium from storage sites, leading to activation of calmodulin-dependent protein kinases. This pathway leads to myosin light chain phosphorylation and platelet contraction. The phospholipase A_2 (PL A_2) pathway releases arachidonic acid (AA) from membrane phospholipids (PL), particularly phosphatidylcholine. Arachidonic acid is then converted into thromboxane A_2 (TxA_2), a potent platelet agonist. Stimulation of these pathways is mediated by G proteins (Gp), which transmit signals from the external surface receptor to the membrane-associated enzyme systems. Cyclic AMP (c-AMP) is an important regulatory factor in the platelet response. Increased levels of c-AMP inhibit the PLC pathway at several points (*dashed line*). The cytoplasmic level of c-AMP is, in turn, regulated by the rate of production (adenylate cyclase) and metabolism (phosphodiesterase, PD'ase). Aspirin (ASA) inhibits platelet function by blocking synthesis of TxA_2.

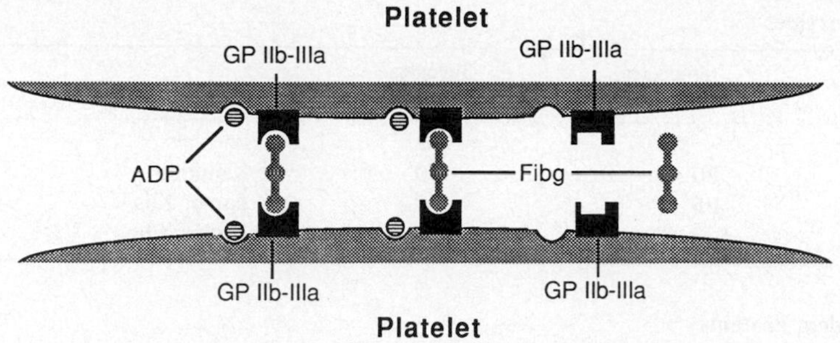

Figure 40.5. Platelet aggregation is mediated by the cross-linking of glycoprotein IIb/IIIa (GP IIb/IIIa) on adjacent platelet membranes. A number of adhesive proteins may mediate this process, but fibrinogen (Fibg) is the major mediator. The structural symmetry of fibrinogen makes it an excellent molecule for this process. Von Willebrand factor may also play an important role in areas of high shear stress. Under resting conditions, the binding site on GP IIb/IIIa for adhesive proteins is not exposed. Upon platelet activation (e.g., by ADP binding to a surface receptor), GP IIb/IIIa undergoes a conformational change, allowing binding of the adhesive protein.

lation of myosin light chain. This pathway is essential for platelet shape change and contraction. Diacylglycerol binds to and activates protein kinase C. Protein kinase C then phosphorylates a number of proteins, including a 45-kd protein essential for platelet secretion. In addition, DG can lead to activation of the phospholipase A_2 pathway.

Activation of phospholipase A_2 leads to the release of arachidonic acid from membrane phospholipids, particularly phosphatidylcholine. Arachidonic acid can be converted into cyclic endoperoxides by cyclooxygenase or metabolized by 12-lipoxygenase. The cyclooxygenase pathway leads to the formation of thromboxane A_2 which itself is a potent stimulator of phospholipase C. Aspirin and other nonsteroidal anti-inflammatory agents have an antiplatelet effect because of their ability to inhibit cyclooxygenase and block formation of thromboxane A_2.

The response of the platelet leads to extension of pseudopodia, secretion of important mediators and proteins, and ultimately contraction of the hemostatic plug. One of the mediators released from the dense granules is ADP, a platelet agonist that can further stimulate surrounding platelets. In addition, it is capable of activating the GP IIb/IIIa complex to mediate the third and final stage of the platelet response, platelet aggregation.

Platelet aggregation is another example of "molecular gluing." GP IIb/IIIa can be cross-linked by a variety of adhesive proteins; the major protein involved in cross-linking platelets in vivo appears to be fibrinogen. Intact fibrinogen is a dimeric molecule that allows reciprocal interaction of its terminal ends (D domains) with GP IIb/IIIa receptors on adjacent platelets. Under resting conditions, the GP IIb/IIIa receptor cannot interact with or bind fibrinogen. However, once a platelet has been activated or exposed to ADP, fibrinogen can bind to and cross-link responding platelets (Fig. 40.5). Thrombospondin, a major component of platelet α granules, appears to stabilize and augment the platelet-platelet interaction mediated by fibrinogen.

In summary, the primary hemostatic response consists of three major stages. Platelet adhesion is the first step and is mediated by vWF interaction with GP Ib and subendothelial receptors. The subsequent shape change and secretion are dependent on activation of multiple biochemical pathways within the platelet. Activation of the platelet leads to expression of GP IIb/IIIa receptors and cross-linking by intact fibrinogen. Defects in various platelet and plasma components of this response mechanism have been described and constitute many of the platelet disorders described in Chapter 41.

SECONDARY HEMOSTASIS

Secondary hemostasis is marked by the conversion of a soluble protein, fibrinogen, into an insoluble gel (1). Formation of the fibrin meshwork results in reinforcement and stabilization of the platelet plug at the site of vascular disruption. The process of fibrin clot formation can be divided into two phases; the first phase consists of formation of the potent procoagulant enzyme thrombin; the second phase consists of the conversion of fibrinogen into fibrin with subsequent polymerization and stabilization.

Thrombin is formed as a result of multiple enzymatic steps, which are known collectively as the coagulation cascade (4–6). Most of the enzymatic steps involve formation of an "enzyme activation complex" composed of an active enzyme, a proenzyme substrate protein, a protein cofactor, and a phospholipid surface that serves to localize the process and concentrate the reactants (Fig. 40.6). The coagulation cascade can be viewed as the formation of a series of these activation complexes. As each enzyme activates many substrate proenzymes, each activation complex represents an amplification step.

The enzymes of the coagulation cascade are serine proteases; that is, they are enzymes that split specific

Table 40.2. Contact System Enzymes

Protein	Molecular Weight	Biological Half-Life	Activated By	Function
	kd	*hr*		
Factor XII (Hageman factor)	80	50	Kallikrein	Activate prekallikrein, factor XI
Prekallikrein (Fletcher factor)	85	50	Factor XIIa	Activate factor XII
Factor XI	160 (dimer)	40	Factor XIIa	Activate factor IX

Table 40.3. Vitamin K-Dependent Proteins

Protein	Molecular Weight	Gla Residues	Biological Half-Life	Activated By	Function
	kd		*hr*		
Factor II (prothrombin)	72	10	60	Factor Xa	Cleave fibrinogen, activates V, VIII, XIII, protein C
Factor VII	48	10	4–6	Factors Xa, IIa	Activates factors IX, X
Factor IX	57	12	25	Factors XIa, VIIa	Activates factor X
Factor X	55	11	24	Factors VIIa, IXa	Activates factor II
Protein C	62	9	6	Thrombin	Inactivates factors Va and VIIIa
Protein S	69	10	Not known	Not activated	No enzymatic activity cofactor for activated protein C

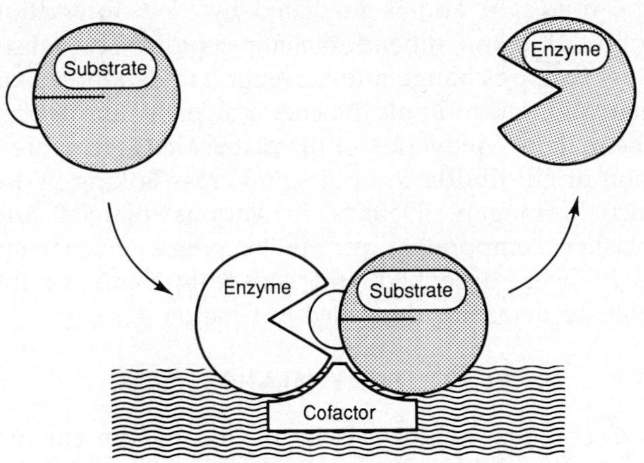

Figure 40.6. The basis of most reactions involving the coagulation cascade is the formation of an enzyme activation complex composed of an active enzyme (serine protease), a substrate that is usually the zymogen of another active enzyme, a cofactor protein that serves to localize the enzyme and substrate to a phospholipid surface, and a phospholipid surface. Thrombin is formed by such a complex in which the active enzyme is factor Xa, the substrate is prothrombin, the cofactor is factor Va, and the phospholipid is provided by a cell surface (e.g., activated platelet).

peptide bonds through the formation of unstable bonds with the reactive serine at the enzyme's active site. Coagulation serine proteases can be divided into two families, the vitamin K–dependent proteins and the contact system proteins (Tables 40.2 and 40.3). The contact system serine proteases share several characteristics: (*a*) the molecular weight of each monomeric unit is 80 to 85 kd; (*b*) they do not require vitamin K for complete synthesis; (*c*) they are not adsorbed by $BaSO_4$ or $Al(OH)_3$; and (*d*) they are not completely consumed during in vitro coagulation of blood. Factor XI is unique among these serine proteases in that it circulates as a dimer linked by disulfide bonds, and it is the only protein of this family that is associated with a bleeding tendency when the factor is absent.

The vitamin K–dependent factors are all characterized by the presence of between nine and 12 γ-carboxyglutamic acid residues near the amino terminal end of the protein. Vitamin K is necessary for the posttranscriptional carboxylation of these glutamic acid residues (Fig. 40.7). In the absence of γ-carboxyglutamic acid residues, these proteins do not bind calcium and do not interact with phospholipid surfaces. These descarboxy forms, which are found in vitamin K deficiency, oral anticoagulant therapy, and liver disease, are thus ineffective at mediating secondary hemostasis. Vitamin K–dependent proteins are heat stable and, with the exception of prothrombin, are not entirely consumed during coagulation in vitro. Some of the proteins (protein C, protein S, factor IX, and factor X) are characterized by an additional posttranscriptional modification, the hydroxylation of an aspartic acid to form β-hydroxyaspartic acid. The functional significance of this modification is still uncertain, but may involve calcium binding by these proteins. Protein S is unique among the vitamin K–dependent proteins in that it has no enzymatic function; rather, it functions as a cofactor for activated protein C.

The remaining coagulation proteins can be grouped into a family designated as thrombin-sensitive proteins and cofactors (Table 40.4). These proteins are all large, with molecular weights greater than 110 kd. Factor V, factor VIII, and high–molecular weight (HMW) kininogen function as cofactors in key enzymatic steps of the coagulation cascade, while fibrinogen functions as a cofactor for the activation of plasminogen by tissue plasminogen activa-

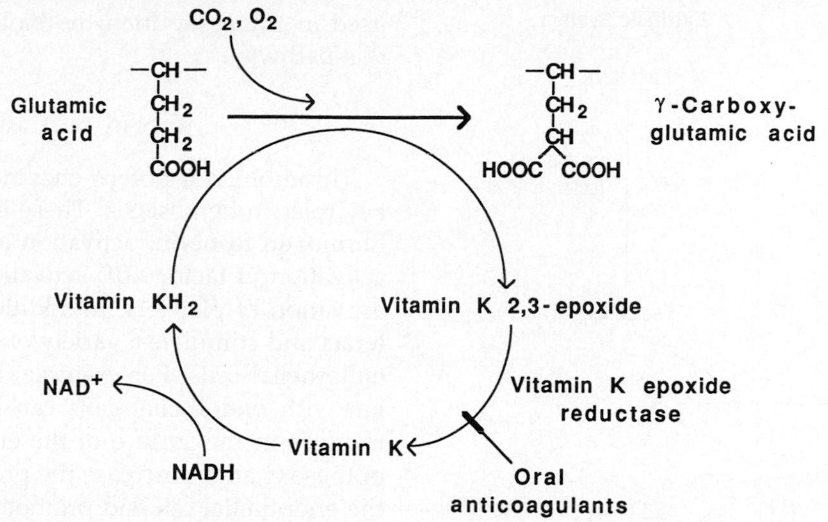

Figure 40.7. Vitamin K is necessary for the posttranslational modification of glutamic acid residues located near the amino terminal end of the vitamin K–dependent proteins. In the presence of reduced vitamin K, these residues are converted to the γ-carboxyglutamic acid residues necessary for calcium binding and interaction with phospholipid surfaces. The vitamin K epoxide formed in this process is then metabolized to regenerate the reduced form of vitamin K. Oral anticoagulants inhibit the regeneration of reduced vitamin K, trapping it in the inactive epoxide form.

Table 40.4. Thrombin-Sensitive Proteins and Cofactors

Protein	Molecular Weight	Biological Half-Life	Activated By	Function
	kd			
Fibrinogen	340	4–5 days	Thrombin	Fibrin clot, cofactor for activation for plasmin
Factor V	330	12–36 hr	Thrombin	Cofactor for activation for prothrombin
Factor VIII	240	12 hr	Thrombin	Cofactor for activation for factor X
High molecular kininogen (Fitzgerald factor)	110	6–7 days	Not known	Cofactor for activation for factor XI, prekallikrein, source of bradykinin
Factor XIII	320	3–5 days	Thrombin	Stabilizes fibrin clot

tor. Factor XIII is the only enzyme in this family; it differs from other coagulation enzymes in that it is a transpeptidase and is responsible for cross-linking and stabilizing the fibrin clot. High–molecular weight kininogen is the only one of these proteins that is not activated by thrombin.

Thrombin Formation

There are at least two mechanisms for initiating thrombin formation; these have been designated the intrinsic and extrinsic pathways. Their names derive from the fact that all components of the intrinsic system are found in circulating blood, while the extrinsic pathway requires the presence of tissue factor, a component not normally present in circulating blood. Recent studies suggest that the extrinsic pathway is the major physiological mechanism for initiating the coagulation cascade; the intrinsic system may be involved in pathological conditions and may also play a role in fibrinolysis.

Activation of the intrinsic system occurs when factor XII binds to negatively charged surfaces, resulting in a conformational change in the molecule and expression of enzymatic activity (Fig. 40.8). Factor XIIa can activate both prekallikrein and factor XI; HMW kininogen serves as a cofactor for both of these activation steps. Kallikrein is a potent activator of factor XII. The initial activation of prekallikrein thus leads to formation of a positive feedback loop, permitting generation of large quantities of factor XIIa in a very short period of time. Calcium is not required during these initial steps involving vitamin K–independent proteins.

Factor XIa activates factor IX in the presence of calcium and phospholipid surfaces, particularly activated platelet membranes. This is the only step for which there is no known protein cofactor. Factor IXa activates factor X in the presence of VIIIa, calcium, and phospholipid. Factor VIII, as it circulates in plasma, has minimal procoagulant activity; however, limited proteolytic cleavage, primarily by thrombin, results in the expression of potent procoagulant cofactor (not enzyme) activity. Factor Xa then converts prothrombin to thrombin in the presence of fac-

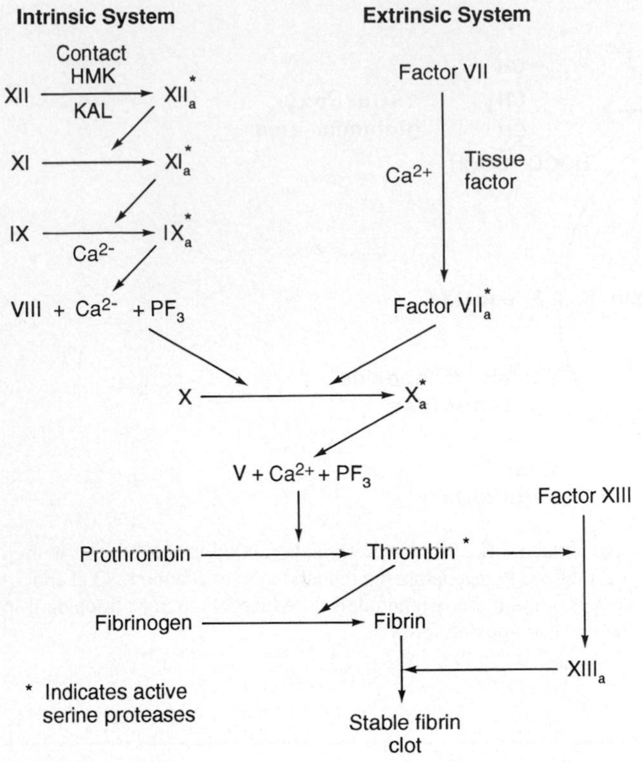

Figure 40.8. The coagulation cascade may be initiated by one of two mechanisms; the contact system, that activates the intrinsic system, and the tissue factor pathway, which initiates the extrinsic system. The intrinsic system begins when factor XII is activated by contact with appropriate negatively charged surfaces. Activated factor XII (XIIa) then activates prekallikrein (Pre K) and factor XI, initiating the enzymatic cascade resulting in thrombin formation. Exposure of blood to tissue factor (TF) leads to VIIa formation. The complex of VIIa, TF, phospholipid (PL) and calcium then activates both factors IX and X, initiating another enzymatic cascade and resulting in thrombin formation. The intrinsic system is measured by the activated partial thromboplastin time (APTT), while the extrinsic system is measured by the prothrombin time (PT).

tor Va, calcium, and phospholipid. Analogous to factor VIII, factor V must be activated by thrombin for full expression of its procoagulant cofactor activity.

The extrinsic pathway begins with exposure of blood to tissue factor. In the presence of tissue factor and calcium, VIIa activates both factor IX and factor X. Factor Xa then converts prothrombin to thrombin, as described previously. Because this step is common to both pathways, it is often designated the "final common pathway." The activation of factor IX by VIIa-tissue factor provides a connection between the intrinsic and extrinsic pathways of coagulation (Fig. 40.8). However, this connection is not evident with the routine tests of hemostasis, namely, the prothrombin time (PT) and activated partial thromboplastin time (APTT). The lack of dependence of the PT on factor VIII and IX concentration is more related to concentration of tissue factor and phospholipid used in the assay than the biological importance of this pathway.

Fibrin Formation

Thrombin is a potent enzyme that serves several key roles in hemostasis. These include conversion of fibrinogen to fibrin, activation of factors V and VIII, activation of factor XIII, activation of protein C, and activation of platelets. In addition, thrombin can interact and stimulate a variety of other cells, including endothelial cells. For example, interaction of thrombin with endothelial cells can lead to fundamental changes in the surface of the endothelial cell. Many of these changes increase the procoagulant activity of the endothelial cell and promote thrombosis. Critical to these functions of thrombin is the fact that conversion of prothrombin is accompanied by separation of the amino terminal, phospholipid-binding portion of the protein from its catalytic (enzymatic) portion. This large fragment is referred to as prothrombin fragment 1.2 ($F_{1.2}$). Thus, thrombin becomes a soluble enzyme in contrast to the other vitamin K–dependent enzymes, which require a phospholipid surface for effective function.

Fibrinogen is a large dimeric protein having a molecular weight of 340 kd. It is composed of six peptide chains: two Aα, two Bβ, and two γ chains. Each half of the fibrinogen molecule is composed of one Aα, one Bβ, and one γ chain linked together by extensive disulfide bonds that are concentrated in the amino and carboxy terminal ends. The extensive cross-linking gives these regions of the molecule a globular structure, while the intervening sequences are arranged in a long helical structure. The two halves of the fibrinogen molecule are linked by disulfide bonds between the amino terminal ends of the γ chains (Fig. 40.9).

Thrombin cleaves a 16–amino acid peptide from the amino terminal end of each Aα chain (fibrinopeptide A) and a 14–amino acid peptide from each amino terminal end of the Bβ chains (fibrinopeptide B). Loss of these peptides from the central domain of the fibrinogen molecule alters the charge distribution and exposes binding sites for the carboxy terminal ends of fibrin, known as the D domains (Fig. 40.9). The fibrin monomers then polymerize in a staggered overlap, with D domains interacting with the central E domain of the adjacent fibrin monomer. Lateral association then leads to gelation of the fibrin.

The fibrin gel is stabilized by factor XIIIa, which covalently cross-links fibrin monomers. Factor XIII is activated by thrombin, but full enzyme activity is expressed only after the active enzymatic subunit (the "a" subunit) separates from its carrier molecule (the

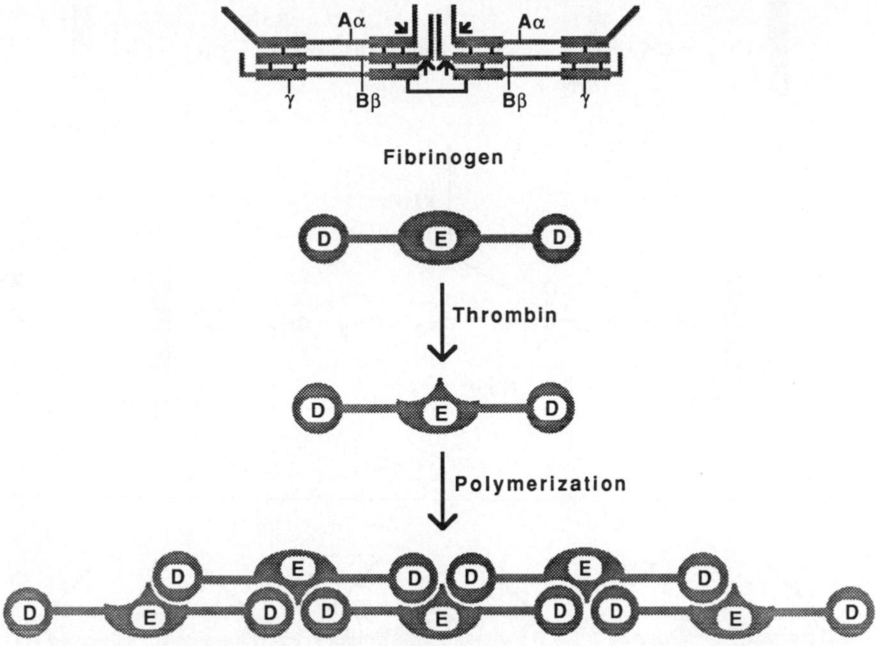

Figure 40.9. Fibrinogen is a large dimeric protein composed of six peptide chains. Each half of the dimer is composed of an Aα, a Bβ, and a γ chain. There are extensive interchain disulfide bonds near the amino termini, resulting in a central nodular region known as the E domain. Interchain disulfide bonds at the carboxy termini also result in nodular regions, known as the D domains. A fibrinogen molecule thus consists of a central E domain linked by helical segments to two D domains. Thrombin removes a short peptide from each Aα and Bβ chain (fibrinopeptides A and B), altering the conformation of the central E domain. This exposes binding sites for D domains within the central E domain and permits polymerization of the fibrin monomers to form the fibrin gel.

"b" subunit), a process that occurs within the fibrin matrix. Factor XIIIa covalently links glutamine to lysine amino acids. The principal sites of cross-linkage are between D domains of adjacent fibrin monomers and between the carboxy terminal ends of the α chains of distant fibrin monomers (Fig 40.10). Covalent cross-linkage greatly stabilizes the fibrin clot and makes it resistant to fibrinolysis.

REGULATION OF HEMOSTASIS

The procoagulant mechanisms described in the previous sections lead to rapid formation of hemostatic plugs at sites of vascular damage (7). Under normal circumstances, coagulation is limited to sites of vascular disruption and is not propagated throughout the vessel. There are multiple systems involved in limiting clot formation to sites of vascular disruption (1). These are known collectively as the regulatory systems. Knowledge about the various systems involved in the regulation of hemostasis has grown tremendously in recent years.

Regulation of the Platelet Response in Hemostasis

A number of factors that contribute to the regulation of the platelet response have been identified; most of these components are derived from intact endothelial cells (Table 40.5). A major inhibitor of the platelet response is prostacyclin, which is formed by metabolism of arachidonic acid through the prostaglandin pathway in endothelial and vascular wall cells. Prostacyclin is a short-lived, but potent inhibitor of platelet aggregation. It stimulates platelet adenylate cyclase, which leads to an increase in cytoplasmic cyclic AMP. Cyclic AMP inhibits the phospholipase C pathway and the release of calcium from storage sites. More recently, a second short-lived metabolite has been found to have profound effects on the platelet response. Endothelial-derived relaxing factor (EDRF) is a potent vasodilator that causes an increase in platelet cyclic GMP levels. The increase in cyclic GMP is associated with inhibition of both platelet adhesion and aggregation. Furthermore, the effect of EDRF and prostacyclin is synergistic; thus, the low basal levels of these two factors may be sufficient to minimize platelet activation under resting conditions.

Endothelial cells also release the enzyme ADPase, which converts ADP into inactive metabolites. ADP is essential for exposure of the GP IIb/IIIa binding sites, which mediate platelet aggregation. Another barrier to platelet activation is the glycocalyx on the surface of intact endothelial cells. The glycocalyx has a negative charge and tends to repulse platelets under resting conditions. In addition, intact endothe-

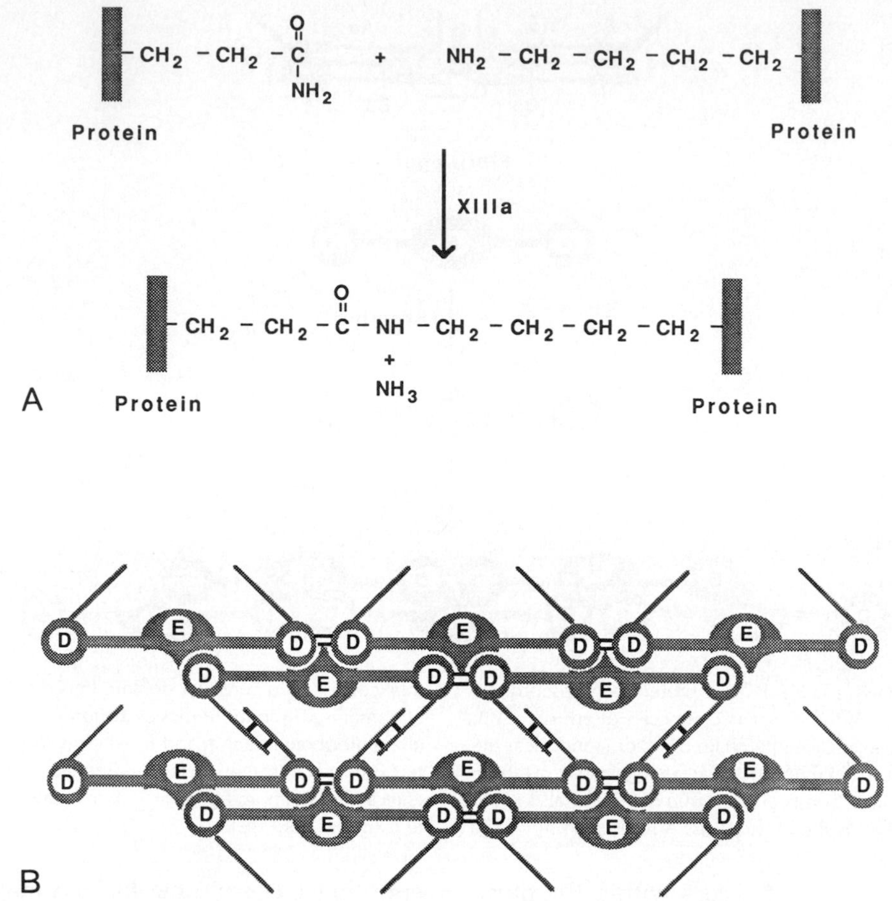

Figure 40.10. Factor XIIIa is a transpeptidase that cross-links peptide chains by inducing covalent linkage between glutamine and lysine amino acids (**A**). There are multiple cross-link sites in fibrin monomers; some are located near the carboxy termini of γ chains and result in cross-linkage of adjacent D domains, while others are located in the carboxy termini of α chains and result in cross-linkage of distant fibrin monomers. The net effect is a highly cross-linked fibrin gel that is resistant to fibrinolysis.

Table 40.5. Regulation of Platelet Response

Component	Action	Effect
Prostacyclin	Increases cyclic AMP	Inhibits aggregation
Endothelial-derived relaxing factor	Increases cyclic GMP	Inhibits aggregation and adhesion
ADPase	Metabolizes ADP	Inhibits aggregation
Endothelial glyocalyx	Electrostatic repulsion	Inhibits platelet adhesion

lial cells serve as a barrier between circulating platelets and any subendothelial vWF. Thus, platelet adhesion is prevented in areas where the endothelium remains intact. Under normal circumstances, these components work in concert to limit platelet activation to sites of endothelial disruption.

Regulation of Fibrin Clot Formations

At least four systems have been identified as having a role in the regulation of fibrin clot formation (Table 40.6). Each of these component mechanisms appears to be critical for effective regulation of hemostasis, and isolated deficiencies of these component systems have been associated with clinical manifestations. Each of the component systems has a unique effect on the formation of fibrin clot, as discussed in the following sections.

TISSUE FACTOR PATHWAY INHIBITOR

Tissue factor pathway inhibitor (TFPI) is the most recently characterized protein involved in the regulation of hemostasis (8). TFPI is a 40-kd protein that has also been called lipid-associated coagulation inhibitor (LACI) and extrinsic pathway inhibitor (EPI). A portion of circulating TFPI is present in the lipoprotein fraction, while the remainder is free in plasma. TFPI is a Kunitz-type inhibitor and rapidly combines with free Xa, inactivating the enzymatic activity of factor Xa. The TFPI-Xa complex then binds to the membrane-associated tissue factor–factor VIIa complex, inhibiting VIIa enzymatic activity (Fig. 40.11). Thus, TFPI is responsible for inhibition of the

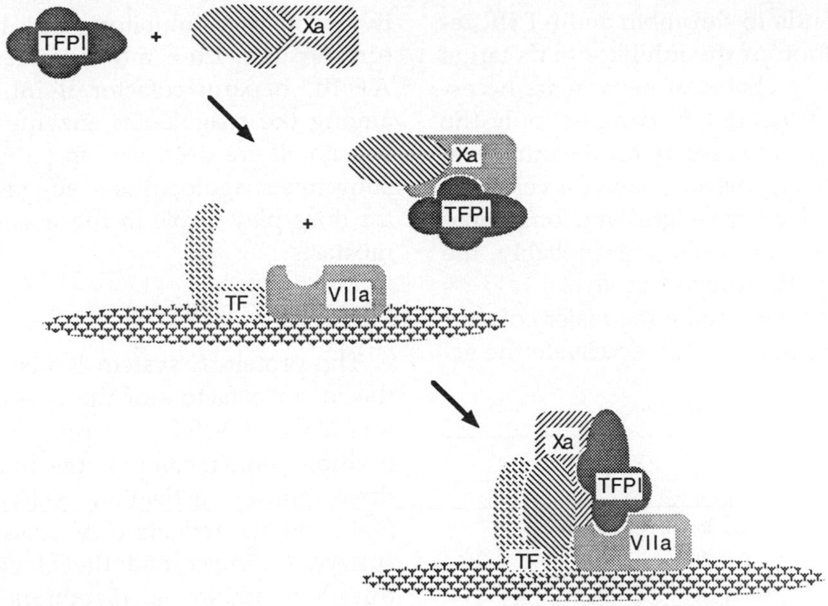

Figure 40.11. Tissue factor pathway inhibitor (TFPI) is a Kunitz-type inhibitor that initially forms a 1:1 complex with factor Xa (Xa). The TFPI-Xa complex then binds to the tissue factor (TF)–factor VIIa(VIIa)–phospholipid complex, inhibiting the activity of VIIa-TF. This provides a mechanism for turning off the tissue factor pathway of initiating the coagulation cascade.

Table 40.6. Regulation of Fibrin Clot Formation

Component	Action	Effect
Tissue factor pathway inhibitor	Inhibits factor VIIa-tissue factor	Inhibits thrombin formation
Serine protease inhibitors	Neutralize thrombin, factor Xa	Inhibit thrombin formation and activity
Protein C system	Proteolysis of factors Va and VIIIa	Inhibits thrombin formation
Fibrinolytic system	Proteolysis of fibrin	Removes excess fibrin clot

major physiological initiator of hemostasis, the factor VIIa–tissue factor complex.

SERINE PROTEASE INHIBITORS

The serine protease inhibitors (SERPINs) are proteins that act as pseudosubstrates for specific enzymes and form covalently linked complexes between the active site serine of the target enzyme and the susceptible bond in the inhibitor (Fig. 40.12). The SERPIN family includes a large number of proteins (Table 40.7). Although most of these proteins are capable of inhibiting multiple enzymes, each is primarily directed toward a few select enzymes.

The major inhibitors involved in the regulation of fibrin clot formation are antithrombin III (AT III) and heparin cofactor II. AT III requires heparin-like molecules for effective neutralization of factor Xa and thrombin. Heparin binds to AT III, inducing a conformational change that results in exposure of the enzyme neutralizing site (Fig. 40.13). In addition, hepa-

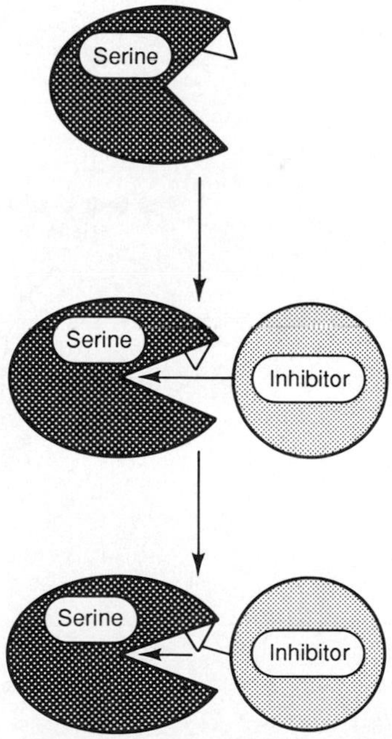

Figure 40.12. The general mechanism of action of serine protease inhibitors is shown schematically. The inhibitors function as pseudosubstrates for the enzyme, which attacks a susceptible peptide bond in the inhibitor. In a typical enzymatic reaction, a transitional bond is formed between the active site serine and the amino acid at the susceptible peptide bond. This transitional bond causes the breakage of the peptide bond, but is unstable. A typical substrate then separates from the enzyme with the altered peptide bond. In the case of an inhibitor, the interaction between the active site serine and the amino acid at the susceptible site results in formation of a stable covalent bond. The inhibitor thus remains covalently coupled to the enzyme, blocking access to the enzymatic pocket.

rin simultaneously binds to thrombin and AT III, resulting in approximation of the inhibitor to its target enzyme. Relatively long chains of heparin are necessary to mediate this function. In contrast, only the conformational change is necessary for the inhibition of factor Xa. Accordingly, this step can be accelerated by both short (low molecular weight) and long heparin polymers. Endothelial cells are probably the source of heparin for this reaction in vivo.

Dermatan sulfate appears to be the major cofactor for heparin cofactor II; heparin can accelerate the activity of this inhibitor, but high concentrations (greater than 1.0 U/ml) are necessary. In contrast to AT III, heparin cofactor II inhibits only thrombin among the coagulation enzymes. Levels of heparin cofactor II are decreased in patients with acute consumptive coagulopathies, suggesting that the inhibitor does play a role in the normal regulation of hemostasis.

Table 40.7. Serine Protease Inhibitors (SERPINs)

Protein	Target Enzymes
Antithrombin III	Factor Xa, thrombin
Heparin cofactor II	Thrombin, chymotrypsin
α_2-Antiplasmin	Plasmin
Protein C inhibitor	Activated protein C, tissue plasminogen activator
Plasminogen activator inhibitor-1	Tissue plasminogen activator, urokinase, activated protein C
C-1-esterase inhibitor	C-1-esterase, factor XIIa, kallikrein
α_1-Antiprotease	Neutrophil elastase, trypsin

PROTEIN C SYSTEM

The protein C system is necessary for regulating the major cofactors of the coagulation cascade, factors Va and VIIIa. The protein C system involves multiple protein components and can be divided into three phases: activation, activity, and regulation (Table 40.8). Activation of protein C occurs on the surface of intact endothelial cells, which express thrombomodulin, a membrane-associated protein that functions as a cofactor for the activation of protein C by thrombin. Thrombin binds to thrombomodulin and undergoes an important conformational change; thrombin associated with thrombomodulin loses its procoagulant activity and no longer

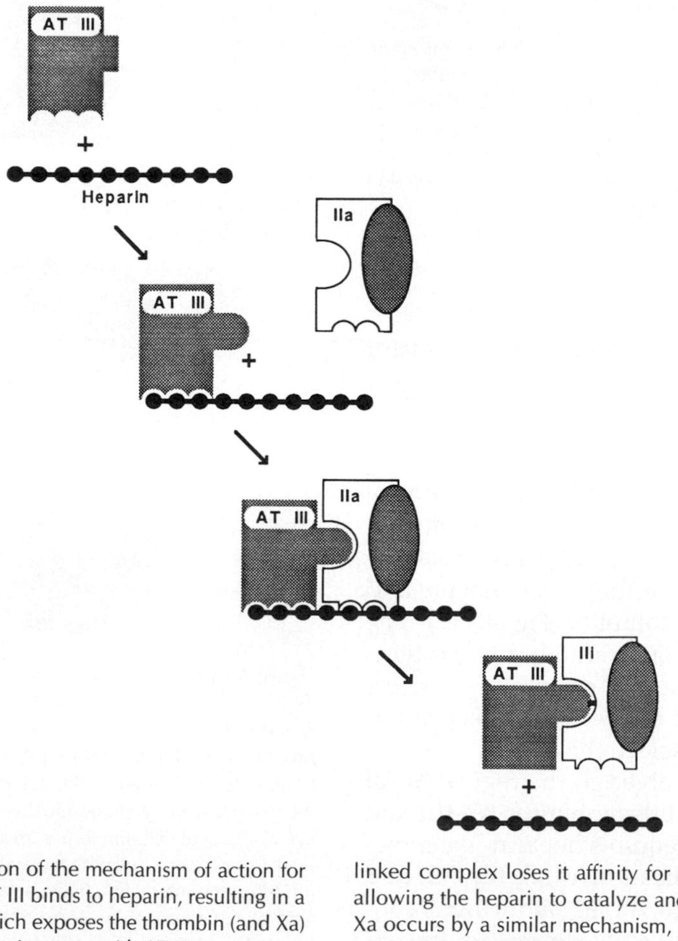

Figure 40.13. A schematic depiction of the mechanism of action for antithrombin III (AT III) is shown. AT III binds to heparin, resulting in a conformational change in AT III, which exposes the thrombin (and Xa) susceptible bond. Thrombin (IIa) then interacts with AT III in a process facilitated by thrombin binding to the heparin chain. The covalently linked complex loses it affinity for and dissociates from the heparin, allowing the heparin to catalyze another reaction. Inhibition of factor Xa occurs by a similar mechanism, except that heparin does not bind to Xa. Thus, Xa inhibition may be mediated by shorter chains of heparin.

Table 40.8. Protein C System

Aspect	Component	Function
Activation	Thrombin	Activates protein C
	Thrombomodulin	Cofactor for activation of protein C by thrombin
	Protein C	Substrate for thrombin-thrombomodulin
Activity	Activated protein C	Proteolytic inactivation of factors Va and VIIIa
	Protein S	Cofactor for activated protein C
	Factors Va and VIIIa	Substrates for activated protein C
Regulation	Protein C inhibitor	Neutralizes activated protein C
	Plasminogen activator inhibitor-1	Neutralizes activated protein C

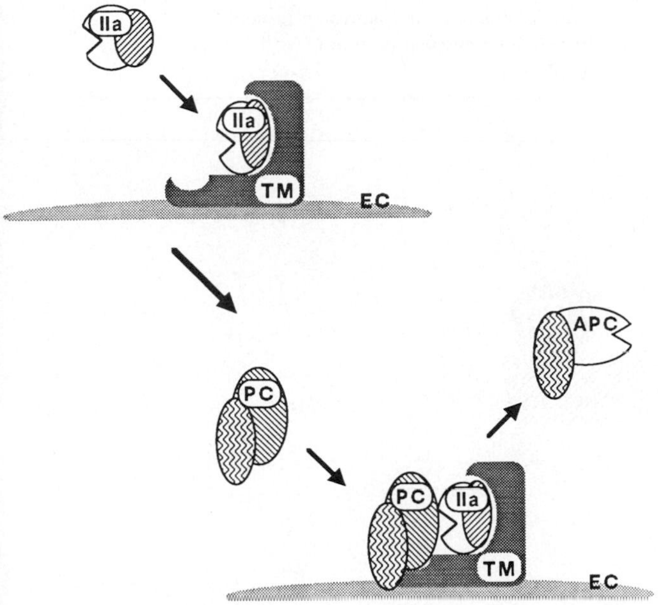

Figure 40.14. Protein C (PC) is activated by an endothelium (EC)-dependent process. Thrombin (IIa) binds to thrombomodulin (TM) on the EC surface and undergoes a conformational change. The IIa-TM complex then activates PC by releasing a short peptide from the heavy chain of PC. The activated protein C (APC) is then released to carry out its functions.

converts fibrinogen to fibrin, activates Va or VIIIa, activates XIII, or activates platelets. Thus, binding of thrombin by endothelial cell surface thrombomodulin is itself an anticoagulant step. The altered thrombin, however, readily activates protein C, a vitamin K–dependent protein (Fig. 40.14), and can still be inhibited by AT III.

Activated protein C (APC) is a proteolytic enzyme which degrades factors Va and VIIIa. This step requires a phospholipid surface, usually supplied by the platelet, and a protein cofactor, protein S (Fig. 40.15). Protein S is another vitamin K–dependent factor; however, it is unique among the vitamin K–dependent coagulation factors in that it is not a serine protease. Protein S is produced by a variety of cells, including hepatocytes, endothelial cells, and megakaryocytes. Thus, protein S is present within platelet α granules and is released in the

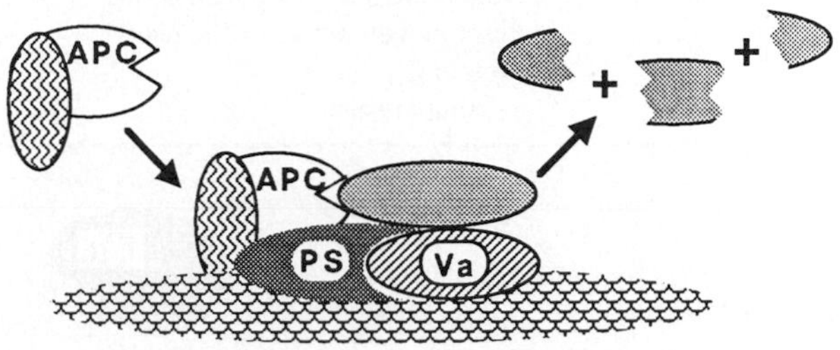

Figure 40.15. Activated protein C (APC) proteolytically inactivates the major cofactors of the coagulation cascade, factors Va and VIIIa. Protein S (PS) serves as a protein cofactor for this phospholipid-dependent process.

environment of a forming hemostatic plug, where it is most needed.

Protein C is inhibited by several SERPINs. The two major inhibitors involved in the regulation of APC appear to be protein C inhibitor, which is identical to plasminogen activator inhibitor-3, and plasminogen activator inhibitor-1. Experimental evidence suggests that APC has profibrinolytic activity. This effect appears to be related to competition between APC and tissue plasminogen activator for these two SERPINs. In the presence of increased amounts of APC, the inhibitors are utilized to neutralize APC, leaving tissue plasminogen activator free to activate plasminogen to plasmin.

FIBRINOLYTIC SYSTEM

The fibrinolytic system is also a complex, multicomponent system (Table 40.9). The major effector enzyme of this system is plasmin, which is derived from plasminogen by limited proteolytic cleavage. Although a number of serine proteases can convert plasminogen to plasmin, the major physiological activator appears to be tissue plasminogen activator (tPA). Urokinase is another important activator of plasminogen, particularly in pathological conditions and within the genitourinary tract. Tissue plasminogen activator requires fibrin for effective activation of plasminogen to plasmin; fibrin appears to function as a cofactor for the activation of plasminogen by tPA (Fig. 40.16). In contrast, urokinase is a direct activator of plasminogen and does not require fibrin as a cofactor.

Table 40.9. Fibrinolytic System

Aspect	Component	Function
Activation	Plasminogen	Substrate for plasminogen activators
	Tissue plasminogen activator (tPA)	Major physiological activator of plasminogen
	Fibrin	Cofactor for activation of plasminogen by tPA
	Urokinase	Direct activator of plasminogen
	Single-chain urokinase	Precursor of urokinase
Activity	Plasmin	Potent proteolytic enzyme
	Fibrin	Major substrate for plasmin
	Fibrinogen	Substrate for free plasmin
	Factors V and VIII	Substrates for free plasmin
	Platelet membrane glycoproteins	Substrates for free plasmin
Regulation	Plasminogen activator inhibitor-1	Inhibits tPA, urokinase and activated protein C
	Protein C inhibitor	Inhibits tPA and activated protein C
	α_2-Antiplasmin	Inhibits plasmin

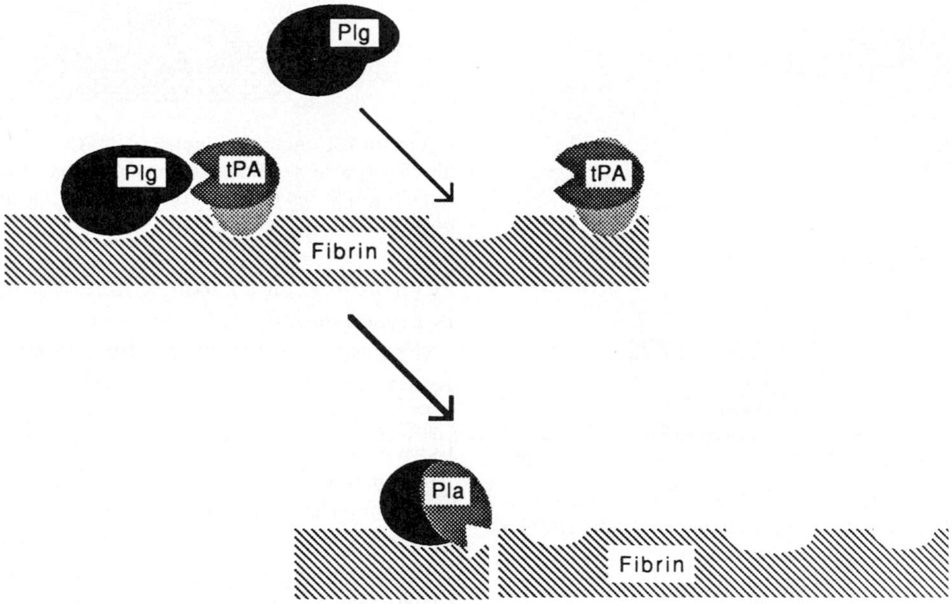

Figure 40.16. Tissue plasminogen activator (tPA) is a serine protease that efficiently activates plasminogen (Plg) to plasmin (Pla) in the presence of fibrin. The locally generated plasmin is then capable of degrading the fibrin clot. tPA is an inefficient activator of plasminogen in the absence of fibrin. Thus, normal plasminogen activation is limited to sites of fibrin formation.

Plasmin is a potent proteolytic enzyme that degrades fibrin clots. Under usual circumstances, plasmin remains bound to the fibrin clot through interaction of lysine binding sites on plasmin with the fibrin matrix. However, if plasmin breaks free of the fibrin clot, it is capable of digesting fibrinogen, factors V and VIII, and platelet membrane glycoproteins. Cleavage of fibrin by plasmin results in the release of adjacent D domains (Fig. 40.17). If these regions have been covalently cross-linked by factor XIIIa, these end products of plasmin digestion are known as D dimers. Antibodies that are specific for D dimers have been developed and can be used to assess fibrinolysis.

Regulation of the fibrinolytic system occurs on at least two levels. Activation of plasminogen to plasmin is regulated by the SERPINs plasminogen activator inhibitor-1 (PAI-1) and protein C inhibitor. As discussed in the section on protein C, these inhibitors also inhibit APC, and their availability for regulation of tPA is dependent on the amount of APC in the environment. The second level of regulation involves the SERPIN α_2-antiplasmin (α_2-AP). α_2-Antiplasmin rapidly inhibits free plasmin. However, it competes with fibrin for the same lysine binding sites on plasmin (Fig. 40.18). Thus, as long as plasmin is bound to the fibrin clot matrix, it is not inhibited by α_2-AP. However, once plasmin breaks free of the fibrin clot, it is instantaneously inhibited by α_2-AP. Pathological fibrinolysis can occur because there is normally twice as much plasminogen as α_2-AP on a molar basis. With marked activation of the fibrinolytic system, the α_2-AP regulatory mechanism is easily overwhelmed. This is one of the key pathological

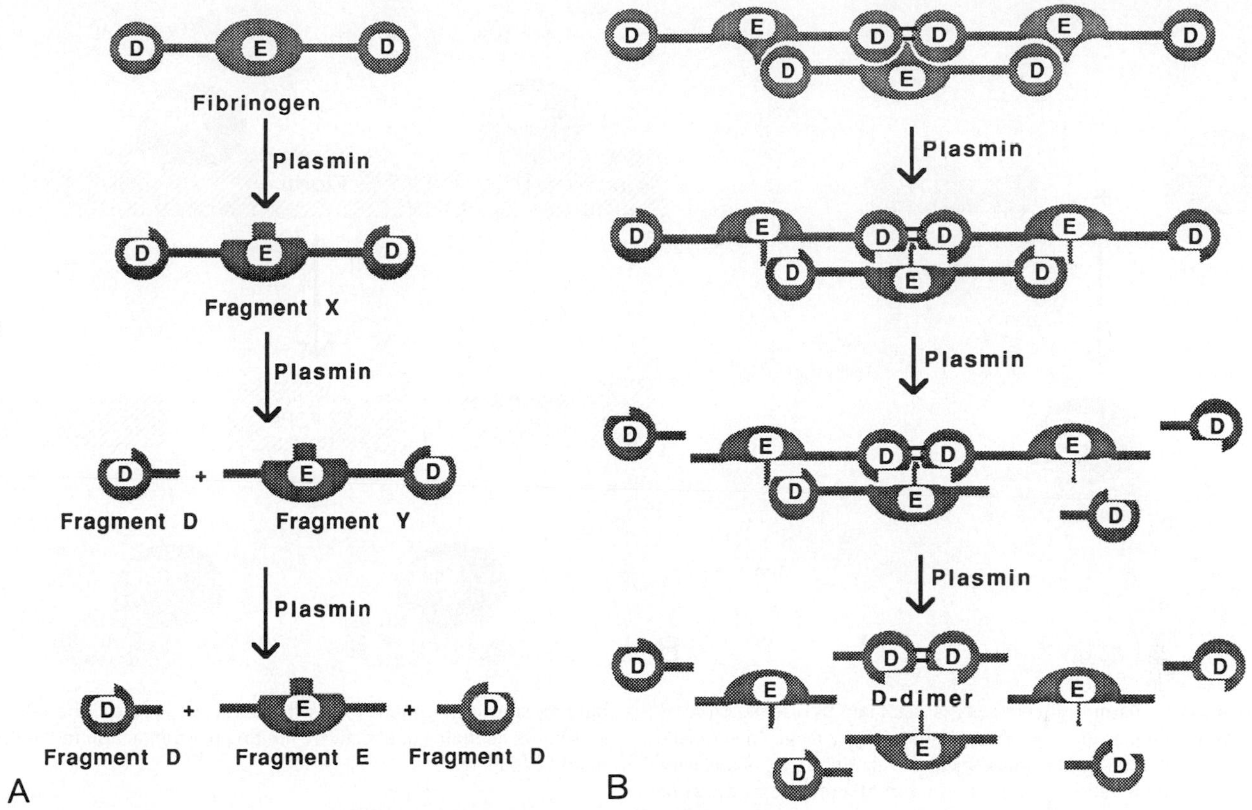

Figure 40.17. Plasmin can degrade either fibrinogen (**A**) or fibrin (**B**) in a stepwise fashion. Plasmin initially attacks the carboxyl terminus of the Aα chain and the amino terminus of the Bβ chain, resulting in the formation of the large degradation product fragment X. Cleavage of an interconnecting helical segment releases a D domain from the residual fragment (fragment Y). Further proteolysis results in the release of fragments D and E. Analogous fragments are released from the degradation of fibrin. However, adjacent D domains covalently linked by factor XIIIa remain cross-linked, forming D-dimers. These D-dimers are thus unique products of plasmin degradation of cross-linked fibrin gels.

changes underlying disseminated intravascular coagulation.

SUMMARY OF THE REGULATORY SYSTEM

Numerous components participate in the downregulation of the hemostatic response. This coordinated effort is normally successful in limiting hemostatic plug formation to sites of vascular disruption. A number of hereditary and acquired defects of the regulatory system have now been described (9, 10). Alterations that result in a decrease in the effectiveness of any one of these regulatory components can lead to increased clot formation in vivo, giving rise to a thrombotic tendency.

AN APPROACH TO HEMOSTATIC DISORDERS

There are a number of reasons why the hemostatic system may be evaluated as part of the clinical management of patients (11, 12). Common reasons include therapeutic drug monitoring, presurgical evaluation of hemostasis, evaluation of a possible bleeding tendency, evaluation of a possible thrombotic tendency, evaluation for the possibility of a circulating lupus anticoagulant, evaluation for the possibility of disseminated intravascular coagulation, and evaluation for other specific disorders. The laboratory plays a key role in monitoring oral anticoagulant and heparin therapy. In contrast, the laboratory has only a minor role in monitoring fibrinolytic therapy (e.g., tPA therapy) or antiplatelet therapy. In general, laboratory parameters measured during these therapeutic regimens provide little useful information, at least currently.

Routine presurgical evaluation of hemostasis remains a controversial topic. Several recent reports have indicated that routine preoperative prothrombin times (PTs) and activated partial thromboplastin times (APTTs) do not predict the risk of bleeding during surgery. Others have suggested that routine evaluation of the hemostatic system may be of use in determining whether or not the patient has an underlying coagulopathy. This controversy highlights the need to distinguish between a test's ability to provide a measure of the risk of bleeding and its ability to detect an abnormality that may or may not place a patient in a somewhat higher risk group. The

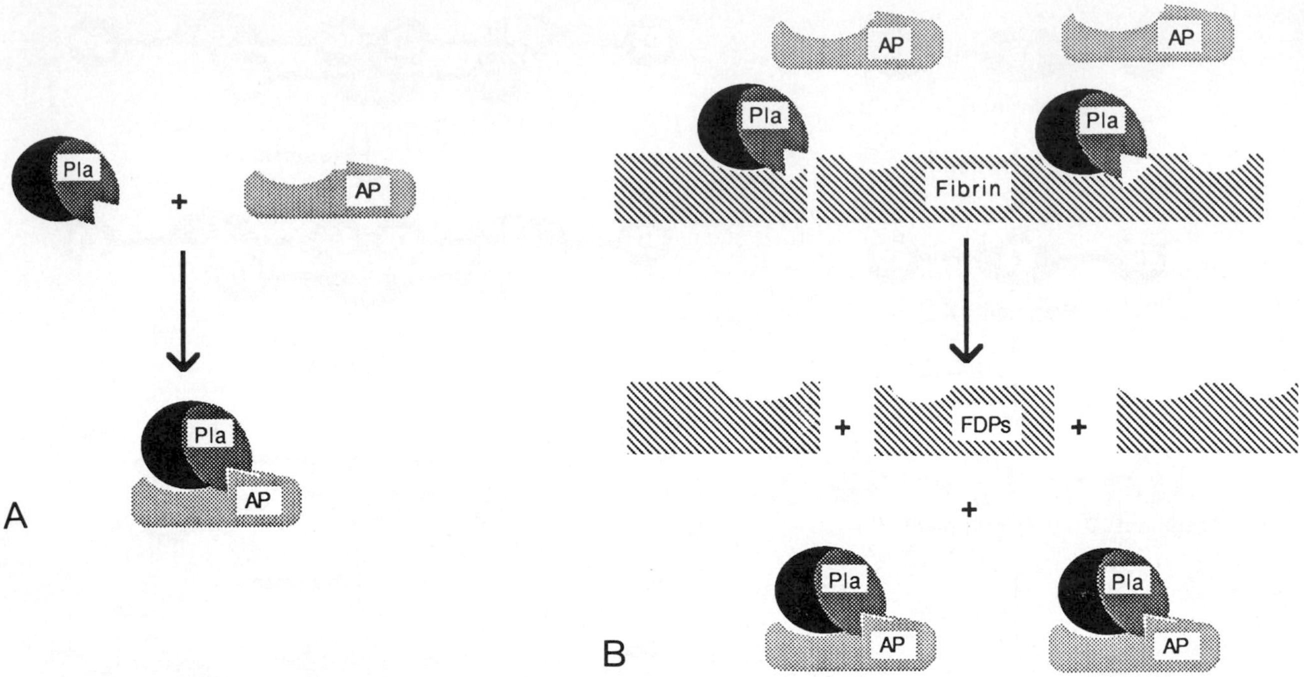

Figure 40.18. Plasmin (Pla) activity is regulated by a serine protease inhibitor, α_2-antiplasmin (AP). Free plasmin is very rapidly neutralized by AP (**A**). In contrast, plasmin associated with a fibrin gel is relatively protected from inhibition because fibrin and AP compete for the same binding sites on plasmin (**B**). As the fibrin gel is lysed, the released plasmin is neutralized, effectively limiting plasmin action to the fibrin matrix exclusively.

following sections outline an approach to the evaluation of patients with apparent bleeding or thrombotic disorders.

Hemostasis is a balanced system with the potent procoagulant mechanisms capable of forming a hemostatic plug at sites of vascular damage and equally potent regulatory systems capable of limiting clot formation to such sites (Fig 40.1). Bleeding or thrombotic disorders can arise whenever this balance is disturbed. Two mechanisms may lead to an increase in bleeding: a decrease or abnormality on the procoagulant side or an increase in regulatory activity. Von Willebrand's disease and hemophilia A provide examples of the first mechanism, whereas heparin therapy provides an example of the second mechanism. Similarly, thrombosis may occur because of defects in the regulatory system (e.g., antithrombin III deficiency) or increased activity on the procoagulant side, as may occur during the course of metastatic carcinoma. As with most problems in medicine, the clinical evaluation of these disorders begins with the clinical history and then moves to the laboratory for identification of specific disorders.

Evaluation of a Potential Bleeding Disorder

The clinical history of a patient with a potential bleeding disorder is used to determine whether the patient truly does have a bleeding problem, whether the problem is likely to be congenital or acquired, and whether the defect is in primary hemostasis, secondary hemostasis, or fibrinolysis. As perceptions of the seriousness of a bleeding problem vary significantly from patient to patient, the clinician must establish the frequency of bleeding, sites of bleeding, and severity of bleeding to determine the actual presence of a significant bleeding diathesis. Age of onset and family history are very helpful in distinguishing between congenital and acquired disorders. An early age of onset is suggestive of a congenital bleeding disorder, whereas the sudden appearance of bleeding in a previously healthy adult suggests an acquired problem. Family history can help establish a pattern of transmission. Some disorders are characterized by sex-linked recessive inheritance; others are characterized by either autosomal dominant or autosomal recessive inheritance.

The pattern of bleeding is very helpful in constructing a differential diagnosis. Mucocutaneous bleeding, characterized by epistaxis, ecchymosis, and genitourinary bleeding, is suggestive of a platelet disorder. Soft tissue bleeding, including hemarthrosis, hematomas, and retroperitoneal bleeding, is more suggestive of a coagulation disorder such as hemophilia A. Delayed bleeding is a classic manifestation of fibrinolytic-type bleeding. The clinical history should include a thorough medical history to document any other medical problems that may predispose to a bleeding diathesis. In addition, a careful

Table 40.10. Common Patterns Associated with Bleeding Disorders

	Platelet Disorders	Coagulation Disorders	Fibrinolytic Disorders
Clinical history	Mucocutaneous bleeding	Soft tissue bleeding	Delayed bleeding
Screening laboratory tests	Long bleeding time and/or low platelet count	Long PT and/or APTT	Normal

medication history, including over-the-counter medications, should be obtained. It is helpful to remember that the most common cause of abnormal platelet function is drug therapy, particularly aspirin therapy.

Following the clinical history, routine screening tests are commonly performed. These include the platelet count and bleeding time to assess platelet function and the PT and APTT to assess fibrin clot formation. Note that these screening tests do not assess fibrin stabilization or fibrinolysis. The bleeding time is a commonly performed test to assess primary hemostasis. A number of techniques for determining the bleeding time have been described, but the most commonly performed method is the template bleeding time using a disposable device. Although this test appears to be simple and straightforward, a number of technical variables can confound results. The bleeding time test is usually performed on the volar surface of the forearm, and the incision is made either perpendicular or parallel to the elbow crease. Those advocating a parallel incision point to the increased sensitivity to platelet defects associated with this type of incision, while those advocating a perpendicular incision point to the diminished scarring with this type of incision. It is important that any one laboratory use only one direction for the incision to obtain consistency in their results. A blood pressure cuff should be applied to the arm, and a constant pressure of 40 mm Hg maintained throughout the procedure. Fluctuation of the venous blood pressure because of a leaky cuff will cause erratic results in the bleeding time. Uniform and consistent pressure must be applied to the bleeding time device to ensure a uniform incision. Excessive pressure can result in a deeper cut and artificial prolongation of the bleeding time, whereas insufficient pressure may lead to a superficial cut and an artificially short time. Blotting is normally performed every 30 seconds and should be done in a manner to prevent disruption of the forming platelet plug. Following the completion of the bleeding time, the wound should be closed with a butterfly-type bandage and covered with a bandage.

The PT and APTT are tests of fibrin clot formation. The PT evaluates the extrinsic system of coagulation, beginning with activation of coagulation by tissue factor–factor VII (Fig. 40.8), and is sensitive to defects in fibrinogen, prothrombin, factor V, factor X, and factor VII. The APTT evaluates the intrinsic system of coagulation and is sensitive to defects in fibrinogen, prothrombin, factor V, factor X, factor VIII, factor IX, factor XI, factor XII, prekallikrein, and HMW kininogen. A number of technical variables can affect performance of the PT and APTT. Among these, specimen acquisition, sample processing, and choice of reagent are key components. Care should be taken to obtain a clean venipuncture sample and to anticoagulate it promptly with an appropriate amount of citrate. The sample should be processed as soon as possible to yield platelet-poor plasma. PT and APTT reagents vary significantly in their sensitivity and responsiveness to various hemostatic disorders. Therefore, the laboratory should be aware of the performance characteristics of their reagents and should carefully construct their own normal range to distinguish normal from abnormal adequately.

Table 40.11. Approximate Frequency of Congenital Bleeding Disorders

Disorder or Deficiency	Frequency per 10^6 Population
Fibrinogen	1
Prothrombin	< 0.5
Factor V	< 0.5
Factor VII	< 0.5
Factor VIII	60–100
Factor IX	10–20
Factor X	< 0.5
Factor XI	1
Factor XIII	< 0.5
α_2-antiplasmin	< 0.5
von Willebrand's disease	> 100
Bernard-Soulier syndrome	< 0.5
Glanzmann's thrombasthenia	< 0.5
Hermansky-Pudlak syndrome	< 0.5

Based on the results of the clinical history and screening laboratory tests, a limited number of patterns emerge (Table 40.10). Platelet disorders are usually characterized by mucocutaneous bleeding and a long bleeding time and/or a low platelet count. In contrast, coagulation disorders are usually characterized by a history of soft tissue bleeding and an abnormality of the APTT or PT. Fibrinolytic disorders are classically characterized by a history of delayed bleeding, often following trauma, and normal screening tests of hemostasis. Based on these initial results, further evaluation for a specific disorder can be undertaken. It is helpful to keep in mind the relative frequency of congenital disorders associated with bleeding (Table 40.11). The three most common are von Willebrand's disease, hemophilia A, and hemophilia B. Specific platelet disorders are reviewed in Chapter 41 and specific coagulation disorders are presented in Chapter 42.

Evaluation of a Potential Thrombotic Tendency

As with the evaluation of bleeding disorders, the evaluation of a potential thrombotic tendency begins with a thorough medical history. One of the primary goals of the history is to determine the likelihood of a congenital defect. In this regard, it is important to note the age of onset of symptoms and any family history of thrombosis. Most congenital defects are associated with onset of symptoms prior to the age of 45, and the family history for most of these disorders is also positive. Congenital thrombophilia is usually associated with recurrent deep venous thrombosis but may, on occasion, be associated with arterial thrombosis. A complete medical history must be obtained to determine if there is an underlying medical illness that may predispose to thrombosis (e.g., metastatic tumor, autoimmune disorders, etc.). A thorough medication history is also important, particularly before prescribing oral contraceptives in young women.

There are no screening assays that assess the regulatory system of coagulation or the degree of activation of the procoagulant mechanisms. Therefore, the laboratory approach to potential thrombotic disorders involves measuring the individual components of the regulatory systems. In general, assays that reflect the biological activity of the protein in question should be selected for use. In practice, such functional assays have been difficult to develop for some components of the system, notably protein C and protein S. In addition, assays for lupus anticoagulant activity and antiphospholipid antibodies may be of use. More recently, a variety of markers of the level of activation of the hemostatic system have been described. These include such peptides as prothrombin $F_{1.2}$, thrombin-antithrombin complexes, protein C activation peptide, and plasminogen-antiplasmin complexes. The usefulness of these assays in determining the risk of thrombosis, however, remains undetermined.

References

1. Bloom AL, Thomas DP. Haemostasis and thrombosis. 2nd ed. Edinburgh: Churchill Livingstone, 1987.
2. Bennett JS. The molecular biology of platelet membrane proteins. Semin Hematol 1990;27:186–204.
3. Kroll MH, Schafer AJ. Biochemical mechanisms of platelet activation. Blood 1989;74:1181–1195.
4. Davie EW, Fujikawa K, Kisiel W. The coagulation cascade: initiation, maintenance and regulation. Biochemistry 1991;30: 10363–10370.
5. Furie B, Furie BC. The molecular basis of blood coagulation. Cell 1988;53:505–518.
6. Mann KG, Nesheim ME, Church WR, Haley P, Krishnaswamy S. Surface-dependent reactions of the vitamin K-dependent enzyme complexes. Blood 1990;76:1–16.
7. Becker RC. Seminars in thrombosis, thrombolysis and vascular biology. 1. The vascular endothelium. Cardiology 1991;78: 13–22.
8. Broze GJ, Girard TJ, Novotny WF. The lipoprotein-associated coagulation inhibitor. In: Coller BS ed., Hemostasis and thrombosis. Philadelphia: WB Saunders, 1991;10:243–268.
9. Mammen EF, Fujii Y. Hypercoagulable states. Laboratory Medicine 1989;20:611–616.
10. Mannucci PM, Tripodi A. Laboratory screening of inherited thrombotic syndromes. Thrombos Haemost 1987;57:247–251.
11. Burns ER. Clinical management of bleeding and thrombosis. Boston: Blackwell Scientific Publications, 1987.
12. Ratnoff OD, Forbes CD. Disorders of hemostasis. 2nd ed. Orlando, FL: Grune & Stratton, 1991.

Suggested Readings

Thomas JH. Pathogenesis, diagnosis and treatment of thrombosis. Am J Surg 1990; 160:547–551.

Weiss HJ. Role of von Willebrand factor in platelet adhesion. In Zimmerman TS, Ruggeri ZM, eds. Coagulation and bleeding disorders: the role of factor VIII and von Willebrand factor. New York: Marcel Dekker, 1989:195–213.

41 Laboratory Evaluation of Platelet Disorders

John T. Brandt

Patients with abnormalities of primary hemostasis (platelet plug formation) typically present with a history of mucocutaneous bleeding. Congenital disorders of platelet function are usually evident early in life, although clinical manifestations may be delayed until adulthood. Acquired abnormalities of primary hemostasis are common causes of clinical bleeding problems and may occur at any age. The combination of mucocutaneous bleeding and a history of a medical problem associated with platelet dysfunction or thrombocytopenia is usually evident in such patients.

This chapter presents a diagnostic approach to congenital and acquired disorders affecting platelet function. The pathogenesis and evaluation of thrombocytopenia, as well as the therapeutic options for various platelet disorders, are briefly reviewed.

EVALUATION OF DISORDERS OF PLATELET FUNCTION

Abnormal platelet function is usually indicated by a history of mucocutaneous bleeding and the combination of an abnormal bleeding time and a normal platelet count. A variety of techniques may be used to further delineate the nature of the platelet defect (Table 41.1), but the most helpful procedures are those necessary for the characterization of von Willebrand factor (vWF) and platelet aggregation studies.

Commonly used procedures to evaluate vWF include vWF antigen (vWF:Ag) concentration (formerly designated VIIIR:ag), ristocetin cofactor activity (vWF:Rcof), platelet aggregation response to ristocetin, vWF crossed immunoelectrophoresis (vWF:CIE) and vWF multimeric analysis by SDS-agarose gel electrophoresis, and Western blotting. Laurell (rocket) immunoelectrophoresis is the most common method used to determine vWF:ag, a measure of the total plasma concentration of vWF that is independent of the multimeric composition of vWF. The aggregation response of formalin-fixed platelets to ristocetin and a limiting concentration of plasma as a source of vWF is the most popular technique for assessing the functional activity of vWF (as vWR:Rcof). A limiting factor of the vWF:Rcof assay is that vWF:Rcof activity does not always correlate with in vivo activity in patients with variant (type II) forms of von Willebrand's disease (vWD).

Crossed immunoelectrophoresis is a relatively simple method for assessing the multimeric composition of vWF. An abnormal distribution of vWF is evident with vWF:CIE in nearly all patients with type II vWD. SDS-agarose gel electrophoresis allows for a more definitive analysis of the multimeric structure and distribution of vWF, and may be of use in characterizing the specific defect in patients with variant vWD.

Platelet aggregation studies are used to assess the response of platelets to a variety of agonists (1). Platelet aggregation is most commonly performed by a turbidimetric method using platelet-rich plasma. More recently, an impedance method that can be used with either whole blood or platelet-rich plasma has been described, although information on performance of this method with congenital disorders of platelet function is limited. Commonly used platelet agonists for in vitro studies include ADP, collagen, epinephrine, arachidonic acid, and ristocetin.

ADP and epinephrine induce a characteristic biphasic wave of aggregation in normal individuals (Fig. 41.1). The initial (primary) wave is due to formation of small aggregates in direct response to agonist interaction with the platelet surface. The second wave is caused by the formation of large aggregates and is dependent on the release of endogenous platelet products. Patients may show a normal biphasic response to these agonists, a primary wave followed by disaggregation (designated a secondary wave defect) or a total lack of response (designated a primary wave defect). The responses to arachidonic acid and collagen are typically monophasic; abnormalities of response to these agonists may include partial, delayed, or absent response.

Normal platelets tend to aggregate to ristocetin when the concentration is greater than 1.0 mg/ml.

Table 41.1. Laboratory Techniques for Evaluation of Platelet Function

Procedure	Property Evaluated	Clinical Uses
Bleeding time	Global platelet function	Screening test of platelet function
Platelet count	Platelet number in peripheral blood	Screening test for platelet disorders
Mean platelet volume	Average platelet size	Assessing platelet mass in peripheral blood; assessing platelet production in response to thrombocytopenia
Platelet aggregation studies	Platelet function	Delineate type of platelet dysfunction; detection of variant von Willebrand's disease (vWD); detection of heparin-induced thrombocytopenia
von Willebrand factor (vWF): antigen	Quantity of vWF protein in blood	Evaluation of possible vWD
von Willebrand factor: ristocetin cofactor assay	Measurement of functional activity of vWF	Evaluation of possible vWD
von Willebrand factor: Multimeric analysis	Measure of vWF polymerization	Evaluation of possible variant vWD
Electron microscopy	Platelet morphology, platelet granules	Evaluation of some congenital platelet disorders
Bone marrow examination	Assessment of platelet production	Evaluation of thrombocytopenia
Platelet antibody determination	Presence or absence of antiplatelet antibodies	Evaluation of possible immune-mediated thrombocytopenia
Platelet survival	Rate of platelet turnover	Determining the mechanism of thrombocytopenia
PF4, βTG	In vivo platelet release	Detection of in vivo platelet activation
Circulating platelet aggregates	In vivo platelet activation	Detection of in vivo platelet activation

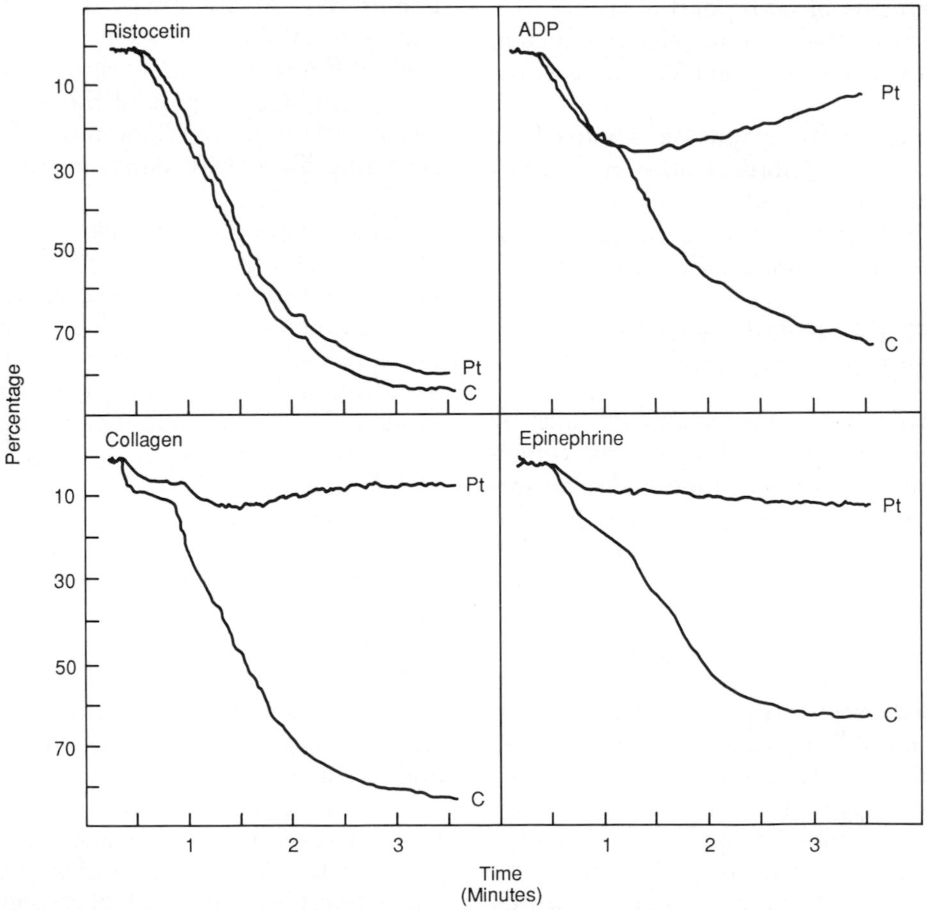

Figure 41.1. Normal (C) and abnormal (Pt) aggregation responses for ADP, collagen, epinephrine, and ristocetin. The normal response to ADP at optimal concentrations is a biphasic wave, with the secondary wave dependent on an intact release response by the responding platelets. An inability to undergo release results in a primary wave of aggregation, followed by disaggregation (Pt); this pattern is designated a secondary wave defect. A total lack of response to ADP would be designated a primary wave defect. Abnormal responses to collagen include a delay in onset of aggregation or, as in this case, a decreased response to collagen. Epinephrine usually results in a biphasic wave of aggregation; abnormalities to this agonist vary from total lack of response to a primary wave followed by disaggregation. Diminished response to ristocetin (not shown) is characteristic of abnormalities of platelet adhesion.

Patients with vWD or Bernard-Soulier syndrome may show a lack of response at these concentrations. Normal platelets do not aggregate at ristocetin concentrations less than 0.8 mg/ml. However, platelet aggregation may be seen at these concentrations in patients with pseudo-vWD and type IIB vWD. Thus, it is important to test with both high (greater than 1.0 mg/ml) and low (less than 0.8 mg/ml) concentrations of ristocetin when performing these assays.

Performance of vWF and platelet aggregation studies play a major role in the evaluation of congenital platelet disorders and possible acquired vWD. In contrast, these studies have only a minor role in the evaluation of other acquired platelet disorders. The clinical history is thus an important aspect of the decision to perform platelet function studies. Congenital disorders of platelet function usually present with a history of mucocutaneous bleeding starting during childhood. These disorders can be classified according to the aspect of platelet function (adhesion, activation, aggregation) that is abnormal and the nature of the specific defect. The laboratory features of disorders of adhesion, activation, and aggregation are sufficiently distinct to permit construction of a flow diagram for their diagnosis (Fig. 41.2).

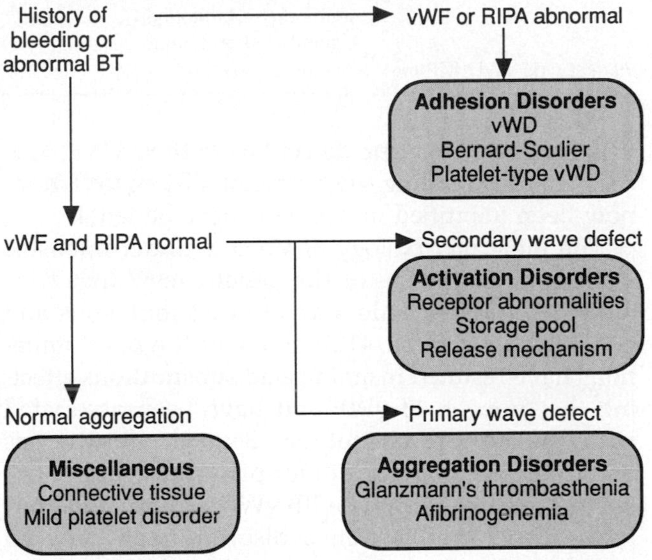

Figure 41.2. Flow diagram for diagnosis of abnormalities of platelet function. Abnormalities of platelet adhesion are characterized by an abnormal aggregation response to ristocetin and/or abnormalities of von Willebrand factor. Abnormalities of platelet activation are usually characterized by a secondary wave type defect with ADP, while abnormalities of platelet aggregation are characterized by a primary wave defect. Occasional patients with mild platelet dysfunction may show a normal response to all the agonists used in routine studies.

CONGENITAL DISORDERS OF PLATELET FUNCTION

Abnormalities of Platelet Adhesion

A number of congenital disorders affecting platelet adhesion have been described (Table 41.2) (2). The most common of these disorders is vWD. The other disorders in this group, although rare, are important for what they teach about the normal process of platelet adhesion and because the therapy of these disorders varies.

VON WILLEBRAND'S DISEASE

Von Willebrand's disease (vWD) is the most common congenital bleeding disorder known, but its actual frequency has not yet been defined accurately (3). Some have estimated the frequency to be as high as 1:100, but clinical experience would suggest a lower incidence. It is typically inherited as an autosomal dominant trait; that is, heterozygotes are clinically symptomatic. Double heterozygous and homozygous forms of the disease have also been described. Patients with vWD have clinical manifestations characteristic of platelet disorders, with the most common complaints related to increased bruising, epistaxis, and menorrhagia. Indeed, the development of iron deficiency anemia in a pubescent female may be an indication of an underlying platelet disorder such as vWD. The family history is usually positive, with male and female relatives being affected with equal frequency.

Table 41.2. Congenital Disorders of Platelet Adhesion

Disorder	Defect	Inheritance
von Willebrand's disease		
Type I	Decreased quantity of all vWF multimers	Autosomal dominant
Type II	Selective decrease of high molecular weight vWF multimers	Autosomal dominant (usually)
Type III	Severe deficiency of all vWF multimers	Autosomal recessive
Hemophilia-type	Defective binding of factor VIII to an abnormal vWF	Autosomal recessive
Platelet-type von Willebrand's disease (pseudo-vWD)	Abnormal platelet GP Ib/IX with increased affinity for normal vWF	Autosomal dominant
Bernard-Soulier syndrome	Deficiency or decreased function of platelet GP Ib/IX	Autosomal recessive
Collagen receptive deficiency	Deficiency of GP Ia	Undetermined
Connective tissue disorders	Decreased platelet adhesion	Autosomal recessive

The bleeding in vWD tends to be mild to moderate, and symptoms often spontaneously improve after adolescence. This disorder is relatively well tolerated, unless the hemostatic system is challenged by trauma or surgery, at which time bleeding may be serious. The postpartum period is another high-risk time for bleeding in women with vWD despite the pregnancy-associated rise in the level of vWF. The level of vWF drops precipitously in the postpartum period, and the patient may begin to bleed seriously. Occasionally, a diagnosis is not established during childhood, and an older patient may present with recurrent gastrointestinal bleeding as the initial manifestation of vWD. These patients are typically over the age of 50. An extensive evaluation of the gastrointestinal tract usually is unrevealing or demonstrates only angiodysplasia.

Homozygous (type III) vWD is usually associated with a more severe hemorrhagic diathesis. The clinical manifestations may mimic those of the hemophilia A due to the very low or absent factor VIII. These patients may be misdiagnosed as having hemophilia A if appropriate laboratory studies are not performed. It is important to discriminate between type III vWD and hemophilia A because the therapy of these two disorders can be different.

Von Willebrand's disease is due to a deficiency or structural abnormality of vWF. Von Willebrand factor is synthesized by endothelial cells and megakaryocytes and is found in subendothelial spaces, plasma, and platelet α granules. Platelet vWF appears to make a significant contribution to platelet plug formation. This is reflected by the relatively shorter bleeding times in those patients who have a low level of plasma vWF and normal platelet vWF.

As indicated in Table 41.2, three major subtypes of vWD have been delineated (3). Type I vWD is characterized by a decrease in the total concentration of vWF with a concordant decrease in all sizes of vWF multimers. Type II vWD is characterized by a selective decrease in high–molecular weight multimers of vWF. The total amount of vWF antigen present in such patients is highly variable and may be within the reference range. A number of subtypes of type II vWD have been described based on the multimeric pattern on high-resolution SDS-agarose gels, ristocetin-induced aggregation at low concentrations of ristocetin, and inheritance. Type III vWD is characterized by absent plasma vWF and represents the homozygous or double heterozygous form of vWD. More recently, a defect in the ability of vWF to bind and transport factor VIII in plasma has been described. Other functions of vWF may be normal or only mildly affected in such patients. As a consequence, these patients may present clinically as mild to moderate hemophilia A with a deficiency of factor VIII; however, the true defect lies in their vWF. Mutations in the binding site for factor VIII on vWF have now been identified in some of these patients.

Table 41.3. Examples of Genetic Defects in von Willebrand's Disease (vWD) and Related Disorders

Clinical Phenotype	Genetic Defects Reported
Type IIA vWD	$Arginine_{834}$ → tryptophan
	$Valine_{844}$ → aspartic acid
	$Serine_{850}$ → proline
	$Glutamine_{875}$ → lysine
	$Valine_{802}$ → leucine
	$Serine_{743}$ → leucine
Type IIB vWD	$Argine_{543}$ → tryptophan
	$Valine_{553}$ → methionine
	$Methionine_{540}$ → duplication
	$Arginine_{545}$ → cysteine
	$Tryptophan_{550}$ → cysteine
	$Proline_{574}$ → leucine
	$Arginine_{578}$ → glutamine
Type III vWD	Gene deletions
	Decreased mRNA expression
	Arginine → stop codons
Hemophilia-type vWD	$Threonine_{28}$ → methionine
	$Arginine_{53}$ → tryptophan
	$Arginine_{91}$ → glutamine
Platelet-type vWD (GP Ibα)	$Glycine_{233}$ → valine

The molecular biology of vWD is under intensive investigation. Defects at the genetic level that have been described include several point mutations and gene deletions (Table 41.3). Some of the point mutations have resulted in amino acid substitutions affecting the function of vWF and have been associated with the type II phenotype. Several substitutions within the binding domain for platelet GP Ib/IX have been associated with type IIB vWD. These mutations have all occurred within a disulfide loop between Cys 509 and Cys 695. Consequently, it has been suggested that these substitutions alter the affinity of vWF for GP Ib/IX. A cluster of amino acid substitutions in the A_2 region (amino acids 717 to 909) of vWF has similarly been associated with the type IIA phenotype. Some of these substitutions are near a protease-susceptible site and may result in increased proteolysis of high–molecular weight multimers of vWF. This hypothesis is supported by the observation that the multimeric composition of vWF is relatively conserved when the plasma from some patients with type IIA vWD is collected into anticoagulants containing protease inhibitors. More recently, amino acid substitutions in the factor VIII binding region of vWF have been identified in patients with pseudohemophilia.

Because of the complex nature of vWF, a number of laboratory procedures must be utilized to evaluate the possibility of vWD when a patient presents with a history of mucocutaneous bleeding. The bleeding time is used as the major screening test

Table 41.4. Typical Laboratory Parameters in von Willebrand's Disease (vWD) and Related Disorders[a]

Parameter	Type I vWD	Type II vWD	Type IIB vWD	Hemophilia-like vWD	Type III vWD	Platelet-type vWD	Bernard-Soulier Syndrome
Bleeding time	↑ or N	↑	↑	N or slight ↑	↑	↑	↑
Platelet count	N	N	↓ or N	N	N	↓ or N	↓
APTT	↑	N or ↑	N or ↑	↑	↑	N or ↑	N
vWF:Ag	↓	↓ or N	N or ↑	N or slight ↓	↓↓	N or ↓	N
vWF:Rcof	↓	↓ or N	↓ or N	N or slight ↓	↓↓	↓ or N	N
VIII	↓	N or ↓	N or ↓	↓	↓↓	N or ↓	N
Aggregation response to ristocetin	↓ or N	↓	↑	N	↓↓	↑	↓↓
vWF multimeric composition	N	Abn	Abn	N	ND	Abn	N

[a]Abbreviations used: APTT, activated partial thromboplastin time; vWF:ag, von Willebrand factor antigen; vWF:Rcof, ristocetin cofactor activity; VIII, factor VIII coagulant activity; N, normal; ND, not done (antigen too low).

and is typically mildly to moderately prolonged in vWD. However, the bleeding time may fluctuate significantly over time and may be within the normal range at any given point. In particular, patients with normal levels of platelet vWF may have only a modest, if any, prolongation of the bleeding time. Therefore, a normal bleeding time in a patient with a history of mucocutaneous bleeding does not rule out vWD, and further laboratory studies are indicated in such patients. The aspirin tolerance test, in which the bleeding time is repeated 2 to 8 hours after a challenge with aspirin (650 mg), may be helpful; patients with mild vWD usually show a marked prolongation of the bleeding time after such an aspirin challenge.

Factor VIII, vWF:ag, and vWF:Rcof assays are used to measure the amount of vWF-factor VIII complex in plasma. Similar levels of these proteins are found when the results of these assays are expressed as percentage of normal plasma in most normal patients and patients with type I vWD. Patients with type II vWD often show a discordance between these parameters; indeed, such a finding should raise the possibility of type II vWD.

SDS-agarose electrophoresis and crossed immunoelectrophoresis are used to assess the multimeric composition of vWF. One of these assays should be performed as part of the routine evaluation of patients suspected of having vWD because the only abnormalities that may be found in some type II vWD patients are a prolonged bleeding time and abnormal vWF multimeric composition.

The diagnosis of vWD depends on the combination of an appropriate clinical history and characteristic laboratory abnormalities (Table 41.4). Patients with type I vWD typically have a prolonged bleeding time, a proportional decrease in vWF:ag, vWF:Rcof and factor VIII, a decreased aggregation response to ristocetin (greater than 1.0 mg/ml), and a normal multimeric composition by either crossed immunoelectrophoresis or SDS–agarose gel electrophoresis. Patients with type II vWD also have a prolonged bleeding time; however, the vWF:ag is variable and may be normal. vWF:Rcof is quite variable and may be normal or increased in some subtypes of type II vWD. Factor VIII activity tends to parallel vWF:ag in these patients and thus may be normal as well. Multimeric analysis demonstrates the characteristic loss of high–molecular weight multimers in these patients. Type III vWD is characterized by very long bleeding times, absent vWF, very low or undetectable factor VIII activity, and absent vWF:Rcof. Multimeric analysis cannot be performed in these patients due to the lack of antigen.

Type IIB vWD is a distinct subgroup; patients with type IIB vWD typically have very long bleeding times and a variable degree of thrombocytopenia. The level of vWF:ag tends to be normal or slightly decreased while vWF:Rcof is usually decreased but may be normal. These patients show an enhanced aggregation response to low concentrations of ristocetin. The molecular defect in these patients appears to be an abnormal binding site for GP Ib/IX on vWF, resulting in enhanced binding of high molecular multimers to normal resting platelets. Apparently the complex of platelet and high–molecular weight multimers of vWF is cleared from the circulation, resulting in the deficiency of higher molecular weight multimers and thrombocytopenia. The synthetic vasopressin analogue desmopressin (DDAVP) may induce further thrombocytopenia, presumably due to release of the abnormal vWF from endothelial cells. These patients should be distinguished from patients with pseudo-vWD, as the latter patients require therapy with platelets rather than cryoprecipitate or factor VIII concentrates.

Many of the bleeding episodes with type I vWD can now be handled with desmopressin. This agent induces a twofold to tenfold increase in the plasma level of vWF, a response that is often adequate to maintain hemostasis during dental procedures or other minor surgical procedures. The fibrinolytic inhibitor, epsilon aminocaproic acid (Amicar), may be a useful adjunct, particularly in procedures involving the oral mucosa. Von Willebrand factor can also be replaced with cryoprecipitate, an excellent source of fully functional vWF. Certain highly purified factor VIII concentrates are also effective in the therapy of vWD. An advantage of the factor VIII concentrates is that they have undergone one or more viral inactivation steps.

PSEUDO–VON WILLEBRAND'S DISEASE

In 1982, a new platelet disorder that mimicked many of the clinical laboratory findings of type II vWD was described. These patients were characterized by a history of mucocutaneous bleeding, prolonged bleeding times, intermittent thrombocytopenia, and decreased concentrations of the high–molecular weight multimers of vWF. Subsequent investigations have indicated that the defect in these patients lies in the platelet receptor for vWF (4). The abnormal GP Ib/IX complex appears to have an increased affinity for vWF in normal plasma. Normal high–molecular weight multimers of vWF bind to these abnormal platelets and cause platelet agglutination and removal of the platelets from the circulation. Because of the clearance of high–molecular weight vWF multimers by the abnormal platelets, multimeric analysis shows a selective decrease in plasma high–molecular weight multimers. Thus, the laboratory picture in these patients resembles that of type IIB vWD (Table 41.4). Analogous to type IIB vWD, platelets from patients with pseudo-vWD also show an enhanced aggregation response to low concentrations of ristocetin.

Pseudo-vWD can be distinguished from type IIB vWD by demonstrating that the defect lies in the patient's platelets and not in the plasma. Platelets from patients with pseudo-vWD have been shown to bind increased amounts of normal vWF at low concentrations of ristocetin. This allows separation of these two disorders, as platelets from patients with type IIB bind normal amounts of vWF. The clinical management of patients with pseudo-vWD differs from those with type IIB vWD; patients with pseudo-vWD should be treated with platelets for the control of bleeding episodes.

BERNARD-SOULIER SYNDROME

The Bernard-Soulier syndrome is a rare autosomal recessive disorder characterized by the onset of mucocutaneous bleeding at an early age, a prolonged bleeding time, and thrombocytopenia with giant platelets. The Bernard-Soulier syndrome is due to a deficiency or functional abnormality of the glycoprotein Ib/IX complex (4). Because of the deficiency of the receptor for vWF, these platelets do not adhere normally to the vessel wall; thus, platelet plug formation is impaired.

Laboratory evaluation of patients with the Bernard-Soulier syndrome usually demonstrates a normal aggregation response to agonists such as ADP, epinephrine, collagen, and arachidonic acid. However, platelets do not aggregate in response to ristocetin. Analysis of vWF shows normal levels of vWF:ag and normal vWF:Rcof activity. The multimeric composition of vWF in patients with Bernard-Soulier syndrome is also normal (Table 41.4).

Therapy of patients with Bernard-Soulier syndrome revolves around transfusion of platelets to control bleeding episodes. Alloimmunization is a problem in these patients due to the frequent transfusion requirements.

COLLAGEN RECEPTOR DEFICIENCY

Recently, congenital deficiency of platelet membrane glycoprotein Ia has been described. These patients have been characterized by a prolonged bleeding time, mild to moderate mucocutaneous bleeding, and defects in platelet aggregation response to collagen; vWF and platelet response to ristocetin are normal. Glycoprotein Ia appears to contribute significantly to normal platelet adhesion and subsequent platelet plug formation through its ability to bind to collagen.

CONNECTIVE TISSUE DISORDERS

Patients who have congenital disorders of connective tissue, such as the Ehlers-Danlos syndrome, may have problems with mucocutaneous bleeding. Bleeding times in such patients are often mildly prolonged. In vitro assessment of platelet function usually shows normal results and normal levels of vWF. The defect in such patients appears to be in the vessel wall receptors that mediate platelet adhesion.

Disorders of Platelet Activation

A number of congenital disorders that affect platelet activation have been described (2). These patients have a clinical history typical of platelet dysfunction, with the onset of mucocutaneous bleeding early on in life. The family history is often positive, suggesting an autosomal dominant pattern of inheritance. However, the precise inheritance pattern for many of these disorders is still poorly defined because only a few kindred have been studied for most of these defects. The bleeding time is typically prolonged, but, as with von Willebrand's disease, may be within the upper range of normal. The aspirin tolerance test can also be used to unmask an underlying platelet defect in this group of patients.

Laboratory studies characteristically show normal levels and multimeric composition of vWF and a nor-

Table 41.5. Congenital Platelet Disorders Associated with Abnormal Platelet Activation

Membrane Receptor Disorders	Storage Pool Disorders	Release Mechanism Disorders
Collagen receptor deficiency	Hermansky-Pudlak syndrome	Cyclooxygenase deficiency
α_2-Adrenergic receptor deficiency	Wiscott-Aldridge syndrome	Thromboxane synthetase deficiency
	Chediak-Higashi syndrome	Defective calcium mobilization
	Idiopathic	Decreased arachidonic acid release
		Abnormal phosphatidyl-inositol metabolism
		Idiopathic

mal platelet response to ristocetin. Platelet aggregation with ADP and epinephrine typically shows a secondary wave defect, characterized by an initial wave of aggregation followed by dissociation of the platelets (Fig. 41.1). The response to arachidonic acid and collagen may be blunted or delayed as well. A number of specific disorders, as briefly described below, have been delineated, but platelet transfusion therapy is the common therapy for all of these disorders. Although the mechanism is unknown, desmopressin has been shown to be effective in some patients and may be a useful adjunct.

Disorders of platelet activation can be divided into platelet membrane receptor disorders, storage pool disorders, and release mechanism disorders (Table 41.5). Deficiency of glycoprotein Ia, a collagen receptor, is associated with an abnormal aggregation response to collagen and defective platelet adhesion. Deficiency of α_2-adrenergic receptors (epinephrine receptors) has been associated with a mild bleeding tendency and failure of platelets to aggregate in response to epinephrine in vitro. In many of these patients, the aggregation response to ADP, collagen, and arachidonic acid has been normal.

Deficiency of platelet granules results in what is known as the storage pool disorders, which have been associated with clinically significant platelet dysfunction. The dense granules, α granules, or both types of granules may be deficient. Deficiency of dense granules has been associated with congenital disorders such as the Hemansky-Pudlak syndrome and the Wiscott-Aldridge syndrome, but may occur independent of such disorders (Table 41.5). Selective deficiency of α granules is designated the gray platelet syndrome due to the pale appearance of platelets on a Wright-Giemsa–stained peripheral blood film.

Several defects affecting platelet metabolic pathways have also been associated with recurrent mucocutaneous bleeding. Deficiency of either cyclooxygenase or thromboxane synthetase results in deficient synthesis of thromboxane A_2. Such patients typically show no aggregation response to arachidonic acid and a secondary wave type defect to ADP. Defects involving mobilization of calcium from storage sites have also been described, but the precise molecular defect has not been delineated in these cases. Release mechanism disorder can be differentiated from storage pool disorders with specialized studies such as electron microscopic evaluation of platelet granules, measurement of serotonin uptake and release, and measurement of ATP release in response to strong agonists such as thrombin. Typically, patients with dense granule deficiency show a decreased uptake of radiolabeled serotonin, a decreased number of granules on electron microscopy, and decreased release of ATP in response to thrombin. Distinction between these types of disorders generally does not affect the clinical management of these patients.

Disorders of Platelet Aggregation

Glanzmann's thrombasthenia is the major disorder affecting platelet-platelet interaction. Glanzmann's thrombasthenia is a rare autosomal recessive disorder characterized by markedly prolonged bleeding times, recurrent mucocutaneous bleeding, and absent aggregation response to ADP, epinephrine, collagen, and arachidonic acid. The aggregation response to ristocetin is often normal in these patients. Glanzmann's thrombasthenia is due to deficiency or abnormality of the glycoprotein IIb/IIIa complex (4). Due to the defect, the platelets cannot bind fibrinogen or other adhesive proteins and thus cannot be cross-linked to accomplish platelet aggregation. The diagnosis is established by the clinical history, a long bleeding time, and the characteristic lack of platelet aggregation with normal fibrinogen levels.

Because of the interaction of glycoprotein IIb/IIIa with the cytoskeleton of the platelet, clot retraction is usually diminished in patients with Glanzmann's thrombasthenia. The platelet antigens PL^{A1}, Bak^a, and Lek^a are located on the glycoprotein IIb/IIIa complex. Patients with Glanzmann's thrombasthenia tend to be negative for these antigens and are thus quite susceptible to alloimmunization. Alloimmunization is a major clinical problem in the management of these patients, because they may become refractory to platelet therapy.

Patients with afibrinogenemia may also have problems with mucocutaneous bleeding and may lack a response to agonists such as ADP, collagen, arachidonic acid, and epinephrine. The defect in

Table 41.6. Acquired Abnormalities of Platelet Function

Medications	Multiple myeloma
Antiplatelet antibodies	Monoclonal proteins
Uremia	Macromolecules
Cardiopulmonary bypass	Hypothyroidism
Consumptive coagulopathies	Liver disease
Acquired von Willebrand's disease	

platelet aggregation in these cases is due to the absence of the fibrinogen as a cross-linking material. The clinical picture in such patients is usually dominated by the major defect in fibrin clot formation. As one would expect, the PT and APTT are basically unmeasurable in such patients.

ACQUIRED DISORDERS OF PLATELET FUNCTION

Acquired abnormalities of platelet function are a more common cause of clinical bleeding than congenital disorders (5). A number of conditions have been associated with abnormal platelet function (Table 41.6). Among these, drug-induced abnormalities are probably the most common cause of abnormal platelet function. In contrast to congenital disorders, in which platelet aggregation studies play a pivotal role in delineating the nature of the platelet defect, platelet aggregation studies have a minor role in evaluating acquired platelet dysfunction. In most patients, the combination of the clinical history and a prolonged bleeding time are sufficient to establish the platelet abnormality; platelet aggregation studies do not add any specific or clinically predictive information in most patients. The major clinical challenge in patients with acquired platelet dysfunction is often devising adequate therapy.

Medications That May Affect Platelet Function

Numerous drugs and foods have been found to have an effect on platelet function either in vivo or in vitro (Table 41.7). Major groups of drugs that affect platelet function include nonsteroidal anti-inflammatory agents, of which aspirin is the most common offender; β-lactam–containing antibiotics; a variety of cardiovascular drugs, particularly β-blockers; psychotropic drugs; anesthetics; antihistamines; and some chemotherapeutic agents. Aspirin is taken by many patients on a routine basis and is also a common ingredient in many over-the-counter medications. Therefore, a history of aspirin ingestion may be difficult to elicit unless detailed questioning is used. Antibiotics are often an overlooked source of impaired platelet function. They can have an adverse effect on in vivo bleeding tendencies.

Uremia

Uremia is associated with a complex coagulopathy dominated by abnormal platelet function. A number of biochemical changes in platelets have been described in patients with uremia, but the precise lesion(s) responsible for the clinical manifestations are still unclear. Anemia contributes significantly to the bleeding associated with uremia, particularly when the hemoglobin is less than 90 to 100 g/liter. Studies have documented that the bleeding time and bleeding tendency both decrease if the hemoglobin concentration is raised by either transfusion or administration of erythropoietin. Other defects that have been reported in uremia include decreased adhesion of platelets to subendothelium, decreased availability of platelet factor 3 (platelet procoagulant activity), increased cytoplasmic c-AMP levels, alterations in cytoplasmic calcium and the rise in calcium following stimulation by a variety of platelet agonists, and alterations in vessel wall prostacyclin synthesis. Platelet aggregation studies in patients with uremia have been variable, with some groups reporting essentially normal aggregation responses and others reporting markedly impaired aggregation responses. In most studies, the aggregation responses observed in vitro have not correlated with clinical bleeding.

Dialysis improves platelet function in patients with uremia and is an important part of the therapeutic approach in these patients. In addition to dialysis and correction of the anemia, a number of other therapeutic options for managing clinical bleeding in these patients have been developed. Cryoprecipitate has been reported to decrease the bleeding time and bleeding severity. The mechanism of action of cryoprecipitate is unclear, but it is relatively rich in vWF, which could promote platelet adhesion. Desmopressin has also been associated with a decrease in the bleeding time and correction of the bleeding tendency in patients with uremia. More recently, conjugated estrogens have been used in these patients with a beneficial effect.

Antiplatelet Antibodies

Antiplatelet antibodies have usually been associated with thrombocytopenia. However, antibodies that bind to the platelet surface can also cause abnormalities of platelet function. Decreased platelet function due to antiplatelet antibodies is most commonly associated with chronic autoimmune thrombocytopenic purpura (ITP). The precise mechanism of abnormal platelet function in these patients is still unclear, but is probably related to interaction of the antibody with platelet surface membrane glycoproteins. Glycoproteins Ib/IX and IIb/IIIa are frequent

Table 41.7. Substances Associated with Abnormal Platelet Function In Vivo or In Vitro

Anti-inflammatory agents	β-Blockers	Miscellaneous
Aspirin	Propranolol	Ethanol
Indomethacin	Labetalol	Dipyridamole
Ibuprofen	Calcium channel blockers	Ticlopidine
Phenylbutazone	Verapamil	Sodium valproate
Sulfinpyrazone	Nifedipine	Hydralazine
Naproxen	Diltiazem	Dextran
Diclofenac	Lipid-lowering drugs	Papaverine
Zompirac	Clofibrate	Suloctidil
Tolmetin	Halofenate	Furosemide
Antibiotics	Cyproheptadine	Ethacrynic acid
Ampicillin	Antihistamines	Acetazolamide
Penicillin	Theophylline	Hydroxychloroquine
Carbenicillin	Aminophylline	Hydrocortisone
Ticarcillin	Chlorpheniramine	Methylprednisolone
Mezlocillin	Diphenhydramine	Daunorubicin
Piperacillin	Foods	Mithramycin
Cephalosporins	Garlic	Chlorpromazine
Tricyclic antidepressants	N-3 fatty acids	Triprolidine
Imipramine	Ginger	Reserpine
Desipramine	Onion	Nitrofurantoin
Amitriptyline	Cumin	Heparin
Nortriptyline	Turmeric	

epitopes for antibodies in chronic ITP. It has been suggested that antibody binding to these critical membrane receptors may impair their physiological function.

Binding of platelet antibodies to the surface of the platelet may also lead to platelet activation and thrombosis. This has been most commonly associated with heparin-induced thrombocytopenia, but has also been noted with heparin-independent antiplatelet antibodies. A potential mechanism for the stimulation of platelets by antibodies has recently been described by Anderson et al. Platelets have Fcγ RII receptors, which have high affinity for immune complexes. Antibody-coated platelets can bind to other platelets via their Fc receptors. Binding of the immune complex (platelet-antibody) to the platelet Fc receptor results in platelet activation and subsequent platelet aggregation.

Myeloproliferative Disorders

A variety of defects have been described in patients with underlying acute or chronic myeloproliferative disorders. In some patients, here is evidence of increased platelet reactivity, as indicated by an increase in circulating platelet aggregates, plasma platelet factor 4β-thromboglobulin, the rate of aggregation and response to ADP. Changes suggesting impaired platelet function are more commonly seen in this group of patients. Such changes include a decrease in the α and dense granules, abnormalities of granule morphology, a decrease in platelet von Willebrand factor and fibrinogen, alteration of platelet membrane glycoproteins, decreased uptake and release of serotonin, decreased aggregation in response to a variety of agonists, and decreased procoagulant activity.

Abnormal platelet function is usually suggested by a discordance between the platelet count and the bleeding time. Clinical manifestations of abnormal platelet function in these patients have included both thrombotic and hemorrhagic complications. Unfortunately, there are no laboratory tests that can determine with accuracy which patient is likely to have thrombotic or hemorrhagic complications. Therefore, there is little use for platelet aggregation studies in evaluating these patients. The one setting in which platelet aggregation studies may be helpful is in assessing a patient with marked thrombocytosis. Many patients with essential thrombocythemia will show abnormal in vitro aggregation studies, whereas patients with reactive thrombocytosis often show normal aggregation studies, unless there is a medication or other medical condition that could affect platelet function.

Fibrinolysis

It has become clear that enhanced fibrinolysis can impair platelet function. Mechanisms for abnormal platelet function with enhanced fibrinolysis include interference of fibrin degradation products (FDPs) with glycoprotein IIb/IIIa binding sites on the platelet and degradation of membrane glycoprotein receptors

Ib/IX and IIb/IIIa by plasmin. Abnormal platelet function resulting from enhanced fibrinolysis is perhaps most commonly seen in patients undergoing cardiopulmonary bypass procedures. The resulting impairment in platelet function probably plays a significant role in postoperative bleeding in such patients. A similar defect may be seen in patients treated with a systemic fibrinolytic agents such as streptokinase or in patients with disseminated intravascular coagulation in which fibrinolysis is a prominent component.

Acquired von Willebrand's Disease

Acquired vWD is an uncommon clinical disorder characterized by the sudden onset of a bleeding diathesis in a previously asymptomatic patient. As with other platelet disorders, the bleeding tends to be mucocutaneous in nature; gastrointestinal bleeding is seen frequently in this disorder. Acquired vWD has been seen in patients with severe congenital vWD, lymphoproliferative disorders, myeloproliferative disorders, other neoplastic disorders, autoimmune disorders, and spontaneously in the elderly. In a large number of these patients, particularly those with underlying malignancies, it has been difficult to demonstrate an inhibitor of vWF. Indeed, in these settings the pathogenesis of the acquired vWD may be enhanced proteolysis or clearance of vWF rather than immune-mediated clearance. In other patients, particularly those with spontaneous onset of bleeding, an antibody to vWF can be demonstrated.

The laboratory findings in acquired vWD are quite variable; most commonly the bleeding time is prolonged, and vWF, as measured by vWF:Ag and vWF: Rcof, is decreased. The factor VIII level is usually concordant with the vWF:Ag level in these patients. Some patients with acquired vWD may show a type II pattern of vWD; in these patients there may be a discordance between vWF:Ag and vWF:Rcof. Multimeric analysis of such patients demonstrates the characteristic decrease in high–molecular weight multimers of vWF.

In patients with an underlying malignancy, therapy of the tumor is often associated with regression of the acquired vWD. In those who have documented inhibitors of vWF, immunosuppression forms the cornerstone of therapy. Various agents have been used to achieve this, including steroids, cytotoxic drugs, and intravenous immunoglobulin. Replacement of vWF with cryoprecipitate is occasionally helpful in such patients.

Other Disorders

Abnormal platelet function has been associated with macromolecules, including high concentrations of monoclonal IgM and high–molecular weight dextrans used for volume expansion. Patients with myeloma and high concentrations of monoclonal IgG occasionally have abnormalities of platelet function as well. On occasion, patients with hypothyroidism or end-stage liver disease may have impaired platelet function.

QUANTITATIVE PLATELET DISORDERS

Evaluation of Quantitative Platelet Disorders

Alterations in the number of circulating platelets is a common clinical finding. Thrombocytopenia is generally of greater clinical concern because of its association with an increased risk of bleeding (6). The major concern with thrombocytosis is distinguishing reactive thrombocytosis from thrombocythemia secondary to myeloproliferative disorders, which may be associated with either bleeding or thrombotic manifestations. Thrombocytopenia is usually classified by the underlying mechanism, whereas thrombocytosis is usually classified in terms of reactive processes and hematologic malignancies.

Platelets are derived by a process of megakaryocytic cytoplasm fragmentation along zones or membranes of demarcation (7). Mature megakaryocytes are derived from the common pluripotent hematopoietic stem cell and undergo a number of maturational steps prior to effective production of platelets. The most primitive precursor committed to megakaryocytic development is referred to as the burst-forming unit megakaryocyte (BFU-MK). A later stage of development is designated the colony-forming unit megakaryocyte (CFU-MK). These two stages differ in their sensitivity to 5-fluorouracil, culture characteristics, and expression of surface antigens, including HLA-DR and platelet membrane glycoproteins. A number of cytokines have been found to affect megakaryopoiesis, but the precise effect and the stage of maturation affected are still uncertain.

The initial bone marrow response to thrombocytopenia is an increase in megakaryocyte cytoplasmic size and nuclear ploidy. This is followed by a gradual increase in the number of CFU-MK. Associated with the increase in megakaryocyte size is an increase in the size of zones of demarcation, resulting in the production of larger platelets. Accordingly, an increase in the mean platelet volume (MPV) is often a hallmark of active thrombopoiesis and may be used as an indicator of the marrow response to thrombocytopenia.

The laboratory approach to the evaluation of alterations in the platelet count begins with a careful review of the clinical history and the peripheral blood morphology, with particular emphasis on platelet

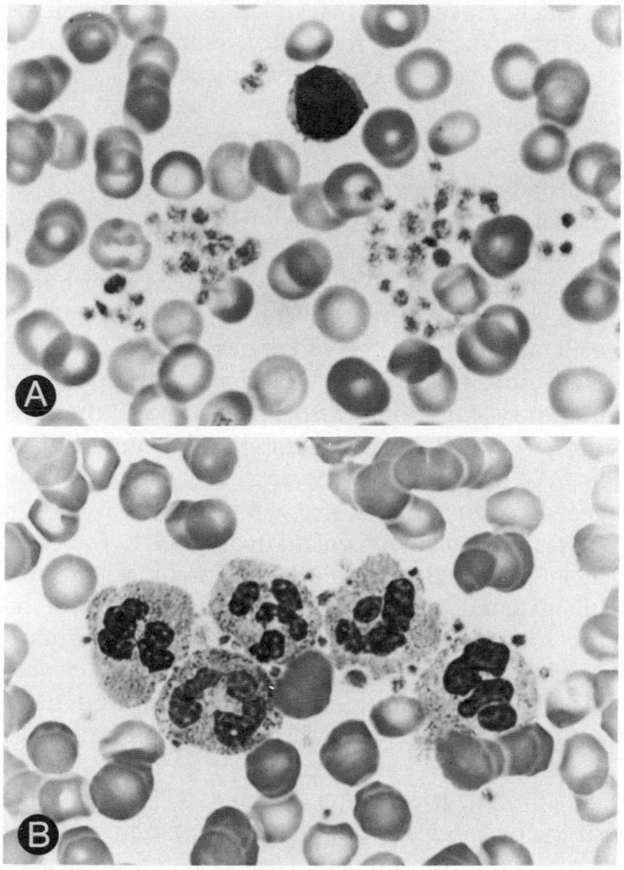

Figure 41.3. Pseudothrombocytopenia may be caused by in vitro agglutination of platelets (A) or platelet satellitosis (B). In vitro platelet agglutination may be EDTA dependent or independent. Both platelet agglutination and platelet satellitosis may affect the accuracy of the white blood cell count as well as the platelet count (original magnification × 500).

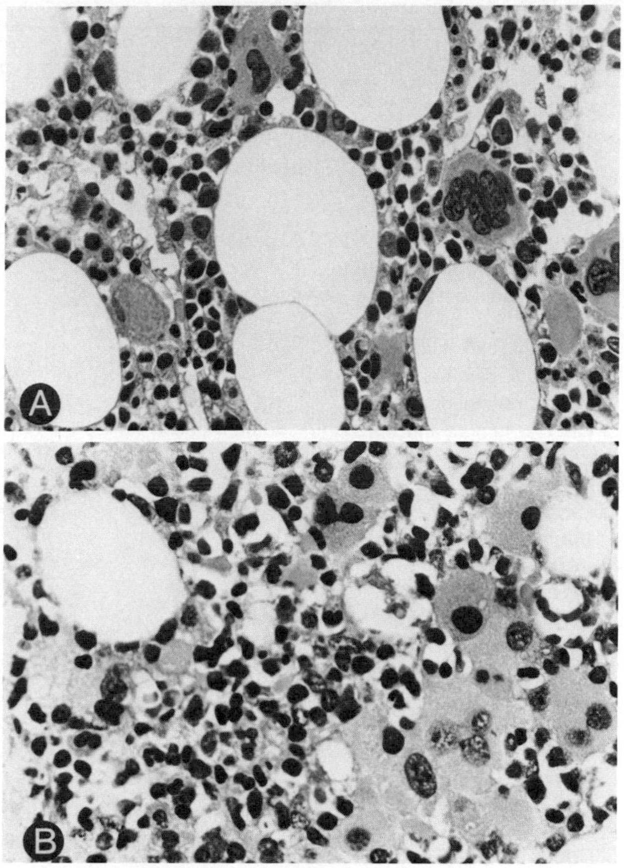

Figure 41.4. Megakaryocytic hyperplasia in reactive conditions is usually characterized by an increase in megakaryocytes throughout the marrow without formation of large clusters (A). In contrast, megakaryocytic hyperplasia associated with myeloproliferative disorders is often characterized by formation of clusters of closely approximated megakaryocytes (B). In addition, megakaryocyte morphology is frequently abnormal in patients with myeloproliferative disorders.

morphology. Analysis of the MPV and platelet volume distribution, and examination of the bone marrow are additional useful steps. The peripheral blood film should be carefully reviewed for evidence of platelet clumps or platelet satellitosis, giant platelets, and the presence of abnormal, hypogranular platelets (Fig. 41.3) (8). Evidence of other hematologic abnormalities such as myelodysplasia, acute leukemia, or the May-Hegglin anomaly, should also be sought. The peripheral blood film findings should be correlated with the MPV determined by the blood counting instrument. In patients who are thrombocytopenic, a low MPV suggests a decreased marrow response to the thrombocytopenia. In contrast, an increased MPV suggests an adequate marrow response to thrombocytopenia and possible increased destruction.

If the cause of thrombocytopenia is not evident from the clinical history and peripheral blood findings, a bone marrow aspirate and biopsy should be examined to determine megakaryocyte number and morphology. Megakaryocyte number and growth pattern are assesssed most accurately by bone marrow biopsy. In reactive conditions associated with an increase in megakaryocytes, the megakaryocytes tend to be randomly spaced throughout the marrow and do not form tight clusters or colonies. In contrast, in patients with myeloproliferative disorders and abnormal megakaryopoiesis, clusters of megakaryocytes that may have a normal or strikingly abnormal morphology are commonly seen (Fig. 41.4). Both the bone marrow biopsy and the bone marrow aspirate can yield useful information regarding megakaryocyte morphology, particularly if a myeloproliferative disorder is suspected. The bone marrow aspirate is particularly useful for assessing whether megakaryocytes are normally shedding platelets. Finally, the bone marrow should be carefully reviewed for evidence of other diseases that may affect platelet production.

Detection of platelet-associated antibodies can be helpful in assessing the possibility of immune-medi-

Table 41.8. Mechanisms of Thrombocytopenia

Increased destruction
Immune-mediated destruction
Autoimmune
Alloimmune (posttransfusion purpura, neonatal)
Drug-dependent antiplatelet antibodies
Immune complex disease
Microangiopathic processes
Thrombotic thrombocytopenic purpura
Hemolytic-uremic syndrome
Disseminated intravascular coagulation
Sepsis
Preeclampsia/eclampsia
Metastatic carcinoma
Malignant hypertension
Vascular tumors and lesions (including artificial valves)
Cardiopulmonary bypass
Major burns
Massive transfusion
Abnormalities of von Willebrand factor
Decreased production
Congenital disorders
Amegakaryocytic thrombocytopenia
Fanconi's anemia
Neonatal rubella
Wiskott-Aldrich
Alport's syndrome
Familial thrombocytopenia
Bone marrow replacement
Metastatic tumor
Leukemia
Storage disorders (e.g., Gaucher's)
Bone marrow failure
Aplastic anemia
Radiation
Chemotherapeutic agents
Drugs
Immune suppression
Viral infections
Ineffective thrombopoiesis
Megaloblastic anemia
Alcoholism
Myeloproliferative and myelodysplastic syndromes
Hypersplenism
Spurious thrombocytopenia
EDTA-dependent antibodies
Temperature-dependent platelet agglutinins
Platelet satellitosis

ated platelet destruction (9). A number of techniques for measuring platelet-associated immunoglobulin have been developed. The most informative assays are those that detect surface-bound immunoglobulin through detection of the Fc component of the antibody. This is because total platelet-associated antibody is equilibrated with plasma, and high plasma levels of IgG are associated with high platelet levels of IgG. In addition, IgG may bind to the platelet through the platelet Fc receptor, leading to a nonspecific increase in platelet-associated IgG.

Additional procedures may be helpful on occasion, depending on the suspected underlying disorder. Such procedures may include electron–microscopy, cytogenetics, bone marrow culture assays, and enzyme assays (e.g., Gaucher's disease).

Thrombocytopenia

Thrombocytopenia may be due to increased destruction, decreased production, artifacts of platelet counting, or splenic sequestration (Table 41.8) (6). Occasionally more than one mechanism may be operative in a given patient. Increased destruction of platelets may be related to congenital abnormalities, for example type IIb vWD and platelet-type vWD, but is more commonly associated with acquired disorders. A number of congenital and acquired disorders may lead to thrombocytopenia secondary to decreased production.

A number of mechanisms may lead to increased platelet destruction (Table 41.8). In clinical practice, antibody-mediated thrombocytopenia is one of the more common mechanisms. Antibodies may induce thrombocytopenia through one or more of several mechanisms, including autoimmune, drug-dependent alloimmune, and immune complex pathways. Thrombotic thrombocytopenic purpura (TTP) and the hemolytic-uremic syndrome (HUS) are characterized by accelerated platelet consumption and microvascular thrombosis. Disseminated intravascular coagulation and sepsis regularly lead to thrombocytopenia. A major side effect of cardiopulmonary bypass is transient thrombocytopenia. Additional mechanisms are listed in Table 41.8.

AUTOIMMUNE THROMBOCYTOPENIA

Autoimmune thrombocytopenia (ITP) is the prototypic example of immune-mediated destruction of platelets. Clinically, ITP is often divided into two forms, acute and chronic ITP (Table 41.9). Acute ITP is often associated with an antecedent viral infection, and it has been suggested that the platelet is an innocent casualty of a cross-reacting antibody that recognizes both the pathogen and platelet membrane. In contrast, chronic ITP appears to be more of a classic autoimmune disorder and is often associated with other immunologic disorders such as systemic lupus erythematosus, rheumatoid arthritis, and auto immune thyroid disease. As indicated in Table 41.9, the clinical course of these two forms of ITP is quite different, with acute ITP having an excellent prognosis and a high rate of spontaneous remission. In contrast, chronic ITP tends to be long-lasting, often requiring long-term immunosuppressive therapy.

In recent years, the target antigens for the antiplatelet antibodies have been identified in many patients with ITP (9). The most frequent antigens involve the glycoprotein Ib/IX and glycoprotein IIb/IIIa

Table 41.9. Comparison of Acute and Chronic Autoimmune Thrombocytopenia

Parameter	Acute ITP	Chronic ITP
Age	All ages; most frequent in childhood	All ages; most frequent in young adults
Gender	F = M	F > M
Onset	Abrupt	Gradual
Platelet count	Often < 50 × 10^9/liter	Often > 50 × 10^9/liter
Platelet-associated IgG	Increased	Increased
Other autoimmune disorders	Usually absent	Often present
Clinical remission	Frequent	Infrequent

complexes. Some patients are characterized by antibodies that react to only one of these membrane proteins, while other patients have antibodies to both proteins. Although antibodies commonly bind to these proteins, they only occasionally cause a clinical picture of acquired Bernard-Soulier (GP 1b/IX) or acquired Glanzmann's thrombasthenia (GP IIb/IIIa).

Typical laboratory features of ITP include moderate to marked thrombocytopenia with a normal to increased MPV. Platelet morphology on peripheral blood smear tends to be normal, except for the shift to slightly larger platelets. Bone marrow examination usually demonstrates normal to increased numbers of megakaryocytes that have a normal morphology. The bleeding time in patients with acute ITP is often proportional to the decrease in platelet count or is even shorter than expected. In contrast, in patients with chronic ITP, the bleeding time may be more prolonged than predicted by the decrease in platelet count, reflecting interference with platelet function by the platelet-associated antibody. Platelet-associated IgG is increased in patients with autoimmune thrombocytopenia, but results of these assays must be interpreted with care because the total platelet IgG is increased in a number of conditions, including those with a high serum concentration of IgG. Characteristically, patients with ITP have an increase in external membrane-associated IgG detected by the recognition of the Fc portion of IgG.

ALLOIMMUNE THROMBOCYTOPENIA

Immune-mediated platelet destruction is also found in posttransfusion purpura, neonatal thrombocytopenia, and thrombocytopenia refractory to random platelet transfusions. The most frequent target antigen in postransfusion purpura is PL^{A1}, an antigen determinate located on glycoprotein IIb/IIIa. Development of HIA-related antibodies and specific antiplatelet antibodies underlies the development of refractoriness as to platelet transfusion. Therapeutic options in such patients include utilization of HLA-matched platelets and actual cross-matching of potential donor platelets with patient antisera. Neonatal thrombocytopenia is usually due to a maternal antibody that crosses the placenta and recognizes the neonatal platelets as foreign. Neonatal thrombocytopenia may also occur in the setting of maternal chronic ITP. Nonimmune neonatal thrombocytopenia is commonly seen in patients with hemolytic disease of the newborn and should be differentiated from these disorders.

DRUG-INDUCED THROMBOCYTOPENIA

Over 100 drugs have been implicated in the development of thrombocytopenia. In most cases, this is due to the development of a drug-dependent antibody that leads to platelet destruction. At least three potential mechanisms for immunologic destruction in this setting have been described. Quinidine-related thrombocytopenia is an example of the mechanism by which drug binds to and alters platelet surface glycoproteins (GPIb/IX), leading to immunologic destruction. Penicillin is an example of the second mechanism, in which the drug serves as a hapten that binds to the platelet surface. IgG then binds to the membrane-associated hapten, leading to premature removal from the circulation. The third mechanism is through stimulation of the Fc receptor on the platelet surface. Heparin-induced thrombocytopenia is an example of this third mechanism.

Heparin-Induced Thrombocytopenia

One of the major side effects of heparin therapy is drug-induced thrombocytopenia. Two forms of heparin-related thrombocytopenia have been identified; the first is characterized by a mild drop in the platelet count (rarely less than 100 × 10^9/liter), while the second is associated with more severe thrombocytopenia. The drop in the platelet count in the mild form usually occurs shortly after heparin therapy is instituted; the platelet count returns to normal whenever heparin therapy is discontinued. In many cases the platelet count will rise toward the preheparin platelet count even if heparin is continued. The mechanism for this form of heparin-related thrombocytopenia is unclear, but no immunologic component has been identified. Patients with this form of heparin-related thrombocytopenia do not appear to be at increased risk of either bleeding or thrombotic complications.

The second form of heparin-related thrombocytopenia caused by an antibody that binds to platelets in the presence of heparin. It remains unclear whether heparin functions as the antigen or whether a neoantigen on a platelet membrane protein is exposed by the binding of heparin to the platelet surface. In either case, the combination of antibody, heparin, and platelet leads to platelet activation and aggregation through stimulation of the platelet Fc receptor. In vivo activation and aggregation are thought to account for the thrombotic complications that may occur with this syndrome. The severe form of heparin-induced thrombocytopenia has been designated by a number of terms, including: heparin-induced thrombocytopenia (HIT), heparin-induced thrombocytopenia-thrombosis (HITT), white clot syndrome, and heparin-associated thrombocytopenia (HAT). In contrast to the first form of heparin-related thrombocytopenia, immune-mediated heparin-induced thrombocytopenia (HIT) usually occurs 7 to 11 days after initiation of heparin therapy, with an average of 9 days. It is associated with moderate to marked thrombocytopenia (less than 100×10^9/liter). The syndrome may occur earlier in the course of heparin therapy if the patient has had a prior exposure to heparin.

The major complication associated with HIT is thrombosis, which may be either venous or arterial. Arterial thrombosis tends to dominate the clinical picture and may involve rather large arteries, including the iliac femoral, popliteal, subclavian, coronary, cerebral, and mesenteric arteries. The thrombotic manifestations may precede the marked drop in the platelet count; therefore, a diagnosis of HIT should be considered in any patient who develops new thromboembolic events while receiving heparin therapy.

The diagnosis of HIT depends on recognizing the temporal association between the drop in platelet count and initiation of heparin therapy or the relationship between new thrombotic events and the institution of heparin therapy. The two most common laboratory methods for evaluating patients with HIT are platelet aggregation studies and platelet release of radiolabeled serotonin. A positive result with either procedure is fairly specific for HIT; a negative result with either procedure does not rule out the syndrome. A prompt rise in the platelet count over 1 to 3 days following cessation of all heparin therapy further substantiates the diagnosis.

The incidence of HIT is currently unknown. Thrombocytopenia was reported to be present in up to 30% of patients receiving heparin in one study. Most other studies have suggested an incidence of less than 1% in patients receiving heparin. Heparin-induced thrombocytopenia may occur when heparin is given by any route, including intravenous, subcutaneous, or intermittently as catheter flushes. HIT has been associated with both bovine and porcine-derived heparins, but a higher incidence of HIT has been associated with bovine heparin. Bovine heparin tends to have a higher negative charge and binds more tightly to platelets.

Therapy of HIT focuses on a discontinuation of all forms of heparin, including heparin-coated catheters. Apparently, sufficient heparin may leak from such catheters to maintain thrombocytopenia in patients who have developed a heparin-dependent antibody. If the patient requires further anticoagulant therapy, oral anticoagulants may be used. If more immediate-acting anticoagulation is needed, low–molecular weight heparins may be tried. However, in a significant number of patients there is cross-reactivity between low– and high–molecular weight heparins. Therefore, before using such agents, it is useful to test this possibility in vitro using either an aggregation or serotonin release study. Another heparinoid (ORG 10172) has been found to be effective in many, but not all patients with HIT. However, in vitro studies should also be performed with this agent to determine if there is cross-reactivity.

THROMBOCYTOPENIA ASSOCIATED WITH HUMAN IMMUNODEFICIENCY VIRUS INFECTION

Thrombocytopenia is a common complication in patients with human immunodeficiency virus (HIV) infection. The mechanism of thrombocytopenia in these patients appears to be multifactorial. In many patients antiplatelet antibodies form, and the thrombocytopenia in these patients is similar to the chronic form of ITP. It has been hypothesized that formation of immune complexes, particularly between viral proteins and antibodies, may also promote thrombocytopenia in these patients. Finally, there is some evidence that the virus may infect megakaryocytes and that thrombopoiesis may be decreased in patients with HIV infection. Substantiating this viewpoint is the increase in platelet count that occurs in many patients following the introduction of ganciclovir therapy.

Thrombotic Thrombocytopenic Purpura and Hemolytic Uremic Syndrome

Thrombotic thrombocytopenic purpura (TTP) and hemolytic uremic syndrome (HUS) are related clinical syndromes characterized by thrombocytopenia, microangiopathic changes on peripheral blood smear, and microvascular thrombosis. The etiology of TTP and HUS remains uncertain. In recent years, epidemiologic evidence has linked the development of HUS to certain infections, particularly specific serotypes of *Escherichia coli*. TTP is most commonly seen 2 to 4 weeks following a viral-like illness. TTP/HUS-like syndromes may also be seen with certain drugs, including mitomycin, cisplatin, and cyclosporin. More recently, TTP/HUS-like manifestations have also been associated with HIV infection.

The classic pentad of clinical findings in TTP are fever, fluctuating neurological deficits, thrombocytopenia, red cell fragmentation, and renal failure. HUS differs in that neurological symptoms tend to be absent and renal failure more pronounced. The diagnosis of TTP/HUS depends on appropriate clinical suspicion and ruling out other causes of microangiopathic hemolytic anemia, particularly acute DIC.

Laboratory parameters typical of HUS and TTP include thrombocytopenia, often with giant platelets, frequent schistocytes and nucleated red blood cells in the peripheral blood, increased reticulocyte count and lactate dehydrogenase (LD), particularly LD1 and normal PT, APTT, fibrinogen, and antithrombin III. Assays for fibrin degradation products are often negative but may show a mild increase. Bone marrow examination shows normal to increased numbers of megakaryocytes. Marrow vessels occasionally show the characteristic microthrombi. As the disease progresses, evidence of a consumptive coagulopathy may emerge. The LD level is useful in monitoring the response to therapy, with a decreasing LD being a favorable sign. A rebound increase in the LD may signify an early relapse of the disorder.

Plasma exchange (apheresis) with fresh frozen plasma appears to be the therapy of choice in these patients. In the absence of prompt therapeutic intervention, the mortality rate approaches 80%; with prompt institution of plasma exchange, the mortality rate is probably less than 20%. Vincristine has been used as an adjunct in some patients who have not responded promptly to plasma exchange. In small series of patients this appears to be an effective additional agent. Steroids, aspirin therapy, and splenectomy remain controversial in these disorders. Relapses occur in up to 25 to 30% of patients who respond to the initial therapy, necessitating continued monitoring of these patients.

OTHER MECHANISMS OF INCREASED PLATELET DESTRUCTION

Increased platelet destruction may be seen in association with a number of other clinical disorders. Sepsis, particularly with Gram-negative bacteria, is one of the more common causes of increased platelet destruction in hospitalized patients. Many of these patients also have a component of acute DIC as well. Diagnosis in these patients depends on recognition of the infectious or consumptive process.

Cardiopulmonary bypass is associated with an acute drop in the platelet count during the procedure. The post–cardiopulmonary bypass platelet count is often 50 to 60% of the prebypass count due to the combination of hemodilution and consumption. The platelet count tends to return to the preoperative level over the first 1 to 2 days following surgery. In most patients, the platelet count following bypass is sufficient to support hemostasis; platelet-type bleeding in these patients is usually due to a qualitative defect rather than a lack of platelets. However, for some patients who start the procedure with borderline platelet counts, the decrease in their platelet count may compromise their ability to form hemostatic plugs in the postoperative period.

A number of venoms from snakes and other biological toxins may lead to a decrease in the platelet count. In these clinical settings, there is often a component of a DIC associated with the envenomation. This may be assessed by measuring fibrinogen, fibrin degradation products, prothrombin time, activated partial thromboplastin time, as well as the platelet count.

A variety of vascular malformations and tumors have been associated with increased platelet consumption due to the abnormal blood flow through the deformed vessels. A classic example of this is the Kasabach-Merritt syndrome, which usually presents in the pediatric age range. Cardiac valve disease and artificial cardiac valves may also lead to a shortened platelet half-life and overt thrombocytopenia in some patients.

Functional hypersplenism is also commonly associated with low peripheral platelet count. The problem in these patients is one of sequestration rather than true thrombocytopenia. Administration of epinephrine or other vasoactive compounds can lead to splenic contraction and release of platelets from the spleen. When this is done, the platelet count often rises to the normal range. Therefore, the total peripheral platelet mass tend to be normal but with an abnormal distribution.

Thrombocytopenia Due to Decreased Production

Decreased platelet production occurs in a variety of clinical settings (Table 41.7). The characteristic findings in these patients are thrombocytopenia with normal to decreased MPV and an abnormal bone marrow. Additional abnormalities evident on the peripheral blood smear often indicate the nature of the underlying disorder.

CONGENITAL DISORDERS ASSOCIATED WITH DECREASED PLATELET PRODUCTION

Thrombocytopenia has been associated with a number of congenital disorders, some of which also demonstrate abnormal platelet function. Amegakaryocytic thrombocytopenia is characterized by nearly total absence of megakaryocytes from the marrow and frequent episodes of leukemoid reactions. This autosomal recessive disorder is frequently associated with skeletal abnormalities, particularly involving the radii (thrombocytopenia with absent radii, TAR syndrome). Platelet size (MPV) tends to be normal to mildly increased; platelet survival is normal; and the bleeding time is proportional to the platelet count.

Fanconi's anemia (congenital aplastic anemia) is an autosomal recessive disorder characterized by severe marrow hypoplasia. Thrombocytopenia may dominate the clinical picture, and death due to hemorrhage is a frequent complication of this disorder. The platelets in Fanconi's anemia have a normal MPV and half-life; the bleeding time is proportional to the platelet count. Megakaryocytes and other hematopoietic elements in the bone marrow are markedly decreased. Fanconi's anemia has been associated with a variety of cytogenetic abnormalities and may terminate as a hematopoietic neoplasm.

The Wiskott-Aldrich syndrome is a sex-linked recessive trait characterized by immunodeficiency, eczema, and thrombocytopenia. The platelet size is significantly decreased in patients with Wiskott-Aldrich syndrome, with the MPV averaging about half of normal. Platelet survival is modestly decreased in this syndrome, but platelet turnover is markedly decreased, indicating ineffective thrombopoiesis. Megakaryocytes are present in normal or mildly increased numbers, consistent with ineffective thrombopoiesis. The bleeding time is disproportionately prolonged for the platelet count, suggesting additional platelet functional abnormalities.

Congenital thrombocytopenia has been described in several families with familial nephritis and deafness (Alport's syndrome). The clinical manifestations have varied between families, some showing the classic association between nephritis and deafness, and others showing only thrombocytopenia and nephritis. This syndrome is inherited as an autosomal dominant trait and has usually been associated with macrothrombocytes (increased MPV). Most often examination of the bone marrow has demonstrated normal numbers of megakaryocytes. There is little information concerning platelet survival in these patients. Platelet function is quite variable between families. Some have a bleeding time proportional to the thrombocytopenia, while others have a relative prolongation of the bleeding time for the degree of thrombocytopenia.

Familial thrombocytopenia is an autosomal dominant trait that has been occasionally reported in the literature. The clinical and laboratory features in these families have been quite variable. Platelet size has varied from normal to increased. Bone marrow examination has shown normal to decreased numbers of megakaryocytes. Platelet survival, when examined, has been quite variable. Usually the bleeding time in affected patients is proportional to the platelet count, suggesting that this is primarily a problem of platelet production.

The May-Hegglin anomaly is an autosomal dominant trait characterized by macrothrombocytes (increased MPV) and the presence of Döhle bodies within neutrophils. The bone marrow in patients with the May-Hegglin anomaly shows a normal number of megakaryocytes, and platelet survival in these patients is also normal. The bleeding time is variable and may be disproportionately prolonged, suggesting additional qualitative platelet defects in some patients. It has been suggested that the total circulating platelet mass is normal in patients with May-Hegglin anomaly due to the increase in the MPV. Indeed, in many of the congenital disorders associated with thrombocytopenia and macrothrombocytes, the problem may be one of production of abnormally sized platelets rather than a decrease in the platelet mass.

The Bernard-Soulier syndrome is an autosomal recessive disorder characterized by deficiency of the GP Ib/IX complex. Thrombocytopenia is frequently observed in these patients and is associated with an increase in the MPV. Bone marrow examination usually demonstrates normal numbers of megakaryocytes; platelet survival is also normal. Two related syndromes also associated with thrombocytopenia are type IIb and platelet-type vWD. Both disorders are inherited as autosomal dominant traits. In, type IIb vWD, the abnormal vWF has an increased affinity for the normal GP Ib/IX receptor, resulting in decreased survival of platelets. In platelet-type vWD, the GP Ib/IX receptor is abnormal and shows an increased affinity for normal vWF, again leading to decreased platelet survival.

Additional platelet functional disorders associated with thrombocytopenia include the Montreal and the gray platelet syndromes. The Montreal platelet syndrome is an autosomal dominant trait characterized by an increase in the MPV, spontaneous aggregation in vitro, and additional functional abnormalities. The gray platelet syndrome appears to be an autosomal recessive disorder characterized by thrombocytopenia, increased MPV, and markedly abnormal mor-

Table 41.10. Conditions Associated With Thrombocytosis

Reactive thrombocytosis
Recovery from acute inflammatory disorders
Chronic inflammation of infections
Hemolytic anemia
Acute hemorrhage
Rebound following suppression (e.g., ethanol chemotherapy, etc.)
Postsplenectomy
Exercise
Iron deficiency
Trauma
Drugs (vincristine, epinephrine)
Malignancy
Neoplastic thrombocytosis (thrombocythemia)
Essential thrombocythemia
Chronic myelogenous leukemia
Polycythemia vera
Myelofibrosis with myeloid metaplasia

phology due to the absence of α granules. The bleeding time in patients with the gray platelet syndrome is often concordant with the degree of thrombocytopenia.

DRUG-INDUCED SUPPRESSION OF PLATELET PRODUCTION

Perhaps the most common cause of decreased platelet production among hospitalized patients today is chemotherapy. Transient thrombocytopenia is a common complication of intensive chemotherapy. Ionizing radiation can also affect platelet production as well as overall hematopoiesis production. A number of other drugs may affect the marrow, leading to hematopoietic hypoplasia and thrombocytopenia. The list of drugs that may cause marrow suppression includes tetracycline, ganciclovir, and chloramphenicol.

OTHER DISORDERS ASSOCIATED WITH DECREASED PLATELET PRODUCTION

A number of viral illnesses have been associated with thrombocytopenia. These include hepatitis, parvovirus, and HIV. It has long been suspected that decreased platelet production can be caused by autoimmune mechanisms, either humoral or cellular. Documentation of the mechanism in such patients has proved to be quite difficult. The bone marrow in these patients usually shows a marked decrease in megakaryocytes, similar to congenital amegakaryocytic thrombocytopenia. Infiltrative processes in the bone marrow may also result in replacement of normal hematopoietic elements and thrombocytopenia. Such infiltrates of the processes may be nonneoplastic, (e.g., Gaucher's disease), or neoplastic (e.g., gacute leukemia). Metastatic tumor may also replace bone marrow, leading to thrombocytopenia; common tumors associated with this problem include breast and prostate carcinoma.

Thrombocytosis

An increase in the peripheral count may occur in a variety of clinical settings (Table 41.10). The mechanism of thrombocytosis in many of these cases is not known. In some cases (e.g., alcohol abuse) the thrombocytosis appears to be a rebound phenomenon following recovery from toxic suppression of thrombopoiesis. The clinical and laboratory evaluation of thrombocytosis revolves around the determination of the associated condition.

Thrombocytosis is a common finding in myeloproliferative disorders. If a myeloproliferative disorder is suspected, a bone marrow examination, cytogenetics, and red blood cell mass determination are helpful. The presence of the Philadelphia chromosome is indicative of chronic myelogenous leukemia, even though the peripheral blood may have the appearance of associated thrombocytopenia.

References

1. Adams GA. Platelet aggregation. In: Longenecker GL, ed. The platelets: physiology and pharmacology. Orlando, FL: Academic Press, 1985:1–14.
2. Hardisty RM, Caen JP. Disorders of platelet function. In: Bloom AL, Thomas DP, eds. Haemostasis and thrombosis. 2nd ed. Edinburgh: Churchill Livingstone, 1987:365–392.
3. Berkowitz SD, Ruggeri ZM, Zimmerman TS. von Willebrand disease. In: Zimmerman TS, Ruggeri ZM, eds. Coagulation and bleeding disorders: the role of factor VIII and von Willebrand factor. New York: Marcel Dekker, 1989:215–259.
4. Bennett JS. The molecular biology of platelet membrane proteins. Semin Hematol 1990;27:186–204.
5. George JN, Shattil SJ. The clinical importance of acquired abnormalities of platelet function. N Engl J Med 1991;324:27–39.
6. Burstein SA, McMillan RM, Harker LA. Quantitative platelet disorders. In: Bloom AL, Thomas DP, eds. Haemostasis and thrombosis. 2nd ed. Edinburgh: Churchill Livingstone, 1987: 333–364.
7. Hoffman R. Regulation of megakaryocytopoiesis. Blood 1989;74:1196–1212.
8. Berkman N, Michaeli Y, Or R, Eldor A. EDTA-dependent pseudothrombocytopenia: a clinical study of 18 patients and a review of the literature. Am J Hematol 1991;36:195–201.
9. George JN. Platelet immunoglobulin G: its significance for the evaluation of thrombocytopenia and for understanding the origin of α-granule proteins. Blood 1990;76:859–870.

Suggested Readings

Kaplan BS, Proesmans W. The hemolytic-uremic syndrome of childhood and its variants. Semin Hematol 1987;24:148–160.

Kroll MH, Schafer AI. Biochemical mechanisms of platelet activation. Blood 1989;74:1181–1195.

Lind SE. The bleeding time does not predict surgical bleeding. Blood 1991;77:2547–2552.

Miller JL. von Willebrand disease. Hematol Oncol Clin North Am 1990;4:107–128.

Nosek-Cenkowska B, Cheang MS, Pizzi NJ, Israels ED, Gerrard JM. Bleeding/bruising symptomatology in children with and without bleeding disorders. Thromb Haemostas 1991;65:237–241.

Pearson TC. Primary thrombocythaemia: diagnosis and management. Br J Haematol 1991;78:145–148.

Randi AM, Rabinowitz I, Mancuso DJ, Mannucci PM, Sadler JE. Molecular basis of von Willebrand disease type IIb. J Clin Invest 1991;87:1220–1226.

Rao AK. Congenital disorders of platelet function. Hematol Oncol Clin North Am 1990;4:65–86.

Shepard KV, Bukowski RM. The treatment of thrombotic thrombocytopenic purpura with exchange transfusions, plasma infusions, and plasma exchange. Semin Hematol 1987;24:178–193.

Warkentin TE, Kelton JG. Heparin-induced thrombocytopenia. In: Coller BS, ed. Progress in hemostasis and thrombosis. Philadelphia: WB Saunders, 1991;10:1–34.

White JG. Inherited abnormalities of the platelet membrane and secretory granules. Hum Pathol 1987;18:123–139.

42 Coagulation Abnormalities

Douglas A. Triplett

Abnormalities of secondary hemostasis (i.e., coagulation proteins) typically present with a different clinical picture than abnormalities of primary hemostasis (1). In classic severe hemophilia the pattern of bleeding will be musculoskeletal and often "spontaneous." In acquired disorders of secondary hemostasis, however, the pattern of bleeding may often have features of mucocutaneous bleeding. This mixed pattern of bleeding reflects the complex pathophysiology of many acquired coagulopathies. Thus, the pure isolated single coagulation factor deficiency that is characteristic of hereditary disorders is rarely seen in acquired states.

This chapter addresses both hereditary and acquired disorders of coagulation proteins. The hereditary abnormalities are discussed initially, followed by the acquired disorders. The laboratory tests used to evaluate secondary hemostasis are reviewed, with special emphasis on interpretation.

HEREDITARY DISORDERS OF COAGULATION PROTEINS

Hemophilia A (Factor VIII Deficiency)

Hemophilia A is an X-linked inherited disorder of factor VIII (antihemophiliac globulin). The incidence is approximately 1:10,000 males. As previously discussed, factor VIII is a critical cofactor in the intrinsic coagulation pathway at the level of factor X activation.

There are variable degrees of factor VIII deficiency, which have been divided arbitrarily into severe, moderate, and mild categories (Table 42.1). Severe hemophilia A is characterized by "spontaneous" musculoskeletal bleeding. This pattern of bleeding is often first evident when the child begins to walk at 9 to 12 months of age. These patients may also present with bleeding following circumcision; however, it is not uncommon for a severely affected child to have minimal bleeding with this procedure. Mild and moderately affected patients may not present until much later in life. Mild hemophilia is often diagnosed when a patient presents with unexplained bleeding following surgery or in association with trauma. Occasionally, very mild hemophilia A patients may complain only of easy bruising or small superficial hematomata.

With the advent of molecular biological techniques, the genetics of hemophilia A have been studies extensively. In 1984, investigators first reported the successful cloning of the human factor VIII gene (2, 3). The entire gene spans 186 Kb (10^3 base-pairs), which comprises approximately 0.1% of the X chromosome. There are a total of 26 exons and 25 introns. The coding DNA is 9 Kb, which codes for 2351 amino acids. The first 19 amino acids are the secretory leader peptide of the nascent factor VIII. The complete amino acid sequence is now established, and the calculated molecular weight is 267,039 daltons. There are three homologous A domains, two C domains, as well as an intervening B domain, which is rich in carbohydrate (Fig. 42.1). Factor VIII may be represented by the following formula: A_1-A_2-B-A_3-C_1-C_2. The A domains show significant homology with similar domains in ceruloplasmin (4).

Both deletions and point mutations have been found in patients with hemophilia A (5). Prior to the availability of molecular biology procedures, it was evident that a significant number of cases of hemophilia A occurred in families with a negative history. Consequently, it was anticipated that "hot spots" would be identified to account for de novo mutations. The "hot spots" appear to be related to CpG dinucleotides (6, 7). The C can be methylated in the 5′ position of the pyrimidine ring and then deaminated to thymine. This leads to the CG → TG and CG → CA mutations. All of these mutations are recognized by TaqI recognition sites.

The laboratory diagnosis of hemophilia A is relatively straightforward. In the majority of cases, the activated partial thromboplastin time (APTT) will be prolonged, while the prothrombin time (PT) and bleeding time (BT) will be within normal limits (Table 42.2) (1). Factor VIII:C assays are necessary to establish the diagnosis. Patients with severe hemophilia A will have factor VIII:C levels that are less than 1% (0.01 unit/ml). Factor assays are relatively easy to perform. However, the laboratory must have a strict quality assurance program to ensure accuracy (8).

Table 42.1. Clinical Classification of Hemophilia A

Severity	Factor VIII Activity (%)	Clinical Picture	Activated Partial Thromboplastin Time	Incidence (%)
Severe	<1	Severe hemarthrosis and spontaneous bleeding	Prolonged	48
Moderate	2–10	Spontaneous bleeding uncommon; serious bleeding from minimal trauma	Prolonged	31
Mild	>10–<30	Spontaneous bleeding rare; unsuspected bleeding after surgical intervention or trauma	Variable	21
Subclinical	>30–<50	Often asymptomatic, will bleed with trauma or surgery	Prolonged/normal	

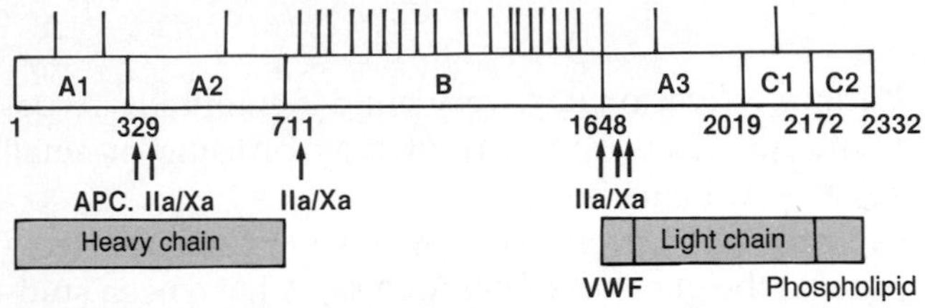

Figure 42.1. Diagram of factor VIII molecule.

Table 42.2. Laboratory Results in Hemophilia A

PT	Normal
APTT	Abnormal[a]
Bleeding time	Normal
Platelet count	Normal
Factor VIII:C assay	Abnormal

[a]The APTT may be borderline or within the reference interval in patients with mild or moderate hemophilia A. This variability is due to both choice of APTT reagent and biological patient variables. For instance, during times of stress, the factor VIII levels may increase, resulting in a normal APTT.

The treatment of hemophilia A has undergone rather dramatic changes in the last 30 years. Prior to the use of cryoprecipitate, the hemorrhaging patient was transfused with either whole blood or fresh frozen plasma. Following the introduction of cryoprecipitate, commercially prepared factor VIII concentrates were introduced in the early 1970s. These concentrates were processed from large pools of plasma that had been obtained from thousands of donors. As a complication of replacement therapy, many hemophiliacs were found to have chronic persistent or chronic active hepatitis (9). In some cases frank cirrhosis was also diagnosed. With the introduction of specific testing for hepatitis B surface antigen and subsequently surrogate testing for non A non B hepatitis virus (hepatitis C-specific ELISA are now available), the incidence of posttransfusion hepatitis decreased. Unfortunately, coincident with the advances of hepatitis screening, transfusion-associated human immunodeficiency virus (HIV) was recognized in the early 1980s (10). This was a particularly devastating finding to all hemophilia A patients who had found greater social and employment opportunities with the use of self-administered factor VIII concentrates.

The late 1980s and early 1990s have been characterized by greater emphasis on increased purity of factor VIII concentrates with enhanced viral attenuation or inactivation. A variety of viral attenuation techniques have been used, including dry heat pasteurization, solvent/detergent treatment, steam treatment, and heating in an organic solvent (11). Also, attempts to increase factor VIII purity were introduced using monoclonal murine antibodies to either human VIII or human von Willebrand factor (VWF) (11). The monoclonal antibodies were used with immunoaffinity chromatography. There are ongoing clinical trials to evaluate the potential of these new products to transmit viral hepatitis and HIV (12). To date, the results are encouraging.

In addition, recombinant human factor VIII is now approved after clinical trials. Of course, the availability of this product would eliminate the concern for viral complications (13).

Factor VIII concentrates should be used to treat an acute bleeding episode or to prepare the patient for surgery. One unit of factor VIII per kilogram of body weight should raise the factor VIII level approximately 2% (0.02 U/ml). The half-life of infused factor VIII is approximately 12 hours. Typically, a bleeding episode is treated with 40 to 50 U/kg with subsequent infusion of 3 to 4 U/kg/hour. In order to monitor response, factor VIII:C assays are recommended on a daily basis. Prophylactic use of factor VIII concentrates may be indicated following a CNS hemorrhage.

In mild/moderate hemophilia A patients, the initial treatment of choice is DDAVP (1-deamino-8-D arginine vasopressin) (14). This synthetic analogue of vasopressin will cause a two- to ten-fold increase in factor VIII:C following an IV infusion of 0.3 to 0.4 μg/kg of body weight. The postulated mechanism of action is release of VWF from endothelial storage sites (Weibel Palade bodies). Repeated doses may lead to diminished response of factor VIII. Side effects of DDAVP include facial flushing, fluid retention due to the antidiuretic effect, and recent reports of thrombosis. The latter complication has been most often identified in older individuals with significant atherosclerotic vascular disease.

One of the most common complications of hemophilia A is the appearance of an alloantibody to factor VIII:C (factor VIII:C inhibitors) (15). Factor VIII:C in-

Table 42.3. Treatment of Factor VIII:C Inhibitors

- High-dose factor VIII concentrates
- Plasmapheresis
- Prothrombin complex concentrates
- Activated prothrombin complex concentrates
- Immunosuppression
- Heterologous factor VIII (porcine)
- Factor VII_a (recombinant)
- Platelet transfusions
- DDAVP
- IV immunoglobulin

hibitors are most commonly seen in severe hemophilia A patients. In the majority of cases they appear prior to the age of 20 years. As part of the annual evaluation of hemophilia A patients it is necessary to screen each patient for factor VIII: C inhibitors. These inhibitors are quantitated utilizing the Bethesda assay system (16). Since most factor VIII:C inhibitors are time- and temperature-dependent, the Bethesda assay involves mixing patient plasma and a source of normal plasma. The mixture is incubated at 37°C. for 2 hours. APTTs are performed at 30, 60, and 120 minutes. By definition, 1 Bethesda unit (BU) is defined as the amount of inhibitor that destroys half the factor VIII:C activity in an equal mixture of patient and normal plasma utilizing the above conditions. It is imperative to quantitate a factor VIII:C inhibitor so proper therapy can be instituted. Patients with high titer inhibitors (e.g., greater than 30 BU) are frequently very difficult to manage. In addition to the Bethesda titer, it is also necessary to obtain a clinical history regarding the patient's anamnestic response. Arbitrarily, the patients have been divided into "low" and "high" responders. "High responders" will demonstrate a marked increase in factor VIII:C inhibitor titer upon exposure to factor VIII concentrates.

A variety of modalities have been used to treat factor VIII:C inhibitors (Table 42.3). Porcine factor VIII is valuable, particularly in patients whose factor VIII inhibitor has little cross-reactivity with porcine VIII (17). Both "activated" and "nonactivated" prothrombin complex concentrates (PCC) (II, VII, IX, X) have been successfully used to treat acute hemorrhage (18). Protein A columns have been used to remove IgG from factor VIII:C inhibitor patients (19, 20). In most cases, factor VIII:C inhibitors are IgG_4. Consequently, the protein A will remove the majority of the intravascular inhibitor compartment.

Hemophilia B (Factor IX Deficiency)

Hemophilia B is also a sex-linked disorder. Christmas disease and factor IX deficiency are frequently used synonyms. The incidence of hemophilia B is approximately 1:40,000 to 1:50,000 population. However, in certain groups such as the Amish and East Indians, hemophilia B occurs as often as hemophilia A. Varying degrees of hemophilia B have been recognized with severe, less than 1 % (0.01 U/ml), moderate, less than 5 % (0.01 to 0.05 U/ml) and mild, greater than 5 % (greater than 0.05 U/ml) phenotypes analogous to factor VIII deficiency. The clinical presentation and genetics of hemophilia B are similar to hemophilia A. Consequently, to make the diagnosis a specific factor IX assay must be done.

Table 42.4. Laboratory Results in Hemophilia B

PT	Normal[a]
APTT	Abnormal[a]
Bleeding time	Normal
Platelet count	Normal
Factor IX assay	Abnormal

[a]In some instances, the prothrombin time may be prolonged, if a bovine brain thromboplastin is used. This has been referred to as the hemophilia B_m variant. The APTT is variable and may be normal in mild hemophilia B patients. This is due to the varying sensitivities of commercial APTT reagents.

With severe and moderate factor IX deficiency, the APTT will be prolonged. However, there appears to be marked variability among the commercial APTT reagents with respect to factor IX sensitivity (21). Mild and moderate hemophilia B patients may therefore have a normal screening APTT. In this case, the family and personal history are extremely important in identifying a bleeding disorder. Typically, the prothrombin time (PT) is normal; however, there is a variant (hemophilia B_m) in which the PT is prolonged if bovine brain thromboplastin is used (Table 42.4). Tests of primary hemostasis (BT and platelet count) are typically normal.

Factor IX is a vitamin K–dependent protein that is produced in the liver. The existence of a second coagulation protein, a deficiency of which was associated with a hemophilia, was first identified by Pavlovsky (22). He demonstrated mutual correction of prolonged clotting times when plasmas from two different hemophiliacs were mixed in vitro. Thus, he demonstrated different coagulation factor deficiencies conclusively. The subsequent study of the various phenotypes of factor IX deficiency was instrumental in emphasizing the marked laboratory heterogeneity in factor-deficient patients despite apparent clinical homogeneity. Utilizing antibodies to factor IX, early investigators found occasional hemophilia B patients who neutralized these antibodies (23). This proved the existence of cross-reacting material (CRM) in patient plasmas with no apparent functional activity. Based on reactivity of patient plasma with heterologous antisera to factor IX, three phenotypic groups have been identified (Table 42.5). The CRM^+ and CRM^R groups have been further characterized by their reactions with XI_a, VII_a, ability to activate factor X, electrophoretic mobility, among

Table 42.5. Phenotypic Classification of Hemophilia B[a]

Type	Factor IX Assays[b]		PT With Bovine Thromboplastin
	Activity	Antigen	
I CRM$^+$	Low	Normal	Normal
CRM$^+$ (Bm)	Low	Normal	Abnormal
CRM$^+$	Low	Normal	Variable
II CRM^R	Low	Intermediate	Normal
III CRM$^-$	Low	Low	Normal

[a]Modified from Giddings JC. Molecular genetics and immunoanalysis in blood coagulation. Chichester, England: Ellis Horwood, 1988:5.

[b]Factor IX deficiency demonstrates a wide variety of phenotypes. Patients may have concordant decrease in both IX activity, as measured by a coagulation assay, and IX antigen, which may be quantitated utilizing various immunologic assays (e.g., ELISA, RIA, Laurell). The variants of factor IX deficiency have variable levels of IX antigen (ranging from normal to reduced) that exceed the activity levels. Some of the variant IX deficiencies also have an abnormal prothrombin time when a bovine thromboplastin is employed.

others (24). Full discussion of these variants is beyond the scope of this text.

The spectrum of clinical symptoms in hemophilia B is similar to those of hemophilia A. With severe factor IX deficiency, patients have recurrent hemarthroses as well as intramuscular hemorrhages. Mild and moderate factor IX deficiency may not be detected until the patient is an adult. Complications are similar to hemophilia A. Recurrent intraarticular hemorrhages may lead to damage of the cartilagenous surfaces of the affected joints and, ultimately, destruction of the joint. Muscle atrophy, nerve injury, contractures, and pseudotumors may also occur.

Alloantibodies to factor IX have been reported in approximately 10% of patients with hemophilia B (15). In most instances, these inhibitors arise in patients with severe hemophilia B. Also, the infectious complications associated with chronic administration of blood products are similar to those of hemophilia A.

Treatment of the severe hemophilia B patient requires the frequent use of prothrombin complex concentrates. These concentrates are made from pools of plasma and initially were prepared by adsorption of plasma by tricalcium phosphate. Subsequently, alcohol fractionation of plasma and DEAE-cellulose adsorption were utilized to prepare more potent concentrates. Recently, heat treatment of PCC has significantly improved the safety of these products with respect to posttransfusion hepatitis and HIV complications. A recombinant factor IX product has been prepared, although its use in clinical trials is still pending. Interestingly, recombinant factor IX has also been produced by transgenetic techniques using sheep milk as a source of human factor IX.

Once transfused, factor IX has an in vivo half-life of approximately 18 to 40 hours. However, the recovery of factor IX following transfusion is only 20 to 40%. This is because of the ready distribution of factor IX to the extravascular compartment (25). Consequently, it is extremely difficult to achieve factor IX levels of greater than 50% following transfusion. In most instances of severe hemorrhage, treatment should be aimed at achieving a factor IX level of 20 to 50%. This is particularly important during the acute episode and the first few days thereafter. Minor hemorrhages usually respond to factor IX levels of approximately 20% (25).

HEMOPHILIA C (FACTOR XI DEFICIENCY)

Factor XI deficiency is an incompletely autosomal recessive hereditary disorder. The majority of factor XI deficiency occurs in individuals of Jewish descent. In an extensive study of Ashkenazi Jews by Seligsohn, the frequency of homozygotes for factor XI deficiency was 0.1 to 0.3%, whereas the heterozygotes were found in 5.5 to 11.0% (26).

Factor XI is a glycoprotein with a molecular weight of 160,000 daltons. Its concentration in plasma is approximately 5 μg/ml. Native factor XI exists as a dimer of two identical subunits linked by disulfide bonds. Factor XI is activated by surface bound factor XIIa (Hageman factor). High molecular weight kininogen (Fitzgerald factor) serves as a cofactor in the activation step of factor XI. The gene for human factor XI has been isolated from a human liver cDNA library. The gene is 25 kb in length and consists of 15 exons and 14 introns. The gene has been located on the distal end of the long arm of chromosome 4. Factor XI is 607 amino acids in length and has significant homology with prekallikrein (Fletcher factor). The major physiological substrate for factor XIa is factor IX, which it cleaves at two sites to yield factor IXa. In contrast to the marked heterogeneity of factor IX deficiency, factor XI-deficient patients typically have levels of factor XI antigen that parallel the factor XI coagulant activity (27).

Two major types of factor XI deficiency have been described. The homozygous patients have factor XI activity below 20% (as related to normal plasma) (28). These patients have a variable history of clinical bleeding and are at risk for significant surgical bleeding. Heterozygous patients have levels of factor XI activity of 30 to 65% and typically have a negative bleeding history. Perhaps the most perplexing aspect of diagnosing factor XI deficiency is the lack of correlation between factor XI assay results and clinical bleeding.

The spectrum of clinical symptoms includes mild mucocutaneous bleeding (epitaxis, menorrhagia) and bleeding following minor surgical procedures such as dental extraction and tonsillectomy. A particularly difficult aspect of management of factor XI deficiency is the variability within an individual patient in response to different surgical procedures. Consequently, it is impossible to predict how an individual patient may respond to a subsequent surgery. Bleeding from organs with excess plasminogen activator activity has frequently been observed (e.g., posttonsillectomy, dental extractions, and transurethral prostate resection). In these instances, the use of Amicar is often helpful.

The management of hemorrhage following surgery or significant trauma involves the use of fresh frozen plasma. The half-life of infused factor XI is approximately 40 to 80 hours. The factor XI level should be maintained above 50%. Arbitrarily, 1 ml of fresh frozen plasma will produce a 2% rise in factor XI activity.

FACTOR VII DEFICIENCY

Deficiency of factor VII is inherited in an autosomal recessive manner. Severe factor VII-deficient patients (homozygotes) may present with a spectrum of clinical bleeding ranging from central nervous system hemorrhage in the neonatal state, hemarthroses, to mild mucocutaneous bleeding (29). The heterozygous patients typically are asymptomatic.

Factor VII is a single chain glycoprotein with an estimated molecular weight of 50,000 daltons. The mature protein contains 406 amino acids, and there are 10 γ-carboxyglutamic acid residues (GLA) located on the amino terminal end. β-hydroxyaspartic acid is also found in the factor VII molecule (30). The activation of factor VII requires cleavage of an arginine isoleucine peptide bond. Factor VII can be activated by several enzymes, including thrombin, factor Xa, factor IXa, and factor XIIa (31).

The gene for factor VII is located on chromosome 13 (Q 34-qter) (32). The complete sequence for the gene spans approximately 12.8 kb of DNA. There are eight exons and seven introns. The gene for factor X is also located on chromosome 13, very close (2.8 Kb) to the factor VII gene (33).

As noted, the spectrum of clinical bleeding in factor VII deficiency is probably the most diverse of any of the hereditary coagulopathies. Paradoxically, some patients with factor VII deficiency have been reported to have thromboembolic episodes (31, 34). Factor VII deficiency has also been described in a variety of hereditary disorders including Dubin-Johnson's, Rotor's, and Gilbert's syndromes (31). Combined factor VII and factor X deficiency has been described with a hereditary form of carotid body tumors.

The diagnosis of congenital factor VII deficiency is established by specific factor VII assays. Typically, the screening coagulation test results include a normal APTT and thrombin time together with a prolonged PT. However, PT results may vary depending on the choice of thromboplastin. Thus, when indicated, it may be appropriate to utilize a panel of thromboplastins to evaluate patients in whom there is a possible factor VII deficiency (human, bovine, and rabbit tissue) (29, 31). Many variant molecules have been identified based on their reactivity with thromboplastins of various species (29, 35). The best predictor of clinical bleeding is the level of factor VII activity obtained with a thromboplastin of human origin (29).

The half-life of factor VII is approximately 6 hours (31). As a result, it is very difficult to obtain levels of factor VII activity of greater than 50%. Transfusion therapy includes the use of fresh frozen plasma or PCC. If prothrombin complex concentrates are used, heat-treated preparations are indicated. Although not available in the U.S., a factor VII concentrate is available in Europe. Interestingly, recombinant factor VIIa has been utilized to treat hemophilia A patients with factor VIII:C inhibitor (36). Factor VIIa leads to direct activation of factor X, thus bypassing the requirement for factor VIII in the coagulation sequence.

Table 42.6. Laboratory Results in Factor X Deficiency[a]

Case	PT	APTT	RVVT	Factor X Antigen	X Assay
Stuart	Abnormal	Abnormal	Abnormal	Low	Low
Prower	Abnormal	Abnormal	Abnormal	Normal	Low
Friuli	Abnormal	Abnormal	Normal	Normal	Low

[a]The table summarizes the more common forms of factor X deficiency. There is a relatively high incidence of CRM^+ variant deficiencies among all of the vitamin K-dependent proteins. Consequently, careful, thorough evaluation is suggested for every case.

HEREDITARY FACTOR X DEFICIENCY (STUART-PROWER FACTOR)

Hereditary factor X deficiency is an autosomal recessive disorder with variable degrees of penetrance. It was originally independently described by two groups who noted there was apparent heterogeneity in patients who were thought to be factor VII-deficient on the basis of a prolonged PT (37, 38). Factor X-deficient patients were first clearly separated from factor VII deficiency on the basis of an abnormal thromboplastin generation time. Subsequently, the Russell viper venom time (RVVT) and APTT were also found abnormal in factor X deficiency (Table 42.6) (39).

Factor X is a glycoprotein with a molecular weight of approximately 59,000 daltons. It is composed of two chains (light chain molecular weight of 16,900 and heavy chain molecular weight of 42,100) (39). Factor X is activated by either the complex of factor

VIIIa, factor IXa, phospholipid and calcium (intrinsic pathway), or tissue factor/VIIa (extrinsic pathway). Activation requires cleavage of a peptide bond on the amino terminal end of the heavy chain.

The gene for human factor X is located on chromosome 13 in the region Q 34-qter (32, 33). It contains an estimated 25 kb of DNA. There are seven introns and eight exons. Location of the introns is analogous to the introns in factor VII, factor IX, and protein C genes.

The spectrum of hereditary factor X deficiency is analogous to that of other hereditary deficiencies of vitamin K-dependent proteins. Patients who have discrepancies between the RVVT and PT results (Friuli defect) have been described (40). In addition, discrepancies between the level of factor X antigen as measured with either radioimmunoassays or antibody neutralization techniques and factor X activity based on clotting assays have been observed (41). Thus, there are CRM^+, CRM^R, and CRM^- variants of hereditary X deficiency (Table 42.6). Hereditary deficiency of factor X may be caused by mutations throughout the gene, resulting in either reduced or absent synthesis and secretion of factor X or the synthesis of an abnormal molecule.

Clinically, patients may present with severe bleeding; however, the most common complaint is easy bruising and hematoma formation (42). Hemarthroses, exsanguinating postoperative hemorrhage, and central nervous system hemorrhage have been reported in the most severely affected patients. Systemic amyloidosis is an important differential diagnostic consideration when isolated factor X deficiency is encountered. Amyloid deposits in these particular cases probably have an increased affinity for factor X, resulting in adsorption of factor X from circulating plasma (43).

The half-life of transfused factor X is approximately 24 to 40 hours with a bimodal survival curve (1). Both fresh frozen plasma and PCC are effective. If concentrates are used, heat-treated products are indicated.

FACTOR V DEFICIENCY (LABILE FACTOR)

Hereditary factor V deficiency is inherited as an aueltosomal recessive trait (44). CRM^+ and CRM^- variants have been described (45, 46). In addition, a disorder referred to as factor V Quebec has been identified (47). In this disorder, there is autosomal dominant inheritance with severe clinical bleeding. However, plasma factor V activity levels are borderline normal with corresponding factor V antigen levels. Paradoxically, platelet factor V activity levels are very low. Thus, as with von Willebrand disease and afibrinogenemia, it may be necessary to evaluate both plasma and platelet factor V to diagnose and characterize factor V deficiency accurately. Several investigators have emphasized the correlation of platelet factor V with clinical bleeding as opposed to a lack of correlation with plasma levels.

The clinical picture in patients with hereditary deficiency of factor V is characterized by a pattern of mucocutaneous bleeding (1). Hemarthroses are relatively uncommon. The differential diagnosis includes combined deficiency of factor V and VIII and acquired factor V deficiency (48, 49). Acquired deficiency of factor V is usually caused by specific antibody inhibitors (49, 50). Inhibitors to factor V are most commonly seen in the postoperative setting or with the administration of certain antibiotics.

Laboratory diagnosis of factor V deficiency is characterized by an abnormal PT and APTT (1). The diagnosis is confirmed with a factor V assay. Approximately one-third of patients will have a prolonged bleeding time (51). As noted previously, factor V is carried within the platelet α granules and also may be associated with the platelet membrane (52). Activated factor V on the surface of the platelet serves as a receptor for factor Xa, thus facilitating the assembly of the prothrombinase complex (53).

Factor V deficiency may be treated with fresh frozen plasma or fresh plasma. The half-life of transfused factor V is approximately 12 hours (54). Platelet concentrates have been used successfully to treat patients with inhibitors to factor V (55).

COMBINED FACTOR V AND FACTOR VIII DEFICIENCY

A combined deficiency of factor V and factor VIII has been reported (48). In most cases this appears to be an autosomal recessive disorder. Thus, there is a history of consanguinity in many of these cases. The plasma levels of factors V and VIII are usually in the range of 15 to 20%. The genetic basis for this disorder is currently unknown.

PROTHROMBIN DEFICIENCY

Hereditary hypoprothrombinemia is an extremely rare autosomal recessive disorder (56, 57). Homozygous patients have levels of prothrombin activity varying from 2 to 25%. Prothrombin is a single-chain glycoprotein with a molecular weight of approximately 71,600. In addition to the γ-carboxyglutamic acid residues that characterize all vitamin K-dependent proteins, there are two kringle structures present. These kringles are analogous to similar structures seen in plasminogen, t·PA, urokinase, and factor XII.

The gene for human prothrombin is located on chromosome 11. It contains approximately 21 kb of DNA and has 14 exons with 13 introns (58).

A number of variants of abnormal prothrombin have been described (59). Defects in factor Xa cleavage site have been identified as well as abnormal calcium binding sites and abnormalities of the thrombin region.

The clinical findings are variable depending on the level of prothrombin activity. Spontaneous hemorrhage and hemarthroses are uncommon, although they have been described in patients with severe deficiency states.

Laboratory findings are characterized by the presence of an abnormal PT and APTT. The PT results may be highly variable depending on the nature of the underlying defect. To establish the diagnosis, a two-stage functional assay of prothrombin is recommended as well as an immunologic assay to detect the presence of prothrombin antigen. In cases of true hypoprothrombinemia, the functional and antigenic assays will be decreased in parallel. In the dysprothrombinemic states, the antigen level will exceed the functional activity.

Treatment consists of the use of fresh-frozen plasma or fresh plasma. In severe clinical bleeding, heat-treated PCC are preferred.

AFIBRINOGENEMIA AND HYPOFIBRINOGENEMIA

Afibrinogenemia is a rare disorder inherited in an autosomal recessive pattern (60). There is often a variable history of clinical bleeding. In many cases, there is bleeding at the time of separation of the umbilical cord or following circumcision. Also, patients may present with intracerebral hemorrhage, spontaneous hematoma formation, or mucocutaneous bleeding. Paradoxically, menorrhagia is uncommon with afibrinogenemia.

Laboratory abnormalities of all of the standard screening tests are present. No endpoint is detected with the PT, APTT, or TT. The bleeding time may be slightly prolonged, and platelet aggregation studies typically show a lack of response to the usual agonists (ADP, epinephrine, and collagen). Although fibrinogen may not be demonstrable in the patient plasma, most patients will have variable amounts of fibinogen within the platelet α granules. Discrepancies between platelet and plasma concentrations of coagulation proteins have also been reported with factor V deficiency and von Willebrand's disease.

Replacement therapy is required to achieve a hemostatic level of fibrinogen between 50 and 100 mg/dl. Cryoprecipitate or fresh frozen plasma are effective. A few cases of antibody formation to fibrinogen have occurred following replacement therapy.

Hypofibrinogenemic patients are characterized by a fibrinogen level that is less than 100 mg/dl (61). Often these patients have a mild bleeding tendency with an autosomal-dominant or, in some cases, an autosomal-recessive pattern of inheritance. In many cases, hypofibrinogenemic patients will have normal PT and APTT results. However, typically the thrombin time will be abnormal. Clottable and immunologic fibrinogen assay results are decreased, thus establishing the diagnosis.

DYSFIBRINOGENEMIA

Hereditary dysfibrinogenemia is inherited in an autosomal-dominant pattern (62). These abnormal fibrinogen molecules are caused by mutations that result in single amino acid alteration in one of the three fibrinogen chains (α, β, or γ chains). Many cases of dysfibrinogenemia have been fully characterized (62–64). The mutations may affect any one of the functional properties of fibrinogen including delayed or absent release of fibrinopeptides A and B, abnormal polymerization, abnormal cross-linking, decreased thrombin binding, abnormal plasmin digestion, and defective secretion by hepatocytes. Clinically, patients may present with hemorrhage, spontaneous abortion, or thromboembolic complications. However, most of these patients are asymptomatic.

Laboratory findings include normal or only minimally prolonged values for PT and APTT. Typically, the TT is prolonged as is the reptilase time. The abnormal TT usually cannot be corrected by the addition of protamine or calcium. Laboratory diagnosis relies on the demonstration of a discrepancy between the level of clottable fibrinogen and antigenic fibrinogen. Specialized studies can be performed including immunoelectrophoresis and SDS polyacrylamide gel electrophoresis to evaluate molecular weights, polypeptide chains, formation of cross-linked γ-chain dimers and α-chain polymers. In addition, polymerization of fibrin monomers may be evaluated by measuring turbidity changes at 305 nm.

Management of patients with dysfibrinogenemia is dependent upon the associated clinical findings. In the case of bleeding, the use of cryoprecipitate is the treatment of choice.

FACTOR XIII DEFICIENCY (FIBRIN STABILIZING FACTOR)

Hereditary deficiency of factor XIII is inherited in an autosomal recessive pattern (65). Factor XIII is a plasma glycoprotein involved in stabilizing the fibrin clot by introducing covalent bonds between fibrin multimers. In addition, factor XIII also cross-links α-2 antiplasmin to the fibrin clot and fibronectin to fibrin or collagen.

Factor XIII circulates in plasma as a tetramer composed of two a-subunits and two b-subunits. The a-subunits are also found in other tissues such as platelets and megakaryocytes, placenta, uterus, and macrophages (66). The a-subunit is responsible for the functional activity of factor XIII.

The gene for the a-subunit is located on the distal end of the short arm of chromosome 6 (67), while the gene for subunit-b is located on the long arm of chromosome 1 (1 q31). In affected individuals, the first evidence of clinical bleeding is often manifested at the time of umbilical cord separation. Patients may also have intracranial hemorrhage as well as intramuscular hematoma formation and easy bruising. Many patients have abnormal wound healing and a history of habitual abortion (65).

The usual screening tests are normal (65). When factor XIII deficiency is suspected, clot solubility in five molar urea or monochloroacetic acid will be abnormal. In addition, a thromboelastogram will also have a markedly abnormal tracing. Subunit-a can be measured using the Laurell technique (68). In a few selected laboratories, factor XIII activity is quantitated using amine incorporation assays (69).

Cryoprecipitate and fresh frozen plasma have been used to treat hereditary factor XIII deficiency. In addition, a concentrate of factor XIII is available in Europe. Since factor XIII has a rather long half-life, and the majority of patients do not become symptomatic until levels of activity are less than 1%, replacement therapy on an intermittent basis is remarkably effective.

HEREDITARY COAGULATION FACTOR DEFICIENCIES NOT ASSOCIATED WITH CLINICAL BLEEDING

Hageman factor (factor XII), Fitzgerald factor (high molecular weight kininogen), and Fletcher factor (prekallikrein) are proteins that are involved in the contact phase of coagulation (Table 42.7) (70). Deficiencies of these proteins are not associated with clinical bleeding. Typically these patients are detected when a screening APTT is found to be markedly prolonged in the presence of a negative clinical history of bleeding. The diagnosis is established by specific factor assays. In the case of Fletcher factor deficiency, prolonged incubation (10 minutes) of the patient plasma with the activator may shorten the prolonged APTT obtained with routine activation (3 to 5 minutes). Similar shortening is not seen with Hageman factor or Fitzgerald deficiencies.

Paradoxically, a number of patients with Hageman factor deficiency and prekallikrein deficiency have been reported with thromboembolic events (71).

III ACQUIRED DISORDERS

Anticoagulant Therapy (Heparin, Coumadin)

The clinical laboratory plays a very important role in monitoring anticoagulant therapy. In fact, monitoring anticoagulant therapy with the PT was the first form of therapeutic drug monitoring.

Heparin is a natural mammalian glycosaminoglycan. The manufacture of heparin involves extraction from bovine lung tissue and porcine or bovine intestinal mucosa. In the U.S., therapeutic use of heparin is limited to unfractionated preparations that are heterogeneous with respect to molecular weights varying from 5000 to 30,000+ daltons (low molecular weight heparin was approved for prophylaxis in 1993). In Europe the introduction of low molecular weight heparins has revolutionized heparin anticoagulant therapy (72). Low molecular weight heparin preparations are manufactured by enzymatic degradation of unfractionated heparins or various other chemical processes. In general, low molecular weight heparins have significant differences in pharmacologic properties as well as their effect on various coagulation assays (Table 42.8).

Heparin requires a naturally occurring plasma constituent to express its anticoagulant activities (73). This plasma protein is antithrombin III, an α-2 globulin produced in the liver (74). Antithrombin III is a member of the SERPIN family of proteins. Thus, the name antithrombin III is something of a misnomer. AT III inhibits all of the serine proteases involved in hemostasis with the exception of factor VIIa. Recent studies suggest AT III may inhibit VIIa when complexed with tissue factor. The inhibitory properties of antithrombin III are timed-dependent in the absence of heparin. With the addition of heparin, the ability of antithrombin III heparin complex to inhibit serine proteases is markedly accelerated (73).

The half-life of injected heparin is in the range of 1 to 2 hours. However, the disappearance and clearance times of heparin are dose-related (75). Higher doses are associated with decreased clearance and longer disappearance times. Heparin may be cleared from the circulation by the kidney and the liver. Endothelial cells also play a role in heparin clearance. Heparin may be neutralized in the circulation by platelet factor 4, which is a platelet-specific protein found in the α granule. Heparin also interacts with other plasma proteins including von Willebrand factor, fibronectin, and vitronectin.

Table 42.7. Hereditary Deficiencies of Contact Factors

	Factor XII	Factor XI	Prekallikrein	HMW-kininogen
Year described	1955	1953	1965	1975
Mode of transmission	Autosomal recessive	Autosomal recessive	Autosomal recessive	Autosomal recessive
Ethnic background	Variable	Predominantly in Jews	Variable	Variable
Bleeding symptoms	None	Mild	None	None
Prothrombin time	Normal	Normal	Normal	Normal
APTT	Prolonged	Prolonged	Prolonged	Prolonged
Intrinsic fibrinolysis	Impaired	Normal	Impaired	Impaired
Kinin formation	Impaired	Normal	Impaired	Impaired
CRM^+ cases	Present	Present	Present	Unknown

Table 42.8. Comparison of Unfractionated and Low Molecular Weight Heparins

Property	Low Molecular Weight Heparin[a]	Unfractionated Heparin
Molecular weight	3,000–5,000	10,000–30,000
Activated partial thromboplastin time	++	++++
Thrombin time	++	++++
Anti-Xa assay	++++	++
Platelet aggregation	+	++++
Binding to endothelium	++	++
Protamine neutralization	+	++++
Lipoprotein lipase	+	++++
Adsorption (sub Q)	+++	++
Clinical bleeding (?)	++	+++
Heparin induced thrombocytopenia	+	+++

[a]Low molecular weight heparin preparations differ from manufacturer to manufacturer.

Although historically heparin was given subcutaneously as well as intravenously (either intermittent or continuous infusion), most patients today receive heparin by continuous infusion. Continuous infusion appears to be the preferred mode of administration, not only because of the ease of obtaining samples for monitoring the heparin effect, but because there appears to be less clinical bleeding. The decrease in clinical bleeding is primarily related to a decrease in the cumulative dose a patient receives over the course of treatment. In the treatment of acute deep vein thrombosis (DVT), usually a loading dose of 5,000 to 10,000 units of heparin is administered immediately followed by approximately 1000 to 1500 units per hour. Dosage may be affected by a variety of factors including the acute nature of the thrombotic process, body weight, and other complicating disease states (e.g., renal and liver disease).

The laboratory monitoring of heparin began with the use of whole blood clotting times (Lee and White) and has progressed to the recent introduction of synthetic substrate assays, which allow quantitation of heparin in units per ml. Based on the College of American Pathology survey program (CAP), most laboratories (greater than 95%) utilize the APTT as a means of monitoring heparin. However, the activated clotting time (ACT) is frequently used in settings where immediate answers are required. This is primarily true in the operating room for patients undergoing bypass procedures. Also, in dialysis units the ACT is a popular means of evaluating the presence of heparin and subsequent neutralization with protamine sulfate.

The APTT is readily available in most laboratories. In addition, because it is part of the ongoing quality control program, the APTT is the preferred test for monitoring heparin therapy. Commercially available partial thromboplastins vary significantly in their sensitivity to heparin (76). When defining an APTT system, it is important for the laboratory to consider the choice of reagent as well as instrumentation. In general, it is best to use instruments and reagents from the same manufacturer. In addition to sensitivity to the presence of heparin, responsiveness is an important property of the APTT system. Responsiveness reflects the degree of prolongation present at a given level of heparin or factor deficiency. Thus, more responsive reagents will yield longer APTT results. It is important to separate the concept of sensitivity and responsiveness in choosing laboratory reagents. An optimal reagent would be both sensitive and responsive.

Historically, the therapeutic target for the prolongation of the APTT was 1½ to 2½ times the upper limit of the normal range. Recently there has been a move to use the patient's baseline APTT to determine the therapeutic range. This provides a more realistic goal and recognizes the frequent occurrence of short APTTs in patients presenting with acute DVT or pulmonary emboli.

Heparin-associated thrombocytopenia (HAT) is one of the most threatening complications of heparin therapy (77). The incidence of HAT has been reported as varying from less than 1% of patients to as high as 30%. There are two types of HAT. Type 1 is seen frequently after the initiation of heparin therapy and consists of a drop in the platelet count into the range of 100,000 to 150,000/ml. This decrease in platelets may persist for several days; however, even though the patient continues to receive heparin, the platelet count subsequently returns to the original value prior to the initiation of heparin therapy. The exact mechanism for this type of HAT is still speculative, although many suggest it is the result of in vivo heparin-induced platelet aggregation with clearance of the aggregates in the liver and spleen.

Type II HAT is associated with antibodies directed against heparin (78). This antibody recognizes a repeating epitope in heparin. The complex of antiheparin and heparin then binds to a platelet membrane Fc receptor. Subsequent immune destruction results in a profound thrombocytopenia (less than 100,000/ml) and often associated thromboembolic events. This form of HAT usually occurs after 6 days of heparin administration; however, it may be seen earlier in patients who have previously been exposed to heparin. Type II HAT is seen regardless of the route of administration or the cumulative dose. Consequently, this form of HAT may be seen in intensive care unit patients who are receiving heparin flushs through indwelling access catheters.

When Type II HAT is suspected, heparin should be discontinued immediately. Typically, in the patient receiving heparin for DVT, oral anticoagulants have already been initiated, and the transition to this form of anticoagulant therapy is relatively easy. In the setting where HAT develops in a patient who requires bypass surgery or renal dialysis, management is considerably more difficult. In some instances it is possible to use a different type of heparin (species of origin) and successfully perform such surgery, provided there is no evidence of cross-reactivity between the patient's antiheparin antibody and the second source of heparin. Other forms of therapy have included the use of dextran, low molecular weight heparin preparations or heparinoids, snake venoms to defibrinate the patient's plasma (Ancrod), and the use of Iloprost, a prostacyclin analog (79, 80). There is no consensus as to the optimal approach.

The laboratory confirmation of the presence of Type II HAT is based on screening assays that are rather crude. Platelet aggregation studies should be performed in the presence of the heparin being utilized for the patient's treatment as well as at least two sources of platelet-rich plasma obtained from normal donors. The aggregation studies consist of heparin, normal platelet-rich plasma, and the patient's platelet-poor plasma mixed in the aggregation cuvette. The presence of aggregation greater than 20% suggests the possibility of HAT. It is important to appreciate that the absence of a positive result does *not* rule out HAT. A more specific test is the serotonin platelet release assay (81, 82). In this assay, complexes of the heparin and IgG bind to the platelet Fc receptor, resulting in the release of serotonin, which can be quantitated. The presence of a positive serotonin release assay is considered diagnostic of HAT (81).

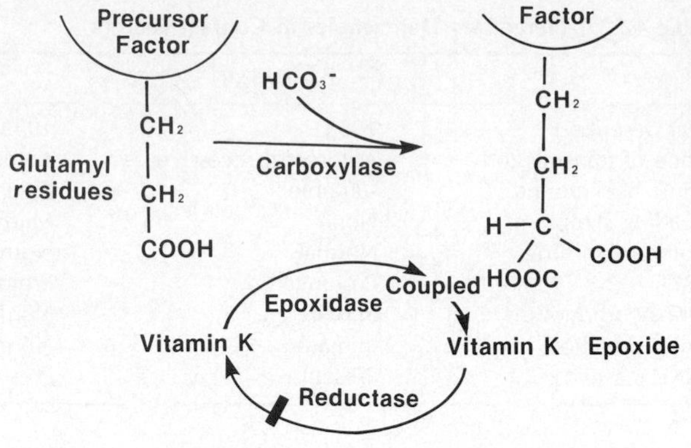

Figure 42.2. Vitamin K pathway.

ORAL ANTICOAGULANT THERAPY

Oral anticoagulant therapy is based on the administration of coumarin or its derivatives. This class of drugs blocks the reductase enzyme in the vitamin K pathway (Fig. 42.2), resulting in increased levels of nonfunctional vitamin K epoxide (83). Vitamin K acts as a cofactor in a posttranslational step converting various vitamin K-dependent protein precursors into functional procoagulant proteins. This vitamin K-driven reaction involves the carboxylation of glutamic acid to give rise to γ carboxyglutamic acid (GLA). These GLA residues function to localize the vitamin K-dependent proteins to phospholipid membrane surfaces. Typically, activated platelets provide this surface; however, other cells such as endothelial cells, monocytes, and tumor cells may function in a similar fashion.

In the presence of oral anticoagulants, formation of GLA residues is impeded. As a result, there is diminished surface localization of the vitamin K-dependent complexes, resulting in an anticoagulant effect. Early reports also suggested that the presence of proteins induced by vitamin K antagonist (PIVKAs) serves an anticoagulant role as well. The PIVKA proteins represent the precursors of the functional procoagulants. Their role in the therapeutic effect of oral anticoagulants remains unresolved.

The monitoring of oral anticoagulant therapy has relied upon the PT and variants of the PT. For many years there has been an international controversy regarding the optimal test system to monitor oral anticoagulants. In the U.S., tissue thromboplastins from various animal species have been used for the PT determination. Today, virtually all of the thromboplastins marketed in the U.S. are of rabbit tissue origin (rabbit brain or rabbit brain/lung). Recombinant human tissue factor preparations are now available in the U.S. However, in Europe a number of differ-

$$\text{INR} = \left[\frac{\text{Pat PT}}{\text{Mean Normal PT}}\right]^{\text{ISI}}$$

Figure 42.3. Derivation of the international normalized ratio (INR). Pat PT, patient's PT result; Mean Normal PT, mean of the normal PT range; ISI, value supplied by reagent manufacturer.

ent types of thromboplastins have been utilized including bovine brain, monkey brain, and human brain. Dr. Leon Poller championed the human brain thromboplastin as a sensitive reagent that would reflect the anticoagulant status of a patient more accurately (84). His efforts resulted in the concept of an international normalized ratio (INR) to express PT (85).

In order to report an INR value, it is necessary to know the international sensitivity index (ISI) for the thromboplastin being used as well as the mean of the PT range (86). The INR merely expresses the ratio of the patient PT to the mean of the normal range raised to the power of the ISI (Fig. 42.3). The INR, therefore, represents the PT that would have been obtained on the patient plasma if the international reference preparation (IRP) of thromboplastin (human brain) had been utilized. Thus, it provides a means of comparing PT results from laboratory to laboratory correcting for the differences in thromboplastin reagents. The concept of the INR has been well received in Europe and is now being implemented in the U.S. Keep in mind that the INR is only appropriate for patients who are *stably* anticoagulated. Patients who are in the early phases of oral anticoagulant therapy or patients in whom the PT is being obtained for other diagnostic purposes should not have their results reported as an INR value.

The introduction of the INR has emphasized the need for lower doses of oral anticoagulants. In the past, when PT results were reported as ratios, the therapeutic range was typically quoted as PT ratios of 1.5 to 2.5. With the use of the INR, the majority of patients are satisfactorily anticoagulated with ratios of 1.3 to 1.6 (87). As a consequence, the incidence of bleeding in patients receiving oral anticoagulant therapy will most likely significantly decrease (87).

FIBRINOLYTIC THERAPY

The use of fibrinolytic agents in the treatment of acute myocardial infarction (AMI) is now well accepted (88). Fibrinolytic agents such as streptokinase (SK) and urokinase (UK) have been available for many years. However, they were only approved for the treatment of pulmonary embolism and massive DVT. Many clinicians were reluctant to use these agents because of unfamiliarity with their dose and the perceived high incidence of hemorrhagic complications. The introduction of tissue plasminogen activator (t·PA) renewed interest in fibrinolytic therapy. With the ready availability of acute coronary angiography, lytic agents were introduced in the treatment of AMI.

One of the primary complications associated with the use of fibrinolytic agents in the treatment of AMI is bleeding. Most commonly, the bleeding is from arterial or venous access sites. The most catastrophic complication is cerebral bleeding.

The nature of the hemorrhagic defect in patients receiving lytic therapy has only recently been studied in detail. Among the alterations induced by lytic agents are a drop in the fibrinogen level with a concomitant rise in fibrin/fibrinogen degradation products. It is well known that fibrin/fibrinogen degradation products will inhibit certain aspects of platelet function and impede the assembly of fibrin monomers in a fibrin clot. Also, plasmin will attack other plasma procoagulant proteins including factors V and VIII. Since plasmin is an indiscriminate serine protease, it will digest certain glycoprotein receptors on both platelets and endothelial cells (glycoprotein IIb/IIIa; glycoprotein Ib). As a result, the administration of lytic agents affects both primary and secondary hemostasis. Furthermore, many patients who are receiving lytic agents are also receiving heparin and antiplatelet medications such as aspirin.

Therefore, the bleeding seen in association with fibrinolytic therapy is multifactoral. Appropriate management of these patients depends upon the individual case. The use of fresh frozen plasma and/or platelets may be indicated in severe circumstances.

ACQUIRED CIRCULATING ANTICOAGULANTS

Circulating anticoagulants may be defined as endogenous substances that interfere with one or more of the in vitro tests of hemostasis. In most cases they are immunoglobulins; however, there are situations in which other substances produce an anticoagulant effect, including the presence of heparin or heparin-like compounds and fibrin/fibrinogen degradation products.

The most commonly encountered circulating anticoagulant is the so-called lupus anticoagulant. A working definition of the lupus anticoagulant is: a circulating immunoglobulin (IgG or IgM; or both) that interferes with one or more of the in vitro phospholipid dependent tests of coagulation (e.g., PT, APTT, dRVVT,) (89). The name lupus anticoagulant is a misnomer because the vast majority of these patients *do not* have systemic lupus erythematosus. In fact, in most hospital settings, this anticoagulant is

Table 42.9. Clinical Conditions Associated with Lupus Anticoagulants

Autoimmune diseases	
	Systemic lupus erythematosus
	Rheumatoid arthritis
	Others, including "overlap" syndromes
Drug exposure	
	Chlorpromazine
	Procainamide
	Hydralazine
	Quinidine
	Antibiotics
	Phenytoin
Infections	
	Bacterial
	Protozoan (*Pneumocystis carinii*)
	Viral
Lymphoproliferative disorders	
	Hairy cell leukemia
	Malignant lymphoma
	Waldenstrom's macroglobulinemia
Miscellaneous disorders	
	Epithelial malignancies
	No underlying disease

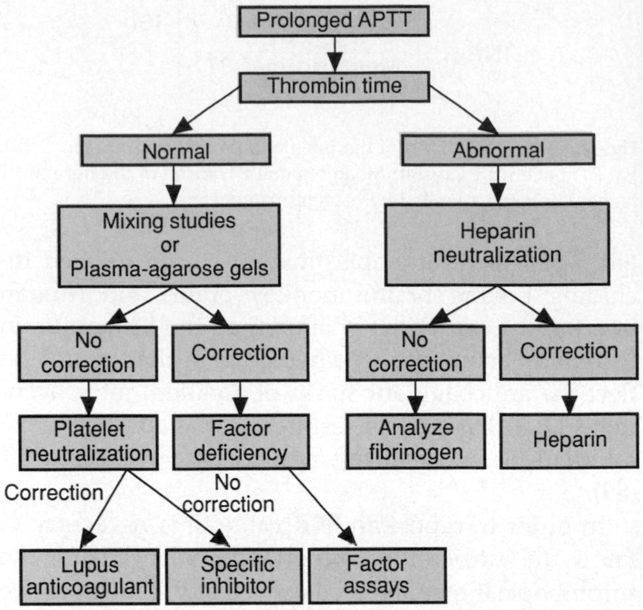

Figure 42.4. Workup of LA.

seen in a variety of other clinical circumstances including the convalescent phase of acute infections, as a result of drugs (chlorpromazine, hydralazine, hydantoin, procainamide, quinidine, and various antibiotics), and in patients in whom there is no apparent underlying disease (Table 42.9). Although most inhibitors of blood coagulation are associated with clinical bleeding, paradoxically, LA seems to be associated with an increased risk of trombosis (90). Clinical bleeding is distinctly uncommon unless there is an additional hemostatic abnormality. Most commonly, the hemostatic abnormalities that may be associated with clinical bleeding in LA patients include thrombocytopenia, qualitative platelet functional defects, and isolated deficiency of prothrombin. The latter appears to be directly related to the LA immunoglobulin, which cross-reacts with prothombin, creating an antigen-antibody complex that is rapidly cleared from the circulation (91).

The laboratory diagnosis of LA requires three distinct steps:

1. Identification of an abnormal screening test;
2. Proof that the abnormal test is caused by an inhibitor; and
3. demonstration that the inhibitor is phospholipid dependent (Fig. 42.4) (89, 92).

In most cases, the abnormal screening test is an unexplained prolonged APTT. In the past this was usually a serendipitous finding that led to further laboratory tests to explain the abnormality. Recently clinicians are asking the laboratory: "Does my patient have an LA?" This question requires a more extensive evaluation. The increased clinical awareness of LA is related to its association with a variety of complications including both arterial and venous thromboembolic events, neurological complications, recurrent spontaneous abortions, and intrauterine fetal death (89, 92–94).

Following the demonstration of an abnormal APTT, mixing studies are indicated to identify the presence of an inhibitor. Although many texts recommend a one-part patient, one-part normal mixture, our experience suggests that the use of four parts patient, one part normal plasma is a more sensitive means of identifying the presence of an inhibitor (89). This is particularly true in cases where the patient's baseline APTT is only minimally prolonged. LA was initially thought to be an immediate inhibitor in contrast to the time dependency seen with factor VIII:C inhibitors. However, recently a number of studies have suggested as many as 30% of LAs are time-dependent (95). Conversely, factor VIII:C inhibitors may be immediate. Thus, the presence or absence of time dependency is not a useful differential diagnostic point to separate factor VIII:C inhibitors from LA. An alternate method to identify the presence of a circulating inhibitor is the use of plasma agarose gels (96).

A variety of test systems have been utilized to identify phospholipid dependence of circulating anticoagulants. Two basic principles have been employed:

1. Decreasing the phospholipid concentration in the test system to enhance the inhibitor effect; and

2. Increasing the amount or changing the configuration of phospholipid in the test system to either "neutralize" or "bypass" the LA (89).

Among the former tests, the tissue thromboplastin inhibition procedure (TTI) is most commonly employed (97). Unfortunately, this test system is not particularly sensitive nor specific. Perhaps the most sensitive test system employing the concept of dilute phospholipid is the dilute Russell viper venom time (dRVVT) (98). The platelet neutralization procedure (PNP) is the most commonly utilized test employing increased amounts of phospholipid (99). In this test, freeze-thawed platelets are added to the patient's platelet-poor plasma and the APTT repeated. In the presence of an LA, there will be significant shortening of the baseline APTT value. As a control, an appropriate buffer is added to the patient plasma.

Occasionally, the confirmatory tests may be misleading or uninterpretable. In this situation it is appropriate to perform factor assays. Typically in the presence of an LA there is nonparallelism of the factor assay curves with an apparent increase in factor activity as the patient plasma is progressively diluted (100).

In addition to the fibrin-based assays to demonstrate LA, many laboratories also utilize an ELISA system to demonstrate the presence of anticardiolipin antibodies (ACA). LA and ACA are often present in the same patient; however, in approximately 30% of cases, there will be a lack of concordance between these two test systems (101). Consequently, when the clinician requests an evaluation of the patient plasma for phospholipid antibodies, it is necessary to perform both fibrin-based assays and the ELISA test system.

Other inhibitors are rarely encountered (Table 42.10). The recent recognition of "nonneutralizing" inhibitors has further compounded the laboratories' difficulties in demonstrating the presence of an inhibitor (Fig. 42.5) (91). With a nonneutralizing inhibitor, the laboratory assays may suggest a factor deficiency because addition of normal plasma to the patient plasma results in correction of abnormal coagulation studies. In these patients it is necessary to demonstrate the presence of an antigen-antibody complex utilizing a variety of techniques such as crossed immunoelectrophoresis (91). The most commonly encountered nonneutralizing inhibitor is that of antiprothrombin antibodies encountered in patients with LA (102).

Table 42.10. Classification of Circulating Anticoagulants

Specific	
Neutralizing	Nonneutralizing
Factor V	Prothrombin
Factor VIII:C	Factor VIII:C
Factor IX	Factor X
Factor XI	VWF
VWF	
Factor XIII	
Nonspecific	
Lupus anticoagulants	
Paraproteins	
FSP	
Global	
Heparin-like activity	

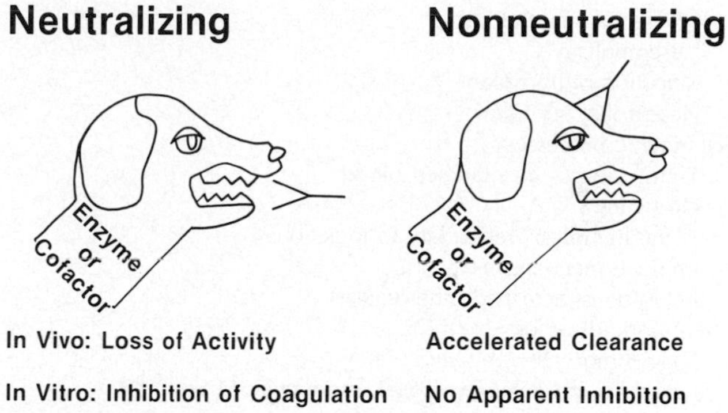

Figure 42.5. Neutralizing and nonneutralizing circulating anticoagulants.

DISSEMINATED INTRAVASCULAR COAGULATION

Disseminated intravascular coagulation (DIC) may be encountered in a variety of different clinical situations (Table 42.11). In most cases it is associated with the exposure of tissue factor or thromboplastin-like material with resulting activation of coagulation pathways at the level of factor X (103). Clinical examples would include amniotic fluid embolus, head injuries, neurosurgery, and certain malignancies. Some tumor cells appear to have a specific enzyme (cysteine protease) that will directly activate factor X. Alternatively, with endothelial injury, there may be activation of the extrinsic pathway, leading to DIC.

It is important to appreciate that DIC is a rapidly evolving pathophysiological response to an underlying disease. Consequently, laboratory testing to establish the diagnosis is often difficult because of the constantly changing balance of underlying mechanisms. In acute DIC with a predominance of thrombin generation and consumption of coagulation factors and activation of fibrinolytic activity, bleeding is the most common clinical manifestation. Typically, acute DIC presents as systemic bleeding with oozing from the sites of venipunctures or recent surgery.

Table 42.11. Classification of Clinical States Associated with Disseminated Intravascular Coagulation

Obstetric complications
Abruptio placentae
Placenta previa
Dead fetus
Amniotic fluid infusion
Placenta accreta
Toxemia of pregnancy
Cesarean section
Abortion
Hydatid mole
Extrauterine pregnancy
Forceps delivery
Normal delivery
Tissue trauma
Major surgery (especially extracorporeal circulation)
Severe trauma and burns
Fat embolism
Rejection of transplant
Heatstroke
Hemolytic processes
Transfusion of mismatched blood
Drowning
Acute hemolysis secondary to infection
Immune mechanisms
Ingestion of acid and other causes
Neoplastic diseases
Solid tumor
Leukemia (promyelocytic M-3, monocytic M-5)
Snakebites
Infections (especially acute forms)
Bacterial: Gram-negative, meningococcal, and pneumococcal septicemia
Rickettsial: Rocky Mountain spotted fever
Viral: hemorrhagic smallpox and hemorrhagic fever (Thai, Korean, and others)
Mycotic: acute histoplasmosis
Parasitic: malaria (blackwater fever)
Miscellaneous
Cirrhosis of the liver
Glomerulonephritis
Acute pancreatitis
Purpura fulminans
Thrombotic thrombocytopenic purpura
Hemolytic uremic syndrome
Shock
Severe progressive stroke
Severe heart failure
Giant hemangioma (Kasabach-Merritt)
Large aortic aneurysm

However, in the subacute and chronic states such as retained dead fetus or underlying disseminated malignancy, the patient may actually present with thrombosis. In this setting, there may be an actual compensatory increase of coagulation factors such as fibrinogen and factor VIII that may exceed the range found in normal subjects.

In acute DIC, the constellation of laboratory findings reflect both the consumption of coagulation proteins as well as the presence of plasmin. Typically, the APTT, PT, and TT will be prolonged. In addition, there is consumption of platelets as well as the regulatory proteins AT III and protein C. Fibrinogen/fibrin degradation products will be increased, and the level of fibrinogen will be decreased. The availability of immunologic assays based on monoclonal antibodies to neoantigens has resulted in test systems that are more specific for fibrin degradation products (104). The D-dimer represents the use of an antibody to such a neoantigen.

In chronic DIC, the platelet count will typically be slightly decreased, whereas the coagulation assays (APTT, PT) may be within normal limits. Fibrin/fibrinogen degradation products and D-dimer will tend to be elevated. There may also be consumption of AT-III.

The treatment of choice for DIC is management of the underlying clinical condition. For instance, in a patient with chronic DIC and retained dead fetus, evacuation of the uterus is the treatment of choice. In a patient with acute DIC secondary to endotoxic shock, appropriate support and antibiotic therapy are treatments of choice.

THROMBOTIC THROMBOCYTOPENIC PURPURA/HEMOLYTIC UREMIC SYNDROME

Thrombotic thrombocytopenic purpura (TTP) and hemolytic uremic syndrome (HUS) are examples of complex disease states that are closely related (105). In TTP there is systemic deposition of intraluminal platelets in the smaller arterioles (106). By contrast, HUS is characterized by involvement of the glomeruli with platelet aggregates (106). Both diseases present as a microangiopathic hemolytic anemia. Typically, there are schistocytes on the peripheral smear together with thrombocytopenia. Recent work would suggest that the etiology of these conditions is variable from case to case. Moreover, the mode of presentation, particularly with TTP, may be characterized by either a single clinical episode, a chronic relaxing form, or an intermittent form (106). Approximately two-thirds of patients with acute TTP appear to have abnormal processing of von Willebrand factor (VWF), which results in the presence of large VWF multimers during periods of remission. It may be difficult to demonstrate these abnormal multimers during the acute episodes. The persistence of large VWF multimers after recovery is sensitive for predicting a relapse. The treatment of choice in TTP is plasma exchange or plasmapheresis plus fresh frozen plasma (107).

LIVER DISEASE

The hemostatic problems encountered in patients with liver disease usually are complex (108). Because the liver plays a key role in the synthesis of the coagulation proteins, regulatory proteins, and factors involved in the fibrinolytic system, the balance between these various components may be altered to varying degrees in any patient with significant compromise of liver function. Also, the liver plays a role in removing activated clotting factors from the circulation as well as fibrinolytic breakdown products. In end-stage liver disease the plasma level of fibrinogen may often be decreased. However, in uncomplicated cirrhosis, obstructive jaundice, chronic hepatitis, and biliary cirrhosis, a high level of fibrinogen may be found. In these latter cases, the thrombin time will often be prolonged because of an acquired dysfibrinogenemia. This is thought to be the result of an increased sialic acid content of fibrinogen.

Levels of the vitamin K-dependent proteins are also decreased in liver disease associated with obstructive jaundice or malabsorption of vitamin K. Factor VII has the shortest half-life of the vitamin K-dependent proteins. Accordingly, the first laboratory abnormality encountered may be an isolated prolongation of the PT.

Patients with liver disease often show a hypofibrinogenemia together with elevation of fibrin/fibrinogen degradation products and thrombocytopenia. This constellation of laboratory findings may be difficult to differentiate from DIC. In the past, many clinicians have relied on the factor VIII:C assay as a means of separating DIC from primary liver disease. Conventional wisdom suggests that DIC will have low levels of factor VIII:C in contrast to the elevated levels seen in liver disease. However, this is *not* a reliable criterion. Often in advanced liver disease there is low-grade intravascular coagulation, making the differential diagnosis of DIC and liver disease an exercise in futility.

Management of hemostatic abnormalities in the setting of liver disease is often frustrating (109). In acute liver failure, replacement of coagulation factors by infusion of fresh frozen plasma may be helpful. In more chronic states, management of the underlying liver disease is the primary objective. The use of fresh frozen plasma and platelets may be helpful to treat acute bleeding episodes. The treatment of bleeding esophageal varices may require a balloon tamponade or surgery.

BLEEDING ASSOCIATED WITH CARDIOPULMONARY BYPASS

Approximately a quarter of a million patients undergo cardiopulmonary bypass (CPB) procedures each year in the U.S. This group of patients utilized approximately 25% of blood products in many institutions. However, there is marked institutional variability in the incidence of bleeding associated with CPB. A variety of risk factors have been identified including time on the extracorporeal system, history of previous cardiac surgery, the nature of the surgery, preoperative medications, and the use and reversal of heparin. As a result of exposure of the circulating blood to a foreign surface, platelet activation with the release reaction occurs. In addition, there is also activation of the fibrinolytic system, which may lead to consumption of fibrinogen, factor V, factor VIII, and other plasma proteins. Also, with activation of the coagulation cascade there may be consumption of the regulatory proteins AT III and protein C.

Consequently, bleeding associated with CPB is multifactoral and requires a systemic approach to the bleeding patient. The first step is to rule out an anatomic defect as a potential explanation of postoperative bleeding. Coagulation tests should include an APTT, TT, heparin assay, and fibrinogen. The TT and heparin assay will provide information as to the possibility of excess heparin or heparin rebound.

Management may require the use of platelets. Occasionally, fresh frozen plasma is indicated for serious coagulopathies. Recently, the use of desmopressin (DDAVP) and aprotinin (Trasylol) have been advocated as a means of controlling bleeding without the use of blood products and their potential complications.

LABORATORY ANALYSIS OF COAGULATION

The most important step in the evaluation of a bleeding patient is a good medical history. Unfortunately, in the clinical laboratory the history is not available unless the laboratory physician takes the initiative to review the patient's chart and talk with the patient. In the majority of cases, the information provided will direct the subsequent laboratory evaluation. The clinical histories of patients with abnormalities of primary and secondary hemostasis differ significantly. Thus, mucocutaneous bleeding should lead to an evaluation of primary hemostasis, while musculoskeletal bleeding would initiate an evaluation of secondary hemostasis.

In most laboratories, six simple procedures can be performed to evaluate a patient with a potential hemostatic abnormality. These six procedures include a review of the peripheral smear, bleeding time, platelet count, APTT, PT, and TT. In virtually all cases, the peripheral smear and platelet count are a byproduct of a CBC and are readily available. The bleeding time is the single best test for evaluating primary hemostasis. In conjunction with the platelet count, it allows a differentiation of qualitative and quantitative platelet disorders.

Table 42.12. Abnormal Thrombin Time

- Heparin
- Fibrin/fibrinogen degradation products
- Paraproteins
- Dysfibrinogenemia
- Hypofibrinogenemia
- Antibodies to thrombin
- Uremia
- Some patients with lupus anticoagulants

The PT and APTT provide an arbitrary dissection of coagulation into the intrinsic (APTT) system and the extrinsic (PT) system. Although in reality this division is artificial, it is very useful from the standpoint of patient evaluation. Isolated prolongation of the prothrombin time is associated with factor VII deficiency, which may be either hereditary or acquired. An abnormal APTT together with a normal PT is indicative of an abnormality in the more proximal part of the intrinsic system (factors XII, XI, VIII, IX, and Fletcher and Fitzgerald). Abnormalities of both test systems are suggestive of a final common pathway defect (factors X, V, II, and I).

The TT is a very useful test and is often overlooked. The TT may be abnormal in a variety of clinical situations (Table 42.12). TT is extremely useful in ruling out the presence of heparin in a patient sample. The finding of a prolonged TT that corrects with the addition of protamine is virtually diagnostic of heparin. Also, the reptilase time may be used to identify heparin as an explanation of prolonged TT. The reptilase time will be normal in the presence of heparin.

Factor assays are indicated in many instances to establish the exact cause for the abnormal screening studies. These assays, depending on the factor, may utilize either the APTT or PT systems. Appropriate attention is necessary to ensure the quality of factor assays. At least two dilutions of the patient's plasma should be used, and the patient's values should be checked to ensure parallelism of the patient's values when compared with the reference curve. Nonparallelism of factor assay results is suggestive of an inhibitor.

Synthetic substrate assays have achieved a greater level of importance in the coagulation laboratory. These assays rely on the use of synthetic oligopeptides (three or four amino acids) that mimic amino acid sequences near the site of enzymatic cleavage in the native substrate (110). For instance, the synthetic substrate utilized to evaluate factor Xa activity consists of the four amino acids, isoleucine-glutamine-glycine-arginine. These four amino acids are located adjacent to the peptide bonds in prothrombin, where factor Xa activates prothrombin to thrombin. An indicator group is attached at the carboxy-terminal end of the oligopeptide. The indicator group may be either a chromogen or a fluorochrome. In most instances, laboratories utilize chromogenic assays.

Among the advantages of synthetic substrate assays are their ready adaptation to automated instrumentation and their basic enzymatic principles. Thus, utilizing synthetic substrates, it is possible to characterize the reactions with greater precision than the classic coagulation assays that rely on a fibrin endpoint. Currently, synthetic substrate assays are most often utilized for the evaluation of the fibrinolytic system. Also, there are commercially available kits for many components of the coagulation system (e.g., factor VIII). In addition, synthetic substrates are extremely useful in the analysis of the regulatory proteins (AT III and protein C).

References

1. Triplett DA. Hemostasis: a case oriented approach. New York-Tokyo: Igaku-Shoin, 1985.
2. Gitschier J, Wood WI, Goralka TM, et al. Characterization of the human factor VIII gene. Nature 1984;312:326.
3. Wood WI, Capon DJ, Simonsen CC, et al. Expression of active human factor VIII from recombinant DNA clones. Nature 1984;312:330.
4. Vehar GA, Keyt B, Eaton D, et al. Structure of human factor VIII. Nature 1984;312:337.
5. Vehar GA, Lawn RM, Tuddenham EGD, Wood WI. Factor VIII and factor V: biochemistry and pathophysiology: In: Scriver CR, Beaudet AL, Sly WS, Valle D, eds. The metabolic basis of inherited disease. 6th ed. New York: McGraw-Hill; 1989:2155–2170.
6. Barker D, Schafer M, White R. Restriction sites containing CpG show a higher frequency of polymorphism in human DNA. Cell 1984;6:131.
7. Youssoufian H, Kazazian HH Jr, Phillips DG, et al. Recurrent mutations in hemophilia A: evidence for CpG dinucleotides as mutation hotspots. Nature 1986;27:380.
8. Maas RL, Triplett DA, Tholen D. Factor VIII assay proficiency assessment: experience in the USA. Scand J Haematol 1984;33 (suppl 41):109.
9. Levine PH, McVerry BA, Attock B, et al. Health of intensively treated hemophiliac with special reference to abnormalities of blood chemistries and splenomegaly. Blood 1977;50:1.
10. Evatt BL, Ramsey RB, Lawrence DN, Zyla LD, Curran JW. The acquired immunodificiency syndrome in patients with hemophilia. Ann Intern Med 1984;100:499.
11. Hrinda ME, Feldman F, Schreiber AB. Preclinical characterization of a new pasteurized monoclonal antibody purified factor VIII:C. Semin Hematol 1990;27 (suppl 2):19–24.
12. Lusher JM, Salzman PM and the Monoclate Study Group. Viral safety and inhibitor development associated with factor VIII C ultra-purified from plasma in hemophiliacs previously unexposed to factor VIII C concentrates. Semin Hematol 1990;27 (suppl 2):1–7.
13. Schwartz RS, Abildgaard CF, Aledort LM, et al. Human recombinant DNA derived anti-hemophiliac factor (Factor VIII) in the treatment of hemophilia A. N Engl J Med 1990;323: 1800–1805.
14. Warrier AI, Luscher JM. DDAVP: a useful alternative to blood components in moderate hemophilia A and von Willebrand's disease. J Pediatr 1983;102:228.

15. Shapiro SS, Hultin M. Acquired inhibitors to blood coagulation factors. Semin Thromb Hemost 1975;1:336–385.
16. Kasper CK, Aledort L, Aronson D, et al. Proceedings: a more uniform measurement of factor VIII inhibitors. Thromb Diath Haemorrh 1975;34:869–872.
17. Brettler DB, Forsberg AD, Levine PE, et al. The use of porcine factor VIII concentrate (Hyate:C®) in the treatment of patients with inhibitor antibodies to factor VIII. Arch Intern Med 1989;149:1381–1385.
18. Lusher JM, Shapiro SS, Palascak JE, et al. Autoplex versus proplex: a controlled double blind study of effectiveness in acute hemarthrosis in hemophiliacs with inhibitors to factor VIII. Blood 1983;62:1135–1138.
19. Kasper CK. Treatment of factor VIII inhibitors. In: Coller BS, ed. Progress in hemostasis and thrombosis. Philadelphia: WB Saunders, 1989:57–86.
20. Nilsson IM, Sundqvest S, Frieburghaus C. Extracorporeal protein A-sepharose and specific affinity chromatography for removal of antibodies. Prog Clin Biol Res 1984;150:225–241.
21. Brandt, JT, Arkin CF, Bovill EG, Rock WA, Triplett DA. Evaluation of APTT reagent sensitivity to factor IX and factor IX assay performance. Results from the College of American Pathologists Survey Program. Arch Pathol Lab Med 1990;114: 135–141.
22. Pavlosky A. Contribution to the pathogenesis of hemophilia. Blood 1947;2:185–191.
23. Denson KWE, Biggs R, Mannucci PM. An investigation of three patients with Christmas disease due to an abnormal type of factor IX. J Clin Pathol 1968;21:160–165.
24. Giddings JC. Molecular genetics and immunoanalysis. In: Williams CE, ed. Blood coagulation. Chichester, England: Ellis Harwood, 1988.
25. Hedner U, Davie EW. Factor IX. In: Colman RW, Hirsh J, Marder VJ, Salzman EW, eds. Hemostasis and thrombosis. 2nd ed. Philadelphia: JB Lippincott, 1987:39–47.
26. Seligsohn U. High gene frequency of factor XI (PTA) deficiency in Ashkenazi Jews. Blood 1978;51:1223.
27. Saito H, Ratnoff OD, Bouma BN, Seligsohn U. Failure to detect variant (CRM^+) plasma thromboplastin antecedent (PTA, factor XI) molecules in hereditary PTA deficiency. A study of 125 patients of several ethnic backgrounds. J Lab Clin Med 1985;106:718.
28. Rapaport SI, Proctor RR, Patch MJ, Yettra M. The mode of inheritance of PTA deficiency: evidence for the existance of major PTA deficiency and minor PTA deficiency. Blood 1961;18:149.
29. Triplett DA, Brandt JT, Batard MA, Schaeffer Dixon JL, Fair DS. Hereditary factor VII deficiency: heterogenecity defined by combined functional and immunochemical analysis. Blood 1985;66:1284.
30. Drakenberg T, Fernlund P, Roepstorff P, Stenflo J. B-Hydoxyaspartic acid in vitamin K dependent proteins. Proc Natl Acad Sci USA 1983;80:182.
31. Triplett DA. The extrinsic system. Clin Lab Med 1984;4:221–244.
32. Ott R, Pfeiffer RA. Evidence that activities of coagulation factors VII and X are linked to chromosome 13 (q34). Hum Genet 1984;66:230.
33. Gilgen-Krantz S, Briquel ME, Andre E, et al. Structural genes of coagulation factors VII and X located on 13 q 34. Ann Genet 1986;29:32.
34. Hall CA, Rapaport RL, Ames SB. A clinical and family study of hereditary proconvertin (factor VII) deficiency. Am J Med 1964;37:172–181.
35. Girolami A. The congenital factor VII abnormalities (dysproconvertinemias). The genetic plot thickens. Folia Haematol 1980;107:131–136.
36. Hedner U, Kisiel W. Use of human factor VIIa in the treatment of two hemophilia A patients with high titer inhibitors. J Clin Invest 1983;71:1836–1841.
37. Telfer TP, Denson KW, Wright DR. A "new" coagulation defect. Br J Haematol 1956;2:308.
38. Houghie C, Barrow EM, Graham JB. Stuart clotting defect. I. segregation of an hereditary hemorrhagic state from the heterogeneous group heretofore called "stable factor" (SPCA, proconvertin, factor VII) deficiency. J Clin Invest 1957;36:485.
39. DiScipio RG, Hermodson MA, Davie EW. The mechanism of activation of bovine factor X (Stuart factor) by a protease from Russell's viper venom. Biochem 1977;16:5253.
40. Girolami A, Lazzarin M, Procidano M, Luzzatto G. A family with heterozygous factor X Friuli defect outside Friuli. Blut 1983;46:149.
41. Fair DS, Edgington TS. Heterogeneity of hereditary and acquired factor X deficiencies by combined immunochemical and functional analyses. Br J Haematol 1985;59:235.
42. Mammen EF. Factor X abnormalities. Semin Thromb Hemostat 1983;9:31.
43. Furie B, Greene E, Furie BC. Syndrome of acquired factor X deficiency in systemic amyloidosis. N Engl J Med 1977;297: 81.
44. Owren PA. Parahemophilia, hemorrhagic diathesis due to the absence of previously unknown clotting factor. Lancet 1947;1:446.
45. Tracy PB, Eide LL, Bowie EJW, Mann KG. Radioimmunoassay of factor V in human plasma. Blood 1982;60:59.
46. Chiu HC, Whitaker E, Colman RW. Heterogeneity of human factor V deficiency: evidence for the existance of an antigen positive variant. J Clin Invest 1983;72:493–503.
47. Giles AR, Tracy PB, Rivard G, Mann KG. Factor V (Quebec): a bleeding diathesis associated with a defective platelet factor V (Abstract 0784). Thromb Haemost 1983;50:250.
48. Seligsohn U, Zivelin A, Zwang E. Combined factor V and factor VIII deficiency among non-Ashkenazi Jews. N Engl J Med 1982;307:1191–1195.
49. Feinstein DI, Rapaport SI, McGehee WG, Patch MJ. Factor V anticoagulants: clinical biochemical and immunological observations. J Clin Invest 1970;49:1578.
50. Fratantoni JC, Hilgartner M, Nachman RL. Nature of the defect in congenital factor V deficiency: study in a patient with an acquired circulating anticoagulant. Blood 1972;39:751.
51. Mammen EF. Factor V deficiency. Semin Thromb Hemost 1983;9:17.
52. Vicic WJ, Lages B, Weiss HJ. Release of human platelet factor V activity is induced by both collagen and ADP and is inhibited by aspirin. Blood 1980;56:448–455.
53. Miletich JP, Jackson CM, Majerus PW. Properties of the factor Xa binding site on human platelets. J Biol Chem 1978;253: 6908–6916.
54. Webster WP, Roberts HR, Penick GD. Hemostasis in factor V deficiency. Am J Med Sci 1964;248:194.
55. Chediak J, Ashenhurst JB, Garlick I, Desser RK. Successful management of bleeding in a patient with factor V inhibitor by blood transfusions. Blood 1980;56:835.
56. Quick AJ, Pisciotta AV, Hussey CV. Congenital hypoprothrombinemic states. Arch Intern Med 1955;95:2.
57. Pool JG, Desai R, Kropatkin M. Severe congenital hypoprothrombinemia in a negro boy. Thromb Diath Haemorrhag 1962;8:235.
58. Degen SJF, Rajput B, Reich E, Davie EW. Coagulation and fibrinolysis characterization of the human prothrombin and human tissue plasminogen activator genes. In: Peeters H, ed. Protides of the biological fluids. Oxford: Pergamon Press, 1985;33:47.

105. Moake JL. Thrombotic thrombocytopenic purpura (TTP) and the hemolytic uremic syndrome (HUS). In: Rakel RE, ed. Conn's current therapy. Philadelphia: WB Saunders, 1989; 339–341.
106. Byrnes JJ, Moake JL. Thrombotic thrombocytopenic purpura and the haemolytic uremic syndrome: evolving concepts of pathogenesis and therapy. Clin Haematol 1986;15:413–442.
107. Shepard KV, Bukowski RM. The treatment of thrombotic thrombocytopenic purpura with exchange transfusions, plasma infusion, and plasma exchange. Semin Hematol 1987;24:178–193.
108. Ratnoff OD. Hemostatic defects in liver and biliary tract disease and disorders of vitamin K metabolism. In: Ratnoff OD, Forbes CD, eds. Disorders of hemostasis. 2nd ed. Philadelphia: WB Saunders, 1991:459–479.
109. Burroughs AK, McCormick PA. Springmans D. Assessment of bleeding risk in chronic liver disease. Fibrinolysis (suppl 3) 2; 1988:56–58.
110. Triplett DA. New developments in diagnostic coagulation testing. In: Beckstein DR, Dixon MR, Blomback B, eds. New advances in hemostasis for transfusion medicine. Arlington, VA: American Association of Blood Banks, 1990:17–25.

43 Regulatory Protein Disorders and Other Thrombotic Abnormalities

Douglas A. Triplett

Thromboembolic disease and its complications are the most common cause of death in the Western world. This chapter focuses on abnormalities of the regulatory proteins and other clinical states associated with thrombotic disorders. Although a number of hereditary abnormalities of regulatory proteins have now been linked to a familial thrombotic tendency, the majority of patients with thrombosis have a complex multifactorial pathophysiology (1–3).

The laboratory contribution to the diagnosis of thrombotic disorders, therefore, is most clearly defined in the case of patients who have a hereditary abnormality. The hereditary disorders are reviewed followed by discussion of various acquired states in which there is a thrombotic predisposition.

HEREDITARY DISORDERS OF REGULATORY PROTEINS

Antithrombin (AT) III is a plasma glycoprotein that is a member of the SERPIN family. AT III inhibits all of the serine proteases involved in hemostasis, with the exception of factor VIIa (1, 4). This inhibition is achieved by forming a 1:1 enzyme-inhibitor complex. The reaction between AT III and serine protease enzymes is greatly accelerated in the presence of heparin or other related glycosaminoglycans (4). Physiologically, the presence of heparin sulfate on the surface of endothelial cells is involved in the down-regulation of hemostasis in conjunction with AT III (5, 6). A number of investigators have utilized activation peptides (fibrinopeptide A, prothrombin fragment 1·2, and factor X activation peptide) to demonstrate that there is an ongoing "tonic" activation of hemostasis (7, 8). This low level of activation is successfully regulated in the normal individual by a variety of regulatory systems, of which the heparin sulfate-AT III component is extremely important (9).

Hereditary deficiency of AT III was the first plasma protein deficiency successfully linked to a thrombotic predisposition (10). In contrast to hereditary disorders of coagulation proteins, AT III-deficient patients were found to have levels of 40 to 50% of normal (9, 11). The association of clinical symptoms with a "borderline" or slight deficiency of this regulatory protein would suggest that the physiological balance of procoagulant/anticoagulant activities is a precarious detente. In contrast, patients with mild hemophilia and levels of factor VIII activity of 5% may be entirely free of bleeding complications unless significantly challenged by trauma or surgery.

AT III deficiency is inherited as an autosomal dominant abnormality (9–11). The AT III gene is located on human chromosome 1 q23–25 (12). The AT III gene consists of six exons and five introns distributed over approximately 19 kb of DNA. There is some homology of the AT III gene with the α_1-antitrypsin gene. The incidence of AT III deficiency in the general population has been estimated at 1:2000 to 1:5000 (13, 14).

Individuals with AT III deficiency are usually symptomatic by the age of 40. Typically, the onset of thromboembolic events occurs in the late teens or 20s (9, 11, 15). On occasion, patients who are in their 50s or 60s with no history of thrombosis may be encountered (11). The majority of the thromboembolic events are venous. In approximately 50% of cases, the initial event is related to some precipitating factor such as surgery, trauma, use of oral contraceptives, or pregnancy (1, 9, 11).

The laboratory evaluation requires specific assays of AT III activity and antigen. The usual screening tests for hemostasis are entirely normal. Antigenic measurement of AT III may utilize a variety of different techniques: radioimmunoassay, radial immunodiffusion, and Laurell rocket immunoelectrophoresis (16, 17). Of these techniques, the Laurell method is most commonly employed. Functional assays may utilize either fibrin endpoint or synthetic substrate systems (18). The most practical functional assay assesses the ability of AT III to inhibit an enzyme in the presence of heparin. Perhaps the most frequently utilized system employs chromogenic substrates (Fig. 43.1). A second functional assay relies on progressive antithrombin III activity. In this assay, the patient's plasma containing AT III is incubated with a

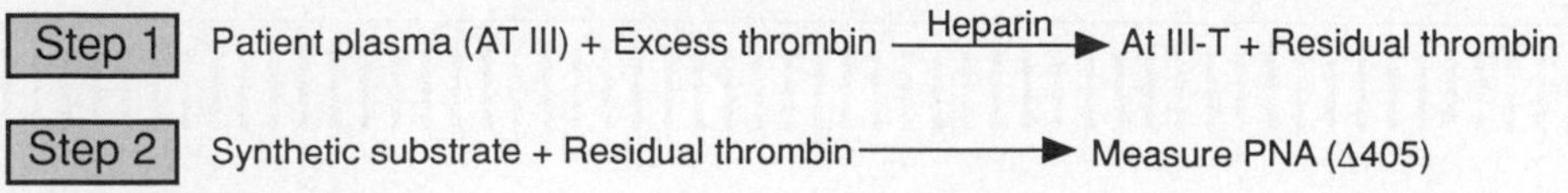

Figure 43.1. Antithrombin III amidolytic assay. The reaction may be measured using a recording spectrophotomer or by an end point method when the reaction is stopped by adding acetic acid. (PNA, paranitroanaline).

Table 43.1. Classification of AT III Deficiency[a]

Type	Antigen	Functional Coagulation	Functional (Heparin)
I	Decreased	Decreased	Decreased
II	Normal	Decreased	Decreased
II (Heparin)	Normal	Normal	Decreased

[a]Type II (heparin) is a dysfunctional AT III with an abnormality at the heparin binding site. The functional coagulation assay is performed in the absence of heparin and evaluates the time-dependent inhibition of either Xa or thrombin. The functional assay in the presence of heparin evaluates both AT III time-dependent inhibition and the ability of heparin to accelerate this inhibition. This assay may be performed using either a coagulation or chromogenic system.

known amount of enzyme (Xa or IIa) in the absence of heparin (18). Discrepancies between these two functional assays have been observed in a number of patient studies (19). Patients with normal progressive AT III activity and decreased activity in the presence of heparin have gene mutations, resulting in abnormalities of AT III heparin binding sites (19–21).

By utilizing both antigenic and functional assays, it is possible to divide inherited AT III deficiency into two distinct types (18). Type I results in reduced synthesis of a biologically normal protein, and type II results in normal antigenic amounts of AT III but decreased functional activity in one of the two aforementioned functional assay systems (22) (Table 43.1). Patients with Type II AT III deficiency secondary to an abnormality in the heparin binding sites often have a milder clinical history and may be asymptomatic in the heterozygous state (20, 21). However, children who are doubly heterozygous for type II AT III deficiency may have significant clinical thrombosis (23, 24).

Acquired AT III deficiency may be seen in a variety of clinical conditions. These include liver disease, nephrotic syndrome, DIC, and acute thrombosis (25, 26). Modest reductions may also be seen in patients using oral contraceptives (25). L-asparaginase is associated with a striking decrease of AT III (27).

The clinical management of patients with AT III deficiency consists of initial treatment with heparin followed by oral anticoagulants (28). Once the diagnosis has been established, many clinicians maintain the patient on life-long oral anticoagulant therapy. With the trend toward lower doses of oral anticoagulants, the complication rate associated with the use of these drugs is anticipated to decrease.

The diagnosis of any of the hereditary disorders of regulatory proteins is often complicated by the initial patient presentation during an acute thrombosis (29, 30). Frequently the patient is already receiving heparin before the laboratory is requested to evaluate the patient for possible regulatory protein deficiencies. In this setting, testing the family may prove to be the best means of establishing a hereditary abnormality.

Protein C Deficiency

Protein C is a vitamin K-dependent protein that is readily converted to active protein C (APC) by a complex of thrombin and thrombomodulin on the surface of endothelial cells. APC will then, in the presence of another vitamin K-dependent protein, protein S, inactivate factor Va and factor VIIIa (3, 31, 32). Thus, the "protein C system" is responsible for the regulation of the two key cofactors in the intrinsic pathway of coagulation. The remaining cofactor, tissue factor, of the extrinsic pathway is regulated by a relatively newly discovered coagulation protein: tissue factory pathway inhibitor (also known as extrinsic pathway inhibitor and as LACI) (33, 34).

Protein S functions in this reaction as a cofactor for APC (3). Protein S binds to both endothelial cells and activated platelets and thus serves as a means of localizing APC to an appropriate cell surface. The complex of APC/protein S will then preferentially inactivate cofactors Va and VIIIa. APC is inhibited by at least two plasma proteins: protein C inhibitor and α-1-antitrypsin (3).

The gene for protein C is found on chromosome 2. The gene contains approximately 11 kb of DNA and has nine exons with eight introns (35). Protein C deficiency is inherited in an autosomal-dominant fashion (36). Heterozygous patients present clinically with either deep or superficial vein thrombosis (37, 38). The time of onset and other related clinical findings are very similar to those of AT III deficiency. In addition, heterozygous protein C deficiency may be first suspected when a patient who presents with DVT is started on a loading dose of oral anticoagulants. As a result, the appearance of coumadin-induced skin necrosis may alert the clinician to the possibility of protein C deficiency (39, 40). Not all patients who develop this complication prove to have hereditary deficiency of protein C. However, any patient with such a history should be evaluated for this possibility.

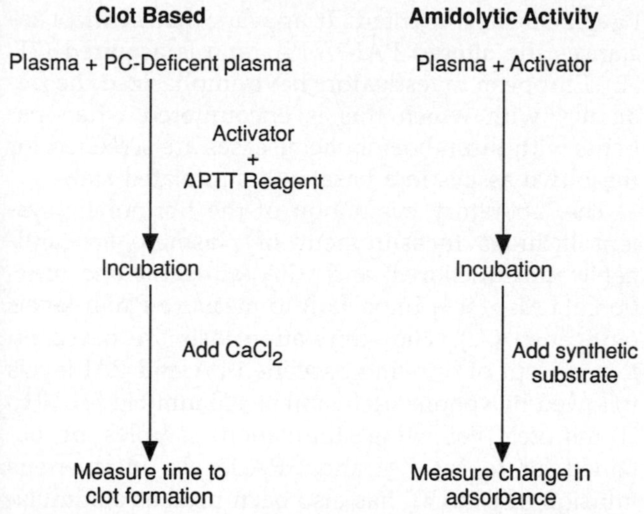

Figure 43.2. Protein C functional assays (venom activation).

Table 43.2. Classification of Protein C Deficiency

Type	Antigen	Functional Coagulation	Functional Chromogenic
Type I	Decreased	Decreased	Decreased
Type IIa	Normal	Decreased	Decreased
Type IIb	Normal	Decreased	Normal

The doubly heterozygous or homozygous protein C deficiency state is associated with purpura fulminans in the newborn (41, 42). This is a particularly devastating presentation characterized by extensive areas of skin necrosis together with cerebral and retinal vein thrombosis. Unless appropriate treatment is initiated immediately, this disorder is fatal (42).

Laboratory evaluation of protein C includes both antigenic and functional assays. The antigenic assays available include Laurell rocket immunoelectrophoresis and ELISA assays (43). Patients with heterozygous protein C deficiency typically have a protein C level of 40 to 50% (reference interval 65 to 130%). These results are similar to values for heterozygous AT III deficiency.

Functional assays for protein C are based on either a fibrin endpoint system or synthetic substrate technology (44, 45). The fibrin endpoint assays rely on an APTT system (Fig. 43.2). The synthetic substrate assays are more direct, requiring less technical time. A number of situations have been described in which the functional coagulation assay is discrepant when compared with the synthetic substrate assay (Table 43.2) (47, 48). Both type I and type II deficiency states have been identified. In type I deficiency, the patient has a decreased plasma level of both functional and antigenic protein C. In type II patients, the antigenic level of protein C is within normal limits, while there is decreased functional coagulation and/or substrate activities.

Once the diagnosis has been established, treatment of protein C deficiency in the heterozygous patient is life-long oral anticoagulation. In the homozygous patient, replacement of protein C using fresh frozen plasma is critical in the initial stages of treatment. Oral anticoagulants are indicated for long-term management. The availability of concentrates of protein C may prove to be valuable in treating these patients.

Protein S Deficiency

The clinical presentation of protein S deficiency patients is similar to AT III and protein C deficiency states (49). In addition to venous thromboembolic events, a number of recent reports have emphasized cerebral vein thrombosis (50, 51). Also, warfarin-induced skin necrosis has been reported with protein S deficiency (52).

Two forms of protein S are present in the circulation: free and bound (3, 53). The free protein S comprises approximately 40% of the plasma compartment and is the functionally active cofactor. In contrast, the bound protein S circulates complexed to a complement component: C4b-binding protein. C4b-binding protein is an acute phase reactant; consequently, a variety of clinical conditions in which acute phase proteins increase will result in some shift in the equilibrium between free and bound protein S (55).

The laboratory evaluation of protein S includes antigenic assays as well as functional assays (53–56). For practical purposes, most laboratories are restricted to the use of antigenic determinations. Total protein S may be assayed with a radioimmunoassay or ELISA assay. Free protein S is based on removing the protein S–C4b-binding protein complex by precipitation with polyethylene glycol. The supernatant is then assayed for residual protein S by either ELISA or radioimmunoassay (3).

Protein S deficiency has been categorized into two types. Type I includes patients in whom there are markedly reduced levels of free protein S but a normal amount of protein S complexed to C4b-binding protein. The type II patients have decreased amounts of both free and bound protein S. The majority of patients described have been type I. Acquired deficiencies of protein S have been described in patients with lupus anticoagulants (57). In addition, protein S has been found to decrease during pregnancy and in the postpartum period (58). Oral contraceptives have also been found to lower both total and free protein S (59). Since protein S is a vitamin K-dependent protein, plasma levels also are decreased in liver disease and vitamin K deficiency.

Treatment of protein S deficiency requires long-term oral anticoagulant therapy.

Heparin Cofactor II Deficiency

Heparin cofactor II is a member of the SERPIN family. It is a single-chain polypeptide with a molecular weight of approximately 66,000 (60). The gene for heparin cofactor II is located on chromosome 22 (61, 62). In contrast to AT III, heparin cofactor II inhibits thrombin but has no inhibitory activity toward other coagulation serine proteases. The ability to inhibit thrombin is greatly accelerated in the presence of high concentrations of heparin. Apparently, physiological activator for heparin cofactor II is dermatan sulfate, which accelerates heparin cofactor II activity approximately 1000-fold (63).

Several patients have been described in whom hereditary deficiency of heparin cofactor II was associated with thrombosis (64–69). In these cases the level of heparin cofactor II was approximately 40 to 60% of normal. Acquired heparin cofactor II deficiency has been seen in patients with DIC, liver disease, and obstetrical complications (69).

Laboratory assays for heparin cofactor II rely on the use of dermatan sulfate as a means of preferentially accelerating the thrombin inhibitory activity of heparin cofactor II (70).

Hereditary Disorders of Fibrinolysis

A variety of hereditary abnormalities of the fibrinolytic system have been linked to a thrombotic predisposition (71–73). Perhaps the most frequently discussed disorders have been dysplasminogenemias and hypoplasminogenemia (74–77). Unfortunately, the family histories in many of these cases have not proved to be as convincing as those seen in the hereditary disorders of AT III, protein C, and protein S (71, 72). Often the propositus is the only symptomatic member of the family, despite the fact that other family members have similar levels of plasminogen or a similar dysfunctional molecule.

Less convincing cases have been reported in which there is possibly a decreased ability to release tissue plasminogen activator (t·PA) from the endothelial cells or alternatively elevated levels of plasminogen activator inhibitor (PAI-1) (78–80). This disequilibrium between t·PA and PAI leads to a hypofibrinolytic state. Again, there are few families in which a hereditary abnormality of this ratio has been documented convincingly (81). In many acquired situations such as hypertriglyceridemia associated with diabetes mellitus and systemic lupus erythematosus, abnormalities of the PAI-1/t·PA ratio have been documented. It appears that in most instances the altered PAI-1/t·PA ratio is acquired (71, 72). European investigators have emphasized the frequency with which this is encountered when patients with thromboembolic diseases are screened for these two assays in a basal and stimulated state.

The laboratory evaluation of the fibrinolytic system includes measurement of plasminogen (antigenic and functional) and t·PA (antigenic and functional). Also, it is important to measure PAI-1 levels (antigenic) (72). The stimulation tests are based on the concept of drawing baseline t·PA and PAI levels followed by venous occlusion at 100 mm Hg for 10 to 20 minutes. Following stimulation, samples are obtained for repeat PAI and t·PA levels. Intravenous infusion of DDAVP has also been used as a stimulatory test.

Dysfibrinogenemia

A number of congenital dysfibrinogenemias have been reported in association with familial thrombosis (82, 83). Both arterial and venous thromboembolic events have been described. In some cases the molecular defect has been identified. It may involve either abnormalities in the thrombin-fibrinogen interaction or plasmin-fibrinogen interaction. In the latter case, the binding of plasminogen to the fibrin clot is impaired, with resulting increased resistance of fibrin to fibrinolysis (72).

ACQUIRED DISORDERS

A variety of acquired conditions are associated with a predisposition to thrombosis. The presence of a lupus anticoagulant (LA) has been linked to thrombotic events. Whether the LA is causative, coincidence, or a consequence is still unresolved. Consequently, patients who present with unexplained thrombosis should be evaluated for the presence of LA (84). This evaluation would include a screening APTT. Also, because LA is merely one member of the family of antiphospholipid antibodies (APA), solid phase assays for anticardiolipin antibodies (ACA) and other antibodies to negatively charged phospholipids should be obtained. In most instances, patients who are LA-positive will also be ACA-positive. In approximately one-third of cases, there will be a lack of concordance between these two assay systems (85).

LA-associated thromboembolic events are both venous and arterial. Consequently, the clinical presentation of these patients may be significantly different from those encountered with hereditary thrombotic disorders. For instance, young adults with cerebrovascular accidents have been frequently found to have LA/ACA (85).

Table 43.3. Laboratory Evaluation of Thrombosis

- APTT
- Anticardiolipin antibody
- Antithrombin III (functional assay—heparin)
- Protein C (functional assay—coagulation)
- Plasminogen (functional)
- Thrombin time
- Protein S (functional assay)
- Heparin cofactor II (functional assay)

Numerous other clinical conditions are associated with thrombotic predispositions. Among these are Trousseau's syndrome, diabetes mellitus, hyperlipidemia, various vasculitides, paroxysmal nocturnal hemoglobinuria, and Kawasaki's syndrome.

Trousseau's syndrome is the presence of recurrent deep or superficial venous thrombosis in association with malignancies. Often the malignancy may be gastrointestinal or pancreatic in origin (86). In many cases the malignancy may be occult, and the patient presents initially with thrombosis. Patients who present with deep vein thrombosis or superficial thrombophlebitis that fails to respond to oral anticoagulant therapy or anti-inflammatory medications should be suspected of possible Trousseau's syndrome. Typically, heparin is the only satisfactory therapy for the management of these patients. The mechanism of increased procoagulant activity in association with malignancy has recently been explored extensively. Initially, it was felt that mucous-secreting tumors produced a substance that directly activated factor X to Xa (87). Also, a tumor cell cysteine protease has been identified (88).

The presence of antiendothelial antibodies has been linked to several thrombotic conditions including Kawasaki's syndrome, hemolytic uremic syndrome, and acute allograft rejection (89).

LABORATORY EVALUATION OF A THROMBOTIC PREDISPOSITION

Candidates for a thrombotic evaluation include young adults with a positive family history of thromboembolic events who present with a thrombosis. There may or may not be a precipitating event. The evaluation of these patients requires assays for AT III, protein C, protein S as well as an evaluation of fibrinogen and the fibrinolytic system (Table 43.3). Despite the availability of these assays, only 15 to 20% of patients with unexplained recurrent thromboembolic events at a young age are found to have identifiable abnormalities (90). Establishing the diagnosis of a hereditary disorder associated with thrombosis is important. This will allow for family counseling and appropriate precautions for family members who are found to be heterozygous for the deficiency with no history of thrombosis. For instance, young women with a family history of AT III deficiency should be cautioned regarding the use of oral contraceptives. Also, management of pregnancy in these patients may require the use of heparin or recently available antithrombin III concentrates.

Because the vast majority of patients with thrombotic events are unexplained, the future exploration of these patients offers the possibility of a number of new assays. For instance, tissue factor pathway inhibitor deficiencies have not, as yet, been described. No doubt a significant number of patients will be found to have abnormalities of endothelial regulatory functions including deficiencies or functional abnormalities of thrombomodulin as well as other regulatory components such as tissue factor expression.

References

1. Bauer KA, Rosenberg RD. The hypercoagulable state. In: Ratnoff OD, Forbes CD, eds. Disorders of hemostasis. 2nd ed. Philadelphia: WB Saunders, 1991:267–291.
2. Rosenberg RD. Regulation of the hemostatic mechanism. In: Stamatoyannopoulos G, Nienhuis AW, Leder P, Majerus PW, eds. The molecular basis of blood diseases. Philadelphia: WB Saunders, 1987:534–574.
3. Esmon CT. Protein C: the regulation of natural anticoagulant pathways. Science 1987;235:1348–1352.
4. Damus PS, Hicks M, Rosenberg RD. Anticoagulant action of heparin. Nature 1973;246:355–357.
5. Marcum JA, Rosenberg RD. Anticoagulantly active heparin like molecules from vascular tissue. Biochemistry 1984;23: 1730–1737.
6. Marcum JA, Rosenberg RD. Heparin like molecules with anticoagulant activity are synthesized by cultured endothelial cells. Biochem Biophys Res Commun 1985;126:365–372.
7. Bauer KA, Brockmans AW, Berticalna RM, et al. Hemostatic enzyme generation in the blood of patients with hereditary protein C deficiency. Blood 1988;71:1418–1426.
8. Bauer KA, Goodman TL, Kass BL, Rosenberg RD. Elevated factor Xa activity in the blood of asymptomatic patients with congenital antithrombin deficiency. J Clin Invest 1985;76:826.
9. Cosgriff TM, Bishop DT, Hershgold EJ, et al. Familial antithrombin III deficiency: its natural history, genetics, diagnosis, and treatment. Medicine (Baltimore) 1983;62:209.
10. Egeberg O. Inherited antithrombin deficiency causing thrombophilia. Thromb Diath Haemorrh 1965;13:516.
11. Thaler E, Lechner K. Antithrombin III deficiency and thromboembolism. Clin Haematol 1981;10:369.
12. Bock SC, Wion KL, Vehar GA, Lawn RM. Cloning and expression of the cDNA for human antithrombin III. Nucleic Acids Res 1982;10:8113–8125.
13. Rosenberg RD. Action and interaction of antithrombin and heparin. N Engl J Med 1975;16:146.
14. Odegard OR, Abildgaard U. Antithrombin III: critical review of assay methods. Significance of variations in health and disease. Haemostasis 1978;7:127.
15. Kitchens CS. Concept of hypercoagulability: a review of its development, clinical application and recent progress. Semin Thromb Hemost 1985;11:293–315.
16. Chan V, Chan TK, Wong V, et al. The determination of antithrombin III by radioimmunoassay and its clinical application. Br J Haematol 1979;41:563–572.

17. Fagerhol MK, Abildgaard U. Immunological studies on human antithrombin III. Scand J Haematol 1970;7:10–17.
18. Bauer KA, Teitel JM, Rosenberg RD. Assays for the quantitation of antithrombin III, thrombin-antithrombin complex and prothrombin activation fragments. In: Colman RW, ed. Disorders of thrombin formation. New York: Churchill Livingstone, 1983:142–155.
19. Wolf M, Boyer C, Lavergne JM, Larrieu MJ. A new familial variant of antithrombin III: antithrombin III Paris. Br J Haematol 1982;51:285–295.
20. Chasse JF, Esnard F, Guitton JD, et al. An abnormal plasma antithrombin with no apparent affinity for heparin. Thromb Res 1984;34:297–302.
21. Owen MC, Borg JY, Soria C, Soria J, Caen J, Carrell RW. Heparin binding defect in a new antithrombin III variant: Rouen 47, Arg to His. Blood 1987;69:1275–1279.
22. Sas G, Blasko G, Banhegyi D, et al. Abnormal antithrombin III (antithrombin III "Budapest") as a course of familial thrombophilia. Thromb Diath Haemorr 1974;32:105–115.
23. Sakuragawa N, Takahashi K, Kondo S, Koide T. Antithrombin III Toyama: a hereditary abnormal antithrombin III of a patient with recurrent thrombophlebitis. Thromb Res 1983;31:305–317.
24. Fischer AM, Cornu P, Sternberg C, et al. Antithrombin III Alger: a new homozygous AT III variant. Thromb Haemost 1986;55:218–221.
25. Von Kaulla E, von Kaulla KN. Antithrombin III and diseases. Am J Clin Pathol 1967;48:69–80.
26. Damus PS, Wallace GA. Immunologic measurement of antithrombin III heparin cofactor and α_2 macroglobulin in disseminated intravascular coagulation and hepatic failure coagulopathy. Thromb Res 1989;6:27–38.
27. Buchanan GR, Holtkamp CA. Reduced antithrombin III levels during L-asparaginase therapy. Med Pediatr Oncol 1980;8:7–14.
28. Kitchens CS. Amelioration of antithrombin III deficiency by coumarin administration. Am J Med Sci 1987;293:403–406.
29. Ansell JE. Hypercoagulability: a conceptual and diagnostic approach. Am Heart J 1987;114:910–91.
30. DeBoer AC, van Riel LAM, den Ottolander GJH. Measurement of antithrombin IIIs, α_2 macroglobulin, and $\alpha_1$antitrypsin in patients with deep venous thrombosis and pulmonary embolism. Thromb Res 1979;15:17–25.
31. Marlar RA, Kliss AJ, Griffin JH. Mechanism of action of human activated protein C, a thrombin dependent anticoagulant enzyme. Blood 1982;59:1067–1072.
32. Walker FJ. Regulation of protein C by protein S: the role of phospholipid in factor Va inactivation. J Biol Chem 1981;256: 11128–11131.
33. Rapaport SI. Inhibition of factor VIIa/tissue factor-induced blood coagulation with particular emphasis upon a factor Xa-dependent inhibitory mechanism. Blood 1989;73:359–365.
34. Broze GJ, Girard TJ, Novotny WF. Regulation of coagulation by a multivalent kunitz-type inhibitor. Biochemistry 1990;29: 7539–7546.
35. Rocchi M, Roncuzzi L, Santamaria R, Archidiacono N, Dente L, Romeo G. Mapping through somatic cell hybrids and cDNA probes of protein C to chromosome 2, factor X to chromosome 13, and alpha 1-acid glycoprotein to chromosome 9. Hum Genet 1986;74:30.
36. Griffin JH, Evatt BL, Zimmerman TS, Kleiss AJ, Wideman C. Deficiency of protein C in congenital thrombotic disease. J Clin Invest 1981;68:1370–1373.
37. Brockmans AW, Veltkamp JJ, Bertina RM. Congenital protein C deficiency and venous thromboembolism: a study of three Dutch families. N Engl J Med 1983;309:340–344.
38. Brockmans AW, Bertina RM. Protein C. In: Poller L, ed. Recent advances in blood coagulation, no. 4. New York: Churchill Livingstone, 1985:117–137.
39. Brockmans AW, Bertina RM, Loeliger EA, Hofmann V, Klingemann HG. Protein C and the development of skin necrosis during anticoagulant therapy. Thromb Haemost 1983;49:251.
40. McGehee WG, Klotz TA, Epstein DJ, Rapaport SI. Coumarin necrosis associated with hereditary protein C deficiency. Ann Intern Med 1984;101:59.
41. Seligsohn U, Berger A, Abend M, et al. Homozygous protein C deficiency manifested by massive venous thrombosis in the newborn. N Engl J Med 1984;310:559–562.
42. Marciniak E, Wilson HD, Marlar RD. Neonatal purpura fulmins: a genetic disorder related to the absence of protein C in blood. Blood 1985;65:15–20.
43. Boyer C, Rothschild C, Wolf M, Amiral J, Meyer D, Larrieu MJ. A new method for the estimation of protein C by ELISA. Thromb Res 1984;36:579–589.
44. Triplett DA, Sandquist DS, Musgrave KA. Clinical application of a functional assay for protein C. Hematol Pathol 1988;1:239–247.
45. Martinoli JL, Stocker K. Fast functional Protein C assay using protac, a novel protein C activator. Thromb Res 1986;43: 253–264.
46. Francis RB Jr, Seyfert U. Rapid amidolytic assay of protein C in whole plasma using an activator from the venom of Agkistrodon Contortrix. Am J Clin Pathol 1987;87:619–625.
47. Barbui T, Finazzi G, Mussoni L, et al. Hereditary dysfunctional protein C (protein C Bergamo) and thrombosis. Lancet 1984;2:819.
48. Tirindelli MC, Franchi F, Tripold A, Mariani G, Mannucci PM. Familial dysfunctional protein C. Thromb Res 1986;44:893.
49. Comp PC, Esmon CT. Recurrent venous tromboembolism in patients with a partial deficiency of protein S. N Engl J Med 1984;311:1525.
50. Engesser L, Brockmans AW, Briet E, Brommer EJ, Bertina RM. Hereditary protein S deficiency: clinical manifestations. Ann Intern Med 1987;106:667–682.
51. Salem HH. The natural anticoagulants. Clin Haematol 1986;15: 371.
52. Friedman KD, Marlar RA, Houston JG, Montgomery RR. Warfarin induced skin necrosis in a patient with protein S deficiency (Abstract). Blood 1986;68:333a.
53. Fair DS, Revak DJ. Quantitation of human protein S in the plasma of normal and warfarin treated individuals by radioimmunoassay. Thromb Res 1984;36:527–535.
54. Malm J, Laurell M, Dahlback B. Changes in the plasma levels of vitamin K dependent protein C and S and of C4b-binding protein during pregnancy and oral contraception. Br J Haematol 1988;68:437–443.
55. Woodhams BJ, Matthews KB, Lee CA, Kernoff PB. Functional protein S assay shows improved correlation with clinical symptoms in hereditary deficiency. Thromb Res 1990;57:651–657.
56. Van de Waart P, Priessner KT, Bechtold JR, Muller-Berghaus G. A functional test for protein S activity in plasma. Thromb Res 1987;48:427–437.
57. Freidman KD, Marlar RA, Gill JC, Endres-Brooks J, Montgomery RR. Protein S deficiency in patients with the lupus anticoagulant. Blood 1986;68:333a.
58. Comp PC, Thurnau GR, Welsh J, Esmon CT. Functional and immunologic protein S levels are decreased during pregnancy. Blood 1986;68:881–885.
59. Boerger LM, Morris PC, Thurnau GR, Esmon CT, Comp PC. Oral contraceptives and gender affect Protein S status. Blood 1987;69:692–694.

60. Tollefsen DM, Majerus DW, Blank MK. Heparin cofactor II. Purification and properties of a heparin-dependent inhibitor of thrombin in human plasma. J Biol Chem 1982;257:2162.
61. Inhorn RC, Tollefsen DM. Isolation and characterization of a partial cDNA clone for heparin cofactor II. Biochem Biophys Res Commun 1986;137:431.
62. Blinder MA, Marasa JC, Reynolds CH, Deaven LL, Tollefsen DM. Heparin cofactor II: cDNA sequence chromosome localization, restriction fragment length polymorphism, and expression in escherichia coli. Biochemistry 1988;27:752.
63. Teien AN, Abildgaard U, Hook M. The anticoagulant effect of heparin sulfate and dermatans sulfate. Thromb Res 1976;8: 859.
64. Sie P, DuPouy D, Pichon J, Boneu B. Constitutional heparin cofactor II deficiency associated with recurrent thrombosis. Lancet 1985;2:414.
65. Tran TH, Marbet GA, Duckert F. Association of hereditary heparin cofactor II deficiency with thrombosis. Lancet 1985;2: 413.
66. Andersson TR, Larsen ML, Abildgaard U. Low heparin cofactor II associated with abnormal crossed immunoelectrophoresis pattern in two Norwegian families. Thromb Res 197;47:243–248.
67. Simioni P, Lazzaro AR, Coser E, Salmistraro G, Girolami A. Hereditary heparin cofactor II deficiency and thrombosis: report of six patients belonging to two separate kindreds. Blood Coagul Fibrinolysis 1990;1:351–356.
68. Weisdorf DJ, Edson JR. Recurrent venous thrombosis associated with inherited deficiency of heparin cofactor II. Br J Haematol 1991;77:125–126.
69. Tollefsen DM, Pestka CA. Heparin cofactor II activity in patients with disseminated intravascular coagulation and hepatic failure. Blood 1985;66:769.
70. Ezenagu LC, Brandt JT. Laboratory determination of heparin cofactor II. Arch Pathol Lab Med 1986;110:1149.
71. Wiman B. The role of the fibrinolytic system in thrombotic disease. Acta Med Scand (Suppl) 1987;715:169–171.
72. Francis CW, Marder VJ. Physiologic regulation and pathologic disorders of fibrinolysis. Hum Pathol 1987;18:263–274.
73. Francis RB. Clinical disorders of fibrinolysis: a critical review. Blut 1989; 59:1–14.
74. Kazama M, Tahara C, Suzuki Z, Gohchi K, Abe T. Abnormal plasminogen, a case of recurrent thrombosis. Thromb Res 1981;21:517–522.
75. Miyata T, Iwanaga S, Sakata Y, Aoki N, Takamatsu J, Kamiya T. Plasminogen Tochigi II and Nagoya. Two additional molecular defects with ala-600-thr replacement found in plasmin light chain variants. J Biochem 1984;96:277–284.
76. Scharrer I, Hach-Wunderle V, Wohl RC, Sinio L, Boreisha I, Robbins KC. Congenital abnormal plasminogen, Frankfurt I, cause for recurrent venous thrombosis. Haemostasis 1988;18(Suppl 1):77–86.
77. Mannucci PM, Kluft C, Traas DW, Seveso P, D'Angelo A. Congenital plasminogen deficiency associated with venous thromboembolism, therapeutic trial with stanozol. Br J Haematol 1986;63:753–759.
78. Wiman B, Ljungberg B, Chmielewska J, Urden G, Blomback M, Johansson J. The role of the fibrinolytic system in deep vein thrombosis. J Lab Clin Med 1985;105:265–270.
79. Brommer EJP, Verheijen JH, Chang GTG, Rijken. Masking of fibrinolytic response to stimulation by an inhibitor of tissue type plasminogen activator in plasma. Thromb Haemost 1985;52:154–156.
80. Gerard RD, Chien KR, Meidell RS. Molecular biology of tissue plasminogen activator and endogenous inhibitors. Mol Biol 1986;3:449.
81. Jorgensen M, Bonnevie-Nielsen V. Increased concentration of the fast acting plasminogen activator inhibitor in plasma associated with familial venous thrombosis. Br J Haematol 1987;65: 175–180.
82. Carrell N, Gabriel DA, Blatt PM, Carr ME, McDonagh J. Hereditary dysfibrinogenemia in a patient with thrombotic disease. Blood 1983;62:439.
83. Al-Mondhiry HAB, Bilezikian SB, Nossel HL. Fibrinogen "New York"—an abnormal fibrinogen associated with thromboembolism: functional evaluation. Blood 1975;45:607.
84. McNeil HP, Chesterman CN, Krilis SA. Immunology and clinical importance of antiphospholipid antibodies. Adv Immunol 1991;49:193–280.
85. Triplett DA, Brandt JT, Musgrave KA, Orr CA. The relationship lupus anticoagulant and antibodies to phospholipid. JAMA 1988;259:550–554.
86. Sick GH, Levin J, Bell WR. Trousseau's syndrome and other manifestations of chronic disseminated coagulopathy in patients with neoplasms: clinical, pathophysiologic and therapeutic features. Medicine (Baltimore) 1977;56:1–37.
87. Pineo GF, Brain MC, Gallus AS, et al. Tumors, mucus production and hypercoagulability. Ann NY Acad Sci 1971;230:262–270.
88. Falanga A, Gordon SG. Isolation and characterization of cancer coagulant: a cysteine protease from malignant tissue. Biochemistry 1985;24:5558–5567.
89. Cines DB. Disorders associated with antibodies to endothelial cells. Rev Infect Dis 1989;(Suppl 4)S705–S711.
90. Mannucci PM, Tripodi A. Inherited factors in thrombosis. Blood Rev 1988;2:27–35.

During the past two decades several major changes in the area of clinical microbiology and infectious diseases have occurred. Advances in medical technology and life-support systems have resulted in [redacted] dramatic increase in the number of patients [redacted] profoundly compromised immune status and/o[redacted] serious underlying diseases. These patients, as [redacted] as persons who are victims of the AIDS epide[redacted]c, are at high risk for infections both from classi[redacted]true" pathogens and from many opportunisti[redacted] pathogens. At the same time, we have witnessed the development and application of new technology [redacted] for the detection and identification of these agents of infection. Developments in immunology, molecular biology, and laboratory automation have both enhanced and complicated the job of the clinical microbiologist. These many changes and advances have placed new demands on the clinical microbiology laboratory. The laboratory must remain flexible enough to develop and offer expanded testing for new and unusual microorganisms as they become recognized as important pathogens in highly immunocompromised patients. The demand for rapid methods and decreased turnaroun[redacted]ime has become particularly acute, underscoring the need for prompt therapeutic intervention in the infected immunocompromised patient. Finally, all of these tasks must be accomplished in a high-quality, cost-effective manner as the laboratory comes under close scrutiny by administrators, third-party payors, and external accreditation agencies.

The increased cost of many diagnostic tests, coupled with severe financial constraints, has caused many laboratories to send out their high-cost, low-volume tests to a reference laboratory. In other instances, simplification of certain tests, such as viral cultures, has allowed laboratories to bring these tests back into the laboratory. Recent developments in immunology and molecular biology have resulted in an increased number of rapid direct testin[redacted]ethods in which the quality of the specimen su[redacted]itted is of utmost importance. In each case, these changes make sample collection, handling, and transportation important considerations.

MICROBIOLOGY

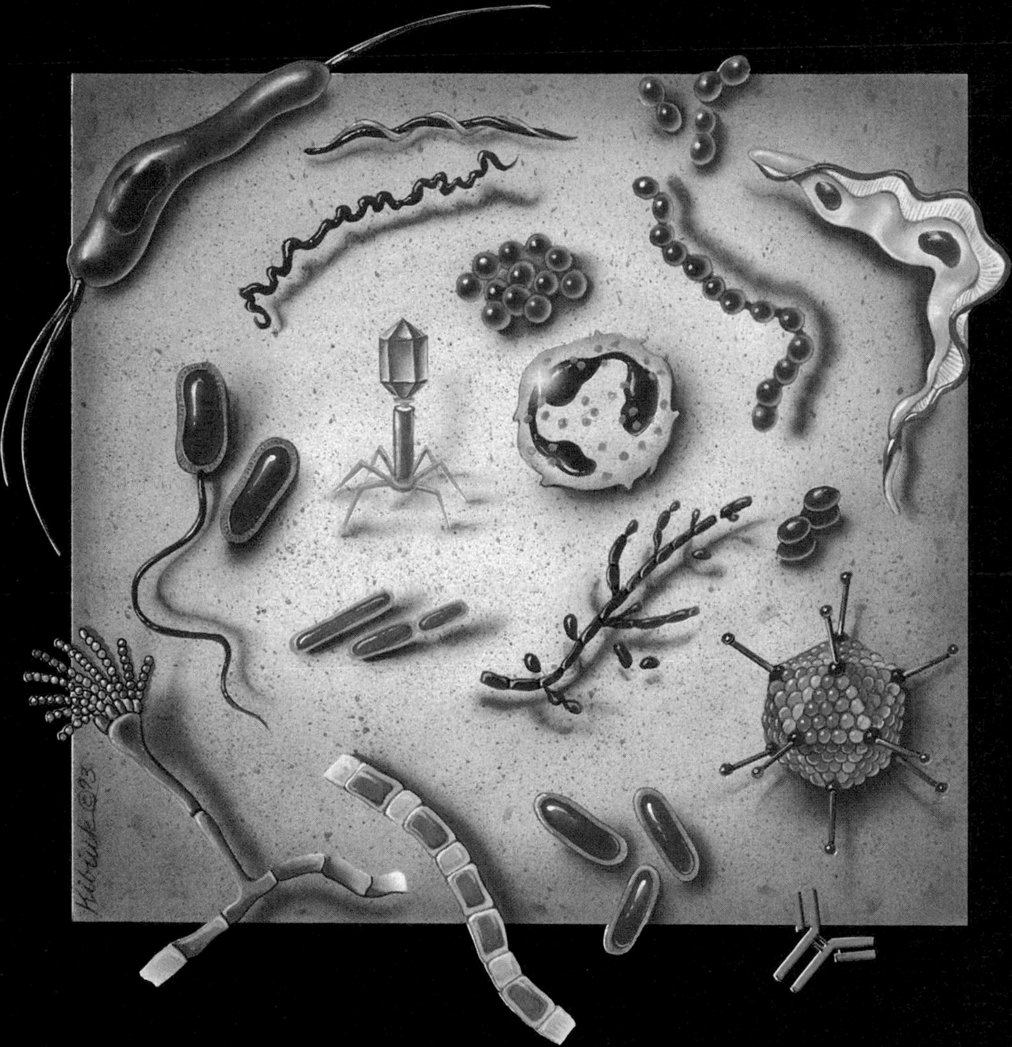

44 Bacteriology

David L. Sewell

The purpose of a clinical microbiology laboratory is (*a*) to provide accurate, timely clinically relevant information about the identity, antimicrobial susceptibility, and significance of microorganisms isolated from a given specimen and (*b*) to help prevent the spread of infection. The issue is complex because of the ubiquitious presence of microorganisms colonizing skin and mucous membranes; the transient presence of organisms in normally sterile sites; the enormous diversity of specimen type and source; the importance of the appropriate selection, collection, and transport of the specimen to the laboratory; and the need to interpret the significance of the recovery of a microorganism on the basis of the patient's history and symptoms. The "routine" workup of a specimen must be flexible enough to accommodate the special situations related to the patient's history and underlying condition. Compounding the problem is the rapidly increasing diversity of methods to perform these tasks, ranging from basic culture technique to miniaturization and automation of conventional identification schemes to monoclonal antibody technology and nucleic acid probes. These techniques must be evaluated in the target population, while remaining cost-effective. The operation of an efficient laboratory requires close communication between the laboratory and the clinician to expedite the early diagnosis and treatment of the patient.

This chapter attempts to address some of these points. The emphasis is on the type of disease produced, the diagnostic procedures used to identify the causative agent, interpretation of clinical significance, and some consideration of antimicrobial therapy. Detailed descriptions of methods are not presented, but the reader is directed to several excellent texts listed as suggested readings.

STAPHYLOCOCCI AND RELATED GENERA

Microbiology

The family Micrococcaceae consists of the four genera *Staphylococcus, Micrococcus, Planococcus,* and *Stomatococcus,* whose members are Gram-positive cocci that are catalase positive and have L-lysine as the diamino acid in the peptidoglycan layer of their cell wall. However, these genera are not closely related based on DNA base composition, nucleic acid hybridization, or 16S ribosomal RNA analysis, and they will probably be moved to other families when additional studies are completed (1). Members of the genus *Planococcus* are infrequently, if ever, isolated from clinical specimens and are not discussed further. Micrococci and *Stomatococcus mucilaginosus* are common inhabitants of the skin and mucous membranes of humans and are sometimes implicated in significant infections.

The genus *Staphylococcus* appears most closely related to the *Bacillus-Lactobacillus-Streptococcus* cluster. According to *Bergey's Manual of Systematic Bacteriology* (1), staphylococci are catalase-positive, Gram-positive cocci, 0.5 to 1.5 μm in diameter, that occur singly, in pairs, and in tetrads, and usually divide in more than one plane to form irregular grape-like clusters. Rare strains may be catalase negative. The cell wall contains peptidoglycan and teichoic acid. Most species are facultative anaerobes, capable of growing in the presence of 10% NaCl and between 18° and 40°C. *Staphylococcus saccharolyticus* grows best anaerobically. Most staphylococci grow well on noninhibitory media, but infrequently some strains may require hemin, menadione, or CO_2 for growth. Staphylococci are susceptible to lysis by lysostaphin but resistant to lysozyme.

Currently, there are 27 species of staphylococci, four of which are coagulase positive (2, 3). Until recently, only *Staphylococcus aureus* was considered pathogenic, and most of the other species were grouped under *Staphylococcus epidermidis.* Based on the work of Kloos, Schleifer, and others (4), 26 species of coagulase-negative staphylococci are now recognized (Table 44.1). *Staphylococcus lugdunensis* and *Staphylococcus schleiferi* are two new species described by Freney et al. (5) that appear to be significant opportunistic pathogens.

Spectrum of Disease

Because of the prevalence of staphylococci on skin and mucous membranes, they are implicated in a va-

Table 44.1. Pathogenic Significance of Staphylococci[a]

Species	Pathogenic Significance
S. aureus	Common
S. epidermidis	Common
S. saprophyticus	Common
S. cohnii	Uncommon
S. haemolyticus	Uncommon
S. hominis	Uncommon
S. saccharolyticus	Uncommon
S. simulans	Uncommon
S. warneri	Uncommon
S. intermedius	Rare/undetermined
S. capitis	Rare/undetermined
S. caprae[b]	Rare/undetermined
S. auricularis	Rare/undetermined
S. xylosus	Rare/undetermined
S. arlettae[b]	Rare/undetermined
S. equorum[b]	Rare/undetermined
S. gallinarum[b]	Rare/undetermined
S. kloosii[b]	Rare/undetermined
S. carnosus[b]	Rare/undetermined
S. sciuri[b]	Rare/undetermined
S. lentus[b]	Rare/undetermined
S. caseolyticus[b]	Rare/undetermined
S. hyicus[b]	Rare/undetermined
S. lugdunensis	Rare/undetermined
S. schleiferi	Rare/undetermined
S. chromogenes[b]	Rare/undetermined
S. delphini[b]	Rare/undetermined

[a]Modified from Pfaller MA, Koontz F. Coagulase-negative staphylococci: rationale for species identification. American Society For Clinical Pathologists Check Sample; 1989;32:1–7.
[b]Isolated from animals or animal products.

riety of infections ranging from skin infections to bacteremia and meningitis. *S. aureus* usually produces a pyogenic exudate or an abscess that may lead to bacteremia and metastatic foci in any organ or site in the body. Most common localized infections involve the skin and soft tissue, including pustules, impetigo, cellulitis, and postsurgical wounds. Dissemination may result in a more serious infection such as bacteremia, endocarditis, meningitis, osteomyelitis, septic arthritis, pneumonia, pericarditis, or renal abscess. Factors predisposing to *S. aureus* infections include impaired integrity of the skin barrier (burns, surgery, ulcers, minor trauma, poor personal hygiene) and underlying conditions (eczema, acne, impaired humoral and cellular immunity, presence of foreign bodies, etc. *Staphylococcus intermedius* (coagulase-positive) is associated with dog-bite infections and may be misidentified as *S. aureus* (6).

In addition to pyogenic infections, *S. aureus* is associated with toxin-induced diseases. The most common form is gastroenteritis. This self-limited disease occurs 2 to 6 hours after the consumption of food containing thermostable enterotoxins produced by *S. aureus* following contamination and improper storage of food. Symptoms consist of acute onset of nausea and vomiting, followed by diarrhea.

The other toxin-mediated diseases, toxic shock syndrome (TSS) and scalded skin syndrome (SSS), are often the result of an asymptomatic focus of infection or colonization. SSS occurs primarily in children and is caused by an exfoliative toxin. TSS results from the in situ production of toxic shock syndrome toxin-1 (TSST-1) and is manifested by high fever, rash, profound hypotension, diarrhea, and shock. Many patients are young menstruating women who use highly absorbent tampons. TSST-1 or other related enterotoxins are involved in nonmenstruation-related TSS linked to local staphylococcal infections.

Coagulase-negative staphylococcal infections are usually indolent, are associated with implanted prosthetic devices, are caused by *S. epidermidis*, and are hospital acquired. The exception is *Staphylococcus saprophyticus*, which causes approximately 15 to 30% of all the urinary tract infections in young sexually active women. Infections by coagulase-negative staphylococci are increasing as the numbers of catheters and indwelling foreign bodies placed in patients increase. Usually these infections are associated with intravenous catheters, peritoneal dialysis catheters, vascular grafts, cerebrospinal fluid shunts, prosthetic joints, and heart valves. Other infections include endocarditis, bacteremia, surgical wound infections, osteomyelitis, peritonitis, infections following ocular surgery, or genitourinary infections associated with catheterization. Over 50% of these infections are caused by *S. epidermidis*.

Epidemiology

Staphylococci are ubiquitous in the human ecosystem, inhabiting the skin, mucous membranes, and gastrointestinal (GI) tract, and are a leading cause of both community and hospital-acquired infections.

S. aureus colonizes the skin, perineal area, umbilical stumps, and sometimes the GI tract of neonates shortly after birth. The anterior nasal vestibule is the primary colonization site in adults. Approximately 20 to 40% of adults in the community are carriers, with much higher rates observed in hospital personnel, patients receiving periodic hemodialysis, and IV drug abusers. Although *S. aureus* can survive for long periods of time on inanimate objects in the environment, person-to-person transmission is the most important route of spread, especially on the hands of the hospital staff. The emergence of methicillin-resistant *S. aureus* is of particular epidemiologic and therapeutic concern throughout the world.

Staphylococcal food poisoning follows the contamination of foodstuffs by food handlers who are either infected or colonized, and the subsequent inadequate refrigeration of the contaminated food. Foods most commonly associated with this disease include meats, dairy products, and salads.

Infections by coagulase-negative staphylococci are usually hospital acquired, caused by *S. epidermidis*, and occur in patients with an indwelling foreign body. Hospital strains are usually multiple antibiotic resistant and colonize the skin and GI tract of hospitalized patients and hospital staff. Most likely, coagulase-negative staphylococci gain access to deeper tissues during the insertion of the foreign body. Although the patient's endogenous flora is the major reservoir for coagulase-negative staphylococci infections, transmission from hospital personnel to the patient has been documented. The highest incidence of nosocomial infections by coagulase-negative staphylococci are observed in the critical care areas, especially the neonatal intensive care unit.

Frequent handwashing and the use of gloves by hospital personnel are the most effective methods for minimizing the spread of staphylococci within the hospital environment.

Of the coagulase-negative staphylococci, *S. epidermidis* is the most frequently isolated from the skin (nares, head, axillae, leg, arms, toe webs) and represents 65 to 90% of all staphylococci recovered (7). *Staphylococcus hominis* is the next most frequently isolated species. Other coagulase-negative staphylococcal species are only occasionally isolated from skin (*Staphylococcus simulans, Staphylococcus xylosus, Staphylococcus cohnii, Staphylococcus warneri, Staphylococcus saccharolyticus, Staphylococcus haemolyticus*) or occupy special niches on the skin (*Staphylococcus capitis*—head; *Staphylococcus auricularis*—ear; *Staphylococcus saprophyticus*—genitourinary skin). The prevalence of *S. lugdunensis* and *S. intermedius* have not yet been determined.

It is often difficult to differentiate infection from colonization and to document transmission and spread of specific strains within the hospital environment. Historically, phage typing, biotyping, or antibiograms were used for identifying an outbreak strain with a unique pattern. These techniques lack sensitivity and specificity for following transmission of coagulase-negative staphylococci. More recently, techniques involving plasmid analysis were found to be useful for studying current outbreaks of coagulase-negative staphylococcal infections but less useful for *S. aureus*, which carries relatively few plasmids. Endonuclease restriction analysis of both plasmid and chromosomal DNA, DNA hybridizatioin, and protein analysis are promising techniques for better understanding the epidemiology of staphylococci.

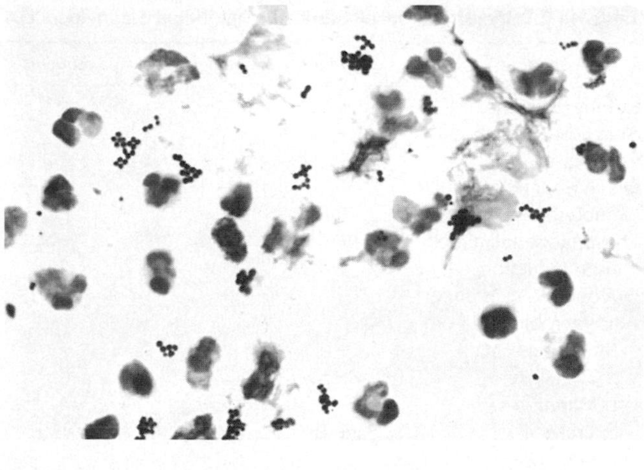

Figure 44.1. Gram stain of material containing polymorphonuclear neutrophils and *S. aureus*.

Diagnostic Procedures

MICROSCOPY

Gram-stained smears of clinical specimens provide rapid and presumptive evidence of staphylococal infection. Staphylococci appear as Gram-positive cocci (0.5 to 1.5 μm in diameter) and occur singly or in pairs or small clusters (Fig. 44.1). These features are not always observed in clinical specimens in which staphylococci have been ingested by phagocytes, have been exposed to cell wall–active antimicrobial agents, or are in the stationary phase of growth. In these situations the bacteria may appear Gram-negative. The Gram stain morphology cannot definitively differentiate staphylococci from other Gram-positive cocci seen in clinical specimens.

CULTURE TECHNIQUES

Most staphylococci grow well on nonselective agar and broth media containing peptone (e.g., sheep blood agar, brain-heart infusion, thioglycollate). On sheep blood agar, growth occurs within 18 to 24 hours at 35° to 37 °C. Colonies are 1 to 3 mm in diameter, usually opaque, smooth, and circular, and have a butyrous consistency. Colonies of *S. aureus* may be pigmented and exhibit β-hemolysis on sheep blood agar, but these observations may also occur with some other staphylococcal species. Colonies of *S. epidermidis* are usually gray-white and nonhemolytic. Nutritionally variant staphylococci require supplementation of the medium with hemin, menadione, thiamine, or pantothenate for growth.

Specimens likely to be contaminated with other bacteria are inoculated onto a selective medium such as colistin-nalidixic acid (CNA) agar, phenylethyl alcohol (PEA) agar, mannitol-salt agar (MSA),

Table 44.2. Identification of Clinically Significant *Staphylococcus* Species[a]

Character	*S. aureus*	*S. epidermidis*	*S. hominis*	*S. haemolyticus*	*S. warneri*	*S. saprophyticus*	*S. simulans*	*S. cohnii*
Colony pigment	+[b]	−	d	d	d	d	−	−
Anaerobic growth	+	+	−	(+)	+	(+)	+	d
Coagulase	+	−	−	−	−	−	−	−
Deoxyribonuclease	+	−	−	−	−	−	±	−
Hemolysis	+	−	−	(+)	(d)	−	(d)	(d)
Phosphatase (alkaline)	+	d	−	−	−	−	(d)	−
Nitrate reduction	+	+	d	d	−	−	+	−
Novobiocin resistance	−	−	−	−	−	+	−	+
Acid (aerobically) from								
Maltose	+	+	+	+	(+)	+	−	(d)
D-Trehalose	+	−	d	+	+	+	d	+
D-Mannitol	+	−	−	d	d	d	+	d
Sucrose	+	+	(+)	+	+	+	+	−
D-Mannose	+	(+)	−	−	−	−	d	(d)

[a]Modified from Jorgensen JH, Kloos WE. Staphylococcal infections. In: Wentworth BB, ed. Diagnostic procedures for bacterial infections. 7th ed. Washington, DC: American Public Health Association, 1987:481.

[b]+, 90% or more strains positive; −, 90% or more strains negative; d, 11–89% of strains positive; ±, 90% or more strains weak positive; ( ), delayed reaction requiring 48 to 72 hr.

Schleifer-Kramer agar, or tellurite-glycine agar. These media inhibit the growth of Gram-negative organisms. On MSA, *S. aureus*, *S. simulans*, and *S. saprophyticus* are differentiated from other species of coagulase-negative staphylococci by their ability to produce acid from mannitol. Selective media should be incubated at least 48 hours for optimal growth.

IDENTIFICATION METHODS

The initial identification of a suspected colony begins with colonial morphology, Gram-stain morphology, and a spot-catalase test to eliminate organisms such as streptococci and corynebacteria. When it is clinically relevant to differentiate between staphylococci and micrococci, seven tests can be used (2). Three of these tests are relatively simple and are recommended for use in the clinical laboratory. They include susceptibility to bacitracin (micrococci), susceptibility to lysostaphin (staphylococci), and the modified oxidase test (negative for most staphylococci). Some clinically significant *Staphylococcus* species are identified by the colony morphology, growth characteristics, enzyme activities, and other biochemical characteristics listed in Table 44.2. In addition to these conventional methods, a number of more rapid commercial identification systems provide nearly all clinical laboratories with the capability of identifying the staphylococci with an accuracy of 70 to 95% (2).

S. aureus, *S. epidermidis*, and *S. saprophyticus* can also be identified with a high degree of accuracy on the basis of colony morphology; coagulase and phosphatase activities; acid production from D-mannitol, D-trehalose, maltose, sucrose, and D-xylose; and novobiocin resistance. *S. aureus* is identified in most cases by the coagulase test. Although *S. intermedius* and *S. hyicus* are also coagulase positive, they are rarely isolated from humans. The standard tube test detects free staphylocoagulase and is the more definitive test, while the slide coagulase test detects bound coagulase (clumping factor). These two tests have been replaced in large part by the commercially available particle agglutination tests that measure bound coagulase and protein A. These systems are quite accurate but may miss some methicillin-resistant *S. aureus* (8).

Stevens and Jones (9) reported that by using a single plate containing trehalose, mannitol, and phenolphthalein, and by testing for novobiocin resistance, they could accurately differentiate *S. epidermidis* and *S. saprophyticus* from other strains of coagulase-negative staphylococci.

DIRECT ANTIGEN OR NUCLEIC ACID DETECTION

Currently, there is no commercially available system for the direct detection of staphylococci in clinical specimens. However, the direct detection of staphylococcal enterotoxins in cultures or foods and the detection of TSST-1 in culture can be performed by using reverse passive latex agglutination or enzyme immununoassay diagnostic kits (10).

SEROLOGIC PROCEDURES

The serologic response to various extracellular products and cell wall components of *S. aureus* has been measured in an attempt to diagnose some forms of staphylococcal disease. The two tests with the most promise are the measurement of antibodies against TSST-1 and teichoic acid (11).

Antibodies to TSST-1, measured by immunodiffusion (ID), radioimmunoassay (RIA), and enzyme immunoassay (EIA), help confirm the diagnosis of TSS.

The patient also has TSS if no antibodies are detected but the strain produces TSST-1, because convalescent antibodies are detected in only about 40% of TSS patients.

Measurement of antibodies to teichoic acid is recommended as an aid in the diagnosis of patients with *S. aureus* endocarditis or bacteremia complicated by metastatic foci. However, inconsistencies in the accuracy of the test, variations in test methodology, poor availability of test reagents, and lack of well-controlled prospective clinical studies have created controversy over the usefulness of this test.

INTERPRETATION OF RESULTS

Staphylococci are some of the most frequently isolated bacteria in the clinical microbiology laboratory because of their ubiquitous presence on the skin and mucous membranes of humans. The isolation of *S. aureus* from an infected site should be considered clinically relevant until proven otherwise.

The isolation of coagulase-negative staphylococci from normally sterile body sites, intravenous catheters, peritoneal dialysates, tissue, and other clinical specimens poses an interpretive challenge to laboratorians and clinicians. Historically, coagulase-negative staphylococci have been dismissed as clinically insignificant contaminants. However, their importance as nosocomial pathogens (in particular *S. epidermidis*) and as a cause of urinary tract infections is now clearly recognized. The clinical relevance of a specific isolate is based on clinical, microbiological, and epidemiologic criteria such as the immune status and presence of a foreign body in the patient, the species of *Staphylococcus* isolated, and the number of specimens from which the identical strain is isolated. Martin et al. (12) recently reported that even a single blood culture containing coagulase-negative staphylococci is likely to be clinically significant in hospitalized patients and suggested that all blood culture isolates be considered significant until proven otherwise.

Therapeutic Considerations

Accurate antimicrobial susceptibility testing must be performed on all clinically significant isolates of staphylococci because of their variable resistance to commonly used antimicrobial agents. Approximately 80 to 90% of strains of *S. aureus* are resistant to penicillin, and 5 to 20% of isolates exhibit resistance to erythromycin, lincomycin, and clindamycin. Gentamicin resistance is also increasing in frequency. Resistance to methicillin and other semisynthetic penicillins is widespread throughout the world. In addition, methicillin-resistant *S. aureus* (MRSA) usually exhibits cross-resistance to other β-lactam antibiotics as well as resistance to macrolides, clindamycin, and tetracycline. Initially, the quinolones demonstrated good activity against MRSA, but increasing resistance is being reported. Most strains are susceptible to rifampin, but this drug cannot be used alone because of the high mutation rate to resistance. Currently, the drug of choice for the empiric treatment of hospital-acquired *S. aureus* infection in institutions with a high prevalence of MRSA is vancomycin until susceptibility to other β-lactam antibiotics can be determined.

Coagulase-negative staphylococci isolated from hospitalized patients are usually resistant to multiple antimicrobial agents, with 60 to 80% of the strains resistant to methicillin. Coagulase-negative staphylococci resistant to methicillin should be considered cross-resistant to all β-lactam antibiotics, regardless of the in vitro susceptibility. Over 50% of coagulase-negative staphylococci exhibit resistance to erythromycin, clindamycin, tetracycline, and chloramphenicol. Resistance to trimethoprim and gentamicin is also increasing. Multiple strains of *S. haemolyticus* have demonstrated resistance to vancomycin. Because of the high incidence of resistance to the penicillinase-resistant penicillins, vancomycin has become the drug of choice for hospital-acquired infections caused by coagulase-negative staphylococci.

Summary and Conclusions

S. aureus, *S. epidermidis*, and *S. saprophyticus* are associated with the majority of staphylococcal infections. *S. aureus* causes infections of skin, soft tissue, bloodstream, and internal organs; staphylococcal food poisoning; and toxic shock syndrome. *S. epidermidis* causes nosocomial infections, especially in patients with indwelling foreign bodies. *S. saprophyticus* causes urinary tract infections in young women.

Staphylococci are usually transmitted person to person with the primary reservoir being the skin and mucous membranes of humans and animals. Most staphylococci are easily isolated on routine media and are identified by morphology, conventional biochemical and metabolic characteristics, and commercial identification kits. Because of the variability of resistance to antimicrobial agents (especially the penicillinase-resistant penicillins), susceptibility testing must be performed.

STREPTOCOCCI, ENTEROCOCCI, AND RELATED GENERA

Microbiology

Historically, the taxonomy of the streptococci and related genera (*Enterococcus*, *Leuconostoc*, *Pediococcus*, *Aerococcus*, *Lactococcus*, and *Gemella*) has been confusing. With the recent application of techniques for the deterimination of genetic relatedness, the taxonomic picture is improving but will continue to change in the coming years.

Leuconostoc and *Pediococcus* (and *Lactobacillus*) have been reported to be resistant to vancomycin and may be confused with viridans streptococci (13). These organisms are opportunisitic pathogens and can be preliminarily differentiated from streptococci based on the morphology of cells grown in broth (*Leuconostoc* are coccobacilli and *Pediococcus* are cocci in pairs and tetrads); gas produced from glucose (positive for *Leuconostoc* and negative for streptococci and *Pediococcus*); and pyrrolidonylarylamidase activity (negative for *Leuconostoc* and *Pediococcus*).

Aerococcus and *Gemella* both resemble viridans streptococci on blood agar. Aerococci tend to form tetrads, while *Gemella* occurs as pairs with adjacent sides flattened (*Gemella haemolysans*) or as pairs and chains (*Gemella morbillorum*; previously *Streptococcus morbillum*). Aerococci are rarely isolated from human disease.

The medically important streptococci are catalase-negative, Gram-positive cocci, are spherical to ovoid (less than 2 μm in diameter), and tend to form pairs or chains. Some species may appear as short rods on initial isolation. Most species are facultative anaerobes (some are obligate anaerobes), exhibit a fermentative metabolism, and have complex but variable nutritional requirements. Growth on solid agar is enhanced by blood, serum, or glucose.

The streptococci are broadly classified according to three different schemes, each of which is partly used in the laboratory. The preliminary classification of streptococci is based on their hemolytic action on blood agar, and differentiates β-hemolytic, α-hemolytic, and nonhemolytic (γ-hemolytic) groups. Further differentiation (especially of the β-hemolytic streptococci) is achieved by serologic classification based on the presence of group-specific antigens and currently performed by commercial particle agglutination kits. With the exception of the group D streptococci, the majority of the α-hemolytic (viridans streptococci) and nonhemolytic species are classified by physiological tests. The interrelationship of these three schemes is depicted in Table 44.3. Historically, the group D streptococci were divided into enterococcal and nonenterococcal strains based on tolerance to salt. Currently, the enterococci are placed in the genus *Enterococcus*, which is composed of 12 species, (14). *Enterococcus faecalis*, *Enterococcus raffinosus*, *Enterococcus avium*, and *Enterococcus gallinarum* are isolated most often from human sources. The nonenterococcal group D isolates, *S. bovis* and *S. equinus*, remain as streptococci.

In addition, a group of streptococci referred to as *Streptococcus milleri* by European and British authors and three separate species (*Streptococcus intermedius*, *Streptococcus constellatus*, and *Streptococcus anginosus*) by American authors are closely related. This group also includes group F and minute hemolytic strains. Coykendall et al. (15) has proposed that they be named *Streptococcus anginosus*. Similarly, the *Streptococcus mutans* group consists of seven species, *Streptococcus mutans*, *Streptococcus rattus*, *Streptococcus cricetus*, *Streptococcus sobrinus*, *Streptococcus ferus*, *Streptococcus macacae*, and *Streptococcus downei* (16). The nutritionally variant streptococci were considered forms of *Streptococcus mitis* or *Streptococcus sangius* but appear to be genetically unrelated and form two species (16).

Spectrum of Disease

Streptococci are part of the normal flora that cause a wide variety of infections, including upper respiratory infections, skin and soft tissue infections, bacteremia, meningitis, urinary tract infections, deep tissue infections, endocarditis, arthritis, and osteomyelitis, as well as nonsuppurative sequelae observed following infection by *Streptococcus pyogenes* (Table 44.3).

Group A streptococcus (*S. pyogenes*) is an important human pathogen and a major cause of upper respiratory and skin infections. Suppurative complications of streptococcal pharyngitis include parapharyngeal space abscesses, otitis media, sinusitus, mastoiditis, and meningitis. Bacteremia may lead to infections in the joints, bones, or other foci. Nonsuppurative sequellae following pharyngitis include acute rheumatic fever (ARF) and acute glomerulonephritis (AGN). Skin infections precede the development of AGN but not ARF. Complications are seen primarily in untreated patients and appear to be increasing in recent years.

Group B streptococcus (*S. agalactiae*) is a major cause of infections in neonates and postpartum women, including neonatal sepsis and meningitis. puerperal sepsis, and chorioamnionitis. The most common adult infections occur in postpartum women and are associated with the genital tract, but a variety of other infections also occur. Age, diabetes mellitus, malignancy, and liver disease are important risk factors.

Group C streptococcus is not a frequent human pathogen but is associated with upper respiratory, skin, and soft tissue infections. Infections caused by group G streptococcus include pharyngitis, otitis media, bacteremia, cellulitis, pneumonia, meningitis, neonatal sepsis, puerperal sepsis, endocarditis, and arthritis.

Table 44.3. Classification of Streptococci Most Frequently Causing Human Infections

Species	Group Antigen	Hemolysis	Sherman Classification	Clinical Features
S. pyogenes	A	β, γ	Pyogenic	Pharyngitis, tonsillitis, otitis media, mastoiditis, sinusitis, scarlet fever, erysipilus, cellulitis, impetigo, pneumonia, endometritus, bacteremia. Nonsuppurative sequelae: acute rheumatic fever, acute glomerulonephritis
S. agalactiae	B	β, γ	Pyogenic	Neonatal sepsis and meningitis, chorioamnionitis, puerperal sepsis, bacteremia, skin and soft tissue infection, urinary tract infection
S. equi (and *zooepidemicus*) *S. dysgalactiae* *S. equisimilis*	C	β	Pyogenic	Upper respiratory, skin and soft tissue infections
S. canis (large colony)	G	β	Pyogenic	Upper respiratory, skin and soft tissue infections, bacteremia, deep tissue infection
E. faecalis (other enterococci)	D	α, β, γ	Enterococci	Endocarditis, urinary tract infection, bacteremia, intra-abdominal abscess, soft tissue infection
S. bovis	D	γ	Nonenterococci	Endocarditis, bacteremia
S. pneumoniae	—	α	—	Pneumonia, bacteremia, meningitis, otitis media, sinusitis
S. anginosus/milleri (*S. intermedius*, *S. constellatus*)	F,A,C,G, None	α, β, γ	Pyogenic viridans	Endocarditis, bacteremia, deep tissue infection
S. mitis, *S. mutans* *S. salivarius* *S. morbillorum*	None or A-O	α, γ	Viridans	Endocarditis (*S. mutans* major cause of caries)
Nutritionally variant *streptococci*	None	α	Viridans	Endocarditis
Other viridans *streptococci*	None	α	Viridans	Rare

Of the enterococci, *E. faecalis* causes disease more frequently than the other species and is implicated in the following infections: endocarditis, intra-abdominal infections, soft tissue infections, urinary tract infections, and bacteremia. It is rarely associated with meningitis or pneumonia.

The group D Streptococcus (nonenterococcal) *S. bovis* causes primarily endocarditis and bacteremia, which is often associated with colonic lesions or instrumentation of the gastrointestinal tract.

Streptococcus pneumoniae is a major respiratory pathogen in adults, especially the elderly or persons with asplenia, sickle cell disease, or immune disorders. It is the most frequent cause of bacterial pneumonia and may cause mastoiditis, sinusitis, otitis media, meningitis, arthritis, and peritonitis.

S. anginosus/milleri is associated with abscesses in various areas of the body (e.g.. skin, brain, liver, abdomen, cervicofacial area, and lung).

The viridans streptococci (including the nutritionally variant streptococci) cause a variety of infections but account for 30 to 50% of all cases of endocarditis in the United States. Some species of viridans streptococci, especially *S. mutans*, cause dental caries.

Epidemiology

The epidemiology of the streptococci is as diverse as the number of species in this group. Group A streptococcal pharyngitis is a common infection of young school-age children, with a peak incidence occurring during the winter and spring. Transmission is ordinarily by person-to-person contact and via nasal or salivary droplets. Outbreaks due to food or water contamination are also documented. Crowding, such as occurs in schools and military barracks, favors transmission. Asymptomatic carriage of group A streptococci occurs in the throats of up to 20% of school-age children. The epidemiology of ARF parallels that of streptococcal pharyngitis.

Streptococcal pyoderma occurs primarily as an endemic disease in children but can occur in epidemics. Crowding, a tropical or subtropical climate, and poor living conditions favor the spread of skin streptococci. AGN may occur following streptococcal pharyngitis or pyoderma.

Group B streptococci colonize the genital and/or lower gastrointestinal tract of pregnant women at a rate ranging from 5 to 40%. Colonization of the newborn occurs either in utero or more commonly during delivery. Nosocomial transmission also occurs, especially in the setting of heavy maternal colonization and crowded nursery conditions.

Enterococci and group D streptococci are found as normal flora in the gastrointestinal tract of humans. Nearly all adults harbor *E. faecalis*. *S. bovis* occurs in 5 to 10% of normal adults but is found more frequently in patients with colon cancer.

S. pneumoniae is part of the normal oropharyngeal flora in 5 to 70% of adults. Transmission is person to

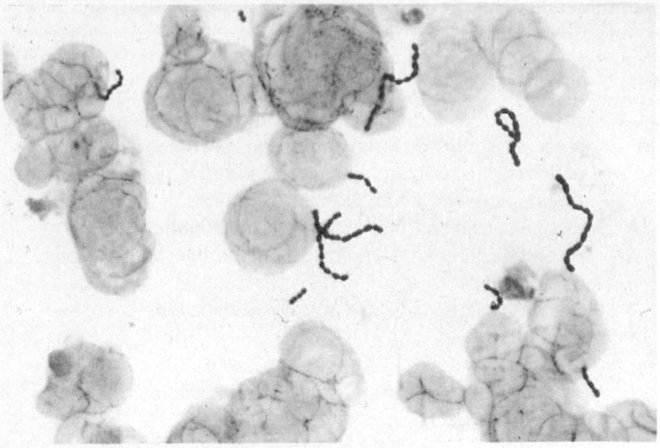

Figure 44.2. Gram stain of blood culture broth positive for streptococci.

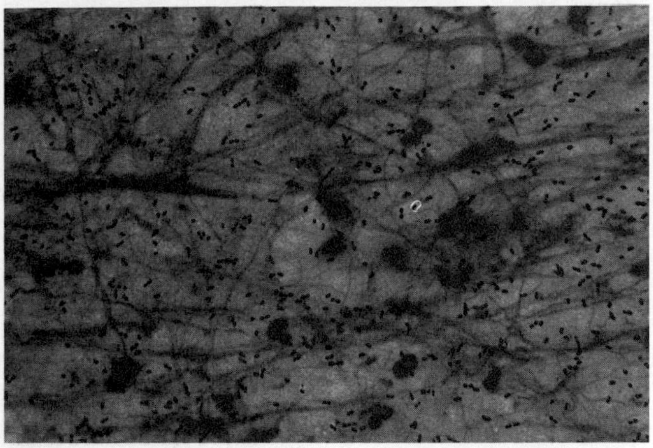

Figure 44.3. Gram stain of *S. pneumoniae* in sputum.

person and is increased by crowding such as occurs in military barracks. Of the 84 capsular serotypes, the majority of infections are caused by the lower-number serotypes.

The viridans streptococci constitute 30 to 60% of the oral flora, with various species residing in different ecological niches of the oropharynx. They also colonize the mucous membranes of the urogenital and gastrointestinal tracts.

Diagnostic Procedures

MICROSCOPY

Streptococci and enterococci are typically ovoid or lancet-shaped, but may elongate to resemble short rods. Most often they occur in pairs or chains when grown in thioglycollate broth (Fig. 44.2). *S. pneumoniae* appears with the adjacent cell wall flattened, lancet shaped, and encapsulated, and occurs predominantly in pairs but may form short chains (Fig. 44.3). It may occasionally appear to be Gram-negative if observed in phagocytes, if the patient is receiving antimicrobial agents, or if the culture is old.

CULTURE TECHNIQUES

Streptococci and enterococci grow well on rich, nonselective broths and agars such as trypticase soy, heart infusion, or Todd-Hewitt, which may be supplemented with blood. Selective agars such as phenylethyl agar (PEA) or colistin-nalidixic acid (CNA) can be used with specimens containing Gram-negative organisms. Trimethoprim-sulfamethoxazol is added to sheep blood agar to improve the recovery of group A streptococci from throat cultures. Nutritionally variant streptococci are recovered by satelliting around a *Staphylococcus* streak, by adding pyridoxal to the growth medium, or by placing a disk containing pyridoxal on the agar plate.

Streptococci and enterococci are facultative anaerobes, often requiring 5 to 10% CO_2 (especially *S. pneumoniae*) for optimum growth. Although it is somewhat controversial, the recovery of group A streptococci appears to be enhanced by anaerobic incubation. All cultures should be incubated at 35° to 37°C.

IDENTIFICATION METHODS

The initial characterization of streptococci and enterococci is based on catalase reaction, hemolysis, colony morphology, and source of the specimen. Streptococci are catalase-negative, but weak reactions may occur, especially with enterococci. The type of hemolytic reaction is usually observed with surface colonies, but the most accurate method uses subsurface colonies. Group A streptococci produce large zones of β-hemolysis with small colonies; group B streptococci produce large colonies with a small zone of β–hemolysis; enterococci usually have large gray colonies with no hemolysis (may be α- or rarely β-hemolytic), and the viridans streptococci are small, raised colonies with α or no hemolysis. *S. pneumoniae* is α-hemolytic with dome-shape colonies that may have a depressed center or appear mucoid.

After the hemolytic reaction has been determined, clinically significant streptococci are presumptively identified by the tests listed in Table 44.4. Group A streptococci are inhibited by bacitracin and hydrolyse L-pyrrolidonyl-β-naphthylamide (PYR). Group B streptococci are hippurate and CAMP positive and PYR negative. Other β-hemolytic streptococci are negative for these tests but are susceptible to trimethoprim-sulfamethoxazole. The β-hemolytic streptococci are definitively identified by detection of the group-specific cell wall carbohydrate antigen by immunofluorescent antibody staining or by any of a

Table 44.4. Presumptive Identification of Streptococci and Enterococci[a]

Category	Hemolysis	*Susceptibility to* Bacitracin	*Susceptibility to* SXT[b]	*Hydrolysis of* Hippucate	*Hydrolysis of* PYR[b]	CAMP	Bile Esculin	Growth In 6.5% NaCl	Optochin and Bile[c]
Group A	β	+	−	−	+	−	−	−	−
Group B	β	−[d]	−	+	−	+	−	+[d]	−
β-hemolytic streptococci (not group A, B, or D)	β	−[d]	+	−	−	−	−	−	−
Group D, enterococcus	α, β, none	−	−	−[d]	+	−	+	+	−
Group D, nonenterococcus	α, none	−	+[d]	−	−	−	+	−	−
Viridans group	α, none	−[d]	+	−[d]	−	−	−[d]	−	−
Pneumococcus	α	±	?	−	−	−	−	−	+

[a]From Howard BJ, Klass J II, Rubin SJ, Weissfeld AS, Tilton RC, eds. Clinical and pathogenic microbiology. St. Louis: CV Mosby, 1987:250.
[b]Symbols: SXT, trimethoprim-sulfamethoxazole; PYR, L-pyrrolidonyl-β-naphthylamide; +, positive reaction or susceptible; −, negative reaction or resistant.
[c]Optochin susceptibility and bile solubility.
[d]Exceptions occasionally occur.

number of commercially available particle agglutination kits.

α-Hemolytic colonies are tested for bile solubility or susceptibility to optochin. *S. pneumoniae* is positive for both tests; other streptococci are negative. The slide bile solubility test is useful for the rapid presumptive identification of *S. pneumoniae* from blood cultures (17). Enterococci and group D streptococci are presumptively identified by hydrolysis of esculin in the presence of bile, growth in 6.5% NaCl, and hydrolysis of PYR. Further identification of enterococci, group D streptococci, and the viridans streptococci can be accomplished by use of the tests listed in Table 44.5, other identification schemes (18), or by using commercial kits. Strains belonging to the *S. anginosus/milleri* group can be presumptively identified by positive reactions for Voges-Proskauer and arginine hydrolysis; esculin hydrolysis; and lack of growth in 6.5% NaCl (19).

DIRECT ANTIGEN OR NUCLEIC ACID DETECTION

A number of commercial particle agglutination kits are available for the direct detection of streptococcal cellular or capsular antigens in body fluids (e.g., CSF, urine, serum) or throat swabs. A wide range of factors affect the sensitivity and specificity of the test, including the type of specimen and the particular kit.

The identification of group A streptococcal antigen from throat swabs is a rapid method to aid in the diagnosis of streptococcal pharyngitis. A positive test is an excellent predictor of infection, but the sensitivity is usually lower than 90%, especially when small numbers of organisms are present. A negative test should be followed with a culture.

Group B streptococcal antigen is detected in CSF, concentrated urine, or urogenital swabs by use of agglutination kits, with a sensitivity approaching 90% and a specificity of greater than 95%.

Detection of pneumococcal antigen in CSF, concentrated urine, sputum, or serum has been attempted by use of particle agglutination kits. The method is most applicable to CSF specimens, in which the sensitivity ranges from 60 to 90%. Lower sensitivity and specificity are observed with urine and serum specimens. The Neufeld capsular swelling reaction (or quellung reaction) is another method to directly detect pneumococci in sputum or CSF. Antiserum is not widely available but can be obtained from the Statens Seruminstitut, Copenhagen, Denmark.

SEROLOGIC PROCEDURES

The detection of antibodies to streptococcal cell wall antigen or extracellular products aids in the diagnosis of recent group A streptococcal infection. These tests are used most frequently for the diagnosis of ARF or AGN in the absence of a recently documented infection. The most helpful tests are antistreptolysin O (ASO), antihyaluronidase (AH), and antideoxyribonuclease B (ADN-B). The lack of significant titers to these three antigens makes the diagnosis of ARF very doubtful. In cases of AGN, ASO titers are usually very low. A slide hemagglutination kit for the detection of five antibodies is best employed as a screening test. Particle agglutination tests for the detection of ASO antibodies are also available.

INTERPRETATION OF RESULTS

The clinical relevance of the isolation of any of the streptococcal species depends on the type of specimen from which the organism was recovered and a knowledge of the spectrum of infections caused by the organism. In addition, one must consider the clinical signs and symptoms of the patient because all of the streptococci are either normal human flora or can be carried asymptomatically. In general, the iso-

Table 44.5. Differentiation of Group D Streptococci, *Enterococcus* Spp., Viridans Streptococci, and Acrococci Found in Human Infections[a]

Test	*E. faecalis*	*E. faeclum*	*E. avium*	*E. durans*	*Aerococci*	*S. bovis*	*S. mutans*	*S. uberis*	*S. intermedius*	*S. bovis* (var.)	*S. constellatus*	*S. equinus*	*S. sanguis* I	*S. salivarius*	*S. mins*	*S. sanguis* II	*S. morbillorum*	*S. acidominimus*
Hemolysis																		
α	+[c]	+	+	+	+	−[b]	−[b]	+	−[b]	−[b]	+	+	+	−[b]	+	+	−[b]	+
β	+	−	−	+	−	−	+	−	−	−	−	−	−	−	−	−	−	−
None	+	+	+	+	−[b]	+	+	+	+	+	−[b]	−	−[b]	+	−[b]	−[b]	+	−[b]
Physiological																		
Bile esculin	+	+	+	+	v	+	−[b]	−	−[b]	+	−[b]	+	−[b]	−[b]	−	−	−	−
Growth in 6.5% NaCl	+	+	+	+	+	−	−	−[b]	−	−	−	−	−	−	−	−	−	−
Growth at 10°C	+	+	−	+	−	−	−	−	−	−	−	−	−	−	−	−	−	−
Pyruvate	+	−	+	−	−	−	−	−	−	−	−	−	−[b]	−	−	−	−	−
Arginine	+[b]	+	−	+	−	−	−[b]	−	+[b]	−	+[b]	−	+	−	−	−[b]	−	−
Esculin	+	+	+	+	v	+	+[b]	+	+	+	+[b]	+	+[b]	+[b]	−	−	−	−
Starch	−	−	−	−	−	+	−	−	−[b]	−[b]	−	−	+[b]	−[b]	−	−[b]	−	−
Hippurate	v	v	−	v	+[b]	−	−	+[b]	−	−	−	−	−	−	−	−	−	+[b]
Sucrose	+[b]	+	+	−[b]	+	+	+	+	+	+	+	+	+	+	+	+	+	+
Lactose	+[b]	+	+	+	+[b]	+	+	+	+	+	−	−	+	+[b]	+	+	−	−
Mannitol	+	+	+	−	v	+	+	+	−	−	−	−	−	−	−	−	−	−
Sorbitol	+[b]	−	+	−	−	−	+	+	−	−	−	−	−[b]	−	−	−	−	−
Arabinose	−[b]	+[b]	+	−	−	−	−	−[b]	−	−	−	−[b]	−	−	−	−	−	−
Sorbose	−	−	+	−	−	−	−	−	−	−	−	−	−	−	−	−	−	−
Insulin	−	−[b]	+[b]	−	−[b]	+[b]	+[b]	+[b]	−	−	−	−	+	+	−	−	−	−
Raffinose	−[b]	+[b]	+	−[b]	v	+[b]	+[b]	+[b]	v	v	−[b]	−[b]	−[b]	+[b]	−	+	−	−
Glucan	N	N	N	N	N	L	D	N	N[b]	N[b]	N	N	D[b]	L[b]	N	D[b]	N	N

[a]From Howard BJ, Klass J II, Rubin SJ, Weissfeld AS, Tilton RC, eds. Clinical and pathogenic microbiology. St. Louis: CV Mosby, 1987;252.
[b]Occasional exceptions occur.
[c]Symbols: +, Positive reactions; −, negative reactions; v, variable reactions; N, no glucans; L, levans; D, dextran.

lation of β-hemolytic streptococci should be interpreted as clinically relevant unless shown otherwise.

Tests for the direct detection of antigens in clinical specimens are particularly helpful when positive but are generally not useful for ruling out the presence of the pathogen when negative. When used for the detection of antigen in fluids other than CSF, there may be nonspecific cross-reactions.

Therapeutic Considerations

The β-hemolytic streptococci remain uniformly susceptible to penicillin and vancomycin and thus do not require routine susceptibility testing. If erythromycin is considered, the isolate should be tested for susceptibility to the drug. The distinction between enterococci and nonenterococcal group D streptococci (*S. bovis*) is important because of differences in susceptibility to antimicrobial agents. Nearly all strains of *S. bovis* are susceptible to penicillin or ampicillin. The enterococcal isolates exhibit resistance or relative resistance to the penicillins, cephalosporins, clindamycin, and aminoglycosides. In addition, the most active agents such as the penicillins and vancomycin are not bactericidal, requiring the use of combination therapy (penicillin plus aminoglycoside) for life-threatening infections. High-level resistance to aminoglycosides is increasing. More disturbing is that some enterococcal strains now exhibit resistance to vancomycin (20).

Although most strains of *S. pneumoniae* are susceptible to penicillin, relatively or highly resistant strains have been detected as well as strains resistant to multiple antibiotics. Because of the increasing resistance, susceptibility tests shouid be performed on all isolates from serious infections or in areas where resistance rates are high.

Most viridans streptococci remain susceptible to penicillin, although strains somewhat resistant or tolerant to penicillin have been reported.

Summary and Conclusions

The streptococci and related genera represent a heterogeneous collection of medically important bacteria that cause a wide spectrum of infections (e.g., pharyngitis, skin and soft tissue infections, deep tissue infections, meningitis, and urinary tract infections). The application of nucleic acid techniques will improve the taxonomy of the streptococci. Most strains can be isolated readily from clinical specimens with the use of enriched laboratory media and can be identified with a combination of serologic, physiological, and biochemical tests. Commercial identification systems are also available as are kits for the direct detection of streptococcal antigen in clinical specimens. Although many of the streptococci remain susceptible to penicillin, increasing resistance to penicillins, cephalosporins, aminoglycosides, and in the case of entercocci, to vancomycin is being observed.

NEISSERIA AND *BRANHAMELLA* (*MORAXELLA*)

Microbiology

The family Neisseriaceae contains four genera, *Neisseria*, *Moraxella*, *Acinetobacter*, and *Kingella*. The latter three genera will be discussed later. In addition to the two commonly recognized pathogens *Neisseriaceae gonorrhoeae* and *Neisseriaceae meningitidis*, the genus *Neisseriaceae* contains a number of usually nonpathogenic species. These include *Neisseria lactamica*, *Neisseria sicca*, *Neisseria subflava*, *Neisseria mucosa*, *Neisseria polysaccharea*, *Neisseria flavescens*, *Neisseria cinerea*, *Neisseria elongata*, *Neisseria canis*, and *Neisseria denitrificans*. *N. canis* is found in the upper respiratory tract of cats and *N. denitrificans* in guinea pigs. *Neisseria kochii* is most likely a subspecies of *N. gonorrhoeae* (21).

The genus *Branhamella* contains four species, of which only *Branhamella catarrhalis* is medically important. Since *Branhamella* has been designated as a subgenus within *Moraxella*, this species is referred to as *Moraxella (Branhamella) catarrhalis* (22). Because of common usage, similar morphology to *Neisseria*, and common identification systems, the terminology *B. catarrhalis* will be used.

Neisseria and *Branhamella* species are Gram-negative, oxidase- and catalase-positive cocci that appear most often in pairs with the adjacent sides flattened (kidney bean shape). *N. elongata* exists as a small coccobacillus and is catalase-negative. These bacteria are aerobic and grow best on enriched media containing blood or serum incubated in a humid atmosphere (5 to 7% CO_2 at 35° to 37°C.

Spectrum of Disease

The clinical spectrum of gonococcal infections involves primarily the mucous membranes of the lower genitourinary tract and less frequently those of the rectum, oropharynx, and conjunctiva. A small proportion of men may be asymptomatic, while up to 80% of women may be asymptomatic or minimally symptomatic.

Gonorrhea in men usually presents as acute urethritis. If untreated, it may progress to prostatitis, epididymitis, or periurethral abscess, but these complications are rare. Anorectal gonorrhea occurs in approximately 40% of homosexual men and pharyngeal infection in about 25%.

Mucopurulent cervicitis is the primary manifestation in women, although involvement of the urethra, rectum, periurethral glands, and the Bartholin gland ducts may occur. The genital infection in 10 to 20% of women progresses to pelvic inflammatory disease (endometritis, salpingitis, tubo-ovarian abscess, peritonitis). Infected mothers may transmit the disease to their babies in utero, during delivery, or postpartum. The conjunctiva is the major site of infection in newborns.

Spread of gonococci from the genitourinary tract, the rectum, or the pharynx to the bloodstream occurs in 0.3 to 5% of infected persons. Disseminated gonococcal infection results in arthritis and dermatitis, with rare complications including meningitis, osteomyelitis, and endocarditis.

N. meningitidis causes bacteremia (meningococcemia), meningitis, chronic meningococcemia (with arthritis and dermatitis), and pneumonia. Rarely, it has been implicated as the cause of pharyngitis and urethritis. The presentation may be subacute to fulminant.

The other *Neisseria* species rarely cause diseases such as meningitis, bacteremia, endocarditis, pericarditis, and ocular infections. *B. catarrhalis* is an important cause of otitis media and sinusitis in children and bronchopulmonary infections in the elderly or persons with underlying pulmonary deficiency, malignancy, or immune deficit. Infrequently, *B. catarrhalis* is the cause of meningitis, septic arthritis, endocarditis, bacteremia, and ocular infections.

Epidemiology

Gonorrhea is a common, worldwide sexually transmitted disease. In 1992, approximately 491,000 cases were reported in the United States (23). An eight to ten times higher incidence exists in the nonwhite populations than in whites. Since *N. gonorrhoeae* colonizes only human mucous membranes, close contact between individuals is required for transmission. Risk factors include young age, urban residence, low educational and socioeconomic background, nonwhite race, prostitution, and multiple sexual partners.

Humans are the only natural host for *N. meningitidis*. The organism resides on the nasopharyngeal mucosal membranes and is transmitted via respira-

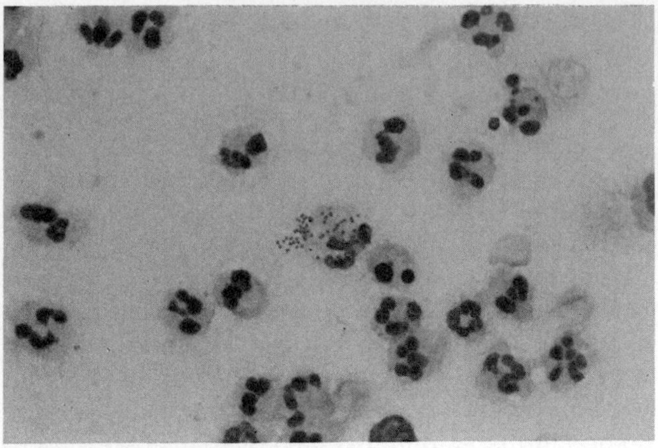

Figure 44.4. Gram stain of *N. gonorrhoeae* in urethral exudate.

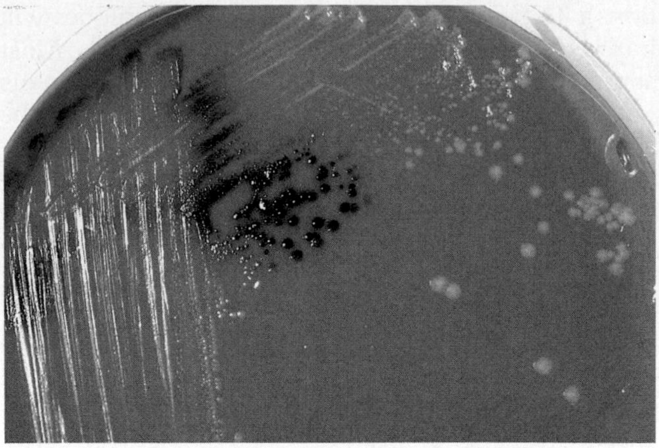

Figure 44.5. Colonies of *N. gonorrhoeae* on Martin-Lewis medium after addition of oxidase reagent. Oxidase-positive colonies turn purple.

tory droplets. The disease predominates in infants and children during endemic periods and shifts to older populations during epidemic periods. Strains belonging to the serogroups A, B, C, and W-135 are most frequently associated with epidemics. The highest incidence occurs in Central Africa.

The other *Neisseria* species are found as part of the oropharyngeal flora in humans. *B. catarrhalis* is not frequently isolated from the oropharynx of adults, but colonization rates appear to be much higher in patients with chronic pulmonary or respiratory tract disease (21).

Diagnostic Procedures

MICROSCOPY

A Gram smear of the appropriate clinical specimen revealing numerous polymorphonuclear leukocytes and many intracellular and extracellular Gram-negative diplococci is nearly diagnostic for *B. catarrhalis* pulmonary infection, gonococcal urethritis and cervicitis, and meningococcal meningitis (Fig. 44.4). The sensitivities of the Gram smear relative to the culture for the detection of gonococci in urethral exudates from symptomatic men, endocervical exudates, and rectal specimens are 95 to 100%, 40 to 60%, and 40 to 60%, respectively (24). The specificity of the smear is 95 to 100% for specimens other than rectal, where an increased prevalence of *N. meningitidis* is observed.

CULTURE TECHNIQUES

Neisseria species and *B. catarrhalis* can be isolated on 5% sheep blood and enriched chocolate agars. *N. gonorrhoeae* requires chocolate agar, *N. meningitidis* grows on blood agar, and the other *Neisseria* species and *B. catarrhalis* grow on media devoid of blood. Optimal growth occurs in 5 to 7% CO_2 at 35° to 37°C. Plates should be incubated for 48 to 72 hours. A selective medium (e.g., modified Thayer-Martin, Martin-Lewis, or New York City medium) is used for the isolation of *N. gonorrhoeae* and *N. meningitidis* from sites that are heavily colonized with other bacterial flora. Some strains of *N. lactamica*, *N. cinerea*, *N. polysaccharea*, and *B. catarrhalis* grow on these selective media, and some strains of *N. gonorrhoeae* are inhibited.

N. gonorrhoeae appears as gray to white opaque glistening colonies of 0.5 to 1.0 mm in diameter (Fig. 44.5). *N. meninitidis* produces a round, translucent blue-gray colony that is approximately 1 mm in diameter. *B. catarrhalis* colonies are grayish-white, opaque, and smooth. The other *Neisseria* species may or may not produce pigmented colonies.

IDENTIFICATION METHODS

The definitive identification of *Neisseria* species and *B. catarrhalis* is based on carbohydrate utilization tests and other physiological characteristics (Table 44.6). *Kingella denitrificans* is included in the table because it grows on the *Neisseria* selective agar and produces acid from glucose. As a result, it may be mistaken for pathogenic *Neisseria*. *N. gonorrhoeae* grows on selective media and produces acid from glucose, while *N. meningitidis* produces acid from both glucose and maltose. *B. catarrhalis*, *N. flavescens*, *N. elongata*, and *N. cinerea* are all asaccharolytic. *B. catarrhalis* is differentiated by the DNase reaction. *N. flavescens* produces polysaccharide in 1% sucrose, while *N. cinerea* does not. *N. elongata* is catalase negative.

Commercial kits are available for the rapid identification of *Neisseria* and *B. catarrhalis* based on reactions with carbohydrate or chromogenic substrates. The accuracy and the number of species identified vary with the system. Confirmation of an isolate as

Table 44.6. Characteristics of Human *Neisseria* spp., *B. catarrhalis,* and *K. denitrificans*[a, b]

Species	Pigment[c]	Superoxol[d]	Acid produced from: Glucose	Maltose	Fructose	Sucrose	Lactose (ONPG)	Polysaccharide from ≥1% sucrose[e]	Reduction of: NO_3	NO_2[f]	DNase	Extra CO_2 needed[g]	Growth on: MTM, ML, or NYC medium	Chocolate, blood agar at 22°C	Nutrient agar at 35°C
N. gonorrhoeae	−	+	+	−	−	−	−	−	−	−	−	VI	+[h]	−	−
N. meningitidis	−	−	+	+	−	−	−	−	−	d	−	I	+	−	+
N. lactamica	−	−	+	+	−	−	+	−	−	d	−	d	+	−	+
N. cinerea	−	−	−[i]	−	−	−	−	−	−	+	−	d	−[j]	−	+
N. polysaccharea	−	−	+	+	−	−	−	+	−	d	−	d	+	−	+
N. kochii	−	+	+	−	−	−	−	−	−	−	−	No	+	−	+
N. flavescens	+	−	−	−	−	−	−	+	−	−	−	I	+	−	+
N. sicca	d	−	+	+	+	+	−	+	−	+	−	No	−	+	+
N. subflava[j,k]															
Biovar *subflava*	+	−	+	+	−	−	−	−	−	+	−	No	−	+	+
Biovar *flava*	+	−	+	+	+	−	−	−	−	+	−	No	−	+	+
Biovar *perflava*	+	−	+	+	+	+	−	+	−	+	−	No	−[l]	+	+
N. mucosa	+	−	+	+	+	+	−	+	+	+	−	No	−	+	+
B. catarrhalis	−	−	−	−	−	−	−	−	+	−	+	No	d	+	+
K. denitrificans	−	−	+	−	−	−	−	−	+	−	−	I	+	−	−

[a]From Knapp JS. Historical perspectives and identification of *Neisseria* and related species. Clin Microbiol Rev 1988;1:417.
[b]ONPG, *o*-Nitrophenyl-β-D-galactopyranoside; DNase, deoxyribonuclease; MTM, modified Thayer-Martin medium; ML, Martin-Lewis medium; NYC, New York City medium. +, Most strains (≥90%) positive; −, most strains (≥90%) negative; d, some strains positive, some strains negative.
[c]Pigment observed in colonies on nutrient agar. Strains of *N. cinerea* and *N. lactamica* are yellow-brown and yellow pigmented when growth is harvested on a cotton applicator or smeared on filter paper.
[d]All *Neisseria* species and *B. catarrhalis* give a positive catalase test with 3% H_2O_2; *N. gonorrhoeae* strains give strong reactions with 30% H_2O_2 (superoxol) whereas other species are negative.
[e]Some strains may be inhibited by 5% sucrose; reactions may be obtained on a starch-free medium containing 1% sucrose. Strains of *N. gonorrhoeae, N. meningitidis,* and *N. kochii* do not grow on this medium.
[f]Results for tests in 0.1% (wt/vol) nitrite; *N. gonorrhoeae* strains and strains of some other species that are negative in 0.1% nitrite can reduce 0.01% (wt/vol) nitrite.
[g]Extra CO_2: VI, very important; I, important for growth; No, not needed for growth.
[h]≥90% of vancomycin-susceptible strains of *N. gonorrhoeae* may not grow on TM or MTM medium.
[i]Some strains of *N. cinerea* may give a weak reaction in glucose in some rapid tests for the detection of acid from carbohydrates.
[j]Some strains of *N. cinerea* have been isolated on gonococcal selective medium, but are colistin susceptible and will not grow when subcultured on selective media. Colistin-resistant mutants of *N. cinerea* have not been described.
[k]Strains of *N. subflava* biovars give consistent patterns of acid production when tested in appropriate media.
[l]Some strains of *N. subflava* biovar *perflava* grow on gonococcal selective media in primary culture, are colistin resistant, and grow on selective media on subculture.

N. gonorrhoeae can be done by fluorescent antibody techniques, particle agglutination tests, enzyme immunoassay (EIA), or by use of nucleic acid probe.

DIRECT ANTIGEN OR NUCLEIC ACID DETECTION

A commercial EIA procedure has been used for the detection of gonococci in genital specimens. The test is as sensitive and specific as the Gram stain for diagnosing urethral gonorrhea in symptomatic men but less sensitive and specific than culture in women (25). Sampling and processing influence the study results. A nucleic acid probe is available for the detection of gonococci in genital specimens. In early studies the sensitivity was greater than 90% and the specificity was excellent. These tests may have a greater role in a sexually transmitted disease clinic, where the prevalence and volume are high, than in a routine clinical microbiology laboratory.

Commercial particle agglutination kits are used for the direct detection of *N. meningitidis* in CSF specimens or concentrated urine. The sensitivity of the procedure (70 to 90%) varies with the concentration of antigen and the kit. Most kits exhibit a high degree of specificity.

SEROLOGIC PROCEDURES

There are no reliable commercially available tests to diagnose gonococcal infections serologically. The serologic determination of an individual's exposure to *N. meningitidis* is primarily of epidemiologic interest.

INTERPRETATION OF RESULTS

The isolation of *N. gonorrhoeae* is always clinically relevant. Since *N. meningitidis* and *B. catarrhalis* are normal flora in the upper respiratory tract, their significance is dependent on the type and quality of the specimen from which they were isolated and the nature of the infectious process. Assessing the clinical significance of the other *Neisseria* species is more difficult, since they rarely cause disease.

The isolation of a Gram-negative, oxidase-positive diplococcus on *Neisseria* selective agar from a genital specimen is presumptively *N. gonorrhoeae*. The identity must be confirmed by additional testing, especially in low-risk patients, because of the implications of a diagnosis of gonorrhea.

Therapeutic Considerations

All clinically relevant isolates of *Neisseria* species and *B. catarrhalis* should be tested for β-lactamase production because of the increasing incidence of plasmid or chromosomally mediated resistance to the penicillins. Ceftriaxone is recommended for the treatment of uncomplicated gonorrhea in adults. Additional consideration should be given for other coexisting sexually transmitted diseases. A follow-up culture should also be obtained after treatment. Penicillin or chloramphenicol is recommended for the treatment of severe meningococcal infections. The third-generation cephalosporins have also been used to treat meningococcal meningitis. Rifampin is recommended for the chemoprophylaxis of household contacts. Nearly all of the other *Neisseria* species are susceptible to penicillin.

β-Lactamase positive strains of *B. catarrhalis* should be considered resistant to penicillin, ampicillin, and amoxicillin (26). Vancomycin, clindamycin, and trimethoprim are inactive, and the penicillinase-resistant penicillins are variably active. The other antimicrobial agents are active and the choice is dependent on the severity of the infection.

Summary and Conclusions

The two clinically important species of *Neisseria* are *N. gonorrhoeae* (causing gonorrhea with all of the varied clinical manifestations) and *N. meningitidis* (causing meningococcemia and meningitis). *B. catarrhalis* is now identified taxonomically with the *Moraxella* genus (*Moraxella* [*Branhamella*] *catarrhalis*) and is an important cause of otitis media and sinusitis in children and bronchopulmonary infections in adults.

The definitive laboratory diagnosis is made by isolation and identification of the etiologic agent. Numerous commercial systems are available for identification of *Neisseria* and *B. catarrhalis*. Direct detection of gonococci by EIA and meningococci by particle agglutination are also possible today.

The emergence of *N. gonorrhoeae* strains resistant to penicillin has resulted in the use of more third-generation cephalosporins for the treatment of infections.

GRAM-POSITIVE AEROBIC TO FACULTATIVELY ANAEROBIC BACILLI

Microbiology

The Gram-positive aerobic to facultatively anaerobic bacilli are a taxonomically diverse group of bacteria that have been grouped together based primarily on cell morphology, endospore formation, and aerobic growth. It is obvious that soon these genera will be rearranged based on cell wall components and genetic relatedness studies.

When a Gram-positive rod is isolated from a clinical specimen, the genera that should be considered include *Bacillus, Listeria, Erysipelothrix, Corynebacte-*

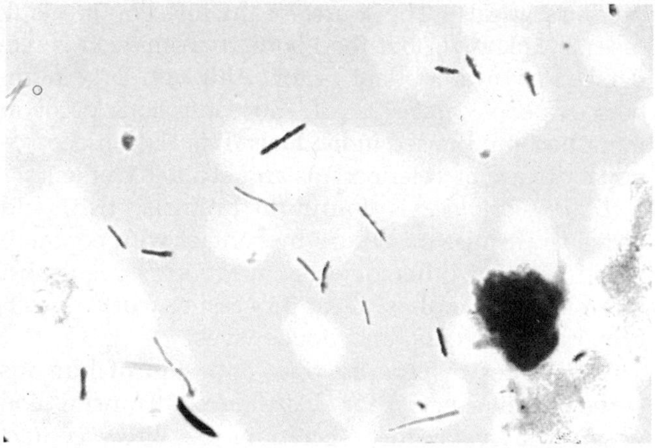

Figure 44.6. Gram stain of blood culture broth containing *Bacillus* species.

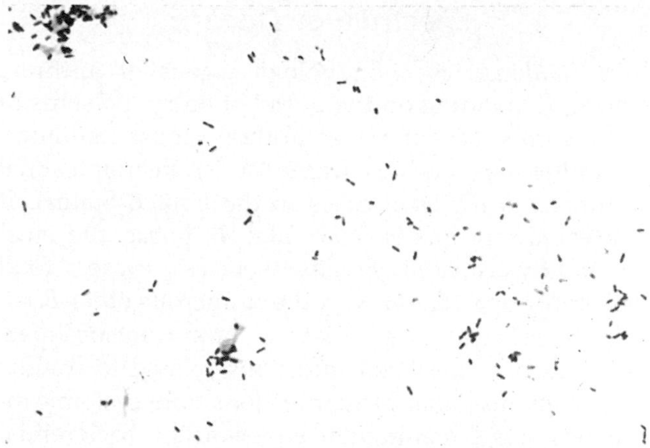

Figure 44.7. Gram stain of blood culture broth containing *Listeria*.

rium, *Mycobacterium*, *Nocardia*, *Lactobacillus*, and occasional strains of *Clostridium*, *Actinomyces*, and *Propionibacterium* because these genera are commonly isolated or associated with infections. *Lactobacillus*, *Clostridium*, *Actinomyces* and *Propionibacterium* are discussed in the anaerobe section. *Mycobacterium* and *Nocardia* are addressed in another chapter. Other genera that need to be considered but are rarely isolated or infrequently associated with human infections include *Arcanobacterium*, (*Clostridium haemolyticum*), *Brevibacterium*, *Kurthia*, *Rothia*, *Arthrobacterium*, *Oerskovia*, and *Rhodococcus*. Most of these organisms are either part of the normal skin or mucous membranes of humans or are found in soil, water, or foodstuffs. For a discussion of these genera, please consult *Bergey's Manual* (1).

The genus *Bacillus* contains over 30 recognized species, of which *Bacillus anthracis* and *Bacillus cereus* are the two most important pathogens. They are Gram-positive straight rods of variable size (2 to 10 μm in length and 0.5 to 2.5 μm in width) that occur singly or in chains (Fig. 44.6). The major characteristic for inclusion in this genus is the formation of endospores (does not always occur on routine laboratory media). The organisms grow on simple media and are facultative anaerobes, catalase positive, oxidase variable, and motile (except *B. anthracis*).

Bergey's Manual (1) recognizes five species of *Listeria* and three organisms of uncertain status. Only *Listeria monocytogenes* and rarely *Listeria ivanovii* are pathogenic for humans. Because species other than *L. monocytogenes* are seldom isolated from clinical specimens, they will not be discussed. *Listeria* is a short Gram-positive rod that occurs singly, in short chains, or in parallel or V forms (Fig. 44.7). It grows on most laboratory media and is facultatively anaerobic, catalase positive, and motile at room temperature.

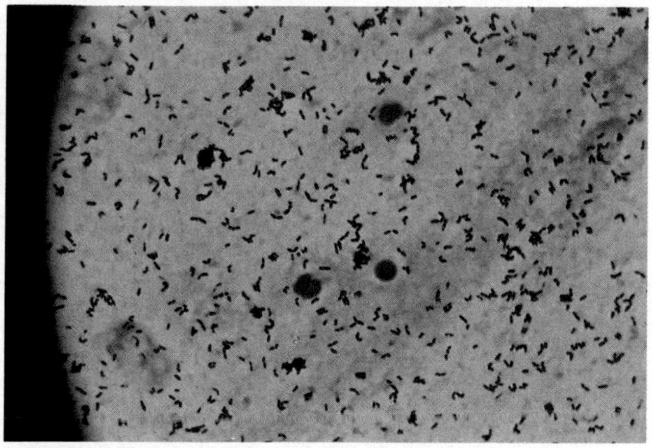

Figure 44.8. Gram stain of *Corynebacterium* in sputum.

Erysipelothrix rhusiopathiae is the only species in the genus. It is a catalase-negative, nonmotile, Gram-positive, straight or slightly-curved rod that occurs singly, in pairs, in short chains, or in filaments.

The genus *Corynebacterium* is most closely related to *Mycobacterium*, *Nocardi*, and *Rhodococcus* based on cell wall and fatty acid composition (1). There are 16 recognized species, but the U.S. Centers for Disease Control (CDC) list "coryneform" groups. Corynebacteria are Gram-positive, straight or slightly curved rods with tapered or club-shaped ends that occur singly or in angular (V or L) forms and palisade arrangements (Fig. 44.8). They are nonmotile, catalase positive, and facultatively anaerobic, and form metachromatic granules. *Arcanobacterium haemolyticum* (*Corynebacterium haemolyticum*) morphologically resembles *Corynebacterium* and is catalase negative and nonmotile.

Rothia dentocariosa is a Gram-positive rod that may appear coccoid, diptheroid, or filamentous. It is catalase positive, facultatively anaerobic, and nonmotile and is part of the normal oropharynegeal flora.

Spectrum of Disease

B. anthracis is the etiologic agent of anthrax, which, depending on the portal of entry, presents in three forms: (*a*) cutaneous anthrax (most common); (*b*) pulmonary anthrax (rare); or (*c*) gastrointestinal anthrax (no reported cases in the United States). If untreated, anthrax is often fatal. *B. cereus*, the most frequently isolated *Bacillus* species, causes food poisoning and, along with the numerous other *Bacillus* species, causes a variety of opportunistic infections such as localized infections related to trauma (especially fulminant eye infections) and systemic infections (e.g., meningitis, endocarditis, bacteremia, and pneumonia).

Listeria monocytogenes causes a mild febrile illness, especially in pregnant women; it also causes severe disease, including meningitis, bacteremia, in utero infections, or localized infections (including skin, ocular, arthritis, abscess, osteomyelitis, and endocarditis), which occur most often in immunocompromised patients.

E. rhusiopathiae infections usually involve localized cutaneous lesions or less frequently a disseminated form that is often associated with endocarditis.

Corynebacterium diphtheriae causes infections of the human upper respiratory tract (diphtheria) and skin. The other corynebacteria, especially *Corynebacterium jeikeium* (CDC group JK), cause a variety of infections in patients who have a prosthesis or who are immunocompromised. The infections include pharyngitis, cellulitis, skin lesions, lymphadenitis, pneumonia, bacteremia, endocarditis, infections of prostheses, abscesses, osteomyelitis, peritonitis in patients receiving continuous ambulatory peritoneal dialysis, and wound infections.

A. haemolyticum is associated with pharyngitis in young adults. *Rothia* strains are associated with endocarditis, abscesses, dental caries, and periodontal disease but are infrequently encountered.

Epidemiology

Anthrax occurs worldwide and is primarily a disease of herbivores. Transmission to humans occurs by contact with infected animals or their products (e.g., wool, hides, goat hair). The reservoir is contaminated soil, where spores can survive for long periods. The other *Bacillus* species are inhabitants of soil and therefore common contaminants of nearly all articles. Contamination of foodstuffs and subsequent improper storage may result in food poisoning.

L. monocytogenes is widespread in nature and has been isolated from the environment (e.g., soil, water, sewage), from animals (e.g., mammals, birds, fish, and humans), and from foodstuffs (e.g., vegetables, dairy products, meats). The source of the infection in many cases is unknown, but food-borne transmission is recognized as an important factor. Although large numbers of people are exposed, most infections occur in immunocompromised individuals. It is also an occupational disease of veterinarians and abattoir workers.

E. rhusiopathiae is found in animals, fish, and birds. Transmission occurs by contact with contaminated meat or other objects. Infection is seen most often in fish handlers, meat processing workers, veterinarians, farmers, and housewives.

The upper respiratory tract and skin of humans serve as the reservoir for *C. diphtheriae*. Transmission occurs via respiratory secretions or direct contact with exudate or contaminated fomites. The incidence of diphtheria is decreasing worldwide, partly related to immunization programs but also to other undefined factors. The other *Corynebacterium* species are common inhabitants of the skin and mucous membranes and are often isolated in the laboratory and dismissed as contaminants. Most infections are nosocomial or occur as the result of contact with animals or their products. *A. haemolyticum* is found in the pharynx and skin of humans.

Diagnostic Procedures

MICROSCOPY

The identification of this heterogeneous group of organisms begins with a Gram stain of the clinical specimen. A predominant single morphology is sought, as well as correlation with the source of the specimen and the signs and symptoms of the patient (Table 44.7).

In suspected cases of diphtheria, growth from the Loeffler's slant is stained with alkaline methylene blue. The typical coryneform morphology and the presence of metachromatic granules suggest *C. diphtheriae*.

Smears can be stained with specific fluorescent antibody reagents for *B. anthracis* through the Centers for Disease Control (CDC). Some strains of *Bacillus* stain Gram-negative as they age. In addition, because they may be oxidase positive, they are sometimes confused with Gram-negative rods. Spores produced by *Bacillus* appear clear with a Gram stain and green with the spore stain.

CULTURE TECHNIQUES

Bacillus species grow well on all noninhibitory blood-containing media and most nutrient media. They produce a variety of colony morphologies and pigments (Fig. 44.9). Phenylethyl alcohol (PEA) agar may be used for contaminated sites. Cultures are incubated at 35°C in air or CO_2. Strict safety precau-

Table 44.7. Microscopic Morphology of Gram-Positive Bacili

Genus	Microscopic Appearance	Comments
Kurthia	Rods in chains, cocci in old cultures	Strict aerobe
Arthrobacter	Marked rod-coccus cycle	Strict aerobe
Brevibacterium	Short rod, cocci in old cultures	Strict aerobe
Bacillus	Medium to large rods	Spores, decolorizes easily
Listeria	Small rods, coccobacilli, short chains	
Oerskovia	Coccoid, extensive branching filaments	
Rothia	Diphtheroid, coccoid, branching filaments	
Mycobacterium	Small to medium rods	Acid-fast, aerobe
Rhodococcus	Rod, coccoid, branching	Pink-coral; sometimes acid fast
Corynebacterium	Diphtheroid, coccobacillus	
C. matruchotii	Rod attached to filament (whip), branching	
Arcanobacterium	Diphtheroid, curved, pleomorphic	
Erysipelothrix	Rods, chains, coccobacillus, pleomorphic	
Nocardia	Branching filaments, short rods	Weakly acid-fast
Lactobacillus	Medium-thick rods, chains	Anaerobe but some grow in CO_2
Propionibacterium	Diphtheroid, some branching	Anaerobe but some grow in CO_2
Actinomyces	Rods, filaments with branching	Anaerobe but some grow in CO_2
Arachnia	Rods, filaments with some branching	Anaerobe but some grow in CO_2
Clostridium	Medium to large rods, some filaments	Anaerobe but some grow in CO_2

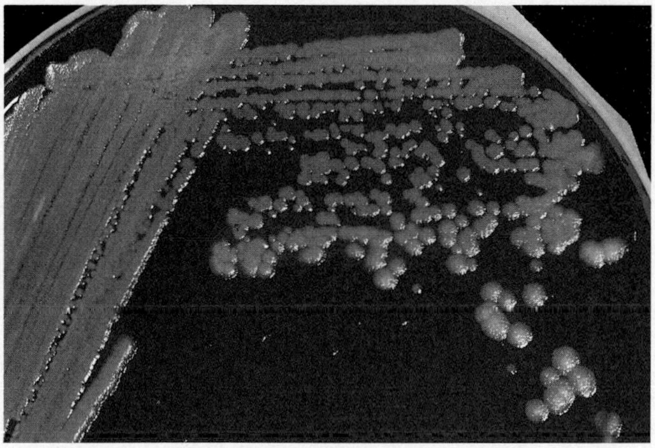

Figure 44.9. Colony of *B. cereus* on sheep blood agar.

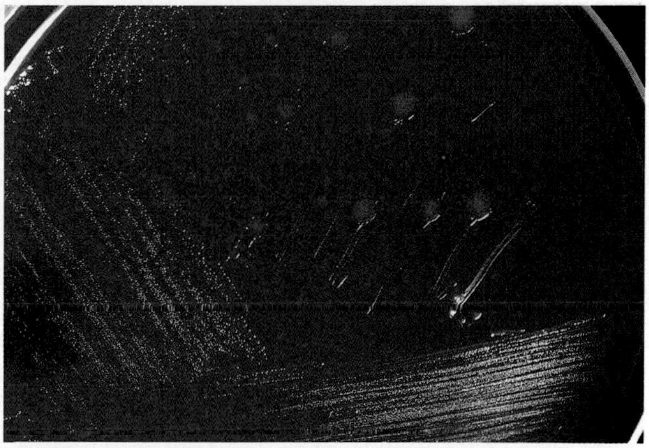

Figure 44.10. Colony of *Listeria* on sheep blood agar after 72 hours' incubation. Note the diffuse zone of β-hemolysis surrounding the colonies.

tions (e.g., biological safety cabinet, gloves) must be used for specimens and cultures suspected of containing *B. anthracis*.

Listeria grows on most laboratory media. After 24 hours' incubation on sheep blood agar, it produces a small (less than 1 mm), translucent, whitish-gray colony with a narrow zone of β-hemolysis, which is best seen after removal of the colony from the medium (Fig. 44.10). Columbia colistin-nalidixic acid (CNA) agar is recommended for isolation from contaminated specimens. New, shortened enrichment procedures have been developed for the isolation of *Listeria* from food and are now recommended for tissues, feces, or environmental cultures (27). *Listeria* grows at 35°C in air or CO_2.

E. rhusiopathie grows on blood-containing media (e.g., blood, chocolate, CNA), but growth in infusion broth containing 1% glucose or trypticase soy broth subcultured at 2 and 7 days may be superior to direct plating. Media should be incubated at 35°C in CO_2 for at least 72 hours.

Corynebacterium grows well on most routine enriched media (e.g., blood, CNA) and produces colonies that are translucent, opaque, white, or gray. In cases of suspected diphtheria, selective agar (e.g., cystine-tellurite agar, modified Tinsdale agar) and Loeffler or Pai agar should be inoculated. Cultures are incubated at 35°C in air or CO_2 for at least 72 hours.

IDENTIFICATION TECHNIQUES

Differential characteristics to presumptively group the different genera of Gram-positive rods are depicted in Table 44.8. Additional testing is usually required for definitive identification.

Overdecolorized *Bacillus* species may be differentiated from Gram-negative rods by spore formation

Table 44.8. Characteristics of Gram-Positive Bacilli[a]

Genus	Catalase	Growth	Motility	Esculin	H_2S (TSI)	TSI s/b[b]	Nitrate Reduction	Urease	Hemolysis	Comments
Kurthia	+	A	+	−	−	−/−	−	+	N	Grows best 20–30°C
Brevibacterium	+	A	−	+	−	+/+	v	−	v	
Bacillus	+	FA	v	+	−	v/v	v	v	v	Easily decolorized spore formation
L. monocytogenes	+	FA	+	+	−	+/+	−	−	B	Motile at room temperature
Oerskovia	+	FA	+	+	−	+/+	v	v	N,A	Yellow pigment
Rothia	+	FA	−	+	−	+/+	+	−	N	Coccoid in broth
Mycobacterium	+	A	−	−	−	−/−	+	v	N	Acid-fast
Rhodococcus	+	FA	−	v	−	−/−	v	v	N	Pink coral pigment
Corynebacterium	+	FA	−[c]	−	−	v/v	v	v	v	
Arcanobacterium	−	FA	−	v	−	+/+	−	−	B	
Nocardia	+	FA	−	+	−	NA	v	v	N	Weakly acid-fast
Erysipelothrix	−	FA	−	−	+	+/+	−	−	N,A	
Lactobacillus	−	AN[d]	−	v	−	+/+	−	−	N,A	
Propionibacterium	+	AN[d]	−	v	−	+/+	−	−	v	
Actinomyces	−[c]	AN[d]	−	+	−	+/+	v	−	N	
Arachnia	−	AN[d]	−	−	−	+/+	−	−	N	
Clostridium	−	AN[d]	v	v	+	v/v	+	v	v	Easily decolorized spore formation

[a]Symbols: +, > 90% of strains positive; −, < 10% of strains positive; v, variable; A, strict aerobe, FA, facultative anaerobe; AN, anaerobe; B, beta; A, alpha; N, nonhemolytic; NA, not available.
[b]s/b = slant/butt, + = acid; −, no change.
[c]Some species positive.
[d]Some species grow in CO_2.

Table 44.9. Identification of *Bacillus* Spp[a]

Species	Width ≥ 1 μm	Penicillin	Motility	Lecithinase	V-P	Nitrate Reduction	Starch Hydrolysis	Anaerobic Growth	Growth in 7% NaCl	Growth at 50°C
B. anthracis	+	s	−	+	+	+	+	+	+	−
B. cereus	+	R	v	+	+	+	+	+	+	−
B. mycoides	+	R	−	+	+	+	+	+	+	−
B. thuringiensis	+	R	v	+	+	+	+	+	+	−
B. megaterium	+	v	v	−	−	v	+	−	+	−
B. subtilis	−	s	+	−	+	+	+	−	+	+
B. pumilus	−	s	+	−	+	−	−	−	+	+
B. licheniformis	−	s	+	−	+	+	+	+	+	+
B. firmus	−	s	v	−	−	+	+	−	+	−
B. coagulans	v	s	+	−	v	v	+	+	−	+
B. circulans	−	NA	v	−	−	v	+	v	v	+
B. polymyxa	−	NA	+	−	+	+	+	+	−	−
B. laterosporus	−	NA	+	+	−	+	−	+	−	+
B. brevis	−	NA	+	−	−	v	−	−	−	+
B. shapaericus	v	NA	+	−	−	+	−	−	v	−
B. alvei	v	NA	+	−	+	+	+	+	−	−
B. macerans	−	NA	+	−	−	+	+	+	−	+

Symbols: +, > 90% of strains positive; −, < 10% of strains positive; v, variable reactions; V-P, Vogues-Proskauer reaction; NA, no data available.

(stimulated on esculin or TSI agar), susceptibility to vancomycin, and resistance to KOH (27). Other tests useful for the identification of clinically relevant isolates are shown in Table 44.9. *Bacillus* species that produce medusa head colonies and are nonmotile, penicillin susceptible, and nitrate positive are presumptively *B. anthracis* and need to be confirmed by the CDC. The laboratory diagnosis of *B. cereus* food poisoning requires quantitative examination of the food, vomitus, or feces.

The misidentification of *Listeria* as an *Enterococcus*, group B *Streptococcus*, or *Corynebacterium* should not occur. All Gram-positive rods or coccobacilli, especially from sterile body fluids, are screened to rule out *Listeria* by positive tests for catalase, tumbling motility at room temperature, esculin hydrolysis, and β-hemolysis on sheep blood (Table 44.8). *L. monocytogenes* can be separated from other *Listeria* species by fermentation of carbohydrates.

E. rhusiopathiae is nonmotile and catalase positive. It is the only Gram-positive rod that produces H_2S in triple sugar iron or Kligler's iron agar slant. Additional characteristics are presented in Table 44.8.

C. diphtheriae (including other strains of *Corynebacterium*, *S. aureus*, and *Listeria*) produces grayish-black colonies on tellurite-containing media and a brown halo on Tinsdale medium. *Corynebacterium ulcerans* and *Corynebacterium pseudotuberculosis*, closely related if not actually strains of *C. diphtheriae*, also form a brown halo. All suspected isolates of *C. diphtheriae* must be identified (Table 44.10) and shown to produce diphtheria toxin by in vivo or in vitro tests. *C. diphtheriae, C. ulcerans*, and *C. pseudotuberculosis* lack pyrazinamidase activity.

The identification of clinically significant *Corynebacterium* species (Tables 44.10 and 44.11) can be difficult because of the heterogeneity and biochemical diversity of the group (28, 29). To promote growth, serum may have to be added to the tests and the tests held for up to 2 weeks. *C. jeikeium* (CDC group JK) exhibits poor growth in routine biochemical tests and multiple resistance to most antimicrobial agents except vancomycin. Various commercial identification kits have been used to identify some of the *Corynebacterium* species.

DIRECT ANTIGEN OR NUCLEIC ACID DETECTION

B. anthracis can be identified directly in specimens by fluorescent antibody stain at the CDC. A fluorescent antibody reagent is also available for the detection of *Listeria* in clinical specimens but it may cross-react with some Gram-positive cocci. Fluorescent antibody techniques have also been described for *C. diphtheriae*. Nucleic acid detection is not commercially available for these organisms.

SEROLOGIC PROCEDURES

B. anthracis can be diagnosed by an indirect hemagglutination procedure performed at the CDC. Serology for *Listeria* infections is of epidemiologic value but is not useful as a diagnostic test.

INTERPRETATION OF RESULTS

The isolation of *Listeria, Erysipelothrix, C. diphtheriae*, or *B. anthracis* is clinically relevant. The significance of any of the other numerous species of Gram-positive rods depends on the type and quality of the specimen, the frequency of isolation, and the nature of the infectious disease process.

Therapeutic Considerations

The drug of choice for the treatment of anthrax is penicillin. The other *Bacillus* species demonstrate variable susceptibility to the penicillins and cephalosporins, but most appear susceptible to aminoglycosides, tetracycline, clindamycin, erythromycin, chloramphenicol, vancomycin, imipenem, and ciprofloxacin (30).

Most of the recommended therapy for listeriosis is based on isolated case reports. Penicillin or ampicillin plus an aminoglycoside administered over a 3- to 6-week period is probably the optimal combination (31). Trimethoprim-sulfamethoxazole is a second choice.

Erysipelothrix is susceptible to penicillin and cephalosporins. Clindamycin can be used in penicillin-allergic patients.

Patients with diphtheria should be given antitoxin and started on penicillin or erythromycin. Clindamycin or rifampin may also be used. Susceptibility of the other *Corynebacterium* species must be determined by testing. *C. jeikeium* (CDC group JK) is susceptible to vancomycin and ciprofloxacin and resistant to most other antimicrobial agents. *A. haemolyticum* is susceptible to penicillin.

Summary and Conclusions

Gram-positive, aerobic to facultatively anaerobic rods describe a heterogeneous group of organisms containing over 20 genera. Most of these organisms are seldom if ever isolated from clinical specimens and are found in the environment (e.g., soil, food) or on the skin and mucous membranes of humans and animals. Because of taxonomic and identification difficulties, many of these species are just now being recognized as important agents of opportunistic infections. *B. anthracis, L. monocytogenes, E. rhusiopathiae*, and *C. diphtheriae* should always be considered clinically significant when isolated.

In general, most of these bacteria are readily isolated on laboratory media containing blood but are difficult to identify definitively. Susceptibility to antimicrobial agents is variable and must be determined for many of these species.

ENTEROBACTERIACEAE

Microbiology

The family Enterobacteriaceae encompasses 28 genera and over 100 species, CDC groups, or biogroups (Table 44.12). Many of the new species are rarely or never found in human specimens. Others are isolated from specimens but seldom cause disease. Most *Salmonella* strains that cause human disease are found in subgroup I, and it is likely that a return to serotype designation for human isolates will occur. *Arizona* is included in the *Salmonella* genus based on genetic relatedness.

The members of this family are generally straight, Gram-negative rods that are catalase positive and oxidase negative, reduce nitrate to nitrite, and are fac-

Table 44.10. Identification of Medically Significant Corynebacteria and Other Coryneforms[a]

Species	Catalase	β-Hemolysis	Nitrate Reduction	Pigment[c]	Urease	Gelatin Hydrolysis	Motility	Esculin Hydrolysis	Carbohydrate Utilization[d]: Glucose	Maltose	Sucrose	Mannitol	Xylose	Response to Serum[e]
C. diphtheriae[f, g]	+	+[f, h]	+[f]	N	–	–	–	–	+	+	–[f]	–	–	d[i]
C. ulcerans[g, j, k]	+	+[h]	–	N	+	–/+[l]	–	–	+	+	–	–	–	–
C. pseudotuberculosis[k, j, m]	+	+[n]	d[n]	y-w	+	–[o]	–	–	+	+	–	–	–	–[p]
C. xerosis[p]	+	–	+	N, y, T	–	–	–	–	+	+[r]	+	–	–	–
C. striatum	+	–	+	N, y-g	–	–	–	–	+	–	+	–	–	–
C. pseudodiphtheriticum	+	–	+	N	+	–	–	–	–	–	–	–	–	–
C. kutscheri	+	d	+	y-w, N	+	–	–	+	+	+	+	–	–	–
C. renale	+	–	–	Y	+	–	–	–	+	–	–	–	–	–
C. pilosum	+	–	+	Y	+	–	–	–	+	+	–	–	–	–
C. cystitidis	+	–	–	N	+	–	–	–	+	+	–	–	+	–
C. matruchotii	+	–	d	N	–	–	–	–	+	d	d	d	–	–
C. minutissimum	+	–	–	N	–	–	–	–	+	+	d	–	–	–
C. bovis	+	–	–	N	–	–	–	–	+	–	–	–	–	–
C. jeikeium (group JK)	+	–	–	N	–	–	–	–	+	d	–	–	–	–
"*C. genitalium*"[s]	+	–	–	N	–	–	–	–	+	wk	–	–	–	–
"*C. aquaticum*"[t]	+	–	–	Y	–	–	+	+	+	+	+	+	+	–

[a]From Coyle MB, Lipsky BA. Coryneform bacteria in infectious diseases: clinical and laboratory aspects. Clin Microbiol Rev 1990;3:227–246.
[b]+, 90% or more positive within 4 days; –, 90% or more negative; d, >10% or <90% positive; wk, weakly positive.
[c]N, White or gray; Y, yellow; y, pale yellow; y-g, yellowish green; y-w, yellowish white; T, tan.
[d]Usually tested in peptone-water with Andrade indicator or in brain heart infusion broth.
[e]Two drops of sterile rabbit serum are required for good growth in peptone-water.
[f]Biotype *mitis* is weakly β-hemolytic; it includes sucrose-positive strains that are rare in the United States and nitrate-negative strains that are subspecies *belfanti*. Biotype *gravis* attacks glycogen and starch and includes a few weakly hemolytic strains and rare isolates that are sucrose-positive. Biotype *intermedius* is not β-hemolytic.
[g]Produces halos on Tinsdale medium and does not hydrolyze pyrazinamide.
[h]Narrow zones of slight hemolysis at 18 to 24 hr.
[i]Biotype *intermedius* is stimulated by serum.
[j]PLD is produced.
[k]Also ferments glycogen and usually starch and trehalose, which should be read for 7 days.
[l]Negative or weak at 37°C; positive at 25°C.
[m]Does not attack glycogen or trehalose and usually not starch.
[n]Usually negative in strains from sheep or goats and positive in those from horses or cattle.
[o]Negative at 35 and 25°C but positive at 30°C after 14 days.
[p]Growth is stimulated by lipid but serum is not added for biochemical tests.
[q]Halos not produced on Tinsdale medium.
[r]In reference 1, this reaction is negative, with occasional strains positive.
[s]Reactions of biotypes 2 (ATCC 33031) and 4 (ATCC 33033).
[t]Glucose oxidizer. Reactions of reference strain ATCC 14655.

Table 44.11. CDC Coryneform Groups and Species That Were Formerly Included with the Corynebacteria[a, b]

Species	Catalase	β-Hemolysis	Nitrate Reduction	Pigment[c]	Urease	Gelatin Hydrolysis	Motility	Esculin Hydrolysis	Carbohydrate Utilization[d]: Glucose	Maltose	Sucrose	Mannitol	Xylose	Response to Serum[e]
Group A-3	+	–	+	N, Y	–	–	+	+	+	+	+	–	+	–
Group A-4	+	–	d	Y, N	–	d	d	+	+	+	+	+	+	–
Group A-5	+	–	d	Y, N	–	d	d	d	+	+	+	+	–	–
B-1	+	–	d	T, N	–	d	–	–	+	d	d	–	–	–
B-3	+	–	–	T, N	–	+	–	–	–	–	–	–	–	–
Group F-1	+	–	d	N	+	–	–	–	+	d	+	–	–	d
Group F-2	+	–	d	N	+	–	–	–	+	+	–	–	–	–
Group G-1[f]	+	–	+	N	–	–	–	–	+ or (+)	d	+ or (+)	–	–	+
Group G-2[f]	+	–	–	N	–	–	–	–	+ or (+)	d	+ or (+)	–	–	+
Group I[g]	+	–	+	N	–	–	–	–	+	d[h]	–	–	–	–
Group E[i]	–	–	–	N	–	–	–	d	+	+	+	–	+	+
Group D-2	+	–	–	N	+	–	–	–	–	–	–	–	–	+
ANF-1	+	–	–	N	–	–	–	–	–	–	–	–	–	–
ANF-3	+	–	+	N	–	–	–	–	–	–	–	–	–	–
Group 1	+	–	+	N	–	–	–	–	–	–	–	–	–	–
Group 2	–	–	–	N	–	–	–	–	+	+	+	+	+	–
Actinomyces pyogenes	–	+	–	N	–	+	–	–	+	+	–	–	–	+
Arcanobacterium haemolyticum[j]	–	+[k]	–	N	–	–	–	–	+	+	d	d	+	+
Oerskovia turbata	+	–	d	Y, N	d	+	+	+	+	+	+	–	+	–
Oerskovia xanthineolytica	+	–	+	Y	d	+	+	+	+	+	+	–	+	–
Rhodococcus equi	+	–	d	P	d	–	–	–	–[m]	–	–	–	–	–

[a]From Coyle MB, Lipsky BA. Coryneform bacteria in infectious diseases: clinical and laboratory aspects. Clin Microbiol Rev 1990;3:227–246.
[b]+, 90% or more positive within 4 days; –, 90% or more negative; + or (+), 90% or more positive, some strains positive after 4 or more days; d, >10% or <90% positive.
[c]N, White or gray; Y, yellow; P, pink (orange to red on glucose-yeast extract agar); T, tan.
[d]Usually tested in peptone-water with Andrade indicator or in brain heart infusion broth.
[e]Two drops of sterile rabbit serum are required for good growth in peptone-water.
[f]Fastidious, but otherwise indistinguishable from *B. matruchotii* in these tests.
[g]Halos not produced on Tinsdale medium.
[h]Group I-2 produces acid from maltose but group I-1 does not.
[i]Fastidious. Major end products are succinic acid and acetic acid.
[j]PLD is produced.
[k]Narrow zones of slight hemolysis after 48 hr on sheep blood.
[l]Growth is stimulated by lipid but serum is not added for biochemical tests due to false-positive xylose reactions.
[m]Weak reaction after 7 days.

Table 44.12. Nomenclature and Classification of the Family Enterobacteriaceae[a]

Genus	No. of Species	Genus	No. of Species
Budvicia	1	*Leminorella*	2
Buttiauxella[b]	1	*Moellerella*	1
Cedecea	3	*Morganella*	1
Citrobacter	3	*Obesumbacterium*[b]	1
		Pragia	1
Edwardsiella	3	*Proteus*	4
Enterobacter	12	*Providencia*	5
Erwinia[b]	~12	*Rahnella*	1
Escherichia	5	*Salmonella*	6 subgroups
Ewingella	1	*Serratia*	9
Hafnia	1	*Shigella*	4
Klebsiella	7	*Tatumella*	1
Kluyvera	2	*Yersinia*	11
Koserella	1	*Xenorhabdus*[b]	2
Leclercia	1		

[a]Modified from Farmer JJ III, Kelly MT. *Enterobacteriaceae*. In: Balows A, Hausler WJ Jr, Herrmann KL, Isenberg HD, Shadomy HJ, eds. Manual of clinical microbiology. 5th ed. Washington, DC: American Society for Microbiology, 1991:360–383.
[b]Not isolated from clinical specimens.

ultatively anaerobic. They are motile by peritrichous flagella or nonmotile, do not form spores, and usually grow on MacConkey agar. They demonstrate a vast heterogeneity in their habitats and pathogenic potential for plants, animals, and humans.

Spectrum of Disease

The members of the Enterobacteriaceae are among the most important bacteria medically and have been associated with infections in every major organ system. Their ubiquitous presence in the environment, in foodstuffs, and on animals and humans; their ability to develop antimicrobial resistance; and the increasing numbers of susceptible patients who are compromised or have prosthetic implants has ensured the involvement of these bacteria in both community- and hospital-acquired infections. Some genera and species such as *Salmonella, Shigella, Yersinia,* and some strains of *E. coli* are primary enteric pathogens causing dysentery, gastroenteritis, enteric fever, and hemorrhagic colitis.

Epidemiology

The members of the family Enterobacteriaceae are widely distributed in the soil, on plants, and in food and colonize the gastrointestinal tract of animals and humans. They also contaminate many types of medical supplies and devices. Community-acquired gastrointestinal disease occurs via consumption of contaminated water or foodstuffs. Bacteria causing nosocomial infections (usually found in the GI or upper respiratory tract of the patient) are transmitted on the hands of hospital personnel or introduced into the patient via contaminated solutions or devices. Numerous techniques are available to track specific strains in food-related outbreaks or in the hospital environment, including serologic typing, biotyping, bacteriocins, antibiograms, and nucleic acid analysis.

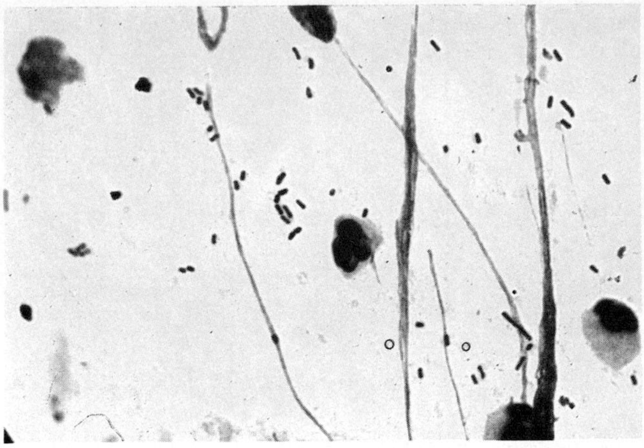

Figure 44.11. Gram stain of *K. pneumoniae* in sputum.

Diagnostic Procedures

MICROSCOPY

On Gram stain, the "enterics" exhibit a characteristic morphology consisting of straight, thick, barrel-shaped rods that may exhibit bipolar staining and are often pleomorphic (Fig. 44.11). *Yersinia pestis* may have a "safety pin" appearance.

CULTURE TECHNIQUES

All members of this group grow luxuriantly within 24 hours in air at 35°C on routine laboratory media such as blood, MacConkey (or eosin methylene blue), or chocolate agar. On blood agar, colonies are usually 1 to 3 mm in diameter, dull, gray, opaque, sometimes muccoid (e.g., *Klebsiella*), sometimes hemolytic (e.g., *E. coli*), and sometimes swarming (e.g., *Proteus*). More selective agars, as well as enrichment broths, are used to isolate enteric pathogens from feces. The characteristic appearances of colonies on these media is listed in Table 44.13. Sorbitol-MacConkey and cefsulodin-irgasan-novobiocin (CIN) agars are used to isolate *E. coli* O:157 and *Y. enterocolica*, respectively. It is recommended that media for the isolation of *Yersinia* be incubated at 22 to 25°C for 48 hours.

IDENTIFICATION TECHNIQUES

With respect to identification, the clinical laboratory has three levels of need: (*a*) a screen for enteric pathogens; (*b*) a presumptive identification of isolates

Table 44.13. Appearance of Commonly Isolated *Enterobacteriaceae* on Various Enteric Media

	MacConkey (MAC) Agar	Eosin-Methylene Blue (EMB) Agar	Hektoen Enteric (HE) Agar	Xylose-Lysine Deoxycholate (XLD) Agar	Salmonella-Shigella (SS) Agar	Deoxycholate Citrate (DC) Agar	Bismuth Sulfite (BS) Agar	Brilliant Green (BG) Agar
Escherichia coli								
Lac +	Flat; red or dark pink; surrounded by zone of precipitated bile	Red black with metallic sheen[b] (Plate 9, A)	Yellow-orange	Yellow	Pink	Deep red-pink	Usually do not grow	Usually do not grow
Lac −	Colorless	Colorless	Yellow-orange or green	Yellow	Colorless	Colorless	Usually do not grow	Usually do not grow
Klebsiella	Pink; mucoid	Purple	Yellow-orange	Yellow	Pink	Pink	Usually do not grown	Usually do not grow
Enterobacter	Pink; not usually as mucoid as *Klebsiella*	Purple	Yellow-Orange	Yellow	Pink	Pink	Usually do not grow	Usually do not grow
Citrobacter, Serratia, Hafnia, Providencia	May appear colorless after 24 hr or slightly pink in 24 to 48 hr	Lavender or colorless	Colorless	Red, yellow, or colorless with or without black centers	Colorless	Colorless	Usually do not grow	Usually do not grow
Proteus, Morganella, Edwardsiella	Colorless[c]	Colorless	Colorless	Red, yellow, or colorless with or without black centers	Colorless	Colorless	Usually do not grow	Usually do not grow
Salmonella	Colorless	Colorless	Green or blue-green	Pink to red with black center	Colorless with black center	Colorless	Green-black	Pink-white opaque: surrounded by brilliant red medium
Shigella	Colorless	Colorless	Green or blue-green	Colorless	Colorless	Colorless	Usually do not grow	Usually do not grow
Yersinia	Colorless to peach	Colorless or purple[d]	Salmon	Yellow	Colorless	Colorless	Usually do not grow	Usually do not grow

[a]From Howard BJ, Klass J II, Rubin SJ, Weissfeld AS, Tilton RC, eds. Clinical and pathogenic microbiology. St. Louis: CV Mosby, 1987:295.
[b]Not all strains produce a metallic sheen; on the other hand, other species of enteric bacilli (for instance, *Yersinia enterocolitica*) may produce a sheen.
[c]*Proteus mirabilis, Proteus vulgaris,* and *Proteus penneri* may swarm.
[d]*Yersinia enterocalitica*, a nonlactose-fermenter that ferments sucrose, produces colorless colonies on Levine EMB agar and purple colonies on the modified Holt-Harris Teague formula, which contains sucrose.

from significant but not life-threatening infections; and (*c*) definitive identification.

Two media (urea and triple sugar iron or lysine iron agar) have been used to screen stool cultures for potential pathogens (Table 44.14). The urease test aids in the detection of *Proteus* and urease-positive *Providencia*. Commercial latex agglutination kits are available to identify colonies of *E. coli* O:157, *Salmonella*, and *Shigella* or to detect their growth in enrichment broth. Screening tests are also being evaluated for the detection of verotoxin-producing *E. coli* (32).

Clinically relevant isolates from non–life-threatening infections can be presumptively identified by colony morphology and a few rapid tests. The identification of the most frequently isolated bacteria is based on lactose fermentation and colony morphology on MacConkey agar, swarming on blood agar, spot indole, motility, and ornithine decarboxylase (Table 44.15). Members of the *Enterobacteriaceae* family are definitely identified by inoculation of numerous conventional biochemical tests, use of commercial manual kits, or by automated systems. All *Salmonella*, *Shigella*, and *E. coli* O:157 isolates should be identified both biochemically and serologically. Biochemicals for the identification of *Yersinia* should be incubated at 22 to 25°C.

DIRECT ANTIGEN OR NUCLEIC ACID TECHNIQUES

Currently, there are no commercially available systems for the direct detection of Enterobacteriaceae in clinical specimens. However, a number of tests are available for the identification of colonies or the detection of virulence factors. As mentioned earlier, *Salmonella*, *Shigella*, and *E. coli* O:157 can be identified by latex agglutination or serotyped by antisera. Also, colonies of *E. coli* can be screened for production of toxins by EIA. Nucleic acid probes are used to identify enterotoxigenic, enteroinvasive, and enteropathogenic *E. coli* (33). Presently, EIA and probes are used primarily for epidemiologic studies by reference centers. Both DNA hybridization and monoclonal antibody systems are being evaluated for the detection of *Salmonella* in food and may become available for use with clinical specimens.

Table 44.14. Typical Reaction Patterns of Enteric Pathogens on Triple-Sugar Iron (TSI) and Urea Agar[a]

Genus	Urea	TSI (Slant/Butt)	H_2S	Oxidase
Salmonella	−	K/A	+ or −	−
Salmonella (rare)	−	A/A	+	−
Shigella	−	K/A	−	−
Edwardsiella	−	K/A	+	
Yersinia	+	A(K)/A	−	−
Aeromonas	−	A(K)/A	−	+
Plesiomonas	−	A(K)/A	−	+

[a]Symbols: A, acid; K, alkaline; +, positive; −, negative; ( ), occasional reactions.

SEROLOGIC PROCEDURES

The febrile agglutination test is used to help diagnose *Salmonella typhi* infections by measuring an antibody response to the O and H antigens. However, numerous factors can produce both false-positive and false-negative reactions, and the test should not be used alone to diagnose typhoid fever.

Serodiagnosis of *Y. enterocolitica* is useful only when one or two serogroups cause the majority of the infections. Serodiagnosis is difficult in the United States because numerous O serogroups cause enteric infections. The criteria for positive and negative tests are also poorly defined.

INTERPRETATION OF RESULTS

The isolation of *Salmonella*, *Shigella*, or *Yersinia* from any site is clinically relevant. The isolation of any member of the Enterobacteriaceae from a normally sterile body fluid or site is significant until proven otherwise. The recovery of these organisms from other specimens (e.g., sputum, urine) must be interpreted considering the patient's underlying condition, prosthesis (including catheters), intubation, type of specimen, and frequency of isolation.

Therapeutic Considerations

Resistance plasmids in members of the Enterobactericeae play a predominant role in antimicrobial

Table 44.15. Presumptive Identification of Common Isolates of Enterobacteriaceae[a]

Characteristic	*E. coli*	*Klebsiella*	*Enterobacter*	*P. mirabilis*	*P. vulgaris*
Colony on MacConkey agar					
Flat, dry	+	NA	NA	NA	NA
Mucoid	NA	+	+	NA	NA
Lactose fermenting	+	+	+	−	−
Swarming on blood agar	NA	NA	NA	+	+
Spot indole	+	−	−	−	+
Ornithine decarboxylase	NA	−	+	+	−
Motility	NA	−	+	NA	NA

[a]Symbols: +, positive; −, negative; NA, not applicable.

resistance. These plasmids often confer resistance to multiple antimicrobial agents and can be transferred to other strains and species. This, combined with the enormous clinical and agricultural use of antimicrobial agents, has led to the rapid emergence of resistance to antimicrobial agents among the Enterobacteriaceae. The R plasmids permit the bacterium to produce enzymes that alter the antimicrobial agent (e.g., β-lactamase), to synthesize metabolic enzymes that resist inhibition by the drug, or to prevent the intracellular accumulation of antimicrobial agents.

Antimicrobial agents in a specific environment select bacteria that are resistant to that particular agent and related compounds. For example, third-generation cephalosporins (compounds that are resistant to many of the β-lactamases found in the Enterobacteriaceae) select bacteria that produce a modified β-lactamase with a much expanded spectrum of activity.

Because of R plasmids and their rapid transfer among bacteria, the optimum antimicrobial therapy for infections caused by members of the Enterobacteriaceae must be determined by in vitro susceptibility test results. Other factors that need to be considered include the pharmacology of the drug, the underlying condition of the patient, and to some degree whether the infection is community- or hospital-acquired.

Summary and Conclusions

The members of the family Enterobacteriaceae are ubiquitous in nature, causing a significant number of gastrointestinal, urinary tract, and nosocomial infections. They are readily isolated on routine media and are identified by numerous manual and commercial methods. Antimicrobial therapy must be based on susceptibility testing of the isolated bacterium.

AEROMONAS AND *PLESIOMONAS*

Microbiology

Aeromonas and *Plesiomonas* are included in the family Vibrionaceae based primarily on polar flagella and the oxidase reaction. Both are Gram-negative, motile, catalase- and oxidase-positive rods that are facultatively anaerobic. The genus *Aeromonas* contains eight species: *Aeromonas hydrophila*, *Aeromonas caviae*, *Aeromonas sobria*, *Aeromonas media*, *Aeromonas veronii*, *Aeromonas schubertii*, *Aeromonas eucrenophila*, and *Aeromonas salmonicida* (not associated with disease in humans). It has been suggested that the *Aeromonas hydrophila* group should be composed of *Aeromonas hydrophila*, *Aeromonas caviae*, *Aeromonas sobria*, and *Aeromonas media* (34).

Spectrum of Disease

Aeromonas causes four types of infections in humans, including diarrhea, cellulitis or wound infections (usually following exposure to water or soil), bacteremia (primarily in the immunocompromised host), and a variety of soft tissue and deep-seated infections (35). *Plesiomonas shigelloides* primarily causes gastrointestinal disease but has been associated with cases of meningitis, bacteremia, wound infections, septic arthritis, and cholecystitis (36).

Epidemiology

Both *Aeromonas* and *Plesiomonas* are found in soil and water, where they cause infections in frogs, reptiles, and fish. Transmission to humans occurs via contaminated water or foodstuffs, and contamination of an injury.

Diagnostic Techniques

MICROSCOPY

There are no available microscopic techniques to detect these bacteria directly in clinical specimens. The morphology on Gram smear is not specific for either genus.

CULTURE TECHNIQUES

Both genera grow well on blood and MacConkey agar and variably on other enteric screening agars. Strains of *A. hydrophila* and *A. sobria* may be β-hemolytic on blood agar. Selective agar is available for recovery from stool specimens.

IDENTIFICATION METHODS

A motile, oxidase- and indole-positive organism can be tentatively identified as *Aeromonas/Plesiomonas/Vibrio*. Vibrios grow in 6% NaCl, whereas *Aeromonas* and *Plesiomonas* do not. Commercial systems will generally identify *Aeromonas* and *Plesiomonas* to the genus level. Key characteristics are listed in Table 44.16. There is no commercial test for the direct detection of antigen or nucleic acid in clinical specimens. Tests are not available for serologic diagnosis.

INTERPRETATION OF RESULTS

The isolation of either *Aeromonas* or *Plesiomonas* from specimens other than stool should be considered significant unless proven otherwise. Isolation from stool is suspicious but may be due to asymptomatic carriage.

Table 44.16. Differential Characteristics of *Aeromonas* and *Plesiomonas*[a]

Organism	DNase	Esculin Hydrolysis	Acid from Mannitol	Vogues-Proskauer	Arginine Dehydrolase	Lysine Decarboxylase	Ornithine Decarboxylase
A. hydrophilia	+	+	+	+	+	+	−
A. caviae	+	+	+	−	+	−	−
A. sobria	+	−	+	+	+	+	−
A. schubertii	+	−	−	+	+	+	−
A. veronii	+	+	+	+	−	+	+
P. shigelloides	−	−	−	−	+	+	+

[a]Symbols: +, positive; −, negative.

Therapeutic Considerations

Aeromonas is resistant to ampicillin and other penicillins, including some of the ureidopenicillins. Isolates are generally susceptible to the third-generation cephalosporins, quinolones, trimethoprim-sulfamethoxazole, and the aminoglycosides. The susceptibility of *Plesiomonas* has not been evaluated extensively. Because both genera can easily acquire resistance to antimicrobial agents, therapy should be based on the results of in vitro susceptibility tests.

Summary and Conclusions

The genera *Aeromonas* and *Plesiomonas* are common inhabitants of the aquatic environment. Infections are seen in both normal and immunocompromised hosts, usually following exposure to or consumption of contaminated water or foodstuffs. Therapy is based on the result of in vitro susceptibility testing.

VIBRIO

Microbiology

The genera *Vibrio*, *Photobacterium*, *Aeromonas*, and *Plesiomonas* are in the family Vibrionaceae. Two new genera (*Listonella* and *Shewanella*) have been proposed for inclusion in this family. Although 34 *Vibrio* species are recognized, only 12 have been associated with infections in humans. In general, *Vibrio* species share the following characteristics: Gram-negative, curved or straight rod, oxidase positive, reduced nitrate to nitrite, sodium required for or stimulates growth, susceptible to vibriostatic compound 0/129, motile by polar flagella, and facultatively anaerobic. *Photobacterium* is not associated with human infections.

Spectrum of Disease

Vibrio cholerae serogroup 01 is the etiologic agent of epidemic cholera. The other pathogenic species are usually associated with food-borne gastroenteritis, soft tissue infections or systemic infections such as meningitis, septicemia, cholecystitis, cellulitis, and a variety of other wound infections. *Vibrio parahaemolyticus* gastroenteritis is the most frequently encountered noncholera *Vibrio* infection. *Vibrio vulnificus* is an especially virulent species associated with primary sepsis (often in patients with preexisting liver disease) or with serious soft-tissue infections in normal hosts.

Epidemiology

Vibrio species inhabit aquatic environments worldwide. Although found primarily in marine ecosystems, some species can live in fresh water. Disease is transmitted via contaminated food (especially shellfish) or water. In epidemic cholera, food and water are usually contaminated by feces of patients and carriers. Gastroenteritis from the noncholera vibrios occurs in sporadic or common source outbreaks following consumption of raw, improperly prepared, or recontaminated seafood. Wounds are infected from exposure to contaminated water. Most infections occur in coastal locations, but more inland cases are being reported because of travel and shipment of contaminated food.

Diagnostic Procedures

MICROSCOPY

Direct examination of stools by wet mount for rapid, darting motility or by Gram smear for Gram-negative curved rods may be helpful in an outbreak situation but is not useful for identification of a sporadic case.

CULTURE TECHNIQUES

Routine primary isolation media such as blood and MacConkey agar are adequate for recovery of vibrios from extraintestinal specimens. Stool specimens are inoculated to thiosulfate-citrate-bile salts-sucrose (TCBS) agar. *Vibrio holisae* grows poorly or not at all on this medium. All cultures should be incubated at 35°C in air or CO_2, where most species form 1- to 2-mm colonies after 24 hours. Alkaline peptone broth can be used for the enrichment of fecal specimens.

Vibrio species may exhibit β-hemolysis on blood agar, are non–lactose fermentors (except *Vibrio vulnificus*) on MacConkey agar, and are differentiated by sucrose fermentation on TCBS. Non–sucrose-fermenting strains produce green colonies, whereas sucrose-fermenting strains form yellow colonies. Oxidase testing should be done from nonselective media.

Table 44.17. Characteristics Useful for Differentiating *Vibrio* from other Oxidase-Positive Genera[a]

Characteristic	*Vibrio*	*Pseudomonas*	*Aeromonas*	*Plesiomonas*
Growth on TCBS	+	−	−	−
Oxidase	+[b]	+	+	+
Fermentative	+	−	+	+
Growth stimulated by NaCl	+	−	−	−
Susceptibility to 0/129 (150 μg)	+	−	−	v

[a]Symbols: +, positive; −, negative; v, variable.
[b]*V. metschnikovii* is oxidase negative.

IDENTIFICATION TECHNIQUES

Initially, *Vibrio* spp. are separated from other genera by the oxidase reaction, fermentative metabolism, requirement of NaCl for growth, and susceptibility to 0/129 (Table 44.17). Identification can be made using routine biochemical tests if the NaCl concentration is increased to 1% (wt/vol) (Table 44.18). Commercial kits identify the more common *Vibrio* species (if the inoculum is prepared in saline) but cannot be used to identify the less common isolates.

DIRECT ANTIGEN OR NUCLEIC ACID DETECTION

Nucleic acid probes have been used in epidemiologic studies but are not commercially available and have not been evaluated as a direct diagnostic test.

Table 44.18. Tests for Differentiation of Members of the Vibrionaceae from Humans[a, b]

Test	*V. cholerae* 01 and non-0	*V. mimicus*	*V. parahaemolyticus*	*V. vulnificus*	*V. alginolyticus*	*V. cincinnatiensis*	*V. fluvialis*	*V. furnissii*	*V. damsela*	*V. hollisae*	*V. metschnikovii*	*Aeromonas* spp.	*Plesiomonas* spp.
Oxidase	+	+	+	+	+	+	+	+	+	+	−	+	+
NO_3-NO_2 + 1% NaCl	+	+	+	+	+	+	+	+	+	+	−	+	+
Indole + 1% NaCl	+	+	+	+	+	−	−	−	−	+/−	−/+	+/−	+
Voges-Proskauer + 1% NaCl	+/−	−	−	−	+/−	+	−	−	+	−	+/−	+/−	−
Urease	−	−	−/+	−	−	−	−	−	+	−	−	−	−
Lysine decarboxylase + 1% NaCl	+	+	+	+	+	+	−	−	+/−	−	+/−	−/+	+
Ornithine decarboxylase + 1% NaCl	+	+	+	+/−	+/−	−	−	−	−	−	−	−	+
Arginine dihydrolase + 1% NaCl	−	−	−	−	−	−	+	+	+	−	+/−	+/−	+
Fermentation of													
Sucrose	+	−	−	−/+	+	+	+	+	−	−	+	+/−	−
Lactose	(+)/−	+/−	−	+	−	−	−	−	−	−	+/−	−/+	+/−
L-Arabinose	−	−	+	−	−	+	+	+	−	+	−	+/−	−
Gas from glucose	−	−	−	−	−	−	−	+	−/+	−	−	−/+	−
Growth in nutrient broth													
0% NaCl	+	+	−	−	−	−	−	−	−	−	−	+	+
3% NaCl	+	+	+	+	+	+	+	+	+	+	+	+	+
6% NaCl	+/−	+/−	+	+/−	+	+	+/−	+/−	+	+/−	+	−	−
8% NaCl	−	−	+	−	+	−	−	−	−	−	−/−	−	−
10% NaCl	−	−	−	−	+/−	−	−	−	−	−	−	−	−
Susceptibility to 0/129													
10 μg	S	S	R	S	R	R	R	R	S	R	S	R	RS
150 μg	S	S	S	S	S	S	S	S	S	S	S	R	S
Growth on TCBS	Y	G	G	G/Y	Y	Y	Y	Y	G	G/−	Y	−	−

[a]From Janda JM, Powers C, Bryant RG, Abbott SL. Current perspectives on the epidemiology and pathogenesis of clinically significant *Vibrio* spp. Clin Microbiol Rev 1988;1:259.
[b]+, Most strains positive; −, most strains negative; +/− or −/+, variable reaction (predominant reaction shown as the numerator; ( ) = delayed reaction; S, susceptible; R, resistant; Y, yellow colonies; G, green colonies.

SEROLOGIC PROCEDURES

V. cholerae is identified as serogroup 01 or non-01 based on somatic antigens tested by a slide agglutination procedure. Serogroup 01 isolates are the cholera strains. A retrospective diagnosis of cholera can be made by a serologic test if the patient has not been vaccinated for cholera.

INTERPRETATION OF RESULTS

The isolation of *V. cholerae* is a reportable event because of the potential public health consequences. The isolation of other *Vibrio* species is clinically relevant, especially in the case of *V. vulnificus*, which has devastating consequences to the patient.

THERAPEUTIC CONSIDERATIONS

Fluid replacement is the primary treatment for epidemic cholera and is sometimes necessary in gastroenteritis caused by other *Vibrio* species. Antimicrobial agents are generally not necessary.

Soft tissue or systemic infections are usually treated with tetracycline. Most strains are also susceptible to chloramphemicol, aminoglycosides, and ciprofloxacin. Antimicrobial susceptibility testing can be performed without added NaCl.

Summary and Conclusions

V. cholerae, *V. parahaemolyticus*, and *V. vulnificus* are the most clinically important species of the pathogenic vibrios. All vibrios inhabit an aquatic environment, primarily a marine ecosystem. Cholera is of worldwide importance, while other noncholera vibrios cause significant gastroenteritis and soft tissue and systemic infections. *Vibrio* species are transmitted to humans through fecally contaminated food and water (*V. cholerae*), contaminated shellfish, or exposure to contaminated water. These bacteria are easily isolated on routine media, but TCBS agar is recommended for stool specimens. Identification is performed by routine biochemical tests containing 1% NaCl or in some cases by commercial kits. The key to the isolation of *Vibrio* is recognition of the colony on the primary isolation plate.

CAMPYLOBACTER AND *HELICOBACTER*

Microbiology

The taxonomy and nomenclature of the genus *Campylobacter* is changing rapidly as old species are renamed and new species identified. Currently, 14 species have been proposed. *Campylobacter pyloridis* has been renamed *Helicobacter pylori* based on RNA analysis (37). *Campylobacter nitrofigilis, Campylobacter concisus, Campylobacter sputorum, and Campylobacter fetus* subsp. *venerealis* are usually not associated with human disease. A number of additional campylobacter-like organisms are awaiting definitive identification.

Campylobacter species are slender, curved, Gram-negative rods (0.5 to 5 μm in length) that may have a "comma," "S," gull wing, or spiral shape, and exhibit a characteristic darting motility (polar flagella) on wet mount. They are oxidase positive, microaerophilic, and capnophilic (5% O_2, 10% CO_2, and 85% N_2) and are inactive toward carbohydrates.

Spectrum of Disease

Campylobacter species are associated with two categories of disease: gastrointestinal and extraintestinal (usually bacteremia). *H. pylori* causes ulcers of the gastric or duodenal mucosa. The majority of gastrointestinal disease is caused by *Campylobacter jejuni* and *Campylobacter coli*. *C. fetus* subsp. *fetus* typically causes extraintestinal infections such as bacteremia, cholecystitis, meningitis, septic abortion, and septic arthritis. Infection is often associated with underlying disorders such as hepatic disease, immunodeficiency, alcoholism, and diabetes.

Epidemiology

Campylobacter species are found in the gastrointestinal tract of wild and domesticated animal species, including cattle, sheep, swine, goats, dogs, cats, rodents, and all fowl. This results in the contamination of food (especially meat), milk, and water that is consumed by humans. Transmission also occurs from direct contact with infected pets (dogs and cats), person-to-person contact, or the sexual practices of homosexual men. Cases occur year-round but with a peak incidence in the summer and fall. *C. jejuni* is isolated more frequently from patients with diarrhea than *Salmonella* or *Shigella*.

Diagnostic Techniques

MICROSCOPY

A presumptive diagnosis of *Campylobacter* enteritis is made by the examination of a stool specimen by Gram stain or wet mount using dark-field or phase-contrast microscopy. *Campylobacter* species will have a very rapid, darting motility on wet mount or have a slender, curved morphology on Gram stain (Fig. 44.12). Safranin should remain on the smear for 2 to 3 minutes to enhance staining.

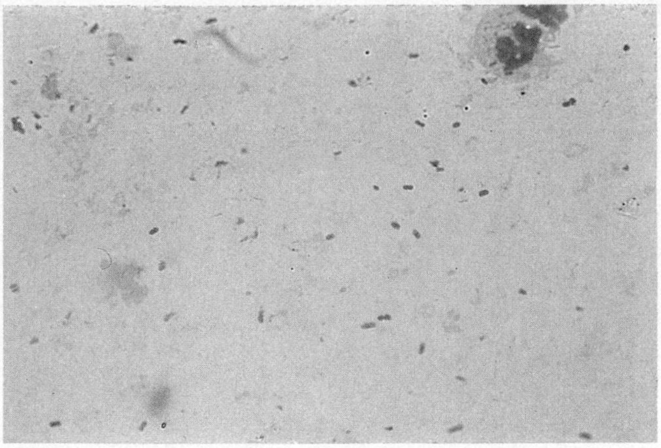

Figure 44.12. Gram stain of *C. jejuni* in stool. Note the curved and S-shaped forms.

CULTURE TECHNIQUES

Campylobacter species grow on most blood-containing media (e.g., blood or chocolate agar). Isolation from stool usually requires direct inoculation to a selective agar (e.g., Campy-BAP, Butzler, or Skirrow medium) or filtration (0.45 to 0.65 μm) and then inoculation to nonselective medium. The latter method is optimal for the recovery of *C. jejuni* and atypical enteric campylobacters. Enrichment broths are not necessary for isolation from stool specimens. All campylobacters grow at 35 to 37°C, but *C. jejuni*, *C. coli*, and *Campylobacter laridis* will also grow at 42°C. Colonies are 1 to 2 mm in diameter, smooth, convex, and translucent after 24 to 48 hours. Enteric campylobacters produce two colony types: round and raised or flat and watery with an irregular edge. Cultures for *C. jejuni* are routinely incubated for 48 hours but may be held up to 5 days for the uncommon campylobacters. Microaerophilic conditions (5% O_2, 10% CO_2, 85% N_2) are required for growth.

H. pylori can be isolated on chocolate agar or a selective medium (38). Cultures are incubated in a microaerophilic, moist environment at 35°C for up to 7 days.

IDENTIFICATION TECHNIQUES

Campylobacter species from stool are presumptively identified by their typical cellular morphology, oxidase-positive reaction, and a rapid, darting motility in broth. Alternatively, suspect colonies can be tested by using a commercial latex agglutination kit. *H. pylori* is presumptively identified by demonstrating a rapid urease reaction (within 30 minutes) after a portion of the gastric biopsy specimen is placed in Christensen's urea broth.

Conventional biochemical and physiological tests are necessary for the definitive identification of *Campylobacter* species (Table 44.19). Guidelines for setting up these tests can be found in reference 39.

DIRECT ANTIGEN OR NUCLEIC ACID TECHNIQUE

Nucleic acid probes have been used to identify suspected colonies or growth in enrichment cultures, but are not commercially available for the direct detection in stool specimens.

SEROLOGIC PROCEDURES

Currently, there are no commercial systems available for the detection of antibodies to *Campylobacter* infection, but the use of serology for the diagnosis of *H. pylori* infection is promising (40).

INTERPRETATION OF RESULTS

The isolation of *C. jejuni*, *C. coli*, or *C. fetus* subsp. *fetus* is considered clinically significant. The isolation of the other *Campylobacter* species should be evaluated with respect to the source and symptoms of the patient. The question of whether *H. pylori* causes gastritis or merely colonizes the gastric mucosa is not completely resolved, but evidence is mounting for its role in the disease.

Therapeutic Considerations

Most cases of gastroenteritis are self limited and do not require antimicrobial therapy unless the patient suffers from severe disease. Septic or bacteremic patients require therapy. *C. jejuni* is susceptible to a number of antimicrobial agents (e.g., erythromycin, tetracyclines, aminoglycosides, quinolones, and clindamycin); erythromycin is the drug of choice for gastroenteritis. Treatment of serious extraintestinal infections should be based on susceptibility testing. *H. pylori* is susceptible to amoxicillin, nitrofurans, metronidazole, and bismuth salts, but relapses often occur.

Summary and Conclusions

Campylobacters are isolated from a variety of animals, are most often transmitted to humans via contaminated food (e.g., meat and milk), and cause significant human disease such as gastroenteritis and disseminated infections. A microaerophilic environment is necessary for their isolation on laboratory media. Selective media or filtration is required for isolation from stool specimens. A limited number of tests are available for the differentiation of the various *Campylobacter* species. When necessary, erythromycin is the drug of choice in gastrointestinal infections. *Campylobacter* species are among the most frequently isolated bacterial agents of diarrheal dis-

Table 44.19. Differential Reactions and Characteristics for Species of the Genus *Campylobacter*[a, b]

Species	Catalase	Nitrate	H_2S (TSI)	Hippurate	Indoxyl Acetate	Growth					Susceptibility[c]	
						25°C	37°C	42°C	1% Glycine	3.5% NaCl	Nalidixic Acid	Cephalothin
C. fetus subsp. *fetis*	+	+	−	−	−	+	+	(−)	+	−	R	S
C. fetus subsp. *venerealis*	+	+	−	−	−	+	+	−	−	−	R	S
C. hyointestinalis	+	+	+	−	−	(+)	+	+	+	−	R	S
C. jejuni subsp. *jejuni*	+	+	−	+	+	−	+	+	+	−	S	R
C. jejuni subsp. *doylei*	d	−	−	+	ND	−	+	(+)	ND	ND	S	S
C. coli	+	+	−	−	+	−	+	+	+	−	S	R
C. laridis	+	+	−	−	−	−	+	+	+	−	R	R
C. upsaliensis	(−)	+	−	−	ND	−	+	+	−	−	S	S
C. cinaedi	+	+	−	−	(−)	−	+	−	+	−	S	I
C. fennelliae	+	−	−	−	+	−	+	−	+	−	S	S
C. cryaerophilia	+	+	−	−	+	+	+	−	−	−	d	R
C. nitrofigilis	+	+	ND	−	−	+	+	−	−	ND	S	S
C. sputorum												
Biovar sputorum	−	+	(+)	−	−	−	+	+	+	−	(S)	S
Biovar bubulus	−	+	+	−	−	−	+	+	+	+	R	S
Biovar fecalis	+	+	+	−	−	−	+	+	+	+	R	S
C. mucosalis	−	+	+	−	−	+	+	+	+	−	R	S
C. concisus	−	+	+	−	ND	−	+	+	+	−	R	R
H. pylori	+	d	−	−	−	−	+	+	d		R	S

[a]Modified from Penner JL. The genus *Campylobacter:* a decade of progress. Clin Microbiol Rev 1988;1:157–172.
[b]+, Positive reaction; −, negative reaction; ND, no test results found; (+), most strains positive but a low percentage negative; (−), most strains negative but some positive or weakly positive; d, different reactions; R, resistant; S, susceptible; I, intermediate zones of inhibition.
[c]Susceptibility to antibiotics was determined with 30-μg disks.

ease. *H. pylori* is associated with ulcers of the gastric or duodenal mucosa.

LEGIONELLA

Microbiology

Legionella is the only genus in the family Legionellaceae and contains more than 30 species and 50 serogroups (41). Most of the species are environmental isolates not associated with human infections.

Legionella species are aerobic, Gram-negative rods that are 0.5 μm in width and 2 to 20 μm in length. The organisms appear coccobacillary in clinical specimens but may be filamentous in some culture media. They stain poorly with safranin, are nutritionally fastidious, and do not grow on routine laboratory media. L-Cysteine is an essential growth component of culture media, while α-ketoglutaric acid and iron stimulate growth. The cellular fatty acids of *Legionella* are primarily branched-chain, and the bacteria contain large amounts of ubiquinones. *Legionella* are catalase positive, urease negative, and oxidase variable. They liquefy gelatin, do not reduce nitrates, and do not metabolize carbohydrates. Some strains produce a pigment that fluoresces yellow-green, blue-white, or red-pink under long-wave ultraviolet light.

Spectrum of Disease

Legionella species cause two clinical syndromes (pneumonia and Pontiac fever, a flu-like illness) and asymptomatic infections. Pontiac fever and asymptomatic infections are diagnosed by an increase in antibody titers to *Legionella*. Extrapulmonary infections are not common but have included bacteremia, sinusitis, pyelonephritis, pericarditis, hepatic and perirectal abscess, endocarditis, peritonitis, and wound infections. Risk factors for the development of pneumonia include cigarette smoking, advanced age, chronic lung disease, and immunosuppression.

Epidemiology

The natural habitat of *Legionella* is aquatic environments, where it exists in symbiosis with other microorganisms. Man-made aquatic reservoirs such as cooling towers and water distribution systems serve as reservoirs for human exposure. Currently, it is believed that potable water systems are the primary reservoir. The mode of transmission from the reservoir to humans remains uncertain but is thought to be primarily airborne. Dissemination from the gastrointestinal tract following ingestion has been proposed but not documented. Epidemic outbreaks are usually associated with institutions such as hospitals, hotels, and resorts.

Diagnostic Techniques

MICROSCOPY

Legionella stains faintly with a routine Gram stain. Visualization is enhanced by staining with safranin

Table 44.20. Phenotypic Properties of *Legionella*[a, b]

Species	Hippurate Hydrolysis	Oxidase	β-Lactamase	Autofluorescence
L. anisa	−[c]	+	+	+/−(BW)
L. birminghamensis	−	+/−	+	+(YG)
L. bozemanii	−	+/−	+/−	+(BW)
L. cherrii	−	−	+	+(BW)
L. cincinnatiensis	−	−	+	−
L. dumoffii	−	−	+	+(BW)
L. erythra	−	+	+	+(RP)
L. feeleii[d]	+/−	−	−	−
L. gormanii	−	−	+	+(BW)
L. hackeliae	−	+	+	−
L. israelensis	−	−	+	−
L. jamestowniensis	−	−	+	−
L. jordanis	−	+/−	+	−
L. longbeachae	−	+	+/−	−
L. maceachernii	−	+	−	−
L. micdadei[a]	−	+	−	−
L. oakridgensis[e]	−	−	+(W)	−
L. parisiensis	−	+	+	+(BW)
L. pneumophilia	+	+/−	+	+(YG)
L. rubrilucens	−	−	+	+(RP)
L. sainthelensi	−	+	+	−
L. santicrucis	−	+	+	−
L. spiritensis	+(W)	+	+	−
L. steigerwaltii	−	−	+	+(BW)
L. wadsworthii	−	−	+	−

[a]Modified from Wilkinson HW. Legionellosis. In: Balows A, Hausler WJ Jr, Ohashi M, Turano A, eds. Laboratory diagnosis of infectious diseases: principles and practice, vol 1. New York: Springer-Verlag, 1988:320–332.
[b]All strains required cysteine to grow except for L. oakridgensis, which required it only when first isolated.
[c]+ = positive; − = negative; +/− = not always positive; W = weakly positive; BW = blue-white; RP = red-pink; YG = yellow-green (not usually observed on charcoal-containing agar for *L. pneumophila*).
[d]Negative for gelatin liquefaction.
[e]Nonmotile.

for 2 to 3 minutes, using carbol-fuschin as the counterstain, or staining only with crystal violet and Gram's iodine without decolorization. The organisms are more difficult to stain in tissue, where the recommended procedure is the Warthin-Starry or Dieterle stain. *Legionella micdadei* may appear acid fast in tissue.

CULTURE TECHNIQUES

The preferred method is to inoculate the specimen to two agar plates, one of which is buffered charcoal yeast extract (BCYE) agar without inhibitory agents. A second medium, BCYE with antimicrobial agents, is recommended for specimens that are likely to be contaminated with other microbial flora. Acid treatment of potentially contaminated specimens may increase the yield (42). *Legionella* have been recovered from blood culture (e.g., biphasic, Bactec, and lysis centrifugation) but may require blind subculture from broth media. BCYE agar is incubated at 35° to 37°C in air or CO_2 (not more than 5%) for up to 2 weeks. Pinpoint growth may be detected in 2 to 3 days. After 5 to 7 days' incubation, colonies are 3 to 4 mm in diameter, gray, convex, and glistening.

IDENTIFICATION METHODS

Suspected colonies on BCYE agar are subcultured to another BCYE plate and to blood agar or preferably to a BCYE plate without added cysteine. Growth on BCYE but not on the other medium is presumptive evidence of a *Legionella* species. *Francisella tularensis* grows on BCYE and may not grow on cysteine-deficient medium.

The isolate is identified at the genus level by commercial immunologic reagents or nucleic acid probes. *Legionella* species can be separated into groups based on a limited number of phenotypic characteristics (Table 44.20) (43). Because therapy is similar for all species, identification to the genus level is adequate for most clinical laboratories.

DIRECT ANTIGEN OR NUCLEIC ACID TECHNIQUES

Kits for the direct detection of antigen in clinical specimens by direct fluorescent antibody (DFA) reagents, nucleic acid probe (NAP), or radioimmunoassay (RIA) (restricted to urine specimens) are commercially available. The sensitivities of the DFA, NAP, and RIA methods are approximately 25 to 80%, 60 to

70%, and 79 to 90%, respectively (44). Specificity for the three methods is 96 to 100%.

SEROLOGIC PROCEDURES

A number of serologic tests are available for the diagnosis of *Legionella* infection. The enzyme immunoassay (EIA) and indirect fluorescent antibody (IFA) tests are the most frequently used. Demonstration of a four-fold rise in titers (IgG and IgM) to 1:128 or greater is considered diagnostic. Between 2 and 8 weeks are sometimes needed to demonstrate an antibody rise. Cross-reactions with other Gram-negative organisms are infrequently observed.

INTERPRETATION OF RESULTS

Since *Legionella* is not part of the normal human flora, the isolation of any species is clinically significant. Culture is the mainstay of diagnosis, with a sensitivity of 50 to 80% from respiratory secretions (44). Direct detection methods are helpful when positive but cannot be used to rule out infection by *Legionella*. A four-fold rise to a 1:128 antibody titer confirms a recent infection. A single high titer is suggestive of recent infection but is not diagnostic.

Therapeutic Considerations

Erythromycin remains the drug of choice for the treatment of *Legionella* infections. Rifampin may be added in some cases because the organism is primarily intracellular. Anecdotal reports suggest that imipenem, ciprofloxacin, trimethoprim-sulfamethoxazole, or tetracycline may be efficacious. Standardized methods for in vitro susceptibility testing of *Legionella* are not available.

Summary and Conclusions

Legionella species are ubiquitous inhabitants of natural and man-made aquatic systems. Transmission is thought to occur from inhalation of aerosolized bacteria. Infections are usually asymptomatic, flu-like in nature, or a pneumonia. Laboratory diagnosis is made by isolation on BCYE agar; direct detection of antigen in clinical specimens by use of a direct fluorescent antibody test, a nucleic acid probe, or radioimmunoassay, or retrospectively by serology. Identification of the isolate to the genus level is sufficient in most instances. Erythromycin is the drug of choice for treatment.

HAEMOPHILUS

Microbiology

The genus *Haemophilus* is one of three genera in the family Pasteurellaceae. Currently, the genus includes 16 species and three species of uncertain status (22). Ten species are associated with humans. *Haemophilus* species are facultatively anaerobic, nonmotile, pleomorphic, coccoid to coccobacillary, Gram-negative rods that require hemin (X factor) or nicotinamide adenine dinucleotide (NAD, V factor) or both for growth. They are usually oxidase and catalase positive, and CO_2 enhances the growth of some species.

Spectrum of Disease

Haemophilus influenzae consists of six capsular serotypes (a to f) and unencapsulated strains. The majority of *Haemophilus* infections in humans are caused by *H. influenzae*, and approximately 95% of invasive disease is due to serotype b. *H. influenzae* type b infections occur primarily in children and include meningitis, bacteremia, epiglottitis, pneumonia and empyema, septic arthritis, cellulitis, pericarditis, osteomyelitis, and a variety of less frequently encountered infections. Encapsulated strains are associated with infections such as chronic bronchitis, otitis media, sinusitis, and conjunctivitis.

The other *Haemophilus* species cause a variety of clinically similar infections. *Haemophilus parainfluenzae*, *Haemophilus aphrophilus*, *Haemophilus paraphrophilus*, and *Haemophilus aegyptius* are the species most frequently isolated from infections. The first three species are most commonly associated with systemic infections, primarily with endocarditis, and *H. aegyptius* with eye infections and Brazilian purpuric fever.

Haemophilus ducreyi is the etiologic agent of the sexually transmitted disease chancroid (soft chancre).

Epidemiology

Haemophilus species are part of the normal flora in the upper respiratory tract (nasopharynx, pharynx, and oral cavity) and the genital tract in women. Unencapsulated strains of *H. influenzae* are isolated from 50 to 90% of the population, whereas serotype b is carried by less than 5%. Transmission of *H. influenzae* is thought to occur via respiratory droplets and is enhanced in crowded conditions (e.g., day care centers). *H. ducreyi* is transmitted by sexual contact. The highest incidence of chancroid is in Asia, Africa, and Central America.

Diagnostic Techniques

MICROSCOPY

The presence of small, Gram-negative coccobacilli in sterile body fluids (e.g., CSF, synovial fluids) or in

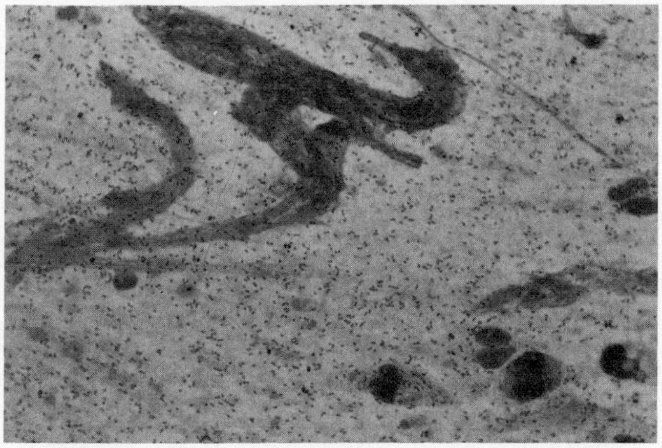

Figure 44.13. Gram stain of *H. influenzae* in sputum.

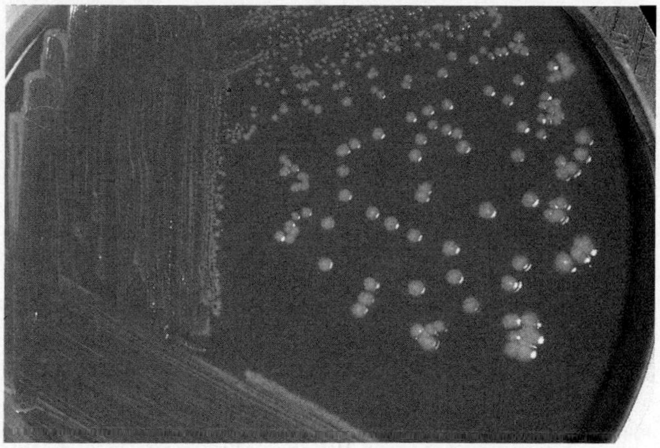

Figure 44.14. Colony of *H. influenzae* on chocolate agar.

respiratory secretions is suggestive of *Haemophilus* (Fig. 44.13).

Gram stain smears of exudate from genital lesions revealing large numbers of Gram-negative coccobacilli occurring in parallel chains (schools of fish) is suggestive of *H. ducreyi*, but smears are usually negative.

CULTURE TECHNIQUES

Specimens should be plated on enriched chocolate agar and incubated in 5% CO_2 at 35° to 37°C for 2 to 3 days. *Haemophilus* may be isolated on blood agar as satelliting colonies around staphylococci or other organisms.

Although *H. ducreyi* can be isolated on enriched chocolate agar, vancomycin (3 μg/ml) should be added to inhibit the growth of contaminating flora. Multiple media (e.g., heart infusion base with 10% fetal bovine serum and 3 μg/ml vancomycin) and multiple cultures are recommended for optimal recovery. Media should be incubated at 33°C in 5% CO_2 in a moist environment for up to 7 days.

Colonies on chocolate agar are usually small (0.5 to 1 mm), grayish, round, translucent, and smooth (Fig. 44.14). *Haemophilus haemolyticus, Haemophilus parahaemolyticus,* and *Haemophilus paraphrohaemolyticus* may be β-hemolytic. Colonies of *H. ducreyi* are small, flat, smooth, and yellow-gray and can be pushed across the agar. *H. aphrophilus* and *H. paraphrophilus* produce larger colonies (1 to 1.5 mm) that are opaque, granular, and yellowish.

IDENTIFICATION METHODS

Most laboratories presumptively identify *Haemophilus* species on the basis of their growth around the disks containing hemin (X factor) or NAD (V factor), or by using the commercially available porphyrin test. Additional testing is necessary for a definitive identification (Table 44.21). *H. influenzae* and *H. parainfluenzae* can be further differentiated into biovars (45). Commercial systems are available for the identification and biotyping of some *Haemophilus* species.

DIRECT DETECTION AND NUCLEIC ACID TECHNIQUES

Particle agglutination kits are available for the direct detection of *H. influenzae* type b capsular antigen in clinical specimens. The systems have the highest sensitivity and specificity when performed on CSF rather than on urine or serum. The sensitivity of the test on CSF specimens varies from 70 to 90%.

SEROLOGIC PROCEDURES

Serologic procedures are not generally useful for assisting in the diagnosis of infection by *Haemophilus* species.

INTERPRETATION OF RESULTS

The isolation of *H. ducreyi*, other *Haemophilus* species from normally sterile body fluids or deep tissues, or *H. influenzae* (*H. aegyptius*) from the eye is clinically relevant. The significance of the isolation of *H. influenzae* (especially serotype b) or other species from respiratory secretions depends on the evaluation of the patient.

Therapeutic Considerations

Empiric treatment for life-threatening infections caused by *H. influenzae* type b consists of third-generation cephalosporins. β-Lactamase activity should be determined on all *Haemophilus* species and susceptibility testing performed on isolates from serious infections.

Table 44.21. Differential Characteristics of the Genus *Haemophilus*[a]

Species	X-Factor Requirement[b]	V-Factor Requirement	Indole	Urease	Hemolysis	Oxidase	Catalase	Glucose	Sucrose	Lactose
H. influenzae	+	+	V[c]	V	−	+	+	+	−	−
H. haemolyticus	+	+	V	−	+	+	+	+	−	−
H. aegyptius	+	+	−	+	−	+	−	+	−	−
H. parainfluenzae	−	+	V	V	−	+	V	+	+	−
H. segnis	−	+	−	−	−	−	V	W[d]	W	−
H. parahaemolyticus[e]	−	+	−	+	+	+	+	+	+	−
H. paraphrophilus	−	+	−	−	−	+	−	+	+	+
H. aphrophilus	−	−	−	−	−	−	−	+	+	+
H. ducreyi	+	−	−	−	−	+	−	−	−	−

[a]Modified from Albritton WL. *Haemophilus influenzae* infections. In: Balows A, Hausler WJ Jr, Ohashi M, Turans A, eds. Laboratory diagnosis of infectious diseases: principles and practice, vol 1. New York: Springer-Verlag, 1988:302–311.
[b]As determined by porphyrin test.
[c]Variable.
[d]Weak.
[e]*H. paraphaemolyticus* and *H. paraphrohaemoyticus* differ only in the requirement for CO_2.

Summary and Conclusions

Haemophilus species are a component of the normal flora of the upper respiratory tract and, in part, the genital tract. *H. influenzae* (especially serotype b) causes the majority of human infections, which range from invasive life-threatening infections (e.g., meningitis) to less serious problems such as bronchitis. The other species are infrequently implicated but can cause similar types of infections, especially endocarditis. *H. ducreyi* is the etiologic agent of chancroid. The requirement of hemin (X factor) and NAD (V factor) for growth helps determine the identity of some species. The increasing resistance of *H. influenzae* has complicated therapy and requires routine susceptibility testing of significant isolates.

NONFERMENTATIVE GRAM-NEGATIVE BACILLI

Microbiology

The group of nonfermentative gram-negative bacilli (NFB) is one of convenience for the clinical microbiologist and describes bacteria that are Gram-negative rods and relatively inert biochemically. On the oxidation-reduction medium of Hugh and Leifson, they may produce an oxidative or alkaline reaction or no reaction. Most species are strict aerobes, are catalase positive (*Eikenella* is catalase negative and facultatively anaerobic), and are oxidase positive (*Acinetobacter*, CDC group Ve-1, Ve-2 are negative; *Pseudomonas cepacia* and *Xanthomonas maltophilia* are weakly positive). *Kingella* and CDC group EF-4 are weak fermentors and may be mistaken for NFB. Most species grow on MacConkey agar (except *Eikenella*, *Moraxella*, some *Flavobacterium* species, and CDC group IIf, IIj, and IVe) at 35°C in air. Some species grow better at 25° to 30°C. The arrangement of the flagella may be useful for the identification of some species.

The classification of the NFB is constantly being revised without a strong consensus from the taxonomists. Table 44.22 lists the current or old name, the proposed name, or a synonym for a limited number of species. The reader is referred to the general references for a more thorough discussion of the classification of NFB (46).

Spectrum of Disease

The NFB comprise approximately 15 to 20% of all the Gram-negative rods that are isolated in the clinical laboratory. *P. aeruginosa* accounts for 70% of the NFB isolates. The next most frequently isolated species are *Acinetobacter*, *P. cepacia*, and *X. maltophilia* (*P. maltophilia*). Infections by the other species are rare, and most isolations are not clinically significant but represent colonization. Infections, when they occur, are usually hospital-acquired necrotizing pneumonia, urinary tract infection, wound infection, bacteremia, and endocarditis. These organisms are not associated with gastrointestinal disease and are seldom isolated from feces.

Pseudomonas aeruginosa is the most frequently isolated NFB. In the hospitalized patient, especially the immunocompromised person, infection by *P. aeruginosa* is often life-threatening and can present as bacteremia, pneumonia, skin and soft tissue infection, urinary tract infection, or gastrointestinal infection. Burn and cystic fibrosis patients are highly susceptible to infection. Commmunity-acquired infections include folliculitis associated with whirlpools; otitis externa in divers, swimmers, and diabetics; osteomyelitis associated with deep puncture wounds; ocular infections associated with wearing contact lenses; and endocarditis and vertebral osteomyelitis in IV drug addicts. *Acinetobacter* is recovered primarily as a colonizer but has caused suppurative infections in

Table 44.22. Taxonomy of Nonfermentative Gram-Negative Bacilli

Current Name	Proposed Name	Synonym
Achromobacter xylosoxidans	*Alcaligenes xylosoxidans* subsp. *xylosoxidans*	*Alcaligenes dentrificans* subsp. *xylosoxidans*
Alcaligenes dentrificans	*Alcaligenes xylosoxidans* subsp. *dentrificans*	*Alcaligenes dentrificans* subsp. *dentrificans*
Alcaligenes odorans	*Alcaligenes faecalis*	*Pseudomonas odorans*
CDC IIe	*Flavobacterium* species IIe	
CDC IIh	*Flavobacterium* species IIh	
CDC IIi	*Flavobacterium* species IIi	
CDC IIb	*Flavobacterium gleum*	
CDC IIf	*Weeksella virosa*	*Flavobacterium genitale*
CDC IIj	*Weeksella zoohelcum*	
CDC Ve-1	*Chryseomonas luteola*	*Chryseomonas polytricha*
CDC Ve-2	*Flavimonas oryzihabitans*	*Pseudomonas oryzihabitans*
CDC IVe	*Oligella ureolytica*	
Moraxella urethralis	*Oligella urethralis*	CDC group M-4
Pseudomonas acidovorans	*Comamonas acidovorans*	
Pseudomonas testosteroni	*Comamonas testosteroni*	
Pseudomonas maltophilia	*Xanthomonas maltophilia*	
Pseudomonas putrefaciens	*Shewanella putrefaciens*	*Alteromonas putrefaciens*

nearly every organ system. It is primarily a nosocomial pathogen, with most infections due to *Acinetobacter calcoaceticus* var. *anitratus*.

Pseudomonas pseudomallei causes melioidosis, a rare infection in North America. Most cases occur in people returning from travel to endemic areas. The disease often presents with acute pneumonia but may occur as a localized infection. A high mortality rate is associated with septicemia and dissemination.

Pseudomonas mallei causes glanders, a disease of horses that may be transmitted to humans. It is rarely seen today.

P. cepacia and *X. maltophilia* are important nosocomial pathogens. Although less virulent than *P. aeruginosa*, these organisms cause similar types of infections in the hospitalized patient. The other pseudomonads are primarily colonizers but have been isolated from documented infections.

Alcaligenes xylosoxidans (*Achromobacter xylosoxidans*) has been reported to cause individual cases of meningitis, pneumonia, peritonitis, urinary tract infection, bacteremia, and endocarditis (prosthetic valve). *Oligella ureolytica* (CDC group Vd) has been recovered from pancreatic abscesses, bacteremia, and urinary tract infections. CDC group IVe has been associated with urinary tract infections in patients with indwelling Foley catheters. *Alcaligenes* has caused external ear infections. The *Flavobacterium* species cause infrequent cases of neonatal meningitis, bacteremia, endocarditis, wound infections, and respiratory tract infections. *Weeksella zoohelcum* (CDC group IIj) is isolated from bites and scratches of dogs and cats and *Weeksella virosa* (CDC group IIf) from urinary tract infections. *Moraxella* (especially *Moraxella lacunata*) causes primarily eye infections. *Eikenella* has been recovered from a variety of infections, including human bites, head and neck infections, skin infections in drug addicts, and a variety of other deep-seated or systemic infections.

Epidemiology

Most NFB can be isolated from soil, water, vegetation, or nearly any moist location. Minimal nutritional requirements and their antimicrobial resistance, particularly of *P. aeruginosa*, have led to their emergence as nosocomial pathogens. Hospital reservoirs include respiratory equipment, disinfectants, sinks, solutions, food, etc., while disease-related reservoirs outside the hospital include whirlpools, hot tubs, and contact lens solution. *P. aeruginosa* colonizes the skin, oropharynx, and gastrointestinal tract in 2 to 10% of healthy persons. The rate of colonization is usually higher in hospitalized patients. Transmission occurs via contaminated solutions, equipment, food, and probably on the hands of hospital personnel. *P. aeruginosa* accounts for approximately 10% of all hospital-acquired infections.

P. pseudomallei inhabits soil and water but is restricted primarily to Southeast Asia and other tropical or subtropical parts of the world. Transmission is primarily through abrasions or cuts but may occur by inhalation or ingestion.

Eikenella and *Moraxella* are common inhabitants of the mucous membranes of the upper respiratory tract. *Eikenella* is also part of the gastrointestinal flora. Infections arise from breaks in the mucous membranes.

Diagnostic Procedures

MICROSCOPY

All of the NFB are Gram-negative rods. In general, *Pseudomonas* species appear as thin rods; *Acinetobacter*

Table 44.23. Characteristics of Genera of Nonfermentative Bacteria[a]

Genus	Catalase	Oxidase	Growth on MacConkey Agar	Motility	Utilization of Glucose
Pseudomonas	+	+[b]	Good	Motile by means of polar flagella	Oxidative
Achromobacter	+	+[c]	Good	Motile by means of peritrichous flagella	Oxidative
Alcaligenes	+	+	Good	Motile by means of peritrichous flagella	Inactive
Acinetobacter	+	−	Good	Nonmotile	Oxidative or inactive
Flavobacterium	+	+	Variable	Nonmotile	Oxidative
Moraxella	+/−	+	Variable	Nonmotile	Inactive
Eikenella	−	+	Negative	Nonmotile	Inactive
Kingella	−	+	Variable	Nonmotile	Delayed fermentative
EF-4	+	+	Variable	Nonmotile	Delayed fermentative

[a]Modified from Oberhofer TR, Howard BJ. Nonfermentative Gram-negative bacteria. In: Howard BJ, Klass J II, Rubin Sj, Weissfeld AS, Tilton RC, eds. Clinical and pathogenic microbiology. St. Louis: CV Mosby, 1987:329–358.
[b]*X. maltophilia* is usually oxidase-negative. *P. cepacia* may be negative.
[c]Symbols: +, Positive; −, Negative; +/−, most strains positive.

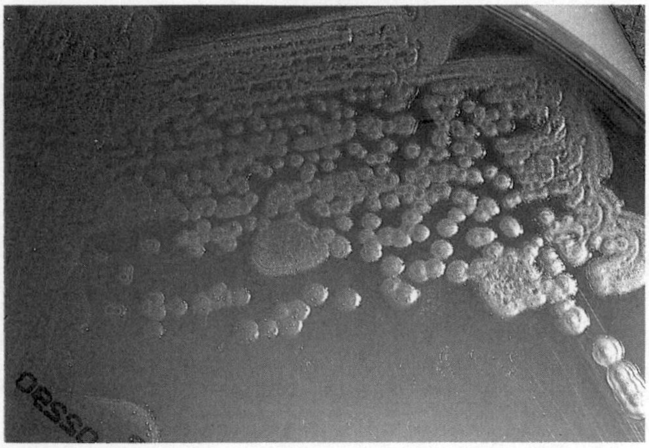

Figure 44.15. Colony of *P. aeruginosa* on Mueller-Hinton agar. Note the blue-green diffusible pigment.

are coccobacillary (may be filamentous); *Moraxella* are fat, short rods; and *Eikenella* are coccobacillary when stained in clinical specimens. The morphology cannot be used for a definitive identification. *Acinetobacter* and *Moraxella* may resemble *Neisseria*.

CULTURE TECHNIQUES

Most NFB are recovered on blood or MacConkey agars after 24 hours at 35°C in air or CO_2. *Eikenella, Moraxella*, and some *Flavobacterium* species and CDC groups do not grow on MacConkey agar, and some NFB grow better at 25° to 30°C.

P. aeruginosa produces a flat colony with a feathered edge; may be β-hemolytic; has a grape-like odor; and may produce a pigment, pyocyanin (blue-green), pyoverdin (fluorescein), pyorubin (red), or pyomelanin (brown) (Fig. 44.15). Pyocyanin pigment production is enhanced by growth on *Pseudomonas* agar (Difco) or Tech agar (BBL); fluorescein by growth on *Pseudomonas* F agar (Difco) or FLO agar (BBL). *P. pseudomallei, Pseudomonas stutzeri*, and CDC group Ve form wrinkled colonies. *Alcaligenes* may produce a fruity odor. The *Flavobacterium* species generally produce a yellow pigment; *Acinetobacter* colonies resemble the Enterobacteriaceae; *Moraxella* colonies are tiny (less than 1 mm) after 24 hours; and *Eikenella* colonies may pit or corrode the agar.

IDENTIFICATION METHODS

The initial characterization of NFB is based on five characteristics: oxidase reaction, catalase reaction, growth on MacConkey agar, motility, and whether the organism uses glucose fermentatively, oxidatively, or not at all (Table 44.23).

The differential characteristics of *P. aeruginosa* and the other pseudomonads are presented in Table 44.24. If pyocyanin is present and the isolate is oxidase positive, it is identified as *P. aeruginosa* without any additional tests. *Pseudomonas* species are motile with polar flagella, grow on MacConkey agar, and are oxidase positive (*X. maltophilia* and *P. cepacia* may be negative), glucose oxidizers, and catalase positive.

Alcaligenes are motile by peritrichous flagella, are oxidase and catalase positive, grow on MacConkey agar, do not oxidize glucose, and are relatively inert. Species of *Acinetobacter* are nonmotile, catalase positive, oxidase negative, and nitrate negative, grow on MacConkey agar, and are either oxidative or inactive toward glucose. *Flavobacterium* species, some *Weeksella*, and some *Sphingobacterium* species are nonmotile, are catalase and oxidase positive, exhibit variable growth on MacConkey agar, produce a yellow pigment, and may be oxidative or inactive toward glucose. The *Moraxella* are nonmotile, inactive toward glucose, oxidase positive, and catalase variable, and exhibit variable growth on MacConkey agar (Table 44.25). *Eikenella corrodens* is oxidase positive, catalase negative, and inactive toward glucose, does not grow on MacConkey agar, is nonmotile, may pit the agar, and has a bleach-like odor (Table 44.25).

A number of commercial systems with variable accuracy are available for the identification of NFB (27). Another commercially available system analyzes cell wall fatty acids by gas-liquid chromatography.

DIRECT ANTIGEN OR NUCLEIC ACID DETECTION

No commercial system is available for the direct detection of NFB in clinical specimens.

SEROLOGIC PROCEDURES

A four-fold rise in titer with the hemagglutination, complement-fixation, or agglutination test aids in the diagnosis of melioidosis. Titers greater than 1:8 (complement fixation) or greater than 1:160 (agglutination) are diagnostic or highly suggestive of infection during the acute illness. These tests are performed only in reference laboratories because of the low incidence of the disease. Serologic tests for the diagnosis of infections caused by the other NFB are not routinely available.

INTERPRETATION OF RESULTS

The isolation of *P. pseudomallei* or *P. mallei* is always clinically significant. Because *P. aeruginosa* is primarily a nosocomial pathogen and is so devastating in the compromised host, its presence in clinical specimens should be considered relevant until proven otherwise. The colonization of the skin and mucous membranes in the compromised patient often precedes systemic infection. *P. aeruginosa* and *P. cepacia* are significant isolates in cystic fibrosis patients. The other NFB are usually colonizers, and the clinical significance of their isolation depends on the underlying condition of the patient, the source of the specimen, the number of other bacterial species isolated, and the need for epidemiologic data.

Therapeutic Considerations

The antimicrobial susceptibility of *P. aeruginosa* and the other pseudomonads is not predictable. Appropriate therapy is dependent on the results of susceptibility testing. Empiric therapy involves one, two, or three agents depending on the severity of the disease and the susceptibility pattern of local isolates. In general, therapy will include an aminoglycoside and an antipseudomonal penicillin or parenteral cephalosporin active against *P. aeruginosa*. The currently recommended treatment for the septicemic form of melioidosis is trimethoprim-sulfamethoxazole plus a third-generation cephalosporin.

Alcaligenes is usually susceptible to trimethoprim-sulfamethoxazole and variable to most other antimicrobial agents. *Moraxella* and *Eikenella* are usually susceptible to penicillin and ampicillin, although isolates containing β-lactamase have been reported. *Eikenella* is resistant to clindamycin.

Summary and Conclusions

The NFB are ubiquitous in soil, water, and most environments. *Eikenella* and *Moraxella* are part of the flora of the mucous membranes in humans and cause endogenously acquired infections. The other NFB, particularly *P. aeruginosa*, are important nosocomial pathogens found in numerous hospital reservoirs (e.g., contaminated solutions, equipment, food, and sinks), and infect nearly every organ system. *P. pseudomallei* and *P. mallei* are the etiologic agents of melioidosis and glanders, respectively. In general, the NFB are easily isolated, growing on most routine media, but difficult to identify by either conventional tests or commercial systems. Pyocyanin pigment is a definitive characteristic of *P. aeruginosa*. The susceptibility of the NFB to antimicrobial agents must be determined by testing. *Eikenella* and *Moraxella* are usually susceptible to penicillin or ampicillin.

MISCELLANEOUS FACULTATIVELY ANAEROBIC GRAM-NEGATIVE BACILLI

Microbiology

The genera and species discussed in this section are usually slow-growing, may not grow on MacConkey agar, and often grow better in a CO_2 enriched atmosphere. They include *Gardnerella*, *Cardiobacterium*, *Chromobacterium*, *Pasteurella*, *Actinobacillus*, *Kingella*, *Capnocytophaga*, *Capnocytophaga canimorsus* (formerly CDC group DF-2), and CDC group EF-4a.

Gardnerella vaginalis was previously classified as *Haemophilus vaginalis* or *Corynebacterium vaginale*. The cell wall is morphologically different from either a Gram-positive or a Gram-negative bacterium, but chemically resembles a Gram-positive organism. *G. vaginalis* is a small (0.5 × 1.5 μm), pleomorphic, fastidious, facultatively anaerobic, nonmotile, oxidase- and catalase-negative Gram-negative to Gram-variable rod that does not grow on MacConkey agar.

Cardiobacterium hominis, the only species in the genus, is a facultatively anaerobic, slow-growing, fastidious, nonmotile, oxidase-positive, catalase-negative, pale-staining Gram-negative rod that appears as pleomorphic and teardrop shaped when grown on yeast extract–deficient medium (47). It may occur in clusters resembling rosettes. It does not grow on MacConkey agar, and growth is enhanced by humidity and CO_2.

The genus *Chromobacterium* contains two species, *Chromobacterium violaceum* and *Chromobacterium fluviatile*, but only *C. violaceum* is isolated from clinical specimens. It is a facultatively anaerobic, motile, oxidase- and catalase-positive, Gram-negative rod that

Table 44.24. Characteristics of Medical *Pseudomonas* Species[a]

Characteristic[b]	*P. aeruginosa* (64)[c]	*P. fluorescens* (96)	*P. putida* (111)	*P. acidovorans* (40)	*P. cepacia* (85)	*P. mallei* (8)	*P. maltophilia* (296)	*P. mendocina* (6)
Acid production								
Fructose	92	98	100	100	100	100	99	100
Galactose	84	99	100	0	100		32	100
Glucose	97	100	100	98	100	100	100	100
Inositol	–	+	–		+	+	–	
Lactose	0	22	23	0	98	0	90	0
Maltose	0	52	32	0	98	0	100	0
Mannitol	67	92	24	98	100	75	0	0
Mannose	83	99	100	0	100		97	100
Rhamnose	27	71	49	0	0	0	0	0
Saccharose	0	56	13	0	80	38	94	0
Xylose	81	98	97	0	100	0	56	100
2-Ketoglutarate	63	71	68	0	12		0	0
ONPG	0	2	3	0	82	0	96	0
Starch hydrolysis	0	0	0	0	0	+/–	0	0
Acylamidase	38	6	1	100	72		0	0
Amino acid attack								
Arginine	98	99	97	0	0	83	0	100
Lysine	0	0	0	0	89	0	100	0
Ornithine	0	0	0	0	42	0	0	0
Phenylalanine	2	2	0	0	0		0	50
Citrate	100	90	90	90	90	0–38	90	
Deoxyribonuclease	13	0	0	0	0		100	0
Esculin hydrolysis	0	0	0	0	72		100	0
Gelatinase, caseinase	58	100	0	3	69	+	100	0
Growth on/at								
1% cetrimide	95	95	86	8	73		0	0
6.5% NaCl	5	3	16	0	0		0	100
1% TTC	75	79	75	3	35		0	0
SS-agar	88	98	97	63	11		0	83
MacConkey	98	100	100	98	89	0	100	100
5°C	0	100	100				0	
42°C	100	0	0				0	
Hemolysis	44	16	1	0	5		0	0
Hydrogen sulfide	0	0	0	0	0	0–25	0	0
Lecithinase	11	92	0	0	28	0	0	0
Lipase	67	42	2	20	100		100	83
Motility	97	100	100	100	99	0	100	100
No. of flagella	1	>1	>1	>1	>1	0	>1	1
Nitrate reductase	36	13	0	93	24	100	46	100
N_2 gas production	59	4	0	0	0	100	0	100
Oxidase	100	100	100	100	84	weak	1	100
PPHB	0	0	0	0	+	+	+	–
Pigments								
Pyocyanin	95	0	0	0	0	0	0	0
Pyoverdin	99	99	99	0	0	0	0	0
Brown	3	0	0					
Orange								
Red	3							
Yellow								
Urease	77	40	50	0	40	50	0	50

[a]From Falcone G, Campa M. Diseases caused by *Pseudomonas*. In: Balows A, Hausler WJ Jr, Ohashi M, Turano A, eds. Laboratory of infectious diseases: principles and practices, vol 1. New York: Springer-Verlag, 1988:438–439.

[b]Abbreviations: ONPG, *o*-nitrophenyl-β-D-galactopyranoside; Arginine, arginine dehydrolase; Lysine, lysine decarboxylase; Ornithine, ornithine decarboxylase; Phenylalanine, phenylalanine deaminase; SS-agar, salmonella-shigella agar; TTC, triphenyltetrazolium chloride; 1, polar monotrichous; >1, polar multitrichous; acid production may be weak or delayed from *P. acidovorans*, *P. pickettii*, *P. pseudoalcaligenes*, *P. putrefaciens*, and *P. vesicularis*.

P. pickettii (12)	P. pseudoalcaligenes (24)	P. pseudomallei (7)	"P." putrefaciens (38)	P. stutzeri (69)	P. vescicularis (3)	P. alcaligenes (28)	P. diminuta (11)	P. testosteroni (7)
100	100	100	18	100	33	0	0	0
100	4	100	3	97	0	0	0	0
100	96	100	61	100	100	0	0	0
		–	–	+		–		
0	0	100	8	0	0	0	0	0
0	21	100	13	100	100	0	0	0
0	0	100	0	78	0	0	0	0
100	4	100	5	93	0	0	0	0
0	0	71	8	49	0	0	0	0
0	0	83	16	0	0	0	0	0
100	17	100	3	100	33	0	0	0
0	0	0	0	4	0	0	0	0
0	0	0	0	0	0	0	0	0
0	0	0	0	91	0	0	0	0
0	8	0	74	0	0	0	0	0
0	21	100	0	1	0	0	0	0
0	0	0	0	0	0	0	0	0
0	0	0	100	0	0	0	0	0
67	25	0	0	36	0	18	0	0
100	0	96	80	90	0		0	
0	0	0	100	0	0	0	55	0
0	0	57	13	0	100	0	0	0
0	0	100	97	0	30	4	73	0
0	46	0	0	0	0	7	0	0
0	4	0	90	99	0	0	0	0
0	0	0	0	0	0	8	0	0
0	0	0	60	84	0	0	0	0
100	92	100	100	100	0	100	100	71
			33					
		100	50	+		71	64	14
0	0	43	0	0	0	14	0	0
0	0	0	100	0	0	0	0	0
0	0	100	0	1	0	0	0	0
100	13	83	100	93	0	39	9	43
100	100	100	100	100	100	100	100	100
1	1	>1	1	1	1	1	>1	1
100	96	83	95	67	0	54	0	86
100	0	100	0	100	0	0	0	0
100	100	100	100	100	100	100	100	100
0	+	0	+	–	+	–	+(–)	+
0	0	0	0	0	0	0	0	0
0	0	0	0	0	0	0	0	0
100	0	43	18	22	0	29	0	0

[c]Numbers in parentheses indicate the number of strains examined. The figures in the body of the table indicate percentage positive reactions. When exact figure is unknown, + indicates presence, and – absence of a character. Carbohydrate acidification refers to concentrations of 1% in OF medium. Motility is examined by microscopy after growth in liquid media at 18–20°C.

Table 44.25. Characteristics of *E. corrodens*, *Moraxella* Species and *Oligella* Species[a]

Characteristic	*E. corrodens*	*M. atlantae*	*M. lacunata*	*M. nonliquefaciens*	*M. osloensis*	*M. phenylpyruvica*	*O. urethralis*
Urease	−	−	−	−	−	+	−
Phenylalanine deaminase	−	−	−/+	−	−	+	−/+
Nitrate reduction	+	−	+	+	+/−	+/−	−
Growth on MacConkey	−	+/−	−	−	−/+	+	+/−
Ornithine decarboxylase	+	NA	NA	NA	NA	NA	NA
Growth in 3% NaCl	NA	NA	+	NA	−	+	+

[a]Symbols: +, >90% of strains positive; −, >90% of strains negative; +/−, most strains positive; −/+, most strains negative; NA, not available.

usually produces a violet pigment. Unlike the other organisms in this section, *C. violaceum* grows on most routine laboratory media in air.

The genus *Pasteurella* contains six recognized species: *Pasteurella multocida*, *Pasteurella pneumotropica*, *Pasteurella ureae*, *Pasteurella gallinarum*, *Pasteurella haemolytica*, and *Pasteurella aerogenes* (22). Five new species have been proposed, *Pasteurella canis* (formerly *Pasteurella* new species 1 or "gas"), *Pasteurella stomatis* (formerly *P. multocida* biotype six), *Pasteurella dagmatis*, *Pasteurella anatis*, *Pasteurella langaa*; and the species *P. pneumotropica*, *P. ureae*, and *P. haemolytica* have been transferred to the genus *Actinobacillus* (48). *P. multocida* is the most common human pathogen of the genus. The other species are only rarely isolated from clinical specimens. *P. multocida* is a facultatively anaerobic, nonmotile, catalase- and oxidase-positive Gram-negative rod that may exhibit bipolar staining and does not grow on MacConkey agar.

The genus *Actinobacillus* contains five species, *Actinobacillus actinomycetemcomitans*, *Actinobacillus lignieresii*, *Actinobacillus equuli*, *Actinobacillus suis*, and *Actinobacillus capsulatus*. The last four species are primarily animal pathogens. It has been proposed that *A. actinomycetemcomitans* be reclassified as a species of *Haemophilus* (49). *A. actinomycetemcomitans* is a facultatively anaerobic, fastidious, slow-growing, small (0.5 × 1.5 μm), nonmotile, catalase-positive, Gram-negative coccobacillary rod that does not grow on MacConkey agar, and grows best in humidity and CO_2.

The genus *Kingella* consists of three species: *Kingella kingae*, *Kingella denitrificans*, and *Kingella indologenes*. *Kingella* species are facultatively anaerobic, nonmotile, catalase-negative, oxidase-positive, Gram-negative rods that do not grow on MacConkey agar.

Three species of *Capnocytophaga* are recognized: *Capnocytophaga ochracea*, *Capnocytophaga gingivalis*, and *Capnocytophaga sputigena*. They are facultatively anaerobic, fastidious, capnophilic, oxidase- and catalase-negative, Gram-negative fusiform rods that may exhibit gliding motility, and do not grow on MacConkey agar.

Capnocytophaga canimorsus (CDC group DF-2) is a weakly oxidase-positive, catalase-positive, nonmotile, fermentative, long, thin, Gram-negative fusiform rod that does not grow on MacConkey agar and grows poorly on other laboratory media (50). *C. canimorsus* shares some characteristics with the genus *Capnocytophaga* but is genetically distinct.

CDC group EF-4a is an oxidase- and catalase-positive, nonmotile, fermentative (for glucose), Gram-negative rod that does not grow on MacConkey agar.

Spectrum of Disease

G. vaginalis is associated with bacterial vaginosis (nonspecific vaginitis), which is characterized by a malodorous vaginal discharge and overgrowth with various anaerobic bacteria. Extragenital infections include bacteremia, vaginal abscesses, neonatal bacteremia, and soft tissue infections. *C. hominis* has been implicated in only a small number of cases of endocarditis and bacteremia (51). *C. violaceum* is associated with urinary tract infections, localized abscesses, and fulminant sepsis with abscesses in multiple organs.

P. multocida is associated with three broad categories of disease: (*a*) localized infection following an animal bite or scratch (usually from a cat); (*b*) chronic respiratory disease, particularly in patients with underlying pulmonary disease; and (*c*) bacteremia with or without metastatic foci. The latter group includes meningitis; brain, liver, and renal abscesses; otitis; mastoiditis; sinusitis; endocarditis; septic arthritis; and peritonitis. Spontaneous peritonitis and septicemia occur most often in patients with cirrhosis.

Actinobacillus is associated with juvenile periodontitis; endocarditis (particularly damaged or prosthetic heart valves); and infrequent reports of meningitis, brain abscess, osteomyelitis, urinary tract infection, pericarditis, and pulmonary infections.

Kingella infections include endocarditis, meningitis, bacteremia, septic arthritis, osteomyelitis, intervertebral disk infections, and infections of the eye. *K. kingae* infections occur primarily in children and young adults; *K. denitrificans* causes endocarditis in adults; and *K. indologenes* has been associated with eye infections and endocarditis.

Capnocytophaga is associated with juvenile periodontitis, bacteremia, endocarditis, osteomyelitis, septic arthritis, sinusitis, pulmonary infections, conjunctivitis, and keratitis. Most infections occur in immunocompromised patients with severe granulocytopenia and oral ulcerations.

C. canimorsus (CDC group DF-2) causes two patterns of disease: (*a*) shock and disseminated intravascular coagulation seen in splenectomized patients, and (*b*) a milder form of disease in patients with a spleen. Infections include septicemia, meningitis, endocarditis, pneumonia, necrotizing wound infections, brain abscess, cellulitis, septic arthritis, corneal ulceration, and glomerulonephritis. Predisposing factors include splenectomy and a history of alcoholism.

CDC group EF-4a causes wound infections and rarely bacteremia.

Epidemiology

G. vaginalis is part of the endogenous flora of the human genital tract. Although bacterial vaginosis is the most common cause of vaginal discharge in sexually active women, the exact role of *G. vaginalis* in this syndrome is poorly understood. Sexual transmission of the disease is not proven, but a high proportion of the male sex partners of women with the syndrome carry *G. vaginalis* on their urethral mucosa.

C. hominis, *A. actinomycetemcomitans*, *Kingella* species, and *Capnocytophaga* species are part of the oropharyngeal flora in humans. Most infections result from endogenous spread of the bacteria, often following dental manipulations or oral disease such as periodontitis.

C. violaceum inhabits soil and water, particularly in warmer climates such as the southeastern United States, Southeast Asia, or South America. Infections generally occur following contamination of wounds with soil or water, or rarely after ingestion of contaminated water.

P. multocida, *C. canimorsus* (CDC group DF-2), and CDC group EF-4a are found in the upper respiratory tract of animals. Groups DF-2 and EF-4a are part of the oropharyngeal flora of dogs, and infections in humans generally follow dog bites or exposure to dog secretions. *C. canimorsus* (DF-2) is occasionally associated with cat bites and scratches. The reservoir for *P. multocida* is the upper respiratory tract of cats, dogs, rabbits, rats, opossums, cattle, sheep, lions, swine, and birds. The frequency of carriage varies with the species but is most common in cats. Transmission to humans occurs following bites, scratches, or exposure to secretions. Of all animal exposure cases, 75% are associated with cats. Approximately 5 to 15% of all cases are not associated with animal exposure, suggesting *P. multocida* may be a minor component of the oropharyngeal flora in humans.

Diagnostic Procedures

MICROSCOPY

Bacterial vaginosis can be presumptively diagnosed by Gram stain of vaginal secretions that demonstrate numerous clue cells (vaginal epithelial cells covered by Gram-variable coccobacilli) associated with a mixed flora of large numbers of Gram-negative to variable coccobacilli in the absence of lactobacilli (52). The syndrome is best diagnosed by clinical criteria and a Gram stain rather than by culture of *G. vaginalis*.

The organisms discussed in this section are Gram-negative rods that cannot be definitely identified by direct examination of the clinical specimen. *C. hominis* is a pale-staining pleomorphic (sometimes teardrop-shaped) rod; *P. multocida* is a small coccobacillus that may exhibit bipolar staining; *A. actinomycetemcomitans* is a small coccobacillus; *Kingella* are small coccobacilli arranged in pairs or chains; *Capnocytophaga* are thin, fusiform rods; and *C. canimorsus* (DF-2) is a filamentous, sometimes curved fusiform rod. Both *C. hominis* and *Kingella* have a tendency to retain the primary stain.

CULTURE TECHNIQUES

G. vaginalis is most easily isolated on human blood bilayer agar with Tween-80 (HBT), on vaginalis agar (V-agar), or on Columbia-colistin-nalidixic agar (CNA). Media is incubated at 35° to 37°C in a humid atmosphere containing 5% CO_2 for 2 days. After 48 hours, colonies are approximately 0.5 mm in diameter, are gray, and exhibit a diffuse β-hemolysis on human but not on sheep blood. On routine sheep blood agar, colonies are pinpoint to barely visible.

C. hominis produces pinpoint colonies on chocolate or blood agar after 2 to 3 days' incubation in a moist, 5% CO_2 atmosphere. A slight green to brown color may develop around the colony.

C. violaceum grows well on blood and MacConkey agar in 24 hours at 35° to 37°C in air. Most colonies exhibit a characteristic violet pigment (produced optimally at 22°C) and often produce an odor of cyanide (almond).

Actinobacillus and *Capnocytophaga* grow best on blood or chocolate agars incubated in high humidity and in a 5 to 10% CO_2-enriched atmosphere. After 2 to 3 days' incubation, colonies of *Actinobacillus* are small (0.5 mm), punctate, and adherent with a mixed morphology. On continued incubation, a star-like, opaque center may be observed under 100× magnification (Fig. 44.16). *Capnocytophaga* produces yellow,

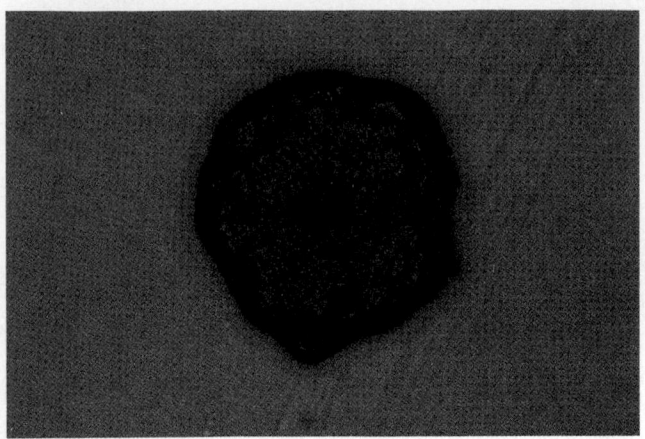

Figure 44.16. Colony of *A. actinomycetemcomitans* on heart infusion agar. Note the central star-shaped structure. (Reprinted with permission from Baron EJ, Finegold SM. Bailey and Scott's diagnostic microbiology. St. Louis: CV Mosby, 1990.)

nonhemolytic colonies with finger-like projections and an almond odor after 2 to 3 days' incubation. Some strains will grow only anaerobically on initial isolation. Colonies may pit the agar.

Kingella grows in air or CO_2 (may enhance growth) but grows poorly under anaerobic conditions. Colonies are 0.5 to 1 mm in diameter after 48 hours' incubation at 35°C and may pit the agar or produce a "fried egg" appearance. *K. denitrificans* grows on Martin-Lewis agar and may be confused with *N. gonorrhoeae*.

Pasteurella grows well on nonselective media such as blood or chocolate agar at 35°C in air or CO_2. Colonies are usually smooth, gray, 1 to 2 mm after 24 hours' incubation, have a musty odor, and may produce a green to brown discoloration on blood agar.

C. canimorsus (DF-2) grows slowly (2 to 4 days) on enriched chocolate agar incubated at 35°C in a humid, CO_2 enriched atmosphere. It also grows on heart infusion agar with 5% rabbit or sheep blood but not on tryptic-soy agar containing blood. Growth is poor under anaerobic conditions.

EF-4a grows well on nonselective media (e.g., blood or chocolate agar) within 24 hours' incubation at 35°C. Colonies are small and yellow-orange and produce a popcorn-like odor.

IDENTIFICATION METHODS

G. vaginalis can be identified presumptively on the basis of negative catalase and oxidase tests, β-hemolytic colonies on HBT agar, and a typical Gram stain morphology. Confirmatory tests include starch and hippurate hydrolysis, α- and β-glucosidase tests, or use of the RIM system (Austin Biological Laboratories).

C. hominis is oxidase positive and catalase negative, and is differentiated from similar organisms (e.g., *Eikenella, Kingella,* and *H. aphrophilus*) by the weak production of indole (must be extracted with xylene) (Table 44.26). Serum may have to be added to carbohydrate tests to ensure growth.

C. violaceum is oxidase and catalase positive, is motile, reduces nitrate, and ferments glucose. It can be distinguished from other genera such as *Aeromonas, Plesiomonas,* and *Vibrio* by negative tests for indole, ornithine and lysine decarboxylase reactions, and lack of fermentation of mannitol and maltose.

Actinobacillus may be differentiated from similar genera with a minimum number of tests (Table 44.26), but the definitive identification of a suspected isolate requires a more comprehensive battery.

Kingella species are catalase negative, oxidase positive, and nonmotile (Table 44.26). *K. kingae* is distinguished from the other two species by β-hemolysis on sheep blood agar and absence of indole production, nitrate reduction, and growth on Martin-Lewis agar. *K. indologenes* produces indole; the other two species do not.

Pasteurella species are catalase and oxidase positive, are nonmotile, and reduce nitrate (Table 44.26). Other characteristic reactions for *P. multocida* include a positive ornithine decarboxylase and negative arginine dehydrolase.

Characteristics useful for the identification of the genus *Capnocytophaga* are listed in Table 44.26. Commercial identification systems are also available.

C. canimorsus (CDC group DF-2) often requires the addition of rabbit serum to obtain adequate growth in the biochemical tests. It is weakly oxidase (positive) and catalase positive; indole, urease, and nitrate-reduction negative; and arginine dehydrolase positive (Table 44.26).

CDC group EF-4a strains are oxidase and catalase positive, reduce nitrate, and are negative for urease and indole production (Table 44.26).

DIRECT ANTIGEN OR NUCLEIC ACID DETECTION

No commercial systems are available for the direct detection of any of these bacteria in clinical specimens.

SEROLOGIC PROCEDURES

No routine serologic tests are available for the diagnosis of infections caused by this group of organisms.

INTERPRETATION OF RESULTS

With the exception of *G. vaginalis*, these bacteria are seldom isolated from clinical specimens. There-

Table 44.26. Differentiation of Selected Genera and Species of Gram-Negative Bacilli[a]

Organism	Fusiform Shape	Catalase	Oxidase	Indole	Motility	Nitrate Reduction	Glucose Fermentation	Growth on MacConkey
C. hominis	−	−	+	+	−	−	+	v
C. violaceum	−	+	v	−[a]	+	+	+	+
Capnocytophaga	+	−	−	−	+	v	+	−
C. canimorsus (DF-2)	+	+	+	−	−	−	v	−
A. actinomycetemcomitans	−	+	v	−	−	+	+	−
P. multocida	−	+	+	+	−	+	+	−
E. corrodens	−	−	+	−	−	+	−	−
Kingella	−	−	+	v	−	v	+	v
H. aphrophilus	−	−	v	−	−	+	+	−
CDC Group EF4a	−	+	+	−	−	+	+	v

[a]Symbols: +, >90% positive; −, >90% negative; v, variable reaction; [a] Some nonpigmented stains are positive.

fore, their isolation is clinically significant until proven otherwise. The isolation of any members of the HACEK group (*Haemophilus, Actinobacillus, Cardiobacterium, Eikenella, Kingella*) from blood is highly suspicious of endocarditis, especially if the patient has oral trauma or poor dentition. The presence of large numbers of *G. vaginalis* in vaginal secretions is suggestive of bacterial vaginosis but does not prove that *G. vaginalis* causes the syndrome.

Therapeutic Considerations

Standardized susceptibility tests are often difficult to perform because of the growth requirements of some of these bacteria. Oral metronidazole is the treatment of choice for bacterial vaginosis. *G. vaginalis* is susceptible to penicillin, clindamycin, vancomycin, metronidazole (4 μg/ml) and its hydroxymetabolite (1 μg/ml), but is resistant to cephalosporins, tetracyclines, sulfadiazine, and quinolones.

C. hominis is susceptible to β-lactam agents, tetracycline, chloramphenicol, and aminoglycosides but variably resistant to clindamycin, erythromycin, oxacillin, and vancomycin.

C. violaceum should be tested for susceptibility to antimicrobial agents. Most isolates are susceptible to tetracycline, chloramphenicol, erythromycin, and trimethoprim-sulfamethoxazole with variable resistance to aminoglycosides. They are often resistant to the β-lactam antibiotics and clindamycin.

P. multocida is susceptible to penicillin, cephalothin, chloramphenicol, and tetracycline. Limited experience is available for the treatment of infections with the newer antimicrobial agents.

Actinobacillus is generally susceptible to chloramphenicol, tetracycline, carbenicillin, and streptomycin, and is variably susceptible to penicillin. In vitro tests indicate susceptibility to the newer cephalosporins, rifampin, trimethoprim-sulfamethoxazole, and ciprofloxacin. Combined penicillin-aminoglycoside therapy has been recommended for endocarditis.

Kingella are generally susceptible to the β-lactams (*K. denitrificans* may be moderately resistant to penicillin), cephalothin, aminoglycosides, tetracycline, chloramphenicol, and sulfonamides.

Capnocytophaga species are susceptible to penicillin, chloramphenicol, tetracycline, erythromycin, clindamycin, and metronidazole, and are resistant to vancomycin and aminoglycosides.

Limited studies of *C. canimorsus* (CDC group DF-2) organisms indicate susceptibility to the penicillins, cephalosporins, tetracycline, chloramphenicol, erythromycin, ciprofloxacin, and clindamycin, and resistance to aminoglycosides. Penicillin is the drug of choice.

CDC group EF-4a organisms appear susceptible to the β-lactams, chloramphenicol, and tetracycline based on limited studies.

Summary and Conclusions

The miscellaneous facultatively anaerobic Gram-negative bacilli discussed in this section are usually inhabitants of the upper respiratory tract of humans (e.g., *Actinobacillus, Kingella, Cardiobacterium,* and *Capnocytophaga*); the genital tract (e.g., *Gardnerella*); the upper respiratory tract of animals (e.g., *Pasteurella, C. canimorsus* [CDC group DF-2], and CDC group EF-4a); or soil and water (e.g., *Chromobacterium*). Infections usually follow the spread of the bacterium from a colonized site or after exposure to animal bites, scratches, or secretions. These species cause a variety of diseases ranging from localized soft tissue infections to systemic life-threatening infections. Most of the organisms are fastidious, do not grow on MacConkey agar; and require increased humidity and CO_2-enriched atmosphere for growth. *Chromobacterium* grows well on most routine media. *C. violaceum* is resistant, *A. actinomycetemcomitans* is moderately resistant, and the other species are susceptible to penicillin.

MISCELLANEOUS GRAM-NEGATIVE BACILLI WITH SPECIAL GROWTH REQUIREMENTS

Microbiology

The microorganisms discussed in this section are not usually isolated on routine laboratory media (e.g., blood and MacConkey agars) after 24 hours' incubation. In general, these bacteria are associated with a specific clinical syndrome of which the laboratory needs to be aware. Many of these organisms pose a considerable challenge regarding their isolation and identification.

The genus *Francisella* contains two species, *Francisella tularensis* and *Francisella novicida* (considered by some to be a biogroup of *F. tularensis*) and the proposed species *Francisella philomiragia* (53). The latter two organisms rarely cause disease in humans. *F. tularensis* is composed of two biovars: type A (biovar *tularensis*) and type B (biovar *palaearctica*). Type A is the most virulent. *F. tularensis* is an aerobic, small (0.2 × 0.2 to 0.7 μm), nonmotile, oxidase-negative, weakly catalase-positive, Gram-negative rod that requires enriched media with added cystine or cysteine for growth.

There are six recognized species of the genus *Brucella*, four of which are pathogenic for humans (*Brucella abortus, Brucella melitensis, Brucella suis,* and *Brucella canis*). *Brucella neotomae* (found in the desert wood rat) and *Brucella ovis* (a pathogen of sheep) have not been shown to cause disease in humans. *Brucella* species are nonmotile, catalase-positive, usually oxidase-positive, Gram-negative coccobacilli or short rods (0.5 × 0.6 to 1.5 μm), and are usually arranged singly but may occur in short chains or groups. The organisms are strict aerobes, often requiring a CO_2-enriched atmosphere on primary isolation. The addition of glucose (1.5 to 2.5%), serum, thiamine, niacin, biotin, and pantothenic acid to the medium promotes growth.

The genus *Bordetella* consists of four species, *Bordetella pertussis, Bordetella parapertussis, Bordetella bronchiseptica,* and *Bordetella avium*. *B. pertussis* is the etiologic agent of whooping cough. *B. parapertussis* may be a variant of *B. pertussis*, although some studies suggest it is more closely related to *B. bronchiseptica*. *B. bronchiseptica* is an animal pathogen (it rarely causes symptomatic disease in humans) and *B. avium*, a bronchiseptica-like organism (formerly *Alcaligenes*), is an avian pathogen. *Bordetella* species are strictly aerobic, small (0.3 × 0.5 to 2.0 μm), Gram-negative coccobacilli that often exhibit bipolar staining and are arranged singly or in pairs. The two human strains are nonmotile. All species require nicotinic acid or nicotinamide and grow best at 35° to 37°C.

Calymmatobacterium granulomatis is the only species in this unassigned genus. It is a nonmotile, encapsulated, Gram-negative coccobacillus (0.5 × 1 to 2 μm) that appears to be antigenically related to *Klebsiella rhinoscleromatis*. It is isolated in chicken embryos, egg yolk slants (Dulaney slants), or special fluid medium.

Streptobacillus moniliformis is one agent of rat-bite fever. It is a pleomorphic, catalase- and oxidase-negative, facultatively anaerobic, Gram-negative rod (0.1 to 0.7 × 1 to 5 μm). Single cells may show beaded central swelling, or chains and filaments (10 to 150 mm in length). The organism grows only on medium containing blood, serum, or ascitic fluid.

The genus *Bartonella* contains only one species, *Bartonella bacilliformis*, which is a motile, aerobic, Gram-negative rod (0.2 to 0.5 × 0.3 to 3 μm) that retains the safranin counterstain poorly. It stains reddish-purple with the Giemsa stain. It grows best at 28° to 30°C on medium containing blood, particularly rabbit blood.

Spectrum of Disease

F. tularensis is the etiologic agent of tularemia, which can present in the following clinical forms: ulceroglandular (80% of cases), oculoglandular, oropharyngeal, glandular (no lesion detected), typhoidal, pleuropulmonary, gastrointestinal, or combinations of these.

Brucellosis is primarily a genitourinary tract infection in animals and affects the reticuloendothelial system in humans. The disease ranges from subclinical to acute infections with the potential to develop relapses or become a chronic infection. Complications may affect almost any organ system but often involve the vertebral bodies. *B. melitensis* and *B. suis* tend to cause more severe infections than *B. abortus* and *B. canis*.

Whooping cough (pertussis) is caused by *B. pertussis* and is characterized by a series of short expiratory coughs followed by an inspiratory gasp that results in the whoop. Complications are primarily due to secondary infections. Rarely, *B. parapertussis* or *B. bronchiseptica* may cause a pulmonary infection or opportunistic infections in compromised hosts.

Granuloma inguinale, donovanosis, and granuloma venereum are synonyms for the disease caused by *C. granulomatis*. The disease begins as single or multiple subcutaneous nodules that progress to open granulomatous lesions that are usually painless. The genitalia are involved in approximately 90% of cases, the rectum in 5 to 10%, and other sites in 1 to 5%.

S. moniliformis is an agent of rat-bite fever that begins with an abrupt onset of fever, chills, rash, and headache. Complications include arthritis, pneumonia, endocarditis, myocarditis, meningitis, and nephritis.

The disease caused by *B. bacilliformis* can present in two forms: Oroya fever (systemic form) and verruga peruana (cutaneous form). The organism grows within and on the surface of erythrocytes as well as in the vascular endothelium.

Epidemiology

Tularemia occurs exclusively in the northern hemisphere. *F. tularensis* is found in wild mammals (e.g., rabbits, muskrats, beavers, deer, bear); domestic animals (e.g., sheep, cats, cattle, dogs); birds; some amphibians and fish; insects (e.g., ticks, deerflies, mosquitoes); and water from streams and wells. The disease is transmitted most often by contact with infected animals, or bites of infected insects; and less frequently by aerosols, consumption of contaminated water or improperly cooked meat, and bites of animals. Tick-borne cases occur primarily in the spring and summer months, while rabbit and muskrat associated cases increase in the winter.

Brucellosis is largely a disease of domestic animals throughout the world, especially in the Mediterranean countries of Europe, Africa, Asia, and Central and South America. The organisms, normal flora of the genital and urinary tracts of animals, are transmitted to humans by direct contact with infected animal tissue, inhalation of aerosols, or consumption of contaminated meat or dairy products. Brucellosis is an occupational disease of persons who handle livestock (e.g., veterinarians, ranchers, abattoir workers).

Pertussis continues to be a problem in populations that are not vaccinated. Humans are the only known reservoir of *B. pertussis*. In the prevaccine era, the disease occurred primarily in children 1 to 5 years of age. Currently in the United States, approximately 50% of the cases occur in children less than 1 year of age and 10 to 15% occur in adults.

C. granulomatis is endemic in New Guinea, India, Australia, the Carribean, and other tropical countries. It is transmitted sexually but may be contracted by other direct contact. The disease is only mildly contagious and has a higher prevalence among individuals of low socioeconomic status and poor personal hygiene.

Wild and laboratory rats and other rodents are the primary reservoir for *S. moniliformis*, although the bacterium has been found in turkeys and milk. Transmission occurs following the bite of a rodent, handling infected tissue, or occasionally after consumption of contaminated food (e.g., milk).

Bartonellosis is restricted to the habitat of the sandfly vector (*Phlebotomus*) in the Andes Mountains of Peru, Equador and Colombia. Asymptomatic human carriers serve as a reservoir.

Diagnostic Procedures

MICROSCOPY

Gram-stained smears of material containing *B. pertussis*, *F. tularensis*, or *Brucella* species may appear negative because the organisms stain poorly and are small. Material should be stained with fluorescent antibody reagents for the detection of *F. tularensis* and *B. pertussis*. These stains are best performed by reference laboratories.

C. granulomatis is usually observed in a Giemsa or Wright stained smear of a scraping of the lesion as clusters of safety pin–shaped rods in the cytoplasm of macrophages (Donovan bodies). The organism appears blue to deep purple with a pink capsule.

S. moniliformis may be directly seen in Giemsa, Wayson, Gram, or acridine orange stained smears of clinical specimens as extremely pleomorphic Gram-negative rods with long filaments, chains, and swollen cells.

The diagnosis of bartonellosis can be made by demonstrating pleomorphic, rod or ring-shaped bacteria on Wright or Giemsa-stained blood smears.

CULTURE TECHNIQUES

Cystine-glucose blood agar is recommended for the isolation of *F. tularensis*, but growth is observed on enriched chocolate, Thayer-Martin, and charcoal yeast extract agars. Occasional strains will grow on sheep blood agar. Growth has also occurred in Bactec blood culture bottles (Johnson Laboratories) inoculated with blood or pleural fluid (54). Colonies are pinpoint, gray, and smooth after 24 to 48 hours at 35°C. *F. tularensis* is highly infectious. Gloves should be worn and cultures worked up in a biological safety hood.

Brucella species can be isolated on sheep blood, chocolate, and charcoal yeast extract (55) agars as well as Farrell's selective medium. Trypticase-soy or brain heart infusion blood culture and Castaneda (biphasic) broths will support growth if the bottles are vented and placed in 5 to 10% CO_2 for up to 4 weeks. Solid media should be incubated in 5 to 10% CO_2 at 35° to 37°C for 3 weeks. After 3 to 4 days, colonies are pinpoint and gray on blood agar.

Bordet-Gengou (BG) and Regan-Lowe (RL) media are used for the initial isolation of *B. pertussis*. The organism produces a small (less than 1 mm), gray, translucent colony with a pearl-like luster on BG agar; and round, shiny colonies on RL medium. Cultures should be incubated at 35 to 37°C for 5 to 7 days in a moist environment.

C. granulomatis can be cultured but requires specialized media or eggs. The laboratory diagnosis is usually based on smear results.

Isolation of *S. moniliformis* requires the use of medium containing blood, serum, or ascitic fluid. It has been recovered on sheep blood and chocolate agars. Cultures are incubated at 35° to 37°C in 5 to 10% CO_2 and high humidity for 1 to 2 weeks. Colonies are round, gray and glistening, and remain viable for 3 to 7 days.

B. bacilliformis is isolated on media containing rabbit, horse, or human blood (e.g., *Leptospira*-enriched medium). Tubes are incubated at 28° to 30°C for 2 to 4 weeks. Morphology is observed by Giemsa stain or dark-field microscopy.

IDENTIFICATION METHODS

The biochemical identification of *F. tularensis* is not recommended because of the highly infectious nature of the organism. Presumptive identification is based on growth characteristics (absence of growth on routine media), morphology (small coccobacillus), oxidase negativity, and catalase positivity (weak). Specific identification is performed by fluorescent antibody or agglutination procedures.

Brucella are glucose oxidizers (or inert), are usually oxidase and catalase positive, and reduce nitrates. Presumptive species identification is based on urease activity (*B. canis* and *B. suis* are positive in less than 30 minutes, *B. abortus* in 1 to 2 hours, and *B. melitensis* is variable); H_2S production (only *B. abortus* is positive); and CO_2 requirement (*B. abortus* usually requires CO_2 for growth). Definitive identification is accomplished by additional tests and agglutination in specific antiserum.

Direct fluorescent antibody test or agglutination with specific antisera for *B. pertussis* can be used for the rapid presumptive identification of suspicious colonies. Some antisera cross-react with *Haemophilus* species.

Differentiation among the *Bordetella* species is accomplished by determinations of the growth rate (fresh isolates of *B. pertussis* take 3 to 5 days; other species 1 to 2 days); urease activity (*B. pertussis* is negative); growth on blood agar (fresh isolates of *B. pertussis* are negative); growth on MacConkey agar (*B. bronchiseptica* is positive); and browning on nutrient agar (*B. parapertussis* is positive). Isolates resembling *B. bronchiseptica* must be differentiated from *Alcaligenes* species.

S. moniliformis is presumptively identified by its growth characteristics and Gram stain morphology. Biochemical tests must be supplemented with serum. *S. moniliformis* does not liquefy gelatin, produce indole, or reduce nitrates; nor does it contain catalase, oxidase, or urease activity.

Calymmatobacterium and *Bartonella* are identified by their characteristic cellular morphology and growth requirements.

DIRECT ANTIGEN OR NUCLEIC ACID DETECTION

Clinical specimens can be examined for *F. tularensis* and *B. pertussis* by the direct fluorescent antibody test, which is available commercially. The interpretation of smears for *B. pertussis* is experience related and should probably be performed in a reference laboratory. Additional methods to directly detect *B. pertussis* antigens or nucleic acids in nasopharyngeal specimens are currently being evaluated (56).

SEROLOGIC PROCEDURES

Tularemia is diagnosed by a standard agglutination test indicating a four-fold rise in titer or a single titer of equal to or greater than 1:160 (indicates current or past infection). The test cross reacts with *Brucella* at low titers.

A variety of tests have been employed for the serologic diagnosis of brucellosis. Antibodies against all *Brucella* species, except *B. canis*, are detected in the standard agglutination test using *B. abortus* antigens. A four-fold rise in titer or a single titre of 1:160 or higher with a compatible illness is diagnostic of brucellosis. Antibodies against *Francisella*, *Yersinia*, and *Vibrio* may cross-react. Complement fixation and indirect hemagglutination titers of 1:64 or higher and 1:100 or higher, respectively, are consistent with the diagnosis. Results with an EIA method suggest that it may be useful for differentiating acute from chronic infection. Populations exposed to *Brucella* (e.g., veterinarians, abattoir workers) often have baseline titers of 1:80 or 1:160.

Serologic tests for *B. pertussis* exposure have been used primarily for epidemiologic purposes, but a recent commercially available EIA system showed promising results for the diagnosis of acute infection.

Patients with rat-bite fever usually have an agglutination titer of 1:80 or higher or demonstrate a four-fold rise in titer. The test is performed only at national reference laboratories. No serologic tests are commercially available for the diagnosis of granuloma inguinale or bartonellosis.

INTERPRETATION OF RESULTS

The isolation or direct identification of any of the aforementioned bacterial species (except *B. parapertussis* and *B. bronchiseptica*) from patients with a compatible illness is clinically significant.

Therapeutic Considerations

The organisms discussed in this section have special growth requirements that make in vitro suscepti-

Table 44.27. Genera of Anaerobic Bacteria

Gram-Negative Rods
Bacteroides
Fusobacterium
Prevotella
Porphyromonas
Anaerorhabdus
Leptotrichia
Bilophilia
Butyrivibrio
Fibrobacter
Succinimonas
Megamonas
Anaerobiospirillum
Mitsuokella
Wolinella
Rikenella
Selenomonas
Ruminobacter
Anaerovibrio
Sebaldella
Desulfomonas
Tissierella
Mobiluncus
Centipeda
Succinivibrio
Gram-Negative Cocci
Veillonella
Acidaminococcus
Megasphaera
Gram-Positive Rods
Clostridium
Actinomyces
Propionibacterium
Bifidobacterium
Eubacterium
Lactobacillus
Gram-Positive Cocci
Peptococcus
Peptostreptococcus
Ruminococcus
Coprococcus
Streptococcus
Staphylococcus
Gemella
Sarcina

bility testing difficult. Therefore, most recommendations for therapy are based on clinical response. Streptomycin is the drug of choice for the treatment of tularemia, although some data suggest that gentamicin may be an alternative. The use of tetracycline or chloramphenicol is associated with a higher relapse rate.

Because brucellosis is difficult to eradicate, some investigators recommend the use of tetracycline plus streptomycin. Aminoglycosides, rifampin, trimethoprim-sulfamethoxazole, chloramphenicol, and ciprofloxacin have also been used, but single-drug therapy is associated with a 10 to 40% relapse rate. Therapy should continue for 3 to 6 weeks.

B. pertussis infections can be treated with erythromycin, trimethoprim-sulfamethoxazole, chloramphenicol, or tetracycline. Treatment can eradicate the organism but may not alter the disease course.

C. granulomatis is susceptible to tetracycline, sulfonamide, trimethoprim-sulfamethoxazole, chloramphenicol, and gentamicin. The drug of choice for the treatment of rat-bite fever and bartonellosis is penicillin. Other alternatives include chloramphenicol, tetracycline, and streptomycin.

Summary and Conclusions

The diseases discussed in this section are infrequently observed, and the laboratory diagnosis is difficult because of the special growth requirements of the etiologic agents. The clinician must alert the laboratory to the possibility of infection by one of these agents so that appropriate isolation procedures will be used. The laboratory must also rule out these bacteria when unusual isolates are seen on Gram smear or isolated.

ANAEROBIC BACTERIA

Microbiology

The classification of anaerobic microorganisms has improved in recent years as better procedures have been developed for the isolation and identification of this group of heterogeneous bacteria. Continued change in nomenclature and recognition of new species can be expected. A list of the medically important genera of anaerobic bacteria based on Gram stain morphology is provided in Table 44.27.

The anaerobic Gram-negative bacilli are straight, curved, or helical; are motile or nonmotile; and are among the most common of the normal flora of the human mucous membranes. Among these genera, *Bacteroides*, *Fusobacterium*, *Prevotella*, and *Porphyromonas* are isolated most frequently from infections.

Of the Gram-negative cocci, only three of the seven *Veillonella* species are occasionally isolated from human infections. *Megasphaera* and *Acidaminococcus* are seldom associated with infections in humans.

The genera of anaerobic Gram-positive bacilli consist of *Clostridium* (spore formers) and five genera of non–spore formers (*Actinomyces*, *Propionibacterium*, *Bifidobacterium*, *Eubacterium*, and *Lactobacillus*). Some species are aerotolerant and vary their morphology with the type of medium and growth conditions,

Table 44.28. Recent Taxonomic Changes of Anaerobic Bacteria

Current Nomenclature	Prior Nomenclature	Current Nomenclature	Prior Nomenclature
Anaerorhabdus furcosus	*Bacteroides furcosus*	*P. micros*	*P. micros*
Bacteroides caccae	*B.* species "3452A"	*P. prevotii*	*P. prevotii*
B. forsythus	New species	*P. tetradius*	New species
B. galacturonicus	New species	*Porphyromonas asaccharolytica*	*B. asaccharolyticus*
B. gracilis	*B. ureolyticus* (in part)	*P. endodontalis*	*B. endodontalis*
B. levii	*B. melaninogenicus* subsp. *levii*	*P. gingivalis*	*B. gingivalis*
B. merdae	New species	*Prevotella bivia*	*B. bivius*
B. pectinophilus	New species	*P. buccae*	*B. buccae*
B. salivosus	New species	*P. buccalis*	*B. buccalis*
B. stercoris	New species	*P. corporis*	*B. corporis*
B. tectum	New species	*P. denticola*	*B. denticoli*
Bilophila wadsworthia	New genus and species	*P. disiens*	*B. disiens*
Centipeda periodontii	New genus and species	*P. heparinolytica*	*B. heparinolyticus*
Clostridium absonum	New species	*P. intermedia*	*B. intermedius*
C. bullosum	*Fusobacterium bullosum*	*P. loescheii*	*B. loescheii*
C. symbiosum	*F. symbiosum*	*P. melaninogenica*	*B. melaninogenicus*
Eubacterium brachy	New species	*P. oralis*	*B. oralis*
E. biforme	New species	*P. oris*	*B. oris*
E. nodatum	New species	*P. oulora*	*B. oulorum*
E. plautii	*F. plautii*	*P. ruminicola*	*B. ruminocola*
E. timidum	New species	*P. veroralis*	*B. veroralis*
Fibrobacter succinogenes	*B. succinogenes*	*P. zoogleoformans*	*B. zoogleoformans*
F. intestinalis	New species	*Rikenella microfusus*	*B. microfusus*
Fusobacterium alocis	New species	*Ruminobacter amylophilus*	*B. amylophilus*
F. periodonticum	Related to *F. nucleatum*	*Sebaldella termitidis*	*B. termitidis*
F. sulci	New species	*Selenomonas artemidis*	New species
F. ulcerans	New species	*S. dianae*	New species
Lactobacillus oris	Resembles *L. brevis*	*S. flueggei*	New species
Megamonas hypermegas	*B. hypermegas*	*S. infelix*	New species
Mitsuokella multiacidus	*B. multiacidus*	*S. noxia*	New species
M. dentalis	New species	*Streptococcus parvulus*	*Peptostreptococcus parvulus*
Peptostreptococcus asaccharolyticus	*Peptococcus asaccharolyticus*	*Tissierella praeacuta*	*B. praeacutus*
		Wolinella curva	New species
P. indolicus	*P. indolicus*	*W. recta*	New species
P. magnus	*P. magnus*	*W. succinogenes*	New species

causing confusion with the aerobic bacilli and streptococci. In general, streptococci produce long chains in broth. In addition, the aerotolerant anaerobes grow better anaerobically (produce larger colonies) than aerobically, and the aerotolerant clostridia (catalase negative) rarely produce spores aerobically. *Bacillus* species are catalase positive and rarely produce spores anaerobically.

The anaerobic Gram-positive cocci are the second most common group of anaerobes encountered in clinical infections. Major taxonomic changes have occurred recently with these genera. All pathogenic strains of *Peptococcus* species (except *Peptococcus niger*) were transferred to the genus *Peptostreptococcus*. Other anaerobic cocci were transferred to the genus *Streptococcus,* and *Peptococcus saccharolyticus* was transferred to the genus *Staphylococcus*. *Peptostreptococcus tetradius* now includes species from the old genus *Gaffkya*.

Some of the numerous nomenclature changes that have occurred in recent years are listed in Table 44.28, and clinically encountered anaerobes are indicated in Table 44.29.

Spectrum of Disease

Anaerobic bacteria are recovered from all types of infections in any organ of the body (57). The most frequently encountered anaerobic infections or toxin-related diseases include pleuropulmonary infection (e .g., pneumonia, abscess, empyema); intra-abdominal infection (e.g., abscess, appendicitis, cholecystitis, peritonitis); antibiotic-associated colitis; and female genital tract infection (e.g., abscess, pelvic inflammatory disease, endometritis, bacterial vaginosis). Other types of infections include head and neck infections (e.g., brain abscess, meningitis, sinusitis, otitis media, dental and periodontal infection), soft tissue infections (cellulitis, myonecrosis), bone and joint infections, bacteremia, endocarditis, bite wounds, botulism (including infant and wound), tetanus, and food poisoning.

Table 44.29. Clinically Encountered Anaerobes[a]

Bacteroides fragilis Group	Anaerobic Gram-positive cocci
B. fragilis	*Peptostreptococcus* group
B. thetaiotaomicron	*P. prevotii*
B. distasonis	*P. anaerobius*
B. ovatus	*P. productus*
B. vulgatus	*P. micros*
B. uniformis	*P. magnus*
B. caccae	*Peptococcus niger*
B. merdae	*Clostridium*
B. stercoris	*C. bifermentans*
B. eggerthii	*C. sordellii*
B. splanchnicus	*C. perfringens*
Prophyromonas and Prevotella	*C. novyi type A*
P. asaccharolytica	*C. sporogenes*
P. gingivalis	*C. cadaveris*
P. endodontalis	*C. septicum*
P. intermedia	*C. difficile*
P. corporis	*C. putrificum*
P. melaninogenica	*C. baratii*
P. denticola	*C. tertium*
P. loescheii	*C. butyricum*
P. bivia	*C. innocuum*
Nonpigmented bile-sensitive	*C. ramosum*
Bacteroides and *Prevotella*	*C. clostridioforme*
P. oris	*C. tetani*
P. buccae	*C. hastiforme*
P. zoogleoformans	*C. subterminale*
P. oralis	*C. histolyticum*
P. buccalis	*C. limosum*
P. veroralis	*C. absonum*
P. oulora	*C. cochlearium*
P. disiens	Gram-positive rods
B. capillosus	*Actinomyces* spp.
B. putredinis	*Propionibacterium propionica*
B. ureolyticus	*Bifidobacterium* spp.
B. gracilis	*Propionibacterium* acnes
Fusobacterium species	*Eubacterium* spp.
F. nucleatum	*Lactobacillus* spp.
F. necrophorum	
F. naviforme	
F. varium	
F. mortiferum	
F. russii	
F. alocis	
Wollinella species	

[a]From Finegold SM, George WL, eds. Anaerobic infections in humans. New York: Academic Press, 1989:33.

Epidemiology

Anaerobic infections caused by non–spore-forming organisms generally arise from the host's indigenous flora following a break in the normal mucosal barrier (e.g., trauma, surgery, implantation of a device). The resulting tissue damage and the presence of obligate aerobes, microaerophiles, or facultative anaerobes act to lower the oxygen tension and redox potential of the affected tissue. This provides the appropriate environment for the growth of anaerobes and explains why most deep-seated abscesses and necrotizing lesions contain multiple species of bacteria.

Infections or intoxications due to spore-forming bacilli (*Clostridium*) are usually transmitted via improperly prepared or stored food (e.g., botulism, *Clostridium perfringens* food poisoning); via contamination of damaged tissue with soil or bowel contents (e.g., clostridial myonecrosis, tetanus); or via contaminated objects or medical personnel in hospitals (e.g., antibiotic-associated colitis due to *Clostridium difficile*).

Diagnostic Procedures

This section provides a limited overview of the procedures that may aid in the isolation or preliminary identification of anaerobic bacteria. The extent to which anaerobes are identified depends on the available facilities, the technical competence of the personnel, and the clinical need for the information (e.g., the detection of the agent or toxin responsible for the disease may indicate a therapy change or the need for an antimicrobial susceptibility test). The selection, collection, and transport of specimens are crucial to clinically relevant laboratory results. The workup of inappropriate or poorly transported specimens is a waste of effort and money. The presence of anaerobes in a specimen is suggested when the material has a foul odor and black discoloration, contains sulfur granules, or fluoresces brick-red under long-wave UV light (366 nm). All laboratories should be able to isolate and presumptively identify anaerobic isolates based on cellular and colony morphology and a few key characteristics. More definitive identification of common isolates can be accomplished with the use of commercial kits, and other significant isolates can be submitted to a reference laboratory for identification.

MICROSCOPY

The Gram stain can provide useful clinical information on the presence of anaerobes and suggest additional media to set up based on the characteristic morphology of some species. The *Bacteroides fragilis* group may be uniform or pleomorphic with a safety-pin appearance (Fig. 44.17), while the pigmented species are often coccobacillary (*Haemophilus*-like) and can be mistaken for Gram-negative cocci (Fig. 44.18). *Fusobacterium nucleatum* is usually very thin with tapered ends (spindle-shaped), often appearing end to end in pairs (Fig. 44.19). *Fusobacterium mortiferum* and *Fusobacterium necrophorum* are filamentous and pleomorphic, with swollen areas and large round bodies. *Actinomyces* appear as thin, branching Gram-positive rods with beaded staining. *Bifidobacterium* species often exhibit clubbing or terminal bifur-

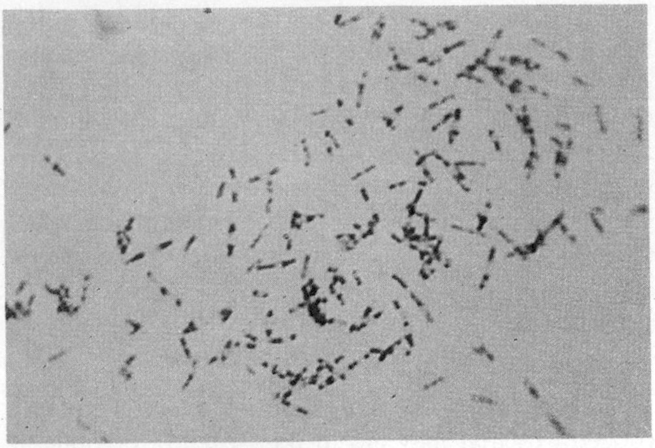

Figure 44.17. Gram stain of *B. fragilis*.

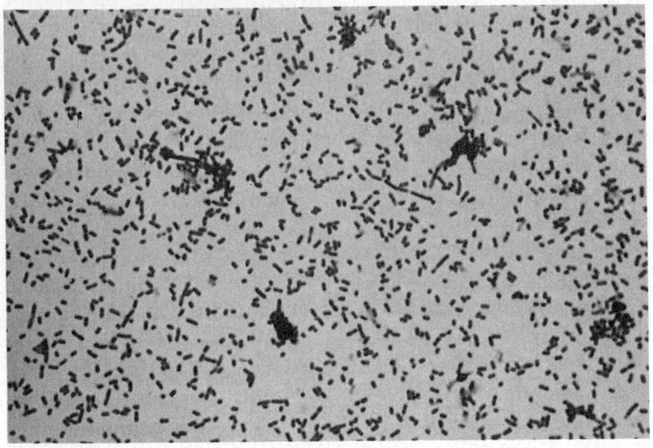

Figure 44.18. Gram stain of pigmented *Prevotella* species.

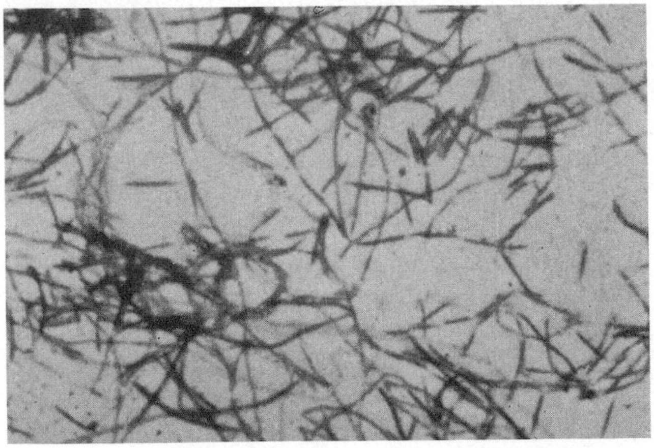

Figure 44.19. Gram stain of *F. nucleatum*. Fusiform shape. (Reprinted with permission from Baron EJ, Finegold SM. Bailey and Scott's diagnostic microbiology. St. Louis: CV Mosby, 1990.)

cation. Peptostreptococci appear as clusters and chains of irregularly stained, somewhat pleomorphic, Gram-positive cocci. *P. magnus* is usually large, and *P. tetradius* occurs in tetrads. *C. perfringens* is a Gram-positive rod (may appear Gram-negative) with

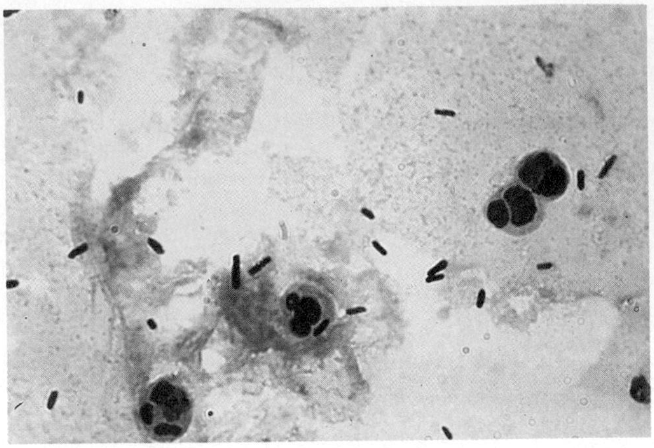

Figure 44.20. Gram stain of body fluid containing *C. perfringens*.

square ends and usually does not contain a spore (Fig. 44.20).

CULTURE TECHNIQUES

A combination of enriched, prereduced, nonselective (e.g., *Brucella* sheep blood agar), selective (e.g., *Bacteroides* bile esculin, kanamycin-vancomycin laked blood, phenylethyl alcohol agars), and enriched thioglycollate media should be used for the recovery and presumptive identification of anaerobes (58). Primary plates are incubated in anaerobic jars at 35°C for 48 hours before examination and are reincubated for 5 to 7 days. In serious infections or suspected actinomycosis, the broth medium should be held for 2 to 4 weeks. During the examination of primary plates and subculture of anaerobic isolates, a holding jar should be used to minimize the exposure of the isolates to oxygen. Colony morphology is examined with a dissecting microscope or a hand-held lens, and each type Gram-stained and subcultured for incubation in CO_2 and anaerobically. Gram-positive cocci that are capnophiles may not grow in CO_2 on initial subculture and require a second subculture to demonstrate growth. The thioglycollate medium should be Gram stained and subcultured if morphologic types appear on smear that are not seen on the primary plates. The cellular and colony morphology on the primary plates can be suggestive of certain groups of organisms (Table 44.30). Cycloserine-cefoxitin-fructose agar (CCFA) is one medium that is recommended for the isolation of *C. difficile* from stool specimens.

IDENTIFICATION METHODS

The preliminary or presumptive identification of anaerobes can be accomplished by using some special tests such as colonial fluorescence; susceptibility to special-potency antibiotic and polyanethol-

Table 44.30. Microscopic and Colonial Morphology of Selected Anaerobes[a]

Organism	Medium[a]	Microscopic Morphology[b]	Colonial Morphology
B. fragilis group	BBE	gnb, pleomorphic	>1 mm ± esculin hydrolysis
Bacteroides spp.	KVLB	gnb	Nonpigmented
Porphyromonas or *Prevotella* spp.	KVLB	cb, gnb	Brown to black or fluorescing brick-red
B. ureolyticus	BA	gnb	Pitting
B. fragilis group	BA	gnb, pleomorphic	Circular, grayish-white translucent to opaque
Pigmenting species	BA	cb, gnb	Circular, darker in center with brown edges
F. nucleatum	BA	Fusiform gnb with pointed ends	Opalescent and speckled
F. necrophorum	BA	pleomorphic gnb, many contain round bodies	Convex to umbonate
A. israelii	BA	branching gpb	Molar tooth
C. perfringens	BA	gpb, square ends	Double zone of β-hemolysis
C. difficile	CCFA	gpb	Yellow colonies that may fluoresce
C. septicum	BA	gpb ± spores	Swarming, β-hemolysis medusa head
C. tetani	BA	gpb, "drumstick"	May swarm, narrow zone β-hemolysis
Peptostreptococcus	BA	gpc	Grow only on BA after 48 hr
Veillonella parvula	BA	gnc	Fluoresce red

[a]Abbreviations: BBE, *Bacteroides* bile esculin-agar; KVLB, kanamycin-vancomycin laked blood agar; BA, *Brucella* blood agar; CCFA, cycloserine-cefoxitin-fructose agar.
[b]Abbreviations: gnb, Gram-negative bacillus; cb, coccobacillus; gpb, Gram-positive bacillus; gpc, Gram-positive coccus.

sulfonate disks; spot indole; and catalase, urease, and nitrate reduction (Table 44.31) (58, 59). Dowell et. al. (60) have devised a modified conventional plate system (presumpto method) that can be used for the preliminary identification of anaerobes.

The definitive identification of anaerobes by reference laboratories includes conventional biochemical tests and gas-liquid chromatographic analysis of fatty acid metabolites (61–63), and is beyond the scope of this discussion. For the nonreference laboratory, a number of commercial systems are available that will correctly identify 70 to 90% of the more commonly encountered isolates (58, 59) and offer a rapid alternative to the conventional method.

DIRECT ANTIGEN OR NUCLEIC ACID DETECTION

Direct analysis methods for the detection of anaerobes in clinical specimens include commercial fluorescent antibody reagents for the identification of the *B. fragilis* and *Prevotella melaninogenica* groups, *Clostridium novyi, Clostridium septicum, Clostridium sordellii,* and *Actinomyces* species. Gas-liquid chromatographic analysis of specimens can presumptively detect the presence of *Bacteroides* or *Fusobacterium* species. Currently, there are no commercial nucleic acid probes for the detection or identification of anaerobes, but a number of probes are being evaluated in research laboratories.

The laboratory diagnosis of antibiotic-associated colitis (AAC) is made by demonstrating the organism, its antigen, or toxins in the stool specimen of a symptomatic patient. The recovery of *C. difficile* by culture is supportive but not definitive evidence for the disease because individuals, particularly infants, may carry the organism in the gastrointestinal tract (64). The detection of *C. difficile* "antigen" by the commercial latex test is rapid, but the test detects both toxigenic and nontoxigenic strains and cross-reacts with some other anaerobes (65, 66). Recently, commercial EIA tests for the detection of toxin A have also become available. At this time, the recommended method is the detection of *C. difficile* toxins by cytopathic effect in tissue culture (64).

The detection of botulinal neurotoxin in the patient's vomitus, serum, feces, or consumed food is done by the mouse bioassay and should be performed by a reference laboratory.

SEROLOGIC PROCEDURES

Serologic procedures are not important tests for the diagnosis of anaerobic infections, but a serum tetanus antitoxin level of 0.01 units/ml or higher makes the diagnosis of tetanus unlikely.

INTERPRETATION OF RESULTS

The significance of the isolation of anaerobes that are a part of the indigenous flora is dependent on the quality of the specimen submitted and the subsequent Gram stain, and must be interpreted in light of the clinical picture. The presence of botulinal neurotoxin is diagnostic of botulism.

The interpretation of the tests used for the laboratory diagnosis of AAC is difficult because the tests lack sensitivity and specificity when compared with the clinical setting of the patient. The use of two tests can often improve the detection of affected patients

Table 44.31. Preliminary Identification of Anaerobes[a]

Group/Species	Antibiotic Disk Pattern K (1 mg)	Co (10 μg)	Va (5 μg)	Characteristics
Bacteroides fragilis group	R[d]	R	R	Bile, R; catalase, V
Pigmenting species	R	V	V	Tan to black colonies[b] Brick-red fluorescence[c]
P. intermedia	R	S	R	Brown to black colonies[b] Brick-red fluorescence[c] Indole, +; lipase, +[b]
Other *Bacteroides* spp.	R	V	R	
Bacteroides ureolyticus group	S	S	R	Colonies pit agar or require formate/fumarate for growth and nitrate, +
B. ureolyticus	S	S	R	Urease +; motile, −
B. gracilis	S	S	R	Urease, −; motile, −
Wolinella spp.	S	S	R	Urease, −; motile, +
Fusobacterium spp.	S	S	R	Colonies generally larger and more opaque than *B. ureolyticus* group
F. nucleatum	S	S	R	Slender cells with pointed end. Indole, +; greens agar; yellow-green fluorescence; three possible colony types
F. necrophorum	S	S	R	Indole, +; lipase, +[b] Umbonate colony[c]
Gram-negative cocci	S	S	R	Three genera; requires GLC, if not Veillonella
Veillonella sp.	S	S	R	Nitrate, + Small coccus
Gram-positive cocci	S	R	S	
P. anaerobius	R	R	S	Sodium polyanethol sulfonate, S
P. asaccharolyticus	S	R	S	Indole, +
Clostridium spp.	V	R	S	Spores present: may appear Gram-negative
C. perfringens	S	R	S	Double-zone β-hemolysis. Cells boxcar shape; spore test, V; reverse CAMP test, +; Nagler test, +
Non–spore-forming bacilli	S	R	S	
Propionibacterium acnes	S	R	S	Indole, +[b], catalase, +[b]; nitrate, +[c]; cells may show short branching
Eubacterium lentum	S	R	S	Cells and colonies small; Arginine required for growth in broth; nitrate, +

[a]Adapted from Edelstein MAC. Laboratory diagnosis of anaerobic infections in humans. In: Finegold SM, George WL, eds. Anaerobic infections in humans. New York: Academic Press, 1989:127.
[b]Not all strains positive; if negative, more tests required.
[c]Not all strains positive.
[d]Symbols: R, resistant; S, susceptible; V, variable; +, positive; −, negative; GLC, gas-liquid chromatography.

(67). Colonoscopy remains the gold standard for the clinical diagnosis of AAC.

Therapeutic Considerations

For most institutions, antimicrobial susceptibility testing of anaerobic isolates should be limited to circumstances related to the seriousness of the infection, lack of response to empiric therapy, lack of established data with a specific agent, or to monitor susceptibility patterns of local isolates. The susceptibility pattern of specific anaerobes cannot always be predicted. This is because of the increasing resistance to penicillin and clindamycin and the differing degrees of effectiveness of the newer agents. Additionally, the several available in vitro test methods (there is no "gold standard") lack comparability, and the results are not always predictive of clinical efficacy. When anaerobic susceptibility tests are performed, the method should conform to the recommendations of the National Committee for Clinical Laboratory Standards (68). A positive β-lactamase test by the nitrocefin method predicts resistance to penicillin G and ampicillin, but not necessarily to other antimicrobial agents. It therefore has limited utility (68).

Metronidazole (inactive against *Propionibacterium* and *Actinomyces*), chloramphenicol, imipenem, and the β-lactam plus β-lactamase inhibitor drugs are active against most anaerobes. Agents that are usually active include clindamycin (increasing resistance among *B. fragilis* group and clostridia); cefoxitin (increasing resistance among *B. fragilis* group and poor activity against clostridia); and antipseudomonal penicillins. Penicillin, cephalosporins (other than cefoxitin, cefotetan, and moxalactam), tetracycline, erythromycin (inactive against most *Fusobacterium* and *B. fragilis*), and vancomycin (active against Gram-positive anaerobes) have variable activity. The aminoglycosides, monolactams, and quinolones have poor activity against anaerobes.

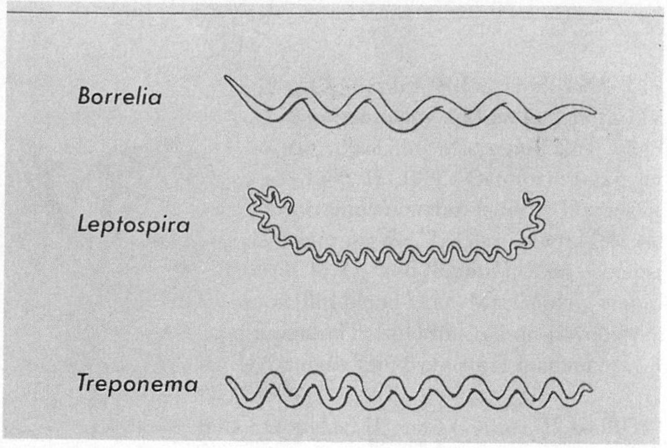

Figure 44.21. Schematic designation of spirochetes based on general morphology. (Reprinted with permission from Baron EJ, Finegold SM. Bailey and Scott's diagnostic microbiology. St. Louis: CV Mosby, 1990.)

Summary and Conclusions

Anaerobic bacteria are common, indigenous organisms found on the mucosal surfaces of humans that cause a variety of infections in any tissue or organ system. The most important aspect of anaerobic microbiology is to ensure the appropriate selection, collection, transport, and inoculation of the specimen. The extent of isolate identification depends on the seriousness of the infection, the clinical need for information, the technical expertise of the laboratory personnel, and the availability of resources.

SPIROCHETES

Microbiology

The order Spirochaetales consists of two families. The family Spirochaetaceae contains the genera *Spirochaeta, Cristispina, Treponema,* and *Borrelia;* and the family Leptospiraceae contains one genus, *Leptospira.* Spirochetes of medical importance are in the genera *Treponema, Borrelia,* and *Leptospira.* The pathogenic species are restricted to a living host and are heterogeneous in their physiology and habitat. Common features include spiral morphology and unique flexuous motility related to axial filaments located in the periplasmic space between the outer membrane and protoplasmic cylinder. In general, the spirochetes are slender, flexible, helical-shaped bacteria that exhibit a corkscrew-like motility and can be loosely grouped into genera by their morphology (Fig. 44.21).

The genus *Treponema* currently contains 13 species. The pathogenic species are 7 to 15 μm in length and 0.1 to 0.2 μm in width with regularly spaced coils and a rotational back-and-forth motility with some bending and snapping.

The treponemes pathogenic for humans can be continuously cultured only by animal passage and consist of two species: *Treponema carateum* (causes pinta) and *Treponema pallidum,* which contains three subspecies: *pallidum* (causes syphilis), *pertenue* (causes yaws) and *endemicum* (causes nonvenereal endemic syphilis or bejel).

The genus *Borrelia* contains 19 species, and these are named according to their arthropod vector. This classification may not be correct, and awaits clarification by genetic relatedness techniques. *Borrelia* are 0.2 to 0.5 × 5 to 20 μm, have 3 to 10 loose coils, and grow well from 30° to 35°C in specialized media.

The genus *Leptospira* contains two species, *Leptospira biflexa,* which is a nonpathogenic free-living spirochete with over 60 serovars, and *Leptospira interrogans,* which causes leptospirosis in animals and humans with over 180 serovars. *Leptospira* are 6 to 20 × 0.1 to 0.2 μm with very tightly wound coils that may be hooked at one or both ends. They are aerobic and require certain nutrients (e.g., long-chain fatty acids) and a specific pH (7.0 to 7.8) for growth at 28° to 30°C.

Spectrum of Disease

T. pallidum subsp. *pallidum* is the etiologic agent of syphilis, which presents in three stages: primary (a chancre at the site of entry); secondary (flu-like illness with generalized rash); and tertiary (lesions in the CNS, cardiovascular system, or any other organ system). Infection of the fetus (congenital syphilis) can occur in untreated women.

Yaws, pinta, and endemic syphilis are distinguished from syphilis based on their clinical manifestations and geographical area of occurrence. Yaws occurs primarily in rural populations of tropical countries; pinta is found in remote rural areas of southern Mexico, Central America, and Colombia; and endemic syphilis primarily affects children in Africa, western Asia, and Australia.

Borrelia recurrentis is the etiologic agent of louse-borne (epidemic) relapsing fever, while other *Borrelia* species cause tick-borne (endemic) relapsing fever. *Borrelia burgdorferi* is associated with Lyme disease.

Leptospirosis is primarily a disease of animals that is occasionally transmitted to humans.

Epidemiology

Syphilis occurs worldwide and is transmitted through sexual contact or transplacentally. Infections may also be acquired through nonsexual contact with lesions or blood. The highest prevalence of the disease is associated with economically deprived individuals engaged in prostitution or sexual activity with multiple partners.

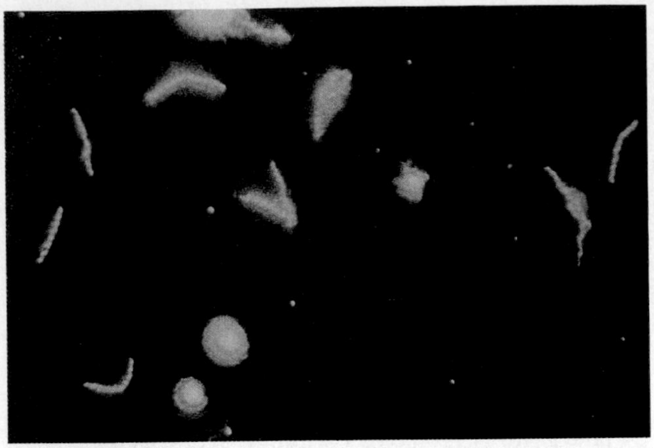

Figure 44.22. Appearance of *T. pallidum* in a dark-field preparation. (Reprinted with permission from Baron EJ, Finegold SM. Bailey and Scott's diagnostic Microbiology. St. Louis: CV Mosby, 1990.)

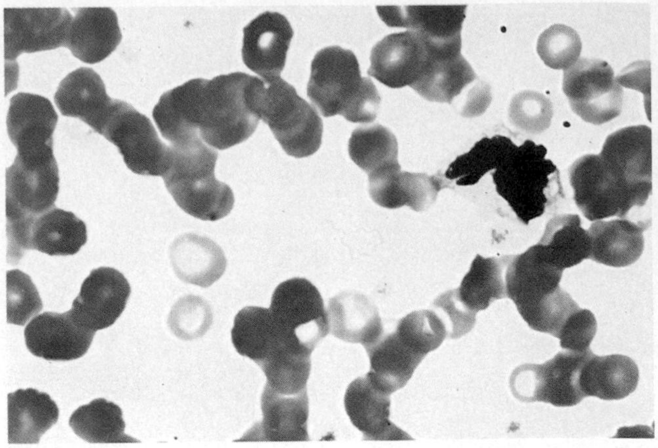

Figure 44.23. Wright-stained peripheral blood smear demonstrating *Borrelia*.

Louse-borne (epidemic) relapsing fever (*B. recurrentis*) is transmitted by the human body louse (*Pediculus humanus*). The infective organisms penetrate intact skin or mucous membranes. Humans are the only hosts. Disease usually occurs from overcrowding such as during famine or wars. The disease is endemic in Central and East Africa and in Bolivia and Peru.

Tick-borne (endemic) relapsing fever (*Borrelia* spp.) is transmitted to humans by infected soft-shelled ticks of the genus *Ornithodorus*. Infection occurs when saliva or coxal secretions are released by feeding ticks. The principal reservoirs are rodents and small animals as well as the ticks that pass the spirochete transovarially.

Lyme disease (*B. burgdorferi*) occurs worldwide and is transmitted primarily by the *Ixodes* species of ticks. The principal reservoirs are rodents and large mammals (e.g., deer). The disease can be spread by the adult, larval, and nymphal stage of the tick.

Leptospirosis is a zoonosis that occurs worldwide and affects many different species of animals. In the United States, the most common sources are dogs, livestock, rodents, wild mammals, and cats. Humans are indirectly infected by contact with urine or with contaminated water and soil, or by direct contact with animals. Leptospirosis is an occupational hazard among farmers, meatpackers, and veterinarians, and is a recreational hazard for campers and swimmers.

Diagnostic Procedures

MICROSCOPY

In primary, secondary, and early congenital syphilis, the treponemes are detected in lesion material by dark-field microscopic examination (Fig. 44.22) or by performance of a direct fluorescent antibody (DFA) test. The dark-field examination cannot be used on oral or rectal lesions because of the presence of morphologically similar nonpathogenic treponemes. The DFA test or silver stain can be used to detect treponemes in tissue.

The diagnosis of borreliosis is made in 70% of cases by examination of blood collected during a febrile episode by dark-field microscopy, Giemsa- or Wright-stained thick and thin smears (Fig. 44.23), or acridine-orange-stained smears. Rarely, spirochetes are detected in the CSF of patients with CNS symptoms. Because of the scarcity of *B. burgdorferi* in clinical specimens, direct examination is not recommended for the diagnosis of Lyme disease.

The direct examination of blood, CSF, or urine by dark-field examination has low sensitivity for the detection of leptospires, as has the DFA test or silver stain on tissue.

CULTURE TECHNIQUES

Isolation of *Borrelia* species in the routine clinical laboratory by in vitro cultivation is not recommended because of the low yield. Although improvements in the cultivation of *B. burgdorferi* from clinical specimens has occurred, the yield remains low and probably should not be attempted by the routine clinical laboratory.

Leptospira is cultivated in two types of media: those supplemented with bovine serum albumin and polysorbate 80 (Ellinghausen, McCullough, Johnson, and Harris—EMJH medium) or those enriched with rabbit serum (Fletcher or Stuart). The EMJH-based formulations are probably the best. Approximately two to three drops of blood (not citrated) or CSF collected during the first week of illness is added to each of three to five tubes of medium. One or two drops of undiluted and 1:10 dilution of urine collected after the first week is added to each of three to five tubes of medium with and without 200 μg/ml of 5-fluorouracil. The cultures are incubated in the dark for 6 weeks at 30°C. Tubes are examined weekly for growth in the form of a ring 1 to 3 cm below the surface, and organisms can be identified by dark-field microscopy.

IDENTIFICATION METHODS

Diagnosis of syphilis depends on the observation of the organisms in lesions by dark-field examination or DFA test, or by the serologic detection of antibodies.

Relapsing fever is diagnosed by the demonstration of organisms in peripheral blood by dark-field examination or by Geimsa- or Wright-stained smears. Lyme disease is recognized by serologic tests.

The isolation of *Leptospira* in culture or the detection of antibodies by serologic tests aids in the laboratory diagnosis. *L. biflexa* and *L. interrogans* can be differentiated by growth at 13°C, growth in presence of purine analogues, or conversion to spheroplasts in 1M NaCl (69).

DIRECT ANTIGEN OR NUCLEIC ACID DETECTION

The DFA test is commercially available for the direct detection of *T. pallidum* in clinical specimens. Other DFA, EIA, and nucleic acid probes are being evaluated in research centers for the direct detection of *Borrelia*, *Leptospira*, and *T. pallidum* but are not commercially available at this time.

SEROLOGIC PROCEDURES

Serologic tests for the diagnosis of syphilis measure two types of antibodies. The nontreponemal (nonspecific) tests measure both IgG and IgM antilipid antibodies formed in response to lipoidal antigen released during infection and/or from the treponemes themselves. The treponemal (specific) tests measure antibodies directed against the organism.

There are four standard nontreponemal tests: (*a*) Venereal Disease Research Laboratory (VDRL) slide; (*b*) rapid plasma reagin (RPR); (*c*) unheated serum reagin (USR); and (*d*) reagin screen test (RST). Of these the RPR test is the most widely used in the United States, and the VDRL is the only accepted nontreponemal test for detection of antibodies in the CSF of patients with suspected neurosyphilis. The nontreponemal tests are used primarily as screening tests and to follow patients on therapy. The sensitivity of the test varies with the stage of the disease (Table 44.32). In the primary stage, patients who have nonreactive tests should have subsequent tests at 1 week, 1 month, and 3 months. In congenital syphilis, a rising titer during a 6-month period is diagnostic, whereas passively transferred antibodies should not be detected after 3 months. The nontreponemal test becomes nonreactive in primary syphilis 1 year after therapy and in secondary syphilis 2 years after treatment. The specificity of these tests is approximately 98% overall but varies with the population. Causes of biological false-positives include a variety of infectious diseases, drug addiction, pregnancy, and autoimmune disease.

Table 44.32. Reactivity of Serologic Tests in Untreated Syphilis

Test	Stage of Disease		
	Primary	Secondary	Latent
Nontreponemal			
(VDRL, RPR)	60–80[a]	99–100	70–90
Treponemal			
FTA–Abs	80–95	99–100	96–100
MHA–TP	70–90	99–100	96–100

[a]Percent reactive.
[b]Abbreviations: VDRL, Venereal Disease Research Laboratory; RPR, rapid plasma reagin; FTA-Abs, fluorescent treponemal antibody absorbed; MHA-TP, microhem-agglutination assay-Treponema pallidum.

There are two principal treponemal tests: (*a*) the fluorescent treponemal antibody-absorbed (FTA-abs); and (*b*) the microhemagglutination assay for *T. pallidum* (MHA-TP). These tests are used primarily to confirm a reactive nontreponemal test and usually remain positive for life. The range of sensitivity of the tests is shown in Table 44.32, and the specificity is 98 to 100%.

A number of different serologic tests have been developed for the serodiagnosis of relapsing fever. Unfortunately, these tests have limited success because of the antigenic variability observed with these organisms.

The methods used to diagnose Lyme disease are the indirect fluorescent antibody (IFA) and EIA tests; the latter test appears to be easier to use and may be more sensitive (70). Both tests can be used to detect antibodies in serum, CSF, or synovial fluid. The problem with both tests is the low sensitivity observed early in the infection (within 3 weeks). Immunoblotting or IgM-capture EIA may be more sensitive in these cases (70). Cross-reactivity among the *Borrelia* species and *T. pallidum* also occurs, but syphilis can be ruled out with a nontreponemal test.

Diagnosis of leptospirosis is usually made by serologic tests that include the microscopic and macroscopic slide agglutination, indirect hemagglutination, and, more recently, EIA and Dot-ELISA tests for the detection of IgM (71). Antibodies usually appear after 1 week and peak after 3 to 4 weeks. Titers may remain elevated for years. The microscopic slide agglutination test is the most sensitive and serovar-specific. In endemic areas, residents will usually have a

tum (histoplasmosis), *Blastomyces dermatitidis* (blastomycosis), and *Paracoccidioides brasiliensis* (paracoccidioidomycosis). Most deep fungal infections result after dissemination of the fungus from the lungs following its inhalation from nature. These infections occur quite regularly in the "normal" host, although, as with most infectious diseases, they are much more rampant and severe when present in the immunocompromised individual, e.g., histoplasmosis and coccidioidomycosis in those with AIDS.

- Opportunistic mycoses: This group of mycoses is, in contemporary medicine, the most significant by far. Opportunistic mycoses are those occurring in the host with abrogated or altered immunity. It is now safe to say that given the right moment, in the correct "living Petri dish," virtually any fungus may incite infectious disease. There are virtually no fungal organisms that cannot cause serious disease in this patient population. These mycoses, more than any other factor, have changed the face of medical mycology and demonstrated the true power of those microbes to render horrific infections. In particular, patients who have neutropenia or leukemia, bone marrow transplant recipients, solid organ transplant patients, burn victims, those with genetic defects in their immune systems, etc., are all susceptible to infection by an ever-growing number of taxonomically diverse fungi. Of course, persons with AIDS have been victims of the opportunistic fungi in escalating numbers. Recognizing that any fungus may incite disease in this patient group, the classic opportunistic mycoses still remain—candidiasis (largely due to *Candida albicans*, but with other species being more and more frequently implicated), cryptococcosis (*Cryptococcus neoformans*, particularly in the AIDS population), aspergillosis (*Aspergillus fumigatus* and *Aspergillus flavus* are the major agents, particularly in neutropenic patients), zygomycosis (mainly due to *Rhizopus arrhizus* in the ketoacidotic diabetic), phaeohyphomycosis (caused by darkly pigmented [dematiaceous] molds and yeasts) and hyalohyphomycosis (caused by lightly pigmented, colorless, or hyaline molds). In large part, modern medical mycology has become the science of infections caused by opportunistic fungi (3–5, 26, 38).

EPIDEMIOLOGY OF MYCOSES

Fungal infections are acquired in a variety of ways, but mainly via acquisition of the etiologic fungus from its site in nature to the human host by accident or happenstance. In most cases, the fungus is living happily in nature, humans intervene through work or play, and the fungal inoculation is acquired. This can be by inhalation (very common), nontraumatic or traumatic inoculation (common), or ingestion (rare). Many of the mycoses are obtained by inhalation of the fungus from a geographic area of the world where the fungus is either wholly endemic or found much more frequently than elsewhere. For example, *Histoplasma capsulatum* variety *capsulatum* and *Blastomyces dermatitidis* are global pathogens, but they are particularly prevalent in the Ohio-Mississippi river valley of the United States. Most cases of histoplasmosis and blastomycosis are diagnosed in individuals who either live or travel in, to, or from these areas. Similarly, *Coccidioides immitis* is endemic only to the lower Sonoran life zone regions of the earth (southwestern United States, parts of Mexico, and Central and South America). Coccidioidomycosis occurs following inhalation of the fungus while in one of the endemic regions. With the abovementioned mycoses, there is no transmission from person to person; these are not communicable, contagious diseases. Another group of human fungal pathogens, the dermatophytic fungi, however, can be transmitted from person to person. With their skin fungal infections, it is possible to implement transmission from one human to another via indirect or direct contact (e.g., acquiring athlete's foot after using a shower stall in bare feet after its previous use by an individual with tinea pedis, or the spread of ringworm of the scalp through a grade-school class when children have used a comb belonging to a classmate with tinea captis). Likewise, humans are frequently infected by dermatophytes after handling their pet cat or dog, or domestic cattle that are infected with various animal dermatophytic pathogens.

As has been mentioned, humans may acquire mycoses following traumatic implantation of the fungal agent from a source in nature. The classic example is rose-handler's or gardener's disease, sporotrichosis, acquired following the handling of rose thorns or sphagnum moss. Many contemporary cases of phaeohyphomycosis occur following traumatic implantation of soil or other materials from nature.

Of growing concern, however, are mycoses obtained in the hospital, often from the same fungi that comprise a part of the normal human flora. The main culprit in this situation is the yeast *Candida albicans*. This fungus is a part of the microbiota of the oral and gastrointestinal tracts of humans and, in women, is often found as normal vaginal flora. Following surgery, antibiotic therapy, chemotherapy, and placement of indwelling devices, *C. albicans* has become a major bloodstream pathogen. The most recent epidemologic figures show this yeast to be the fourth most prevalent cause of hospital-acquired bloodstream infection (7, 26, 38). In surgical and medical intensive care units, this yeast is a matter for critical concern in modern medicine. In fact, without question, candidiasis is the most prevalent and significant mycosis of humans (7, 8, 11, 24, 26, 27, 37, 38, 42, 46, 53).

Finally, in the setting of the neutropenic patient, fungi from among the environmental flora—found everywhere at all times—have become major killers. For example, in bone marrow and liver transplant services, the aspergilli are of grave concern (9, 35, 43). The mortality rate from invasive asperigillosis is unacceptably high, approximately 80 to 100% in most published studies (9, 35). Often, outbreaks follow periods of hospital construction or renovation when the asexual spores (conidia) of aspergilli are prevalent in the air. Another opportunistic fungus that is widely dispersed in nature is *Fusarium*. Fusaria are among the most frequent of plant pathogenic fungi but now cause a higher rate of mortality in granulocytopenic patients than aspergilli (3, 4, 19, 31, 43). Such nosocomial opportunistic pathogenic fungi are on the rise, and constant vigilance must be exercised if mortality is to be minimized in the susceptible patient populations.

DIAGNOSTIC PROCEDURES (BY DISEASE TYPE)

Superficial Mycoses

Agents of superficial mycosis are organisms that attack the keratinized outer layers of the skin, hair, and nails (54). Infections of this sort are usually of cosmetic concern only and cause little if any discomfort to the patient.

Malassezia furfur

Malassezia furfur is responsible for the condition known as pityriasis versicolor and can be found worldwide. Pityriasis versicolor presents as a series of darkened patches in very light-skinned individuals or as nonpigmented patches on individuals with darker skin. These areas will fluoresce yellow under a Wood's lamp. KOH examination reveals a characteristic "spaghetti and meatballs" appearance due to the fragments of hyphae mixed with round yeast cells. *M. furfur* has also recently been implicated in fungemia in neonates and some adult patients receiving intralipid intravenously (4, 27, 42). Fungemic episodes usually resolve once the indwelling catheter is removed.

M. furfur can easily be seen on Gram stain of positive blood culture broths but will not grow on Sabouraud agar when subcultured. The simple overlaying of the culture plate with olive oil will result in abundant growth within 48 hours. Any time a yeast is suspected but is not recovered this simple method should be employed. At present, there are no direct antigen or DNA methods nor serologic procedures useful for detection of this yeast. The characteristic appearance of yeast cells resembling small bottles (this fungus was originally termed the "bottle bacillus") seen in blood from patients receiving parenteral nutritional support with products containing oleic acid, coupled with lack of growth on routine laboratory media, should present a high index of suspicion to both the clinician and laboratorian for *M. furfur* fungemia.

Phaeoannellomyces werneckii

Phaeoannellomyces werneckii, previously called *Cladosporium werneckii*, is responsible for the superficial phaeohyphomycotic condition of tinea nigra. Tinea nigra appears as a dark brown to black patch, most often on the palms of the hands and soles of the feet. Although tinea nigra is also mainly of cosmetic concern it must be differentiated from malignant melanoma prior to any treatment. Often extensive surgery can be avoided with a KOH examination of the affected area.

Once fungal elements are determined to be present, skin scrapings should be placed on mycological media with antibiotics. A dematiaceous yeast-like colony should appear within 3 weeks and may become velvety with age. The degree of hyphal growth depends heavily on the media and conditions under which the colony grows. Microscopic examination reveals two-celled cylindrical yeast-like cells and, depending on the age of the colony, toruloid hyphae.

Phaeoannellomyces werneckii is identified microscopically by seeing characteristic darkly pigmented annelloconidia (condidia possessing annellides or rings), which often slide down the sides of the conidiophore (Fig. 45.1) (27, 42, 54). Because no additional means, e.g., serological tests, are currently available to identify this fungus or this disease, microscopic morphology, coupled with the characteristic lesions on the patient's skin, is the only satisfactory identification procedure.

White Piedra

Trichosporon beigelii (formerly *Trichosporan cutaneum*) is the causative agent for the condition called white piedra which affects the hair of the head, beard, and body. This fungus surrounds the hair shaft and forms a white to brown swelling along the hair strand. By running a section of hair between the thumb and forefinger, the nodules can easily be removed. This condition is related to poor hygiene. Once infected, the hair should be cut or shaved and

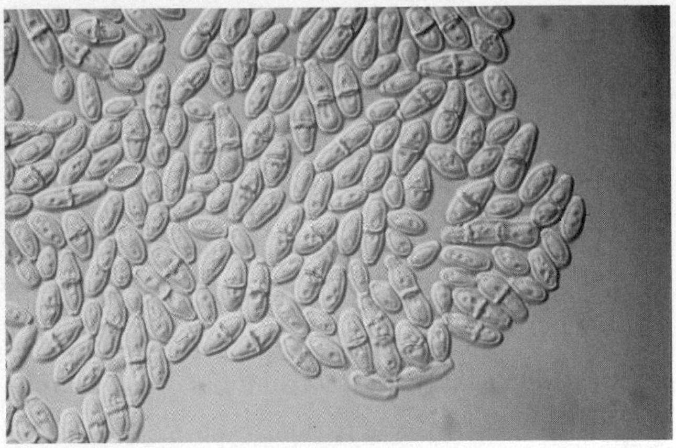

Figure 45.1. Microscopic appearance of *Phaeoannellomyces werneckii* (Nomarski optics, ×1250).

kept clean. These steps usually negate the necessity of medical treatment.

When microscopic examination reveals hyphal elements or arthroconidia and/or budding yeast cells, infected hair may be placed on mycological media without cycloheximide. Cream-colored, dry, wrinkled colonies should form within 48 to 72 hours at room temperature.

T. beigelii can be identified in the same manner as other yeast isolates. Sugar assimilations, KNO_3 assimilation, urease production, and morphology on corn meal should be determined. *T. beigelii* is KNO_3 negative and urease positive and grows at 37°C.

A most important microscopic characteristic is production of both arthroconidia (rectangular cells resulting from the fragmentation of hyphal cells) and blastoconidia (budding yeast cells). In *T. beigelii* one can see the arthroconidia and blastoconidia concurrently (27, 42, 53, 54).

Black Piedra

Another condition affecting the hair, most often that of the scalp, is black piedra. The causative agent of black piedra is *Piedraia hortae*. Black piedra presents as dark, rock-like hyphal masses that surround and penetrate the hair shaft. Examination of the hyphal masses reveals branched hyphae tightly held together with a cement-like substance. Black piedra is also a condition of poor hygiene and is easily resolved with a haircut and proper regular washings.

Piedraia hortae can be cultured on routine mycological media. Very slow growth may be observed at 25°C and may begin as a yeast-like colony, later becoming velvety as hyphae develop. Asci may be observed microscopically, usually ranging from 4 to 30 μm and containing up to eight ascospores. The characteristic "cement-like" material holding all the above-mentioned structures in place around hair shafts, is typical of the group of fungi in which *Piedraia hortae* is classified, namely the Loculoascomycetes (27, 42).

Cutaneous Mycoses

There are many species of dermatophytic fungi possessing the ability to cause disease in humans and animals. All have in common the ability to invade the skin, hair, or nails. In each case, these fungi are keratinophilic and keratinolytic, being able to break down the keratin surfaces of these structures. In the case of skin infections, the dermatophytes invade only the upper, outermost layer of the epidermis, the stratum corneum. Likewise with hair and nails, being part of the skin, only the keratized layers are invaded. Often the growth of dermatophytes in the skin per se is not the major reason for skin symptoms, but rather the host immune response to the presence of the fungal elements. The outcome of acute versus chronic dermatophytoses is mainly the result of the host immune response rather than the invasiveness of the fungi.

The various forms of dermatophytosis are often referred to as "tinea", e.g., tinea capitis (scalp infection), tinea corporis (infection of the trunk), tinea cruris (infection of the groin), tinea pedis (infection of the feet), etc. A major clinical manifestation of dermatophytoses is infection of the nails (onychomycosis or tinea unguinum). Three genera of dermatophytes are known (27, 42, 54): *Microsporum*, *Trichophyton*, and *Epidermophyton*. Without question the most common pathogenic species observed by clinicians is *Trichophyton rubrum*. This species incites the bulk of athlete's foot and nail infection seen by dermatologists and other clinicians. Other species of *Trichophyton* frequently causing human diseases are *Trichophyton tonsurans* (infection of the hair and scalp) and *Trichophyton mentagrophytes*. Of the species of *Microsporum*, *Microsporum canis* and *Microsporum gypseum* are most often seen in the United States. Infection due to *M. canis* most often follows handling of cats and dogs, where the fungus resides naturally. Infections caused by *Epidermophyton floccosum* most often affect the feet and the groin.

Dermatophytosis can manifest clinically in diverse ways, but most diagnoses are made based on clinical appearance and patient history. Cultures are always desirable and can be obtained from scraping the affected areas and placing the skin, hair, or nail tissue on any number of laboratory media such as Sabouraud agar, with and without antibiotics, or dermatophyte test medium (DTM). An alternative is employment of potato flakes agar, containing the color indicator bromthymol blue (41). With this medium,

Table 45.3. Characteristic Features of Macroconidia and Microconidia of Dermatophytes

Genus	Macroconidia	Microconidia
Epidermophyton	Smooth-walled, borne in clusters of two or three	Absent
Microsporum	Numerous, large, thick- and rough-walled[a]	Rare
Trichophyton	Rare, smooth, thin-walled	Numerous, spherical, teardrop- or peg-shaped[b]

[a]Except *M. audouinnii*.
[b]Except *T. schoenleinii*

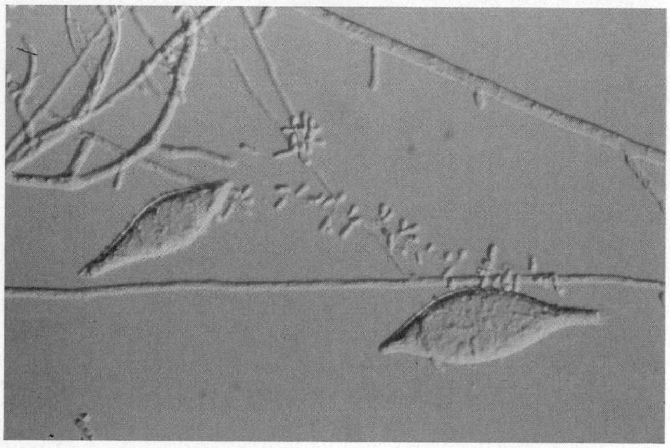

Figure 45.2. Macroconidia and microconidia of *Microsporum canis* (Nomarski optics, ×625).

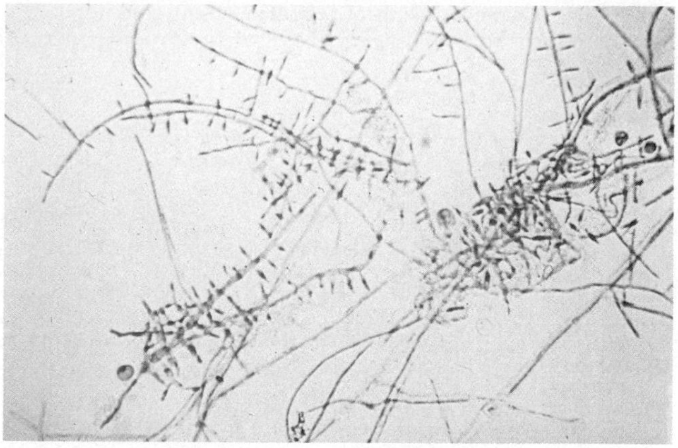

Figure 45.3. Microconidia of *Trichophyton tonsurans* (×600).

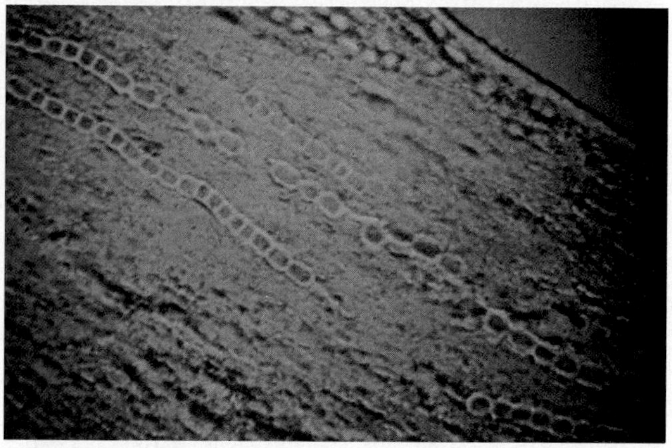

Figure 45.4. Potassium hydroxide preparation demonstrating hyphal elements characteristic of dermatophytes. *Trichophyton tonsurans* in hair shaft (×600).

the dermatophytic fungi change the medium from yellow to blue but do not obscure the pigments produced by various dermatophytes that are often useful as adjuncts in identification. Also, this medium promotes sporulation of dermatophytes to enhance microscopic identification. As with DTM, many nondermatophytic fungi also grow on potato flakes agar and may turn the medium blue. The final identification lies with examination of the fungus under the microscope.

Microscopically, the genus *Microsporum* is identified by observation of its macroconidia, while with the genus *Trichophyton*, microconidia are the characteristic structures (Table 45.3). *Epidermophyton floccosum* produces no microconidia, but its smooth-walled macroconidia borne in clusters of two or three are most distinctive. *Microsporum canis* produces characteristic large, thick- and rough-walled macroconidia (Fig. 45.2). Its macroconidia are multicellular (five to eight cells per conidium). *Trichophyton rubrum* produces microconidia that are teardrop- or peg-shaped borne rough along the sides of hyphae, while *T. mentagrophytes* produces both single cigar-shaped macroconidia and grape-like clusters of spherical microconidia. *T. tonsurans* produces variably sized and shaped microconidia, with relatively large spherical conidia often being right alongside of small, parallel-walled conidia and other microconidia of various sizes and shapes (Fig. 45.3).

Skin scraping, nail scraping, and observation of hairs directly by microscopy are also most helpful in diagnosing dermatophytic infections. Employing a drop of potassium hydroxide (15% KOH) on a glass slide over the surface of the specimen will often reveal filamentous, clear hyphal elements characteristic of dermatophytes (Fig. 45.4). Most recently, the use of calcofluor white has been employed in examining specimens for fungal elements and has demonstrated excellent results.

Identification of dermatophytes to genus is relatively straightforward, but species-level identification may be considerably more difficult.

Subcutaneous Mycoses

Many fungal pathogens can produce subcutaneous manifestations as part of their disease process; however, certain fungi are commonly introduced traumatically through the skin and have a propensity

Table 45.4. Common Agents of Subcutaneous Mycoses

Disease	Organism	Growth		
		Tissue	Culture (25°C)	Culture (37°C)
Sporotrichosis	*Sporothrix schenckii*	Yeast (rare, cigar shaped)	Mold	Yeast
Chromoblastomycosis	*Cladosporium*	Hyphae[a]	Mold	Mold
	Fonsecaea	Hyphae[a]	Mold	Mold
	Phialophora	Hyphae[a]	Mold	Mold
Mycetoma	*Pseudallescheria*	Hyphae[b]	Mold	Mold
	Madurella	Hyphae[b]	Mold	Mold

[a]Dematiaceous, often blunted to form oval sclerotic bodies.
[b]May be in the form of microcolonies or granules.

to involve the deeper layers of the dermis, subcutaneous tissue, and bone. Although they may ultimately be expressed clinically as lesions on the skin surface, they rarely spread to distant organs. In general, the clinical course is chronic and insidious, and, once established, the infections are refractory to most antifungal therapy. The most common subcutaneous mycoses are lymphocutaneous sporotrichosis, chromoblastomycosis, and eumycotic mycetoma (Table 45.4). Although lymphocutaneous sporotrichosis is caused by a single fungal pathogen, *Sporothrix schenckii*, the other subcutaneous mycoses are clinical syndromes caused by multiple fungal etiologies (27, 34, 42). The causative agents of subcutaneous mycoses are generally considered to have low pathogenic potential and are commonly isolated from soil or decaying vegetation. Exposure is largely occupational or related to hobbies (e.g., gardening, wood gathering). Infected patients generally have no underlying immune defect.

Lymphocutaneous Sporotrichosis

Lymphocutaneous sporotrichosis is caused by *Sporothrix schenckii*, a dimorphic fungus that is ubiquitous in soil and decaying vegetation (27, 29, 42). Infection with this organism is chronic and is characterized by nodular and ulcerative lesions that develop along lymphatics that drain the primary site of inoculation. Dissemination to other sites such as bones, eyes, lungs, and central nervous system is extremely rare, occurring in less than 1% of all cases (27, 42). Histopathologically the organism stimulates both acute pyogenic and granulomatous inflammatory reactions. In tissues, the organism appears as a 3- to 5-μm cigar-shaped yeast (Fig. 45.5), but is rarely observed in human lesions. Thus, direct microscopic examination of infected material is usually unrewarding. Definitive diagnosis usually request culture of infected pus or tissue. *S. schenckii* grows within 2 to 5 days on a variety of mycological media and appears as a budding yeast at 37°C and as a mold at 25°C. The colonies at 25°C are initially white and moist, turning brown to black with prolonged incubation. Microscopically, the mold appears as delicate branching hyphae with numerous conidia developing in a rosette pattern at the ends of conidiophores (Fig. 45.6). Laboratory confirmation is established by converting the mycelial growth to the yeast form by subculture at 37°C. Alternatively, the organism may be identified immunologically through the use of exoantigen test. Treatment usually consists of the oral administration of a saturated solution of potassium iodide.

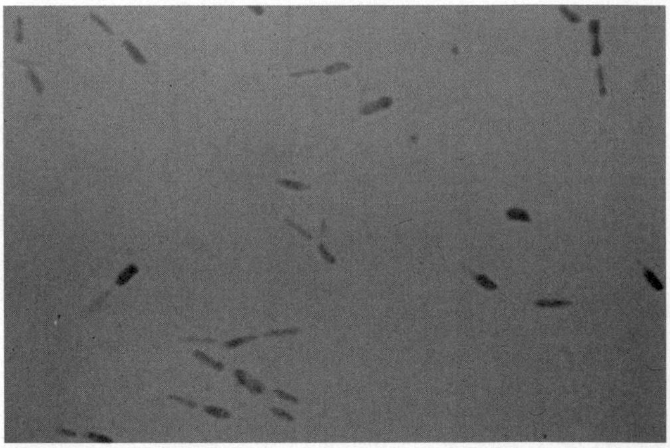

Figure 45.5. Microscopic appearance of *Sporothrix schenckii* yeast (×1200).

Chromoblastomycosis

Chromoblastomycosis is most commonly seen in the tropics, when the warm, moist environment coupled with the lack of protective footwear and clothing predisposes individuals to direct inoculation with infected soil or other organic matter. The organisms most often associated with chromoblastomycosis are dematiaceous (pigmented) fungi of the genera *Fonsecaea*, *Cladosporium*, and *Phialophora* (27, 29, 42). Multiple species of these genera have been implicated in this disease process. These organisms are identified according to the pattern and type of sporulation, and in many cases more than one pattern may be observed for a given isolate. For this reason, there remains considerable confusion and controversy regarding the taxonomic placement of many of the

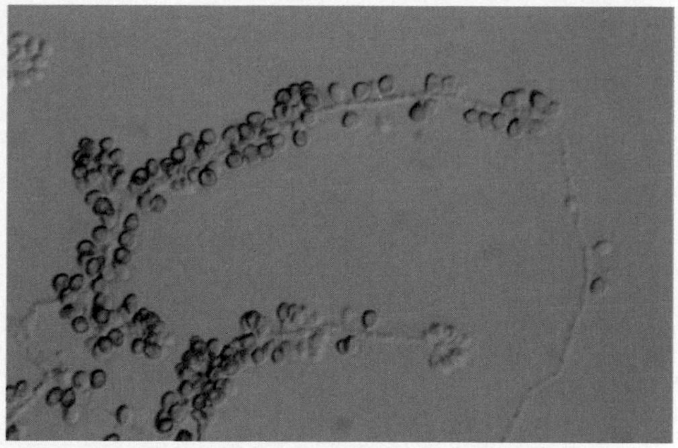

Figure 45.6. Microscopic appearance of the mold phase of *Sporothrix shenckii* demonstrating the rosette pattern of conidia at the end of a conidiophore, and dark sessile conidia along the hyphae (Nomarski optics ×1250).

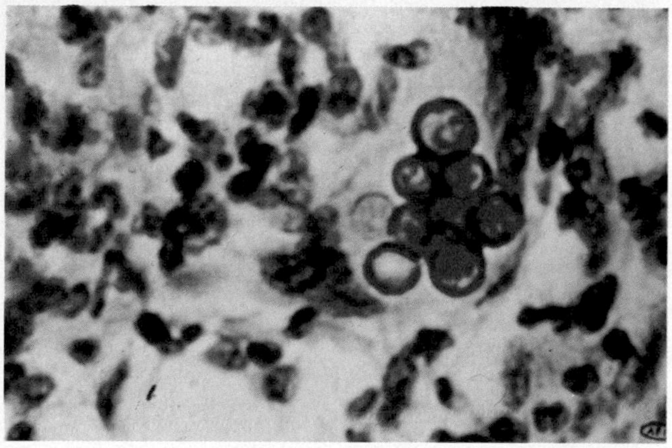

Figure 45.7. Histopathologic section of a lesion of chromoblastomycosis demonstrating the presence of sclerotic or Medlar bodies (×1200).

dematiaceous fungi that cause chromoblastomycosis. Clinically, the disease is characterized by warty, cauliflower-like lesions, which develop slowly and extend via satellite lesions (27, 29, 42). The lymphatics are usually not involved and the lesions are painless unless they are involved with secondary bacterial infection. The diagnosis of chromoblastomycosis is generally made by histopathologic examination of infected tissue. Typical lesions demonstrate pseudoepitheliomatous hyperplasia and characteristic brown or copper-colored spherical cells or hyphae known as sclerotic or Medlar bodies (Fig. 45.7). These are the tissue forms of the fungus. The cultures grow as dematiaceous molds but may take weeks to appear and longer to develop the characteristic conidia. Treatment consists of surgery and antifungal therapy. Unfortunately, because most individuals present with advanced disease, therapy is frequently unsuccessful.

Eumycotic Mycetoma

As with chromoblastomycosis, most mycetomas are seen in the tropics. A mycetoma is defined clinically as a localized chronic granulomatous infectious process involving cutaneous and subcutaneous tissues (34). The process may be quite extensive and deforming with destruction of local bony structures. Most commonly mycetomas are localized to the feet and hands but may also involve other parts of the body such as the back, shoulders, and buttocks. The lesions consist of multiple granulomas and abscesses that suppurate and drain through sinus tracts. The etiologic agents of eumycotic mycetomas encompass a wide range of fungi, including *Pseudallescheria boydii* and *Madurella grisea* (27, 34, 42). Examination of the drainage from sinus tracts may reveal small granules or microcolonies of mycelial filaments. These granules may range from microscopic to 2 mm in diameter and vary according to the infecting species. Histopathologic examination of tissue may reveal hyphal elements and granules (Fig. 45.8). The precise microbiological features depend on the organism involved. Identification of the fungi causing eumycotic mycetomas is by morphology of the asexual conidia formed in culture. It is important to establish the etiology of the infection by culturing specimens, since the clinical management will depend on the causative organism. An identical picture to eumycotic mycetoma may be caused by various actinomycetes belonging to the genera *Actinomyces*, *Nocardia*, *Streptomyces*, and *Actinomadura* (34, 42). These infections, known as actinomycotic mycetoma, may be treated with antibacterial agents, whereas eumycotic mycetomas respond poorly to antifungal therapy and frequently require excision or amputation.

Systemic Mycoses Due to Dimorphic Fungal Pathogens

The dimorphic fungal pathogens are organisms that exist in a mold form in the natural environment or in the laboratory at 25° to 30°C and in the yeast or spherule form in tissues or when grown on enriched medium in the laboratory at 37°C (27, 42, 50). The organisms in this group are considered primary or systemic pathogens and include *Histoplasma capsulatum* var. *capsulatum*, *Histoplasma capsulatum* var. *duboisii*, *Blastomyces dermatitidis*, *Coccidioides immitis*, and *Paracoccidioides brasiliensis* (Table 45.5). These organisms have also been termed endemic pathogens, because susceptibility to infection with each organism is generally acquired by living in a geographic area constituting the natural habitat of the particular fungus. In the environment or at 25° to 30°C, these

Table 45.5. The Dimorphic Endemic Fungal Pathogens

Disease	Organism	Geographic Distribution	Tissue	Growth Culture (25°C)	Growth Culture 37°C)
Histoplasmosis	*Histoplasma capsulatum* var. *capsulatum*	Ohio and Mississippi River valleys	Intracellular yeast	Mold	Yeast
	Histoplasma capsulatum var. *duboisii*	Africa	Intracellular yeast	Mold	Yeast
Blastomycosis	*Blastomyces dermatitidis*	Ohio and Mississippi River valleys	Large, broad-based budding yeast	Mold	Yeast
Coccidioidomycosis	*Coccidioides immitis*	Southwestern U.S. Mexico, Central and South America	Spherule	Mold	Spherules
Paracoccidioidomycosis	*Paracoccidioides brasiliensis*	Central and South America	Multipolar budding yeast	Mold	Yeast

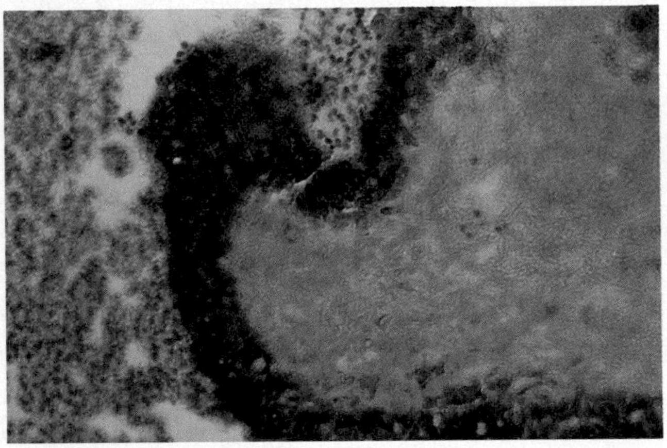

Figure 45.8. Tissue section taken from an eumycotic mycetoma illustrating a granule or microcolony (×300).

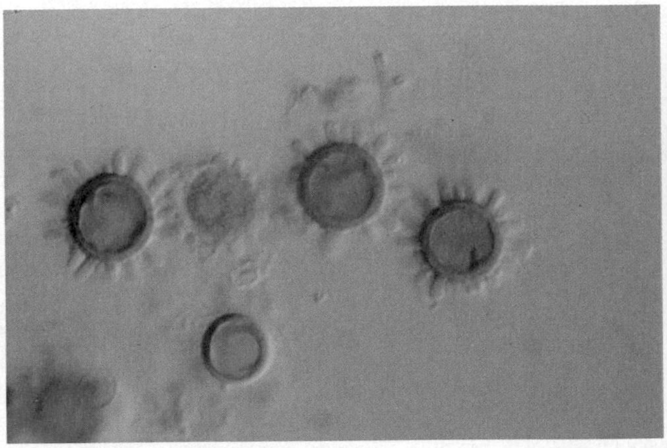

Figure 45.9. Microscopic appearance of the mold phase of *Histoplasma capsulatum* var. *capsulatum* demonstrating tuberculate macroconidia (Nomarski optics, ×1250).

organisms all produce a mycelial form with hyaline, branching, septate hyphae. The tissue form of *H. capsulatum*, *B. dermatitidis*, and *P. brasiliensis* is a bubbling yeast, which may be reproduced on enriched media at 37°C. *C. immitis* forms spherules in tissue or in vitro under appropriate conditions. Infection due to these agents is usually acquired by inhalation of conidia from an environmental source. In recent years, infections with *H. capsulatum* and *C. immitis* have emerged as major opportunistic pathogens in individuals with AIDS (16, 50). These infections are generally thought to be due to reactivation of previous infection in these highly immunosuppressed individuals.

Histoplasmosis

In 1905, Darling described the causative agent of histoplasmosis as a parasite, then later placed it in the fungal family (27, 42). Histoplasmosis is distributed worldwide but is most noted from its endemic regions of the Mississippi and Ohio river valleys. Human disease can be linked to either *Histoplasma capsulatum* var. *capsulatum* (United States) or *H. capsulatum* var. *duboisii* (Africa). Disease ranges from slight pulmonary involvement to disseminated disease and is known for its intracellular nature.

H. capsulatum var. *capsulatum* is most often recovered from respiratory secretions or from blood or bone marrow. Appropriate specimens should be collected and transported to the laboratory as rapidly as possible. It is recommended that the specimen be placed directly on brain-heart infusion medium with chloramphenicol and gentamicin to eliminate overgrowth by normal bacterial flora. Once an organism is isolated, it should be transferred to potato flakes, Sabhi, or Gorman's media, which is specially formulated to enhance the growth of systemic pathogens and may provide optimum conditions for growth. Cultures incubated at 25°C grow very slowly, resulting in cottony white colonies in 7 to 28 days. The mold phase of *H. capsulatum* is characterized by thin, branching, septate hyphae that produce tuberculate macroconidia and microconidia (Fig. 45.9).

When *Histoplasma capsulatum* is suspected, further laboratory testing is required to differentiate it from saprobic fungi. *H. capsulatum* grows well on cycloheximide-containing medium. Conversion to the yeast form is achieved by incubating the culture

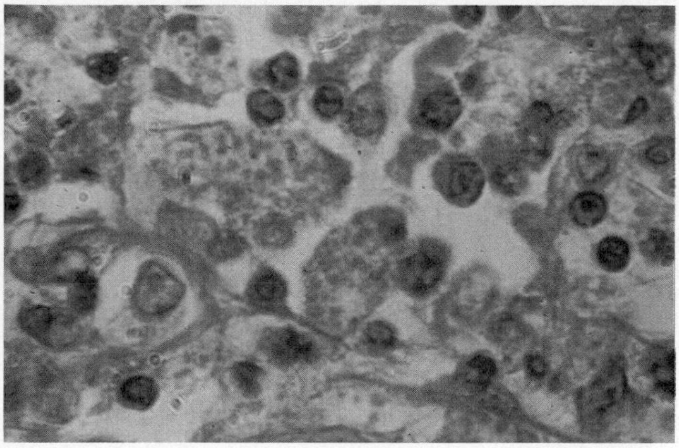

Figure 45.10. Microscopic appearance of the tissue phase of *Histoplasma capsulatum* var. *capsulatum* demonstrating intracellular yeast forms (×1000).

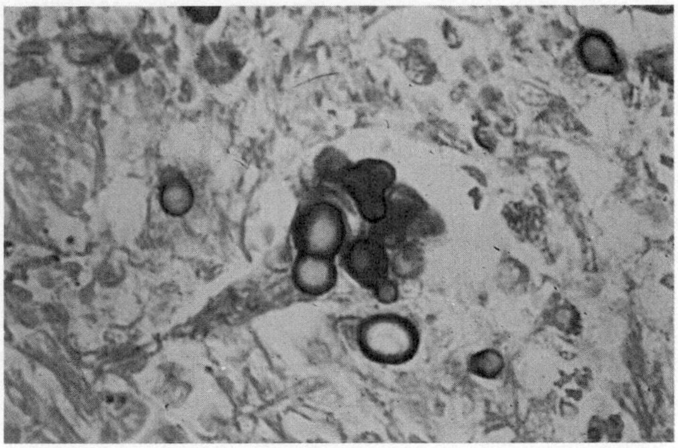

Figure 45.11. Microscopic appearance of the tissue phase of *Blastomyces dermatitidis* demonstrating a large, broad-based budding yeast (×600).

at 37°C on brain-heart infusion agar. This process may take several weeks before conversion is observed. Saprobic fungi will not convert to yeast form. Other more rapid means of identifying *H. capsulatum* from culture includes the exoantigen test and the use of DNA probes (25, 27, 50). In the exoantigen test, antigens are extracted from culture material and reacted against antihistoplasma antibody in an immunodiffusion test. In the DNA probe test, nucleic acids are extracted from culture material and reacted against a probe specific for *H. capsulatum* ribosomal RNA. With these methods, definitive identification may be made in 2 hours (DNA probe) to 3 days (exoantigen) (25, 27, 50).

Additional means of diagnosing histoplasmosis includes histopathologic examination of infected tissue and serology. The tissue phase of *H. capsulatum* is a small budding yeast cell 2 to 5 mm in diameter found almost exclusively within macrophages (Fig. 45.10). It may be visualized with Giemsa or silver stains. Serologic diagnosis employs both immunodiffusion and complement fixation tests and has been quite useful (50). An assay to detect antigen in urine has also been developed that has excellent sensitivity and specificity (27, 42, 50). Unfortunately, its availability is limited to a single laboratory.

Blastomycosis

Blastomyces dermatitidis is another of the systemic fungi that become infective upon inhalation of conidia. Like other systemic pathogens, *B. dermatitidis* is found in a specific region of the United States, most notably the Ohio and Mississippi river valley region. Disease begins with granulomatous lung involvement but may disseminate to other body sites. The most common form of dissemination is the appearance of cutaneous pustular lesions. Yeast cells can be recovered from biopsies and aspirates of the lesions. Less common involvement may be seen in bone and subcutaneous tissue.

When blastomycosis is suspected, clinical material (e.g., sputum, pus) should be placed on inhibitory media, without cycloheximide, such as brain-heart infusion (BHI) agar with chloramphenicol and gentamicin and incubated at 25°C for 7 to 28 days (27, 42, 50). Growth is very slow and ranges in appearance from a white to a tan fluffy mold. Microscopic examination at this point is not diagnostic. Probable *Blastomyces* isolates must be converted to the yeast phase by subculturing the isolate to a BHI blood agar slant and incubating at 37°C in CO_2 (a candle jar is sufficient). Yeast forms should be visible within a week. Microscopic examination at this point reveals characteristic broad-based budding yeasts.

Although microscopic examination of the yeast gives valuable information, a definitive identification may be made from mycelial phase cultures using the exoantigen test as described for *H. capsulatum*. A commercially available DNA probe assay also allows the identification of *B. dermatitidis* from either yeast or mycelial phase cultures in 2 hours or less (27). Additional means of diagnosing blastomycosis includes histopathologic examination of infected tissue. The tissue phase of *B. dermatitidis* is a large yeast with broad-based buds (Fig. 45.11). Serologic tests for diagnosing blastomycosis have not been particularly useful. Antigens for complement fixation tests are available, but complement fixing antibodies are absent in up to 50% of cases.

Coccidioidomycosis

Coccidioidomycosis (Posadas' disease, coccidioidal granuloma, Valley fever, desert rheumatism, Valley bumps, California disease) is commonly a self-limiting, mild to sometimes moderately severe respiratory disease, resulting from the inhalation of

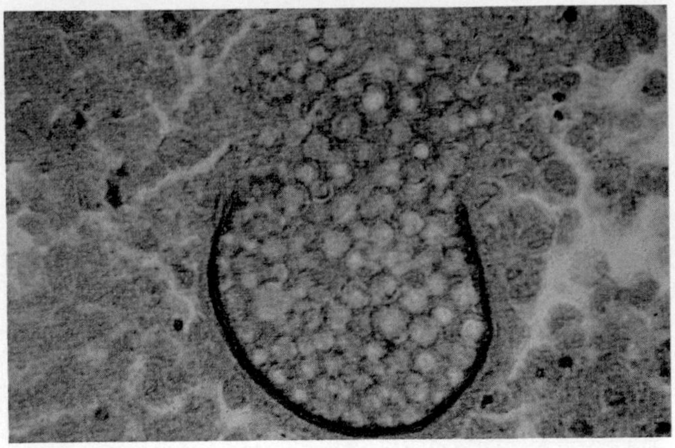

Figure 45.12. Tissue section taken from an individual with coccidioidomycosis demonstrating a spherule containing multiple endospores (×600).

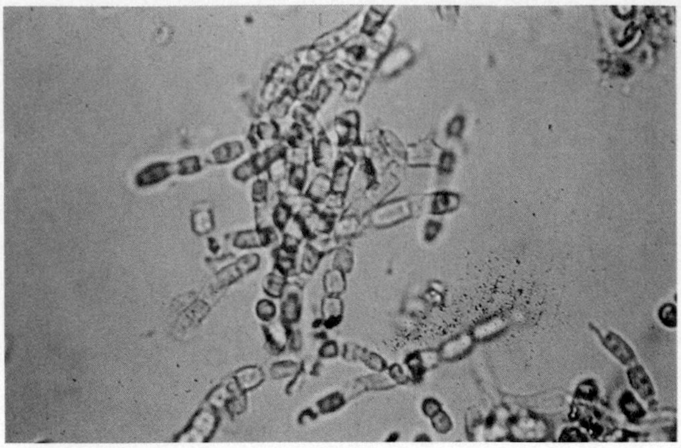

Figure 45.13. Microscopic appearance of the mold phase of *Coccidioides immitis* demonstrating arthroconidia (×600).

arthroconidia produced by the etiologic agent *Coccidioides immitis* (1, 16, 27, 42, 50). The organism resides in a narrow ecological niche known as the Lower Sonoran Life Zone, characterized by low rainfall and semi-arid conditions. Highly endemic areas include the San Joaquin Valley in California, Maricopa and Pima counties in Arizona, and southwestern Texas. Outside the United States, areas of high endemicity are found in northern Mexico, Guatemala, Honduras, Venezuela, Paraguay, Argentina, and Colombia.

Since *C. immitis* is probably the most virulent of all human mycotic agents, the inhalation of only a few arthroconidia produces primary coccidioidomycosis, which may include asymptomatic pulmonary disease, allergic manifestations (toxic erythema, erythema nodosum or "desert bumps," and erythema multiforme or "valley fever" and arthritis ("desert rheumatism"). Primary disease usually resolves without therapy and confers a strong, specific immunity to reinfection, which is detected by the coccidioidin skin test. In patients symptomatic for 6 weeks or longer, the disease progresses to secondary coccidioidomycosis, which may include nodules, cavitary disease, or progressive pulmonary disease; single or multisystem dissemination follows in approximately 1% of this population. Filipinos and blacks run the highest risk of dissemination, with meningeal involvement a common sequela. The sex distribution for clinically significant disease is approximately 9:1 (male:female). The exception is in pregnant women among whom the dissemination rate equals or exceeds that for men.

After inhalation, barrel-shaped arthroconidia (2.5 to 4 by 3 to 6 μm) become more rounded as they convert to spherules (Fig. 45.12). At maturity, the spherules (30 to 60 μm in diameter) produce endospores by a process known as "progressive cleavage." Rupture of the spherule walls releases the endospores, which in turn form new spherules. Caution must be exercised with making a diagnosis by histopathology only, as small, empty spherules may resemble the yeast cells of *Blastomyces dermatitidis*, and endospores (2 to 5 μm in diameter) can be confused with cells of *Crypotcoccus neoformans*, *Histoplasma capsulatum* var. *capsulatum*, and *Paracoccidioides brasiliensis*.

Coccidioides immitis (Rixford ezt Gilchrist, 1896,) is a dimorphic fungus with a variety of mold morphologies at 25°C. Initial growth is white to gray, moist, and glabrous, and occurs within 3 to 4 days. It rapidly develops abundant aerial mycelia, and the colony appears to enlarge in a circular "bloom." Mature colonies usually become tan to brown to lavender.

Microscopically, fertile hyphae arise at right angles to the vegetative hyphae and produce alternating (separated by a disjunctor cell) hyaline arthroconidia (Fig. 45.13). When released, conidia have an annular frill at both ends. As the culture ages, the vegetative hyphae also fragments into arthroconidia. Some taxonomists classify *C. immitis* as the *Malbranchea* state of *Coccidioides immitis*. *Malbranchea* differs from *C. immitis* by not converting to endosporulating spherules at 37° to 40°C in infected animals or special culture media; it also fails to produce lines of identity in the exoantigen test that is specific for *C. immitis*.

Identification of *C. immitis* from culture may be accomplished by using the exoantigen or DNA probe tests (25, 27, 50). Additional means of diagnosing coccidioidomycosis include histopathologic examination of infected tissue for the presence of spherules and serologic testing. Several serologic procedures exist for initial screening, confirmation, and prognostic evaluation (1, 14, 16, 27, 42, 50). For initial diagnosis, the combined use of the immunodiffusion (ID) test and the latex particle agglutination

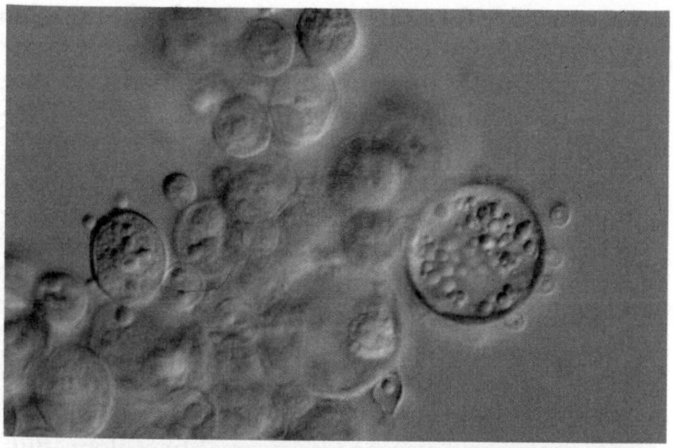

Figure 45.14. Microscopic appearance of the tissue phase of *Paracoccidioides brasilensis* demonstrating multipolar budding yeast forms (Nomarski optics, ×1250).

test (LPA) detects approximately 93% of cases. The complement fixation (CF) and tube preciptin (TP) tests may also be employed for diagnosis as well as for confirmation. Prognostic studies frequently employ serial CF titers.

Paracoccidioidomycosis

Paracoccidioidomycosis (South American blastomycosis, Brazilian blastomycosis, Lutz-Spendore-Almeida disease, paracoccidioidal granuloma) is a chronic, progressive fungal disease endemic to Central and South America (12, 27, 42, 50). Geographic areas of highest incidence (Holdridge plant classification zone) are typically humid, high-rainfall areas with acidic soil conditions. As with other systemic mycoses, the sex distribution for clinically significant disease is approximately 9:1 (male:female).

While the primary route of infection is pulmonary (usually inapparent and asymptomatic), subsequent dissemination leads to the formation of ulcerative granulomatous lesions of the buccal, nasal, and, occasionally, gastrointestinal mucosa; concomitant striking lymph node involvement is also evident. Although the causative agent, *Paracoccidioides brasiliensis*, has a rather narrow range of temperature tolerance (as evidenced by its predilection for growth in cooler areas of the body [nasal and oropharyngeal], dissemination to other organs (particularly the adrenals) occurs with diminished host defenses.

Cutaneous and mucosal lesions typically show a pseudoepitheliomatous hyperplasia accompanied by a marked pyogenic and granulomatous response. As a similar tissue reaction is also seen in coccidioidomycosis, and, particularly, blastomycosis, a definitive diagnosis depends upon the demonstration of characteristic yeast cells.

The typical budding yeast cells measure 12 to 40 μm in diameter, with multipolar budding around the periphery, resembling a "mariner's wheel" (Fig. 45.14). These "daughter" cells (2 to 5 μm in diameter) are connected by a narrow base, as contrasted with the broad base attachment in blastomycosis. Many buds of various sizes may occur, or there may be only a few large buds, giving the appearance of a "Mickey Mouse cap" to the yeast cell. Caution must be exercised when making a diagnosis by histopathology only, as the cells in their various sizes and configurations may mimic young spherules of *Coccidioides immitis*, the budding cells of *Blastomyces dermatitidis*, or the small yeast cells of *Histoplasma capsulatum* var. *capsulatum*.

Paracoccidioides brasiliensis is a dimorphic fungus that produces a variety of mold morphologies when grown at 25°C (12, 27, 42, 50). Flat colonies are glabrous to leathery, wrinkled to folded, floccose to velvety, pink to beige to brown, with a yellowish-brown reverse, and resemble those of *Blastomyces dermatitidis*. On BHI blood agar at 37°C, the mycelial phase rapidly converts to the yeast phase.

Microscopically, the mold form produces small (2 to 10 μm in diameter, one-celled conidia, generally indistinguishable from those observed with the mold phase of *Blastomyces dermatitidis* or the microconidia of *Histoplasma capsulatum* var. *capsulatum*. When mycelial fragments are transferred to an enriched medium at 37°C, conversion to the characteristic yeast phase occurs.

Diagnosis may be made by culture, histopathologic examination of infected tissues, and serology (12, 27, 42, 50). Both complement fixation (CF) and agar gel immunodiffusion (ID) procedures are available for serodiagnosis. The CF test, using yeast-derived antigen, is positive in 80% of active disease. Titers of 1:64 or higher are generally considered diagnostic. While the CF titer usually decreases with therapy, it may persist in the range of 1:8 to 1:32. The immunodiffusion test is positive in approximately 95% of active cases, has low cross-reactivity, and diminishes with successful therapy.

Opportunistic Mycoses

The opportunistic mycoses occur primarily in immunocompromised individuals, particularly those with malignancies and AIDS, and after major surgery, severe burn injury, and bone marrow and solid organ transplantation. The number and type of fungal pathogens included in this category is increasing rapidly (3–5, 19, 22, 26, 31, 38). The most well-known causes of opportunistic mycoses include *Candida* and other opportunistic yeasts (including *Cryptococcus neoformans*), *Aspergillus* species, and the Zygo-

Table 45.8. Differential Characteristics of Some Clinically Significant *Aspergillus* Species

Species	Colonial Morphology	Microscopic Morphology
A. fumigatus	White to gray-green; slate gray with age; reverse yellow to variable; growth at 45–50°C	Smooth-walled conidiophore terminates in dome-shaped vesicle bearing uniseriate phialides from the upper portion only; conidial heads strongly columnar; conidia echinulate
A. flavus	Yellow to lime-green; reverse pinkish; brown to black sclerotia may be present	Rough; thick-walled conidiophores bear globose vesicles; uniseritate or biseriate phialides cover the majority of the vesicle; conidial heads radiate; conidia echinulate
A. nidulans	Dark green to yellow-green; reverse pinkish	Short, sinuous, pale brown conidiophores bearing hemispherical vesicles; biseriate phialides cover upper half of vesicle; globose, rough-walled conidia form short columns; cleistothecia and Hulle cells present
A. niger	White to carbonaceous black; reverse pale yellow	Large, smooth, thick-walled conidiophores bearing globose vesicles; biseriate phialides cover entire vesicle; conidial heads are radiate; conidia thick-walled, echinulate
A. terreus	Cinnamon-buff to brown; reverse dull yellow to brown	Delicate fruiting head when compared to above species; short, flexous conidiophores terminate in small, domelike vesicles; biseriate phialides cover most of the vesicle; small conidia to elliptical; single aleurioconidia formed on submerged hyphae; conidial heads columnar

and (*e*) in the host with abrogated immunity, systemic and fatal disseminated disease (9, 27, 42, 43).

Clinical manifestations, apparently related to the immune status of the host and fungal exposure, are ear infections (incited primarily by *Aspergillus niger*), mycotic keratitis (keratomycosis), sinusitis, cutaneous aspergillosis (often sequela of disseminated disease), pulmonary aspergillosis, central nervous system involvement, bone disease, endocarditis, and fatal disseminated aspergillosis (in organ transplant and leukemic patients) (9).

As with other ubiquitous fungi, the diagnosis of aspergillosis necessitates caution when evaluating the isolation of an *Aspergillus* species from clinical specimens. Recovery from surgically removed tissue or sterile sites, accompanied by positive histopathology (monilaceous, septate, dichotomously branching hyphae) should always be considered significant; isolation from normally contaminated sites requires closer scrutiny.

Although approximately 19 species of aspergilli have been documented as agents of human disease, the major clinical entities are caused by *Aspergillus fumigatus*, *A. flavus*, *A. niger*, and *Aspergillus terreus* (Table 45.8). The increased, clinically significant isolation of *Aspergillus nidulans* merits its recognition as a possible emerging pathogen.

Culture Methods and Identification. Most etiologic agents of aspergillosis grow readily on routine mycologic media lacking cycloheximide, at both 25° and 35°C; *A. fumigatus*, a thermotolerant species, has a maximum growth temperature of 45° to 50°C. Species-level identification of the major human pathogens can usually be made by observing cultural and microscopic characteristics from growth on potato dextrose agar, while the less commonly seen isolates require standardized media (Czapek-Dox and 2% malt agar) to utilize identification keys (27, 42, 53). Microscopic morphology (conidiophores, vesicles, metulae, conidiogenous cells [phialides], conidia) is best observed with the aid of a slide culture (Table 45.8 and Fig. 45.18).

Serologic Diagnosis. Both immunodiffusion (ID) and countercurrent immunoelectrophoresis (CIE) tests are available for the detection of antibodies to aspergillal antigens, as these antibodies are generally uncommon in sera from healthy individuals (9, 14, 27, 42, 53). They have limitations, however, in the setting of the immunocompromised host, who is frequently unable to mount an antibody response. Recent efforts for serodiagnosis have been directed toward demonstration of the *Aspergillus* antigen, galactomannan, employing countercurrent immunoelectrophoresis (CIE), radioimmunoassay (RIA), latex agglutination, and enzyme immunoassay (EIA) methodologies (9, 13, 27). While antigen detection appears promising, further evaluation is needed to establish its utility in diagnosing invasive disease early enough to permit efficacious therapy.

Zygomycosis

Zygomycetes causing human disease encompass several genera in the division of Zygomycota (Table 45.9). The principal human pathogens in the class Zygomycetes are encompassed by two orders: the Mucorales and the Entomophthorales. In the order Mucorales, pathogenic genera include *Rhizopus*, *Mucor*, *Absidia*, *Rhizomucor*, *Saksenaea*, *Cunninghamella*, *Syncephalastrum* and *Apophysomyces* (20, 27, 42). As with other saprobic mold-fungi, immunosuppression and trauma are frequent predisposing factors in zygomycosis. Metabolic acidosis, induced by several conditions, appears to be the foremost predisposing factor in classic rhinocerebral zygomycosis caused primarily by *Rhizopus arrhizus*. The predilection of these fungi for the vascular system with resulting in-

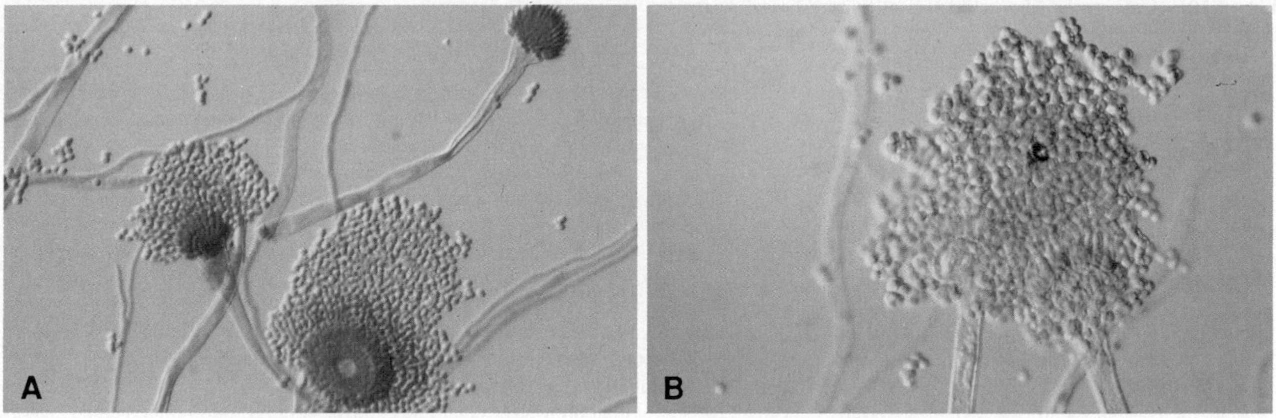

Figure 45.18. Microscopic appearance of *Aspergillus* species (Nomaski optics, ×625). **A**, *Aspergillus fumigatus*. **B**, *Aspergillus flavus*.

Table 45.9. Predominant Agents of Zygomycosis

Superkingdom:	Eukaryota
Kingdom:	Fungi
Division:	Zygomycota
Class:	Zygomycetes
Order:	Mucorales
Family:	Mucoraceae
Genera/species:	*Rhizopus arrhizus*
	Rhizopus rhizopodiformis
	Mucor circinelloides
	Absidia corymbifera
	Rhizomucor pusillus
	Rhizomucor miehei
	Apophysomyces elegans
Family:	Syncephalastraceae
	Syncephalastrum racemosum
Family:	Mortierellaceae
	Mortierella molfii
Family:	Cunninghamellaceae
	Cunninghamella bertholletiae
Family:	Saksenaeaceae
	Saksenaea vasiformis
Family:	Thamnidiaceae
	Cokeromyces recurvatus
Order:	Entomophthorales
Family:	Ancylistaceae
	Conidiobolus coronatus
Family:	Basidiobolaceae
	Basidiobolus ranarum

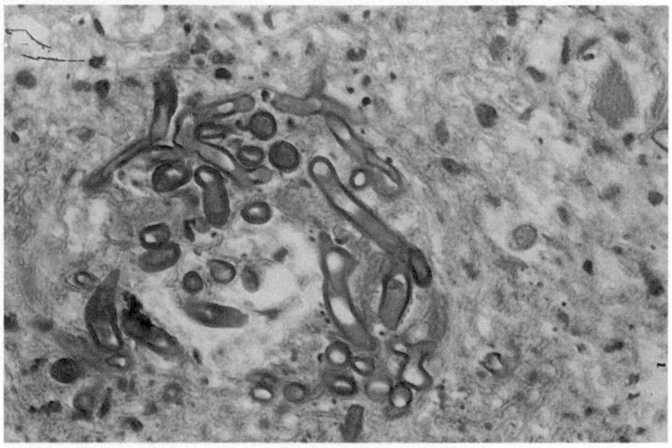

Figure 45.19. Tissue section from an individual with zygomycosis demonstrating ribbon-like, aseptate hyphae (×600).

farction and necrosis, combined with their rapid growth rate, makes them some of the most fulminant agents of mycotic disease. The order Entomophthorales contains two pathogenic genera, *Conidiobolus* and *Basidiobolus*. These agents generally incite a more chronic, granulomatous infection of subcutaneous tissues.

Histopathology. Histopathologically, fungi in the order Mucorales are seen as ribbon-like, aseptate or sparsely septate moniliaceous hyphae (Fig. 45.19). In contrast to hyphomycetes, their diameter often exceeds 10 μm. As the zygomycetes are an extremely ubiquitous group of fungi, demonstration of characteristic fungal elements in tissue merits considerably more importance than the mere isolation of a mucoraceous fungus. The tissue presentation seen by members of the Entomophthorales is that of more regularly septate hyphae, often, but not consistently, accompanied by an eosinophilic halo termed the Splendore-Hoeppli phenomenon. The isolation of these agents always merits attention, as they have not been incriminated as laboratory contaminants.

Culture Methods. Specimens for culture may be obtained from various sites, but biopsies at the edges of necrotic sites are the most rewarding. As hyphal elements are fragile, tissue should be minced, rather than ground, and processed immediately. If a delay in transport is unavoidable, store at room temperature, as zygomycetes rapidly lose viability when refrigerated.

Growth of most genera of pathogenic Mucorales is readily visible (within 12 to 18 hours) on standard mycological media lacking cycloheximide, and occurs at either 25° or 37°C. It is easily recognized by the

Table 45.10. Differential Characteristics of Some Clinically Significant Zygomycete Genera[a]

Genus	Colonial Morphology	Microscopic Morphology
Rhizopus	Rapid growth, cottony, white; becoming gray to brown	Long, unbranched sporangiophores, solitary or in clusters arising from rhizoids; sporangia dark, globose, containing mostly angulated, striated sporangiospores; columella hemispheric
Mucor	Rapid growth, cottony, white; becoming gray to brown	Rhizoids absent; branched or simple sporangiophores arise from hyphae; sporangia globose; sporangiospores globose to cylindrical; columella variable
Absidia	Rapid growth, cottony, gray to olive	Finely branched sporangiophores arise from stolons between rhizoids; pear-shaped sporangia contain globose sporangiospores; conspicuous apophysis merges with round columella; septum usually present in sporangiophore below apophysis
Rhizomucor	Rapid growth, white, becoming gray-brown, low aerial mycelium	Sporangiophores arise from branched aerial hyphae or stolons; rhizoids poorly developed; globose sporangia contain small, round sporangiospores; thermotolerant, growth at 50°–55°C
Cunninghamella	Rapid growth, white, becoming dark gray	Erect sporangiophores terminate in globose vesicles; additional smaller, whorled branches of sporangiophores occur beneath primary vesicle; vesicles bear one-spored sporangiola on short stalks (denticles)
Syncephalastrum	Rapid growth, white, becoming gray to black	Branched sporangiophores terminate in globose vesicles; tubular sporangia (merosporangia) contain single row of globose sporangiospores; rhizoids usually present
Saksenaea	Rapid growth, white, woolly	Induce sporulation on nutritionally deficient media; flask-shaped sporangia on short sporangiophores; rhizoids at base of sporangiophore
Apophysomyces	Rapid growth, white, cottony	Induce sporulation on nutritionally deficient media; sporangiophores arise from hyphae, with supporting "foot-cells"; pear-shaped sporangia, pronounced dark apophysis; sporangiospores oblong
Mortierella	Rapid growth, white, cottony, garlic-like odor; colonies appear as overlapping "rosettes"	Short tapering sporangiophores arise from rhizoids; small, multispored sporangia rapidly deliquesce; sporangiospores kidney-shaped with double wall
Cokeromyces	Moderate growth, tan, flat, tenacious, becoming brown-gray	Dimorphic; yeast at 37°C; sporangiole stalks arise from vesicle and recurve backward, terminating in multispored sporangiola; zygospores abundant

[a]Reproduced from Goodman NL, Rinaldi, MG. Agents of zygomycosis. In: Balows A, Hausler WJ Jr, Herrmann K, Isenberg HD, Shadomy HJ, eds. Manual of clinical microbiology. 5th ed. Washington, DC: American Society for Microbiology, 1991:674–692.

rapid growth rate (filling the tube or Petri dish in a matter of days) and gray to brown woolly colonies. Further identification to the genus and species level is based primarily upon microscopic morphology (Table 45.10 and Fig. 45.20), as no practical biochemical or serological methods exist (20, 27, 42).

The Entomophthorales generally require 3 to 4 days before growth is apparent, and are characterized by thin, flat, gray to pale yellow waxy colonies adhering to the agar. As they mature, conidia are forcibly expelled onto the Petri dish lid, giving it a "ground-glass" appearance.

Hyalohyphomycosis

The term hyalohyphomycosis includes all infections due to nondematiaceous molds that appear as colorless, septate, branched or unbranched hyphal elements in tissue (Fig. 45.21) (2–4, 27, 42, 43). Numerous genera of moniliaceous (hyaline) hyphomycetes are documented agents of hyalohyphomycosis, and the list continues to grow (Table 45.11).

Although infections caused by most of these fungi are relatively rare, they appear to be increasing in incidence (3, 4). Most disseminated infections are thought to be acquired by the inhalation of spores or by the progression of previously localized cutaneous lesions. In this chapter, the discussion of specific genera is limited to selected clinically important hyaline mold-fungi, including *Fusarium*, *Pseudallescheria*, *Scedosporium*, and *Scopulariopsis*.

Histopathology. Most agents of hyalohyphomycosis have the same tissue morphology and elicit a similar pathologic response (Fig. 45.21). Consequently it is impossible to make a correct diagnosis of the etiologic agent on the basis of histopathology alone, and all suspected material should be submitted for fungal culture and identification (27, 42, 43).

Culture Methods and Characteristics of Selected Medically Significant Hyphomycetes. The common etiologic agents of hyalohyphomycosis grow readily on routine mycologic media at both 25° and 35°C. Growth on cycloheximide-containing media shows considerable variability, and this criterion should not be used when determining the potential pathogenicity of an isolate. While the isolation of moniliaceous agents presents few problems, their identification is occasionally hampered by lack of the production of characteristic structures; e.g., asexual propagules. Growth on potato dextrose agar (PDA) or potato flakes agar generally promotes profuse conidiation and produces the characteristic macroscopic mor-

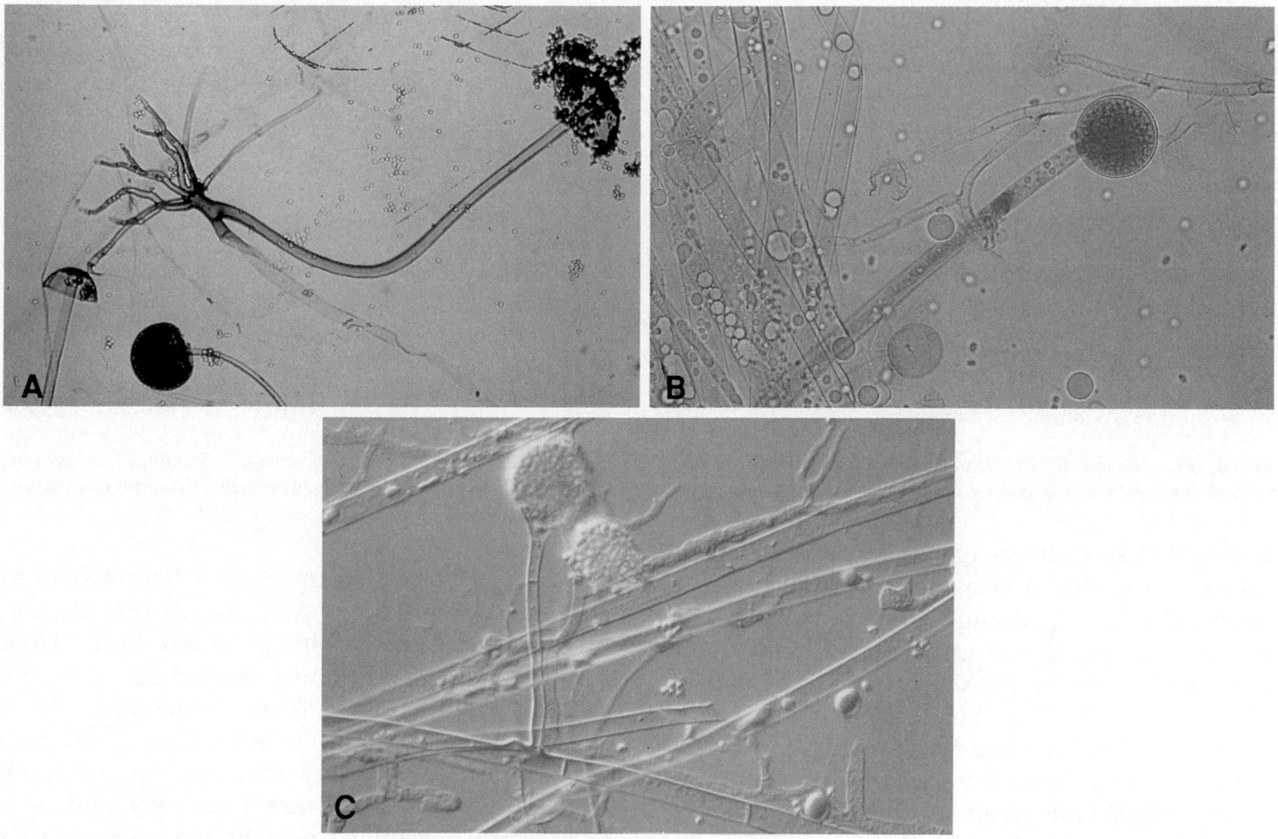

Figure 45.20. Microscopic appearance of selected zygomycetes. **A**, *Rhizopus* spp. (×300). **B**, *Mucor* spp. (×600). **C**, *Absidia* spp. (Nomarski optics, ×625).

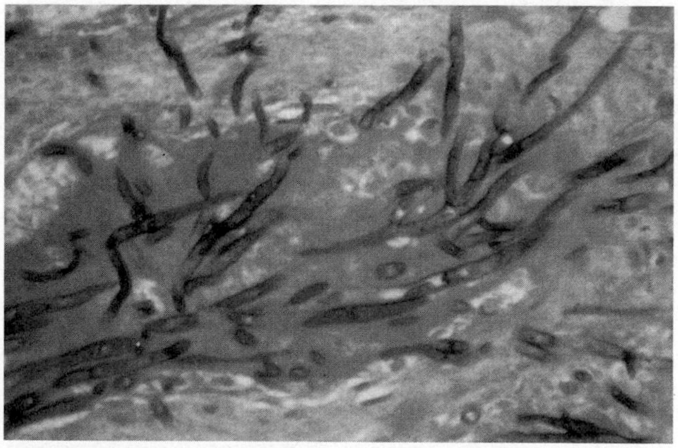

Figure 45.21. Tissue section from an individual with hyalohyphomycosis due to *Fusarium* spp. (×600)

phologies necessary for separation of genus- or species-level identification. Microscopic morphology is best observed with the aid of a slide culture.

Fusarium species have been recognized with increased frequency as causes of disseminated infection in immunocompromised patients (3, 4, 19, 31). The most common species isolated from clinical specimens include *Fusarium moniliforme*, *Fusarium oxysporum*, and *Fusarium solani* (33, 43). The hallmark of disseminated fusariosis is the appearance of multiple purpuric cutaneous nodules with central necrosis. Biopsy of these nodules generally reveals branching, hyaline, septate hyphae invading dermal blood ves-

Table 45.11. Documented Agents of Hyalohyphomycosis[a]

Acremonium	*Graphium* species
falciforme	*Lecythophora*
kiliense	*hoffmannii*
recifei	*mutabilis*
restrictum	*Paecilomyces*
Beauveria bassiana	*variotii*
Chrysosporium species	*Penicillium*
Cylindrocarpon species	*chrysogenum*
Fusarium	*citrinum*
chlamydosporum	*commune*
dimerum	*expansum*
moniliforme	*lilacinum*
napiforme	*marneffei*
oxysporum	*spinulosum*
proliferatum	*Scedosporium*
semitectum	*apiospermum*
solani	*inflatum*
sporotrichoides	*Scopulariopsis*
Geotrichum	*brevicaulis*
candidum	*candida*
penicillatum	

[a]This list is not all-inclusive.

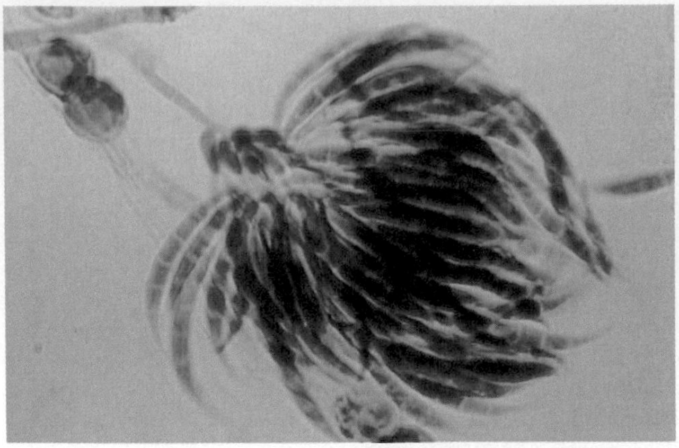

Figure 45.22. Microscopic appearance of *Fusarium* spp. demonstrating characteristic sickle-shaped macroconidia (×600).

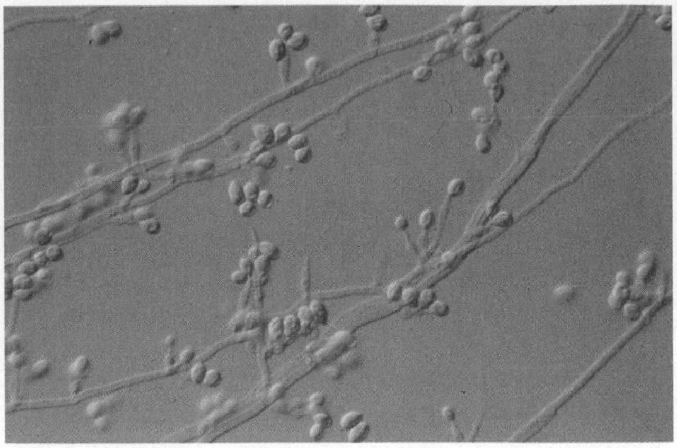

Figure 45.23. Microscopic appearance of *Scedosporium prolificans* demonstrating characteristic annellides with swolen bases (Nomarski optics, ×625).

sels (Fig. 45.21). Cultures of the biopsy material and of blood are useful in establishing the diagnosis of *Fusarium* infection. Although blood cultures are virtually always negative in invasive infections due to *Aspergillus* species, approximately 75% of patients with fusariosis will have positive blood cultures. In culture, colonies of *Fusarium* species are rapidly growing, cottony to woolly, flat, and spreading. Colors may include blue-green, beige, salmon, lavender, red, violet, and purple. Macroscopic identification should only be made from colonies grown on PDA, as color may be quite variable and is highly medium dependent (27, 33, 42, 43). Microscopically, *Fusarium* species are characterized by the production of both macroconidia and microconidia (Fig. 45.22) (27, 33, 42, 43). Microconidia are single- or double-celled, ovoid to cylindrical, and generally borne as mucous balls or short chains. Macroconidia are fusiform or sickle-shaped and many-celled (Fig. 45.22). *Fusarium* species may be misidentified as *Acremonium* when macroconidia are not observed.

Pseudallescheria boydii may be readily isolated from soil and is an occasional cause of mycetoma worldwide; however, it is also the cause of serious disseminated and localized infection in immunocompromised patients (3, 4, 27, 42). In addition to widespread disseminated disease, *P. boydii* has been reported to cause corneal ulcers, endophthalmitis, sinusitis, pneumonia, endocarditis, meningitis, arthritis, and osteomyelitis. *P. boydii* is indistinguishable from *Aspergillus* species and other agents of hyalohyphomycosis on histopathologic examination. Such distinction is important clinically, as *P. boydii* is resistant to amphotericin B and susceptible to miconazole (27, 42). Thus, appropriate cultural and mycologic identification is necessary for optimal therapy. The taxonomy and nomenclature of this fungus have caused a tremendous amount of confusion. *Pseudallescheria boydii* (earlier names are *Allescheria boydii and Petriellidium boydii*) is a homothallic fungus; i.e., it does not require two mating strains to produce the teleomorph, or sexual form. Hence, some strains may produce cleistothecia containing ascospores in culture. More commonly, the anamorph (asexual form) is seen (i.e., *Scedosporium apiospermum*). Macroscopically, colonies are moderately rapidly growing, woolly to cottony, and are initially white, becoming smoky brown to green. Microscopically, conidia are one-celled, elongate, and pale brown and are borne singly or in balls on either short or long conidiophores (27, 42).

Scedosporium prolificans (formerly *Scedosporium inflatum*) is a potentially virulent and highly aggressive emerging agent of hyalohyphomycosis (27, 44). Although far less important than *Fusarium* or *P. boydii*, infections due to *S. prolificans* are associated with soft tissue trauma and are characterized by widespread local invasion, tissue necrosis, and osteomyelitis (44). *S. prolificans* resembles *P. boydii* (*S. apiospermum*) in macroscopic and microscopic morphology. The formation by *S. prolificans* of annelloconidia in wet clumps at the apices of annellides with swollen bases is the most useful characteristic in differentiating this organism from *P. boydii* (*S. apiospermum*) (Fig. 45.23).

Scopulariopsis species are ubiquitous soil saprobes that have been rarely implicated in invasive human disease. *Scopulariopsis brevicaulis* is the most frequently isolated species. Infection is usually confined to the nails; however, serious deep infection has been noted recently in neutropenic leukemia patients and following bone marrow transplantation (7, 42, 43). Both local and disseminated infections have been described with involvement of the nasal septum, skin and soft tissues, blood, lungs, and brain. Diagnosis is made by culture and histopathology. *Scopulariopsis* species grow moderately to rapidly at room temperature on virtually all laboratory media.

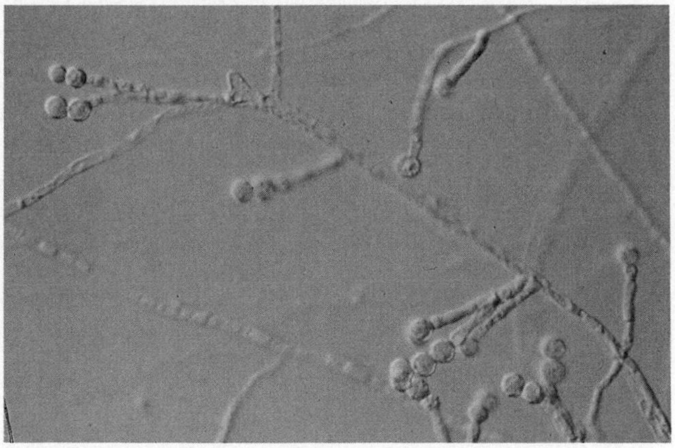

Figure 45.24. Microscopic appearance of *Scopulariopsis* spp. showing anneloconidia in basipetal chains (Nomarski optics, ×625).

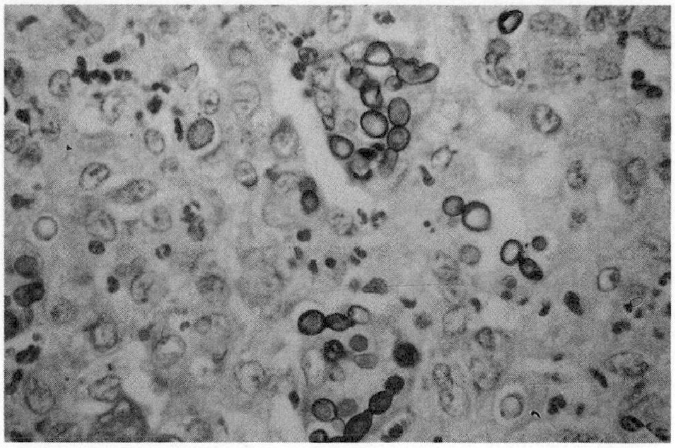

Figure 45.25. Tissue section from an individual with phaeohyphomycosis caused by *Bipolaris spicifera*. Stains for melanin, such as Fontana-Masson, may be used to accentuate and confirm the presence of melanin in the fungal cell walls (Fontana-Masson stains, ×260).

Colonies are initially glabrous (smooth), becoming granular to powdery. Young colonies are white, and become very pale buff to buff brown depending on the species. Conidiophores are simple or branched; the conidiogenous cells are annellides that form solitarily or in clusters, or may form a scopula; e.g., a "broom-like" structure similar to that seen with *Penicillium* species. Annelloconidia are smooth initially, become rough at maturity, are shaped like light bulbs, and form in basipetal chains (Fig. 45.24).

Phaeohyphomycosis

Phaeohyphomycosis is defined as tissue infection caused by dematiaceous (pigmented) hyphae and/or yeasts (2, 27, 42). Infections due to dematiaceous fungi constitute a significant and increasingly prevalent group of opportunistic fungal diseases and may take the form of disseminated disease or become localized to the lung, paranasal sinuses, or central nervous system (27, 29, 42). Primary inoculation, resulting in a localized subcutaneous infection, occurs commonly in underdeveloped countries. The dematiaceous fungi that have been documented to cause human and animal infection encompass a large number of different species; however, the majority of human infections have been caused by *Alternaria*, *Bipolaris*, *Cladosporium*, *Curvularia*, and *Exserohilum* species (27, 29).

Histopathology. In tissue, hyphae with or without yeast forms are present. Because the pigmentation (due to the presence of melanin in hyphal walls) may not be readily apparent, these fungi may be confused with *Aspergillus* species on histopathologic examination. Staining with the Fontana-Masson technique (a melanin-specific stain) may help visualize the dematiaceous elements (Fig. 45.25). Alternatively, the pigmented hyphae/yeasts may be detected by examining an unstained tissue section by brightfield microscopy (29).

Clinical and Mycologic Characteristics of Selected Medically Important Phaeohyphomycetes. The dematiaceous fungi differ considerably in the clinical spectrum of infection and response to therapy (27, 29). Furthermore, the different genera are not readily distinguished on histopathologic examination. Thus, an accurate microbiologic diagnosis based on culture of the infected tissue is important for optimal clinical management of infections due to these fungi.

Alternaria species are important causes of paranasal sinuisitis in both healthy and immunocompromised patients. Other sites of infection include skin and soft tissue, cornea, lower respiratory tract, and peritoneum. *Alternaria alternata* is the best documented human pathogen in this genus. In culture, *Alternaria* colonies are rapidly growing, cottony, and gray to black. The conidiophores are usually solitary and simple or branched. The conidia develop in branching chains and are dematiaceous, muriform, and smooth or rough and taper toward the distal end with a short beak at their apices (Fig. 45.26) (27, 29).

Cladosporium species are occasionally isolated from cutaneous, eye, and nail infections. These fungi are rapidly growing with a velvety, olive gray to black colony. The conidiophores arise from the hyphae and are dematiaceous, tall, and branching. The conidia may be smooth or rough and single- to several-celled and form in branching chains at the apex of the conidiophore (27, 29). The conidia at the branch points of the chains may have a shield-like shape and are referred to as shield cells.

Curvularia species are ubiquitous inhabitants of the soil and have been implicated in both disseminated and local infection. Sites of infection include

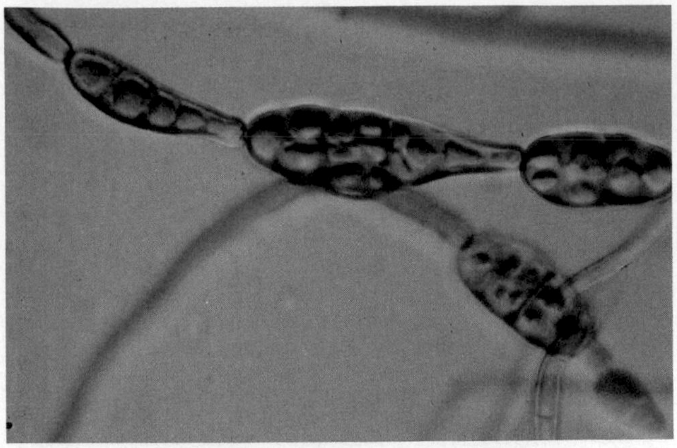

Figure 45.26. Microscopic appearance of *Alternaria alternata* (Nomarksi optics, ×1250).

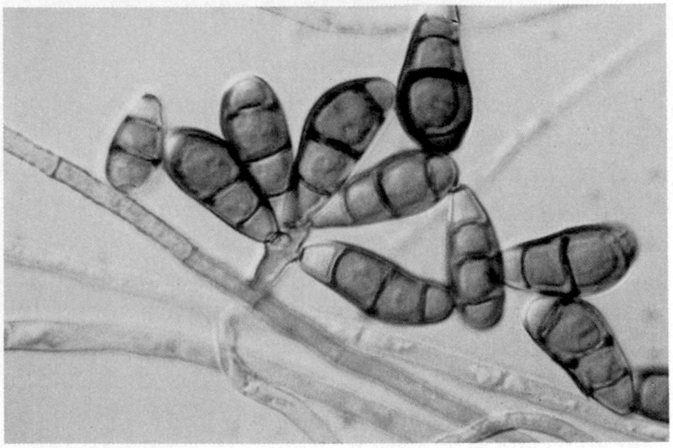

Figure 45.27. Microscopic appearance of *Curvularia* spp. demonstrating conidia and geniculate conidiophore (Nomarski optics, ×1250).

endocarditis, local catheter infection, nasal septum and paranasal sinuses, lower respiratory tract, skin and subcutaneous tissue, bones, and cornea (27, 29, 42). In clinical specimens, the hyphae may appear nonpigmented (hyaline). Common species causing disease in humans are *Curvularia geniculata*, *Curvularia lunata*, *Curvularia pallescens*, *Curvalaria senegalensis*, and *Curvularia verruculosa*. In culture, *Curvularia* colonies are rapidly growing, woolly, and gray to grayish black or brown. Microscopically, the conidia are dematiaceous, two- to several-celled, and curved (Fig. 45.27). The conidiophores are dematiaceous, solitary or in groups, septate, simple or branched, sympodial, and geniculate (27, 29).

Infections caused by the genera *Biopolaris* and *Exserohilum* present similarly to those due to *Aspergillus* species, except that disease progresses more slowly. Clinical presentations include dissemination with vascular invasion and tissue necrosis, involvement of the central nervous system and paranasal sinuses, and association with allergic bronchopulmonary disease. Most commonly, these organisms cause sinusitis in "normal" (atopic/asthmatic) hosts and more invasive disease in immunocompromised hosts. Marijuana smoking may be a risk factor for infection with these organisms. In culture, *Bipolaris* and *Exserohilum* both form rapidly growing, woolly, gray to black colonies. Microscopically, the conidiophores are sympodial and geniculate. The conidia are dematiaceous, oblong to cylindrical, and multicelled.

THERAPY

The emergence of fungal pathogens as important agents of human infection has resulted in an increase in the use of systemic antifungal agents worldwide and the introduction of a number of new antifungal agents with systemic activity (6, 10, 17, 21, 28, 47, 48, 52). A variety of antifungal agents are now available for the treatment of fungal infections. Ten of these compounds are discussed briefly in this chapter (Table 45.12). They include representatives of the polyene macrolide class (amphotericin B, amphotericin B lipid complex, liposomal amphotericin B, and amphotericin B cholesterol dispersion), the azoles (miconazole, ketoconazole, fluconazole, itraconazole, and saperconazole), and an inhibitor of pyrimidine synthesis (5-fluorocytosine). In addition, the rationale for, and limitations of, in vitro susceptibility testing are discussed with a description of the current efforts to develop a standardized in vitro testing method and to establish clinical correlations for in vitro test results.

Antifungal Agents

Amphotericin B and the liposomal and lipid complex formations of amphotericin B are polyene macrolide antibiotics used primarily in the treatment of systemic and life-threatening fungal infections. These compounds act by binding to ergosterol in the fungal cell membrane, causing loss of membrane integrity and osmotic instability (28). Amphotericin B is the drug of choice for the treatment of aspergillosis, disseminated candidiasis, cryptococcosis, and zygomycosis (6, 28, 47). It is also effective in the treatment of coccidioidomycosis, histoplasmosis, and blastomycosis (Table 45.13). Unfortunately, the therapeutic efficacy of amphotericin B is limited by significant toxicity, specifically nephrotoxicity. The liposomal and lipid complex formulations of amphotericin B were designed to increase the therapeutic index (increase efficacy and decrease toxicity) for amphotericin B therapy and to maximize the delivery of amphotericin B to patients with deep-seated fungal infections such as hepatosplenic candidiasis and invasive pulmonary aspergillosis (6, 21). Three different formulations are under investigation. Ampho-

Table 45.12. Antifungal Agents with Systemic Activity

Drug	Route	Mechanism	Comments
Amphotericin B	IV	Binds to ergosterol, causing direct membrane damage	Established agent. Broad spectrum. Toxic.
Amphotericin B lipid complex	IV	Binds to ergosterol, causing direct membrane damage	Investigational agent. Less toxic than amphotericin B.
Liposomal amphotericin B	IV	Binds to ergosterol, causing direct membrane damage	Investigational agent. Less toxic than amphotericin B.
Amphotericin B cholesterol dispersion	IV	Binds to ergosterol, causing direct membrane damage	Investigational agent. Less toxic than amphotericin B.
Miconazole	IV	Inhibits membrane sterol synthesis	Toxic agent with modest activity against *Candida* and other yeasts. Active against *Pseudallescheria boydii*.
Ketoconazole	Oral	Inhibits membrane sterol synthesis	Established agent with modest broad-spectrum activity.
Fluconazole	Oral, IV	Inhibits membrane sterol synthesis	Triazole with broad-spectrum activity. Good central nervous system penetration. Good in vivo activity against *Candida* and *Cryptococcus neoformans*.
Itraconazole	Oral	Inhibits membrane sterol synthesis	Triazole with broad-spectrum activity, including *Aspergillus*. Excellent in vivo activity against endemic mycoses.
Saperconazole	Oral	Inhibits membrane sterol synthesis	Investigational triazole with broad-spectrum activity. Good in vivo activity against endemic mycoses.
Flucytosine	Oral	Inhibits DNA and RNA synthesis	Toxicity and resistance are problems. Used in combination with amphotericin B.

Table 45.13. Antifungal Therapy for Deep Mycoses

Infection	Agents: First Choice	Agents: Alternatives[a]
Aspergillosis	Amphotericin B (±5-FC)	Itraconazole
Blastomycosis	Amphotericin B Itraconazole[b]	Ketoconazole[b]
Candidiasis	Amphotericin B (±5-FC)	? Fluconazole
Chromoblastomycosis	Itraconazole	5-FC
Coccidiodomycosis	Amphotericin B	Ketoconazole[b] Itraconazole[b] Fluconazole[c] Intrathecal amphotericin B[c]
Cryptococcosis	Amphotericin B (±5-FC)	Fluconazole
Fusariosis	Amphotericin B	Itraconazole
Histoplasmosis	Amphotericin B Itraconazole[d]	Ketoconazole[d] Fluconazole[d]
Phaeohyphomycosis	Amphotericin B	Itraconazole
Pseudallescheriosis	Itraconazole	Miconazole or Ketoconazole
Sporotrichosis	Oral iodides[e] Amphotericin B[f]	Itraconazole[e]
Trichosporonosis	Amphotericin B	None established
Zygomycosis	Amphotericin B	None established

[a]Limited data exist for most alternative agents.
[b]Indolent, nonmeningeal.
[c]Meningeal.
[d]Chronic pulmonary or indolent, nonmeningeal disseminated infection.
[e]Lymphocutaneous.
[f]Extracutaneous.

tericin B lipid complex, a 1:1 molar complex of phospholipids and drug; Ambisome, a phospholipid/cholesterol liposome formation; and Amphocil, a 1:1 molar complex of cholesterol sulfate and amphotericin B. The resultant liposomal and lipid complex preparations have selective toxicity for fungal cells but not for mammalian cells and theoretically promote delivery of the drug to the site of infection, while avoiding the toxicity of supramaximal doses of amphotericin B. The available clinical data indicate that these formulations allow the administration of higher doses of amphotericin B with no increase in acute toxicity and no chronic toxicity (6, 21). Importantly, there is no evidence of dose-limiting nephrotoxicity. The therapeutic efficacy of these formulations remains to be established, but preliminary clinical data are promising.

The azole class of antifungal compounds consists of a large number of agents with systemic antifungal activity, including the imidazoles (miconazole and ketoconazole) and the newer triazoles (itraconazol, fluconazole, and saperconazole) (Table 45.12) (10, 17, 52). The azole antifungals interact with cytochrome P-450–dependent enzymes with resulting impairment of ergosterol synthesis and depletion of ergosterol in the fungal cell membrane (28). This results in inhibition of fungal cell growth. The imidazoles, miconazole and ketoconazole, are established broad-spectrum agents active against a variety of fungal pathogens, including yeasts, dimorphic organisms, dermatophytes, and opportunitistic pathogens (Tables 45.12 and 45.13). The triazoles, itraconazole, fluconazole, and saperconazole all show promise as broad-spectrum, orally active, systemic agents with less potential for toxicity than the currently available imidazoles (10, 52). Both fluconazole and itraconazole currently have important roles as agents of first choice or as major alternatives in the treatment of deep mycoses (Table 45.13) (10, 21, 52). Ongoing and future clinical trials will more clearly define the specific roles of the triazoles in the treatment of systemic mycoses (6, 10, 21, 30, 51, 52, 57).

5-fluorocytosine (5-FC) is a water-soluble fluorinated pyrimidine antimetabolite used orally (intravenous formulation is investigational) in the treatment of systemic infections caused by susceptible pathogenic or opportunistic yeasts and fungi. The spectrum of susceptible fungal pathogens is narrow and includes *Candida* species, *Cryptococcus neoformans*, and some agents of chromoblastomycosis (Table 45.13). 5-FC acts as a competitive antimetabolite for uracil in the synthesis of fungal RNA, and it also inactivates thymidylate synthetase (28). These activities can be antagonized by a variety of purine and pyrimidine bases and nucleosides.

Antifungal Susceptibility Testing

In vitro susceptibility tests with antifungal agents are performed for the same reasons that tests with antibacterial agents are performed (28, 45). Ideally, in vitro susceptibility tests will (*a*) provide a reliable estimate of the relative activities of two or more antifungal agents, (*b*) correlate with in vivo antifungal activity and predict the likely outcome of therapy, (*c*) provide a means by which to monitor the development of resistance among a normally susceptible population of organisms, and (*d*) predict the therapeutic potential of newly discovered investigational agents. Unfortunately, there is little evidence to support the correlation of antifungal susceptibility test results with clinical outcome. Although recent studies suggest some correlation with in vitro susceptibility test results for amphotericin B and clinical outcome (15, 40), the general applicability of these results remains confused by the retrospective nature of the studies, the documented variability of the nonstandardized in vitro test methods used, and the difficulty in defining fungal diseases and their responses to therapy (28, 45).

Given the increasing number of antifungal agents and the perceived need for in vitro susceptibility testing to aid in their clinical application, it has become apparent that efforts are needed to standardize antifungal susceptibility testing just as they were previously for antibacterial testing (18, 28, 39, 45). In addressing this issue, the National Committee for Clinical Laboratory Standards (NCCLS) has established a subcommittee to coordinate work on antifungal susceptibility tests with a goal of developing a reliable reference method for in vitro susceptibility testing of yeasts and other fungi and ultimately to correlate the results of this method with clinical effectiveness.

Several multicenter studies conducted by the NCCLS subcommittee have identified a number of important technical issues affecting the precision and intralaboratory and interlaboratory reproducibility of in vitro susceptibility test procedures with yeasts and several commonly used antifungal agents, including amphotericin B, 5-FC, ketoconazole, and fluconazole (18, 39, 45). To date, significant progress has been made in developing a standardized method for in vitro susceptibility testing of antifungal agents (18, 39). The results of these studies have been incorporated into a reference method that has been recently published (32). Despite this progress, the clinical relevance of in vitro antifungal susceptibility testing remains unclear. Obviously this issue must be resolved before fungal susceptibility testing can be offered routinely in the clinical microbiology laboratory.

SUMMARY AND CONCLUSIONS

Our understanding of the epidemiology and pathogenesis of fungal infections has improved considerably over the past decade. By weight of sheer numbers, we have the best understanding of candidal infections; however, there is little doubt that newer fungi previously considered nonpathogens have now emerged as significant human pathogens, particularly in the immunocompromised host. Recognition of these emerging fungal pathogens has resulted in improved understanding of their clinical presentation and response to available therapeutic measures. Clearly, additional efforts are necessary to improve diagnosis and management and to better understand the pathogenesis of infection due to this diverse group of fungal pathogens. Future studies should include clinical trials of prophylactic agents to prevent colonization, of empiric agents for early treatment of suspected infections, and of therapeutic agents to treat documented infections. Advances in diagnostic methods may provide earlier diagnosis and thus encourage earlier and potentially more effective therapeutic interventions. Finally, epidemiological studies documenting the rates of colonization and infection due to these emerging fungal pathogens, as well as studies of the effectiveness of various components of infection control and antibacterial drug use, and optimal guidelines for insertion and management of vascular catheters are urgently needed.

References

1. Ajello L, ed. Coccidiodomycosis: current clinical and diagnostic status. New York: Stratton Intercontinental, 1977.
2. Ajello L. Hyalohyphomycosis and phaeohyphomycosis: two global disease entities of public health importance. Eur J Epidemiol 1986;2:243–251.

3. Anaisse EJ, Bodey GP, Kantarjian H, Ro J, Vartivarian SE, Hopfer R, Hoy J, Rolston K. New spectrum of fungal infections in patients with cancer. Rev Infect Dis 1989;11:369–378.
4. Anaisse EJ, Bodey GP, Rinaldi MG. Emerging fungal pathogens. Eur J Clin Microbiol Infect Dis 1989;8:323–330.
5. Anaisse E, Bodey GP. Disseminated trichosporonosis: meeting the challenge. Eur J Clin Microbiol Infect Dis 1991;10:711–713.
6. Armstrong D. Treatment of opportunistic fungal infections. Clin Infect Dis 1993;16:1–9.
7. Banerjee SN, Emori TG, Culver DH, Gaynes RP, Jarvis WR, Horan T, Edwards JR, Tolson J, Henderson T, Martone WJ. Secular trends in nosocomial primarly blood stream infections in the United States, 1980–1989. Am J Med 1991;91(Suppl 3B): 865–895.
8. Barnett J, Payne R, Yarrow D. Yeasts: characteristics and identification. 2nd ed. Cambridge: Cambridge University Press, 1990.
9. Bennett JE. *Aspergillus* species. In:Mandell GL, Doublas RG Jr, Bennett JE, eds. Principles and practice of infectious diseases. 2nd ed. New York: John Wiley & Sons, 1985:1447–1451.
10. Bodey GP. Azole antifungal agents. Clin Infect Dis 1992; 14(Suppl 1):S161–S169.
11. Bross J, Talbot GH, Maislin G. Hurwitz S. Risk factors for nosocomial candidemia: a case-control study in adults without leukemia. Am J Med 1989;87:614–619.
12. Brummer E, Castaneda E, Restrepo A. Paracoccidioidomycosis: an update. Clin Microbiol Rev 1993;6:89–117.
13. deRepentigny L, Boushira M, Ste-Marie L, Bosisio G. Detection of galactomannan antigenemia by enzyme immunoassay in experimental invasive aspergillosis. J Clin Microbiol 1987;25:863–867.
14. deRepentigny L. Serological techniques for diagnosis of fungal infection. Eur J Clin Microbiol Infec Dis 1989;8:362–375.
15. Dick JD, Merz WG, Saral R. Incidence of polyene-resistant yeasts recovered from clinical specimens. Antimicrob Agents Chemother 1980;18:158–163.
16. Einstein HE, Johnson RH, Coccidioidomycosis: New aspects of epidemiology and therapy. Clin Infect Dis 1993;16:349–354.
17. Fromtling RA. Overview of medically important antifungal azole derivatives. Clin Microbiol Rev 1988;1:187–217.
18. Fromtling RA, Galgiani JN, Pfaller MA, Espinel-Ingroff A, Bartizal KF, Bartlett MS, Body BA, Frey C, Hall G, Roberts GD, Nolte FB, Odds FC, Rinaldi MG, Sugar AM, Villareal K. Multicenter evaluation of a broth macrodilution antifungal susceptibility test for yeast. Antimicrob Agents Chemother 1993;37: 39–45.
19. Gamis A, Gudnason T, Giebink GS, Ramsey NKC. Disseminated infection with *Fusarium* in recipients of bone marrow transplants. Rev Infect Dis 1991;13:1077–1088.
20. Goodman NL, Rinaldi MG. Agents of zygomycosis. In: Balows A, Hausler WJ Jr, Herrmann K, Isenberg HD, Shadomy HJ, eds. Manual of clinical microbiology. 5th ed. Washington DC: American Society for Microbiology, 1991: 674–692.
21. Graybill JR. Future directions of antifungal chemotherapy. Clin Infect Dis 1992;14(Suppl 1):S170–S181.
22. Harvey RL, Myers JP, Nosocomial fungemia in a large community teaching hospital. Arch Intern Med 1987;147:2117–2120.
23. Hopwood V, Warnock DW. New developments in the diagnosis of opportunistic fungal infection. Eur J Clin Microbiol 1986;5:379–388.
24. Jones JM. Laboratory diagnosis of invasive candidiasis. Clin Microbiol Rev 1990;3:32–45.
25. Kaufman L, Standard P. Improved version of the exoantigen test for identification of *Coccidioides immitis* and *Histoplasma capsulatum* cultures. J Clin Microbiol 1978;8:42–45.
26. Komshian SV, Uwaydak AK, Sobel JD, Crane LR. Fungemia caused by *Candida* species and Torulopsis glabrata in the hospitalized patient: frequency, characteristics, and evaluation of factors influencing outcome. Rev Infect Dis 1989;11:379–390.
27. Kwon-Chung KH, Bennett JE. Medical mycology. Philadelphia: Lea & Febiger, 1992.
28. McGinnis MR, Rinaldi MG. Antifungal drugs: mechanisms of action, drug resistance, susceptibility testing, and assays of activity in biological fluids. In: Lorian V, ed. Antibiotics in laboratory medicine. 3rd ed. Baltimore: Williams & Wilkins, 1991: 198–257.
29. McGinnis MR, Salkin IF, Schell WA, Pasarell L. Dematiaceous fungi. In: Balows A, Hausler WJ Jr, Herrmann K, Isenberg HD, Shadomy HJ, eds. Manual of clinical microbiology. 5th ed. Washington, DC: American Society for Microbiology, 1991:644–658.
30. McIlroy MA. Failure of fluconazole to suppress fungemia in a patient with fever, neutropenia, and typhlitis. J Infect Dis 1991;163:420–421.
31. Minor RL Jr, Pfaller MA, Gingrich RD, Burns LJ. Disseminated *Fusarium* infections in patients following bone marrow transplantation. Bone Marrow Transplant 1989;4:653–658.
32. National Committee for Clinical Laboratory Standards. Reference method for broth dilution antifungal susceptibility testing for yeasts. Proposed standard. Document M27-P. Villanova, PA: National Committee for Clinical Laboratory Standards, 1992.
33. Nelson PA, Toussoun TA, Marasas WFO. *Fusarium* species. University Park, PA: The Pennsylvania State University Press, 1983.
34. Padhye AA, Ajello L. Fungi causing eumycotic mycetomas. In: Balows A, Hausler WJ JR, Herrmann K, Isenberg HD, Shadomy HJ, eds. Manual of clinical microbiology. 5th ed. Washington, DC: American Society for Microbiology, 1991: 693–700.
35. Pannuti CS, Gingrich RD, Pfaller MA, Wenzel RP. Nosocomial pneumonia in adult patients undergoing bone marrow transplantation: a 9-year study. J Clin Microbiol 1991;9:1–5.
36. Pincus D, Salkin I, Hurd N, Levy I, Kemna M. Modification of potassium nitrate assimilation test for identification of clinically important yeasts. J Clin Microbiol 1988;26:366–368.
37. Pfaller MA. Laboratory aids in the diagnosis of invasive candidiasis. Mycopathologia 1992;120:65–72.
38. Pfaller M, Wenzel R. Impact of the changing epidemiology of fungal infections in the 1990's. Eur J Clin Microbiol Infect Dis 1992;11:287–291.
39. Pfaller MA, Rinaldi MG, Galgiani JN, Bartlett MS, Body BA, Espinel-Ingroff A, Fromtling RA, Hall GS, Hughes CE, Odds FC, Sugar AM. Collaborative investigation of variables in antifungal susceptibility testing of yeasts. Antimicrob Agents Chemother 1990;34:1648–1654.
40. Powderly WG, Kobayashi GS, Herzig GP, Medoff G. Amphotericin B-resistant yeast infection in severely immunocompromised patients. Am J Med 1988;84:826–832.
41. Rinaldi MG. Use of potato flakes agar in clinical mycology. J Clin Microbiol 1982;15:1159–1160.
42. Rippon JW. Medical mycology: the pathogenic fungi and the pathogenic actinomycetes. 3rd ed. Philadelphia: WB Saunders, 1988.
43. Rogers AL, Kennedy MJ. Opportunistic hyaline hyphomycetes. In: Balows A, Hausler WJ Jr, Herrmann K, Isenberg HD, Shadomy HJ (eds). Manual of clinical microbiology. 5th ed. Washington, DC: American Society for Microbiology, 1991:659–673.
44. Salkin IF, McGinnis MR, Dykstra MH, Rinaldi MG. *Scedosporium inflatum*, an emerging pathogen. J Clin Microbiol 1988;26:498–503.

45. Shadomy S, Pfaller MA. Laboratory studies with antifungal agents: susceptibility tests and quantitation in body fluids. In: Balows A, Hauser WJ Jr, Herrmann K, Isenberg HD, Shadomy HJ, eds. Manual of clinical microbiology. 5th ed. Washington, DC: American Society for Microbiology, 1991:1173–1183.
46. Tollemar J. Ringden O, Bostrom L, Nilsson B, Sundberg B. Variables predicting deep fungal infections in bone marrow transplant recipients. Bone Marrow Transplant 1989;4:635–641.
47. Walsh TJ, Pizza A. Treatment of systemic fungal infections: recent progress and current problems. Eur J Clin Microbiol Infect Dis 1988;7:460–475.
48. Walsh TJ, Jarosinski PF, Fromtling RA. Increasing usage of systemic antifungal agents. Diagn Microbiol Infect Dis 1990;13:37–40.
49. Walsh TJ, Melcher GP, Rinaldi MG, Lecciones J, McGough DA, Kelly P, Lee J, Callender D, Rubin M, Pizzo PA. *Trichosporon beigelii*, an emerging pathogen resistant to amphotericin B. J Clin Microbiol 1990;28:1616–1622.
50. Walsh TJ, Mitchell TG. Dimorphic fungi causing systemic mycoses. In: Balows A, Hausler WJ Jr, Herrmann K, Isenberg HD, Shadomy HJ, eds. Manual of clinical microbiology. 5th ed. Washington, DC: American Society for Microbiology, 1991:630–643.
51. Warnock DW, Burke J, Cope JJ, Johnson EM, von Fraunhofer NA, Williams EW. Fluconazole resistance in *Candida glabrata*. Lancet 1988;2:1310.
52. Warnock DW. Itraconazole and fluconazole: new drugs for deep fungal infections. J Antimicrob Chemother 1989;24:275–277.
53. Warren NG, Shadomy HJ. Yeasts of medical importance. In: Balows A, Hausler WJ Jr, Herrmann K, Isenberg HD, Shadomy HJ, eds. Manual of clinical microbiology. 5th ed. Washington, DC: American Society for Microbiology, 1991:617–629.
54. Weitzman I, Kane J. Dermatophytes and agents of superficial mycoses. In: Balows A, Hausler WJ Jr, Hermann K, Isenberg HD, Shadomy HJ, eds. Manual of clinical microbiology. 5th ed. Washington, DC: American Society for Microbiology, 1991:601–616.
55. Wey SB, Mori M, Pfaller MA, Woolson RF, Wenzel RP. Hospital acquired candidemia: the attributable mortality and excess length of stay. Arch Intern Med 1988;148:2642–2645.
56. Wey SB, Mori M, Pfaller MA, Woolson RF, Wenzel RP. Risk factors for hospital acquired candidemia: a matched case-control study. Arch Intern Med 1989;149:2349–2353.
57. Willocks L, Leen CLS, Brettle RP, Urquhart D, Russell TB, Milne LJR. Fluconazole resistance in AIDS patients. J Antimicrob Chemother 1991;28:937–939.
58. Wingard JR, Merz WG, Rinaldi MG, Johnson TR, Karp JE, Saral S. Increase in *Candida krusei* infections among patients with bone marrow transplantation and neutropenia treated prophylactically with fluconazole. N Engl J Med 1991;325:1274–1277.

46 Chlamydia, Mycoplasma, and Rickettsia

Stephen G. Jenkins

CHLAMYDIA

Chlamydiae are obligate intracellular bacterial parasites of eukaryotic cells. Once called *Bedsonia* species (for Sir Samuel Bedson, who first isolated and described the causative agent of psittacosis), trachoma-inclusion conjunctivitis, (TRIC) agents, and *Miyagawanella* species, these organisms were once considered viruses because of their inability to synthesize ATP or to grow on artificial media. They are dissimilar to the viruses, however, in that they contain both RNA and DNA, are susceptible to antibacterial agents, have cell walls similar to Gram-negative bacteria, synthesize protein utilizing their own ribosomes, and divide by binary fission. First isolated in embryonated eggs in 1957 and in cell culture in 1963, these organisms have been described as "energy parasites" (1).

Because of their unique developmental cycle, the chlamydiae are taxonomically classified in a separate order, *Chlamydiales* (from the Greek *chlamys*, a cloak draped around the shoulder, in reference to the intracytoplasmic inclusions "draped" around the infected cell's nucleus). The order contains one genus, *Chlamydia*, which in turn currently contains three species: *Chlamydia psittaci*, with several poorly characterized serotypes, *Chlamydia trachomatis* (15 serotypes: A, B, B_a, to K, L_1, L_2, and L_3), and the TWAR agent (*Chlamydia pneumoniae*) (2). Several distinct clinical syndromes are caused by the specific chlamydial serotypes (Table 46.1). *C. trachomatis* can be differentiated from *C. psittaci* based on its ability to form glycogen inclusions detectable in infected cell cultures with an iodine staining technique and its susceptibility to sulfonamides. Laboratory properties differentiating the chlamydial species are outlined in Table 46.2. Cellular infection with *C. trachomatis* results in a single inclusion that tends to displace the nucleus, whereas the inclusions of *C. psittaci* typically rupture early, resulting in a perinuclear distribution that fails to displace the nucleus. In addition, species can be definitively distinguished using monoclonal antibody stains.

C. trachomatis and *C. psittaci* possess a common group-reactive lipopolysaccharide antigen (3), have a similar small genomic size, and demonstrate approximately 10% DNA homology. *C. pneumoniae*, by comparison, lacks significant DNA homology with either of the other species, has different restriction endonuclease patterns, and appears to generally lack extrachromosomal DNA as is typically demonstrable in strains of *C. trachomatis* and the majority of *C. psit-*

Table 46.1 Human Clinical Disease Caused by Chlamydial Species

Species	Serotypes	Disease	Major Symptoms	Infection Site	Mode of Transmission
C. pneumoniae	One	Pneumonia	Diffuse lung disease	Pulmonary	Person to person
C. psittaci	Several	Psittacosis (ornithosis)	Subclinical; mild respiratory illness or overt pneumonia	Pulmonary	Birds (including fecal droppings) to man; rarely human to human
C. trachomatis	A, B, Ba, C	Endemic trachoma	Chronic conjunctivitis; may result in blindness	Ocular	Human to human
	L1, L2, L3	Lymphogranuloma venereum	Transient genital ulcers, inguinal (males), pelvic or retroperitoneal (women) lymphadenopathy	Lymph nodes, rectum	Sexual
	D–K	Adult inclusion conjunctivitis	Acute follicular conjunctivitis	Ocular	Genital to eye
		Genital tract infection	Nongonococcal urethritis, cervicitis, epididymitis, proctitis, salpingitis	Genital tract, rectum	Sexual
		Inclusion conjunctivitis of the newborn	Acute mucopurulent conjunctivitis	Ocular	Genital to eye during passage through birth canal
		Pneumonitis/pneumonia of the newborn	Afebrile, chronic diffuse pulmonary disease; pneumonia	Pulmonary	Aspiration during passage through birth canal

Table 46.2. Laboratory Characteristics of Human Chylamydial Species

Characteristic	*C. Trachomatis* LGV Biovar	*C. Trachomatis* Trachoma Biovar	*C. Psittaci*	*C. Pneumoniae*
Inclusions				
Refractile, vacuolar	+	+	0	0
Iodine staining glycogen	+	+	0	0
Intracerebral injection lethal for mice	0	+	+	0
Sulfadiazine susceptibility	+	+	0	0
Cell culture				
L-cell plaques	0	+	+	0
Enhanced recovery following				
Cell treatment with diethylaminoethyl-dextran	+	0	0	+
Centrifugation	+	0	0	+

taci isolates (4, 5). DNA homology is generally high within each species.

All three recognized chlamydial species exhibit two distinct forms during their unique developmental cycle. The 300-nm elementary body is especially adapted for extracellular survival and represents the infectious form in the life cycle. The elementary bodies of *C. pneumoniae* are described as pleomorphic but typically pear-shaped (6), whereas those of *C. trachomatis* and *C. psittaci* are usually round. Upon contact with and attachment to a susceptible cell, the elementary body is actively taken into a phagosome by endocytosis, where the entire replication cycle takes place. Lysosomal fusion, however, fails to occur. Over the next 6 to 8 hours, the elementary body undergoes reorganization into the metabolically active but noninfectious reticulate or initial body. For 18 to 24 hours, the reticulate body synthesizes new material and divides continuously by binary fission within a membrane-bound vacuole. Adapted for intracellular functions, reticulate bodies cannot survive in the extracellular milieu and are incapable of infecting other cells. After this period of synthesis and division, the reticulate bodies reorganize and condense into compact elementary bodies still bound within the phagocytic vesicle. Depending on the strain, somewhere between 48 and 72 hours after the cellular infection was initiated, the vacuoles release their contents and the cell lyses, releasing infectious elementary bodies.

Chlamydia trachomatis

SPECTRUM OF DISEASE

Once designated the lymphogranuloma-venereum-trachoma inclusion conjunctivitis (LGV-TRIC) agent, *C. trachomatis* is now recognized as an important cause of cervicitis and pelvic inflammatory disease in women, nongonoccocal urethritis (NGU) and epididymitis in men, and inclusion conjunctivitis and interstitial pneumonia in neonates. The host range of *C. trachomatis* is restricted to humans except for the mouse neumonitis agent. *C. trachomatis* is reportedly the most common sexually transmitted disease in developed countries (7), causing an estimated 4 million infections per year in the U.S. alone, with resulting annual estimated direct and indirect costs totaling $1.4 billion (8).

Inclusion Conjunctivitis

Ocular infections have been documented in approximately one-third of neonates treated prophylactically with silver nitrate whose mothers were infected with *C. trachomatis* at parturition (9). Therefore, neonatal chlamydial conjunctivitis may be seen in up to 2 to 6% of infants born in areas where the prevalance of sexually transmitted infection is high. Typically appearing 2 to 25 days after delivery (earlier in the setting of premature rupture of membranes), inclusion conjunctivitis is characterized by edematous, inflamed conjunctivae with a copious mucopurulent discharge. In cases of chronic or relapsing infection, conjunctival follicles may develop. The infection is usually self-limited, resolving spontaneously over a period of several months with no significant sequelae even without antimicrobial therapy. Inclusion conjunctivitis in the adult, albeit relatively rare, presents acutely with a foreign body sensation, mucopurulent discharge, photophobia, and follicular conjunctivitis with or without keratitis. Except in cases of reinfection, symptoms disappear spontaneously over a period of several months to 2 years. Adult ocular infection usually occurs in patients whose sexual partner(s) show signs of genital chlamydial infection (10).

Trachoma

Endemic trachoma is a chronic disease characterized by recurrent corneal and conjunctival infection with *C. trachomatis*. Pannus formation and conjunctival scarring occur as sequelae to the chronic follicular keratoconjunctivitis. Historically, trachoma represented the single greatest cause of blindness in the world and probably remains today the single most common cause of preventable blindness (11). In 1973, approximately 400,000,000 people worldwide were afflicted with trachoma, which resulted in blindness in 2,000,000 (12). Although the number and size of endemic areas have been significantly reduced since 1950, trachoma continues to occur, mainly among the impoverished, in less developed regions of the world, especially of northern Africa, the Middle East, and northern India. It is still occasionally seen in Native Americans in the southwestern United States. In endemic areas, children are often infected with serotypes A to C of *C. trachomatis* during the first 3 months of life. Transmission is not genital but by close contact with infected persons or from flies carrying infectious ocular material from eye to eye (13). Although relatively unusual, acute disease in adults over 20 years of age is much more common in women than in men, apparently due to closer contact with children.

Typically, trachoma begins acutely with inflammation of the bulbar and palpebral conjunctivae. Although initially a mixed cellular response is seen in the ocular exudate, macrophages and lymphocytes coalesce within a few weeks, forming soft, necrotic subconjunctival follicles. At this stage the disease may resolve spontaneously, unless reinfection occurs. Upon repeated infection, however, corneal vascularization begins and progresses concomitantly with conjunctival scarring. Repeated bacterial superinfections contribute to this process. The synergistic combination of bacterial infection, corneal vascularization, and conjunctival scarring results in blindness.

Lymphogranuloma venereum

C. trachomatis serotypes L_1, L_2, and L_3 cause a venereally transmitted disease, lymphogranuloma venereum (LGV), endemic to regions of South America, Africa, and Asia. Climatic bubo, tropical bubo, and estiomene are all synonyms for this disease referred to on occasion in 18th century literature (14). Although uncommon in the United States, with fewer than 500 cases typically reported yearly to public health departments, it is seen more frequently in the warmer, more humid regions of the country, especially the southeast, in people of lower socioeconomic status, in male homosexuals, and in individuals returning from other endemic regions. The disease is reported three times more frequently in men than in women. Transmission following laboratory accidents during aerosolization of the agent without appropriate biosafety measures and through fomites has reportedly occurred and resulted in pulmonary infection with pleural effusion, pneumonitis, and hilar and/or mediastinal lymphadenopathy. Probable reservoirs in the population include persons ignoring symptoms of cervical, urethral, or anorectal infection and individuals with asymptomatic disease.

LGV is the only chlamydial infection resulting in multisystem disease and causing constitutional symptoms. During the primary phase of the illness, 3 days to 3 weeks following exposure, a small painles herpetiform vesicle or ulcer develops, which heals without scarring. The lesions are only infrequently noticed by infected individuals on the affected sexual organ. In gay men and sometimes in women, the primary lesion may be an anorectal ulcer with associated symptoms of diarrhea, tenesmus, and a bloody, mucopurulent rectal discharge resulting from ulceration of the rectosigmoid colon. In such cases, fever and other constitutional symptoms are frequent, and perirectal or inguinal lymphadenopathy may result. A diffuse inflammatory response with mucosal ulceration, crypt abscesses, and granuloma formation is seen upon histologic examination of a rectal biopsy during this stage of the disease.

The primary phase of illness is followed 2 to 6 weeks later by a secondary stage characterized by suppurative regional lymphadenopathy and pronounced constititional symptoms, including chills, fever, anorexia, headache, and arthralgias. Characteristic small, stellate abscesses surrounded by histiocytes are noted upon histologic examination of affected nodes. Other laboratory abnormalities commonly seen during this period include a leukocytosis, an elevated erythrocyte sedimentation rate, and abnormal liver function tests. During this phase, sequelae resulting from anorectal infection may include perirectal abscesses and rectovaginal or ischiorectal fistulas. Less frequently observed symptoms include hepatitis, erythema nodosum, "aseptic" meningitis, meningoencephalitis, and arthritis with a culture-negative effusion.

The late phase of the disease results from the sequelae caused by fibrotic changes and interference with normal lymphatic drainage. Chronic and progressive, infiltrative or ulcerative involvement of the scrotum, penis, or urethra with fistula development, ulcers, and posterior urethral strictures is not uncommon in men with untreated genital infection. Rectal strictures may result in "pencil stools." Rarely, lymphedema may cause genital elephantiasis, with vulvar or penile enlargement and disfigurement. Chronic ulceration of the vulva and pedunculated perianal protrusions (lymphorrhoids) may also occasionally occur.

Nongonococcal Urethritis and Prostatitis

Isolated in 30 to 50% of all cases, *C. trachomatis* serotypes D to K are the microorganisms, most commonly associated with male nongonococcal urethritis (NGU). Up to one-third of men with urethral chlamydial infection may be without symptoms, and the organism can be isolated from a significant percentage of asymptomatic sexually active males. Although the symptoms of NGU are generally less acute than in cases of gonorrhea, the two cannot be reliably differentiated based on symptomology alone. In NGU, the urethral discharge is typically less purulent and smaller in volume than in gonococcal infection and results in less dysuria. Signs of NGU include erythema and tenderness of the meatus and a urethral exudae often demonstrable only upon urethral stripping in the morning prior to urination. One to two percent of chlamydial urethral infections have been reported to evolve into epididymitis. *C. trachomatis* is the most frequently isolated agent in young heterosexual men with this disease in whom structural genitourinary tract abnormality is absent (15). *C. trachomatis* has also been reported to be associated with "venereal" Reiter syndrome (16) and has been isolated in up to 80% of cases of postgonococcal urethritis. Among homosexual men, it may cause proctitis or proctocolitis, depending on the serotype of the infecting strain.

Gynecological Infections

Genital infection with *C. trachomatis* is more prevalent in women than in men, but often escapes clinical detection. The adult female may have asymptomatic endocervical infection (17) or may present with mucopurulent cervicitis with vaginal discharge, urethritis, bleeding cervical erosions, proctitis, pelvic inflammatory disease, and/or salpingitis. Vaginitis does not occur. *C. trachomatis* has been isolated from the cervix of 30 to 60% of women with a history of sexual contact with a partner with NGU or gonorrhea or who diagnosed themselves with gonococcal infection, from 10 to 20% of women presenting to sexually transmitted disease (STD) clinics without a history of contact with parties with urethritis, and from 5 to 10% of young women visiting family planning centers, prenatal clinics, or gynecologic clinics (18). Detection rates are higher in sexually active teenagers, particularly those who are pregnant and those attending STD clinics. The prevalence of infection with *C. trachomatis* is also higher in those of lower socioeconomic status, of black race, residing in urban areas, of divorced marital status, and with increased numbers of sexual partners. It also appears to be higher in users of oral contraceptives (19). In most studies, *C. trachomatis* is several times more prevalent than *Neisseria gonorrhoeae*.

The consequences of chlamydial infection in young women are significant. Up to 10% of women with genital infection show signs and symptoms of acute salpingitis. Among women with ascending infection, important sequelae include chronic pelvic pain, infertility resulting from occlusion of the fallopian tubes, and ectopic pregnancy. Asymptomatic cervical infection is common, and most women with involuntary infertility resulting from bilateral tubal damage fail to give a history of prior pelvic infection. Accordingly, it is highly probable that the proportion of women with ascending chlamydial infection is much higher than 10%. *C. trachomatis* has been detected in approximately two-thirds of women with mucopurulent cervicitis. Over 80% of women with chlamydial genital infection demonstrate this syndrome upon gynecologic examination (20).

Acute endometritis due to *C. trachomatis* can progress to salpingitis following insertion of an intrauterine device, dilatation and curettage, hysterosalpingography, and subsequent to abortion or parturition. In a number of reported studies, *C. trachomatis* has been isolated from the urethra or cervix or approximately one-third of women with laparoscopically documented acute pelvic inflammatory disease and from a comparable portion of women with clinical evidence of salpingitis, symptoms of which include low abdominal pain, discomfort during sexual intercourse, and abnormal vaginal bleeding. Serologic studies have demonstrated that *C. trachomatis* infection has occurred in up to 60% of women with salpingitis. In addition, the agent can be isolated more frequently than *N. gonorrhoeae* from women with this disease, although symptoms typically appear to be less severe. Serologic detection of IgM or high titers of IgG antibodies to *C. trachomatis*, both suggestive of recent or active infection, have been reported in up to 87% of women with acute perihepatitis or peritonitis (Fitz-Hugh Curtis syndrome) (21). Related intraperitoneal disease reportedly associated with chlamydial infection include periplenitis and periappendicitis.

The risk for developing involuntary infertility as a result of tubal occlusion increases with the severity and number of episodes of salpingitis. The overall risk of infertility reportedly approximates 10% following a single episode of salpingitis, 30% with two episodes, and over 50% following infection on three or more occasions. Supporting this association, *C. trachomatis* has been isolated from a large porportion of peritubal and tubal specimens cultured from infertile women with tubal obstruction (22).

The dysuria-pyuria (urethral) syndrome has also been ascribed to *C. trachomatis* (23). In young women with frequency and dysuria, *C. trachomatis* can often be isolated. The agent has also been detected in pus expressed from the Bartholin's gland in cases of bartholinitis and occasionally from the rectum in women with chlamydial genital infection. Conflicting evidence exists on the importance of *C. trachomatis* as a cause of chorioamnionitis, premature rupture of membranes, premature delivery, spontaneous abortion, and stillbirth and on the influence of prior infection on the success of in vitro fertilization procedures.

Neonatal Pneumonia

Onset of classic chlamydial interstitial pneumonia in infants is gradual, with a range from 2 weeks to 3 months. The majority of cases are detected within 3 to 6 weeks of birth. Although the course of illness is protracted, the majority of infants remain consistently afebrile. In most cases, serum IgG and IgM levels are elevated, and the peripheral blood eosinophil count exceeds 300/mm^3 (24). Precedent conjunctivitis and/or ear abnormalities have been noted in many cases (25). Rhinitis with nasal obstruction, typically without nasal discharge, often represents the initial clinical manifestation.

A sequence of closely spaced staccato coughs each separated by a brief inspiration, tachypnea, hyperinflation, and rales with diffuse interstitial involvement typify the illness. Roentgenographic findings usually include pulmonary infiltrates, peribronichial thickening, and focal consolidation. A specific antibody response to the infecting strain of *C. trachomatis* is often demonstrable. A pronounced eosinophilic exudate is observed upon examination of tracheal secretions. Clinical illness usually lasts for several weeks, but rales and radiologic abnormalities may persist for months.

EPIDEMIOLOGY

The basic epidemiology of *C. trachomatis* infection was defined early in this century. The associaton between neonatal conjunctival infection, the maternal cervix, and infection among siblings, suggesting transmission by mucous membrane contact, was described as early as 1942 (26). Although the etiologic agent was thought to be a virus, the full spectrum of disease including female cervical infection, neonatal inclusion conjunctivitis, urethritis, and ophthalmitis in adults was comprehensively delineated prior to the advent of the antibiotic era. Although the role of *C. trachomatis* in NGU is still unclear, the agent can be isolated from a large proportion of men with this syndrome as well as from a significant number of female contacts with these men. Likewise, the majority of fathers of infants with inclusion conjunctivitis are positive for *C. trachomatis* upon urethral culture. Concomitant chlamydial infection at several body sites is also relatively common, and the majority of individuals with chlamydial conjunctivitis have simultaneous pharyngeal or genital colonization and/or infection.

Several conditions are associated with an increased prevalence of female chlamydial infection. These include cervical anomalies such as cervicitis. Women with cervical dysplasia have a high antibody positivity rate to *C. trachomatis,* but it is unclear whether chlamydial infection has caused the dysplasia or, alternatively, whether *C. trachomatis* preferentially colonizes dysplasitc sites. *C. trachomatis* cervical infection also appears to be more common in women with a history of other sexually transmitted disease. In addition, there appears to be an increased culture recovery rate from specimens collected during the first and fourth weeks of the female menstrual cycle. Risk factors in adolescent women include a younger age at first sexual intercourse, increased number of years of sexual activity, and use of oral contraceptives.

Although contact with infected mucosal membranes represents the most common route of exposure, ocular trachoma may be acquired via fomite inoculation and by swimming in contaminated water. Trachoma has also been acquired during ocular tonometry from equipment improperly sterilized between each procedure.

C. trachomatis can also cause sexually transmitted disease in children. When vaginal, rectal, or pharyngeal chlamydial infection occurs in children outside of the neonatal period, an investigation should be conducted to determine whether sexual abuse has occurred. Although infection with *C. trachomatis* in children does not prove that they are victims of sexual abuse, it should alert caretakers to the possibility of such a problem. Similarly, children undergoing medical evaluation for sexual abuse should be cultured for chlamydiae from pharyngeal, rectal, and vaginal sites, as appropriate.

DIAGNOSTIC PROCEDURES

Specimen Selection Collection

Specimens collected for the detection of chlamydiae should be handled with care. Such specimens may contain other agents of potential risk to the health care worker. Following aerosolization and inhalation of LGV strains of *C. trachomatis* in a laboratory setting, accidental infection resulting in pneumonitis and mediastinal lymphadenitis has been reported (27).

All samples collected for chlamydial isolation should be stored at refrigerator temperature prior to processing and inoculated to appropriate cell lines within 48 hours. If specimen processing is expected to be delayed for more than 48 hours after collection, specimens should be frozen at −70°C or below.

Although LGV strains of *C. trachomatis* have been isolated from clotted whole blood, blood culture is not recommended for routine diagnosis of infection. The specimen most frequently submitted to the laboratory for chlamydial isolation is the genital swab. Scrapings are preferred, but specimens from the conjunctivae and the genital tract are most easily collected with a swab. Cervical specimens may also be collected with a cytologic sampling brush. Materials utilized for some swabs have been shown to be toxic to the cell lines used to support the in vitro replication of chlamydiae and to inhibit chlamydial multiplication. Swabs prepared with dacron, rayon, or cotton fibers should be used for specimen collection. Likewise, swabs with plastic or metal shafts are superior to toxic wooden-shaft varieties. Confusing artifacts may result with some dacron swabs when iodine staining techniques are used to demonstrate *C. trachomatis* inclusions. Similarly, alginate swabs can result in the formation of confusing artifacts when dark-field microscopy is utilized to reveal chlamydial inclusions by Giemsa stain.

Removal of mucus and pus prior to obtaining an endocervical sample reduces the rate of bacterial contamination and the frequency of cytotoxicity in inoculated cell cultures and results in better smears for direct fluorescent antibody staining. Infected cells, required for the detection of chlamydiae by cell culture techniques, are also increased in number in samples collected following removal of excess cervical mucus. Concomitant culture of the cervix and the urethra with subsequent specimen pooling increases the culture positivity rate substantially at minimal added expense.

Specimens submitted for diagnosis of chlamydial infection include scrapings or swabs from the conjunctivae, urethra, cervix, and rectum, bubo pus, sputa, throat washings, and tissue. Because epithelial cells, as opposed to mucus or pus, must be collected, vigorous rubbing of the swab against the involved site is required for optimal specimen acquisition. When collecting eye specimens, the eyelid should be everted and the swab rolled directly over the surface of the conjunctivae. In cases of urethritis in the male, the swab should be inserted 3 to 5 cm into the urethra and withdrawn using a rotating motion. In cases of cervicitis in the female, the endocervical specimen should always be collected from the squamocolumnar junction.

Deep posterior nasopharyngeal specimens are required for the diagnosis of chlamydial respiratory tract infection. Techniques used for the collection of samples for the detection of *Bordetella pertussis* are appropriate for this purpose. In suspected cases of lymphogranuloma venereum, pus from an affected lymph node should be apsirated with a syringe needle following insertion through apparently healthy tissue rather than directly into the bubo. Infected fluctuant nodes usually contain frank pus. If none is aspirated, sterile nonbacteriostatic saline should be injected into the node and drawn back into the same syringe in an attempt to collect material for diagnostic testing. Collection of specimens in cases of proctitis or lower gastrointestinal tract infection is best accomplished using direct anoscopic visualization of the suspected sites, optimally from ulcerative or hypertrophic lesions. Isolation of chlamydiae from the upper genital tract represents the only valid technique for documenting *C. trachomatis* involvement in cases of endometritis and acute salpingitis. Optimal gynecologic techniques for the collection of clinical specimens include laparoscopically directed fallopian tube biopsy or needle aspiration and/or guarded endometrial biopsy or washing (28).

No single transport medium has yet been accepted as optimal for the recovery of *C. trachomatis* from clinical specimens. Although labile at temperatures above 6°C, the organism is relatively stable at refrigeration temperatures. A single freeze-thaw cycle results in at least a 1-log loss in infectivity. If a specimen requires storage for less than 72 hours, it is therefore recommended that the sample be maintained at 4 to 6° rather than be frozen. Some laboratorians, however, recommend that all specimens be frozen at less than or equal to −70°C until processing. Two commonly employed transport media are a sucrose-phosphate-glutamate medium and a cell culture medium supplemented with 10% fetal bovine serum. Most chlamydial infections occur in body sites normally colonized with bacterial flora. As a result, specimens collected for the isolation of *C. trachomatis* must usually be treated with antibiotics prior to cell culture inoculation. Antibiotics without chlamydial activity but active against the organisms commonly encountered at the collection site are usually incorporated into the transport medium itself. Aminoglycosides such as gentamicin, uniformly inactive against chlamydiae, have proven to be particularly useful for this purpose. Formulations commonly include vancomycin (100 μg/ml) and gentamicin (10 μg/ml) as antibacterial agents and nystatin (25 to 50 μg/ml) or amphotericin B (2.5 to 4.0 μg/ml) to suppress the growth of yeasts. Tetracyclines, erythromycins, and penicillins should not be used because they interfere with chlamydial isolation procedures. Specimens such as homogenized tissue, semen, and bubo aspirates should be diluted 1:10 and 1:100 in cell culture medium prior to shell vial

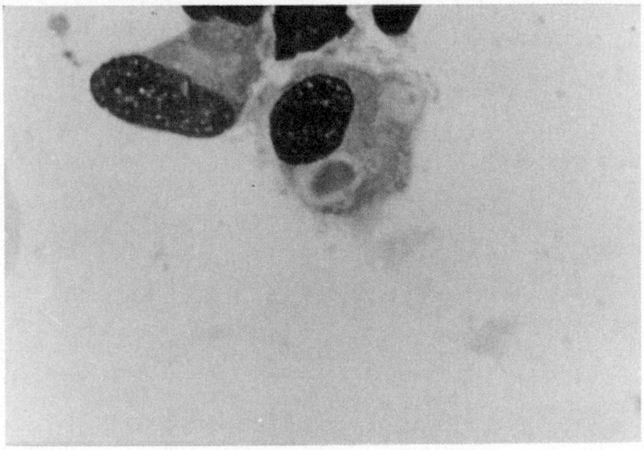

Figure 46.1. Giemsa-stained chlamydial inclusion in cell scraping from a case of neonatal conjunctivitis.

inoculation because they are often toxic to cells in culture.

Direct Microscopy

An adequate specimen for cytologic examination should include at least 1000 epithelial cells spread evenly over the surface of the slide such that the cells can be examined individually. Although historically the Giemsa stain proved useful for the detection of chlamydial inclusions, the technique is no longer recommended for routine diagnosis of *C. trachomatis* infection because direct fluorescent antibody and culture systems have proven to be significantly more sensitive. The Giemsa-stained smear may still represent the diagnostic technique of choice in cases of inclusion conjunctivitis of the neonate when large numbers of infected inclusion- containing cells can usually be detected in a rapid and cost-effective manner (Fig. 46.1).

Direct visualization of chlamydial elementary bodies using fluorescein-conjugated monoclonal antibodies on urethral, endocervical, conjunctival, and rectal specimens and in respiratory tract or nasopharyngeal aspirates from infants with pneumonitis has proven to be a rapid and sensitive technique for the diagnosis of *C. trachomatis* infection. This technique obviates the need for transport media, and fixed slides are stable for up to 1 week at either room or refrigeration temperature. Although relatively time-consuming in the laboratory, the method is especially useful in low-volume settings and when specimens must be transported from distant collection sites prior to testing. A distinct advantage of direct fluorescent antibody testing over antigen detection and culture techniques is the capability to evaluate the adequacy of the specimen during slide examination. Cuboidal columnar epithelial cells attest to the fact that the sample was collected properly, whereas excessive cervical mucus and/or a preponderance of squamous epithelial cells indicate inadequate site preparation or specimen collection. Murine monoclonal antibodies directed against the major outer membrane proteins (MOMP) of all 15 known human serovars of *C. trachomatis* and in both forms of the organism (the infectious elementary body and the replicating, metabolically active reticulate body) are generally felt to be superior to antibody preparations specific for chlamydial lipopolysaccharide (LPS) because the fluorescence is more intense with MOMP preparations. Bacteria other than chlamydiae, however, may sometimes stain with anti-MOMP antibodies either through nonspecific immunoglobulin binding or from cross-reactivity with shared epitopes. This phenomenon is frequently observed with rectal specimens, possibly because of the large numbers of bacteria normally present in such specimens or resulting from cross-reacting antigens in *Peptostreptococcus productus* (29). In specimens from other body sites, cross-reacting bacterial species are less common and can reliably be differentiated from fluorescing elementary bodies on a morphologic basis. Because common epitopes exist between chlamydial and other Gram-negative bacterial lipopolysaccharides, direct fluorescent antibody reagents directed against chlamydial LPS have the potential for cross-reactivity with bacterial species. This would not be expected with antibody preparations directed against the chlamydial MOMP.

A high-quality fluorescence microscope is essential for proper examination of clinical specimens using direct fluorescent antibody (DFA) techniques. Differences in optical alignment, illumination power, and filter quality and wavelength will result in significant variability in the fluorescent intensity of elementary bodies. To control for these variables, known positive and negative specimens should be run routinely along with patient tests to substantiate satisfactory reagent and microscope performance. Slides are typically scanned under 400× total magnifiication, and suspicious structures are confirmed using a 1000× oil immersion objective. The sensitivity of DFA methods when compared with culture is a function of the sensitivity of the comparative cell culture technique, the patient population examined, and the number of elementary bodies required for interpretation of a smear as positive. The sensitivity of DFA techniques in studies of female cervical specimens has reportedly range from 70 to 100%, whereas the specificity typically exceeds 95% for both men and women. In studies that have employed a third technique to resolve discrepant results between DFA and culture methodologies for the diagnosis of chlamydial infection in women, false-negative cultures have been reported for endocervical specimens. The DFA test appears to be more sensitive for the detection of elementary bodies in female endocervical samples than in male urethral specimens (approximately 70%), probably because of the discomfort associated with specimen collection. Because lower numbers of elementary bodies are typically observed in urethral samples than in endocervical specimens, the number required for the interpretation of a test as positive may have to be lowered for urethral specimens to achieve adequate test sensitivity.

Culture Techniques

The McCoy cell, a heteroploid mouse cell of uncertain origin, is the cell line most frequently used for the isolation of chlamydiae from clinical specimens. Although a number of other cell lines have proven satisfactory for this purpose, extensive research has been done, and all standard procedures have been developed using this line. Regardless of the cell line used, the most critical step in enhancing chlamydial replication is increased contact between the infectious elementary bodies and the cell monolayer. This can be accomplished mechanically (centrifugation) or by changing the surface charge of the cell (treating with DEAE-dextran). Cell irradiation or treatment with an antimetabolite (5-iodo-2-deoxyuridine, cytochalasin B, or cycloheximide) further enhances chlamydial replication. Specimen centrifugation onto cycloheximide-treated McCoy cell monolayers, either on coverslips in 1-dram shell vials or in microtiter wells, at this time, represents the method of choice for the culture of chlamydiae.

To process the specimen for cell culture inoculation, all cell-containing fluid should be expressed from the swab into the transport medium container, the swab discarded, and the specimen vortexed in a centrifuge tube containing glass beads. Coarse debris may be removed from the specimen by centrifuging at a low speed for a brief period of time. Cell monolayers should then be challenged with the clinical specimen by centrifuging at 2500 to 3000*g* (centrifugation of microtiter plates is limited to approximately 1500*g*) for 1 hour at 30° to 35°C. Controlled temperature centrifuges assist in maintaining a constant acceptable temperature during this centrifugation process. The clinical inoculum should be removed after a 1- to 2-hour incubation period (immediately following centrifugation for specimens likely to be toxic to the McCoy cells), and fresh medium containing 1 μg/ml of cycloheximide should then be added.

Cells should then be incubated at 35° to 37°C in air with 5% CO_2 (CO_2 is unnecessary for stoppered vials) and stained to detect chlamydial inclusions at times appropriate for the staining system employed.

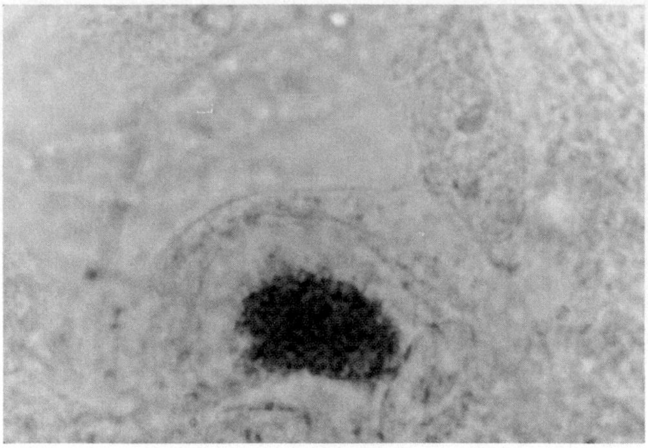

Figure 46.2. Iodine-stained *Chlamydia trachomatis* inclusion in infected MyCoy cell culture.

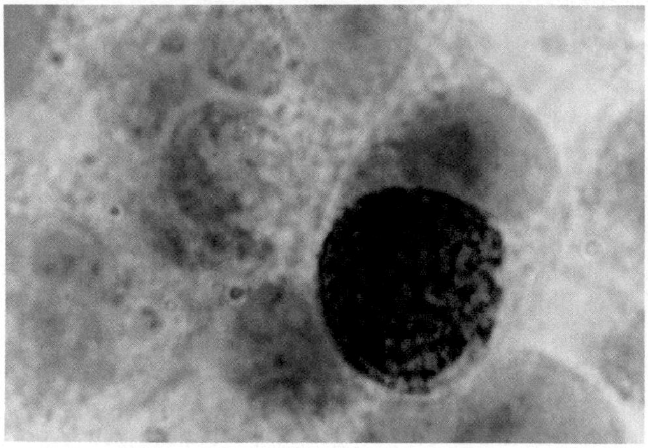

Figure 46.3. Immunoperoxidase-stained chlamydial inclusion in infected McCoy cell culture.

Cells should be methanol-fixed prior to staining. The optimal culture incubation time for both the Giemsa and the iodine (Fig. 46.2) staining techniques is from 60 to 72 hours, when glycogen concentrations are at a maximum. Immunofluorescent and immunoperoxidase (Fig. 46.3) procedures are capable of detecting chlamydial inclusions as early as 18 hours after cell culture challenge, but cultures inoculated in duplicate are typically incubated and stained after 24 hours' and after 48 hours' incubation. Immunoperoxidase and immunofluorescent staining techniques also appear to be more sensitive than the iodine stain and result in increased isolation rates, but are more expensive to perform and require more attention to staining.

The use of 96-well microdilution plates for the isolation of chlamydiae affords considerable cost savings both for media and plastic disposables and expedites the simultaneous processing of multiple specimens. Two possible problems with this technique are the potential for cross-contamination due to the proximity of the microtiter wells and the possibility that the decreased cell surface may result in lower isolation rates. Equivalent isolation rates are seen with vials and microtiter plates when specimens are collected from symptomatic individuals. When asymptomatic populations are screened, however, shell vials are clearly superior. Blind passage is required in this setting for maximal recovery rates (approximately 25% of asymptomatic individuals and 10% of symptomatic persons will be positive only when specimens are tested by this technique), and subculture from microtiter wells is considerably more difficult and less efficient than from shell vials. To accomplish the passage, an inoculated cell culture incubated for 72 to 96 hours should be homogenized and the suspended cells used to challenge a second cell monolayer.

Enzyme-linked Immunoassays

Screening tests based on enzyme-linked immunosorbent assay (EIA) technology were introduced shortly after the commercial availability of DFA tests. The first EIA kit commercially available was Chlamydiazyme (Abbott Diagnostics, North Chicago, Illinois). The performance of this assay has been evaluated by a number of investigators (30–36). Most studies have found Chlamydiazyme to be highly useful in the screening of both symptomatic and asymptomatic women in high- and moderate-risk groups. The assay appears, however, to suffer a lack of sensitivity for screening women in low-risk populations. Likewise, the assay is satisfactory for screening symptomatic males for chlamydial infection but demonstrates relatively low positive and negative predictive values when asymptomatic men are tested (37). Since considerable discomfort is associated with specimen collection in men, the assay may also prove useful for the screening of male urine specimens to establish the diagnosis of chlamydial infection. In a multicenter study, this procedure showed an 87.2% sensitivity and 98.9% specificity compared to urethral swabs tested by cell culture. When screening female urine specimens, however, the current assay appears to lack specificity.

Although the number of published studies examining the performance of other EIA tests is limited, results similar to those reported for Chlamydiazyme have, for the most part, been observed. Investigators have also generally found EIA to perform in a satisfactory manner when testing ocular specimens, but limited data suggest that EIA may not perform as well when examining specimens from the respiratory tract (38, 39). Studies have also shown that false-positive results occur when testing clinical specimens for chlamydiae using EIA tests, particularly with samples from the lower gastrointestinal tract. As a result, commercially available EIA kits are not currently approved for the testing of rectal specimens.

Other available techniques include filtration EIA procedures. In these assays, chlamydiae are trapped in nitrocellulose membranes and detected using monoclonal antibodies directed against the chlamydial LPS using a radiometric or colorimetric antibody detection technique. These tests may offer increased sensitivity over earlier assays and clearly decrease the time required to test an individual specimen. Relatively inexpensive, these procedures also lend themselves to rapid nonbatch testing of multiple specimens as they are received into the laboratory.

Nucleic Acid Probes

Because of the inherent high degree of specificity with nucleic acid probes, these techniques are actively being investigated and developed as tools for the detection of chlamydiae in clinical specimens. Problems observed in early studies were a function of the relatively low amounts of ribosomal ribonucleic acid (rRNA) present in chlamydial elementary bodies and the small number of organisms typically present in many clinical specimens. Although early studies indicated that chlamydial probes lacked the sensitivity required for diagnostic reagents (40, 41), more recent work suggests that, with appropriate modifications, these tests may be as sensitive as culture (42). A commercially produced kit (PACE; Gen-Probe, San Diego, CA) utilizing a chemiluminescent probe complementary to chlamydial rRNA is reported to be somewhat less sensitive than either culture or Chlamydiazyme (43), but additional studies are necessary before a valid conclusion can be drawn regarding the clinical utility of this particular assay. Although technically less demanding than in the earlier stages of development, nucleic acid probes are still relatively expensive, and their usefulness in the clinical setting for the diagnosis of chlamydial infection remains to be determined.

Serology

Serologic techniques are infrequently used to diagnose chlamydial genital tract infection. Although most individuals with documented chlamydial infection have detactable antibodies to *C. trachomatis,* there also appears to be a high prevalence of antibody positivity in uninfected individuals in sexually active populations. This is because chlamydial genital and respiratory tract infection is common, and antibodies to chlamydiae persist following the resolution of infection. In addition, considering the chronic nature of the disease, it is often difficult to demonstrate a diagnostic fourfold rise in antibody titer in persons with active infection.

Skin tests for the diagnosis of LGV, however, have been available since 1938 (44). Originally, skin test antigen was prepared from sterilized bubo or genital exudate material collected from individuals with LGV. The widespread application of the "Frei test" became possible when it was found that large quantities of LGV antigen could be prepared in the yolk sac of developing chick embryos (45). Because the test lacks acceptable sensitivity and specificity (46), serologic techniques have, for the most part, supplanted it. A single titer of 256 or higher by complement fixation is generally considered diagnostic of infection with LGV. This technique lacks sensitivity for diagnosing other infections caused by *C. trachomatis.*

The microimmunofluorescence test (MIF) for the detection of antibodies to chlamydiae was developed in the early 1970s. It is highly reliable in detecting IgG-class antibodies in individuals previously infected with chlamydiae, and, as a result, has proven useful for epidemiologic investigations examining rates of infection with *C. trachomatis* (47, 48). The MIF test also detects IgM antibodies in women with primary chlamydial genital tract infection with a high degree of sensitivity. Its primary use, however, has been in the clinical diagnosis of chlamydial pneumonitis in neonates. Detection of antichlamydial IgM has been shown to be a highly sensitive and specific method for diagnosing this syndrome. The MIF test may be the method of choice for establishing this diagnosis. Although the MIF test primarily detects serotype-specific antibody, chlamydial genus reactivity can be measured if reticulate body antigen is incorporated into the test reagent (49).

Whole inclusion immunoperoxidase and immunofluorescent tests represent additional techniques for the detection of antibodies to chlamydiae. Since lipopolysaccharaide is found in high concentrations in chlamydial inclusions, whole inclusion antibody testing measures reactivity with chlamydial genus antigens. Likewise, ELISA tests utilizing broadly cross-reactive elementary or reticulate body antigen from LGV serotypes usually detect genus antibodies. Although sensitive, both test types appear to detect cross-reacting *C. pneumoniae* antibodies, thus limiting their utility for the diagnosis of infection with *C. trachomatis.* ELISA techniques have also been used to detect IgM-class antibodies to diagnose neonatal chlamydial pneumonia. Elevated IgM titers are seen in infants with chlamydial pneumonia, but not in infants with chlamydial conjunctivitis who are often colonized in their upper airways with *C. trachomatis.* Detection of IgM antibodies may, therefore, represent a more specific means of diagnosing this syndrome than culture or antigen detection.

INTERPRETATION OF LABORATORY RESULTS

Most currently available laboratory tests for the diagnosis of *C. trachomatis* infection are relatively expensive and labor-intensive. The frequency of *C. trachomatis* infection in the population mandates that reliable diagnostic testing be generally available. The U.S. Centers for Disease Control and Prevention (CDCP) recommended in 1985 that symptomatic individuals at high risk for sexually transmitted chlamydial infection be treated with appropriate antibiotics empirically (18). This approach is both cost-effective and rational in clinical settings serving high-risk populations for patients willing to acquiesce to treatment for an unproven infection. Nonculture techniques for the diagnosis of *C. trachomatis* infection are generally highly sensitive but lack specificity, particularly in low-risk populations. As a result, until proven otherwise, positive screening tests in low-risk patients with nonspecific symptoms should be confirmed with more specific tests, such as culture, before initiation of antimicrobial therapy.

Specific test selection for the diagnosis of infection with *C. trachomatis* is usually based on cost, public health, and laboratory expertise factors. Culture techniques are generally considered cost-effective for the diagnosis of chlamydial infection in high-risk women presenting to STD clinics, whereas empiric antibiotic therapy appears to be more cost-effective for men in the same setting (50). In populations with chlamydial cervical infection prevalences from 2 to 7%, antigen detection tests have proven cost-effective for screening purposes (51, 52).

Because of the limitations of all of the current testing techniques, the selection of specific test methods for the diagnosis of chlamydial infection by the laboratory should take into account the test cost, the projected number of tests to be performed, personnel requirements, potential problems with specimen transport, and the patient population to be examined. Cell culture techniques are 100% specific, allow for characterization of isolated strains, and are applicable to all types of clinical specimens. They currently represent the methods of choice when unequivocal specificity is required by the diagnosing clinician. Demanding somewhat less technical expertise, antigen detection procedures, by comparison, offer the advantages of ease of specimen transport, decreased hazard to the laboratory worker, and are generally less labor-intensive. DFA, ELISA, and culture methodologies appear to be fairly comparable in terms of sensitivity. The lower specificities of direct antigen detection tests in low-risk populations generally preclude their use for screening purposes in such settings. Considerable social stigma is still attached to the presence of sexually transmitted disease. To minimize the emotional cost associated with a report of a positive result, clinicians should communicate to their patients the predictive value of a positive test with the specific technique employed by the laboratory.

THERAPEUTIC CONSIDERATIONS

Sulfonamides, erythromycin, rifampin, and tetracyclines are all highly active in vitro against *C. trachomatis*. In cases of inclusion conjunctivitis, topical therapy with tetracycline or sulfonamide for 2 to 3 weeks will often suppress signs of infection but will not necessarily eradicate the infecting agent from the nasopharynx or conjunctiva. This is of particular import in infants at risk for the development of chlamydial pneumonia. *C. trachomatis* colonization of the conjunctivae has been shown to persist for up to 40 weeks and nasopharyngeal carriage up to 18 months or more in the face of topical therapy. Therefore, systemic treatment of neonatal inclusion conjunctivitis with erythromycin, or, in older infants, with sulfonamides is indicated to eradicate the ocular infection as well as to prevent pneumonia. Systemic therapy with a tetracycline is recommended for adult disease. In chronic trachoma, therapy is more difficult. Extended treatment with doxycycline appears to be the most effective regimen. Surgical correction of trachoma-associated lid deformities reduces the incidence of blindness.

The best approach to the prevention of neonatal chlamydial infection is prenatal diagnosis and treatment of infected parents. Ocular prophylaxis with silver nitrate does not prevent the establishment of chlamydial infection in the infant, whereas prophylaxis with erythromycin appears to be at least somewhat effective. It does not, however, decrease the overall acquisition of *C. trachomatis* (53) and is ineffective if application to the infant's eyes is delayed.

The recommended antimicrobial agent for the treatment of LGV is tetracycline. Alternative regimens include courses of erythromycin, doxycycline, or sulfamethoxazole. All of these regimens rapidly improve constitutional symptoms, but have little impact in the duration of healing buboes (54). Late complications are not generally affected by antibiotic therapy. Surgical intervention is often required to repair strictures and fistulas and to address elephantiasis.

The most effective agents for the treatment of genital tract infection with *C. trachomatis* are the tetracyclines. Although relatively resistant chlamydial strains have been described, erythromycins have generally been shown to be efficacious for therapy of genital infections caused by *C. trachomatis*, and represent the alternative drugs of choice (18). No such resistance has been reported to the tetracyclines. Chloramphenicol, rifampin, and oral ampicillins (administered in high doses) and the newer fluoroquinolones such as ofloxacin have all been reported to be effective for treatment of infection with *C. trachomatis* (55–57), but they are not recommended as first-line agents for chlamydial infection. Optimal treatment during pregnancy for *C. trachomatis* infection has not been established. A regimen of erythromycin (stearate, base or ethylsuccinate; not estolate) or azithromycin is probably the best approach.

With the exception of the neo-azalide compound azithromycin, single-dose therapy with any antibiotic does not reliably eradicate *C. trachomatis* from genital tract sites. Therapy for an extended period of time, at least 10 days, is recommended for complicated infections. All attempts to treat pelvic inflammatory disease on an outpatient basis should include intramuscular injection of a third-generation cephalosporin (such as cefotaxime or ceftriaxone) to provide coverage for *N. gonorrhoeae* as well as tetracycline for chlamydiae. The fluoroquinolones as a group have significant activity against gonococci and some, especially ofloxacin, are highly active against *C. trachomatis*. Further clinical trials will help define the role of these agents for the treatment of chlamydial genital tract infections.

Chlamydia psittaci

Psittacosis (parrot fever, ornithosis) is a zoonotic disease primarily infecting birds that is accidentally transmitted to man. First described in psittacine birds (parrots and parakeets), *C. psittaci* has been shown to infect most avian species as well as many nonprimate mammals, causing varying degrees of illness. In Switzerland in 1879, Ritter described several human cases of unusual pneumonia associated with tropical bird exposure. Morange named the disease (from the Greek word for parrot, *psiittakos*) following an outbreak in 1894 in which he attributed the source of the disease to parrots. Meyer chronicled outbreaks in several countries from 1929 to 1930 following large-scale importation of infected South American parrots to the U.S. and Europe (58). During the investigation of an outbreak at the London Zoo in 1930, Bedson isolated the causative agent from avian and human tissues. Rivers and his associates explained that the probable route of transmission to man was via the upper respiratory tract following inhalation of dried excreta from birds shedding the agent. During ecologic studies on infection in Australian wild birds, Burnet proved that fledglings acquired the infection in the nest from asymptomatic parents. Between 1965 and 1980, from 40 to 160 human cases were reported annually in the U.S. (59) with a 1 to 5% mortality rate.

PATHOGENESIS AND SPECTRUM OF DISEASE

In man, following inhalation into the respiratory tract, *C. psittaci* migrates to the reticuloendothelial cells of the spleen and liver, where it replicates intracellularly, resulting in chlamydia-laden macrophages. Invasion of the lung and other organs then follows by hematogenous seeding. This two-step process explains the relatively long incubation period (from 7 to 15 days or longer) observed in this disease. A predominantly lymphocytic inflammatory response occurs in both the alveolar and interstitial spaces of the lungs, particularly in the dependent lobes. This results in alveolar wall thickening, edema, and sometimes necrosis. Small hemorrhages may occur, accounting for the hemoptysis sometimes seen clinically. Mucus plugging of the brochioles contributes to the dyspnea and cyanosis often observed in severe disease. The epithelial lining of the bronchial tree typically remains intact. Liver, spleen, and hilar node enlargement may occur, and focal splenic and hepatic necrosis can result. In fatal cases, meningeal, pericardial, brain and adrenal changes have been noted upon histologic examination of tissues collected at autopsy.

Although the lung is the organ most prominently involved, *C. psittaci* causes a systemic illness in man. The course of clinical disease, however, varies widely. The infection generally manifests itself with sudden onset of chills and high fever (38° to 40.5°C), but may present insidiously with slowly increasing malaise and fever over a 2- to 4-day period. Severe headache is often the patient's major complaint. Arthralgias and painful myalgias (especially in the back of the neck), anorexia, and malaise are other common symptoms. A pale macular rash (Horder spots) has been described. Jaundice is noted only in very severe cases.

A persistent dry hacking cough, which can appear at any time during the course of infection, is a prominent feature of the disease. Small amounts of mucoid, occasionally blood-streaked sputum may be produced. Gastrointestinal symptoms are experienced by only a minority of patients and, when present, include diarrhea, nausea, vomiting, and abdominal bloating. Other uncommon complaints include epistaxis and mild sore throat. Changes in mental status, associated with hypoxia, may be observed toward the end of the first week of illness and occasionally progress to lethargy, delirium, and even coma.

EPIDEMIOLOGY

Virtually any species of bird can serve as a host to *C. psittaci*. As a result, psittacosis is truly a cosmopolitan disease. Although psittacine birds remain the major reservoir for human infection, cases associated with exposure to infected ducks, cockatiels, sparrows, canaries, pigeons, and occasionally, various mammalian species have all been reported. Many cases in recent years have occurred in persons processing carcasses of domestic fowl, especially turkeys (60). Usually a sporadic disease, approximately one-half of all cases occur in pet bird owners. The disease is considered an occupational hazard for pet shop employees, zoo workers, veterinarians, and others who capture or raise psittacine birds for sale and profit.

A dramatic drop in the incidence of cases of psittacosis in the United States has been noted over the past few decades. Factors contributing to this decline include the use of tetracycline-containing poultry feed and the federal requirement that all commerically imported psittacine birds be treated for 30 days with antichlamydial drugs prior to transport into the country. Although antibiotics do not totally eradicate the agent from infected birds, they greatly reduce the transmission rate of the organism. Imported and domestic birds are often housed together or in close proximity in commercial settings. Since birds rapidly become infectious under stressful and crowded conditions, the potential for the spread of the organism in such settings always remains a real possibility.

C. psittaci is found in relatively high titer in the excreta, feathers, blood, and tissues (particularly the kidneys, spleen, and liver) of infected birds. Although birds can show signs of overt illness and die from infection, more frequently they demonstrate only minor symptoms such as lethargy, diarrhea, failure to feed, and ruffled feathers. This often results in close contact with the owner investigating the cause for the bird's altered behavior. Asymptomatic birds and those that have recovered from illness often continue to shed the organism for several months.

The agent can survive in dried bird excreta for long periods of time, and aerosolization of such contaminated materials with subsequent inhalation usually results in human infection. Bird bites, mouth-to-beak intimate contact, and manipulation of contaminated tissues and feathers have also led to infection. Prolonged, close contact with infected birds is not required for acquisition of the organism. Well-documented cases in which individuals have had only momentary contact with potentially contaminated environments have been reported. This may explain why approximately 20% of cases have no known route of exposure. No documented cases exist from ingestion or handling of dressed, eviscerated poultry.

Several reported instances of direct person-to-person transmission, primarily involving hospital personnel, have been recorded. Disease in these cases has reportedly been more severe than that following exposure to infected avians. The reasons for these observations are speculative, but include theoretical alterations in strain virulence following human passage and a dose effect.

DIAGNOSTIC PROCEDURES

Culture

Although the diagnosis of psittacosis can be confirmed by isolation of the organism, attempts to isolate *C. psittaci* from clinical or animal specimens may be hazardous to laboratory personnel, and such procedures should be offered only by facilities with specialized training in the handling of the etiologic agent under laboratory conditions. Strains of *C. psittaci* can be successfully recovered from experimental laboratory animals following challenge with clinical materials, but cell culture and embryonated egg techniques are probably more sensitive for primary isolation of these agents. Several cell lines have been used to cultivate *C. psittaci*. L cells efficiently support the growth of the agent, most strains forming cytopathic plaques that result in additional cycles of chlamydial replication, and eventually infecting the entire monolayer. Specific identification can be made by staining infected cells with commercially available genus-specific immunofluorescent antibody reagents. *C. trachomatis* can be differentiated from *C. psittaci* with species-specific immunofluorescent antibody preparations or based on the failure of *C. psittaci* intracellular inclusions to stain with iodine.

Serology

Because of the high titers of complement-fixing antibody produced in cases of psittacosis, complemented fixation tests are widely used by public health laboratories to confirm the diagnosis of the disease. Although a single titer of 32 or higher is consistent with a presumptive diagnosis of psittacosis, a fourfold rise in titer between acute and convalescent serum specimens collected a minimum of 3 weeks apart is interpreted as definitive evidence of *C. psittaci* infection. Antibody titers generally rise by the second week of illness. Antimicrobial therapy inititated early in the disease can delay or diminish production of complement-fixing antibodies and, as a result, decrease the sensitivity of the test (61). Technically demanding, the accuracy of the complement fixation test is highly dependent upon the quality of available test antigen. Unfortunately, satisfactory reagents are not always available commercially. Because *C. psittaci* is a common cause of inclusion conjunctivitis in guinea pig colonies, all lots of guinea pig-derived complement must be carefully tested for the presence of interfering chlamydial antibody before being placed in service (62).

INTERPRETATION OF LABORATORY RESULTS

Routine laboratory tests are usually of little value in establishing diagnosis of psittacosis. White blood cell counts typically fall within the normal range, although an unremarkable leukocytosis or leukopenia may be observed. Occasionally, patients become anemic during the course of the disease. During acute stages of the illness, protein may be detectable in the urine. Despite the fact that hepatomegaly is common, results of liver function tests are usually within normal limits. Analysis of cerebrospinal fluid is unrewarding. Microscopic examination of a Gram-stained smear reveals few bacteria and occasional white cells.

The diagnosis, therefore, is usually dependent upon the results of serologic testing. False-positive rises in antibody are rare, but have been reported in some patients with legionellosis. Although infrequently necessary, clinical specimens may be shipped, upon approval of the state public health laboratory, to the CDCP for attempts to isolate the agent.

THERAPEUTIC CONSIDERATIONS

The tetracyclines are extremely effective agents for the treatment of psittacosis. Following initiation of antimicrobial therapy, clinical improvement can usually be observed within 48 to 72 hours. Relapses, however, are common unless treatment continues for 10 days to 2 weeks after defervescence. Case fatality rates ranged from 20 to 40% in the preantibiotic era, but today the prognosis is good with appropriate therapy. All suspected cases should be reported promptly to public health authorities.

Chlamydia pneumoniae

SPECTRUM OF DISEASE

C. pneumoniae was originally designated the TWAR agent, a name constructed by combining the laboratory identifiers from the first two isolates, TW-183 and AR-39. It has been shown to cause both upper and lower respiratory tract infections including pneumonia. Initially considered a strain of *C. psittaci*, the agent has been shown to be distinct from other chlamydiae by restriction endonuclease and DNA-

DNA hybridization analyses (63). Unlike *C. psittaci*, where human infection usually follows exposure to infected birds, *C. pneumoniae* is transmitted from human to human. The organism generally causes a mild self-limited pneumonia in teenagers and young adults. Early symptoms including pharyngitis, with or without laryngitis, may represent the only clinical evidence of infection. Other individuals may develop bronchitis, which in turn may further progress to a pneumonia lacking any distinguishing clinical or roentgenographic characteristics. The organism is increasingly being recognized as a cause of serious respiratory infection in persons with AIDS (64) and in other immunocompromised individuals. Fever, cough, and sore throat are the most common symptoms. Young individuals with mild pneumonia typically fail to show abnormalities in white blood cell counts or leukocyte differentials. In older adults with other chronic illnesses, disease is often more severe and may result in hospitalization. Such patients are more apt to show a leukocytosis. The erythrocyte sedimentation rate is typically elevated. Some patients have a biphasic illness where an initial episode of pharyngitis and laryngitis resolves spontaneously, but is followed in 2 to 3 weeks by bronchitis and pneumonia. Although the first isolate of *C. pneumoniae* was recovered from a conjunctival specimen, no further association with ophthalmic infection has been reported. One study has reported increased levels of antibody to *C. pneumoniae* with seroconversion in patients with acute myocardial infarction and chronic coronary heart disease, when compared with healthy controls, suggesting that the organism might be a factor in the pathogenesis of cardiovascular disease (65).

EPIDEMIOLOGY

Unlike *C. psittaci*, no avian or other animal reservoirs have been identified for *C. pneumoniae*. Human-to-human transmission appears to be the only significant mechanism for spread of the agent. Although the mode of transmission has not been specifically identified, it is presumed to be via a respiratory route. *C. pneumoniae* does not appear to be sexually transmitted (66). Antibody prevalence is generally low during the childhood years, rising rapidly in teenagers. In adults, the prevalence of *C. pneumoniae* antibodies reportedly ranges from 25 to 50%. Antibody persistance in the elderly suggests repeated infection with resulting periodic boosts in titer. The prevalence of antibody is reportedly higher in males than in females. In several outbreaks among military recruits, boarding school students, and in the general population, retrospective serologic studies have demonstrated that *C. pneumoniae* was the cause of pneumonia. Prospective studies have since incriminated *C. pneumoniae* in similar outbreaks among college students. One recent investigation indicated that *C. pneumoniae* was an important cause of hospital-acquired pneumonia in intubated patients having undergone some type of surgical procedure (67). Reported outbreaks have occurred throughout the world during all seasons of the year.

DIAGNOSTIC PROCEDURES

Culture

HeLa-229 cells are more susceptible to infection with *C. pneumoniae* than the McCoy cells utilized in most laboratories for the isolation of other species of chlamydia. Multiple cell passage may be required to successfully recover the organism. Egg cultivation, however, may be required for the isolation of the agent from some specimens. If HeLa-229 cells are used for the isolation of *C. pneumoniae*, pretreatment of the monolayers with diethylaminoethyl-dextran increases the susceptibility of the cells to infection.

Serology

Two patterns of antibody response to *C. pneumoniae* are seen. During primary infection, complement-fixing antibodies appear early, followed in 10 days to a month by IgM antibodies measurable by microimmunofluorescence techniques. Typically, IgG-class antibodies are not detected until 6 to 8 weeks after onset of illness. In the second pattern, attributed to reinfection, complement-fixing antibody is not detectable, and IgM antibody occurs in low titer or cannot be detected at all. A rapid anamnestic IgG antibody response occurs upon reinfection. Whole inclusion immunofluorescent testing and ELISA tests utilizing broadly cross-reactive LGV antigen appear to be of limited value because of cross-reactivity with *C. trachomatis*.

THERAPEUTIC CONSIDERATIONS

Few comparative antibiotic trials have been conducted to determine clinical efficacy in the treatment of *C. pneumoniae* infection. In vitro, clarithromycin has been reported to be more active on a weight basis than other macrolides, tetracyclines, and ciprofloxacin. Limited clinical experience suggests that eryhthromycin may be inadequate for the treatment of serious infection, resulting in prolonged symptoms or relapse. Based on clinical experience in other types of chlamydial infections, tetracyclines currently appear to represent the drugs of choice.

MYCOPLASMA

Mycoplasmas, the smallest organisms capable of self-replication, were first isolated by Roux and Nocard from cattle with contagious bovine pleuropneumonia in 1898. Subsequent isolates from other sources were termed pleuropenumonia-like organisms. Members of the class *Mollicutes* (Latin: *mollis,* soft; *cutis,* skin), they are characterized by the absence of a cell wall and are, therefore, refractory to treatment with β-lactam class antibiotics. All mycoplasmas require lipids and lipid precursors for plasma membrane synthesis. Like viruses, they pass through filters that retain bacteria but, except for cell wall, possess all other cellular constituents of bacteria. Unlike cell wall-deficient bacteria (L forms), they fail to revert to bacteria when cultured under appropriate conditions.

Microbiology and Taxonomy

Despite superficial cultural similarities, the mycoplasmas comprise a heterogenous group of microorganisms differing from each other in DNA composition, metabolic reactions, nutritional requirements, antigenic composition, and host species specificity. The differentiating characteristics of the various human mycoplasmas are outlined in Table 46.3. They are divided into three taxonomic families: The *Mycoplasmataceae* and *Spiroplasmataceae* (both requiring cholesterol for growth), and the non-cholesterol-dependent *Acholeplasmataceae.* Included in the family *Mycoplasmataceae* are the *Mycoplasma* species which do not hydrolyze urea, and the genus *Ureaplasma,* strains of which produce abundant quantities of urease. There are 51 recognized species in the genus *Mycoplasma* and two, *Ureaplasma urealyticum* and *Ureaplasma diversum,* in the genus *Ureaplasma.* Ten *Mycoplasma* species have been detected in the clinical laboratory. *Mycoplasma pneumoniae* is the cause of primary atypical pneumonia. *Mycoplasma salivarium* and *Mycoplasma orale* are common inhabitants of the oropharynx, particularly in individuals with poor oral hygiene, whereas *Mycoplasma buccale, Mycoplasma faucium, Mycoplasma primatum,* and *Mycoplasma lipophilum* are less frequent oropharyngeal colonizers. *Mycoplasma fermentans* is a rare isolate from genital tract and oropharyngeal specimens. *Mycoplasma hominis,* generally considered a genital tract mycoplasma, can also cause infection at other body sites. *Mycoplasma genitalium,* which may cause some cases of nonspecific urethritis, and *U. urealyticum* are also isolated from genital tract specimens. An additional, probably pathogenic, mycoplasma has recently been identified and is tentatively termed *Mycoplasma incognitus* (68).

Mycoplasmas are ubiquitous in nature as saprophytes and/or parasites of plants and animals. Several plant and animal diseases are caused by mycoplasmas, and many have served as models for evaluating the role of mycoplasmas in human disease. *Mycoplasma* species also cause contamination of cell cultures used for research and diagnostic purposes, interfering with their metabolic processes and slowing their rate of growth. The spiroplasmas that infect insects and plants have a helical structure, whereas most other mycoplasmas are spherical. The morphology of individual organisms, however, varies based on differences in growth conditions and the stage of the cell cycle. Some mycoplasmas form branching filaments 0.3 to 0.4 μm in diameter and up to 1500 μm long, which divide to form new spherical bodies. Most mycoplasmas are facultative anaerobes. Strains isolated from cattle and sheep rumen that grow only under strict anaerobiosis, however, are termed anaeroplasmas. Most mycoplasmas divide by binary fission. The genomes of ureaplasmas and mycoplasmas approximate 500 kd, whereas those of the acholeplasmas and the spiroplasmas are about 1000 kd. The morphology of four species of mycoplasmas, *M. pneumoniae, M. genitalium, M. pulmonis,* and *M. gallisepticum,* is characterized by specialized structures at one or both poles of the organisms. *M. genitalium* and *M. pneumoniae* have a tapered, filamentous tip containing a dense, central rod-like core. Specialized structures have also been observed in strains of *M. pulmonis,* and pear-shaped polar blebs have been reported in *M. gallisepticum.* These structures may assist the organisms in attachment to the respiratory or genital mucosa, as they usually represent the points of intimate contact by the mycoplasmas with the membranes of the host cells. They may also be involved in locomotion because these four mycoplasmas demonstrate a gliding motility in which the organisms move tip first.

Mycoplasmal cells do not Gram stain, but may be stained, albeit poorly, with a Giemsa technique. Because of their plasticity, mycoplasmas all have a tendency to grow down into solid media. This may result in the production of colonies with a characteristic "fried egg" appearance (an opaque central zone of growth in the agar surrounded by a translucent peripheral surface zone). These "typical" colonies, however, do not always develop. Colonial morphology is a function of the medium constituents and degree of hydration, and atmospheric conditions. Mycoplasma colonies vary in size from 50 to 600 μm and consequently are best visualized through a clear medium with a dissecting microscope. On primary isolation, colonies of *M. pneumoniae* typically appear mulberry-like without translucent peripheral growth, although larger colonies with the characteristic zone

Table 46.3. Characteristics of Human Mycoplasmas

Species	Frequency of Isolation	Usual Site of Isolation	Nature of Disease	Metabolic Activity			Optimum pH	Growth-Enhanced in Gaseous Environment			Days to Detection of Colonial Growth
				Arginine	Urea	Glucose		Aerobic	Anaerobic	CO_2	
M. orale	Frequent	Oropharynx	Unknown	+	0	0	7.0	+	+ +	LD[a]	3–10
M. salivarium	Frequent	Oropharynx	Unknown	+	0	0	6.0–7.0	+	+ +	+	2–5
M. buccale	Rare	Oropharynx	Unknown	+	0	0	7.0	+	+ +	LD	3–10
M. faucium	Rare	Oropharynx	Unknown	+	0	0	7.0	+	+ +	LD	3–10
M. lipophilium	Rare	Oropharynx	Unknown	+	0	0	7.3	LD	LD	LD	LD
Acholeplasma laidlawii	Extremely rare	Oropharynx	Unknown	0	0	+	6.0–8.0	+ +	+ +	+ +	1–5
M. fermantans	Infrequent	Genitourinary tract	Unknown	+	0	+	7.3	+	+ +	LD	3–20
M. primatum	Rare	Genitourinary tract	Unknown	+	0	0	LD	LD	LD	LD	LD
M. genitalium	Rare	Genitourinary tract	Nongonococcal urethritis	0	0	+	7.3	LD	0	+ +	slow
M. hominis	Frequent	Genitourinary tract	Septicemia, abscesses, arthritis, endometritis, other reproductive disorders	+	0	0	5.5–8.0	+ +	+ +	+ +	1–4
Ureaplasma urealyticum	Frequent	Genitourinary tract	Nongonococcal urethritis, arthritis, other reproductive disorders	0	+	0	5.5–6.5	+ +	+ +	+ +	1–4
M. pneumoniae	Frequent	Oropharnyx, respiratory tract	Tracheobronchitis, pneumonia	0	0	+	6.5–7.5	+ +	0	+ +	3–20

[a]LD—limited data

of peripheral growth do sometimes develop. Ureaplasmas usually produce small colonies (15 to 30 μm in diameter), but on media buffered to pH 6.0, colonies up to 300 μm in size often develop. Because of the tiny colonies characteristically produced in culture, ureaplasmas were originally designated T strains or T mycoplasmas.

Mycoplasmas are highly fastidious organisms, requiring enriched media, typically containing peptones, yeast extract (supplying preformed nucleotide precursors), and animal sera (10 to 20%). The serum provides a complex of lipoprotein and cholesterol, which is incorporated into the lipid membrane of sterol-requiring mycoplasmas. Because acholeplasmas synthesize saturated long-chained fatty acids and carotenoids, which substitute for cholesterol in the plasma membrane, they have no need for exogenous cholesterol. Multiplication rates for mycoplasmas are generally lower than those for bacteria, ranging from as short as 1 hour to as long as 6 to 9 hours *(M. pneumoniae).* The microbial yield from broth cultures is low (1 to 20 mg of protein/liter). Cells are best visualized in broth culture using phase-contrast or dark-field microscopy. *Mycoplasma* species usually utilize either glucose or arginine as a major energy source, although some strains are capable of using both. The carbohydrate-metabolizing species break down glucose by glycolytic pathways, mainly to lactic acid. In most mycoplasmas, the respiratory pathways are flavin-terminated, and heme compounds, catalase, and cytochromes are therefore absent. Species that metabolize arginine use a three-enzyme system to convert it to ammonia via ornithine, the process providing the organism with ATP. By comparison, the ureaplasmas utilize neither glucose nor arginine, but convert urea to ammonia by means of urease, although their requirement for urea as an energy source has not been proven.

Mycoplasma pneumoniae

SPECTRUM OF DISEASE

M. pneumoniae (once termed the Eaton agent) is a human pathogen that primarily causes acute respiratory disease including pneumonia. Tracheobronchitis is the most common clinical syndrome resulting from *M. pneumoniae* infection. The organism also accounts for as much as 10% of radiographically proven pneumonia. Serious disease is seen principally in older children and young adults, whereas milder disease typically occurs in infants and young children. Although it occurs sporadically in all seasons and in epidemics, lasting months to years, some reports indicate that infection is more common in the fall and winter months. Following exposure, the incubation period to illness is approximately 3 weeks, with the majority of cases occurring within 15 to 25 days. Onset of disease is typically insidious, and constitutional symptoms including headache, fever, and malaise are usually noted 2 to 4 days before disease localization. Pneumonia, pharyngitis, and tracheobronchitis are all clearly caused by infection with this organism. A variety of complications associated with these syndromes have also been described. It has been further suggested that even in the absence of respiratory disease, some cases of otitis media, erythema multiforme and other skin diseases, pericarditis and myocarditis, and neurological disease may result from *M. pneumoniae* infection. Clinical manifestations attributed to *M. pneumoniae* infection are outlined in Table 46.4.

Although in cases of tracheobronchitis, tracheitis with frequent bouts of paroxysmal coughing and substernal pain may be conspicuous, basic bronchitis with frequent cough is more commonly noted. Respiratory illness in infants or older children accompanied by wheezing suggest the presence of bronchiolitis. Diagnosis is complicated by the high proportion of tracheobronchitis cases caused by viral agents. Bronchitic patients tend to have fewer and milder systemic symptoms, a shorter duration of cough and fever, and a lower frequency of high-titered serum cold agglutinins than patients with pneumonia. Complications described following pneumonia with *M. pneumoniae* are also seen in cases of tracheobronchitis, but appear to occur at a lower frequency.

Pharyngitis often accompanies lower respiratory tract infection with *M. pneumoniae,* but it may be the predominant symptom in the disease (69). In such cases, the onset is usually insidious with headache and fever, but sore throat appears early and becomes the chief complaint. Coryza and cough may also be present. The posterior pharynx is usually diffusely erythematous, and tonsillar and pharyngeal exudates may be observed. Tender anterior cervical nodes are usually noted. A clinical diagnosis of pharyngitis due to *M. pneumoniae* is not possible because symptoms are usually indistinguishable from those caused by bacterial and viral agents. Likewise, isolation of the organism from respiratory secretions in such cases does not necessarily establish *M. pneumoniae* as the cause of the pharyngitis. Two recent pediatric studies have shown that *M. pneumoniae* may be isolated as frequently from asymptomatic children as from those with pharyngitis and that a rise in antibody titer only rarely correlates with organism isolation and/or clinical pharyngitis (70, 71). Rhinitis is reported to be the major clinical finding in children less than 1 year of age with *M. pneumoniae* infection. Isolated cases of bullous myringitis, with

Table 46.4. Clinical Illness Attributed to *Mycoplasma pneumoniae* Infection

Primary Illness			Complications	
Definite Causation	Possible Association	Reported Association	Definite or Probable Association	Reported
Pneumonia	Otitis media	Arthritis	Pleural effusion	Pleuritis
Tracheobronchitis	Myringitis	Pancreatitis	Atelectasis	Pneumatocele
Bronchiolitis	Erythema multiforme (major and minor)	Fever of unknown origin	Respiratory insufficiency	Lung abscess
Pharingitis	Myocarditis		Relapse	Bronchiectasis
Rhinitis	Pericarditis		Sinusitis	Bronchiolitis obliterans
	Meningoencephalitis		Otitis media	Bacterial superinfection
	Neuritis		Myringitis	Cavitary disease
	Meningitis		Maculopapular rash	Nephritis
			Vesicular rash	Hepatitis
			Urticaria	Pancreatitis
			Erythema nodosum	IgA nephropathy
			Erythema multiforme	Pediatric nephrotic syndrome
			Intravascular erythrocytic hemolysis	Thrombocytopenic purpura
			Intravascular coagulation	Pelger-Huet anomaly
			Raynaud's syndrome	Hemophagocytosis
			Myocarditis	Transverse myelitis
			Pericarditis	Leukencephalitis
			Arthritis	Optic neuritis
			Meningoencephalitis	Cerebrovascular accident
			Neuritis	Hearing loss
			Meningitis	Polymyositis
			Cerebellar ataxia	Pediatric benign myositis
			Changes in mentation	

associated severe ear pain, may result as a complication of *M. pneumoniae* respiratory tract infection, but the previously held theory that most isolated cases of bullous myringitis are caused by this organism is probably invalid.

Lower respiratory illness caused by *M. pneumoniae*, once called "walking pneumonia," is usually mild. Hospitalization generally is not required; only about 2% of children and 10% of adults with *M. pneumoniae* illness are admitted to hospitals. Prodromal headache is more common in teenagers and adults than in children. Before cough appears, headache, fever, and malaise increase in severity over a 2- to 4-day period. A cough (nonproductive) then becomes the major manifestation of illness, and its absence makes the diagnosis of *M. pneumoniae* infection unlikely. Diffuse or substernal soreness in the chest that increases on inspiration is common. Frank pleuritic pain, however, is rare. Mild sore throat, laryngitis, coryza, and earache may be seen. Fever is sustained unless altered by antipyretics, and maximum temperature may reach 104°F, but is typically less than 102°F. Frank shaking chills are uncommon. Tender anterior cervical nodes are often reported. Muscle tenderness is common, and nausea, vomiting, anorexia, and arthralgias may occur. Skin rash is seen in approximately 15% of cases a few days after onset. Usually maculopapular in nature, it may also be vesicular or bullous. Clinically inapparent sinusitis is common.

Although the course of pneumonia is variable, recovery is the rule. Death has been reported, but is rare. In untreated cases, fever lasts from 2 days to 2 weeks. Slow progressive symptomatic improvement is typical. Cough, malaise, and radiographic abnormalities frequently persist for 2 to 6 weeks. The most common complications of *M. pneumoniae* infection are pulmonary in nature. Extensive lung involvement with lobar consolidation may result in respiratory insufficiency. In mild cases, significant pleural effusion and transient atelectasis may occur. In patients with sickle cell disease, severe illness with significant pleural effusion is common.

Clinical relapse occurs within 2 to 3 weeks of the initial illness in approximately 10% of all cases and may be accompanied by a radiographically confirmed infiltrate in the lung segment initially involved or in another segment of the same or opposite lung. Residual pleural abnormality and subsequent pneumatocele development, lung abscess, cavitation, bronchiolitis obliterans, secondary bacterial infection, and bronchiectasis have all been reported following pneumonia caused by *M. pneumoniae*, although the role of the organism in these sequelae is unclear. Myringitis may be seen, and secondary bacterial ear infections in children are not uncommon.

Illness caused by *M. pneumoniae* may be complicated by urticaria, erythema nodosum, or more commonly by erythema multiforme or Stevens-Johnson syndrome. Erythema multiforme major may be primarily caused by *M. pneumoniae* and, although a history of preceding illness usually exists, it can occur in the absence of associated respiratory disease. The organism has been cultured from vesicular fluid of these patients. Significant intravascular hemolysis can occur in association with high-titer cold agglutinins, but clinically inapparent hemolysis is probably more common. In patients with clinical hemolysis titers in excess of 1:500 are typically seen and hemagglutinins are also usually demonstrable at 37°C. Intravascular hemolysis usually occurs late in the illness and may coincide with return of the body temperature to normal. Other occasionally reported hematologic complications include Raynaud's phenomenon and disseminated intravascular coagulation.

Neurological complications of *M. pneumoniae* infection have been reported in up to 10% of hospitalized patients (72, 73). The most commonly described syndromes are meningitis, encephalitis, meningoencephalitis, and mono- or polyneuritis. Less commonly reported complications include cerebrovascular accident, "toxic" psychosis, cerebellar ataxia, transverse myelitis, and several types of mononeuropathy including cranial nerve palsy, phrenic nerve paralysis, and sudden deafness. *M. pneumoniae* has been reported to be the possible cause of up to 6 to 8% of all cases of aseptic meningitis (74) and many cases of meningitis, neuritis, and meningoencephalitis attributed to *M. pneumoniae* are not associated with antecedent respiratory illness. Although the course of such infections has not been well characterized, residual neurological deficits and death have been described, and isolation of *M. pneumoniae* from the cerebrospinal fluid has been accomplished. In cases of meningitis and meningoencephalitis, various types of leukocytic CSF responses have been observed, but mononuclear cells usually predominate. The CSF protein level is usually elevated, and the glucose concentration is normal or low.

Reported cardiac complications range from clinically inapparent changes in electrocardiograms to significant peri- and myocarditis with prominent pericardial effusion. Marked arthralgia is common, but overt arthritis is rare. Other reported complications include juvenile benign myositis, polymyositis, hepatitis, thrombocytopenic purpura, hemophagocytosis, Pelger-Huët abnormalities, pancreatitis, nephritis, IgA nephropathy, and nephrotic syndrome in children (75).

EPIDEMIOLOGY

M. pneumoniae is a cosmopolitan cause of respiratory disease, but epidemics have been best documented in temperate climates. In large urban areas, the organism is endemic, and infection and disease occur year-round. During the summer months, it may cause up to 50% of all pneumonias. Some evidence suggests that epidemics occur at 4- to 8-year intervals both in military and civilian populations and, during such periods, disease is most prevalent in the late summer and early fall months. Typical epidemics start in the fall, are slow in onset, and may persist in the community for as long as 2 years. Infection during epidemic periods is three to five times more frequent than in nonepidemic years, with overt disease being most common in older children and young adults. Smaller outbreaks, however, can be observed at any time. The proportion of all pneumonias attributable to *M. pneumoniae* varies with the population studied. Frequencies have ranged from 4% in an indigent civilian population to 44% in a population of military personnel. In a large community study in Seattle, Washington, approximately 15% of all documented pneumonias were attributed to *M. pneumoniae* (76). This is probably representative of communities throughout the developed world. The relatively mild nature of typical *M. pneumoniae* infection is underscored by the fact that less than 5% of resultant pneumonia cases are severe enough to require hospitalization.

M. pneumoniae infection rates are highest in school-age children and young adults. It is the most common etiologic agent of pneumonia in children 5 to 15 years of age. In the Seattle survey, this organism was responsible for 30 to 60% of all pneumonias in the 5- to 20-year-old age group. Although pneumonia attributable to *M. pneumoniae* is less common in adults, it remains a significant pulmonary pathogen throughout life. In addition, *M. pneumoniae* is reported to be the most common cause of tracheobronchitis and lower respiratory disease, with wheezing in children 5 to 15 years of age (77). Pneumonia appears to be somewhat more common and illness more severe in young males than in young females. Higher infection rates are seen, however, in women 30 to 39 years old than in men of comparable age, probably reflecting increased exposure to school-aged children. Although data are somewhat conflicting, both day care center and family studies have shown that symptomatic *M. pneumoniae* infection is also common in children less than 5 years of age, although the disease is typically mild (78–80). Despite common complaints of coryza and wheezing, most children with *M. pneumoniae* infection remain afebrile.

M. pneumoniae transmission between school-aged children is frequently followed by introduction into and slow but extensive spread within families. The limiting factor determining whether an exposed family member will acquire the organism appears to be immunity resulting from previous infection. Transmission in institutionalized and school populations is generally slow, requiring close contact with an infected individual. Spread between playmates appears to be more efficient than among classmates in a schoolroom setting. High transmission rates have also been observed in college populations and in military recruits where close contact in dormitories and barracks appears to play an important role (81–84). Transmission by individuals with asymptomatic infection has not been documented. Because of the evidently low communicability, the requirement for close contact for efficient transmission, and the relatively long incubation period, the spread of *M. pneumoniae* in the community is slow, and infections appear endemic in nature. Epidemics, however, have occurred, and point-source outbreaks lacking characteristics of prolonged close contact have been reported, implying that small-particle aerosol transmission may occur. Risk of clinical disease from *M. pneumoniae* infection is low among children less than 5 years of age, high for those in the 5 to 20-year-old range, and, again, lower among adults over 20 years of age. When it occurs, though, illness is usually more severe in middle-aged and elderly individuals.

DIAGNOSTIC PROCEDURES

Specimen Selection/Collection

M. pneumoniae infects the entire respiratory tract and, as a result, may be isolated from throat swabs or washings, nasopharyngeal swabs, tracheal aspirates, lung biopsies, and sputum. Since the organisms attach to epithelial cells of the respiratory mucosa, specimens should contain cellular material for optimal yield. *M. pneumoniae* has, on rare occasions, also been isolated from nonrespiratory sites including blood, cerebrospinal fluid, and internal abdominal organs. Because the natural course of infection lasts for 6 to 8 weeks, the collection time is not critical. Patients typically present to a physician only after being symptomatic for several days to a week. Antibiotics often eradicate *M. pneumoniae* slowly, so the organism can often be recovered from clinical specimens during therapy, but specimen collection prior to initiation of antimicrobial therapy should be accomplished whenever possible. Because *M. pneumoniae* is relatively fastidious and very susceptible to drying, direct specimen inoculation onto growth media as soon as possible after acquisition of the specimen is strongly encouraged. Vials of liquid SP-4 medium or trypticase soy broth with 0.5% bovine albumin may be inoculated at the patient's bedside with swab specimens and transported expeditously to the laboratory at room temperature. Antibiotics, such as penicillin, are usually incorporated in transport media to suppress bacterial overgrowth. Sputum, throat washings and other liquid specimens, and tissue samples can be transported to the microbiology laboratory in sterile leak-resistant containers, preferably on ice, for processing. If delay in processing (more than 24 hours) is anticipated, specimens should be frozen at $-70°C$ or below. Organisms survive indefinitely under these storage conditions. Likewise, if specimens are to be transported over long distances, shipment on dry ice is recommended. Containers placed on dry ice should be tightly sealed to prevent absorption of CO_2 by specimens. Short-term storage of specimens at $-20°C$ is acceptable, but longer-term storage at this temperature (more than a few weeks), results in loss of *M. pneumoniae* viability. Provided the medium contains protein, mycoplasmas are unique in their ability to withstand repeated episodes of freezing and thawing.

Currently, there are no useful staining techniques for the direct microscopic detection of *M. pneumoniae* in clinical specimens. Although mycoplasmas grown in culture appear Gram-negative, individual organisms are too small and take up safranin too poorly to be detected on microscopic examination of Gram-stained clinical specimens. As a result, laboratory diagnosis of mycoplasmal infection usually depends upon recovery of the organism in culture, detection of its presence using genetic probes, or on the results of serologic assays. An indirect immunofluorescent method that demonstrates mycoplasma-specific antigen associated with epithelial cells in sputum has, however, been described (85). *M. pneumoniae* can also be detected in sputum samples using electron microscopic methods. Characteristic filamentous shaped organisms can be observed attached to epithelial cell membranes by specialized terminal organelles (86).

Culture Techniques

Media for the isolation of mycoplasmas usually contain a base of soybean or beef protein supplemented with serum (10 to 20%) as a source of mandatory sterols and yeast extract to provide peptides and other growth factors including preformed nucleic acid precursors. Because *M. pneumoniae* replicates more slowly than most bacteria and many fungi commonly encountered in clinical specimens, antimicrobial agents are generally added to make the media selective, preventing overgrowth by more rapidly growing microorganisms. Exploiting the fact that mycoplasmas lack the cell walls characteristic of most bacteria and are therefore intrinsically resistant to cell wall active agents, β-lactam antibiotics such as penicillin and polymyxins (typically active against most Gram-negative species) are commonly employed for the inhibition of contaminating bacteria. Thallium acetate is also sometimes used to inhibit the growth of contaminating bacteria. Because it interferes with the growth of *U. urealyticum* and *M. genitalium,* it should be avoided when attempting to isolate these species. Care should be taken when handling this compound because it is also toxic to humans. Likewise, the addition of antifungal agents such as amphotericin B (1:2000) is useful in preventing overgrowth by contaminating yeasts. Methylene blue is also sometimes utilized as a medium supplement to inhibit other species of mycoplasma.

Careful quality control of all media components is essential for optimal mycoplasma recovery rates. Some lots of yeast extract fail to provide essential growth factors. A high-quality yeast extract can be easily prepared using techniques described by Kenny (87). Some lots of horse serum contain antibodies that inhibit *M. pneumoniae* replication. Use of γ-globulin-free horse serum prevents this problem, but "agamma" sera are generally less effective than whole sera in supporting the replication of mycoplasmas. Many commercial lots of sera are essentially dialyzed and, therefore, lack bicarbonate. Although this results in a more favorable pH for the growth of *M. pneumoniae,* these sera are otherwise deficient in factors promoting the organism's replication. Because some lots have been shown to be contaminated with animal strains of mycoplasmas, horse and other sera for use in culture media should only be purchased from vendors testing for their presence and guaranteeing their sterility.

Because the *Mycoplasmatales* represent a heterogeneous group of organisms, no single medium will provide optimal conditions to accomplish the isolation of all species. As outlined in Table 46.2, media with different pHs are necessary. A pH of 6.0 is required by *U. urealyticum* for optimal replication, and little growth is observed above pH 7.0. By contrast, most other species grow well in media with a 7.0 pH. *M. pneumoniae* is the most pH-tolerant species, growing in media with a pH range from 5.5 to 8.0. For pH to be monitored visually, inclusion in the medium of a pH indicator, such as phenol red, is recommended. The incubation atmosphere is also an important growth factor. *M. genitalium* and *M. pneumoniae,* both obligate aerobes, are stimulated by atmospheric CO_2. Growth stimulation by atmospheric CO_2 may actually be a function of pH change in the bicarbonate-containing medium. *M. salivarium, M. orale, M. buccale,* and *M. faucium* grow best under anaerobic conditions and grow poorly on H agar aerobically. *M. fermentans, U. urealyticum,* and *M. hominis* appear to be minimally affected by incubation atmosphere.

Quality control testing should be performed on all prepared media to demonstrate that optimal growth of mycoplasmas can be achieved. For this purpose, it is highly recommended that laboratories use *recent* clinical isolates of all species being sought in culture. Stock strains adapted to culture conditions often grow readily on media that fail to support the growth of organisms from clinical specimens. Artifacts are also a major problem in the detection of mycoplasmas in clinical materials because debris and host cells can resemble fried-egg colonies. It is therefore imperative that all laboratories prove that observed colonies represent transferable entities with specific properties before issuing a report indicating that a mycoplasma has been isolated from a clinical specimen. Some lots of serum induce the formation of pseudocolonies, whorls of magnesium and calcium soap crystals appearing on the surface of agar plates. Although transferable, these crystals can be differentiated from true colonies of mycoplasmas because they fail to produce metabolic products.

To isolate *M. pneumoniae,* a 0.1-ml volume of transport medium in which a swab has been extracted should be simultaneously inoculated onto a solid medium, such as H agar or SP-4 medium, and into a biphasic broth medium. A combination of both SP-4 (88) and a biphasic system (89) appears to be the most sensitive currently available approach for the recovery of *M. pneumoniae.* Isolation of the agent is best accomplished from sputum or tracheal aspirate, but nasopharyngeal and oropharyngeal swab specimens also often prove fruitful. Body fluids, sputa, and disrupted tissue specimens should be diluted 1:10 and 1:100 before media inoculation to lower the concentration of inhibitory substances commonly found in tissue samples. Agar plates should be incubated aerobically at 35° to 37°C in a sealed container and examined for the presence of characteristic colonies with a stereoscopic microscope under oblique light at 20× to 40× total magnification after 2, 10, 15, and 21 days' incubation. This provides the best working distance and resolution for observation of colonies on an agar surface through the bottom of an unopened plate. This rapid technique prevents contamination of the media surface with microorganisms, including mycoplasmas, during the multiple-plate examinations. Biphasic cultures should be observed for a pH decrease as indicated by a color change of the phenol red indicator from red to yellow-green due to acid production by *M. pneumoniae* resulting from glucose fermentation. They should also be examined microscopically by viewing the broth through the side of the container for the presence of spherules, fluid medium colonies appearing as early as 5 days after medium inoculation. *M. pneumoniae* does not produce turbidity in liquid me-demonstrate a significant rise in antibody titer. Reportedly, the best antigen preparation is a chloroform-methanol extract of whole organisms containing a glyceroglycolipid hapten (96). These *M. pneumoniae* lipid antigens are a mixture of relatively simple glycolipids widely distributed in nature (detected in human cardiac muscle, brain tissue, certain streptococci, and even in some leafy vegetables). These antigens have also been shown to cross-react with those of *M. genitalium*, a cause of urethritis. The potential for false-positive results is, therefore, a concern with these assays, and problems have in fact been demonstrated. Patients with documented bacterial meningitis have been reported to manifest clearly false-positive, yet significant antibody increases to *M. pneumoniae* antigens (97) and false-positives are also known to occur in some cases of acute pancreatitis. Reports based on CF tests that implicate *M. pneumoniae* in various neurological syndromes must, therefore, be interpreted with caution as they may be the result of these cross-reacting antibodies. Although such serologic overlap may be seen, the diseases for which a serologic diagnosis might be attempted are dissimilar. Thus, except in the unlikely event of concomitant infection with two cross-reacting agents, confusion in the interpretation of serologic results should be uncommon.

The metabolic inhibition test, reportedly more sensitive than CF, measures the ability of the patient's serum to inhibit growth of *M. pneumoniae*. Antibiotics in the patient's blood, however, may result in false-positive results. The test requires experience in mycoplasma culture techniques and, as a result, is not generally available. Likewise, immunofluorescent staining of infected chick embryo lung tissue is both sensitive and specific, but technically difficult and not available in laboratories outside of a research setting. Both immunofluorescent and ELISA techniques, comparable in sensitivity and specificity to CF assays, offer the advantage of permitting separate detection of IgG and IgM class antibodies. ELISA techniques using solubilized whole organisms and unfractionated extracts lack sensitivity because the active components are represented in such small quantities in the antigenic mixture that they are undetectable. By comparison, the use of purified adhesion P1 protein in ELISA system appears to offer acceptable levels of sensitivity while increasing the specificity of the test significantly over techniques using whole lysed *M. pneumoniae* organisms.

Interpretation of Diagnostic Test Results

Roentgenographic chest examination typically reveals a unilateral segmental lower lobe bronchopneumonia. Multilobe involvement, however, is not unusual, and lobar consolidation may be observed. Although small pleural effusions are noted in approximately 25% of cases, significant pleural effusion is rare. Peripheral white blood cell counts are typically within normal range, but counts greater than $10{,}000/mm^3$ are seen in approximately 25% of cases of bronchopneumonia, and counts greater than $15{,}000/mm^3$ may be reported. Leukocyte differentials usually demonstrate 60 to 85% polymorphonuclear leukocytes with occasional bands. Erythrocyte sedimentation rates are typically strikingly elevated. Gram-stained sputum specimens usually reveal large numbers of leukocytes, but no predominant bacterium. Usual upper respiratory flora is generally reported on sputum culture. Standard blood cultures are negative. Urinalyses are likewise typically reported as within normal limits except for the occasional detection of albuminuria, usually attributed to fever. Some patients develop antinuclear antibodies.

In the setting of a compatible clinical syndrome, isolation of *M. pneumoniae* in culture or detection of the agent using a nucleic acid probe from a respiratory tract specimen should be considered diagnostic. The organism is not usually a member of the normal respiratory tract microflora. Because carriage of *M. pneumoniae* can often be demonstrated for 6 to 8 weeks after recovery from illness, the potential for confusion does exist in cases of subsequent but unrelated illness. Since asymptomatic infections are fairly common, detection of the organism during an illness caused by another agent might likewise confound the diagnosis. Under optimal conditions, only 85% of patients demonstrating a four-fold rise in antibody titer to *M. pneumoniae* are typically culture-positive. The precise value of a negative probe or culture, therefore, is not known. Some combination of culture, nucleic acid probe, and serology would be expected to result in the fewest missed diagnoses.

Therapeutic Considerations

M. pneumoniae is susceptible in vitro to many broad-spectrum antimicrobial agents including tetracyclines, erythromycins, chloramphenicol and the aminoglycosides but are resistant to inhibitors of cell wall syntheseis such as the β-lactams, because they lack typical bacterial cell walls. Although in vitro susceptibility testing of *M. pneumoniae* is usually not performed and standardized procedures for such testing have not been developed, erythromycin-resistant strains have been reported. Untreated, illness caused by *M. pneumoniae* typically resolves in 2 to 3 weeks, but symptoms resolve more rapidly with appropriate antimicrobial therapy. Antibiotics effective in the treatment of pneumonia caused by *M. pneumoniae* include tetracycline and its analogues as well as erythromycin. In controlled clinical trials, both have been shown to shorten the duration of clinical symptoms and to accelerate the clearing of infiltrates observed on chest roentgenographs. Because tetracyclines result in discoloration of teeth in children, the finding that standard doses of erythromycin diffuse well into respiratory secretions and result in higher blood levels than tetracyclines, and because the organism is more sensitive in vitro, erythromycins are considered by many clinicians to be the drugs of choice for the treatment of *M. pneumoniae* pneumonia. The two antimicrobial agents have, however, proven comparable in clinical trials. Whereas tetracyclines have the advantage of proven efficacy against some other organisms associated with "atypical" pneumonia including *C. psittaci, Coxiella burnetii,* and *C. pneumoniae,* erythromycins have proven effective in the treatment of Legionnaire's disease. Clinical failures with tetracyclines that have responded to erythromycin and clinical resistance to erythromycin responding to tetracyclines have both been reported. With these factors in mind, a 2- to 3-week course of therapy with either agent is recommended for treatment of *M. pneumoniae* pneumonia. Despite in vitro susceptibility, clindamycin does not appear to be clinically effective. Use of other therapeutic modalities including antitussives, antipyretics, assisted ventilation, and oxygen therapy should be based on assessment of individual patient needs. Because illness is clinically indistinguishable from that caused by any number of viruses, routine treatment of individuals with pharyngitis and tracheobronchitis is not recommended unless a specific diagnosis has been made based on laboratory findings. If, however, prolonged illness is observed and *M. pneumoniae* has been established as the etiologic agent, either tetracycline or erythromycin therapy may be indicated. Because antibiotic-treated individuals continue to harbor organisms in the posterior pharynx for up to 2 to 3 months, antimicrobial therapy does not appear to decrease transmission rates to close contacts.

No method has proven uniformly effective in preventing infection and disease with *M. pneumoniae.* As a result, patients should probably be isolated, and attempts should be made in home settings to discourage close contact with infected individuals. One study in exposed family members examined the chemoprophylactic use of oxytetracycline for 10 days for prevention of subsequent cases of disease. A significantly lower illness rate was reported in those receiving treatment, but no difference in infection rates was demonstrable between treatment and placebo groups (98). These results suggest that this approach is ineffective in preventing the establishment of colonization with *M. pneumoniae* in such settings. It may have some role in the prevention of clinical illness, however. Alternatively, because antibiotics were given early during the incubation period of the disease, such therapy may have actually constituted early treatment. Further studies are needed to determine whether such an approach may prove useful in a wider setting.

Vaccine trials using both live attenuated and killed organisms have failed to result in protection rates greater than 30 to 50%, despite significant antibody responses in recipients to vaccine antigens. Because symptoms in the disease appear to be mediated by the immune response and because immunity is short-lived, research into the use of live vaccines for the prevention of serious *M. pneumoniae* disease has slowed. Research continues, however, on the potential use of purified subunit materials, such as the adhesin protein that mediates attachment to cell membranes, for vaccine purposes.

Mycoplasma hominis and *Ureaplasma urealyticum*

SPECTRUM OF DISEASE

Mycoplasma hominis

M. hominis colonizes both the genitourinary tract (20 to 40% of women and a smaller percentage of adult males) and, occasionally, the oropharynx. It has, however, been reported in infections following facial and transpharyngeal oral surgery (99) and in cases of exudative pharyngitis (100–102). In addition, it has been isolated sometimes in pure culture, from the upper urinary tract of patients with acute pyelonephritis. In many such infections, antibody to *M. hominis* has been demonstrable in both urine and serum. Data from several studies suggest that the organism is an infrequent cause of acute pyelonephritis and acute exacerbations of chronic pyelonephritis. Likewise, *M. hominis* is frequently recovered, when appropriate culture procedures are utilized, from tubo-ovarian and pelvic abscesses as well as from inflamed fallopian tubes. In both Swedish and British studies (103), the organism was isolated directly from the fallopian tubes of approximately 10% of women with acute salpingitis using laparoscopic techniques to collect specimens and to establish the diagnosis. In these studies, antibody was detectable in the serum of approximately 50% of patients with salpingitis compared to 10% of healthy women. Seroconversion was also demonstrable in approximately one-half of women from whom *M. hominis* was isolated from the lower genital tract. Other studies, however, have reported that women with gonococcal pelvic inflammatory disease were not more likely to demonstrate detectable serum antibodies to *M. hominis* than those result in premature delivery (126). Infants delivered vaginally are much more frequently colonized with these agents than babies delivered by cesarean section. *U. urealyticum* has been isolated from at least one body site in 30 to 62% of all infants born to women positive by cervical culture for the agent and, likewise, *M. hominis* can be recovered from 18 to 45% of babies born to women harboring the organism (127, 128). Ureaplasmas have been recovered in culture from genital specimens of approximately one-third of infant females. *M. hominis* is isolated somewhat less often from these same specimens. These organisms are recovered significantly less frequently from genital specimens of infant boys. This is probably because of the decreased exposure of their genital mucosal surfaces. The finding that genital mycoplasmas can be isolated from nose and throat cultures of approximately 15% of infants of both sexes supports this premise. Persistence of neonatal colonization with genital mycoplasmas generally ends by 2 years of age (129), although the organisms occasionally persist to puberty in young girls. In one reported study, up to 20% of prepubertal females remained colonized with *U. urealyticum* and approximately 6% with *M. hominis*. Genital mycoplasmas have only rarely been isolated from prepubertal males outside of the neonatal period. Both organisms are found considerably more often in sexually abused children (130).

DIAGNOSTIC PROCEDURES

Specimen Selection/Collection

With appropriate collection and culture techniques, genital mycoplasmas can often be recovered from the urine and from cervical, vaginal, or urethral swabs of asymptomatic individuals. *U. urealyticum* has also been isolated in pure culture from several usually noncolonized sites including (*a*) the blood of patients with low-grade temperature elevations; (*b*) lung tissue of infants with neonatal pneumonia; (*c*) prostatic secretions of patients with prostatitis; (*d*) the upper urinary tract of patients with renal calculi and upper urinary tract disease; (*e*) fluid from arthritic joints of hypogammaglobulinemic individuals; and (*f*) fetal membranes or tissues. *M. hominis* has likewise been isolated from several normally noncolonized body specimens including the blood of postpartum patients with fever, the CSF of neonates with signs and symptoms of meningitis and sepsis, surgical drainage, mediastinal and abdominal fluids, joint fluid of arthritic persons with hypogammaglobulinemia, bronchoalveolar lavage, throat swabs, abscesses, prostatic secretions, semen, and tissue specimens.

These organisms appear to represent usual flora in the female genital tract. As a result, care must be exercised when collecting samples from internal sites not to contaminate specimens with cervical, vaginal, or urethral secretions. Swabs should be suspended in a suitable transport medium (such as 0.5% albumin in 2 ml of soybean-casein digest broth containing 200 to 400 U.S. units of penicillin per milliliter). Transport media should contain both protein and a peptone to provide maximum protection to the cell wall-deficient mycoplasmas. A transport medium is not required for submission of fetal tissues and membranes, but such specimens should be maintained in a moist environment until culture inoculation can be accomplished. Although swabs with wooden shafts should not be used for specimen collection (plastic and aluminum are acceptable), the tip composition (cotton, rayon, or calcium alginate) does not appear to be a factor in the recovery of these organisms. Ideally, specimens should be transported to the laboratory without delay and inoculated to an appropriate culture system. Specimens may, however, be held up to 24 hours at 4°C without significant loss of organism viability. For longer delays, specimens should be frozen at −70°C. Successful recovery of these organisms can still be accomplished years after freezing at this temperature, provided the transport medium contains a protein additive. Urine specimens should be transported to the laboratory on ice (specimen transport devices containing boric acid preservatives are not recommended) and centrifuged at 600 × g to sediment epithelial cells and other debris. The pellet from the centrifuged urine specimen should be diluted 1:2 in transport medium prior to culture inoculation. Because urine protein concentrations are typically low, a urine sample submitted for recovery of mycoplasmas should not be frozen unless the specimen pellet is reconstituted with transport media containing a protein supplement. Body fluids, sputa, and tissues should be diluted 1:10 or 1:100 in transport media prior to culture inoculation to remove inhibitory substances. Specimen storage for more than several days at −20°C is not recommended because the organism is known to lose viability at this temperature.

Blood specimens for the isolation of genital mycoplasmas should be collected in a syringe without anticoagulant because *M. hominis* and *U. urealyticum* are inhibited to some degree by these compounds. Blood should be inoculated into an appropriate blood culture medium at the patient's bedside. Since *M. hominis* will replicate in most blood culture systems (but does not alter the appearance of the media), blood for the isolation of this organism can be inoculated directly into routine blood culture bottles, but must be subcultured blindly on a daily basis for 5 days to detect growth of the organism. Alternatively, a medium specifically formulated for isolation of *M. hominis* from blood (28) may be used. Blood should be diluted at least 1:10 in medium to prevent inhibition by factors normally present in clinical specimens. In blood cultures tested using radiometric techniques, the instrument may detect the organism's metabolism and respond with a positive growth signal (131). Although Gram stains of the media will be negative, the organism can be visualized using the acridine orange staining procedure, and the organism can be recovered upon subculture of the broth medium. No commercially available methods currently exist for the accurate direct detection of genital mycoplasmas in clinical specimens.

Culture Techniques

The four mycoplasmas commonly encountered in genital tract specimens have substantially different growth properties. *M hominis* and *U. urealyticum,* the two most important clinically, grow rapidly and can be readily isolated. *M. fermentans* and *M. genitalium* are more difficult to detect in culture. Because *M. hominis* tends to overgrow *U. urealyticum* when isolated concomitantly, separate culture systems are required for the recovery of the two organisms. Whereas *M. hominis* grows over a pH range from 6 to 8, *U. urealyticum* fails to grow at a pH greater than 7.0 and multiplies optimally in a pH range from 5.5 to 6.5. As a result, *M. hominis* can replicate in media designed for the isolation of *U. urealyticum* but the converse is not generally true. *M. hominis* is susceptible to lincomycin, whereas *U. urealyticum* is not. Thus, inclusion of 20 to 50 μg/ml of lincomycin in the medium effectively selects for *U. urealyticum.* Erythromycin has likewise been used successfully as a selective agent in media designed to recover *M. hominis.* Two media systems commonly used are U agar and U broth for the isolation of *U. urealyticum* and H agar and H broth for the recovery of *M. hominis.* Because the final pH of both H agar and H broth is greater than 7.0, they effectively select for *M. hominis.* A number of other media used successfully for isolation of these organisms have been described (132–134). Another reported effective approach for the isolation of these organisms combines A-7 agar with a modified SP-4 broth containing arginine and SP-4 broth supplemented with urea (135).

Because of the steep death phase resulting from exhaustion of urea and the elevated pH of the medium from urease activity, *U. urealyticum* presents unique problems during isolation attempts. In both broth and solid media it is essential that the culture system be properly buffered and that a sufficient, yet not excessive, quantity of urea be supplied. After a color change in broth medium, *U. urealyticum* may remain viable for as few as 12 hours, whereas colonies survive for approximately 2 days after detection on solid media. 2-(N-morpholino)ethanesulfonic acid (MES) at a pH of 6.3 is a very effective buffer for this purpose. Molar ratios of buffer to urea for broth cultures are 2:1 to 4:1. In agar, a 10:1 buffer to urea ratio can prevent inhibitory pH increases at the site of colonial growth, preventing resulting loss of organism viability. In broth systems the addition of a reducing agent, such as 1mM sodium sulfite, reduces the lag phase for many strains of *U. urealyticum.* The organism is detected in culture by its production of a readily recognizable pH change resulting from urea hydrolysis.

Of the potentially pathogenic mycoplasmas, *M. hominis* is the least fastidious. In addition to H agar and H broth, nonhemolytic colonies may be observed on many routine blood-containing bacteriologic media. The most productive are those with an enriched base such as Columbia CNA, supplemented anaerobic blood agar, and chocolate agar. Growth on standard sheep blood agar is inconsistent. On these media, *M. hominis* grows fastest under conditions of anaerobiosis and somewhat slower under hypercapneic incubation. Colonies are so small that they are usually only detectable when present in large numbers on these media and when plates are carefully examined. The organism may be observed on anaerobic plates after 48 hours' incubation, but some isolates may require 72 hours before detection is possible. Growth is typically noted 24 hours later with cultures incubated in 5% CO_2. In either environment, *M. hominis* colonies are extremely small (approximately) 0.05 mm in diameter) and may be interpreted as specimen debris or water condensation when plates are examined with the unaided eye. Debris, however, is seldom observed outside of the area of primary inoculation. Strong light assists in plate examination. Colonies may be noted only when media are examined under light at an oblique angle. Plate examination under a dissecting microscope also assists in colony recognition. Whereas *U. urealyticum* produces no discernible turbidity in broth culture, *M. hominis* can cause a faint, yet distinct haze.

For optimal isolation of both organisms, 0.1-ml aliquots of the clinical specimen should be inoculated with a loop or pipette to both agar and broth media. Both U and H agar plates should be streaked for isolation so that the plane of focus may be easily identified. Plates may be incubated at 35° to 37°C under aerobic, anaerobic, or hypercapneic conditions, provided an optimum pH is maintained in the test system. Anaerobic incubation of these media does not appear to increase recovery rates for either *M. hominis* or *U. urealyticum* per se, but such conditions may discourage the growth of aerobic bacteria and fungi. Strict anerobic conditions do appear to enhance growth of *M. fermentans* and prevent the growth of *M. genitalium*. Care should be exercised to avoid drying of agar plates under all incubation conditions. Aliquots of specimen (0.1 ml) should also be inoculated into a tube of H broth as well as a U diphasic medium system and incubated under aerobic conditions. After culture inoculation, the remaining specimen should be stored frozen at −70°C. Plates should be examined for growth after 1, 2, 3 and 4 days' incubation with a stereoscopic microscope at 40 to 60× total magnification, with the agar surface viewed through the bottom of the plate to avoid media contamination. Oblique lighting enhances colony visibility. Standard compound microscopes work poorly because of the short working distance of the lenses and poor contrast. The U broth must be examined twice daily to detect a color change indicative of mycoplasmal growth. Nearly all isolates of both *M. hominis* and *U. urealyticum* will be detected within 5 days of inoculation in broth media. Both organisms grow rapidly in broth, with doubling times from 1 to 3 hours. Cultures rapidly decline in viability after peak growth, which occurs prior to any observable pH shift. This complicates choosing an optimal time for subculture.

Aliquots from all positive broth cultures should be immediately subcultured to both a fresh U broth and a U agar plate. *U. urealyticum* colonies can be identified using a $CaCl_2$ staining technique (0.1 M $CaCl_2$ and 0.1 M urea) or with the single-reagent test of Shepard (136, 137). Upon addition of a drop of reagent to the plate, colonies of *U. urealyticum* produce a brown halo discernible under transmitted light within 1 to 5 minutes, whereas colonies of *M. hominis* demonstrate no such reaction. Positively staining transferable isolates that hydrolyze urea may be definitively reported as *U. urealyticum*. Although there are at least 14 serotypes of *U. urealyticum* (138), antisera are not commercially available at this time for further characterizing clinical isolates.

M. hominis produces relatively large colonies (200 to 300 μm in diameter) on both U and H agars, unless lincomycin is included in the medium as a selective agent. Although most large-colony isolates recovered on H agar are *M. hominis*, bacteria-producing colonies similar to *M. hominis* are sometimes recovered. *M. hominis* can be distinguished from cell-walled bacteria based on its failure to Gram stain. *M. hominis* colonies recovered on blood-containing media will stain, however, using the traditional Dienes technique. Subculture to a penicillin-containing medium, such as A-7 agar, which inhibits some bacteria, may in some case clarify whether an isolate is indeed a mycoplasma. Large-colony isolates may be presumptively identified as *M. hominis* if they are transferable entities that utilize arginine (in H broth supplemented with 50 mM arginine). A commercially available arginine broth containing penicillin, erythromycin, polymyxin, and amphotericin (Remel, Lenexa, Kansas) originally formulated for the isolation of *M. hominis* from contaminated urogenital specimens, prevents false-positive reactions that can occur if organisms being tested are arginine-utilizing bacteria other than mycoplasmas. The medium can be inoculated with a few drops of a saline suspension of growth from either the primary or the subculture plates. The inoculum can be prepared by transferring a small block of colony-bearing agar to a tube of saline and vortexing the tube vigorously. Both the inoculated tube and an uninoculated control should be incubated overnight and read for a color change from salmon to red, indicating arginine hydrolysis. A final examination of a Gram-stained smear of positive arginine broths assures that the reaction is not the result of contaminating bacteria. Isolates may be definitively identified using growth inhibition techniques similar to those described above for *M. pneumoniae*.

Colonies may be transferred with an inoculating needle, but an agar block method is generally considered more convenient. With this technique, a small piece of medium bearing the colonies is cut from the agar plate and transferred face down to the medium of choice. The block is then rubbed over the first quadrant of the plate to transfer the colonies, and the remainder of the plate is streaked in a conventional manner using a needle or loop. The inoculated medium is incubated and examined after 24 and 48 hours. Colonies should have the characteristic "fried-egg" appearance commonly associated with mycoplasmas. Upon subculture, colonies are typically larger than on primary isolation media, and, as a result, more easily detectable with the unaided eye. Attempts to isolate *Mycoplasma* and *Ureaplasma* species are, unfortunately, commonly hampered by the presence of confounding artifacts on culture media. Mammalian cellular debris may closely resemble colonies on agar plates. Debris, however, does not transfer. This represents the rationale for the requirement that all isolates suspected of being mycoplasmas be transferable entities.

Serology

Research attempts to detect antibody responses to ureaplasmal infection have generally been nonproductive. Responses have been detected, however, in about 50% of patients through the use of multiple serotypes in the metabolic inhibition test and by ELISA (139). Assays are not currently commercially available to routine clinical laboratories for detection of antibodies to either *U. urealyticum* or *M. hominis.* However, an ELISA technique that measures both IgG and IgM serum antibodies to *M. hominis* is performed by some reference laboratories (140). This assay has proven useful only when testing paired sera collected from patients with culture-documented infection. Because of the relative ubiquity of *M. hominis,* an elevated titer in a single serum specimen is difficult to interpret. An immunofluorescent technique has also been described and shows some promise for serodiagnosis of infection with these organisms, but antigens are available to date only in research settings. A microimmunofluorescent procedure has been utilized to detect antibodies to *M. genitalium* (141).

Interpretation of Laboratory Results

Interpretation of the significance of recovery of either *U. urealyticum* or *M. hominis* from a clinical specimen is sometimes difficult. Under most circumstances, isolation of *U. urealyticum* from cervical specimens has little significance because of the high colonization rate in apparently healthy women. Although reported colonization rates with *M. hominis* are somewhat lower, its recovery from cervical specimens must likewise be interpreted with caution. Isolation of either organism from usually sterile specimens and locations such as blood, amniotic fluid, fallopian tube, upper urinary tract, and other internal sites has greater significance. Recovery of *U. urealyticum* in large numbers from the urethra of a male with nongonococcal urethritis is probably significant. Cultures for other pathogenic microorganisms should be concomitantly performed on all specimens submitted for culture of these agents. Positive serologic and cultural results should be interpreted only in conjunction with other laboratory results and clinical findings.

THERAPEUTIC CONSIDERATIONS

Mycoplasmas lack a typical bacteria cell wall. They are, therefore, resistant to β-lactam class antibiotics and other inhibitors of cell wall synthesis. These organisms are, however, characteristically susceptible to many broad-spectrum antibiotics including fluoroquinolones such as ciprofloxacin and protein synthesis inhibitors such as chloramphenicol, tetracycline, and clindamycin. At clinically achievable levels, tetracycline inhibits most strains of *M. hominis* and *U. urealyticum.* By comparison, erythromycin demonstrates only moderate activity against *U. urealyticum* and lacks activity against *M. hominis.* Characteristically, both organisms are susceptible to spectinomycin, an antibiotic sometimes used for the treatment of infections caused by penicillinase-producing strains of *N. gonorrhoeae.* In part because standardized procedures are not currently available, in vitro susceptibility testing is not usually performed on clinical isolates of these organisms. Modifications of standard disc diffusion as well as broth and agar dilution methods have, however, been attempted. A broth disc test method using urine sediment as an inoculum has been developed for *U. urealyticum* (142, 143). This technique has also proven useful for susceptibility testing of *M. hominis.* The principal difference between the broth-disk test sometimes used for anaerobes and that used for mycoplasmas is the procedure utilized for determining the endpoint. Instead of examining media for the presence or absence of turbidity as a growth indicator, the procedure is scored by testing for arginine hydrolysis. An appropriate number of antimicrobial susceptibility test disks are added to tubes of arginine broth, and the medium is inoculated with several drops of a suspension of the clinical isolate. Evidence of growth inhibition is based on the failure of the indicator to change color, whereas resistance (growth) results in arginine hydrolysis with a resulting color change of the medium.

Both *C. trachomatis* and *U. urealyticum* apparently cause NGU. A 100-mg dose of a tetracycline, such as doxycycline, given twice daily for 7 days, represents standard therapy for this syndrome. About 10% of ureaplasmas are resistant to tetracyclines, however, and patients with infections caused by such strains typically fail to respond to treatment with a tetracycline. If laboratory capabilities exist, these patients should be tested for tetracycline-resistant ureaplasmas and treated with a half-gram of erythromycin four times daily for a week, as most strains of tetracycline-resistant *U. urealyticum* appear to be susceptible to this agent.

Since most strains of *M. hominis* and *C. trachomatis* are susceptible to the tetracyclines, in localities where a significant proportion of PID is nongonococcal, it is likewise advisable to treat this syndrome with a tetracycline. However, because of the emergence of tetracycline-resistant strains of *M. hominis,* other antibiotics such as clindamycin may be required for effective treatment of this disease. When cases of prolonged postabortal or postpartum fever are presumed to be caused by *M. hominis,* treatment with a tetracycline should be considered, again realizing that tetracycline-resistant strains may be involved. In other more serious illnesses in which *M. hominis* is thought to be responsible, such as arthritis in a hypogammaglobulinemic person and neonatal infections, tetracycline resistance should always be considered.

For conditions in which a mycoplasmal etiology has not been definitively established, such as spontaneous abortion, infertility, and low birth weight, examination for these organisms or specific therapy directed against them, is not, except in a research setting, currently justifiable on a routine basis, and treatment before conception does not necessarily eliminate the genital mycoplasmas for the duration of pregnancy. Likewise *M. hominis* and/or *U. urealyticum* can be cultured from approximately half of all adults with nonspecific urogenital conditions. Thus, neither ascribing these organisms a causative role in such syndromes nor prescribing specific antibiotic therapy directed against them is currently warranted.

AIDS-Associated Mycoplasma (*Mycoplasma incognitus*)

A previously unrecognized pathogenic human *mycoplasma* tentatively designated *M. incognitus* was first recognized by Lo and coworkers (144). The organism, originally identified as a virus-like infectious agent (VLIA), was initially thought to be a large DNA virus. The organism was isolated as the result of an experiment in which purified DNA derived from Kaposi's sarcoma tissues of persons with AIDS was introduced into NIH3T3 cells by transfection. Cells were monitored for transforming foci, and a transformant, designated sb_{51}, was recovered.

The agent, which passed through a 0.22-μm-pore-size filter, was subsequently shown to infect normal cells. Electron microscopic examination of infected cells demonstrated nearly spherical virus-like particles 140 to 280 nm in diameter. The agent detected in the cytoplasm, along the cell membrane, and occasionally in the nuclei of infected cells, showed minimal or no cytopathic effect. The small size of the membrane-bound intracellular particles, their capability to result in persistent cell infection, and their ability to transfect susceptible cells resulted in the conclusion that the particles were viral in nature. Southern blot analysis, however, revealed that no cross-hybridization existed with any known virus tested. Ribosomal RNA analysis, using *Escherichia coli* probes, revealed significant homology, suggesting that the VLIA particles were procaryotic in nature. Because the agent were filterable, subsequent testing with DNA from several *Mycoplasma* species was attempted. Results indicated that the particles were related to mycoplasmas.

Biochemical, antigenic, and DNA analysis demonstrated that *M. incognitus* was distinct from all other recognized human *Mycoplasma* species, but very closely related to *M. fermentans*. The organism can be grown in SP-4, a cell-free medium designed to support the growth of fastidious mycoplasmas. Antigenic cross-reactivity can also be demonstrated between the VLIA particles and *M. fermentans*. It is also similar to *M. fermentans* in that it utilizes glucose both anaerobically and aerobically, metabolizes arginine, and is susceptible to tetracycline, but resistant to erythromycin (145).

Several differences between the "Lo mycoplasma" and *M. fermentans*, however, do exist and may justify assigning the organism to a new species, *M. incognitus*. The organism is capable of intracellular parasitism, a trait not reported with *M. fermentans*, and individual colonies and particles are smaller than those of *M. fermentans*. It also appears to be somewhat more fastidious than *M. fermentans* and has not been isolated directly from infected human or experimental animal body fluids or tissues. In addition, monoclonal antibodies directed against the VLIA particles fail to cross-react with *M. fermentans*. Restriction enzyme digests also differ between the two organisms. Finally, the pathogenic properties of the organism are quite different from those described for *M. fermentans*.

The Lo mycoplasma was originally detected in peripheral blood mononuclear cells and autopsy tissues of persons with AIDS. The organism has since been visualized in brain, liver, and spleen tissues of infected patients using electron microscopy. Histopathologic tissue examination reveals a variety of results ranging from little change to occasional extensive necrosis, with or without evidence of an inflammatory response. No other known infectious agents were demonstrable in the lesions. Whether *M. incognitus* represents a cofactor, an opportunist, or a primary etiologic agent in the lesions described in these immunocompromised patients remains unclear. The organism is clearly infectious, though, and is apparently responsible for disease progression in some individuals. In one recent report, six geographically separated, previously healthy non–HIV-positive patients with acute influenza-like symptoms died with fulminant *M. incognitus* infection with multisystem involvement 1 to 7 weeks after onset of illness. The organism was found extracellularly and intracellularly in necrotizing lesions of spleen, lung, liver, and adrenal gland tissues in all six patients, as demonstrated by electron microscopic, immunoserologic, in situ hybridization, and polymerase chain reaction techniques. No other potential infectious agents were demonstrable. A minimal cellular immune response with few inflammatory cells suggested that the organism may have immunosuppressive properites or, alternatively, that it is capable of avoiding immune defenses by antigenic mimicry.

Monoclonal antibodies directed against epitopes of *M. incognitus* have also been used to immunohistochemically demonstrate the organism in liver, spleen, lymph node, thymus, or brain in 22 patients with AIDS, as well as in two placentas delivered by patients with AIDS. A ^{33}S-labeled DNA probe specific for *M. incognitus* and an in situ hybridization technique have also detected *M. incognitus*-specific genetic material in these tissues. Likewise, ultrastructural analysis of the specific areas of tissue highly positive for *M. incognitus* antigens has revealed characteristic VLIA particles both intracellulary and extracellularly. The organism is, therefore, apparently cytopathic and cytocidal. *M. incognitus* has also been shown to cause fatal systemic infection in experimental silver leaf monkeys. Experimentally infected animals showed only a transient immune response and developed wasting syndromes, resulting in death within 7 to 9 months. Progressive weight loss, tissue necrosis, and a minimal inflammatory cellular and antibody response were noted in all infected animals. The organism was found in the nuclei and the cytoplasm of infected tissues in the absence of other possible etiologic agents. The organism apparently has little specific tissue tropism.

Neither the prevalence nor the significance of *M. incognitus* in human disease is known. The organism appears to be invasive in some immunocompromised patients and capable of inducing immunosuppression in previously healthy persons. The functional deficit of various organ systems, in the absence of other etiologic agents, is apparently associated with cryptic infection with *M. incognitus*, therein the proposed species name. The high prevalance of VLIA infection in persons with AIDS has led to conjecture that *M. incognitus* may play a significant disease-promoting role in HIV-infected individuals. Independently, French investigators have reported that tetracycline analogs inhibit the cytopathic effects of HIV in T-lymphoblastoid tumor cell lines without suppression of virus production (146). Consistent with this theory, *M. incognitus* infection has been shown to accentuate the cytocidal effects of HIV in CD_4-positive human cell lines (147). Because the Lo mycoplasma is potentially amenable to antimicrobial therapy, this possibility warrants in-depth investigation. In vitro, ciprofloxacin appears to be the most active antibiotic against *M. incognitus*. Carefully controlled and matched clinical trials in appropriate persons with AIDS using antibiotics to which the Lo mycoplasma is highly susceptible in vitro should help to clarify this issue.

The suggestion that a procaryotic cell can be generated by transfection of a eucaryotic cell is highly controversial. Other plausible explanations exist for this reported finding, including contamination of the cell line with the Lo mycoplasma during laboratory manipulations or introduction of the organism from an unidentified source during routine passage of the cells in culture or during early transfection cycles. Alternatively, *M. incognitus* may have been present in the Kaposi's sarcoma cells that served as the source of transfecting DNA. This process would involve the transcription and translation of the entire *M. incognitus* genome (approximately 500 megadaltons) by the genetic apparatus of a eucaryotic cell and the final assembly of a functional procaryotic cell. Although highly unlikely, further research is likewise justified to investigate this possibility.

RICKETTSIAE

Rickettsiae are fastidious obligate intracellular bacterial parasites (except *Rochalimaea*) causing a variety of clinical illnesses in humans. The family Rickettsiaceae contains three genera (*Coxiella, Rochalimaea,* and *Rickettsia*), and each species has only one immunotype, except for *Rickettsia tsutsugamushi,* which has eight. The genus name honors the early 20th century American physician, Dr. H. T. Ricketts, who discovered and ascertained the life cycle of *Rickettsia rickettsii,* the causative agent of Rocky Mountan spotted fever, and who in 1910 contracted and died of typhus while studying the disease in Mexico. The organisms are pleomorphic coccobacilli measuring approximately 0.3 μm in diameter and ranging from 0.3 to 2.0 μm in length. Because of their size and lack of contrast with host tissues, they are visualized poorly on Gram stain, but can be demonstrated in clinical specimens using Gimenez, Giemsa, and Machiavello techniques. Despite their dependence on the intracellular milieu of animal cells for growth and reproduction, they are clearly bacterial in nature. They contain both DNA and RNA, multiply by transverse binary fission, possess synthetic and energy-generating enzyme systems, are inhibited by several antibacterial agents, and at least one species contains muramic acid. Both typhus and spotted fever group rickettsial agents (except *R. tsutsugamushi,* the causative agent of scrub typhus) also contain lipopolysaccharides characteristic of other Gram-negative bacteria.

With the exception of *Coxiella burnetii* (the etiologic agent of Q fever) rickettsiae survive for only short periods of time outside of an animal host. Transmitted primarily by the airborne route, *C. burnetii* is stable to many harsh environmental conditions including desiccation, sunlight, and heat. Because of the contagious and fastidious nature of these organisms, if isolation attempts are considered, specimens should be processed only in experienced laboratories with equipment appropriate for their safe manipulation. Blood specimens are generally adequate for rickettsial isolation. Serum should be separated from clotted blood as soon as possible after collection, and the clot should be frozen quickly in dry ice and alcohol, and continuously stored at −70°C or below (including during transport) until thawed for laboratory animal injection.

Rickettsial diseases share several features in common including (*a*) a small blood vessel vasculitis as a common pathological lesion (except for Q fever, in which pulmonary disease plays an equally important role); (*b*) acute clinical illness characterized by headache, fever, and rash (again, except Q fever, which typically does not result in a rash); (*c*) response to a number of broad-spectrum antimicrobials; (*d*) causative organisms stain a characteristic red color with Gimenez staining techniques; (*e*) serum agglutinins are produced to either OX-K, OX-2, or OX-19 strains of *Proteus vulgaris* (the Weil-Felix reaction), except in Q fever and rickettsialpox; and (*f*) etiologic agents are transmitted under natural conditions to mammalian hosts either by insects (fleas and lice) or arachnids (mites and ticks), except Q fever, where inhalation of aerosols represents the major mechanism of transmission. Aerosol transmission of any agent may, however, be an efficient mode of transmission in laboratory settings where high concentrations of rickettsia are used, if proper safety precautions are not employed. All rickettsiae, except heterogeneic strains of *R. tsutsugamushi*, induce complement-fixing antibodies in infected vertebrate hosts and produce immunity to reinfection of long duration. Infection with a strain causing one of the four major groups of rickettsial illnesses confers partial or complete protection against infection by any other rickettsia belonging to the same disease group. There is little cross-protection, however, between strains causing different types of disease. Although immunization does not confer protection as long-lasting as natural infection, it has been successfully employed to reduce mortality rates in specific populations. With the exception of typhus caused by *Rickettsia prowazekii*, all other rickettsial infections represent zoonoses in which humans are merely an incidental and accidental blind end host. Characteristics differentiating the various rickettsial agents that infect humans are outlined in Table 46.5.

Rickettsia rickettsii

Rocky mountain spotted fever (RMSF), caused by *Rickettsia rickettsii*, was first recognized at the turn of the 20th century in parts of Montana and Idaho. At first thought to be limited to the Rocky Mountain area, the disease began to be recognized in the eastern United States in the 1930s. Today, RMSF is the most frequently diagnosed rickettsial illness in the U.S., and has been reported to occur in all regions of the country, with the possible exception of Vermont. Nearly two-thirds of all patients diagnosed with RMSF are under 15 years of age. Despite the clinical efficacy of both chloramphenicol and tetracycline in treating this disease, the mortality rate remains between 5 and 7%. Deaths are usually attributable to failure to include RMSF in the initial differential diagnosis of the illness early on when antimicrobial therapy would be expected to be curative.

EPIDEMIOLOGY

Because *R. rickettsii* is primarily a parasite of ticks, the epidemiology of RMSF in humans is closely associated with the biology of the ticks that transmit it. The dog tick (*Dermacentor variabilis*), in the East, the wood tick (*Dermacentor andersonii*) in the West, and the Lone Star tick in the Southwest are all natural carriers and vectors of the organism. *R. rickettsii* do not kill their arthropod hosts, but are passed transovarially from one tick generation to the next. Congenitally acquired *R. rickettsii* in tick ova persist through larval and nymphal stages of development and ultimately to the adult over a 2-year cycle. Infected adult ticks can further survive for as long as 4 years without a blood meal. Larval and nymphal stages of the tick both require a blood meal from a small mammal for development to the next stage of its life cycle. Adult females also require a blood meal, but from a larger mammal such as a horse, sheep, or dog, for oviposition. As a result, many small wild animals as well as some domestic animals possess RMSF antibodies, suggesting their importance in the tick-mammal-tick cycle. RMSF is seasonal in nature, most cases occurring during the period of greatest tick activity from April through September. Like other rickettsial diseases, RMSF can also be acquired by the respiratory route in laboratory settings where manipulation of highly concentrated rickettsial preparations may occur. A case of RMSF acquired from blood transfusion has also been reported (148).

SPECTRUM OF DISEASE

Following the bite of an infected tick, the primary lesion of RMSF is a vasculitis. The organism multiplies within the endothelial cells lining small blood vessels and disseminates widely via the bloodstream. *R. rickettsii* can be visualized both in the nucleus and the cytoplasm of infected cells. Focal areas of endothelial proliferation and perivascular mononuclear cell infiltration result in thrombosis and erythrocyte leakage into surrounding tissues. These vascular lesions account for the more prominent clinical features of the disease, including headache, rash, and mental confusion as well as, in severe cases, heart failure and shock. Vascular lesions can occur anywhere in the body, but are most easily appreciated in the skin, gonads, and adrenals. Inflammation of car-

Table 46.5. Characteristics of Selected Rickettsial Agents Infecting Humans

Disease	Etiologic Agent(s)	Geographic Location	Arthropod Vector	Mammalian Reservoir	Mode of Transmission	Weil-Felix Results OX-2	OX-K	OX-19	Type and Distribution of Rash	Eschar
Spotted fever group										
Rocky Mountain spotted fever	*R. rickettsii*	Western hemisphere	Ixodid tick	Foxes, dogs, rodents	Tick bite	1+	0	3+	Extremities to trunk	No
Boutonneuse fever	*R. conorii*	Mediterranean, Black Sea, Caspian Sea, Middle East, India, Africa	Ixodid tick	Rodents, dogs	Tick bite	3+	0	1+	Trunk, face, extremities	Yes
Rickettsial pox	*R. akari*	N. America, U.S.S.R., Southern Africa, Korea	Mites	House mice, commensal rodents	Mite bite	0	0	0	Vesicular; trunk, face, extremities	Yes
Siberian tick typhus	*R. sibirica*	Armenia, Central Asia, Siberia, Mongolia, Central Europe	Ixodid tick	Rodents	Tick bite	3+	0	1+	Trunk, face, extremities	Yes
Queensland tick typhus	*R. australis*	Australia	Ixodid tick	Marsupials	Tick bite	3+	0	1+	Trunk, face, extremities	Yes
Typhus group										
Epidemic typhus	*R. prowazekii*	Cosmopolitan	Human body louse, squirrel ectoparasites	Humans, flying scuirrels	Scratching infected louse feces into skin lesion	1+	0	3+	Trunk to extremities	No
Brill-Zinsser	*R. prowazekii*	N. America, Europe, Africa	Recrudescence of latent epidemic typhus years after primary illness			0	0	0	Trunk to extremities (sometimes absent)	No
Murine typhus	*R. typhi (mooseri)*	Cosmopolitan	Flea	Rodents	Scratching infected flea feces into skin lesion	1+	0	3+	Trunk to extremities	No
Scrub typhus	*R. tsutsugamushi*	Asia, India, Australia, Pacific Islands	Trombiculid mite	Rodents	Chigger bite	0	3+	0	Trunk to extremities	Yes
Q fever	*Coxiella burnettii*	Cosmopolitan	Ixodid tick	Rodents, goats, sheep, cattle	Inhalation of contaminated aerosol; possibly tickbite	0	0	0	None	No
Trench fever (cat-scratch disease?)	*Rochalimaea quintana*	Europe, Africa, N. America	Human body louse	Humans (housecats?)	Scratching louse feces into skin lesion; cat-scratch?	0	0	0	Transient or none; lymphadenopathy?	No
Ehrlichiosis	*Ehrlichia canis, Ehrlichia sennetsu*	Japan, U.S.	Ixodid tick? brown dog tick?	dogs, domestic animals; foxes? coyotes?	tick bite	0	0	0	Usually absent	No

diac and central nervous system parenchyma can accompany vaculitis in these tissues, and patch interstitial myocarditis can be routinely demonstrated in fatal cases. Upon histopathological examination, interstitial edema and inflammation with relative preservation of cardiac myofibrils is characterisically noted. In neural tissues, mononuclear infiltrates and focal proliferative glial nodules may be observed. In most cases with kidney involvement, inflammation involves both renal interstitium and blood vessels, and acute tubular necrosis frequently occurs.

Onset of disease in humans, which may be either gradual or abrupt in nature, usually occurs 2 to 8 days after a bite from an infected tick. Fever characteristically rises rapidly to 104° to 105°F (40° to 40.6°C) and remains persistently high. Some patients, however, demonstrate graphic temperature oscillations of 3° to 5°F (1.8° to 2.8°C) over a few hours. The rash in RMSF typically appears by the second or third day, but may be delayed until the sixth day or later in some patients. Characteristically, the initial small erythematous macules blanch on pressure and as a rule progress relatively rapidly, becoming maculopapular or petechial in nature. In untreated patients, lesions may become confluently hemorrhagic and, on rare occasions, result in massive dermal necrosis. In most cases, the rash initially appears peripherally on the wrists and ankles, spreading within hours up the extremities to the trunk. A highly useful diagnostic feature of the rash is its regular appearance on the soles and palms. Eschars, characteristic of several other rickettsial infections, have only rarely been reported in RMSF. The absence of a rash in a patient with appropriate clinical symptoms and a suggestive epidemiologic history should not preclude initiation of antimicrobial therapy.

The characteristic headache in older children and adults is intense, persistent, and refractory to all analgesic efforts. Younger children may not complain of headache. Toxicity and signs of meningoencephalitis are common features of the disease. Initial symptoms including restlessness, apprehension, and irritability, may progress quickly to mental confusion, delirium, and sometimes, coma. Meningismus is not always accompanied by abnormalities of CSF laboratory parameters. Grand mal or focal seizures may occur. Both cortical blindness and central deafness (transitory or permanent) may be noted. Other neurological symptoms (usually of short duration) may include spastic paralysis, ataxia, and sixth nerve palsy. Children with RMSF sometimes show residual deficits in cognitive function, which may result in learning disability.

Pulmonary involvement reportedly occurs in 10 to 40% of patients. Rales as well as abnormalities in chest radiographs and arterial blood gas measurements may be noted. Focal infiltrates or pulmonary edema and cardiomegaly may be seen on chest x-ray. Congestive heart failure and arrhythmias are frequently reported. Arthralgia and muscle tenderness, particularly of the calf or thigh muscles, are common complaints. Other signs include edema of the face or extremities, torticollis, and conjunctival suffusion. Profound hyponatremia is frequently noted. As reported with other rickettsial illnesses, persons with glucose-6-phosphate dehydrogenase (G6PD) deficiency may be at increased risk of severe morbidity and mortality from RMSF infection.

DIAGNOSTIC PROCEDURES

No laboratory test is currently commercially available to diagnose RMSF early in the course of disease. *R. rickettsii* may be identified in skin biopsies using immunofluorescent techniques, but reagents are not readily available, and considerable subjectivity is employed in the interpretation of smears. Serologic studies infrequently are positive before the 10th to 12th day of illness. Serologic tests are important for epidemiologic purposes and to confirm a diagnosis of RMSF. During the first 4 to 5 days of illness, the leukocyte count is normal or slightly below normal. As the disease progresses, secondary bacterial infection may occur, inducing a significant leukocytosis. Mild to severe thrombocytopenia is the rule.

The Weil-Felix test can be performed rapidly, is available in most clinical laboratories, and may be positive as early as more specific rickettsial tests. In the appropriate clinical setting, therefore, the test may provide useful supporting information in establishing a diagnosis of RMSF. Because it is based on the production of nonspecific cross-reacting antibodies to strains of *Proteus vulgaris*, the test, by definition, lacks specificity. *Proteus* infections in humans are fairly common, and as a result, low-titered antibodies (1:20 to 1:80) to *Proteus* OX strains are frequently noted in normal human serum. A rising titer to *Proteus* OX-19 or OX-2 or a single titer of 1:160 or higher may have diagnostic significance in individuals with symptoms consistent with *R. rickettsii* infection.

Other serologic tests that have been used for diagnostic purposes in cases of RMSF include complement fixation (CF), indirect hemagglutination (IHA), microagglutination (MA), latex agglutination (LA), and microimmunofluorescence (MIF). All have limitations, and initiation of appropriate antibiotic therapy early in the course of disease sometimes interferes with antibody production, as measured by these assays. The CF and MA tests are highly specific but lack sensitivity. Because short-lived IgM class antibodies are detected, IHA and LA are sensitive and specific, but of little value in seroepidemiologic studies. Both specific and sensitive, IF assays are subject to bias on the part of the examiner. With both the CF and IF techniques, antigenic crossreactivity can occur between the typhus and spotted fever groups, but epidemiologic, clinical, and geographic features of the diseases should clearly differentiate them. ELISA techniques show promise for the detection of both IgG- and IgM-class antibodies, but reagents are currently not available from commercial sources.

Sera from patients with RMSF have been reported to demonstrate a unique profile when tested by frequency-pulsed electron capture gas liquid chromatographic techniques (149). Characteristic profiles reportedly can be detected as early as 1 day after onset of clinical disease, long before antibody is typically detectable. Unfortunately, such techniques are expensive and are not available to most clinical laboratories, particularly in rural settings where many cases of RMSF occur.

Diagnosis of RMSF can be confirmed by isolation of *R. rickettsii* from blood collected during the first few days of illness, prior to production of specific antibody. Cell culture, embryonated hens' eggs, and guinea pig inoculation have all been used successfully for this purpose. These procedures are expensive and inherently dangerous, and because of the availability of specific serologic assays, culture techniques are infrequently employed.

THERAPEUTIC CONSIDERATIONS

Prior to the advent of specific antimicrobial therapy, the overall mortality rate from RMSF approached 25%. Both chloramphenicol and tetracycline, however, are highly effective antibiotics for the treatment of RMSF when administered early in the course of illness at maximum recommended doses. β-lactam class drugs and streptomycin have little or no activity against rickettsial agents. Sulfonamides may actually have a deleterious effect in cases of RMSF and are contraindicated. Since both tetracycline and chloramphenicol are rickettsiostatic, host defenses play a critical role in the recovery of patients infected with *R. rickettsii.*

The major strategy for the prevention of RMSF is personal avoidance or reduction of tick contact. Wearing trousers tucked into boots or shoes and limiting access to exposed skin around the neck and wrists alleviates inspection for ticks. Frequent removal of ticks is also important because ticks must be attached and feeding for 4 to 6 hours or more before disease transmission occurs. Application of repellents such as dimethyl pthalate to clothes and exposed parts of the body further reduces the risk of disease transmission. Tick control in field settings with malathion or lindane is not practical on a large scale.

Other Spotted Fever Group Rickettsial Diseases

Three other spotted fever group rickettsial species recognized as human pathogens (*Rickettsia sibirica, Rickettsia conorii,* and *Rickettsia australis*) are transmitted by tick bite. *R. conorii* illness has taken on many different geographic names including Mediterranean spotted fever, Kenya tick typhus, Marseilles fever, South African tick bite fever, Israel tick typhus, and Indian tick typhus. A typical spotted fever group rickettsia, *R. conorii* shows more than 90% DNA homology with *R. rickettsii.* Cross-reacting lipopolysaccharide and protein antigens have been described with these two species, and cross-protection is shared among *R. rickettsii, R. conorii,* and *R. sibirica. R. australis* causes Queensland tick typhus, and *R. sibirica* is the etiologic agent of Siberian tick typhus.

EPIDEMIOLOGY

During the 1970s and 1980s, an increased incidence of spotted fever rickettsioses was observed in many parts of the world, especially in Israel, France, and Spain. Spotted fever rickettsial illnesses have also been reported from Japan and China (150, 151). Boutonneuse fever (fièvre boutonneuse) was first described by Conor and Bruch in Tunisia in 1909. *R. conorii* infection has since been described in Ethiopia, Kenya, India, Pakistan, Morocco, South Africa, and southern Europe. Documented infection with *R. sibirica* has been reported from China, Mongolia, the USSR, and Pakistan. *R. australis* is limited geographically to northern Australia. The spotted fever rickettsial agent of Japan appears to be a separate species, whereas the spotted fever group rickettsial agent of southern Asia has yet to be fully characterized. The epidemiology of boutonneuse fever is closely related to tick ecology, especially *Rhipicephalus sanguineus* as well as other species including *Ixodes, Haemaphysalis, Dermacentor, Amblyomma,* and *Hyalomma. R. conorii,* transmitted to humans via tick bite, is maintained in ticks transovarially. Likewise, transovarial transmission of *R. sibirica* establishes an important reservoir of the organism in nature. Most cases occur during the summer months, the peak feeding season for infected ticks. A significant number of cases are imported in travelers returning to the United States and northern Europe from southern Europe and Africa. *R. sibirica* has been recovered from both ticks and humans in northern China. Spotted fever group rickettsial agents have also been isolated from six tick species as well as from wild mammals in northern Asia.

SPECTRUM OF DISEASE

In 1923, in Marseille, Pieri and Olmer described a distinctive lesion of the disease, the "tache noire" or "black spot." Initially a small indurated lesion that develops at the tick bite site, it becomes necrotic at its center, progresses to an eschar, and induces regional lymphadenopathy. If biopsied early in the course of the illness, rickettsia can be visualized in the lesion by immunofluorescence. The pathogenesis of the tissue injury in boutonneuse fever has been well characterized through study of this eschar. Perivascular edema as well as dermal and epidermal necrosis result from endothelial damage by *R. conorii*. Autopsies of fatal cases of boutonneuse fever show disseminated vascular infection and damage by *R. conorii*, including vascular lesions in lung, kidney, pancreas, heart, liver, spleen, gastrointestinal tract, and skin as well as a meningoencephalitis. Liver biopsy reveals focal hepatocellular necrosis. Although boutonneuse fever has historically been described as a benign illness, analysis of recent data from Israel, France, and Spain indicates a mortality rate of from 1.4 to 5.6% (152), not dissimilar from the reported rate for RMSF. Following a mean incubation period of 7 days, myalgias, fever, and headache herald the onset of illness. Observation of a tache noire facilitates the clinical diagnosis. Disease is typically more severe in individuals with underlying conditions such as alcoholism, cardiac insufficiency, diabetes, older age, and G6PD deficiency. Typically, illness is milder in children than in adults.

DIAGNOSIS AND THERAPY

Diagnosis of boutonneause fever may be established by immunofluorescent staining of *R. conorii* in skin biopsies of involved areas. Antibodies to *R. conorii* may be demonstrable during the convalescent period by latex agglutination, complement fixation, or microimmunofluorescence techniques. Chloramphenicol, tetracycline, doxycycline, and ciprofloxacin (153) have all proven to be effective therapeutic agents for the treatment of boutonneuse fever.

Rickettsia akari

Rickettsialpox is a zoonotic, nonfatal febrile illness caused by *R. akari*. First described in New York City in 1946, it has been reported from other urban areas of the United States and South Africa, from Ukranian and other Soviet cities, and from Korea. The organism, like many other rickettsia, is a small, coccobacillary obligate intracellular parasite that stains best in tissues with Giemsa stain. The organism, like *R. rickettsii*, replicates both in the nucleus and the cytoplasm of infected cells. *R. akari* demonstrates significant serologic cross-reactivity with other agents in the spotted fever group of rickettsia.

EPIDEMIOLOGY

The house mouse represents the natural host of the mite that transmits rickettsialpox in the United States, whereas, in the U.S.S.R., commensal rats have been shown to carry the organism, and wild rodents are suspected of carrying the disease in South Africa. The organism cycles naturally between the mite vector (*Alodermanyssus sanguineus*) and the house mouse (*Mus musculus*). The mite, which passes *R. akari* transovarially, represents both the reservoir and the vector for the disease. Humans acquire infection when insufficient mouse hosts are available to the ectoparasite, necessitating search for alternative sources of a blood meal. Humans, therefore, represent incidental and accidental hosts of the agent. The disease affects persons of all ages and females and males appear to be equally susceptible to infection.

SPECTRUM OF DISEASE

Because of the nonfatal nature of the illness, comprehensive pathological data are unavailable. After the mite bite, however, *R. akari* appears to multiply locally in the skin. Rickettsemic dissemination of the organism occurs later, near the time that clinical symptoms present. Histopathological examination of skin biopsies have revealed capillary fibrinous thrombosis and necrosis with mononuclear cell infiltrates, similar to the angiitis reported for other rickettsial infections. Organisms have not been visualized in biopsied tissues by either light or electron microscopy. Although histologic features are sufficiently characteristic to assist in the diagnosis of the disease, skin biopsies are usually not necessary to establish a diagnosis of rickettsialpox. The value of immunofluorescent techniques for examination of tissue biopsies has not been established.

Because most infected patients have continuous exposure to the vector in their domiciles and are usually not aware of the mite bite (the mite is extremely small, colorless, and its bite is painless), the exact incubation period of rickettsialpox has not been precisely determined, but probably ranges from 9 to 14 days. A red papule characteristically forms at the mite bite site, slowly progressing to a papulovesicle and further to a black scab or eschar 0.5 to 3.0 cm in diameter, at or about the time of fever onset. A single eschar is usually observed, but patients with two or more lesions have been reported. Nontender lymphadenopathy is typically present. Onset of symptoms is sudden. Fever is irregular, typically fluctuates between 100° and 103°F (37.8° to 39.5°C), infrequently lasts longer than 1 week, and is usually accompanied by chills and the headache characteristic of rickettsial illnesses. Because of the hectic nature of the fever, most patients have rigors and sweat profusely. Nausea, vomiting, abdominal pain, myalgia (especially of the back), photophobia, pharyngitis, and/or rhinorrhea are sometimes noted. The rash, the most distinctive characteristic of the illness, usually develops within several days of fever onset (range, hours to 9 days). Scattered nonpruritic macules progress rapidly to become firm maculopapules 2 to 10 mm in diameter and, within 2 additional days, form suprapapular vesicles that heal by crusting. Lesions usually appear on the trunk, face, and extremities, but may also emerge on the soles, palms, and mucous membranes. The number of lesions ranges from as few as five or six to over 100. In adults, the haphazard vesicular distribution mimics a chickenpox rash.

DIAGNOSTIC AND THERAPEUTIC CONSIDERATIONS

Early in the illness, a mild leukopenia is frequently seen. Serologic diagnosis can be made with complement fixation or immunofluorescence using either *R. akari* or *R. rickettsii* antigens. Weil-Felix tests are of no value because agglutinins are not produced to *Proteus* antigens. Complications are rare, and mortality has not been reported. Untreated, illness lasts for 2 to 3 weeks, but residual lassitude and headache may persist for 1 to 2 weeks. Relapse is rare. Tetracyclines and chloramphenicol are the drugs of choice. As in other rickettsial illnesses, antibiotic therapy interferes with antibody production and detection. Convalescent specimens should be collected 6 to 8 weeks after onset of symptoms in treated patients if initial serologic assays are negative. Because of the mild nature of the illness in young children, antibiotic therapy may be withheld.

The disease may be used as a flag or marker for excessive proliferation of mice and mites in a neighborhood or building. Control of mice and their ectoparasites effectively prevents human infection.

Coxiella burnetii

C. burnetii is the etiologic agent of Q fever, a cosmopolitan acute (occasionally chronic) febrile illness characterized in humans by headache, fever, and, in more than 50% of cases, a pneumonitis. The most frequently infected animal reservoirs for this zoonosis are sheep, goats, and cattle. Domestic ungulates, these animals, when infected, shed the agent in feces, urine, milk, and, in particularly high titer, in products of conception. The placenta of infected sheep may contain as many as 10^9 organisms/g of tissue. Humans are usually infected by inhalation of contaminated aerosols. Following an incubation period of approximately 20 days (range, 14 to 39 days), persons develop fever, chills, severe headache, fatigue, and myalgia. Other symptoms reflect the organs involved in the infection. Unlike other rickettsial infections, rash is extremely rare in patients with Q fever. The rash seen in cases of chronic Q fever and endocarditis results from an immune complex vasculitis, and is described as a palpable purpura. *C. burnetii* does not induce cross-reacting antibodies to *Proteus* OX strains. Patients are, therefore, negative by the Weil-Felix test.

The organism is a highly pleomorphic coccobacillus with components of a Gram-negative cell wall, measuring 0.3 × 1 μm in size. Unlike other rickettsiae, it enters the cell by a passive mechanism, where it survives in the phagolysosome. The low pH of this milieu appears to be essential for metabolic activity by *C. burnetii.* Extremely infectious for humans, a single cell of *C. burnetii* appears to be sufficient to cause infection. Both small and large cell variants have been described, and a spore stage has been reported (154), possibly explaining its striking resistance to desiccation and its ability to withstand other harsh environmental conditions. It survives for up to 10 months on wool at 15° to 20°C, for more than 40 months in skim milk at ambient temperature, and for longer than 1 month in fresh meat in cold storage. Although it is destroyed by 2% formaldehyde, *C. burnetii* has been recovered from infected tissues preserved in formaldehyde for as long as 5 months and has been isolated from fixed paraffin-embedded tissue. Disinfectants that effectively destroy *C. burnetii* include 5% hydrogen peroxide and 1% lysol.

EPIDEMIOLOGY

C. burnetii infection occurs worldwide, and has been reported from at least 51 countries on five continents (155). Although the organism has been isolated from a variety of animals including fish, pigeons, ducks, geese, turkeys, several species of wild birds, camels, hogs, deer mice, harvest mice and other rodents, rabbits, marsupials, dogs, cats, camels, squirrels, water buffalo, and a variety of farm animals including cattle, sheep, and goats, as well as from arthropods, humans are the only animals in which clinical illness regularly occurs. The epidemiology of Q fever varies from one geographic location to another. Humans become infected with *C. burnetii* following inhalation of small-particle aerosols harboring the organism. In 1935, Derrick, a medical health officer in Queensland, Australia, investigated an outbreak of febrile illness affecting 20 employees of a Brisbane abbatoir, coining the term Q (query) fever for the disease (156). Freeman and Burnet (157) were the first to demonstrate that the organism recovered from the urine and blood of infected patients was a rickettsia. Almost simultaneously, Cox and Davis (158) isolated an organism from *Dermacentor andersonii* ticks collected near Nine Mile Creek, Montana and named the agent, *R. diaporica*. Dyer was later able to prove that *R. burnetii* (Burnet and Freeman's isolate) and *R. diaporica* were one and the same (159).

Q fever is characteristically an occupational disease, affecting individuals with direct animal contact, such as veterinarians, farmers, and abbatoir employees. Indirect contact with infected animals, however, has also resulted in outbreaks of the disease. In one such outbreak in Switzerland, over 350 individuals living along a road over which infected sheep traveled, developed the disease (160). Similarly, an outbreak occurred among persons living along a road in England following exposure to contaminated straw, dust, or manure from farm vehicles (161). A cluster of cases has been reported in laundry workers following handling of contaminated clothing (162). Laboratory exposure to *C. burnetii* (163) and transport of infected sheep through hospital corridors (164) to research laboratories have also resulted in significant Q fever outbreaks. In addition, ingestion of contaminated raw milk (165), skinning infected wild animals, and exposure to infected parturient cats (166) have been shown to be associated with Q fever transmission.

C. burnetii has been isolated from mothers' milk (167) and from human placental tissues (168). It has also been transmitted by blood transfusion, albeit rarely (169). Although documented infection has not been reported as a result of providing patient care to infected persons, transmission has apparently occurred during the performance of a postmortem examination (170). Person-to-person transmission has also been reported among close household contacts in a family setting (171).

The transmission cycle of *C. burnetii* to man involves environmental maintenance of the agent within arthropod vectors, particularly ticks. These ectoparasites transmit the organism to a variety of vertebrates, large and small, wild and domestic. Infected domesticated ungulates are typically asymptomatic, but infection may result in stillbirth or abortion, the heavily infected placenta contaminating the environment at parturition. In such contaminated areas, air samples yield the organism for up to 2 weeks following parturition, and viable organisms can be recovered from the soil for as long as 150 days. Humans may then be infected by inhalation of contaminated aerosols.

SPECTRUM OF DISEASE

Following proliferation of the organism in the pulmonary tract, rickettsemia occurs, resulting in onset of systemic symptoms. A variety of clinical syndromes may be seen including a self-limited febrile illness, pneumonia, endocarditis, osteomyelitis, hepatitis, encephalitis, "aseptic" meningitis, and others. Self-limited febrile illness probably represents the most frequent manifestation of infection with *C. burnetii*. In highly endemic areas, significant proportions of the population may be seropositive, but individuals fail to recall pneumonia or other serious illness potentially attributable to infection with the organism. The severity of symptoms and extent of disease is a function of the aerosol inoculum size, the characteristics of the infecting strain, and the age at which infection takes place. Although the proportion of all Q fever infections that are asymptomatic is not known, individuals totally devoid of symptoms have been reported (172).

Pneumonia

Patients with Q fever may present with any one of three distinct types of pneumonia. In young adults, the most frequent form is described as an atypical pneumonia with a dry nonproductive cough. Sputum and blood cultures are negative for usual respiratory pathogens. Rapidly progressive pneumonia with pulmonary consolidation resembling Legionnaire's disease occurs, but is uncharacteristic. The most common presentation is pneumonia as an incidental finding in a patient with fever of unknown origin. Symptomatic cough and/or pleuritic chest pain are noted in only approximately one-fourth of all patients with roentgenographically confirmed Q-fever pneumonia. Diverse radiographic findings have been reported in cases of Q-fever pneumonia. Segmental and subsegmental pleural-based opacities are frequently noted. Although occasionally substantial, pleural effusion is characteristically minimal. Nonspecific increases in reticular markings, hilar lymphadenopathy, and atelectasis may all be seen. Rare fatalities due to *C. burnetii* pneumonia have been reported, but coexisting conditions usually played a significant contributory role in the deaths. Limited information exists regarding histopathological findings in human *C. burnetii* pneumonia. Small coccobacillary organisms have been observed with alveolar macrophages in specimens obtained by transbronchial biopsy. Severe focal, intra-alveolar hemorrhagic and necrotizing pneumonia with associated necrotizing bronchitis was reported in one fatal case in a 43-year-old male. Organisms consistent with *C. burnetii* as well as intra-alveolar histiocytes, plasma cells and lymphocytes were observed using a modified Giemsa staining technique (173). A resolving lesion in one case of Q-fever pneumonia was characterized as an inflamamtory pseudotumor composed of foamy macrophages, lymphocytes, and plasma cells in which the bronchiolar epithelial lining was variably focally denuded, regenerated, or hyperplastic (174). Although resolution of roentgenographic abnormalities are typically noted within 1 month following initiation of antimicrobial therapy, as many as 70 days may be required.

Onset of illness may be insidious or sudden. Major complaints include fever (98% of patients), chills (88%), diaphoresis (84%), severe headache (75%), myalgia (68%), nausea (50%), and vomiting (25%). Approximately one-fifth of all patients with Q fever present with diarrhea. Splenomegaly is noted in about 5% of patients. Because severe headache and fever suggest infection of the central nervous system, lumbar punctures are often performed on patients with Q fever. Results of laboratory analyses performed on cerebrospinal fluid are usually within normal limits, although *C. burnetii* may be isolated if CSF is cultured appropriately. Although approximately one-third of patients demonstrate a leukocytosis, white blood cell counts are typically normal. Although serum bilirubin levels are usually within normal limits, most patients have levels of hepatic transaminases two to three times above the normal range. Inappropriate secretion of antidiuretic hormone occurs on rare occasions (175).

Because most laboratories are not equipped to isolate *C. burnetii*, the diagnosis of Q-fever pneumonia is usually confirmed serologically by demonstrating a four-fold rise in antibody titer between acute and convalescent specimens. ELISA, microagglutination, CF (the most frequently used technique), and microimmunofluorescence procedures have all been successfully employed for this purpose. Cross-reacting antibodies between *C. burnetii* and other potential pathogens have not, to date, been reported. Although use of the IFA test to detect IgM-class antibodies may facilitate the rapid diagnosis of Q fever, IgM antibodies have been reported to persist in some cases for as long as 678 days (176) and, in one study, 3% of persons continued to show significant IgM titers 1 year after primary infection (177).

Tetracyclines represent the current drugs of choice for treatment of Q-fever pneumonia. Chloramphenicol has also proven to be clinically useful, whereas results with erythromycin have been variable. Evidence exists that discrete strains of *C. burnetii* are responsible for the distinct disease syndromes observed clinically and that these distinct isolates have different antibiotic susceptibility profiles. In vitro susceptibility studies using infected L-929 cells demonstrated that an isolate from a patient with chronic Q fever was significantly more resistant to rifampin, doxycycline, and three fluoroquinolones: ofloxacin, ciprofloxacin, and norfloxacin than strains from persons with acute infection (178). In vitro susceptibility studies by the same investigators have also indicated that, in general, the quinolones and rifampin are more effective than doxycycline, chloramphenicol, and trimethoprim. Polymyxin B, penicillin G sulfamethoxazole, streptomycin, erythromycin, gentamicin, and tetracycline have minimal or no in vitro activity (179).

Endocarditis

The major clinical manifestation of "chronic" Q fever is endocarditis, usually involving abnormal or prosthetic cardiac valves. In patients with a defective cell-mediated immune response to *C. burnetii*, any part of the cardiovascular system may, however, become infected. Rare in children, the disease presents clinically as culture-negative endocarditis, frequently without fever. Hypergammaglobulinemia and clubbing of the fingers is often noted. More than 50% of patients display hepatomegaly and splenomegaly. About 20% of patients have a pruritic rash resulting from a leukocytoclastic vasculitis. An elevated erythrocyte sedimentation rate, characteristically greater than 100 mm/hr, anemia, and microscopic hematuria are also frequently found. The course of disease is complicated by arterial emboli in approximately one-third of patients. In most cases the diagnosis is confirmed serologically. A CF titer of 1:200 or higher to phase I antigen is usually seen in patients with Q-fever endocarditis, whereas patients with acute Q fever rarely demonstrate antibody titers of this magnitude to phase I antigen. Similar results are seen with microimmunofluorescent assays, but specific titers considered diagnostic of Q-fever endocarditis have not been suggested. IgA antibodies to phase I antigen have been reported in both chronic and acute Q fever, although titers were lower in the latter disease (176).

Specific recommendations for the treatment of Q-fever endocarditis are lacking, but combination therapy with tetracycline and either rifampin or trimethoprim/sulfamethoxazole has been used for this purpose. Many experts feel that therapy should be lifelong. One recent study found that addition of a quinolone to doxycycline was statistically more effective than doxycycline alone in preventing mortality in cases of Q-fever endocarditis. Based on clinical, serologic, and valve tissue culture findings that no treatment was able to cure these patients within 2 years, a minimum of 3 years of therapy with this combination of antibiotics was recommended (180). Antibody levels decline slowly during therapy, and titers should be monitored every 6 months during treatment and every 3 months for the 2 years following completion of therapy. Improvement of anemia, correction of the hypergammaglobulinemia, and a decline in the erythrocyte sedimentation rate are noted with successful treatment. Cardiac valve replacement is frequently necessary.

Hepatitis

Q-fever hepatitis may present in any one of three ways: as an incidental finding in a patient with Q-fever pneumonia, as an infectious hepatitis-like syndrome, or as a fever of unknown origin with characteristic "doughnut" granulomata (dense fibrous rings surrounded by a central lipid vacuole) on liver biopsy. "Doughnut" granulomata may also be seen upon histopathological examination of liver tissue in patients with infectious mononucleosis or Hodgkin's lymphoma. Although the organism has not been seen with hepatic parenchyma, *C. burnetii* has been isolated from the liver tissue of patients with Q-fever hepatitis. Two weeks of antibiotic therapy appears to be sufficient for successful treatment of Q-fever hepatitis.

Central Nervous System Infection

Although little evidence exists of serious brain involvement in acute Q fever, the severe headache manifested in the disease probably results from CNS infection. Aseptic meningitis, encephalitis, and vertebral osteomyelitis (181) have also been reported, albeit rarely. Q fever may also occur in neonates causing malaise, fever of unknown origin, febrile seizures, pneumonia, and/or meningeal irritation. Reported hematologic manifestations include bone marrow necrosis, hemolytic anemia, histiocytic hemophagocytosis, transient aplastic anemia, reactive thrombocytosis, and, on rare occasions, thrombocytopenia. The disease may, on occasion, resemble lymphoma. Erythema nodosum and optic neuritis have also reportedly occurred in association with Q fever.

PREVENTION

Prevention of Q fever is based on limiting exposure to potentially infected animals and their excreta. Use of seronegative sheep in research facilities should prevent outbreaks in those settings. Isolation procedures, other than universal blood and body fluid precautions, for hospitalized patients is not warranted because person-to-person spread is not a concern. Consumption of pasteurized versus raw milk effectively prevents the spread of Q fever by this route. Control of ectoparasites on domesticated ungulates is also important in preventing cases of Q fever.

Rickettsia prowazekii

Epidemic or louse-borne typhus, the prototypic typhus group rickettsial disease, is caused by *R. prowazekii,* as is its recrudescent form, Brill-Zinsser disease. The disease has also been called jail fever, fleckfieber, tarbardillo, typhus exanthematicus, and classic typhus. The primary illness was first differentiated from typhoid fever by Gephard in 1836. Brill, in 1910, described an illness similar to typhus, but milder and unaccompanied by the presence of body lice. In 1934, Zinsser postulated that it represented recrudescent louse-borne typhus, a theory subsequently confirmed.

EPIDEMIOLOGY

Epidemics of typhus in the 20th century have paralleled the history of famine and war. An estimated 30 million cases, with 3 million resultant deaths, occurred in eastern Europe and the Soviet Union from 1918 to 1922. During the World War II, typhus was epidemic in concentration camps in North Africa and eastern Europe. Its reputation as a medical problem in the miltary was used cunningly to protect residents of German-occupied areas of Europe from deportation to concentration camps for forced labor. To avoid areas of epidemic typhus, the German military used the Weil-Felix test for diagnosis. Taking advantage of the scenario to artificially create areas of apparent epidemics in regions of Poland, certain physicians vaccinated persons with any symptom even remotely suggestive of typhus with formalin-killed strains of *Proteus vulgaris,* OX-19. Thinking that they were receiving a "rejuvenating protein suspension," persons so vaccinated were unknowingly effectively protected from arrest by German authorities (182).

R. prowazekii, the etiologic agent of epidemic typhus, is an obligate intracellular bacterial parasite that replicates by binary fission. Antigenically it is closely related to the causative agent of murine typhus, *R. typhi.* Although usually coccobacillary, the organism may be highly pleomorphic. Using Giemsa, Gimenez, or other special stains, the organism is easily visualized in the cytoplasm of infected cells upon histopathological examination of tissue sections. Because of the inherent danger of infection with the organism, isolation attempts should only be made by experienced personnel in appropriately equipped laboratory facilities. The organism will remain viable and can be isolated for several days at refrigeration temperature and for years in blood clots collected from infected persons.

The human body louse, *Pediculus humanus corporis,* is responsible for person-to-person transmission of *R. prowazekii.* The cycle is initiated when a louse feeds on a newly introduced infected, rickettsemic person with primary louse-borne typhus or an individual with recrudescent typhus. The organism infects the alimentary canal of the louse, resulting in production of large numbers of organisms in its feces within 7 days. Transmission of lice from person to person requires close personal contact with infested individuals or their clothing. Conditions that promote proliferation of lice exist during colder months, during wars, and following natural disasters when clothing is infrequently changed, crowded conditions occur, and bathing is uncommon. Lice defecate as they take a blood meal and irritation, resulting from the bite, causes the host to scratch the site, contaminating the bite wound with the feces of the louse. Human infection may also occur following mucous membrane exposure to contaminated louse feces.

Infected lice die 1 to 3 weeks after infection with *R. prowazekii* because of alimentary canal obstruction. Transovarial transmission from louse to its progeny does not occur. In addition to humans, an *R. prowazekii* reservoir apparently exists in the southern flying squirrel, *Glaucomys volans* (183). The ecologic distribution of the squirrel ranges over the entire eastern U.S. from southern Maine to Florida and westward to the central states from eastern Texas to Minnesota. Transmission presumably occurs among these rodents via their ectoparasites, squirrel fleas and lice. Indigenously acquired cases of epidemic typhus in the eastern U.S., diagnosed serologically, have been attributed to exposure to these animals, although the mechanism of transmission is not clear (184, 185). In these cases no evidence existed for person-to-person transmission.

SPECTRUM OF DISEASE

In humans, following local multiplication at the bite site, the organism disseminates hematogenously. Like most other rickettsiae, *R. prowazekii* infects the endothelial cells lining capillaries, venules, and arterioles. This results in a vasculitis, intraluminal deposition of platelets and fibrin, and vascular occlusion. Perivascular infiltrates of histiocytes, plasma cells, lymphocytes, and polymorphonuclear leukocytes with or without overt vascular necrosis may occur. Angiitis is most pronounced in the skin, kidneys, heart, central nervous system, and skeletal muscle. When local thrombosis is extensive, gangrenous changes of the skin, digits, and distal portions of the extremities may occur.

Following an incubation period of about 1 week, typhus presents abruptly with intense headache, fever, chills, and myalgia. No eschar is noted. Fever increases rapidly to 102° to 104°F and becomes unremittent. Prostration results. On or about the fifth day of illness, a nonconfluent rash that blanches on pressure appears in the axillary folds and on the upper part of the trunk, and spreads centrifugally. During the following several days, the rash becomes maculopapular, darker, petechial and confluent and covers the entire body, except for the soles, palms, and face. Less common findings include a nonproductive cough with radiologic evidence of pulmonary infiltrates, tinnitus, and deafness. Although symptoms in cases of indigenously acquired epidemic typhus are usually milder than those of louse-borne typhus, life-threatening illness has been reported.

In uncomplicated, untreated cases of epidemic typhus, persons defervesce after 2 weeks of illness. Recovery of normal mentation is rapid, but a prolonged convalescent period of 2 to 3 months is typically required before strength is fully recovered. Although the overall fatality rate is quite variable, it has been reported to be as high as 40% under adverse conditions and is highest in individuals over 60 years of age. Disease is characteristically milder in children. Specific antimicrobial therapy results in prompt recovery.

Appropriate clinical symptoms in a congruous environmental setting usually dictates a diagnosis of louse-borne typhus. The progression of the rash assists in differentiating the disease from RMSF, in which the rash spreads centripetally from the ankles and wrists. Because the disease is rare and due to its protean clinical symptoms, diagnosis of the illness in the U.S. requires a high index of suspicion. Reactions in the Weil-Felix test are identical to those seen in cases of murine typhus. Thus, specific serologic tests may be required to differentiate the two diseases.

PREVENTION AND THERAPY

Both tetracyclines and chloramphenicol are effective therapeutic agents for the treatment of typhus. In louse-borne typhus, a single 100-mg oral dose of doxycycline is curative, whereas multidose therapy is recommended for the treatment of indigenously acquired and murine typhus. Inititation of therapy early in the course of illness, before serious complications occur, virtually eliminates fatal disease. If treatment is started very early on in the disease, within the first 48 hours, occasional patients will relapse.

Such patients respond well to a second course of antibiotic therapy.

Prevention of epidemic typhus is based on control of the human body louse and conditions that promote its proliferation. Although a vaccine is available, delousing an affected population with a lousicidal insecticide is the primary approach to the prevention of infection. Lindane and dichlorodiphenyltrichlorethane (DDT) in powder form are usually effective, but malathion or carbamyl may be necessary if lice do not respond to these agents. The typhus vaccine is prepared from formaldehyde-inactivated *R. prowazekii* propagated in embryonated eggs. Vaccination is recommended only for high-risk individuals including certain scientific researchers such as anthropologists, archaeologists, or geologists; oil field and certain construction workers; missionaries, some government employees who live, work, or travel in foreign countries where the disease is still endemic and who have close personal contact with the indigenous population; medical pesonnel who provide patient care in areas in which louse-borne typhus occurs; and laboratory workers who handle *R. prowazekii.*

BRILL-ZINSSER DISEASE

Brill-Zinsser disease represents recrudescent illness in a person previously infected with *R. prowazekii.* In the United States, it occurs primarily in eastern European immigrants who were initially infected during the World War II. Although its pathogenesis is unclear, it is presumed to be precipitated by stressful conditions and/or a waning immune response to the organism. Although similar to primary louse-borne typhus, symptoms are typically milder, and the disease more closely resembles murine typhus. The Weil-Felix test is usually negative, but low-titered antibody to *Proteus* OX-19 may be present. Detection of IgM antibodies specific for *R. typhi* or *R. prowazekii* helps to differentiate murine typhus and primary epidemic typhus from Brill-Zinsser disease, in which only IgG antibodies to *R. prowazekii* are detectable. Treatment is identical to that for primary louse-borne typhus. No recognized method exists for prevention of recrudescent *R. prowazekii* disease other than prevention of primary infection.

Rickettsia typhi

EPIDEMIOLOGY

Based on an analysis of epidemiologic studies, Maxcy, in 1926, proposed that the reservoir for typhus in the United States was the rat and that its transmission to humans resulted from exposure to the rat's ectoparasites. In 1931, Dyer and collaborators substantiated Maxcy's theory, isolating *R. typhi* from rat brain and from rat fleas. *R. typhi,* previously designated *R. mooseri,* is the causative agent of murine or endemic typhus. Like *R. prowazekii,* it is an obligate intracellular bacterial parasite, and the two organisms share common soluble antigens. Mainly coccobacillary in nature, *R. typhi* is somewhat less pleomorphic than *R. prowazekii* when visualized in the cytoplasm of infected cells with Gimenez or Giemsa stain.

Murine typhus is a cosmopolitan zoonosis, affecting individuals whose occupation or living conditions bring them into close contact with rats and their fleas. *Xenopsylla cheopis,* the rat flea, is the primary vector responsible for transmission of the organism to humans. The decline in cases of endemic typhus reported in the Unted States is a function of intensive efforts made to reduce the numbers of rats and their ectoparasites, particularly in urban areas. The majority of recently reported cases in the U.S. have been from the southeastern and Gulf Coast port states. Although primarily an urban disease, rural cases can and do occur, especially in individuals working in food storage areas and in granaries. Worldwide, both sporadic cases and outbreaks occur in areas where conditions favor rat proliferation and where inadequate ectoparasite control measures are utilized.

The disease is not fatal to the infected rat. The organism is transmitted from rat to rat by *X. cheopis,* the rat flea, and possibly by the rat louse, *Polypax spinulosis,* as well as by other biting insects. The organism multiplies in the alimentary canal of the infected flea and, unlike *R. prowazekii,* fails to cause harm to the transmitting vector. The organism appears to be transmitted transovarially in the flea (186). As the infected flea takes a blood meal, it defecates. Heavily contaminated with *R. typhi,* the feces result in human infection when soiling of the bite wound occurs, frequently by scratching a pruritic lesion. Infection may also occur following mucous membrane exposure (conjunctival or nasal) to contaminated rat flea feces. Human infection in a laboratory setting following an aerosol exposure has also been reported (187).

SPECTRUM OF DISEASE

Because the disease is rarely fatal, descriptions of histopathological changes in tissues of persons infected with *R. typhi* are limited. In one reported fatal case in an 81-year-old woman from Texas, postmortem examination showed interstitial pneumonia, alveolar hemorrhage, cerebral petechiae, multifocal interstitial nephritis with hemorrhage, splenomegaly, interstitial myocarditis, portal triaditis, and hemorrhages of the urinary tract mucosa. The organism was demonstrated in lung, liver, cardiac, brain, and renal tissues. Microscopic changes were reportedly similar to those seen in fatal cases of epidemic typhus (188).

Following a 1 to 2 week incubation period, clinical symptoms of murine typhus typically present insidiously with fever, myalgia, headache, and a nonproductive cough. Onset may, however, be sudden. No eschar is noted. Rash, which occurs in 60 to 80% of patients, first becomes evident 3 to 5 days after onset of fever and usually lasts for 4 to 8 days. The intensity and duration of the rash is quite variable, however, and in some cases it is evanescent. Initially macular in nature, the rash becomes maculopapular over time. Remaining central in distribution, it is concentrated mainly on the abdomen and upper thorax. This compares to the peripheral distribution of the rash characteristically seen in RMSF. In untreated adult patients, temperature usually ranges between 38.9° and 40°C (102° to 104°F) and lasts for 12 to 16 days.

DIAGNOSTIC PROCEDURES

The diagnosis of endemic typhus is usually made serologically. Patients demonstrate antibodies to *P. vulgaris* OX-19 in the Weil-Felix reaction. A presumptive diagnosis may be based on a single titer of 1:320 or higher during the second week of illness or demonstration of a four-fold rise in titer between acute and convalescent samples collected 10 days to 2 weeks apart in a patient with a compatible history and clinical picture. On occasion, low-level antibody to *Proteus* OX-2 may also be detected; antibodies to *Proteus* OX-K are not demonstrable. CF antibodies become detectable several days after the Weil-Felix test is positive. The soluble antigen used in the CF test cross-reacts with antibody to *R. prowazekii* in essentially all cases. Differentiation of the two diseases is based on history and, when necessary, by culture of the organism or use of an IFA technique after cross-absorption of the test patient's serum with defined antigens of *R. typhi* and *R. prowazekii.* As with other rickettsiae, isolation of *R. typhi* in culture is hazardous and should be attempted only by experienced personnel in a suitably equipped laboratory. If culture is to be attempted, a blood specimen should be collected prior to initiation of antimicrobial therapy, allowed to clot, the serum decanted, and the clot frozen at −70°C or below until shipment on dry ice can be arranged to an appropriate reference laboratory. Alternatively, if storage is to be for less than 48 hours, the clot may be held at refrigerator temperature.

THERAPEUTIC CONSIDERATIONS

Both chloramphenicol and the tetracyclines have proven effective for the treatment of murine typhus. Patients typically defervesce within 48 hours after initiation of antibiotic therapy. As with epidemic typhus, patients treated very early on in the disease may relapse, albeit rarely, and characteristically respond well to a second course of antibiotics.

Cases of endemic typhus should serve as a flag to public health officials that rodent and ectoparasite control in the community is ineffective. Such conditions have the potential to facilitate transmission of other diseases in which rodents and their ectoparasites serve as reservoirs and vectors, such as rat bite fever and plague. It is critically important to coordinate rodent and ectoparasite eradication efforts. Eradication of the rodent population alone encourages ectoparasite transfer to alternative blood meal sources, including humans.

Rickettsia tsutsugamushi

R. tsutsugamushi (R. orientalis) is the etiologic agent of scrub typhus, an acute human febrile zoonotic illness transmitted via the bite of larval-stage trombiculid mites (chiggers). Endemic in the Far East, cases imported into the United States have been reported. The organism is an obligate intracellular bacterial parasite that replicates in the cytoplasm of infected cells. Giemsa stain is quite effective for visualization of the agent, and a minor modification of the Gimenez technique results in bright red staining of the organism in infected tissues. Although many serotypes exist, three (Kato, Karp, and Gilliam) demonstrate sufficient cross-reactivity with other strains to serve as effective antigens for serodiagnostic IFA testing procedures (189).

EPIDEMIOLOGY

Geographically, the endemic area for scrub typhus ranges from eastern Asia to the western Pacific including portions of Korea, Australia, Japan, India, and Pakistan. The disease acquired its name from the nature of the vegetation harboring the vectors, *Leptotrombidium deliense,* and others. These parasites frequently inhabit areas with scrub or secondary vegetation in transitional terrain between meadows and forests. The scrub designation is not totally accurate, however, because vector chiggers infected with the rickettsia have also been found in semiarid and sandy beach locales. In many parts of the Far East, the disease is endemic in rural settings, most cases occurring as a result of occupational exposure. Scrub typhus is also a source of concern to military and local resident populations in endemic areas. During the Vietnam conflict, a number of American soldiers developed scrub typhus, although frequently cases were initially misdiagnosed as infectious mononucleosis.

Trombiculid mites also probably represent the major reservoir of *R. tsutsugamushi* in nature. Most chiggers feed only once, regardless of the mammalian source of their blood meal, and efficiently transmit the agent transovarially to essentially all of their progeny. The organism may also be transmitted to small rodents on which the trombiculid mites feed. Of the four stages in the life cycle of trombiculid mites, only one, the six-legged larval form, feeds on mammals, including humans, who traverse or camp in areas where the mites live and breed. All other stages of the mite are spent in the ground, where they feed on decaying organic matter. Chiggers and mites characteristically remain within a several meter area of where they hatch, creating highly focal "islands of infection" in endemic areas (190). *R tsutsugamushi* is inoculated into the host when the infected trombiculid mite feeds, usually on a lower limb following a walk-through vector-laden brush. Multiplication of the organism at the bite site results in a papule that subsequently ulcerates and eventually forms a black crust, the eschar. The characteristic eschar forms, however, in only about 50% of all persons infected with *R. tsutsugamushi*. Over the next 4 to 5 days, regional lymphadenopathy occurs and progresses to generalized lymphadenopathy, particularly in the axilla, neck and inguinal areas. This is followed by rickettsemia, which begins before the onset of systemic clinical symptoms.

SPECTRUM OF DISEASE

Analogous to other rickettsial infections, the basic pathological lesion in scrub typhus is a perivasculitis of the small blood vessels. Clinical manifestations of infection are first noted from 6 to 18 days, usually 10 to 12 days, after the bite of an infected chigger. Onset of symptoms is usually sudden with severe headache, fever, and myalgia. In the region of the bite wound or eschar, tender lymphadenopathy is usually noted. During the first several days of illness, temperature typically rises quickly to 104° to 105°F (40° to 40.5°C). A relative bradycardia is usually observed early in the course of disease. Other symptoms sometimes encountered during this stage of the illness include conjunctival injection, ocular pain, a nonproductive cough, and apathy. Depending on the virulence of the infecting strain and the host susceptibility, severity of symptoms can vary considerably. Approximately 5 days into the illness, a rash appears on the trunk, spreading to the extremities. Sometimes evanescent, the rash is at first macular in nature, but may become papular. Hepatosplenomegaly and generalized lymphadenopathy, rare in other rickettsial diseases, also typically occur at this time.

In the second week of illness, a small fraction of persons may develop slurred speech, nervousness, delirium, nuchal rigidity, tinnitus, or deafness. Laboratory parameters of CSF collected from such individuals usually remain within normal limits, although a slight increase in mononuclear cells may be observed. Myocarditis and disseminated intravascular coagulation have both been reported. In untreated patients, fever usually subsides after about 2 weeks of illness, but mortality rates of from 1 to 60% have been reported. When death occurs, it is usually due to pneumonia, circulatory collapse, or cardiac failure. Specific antibiotic therapy shortens the length of illness considerably and prevents fatalities. Because of the large number of strains of *R. tsutsugamushi*, reinfection can occur. Although immunity to homologous serotypes is essentially lifelong, protection from infection with heterologous strains is short-lived. The prolonged persistence of *R. tsutsugamushi* in the human host suggests that transplacental transmission of the organism occurs, although isolation of the organism from human placental tissue has not been accomplished.

DIAGNOSTIC PROCEDURES

Routine laboratory tests are of limited value in diagnosing scrub typhus. Leukopenia may occur early, but a leukocytosis is characteristically noted as the disease progresses. Albuminuria is sometimes noted, but results of liver function tests usually remain within the normal range. Despite its poor sensitivity, Weil-Felix testing, because of its ease and availability, remains the most frequently used laboratory test for diagnosing scrub typhus. Antibodies to *P. vulgaris* OX-K are detectable in approximately half of all patients during the second week of the disease. Tests for antibodies to *Proteus* OX-19 and OX-2 are negative. A single antibody titer of 1:320 or higher or a fourfold rise in titer from 1:50 is generally considered significant. Although the test is relatively specific, patients with leptospirosis may show cross-reacting antibody to *Proteus* OX-K, resulting in misdiagnosis. Indirect IFA and immunoperoxidase procedures reportedly are more reliable than Weil-Felix testing, but, because of the heterogeneity of the genus, eight or more antigenic strains must be included in the assays. As a result, these procedures are available in a very limited number of laboratories. A single antibody titer of 1:400 or higher with the IFA procedure is reportedly 95% accurate in correctly diagnosing scrub typhus infection (191). High IFA titers are also seen in persons repeatedly infected with the organism. Initiation of appropriate antimicrobial therapy early on in the illness may interfere with antibody production. *R. tsutsugamushi* antibody, as measured by IFA techniques, is short-lived. Seroepidemiologic studies based on IFA procedures have, as a result, probably understated the incidence of the disease in endemic areas. The organism has been successfully cultured from the blood of infected patients following intraperitoneal injection of white mice. Subsequent examination of mouse tissues reveals rickettsia on Giemsa stain. CF testing is only infrequently used for diagnostic purposes in this disease.

THERAPEUTIC CONSIDERATIONS

Chloramphenicol and tetracycline are both effective agents for the treatment of scrub typhus, but symptoms reportedly dissipate more quickly with tetracycline (192). Fluoroquinolones including ciprofloxacin also appear to be active against *R. tsutsugamushi* (193). Patients usually defervesce within 24 hours after initiation of appropriate therapy. Relapse and reinfection, rare in other rickettsial disease, can occur, particularly if therapy is initiated before the fourth or fifth day of illness. Because both chloramphenicol and tetracycline are rickettsiastatic, antibiotic therapy for up to 2 weeks may be necessary with these agents to prevent relapse. Some reports indicate that single-dose doxycycline may be effective for the treatment and prevention of recurrent disease (194, 195).

PREVENTION

To prevent infection with *R. tsutsugamushi*, persons spending time outdoors in endemic areas should wear protective clothing impregnated with insect repellents. They should also cover exposed skin surfaces with repellents, such as dimethyl- or dibutylphthalate, to avoid chigger bites. Short-term vector control of camp grounds may be accomplished by cutting, burning, or otherwise eliminating scrub vegetation, as well as by spraying heavily with insecticides such as dieldrin or lindane. Because of the serotypic heterogeneity of the organism, an effective vaccine has not yet been developed. Chemoprophylaxis with both doxycycline and chloramphenicol (196) have been reported with some success in military populations, but in larger settings its practicality seem problematic. Doxycycline has, however, been shown to be an effective prophylactic agent when initiated prior to exposure in endemic areas and continued for 6 weeks after such exposure.

Ehrlichia Species (Human Ehrlichiosis)

Ehrlichia spp. are intraleukocytic bacteria accidentally transmitted to humans following the bite of an infected tick. Of the five recognized species, *Erlichia canis* and *Erlichia sennetsu* are the two proven to cause zoonotic illness in man. Isolation of *E. sennetsu*, as a human pathogen, was first accomplished in Japan in 1954 from a patient with clinical illness similar to infectious mononucleosis (197). *E. sennetsu* infection results in an acute febrile illness with a lymphocytosis as well as postauricular and posterior cervical lymphadenopathy. To date, the disease has only been reported from Malaysia and Japan, although serologic evidence indicates that the disease may also occur in the Philippines. The first human infection with *E. canis* was described in the United States in Arkansas in 1986 (198).

Ehrlichia spp. are obligate intracellular organisms that parasitize peripheral blood mononuclear and polymorphonuclear leukocytes. Like chlamydiae, they form intracellular inclusion bodies or morulae, measuring 2 to 5 μm in size. These inclusion bodies, best demonstrated with Giemsa or Leishman stain, are themselves made up of elementary bodies measuring 0.2 to 0.8 μm in diameter. Parasitized cells include lymphocytes, band and segmented neutrophils, and monocytes. Electron microscopic study of inclusions reveals structures compatible with rickettsia. Detection of inclusion bodies during examination of peripheral blood smears in the dog is uncommon. Electron micrographs have demonstrated that *E. sennetsu* resides within intracytoplasmic vesicles, unlike other rickettsiae that lie free in the cytoplasm.

EPIDEMIOLOGY

E. canis, first isolated from dogs in Algeria, is a cosmopolitan tick-borne illness of wild canids and, occasionally, domesticated dogs characterized by acute and chronic phases of disease. Following a 10- to 14-day incubation period, dogs develop an acute febrile illness. Symptoms may include anorexia, lethargy, depression, lymphadenopathy, splenomegaly, hematuria, hypoalbuminemia, lymphopenia, and thrombocytopenia (199). The organism has been successfuly cultivated in vitro in canine blood monocytes. The frequently fatal chronic phase of the disease is further characterized by bone marrow hypoplasia and pancytopenia. First discovered in the United States in 1963, serologic evidence of infection with *E. canis* has now been reported among dogs in at least 34 states (200). During the Vietnam conflict, a severe epizootic of canine ehrlichiosis occurred. Because of the severe and frequently fatal hematologic manifestations of the disease, including hemorrhage resulting from the significant thrombocytopenia, the disease became known as tropical canine pancytopenia. In canines, pathology in fatal cases is characterized by hemorrhage and invasion of internal organs by plasma cells as well as perivascular cuffing by plasmacytes in the meninges, lungs, spleen, and kidneys. Transovarial transmission of *E. canis* in the vector for dogs, *Rhipicephalus sanguineus* (the brown dog tick) does not apparently occur. The reservoir in nature for continued tick infection is not clear. The potential tick vectors include *Ixodes dammini* and *Amblyomma americanum* (201). No evidence exists that human ehrlichiosis is transmitted directly from dogs to humans.

Erlichia risticii and *Erlichia equi* are the etiologic agents of equine monocytic ehrlichiosis (Potomac horse fever) and equine ehrlichiosis, respectively. *E. risticii* infections are characterized by fever, leukopenia, anorexia, laminitis, and/or diarrhea. Initially discovered in Maryland, the disease is now thought to be endemic in Connecticut, New Jersey, New York, Pennsylvania, Ohio, and Idaho.

SPECTRUM OF DISEASE

In a review coordinated by the CDCP (202), cases of human ehrlichiosis were reported from 11 states, most in the southeastern and south central regions of the country. Illness developed between the months of March and October. The incubation period for the disease appears to be from 12 to 14 days. Because *R. sanguineus* does not ordinarily feed on humans, some confusion exists over the vector of *E. canis* to humans. In humans, a prodrome of lower back pain, nausea, and vomiting has been reported (203). Almost all patients have sudden onset of high fever, often accompanied by a relative bradycardia of less than 90 beats per minute. Severe headache is typically present, and renal failure has been reported. Otherwise, most other clinical findings are normal. The epidemiology, history of tick attachment (in some cases), and clinical findings suggest a diagnosis of RMSF, but rash, in cases of human ehrlichiosis, is present in only approximately 20% of all patients. Most cases have been detected by testing serum samples from patients suspected of having RMSF, but who failed to demonstrate antibodies to *R. rickettsii*. Most reported patients have been males (approximately 70%) between the ages of 30 and 60, implying, in many cases, occupational exposure to vector ticks. Over 80% of patients report a history of tick exposure in the 4-week period prior to onset of symptoms, most within 1 to 3 weeks. Although approximately two-thirds of all reported cases have been hospitalized, all have recovered without residual problems.

DIAGNOSTIC PROCEDURES

In Fishbein's study, the most common hematologic abnormality at presentation was an absolute lymphopenia, wth a median lymphocyte count of 408/mm^3 and a range from 234 to 1365 cells/mm^3. The median reported total leukocyte count was 3000/mm^3. Thrombocytopenia also appeared to be a significant finding in this series. The median platelet count during the first week of hospitalization was 68,000/mm^3 with a range from 49,000 to 75,000/mm^3. Abnormalities in liver function tests including aspartate aminotransferase (AST) and alanine aminotransferase were also common. AST levels peaked approximately 1 week after onset of illness, with a median value of 335 units/dl and a range from 90 to 538 units/dl (202).

Ehrlichia species demonstrate a high degree of antigenic relatedness. As a result, considerable cross-reactivity is encountered in seroepidemiologic studies of animals. IFA is the technique of choice for diagnosing human *E. canis* infection. The test, a modification of the IFA procedure developed for diagnosing canine ehrlichiosis, is performed at the CDCP as well as by some reference laboratories. When necessary, testing at the CDCP should be coordinated through local and state public health authorities. Concomitant submission of both acute and convalescent serum specimens, collected 2 to 4 weeks apart, is required.

THERAPEUTIC CONSIDERATIONS

Tetracycline and its analogues, such as doxycyline, appears to be active against *Ehrlichia* species in humans and in canines (in both acute and chronic stages of the disease), shortening the duration of fever and accelerating recovery. Therapy should be continued for a minimum of 3 days after defervescence. Because hematologic abnormalities are salient features of this disease and because efficacy in the treatment of human infection has not been demonstrated, chloramphenicol is not recommended. Physicians should consider the possibility of ehrlichiosis when patients present with fever and a history of recent tick exposure.

As with other tick-borne rickettsioses, prevention is best accomplished by wearing protective clothing when spending time outdoors in endemic areas, using insect repellents on exposed skin surfaces, and checking for and removing ticks on a frequent basis.

Rochalimaea quintana

R. quintana, the etiologic agent of trench fever, was discovered in the course of studies undertaken to determine the cause of epidemic typhus during World War I. It was initially thought to represent

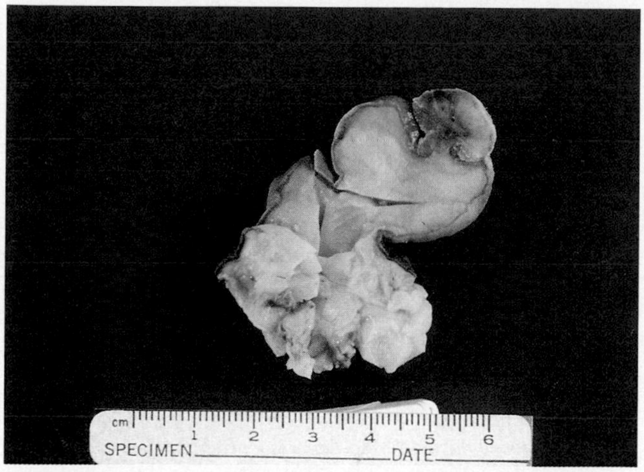

Figure 46.4. Bacillary angiomatosis; gross histologic appearance of a leg lesion in a person infected with the human immunodeficiency virus (courtesy of Salvador Castro, M.D.)

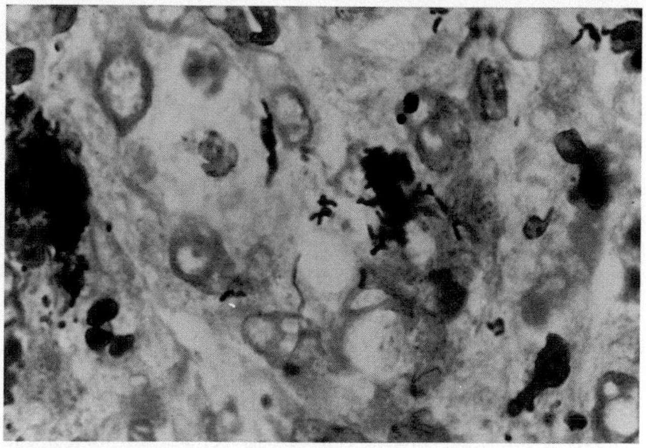

Figure 46.5. Microscopic appearance of bacilli demonstrable by Warthin-Starry stain in a case of bacillary angiomatosis (1000 × total magnification).

part of the normal gut flora of the human body louse. Although usually considered with the rickettsiae, it is a member of a distinct genus. Unlike rickettsiae, it is usually located extracellularly and can be cultivated on artificial media. The organism is named after one of the early investigators of rickettsial diseases, the Brazilian scientist H. da Rocha-Lima, and for the nature of the illness, in which febrile episodes recur after each fifth (quintana) afebrile day.

Isolates of *R. quintana* resemble rickettsiae in size, cell structure, cell wall composition, mode of replication (binary fission), metabolism (utilize succinate and glutamate, but not glucose), and tinctorial properties (stain with Gimenez and Macchiavello techniques). The organism is susceptible to inactivation by usual disinfectants, but, like *R. prowazekii*, survives for months in dried louse feces. *R. quintana* is distinct from *Rickettsia* species in its guanine plus cytosine content (38.5%) and in its ability to grow on artificial (cell-free) media. The organism was first isolated by Vinson in 1966 on a blood agar base medium supplemented with both 6% horse serum (inactivated at 56°C for 30 minutss) and 4% washed, hemolyzed horse red blood cells incubated at 37°C in a moist atmosphere of 5% CO_2 in air. Following 12 to 14 days of incubation, colonies, which develop only on the medium surface, are round, lenticular, mucoid, translucent, and measure 65 to 200 μm in size. The organism will not replicate under anaerobiosis or without supplemental carbon dioxide, demonstrates an absolute requirement for hematin for synthesis of heme-proteins, and does not produce H_2O_2 or catalase.

The only experimental animal model thus far described for *R. quintana* is the rhesus monkey. Several serologic techniques have been used to detect antibodies to the organism in humans, including CF, passive hemagglutination, ELISA, and radioimmunoprecipitation. *R. quintana* appears to share common antigens with certain rickettsiae, however, resulting in cross-reactions that may obfuscate determinations of the true incidence of the disease when analyzing data from seroepidemiologic studies.

Recent studies using polymerase chain reaction techniques suggest that the etiologic agent of bacillary angiomatosis (204) is a rickettsia-like organism, closely related to *R. quintana*. This disease, which results in proliferation of small blood vessels in the skin and visceral organs, affects primarily individuals with human immunodeficiency virus infection and other immunocompromised hosts. The agent can be visualized in tissue sections of lesions with a Warthin-Starry silver stain (Figs. 46.4 and 46.5) but have not, as of yet, been successfully cultivated. Some evidence exists that this same organism, or one closely related, may cause bacillary peliosis hepatis (205) and/or cat-scratch disease. The organism putatively responsible for these syndromes has tentatively been named *Rochalimaea henselae*. Distinguishing between cat-scratch disease and disseminated bacillary angiomatosis in the immunocompromised host can be difficult. The causative agent of cat-scratch disease, however, has been isolated in culture (206) and has for now been named *Afipia felis*. The organism is reportedly a Gram-negative bacterium that grows preferentially at 30 to 32°C in a biphasic brain-heart infusion agar system. Additional nucleic acid analyses will help to further clarify the relationship beween these organisms and *R. quintana*.

References

1. Moulder JW. A primer for chlamydiae. In: Mardh PA, Holmes KK, Oriel JD, et al., eds. Chlamydial infections. Amsterdam: Elsevier Biomedical, 1982: 3–14.
2. Kuo CC, Chen HH, Wang SP, et al. Characterization of TWAR strains, a new group of *Chlamydia psittaci*. In: Oriel D. Ridgway G, Schachter J, et al., eds. Chlamydial infections. Cambridge: Cambridge University Press, 1986:321–324.
3. Dhir SP, Hakamori S. Kenny GE, et al. Immunochemical studies on chlamydial group antigen. (Presence of a 2-keto-3-deoxycarbohydrate as immunodominant group). J Immunol 1972:109:116–122.
4. Grayston JT, Kuo CC, Wang SP, et al. A new *Chlamydia psittaci* strain, TWAR, isolated in acute respiratory tract infections. N Engl J Med 1986; 315:161–168.
5. Campbell LA, Kuo CC, Grayston JT. Characterization of the new *Chlamydia* agent, TWAR, a unique organism by restriction endonuclease analysis and DNA-DNA hybridization. J Clin Microbiol 1987;25:1911–1916.
6. Chi EY, Kuo CC, Grayston JT. Unique ultrastructure in the elementary body of *Chlamydia* sp. strain TWAR. J Bacteriol 1987;169:3757–3763.
7. Thompson SE, Washington AE. Epidemiology of sexually transmitted *Chlamydia trachomatis* infections. Epidemiol Rev 1983;5:96–123.
8. Washington AE, Johnson RE, Sanders LL Jr. *Chlamydia trachomatis* infections in the United States: what are they costing us? JAMA 1987; 257:2070–2072.
9. Bowie WR, Holmes KK. *Chlamydia trachomatis* (trachoma, perinatal infections, lymphogranuloma venereum, and other genital infections). In: Mandell GL, Douglas RG Jr., Bennett JE, eds. Principles and practice of infectious diseases. 3rd ed. New York: Churchill Livingstone, 1990:1426–1440.
10. Ronnerstam R, Perrson K. Chlamydial conjunctivitis in a Swedish population. In: Mardh PA, Holmes KK, Oriel JD, et al, eds. Chlamydial infections. Amsterdam: Elsevier Biomedical, 1982:87–90.
11. Barnes RC. Laboratory diagnosis of human chlamydial infections. Clin Microbiol Rev 1989;2:119–136.
12. Tarizzo M, ed. Field methods for the control of trachoma. Geneva: World Health Organization, 1973:9.
13. Rubin SJ. Chlamydiae. In: Howard BJ, Klaas J, Rubin SJ, Weissfeld AS, Tilton RC, eds. Clinical and pathogenic microbiology. St. Louis: CV Mosby, 1987:835–842.
14. Wilfert C, Gutman L. Chlamydial infections. In: Feigin RD, Cherry JD, eds. Textbook of pediatric infectious diseases. 2nd ed. Philadelphia: WB Saunders, 1987:1867–1877.
15. Berger RE, Alexander ER, Monda GD, Ansell J, McCormick G, Holmes KK. *Chlamydia trachomatis* as a cause of "idiopathic" epididymitis. N Engl J Med 1978;298:301–304.
16. Keat A, Thomas BJ, Taylor-Robinson D. Chlamydial infection in the aetiology of arthritis. Br Med Bull 1983;39:168–174.
17. Paavonen J, Kiviat N, Brunham RC, et al. Prevalence and manifestations of endometritis among women with cervicitis. Am J Obstet Gynecol 1985;152:280–286.
18. Centers for Disease Control. *Chlamydia trachomatis* infections: policy guidelines for prevention and control. MMWR 1985;34 (Suppl 3):53–74.
19. Washington AE, Gove S, Schachter J, Sweet RL. Oral contraceptives, *Chlamydia trachomatis* infection, and pelvic inflammatory disease: a word of caution. JAMA 1985;253:2246–2250.
20. Brunham RC, Paavonen J, Stevens CE, et al. Mucopurulent cervicitis: the ignored counterpart of urethritis in men. N Engl J Med 1984;311:1–6.
21. Wang SP, Eschenbach DA, Holmes KK, Wager G, Grayston JT. *Chlamydia trachomatis* in the Fitz-Hugh-Curtis syndrome. Am J Obstet Gynecol 1980;138:1034–1038.
22. Henry-Suchet J, Catalan F, Loffredo V, et al. *Chlamydia trachomatis* associated with chronic inflammation in abdominal specimens from women selected for tuboplasty. Fertil Steril 1981;36:599–605.
23. Stamm WE, Wagner KF, Amsel R, et al. Causes of the acute urethal syndrome in women. N Engl J Med 1980;303:409–415.
24. Beem MO, Saxon EM. Respiratory-tract colonization and a distinctive pneumonia syndrome in infants infected with *Chlamydia trachomatis*. N Engl J Med 1977;296:306–310.
25. Tipple MA, Beem MO, Saxon EM. Clinical characteristics of the afebrile pneumonia associated with *Chlamydia trachomatis* infection in infants less than 6 months of age. Pediatrics 1979;63:192–197.
26. Thygeson P, Stone W. Epidemiology of inclusion conjunctivitis. Arch Ophthalmol 1942;27:91–122.
27. Bernstein DI, Hubbard T, Wenman WM, et al. Mediastinal and supraclavicular lymphadenitis and pneumonitis due to *Chlamydia trachomatis* serovars L1 and L2. N Engl J Med 1984;311:1543–1546.
28. Clyde WA, Kenny GE, Schachter J. Laboratory diagnosis of chlamydial and mycoplasmal infections. In: Drew WL, ed. Cumitech 19. Washington, DC: American Society for Microbiology, 1984.
29. Cles LD, Bruch K, Stamm WE. Staining characteristics of six commercially available monoclonal immunofluorescent reagents for direct diagnosis of *Chlamydia trachomatis* infections. J Clin Microbiol 1988;26:1735–1737.
30. Amortegui AJ, Meyer MP . Enzyme immunoassay for detection of *Chlamydia trachomatis* from the cervix. Obstet Gynecol 1985;65:523 – 526.
31. Chernesky MA, Mahony JB, Castriciano M, et al. Detection of *Chlamydia trachomatis* antigens by enzyme immunoassay and immunofluorescence in genital specimens from symptomatic and asymptomatic men and women. J Infect Dis 1986;154:141–148.
32. Howard LV, Coleman PF, England BJ, Herrmann JE. Evaluation of Chlamydiazyme for the detection of genital infections caused by *Chlamydia trachomatis*. J Clin Microbiol 1986;23:329–332.
33. Van Ulsen J, Van Zuuren-van der Horst A, Tjiam KH, et al. Solid-phase enzyme immunoassay for detection of *Chlamydia trachomatis*. Eur J Clin Microbiol 1985;4:397–399.
34. Taylor-Robinson D, Thomas BJ, Osborn MF. Evaluation of enzyme immunoassay (Chlamydiazyme) for detecting *C. trachomatis* in genital tract specimens. J Clin Pathol 1987;40: 194–199.
35. Hipp SS, Yangsook H, Murphy D. Assessment of enzyme immunoassay and immunofluorescence test for detection of *Chlamydia trachomatis*. J Clin Microbiol 1987;25:1938–1943.
36. Pothier P, Kazmierczak A. Comparison of cell culture with two different chlamydia tests using immunofluorescence or enzyme-linked immunosorbent assay. Eur J Clin Microbiol 1986;5:569–572.
37. Ryan RW, Kwasnik I, Steingrimsson O, Gudmundsson J, Thorarinsson H, Tilton RC. Rapid detection of *Chlamydia trachomatis* by an enzyme immunoassay method. Diagn Microbiol Infect Dis 1986;5:225–234.
38. Mabey DCW, Robertson JN, Ward ME. Detection of *Chlamydia trachomatis* by enzyme immunoassay in patients with trachoma. Lancet 1987;2:1491–1492.
39. Hammerschlag MR, Roblin PM, Cummings C, Williams TH, Worku M, Howard LV. Comparison of enzyme immunoassay and culture for diagnosis of chlamydial conjunctivitis and

respiratory infections in infants. J Clin Microbiol 1987;25: 2306–2308.
40. Hyypia T, Jalava A, Larsen SH, Terho P, Hukkanen V. Detection of *Chlamydia trachomatis* in clinical specimens by nucleic acid spot hybridization. J Gen Microbiol 1985;131:975–978.
41. Palva A, Jousemier-Somer H, Saikku P, Vaananen P, Soderlund H, Ranki M. Detection of *Chlamydia trachomatis* by nucleic acid sandwich hybridization. FEMS Microbiol Lett 1984;23:83–89.
42. Pao CC, Lin SS, Yang TE, Soong YK, Lee PS, Lin JY. Deoxyribonucleic acid hybridization analysis for the detection of urogenital *Chlamydia trachomatis* infections in women. Am J Obstet Gynecol 1987;156:195–199.
43. Peterson EM, Oda R, Alexander R, Greenwood JR, De La Maza LM. Molecular techniques for the detection of *Chlamydia trachomatis.* J Clin Microbiol 1989;27:2359–2363.
44. Frei W. On the skin test in lymphogranuloma inguinale. J Invest Dermatol 1938;1:367–377.
45. Rake G, McKee CM, Shaffer MF. Agent of lymphogranuloma venereum in the yolk sac of the developing chick embryo. Proc Soc Exp Biol Med 1940;43:332–334.
46. Schachter J, Smith DE, Dawson CR, et al. Lymphogranuloma venereum. I . Comparison of the Frei test, complement fixation test, and isolation of the agent. J Infect Dis 1969;120:372–375.
47. Wang SP, Grayston JT. Immunologic relationship between genital TRIC, lymphogranuloma venereum, and related organisms in a new microtiter indirect immunofluorescence test. Am J Ophthalmol 1970;70:367–374.
48. Wang SP, Grayston JT, Alexander ER, Holmes KK. Simplified microimmunofluorescence test with trachoma-lymphogranuloma venereum (*Chlamydia trachomatis*) antigens for use as a screening test for antibody. J Clin Microbiol 1975;1:250–255.
49. Yong EC, Chinn SJ, Caldwell HD, Kuo CC. Reticulate bodies as single antigen in *Chlamydia trachomatis* serology with microimmunofluorescence. J Clin Microbiol 1979;10:351–356.
50. Nettleman MD, Jones RB, Roberts SD. Cost-effectiveness of culturing for *Chlamydia trachomatis.* A study in a clinic for sexually transmitted diseases. Ann Intern Med 1986;105:189–196.
51. Phillips RS, Aronson MD, Taylor WC, Safran C. Should test for *C. trachomatis* cervical infection be done during routine gynecologic visits? An analysis of the costs of alternative strategies. Ann Intern Med 1987;107:188–194.
52. Trachtenberg Al, Washington AE, Halldorson S. A cost-based decision analysis for chlamydia screening in California family planning clinics. Obstet Gynecol 1988;71:101–108.
53. Hammerschlag MR, Chandler JW, Alexander ER, et al. Erythromycin ointment for ocular prophylaxis of neonatal chlamydial infection. JAMA 1980;244:2291–2293.
54. Greaves AB, Hilleman MR, Taggart SRT, et al. Chemotherapy in bubonic lymphogranuloma venereum. Clinical and serological evaluation. Bull WHO 1957;16:277–289.
55. Bowie WR. Treatment of chlamydial infections. In: Mårdh PA, Holmes KK, Oriel JD, et al., eds. Chlamydial infections. Amsterdam: Elsevier Biomedical Press, 1982:231–244.
56. Handsfield HH, Alexander ER, Wang SP, et al. Differences in the therapeutic response of chlamydia-positive and chlamydia-negative forms of nongonococcal urethritis. J Am Vener Dis Assoc 1975;2:5–9.
57. Bowie WR, Alexander ER, Floyd JF, et al. Differential response of chlamydial and ureaplasma-associated urethritis to sulfafurazole (sulfixoxazole) and aminocyclitols. Lancet 1976;2:1276–1278.
58. Meyer KF. The ecology of psittacosis and ornithosis. Medicine 1942;21:175–206.
59. Potter ME, Kaufmann AF, Plikaytis BD. Psittacosis in the United States 1979. CDC Surveillance Summaries. MMWR 1983;32 (suppl 1):27–31.
60. Centers for Disease Control. Psittacosis associated with turkey processing–Ohio. MMWR 1982;30:638–640.
61. Meyer KF, Eddie B. The influence of tetracycline compounds on the development of antibodies in psittacosis. Am Rev Tuberc 1956;74:566–571.
62. Schachter J. Chlamydiae. In: Rose NR, Friedman H, eds. Manual of clinical immunology, 2nd ed. Washingon, DC: American Society for Microbiology, 1980;701–706.
63. Campbell LA, Kuo CC, Grayston JT. Characterization of the new *Chlamydia* agent, TWAR, as a unique organism by restriction endonuclease analysis and DNA-DNA hybridization. J Clin Microbiol 1987;25:1911–1916.
64. Augenbraun MH, Roblin PM, Chirgwin K, Landman D, Hammerschlag MR. Isolation of *Chlamydia pneumoniae* from the lungs of patients infected with the human immunodeficiency virus. J. Clin Microbiol 1991;29:401–402.
65. Saikku P, Leinonen M, Mattila K, et al. Serological evidence of an association of a novel *Chlamydia,* TWAR, with chronic coronary heart disease and acute myocardial infarction. Lancet 1988;2(8618):983–986.
66. Li DK, Daling JR, Wang SP, Grayston JT. Evidence that *Chlamydia pneumoniae,* strain TWAR, is not sexually transmitted. J Infect Dis 1989;160:328–331.
67. Grayston JT, Diwan VK, Cooney M, Wang SP. Community- and hospital-acquired pneumonia associated with *Chlamydia* TWAR infection demonstrated serologically. Arch Intern Med 1989;149:169–173.
68. Lo SC. A newly identified human *Mycoplasma* disease. Infect Dis News 1990;9:73–75.
69. McMillan JA, Sandstorm C, Weiner LB, et al. Viral and bacterial organisms associated with acute pharyngitis in a school-aged population. J Pediatr 1986;109:747–752.
70. Gerber MA, Randolph MF, Chanatry J, Mayo DR, Schachter J, Tilton RC. Role of *Chlamydia trachomatis* and *Mycoplasma pneumoniae* in acute pharyngitis in children. Diagn Microbiol Infect Dis 1987;6:263–265.
71. Huovinen P, Lahtonen R, Ziegler T, et al. Pharyngitis in adults: the presence and coexistence of viruses and bacterial organisms. Ann Intern Med 1989;110:612–616.
72. Cassell GH, Cole BC. Mycoplasmas as agents of human disease. N Engl J Med 1981;304:80–89.
73. Ponka A. The occurrence and clinical picture of serologically verified *Mycoplasma pneumoniae* infections with emphasis on central nervous system, cardiac, and joint manifestations. Ann Clin Res 1979;24:1–60.
74. Sköldenberg B. On the role of viruses in acute infectious diseases of the central nervous system. Clinical and laboratory studies on hospitalized patients. Scand J Infect Dis 1972;3(suppl):1–96.
75. MacDonald NE, Wolfish N, McLaine P, Phipps P, Rossier E. Role of respiratory viruses in exacerbations of primary nephrotic syndrome. J Pediatr 1986;108:378–382.
76. Foy HM, Kenny, GE, Cooney MK, Allan ID. Long-term epidemiology of infections with *Mycoplasma pneumoniae.* J Infect Dis 1979;139:681–687.
77. Chapman RS, Henderson FW, Clyde WA Jr. Collier AM, Denny FW. The epidemiology of tracheobronchitis in pediatric practice. Am J Epidemiol 1981;114:786–797.
78. Henderson FW, Clyde WA Jr, Collier AM, et al. The etiologic and epidemiologic spectrum of bronchiolitis in pediatric practice. J Pediatr 1979;95:183–190.
79. Foy HM, Grayston JT, Kenny GE, Alexander ER, McMahan R. Epidemiology of *Mycoplasma pneumoniae* infection in families. JAMA 1966;197:859–866.

169. Editorial comment on Q fever transmitted by blood transfusion—United States. Can Dis Wkly Rep 1977;3:210.
170. Harman JB. Q fever in Great Britain. Lancet 1949;2:1028–1030.
171. Mann JS, Douglas JG, Inglis JM, Leitch Ag. Q fever: person to person transmission within a family. Thorax 1986;41:974–975.
172. Luoto L, Casey ML, Pickens EG. Q fever studies in Montana. Detection of asymptomatic infection among residents of infected dairy premises. Am J Epidemiol 1965;81:356–369.
173. Urso FP. The pathologic findings in rickettsial pneumonia. Am J Clin Pathol 1975;64:335–342.
174. Janigan DT, Marrie TJ. An inflammatory pseudotumor of the lung in Q fever pneumonia. N Engl J Med 1983;30:86–88.
175. Biggs BA, Douglas JG, Grant IW, Crompton GK. Prolonged Q fever associated with inappropriate secretion of anti-diuretic hormone. J Infect 1984;8:61–63.
176. Worswick D. Marmion BP. Antibody repsonses in acute and chronic Q fever and in subjects vaccinated against Q fever. J Med Microbiol 1985;19:281–296.
177. Dupuis G Péter O, Peacock M, Burgdorfer W, Haller E. Immunoglobulin responses in acute Q fever. J Clin Microbiol 1985;22:484–487.
178. Yeaman MR, Baca OG. Unexpected antibiotic susceptibility of a chronic isolate of *Coxiella burnetii*. Ann NY Acad Sci 1990;590:297–305.
179. Yeaman MR, Mitscher LA, Baca OG. In vitro susceptibility of *Coxiella burnetii* for antibiotics including several quinolones, Antimicrob Agents Chemother 1987;31:1079–1084.
180. Levy PY, Drancourt M, Etienne J, et al. Comparison of different antibiotic regimens for therapy of Q fever endocarditis. Antimicrob Agents Chemother 1991;35:533–537.
181. Ellis ME, Smith CC, Moffatt MAJ. Chronic or fatal Q-fever infection: a review of 16 patients seen in north-east Scotland (1967–1980). Q J Med 1983;205:54–66.
182. Lazowski ES, Matulewicz S. Serendipitous discovery of artificial Weil-Felix reaction used in "private immunological war". ASM News 1977;43:300–302.
183. Bozeman FM, Masiello SA, Williams MS, et al. Epidemic typhus rickettsiae isolated from flying squirrels. Nature 1975;255:545–547.
184. McDade JE, Shephard CC, Redus MA, Newhouse VF, Smith JD. Evidence of *Rickettisa prowazekii* infections in the United States. Am J Trop Med Hyg 1980;29:277–284.
185. Duma RJ, Sonenshine DE, Bozeman FM, et al. Epidemic typhus in the United States associated with flying squirrels. JAMA 1981;245:2318–2323.
186. Farhang-Azad A, Traub R, Baqar S. Transovarial transmission of murine typhus rickettsiae in *Xenopsylla cheopis* fleas. Science 1985;277:543–544.
187. Centers for Diseases Control. Laboratory-acquired endemic typhus—Maryland. MMWR 1978;27:215–216.
188. Walker DH, Betz TG, Taylor JP, et al. Histopathology and immunohistologic demonstration of the distribution of *Rickettsia typhi* in fatal murine typhus. Seventh national meeting of the American Society for Rickettsiology and Rickettsial Diseases, Santa Fe, NM, April 16, 1988.
189. Robinson DM, Brown GW, Gan E, et al. Adaptation of microimmunofluorescent test to the study of human *Rickettsia tsutsugamushi* antibody. Am J Trop Hyg 1976;25:900–905.
190. Saah AJ. Rickettsia tsutsugamushi (Scrub typhus). In: Mandell GL, Douglas RG Jr, Bennett JE, eds. Principles and practice of infectious diseases. New York: Churchill Livingstone, 1990:1480–1482.
191. Brown GW, Shirai A, Rogers C, et al. Diagnostic criteria for scrub typhus: probability values for immunofluorescent antibody and proteus OXK agglutinin titers. Am J Trop Med Hyg 1983;32:1101–1110.
192. Sheehy TW, Hazlett D, Turk RE. Scrub typhus, a comparison of chloramphenicol and tetracycline in its treatment. Arch Intern Med 1973;132:77–80.
193. McClain JB, Joshi B, Rice R. Chloramphenicol, gentamicin, and ciprofloxacin against murine scrub typhus. Antimicrob Agents Chemother 1988;32:285–286.
194. Brown GW, Saunders JP, Singh S, et al. Single dose doxycycline therapy for scrub typhus. Trans R Soc Trop Med Hyg 1978;72:412.
195. Olson, JG, Fang RCY, Dennis DT. Risk of relapse associated with doxycycline therapy for scrub typhus. In: Burgdorfer W, Anacker, eds. Rickettsiae and rickettsial diseases. New York: Academic Press, 1981:201.
196. Olson JG, Bourgeois AL, Fang RCY, et al. Prevention of scrub typhus, prophylactic administration of doxycycline in a randomized double blind trial. Am J Trop Med Hyg 1980;29:989–997.
197. Misao T, Kobayashi. Studies on infectious mononucleosis (glandular fever). I. Isolation of etiologic agent from blood, bone marrow, and lymph node of a patient with infectious mononucleosis by using mice. Kyushu J Med Sci 1955;6:145–152.
198. Maeda K, Markowitz N, Hawley RC, Ristic M, Cox D, McDade JE. Human infection with *Ehrlichia canis*, a leukocytic rickettsia. N Engl J Med 1987;316:853–856.
199. Kuehn NF, Gaunt SD. Clinical and hematologic findings in canine ehrlichiosis. J Am Vet Med Assoc 1985;186:355–358.
200. Keefe TJ, Holland CJ, Salyer PE, Ristic M. Distribution of *Ehrlichia canis* among military working dogs in the world and selected civilian dogs in the United States. J Am Vet Med Assoc 1982;181:236–238.
201. Magnarelli LA. Ehrlichiosis: a veterinary problem with growing epidemiologic importance. Clin Microbiol News 1990;12:145–147.
202. Centers for Disease Control. Human ehrlichiosis—United States. MMWR 1988;37:270–277.
203. Fishbein DB, Sawyer LA, Holland CJ, et al. Unexplained febrile illnesses after exposure to ticks. Infection with an *Ehrlichia?* JAMA 1987;257:3100–3104.
204. Relman DA, Loutit JS, Schmidt TM, et al. The agent of bacillary angiomatosis: an approach to the identification of uncultured pathogens. N Engl J Med 1990;323:1574–1580.
205. Perkocha LA, Geaghan SM, Yen TSB, et al. Clinical and pathological features of bacillary peliosis hepatis in association with human immunodeficiency virus infection. N Engl J Med 1990;323:1581–1586.
206. English CK, Wear DJ, Margileth AM, Lissner CR, Walsh GP. Cat-scratch disease: isolation and culture of the bacterial agent. JAMA 1988;259:1347–1352.

47 Aerobic Actinomycetes

Michael A. Saubolle

The order Actinomycetales includes a vast array of taxonomically heterogeneous genera and species, of which the majority are saprophytic and only a small minority pathogenic for humans. In most instances, actinomycetes may be found universally in the environment or as an integral part of the normal human and animal microbiota. Human infection by this group of organisms is uncommon, and when it occurs, it is most often "opportunistic." Nevertheless, there has been a recent increase in recognizable infections due to aerobic actinomycetes. This increase may in part be the result of shifts in population dynamics, including increasing age and centralization in urban areas, and to the increasing prevalence of chronic obstructive lung disease and immunocompromising conditions.

The aerobic actinomycetes cause a wide spectrum of diseases in humans, which require very different therapeutic approaches depending on the specific infecting organism. In some instances, such as with tuberculosis and leprosy, the role of the aerobic actinomycetes is well known. In others, their role is less well appreciated and their incidence may be greater than suspected. Clinical manifestations span from localized infection to disseminated disease, from acute to chronic presentation, and from tissue invasion to tissue reaction to allergens. Clinical characteristics and histopathology may vary greatly between taxa, although presentations often overlap significantly. Sometimes, arrival at the true etiology may be possible only by cultural or other techniques. Initial infection, however, almost always occurs from exogenous sources because these organisms are rarely found as normal microbial flora of humans.

With the exception of *Mycobacterium leprae*, *Mycobacterium tuberculosis* complex, and the genus *Dermatophilus*, most aerobic actinomycetes exist predominantly as saprophytes. Their presence has been noted in a wide variety of natural as well as manmade environments. Wide variation in the geographic prevalence between species contributes to their diverse epidemiology.

The large number of species present within Actinomycetales, together with the confusion and difficulty often associated with their identification, add importance to the laboratory's familiarization with more commonly isolated species. The laboratory should be able to differentiate quickly between probable saprophytes and possible pathogens, and to provide guidance to the clinician in interpreting findings and in choosing therapeutic modalities.

GENERAL ASPECTS

Microbiology (Classification)

Actinomycetes are prokaryotic bacteria that often elongate or form filaments with tendency toward some degree of true branching. Morphologic and chemical characteristics help separate these organisms into broad groups and are useful for classification and identification purposes.

Aerobic actinomycetes that produce hyphae, which later fragment into coccal elements to renew the growth cycle, can be considered as "nocardioform." The term does not, however, imply a close relationship between members of the group. Specifically, the nocardioform actinomycetes show a tendency to produce mycelia that are often transitory or fleeting and that break up quickly into coccoid or bacillary forms. Some genera in this group (*Nocardia*, *Streptomyces*, *Oerskovia*) produce thin substrates or aerial mycelia and may resemble fungi, while other genera (*Mycobacterium*, *Rhodococcus*) have rudimentary or absent mycelia, remaining most commonly in coccoid or short bacillary form (1–6). Actinomycetes that produce spores in or on their mycelia may be considered as a second group, referred to as sporoactinomycetes (the actinomadurae and streptomycetes). The genus *Dermatophilus* belongs to yet another group of actinomycetes that form mycelia and show division both transversely and longitudinally, producing multilocular, primitive sporangia (1–3).

The amino acids, carbohydrates, and lipids found in the cell wall seem to be stable in many genera, and their analysis is often helpful for organism identification. The presence of diaminopimelic acid (DAP) and its stereoisomeric configuration (meso or L-form) in clinically significant aerobic actinomycetes may be an important step in their classification and differentia-

Table 47.1. Selected Differential Characteristics of Aerobic Actinomycetes Encountered in Clinical Specimens[a,b]

Characteristic or Feature	Genus					
	Oerskovia	Nocardia	Rhodococcus	Actinomadura	Nocardiopsis	Streptomyces
Cell wall type	VI	IV	IV	III	III	I
Cell wall sugars	Galactose	Arabinose Galactose	Arabinose Galactose	Madurose	No characteristic sugars	No characteristic sugars
Size of mycolic acids (number of carbons)		40–60	34–64			
Acid-fastness[c]: weak	–[d]	+	V[e]	–	–	–
strong	–	–	–	–	–	–
Lysozyme resistance		+	V	–	–	–
Hyphal fragmentation	+ (motile)	+	+	–	–	V
Decomposition of:						
Urea	–	+	+	–	–	Somaliensis – griseus +
Casein	+	SP[e]	–	+	+	+
Tyrosine	–	SP	SP	+	+	+
Xanthine	SP	SP	?[e]	–	+	SP
Hypoxanthine	SP	SP	?	+	+	?

[a]*Mycobacterium* and *Dermathophilus* are not listed because the former is characterized in Table 47.4, and the latter is easily differentiated and rarely encountered in clinical specimens.
[b]Compiled from references 1, 6, 14, 18.
[c]Acid-fastness: weak—0.5 to 1% sulfuric acid in decolorizer; strong—3% hydrochloric acid in decolorizer.
[d]Plus and minus signs designate presence or absence, respectively, of a feature or characteristic in the majority of strains (>80 to 85%)
[e]V indicates variability; SP indicates species-dependent; ? indicates data not available.

tion from the genus *Oerskovia* and certain other saprophytic genera (1–3). The cell wall chemotype allows for further differentiation within the clinically significant actinomycetes. Cell wall type I consists of the L-isomer of DAP (*Streptomyces*); cell wall type II, of meso-DAP and glycine; cell wall type III, of meso-DAP and madurose (*Actinomadura* and *Dermatophilus*); and cell wall type IV, of meso-DAP, arabinose, and galactose (*Mycobacterium*, *Nocardia*, and *Rhodococcus*). Cell wall type VI lacks DAP but has galactose and variable amounts of aspartate (*Oerskovia*; Table 47.1) (1–3).

Mycolic acids are present in the majority of genera of clinically significant aerobic actinomycetes (e.g., the corynebacteria, mycobacteria, nocardia, and rhodococci), whereas they are absent in genera considered saprophytic (e.g., the *Faenia* aggregate including *Faenia*, *Pseudonocardia*, *Saccharomonospora*, *Saccharopolyspora*, and *Actinopolyspora*), as well as in *Oerskovia* (1–3). The mycolic acid–containing genera can be differentiated further by the overall size (number of carbons) of the mycolates into the corynebacteria (containing small corynomycolates), the nocardia (medium nocardomycolates), and the mycobacteria (large mycolates) (Table 47.1). Additionally, mycobacteria, nocardia, and rhodococci may be differentiated from corynebacteria by the absence of tuberculostearic acid in the latter organisms (1–3).

Traditionally, initial identification of the aerobic actinomycetes requires recognition of their individual colonial and microscopic morphologies and staining characteristics. Unfortunately, some of the genera frequently resemble each other, and at times it may be hard to differentiate them. Evaluation of growth rates and patterns, delineation of antibiograms, and limited biochemical studies may provide further information as to an isolate's identity. More definitive identification requires analysis of whole cell hydrolysates for characteristic components such as sugars and lipids, together with more extensive biochemical testing. Recently, newer techniques such as nucleic acid probes, immunoassay, gas liquid chromatography, and high-pressure liquid chromatography have been applied with some success for the identification of some genera and species (7–13).

Diagnostic Procedures

LABORATORY SAFETY CONSIDERATIONS

Laboratories processing specimens for the detection, isolation, and identification of aerobic actinomycetes and especially of mycobacteria should ensure that safety measures are in place and that safety procedures are appropriately implemented and enforced. Biosafety level 2 practices, equipment, and facilities are suggested for processing specimens for inoculation to isolation media and the preparation of smears. Biosafety level 3 conditions are suggested for performing identification studies and working with large inocula of isolated mycobacteria (6, 14, 15).

Appropriate facilities must be available for working with mycobacterial cultures and should include a separate, dedicated room maintained at negative pressure to the rest of the laboratory. The room should contain a laminar-flow biological safety cabinet equipped with a high-efficiency filtration system, an adequate air draw across the front, and an ultraviolet light for surface decontamination. An autoclave should be present in an adjacent area to decontaminate infectious waste prior to transport to disposal areas. High-speed centrifuges should be equipped with bucket covers and domes to contain possible broken tubes. Electric incinerators rather than Bunsen burners should be utilized to avoid splatters. A container of sand and 95% alcohol or a 5% phenol solution should also be available to clean wires, spades, or loops prior to their insertion in the incinerator.

Gloves, masks, caps, and gowns should be worn when working with cultures. All procedures should minimize aerosol production while maximizing protection from infection by droplet nuclei. All personnel working in the laboratory should be given tuberculin skin tests biannually to elucidate any conversions.

LABORATORY PROFICIENCY CONSIDERATIONS

Not all laboratories can be expected to have the facilities, volume, or expertise to work with the aerobic actinomycetes, and especially with the mycobacteria, within adequate safety or proficiency parameters. The College of American Pathologists (CAP) and the American Thoracic Society (ATS) have recommended progressive extents (CAP) and levels (ATS) of proficiency of services rendered by laboratories for the diagnosis of mycobacterial diseases (7, 8, 14, 16).

CAP

Four extents of services are recognized. *Extent 1* laboratories perform no mycobacteriologic procedures, referring all such work to reference laboratories. *Extent 2* laboratories may perform direct acid-fast stains and initial inoculations onto isolation media with referral of any isolates to a reference laboratory for identification. *Extent 3* laboratories should be able to isolate and separate *M. tuberculosis* (MTB) from the nontuberculous mycobacteria (NTM). They should be capable of identifying the former while providing preliminary group identities for the latter (e.g., photochromogens, scotochromogens, rapid growers). Antimicrobial susceptibility studies may or may not be performed by extent 3 laboratories. *Extent 4*, the last level recognized, refers to laboratories capable of definitive mycobacterial identification to the extent necessary for establishing a correct diagnosis and for selecting appropriate therapy. Susceptibility studies, however, may or may not be performed.

ATS

Three levels of proficiency of laboratory service are recognized. *Level 1* laboratories should be proficient at accepting adequate clinical specimens and transferring them to an appropriate level laboratory; direct acid-fast smears may be prepared and examined if a volume of 10 to 15 specimens a week is available. Otherwise, smears should be referred to a level 2 laboratory. *Level 2* laboratories may additionally process specimens for culture, identify *M. tuberculosis*, and perform susceptibility studies. They may be expected to retain isolates for 6 months in case other studies are necessary; a volume of 20 specimens a week is suggested to maintain proficiency. *Level 3* laboratories should be capable of all studies performed by level 1 and 2 laboratories. In addition, they should be able to identify mycobacterial species, perform susceptibility studies, and provide training while conducting research.

PRIMARY ISOLATION

In most instances, isolation of an agent causing disease is necessary to provide definitive identification and to perform antimicrobial susceptibility studies when such are available. Specific isolation methods for individual groups of aerobic actinomycetes vary widely. Methods that are optimal for the recovery of groups such as the mycobacteria may not be suitable for groups such as the actinomadura or streptomyces. For some actinomycetes (e.g., *Mycobacterium leprae*), isolation methods are not routinely available, while for others, isolation methods may require selective concentration, decontamination, and/or culture onto specialized media for optimal recovery.

Methods of specimen collection and transport to the laboratory directly influence the detection and isolation of the aerobic actinomycetes. Not all laboratories should be capable of isolation or detection of all genera of actinomycetes. Still, they should be able to provide information to enhance collection techniques and to expedite specimen transportation with minimum delay and maximum quality assurance.

Many different types of specimens may be submitted for isolation and/or detection of aerobic actinomycetes. The exact types of specimens to be evaluated are usually predicated on the clinical presentation of the patient, the organ system or tissue involved, and the suspected etiology.

The majority of specimens from mycobacterial or nocardial infections are from the respiratory tract, followed by lymph node tissue, urine, other tissue, and normally sterile body fluids. Specimens from patients with the acquired immunodeficiency syndrome (AIDS) may include blood and stool. Specimens from actinomycotic mycetomas may include pus, serosanguinous fluid, sinus scrapings, or other biopsy material.

The slower growth of the actinomycetes becomes a problem when other rapidly growing organisms are present in the specimen; such normal or contaminating flora may overgrow the etiologic agent. Collection methods should therefore bypass areas of contamination. In some instances, specimens containing mixed flora should be processed to eliminate the contamination or be inoculated onto selective media to allow the pathogens a chance to grow. All specimens should be refrigerated if not processed within a few hours.

Mailing

The packaging of specimens or cultures to be mailed to reference laboratories must adhere to the Code of Federal Regulations. Screw-cap, watertight tubes must be used. These must be placed within a second watertight container (usually metallic) with enough absorbent material capable of taking up liquid in case of breakage. One or more of these can be packed into containers made of paperboard wood and mailed only after appropriate warning labels are attached (7, 8, 15, 17).

DIRECT DETECTION

Microscopic evaluation of specimens can provide rapid information on the presence or absence of (*a*) the possible etiologic agent, (*b*) infected material characterized by polymorphonuclear or mononuclear leukocytes, or (*c*) contamination characterized by squamous epithelial cells. A variety of wet-mount, Gram-stain, or other special stains may be used to detect the aerobic actinomycetes either directly from specimens (sputum, pus, tissue, stool, etc.) or after their decontamination and/or concentration (e.g., specimens for mycobacteria, normally sterile body fluids). Newer molecular-based technologies offer promise for alternative, more sensitive direct detection methods and will soon become more generally available.

Serologic Procedures

The complexity, heterogeneity, and cross-reactivity of antigens among the aerobic actinomycetes have historically precluded the routine use of serologic techniques for diagnosis. Available reagents and immunoassays are currently neither adequately sensitive nor specific for clinical applications. Recent methods based on enzyme-linked immunosorbent assays provide some hope that production and purification of antigens may in the future lead to clinically useful serologic studies for mycobacteria and nocardia. Preparation of such antigens is feasible, as was shown by the isolation of a 55-kd protein of nocardia, which, when used in enzyme immunosorbent assay, was found to provide adequate test sensitivity and specificity. Such applications, however, are only in their initial stages. More information will be necessary to provide standard, interpretable serologic tests (10, 18–22).

Skin tests may be of value, both in mycobacteriosis and in actinomycotic mycetoma. Reviews of skin tests and their interpretation and significance can be found elsewhere and are not discussed in this chapter (8, 19, 23).

Interpretation of Data

The presence of some genera of aerobic actinomycetes in clinical material is highly associated with an active disease process. Thus, identification of MTB, *M. leprae*, or *Dermatophilus congolensis* in patients is always considered significant. Correlation of other groups of actinomycetes, such as the NTM and nocardia, with disease is more difficult. The environmental prevalence of many actinomycetes, coupled with their low virulence, increases the difficulty of interpreting their causal role in an infectious process.

Therapeutic Considerations

Therapeutic regimens for aerobic actinomycetes vary considerably according to the infecting species, the disease process, and the immunocompetency of the patient. Surgical intervention supplements or supplants antimicrobial therapy in some instances. Although standardized procedures for susceptibility studies do not exist for all genera or species, methods for a few have been developed adequately enough to provide guidance (e.g., the nocardia and mycobacteria). In other cases, the disease is self-limited, and therapeutic intervention is not normally required (e.g., dermatophilosis).

This chapter focuses on the characteristics of the genera *Mycobacterium*, *Nocardia*, and *Rhodococcus*. The genera *Actinomadura*, *Nocardiopsis*, *Streptomyces*, *Oerskovia*, and *Dermatophilus* are briefly reviewed (Table 47.2). The corynebacteria and the anaerobic and thermophilic actinomycetes are not discussed.

Table 47.2. Clinically Significant Aerobic Actinomycetes

Genus	Species	More Commonly Associated Infections
Actinomadura	*A. madurae* and *A. pelletieri* most significant; soil organisms	Mycetoma
Dermatophilus	*D. congolensis* the only sp.; obligate animal parasite	Pustular, exudative dermatitis
Mycobacterium	*M. leprae, M. tuberculosis, M. africanum* and *M. bovis* obligate pathogens	*M. leprae*: leprosy, *M. tuberculosis, M. africanum, M. bovis*: tuberculosis
	Other spp. of nontubercular mycobacteria (NTM) are only potential pathogens	NTM: pulmonary, abscesses, systemic
Nocardia	Of nine presently recognized spp., only *N. asteroides* complex (common), *N. brasiliensis* (uncommon), *N. otitidiscaviarum* (rare), and *N. transvalensis* (very rare) are associated with disease; found in soil and organic debris	*N. asteroides*: lungs, abscesses, systemic *N. brasiliensis, N. otitidiscaviarum*: localized abscess, mycetoma
Nocardiopsis	*N. dassonvillei* significant but rare	Mycetoma
Oerskovia	Two spp.: *O. turbata* and *O. xanthineolytica*; associated with soil	Bacteremia, endocarditis, peritonitis; associated with foreign bodies
Rhodococcus	*R. equi* most commonly associated with disease; some other incertae sedis and unidentified species have been implicated	Bacteremia, pneumonia, endophthalmitis, peritonitis
Gordona	*G. bronchialis* and *G. terrae* are potentially significant	Skin and pulmonary
Tsukamurella	*T. paurametabolum* to replace *R. aurantiacus*	Abscesses, synovitis
Streptomyces	Over 700 spp., but only *S. somaliensis* and *S. griseus* commonly asscoiated with disease; soil organisms	Abscess, mycetoma

MYCOBACTERIUM

Microbiology (Classification)

The genus *Mycobacterium* consists of a diverse group of strongly acid-fast bacilli (AFB) with high lipid content. The lipids in the cell and its wall include waxes with characteristic long-chain (60- to 90-carbon) mycolic (fatty) acids.

The diversity in the genus *Mycobacterium* is manifested by variability in morphology, growth rate characteristics, nutritional and temperature requirements, as well as pathogenicity. There are over 54 species of mycobacteria currently recognized, but fewer than 25 species are more commonly associated with human infections (Table 47.3) (3, 7, 24). *M. tuberculosis* (MTB), *M. bovis*, *M. africanum*, and *M. leprae* have a high propensity for causing disease and are always considered as pathogens. With the exception of *M. leprae*, the causative agent of leprosy, they all cause classic tuberculosis and form the *M. tuberculosis* complex. There is presently some doubt as to the individual status of the genus *M. africanum*, which biochemically and by DNA relatedness studies may be indistinct from MTB (24).

Mycobacteria that do not belong to the MTB complex have been designated by several terms, including "anonymous," "atypical," "mycobacteria other than tuberculosis" (MOTT), "opportunistically pathogenic mycobacteria," and "nontuberculous mycobacteria" (NTM).

Originally, colonial morphology and chromogenicity (carotenoid pigmentation) were used to categorize species of NTM. Additionally, growth rates of species were incorporated into the categorization method to delineate divisional units referred to as Runyon groups (Table 47.3). The Runyon groups included the pigmented photochromogens (group I: yellow to orange pigment development after exposure to light; Fig. 47.1) and scotochromogens (group II: pigment development in the dark), the normally colorless nonphotochromogens (group III; Fig. 47.2) and the rapid growers (group IV). This classification was useful, but not completely accurate, because some species' characteristic chromogenicity and growth rates are influenced by other environmental factors such as temperature (7, 8, 14, 16, 24, 25).

The spectrum of biochemical activity of culturable mycobacterial species also provides a useful tool for classification and identification. Species of NTM that biochemically and pathogenically resemble each other may be considered as complexes, and further differentiation is not normally clinically required. Because it is difficult to differentiate biochemically between *Mycobacterium avium* and *Mycobacterium intracellulare*, the two may be grouped together as the *M. avium* complex (MAC). However, the previously suggested Mycobacterium fortuitum complex should not be used to group the rapid growers *M. fortuitum* and *M. chelonae*, because they can be easily differentiated biochemically and have differences in antimicrobial susceptibility profiles (14, 24).

The genus *M. fortuitum* itself is heterogeneous, being composed of at least two biovars and a third biovariant complex. *M. chelonae* comprises two easily separable subspecies, *chelonae* and *abscessus*, as well as a group of *chelonae*-like organisms that have not

Table 47.3. Mycobacterial Species More Commonly Encountered in Clinical Specimens in the United States[a]

Group (Characteristic)	Species: Obligately Pathogenic	Species: Probably or Potentially Pathogenic[b]	Species: Probably Saprophytic/ Rarely Pathogenic[c]
Tuberculosis complex (slow growth; nonpigmented)	*M. tuberculosis* *M. bovis* *M. leprae*		
I. Photochromogens (slow growth; light stimulated pigment)		*M. kansasii* *M. simiae* *M. marinum*	
II. Scotochromogens (slow growth; pigmented irrespective of light)		*M. scrofulaceum* *M. xenopi* *M. szulgai*[d]	*M. flavescens* *M. gordonae*
III. Nonphotochromogens (slow growth; nonpigmented)		*M. avium* *M. intracellulare* *M. haemophilum*	*M. gastri* *M. terrae* *M. triviale*
IV. Rapid growers (growth within 7 days; nonpigmented)		*M. fortuitum* *M. chelonae*	*M. smegmatis*

[a]Compiled from 24, 28.
[b]Other potentially pathogenic species include *M. malmoense, M. asiaticum,* and *M. ulcerans* (obligate pathogen).
[c]Other rarely pathogenic, commonly saprophytic species: *M. neoaurum, M. nonchromogenicum, M. parafortuitum* complex, *M. paratuberculosis, M. phlei, M. thermoresistibile,* and *M. vaccae*.
[d]Photochromogenic at 25°C, but scotochromogenic at 35°C.

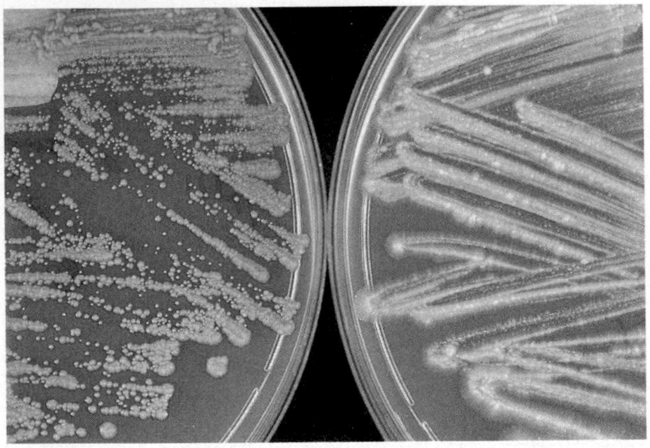

Figure 47.1. Colonies of the photochromogen *Mycobacterium kansasii* showing typical formation of carotenoid pigmentation only after exposure to light (*left*) and not when kept in the dark (*right*).

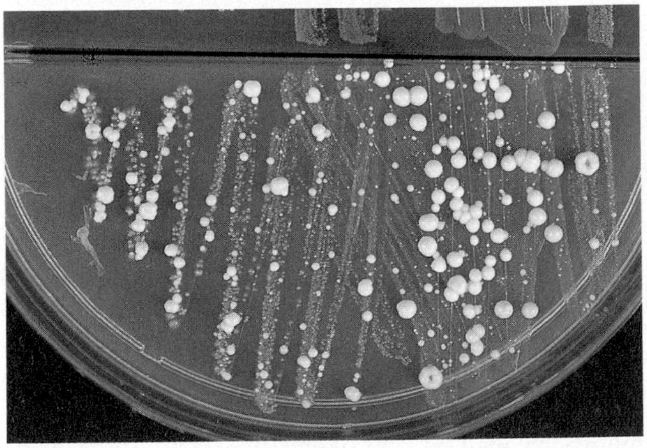

Figure 47.2. Nonpigmented colonies of members of the *Mycobacterium avium-intracellulare* complex.

yet been completely taxonomically characterized. It is significant that these groupings are supported by a variety of classification methods, including biochemical, immunologic, numerical taxonomic, and DNA homology methods, as well as by clinical response to various antimicrobial agents.

Recently, applications of DNA/DNA hybridization techniques for species relatedness and high-performance liquid chromatography for mycolic acid patterns have facilitated the differentiation of species (7, 8). Results of some of these studies have reaffirmed or cast doubt upon the status of some mycobacterial species. Thus, the separate species status of *M. avium* and *M. intracellulare* was reaffirmed, while that of *M. africanum* was deemed as probably unjustified. Such methods have only recently become more commonly available to clinical laboratories, and their routine application is becoming feasible for cost-effective identification in clinical practice.

Esoteric identification methods such as bacteriophage typing and serotyping may at times be useful for epidemiologic study (7). However, their poor reproducibility and specificity, together with the difficulty of standardizing of test systems, have made them unsuccessful as routine tools for mycobacterial classification.

Spectrum of Disease

M. leprae, a pathogenic member of the mycobacteria, is the causative agent of leprosy. The clinical phases of leprosy are broad, ranging from the primary silent (replication of organisms in skin macrophage) and indeterminate (replication in peripheral nerves) phases to the more severe tuberculoid and lepromatous states. Erythematous or hypopigmented skin lesions and damage to peripheral nerves are characteristic and may be progressive, depending on the stage of the disease process (26).

Members of the MTB complex, primarily transmitted person to person via droplet nuclei and the respiratory tract, produce the well-known clinical entity of tuberculosis. In the normal host, MTB remains the primary etiology of pulmonary (85% of cases) as well as of extrapulmonary (15% of cases) tuberculosis in the United States. There is an increased risk of dissemination in the immunocompromised patient (8). The risk of patients developing clinical disease within the first year of being infected is approximately 5%, but declines thereafter. However, risk of reactivation increases with the decrease of cellular immunity in the elderly.

Primary tuberculosis may be considered an infection of the reticuloendothelial system. The organisms are ingested but not inactivated by alveolar macrophage and polymorphonuclear cells, pass through the lymphatics, and finally enter the bloodstream to reseed the lungs or other sites. Extrapulmonary sites may include lymph nodes (28%), spinal column, as well as meninges (5%), genitourinary tract (13%), bone and joint (10%), peritoneal cavity (4%), and bone marrow. Miliary tuberculosis includes the simultaneous infection of several sites and is seen in approximately 10% of extrapulmonary cases. Pulmonary disease may be acute and rapidly progressive or chronic with cavitation (8).

The NTM, unlike the obligately pathogenic members of the mycobacteria, are far less invasive and require an underlying factor present in the patient to be able to successfully colonize and cause progressive disease. Members of MAC and, to a lesser extent, *Mycobacterium kansasii* have a predilection for patients having been immunocompromised by AIDS or malignancy, or for those having chronic pulmonary disease with parenchymal lung damage. Percutaneous trauma (surgery, catheterization, accidental puncture) increases the risk for infection with *M. fortuitum* and *M. chelonae* (23, 25, 27).

Clinical presentation with infection due to the NTM primarily includes pulmonary (81%), lymph (7%), and cutaneous/soft tissue (2%) sites, but may also involve peritoneal, joint/bone, ocular, gastrointestinal, heart valve, meningeal, and urogenital sites. Dissemination may also occur, especially in the severely immunocompromised host; members of MAC account for the majority of disseminated cases (96%), but other species may also disseminate (24, 25, 28).

Members of MAC and *M. kansasii* are the most commonly encountered mycobacterial pathogens causing chronic pulmonary disease in the United States. Indistinguishable, indolent but potentially progressive lung disease may occasionally be caused by *M. chelonae*, *M. fortuitum*, *M. xenopi*, *M. simiae*, *M. malmoense*, and *M. szulgai*. Recently, members of MAC have become implicated in the invasion of the gastrointestinal mucosa and dissemination into blood of patients with AIDS; in such patients, the respiratory tract may not be as commonly involved. Interestingly, *M. avium* may be more virulent than *M. intacellulare*, accounting for the majority of infections.

Cervical lymphadenopathy, often encountered in immunocompetent pediatric patients, is commonly caused by NTM. Members of MAC are again the most common cause, although *Mycobacterium scrofulaceum* may also be encountered in this setting. Other reported etiologies include *M. kansasii* and, more recently, *Mycobacterium haemophilum* (24, 25).

Several species of NTM favor reduced growth temperatures and characteristically infect cooler cutaneous or subcutaneous areas. Localized papulonodular skin lesions at sites contacting unchlorinated fresh or salt water are caused by *Mycobacterium marinum*. *Mycobacterium ulcerans*, encountered primarily in Australia, Africa, and Mexico, causes a subcutaneous infection that can progress to ulceration. *M. haemophilum* has been associated with chronic skin lesions in immunocompromised patients as well as with cervical lymphadenopathy in immunocompetent patients (24, 25, 28).

M. chelonei and *M. fortuitum* have emerged as major opportunistic pathogens infecting previously traumatized soft tissue such as that associated with penetrating wounds, sternotomies, mammoplasties, percutaneous catheter insertions, and keratitis/corneal ulcerations. These species have also been reported in association with cases of prosthetic valve endocarditis, osteomyelitis, synovitis, meningitis, and disseminated disease (28).

Other species of NTM (e.g., *Mycobacterium gordonae*, *Mycobacterium flavescens*, *Mycobacterium terrae*, *Mycobacterium asiaticum*, *Mycobacterium gastri*, *Mycobacterium thermoresistibile*, *Mycobacterium neoaurum*) are commonly considered contaminants in culture and are rarely associated with human disease. Occasional associations with infections in immunocompromised patients, however, have been documented. Evidence for other causal associations between NTM and certain syndromes (e.g., between *Mycobacterium paratuberculosis* and some cases of Crohn's disease) has been accumulating, but has not yet been adequately verified (25).

Epidemiology

The mycobacteria commonly associated with disease in humans and considered always to be pathogenic, are not found free-living in nature, but remain obligate animal parasites. Leprosy and tuberculosis occur worldwide. The former, caused by *M. leprae*, afflicts over 10 million people, especially in third-world or underdeveloped countries. Person-to-person transmission through contact with intact or abraded skin, as well as by deposition on the nasal mucosa through inhalation is increased by crowded conditions and close contact (26).

Tuberculosis, caused by MTB, *M. bovis*, and, in Africa, by *M. africanum*, causes approximately 2 to 3 million deaths and 8 to 10 million new cases each year. In the United States, infection caused by *M. bovis* has been almost eradicated by curtailment of its presence in cattle and by control of its transmission in raw milk using pasteurization. Control of dissemination of *M. tuberculosis* is more problematic, although mortality due to tuberculosis had begun to decline in the western world as a result of improved living conditions and efficacious therapeutic modalities introduced in the 1940s. That trend, however, was slowed and even reversed in the United States within the past decade. The highest number of cases were reported in the larger metropolitan areas such as New York, Los Angeles, Miami, Dallas, and San Francisco. Possible reasons for this increased number of cases include reactivation of organisms or rapid progression of new infection in patients with AIDS, the influx of immigrants from abroad, a growing homeless population, and an elevation in the ages of the elderly. To reverse the present trend, it will be necessary to improve case and contact finding through screening programs, together with the use of chemoprophylaxis, especially in high-risk groups (8).

Unlike members of the *M. tuberculosis* complex, the NTM are easily found in the environment, being isolated from soil, water, sewage, house dust, air, and raw milk. Infection of humans occurs by normally unpreventable ingestion, inhalation, or inoculation from environmental sources, and person-to-person spread does not occur. Control of the acquisition of infection is extremely difficult (23–25, 28).

The NTM inhabit a wide variety of ecological niches. Sometimes, their presence in some locations may bring them in closer proximity to a human population and to increased isolation from clinical specimens. Thus, the isolation of members of MAC from water supplied to large metropolitan areas and specific sources in hospitals as well as homes may have clinical implications. These organisms have also been noted in air, water, dust, soil, plants, and animals.

Other members of NTM have been isolated from environmental sources such as soil, water, and dust (*M. fortuitum*, *M. chelonae*), soil, water, milk, and oysters (*M. scrofulaceum*), untreated fresh or salt water (*M. marinum*), and water as well as animals (*M. xenopi*, *M. simiae*). *M. xenopi* has also been isolated from birds, coastal areas, and human tonsils, while *M. simiae* has been isolated from monkeys. Although *M. kansasii* has, on several occasions, been isolated from water, its overall ecological habitat is not known. Environmental sources for *M. haemophilum*, *Mycobacterium szulgai*, *Mycobacterium malmoense*, *Mycobacterium ulcerans*, and the more fastidious mycobacteria also remain unknown (23, 25).

The incidence of members of MAC is highest in the southeastern part of the United States, although high isolation rates have been reported from the southwest, Hawaii, Kansas, several states bordering Canada, the Gulf of Mexico, and along the Atlantic coast. This pattern is probably related to the association of *M. avium* with coastal plains and surface waters rather than mountainous areas and groundwater sources. *M. kansasii* has a characteristic incidence pattern that includes west-south-central areas and extends along the southern border of the United States between California and Florida.

In terms of isolation rates, members of MAC have the greatest incidence, followed by *M. kansasii*. Together, the two genera may make up 75 to 85% of all significant isolates of NTM in the clinical laboratory. Members of MAC are less likely to be considered clinically significant (45 to 47%) than *M. kansasii* (72 to 75%). Isolation rates of other NTM drop off sharply with *M. fortuitum* and *M. chelonae*, making up 12 to 15%; and the remaining species, in aggregate, less than 10% of all isolates (25, 28). Whereas previously the NTM were typically isolated from middle-aged, white males residing in rural areas, several epidemiologic changes have recently been noted with the incidence of infection having increased as a whole.

Diagnostic Procedures

SPECIMEN COLLECTION

Respiratory Tract

Normally, three to five expectorated sputum samples collected on several different early mornings are sufficient to detect mycobacteria. Additional samples do not improve recovery. Specimens pooled over a 24-hour period are not acceptable because of their increased contamination and slower recovery rate.

Sputum should originate from deep in the lung, and the patient should be advised on how to cough appropriately. Rinsing the mouth with water may decrease contamination. Screening for upper respiratory tract contamination is not necessary, but there should be evidence of lower tract secretions in the specimen provided (7, 15, 17).

Specimens from patients unable to produce sputum on their own may be collected by including coughing by nebulization of 5 to 10% saline or by bronchoscopy. Frequently, several expectorated sputum specimens collected a day or two after bronchoscopy enhance the detection of mycobacteria. In some difficult patients, transthoracic needle or open-lung biopsies may be attempted, with the latter method having the best yield. In all cases, the method of collection should be noted on the requisition.

Each specimen should be 5 to 10 ml and may be collected or transported in 50-ml centrifuge tubes. If specimens are to be mailed to a reference laboratory, 1% cetylpyridinium chloride with 2% sodium chloride may be added to the sputum as an initial decontamination step prior to shipping; AFB may survive up to 8 days in transit using this technique.

Gastric Washings

Aspiration of swallowed sputum from the stomach is reserved for patients unable to provide sputum by other means, usually the obtunded or the young. The procedure is performed early in the morning and on an empty stomach. Gastric aspirations should be processed rapidly, or 100 mg of sodium bicarbonate should be added as a buffer.

Normally Sterile Body Fluids

Specimens in this category may include 2 to 5 ml of cerebrospinal fluid (CSF), pericardial or synovial fluids, 10 to 15 ml of peritoneal, bile, paracentesis, dialysis fluid, or pleural fluid, and 3 to 5 ml of exudates. Such specimens should be collected in sterile screw-cap containers. Body fluids may be diluted in saline or a buffer to allow the relatively buoyant acid-fast bacilli to sediment adequately during centrifugation.

Tissue

Surgical biopsies should be submitted in sterile nonbacteriostatic saline to keep them from dehydrating. Larger pieces can be cut up and homogenized in a mechanized tissue grinder or ground in a mortar and pestle. Specimens that cannot be processed immediately may be frozen at −20°C for transport.

Urine

Appropriate cleansing of genitalia should precede collection of the first morning voided urine specimens. Each specimen should have a minimum of 15 ml, and the entire voided volume is preferable. Three to five specimens collected over as many days are normally adequate. Twenty-four–hour pooled specimens are not acceptable because acid-fast bacilli may be harmed by long-term exposure to urine. Specimens may be stored for short periods at 4°C.

Sinus Tracts

Caution must be used in collecting drainage material from sinus tracts, which are notorious for being easily contaminated or colonized. Attempts at collecting by needle aspiration or biopsy are preferable. Swabs are poor substitutes for exudates or biopsies, and often will decrease yields. When used, swabs should be inoculated directly to solid or broth media.

Blood

Isolation of mycobacteria, nocardia, or rhodococci from blood is possible, primarily in immunocompromised patients, and such attempts should be reserved for such patients. Mycobacteria are especially prevalent in patients with AIDS. Blood should be collected in the Isolator lysis-centrifugation (E. I. du Pont de Nemours) system or inoculated into the Bactec (Johnston Laboratories) blood culture system for mycobacteria.

Stool

Stool specimens are recommended only for the detection of mycobacterial involvement of the gastrointestinal tracts of patients with AIDS. Swabs are not acceptable. Rather, stool specimens should be submitted in clean containers or in stool transport systems. Some workers suggest culturing stool only if their smears show the presence of acid-fast bacilli. The stool can be emulsified in 5 ml of Dubos albumin broth and processed like a sputum sample after overnight incubation at 35°C. Fresh specimens not processed immediately may be frozen at −20°C.

PRIMARY ISOLATION

Specimens considered to contain normal or superinfecting bacterial flora that can overgrow the much slower growing mycobacteria must be processed to remove or decrease the contaminants. Methods for decontamination include strong alkali, acid, or other chemicals to which the lipid-rich mycobacteria are more resistant than other bacteria. However, mycobacteria are also influenced by the decontamination procedure, with only 10 to 20% of their numbers surviving in clinical specimens. Therefore, the most gentle decontamination methods are used as necessary, with harsher methods being reserved for highly contaminated specimens containing organisms such as the pseudomonads, which are more resistant to normal procedures. Procedural steps must be followed carefully to prevent decreased survival of mycobacteria. The high lipid content of mycobacteria is responsible for their greater buoyancy in clinical specimens and especially in liquids and body fluids. Therefore, mucoid specimens such as sputum, or those with high specific gravity or density, must be digested, liquefied, and/or diluted prior to concentration of AFB. Centrifugation must be performed for 15 to 30 minutes at a minimum relative centrifugal force of 2000*g* and preferably at a force approaching 3000 to 4000*g* (7, 8, 14–16).

Most concentration procedures employ combinations of mucolytic agents together with decontaminating agents. The most commonly used agents include *N*-acetyl-L-cysteine or alternatively, dithiothreitol (Sputolysin) as mucolytic agents, combined with 2% sodium hydroxide as a decontaminant. Another acceptable decontamination method incorporates benzalkonium chloride (Zephiran) with trisodium phosphate. Use of oxalic acid combined with a mucolytic agent is beneficial for specimens that are heavily contaminated with Gram-negative rods. Specimens requiring decontamination and concentration normally include sputum (inclusive of specimens collected by bronchoscopy), urine, gastric aspirates, stool, and contaminated tissue or swabs of pus. Heavy contamination with Gram-negative rods and especially pseudomonads may be expected in sputum from patients with cystic fibrosis or bronchiectasis due to other etiologies.

Decontamination is unnecessary for specimens such as normally sterile body fluids or tissue biopsies that are not expected to be contaminated by normal bacterial flora. If any question as to sterility status of a specimen exists, it may be advisable to first culture a portion of the specimen overnight in nutrient broth or agar to detect bacterial overgrowth prior to processing for AFB.

Primary isolation media may include nonselective egg-based media, agar-base media, and liquid media or modifications of these to formulate selective media. Egg-based media such as Lowenstein-Jensen, Petragnani, and American Thoracic Society usually contain products that make them opaque. Although all three media maximize recovery of mycobacteria, Lowenstein-Jensen media are commonly preferred for optimal performance. Agar-base media such as Middlebrook, Cohn, 7H10, and 7H11, are clear and therefore help in visualization of early mycobacterial growth; such early detection of colonies is enhanced by using a dissecting microscope. Liquid media include formulations such as the 7H9 broth and Dubos broth (16).

Selective media normally contain antimicrobial agents to inhibit bacterial and fungal contamination. These may include modifications of Lowenstein-Jensen media (Gruft modification and mycobactosel) or of 7H10 (Middlebrook medium) and 7H11 (Mitchison's medium). Recently, a liquid 7H12 broth medium was introduced that had the same characteristics as the modified, selective 7H11 medium, but with an added ^{14}C radiolabeled fatty acid component (Bactec; Johnston Laboratories). Growth in this medium is detected radiometrically by measuring the release of CO_2 and following a growth index. The new Bactec mycobacterial media and detection system has increased recovery of members of MAC and has reduced the overall time to recovery of mycobacteria by 1 to 3 weeks (7, 9, 16). It has also allowed the recovery of the more fastidious mycobacteria.

To maximize recovery, use of at least two primary solid media is recommended. Additionally, normally sterile specimens should be inoculated to a broth medium such as 7H9 broth. When the Bactec system is being used, one of the agar media may be omitted. A popular combination includes a Bactec 12B medium with two Lowenstein-Jensen egg-based agar slants. 7H10 or 7H11 media are not normally recommended for primary isolation, but may be very useful for evaluation of susceptibilities or of colonial morphologies, as well as being excellent primary media when modified to become selective. Isolation of *M. haemophilum* requires the additional use of chocolate or blood agars, or media containing hemin or 1% ferric ammonium citrate.

Cultures should be incubated at 35° to 37°C in 5 to 10% CO_2 in the dark. Glass bottles or tubes should initially be kept at a slant with caps loosened to allow CO_2 entry. Plates may be placed in CO_2-permeable polyethylene bags and incubated inverted. Cultures may be incubated in ambient air after the first 2 to 3 weeks. Specimens from topical skin lesions, lymph nodes, and the environment should be incubated at both 30°C and 35° to 37°C to enhance growth of mycobacteria preferring lower temperatures (*M. marinum*, *M. haemophilum*, and *M. ulcerans*). Cultures should be held for 8 weeks, although some workers feel that 6 weeks is adequate if a Bactec system is also used. Examination for growth should occur twice weekly for the first 4 weeks and once weekly thereafter (7, 8, 14, 16, 17).

IDENTIFICATION METHODS

The mycobacteria are generally straight or slightly curved rods measuring 0.3 to 0.6 μm × 1 to 4 μm. Mycelia are rarely observed, and when produced, fragment easily into coccobacillary units.

On traditional agar media, growth rate differentiates the mycobacteria: rapid growers require less than 7 days for visual recognition under optimal conditions; slow growers require more than 7 days. With additional use of pigmentation and some key bio-

Table 47.4. Major Differentiating Tests for More Common Mycobacterial Isolates[a]

Runyon Group	*Mycobacterium* Species	Niacin	Nitrate Reduction	Catalase: Semiquantitative (>45 mm)	Catalase: Heat-Stable	Tween 80 Hydrolysis (5-day)	Tellurite Reduction	Urease	Arylsulfatase (3-day)
	tuberculosis	+[b]	+	−	−	−	V(−)	V(+)	−
	bovis	−	−	−	−	−	V(+)	V(+)	−
I.	*kansasii*	−	+	+	+	+	V(−)	V(−)	−
	simiae	V(+)	−	+	+	−	+	V(+)	−
	marinum	−	−	−	−	+	V(−)	+	V(−)
II.	*scrofulacium*	−	−	+	+	−	V(−)	V(+)	−
	xenopi	−	−	−	V(−)	−	V(−)	−	V(−)
	szulgai	−	+	+	+	V(−)	V(+)	+	V(−)
	gordonae	−	−	+	+	+	−	V(−)	−
	flavescens	−	+	+	+	+	V(−)	+	−
III.	*avium-complex*	−	−	−	V(+)	−	+	−	−
	gastri	−	−	−	−	+	V(+)	V(−)	−
	terrae-complex	−	+	+	+	+	V(−)	−	−
IV.	*fortuitum*	−	+	+	+	V	V(+)	+	+
	chelonae	V(−)	−	+	V(+)	V(−)	V(+)	+	+
	smegmatis		+	+	+	+	+		−

[a]Compiled from references 15, 16, 24.
[b]Plus signs and minus signs designate the presence or absence, respectively, of a feature or capability in the majority (>80 to 85%) of strains; V indicates variability, while the (+) or (−) signs following the V indicate a greater or lesser percent, respectively, of strains having a feature or capability.

chemical studies, it is possible to identify most of the more common clinical isolates (Table 47.4).

Members of the strictly pathogenic MTB complex are slow growers and, having buff-colored colonies, are considered nonpigmented. Selection of key tests for this group of organisms should include production of niacin and heat-stable catalase as well as evaluation for nitrate reduction (Table 47.4). Susceptibility to thiophen-2-carboxylic acid hydrazide (TCH) further differentiates *M. bovis* from MTB (7, 8, 14–16).

Nontuberculous mycobacteria may be differentiated by growth rate and pattern of pigment production into the four Runyon groups. *M. chelonae* and *M. fortuitum* are not pigmented, but these rapid growers may have carotenoid pigments. A few species of NTM may have varying characteristics of pigment production, thereby limiting the usefulness of the Runyon classification. Thus, on occasion, *M. szulgai* may slow scotochromogenicity at 35°C and photochromogenicity at 25°C; rarely, scotochromogenic strains of the normally photochromogenic *M. kansasii*, as well as slightly pigmented strains of nonphotochromogens, may be encountered.

Identification of species may be accomplished using the following key biochemical tests: photochromogens—nitrate reduction, Tween 80 hydrolysis, arylsulfatase, and growth at 30°C and 35°C; scotochromogens—nitrate reduction, semiquantitative catalase, Tween 80 hydrolysis, urease, arylsulfatase, and tolerance to 5% sodium chloride; nonphotochromogens—nitrate and tellurite reduction, semiquantitative and heat-stable catalase, and Tween 80 hydrolysis; rapid growers—nitrate reduction and tolerance to 5% sodium chloride. Thorough descriptions of test methods and extensive biochemical reaction keys have recently been published (7, 8, 14, 16, 17).

Susceptibility profiles may be helpful in differentiating the clinically significant rapid growers to biovariant (*M. fortuitum* biovars *fortuitum*, *peregrinum*, and an unnamed complex) and subspecies (*M. chelonae* subspecies *chelonae*, *abscessus*, and chelonae-like organisms) levels. As a whole, members of the species *fortuitum* are commonly susceptible to ciprofloxacin and to pipemidic acid, although biovariants in *peregrinum* and in the unnamed complex have higher minimal inhibitory concentrations (MICs) with ciprofloxacin, and 30 to 50% of them may also be resistant to pipemidic acid. Members of the species *M. chelonae* may be differentiated to subspecies *chelonae* and *abscessus* by the former's high MIC with cefoxitin (greater than 64 μg/ml) and susceptibility to tobramycin in contrast to the latter's lower MICs with cefoxitin and resistance to tobramycin (29).

The Bactec system has also been used to successfully differentiate between members of the MTB complex and the NTM. The NAP (*p*-nitro-α-acetylamino-β-hydroxy-propiophenone) differentiation test uses the characteristic inhibitory capacity of NAP against isolates of MTB complex and its incapability to inhibit the NTM. Using this system, the two groups can be differentiated within 5 days of isolation (7).

Introduction of genetic probes has allowed for rapid and specific identification of many mycobacteria. Currently, chemiluminescent-labeled probes are becoming more readily available and easier to use in the clinical setting. These probes are directed at mycobacterial ribosomal RNA and are commercially available for specific identification of members of the MTB complex as a whole, of *M. avium*, *M. intracellulare*, *M. kansasii* and *M. gordonae*. Reported sensitivities and specificities of the probes for isolate identifications are greater than 95%. They can be used on isolates grown in broth or on solid culture media and their use in conjunction with the Bactec isolation system has significantly reduced the time to detection and identification of the mycobacteria. However, poor sensitivity and specificity precludes their use for direct mycobacterial detection in specimens at this time (7–9).

Immunologic probes, using radioimmunoassay, ELISA, and immunoblot technology, have also been recently developed. These systems, directed against fairly crude preparations of mycobacterial antigens, show promise for potentially becoming inexpensive alternatives for rapid identification of mycobacteria in cultures (7, 8).

Although gas-liquid chromatography has shown itself to be a promising tool for mycobacterial identification, the use of high-performance liquid chromatograph for analysis of mycolic acids as bromophenacyl esters provides the most distinct patterns for individual species identification (12). The latter method is especially useful for the identification of the NTM.

DIRECT DETECTION

Microscopy

For direct microscopic detection of mycobacteria, centrifugation of specimens such as CSF, urine, and homogenized sputum at a minimal 2000*g* to 4000*g* is recommended to increase yield. Pellicles found on CSF specimens should be cut up and a portion smeared for staining. However, routine direct staining of urine, CSF, and bone marrow specimens may not be necessary and is not recommended (unless perhaps if the patient is suspected of having AIDS), because the yield in such specimens is negligible (7, 8, 14–17).

All smears may be air dried and heat fixed, either by passing them through a flame rapidly several times or by allowing them to fix on an electric hot plate at 50°C for approximately 30 minutes. In most instances, light (thin) smears should be prepared, as material from these has a lower tendency to flake off during staining. Care must be exercised with all unstained slides because any AFB present may still be viable.

The high lipid content of the mycobacteria allows them to retain certain basic dyes better than other bacteria even after treatment with acid-alcohol. This characteristic provides the mycobacteria with the trait of being "acid-fast" (Fig. 47.3). Although they share acid-fastness to some degree with nocardia and rhodococci, the latter two show much less ability to retain the dyes.

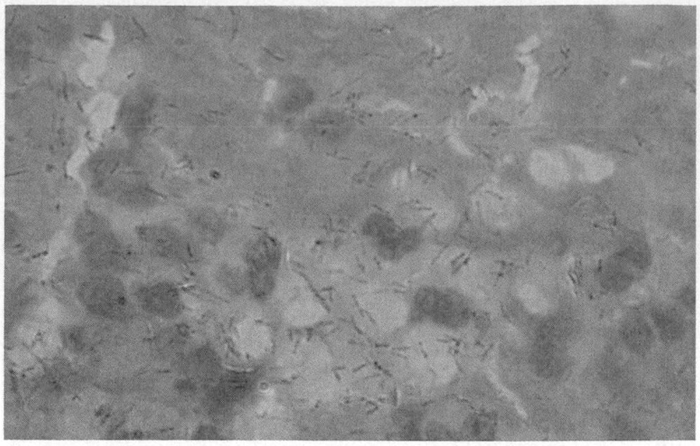

Figure 47.3. Acid-fast bacilli in a direct Kinyoun stain of synovial fluid yielding *Mycobacterium haemophilum*.

Several staining methods are available, including those using the aniline dye, carbolfuchsin (Ziehl-Neelsen and Kinyoun stains) or a fluorochrome dye, auramine O. The last is often used in conjunction with a counterstaining fluorochrome, rhodamine. The auramine fluorochome stain has the same specificity as those using aniline dyes, but is probably more sensitive. Using this system, smears may be scanned for brightly fluorescing rods against a dark background at lower power (25× or 40× objectives). A mercury vapor or a halogen lamp (in an epifluorescent microscope) may be used as light sources in conjunction with appropriate filters. Although useful for scanning smears, the fluorochrome method has several problems, including inability to provide morphologic detail or to stain some isolates of rapidly growing mycobacteria (7, 8, 14–16).

Of the two methods using carbolfuchsin, Kinyoun's method is simpler to perform because constant heating of the smear is not required. Otherwise, Kinyoun's cold stain and the Ziehl-Neelsen stain are comparable, decolorizing with a strong acid-alcohol (e.g., 95% ethanol and 3% hydrochloric acid). Examination of smears prepared by both methods requires use of 100× objectives and oil immersion.

The same characteristics that afford the mycobacteria acid-fast properties contribute to the difficulty of staining them by other stains, especially by the Gram method. Gram-stained preparations do not usually detect mycobacteria. However, in smears with heavy concentration of organisms, the rods may appear as poorly stained, beaded bacilli, or as "ghost" outlines that have taken up neither crystal violet nor safranin.

When scanning smears, at least 100 fields should be examined prior to labeling them negative. Smears positive by the fluorochrome method should be restained by the Kinyoun or Ziehl-Neelsen stains to confirm morphology. The immersion oil objective lens should be wiped clean after viewing a positive slide to avoid the chance of contamination of negative smears by carryover of AFB in the oil from the positive slide. Members of the MTB complex will typically be 2 to 8 μm long and may be slightly curved, whereas members of the NTM may have a banded appearance (*M. kansasii*) or have a pleomorphic morphology (*M. avium*). However, definitive identification cannot be made on microscopic morphology alone. Reporting of positive slides should include some form of quantitation to allow interpretation of the smears (e.g., 1 to 2 AFB/smear: not considered positive/additional specimens suggested; 3 to 9 AFB/smear: rare; greater than 10 AFB/smear: few; greater than 1 AFB/oil immersion field: many) (15, 16).

Other Means of Detection

Newer methods for the recognition of mycobacteria in specimens include immunoassay for antigens, frequency-pulsed electron-capture gas liquid chromatography (FPEC-GLC) for tuberculostearic acid (TSA), nucleic acid probes for specific DNA or RNA base sequences, and genome amplification using the polymerase chain reaction (PCR) or other molecular assays (7–10).

Detection of mycobacterial antigens by immunoassay or of species-specific DNA or RNA sequences by gene probes are presently not adequately sensitive to recommend their routine application. These methods are no more sensitive than direct microscopy (8, 10).

Approaches using the PCR assay to amplify genetic targets followed by specific probes for recognizing specific gene sequences have recently been described. These methods are reported to have much greater sensitivity than do direct probes. With more such advances, there will be a great impact on direct detection and therefore on rapid diagnosis of mycobacterial diseases, including tuberculosis and leprosy (30).

Fatty acid profiles and detection of free TSA by FPEC-GLC in serum and CSF for diagnosis of tuberculous meningitis may also be useful. Recognition of TSA in sputum, however, is less easily accomplished and less diagnostic because of its poor distribution in the specimen and its lack of specificity for tuberculosis (8).

INTERPRETATION OF RESULTS

Criteria to ascertain the role of less pathogenic mycobacterial isolates include (*a*) clinical and roentgenographic evidence of disease; (*b*) repeated isolation from the same site over an extended time period; (*c*) increased number of organisms in direct smears or on semiquantitative culture; (*d*) presence of organisms in a normally sterile site; and (*e*) species identity of the organism. Risk factors in the host, together with failure to identify other pathogenic etiologies, may provide additional clues. The usefulness of the histopathological evaluation of a specimen for documentation and correlation of the infectious process cannot be overstressed. Although these criteria were created to facilitate diagnosis of infections caused by the NTM, they are also useful for suspected nocardial and other actinomycotic infections (23, 25, 27).

Care must be exercised in interpreting results of direct smears of specimens and culture. Sensitivity and specificity of procedures are less important on the whole than are their accuracy for positive and negative prediction. The overall sensitivity and specificity of direct detection of AFB in sputum of patients with tuberculosis has been reported to be 22 to 43% and greater than 99%, respectively. Although good, the predictive value of a positive smear depends on the prevalence of disease. Furthermore, it is often difficult to microscopically differentiate between organisms belonging to the MTB complex and the NTM. Sensitivity and the capability of acid-fast smears to predict the absence of AFB in specimens is notoriously poor. Sensitivity can be increased by using auramine-rhodamine, by concentrating specimens, and by examining multiple specimens (7, 10, 15).

Multiple species may be present in a few infectious cases. Thus, isolation of an NTM identified by the Bactec NAP test does not absolutely negate the potential presence of MTB. The latter may grow out on subculture of the primary Bactec vial or be later recognized on primary agar slants. Thus, great care must be taken to ascertain that multiple morphologies are not present in primary broth cultures.

Cross-contamination of culture tubes has also been known to occur, and care must be exercised to reduce or discover such a possibility. Inoculation order of tubes should be documented and positivity of consecutive (or closely following) specimens evaluated carefully for the possibility of carryover contamination. All information derived from laboratory studies must be correlated to patient and clinical considerations (7, 8).

Therapeutic Considerations

Leprosy, tuberculosis, and the nontubercular mycobacterioses require different treatment protocols. On one side of the spectrum, disease may be localized and self-limited (e.g., localized granuloma caused by *M. marinum*) or may require surgical excision alone (e.g., cervical lymphadenitis caused by *M. avium* or *M. scrofulacium*). On the other side, they may require multiple drug regimens over an extended period of time (e.g., extensive pulmonary disease caused by resistant MTB or *M. avium*).

Treatment of leprosy depends on the stage of the disease. Dapsone and rifampin remain the primary agents for the tuberculoid stage (paucibacillary), while clofazimine is added during the lepromatous stage (multibacillary). Ethionamide or prothionamide may be used in place of clofazimine (26).

Antituberculosis therapy is dependent on susceptibility of the isolate and on the state of the disease process. Resistance, especially to isoniazid (INH), is increasing. Variables associated with increased predictability of resistance include prior antituberculous therapy, patient's original country of residence, and his or her duration of stay in the United States. An increased incidence of resistance has been especially prominent in asiatics and hispanics and in several inner-city locations in the United States (7, 8, 15).

Recently, the combination of INH and rifampin administered for a relatively short course of 9 months has been found to be as efficacious as the old 2-year courses in uncomplicated tuberculosis. The addition of pyrazinamide to this battery for the first 2 months allows the use of INH and rifampin to be shortened to 6 months (31).

Resistant isolates of MTB require the use of additional antimicrobial agents. The older agents include ethambutol (as the agent of choice of INH-resistant isolates) and streptomycin, ethionamide, capreomycin, kanamycin, cycloserine, and *p*-aminosalicylic acid. Newer agents that may play a part in therapy in the near future include the fluoroquinolones, clarithromycin, and combinations of β-lactam drugs with β-lactamase inhibitors. INH is recommended for a 6-month preventive protocol for appropriate patients with positive skin tests who otherwise have no evidence of disease (7, 8, 31).

The final choice of agents of MTB is aided by in vitro susceptibility studies. Methods for such studies have been well established and determine the proportion of bacilli in a population that are resistant to an agent. A poor clinical outcome is predictable with an agent to which more than 1% of bacilli in any single population are resistant. Thus, the proportional susceptibility method determines the percent of resistant organisms within a population being studied. Middlebrook 7H10 or 7H11 agar, impregnated with antituberculous agents at specific concentrations, is overlaid with inocula of known size. The plates are read quantitatively after an appropriate incubation period, with resistance being defined as growth of more than 1% of the initial inoculum as measured on the control plate (32).

The Bactec radiometric system has also been applied to study in vitro susceptibilities of MTB against INH, rifampin, ethambutol, streptomycin, and pyrazinamide with good results. The system is a modification of the conventional proportion method. Instead of an agar base, the test uses Middlebrook 7H12 broth with a radiolabeled fatty acid in the substrate. As in the Bactec culture method, growth of AFB in the media releases radioactive CO_2 in the bottle, which is then measured radiometrically. The amount of growth (as indicated by changes in the growth index) in the media with known drug concentrations compared with that in the control bottle has been correlated to the presence or absence of resistance in 1% of the inoculum. Thus, if an isolate grows beyond a specific growth index compared with the control, it is considered resistant to that specific agent. This method of testing has a very rapid turnaround time, with results being normally available in under a week. Unfortunately, the method cannot presently be used to study other agents (7, 32).

The conventional studies, as well as those using the radiometric system, may be performed on culture isolates (indirect method) or directly on concentrated specimens (direct method) in which AFB have been seen on smear. Care must be used in interpreting direct tests because of variables present, and results should be verified by indirect studies (7, 32).

Many of the nontuberculous mycobacterioses are not amenable to antimicrobial therapy. Most clinically significant NTM are resistant to the first-line antituberculous agents. *M. kansasii*, alone, being commonly treatable with protocols using rifampin together with INH and ethambutol or streptomycin, is only slightly more difficult to treat than MTB (8, 23, 25).

Members of MAC, however, are notoriously resistant and often require regimens combining more than four agents. Ethionamide, streptomycin, capreomycin, and kanamycin have often been used in various combinations with agents already mentioned. Clofazimine and rifabutin have been disappointing in some regimens for patients with AIDS. Surgical intervention is often recommended for localized disease (23, 25).

The rapidly growing mycobacteria are also difficult to treat, being primarily resistant to conventional antituberculous agents. Approaches to therapy often include surgical intervention and debridement of localized infection together with antimicrobial therapy consisting of multiple agents. Amikacin, doxycycline, cefoxitin, sulfonamides, and imipenem may improve outcome when used in various combinations with conventional drugs. Ciprofloxacin has good activity against *M. fortuitum* but not against *M. chelonae*. The agent should not be used alone, however, as resistance may surface during therapy (29).

Historically, conventional in vitro susceptibility studies of NTM have had poor predictive value because antimicrobial concentrations for the evaluation of clinical usefulness have not been established. Recent evidence, however, indicates that such studies can be helpful in drug selection, with bacteriologic clearance occurring more frequently when regimens include more agents to which the isolate is susceptible (33).

The Bactec system may play a major role in the near future in elucidating minimal inhibitory concentrations (MICs) of various antimicrobial agents for the NTM. Such studies seem to have a greater predictive value for outcome and have the capability for determination of synergy between certain agents.

NOCARDIA

Microbiology (Classification)

The genus *Nocardia* has historically contained a very heterogeneous group of organisms, primarily because species identification was based solely on morphologic criteria. Presently, the definition of the genus is based on the lipid content of the cell wall and on peptidoglycan composition. The nocardia possess a type IV cell wall, but may be differentiated from the mycobacteria by the former's shorter chained (40- to 60-carbon) mycolic acids. Thus, many species originally lumped under the nocardia have been reassigned to new or other genera (*Actinomadura, Nocardiopsis, Oerskovia,* and *Rhodococcus*) (1, 2).

The genus *Nocardia* has only nine recognized species (*N. asteroides, N. farcinica, N. brasiliensis, N. otitidiscaviarum, N. amarae, N. brevicatena, N. carnea, N. vaccinii,* and *N. transvalensis*). Characterization of the recognized species is based on a multitude of morphologic and physiological determinants. The species *N. farcinica*, which resembles *N. asteroides*, has an uncertain status (34). The species *N. asteroides* is itself very heterogeneous, based on numerical taxonomic and DNA homology studies (see Addendum). Seven immunotypes and isolates with other variable characteristics may still be found grouped in this species (1, 2, 6, 18, 35).

Spectrum of Disease

In the United States, the nocardia are commonly considered to be opportunistic pathogens seen primarily in immunocompromised patients, in those receiving long-term corticosteroid therapy, or in those who have undergone traumatic percutaneous abrasions. Nocardial infections are especially prevalent in patients with parenchymal lung damage due to chronic lung disease. Although *N. asteroides, N. brasiliensis,* and *N. otitidicaviarum* are the species commonly associated with human infection, the controversial *N. farcinica*, being normally misidentified as *N. asteroides*, may play a larger role than presently recognized (34). *N. asteroides* (and in instances misidentified *N. farcinica*) is the most common cause of nocardiosis (90%) in the United States, with *N. brasiliensis* being encountered in a significantly smaller number of cases (7%), and *N. otitidiscaviarum* being rarely implicated. Their primary manifestation is either pulmonary or systemic disease or localized cutaneous/subcutaneous infection. Outside the United States the nocardia, especially *N. brasiliensis* and *otitidiscaviarum*, are commonly associated with actinomycotic mycetoma, a localized, progressive, yet chronic infection of skin and soft tissue (6, 18, 34, 36–38).

Infection with *N. asteroides* most commonly originates in the pulmonary tract. The infection may be transient or subclinical, or it may progress to an acute or chronic respiratory illness. Inapparent infections may be more common than previously suspected. It has been suggested that colonization of the respiratory tract in some patients with underlying conditions (cystic fibrosis, asthma, bronchitis, tuberculosis, malignancy) may be encountered frequently. Up to 53% of some reported patients with nocardia isolated from sputum were considered to be only colonized. However, nocardial infections are also commonly manifested as progressive disease in patients with underlying immunocompromising conditions. Common predisposing factors include long-term corticosteroid therapy, chronic pulmonary disease, organ transplantation, and lymphoreticular neoplasms. In many of these patients, nocardiosis carries a high mortality rate and recurrence rate despite prolonged and aggressive therapy (39, 40).

N. asteroides has a propensity to disseminate from the pulmonary tract to other sites via the bloodstream, although an estimated rate of 30 to 45% may be overly high. When dissemination occurs, the areas associated with the central nervous system (brain, meninges, spine) are frequently targeted, although other sites—including lymph nodes, skin, pleura, and eyes—may become involved (18, 24, 40).

Unlike the mycobacteria, nocardial lesions are typically suppurative in nature, with progression to acute necrosis and abscess formation. Granulomatous lesions are rarely formed.

N. asteroides is most commonly associated with pulmonary and disseminated disease, and less frequently with direct soft tissue infection. In contrast,

N. brasiliensis and *N. otitidiscaviarum* are frequently found involving soft tissue. The organisms are probably introduced into subcutaneous tissue through traumatic inoculation via thorns or splinters, with extremities being involved most frequently. Infected sites tend to swell, and lesions may progress to form draining sinus tracts; small white granules may often be present in the draining material, representing masses of nocardial cells compacted together. Such mycetomas are characteristically seen in older soft tissue infections. However, both species may occasionally cause systemic disease and involve the pulmonary tract. Lymphocutaneous "sporotrichoid" infections may also be encountered, especially with *N. brasiliensis* (24, 38, 41).

Epidemiology

The clinically significant nocardial species normally reside as saprophytes in soil and may be associated with plant material as well as water, air, and dust. Their geographic distribution is probably responsible for the variation in species' prevalence in association with disease. The most common species, *N. asteroides*, is prevalent in more temperate climates, while *N. brasiliensis* is more commonly associated with tropical areas. *Nocardia otitidiscaviarum* is an infrequent isolate from soil throughout the world (1).

The majority of *N. asteroides* infections in the United States are acquired via the respiratory tract, although traumatic inoculation may also occur. Person-to-person transmission of nocardiosis is uncharacteristic, but acquisition in small clusters of patients in close proximity to each other suggests that possibility (42).

The epidemiology of nocardiosis from *N. asteroides* seems to have changed from being a primary infection in the normal host to one associated increasingly with debilitated patients. *N. brasiliensis* is primarily acquired percutaneously, although respiratory acquisition is possible. Infection with this genus, as with *N. otitidiscaviarum*, is usually primary and is most frequently seen in the normal host.

Diagnostic Procedures

SPECIMEN COLLECTION

The same principles used for mycobacteria specimen collection can be used for nocardia specimens. Respiratory specimens are the most common, but tissues, other normally sterile body fluids, as well as pus, exudates, and even blood may yield nocardia in the right clinical setting.

PRIMARY ISOLATION

Nocardia are able to grow on most readily available routine media such as 5% sheep blood and chocolate agars, Mueller-Hinton agar, tryptic soy agar, various broths, Sabouraud dextrose agar, brain-heart infusion agar, and Lowenstein-Jensen agar. Unfortunately, overgrowth of the nocardia by more rapidly growing bacteria and fungi in heavily contaminated clinical specimens is a common problem. Thus, repeated isolation attempts are necessary before infection can be considered unlikely (6, 17, 18).

Because of the overgrowth problem, several primary plating media should be used to optimize isolation. Sabouraud dextrose agar, selective buffered charcoal yeast extract agar, as well as Thayer-Martin agar and Lowenstein-Jensen agar may be used in conjunction with routine blood or chocolate agar plates to isolate nocardia selectively. Selective media may be inhibitory to some nocardia and should not be used alone.

A paraffin-baiting technique, using sterile carbon-free broth and a paraffin-coated glass rod, has been described and is reported to almost double isolation rates for nocardia. The method relies on the propensity of nocardia to invade and use the paraffin on the glass rod as a growth medium. However, the technique has not been popular in clinical laboratories because of its cumbersome nature and longer time to recovery (17, 18).

Pretreatment and processing of contaminated specimens with *N*-acetyl-L-cysteine or other decontaminating methods used for the mycobacteria are deleterious to the nocardia. Such treatment can significantly decrease viability and should not be used as a primary isolation method. However, isolates can survive in some instances, and nocardia can be isolated in the mycobacterial section of the laboratory.

Primary media should be incubated aerobically at 35° to 37°C for up to 2 to 3 weeks. Cultures may also be set up simultaneously at 26°C, especially if the identity of the potential pathogen is not suspected. Although CO_2 enhancement of nocardial growth has been reported, experience has shown that CO_2 is not necessary for initial isolation of fresh isolates. Cultures should be examined every 2 days for the first week and at least twice weekly thereafter. Clear media are superior for early microscopic recognition of nocardial colonies, which can often be distinguished by their filamentous appearance and possible aerial mycelia. Colonies most frequently are chalky white, turning yellow-orange with age.

IDENTIFICATION

Nocardial isolates may be recognized once the colonies reach a size that will show their chalky aerial mycelia. These are best observed under a dissecting microscope. Commonly, young colonies are pure white, turning to an orange color with age. Staining will show Gram-positive to stippled, branching rods, or occasionally coccobacilli indicative of hyphal fragmentation. A certain percentage of the population of organisms from a colony will stain acid-fast when a weak acid decolorizing solution (0.5 to 1% sulfuric acid) is used with the modified Kinyoun stain.

Resistance of nocardial isolates to lysozyme differentiates them from other streptomycetes. Although the rhodococci have a variable response to lysozyme, they are normally less acid-fast than nocardia, and their colonies often have a salmon-pink color. The nocardia and rhodococci can further be presumptively differentiated by their susceptibility profiles with vancomycin and erythromycin (6, 18, 43, 44).

The three major clinically significant species may be identified by their patterns of hydrolysis of casein, tyrosine, hypoxanthine, and xanthine (see Addendum). *N. brasiliensis* hydrolyzes casein and tyrosine, being variable with hypoxanthine, while *N. otitidiscaviarum* hydrolyzes hypoxanthine and xanthine alone, and *N. asteriodes* is inert (2, 6, 18, 34). These common studies cannot differentiate between *N. asteroides* and *N. farcinica*. Recently, Wallace suggested that the two species may be separated by the latter being able to grow at 45°C (3 days), to produce acid from rhamnose and to utilize acetamide, while being resistant to tobramycin and cefamandole (34).

More definitive identification to the generic level requires evaluation of whole cell hydrolysates and analysis for characteristic mycolic acid or lipid patterns. Utilizing a variety of organic compounds can also provide more specific information as to species. These more definitive studies are not commonly available and are not normally needed for most identifications, but are reviewed elsewhere (17).

DIRECT DETECTION

The nocardia may frequently be detected in routine Gram-stained smears of specimens as long, delicate, branched, beaded to Gram-positive filaments (Fig. 47.4). Shorter rods and coccal forms are also possible. The Gram stain is probably the most sensitive stain for the detection of these organisms. Although the nocardia have "weak" acid-fast properties, they do not complex the basic dyes as tenaciously as the mycobacteria, and they require a milder acid-alcohol wash. Thus, a modified Kinyoun stain using 0.5% sulfuric acid decolorizer will stain 60 to 90% of nocardia in specimens. Not all nocardia within a single population or specimen will stain acid-fast (partial acid-fastness), and the property may be lost through aging of cultures. A modified

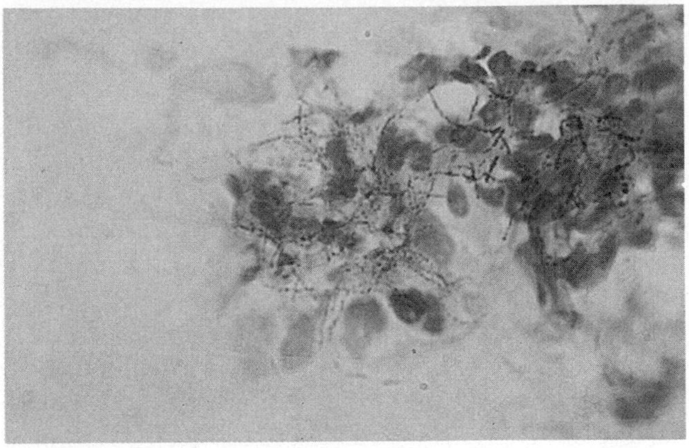

Figure 47.4. Direct Gram stain of sputum showing delicate, branched, beaded to Gram-positive filaments characteristic of *Nocardia* species (magnification × 1000).

auramine-rhodamine stain may also be used to provide an opportunity for detection by fluorescent microscopy.

Unlike material from actinomycetomas, specimens from respiratory, cutaneous, and systemic nocardiosis usually do not contain actinomycotic sulfur granules. When present, granules may be crushed between two slides and observed by wet mount or by Gram stain for typical branching filaments. A modified acid-fast stain may then be performed for identification of the organisms as "presumptive" *Nocardia* species, if positive. Negative stains, however, cannot rule out nocardial organisms. The Gram-Weigert, Brown and Brenn, and modified acid-fast stains may all detect actinomycetes in tissue and sulfur granule preparations, whereas the hematoxylin and eosin stain will not (6, 17, 19).

Therapeutic Considerations

Sulfamethoxazole-trimethroprim (SXT) and the sulfonamides remain the drugs of choice for nocardiosis. Treatment should be prolonged for a minimum of 3 to 12 months, with recovery or improvement being best in pulmonary or localized soft tissue infections (80 to 97%) and worst in disseminated disease (50 to 63%) (6, 18).

Alternative agents include minocycline, amikacin, the third-generation cephalosporins, the amoxicillin-clavulanic acid combination, and imipenem. These agents, however, have variable activity against *N. asteroides* in vitro. *N. farcinica* may show increased resistance and is usually resistant to cefotaxime, ceftriaxone, and cefamandole (34). *N. brasiliensis* and *N. otitidiscaviarum* have a less variable response to β-lactam antimicrobials, and the aminoglycosides. Synergism against the nocardia has been suggested for the combinations of imipenem with both cefotaxime and

SXT. Aztreonam has poor activity against these organisms, while erythromycin, chloramphenicol, and vancomycin are inactive (6, 18, 39, 40, 45, 46).

The variable response of *N. asteroides* to a number of antimicrobials suggests that isolates be tested in vitro for specific guidelines. Although methods for susceptibility studies of the nocardia have not officially been promulgated, broth and agar dilution determinations of MICs as well as disk diffusion qualitative methods have been studied. The disk diffusion method described by Wallace can be used effectively to screen isolates. Studies can be performed using organisms suspended to a 0.5 McFarland barium standard to inoculate the surface of Mueller-Hinton agar plates, dropping commercial disks containing antimicrobials desired, incubating the plates for 48 to 72 hours at 35°C in air, and measuring zone diameters. Isolates that provide poor growth on Mueller-Hinton agar can be studied on 5% sheep blood or chocolate Mueller-Hinton agars. Preliminary interpretations of the diameters of zone of inhibition have been suggested by Wallace (47).

The broth-microdilution test system using cation-supplemented Mueller-Hinton broth has been preliminarily shown to correlate with the disk diffusion method and is practical for many laboratories. Further study is needed to confirm clinical applications.

Screening of *N. asteroides* for β-lactamase is not recommended, since the majority of isolates will be positive; the production of the enzyme does not correlate with response to β-lactams (47).

RHODOCOCCUS, GORDONA, AND *TSUKAMURELLA*

Microbiology (Classification)

Members of this group of organisms are diverse in their morphology and growth patterns. Their grouping and identification are based primarily on cell wall constituents (being those of type IV, with mycolic acid sizes ranging from 32 to 66 carbons in length) as well as biochemical criteria. Considered originally as *rhodochrous* strains of the genus *Mycobacterium*, the rhodoccocci were given their own genus status in the 1970s and are currently made up of 20 recognized species (4). Recently, there has been a redefining of the genus *Rhodococcus*, with removal of several species to the genus *Gordona* and renaming of one species as *Tsukamurella* (see Addendum).

Spectrum of Disease

Rhodococci and related genera are rarely involved in human disease, but recent reports and observations may indicate their increasing role as opportunistic pathogens in the immunocompromised host. Primarily a pathogen of livestock, *R. equi* is the species most commonly associated with human infections. The organism has been implicated with pulmonary disease, including lung abscess and cavitation, often concomitantly with bacteremia in patients with neoplastic disease or on immunosuppression (2, 43). Separate reports have implicated *R. equi* in localized infection of a cervical lymph node as well as in endophthalmitis (44). The organism may also cause bacteremia and disease in patients with implanted Hickman catheters (unpublished personal observation) or AIDS.

Epidemiology

The rhodococci may be found in a number of environmental locations, and especially in soil. They have been isolated as well from fresh water, marine habitats, and the gut of some arthropods. They also have been associated with feces of herbivores and swine. The presence of fecal contamination significantly increases the multiplication of the organisms in the soil. Isolation of the organism from sputum and central lines suggests its acquisition from air or dust, which may be inhaled or may contaminate medical devices. Corticosteroids and immunocompromising conditions enhance patient susceptibility to clinically manifested infection (1, 44).

Diagnostic Procedures

SPECIMEN COLLECTION

Follow the same guidelines given for the nocardia.

PRIMARY ISOLATION

On culture plates, rhodococci may originate as clear to white, nonhemolytic, rounded, and frequently mucoid colonies that may turn salmon-pink to red within 2 to 5 days (Fig. 47.5.). Pigmentation may vary from red to cream. Growth is good between 15° and 40°C, but is slow, often requiring several days for visual observation. Microscopically, the organisms are Gram positive and coccobacillary, resembling other coryneform bacteria. A small number of cells within a population may be stained by the modified Kinyoun weak acid-fast stain, contributing to their being confused with fragmented nocardial cells. Unlike the nocardia, however, rhodococci are susceptible to vancomycin and erythromycin.

In addition to colonial and microscopic recognition, the rhodococci may be preliminarily recognized and identified by their production of catalase, hydrolysis of urea, and reduction of nitrate. They are otherwise quite inert and unable to produce acid from carbohydrates. Definitive identification is diffi-

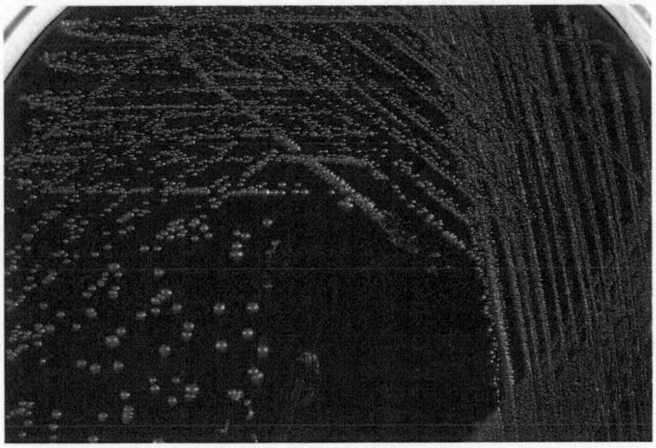

Figure 47.5. Colonies of *Rhodococcus* species with typical salmon-pink to red pigmentation (shown on sheep blood agar).

cult and may require cell analysis for meso-DAP, arabinose, and galactose, as well as more extensive physiological and molecular testing (1, 2, 4, 43, 44).

DIRECT DETECTION

The rhodococci are typically seen as Gram-positive short rods or coccobacilli and are frequently confused with the diphtheroids. Although having partially acid-fast properties, these organisms are less frequently seen as being acid-fast than the nocardia. The organisms do not have characteristic morphologies that would lead one to suspect them as being rhodococci on direct Gram stain.

Therapeutic Considerations

The rhodococci, unlike the nocardia, are normally susceptible to erythromycin, rifampin, and vancomycin, as well as to the aminoglycosides, penicillin G, and doxycycline. The combination of erythromycin and rifampin seems to act synergistically against the intracellular rhodococci. Duration of therapy is uncertain, although many weeks may be required because relapses may occur after shorter periods. Surgical intervention may also be necessary in instances. Standardized susceptibility tests are not available, although methods applied for the nocardia may provide insight into susceptibility patterns when necessary (4, 44, 49).

ACTINOMADURA, NOCARDIOPSIS, AND *STREPTOMYCES*

Microbiology (Classification)

The genus *Actinomadura* is a member of an aggregate of sporoactinomycetes called maduromycetes. The organisms in this artificial group are not necessarily genetically related, but share the characteristic of having a chemotype III cell wall and containing the sugar madurose. They can be easily distinguished from *Dermatophilus* morphologically. Originally classified in the genus *Nocardia*, the *Actinomadura* were later given individual genus status. Currently, only two species (*Actinomadura madurae* and *Actinomadura pelletieri*) have clinical importance. Previous members such as the species *dassonvillei* were found to lack madurose and were transferred to the genus *Nocardiopsis* (1, 2).

The genus *Streptomyces* consists of over 700 poorly defined species of sporoactinomycetes with cell-wall type I (L-DAP, glycine but no sugar). Of all the species present in this genus, only *Streptomyces somaliensis*, *Streptomyces griseus*, and *Streptomyces paraguayensis* are commonly associated with human disease (1, 2, 35).

Spectrum of Disease

Infectious manifestations of members of the genera *Actinomadura*, *Nocardiopsis*, and *Streptomyces* are primarily limited to the formation of localized, suppurative, mostly chronic lesions. These mycetomas occur commonly in parts of the body coming into frequent contact with soil or that may be abraded or traumatized. The more common causative species of actinomycetes include *A. madurae*, *A. pelletieri*, and *S. somaliensis*, and, less frequently, *S. griseus*, as well as *N. dassonvillei*. The organisms gain entry into subcutaneous tissues through slight or imperceptible breaks in the skin. A painless nodule forms, becomes fluctuant, and usually forms a sinus tract through which pus is discharged. Draining pus often contains pigmented granules made up of filamentous, compacted microcolonies of the organism and ranging in color from white to yellow (*A. madurae* and *S. somaliensis*) or red to pink (*A. pelletieri*). Additional nodules and sinus tracts form over time, with fibrous tissue eventually deforming the areas involved. Unchecked, progression of the lesions may involve connective tissue, muscle, and bone. Unlike the fungal mycetomas, the granulomatous response to actinomycotic infections does not normally occur, and the response characteristically remains pyogenic. The disease remains localized. Hematogenous spread is rarely encountered (except with nocardia), although spread via the lymphatics to involve lymph nodes is possible (37, 38).

Epidemiology

The clinically significant species of *Actinomadura*, *Nocardiopsis*, and *Streptomyces*, primarily soil inhabitants, have diverse geographic prevalences, although none is common in the United States. Mycetomas caused by *A. madurae* are cosmopolitan, although tending to be more frequent in tropical or subtropical regions. The organism is isolated frequently in North and South America, Africa, and Asia. *A. pelletieri* has a predilection for areas with heavy rainfall and is more restricted to areas of Africa and South America (19, 37).

S. somaliensis prefers arid regions, sandy soil, with vegetation consisting of thorny plants. It therefore causes mycetomas most frequently in Africa, Mexico, and portions of South America, although it may be found in other continents as well.

Diagnostic Procedures

SPECIMEN COLLECTION

Biopsy of deeper tissue is preferred for the evaluation of actinomycotic mycetomas, because surface material may be contaminated or colonized. Other specimens may include pus, drainage fluid, or sinus scrapings either from open lesions or from aspirates.

PRIMARY ISOLATION

Culture methods for the actinomadurae, the nocardiopses, and the streptomycetes are similar to those for the nocardia. The actinamadurae may at times be difficult to isolate from clinical specimens. The former, together with the streptomycetes, may not grow on all of the media described for the nocardia, but may produce small colonies on noncardia selective agars. Thus, such media should be supplemented by other routine media as outlined for the nocardia, as well as by Sabouraud dextrose agar, both with and without chloramphenicol (0.05 mg/ml). Incubation should be at 26°C as well as at 35° to 37°C for up to 3 weeks (17).

IDENTIFICATION

Members of the genus *Actinomadura* are normally slow-growing, with colonies that are glabrous or waxy, heaped, and either white to cream (*A. madurae*) or pink to coral red (*A. pelletieri*) in color. Microscopically, they are Gram-positive, non–acid-fast, bacillary organisms with branching vegetative mycelia. The mycelia of the two clinically important species only rarely fragment and do not usually produce aerial forms. Streptomycetes, on the other hand, are fast-growing and produce colonies similar to those of the actinomadurae.

Simplified differential identification schemes may include cell wall analysis for the presence of meso-DAP and madurose in the actinomadurae, of meso-DAP without characteristic sugars in nocardiopsis, and of L-DAP in the streptomycetes. *A. madurae* and *A. pelletieri* can be differentiated by the red coloration of the latter's colony (17, 19).

DIRECT DETECTION

In cases of mycetoma, biopsy or drainage material should be examined for the presence of granules. Granules, which are usually hard and of variable sizes, should be washed in sterile saline several times and examined for filaments (17, 19). The granules may be examined microscopically after emulsification in a drop of 10% potassium hydroxide or after crushing between two slides. They can also be stained by the Gram method to visualize the tangled filamentous forms of the actinomycetes, thereby differentiating them from the broader, cross-walled mycelia of the fungi. A positive modified acid-fast stain can also differentiate between the nocardia and the actinomadura and streptomyces; however, negative stains may also occur with the nocardia. As with the nocardia, the Brown and Brenn's modification of the Gram stain and the Gram-Weigert stain will detect the aerobic actinomycetes in tissue (17, 19).

Therapeutic Considerations

Actinomycotic mycetoma responds to antimicrobial therapy, although regimens of several months' duration are necessary to curb relapse. Surgical debridement may enhance healing. Streptomycin sulfate, usually combined with another agent, is most commonly suggested. The second agents recommended may be dapsone for *A. madurae* and *S. somaliensis*, and SXT for *A. pelletieri*. SXT has also been suggested for streptomycetes not initially responding to dapsone. Susceptibility studies are not routinely recommended (19, 37).

OERSKOVIA AND *DERMATOPHILUS*

Microbiology (Classification)

The genus *Oerskovia*, closely related to *Cellulomonas*, consists of two species, *Oerskovia turbata* and *Oerskovia xanthineolytica*. Classification of the oerskoviae has been difficult, and until recently they had been placed in many genera, including *Nocardia*. Morphologic characteristics, absence of DAP and mycolates, and presence of type VI cell wall constituents, with lysine and galactose as major components, separate the oerskoviae from other aerobic actinomycetes. Other characteristics of oerskoviae include their being facultative anaerobes and having the ability to fragment into motile bacillary elements (2).

The genus *Dermatophilus* contains but a single species, *Dermatophilus congolensis*, an obligate animal pathogen with meso-DAP and madurose as major cell-wall components. The organism characteristically divides by transverse, longitudinal, and horizontal septation of the mycelium, leading to the formation of motile zoospores. A tough, gelatinous capsule is formed surrounding the branching vegetative mycelium at points of division where zoospores mature, representing a multilocular sporangium.

Spectrum of Disease

Members of the genus *Oerskovia* have rarely been implicated in human disease, although the number of cases may be rising and may be greater than had been suspected. Fewer than 40 isolates were submitted for identification to the U.S. Centers of Disease Control and Prevention in Atlanta prior to 1977. Of those submitted, original sites of isolation included blood, heart, CSF, and others. Recently published reports have implicated the oerskoviae in endocarditis, bacteremia, peritonitis, endophthalmitis, meningitis, and pyonephrosis. The organisms are associated with foreign body infections (e.g., Hickman/Tenkhoff catheters, prosthetic heart valves) or with infections caused by penetrating injuries (49).

D. congolensis, the only species in the genus, causes streptotrichosis in animals; this dermatophilosis is a pustular, exudative dermatitis affecting many wild and domestic animals, especially sheep, cattle, and horses. The organism is found obligately on animals, never having been isolated from the environment. It may be transmitted to humans, either directly through contact with infected animals or possibly through bites by arthropods that may carry infective zoospores. Infection, however, probably requires some form of dermal abrasion because Dermatophilus is not invasive. Presenting either as multiple pustules or as a desquamative keratitis of the hands and forearms, the infection is usually self-limiting in humans (1).

Epidemiology

The oerskoviae are primarily found in soil, although they may also contaminate grass clippings and possibly other plant debris. Human infections are associated with contamination of indwelling foreign bodies or with traumatic inoculation from the natural reservoir (2, 49).

Dermatophilus is an obligate parasite associated with livestock and other feral animals. Direct contact of abraded skin with material such as skin or hair of diseased animals carrying infective zoospores is the normal route of transmission. The disease is uncommon in the United States (1).

Diagnostic Procedures

SPECIMEN COLLECTION

Blood, CSF, or other normally sterile body fluids (depending on the patients presenting condition) readily yield the oerskoviae, while recommended specimens for *Dermatophilus* include material from unopened pustules, exudates, biopsies, scrapings, and scabs. Specimens for the latter should be submitted in sterile tubes or in adequate volume on premoistened sterile swabs and should be kept at room temperature (17).

PRIMARY ISOLATION

Isolation of the oerskoviae is readily achieved on most routine bacterial agar or broth-based media, including sheep blood and chocolate agar. The organisms may fail to grow, however, on fungal media such as Sabouraud dextrose agar. Cultures may be incubated at 35°C aerobically in CO_2 or anaerobically. Growth is normally evident after 24 to 48 hours of incubation (49).

Isolation of *Dermatophilus* may be accomplished by inoculating the specimens onto beef infusion-blood agar and incubating for up to a week aerobically at 35° to 37°C. Plates may also be incubated in the presence of 5 to 10% CO_2. Specimens with heavy contamination may require selective processing, employing either animal passage or the predilection of zoospores for CO_2.

IDENTIFICATION

Members of the genus *Oerskovia* produce bright yellow colonies after 48 hours of incubation. Microscopically, they may show extensively branching mycelia that fragment into short, motile, rodlike bacilli; aerial mycelia, however, are not seen. Characteristically, younger filaments are Gram positive and non–acid fast. The organisms are oxidase negative, and catalase positive if grown aerobically. Susceptibility to vancomycin readily separates the oerskoviae from the nocardia and rapid-growing NTM, while colony pigmentation separates them from the coral red colonies of the rhodococci (2, 49). The oerskoviae are active biochemically, producing acid from glucose, lactose, sucrose, maltose, and xylose. Identification to species level may be achieved by hydrolysis studies. *O. xanthineolytica* hydrolyzes casein, xanthine, hypoxanthine, and esculin, but not tyrosine, whereas *O. turbata* does not normally hydrolyze xanthine or hypoxanthine (49).

Dermatophilus may be recognized as tiny, pitting colonies after a days incubation, turning orange within 2 to 5 days with β-hemolysis evident in areas of heavy growth (17).

The single species in this genus can be identified by the characteristic microscopic morphology, which is similar to that seen in clinical specimens. Colonial growth is optimal at 37°C when enriched media are used, and production of aerial mycelium is promoted by 10% CO_2. Older colonies (2 to 5 days) become orange and begin to show β-hemolysis in areas of heavy growth. Whole-cell hydrolysate analysis for DL-DAP and madurose, together with casein and starch hydrolysis may help in furthering identification of a few strains, but such studies are rarely needed (17).

DIRECT DETECTION

The oerskoviae may readily be detected in specimens as Gram-positive rods when stained by routine methods (49). Concentration of normally sterile body fluids such as CSF may be helpful.

Direct detection of *Dermatophilus* is best accomplished using the Giemsa stain of submitted smears or tissue. The Gram-stain and methylene blue wet mount may also be useful. The organisms typically show 2 to 5 μm wide, branched filaments with transverse and longitudinal division. Packets containing coccoid cells may be present (17).

Therapeutic Considerations

Although experience is limited, infections caused by members of the genus *Oerskovia* are often difficult to treat because of their common association with foreign bodies. Effective antimicrobial agents have included ampicillin, penicillin, rifampin, the aminoglycosides, and vancomycin. However, the refractory nature of such infections to therapy is evidenced by reports of failure of treatment with effective agents unless the foreign body was first removed (49). Although in vitro susceptibility studies are not standardized and should not be relied on heavily, methods used for the rhodococci or nocardia may provide some information.

Infection with *Dermatophilus* is normally self-limited, and systemic therapy is not usually required.

SUMMARY AND CONCLUSIONS

Many of the aerobic actinomycetes have gained increased prominence as pathogens at a time when the number of patients with immunocompromising conditions is also on the rise. Sophisticated medical technology together with newer diseases that induce immunodeficiency are at least partially to blame.

Added recognition of the infective capability of the aerobic actinomycetes and better understanding of their epidemiology, clinical course, and susceptibilities to antimicrobial agents are paramount to rapid diagnosis and better patient care. More sensitive and specific methods for serologic diagnosis, together with more rapid recovery systems and identification methods will also be necessary. Invariably, clinical laboratories must become aware of the role played by the aerobic actinomycetes in disease and must recognize when identification, susceptibility testing, and therapeutic or surgical interventions are necessary.

ADDENDUM

Several newer species of mycobacteria have recently been more frequently implicated as etiologies of systemic disease in immunocompromised patients, especially in those with AIDS. Included in this group are a number of clinically significant isolates resembling *M. xenopi* but with distinctly different HPLC profiles; these have tentatively been given the name *Mycobacterium celatum* (50). Additionally, a second number of isolates characterized by slow growth and a fastidious nature (originally growing only in broth cultures and often taking more than 4 to 6 weeks to recover) have also been implicated in disease in the immunocompromised patient. Some of these isolates, with unique 16S rRNA, resemble but are distinct from *Mycobacterium simiae* and *Mycobacterium malmoense*, being tentatively named *Mycobacterium genavense* (51).

Recent evidence suggests that the clinically relevant organisms traditionally identified in the laboratory as *N. asteroides* include isolates with very heterogeneous, yet stable phenotypic characteristics. In reality, this group can be thought of as a complex and includes at least the species *N. asteroides* in the strict sense, the previously clinically misidentified *N. farcinica*, and the newly proposed species *N. nova* (52, 53). The latter two species probably account for a larger proportion of human clinical isolates than previously thought, with *N. farcinica* making up almost 30% of isolates in some collections. The three species can be differentiated by several tests and susceptibility profiles (Table 47.5); laboratories should at least be able to differentiate between *N. farcinica* and the other species because it has a greater resistance profile and may be more invasive (52, 53).

The rhodococci have also recently undergone a reorganization. Previously, they consisted of a large group of organisms that could be further divided into two stable groups based on chemical constituents. One group is made up of 34- to 52-carbon mycolic acids, no mycobactins, and eight isoprene dehydrogenated menaquinones (IDMs), while the second group has 48- to 66-carbon mycolic acids, no myco-

Table 47.5. Differentiation of *Nocardia asteroides, N. farcinica,* and *N. nova*[a]

Test	% Positivity (P) or Susceptibility (S)		
	N. asteroides	*N. farcinica*	*N. nova*
Growth at 45°C (3 days)	43 P	100 P	5 P
Rhamnose	10 P	80 P	5 P
Acetamide	17 P	80 P	0 P
Arylsulfatase	5 P	0 P	75 P
Cefamandole (S:>20 mm)	95 S	7 S	100 S
Tobramycin (S:>20 mm)	83 S	0 S	17 S
Erythromycin (s:>30 mm)	2 S	0 S	100 S

[a]Data from Wallace RJ, Brown BA, Tsukamura M, et al. Clinical and laboratory features of *Nocardia nova*. J Clin Microbiol 1991; 29:2407–2411. and Schiff TA, McNeil MM, Brown JM. Cutaneous *Nocardia farcinica* infection in nonimmunocompromised host. Clin Infect Dis 1993;16:756–760.

bactins, and nine IDMs (54). The redefinition of this group of organisms removed those members of the second group to the genus *Gordona* (*Gordona bronchialis, Gordona terrae*) and left those in group one in the genus *Rhodococcus*, with the most common isolate being *Rhodococcus equi* (54, 55). Furthermore, *Rhodococcus aurantiacus*, a rare cause of abscesses and synovitis, have been renamed as *Tsukamurella paurometabolum*.

References

1. Goodfellow M, Cross T. Classification. In: Goodfellow M, Mordarski M, Williams ST, eds. The biology of the actinocetes. London: Academic Press, 1984:7–164.
2. Lechevalier HA, Goodfellow MA, Lechevalier MP, Prauser H. Nocardioform actinomycetes. In: Williams ST, Sharpe ME, Holt JG, eds. Bergey's manual of systematic bacteriology. Baltimore: Williams & Wilkins, 1989;4:2348–2382.
3. Wayne LG, Kubica GP. Genus *Mycobacterium*. In: Holt JG, ed. Bergey's manual of systematic bacteriology. Baltimore: Williams & Wilkins, 1986;2:1436–1457.
4. Coyle MB, Lipsky BA. Coryneform bacteria in infectious diseases: clinical and laboratory aspects. Clin Microbiol Rev 1990;3:227–246.
5. Tisdall PA, Roberts GD. Aerobic actinomycetes and the clinical microbiology laboratory. Clin Microbiol Newsl 1979;1:1–3.
6. Hoeprich PD. Nocardiosis. In: Hoeprich PD, Jordan MC, eds. Infectious diseases. 4th ed. Philadelphia: JB Lippincott, 1989: 449–457.
7. Musial CE, Roberts GD. Tuberculosis and other mycobacterioses. In: Wentworth BB, ed. Diagnostic procedures for bacterial infections. 7th ed. Washington, DC: American Public Health Association, 1987:537–580.
8. Good RC. Tuberculosis. In: Balows A, Hausler WJ Jr, Ohashi M, Turano A, eds. Laboratory diagnosis of infectious diseases, principles and practice. New York: Springer-Verlag, 1988:504–518.
9. Ellner PD, Kiehn TE, Cammarata R, Hosmer M. Rapid detection and identification of pathogenic mycobacteria by combining radiometric and nucleic acid probe methods. J Clin Microbiol 1988;26:1349–1352.
10. Daniel TM. Rapid diagnoisis of tuberculosis: laboratory techniques applicable in developing countries. Rev Infect Dis 1989;11(suppl 2):S471–S478.
11. Friedman LN, Filderman AE, D'Aquila TG, Reynolds HY. ELISA analysis of BACTEC bottles for earlier diagnosis of tuberculosis. Am Rev Respir Dis 1989;140:668–671.
12. Butler WR, Kilburn JO. High-performance liquid chromatography patterns of mycolic acids as criteria for identification of *Mycobacterium chelonae, Mycobacterium fortuitum*, and *Mycobacterium smegmatis*. J Clin Microbiol 1990:28:2094–2098.
13. Brownell GH, Belcher KE. DNA probes for the identification of *Nocardia asteroides*. J Clin Microbiol 1990;28:2082–2086.
14. Sommers HM, Good RC. *Mycobacterium*. In: Lennette EH, Balows A, Hausler WJ Jr, Shadomy HJ, eds. Manual of clinical microbiology. 4th ed. Washington, DC: American Society for Microbiology, 1985:216–248.
15. Berlin OGW. Mycobacteria. In: Baron EJ, Finegold SM, eds. Diagnostic microbiology. 8th ed. St. Louis: CV Mosby, 1990: 597–640.
16. Sommers HM, McClatchy JK. Laboratory diagnosis of the mycobacterioses. In: Morello JA, ed. Cumulative techniques and procedures in clinical microbiology, number 16. Washington DC: American Society for Microbiology, 1983.
17. Schaal KP. Laboratory diagnosis of actinomycete diseases. In: Goodfellow M, Mordarski M, Williams ST, eds. The biology of the actinomycetes. London: Academic Press, 1984:441–456.
18. Hollick GE. Nocardiosis. Clin Microbiol Newsl 1988; 10:105–109.
19. Venugopal TV, Venogopal PV. Mycetoma. In: Braude AI, ed. Medical microbiology and infectious disease. Philadelphia: WB Saunders, 1981:1762–1775.
20. Good RC. Editorials: serologic methods for diagnosing tuberculosis. Ann Intern Med 1989;110:97–98.
21. Daniel T, Debanne SM. The serodiagnosis of tuberculosis and other mycobacterial diseases by enzyme-linked immunosorbent assay. Am Rev Respir Dis 1987;135:1137–1151.
22. Lind A, Ridell M. Immunologically based diagnostic tests: humoral antibody methods. In: Kubica GP, Wayne LG, eds. The mycobacteria: a sourcebook. New York; Marcel Dekker, 1984: 221–248.
23. Woods GL, Washington II JA. Mycobacteria other than *Mycobacterium tuberculosis*: review of microbiologic and clinical aspects. Rev Infect Dis 1987;9:275–294.
24. Good RC. Opportunistic pathogens in the genus *Mycobacterium*. Annu Rev Microbiol 1985;39:347–369.
25. Saubolle MA. Nontuberculous mycobacteria as agents of human diseases in the United States. Clin Microbiol News 1989;11:113–117.
26. Hastings RC, Gillis TP, Krahenbuhl JL, Franzblau SG. Leprosy. Clin Microbiol Rev 1988;1:330–348.
27. Wolinsky W. Nontuberculous mycobacteria and associated diseases. Am Rev Respir Dis 1979;119:330–348.
28. O'Brien RJ, Geiter LJ, Snider DE Jr. The epidemiology of nontuberculous mycobacterial diseases in the United States. Results from a national survey. Am Rev Respir Dis 1987;135: 1007–1014.
29. Wallace RJ Jr, Bedsole G, Sumpter G, et al. Activities of ciprofloxacin and ofloxacin against rapidly growing mycobacteria with demonstration of acquired resistance following single-drug therapy. Antimicrob Agents Chemother 1990;34:65–70.
30. Boddinghaus B, Rogall T, Flohr T, Blocker H, Bottger EC. Detection and identification of mycobacteria by amplification of rRNA. J Clin Microbiol 1990;28:1751–1759.
31. Parenti F. New experimental drugs for the treatment of tuberculosis. Rev Infect Dis 1989; 11(suppl. 2):S479–S483.
32. Nolte FS. Antimicrobial susceptibility test procedures for mycobacteria. In: Wentworth BB, ed. Diagnostic procedures for bacterial infections. 7th ed. Washington, DC: American Public Health Assocation, 1987;669–678.
33. Horsburgh CR, Mason UG, Heifets LB, Southwick K, Labrecque J, Iseman M. Response to therapy of pulmonary *Mycobacterium avium-intracellulare* infection correlates with results of *in*

vitro susceptibility testing. Am Rev Respir Dis 1987;135:418–421.

34. Wallace RJ Jr, Tsukamura M, Brown BA, et al. Cefotaxime-resistant *Nocardia asteroides* strains are isolates of the controversial species *Nocardia farcinica*. J Clin Mircobiol 1990;28:2726–2732.
35. Mishra SK, Gordon RE, Barnett DA. Identification of nocardiae and streptomycetes of medical importance. J Clin Microbiol 1980;11:728–736.
36. Beaman BL, Burnside J, Edwards B, Causey W. Nocardial infections in the United States, 1972–1974. J Infect Dis 1976;134:286–289.
37. Mahgoub ES. Agents of mycetoma. In: Mandell GL, Douglas GL Jr, Bennett JE, eds. Principles and practice of infectious diseases. 3rd ed. New York: Churchill Livingstone, 1990:1977–1980.
38. Tight RR, Barlett MS. Actinomycetoma in the United States. Rev Infect Dis 1981;3:1139–1150.
39. Berkey P, Bodey GP. Nocardial infection in patients with neoplastic disease. Rev Infect Dis 1989;11:407–412.
40. Wilson JP, Turner HR, Kirchner KA, Chapman SW. Nocardial infections in renal transplant recipients. Medicine 1989;68:28–57.
41. Smego RA Jr, Gallis HA. The clinical spectrum of *Nocardia brasiliensis* infection in the United States. Rev Infect Dis 1984;6:164–180.
42. Houang ET, Lovett IS, Thompson FD, Harrison AR, Jockes AM, Goodfellow M. Nocardia asteroides infection—a transmissible disease. J Hosp Infect 1980;1:31–40.
43. Van Etta LL, Felice GA, Ferguson RM, Gerding DN. *Corynebacterium equi*: a review of 12 cases of human infection. Rev Infect Dis 1983;5:1012–1018.
44. Ebersole LL, Paturzo JL. Endophthalmitis caused by *Rhodococcus equi* Prescott serotype 4. J Clin Microbiol 1988;26:1221–1222.
45. Southern PM Jr, Kutscher AE, Ragsdale R, Luttrell B. Susceptibility in vitro of *Nocardia* species to antimicrobial agents. Diagn Microbiol Infect Dis 1987;8:111–122.
46. Dewsnup DH, Wright DN. In vitro susceptibility of *Nocardia asteriodes* to 25 antimicrobial agents. Antimicrob Agents Chemother 1984;25:165–167.
47. Wallace RJ, Steele LC. Susceptibility testing of *Nocardia* species for the clinical laboratory. Diagn Microbiol Infect Dis 1988;9:155–166.
48. Woolcock JB, Mutimer MD. *Corynebacterium equi*: in vitro susceptibility to twenty-six antimicrobial agents. Antimicrob Agents Chemother 1980:1976–1977.
49. Rihs JD, McNeil MM, Brown JM, Yu VL. *Oerskovia xanthineolytica* implicated in peritonitis associated with peritoneal dialysis: case report and review of *Oerskovia* infections in humans. J Clin Microbiol 1990;28:1934–1937.
50. Butler WR, O'Connor SP, Yakrus MA, et al. *Mycobacterium celatum* sp. nov. Int J Syst Bacteriol 1993;43:539–548.
51. Coyle MB, Carlson LDC, Wallis CK, et al. Laboratory aspects of "*Mycobacterium genavense*," a proposed species isolated from AIDS patients. J Clin Microbiol 1992;30:3206–3212.
52. Wallace RJ, Brown BA, Tsukamura M, et al. Clinical and laboratory features of *Nocardia nova*. J Clin Microbiol 1991;29:2407–2411.
53. Schiff TA, McNeil MM, Brown JM. Cutaneous *Nocardia farcinica* infection in nonimmunocompromised host. Clin Infect Dis 1993;16:756–760.
54. Prescott JF. *Rhodococcus equi*: an animal and human pathogen. Clin Microbiol Rev 1991;4:20–34.
55. Lasker BA, Brown JM, McNeil MM. Identification and epidemiological typing of clinical and environmental isolates of the genus *Rhodococcus* with use of a digoxigenin-labeled rDNA gene probe. Clin Infect Dis 1992;15:223–233.

48 Instrumentation and Automation in Clinical Microbiology

Michael A. Pfaller and Marie Pezzlo

The many changes that have taken place in the field of infectious diseases over the past 20 years have provided a formidable challenge to the clinical microbiology laboratory. The increase in serious bacterial, fungal, and viral infections in the immunocompromised host, the development of new antimicrobial agents and drug-resistant microbes, and the need to define the epidemiology of nosocomial infections all require that the laboratory provide not only accurate, but rapid, identification and antimicrobial susceptibility testing of clinical isolates (1–4). In addition to these concerns, the current economic climate also requires that the laboratory perform these tasks in a cost-effective manner.

Although the conventional macrotube methods of microbial (largely bacterial) identification and antimicrobial susceptibility testing are still used in microbiology laboratories, the state-of-the-art is the systems approach, which emphasizes standardization, speed, reproducibility, and in the last 10 to 15 years, mechanization and automation (1, 3–26). Thus, the conventional methods have been adapted or streamlined into miniaturized test systems that use numerical coding systems, computer-generated data bases, and reaction endpoints that can be reached after 2 to 6 hours of incubation (5–7, 9–15, 17–22, 26).

These advances in microbial identification and antimicrobial susceptibility testing have resulted in commercial systems that are more reproducible and rapid than their conventional counterparts (3–5, 7, 10, 11, 16). One of the more recent advances in the rapid identification of pathogenic microorganisms is the use of chromogenic or fluorogenic substrates to assess preformed enzyme activity. By detecting preformed enzymes, these systems provide a rapid means of identifying clinically important organisms within 2 to 4 hours of inoculation (12, 13, 15, 18, 19). The use of chromogenic or fluorogenic substrates has also been employed as a rapid and sensitive means of assessing the in vitro susceptibility of bacteria to several antimicrobial agents (21, 22). However, the advantages of these advances may be lost if the tests cannot be read consistently. Several of the commercially available systems offer a variety of biochemical and antimicrobial susceptibility tests, systematic coding systems, and broad computer-generated data bases; however, they are potentially subject to reader bias (4, 12, 13, 16, 24). Fortunately, this problem has largely been circumvented with the development of microprocessor-based instrumentation that can both read and interpret the tests in an identification or antimicrobial susceptibility testing system, thus providing excellent standardization, accuracy, and reproducibility (1, 4–6, 16–18, 20, 24).

There are several instrument-assisted approaches available for microbial identification and antimicrobial susceptibility testing (Table 48.1); however, these systems usually require several manual steps and cannot be considered as truly automated. Currently, there are only three microbiology systems that are sufficiently automated to justify the term "walkaway" systems (Table 48.2). In each case, some initial manual set-up time is required, but once the inoculated tray or card is placed into the instrument, all subsequent incubation, addition of reagents, reading, interpretation, and reporting of test results is accomplished automatically. The availability of the results is not dependent upon the presence of the laboratory staff, and the results are often available within a few hours. These systems require the least amount of technical time and, therefore, may provide a decreased labor cost.

Although the majority of the automated and semiautomated microbiology systems currently available are designed to function optimally on pure isolates of bacteria or fungi, several instrument systems have been designed for the direct detection of organisms in clinical samples of blood, respiratory secretions, and urine (Table 48.3). This chapter describes these direct detection methods as well as the automated and semiautomated methods for microbial identification and antimicrobial susceptibility testing. Specifically, the advantages and disadvantages of each approach are given, as well as suggested potential directions for future development and improvement. Because of the rapid in-

Table 48.1. Features of Specific Semiautomated MIC-ID Systems

Features	FOX	MicroSCAN	Pasco	Sceptor	Sensititre	UniScept	Autobac	Avantage
Inoculation of panels	Manual	Manual	Manual	Manual or automatic	Manual or automatic	Manual or automatic	Manual	Manual
Incubation	Off-line	Off-line	Off-line	Off-line	Off-line	Off-line	Off-line	MIC:on-line IDP:off-line
Test interpretation	Manual or automatic	Manual or automatic	Manual	Manual or automatic	Manual or automatic	Manual or automatic	Automatic	Automatic
Identification capabilities (ID)								
Gram-negative	x	x	x	x	x	x	x	x
Gram-positive		x		x		x		
Anaerobes		x		x		x		
Haemophilus-Neisseria	x	x				x		
Yeast		x				x		x
Antimicrobial susceptibility testing capabilities (AST)								
Gram-negative	x	x	x	x	x	x	x	x
Gram-positive	x	x	x	x	x	x	x	x
Anaerobes				x				

Table 48.2. Features of Fully Automated Walkaway Microbiology Systems

Features	Vitek AMS	AutoSCAN W/A	ALADIN
Inoculation of panels	Automatic	Manual	Manual or automatic
Incubation	Bacteria:on-line yeast:off-line	On-line	On-line
Principle of detection	Photometry	Photometry and fluorescence	Video image analysis
Incubation time (hours)	Bacteria:4–15 hours yeast:22–24 hours	Rapid:2–7 hours conventional:18–24 hours	Rapid:2–5 hours conventional:18–24 hours
Test interpretation	Automatic	Automatic	Automatic
Identification capabilities (ID)			
Gram-negative	x	x	x
Gram-positive	x	x	x
Anaerobes	x		x
Haemophilus-Neisseria	x	x	x
Yeast	x	x	x
Antimicrobial susceptibility testing capabilities (AST)			
Gram-negative	x	x	x
Gram-positive	x	x	x
Anaerobes			

troduction of microbiology products and instrumentation and the frequent modification of existing systems, we have not attempted to provide a detailed description of each of the individual microbiology systems. Rather, we have provided a general overview of the use of automation and instrumentation as applied to the detection, identification, and antimicrobial susceptibility testing of microbial pathogens.

AUTOMATED MICROBIOLOGY SYSTEMS

Instrument-Assisted Identification and Antimicrobial Susceptibility Testing Systems

Currently, there are many instrument-assisted or semiautomated microbiology systems available for performing microbial identification and antimicrobial susceptibility testing functions (Table 48.1). The vast majority of these systems employ either frozen or dried microdilution panels. A variety of microdilution formats are available, including identification only, antimicrobial susceptibility testing only, and combination panels that allow identification and susceptibility testing to be performed simultaneously on the same panel. In addition to identification (ID) and antimicrobial susceptibility testing (AST) of the more common aerobic and facultative Gram-negative and Gram-positive bacterial pathogens, systems are available for testing anaerobes (ID and AST), the more fastidious Gram-negatives such as *Neisseria*, *Haemophilus*, and *Moraxella* (*Branhamella*) species (ID only), and yeasts (ID only) (Table 48.1) (17, 18, 20).

The extent to which instrumentation is applied to these systems ranges from manual inoculation and incubation aided by simple light box readers and manual entry of data into a computer system,

Table 48.3. Instrumentation for Detection of Microorganisms in Clinical Specimens[a]

Specimen	Instrument	Principle	Detection	Automation	Time to Detection
Blood	Bactec 460	Radiometric CO_2	GD	Semi	Hours to days
	Bactec NR 660	Infrared CO_2	GD	Semi	Hours to days
	Bact/Alert	Colorimetric CO_2	GD	Auto	Hours to days
Urine	Bac-T-Screen	Colorimetric Filtration	GI	Semi	1 minute
	UTIScreen	Bioluminescence	GI	Semi	45 minutes
	ARx Avantage	Photometry	GD	Auto	1–5 hours
	Autobac	Photometry	GD	Auto	1–5 hours
	Vitek	Photometry	GD	Auto	4–13 hours[b]
Respiratory	Bactec 460TB	Radiometric CO_2	GD	Semi	Days to weeks

[a]Abbreviations: GD, growth-dependent; GI, growth-independent; semi, semiautomated; auto, automated.
[b]Includes detection and identification.

to highly sophisticated semiautomated reconstitution-inoculation stations coupled with highly refined manual or automated readers and state-of-the-art computers. Inoculation systems may employ manual multiwell inoculators (multichannel pipettes or multipin inoculators) or automatic microprocessor-controlled dispensers that will dispense an inoculum suspension into all wells of a microdilution panel within 30 to 60 seconds. Although in some laboratories the automated dispensing of antibiotic solutions is necessary to prepare custom MIC panels, this is becoming less common because of the wide availability and variety of commercially prepared panels. These panels are available in a variety of formats that incorporate a wide choice and number of antibiotics and can accommodate the needs of most customers.

Once inoculated, the ID and/or MIC microdilution panels are generally incubated off-line in a standard incubator, although some of the larger systems such as the Autobac Series II (Organon Teknika, Durham, NC) and ARx Avantage (Abbott Laboratories, Irving, TX) may utilize dedicated incubator-shaker modules. In most instances, the panels may be read either manually or by instrument following incubation periods ranging from 2 to 24 hours. Visual interpretation of test results is usually aided by a light box designed to enhance visualization, and entry of test results into the system is facilitated by the use of a keyboard, light pen, and LED indicator lights, or a sonic stylus. The more automated reading systems employ the principles of photometry (turbidimetry and colorimetry) or fluorescence to read individual test wells and automatically transfer the test results to a computer that records, interprets, and reports the ID and MIC results. The automated reading systems frequently employ readings at multiple wavelengths in order to facilitate discrimination of weak or borderline reactions. The system utilizing fluorescence-based tests (Sensititre, Gibco Laboratories) has taken advantage of the high degree of sensitivity inherent in fluorescence technology to provide ID and MIC results in an extremely rapid (2 to 5 hours) time frame (18, 21, 22).

Regardless of whether the tests are read visually or automatically, the results are entered into some sort of data management system. At the very simplest level, this may merely be a system for recording and printing results. The user must obtain the identification of an organism by manually looking up the biochemical profile in a code book and then entering the identification into the system. Increasingly, however, microbiology systems provide true data management capabilities that allow the test results to be automatically compared to a large data base. Thus, the user is provided with the organism identification as well as the biochemical and antibiotic susceptibility profile. The modern systems provide total microbiology laboratory data handling with minimal clerical activity and include patient reports, data storage, and data retrieval for epidemiologic and quality assurance purposes.

The obvious advantages of using instrumentation in clinical microbiology are the standardization of microbiology test procedures and the simplification of many tedious, labor-intensive steps, thus allowing many more procedures to be performed in a wider variety of laboratories. In addition, those systems employing automatic test reading have taken advantage of the enhanced sensitivity and precision of photometric and fluorometric measurements to provide test results in a more rapid fashion. In general, the performance of most of the instrument-assisted and semiautomated identification and antimicrobial susceptibility testing systems is at least as good as the more manual conventional methods. Accuracies of 90 to 95% relative to conventional methods are reported routinely for both identification and susceptibility testing systems (5, 7, 9, 12, 13, 17, 18, 20–22). The widespread availability of these systems provides an improved level of performance and standardization among laboratories and allows many laboratories to perform microbiology testing that otherwise would have to be sent out to reference laboratories.

Automated Walkaway Identification and Antimicrobial Susceptibility Testing Systems

Although many of the instrument-assisted microbiology systems described in the previous section offer significant advances in the performance of identification and antimicrobial susceptibility testing procedures, they still require constant interactive operator interface to inoculate panels, transfer them to an incubator, and return them to the instrument for reading, usually one at a time (23, 25). Thus, these systems must be considered to be largely "mechanized" or semiautomated rather than fully automated. Even the more complex and highly instrument-dependent systems such as the Autobac Series II and the ARx Avantage cannot be considered truly automated because these systems require off-line incubation for a large portion of their testing and thus are not true "walkaway" systems.

Advances in engineering and automation have provided microbiology laboratories with systems that may be referred to as walkaway systems (Table 48.2). These systems still require manual transfer of inoculated panels into an incubator/reader; however, the instrument then automatically incubates, reads, and interprets the biochemical and antimicrobial susceptibility tests and provides a printout of the final test results at the appropriate time. The microbiological analyses may be performed in either a batch or interactive mode, and the availability of the results are not dependent upon the presence of the laboratory staff. These systems provide the highest level of automation and the greatest potential advantage to the diagnostic laboratory.

Presently, there are only three microbiology systems that may be considered walkaway systems (Table 48.2). These systems include the Vitek AutoMicrobic System (Vitek Systems, Hazelwood, MO), the autoSCAN W/A (W/A, Baxter MicroScan, West Sacramento, CA), and the Automated Laboratory Diagnostic Instrument or ALADIN (Analytab Products, Plainview, NY). In addition to providing a high level of automation with its attendant labor-saving potential, these systems are highly flexible, offering a wide range of testing capabilities and employ sophisticated optical detection mechanisms that provide sensitive, specific, and rapid reading and interpretation of reaction endpoints.

The Vitek system was one of the first truly automated identification and antimicrobial susceptibility testing systems in microbiology. The system consists of several modules, including a manual diluent dispenser, a filling and sealing unit that inoculates and seals up to 10 multiwell test cards simultaneously, a reader/incubator module with a capacity for 30 to 240 test cards, a computer control module, data terminal, and multicopy printer. The data handling capabilities of the system can be expanded considerably by the addition of a data management system to provide epidemiologic analysis of demographic and test data. Once inoculated, the test cards are inserted into the reader/incubator module, and the system employs a series of light emitting diodes (LEDs) and phototransistor detectors to automatically scan the cards at 20- to 60-minute intervals and measure the extent of light transmission through the individual test wells. The information is stored in the computer module, and the percent change in light transmission for each well is compared with a threshold value to determine whether or not a reaction is considered positive. Although originally designed to enumerate and identify common urinary tract pathogens, the Vitek system has undergone extensive modification over the years. Its capabilities now include the identification and antimicrobial susceptibility testing of aerobic and facultative Gram-negative and Gram-positive bacteria in 4 to 8 hours, the identification of anaerobes, *Neisseria,* and *Haemophilus* species in 4 hours, and yeast identification in 22 to 24 hours as well as the detection, enumeration, and identification of common pathogens in urine in 1 to 13 hours (3–5, 11–14, 17–19, 26). The performance of the Vitek system in the detection and identification of urinary pathogens and the identification and antimicrobial susceptibility testing of common clinical pathogens has been evaluated extensively (5, 11–14, 17–19, 26). In general, the system compares quite favorably with conventional and semiautomated methods, and accuracies well in excess of 90 to 95% are reported routinely. The popularity of the Vitek system in the United States is evidenced by the fact that it is the single most common automated or semiautomated system employed by participants in the College of American Pathologists (CAP) proficiency testing program (27).

The remaining two walkaway systems, the autoSCAN W/A and the ALADIN, represent what some consider to be a new generation of automated microbiology systems (23). Like the Vitek system, the W/A and ALADIN still require inoculation and transfer of the appropriate panels into the incubator/reader and essentially eliminate operator interface after this step. In contrast to the Vitek system, however, these two systems employ several more highly automated techniques to detect conventional microbiological reactions. Both systems utilize new liquid handling techniques and robotics to add reagents and move inoculated panels from one station to the next for automatic processing (6, 15, 19, 20, 23). These systems also use more elaborate optical systems such as fiber optics, video image analysis, fluorescence, and other more sensitive photodetection methods as well as bar code readers and more complex computers (6, 15, 19, 20, 23). This newer automated technology, coupled with reagent systems that utilize the hydrolysis of enzymatic substrates to profile and identify microorganisms in 2 to 5 hours, can provide more hands-off microbiology and more same-day identification and antimicrobial susceptibility testing than is currently available with the Vitek and the many semiautomated systems.

The autoSCAN W/A is an automated microbiology system that employs simple robotics, fiber optics, and both colorimetric and fluorometric detection to automatically incubate, add reagents, and read both conventional (overnight) and rapid (2 to 7 hours) identification and antimicrobial susceptibility test panels (15, 19). Data management is accomplished by a sophisticated computer system that automatically analyzes and prints the final results and can be interfaced directly with larger laboratory and hospital computer systems. The capabilities of the W/A include rapid fluorogenic identification (2 hours) and antibiotic susceptibility testing (3 to 7 hours) of both Gram-negative and Gram-positive bacteria, rapid chromogenic identification (4 hours) of yeasts, anaerobic bacteria, and *Haemophilus* and *Neisseria* species, and conventional (overnight) identification and antimicrobial susceptibility testing of these organisms using dried or frozen microdilution panels. To date, few comparative evaluations of the W/A have been performed; however, those that have been completed indicate that the system compares favorably with both conventional and automated (Vitek) systems for the identification and antimicrobial susceptibility testing of clinical isolates (15, 19).

The ALADIN is another highly automated microbiology system that utilizes more advanced liquid handling techniques, robotics, and analysis of reaction endpoints through video imaging and subsequent computer-assisted interpretations to automatically incubate, add reagents, read, and dispose of both conventional (overnight) and rapid (2 to 5 hours) identification and antimicrobial susceptibility panels (6, 20). The ALADIN permits various combinations of inoculated identification and antimicrobial susceptibility testing panels produced by Analytab Products to be introduced into an incubation chamber on a common carrier. It employs an elevator and mechanical arm to transfer the carrier, at intervals determined by the computer software, to and from an illuminated reading station or a reagent dispensing station as needed (6). The reaction endpoints in each microtube are detected using a video camera and appropriate filters selected by the computer on the basis of the analytical requirements of each test and the need to establish the results using chromogenic, turbidometric, or colorimetric endpoints (6, 20). The camera is programmed to focus on the area of interest for a specific microtube (e.g., top portion of the indole well or bottom portion of the fermentation wells) where color changes or growth are anticipated (6, 20). For antimicrobial susceptibility tests, the video imaging can interpret subtle variations and complications such as fading endpoints, bacterial aggregates, pellicles, sediments, and bubbles (6, 20). The video image of each microtube is transmitted to the image processor, and the raw data are analyzed, interpreted, and reported automatically. The ALADIN automatically discards all tests upon completion and allows the insertion of a new carrier into the vacated slot. The capabilities of the ALADIN include breakpoint (Kirby-Bauer) and quantitative (MIC) antimicrobial susceptibility testing of Gram-negative and Gram-positive bacteria as well as conventional (overnight) and rapid (2 to 5 hours) identification of aerobic and facultative Gram-negative and Gram-positive bacteria, anaerobes, fastidious Gram-negatives (*Neisseria, Moraxella* [*Branhamella*]), and yeasts. Clinical evaluations of the ALADIN have been limited.

One recent multicenter study demonstrated excellent (greater than 95%) agreement between video-generated results and visually determined findings for both biochemical and antimicrobial susceptibility tests (6). More extensive clinical trials will be necessary to establish the role of the ALADIN system in the clinical microbiology laboratory. Still, video image analysis and newer advances in robotics, microprocessor, and cell-sorting technologies represent an exciting and powerful automated analytical approach to studying structural and biochemical parameters of microbial cells (23). The application of this technology will likely extend the capabilities of the clinical microbiology far beyond those that are possible using current conventional methods.

DETECTION SYSTEMS

Blood

A great deal of time and effort have been spent in developing and improving techniques for the detection and processing of microorganisms found in blood (4, 28–35). Unfortunately, efforts at automation in this area have been hindered by the low numbers of organisms present in the blood of infected patients. To a large degree, this has made the rapid detection of septicemia impractical, and microbiologists must rely on the detection of microbial growth with its inherent delays.

In considering the automation of growth-dependent culture systems, few options are available. Until recently, the only automated blood culture technique available was the radiometric Bactec 460 (Becton Dickinson Diagnostic Instrument Systems, Sparks, MD). With this system, the detection of microorganisms present in blood culture bottles is accomplished with the Bactec instrument, the principle of which is based on the measurement of ^{14}C-labeled CO_2 in the head-space air of blood culture bottles containing broth, various growth supplements, and ^{14}C-labeled growth substrates. The ^{14}C-labeled CO_2 is produced by the metabolism of microorganisms and thus is an indirect marker for the presence of bacteria or fungi in the blood inoculated into the system. The advantage of this approach is the elimination of the necessity of examining blood culture broth microscopically (Gram stain) and by blind subculture in order to detect the presence of low numbers of microorganisms. Through the effective use of instrumentation, the radiometric Bactec 460 system permits the performance of blood cultures in much less time and with the possibility for convenient and extensive data analysis. The rate of detection of bacteremia and fungemia as well as the length of time to detection achievable with the Bactec 460 system are at least equivalent to those expected with conventional nonradiometric broth blood culture procedures (28, 31, 33). The radiometric Bactec 460 system has been successfully adapted to detect the presence of *Mycobacterium* species in respiratory secretions and blood (see below). Further refinements of the Bactec system have led to the development of a nonradiometric blood culture system, the Bactec NR 660.

The Bactec NR 660 was developed to address concerns over the handling and disposal of isotopes in the diagnostic laboratory. This system, like the Bactec 460, is based on the detection of CO_2 as a marker for microbial growth; however, the Bactec NR 660 employs infrared spectroscopy, rather than a radiometric method, as a means of detecting CO_2 in the head space of the blood culture bottles (28, 32, 34, 35). The Bactec NR 660 system, although more expensive and bulkier than the 460, offers advantages of no isotope, a shorter cycle time for examination of bottles, and because it may be purchased as a self-contained system (including incubator), less manual handling of bottles. In clinical laboratory comparisons of the Bactec NR 660 versus the Bactec 460 (28, 32, 34) and other blood culture systems (35), the Bactec NR 660 was shown to have comparable or even superior rates of detection and time to positivity. The recent development of blood culture bottles containing antibiotic-adsorbing resins and a 10-ml blood specimen capacity (versus 5 ml for the Bactec 460) and the development of a fully automated blood culture system (Bactec NR 860) promise to further enhance the performance of the Bactec NR 660 system (34).

The success of the Bactec system has stimulated the development of several alternative instrumented approaches to performing blood cultures. These include techniques based on a variety of physicochemical principles, including microcolorimetry, pH, flow cytometry, filtration bioluminescence, electrochemical detection, and colorimetry (28–30). Of these, only colorimetry has been developed to the extent that commercially available instrumentation employing this technique is now, or will soon be, available for the routine detection of bacteremia and fungemia in the clinical laboratory (Table 48.3).

The BacT/Alert (Organon Teknika, Durham, NC) is a modular walkaway blood culture system that employs colorimetric sensors in each bottle to detect CO_2 production by aerobic and anaerobic organisms. Because the blood cultures are continuously monitored in their own incubator module, this system should require even less "hands-on" time than the Bactec system, resulting in further simplification of the blood culture process. The clinical usefulness of this system is currently being assessed in comparative trials.

The usefulness of instrumented blood culture systems has been well established by the widespread use of the Bactec system. Although innovative new systems such as the BacT/Alert may offer important labor-saving advantages to the clinical laboratory, they are unlikely to improve significantly on the sensitivity and time to detection offered by the Bactec system. This is partly because all of these systems are growth-dependent. It is unlikely that any *clinically significant* improvement in the timely detection of microorganisms in the blood will result from further refinements of new or existing technology that requires microbial growth. Instrumentation may streamline this process and make it more efficient for the laboratory, but true clinical advances await the successful adaptation of growth-independent detection methods, such as the amplification and detection of bacterial nucleic acids that can provide detection and identification within 1 to 2 hours.

Urine

Urine specimens represent the most common specimen type sent to the clinical microbiology laboratory for culture. For this reason, considerable time and effort have been expended over the last decade in developing instrumentation to more efficiently process urine specimens within the clinical laboratory. Work in this area has been complicated by great confusion and controversy over the definition of significant bacteriuria (36–40). The gold standard regarding the definition of a urinary tract infection (UTI) in an asymptomatic patient has long been greater than 10^5 colony-forming units (CFU)/ml of urine; however, consideration of as few as 10^2 CFU/ml of coliforms and the presence of pyuria may be appropriate for the diagnosis of UTI in young, symptomatic females (36, 37).

Many methods have been evaluated for screening urine specimens for bacteriuria. These include microscopic, enzymatic, culture, and automated techniques. Semiautomated and automated methods have been developed to meet the increased interest in rapid screening for bacteriuria. Urine screening allows the rapid identification of urine specimens that are positive for bacteriuria, making laboratory processing more efficient and providing rapid results for clinical decision making. At present, it appears that, although we have a rather large number of systems for screening and processing urine specimens, none is sufficiently sensitive to allow the complete abandonment of the conventional urine culture for certain patient groups (4, 36, 38–40). Nevertheless, several of the available semiautomated and automated methods have the potential to provide useful information in a rapid fashion on a large percentage of urine specimens submitted to the clinical laboratory (36, 38–40).

The instrument-assisted bacteriuria screening techniques that are available for use in the diagnostic laboratory include both semiautomated growth-independent screening techniques and more fully automated screening and processing systems (Table 48.3). The growth-independent methods include the Bac-T-Screen (Vitek Systems, Hazelwood, MO), a colorimetric filtration device, and a system based on bioluminescent detection of bacterial adenosine triphosphate (ATP), the UTIscreen (Los Alamos Diagnostics, Los Alamos, NM). Because they do not depend upon bacterial growth, these screening tests are rapid, with processing times ranging from 1 to 2 minutes for the Bac-T-Screen up to 45 minutes for the UTIscreen. The sensitivity of these assays is comparable and in the range of 80 to 90% at the 10^4 CFU/ml breakpoint (4, 36, 38–40).

The growth-dependent assays include the larger automated microbiology instruments, the Vitek System, the Autobac Series II, and the ARx Avantage. All of these systems use light transmission photometry as the basis for detecting bacteriuria (Table 48.3). The Avantage and Autobac are both screening systems, providing results in 1 to 6 hours (36, 38). The Vitek provides detection, enumeration, and identification of the most common urinary pathogens in 4 to 13 hours, with most specimens containing greater than 10^5 CFU/ml identified in 5 to 9 hours (36, 38, 39). These systems have a sensitivity for detection of greater than 10^4 CFU/ml in the range of 85 to 90%, which is similar to that seen with the growth-independent systems (36, 38, 39).

Although most of these instrument-oriented approaches appear to offer some advantages for the processing of urine specimens, including a rapid turnaround time and a high predictive value of a negative (4, 36, 38–40), many clinicians and laboratorians believe that they are not sufficiently sensitive to be used in deciding whether or not a specimen should be cultured (4, 36, 38–40). Several alternative strategies involving combinations of one or more rapid screening tests with one of the rapid automated identification and antimicrobial susceptibility testing systems have been employed in an effort to further streamline urine processing (4, 36, 39). However, these approaches are not widely practiced, and the routine urine culture remains the method of choice for most clinical laboratories.

Respiratory Specimens

Aside from Gram staining, the direct processing of respiratory specimens has been difficult. Although the detection of viral and bacterial antigens in respiratory specimens by either indirect or direct immunofluorescence has been quite successful (41, 42), these approaches are largely manual and labor intensive. Likewise, the use of DNA probes to detect *Legionella* (42, 43) and *Mycoplasma pneumoniae* (44) employs a scintillation counter and is potentially automatable, but presently it must be considered an instrument-assisted *manual* approach to the processing of respiratory specimens.

Undoubtedly, the most significant impact of automation regarding respiratory specimens has taken place in the diagnosis of mycobacterial infection. The adaptation of the Bactec 460 radiometric system for the detection, identification, and susceptibility testing of *Mycobacterium tuberculosis* and other mycobacterial species has been shown by several investigators to be extremely useful in the direct processing of respiratory specimens (4, 45–48). The system employs standard sputum concentration techniques and a combination of polymyxin B, amphotericin B, carbenicillin, and trimethoprim to minimize contamination by nonmycobacterial organisms. This decontamination treatment allows the specimen to be inoculated directly into Middlebrook 7H12 broth medium containing ^{14}C-labeled palmitic acid. Mycobacterial growth is detected by routine monitoring on the Bactec 460 instrument.

In a large, multicenter collaborative study, Roberts and coworkers (47) demonstrated that 94.6% of all smear-positive specimens were detected as culture positive with the Bactec compared to 90.8% with conventional culture methods. The mean time to detection with the Bactec was 8.3 days for *M. tuberculosis* and 5.2 days for other mycobacterial species. In contrast, detection times using conventional culture methods were 19.4 and 17.8 days, respectively. Antimicrobial susceptibility testing results for *M. tuberculosis* showed excellent (95 to 100%) agreement between Bactec and conventional methods. The mean reporting time for antimicrobial susceptibility results ranged from 4.2 to 6.9 days for the Bactec method and from 13.7 to 32 days for conventional methods. The mean total time required for the detection and antimicrobial susceptibility testing of *M. tuberculosis* was 18 days for the Bactec method and 38.5 days for the conventional methods. In contrast to the findings with smear-positive specimens, the Bactec system performed less well on smear-negative specimens. Only 71.8% of these specimens were detected by the Bactec versus 88.7% detected by the conventional culture procedures (46).

In addition to the detection and antimicrobial susceptibility testing of mycobacteria, the Bactec system is also useful in the identification of *M. tuberculosis* using the specific inhibitor *p*-nitro-α-acetylamino-β-hydroxypropiophenone (NAP) (45, 48). Morgan et al. (48) demonstrated that the NAP differential procedure was a rapid and reliable method for identifying *M. tuberculosis*, providing correct classification of 99 to 100% of isolates within 5 days. More recently, the Bactec detection system has been coupled with the use of DNA probes specific for *M. tuberculosis*, *M. avium*, and *M. intracellulare* to provide both detection and identification of these species within 2 to 4 weeks, compared to the 9 to 11 weeks usually required with conventional culture and biochemical identification methods (49). Thus, the combined approach of semiautomated culture, DNA probe technology for the detection identification, and antimicrobial susceptibility testing of mycobacteria is quite effective. It provides the physician with accurate and clinically useful results and is much more efficient than conventional methods of growth detection and biochemical testing.

ADVANTAGES AND LIMITATIONS OF AUTOMATION AND INSTRUMENTATION IN CLINICAL MICROBIOLOGY

Several of the more obvious advantages of automation and instrumentation in clinical microbiology have been mentioned in previous sections of this chapter. These include improved turnaround time for most microbiological analyses, standardization of test performance and interpretation, and with the more highly automated systems, significant labor-saving potential. The instrument approaches discussed in this chapter can accomplish many of the more commonly performed functions in the microbiology laboratory, namely detection, identification, and antimicrobial susceptibility testing of common clinical pathogens. Thus, the potential exists to automate a sizable portion of the laboratory workload using one or more of these instruments (4, 16, 17, 23). With newer data management systems and the ability to interface these systems directly to laboratory or hospital computer systems, on-line reporting of microbiological data is possible. In many cases, the use of instrumentation and automation may significantly expand and enhance the microbiological testing capabilities of the clinical laboratory.

In addition to these well-defined and well-documented advantages, there are several less obvious advantages of automation in clinical microbiology. These include improvements in cost-effectiveness, accuracy of microbiological analyses, and overall patient care. It has been difficult to illustrate the impact of automation in each of these areas; however, there are recent examples in the literature supporting each of these potential advantages (10, 11, 12, 16–19, 50, 51). Additional studies are necessary to document more clearly the advantages of automation in the care of patients with infectious diseases.

Despite the many advantages of instrumentation and automation, there are several significant limitations that must be considered when introducing instrumentation into the diagnostic clinical microbiology laboratory (17, 25). Although the level of automation in clinical microbiology is clearly increasing, it is notable that the entire procedure of specimen handling, organism detection, identification, and antimicrobial susceptibility testing is not completely automated for any given specimen submitted for microbiological analysis. The microbiologist must still process each specimen, usually manually, in a manner sufficient to isolate the organism of interest in pure culture. It is only after this primary isolation procedure and manual preparation of an inoculum suspension that the automated aspects of testing can actually begin. Thus, there is a need for further automation of the handling and processing of specimens submitted for microbiological analysis. Specifically, there is a need for detection and identification of microorganisms *directly* in patient samples. The ability to detect antibiotic-resistant organisms rapidly and directly in patient samples such as blood or other normally sterile body fluids would likely have a major impact on the delivery of care to these infected patients.

Although the accuracy of many of the automated and semiautomated systems is generally comparable to conventional methods for tests employing overnight incubation, this is not always true for rapid test instruments employing short (3 to 5 hours) incubation times (15, 17, 25, 52–54). This problem is particularly notable when considering instruments performing rapid antimicrobial susceptibility testing. Although overall most of the rapid semiautomated and automated susceptibility testing systems are reported to be at least 90 to 95% accurate when compared to conventional methods, significant problems and concerns remain with respect to certain organism-drug combinations. In general, these involve organisms that display heteroresistance (52, 53), inducible resistance mechanisms (17, 53, 54), or high mutation rates to drug resistance (53, 54). In each case, these resistance mechanisms may become apparent only after an incubation period in excess of the 3- to 5-hour target period employed by the rapid test system. These concerns of decreased accuracy are somewhat less when considering the rapid automated identification systems; however, these systems have been unable to identify isolates that also cause problems for other commercial and conventional systems that employ longer incubation times (14, 15, 18, 25).

Additional limitations of automated systems include the lack of standardized quality control (QC) procedures sufficient to detect subtle deterioration in test antibiotic potencies (53, 55) and the lack of flexibility of the systems, particularly with regard to manual back-up in the case of mechanical failure (17, 18, 25). Although manufacturers may have detailed QC and preventive maintenance procedures, concern has been expressed because QC organisms used to verify antimicrobial susceptibility test performance are usually either highly susceptible or resistant to the test agents and thus are off-scale (53, 55). Such off-scale test results do not serve a useful QC function.

The lack of flexibility in laboratories wedded to a single piece of instrumentation has long been a concern of microbiologists. This is most notable with regard to the selection of antimicrobial agents for susceptibility testing. Although manufacturers have made great progress in providing a wide range of panel designs and custom panels, this remains a problem for most commercial systems. Another concern related to the flexibility of microbiology instrumentation is the ability, or lack thereof, to manually read test results in the case of mechanical failure. When a mechanical failure does occur, most of the instrument methods cannot be performed using manual interpretation because subtle and varying definitions of growth or reaction endpoints are employed by the instruments (17). Certainly, some of the less highly automated microdilution methods that employ overnight incubation can be incubated off-line and read manually; however, this is not the case with the newer rapid identification and antimicrobial susceptibility testing systems. Therefore, laboratories employing rapid automated or semiautomated systems such as Vitek, Autobac, Avantage, ALADIN, or autoSCAN W/A must always maintain an additional manual back-up testing procedure for times of mechanical failure or when an organism fails to grow in the automated system.

Finally, the cost of microbiology instrumentation remains an issue, particularly in the case of the larger, more highly automated systems. Reagent costs are rarely lower than those for manual tests, particularly for low-volume laboratories. Likewise, instrumentation costs of $30,000 to greater than $100,000 make it almost impossible for many laboratories to implement instrumentation in microbiology. Although reagent-rental or lease-purchase agreements may provide a flexible means by which laboratories can acquire newer instrumentation and avoid a large capital expenditure, this type of arrangement does not always meet with the approval of laboratory and hospital administration. It is likely that the major cost justification for the use of the more expensive, highly automated microbiology instruments can be derived from labor savings within the laboratory and demonstration of the positive impact of rapid testing and reporting on patient care. Documentation of these positive cost-effective aspects of automation has been difficult, but published data do exist and provide the framework for rational application and evaluation of automation in clinical microbiology (16, 39, 45, 49–51).

FUTURE DEVELOPMENTS

Automation of microbiological testing has progressed considerably over the last 20 years. Currently, new technology with the potential for further automating and revolutionizing the diagnosis of infectious diseases is being developed at a remarkable rate. We are already beginning to see the application of robotics, more sophisticated liquid handling techniques, and advanced optical detection methods that allow many routine microbiological analyses to be performed in a completely automated fashion. These systems will soon be linked with amplification and detection systems employing DNA probes, monoclonal antibodies, and flow cytometry to provide a sensitive and highly automated means of detecting and characterizing microbial pathogens that extends well beyond the simple growth–no growth types of analyses currently dominating clinical microbiology. It is too early to tell, but it is likely that systems will begin to employ more highly sophisticated physicochemical means of characterizing microorganisms such as circular intensity differential light scattering, mass spectrometry, and nuclear magnetic resonance spectroscopy. The polymerase chain reaction (PCR) has already been used to amplify 16S ribosomal RNA gene fragments directly from tissue samples and thus simultaneously detect and identify preliminarily a previously uncultured and uncharacterized pathogen causing infection in immunocompromised patients (56). PCR coupled with nucleic acid sequence analysis is already highly automatable and will be applicable to the diagnosis of infectious disease of both known and unknown causes.

Regardless of the technology employed, the microbiological instrumentation of the future must be multifunctional in order to be cost-effective and to maximize the impact on testing performed in the clinical microbiology laboratory. This means that a single instrument must provide detection, identification, and susceptibility testing capabilities and that it must perform these functions on a single patient sample. This may not be possible for certain types of specimens, but it certainly should be a goal for specimens such as blood and normally sterile body fluids. Thus, the developers and manufacturers of microbiological instrumentation should take note of the progress made in other areas of laboratory medicine such as clinical chemistry where multifunctional, random-access instrumentation has been in place for at least a decade.

SUMMARY AND CONCLUSIONS

Automation in clinical microbiology has lagged behind other areas of laboratory medicine. Recent progress in applying established technology to microbiological analysis has resulted in the development of several hands-off or walkaway approaches to the detection, identification, and antimicrobial susceptibility testing of microorganisms. These systems will certainly streamline the operation of many microbiology laboratories; however, their ability to impact on patient care will be limited as long as they remain dependent upon microbial growth. Recent developments in molecular biology have provided clinical microbiologists with the tools whereby automated detection and identification of microbial pathogens directly in patient samples are possible. Although these advances do not yet address the problem of determining the antimicrobial susceptibility profile of an organism once detected, they are nevertheless significant improvements in our ability to diagnose infectious diseases. It is clear that significant advances in our diagnostic capabilities will require the application of techniques that are radically different from the standard agar and broth-based, growth-dependent methods familiar to all clinical microbiologists. The unwillingness of microbiologists to depart from the tried and true conventional methods is understandable; however, this approach has likely impeded the progress of diagnostic microbiology. The challenge facing the clinical microbiologist at present is to become integrally involved in the development, evaluation, and application of this new technology for the diagnosis of infectious diseases. The overriding goal is to bring diagnostic microbiology into a clinically relevant time frame, thereby providing a real impact on patient care.

References

1. D'Amato RF, Holmes B, Bottone ES. The systems approach to diagnostic microbiology. Crit Rev Microbiol 1981;9:1–44.
2. Isenberg HD. Microbiology and the ailing patient. In: Lorian V, ed. Significance of medical microbiology in the care of patients. 2nd ed. Baltimore: Williams & Wilkins, 1982:1–11.
3. Malloy PJ, Miceika BG, Ducate MJ. Automated methods in microbiology. II. Identification and susceptibility testing. Am J Med Technol 1983;49:313–321.
4. Pfaller MA. Automated instrument approaches to clinical microbiology. Diagn Microbiol Infect Dis 1985;3:15S–23S.
5. Barry AL, Gavan TL, Badal RE, Telenson MJ. Sensitivity, specificity, and reproducibility of the AutoMicrobic System (with the Enterobacteriaceae-plus Biochemical Card) for identifying clinical isolates of gram-negative bacilli. J Clin Microbiol 1982;15:582–588.
6. D'Amato RF, Isenberg HD, McKinley GA, Baron EJ, Tepper R, Shulman M. Novel application of video image processing to biochemical and antimicrobial susceptibility testing. J Clin Microbiol 1988;26:1492–1495.
7. DiPersio JR, Dyke JW, Vannest RD. Evaluation of the updated MS-2 bacterial identification system in comparison with the API 20E system. J Clin Microbiol 1983;18:128–135.
8. Edberg SC, Edberg MK. Comparison of identification systems for Enterobacteriaceae. J Clin Lab Auto 1982;2:263–265.
9. Gavini F, Husson MO, Izard D, Bernigaud A, Quiviger B. Evaluation of Auto-Scan-4 for identification of members of the family Enterobacteriaceae. J Clin Microbiol 1988;26:1586–1588.
10. Jorgensen JH, Johnson JE, Alexander GA, Paxson R, Alderson GL. Comparison of automated and rapid manual methods for the same-day identification of Enterobacteriaceae. Am J Clin Pathol 1983;79:683–687.
11. Kelly MT, Latimer JM. Comparison of the AutoMicrobic System with API, Enterotube, Micro-ID, Micro-Media Systems, and conventional methods for identification of Enterobacteriaceae. J Clin Microbiol 1980;12:659–662.
12. Pfaller MA, Bale MJ, Schulte KR, Koontz FP. Comparison of the Quantum II Bacterial Identification System and the AutoMicrobic System for the identification of gram-negative bacilli. J Clin Microbiol 1986;23:1–5.
13. Pfaller MA, Preston T, Bale M, Koontz FP, Body BA. Comparison of the Quantum II, API Yeast Ident, and AutoMicrobic Systems for identification of clinical yeast isolates. J Clin Microbiol 1988;26:2054–2058.
14. Plorde JJ, Gates JA, Carlson LG, Tenover FC. Critical evaluation of the AutoMicrobic System Gram-Negative Identification Card for identification of glucose-nonfermenting gram-negative rods. J Clin Microbiol 1986;23:251–257.
15. Tenover FC, Mizuki TS, Carlson LG. Evaluation of autoSCAN-W/A Automated Microbiology System for the identification of non-glucose-fermenting gram-negative bacilli. J Clin Microbiol 1990;28:1628–1634.

16. Pezzlo M. Accomplishments of current automated microbiology instruments. In: Jorgensen JH, ed. Automation in clinical microbiology. Boca Raton, FL: CRC Press, 1987:191–195.
17. Jorgensen JH. Instrument systems which provide rapid (3- to 6-hr) antibiotic susceptibility results. In: Jorgensen JH, ed. Automation in clinical microbiology. Boca Raton, FL: CRC Press, 1987;85–97.
18. Murray PR. Rapid automated identification systems. In: Jorgensen JH, ed. Automation in clinical microbiology. Boca Raton, FL: CRC Press, 1987:53–67.
19. Pfaller MA, Sahm D, O'Hara C, et al. Comparison of the autoSCAN-W/A Rapid Bacterial Identification System and the Vitek AutoMicrobic System for the identification of gram-negative bacilli. J Clin Microbiol 1991;29:1422–1428.
20. Murray PR. Overnight automated identification systems. In: Jorgensen JH, ed. Automation in clinical microbiology. Boca Raton, FL: CRC Press, 1987:41–51.
21. Staneck JL, Allen SD, Harris EE, Tilton RC. Automated reading of MIC microdilution trays containing fluorogenic enzyme substrates with the Sensititre Autoreader. J Clin Microbiol 1985;22:187–191.
22. Doern GV, Staneck JL, Needham C, Tubert T. Sensititre Autoreader for same-day breakpoint broth microdilution susceptibility testing of members of the family Enterobacteriaceae. J Clin Microbiol 1987;25:1481–1485.
23. Goldstein J. Future development of automated instruments for microbiology. In: Jorgensen JH, ed. Automation in clinical microbiology. Boca Raton, FL: CRC Press, 1987:215–220.
24. O'Hara CM, Rhoden DL, Smith PB. Agreement between visual and automated UniScept API readings. J Clin Microbiol 1990;28:452–454.
25. Staneck JL. The shortcomings of current automation in clinical microbiology. In: Jorgensen JH, ed. Automation in clinical microbiology. Boca Raton, FL: CRC Press, 1987:197–208.
26. Isenberg HD, Gavan T, Smith P, et al. Collaborative investigation of the AutoMicrobic System *Enterobacteriaceae* biochemical card. J Clin Microbiol 1980;11:694–702.
27. Jones RN, Edson DC. Antimicrobial susceptibility testing (AST) trends and accuracy in the United States: a review of the College of American Pathologists microbiology surveys 1972–1989. Arch Pathol Lab Med (in press).
28. Doern GV. Instrumented approaches to performing blood cultures. In: Jorgensen JH, ed. Automation in clinical microbiology. Boca Raton, FL: CRC Press, 1987:7–13.
29. Kagan RL, Schuette WH, Zierdt CH, MacLowry JD. Rapid automated diagnosis of bacteremia by impedence detection. J Clin Microbiol 1977;5:51–57.
30. Wallis C, Melnick JL. Rapid, colorimetric method for the detection of microorganisms in blood culture. J Clin Microbiol 1985;21:505–508.
31. Reimer LG, McDaniel JD, Mirrett S, Reller LB, Wang WLL. Controlled evaluation of supplemented peptone and Bactec blood culture broths for the detection of bacteremia and fungemia. J Clin Microbiol 1985;21:531–534.
32. Junkind D, Millan J, Allen S, Dyke J, Hill E. Clinical comparison of a new automated infrared blood culture system with the BACTEC 460 system. J Clin Microbiol 1986;23:262–266.
33. Wasilauskas B, Gay R, Zwadyk P, Pfaller M, Koontz F. Multicenter comparison of MicroScan and BACTEC blood culture systems. J Clin Microbiol 1987;25:2355–2358.
34. Courcol RJ, Durocher AV, Roussel-Delvallez M, Fruchart A, Martin GR. Routine evaluation of BACTEC NR-16A and NR-17A media. J Clin Microbiol 1988;26:1619–1622.
35. Schwabe LD, Randall EL, Miller-Catchpole R, Squires CI, Gottschall RL. A comparison of Oxoid Signal with nonradiometric BACTEC NR-660 for detection of bacteremia. Diagn Microbiol Infect Dis 1990;13:3–8.
36. Pezzlo M. Detection of urinary tract infections by rapid methods. Clin Microbiol Rev 1988;1:268–280.
37. Pfaller M, Ringenberg B, Rames L, Hegeman J, Koontz F. The usefulness of screening tests for pyuria in combination with culture in the diagnosis of urinary tract infection. Diagn Microbiol Infect Dis 1987;6:207–215.
38. Pezzlo M. Instrument methods for detection of bacteriuria. In: Jorgensen JH, ed. Automation in clinical microbiology. Boca Raton, FL: CRC Press, 1987:15–29.
39. Pfaller MA, Koontz FP. The use of rapid screening tests in conjunction with the AutoMicrobic System: a time and cost-effective approach. J Clin Microbiol 1985;21:783–787.
40. Pfaller MA, Baum CA, Niles AC, Murray PR. Clinical laboratory evaluation of a urine screening device. J Clin Microbiol 1983;18:674–679.
41. Ahluwalia G, Embree J, McNicol P, Law B, Hammond GW. Comparison of nasopharyngeal aspirate and nasopharyngeal swab specimens for respiratory syncytial virus diagnosis by cell culture, indirect immunofluorescence assay and enzyme-linked immunosorbent assay. J Clin Microbiol 1987;25:763–767.
42. Doebbeling BN, Bale MJ, Koontz FP, Helms C, Wenzel RP, Pfaller MA. Prospective evaluation of the Gen-Probe assay for detection of Legionellae in respiratory secretions. Eur J Clin Microbiol Infect Dis 1988;7:748–752.
43. Pasculle AW, Veto GE, Krystofiak S, McKelvey K, Vrsalovic K. Laboratory and clinical evaluation of a commercial DNA probe for the detection of *Legionella* spp. J Clin Microbiol 1989;27:2350–2358.
44. Kleemola SRM, Karjalainen JE, Räty RKH. Rapid diagnosis of *Mycoplasma pneumoniae* infection: clinical evaluation of a commercial probe test. J Infect Dis 1990;162:70–75.
45. Morgan MA, Roberts GD. Radiometric detection, identification, and antimicrobial susceptibility testing of mycobacteria. In: Jorgensen JH, ed. Automation in clinical microbiology. Boca Raton, FL: CRC Press, 1987:31–38.
46. Morgan MA, Horstmeier CD, DeYoung DR, Roberts GD. Comparison of a radiometric (BACTEC) and conventional culture media for recovery of mycobacteria from smear-negative specimens. J Clin Microbiol 1983;18:384–388.
47. Roberts GD, Goodman NL, Heifets L, et al. Evaluation of the BACTEC radiometric method for recovery of mycobacteria and drug susceptibility testing of *Mycobacterium tuberculosis* from acid-fast smear-positive specimens. J Clin Microbiol 1983;18:689–696.
48. Morgan MA, Doerr KA, Hempel HO, Goodman NL, Roberts GD. Evaluation of the *p*-nitro-α-acetylamino-β-hydroxypropiophenone differential test for identification of *Mycobacterium tuberculosis* complex. J Clin Microbiol 1985;21:634–635.
49. Ellner PD, Kiehn TE, Cammarata R, Hosmer M. Rapid detection and identification of pathogenic mycobacteria by combining radiometric and nucleic acid probe methods. J Clin Microbiol 1988;26:1349–1352.
50. Matsen J. Rapid reporting of results—impact on patient, physician, and laboratory. In: Tilton RC, ed. Rapid methods and automation in microbiology. Washington, DC: American Society for Microbiology, 1982:98–102.
51. Trenholme GM, Kaplan RL, Karakusis PH, et al. Clinical impact of rapid identification and susceptibility testing of bacterial blood culture isolates. J Clin Microbiol 1989;27:1342–1345.
52. Aldridge KE, Janney A, Sanders CV, Marier RL. Interlaboratory variation of antibiograms of methicillin-resistant and methicillin-susceptible *Staphylococcus aureus* strains with conventional and commercial testing systems. J Clin Microbiol 1983;18:1226–1236.
53. Thornsberry C. Automated procedures for antimicrobial susceptibility tests. In: Lennette EH, Balows A, Hausler WJ JR,

Shadomy HJ, eds. Manual of clinical microbiology. 4th ed. Washington, DC: American Society for Microbiology, 1985: 1015–1018.

54. Lampe MF, Aitken CL, Dennis PG, et al. Relationship of early readings of minimal inhibitory concentrations to the results of overnight tests. Antimicrob Agents Chemother 1975;8:429–433.

55. Kellogg JA. Inability to adequately control antimicrobial agents on AutoMicrobic System gram-positive and gram-negative cards. J Clin Microbiol 1985;21:454–456.

56. Relman DA, Loutit JS, Schmidt TM, Falkow S, Tompkins LS. The agent of bacillary angiomatosis—an approach to the identification of uncultured pathogens. N Engl J Med 1990;23: 1573–1580.

49 Antimicrobial Susceptibility Testing

Carl L. Pierson

Antimicrobial susceptibility test results are regarded by most clinicians as vital information for the selection of antimicrobics to treat an established infection or to prevent an infection. Requests for susceptibility testing are so common that it is routine for clinicians to ask for this test in conjunction with culture prior to knowing the outcome of the culture. This results in either excessive testing or places the decision of which organisms to test on the microbiologist based primarily on culture results alone. The very fact that a susceptibility test was done on an isolate tends to enhance suspicion on the part of the clinician that the tested organism is a pathogen.

Unfortunately, few clinicians who use susceptibility test results understand the methods used to generate them and, more importantly, the limitations of using such in vitro procedures to predict efficacy in their patients. With the addition of the numerous antimicrobics being added yearly to the physician's armamentarium with their varied antimicrobial profiles and pharmacokinetics, the complexity of choosing an appropriate therapeutic agent has increased dramatically. Therefore, clinical pathologists and microbiologists must work closely with the infectious disease specialists and pharmacists within a medical care setting to provide meaningful reports and interpretations to assist in this selective process. Quality assurance indicators that are designed to monitor how clinicians use laboratory information often reveal where false assumptions are being made from a laboratory report. Clinical pathologists and microbiologists must continue to stay abreast of the laboratory testing methods being used and their clinical relevance, and must interact with the clinicians using this information to produce useful reports leading to appropriate drug utilization.

The clinical relevance of in vitro susceptibility results is not altogether clear in many instances. Bacterial pathogens that test "susceptible" to an antimicrobic selected for therapy may be effectively treated in an immunocompetent patient, but the drug may be ineffective in an immunocompromised patient. Most studies that attempt to correlate treatment success with in vitro susceptibility fail to show a positive correlation; however, there frequently is a positive correlation between organisms that test resistant and treatment failure (1–4). Therefore, the apparent value of the susceptibility test is to monitor for organism resistance to selected antimicrobics.

The developmental history of susceptibility test methods was recently reviewed (5). Much effort has gone into developing testing standards so that interlaboratory results are more consistent. Drs. Hans Ericsson and John Sherris worked with an international team to publish the International Collaborative Study report in 1971 (6). These remarkable studies laid the groundwork upon which most subsequent work on test standardization for disk diffusion and broth dilution techniques was done. In the U.S., this continuing task has been taken up by the National Committee for Clinical Laboratory Standards (NCCLS) subcommittee on antimicrobial susceptibility tests, which publishes testing standards and supplemental updates for these standards on a periodic basis. Other subcommittees have been formed to develop methods for testing antifungal agents and to perform other special tests such as the minimum bactericidal concentration (MBC) test and the serum bactericidal test (SBT), which, by consensus approval, could become standards.

The areas of responsibility for the performance of susceptibility testing that rest with the microbiology laboratory are listed in Table 49.1. Microbiology specimens submitted for routine bacteriologic culture usually arrive in the laboratory accompanied by a requisition for "culture and susceptibility." This implies that a susceptibility test is to be done if a possible pathogen is isolated that is known to vary in its susceptibility to antimicrobics commonly used for treatment, and methods exist to perform and interpret the test. Organisms that typically show no variation in susceptibility to the recommended drugs of choice need not be tested, e.g., *Streptococcus pyogenes* has always tested susceptible to penicillin when done appropriately. Other pathogens must be treated empirically without the benefit of susceptibility testing either because the in vitro results are known not to reflect the clinical response to therapy with a drug or because the laboratory has no way of interpreting the results obtained from such a test. An

Table 49.1. Laboratory Responsibilities for Performing Antimicrobial Susceptibility Tests

Selection of isolates to be tested
Selection of antimicrobics to test
Perform tests using standardized procedures whenever possible
Assist with interpretation of nonstandardized tests
Reporting of results
  Accurately
  Timely
  Selectively

example of the former would be the activity of cefamandole on oxacillin-resistant *Staphylococcus aureus;* an example of the latter would be the activity of ceftriaxone against *Streptococcus pneumoniae.*

With the rapidly increasing number of antimicrobics available for clinical use, a method of determining which agents need to be tested and/or reported against appropriate bacteria had to be developed. The NCCLS documents M2-A4 (standards for the disk diffusion method) and M7-A2 (standards for dilution methods) offer suggested groupings that can be used to limit the number of drugs requiring testing based on drug class and probability of obtaining like results (7, 8). Suggestions are also offered for selective reporting of results to encourage the use of less expensive yet effective antimicrobics. If an organism shows resistance to a first-tier antimicrobic, another one of a similar class that shows good activity can be reported from a secondary tier. Antimicrobics approved for use by the hospital formulary committee should be used as a guide for drug selection. Consultation with local infectious disease specialists who utilize the laboratory can also offer valuable assistance on drug selection and drug concentrations to test, but NCCLS standards should be followed unless there are overriding local circumstances to the contrary. Whenever an alternative method is used, it should be justified, and the clinician should be notified that a nonstandardized method was used. Under such circumstances, NCCLS interpretations should not be used, and it may be necessary to report the result without an interpretation.

COMMON IN VITRO ANTIMICROBIAL SUSCEPTIBILITY TESTS

There are perhaps a dozen different laboratory tests in use to determine organism susceptibility to various antimicrobics (Tables 49.2 and 49.3) but only a few are used with any frequency in most laboratories doing such testing on a routine basis. In addition, special reference laboratories may also perform susceptibility tests for mycobacteria, fungi, and certain viruses.

Table 49.2. Frequently Used In Vitro Susceptibility Tests

Dilution tests
  Broth microtiter
  Agar
  Semiautomated
Disk diffusion ("Kirby-Bauer")
Spot tests (β-lactamase)

Table 49.3. Infrequently Used In Vitro Susceptibility Tests

Minimum bactericidal concentration (MBC)
Serum Bactericidal test (SBT, "Schlichter test")
Time-kill kinetic assay
Drug synergy tests
  "Checkerboard"
  Time-kill kinetic assay

To date, there are only three susceptibility testing standards issued by the NCCLS:

- M7-A2 *Methods for Dilution Antimicrobial Susceptibility Tests for Bacteria that Grow Aerobically*—2nd ed. (1990);
- M2-A4 *Performance Standards for Antimicrobial Disk Susceptibility Tests.* 4th ed. (1990); and
- M11-A2 *Methods for Antimicrobial Susceptibility Testing of Anaerobic Bacteria.* 2nd ed. (1990).

NCCLS publications for other susceptibility testing procedures are available but have not been given standard status to date. Still, they contain valuable information regarding the state of the art. These publications include:

- M21-P *Methodology for the Serum Bactericidal Test* (1987);
- M23-T *Development of In Vitro Susceptibility Testing Criteria and Quality Control Parameters* (1990);
- M24-P *Antimycobacterial Susceptibility Testing* (1990);
- M26-P *Methods for Determining Bactericidal Activity of Antimicrobial Agents* (1987); and
- M27-P *Reference Method for Broth Dilution Antifungal Susceptibility Testing of Yeasts* (1992).

Microdilution Minimum Inhibitory Concentration Test

The microdilution minimum inhibitory concentration (MIC) provides a quantitative measurement (in μg/ml) of the lowest concentration of antimicrobial agent that inhibits the growth of a bacterium. The reader is advised to consult the NCCLS standard M7-A2 for a detailed description of procedures for this test method (8).

Selected antimicrobics can be obtained either from the pharmaceutical manufacturer or a commercial distributor. Only standardized powders or liquids specifying specific activity are to be used. The agents are dissolved in appropriate solvents and finally diluted to appropriate concentrations and distributed into the wells of molded microtiter plates. The filled plates can be either frozen at −70°C or dessicated and stored at room temperature. The concentrations selected for each agent are determined by the achievable blood (or urine) concentrations obtained with recommended dosage schedules and routes of administration. Traditional MIC panels contain a twofold dilutional series of concentrations for each agent, ranging from easily achievable concentrations (susceptible) to those that are usually unachievable (resistant) in blood (or urine). As a result of the large number of antimicrobics available for testing, some panels are designed as "breakpoint panels" that limit the number of dilutions used to the minimum necessary to provide interpretive information. This allows for more drugs to be tested per panel. Other drugs are present in single concentrations and are used primarily for screening for one-point levels of resistance.

Prior to use, frozen panels must be defrosted and subsequently inoculated with the test organism, making sure that the inoculum volume does not exceed more than 10% of the final volume in each well. Usually 1 to 5 μl of inoculum is added to 100 μl of diluted antimicrobic solution in each well. Dessicated panels are usually rehydrated and inoculated simultaneously by suspending the appropriate number of organisms directly in the rehydrating growth medium.

Several different growth media have been used to assess antimicrobic activity. Some nutritionally fastidious bacteria (e.g., *Haemophilus influenzae*) require the presence of supplementary growth factors (9). Others may require higher concentrations of cations to express resistance characteristic not seen otherwise (10–12). Serum or serum components may be added to show the effect of additional protein on antimicrobic activity (13–15). For routine testing, however, the growth medium selected for use in MIC testing in the United States is Mueller-Hinton broth (MHB) that contains a final concentration of 20 to 25 mg/l of Ca^{2+} and 10 to 12.5 mg/l of Mg^{2+}cation-adjusted Mueller-Hinton broth (CAMHB). This cation concentration is especially important when testing the activity of certain aminoglycosides against *Pseudomonas aeruginosa* (11). To enhance the expression of resistance to oxacillin in staphylococci, the CAMHB must also contain 2% NaCl (12). The pH of the medium must fall within the range of 7.2 to 7.4 (16).

Bacteria to be used can be harvested from either solid media or broth culture. The phase of growth that the organism is in appears to have little effect on the results, but it is important to have a relatively fresh culture to assure that a high percentage of the bacterial cells are viable. Initially, a portion of four to five similar colonies from a pure culture or from colonies well isolated on a plate are to be harvested and suspended in water and the turbidity adjusted to match that of a 0.5 McFarland turbidity standard or an O.D. of approximately 0.08 @ 625 nm. This provides an approximate concentration of 10^8 viable cells/ml. This suspension must be further diluted in CAMHB to achieve a concentration such that the final concentration in the microdilution well will be about 5×10^5 CFU/ml. Although this concentration is somewhat arbitrary, it has been determined that when inoculum concentrations substantially higher than this are used, e.g., 10^7 CFU/ml, false-resistant results can be obtained; lower inoculum concentrations can yield false-susceptible results (17). It is advisable to periodically (weekly) remove a sample from the growth control well of an inoculated MIC panel and perform a colony count to document that the inoculum concentration is within the correct range.

Inoculated panels are to be incubated 18 to 24 hours at 35°C in a room air incubator. CO_2 incubators are not to be used because the CO_2 increases the acidity of the growth medium, which can significantly alter the activity of certain antimicrobics. A full 24-hour incubation time is recommended when testing staphylococci for oxacillin resistance. These resistant organisms are slow-growing, and "heteroresistant" strains are present in low numbers, i.e., only one out of 10^6 cells may express resistance (12). It may be necessary to incubate coagulase-negative staphylococci up to 48 hours to detect oxacillin resistance. Rapid-growing mycobacteria may also be tested for susceptibility using this method, but they usually require 3 to 4 days of incubation prior to reading (18).

The panels are read by holding them over a light source that provides indirect background lighting. This type of illumination is optimal for detecting faint buttons of growth at the base of the wells. All panels are to have a growth control well that contains no antimicrobic, and a sterility well that contains no antimicrobic and was not inoculated. Both control wells should be examined prior to assessing the rest of the panel. The sterility well should show no evidence of growth, and the growth control well should show obvious growth that is consistent with the pattern of growth expected for the organism type inoculated. Gram-positive cocci usually form a discrete button at the bottom of the well, whereas Gram-negative bacilli frequently grow in a more diffuse pattern, although neither of these characteristics are absolute. If the control wells do not appear as expected, the reading for the panel should be aborted and the isolate retested. If the control wells are acceptable, each series of dilutions of an antimicrobic should be examined for an endpoint where the lowest concentration in the antimicrobic series has completely inhibited the growth of the inoculated organism. This concentration is recorded for each antimicrobic tested. Most endpoints are quite easy to determine; some, especially certain bacteriostatic drugs, may not produce a sharp endpoint, and exhibit a "trailing effect." With experience, an endpoint can usually be determined where there is a sharp (80% or more) decrease in the amount of growth seen.

Specific control strains must be tested at least weekly to monitor drug concentrations in the panels and to assure that the technique being used to set up the panels is adequate to obtain accurate results. Quality control (QC) guidelines are available from the NCCLS (M23-T). Currently, there are four strains that are recommended for routine quality control of MIC panels:

- *Staphylococcus aureus,* ATCC 29213 (β-lactamase positive);
- *Enterococcus faecalis,* ATCC 29212;
- *Escherichia coli,* ATCC 25922; and
- *Pseudomonas aeruginosa,* ATCC 27853.

Additional strains should be tested when certain drugs or specific bacteria are to be tested:

- *E. coli,* ATCC 35218 when β-lactam/β-lactam inhibitor combinations are being tested (β-lactamase positive);
- *Haemophilus influenzae,* ATCC 49247 or 49766 when testing an *H. influenzae* isolate; and
- *Neisseria gonorrhoeae,* ATCC 49226 when testing an isolate of *N. gonorrhoeae.*

All of the above strains are available from the American Type Culture Collection (ATCC), Rockville, MD. The ideal control strain would yield an MIC that is in the intermediately susceptible range for the drug being monitored. Unfortunately, many of the new broad-spectrum antimicrobics are highly active against the older control strains and produce MICs that are much lower than the lowest concentration being tested. New, stable, resistant control strains are needed for these drugs to provide adequate QC.

The MIC results are to be reported in μg/ml and an interpretation given for each drug as to whether the MIC falls within the range considered by the NCCLS standard to be susceptible, intermediately susceptible, or resistant. Infections caused by organisms that yield intermediately susceptible results may still be treated effectively by the drug if higher dosages can be administered or if the drug is known to concentrate within the infected locus such as in urine or bile. When organism-drug combinations are tested and no interpretations are available, no interpretations should be given until there is enough clinical evidence to show that an interpretation is justified. As mentioned previously, attempts should be made to limit the number of drugs reported to those that offer a more limited yet good spectrum of activity and are less expensive to purchase and administer.

Disk Diffusion Method

This method, commonly referred to as the Kirby-Bauer test, provides a qualitative measure of the ability of an antimicrobic to inhibit the growth of a rapidly growing bacterium. The disk diffusion method was the first standardized susceptibility method available and remains a very useful method despite the continuing shift of laboratories to either the microdilution MIC method or a semiautomated procedure.

Disks containing a given concentration of an antimicrobic are placed on a confluently inoculated agar plate and incubated for 16 to 24 hours. At the end of the incubation period, zones of growth inhibition are measured across the disk diameter and recorded to the nearest millimeter. The results are interpreted as susceptible, intermediately susceptible, or resistant by using the interpretive tables provided in the NCCLS standard M2-A4 (7). No quantitative results can be given with this method.

For routine disk diffusion testing, most clinical laboratories use plastic culture dishes with diameters of 150 mm that have been filled with Mueller-Hinton agar to a depth of 4 mm. Cation supplementation is usually unnecessary because the agar itself contributes adequate amounts of Ca^{2+} and Mg^{2+}, and the companies providing the media now monitor their products and supplement them when necessary. The media can be supplemented with other products such as horse blood, which supplies thymidine phosphorylase and allows for more accurate measurement of trimethoprim and sulfamethoxazole activity, which are inhibited by the presence of thymidine (20). Blood-supplemented plates are often necessary to obtain adequate growth of some fastidious organisms such as some streptococci and diphtheroids (9). To test *N. gonorrhoeae,* the NCCLS standards recommend the use of GC agar instead of Mueller-Hinton agar. The 150-mm plates can accommodate about 12 individual susceptibility disks; the actual number depends on the anticipated size of the zones of inhibition, which should not overlap. This size is partly dependent on the concentration of the drug in the disk and the diffusion characteristics of the drug through the agar. Drugs such as penicillin can produce very

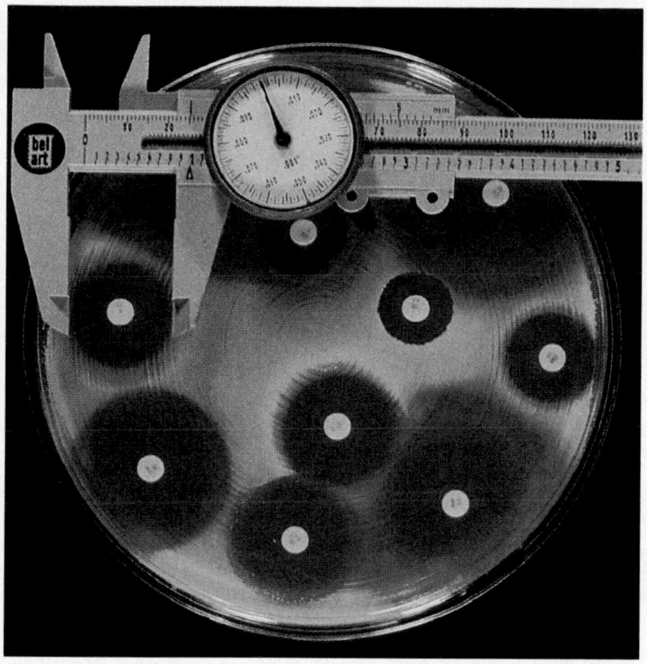

Figure 49.1. Measuring zones of inhibition around antimicrobic disks using a micrometer.

large zones of inhibition when testing very susceptible organisms, whereas others such as most aminoglycosides produce relatively small zones but can still be considered clinically effective. The agar plates can be maintained at 4°C for up to the given expiration date. Regardless of the date, however, the agar surface should be smooth, level, and of the correct depth (4 mm) prior to placing a plate into service. No condensation should be apparent on the plate surface after the plate has been allowed to reach room temperature.

Inoculum preparation is similar to the previously described MIC preparation. The tops of four to five well-isolated uniform colonies are touched with an inoculating loop and used to inoculate 4 to 5 ml of a nutrient broth (e.g., TSB or BHI). The broth is incubated at 35° to 37° C for sufficient time to allow the growth to reach a tubidity equal to or greater than a 0.5 McFarland turbidity standard and subsequently diluted if necessary with broth to be equivalent to this standard. An acceptable alternative method is to remove sufficient fresh growth from a nonselective agar medium to obtain adequate tubidity. A nontoxic swab is immersed into the broth, swirled to eliminate air bubbles, and the excess fluid pushed out of the swab by rotating it against the wall of the tube above the fluid level. The swab is used to streak the agar plate for confluent growth. Care must be taken not to over- or underinoculate the plate because this can alter the resulting zone of inhibition (21). A correctly inoculated plate will reveal individual but closely packed colonies with careful inspection of the plate after incubation.

Filter paper disks containing designated amounts of an antimicrobic can be obtained from either the manufacturer or several commercial supply firms. They are usually supplied in sealed cartridges with a dessicating agent to assure dryness. Moisture can decrease potency. It is necessary to put the disks in a non-self-defrosting freezer for long-term storage and keep a working supply in a refrigerator under dessication. The disks should be allowed to warm to room temperature prior to opening them for use.

The disks must be placed onto the surface of the inoculated agar plate no later than 15 minutes after inoculation. Once applied, they cannot be repositioned because the antimicrobic begins to diffuse immediately. The plates are to be incubated in a non-CO_2 incubator at 35°C for 16 to 18 hours unless otherwise specified. After this time, the zone of inhibition can be measured to the nearest mm and the results interpreted following the appropriate NCCLS Standard table. Figure 49.1 illustrates the use of this technique.

Generally, supplements should be added only when necessary to obtain adequate growth. Certain fastidious organisms such as *H. influenzae, N. gonorrhoeae,* and *S. pneumoniae* will require blood supplements and a 5 to 7% CO_2 atmosphere to grow. Whenever media supplements are used, appropriate control strains must be tested to assure proper test function and interpretation of results.

The determination of disk diffusion interpretation is based on correlating MIC results with corresponding zone diameters. These are inversely proportional; i.e., as the MIC increases, the zone diameter of inhibition decreases. When a variety of organisms with varying susceptibilities to an antimicrobic are tested by both methods and the results plotted with the increasing MIC results on the y axis and the increasing zone sizes in millimeters plotted on the x axis, a regression curve with a negative slope is obtained (Fig. 49.2). Depending in large part on the pharmacokinetics of the drug, interpretive zone sizes can be determined that correspond to those used for interpreting MIC results. For various reasons, this correlation does not alway exist and discrepant results can occur.

Recently, a new test method has been developed called the E Test (AB Biodisk, North America, Inc., Piscataway, NJ), which is a modification of the disk diffusion test but provides an MIC result (22). This test is set up in the same way as the disk diffusion test except that, in place of the disks, one uses 5- × 50-mm plastic strips having a continuous gradient of antimicrobic immobilized on one side and an MIC interpretive scale corresponding to 15 two-fold MIC di-

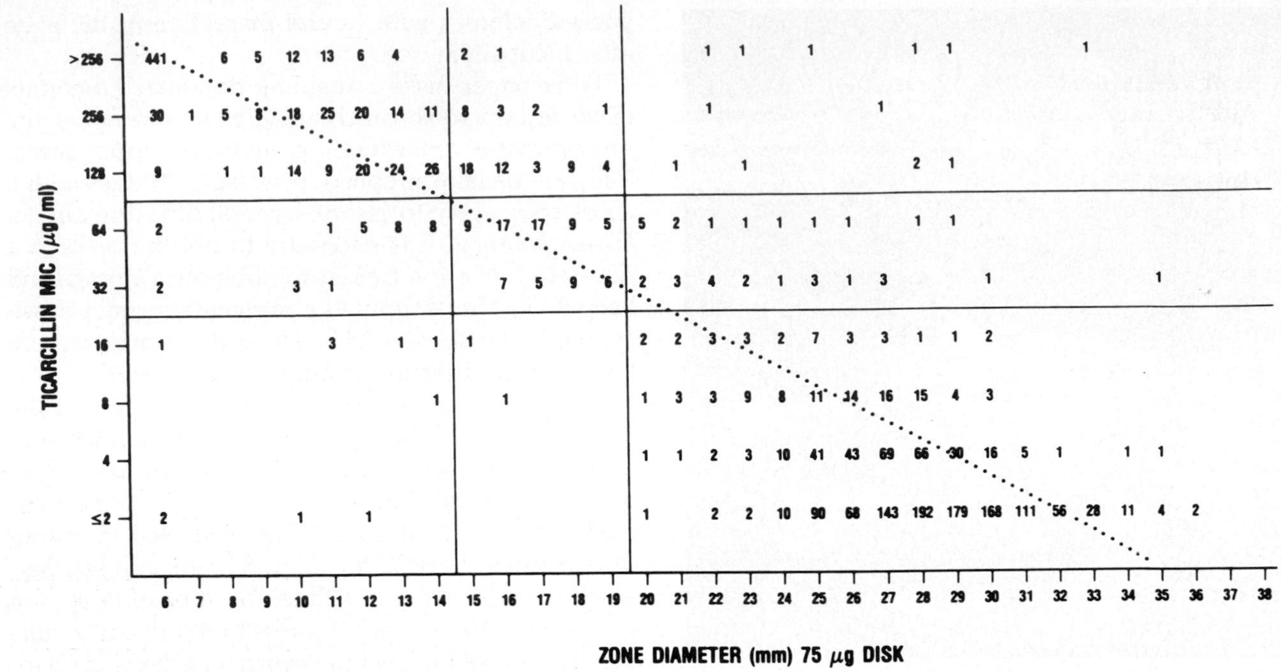

Figure 49.2. Regression analysis of *Enterobacteriaceae* susceptibility to ticarcillin. Broth microdilution MICs (*y* axis) are plotted against zones of inhibition (*x* axis) obtained by disk diffusion. Horizontal and vertical lines represent current breakpoints for interpretation of test results. (Reprinted with permission from Barry A, Fuchs P, Gerlach E, et al. Antimicrob Agents Chemother 1992;36:139.)

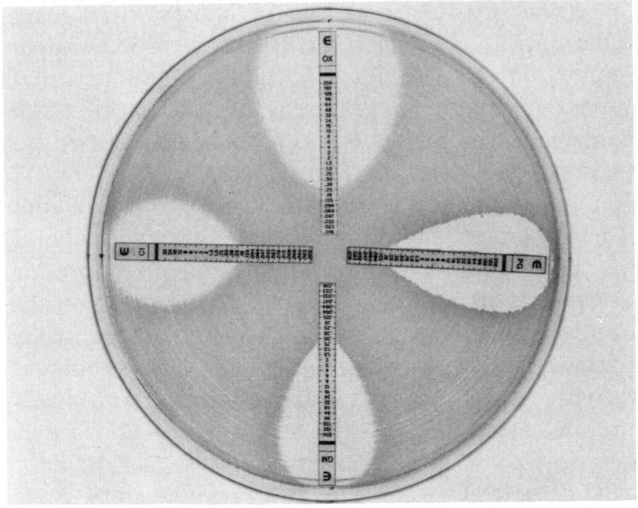

Figure 49.3. The E-test. Elliptical zones of inhibition around antimicrobic-impregnated strips. The MIC is read from the on-strip scale where the zone touches the side of the strip.

lutions on the other side. After incubation, the zone of inhibition takes the shape of an ellipse. The MIC is read at the point where the zone intersects the MIC scale on the strip (Fig. 49.3). Studies show this method to give greater than 95% agreement with the standardized microbroth dilution method. To date, this method has not received approval by the FDA, but it is being used clinically in Europe.

Again, most testing laboratories are opting to use methods that provide an MIC result, rather than the disk diffusion test. It should be noted that both methods provide clinically useful information. Under most clinical situations, the interpretive result is all that is needed for the choice of antimicrobic. There are also advantages to the use of each method. With the disk diffusion method, it is easy to substitute one disk for another. Unless you prepare your own MIC trays, you are dependent on a commercial provider for the drug profiles available. It is also easier to spot contamination and low-level resistance than it is with the microbroth dilution method. However, the disk diffusion method is approved for use only with rapid growing organisms, whereas the microbroth dilution method can be incubated for longer periods of time and, therefore, can be used to test slower growing nonfermenters, anaerobes, and even the rapid-growing mycobacteria (18). It also lends itself more readily to automation with prepared trays having long outdates. MBCs cannot be done using agar diffusion techniques.

Susceptibility Testing of Anaerobic Bacteria

Although testing standards exist for anaerobes (NCCLS M11-A2), it is now recommended that most clinical laboratories severely limit the frequency of such testing (22). Empiric choice of agents shown by clinical trials to be effective against pathogenic anaerobes is usually sufficient. Susceptibility testing of anaerobes is indicated primarily in situations where the infection did not respond to recommended therapy or for periodic screening of local isolates to assess the relative activity of recommended antimicrobics.

Various methods have been used, but none appear totally adequate for the testing of all pathogenic anaerobes. An agar dilution method has been chosen as the reference method, but it is not a convenient method for most clinical laboratories to use. The reader is referred to the M11-A2 standard for details on this method. In brief, antimicrobics are made up from standard powders, as mentioned earlier, and added to melted Wilkins-Chalgren agar supplemented with hemin and vitamin K_1 to achieve the desired concentration. The molten agar is immediately poured into Petri plates and allowed to solidify and the surface to dry after reaching room temperature before inoculation. An alternative medium, Wadsworth *Brucella* blood agar using 5% laked sheep blood, has been suggested as an alternative and appears to support the growth of a broader range of anaerobes. MICs may average about one dilution higher with this medium. Thioglycollate broth enriched with hemin and vitamin K_1 is inoculated with a fresh isolate taken from an anaerobic blood agar plate and incubated to obtain turbid growth. The growth is adjusted to obtain a concentration such that 10^5 CFU are deposited onto the surface of the agar in the form of a spot. Several organisms can be tested on each plate containing a specific antimicrobic concentration. The concentrations recommended for testing for each agent are given in the Standard but should span the physiologically achievable range with maximum dosage. The aforementioned procedures can be done under aerobic conditions, but following inoculation, the plates must be incubated at 35° to 37°C under anaerobic conditions for 48 hours before determining endpoints. The endpoint is the lowest concentration tested that inhibits growth of the isolate. Some inoculum spots may show a haze or one to two colonies of reduced size compared to the growth control, but should be ignored. If trailing occurs, the endpoint is read at the concentration where a major decrease in colony count or size occurs. The result is interpreted as either susceptible or resistant. No intermediate or moderately susceptible catagories exist, because the maximum dosage is recommended for the treatment of anaerobic infections.

Most laboratories testing anaerobes use a microdilution broth method. The methodology is quite similar to that described for testing organisms that grow aerobically; however, some significant differences exist. Various test media have been used including Schaedler's, West-Wilkins, brain heart infusion, and Wilkins-Chalgren broth. None are capable of supporting the growth of all anaerobes that one may want to test. Any of these can be used so long as the control strains respond appropriately. The recommended control strains are:

- *Bacteroides fragilis*, ATCC 25285;
- *Bacteroides thetaiotaomicron*, ATCC 29741;
- *Clostridium perfringens*, ATCC 13124; and
- *Eubacterium lentum*, ATCC 430555.

It is recommended that at least two of these control strains be run with each batch of tests or at least weekly. The inoculum is prepared as described for the standard agar dilution, but the final concentration should be about 10^6 CFU/ml in each dilution well. The inoculum volume should not exceed 0.01 ml, and the final volume in each well should not be less than 0.1 ml. The incubation time should be 48 hours under anaerobic conditions. The endpoint should be the lowest concentration of each drug dilutional series that shows either no growth or significantly reduced growth compared to the growth control well. It has been noted that the MICs obtained by microtiter broth dilution usually run about one dilution lower than those obtained by agar dilution.

Older studies refer to a disk elution technique where disks containing a given concentration of an antimicrobic were added to a given volume of test medium and time was allowed for the antimicrobic to elute into the medium (23). Usually, only one concentration was tested, and the isolate was considered either sensitive or resistant depending on whether or not it was inhibited. This technique is no longer recommended by the NCCLS, especially when testing cephalosporins.

The β-Lactamase Test

The β-lactamase test is a rapid, sensitive procedure for screening isolates for resistance to β-lactamase-susceptible antimicrobics. The genetic ability of bacteria to produce β-lactamase is universal because it appears to be needed for cell wall growth. However, certain bacteria are capable of producing sufficient quantities of these enzymes to effectively neutralize the killing capacity of certain β-lactam antimicrobics before they can reach vulnerable "penicillin-binding proteins" that serve as their primary targets. The genetic information coding for these enzymes can be carried on plasmids or integrated into the chromosome. Some β-lactamases are produced constitutively and others must be induced to produce detectable amounts (24, 25). Irrespective of the method of production, if a β-lactamase is detected, all susceptible β-lactam antimicrobics are considered to be ineffective against the organism. This type of resistance spawned the development of many new β-lactam drugs that either are inherently resistant to

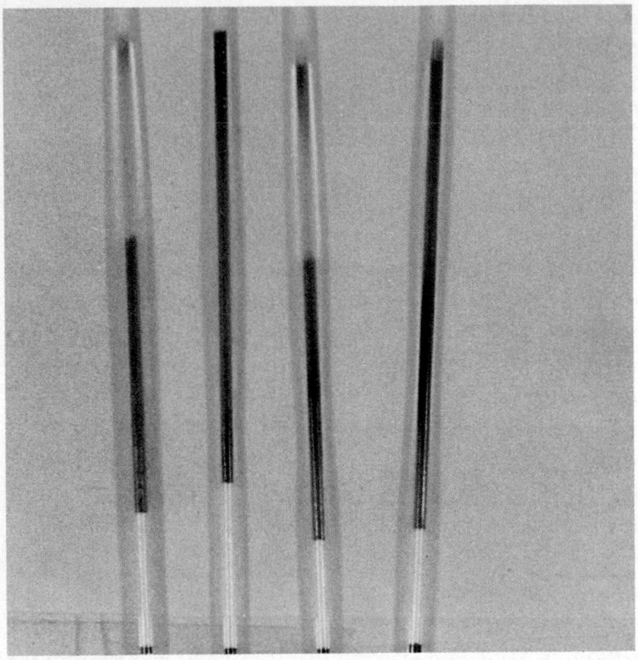

Figure 49.4. Detection of penicillinase production by the acidometic method. The production of penicilloic acid from the action of penicillinase on penicillin is indicated by the change of the pH indicator from red to yellow.

the enzyme's action or are coupled with specific enzyme inhibitors that irreversibly bind with the enzyme to render it inactive.

Three methods have been used in the clinical laboratory for the detection of β-lactamases: acidometric, chromogenic cephalosporin, and iodometric.

The acidometric method takes advantage of the enzyme's hydrolytic action on the β-lactam ring, producing penicilloic acid, which has an additional carboxyl group. This causes the pH of the medium to decrease sufficiently to cause the pH indicator to change color. A convenient technique is to draw a solution containing penicillin and a pH indicator into a capillary tube and subsequently to stab one or more colonies with the end of the tube, creating an organism plug that makes contact with the solution. If β-lactamase is produced, the solution adjacent to the plug will begin to become acidic (Fig. 49.4). This method is easy and quite inexpensive but may not react with certain enzymes that are more specifically active against cephalosporins than against penicillins.

The chromogenic cephalosporin method is currently considered the optimal method because it appears to react with all classes of β-lactamases known to date. This method takes advantage of the chromogenic properties of specific cephalosporins that change color when hydrolyzed. A disk containing the chromogenic cephalosporin is wetted with water or saline and the test organism is removed from an agar plate and streaked onto the disk surface. If an isolate is a β-lactamase producer, it will cause a color change, usually within 15 minutes. Impregnated disks are available from commercial sources.

The iodometric method is seldom used in clinical laboratories but can be a very sensitive method for detecting penicillinases. The method relies on the ability of penicilloic acid to function as a reducing agent, converting iodine to iodide. When a solution containing penicillin, iodine and starch is inoculated with a penicillinase-producing bacterium, the iodine is reduced to iodide and the starch solution changes from a blue-black color to colorless.

Organisms that are routinely tested for β-lactamase production are *H. influenzae, Moraxella catarrhalis, N. gonorrhoeae, Bacteroides* spp., and *Fusobacterium* spp. The vast majority of staphylococci also produce a penicillinase that is readily detected following induction, but the incidence is so high that few laboratories bother testing for the few isolates that are nonproducers. Certain Gram-negative facultative anaerobes also produce β-lactamases that render specific antimicrobials inactive. Such activity results in high MICs, and it is usually not necessary to test such isolates for β-lactamase production. This is because the enzyme-labile antimicrobics are not usually used against these organisms. Certain Gram-negative bacilli such as *Enterobacter cloacae* may only produce a β-lactamase following induction with a specific β-lactam antimicrobic such as cefoxitin or imipenem. The clinical significance of this is uncertain at present; however, certain strains may convert to constitutive enzyme production, which is clinically significant.

Inducible strains can be detected using a modification of the disk diffusion test (26). At the time of inoculation, a disk containing a low (noninhibiting) concentration of an inducing antimicrobic is placed just outside the zone of inhibition normally obtained with an enzyme-susceptible antimicrobic. After incubation, the shape of the zone of inhibition is noted. If no enzyme is induced, the shape of the zone will remain circular; however, if induced β-lactamase is produced in the presence of the inducing agent, the zone will become flattened at the side adjacent to the inducing disk (Fig. 49.5). Such a test is usually only necessary when an appropriate organism appears to be susceptible in vitro but resistant in vivo and a potentially inducing antimicrobic is being administered in addition to the β-lactamase-susceptible drug.

Other Tests to Detect Drug-Inactivating Enzymes

Relatively rare isolates of *H. influenzae* produce choramphenicol acetyltransferase, which renders

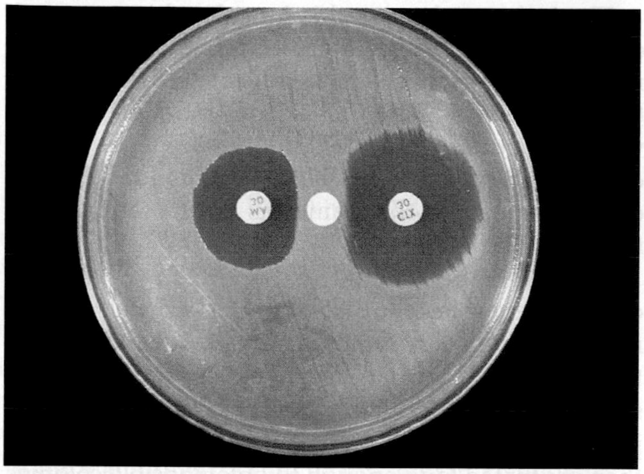

Figure 49.5. Evidence of the induction of β-lactamase by the disk-diffusion technique. The zones of inhibition are flattened adjacent to the central disk containing an inducing agent.

them resistant to chloramphenicol (27). A 10-minute disk or tube test is available to detect this enzyme. Most laboratories do not perform this test unless a strain of *H. influenzae* capable of producing this enzyme has been detected in the community or there is a treatment failure.

Aminoglycoside modifying enzymes can be detected by testing for enzyme-substrate activity or, more recently, by specific DNA probes but, to date, these tests are performed only in research settings (28, 29).

Semiautomated Susceptibility Testing

Several instruments have recently been introduced that facilitate susceptibility testing; a few approach full automation and usually perform organism identification procedures as well (30, 31). Briefly, each system is composed of three major components: a module that serves as an incubator/reader; a computer with a keyboard that allows data/command entry and controls all system functions; and a printer to provide hard copy. Prepared susceptibility test panels, usually provided in the dried form for longer shelf life, are packaged to be run only on the designated system. Most companies provide several different formats to choose from, or they can customize panels at extra cost. The test isolate is prepared by diluting the suspension in an inoculating medium to obtain a designated turbidity. This inoculum is used to simultaneously hydrate and inoculate the panels. This is done either by hand-held disposable transfer devices, mechanical inoculators or a vacuum unit. Once inoculated, the panels are appropriately labeled and accessioned in the computer for subsequent tracking. The panels are then loaded into the incubator/reader. The panels are "read" by the instrument at periodic intervals using light emitting diodes or fiberoptics as light sources, coupled with detectors to monitor changes in turbidity in each well. One system (API ALADIN, Analytab Products) employs a video imaging system to read each well. Incubation times vary, depending on the system, from 3.5 hours using fluorogenic substrates to 18 hours with conventional substrates. As each test is finalized, the position becomes available for another panel. Systems in clinical use have been evaluated for accuracy by comparing results with the standardized reference methods (32, 33).

Testing errors have been catagorized as very major, major, or minor. A very major error occurs when the test system calls an isolate susceptible to an antimicrobic, but the reference system calls it resistant (false-susceptible). A major error occurs when the test system calls an isolate resistant, and the reference method calls it susceptible (false-resistant). Minor errors result when the interpretation varies between susceptible and intermediately susceptible or between resistant and intermediately susceptible relative to the reference method. The FDA requires the manufacturer to recommend to the user of a system that an alternative method should be used whenever a drug/bug combination produces a very major error more than 1.5% of the time or a major error more than 3% of the time. Through software modifications, most approved systems now produce acceptable and reproducible results, but some problems still occur, especially with slow-growing and fastidious bacteria, oxacillin-heteroresistant staphylococci, and gentamicin-resistant enterococci. Systems that report results within 5 to 6 hours may have difficulty detecting resistance in isolates that produce inducible β-lactamase.

Sites using such systems report improved reproducibility of results and a modest savings in personnel time, although usually not enough to free up a technologist for other duties. Two-way interfaces help to limit the amount of data input necessary during accessioning. The system's computer is able to generate useful summary reports and susceptibility trend analyses.

To date, these systems are not fully automated. The inoculum must still be prepared by hand and the panels inserted into the system. No system has been free of major error; therefore, each testing site must maintain a backup system or use a reference laboratory to obtain results for specified bug/drug combinations. Some panels cannot be read manually in the event of a system malfunction. The primary motive for going to an automated system is to increase efficiency and to realize a cost savings; to date, these systems have had minimal favorable impact. Yet, the

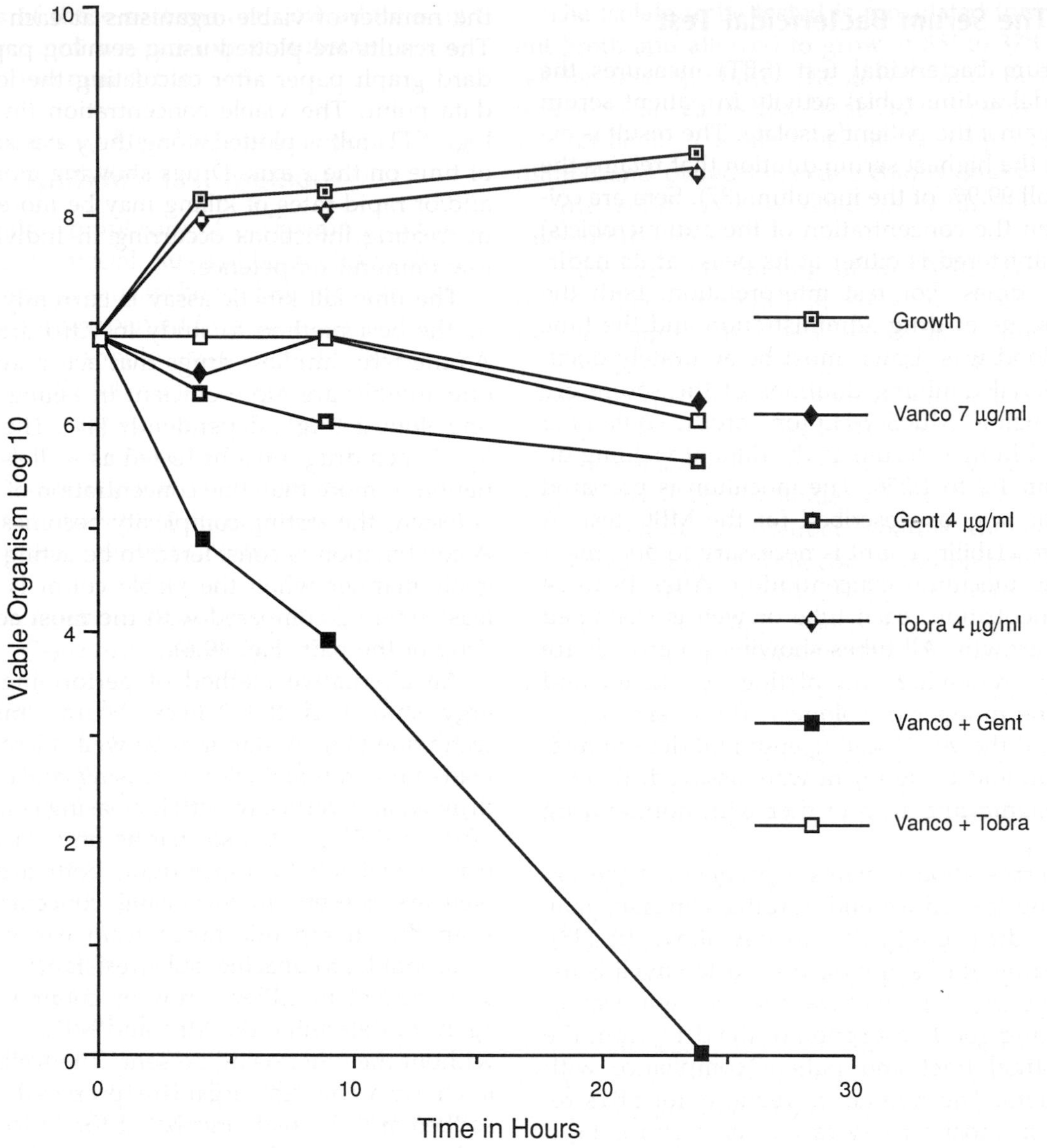

Figure 49.6. Time-kill kinetics. Rate of bactericidal activity of single and combined agents on *Enterococcus faecium*. Synergistic killing is occurring with the combination of vancomycin plus gentamicin.

centration (FIC) of drug A (FIC_A). The same is done for drug B to obtain the FIC_B. The two factional concentrations are added together to obtain the fractional index.

$$\frac{A}{MIC_A} + \frac{B}{MIC_B} = FC_A + FC_B = FI$$

There are several possible choices of combinations to choose for calculating the index. Thus, the logical choice is to select those concentrations that are within the lower physiological range for each drug. If the index is 0.5 or less, the drugs are acting with synergy. As the index increases, the drug interactions progress from additive to indifferent to antagonistic.

SUSCEPTIBILITY TESTING OF MYCOBACTERIA

It is recommended that mycobacterial isolates be tested for susceptibility to antimycobacterial agents in the event that initial therapy fails or when there is a high suspicion that an organism may be resistant due to isolation of other resistant isolates within a region. Although a number of susceptibility techniques have been used, most laboratories use one of two techniques for testing slow-growing mycobacteria, primarily *Mycobacterium tuberculosis* complex organisms: the modified proportion method for which the NCCLS has issued a proposed standard (M24-P) and the more rapid radiometric method.

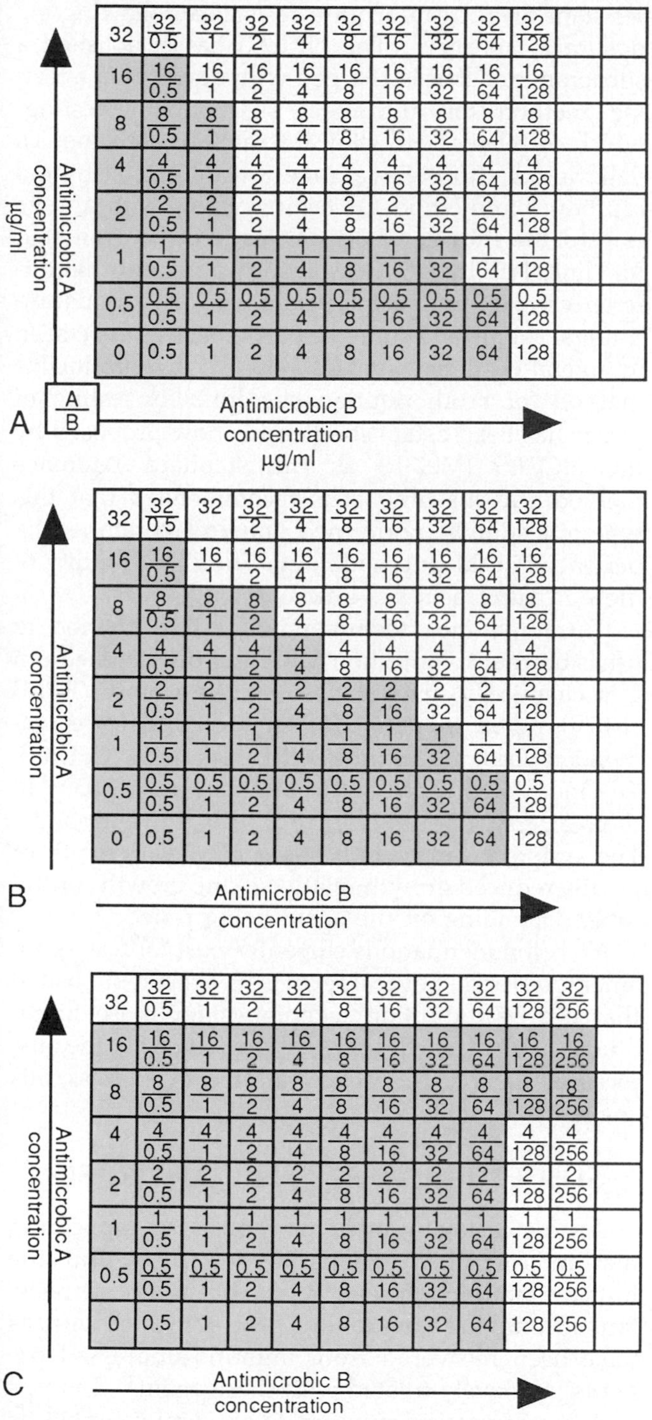

Figure 49.7. "Checkerboard" technique for determining antimicrobic interaction. **A,** Drug synergy. **B,** Additive effect. **C,** Drug antagonism.

Modified Proportion Method

This technique is much like the agar dilution method in that selected drugs are added to molten agar growth medium to obtain a set concentration prior to inoculation with the mycobacterial isolate. After 3 weeks of incubation, the amount of growth on the surface of the medium containing the drug is compared to the growth seen on the medium without any drug. If the number of colonies on the drug-containing medium exceeds 1% of the number counted on the drug-free medium, the organism is considered resistant to the drug. The medium of choice is Middlebrook and Cohn 7H10 agar supplemented with oleic acid, albumin, dextrose, and catalase (OADC). The 7H10 agar medium is cooled to 50°to 56°C, the OADC supplement and antimicrobic added, and each antimicrobic mixture poured into a quadrant of a divided plastic Petri dish to an agar depth of 3 to 4 mm and allowed to solidify and the surface to dry prior to inoculation. Instead of adding the antimicrobic directly to the molten agar, a more convenient method is to place enough elution disks containing a designated amount of the agent into the plate and pour drug-free agar medium over the disks to obtain the correct concentration.

The drugs recommended for testing against *M. tuberculosis* are divided into primary and secondary panels. The primary panel includes isoniazid, rifampin, streptomycin, and ethambutol. If the isolate shows resistance to isoniazid or rifampin, the secondary panel should be tested, which includes ethionamide, capreomycin, cycloserine and kanamycin. More acidic conditions are required for testing pyrazinamide.

The inoculum can be prepared directly from the concentrated specimen if acid-fast bacilli (AFB) are seen by direct microscopic examination or from the colonies obtained on growth media. For direct inoculation, the specimen may have to be diluted with sterile water, depending on the number of AFB seen per microscopic field. For example, if one sees 4 to 36 AFB/field on an auramine-stained smear using ×450 magnification, it is recommended that the specimen be diluted 1:10 and 1:100. Three drops of each dilution are added to separate quadrants of each drug concentration being tested plus a drug-free quadrant. Colonies removed from growth media can be suspended in a tube of Middlebrook 7H9 broth containing glass or plastic beads and carefully vortexed to dispense the clumps. The suspension is then adjusted to an optical density equivalent to a McFarland standard #1 and further diluted to yield 1:100 and 1:10,000 dilutions. Three drops (or 0.1 ml) of each dilution are added to each quadrant, as before. The inoculated plates are incubated medium side down in 5 to 10% CO_2 at 35° to 37°C for 3 weeks. At least one of the dilutions should yield a countable number of colonies of sufficient quantity so that a meaningful percentage can be calculated. If more than 1% of the population seen on the drug-free control quadrant grow in a quadrant containing a drug, the isolate is to be reported as resistant at that concentration. Drug-susceptible (e.g., ATCC 27294) and moderately resistant control strains should be run with each new batch of prepared plates or weekly to monitor drug activity.

Radiometric Testing Method

This method requires the use of the BACTEC TB system (Becton Dickinson Diagnostic Instrument Systems, Sparks, MD), which is the BACTEC 460 blood culture system fitted with an exhaust hood to prevent contaminated aerosols from being discharged into the atmosphere. Glass vials containing a Middlebrook broth formulation and ^{14}C palmitic acid (BACTEC 12B medium) with and without a selected antimicrobic are inoculated with the test mycobacterium and incubated. Growth of mycobacteria is monitored by the instrument, which measures the amount of $^{14}CO_2$ released into the vial headspace from the microbial catabolism of the ^{14}C-labeled palmitic acid. The measurement is provided as a growth index (GI). GI measurements are taken every 24 hours for at least 4 to 5 days and until the control vial's GI reaches at least 30. The GI of the drug-containing vial is compared to that of the drug-free control vial, which receives a 100-fold more dilute inoculum. If the magnitude of change of the GI of the drug-containing vial (ΔGI) exceeds that of the ΔGI of the growth control, the isolate is said to be resistant to the drug.

Because of the speed with which susceptibility results can be generated with the radiometric method, it has become a very popular method for those having the BACTEC TB System.

The aforementioned methods have been designed and recommended for testing the susceptibility of *M. tuberculosis* complex organisms only, but these methods, with some modifications, have also been used to test the susceptibility of other slow-growing *Mycobacterium* species. Such testing should be done only by experienced reference laboratories with high testing volumes.

Testing the susceptibility of rapid-growing mycobacteria can be done using the standard microdilution method with extended incubation time or by the agar dilution or disk elution method using cation-supplemented Mueller-Hinton broth with or without OADC. These organisms are usually not affected by the primary drugs active against the slow-growing mycobacteria at useful concentrations; therefore, more conventional drug panels should be used to test these organisms.

SUSCEPTIBILITY TESTING OF YEASTS

As more antifungal agents become available, there is a natural tendency to see if an isolate is naturally resistant or if it can acquire resistance following exposure to an agent. The NCCLS has established a subcommittee that is charged with developing a testing method for antifungal susceptibility testing, which correlates with clinical treatment outcome. To date, initial efforts have gone toward establishing a reproducible method for testing yeasts with an eye toward the future, when the test will be evaluated for clinical utility (43). It is already apparent that differences exist in yeast susceptibility to various antifungal agents and that such differences can be seen in animal challenge studies (44, 45). A reproducible method for broth dilution susceptibility testing of yeasts has been established and is now proposed by the NCCLS (M27-P) as the standard reference method. At this time, it is recommended that this type of testing be performed only in laboratories experienced in this methodology. The clinical utility of these in vitro results is unknown.

Currently, the recommended testing method to use is broth macrodilution MIC, and the test medium is a chemically defined tissue culture broth, RPMI 1640 buffered to pH 7.0 with MOPS. The recommended yeast inoculum size is 1 to 5 × 10^3 CFU/ml. The inoculated tubes are to be incubated at 35°C in room air for 24 hours prior to reading the endpoints. The endpoint can be either lack of visual growth or greatly reduced growth relative to the growth control tube, depending on the agent being tested.

No recommendations currently exist for testing filamentous fungi. Several reports have been published that use agar dilution techniques for these fungi. Studies are currently being conducted under the auspices of the NCCLS subcommittee to address this challenging problem.

SUSCEPTIBILITY TESTING OF VIRUSES

An increasing number of reports are appearing that indicate that various herpesviruses and the human immunodeficiency virus 1 can become resistant to antiviral compounds (46, 47). Such viruses have been recovered from immunosuppressed patients previously treated with these agents. Coupled with the increasing number of antiviral compounds becoming available, clinical virology laboratories are being pressured to develop methods to determine viral resistance. No recommended method currently exists, but several have been used experimentally. The more popular method to test for resistance in herpesviruses, primarily in HSV and CMV isolates, is the plaque reduction assay. Cell monolayers are inoculated with a countable number of viral plaque-forming units followed by the addition of the antiviral compound to be tested at various concentrations. Following incubation, the reduction in the number of plaques produced compared to drug-free controls is determined and the result is expressed as the drug concentration capable of reducing the number of plaque-forming units by 50% (ID_{50}).

Another method useful for testing large numbers of isolates is the dye uptake assay. The cell culture is inoculated with the test virus and exposed to the antiviral agent in various concentrations. Following incubation, neutral red dye is added that is taken up by the remaining viable cells. The amount of retained dye is measured spectrophotometrically by eluting the dye from washed cells into a phosphate-alcohol solution. The concentration of drug that increases the amount of dye retained by 50% is the ID_{50}.

Other methods that measure the relative amounts of viral protein or nucleic acid produced have also been used to assay antiviral activity.

SUMMARY

The value of the in vitro antimicrobic susceptibility test is dependent on how well it can predict efficacy of the drug in vivo. The outcome of an infection is dependent on numerous host defense mechanisms. If critical mechanisms are impaired to a significant degree, the outcome may not be influenced by the administration of an appropriate antimicrobic, resulting in what may appear to be drug failure. It is, therefore, imperative that the immunologic status of the patient be considered when selecting antimicrobics and when interpreting the results of their use. In spite of these restrictions, the susceptibility test has proven to be of value to the clinician.

Much effort has gone into the development of these tests to make them applicable and consistent. Obviously, one cannot accurately simulate the in vivo environment; therefore, compromises have to be made that may affect the susceptibility results, but much effort has gone into minimizing these variables. The testing media, atmosphere, inoculum density, and drug concentrations have all been standardized for testing most clinically significant bacteria. However, this is not a static situation. The NCCLS subcommittees are continually facing changes in available antimicrobics, their pharmacokinetics and their approved applications, infectious agents, and advances in our knowledge regarding microbial resistance mechanisms, and also in our knowledge of altered host defenses and the various effects that available forms of chemotherapy have on these defenses.

Routine susceptibility tests measure microbial inhibition, not bactericidal activity, and as clinicians institute the use of drugs that compromise host defenses, the measurement of bactericidal activity may become vital for such individuals. The measurement of bactericidal activity adds an additional level of complexity and expense to the standard tests that must be considered. To date, no standards exist for this procedure nor are there standard interpretations for the results obtained.

Another complex issue is the testing of multidrug interaction. More than one antimicrobic is frequently used to treat life-threatening infections, whereas the standard susceptibility tests test the activity of solitary agents. Because the interaction of various antimicrobials is not predictable against many bacteria, such information may be of great importance for drug selection.

As the list of fungi and viral agents known to cause infectious disease continues to expand and as the number of antifungal and antiviral agents available to treat these infectious agents increases, the need to test these agents may soon be necessary. Methods currently being used indicate that both intrinsic and acquired resistance exists in the eukaryotic fungi and in several viral groups. To this end, appropriate NCCLS subcommittees are working to establish procedures that will meet this clinical need and be practical for microbiology laboratories to implement.

CONCLUSION

Methods currently in use to test pathogenic bacteria for their susceptibility to selected antimicrobial agents appear to be of value in assisting the clinician in the appropriate selection of an antimicrobic. However, the role of the clinical pathologist or microbiologist does not end at this point. In many institutions, these individuals are called upon to participate in decision-making sessions ranging from direct patient care to institutional infection control procedures. An important aspect of this role is to know what effect the selection of one or more antimicrobics may be on an individual or on the population in a health care environment. A thorough knowledge of the activity of antimicrobics, the infectious agents to which they are directed, and the patient population being treated is necessary to be effective in this role. Such individuals must serve as a liaison between the clinical laboratory and the rest of the medical community, who depend on these results and their interpretation for patient care.

References

1. Washington JA II. Discrepancies between in vitro activity of and in vivo response to antimicrobial agents. Diagn Microbiol Infect Dis 1983;1:25–31.
2. Williams JD. The correlation of in vitro susceptibility tests with in vivo results of antibiotic treatment. Scand J Infect Dis 1978;13(suppl):64–66.

3. Greenwood D. In vitro *veritas*? Antimicrobial susceptibility tests and their clinical relevance. J Infect Dis 1981;144:380–385.
4. Snydman DR, Cuchural GJ Jr, McDermont L, Gill M. Correlation of various in vitro testing methods with clinical outcomes in patients with *Bacteroides fragilis* group infections treated with cefoxitin: a retrospective analysis. Antimicrob Agents Chemother 1992;36:540–544.
5. Sherris JC. Antimicrobic susceptibility testing: a personal perspective. Clin Lab Med 1989;9:191–202.
6. Ericsson HM, Sherris JC. Antibiotic sensitivity testing—report of an International Collaborative Study. Acta Pathol Microbiol Scand [B]1971;217(suppl):1–90.
7. National Committee for Clinical Laboratory Standards. Performance standards for antimicrobial disk susceptibility tests. 4th ed. Standard M2-A4. Villanova, PA: National Committee for Clinical Laboratory Standards, 1990.
8. National Committee for Clinical Laboratory Standards. Methods for dilution antimicrobial susceptibility tests for bacteria that grow aerobically. 2nd ed. Standard M7-A2. Villanova, PA: National Committee for Clinical Laboratory Standards, 1990.
9. Thornsberry C, Swenson JM, Baker CN, et al. Methods for determining susceptibility of fastidious and unusual pathogens to selected antimicrobial agents. Diagn Microbiol Infect Dis 1988;9:139–153.
10. D'Amato RF, Thornsberry C. Calcium and magnesium in Mueller-Hinton agar and their influence on disk diffusion susceptibility results. Curr Microbiol 1979;2:135–138.
11. Barry AL, Reller LB, Miller GH, et al. Revision of standards for adjusting the cation content of Mueller-Hinton broth for testing susceptibility of *Pseudomonas aeruginosa* to aminoglycosides. J Clin Microbiol 1992;30:585–589.
12. Pfaller MA, Wakefield DS, Stewart B, et al. Evaluation of laboratory methods for the classification of oxacillin-resistant and oxacillin-susceptible *Staphylococcus aureus*. Am J Clin Pathol 1988;89:120–125.
13. Reimer LG, Stratton CW, Reller, LB. Minimum inhibitory and bactericidal concentrations of 44 antimicrobial agents against three standard control strains in broth with and without human serum. Antimicrob Agents Chemother 1981;19:1050–1055.
14. Traub WH, Spohr M, Bauer D. *Pseudomonas aeruginosa*: Invitro susceptibility to antimicrobial drugs, single and combined, with and without defibrinated human blood. Chemother. 1988;34:284–297.
15. Pruul H, McDonald PJ. Potentiation of antibacterial activity of azithromycin and other macrolides by normal human serum. Antimicrob Agents Chemother 1992;36:10–16.
16. Bulger RR, Washington JA II. Effect of inoculum size and β-lactamase production on in vitro activity of new cephalosporins against *Haemophilus* species. Antimicrob Agents Chemother 1980;17:393–396.
17. Hwang JMD, Piccinini TE, Lammel CL, et al. Effect of storage temperature and pH on the stability of antimicrobial agents in MIC trays. J Clin Microbiol 1986;23:959–961.
18. Gay JD, DeYoung DR, Roberts GD. In vitro activities of norfloxacin and ciprofloxacin against *Mycobacterium tuberculosis, M. avium, M. chelonei, M. fortuitum* and *M. kansasii*. Antimicrob Agents Chemother 1984;26:94–96.
19. Ferguson RW, Weissfield AS. Comparison of the suitability of three common bacterial media for susceptibility testing of trimethoprim-sulfamethoxazole. J Clin Microbiol 1984;19:85–86.
20. Flournoy DJ, Shirley RA. Influence of inoculum concentration on zone size in disk diffusion testing. Lab Med 1985;16:616–618.
21. Baker CN, Stocker SA, Culver DH, Thornsberry C. Comparison of the E-Test to agar dilution, broth microdilution, and agar diffusion susceptibility testing techniques by using a special challenge set of bacteria. J Clin Microbiol 1991;29:533–538.
22. Finegold SM. Susceptibility testing of anaerobic bacteria. J Clin Microbiol 1988;26:1253–1256.
23. Wilkins TD, Thiel T. Modified broth-disk method for testing the antibiotic susceptibility of anaerobic bacteria. Antimicrob Agents Chemother 1973;3:350–356.
24. Sanders WE, Sanders CC. Inducible β-lactamases: clinical and epidemiologic implications for use of newer cephalosporins. Rev Infect Dis 1988;10:830–838.
25. Bush K. Beta-lactamase inhibitors from laboratory to clinic. Clin Microbiol Rev 1988;1:109–123.
26. Sanders CC, Sanders WE. Microbial resistance to newer generation of β-lactam antibiotics: clinical and laboratory implications. J Infect Dis 1985;151:399–406.
27. Walker CW, Brown DFJ. The reliability of methods for detecting chloramphenicol resistance in *Haemophilus influenzae*. J Antimicrob Chemother 1988;22:905–910.
28. Courvalin P. Genotypic approach to the study of bacterial resistance to antibiotics. Antimicrob Agents Chemother 1991;35:1019–1023.
29. Tenover FC. Studies of antimicrobial resistance genes using DNA probes. Antimicrob Agents Chemother 1986;29:721–725.
30. Pierson CL, McClatchey KD. Automation in clinical microbiology. In: Lederberg J, ed. Encyclopedia of microbiology. New York: Academic Press 1992;1:171–179.
31. Jorgenson J. Automation in clinical microbiology. Boca Raton, FL: CRC Press, 1987.
32. Cherubin CD, Eng R, Appleman M. A critique of semiautomated susceptibility systems. Rev Infect Dis 1987;9:655–659.
33. Kiehlbauch J, Kendle JM, Carlson LG, et al. Automated antibiotic susceptibility testing: comparative evaluation of four commercial systems and present state. Clin Lab Med 1989;9(2):319–340.
34. Sherris JC. Problems in in vitro determination of antibiotic tolerance in clinical isolates. Antimicrob Agents Chemother 1986;30:633–637.
35. Murray BE. The life and times of the enterococcus. Clin Microbiol Rev 1990;3:46–65.
36. Eagle H, Musselman AD. The rate of bactericidal action of penicillin in vitro as a function of its concentration, and its paradoxically reduced activity at high concentrations against certain organisms. J Exp Med 1948;88:99–131.
37. Schlichter JG, MacLean H. A method of determining the effective therapeutic level in treatment of subacute bacterial endocarditis with penicillin. Am Heart J 1947;34:209–211.
38. Reller LB. The serum bactericidal test. Rev Infect Dis 1986;8:803–808.
39. Standiford HC, Tatem BA. Technical aspects and clinical correlations of the serum bactericidal test. Eur J Clin Microbiol Infect Dis 1986;5:79–87.
40. Eliopoulos GM, Moellering RC Jr. Antimicrobial combinations. In: Lorian V, ed. Antibiotics in laboratory medicine. 3rd ed. Baltimore: Williams & Wilkins, 1991;432–492.
41. Blaser J. Interactions of antimicrobial combinations in vitro: the relativity of synergism. Scand J Infect Dis 1991;74(suppl):71–79.
42. Van der Auwera P. Synergistic, additive, and antagonistic activity of antimicrobial agents: How to measure? What are the clinical consequences? Applications to the new fluoroquinolones. Infect Dis Newsl 1992;11:49–54.
43. Pfaller MA, Rinaldi MG, Galgiani JN, et al. Collaborative investigation of variables in susceptibility testing of yeasts. Antimicrob Agents Chemother 1990;34:1648–1654.
44. Powderly WG, Kobayashi GS, Herzig GP, et al. Amphotericin B-resistant infection in severely immunocompromised patients. Am J Med 1988;84:826–832.

45. Stiller RL, Bennett JE, Scholer HJ, et al. Correlation of in vitro susceptibility test results with in vivo response: flucytosine therapy in systemic candidiasis model. J Infect Dis 1983;147: 1070–1077.
46. Drew LW, Matthews TR. Susceptibility testing of Herpes viruses. Clin Lab Med 1989;9:279–286.
47. Birch CJ, Tachedjian G, Doherty RR, et al. Altered sensitivity to antiviral drugs of Herpes simplex virus isolates from a patient with the acquired immunodeficiency syndrome. J Infect Dis 1990;162:731–734.

Suggested Readings

Lorian V. Antibiotics in laboratory medicine. 3rd ed. Baltimore: Williams & Wilkins, 1991.

Schoenknecht FD, Tenover FC, ed. Antimicrobial susceptibility testing. Clin Lab Med 1989;9:1–348.

Thornsberry C. Antimicrobial agents and susceptibility tests. In: Balows A, Hausler WJ, Jr, Herrmann KL, Isenberg HD, Shadomy HJ, eds. Manual of clinical microbiology. 5th ed. Washington DC: American Society for Microbiology, 1991.

50 Diagnostic Nucleic Acid Probes for Infectious Agents

Fred C. Tenover

Nucleic acid hybridization techniques are available to aid microbiologists in the detection and identification of infectious agents. Many nucleic acid probes are now available from commercial sources and come packaged in kit form to facilitate use. This chapter explores the types of probes available and the advantages and disadvantages using this technology in the clinical microbiology laboratory.

DEFINITIONS

Nucleic acid probes are pieces of DNA or RNA, labeled with radioisotopes, enzymes, or chemiluminescent reporter molecules, that can bind to complementary sequences of nucleic acid with high specificity (Fig 50.1). Probes can be composed of DNA or RNA, can be directed to DNA or RNA targets, and can be 15 to thousands of bases in length. Oligonucleotide probes (often defined as probes under 50 base pairs in length) can be chemically synthesized in large quantities with high fidelity. This is the type of probe most frequently incorporated into commercial kits. Oligonucleotide probes hybridize rapidly to target molecules; however, each can carry only one or two reporter molecules. Therefore, they may be slightly less sensitive than longer probes unless some means of signal amplification is used.

Hybridization reactions must be carried out under carefully controlled conditions of temperature, salt concentration, and pH. Changes in any of these variables can affect the outcome of the analysis by changing the number of mismatched base pairs that can be tolerated when two molecules come together to form a hybrid. Taken together, these variables constitute the stringency of the reaction. The higher the stringency, the fewer the number of mismatched base pairs that can be tolerated and still have the two strands of nucleic acid form a stable, double-stranded molecule (1). At low stringency, for example, a probe directed against DNA from *Neisseria gonorrhoeae* may react with other species of *Neisseria* as well, resulting in a positive hybridization signal. Under conditions of high stringency, however, only gonococcal DNA would be recognized and bound by the probe.

Reporter Molecules

Radioactive isotopes, enzymes, antigenic moieties, and chemiluminescent molecules have all been used to label probes so that the binding of the probe to the target molecules can be detected. The labels are collectively referred to as reporter molecules, and each has advantages and disadvantages.

^{32}P is the radioisotope that has been used most extensively for labeling probes. It has a very high specific activity but a half-life of only 2 weeks. Thus, it imparts to probes a very high level of sensitivity, but it requires probes to be labeled frequently, which is time consuming. Also, use of this isotope in the clinical laboratory necessitates additional safety and control measures that can be costly and burdensome. Nevertheless, at least one commercial kit employs a ^{32}P label on its probe. Probes labeled with ^{32}P can be detected by autoradiography or by scintillation counting.

Another radioisotope that has been used in commercially prepared kits is ^{125}I. The amount of the isotope used in the kits is sufficiently low that disposal is not problematic. However, the relatively short half-life of this isotope usually results in a kit shelf life of only 4 to 6 weeks. Thus, ^{125}I also has some disadvantages.

The direct labeling of oligonucleotide probes with enzymes such as alkaline phosphatase has been accomplished using carbon chain linker arms that vary from 8 to 16 units in length (2). While the sensitivity of the alkaline phosphatase–labeled probes is lower than that of ^{32}P, the ease of use of enzyme-labeled probes is a considerable advantage.

Recently, a series of antigenic moieties have been used to label DNA or RNA probes. After the hybridization reaction is completed, an enzyme linked to an antibody is used to find the antigenic moiety attached to the probe. Substrates such as acetylaminofluorine and digoxigenin have been incorporated into kits for labeling nucleic acid. Both are effective, although acetylaminofluorine is more toxic than digoxigenin, which is now widely used.

Finally, some commercial kits employ probes with chemiluminescent labels. These reporter groups release light when reacting with specific substrates after the hybridization reaction is complete. Chemiluminescent reporters show high sensitivity but require additional instrumentation for detection.

Hybridization Formats

Hybridization reactions can be carried out with both the target and the probe in liquid phase; with the target immobilized on a solid support, such as a nylon or nitrocellulose membrane; in a sandwich format, in which one probe is immobilized on a membrane or in a microtiter plate well to capture the target sequence, while another probe is used for detection; or in an in situ format, in which probes are used to find infectious agents in fixed tissues on slides. The advantages of liquid hybridization include the speed of the reaction and the relatively small sample size required. Solid-phase reactions have the advantage of being able to screen multiple specimens simultaneously and are more cost effective than liquid formats; the capture formats offer, at least theoretically, increased specificity through the use of a dual-probe system. In situ hybridization techniques are used infrequently in the clinical microbiology laboratory but have frequent application in histology and cytopathology.

Table 50.1. Reasons for Using Probes in the Laboratory

1.	Reduce time necessary to identify organisms
2.	Broaden range of organisms that can be identified
3.	Reduce number of tests sent to reference laboratories

Indications for Using Probe-based Tests in the Laboratory

Three reasons to use nucleic acid hybridization tests in the laboratory are (*a*) to speed the identification of fastidious microorganisms; (*b*) to broaden the range of microorganisms that can be detected and identified by the laboratory; and (*c*) to reduce the costs associated with sending tests to reference laboratories (Table 50.1) (3).

Although probe tests may be more expensive than traditional biochemical tests, the rapid turnaround time of probe technology often translates into an overall savings to the hospital and patient by providing a timely diagnosis. This can preclude costly additional tests, unnecessary therapeutic regimens, or stays in expensive isolation rooms (e.g., in cases of suspected tuberculosis).

The addition of probe-based tests may allow laboratories to screen for pathogens, such as human papillomavirus (4, 5) or the enterohemorrhagic

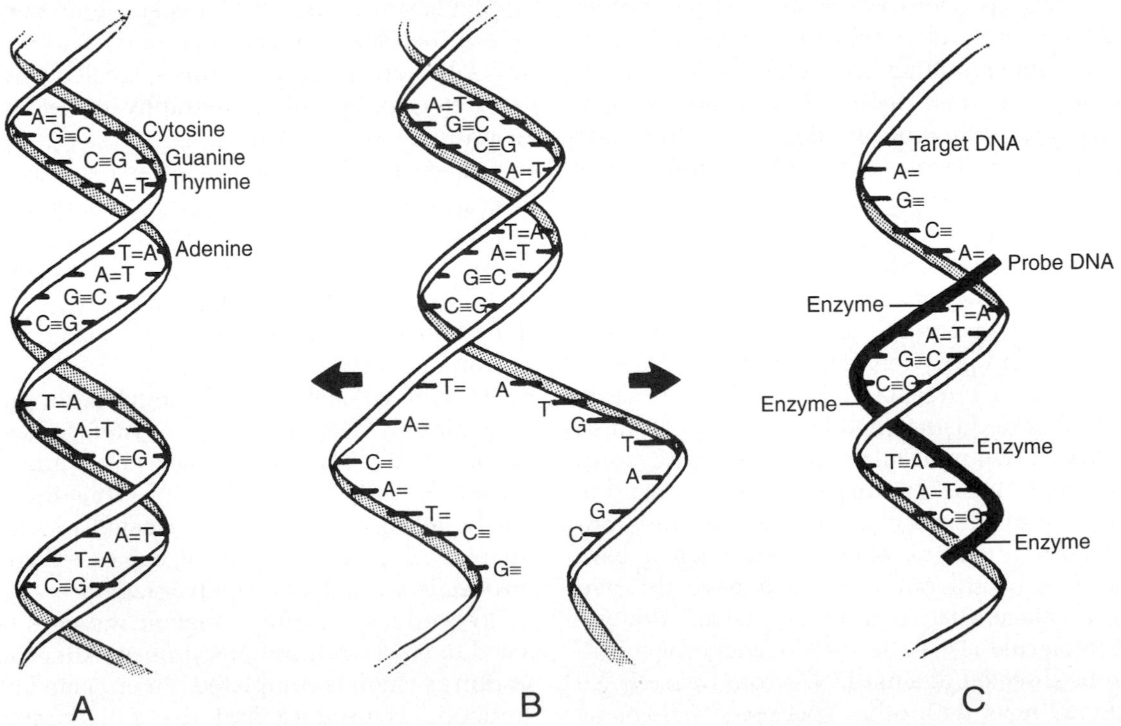

Figure 50.1. Structure of deoxyribonucleic acid, effects of denaturation and binding of probe for target DNA. **A.** Native DNA; **B.** Denature DNA to single strands; **C.** Binding of labeled probe to target DNA. (From Tenover FC. Clin Microbiol Rev 1988;1:83.)

Table 50.2. Commercially-Prepared Probes Available for Diagnostic Laboratory Use

Organism	Company	Detection Method
CULTURE CONFIRMATION ASSAYS		
Bacteria		
Campylobacter[a]	Gen-Probe	C[b]
Enterococci	Gen-Probe	C
Group B streptococcus	Gen-Probe	C
Escherichia coli	Gen-Probe	C
Haemophilus influenzae	Gen-Probe	C
Listeria monocytogenes	Gen-Probe	C
Mycobacterium tuberculosis complex	Gen-Probe	C
Mycobacterium avium	Gen-Probe	I
M. avium complex	Gen-Probe	C
Mycobacterium intracellulare	Gen-Probe	C
M. intracellulare	SynGene	AP
Mycobacterium gordonae	Gen-Probe	C
Mycobacterium kansasii	Gen-Probe	C
Neisseria gonorrhoeae	Gen-Probe	C
Fungi		
Cryptococcus neoformans	Gen-Probe	C
Histoplasma capsulatum	Gen-Probe	C
Blastomyces dermatitidis	Gen-Probe	C
Coccidiodes immitis	Gen-Probe	C
Viruses		
Human papilloma virus[c]	Digene	P
DIRECT DETECTION IN CLINICAL SAMPLES		
Chlamydia trachomatis	Gen-Probe	C
Legionella pneumophila	Gen-Probe	I
Neisseria gonorrhoeae	Gen-Probe	C
Viruses		
Human papilloma virus[d]	Digene	P

[a]Thermophilic campylobacters including *C. jejuni*, *C. coli*, and *C. lari*.
[b]C, chemiluminescent; I, ^{125}I; AP, alkaline phosphatase; P, ^{32}P.
[c]Typing of isolates detected with ViraPap test.
[d]Direct detection of human papilloma virus in samples.

strains of *Escherichia coli* (e.g., O157:H7 strains) (6), for which traditional culture techniques are either not available or not practical, thus broadening the scope of pathogens that can be detected by the laboratory. This is a key area that microbiologists should consider. However, the sensitivity, specificity, and positive and negative predictive values of such probes should be carefully evaluated before these tests are placed on line. Probe tests without doubt will be very costly to use in low-prevalence situations.

Probe kits for pathogens such as *Chlamydia trachomatis* or other sexually transmitted diseases may also allow smaller laboratories to perform testing for these organisms in house, avoiding the expense of sending tests to reference laboratories. This presumes that the smaller laboratory has the staffing to perform such testing. If the staffing is available, laboratories may even market these tests, particularly to outpatient clinics or physicians' offices, thereby generating a new source of income (7). A laboratory considering such an undertaking, however, should recognize the standards of quality control and proficiency testing required to maintain and operate a reference laboratory, even when undertaken on a small scale.

Table 50.2 lists the probe kits that were commercially available at the time this chapter was written. The individual areas of use are summarized in the following sections.

PROBES FOR ENTERIC PATHOGENS

At present, laboratories often use a multifaceted approach to the diagnosis of enteric pathogens. This usually includes direct microscopy, bacterial cultures on a variety of differential and selective media, enrichment broths followed by examination with latex agglutination assays, enzyme-linked immunosorbent assays (ELISAs) (particularly for rotaviruses), and cell culture assays for detection of *Clostridium difficile* toxin. It would be highly desirable to process stool samples using a single protocol without losing the ability to screen for the wide variety of pathogens now being sought in fecal samples.

DNA probes offer a potential solution to this problem. There are few enteric pathogens—bacterial, viral, or protozoan—for which probes have not been described (8). The list of probes includes *Clostridium difficile, Entamoeba histolytica* (9), species of *Giardia* (10), *Salmonella, Shigella, Campylobacter, Yersinia,* and *Vibrio*; rotaviruses, enteric adenoviruses, and a number of other organisms, including the enterotoxigenic, enteroinvasive, enteroadherent, enteropathogenic, and enterohemorrhagic strains of *E. coli*. However, only the probe for the thermophilic *Campylobacter* species is available in a commercially prepared kit, and it is a culture confirmation assay that cannot be used to detect organisms directly in fecal samples (11).

The difficulty in developing probe assays for enteric pathogens is the relatively small numbers of organisms that are often present in the stool of an infected patient. This may necessitate the use of a rapid DNA extraction technique to isolate nucleic acid from the stool specimen as a first step in probe analysis. Several nucleic acid extraction systems have been described (12, 13). Alternatively, amplification techniques, such as the polymerase chain reaction, could be used in combination with probes to detect enteric pathogens. The use of multiple primer pairs in conjunction with PCR assays performed directly on stool samples to amplify both the heat-labile and heat-stable enterotoxin genes of *E. coli*, as well as the *ial* locus on the *Shigella* virulence plasmid, has been reported (14).

One additional issue yet to be resolved is what to do with samples that are positive with a probe test. Presumably, most hospital laboratories would culture the specimen to recover the pathogen for susceptibility testing or strain typing. Depending on the pathogen, these could be potentially important for patient management or for epidemiological studies. However, the use of the probe will increase the cost of doing stool cultures because, in this instance, it is being used as a culture enhancement, not as a culture replacement. One presumes that the small number of positive stool cultures would still make this an effective screening procedure. Yet, this would need to be proved in field studies. Recent articles suggest that many of the stool cultures currently submitted on hospital inpatients are of no clinical value (15).

PROBES FOR RESPIRATORY PATHOGENS

Probe technology has made a major contribution to the detection and identification of respiratory pathogens. Probe kits to detect *Legionella* species (16, 17) directly in respiratory samples have been available for a number of years. Kits for the identification of *Mycoplasma pneumoniae* (18, 19) are no longer available. In addition, the use of probes for the identification of mycobacteria grown in vitro has been widely accepted. Currently, probes to identify colonies of *Mycobacterium tuberculosis, Mycobacterium avium, Mycobacterium intracellulare*, and *Mycobacterium gordonae* and *Mycobacterium kansasii* are available (20, 21). The latter probes can be used in conjunction with the BACTEC (Becton Dickinson Diagnostic Instrument System) radiometric broth detection system to enhance the speed of detection of mycobacterial infections (22) and are particularly helpful in documenting mixed mycobacterial infections (23).

The probes for *Legionella* species are a prime example of the strengths and weaknesses of this technology. On the one hand, the probe is capable of detecting all species of *Legionella* (24) rather than just *Legionella pneumophila*, the most common pathogen of the species. However, the sensitivity of the probe assay, which is comparable to or perhaps slightly better than direct fluorescent antibody assays, is not high enough to justify discontinuation of cultures for *Legionella* (17). Thus, the probe becomes an ancillary test rather than the primary test. One report of false-positive results without culture was likely due to *Legionella birminghamensis*, a species described sometime later (25).

The other probes directed against respiratory pathogens that have been widely used are those for cytomegalovirus (CMV) (26). While none of those produced commercially are yet approved for diagnostic use, there is a considerable body of literature that has developed in this area. Of primary importance has been the use of probes for in situ hybridization analysis of fixed lung tissue sections (27). While this application of probes is not germane to the clinical microbiology laboratory per se, it is a significant development that is finding widespread appeal among pathologists, many of whom look to the microbiology or virology laboratory for evidence of the growth of the virus in cell culture. The use of probes as culture confirmation assays for CMV grown in cell culture has also been reported, although it appears to be no more sensitive than monoclonal antibody assays, which are less expensive.

PROBES FOR SEXUALLY TRANSMITTED PATHOGENS

Probes can be useful for the rapid detection of sexually transmitted agents directly in clinical samples. A probe for *N. gonorrhoeae* was first described by Totten et al. (28). They demonstrated that direct detection of gonococcal DNA in urethral exudates of males, using a probe derived from the cryptic plasmid of *N. gonorrhoeae*, was about 95% sensitive compared to culture (28). Commercially prepared probes for *N. gonorrhoeae* and *Chlamydia trachomatis* that can be used in tandem to test a single patient sample are now available.

The fact that both the gonococcal and chlamydial assays can be run from material collected from a single swab is a distinct advantage, as long as the sample collection is adequate. However, unlike the direct fluorescent antibody assay, these assays do not allow the quality of the sample to be assessed before performing the assay. For sexually transmitted disease clinics or other high-volume outpatient facilities, such a combination of tests, given acceptable levels of sensitivity and specificity and an area of moderately high prevalence, are cost effective and justifiable from the standpoint of predictive values. For other hospital laboratories or clinics in areas of low prevalence that receive relatively few samples, such combinations are probably not warranted because the predictive value of the test will be low. Culture tests for *N. gonorrhoeae* and *C. trachomatis* or the direct fluorescent antibody test for the latter will be more cost effective.

Before using probes for sexually transmitted diseases, the price of false-positive and false-negative tests must be considered (29, 30). Because of the social and public health implications of false-positive and false-negative tests, the laboratory must have considerable confidence in the tests used. In addition, the critical issues of strain typing and susceptibility testing need to be considered when using probes for detecting *N. gonorrhoeae*. Without a colony of the organism with which to work, serotyping will not be available for epidemiological studies of disease transmission. It also will not be possible to perform susceptibility testing of isolates. Thus, the recognition of ceftriaxone-resistant organisms may be significantly delayed, and this may have a disastrous outcome if the resistant strains are widely disseminated before recognition. On the other hand, probe assays may be much more reliable than the culture techniques available in some laboratories for these pathogens. These points need to be considered before this technology is widely implemented in these settings. Probes may not be appropriate for cases involving legal issues such as rape or child abuse. Without cultures, additional tests to confirm the identity of the organism cannot be performed if needed.

The other sexually transmitted agents for which probes have become important are the human papillomaviruses (4, 5). Because cell culture examination of samples is not feasible for these viruses, probe tests have become an important diagnostic tool. Several different kits, both to detect the presence of the virus and to type the viruses present, are now commercially available. Whether the use of the probe assays will become commonplace has yet to be determined.

Probes for other sexually transmitted agents, such as *Treponema pallidum*, *Haemophilus ducreyi*, and *Ureaplasma urealyticum* have been described, but they have not been used to any great degree in clinical laboratories.

PROBES FOR BLOOD-BORNE PATHOGENS

A number of different pathogens, including bacterial, viral, and protozoan agents, can infect the bloodstream. In some cases, probes have been used in conjunction with other diagnostic systems, such as the Isolator blood culture system, to detect bloodstream infections of *Salmonella typhi* (31). In other cases, e.g., in diagnosing malaria (32) and *Babesia* infections (33), the probe is used as the primary diagnostic tool. Probes have also been used to detect viral agents in blood, including the human immunodeficiency virus (34) and hepatitis B virus (35). There is considerable potential for using probes to decrease the time necessary to detect pathogens of many varieties in the blood stream. Once again, as with stool pathogens, the critical factor is the number of organisms present in the sample. Because the concentration of bacteria present in the bloodstream may frequently be less than 10 organisms per milliliter, the detection of such infections without some means of either biological or nucleic acid amplification would be difficult. Yet, if an amplification method, such as the polymerase chain reaction, was available, the time required for the detection and identification of blood-borne pathogens could be dramatically reduced.

PROBES FOR VIRAL AGENTS

Probes for a wide variety of viral agents have been described (33). As with probes for bacterial pathogens, probes have been used to identify viruses grown in cell culture as well as to identify the presence of viral DNA directly in clinical specimens. In this regard, in situ hybridization techniques for detecting viruses in histologic samples have been particularly successful (36, 37). However, such techniques are not carried out in clinical microbiology laboratories.

One development of particular interest in clinical virology has been the introduction of probes for the human papillomaviruses (HPVs) for screening genital specimens. Because HPV cannot be readily propagated in vitro, this test, which is available commercially, has broadened the spectrum of infectious agents that can be detected by the laboratory. Use of the polymerase chain reaction to enhance the sensitivity of detection of HPV, however, has shown that many women carry this virus in the absence of histopathologic changes (38). The use of these methods in this situation requires further study to define the clinical utility of the data.

PROBES FOR FUNGI, PROTOZOA, AND HELMINTHS

The availability of probes for the identification of fungi would be of significant value to many diagnostic laboratories. While probes that hybridize to fungal DNA have been reported, they have been used primarily for epidemiologic studies and not for primary identification (39). Lysis techniques to release DNA reliably from fungal cells have been difficult to develop (40). This has been a considerable stumbling block in the advancement of hybridization technology in the field of mycology. However, commercially available tests for culture confirmation of several dimorphic fungi, which rely on sonication of the organism with glass beads to break the cell wall, have been used successfully.

Probes that recognize protozoa and helminths other than the diarrheal pathogens include those for Leishmania (41) and *Trypanosoma* (42) species and the filarial worm *Brugia malayi* (43). All have been described, but none are commercially available.

PROBES FOR ANTIMICROBIAL RESISTANCE GENES

Although over 50 probes for antimicrobial resistance genes have been described, hybridization technology for the direct detection of resistance genes in organisms has not been widely used in clinical laboratories. One problem is the number of potential classes of resistance genes that are unrelated by DNA-DNA homology but that could mediate resistance to a drug such as ampicillin is quite large. Some of these genes encode β-lactamases; others result in altered porins that reduce access of the drug to the site of action. It would be a difficult task to make a cocktail of probes that would detect each of the known mechanisms of resistance to ampicillin that could potentially be present in a given clinical sample. On the other hand, there are some organism-drug combinations in which an organism infects a normally sterile body site and has relatively few modes of antimicrobial resistance that are clinically relevant (e.g., penicillinase-producing *N. gonorrhoeae* in urethral samples from males or the methicillin resistance gene from *Staphylococcus aureus*.) For a limited number of these cases, it is possible that the combination of a diagnostic probe and a susceptibility testing probe could be successfully applied (45).

The possibility of using hybridization assays and probes as a means of determining the susceptibility of viruses or parasitic agents to drugs is also feasible. Antiviral susceptibility testing using hybridization assays in place of plaque reduction assays has been applied to studies of acyclovir resistance in herpes simplex virus (46). In addition, probes also have been used to detect chloroquin resistance in *Plasmodium falciparum* (47). Both antiviral and antiparasitic assays may find greater usage in the future.

FUTURE DIRECTIONS

The use of probe-based assays in the clinical laboratory will in all likelihood continue to increase. Procedures for automating hybridization assays are also in various stages of development (48), although at present such machines are directed toward in situ hybridization assays rather than the processing of routine microbiological samples. New hybridization methods that do not require the separation of the nascent probe-target complexes from the reaction mixture for detection are now commonplace (homogeneous assays). These assays are fast (often less than 30 minutes) and highly accurate.

While the number of commercially prepared probe kits continues to increase, so does the recognition of the power of amplification-based assay systems, such as the polymerase chain reaction, for the detection of low numbers of organisms in clinical samples (49, 50). This technology is covered in detail elsewhere in this volume, yet it is important to note that this technology must be approached with caution by the clinical laboratory for three reasons. Currently, the major drawback to this technique is the problem of contamination that arises when millions of copies of target sequences are being produced in a laboratory over long periods of time (51). In addition, the technology is costly. Finally, the significance of finding a few copies of a particular agent present in a particular body site is not well established for most pathogens. While the finding of human immunodeficiency virus in the blood of a patient is indicative of infection, would the same concern be raised with the finding of small quantities of cytomegalovirus or enterovirus in nonimmunocompromised patients? Such questions require more data before these techniques should be introduced into the laboratory.

References

1. Britten RJ, Davidson EH. Hybridization strategy. In: Hames BD, Higgins SJ, eds. Nucleic acid hybridization: a practical approach. Oxford: IRL Press, 1985:3–14.
2. Jablonski E, Moomaw EW, Tullis RH, Ruth JL. Preparation of oligodeoxynucleotide-alkaline phosphatase conjugates and their use as hybridization probes. Nucleic Acids Res 1986;14: 6115–6121.
3. Tenover FC. Diagnostic deoxyribonucleic acid probes for infectious diseases. Clin Microbiol Rev 1988;1:82–101.
4. Beckmann AM, Myerson D, Daling JR, Kiviat NB, Fenoglio C, McDougall JK. Detection and localization of human papillomavirus DNA in human genital condylomas by in situ hybridization with biotinylated probes. J Med Virol 1985;16:265–273.
5. Caussy D, Orr W, Daya AD, Roth P, Reeves W, Rawls W. Evaluation of methods for detecting human papillomavirus deoxyribonucleic acid sequences in clinical specimens. J Clin Microbiol 1988;26:236–243.
6. Levine MM, Xu JG, Kaper JB, et al. A DNA probe to identify enterohemorrhagic *Escherichia coli* of O157:H7 and other serotypes that cause hemorrhagic colitis and hemolytic uremic syndrome. J Infect Dis 1987;156:175–182.
7. Hallam K. The rising trend in outpatient testing. Med Lab Observer 1986;18:24–28.
8. Tenover FC. DNA probes for bacterial stool pathogens. In: Tenover FC, ed. DNA probes for infectious diseases. Boca Raton, FL: CRC Press, 1989:53–64.
9. Samuelson J, Acuna-Soto R, Reed S, Biagi F, Wirth D. DNA hybridization probe for clinical diagnosis of *Entamoeba histolytica*. J Clin Microbiol 1989;27:671–676.
10. Meloni BP, Lymbery AJ, Thompson RCA. Characterization of *Giardia* isolates using a non-radiolabeled DNA probe, and correlation with the results of isoenzyme analysis. Am J Trop Med Hyg 1989;40:629–637.
11. Tenover FC, Carlson L, Barbagallo S, Nachamkin I. DNA probe culture confirmation assay for identification of thermophilic *Campylobacter* species. J Clin Microbiol 1990;28:1284–1287.
12. Olive DM. Detection of enterotoxigenic *Escherichia coli* after polymerase chain reaction amplification with a thermostable DNA polymerase. J Clin Microbiol 1989;27:261–265.
13. Coll P, Phillips K, Tenover FC. Evaluation of a rapid method of extracting DNA from stool samples for use in hybridization assays. J Clin Microbiol 1989;27:2245–2248.
14. Frankel G, Giron JA, Valmassoi J, Schoolnik GK. Multi-gene amplification: simultaneous detection of three virulence genes in diarrhoeal stool. Molec Microbiol 1989;3:1729–1734.

15. Siegel DL, Edelstein PH, Nachamkin I. Inappropriate testing for diarrheal diseases in the hospital. JAMA 1990;263:979–982.
16. Edelstein PH, Bryan RN, Enns RK, Mohne DE, Kacian DL. Retrospective study on Gen-Probe rapid diagnostic system for detection of *Legionellae* in frozen clinical respiratory tract samples. J Clin Microbiol 1987;25:1022–1026.
17. Doebbeling BN, Bale MJ, Koontz FP, Helms CM, Wenzel RP, Pfaller MA. Prospective evaluation of the Gen-Probe assay for the detection of Legionellae in respiratory specimens. Eur J Clin Microbiol Infect Dis 1988;7:748–752.
18. Dular R, Kajioka R, Kasatiya S. Comparison of Gen-Probe commerical kit and culture technique for the diagnosis of *Mycoplasma pneumoniae* infection. J Clin Microbiol 1988:26: 1068–1069.
19. Kleemola SRM, Karjalainen JE, Räty RKH. Rapid diagnosis of *Mycoplasma pneumoniae* infection: clinical evaluation of a commercial probe test. J Infect Disc 1990;162:70–75.
20. Gonzalez R, Hanna BA. Evaluation of Gen-Probe DNA hybridization systems for the identification of *Mycobacterium tuberculosis* and *Mycobacterium avium-intracellulare*. Diagn Microbiol Infect Dis 1987;8:69–73.
21. Drake TA, Hindler JA, Berlin OGW, Bruckner D. Rapid identification of *Mycobacterium avium* complex in culture using DNA probes. J Clin Microbiol 1987;25:1442–1445.
22. Conville PS, Keiser JF, Witebsky FG. Comparison of three techniques for concentrating positive BACTEC 13A bottles for mycobacterial DNA probe analysis. Diagn Microbiol Infect Dis 1989;12:309–313.
23. Conville PS, Keiser JF, Witebsky FG. Mycobacteremia caused by simultaneous infection with *Mycobacterium avium* and *Mycobacterium intracellulare* detected by analysis of a BACTEC 13A bottle with the Gen-Probe kit. Diagn Microbiol Infect Dis 1989;12:217–219.
24. Wilkinson HW, Sampson JS, Plikaytis BB. Evaluation of a commercial gene probe for identification of *Legionella* cultures. J Clin Microbiol 1986;23:217–220.
25. Laussucq S, Schuster S, Alexander WJ, Thacker WL, Wilkinson HW, Spika JS. False-positive DNA probe test for *Legionella* species associated with a cluster of respiratory illnesses. J Clin Microbiol 1988;26:1442–1444.
26. Spector SA, Danker WM, Denaro F, Spector DH. DNA probes for detection of human cytomegalovirus. In: Tenover FC, ed. DNA probes for infectious diseases. Boca Raton, FL: CRC Press, 1989:135–144.
27. Beckmann AM, Myerson D. Diagnosis of human papillomavirus and human cytomegalovirus by hybridization histochemistry. In: Tenover FC, ed. DNA probes for infectious diseases. Boca Raton, FL: CRC Press, 1989:145–162.
28. Totten PA, Holmes KK, Handsfield HH, Knapp JS, Perine PL, Falkow S. DNA hybridization technique for the detection of *Neisseria gonorrhoeae* in men with urethritis. J Infect Dis 1983;148:462–471.
29. Schachter J. Rapid diagnosis of sexually transmitted diseases—speed has its price. Diagn Microbiol Infect Dis 1986;4: 185–189.
30. Corey L. Laboratory diagnosis of herpes simplex virus. Principles guiding the development of rapid diagnostic tests. Diagn Microbiol Infect Dis 1986;4:111S–119S.
31. Rubin FA, McWhirter PD, Punjabi NH, et al. Use of a DNA probe to detect *Salmonella typhi* in the blood of patients with typhoid fever. J Clin Microbiol 1989;27:1112–1114.
32. Barker RH, Suebsaeng L, Rooney W, Alecrim GC, Dourado HV, Wirth DF. Specific DNA probe for the diagnosis of *Plasmodium falciparum* malaria. Science 1986;231:1434–1436.
33. McLaughlin GL, Edlind TD, Ihler GM. Detection of *Babesia bovis* using DNA hybridization. J Protozool 1986;33:125–128.
34. Richman DD, McCutchen JA, Spector SA. Detecting human immunodeficiency virus RNA in peripheral blood mononuclear cells by nucleic acid hybridization. J Infect Dis 1987;156: 823–827.
35. Blum HE, Figus A, Haase AT, Vyas GN. Laboratory diagnosis of hepatitis B infection by nucleic acid hybridization analyses and immunohistologic detection of gene products. Dev Biol Stand 1985;59:125–139.
36. Blum HE, Haase AT, Vyas GN. Molecular pathogenesis of hepatitis B virus infection: simultaneous detection of viral DNA and antigens in paraffin-embedded liver sections. Lancet 1984;2:771–775.
37. Unger ER, Budgeon LR, Myerson D, Brigatti DJ. Viral diagnosis by in situ hybridization. Description of a rapid simplified colorimetric method. Am J Surg Pathol 1986;10:1–8.
38. Tidy JA, Parrt GCN, Ward P, et al. High rate of human papillomavirus type 16 infection in cytologically normal cervices. Lancet 1989:1:434–437.
39. Fox BC, Mobley HLT, Wade JC. The use of a DNA probe for epidemiological studies of candidiasis in immunocompromised hosts. J Infect Dis 1989;159:488–494.
40. Crowley P, Oliver SG. A microculture hybridization technique for the detection of specific DNA sequences in filamentous fungi. Exp Mycol 1987;11:70–73.
41. Wirth DF, Pratt DM. Rapid identification of *Leishmania* species by specific hybridization of kinetoplast DNA in cutaneous lesions. Proc Natl Acad Sci USA 1983;79:6999–7003.
42. Gonzalez A, Prediger E, Huecas ME, Nogueira N, Lizardi PM. Minichromosomal repetitive DNA in *Trypanosoma cruzi*: its use in a high-sensitivity parasitic detection assay. Proc Natl Acad Sci USA 1984;81:3356–3360.
43. Sim BKL, Mak JW, Cheong WH, et al. Identification of *Brugia malayi* in vectors with a species-specific DNA probe. Am J Trop Med Hyg 1986;35:559–564.
44. Tenover FC. Studies of antimicrobial resistance genes using DNA probes. Antimicrob Agents Chemother 1986;29:721–725.
45. Perine PL, Totten PA, Holmes KK, et al. Evaluation of a DNA hybridization method for the detection of African and Asian strains of *Neisseria gonorrhoeae* in men with urethritis. J Infect Dis 1985;152:59–63.
46. Swierkosz EM, Scholl DR, Brown JL, Jollick JD, Gleaves CA. Improved DNA hybridization method for detection of acyclovir resistant herpes simplex virus. Antimicrob Agents Chemother 1987;31:1465–1469.
47. McLaughlin GL, Deloron P, Huong AY, Sezibera C, Campbell GH. DNA hybridization for assessment of response of *Plasmodium falciparum* to chloroquin therapy. J Clin Microbiol 1988;26: 1704–1707.
48. Unger ER, Brigati DJ. Colorimetric in-situ hybridization in clinical virology: development of automated technology. Curr Top Microbiol Immunol 1989;143:21–31.
49. Saiki RK, Gelfand DH, Stoffel S, et al. Primer-directed enzymatic amplification of DNA with a thermostable DNA polymerase. Science 1988;239:487–491.
50. Kwoh DY, Davis GR, Whitfield KM, Chappelle HL, DiMichele LJ, Gingeras TR. Transcription-based amplification system and detection of amplified human immunodeficiency virus type 1 with a bead-based sandwich hybridization format. Proc Natl Acad Sci USA 1989;86:1173–1177.
51. Kwok S, Higuchi R. Avoiding false positives with PCR. Nature 1989;339:237–238.

51 Quality Control and Quality Assurance

Ron B. Schifman

A good quality assurance program continuously improves the reliability, efficiency, and utilization of laboratory services. The elements of quality assurance consist of structure, process, and outcome (1). Structure is the aspect related to adequacy of the workplace and the provisions required to do the job. Process describes the proficiency with which the work is done, while outcome reflects the consequences of work performed. Quality can be measured by specifying indicators and setting thresholds for acceptable performance. This spans a wide spectrum from monitoring reagent performance to assessing test usage. Limits may be set so that action is taken only when the number of deficiencies exceeds a specified threshold, or may be defined as sentinel events that require review and action whenever they are encountered. Although monitoring is important, the most effective results are achieved by employing strategies to prevent problems rather than by detecting and correcting defects after they have occurred (2).

A clear understanding of quality assurance objectives is a prerequisite for developing a worthwhile program. In the broadest sense, the goal is to examine what is done and use this information to improve upon the process in the most effective way possible. Quality assurance includes the complementary elements of quality control and quality improvement. Quality improvement objectives are achieved by deliberately designing reliability into the system. It is a method for anticipating and preventing problems before they happen, while the aim of quality control is to find defects and correct them (Fig. 51.1) (3-5).

Passage of the 1967 Clinical Laboratory Improvement Act marked the beginning of systematic laboratory quality assurance. Since then, most attention has focused on quality control (6). This includes monitoring the dependability of reagents, procedures, and equipment by internal and external proficiency testing. Less consideration has been given to other components of quality that deal with issues of how and why tests are ordered and how results are utilized. With the growth of new requirements from regulatory and accreditation bodies, the latter issue will gain more importance. In addition, the idea that quality is ultimately determined by how laboratory practice affects patient outcome is becoming more widely accepted.

QUALITY CONTROL

Basic Elements

Documentation is an essential requirement. All methods, policies, quality control results, and corrective actions need to be described in writing and available to those working in the microbiology laboratory or responsible for its management.

PROCEDURE MANUAL

The procedure manual is a reference document describing all established methods, materials, and policies. Its purpose is to standardize the performance of laboratory operations. It includes procedures for collecting, transporting and rejecting specimens, methods for processing samples and reporting results, quality control procedures for reagents, media, and equipment, as well as procedures to follow when quality control data indicate unacceptable performance. Pertinent hospital and laboratory policies, including guidelines for safety and waste disposal, are also included. The manual should have a consistent format for method descriptions and should include appropriate citations. Another manual describing specimen and requisition requirements, storage and transport conditions, laboratory policies, and safety precautions must be available to physicians, nurses, and anyone else who is responsible for ordering tests or collecting specimens.

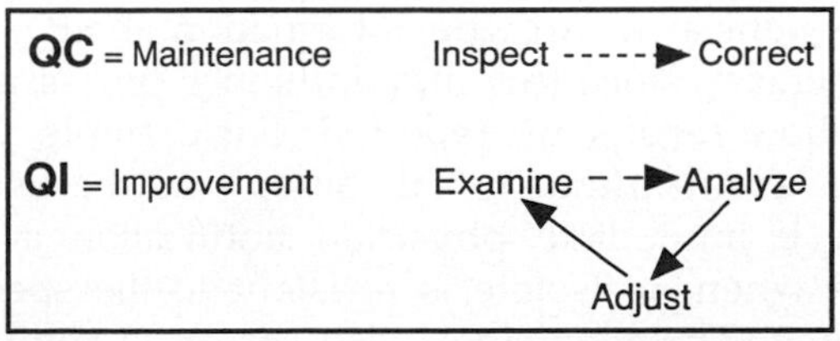

Figure 51.1. Differences between quality control (QC) and quality improvement (QI).

QUALITY CONTROL LOGS

The quality control (QC) log is a form for documenting quality control results and corrective actions. It contains the date and time that testing is performed, the person doing the test, the test results, acceptable limits, interpretation of results (pass or fail), and, when necessary, comments on corrective actions. A place to document periodic review and a description of procedures to follow when deficiencies are identified should also be included.

WORKSHEETS

Worksheets are used to document observations made during specimen processing. Documentation includes specimen descriptions, growth on specific media and flow diagrams of biochemical results, and susceptibility tests. The worksheet can be employed to evaluate potential problems after specimens and culture plates are discarded. It also organizes the evaluation of culture findings and helps with processing partially completed examinations with pending tests.

Quality Control of the Microbiology Specimen

Quality microbiology results are achieved when proper specimens are collected for appropriate reasons. Examining an unsuitable specimen or responding to a clinically inappropriate request is not only inefficient, but the results can be misleading (7). Ongoing instruction of those collecting and ordering tests is the most effective method for reducing this source of error. In addition, specific monitors of specimen quality and test usage are useful for identifying distinct problem areas requiring more intensive control (see Quality Improvement section below).

TEST ORDERING AND THE REQUISITION FORM

The microbiology requisition should provide enough information to evaluate a specimen's suitability for processing. It needs to include the patient's name and identification, requesting physician, date and time of collection, examination requested (including special requests), and specimen source. It is also beneficial to provide information about antibiotic therapy, since this may influence processing or affect how results are reported. For example, information about antimicrobial therapy can be used to decide if immediate physician notification is warranted when an isolate is resistant to the specified antibiotic. The requisition also serves to communicate information from the laboratory about specimen requirements. This may include a statement about specimen transport, container requirements, volume for blood cultures, or the need to submit multiple specimens (e.g., sputum specimens for *Mycobacterium* spp. culture).

The clinical relevance of examining a specimen must also be considered. Material from a decubitus ulcer, periodontal lesion, nose, perirectal abscess, or foley catheter tip rarely provides clinically useful information, and these specimens should be processed only after consultation with the requesting physician, or not at all (7). Communication is important when a poor-quality specimen is determined to be unsuitable for processing. The reasons for rejecting the sample are explained and, when possible, an alternative procedure or corrective action is recommended. Since opinions about specimen quality differ, the rejected specimen should be held at 4°C until a final decision is made. A low threshold for processing poor-quality specimens should be maintained when another would be difficult to collect (i.e., cerebral spinal fluid). However, a comment about the apparent problem must be included on the final report to avoid the possibility of a misinterpretation.

It is important to establish guidelines for rejecting a specimen or questioning its value when there is incomplete information (e.g., swab from unknown site), an improper submission (e.g., delayed specimen transport), an inappropriate test request (e.g., anaerobic urine culture), or poor-quality collection (e.g., expectorated sputum containing numerous epithelial cells) (8).

Specimen Processing

Evaluation of a microbiology specimen is technically complex and labor intensive. The extent of processing depends on evaluating the probable clinical significance of information obtained from the examination and affects the interpretation of final results.

GROSS AND MICROSCOPIC EXAMINATION

Gross examination helps determine a specimen's suitability for processing. Inadequate sample volume, use of a nonsterile container, or improper collection technique are grounds for rejection. However, a sample should not be rejected on the basis of its gross appearance alone (e.g., sputum specimen that macroscopically appears like saliva). Gross examination is also useful for sampling the most promising portions of sputum or wound specimens containing mucus, pus, or blood. The sample's description or volume in the case of blood or fluid should be indicated on the worksheet and report.

Examination and quantitative evaluation of direct smears is beneficial for assessing specimen quality, checking culture results, and establishing a preliminary diagnosis (8). An expectorated sputum sample containing excessive epithelial cells indicates oropharyngeal contamination and has dubious value, while enteric pathogens may be expected in a stool specimen containing white cells. Correlations between quantitative smear and culture results can be used to maintain consistency and as an internal check on the accuracy of processing and interpretation. For example, quantitative culture results that are consistently higher than the amount of bacteria seen on smear examinations suggest a problem related to sampling, interpretation, or processing (i.e., overstreaking of the primary inoculum).

PREPARATION OF THE PRIMARY CULTURE

Guidelines for preparing primary cultures are based on the specimen source. Instructions should specify media and incubation requirements. Streaking agar plates should be standardized to include the number of times the loop is struck back into the primary inoculum. This improves the reproducibility of quantitative interpretations and is monitored simply by examining primary culture plates.

The accuracy of delivering specific sample volumes with a calibrated loop is affected by the angle at which the tip is withdrawn from a sample as well as the diameter of the container being sampled. It is important that these variables be standardized, since error rates may approach 100%. Accuracy and reproducibility of the calibrated loop method can be determined by absorption spectroscopy or weight determination tests.

EVALUATION AND REPORTING OF CULTURE RESULTS

A worksheet is used to document all culture and smear observations and test results. Culture plates should be retained for at least several days in the event that reexamination is necessary after the final report has been submitted. This can happen when there is a concern that results are erroneous or when additional assessments are needed. Likewise, it is worthwhile to save isolates from high-quality specimens since they may occasionally be needed for epidemiologic evaluations. Most bacteria can be stored for a prolonged period of time in bovine serum at −40°C.

QUALITY ASSURANCE OF THE FINAL REPORT

Decisions about what to report depend on the specimen source, clinical relevance, direct smear, identification and quantity of isolates, and sometimes communication (directly or via the requisition) with the physician. Work performed to reach the final result may be reliable but of poor quality if the report's significance is misunderstood. Making decisions about the extent of work to perform on specimens obtained from nonsterile sites that yield mixed flora of undetermined significance presents a challenge, since in many cases the results provide no useful information. Complete testing and susceptibility of all isolates is unnecessary, misleading, and inefficient (8). Microbiologists should not be compelled to identify and report every isolate detected in mixed cultures. For example, reporting all organisms detected in an expectorated sputum sample that is ordinarily contaminated with upper respiratory flora can be misinterpreted and is not appropriate. In this circumstance it is better to report predominant growth or simply indicate the presence of mixed flora. Similarly, decisions about performing susceptibility tests on isolates from mixed cultures should be given careful consideration because susceptibility testing of all isolates is wasteful and may result in unnecessary antibiotic usage (7). The direct smear and clinical circumstance help guide the evaluation of specimens with mixed flora.

Daily review of final reports is an important quality control procedure. Direct microscopic examinations should be qualitatively and quantitatively compared with culture results. Poor correlation between smear and culture results occurs from inaccurate readings, poor technique, unsatisfactory media, inappropriate growth conditions, or the presence of dead organisms. The smear, culture, and worksheet should be reviewed when discrepancies are detected. Results should also correlate with specimen source. For example, *Enterococcus* spp. are generally not recovered from sputum specimens, while *Streptococcus pneumoniae* is not an expected urinary tract pathogen. Susceptibility results should be consistent with the organism's identification (Table 51.1). A mismatch can indicate errors in either test and should be investigated before the final report is issued.

When an error is detected after the final report goes out, a revised report should describe corrections but must not be modified in a way that conceals the initial erroneous result. An ongoing system should be in place for actively searching for errors in reported results. This can be done by retrospective comparison of results on worksheets, instrument logs, etc., with results reported on the chart. The clinical significance of errors discovered after the report is available for patient care should be classified and periodically reviewed to determine if modifications in procedures or policies are needed (see Quality Improvement section) (Fig. 51.2).

Section: General (Section Specific)

1. Responsibility: Laboratory Director, Section Supervisor
2. Scope of care: Verified and reported results that are discovered to contain an error.
3. Aspects of care: Wide spectrum—from no complication to potential for adverse outcome.
4. Clinical indicators: Any change made in a laboratory report after it has been finalized, verified and made available for patient care. Errors are divided into three categories based on the impact on patient care.

   Category A error—The primary provider has responded to the result by ordering the next test, repeating the test, changing treatment or diagnosis.

   Category B error—A serious error but unlikely to affect patient care—similar to category A error but primary care provider has not yet been notified or acted on the reported erroneous error.

   Category C error—Minor clerical error in reporting and "cosmetic" corrections to report.
5. Threshold for evaluation: All category A errors are brought to the attention of the Laboratory Director for evaluation as soon as possible. All Category B errors must be expeditiously reviewed by the section supervisor. Category C errors require no immediate action unless the monthly number exceeds twice the average monthly rate during the preceeding 12 months.
6. Data collection and evaluation:

   Data source(s): Complaints, delta checks. Comparative review between instrument logs and computer reports on random sample of at least 100 results should be performed weekly for results that are manually entered.

   Data collection: Record each incident on error reporting worksheet.

   Sample: All identified errors.

   Frequency: Continuous.

   Mode: Concurrent
7. Data evaluation: Calculate error rates by category and section. Calculate frequency of errors detected by random review. Appropriate written documentation should accompany each Category A and B error. This should include a review of findings after investigation of the problem, circumstances related to the cause and effect of error. A plan should be developed for corrective actions to prevent or reduce recurrence of errors that are critical or repeat.
8. Action: Category C errors that exceed the threshold should prompt a review of the section's clerical and analytical procedures with development of a plan to improve performance. Category A or B errors requiring corrective action should address the cause and severity of the problem. The primary care physician should be directly contacted by phone or written communication for all category A errors; this may also be necessary for some category B errors. Any error that requires a change in the medical record must be properly identified as a changed report.
9. Evaluation of effectiveness and documentation of improvement: Effectiveness is measured by the extent with which errors can be reduced in number and their recurrence limited. Use error reporting data to monitor trends, identify source of problems and educate technologists and clerical support staff. Document all changes in procedures that may impact error reduction or prevention.
10. Communication of relevant information: Error reporting data, significant findings, plans of action and resolution of problems are presented in Service minutes and to the Laboratory Utilization Review Subcommittee.

Figure 51.2. Error reporting procedure.

Quality Control of Materials and Procedures

Accurate and reproducible results are obtained when tests are performed in a consistent manner with dependable materials. Reaching a final result generally involves numerous procedural steps and the interpretation of many pieces of information. While this creates a challenge to ensure that all materials are in control, it also provides an opportunity to evaluate the consistency and interrelationships of method results. A single unexpected or inappropriate finding may identify a problem without necessarily producing an inaccurate result. Thus, each microbiological study provides its own internal quality control checks to identify procedural errors and material defects.

REAGENTS AND STAINS

Reagents must be dated when received and when first used. Expiration dates and storage requirements must be indicated on all reagent containers. A standardized label and log helps ensure consistency.

The performance of reagents and stains is evaluated by demonstrating appropriate reactivity by stock control organisms. There is generally a wide tolerance for errors since most reactions are interpreted as positive or negative. Furthermore, a single discrepancy may not affect the accuracy of a final result since bacterial identifications are usually determined by multiple tests with variable reactivities. Errors are detected when a reagent does not show an expected reaction when compared with other test results. For example, a reagent defect is suggested when an isolate of *Escherichia coli* demonstrates a negative indole reaction.

Regulatory and accreditation agencies specify how the performance of certain reagents and stains are to be evaluated (9). However, these expectations have been challenged as excessive and inefficient because there is inconsistency between checklists (Table 51.2), requirements often fail to consider the wide variability in performance between materials, and they do not always conform with published state-of-the-art consensus recommendations. The frequency and methods for monitoring reagent reliability should depend on their performance characteristics, manufacturers' recommendations, frequency of use, and user's experience. As a general rule, reagent performance is evaluated when first prepared or whenever a new lot is placed in service. The need for additional monitoring can be determined by assessing the frequency of deficiencies found with regular use. Reagents that demonstrate a potential to fail or are seldom employed should be monitored with each use. Likewise, reagents that prove to always perform as expected can be evaluated with less intensity (10). Interpretation of reagent performance by review of quality control documentation provides a rationale for accepting or modifying procedures and helps demonstrate compliance with regulatory agency expectations (11).

MEDIA

All media must be labeled with lot number, preparation date, expiration date, and constituents or media name. It should be marked with the date when first placed into service and stored according to manufacturer's recommendations. The performance of each new lot or shipment of media must be evaluated before it is used. This includes visual inspection, sterility checks, and performance characteristics.

Culture media must be tested for contamination before being placed into service by incubating a proportion of each new lot overnight. Appropriate stock control organisms are employed to check for expected positive and negative reactions and growth requirements. Examples of expected growth patterns and reactions with control organisms is shown in Table 51.3. Refer to references 6, 12, 13, and 14 for a complete listing.

Table 51.1. Common Predictable Susceptibility Patterns

Susceptibility Result	Organism
Ampicillin sensitive	*Proteus mirabilis* (tetracycline resistant) *E. coli* (tetracycline sensitive)
Ampicillin and carbenicillin resistant	*Klebsiella* spp., *Citrobacter diversus*
Ampicillin and cephalothin resistant	*Enterobacter* spp. *Citrobacter freundii* *Serratia* spp.
Ampicillin, cephalothin and tetracycline resistant	*Providencia* spp. *Proteus vulgaris* *Morganella morganii*

Table 51.2. Checklist Requirements by Inspection and Accreditation Organizations

Procedure	Joint Commission for Accreditation of Healthcare Organizations	College of American Pathologists
Quality control of reagents and stains	On each day of use	For each new batch and at least weekly
Quality control of media	Each batch is tested before or concurrently with its use with selected organisms	Some media exempted from testing with reference strains if this has been done by manufacturer

Table 51.3. Examples of Performance Standards for Media[a]

Medium	Test Organisms[b]	Incubation Conditions	Expected Results
Transport media			
Culturette swab	*Haemophilus influenzae* 10211	Pick one colony on swab. Reinsert swab into tube and crush vial. Hold tube at room temperature for 24 hr. Use swab to inoculate chocolate agar. Incubate plate at 35°C in CO_2 for 24 hr.	Good growth
	Streptococcus pneumoniae 6305	Pick one colony on swab. Reinsert swab into tube and crush vial. Hold tube at room temperature for 24 hr. Use swab to inoculate sheep blood agar. Incubate plate at 35°C aerobically for 24 hr.	Good growth
Growth and selective/differential media			
Sheep blood agar	*Streptococcus pyogenes* 19615	35°C / aerobic or CO_2 / 24 hr	Good growth, β-hemolysis
	Staphylococcus aureus 25923		Good growth
	Streptococcus pneumoniae 6305		Good growth, α-hemolysis
	Escherichia coli 25922		Good growth, β-hemolysis
MacConkey agar	*Escherichia coli* 25922	Aerobic, 24 hr	Good growth, rose-red colonies
	Proteus mirabilis 12453		Good growth, colorless colonies, inhibition of swarming
	Salmonella typhimurium 14028		Good growth, colorless colonies
	Enterococcus faeculis 29212		Inhibition, partial
Biochemical differential media[c]			
Triple sugar iron agar (TSI)	*Salmonella typhimurium*	35°C / aerobic / 24 hr	Alkaline slant, acid butt, with gas, H_2S positive
	Shigella flexneri		Alkaline slant, acid butt
	Pseudomonas aeruginosa		Alkaline slant, no change in butt
	Escherichia coli		Acid slant, acid butt, with gas

[a]Full listing of performance standards may be found in references 9 and 13.
[b]Number is ATCC identification.
[c]Standardized reference strains have not been established.

Deficiencies may also be detected during routine processing. For example, sheep blood agar may support the growth and show expected hemolytic reactions for *Streptococcus pneumoniae* and *Streptococcus pyogenes* in control tests, but fail to produce an accurate cAMP test. This type of problem will only be identified if a high index of suspicion is maintained and media performance is continuously cross-checked with expected culture and identification findings.

Many types of commercially available media are consistently reliable because extensive quality control testing is performed before distribution, and it has been shown that reevaluation in the clinical laboratory is unnecessary. Regulatory agencies accept a recent consensus recommendation from the National Committee for Clinical Laboratory Standards (NCCLS) that certain types of bacterial and fungal media do not require intensive monitoring if sterility (less than 5% contamination) and performance has been checked and documented by the manufacturer (Table 51.4) (14).

Table 51.4. Commercially Prepared, Ready-to-Use Media That Do Not Require Retesting if Manufacturers Can Document Reliability by Meeting NCCLS Performance Criteria

Solid Media	Liquid Media
Blood, aerobic and anaerobic	Thioglycolate
MacConkey	Tryptic digest casein soy
Eosin-methylene blue	Gram-negative (GN)
Colistin-nalidixic acid (aerobic)	Enterococcus, selective
Lowenstein-Jensen	Thiol
Phenylethyl alcohol (aerobic)	Brain-heart infusion
Hektoen enteric	Selenite
Sabouraud dextrose	
Xylose lysine deoxycholate	
Mannitol salt	
Middlebrook	
Mycology, selective	
Salmonella-Shigella	

ANTISERA AND ANTIGENS

Monitoring the performance of serologic tests with positive and negative controls is similar to quality control practices described for other reagents. However, these materials tend to be more labile and susceptible to contamination. Exposure to room temperature for prolonged periods should be avoided. Antisera should be grossly inspected before tests are performed and contamination suspected when a clear solution becomes turbid. It is generally necessary for antisera to be monitored each time a test is performed. Controls not only ensure proper reactivity but also aid in the interpretation of reactions. Before a new lot is placed into service, its performance should be tested in parallel with the expiring lot to check for between test consistency.

Quality Control of Antimicrobial Susceptibility Tests

In the late 1960s, the U.S. Food and Drug Administration began to monitor and regulate the production of antibiotic-containing disks utilized for susceptibility testing. In the early 1970s, progress was made in standardizing susceptibility test procedures, and since 1975, the NCCLS has published a series of ongoing recommendations for the performance, surveillance, and interpretation of broth dilution and agar diffusion procedures.

The quality control of antimicrobial susceptibility tests consists of monitoring the precision and accuracy of results, performance of materials, and execution of manual and automated procedures. Monitoring is done by testing genetically stable reference strains with the same materials and procedures that are employed for routine testing. While this practice eliminates the need to evaluate each component of the assay separately, it has the potential to fail if two deficiencies occur that simultaneously cancel each other out and provide apparently accurate results (e.g., light inoculum tested against low-potency antibiotic disks). Furthermore, this method is not as effective for testing the performance of broth dilution methods.

Quality assurance of susceptibility testing should extend beyond the limits of methodological performance. Susceptibility results may have a profound impact on therapy and outcome. Procedures for ensuring that susceptibility results are reported in a sufficiently timely fashion and are appropriately utilized are important additional considerations.

SELECTION OF ANTIBIOTICS AND METHOD OF REPORTING

A decision to perform susceptibility testing should be based on the clinical relevance of culture findings. Testing is usually unnecessary for organisms that have predictable susceptibility patterns (e.g., *Streptococcus pyogenes* against penicillin G). In some cases one test result will influence the interpretation of another. Methicillin-resistant *Staphylococcus* spp. may show false susceptibility to cephalothin and should always be reported as resistant to this antibiotic. Tests for certain antibiotic-organism combinations are unreliable with routine methods (e.g., erythromycin/*Haemophilus influenzae, Enterococcus* spp./cephalosporin) or do not reliably predict clinical outcome (e.g., cefamandole susceptibility in *Haemophilus influenzae* meningitis). The choice of antibiotics to test depends on the bacterial isolate and culture site. Recommendations for selecting the proper combination are published, but the final decision should be made after consultation with the pharmacy, medical staff, infectious disease specialist, and other interested parties.

Routine susceptibility tests should be performed only on rapidly growing aerobic organisms. Methods for testing slow-growing, fastidious organisms, with the exception of *Haemophilus influenzae, Neisseria gonorrhoeae,* and *Streptococcus pneumoniae,* are not standardized and may yield invalid results. In these cases therapy is guided by expected results based on published studies from reference laboratories.

CONTROL STRAINS

Quality control reference organisms must be available to monitor the precision and accuracy of susceptibility tests (15, 16). They may be stored for long periods at 40°C in 50% calf serum. Tests should be performed from fresh subcultures that have been incubated for at least 18 hours. Subcultures should be checked for contamination and good growth before use. Tests performed directly from stored stock cultures may produce unreliable results.

E. coli ATCC 25922, *Staphylococcus aureus* ATCC 25923, *Pseudomonas aeruginosa* ATCC 27853, and *N. gonorrhoeae* ATCC 49226 are recommended for monitoring (15, 16). *S. aureus* ATCC 29213 is a weak β-lactamase producer that is specifically recommended for broth dilution assays. *P. aeruginosa* ATCC 27853 may spontaneously develop resistance to carbenicillin when repeatedly subcultured. A new subculture should be prepared from stock cultures when this occurs. High levels of thymidine in Mueller-Hinton medium that may adversely affect trimethoprim-sulfamethoxazole susceptibility testing can be detected by *S. faecalis* ATCC 29212 or 33186. β-lactamase producing *E. coli* ATCC 35218 has been selected to test the performance of disks with a combination of β-lactam antibiotic and β-lactamase inhibitor (e.g., clavulinic acid). Additional control organisms may be selected by individual laboratories for specific purposes. For example, methicillin resistance in some strains of *Staphylococcus aureus* may be difficult

Table 51.5. Control Limits for Monitoring Antimicrobial Disk Susceptibility Tests[a]

Antibiotic (Disk Content)	*E. coli* ATCC 25992		*S. Aureus ATCC 25923*	
	Zone Diameter Limits (mm)[b]	Maximum Zone Diameter Range (mm)[c]	Zone Diameter Limits (mm)	Maximum Zone Diameter Range (mm)
Amikacin (30 μg)	19–26	6	20–26	6
Cefazolin (30 μg)	23–29	8	29–35	8
Chloramphenicol (30 μg)	21–27	10	19–26	10
Trimethoprim/sulfamethoxazole (1.25/23.75 μg)	24–32	10	24–32	10

[a]Partial list, see reference 13.
[b]*Daily quality control*: Corrective action is required when: (*a*) more than one of 20 consecutive tests exceed zone diameter limits; (*b*) any single value is above or below 4 standard deviations (i.e., midpoint ± maximum minus minimum zone diameter limits), or (c) any consecutive series of 5 tests exceed the allowable zone diameter range (largest minus smallest zone diameter).
[c]*Weekly quality control:* To perform weekly quality control: (a) no more than three consecutive tests must be outside zone diameter limits during 30 test periods; (*b*) none exceed 4 s.d.; and (c) none in each group of six zone diameter ranges (of 30 performed) exceed allowable maximum range. When these conditions are satisfied, quality control can be performed weekly until a test fails by exceeding allowable zone diameter limits. When a deficiency is detected, weekly quality control may continue after five consecutive tests of the organism/ antibiotic combination that failed show no value beyond the allowable zone diameter limits, and the range of the five tests is within the maximum zone diameter range.

to detect by standard and automated methods. Laboratories that encounter these stains may wish to periodically test a well-characterized strain of methicillin-resistant *S. aureus* as part of routine quality control activities.

ANTIBIOTICS

Substantial variability may occur from inactivation of antibiotics during transport and normal use. β-Lactam antibiotics are especially labile in the presence of excess humidity and high temperatures. Antibiotic disks must be periodically evaluated. This is done by monitoring zone diameters produced by reference strains that indicate antibiotic potency. Recommended control limits are established for these strains from collaborative studies. A precision control value for disk diffusion tests is calculated from the five previous susceptibility determinations performed on reference strains. A maximum range of allowable values as well as cumulative mean zone diameters are used to monitor intra-assay precision (Table 51.5) (12). A single value that significantly deviates below the control range suggests deterioration of antibiotic, and the batch of disks should be discarded. Values that are consistently above or below the control means suggest a deficiency in inoculum preparation or inoculation technique. A deteriorating lot of antibiotic disks may be detected by a trend toward declining control zone diameters. Control values that deviate in opposite directions when testing aminoglycosides and tetracycline suggest unsatisfactory medium pH.

Quality control limits for broth dilution procedures are also established for control reference strains. However, these tests are often not configured to contain appropriate dilution schemes to properly check accuracy and precision. This is because the lowest dilution is higher than the minimum inhibitory concentration of the reference strain.

Expected precision for broth dilution tests is plus or minus one twofold dilution from the modal minimal inhibitory concentration (MIC) level (16). The precision of automated and commercially prepared broth dilution methods tends to be better than the reference broth dilution assay. Because broth dilution control ranges may vary between commercial methods, control limits determined from reference methods may not conform when commercial and automated dilution assays are monitored.

INOCULUM

The preparation of standardized inoculum is a critical component of susceptibility methods and must be precise. Bacterial suspensions should be made with the aid of a light box or photometer. Inoculum preparation without comparison to a turbidity standard is discouraged. The accuracy of inoculum preparation techniques should periodically be determined by performing quantitative colony counts from standardized inocula. Accurate susceptibility results can be obtained with inoculum in either stationary or log phase growth.

Broth dilution tests must include a growth control (inoculation of broth media without antibiotics) to determine inoculum viability and as a control to interpret endpoints. The inoculum for broth dilution and automated susceptibility tests should also be tested for purity by making a subculture from the bacterial suspension and observing for pure growth after overnight incubation.

MEDIA

Mueller-Hinton medium is recommended for the susceptibility testing of aerobic organisms. Three major variables have been identified that influence the test including cation concentration, pH, and thymidine concentration. These factors must be carefully monitored and adjusted when necessary to obtain satisfactory results.

Mueller-Hinton medium must have adequate levels of magnesium (25 mg/liter) and calcium (50 mg/liter) to detect aminoglycoside resistance in some strains of *Pseudomonas aeruginosa*. The calcium and magnesium concentration of each batch of Mueller Hinton media should be specified by the manufacturer or determined in the laboratory. Alternatively, a control strain of *P. aeruginosa* with a moderately resistant MIC (8–16 μg/ml) may be tested with each new lot of media. A cation deficiency should be suspected if this organism fails to demonstrate aminoglycoside resistance.

The pH of Mueller-Hinton medium should range between 7.2 and 7.4. This should be documented by the manufacturer or measured in the laboratory. Unsatisfactory pH may be suspected when mean zone diameters of control organisms tested against tetracycline and gentamicin deviate in opposite directions.

The thymidine concentration in Mueller-Hinton medium affects susceptibility tests with trimethoprim and sulfa antibiotics. Excess thymidine and thymine levels may produce falsely resistant results. A decreased zone diameter and inner colonies, or increased MIC observed when testing *Streptococcus faecalis* ATCC 29212 against trimethoprim-sulfamethoxazole suggests an inappropriately high level of thymidine.

PERFORMANCE AND INTERPRETATION

Unsatisfactory technical performance is the most common source of error associated with susceptibility testing. In one study, 3.9% of diffusion susceptibility results performed with control strains were inaccurate (10). In nearly all cases, errors were linked with performance failures, while material deficiencies were detected in only 0.06% of all control tests. Technical problems included unsatisfactory inoculum (most common), improperly placed disks, and rarely, misreading of zone diameters. Errors may also occur when tests are correctly performed but results are misinterpreted or inaccurately reported. This problem is well illustrated by an interlaboratory proficiency survey conducted to assess the accuracy of detecting a strain of penicillin-resistant *Streptococcus pneumoniae*. Nearly all participants performed the test accurately, but less than 15% reported a correct result because proper criteria for interpreting the result were not applied.

FREQUENCY OF QUALITY CONTROL TESTING

Guidelines for diffusion susceptibility testing include daily quality control with reference strains. However, it is apparent that many laboratories can achieve acceptable results with less frequent testing. Weekly quality control testing is acceptable if a laboratory can document adequate daily performance for 30 days. This is accomplished by observing no more than three values outside of control limit for each antibiotic during this time period. Daily quality control testing must resume when weekly surveillance demonstrates an accuracy control problem, and continue until the problem is identified and corrected. While this approach appears to be more efficient than daily checks, it may be unrealistic for testing multiple antibiotics. It becomes impractical to isolate one antibiotic from all the others for daily QC checking since disks are generally dispensed as a group onto plated media, and when testing many different antibiotics there is a high probability of frequent quality control problems. For these reasons, some laboratories find it as convenient to perform daily QC. Nevertheless, reference strains should always be tested with all new lots of media and antibiotics. Daily quality control with reference strains is recommended for broth dilution and automated methods.

Reference Laboratory

A referral clinical laboratory is a valuable resource for checking the accuracy of results and is essential for providing assistance when difficult culture, identification, susceptibility, or serologic problems are encountered. This is particularly important if an unusual result is obtained or a test is infrequently performed. Confirmation of results provides confidence in the laboratory's procedures and materials. New findings or discrepancies serve to resolve potential problems and enhance the education and experience of laboratory personnel.

External Quality Assurance Programs

PROFICIENCY TESTING

An important component of quality control in the microbiology laboratory is the processing of unknown specimens with defined constituents (17). Results obtained from these specimens are compared with expected results to evaluate the quality of laboratory performance. Internal proficiency testing is conducted by processing test specimens that are disguised as routine samples. This exercise has the advantage of evaluating all procedures and materials that are routinely employed to process specimens (i.e., transport, smear, culture, timeliness of reporting, etc.). More commonly, external proficiency testing is conducted by outside laboratories and agencies to evaluate interlaboratory performance. The largest clinical microbiology proficiency survey is conducted by the College of American Pathologists (CAP) to evaluate identification and susceptibility procedures. This program has important benefits for assessing the performance of specific methods. These include identification of individual laboratory deficiencies, detection of inadequate or improved methods, continuing education, and standardization of methods and materials. External proficiency challenges have demonstrated that most laboratories can achieve acceptable results with standardized disk diffusion methods. Q-Probes is another CAP program, oriented toward interlaboratory assessment of other quality assurance standards.

Quality Control of Equipment and the Environment

The performance of laboratory equipment must be properly monitored to identify problems that will affect test results. This should include written instructions for preventive maintenance, performance checks, and calibration procedures. All maintenance and performance activities as well as equipment failures and repairs must be documented and periodically reviewed. Suggested performance monitoring schedules for general laboratory equipment and tolerance limits for common laboratory equipment are published elsewhere (12, 13).

The laboratory environment must be kept clean and well ventilated. A minimum of at least 100 square feet should be available per full time equivalent employee. Incandescent lighting should be used, when possible, for reading culture plates and tubes. Cultures should be processed in one area to avoid the potential hazard of transporting potentially harmful pathogens. Policies for handling infectious and hazardous waste should be developed (18).

QUALITY MANAGEMENT

Quality assurance (QA) is a process for monitoring the functional components of a system and for correcting defects when unacceptable performance is identified. Quality is typically assessed by specifying performance indicators and setting targets (thresholds) for acceptable proficiency. Limits may be set so that action is taken only when the number of deficiencies exceeds a specified threshold, or they may be defined as sentinel events that require review and action whenever encountered.

Quality management also entails *quality improvement* (QI) objectives, which address methods to continuously improve reliability, efficiency, and utilization of laboratory services (Fig. 51.1). (5, 19, 20). Experience in other service industries has shown that the most effective and long-lasting improvements are achieved by adopting strategies to anticipate and prevent problems rather than by only identifying and correcting defects after they have occurred (21).

Table 51.6. Principles of Continuous Quality Improvement in Health Care

- Emphasis on examining processes
- Coordination and integration between clinical and administrative functions.
- Opportunities to improve health service processes are more frequent than opportunities to correct mistakes and errors.
- The management goal is to help individuals improve processes in which they are involved.

Table 51.7. Shift of Emphasis in Joint Commission Standards

Old	New
Primary focus on clinical aspects of care.	Focus on interrelated processes (management, support, and clinical) that in combination affect patient outcomes.
Compartmentalization of QA activities by hospital structure (e.g., department, service, discipline).	Integrated, cross-disciplinary, and cross-departmental QI activities organized around flow of patient care.
Focus on individual performance, especially problem performance.	Focus on coordination and integration to improve processes.
Identify and correct problems.	Improve processes to prevent problems.
Segregation of appropriate ("Was the right thing done?") and effective ("Was it done right?") care from efficiency (value) of care.	Linking the goals of improving patient outcomes with efficiency of care.

Beginning in 1992, the Joint Commission for Accreditation of Healthcare Organizations (JCAHO), has been incrementally revising accreditation standards to embrace the principles and goals of continuous quality improvement (22). This change represents a gradual evolution from monitoring and evaluating departmental activities to a general examination of how the system manages the flow of patient care in order to reveal opportunities for improvement. As a result, there will be an expanding emphasis on coordinating and integrating interdepartmental activities, and more attention will be given to improving processes and preventing problems (Tables 51.6 and 51.7).

Because quality management is an information-driven process, substantial attention has focused on choosing indicators. A clinical indicator (or monitor) is a measurable variable related to some aspect of care (23). It is tempting to begin the process of establishing a quality assurance procedure by first specifying indicators, before actually defining how the information will be used. However, this approach will limit the chance for success.

Objectives for quality improvement should be clearly established *before* determining the sources of data to be used for monitoring and evaluation. This

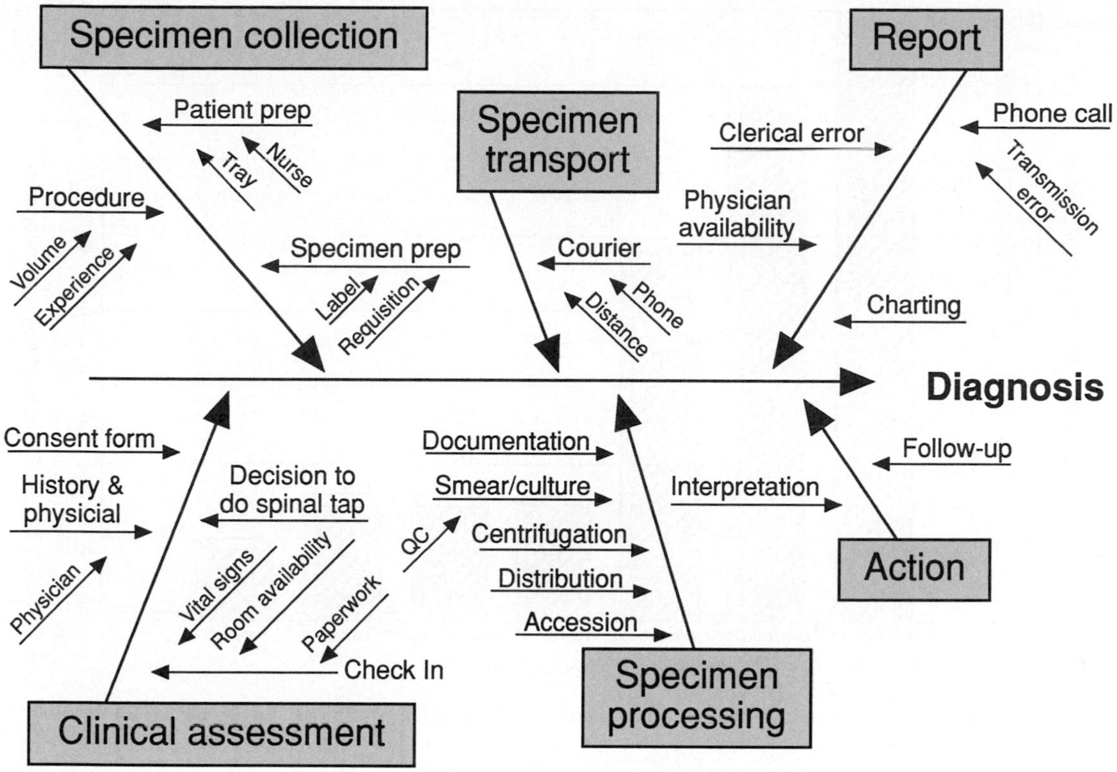

Figure 51.3. Fishbone diagram of bacterial meningitis diagnosis describing multiple interdepartmental factors influencing the timeliness of testing.

avoids the trap of developing a procedure based on ease of data collection rather than pertinence to a specific quality improvement issue. It is important to understand that useful indicators may require access to sources of information (such as chart review and contact with clinical staff) that are not readily available from the laboratory database. Under these circumstances, data collection can be labor intensive and drain limited resources. It is therefore important to start with a carefully defined goal that considers how the information will be used to improve care.

For quality improvement purposes, information is not used to show that everything is all right or as an end in itself. Its purpose is to analyze a process in order to find the cause of expected or unexpected deficiencies and to determine how the process affects clinical outcome. This knowledge is used to make adjustments that will prevent future deficiencies, and by doing so, create sustained improvement.

DEVELOPING A QUALITY IMPROVEMENT PROCEDURE

The following outline lists the steps that should be considered for developing a quality improvement procedure. Specific examples follow.

1. *Define the process.* First ask the question, "What is the quality improvement goal?" This can be based on suggestions from the medical staff, a perceived deficiency noted in the laboratory, or a generally accepted pattern of appropriate laboratory practice. General categories to be considered may include specimen collection and transport, patient preparation, test selection, and utilization of results. During the planning stage, it may be useful to create a fishbone chart that explains specific aspects of the process. This may direct attention to specific, problem-prone areas (Fig. 51.3). At this point, establish a proposal containing an analysis of the process and the basis for undertaking the quality improvement procedure.

2. *Get consensus.* Quality improvement requires everyone involved in the process to understand the objectives and have a commitment to improve. Leaders must first "buy in" to the quality improvement process before progress is made (2–5). Physicians, nurses, and other health care workers have a stake in laboratory quality objectives because it has an impact on the quality of their practice. Openness and communication are the key ingredients for developing constructive attitudes toward change and improvement. Everybody must be constantly informed and understand each other's needs and goals. Most importantly, everyone must agree on what is appropriate and endorse the plan. Without interdepartmental support, the plan is unlikely to succeed.

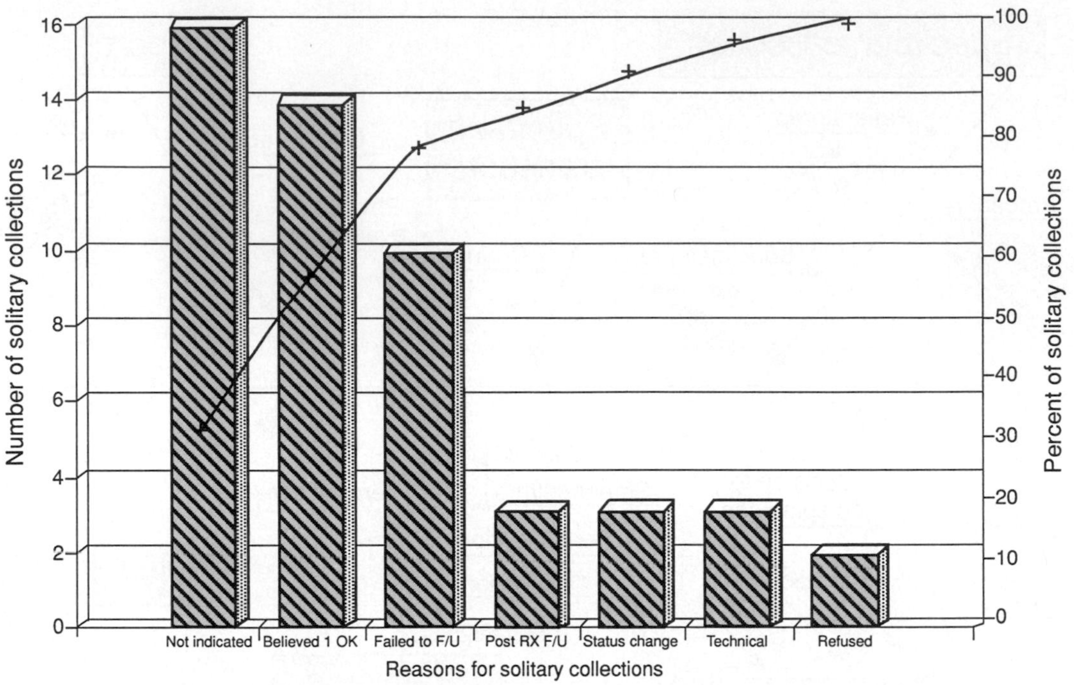

Figure 51.4. Pareto chart of solitary blood cultures. (From Schifman RB, Bachner P. Blood culture utilization (Q-Probes). Northfield, IL: College of American Pathologists, 1990.)

3. *Establish data indicators to monitor improvement.* Select data elements that can help discriminate between a system that is operating appropriately and one that is flawed. Data should be used to describe how the system is operating, and its analysis should be used to suggest adjustments that will lead to sustained improvement. Solicited feedback from people involved with using laboratory services is a data element often overlooked. This serves two purposes. First, it may point out a problem that is more effectively remedied by the user. Furthermore, it can provide additional perspective to help the laboratory understand the origins of possible shortcomings in the system.

The Pareto chart (Fig. 51.4) is a useful format for examining quality assurance data because it is goal oriented. The Pareto chart provides a display on the x axis of specific categories or groupings. It begins with the category having the greatest number of events, followed consecutively by the others in descending order. The absolute amount in each specific group is shown on the left y axis and a cumulative distribution (from 0 to 100%) for each is shown on the right y axis. This type of presentation displays quantitative relationships between groups and helps set priorities for action. Making a change in the most prevalent category is expected to have the greatest impact on overall improvement. Presenting data in this way helps anticipate the most likely sources of difficulty and sets priorities for improvement. During the planning stages, if the expected results can be plotted as a Pareto chart, it is likely that the information will be useful for quality improvement. It becomes easier to implement corrective strategies when the sources of error and their prevalence are known.

4. *Data analysis and system/process modification.* First, it is necessary to know when and how to make modifications. Specifications for meeting quality assurance goals (also referred to as thresholds) are established during the planning stages but often require adjustment as data are collected. In some circumstances the goals are clear. For example, no institution should accept a rate greater than 0% for losing a CSF specimen. However, does this threshold also apply to unlabeled CSF specimens? That is, should there be a procedure for investigating the source of the problem whenever an unlabeled CSF specimen is received (referred to as a sentinel event), or can a certain, low percentage (or threshold) of such events be tolerated?

This concern is where the JCAHO recommendations and industrial quality improvement models differ. The industrial model suggests that the goal should be zero defects with emphasis on prevention. The JCAHO approach, using thresholds, implies that an acceptable number of apparent discrepancies can occur, but when a certain level is noted, corrective action is taken. In practice, both approaches are useful, depending on the circumstances. In some cases a zero-defect approach may be unnecessarily restrictive and wasteful based on the clinical situation. For example, it may be inefficient to track down the

Category: Urine specimens

Objective	*Indicator*	*Standard*	*Threshold*	*Action contact*
Improve test interpretation	Concomitant urinalysis	No. and % with concomitant urinalysis	< 90%	Ward secretaries
Improve specimen collection	Mixed positive culture	Positive cultures: No. and % with mixed results	< 20%	Nursing staff
Improve patient treatment (inpatients)	Positive culture with no therapy one day after report	No. and % with no therapy given one day after positive result	0%	Clinical pharmacist

	Test interpretation	*Specimen collection*	*Patient therapy*
Cum 1989	1521 (94%)	321 (13%)	279 (8%)
Jan	134 (92%)	40 (10%)	36 (9%)
Feb	120 (84%)	34 (12%)	30 (0%)
Mar	166 (98%)	51 (10%)	Not done
Apr	111 (94%)	28 (7%)	26 (0%)
May	133 (95%)	30 (14%)	26 (0%)
June			

Notes

Jan: Pharmacist forgot to review weekend lab reports. One patient became septic, the other two were urinary catheter nosocomial infections that were eventually treated. All on urology service. Physicians on this service were reminded about how to review culture and sensitivity results using computer terminal.

Feb: Ward secretaries reminded to order UA whenever urine culture ordered.

Mar: Improvement in UA's done. Pharmacist on vacation.

Apr: Threshold for specimen collection will be decreased to 15%.

May: Review, no action.

Figure 51.5. Sample QA log sheet.

cause of excessive urine cultures on a single patient if this happens infrequently, particularly when such an incident would be unlikely to result in a detrimental outcome for the patient. On the other hand, setting thresholds too high can lead to a false sense of confidence or conceal potential avenues for quality improvement.

Without standards, how are criteria for quality assurance goals established? They should not be set by the laboratory based on convenience, anticipation of clinical need, or in response to complaints. Those who use laboratory information have the greatest stake in these criteria and should be primarily responsible for establishing specifications based on rational medical requirements, scientific data, and in the future, practicing guidelines (24, 25).

When specific flaws or problem-prone areas in the system are understood, actions either to anticipate and prevent problems or to make corrections that lead to permanent enhancements can be attempted. This is done by working in conjunction with other members of the health care team to adjust the system to facilitate more efficient or appropriate use of laboratory services on the basis of knowledge gained from the data collection and analysis.

5. *Documentation.* Findings and actions should be documented. This can take the form of a log sheet that specifies the indicator, results, criteria for analyzing data (e.g., thresholds), and actions. It must be emphasized again that documentation is not an end in itself. Data should not be collected for documentation purposes only. It should be used to understand how the system works so that appropriate adjustments can be made for improvement. Requiring that the monitor's quality improvement objective be specified helps direct attention toward its purpose. An example of a documentation worksheet is shown in Figure 51.5 with a short list of possible indicators.

6. *Evolution toward an ongoing activity.* It is important to recognize that quality assurance endeavors are continuous. Monitoring, adjusting, and reevaluating the structure, process, and outcome of labora-

Table 51.8. Representative QA Monitors

Procedure	Objective	Indicator	Analysis
Blood culture	Appropriate utilization	Solitary or >3 collections per 24 hr	Determine prevalence and reasons for solitary and excessive blood cultures.
	Adherence to aseptic collection and processing	Contaminated cultures	Percent of contaminants; overall rates and per phlebotomist, ward, etc. Review procedures when high rate identified.
Sputum specimens	Appropriate collections	Specimens with >25 epithelial cells/low power field (smear)	Percent of specimens; overall rates and per specific location. Educational intervention when high rates identified.
	Appropriate utilization	Solitary collections for acid fast bacilli	Percent of specimens; overall rates and per specific location. Determine reasons for solitary collections.
		Repeated cultures on same patient	Reasons for greater than two specimens per week. Pneumonia suspected?
	Accuracy of smear interpretation	Correlation of smear and culture results	Review discrepancies and reasons for misinterpretation of smear results.
Stool specimens	Appropriate utilization	Ova & parasite exams or bacterial cultures ordered after ≥3 hospital days	Percentage of positive results (should be very low or 0). Reasons for requests. Determination of *C. difficile* etiology was considered.
Cerebral spinal fluid specimens	Appropriate collection	Sufficient volume for requested tests	Number with insufficient volume; overall and by service/location. Review procedures and reasons when high rate identified.
		Contaminated cultures	Number of contaminants; overall and by service/location. Review on increasing trend (laboratory or collection deficiency?)
	Appropriate utilization	Orders for syphilis serology, cryptococcal antigen or mycobacterial cultures with otherwise normal findings	Percent of positive results. Reasons for test selection. Development of algorithms for testing.
	Result utilization	Therapeutic response to preliminary gram smear report	Percent of patients treated with antibiotics after positive Gram smear reported. Should be 100% in unambiguous cases.
Urine specimens	Appropriate collection	Number of mixed (≥3 different organisms	Percent of specimens; overall and by location. Determine reasons (delayed transport, collection problem, patient selection, etc).
	Appropriate utilization	Number of urine cultures without concomitant urinalysis (for pyuria determination).	Percent of specimen; overall and by location. Determine reasons why urinalysis was not ordered. Urine culture indicated?
		Repeated cultures on same patient.	Reasons for greater than 2 specimens per week. UTI suspected or confirmed?
Reporting errors	Accuracy of reports	Random review of worksheets with final, charted results.	Review all discrepancies. Reasons for clerical errors, affect on patient outcome.
Susceptibility tests	Utilization of results	Correlation of antimicrobial therapy with susceptibility	Record percent of appropriate and discrepant treatments. Physician should be immediately notified of discrepancies.
	Antibiotic utilization	Calculate cumulative susceptibility rate	Publish data for empiric therapy decisions and review for endemic resistance trends.

tory services is an ongoing activity that should be a routine part of laboratory practice. Experience has shown that improvement often occurs in small increments. Therefore, expectations for rapid progress should not be set too high, nor should efforts abate when accomplishments appear to be meager in relation to goals.

Specific Examples

As a means to illustrate and amplify the previous discussion, specific examples of quality assurance procedures are described in this section. It is impossible to provide an exhaustive list of quality assurance procedures because they must be individualized for the needs and resources of each institution. In general, it is worthwhile to evaluate specimen collection and transport, test selection, and result utilization for each major category of microbiology test, which, because of the nature of testing, can be conveniently stratified by specimen source (Table 51.8). The procedures are developed using the JCAHO 10-step model to illustrate the principles of this ap-

Survey of sputum quality, first quarter 1989

Ward with 4+ EPIs	*Sputum Samples Submitted*	*No. with 4+ EPIs*	%
A	12	2	17
B	29	7	24
C	6	3	50*
D	71	18	25
E	33	4	12
F	9	7	78*
G	11	1	9
Total	171	41	24.6

*These wards may need more intensive instruction on specimen collections or indications for sputum culture.

Figure 51.6. Example of data from sputum quality monitor.

proach. However, this should not be viewed as a standard method for quality assurance procedures. There is no standard.

SPECIMEN COLLECTION AND TRANSPORTATION

Adherence to standard collection and transportation procedures improves specimen quality. It is helpful to structure collection guidelines by anatomic site and pathogen. Indications for obtaining a specimen should be described. Instructions for transporting specimens to the laboratory should specify time limits, transport medium, and type of container. Materials for transporting specimens should be specified by the laboratory.

The most effective approach for getting good specimens is to prevent problems before they happen. It is beneficial to schedule regular meetings with medical and nursing staffs to review procedures and address concerns. Written instructions need to be readily available in all clinical areas, and direct communication with the microbiology laboratory should be encouraged. Monitoring tends to be most effective when data are stratified by specific hospital location. Hospital wards are generally restricted to certain medical specialties with dissimilar needs and problems, and are likely to have the same nursing and support staff who are responsible for collecting specimens. Examples of indicators include transport times and sputum quality. When monitoring is done, it becomes easy to spot wards that show a greater than average specimen transport time or that submit proportionately large numbers of sputum samples with excessive epithelial cells (Fig. 51.6). In these circumstances, more intensive educational activities or other corrective measures are warranted. Likewise, continued monitoring will demonstrate the success or failure of attempts to correct the problem (Fig. 51.7).

TURNAROUND TIME

Laboratory turnaround time is necessarily longer for the microbiology laboratory because of inherent delays required to complete cultures. For example, the median turnaround time for negative urine cultures is 24.6 hours (26). Moderate preanalytic factors that may delay specimen collection for culture for even a few hours are not particularly important, since cultures are typically evaluated once or at most twice per day. However, delays in specimen transport should be prevented to avoid compromising the specimen (e.g., overgrowth of bacteria in urine specimens). Direct monitoring of the period between specimen collection and laboratory arrival can be difficult to do reliably. Indirect measurements such as the number of mixed urine specimens can serve as a coarse indicator. Ideally, commitment to provide a short turnaround time by those who are responsible for collection and transport is the best possible solution. This may be accomplished by involving the laboratory in repeatedly emphasizing the importance of rapid transport for diagnostic reliability. Many rapid methods for reducing the lag associated with identification and sensitivity testing have been evaluated for reliability, although it still remains to be determined if these methods truly affect patient outcome. A more important factor may be the lag between result reporting and physician actions. (See later discussion on Test Utilization.)

Smear examinations and perhaps direct testing for the presence of antigen (e.g., latex agglutination tests on CSF) are the only genuine stat tests in microbiology. A rapid presumptive etiologic diagnosis in life-threatening infections is critical. In this setting, factors that affect preanalytic delays are important to understand to streamline the process (27). Figure 51.2 is a fishbone diagram illustrating the many components of this process. When turnaround time is unacceptable, data presented in this fashion

Section: Microbiology

1. Responsibility: Microbiology Supervisor and Laboratory Director
2. Scope of care: All patients having sputum cultures.
3. Aspects of care: High volume, problem prone.
4. Clinical indicators: Excessive number of epithelial cells on gram smear.
5. Threshold for evaluation: Any month in which total number of sputum samples having 4+ (>25/LPF) epithelial cells exceeds 20% or any ward or outpatient location in which epithelial cells exceed 33% on two successive months, or four times per year.
6. Data collection and evaluation:
   Data source(s): Patient's microbiology report
   Data collection: Computer print out of gram smear results on all sputum cultures.
   Sample: All patients in whom sputum cultures are requested.
   Frequency: Monthly collection and evaluation
   Mode: Concurrent, ongoing
7. Data evaluation: The percentage of specimens having 4+ epithelial cells, stratified by ward or outpatient location.
8. Action: Targeted educational activities are performed at each location showing poor sputum quality based on thresholds for evaluation. Global educational activities are conducted when hospital-wide threshold is exceeded. Solicit feedback from nursing staff and Pulmonary section about how to improve specimen collections.
9. Evaluation of effectiveness and documentation of improvement: The number of occurrences that exceed guidelines serves as an indicator of sputum quality. Document any changes in procedures or recommendations from nursing staff or other departments. Improvement is documented by observing a decline in epithelial cell counts after intervention.
10. Communication of relevant information: Summarized reports, trend analysis, modification of criteria, exceptions, problem identification and problem resolution are discussed at the laboratory's monthly QA meeting and reported to the nursing service QA committee.

Figure 51.7. Sputum quality procedure.

Table 51.9. Mean CSF Turnaround Time (1989 Q-Probe)[a]

	n	Median (min)	Percentile 90%	Percentile 10%
Cell count	451	32	64	15
Glucose	436	34	62	17
Protein	433	37	68	20
Gram's stain	406	45	85	24

[a]From Steindel S. Analytical turn-around time. Northfield, IL: College of American Pathologists, 1989.

can provide a useful tool for brainstorming sessions to evaluate different parts of the problem.

A survey of over 400 clinical laboratories conducted as part of the College of American Pathologists Q-Probe quality assurance program showed that the median turnaround time for processing, examining, and reporting CSF Gram smears was 45 minutes (Table 51.9) (28). The target turnaround time that laboratories established for this procedure was set at less than 60 minutes for 45%, 60 minutes for 47%, and more than 60 minutes for 8%. The Q-Probe survey demonstrated that these goals were met on average 62% of the time, and 15.3% met the goal 100% of the time.

Another important quality assurance goal that is not yet a routine part of laboratory practice is making sure that smear results are properly reported, interpreted, and utilized in serious infections. Although microbiologists are not accustomed to pursuing this objective, a plausible monitor would involve checking for an appropriate clinical response to the report. For example, reporting "pleomorphic Gram-negative rods with numerous inflammatory cells" in a CSF specimen would invoke a procedure to verify that the patient is receiving appropriate therapy. Quality improvement means preventing problems and taking responsibility rather than claiming, "it's somebody else's problem."

Test Utilization

Evaluating the appropriateness of test ordering is an important quality assurance task. Sometimes, distinctive clinical circumstances other than the specimen's characteristics prevail when making this decision. For instance, ova and parasite examinations on inpatients or tests for *Clostridium difficile* toxin in patients not receiving antibiotics are usually non-

Table 51.10. Solitary Blood Culture Q-Probe, 1989[a]

Category	Blood Culture sets	Solitary Blood Cultures (Median)
		%
Outpatient	25,210	25.0
Inpatient	124,033	9.8
Pediatrics	20,636	88.8
Total	169,879	21.5

[a]Schifman RB, Bachner P. Blood culture utilization (Q-Probes). Northfield, IL: College of American Pathologists, 1990.

productive. However, clinical correlations for evaluating test usage usually require information from outside sources (e.g., chart audits). This is a formidable challenge, since monitoring is labor intensive. Also, intervention to modify test usage when standards are not met requires multidepartmental cooperation, is difficult to implement, and its effectiveness is transient without continuous effort.

Microbiology testing is done primarily for diagnosis, as opposed to its purpose in other laboratory sections, where testing is done primarily for monitoring. This makes it easier to assess the appropriateness of test usage because outcome directly relates to the timeliness and accuracy of diagnosis. An interesting consequence of this is that test underutilization is often identified. For example, although it is well established that two or more separate blood culture specimens per febrile episode are needed to achieve maximum sensitivity and to interpret results properly, approximately 25% of blood cultures collected nationwide are solitary (Table 51.10 and Fig. 51.4) (29). This may have serious consequences if the diagnosis of bloodstream infection is missed.

Information about the percentage of solitary blood cultures is easy to collect from laboratory accession logs. However, this in itself does not fulfill quality improvement objectives since the data do not reveal *why* solitary blood cultures are obtained. To improve blood culture practice, information about the proportion of solitary blood culture procedures is useless unless there is some understanding about why this occurs. A solitary blood culture is a sentinel event that triggers an attempt to obtain physician feedback about the apparent problem (Figs. 51.8 and 51.9). Modifications in the specimen collection process can more readily be made when specific reasons for correctable solitary collections are known. Procedures to resolve this problem include sending reminders to physicians or giving instructions to a phlebotomy team to collect multiple specimens when a blood culture is ordered (30).

Other examples of underutilization include failing to obtain sufficient sputum samples when tuberculosis is suspected (31), ordering blood cultures in cases of suspected pneumonia, or obtaining urine cultures in patients with nosocomial urinary tract infections (32). Excessive culturing can also be a problem (33, 34). Most laboratories are not aware of these utilization problems because they are not monitored, and even when problems are detected, solutions are difficult to achieve.

When considering the value of assessing test utilization, the first response that may come to mind is cost containment. Since testing is, to a certain extent, discretionary and accounts for nearly a quarter of all health care expenditures, it is an obvious target for cost reduction (35). Improper test utilization is often equated with excessive testing. The corollary to this presumption is that health care costs will decline in proportion to the volume of testing that is reduced (36). However, this notion overlooks the substantial indirect costs of clinical laboratory operations. For example, it has been shown that a 10% reduction in utilization would reduce true costs by less than 2%, while a massive 50% reduction would save no more than 20% of costs (37). As shown by the solitary blood culture example, it is sometimes necessary to do *more* tests to improve test utilization. Additionally, test costs rather than number of tests done is the most important determinant of laboratory expense (33). In some cases, however, inappropriate testing adds to potential costs when associated with unwarranted clinical assessment of false-positive results (38). What other benefits might be gained by improving test utilization? The most important goal should be to optimize the contribution that laboratory services make toward patient care while avoiding harmful effects. This is done by striving to assure that testing is purposeful and efficient.

Although there is substantial information in the literature dealing with test utilization, it should be noted that nearly all of this work has been conducted at teaching institutions where the housestaff are primarily responsible for ordering tests. This naturally biases the literature's view of test utilization toward physicians in training, making conclusions and recommendations difficult to extrapolate to other localities. Physicians in training are naturally expected to have less knowledge and experience with using laboratory tests, but this probably does not represent what happens in various other health care settings.

Improvement in test utilization is typically measured by the degree to which the volume of testing is reduced; i.e., the best utilization is less utilization. However, an association between reduced testing and clinical outcome has never been demonstrated. Until there is more evidence, one might just as convincingly argue that it is better to test a little too much than risk missing an important clinical finding

Section: Microbiology

1. Responsibility: Laboratory Director, Microbiology supervisor, patient's attending physician
2. Scope of care: All patients for whom a blood culture is performed.
3. Aspects of care: Critical and problem prone test.
4. Clinical indicators: It is standard practice to obtain at least two separate blood cultures, at different times to achieve acceptable sensitivity and to properly interpret results. (Aronson MD, Bor DH. Blood cultures. Ann Intern Med 1987;106:246–253). A solitary blood culture may signify an improper procedure.
5. Threshold for evaluation: Solitary blood culture—defined as one collection per 24 hours.
6. Data collection and evaluation:
   Data source(s): Blood culture log.
   Data collection: Computer printout.
   Sample: All patients having a blood culture.
   Frequency: Weekly
   Mode: Concurrent, ongoing
7. Data evaluation: Log is reviewed by Clinical Pathologist for solitary blood cultures. These are flagged for necessary action. Solitary blood cultures as percent of total blood cultures are calculated.
8. Action: Laboratory Director sends memorandum to Attending physician for review and response.
9. Evaluation of effectiveness and documentation of improvement: Flagged cases and responses are recorded and stratified by Attending physician and Service. Use data to monitor trends, identify source of problem and educate physicians. Document all procedure/policy changes that may impact improvement in blood culture collections.
10. Communication of relevant information: Percent solitary blood cultures, responses, trend analysis, modification of criteria, exceptions, problem identification and problem resolution are presented in Service minutes and at Laboratory Utilization Review Subcommittee.

Figure 51.8. Blood culture utilization procedure.

(39). The best approach is to order just the right number of tests, but nobody knows what that is.

Many hospital pharmacies restrict certain medications to specific indications or require special approval to limit the use of agents that may be expensive, toxic, or of limited benefit. Laboratories can use the same approach. Certain tests that are costly or have limited value may be restricted by requiring consultation or justification (40, 41). For example, a recent report suggests restricting routine stool specimens for bacterial culture and parasite examinations to outpatients or within 3 days of hospitalization, since the positive yield in other hospitalized patients is exceedingly small (42). Stool examination for *C. difficile* may likewise be restricted only to patients who have received antibiotics within a certain period of time. However, some restriction policies, such as requiring justification for each test or limiting the number of tests ordered per day, are perhaps only applicable for teaching institutions (40). Several studies have made the interesting observation that simply displaying the costs of tests while ordering, or providing daily feedback of inpatient charges, significantly reduces the number of tests ordered (43, 44).

Although restriction policies and financial incentives may help cut down unnecessary testing (and workload), they probably provide little direct benefit to the patient. On the other hand, methods to ensure that appropriate tests are ordered when indicated (as opposed to preventing inappropriate tests from being ordered when they are not indicated) as well as proper use of test results are factors that will more likely improve "quality and appropriateness of services provided." Additionally, if corrective action can be concurrently linked to the monitoring and evaluation process, the patient receives the benefit immediately.

Perhaps one of the most potentially rewarding techniques for evaluating test utilization involves using another test, test result, or other readily available piece of information. The impact on patient care can be substantial if insufficient testing or misapplication of a result can be identified and corrected. For example, because of the importance of pyuria in interpreting the results of urine culture, a urinalysis should probably be done at the same time (Fig. 51.5). How many urine cultures done at your institution are not accompanied by a urinalysis?

RE: Solitary blood culture

TO: Dr.

A solitary blood culture was ordered on the patient listed below. It is generally considered appropriate practice to collect at least two separate blood cultures per febrile or septic episode, to achieve acceptable sensitivity and to properly interpret results. As part of our quality assurance program this matter is brought to your attention. I would be grateful for your assessment and response. Thank you.

Patient: ______________________________

Specimen collection date: __________

RESPONSE:

The blood culture was indicated, but a solitary blood culture was obtained because:

[ ] I believed that one was sufficient.
[ ] Technical or procedural problem prevented a second collection.
[ ] There was a change in the patient's clinical status, changing the indication.
[ ] The diagnostic plan was to collect another culture, but was not carried through.
[ ] Patient refused another phlebotomy, or left before another could be performed.
[ ] Incorrect collection procedure (i.e. two tubes collected, or bottle filled simultaneously, rather than by separate venipuncture).
[ ] Multiple blood cultures obtained in the past—solitary blood culture performed as follow up procedure to monitor patient's response to therapy.
[ ] Other reason (please specify).
[ ] Blood culture was not indicated

Laboratory Director

Figure 51.9. Solitary blood culture memorandum.

Consider the patient who is admitted to the hospital with suspected pyelonephritis. The following day, *E. coli* is isolated from the patient's blood and urine, and by that evening, susceptibility results are available. Ask any laboratory worker what the quality assurance goals are in this case, and the likely reply will focus on specimen collection, media performance, incubator temperatures, and reliability of the susceptibility method. An astute observer also might comment on the merits of completing the test in less than 24 hours. Do these components fulfill quality improvement goals?

Unfortunately, when a result is produced, its clinical significance is rarely appreciated because information about the patient's therapy and clinical condition is unavailable. Nevertheless, the microbiology laboratory is often the earliest source of critical diagnostic information. What if the susceptibility test results indicate that therapy is inadequate for the case described above? It is likely that there would be a significant delay in adjusting therapy. Although all the necessary information is available to the "system," the patient does not benefit because the data are not integrated in a timely and effective fashion.

Since the turnaround time for culture and susceptibility testing is long, antimicrobial therapy is given empirically until laboratory results either support the therapeutic decision or suggest alternative antibiotic choices. Assuming that culture and susceptibility results are a valid guide to therapeutic response, any further lag in applying this information can compromise use of these tests in several ways. First, an extended lapse between the time a test is reported and when it is evaluated by a physician can have serious consequences if it delays recognition of a serious infection or delays treatment modification. In addition, physicians are reluctant to change therapy when a patient shows improvement, even when test results indicate that less costly or less toxic agents could be used. This becomes even more likely as the time between specimen collection and evaluation of results by the physician lengthens. One study demonstrated that the mean interval between reporting a final culture result and action on the result could be reduced from 26 hours to 2.4 hours when a data monitoring and feedback system was implemented by a pharmacist (45). In another study, rapid reporting to physicians of blood culture susceptibility results by an infectious disease specialist with knowledge of the patient's antibiotic therapy significantly improved antibiotic utilization (46). These results and other studies (47) indicate that antibiotic usage can be substantially improved when pharmacy data are available at the time microbiology tests are completed,

and/or discharge diagnoses to determine which charts merit further review.

The clinical microbiology laboratory provides important culture and antibiotic susceptibility data for this surveillance effort. Review of microbiology reports may be the single most common case-finding method employed routinely for nosocomial infection surveillance. Wenzel et al. (15) and Gross et al. (16) have found that daily review of positive culture reports was nearly as effective as a ward-based, comprehensive surveillance for identifying nosocomial infections. Laboratory-based surveillance allows large amounts of data to be easily collected and reviewed, facilitating early recognition and investigation of outbreaks or clusters of nosocomial infections. This process may be enhanced by the use of the hospital computer system to collect and process data from many sources, including the microbiology laboratory, pharmacy, and radiology. The value of computer-assisted surveillance was documented by Schifman and Palmer (17), who used computer analysis of culture and antibiotic susceptibility data, coupled with epidemiologic investigation, to detect 19 clusters of cross-infection in a 6-month period of time.

It should be emphasized that microbiology reports alone may not provide enough information to identify all infections or all outbreaks. Both the frequency of culturing and the manner in which the cultures are obtained and transported to the laboratory strongly influence the sensitivity and specificity of laboratory-based surveillance. Thus, a combined approach employing initial screens such as data from the microbiology laboratory and nursing Kardex may provide optimal surveillance. The use of this approach has been validated at the University of Iowa and shown to have a sensitivity of 81% and a specificity of 98% for detection of nosocomial infections (18).

Continuing Education

An important component of a successful infection control program is communication. Thus, it is essential for infection control personnel, most of whom have little or no laboratory background, to have a working knowledge of clinical microbiology. Likewise, it is important for the microbiologist to learn the fundamental concepts of the epidemiologist. The continuing education and improved communication between these two groups can be accomplished by regular laboratory rounds to review culture results, ask questions, and discuss current problems and issues relevant to infection control activities. In addition, weekly conferences to discuss ongoing infection control issues and epidemiologic principles are also useful. Inclusion of the infectious disease consult service and other interested clinicians in these activities will also enhance communication and provide additional clinical insight into such discussions.

ROLE OF THE CLINICAL MICROBIOLOGY LABORATORY IN INFECTION CONTROL

In addition to the broad, committee-related activities described above, the clinical microbiology laboratory provides certain laboratory services and expertise, frequently beyond routine laboratory practice, that are essential to the detection and investigation of nosocomial infection. In short, investigation of a potential epidemic of nosocomial infection is impossible without prompt, accurate, and reproducible microbiological support. The areas of concern that will be discussed include the accurate identification of nosocomial pathogens, timely reporting of laboratory data, specialized studies for outbreak investigation, and appropriate culture of hospital personnel and environment.

Accurate Identification of Nosocomial

The results of routine culture and identification procedures performed in the clinical microbiology laboratory are usually the first indication of a nosocomial infection and thus are as important to the infection control practitioner as they are to the clinician caring for the patient. The standard procedures employed routinely in the laboratory are usually sufficient; however, the clinical microbiology laboratory must realize that culture results suggestive of colonization as well as infection may be important to infection control personnel.

The adequacy and quality of a specimen sent for microbiological examination are important for infection control as well as for diagnostic purposes. All specimens should be examined upon receipt in the laboratory, and those that are inappropriate (e.g., swab of an abscess for anaerobes) or in which problems (lack of adequate transport media, leakage of specimen container) or delays (> 1hr for most specimens) in transport have occurred should not be processed further. Whenever possible, specimens should be examined microscopically not only to provide rapid diagnostic information but also to ensure that the specimen is of sufficient quality to merit processing further. For example, the application of rapid, nonculture methods for detection of pathogens such as respiratory syncytial virus (RSV), *Legionella pneumophila*, or rotavirus may be extremely useful for clinical and epidemiologic purposes, but only if the specimen is adequate. Thus, the lack of cellular material in a nasopharyngeal wash specimen submitted for detection of RSV antigen indicates inadequate specimen collection and a high probability of a false-negative test result in an infected patient. Likewise, microscopic examination of Gram stain of sputum specimens remains an excellent means of determining whether or not these specimens are contaminated by oropharyngeal secretions (19). Rigorous monitoring of specimen handling and enforcement of strict criteria for acceptance of clinical specimens will ensure specimen quality and provide accurate microbiological data to both clinician and epidemiologist.

Perhaps the most useful and widely available rapid diagnostic test is the microscopic examination of Gram-stained material. The importance of the Gram stain in the detection of nosocomial pathogens cannot be overemphasized. This procedure provides information rapidly and may detect and identify organisms of epidemiologic importance that may not be apparent on culture. Thus, the microbiology laboratory should make sure that infection control personnel are aware of the results of the Gram stain, as well as culture, of epidemiologically important specimens.

In recent years, several additional, rapid, culture-independent diagnostic tests have been made available for the detection of infectious agents of nosocomial importance. For example, the application of immunological or DNA probe-based assays allows the diagnosis of infections due to RSV, *Legionella* species, and rotavirus to be made within 1 to 2 hours of specimen collection (20–22). The speed and accuracy of these detection methods allow infection control personnel to identify infected patients rapidly and to adopt appropriate measures to control and prevent the spread of these agents to susceptible patients and hospital personnel. Although inappropriate application of these newer diagnostic tests may create problems, such as pseudoepidemics of *Legionella* infections (23), the overall effect should be to enhance the effectiveness of diagnostic methods and infection control efforts.

Although many nosocomial infections continue to be caused by easily detected and identified bacterial pathogens such as the Enterobacteriaceae, *P. aeruginosa*, and *S. aureus*, the spectrum of nosocomial pathogens is expanding as advances in medical care result in increased survival of severely ill and immunocompromised patients. In the past decade, we have seen an increase in nosocomial infections due to agents thought of as "normal flora," such as coagulase-negative staphylococci, *Candida* species, and *Enterococcus* species as well as an increasing array of unusual or fastidious bacterial (*Pseudomonas* species, *Xanthomonas maltophilia*, *Legionella* species, *Acinetobacter* species), fungal (*Aspergillus* species, *Fusarium* species, demateaceous fungi), viral (RSV, rotavirus, cytomegalovirus), and parasitic (*Pneumocystis carinii*, *Cryptosporidium*) pathogens. This ever expanding spectrum of nosocomial pathogens requires that the clinical microbiology laboratory continually update its approach to nosocomial infections, including knowledge of the important pathogens as well as appropriate methods for detection, identification, and antimicrobial susceptibility testing.

Most laboratories have the capability of identifying microorganisms to species level and performing antimicrobial susceptibility testing. The use of one or more of the commercially available biochemical test panels, such as those manufactured by API (Analytab, Plainview, NY), Vitek (Vitek Systems, Hazelwood, MO), or MicroScan (Baxter MicroScan, West Sacramento, CA), provide a reasonably accurate means of identifying both common and uncommon organisms to species level. This level of identification is essential for the epidemiologist to detect potential nosocomial transmission of a given organism. The failure of a laboratory to identify major nosocomial pathogens such as coagulase-negative staphylococci, *Candida* spp., or *Pseudomonas* spp. to species level may obscure real problems and make retrospective epidemiologic investigation impossible. Similarly, the performance of careful, standardized antimicrobial susceptibility testing is of major importance in nosocomial infection surveillance. The identification of specific antimicrobial resistance patterns may be invaluable in tracing the spread of particular nosocomial pathogens. The laboratory must ensure that the susceptibility testing methods employed are adequate to detect resistance of nosocomial pathogens to certain antimicrobial agents. For example, it is now well established that certain test methods fail to detect methicillin-resistant *S. aureus* (MRSA) (24). Given the importance of MRSA as a nosocomial pathogen, it is imperative that laboratories be aware of these limitations in susceptibility testing and employ methods that have been proven reliable in detecting MRSA.

In addition to routine identification and susceptibility testing, the microbiology laboratory must also maintain flexibility in order to adapt to newer techniques and the emergence of specific nosocomial pathogens. For example, the availability of rapid, culture-independent methods of detection of viral and bacterial pathogens may be critical to the detection and control of infection due to pathogens such as RSV and *Legionella* spp. Likewise, the emergence of high-level resistance to aminoglycosides among *Enterococcus* spp. may require that the laboratory provide screening of clinical isolates of enterococci for high-level resistance to gentamicin and streptomycin (25). Quantitative or semiquantitative cultures of intravascular catheters (26) or bronchoalveolar lavage fluid (27), although more labor intensive, may be essential for the accurate diagnosis of catheter-related infection or nosocomial pneumonia. Thus, the laboratory must constantly consider whether techniques in addition to those employed for routine detection and identification can aid infection control goals.

Reporting of Laboratory Data

The results of cultures and antimicrobial susceptibility testing generated routinely by the clinical microbiology laboratory are an extremely important source of data for nosocomial infection surveillance. These results are usually reviewed by infection control personnel on a daily basis. Direct communication between laboratory and infection control personnel during laboratory rounds is highly desirable and effective and may serve to clarify issues of colonization versus infection and to focus laboratory efforts to support the goals of infection control optimally.

Reports of certain culture results may warrant a phone call from the laboratory to infection control personnel in order to ensure that control measures are implemented as soon as possible. Examples include positive blood and normally sterile body fluid cultures, smears and cultures positive for acid-fast bacilli, isolation of enteric pathogens such as *Shigella* or *Salmonella*, and isolation of multiply antibiotic-resistant organisms such as MRSA. In addition, detection of new or unusual pathogens (*Legionella* spp., vancomycin-resistant Gram-positive organisms) should be related promptly to infection control personnel. The rapid reporting of nosocomial pathogens is essential for designing and implementing effective control measures. The availability of some of the newer rapid methods for detection and characterization of microorganisms may greatly facilitate this process. In many cases, the early reporting of preliminary data is preferable to a delayed "final report" in dealing effectively with nosocomial infection problems.

The microbiology laboratory results should be readily accessible to both laboratory personnel and clinical and infection control workers. In many cases, the results are stored on a computer, thus facilitating data retrieval and analysis. In the absence of computer storage, laboratory data may be maintained in bound log books organized by date, specimen type, and organism identification. Laboratory records should include the microbiology work cards and should be kept on file for at least 2 years. The information stored should include specimen type, date of collection, patient identification, hospital number, hospital service, wards, and organisms identified, including antimicrobial susceptibility patterns and the results of any specialized identification or typing procedures. This information should also include the dates and other details of technical and/or taxonomic changes that may affect the results and reporting of microbiological data. Such information supplies infection control personnel with a baseline, which is essential in the analysis of trends or patterns of infection.

Both clinicians and infection control workers may benefit greatly from periodic summaries of selected microbiology results. It may be very useful to tabulate the frequency of isolation of particular nosocomial pathogens by anatomical site and hospital service. Likewise, tables summarizing the antimicrobial susceptibility profiles of the most commonly isolated nosocomial pathogens and selected fastidious or slow-growing (difficult to test) isolates by anatomical site are very useful in guiding empirical therapy and in following general trends in antibiotic resistance within the hospital (28). Care should be taken to exclude repeat cultures of the same organism from the same patient in order to avoid introducing biases to the data. Inclusion of antibiotic cost information may also be appropriate to aid in the reduction of the expenses of antimicrobial therapy.

Specialized Studies for Outbreak Investigation

The detection of a cluster or outbreak of nosocomial infections requires prompt, efficient action by the infection control team in order to define the extent of the outbreak and to design and implement effective control measures. The clinical microbiology laboratory, as an important component of the infection control team, may be called upon to provide rapid, intensive laboratory support throughout the epidemic period. The demands placed upon the laboratory may be great and may require communication and advance preparation in order to deal effectively with an outbreak situation. Advance preparation may be based on the types of outbreaks that have occurred most frequently in the past in a given hospital. Communication between laboratory and infection control personnel facilitates such planning and allows the laboratory to anticipate the need for personnel, materials, and space required for a "typical"

Table 52.1. Culture of Potential Sources of Cross-Infection in Nosocomial Infection Outbreak[a]

Source	Culture Method	Comment
Blood products	Broth culture incubated aerobically and anaerobically at 30 to 32°C for 10 days	Following transfusion reaction; obtain simultaneous blood culture by venipuncture
Parenteral fluids and IV devices	Broth or membrane filter method	Culture needle, catheter, administration set, fluid, closure. Obtain blood culture.
Environmental surfaces	Swab-rinse or impression plate	No evidence that any particular level of contamination correlates with nosocomial infection.
Tubes and containers	Broth-rinse or swab-rinse with semiquantitative plating	At least two colonies of each morphological type should be picked for identification.
Disinfectants and antiseptics	Plating of serial dilutions of the product with and without specific neutralizers	Organisms usually nonfermenting, gram-negative, aerobic bacilli.
Respiratory therapy equipment	Broth-rinse or swab-rinse	Only in situations of high endemic or epidemic levels of nosocomial respiratory infection.
Air	Mechanical air sampler (preferred). Settling plates (poor)	No uniform agreement on acceptable levels of contamination. Lack of correlation with infection.
Water and ice	Membrane filter	Poor correlation of culture findings with illness.
Personnel hands	Broth-bag: 10 to 20 ml nutrient broth in sterile plastic bag. Wash hands in broth and plate semiquantitatively.	May confirm the mechanism of cross-infection. Impress the importance of handwashing.

[a] Cultures to be performed only if clearly indicated by available epidemiologic data.

outbreak situation. The extra costs associated with outbreak investigation should also be anticipated by the hospital's administration, and they should not be borne by the laboratory or charged to the individual patients involved in the outbreak. These are all important issues that should be clarified by the infection control committee or appropriate governing body prior to a crisis situation.

The investigation of an outbreak of nosocomial infection may require the performance of large numbers of cultures of specimens obtained from patients, hospital personnel, and the environment. Whenever possible, selective or differential media, or both, should be employed in order to reduce the workload in the laboratory and to expedite the processing of specimens. Likewise, enrichment cultures, alone or in combination with selective media, may be necessary to optimize conditions for detection of specific nosocomial pathogens, such as methicillin-resistant staphylococci, that are present in low numbers (29). Given the resources (personnel and materials) required to process these cultures and identify the organisms isolated, it is imperative that the cultures specifically address epidemiologic findings.

Depending upon the epidemiologic data available and the nosocomial pathogen(s) of interest, the infection control and laboratory workers may also need to employ specialized methods for sampling and culturing potential vehicles of cross-infection (Table 52.1). The details of these methods are beyond the scope of this chapter and have been summarized extensively in review articles and reference texts (30–32).

Epidemiologists frequently rely upon the laboratory for identification and typing of nosocomial pathogens and for providing evidence for the biological and genetic relatedness of these organisms as an aid in the epidemiologic investigation. As mentioned previously, the species identification and antimicrobial susceptibility pattern (antibiogram) are often sufficient to confirm the epidemiologic relationship between different isolates; however, there is an increasing need for more detailed subspecies delineation or typing of nosocomial pathogens. The rationale for such strain delineation is that repeated isolation of an organism with identical markers from one or more patients suggests that the organism may have originated from a single clone and therefore is more likely to represent infection (individual patient) or transmission from patient-to-patient from a common source or by a common mechanism. When a species of bacteria or fungi that appears to be the cause of infection is a frequent member of the normal flora or environment, simple species identification is no longer useful in distinguishing between infection and colonization or in tracing the source of the infecting organism. The ubiquitous nature of many important nosocomial pathogens such as *Staphylococcus epidermidis*, *S. aureus*, *Candida albicans*, *Enterococcus faecalis*, and *Pseudomonas aeruginosa* has necessitated the development of additional methods of strain delineation within species for use as epidemiologic tools.

The intelligent, cost-effective application of epidemiologic typing methods requires that typing only be performed with well-defined epidemiologic objectives in mind. Most commonly, these objectives include: (*a*) determination of the extent of an outbreak; (*b*) determination of the mode of transmission of nosocomial infections; (*c*) evaluation of the efficacy of preventative measures; and (*d*) monitoring of infection in special areas, such as intensive care units, where cross-infection is a particular hazard. Each of these objectives places different demands on a typing system and may not be fulfilled by one typing method.

The ideal typing system should be standardized, reproducible, stable, sensitive, broadly applicable, readily available, inexpensive, and of proven value based on epidemiologic investigation (33, 34). A review of the currently available typing methods indicates that no single method is ideal and that many epidemiologic investigations may require more than one typing method for optimal strain delineation (30, 33, 34). Regardless of the methods employed, the indiscriminate application of typing methods without sound epidemiologic backing is wasteful and may provide conflicting and confusing information.

Several different epidemiologic typing methods have been applied in studies of nosocomial pathogens (Tables 52.2 and 52.3). These include various traditional nonmolecular methods such as antimicrobial susceptibility profiles (antibiogram), biochemical profiles (biotype), serological typing, bacteriocin typing, and bacteriophage susceptibility patterns (phage typing). In recent years, molecular typing methods such as plasmid pattern analysis, restriction endonuclease analysis of plasmid and genomic DNA, Southern hybridization analysis, immunoblot fingerprinting, outer membrane protein profiling, and multilocus enzyme electrophoresis (isoenzyme analysis) have been used to type nosocomial pathogens (30, 31, 33–35). Each of these typing methods has advantages and disadvantages when applied to a specific situation. In addition to the ability to define strains within species, of major importance to the clinical laboratory is the ease of performance and interpretation of the test and the availability of reagents. The usefulness of the typing systems may vary with the specific nosocomial pathogen of interest (Table 52.3); however, all of these typing systems have been helpful in understanding the epidemiology of nosocomial infections. Although many hospital laboratories may not have the facilities necessary to perform specialized typing procedures, they should be aware of those organisms that can and cannot be typed and be willing to assist the epidemiologist in identifying centers where such typing can be performed, if indicated, during the course of an epidemiologic investigation. A more detailed discussion of the advantages, disadvantages, and availability of the various typing methods listed in Table 52.2 may be found in several recent reviews (30, 31, 33–35).

Table 52.2. Traditional (Nonmolecular) and Molecular Methods for Epidemiologic Typing of Nosocomial Pathogens

Traditional Typing Methods	Molecular Typing Methods
Antimicrobial susceptibility profile (antibiogram, resistotype)	Immunoblot fingerprinting
Bacteriocin production or susceptibility (bacteriocin type)	Multilocus enzyme electrophoresis
	Outer membrane protein profiling
Bacteriophage susceptibility (phage type)	Plasmid pattern analysis
Biochemical profile (biotype)	Pulsed-field electrophoresis (electrophoretic karyotype)
Colony morphology (morphotype) Dienes reaction	Restriction endonuclease analysis of plasmid and genomic DNA
Serological typing (serotype)	Southern hybridization analysis (DNA probe)

Regardless of the typing system employed, one basic principle to remember is that a valid comparison between two or more isolates is difficult to make unless all isolates are tested under identical conditions. This usually means performance of the test by the same person, on the same day, using the same lot of reagents. In addition, it is not sufficient to show that isolates from a nosocomial outbreak have identical epidemiologic markers. In order to make valid conclusions concerning the epidemic strain, it must be shown that control isolates from epidemiologically unrelated patients and environmental sources (where appropriate) are different from the outbreak strain (34, 35). Judicious application of the available typing methods in concert with careful epidemiologic investigation will provide insight into important epidemiologic questions such as the site of origin (reservoir) of organisms causing nosocomial infections and the frequency and mechanism of nosocomial transmission of hospital pathogens.

Although supplemental testing may be valuable in clarifying the epidemiologic relationships among nosocomial pathogens, it is impossible to accomplish unless the appropriate isolates have been saved in the laboratory. The laboratory, in cooperation with infection control personnel, should identify and save epidemiologically important isolates. The number and type of isolates to be saved and the duration of

Table 52.3. Epidemiologic Typing Methods for the Eight Most Frequently Reported Nosocomial Bloodstream Isolates in the United States[a]

Pathogen	Typing Method
Coagulase-negative staphylococci	Plasmid and restriction endonuclease analysis, biotype, antibiogram, phage type
Staphylococcus aureus	Plasmid and restriction endonuclease analysis, multilocus enzyme electrophoresis, phage typing, immunoblot fingerprinting, antibiogram, biotype, serotype, bacteriocin type
Enterococci	Plasmid and restriction endonuclease analysis, antibiogram, biotype
Candida species	Restriction endonuclease analysis, electrophoretic karyotype, multilocus enzyme electrophoresis, immunoblot fingerprint, biotype, killer toxin type, serotype
Escherichia coli	Plasmid and restriction endonuclease analysis, antibiogram, serotype, biotype, phage type, bacteriocin type, multilocus enzyme electrophoresis
Enterobacter species	Plasmid and restriction endonuclease analysis, antibiogram, biotype, bacteriocin type, phage type, multilocus enzyme electrophoresis, serotype
Pseudomonas aeruginosa	Restriction endonuclease analysis, serotype, bacteriocin type, antibiogram, biotype, phage type, plasmid analysis
Klebsiella pneumoniae	Plasmid and restriction endonuclease analysis, antibiogram, serotype, biotype, phage type, bacteriocin type, multilocus enzyme electrophoresis

[a]Data Horan T, Culver D, Jarvis W, et al. Pathogens causing nosocomial infections: preliminary data from the National Nosocomial Infections Surveillance System. Antimicrob Newsletter 1988;5:65–67.

storage will vary from hospital to hospital depending on the space and resources available. One approach might be to save, at least temporarily, all isolates from blood and other normally sterile body fluids, multiply antibiotic-resistant Gram-negative bacilli, and methicillin-resistant strains of *S. aureus* (36). The isolates may be stored for several months on agar slants or on a more permanent basis by freezing (−70°C) or lyophilization. Regardless of the laboratory policy on saving organisms, a system for reviewing and periodically discarding stored isolates should also be established.

Cultures of Hospital Personnel and Environment

Cultures of hospital personnel should be performed rarely and only when epidemiologic evidence suggests that an individual may be involved in the transmission of a nosocomial pathogen. The anatomical site to be cultured depends on the pathogen's reservoir and the suspected mode of transmission. Because the hands of hospital personnel may be important vehicles in the transfer of nosocomial pathogens from patient-to-patient, hand cultures may be useful in confirming the mechanism of cross-infection as part of an outbreak investigation. In addition, hand cultures of hospital personnel may serve as an important educational exercise to underscore the importance of handwashing in preventing nosocomial infection (36). A sensitive method of culturing hands to detect transient or resident flora is the broth-bag technique (Table 52.1). With this technique, the subject vigorously washes his or her hands in 10 to 20 ml of nutrient broth that has been supplemented with Tween 80, sodium thiosulfate, and/or lecithin in order to neutralize any residual antiseptics (37). An aliquot of the broth is then plated onto selective and nonselective media and observed for growth of the pathogen of interest.

As a general rule, routine cultures of hospital personnel and the environment should not be performed. Nevertheless, routine monitoring of sterilization, infant formula and other hospital-prepared products, blood components prepared in an "open" system, dialysis fluid, and disinfected equipment may still be indicated (30, 38). Sampling activities that have been specifically singled out as unnecessary due to high cost and lack of clinical or epidemiologic benefit include routine culturing of patients or hospital personnel, routine sampling of commercial patient-care items, in-use testing of antiseptics and disinfectants, random culturing of blood units to ensure sterility, routine culturing of respiratory therapy equipment, routine culture of peritoneal dialysate, and routine culture of air (30, 38). Routine cultures of the environment and hospital personnel are a burden to the laboratory and seldom, if ever, provide useful information or lead to specific interventions. In the rare instances when such cultures are performed, they should be done in association with patient illnesses, with appropriate epidemiologic indications, or as part of an educational program.

CONCLUSION

The clinical microbiology laboratory is an essential component of the hospital infection control program. The continual evolution of the spectrum of nosocomial pathogens and the rapid development and application of new technologies in the diagnostic laboratory require ongoing cooperation and collaboration between the laboratory and infection control personnel. A good working relationship between the clinical microbiologist and hospital epidemiologist has a positive influence on both laboratory and infection control operations and facilitates the investigation and control of nosocomial infection problems.

References

1. Horan T, Culver D, Jarvis W, et al. Pathogens causing nosocomial infections: preliminary data from the National Nosocomial Infections Surveillance System. Antimicrob Newsletter 1988;5:65–67.
2. Pfaller MA, Herwaldt LA. Laboratory, clinical and epidemiologic aspects of coagulase-negative staphylococci. Clin Microbiol Rev 1988;1:281–291.
3. Martin MA, Pfaller MA, Wenzel RP. Mortality and hospital stay attributable to coagulase-negative staphylococcal bacteremia. Ann Intern Med 1989;110:9–16.
4. Wey SB, Mori M, Pfaller MA, Woolson RF, Wenzel RP. Hospital acquired candidemia: attributable mortality and excess length of stay. Arch Intern Med 1988;148:2642–2645.
5. Pfaller MA. Opportunistic fungal infections: the increasing importance of *Candida* species. Infect Control Hosp Epidemiol 1989;10:270–273.
6. Spengler RF, Greenough WE III. Hospital costs and mortality attributed to nosocomial bacteremias. J Am Med Assoc 1987;240:2455–2458.
7. Gross PA, Neu HC, Aswapokee P, Van Antwerpen C, Aswapokee N. Deaths from nosocomial infections: experience in a university hospital and a community hospital. Am J Med 1980;68:219–223.
8. Wenzel RP. The mortality of hospital-acquired bloodstream infections: need for a new vital statistic? Internatl J Epidemiol 1988;17:225–227.
9. Hughes JM, Jarvis WR. Epidemiology of nosocomial infections. In: Lennette EH, Balows A, Hausler WJ Jr, Shadomy HJ, eds. Manual of clinical microbiology. 4th ed. Washington, DC: American Society for Microbiology, 1985:99–104.
10. Bross J, Talbot GH, Maislin G, Hurwitz S, Strom BL. Risk factors for nosocomial candidemia: a case-control study in adults without leukemia. Am J Med 1989;87:614–620.
11. Wakefield DS, Helms CM, Massanari RM, Mori M, Pfaller M. The cost of nosocomial infection: relative contributions of laboratory, antibiotic, and per diem costs in serious *S. aureus* infections. Am J Infect Cont 1988;16:185–192.
12. Haley RW, Culver DH, White JW, et al. The efficacy of infection control surveillance and control programs in preventing nosocomial infections in U.S. hospitals. Am J Epidemiol 1985;121:182–205.
13. Cruse PJE. Surgical wound sepsis. Cand Med Assoc J 1970;102:251–258.
14. Emori TG, Haley RW, Garner JS. Technique and use of nosocomial infection surveillance in U.S. hospitals. Am J Med 1981;70:933–940.
15. Wenzel RP, Osterman CA, Hunting KJ, Gwaltney JM Jr. Hospital-acquired infections. I. Surveillance in a university hospital. Am J Epidemiol 1976;103:251–160.
16. Gross PA, Beaugard A, Van Antwerpen C. Surveillance for nosocomial infections: can the sources of data be reduced? Infect Control 1980;1:233–236.
17. Schifman RB, Palmer RA. Surveillance of nosocomial infections by computer analysis of positive culture rates. J Clin Microbiol 1985;21:493–495.
18. Broderick A, Mori M, Nettleman MD, Streed SA, Wenzel RP. Nosocomial infections: validation of surveillance and computer modeling to identify patients at risk. Am J Epidemiol 1990;131:734–742.
19. Wong LK, Barry AL, Horgan SM. Comparison of six different criteria for judging the acceptability of sputum specimens. J Clin Microbiol 1982;16:627–631.
20. Ahluwalia G, Embree J, McNicol P, Law B, Hammond GW. Comparison of nasopharyngeal aspirate and nasopharyngeal swab specimens for respiratory syncytial virus diagnosis by cell culture, indirect immunofluorescence assay and enzyme-linked immunosorbent assay. J Clin Microbiol 1987;25:763–767.
21. Doebbeling BN, Bale M, Koontz FP, Helms CM, Wenzel RP, Pfaller MA. Prospective evaluation of the Gen-Probe DNA probe assay for detection of Legionellae in respiratory specimens. Eur J Clin Microbiol Infect Dis 1988;7:748–752.
22. Arens M, Swierkosz EM. Detection of rotavirus by hybridization with a nonradioactive synthetic DNA probe and comparison with commercial enzyme immunoassays and silver-stained polyacrylamide gels. J Clin Microbiol 1989;27:1277–1279.
23. Laussucq S, Schuster D, Alexander WJ, Thacker WL, Wilkinson HW, Spika JS. False-positive DNA probe test for *Legionella* species associated with a cluster of respiratory illnesses. J Clin Microbiol 1988;26:1442–1444.
24. Pfaller MA, Wakefield DS, Stewart B, Bale M, Hammons GT, Massanari RM. Evaluation of laboratory methods for the classification of methicillin-resistant and methicillin-susceptible *Staphylococcus aureus*. Am J Clin Pathol 1988;89:120–125.
25. Murray BE. The life and times of the enterococcus. Clin Microbiol Rev 1990;3:46–65.
26. Maki DG, Weise CE, Safafin HW. A semi-quantitative culture method for identifying intravenous-catheter-related infection. N Engl J Med 1977;296:1305–1309.
27. Kahn FW, Jones JM. Diagnosing bacterial respiratory infection by bronchoalveolar lavage. J Infect Dis 1987;155:862–869.
28. Martin MA, Pfaller MA, Rojas PB, Woolson RF, Wenzel RP. In vitro susceptibility of nosocomial gram negative bloodstream pathogens to quinolones and other antibiotics—a statistical approach. J Antimicrob Chemother 1989;23:353–361.
29. Kernodle DS, Barg NL, Kaiser AB. Low-level colonization of hospitalized patients with methicillin-resistant coagulase-negative staphylococci and emergence of the organisms during surgical antimicrobial prophylaxis. Antimicrob Agents Chemother 1988;32:202–208.
30. McGowan JE Jr. Role of the microbiology laboratory in prevention and control of nosocomial infections. In: Lennette EH, Balows A, Hausler WJ Jr, Shadomy HJ, eds. Manual of clinical microbiology. 4th ed. Washington, DC: American Society for Microbiology, 1985:110–122.
31. Restuccia PA, Cunha BA. Microbiological aspects of infection control. In: Wenzel RP, ed. Prevention and control of nosocomial infections. Baltimore: Williams & Wilkins, 1987: 205–207.
32. Simmons BP. Centers for Disease Control guidelines for hospital environmental control—microbiologic surveillance of the environment and of personnel in the hospital. Infect Control 1981;2:145–146.
33. Aber RC, Mackel DC. Epidemiologic typing of nosocomial microorganisms. Am J Med 1981;70:899–905.
34. Pfaller MA. Typing systems for epidemiology. In: Balows A, Hausler WJ Jr, Herrman K, Isenberg HD, Shadomy HJ, eds.

Manual of clinical microbiology. 5th ed. Washington, DC: American Society for Microbiology, 1991:171–182.
35. Mayer LW. Use of plasmid profiles in epidemiologic surveillance of disease outbreaks and in tracing the transmission of antibiotic resistance. Clin Microbiol Rev 1988;1:228–243.
36. Goldmann DA. Microbiologic aspects of infection control. In: Donowitz LG, ed. Hospital acquired infection in the pediatric patient. Baltimore: Williams & Wilkins, 1988:369–385.
37. Doebbeling BN, Pfaller MA, Houston AK, Wenzel RP. Removal of nosocomial pathogens from the contaminated glove: implication for glove reuse and handwashing. Ann Intern Med 1988;109:394–398.
38. McGowan JE Jr, Weinstein RA, Mallison GF. The role of the laboratory in control of nosocomial infection. In: Bennett JV, Brachman PS, eds. Hospital infections. 2nd ed. Boston: Little, Brown, 1986:113–134.

53 Autopsy Microbiology

Mary J. Reznicek and Franklin P. Koontz

Autopsies are one of the most powerful learning tools the field of medicine has in its armamentarium for understanding disease. They are performed for a variety of reasons: to gain additional information into the pathogenesis of disease, to identify clinically unsuspected disease processes and to correlate premortem clinical diagnoses with postmortem diagnoses. The autopsy is a valuable teaching tool and quality control measure that works most efficiently when there is open communication between the primary physician and the pathologist. This ensures that valuable information is exchanged between both parties to facilitate a greater understanding of disease processes.

Despite the advent of the antibiotic era, infection has remained a significant cause of death in the United States. Therefore, the ability to identify an infectious process at autopsy is crucial. The diagnosis of an infectious disease at autopsy, like the diagnoses made in living patients, can be accomplished by positive cultures, tissue histology, and serologic procedures. These tests can be utilized singly or in combination.

Postmortem cultures can be a very useful component of the postmortem examination. They can be utilized to detect infections not suspected clinically, such as mycobacterial or fungal infections. They can also be useful in pinpointing the source of a known sepsis. For example, the discovery at autopsy of a *Staphylococcus aureus* psoas muscle abscess in a patient with known *S. aureus* sepsis and no other potential sites of bacterial seeding would certainly make the abscess the most likely source. Culturing can also be useful as a quality control measure to assess the effectiveness of antimicrobial therapy. As a quality control measure, the identification of an unsuspected infectious process can also help clinicians identify, in a retrospective fashion, other tests that might have aided in the premortem identification of an infection.

All of the knowledge gained by postmortem culturing is dependent on the utilization of proper methods to collect and process samples. This would include proper cooling of the body after death, avoiding lengthy delays in the performance of an autopsy, the use of sterile culturing techniques, and the use of good interpretive skills to correlate the clinical history, culture results, and the gross and histologic findings.

MICROBIOLOGY OF AUTOPSY TISSUE

The use of cultures in autopsy microbiology is controversial, and opinions vary on its usefulness. Several basic questions concerning the validity of postmortem cultures have been discussed in the literature. Most of these questions center around the basic question of whether a dead human body with its own inherent normal bacterial flora is suitable for culturing. More specifically, these questions are:

1. Does agonal or postmortem bacterial invasion occur?
2. What effect does the postmortem interval have on culture results?
3. Are human viscera sterile?

Two theories exist that support the idea that autopsy material is unsuitable for culture: the theories of *agonal invasion* and *postmortem invasion*. The theory of agonal invasion states that the diminished vitality of the dying body predisposes it to disseminated infection. The theory of postmortem invasion suggests that bacteria multiply and migrate throughout the body after death. Potential sites of dissemination include the normal flora of the oropharynx, which can seed the lung and blood, and normal GI tract flora, which can seed the liver, spleen, and blood.

Both these theories promote the concept that increasing numbers and types of organisms would be seen after death. Similarly, one would expect that the number of positive cultures would increase in direct proportion to the postmortem time interval. However, this concept does not appear to be valid if one considers several studies that illustrate that the postmortem interval has no effect on the number of positive cultures at autopsy (1–7). The postmortem interval in these studies ranged from 14–48 hours, and bodies were placed in a cooler at 4° to 5°C soon after death. There was no increase in positive autopsy cultures as the postmortem interval increased. In contrast, Carpenter and Wilkins (8) conducted a retrospective study of 2033 autopsy cases that showed a rise in postmortem positive cultures with increasing postmortem intervals up to 18 hours. Unfortunately, because the distribution of cases between short and long delay intervals was not provided, the conclusions of this study are open to question. Overall, the majority of the published evidence suggests that, if proper cooling of the body takes place and the autopsy is performed in a timely manner, agonal or postmortem invasion (if either exists) should not produce false-positive culture results.

The high frequency with which positive cultures are isolated from autopsy tissues that clinically and pathologically appear normal has raised the question of whether human viscera are sterile. This question has sparked controversy about the increasing numbers of cadaver organs harvested for transplant. A study of 148 surgical biopsies (excluding skin and GI tract) showed that approximately 28% were culture-positive (2). Because the samples were surgical biopsy specimens, one cannot argue that agonal or postmortem invasion played any role. Considering the transient bacteremias that are known to occur in individuals undergoing dental or urologic procedures, it is not surprising that human viscera may not be sterile at any given time. In healthy individuals, these numbers of circulating bacteria are likely to be too small to result in clinical disease. In interpreting a positive postmortem culture result, one must be careful not to equate a positive culture with disease without first correlating the culture results with the clinical history and histologic findings. A positive culture result may be *valid* in light of the above discussion, but the determination of its *clinical significance* is of major importance in ascertaining its contribution to the cause of death.

Knapp and Kent (1) addressed this issue and suggested that low levels of bacteria may be present in noninfected organs at the time of autopsy. They showed by quantitative cultures that less than 10^5 organisms per milliliter in lung tissue correlated with the absence of pulmonary disease by autopsy histology and, conversely, more than 10^5 organisms per milliliter in lung tissue correlated with clinical and pathological pneumonia.

It is imperative to understand that the data and concepts expressed in the above discussion are totally dependent upon proper culturing techniques at the time of autopsy. Although the "sterile autopsy technique" suggested by O'Toole et al. (4) is impractical for routine use, DeJongh et al. (3) have described a more practical technique. This technique is described in detail elsewhere in this chapter (see Specimen Collection and Transport, below).

Avoiding contamination of tissues with fluids introduced into the body cavities at the time of dissection is an important aspect of culturing. One study by Silva and Sonnenwirth (7) reported that blood cultures obtained from the heart through a closed chest were more likely to yield significant results than those obtained from an exposed right atrium. They also showed that bowel manipulation increased the number of positive cultures. Contamination of postmortem cultures with normal flora from the bowel or nasopharynx can lead to significant problems. However, these can be controlled by strict adherence to protocols or procedures adapted for the care and handling of the cadavers from the moment of death to the completion of the autopsy.

SPECIMEN COLLECTION AND TRANSPORT

Preparation

Before beginning the autopsy, it is imperative to fully review the patient's chart. The value of the autopsy is directly proportional to the preparation by the prosector. The information contained in the patient's chart can be used to ascertain the clinical questions that need to be answered by the autopsy. Areas of the hospital record that are particularly helpful include current hospital notes, transfer notes, and past discharge notes, which often provide an excellent review of the patient's medical history. Radiology examinations such as x-rays, CT scans, and WBC scans will often point out areas of suspected infections. For example, when the clinical note states "suspected pancreatic pseudocyst," the CT scan may be helpful in describing the exact location of the cyst and the size. If the prosector is unsure of the clinical questions, it can be extremely helpful to consult with the physician who managed the patient. This is strongly recommended in every autopsy case and can often provide more recent data that may not be evident in the chart.

In reading the patient's record, it is important to delineate those cases in which infection was thought to play a clinically important role and those cases in which the cause of death is unknown and infection is a possible cause. In the former situation, the prosector should study clinically suspicious areas of infection by gross and microscopic examination and possibly by culture. Autopsy data, whether gleaned from gross observation, histologic examination, or microbiological culture, serve as quality control mechanisms for antemortem concepts. The autopsy can clarify these concepts regardless of whether the findings are positive or negative. For example, the clinicians and the radiologist may suspect a right lower lobe pneumonia in a patient who dies a few days later. The prosector, by reading the chart, knows this information and, despite the gross findings of dependent congestion and a lack of consolidation in the right lung, can obtain samples of that area for microbiological culture and histologic examination. By doing so, the prosector can adequately address the antemortem diagnosis of pneumonia. Additional information can be gleaned from the hospital record relative to the use of antimicrobial therapy. This information could be critical in evaluating the effectiveness of specific antimicrobial therapy.

Diagnosing an unsuspected infection when the cause of death is unknown is also a responsibility of the prosector. It is important to consider doing cultures in this situation. It is relatively easy to culture during the autopsy; however, the chance is lost after the tissue has been placed in formalin and the cadaver has been taken to the funeral home. For example, a 35-year-old male is admitted to the hospital with severe congestive heart failure, and he dies before a workup is performed. No definite etiology for the congestive failure is known. The clinical differential includes cardiomyopathy, myocardial infarction, cor pulmonale, and myocarditis. Histologic sections of the heart show scattered inflammatory cells indicative of a myocarditis. In this case, confirmatory viral cultures would not only add strength to the diagnosis of myocarditis but would also give valuable epidemiologic information. Similar information can also be supplied by specific serologic tests. If antemortem tests were performed for specific antibodies, postmortem serum should be submitted for convalescent titers.

In reviewing the hospital record, it is important to ascertain whether the patient may have had an infectious disease that would place individuals present at the autopsy at risk, such as tuberculosis, hepatitis, and AIDS. In cases of suspected tuberculosis, PPD results and sputum culture results may be informative. For hepatitis, elevated liver function tests or a previous history of transfusion or drug abuse should be noted. If AIDS is suspected, the patient's HIV status and personal risk history should be determined. The presence of multiple opportunistic infections, such as *Pneumocystis carinii* pneumonia and/or atypical mycobacterial infection, in an otherwise normal host, or an unknown cause of death, should also arouse suspicions. Although universal precautions are recommended for all autopsies, particular caution should be exercised in instances where infectious diseases are suspected. In such cases, it is best to limit the number of people in the autopsy suite, thereby decreasing the number of people possibly exposed. In addition, consideration might be given to limiting the autopsy to areas of clinically suspected disease. For example, in a patient who died of fulminant hepatitis, there may be no reason to examine the brain except for completeness. In these cases, limiting the autopsy may be indicated.

Culturing

The extent of postmortem culturing is a problem that has never been specifically addressed. If only one area is to be cultured, the spleen and heart blood are favored as reliable sites. However, additional cultures from other areas such as lungs and kidneys will more accurately reflect the spectrum of bacteria affecting the patient. The clinical history and the gross appearance of the organs at autopsy can also help the prosector to decide how many postmortem cultures are necessary. For example, in a patient with a clinical history of sepsis, cultures of heart blood and spleen should be taken even if gross organ appearance is normal. If both sites grow identical organisms, a diagnosis of sepsis is supported.

In transplant patients and other immunocompromised hosts, special diligence must be shown. In the event of an established disseminated infection, it is clinically important to identify the site of entry of the infection and/or the primary organ of involvement that may be seeding the rest of the body. Entry sites other than the typical respiratory route include indwelling catheters, Hickman catheters, skin wounds, and nasal lesions. Extensive culturing in these patients is recommended to document the dissemination of the infection and to identify possible sources of infections.

The extent of culturing not only refers to the number of cultures but to the types of cultures as well. In immunocompromised patients, the use of special viral, fungal, or mycobacterial cultures in addition to routine bacteriology should be considered. These special cultures must be clearly requested on the test requisition form because they are not routinely performed on autopsy specimens in most laboratories.

The use of cultures should not be discounted because of antemortem antimicrobial therapy (8–12). Some studies have shown that antibiotics per se do not influence the number of positive cultures at autopsy. In addition, the availability of resin bottles or other antibiotic removal devices for blood cultures may also help increase this yield. In patients who have received antimicrobial therapy, postmortem cultures can assess the effectiveness of the drug.

As previously discussed, the techniques employed in obtaining postmortem cultures clearly affect the usefulness of the results. A more practical technique, described by DeJongh et al. (3), compares very favorably with those used in autopsies performed under strict sterile operative conditions. This technique, as it applies to blood, urine, CSF, and tissue, includes the following steps:

1. After making the initial incisions, visually inspect the cavities for fluid accumulations that can be cultured immediately before manipulation. Gently inspect organs for areas suspicious for infection. Consider culturing organs that are *clinically* suspected of harboring infection.
2. Dry the area to be cultured by searing with a hot steel spatula while keeping the organ elevated away from any secretions. Avoid dripping gloves that may contaminate the surface after it has been sterilized.
3. For tissue culture, remove a 1 cm^3 portion of tissue with a sterile forceps and blade and place it in a sterile Petri dish that has been properly identified with the patient's name, the culture site, and the specific type of culture desired (e.g., viral and fungal).
4. For blood culture, aspirate blood from the right atrium with a sterile syringe and inject 10 ml into aerobic and anaerobic blood culture bottles whose surfaces have been sterilized. Consider using a resin culture bottle if the patient has been on antibiotics. In cases of suspected fungemia, centrifugation lysis blood tubes (Isolator, DuPont) may be used.
5. To obtain urine for culture, aspirate urine directly from the bladder with a sterile syringe and inject it into a sterile tube.
6. CSF fluid for culture can be obtained from the lateral ventricle through the corpus callosum after the skull cap is removed or by cisternal tap through the skin. Both methods are adequate when performed aseptically.
7. Cultures of abscesses and granulomata should be obtained from both the center and the peripheral wall of the lesions. Depending on the disease, the organisms can be in either location.
8. Use different sets of sterile instruments for each culture/site.
9. If the microbiology laboratories are not all in one location, divide the specimens aseptically for the bacteriology, mycology, TB, and virology laboratories. The specimens should be delivered promptly to the microbiology laboratory.

Thus, by careful sampling, surface decontamination, and handling of tissues, one can obtain postmortem cultures that are useful in assessing the importance of infection in the death of a given patient.

It is very important to adequately fill out the laboratory requisitions. Tissue from surgical specimens may be automatically plated for bacteriology, anaerobes and fungi; however, autopsy cultures, because of their low yield, may not get the same treatment. It is important to let the microbiology laboratory know what is suspected. For example, if you clinically suspect an organism that has special growth requirements, like *Haemophilus*, that information must be relayed to the laboratory to ensure proper handling of the specimen.

Table 53.1. Specific Body Sites for Viral Culturing

Syndrome	Specimens
Respiratory	Lung, tracheal swab
CNS	Brain, spinal cord, CSF, feces
Cardiac	Heart, nasopharyngeal swab, feces, pericardial fluid
Liver	Liver, nasopharyngeal swab, feces, blood
GI	Feces, GI tract

Tissue specimens for viral culture should be placed in transport media and kept at 4°C if any delay in transport to the laboratory is anticipated. If a longer delay (more than 48 hours) is anticipated, the specimen should be snap frozen in liquid nitrogen. Slow freezing may kill some unstable viruses. In suspected viral syndromes, the virus may be excreted in body fluids and thus may be present in urine and feces as well as in the organ of primary interest. Culturing multiple areas may result in higher yield (see Table 53.1).

One procedure that can be performed immediately in the morgue is a touch preparation of the infected organ. A Diff-Quick (Fisher Scientific) or Giemsa stain set-up and a microscope can be kept in the morgue. This procedure can permit the rapid identification of yeast, molds, or granulomatous inflammation and thereby help direct the extent and type of culturing (see Fig. 53.6). It also presents the opportunity to give rapid feedback to the clinician while the clinical situation is still fresh in his or her mind.

Specimen Processing

Autopsy culture specimens should be processed by the laboratory in much the same way as clinical specimens. These techniques have already been described in previous chapters. However, in processing these specimens, the general philosophy is to avoid picking up less meaningful data. Broth cultures can be avoided because the low levels of organisms at autopsy are unlikely to be clinically significant. Culture plates that grow multiple organisms are also unlikely to be significant in most clinical situations.

Additional microbiological methods that can be applied include print culture (13), immunofluorescence, DNA probes, and polymerase chain reaction (PCR) (14). In general, these methods involve additional laboratory time and expensive reagents. Print cultures involve pressing culture media directly against the block of tissue to be cultured. The print cultures can then be directly correlated to the presence of an inflammatory response in the tissue section, allowing a rough quantitation of organisms to be made. A similar principle was advocated by Knapp and Kent (1) 12 years earlier when they compared quantitative cultures of lung tissue with Gram stains of tissue imprints and histologic sections. The advantage of this technique is the ability to directly correlate culture information to histologic sections. In both studies, contaminants were readily identified by the low numbers of organisms grown in culture (1) or by the pattern of growth. For example, in the print culture method, contaminating bacteria are generally restricted to the edges of the culture imprint (13).

At present, rapid diagnostic methods such as DNA probes and immunofluorescence should be reserved for autopsy cases in which an organism is suspected clinically and pathologically despite negative routine laboratory cultures and tissue sections. Special techniques may also be necessary for organisms that cannot be easily cultured or identified by routine histologic stains, such as *Rickettsia*.

Special histologic stains on formalin-fixed autopsy tissue can also be performed alone or in combination with cultures to diagnose an infectious process. Which special stains to order can often be determined by the routine hematoxylin and eosin (H&E) stain, which provides information as to the type and degree of cellular host response. These host responses can be divided into the broad categories of acute inflammation, chronic inflammation, and granulomatous inflammation, and the identification of one of these can alert the prosector to search for the presence of an organism that characteristically elicits that type of host response (Table 53.2).

Several characteristic host reactions can be identified. Infection with *Pneumocystis* can produce honeycombed, intra-alveolar material seen in immunocompromised patients as well as the interstitial plasma cell infiltrates seen in patients with intact immune systems. Viruses such as *cytomegalovirus* and *herpes simplex*, when they occur on a mucosal surface, may cause necrosis and ulceration with acute inflammation. Other viruses may only elicit chronic inflammation. Areas of infarction with vascular thrombosis should suggest the possibility of *Aspergillus* or Zygomycetes.

In general, the host response is a reflection of the status of the patient's immune system. For example, a patient with a competent immune system forms a caseous granuloma around an organism such as *Mycobacterium tuberculosis*. Few organisms, if any, can be identified in these lesions. In patients with AIDS or chronic immunosuppression, well-formed granulomata are usually not found. The response may range from ill-formed collections of histiocytes to only scattered histiocytes. In these cases, abundant organisms are usually seen within histiocytes.

After developing a differential diagnosis as to the type of infectious process, the proper histologic stain can be selected. Table 53.3 lists the most commonly

Table 53.2. Host Tissue Reactions to Organisms

Host Tissue Reaction	Organisms
Acute inflammation	Routine bacteria, actinomyces, *Nocardia*, blastomyces, *Candida*, and herpes virus
Chronic inflammation	Viruses, *Pneumocystis*
Granulomatous inflammation	Mycobacteria, *Cryptococcus, Histoplasma, Coccidioides, Candida*
Caseous necrosis	Mycobacteria, *Histoplasma, Coccidioides*
Thrombosis	*Aspergillus*, Zygomycetes, *Fusarium*

Table 53.3. Commonly Used Histological Stains to Demonstrate Organisms in Tissues

Stain	Organism	Example
Hematoxylin and eosin	Viral inclusions (specifically CMV, *herpes*, adenovirus, rabies); *Toxoplasma*; dematiaceous (pigmented) fungi; other fungi (*Aspergillus*, Zygomycetes) Demonstrates cellular response	CMV (Fig. 53.1*A*) *Herpes* (Fig. 53.1*B*) Adenovirus (Fig. 53.1*C*) *Toxoplasma* (Fig. 53.1*D*) *Aspergillus* (Fig. 53.1*E*)
Gomori's methenamine silver nitrate (GMS)	Fungi (yeast and mycelial forms); *Pneumocystis*	*Histoplasma* (Fig. 53.2*A*) *Candida* (Fig. 53.2*B*) *Aspergillus* (Fig. 53.2*C*) *Blastomyces* (Fig. 53.2*D*)
Periodic acid–Schiff (PAS)	Fungi (yeast and mycelial forms), especially good for sporotrichosis, *Blastomyces*, and Zygomycetes	*Blastomyces* (Fig. 53.3*A*) Zygomycosis (Fig. 53.3*B*) *Coccidiodes* (Fig. 53.3*C*)
Acid fast stains (AFB, Fite, Kinyoun)	Mycobacteria, Nocardia, (Fite—*Mycobacterium leprae*)	Mycobacteria (Fig. 53.4)
Gram	Most bacteria, including Actinomycetes Also stains fungi, especially on touch preparations	*Nocardia* (Fig. 53.5)
Giemsa (Diff-Quick)	*Ricksettsia, Pneumocystis* (will stain internal structure), fungi	*Histoplasma* (Fig. 53.6*A*) *Pneumocystis* (Fig. 53.6*B*) *Candida* (Fig. 53.6*C*)
Mucicarmine	*Cryptococcus* (mucin positive capsule)	*Cryptococcus* (Fig. 53.7)
Warthin-Starry	Spirochetes, cat-scratch fever organism	

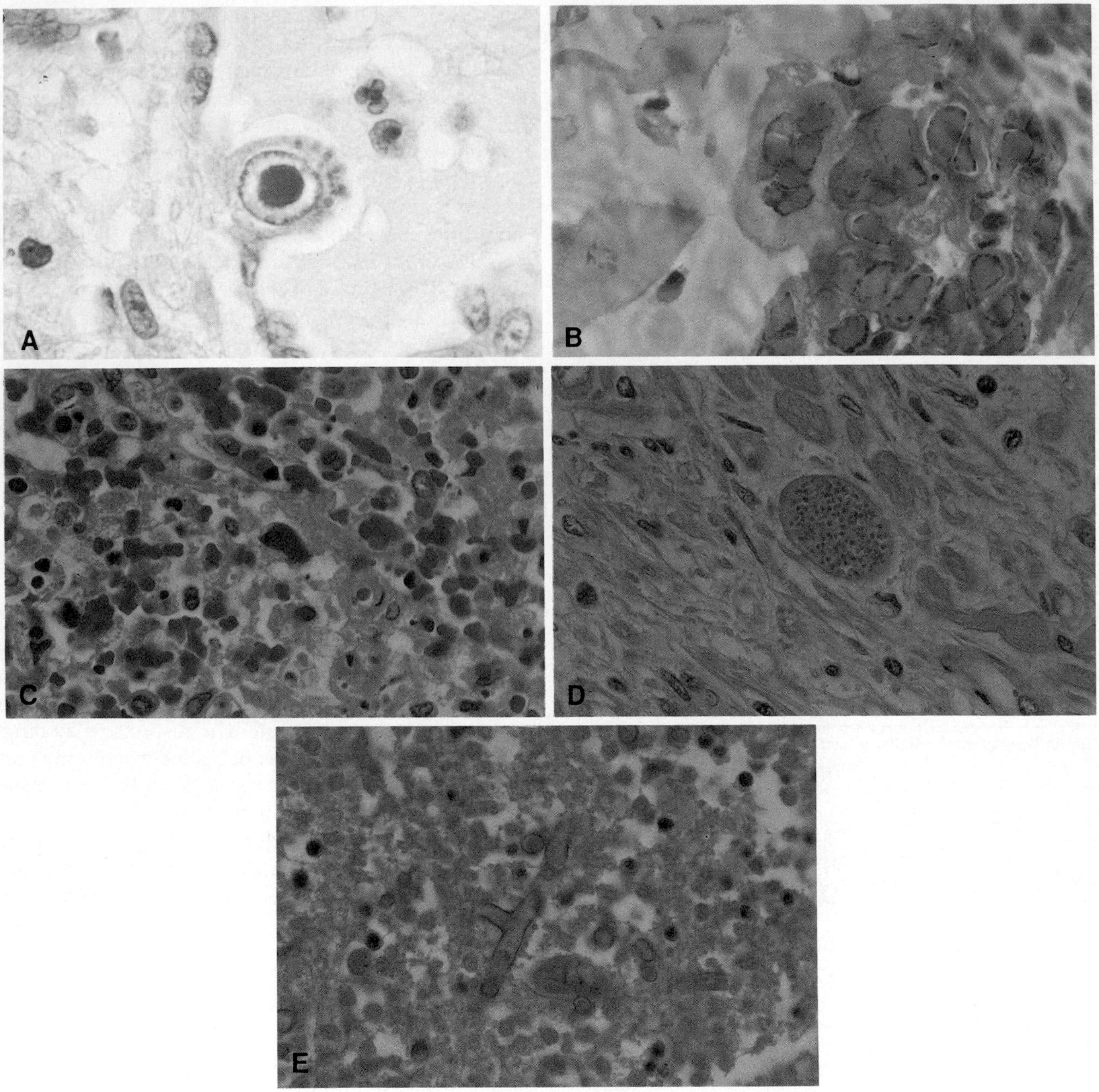

Figure 53.1. **A**, Lung tissue with characteristic "owl's-eye" *cytomegalovirus* nuclear inclusion and cytoplasmic inclusions (H&E, ×1000, oil). **B**, Esophageal tissue with *herpes* virus intranuclear inclusions with multinucleation (H&E, ×1000, oil). **C**, Lung tissue with a "smudged" intranuclear inclusion characteristic of adenovirus (center H&E, ×1000, oil). **D**, Heart tissue with an intramyocardial *Toxoplasma* cyst (H&E, ×1000, oil). **E**, Lung tissue with invasive *Aspergillus* (H&E, ×1000, oil).

employed histologic stains and the organisms they demonstrate (Figs. 53.1 to 53.7). Under ideal circumstances, these results can be correlated to positive culture results.

It is important to remember that histological stains complement each other. The H&E stain provides information about the type of host response, and the Gomori methenamine silver (GMS) stain acts as a good screening tool for the presence of fungi. With the GMS stain, the fungus stains black on a green background, but host response is not demonstrated. Therefore, correlation between the GMS and H&E stains will provide information about both host response and the presence of organisms. A combination stain utilizing GMS with an H&E counterstain will provide both sets of information and, coincidentally, photographs well (Fig. 53.8).

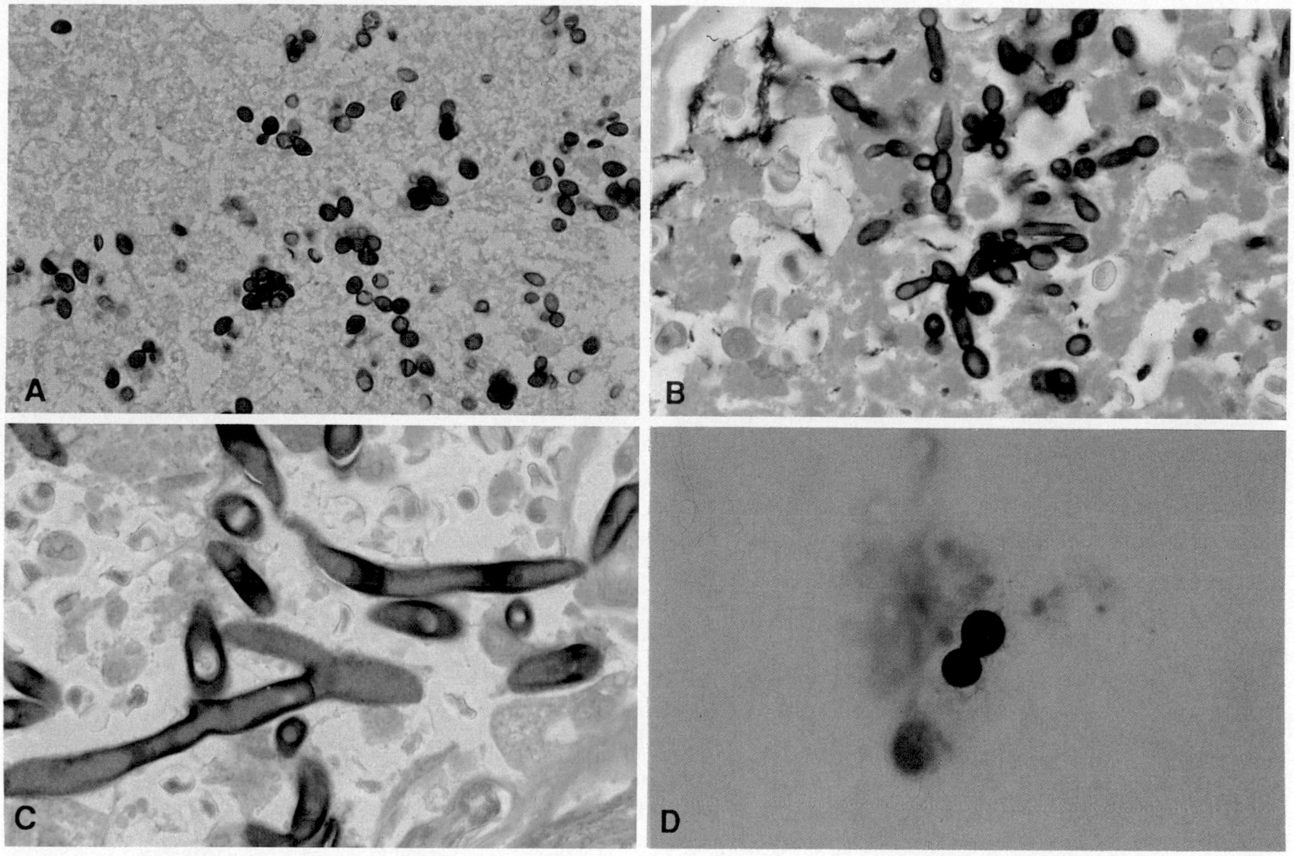

Figure 53.2. **A**, Lung granuloma with *Histoplasma* organisms (GMS, ×1000, oil). **B**, Lung tissue with invasive *Candida* and characteristic pseudohyphae with pinching at the septae (GMS, × 1000,oil). **C**, Lung tissue with invasive *Aspergillus* and characteristic true septae (no pinching) and 45° angle branching (GMS, ×1000, oil). **D**, Cytology bronchial specimen with broad-based bud of *Blastomyces* (GMS, ×1000, oil).

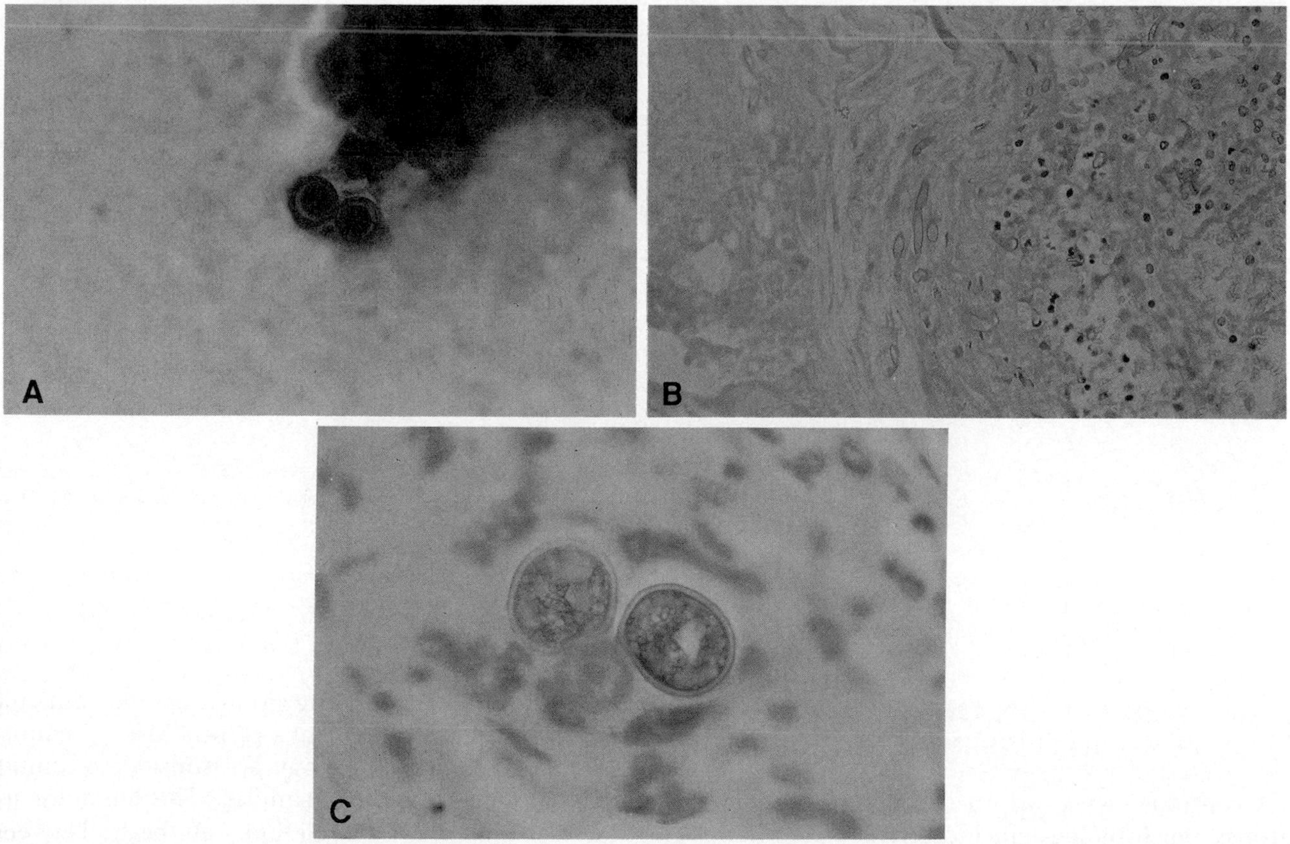

Figure 53.3. **A**, Cytology bronchial specimen with internal structure of *Blastomyces* (PAS, ×1000, oil). **B**, Sinus vessel wall containing characteristic pleomorphic ribbon appearance and absence of septae in zygomycosis (PAS, ×2000). **C**, Lung granuloma with *Coccidiodes* spherule (PAS, ×1000, oil).

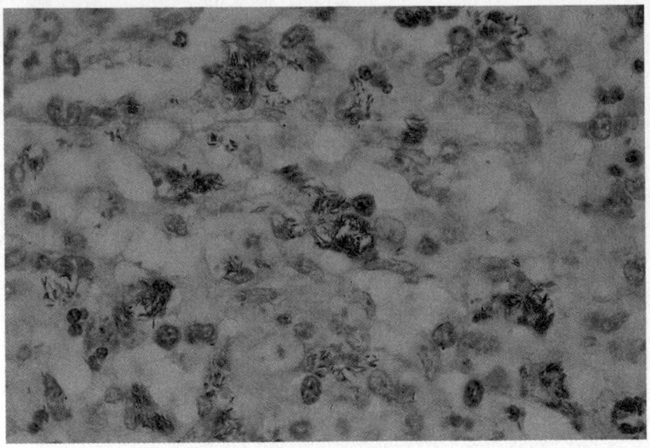

Figure 53.4. Lymph node tissue with acid-fast positive rods within histiocytes characteristic of *Mycobacterium avium-intracellulare* (AFB, ×1000, oil).

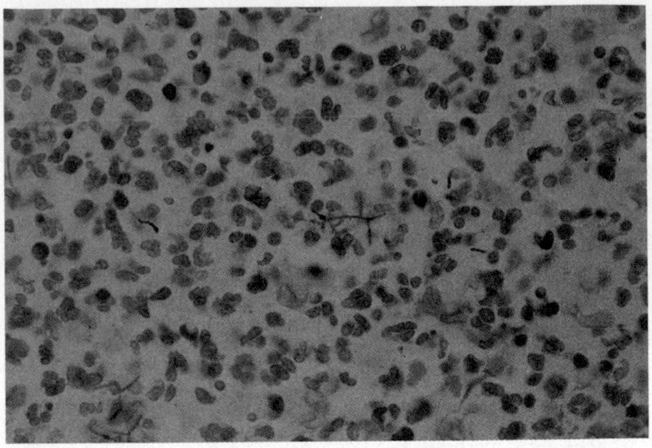

Figure 53.5. Skin abscess tissue with Gram-variable, right-angle branching, filamentous bacteria characteristic of *Nocardia* (Gram, ×1000, oil).

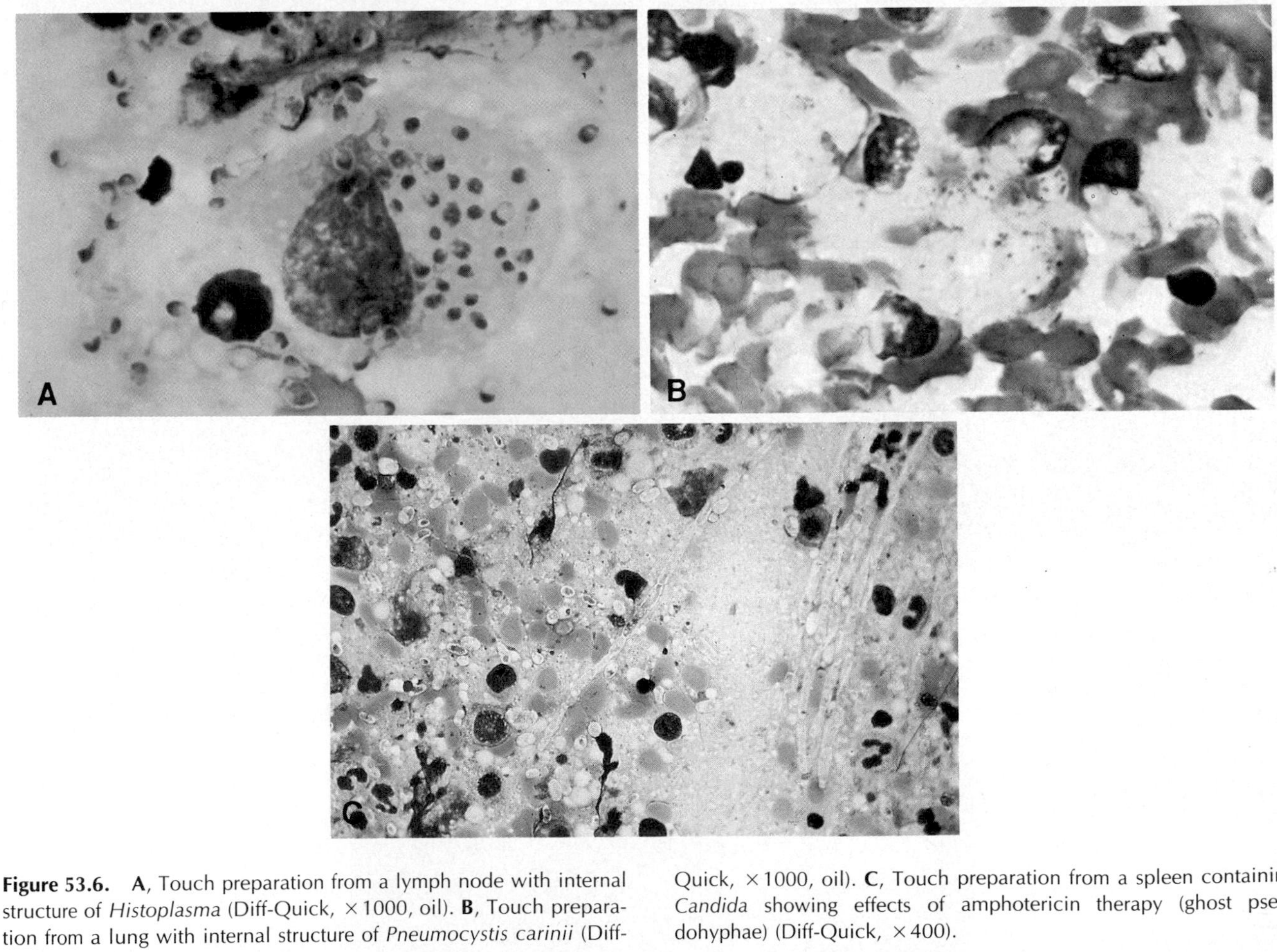

Figure 53.6. **A**, Touch preparation from a lymph node with internal structure of *Histoplasma* (Diff-Quick, ×1000, oil). **B**, Touch preparation from a lung with internal structure of *Pneumocystis carinii* (Diff-Quick, ×1000, oil). **C**, Touch preparation from a spleen containing *Candida* showing effects of amphotericin therapy (ghost pseudohyphae) (Diff-Quick, ×400).

INTERPRETATION OF POSTMORTEM CULTURE RESULTS

A common sense approach to the evaluation of autopsy microbiology includes the correlation between clinical history, culture results, and tissue histology. Determining which results represent contamination versus true infections can be difficult; however, when the patient's clinical history, culture results, and tissue histology are considered jointly, this job becomes much simpler. The literature indicates only fair correlation, at best, between premortem and postmortem cultures. In a study by Wood et al. (12), a positive correlation of 76% was noted when antemortem and postmortem blood cultures were compared with anatomical evidence of infection in 62 autopsy cases. In a study by Koneman and Davis (10) comparing only antemortem and postmortem cultures, the results were less inspiring; no correlation was demonstrated between antemortem and postmortem cultures in 42, 63, and 52% of sputum-lung, urine-kidney, and blood-heart cultures, respectively. In practice, the degree of correlation is largely dependent on the ability of the prosector to select the correct areas to sample for culture, to use the correct technique to procure the samples, and to delineate the insignificant results from the clinically important ones. The following sections suggest an approach to the interpretation of positive culture results from blood, tissues, and fluids.

Positive Blood Cultures

1. Interpret positive cultures carefully. Could the organism be a contaminant? Some of the common contaminants in morgues include *Staphylococcus epidermidis*, *Streptococcus* species, *Corynebacterium* species, *Pseudomonas fluorescens/putida*, and other environmental organisms, such as *Flavobacterium* species. Contamination is also indicated if an excessive number of days (more than 5 to 7) is required for the blood culture bottle to become positive or if only one of two bottles is positive.
2. Did the spleen culture or other tissue cultures grow the same organism as the blood culture? Having the same organism cultured from multiple sites certainly strengthens an argument for sepsis.
3. Could the antemortem clinical course be consistent with sepsis? Patients with sepsis often have a rapid downward course with fever and hypotension.

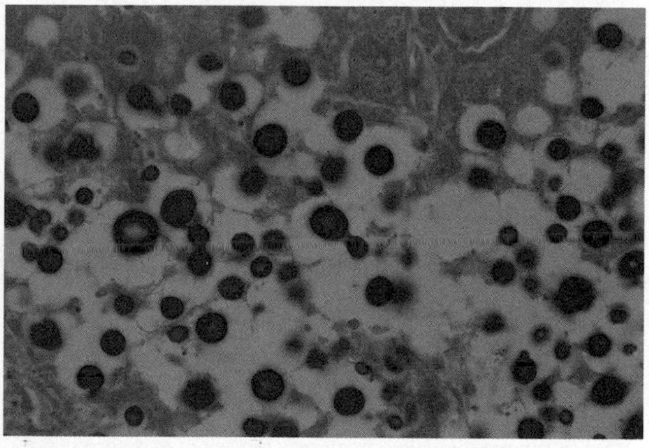

Figure 53.7. Liver granuloma with characteristic variably sized budding yeasts surrounded by a mucoid capsule (mucicarmine positive) characteristic of *Cryptococcus* (mucicarmine, ×1000, oil).

Positive Tissue or Fluid Cultures

1. Were organisms demonstrated on tissue sections or on Gram stains of homogenized tissue at the time of culture? Given the large number of organisms required to be able to demonstrate even one organism histologically per high power field, it is not surprising that one is frequently unable to demonstrate organisms in tissue stains. However, if organisms that are detected in tissue or on a Gram stain from culture material correlate with the culture results, it will significantly strengthen a diagnosis of infection.
2. Is a host response present that is consistent with the proposed infection? Growth of multiple organisms in a lung culture that is confirmed by tissue Gram stain without evidence of tissue reaction or inflammation most likely indicates agonal aspiration of stomach contents and not a pneumonia. Gross findings of a consolidated lobe of lung with microscopic findings of an acute intra-alveolar inflammatory infiltrate and a positive culture of *Streptococcus pneumoniae* are classic findings typ-

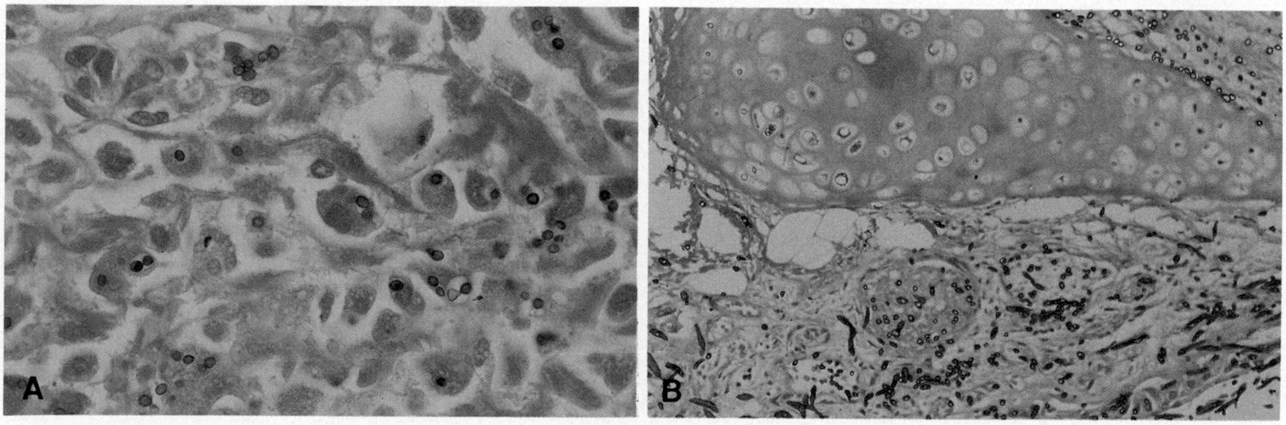

Figure 53.8. GMS with H&E counterstain preparation showing: **A**, *Histoplasma* organisms within histiocytes (×400). **B**, *Aspergillus* invading through bronchial cartilage (×200).

ical of pneumonia. Limited inflammatory responses may occur in immunosuppressed patients; in these cases, tissue responses such as cell necrosis, fibrinous exudate, and cellular atypia may be indicative of infection.

3. How well do the autopsy findings correlate with the antemortem diagnosis? For example, the isolation of poliovirus from the stool of a patient who died at age 2 of congenital heart disease may raise the question of premortem administration of polio vaccine rather than actual infection. Polio vaccine is a live attenuated vaccine, and virus can be cultured from stool for several weeks in patients receiving the oral vaccine.

By correlating the clinical findings, the autopsy histology findings, and the results of microbiological cultures, under- or overinterpretation of the findings can be avoided. Items that should definitely be addressed in the autopsy report include the confirmation of clinically suspected infections, the adequacy of antemortem antimicrobial therapy, the findings of a clinically unsuspected infection, and the inability to demonstrate a clinically suspected infection.

Methods to determine the adequacy of antimicrobial therapy may include susceptibility testing of the postmortem isolate to the antibiotic given antemortem. This information may be very important epidemiologically, especially in an intensive care unit situation in which multiple patients may be colonized or may later develop infections with the same organisms.

CONCLUSIONS

The use of microbiological techniques in autopsy pathology can be an important part of the postmortem examination. Infections continue to play a major role in causing significant morbidity and mortality. The confirmation or discovery of infections at autopsy is an important duty of the pathologist. While it can be argued that at times the results of microbiological studies are more confusing than helpful, careful correlation with the patient's clinical history and microscopic pathology often clarifies difficult cases. It is important to recall that postmortem culturing is affected by many variables, including culturing techniques, gross observational skills, adequate tissue sampling, antimicrobial therapy, possible contamination by normal flora, and the possibility that viscera may not be sterile. Thus, the finding of positive cultures should not be equated with infection unless supported by clinical and histopathological evidence. Understanding the strengths and weaknesses of postmortem culturing will help ensure that results are interpreted correctly. Although postmortem culturing has certain limitations, this should not preclude its use by pathologists.

Acknowledgment

The authors wish to thank Ms. Linda Schneekloth for her excellent secretarial assistance.

References

1. Knapp BE, Kent TH. Postmortem lung cultures. Arch Pathol 1968;85:200–203.
2. Minckler TM, Newell GR, O'Toole WF, Niwayama G, Levine PH. Microbiology experience in collection of human tissue. Am J Clin Pathol 1966;45:85–92.
3. DeJongh DS, Loftis JW, Green GS, Shively JA, Minckler TM. Postmortem bacteriology. Am J Clin Pathol 1968;49:424–428.
4. O'Toole WF, Saxena HM, Golden A, Ritts RE. Studies of postmortem microbiology using sterile autopsy technique. Arch Pathol 1965;80:540–547.
5. Kurtin JJ. Studies in autopsy bacteriology. Am J Clin Pathol 1958;30:239.
6. Wilson WR, Dolan CT, Washington JA, Brown AL, Ritts RE. Clinical significance of postmortem cultures. Arch Pathol 1972;94:244–249.
7. Silva H, Sonnenwirth AC. A practical and efficacious method for obtaining significant postmortem blood cultures. Am J Clin Pathol 1969;52:433–437.
8. Carpenter HM, Wilkins RM. Autopsy bacteriology: review of 2,033 cases. Arch Pathol 1964;77:73–81.
9. Koneman EW. Postmortem bacteriology. Crit Rev Clin Lab Sci 1970;1:5–23.
10. Koneman EW, Davis MA. Postmortem bacteriology. III. Clinical significance of microorganisms recovered at autopsy. Am J Clin Pathol 1974;61:28–40.
11. Roberts FJ. A review of postmortem bacteriological cultures. Can Med Ass J 1969;100:70–74.
12. Wood WH, Oldstone M, Schultz RB. A re-evaluation of blood culture as an autopsy procedure. Am J Clin Pathol 1965;43: 241–247.
13. Zanen-Lim OG, Zanen HC. Postmortem bacteriology of the lung by print culture of frozen tissue. J Clin Pathol 1980;33: 474–480.
14. DuMoulin GC, Paterson DG. Clinical relevance of postmortem microbiologic examination: a review. Hum Pathol 1985;16:539–548.

54 Diagnostic Virology

James C. Overall, Jr.

Common complaints from physicians about diagnostic virology include: "Even if you get an answer back from the virology laboratory, it's too late to be useful clinically; the patient is either dead or recovered from his illness." "Why bother finding out what virus is causing the illness? You can't treat it anyway." However, with the technological advances in rapid viral diagnosis and the development of a number of effective and safe antiviral drugs in recent years, neither of these complaints is valid any longer.

Shown in Table 54.1 are the results of 7,855 specimens submitted for viral culture or antigen detection to the diagnostic virology laboratory at the Associated Regional and University Pathologists, University of Utah Medical Center. Sixteen percent were positive, with a mean *turnaround time* of positive results of 1.3 days. The 14% of specimens positive for a virus, compares favorably with the 5% reported rate for positive blood cultures (1). The 1.3-day mean time to positive test results includes confirmed specific identification of herpes simplex virus (HSV), cytomegalovirus (CMV), influenza A and B viruses, respiratory syncytial virus (RSV), adenoviruses, and varicella zoster virus (VZV), and presumptive identification of an enterovirus. The particular methods used to detect and identify these viruses will be described below. For more technical detail about specific viruses, please see recent reviews (2–5b), chapters (6, 7, 9), or textbooks (8–11).

Table 54.2 lists the *antiviral agents* licensed for use in 1992 and the viruses against which the drugs are active. Note that the drugs are very selective, i.e., clinically active against only one or a few viruses. Therefore, a *specific viral diagnosis* must be made to select the proper drug. For more detailed information about the antiviral drugs, consult several recent textbooks (12, 13), or reviews (14, 15, 16).

VALUE OF SPECIFIC VIRAL DIAGNOSIS

There is value in making a specific virologic diagnosis, not only for the individual patient, but also for the community and hospital. For *the patient*, assistance in the decision to initiate antiviral therapy has already been mentioned. In addition, identification of a particular virus in a patient can result in the discontinuation of unnecessary antibiotic therapy and shorten the duration of hospitalization. For example, in the infant admitted with a diagnosis of meningitis and given oral antibiotic therapy prior to admission, culture of an enterovirus from the CSF can discriminate between: (*a*) partially treated bacterial meningitis requiring 10 days of hospitalization and intravenous antibacterial therapy, and (*b*) viral meningitis, where patients can be managed symptomatically and often discharged after a few days (17, 18). Identification of a viral agent can often enable cessation of unnecessary diagnostic tests (e.g., in a patient with a fever of unknown origin) and allow provision of a more accurate prognosis, both acute and long term.

At the *community* level, identification of a specific viral disease (e.g., measles) can aid in the recognition of illness in subsequent patients and in the institution of preventive measures (e.g., vaccine). In the *hospital* setting, detection of a particular virus can allow more rational use of infection control measures. For example, influenza virus is known to be transmitted by small particle aerosol and requires separate room respiratory isolation (19). In contrast, RSV is transmitted by direct contact or large droplet aerosol and needs only good handwashing (20), gloves and gown (21), and perhaps mask to prevent spread. Finally, diagnosis of a particular virus will enable rational use of antiviral prophylaxis in selected situations. For example, if an index case of influenza A

Table 54.1. Diagnostic Virology Laboratory—Specimens[a]

Pathogen/Test	Specimens		Positive		Time to Positive
	Number	Percent	Number	Percent	
HSV culture	4168	35.8	918	22.0	16 hr
CMV culture	2759	23.7	180	6.5	2.1 days
Respiratory virus culture	1703	14.6	54	3.2	7.1 days
Enterovirus culture	1660	14.2	90	5.4	5.6 days
Rota, adenovirus antigen	772	6.6	205	26.6	2 hr
RSV antigen	420	3.6	115	27.4	3 hr
VZV culture	172	1.5	19	11.0	5 days
Total	11,654	100.0	1581	13.6	1.3 days

[a]From July 1990–June 1991, Associated Regional and University Pathologists (ARUP), Salt Lake City, UT.

Table 54.2. Licensed Antiviral Agents—1992

Generic Drug	Brand Name	Virus
Amantadine	Symmetrel	Influenza A
Acyclovir	Zovirax	HSV, VZV[a]
Ribavirin	Virazole	RSV
Ganciclovir	Cytovene	CMV
Zidovudine	Retrovir	HIV
Dideoxyinosine	Videx	HIV
r Interferon alpha, gamma	Several	HPV warts, chronic viral hepatitis

[a]Abbreviations: HSV, herpes simplex virus; VZV, varicella zoster virus; RSV, respiratory syncytial virus; CMV, cytomegalovirus; HIV, human immunodeficiency virus; HPV, human papilloma virus.

is identified in a nursing home patient, use of amantadine in the other residents and staff of the facility for a 2- to 3-week period can prevent serious illness (22).

APPROACH TO VIRAL DIAGNOSIS

There are two major approaches to the diagnosis of a viral infection: virologic and serologic. The *virologic approach* includes (*a*) isolation of infectious virus in cell culture or in laboratory animals; (*b*) detection of viral antigen by immunologic methods such as immunofluorescence (FA) or enzyme immunoassay (EIA); (*c*) identification of viral particles by electron microscopy (EM); and (*d*) detection of viral nucleic acid by labeled complementary DNA probes. The *serologic approach* includes (*a*) demonstration of a 4-fold or greater rise in antiviral antibody using acute and convalescent sera and a variety of methods that measure predominantly IgG antibody; and (*b*) demonstration of virus-specific IgM antibody in a single late acute or early recovery phase serum.

As is true for any diagnostic test, the timing, quality, and handling of the specimen are critical for an accurate diagnosis. For the virologic approach to diagnosis, it is important to obtain specimens during the *acute infection* from the *site of disease*. For example, samples collected after bacterial and fungal cultures have returned negative and the patient has begun to recover are unlikely to yield infectious virus. And a positive viral culture from a stool specimen in a patient with suspected viral meningitis (instead of CSF) may provide misleading results.

SPECIMEN COLLECTION AND TRANSPORT

The *optimal specimens* vary depending on the site of disease. *Lesions* that can be sampled with a *swab* include vesicles or ulcers on the skin or mucous membranes, the pharynx, the conjunctiva, the urethra, and the cervix. Several different cotton or dacron swabs with an accompanying transport tube are commercially available (23). For culture of infectious virus, calcium alginate swabs should be avoided, particularly if the swab is left in the transport media, since the alginate can destroy infectivity (23, 24).

For pediatric *respiratory illnesses*, several investigations have shown that the nasopharyngeal (NP) aspirate or nasal wash provide a better yield of virus than a NP swab (25–27). The NP aspirate is obtained by passing a suction catheter into the posterior nasopharynx, a procedure that usually elicits coughing up secretions from the lower respiratory tract. Gentle suction is applied with a device that allows the respiratory secretions to be delivered into a suction trap vial or tube. If insufficient respiratory secretions are obtained, 2 ml of nonpreservative saline can be instilled in the opposite nostril, and the suction process repeated. Nasal wash specimen collection is accomplished by aspirating 3 ml of saline into a suction bulb with a snout. The saline is instilled into one nostril and immediately aspirated back into the suction bulb. In adults, the usual recommended specimens for respiratory viruses are a throat swab or a throat wash with viral transport media (28). It might be, however, that an NP aspirate or nasal wash are the preferred specimens in adults also, since most respiratory viruses replicate preferentially in columnar epithelial cells located primarily in the posterior NP and in the lower respiratory tract.

For stool specimens, fresh stool is preferred over a rectal swab (28). Urine specimens should be obtained using sterile procedures, just as one would do for bacterial cultures.

A number of viruses are present in the *blood* during acute infection, and isolation/detection of virus from this body fluid can be an important indicator of disease. Several viruses are associated with white cells, including CMV, HSV, human immunodeficiency virus (HIV), and the enteroviruses (coxsackie, echo, polio). HIV is found in lymphocytes and macrophages (29), while CMV is associated with neutrophils, and to a lesser extent macrophages (30). The enteroviruses can be isolated from plasma, as well as from white cells (31). The optimal blood fraction for HSV has not been well delineated. Since the particular virus being sought may not be clearly known, it may be optimal to process blood specimens to obtain both neutrophil and mononuclear cell fractions by gravity sedimentation or by separation techniques that provide both fractions (30). There is limited direct information on the optimal anticoagulant for blood specimens: heparin, ethylenediaminetetraacetic acid (EDTA), or acid citrate dextrose (ACD). One investigation demonstrated no difference between heparin and EDTA-anticoagulated blood in the recovery of CMV (32). Recovery rates of HIV from blood were higher with EDTA than heparin anticoagulated blood (33). Since it is also known that heparin can inactivate the herpesviruses in vitro (34), it seems reasonable to recommend the use of EDTA (purple top) tubes.

For critical specimens such as biopsies of tissues, or where there is concern about labile infectivity for particular viruses (e.g., RSV or VZV), there are commercially available tubes or vials with transport media containing albumin or serum as a stabilizer (e.g., m4 transport media from Microtest).

The optimal temperature for *storage* and *transport* of specimens for viral culture is 4°C (refrigerator, or wet ice temperature). Most viruses will be stable for 2 to 5 days at this temperature (35–37). Freezing at −20°C (ordinary freezer temperature) destroys or significantly reduces infectivity of virtually all viruses. Since freezing may also alter the ability to detect viral antigen with some commercially available kits, all viral specimens should be stored and transported at 4°C. If specimens need to be stored for longer than 3 to 4 days, an ultralow-temperature freezer (−70°C) should be used, and the specimen transported to the virology laboratory on dry ice.

VIROLOGIC METHODS IN VIRAL DIAGNOSIS

Viral Isolation

Isolation of infectious virus in cell cultures is the method most commonly used to detect most viruses. Since not all culturable viruses will grow in a single cell line, several different cells are used. The cells used during the winter season to isolate respiratory viruses include: primary rhesus monkey kidney (RMK), Madin-Darby canine kidney, Hep-2 (a human epithelial carcinoma cell line), buffalo green monkey kidney (BGMK) continuous cell line, and a human fibroblast cell. These are different from the cells used for the summer/fall enterovirus season: primary RMK, Hep-2, BGMK, RD (a human rhabdomyosarcoma cell line), and a human fibroblast cell. Many viruses will demonstrate a cytopathic effect (CPE) within a few days, while some may take as long as a week or two. Some viruses do not cause typical CPE and are identified by the adsorption of red cells to the surface of virus-infected cells in the culture (e.g., hemadsorption for the influenza and parainfluenza viruses). For some viruses, such as several of the coxsackie A viruses and Colorado tick fever virus, mouse inoculation is required.

With cell culture systems, *presumptive identification* of a particular virus or virus group (e.g., HSV or RSV or an enterovirus) can be performed within a few or several days based on the CPE: characteristics, time of onset, cell type in which it occurs. This presumptive identification can be greatly facilitated if the test request slip contains the important information requested: source of the specimen (e.g., swab of a genital ulcer or a conjunctival swab, rather than just a swab source not identified), and clinical diagnosis (e.g., genital herpes, influenza, aseptic meningitis).

Confirmation of a specific virus or serotype of a virus (e.g., HSV type 2, influenza A H3N2, echovirus 11) requires use of immunologic methods with antibody of known specificity. In recent years, fluorescein or peroxidase-conjugated monoclonal antibodies (McAb) have become available commercially to detect viral antigen in cell cultures: e.g., HSV (38–42), CMV (43–46), VZV (47), RSV (48–50), influenza A and B (51), the parainfluenza viruses (52), and the adenoviruses (53). To identify the specific serotype of influenza A or B, inhibition of hemagglutination by specific serotype antisera is used (28). For confirmation of a specific coxsackie or echovirus serotype, neutralization of CPE with pools of antisera and then individual antisera is still required (54).

In recent years, the technique of *centrifugation* of the patient specimen onto the cell monolayer on a coverslip in the bottom of a *shell vial* followed by staining for *viral antigen* with McAb after 1 or 2 days of incubation has significantly reduced the time required to detect and confirm a number of viruses (42, 45, 50, 51, 53). The centrifugation step shortens the time required for replication of the virus and production of viral antigen in cell cultures. For more slowly growing viruses such as CMV, the use of McAb against nonstructural proteins produced early in the replication cycle (i.e., immediate early antigen or early antigen) allows detection of virus even before CPE can be observed (45). Table 54.3 compares the times to detection for several viruses using the shell vial centrifugation/viral antigen staining (SVC/VAS) method vs. conventional CPE. The time to detection and confirmation is much faster with the SVC/VAS method with every virus listed. For example, with CMV the SVC/VAS method detects 50% of the total positives in 1 day and 90% in 2 days, while it requires 10 days to detect 50% with conventional CPE. Many diagnostic virology laboratories, therefore, use the SVC/VAS technique, particularly for detection of CMV.

The major *viruses detected* by isolation in *cell culture* include HSV, CMV, RSV, influenza A and B, the parainfluenza viruses, the adenoviruses, the enteroviruses (coxsackie A and B, echo, polio), and VZV. Although animal isolation is rarely done at commercial diagnostic virology laboratories, this may be required to isolate some viruses (e.g., Colorado tick fever and many of the coxsackie A viruses). Animals for isolation of viruses are available at many state health laboratories.

Table 54.3. Virus Identification: Centrifugation Plus Stain versus Conventional Cytopathic Effect

Virus	Centrifugation + Stain		Conventional CPE	
	Days in Culture	Percent Detected	Days in Culture	Percent Detected
HSV	1	96–99[a,c]	1	50[b]
CMV	1	55[c]	10	50[c]
CMV	2	95[c]		
VZV	2	90[d]	5	50[d]
Adenovirus	2	97[e]	4	50[e]
Influenza	2	60[f]	4	50[f]

[a]Salmon VC, Speranza MJ, Turner RB, et al. J Clin Microbiol 1986;23:683.
[b]Salmon VC, Stanberry LR, Overall JC, et al. Diagn Microbiol Infect Dis 1984; 2:317.
[c]Salmon VC, Overall JC. Unpublished observations.
[d]Landry ML. VA Practitioner, 1988;35.
[e]Espy MJ, Hierholzer JC, Smith TF. Am J Clin Path 1987;88:358.
[f]Espy MJ, Smith TF, Harmon MW, et al. J Clin Microbiol 1986;24:677.

There are several *advantages* to using isolation of infectious virus as the method of diagnosis. First, a broad range of viruses can be isolated. For example, from a respiratory secretion specimen a number of different respiratory viruses can be isolated, while an antigen detection test may identify only one virus (e.g., RSV). Second, isolation of infectious virus makes the agent available for further characterization. For example, demonstration that a strain of HSV isolated from an AIDS patient responding poorly to acyclovir (ACV) therapy is resistant to ACV but sensitive to foscarnet can be a helpful guide for change in treatment (55). Third, viral isolation is often considered the gold standard since there are no false-positive results (100% specificity) and culture is often more sensitive than antigen detection. It should be emphasized, however, that there may be true antigen-positive, culture-negative specimens. Samples may have been obtained late in the course of illness or collected/transported improperly; this could result in loss of viral infectivity but stability of antigen.

There are also several *disadvantages* to viral isolation. It requires the availability of a cell culture laboratory, with the need for specialized equipment and supplies and trained personnel. Second, isolation is slower than antigen detection, with results in days rather than hours. Finally, specimen collection and transport conditions are more critical for isolation than antigen tests.

Viral Antigen Detection

There are two major kinds of specimens on which viral antigen detection tests are performed. First, tests can be performed on cell cultures for early detection/confirmation of viral antigen, such as with the SVC/VAS technique mentioned above. Second, tests can be done on specimens directly from patients: nasal or nasopharyngeal secretions, bronchoalveolar lavage (BAL) specimens, scrapings of vesicles or conjunctivae, swabs of the cervix or urethra, stool samples, or tissue biopsies. Since viral antigen is present in cells, it is important that specimens from patients contain a sufficient number of cells. Methods to detect viral antigen may be either direct or indirect. With direct methods, fluorescein or an enzyme or a radiolabel (the indicator system) is conjugated to the antibody used to detect the virus (primary antibody). With indirect methods, the indicator system is conjugated to a secondary antibody (e.g., rabbit anti-mouse) which is in turn directed against the primary antibody (e.g., mouse McAb). The indirect method can be constructed to react with human IgG or IgM molecules for use in antibody assays. The major indicator systems include immunofluorescence assay (FA), enzyme immunoassay (EIA), and radioimmunoassay (RIA).

In the EIA procedure, an enzyme (e.g., peroxidase) conjugated to the detector antibody results in the change of a colorless substrate to a colored product which can be read by the naked eye or quantitated in an automated spectrophotometer. The EIA procedure can be adapted to perform (*a*) an enzyme-linked immunosorbent assay (ELISA) where an unlabeled antibody (the capture antibody) is bound to a solid phase (e.g., a latex bead or the bottom of a microtiter plate well) to "capture" the antigen and a second enzyme-labeled antibody is added to detect the captured antigen; or (*b*) immunoperoxidase (IP) methods to demonstrate specific viral antigen by light microscopy in tissues from biopsy or autopsy specimens or cells from viral cell cultures. Many commercial ELISA and FA kits are available to detect viral antigen in patient specimens or cell cultures or IgG or IgM antiviral antibody.

The major viral antigens that can be detected in direct patient specimens include (*a*) rotavirus and enteric adenovirus in stool specimens; (*b*) RSV, influenza A and B, the parainfluenza viruses, and the adenoviruses in respiratory specimens; (*c*) hepatitis B surface antigen (HBsAg) and HIV p24 antigen in serum; (*d*) HSV and VZV in vesicle/ulcer swab specimens; and (*e*) CMV in BAL specimens. The major viruses detected by the SVC/VAS method include CMV, HSV, RSV, and the influenza viruses and adenoviruses.

There are several *advantages* to viral antigen detection. First, specimen collection and transport conditions are less critical than for viral isolation. Second, antigen detection test results are available sooner than viral isolation, usually within hours. Third, the antigen tests can detect viruses that will not grow in commercially available cell culture systems (e.g., rotavirus, enteric adenovirus, HBV, HIV). Fourth, the antigen detection tests do not require cell culture laboratory equipment and trained personnel for performance. And finally, as mentioned above, there may be specimens in which viral infectivity has been lost (negative viral isolation results) but antigenicity has been preserved (true antigen-positive test).

There are also several *disadvantages* to viral antigen detection. First, there must be a good antiserum and test kit commercially available for the virus sought in the specimen. Examples of medically important viruses for which antigen detection systems are not yet available are Epstein-Barr virus (EBV), hepatitis A and C viruses, the enteroviruses, rubella, mumps, the arboviruses, and parvovirus B19. Second, a separate antigen detection test must be performed for each virus being sought. For example, with respiratory secretions, one test must be performed for RSV, another for influenza A, still another for influenza B, and so on. Finally, depending on the particular virus and antigen detection system available, the antigen test may be less sensitive and is always less specific than viral isolation.

Electron Microscopy

The initial identification of all the agents causing viral gastroenteritis involved electron microscopy (EM) (56–62). Antigen detection tests are available for two of the three most common causes of viral diarrhea: rotavirus (63, 64) and enteric adenovirus (65). The other agents require either EM or research laboratory serologic tests: Norwalk virus, astrovirus, calicivirus, or small round virus (57, 59). Other uses for EM include detection of herpesvirus particles in vesicle fluid (HSV or VZV) (66) or in brain tissue (HSV, CMV, EBV) (67). Although EM allows detection of viral particles within hours, there are several disadvantages. A large enough concentration of particles must be present in the specimen to allow detection, and the procedure is expensive and not widely available. In general, EM has been used where no other viral diagnostic method is available, and/or in institutions where there is someone with a particular interest in EM viral diagnosis.

DNA Probes

DNA probes are discussed in other chapters, thus aspects related to viral diagnosis are not covered in great depth here. Since single-stranded (ss) DNA binds only to its complementary DNA strand, DNA probes labeled with a detector (^{32}P, ^{131}I, an enzyme, or a potent antigen) should be *highly specific* in identifying DNA viruses (68–71). And through the use of the enzyme RNA-dependent DNA polymerase (reverse transcriptase or RT), double-stranded (ds) DNA for detection by DNA probes can be synthesized from RNA viruses. For some viruses, such as the *human papilloma viruses* (HPVs), growth in conventional cell culture systems is not possible, and antigen detection kits are not available (72–74). Detection of HPV DNA in cell smears or tissue biopsies from patients by in situ hybridization or dot blots (74) is the only method currently available for diagnosis.

With other viruses, such as *human immunodeficiency virus* (HIV), the traditional diagnostic virology methods are not optimal. Virus isolation must be done using lymphokine-stimulated lymphocyte cultures and may require 2 to 3 weeks for completion (75). Detection of HIV p24 antigen in serum appears to be insensitive in the early diagnosis of perinatally or postnatally-acquired AIDS (76–78). The antibody response to AIDS in children and adults may not occur for several months after the acute illness (77, 79), and maternal transplacental antibody may confound the serologic diagnosis of perinatal AIDS for up to 15 months (80). Detection of the viral genome offers several advantages for early and specific diagnosis. Unfortunately, the concentration of HIV proviral DNA in peripheral white cells is insufficient to detect by conventional DNA probe methods (75). The remarkable development of *polymerase chain reaction* (PCR) technology (81–84), has allowed 10^5- to 10^6-fold amplification of a defined segment of viral DNA (the target) so that DNA probes can then be used for detection. The use of PCR/DNA probe for HIV-specific DNA is ideal since accurate identification of the virus in a patient's white cells enables definitive diagnosis of a disease that has many implications for personal health, antiviral therapy, and transmission to exposed contacts. The major disadvantage of PCR for the diagnosis of HIV infections is the possibility of false-positive results, largely from cross-contamination between specimens or amplified product.

DNA probe kits are also commercially available for detection of HSV (38, 85–87), CMV (88–90) and HBV (91). However, there are some *problems* and *deficiencies* with PCR and DNA probe technology. In the absence of some form of amplification such as PCR, the concentration of viral genomes in direct patient specimens is too low to allow detection with adequate sensitivity. For example, the commercially available probes for HSV and CMV detected only 70 to 90% of virus isolation positive specimens (38, 86). One could logically assert that PCR amplification of the genome in patient samples could circumvent such low genome concentration and low sensitivity problems. However, this raises another issue in the accurate diagnosis of viral *disease*. With viruses such as HSV or CMV that are known to cause latent infection with periodic reactivation, it is important to distinguish between latency, asymptomatic shedding, and true viral disease. One could next argue that quantitation of the amount of virus in direct patient specimens would be of assistance: more virus in disease and less in asymptomatic shedding (92, 93). But currently it is technically difficult and demanding to perform *quantitative* PCR.

Since PCR results in 10^5 to 10^6 levels of amplification, even minor degrees of *cross-contamination* in the laboratory can cause *false-positive* results (81)—a significant concern in the accurate diagnosis of AIDS. Reducing the likelihood of contamination can be achieved by scrupulous attention to clean laboratory practices and by detection of the amplified product in a different location than the PCR amplification step and the preparation of reagents in still another location. However, the possibility of cross-contamination causing false-positive results still remains a concern.

Methods in addition to PCR that are under evaluation to improve the sensitivity and/or specificity of DNA probe detection include (*a*) target cycling or binding of the DNA target/probe complex to magnetic beads to decrease background noise, and (*b*) Q-β replicase amplification of MDV-1 (a special RNA molecule bound to the probe) to amplify the detector probe (69). Alternatives to PCR for nucleic acid amplification include ligase chain reaction (LCR) and self-sustained sequence replication (3SR) (69a).

It is hoped that continued technological advances will circumvent or substantially reduce many of the problems mentioned. If so, it may well be that detection of viral genomes in patient specimens with a high degree of sensitivity and specificity will become an important wave of the future in diagnostic virology.

Choice of Virus Detection Method

What are the important issues to be considered when choosing a particular method for detection of a given virus in clinical specimens? The use of an antigen detection system such as DFA or EIA can produce results within hours. But there may be problems with sensitivity and specificity of commercially available detection kits for low concentrations of viral antigen in direct patient specimens. In addition, there need to be reagents and a kit to detect the particular virus in question. The use of labeled DNA probes plus amplification of the targeted portion of the viral genome in clinical specimens offers many theoretical advantages for exquisite sensitivity and specificity, but this has not yet been translated into generally available commercial kits for use in the routine diagnostic virology laboratory. In addition, for probe technology to compete successfully with viral antigen detection and isolation of viruses in cell culture, such issues as turnaround time (TAT) for results and cost (both expense of reagents/kits and technical hands-on time) must be considered.

The major advantages to viral isolation include 100% specificity and availability of the live virus for further biological characterization (e.g., serotyping, antiviral resistance). The major disadvantages include the need for optimal storage and transport conditions and slower TAT. The use of the SVC/VAS methods has considerably shortened TATs to one to two days for many viruses, but this is still longer than antigen detection methods.

The particular method chosen may vary with the given virus, and it is likely that a combination of methods may need to be used. For example, it may be that an antigen detection method with less than optimal sensitivity and specificity but short TAT will be used for initial presumptive diagnosis, followed by definitive confirmation by viral isolation or DNA probe technology.

SEROLOGIC METHODS IN VIRAL DIAGNOSIS

There are *two major uses* for serologic methods in viral diagnosis: (*a*) to *diagnose* a current or recent acute viral infection; and (*b*) to determine *susceptibility* or *immunity* to a particular virus (e.g., VZV in a history negative health care worker exposed to a patient with chickenpox). Measurement of IgG antiviral antibodies is used to determine immunity, while quantitation of IgG or IgM antibodies can diagnose current or recent infection. Older serologic methods, such as neutralization (neut), complement fixation (CF), or hemagglutination inhibition (HI), measure only IgG or "total" antibodies, while the newer techniques, such as IFA or ELISA, can be modified to detect either IgG or IgM.

From a clinical or virologic standpoint, there are several situations where a *serologic diagnosis* is necessary or more *useful* than the virologic approach. First, the infectious virus or viral product (antigen, nucleic acid) is not readily available from the patient. A good example would be arbovirus infections of the CNS, where viremia has cleared by the time the patient presents with encephalitis, and clinicians would not want to perform a brain biopsy to define the etiologic agent. Second, specimens from the patient containing virus are available but the virus won't grow or is difficult to grow in cell culture and tests for viral antigen or nucleic acid are not available. Good examples here include EBV, hepatitis A and C, rubella, and parvovirus B19. Finally, serologic tests are more useful when the incubation period is prolonged (e.g., 3 to 6 weeks) and antibody is already present in the circulation when the patient presents with illness.

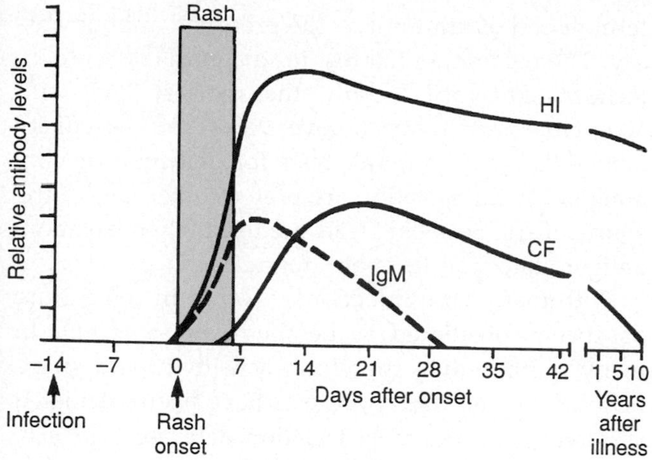

Figure 54.1. Antibody responses during acute measles. *HI*, hemagglutination inhibition antibody; *CF*, complement fixation antibody. (Centers for Disease Control. Measles: United States. MMWR 1982;31:402.)

Examples here include EBV and CMV mononucleosis and viral hepatitis.

Figure 54.1 shows a *typical antibody response* to acute measles. A similar response would be expected with virtually any acute, short incubation period (i.e., several days to 2 weeks), viral illness. At the onset of the rash or other illness, antibody is undetectable or low titer. Within 10 days to 2 weeks, appreciable titers of antibody are detectable. With older serologic assays that measure IgG antibody, such as hemagglutination inhibition (HI) or complement fixation (CF), a 4-fold or greater rise in titer between acute and convalescent sera (e.g., < 1:8 to 1:256) enables a diagnosis of measles.

With IgG antibody assays, a 4-fold fall in titer is presumptive evidence of a relatively recent infection, while unchanging low titers would be evidence against recent infection and indicate infection in the past (immunity). The presence of high titer antibody in a single convalescent phase serum specimen is not usually sufficient to enable a definitive diagnosis. Note that CF antibody titers rise later, reach lower levels, and may disappear several years after the acute illness. Alternatively, the presence of measles-specific IgM antibody in a single serum obtained 1 to 2 weeks after onset of illness also enables a diagnosis of measles. Typically, the IgM antibody disappears from the serum within a few weeks to a few months after the acute illness.

Many laboratories are now using ELISA kits to measure antibody titers. Results are reported in *optical density* (OD) units, rather than dilutions of serum (e.g., 1/8, 1/256, etc.). The OD units may vary, depending on the particular ELISA kit used and the given virus. In order to interpret results, therefore, reference range units must be provided by the performing laboratory: no detectable antibody or negative; low-, mid-, or high-positive.

The traditional dogma about the *IgM test* is that a positive result on a single serum specimen obtained during convalescence is diagnostic of a current or recent infection. Importantly, however, there can be false-positive and false-negative results. *False-positive* results can occur when there is cross-reactivity, particularly among the herpesviruses (94). Another major factor causing false-positive results is the presence of rheumatoid factor (RF) in the serum (95, 96). RF is an IgM antibody that binds to the Fc portion of IgG. So if RF and specific IgG antibody are present in the same serum sample, the IgG binds to the viral antigen and the IgM RF to the IgG, giving a positive test result. Because of the known false-positive IgM test results from RF, a number of the commercially available kits either contain or offer reagents which will remove IgG from the serum. With certain viruses (e.g., EBV), IgM antibody can persist in the serum of some patients for several months after the acute illness (97). Finally, with viruses that are known to cause latent infection (e.g., HSV and CMV), reactivation can result in the production of IgM antibody (98, 99). So, in these latter two examples, presence of IgM antibody can represent acute infection months earlier or reactivated latent infection, rather than an acute, recent, primary infection.

False-negative IgM tests can occur because of no or a low IgM response or a delay in the IgM response, particularly in the immunologically immature host (e.g., the neonate with congenital CMV or HIV infection) or in immunosuppressed patients (e.g., AIDS patients) (99–101). False-negative IgM tests can also occur when high-titer IgG antibody in the serum binds to all the viral antigen sites in the kit and prevents adsorption of IgM molecules (competitive inhibition) (95). In summary, although IgM tests may be very useful in the diagnosis of an acute viral infection, both positive and negative results must be interpreted with caution.

The major viruses where serologic tests provide the most useful or only means for diagnosis of acute infection are listed in Table 54.4.

When using IgG antibody tests to determine susceptibility or *immunity* to a particular virus, it is important to use the *most sensitive method* to detect antibody. As shown in Figure 54.1, CF antibody titers are much lower than HI levels, and may disappear after several years. Therefore, no detectable CF antibody may not indicate susceptibility. Studies on patients with VZV infections (102) demonstrated this finding.

The major *advantages* to serologic diagnosis of viral infections include (*a*) the serum is easy to obtain; (*b*) serologic tests are widely available; and (*c*) the specimen can be transported easily. The major *disadvantages* include (*a*) tests for IgG antibody require acute and convalescent sera; (*b*) tests for IgM antibody can have false-positive and false-negative results; and (*c*) most importantly, there is usually a delay of 2 to 3 weeks before a diagnosis can be made with short incubation period infections.

OPTIMAL TESTS FOR SPECIFIC VIRUSES

Table 54.5 lists the medically important viruses, together with the recommended tests for viral diagnosis: (*a*) for acute infection diagnosis—proper specimens, the optimal test for rapid and accurate results, and the usual turnaround time (TAT); and (*b*) for determination of immunity—the preferred antibody assay. The recommended test for diagnosis of acute infection takes into account the shortest TAT with acceptable sensitivity (above 90%) and specificity (above 95%). In general, tests for detection of viral antigen or viral isolation are preferred because of the shorter TAT. Serologic tests are used when isolation/antigen detection tests are not available.

With many viral infections, *isolation* in cell culture has been considered to be the *"gold standard."* In many publications, therefore, sensitivity and specificity of antigen detection tests have been calculated assuming that the viral isolation data are "correct" (100% sensitive and 100% specific). However, this may not always be the case, since specimen collection, storage, and/or transport conditions may not have been optimal with resultant loss in viral infectivity but preservation of antigenicity. Assuming viral isolation results are the gold standard, therefore, would overestimate the sensitivity of isolation but underestimate the sensitivity of antigen detection. In the results summarized for individual viruses below, there has been an attempt (where the reporting of the data allows) to determine *total true positive* specimens: virus isolation positive, plus virus isolation negative but two antigen detection tests positive (e.g., DFA and ELISA). True negative specimens

Table 54.4. Major Viruses—Serologic Diagnosis

Virus	Test	Comment
EBV	Mono spot VCA IgM	DNA probe in research labs
Hepatitis A, B, C, D	ELISA tests IgG, IgM	Antigen tests for B, D
Measles Rubella Mumps	ELISA tests IgG, IgM	Culture available but tedious, long delay
Arbovirus encephalitis	IgG tests	Brain not available, for culture, antigen
Parvovirus B19	IgG, IgM tests	DNA probe in research labs
Respiratory viruses	IgG tests	Useful when antigen, culture negative

Table 54.5. Most Rapid, Expedient, Sensitive, and Specific Test for Viral Diagnosis

Virus Group, Virus	Diagnose Acute Infection: Specimen	Test	Time[a]	Determine Immunity[b]	Comments
Herpesviruses					
Herpes simplex virus (HSV)	Vesicle/ulcer/eye/ NP/mouth swab, CSF, Periph WBCs[e], Tissue biopsy	Culture in shell vial	16 hr	ELISA[c] FA[d]	Encephalitis a special problem in diagnosis
Cytomegalovirus (CMV)	Urine, BAL[f], NP aspirate, Periph WBCs, Tissue biopsy	Culture in shell vial	24–48 hr to 10 days	ELISA FA	Asymptomatic shedding vs. true infection
Epstein-Barr virus (EBV)	Serum	Monospot VCA IgM	1–2 days	VCA[g]	May need to repeat test
Varicella-zoster virus (VZV)	Vesicle/ulcer swab	Culture in shell vial	3 days	ELISA FAMA[h]	CF antibody low sensitivity to determine immunity
Human herpes virus type 6 (HHV-6)	Serum	Anti-HHV-6 IgM	1–3 days	ELISA	
Respiratory viruses					
Respiratory syncytial virus (RSV)	NP aspirate Trach. asp. Throat swab	Antigen ELISA DFA Culture	4 hr 6 days	ELISA	For all respiratory viruses, may diagnose acute infection by acute and convalescent sera for IgG antibody titers
Influenza A, B	NP aspirate Trach. asp. Throat swab	Antigen DFA Culture	3 hr 7 days	ELISA HI[i]	
Parainfluenza 1, 2, 3	NP aspirate Trach. asp. Throat swab	Antigen DFA Culture	3 hr 7 days	ELISA HI	

Table 54.5.—*continued*

Virus Group, Virus	Diagnose Acute Infection: Specimen	Test	Time[a]	Determine Immunity[b]	Comments
Respiratory viruses—*continued*					
Adenovirus	NP aspirate Trach. asp. Throat/eye swab	Culture Antigen DFA ELISA	7 days 3 hr	ELISA	
Hepatitis viruses					
Hepatitis A	Serum	Anti-HAV IgM	2 days	Anti-HAV IgG	Culture not available for any of the hepatitis viruses
Hepatitis B	Serum	HBsAg Anti-HBc IgM	2 days	Anti-HBs	
Hepatitis C	Serum	Anti-HCV ELISA Confirmatory Immunoblot	2 days 10 days	Unknown	
Hepatitis D	Serum	HDag Anti-HDV IgM	2 days	Unknown	
Gastroenteritis viruses					
Rotavirus	Stool	Antigen ELISA LATEX	3 hr	Research	Culture not available for these GE viruses
Enteric adenovirus	Stool	Antigen ELISA	3 hr	Research	
Enteroviruses Coxsackie Echo Polio	NP/throat swab, CSF, Peripheral WBCs, Stool	Culture	6 days	Neutral antibody	Neutralizing antibody test not widely available
Measles	Serum: acute, 10 days–2 wk post onset	Anti-measles IgG IgM	2 days	ELISA IFA	Culture available but time consuming
Rubella	Serum: acute, 10 days–2 wk postonset	Anti-rubella IgG IgM	2 days	ELISA IFA	Culture difficult and time consuming
Mumps	Serum: acute, 10 days–2 wk postonset	Anti-mumps IgG IgM	2 days	ELISA IFA	Culture available but time consuming
Human immunodeficiency virus (HIV)	Serum	Anti-HIV ELISA Western immunoblot p24 antigen	2 days 2 days 2–4 days	Unknown	
	Peripheral WBCs	Culture for HIV PCR,DNA probe	3 wk 5 days		
Arbovirus encephalitis	Acute and convalesent sera	Antibody CF	2–5 days	IFA CF	
Colorado tick fever	Blood clot	Culture: mouse inoculation	2 wk	Research	Available in state health labs
Parvovirus B19	Serum	Anti-parvo IgM	2–3 days	ELISA RIA	Not widely available
	Periph WBCs	PCR[j]	2 wk		

[a]Mean time from receipt of specimen in the laboratory to positive test results.
[b]Serum specimen for IgG antibody, using the test method indicated.
[c]ELISA, enzyme-linked immunosorbent assay.
[d]FA, immunofluorescence assay. DFA, direct FA. IFA, indirect FA.
[e]EDTA, anticoagulated peripheral blood for culture of white cells (buffy coat).
[f]BAL, bronchoalveolar lavage.
[g]VCA, viral capsid antigen.
[h]FAMA, immunofluorescence assay against membrane antigen.
[i]hemagglutination inhibition.
[j]PCR, polymerase chain reaction.

would be the remainder of the samples. Sensitivity and specificity calculations are based on the true positive and true negative specimens.

Herpes Simplex Virus

The major illnesses associated with herpes simplex virus (HSV) are herpes gingivostomatitis (primary oral), herpes labialis (recurrent oral), primary and recurrent genital herpes, primary and recurrent herpes conjunctivitis/keratitis, herpes encephalitis, and neonatal herpes. Most lesions can be sampled with a swab: vesicles or ulcers on the skin or mucous membranes, inflammation of the conjunctiva, cervix, or urethra. Other samples include buffy coat when viremia is suspected (e.g., neonatal herpes, disseminated disease in immunosuppressed hosts), CSF in meningitis complicating primary genital herpes and in neonatal herpes, and tissue biopsies in selected situations. With mucocutaneous vesicles or ulcers, it is important to sample lesions as early as possible in the course of the lesion (103). In our diagnostic virology laboratory, use of the SVC/VAS method in mink lung cell enables detection by the next day (16 to 24 hours), of 96% of the culture positives, with 100% specificity, compared with total cultures positive by CPE over 5 days (42, author's unpublished observations). Routine CPE in a sensitive cell line detects 50% of the positives in 24 hours; 80% in 48 hours; and 95% at 72 hours (104). Importantly, culture is not 100% sensitive. In a study of genital herpes lesions, culture was 80% sensitive, while DFA on cells scraped from the base of lesions was 79% sensitive (105). Both were 100% specific.

Recently, two promising *antigen detection* systems that can provide results within hours have been marketed. Sensitivity is approximately 80% and specificity 100% as compared with culture (106, 107). Unfortunately, results with asymptomatic shedding and resolving lesions that contain less virus are not as promising (sensitivity 60 to 75%), so these kits would be less useful in situations where there is a genuine need for rapid and accurate testing for HSV. For example, sampling vaginal secretions at the time of labor assists in decisions about cesarean section to prevent neonatal herpes.

Herpes encephalitis presents a particular diagnostic problem. In untreated patients, mortality is 70%, and severe neurologic sequelae occur in over 95% of survivors (108–110). Intravenous acyclovir (ACV) therapy has reduced mortality to 30% with 50% of survivors recovering normally (108). Patients with herpes encephalitis typically have focal neurologic clinical features or evidence of focal temporal lobe lesions on neurodiagnostic studies. However, approximately 50% of patients who present with focal disease have diagnoses other than herpes encephalitis (e.g., stroke, brain tumor, enteroviral meningoencephalitis, tuberculous meningitis, etc.) (111, 112). The current definitive means for establishing a diagnosis of herpes encephalitis is a brain biopsy of the involved site, with isolation of infectious virus or demonstration of viral antigen (67).

Although current management of patients with focal encephalitis remains controversial (113–115), most clinicians will initiate ACV therapy without a biopsy and progress to invasive diagnostic procedures only in patients who worsen on therapy or whose clinical course and/or neurodiagnostic studies are atypical. Clearly, this is a situation where an accurate, noninvasive, diagnostic test would be preferable. Routine virologic studies of CSF have not been rewarding. HSV has been isolated from only 4% of CSF specimens from biopsy-proven cases (67). Studies examining altered CSF/serum anti-HSV antibody ratios (67, 116–119), HSV-specific IgM in the CSF (118), antibody against HSV-1 glycoprotein B in CSF (120, 121), and HSV-1 antigen in CSF (122) have yielded results diagnostic of HSV infection of the CNS, but CSF specimens obtained very early in the course of illness were unlikely to be positive. In general, CSF samples obtained 10 days to 2 weeks into the illness were required to have positive results in the majority of patients. Recently, however, promising results have been obtained on CSF samples obtained in the first several days of illness by using PCR to amplify the HSV genome and a labeled DNA probe for detection (123–123c). The PCR/DNA probe results were obtained in a research laboratory, and it is hoped that such testing will become commercially available in the near future.

Although *HSV antibody* can be demonstrated in the serum of patients who have recovered from primary infection, it has little relevance as a measure of immunity because of latency and reactivation in recurrent lesions of the lips, genitalia, eyes, and other skin sites (124). On the other hand, studies of HSV-2 type specific antibody (directed against glycoprotein G, a type-specific antigen) have provided important information about the frequency of and risk factors for infection with this virus, and the likely occurrence of asymptomatic primary infections (125). Importantly, commercially available FA and ELISA antibody assays, even when tested against HSV-1 and HSV-2 antigens, do not discriminate cleanly among individuals infected with HSV-1 only, HSV-2 only, or both viruses (126, 126a). HSV-2 type specific antibody assays could be used to screen at-risk pregnant women; those seropositive could be tested at the time of labor for shedding of HSV-2 in vaginal secretions (125).

Cytomegalovirus (CMV)

Significant clinical disease with CMV usually occurs only in immunologically immature hosts (congenital CMV disease) or in immunosuppressed patients (pneumonitis, chorioretinitis, colitis, hepatitis) (127, 128). Since CMV can be shed asymptomatically for months to years after primary infection (127), and can be reactivated asymptomatically during periods of immunosuppression (129), it is important to be able to distinguish between such asymptomatic shedding and true CMV disease. The major sites for asymptomatic shedding are urine, cervical secretions, semen, and, to a lesser extent, saliva and respiratory secretions (130). Although higher titers of virus are generally present during disease than during asymptomatic shedding, there may be considerable overlap. So quantitation or semiquantitation of the amount of CMV present in clinical specimens can be helpful (but not absolute) in the diagnosis of CMV disease (131).

The only situation where isolation of CMV from *urine* is of undisputed diagnostic value is specimens obtained from neonates during the first several days of life as evidence of congenital infection. In virtually all other situations, it is not possible to be certain whether CMV in urine represents primary infection, reactivation disease, or asymptomatic shedding. Hence, other types of clinical samples have been assessed to determine suitability for predicting CMV disease: bronchoalveolar lavage (BAL) specimens and peripheral white cells (buffy coat).

In *immunosuppressed patients*, such as organ transplant recipients or AIDS patients, diffuse *pneumonitis* is a frequent opportunistic infection associated with appreciable mortality and morbidity (132, 133). Etiologic agents include CMV, *Pneumocystis carinii*, HSV, the respiratory viruses, *Legionella pneumophila*, and a number of other bacterial and fungal agents. Since each agent requires different antimicrobial therapy, it is important to define etiology. Ganciclovir (GCV) has been licensed for treatment of CMV disease in immunosuppressed patients (134, 135), and therapy of CMV pneumonitis with GCV in combination with CMV hyperimmune intravenous immune globulin (IVIG) has been very promising (136–139). Since GCV has significant adverse effects (140), it is important to determine whether CMV in respiratory secretions represents lung disease or asymptomatic shedding.

Most medical centers perform BAL as the diagnostic procedure of first choice in defining the etiology of pneumonitis in immunosuppressed patients. There are differences of opinion on the accuracy of detection of CMV from BAL specimens in the diagnosis of *CMV pneumonitis*. Among three studies that compared results from BAL specimens with lung biopsy virologic and histopathologic evidence of CMV pneumonitis, one found virus isolation from BAL to be 95% sensitive (141), and the other two only 71 to 77% sensitive (131, 142). Two of the three found virus isolation to be 95 to 100% specific (141, 142) while the other demonstrated a specificity of only 50% (142). Of the two studies that examined CMV antigen in cells of BAL specimens by FA and McAb, one found an excellent correlation with CMV lung disease (100% sensitivity and specificity when more than 0.5% of cells demonstrated antigen) (131), while the other did not (59% sensitivity, 100% specificity) (141).

Whether other methods to measure the amount of CMV in BAL fluids will improve diagnostic accuracy remains to be determined. As a practical matter, clinicians will administer GCV to severely immunosuppressed patients (such as bone marrow transplant recipients) with pneumonitis and positive CMV cultures from BAL specimens, because the adverse consequences of withholding therapy in the presence of true CMV disease are unacceptable.

In several studies, isolation of *CMV* from *buffy coat* has been useful in the diagnosis of current CMV disease (130, 143–147) or as a predictor of future CMV pneumonitis in organ transplant recipients (129, 148). However, there may be both false-negative and false-positive results. For example, in renal transplant recipients, viremia was present in only 67% of patients with CMV disease, and was found in 12% of subjects without disease (149). Certainly the correlation of CMV isolation from blood with disease is much better than from throat swabs or urine (129), and the association may be stronger in patients with more severe immunosuppression (e.g., bone marrow and cardiac transplant recipients, AIDS) (128, 129, 146). Since CMV is found mainly in neutrophils, and to a lesser extent in monocytes (30), it is important to use leukocyte separation procedures that recover both neutrophils and mononuclear cells (32) in efforts to isolate CMV from the buffy coat.

The preferred method of culturing CMV from clinical specimens is *SVC/VAS*. In our diagnostic virology laboratory, 50% of ultimately positive specimens were detected in SVC/VAS system in 24 hours, and an additional 40% by 48 hours. The remaining 10% required a mean of 10.6 days to detect by conventional CPE, while the SVC/VAS positive specimens were detected in a mean of 7.7 days. A number of publications have demonstrated the superiority of the SVC/VAS system over conventional CPE in cell culture for urine and BAL specimens (45, 150, 151). However, with buffy coat specimens, use of the SVC/VAS system alone will miss 25 to 30% of positives

(150–153), so conventional tube culture must be used also with examination for CMV CPE for 3 to 4 weeks.

Investigators in Europe have demonstrated the diagnostic value of staining with McAb for CMV immediate early antigen (IEA) in polymorphonuclear neutrophils (PMNs) from the peripheral blood of immunosuppressed patients (152–156). CMV IEA was demonstrated either in cytospin preparations of PMNs harvested directly from patients blood (*CMV antigenemia*), or in shell vial culture inoculated with PMNs and stained after 2 days (154) or 4 to 6 days (152, 155, 156) in culture (*CMV viremia*). Tests for CMV antigenemia were positive in more specimens than CMV viremia. But antigenemia seemed to be specific for CMV infection, since positive specimens occurred only in patients with other laboratory evidence of CMV infection: isolation of CMV in urine or other blood specimens from the same patient, or demonstration of a CMV antibody response (155, 156). The CMV antigenemia was an earlier indicator of CMV infection than CMV viremia or viruria, or antibody response (155). A major disadvantage of the CMV antigenemia test is that blood samples should be processed shortly after collection for optimal results (156a), as this limits performance of the test to institutions that are in close proximity to a diagnostic virology laboratory that does the test. CMV antigenemia has not been explored extensively as a diagnostic method in the United States, but should be further evaluated.

Testing for CMV IgG antibody has not been particularly useful in the diagnosis of acute or reactivation infection because of the delay in results: seroconversion several days to a few weeks after onset of illness (155). In immunologically immature hosts or in immunosuppressed patients, the CMV IgM response during acute infection may also be delayed or may not occur at all. For example, CMV IgM antibody was present in the serum of only 70% of neonates proven to be congenitally infected by demonstration of viruria during the first few days of life (99).

The major uses of *CMV serology* in diagnostic virology laboratories, therefore, appear to be (*a*) to determine susceptibility or immunity in exposed or potentially exposed health care workers (157) or day care center personnel (158); (*b*) to identify CMV seronegative blood donors for high risk patients (e.g., premature neonates, organ transplant recipients); and (*c*) to diagnose CMV infections in organ transplant recipients who were seronegative prior to transplant (159, 160). Several of the commercially available ELISA or fluorescence-based IgG tests have acceptable sensitivity and specificity for this use (161–164).

Epstein-Barr Virus

The mainstay in the diagnosis of Epstein-Barr virus (EBV) infections is the Davidsohn modification (165) of the original Paul-Bunnell *heterophil antibody* test (166). During recovery from EBV infectious mononucleosis (IM), IgM antibodies are produced, which react with sheep red cells and cause agglutination. The Davidsohn modification was to demonstrate differential absorption: IM-associated heterophil antibodies are adsorbed by beef red cells but not guinea pig kidney cells. More recent modifications of the heterophil antibody test employ horse or beef red blood cell antigens, which are more sensitive and specific (97), and are attached to latex or other particles and constructed in a slide or card test format (167, 168).

Heterophil antibodies occur in approximately 85% of patients with the mononucleosis syndrome (169, 170) and usually disappear in a few weeks to a few months. Responses may be delayed in some individuals (169), so repeat testing may be required to confirm the diagnosis. Importantly, the heterophil test is negative in 70 to 80% of EBV infections in children under 4 years of age (171, 172), so EBV-specific antibody tests are required for accurate diagnosis in this age group. Also important is the fact that sheep or horse red blood cell heterophil antibodies may persist for over a year after acute illness in 20 to 70% of patients (97). This persistence of heterophil positivity can result in the erroneous diagnosis of recurrent or "chronic" IM. In cases of *heterophil-negative* mononucleosis, CMV is the cause in 70% and EBV (proven by EBV-specific serology) in 16%, while rubella, toxoplasma, and adenovirus are rare causes (173).

In several situations, EBV-specific serologic tests may need to be performed: (*a*) when heterophil antibody testing is negative in patients with clinical mononucleosis and EBV disease is strongly suspected; (*b*) in children under 5 with IM, where the heterophil test is insensitive; and (*c*) where the clinical picture of IM is atypical (169, 174).

The following EBV-specific antibody tests are commercially available: IgG and IgM against viral capsid antigens (VCA), anti–early antigen (EA), and anti–Epstein-Barr nuclear antigen (EBNA). The kinetics of the response to these antigens are shown in Figure 54.2. The most useful test in the diagnosis of acute IM is VCA IgM; it appears soon after the onset of symptoms, disappears after a few weeks to months, and is 91 to 98% sensitive and 99% specific in the diagnosis (97, 169). VCA IgG antibody titers are already elevated when patients become ill and persist for life, so are less useful for diagnosis of acute infection. Anti-EA antibodies rise early and disappear in a few months, while anti-EBNA appear late and per-

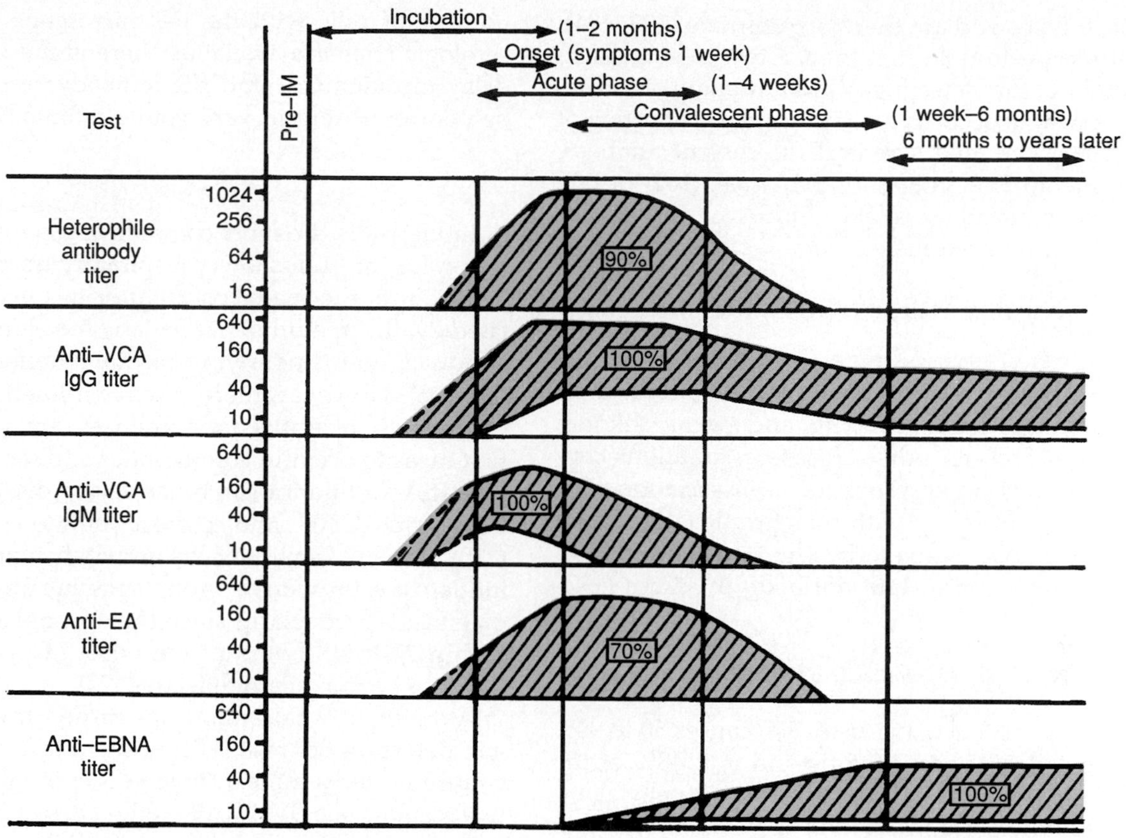

Figure 54.2. Antibody responses during EBV-induced infectious mononucleosis. (Modified from Sullivan JL. Epstein-Barr virus and the x-linked lymphoproliferative syndrome. Adv Pediatr 1983;30:365.)

sist for life in individuals who recover. In the individual who recovers from IM and is several months postacute illness, therefore, there would be moderate antibody titers to VCA IgG and EBNA, but low to absent titers against VCA IgM and EA (175).

In 1985 two papers were published describing what was called the chronic mononucleosis syndrome (176, 177). EBV was implicated as a cause based on (*a*) very high VCA IgG titers; (*b*) absent to low VCA IgM; (*c*) high anti-EA, and (*d*) absent to low anti-EBNA. Subsequent studies have demonstrated that EBV plays little or no etiologic role in this syndrome (178–182), and the name has been changed to the more appropriate "*chronic fatigue syndrome*" (CFS) (183, 184, 185). Many otherwise normal individuals have EBV antibody titers similar to those originally described in "chronic mononucleosis" (178), and most individuals with CFS do not have the "classic" chronic EBV titers (180). The cause(s) for the CFS remain(s) elusive (181, 183, 184). There is no specific diagnostic test, so the diagnosis remains one of exclusion (184).

Direct tests for EBV, such as cultivation in cord blood leukocytes (186) or detection of the genome by DNA probe (187), are performed in research laboratories, but are not yet available in a commercial kit.

EBV may rarely cause or contribute to acute fulminant disease: the X-linked lymphoproliferative syndrome (188) and the virus-associated hemophagocytic syndrome (189). Heterophil and EBV antibodies may be absent, so diagnosis depends on demonstration of the virus by culture or DNA probe.

Varicella Zoster Virus

The diagnosis of chickenpox or herpes zoster can usually be made clinically. In the selected instances where laboratory diagnosis is important, virus can be cultured from vesicle fluid and viral antigen can be demonstrated in cells scraped from the base of lesions (47). Infectious virus is quite labile. As much *clear* vesicle fluid should be aspirated as possible, mixed with a small volume of cell culture media (0.5 to 1.0 ml), and transported to the virology laboratory quickly. Isolation of the virus requires about 4 to 6 days. The DFA with McAb to varicella zoster virus (VZV) antigen is 92% sensitive (47).

VZV serologic tests are used usually to determine susceptibility or immunity: e.g., in a health care worker with no history of varicella, who is exposed to a patient with chickenpox or who wants to receive the varicella vaccine (190–192). Interestingly, 90% of such history-negative health care workers do have

VZV antibodies and are therefore immune (193, 194). It is important to note that the CF test is an insensitive method for detecting VZV antibody, as false-negative results occur in an appreciable proportion of cases (102). The gold standard fluorescent antibody against membrane antigen (FAMA) test (102) or one of the commercially available ELISA or IFA assays (195) should be used instead.

Human Herpesvirus Type 6

Human herpesvirus type 6 (HHV-6) is now known to cause *roseola* or exanthem subitum, a febrile illness with rash in infants and young children (196). The search for other disease associations continues. There is no evidence for an association with Kawasaki syndrome or with the chronic fatigue syndrome. Diagnosis is made by the demonstration of IgG seroconversion or IgM antibody in serum (197–200).

Respiratory Syncytial Virus

Respiratory syncytial virus (RSV) causes 50 to 90% of the episodes of bronchiolitis and 5 to 40% of the cases of pneumonitis in infants (201). Virtually all infants or toddlers are infected by 2 years of age, and approximately 1% of infants are hospitalized during the first year of life because of RSV-related disease (201). Infants with cyanotic congenital heart disease (CHD), particularly if they are on cardiac medications, and infants with chronic lung disease such as bronchopulmonary dysplasia (BPD), particularly if they are oxygen dependent, are at much greater risk for mortality and serious morbidity from RSV bronchiolitis or pneumonitis (202). The availability of aerosol ribavirin antiviral therapy for RSV has stimulated the need for rapid viral diagnosis (203, 204).

Since culture for RSV requires a mean of 5 to 7 days to positive results, attention has focused on rapid detection of *viral antigen* in respiratory secretions obtained by NP aspirate or nasal wash specimens. Two major approaches are available commercially: ELISA and DFA. For the most recently developed or modified ELISA kits, sensitivity is 71 to 94% and specificity 80 to 97%, while for DFA the figures are 83 to 92% and 95 to 97%, respectively (26, 48, 49, 50). The major advantages to ELISA include automation, objective end points that do not require a trained microscopist, and more efficient processing of a large number of specimens. There are membrane filter ELISA kits with individual tests for processing small numbers of specimens that have reported sensitivities of 86 to 91% and specificities of 91 to 96% (205, 206). The major advantages to DFA include greater sensitivity and specificity, and an ability to assess quality of the specimen by determining the number of cells with the FA microscope. Although serologic tests are available, there is the problem of delay in diagnosis, and the antibody response may be poor or absent in very young infants (207).

Influenza Viruses

Influenza is the most common cause for hospitalization for infectious lower respiratory tract disease in adults. It is the major contributor to pneumonia-related deaths in adults, particularly the elderly and individuals with underlying cardiopulmonary disease (19, 208). However, more cases of influenza occur in children than adults, and children are usually the first cases to occur in communities and families (209). Like RSV, influenza can cause severe disease in children with CHD and chronic pulmonary disease (210). The availability of the antiviral amantadine for influenza A provides a strong stimulus for rapid viral diagnosis, particularly since therapy must be begun within 24 to 48 hours of the onset of symptoms in order to be maximally effective (22).

As with RSV, attention has turned towards antigen detection for rapid diagnosis of influenza, since culture requires a mean time of 3 to 5 days for positive results. The SVC/VAS method has shortened the time for detection of influenza to 48 hours, but this procedure was only 37 to 60% sensitive compared with culture (51, 211). Initial evaluation of a rapid membrane-bound ELISA indicated a sensitivity of 100% and a specificity of 92% compared with culture and DFA (212). More recent results indicated sensitivity of only 50 to 70%, but similar specificity (212a, author's unpublished observations). Most studies of DFA using commercial reagents for influenza antigen in respiratory secretion cells have demonstrated low sensitivity (9 to 52%), but specificity 95% or greater (52, 211, 213, 214). Again, serology is available but results in a delay in diagnosis (19, 208).

Other Respiratory Viruses

There are less urgent needs to make a rapid diagnosis of parainfluenza or adenovirus infections, because of the lack of proven effective antiviral therapy. The time required for positive culture results is 4 to 6 days (53, 215, 216). DFA is available, but the sensitivity is low: 50 to 60% for the parainfluenza viruses and only 10 to 20% for the adenoviruses (52, 213).

Hepatitis Viruses

There are now five known hepatitis viruses—A, B, C, D, and E—a veritable alphabet soup of agents encompassing both DNA and RNA viruses. Only the first four are known to cause disease in the United

States. Hepatitis E virus (HEV), also known as epidemic or enteric-transmitted non-A, non-B hepatitis, is likely a member of the enterovirus group that causes outbreaks of fecal-oral spread hepatitis in developing countries (217, 218).

The annual number of cases of hepatitis reported to the CDC in 1989 were: A, 28,500, B, 23,200, and non-A, non-B (mostly C) hepatitis, 2,600 (219). The actual number of cases may be 5- to 10-fold higher. Hepatitis A virus (HAV) is the major cause of fecal-oral spread hepatitis in the United States (220), with outbreaks known to occur from contaminated food or water (221), or in closed settings such as day care centers (222). Most infections occur in young children, but these are usually asymptomatic. For hepatitis B and C, the major risk factors are similar: intravenous drug abuse (IVDA), homosexuality, sexual partner of a known chronic carrier, multiple sexual partners, recipient of blood or blood products, and health care workers exposed to blood (219). Hepatitis B virus (HBV) is a very important cause of perinatal transmission (223), but the frequency of maternal-fetal/neonatal transmission with hepatitis C virus (HCV) is not yet defined clearly (224). Prior to implementation of universal screening of blood donors for HCV, this virus was demonstrated to be the cause of 80% of posttransfusion hepatitis cases (225). Since hepatitis D virus (HDV) is known to infect only individuals with acute or chronic HBV infection, the risk factors for infection with HDV are very similar to those for HBV (226).

Chronic hepatitis is known to occur with B, C, and D, but not A (219). Cirrhosis is a known sequela of chronic hepatitis with all three viruses (219), but so far only B and C have been associated with hepatocellular carcinoma (227–230). Chronic B and C hepatitis have responded to therapy with human interferon (231, 232).

Table 54.5 lists the tests to diagnose acute hepatitis and to determine immunity for each of the four hepatitis viruses seen in the United States. In both acute and chronic hepatitis B, HBsAg and total anti-HBc are both present. Anti-HBc IgM is generally present in acute hepatitis, but absent in chronic disease. Presence of HBeAg and absence of anti-HBe antibody are markers of greater infectivity (increased likelihood of perinatal, sexual, and blood transfusion transmission) and a worse prognosis (greater risk of progression to chronic hepatitis, cirrhosis, and hepatocellular carcinoma) (233–235).

The remarkable effort to isolate and clone the gene of the major non-A, non-B hepatitis virus (236) and to express the nonstructural protein c100-3 in a bacterial vector (237) led to the identification and characterization of HCV and to the demonstration that this virus was the causative agent in the vast majority of cases of posttransfusion hepatitis (238). The c100-3 protein was used to develop a first-generation anti-HCV antibody assay. As this assay became more widely used, several limitations became apparent. Often the antibody could not be detected for months up to a year after the initial infection (225). Anti-HCV usually persisted in cases of chronic hepatitis, but often disappeared in individuals who experienced acute hepatitis with recovery (225). Finally, false-positive results were shown to occur in individuals with active autoimmune chronic liver disease (239). Development of the confirmatory immunoblot test for HCV antibody significantly reduced the problem of false-positive test results (239), but the other problems remained: delay in seroconversion and loss of antibody in individuals who recover (225, 240). Recently developed second-generation ELISA and immunoblot assays which incorporate HCV structural proteins appear to be more sensitive and specific, and antibody is detectable sooner after initial infection (240a). Finally, reverse-transcriptase PCR for HCV RNA in serum appears to be the most sensitive and specific test (240b, 240c), but commercial assays are not yet available.

Gastroenteritis Viruses

Viruses are the major cause of diarrheal disease worldwide. The most common agents are rotavirus, accounting for 30 to 40% of cases, Norwalk virus, 20 to 30%, and enteric noncultivatable adenoviruses, 5 to 15% (56–59, 62, 241). In the United States, rotavirus causes disease primarily in the infant/toddler age group during the winter months (242), while adenoviruses 40–41 involve the same age group year round (243). Norwalk virus is the most common cause of outbreak-associated gastroenteritis (GE) in older children and adults (58).

None of the GE viruses grow in conventional cell cultures, but all can be detected by EM (57). Commercial ELISA tests with over 95% sensitivity and specificity (56, 63, 64) are available to detect both rotavirus and enteric adenovirus.

Enteroviruses

Nonpolio enteroviruses (coxsackie A and B, echo) are the most common cause of hospitalization for febrile illness in infants under 2 months of age (244–246), and the most common cause of aseptic meningitis in older infants, children and adults (18, 247). Although there are not currently licensed antiviral agents for enteroviral infections, the ability to differentiate between bacterial sepsis/meningitis and enteroviral disease may allow the discontinuation of unnecessary diagnostic tests and antibiotic therapy and shortening of the duration of hospitalization (18, 248).

A group antigen common to all the enteroviruses has been sought (249, 250), and intensive efforts have been made to develop DNA probes to a conserved portion of the enteroviral genome (251–256), However, such methods for rapid diagnosis have not yet achieved sufficient sensitivity, specificity, and practicality for the usual diagnostic virology laboratory. The major means for laboratory diagnosis of enteroviral infections, therefore, remains isolation of virus in cell culture by examining for viral CPE. By using four different cell lines for isolation, presumptive diagnosis of coxsackie A versus coxsackie B versus echovirus can be made more quickly (257–259). The coxsackie B viruses grow best in buffalo green monkey cells, and coxsackie A and echo, in human rhabdomyosarcoma (RD) cells (259). The usual time for presumptive diagnosis by CPE is 4 to 7 days. Antibody titers are not usually performed for the enteroviruses, unless there is a need to prove an etiologic role with an isolate from the stool of a patient. In this instance, one must demonstrate a 4-fold or greater antibody titer rise in acute and convalescent sera that bracket the illness. At our diagnostic virology laboratory, however, we do offer two sets of neutralizing antibody titers against the enteroviruses: (*a*) the coxsackie B group (1–6), for use when there are illnesses typically caused by these viruses (e.g., myocarditis, pericarditis, pleurodynia); and (*b*) the four to five most frequent echovirus serotypes currently causing disease in the community. Again, acute and convalescent sera bracketing the illness are necessary for optimal diagnosis.

In recent studies of enteroviral infections in young infants, the following isolation rates were obtained from clinical specimens: stool, 80 to 85%; throat swab, 50 to 60%; CSF, 40 to 70%; and buffy coat 40 to 50% (260, 261). Although at first glance it would appear that stool is the preferred clinical specimen, there are two major problems. First, enteroviruses may be shed asymptomatically in the stool for weeks after an illness, so isolation from stool alone does not establish an etiologic role for current illness. One must also demonstrate seroconversion in acute and convalescent sera bracketing the illness. Second, live oral polio vaccine (OPV) can be shed in the stool for days to weeks after vaccine administration, and can result in a positive enterovirus isolation from a stool specimen (262). Stools should be avoided as clinical specimens for enterovirus culture in infants around the OPV administration ages (2, 4, 15–18 months, and school entry) (262). Isolation of an enterovirus from the throat is almost always associated with disease, and clearly recovery from CSF or blood is proof of an etiologic role.

Measles, Mumps, Rubella

Although each of these viruses can be cultured in conventional cell lines, it requires 7 to 10 days for measles and mumps and over 3 weeks for rubella (263–268). With measles virus, the use of the SVC/VAS method with commercially available mouse McAb has resulted in a sensitivity compared to routine culture of 78% at 1 to 2 days and 100% at 5 days (269). Direct staining for measles virus antigen with this same McAb was 100% sensitive compared with culture for NP swab specimens, but only 67% sensitive for throat swab and 85% for urine specimens (269).

The usual means for laboratory diagnosis of acute measles, mumps, and rubella is serologic: 4-fold or greater rise in IgG antibody in sera bracketing the illness or presence of virus-specific IgM antibody in a single early convalescent serum. Although the traditional serologic test is hemagglutination inhibition (HI) for IgG antibody, a number of FA and ELISA IgG and IgM kits are commercially available (266, 268, 270–274). Care must be used in interpreting positive IgM tests. The IgM antibody response may be delayed, so a negative test result does not rule out recent infection. If the diagnosis is strongly suspected, a repeat test should be performed 1 to 2 weeks later. False-positive results may also occur. Mumps IgM antibody has persisted for months after acute illness (275). IgM antibodies that cross-react with rubella have been found in patients with infectious mononucleosis (276), parvovirus B19 infection (277), and CMV infection (278). False-positive rubella IgM tests can be a particular concern in pregnant women (279). It may be wise, therefore, to confirm critical IgM positive results with (*a*) an IgM assay from another manufacturer; or (*b*) a 4-fold rise in IgG antibodies (278, 279).

Human Immunodeficiency Virus

Human immunodeficiency virus type 1 (HIV-1) is the cause of the acquired immune deficiency syndrome (AIDS) in the United States. The major diagnostic tests for AIDS are both serologic and virologic: ELISA and Western immunoblot for HIV antibody, ELISA for p24 antigen, culture of peripheral blood mononuclear cells (PBMC) for infectious virus, and use of PCR/DNA probes to detect HIV proviral DNA in PBMC (75, 280). Different laboratory diagnostic strategies are needed for the three most common situations where HIV infection is considered: (*a*) the adult or older child who presents with clinical features of AIDS or AIDS-related complex (ARC): weight loss or failure to thrive, persistent mucosal candidiasis, opportunistic infection or malignancy, etc.; (*b*) the infant with suspected AIDS, sometimes with knowledge that the mother is HIV seropositive; and (*c*) the individual exposed to someone infected with HIV, who wants to know if he or she has been infected (e.g., health care worker with needle-stick or blood exposure, individual with high-risk sexual contact).

The adult or older child who presents with features of AIDS or ARC has been infected with HIV for weeks to months and already has antibody to the virus in serum. The traditional approach in this situation is to order a screening ELISA, with a repeat ELISA in those positive, and for those with repeat positive ELISAs, a confirmatory Western blot (75, 280, 281). The sensitivity and specificity of the screening ELISA with confirmatory immunoblot test sequence are influenced by the type of patient population examined. In populations with a moderate to high prevalence of infection, the current ELISAs have excellent sensitivity (97 to 99%) and specificity (90 to 99%), and are quite reliable in the diagnosis of HIV infection (280). But in low-risk populations, such as blood donors with an expected prevalence of infection of 0.3%, up to 90% of positive results may be false-positive (280). The Western immunoblot measures the antibody response to nine HIV proteins or glycoproteins: gp160, gp120, p66, p55, p51, gp41, p31, p24, and p17 (280). Recent CDC criteria indicate that HIV infection is confirmed if there is a response to any two of the following: p24, gp41, or gp120/160 (282). A response to none of the HIV bands, of course, represents a negative test. If there is a response to some, but not all of the HIV antigen bands necessary to satisfy the CDC criteria, the result is said to be indeterminate, and repeat testing over the next 6 months is recommended. If a person's Western blot results remain indeterminate over a 6-month period, he or she should be considered *not* infected with HIV-1 (282). In low-risk populations, patients with screening ELISA positive and indeterminate Western blot results are rarely, if ever, infected with HIV on follow-up serum testing (283).

If the results of serologic testing are not definitive on a suspected AIDS or ARC patient where it is important to make a diagnosis quickly (e.g., to institute anti-HIV therapy), there are two additional approaches: testing for surrogate markers or testing for the virus directly. In the patient with high-risk behavior (e.g., intravenous drug abuse, sexual contact with a known HIV-positive person, etc.) and with clinical features strongly suggestive of ARC or AIDS, the presence of surrogate laboratory markers may help to make a presumptive diagnosis: low CD4 counts, lymphopenia, elevated β_2-microglobulinemia, neutropenia or thrombocytopenia not explained on any other basis, or hypergammaglobulinemia (280, 281). However, if surrogate markers are used, it is important to confirm the diagnosis with HIV-specific tests as soon as possible. Second, tests may be undertaken for p24 antigen, the HIV genome by PCR and DNA probes, or culture of PBMC for the virus (75). In the setting of the high-risk patient with clinical features of ARC or AIDS, the p24 antigen test is 99% specific (75, 280). The sensitivity of the antigen test varies according to the clinical disease status: 4% in asymptomatic patients, 56% in ARC patients, and 76% in AIDS patients (284). The tests for HIV genome and culture of virus are available only in research or tertiary referral commercial laboratories and take several days to a few weeks to perform (75), so results are not readily available for patient management.

In the infant with suspected AIDS whose mother is HIV seropositive, the presence of maternal transplacentally transmitted antibody confounds the interpretation of the screening ELISA or the Western immunoblot up to 15 months of age (281). In the *symptomatic* infant over 4 to 6 months of age, detection of p24 antigen (76) or the HIV genome by PCR (285), or culture of the virus from PBMC (286) are quite useful in making a definitive diagnosis. However, none of these three virologic tests is reliably positive in the 1- to 2-month-old *asymptomatic* infant born to a HIV seropositive mother (76, 285, 286). In the older infant or child born to a seropositive mother with clinical features strongly suggestive of AIDS (e.g., failure to thrive, developmental delay or loss of milestones, persistent oral or esophageal candidiasis, chronic diarrhea, acute systemic bacterial infection, opportunistic pneumonitis), the surrogate tests may strongly support the diagnosis: low CD4 cell counts that must be compared to norms for age (287), neutropenia or thrombocytopenia without another explanation, and hypergammaglobulinemia (281).

In the individual with a known HIV exposure, antibody to the virus may not be detectable for months (288), so serial testing will be required. Almost all immunocompetent individuals will be seropositive 6 months after exposure (77). Up to 50% of individuals may develop a mononucleosis-like syndrome 2 to 4 weeks after infection (289). P24 antigenemia may be present during the mononucleosis-like illness before the appearance of antibody (289, 290), but this disappears as antibody develops.

Arbovirus Encephalitis

The major arboviruses causing encephalitis in the United States are St. Louis encephalitis virus, accounting for 66% of total cases, California encephalitis, 19%; western equine encephalitis, 2%; and eastern equine encephalitis virus, < 1%, (291). The majority of cases of arbovirus encephalitis occur in the states with the largest mosquito populations: the coastal states, the Great Lakes regions, and the states bordering the Mississippi and Missouri rivers (292). As the names of the viruses suggest, there is great regional variation in the number of cases and the particular viruses causing disease.

Since viremia has usually cleared by the time patients come for medical attention and since brain biopsy is rarely indicated or performed, the virus or viral product is not available for direct detection. The diagnosis is made by demonstrating seroconversion on acute and convalescent sera bracketing the illness. Available assays include traditional CF tests and ELISA kits (293, 294).

Colorado Tick Fever Virus

Colorado tick fever (CTF) is limited to the Rocky Mountain states, and, as the name suggests, is transmitted by the wood tick *Dermacentor andersoni* (295). Typical features include a biphasic flu-like illness without respiratory symptoms, and an associated leukopenia. Viremia is prolonged and the virus is associated with red cells (296). Diagnosis is usually confirmed by mouse inoculation of disrupted blood clot material (297).

Parvovirus B19

This virus causes erythema infectiosum (EI or fifth disease) (298), aplastic crisis in patients with hemolytic anemia syndromes (299), persistent anemia in immunosuppressed patients (300), and abortion and fetal hydrops in pregnant women (301). The virus is not cultivatable with routine methods. Diagnosis of acute infection is made by detection of parvovirus DNA in serum or peripheral white cells (302, 303), or demonstration of IgG seroconversion or IgM antibody in serum (304). Post infection or immunity is determined by the presence of IgG antibody. Commercial kits have recently become available for parvovirus antibody titers (304a).

Perinatal Viral Infections

The major viruses infecting the fetus and newborn infant are CMV, rubella, HSV, enteroviruses, HIV, and HBV. HIV has already been discussed above, and HBV rarely results in acute disease in young infants. If we consider the four remaining viruses and the situations where infection results in *disease* in the fetus or newborn, CMV and rubella are usually acquired congenitally by transplacental transmission with symptoms present at birth; while HSV and enteroviruses are usually acquired during the birth process or postnatally with onset of symptoms several days to a few weeks after birth. Clinicians faced with a suspected perinatal viral infection in a neonate often request TORCH titers (T = toxoplasma, O = other, R = rubella, C = CMV, H = HSV) on the infant and mother. However, this is *not* an effective means to establish a rapid diagnosis. Routine TORCH titers measure IgG antibody that is passed transplacentally from mother to fetus. Since this is an active transport mechanism, the titer of virus-specific IgG antibody in the neonate may be 2-fold and occasionally 4-fold higher than in the mother. Antibody present in neonatal serum, therefore, could represent an infection in the mother during this pregnancy or months to years earlier. So mere presence of antiviral IgG antibody in the serum of a neonate or the mother after birth does not prove current active infection. Only when IgG antiviral antibody persists beyond 4 to 6 months of age in the infant (the usual time for maternal transplacental antibody to disappear), can one assume active infection in the fetus or neonate. The IgG TORCH titer approach, therefore, cannot make a diagnosis for 4 to 6 months.

The virologic approach or culture of virus is the most direct and rapid method for CMV, HSV, and enteroviruses. Suggested specimens include (*a*) for CMV, urine and buffy coat obtained in the first several days of life; (*b*) for HSV, swabs of mucocutaneous vesicles or ulcers or conjunctival lesions, CSF, and buffy coat; and (*c*) for enteroviruses, throat swab, CSF, buffy coat, and stool. Although rubella can be recovered from throat swabs and occasionally CSF (305), the virus isolation process is tedious and can require 3 to 4 weeks for confirmation.

An alternative approach to the diagnosis of congenital viral infections is the demonstration of IgM antiviral antibody in neonatal serum. IgM is not normally passed transplacentally, and its presence indicates current or recent infection in the neonate. As mentioned above, commercial tests for rubella, CMV, and HSV IgM are available. Since culture of rubella virus is delayed, the demonstration of rubella IgM in a neonate with features consistent with congenital rubella (e.g., small for gestational age, hepatosplenomegaly, petechiae, jaundice, cataracts, abnormal heart sound) would confirm the diagnosis. However, the anti-CMV IgM is positive in only 50 to 70% of neonates with congenital infection proven by isolation of virus from urine obtained within the first few days of life (99, 306). The use of IgM serology for rapid diagnosis of neonatal HSV infections is inappropriate, since it may be 2 to 3 weeks after infection before a response is detected (307).

SUMMARY

Rapid diagnosis of infections with all the viruses listed in Table 54.5 requires the use of a variety of virologic and serologic techniques. In general, virologic methods are used when clinical specimens readily available from the patient contain the virus. Serologic methods are used when virologic methods do not provide timely results or are not available and when the incubation period is long so that the patient already has antibody when presenting with illness. Among the virologic methods, antigen detection tests are preferred since results can be available within hours, but sensitivity and specificity must be sufficiently high to allow accurate conclusions. Finally, isolation of infectious virus is 100% specific and enables further biological characterization of the agent, and, if shell vial culture/viral antigen stain methods are available, can provide results within 1 to 3 days. Although it is the responsibility of the diagnostic virology laboratory personnel to choose the best test for diagnosis of each virus, it is also important for the clinician to understand the advantages and limitations of the methods used so that results can be properly interpreted.

References

1. Roberts FJ, Geere IW, Colman A. A three-year study of positive blood cultures with emphasis on prognosis. Rev Infect Dis 1991;13:34–46.
2. Dennehy PH. Rapid diagnosis of pediatric viral infections. Contemp Pediatr 1990;7:80–96.
3. Drew WL. Controversies in viral diagnosis. Rev Infect Dis 1986;8:814–824.
4. Richman DD. Developments in rapid diagnosis. Infect Dis Clin North Am 1987;1:311–322.
5. Spector S, Dankner WM. Rapid viral diagnostic techniques. Advan Pediatr Infect Dis 1986;1:37–59.
5a. Storch GA. The diagnosis of viral infections (review). Infect Dis Clin Pract 1993;2:1–20.
5b. Overall JC Jr. Is it bacterial or viral? Laboratory differentiation. Pediatr Rev 1993;14:251–261.
6. Menegus MA, Douglas RG Jr. Viruses, rickettsiae, chlamydiae, and mycoplasmas. In: Mandell GL, Douglas RG Jr, Bennett JE, eds. Principles and practice of infectious diseases. New York: Churchill Livingstone, 1990:193–205.
7. Yolken RH. Laboratory diagnosis of viral infections. In: Galasso GJ, Whitley RJ, Merigan TC, eds. Antiviral agents and viral diseases of man. New York: Raven Press, 1990: 141–181.
7a. Sokol DM, Demmler GJ. Rapid viral diagnosis. In: Feigin RD, Cherry JD, eds. Textbook of pediatric infectious diseases. 3rd ed. Philadelphia: WB Saunders, 1992:2369–2384.
8. Balows A, Hausler WJ Jr, Herrmann KL, Isenberg HD, Shadomy HJ. Manual of clinical microbiology. Washington, DC: American Society for Microbiology, 1991.
9. Lennette EH. Laboratory diagnosis of viral infections: principles and practice. New York. Marcel Dekker, 1992.
10. Schmidt NJ, Emmons RW. Diagnostic procedures for viral, rickettsial and chlamydial infections. Washington, DC: American Public Health Association, 1989.
11. Specter S, Lancz GJ. Clinical virology manual. 2nd ed. New York: Elsevier, 1992.
12. Galasso GJ, Whitley RJ, Merigan TC. Antiviral agents and viral diseases of man. New York: Raven Press, 1990.
13. Lietman PS, Fiddian P, Chapman SK. The Wellcome International Antiviral Symposium. Am J Med 1988;85:1–213.
14. Balfour HH Jr, Englund JA. Antiviral drugs in pediatrics. Am J Dis Child 1989;143:1307–1316.
15. Crumpacker CS II. Molecular targets of antiviral therapy. N Engl J Med 1989;321:163–172.
16. Montgomery JA. Approaches to antiviral chemotherapy. Antiviral Res 1989;12:113–132.
17. Chonmaitree T, Menegus MA, Powell KR. The clinical relevance of "CSF viral culture": a two-year experience with aseptic meningitis in Rochester, NY. JAMA 1982;247: 1843–1847.
18. Wildin S, Chonmaitree T. The importance of the virology laboratory in the diagnosis and management of viral meningitis. Am J Dis Child 1987;141:454–457.
19. Glezen WP, Couch RB. Influenza viruses. In: Evans AS, ed. Viral infections of humans: epidemiology and control. New York: Plenum, 1989:419–449.
20. Hall CB, Douglas RG Jr. Modes of transmission of respiratory syncytial virus. J Pediatr 1981;99:100–103.
21. Leclair JM, Freeman J, Sullivan BF, Crowley CM, Goldmann DA. Prevention of nosocomial respiratory syncytial virus infections through compliance with glove and gown isolation precautions. N Engl J Med 1987;317:329–334.
22. Tominack RL, Hayden FG. Rimantadine hydrochloride and amantadine hydrochloride use in influenza A virus infections. Infect Dis Clin North Am 1987;1:459–478.
23. Johnson FB. Transport of viral specimens. Clin Microbiol Rev 1990;3:120–131.
24. Bettoli EJ, Brewer PM, Oxtoby MJ, Zaidi AA, Guinan ME. The role of temperature and swab materials in the recovery of herpes simplex virus from lesions. J Infect Dis 1982;145:399.
25. Ahluwalia G, Embree J, McNicol P, Law B, Hammond GW. Comparison of nasopharyngeal aspirate and nasopharyngeal swab specimens for respiratory syncytial virus diagnosis by cell culture, indirect immunofluorescence assay, and enzyme-linked immunosorbent assay. J Clin Microbiol 1987;25: 763–767.
26. Masters HB, Weber KO, Groothuis JR, Wren CG, Lauer BA. Comparison of nasopharyngeal washings and swab specimens for diagnosis of respiratory syncytial virus by EIA, FAT, and cell culture. Diagn Microbiol Infect Dis 1987;8: 101–105.
27. Treuhaft MW, Soukup JM, Sullivan BJ. Practical recommendations for the detection of pediatric respiratory syncytial virus infections. J Clin Microbiol 1985;22:270–273.
28. Lennette DA. Collection and preparation of specimens for virological examination. In: Lennette EH, Balows A, Hausler WJ Jr, Shadomy HJ, eds. Manual of clinical microbiology. Washington, DC: American Society for Microbiology, 1985: 687–693.
29. McSharry JJ, Costantino R, Robbiano E, Echols R, Stevens R, Lehman JM. Detection and quantitation of human immunodeficiency virus-infected peripheral blood mononuclear cells by flow cytometry. J Clin Microbiol 1990;28:724–733.
30. Dankner WM, McCutchan JA, Richman DD, Hirata K, Spector SA. Localization of human cytomegalovirus in peripheral blood leukocytes by in situ hybridization. J Infect Dis 1990;161:31–36.
31. Prather SL, Dagan R, Jenista JA, Menegus MA. The isolation of enteroviruses from blood: a comparison of four processing methods. J Med Virol 1984;14:221–227.

32. Paya CV, Wold AD, Smith TF. Detection of cytomegalovirus from blood leukocytes separated by Sepracell-MN and Ficoll-Paque/Macrodex methods. J Clin Microbiol 1988;26:2031–2033.
33. Bayliss GJ, Jesson WJ, Mortimer PP, McLean KA, Evans BA. Cultivation of human immunodeficiency virus from whole blood: effect of anticoagulant and inoculum size on virus growth. J Med Virol 1990;31:161–164.
34. Vaheri A, Cantell K. The effect of heparin on herpes simplex virus. Virology 1963;21:661–662.
35. Johnson FB, Leavitt RW, Richards DF. Evaluation of the Virocult transport tube for isolation of herpes simplex virus from clinical specimens. J Clin Microbiol 1984;20:120–122.
36. Stagno S, Pass RF, Reynolds DW, Moore MA, Nahmias AJ, Alford CA. Comparative study of diagnostic procedures for congenital cytomegalovirus infection. Pediatr 1980;65: 251–257.
37. Yeager AS, Morris JE, Prober CG. Storage and transport of cultures for herpes simplex virus, type 2. Am J Clin Pathol 1979;72:977–979.
38. Fung JC, Shanley J, Tilton RC. Comparison of the detection of herpes simplex virus in direct clinical specimens with herpes simplex virus-specific DNA probes and monoclonal antibodies. J Clin Microbiol 1985;22:748–753.
39. Johnson FB, Leavitt RW, Richards DF. Comparison of the Scott Selecticult-HSV kit with conventional culture and direct immunoperoxidase staining for detection of herpes simplex virus in cultures of clinical specimens. J Clin Microbiol 1985;21:438–441.
40. Lipson SM, Schutzbank TE, Szabo K. Evaluation of three immunofluorescence assays for culture confirmation and typing of herpes simplex virus. J Clin Microbiol 1987;25:391–394.
41. Peterson EM, Hughes BL, Aarnaes SL, De La Maza LM. Comparison of primary rabbit kidney and MRC-5 cells and two stain procedures for herpes simplex virus detection by a shell vial centrifugation method. J Clin Microbiol 1988;26: 222–224.
42. Salmon VC, Turner RB, Speranza MJ, Overall JC Jr. Rapid detection of herpes simplex virus in clinical specimens by centrifugation and immunoperoxidase staining. J Clin Microbiol 1986;23:683–686.
43. Ashley R, Peterson E, Abbo H, Gold D, Corey L. Comparison of monoclonal antibodies for rapid detection of cytomegalovirus in spin-amplified plate cultures. J Clin Microbiol 1989;27:2858–2860.
44. Gleaves CA, Lee CF, Kirsch L, Meyers JD. Evaluation of a direct fluorescein-conjugated monoclonal antibody for detection of cytomegalovirus in centrifugation culture. J Clin Microbiol 1987;25:1548–1550.
45. Gleaves CA, Smith TF, Shuster EA, Pearson GR. Rapid detection of cytomegalovirus in MRC-5 cells inoculated with urine specimens by using low-speed centrifugation and monoclonal antibody. J Clin Microbiol 1984;19:917–919.
46. Randazzo DN, Michalski FJ. Comparison of antibodies for rapid detection of cytomegalovirus. J Clin Microbiol 1988;26: 369–370.
47. Gleaves CA, Lee CF, Bustamante CI, Meyers JD. Use of murine monoclonal antibodies for laboratory diagnosis of varicella-zoster virus infection. J Clin Microbiol 1988;26: 1623–1625.
48. Freymuth F, Quibriac M, Petitjean J, et al. Comparison of two new tests for rapid diagnosis of respiratory syncytial virus infections by enzyme-linked immunosorbent assay and immunofluorescence techniques. J Clin Microbiol 1986;24: 1013–1016.
49. Halstead DC, Todd S, Fritch G. Evaluation of five methods for respiratory syncytial virus detection. J Clin Microbiol 1990;28:1021–1025.
50. Johnston SLG, Siegel CS. Evaluation of direct immunofluorescence, enzyme immunoassay, centrifugation culture, and conventional culture for the detection of respiratory syncytial virus. J Clin Microbiol 1990;28:2394–2397.
51. Espy MJ, Smith TF, Harmon MW, Kendal AP. Rapid detection of influenza virus by shell vial assay with monoclonal antibodies. J Clin Microbiol 1986;24:677–679.
52. Stout C, Murphy MD, Lawrence S, Julian S. Evaluation of a monoclonal antibody pool for rapid diagnosis of respiratory viral infections. J Clin Microbiol 1989;27:448–452.
53. Espy MJ, Hierholzer JC, Smith TF. The effect of centrifugation on the rapid detection of adenovirus in shell vials. Am J Clin Pathol 1987;88:358–360.
54. Lim KA, Benyesh-Melnick M. Typing of enteroviruses by combinations of antiserum pools. Application to typing of enteroviruses (coxsackie and echo). J Immunol 1960;84: 309–317.
55. Chatis PA, Miller CH, Schrager LE, Crumpacker CS. Successful treatment with foscarnet of an acyclovir-resistant mucocutaneous infection with herpes simplex virus in a patient with acquired immunodeficiency syndrome. N Engl J Med 1989;320:297–300.
56. Centers for Disease Control. Viral agents of gastroenteritis. MMWR 1990;39:1–24.
57. Christensen ML. Human viral gastroenteritis. Clin Microbiol Rev 1989;2:51–89.
58. Dolin R, Treanor JJ, Madore HP. Novel agents of viral enteritis in humans. J Infect Dis 1987;155:365–376.
59. Fairchild PG, Blacklow NR. Viral diarrhea. Infect Dis Clin North Am 1988;2:677–684.
60. Flewett TH. Diagnosis of enteritis virus. Proc R Soc Lond [Biol] 1976;69:693–696.
61. Middleton PJ, Szymanski MT, Petric M. Viruses associated with acute gastroenteritis in young children. Am J Dis Child 1977;131:733–737.
62. Rodriguez WJ. Viral enteritis in the 1980s: perspective, diagnosis and outlook for prevention. Pediatr Infect Dis J 1989;8: 570–578.
63. Dennehy PH, Gauntlett DR, Tente WE. Comparison of nine commercial immunoassays for the detection of rotavirus in fecal specimens. J Clin Microbiol 1988;26:1630–1634.
64. Mathewson JJ, Winsor DK, DuPont HL, Secor S. Evaluation of assay systems for the detection of rotavirus in stool specimens. Diagn Microbiol Infect Dis 1989;12:139–141.
65. Herrmann JE, Perron-Henry DM, Blacklow NR. Antigen detection with monoclonal antibodies for the diagnosis of adenovirus gastroenteritis. J Infect Dis 1987;155:1167–1171.
66. Kimura A, Tosaka K, Nakao T. An electron microscopic study of varicella skin lesions. Archiv Gesamte Virusforsch 1972;36:1–12.
67. Nahmias AJ, Whitley RJ, Visintine AN, Takei Y, Alford CA, Collaborative Antiviral Study Group. Herpes simplex virus encephalitis: laboratory evaluations and their diagnostic significance. J Infect Dis 1982;145:829–836.
68. Engleberg NC. Nucleic acid probe tests for clinical diagnosis—where do we stand. ASM News 1991;57:183–186.
69. Siegler N. DNA-based testing: a progress report. ASM News 1989;55:308–312.
69a. Wolcott MJ. Advances in nucleic acid-based detection methods. Clin Microbiol Rev 1992;5:370–386.
70. Tenover FC. Diagnostic deoxyribonucleic acid probes for infectious diseases. Clin Microbiol Rev 1988;1:82–101.
71. Warford AL, Levy RA. Use of commercial DNA probes. Clin Lab Sci 1989;2:105–108.

72. Cripe TP. Human papillomaviruses: pediatric perspectives on a family of multifaceted tumorigenic pathogens. Pediatr Infect Dis J 1990;9:836–844.
73. Howley PM, Schlegel R. The human papillomaviruses: an overview. Am J Med 1988;85(suppl 2A):155–158.
74. Roman A, Fife KH. Human papillomaviruses: are we ready to type. Clin Microbiol Rev 1989;2:166–190.
75. Jackson JB, Balfour HH Jr. Practical diagnostic testing for human immunodeficiency virus. Clin Microbiol Rev 1988;1: 124–138.
76. Borkowsky W, Krasinski K, Paul D, et al. Human immunodeficiency virus type 1 antigenemia in children. J Pediatr 1989;114:940–945.
77. Horsburgh CR Jr, Jason J, Longini IM Jr, et al. Duration of human immunodeficiency virus infection before detection of antibody. Lancet 1989;2:637–640.
78. Schneweis KE, Ackermann A, Friedrich A, et al. Comparison of different methods for detecting human immune deficiency virus in human immunodeficiency virus-seropositive hemophiliacs. J Med Virol 1989;29:94–101.
79. Allain JP, Paul DA, Laurian Y, Senn D. Members of the AIDS-Haemophilia French Study Group. Serological markers in early stages of human immunodeficiency virus infection in haemophiliacs. Lancet 1986;2:1233–1236.
80. Falloon J, Eddy J, Wiener L, Pizzo P. Human immunodeficiency virus infection in children. J Pediatr 1989;114:1–30.
81. Eisenstein BI. The polymerase chain reaction: a new method of using molecular genetics for medical diagnosis. N Engl J Med 1990;322:178–181.
82. Mullis KB, Faloona FA. Specific synthesis of DNA in vitro via a polymerase catalyzed chain reaction. Methods Enzymol 1987;155:335–350.
83. Oste C. Polymerase chain reaction. Biotechniques 1988;6: 162–167.
84. Schochetman G, Ou C-Y, Jones WK. Polymerase chain reaction. J Infect Dis 1988;158:1154–1157.
85. Espy MJ, Smith TF. Detection of herpes simplex virus in conventional tube cell cultures and in shell vials with a DNA probe kit and monoclonal antibodies. J Clin Microbiol 1988;26:22–24.
86. Langenberg A, Smith D, Brakel CL, et al. Detection of herpes simplex virus DNA from genital lesions by in situ hybridization. J Clin Microbiol 1988;26:933–937.
87. Qadri SMH, Qadri SGM, Khan GY, McGarry TJ, Al-Ahdal MN. Detection of herpes simplex virus by biotinylated DNA probes. Diagn Microbiol Infect Dis 1988;11:145–149.
88. Gleaves CA, Hursh DA, Rice DH, Meyers JD. Detection of cytomegalovirus from clinical specimens in centrifugation culture by in situ DNA hybridization and monoclonal antibody staining. J Clin Microbiol 1989;27:21–23.
89. Hilborne LH, Nieberg RK, Cheng L, Lewin KJ. Direct in situ hybridization for rapid detection of cytomegalovirus in bronchoalveolar lavage. Am J Clin Pathol 1987;87:766–769.
90. Robey SS, Gage WR, Kuhajda FP. Comparison of immunoperoxidase and DNA in situ hybridization techniques in the diagnosis of cytomegalovirus colitis. Am J Clin Pathol 1988;89:666–671.
91. Valentine-Thon E, Steinmann J, Arnold W. Evaluation of the commercially available HepProbe kit for detection of hepatitis B virus DNA in serum. J Clin Microbiol 1990;28:39–42.
92. Brown ZA, Kern ER, Spruance SL, Overall JC. Clinical and virologic course of herpes simplex genitalis. West J Med 1979;130:414–421.
93. Guinan ME, MacCalman J, Kern ER, Overall JC Jr, Spruance SL. The course of untreated recurrent genital herpes simplex infection in 27 women. N Engl J Med 1981;304:759–763.
94. Nielsen CM, Hansen K, Andersen HMK, Gerstoft J, Vestergaard BF. An enzyme labeled nuclear antigen immunoassay for detection of cytomegalovirus IgM antibodies in human serum: specific and nonspecific reaction. J Med Virol 1987;7: 111–113.
95. Champsaur H, Fattal-German M, Arranhado R. Sensitivity and specificity of viral immunoglobulin M determination by indirect enzyme-linked immunosorbent assay. J Clin Microbiol 1988;26:328–332.
96. Salonen EM, Vaheri A, Suni J, Wager O. Rheumatoid factor in acute viral infections: interference with determination of IgM, IgG, and IgA antibodies in an enzyme immunoassay. J Infect Dis 1980;142:250–255.
97. Evans AS, Niederman JC, Cenabre LC, West B, Richards VA. A prospective evaluation of heterophile and Epstein-Barr virus-specific IgM antibody tests in clinical and subclinical infectious mononucleosis: specificity and sensitivity of the tests and persistence of antibody. J Infect Dis 1975;132:546–554.
98. Kuhn JE, Dunkler G, Munk K, Braun RW. Analysis of the IgM and IgG antibody response against herpes simplex virus type 1 (HSV-1) structural and nonstructural proteins. J Med Virol 1987;25:135–150.
99. Stagno S, Tinker MK, Elrod C, Fuccillo DA, Cloud G, O'Beirne AJ. Immunoglobulin M antibodies detected by enzyme-linked immunosorbent assay and radioimmunoassay in the diagnosis of cytomegalovirus infections in pregnant women and newborn infants. J Clin Microbiol 1985;21:930–935.
100. Frickhofen N, Abkowitz JL, Safford M, et al. Persistent B19 parvovirus infection in patients infected with human immunodeficiency virus type 1 (HIV-1): a treatable cause of anemia in AIDS. Ann Intern Med 1990;113:926–933.
101. Kahlon J, Whitley RJ. Antibody response of the newborn after herpes simplex virus infection. J Infect Dis 1988;158: 925–933.
102. Gelb LD. Varicella-zoster virus. In: Fields BN, Knipe DM, eds. Fields virology. New York: Raven Press, 1990:2011–2054.
103. Webb DH, Fife KH. Genital herpes simplex virus infections. Infect Dis Clin North Am 1987;1:97–122.
104. Salmon VC, Stanberry LR, Overall JC Jr. More rapid isolation of herpes simplex virus in a continuous line of mink lung cells than in vero or human fibroblast cells. Diagn Microbiol Infect Dis 1984;2:317–324.
105. Lafferty WE, Krofft S, Remington M, et al. Diagnosis of herpes simplex virus by direct immunofluorescence and viral isolation from samples of external genital lesions in a high-prevalence population. J Clin Microbiol 1987;25:323–326.
106. Dorian KJ, Beatty E, Atterbury KE. Detection of herpes simplex virus by the Kodak SureCell herpes test. J Clin Microbiol 1990;28:2117–2119.
107. Verano L, Michalski FJ. Herpes simplex virus antigen direct detection in standard virus transport medium by DuPont Herpchek enzyme-linked immunosorbent assay. J Clin Microbiol 1990;28:2555–2558.
108. Whitley RJ, Alford CA, Hirsch MS, et al. Vidarabine versus acyclovir therapy in herpes simplex encephalitis. N Engl J Med 1986;314:144–149.
109. Whitley RJ, Soong SJ, Dolin R, et al. Adenine arabinoside therapy of biopsy-proved herpes simplex encephalitis. N Engl J Med 1977;297:289–294.
110. Whitley RJ, Soong SJ, Hirsch MS, et al. Herpes simplex encephalitis: vidarabine therapy and diagnostic problems. N Engl J Med 1981;304:313–318.
111. Whitley RJ, Cobbs G, Alford CA, et al. Diseases that mimic herpes simplex encephalitis. JAMA 1989;262:234–239.
112. Whitley RJ, Soong SJ, Linneman C Jr, et al. Herpes simplex encephalitis: clinical assessment. JAMA 1982;247:317–320.

113. Fishman RA. No, brain biopsy need not be done in every patient suspected of having herpes simplex encephalitis. Arch Neurol 1987;44:1291–1292.
114. Hanley DF, Johnson RT, Whitley RJ. Yes, brain biopsy should be a prerequisite for herpes simplex encephalitis treatment. Arch Neurol 1987;44:1289–1290.
115. Wasiewski WW, Fishman MA. Herpes simplex encephalitis: the brain biopsy controversy. J Pediatr 1988;113:575–578.
116. Klapper PE, Laing I, Longson M. Rapid non-invasive diagnosis of herpes encephalitis. Lancet 1981;2:607–608.
117. Koskiniemi ML, Vaheri A. Diagnostic value of cerebrospinal fluid antibodies in herpes simplex virus encephalitis. J Neurol Neurosurg Psychiatry 1982;45:239–242.
118. Koskiniemi M, Vaheri A, Taskinen E. Cerebrospinal fluid alternations in herpes simplex virus encephalitis. Rev Infect Dis 1984;6:608.
119. Levine DP, Lauter CB, Lerner M. Simultaneous serum and CSF antibodies in herpes simplex virus encephalitis. JAMA 1978;240:356–360.
120. Grimaldi LME, Roos RP, Manservigi R, Spear PG, Lakeman FD, Whitley RJ. An isoelectric focusing study in herpes simplex virus encephalitis. Ann Neurol 1988;24:227–232.
121. Kahlon J, Chatterjee S, Lakeman FD, Lee F, Nahmias AJ, Whitley RJ. Detection of antibodies to herpes simplex virus in the cerebrospinal fluid of patients with herpes simplex encephalitis. J Infect Dis 1987;155:38–44.
122. Lakeman FD, Koga J, Whitley RJ. Detection of antigen to herpes simplex virus in cerebrospinal fluid from patients with herpes simplex encephalitis. J Infect Dis 1987;155: 1172–1178.
123. Rowley AH, Whitley RJ, Lakeman FD, Wolinsky SM. Rapid detection of herpes-simplex-virus DNA in cerebrospinal fluid of patients with herpes simplex encephalitis. Lancet 1990;335: 440–441.
123a. Aurelius E, Johansson B, Sköldenberg B, Staland A, Forsgren M. Rapid diagnosis of herpes simplex encephalitis by nested polymerase chain reaction assay of cerebrospinal fluid. Lancet 1991;337:189–192.
123b. Rozenberg F, Lebon P. Amplification and characterization of herpes virus DNA in cerebrospinal fluid from patients with acute encephalitis. J Clin Microbiol 1991;29:2412–2417.
123c. Aurelius E, Johansson B, Sköldenberg B, Forsgren M. Encephalitis in immunocompetent patients due to herpes simplex virus 1 or 2 as determined by type-specific polymerase chain reaction and antibody assays of cerebrospinal fluid. J Med Virol 1993;39:179–186.
124. Overall JC. Dermatologic viral diseases. In: Galasso GJ, Buchanan RA, Merigan TC, eds. Antiviral agents and viral diseases of man. New York: Raven Press, 1984:247–300.
125. Johnson RE, Nahmias AJ, Madger LS, Lee FK, Brooks CA, Snowden CB. A seroepidemiologic survey of the prevalence of herpes simplex virus type 2 infection in the United States. N Engl J Med 1989;321:7–12.
126. Ashley RL, Militoni J, Lee F, Nahmias A, Corey L. Comparison of western blot (immunoblot) and glycoprotein G-specific immunodot enzyme assay for detecting antibodies to herpes simplex virus types 1 and 2 in human sera. J Clin Microbiol 1988;26:662–667.
126a. Ashley R, Cent A, Maggs V, Nahmias A, Corey L. Inability of enzyme immunoassays to discriminate between infections with herpes simplex virus types 1 and 2. Ann Intern Med 1991;115:520–526.
127. Demmler GJ. Infectious Diseases Society of America and Centers for Disease Control: summary of a workshop on surveillance for congenital cytomegalovirus disease. Rev Infect Dis 1991;13:315–329.
128. Jacobsen MA, Mills J. Serious cytomegalovirus disease in the acquired immunodeficiency syndrome (AIDS). Ann Intern Med 1988;108:585–594.
129. Dummer JS, White LT, Ho M, Griffith BP, Hardesty RL, Bahnson HT. Morbidity of cytomegalovirus infection in recipients of heart or heart-lung transplants who received cyclosporine. J Infect Dis 1985;152:1182–1191.
130. Drew WL. Diagnosis of cytomegalovirus infection. Rev Infect Dis 1988;10(suppl 3):S468–S476.
131. Emanuel D, Peppard J, Stover D, Gold J, Armstrong D, Hammerling U. Rapid immunodiagnosis of cytomegalovirus pneumonia by bronchoalveolar lavage using human and murine monoclonal antibodies. Ann Intern Med 1986;104: 476–481.
132. Masur H, Shelhamer J, Parrillo JE. The management of pneumonias in immunocompromised patients. JAMA 1985;253: 1769–1773.
133. Rosenow E, Wilson WR, Cockerill FR. Pulmonary disease in the immunocompromised host. Mayo Clin Proc 1985;60: 473–487, 610–631.
134. Merigan TC, Lane HC. Cytomegalovirus infection and treatment with ganciclovir. Rev Infect Dis 1988;10(suppl 3):S457–S572.
135. Balfour HH Jr. Management of cytomegalovirus disease in antiviral drugs. Rev Infect Dis 1990;12(suppl 7):S849–S860.
136. Emanuel D, Cunningham I, Jules-Elysee K, et al. Cytomegalovirus pneumonia after bone marrow transplantation successfully treated with the combination of ganciclovir and high-dose intravenous immune globulin. Ann Intern Med 1988;109:777–782.
137. Frank I, Friedman HM. Progress in the treatment of cytomegalovirus pneumonia. Ann Intern Med 1988;109:769–770.
138. Reed EC, Bowden RA, Dandliker PS, Lilleby KE, Meyers JD. Treatment of cytomegalovirus pneumonia with ganciclovir and intravenous cytomegalovirus immunoglobulin in patients with bone marrow transplants. Ann Intern Med 1988;109:783–788.
139. Snydman DR. Cytomegalovirus immunoglobulins in the prevention and treatment of cytomegalovirus disease. Rev Infect Dis 1990;12(suppl 7):S839–S848.
140. Buhles WC, Mastre BJ, Tinker AJ, Strand V, Koretz SH, Syntex Collaborative Ganciclovir Treatment Study Group. Ganciclovir treatment of life- or sight-threatening cytomegalovirus infection: experience in 314 immunocompromised patients. Rev Infect Dis 1988;10(suppl 3):S495–S506.
141. Crawford SW, Bowden RA, Hackman RC, Gleaves CA, Meyers JD, Clark JG. Rapid detection of cytomegalovirus pulmonary infection by bronchoalveolar lavage and centrifugation culture. Ann Intern Med 1988;108:180–185.
142. Erice A, Hertz MI, Snyder LS, Englund J, Edelman CK, Balfour HH Jr. Evaluation of centrifugation cultures of bronchoalveolar lavage fluid for the diagnosis of cytomegalovirus pneumonitis. Diagn Microbiol Infect Dis 1988;10:205–212.
143. Armstrong D, Balakrishnan SL, Steger L, Yu B, Stenzel KH. Cytomegalovirus infections with viremia following renal transplantation. Arch Intern Med 1971;127:111–115.
144. Cheeseman SH, Rubin RH, Stewart JA, et al. Controlled clinical trial of prophylactic human-leukocyte interferon in renal transplantation. N Engl J Med 1979;300:1345–1349.
145. Fiala M, Payne JE, Berne TV, et al. Epidemiology of cytomegalovirus infection after transplantation and immunosuppression. J Infect Dis 1975;132:421–433.
146. Meyers JD, Flournoy N, Thomas ED. Risk factors for cytomegalovirus infection after human marrow transplantation. J Infect Dis 1986;153:478–488.

147. Vilmer E, Mazeron MC, Rabian C, et al. Clinical significance of cytomegalovirus viremia in bone marrow transplantation. Transplantation 1985;40:30–35.
148. Meyers JD, Reed EC, Shepp DH, et al. Acyclovir for prevention of cytomegalovirus infection and disease after allogeneic marrow transplantation. N Engl J Med 1988;318:70–75.
149. Pass RF, Whitley RJ, Diethelm AG, Whelchel JD, Reynolds DW, Alford CA. Cytomegalovirus infection in patients with renal transplants: potentiation by antithymocyte globulin and an incompatible graft. J Infect Dis 1980;142:9–17.
150. Paya CV, Wold AD, Smith TF. Detection of cytomegalovirus infections in specimens other than urine by the shell vial assay and conventional tube cell cultures. J Clin Microbiol 1987;25:755–757.
151. Rabella N, Drew WL. Comparison of conventional and shell vial cultures for detecting cytomegalovirus infection. J Clin Microbiol 1990;28:806–807.
152. Schirm J, Timmerije W, van der Bij W, et al. Rapid detection of infectious cytomegalovirus in blood with the aid of monoclonal antibodies. J Med Virol 1987;23:31–40.
153. Wunderli W, Kagi MK, Gruter E, Auracher JD. Detection of cytomegalovirus in peripheral leukocytes by different methods. J Clin Microbiol 1989;27:1916–1917.
154. Revello MG, Percivalle E, Zavattoni M, Parea M, Grossi P, Gerna G. Detection of human cytomegalovirus immediate early antigen in leukocytes as a marker of viremia in immunocompromised patients. J Med Virol 1989;29:88–93.
155. van der Bij W, Schirm J, Torensma R, van Son WJ, Tegzess AM, The TH. Comparison between viremia and antigenemia for detection of cytomegalovirus in blood. J Clin Microbiol 1988;26:2531–2535.
156. van der Bij W, Torensma R, van Son WJ, et al. Rapid immunodiagnosis of active cytomegalovirus infection by monoclonal antibody staining of blood leukocytes. J Med Virol 1988;25:179–188.
156a. The TH, van der Ploeg M, van den Berg AP, Vlieger AM, van der Giessen M, van Son WJ. Direct detection of cytomegalovirus in peripheral blood leukocytes—a review of the antigenemia assay and polymerase chain reaction. Transplantation 1992;54:193–198.
157. Balcarek KB, Bagley R, Cloud GA, Pass RF. Cytomegalovirus infection among employees of a children's hospital. JAMA 1990;263:840–844.
158. Pass RF, Hutto C. Group day care and cytomegalovirus infections of mothers and children. Rev Infect Dis 1986;8:599–605.
159. Adler S. Transfusion-associated cytomegalovirus infections. Rev Infect Dis 1983;5:977–993.
160. Bowden RA, Sayers M, Flournoy N, et al. Cytomegalovirus immune globulin and seronegative blood products to prevent primary cytomegalovirus infection after marrow transplantation. N Engl J Med 1986;314:1006–1010.
161. Gleaves CA, Wendt SF, Dobbs DR, Meyers JD. Evaluation of the CMV-CUBE assay for detection of cytomegalovirus serologic status in marrow transplant patients and marrow donors. J Clin Microbiol 1990;28:841–842.
162. Hursh DA, Abbot AD, Sun R, Iltis JP, Rice DH, Gleaves CA. Evaluation of a latex particle agglutination assay for the detection of cytomegalovirus antibody in patient serum. J Clin Microbiol 1989;27:2878–2879.
163. Leland DS, Barth KA, Cunningham EB, Jansen J, Tricot GJ, French MLV. Evaluation of four methods for cytomegalovirus antibody detection for use by a bone marrow transplantation service. J Clin Microbiol 1989;27:176–178.
164. Schaefer L, Cesario A, Demmler G, et al. Evaluation of Abbott CMV-M enzyme immunoassay for detection of cytomegalovirus immunoglobulin M antibody. J Clin Microbiol 1988;26:2041–2043.
165. Davidsohn I. Serologic diagnosis of infectious mononucleosis. JAMA 1937;108:289–295.
166. Paul JR, Bunnell WW. The presence of heterophile antibodies in infectious mononucleosis. Am J Med Sci 1932;183:90–104.
167. Kim M, Wadke M. Comparative evaluation of two test methods (enzyme immunoassay and latex fixation) for the detection of heterophil antibodies in infectious mononucleosis. J Clin Microbiol 1990;28:2511–2513.
168. Tilton RC, Dias F, Ryan RW. Comparative evaluation of three commercial tests for detection of heterophile antibody in patients with infectious mononucleosis. J Clin Microbiol 1988;26:275–278.
169. Fleisher GR, Collins M, Fager S. Limitations of available tests for diagnosis of infectious mononucleosis. J Clin Microbiol 1983;17:619–624.
170. Henle W, Henle GE, Horwitz CA. Epstein-Barr virus specific diagnostic tests in infectious mononucleosis. Hum Pathol 1974;5:551–565.
171. Sumaya CV, Ench Y. Epstein-Barr virus infectious mononucleosis in children: I. Clinical and general laboratory findings. Pediatrics 1985;75:1003–1010.
172. Sumaya CV, Ench Y. Epstein-Barr virus infectious mononucleosis in children. II. Heterophil antibody and viral-specific responses. Pediatrics 1985;75:1011–1019.
173. Horwitz CA, Henle W, Henle G, et al. Heterophil-negative infectious mononucleosis and mononucleosis-like illnesses. Am J Med 1977;63:947–951.
174. Sumaya CV. Epstein-Barr virus serologic testing: diagnostic indications and interpretations. Pediatr Infect Dis 1986;5: 337–342.
175. Schleupner CJ, Overall JC Jr. Infectious mononucleosis and Epstein-Barr virus. Postgrad Med 1979;65:83–89, 95–105.
176. Jones JF, Ray CG, Minnich LL, Hicks MJ, Kibler R, Lucas DO. Evidence for active Epstein-Barr virus infection in patients with persistent, unexplained illnesses: elevated anti-early antigen antibodies. Ann Intern Med 1985;102:1–7.
177. Straus SE, Tosato G, Armstrong G, et al. Persisting illness and fatigue in adults with evidence of Epstein-Barr virus infection. Ann Intern Med 1985;102:7–16.
178. Buchwald D, Sullivan JL, Komaroff AL. Frequency of "Chronic active Epstein-Barr virus infection" in a general medical practice. JAMA 1987;257:2303–2307.
179. Hellinger WC, Smith TF, Van Scoy RE, Spitzer PG, Forgacs P, Edson RS. Chronic fatigue syndrome and the diagnostic utility of antibody to Epstein-Barr virus early antigen. JAMA 1988;260:971–973.
180. Holmes GP, Kaplan JE, Stewart JA, Hunt B, Pinsky PF, Schonberger L. A cluster of patients with a chronic mononucleosis-like syndrome: is Epstein-Barr virus the cause? JAMA 1987;257:2297–2302.
181. Straus SE. The chronic mononucleosis syndrome. J Infect Dis 1988;157:405–412.
182. Tobi M, Straus SE. Chronic Epstein-Barr virus disease: a workshop held by the National Institute of Allergy and Infectious Diseases. Ann Intern Med 1985;103:951–953.
183. Gold D, Bowden R, Sixbey J, et al. Chronic fatigue: a prospective clinical and virologic study. JAMA 1990;264:48–53.
184. Holmes GP, Kaplan JE, Nelson MG, et al. Chronic fatigue syndrome: a working case definition. Ann Intern Med 1988;108:387–389.
185. Katz BL, Andiman WA. Chronic fatigue syndrome. J Pediatr 1988;113:944–947.
186. Niederman JC, Miller G, Pearson HA, Pagano JS, Dowaliby JM. Infectious mononucleosis: Epstein-Barr virus shedding in saliva and the oropharynx. N Engl J Med 1976;294:1355–1359.

187. Miller G, Katz BZ, Niederman JC. Some recent developments in the molecular epidemiology of Epstein-Barr virus infections. Yale J Biol Med 1987;60:307–316.
188. Grierson H, Purtillo DT. Epstein-Barr virus infections in males with X-linked lymphoproliferative syndrome. Ann Intern Med 1987;106:538–545.
189. McClain K, Gehrz R, Grierson H, Purtilo D, Filipovich A. Virus-associated histiocytic proliferations in children: frequent association with Epstein-Barr virus and congenital or acquired immunodeficiencies. Am J Pediatr Hematol Oncol 1988;10:196–205.
190. Gershon AA. Live attenuated varicella vaccine. Annu Rev Med 1987;38:41–50.
191. Gershon AA, Steinberg SP, LaRussa P, et al. Immunization of healthy adults with live attenuated varicella vaccine. J Infect Dis 1988;158:132–137.
192. Starr SE. Status of varicella vaccine for healthy children. Pediatrics 1989;84:1097–1099.
193. Krasinski K, Holzman RS, LaCouture R, Florman A. Hospital experience with varicella-zoster virus. Infect Control 1986;7: 312–316.
194. McKinney WP, Horowitz MM, Battiola RJ. Susceptibility of hospital-based health care personnel to varicella-zoster virus infections. Am J Infect Control 1989;17:26–30.
195. LaRussa P, Steinberg S, Waithe E, Hanna B, Holzman R. Comparison of five assays for antibody to varicella-zoster virus and the fluorescent-antibody-to-membrane-antigen test. J Clin Microbiol 1987;25:2059–2062.
196. Yamanishi K, Shiraki K, Kondo T, et al. Identification of human herpesvirus-6 as a causal agent for exanthem subitum. Lancet 1988;1:1065–1067.
197. Niederman JC, Kaplan MH, Liu CR, Brown NA. Clinical and serological features of human herpesvirus-6 infection in three adults. Lancet 1988;2:817–819.
198. Okuno T, Takahashi K, Balachandra K, et al. Seroepidemiology of human herpesvirus 6 infection in normal children and adults. J Clin Microbiol 1989;27:651–653.
199. Ueda K, Kusuhara K, Hirose M, et al. Exanthem subitum and antibody to human herpesvirus-6. J Infect Dis 1989;159: 750–752.
200. Yoshikawa T, Suga S, Asano Y, Yazaki T, Kodama H, Ozaki T. Distribution of antibodies to a causative agent of exanthem subitum (human herpesvirus-6) in healthy individuals. Pediatrics 1989;84:675–677.
201. Hall CB. Respiratory syncytial virus. In: Feigin RD, Cherry JD, eds. Textbook of pediatric infectious diseases. Philadelphia: WB Saunders, 1987:1653–1676.
202. MacDonald NE, Hall CB, Suffin SC, Alexson C, Harris PJ, Manning JA. Respiratory syncytial viral infection in infants with congenital heart disease. N Engl J Med 1982;307: 397–400.
203. Hall CB, McBride JT, Gala CL, Hildreth SW, Schnabel KC. Ribavirin treatment of respiratory syncytial viral infection in infants with underlying cardiopulmonary disease. JAMA 1985;254:3047–3051.
204. Hall CB, McBride JT, Walsh EE, et al. Aerosolized ribavirin treatment of infants with respiratory syncytial viral infection. N Engl J Med 1983;308:1443–1447.
205. Thomas EE, Book LE. Comparison of two rapid methods for detection of respiratory syncytial virus (RSV) (TestPack RSV and Ortho RSV ELISA) with direct immunofluorescence and virus isolation for the diagnosis of pediatric RSV infection. J Clin Microbiol 1991;29:632–635.
206. Waner JL, Whitehurst NJ, Todd SJ, Shalaby H, Wall LV. Comparison of Directigen RSV with viral isolation and direct immunofluorescence for the identification of respiratory syncytial virus. J Clin Microbiol 1990;28:480–483.
207. Welliver RC. Detection, pathogenesis, and therapy of respiratory syncytial virus infections. Clin Microbiol Rev 1988;1: 27–39.
208. Betts RF, Douglas RG Jr. Influenza virus. In: Mandell GL, Douglas RG Jr, Bennett JE, eds. Principles and practices of infectious diseases. New York: Churchill Livingstone, 1990: 1306–1325.
209. Glezen WP, Decker M, Joseph SW, Mercready RG Jr. Acute respiratory disease associated with influenza epidemics in Houston, 1981–1983. J Infect Dis 1987;155:1119–1126.
210. Glezen WP, Decker M, Perrotta DM. Survey of underlying conditions of persons hospitalized with acute respiratory disease during influenza epidemics in Houston, 1978–1981. Am Rev Respir Dis 1987;136:550–555.
211. Johnston SLG, Siegel CS. A comparison of direct immunofluorescence, shell vial culture, and conventional cell culture for the rapid detection of influenza A and B. Diagn Microbiol Infect Dis 1991;14:131–134.
212. Waner JL, Todd SJ, Shalaby H, Murphy P, Wall LV. Comparison of Directigen FLU-A with viral isolation and direct immunofluorescence for the rapid detection and identification of influenza A virus. J Clin Microbiol 1991;29:479–482.
212a. Ryan-Poirier KA, Katz JM, Webster RG, Kawaoka Y. Application of directigen FLU-A for the detection of influenza A virus in human and nonhuman specimens. J Clin Microbiol 1992;30:1072–1075.
213. Salomon HE, Grandien M, Avila MM, Pettersson CA. Comparison of three techniques for detection of respiratory viruses in nasopharyngeal aspirates from children with lower acute respiratory infections. J Med Virol 1989;28:159–162.
214. Takimoto S, Grandien M, Ishida MA, et al. Comparison of enzyme-linked immunosorbent assay, indirect immunofluorescence assay, and virus isolation for detection of respiratory viruses in nasopharyngeal secretions. J Clin Microbiol 1991;29:470–474.
215. Landry ML. Rapid viral diagnosis: the use of centrifugation cultures. VA Practitioner 1988;35–42.
216. Waner JL. Parainfluenza viruses. In: Balows A, Hausler WJ Jr, Herrmann KL, Isenberg HD, Shadomy HJ, eds. Manual of clinical microbiology. Washington, DC: American Society for Microbiology, 1991:878–882.
217. Krawczynski K, Bradley DW. Enterically transmitted non-A, non-B hepatitis: Identification of virus-associated antigen in experimentally infected cynomolgus macaques. J Infect Dis 1989;159:1042–1049.
218. Velazquez O, Stetler HC, Avila C, et al. Epidemic transmission of enterically transmitted non-A, non-B hepatitis in Mexico, 1986–1987. JAMA 1990;263:3281–3285.
219. Centers for Disease Control. Protection against viral hepatitis. MMWR 1990;39:1–26.
220. Pavia AT, Nielson L, Armington L, Thurman DJ, Tierney E, Nichols CR. A community-wide outbreak of hepatitis A in a religious community: impact of mass administration of immune globulin. Am J Epidemiol 1990;131:1085–1093.
221. Kosatsky T, Middaugh JP. Linked outbreaks of hepatitis A in homosexual men and in food service patrons and employees. West J Med 1986;144:307–310.
222. Hadler SC, McFarland L. Hepatitis in day care centers: epidemiology and prevention. Rev Infect Dis 1986;8:548–557.
223. Schalm SW, Mazel A, de Gast GC, et al. Prevention of hepatitis B infection in newborns through mass screening and delayed vaccination of all infants of mothers with hepatitis B surface antigen. Pediatrics 1989;83:1041–1047.
224. Centers for Disease Control. Public Health Service interagency guidelines for screening donors of blood, plasma, organs, tissues, and semen for evidence of hepatitis B and hepatitis C. MMWR 1991;40:1–17.

225. Alter HJ, Purcell RH, Shih JW, et al. Detection of antibody to hepatitis C virus in prospectively followed transfusion recipients with acute and chronic non-A, non-B hepatitis. N Engl J Med 1989;321:1494–1500.
226. Chatzinoff M, Friedman LS. Delta agent hepatitis. Infect Dis Clin North Am 1987;1:529–545.
227. Alward WLM, McMahon BJ, Hall DB, Heyward WL, Francis DP, Bender TR. The long-term serological course of asymptomatic hepatitis B virus carriers and the development of primary hepatocellular carcinoma. J Infect Dis 1985;151:604–609.
228. Beasley RP, Lin CC, Hwang LY, Chien CS. Hepatocellular carcinoma and hepatitis B virus. Lancet 1981;2:1129–1133.
229. Ellis JC. Screening for hepatocellular carcinoma. West J Med 1988;149:183–187.
230. Kaklamani E, Trichopoulos D, Tzonou A, et al. Hepatitis B and C viruses and their interaction in the origin of hepatocellular carcinoma. JAMA 1991;265:1974–1976.
231. Di Bisceglie AM, Martin P, Kassianides C, et al. Recombinant interferon alfa therapy for chronic hepatitis C. N Engl J Med 1989;321:1506–1510.
232. Perrillo RP, Schiff ER, Davis GL, et al. A randomized, controlled trial of interferon alfa-2b alone and after prednisone withdrawal for the treatment of chronic hepatitis B. N Engl J Med 1990;323:295–301.
233. Cappel R, De Cuyper F, Van Beers D. e Antigen and antibody, DNA polymerase, and inhibitors of DNA polymerase in acute and chronic hepatitis. J Infect Dis 1977;136:617–622.
234. Fay O, Tanno H, Roncoroni M, Edwards VM, Mosley JW, Redeker AG. Prognostic implications of the e antigen of hepatitis B virus. JAMA 1977;238:2501–2503.
235. Okada K, Kamiyama I, Inomata M, Imai M, Miyakawa Y, Mayumi M. e Antigen and anti-e in the serum of asymptomatic carrier mothers as indicators of positive and negative transmission of hepatitis B virus to their infants. N Engl J Med 1976;294:746–749.
236. Choo QL, Kuo G, Weiner AJ, Overby LR, Bradley DW, Houghton M. Isolation of a cDNA clone derived from a blood-borne non-A, non-B viral hepatitis genome. Science 1989;244:359–362.
237. Kuo G, Choo QL, Alter HJ, et al. An assay for circulating antibodies to a major etiologic virus of human non-A, non-b hepatitis. Science 1989;244:362–364.
238. Esteban JI, Gonzalez A, Hernandez JM, et al. Evaluation of antibodies to hepatitis C virus in a study of transfusion-associated hepatitis. N Engl J Med 1990;323:1107–1112.
239. Martin P. Hepatitis C: from laboratory to bedside. Mayo Clin Proc 1990;65:1372–1376.
240. Alter MJ, Hadler SC, Judson FN, et al. Risk factors for acute non-A, non-B hepatitis in the United States and association with hepatitis C virus infection. JAMA 1990;264:2231–2235.
240a. Aach RD, Stevens CE, Hollinger FB, et al. Hepatitis C virus infection in post-transfusion hepatitis. N Engl J Med 1991;325:1325–1329.
240b. Farci P, Alter HJ, Wong D, et al. A long-term study of hepatitis C virus replication in non-A, non-B hepatitis. N Engl J Med 1991;325:98–104.
240c. Lau JYN, Davis GL, Kniffen J, et al. Significance of serum hepatitis C virus RNA levels in chronic hepatitis C. Lancet 1993;341:1501–1504.
241. Lew JF, Glass RI, Petric M, et al. Six-year retrospective surveillance of gastroenteritis viruses identified at ten electron microscopy centers in the United States and Canada. Pediatr Infect Dis J 1990;9:709–714.
242. LeBaron CW, Lew J, Glass RI, Weber JM, Ruiz-Palacios GM, the Rotavirus Study Group. Annual rotavirus epidemic patterns in North America. JAMA 1990;264:983–988.
243. Kotloff KL, Losonsky GA, Morris JG Jr, Wasserman SS, Naz-Singh N, Levine MM. Enteric adenovirus infection and childhood diarrhea: an epidemiologic study in three clinical settings. Pediatrics 1989;84:219.
244. Jenista JA, Powell KR, Menegus MA. Epidemiology of neonatal enterovirus infection. J Pediatr 1984;104:685–690.
245. Krober MS, Bass JW, Powell JM, Smith FR, Seto DSY. Bacterial and viral pathogens causing fever in infants less than 3 months old. Am J Dis Child 1985;139:889–892.
246. Modlin JF. Perinatal echovirus infection: insights from a literature review of 61 cases of serious infection and 16 outbreaks in nurseries. Rev Infect Dis 1986;8:918–926.
247. Wilfert CM, Lehrman SN, Katz SL. Enteroviruses and meningitis. Pediatr Infect Dis 1983;2:333–341.
248. Dagan R, Hall CB, Powell KR, Menegus MA. Epidemiology and laboratory diagnosis of infection with viral and bacterial pathogens in infants hospitalized for suspected sepsis. J Pediatr 1989;115:351–356.
249. Beck MA, Tracy SM. Evidence for a group-specific enteroviral antigen(s) recognized by human T cells. J Clin Microbiol 1990;28:1822–1827.
250. Yousef GE, Mann GF, Brown IN, Mowbray JF. Clinical and research application of an enterovirus group-reactive monoclonal antibody. Intervirol 1987;28:199–205.
251. Chapman NM, Tracy S, Gauntt CJ, Fortmueller U. Molecular detection and identification of enteroviruses using enzymatic amplification and nucleic acid hybridization. J Clin Microbiol 1990;28:843–850.
252. Chatterjee NK, Kaehler M, Deibel R. Detection of enteroviruses using subgenomic probes of coxsackie virus B4 by hybridization. Diagn Microbiol Infect Dis 1988;11:129–136.
253. Petitjean J, Quibriac M, Freymuth F, et al. Specific detection of enteroviruses in clinical samples by molecular hybridization using poliovirus subgenomic riboprobes. J Clin Microbiol 1990;28:307–311.
254. Rotbart HA. Enzymatic RNA amplification of the enteroviruses. J Clin Microbiol 1990;28:438–442.
255. Rotbart HA, Eastman PS, Ruth JL, Hirata KK, Levin MJ. Nonisotopic oligomeric probes for the human enteroviruses. J Clin Microbiol 1988;26:2669–2671.
256. Rotbart HA, Levin MJ, Villarreal LP, Tracy SM, Semler BL, Wimmer E. Factors affecting the detection of enteroviruses in cerebrospinal fluid with coxsackievirus B3 and poliovirus 1 cDNA probes. J Clin Microbiol 1985;22:220–224.
256a. Rotbart HA. Nucleic acid detection systems for enteroviruses. Clin Microbiol Rev 1991;4:156–168.
257. Chonmaitree T, Ford C, Sanders C, Lucia HL. Comparison of cell cultures for rapid isolation of enteroviruses. J Clin Microbiol 1988;26:2576–2580.
258. Dagan R, Menegus MA. A combination of four cell types for rapid detection of enteroviruses in clinical specimens. J Med Virol 1986;19:219–228.
259. Menegus MA, Hollick GE. Increased efficiency of group B coxsackievirus isolation from clinical specimens by use of BGM cells. J Clin Microbiol 1982;15:945–948.
260. Dagan R, Jenista JA, Menegus MA. Clinical, epidemiological and laboratory aspects of enterovirus infection in young infants. In: de la Maza LM, Peterson EM, eds. Medical virology IV. Hillsdale, NJ: Lawrence Erlbaum Associates, 1985:123–151.
261. Dagan R, Jenista JA, Prather SL, Powell KR, Menegus MA. Viremia in hospitalized children with enterovirus infections. J Pediatr 1985;106:397–401.
262. Peter G, Lepow ML, McCracken GH, Phillips CF. Report of the Committee on Infectious Diseases. 22nd ed. Elk Grove Village, IL: American Academy of Pediatrics, 1991:1–670.

263. Fuccillo DA, Sever JL. Measles, mumps, and rubella. In: Specter S, Lancz GJ, eds. Clinical virology manual. New York: Elsevier, 1986:437–449.
264. Herrmann KL. Rubella. In: Lennette EH, ed. Laboratory diagnosis of viral infections. New York: Marcel Dekker, 1985: 481–497.
265. Kleiman MB. Mumps virus infections. In: Lennette EH, ed. Laboratory diagnosis of viral infections. New York: Marcel Dekker, 1985:369–384.
266. Salmi AA. Measles virus. In: Balows A, Hausler WJ Jr, Herrmann KL, Isenberg HD, Shadomy HJ, eds. Manual of clinical microbiology. Washington, DC: American Society for Microbiology, 1991:904–911.
267. Schiff GM. Measles (rubeola). In: Lennette EH, ed. Laboratory diagnosis of viral infections. New York: Marcel Dekker, 1985:359–367.
268. Swierkosz EM. Mumps virus. In: Balows A, Hausler WJ Jr, Herrmann KL, Isenberg HD, Shadomy HJ, eds. Manual of clinical microbiology. Washington, DC: American Society for Microbiology, 1991:912–917.
269. Minnich LL, Goodenough F, Ray CG. Use of immunofluorescence to identify measles virus infections. J Clin Microbiol 1991;29:1148–1150.
270. Chernesky MA, Mahony JB. Rubella virus. In: Balows A, Hausler WJ Jr, Herrman KL, Isenberg HD, Shadomy HJ, eds. Manual of clinical microbiology. Washington, DC: American Society for Microbiology, 1991:918–924.
271. Field PR, Ho DWT, Cunningham AL. Evaluation of rubella immune status by three commercial enzyme-linked immunosorbent assays. J Clin Microbiol 1988;26:990–994.
272. Linde GA, Granstrom M, Orvell C. Immunoglobulin class and immunoglobulin G subclass enzyme-linked immunosorbent assays compared with microneutralization assay for serodiagnosis of mumps infection and determination of immunity. J Clin Microbiol 1987;25:1653–1658.
273. Neumann PW, Weber JM, Jessamine AG, O'Shaughnessy MV. Comparison of measles antihemolysin test, enzyme-linked immunosorbent assay, and hemagglutination inhibition test with neutralization test for determination of immune status. J Clin Microbiol 1985;22:296–298.
274. Shankaran P, Reichstein E, Khosravi MJ, Diamandis EP. Detection of immunoglobulins G and M to rubella virus by time-resolved immunofluorometry. J Clin Microbiol 1990;28:573–579.
275. Benito RJ, Larrad L, Lasierra MP, Benito JF, Erdociain F. Persistence of specific IgM antibodies after natural mumps infection. J Infect Dis 1987;155:156–157.
276. Morgan-Capner P, Tedder RS, Mace JE. Rubella specific IgM reactivity in sera from cases of infectious mononucleosis. J Hyg (Camb) 1983;90:407–413.
277. Kurtz JB, Anderson MJ. Cross-reactions in rubella and parvovirus specific IgM tests. Lancet 1985;2:1356.
278. Morgan-Capner P. Diagnosing rubella. Br Med J 1989;299: 338–339.
279. Bellin E, Safyer S, Braslow C. False positive IgM-rubella enzyme-linked immunoassay in three first trimester pregnant patients. Pediatr Infect Dis J 1990;9:671–672.
280. Schleupner CJ. Detection of HIV-1 infection. In: Mandell GL, Douglas RG Jr, Bennett JE, eds. Principles and practice of infectious diseases. New York: Churchill Livingstone, 1990: 1092–1102.
281. Husson RN, Comeau AM, Hoff R. Diagnosis of human immunodeficiency virus infection in infants and children. Pediatrics 1990;86:1–10.
282. Association of State and Territorial Public Health Laboratory Directors and AIDS Program, Centers for Disease Control. Interpretation and use of the Western blot assay for serodiagnosis of human immunodeficiency virus type 1 infections. MMWR 1989;38(suppl S-7):1–7.
283. Jackson JB, MacDonald KL, Cadwell J, et al. Absence of HIV infection in blood donors with indeterminate Western blot tests for antibody to HIV-1. N Engl J Med 1990;322:217–222.
284. Kenny C, Parkin J, Undershill G, et al. HIV antigen testing. Lancet 1987;1:565–566.
285. Rogers MF, Ou CY, Rayfield M, et al. Use of the polymerase chain reaction for early detection of the proviral sequences of human immunodeficiency virus in infants born to seropositive mothers. N Engl J Med 1989;320:1649–1654.
286. Edwards JR, Ulrich PP, Weintrub PS, et al. Polymerase chain reaction compared with concurrent viral cultures for rapid identification of human immunodeficiency virus infection among high-risk infants and children. J Pediatr 1989;115: 200–203.
287. Centers for Disease Control. Guidelines for prophylaxis against *Pneumocystis carinii* pneumonia for children infected with human immunodeficiency virus. JAMA 1991;265: 1637–1644.
288. Imagawa DT, Lee MH, Wolinsky SM, et al. Human immunodeficiency virus type 1 infection in homosexual men who remain seronegative for prolonged periods. N Engl J Med 1989;320:1458–1462.
289. Tindall B, Cooper DA, Donovan B, Penny R. Primary human immunodeficiency virus infection: clinical and serologic aspects. Infect Dis Clin North Am 1988;2:329–341.
290. Goudsmit J, Paul DA, Lange JMA, et al. Expression of human immunodeficiency virus antigen (HIV-Ag) in serum and cerebrospinal fluid during acute and chronic infection. Lancet 1986;1:177–180.
291. Centers for Disease Control. Human arboviral encephalitis—United States, 1982. MMWR 1983;32:160–167.
292. Whitley RJ. Viral encephalitis. N Engl J Med 1990;323: 242–250.
293. Calisher CH, Berardi VP, Muth DJ, Buff EE. Specificity of immunoglobulin M and G antibody responses in humans infected with eastern and western equine encephalitis viruses: application to rapid serodiagnosis. J Clin Microbiol 1986;23: 369–372.
294. Calisher CH, Pretzman CI, Muth DJ, Parsons MA, Peterson ED. Serodiagnosis of a crosse virus infections in humans by detection of immunoglobulin M class antibodies. J Clin Microbiol 1986;23:667–671.
295. Spruance SL, Bailey A. Colorado tick fever. Arch Intern Med 1973;131:288–293.
296. Goodpasture HC, Poland JD, Francy DB, Bowen GS, Horn KA. Colorado tick fever: clinical, epidemiologic, and laboratory aspects of 228 cases in Colorado in 1973–1974. Ann Intern Med 1978;88:303–310.
297. Shope RE. Arboviruses. In: Balows A, Hausler WJ Jr, Kerrman KL, Isenberg HD, Shadomy HJ, eds. Manual of clinical microbiology. Washington, DC: American Society for Microbiology, 1991:930–938.
298. Plummer FA, Hammond GW, Forward K, et al. An erythema infectiosum-like illness caused by human parvovirus infection. N Engl J Med 1985;313:74–79.
299. Serjeant GR, Mason K, Topley JM, Serjeant BE. Outbreak of aplastic crises in sickle cell anaemia associated with parvovirus like agent. Lancet 1981;2:595–597.
300. Kurtzman GJ, Ozawa K, Hanson G, Oseas R, Young NS. Chronic bone marrow failure due to persistent B19 parvovirus infection. N Engl J Med 1987;317:287–294.

301. Anand A, Gray ES, Brown T, Clewley JP, Cohen BJ. Human parvovirus infection in pregnancy and hydrops fetalis. N Engl J Med 1987;316:183–186.
302. Koch WC, Adler SP. Detection of human parvovirus B19 DNA by using the polymerase chain reaction. J Clin Microbiol 1990;28:65–69.
303. Mori J, Field AM, Clewley JP, Cohen BJ. Dot blot hybridization assay of B19 virus DNA in clinical specimens. J Clin Microbiol 1989;27:459–464.
304. Anderson LJ, Tsou C, Parker RA, et al. Detection of antibodies and antigens of human parvovirus B19 by enzyme-linked immunosorbent assay. J Clin Microbiol 1986;24:522–526.
304a. Erdman DD, Usher MJ, Tsou C, et al. Human parvovirus B19 specific IgG, IgA, and IGM antibodies and DNA in serum specimens from persons with erythema infectiosum. J Med Virol 1991;35:110–115.
305. Korones SB, Ainger LE, Monif GRG, Roane J, Sever JL, Fuste F. Congenital rubella syndrome: new clinical aspects with recovery of virus from affected infants. J Pediatr 1965;67:166–181.
306. Thomson RB Jr, Benedict ML, Blaise LC. Evaluation of a commercially available cytomegalovirus-specific IgM test for the diagnosis of cytomegalovirus infection in the symptomatic newborn. Diagn Microbiol Infect Dis 1987;7:211–214.
307. Kohl S. The neonatal human's immune response to herpes simplex virus infection: a critical review. Pediatr Infect Dis J 1989;8:67–74.

55 Parasitology

Larry G. Reimer, DeVon Hale, and Michael A. Pfaller

Medical parasitology is the study of invertebrate animals capable of causing disease in humans. In the context of this chapter, the term parasite refers to organisms belonging to three major subdivisions or taxonomic groups. These include the Protozoa (amebas, flagellates, ciliates, sporozoans, coccidia, microsporidians), the Platyhelminthes or flatworms (cestodes, trematodes), and the Nematodes or roundworms (Table 55.1). The Protozoa are rather simple microscopic unicellular eukaryotic organisms, whereas the Platyhelminthes and Nematoda are highly complex macroscopic multicellular worms possessing differentiated tissues and complex organ systems.

Although parasitic diseases are frequently considered "tropical" and thus of little relevance to physicians practicing in the more temperate, developed countries of the world, it is clear that the world has become a very small place and that it is essential for physicians to have knowledge of parasitic diseases. By any estimation the numbers of parasitic infections and of parasite-associated deaths are staggering and must be of concern to all health care workers (Table 55.2). Increasingly, tourists, missionaries, Peace Corps volunteers, and others are visiting and working for extended periods of time in exotic, remote parts of the world and thus are at risk for parasitic and other infections that are rare in the United States. Another source of infected patients is the ever-increasing population of refugees from developing countries. Finally, the profound immunosuppression accompanying advances in medical therapy as well as that associated with infection with the human immunodeficiency virus (HIV) places an increasing number of individuals at risk for developing infections due to certain parasites. Given these considerations, clinicians and laboratory workers should certainly be aware of the possibility of parasitic disease and should be trained in the ordering, performance, and interpretation of the appropriate laboratory tests to aid in diagnosis and therapy.

Although the mainstay of diagnostic clinical microbiology is the isolation of the causative pathogen in culture, diagnosis of parasitic diseases is almost entirely accomplished by morphologic (usually microscopic) demonstration of parasites in clinical material. Occasionally serodiagnosis is helpful in establishing the diagnosis. Proper diagnosis requires that (*a*) the physician consider the possibility of a parasitic infection, (*b*) appropriate specimens are obtained and transported to the laboratory in a timely fashion, (*c*) the laboratory competently performs the appropriate

Table 55.1. Classification of Human Parasites

PROTOZOA	NEMATODES
Amebas	*Ascaris lumbricoides*
Entamoeba histolytica	*Enterobius vermicularis*
Entamoeba coli	*Ancylostoma duodenale*
Entamoeba polecki	*Necator americanus*
Entamoeba hartmanni	*Strongyloides stercoralis*
Endolimax nana	*Trichuris trichiura*
Iodamoeba bütschlii	*Trichinella spiralis*
Naegleria fowleri	*Toxocara canis*
Acanthamoeba culbertsoni	*Ancylostoma braziliense*
Flagellates	*Wuchereria bancrofti*
Giardia lamblia	*Brugia malayi*
Chilomastix mesnili	*Loa loa*
Dientamoeba fragilis	*Onchocerca volvulus*
Trichomonas hominis	*Mansonella ozzardi*
Trichomonas vaginalis	*Mansonella streptocerca*
Leishmania tropica	*Mansonella perstans*
Leishmania mexicana	*Dirofilaria* spp.
Leishmania braziliensis	TREMATODES
Leishmania donovani	*Fasciolopsis buski*
Trypanosoma gambiense	*Heterophyes heterophyes*
Trypanosoma rhodesiense	*Metagonimus yokogawai*
Trypanosoma cruzi	*Opisthorchis sinensis*
Ciliates	*Opisthorchis viverrini*
Balantidium coli	*Fasciola hepatica*
Sporozoa	*Paragonimus westermani*
Plasmodium vivax	*Schistosoma mansoni*
Plasmodium malariae	*Schistosoma japonicum*
Plasmodium ovale	*Schistosoma haematobium*
Plasmodium falciparum	CESTODES
Babesia microti	*Diphyllobothrium latum*
Pneumocystis carinii	*Dipylidium caninum*
Coccidia	*Hymenolepsis nana*
Cryptosporidium sp.	*Hymenolepsis diminuta*
Isospora belli	*Taenia solium*
Blastocystis hominis	*Taenia saginata*
Toxoplasma gondii	*Echinococcus granulosus*
Microsporidia	*Echinococcus multilocularis*
Encephalitozoon	*Multiceps multiceps*
Nosema	
Pleistophora	
Enterocytozoon	

procedures for recovery and identification of the etiologic agent, (*d*) the laboratory results are effectively communicated to the physician, and (*e*) the results are correctly interpreted by the physician and applied to the care of the patient. For most parasitic diseases, appropriate test selection and interpretation is based on an understanding of the life cycle of the parasite as well as the pathogenesis of the disease process in humans. For example, although *Ascaris* is usually considered an intestinal nematode, early and profound clinical symptoms may be caused by larval migration through tissues weeks before eggs are present in feces.

In this chapter we attempt to provide an overview of the basic parasitology, epidemiology, clinical disease, and pathology of the major protozoan and helminthic parasites infecting humans. Individual organisms and disease processes are discussed under the major headings of blood and tissue protozoa, intestinal and urogenital protozoa, nematodes, trematodes, and cestodes. The reader is referred to several excellent reference texts for more detailed information (1–3).

Table 55.2. Estimated Worldwide Prevalence of Parasitic Infections

Infection	Number Infected	Annual Deaths
Amebiasis	10% of world population	40,000–110,000
Malaria	400–490 million	2.2–2.5 million
African trypanosomiasis	100,000 new cases/year	5,000
American trypanosomiasis	24 million	60,000
Leishmaniasis	1.2 million	
Schistosomiasis	>200 million	0.5–1 million
Opisthorchiasis	19 million	
Paragonimiasis	3.2 million	
Fasciolopsiasis	10 million	
Filariasis	85–100 million	
Onchocerciasis	>30 million	
Dracunculiasis	10 million	
Ascariasis	1 billion	1550 (intestinal obstruction)
Hookworm	900 million	
Trichuriasis	500–800 million	
Strongyloidiasis	35 million	
Cestodiasis	65 million	

BLOOD AND TISSUE PROTOZOA

The protozoa of blood and tissues include the sporozoan parasites *Plasmodium*, *Babesia microti*, and *Toxoplasma gondii*; the hemoflagellates *Leishmania* and *Trypanosoma*; and the free-living amebae *Naegleria* and *Acanthamoeba*. For purposes of this chapter we also include *Pneumocystis carinii* as a sporozoan tissue parasite, although it will likely be reclassified as a fungus based on recent studies of ribosomal RNA sequences (4). The major clinical manifestations of the protozoa causing bloodstream infection (malaria and babesia) are secondary to the destruction of red blood cells or sludging of infected red blood cells in the microvasculature of the brain and other organs. The protozoa causing tissue infection may cause significant damage to specific organs such as the eyes (toxoplasmosis, acanthamoeba keratitis), the brain (toxoplasmosis, amebic meningoencephalitis, African sleeping sickness), the heart (toxoplasmosis, Chagas' disease), or the gastrointestinal tract (Chagas' disease). *Pneumocystis carinii* primarily causes pneumonia; however, invasion of other sites such as the eye have been reported (5–7) (Table 55.3).

Malaria

Malaria is the most important of all protozoan diseases; it annually infects over 250 million individuals and is a leading cause of illness and death in the developing world (Table 55.2). Efforts at eradication have failed due to the ability of both the anopheline mosquito vector and the parasite to develop resistance to various eradication and treatment options.

Table 55.3. Major Blood and Tissue Protozoa

Organism	Disease	Vector	Location	Laboratory Diagnosis
Plasmodium	Malaria	*Anopheles* mosquito	Blood	Giemsa-stained blood film
Babesia	Babesiosis	*Ixodes* tick	Blood	Giemsa-stained blood film
Toxoplasma gondii	Toxoplasmosis	None; foodborne, fecal-oral	Reticuloendothelial system	Parasites in biopsy, serology
Leishmania	Leishmaniasis	*Phlebotomus* sandfly	Skin Mucosa Reticuloendothelial system	Parasites in Giemsa-stained smears, biopsy
Trypanosoma cruzi	Chagas' disease American trypanosomiasis	Reduviid bug	Blood Reticuloendothelial system	Trypanosomes in blood, biopsy
Trypanosoma brucei gambiense or *rhodesiense*	Sleeping sickness African trypanosomiasis	Tsetse fly	Blood Lymphatics CNS	Trypanosomes in blood, CSF
Pneumocystis carinii	Pneumocystosis	None ? airborne	Lung tissue Extrapulmonary tissue	Parasites in biopsy, lung aspirate

Table 55.4. Selected Clinical Characteristics of Four Types of Malaria

Characteristic	*P. falciparum*	*P. vivax*	*P. ovale*	*P. malariae*
Usual incubation period (days)	8–11	10–17 or longer	10–17 or longer	18–40 or longer
Severity of primary attack	Severe in nonimmune	Mild to severe	Mild	Mild
Periodicity (hours)	None	48	48	72
Duration of untreated primary attack (weeks)	2–3	3–8	2–3	3–24
Duration of untreated infection	6–17 months	5–7 years	12 months	20+ years
Average parasitemia (per mm^2)	20,000 or greater	10,000	9,000	6,000
Anemia	Frequent and severe	Mild	Mild	Mild
CNS involvement	Yes, severe	Rare	Rare	Rare
Nephrotic syndrome	Rare	Rare	No	Frequent

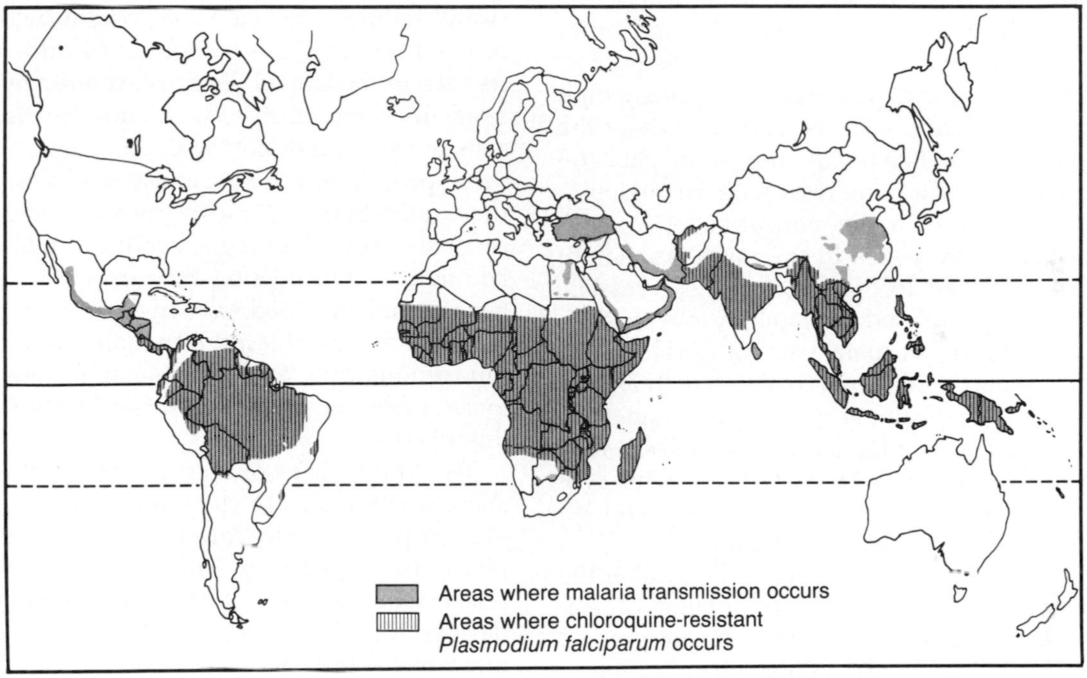

Figure 55.1. World distribution of malaria. (From Markell EK, Voge M, John DT. Medical parasitology. Philadelphia: WB Saunders, 1992.)

In the United States malaria is well controlled, although it remains the most common acute febrile illness imported into the country.

Classification

Malaria is caused by blood-borne pathogens of the genus *Plasmodium*. There are four species that can infect humans and that are associated with somewhat different clinical presentations, laboratory characteristics, and geographic distribution (Table 4). These four species include *Plasmodium vivax, Plasmodium ovale, Plasmodium malariae*, and *Plasmodium falciparum*. *Plasmodium vivax* is the most common species worldwide, being found in India, Pakistan, Southeast Asia, South and Central America, and rarely in Africa. *P. ovale* is limited in distribution primarily to Africa. *P. malariae* is found in all countries with malaria, although it is much less prevalent than either *P. vivax* or *P. falciparum*. *P. falciparum* ranks second in prevalence to *P. vivax* and is primarily a tropical species. It is found most often in individuals from Africa, Haiti, and New Guinea, but is also seen in Southeast Asia, South America, and the Pacific Islands. Clinically, *P. falciparum* infections are the most serious among the four species of plasmodia. Figure 55.1 depicts the distribution of malaria transmission, including that of drug-resistant strains.

Clinical Manifestations

Malaria is characterized by acute cyclical periods (paroxysms) of high fever and shaking chills. After several replicative cycles of the parasite within the patient, a classic pattern of illness occurs. Patients develop a dull headache and generalized malaise followed by severe chills, peripheral vasoconstriction, and polyuria. Within a few hours patients have high fever, flushing, and, after 2 to 6 hours, a drenching sweat that resolves the episode but leaves the patient exhausted. Complete cycles occur in a tertian (48-hour) pattern in *P. vivax* and *P. ovale* and in a quartan

(72-hour) pattern in *P. malariae* infections. A definite pattern frequently cannot be identified in *P. falciparum* infections; however, sometimes pronounced synchronization may be seen with a 36- to 48-hour periodicity. In addition to fever and chills, patients may also have flu-like symptoms with myalgias, arthralgias, nausea, vomiting, abdominal pain, and headache. On physical examination patients may have splenomegaly, hepatomegaly, or jaundice, although none of these is seen often. The most common laboratory abnormality associated with malaria is hemolytic anemia and hyperbilirubinemia. Elevated liver function tests, hyponatremia, and other nonspecific laboratory abnormalities may also occur.

The density of parasitemia may be extremely high in *P. falciparum* malaria, with as many as 50% of the red cells being parasitized. This degree of parasitemia can lead to severe hemolysis with hemoglobinuria and severe anemia. Sequestration of *P. falciparum*–infected erythrocytes in the microvasculature of the body may lead to occlusion of these vessels, causing symptoms related to capillary obstruction. With severe disease, virtually always caused by *P. falciparum*, evidence of cerebral infection with altered consciousness, encephalopathy, seizures, and focal neurologic deficits or intravascular hemolysis with renal failure (blackwater fever) may occur. This syndrome is considered a medical emergency and requires immediate and aggressive therapy.

There are several genetic factors that may alter the susceptibility to, and the clinical presentation of, malaria. The development of *P. falciparum* is suppressed by the presence of fetal hemoglobin, hemoglobin S, and perhaps other abnormal hemoglobins as well (8). Persons with sickle cell trait have less severe infections with *P. falciparum* and do not suffer from lethal sickle cell disease. The high frequency of hemoglobin S in certain parts of Africa is due to the selective advantage of this balanced polymorphism. Likewise, persons with the Duffy-negative blood type (Fy^a- and Fy^b-negative) are resistant to infection with *P. vivax*. The Duffy blood group antigen is the specific receptor for invasion of red cells by *P. vivax* merozoites (8). The low incidence of *P. vivax* in Africa is explained by the fact that most African blacks are Duffy-negative.

The course of untreated malaria depends greatly on the infecting species. As noted above, most fatal cases of malaria are caused by *P. falciparum*. In nonfatal cases, the febrile paroxysms become less severe over time and the disease gradually subsides. Clinical and parasitologic relapses may occur after months or years in individuals with *P. vivax* or *P. ovale* infection. These relapses are due to the emergence of latent exoerythrocytic forms present in the liver (hypnozoite; see Life Cycle below). *P. malariae* frequency causes an extremely low-grade parasitemia, and individuals with *P. malariae* infection may be asymptomatic with recrudescences occurring sporadically. It is thought that relapses or recrudescences may be associated with changes in the host's defense mechanisms or possibly with antigenic variation in the infecting organism.

Life Cycle

Malaria is transmitted to humans by the bite of the female *Anopheles* mosquito. Between 65 and 70 species of naturally infected *Anopheles* mosquitoes have been found in various parts of the world. Most malaria seen in the United States is acquired by visitors or residents from countries with endemic disease and is considered "imported" malaria. However, because the appropriate vector *Anopheles* mosquito is found in the United States, domestic transmission of the disease has been observed (introduced malaria) (8). In addition to transmission by mosquitos, malaria can be acquired by blood transfusions from an infected donor or by the sharing of needles and syringes by intravenous drug users. Congenital transmission of malaria from an infected mother to the fetus is also described.

The four species of *Plasmodium* infecting humans share a common life cycle (Fig. 55.2) involving an asexual phase (schizogony) in humans and a sexual phase (sporogony) in the mosquito. The sexual phase requires a developmental period of 8 to 12 days in the mosquito and results in the production of infectious sporozoites.

The infective sporozoites are injected into the subcutaneous capillaries of the vertebrate host as the mosquito feeds. The sporozoites penetrate the parenchymal cells of the liver, where they multiply asexually (exoerythrocytic schizogony) to produce thousands of uninucleate merozoites and form a tissue schizont. This growth of parasites in the liver is called the exoerythrocytic phase.

Following a period of development (8 to 25 days depending on the species), the merozoites rupture from the hepatic cell and are released into the circulation, where they invade red blood cells. In infection due to *P. falciparum* and *P. malariae*, the tissue schizonts all rupture simultaneously, and none persist in the liver. In contrast, *P. vivax* and *P. ovale* produce two types of exoerythrocytic forms: a primary type that develops and ruptures within 6 to 9 days and a secondary type called a hypnozoite that may remain dormant in the liver for weeks, months, or years. The hypnozoite form is responsible for relapses of erythrocytic infection observed with *P. vivax* and *P. ovale*.

Although relapses of *P. vivax* and *P. ovale* malaria may occur due to the persistent exoerythrocytic

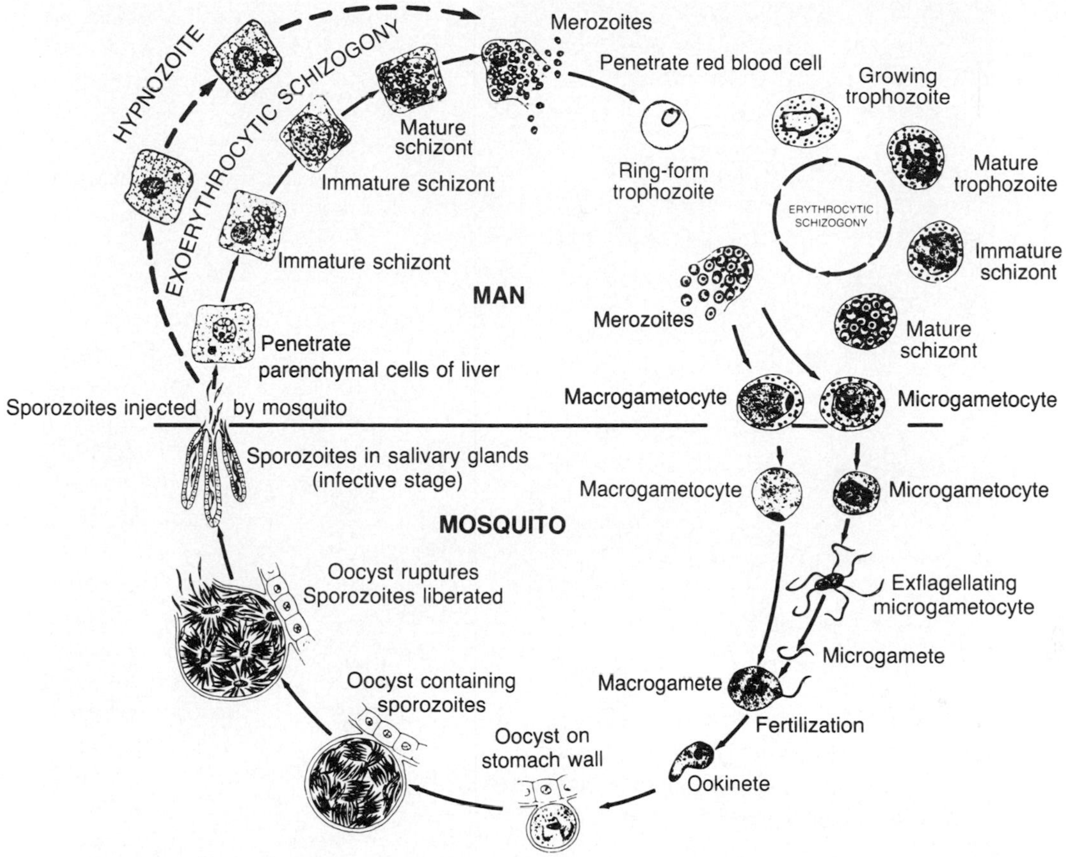

Figure 55.2. Life cycle of malaria (From Strickland GT. Tropical medicine. 7th ed. Philadelphia: WB Saunders, 1991).

(hypnozoite) phase, this is not the case with *P. falciparum* and *P. malariae,* which lack a dormant hepatic stage. Recurrent parasitemia with these species is due to proliferation of persistent erythrocytic forms and is known as recrudescence. The prolonged delayed recrudescences occasionally seen with *P. malariae* are due to erythrocytic parasites that have persisted in the tissue microcirculation.

The merozoites released from tissue schizonts invade circulating red blood cells and initiate the erythrocytic phase of infection. It is the erythrocytic phase that is responsible for the clinical manifestations of malaria and on which laboratory diagnosis is based (Fig. 55.3). The different species of plasmodia selectively infect red blood cells of different ages. *P. vivax* and *P. ovale* preferentially infect young red blood cells, *P. malariae* infects only older circulating red cells, and *P. falciparum* can infect red cells of any age. The merozoites infecting red cells become small, rounded trophozoites or ring forms. Over time, the parasites develop into irregular ameboid trophozoites that utilize hemoglobin and produce an iron-containing pigment known as hematin or hemozoin. The mature trophozoite undergoes nuclear division and segmentation to form a mature schizont containing up to 24 merozoites in a process known as erythrocytic schizogony. The erythrocytes containing the mature schizont rupture, liberating merozoites, which then go on to invade new red blood cells. This erythrocytic cycle is repeated over and over with a periodicity that differs according to the species of *Plasmodium*.

Subpopulations of merozoites may also differentiate into sexual forms or gametocytes. The female form is called the macrogametocyte and the male form is called the microgametocyte. The gametocytes are ingested in the blood meal of a mosquito, sexual reproduction takes place, and the life cycle of the parasite is completed within the gastrointestinal tract of the mosquito with the production of new sporozoites.

Diagnosis

Malaria should be considered in any patient with an acute febrile illness and recent travel to or migration from an endemic area. The diagnosis is generally made by demonstration of the parasite within red blood cells. Organisms are easily seen in capillary blood obtained by fingerstick, although venous blood may also be used. Blood does not have to be obtained during the febrile period of infection; parasites may be present in blood even during the asympto-

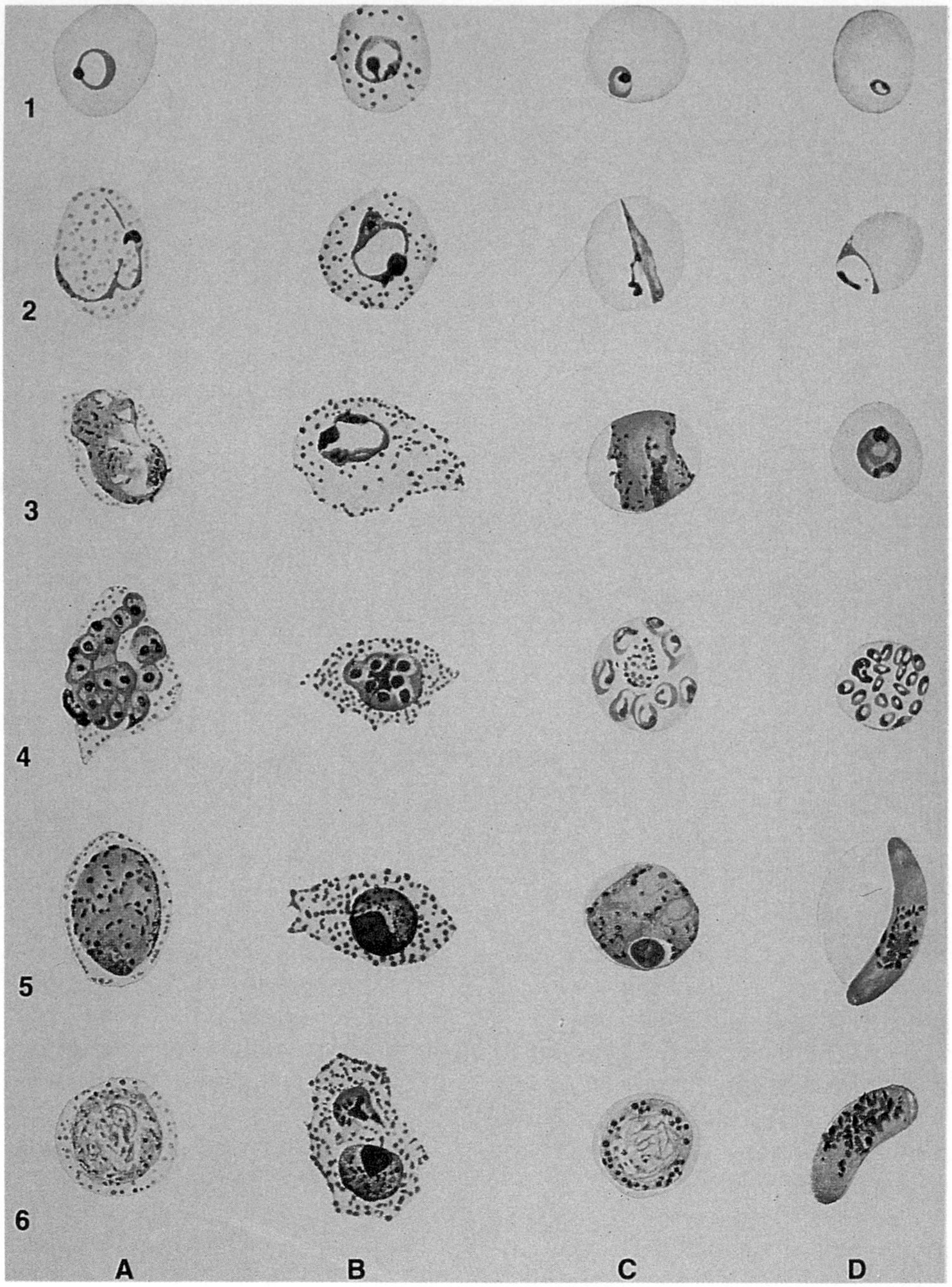

Figure 55.3. Developmental forms of four species causing human malaria. Columns: **A**, *Plasmodium vivax*; **B**, *P. ovale*; **C**, *P. malariae*; **D**, *P. falciparum*. Rows: *1*, young trophozoites; *2*, growing trophozoites; *3*, mature trophozoites; *4*, mature schizonts; *5*, macrogametocytes; *6*, microgametocytes. (From Wilcox A: Manual for the microscopical diagnosis of malaria in man. Bulletin No. 180. Bethesda, MD: National Institutes of Health, 1942).

matic periods. The level of parasitemia may be low enough, however, that multiple attempts may be necessary to detect organisms within red cells.

Two types of blood films are prepared and examined for the laboratory diagnosis of malarial infections: thin films, with the blood spread over the slide in a thin layer, and thick films, with the blood concentrated in a small area. In the thick film preparation, the red blood cells are lysed, and only white blood cells, platelets, and parasites (if present) are visible. The thick film is preferred for diagnosis, since it permits the examination of a relatively large amount of blood and may be a more sensitive means of detecting low-grade parasitemias that may be missed with thin films. However, morphologic features of parasites are more distinct and typical in thin films, and thus both types of blood films should be prepared.

The preferred stain for malarial parasites in both thick and thin films is Giemsa buffered to pH 7.0. Al-

Table 55.5. Comparative Morphologic Features of Malarial Parasites in Stained Thin Blood Films

Characteristics	*P. falciparum*	*P. vivax*	*P. ovale*	*P. malariae*
Infected erythrocyte				
enlarged[a]	−	+	±	−
oval, fimbriated	±	±	+	−
Schüffner's dots[a]	−	+	+	−
Maurer's dots	+	−	−	−
Parasite				
Multiple in single erythrocyte	+	±	−	−
Multiple forms	−	+	+	+
Only ring forms[a]	+	−	−	−
Large ameboid rings	−	+	+	+
Double chromatin dots	+	±	−	−
Peripheral location in erythrocyte	+	±	−	−
Band forms	−	−	−	+
Banana-shaped gametocytes[a]	+	−	−	−
Number of merozoites	8–24	12–24	8–12	6–12

[a]Reliable criteria.

though Wright's stain is commonly used to stain peripheral smears for hematologic examination, neither Wright's nor other Romanowsky stains produce the critical differentiation of morphologic features obtained with a Giemsa stain.

Identification of malarial parasites to species level is critical. Patients with falciparum malaria are likely to have more severe disease, including severe hemolysis and cerebral involvement that can result in death in a matter of hours if not appropriately treated. Patients with infections due to *P. vivax* or *P. ovale* require treatment for both erythrocytic and exoerythrocytic forms to avoid relapsing infection.

Identification to species level is accomplished by a combination of epidemiologic, clinical, and morphologic criteria (Tables 55.4 and 55.5). As noted above, certain malarial species are seen more frequently in various geographic locations. The periodicity of clinical signs and symptoms is helpful, and patients with high levels of parasitemia or profound symptoms are more likely to have *P. falciparum* infection. When examining blood smears there are three major factors to be considered (Table 55.5 and Fig. 55.3): appearance of erythrocytes, appearance of parasites, and developmental stages found. For falciparum malaria (Figs. 55.3 to 55.5), infected red blood cells are normal in size; multiple parasites may be present per cell; the trophozoite stage is a small ring form with double chromatin dots sometimes peripherally located against the wall of the cell in an "appliqué" pattern; schizonts or other mature forms are seldom seen; and the gametocyte is banana shaped. In infections due to *P. vivax* and *P. ovale* (Figures 55.3 and 55.5 to 55.7), infected red blood cells are usually enlarged and contain numerous pink granules or Schüffner's

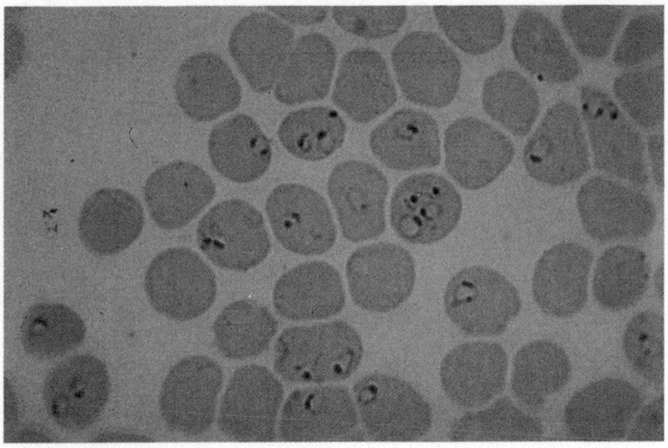

Figure 55.4. *Plasmodium falciparum:* ring forms in film of peripheral blood. (From Smith JW, et al. Diagnostic medical parasitology: blood and tissue parasites. Chicago: American Society of Clinical Pathologists, 1976.)

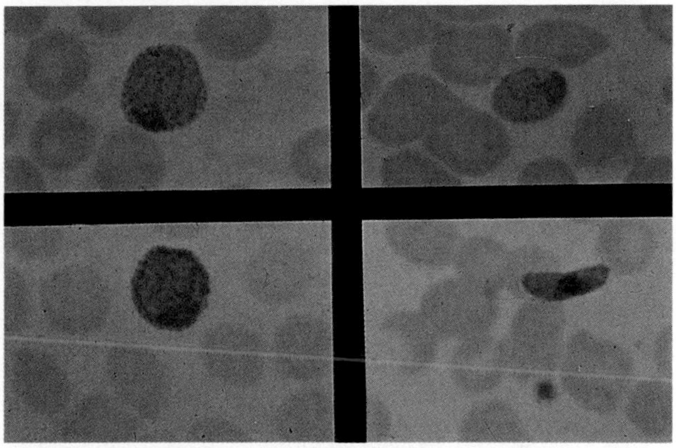

Figure 55.5. Macrogametocytes of *Plasmodium vivax* (*top left*), *P. malariae* (*top right*), *P. ovale* (*bottom left*), and *P. falciparum* (bottom right). (From Smith JW, et al. Diagnostic medical parasitology: blood and tissue parasites. Chicago: American Society of Clinical Pathologists, 1976.)

dots; the trophozoite is ring shaped but ameboid in appearance; more mature trophozoites and erythrocytic schizonts containing up to 24 merozoites are present; and the gametocytes are round. The erythrocytes infected with *P. ovale* are often oval or fimbriated (more than 30% of infected red blood cells). Infections due to *P. malariae* (Figs. 55.3, 55.5, 55.7, and 55.8) are characterized by parasitized red cells that are normal to small in size, trophozoites with dense cytoplasm and occasional band forms, schizonts with 6 to 12 merozoites occasionally arranged in a "rosette" pattern around a pigment clump, and round gametocytes.

Although mixed infections with more than one species of *Plasmodium* can occur, documentation is rare and caution should be used in making such a diagnosis unless there is definitive evidence of two species. The most common mixed infection is due to

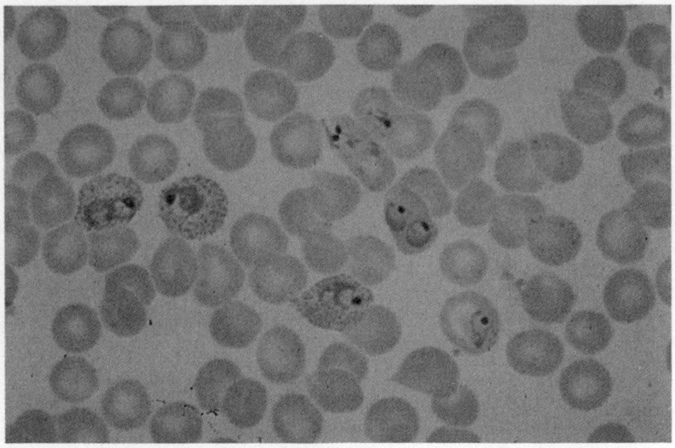

Figure 55.6. *Plasmodium vivax*: young growing trophozoites and ring forms (×1000). (From Smith JW, et al. Diagnostic medical parasitology: blood and tissue parasites. Chicago: American Society of Clinical Pathologists, 1976.)

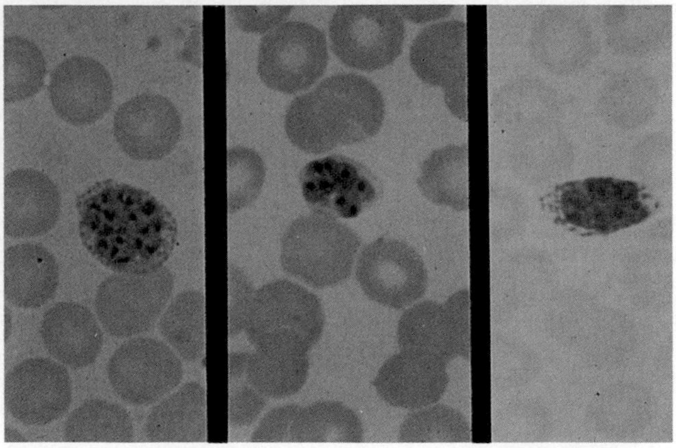

Figure 55.7. Mature schizonts of *Plasmodium vivax* (*left*), *P. malariae* (*center*), and *P. ovale* (*right*) (×1000). (From Smith JW, et al. Diagnostic medical parasitology: blood and tissue parasites. Chicago: American Society of Clinical Pathologists, 1976.)

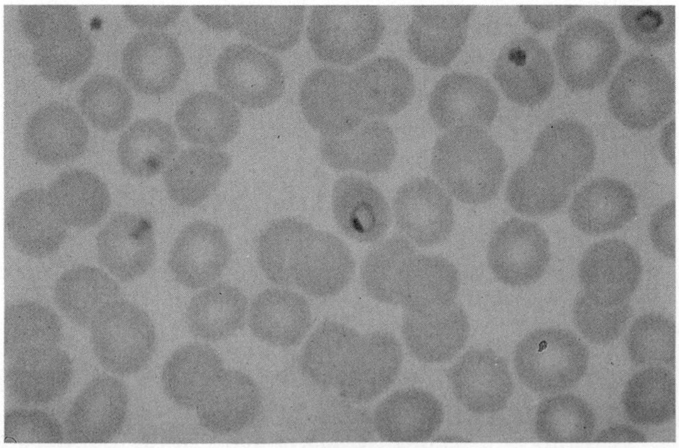

Figure 55.8. *Plasmodium malariae*: ring forms in thin film of peripheral blood. (From Smith JW, et al. Diagnostic medical parasitology: blood and tissue parasites. American Society of Clinical Pathologists, 1976.)

a combination of *P. falciparum* and *P. vivax*. The presence of characteristic *P. falciparum* gametocytes in a patient otherwise infected with *P. vivax* (enlarged red blood cells, multiple developmental forms present) is considered diagnostic. If only ring forms are present the diagnosis of dual infection must be considered tentative at best.

Several serodiagnostic tests have been developed for malaria; however, they are primarily used for seroepidemiologic studies and are rarely necessary to diagnose clinical infections. Newer methods include antigen detection by enzyme-linked immunosorbent assay (ELISA) or radioimmunoassay, nucleic acid detection by DNA probe polymerase chain reaction (PCR), and detection of sporozoite- and merozoite-specific antibodies by ELISA or indirect immunofluorescence (8, 9).

Treatment

Chloroquine is the drug of choice for both prophylaxis and treatment of infection due to *P. vivax, P. ovale, P. malariae*, and susceptible strains of *P. falciparum* (8, 10). Only *P. falciparum* is known to develop resistance to chloroquine; however, recent reports suggest the presence of chloroquine-resistant *P. vivax* in Papua New Guinea (1, 10). Chloroquine-resistant strains of *P. falciparum* exist in virtually all malarious areas of the world except Central America, Haiti, North Africa, and parts of the Middle East, and their existence clearly complicates the prophylaxis and treatment of malaria. Updates on the prevalence of chloroquine-resistant *P. falciparum* and recommendations for antimalarial prophylaxis are published annually by the U.S. Centers for Disease Control and Prevention and by the World Health Association.

Patients infected with chloroquine-resistant *P. falciparum* (or *P. vivax*) may be treated with other agents, including mefloquine, quinine, quinidine, Fansidar (pyrimethamine-sulfadoxine), or doxycycline. Since quinine and Fansidar are potentially toxic, they are used more often for treatment rather than prophylaxis. Amodiaquine, an analogue of chloroquine, is effective against chloroquine-resistant *P. falciparum*; however, toxicity (agranulocytosis and hepatitis) limits its use.

Chloroquine and other blood schizonticides (quinine, quinidine, mefloquin, Fansidar, doxycycline) are not effective against the exoerythrocytic phase (hypnozoite) of *P. vivax* or *P. ovale*. To obtain a radical cure with these infections primaquine is used to eradicate the hypnozoite and prevent its development to the tissue schizont stage and the subsequent release of infectious merozoites. Primaquine is not indicated for either *P. falciparum* or *P. malariae* infections because these parasites do not produce a hypnozoite stage in the liver. Use of primaquine may be dangerous in individuals with glucose-6-phosphate dehydrogenase (G6PD) deficiency and in whom the drug may cause hemolysis of older erythrocytes.

Prevention of malaria by vector control (insecticides, drainage of breeding sites) and personal protection measures against mosquito bites (mosquito netting, screening, insect repellents) are adjunctive measures to specific chemoprophylaxis and treatment regimens. The development of vaccines to protect individuals living in or traveling to endemic areas is under investigation, although results have been disappointing thus far.

Babesia

Babesiosis is a zoonosis infecting a variety of animals, including deer, cattle, and rodents. Humans are accidental hosts. Babesiosis is transmitted in nature by ixodid, or hard-bodied, ticks.

Classification

Babesiosis is caused by intraerythrocytic sporozoan parasites of the genus *Babesia*. Morphologically, *Babesia* resemble malaria parasites but can be distinguished from them by the absence of pigment within infected erythrocytes. Over 70 different species of *Babesia* have been described, including *Babesia bigemina, Babesia argentina*, and *Babesia divergens* in cattle; *Babesia caballi* and *Babesia equi* in horses; *Babesia canis* in dogs; and *Babesia microti* and *Babesia rodhani* in rodents. Identification of the different species is based on morphology and the vertebrate host in which the parasite is found.

Babesiosis is a zoonotic disease occurring in Europe and the United States. The tick vector responsible for transmitting babesiosis, *Ixodes dammini*, is found throughout much of the United States. The natural reservoir hosts are field mice, voles, and other small rodents. Babesiosis is endemic in the United States, particularly on the East Coast. *Babesia microti*, the usual cause of babesiosis in the United States, generally causes a mild disease and is rarely fatal. *B. divergens*, which has been reported more frequently from Europe, causes severe, often fatal infections in individuals who have undergone splenectomies. Although most infections follow tick bites, transfusion-related infections have been reported.

Clinical Manifestations

Human babesiosis ranges in severity from asymptomatic to prolonged severe illness. For the most part infection is self-limited and is characterized by general malaise, fever without periodicity, headache, chills, sweating, fatigue, and weakness (11). The incubation period varies from 1 to 4 weeks. Mild to moderately severe hemolytic anemia and hepatosplenomegaly may develop secondary to red cell destruction by the parasite. In severe cases, renal failure and a picture of acute disseminated intravascular coagulation have been observed. The illness may last from a few weeks to several months. Low-grade parasitemia, with or without symptoms, may persist for up to 4 months. Splenectomy or functional asplenia, as well as immunosuppression and advanced age, appear to increase individual susceptibility to infections, as well as more severe disease.

Life Cycle

Human babesiosis follows contact with an infected ixodid tick. The infectious forms are introduced into the bloodstream by the bite of the tick and infect erythrocytes. There is no evidence for an exoerythrocytic cycle such as that occurring in malaria. *Babesia* multiplies by budding within the red cell to form two to four daughter parasites. The red cells lyse, releasing merozoites that can then infect other red cells and maintain the infection. The major clinical features of babesiosis, including hemolytic anemia, jaundice, and renal failure, are the result of multiplication within the red cells and their subsequent destruction.

The infected red blood cells can also be ingested by feeding ticks, in which additional replication can take place. Transovarial transmission from adult to larval tick also serves to maintain the infection within the tick population.

Diagnosis

As with malaria, the diagnosis of babesiosis requires the identification of characteristic intra-erythrocytic parasites on Giemsa-stained thin or thick blood films (Fig. 55.9). Laboratory personnel must be experienced in differentiating *Babesia* and *Plasmodium* species. The morphologic characteristics of *Babesia* parasites are variable; however, *B. microti* usually appears as a small ring form indistinguishable from young trophozoites of *P. falciparum*. In contrast to *Plasmodium* species, no pigment is produced in erythrocytes infected with *Babesia*. Although characteristic, the tetrad form is rarely seen in human blood films. *Babesia* infections can also be diagnosed by animal (hamster) inoculation. Serologic tests are also available.

Treatment

Human infections due to *B. microti* are generally self-limited and thus the effectiveness of treatment regimens has been difficult to evaluate. Symptomatic

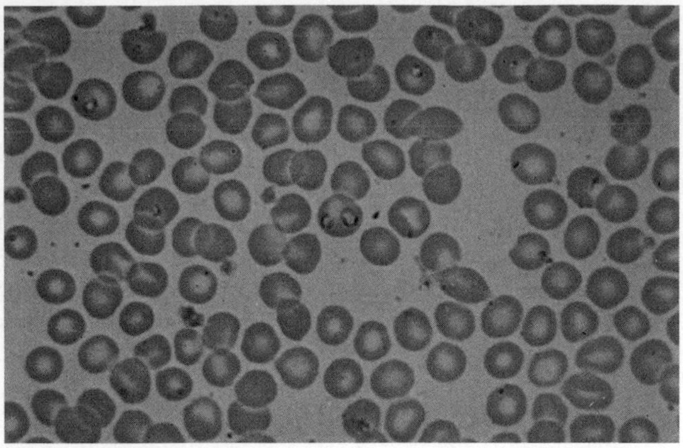

Figure 55.9. *Babesia microti* ring forms (Giemsa stain, ×1000). (From Smith JW, et al. Diagnostic medical parasitology: blood and tissue parasites. Chicago: American Society of Clinical Pathologists, 1976.)

therapy is probably adequate for most patients. Various antiprotozoal regimens including chloroquine and pentamidine have been used with variable results. Severely ill (usually asplenic) patients have been treated successfully with quinine and clindamycin. Exchange blood transfusion has also been successful in splenectomized patients with severe infections due to *B. microti* or *B. divergens* (11).

Preventive measures in endemic areas include wearing protective clothing and using insect repellents to minimize tick exposure. Because ticks must feed on humans for several hours before transmission occurs, prompt removal of ticks may also be protective.

Hemoflagellates

The blood and tissues of humans may be infected by one of several species of flagellate protozoa belonging to the family Trypanosomatidae. All belong to the genera *Leishmania* or *Trypanosoma*. All of these organisms have developmental stages in bloodsucking arthropods (intermediate host) and in humans (definitive host), and many have a nonhuman mammalian reservoir host. *Leishmania* species are transmitted by sandflies (*Phlebotomus, Lutzomyia*), and the trypanosomes are transmitted by either the tsetse fly (*Glossina*) (African trypanosomes) or triatomid bugs (American trypanosomes).

The hemoflagellates may occur in a variety of stages in the human host and the insect vectors (Fig. 55.10). The amastigote form is an intracellular form that is small (2 to 5 μm) and round or oval in shape with a postcentral nucleus, anterior to which are the rodlike kinetoplast and an intracytoplasmic remnant of the flagellum called the axoneme. The promastigote is an extracellular form present in culture and in the arthropod host. It is elongate and slender with a free flagellum. The kinetoplast is located at the anterior (flagellar) end of the parasite. The trypomastigote is the mature extracellular form that may be found in both the arthropod and the blood of the human host. It is long (17 to 30 mm) and slender with a centrally located nucleus and a subterminal kinetoplast. The axoneme forms the outer edge of the undulating membrane and extends anteriorly. The free flagellum projects from the anterior end of the parasite. The flagellum and the undulating membrane serve as a means of locomotion.

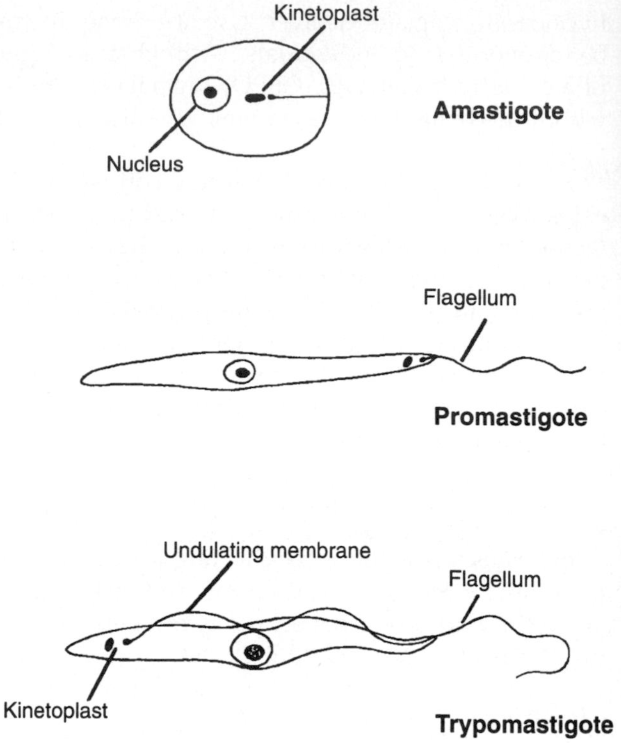

Figure 55.10. Morphological types seen in various hemoflagellates of humans (From Markell EK, Voge M, John DT. Medical parasitology, 7th ed. Philadelphia: WB Saunders, 1992.)

The number of stages present in the life cycle of the parasite varies with the genus and species. The amastigote form is present in the reticuloendothelial cells of individuals infected with *Leishmania* species and in cardiac muscle and other tissues of patients with American trypanosomiasis (Chagas' disease). The trypomastigote form occurs in the blood stream, lymphatics, and cerebrospinal fluid in both Gambian and Rhodesian forms of African trypanosomiasis and in the blood stream in Chagas' disease. Nonflagellate, cryptic forms have also been observed in the choroid plexus of individuals with African trypanosomiasis. The promastigote form is the developmental stage present in the midgut and pharynx of the arthropod vector of leishmaniasis. An epimastigote form (not shown), having a free flagellum and partial undulating membrane, is found in the salivary glands of the tsetse fly vector of African trypanosomiasis. Both promastigote and epimastigote forms may be present in the triatomid vector of Chagas' disease.

LEISHMANIA

Classification

Leishmaniasis is caused by a group of protozoan parasites transmitted by species of sandflies (*Phlebotomus, Lutzomyia*). There are three general forms of leishmaniasis: cutaneous, mucocutaneous, and visceral. Individual members of this group have unique geographical distributions and propensities to cause disease. The *Leishmania tropica* group causes cutaneous disease in the Old World (around the Mediterranean Sea, North and East Africa, the Near East, southern Russia, the Middle East, Afghanistan, India, and China); the *Leishmania mexicana* and *Leishmania braziliensis* groups cause cutaneous and mucosal disease in the New World (from Mexico south through Central and South America, especially Colombia, Ecuador, Venezuela, Peru, and Brazil); and the *Leishmania donovani* group causes visceral disease in both the Old and New World (12).

Leishmania live as amastigotes within the reticuloendothelial cells of the skin, mucous membranes, and viscera. Multiplication is by binary fission. The different species of *Leishmania* cannot be distinguished morphologically. Separation into species and subspecies has been based on unique clinical syndromes, geographic distribution, specific animal reservoirs, and species of sandfly associated with transmission. Recently the application of newer taxonomic and genetic techniques such as restriction analysis of kinetoplast DNA, isoenzyme patterns, and serologic testing has led to some changes in classification and will likely lead to additional changes in the future.

Clinical Manifestations

Visceral Leishmaniasis. Visceral leishmaniasis or kala-azar is caused by *L. donovani* and is endemic in some parts of South America, Africa, China, India, and the Mediterranean area. Infection ranges from asymptomatic in the majority of individuals to an overwhelming systemic illness with death in some. The disease may begin with a skin lesion but primarily is a disease involving the reticuloendothelial system of the visceral organs. The incubation period is variable, but clinical manifestations generally occur 3 to 8 months after exposure. The disease tends to be most pronounced in small children.

Although clinical symptoms may arise quickly with an acute illness, most patients have the insidious development of fever, lassitude, abdominal discomfort and distention secondary to massive hepatosplenomegaly, and progressive emaciation. Fever may be high and intermittent, similar to malaria, or may be continuous and low-grade with night sweats. Symptoms are generally present for weeks to months before patients seek medical attention. These long delays are responsible for the high complication and fatality rates (up to 75%) that have been reported in many studies.

On physical examination the major findings include pallor, jaundice, and hepatosplenomegaly. Both liver and spleen can become massively enlarged but remain soft. The skin becomes thin and dry and may acquire an earth-gray color. Laboratory abnormalities include anemia, leukopenia, and thrombocytopenia. A polyclonal hypergammaglobulinemia is common, and circulating immune complexes may lead to glomerulonephritis.

The pathogenesis of the disease is a mixture of the direct effects of the organism on infected cells and the host response to the infectious process. *L. donovani* disseminates throughout the reticuloendothelial system after ingestion by macrophages. Multiplication of the parasites within the liver, spleen, and bone marrow leads to the clinical syndrome of kala-azar.

Although most infected patients mount an immune response based on production of antibody, T cells appear to be necessary for activation of macrophages to phagocytize and kill the organism. Patients with the most severe disease, usually the young or malnourished, have an inadequate T-cell response to infection.

Visceral leishmaniasis is usually a sporadic disease occurring in endemic areas. Outbreaks have also been described. For example, in the State of Bihar, India in 1977, 70,000 to 100,000 cases with 4,000 deaths were reported (13).

Cutaneous and Mucocutaneous Leishmaniasis. Cutaneous leishmaniasis is caused by several species of *Leishmania* and occurs in both the Old and New World. Cutaneous leishmaniasis of the Old World is an infection characterized by nodular and ulcerative skin lesions caused by *Leishmania tropica, Leishmania major*, and *Leishmania aethiopica*. It is also known as Oriental sore, Baghdad boil, and Delhi boil, among other names.

Cutaneous leishmaniasis of the Old World usually begins as a small papule that develops between 2 weeks and 6 months following the bite of an infected sandfly. This papule slowly enlarges and ulcerates. The ulcer remains shallow and has a well-defined, slightly raised margin. The lesion may be dry or moist and may be single or develop multiple satellite lesions. Regional adenopathy may be present. The

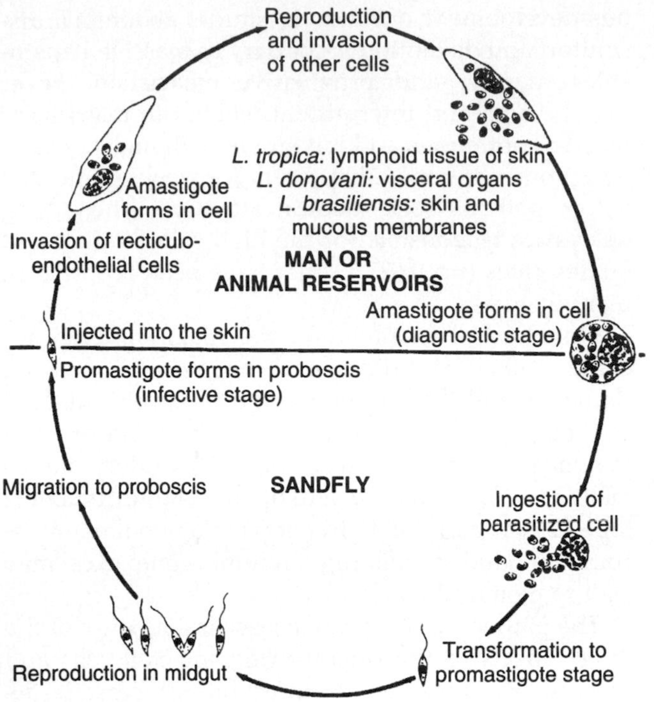

Figure 55.11. The life cycle of *Leishmania*. (From Strickland GT. Hunter's tropical medicine. 7th ed. Philadelphia: WB Saunders, 1991.)

ulcer is usually painless and heals spontaneously after several months unless it is secondarily infected with bacteria. Alternative presentations include papules that do not ulcerate but that disseminate to distant sites and remain active for years, or leishmaniasis recidivans, a relapsing disease with lesions that heal in the center but continue to advance at the periphery and may spread to involve mucous membranes, leading to local destruction of nasal tissue.

Cutaneous leishmaniasis of the New World is also characterized by ulcerative skin lesions. The organism complex causing infection in Central America and southern Mexico is referred to as the *L. mexicana* complex. *L. mexicana* causes a lesion known as chiclero ulcer. The characteristic lesions of the ear occur in 40% of patients and are chronic, lasting many years. *L. braziliensis* causes cutaneous and mucocutaneous infections in humans occurring mainly in Brazil but also seen in other parts of South America. Simple cutaneous lesions caused by *L. braziliensis* generally heal spontaneously within 6 to 18 months but may persist much longer. Persons infected with *L. braziliensis* may develop metastatic spread of the disease to the nasal, pharyngeal, and buccal mucosa. This mucocutaneous form of infection is known as espundia. The mucosal lesions may develop months to years after the onset of cutaneous lesions. Lesions of mucous membranes are slow healing and progressive and may result in massive destruction of the nasal septum, palate, lips, pharynx, and larynx. If untreated this form of the disease may result in death due to aspiration, secondary bacterial infection, or progressive malnutrition.

Life Cycle and Transmission

The life cycle of *Leishmania* is relatively simple and is generally shared by all species (Fig. 55.11). Sandflies feeding on infected individuals ingest free amastigotes or parasitized macrophages. Upon reaching the midgut of the insect, the amastigotes transform into flagellated promastigotes which multiply in the gut and migrate to the proboscis, where they are introduced into the skin of a vertebrate host during a blood meal. Promastigotes injected into the host invade the reticuloendothelial cells, transform into amastigotes, multiply within the phagolysosome and destroy the cell. The liberated amastigotes then invade other cells, continuing the cycle.

Leishmania live in a variety of canine and rodent reservoirs throughout the world. These reservoir hosts may have mild or asymptomatic disease, cutaneous lesions only, or severe visceral disease. Humans may also serve as the reservoir host, particularly in epidemic situations. Rare cases of transmission by blood transfusion or parenteral contact in laboratory settings has been described.

Since there is no animal reservoir of infection in North America, cases of leishmaniasis that occur in the United States occur in individuals who have traveled to endemic areas and who have had exposure to the insect vector. Visceral leishmaniasis is most commonly seen in infants and small children in South America and the Mediterranean region and in older children and adults elsewhere. The immunological mechanism for the predisposition of certain age groups to infection is poorly understood.

Diagnosis

The diagnosis of leishmaniasis is usually made by demonstration of amastigotes in reticuloendothelial cells. Cutaneous and mucocutaneous infection may be diagnosed by examination of material scraped or aspirated from the margin of the ulcer. The material is smeared on a slide and stained with Wright's or Giemsa stain. Biopsies from the edge of the lesion may also be obtained and stained by standard histological methods. Visceral leishmaniasis may be diagnosed by microscopic examination of Giemsa-stained aspirates of bone marrow or spleen. The amastigote stage of the parasite may be found within macrophages or spread out from ruptured cells (Fig. 55.12). The kinetoplast of the organism stains well with Giemsa stain and provides a means of differentiating *Leishmania* from fungal pathogens such as *Histo-*

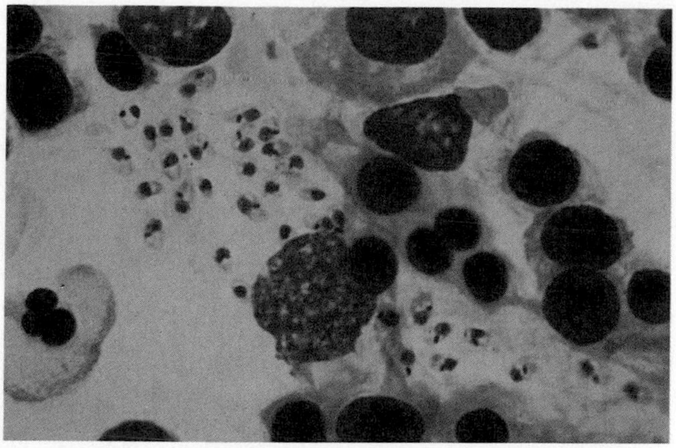

Figure 55.12. *Leishmania donovani*: amastigote in human bone marrow smear (Giemsa stain, ×1280). (From Smith JW, et al. Diagnostic medical parasitology: blood and tissue parasites. Chicago: American Society of Clinical Pathologists, 1976.)

plasma. Although culture of promastigotes on artificial media may also establish the diagnosis, it is not widely available. A skin test, the Montenegro test, is frequently positive in cutaneous or mucocutaneous disease; however, it is usually negative in visceral infection. A variety of serologic tests are available and may be useful in diagnosis or epidemiological studies. Recently, DNA probes have been developed for direct examination of cutaneous lesions. There are no commercially available products for these tests, and careful studies to determine the accuracy of testing procedures have not yet been performed.

Treatment

Visceral leishmaniasis is treated with pentavalent antimonial compounds. Pentostam (stibogluconate sodium) is the agent most commonly employed and readily available. Therapy is not uniformly successful, and relapse rates of 2 to 8% are seen. Repeat therapy with the same compound for extended periods of time may ultimately prove successful in difficult cases. Alternative approaches include the addition of allopurinol or treatment with pentamidine, amphotericin B, or one of a number of alternative oral agents (12, 14). There is some toxicity associated with treatment with any of these compounds, and data on their effectiveness are limited.

Since simple cutaneous infection is usually self-limited, treatment is generally not administered. Treatment is considered for large lesions, for patients with potential or ongoing mucosal disfigurement, and occasionally for cosmetic reasons.

TRYPANOSOMA

The trypanosomes infecting humans cause two distinctly different forms of disease: African trypanosomiasis (sleeping sickness) caused by *Trypanosoma brucei gambiense* and *Trypanosoma brucei rhodesiense* and American trypanosomiasis (Chagas' disease) caused by *Trypanosoma cruzi*. All of these species utilize bloodsucking arthropods as intermediate hosts and vectors for the transmission of infection.

African Trypanosomiasis

Classification. The African trypanosomes, *T. brucei gambiense* and *T. brucei rhodesiense*, are transmitted by species of *Glossina* (tsetse fly). Transmission is limited to the tsetse fly belt in central Africa. The two subspecies are indistinguishable morphologically but differ in the severity and rapidity of disease progression. In both *T. brucei gambiense* and *T. brucei rhodesiense*, the individual trypanosomes vary considerably in size and shape, ranging from delicate, spindle-shaped organisms with a free flagellum to broad, stumpy forms in which a free flagellum is not evident. Parasites may range from 14 to 22 μm in length and from 1.5 to 3.5 μm in breadth. The nucleus is usually centrally located or slightly posterior, and the posterior end of the organism is blunted rather than pointed.

Clinical Manifestations. Infection with the two subspecies results in different but overlapping clinical syndromes separated primarily by the rapidity with which the infection progresses. *T. brucei gambiense* is endemic in the Central African area, extending from the west coast through the central and equatorial zone as far east as Lake Victoria and Tanzania. It produces chronic disease, often ending fatally, with central nervous system involvement after several years' duration. *T. brucei rhodesiense* is generally limited to the savannah areas of East Africa. Rhodesian sleeping sickness is characterized by a more fulminant course with the rapid onset of severe symptoms frequently resulting in the death of the patient within a few months. Both varieties of African trypanosomiasis are associated with a mortality rate approaching 100% in untreated patients.

Infection with *T. brucei gambiense* and *T. brucei rhodesiense* occurs following the bite of a tsetse fly. At the site of the bite a painless nodule develops known as the trypanosomal chancre. This lesion becomes firm and rubbery and resolves after about 2 weeks. Headache, fever, arthralgias, insomnia, edema, and lymphadenopathy accompany the early skin lesion as the parasite enters the bloodstream. Swelling of the posterior cervical lymph nodes is characteristic of Gambian disease and is called Winterbottom's sign. Eventually the organism enters the central nervous system, resulting in a variety of signs and symptoms, including irritability, tremors, ataxia, convulsions, meningoencephalitis, personality change, daytime

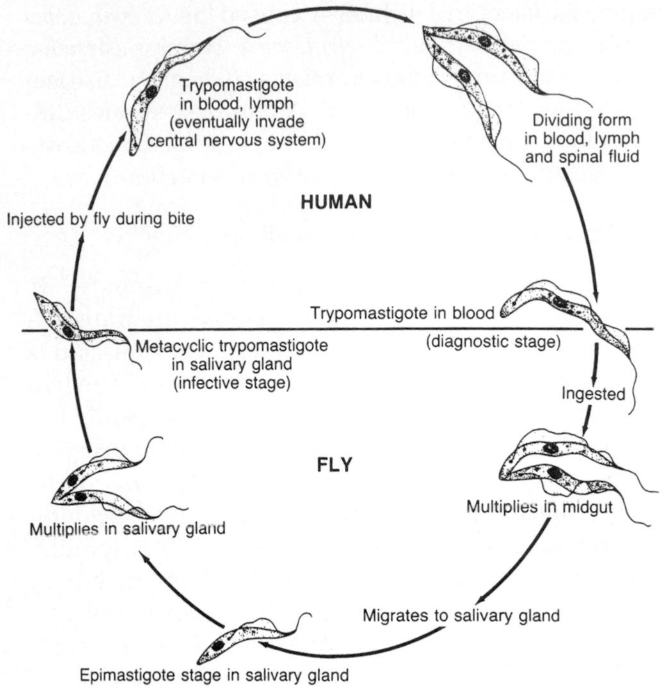

Figure 55.13. Life cycle of *Trypanosoma brucei gambiense* and *T. brucei rhodesiense*. (From Strickland GT. Hunter's Tropical Medicine, 7th ed., WB Saunders, 1991.)

somnolence, pronounced wasting, and eventually coma. Death is the result of central nervous system damage, combined with other infections such as malaria or pneumonia.

Infection with the more virulent *T. brucei rhodesiense* results in greater numbers of organisms in the blood and is generally without lymphadenopathy. Central nervous system invasion occurs early in the infection. The chronic stages of infection are not often seen with Rhodesian disease because, in addition to rapid central nervous system involvement, the organism produces kidney damage and myocarditis, leading to death. Persons with the Rhodesian form of sleeping sickness are usually dead within 9 to 12 months if untreated (15).

Life Cycle. The two African trypanosomes have similar life cycles (Fig. 55.13). Humans and other animals serve as hosts for the trypomastigote form, which lives and multiplies in the blood, lymph nodes, spleen, and cerebrospinal fluid. Tsetse flies become infected during meals on either humans or other infected animals, including a variety of wild and domestic animals. Within the fly, the trypomastigotes multiply within the lumen of the gut, migrate to the salivary glands where they metamorphose into epimastigote forms, and eventually transform into metacyclic trypomastigotes that enter mammalian hosts during feeding. Upon entering the human host, the infective trypomastigotes remain in the tissues at the site of entry, often causing an interstitial

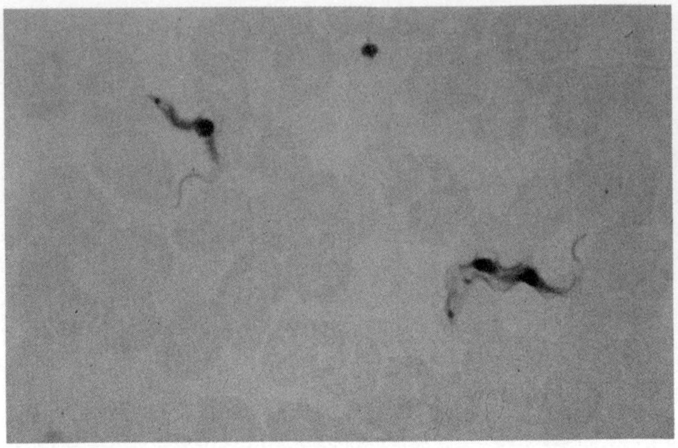

Figure 55.14. *Trypanosoma rhodesiense*: trypomastigotes in thin blood film (Giemsa stain, × 1280). (From Smith JW, et al. Diagnostic medical parasitology: blood and tissue parasites. Chicago: American Society of Clinical Pathologists, 1976.)

inflammatory reaction. After several days they gain entry into the bloodstream, where they multiply and then invade the lymphatics and central nervous system. Although they do not typically invade cells, they elicit an inflammatory response and hyperplasia of the vascular endothelium and produce injurious effects in every organ and tissue in the body.

Diagnosis. Definitive diagnosis of African trypanosomiasis is made by demonstration of the parasite in Giemsa-stained blood films during febrile periods and in lymph node aspirates at other times. Examination of cerebrospinal fluid may be useful in individuals infected with *T. brucei gambiense*; however, patients with *T. brucei rhodesiense* infection rarely survive long enough for the parasites to invade the central nervous system in large numbers. Parasites may be seen on wet preparations of blood and other fluids, but are most easily detected in thick films of blood stained with Giemsa (16). Ideally, both thick and thin films should be examined, as the characteristic morphology of the trypomastigote is best seen in thin smears (Fig. 55.14). Methods for concentrating parasites in blood may also be helpful. Approaches include centrifugation of heparinized samples or DEAE-cellulose anion-exchange chromatography. Levels of parasitemia vary widely, and several attempts to detect the organism over a number of days may be necessary. Since trypomastigotes disintegrate rapidly upon removal from tissues, preparations should be fixed and stained almost immediately. In vitro culture methods or inoculation of blood into suckling mice with subsequent detection of the parasite in tissue are available but not generally used in the diagnosis of African trypanosomiasis.

Serologic tests are also useful diagnostic techniques. Immunofluorescence, ELISA, precipitin, and direct and indirect agglutination methods have been used. Most reagents for such tests are not available commercially. One difficulty in performing and applying serologic tests is the marked variability of the surface antigens of trypanosomes. Such antigens change over time for parasites infecting individual patients, thus antibody reactions may change over time unless antibody reagents identify more constant regions of the parasite surface.

Treatment. Therapy has generally been with suramin or pentamidine, although these drugs do not penetrate the central nervous system well. Arsenicals like melarsoprol have been used to treat more advanced central nervous system disease, although these agents are quite toxic. DL-α-Difluoromethylornithine (DFMO, eflornithine) has recently been introduced and holds promise for treatment of all stages of disease, especially in Gambian trypanosomiasis. Alternative approaches to the control of trypanosomiasis have been to administer pentamidine as prophylaxis every 6 months in endemic areas, or to attempt to eradicate fly vectors. Neither of these approaches has met with great success.

American Trypanosomiasis

Classification. American trypanosomiasis or Chagas' disease, although caused by a similar-appearing parasite, is different clinically and epidemiologically from African trypanosomiasis. Chagas' disease is caused by *Trypanosoma cruzi*, an organism that differs from other trypanosomes infecting humans in that it has an intracellular amastigote stage in cardiac muscle and other tissues, as well as trypomastigote forms circulating in the blood. Unlike other trypanosomes, *T. cruzi* does not multiply in the blood. The amastigote stage replicates intracellularly within the tissues. *T. cruzi* is found in most of Central and South America and is transmitted to humans by the bite of reduviid bugs.

Clinical Manifestations. Chagas' disease may present clinically as an asymptomatic, acute, or chronic disease process. Some individuals may manifest all three stages of the disease. The disease is most severe in children under 5 years of age and frequently presents as an acute process with central nervous system involvement. The disease is usually more subacute or chronic in older children and adults. Following the bite of the vector insect the organisms proliferate locally in the tissues, producing an erythematous indurated area called a chagoma. These lesions frequently appear on the face and if present around the eye are known as Romaña's sign.

Acute infection is characterized by fever, chills, malaise, myalgia, and fatigue. Parasites may be present in the blood during the acute phase; however, they are sparse in patients older than 1 year. An acute attack may terminate in a few weeks in death or recovery, or the patient may enter the chronic stage of infection. Infected young children may develop central nervous system involvement and die within a few days or weeks.

In the chronic phase of disease organisms proliferate as amastigotes in cardiac, skeletal, smooth muscle, and neurological cells as well as the cells of the reticuloendothelial system. Damage to the autonomic nervous system of the heart and digestive tract as well as to the musculature of these organs produces the characteristic cardiac conduction and esophageal and colonic motility defects seen in chronic Chagas' disease. The chronic phase of disease commonly presents with myocarditis, megacardium, and electrocardiographic changes. Less commonly patients may suffer from impaired esophageal and gastrointestinal motility and massive enlargement of the digestive tract, particularly the esophagus and colon (megaesophagus and megacolon). Hepatosplenomegaly is also apparent. Involvement of the central nervous system may produce a meningoencephalitis. Death from chronic Chagas' disease results from heart failure, cardiac arrhythmias, and other complications secondary to tissue destruction in the many areas invaded by the organisms.

Life Cycle. In the vertebrate host, *T. cruzi* occurs in the blood as a nondividing trypomastigote form. The life cycle of *T. cruzi* (Fig. 55.15) differs from that of the other *Trypanosoma* species with the development of an intracellular amastigote form within the tissues. The amastigote multiplies within the parasitized cells by binary fission, thus causing disruption of the cell. The released amastigotes then invade other cells and multiply within them. After a period of growth within the tissues, the amastigotes transform into trypomastigotes and are released into the circulating blood, where they may be ingested by new insect vectors. Within the reduviid bug, the organism transforms into the epimastigote stage and then back into the infective trypomastigote. The infective trypomastigotes pass out of the bug in its feces, and are deposited on the skin during feeding, and then may be rubbed into the bite or a skin abrasion. The infective stages are almost immediately ingested by macrophages and transformed into amastigotes.

Diagnosis. The diagnosis of Chagas' disease is based on the visualization of trypomastigotes in blood during the initial acute phase or during febrile periods during the chronic stage. The highest yield occurs during the early acute phase; latent or chronic disease is seldom associated with enough parasitemia to make direct detection possible. Amastigote forms may be found in biopsies of affected tissue

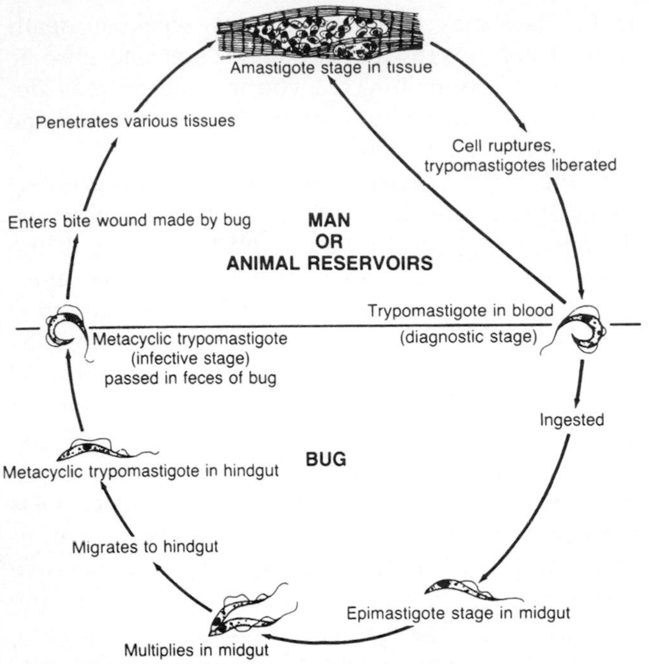

Figure 55.15. Life cycle of *Trypanosoma cruzi*. (From Strickland GT. Hunter's Tropical Medicine, 7th ed., WB Saunders, 1991.)

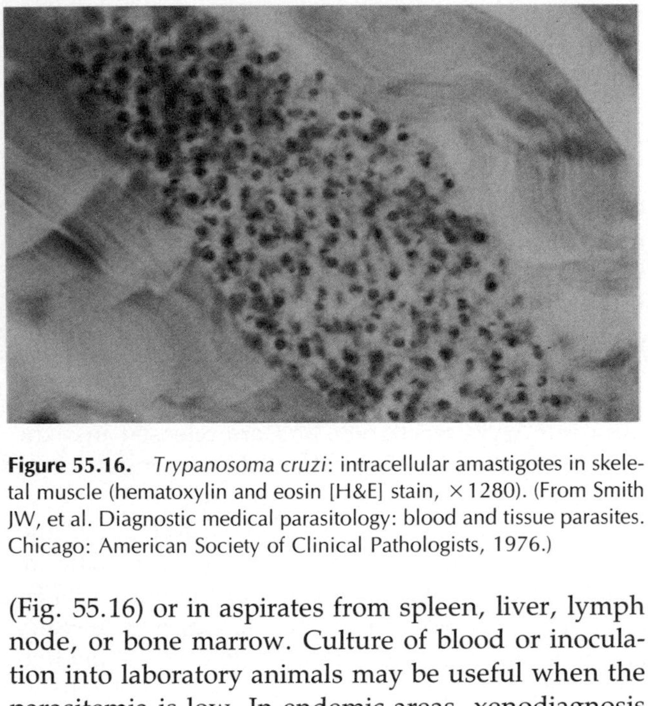

Figure 55.16. *Trypanosoma cruzi*: intracellular amastigotes in skeletal muscle (hematoxylin and eosin [H&E] stain, ×1280). (From Smith JW, et al. Diagnostic medical parasitology: blood and tissue parasites. Chicago: American Society of Clinical Pathologists, 1976.)

(Fig. 55.16) or in aspirates from spleen, liver, lymph node, or bone marrow. Culture of blood or inoculation into laboratory animals may be useful when the parasitemia is low. In endemic areas, xenodiagnosis is widely used. Trypanosome-free reduviid bugs are allowed to feed on the patient suspected to be suffering from Chagas' disease, and the feces of the bug are examined for the appearance of parasites over a period of about 10 days.

Diagnosis of chronic disease is largely based on serologic testing. A variety of serologic tests are available, including direct hemagglutination, complement fixation, immunofluorescence assays, and ELISA. No single method is felt to be adequate, and most patients are evaluated by multiple assays before making a final diagnosis.

Treatment. Treatment of Chagas' disease is limited by the lack of reliable agents. The current drug of choice is nifurtimox, a nitrofuran derivative. While it has some activity against the acute phase of disease, it has little activity against tissue amastigotes and has a number of side effects. Alternative agents include allopurinol and benznidazole, an imidazole compound. Another imidazole, the antifungal agent ketoconazole, has been shown to inhibit the intracellular multiplication of *T. cruzi* amastigotes and to afford protection to mice infected with *T. cruzi* (17).

Prevention of infection is also important. Vector control through the use of insecticide treatment of reduviid bug–infected dwellings, eradication of nests, and construction of homes to prevent nesting of bugs is essential. Screening of blood by serological means or excluding blood donors from endemic areas prevents some infections that would otherwise be associated with transfusion therapy.

Toxoplasma gondii

Classification

Toxoplasma gondii is a typical coccidian parasite related to *Plasmodium*, *Babesia*, *Isospora*, and other members of the phylum Apicomplexa. *T. gondii* is an intracellular parasite and is found in a wide variety of animals, including birds and humans. There is only one species and there appears to be little strain-to-strain variation. Human infection with *T. gondii* is ubiquitous; however, it is increasingly apparent that certain immunocompromised patients are more likely to have severe manifestations. The essential reservoir host of *T. gondii* is the common house cat and other felines.

Clinical Manifestations

Multiple clinical syndromes have been described for infection with *T. gondii*. Most common, however, is asymptomatic infection in normal hosts (18). When symptomatic disease occurs, the infection is characterized by intracellular replication of the organisms, cell destruction, and eventual cyst formation.

A small percentage of otherwise normal individuals on first exposure to the organism will develop an acute illness with cervical or generalized adenopathy. The adenopathy is typically nontender and nonfluctuant; however, occasionally the nodes can be quite tender. In certain individuals the acute infection may resemble infectious mononucleosis with fever, malaise, headache, night sweats, myalgias, sore throat, maculopapular rash, and hepatosplenomegaly (18). Atypical lymphocytes may be present on peripheral smear. A small percentage of these patients can have major complications, including retroperitoneal adenopathy with severe abdominal pain, chorioretinitis, myocarditis, pneumonia, or encephalitis. Most individuals with acute infection, however, have a benign course with spontaneous recovery in days to weeks.

Congenital infection with *T. gondii* also occurs in infants born to mothers who are infected during pregnancy. The likelihood of transmission of the organism from mother to infant increases during the course of gestation, with infection occurring in about 25% of infants exposed in the first trimester, 54% in the second, and 65% in the third. If infection occurs in the first trimester the result is spontaneous abortion, stillbirth, or severe disease. Manifestations of infection in the infant infected after the first trimester include epilepsy, encephalitis, microcephaly, intracranial calcifications, hydrocephalus, psychomotor or mental retardation, chorioretinitis, strabismus, blindness, anemia, jaundice, rash, pneumonia, diarrhea, and hypothermia (19).

Infants may be asymptomatic at birth only to develop disease months to years later. Most often these children develop chorioretinitis with or without blindness, or develop other neurological problems, including retardation, seizures, microcephaly, or hearing loss.

In immunocompromised older patients a different spectrum of acquired disease is seen. Reactivation of latent toxoplasmosis is a special problem in these individuals. The presenting symptoms of *Toxoplasma* infection in immunocompromised patients are usually neurologic, most frequently consistent with diffuse encephalopathy, meningoencephalitis, or cerebral mass lesions. Reactivation of cerebral toxoplasmosis has emerged as a major cause of encephalitis in patients with AIDS (20). The disease is usually multicentric, with more than one mass lesion appearing in the brain at the same time. Symptoms are related to the location of the lesions and may include hemiparesis, seizures, visual impairment, confusion, and lethargy. Other sites of possible infection include the eye, lung (21), and testes (22). Although disease is seen predominantly in patients with AIDS, it may also occur with similar manifestations in other immunocompromised patients, in particular in those undergoing organ transplantation.

Life Cycle and Epidemiology

The life cycle of *T. gondii* is shown in Figure 55.17. The complete life cycle (both asexual and sexual reproduction) occurs, as far as it is known, only in the cat. Humans and other animals are considered to be

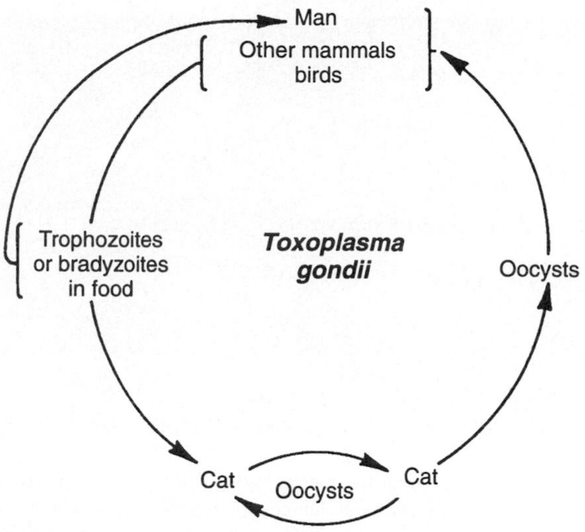

Figure 55.17. Life cycle of *Toxoplasma gondii*. (From Markell EK, Voge M, John DT. Medical parasitology. 7th ed. Philadelphia: WB Saunders, 1992.)

intermediate hosts in which only asexual reproduction, characterized by proliferative forms and cysts, has been observed. Felines ingest oocysts from the environment and cysts (bradyzoites) from tissues of other species. Organisms develop within the intestinal cells of the cat to form oocysts, which are passed in the feces. Oocysts shed in the feces are immature, becoming infective in 1 to 5 days. Intermediate hosts become infected by ingesting mature oocysts or by ingesting cyst-containing meat from other infected animals. Once ingested by the intermediate host the organism develops into the rapidly multiplying tachyzoite form that is responsible for the initial spread of infection. The tachyzoites disseminate via the bloodstream to many organs and tissues, where they undergo intracellular replication. Multiplication of the parasites within an infected cell usually leads to death and rupture of the cell, releasing the tachyzoites to infect new cells, or it may lead to formation of a cyst within the infected tissue. The cyst form predominates in chronic or latent toxoplasmosis. Individual cysts contain the slowly developing bradyzoites and measure up to 0.1 mm in diameter. Disease manifestations in chronic toxoplasmosis are primarily the result of the mechanical presence of the enlarging cyst.

Human infection occurs after ingestion of viable cysts or trophozoites in undercooked meat or infective oocysts from cat fecal contamination. Since oocysts require several days outside the feline host to mature, infection will generally occur only if there is exposure to soil previously contaminated or to cat feces in a litter box that has not been cleaned for several days. Transmission of infection from contaminated beef, pork, lamb, and goat's milk has been

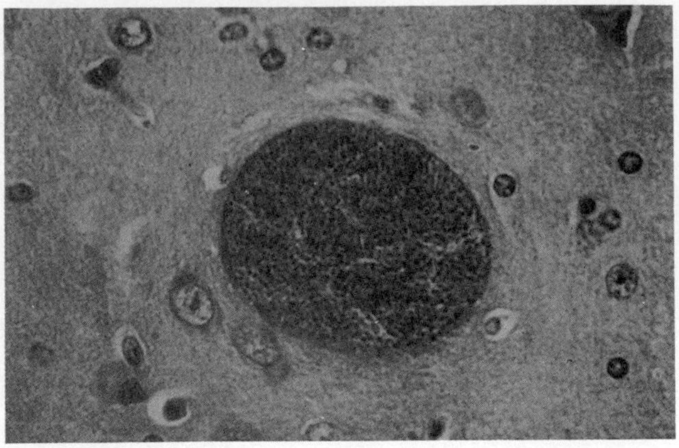

Figure 55.18. *Toxoplasma gondii*: cyst in brain section (H&E stain, × 560). (From Smith JW, et al. Diagnostic medical parasitology: blood and tissue parasites. Chicago: American Society of Clinical Pathologists, 1976.)

described. Fresh fruit and vegetables may also be a source of infection if the soil they are grown in is contaminated with oocysts. Aside from congenital infection, transmission of infection from person to person has been described only rarely via blood transfusion or solid organ transplantation.

Seroprevalence rates vary from place to place for reasons that remain obscure; however, studies indicate that populations with greater consumption of rare or uncooked meat are more likely to be seropositive. For example, the highest recorded rate (93%) has been reported in Parisian women who prefer undercooked or raw meat (1, 20). Rates may also vary by climate, as oocysts do not survive well in colder regions.

Although the rate of seroconversion is similar for individuals within a geographic location, that of severe infection is dramatically affected by the immune status of the individual. Patients with defects in cell-mediated immunity, especially those with HIV infection or following organ transplantation (on immunosuppressive therapy), are most likely to have disseminated or central nervous system disease. Illness in this setting is generally felt to be caused by reactivation of previously latent infection rather than new exposure to the organism.

Diagnosis

There are several possible approaches to the diagnosis of toxoplasmosis. The diagnosis may be established by laboratory tests, including direct visualization of the organism in tissue, growth in culture, or more commonly by serologic methods. In immunocompromised individuals the diagnosis is often presumptive based on typical findings and clinical impression.

Direct examination of tissue suspected of infection is the definitive method of diagnosis (Fig. 55.18). Biopsy specimens from lymph nodes, brain, liver, myocardium, or other suspected tissue or from body fluids—including cerebrospinal fluid, amniotic fluid, bronchoalveolar lavage fluid, or peritoneal fluid—can be examined directly for the organisms. The most useful stains appear to be direct fluorescent antibody stains and peroxidase-antiperoxidase stains using antibodies to *T. gondii*. The fluorescent antibody stains available to date have not been as sensitive and specific as the immunoperoxidase stain. Newer monoclonal antibody–based fluorescent stains may prove to be better than the older polyclonal versions. In addition, Wright-Giemsa stains of tissue specimens can be utilized to see the organism.

Culture methods for *T. gondii* are largely experimental and are not usually available in clinical laboratories. The two methods available are to inoculate potentially infected material into either mouse peritoneum or tissue culture. Tissue cultures are more readily available, may grow organisms more quickly, and are easier to process because identification simply requires microscopic examination of the culture vial. Mouse inoculation may be more sensitive, however.

Serologic testing is commonly employed for the diagnosis of toxoplasmosis. As with other infectious serologies, attention to increasing IgG titers in serially collected blood samples or a positive IgM titer is essential to differentiate acute, active infection from previous asymptomatic or chronic infection. Although the Sabin-Feldman dye test is considered the reference method for serologic testing, it is not widely employed in clinical laboratories due to the requirement for live organisms as the antigen source. Several alternative methods are available, including indirect fluorescent antibodies, indirect hemagglutination, complement fixation, and ELISA methods for both IgG and IgM antibodies. Currently the ELISA tests for IgG and IgM are the most widely used because of their simplicity and rapidity in documenting acute infections. These tests are not generally satisfactory in immunocompromised individuals with latent or reactivated infections, because these patients frequently fail to produce an IgM response or an increasing IgG titer.

Treatment

Therapy of toxoplasmosis depends on the nature of both the infectious process and the immunocompetence of the host. Most mononucleosis-like infections in normal individuals resolve spontaneously without intervention. On the other hand, disseminated or central nervous system infection in compromised patients must be treated. Prior to its association with HIV infection, immunocompromised patients with toxoplasmosis were treated for 4 to 6 weeks. In the setting of HIV infection the rate of relapse when therapy is discontinued is about 25%. Such patients are now treated with an initial high-dose regimen of pyrimethamine and sulfadiazine, and then continued on lower doses of both drugs indefinitely (23). Although pyrimethamine and sulfadiazine are the agents of choice, side effects, in particular rash and bone marrow suppression, often require changes to alternative agents. Unfortunately, alternatives have not been tested in any large-scale trials, and their effectiveness is not established. The alternative regimens include clindamycin plus pyrimethamine and trimethoprim-sulfamethoxazole. Response to therapy occurs in 80 to 90% of patients, with improvement most likely to occur in patients with milder disease. Ocular infections generally respond well to pyrimethamine and sulfadiazine, with treatment periods lasting approximately 1 month.

Infection in the first trimester of pregnancy has been difficult to manage because pyrimethamine is teratogenic in laboratory animals. Both clindamycin and spiramycin have been substituted with apparent success. Spiramycin does not appear to be effective therapy for toxoplasmosis in immunocompromised individuals.

The use of corticosteroids in treatment of toxoplasmosis remains controversial. It is definitely believed to be of benefit in ocular infections that involve or threaten the macula. The use of steroids for central nervous system infections, even when brain edema is evident on computed tomographic scan, is not accepted as beneficial. Steroids are generally added in such cases only when progression of clinical symptoms continues despite appropriate antimicrobial therapy.

As more immunocompromised patients at risk for disseminated toxoplasmosis are identified, greater emphasis is being placed on preventive therapy. Routine serologic screening of patients is now being performed prior to organ transplantation and early in the course of HIV infection. Those with positive serologies are at much higher risk for development of disease and are now being considered for prophylaxis. Trimethoprim-sulfamethoxazole, which is also used as prophylaxis to prevent *Pneumocystis* infections, also appears to be effective at preventing or limiting infections with *Toxoplasma*. Additional preventive measures for pregnant women and immunocompromised hosts should include avoiding both consumption of raw or undercooked meat and exposure to cat feces.

Pneumocystis carinii

Classification

Pneumocystis carinii has long been considered a sporozoan parasite based on morphologic characteristics, response to antiparasitic drugs, and failure to grow on bacterial or fungal media. More recently, the sequence of *P. carinii* ribosomal RNA suggests that the organism is more closely related to the fungi than to the protozoa (4). *P. carinii* causes pulmonary infections in a variety of domestic and wild animals as well as humans.

Clinical Manifestations

Pneumocystis most often causes an interstitial pneumonitis with plasma cell infiltrates. Subclinical infections in healthy individuals are probably frequent, and the organism may remain latent for long periods of time. It has been suggested that the organism maintains a commensal relationship with the healthy host, proliferating and causing disease only when the host's resistance is lowered. Infection almost always occurs in immunocompromised hosts, and *P. carinii* pneumonia is the most common opportunistic infection seen in patients with AIDS. Pneumocystosis is also seen frequently in premature and malnourished children. Clinical manifestations include the insidious onset of dry cough, dyspnea, and fever. Symptoms may develop over a period of 2 to 3 weeks before they become severe enough for the patient to seek medical attention.

At the time of initial evaluation patients may have minimal evidence to suggest the presence of pneumonia. Although chest radiographs usually show bilateral interstitial infiltrates, the x-ray may be entirely normal. Additional parameters that help suggest the diagnosis include hypoxia or decreased oxygen saturation, and increased pulmonary uptake on gallium scans.

In the past few years extrapulmonary infections with *P. carinii* have been described in patients with AIDS. Multiple sites of involvement have been observed, including ear, eye, liver, and bone marrow (5–7). Most such patients have received aerosolized pentamidine as prophylaxis to prevent *P. carinii* pneumonia.

Life Cycle and Epidemiology

P. carinii is a ubiquitous organism, with infections reported worldwide. Entry of the organism into the host appears to be by the respiratory route from the environment. There appears to be little person-to-person transmission, although the mechanism by

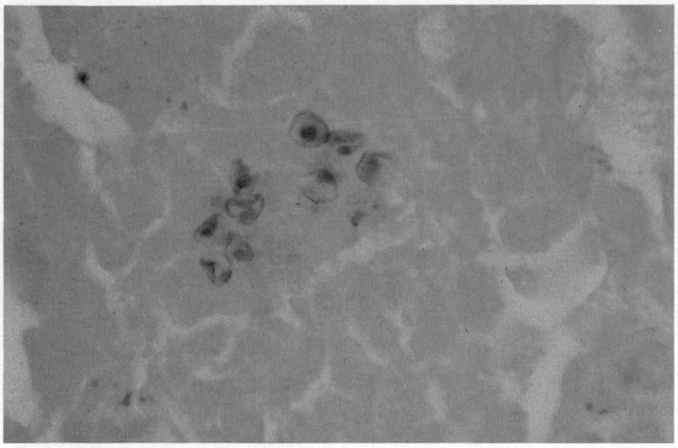

Figure 55.19. *Pneumocystis carinii* cysts in lung impression smear (silver stain, ×1200). (From Smith JW, et al. Diagnostic medical parasitology: blood and tissue parasites. Chicago: American Society of Clinical Pathologists, 1976.)

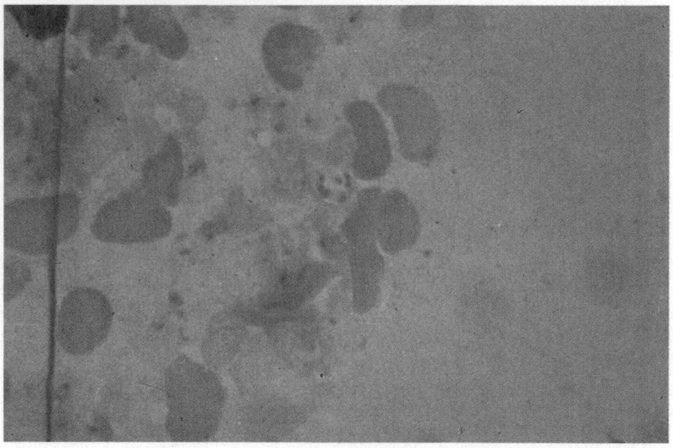

Figure 55.20. *Pneumocystis carinii* cysts and sporozoites in lung impression smear (Giemsa stain, ×1200). (From Smith JW, et al. Diagnostic medical parasitology: blood and tissue parasites. Chicago: American Society of Clinical Pathologists, 1976.)

which patients acquire the organism and its natural habitat in the environment are unknown.

The life cycle of *P. carinii* includes a resistant cyst stage, intracystic sporozoites, and free trophozoite forms (Figs. 55.19 and 55.20). Cysts are round, ovoid, or cup-shaped, are 5 to 12 μm in diameter, and contain four to eight intracystic bodies or sporozoites. The sporozoites are released from the mature cyst and become trophozoites. The extracystic or trophozoite form is pleomorphic, 1 to 4 μm in diameter, with a red nucleus and blue cytoplasm on Giemsa stain. The trophozoite does not invade the pulmonary epithelial cells but rather adheres to the surface of the alveolar epithelium, where it in turn develops into the cyst stage producing additional sporozoites. Masses of cysts and trophozoites are seen in pulmonary specimens obtained from patients with *P. carinii* pneumonia.

Diagnosis

Diagnosis of *P. carinii* pneumonia is established by demonstrating organisms in lung tissue, bronchoscopy specimens, or sputum (Figs. 55.19 and 55.20). Bronchoalveolar lavage fluid alone is adequate for demonstration of the organism in over 90% of AIDS patients. The yield is somewhat lower in patients with other underlying immune deficiencies. Induced sputum specimens may also be useful in AIDS patients due to the tremendous organism burden. Percutaneous lung aspirates, transbronchial biopsies, and open lung biopsies are occasionally needed for diagnosis but are not performed unless bronchial lavage results are negative.

The parasites can be stained with methenamine silver or Giemsa stain, or with specific fluorescein-labeled antibodies (24). In Giemsa-stained preparations, the individual sporozoites within the cysts as well as the free trophozoites can be seen. Methenamine silver stains the cyst wall black but will not reveal trophozoites. The recently available fluorescent antibody stains appear to be at least as sensitive and specific as the silver or Giemsa stains (24).

P. carinii does not grow well in culture and this is not a viable diagnostic approach. Serologic tests are not available.

Treatment

Therapy of acute *P. carinii* pneumonia is usually with parenteral trimethoprim-sulfamethoxazole. For patients who cannot tolerate this combination or in patients who have not responded after several days of treatment, the alternative agent is intravenous pentamidine. In mild infections lower doses of trimethoprim-sulfamethoxazole, aerosolized pentamidine, or dapsone may be used with good success. Alternative agents are being studied to both improve patient outcome and reduce the toxicity associated with these therapies. The addition of corticosteroids to the treatment regimen has been controversial, but recent studies have shown that the addition of steroids does improve outcome for patients with severe disease.

Equally as important as treatment of acute infection is the institution of prophylactic therapy to prevent recurrences of infection or primary infection in high-risk patients. Up to 85% of AIDS patients will develop *Pneumocystis* pneumonia in the absence of prophylaxis. Agents employed for prophylaxis include oral trimethoprim-sulfamethoxazole, dapsone, and aerosolized pentamidine. Although recommendations continue to change, it appears that trimethoprim-sulfamethoxazole or dapsone is preferred and that these agents are associated with fewer breakthrough infections and less chance for extrapulmonary infection.

Free-living Amebae

Classification

Free-living amebic infections are caused by organisms belonging to the genera *Naegleria* and *Acanthamoeba*. These organisms are ubiquitous in nature and are free-living in soil or water. *Naegleria* species are classified as ameboflagellates and are able to exist temporarily in a flagellate form as well as in an aflagellar ameboid form. *Acanthamoeba* organisms never produce flagella. Both organisms may undergo cyst formation outside the host, but only *Acanthamoeba* forms cysts in infected tissue.

Clinical Manifestations

Both *Naegleria* and *Acanthamoeba* organisms are opportunistic pathogens. Infections range from acute fulminating primary amebic meningoencephalitis to the more chronic granulomatous encephalitis and amebic keratitis. In most cases it is thought that the infection was acquired from the environment either by swimming in contaminated water, inhalation of cysts in dust, or direct implantation on the surface of the cornea either by dust or contaminated contact lens material.

Acute primary amebic meningoencephalitis is most commonly caused by *Naegleria fowleri* and occurs when amebae present in water invade the nasal mucosa and extend into the brain. Acute amebic meningoencephalitis may be indistinguishable from bacterial meningitis and is marked by fever, severe frontal headache, stiff neck, nausea, and vomiting. Abnormalities of taste and smell may be present and seizures are common. The process is rapid and may progress to coma within 48 hours. The cerebrospinal fluid is purulent and may contain many erythrocytes and motile amebae. The vast majority of cases are fatal.

In contrast to *Naegleria*, central nervous system involvement with *Acanthamoeba* is generally a more subacute or chronic process with a granulomatous encephalitis and single or multiple brain abscesses. Headache and fever are present but are more insidious and low grade. A wide variety of neurologic signs eventually appear depending on the area of the brain involved. The cerebrospinal fluid may contain both neutrophils and mononuclear cells, but amebae are rare. This form of amebic meningoencephalitis occurs more commonly in immunosuppressed individuals and is uniformly fatal.

Other forms of infection with free-living amebae are usually due to *Acanthamoeba* and include ocular, cutaneous, pulmonary, and sinus involvement. The most common of these infections is amebic keratitis. The keratitis is usually associated with corneal trauma followed by contact with contaminated soil or water. In recent years the most common form of amebic keratitis has been associated with improper use of contact lenses, particularly extended-wear lenses. Cases of apparent disseminated cutaneous and subcutaneous infection with *Acanthamoeba* have been described in AIDS patients (25). These infections present with multiple soft tissue nodules which on biopsy contain *Acanthamoeba*. Central nervous system or deep tissue involvement may also be present with this form of infection.

Life Cycle

The life cycle of the free-living amebae is relatively simple, involving both cyst and motile trophozoite forms. In addition, *Naegleria* has a flagellate stage that alternates with the ameboid trophozoite phase. Free-living forms of the amebae come into contact with nasal or respiratory mucosa following exposure to contaminated water or dust. Following multiplication locally, invasion of the central nervous system and other tissues occurs by hematogenous spread. In *Naegleria* infection only the ameboid trophozoites are found within the tissue, whereas with *Acanthamoeba* infection both trophozoites and cysts are found in tissues. Amebic keratitis occurs by direct contact of the cornea with amebae, which may be introduced through mild corneal trauma or by exposure to contaminated water or contact lens material or solutions. Trophozoites and cysts of *Acanthamoeba* are found in infected corneal tissue.

Diagnosis

Diagnosis of free-living amebic infections is established by demonstrating the organisms in cerebrospinal fluid, nasal discharge, or tissue (corneal scrapings, biopsy) by light or phase microscopy, by culture, or by animal inoculation. *Naegleria* and *Acanthamoeba* may be difficult to differentiate in tissue. Isolation in culture may be accomplished by growing the organism on plain agar plates seeded with Gram-negative enteric bacilli. *Naegleria* measure 8 to 15 μm in diameter and have blunt pseudopodia, whereas *Acanthamoeba* are 10 to 15 μm and have spinelike pseudopodia. Additional differentiating features are the presence of a flagellate stage with *Naegleria* and the production of a cyst form in tissue with *Acanthamoeba*. Immunofluorescent staining has been used to differentiate these organisms in tissue.

Treatment

Treatment of free-living amebic infections is largely ineffective. Amebic meningoencephalitis due to either *Naegleria* or *Acanthamoeba* is unresponsive to antibacterial and antiamebic drugs. Amphotericin B,

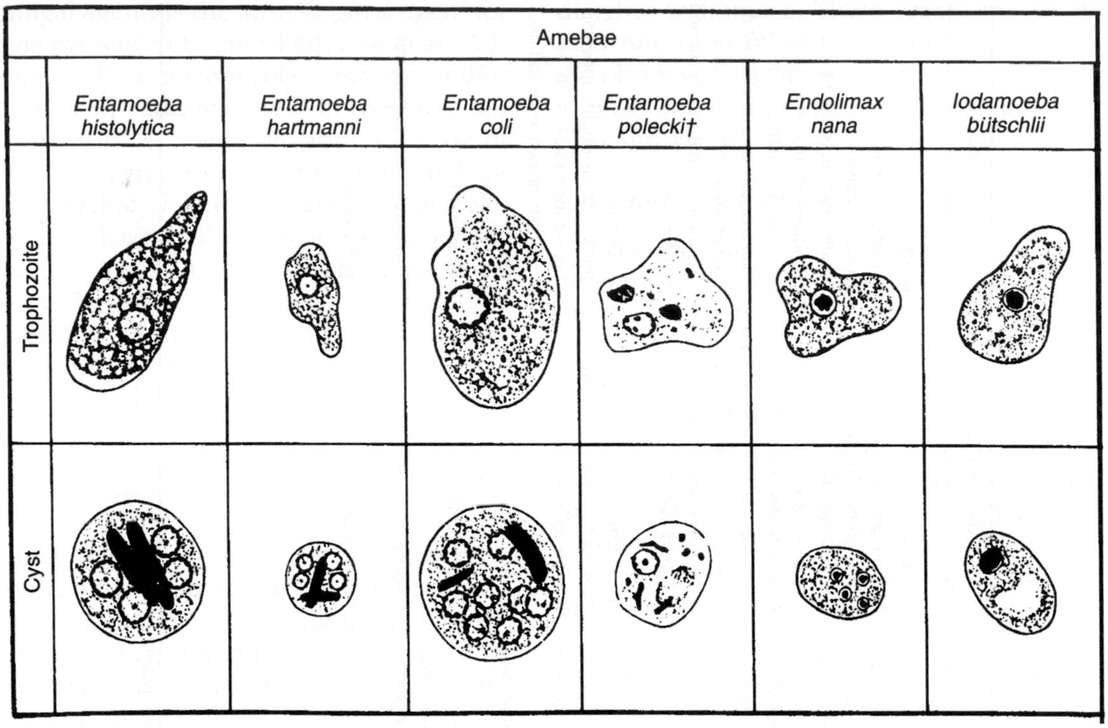

Figure 55.21. Amebae found in stool specimens of humans. *Entamoeba polecki* is rare, probably of animal origin. (From Smith JW, et al. Diagnostic medical parasitology: intestinal protozoa. Chicago: American Society of Clinical Pathologists, 1976.)

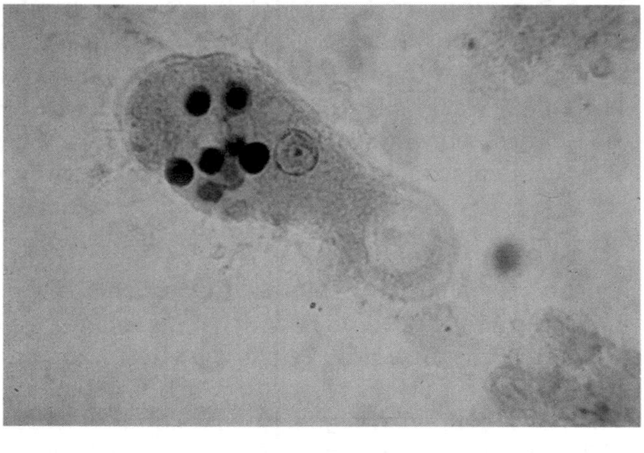

Figure 55.22. *Entamoeba histolytica* trophozoite with ingested erythrocytes in fecal smear (trichrome stain, ×1125). (From Smith JW, et al. Diagnostic medical parasitology: intestinal protozoa. Chicago: American Society of Clinical Pathologists, 1976.)

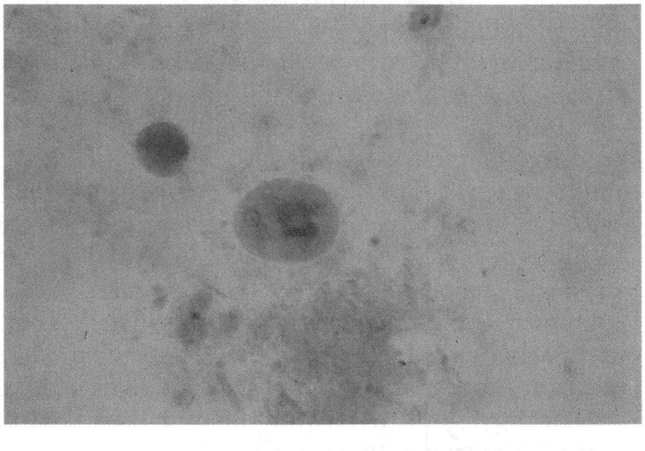

Figure 55.23. Mature cyst of *Entamoeba histolytica* containing chromatoidal bodies (trichrome stain of fecal smear, ×1200). (From Smith JW, et al. Diagnostic medical parasitology: intestinal protozoa. Chicago: American Society of Clinical Pathologists, 1976.)

gestion of infective cysts in contaminated food or water, the cysts pass through the stomach, where exposure to gastric acid stimulates excystation and release of the pathogenic trophozoite in the duodenum. The number of trophozoites produced varies with the number of nuclei in the cyst stage. The trophozoites become established and proliferate by binary fission in the large intestine, where they produce extensive local necrosis. Under certain conditions encystation occurs. The resulting cysts are passed in the feces, thus perpetuating the cycle.

E. histolytica has a worldwide distribution; however, its highest incidence is in underdeveloped tropical and subtropical regions with poor sanitation and contaminated water. Many of the infected individuals are asymptomatic carriers and represent a reservoir for the spread of *E. histolytica* to others. Both symptomatic and asymptomatic individuals infected with *E. histolytica* may pass infectious cysts, as well as noninfectious trophozoites, in their stools. The trophozoites are unable to survive for prolonged periods in the environment and are destroyed by gas-

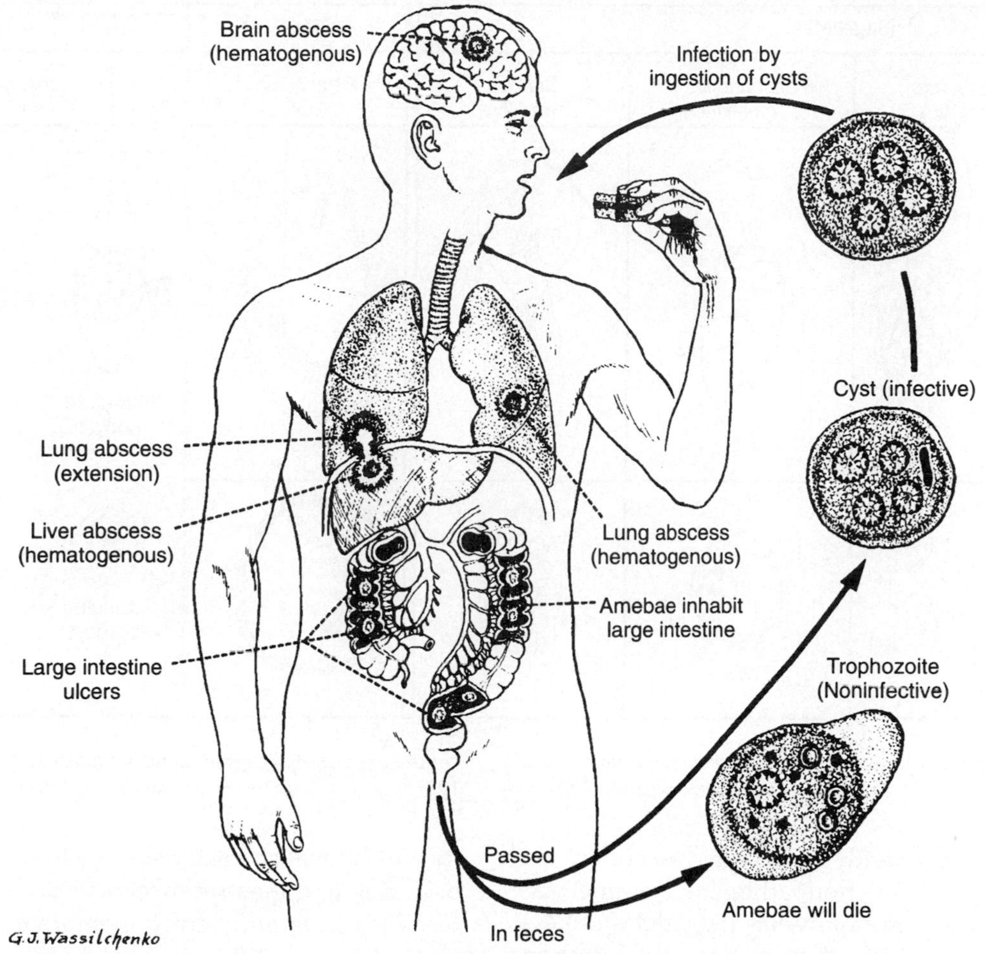

Figure 55.24. Life cycle of *Entamoeba histolytica*. (From Markell EK, Voge M, John DT. Medical parasitology. 7th ed. Philadelphia: WB Saunders, 1992.)

tric acid if ingested. Contamination of food and water with infectious cysts is a particular problem in hospitals for the mentally ill, military and refugee camps, prisons, and crowded day-care facilities. Sexual transmission of cysts by oral-anal sexual practices is an important means of transmission of amebiasis in homosexual populations.

Diagnosis. Examination of stool specimens will usually allow the diagnosis of intestinal amebiasis. The identification of *E. histolytica* trophozoites and cysts in stools and trophozoites in tissue is diagnostic of amebic infection. Microscopic examination of stool specimens is insensitive and diagnosis may require collection and examination of multiple stool specimens or a purged series. False-negative stool examinations are due to the fact that the parasites are not usually distributed homogeneously in the specimen and are concentrated in the intestinal ulcers and at the margins of abscesses, rather than in the stool or the necrotic center of the abscess. False-positive microscopic examinations may be due to failure to distinguish *E. histolytica* from other nonpathogenic amebae (see Table 55.6 and Fig. 55.21), as well as polymorphonuclear leukocytes. Extraintestinal amebiasis may be diagnosed using radiographic scanning procedures for the liver, lung, or brain. Specific serologic tests are frequently positive in individuals with extraintestinal or symptomatic intestinal disease and are negative in asymptomatic carriers and uninfected individuals.

Treatment. Treatment of amebiasis varies with the clinical stage of the infection. Asymptomatic carriage may be eradicated with iodoquinol, diloxanide furoate, or paromomycin. Acute amebic colitis is treated with metronidazole plus iodoquinol. Amebic dysentery may be treated with emetine, dehydroemetine, or metronidazole followed by iodoquinol. Metronidazole is generally considered the agent of choice in the treatment of extraintestinal amebiasis. Drainage of large amebic abscesses may occasionally be necessary.

Other Intestinal Amebae

Other amebae can parasitize the oral and gastrointestinal tract of humans. These include *Entamoeba coli*, *Entamoeba gingivalis*, *Entamoeba hartmanni*, *Entamoeba polecki*, *Endolimax nana*, and *Iodamoeba bütschlii*.

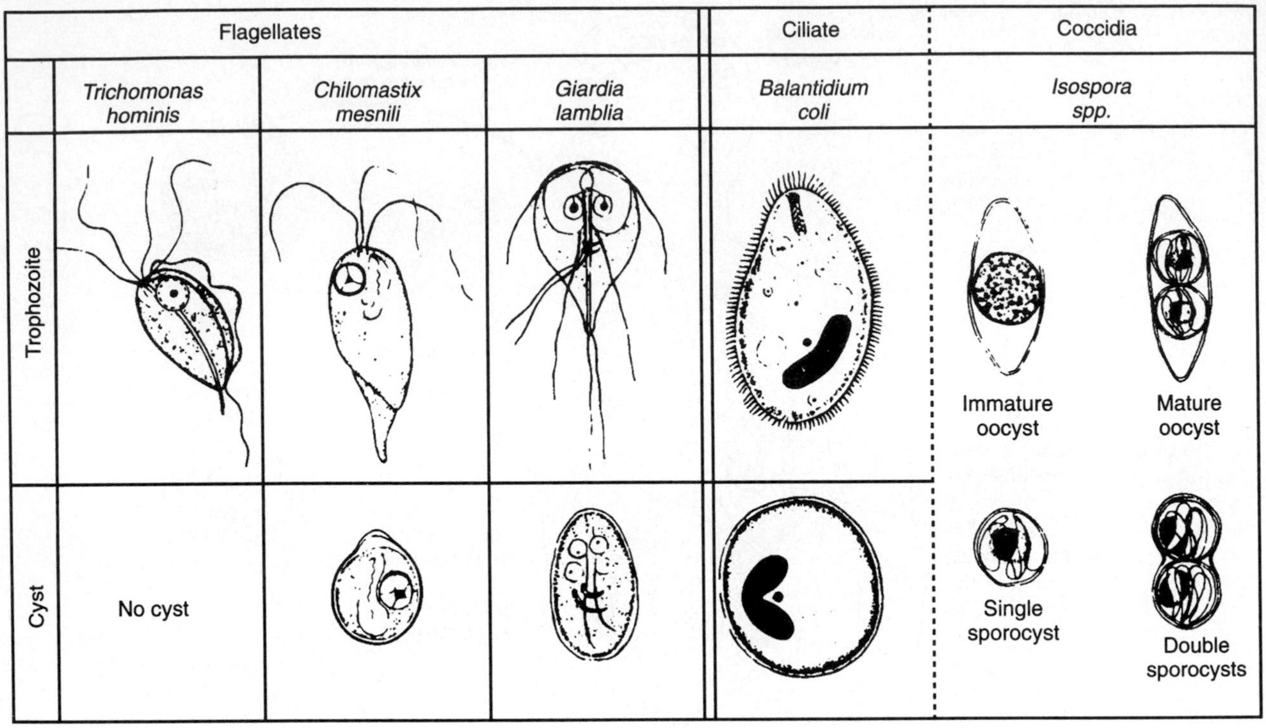

Figure 55.25. Protozoa found in human feces (flagellates, ciliate, coccidia). (From Smith JW, et al. Diagnostic medical parasitology: intestinal protozoa. Chicago: American Society of Clinical Pathologists, 1976.)

All of these amebae, with the possible exception of *E. polecki*, are considered nonpathogenic commensals. *E. polecki* most commonly infects pigs and monkeys, but may cause mild diarrhea in humans. Infections due to *E. polecki* are confirmed microscopically and are treated in a manner similar to amebiasis caused by *E. histolytica*.

The nonpathogenic amebae must be differentiated microscopically from *E. histolytica*. This is particularly true for *E. coli*, which is similar in size to *E. histolytica* and is frequently found in stool specimens from patients exposed to contaminated food or water. Careful microscopic examination of trophozoite and cyst forms present in stained and unstained specimens is essential for the accurate identification of intestinal amebae (see Table 55.6 and Fig. 55.21).

Flagellates

There are three clinically significant species of flagellates found in humans, *Giardia lamblia*, *Trichomonas vaginalis*, and *Dientamoeba fragilis*. Nonpathogenic commensal flagellates include *Chilomastix mesnili*, *Trichomonas hominis*, *Trichomonas tenax*, *Enteromonas hominis*, and *Retortamonas intestinalis*.

The trichomonads and *D. fragilis* have only trophozoite stages in their life cycle, whereas the other flagellates have both trophozoite and cyst stages (Fig. 55.25). The flagellates other than *D. fragilis* are easily recognized by their characteristic rapid motility. Additional characteristics include shape, number of nuclei, and the presence of fibrils and other structures, such as undulating membrane, sucking disk, and cytostome (Table 55.7).

Diseases produced by flagellates are primarily the result of mechanical irritation and inflammation of intestinal and/or urogenital mucosa. The tissue invasion and destruction seen with *E. histolytica* is rare with flagellates.

Giardia lamblia

Classification. *G. lamblia* is characterized by the presence of both actively motile trophozoites and sessile cyst forms in the same specimen. *Giardia* is one of the most easily recognized intestinal parasites. The pear-shaped trophozoite is bilaterally symmetrical containing two nuclei and eight flagellae (Figs. 55.25 and 55.26). The trophozoite ranges from 10 to 20 μm in length and contains a large ventral sucking disk, which occupies the anterior half to three-fourths of the body. Division is by longitudinal binary fission. The mature cyst form ranges from 8 to 19 μm in length and contains four nuclei. The nuclei are concentrated toward the anterior end and are not distinct in unstained preparations. *Giardia* cysts are recognized by their oval shape, by the fibrils present in the cytoplasm, and by the anteriorly located nuclei (Figs. 55.25 and 55.27).

Table 55.7. Morphology of Intestinal and Urogenital Flagellate Trophozoites and Cysts

	Giardia lamblia	*Dientamoeba fragilis*	*Trichomonas vaginalis*
Trophozoites			
Size	10–20 μm	5–15 μm	5–30 μm
Shape	Pear-shaped	Oval to round	Pear-shaped
Motility	"Falling leaf" motility in very diluted preps, otherwise motility is "back-and-forth" beating of flagella	Ameboid	Jerky, nondirectional
Nuclei	Two	Two, no chromatin, small karyosome divided into four to six distinct granules	One
Characteristic features	Sucking disk on ventral surface	Cytoplasm is finely granular, vacuolated with bacteria inclusions	Short undulating membrane, no free posterior flagellum; axostyle protruding posteriorly.
Cysts			
Size	8–19 μm	No cyst form exists	No cyst form exists
Shape	Oval or elliptical		
Nuclei	Four, usually located on one end		
Characteristic features	Flagella and fibrils are positioned longitudinally in cysts, others lie laterally in cyst		
Clinical manifestations	Acute: Irritation of mucosal lining, increased mucus secretion, dehydration, and epigastric pain, diarrhea, weight loss, and flatulence Chronic: epigastric pain, flatulence, diarrhea, weight loss and malabsorption	Diarrhea, abdominal pain, nausea, anorexia, malaise, and fatigue	Vaginal irritation and discharge, urethritis, prostatitis
Diagnostic methods[a]	O&P exam, DFA stain, ELISA, Entero-Test (String Test)	O&P exam with permanent stain	Direct, wet mount, culture, DFA stain

[a]Abbreviations: DFA, direct fluorescent antibody; ELISA, enzyme-linked immunosorbent assay; O&P exam, ova and parasites examination.

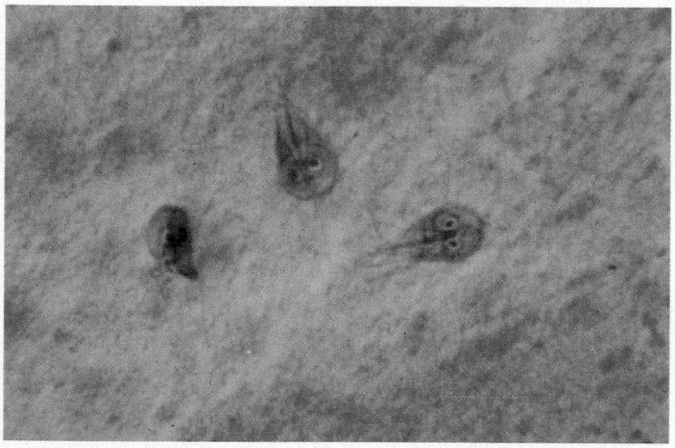

Figure 55.26. *Giardia lamblia* trophozoites in fecal smear (Kohn's chlorazol black E stain, ×1125). (From Smith JW, et al. Diagnostic medical parasitology: intestinal protozoa. Chicago: American Society of Clinical Pathologists, 1976.)

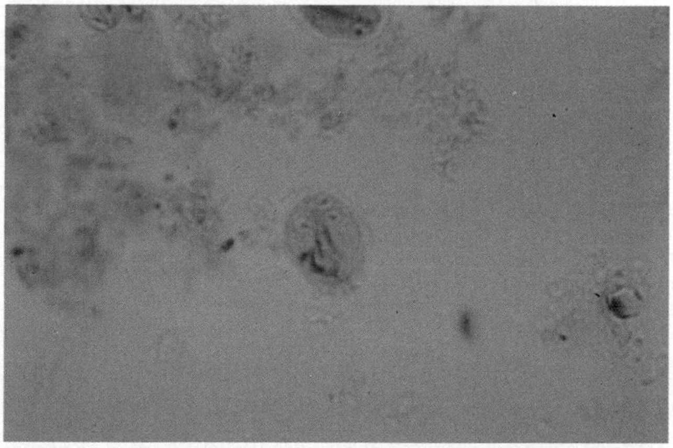

Figure 55.27. *Giardia lamblia* cysts in fecal smear (trichrome stain, ×1600). (From Smith JW, et al. Diagnostic medical parasitology: intestinal protozoa. Chicago: American Society of Clinical Pathologists, 1976.)

Clinical Manifestations. *Giardia lamblia* causes an infection of the small intestine (Fig. 55.28). Infection can be asymptomatic (in up to 50% of individuals) or symptomatic. Symptomatic disease may range from mild diarrhea to a full malabsorption syndrome with diarrhea and steatorrhea. The disease may be accompanied by abdominal bloating, cramps, and flatulence; however, blood and pus are rarely present in stools. The organisms appear to cause disease by both mechanical blockage of the absorptive surface of the small bowel and damage to the mucosal epithelium (27). Frank tissue necrosis as seen in amebiasis does not occur, and spread beyond the gastrointestinal tract is rare. Although spontaneous recovery gener-

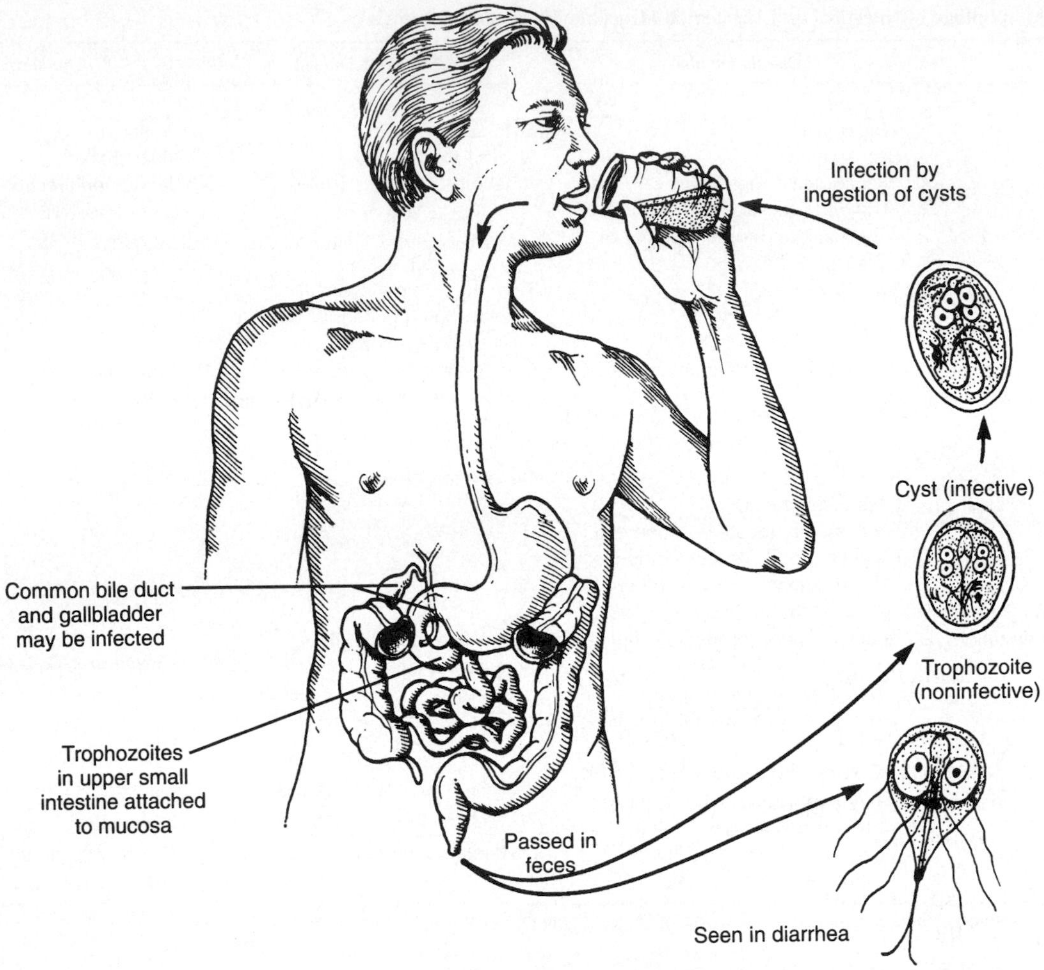

Figure 55.28. Life cycle of *Giardia lamblia*. (Modified from Markell EK, Voge M, John DT. Medical parasitology. 7th ed. Philadelphia: WB Saunders, 1992.)

ally occurs after 10 to 14 days, a more chronic disease with multiple relapses may develop. Individuals with IgA deficiency are particularly prone to developing chronic giardiasis.

Diagnosis. The predominant form seen on stool examination is the cyst form (Fig. 55.28). Trophozoites may be present in diarrheal stools or duodenal aspirates. Organisms may be visualized on a direct wet preparation with or without iodine staining. The use of stool concentration techniques and permanently stained (trichome) fecal smears are necessary for complete stool workup (27). In addition to conventional microscopy, several immunologic tests for detection of fecal antigen are available commercially. These tests include counterimmunoelectrophoresis, enzyme immunoassay, and indirect immunofluorescent staining. Reported sensitivities range from 88 to 98% and specificities from 87 to 100% (27).

Treatment. Treatment of both asymptomatic cyst passers as well as symptomatic individuals is necessary to interrupt the transmission of *G. lamblia*. The drug of choice is quinacrine hydrochloride (Atabrine). Metronidazole is also effective and may be less toxic. More than one course of therapy may be necessary in certain individuals. Prevention and control of giardiasis involves avoidance of contaminated food and water.

Dientamoeba fragilis

Classification. *Dientamoeba fragilis*, originally classified as an ameba, is now considered an ameba-like flagellate more closely related to the genus *Trichomonas*. The organism lacks a cyst stage and is frequently binucleate. Electron microscopic studies have revealed internal structures typical of a flagellate.

Clinical Manifestations. Many individuals infected with *D. fragilis* are asymptomatic. In certain individuals the organism may cause mucosal irritation of the cecum and upper colon with accompanying symptoms of abdominal discomfort, flatulence, diarrhea, anorexia, and weight loss (28). The organism

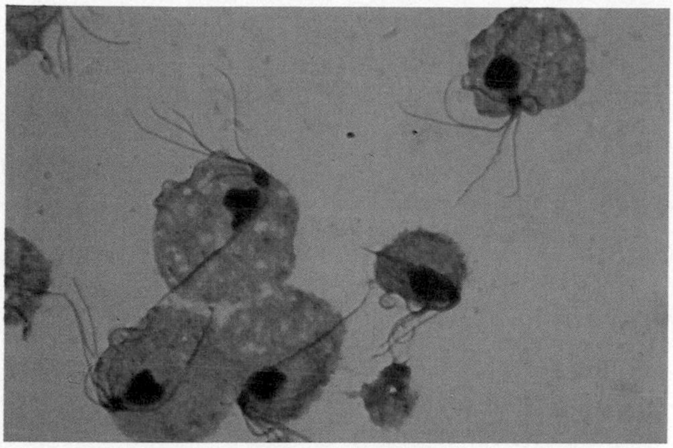

Figure 55.29. *Trichomonas vaginalis* trophozoites (Giemsa stain, ×2400). (From Smith JW, et al. Diagnostic medical parasitology: intestinal protozoa. Chicago: American Society of Clinical Pathologists, 1976.)

has been found in human bile ducts; however, its role in biliary tract disease is unknown.

Life Cycle and Epidemiology. *D. fragilis* resides in the mucosal crypts. The mode of transmission remains uncertain but most likely is fecal-oral in nature. It is postulated that the delicate trophozoite is transported from person to person inside the protective shell of helminth eggs such as the pinworm *Enterobius vermicularis*.

Diagnosis. Infection with *D. fragilis* is documented by detecting the labile trophozoites in appropriately preserved and stained stool specimens. The excretion of the parasite may fluctuate markedly from day to day, and thus collection of several stool samples may be necessary. Examination of a purged stool sample may also be useful.

Treatment. The antiamebic drugs iodoquinol and tetracycline are often stated to be the drugs of choice for *D. fragilis* infections; however, the cure rates are not high with these drugs (28). A more effective agent appears to be paromomycin. Metronidazole, furazolidone, and diloxanide furoate may also be effective against *D. fragilis* but require additional investigation.

Trichomonas vaginalis

Classification. *Trichomonas vaginalis* is a parasite of the urogenital system. *T. vaginalis* exists only as a trophozoite and is found in the urethras and vaginas of women and in the urethras and prostates of men. The organism is oval, is 5 to 30 μm wide, and possesses four flagella and a short undulating membrane that are responsible for motility (Fig. 55.29). There is a single large nucleus and an axostyle, composed of microtubules, that projects from the posterior end. The organism is actively phagocytic and grows optimally under anaerobic conditions.

Clinical Manifestations. Infection with *T. vaginalis* may be asymptomatic in both women and men. Symptomatic infection in women may range from a mild watery discharge to severe vaginitis with extensive inflammation and erosion of the epithelial lining, associated with burning, itching, and dysuria. Infection in men may involve the urethra, prostrate, and/or seminal vesicles. A urethral discharge accompanied by dysuria, nocturia, and prostatic tenderness may be observed.

Life Cycle and Epidemiology. *T. vaginalis* is strictly a parasite of the urogenital system, where it exists as a motile trophozoite. Transmission is due primarily to sexual contact or, less commonly, by contaminated fomites (toilet articles, clothing). Perinatal acquisition of disease is reported secondary to passage through the mother's infected birth canal.

Diagnosis. Diagnosis of infection with *T. vaginalis* is usually made by examining wet mounts of vaginal discharge or prostatic secretions, or by examination of urine from both men and women. Stained or unstained smears may be examined (Fig. 55.29). The diagnostic yield may be improved by culturing the organism (93% sensitivity) or using monoclonal fluorescent antibody staining (86% sensitivity). Serologic tests may be useful in epidemiologic surveillance.

Treatment. The treatment of choice is metronidazole; however, resistance has been reported, and retreatment with higher doses may be required. Both male and female sexual partners should be treated to avoid reinfection.

Ciliates

Balantidium coli is the only ciliate known to cause infection in humans. The organisms inhabit the large intestine, cecum, and terminal ileum where they may cause extensive ulceration.

Balantidium coli

Classification. *B. coli* is a large ciliated protozoa ranging in size from 40 to over 200 μm in greatest dimension. The trophozoite is covered uniformly with rows of hair-like cilia that aid in motility. The organism is structurally more complex than an ameba, with both macronuclei and micronuclei, a cytostome, and numerous cytoplasmic contractile and food vacuoles (Fig. 55.30). The organism may exist in both trophozoite and cyst stage. Reproduction is by binary fission, although conjugation may occur.

Clinical Manifestations. Infection with *B. coli* may be asymptomatic or present with a picture of severe intestinal involvement that can mimic the intestinal phase of amebiasis. Symptomatic disease is characterized by abdominal pain, cramping, and ten-

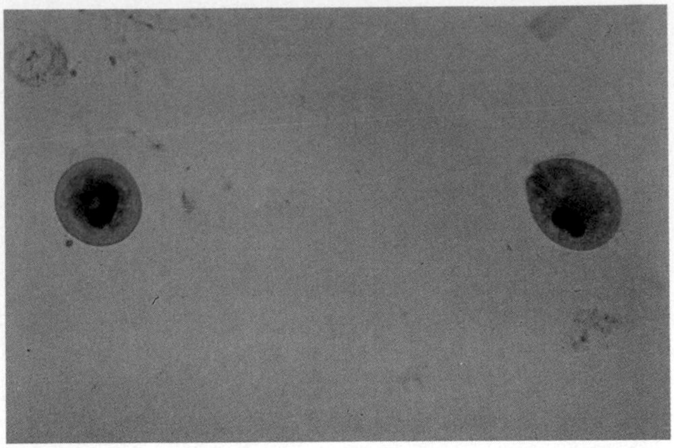

Figure 55.30. *Balantidium coli* cyst and trophozoite in fecal smear (trichrome stain, ×180). (From Smith JW, et al. Diagnostic medical parasitology: intestinal protozoa. Chicago: American Society of Clinical Pathologists, 1976.)

derness accompanied by nausea, tenesmus, and watery stools with blood and pus. Intestinal ulceration may be extensive, but metastatic (extraintestinal) spread is rare.

Life Cycle and Epidemiology. The life cycle of *B. coli* is simple, involving ingestion of cysts in contaminated food or water, excystation, and invasion of trophozoites into the mucosa of the large bowel. *B. coli* is distributed worldwide, but infection is rare. In the United States, epidemics have occurred in mental hospitals. Swine constitute an important reservoir in other parts of the world. Risk factors for human disease include contact with swine and substandard hygienic conditions.

Diagnosis. As in other intestinal infections caused by protozoa, the diagnosis of balantidiasis is confirmed by detection of the large cysts and trophozoites on microscopic examination of an appropriately collected stool specimen (Fig. 55.30). The organism is detected early in fresh, wet microscopic preparations.

Treatment. The treatments of choice are tetracycline and iodoquinol. Metronidazole and paromomycin are alternative antimicrobials; however, mixed results have been reported with metronidazole. Preventive measures include appropriate personal hygiene and maintenance of sanitary conditions.

Coccidia

Coccidia are intracellular parasites that are part of a large group called Apicomplexa. This group includes intestinal parasites such as *Isospora*, *Cryptosporidium*, and *Blastocystis* as well as the blood and tissue parasites discussed earlier (*Plasmodium*, *Babesia*, *Toxoplasma*). All coccidia demonstrate both sexual (sporogonic) and asexual (schizogonic) reproductive cycles.

Isospora

Classification. Isosporiasis is caused by *Isospora belli*, a coccidian parasite of the intestinal epithelium. The organism is present in the stool in the form of oocysts, which average 30 μm in length by 12 μm in width. The mature oocyst contains two sporocysts, each with up to four sausage-shaped sporozoites (Fig. 55.25).

Clinical Manifestations. Infections range from asymptomatic to significant gastrointestinal disease resembling giardiasis or cryptosporidiosis. Symptoms include diarrhea, abdominal pain and cramping, flatulence, malaise, anorexia, weight loss and low-grade fever. Symptomatic disease is usually self-limited; however, illness may persist for months or years, particularly in immunocompromised individuals such as those with AIDS.

Life Cycle and Epidemiology. Infection with *I. belli* is initiated with the ingestion of mature oocysts in contaminated food or water. Following ingestion, excystation occurs in the small bowel releasing sporozoites, which in turn invade intestinal epithelial cells and become rounded trophozoites. The trophozoites undergo schizogony and produce merozoites, which ultimately rupture the host cell and are released to invade other epithelial cells. Some merozoites become sexual gametocytes. The product of sexual reproduction is the oocyst, which is released into the bowel lumen and eliminated in the feces. Fecal oocysts mature within 48 hours and are then infective.

Isospora is distributed worldwide, but is rarely reported in humans. In recent years, *I. belli* has been recognized as an important opportunistic pathogen in individuals suffering from AIDS. Infection follows ingestion of contaminated food or water, or oral-anal sexual contact. There is no evidence of an animal reservoir of *I. belli*.

Diagnosis. The presence of oocysts in stool may be difficult to detect without a concentration procedure. Zinc sulfate or sugar flotation is the most sensitive stool concentration technique. Stool concentrates may be stained with either iodine or a modified acid-fast procedure. Intestinal mucosal biopsy may be necessary to establish the diagnosis when stool specimens are negative.

Treatment. The treatment of choice is combined therapy with pyrimethamine and sulfadiazine or trimethoprim-sulfamethoxazole. Prevention and control are accomplished by adequate sanitation and avoidance of oral-anal sexual contact.

Cryptosporidium

Classification. *Cryptosporidium* species are coccidian parasites closely related to *Isospora belli* and

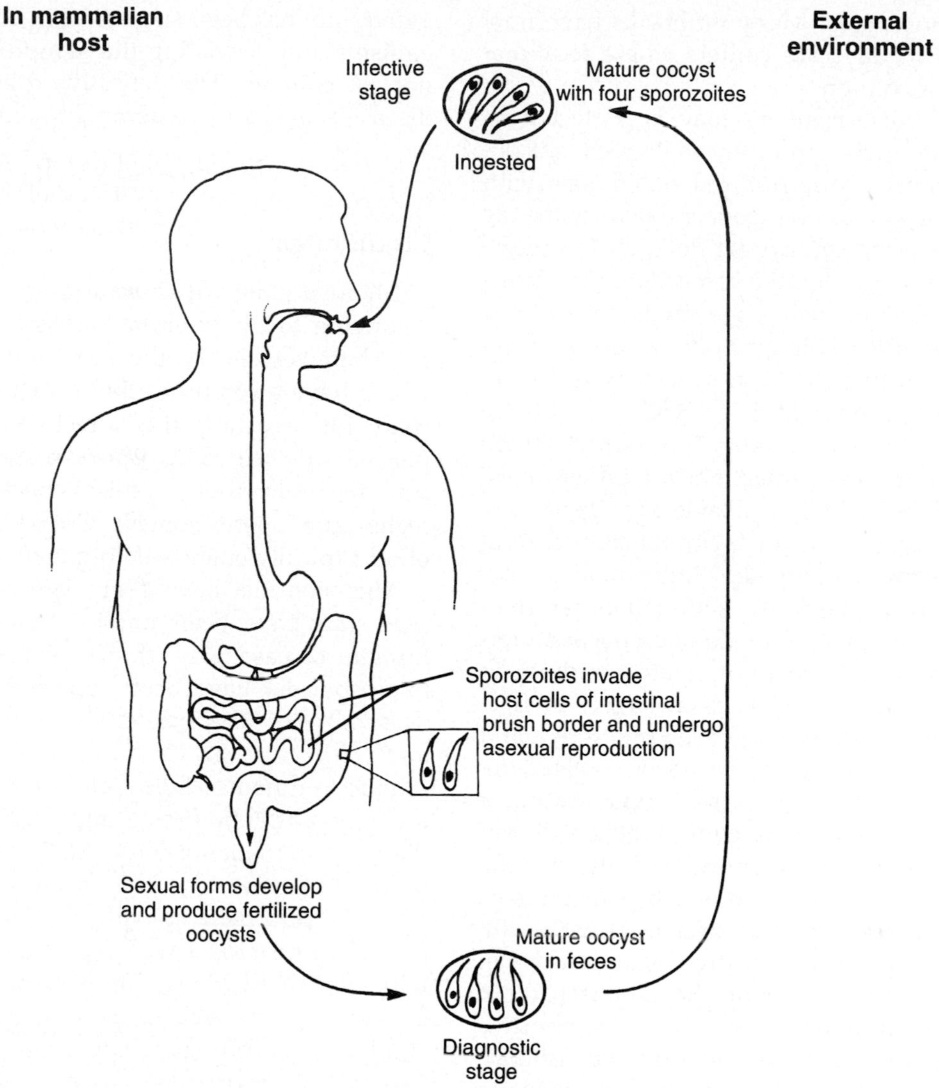

Figure 55.31. Life cycle of *Cryptosporidium* species.

Toxoplasma gondii. *Cryptosporidium parvum* is the species associated with all well-documented cases of cryptosporidiosis in mammals (29). *Cryptosporidium* has an apical complex but produces neither cilia nor flagella. The parasite is characterized by an oocyst without sporocysts and containing four sporozoites. Development of the oocyst takes place intracellularly just beneath the surface membrane of the intestinal epithelial cell and is thus extracytoplasmic.

Clinical Manifestations. Infection with *C. parvum* is usually asymptomatic or a mild, self-limited enterocolitis characterized by watery diarrhea without blood. Immunocompromised individuals may have severe diarrhea characterized by 50 or more stools per day with marked fluid loss, abdominal discomfort, nausea, anorexia, fever, and weight loss. Infection in these individuals may persist for months to years. In patients with AIDS, *Cryptosporidium* has been found in sputum, lung biopsy specimens, and the biliary tract (29).

Life Cycle and Epidemiology. The life cycle of *Cryptosporidium* resembles that of other coccidian parasites (Fig. 55.31). Mature oocysts containing sporozoites are the infective stage. Infection is initiated with the ingestion of oocysts in contaminated food or water. After excysting from oocysts in the lumen of the intestine, sporozoites invade host cells within the brush border of the intestinal epithelium and develop into trophozoites. Both asexual and sexual reproduction occurs in the epithelial cells. Sporulated oocysts are released in the feces and serve to transmit the infection from one host to another.

Cryptosporidiosis is a zoonosis and can be spread from animal reservoirs to humans, as well as from person to person. The most common means of infection are the fecal-oral and oral-anal routes. Individuals at high risk include veterinarians, animal handlers, and homosexuals. Many outbreaks have now been described in day care centers where fecal-oral transmission is common.

Diagnosis. *Cryptosporidium* may be detected in large numbers in unconcentrated stool specimens obtained from immunocompromised individuals with diarrhea. Oocysts may be concentrated with the modified zinc sulfate centrifugal flotation technique or by Sheather's sugar flotation procedure (29). Specimens may be stained using the modified acid-fast method or by an indirect immunofluorescence assay. The number of oocysts shed in stool may fluctuate; therefore it is recommended that a minimum of three specimens be examined. Serologic procedures for diagnosing and monitoring infections are under investigation but are not widely available at present.

Treatment. Treatment of symptomatic cryptosporidiosis in immunocompetent individuals is usually not undertaken due to the self-limited nature of the disease and the lack of a safe and effective therapy. Unfortunately, treatment of cryptosporidiosis in immune deficient persons has been largely ineffective. No controlled studies have been published, and all therapeutic information is based on isolated reports and anecdotal information. Spiramycin, a macrolide antibiotic, may help control the diarrhea in some patients with cryptosporidiosis during the early stages of AIDS, but is ineffective in patients who have progressed to the later stages of AIDS (29). Spiramycin was no more effective than placebo in treating cryptosporidial diarrhea in infants (29). In the absence of an effective treatment, supportive measures to restore the fluid loss from watery diarrhea appears to be the only intervention available to most clinicians.

Blastocystis hominis

Blastocystis hominis is a common inhabitant of the human intestinal tract and the subject of considerable controversy concerning its taxonomy and pathogenicity. Previously, *B. hominis* was regarded as a nonpathogenic yeast; however, more recent studies confirm its identity as a protozoan and place it in the family Sporozoa (30). The organism is found in stool specimens obtained from asymptomatic individuals as well as those with persistent diarrhea. Although it has been suggested that the finding of large numbers of *B. hominis* (5 or more organisms per oil immersion field) in the stool of symptomatic patients is consistent with its role in disease (30), other investigators have concluded that "symptomatic blastocystosis" was attributable to either an undetected pathogen or functional bowel problems. The organism may be detected in wet mounts or trichrome-stained smears of fecal specimens. Treatment with metronidazole or iodoquinol has been successful in eradicating the organisms and alleviating the symptoms in some, but not all, patients. The definitive role of *B. hominis* in disease remains to be demonstrated.

Microsporidia

Classification

Microsporidia are obligate intracellular pathogens belonging to the phylum Microspora. The parasites are characterized by the structure of their spores, which have a complex tubular extrusion mechanism used for injecting the infective material (sporoplasma) into cells. Microsporidia are considered to be primitive eukaryotic organisms because they lack mitochondria, peroxisomes, Golgi membranes, and other typically eukaryotic organelles.

Microsporidia have been detected in human tissues and have been implicated as participants in human disease (31–34). To date, five genera of microsporidia have been reported in humans: *Encephalitozoon*, *Pleistophora*, *Nosema*, *Microsporidium*, and *Enterocytozoon*. Of these, only *Enterocytozoon* is unique to humans. *Enterocytozoon bieneusi* has gained increasing attention as an important cause of chronic diarrhea in patients with AIDS (31, 32); *Encephalitozoon*-like organisms have been reported in the tissues of AIDS patients with hepatitis and peritonitis (31, 33); *Pleistophora* was the cause of myositis in a patient with AIDS (31, 33); *Nosema* has caused localized keratitis as well as disseminated infection in a child with severe combined immunodeficiency (31, 33); and *Microsporidium* has caused infection of the human cornea (31, 33).

Clinical Manifestations

Clinical signs and symptoms of microsporidiosis are quite variable in the few human cases reported. Intestinal infection due to *E. bieneusi* in AIDS patients resembles that which occurs in patients with cryptosporidiosis and isosporiasis. Patients experience chronic watery diarrhea without blood or mucus. The diarrhea is persistent and debilitating, leading to dehydration and extreme wasting. The clinical presentation of infection with other species of Microspora is dependent on the organ system involved and ranges from localized ocular pain and loss of vision (*Microsporidium* and *Nosema* species) to neurologic disturbances and hepatitis (*Encephalitozoon cuniculi*) to a more generalized picture of dissemination with fever, vomiting, diarrhea, and malabsorption (*Nosema*). In the latter disseminated infection with *Nosema connori*, the organism was seen involving the muscles of the stomach, bowel, arteries, diaphragm,

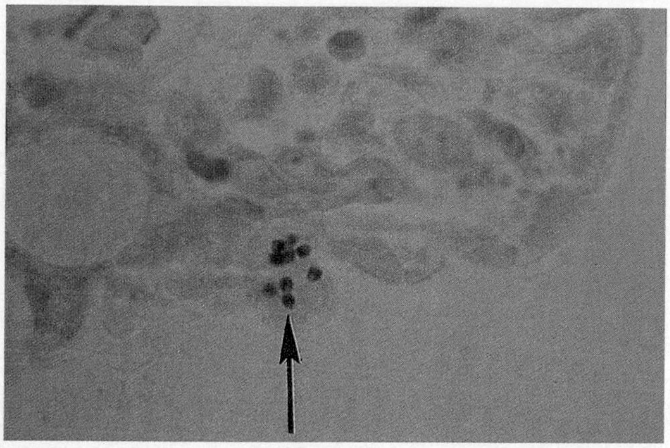

Figure 55.32. Gram-positive spores of microsporidia (*arrow*) in jejunal biopsy (Brown-Brenn stain, ×1750). (From Weber R, Bryan RT, Owen RL, et al. Improved light-microscopical detection of microsporidia in spores and stool and duodenal aspirates. N Engl J Med 1992;326:161–166.)

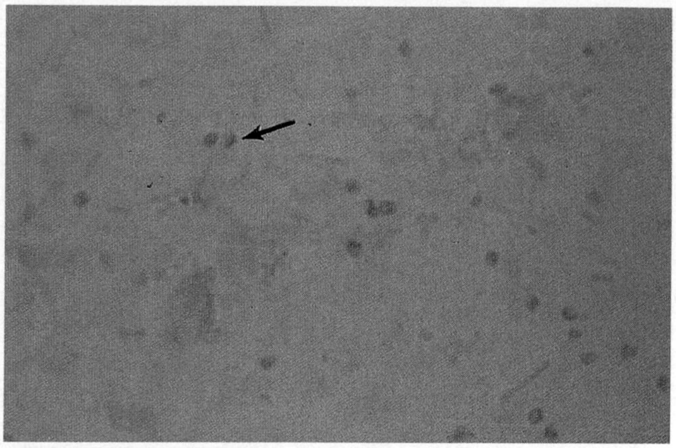

Figure 55.33. Smear of formalin-fixed stool specimen, showing pinkish red–stained microsporidia spores, some with a distinct pinkish belt-like stripe (*arrow*). Bacteria are stained faint green (chromotrope-based stain, ×1800). (From Weber R, et al. N Engl J Med 1992;326: 161–166.)

and heart and the parenchymal cells of the liver, lungs, and adrenals (33).

Life Cycle

Microsporidia are obligate intracellular parasites with a wide host range among invertebrate and vertebrate animals. Transmission is accomplished by ingestion of spores that have been shed in the urine and feces of infected animals. Following ingestion by a new host, pressure builds up inside the spore, causing the polar filament to evert and injecting the sporoplasm with its nuclear material into an adjacent cell in the intestine, where it multiplies and is disseminated (33). Although some species are highly selective in the cell type that they invade, collectively the microspora are capable of infecting every organ of the body.

Once inside a suitable host cell the microsporidia multiply extensively, either within a parasitophorous vacuole or free within the cytoplasm of the host cell. The intracellular multiplication includes a phase of repeated divisions by binary fission (merogony) or multiple fission (schizogony) and a phase culminating in spore formation (sporogony). Parasites spread from cell to cell to continue merogony, which may overlap sporogony. During sporogony, sporonts divide into sporoblasts and sporoblasts mature into spores containing the infective sporoplasm. The mature spores are then excreted into the environment and the cycle continues.

Diagnosis

There are several techniques that have been useful for recognizing microsporidia in human material. Diagnosis is frequently made by identification of the organisms in biopsy material and by light microscopic examination of cerebrospinal fluid and urine. Spores measuring between 1.0 and 2.0 μm may be visualized by Gram (Gram-positive), acid-fast, periodic acid–Schiff, and Giemsa staining techniques (Fig. 55.32). Giemsa-stained organisms are easier to see in histologic sections than those stained with hematoxylin and eosin. Immunohistochemical techniques may also be useful. Electron microscopy is considered the gold standard for diagnostic confirmation of microsporidiosis; however, its sensitivity is unknown. Species identification requires transmission electron microscopy.

Recently a new chromotrope-based staining technique for light-microscopic detection of *E. bieneusi* spores in stool and duodenal aspirates was described (34). The chromotrope-based technique prospectively detected microsporidia spores on light microscopy of unconcentrated formalin-fixed fecal material from four patients in whom the diagnosis was subsequently confirmed by biopsy. The spores showed a characteristic pinkish-red staining pattern and could be distinguished easily from bacteria, yeasts, and fecal debris (Fig. 55.33). This new technique may serve as a practical noninvasive means of diagnosing microsporidiosis.

Additional diagnostic techniques, including culture and serologic testing, are currently under investigation. These techniques are not considered reliable enough for routine diagnosis at the present time.

Treatment

There is no known effective treatment for microsporidium infections. Treatment with metronidazole has resulted in temporary improvement in patients with intestinal microsporidiosis. Likewise, some patients have been treated with sulfa drugs and sur-

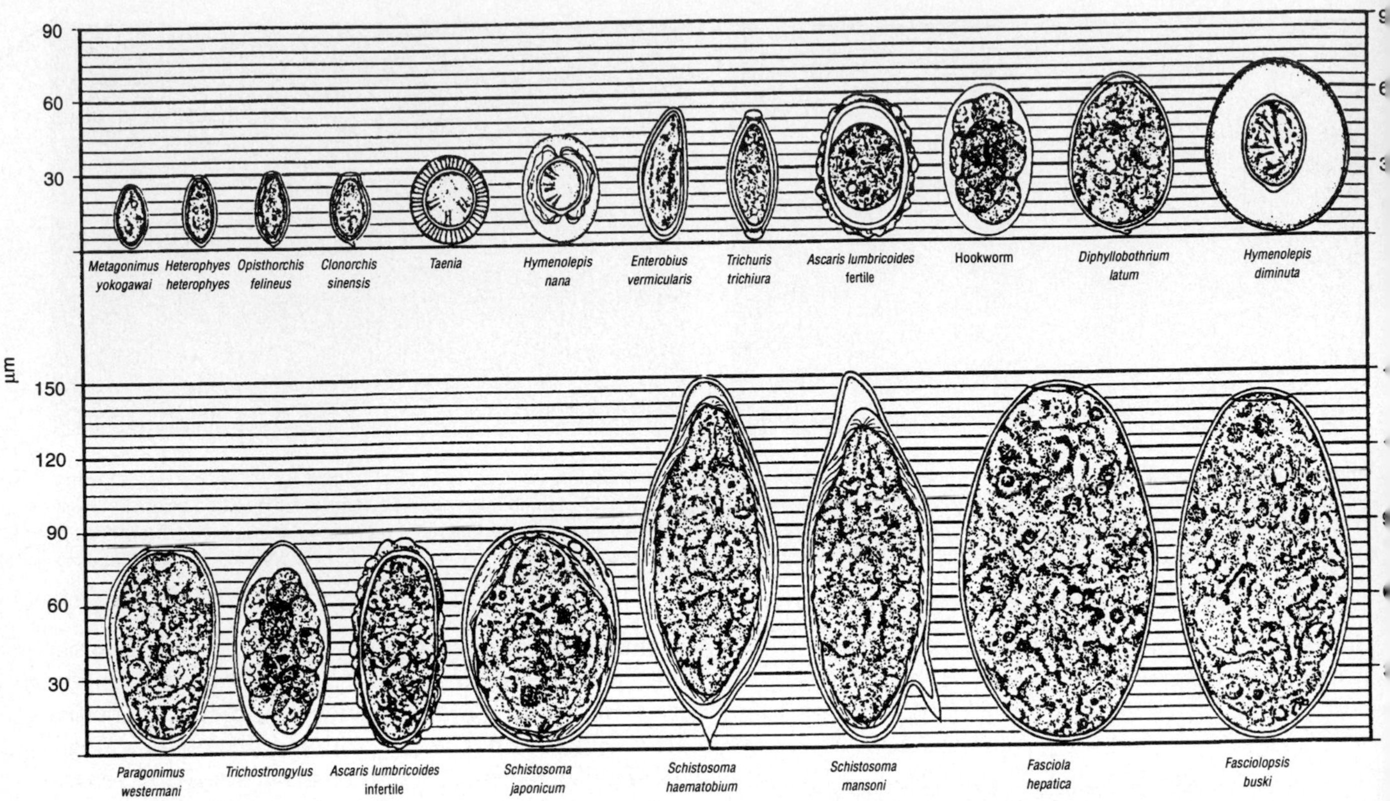

Figure 55.34. Helminths found in human specimens: relative sizes. (From Smith JW, et al. Diagnostic medical parasitology: intestinal helminths. Chicago: American Society of Clinical Pathologists, 1976.)

vived. In vitro studies have demonstrated activity of trimethoprim-sulfisoxazole and the antibiotic fumagillin against *E. cuniculi*, but these results have not been confirmed in vivo.

HELMINTHS

Helminths may assume both free-living and parasitic life forms and are classified into nematodes (roundworms) and platyhelminths (flatworms). The helminths are generally macroscopic, and the adult worms may vary tremendously in size from barely visible to 10 meters in length.

Appropriate and timely diagnosis of a helminthic infection is dependent on a clear understanding of the life cycles of the parasites, the tissues likely to be involved, and the geographic distribution of the organisms. The life cycles of helminths may be quite complex and include both direct and indirect cycles. The direct cycle requires only the definitive host, whereas indirect cycles require an intermediate host in which larval stages develop as well as definitive hosts, which harbor the adults.

The clinical signs and symptoms of helminthic infections depend on the location of the organisms and may be caused by adults, larvae, or eggs. The host response to the presence of organisms may be prominent and often includes eosinophilia, especially in the early stages of infection when the parasites are in tissue.

The final diagnosis is usually dependent on detection and identification of a mature or developmental (larvae, embryo, egg) stage of the parasite. Occasionally the diagnosis must be made clinically or serologically.

The majority of helminths produce characteristic eggs that are passed in the feces and serve as the chief means of diagnosing the infections. The identification of eggs should be approached in a systematic manner taking into account the size and shape of the egg, the thickness of the shell, and the presence or absence of specialized structures such as spines, knobs, or opercula (Fig. 55.34). The presence and characteristics of larvae present within the eggs may also be useful.

Nematodes

Nematodes are the most common helminths parasitizing humans and include intestinal nematodes as well as blood and tissue nematodes. The most common nematodes of medical importance are those inhabiting the intestinal tract (Table 55.8). Most of these organisms have a direct life cycle and their presence may be confirmed by detecting the characteristic eggs in feces.

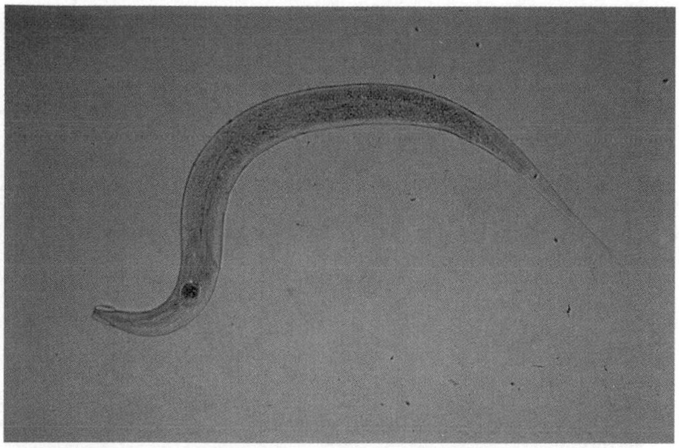

Figure 55.35. *Enterobius vermicularis*, adult female (whole mount). (From Smith JW, et al. Diagnostic medical parasitology: intestinal helminths. Chicago: American Society of Clinical Pathologists, 1976.)

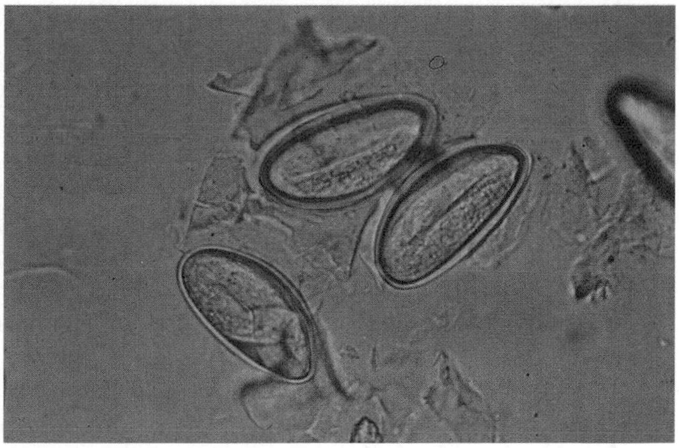

Figure 55.36. *Enterobius vermicularis*, embryonated eggs (low power). (From Smith JW, et al. Diagnostic medical parasitology: intestinal helminths. Chicago: American Society of Clinical Pathologists, 1976.)

The filariae are among the most important of the blood and tissue nematodes. The filariae are long, slender roundworms that parasitize the blood, lymph, and subcutaneous and connective tissues of humans. All of the filariae are transmitted by insect vectors and most produce larvae called microfilariae that may be demonstrated in the blood, lymph, or connective tissue of the human host.

Enterobius vermicularis

Infection with *E. vermicularis*, the common pinworm, is the most common helminthic infection in North America. Both female and male worms inhabit the cecum and large bowel. The female worm measures up to 13 mm in length, is cream-colored with bilateral ridges or alae, and a sharply pointed tail (Table 55.8 and Fig. 55.35). The male is smaller and rarely seen.

The gravid female migrates from the cecum to the perianal area, where as many as 20,000 eggs are deposited on the perianal skin. The eggs may be transmitted from hand to mouth or inhaled as fomites. The ingested eggs hatch in the small intestine and migrate to the cecum, where they mature into adults in 2 to 6 weeks, thus completing the cycle.

Clinical signs and symptoms of pinworm infection are generally mild. Intestinal pathology is rare; however, inflammation and granuloma formation around eggs has been reported. The role of the worm in appendicitis is questionable despite its occasional presence in the lumen of the resected appendix.

The most common clinical presentation is that of anal pruritus caused by the secretions of the migrating worms. Scratching may lead to further irritation and excoriation, occasionally complicated by secondary bacterial infection. Migration of the worms into the vagina or urinary bladder may produce genitourinary problems and granulomas.

The diagnosis of enterobiasis is usually suggested by the clinical manifestations and confirmed by detection of the characteristic eggs (Fig. 55.36) on the anal mucosa. Detection of the eggs is accomplished by applying the sticky surface of a piece of cellophane tape to the mucocutaneous junction of the anus, applying the tape to the surface of a microscope slide and examining the slide under low power. Multiple samplings may be required to detect the eggs. Occasionally the female worm may be observed on the surface of the stool or on the perianal skin. Sampling should be obtained at night or in the morning prior to bathing. Systemic signs of infection such as eosinophilia are rare.

The treatment of choice is pyrantel pamoate with mebendazole as an alternative. Due to the potential for cross-infection in the family environment, it is recommended that all members of the family group be treated simultaneously. Although cure rates are high, reinfection is common.

Trichuris trichiura

Trichuris trichiura is the causative agent of whipworm infection. The worm is characterized by a long, thin, threadlike anterior portion and a bulbous posterior portion. The adult whipworm is 30 to 50 mm in length, and the female worm may produce 3,000 to 10,000 eggs per day. The adult worms reside in the cecum and large intestine and may persist for up to 8 years. The whipworm is a cosmopolitan parasite and may infect up to half a billion people worldwide.

Trichuris is one of the soil-transmitted helminths with a simple life cycle. The distinctive eggs (Fig. 55.37) are passed in the stool and are deposited on soil, where they must mature for at least 10 days before they contain infective larvae. When ingested by the appropriate host, larvae are released in the

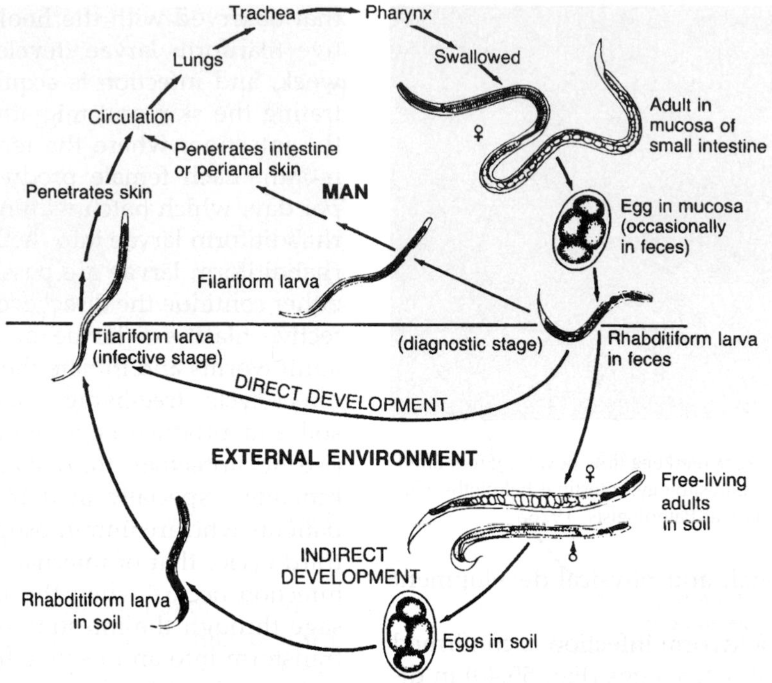

Figure 55.41. Life cycle of *Strongyloides stercoralis*. (From Strickland GT. Hunter's tropical medicine. 7th ed. Philadelphia: WB Saunders, 1991.)

tions, eggs are generally not present in the feces of patients with strongyloidiasis. When absent from the stool, larvae may be detected in duodenal aspirates or in sputum in cases of massive infection. Serologic tests are not generally available.

All infected patients should be treated to prevent autoinfection and potential dissemination (hyperinfection) of the parasite (35). The drug of choice for both mild and severe infection is thiabendazole. Stools should be checked after therapy to ensure adequate treatment. Patients in endemic areas should be examined thoroughly for the presence of this parasite both before and during steroid treatment or immunosuppressive therapy. Strict infection control measures should be enforced when caring for individuals with hyperinfection syndrome, as stool, saliva, vomitus, and body fluids may contain infectious filariform larvae. Similar to hookworm, *Strongyloides* control requires education, proper sanitation, and prompt treatment of existing infections.

Trichinosis

Trichinosis is caused by *Trichinella spiralis*, the adult form of which lives in the duodenal and jejunal mucosa of flesh-eating mammals worldwide. The larval form of *T. spiralis* is present in undercooked or contaminated meat. Among domestic animals, swine are most frequently involved. Humans become infected by ingestion of inadequately cooked meat that contains the encysted larval form of the organism. Upon ingestion, the encysted larvae are freed by gastric digestion, penetrate the mucosa of the intestine, and mature just above the lamina propria. The adult male and female worms mate in the intestinal mucosa and the female produces new larvae, which enter the vascular system and are eventually deposited in skeletal muscle. A single female worm may produce larvae over a period of 4 to 16 weeks, generating up to 1500 larvae, each measuring 6 by 100 μm. Larvae penetrating striated muscle continue to grow and molt and are eventually enclosed in a fibrous capsule, which may calcify over a period of 6 to 18 months. The muscles invaded most frequently include the extraocular muscles of the eye; the tongue; the deltoid, pectoral, and intercostal muscles; the diaphragm; and the gastrocnemius. The encysted larvae remain viable for many years and would be infectious if ingested by a new animal host.

Trichinosis is one of the few tissue parasitic diseases still seen in the United States. As with other parasitic infections, most patients have minimal or no symptoms. The clinical presentation depends largely on the tissue burden of organisms and the location of the migrating larvae. Patients in whom 10 or fewer larvae are deposited per gram of tissue are usually asymptomatic; those with 100 or more generally have significant disease; and those with 1000 to 5000 have a very serious course that occasionally ends in death. The most common clinical manifestations of trichinosis are fever, myalgias, weakness, malaise, periorbital edema, and headache. Less frequent manifestations include skin rash, generalized edema, diarrhea, nausea, splinter hemorrhages, and subconjunctival bleeding. Symptoms generally appear around 2 weeks after initial infection and persist for several weeks. Diarrhea, if it occurs at all, tends to be early in infection when adult worms are still in the intestinal tract. Weakness occurs late as an end-stage manifestation of the presence of the calcifying larvae in the muscle tissue.

Trichinosis occurs throughout most of the world except Australia and the Pacific Islands. In the United States infections are becoming less frequent due to decreased consumption of pork and pork products, federal guidelines for the commercial preparation of pork products, and federal legislation regarding the preparation and composition of livestock feed to avoid inclusion of infected meat. Nevertheless, it is estimated that more than 1.5 million Americans carry live *Trichinella* cysts in their musculature and that 150,000 to 300,000 acquire new infection annually (36).

The diagnosis of trichinosis is confirmed by performing a muscle biopsy and visualizing the encysted larvae. Key to making the diagnosis is clinical suspicion of the disease and pursuit of the biopsy. The deltoid or gastrocnemius muscle will usually provide the best yield. Often several individuals are infected because of a common exposure to the same poorly prepared meat product. Along with the wide variety of clinical symptoms that are seen, patients usually have an eosinophilia ranging from 15 to 50% of the peripheral white cell count. Together, these epidemiologic, clinical, and laboratory features should lead to suspicion of the disease.

A serologic test using bentonite flocculation is a possible approach to confirming infection. Significant antibody titers are usually absent before the third week of illness, but then may persist for years. ELISA tests are also under development, and one such test has been used as a screening method to detect infection in animals as part of the inspection process prior to the sale of meat products (37).

Treatment of trichinosis is primarily symptomatic since there are no good antiparasitic agents for the tissue larvae. Patients with severe infections may be treated with corticosteroids. Treatment of the adult worms in the intestine with mebendazole may halt the production of new larvae. Prevention is based on thorough cooking of pork and other meat.

Toxocariasis

Toxocariasis or visceral larval migrans (VLM) is caused by *Toxocara canis*, a large intestinal ascarid of canines. The complete life cycle of this parasite occurs in dogs and is similar to that of the human *Ascaris*. Canines ingest *Toxocara* eggs, which hatch into larvae in the small intestine. These larvae migrate to liver, lung, and trachea, are swallowed again, and mature into adult worms. Each female worm discharges approximately 200,000 eggs daily into the feces. Passage of larvae from pregnant females to fetuses can also occur and leads to ongoing infection when puppies are born. After reaching the soil, the eggs must embryonate for 2 to 3 weeks and thereafter are infectious for both canines and humans. The eggs may remain viable in soil for months to years.

Human infection occurs upon ingestion of infectious eggs. The eggs hatch in the small intestine and the liberated larvae pass through the pulmonary capillaries and reach the systemic circulation. The larvae continue to grow, penetrate the vascular walls, and migrate through various tissues. Rarely, if ever, do the larvae reach the intestine and complete the maturation to adulthood in the human host.

The clinical manifestations of toxocariasis in humans are related to the migration of the larvae through tissues. The larvae may invade any tissue of the body, where they can induce necrosis, bleeding, and the formation of eosinophilic granulomas. Patients may be asymptomatic or have only eosinophilia, but can also have serious disease that is directly related to the number and location of the lesions caused by the migrating larvae and the degree to which the host is sensitized to the larval antigens. The organs most frequently involved include the lungs, heart, kidney, liver, skeletal muscles, eye, and central nervous system. Signs and symptoms include cough, wheezing, fever, rash, anorexia, seizures, fatigue, and abdominal discomfort. On examination, patients may have hepatosplenomegaly as well as nodular, pruritic skin lesions. Death may result from respiratory failure, cardiac arrhythmia, or brain damage. Ocular disease can also occur with the movement of larvae through the eye and may be mistaken for malignant retinoblastoma. Prompt diagnosis is required to avoid an unnecessary enucleation.

T. canis is a cosmopolitan parasite. Wherever infected canines are present, the eggs are a threat to humans. The incidence of infection appears to be higher in the southeastern sections of the United States. Seroprevalence studies indicate that approximately 4 to 20% of the population has ingested *T. canis* eggs at some time. Children are particularly susceptible to infection, presumably due to more frequent exposure to contaminated soil and the tendency to put objects in their mouth.

Diagnosis of visceral larval migrans is based on clinical findings, the presence of eosinophilia, known exposure to dogs, and serologic confirmation. ELISA assays are readily available and appear to offer the best serologic marker for disease. Examination of feces from infected patients is not useful, as egg-laying adults are not present. Tissue examination for larvae may provide a definitive diagnosis but may be negative due to sampling error.

Treatment is primarily symptomatic since antiparasitic agents are not of proven benefit. Agents including diethylcarbamazine, thiabendazole, and mebendazole have been tried. Corticosteroid therapy may be lifesaving if the patient has serious pulmonary, myocardial, or central nervous system involvement, since a major component of the infection is an inflammatory response to the organism.

Cutaneous Larva Migrans

Cutaneous larva migrans is an infection of the skin caused by the dog and cat hookworm *Ancylostoma braziliense*. This species of hookworm naturally infects dogs and cats and accidentally infects humans. Eggs discharged in the feces are deposited on warm, moist, sandy soil, where they develop into filariform larvae capable of penetrating skin on contact. The larvae can penetrate intact human skin but can develop no further in the human host. The larvae remain trapped in the skin and subcutaneous tissue for weeks to months, during which time they continue to migrate, creating serpentine tunnels and provoking a severe erythematous and vesicular reaction. Clinically, the patient notes a pruritic, raised, red, linear lesion approximately 10 to 20 cm long. Scratching of the irritated skin may lead to secondary bacterial infection. About half of the patients will develop transient pulmonary infiltrates with peripheral eosinophilia (Löffler's syndrome), presumably due to pulmonary migration of the larvae. Larvae are rarely found in sputum or skin biopsies and the diagnosis must be made on clinical grounds.

The infection is treated adequately with thiabendazole. Antihistamines may be helpful in controlling the pruritus. Preventive measures include the wearing of shoes, the deworming of pets, and the improvement of sanitation.

Filariasis

The filariae are nematodes that are widely distributed in nature. The adults are long and slender, measuring many centimeters in length, and may inhabit virtually any tissue, including blood and lymphatic vessels, pleural and peritoneal cavities, subcutaneous tissue, heart, and brain. Some species migrate in tissues and others remain localized and may become encased in a fibrous tissue reaction. The adults mate in the tissues, producing many progeny called microfilariae. The microfilariae are small (200 to 300 μm), slender, motile forms, which may be found in the circulating blood or migrating in the subcutaneous tissues, depending on the species.

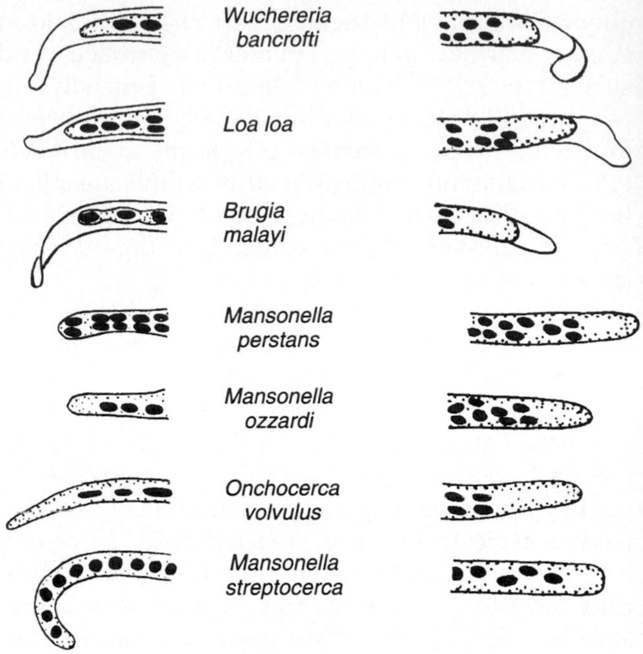

Figure 55.42. Differentiation of microfilariae, on the basis of posterior ends (*left*) and anterior ends (*right*) of the microfilariae. Note the distribution of nuclei, their presence or absence in the extreme caudal portion, and the presence or absence of a sheath. (From Markell EK, et al. Medical parasitology. 7th ed. Philadelphia: WB Saunders, 1992.)

Microfilariae are classified by morphological characteristics, geographic location, and type of clinical infection seen. The major division of microfilaria is by the presence or absence of a sheath surrounding the parasite (Fig. 55.42). Unsheathed microfilaria include *Onchocerca volvulus, Mansonella ozzardi, Mansonella perstans,* and *Mansonella streptocerca*. The sheathed microfilaria include *Wuchereria bancrofti, Brugia malayi,* and *Loa loa*. Definitive identification to species is based on the presence and number of nuclei seen in the tail of the microfilaria. Alternatively, these parasites can be divided as causes of cutaneous, lymphatic, or body cavity infection. Species identification of blood microfilariae is particularly important, because some may cause serious disease while others rarely do.

Onchocerciasis

Onchocerciasis, a major cause of blindness worldwide, is caused by the skin filaria *Onchocerca volvulus*. Humans become infected by the bite of black flies of the genus *Simulium*. The filariform larvae of the parasite are injected by the bite of the fly into the skin and migrate to subcutaneous connective tissue, where they develop into adult worms. The 20- to 30-mm adults become encased in fibrous subcutaneous nodules within which they may remain viable for up

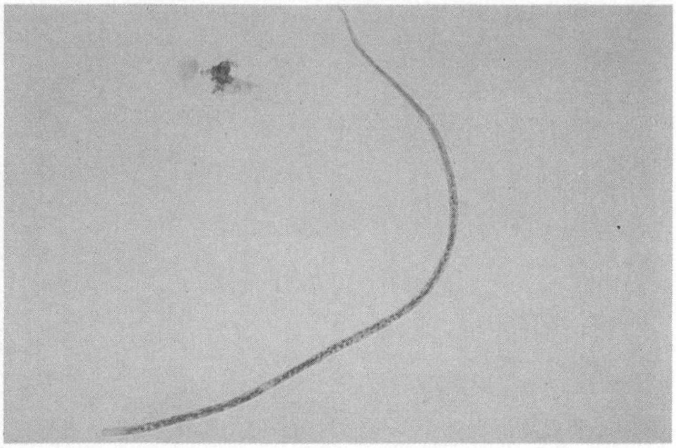

Figure 55.43. *Onchocerca volvulus:* microfilaria teased from skin snip (H&E stain). (From Smith JW, et al. Diagnostic medical parasitology: blood and tissue parasites. Chicago: American Society of Clinical Pathologists, 1976.)

to 15 years. The female worm gives birth to up to 2000 microfilariae each day. These larval forms exit the capsule to migrate for up to 2 years in the subcutaneous tissues, skin, and eye. The life cycle is completed by ingestion of the microfilaria by new black flies in which the microfilaria transform into infectious filariform larvae.

Clinical onchocerciasis is characterized by infection involving the skin, subcutaneous tissue, lymph nodes, and eyes. Patients present with pruritus, subcutaneous nodules, or visual impairment. The clinical manifestations of the infection are due to the acute and chronic inflammatory reaction to antigens released by the microfilariae as they migrate through the tissues. Within the skin this inflammatory process results in loss of elasticity and areas of depigmentation, thickening, and atrophy. Subcutaneous inflammation may produce fibrosing, obstructive lymphadenitis, which may result in elephantiasis. Firm, nontender, mobile nodules may develop, especially over bony prominences.

Onchocerciasis affects over 50 million people in tropical Africa and Central and South America, and causes blindness in approximately 5% of infected individuals. The mechanisms for development of eye disease is thought to be a combination of both direct invasion by the microfilaria and antigen-antibody complex deposition within the ocular tissues (38). Patients progress from conjunctivitis with photophobia to punctate and sclerosing keratitis. Internal eye disease with anterior uveitis, chorioretinitis, and optic neuritis may also occur. The disease is one of the leading causes of blindness worldwide. In certain communities in West Africa, up to half of the adult male population is blind due to this infection.

Diagnosis of onchocerciasis is made by demonstration of microfilaria in skin snip preparations from the infrascapular or gluteal region. A sample is obtained by raising the skin with a needle and shaving the epidermal layer with a razor. The specimen is incubated in saline for several hours, then inspected with a dissecting microscope for the presence of nonsheathed microfilaria (Fig. 55.43). In patients with ocular disease, the organism may also be seen in the anterior chamber with the aid of a slit lamp. Serologic and culture methods are not helpful, although efforts to develop serological detection methods are ongoing.

Treatment includes the use of diethylcarbamazine to eradicate the microfilariae and either surgical excision of nodules or administration of suramin for the adult worms. Recently, ivermectin has been demonstrated to be more effective than diethylcarbamazine in eradicating the microfilariae and does not appear to induce the allergic manifestations seen with the latter agent (39).

Mansonella

Filarial infections caused by *Mansonella* species (*M. perstans*, *M. ozzardi*, and *M. streptocerca*) are generally asymptomatic, but may cause dermatitis, lymphadenitis, hydrocele, and rarely lymphatic obstruction resulting in elephantiasis. All of the *Mansonella* species produce nonsheathed microfilariae (Fig. 55.42) in blood and subcutaneous tissues, and all are transmitted by biting midges (*Culicoides*) or black flies (*Simulium*). These filaria are found in South America and Central Africa. All are treatable with diethylcarbamazine. Species identification, if desired, can be accomplished with blood smears noting the structure of the microfilariae. Serologic tests are also available.

Lymphatic Filariasis

Lymphatic filariasis constitutes a group of diseases characterized by lymphatic obstruction that results in a condition known as elephantiasis. The two species of filaria most commonly involved are *Wuchereria bancrofti* and *Brugia malayi*. The adult forms of these filariae parasitize the lymphatic vessels, primarily in the arms, legs, or groin, where they may exist for as long as 10 years. The female worms produce sheathed microfilariae (Fig. 55.42) that enter the bloodstream of the host and circulate with a nocturnal periodicity. The microfilariae may be found in greatest numbers in the peripheral circulation between 9:00 PM and 2:00 AM, a time period that corresponds to the peak feeding time of the mosquito vectors (*Culex*, *Aedes*, *Anopheles*, or *Mansonia*). The microfilariae that are ingested by the mosquito vector transform first into rhabditiform and then into filariform larvae within the mosquito. The infective filariform larvae actively penetrate the feeding site when the mosquito takes

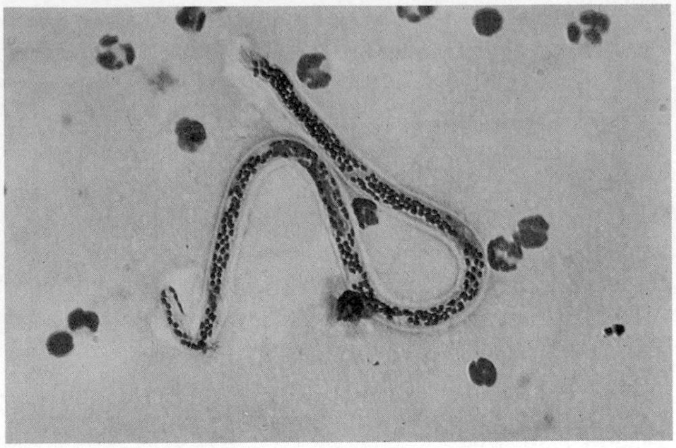

Figure 55.44. *Wuchereria bancrofti*: microfilaria in thick film (Giemsa stain). (From Smith JW, et al. Diagnostic medical parasitology: blood and tissue parasites. Chicago: American Society of Clinical Pathologists, 1976.)

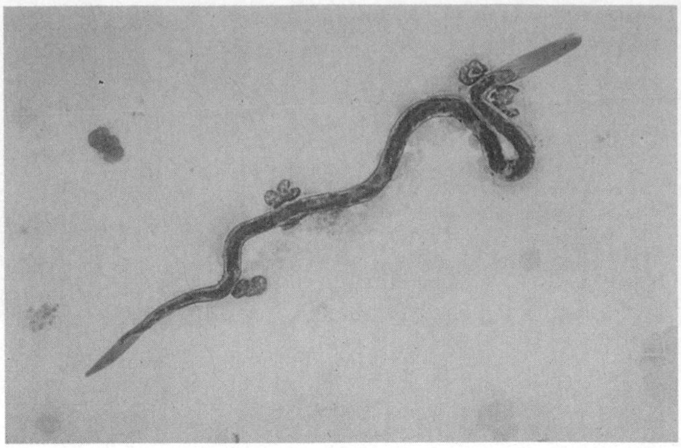

Figure 55.45. *Brugia malayi*: microfilaria in thin film (Giemsa stain). (From Smith JW, et al. Diagnostic medical parasitology: blood and tissue parasites. Chicago: American Society of Clinical Pathologists, 1976.)

its next meal and migrate to the lymphatic vessels, where they reach adulthood in 6 to 12 months.

Clinical manifestations of infection with *W. bancrofti* and *B. malayi* vary from asymptomatic infection with positive serology but no detectable microfilariae to lymphatic inflammation and chronic lymphatic obstruction with development of lymphoceles, lymphangitis, and elephantiasis. Acute symptoms may include fever, headache, and back pain in association with lymphangitis. The acute presentation is thought to be due to the inflammatory response to the presence of molting adolescent worms and dead or dying adults within the lymphatic vessels. The acute response is followed by the formation of granulomas, fibrosis, and permanent lymphatic obstruction. With repeated exposure over many years individuals develop heavy infections and massive lymphatic blockade. The resultant lymphedema and fibrosis may be complicated by recurrent bacterial infections, which contribute to the tissue damage. Continuation of this process over a period of decades results in elephantiasis, usually most severe in the lower extremities and genitalia (40). Occasionally ascites and pleural effusions secondary to rupture of enlarged lymphatics into the peritoneal or pleural cavities may be observed.

It is estimated that lymphatic filariasis currently infects between 80 and 100 million individuals in Africa, Latin America, the Pacific Islands, and Asia. *W. bancrofti* is distributed throughout these areas, whereas *B. malayi* is limited to Southeast Asia and Indonesia.

Eosinophilia is usually present during acute inflammatory episodes; however, demonstrations of microfilariae in blood is required for definitive diagnosis. Microfilariae can be demonstrated in Giemsa-stained blood films as for malaria (Figs. 55.44 and 55.45). If the parasitemia is scant, the blood specimen may be concentrated before it is examined (40). Given the nocturnal periodicity of the microfilaremia, it is recommended that blood specimens be obtained between 9:00 PM and 2:00 AM.

Both *W. bancrofti* and *B. malayi* produce sheathed microfilariae. Further identification is based on the study of head and tail structures (Fig. 55.42). Clinically, an exact species identification is not critical, as the treatment for all filarial infections is identical (diethylcarbamazine), with the possible exception of *O. volvulus* (ivermectin plus suramin).

Serologic testing is available but may lack sensitivity and specificity. Detection of circulating filarial antigens is promising but not widely available as a diagnostic test.

Treatment is of little benefit in most cases of lymphatic filariasis. Diethylcarbamazine has been used but has little apparent effect on adult worms. Ivermectin appears promising, although controlled studies have not yet been performed. Supportive and surgical therapy for lymphatic obstruction may be of some cosmetic help. Control programs combine mosquito control with mass treatment of the entire population.

Loa loa

Loiasis is a filarial disease found primarily in the rain forests of Africa, where *L. loa* is transmitted by biting flies of the genus *Chrysops*. The adult worms can persist in the human host for 17 years or more and migrate continuously through the subcutaneous tissues. During migration, the parasites elicit an intense eosinophilia and produce localized areas of allergic subcutaneous inflammation known as Calabar swellings. These swellings reach 10 to 20 cm in diameter, last 2 to 3 days, and may be accompanied by fever, pruritus, and pain. Occasionally, the adult worm may migrate across the eye subconjunctivally, producing tearing, pain, edema, and impaired vision.

The adult female produces sheathed microfilariae, which may be detected in the bloodstream during daytime hours. The sheath of the microfilariae does not stain with Giemsa and the tail has nuclei extending to the rounded tip (Fig. 55.42).

The diagnosis of loiasis may be made by recovering the adult worm from the eye or by detecting microfilariae in the blood or from aspirates of Calabar swellings. Eosinophilia is constant and may constitute 50 to 70% of the peripheral white count. Diethylcarbamazine is effective against both adults and microfilariae; however, destruction of the parasites may induce severe allergic reactions, which require treatment with corticosteroids. The role of ivermectin remains undefined for this infection.

Dirofilaria immitis

Dirofilaria immitis, the canine heartworm, is endemic in the Southeastern United States. It is transmitted by mosquitoes and has a typical filarial life cycle, with the dog serving as the definitive host. Accidental infections in humans may be acquired by the bite of the mosquito vector, resulting in one or more worms becoming lodged in the right heart or pulmonary artery. Since humans are unsuitable hosts for *Dirofilaria*, the parasite dies before maturing and is embolized to smaller branches of the pulmonary vasculature, where it may cause a small area of infarction that heals and may appear as a coin lesion on a chest radiograph. Throughout this process most patients remain asymptomatic. The pulmonary coin lesion may pose a problem because it resembles a malignancy requiring surgical removal. A definitive diagnosis is made when a thoracotomy specimen is examined microscopically, revealing the typical cross-sections of the parasite (41).

Unfortunately, no laboratory test currently available can provide an accurate diagnosis of dirofilariasis (42). Peripheral eosinophilia is rare and the radiographic features are insufficient to allow one to distinguish pulmonary dirofilariasis from bronchogenic carcinoma. Serologic tests are not sufficiently sensitive or specific to be clinically useful (43).

Dracunculus medinensis

Dracunculiasis is a chronic subcutaneous infection caused by the tissue-invading nematode *Dracunculus medinensis*. *D. medinensis* has a simple life cycle depending on fresh water and a copepod of the genus *Cyclops*, which serves as the intermediate host. The infection in humans is initiated when a copepod infected with the larval stage of *D. medinensis* is ingested in drinking water. Following ingestion, the larvae are released from the copepods in the stomach and small intestine, penetrate the wall of the digestive tract, and migrate to the retroperitoneal space, where they mature. Male and female worms mate in this location. The gravid female then migrates to the subcutaneous tissues, usually in the extremities, where a vesicle is formed in the host tissue. The vesicle ulcerates and the worm protrudes a loop of uterus through the ulcer. Upon contact with water, the larval worms are released. The larvae are then ingested by the *Cyclops* in fresh water, where they may in turn infect another mammalian host. Once the female has discharged all the larvae, it may retreat into deeper tissue where it is gradually absorbed, or may simply be expelled from the site.

Dracunculiasis is generally asymptomatic until the gravid female creates the vesicle and the ulcer in the skin for the liberation of larvae. The time between initial exposure and ulceration is usually about 1 year. The site of the ulceration is painful and erythematous and the adult worm may be visible in the center of the lesion. At the time of ulceration, the patient may develop local or generalized pruritus, nausea, diarrhea, and shortness of breath. Fluid present at the site of ulceration may contain many visible larvae. Patients with multiple adult worms may have several ulcerations occur simultaneously. Occasionally the site may become secondarily infected with bacteria, leading to abscess formation and further tissue destruction.

D. medinensis occurs in many parts of Asia and equatorial Africa, infecting an estimated 10 million individuals. Reservoir hosts include dogs and other mammals. Humans perpetuate the cycle when infected individuals bathe or stand in the wells or ponds from which drinking water is obtained. Larvae are discharged from the lesions on the arms, legs, feet, and ankles to infect the copepods in the water, which are in turn collected with the drinking water.

Diagnosis of this infection is usually straightforward clinically, with the adult worm present in the ulcerated skin lesion. Larvae can also be detected under the microscope in samples of fluid from the ulcer site.

Treatment may be accomplished by administration of niridazole, metronidazole, or thiabendazole. Alternatively, the worm may be removed surgically. The ancient method of slowly wrapping the worm on a twig, thus extracting it from the ulcer, is still used in many endemic areas. This process may be complicated by infection and/or toxic reactions if the worm is broken during removal.

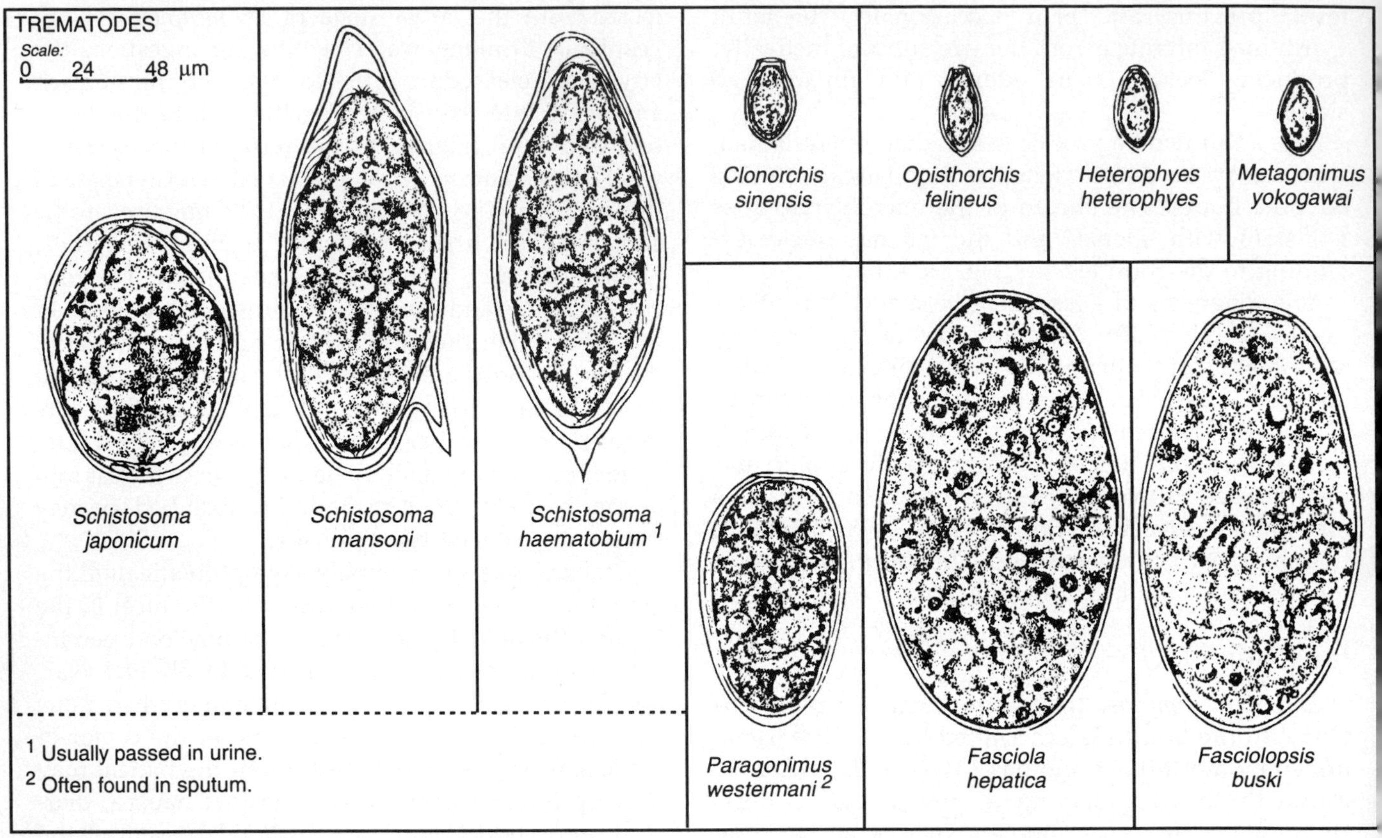

Figure 55.46. Trematode eggs found in human feces. (From Smith JW, et al. Diagnostic medical parasitology: intestinal helminths. Chicago: American Society of Clinical Pathologists, 1976.)

Prevention requires education concerning the life cycle of the parasite and avoidance of water contaminated with *Cyclops*. Ideally, adequate treatment of water supplies would result in elimination of this infection.

Trematodes

The trematodes or flukes are members of the Platyhelminthes and are generally flat, fleshy, leaf-shaped worms. They vary in length from a few millimeters to several centimeters and possess two muscular suckers: one oral, surrounding the opening to the primitive digestive tract, and one ventral for attachment. The digestive system consists of a muscular pharynx and esophagus and bilateral ceca that end blindly near the posterior aspect of the worm.

The flukes may be divided into two major categories based on their reproductive systems. The majority of flukes are hermaphrodites. The adult hermaphrodite contains both male and female gonads and produces operculate eggs (Fig. 55.46). The schistosomes constitute the second major category and include organisms with separate sexes. The female schistosome deposits only nonoperculated eggs. Schistosomes also have more rounded bodies than do the hermaphroditic flukes. Both schistosomes and hermaphroditic flukes have similar life cycles that include one or more intermediate hosts. Mollusks (snails or clams) are essential, first intermediate hosts for all trematodes. The mollusks are infected by ciliated larvae, or miracidia, which are released from eggs that have been deposited into fresh water. Within the first intermediate host the miracidia undergo asexual reproduction to produce thousands of motile cercariae, which are released into the water where they actively swim about in search of their next host. In the case of schistosomes, the cercariae directly penetrate the skin of humans and produce infection. The cercariae of the hermaphroditic flukes encyst in or upon an aquatic plant or animal (crustacean or fish), where they develop into infective metacercariae. Their cycle is completed when the second intermediate host is ingested by a human.

Another means of classifying the trematodes that cause human infection is by the anatomic location of the parasite in the human host. Thus we have the intestinal trematodes (Table 55.9), the liver and lung trematodes (Table 55.10), and the blood trematodes (Table 55.11). Of the many trematodes infecting humans, only seven representative agents will be

Table 55.9. Morphology of Intestinal Trematodes

	Fasciolopsis buski	*Heterophyes heterophyes*	*Metagonimus yokogawai*
Method of infection	Ingestion of water chestnut, bamboo shoots	Ingestion of freshwater fish	Ingestion of freshwater fish
Location in host	Attached to wall of the small intestine	Crypts and lumen of the small intestine	Crypts and lumen of the small intestine
Reservoir host	Dogs, pigs, rabbits	Fish-eating mammals	Fish-eating mammals
Intermediate host	*Segmentina* or *Hippeutis* snails	*Pironella* and *Cerithidea* snails	*Semisulcospira* snails
Adult worm	Large, up to 75 mm long × 20 mm wide	Small, pyriform-shaped, 1.–2.5 mm long × 0.3–0.7 mm wide, single ovary is situated anterior to the posterior testes	Small, pyriform-shaped, 1.–2.5 mm long + 0.3–0.7 mm wide, single ovary is situated anterior to the posterior testes
Egg morphology	Ellipsoidal, unembryonated, operculated, 130–150 μm × 63–90 μm	Ovoid, operculated, 20–30 μm × 15–17 μm, contain a miracidium when discharged	Ovoid, operculated, 20–30 μm × 15–17 μm, contain a miracidium when discharged
Clinical manifestations	Attachment of worm may cause hypersection of mucus, hemorrhage, ulcerations, abscess, bowel obstruction, acute ileus, eosinophilia, leukocytosis, malabsorption	Abdominal pain, mucous diarrhea, ulceration of intestinal wall, may invoke pathologic lesions in the brain and heart	Abdominal pain, mucous diarrhea, ulceration of intestinal wall, may invoke pathologic lesions in the brain and heart
Diagnostic methods[a]	O&P exam	O&P exam	O&P exam
Specimen	Feces	Feces	Feces
Common name	Large intestinal fluke	Heterophid fluke	Heterophid fluke

[a]O&P exam, ova and parasites examination.

discussed: the blood flukes, all of which are members of the genus *Schistosoma* (*Schistosoma mansoni, Schistosoma haematobium*, and *Schistosoma japonicum*), the liver flukes (*Fasciola hepatica* and *Opisthorchis sinensis*), the lung fluke (*Paragonimus westermani*), and the intestinal fluke (*Fasciolopsis buski*). The other flukes causing infection in humans are similar to these representative agents in terms of epidemiology, clinical syndromes, and therapy. Basic details of additional intestinal and tissue flukes are provided in Tables 55.9 and 55.10.

Intestinal Trematodes

A number of intestinal trematodes are recognized, including *Fasciolopsis buski, Heterophyes heterophyes*, and *Metagonimus yokogawai* (Table 55.9). *F. buski* is the largest, most prevalent, and important intestinal fluke. *F. buski* is a large (75 mm long by 20 mm wide) fleshy worm (Fig. 55.47) that is a common parasite of pigs and humans in China and Southeast Asia. It is estimated that approximately 10 million individuals are infected with this intestinal parasite.

F. buski demonstrates a life cycle typical of hermaphroditic trematodes. In this case the metacercariae are encysted on aquatic plants, which serve as the second intermediate host. Ingestion of the metacercariae along with the freshwater vegetation results in establishment of the infection in the small intestine. The flukes live attached to the mucosa of the duodenum and jejunum by means of the ventral sucker. Self-fertilization occurs and egg production begins 3 months after the initial infection with the metacercariae. The eggs are broadly ellipsoidal, 130 to 150 μm by 60 to 90 μm, are unembryonated, and have a small, indistinct operculum (Figs. 55.46 and 55.48). The eggs are passed in the feces and gain access to fresh water, where they require a prolonged maturation period. Following maturation, the eggs release a ciliated, free-swimming larval stage (miracidium) that seeks a particular species of snail for further development.

The symptomatology of *F. buski* infection is directly related to the worm burden in the small intestine. Ulceration of the superficial mucosa may occur, accompanied by inflammation and hemorrhage. Diarrhea and epigastric pain similar to that of a duodenal ulcer are the main presenting symptoms. Anorexia, nausea, and vomiting can occur, accompanied by eosinophilia. A malabsorption syndrome similar to giardiasis is common, and intestinal obstruction may occur if there are enough worms.

The diagnosis is made by finding the large, oval, bile-stained, operculate eggs in the stool (Fig. 55.48). The measurements and appearance of *F. buski* eggs are similar to those of the liver fluke *Fasciola hepatica*, and differentiation of the eggs of these species alone is not usually possible. The large adult flukes can rarely be found in feces or specimens collected at surgery.

The treatment of choice is praziquantel. Alternatively, niclosamide may also be used. Prompt treatment of infected humans may minimize the spread of infection. Prevention may also include proper san-

Table 55.10. Morphology of Liver and Lung Trematodes

	Opisthorchis sinensis	*Opisthorchis viverrini*	*Fasciola hepatica*	*Paragonimus westermani*
Method of infection	Ingestion of raw fish	Ingestion of raw fish	Ingestion of raw water plants	Ingestion of crabs, crawfish
Location in host	Bile ducts of the liver	Bile ducts of the liver	Bile ducts of the liver	Encapsulated in parenchyma of the lung
Reservoir host	Dogs, cats, fish-eating mammals	Dogs, cats, fish-eating mammals	Herbivores	Dogs, cats, tigers, lions
Intermediate host	1st: *Parafossarulus, Bulinus, Semisulcospira, Alocinma,* and *Melanoides* snails	1st: *Bithynia* snail 2nd: Freshwater fish	1st: *Parafossarulus, Bulinus, Semisulcospira, Alocinma,* and *Melanoides* snails	1st: *Semisulcospira* and *Brotia* snails 2nd: Crabs, crawfish
Adult worm	Flattened, spatulate, 10–25 mm long, × 3–5 mm wide, hermaphroditic with single round ovary anterior to testes	10–25 mm long, 2 testes lying one behind the other in posterior end, ovary anterior to testes	Large, fleshy, up to 30 mm long × 14 mm wide, anterior end is cone-shaped, all internal organs are branched	Ovoid, 7.5–12 mm × 4–6 mm, hermaphroditic, lobed ovary located anterior to testes, testes lie side by side in posterior part of body
Egg morphology	Ovoid, thick-shelled, seated operculum, 27–35 μm × 12–19 μm, knob at abopercular end, prominent shoulders, contains miracidium	19–29 μm × 12–17 μm, operculated, prominent shoulders, contains miracidium	Large, ellipsoidal, unembryonated, operculated 130–150 μm × 63–90 μm, operculum is small	Ovoid, large, thick-shelled, unembryonated when passed in sputum or feces, 80–120 μm × 45–70 μm, thickened at abopercular end
Clinical manifestations	Biliary tract obstruction, bile retention, acute pancreatitis, cholecystitis, cholelithiasis, fever, chills, diarrhea, epigastric pain, enlarged tender liver, jaundice	Infection confined to biliary tract system, weakness, pain in right upper quadrant, elevated serum IgE levels (3 or 4 times)	Fever, right upper quadrant pain, eosinophilia associated with migratory phase, biliary obstruction, cholangitis, acute epigastric pain, fever, jaundice, enlarged liver, eosinophilia	Cough with increased production of blood-tinged sputum, chest pain, dyspnea with chronic bronchitis, fever, headache, nausea, vomiting, visual disturbances, motor weakness, localized or general paralysis
Diagnostic methods[a]	CF, HAI, O&P exam	O&P exam	CF, HAI, IIF, immunodiffusion, immunoelectrophoresis, countercurrent electrophoresis, O&P exam	CF, O&P exam
Specimen	Feces	Feces	Feces	Feces
Common name	Chinese liver fluke		Sheep liver fluke	Oriental lung fluke

[a]Abbreviations: CF, complement fixation; HAI, hemagglutination inhibition; IIF, indirect immunofluorescence; O&P exam, ova and parasites examination.

Table 55.11. Morphology of Blood Trematodes

	Schistosoma mansoni	*Schistosoma japonicum*	*Schistosoma haematobium*
Method of infection	Cercaria penetrates skin of humans, loses tail, becomes a schistosomulum and migrates to blood vessel where it develops to an adult	Cercaria penetrates skin of humans, loses tail, becomes a schistosomulum and migrates to blood vessel where it develops to an adult	Cercaria penetrates skin of humans, loses tail, becomes a schistosomulum and migrates to blood vessel where it develops to an adult
Location in host	Venous plexus of colon and lower ileum; portal system of liver	Venous plexus of small intestine	Plexus of bladder, rectum
Reservoir host	Humans, nonhuman primates	Dogs, cats, cattle, water buffalo, pigs	Humans
Intermediate host	*Biomphalaria* snail	*Oncomelania* snail	*Bulinus* snail
Adult worm	Sexes are separate, males 6.4–12 mm long, 6–9 testes in anterior half of body, females 7.2–17 mm long	Sexes are separate, sizes are comparable, contains more eggs in utero than *S. mansoni* or *S. haematobium*	Sexes are separate, males 10–15 mm long, females 20 mm long, tegument has minute tuberculations, female may contain between 20–100 eggs in uterus
Egg morphology	114–175 μm × 45–70 μm, nonoperculated, transparent shell, prominent lateral spine, contain miracidium when passed in feces	Round, large, nonoperculated, 70–100 μm × 55–65 μm, transparent shell, small inconspicuous spine	Large, nonoperculated, transparent shell, prominent terminal spine, 112–170 μm × 40–70 μm
Clinical manifestations	Cercarial dermatitis, high fever, hepatosplenomegaly, lymphadenopathy, eosinophilia, dysentery, abdominal pain, liver tenderness, urticaria, general malaise, blood and mucus in stools	Cercarial dermatitis, high fever, hepatosplenomegaly, lymphadenopathy, eosinophilia, dysentery, abdominal pain, liver tenderness, urticaria, general malaise, blood and mucus in stools	Cercarial dermatitis, high fever, hepatosplenomegaly, lymphadenopathy, eosinophilia, dysentery, abdominal pain, liver tenderness, urticaria, general malaise, hematuria, dysuria
Diagnostic methods[a]	CF, HAI, IIF, immunoelectrophoresis, enzyme-linked immunoassay, O&P exam	CF, HAI, IIF, immunoelectrophoresis, enzyme-linked immunoassay, O&P exam	CF, HAI, IIF, immunoelectrophoresis, enzyme-linked immunoassay, O&P exam
Specimen	Stool, rectal biopsy, serology	Stool, rectal biopsy, serology	Urine, serology
Common name	Manson's blood fluke	Blood fluke	Bladder fluke

[a]Abbreviations: CF, complement fixation; HAI, hemagglutination inhibition; IIF, indirect immunofluorescence; O&P exam, ova and parasites examination.

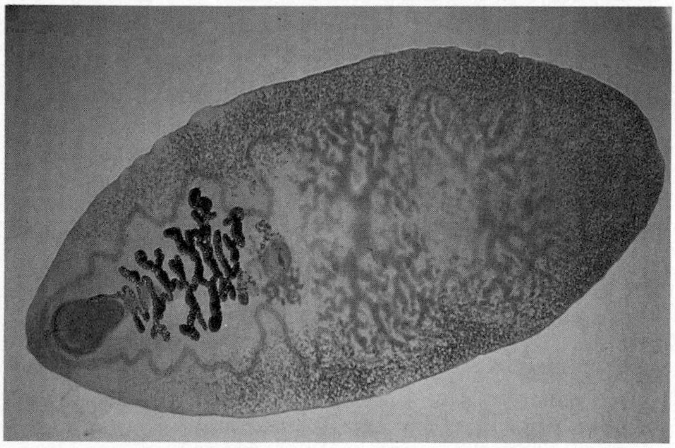

Figure 55.47. *Fasciolopsis buski*, adult worm (carmine stain, whole mount). (From Smith JW, et al. Diagnostic medical parasitology: intestinal helminths. Chicago: American Society of Clinical Pathologists, 1976.)

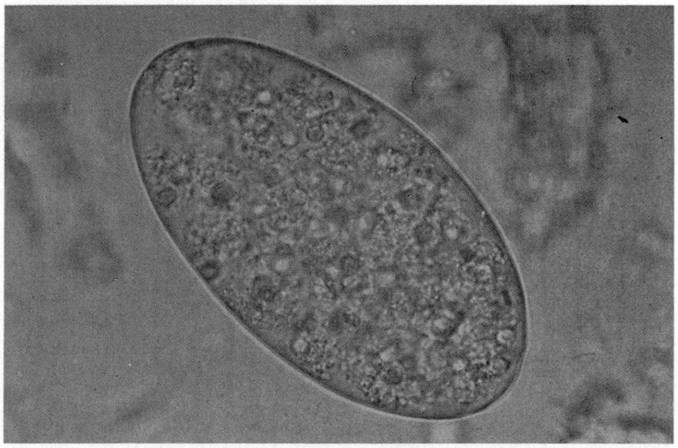

Figure 55.48. *Fasciolopsis buski*, egg (high power). (From Smith JW, et al. Diagnostic medical parasitology: intestinal helminths. Chicago: American Society of Clinical Pathologists, 1976.)

itation and elimination of the reservoir hosts through the use of molluscasides.

Liver Trematodes

There are several liver flukes in various geographic regions that parasitize the biliary passages of humans. These include *Fasciola hepatica, Opisthorchis sinensis, Opisthorchis viverrini, Opisthorchis felineus,* and *Dicrocoelium dendriticum* (Table 55.10). The most important of these, *F. hepatica* and *O. sinensis* are discussed in this chapter.

Fasciola hepatica. The largest of the liver flukes is *F. hepatica,* a common parasite of sheep and cattle. *F. hepatica* has a worldwide distribution.

The large (30 mm by 13 mm), fleshy adult flukes live in the biliary tree, where they lay eggs that are passed in the feces. The eggs develop in water and follow a life cycle similar to that of *Fasciolopsis buski*, with human infection resulting from ingestion of freshwater vegetation that harbors the encysted metacercariae. When ingested, the infective larvae are released from their cysts and migrate through the duodenal wall, across the peritoneal cavity, and into the bile ducts (via the liver), where they become adult worms. As with *F. buski*, self-fertilization occurs and egg production begins approximately 3 to 4 months after the initial infection. The large (130 to 150 μm by 60 to 90 μm), operculated eggs (Fig. 55.46) are excreted in the stool.

Early clinical signs and symptoms are due to the migration of the larvae through the liver. Right upper quadrant pain and tenderness, hepatomegaly, chills and fever, with marked eosinophilia may be observed. The presence of the adult worms in the biliary tree elicits an inflammatory response with resultant hyperplasia of the epithelium and eventual fibrosis. Biliary obstruction due to bile duct fibrosis and stone formation may occur. Penetration of adult worms into the liver parenchyma occurs rarely but may result in necrotic foci and abscess formation known as "liver rot."

The diagnosis is established by detecting the characteristic eggs in stools. The unembryonated, operculate eggs cannot be distinguished from those of *F. buski* (Figs. 55.46 and 55.48). Distinction between the two flukes is necessary for therapeutic purposes, as *F. buski* responds favorably to praziquantel whereas *F. hepatica* does not. The two species may be distinguished by sampling the patient's bile to detect the eggs of *F. hepatica*. Care must be taken to differentiate true infection from the spurious presence of eggs resulting from the ingestion of infected liver. Several stool samples should be examined to rule out such spurious observations and ensure that there is a true infection.

F. hepatica responds poorly to praziquantel. Treatment with bithionol or triclabendazole has been effective. Control measures are similar to those for *F. buski*.

Opisthorchis sinensis. The Chinese liver fluke, *O. sinensis*, is the most common liver fluke that infects humans. *O. sinensis* infects approximately 19 million individuals in China, Japan, Korea, and Vietnam (44). It is also seen among residents of the United States and can be traced to the consumption of raw, pickled, smoked, or dried freshwater fish harboring viable metacercariae. Cats and dogs serve as important reservoir hosts.

The adult fluke is small and delicate, measuring 10 to 25 mm long by 3 to 5 mm wide (Fig. 55.49). *O. sinensis* may survive in the biliary tract for up to 50 years producing approximately 2000 eggs per day. The tiny (15 × 30 μm), urn-shaped eggs enter the duodenum with the bile and are discharged in the feces. On reaching fresh water, the eggs are ingested by the molluscan first intermediate host, transformed into cercariae, and released to penetrate the tissues of freshwater fish, in which they encyst to become infective metacercariae. Infection is acquired by ingestion of uncooked fish. The ingested larvae excyst in the duodenum and migrate via the ampulla of Vater and the common bile duct into the bile ducts of the liver, where they mature and live.

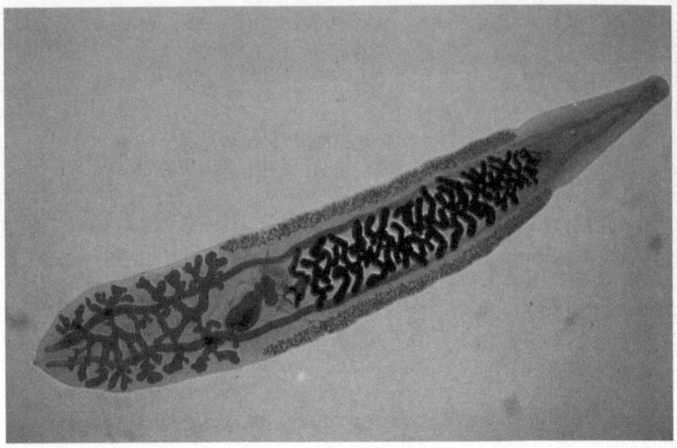

Figure 55.49. *Opisthorchis sinensis*, adult worm (carmine stain, whole mount). (From Smith JW, et al. Diagnostic medical parasitology: intestinal helminths. Chicago: American Society of Clinical Pathologists, 1976.)

Infection in humans is usually mild and asymptomatic. Severe infections involving large numbers of flukes may produce fever, diarrhea, epigastric pain, hepatomegaly, anorexia, and occasionally jaundice. Biliary obstruction may occur, and individuals with severe longstanding infection may develop bile duct carcinoma. Invasion of the gallbladder or pancreatic ducts may occur, causing cholecystitis and pancreatitis.

The diagnosis is made by recovering the distinctive eggs from stools. The eggs measure 27 to 35 μm by 12 to 19 μm and are characterized by a distinct operculum with prominent shoulders and a tiny knob at the posterior (abopercular) pole (Fig. 55.50). In mild infections, repeated examinations of stool or duodenal aspirates may be necessary. In acute symptomatic infection, there is usually an eosinophilia and elevation of serum alkaline phosphatase levels. Radiographic imaging procedures may detect abnormalities of the biliary tract.

Effective treatment may be accomplished with praziquantel. Prevention requires avoidance of improperly cooked fish and the implementation of proper sanitation policies.

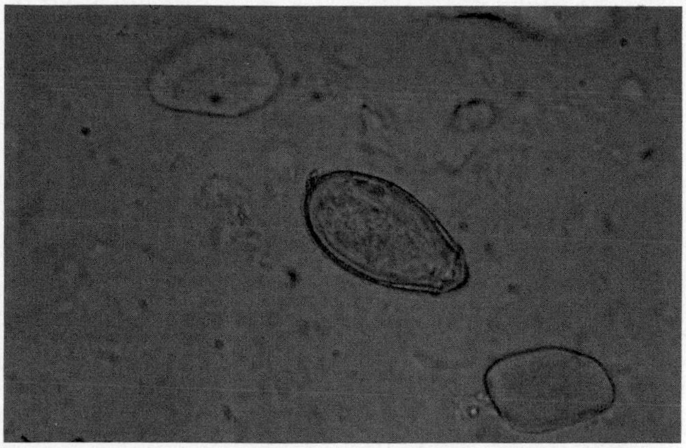

Figure 55.50. *Opisthorchis sinensis*, egg (oil immersion). (From Smith JW, et al. Diagnostic medical parasitology: intestinal helminths. Chicago: American Society of Clinical Pathologists, 1976.)

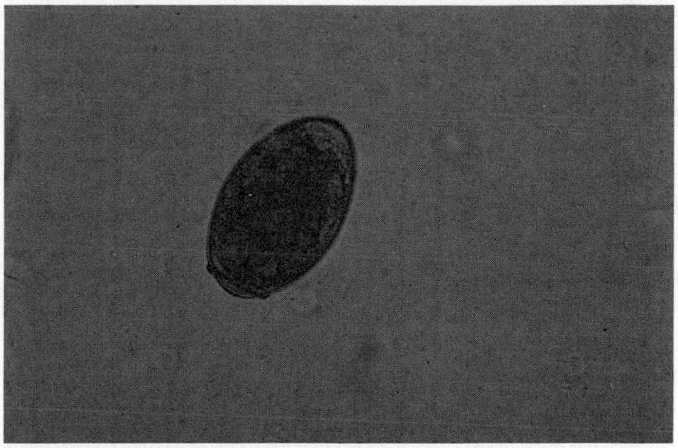

Figure 55.51. *Paragonimus westermani*, egg (high power). (From Smith JW, et al. Diagnostic medical parasitology: intestinal helminths. Chicago: American Society of Clinical Pathologists, 1976.)

Lung Trematodes

The principal lung fluke of humans is *Paragonimus westermani*, which is found in the Orient; however, several additional species of *Paragonimus* have been described parasitizing humans and other animals in Africa and South, Central, and North America. *P. westermani* is a small (10 mm by 5 mm), reddish-brown worm that is a common parasite of shore-feeding animals (pigs, wild boars, monkeys) as well as humans in China, Japan, and Southeast Asia. Its prevalence is directly related to the consumption of uncooked freshwater crabs and crayfish. It is estimated that approximately 3 million individuals are infected with this lung fluke. As many as 1% of all Indochinese immigrants to the United States are infected with *P. westermani* (45).

The adult worms are usually found encysted in the pulmonary parenchyma of their definitive host. Infection is acquired by the ingestion of raw or partially cooked crabs or crayfish containing encysted metacercariae in their tissues. Once ingested, the metacercariae excyst in the duodenum and migrate through the intestinal wall into the peritoneal cavity, through the diaphragm, and finally reach maturity in the lungs 5 to 6 weeks later. Occasionally organisms undergo aberrant migration and are retained in the intestinal wall and mesentery or migrate to other ectopic foci such as the liver, pancreas, skeletal muscle, subcutaneous tissue, or the central nervous system.

Upon reaching the pulmonary parenchyma, the flukes become encapsulated by the host's fibrous reaction. The adult worms deposit operculate, golden-brown eggs within the fibrous capsule. The capsule ultimately erodes into a bronchiole and discharges the eggs into the respiratory tree. The eggs may then be coughed up and spat out or swallowed and passed in the stool.

The clinical manifestations of paragonimiasis may be due to larvae migrating through tissues or to adults established in the lungs or other ectopic sites. The onset of the disease coincides with larval migration and is associated with fever, chills, and high eosinophilia. Once established in the lungs, the adult worms stimulate an inflammatory reaction that results in fever and a chronic cough with increased sputum production and occasional hemoptysis. Evacuation of the capsule or cyst containing the adult worms and eggs produces a cavity, which may become secondarily infected with bacteria. The expectorated sputum is blood-tinged and contains numerous gold-brown eggs. Severe infections produce a chronic pneumonia with abscess formation and pulmonary fibrosis. Dyspnea, severe chest pain, and pleural effusion may be seen. Location of larvae, adults, and eggs in ectopic sites may produce severe clinical symptoms depending on the site involved. Cerebral paragonimiasis occurs in approximately 1% of Oriental cases and may produce a severe neurologic disease including seizures, paralysis, and visual disturbances.

The laboratory diagnosis of paragonimiasis is dependent on the detection of the golden-brown, operculated eggs in sputum and feces (Fig. 55.51). Pleural effusions, when present, should also be examined for eggs. Marked eosinophilia is common and chest radiographs often show nodular shadows, calcifications, or patchy infiltrates. Serologic procedures are available through reference laboratories and may be useful, particularly in cases with extrapulmonary (e.g., central nervous system) involvement.

The disease responds adequately to treatment with either praziquantel or bithionol. Control requires adequate cooking of freshwater crustaceans before ingestion.

Blood Trematodes (Schistosomiasis)

Schistosomiasis is a major parasitic infection of tropical areas with some 200 million infections worldwide (46–48). The three schistosomes most frequently associated with human disease are *Schistosoma mansoni*, *S. japonicum*, and *S. haematobium*. As discussed previously, schistosomes differ from the hermaphroditic flukes in body structure, in having separate sexes, in having nonoperculated eggs, and in having a life cycle that includes only one intermediate host. They are also obligate intravascular parasites inhabiting the venules of the intestine (*S. mansoni* and *S. japonicum*) and the bladder (*S. haematobium*) rather than the cavities, ducts, and other tissues parasitized by the hermaphroditic flukes.

Infection with schistosomes is acquired by exposure to fresh water containing ciliated, free-swimming cercariae. The cercariae penetrate intact skin, causing intense pruritus; enter the circulation; and develop in the intrahepatic portal circulation. Adult male and female worms pair up early in development. The flat 1- to 2-cm male has a longitudinal (gynecophoral) canal resulting from folding the lateral aspects of the body toward the center. The long, slender, cylindrical female resides in the canal and the two worms stay together in this fashion for the rest of their lives. After mating in the portal vein, the paired adult worms migrate to their final location in the small venules of the mesentery (*S. mansoni* and *S. japonicum*) and venous plexuses of the bladder (*S. haematobium*). In general, *S. japonicum* resides in the venous radicals of the small intestine, *S. mansoni* resides in the vicinity of the descending colon and rectum, and *S. haematobium* resides in the veins of the bladder and other pelvic organs. On reaching the submucosal venules, the worms initiate oviposition, which may continue at the rate of 300 to 3000 eggs daily for 4 to 35 years. Although the host inflammatory response to the adult worms, which are coated with host proteins, is minimal, the eggs elicit an intense inflammatory reaction with both mononuclear and polymorphonuclear cellular infiltrates and the formation of microabscesses. In addition, the larvae inside the eggs produce enzymes that aid in tissue destruction and allow the eggs to pass through the mucosa and into the lumen of the bladder and bowel, where they are passed to the external environment in the urine and feces, respectively.

The eggs are fully embryonated when they are passed to the environment and hatch quickly upon reaching fresh water to release motile miracidia. The miracidia then invade the appropriate snail host, where they develop into thousands of infectious cercariae. The free-swimming cercariae are released into the water, where they are immediately infectious for humans and other mammals.

The infection is similar in all three species of human schistosomes in that disease results primarily from the host immune response to the eggs rather than from the adult worms. As noted above, the very earliest signs and symptoms of infection are due to the penetration of the cercariae through the skin. Immediate and delayed hypersensitivity to parasite antigens results in an intensely pruritic papular skin rash.

The onset of oviposition, 1 to 2 months after primary exposure, results in a symptom complex known as the Katayama syndrome, which is marked by fever, chills, cough, urticaria, arthralgias, lymphadenopathy, splenomegaly, and abdominal pain. Laboratory abnormalities include leukocytosis, eosinophilia, and a polyclonal gammopathy with elevated levels of IgG, IgM, and IgE. This symptom complex may persist for 3 months or more and is thought to be due to the massive release of parasite antigens with subsequent immune complex formation.

The more chronic and significant phase of schistosomiasis is due to the presence of the eggs in the various tissues and the resulting formation of granulomas and fibrosis (46). The retained eggs induce extensive inflammation and scarring, the clinical significance of which is directly related to the location and number of eggs. In *S. haematobium* infection, egg deposition in the walls of the bladder results in hematuria and dysuria and eventually may result in scarring and loss of bladder capacity, obstructive uropathy, and bladder carcinoma. Infections with *S. mansoni* and *S. japonicum* may produce hepatic and intestinal abnormalities. Deposition of eggs in the bowel mucosa results in inflammation and thickening of the bowel wall with associated abdominal pain, diarrhea, and blood in the stool. Importantly, eggs of *S. mansoni* and *S. japonicum* may be carried by the portal vein to the liver, where the resulting inflammation can lead to periportal fibrosis and eventually to portal hypertension with its associated manifestations. Although *S. mansoni* and *S. japonicum* eggs are primarily deposited in the intestine, eggs may appear in the brain, spinal cord, lungs, and other sites. Deposition of eggs in the central nervous system (brain and spinal cord) occurs more commonly with *S. japonicum* and may produce severe neurologic problems.

The geographic distribution of the various species of *Schistosoma* is dependent on the availability of a suitable snail host. *S. mansoni* is the most widespread

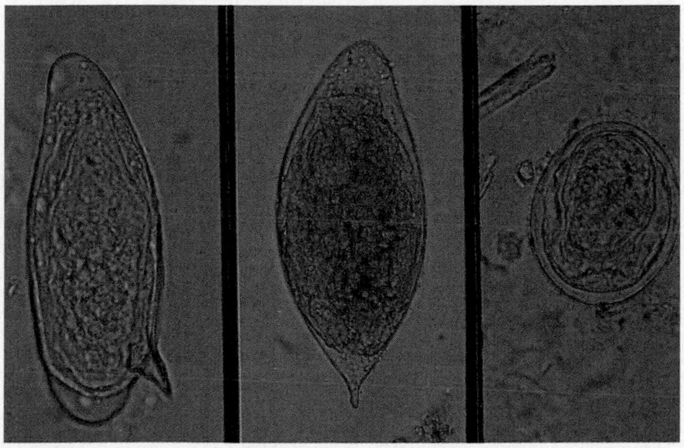

Figure 55.52. Eggs of *Schistosoma mansoni* (*left*), *S. haematobium* (*center*), and *S. japonicum* (*right*) (high power). (From Smith JW, et al. Diagnostic medical parasitology: intestinal helminths. Chicago: American Society of Clinical Pathologists, 1976.)

of the blood flukes, occurring in Africa and the Middle East as well as in South America, Puerto Rico, and several Caribbean islands. *S. haematobium* is largely confined to Africa and the Middle East, where its distribution overlaps that of *S. mansoni*. *S. japonicum* is known as the Oriental blood fluke and is found only in Japan, China, the Philippines, and the Celebes. Schistosomiasis may be considered a disease of economic progress, as the development of massive land irrigation projects in desert and tropical areas has resulted in the dispersion of infected humans and snails to previously uninvolved areas.

The diagnosis of schistosomiasis is usually established by the demonstration of characteristic eggs in urine or feces. Concentration techniques may be necessary in light infections. Biopsy of bladder or rectal mucosa may be positive when repeated examination of urine and stool specimens are negative. In general, the three species of *Schistosoma* may be readily differentiated by their characteristic egg morphology (Table 55.11 and Figs. 55.46 and 55.52). The eggs of *S. mansoni* are oval, possess a sharp lateral spine, and measure 114 to 175 μm by 45 to 70 μm. Those of *S. haematobium* differ primarily in the terminal location of the spine. The eggs of *S. japonicum* are more nearly circular, possess a minute lateral spine, and measure 70 to 100 by 55 to 65 μm.

Examination of eggs for viability is necessary to confirm the presence of active infection. This is accomplished most easily by the detection of movement of flame cell cilia within the egg upon microscopic examination. Alternatively, the eggs may be hatched in water. Quantitation of egg output in stool or urine is useful in estimating the severity of infection and in following the response to therapy.

Serologic testing is available but is largely of epidemiologic interest only. The development of newer tests using stage-specific antigens may allow the distinction of active from inactive disease and thus have greater clinical utility.

Specific therapy with praziquantel may be indicated for individuals with moderate or severe active infections. Anthelmintic therapy may terminate oviposition but will not affect lesions caused by eggs already deposited in tissues. Schistosomal dermatitis and the Katayama syndrome may be treated with the administration of antihistamines and corticosteroids.

Prevention of schistosomiasis has been difficult (47, 48). Proper sanitation and the use of molluscicides are necessary steps in interrupting the transmission of the parasite. Vaccine development is an area of intense research interest but a candidate vaccine is not available for human use at this time.

Cestodes

The cestodes or tapeworms are members of the Platyhelminthes and are generally long, flat, segmented, ribbon-like intestinal parasites. They vary in length from species in which adults are barely visible to the naked eye to species 20 to 25 feet long. The adult tapeworms are divided into three distinct body parts: the anterior portion or scolex, a generative neck, and a long, segmented body, the strobila. The head or scolex is equipped with various structures for attachment to the intestinal mucosa. These attachment structures vary with species but usually include muscular suckers (*Taenia* species), long, lateral grooves or bothria (*Diphyllobothrium latum*), and a retractable rostellum armed with a crown of chitinous hooks (*Taenia solium*) (Fig. 55.53). Posterior to the scolex is the neck, which gives rise to the strobila, consisting of individual body segments or proglottids.

All tapeworms are hermaphroditic, and each proglottid contains both male and female reproductive organs. Proglottids develop from immature to mature to egg-producing, with the most developed segments located farthest from the neck. Each self-contained proglottid is joined to the rest of the worm by a common cuticle, nerve trunks, and excretory canals. Tapeworms have no digestive system, and nutrients are absorbed from the host intestine through the complex cuticle of the worm. Gravid proglottids release their eggs by rupturing, disintegrating, or passing the eggs through a uterine pore. In some species (*T. solium* and *Taenia saginata*), eggs are not released from intact proglottids; instead, gravid proglottids separate from the remainder of the worm and are passed intact in the feces. The eggs of most cestodes are nonoperculated and contain a fully developed, six-hooked (hexacanth) embryo. In contrast, the eggs of the fish tapeworm, *D. latum*, are

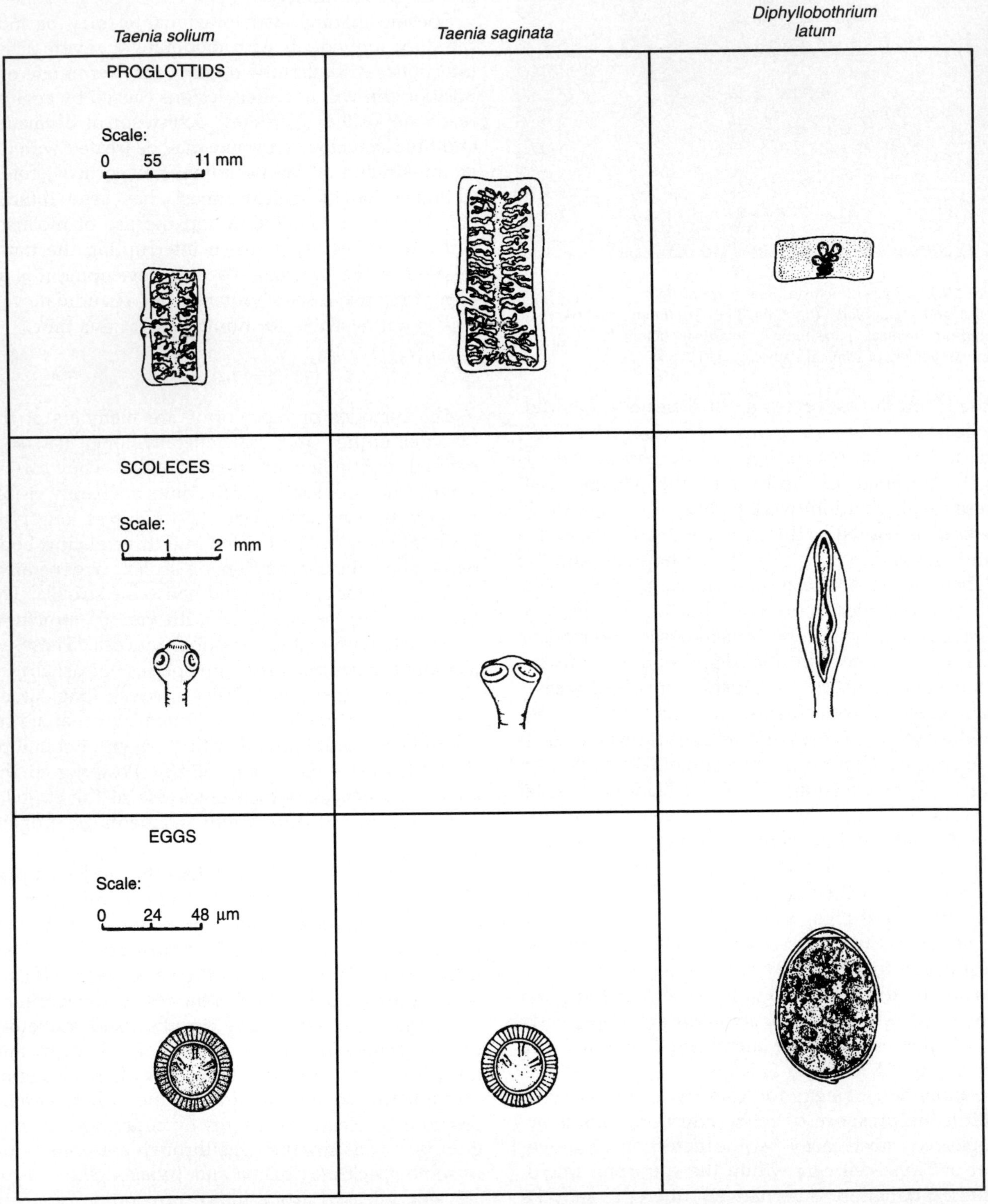

Figure 55.53. Diagnostic features of *Taenia solium, T. saginata,* and *Diphyllobothrium latum*. (From Smith JW, et al. Diagnostic medical parasitology: intestinal helminths. Chicago: American Society of Clinical Pathologists, 1976.)

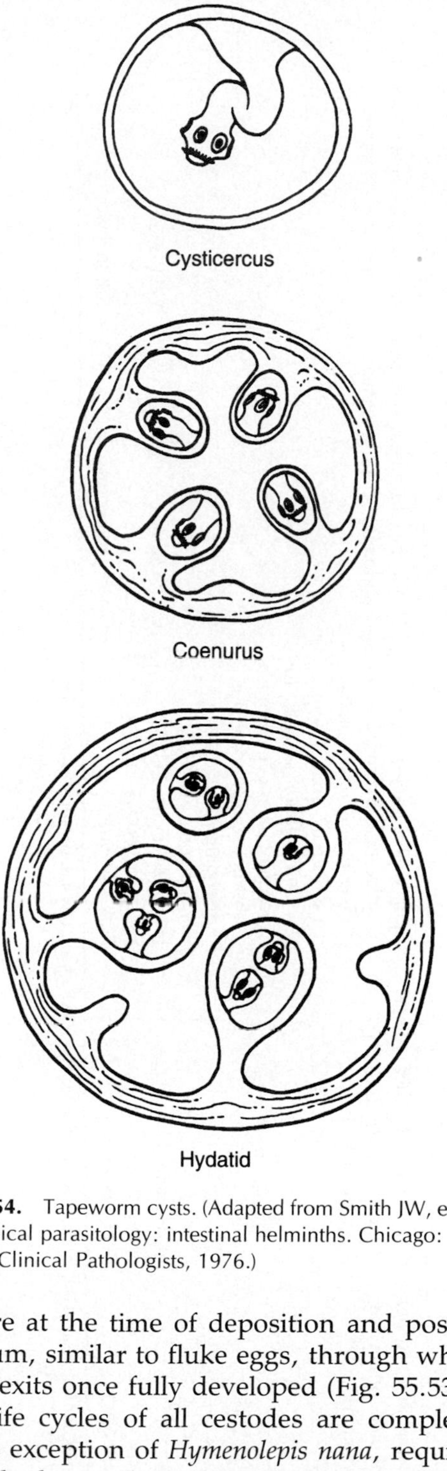

Figure 55.54. Tapeworm cysts. (Adapted from Smith JW, et al. Diagnostic medical parasitology: intestinal helminths. Chicago: American Society of Clinical Pathologists, 1976.)

immature at the time of deposition and possess an operculum, similar to fluke eggs, through which the embryo exits once fully developed (Fig. 55.53).

The life cycles of all cestodes are complex and, with the exception of *Hymenolepis nana*, require passage of the larvae through one or more intermediate hosts. For most cestodes, the eggs are ingested by the specific intermediate host and hatch within its gut. The released larvae then penetrate the intestinal mucosa and migrate to the tissues where they encyst and develop to the infective stage. The life cycle is completed when infective larvae are ingested by the appropriate definitive host. *D. latum*, whose eggs are immature upon release, requires two intermediate hosts to complete its larval development: aquatic invertebrates (copepods) and fish. The larval stages present in the tissues of intermediate hosts vary with the different species of cestode and include cysts with a single immature scolex or protoscolex (cysticercus; *Taenia* species), cysts with multiple protoscolices (coenurus; *Multiceps* species), and cysts containing multiple daughter cysts, each with multiple protoscolices (hydatid cyst; *Echinococcus* species) (Fig. 55.54). In some instances humans serve as a form of intermediate host that harbors larval stages. These extraintestinal larval infections are named according to the larval stage found in tissue (cysticercosis, coenurosis, hydatid disease) and are usually more serious than the presence of adult worms in the intestine.

There are numerous cestodes known to infect humans, including *Taenia saginata, T. solium, Diphyllobothrium latum, Echinococcus granulosus, Echinococcus multilocularis, Hymenolepis diminuta, H. nana, Dipylidium caninum*, and *Multiceps multiceps*. Together they infect approximately 65 million individuals, producing embarrassment, discomfort, anemia, and occasionally death. Of the many cestodes causing intestinal and tissue infections in humans, only four representative agents will be discussed: the pork tapeworm and cause of cysticercosis, *T. solium*; the beef tapeworm, *T. saginata*; the fish tapeworm, *D. latum*; and *E. granulosus*, the agent of hydatid disease. Basic details of the common intestinal cestodes of medical importance are provided in Table 55.12.

Taenia solium

Taenia solium, the pork tapeworm, inhabits the human jejunum, where it may survive for decades and grow to a maximum length of 3 to 5 meters. Its small scolex is armed with four sucking disks and a rostellum with a double row of hooklets (Fig. 55.53). Differentiation of *T. solium* from *T. saginata* may be accomplished by examination of the scolex and proglottids (Fig. 55.53). Gravid proglottids of *T. solium* are smaller than those of *T. saginata* and contain only 7 to 13 lateral uterine branches versus 15 to 30 for the beef tapeworm. *T. solium* is widely distributed throughout much of the world and is particularly common in eastern Europe, Asia, Africa, and Latin America. It is seen infrequently in the United States.

As indicated previously, the gravid proglottids of *Taenia* species become detached from the strobila and either rupture—releasing the characteristic eggs within the intestine—or are passed intact in the feces (Fig. 55.55). The eggs are spherical, 30 to 40 μm in diameter, and possess a thick, radially striated shell containing a six-hooked hexacanth embryo (Fig. 55.56). Both pigs and people may become intermedi-

Table 55.12. Morphology of Cestodes

	Diphyllobothrium latum	*Taenia saginata*	*Taenia solium*	*Hymenolepis nana*	*Hymenolepis diminuta*
Method of infection	Ingestion of raw fish	Ingestion of undercooked beef	Ingestion of undercooked pork and ova	Ingestion of cysticeroid in infected arthropod, ingestion of egg, autoinfection	Ingestion of cysticercoid in infected arthropod
Location in host	Adult in small intestine	Adult in small intestine	Adult in small intestine	Adult in small intestine; larvae in volli of small intestine	Adult in small intestine
Intermediate hosts	Copepods and fish	Cattle	Hog	Arthropods (beetles, fleas), rats, mice	Arthropods (beetles, fleas), rats, mice
Adult worm	4–10 m in length, gravid proglottids 3× 11 mm, rosette-shaped central uterus, genital pore on mid-ventral surface	4–8 m in length, no rostellum or hooklets, mature proglottids, the ovary has 2 lobes and a vaginal sphincter muscle, gravid proglottids 18–20 mm × 5–7 mm, 15–30 lateral branches on each side of central uterine stem	3–5 m in length, mature proglottids, the ovary has 2 lobes and an accessory lobe, vaginal sphincter muscle is absent, gravid proglottids 11 × 5 mm, 7–13 lateral branches on each side of the central uterine stem	Small, 2.5–4 cm long, proglottids are wider than they are long	20–60 cm long, proglottids are wider than they are long
Scolex	Small, 3 × 1 mm, spatulate with 2 shallow grooves	Small, 1–2 mm in diameter with 4 suckers	Small, 1 mm in diameter, 4 suckers, rostellum with 2 rows of hooklets	Small, knob-like with 4 suckers, rostellum and hooklets	Knob-like, 4 suckers, rostellum, no hooklets
Egg morphology	Ovoid, operculated, thick-shelled, 58–75 μm × 40–50 μm	Spherical, 31–43 μm, thick, radially striated, contains 6-hooked embryo (oncosphere)	Spherical, 31–43 μm, thick, radially striated, contains 6-hooked embryo (oncosphere)	Spherical, thin, hyaline shell 30–47 μm in diameter, 6-hooked oncosphere, polar filaments	Spherical, thick-shelled, 70–85 μm × 60–80 μm, 6-hooked oncosphere, no polar filaments
Clinical manifestations	Intestinal obstruction, diarrhea, abdominal pain, or anemia, possible vitamin B_{12} deficiency	Obstruction, diarrhea, hunger pains, weight loss, appendicitis	Adult worm: hunger pains, indigestion, diarrhea, constipation, eosinophilia Cysticercus: epileptiform seizures, abnormal behavior, transient paresis, intermittent obstructive hydrocephalus, disequilibrium, meningoencephalitis	Headache, dizziness, anorexia, abdominal pain, diarrhea	Infection is usually tolerated; very few symptoms
Diagnostic methods[a]	O&P exam	O&P exam, HAI, ELISA	HAI, O&P exam, ELISA	O&P exam	O&P exam
Specimen	Feces	Feces, proglottids, scolex	Feces, proglottids, scolex	Feces	Feces
Common name	Broad fish tapeworm	Beef tapeworm	Pork tapework	Dwarf tapeworm	Rat tapeworm

[a]Abbreviations: ELISA, enzyme-linked immunosorbent assay; HAI, hemagglutination inhibition; O&P exam, ova and parasites examination.

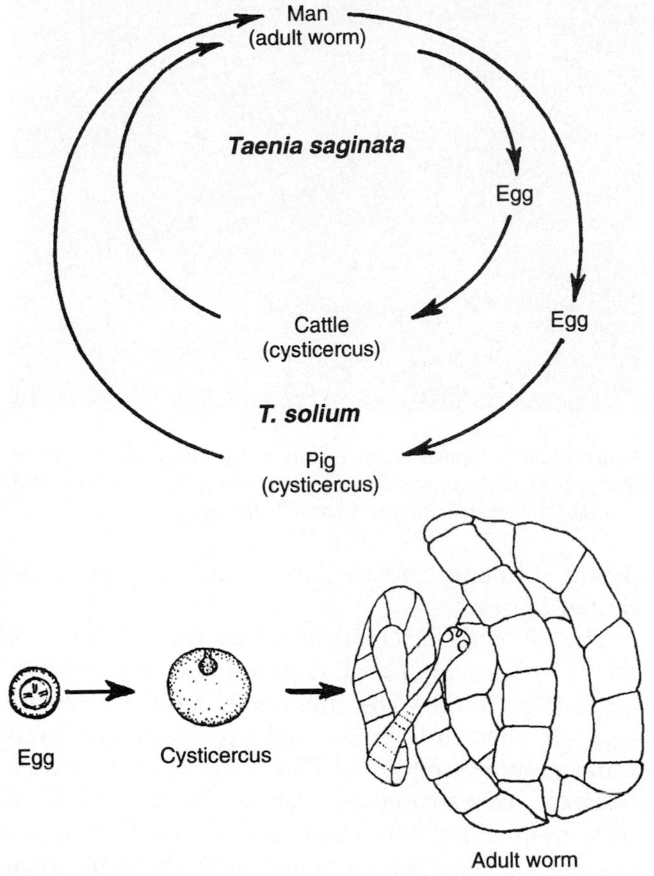

Figure 55.55. Life cycles of *Taenia saginata* and *Taenia solium*. (From Markell EK, Voge M, John DT. Medical parasitology. 7th ed. Philadelphia: WB Saunders, 1992.)

ate hosts when they ingest food contaminated with viable eggs. Autoinfection may occur when eggs are transferred from the perianal area to the mouth on contaminated fingers. Once ingested, the eggs hatch in the stomach of the intermediate host, releasing the hexacanth embryo or onchosphere. The onchosphere penetrates the intestinal wall and migrates in the circulation to the tissues, where it develops into a cysticercus over 3 to 4 months. The cysticerci may develop in muscle, connective tissue, brain, lung, and eyes and remain viable for up to 5 years. Humans may become the definitive host for this parasite when they ingest inadequately cooked pork containing cysticerci. Digestion of the infected meat releases the cysticercus, which then everts, exposing the scolex, attaches to the intestinal mucosa, and develops into an adult worm, thereby completing the cycle.

The symptoms produced by the presence of the adult *T. solium* in the intestine is minimal. Most patients are asymptomatic and become aware of the infection only when they see proglottids in their feces. Occasionally individuals report abdominal discomfort, nausea, diarrhea, and weight loss.

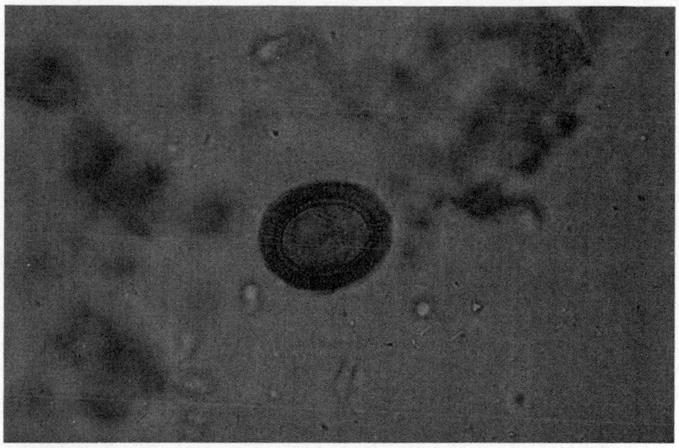

Figure 55.56. *Taenia* species, egg (high power). (From Smith JW, et al. Diagnostic medical parasitology: intestinal helminths. Chicago: American Society of Clinical Pathologists, 1976.)

An entirely different clinical picture may present when humans serve as the intermediate host. Cysticercosis may be of little consequence if the larvae lodge in the muscles or subcutaneous tissues; however, serious disease may follow as cysticerci develop in vital areas such as the brain or eyes (49). In the brain they may produce seizures, meningoencephalitis, hydrocephalus, and cranial nerve damage. In the eye, loss of visual acuity and visual field defects may occur. Tissue reaction to viable larvae may be only moderate, thus minimizing symptoms; however, the death of the larvae stimulates a marked inflammatory reaction with exacerbation of symptoms and resulting fever, muscle pains, and eosinophilia.

The laboratory diagnosis of intestinal infection is made by finding eggs or proglottids in the stool. As the eggs of *T. solium* and *T. saginata* are identical (Fig. 55.56), it is necessary to examine a proglottid to identify the species correctly (Fig. 55.53). The diagnosis of cysticercosis is usually established by detection and surgical removal of soft-tissue nodules, the appearance of calcified cysticerci in soft-tissue roentgenograms, and detection of cysts in the eye. Central nervous system lesions may be detected by computed tomography, radioisotope scanning, or ultrasonography. Serologic studies may be useful, but false positives may occur in individuals with other helminthic infections.

The treatment of choice for intestinal infection is niclosamide, which acts directly on the worm. Praziquantel, paromomycin, and quinacrine are effective alternatives. The drug of choice for cysticercosis is praziquantel (50). Concomitant steroid administration may be useful in minimizing the inflammatory response to the dying larvae. Surgical removal of cerebral and ocular cysts may be necessary. Preventive measures include proper sanitation, adequate cooking of all pork products, and prompt treatment of all human cases of *T. solium* infection to minimize egg transmission.

Taenia saginata

Taenia saginata, the beef tapeworm, closely resembles *T. solium* and may parasitize the jejunum and small intestine of humans for up to 25 years, attaining a length of 10 meters. *T. saginata* bears a scolex armed with four muscular suckers but no hooklets, and its proglottids contain 15 to 30 uterine branches. *T. saginata* is rare in the United States but is highly prevalent in Africa, the Middle East, eastern Europe, and South America.

The life cycle of *T. saginata* is virtually identical to that described for *T. solium* (Fig. 55.55). A major difference is that humans rarely, if ever, act as intermediate hosts for *T. saginata*. As with *T. solium*, humans are infected when they ingest inadequately cooked meat containing cysticerci.

The clinical syndrome associated with *T. saginata* is similar to intestinal infection with *T. solium*. Patients are generally asymptomatic or may complain of vague abdominal pains, chronic epigastric discomfort, and weakness.

As with *T. solium*, the diagnosis is made by detection of eggs and proglottids in feces. Motile proglottids may be observed in freshly passed stool. Differentiation of *T. saginata* from *T. solium* is made by examination of mature proglottids or recovery of the entire worm with a scolex lacking hooklets.

Treatment is identical to that described for the intestinal phase of *T. solium*. A single dose of niclosamide is highly effective in elimination of the adult worm. Prevention is dependent on proper sanitation and adequate cooking of beef.

Diphyllobothrium latum

Diphyllobothrium latum, the fish tapeworm, inhabits the human jejunum and ileum, where it may survive for many years and grow to a maximum length of 4 to 20 meters. Its elongated, fusiform scolex is armed with two lateral sucking grooves or bothria (Fig. 55.53). Unlike the *Taenia* species, the proglottids are uniformly wider than they are long and contain a centrally positioned, rosette-shaped uterus. The large (58 to 75 by 40 to 50 μm), ovoid, operculated eggs (Figs. 55.53 and 55.57) are discharged through the uterine pore of the proglottid. Over 1 million eggs are released per day into the fecal stream. *D. latum* is found worldwide, most prevalently wherever raw, picked, or undercooked freshwater fish (including salmon) is eaten by humans. Human infections are found in central and northern Europe, Scandinavia, Siberia, China, and Japan. In North America, endemic foci have been described in Alaska, Canada, and the Great Lakes region of the United States.

Figure 55.57. *Diphyllobothrium latum*, egg (low power). (From Smith JW, et al. Diagnostic medical parasitology: intestinal helminths. Chicago: American Society of Clinical Pathologists, 1976.)

The life cycle of *D. latum* differs from that of the *Taenia* species in that it requires two intermediate hosts (Fig. 55.58). The unembryonated, operculate eggs are shed in the feces and upon reaching fresh water require a period of 2 to 4 weeks to develop a ciliated, free-swimming larval form called a coracidium. The fully developed coracidium leaves the egg via the operculum and is ingested by small freshwater crustaceans (e.g., *Cyclops* and *Diaptomus*), where it develops into a procercoid larval form. The crustacean is then eaten by a fish and the infectious plerocercoid larvae develop in the musculature of the fish. Humans are infected when they eat raw or undercooked fish containing the plerocercoid larval forms.

Clinically, as is the case with most tapeworm infections, most *D. latum* infections are asymptomatic. Occasionally individuals complain of epigastric pain, abdominal cramping, nausea, vomiting, and weight loss. As many as 40% of *D. latum* carriers may have low serum levels of vitamin B_{12}, presumably as a result of the competition between the host and the worm for dietary vitamin B_{12}. A small percentage (0.1 to 2%) of individuals infected with *D. latum* develop clinical signs of vitamin B_{12} deficiency, including megaloblastic anemia and neurologic manifestations such as numbness, paresthesia, and loss of vibration sense.

The diagnosis of *D. latum* infection is made by detection of the bile-stained operculated egg (Fig. 55.57) or typical proglottids in stool. Concentration techniques are usually not necessary, as the worms produce large numbers of ova.

Treatment is similar to that described for *T. saginata* infections: single-dose therapy with niclosamide is highly effective. Vitamin B_{12} supplementation may

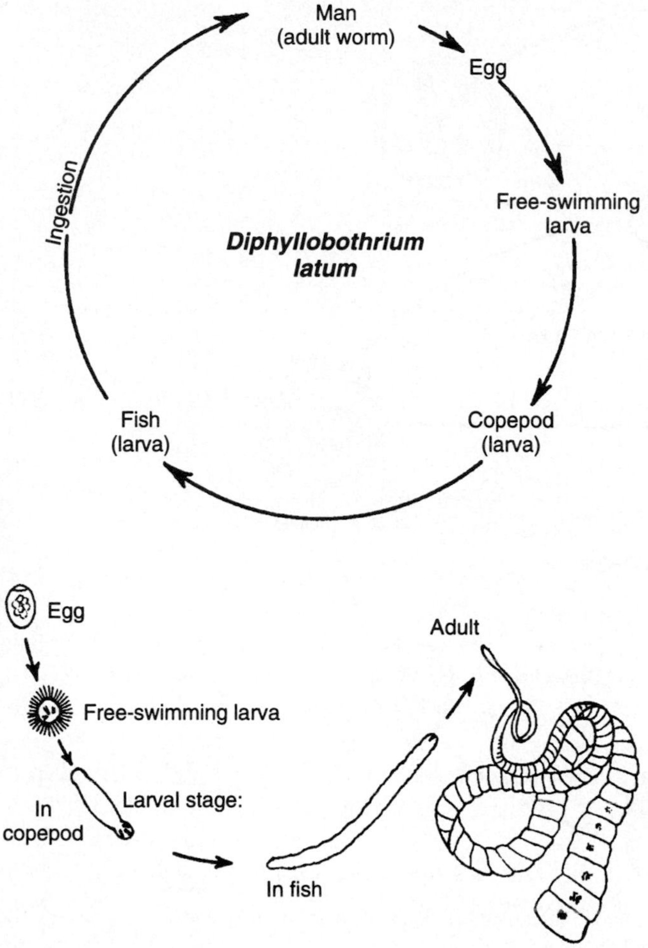

Figure 55.58. Life cycle of *Diphyllobothrium latum*. (From Markell EK, Voge M, John DT. Medical parasitology. 7th ed. Philadelphia: WB Saunders, 1992.)

be necessary in individuals with evidence of clinical vitamin B_{12} deficiency (e.g., anemia and neurologic symptoms). Thorough cooking of all salmon and freshwater fish and attention to proper sanitation are necessary preventive measures.

Echinococcus granulosus

Echinococcosis or hydatid disease is a tissue infection of humans caused by the larvae of the cestode *Echinococcus granulosus*. The adult *E. granulosus* is a small (5 mm) intestinal parasite of canines (dog, fox, wolf, coyote, etc). The worm consists of a *Taenia*-like scolex with four sucking disks and a double row of hooklets, and a strobila containing three proglottids: one immature, one mature, and one gravid. The eggs, which are identical in appearance to those of *Taenia* species (Fig. 55.56), are released from the terminal gravid proglottid and are shed in the feces, where they may be ingested by one of a number of mammalian intermediate hosts, including sheep, goats, deer, moose, and humans (Fig. 55.59). The ingested eggs hatch and the embryos penetrate the intestinal mucosa and are carried by the circulation to lodge in the liver, lungs, brain, heart, bone, and other tissues. Within the tissues the larvae form hydatid cysts characterized by a laminated germinative membrane from which daughter cysts or brood capsules arise, each containing multiple inverted protoscolices (Fig. 55.54). The cysts expand slowly, accumulating fluid and hydatid sand composed of scoleces, hooks, and calcareous corpuscles from disintegrating brood capsules. Cysts generally reach a diameter of 1 cm over 6 months and ultimately may attain a size of 5 to 20 cm over a period of several years. Spillage of cyst contents may lead to the development of cysts in other sites, as the protoscolices have the germinative potential to form new cysts. When hydatid-containing tissues of the intermediate host are ingested by a canine, thousands of scolices are released in the intestine to develop into adult worms. Humans and herbivores do not become infected with the adult worm.

Human infection with *E. granulosus* is most commonly seen in countries where domestic herbivores such as sheep, cattle, and goats are raised in close contact with dogs (51). The highest incidence of hydatid disease is seen in Australia, New Zealand, South America, South and East Africa, Central Europe, and the Middle East. It also occurs in Alaska, Canada, and in the sheep farming regions of the United States (Utah, New Mexico, Arizona, California). Humans become infected following ingestion of contaminated food and water, as well as from hand-to-mouth transmission of eggs as a result of handling dogs infected with the adult worm.

Human infection is typically asymptomatic for as long as 5 to 20 years following acquisition of the infection. The clinical manifestations of hydatid disease are due to the space-occupying nature of the slowly expanding cyst and thus are directly related to the number, anatomic location, and rate of growth of the cysts. In the majority of cases the cysts are located in the lung or the liver and present with cough, hemoptysis, chest pain, or abdominal pain and tenderness. Rupture of the cysts may occur in 20% of cases, producing fever, urticaria, and occasionally anaphylactic shock and death due to the release of antigenic cyst contents. Cyst rupture may also lead to dissemination of infection due to the release of thousands of protoscolices. Cysts present in bone may result in pathologic fractures, whereas those in the brain present as tumorlike space-occupying lesions with seizures, visual disturbances, and hydrocephalus. Over time the cyst may die and become calcified.

Diagnosis of hydatid disease is difficult and depends primarily on clinical, radiographic, and serologic findings. Cysts may be observed on routine roentgenograms or by computed tomographic or ul-

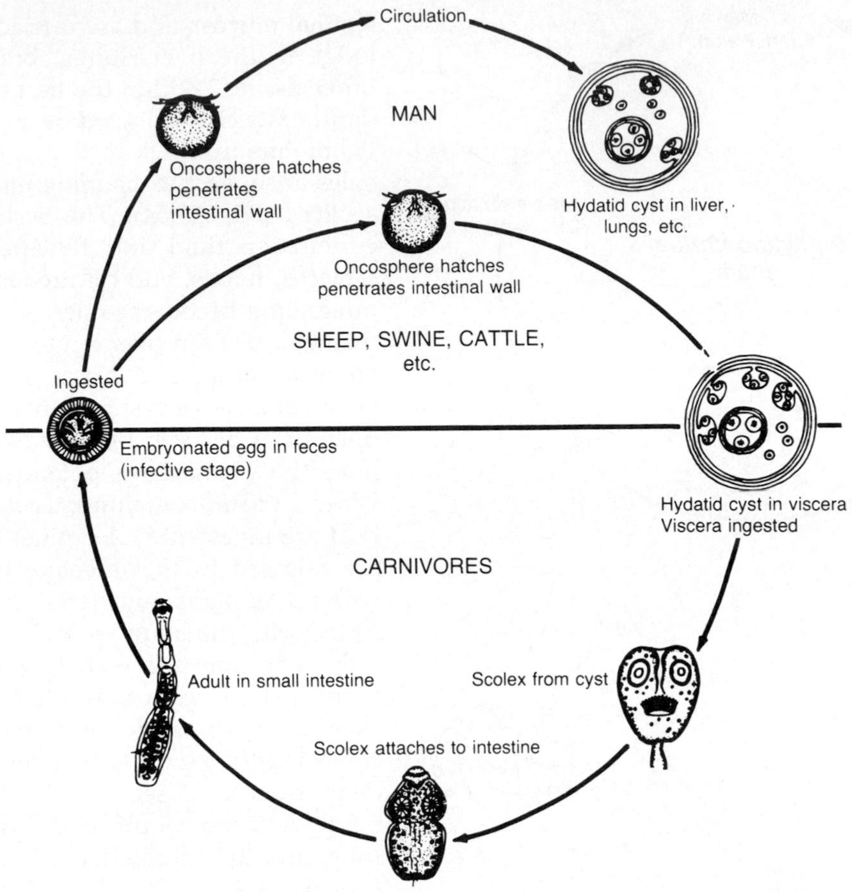

Figure 55.59. Life cycle of *Echinococcus granulosus*. (From Strickland GT. Hunter's tropical medicine. 7th ed. Philadelphia: WB Saunders, 1991.)

trasonic scanning procedures. Although aspiration of cyst contents and demonstration of hydatid sand (scolices, hooks, etc.) may be diagnostic, it is contraindicated due to the risk of anaphylaxis and dissemination of infection. Serologic testing may be useful but is negative in 10 to 40% of infections (52).

Surgical excision of hydatid cysts is the therapy of choice for symptomatic patients. Aspiration of cyst contents and instillation of formalin, hypertonic saline, silver nitrate, or cetrimide to kill the protoscolices and detoxify the remaining fluid may be indicated. If surgery is contraindicated, medical therapy with high-dose albendazole or praziquantel may be considered. Preventive measures include attention to personal hygiene and handwashing and deworming of infected dogs. Dogs should never be allowed to feed on the viscera of slain animals.

References

1. Markell EK, Voge M, John DT, eds. Medical parasitology. 7th ed. Philadelphia: WB Saunders, 1992.
2. Sherris JC, ed. Medical microbiology: an introduction to infectious diseases. 2nd ed. New York: Elsevier, 1990.
3. Strickland GT, ed. Hunter's tropical medicine. 7th ed. Philadelphia: WB Saunders, 1991.
4. Edman JC, Kovacs JA, Masur H, et al. Ribosomal RNA sequence shows *Pneumocystis carinii* to be a member of the fungi. Nature 1988;334:19–22.
5. Northfelt D, Clement MJ, Safrin S. Extrapulmonary pneumocystosis: clinical features in human immunodeficiency virus infection. Medicine 1990;69:392–398.
6. Raviglione MC. Extrapulmonary pneumocystosis: the first 50 cases. Rev Infect Dis 1990;12:1127–1138.
7. Telzak EE, Cote RJ, Gold JWM, et al. Extrapulmonary *Pneumocystis carinii* infections. Rev Infect Dis 1990;12:380–386.
8. Strickland GT. Malaria. In: Strickland GT, ed. Hunter's tropical medicine. 7th ed. Philadelphia: WB Saunders, 1991:586–602.
9. Maddison SE. Serodiagnosis of parasitic diseases. Clin Microbiol Rev 1991;4:457–469.
10. Rieckmann KH et al. *Plasmodium vivax* resistance to chloroquine? Lancet 1989;2:1183–1184.
11. Gombert ME et al. Human babesiosis: clinical and therapeutic considerations. JAMA 1982;248:3005–3007.
12. Marsden PD. Selective primary health care: strategies for control of disease in the developing world. XIV. Leishmaniasis. Rev Infect Dis 1984;6:736–744.
13. Anonymous. Problems with leishmaniasis. Br Med J 1978;2:1179–1180.
14. Berman JD. Chemotherapy for leishmaniasis: biochemical mechanisms, clinical efficacy, and future strategies. Rev Infect Dis 1988;10:560–586.
15. Molyneux DH. Selective primary health care: strategies for control of disease in the developing world. VII. African trypanosomiasis. Rev Infect Dis 1983;5:945–956.

16. Van Meirvenne N, LeRay D. Diagnosis of African and American trypanosomiasis. Br Med Bull 1985;41:156–161.
17. McCabe RE et al. Ketoconazole protects against infection with *Trypanosoma cruzi* in a murine model. Am J Trop Med Hyg 1983;32:960–962.
18. Krick JA, Remington JS. Current concepts in parasitology. Toxoplasmosis in adults—an overview. N Engl J Med 1978;298:550–558.
19. Desmonts G, Couvreur J. Congenital toxoplasmosis: a prospective study of 378 pregnancies. N Engl J Med 1974;290: 1110–1116.
20. Luft BJ, Remington JS. Toxoplasmic encephalitis. J Infect Dis 1988;157:1–6.
21. Oksenhendler E, Cadranel J, Sarfati C, et al. *Toxoplasma gondii* pneumonia in patients with the acquired immunodeficiency syndrome. Am J Med 1990;88(Suppl 5):18N–21N.
22. Crider SR, Horstman WG, Massey GS. *Toxoplasma* orchitis: report of a case and a review of the literature. Am J Med 1988;85: 421–424.
23. Pedrol E, Gonzalez-Clemente JM, Gatell JM, et al. Central nervous system toxoplasmosis in AIDS patients: efficacy of an intermittent maintenance therapy. AIDS 1990;4:511–517.
24. Cregan P, Yamamoto A, Lum A, et al. Comparison of four methods for rapid detection of *Pneumocystis carinii* in respiratory specimens. J Clin Microbiol 1990;28:2432–2436.
25. May LP, Sidhu GS, Buchness MR. Diagnosis of *Acanthamoeba* infection by cutaneous manifestations in a man seropositive to HIV. J Am Acad Dermatol 1992;26:352–355.
26. Kappus KK, Juranek DD, Roberts JM. Results of testing for intestinal parasites by state diagnostic laboratories, United States, 1987. Morbid Mortal Reports 1991;40:25–45.
27. Wolfe MS. Giardiasis. Clin Microbiol Rev 1992;5:93–100.
28. Yang J, Scholten TH. *Dientamoeba fragilis*: a review with notes on its epidemiology, pathogenicity, mode of transmission, and diagnosis. Am J Trop Med Hyg 1977;26:16–22.
29. Current WL, Garcia LS. Cryptosporidiosis. Clin Microbiol Rev 1991;4:325–358.
30. Zierdt CH. *Blastocystis hominis*—past and future. Clin Microbiol Rev 1991;4:61–79.
31. Canning EU, Hollister WS. *Enterocytozoon bieneusi* (*Microspora*): prevalence and pathogenicity in AIDS patients. Trans R Soc Trop Med Hyg 1990;84:181–186.
32. Orenstein JM, Chiang J, Steinberg W, Smith PD, Rotterdam H, Kotler DP. Intestinal microsporidiosis as a cause of diarrhea in human immunodeficiency virus-infected patients: a report of 20 cases. Hum Pathol 1990;21:475–481.
33. Shadduck JA, Greeley E. Microsporidia and human infections. Clin Microbiol Rev 1989;2:158–165.
34. Weber R et al. Improved light-microscopical detection of microsporidia spores in stool and duodenal aspirates. N Engl J Med 1992;326:161–166.
35. Irga-Siegman Y, Kapila R, Sen P, et al. Syndrome of hyperinfection with *Strongyloides stercoralis*. Rev Infect Dis 1981;3: 397–407.
36. Plorde JJ. Tissue nematodes. In: Sherris JC, ed. Medical microbiology: an introduction to infectious diseases. 2nd ed. New York: Elsevier, 1990:765–775.
37. Waldrop MM. Testing for trichinosis. Science 1985;227:621–624.
38. MacKenzie CD, Williams JF, Sisley BM, et al. Variations in host responses and the pathogenesis of human onchocerciasis. Rev Infect Dis 1985;7:802–808.
39. Pacque M, Munoz B, Greene BM, et al. Community-based treatment of onchocerciasis with ivermectin: safety, efficacy, and acceptability of yearly treatment. J Infect Dis 1991;163:381–385.
40. Nanduri J, Kuzura JW. Clinical and laboratory aspects of filariasis. Clin Microbiol Rev 1989;2:39–50.
41. Ro JY, Tsakalakis PJ, White VA, et al. Pulmonary dirofilariasis: the great imitator of primary or metastatic lung tumor. Hum Pathol 1989;20:69–76.
42. Fleisher AG, Messina JJ, Ryan SF, Hopkins KS. Human pulmonary dirofilariasis: does diagnosis require thoracotomy? Ann Thorac Surg 1988;45:447–448.
43. Glickman LT, Grieve RB, Schantz PM. Serologic diagnosis of zoonotic pulmonary dirofilariasis. Am J Med 1986;80:161–164.
44. Rim HJ. The current pathology and chemotherapy of clonorchiasis. Korean J Parsitol 1986;24(Suppl 3):1–141.
45. Johnson RJ, Jong EC, Dunning SB, Carberry WL, et al. Paragonimiasis, diagnosis and the use of praziquantel in treatment. Rev Infect Dis 1985;7:200–206.
46. Nash TE, Cheever AW, Ottesen EA, Cook JA. Schistosoma infection in humans: perspectives and recent findings. Ann Intern Med 1982;97:740–754.
47. Strickland GT. Schistosomiasis: eradication or control? Rev Infect Dis 1982;4:951–954.
48. Warren KS. Selective primary health care: strategies for control of disease in the developing world. I. Schistosomiasis. Rev Infect Dis 1982;4:715–726.
49. Grisolia JS. Cysticercosis update. West J Med 1984;140:901–904.
50. Moodley M, Moosa A. Treatment of neurocysticercosis: is praziquantel the new hope? Lancet 1989;1:262–263.
51. McManus DP, Smyth JD. Hydatidosis: changing concepts in epidemiology and speciation. Parasitol Today 1986;2:163–168.
52. Craig PS, Zeyhle E, Romig T. Hydatid disease: research and control in Turkana. II. The role of immunological techniques for the diagnosis of hydatid disease. Trans R Soc Trop Med Hyg 1986;80:183–192.

Section X

Section Chief: *David F. Keren*

The field of diagnostic immunology has become considerably broader in the past decade. The advent of flow cytometry, monoclonal reagents, and chemiluminescent probes, and the development of a clearer understanding of the immunopathology of autoimmune diseases have resulted in a tremendous increase in the number and types of diagnostic tests that are available. This section deals with the exploitation of immunologic techniques for clinical diagnosis.

Each chapter reviews features of diseases relevant to diagnostic immunology and discusses the techniques involved in the pathologic diagnosis. There is necessarily a modest degree of redundancy between some chapters within this section and those within other sections. For instance, some of the serology discussed here may also be relevant in the infectious disease sections. Some of the ligand assays discussed by Dr. England and Dr. Smart are complementary to information on radioimmunoassay in the chemistry section. Nonetheless, each chapter stands on its own with regard to the utility of the procedures discussed for making clinical diagnoses.

An attempt has been made to coordinate the chapters in this section to cover the field of diagnostic immunology as it relates to the diagnostic world today. Only minimal attention has been paid to the more historic aspects of the field. This is for the sake of readability and relevance to today's diagnostic procedures, and is not meant to suggest that earlier techniques were not useful.

In each chapter, authors express their own opinions about the particular procedures being discussed. This gives the reader important viewpoints from experts in the field.

MMUNOPATHOLOGY

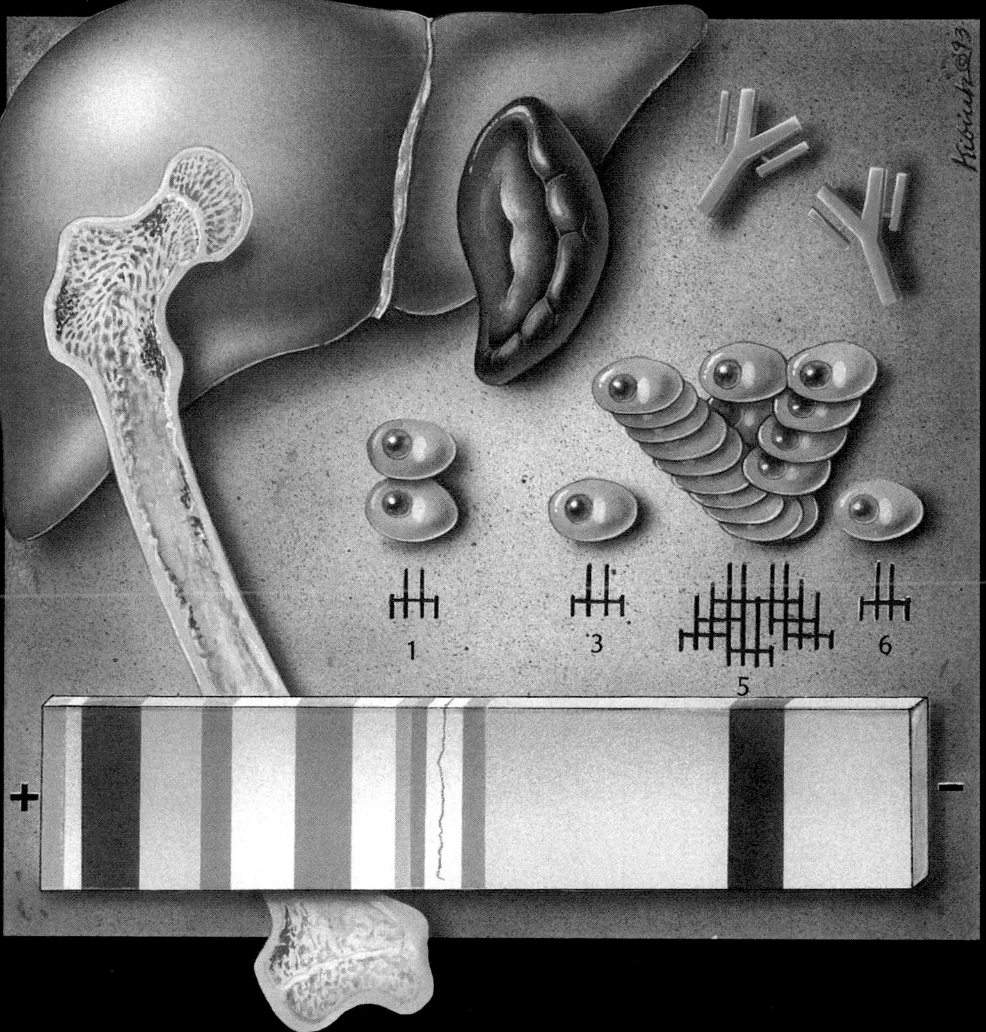

56 Basic Principles of Immunodiagnosis

Roger S. Riley

The immune system is part of the body's defense against environmental agents (viruses, bacteria, fungi, etc.) and against our own cells that turn cancerous or learn to react against us. During the process of evolution, the immune system has acquired an impressive array of capabilities that are essential for its normal function. More than one trillion cells of various types constitute the immune system. Many of these cells are capable of differentiating "self" from "non-self," rapidly destroying or disabling an invading organism, and "remembering" the encounter, so that an infectious organism is prevented from ever causing harm again. During the defense process, immune cells are constant and effective communicators through direct cell-to-cell contact, or through the production of a wide variety of chemical intermediaries.

Scientists have applied an increasingly sophisticated array of tools and techniques to the investigation of the immune system. As a result, cells and cell products (antibodies, biological modifiers) with specific reactivity can be produced through laboratory manipulation of the immune response. These developments have greatly increased our understanding of the immune system and offer the promise of a natural, effective therapy for many immune and nonimmune diseases. In addition, immunologic products have been applied to medical diagnosis in a variety of imaginative ways, and have became fundamental reagents in the clinical laboratory.

The term "immunoassay" refers to a biological test system that utilizes one or more immunologic products or reagents. The basis for most immunoassays is the binding of an immunoglobulin molecule (antibody) to an antigen. However, other immunologic reagents, such as complement, are used in some immunoassays, and cell-to-cell interactions are the basis for others. In an immunoassay, the antigen may be another immunoglobulin molecule, a component of the cell membrane, or any other substance against which a specific antibody can be generated. The great specificity of the antigen-antibody reaction, and the development of techniques allowing the large-scale production of antibodies have contributed to the clinical popularity of the immunoassay. To be useful in diagnosis, the product of an antigen-antibody interaction (immune complex) must be visualized and quantitatively measured by some means. Direct visualization with the naked eye is possible if the antigen is attached to cells or particles that clump together, or "agglutinate" upon interaction with the antibody. Although this simple interaction was the basis for early immunoassays, and is still being used today, precise measurement of the antigen-antibody interaction requires that one or the other be labeled or "tagged" by some means.

BASIC IMMUNOLOGY

The Immune Response

Animals respond to foreign substances (e.g., viruses or bacteria) by producing protein molecules in the blood, called antibodies. Antibodies bind to the foreign substance as a part of the body's efforts to counteract it. Antibodies have the property of being highly specific, that is, they will bind only to the foreign substance that caused them to be produced. Thus, any substance recognized by an animal as "foreign" and causing that animal to make antibodies is designated by the general term antigen.

The biological phenomenon of antibody production has been used in laboratory tests to identify substances found in human tissue. Since antibodies are highly specific for the antigen that caused them to be formed, they can be used to chemically locate that antigen in tissue. This is generally accomplished by the following method:

1. A sample of the human substance (e.g., protein, enzyme, hormone) is injected into an animal (e.g., a rabbit). Since the substance is of human origin, the animal recognizes it as "foreign" and makes antibodies against it. The human substance is the antigen causing the animal to produce antibodies. This process is known as immunization.
2. A blood sample is then withdrawn from the animal, and the "antihuman" antibodies are isolated and retrieved from the serum. These antibodies are highly specific for the human sub-

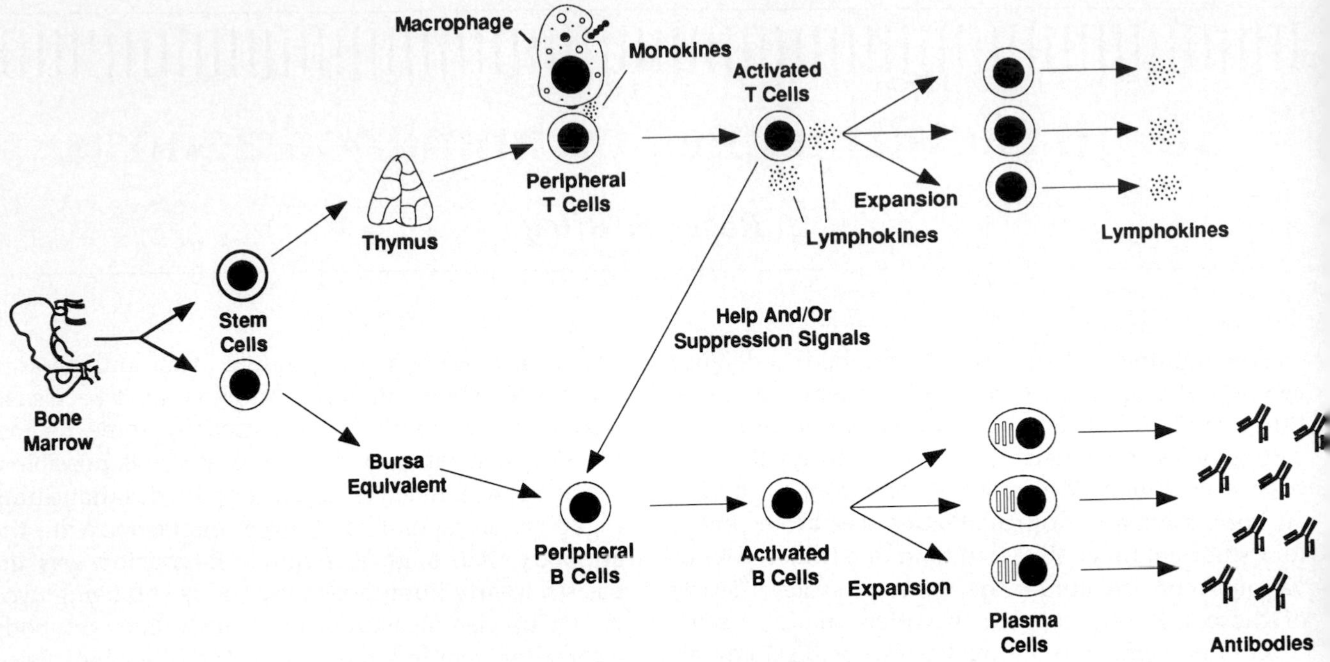

Figure 56.1. A schematic representation of the immune response.

stance (antigen) that caused them to be formed and will not chemically bind with any other antigen in the tissue.

3. In a laboratory situation, the antibodies can be applied to patient cell or tissue preparations. The antibody molecules will react with the type of human antigen that caused them to be made if it is present in the tissue. If the antigen is not present, no specific reaction will occur.

A new (de novo) immune response begins with phagocytosis of the foreign invader, digestion and "processing" of the material, and "presentation" of some of the processed antigen on the cell surface (1). In conjunction with the self-HLA markers on the phagocyte and chemical mediators released from the phagocyte ("monokines"), the processed antigen is recognized by one kind of T lymphocyte (T-helper cell). These "activated" T-helper lymphocytes secrete a number of soluble substances (lymphokines, immune system hormones), which stimulate other immune cells, including "suppressor T lymphocytes," which have a negative regulatory effect on the immune system. Another type of lymphocyte (B lymphocyte) produces soluble proteins, termed antibodies (immunoglobulins). Each B cell is programmed to produce an antibody molecule which is highly specific for a single antigenic substance. Once activated by lymphokines or by encounter with its antigen, a B cell rapidly reproduces. Each of these identical B cells differentiates into an antibody-producing factory (plasma cell) that can release thousands of antibody molecules a second (Fig. 56.1).

Most T and B lymphocytes involved in an immune response die within several days. However, after each encounter, clones of "memory" cells persist in the body for life. If the offending antigen is ever encountered again, these cells are primed to quickly go into action without the delay faced during the first encounter.

A group of peptides termed cytokines are extremely important for immunoregulation and intracellular communication within the immune and inflammatory systems. These substances include the interleukins (IL), interferons (IFN), tumor necrosis factors (TNFs), and hemopoietic growth factors (colony stimulating factors, CSF) (2, 3). Most of these substances were initially identified on the basis of a single biological effect, but many have been subsequently found to have diverse local, and even systemic effects. At the cellular level, cytokines interact through high-affinity surface receptors. The intracellular mechanism of action of many cytokines is presently unknown, although several cytokine receptors initiate the activation of phosphoinositase C, adenylate cyclase, protein kinase C, tyrosine kinase, or other enzymes. Because of the availability of immunoassays for the accurate measurement of cytokines in normal and diseased individuals, and the discovery of recombinant DNA techniques to produce these substances in virtually unlimited quantity, there is great interest in their potential diagnostic and therapeutic applications.

Polyclonal Antibodies

The natural immune response to an antigen is the generation of antibodies. Multiple clones of plasma cells respond to an antigenic challenge, and each produces antibodies that differ in antibody class, light-chain isotypes, idiotypic specificity, and combining ability (avidity). The number of antibody specificities generated depends upon the complexity of the antigen. While synthetic materials with repetitive epitopes may produce antibodies of a single specificity, hundreds to thousands of different antibodies are usually released in response to a large protein or cellular structure with multiple epitopes. Commercially, these "polyclonal antibodies" are usually obtained from animal sources. However, some antibodies, such as those with specificity for the HLA antigens, are commonly obtained from the serum of multiparous females or patients who have received multiple transfusions.

The commercial production of polyclonal antibodies from animals comprises a large industry that is closely protected by trade secrets. As a result, few details have been published in the literature (4). One exception is a review by Ritchie (5), who has published his experience gained from more than 10,000 animal bleedings.

The major considerations in the production of antibodies to an antigen (immunogen) include:

- Size and chemical composition of the immunogen;
- Animal species used as the host;
- Age and general health of the animal host;
- Route of immunization;
- Dose of immunogen; and
- Immunization schedule.

A wide variety of animal species have been utilized for the preparation of polyclonal antibodies. The choice of animal depends on many factors, including the size of the animal, the cost and ease of maintenance, the phylogenetic similarity of the animal to the species from which the immunogen is recovered, and the absence of native materials antigenically similar to the immunogen (5). Goats are the best host for the production of large volumes of polyclonal antibodies because of the hardiness of the goat and the ease and relatively low cost of maintaining goat herds for long periods of time (5). Rabbits are an excellent source of quality antibodies, but their smaller size and higher maintenance cost are problematic. Guinea pigs have been used for the production of anti-insulin antibodies because their native insulin is significantly different from human insulin, while fowl, fish, and reptiles produce antibodies that do not fix complement (5). The immunogen dosage and schedule of administration are important considerations in determining the quality and potency of antibody produced (5). The immunogen is commonly injected at 1- to 2-week intervals for periods of several weeks, followed by a challenge dose after a month's rest; however, each investigator uses a different schedule. If a good response is obtained, antibody titers may continue to rise with additional immunizing doses for 6 months or more. The animal is bled on a regular schedule until the antibody titer begins to drop, at which time reimmunization is attempted. Some immunogens are given with an adjuvant (Freund's adjuvant, mineral oil), which enhance antibody production by producing an inflammatory response at the site of injection. The dose of the immunogen is the most difficult factor to control, since a subliminal dose may cause tolerance, while an excessive dose can produce immune paralysis (5). Administration of the immunogen over a wide range (5-log or greater) may be required to produce immunization.

After immunization has taken place, the antibody concentration, reactivity, and other properties are measured (6). Undiluted serum can generally be stored at −20°C to −70°C for several years without loss of potency. However, in many cases, the immunoglobulin fraction of the serum is isolated and further purified. Purified antibody preparations can also be lyophilized and stored for years at room temperature. Immunoglobulin of the IgG class is usually preferred over IgM for immunoassays, since it is more stable, easier to purify, and is produced in the highest concentration (5).

The major disadvantage of polyclonal antibodies for diagnostic testing is lot-to-lot variation in specificity and avidity, so that quality control becomes difficult. In addition, the antigen must exist in a highly purified state to generate a polyclonal antibody preparation that does not cross-react with other substances. Also, many antigens are poorly immunogenic or nonimmunogenic. Nevertheless, until recently, polyclonal antibody preparations were the only ones available, and they have been applied very successfully for diagnostic purposes, especially in radioimmunoassay techniques and immunoperoxidase staining.

Monoclonal Antibodies

A clone of plasma cells derived from a single B lymphocyte produces immunoglobulin molecules that are specific for a certain antigen (monoclonal antibodies). Plasma cells represent the end stage of the B-cell maturation process and cannot be stimulated to divide further. Therefore, until the mid-1970s, the only source of monoclonal antibodies in large quantity was body fluids and effusions from patients with malignant plasma cell tumors. Monoclonal antibodies from this natural source were essential for the elucidation of antibody structure and function, but were of no value for other research or clinical applications. However, in 1975 Kohler and Milstein devised a practical method of immune manipulation that allowed the production of unlimited quantities of monoclonal antibodies specific for any immunogenic substance (7). This discovery was one of the most important in the history of science since it has lead to innumerable discoveries in the immunologic sciences, to numerous improvements in medical diagnosis, and to a large industry devoted to the commercial production of monoclonal antibodies (7–14).

PRODUCTION OF MONOCLONAL ANTIBODIES

Kohler and Milstein devised a technique to "fuse" nonimmortalized antibody-producing plasma cells from an immunized animal with immortalized myeloma tumor cells that produced either no antibody or antibody with an irrelevant specificity. The resulting "hybridoma" rapidly reproduced in culture while retaining the ability to synthesize immunoglobulin with the specificity of the original plasma cell. The hydridoma cells could be grown in culture or in the peritoneal cavity of an animal to obtain large quantities of monoclonal antibody.

Hybridoma production begins with the immunization of a mouse with a specific antigen (11, 13, 15–19). Plasma cells from the spleen of the mouse are then isolated and brought into contact with cells from a non–antibody-producing mutant murine malignant myeloma cell line that is deficient in the enzyme hypoxanthine guanine phosphoribosyl transferase (HPRT). Cellular interaction takes place in the presence of polyethylene glycol or another fusing (surface active) agent such as the Sendai virus. Under these conditions, fusion of the cell membranes of some of the cells occurs, and later the nuclear membranes fuse together as well. Many hybrid cells lose chromosomes in the process of fusion, but some retain most of the genetic information from both parents. The next step is to separate proliferating cells that produce antibody of the desired specificity from non–antibody-producing cells, hybridomas producing antibody of undesired specificity, and from parental myeloma and plasma cells. A special culture medium containing hypoxanthine, aminopterin, and thymidine (HAT medium) is used to separate hybridomas from the cell mixture. The plasma cells cannot divide, and the HAT medium prevents growth of the mutant myeloma cells, since they are deficient in HPRT and cannot use the hypoxanthine and thymidine in the culture media. Therefore, only the hybridoma cells survive and grow in the culture. Each hybrid, antibody-producing cell is isolated and cultured, and the antibody produced is studied for its specificity. If a desired antibody is found, large quantities can be produced by growth of the hybrid cells in conventional tissue culture systems, in the peritoneal cavities of immunodeficient mice or nude rats, or in recently developed hollow fiber culture systems. The hybridoma cells continuously produce monoclonal antibody as long as they retain the necessary genes (Fig. 56.2).

CLINICAL APPLICATIONS OF MONOCLONAL ANTIBODIES

Monoclonal antibodies are highly specific for a desired antigen and can be produced in almost unlimited quantities. In addition, monoclonal antibodies can be generated from relatively impure antigen preparation and show consistent sensitivity and specificity from lot to lot. For in vivo applications, the relatively small amounts of monoclonal antibodies that are utilized do not often lead to the development of heterophile (interspecies specific) antibodies in the host. However, the production of a monoclonal antibody with the desired specificity does not always lead to a useful product, since the avidity (combining ability) of the antibody may be low, or the antigen may be sparse on some cells and difficult to detect. For these and other reasons, polyclonal antibodies are still preferred over monoclonal antibodies for some applications.

Monoclonal antibodies have become essential reagents for a wide variety of in vivo and in vitro diagnostic and therapeutic purposes (20–30). These applications can be classified as follows:

- In vitro diagnosis
  - Monoclonal antibodies specific for leukocyte antigens
  - Monoclonal antibodies specific for non-leukocyte antigens
- In vivo imaging
- Immunotherapy
  - Organ transplantation
  - Malignant neoplasms

Monoclonal Antibodies Specific for Leukocyte Antigens

Monoclonal antibodies specific for lymphoid antigens have been the most widely utilized of all monoclonal antibodies. Since the differentiation of T and B lymphocytes by rosetting and other techniques was tedious, time-consuming, and inaccurate, the development of a series of monoclonal antibodies specific

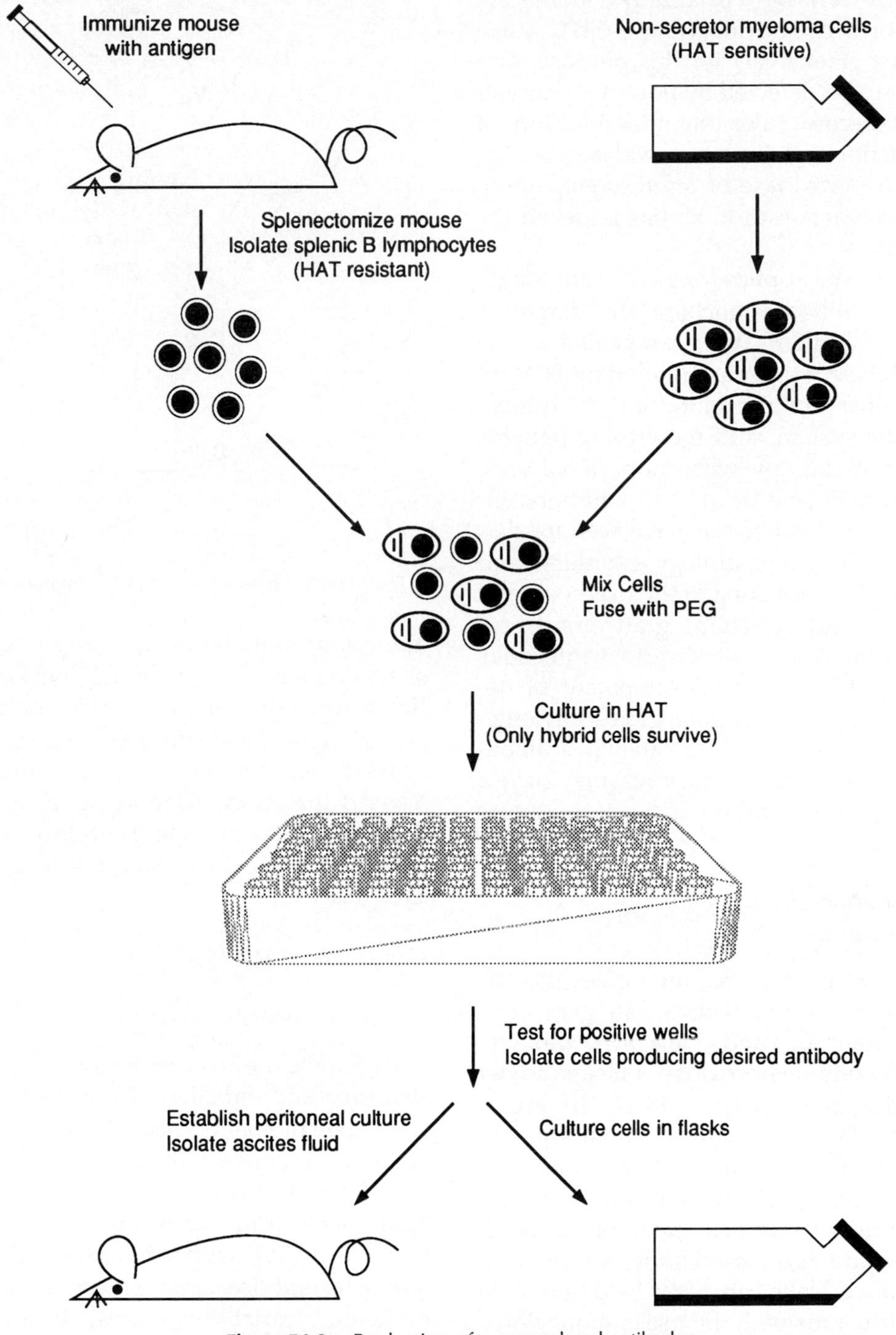

Figure 56.2. Production of a monoclonal antibody.

for T lymphocyte antigens in the late 1970s was a revolutionary event. These monoclonal antibodies (the OKT series) were rapidly applied in the diagnostic immunology laboratory for studying the phenotype of lymphoproliferative disorders and for the care of patients infected with the human immunodeficiency virus (HIV). Unfortunately, the rapid availability of numerous monoclonal antibodies, often with similar or identical reactivity, lead to much confusion among immunologists. Fortunately, the World Health Organization (WHO) sponsored a series of workshops to compare and classify the reactivity of antileukocyte antibodies supplied from laboratories around the world. It was decided to group antileukocyte antibodies with similar reactivity into "clusters." In addition, a "cluster designation" (CD) number was assigned to each of these groups.

Cellular identification and quantitation with a monoclonal antibody requires that the antibody be labeled or "tagged" by some means so that the antibody-cell complex can be visualized. Fluorescent dyes such as fluorescein isothiocyanate (FITC) have been utilized most extensively for this purpose, and the labeled cells can be detected by flow cytometry or fluorescence microscopy. For the identification of cells in tissue sections, immunoperoxidase staining using horseradish peroxidase or another enzyme to produce a colored reaction product has achieved the widest utilization.

The major diagnostic applications of the antileukocyte monoclonal antibodies include the diagnosis and monitoring of patients with congenital or acquired immunodeficiency disease (including HIV infection), the classification and monitoring of tumors of the hemopoietic system, and monitoring patients undergoing in vivo therapy with monoclonal antibodies such as anti-T_3 (see below). In addition, antileukocyte monoclonal antibodies have been used as reagents for automated hematology counters, and have great potential for assisting in the diagnosis and monitoring of allograft rejection, graft-versus-host disease, autoimmune disease, and various infectious diseases. However, the recent development of designer antibodies (immunoglobulins genetically engineered for a specific purpose) and catalytic antibodies (antibodies that behave like enzymes) may have a dramatic impact upon the immunoassay of the future (14, 31).

Monoclonal Antibodies Specific for Nonleukocyte Antigens

The availability of monoclonal antibodies specific for a multitude of nonleukocyte antigens has changed both anatomic and clinical pathology. Hybridoma technology has provided a means to detect substances that previously could not be evaluated. Armed with the technique of immunoperoxidase staining and an armamentarium of monoclonal antibodies, the surgical pathologist can differentiate between lesions that were impossible to precisely diagnose only a decade ago. In addition, small numbers of human cancer cells can often be detected in body fluids and effusions with the use of monoclonal antibodies. Examples of some of the nonleukocyte monoclonal antibodies utilized in surgical pathology include those directed against epithelial cell antigens (epithelial membrane antigen), intermediate filaments (keratins, desmin, vimentin, neurofilament, glial fibillary acidic protein), hormones (serotonin, synaptophysin), infectious agents (CMV), and tumor-specific antigens (prostatic-specific antigen).

In the clinical pathology laboratory, monoclonal antibodies have also provided a means to quantitate a wide variety of soluble biological products such as antibodies, hormones, and enzymes. In addition,

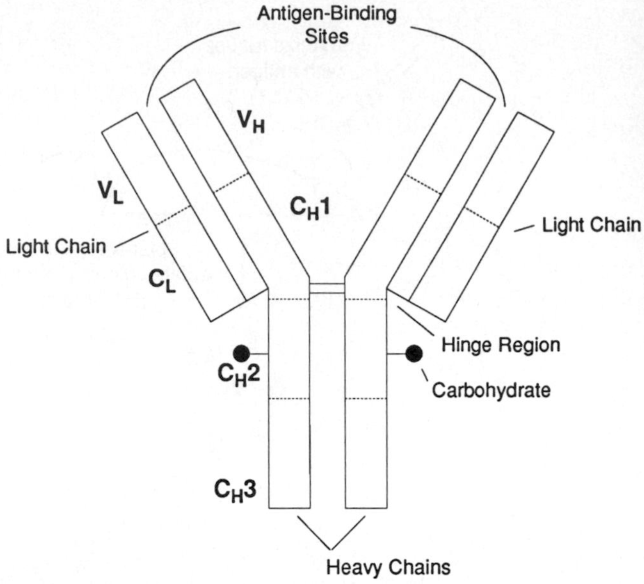

Figure 56.3. Basic structure of the immunoglobulin molecule.

monoclonal antibodies have improved the specificity of assays that were previously performed with polyclonal antibodies or colorimetric methods. For example, a monoclonal antibody–based enzyme immunoassay for carcinoembryonic antigen has been devised that is much more specific than the earlier radioimmunoassay (32). Therefore, fewer false-positives occur due to inflammatory bowel disease or liver disease.

GENERAL PRINCIPLES OF IMMUNOASSAYS

Immunoglobulin Structure

Antibodies are protein molecules with a specific structure and function. Each molecule consists of two types of chains (heavy and light). The primary amino acid sequence of each chain is specified by the genetic code. Sequence analysis of the heavy and light chains from many immunoglobulin molecules revealed regions with similar (homologous) composition (constant domains), and other regions with little homology (variable domains). In addition, selective areas within the variable regions showed extreme variability (hypervariable regions) (Fig. 56.3). Five immunoglobulin classes (IgA, IgG, IgM, IgE, IgD) have been defined on the basis of sequence identities in the constant domains.

The spatial conformation of the heavy and light chains of the immunoglobulin molecule is determined by hydrogen bonding between portions of the amino acid chains (secondary structure). Hydrogen and hydrophobic bonds between the polypeptide chains result in a complex globular configuration of the molecule (tertiary structure), while associations between the heavy and light chains define the quaternary structure.

The specific biological function of each immunoglobulin class is determined by the tertiary structure of the constant domains (Fc region), while the antigen combining regions (Fab regions) of the molecule are formed by spatial associations between the variable regions of the heavy and light chains. In each antigen combining site, the hypervariable regions of one heavy chain and one light chain are brought in close proximity by tertiary folding to define an area complementary to the structure of an antigen. The number of antigen combining sites determines the valence of the immunoglobulin molecule. IgG, IgD, and IgE exist as monomers, with a valence of 2, while the IgM molecule is a pentamer, with a valence of 10. Both monomeric and dimeric forms of IgA have been defined, with respective valences of 2 and 4. Binding sites for complement, the phagocyte and bacterial Fc receptor, staphylococcal protein A, and rheumatoid factor are present in the Fc receptor of the molecule (33).

Antigen-Antibody Interactions

Antigen-antibody interactions can be classified as primary, secondary, and tertiary. Primary reactions involve antigen binding and the formation of the antigen-antibody (immune) complex; secondary reactions involve interactions between antigen-antibody complexes (i.e., agglutination, precipitation, complement fixation); and tertiary reactions arise as an in vivo consequence of the interaction of immune complexes with immune cells and other immune products (i.e., opsonization, chemotaxis).

The antigen-binding region is a shallow cleft (approximately 30Å × 14Å × 6Å) at the distal end of the Fab region. The binding of an antigen to an antibody is an event determined by the complementary geometric fit of the antigen in the binding groove, and by other factors, such as the temperature, pH, and ionic strength. The antigen binding site accommodates approximately four to five peptides of a protein antigen, or three to five residues of other types of antigens. Binding involves noncovalent forces, including hydrogen bonds, as well as electrostatic, hydrophobic, and van der Waals forces. In chemical terms, the interaction of an antigen and antibody is a reversible reaction governed by the law of mass action, such that:

$$\text{Free Ag} + \text{Free Ab} \underset{k_2}{\overset{k_1}{\rightleftharpoons}} \text{Ag}\cdot\text{Ab Complex}$$

where k_1 of k_2 are the respective rates for the formation and dissociation of the antigen-antibody complex. At equilibrium, the formation of a stable immune complex is determined by the ratio between the rate constants:

$$K = \frac{k_1}{k_2} = \frac{(\text{Ag}\cdot\text{Ab})}{(\text{Ag})(\text{Ab})}$$

where K is the equilibrium constant (affinity constant) of the reaction. The association constant of an antigen and antibody is also influenced by other factors, including the valence of the antibody, and the valence and epitopic density of the antigen. The term avidity is used in reference to the overall stability of an antigen-antibody complex. Although the kinetics of the antigen-antibody reaction can be precisely defined for reactions involving monoclonal antibodies, polyclonal antibody preparations are more difficult to characterize, since they consist of heterogenous mixtures of antibodies of different class, valence, specificity, and affinity. In this circumstance, the average affinity (K_0) is defined by the reciprocal of the free antigen concentration when 50% of the binding sites are occupied:

$$K_0 = \frac{1}{(\text{Ag Free})}$$

Cross-reactivity occurs when antibodies react with heterologous antigens that are similar in structure, but not identical to the original (homologous) antigen. Cross-reactivity is partly due to the heterogeneous nature of the humoral immune response against an immunogenic substance, and by the presence of multiple antigenic determinants on most complex natural antigens. In addition, an antibody will bind substances that are structurally similar to the homologous antigen, although usually with less affinity. The phenomenon of cross-reactivity is an important practical consideration in the design and clinical utilization of immunoassays, since the sensitivity of the assay can be reduced, false interpretations can be made, and inappropriate therapy initiated.

A number of different consequences can result from the interaction of antigen-antibody complexes with each other, and with other immune substances such as complement. These secondary immune reactions are influenced by the nature, valence, and concentration of the antigen, and by the valence, concentration, avidity, and immunoglobulin class of the antibody. Generally, multivalent antigens and antibodies are required for the induction of a secondary immune reaction. In the past, detection of the secondary immune reaction was the only means available for the detection and analysis of immune components. As a result, antisera were often classified by their ability to cause precipitation (precipitins), the hemolysis of red blood cells (hemolysins), the agglutination or precipitation of particulate antigens (agglutinins, precipitins), and other reactions. In addition, the suffix *-ogen* was attached to an antigen that elicited a secondary immune response (agglutinogen, precipitogen, etc.). The in vivo, or tertiary consequences of the immune reaction are complex, and generally involve the interaction of antigen-antibody complexes with cells and other immune products.

Clinical Utilization of the Antigen-Antibody Interaction

The humoral and cellular products of the immune system have achieved widespread utilization as reagents for medical diagnosis. In this regard, the unique specificity of the antibody has proven invaluable for the detection and quantitation of immune-related substances (other antibodies, immune products, cells), as well as a wide variety of substances unrelated to the immune system (hormones, drugs, tumor antigens, red blood cell antigens, etc.). Therefore, antibodies and other immune products are standard reagents not only in the clinical immunology laboratory, but in surgical pathology, immunohematology, hematology, microbiology, and clinical chemistry.

CLASSIFICATION OF IMMUNOASSAYS

Immunoassays are studies of the antigen-antibody reaction performed to detect the presence of an antigen, antibody, or immune complex (qualitative immunoassay), or to measure the concentration of one of the components of an antigen-antibody reaction (quantitative immunoassay).

PRACTICAL CONSIDERATIONS IN IMMUNODIAGNOSIS

The diagnostic relevancy of an immunoassay depends on the choice of the proper assay, adequate specimen collection and transportation, prompt and accurate laboratory analysis, and rapid reporting of the results of the assay in a format relevant to the clinician. For substances that are normally present in relatively large concentrations in the body (i.e., many serum proteins, some antibodies), or that undergo large changes in concentration in response to a disease process, relatively insensitive methods such as passive agglutination may suffice for diagnosis. However, for the detection of small but diagnostically relevant changes in the concentration of a substance, or to quantitate hormones, immunoregulatory substances, and other substances that are present in minute quantities, the most sensitive immunoassays available (i.e., radioimmunoassay, enzyme immunoassay) may be required.

In practice, an immunoassay is performed in a system of defined volume under controlled reaction conditions and with precisely measured volumes of test specimen and reagents. Under these conditions, the signal strength of the parameter is proportional to the concentration of the measured variable. Dilutions of a purified preparation of the test substance are used to prepare a standard curve, and the concentration of the variable in an unknown specimen is determined from the standard curve. The results of these assays may be reported as quantitative, semiquantitative, or dichotomous (binary, positive/negative). In many immunoassay systems, especially for the presence of serum antibodies, serial dilutions of the specimen are tested, and the end result is taken as the highest specimen dilution that produces an arbitrary defined signal strength (titer). In these circumstances, it is common to first assay a single fixed dilution of the specimen. If the signal strength of the "screening assay" is below a predefined limit, the assay is reported as negative and no additional testing is performed. However, if the signal strength of the screening assay is above the predefined limit (positive), additional dilutions are tested until the minimal signal strength is reached. The serum titer required to produce this result is reported as the endpoint.

Ultimately, immunoassay results are used to determine whether an individual patient is diseased or nondiseased. Unfortunately, in any large population there are small numbers of diseased individuals with normal assay results (false-negative results), and another population of nondiseased people with abnormal values (false-positive results). Causes of false-positive and false-negative immunoassays include cross-reactivity of the test reagents with an unrelated disease product, the presence of substances that interfere with the formation of the antigen-antibody complex, errors in test performance, and other factors. Under these circumstances, the correct clinical interpretation of the results of an immunoassay requires up-to-date information about the overall performance of the immunoassay procedure under consideration (reproducibility, diagnostic accuracy, etc.), as well as knowledge of disease pathogenesis and the immune response to the disease process.

NONCELLULAR IMMUNOASSAYS

Agglutination

Agglutination is a secondary immune phenomenon that occurs when insoluble or particulate antigens (cells or other particles) are cross-linked by an immune reaction (Fig. 56.4). Agglutination occurs because antibodies have two or more antigen recognition sites (bi-valency or multivalency). If multiple antigenic recognition sites are present on a particle, lattices can be formed that grow in size and eventually become a mass that is macroscopically visible. The major factors affecting the agglutination reaction include the class, affinity, and avidity of the antibody, the proximity and number of binding sites on the particle, the relative concentrations of antibody and particles, electrostatic interactions ("zeta potential"), and the viscosity of the medium. Antibodies of the IgM class, with 10 antigen-combining sites, are usually the best "agglutinins," and have been said to be more than 750 times more efficient than IgG in agglutination (34). Since particles in suspension often possess negative charges and repel each other, it may be necessary to overcome the "zeta potential" by the addition of protein or inorganic salts to permit particle cross-linking. Antibody excess may prevent agglutination by coating all of the binding sites, while inadequate antibody may not provide sufficient cross-linking for agglutination. In practice, this "prozone" phenomenon may require adjustment of particle or antibody concentration, or performing an assay at a number of different concentrations. Interference with agglutination by any of these factors after a primary immune reaction is termed "incomplete agglutination."

Agglutination tests can be classified as direct or indirect, depending on whether the analyte is present in its native state, or linked to a particle to allow detection of the antigen-antibody reaction. Mixed agglutination and hemagglutination inhibition are other variations of this type of immunoassay.

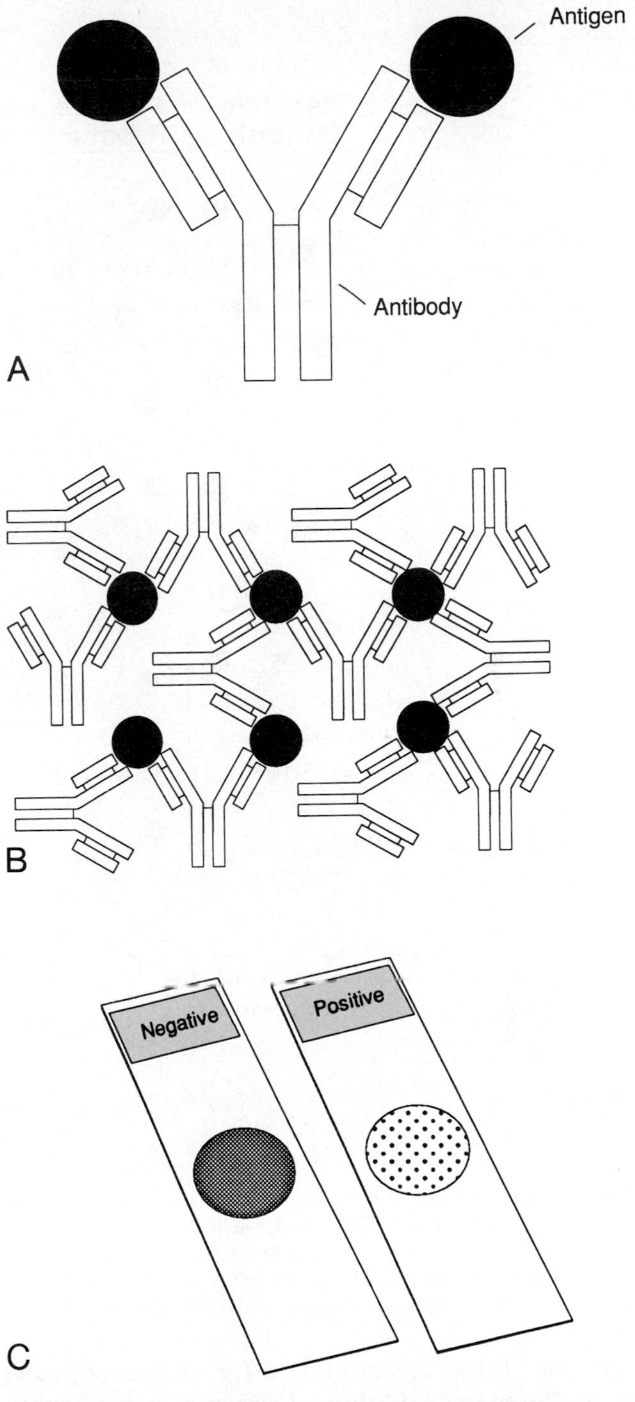

Figure 56.4. The agglutination reaction. Schematic illustration of the interaction of an antibody with an insoluble antigen, resulting in agglutination. **A**, The formation of antigen-antibody complexes. **B**, Cross-linking of the antigen-antibody complexes to form a lattice. **C**, Schematic illustration of the visual appearances of positive and negative agglutination reactions. The appearance of the reaction is greatly influenced by whether the assay is performed on a flat surface or in a vessel, such as a test tube or microtiter plate. The physical characteristics of the vessel (round bottom or V-bottom) are also important.

DIRECT AGGLUTINATION

Direct agglutination occurs when a suspension of particles is mixed with a specific antibody solution. If specific antibody with two or more antigen recognition sites is present, the particles may rapidly link together to form visible clumps (34) (Fig. 56.5). The classic example of the application of direct agglutination reaction is the Widal test for the diagnosis of typhoid fever. In this test, specific anti-*Salmonella* antibodies are detected by adding a constant amount of a *Salmonella typhi* cell suspension to serum that has been serially diluted. After appropriate incuba-

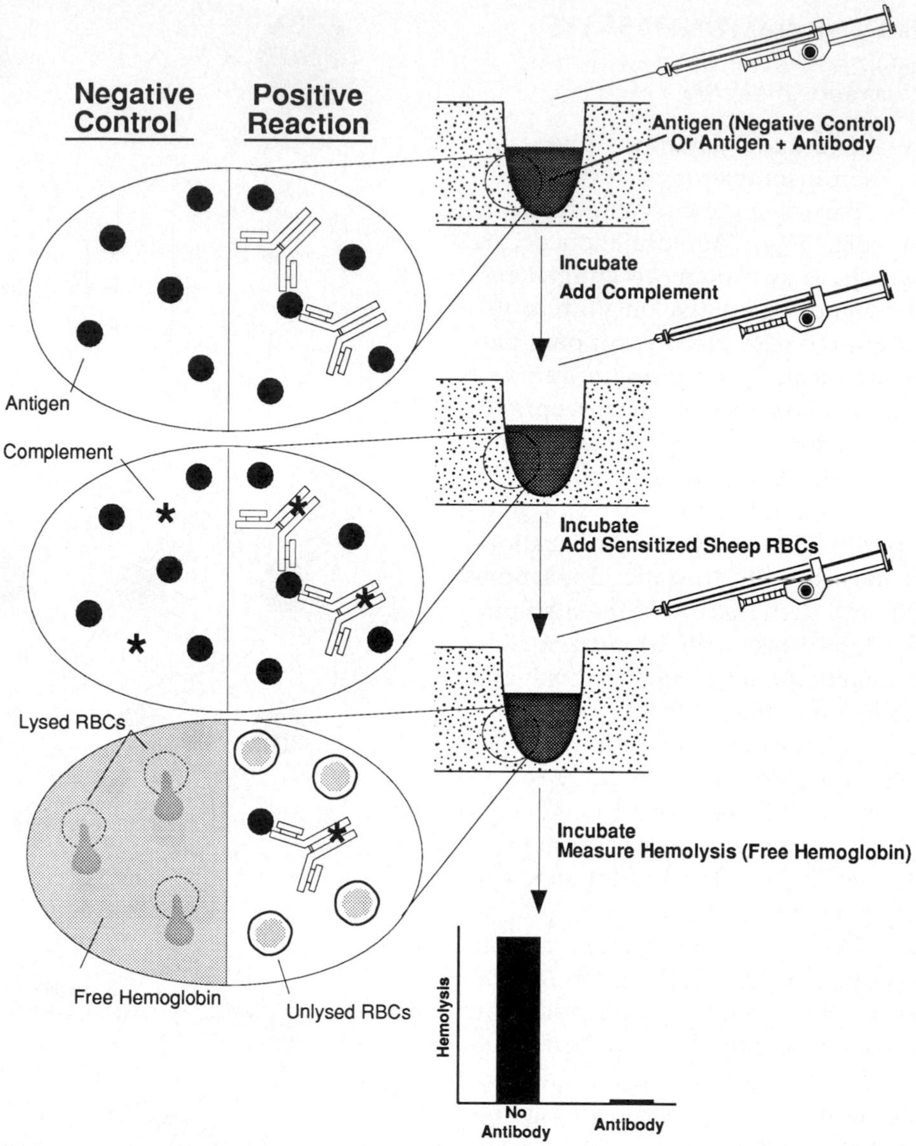

Figure 56.5. Principle of the complement fixation assay. In this assay, antigen and antibody are allowed to interact in solution, and complement is then added. In the presence of an antigen-antibody complex, complement binds to the Fc portion of the antibody molecule. If there is no antigen-antibody complex, complement exists free and unbound in the reaction solution. Sensitized sheep red blood cells are added as an indicator for the presence of unbound complement. The sheep red blood cells are lysed only in the solutions with free complement and an absence of antigen-antibody-complement complexes.

tion, the tubes are examined for visible agglutination. The highest dilution of serum showing agglutination is the titer of the antibody.

The agglutination of red blood cells by antibodies directed against natural components of the cell surface is a type of direct agglutination termed hemagglutination. In immunohematology, direct hemagglutination is the principal method for the detection of antibodies specific for erythrocytic antigens.

Interspecies hemagglutinins (heterophil antibodies) can lead to false-positive results in agglutination tests that utilize nonhuman erythrocytes. Heterophil antibodies can be produced in the sera of some normal individuals, as well as patients with serum sickness, autoimmune diseases, and some infectious diseases. However, in infectious mononucleosis, the presence of sheep red blood cell agglutinins in high titer is highly characteristic of the disease.

INDIRECT AGGLUTINATION

Indirect agglutination techniques utilize particles as passive carriers of an antigen (direct passive agglutination) or antibody (reverse passive agglutination) (34). Although coated red blood cells (passive hemagglutination) were initially utilized in the clinical applications of the indirect agglutination principle (35, 36), inert particles (charcoal, bentonite clay, inorganic colloidal particles) have proven more versatile for many applications. More recently, the use of coated latex microspheres, colloidal gold, dye particles, and other substances has permitted the development of simple, cost-efficient assays for a wide range of clinically important substances (37). The sensitivity of these assays does not approach that of enzyme immunoassay, radioimmunoassay, and other techniques, but is adequate for many purposes. Particle inhibition tests have also been described, in which the presence of an antigen in the serum prevents the attachment of an antibody to an antigen on the surface of a particle. The term "particle immunoassay" has been applied to agglutination tests in which particles are used as a label for an antigen or antibody (38).

The coating or "sensitization" of a particle for use in an immunoassay is accomplished by three techniques. Untreated erythrocytes spontaneously adsorb many proteins to their surface (thyroglobulin and other hormones, purified protein derivative, serum proteins, bacterial products). Other substances are adsorbed after treatment of the erythrocyte with tannic acid ("tanned" red blood cells) or enzymes (39). Covalent attachment has been used for substances that cannot be adsorbed by these techniques. Sensitized erythrocytes are usually fixed with formaldehyde, glutaraldehyde, or another compound to increase the shelf life. The use of latex particles for immunoassay was first reported by Singer and Plotz in 1956 (40). Latex particles are usually coated by passive means, with the quantity of the adsorbed protein adjusted to provide agglutination of the analyte in its biological range. In addition, the use of latex particles avoids much of the variability encountered with red blood cells. Even so, the prozone phenomenon can still be significant, and careful adherence to the manufacturer's instructions is necessary during the performance of clinical assays utilizing coated microspheres.

Examples of substances routinely detected by passive agglutination include rheumatoid factor, antinuclear antibodies, C-reactive protein, human chorionic gonadotropin (hCG), parasitic, fungal, and bacterial antigens, and antibodies specific for some infectious agents. Special variations of the passive agglutination technique include microhemagglutination, the Rose-Waaler test, the VDRL and RPR, and the Paul-Bunnell test.

Microhemagglutination techniques are used in a popular confirmatory test for syphilis (microhemagglutination assay–treponema pallidum, MHA-TP), and in the detection of antithyroid antibodies specific for microsomal and thyroglobulin antigens. These assays utilize small quantities of tanned, coated red blood cells that are reacted with the test serum in a special plastic microtiter tray. The reaction is read with a magnifying mirror or microscope with a low-power objective. Agglutination results in the formation of a diffuse matrix coating the bottom of the tube, while nonagglutinated cells settle to form a compact button at the bottom of the tube. The Rose-Waaler test is an assay for rheumatoid factor that utilizes sheep red blood cells sensitized with subagglutinating amounts of rabbit antisheep erythrocyte IgG (34). Agglutination results when these cells are mixed with serum containing anti-IgG (rheumatoid factor). The VDRL and RPR (rapid plasma reagin) are tests for antisyphilitic antibodies. These tests utilize the natural cross-reactivity of these antibodies with a lipid (cardiolipin) found in high concentrations in neural tissue and cardiac muscle. In the VDRL, particles of purified cardiolipin are mixed with a dilution of the test specimen (serum or CSF) under defined conditions, and examined for macroscopically visible aggregates. The RPR is an improved modification of the VDRL that utilizes charcoal particles coated with a stabilized mixture of cholesterol and cardiolipin. Serum dilutions are used to "titer" positive specimens. However, all states have enacted laws requiring confirmation of a positive RPR or VDRL by a confirmatory test utilizing antigens isolated from *Treponema pallidum* (MHA-TP or FTA-ABS).

The utilization of differently colored latex particles for the simultaneous detection and identification of more than one antigen has been reported. In the system described by Hadfield, Lane, and McIllmurray (1987) (41), three different *Salmonella* serogroup antigens were detected by the use of separately labeled colored latex particles, while a two-color system was used for the detection of Group A streptococci.

Several techniques have been used to increase the sensitivity of agglutination assays. Immunoassay by particle counting (IMPACT) has a sensitivity of 10 to 1000 times that of slide-based latex agglutination assays (42). In this technique, a standard number of coated latex particles are incubated with the specimen, and the reaction mixture is passed through an automated particle counter. Agglutinated and unagglutinated particles are differentiated on the basis of light scatter, and the number of unagglutinated particles is used to construct a dose-response curve. The concentration of an unknown specimen is determined from the dose-response curve. Although these assays are rapid, fully automated, and do not require a separation step, they require expensive equipment and do not have the sensitivity of radioimmunoassay or enzyme immunoassay. Latex agglutination on microtiter plates has also been described, with the quantification of agglutination by turbidimetric measurement at 405 nm (43).

Particle assays utilizing inorganic colloid particles (sols) are referred to as sol particle immunoassays (SPIAs) (38). Colloidal gold particles are used most often in SPIAs, although the use of other colloidal substances has been reported. Gold sols have a red color that is not affected by the adsorption of antibodies, but is changed by aggregation. In practice, the agglutination of sensitized 50-nm gold particles is determined by measuring a decrease in absorbance at 540 nm. Alternatively, the color change may be determined visually.

Hydrophobic colloidal dye particles have been utilized in agglutination immunoassays (disperse dye immunoassay, DIA). In these immunoassays, the dye particle aggregates can be directly measured, or the dye can be extracted into organic solvents and quantitated colorimetrically (38). Foron Brilliant Blue SR (Sandoz), Terasil Brilliant Flavin 8GFF (Ciba-Geigy), Palanil Luminous Red G, and Palanil Yellow 3GE (BASF) have been used as dye sols (38). Colloidal dyes are most effective in sandwich-type immunoassays, which allows amplification of the signal to occur. Sandwich DIAs are performed with antibody-coated microtitration plates. The sample is incubated in the plates, followed by the addition of the bound dye label. After a second incubation and washing, the dye is extracted into an organic solvent and the absorbance is read in a spectrophotometer.

AGGLUTINATION INHIBITION

Agglutination inhibition reactions are based on the competition for antibody-binding sites between antigens in solution and the same or similar antigens localized on indicator cells or particles. These assays are normally performed by reacting the test solution with an antibody preparation, followed by reaction with the indicator cells or particles. Antigen in the test solution, if present, reacts with the antibody, and subsequently prevents, or decreases, agglutination of the indicator. Therefore, lack of agglutination is indicative of a positive test (34).

Agglutination inhibition is widely utilized for the detection of human chorionic gonadetropin (HCG) in the urine. In the assay, test urine is reacted with anti-HCG antibody, and then with HCG-coated latex particles. Another application of agglutination inhibition is for the detection of antibodies specific for rubella, influenza, and other viruses. This assay is based on the presence of specific viral receptors on erythrocytes, so that hemagglutination can result from the presence of viral particles or viral antigens (viral hemagglutination). Inhibition of hemagglutination by antiviral antibodies is used in the practical application of this phenomenon.

Cell Lysis

An antigen antibody reaction on a cell membrane can result in lysis of the cell if complement is present. If the cells are red blood cells, hemolysis takes place. Cell lysis forms the base for the complement fixation test, which is a very sensitive method for the detection and quantitation of antigens or antibodies. The serum specimen is first heated to 56°C to inactivate native complement. Measured amounts of antigen and complement are then added. If antibody specific for the added antigen is present in the serum, antigen-antibody complexes will form, and these will bind or fix all of the complement. The reaction mixture is then checked for the presence of free complement. The indicator system for complement consists of sheep red blood cells plus an antibody specific for sheep red blood cells. If all of the complement has been fixed, none will be free to lyse the sheep red blood cells, and the test is positive. If no antibody was present in the patient's serum, then the complement is not fixed and is free to interact with the indicator system and lyse the red cells. Under these circumstances, the test is negative (Fig. 56.5). Properly conducted complement fixation tests require the use of appropriate controls to ensure that the results will not be adversely affected by the presence of anticomplement compounds, such as denatured immunoglobulins, heparin, chelating agents, or microbial contaminants. The complement fixation test is useful in measuring antiviral activity to a number of viruses, as well as many bacteria, fungi, and parasites.

A completely different procedure utilizing lytic reactions is the viral neutralization test. This method is based on the fact that certain viruses, such as herpes simplex, produce effects (cytopathic effects) when added to target cells growing in tissue cultures. This phenomenon can be used to search for virus-neutralizing antibodies in a serum sample. This is done by adding the serum suspected of containing the antibody to a virus suspension and then adding this mixture to a susceptible cell culture. If the cells fail to show any change, then antibodies present in the serum sample "neutralized" the cytopathic effect of the virus. If cytopathologic effects develop, then neutralizing antibodies were not present.

Immunoprecipitation

Immunoprecipitation is a secondary immunologic phenomenon that results from the reaction of an antibody and soluble antigen in the proper proportions, with the formation of an insoluble immune complex. Immunoprecipitation has been utilized since the 1920s for the quantitation of antigens and antibodies.

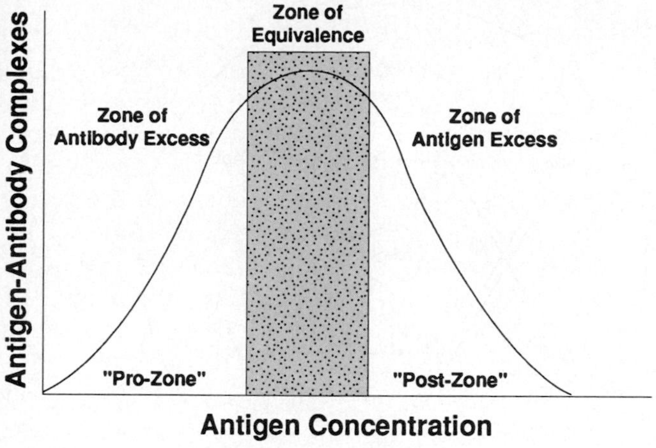

Figure 56.6. The precipitation curve and a schematic depiction of the phenomenon of immunoprecipitation.

BASIC PRINCIPLES OF IMMUNOPRECIPITATION

Immunoprecipitation, as a manifestation of the antigen-antibody reaction, was first described by Heidelberger and Kendall in 1935. Immunoprecipitation requires the presence of bivalent or multivalent antibodies, and an antigen with at least two antigenic determinants per molecule. Cross-linking of antigen molecules results in the formation of a lattice, which gradually grows in size. Eventually, the lattice may become insoluble and precipitate from the solution. If immunoprecipitation is studied as a function of antigen concentration, with the same concentration of antibody, three phases can be delineated. During the initial phase of antibody excess (prozone), the number of antigenic determinants is small relative to the antibody concentration, and lattice formation is prohibited. As the amount of antigen is increased, the zone of equivalence is reached, where the reactants are at their "optimal proportions," and maximum precipitation occurs. At this point, hydrophobic and ionic interactions between smaller complexes increases the size of the aggregates. The final phase is one of antigen excess (postzone), where all of the antibody binding sites are saturated, cross-linking of antibody molecules cannot occur, and lattice formation is prohibited (Fig. 56.6).

The time course of an immunoprecipitation reaction can vary from hours to days, depending on the affinity, avidity, and valence of the antibody; the size and number of antigenic determinants of the antigen; the reaction temperature, ionic strength, and viscosity of the medium; interactions between the medium and reactants; and other factors. The time course can be greatly accelerated by assisting the migration of the reactants through the use of an electric field. However, immunoprecipitation reactions generally lack the speed and sensitivity of many other immunoassay techniques, and the use of this type of analysis in the clinical laboratory is declining.

Table 56.1. Classification of Immunoprecipitation Assays

Passive immunodiffusion assays
Ouchterlony double diffusion
Radial immunodiffusion
Active immunodiffusion assays
Countercurrent immunoelectrophoresis
Rocket immunoelectrophoresis
Combined immunodiffusion assays
Immunoelectrophoresis
Immunofixation electrophoresis

Immunoprecipitation reactions can be classified according to whether the interaction of the antigen and antibody is allowed to occur passively or actively (under the influence of an electric field) (44). Passive immunoprecipitation can be further classified according to the nature of the reaction medium (fluid or gel) (Table 56.1).

A support medium composed of a substance extracted from seaweed (agarose) has been found to provide much better resolution than the gels used in the past. In passive immunodiffusion techniques utilizing gels, antigen and antibody solutions are usually placed in separate regions of the gel and the molecules diffuse radially outward through pores in the gel. When equilibrium is reached, a concentration gradient is formed for each reactant. The concentration is highest near the well and decreases geometrically with distance from the well. At the point in the region between the reactants where their concentrations fall into the zone of equivalence, an immunoprecipitate appears as a narrow band ("precipitin band"). Multiple precipitin lines are formed if more than a single antigen and/or antibody with different rates of diffusion are present. An alternative method of passive immunoprecipitation utilizes gels in which one of the reactants (antibody or antigen) is dissolved during the preparation of the gel. The rate of diffusion is dependent on the molecular weight and size of the antigen(s) and antibody(s), the pore size, degree of hydration and other properties of the support medium, the ionic strength and composition of buffer, and the interaction between the reactants and the support medium. In the preparation of a gel for passive immunoprecipitation, agarose (usually 1% wt/vol) is completely dissolved in distilled water or saline by heating with frequent stirring at temperatures of 100° to 110°C. If antisera is added, the solution is first cooled to approximately 50°C to prevent protein denaturation (44). Gels are cast in Petri dishes or on glass plates or Mylar sheets using gel-molding frames. Wells are added at the time the gel is cast,

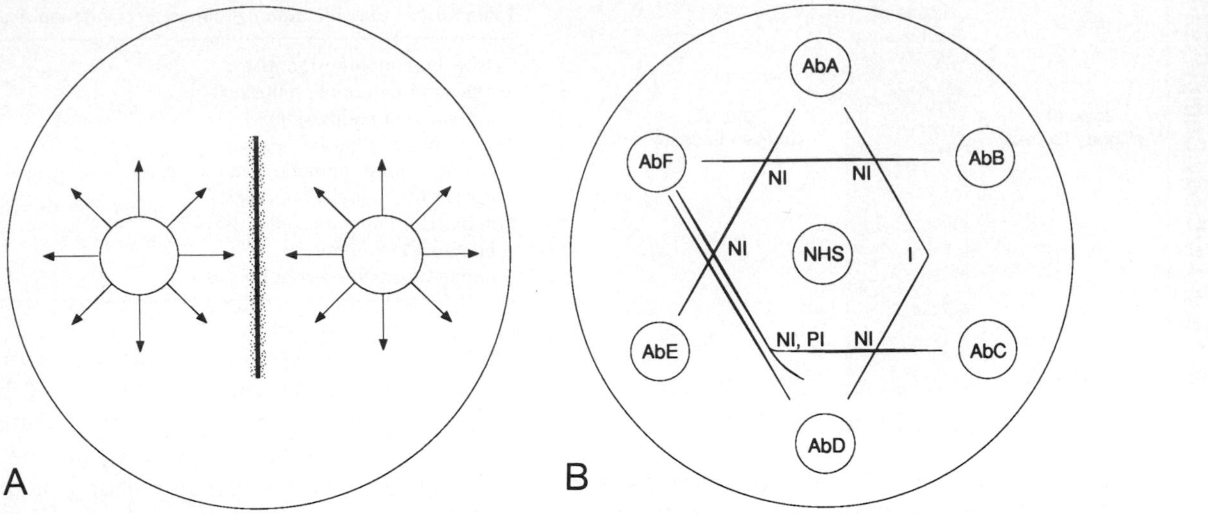

Figure 56.7. Principle of double (Ouchterlony) immunodiffusion. In this adaptation of the immunoprecipitation reaction, antigen and antibody are placed in wells punched in agarose gel (**A**). The reactants diffuse through the gel, and a visible line forms at the point of equilibrium, where an antigen-antibody reaction occurs. **B**, In this example, normal human serum was placed in the center well, and various antibody solutions in the six surrounding wells. If an antigen-antibody reaction occurs, the identity (I), nonidentity (NI), or partial identity (PI) of the reactants can be ascertained by the characteristics of the precipitin line. For example, the cross-lines (NI) indicate that antibody A (AbA) and antibody B (AbB) react with different antigenic determinants, while antibody B and antibody C (AbC) react with the same antigenic determinant (reaction of identity). Antibody D (AbD) and antibody E (AbE) react with the same antigenic determinant, but the spur indicates the presence of an additional antigenic determinant recognized by AbD but not AbE. The double precipitin line indicates the presence of an antigen recognized by AbE but not by AbD or AbF.

or at a later time, using a variety of templates. Precipitin lines may be directly visible if the concentration of antigen and antibody was high enough. Alternately, it may be necessary to stain the gel with dyes such as Coomassie Brilliant Blue R2500 or amido black to visualize the faint precipitin lines or to clarify the pattern of precipitation. Gels may be stored in a preservative, or dried and stored.

PASSIVE IMMUNODIFFUSION IMMUNOASSAYS

Ouchterlony Double Diffusion

The two basic passive immunodiffusion techniques include double (Ouchterlony) immunodiffusion and single diffusion radial immunodiffusion (RID). In the Ouchterlony procedure, antigen and antibody preparations are placed in separate wells cut in a thin layer of agar in a Petri dish. Typically, an antibody solution is placed in a center well, while antigen controls and test solutions are placed in wells around the outside of the gel. The reactants diffuse through the agar until they meet at optimal proportion, where bands of precipitation are formed. The antigenic relationships of the reactants are reflected in the precipitation pattern. The three basic patterns of reaction include identity, nonidentity, and partial identity. In reactions of identity, the two precipitation bands merge into a solid line. In reactions of nonidentity, the lines of precipitation cross. Partial identity is indicated by spur formation indicating that one of the antigens is cross-reactive with, but not identical to, the other (Fig. 56.7).

Double immunodiffusion assays are simple and inexpensive to perform, and do not require elaborate equipment. However, the precipitin reactions require a day or more for completion, and the results are qualitative and not quantitative. Also, the reaction patterns may be time-consuming and difficult to interpret. For these reasons more rapid, quantitative methods of immunochemical analysis have replaced double immunodiffusion for most high-volume clinical applications. One exception is in the identification of patients with some autoimmune antibodies, such as those directed against the Smith (Sm) antigen and ribonucleoprotein (RNP). Problems can arise from the presence of irregular wells, overfilling of the wells, incubation on a nonlevel surface, or at an improper temperature. False-negative results can theoretically result from antigen or antibody excess, and the gels and antigen or antibody reagents may have a limited shelf life. Other potential problems include bacterial or fungal contamination, and drying of the gels during incubation (44).

Radial Immunodiffusion

Radial immunodiffusion (RID) is a gel-based quantitative immunoprecipitation method. In this procedure, a monospecific antibody with high affinity and excellent precipitating ability is added to an agarose

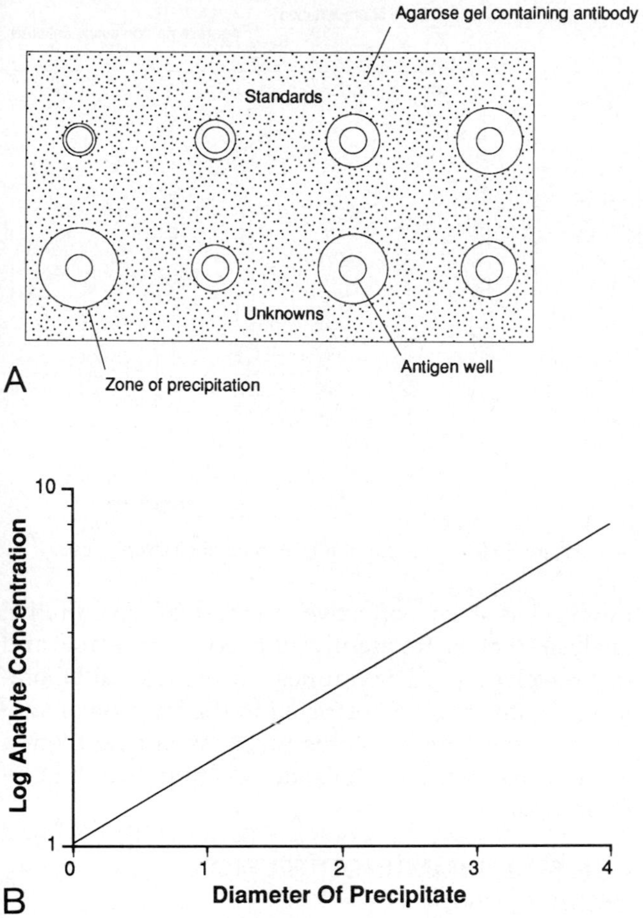

Figure 56.8. Radial immunodiffusion.

solution before gels are cast. Wells are punched into the gel, antigen solution is added to the wells, and the gels are incubated. Under these circumstances, the antigen diffuses radially outward, resulting in a "ring" of precipitation around each well at the zone of equivalence (45–47). The diameter of the ring is proportional to the concentration of antigen in the well (Fig. 56.8).

The molecular weight of the antigen is the major determinant of the time required for performance of a radial immunodiffusion assay. Generally, this varies from 24 hours for small proteins like α_1-antitrypsin to as long as 72 hours for high–molecular weight proteins such as IgM. In practice, at least three antigen solutions of known concentrations ("standards") are included with each assay, and their ring diameter is used to construct a standard curve, from which the concentrations of unknown solutions are determined. Ring diameters can be measured with the use of a ruler and magnifying glass, although more accurate measurements require a special reading device. To compensate for irregularities in the wells, it is customary to measure each ring diameter twice at right angles and to calculate the average of the measurements (44). Measurements of ring diameter may be taken at the endpoint of the reaction (Mancini or endpoint diffusion method), or at a fixed time prior to the endpoint (usually 18 hours) (Fahey or kinetic diffusion method). In the endpoint diffusion method, the standard curve is prepared on linear graph paper by plotting the concentration of antigen on the x axis and the diameter squared of the precipitin ring diameter on the y axis. If the standard curve is nonlinear, a line of best fit is drawn. The antigen concentration of an unknown solution is usually determined directly from the standard curve, although mathematical interpolation can also be used. In the less precise kinetic diffusion method, precipitin ring diameter is plotted on the x axis of semilogarithmic graph paper, and the concentration of the reference solutions is plotted on the y axis. Standard curves are not extended beyond the range of the standards. Specimens whose precipitin ring diameters exceed that of the reference solutions are diluted and reassayed, while specimens with precipitin rings smaller than the most dilute standard are reassayed with a more sensitive system, or reported as being "less than" the value of the reference standard. Potential causes of inaccurate results include overfilling of the wells, damage to the wells during pipetting, inappropriate incubation time or temperature, and errors in reading precipitin diameters, preparing the standard cure, and determining unknown concentrations.

ACTIVE IMMUNODIFFUSION IMMUNOASSAYS

The movement of a substance through a gel is greatly accelerated by an electric field. "Active" methods of immunodiffusion utilize this modification to decrease the time required for the formation of an immune complex. In addition to the properties of gels described above, reverse buffer flow or electroendosmosis (EEO) is important in the consideration of gel electrophoresis. Gels with high reverse buffer flow are used in applications where immunoglobulins move cathodically (i.e., countercurrent immunoelectrophoresis), while medium- or low-EEO gels are used for other applications (44).

Countercurrent Immunoelectrophoresis

In countercurrent immunoelectrophoresis (CIEP, electroimmunodiffusion) antigen and antibody solutions are located into parallel wells placed on opposite sides of an agarose gel. In the presence of an electric field at pH 8.6 (cathode on side of antigen wells, anode on side of antibody wells), the antibody molecules migrate toward the cathode, and the antigen toward the anode. After electrophoresis, precipitin lines will form between the wells at the zone of equivalence (44). The position of the precipitin line relative to the wells is dependent on the relative antigen and antibody concentrations, their ability to move through the pores of the gel, and the migration of these substances in an electric field. If the concentration of antibody is maintained constant, CIEP becomes semiquantitative, since the migration distance of the precipitin line from the antigen well increases with the ratio of antigen/antibody concentration. In practice, serial dilutions of antigen are used as a reference for the concentration of an unknown solution. CIEP was first utilized clinically for the detection of hepatitis B antigen, and has since been utilized for the detection of a variety of other microbial antigens, as well as autoantibodies and antibodies directed at infectious agents (i.e., influenza type A virus, adenovirus, cytomegalovirus, and *Haemophilus influenzae*).

Rocket Immunoelectrophoresis

Rocket immunoelectrophoresis (electroimmunoassay) is a technique in which an electric force is used to drive an antigen into a gel containing an antibody. Immune complex formation results in the formation of a triangular or "rocket-shaped" precipitate (48). The total area, or even the height of the immunoprecipitate, is proportional to the concentration of antigen. Low-EEO agarose is utilized in rocket immunoelectrophoresis, with the goal of minimizing migration of the antibody in the electric field. Since antigens may migrate either anodally or cathodally in the electric field, the wells must be placed to maximize use of the gel. Since the majority of plasma proteins migrate anodally in such a system, wells are usually placed near the cathode. Technical skill is required to perform rocket immunoelectrophoresis, since the samples must be applied to the gel rapidly to avoid lateral diffusion of the antigens, widening of the immunoprecipitin arcs, or even mixing of antigens in adjacent wells (44). A low-voltage field across the gel during sample application is used to minimize application artifacts. The voltage is then increased and maintained until the end of the reaction (usually several hours). Following electrophoresis, the gel is washed and stained, and the distance from the middle of each well to the top of the corresponding peak is measured with a precision of 0.1 mm. Standards spanning a wide range of concentration are assayed with the test specimens, and a curve is plotted from the peak heights of the standard (x axis—peak height; y axis—concentration of standard). The concentration of the test specimens can be extrapolated from the standard curve, or calculated mathematically (Fig. 56.9). Rocket immunoelectrophoresis is a cost-effective method of quantitative analysis that is frequently utilized in research and test development laboratories. In the clinical laboratory, its utilization is restricted to the analysis of substances where high-volume methods of quantitation are not feasible, such as some clotting factors or α-fetoprotein.

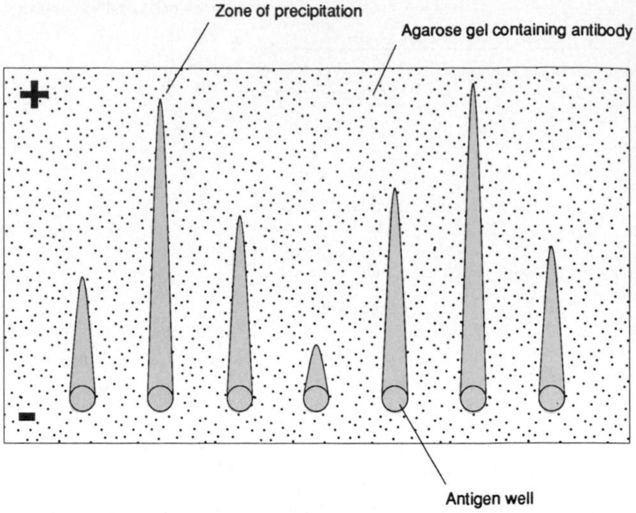

Figure 56.9. Principle of rocket immunoelectrophoresis.

COMBINED IMMUNODIFFUSION TECHNIQUES

Techniques in which active and passive immunodiffusion are combined (immunoelectrophoresis, immunofixation electrophoresis) are useful in resolving complex mixtures of antigens.

Immunoelectrophoresis

Immunoelectrophoresis (IEP) is a technique for the separation and analysis of serum proteins. It was first introduced by Grabber and Williams in 1953 and modified by Scheidegger in 1955. IEP is a two-stage procedure in which proteins are first separated electrophoretically, and then identified by immunoprecipitation (49–51) (Fig. 56.10). IEP is performed as follows:

1. The test solutions (serum, urine, CSF, etc.) are pipetted into cylindrical wells in a buffered agarose gel;
2. Electrophoretic separation of the proteins is performed;
3. Antisera is placed in troughs that run parallel to the path of electrophoretic migration and span most of the width of the gel;
4. The gel is placed into a humidity chamber for 10 to 15 hours. During this time proteins and antibodies diffuse into the gel and precipitin arcs form

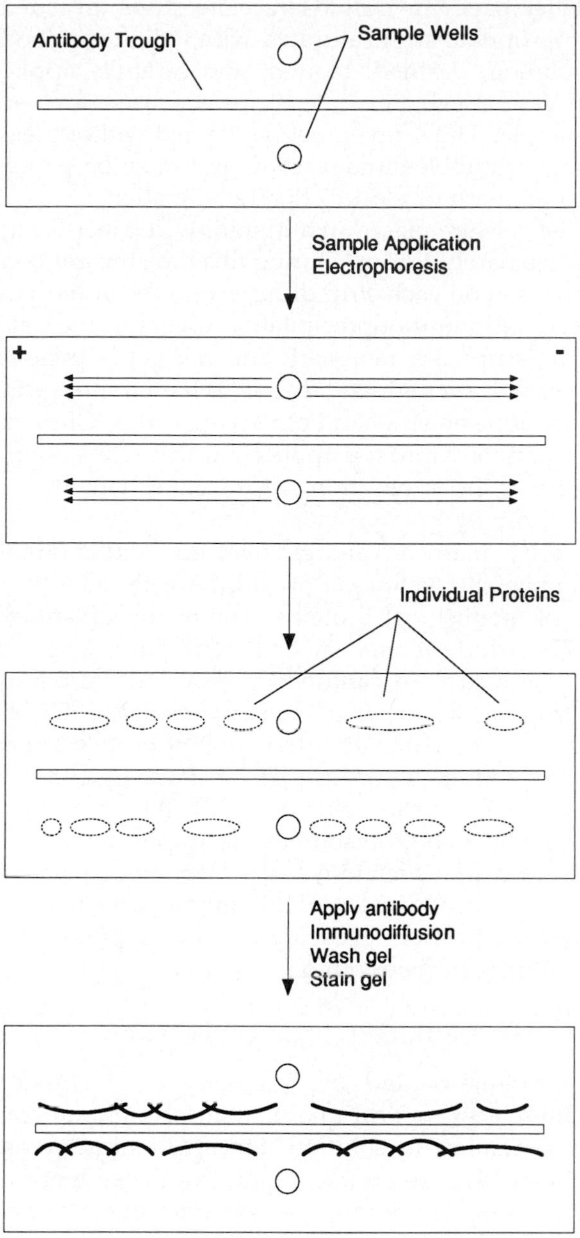

Figure 56.10. Theory and technique of immunoelectrophoresis. In immunoelectrophoresis, electrophoresis and immunodiffusion are sequentially applied to separate and identify protein antigens. The antigen is first applied to wells in an agarose or cellulose acetate gel, followed by electrophoresis. After electrophoretic separation of the proteins, an antibody solution is placed in the center trough, and immunodiffusion is allowed to occur. Arcs of immunoprecipitation indicate an antigen-antibody reaction. The gel is then washed and stained with a protein-specific dye to clarify the reaction pattern. In clinical practice, antibodies against human immunoglobulin heavy and light chain immunoglobulins are commonly used with immunoelectrophoresis to identify abnormal proteins.

in the equivalence region between each well and trough; and

5. The gel is stained, dried and visually inspected and interpreted.

During IEP, a separate precipitin arc is formed for each antigenic component against which a corresponding antibody is present. Patterns of identity, nonidentity, and partial identity are formed that are identical to those formed during Ouchterlony immunodiffusion and other immunodiffusion techniques. Although a complex pattern of arcs results if a polyspecific antiserum is utilized, monospecific antisera are usually employed for the identification of individual serum proteins. In the usual clinical laboratory application of IEP (the identification of monoclonal gammopathies), the aforementioned gel setup is customary.

The major advantages of IEP include small sample requirements, sensitivity, and specificity. However, the technique is time-consuming, labor-intense, and requires skill and experience to perform and interpret. In addition, the results are only semiquantitative, and are greatly affected by variations in the antigen-antibody ratio, antibody titer, and by the specificity, avidity, and affinity of the antisera utilized. Problems of antigen or antibody excess are most frequently encountered. Under conditions of antigen excess, the precipitin arc moves closer to the antibody trough, and becomes thickened and elongated. The precipitin arc often has a diffuse appearance on the trough side, and can even disappear in situations of extreme antigen excess, in which the precipitin reaction is in the prozone. With antibody excess, the precipitin arc moves closer to the antigen well, and assumes an increasingly diffuse appearance. A similar problem of indistinct precipitin arcs is encountered with a low antigen concentration, and in the presence of a weak antigen-antibody reaction.

Immunofixation Electrophoresis

Immunofixation electrophoresis (IFE, IFX) was introduced by Alper and Johnson for the identification of genetic variants of proteins, and was subsequently modified by Ritchie and Smith, and by Arnaud and collaborators (52–54). However, since IFE has many advantages over IEP for the identification of monoclonal proteins, it has achieved increasing utilization in the clinical laboratory in recent years (55–59).

IFE, like IEP, is a two-step procedure requiring electrophoretic separation of proteins followed by immunoprecipitation. However, in IFE the antibody is applied directly to the surface of the gel over the electrophoretically separated proteins, rather than in a trough parallel to the axis of electrophoretic migration (Fig 56.11). The technique is performed as follows:

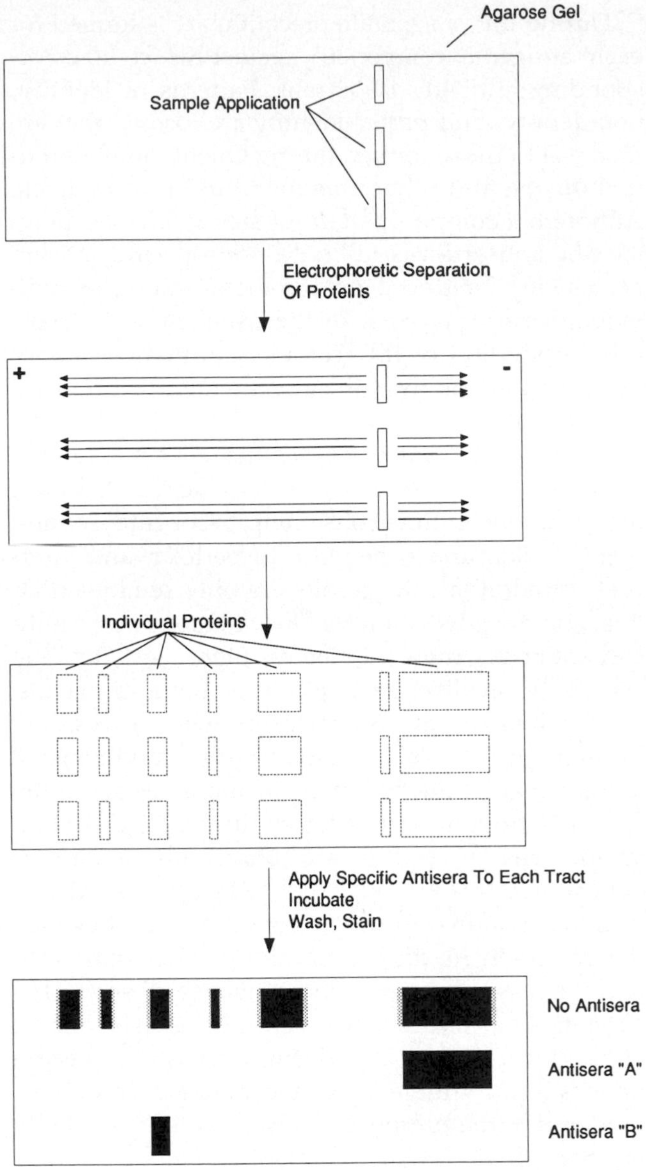

Figure 56.11. Technique of immunofixation electrophoresis. In this technique, strips of filter paper or cellulose acetate are soaked with antisera and placed on the surface of an agarose gel containing proteins first separated by electrophoresis. Immunodiffusion of the antisera into the agarose gel occurs, and a band of immunoprecipitation occurs at the site of each antigen-antibody reaction. The gel is washed and then stained with a protein-specific dye.

1. Samples are applied to agarose gel and separated electrophoretically, using conventional techniques. Protein solutions should be diluted to a concentration of 50–100 mg/dl before application. During application, each specimen must be clearly separated from the adjoining specimens to avoid cross-contamination, and care must be taken to place the electrodes so that the path of migration is parallel to the short axis of the gel. The gel must not be fixed after electrophoresis.
2. Filter paper or cellulose acetate strips are cut to appropriate size, saturated with a dilute antibody solution, drained, blotted, and carefully applied over the gel. Separate strips are used for each sample. The strips must be applied without leaving air bubbles underneath, and must be parallel to the path of electrophoretic migration.
3. The gels are placed in a humidity chamber for approximately 1 hour. During this time the antibody solution on each strip diffuses into the underlying gel, and immunoprecipitation occurs in the gel.
4. The strips are removed, and the gel is pressed, washed, stained, and dried. Each immunoprecipitate appears as a band of varying width. Diffusion of antibody into the application strips also occurs, so that the application strips can be stained.

IFE has many advantages over IEP, and is rapidly becoming the technique of choice for the identification of monoclonal proteins. The major advantages of IFE include its speed, high sensitivity, and relatively low cost. In conjunction with high-resolution electrophoresis and nephelometric analysis, IFE permits accurate, complete evaluation of protein abnormalities within hours instead of days. In addition, the precipitin bands obtained with IFE are directly comparable to high-resolution electrophoresis, which aids in the interpretation of electrophoretic patterns. The major disadvantage of IFE, in comparison to IEP, is that the precipitin reaction is more dependent on the antigen/antibody ratio.

Turbidimetry and Nephelometry

Turbidimetry and nephelometry are techniques for the electro-optical quantitation of immune complex formation in solution. Since turbidimetry and nephelometry are precise, rapid, automated methods of immunoquantitation, they are extensively utilized in the clinical laboratory for the quantitation of a large number of medically important substances.

LIGHT SCATTERING

The interaction of light with a particle can result in reflection, refraction, absorption, or scatter of the beam. When an immune complex is formed under carefully controlled conditions, measurement of these parameters can provide information regarding the quantity of antigen or antibody that is present. Turbidimetric techniques determine the reduction in the intensity of incident light from all interactions of an immune complex with a light beam, while nephelometric techniques measure light scattered at a specific angle to the incident beam. Although the ability of both systems to measure particles is highly dependent upon the design and quality of the optical

Condition	In $Ag_x^{(m)}\ Ab_y^{(2)}$	Result
Extreme antibody excess	$\frac{y}{x} \geq m$	No steps (2), (3)
Antibody excess	$m > \frac{y}{x} > \frac{m}{2}$	Scatter ↑ as $\frac{y}{x}$ ↓
Equivalence	$\frac{y}{x} = \frac{m}{2}$	Maximum scatter
Antigen excess	$\frac{m}{2} > \frac{y}{x} > \frac{1}{2}$	Scatter ↓ as $\frac{y}{x}$ ↓
Extreme antigen excess	$\frac{y}{x} < \frac{1}{2}$	No steps (2), (3)

Figure 56.12. Light scatter during immunoprecipitation. The initial antigen concentration (*x*), antibody concentration (*y*) and antigen valency (*m*) are denoted as indices for various regions of the "kinetic Heidelberger curve." The antibody concentration is fixed, and the antibody is assumed to have a valence of 2. The regions of the kinetic Heidelberger curve include: (1) Primary immunochemical formation of antigen-antibody complexes; (2) secondary immunochemical linking of complexes; and (3) rapid buildup of scattering centers due to subsequent hydrophobic and charge-based interactions among complexes. (Adapted with permission from Sternberg JC. Rate nephelometry. In: Rose HR, Friedman H, Fahey JL, eds. Manual of clinical laboratory immunology. 3rd ed. Washington, DC: American Society for Microbiology, 1986:34.)

and electronic instrumentation utilized, nephelometry is more sensitive to small particles than turbidimetry, while turbidimetry more accurately quantitates large complexes (60).

Thus, for the interaction of light of wavelength λ and intensity I_0 with a particle of polarizability α, the intensity of emitted radiation (I_θ) at distance *r* from the particle is defined by the following relationship:

$$I_\theta = \frac{8\pi^4\alpha^2 I_0}{\lambda^4 r^2}$$

There are several consequences of this relationship (60). For example, since light scatter is proportional to $1/\lambda^4$, blue light (λ 450 nm) is scattered more than red light (λ 650 nm). In addition, white light scattered at an angle of 90° appears blue, while transilluminated white light appears red because of removal of the blue wavelengths.

The formation of immunochemical aggregates, as depicted by the Heidelberger curve, involves the formation of small immune complexes through a primary immunochemical reaction, secondary interlinking of the complexes, and the tertiary formation of large aggregates through hydrophobic and charge-based interactions (61). Rayleigh scatter predominates during the primary and secondary immunochemical interactions, but large scatter complexes formed during the tertiary reaction may exceed the threshold for Rayleigh-Deybe scatter (Fig. 56.12).

In the region of antibody excess, light-scattering immune complexes form most rapidly during the first 20 seconds of the reaction (60). However, the formation of additional light-scattering complexes continues for several minutes, reaches a plateau (equilibrium phase), and then decreases as intraparticle destructive interactions occur, and an insoluble immunoprecipitate is formed. In conditions of antibody excess, both the peak rate of the formation of light-scattering complexes, and the amount of complexes that exist at the plateau region are dependent on the antigen concentration. "Endpoint" nephelometric or turbidimetric systems measure the curve at the plateau phase to determine antigen concentration, while "rate," or "kinetic" immunoprecipitation methods utilize the portion of the curve where the peak rate of reaction is maximal.

A problem faced by all quantitative immunoassay systems, but particularly by turbidimetric and nephelometric systems, is the symmetric shape of the Heidelberger curve. Thus, a constant mass of immune complex can represent two distinct concentrations of antigen, one in the antibody excess zone, and one in the region of antigen excess (61). In turbidimetry and nephelometry, this problem is avoided by measuring immune complex formation in the region of antibody excess. This permits the formation of complexes of a constant size and provides a reproducible, stoichiometric relationship between the number of complexes formed at a given antigen concentration (61).

In addition to antigen concentration, the formation of immune complexes is influenced by antibody avidity, ionic strength, pH, the presence of molecules with hydrophilic or hydrophobic properties, and the nature and concentration of anions (60). Antichaotropic ions with a high charge density (PO_4^{3-}, HPO_3^-, SO_4^{2-}) decrease solvation effects and promote immune complex formation, while chaotropic ions (SCN^-, ClO_4^-, NO_3^-) increase the availability of solvent ions and reduce immune complex formation. The use of polymers, such as dextran and the polyethylene glycols (PEG), to enhance immunoprecipitation was first reported by Hellsing and Laurent in 1964 and is commonly used in both turbidimetry and nephelometry (62). The immunoenhancing effect of polymers is probably due to steric exclusion, which has the effect of decreasing the solubility of protein molecules, driving the antigen-antibody interaction toward immune complex formation, increasing the slope of the antibody excess part of the precipitin curve, and displacing equivalence towards higher antigen concentrations (60). PEG with a molecular weight of 6000 daltons (PEG 6000) is one of the most effective immunoenhancers, leading to a markedly decreased reaction time and marked increases in peak rate (60). PEG also precipitates lipoproteins, leading to increased optical clarity and decreased background scattering.

TURBIDIMETRIC IMMUNOASSAYS

Turbidimetry has been used since the early 1950s as a method of quantitative analysis. In this technique, the reduction in light intensity caused by interaction of a light beam with a suspension of particles is determined spectrophotometrically. The ratio of the incident and transmitted light is determined and expressed in absorbance units (*A*):

$$A = 2 - \log_{10} \cdot T$$

where T is the percent turbidity. In the clinical laboratory, the major advantage of turbidimetry is that it can be performed with automated spectrophotometers, centrifugal analyzers, and other common, multipurpose instruments. The major disadvantage of turbidimetry is the requirement for a relatively high particle concentration, and the relatively small change in light intensity caused by particle absorbance. As a result, optical quality and alignment are extremely important for accurate turbidimetric quantitation, and the results can be affected by extraneous factors, such as the presence of dust or dirt particles. Light with a wavelength in the near-ultraviolet (290 to 410 nm) is usually utilized for illumination, while the photodetector must be aligned with the incidence source, and detect light over a narrow angle (63). The optical clarity of the reagents and the reaction cuvettes or cells is important, and the system must be able to rapidly mix reagents for analysis. The antisera must have high avidity and specificity, and show optical clarity. The IgG fraction is generally the most suitable for turbidimetric analysis. An immunoenhancer, such as dextran or polyethylene glycol, is frequently added to the reaction mixture to facilitate immune complex formation, and this must not cause turbidity when mixed with the antisera. The presence of turbid substances (i.e., chylomicrons and other lipoproteins, endogenous immune complexes, monoclonal proteins, etc.) in the samples is a problem that is difficult to compensate with reagent blanks or other means.

NEPHELOMETRIC IMMUNOASSAYS

Nephelometric techniques have been applied very successfully to the immunochemical measurement of specific proteins, drugs, and other substances (60, 64). In nephelometry, a known amount of specific antibody is added to a solution containing the antigen being measured. The intensity of light scattered from the large antigen-antibody complexes formed during the reaction is measured, and the rate signal is transmitted to a microcomputer, where concentration units are determined.

Techniques of rate nephelometry are almost exclusively utilized in commercial nephelometers for clinical laboratory applications. In rate nephelometry, a fixed antibody concentration is utilized, and measurements of light scatter are made under conditions of antibody excess region, where antigen concentration can be determined from measurements of light scatter. The course of a nephelometric reaction has the complex shape shown in Fig. 56.13. A small amount of Rayleigh scatter is initially present, and this increases slightly when the sample, and then the antisera are added. Scatter intensity then undergoes a sigmoidal increase with the progression of primary and secondary immunochemical reactions and the formation of large scattering centers. There is no real endpoint, but the scatter intensity gradually reaches a maximum and then decreases as large complexes settle out. The reaction conditions are adjusted so that the maximum rate (scatter versus time) occurs during the first minute of the immunochemical reaction.

Commercial nephelometric systems monitor scatter and the rate of change of scatter at a forward angle of 70° in a stirred reaction cell. The reaction is performed in a phosphate-buffered saline solution, and polyethylene glycol is used as an immunoenhancer. Other nephelometric systems, including a particle-enhanced turbidimetric inhibition immunoassay (PETINIA), have been described. PETINIA is a competitive binding assay utilizing hapten-coated latex particles. Agglutination, measured by a change in turbidity at 340 nm, is inhibited by binding of the unlabeled hapten to the antibody (65).

LIGAND IMMUNOASSAYS

General Principles of Ligand Assays

A ligand is a substance that will bind to another substance. In a ligand assay, one component of the reaction ("label," "tracer") is tagged in some manner, so that the reaction can be measured. The substance to be measured (ligand, analyte, or hapten) can be an immunoglobulin, drug, tumor marker, hormone, infectious agent, autoantigen, lipoprotein, oncoprotein, or other substance. The substance that binds the ligand (binding substrate) is usually an antibody (immunoassay), but can be a receptor (receptor assay), carrier protein (protein-binding assay), or any substance that specifically binds the ligand with a high affinity. The labeled reagent can exist in a solubilized form, or it can be immobilized (bound) to a solid surface such as a test tube, the sides of the wells of a microtitration plate, a latex particle, or a plastic bead. In addition to the analysis of soluble substances in body fluids, the principle of ligand

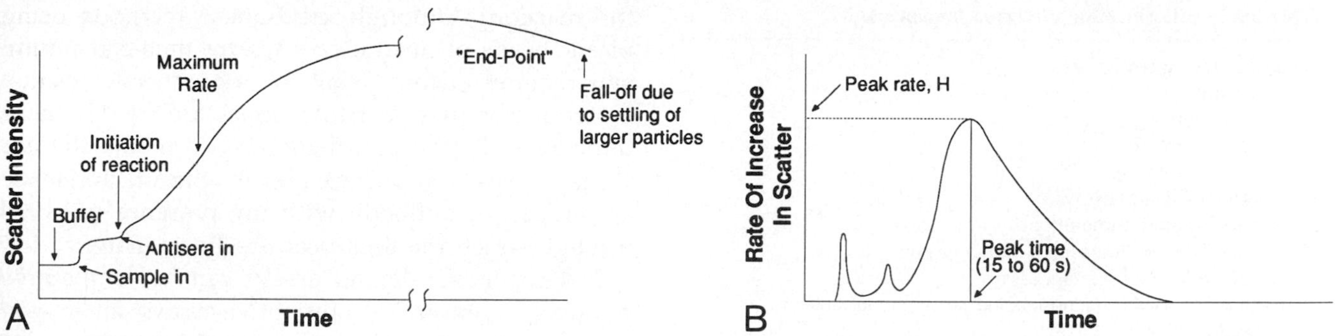

Figure 56.13. Time course of the nephelometric signal produced during an immunoprecipitation reaction. **A**, Variation in the *t* versus time. **B**, Rate of increase of scatter versus time. (Reprinted with permission from Sternberg JC. Rate nephelometry. In: Rose NR, Friedman H, Fahey JL, eds. Manual of clinical laboratory immunology. 3rd ed. Washington, DC: American Society for Microbiology, 1986:34.)

analysis is also utilized in tissue-based assays such as direct and indirect immunofluorescence, flow cytometry, and immunoperoxidase staining.

Kinetic Aspects of Ligand Analysis

The amount of ligand that binds to a substrate is defined by the number of binding sites and by the affinity of the binding substrate. The affinity is the sum of the strength of the hydrogen binding, van der Waals forces, ionic interactions, and other forces which influence the reaction. Thus, by the law of mass action,

$$Ag + Ab \underset{K_2}{\overset{K_1}{\rightleftharpoons}} Ag{\cdot}Ab$$

where K_1 and K_2 are the equilibrium constants for the reaction.

At equilibrium, the rates of the forward and reverse reactions are equal ($K_1 = K_2$) and the proportions of bound and unbound ligand become constant. The equilibrium constant (K_a) for this reaction is represented by the equation:

$$K_a = \frac{K_1}{K_2} = \frac{(Ag{\cdot}Ab)}{(Ag)(Ab)}$$

When 50% of the binding sites are occupied, K_a is equal to the reciprocal of the free ligand concentration. K_a is expressed in liters per mole or moles per liter^{-1} and has a magnitude in the range of 10^7 to 10^{11}liters/mole in most clinical laboratory assays.

Multiple ligand assays are utilized in the clinical laboratory for the quantitation of a wide variety of substances of medical importance. Basically, these assays differ in the labeling substance (radioisotope, enzyme, fluorescent dye, chemiluminescence precursor, bioluminescent substance, metal atom, bacteriophage, liposome, metal sols, latex particles, etc.), binding substrate (antibody, receptor, transport protein), reaction kinetics (reagent excess, competitive binding), and the requirement for separation of the free and bound label (heterogeneous, homogeneous).

Unfortunately, the diversity of methodology has led to practical problems in the classification and nomenclature of the ligand assay systems (66). By convention, the type of label appears first in competitive assays (i.e., radioimmunoassay, radioreceptor assay), while the binding substrate appears first in the name of a reagent excess assay (i.e., immunoradiometric assay). All reagent excess antigen assays utilizing an antibody-binding substrate can be referred to as immunometric assays. The acronym ELISA (enzyme-linked immunosorbent assay) is commonly, and incorrectly, utilized to refer to all types of enzyme immunoassays and immunoenzymometric assays. The classification system utilized below (Table 56.2) is based on the classic differentiation of heterogenous and homogenous assays and a new classification system proposed by Gosling (1990) (66).

Heterogenous Ligand Assays

Heterogenous ligand assays require physical separation of the free label from the label bound to the substrate. Techniques for this purpose rely on differences in the size or chemical composition of the bound and free label. The development of techniques that allow complete separation of the bound and free components has been one of the most challenging aspects of ligand assay techniques. In general, the relatively nonspecific separation methods utilized in the past (adsorption, chemical precipitation) have been replaced by more specific techniques (immune precipitation, solid-phase techniques).

Adsorption is based on the difference in size between the free label and the label-substrate complex. Porous materials (charcoal, silica, ion exchange

Table 56.2. Classification of Ligand Immunoassays

Heterogeneous ligand assays
Competitive
Noncompetitive
Antigen capture
Antibody capture
Homogeneous ligand assays
Enzyme-multiplied immunoassays
Substrate-labeled fluorescent immunoassay
Coenzyme labeled immunoassays
Immunoassays with ligand-labeled prosthetic groups and ligand-labeled modulators
Enzyme-enhancement immunoassay
Enzyme immunochromatography
Fluorescence polarization immunoassay

resins, sephadex, etc.) adsorb small molecules (free label) but not larger particles (label-substrate complex). The adsorbent, with attached free label, can be removed from the reaction mixture by centrifugation or other techniques, leaving the substrate in the supernatant. In practice, a mixture of charcoal and cross-linked dextran is the most widely utilized adsorbent. The dextran prevents nonspecific adsorption of protein and also determines the size of the free label that can be adsorbed. The properties of the adsorbing particles such as sephadex can be also modified to maximize the specificity of the separation process. Chemical agents (ammonium sulfate, ethanol, sodium sulfate, polyethylene glycol) alter the solubility of proteins in solution, causing precipitation. Following centrifugation, the free label remains in the supernatant, where it can be measured. The action of these agents is nonspecific, since both free and bound proteins are precipitated. Immune precipitation ("second antibody," "double antibody") methods utilize a precipitating antibody specific for the primary antibody. Insoluble complexes are produced that can be removed by centrifugation, leaving the free label. These methods are similar to chemical precipitation in that all free and bound (labeled and unlabeled) substrate is removed from the reaction mixture. In solid-phase separation, either the ligand or primary antibody is immobilized to an inert physical surface. Since the antigen-antibody reaction occurs on the surface, the free and bound ligand can easily be separated. A variety of imaginative solid-phase methods have been devised, first utilizing coated paper or polystyrene (test tubes, beads, microtiter trays, paddles, etc.), and more recently membranes (nitrocellulose, nylon, polymers). The major requirements for solid-phase immobilization are complete and uniform coating of the surface and linkage of the antigen or antibody to the solid phase by a technique that neither alters binding interactions nor permits spontaneous release during the reaction. Although solid-phase methods using plastic beads or microtiter trays are time-consuming and require technical skill for reproducible results, most membrane-based techniques are free of these difficulties. Permeable membranes combine the advantages of a large surface area for the attachment of an antigen or antibody with the presence of pores through which the liquid can freely circulate.

Heterogeneous ligand assays can be competitive or noncompetitive. In competitive assays, a constant amount of binding substrate and labeled ligand is utilized, and the amount of unlabeled ligand is the variable that is measured (Fig. 56.14). The labeled ligand is present in relatively large quantities, and a smaller amount of unlabeled ligand is allowed to compete for the available binding sites. The larger the quantity of unlabeled ligand present, the more labeled ligand will be displaced from the binding substrate. Following separation, the amount of free or bound labeled ligand can be determined.

Noncompetitive (reagent excess) assays are usually of the "sandwich" type, in which either an antigen or antibody is immobilized to an inert support. "Antigen capture" assays require an immobilized antibody. The analyte or ligand control is added and binds to the available substrate sites. Labeled antibody is then added, and a sandwich is formed with the antigen in the middle. Following a wash step to remove unbound labeled antibody, the bound antibody is measured, and is directly proportional to the quantity of unlabeled antigen present. The "antibody capture" is similar, but requires a ligand linked to the solid phase. Following reaction with an antibody-containing specimen or control, and a wash step to remove unbound antibody, the presence of bound antibody is detected by the use of labeled antihuman globulin. The amount of bound label is directly proportional to the quantity of specific antibody (Fig. 56.15).

Homogeneous Ligand Assays

Homogeneous ligand assays do not require separation of the free and bound fractions. Many of these assays have grown in popularity in the clinical laboratory in recent years because of their speed, sensitivity, and overall technical simplicity. There are numerous types of homogeneous ligand assays utilizing enzyme and fluorescent labels. Examples include the enzyme-multiplied immunoassay technique (EMIT), enzyme immunochromatography, substrate-labeled fluorescent immunoassay (SLFIA), and fluorescent polarization immunoassay (FPIA). These and other homogeneous ligand assays are described in the sections below.

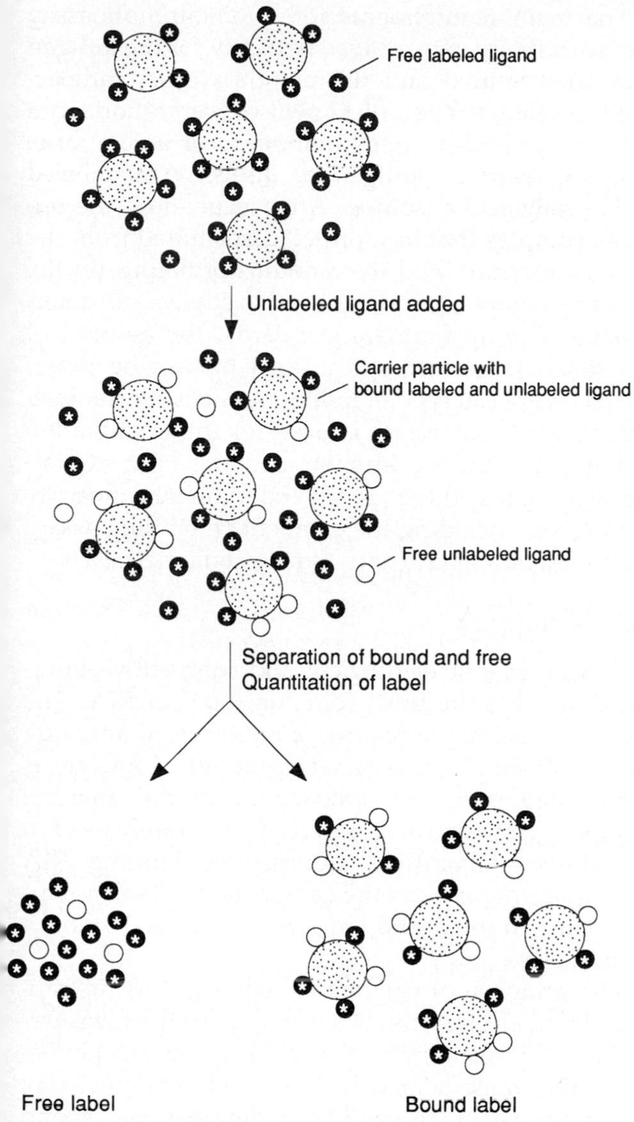

Figure 56.14. Principle of competitive binding immunoassays. An unlabeled ligand is added to a mixture containing measured amounts of free labeled ligand and carrier particles with bound labeled ligand. The label is usually a monoclonal antibody or a radioactive isotope. Displacement of some of the bound labeled ligand by the unlabeled ligand results in a mixture of free labeled ligand, free unlabeled ligand, and carrier particles with labeled and unlabeled ligand. The carrier particles are then separated from the mixture, and the amount of free or carrier-bound ligand is determined by the appropriate assay procedure. If standard curves are prepared using known amounts of unlabeled ligand, the amount of analyte in an unknown solution can be determined from the curves.

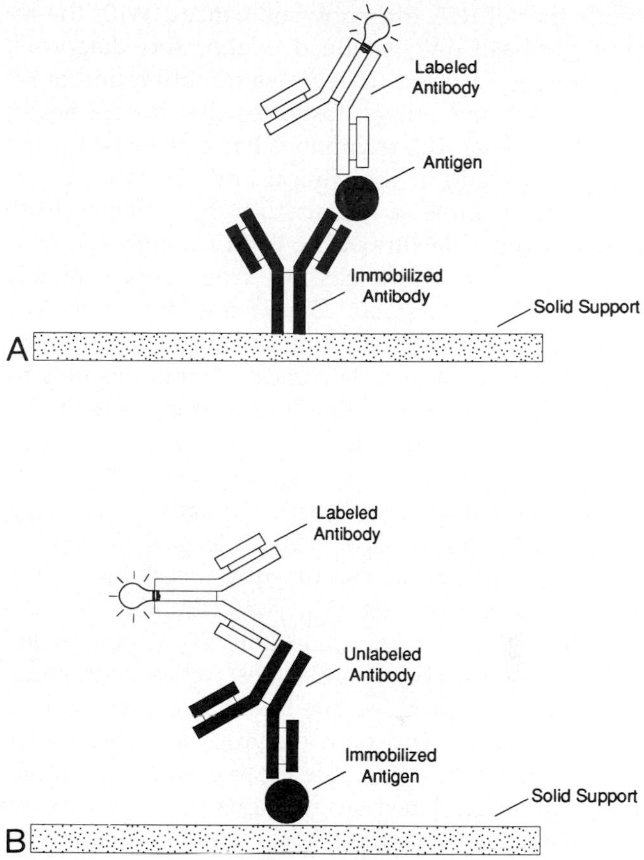

Figure 56.15. Principle of noncompetitive immunoassays. **A**, Antigen capture. **B**, Antibody capture. Antigen capture assays utilize an antibody immobilized to an inert support (usually a plastic test tube or plastic microtiter tray). Antigen (control ligand or analyte) is added, and an immune complex forms on the inert support. After incubation and washing, a labeled antibody specific for the antigen is added. The reaction mixture is incubated, washed, and the amount of bound antibody is measured. The concentration of analyte in an unknown solution can be determined from a standard curve prepared with known amounts of antigen. In antibody capture assays, a similar principle is used to measure the concentration of an antibody.

Isotopic and Nonisotopic Labels

The choice of "label" is one of the most important considerations in ligand assays. In this regard, the sensitivity of the assay is largely dependent upon the specific activity (number of detectable events per label molecule per unit time) of the label. However, other factors, such as the ease and sensitivity of detection, freedom from background activity or environmental influences, ease of conjugation to a ligand, cost, and other factors are important.

Since the introduction of the radioimmunoassay 30 years ago, ^{125}I and other radioactive nuclides have been widely utilized as labels in immunoassay procedures. The popularity of radioisotopes as a label has grown because of their sensitivity, measurement precision, lack of background, and freedom from environmental influences. However, these compounds are expensive, pose a significant health risk to the laboratory technologist, require special handling and disposal, and have a limited shelf life. In addition, specialized, expensive instrumentation is required for the measurement of radioactivity, automation is difficult, licensing is required, and strict compliance with national, state, and local laws is required for their use (67). Fortunately, the sensitivity of the nonisotopic label immunoassays approaches or exceeds that of RIA for many substances. With the recent emphasis on cost-effective laboratory diagnosis, and the urgent need to decrease the utilization of radioisotopes and other substances that pose a health risk, the use of RIA techniques has decreased during the past decade in the clinical and research laboratory. For example, a recent study by Gosling (1990) (66) showed a decline in the use of radioisotopes as labels in new immunoassays from approximately 50% in 1980 to a stable 25% in the late 1980s. The major reason for the continued use of the radioimmunoassay in large-scale clinical laboratories may be the widespread belief that these assays are inherently stable and have low between-assay variability (66).

The advantages and disadvantages of radioisotopes with nonisotopic labels (enzymes, fluorochromes, chemiluminescent substances) have been studied extensively (68–72). For example, ^{125}I has a specific activity of one detectable event per second per 7.5×10^6 labeled molecules, while chemiluminescent labels produce one detectable event per labeled molecule, and both enzymes and fluorescent labels can produce many detectable events per molecule. Although detection problems limit the superior sensitivity of fluorescent and chemiluminescent labels, newer methods of application have resolved many of these problems. In one comparative review of the sensitivity of various commercial methods for the detection of serum thyrotropin, the time-resolved fluorescence immunoassay technique appeared to have the highest sensitivity (0.02 mIU/liter), followed by enhanced luminescence immunoassay (0.04 mIU/liter), enzyme immunoassay (0.1 mIU/liter), immunoradiometric assay (0.02–0.25 mIU/liter), and radioimmunoassay (0.7 mIU/liter) (67). The search continues for even more sensitive methods that are cost-effective and can easily be applied in a clinical laboratory setting.

Radioimmunoassay

RIA techniques are among the most sensitive laboratory procedures available. As a result, RIA has been the principal method for the detection of substances that are present in very low concentration in biological fluid (10^{-6}–10^{-9} g/ml). In clinical medicine, the radioimmunoassay was introduced in 1960 by Yalow and Berson for the measurement of plasma insulin levels (73). It was quickly applied to the measurement of other peptide hormones, and has subsequently been used for the determination of hundreds of substances, including drugs and toxins, infectious agents, tumor antigens, tissue peptides, and other substances.

The main requirements for a radioimmunoassay are an antibody with a high specificity for the antigen being determined and the use of a pure, radioactively labeled antigen of known concentration. In a radioimmunoassay, one component of an immune complex reaction (antigen or antibody) is labeled with a radioactive isotope. After incubation, the immune complex that has formed is separated from the reaction mixture, and the amounts of bound (in the immune complex) and free radioactivity are determined. With appropriate standards, the amount of the substance under study (analyte) can be determined. A special type of radioimmunoassay (radioallergosorbent technique) is used for the quantitation of antigens that are immunoglobulins. For nonimmunoglobulins, there are several radioimmunoassay techniques, including the competitive binding assay, excess-reagent assay, and immunoradiometric assay.

RIA Techniques

Excess-reagent (sandwich) and competitive binding assays are the most common types of RIA. The sandwich technique requires a radiolabeled antibody that is utilized in excess. The amount of analyte is determined from the radioactivity in the immune complex. This type of RIA procedure is rarely used in the clinical laboratory. Competitive binding RIA techniques depend on the competition between radiolabeled and unlabeled antigen for a limited amount of antibody.

The principle of competitive binding was first applied in an electrophoretic technique for the measurement of thyroxine in human plasma, but quickly became the most widely utilized radioimmunoassay technique (74). Competitive binding assays depend on the competition between radiolabeled and unlabeled antigen for the binding sites on a limited amount of antibody. In this procedure the unlabeled analyte is allowed to compete with a highly purified radiolabeled antigen (radiolabeled ligand) for binding to a limited amount of antibody, under conditions of antigen excess. After incubation under appropriate conditions, the antibody-bound (B) and unbound (free, F) analytes are separated and the amount of radioactivity is determined in each. These values are used to calculate the ratio of bound to free analyte (B/F). The more unlabeled analyte present, the lower the B/F ratio, since more labeled analyte will be displaced from the antibody. A sigmoidal curve results if the B/F ration is plotted against the ligand concentration. This is usually avoided by plotting the logit against the log of the ligand concentration. The logit is calculated by the following equation:

$$\frac{Y}{1 - Y}$$

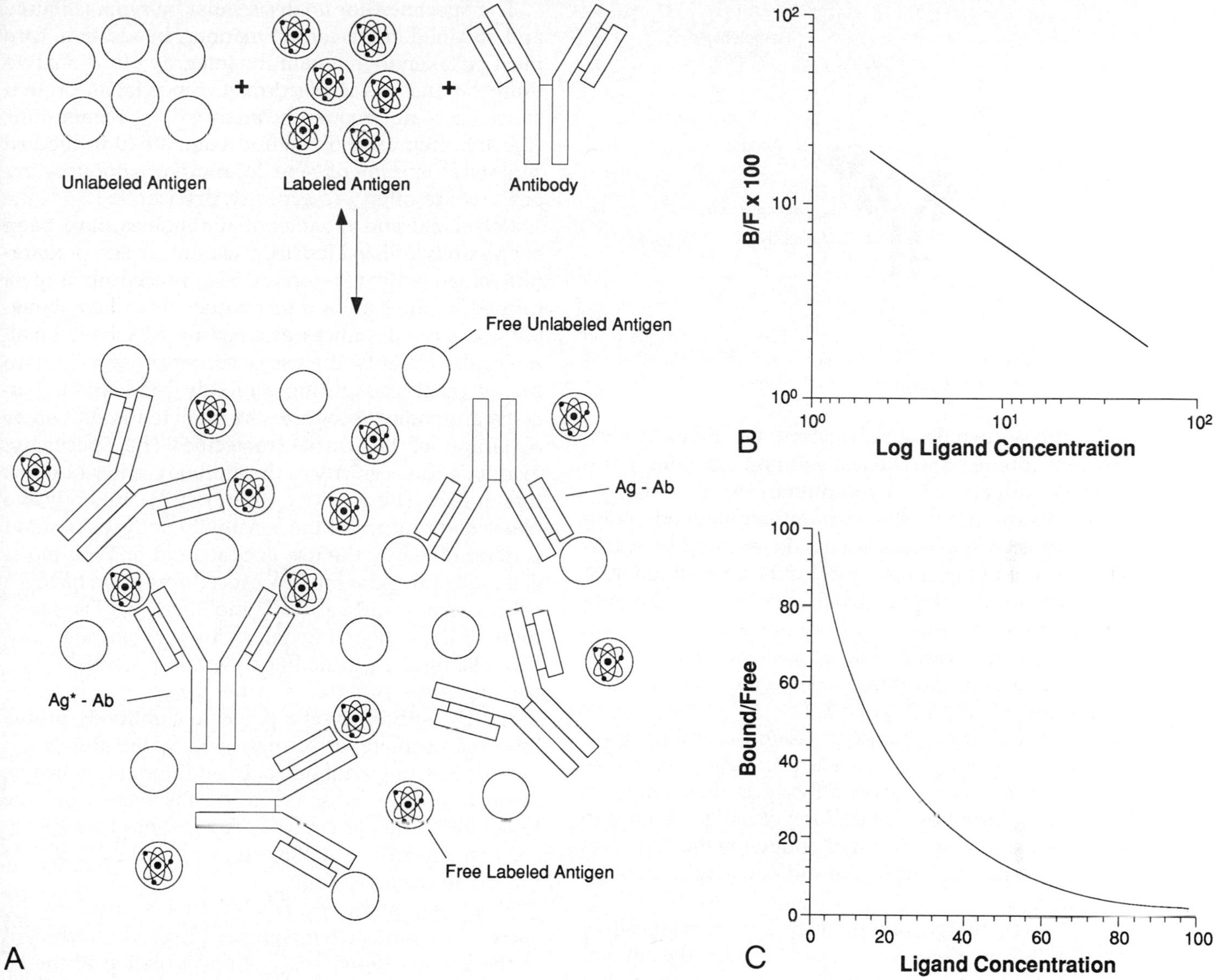

Figure 56.16. Radioimmunoassay by competitive binding. **A**, Schematic illustration of the theory of competitive binding. **B**, Graphic analysis by logit plot. **C**, Graphic analysis by a plot of B/F vs. ligand concentration.

where

$$Y = \frac{B/F}{B_0/F_0}$$

where B is the counts per minute of bound radioligand, F is the counts per minute of free radioligand, B_0 is the counts per minute of bound ligand determined in a system with no unlabeled ligand (zero value), and F_0 is the counts per minute of free radioligand in a system with no unlabeled ligand (Fig. 56.16).

In practice, the concentration of an unknown analyte is determined by reference to a standard curve prepared from the reaction of a serially diluted solution of purified unlabeled antigen. It is necessary that the unknown specimen be analyzed under precisely the same conditions as the standard curve.

The labeled and unlabeled antigen are not required to be chemically or biologically identical, but must follow the law of mass action.

A similar principle of competitive binding is also utilized in the radioreceptor assay. In the radioreceptor assay, the receptor is not an antibody, but a purified preparation of a circulating binding protein (thyroid binding globulin, cortisol binding protein, intrinsic or for vitamin B_{12}, etc.), membrane receptor, or cytoplasmic receptor.

The excess reagent, ("two-site," "double-antibody") radioimmunoassay is a "sandwich" technique in which two antibodies are utilized in excess. One antibody, which is unlabeled, is attached to a

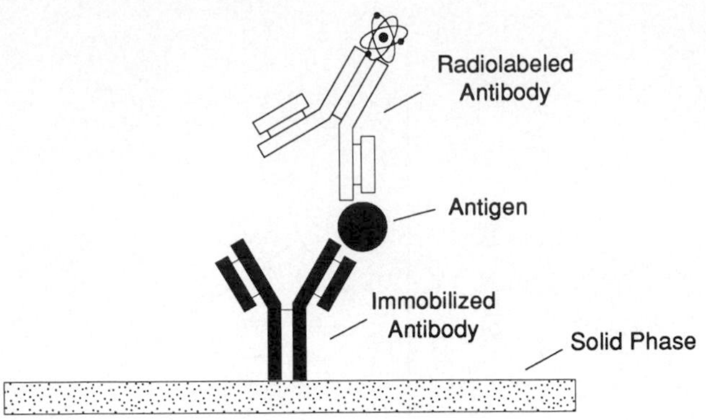

Figure 56.17. "Principle of "sandwich" RIA. This technique is an antigen capture immunoassay in which a radiolabeled antibody is used to measure the concentration of an antigen.

solid phase (usually a polystyrene test tube) by electrostatic interaction. The test solution, containing unlabeled antigen (with two antibody binding sites) is added to the tube, where an antigen-antibody complex forms. After excess antigen is removed by washing, the second (radiolabeled) antibody is added, and the formation of the sandwich is completed. Following another washing step to remove unlabeled antibody, the amount of bound radioactivity is measured, and is proportional to the amount of antigen in the test solution (Fig. 56.17).

In the immunoradiometric assay, the antigen is reacted in the liquid phase with an excess of radiolabeled antibody. Excess antibody is then removed from the solution by the addition of antigen bound to a solid phase. The amount of antigen in the test solution is determined from the radioactivity remaining in solution.

The radioallergosorbent technique is a sensitive method for the detection of specific antibodies in biological fluids. It is a sandwich technique utilizing a purified antigen bound to a solid support. The immobilized antigen is incubated with the test solution, resulting in the formation of an immune complex on the solid support. The formation of the sandwich is completed by the addition of radiolabeled antiglobulin, and the amount of bound radioactivity is determined after a final wash. Under these circumstances, the measured radioactivity is directly proportional to the amount of antibody present.

Practical Considerations in RIA Analysis

The major considerations in an RIA are an antibody with a high specificity for the analyte being determined, a highly purified, radioactively labeled preparation of the analyte, and an efficient method for separating antibody-bound and free components after the reaction. Other considerations include specimen adequacy, measurement of radioactivity, and the appropriate utilization of standards.

The specimen for analysis must be representative and obtained in the correct manner. In addition, care must be taken to maintain the integrity of the analyte until the analysis is performed. Since labile protein substances are frequently analyzed, specimens for RIA are often centrifuged and maintained in the frozen state. Specimens sent to another laboratory for analysis are often preserved in dry ice.

Polyclonal and monoclonal antibodies have been successfully utilized in RIA procedures. The preparation of an antibody for an RIA procedure is performed by the standard techniques described above. Since many substances assayed by RIA have small molecular weights, the use of carrier proteins is commonly employed during antibody production, and some antibodies recognize the analyte in addition to a portion of the carrier molecule. The specificity, avidity, and specificity of the antibody are critical factors in RIA. The avidity (affinity) of the antibody is a major determinant of the sensitivity of the assay, and is determined by the use of Scatchard or Wolf plots. Generally, antisera for RIA procedures must have Ka values between 10^{-2} and 10^{-9} mol/liter (75). The sensitivity of the antibody is determined by binding studies utilizing the purified analyte and potential cross-reacting substances at a wide range of concentrations. The specificity of a polyclonal antibody preparation can sometimes be improved by the absorption of cross-reacting antibodies. In addition, steps can be taken to remove cross-reacting substances from the test solution before analysis. An antisera titer is chosen (usually 1:105 to 1:106) that will bind 30 to 50% of the labeled analyte (75).

The preparation of a labeled analyte involves the choice of a radioactive isotope, physical attachment of the isotope to the analyte, and isolation of the labeled analyte in a highly purified form. The choice of radiolabel depends on its ease of conjugation, specific activity, radioactive half-life, and emission characteristics. The specific activity (activity per unit weight of isotope) determines the amount of radiolabeled ligand that must be present to produce an adequate sensitivity. The half-life of the radioisotope must be sufficient to give an adequate shelf life. Generally, ^{125}I is utilized as a label for proteins, peptides, and hormones, since it has a relatively long half-life (60 days), emits a large number of disintegrations per minute, and emits γ radiation of relatively low energy. ^{3}H is often utilized to label steroids, but its long half-life, β emission, and relatively low number of disintegrations per minutes are disadvantages. Other radioisotopes used in RIA include ^{14}C and ^{131}I. For the measurement of vitamin B_{12}, ^{57}Co or ^{60}Co is used to substitute for the cobalt that is naturally present. The characteristics of these radioisotopes are listed in Table 56.3.

Table 56.3. Properties of Selected Radioisotopes Used in Patient Care[a]

			Beta Emission				
				Energy (MeV)		Gamma Emission	
Element	Isotope	Half-life	Abund %	Max	Mean	Abund %	Energy (MeV)
Hydrogen	^{3}H	12.3 a	100%	0.0186	0.0057	None	—
Carbon	^{14}C	5730 a	100%	0.1561	0.0493	None	—
Phosphorus	^{32}P	14.3 d	100%	1.710	0.6948	None	—
Chromium	^{51}C	27.8 d	ec-1	—	—	9	0.3198
			ec-2	—	—		
Iron	^{59}Fe	45 d	53	0.4750	0.1527	56	1.0950
			45	0.02730	0.0808	43	1.2920
			1.1	0.1300	0.0355	2.8	0.1925
Cobalt	^{57}Co	270 d	ec-1	—	—	89.2	0.0144
			ec-2	—	—	89.0	0.1219
						11.0	0.1363
Cobalt	^{60}Co	5.26 d	99.8%	0.313	0.0941	100	1.3325
						99.8	1.1732
Technetium	^{99m}Tc	6.0 h		Isometric level decay		98.6	0.0022
						98.6	0.1405
						1.4	0.1427
Iodine	^{125}I	60 d	ec	—	—	100	0.0355
Iodine	^{131}I	8.05 d	90.4	0.0606	0.1917	85.3	0.3645
			6.9	0.33	0.0955	6.9	0.6370
			1.6	0.25	0.0701	5.1	0.0802
						5.1	0.2843
						1.6	0.7229
Cesium	^{137}Cs	30.0 a	93.5	0.514	0.1749	93.5	0.6616
			6.5	1.176	0.4272		

[a]From Holden NE, Walker FW. Chart of the nuclides. 10th ed. U.S. Atomic Energy Commission, 1968.

Chemical methods are utilized to attach the radiolabel to the analyte. It is essential that this be done in such a way as to achieve a uniformly labeled product with maximal utilization of the reactants, and with minimal chemical damage to the analyte. For peptides and proteins containing tyrosine residues and labeled with ^{125}I, an iodination reaction catabolized by lactoperoxidase or chloramine-T is often used (75). Lactoperoxidase catalyzes the reaction of H_2O_2 and $Na^{125}I$ to form active iodine (I^+), which in turn reacts with the tyrosyl residue of proteins. Chloramine-T is a derivative of ρ-toluene sulfonamide that produces a similar incorporation of iodine into the aromatic ring of tyrosine. Enzymatic iodination with lactoperoxidase is preferable because it causes fewer reactions with other amino acid residues than chloramine-T. A conjugation method utilizing an iodinated ester is utilized to label proteins lacking tyrosine residues.

Once the labeling process has taken place, the labeled analyte is separated from free label and from damaged analyte by chromatographic or electrophoretic procedures. The product is thoroughly evaluated for nonspecific binding and immunoreactivity under a number of conditions (75). In addition, a high specific activity (large amount of radioisotope per quantity of analyte) is desirable. The specific activity is commonly expressed as microcuries per microgram (μCi/μg) or disintegrations per minute per micromole (dpm/μM). For routine RIA procedures, an amount of label producing 10,000 to 25,000 dpm per assay tube (generally 0.01 μCi) is used, although maximum sensitivity is achieved with a high-affinity antibody and minimal quantities of label (often producing only 1,000 to 2,000 dpm/tube) (75).

Separation of the free and bound analyte is the least precise part of the radioimmunoassay. Since the antigen-antibody complex is larger than the free antigen, this size difference is the basis of most separation methods. Although a variety of separation methods have been employed, solid-phase separation, immunoprecipitation, and chemical precipitation are the most widely used. Absorption with dextran-coated charcoal particles is a solid-phase separation technique that is commonly employed in the RIA analysis of steroids and many other substances (76). In this technique, the smaller unbound antigen particles are bound, while the larger complexes remain in the supernatant. Unfortunately, it is difficult to prepare a uniform suspension of charcoal particles for pipetting, and the absorption process can be interfered with by ionic factors, protein concentrations, and many other factors. Adsorption with silicates and chalk has also been utilized. Chemical substances such as saturated ammonium sulfate solution, ethanol, or polyethylene glycol (Carbowax) precipitate the antigen-antibody complex, which can be removed from the reaction mixture by centrifugation

(77). Immunoprecipitation (double-antibody precipitation) methods utilize an antibody (secondary antibody) from a different animal species, which is directed against epitopes of the antibody (primary antibody) binding the analyte. Under the proper reaction conditions and antibody concentrations, precipitates are formed that can be separated by centrifugation, electrophoresis, or chromatography (sephadex, polyacrylamide, ion-exchange). Although simple in theory, in practice it is difficult to achieve precision with immunoprecipitation. A combination of immunoprecipitation and chemical separation with polyethylene glycol has been used to increase turn-around time in RIA testing. Recently, coated magnetized particles have been successfully utilized in some assays.

Enzyme Immunoassay

The enzyme immunoassay (EIA) is a type of nonisotopic immunoassay in which enzymes, coenzymes, fluorigenic substrates, or enzyme inhibitors are used as labels (78).

Enzymes are utilized as labels in both heterogeneous and homogeneous assay systems and are used to assay both antigens and antibodies. The major prerequisite is that the antigen or antibody must be linked to an enzyme or other nonisotopic label without destroying the immunologic or enzymatic activity of the antigen-antibody complex. In addition, in heterogeneous enzyme immunoassays requiring a solid phase, the antigen or antibody under study must be attached to the solid-phase support in a manner that does not alter immunologic activity.

Enzymes utilized in immunoassay systems must be stable, available in a highly purified state, have a high turnover rate, undergo minimal interference by substances likely to be in the test solution, and be specific for the substrate. The final reaction product should be detected by a convenient means with a low detection limit. The most widely utilized enzyme in enzyme immunoassay is horseradish peroxidase (HRP). The substrate of HRP is hydrogen peroxide (H_2O_2), and the product is oxygen. This oxygen produced during the reaction is used to oxidize a reduced, colorless chromogen (usually reduced orthophenylenediame, OPD). The final product, oxidized OPD, has a brown color. Gosling found horseradish peroxidase to be presently utilized as a label in approximately 50% of new assays, while alkaline phosphatase was used in about 25% (66). Glucose oxidase, β-D-galactosidase, and a wide variety of other enzymes have also been used. Utilizing fluorimetric techniques, the respective detection limits for HRP, β-galactosidase, and alkaline phosphatase were 5, 0.2, and 10 amol. Utilizing alkaline phosphatase in an amplified immunoassay system with colorimetric detection, Johannsson et al. (79) reported a detection limit of 0.01 amol. In this amplified technique, $NADP^+$ was used as the substrate for alkaline phosphatase, and the product (NAD^+) served as the coenzyme for a secondary dehydrogenase enzyme present in excess. Since hundreds of NAD^+ molecules are produced by alkaline phosphatase, and each NAD^+ molecule can serve as the enzyme for hundreds of dehydrogenase reactions, the original reaction is greatly amplified. Ishikawa et al. reported a new technique (immune complex transfer enzyme immunoassay) that permitted the detection of 0.02 amol of TSH (80).

In addition to horseradish peroxidase, alkaline phosphatase and other enzymes have been employed in immunoassay (Fig. 56.18).

The coupling of an enzyme to an antibody or protein antigen must be performed in a manner that minimally alters immunoreactivity and enzyme activity. In addition, the coupling reaction must result in efficient incorporation of the label, and the conjugate should be stable, with a long shelf life (78). Chemical reactions resulting in the activation of a carboxyl group are commonly utilized for the formation of hapten-enzyme conjugates. The mixed anhydride, carbodiimide, and *N*-hydroxysuccinimide ester coupling methods utilize this reaction. Other methods of hapten-enzyme coupling include periodate cleavage, or the use of heterobifunctional active esters such as *m*-maleimidobenzoic acid *N*-hydroxysuccinimide ester (MBSE) or related compounds (81). Methods for protein-protein coupling include glutaraldehyde cross-linking, periodate coupling, dimaleimide coupling, the use of homobifunctional reagents such as 4,4′-difluoro-2,2′-dinitrophenyl sulfone (FNPS), toluene-2,4-diisocyanate (TDIC), or benzoquinone, and the use of MBSE. Although coupling reactions that involve sites of antigen-antibody combination usually result in a reduction in avidity, coupling can result in an increased affinity and avidity in some circumstances. After the coupling reaction, the conjugate must be purified, and then characterized in terms of the hapten to enzyme ratio, enzyme activity, and immunoreactivity (81).

Classification of Enzyme Immunoassays

Enzyme immunoassays are usually classified on the basis of the requirement for separation of the free and bound reactants. In heterogeneous enzyme immunoassays, enzyme activity is not affected by the interaction of antigen and antibody, and a separation step is required. The term ELISA is widely used as a general term for the heterogeneous enzyme immunoassays (82). In homogeneous EIA, there is no need

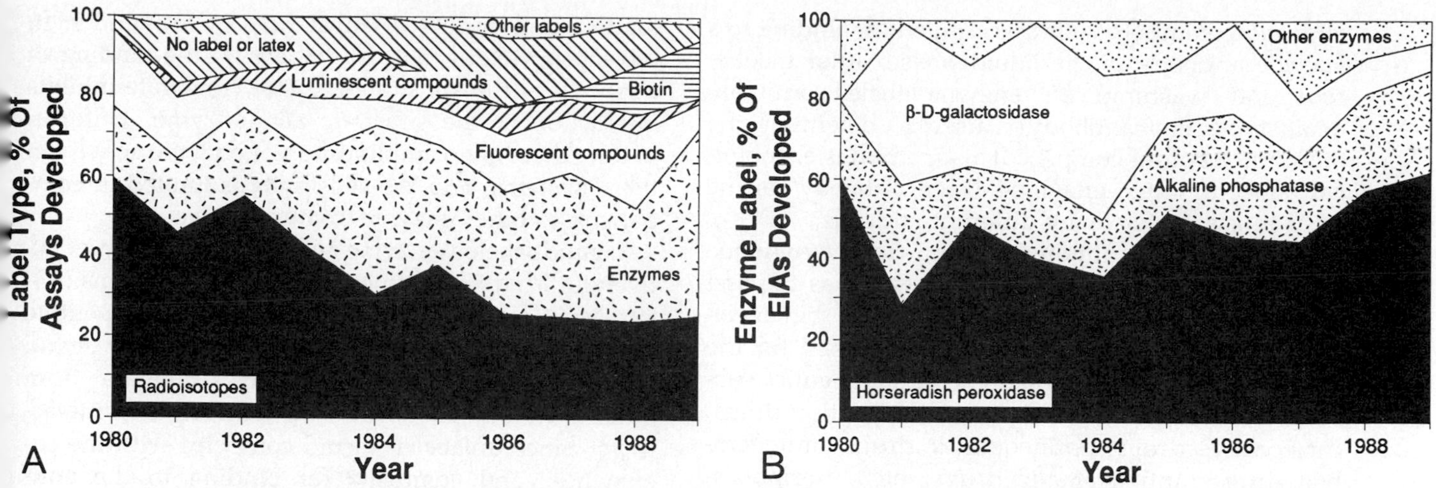

Figure 56.18. Recent trends in the use of enzyme labels in immunoassay. **A**, The popularity of the five most popular labeling substances (radioisotopes, enzymes, fluorochromes, and biotin) is shown, together with the utilization of "no label" or latex assays (nephelometric, latex agglutination, and particle-counting assays). **B**, Trends in the use of the three major enzymes (horseradish peroxidase, alkaline phosphatase, β-D-galactosidase). (Reprinted with permission from Gosling JP. A decade of development in immunoassay methodology. Clin Chem 1990;36:1408.)

for a separation step, since enzyme activity is modulated by the antigen-antibody interaction.

The separation techniques that can be utilized in heterogeneous enzyme immunoassays are limited by the large size of most enzyme molecules. As a result, solid-phase techniques (i.e., antigen- or antibody-coated polystyrene test tubes or microtiter trays; polystyrene, latex, or agarose beads or particles, magnetized beads, etc.) have been principally utilized for separation of the bound and free enzyme conjugate. Immunoprecipitation with polyethylene glycol, a second antibody, or a preprecipitated complex of two antibodies has also been utilized in some cases.

Competitive EIA techniques are similar to RIA. In these techniques, a limited amount of specific antibody is attached to a solid phase. Unlabeled ligand (unknown sample, control, or standard) and a known amount of labeled antigen are incubated with the solid phase. After washing, the enzyme substrate is added and the end product is quantitated by colorimetry or another technique. As in RIA, the amount of bound enzyme-labeled ligand is inversely proportional to the concentration of unlabeled antigen. The major disadvantages of this method include the need for relatively large amounts of pure antigen, and the requirement that each different antigen be coupled to an enzyme. Variations of the standard competitive EIA have been described. For example, an "antibody masking enzyme tag immunoassay" (AME-TIA) has been described (83). In this procedure enzyme is conjugated to both a ligand and a second compound ("tag"). A solid phase is coated with an insolubilized receptor specific for the tag. In the assay unlabeled ligand and the ligand-enzyme-tag conjugate compete for binding to an antibody. Since the tag is masked when the enzyme conjugate is bound to the enzyme, the amount of final product is directly proportional to the quantity of free ligand. In the initial description of the assay, biotin was utilized as the tag, and avidin as the insoluble receptor.

Immunoenzymometric assays are noncompetitive (i.e., excess reagents are utilized). The antigen is first reacted with an excess of enzyme-labeled antibody, and a solid-phase antigen is then added in excess to remove unreacted enzyme-labeled antibody. After washing, the substrate is added. The amount of final product is inversely proportional to the concentration of free antigen. The major advantages of this technique include the lack of a requirement for a purified antigen and the ability to detect small haptens, which are difficult to quantitate by other means.

Several "sandwich" modifications of the enzyme immunoassay to quantitate antigen have been described. The two-site immunoenzymometric assay utilizes a solid phase coated with specific antibody in excess. The test solution containing antigen is added to the solid phase and incubated, permitting the antigen to bind to the immobilized antibody. After washing to remove unreacted antigen, the solid phase is incubated with an excess amount of enzyme-labeled antibody in the liquid phase. The enzyme substrate is added after a second wash, and the amount of end product is directly proportional to the amount of antigen in the test solution. Since the antigen must be able to bind to two different antibodies simultaneously, this procedure is best utilized to detect large, complex antigens with two or more antigenic sites. A competitive sandwich assay for antigen detection (double antibody immunoenzymometric assay) utilizes solid phase antigen. The solid phase is allowed to compete with free antigen for binding to a specific antibody in the liquid phase. After incubation and washing, an enzyme-labeled antibody against the first antibody is used to determine the amount of bound complex. This method is economical, since a single enzyme-labeled antibody can be used in assays for many different antigens.

The enzyme multiplied immunoassay technique (EMIT, Syva Company, Palo Alto, CA) was the first homogeneous enzyme immunoassay to be developed, and has since been extensively used for the quantitation of numerous chemotherapeutic substances (drugs of abuse, antiepileptic drugs, cardioactive drugs, antineoplastic drugs, antimicrobial drugs, antihistamatic drugs, etc.), hormones, and other substances. In the EMIT assay system the ligand (usually a hapten) is covalently linked to an enzyme (usually NAD-dependent glucose-6-phosphate dehydrogenase). In most EMIT assays, the binding of an antihapten antibody inhibits enzyme activity, probably by interfering with the molecular conformational changes which take place during the enzyme reaction or by direct steric exclusion of substrate binding (84). Since free hapten competes with the antibody for binding to the enzyme immobilized hapten, the quantity of end product is directly proportional to the concentration of free hapten. In a few EMIT assays, enzyme activity is increased by the binding of antibody to the bound hapten. For example, in the EMIT assay for thyroxine, the enzyme-hapten (malate dehydrogenase-thyroxine) complex is inactive until antibody binding occurs. It is believed that the bound thyroxine occupies the active site of the enzyme, but is removed from this area during the steric rearrangements which take place upon antibody binding (85). In the standard EMIT assay, 50 μl of the specimen is diluted with buffer, and the enzyme substrate is added, followed by the enzyme-hapten conjugate. The reaction mixture is aspirated into the flow cell of a spectrophotometer, which is maintained at 30° C, and the change in absorbance is determined over a 30-second interval. The assay for some substances requires different specimen volumes, reading times, or pretreatment of the specimen to improve sensitivity. Although the basic equipment for an EMIT assay consists of a spectrophotometer and pipetter-diluter, numerous adaptations have been made for utilization in automated analyzers such as continuous flow systems, discrete analyzers, centrifugal analyzers, the DuPont ACA, etc. The NAD-dependent reaction can be measured fluorimetrically as well, and this detection method has been utilized to increase the sensitivity of the reaction.

A homogeneous substrate-labeled fluorescent immunoassay (SLFIA) has been described for the quantitation of a variety of substances of low and high molecular weight (86). In this assay, the binding of antibody to the substrate-enzyme conjugate inhibits interaction of the substrate and enzyme. Unfortunately, there is no amplification of enzyme activity in these systems, and the sensitivity is limited in comparison to other enzyme immunoassays.

Ligand-labeled enzyme cofactors have been effectively utilized in enzyme immunoassay systems (87–89). Most commonly, these systems are competitive in nature, with a specific antibody against the ligand preventing the coenzyme-ligand conjugate from binding to the apoenzyme and reducing enzyme activity. Since unlabeled ligand competes with the coenzyme-ligand conjugate for binding to the antibody, enzyme activity is directly proportional to the amount of unlabeled antigen. Nicotinamide adenine dinucleotide (NAD) is a cofactor for many enzymes (lactic dehydrogenase, malic dehydrogenase, etc.), and has been used as the cofactor in several of these assays. The major disadvantage of coenzyme-labeled immunoassays is their susceptibility to endogenous cofactors and other enzymes.

Immunoassays utilizing ligand-labeled prosthetic groups are similar to those using enzyme cofactors. The ligand-prosthetic group (usually flavin adenine dinucleotide, FAD) competes with unlabeled ligand for a limited amount of specific antibody. The free, but not the antibody-bound conjugate can interact with an apoenzyme, such as apoglucose oxidase, to generate the active enzyme (87). Similar assays with ligand-labeled modulators (antibody, inhibitor, receptor) have been reported (90).

The enzyme-enhancement immunoassay (EEIA) is one manner in which enzyme-labeled antibodies have been utilized (91). In this system an enzyme-labeled antibody (E-AB_1) and a succinylated antibody (AB_2) are utilized. These antibodies form a complex with a polyvalent antigen in the reaction mixture to form a negatively charged microenvironment. Under these circumstances, the substrate is converted into a product (P_2) that alters the light-scattering properties of the complex. The free-enzyme conjugate forms a product (P_1) that remains soluble. The reaction is measured by turbidimetry. Wei and Reibe (92) described an enzyme-labeled immunoassay utilizing phospholipase C conjugated to rabbit antihuman IgG.

Recent Advances in Enzyme Immunoassay

Numerous innovative modifications of enzyme immunoassay techniques have been described utilizing microparticles, liposomes, recombinant enzyme fragments, biosensors, flow cytometry, and other materials and techniques. For example, Wilkins et al.

(93) developed a highly sensitive homogeneous assay for thyrotropin using 800-nm particles and a new modular immunoassay system (Multipact). The assay was also the first to use fragmented monoclonal antibodies, to avoid serum interference. The accuracy and precision of the assay were comparable to a highly sensitive commercial immunoradiometric assay (IRMA) for TSH. Two novel phase-separation immunoassays were described by Auditore-Hargreaves (94). In one system, the solid phase is generated in situ, after specific binding has occurred. This technique (de novo polymerization) was developed to minimize nonspecific binding and to enhance reaction kinetics. Thermal precipitation was used in the second system, which incorporated water-soluble polymers temperature-dependent solubility.

The use of liposomes in immunoassay systems has also been described. For example, in the technique reported by Litchfield, Freytag, and Adamich (95), alkaline phosphatase was incorporated into liposomes. In a competitive assay, lysis of the liposomes and enzyme release by a hapten-cytolysin conjugate was prevented by conjugation with an antihapten antibody.

An enzyme immunoassay system utilizing recombinant enzyme fragments has recently been described (96, 97). In this system, termed CEDIA, two separate *Escherichia coli* genes for β-galactosidase are engineered to produce separate, enzymatically inactive fragments that can spontaneously recombine to form an active β-galactosidase enzyme. An antiligand antibody is attached to one fragment (enzyme acceptor, EA), while the second fragment (enzyme donor, ED) is labeled with ligand conjugate and enzyme substrate. The degree of recombination of the two fragments to form an active enzyme is regulated by the binding of antibody to the enzyme donor-ligand conjugate. In practice, a competitive system is used, in which there is competition between the ligand in the specimen and the ED-ligand conjugate for a limited amount of antibody. Variations of the assay include a three-reagent system with enhanced sensitivity, and a single reagent system suitable for on-site testing. The advantages of CEDIA in comparison to other homogeneous immunoassays include high sensitivity, linear standard curves, and low endogenous enzyme activity. The assay has been adapted for use in several commercial automated clinical laboratory analyzers.

Immunosensors have been utilized for a variety of in vivo and in vitro applications. Although most immunosensors are based on electrochemical detection, potentiometric, voltampermetric, thermometric, optoelectronic, acoustoelectronic and other methodologies have been described (98–106). Another immunoassay detection system monitors antigen or antibody binding on a surface by surface plasmon oscillations (107).

A variety of new membranes, fibers, and other materials are being used as solid phases in immunoassays. In radial partition immunoassays, antibodies are immobilized to glass fiber paper, and enzyme activity is measured fluorometrically (108). In one assay for the detection of human choriogonadotropin, the capture antibody is immobilized to a nylon membrane in contact with an absorbent material (109). Both reference and test zones are included. Another popular assay for pregnancy detection uses the novel approach of microparticle-capture on glass-fiber membranes. This technique is based on the principle that coated polystyrene microparticles irreversibly adhere to the surface of glass fibers or glass-fiber membranes. Microparticles coated with anti-choriogonadotropin antibodies are applied to a glass filter along a narrow line (test line), while choriogonadotropin-coated microparticles are fixed along an intersecting horizontal line at right angles to the first (reference line). The sample is first passed through the filter, followed by the enzyme-antibody conjugate and substrate. If the reagents are functional, color is formed along the reference line to give a minus sign. If choriogonadotropin was present in the sample, the test line is also colored, giving a plus sign.

Fluorescence and Chemiluminescence

Coon and associates were the first to use fluorescent dyes (fluorochromes) as a label for an antibody molecule. Since that time, these dyes have proven to be sensitive and versatile labels for the detection and quantitation of antigens and antibodies in body fluids and tissues. Fluorochromes are easily conjugated to most substances of biological importance, and are easily measured in the laboratory. In addition, some fluorescent probes can be coupled to other excited states or chemical species by energy transfer or chemical reactions.

Fluorescence and Phosphorescence

The emission of light is one possible outcome of the interaction of a molecule with light or other electromagnetic radiation. In response to the absorption of energy, fluorochromes enter an "excited state," during which changes in electron configuration occur. However, the molecules are unstable in the excited state, and undergo a rapid return to the stable or "resting" state. During this transition, most of the absorbed energy is dissipated in the form of heat, but some may be released (emitted) as a photon of light (luminescence). There are two types of lumines-

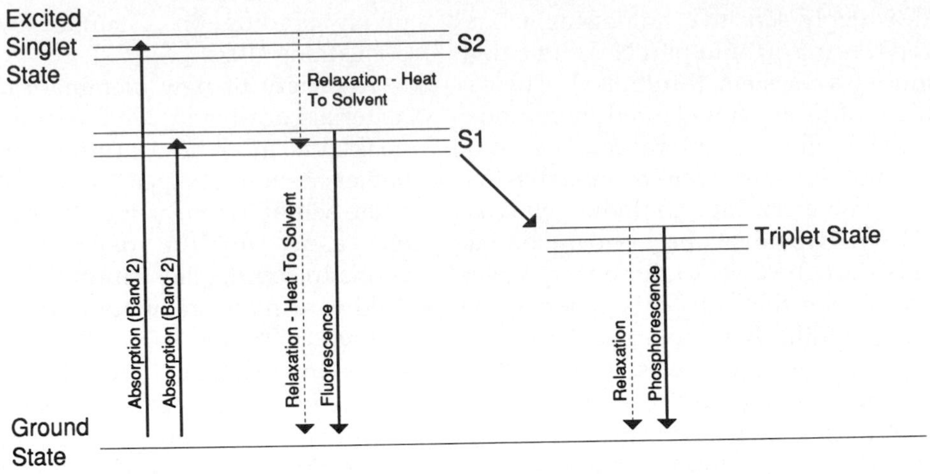

Figure 56.19. Energy transitions during fluorescence and phosphorescence. The absorption of light causes a transition of the molecule from its ground state singlet (S0) to one of a number of excited singlet states (S1, S2, etc.). The molecule is electronically unstable in the excited state, and the excess energy is dissipated by nonradiative means (heat) or radiative energy transfer (luminescence) during a return to the ground state. Fluorescence occurs if the molecule undergoes a direct radiative transition to the ground state, while phosphorescence results in cases where the transition involves a series of semistable triplet states (T1, T2, etc.). Nonradiative transitions are indicated by straight arrows, and radiative transitions by dotted lines. (Reprinted with permission from Hemmila I. Fluoroimmunoassays and immunofluorometric assays. Clin Chem 1985;36:360.)

cence, depending on whether the time between excitation and emission is short (less than 10^{-8} second, fluorescence) or long (more than 10^{-4} second, phosphorescence). Since some energy is lost as heat, the wavelength of the emitted energy is longer (lower energy) than that of the wavelength of the excitation source (higher energy) (Fig. 56.19).

Each fluorochrome is characterized by a number of parameters, including the maximum wavelengths of maximal excitation (λ^{Abs}_{Max}) and emission (λ^{Fluor}_{Max}), the Stoke's shift, the extinction coefficient (ϵ) in the region of excitation, the quantum yield (Q), and the decay rate of the excited-state (τ). The Stokes's shift is the difference between λ^{Abs}_{Max} and λ^{Fluor}_{Max}. It is usually 20 to 50 nm for most fluorescent compounds, but may be as great as 200 nm for certain phosphorescent compounds (Table 56.5). The maximum intensity of fluorescent emission occurs when a fluorochrome is excited with light at the wavelength of the excitation maximum. Decreases in fluorescent intensity occur at wavelengths above and below the maximum excitation wavelength. In practice, the excitation maximum cannot be utilized in two circumstances: (*a*) if the light source does not provide an emission line of the proper wavelength; or (*b*) if two or more fluorochromes with different excitation maxima are simultaneously used with a single monochromatic excitation source. In these circumstances, compromises can be made as long as the intensity of the signal emitted is adequate for particle detection. Fortunately, the intensity of the fluorescent emission is always proportional to an amount of fluorochrome present at a fixed wavelength. Optical filters are utilized in laboratory instruments to maximize parameters for a particular fluorochrome or combination of fluorochromes.

The chemical and biological properties of a fluorochrome are influenced by the chemical composition of the substance, the physical and chemical environment in which the substance is placed, and a variety of other factors. In addition to a large extinction coefficient (ϵ) in the region of excitation, high quantum yield, an optimal excitation wavelength, and a proper excited state lifetime, fluorochromes must be photostable, biologically inert, and undergo minimal interference by other substances that may be present ("quenching") (110). The compound must also possess functional groups for binding to an antigen or antibody. Isothiocyanates, chlorotriazinyl derivatives, or hydroxysuccinimido active esters covalently bind to the primary amino group of proteins, while iodoacetamido and maleimido groups attach to sulfhydryl groups (110). In conjugates of a fluorochrome with a protein antigen or antibody, the molar fluorescein to protein ratio (F/P ratio) is important. The F/P ratio is an indication of the relative number of fluorochrome molecules per protein molecule. Staining sensitivity is reduced if the F/P ratio is too small, while nonspecific fluorescence can be caused by an F/P ratio which is too high.

Although no single substance has all of the properties of an "ideal" fluorochrome, fluorescein isothiocyanate, rhodamine, and phycoerythrin are employed for most applications at present. The properties of these and other fluorochromes of biological interest are summarized in Table 56.4.

Table 56.4. Properties of Fluorochromes

Type of Probe/ Name of Probe	Absorption Maximum	Emission Maximum	Extinction Maximum	Quantum Yield
Covalent labels	*nm*	*nm*		
FITC-NH-CH3	490	520	67	0.71
FITC-NH-Ab	490	520	67	0.1–0.4
Phycoerythrin-R	480–565	578	1960	0.68
Allophycocyanin	650	660	700	0.68
Peridinin-chlorophyll	470	677	—	—
TRITC-amines	554	573	85	0.28
XRITC-NH-CH3	582	601	79	0.26
XRITC-NH-Ab	580	604		0.08
Texas Red-amines	596	620	85	0.51
Texas Red-NH-Ab	596	620	85	0.01
Extrinsic RNA/DNA probes				
Propidium iodide	536	623	6.4	0.09
Ethidium bromide	510	595	3.2	—
Hoechst 33342	340	450	120	0.83
DAPI	350	470	—	—
Acridine orange (DNA)	480	520	—	—
Acridine orange (RNA)	440–470	650	—	—
Pyronine Y (dsDNA)	549–561	567–574	67–84	0.04–0.26
Pyronine Y (dsRNA)	560–562	565–574	70–90	0.05–0.21

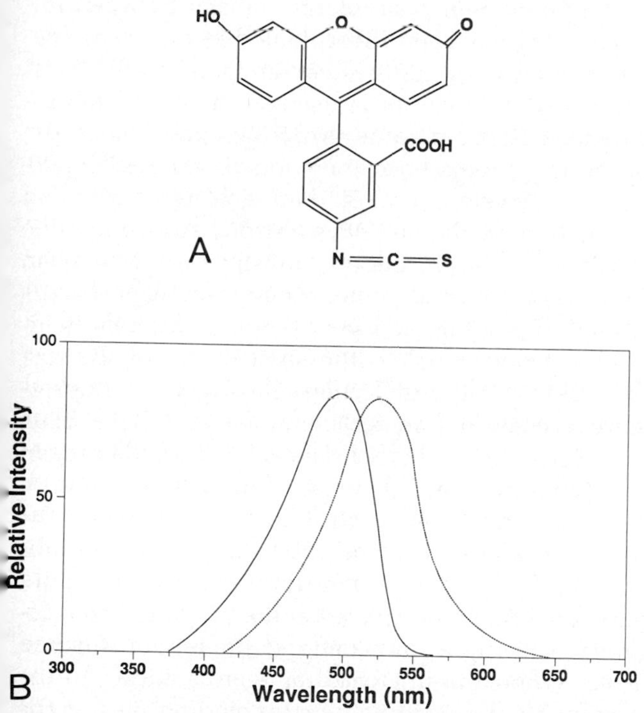

Figure 56.20. Molecular structure (**A**) and fluorescence spectra (**B**) of fluorescein isothiocyanate.

Fluorescein isothiocyanate (FITC) is the most widely used fluorochrome. FITC is excited at a wavelength of 492 nm and emits light at a wavelength of 510 nm (Fig. 56.20). This substance binds neutral amino acids, and has been used as a tag for antibodies, hormones, lipids, lectins, and a wide variety of other biological molecules. The advantages of FITC are its solubility in water, high quantum efficiency, and large extinction coefficient, while its disadvantages include a pH dependence of fluorescent emission, moderate photoinstability, and an excitation wavelength less than 500 nm (110). Between two and five fluorescein molecules can usually be attached to most biological molecules before quenching limits fluorescent intensity. Covalent binding requires an alkaline pH (pH 8.5 to 9.0) where the pH amino groups are in a reactive form.

Rhodamine derivatives (rhodamine isothiocyanate, Texas red, etc.) have higher fluorescent excitation and emission wavelengths than FITC, and are often used in conjunction with FITC for multiparametric analysis. Most of these compounds are less water soluble than FITC, but are photostable and have fluorescent properties that are independent of pH (110).

Research in the early 1980s led to the development of a new class of fluorochromes, which have been termed phycofluors (110–114). The major phycobiliproteins include the phycoerythrins (R-phycoerythrin, B-phycoerythrin), R-phycocyanin, and allophycocyanin. The advantages of these compounds include extremely high absorbance coefficients over a wide spectral range, very high quantum yields, constant fluorescence over a broad pH range, solubility in aqueous solution, and environmental stability. In addition, phycobiliproteins contain numerous lysyl side chains, which permit easy conjugation to biological molecules, and which can confer binding specificity (immunoglobulins, lectins, protein A, avidin) (112, 113).

Fluorescent Immunoassays

The utilization of fluorochromes for the identification and localization of antigen, antibodies, and immune complexes in histochemical, cytochemical, and cellular assays is described below. More recently, fluorochromes have been used in the clinical laboratory to quantitate antigens and antibodies in a manner analogous to radioimmunoassay and enzyme immunoassay (115, 116). Unfortunately, these assays have achieved limited application because of the need for specialized instrumentation, as well as extensively purified and well-characterized reagents. In addition, inherent limitations in the detection of fluorescent emissions limit the sensitivity of conventional fluorometric methods to the nanomolar range and above (67). These limitations include background fluorescence (particularly from autofluorescent substances normally present in serum), nonspecific binding of the reagents, fluorescence "quenching," difficulties in differentiating the excitation and emission signals, and the light-scattering phenomenon. Fortunately, new fluorescent reagents and new techniques of applying these labels have alleviated many of these problems. Particularly important has been the use of certain heavy metal compounds (i.e., lanthanide complexes) in conjunction with techniques such as time-resolved fluorescence immunoassay. In addition, the ability to chemically alter the properties of fluorochromes has resulted in great interest in the adaptation of fluorescent compounds for clinical laboratory diagnosis. Various biological dyes and even dyes utilized in the textile industry have been targets for these investigations as the parent compounds for synthesis of new fluorochromes. Since fluorochromes can act as substrates in biochemical reactions, these "fluorogenic substrates" have been extremely useful in the study or quantitation of cellular properties (pH, membrane potential) or biological activity (enzyme activity, activation). The utilization of a compound as a fluorogenic substrate requires that it undergo a change in fluorescent properties (gain or loss of fluorescence, change in λ^{Fluor}_{Max}, etc.) with a change in the biological property or substance being studied.

Analytical fluorescence assays are most commonly classified as heterogeneous or homogeneous, based on the need for separation of the bound and free reagent. Other considerations include the type of reaction mechanism (competitive or noncompetitive) and labeled component (ligand or antibody).

A solid phase is utilized in most heterogeneous fluorescent immunoassays for separation of the labeled and unlabeled reagents. Both competitive and noncompetitive reaction mechanisms have been described. Quantitation of the reaction mechanism is usually performed with a fluorimeter.

Homogeneous immunoassays are rapid and easy to perform, although their sensitivity is limited in comparison to heterogeneous assays unless special instrumentation is utilized (typically 10^{-10} molar of analyte per liter) (117). In addition, these assays require highly purified labeled antigen and specific antibody.

The quenching or enhancement of fluorescence of a ligand-labeled chromophobe caused by the binding of an antibody has been used to quantitate some substances. The enhancement fluoroimmunoassay for thyroxine (T_4) described by Smith (118) utilizes a fluorescent derivative of thyroxine that undergoes an enhancement in fluorescent intensity upon the binding of an anti-T_4 antibody. In a competitive binding assay, unlabeled T_4 in the reaction mixture competes for the antibody. With a sensitive fluorimeter (Aminco Bowman SPF fluorimeter), the assay had sensitivity equivalent to the standard radioimmunoassay for T_4.

The phenomenon of energy transfer between fluorochromes has been incorporated into clinical analytical assays for multivalent antigens (119). Most commonly, fluorescein is used as the donor fluorochrome, and rhodamine is the acceptor. Since the maximum fluorescence emission of fluorescein occurs at a wavelength of 525 nm, and tetraethyl- and tetramethyl-rhodamine have a strong absorption line at this wavelength, energy transfer can occur from fluorescein to rhodamine. Energy transfer occurs through dipole-dipole interaction at a rate that is inversely proportional to the sixth power of the distance between the molecules. Two types of fluorescence excitation transfer immunoassays have been described. The antibody is labeled with rhodamine in both types of assays. However, in one type the antigen is directly labeled with fluorescein, while in the other type an indirect label (FITC-labeled antibody) is used. In the direct assay, the fluorescein-labeled antigen and rhodamine-labeled antibodies are mixed together, causing a quenching of fluorescein fluorescence. When the unlabeled antigen is added to the reaction mixture, competition for binding sites on the antibody occurs, resulting in liberation of some of the fluorescein-labeled antigen, decreased quenching, and increased fluorescein fluorescence. The principle of the indirect assay is similar.

A fluorescent protection assay has been described for the analysis of protein antigens (immunoglobulin, hormones, serum proteins) or antibodies. In the assay for an antigen, the reactants include a fluorescein-labeled protein antigen, an antibody specific for the antigen, and a second antibody specific for fluorescein. The principle of the assay is that (*a*) binding of the antifluorescein antibody to the labeled protein results in the quenching of fluorescence; (*b*) the antigen-specific antibody sterically inhibits binding of the antifluorescein antibody; and (*c*) unlabeled antigen competes with the fluorescein-labeled antigen for antibody-binding. Thus, fluorescence intensity is proportional to the quantity of unlabeled antigen.

The substrate-labeled fluorescent immunoassay (SLFIA) has been utilized for the quantitation of haptens (including many therapeutic drugs), as well as immunoglobulins and other proteins. A complex of antigen and a fluorogenic substrate of an enzyme forms the basis of this assay. The progression occurs as follows: (*a*) the antigen is cleaved from the substrate complex by an appropriate enzyme, resulting in the formation of a fluorescent product; (*b*) the presence of an antibody to the antigen inhibits enzymatic cleavage; (*c*) free antigen inhibits antibody binding; (*d*) the rate of production of fluorescence is proportional to the free antigen concentration. In practice, umbelliferyl-β-galactoside is usually utilized as the labeled enzyme substrate, and β-galactosidase is the enzyme. For many antigens, the sensitivity of this assay is comparable to radioimmunoassay.

Particle concentration fluorescence immunoassays use small polystyrene beads as the solid phase. The reaction is performed in microtitration plates in which a 2 mm–diameter porous membrane forms the bottom of each well. Specimens and reagents are removed from the wells by the use of suction. Total particle fluorescence is determined by front surface fluorescence. This system has been used for the quantitation of serum immunoglobulins and antibodies (120).

Fluorescence Polarization Immunoassays

Fluorescence polarization is a special property of fluorochromes that was first applied to an analytical assay by Dandliker et al. (121, 122). Light is composed of electric and magnetic fields (vectors), and polarization is defined by the orientation in time and space of the electric vector (123). If the electric vector can be considered to consist of two orthogonal components, the state of polarization of a light beam is defined by the relative amplitudes and phases of the orthogonal components. The orthogonal components are of equal magnitude and have no fixed relationship in the case of unpolarized (incoherent) light. In contrast, perfectly polarized light is coherent, and the orthogonal components are fixed in their relationship to each other (123).

Light produced from fluorescence emission is noncoherent, since it arises from the summation of uncorrelated individual emission events (123). However, polarized light is absorbed by a chromophore in the same manner as nonpolarized light, provided the "absorption transition moment" of the chromophore is in the same direction as the plane of polarization. The rate of depolarization can be determined by measuring the sample with detectors parallel and perpendicular to the plane of polarization (123, 124).

The degree of polarization increases with restricted motion of a chromophore due to increased viscosity of the medium or decreased fluidity of the membrane or other structural component. Therefore, small fluorochrome-labeled molecules in an aqueous solution have unrestricted motion and exhibit low polarization. However, when combined with an antibody, the molecular motion of the fluorochrome is decreased, and the degree of fluorescence polarization increases.

Fluorescence polarization assays have been primarily utilized in the clinical laboratory for the analysis of small molecular weight substances, such as drugs and hormones. In one technique, polarization fluoroimmunoassay (PFIA), the increased signal associated with binding of an antibody to a fluorophore-labeled antigen is measured (122). Assays for gentamicin, phenytoin, amphetamine, and other substances have been described (125–128). The newly developed simpler, less expensive instrumentation for the laboratory may increase the utilization of fluorescence polarization.

The excited state life-time of a fluorescent compound has been applied in a type of fluorescent immunoassay termed "'time-resolved fluorescence immunoassay (TR-FIA)." These assays use fluorochromes with relatively long decay times, especially the rare earth metal chelates (10–10,000 μsec). In TR-FIA a rapidly pulsing excitation source is used, and fluorescence intensity is measured at a fixed interval after excitation. Since the decay time of substances that may cause background fluorescence is usually less than 10 nanoseconds, the inherent sensitivity of these methods is much greater than conventional fluorescent immunoassays (67, 129). The rare earth metal europium (Eu) has been used most extensively as a label in time-resolved immunoassays, although other trivalent lanthanide ions, such as terbium (Tb^{3+}) and samarium (Sm^{3+}) have been used as well (130). Fluorometers for time-resolved fluorescence immunoassays are modified to measure only a portion of the emission cycle.

Particle-based flow cytometric fluorescence immunoassays have been described. For example, fluorescence quantitation by flow cytometry has been applied in an equilibrium-type competitive-binding fluorescence immunoassay (131). In this assay, relatively large (10 μm diameter) antibody-coated nonfluorescent particles were used with very small (0.10 μm diameter) antigen-coated fluorescent latex particles. During incubation with the sample, soluble unlabeled antigen competes with the small, antigen-labeled particles for binding to the larger spheres. The fluorescence distribution of 5000 of the large spheres is determined by flow cytometry, and read against a standard curve prepared with known concentrations of antigen. The sensitivity of this technique was 10^{-12} mol/liter, for quantitation of the antigen horseradish peroxidase, and the sensitivity was increased to 10^{-12} mol/liter in a double-antibody "sandwich" assay. Lindmo et al. described a different flow cytometric technique using two particle types coated with antibody of the same specificity but different affinity (132).

Chemiluminescent Immunoassays

Chemiluminescence is the emission of light from a chemical reaction (133). Chemiluminescence and chemiluminescence energy transfer have been utilized for the detection of a variety of substances in the 10^{-18} to 10^{-21} mol range (98, 134–139). Most of these assays utilize synthetic chemiluminescent compounds such as luminol (3-amino-phthalhydrazine), luminol derivatives such as isoluminol, or acridinium ester derivatives as labels for antigens or antibodies. Photon emission is measured in a luminometer or liquid scintillation counter after the addition of an oxidizing agent (i.e., H_2O_2) and a catalyst (i.e., hemin, lactoperoxidase, copper or cobalt ions). Although the low efficiency (less than 1%) of photon emission limits the sensitivity of assays based on chemiluminescence, the stability of the reagents and the low background activity are advantages. Chemiluminescence energy transfer has been used to increase the sensitivity of the assay (137).

CELLULAR IMMUNOASSAYS

The development of assays for the identification and enumeration of immune cells and for the assessment of cell function has been essential for the understanding of the immune system. In addition to applications in organ transplantation, these assays have been useful in the diagnosis and treatment of patients with malignant neoplasms, autoimmune diseases, and infectious diseases. The major technical developments in cellular immunology have included:

- In vitro cytotoxicity assays;
- The discovery and utilization of anti-HLA antisera from multiparous women in histocompatibility testing;
- Cryopreservation and thawing of lymphocytes;
- Assays of cell-mediated immune function (mixed lymphocyte culture, antibody-dependent cell-mediated cytotoxicity);
- Cellular typing utilizing cell-mediated lympholysis (CML), homozygous typing cells (HTC), and primed lymphocyte typing (PLT);
- Miniaturization, automation, standardization, and improved quality control;
- Monoclonal antibody technology; flow cytometry; and immunochemical analysis; and
- Gene cloning, DNA sequence analysis, and recombinant DNA technology.

Basic Techniques in Cellular Immunoassay

SPECIMEN COLLECTION AND CELL PREPARATION

Specimen Collection and Transportation

A successful cellular assay begins with the procurement of the proper specimen in the correct manner with prompt transportation of the specimen to the clinical laboratory. Care must be taken that the person obtaining the specimen is correctly informed about specimen requirements for the assay that has been ordered, and that any special instructions for obtaining the specimen are followed. For most cellular immunoassays, 5–10 ml of anticoagulated venous blood is required, although cellular immunoassays may require serum or plasma, other body fluids, or lymphoid tissue. Since immune cells and many immune substances are labile, the specimen should be received within the laboratory and processed within 24 hours. Most specimens are maintained at room temperature during transportation.

Cell Separation and Purification

The peripheral blood, lymph nodes, spleen, and other components of the immune system consist of a heterogenous mixture of cell types (lymphocytes, monocytes, granulocytes, macrophages, red blood cells, and platelets). However, most cellular assays assess the properties or function of one particular cell type, and cannot be performed in the presence of large numbers of contaminating cells. Purified lymphocyte preparations are preferred in many cellular assays because they strongly express HLA Class I and Class II antigens, while monocyte cell preparations are utilized for many cellular assays, but other assays require isolated granulocytes, platelets, or even a purified subset of a particular cell type. Some techniques for the isolation and purification of cells are based on differences in basic physical properties (size, density, granularity, etc.), while others rely

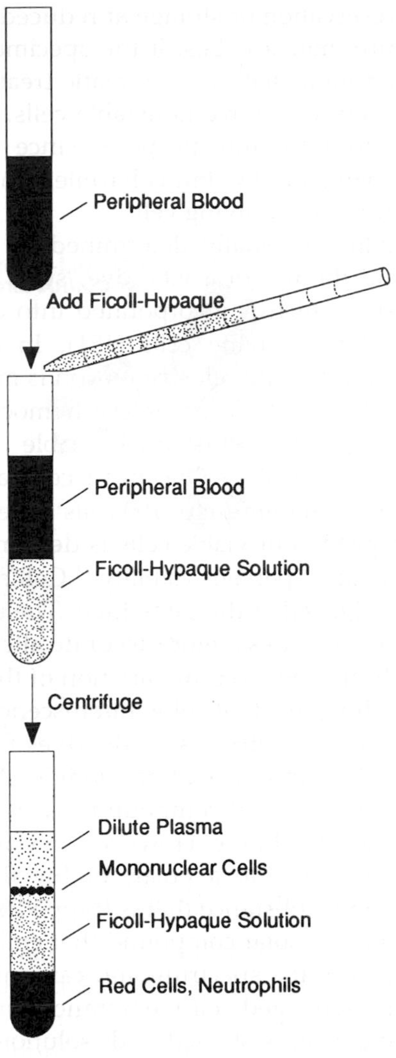

Figure 56.21. Technique of Ficoll-Hypaque density isolation of mononuclear cells. Whole blood is layered into a Ficoll-Hypaque mixture (specific gravity 1.007), and the test tube is centrifuged. During centrifugation, the lymphocytes are separated from the other formed elements of the blood and form a discrete layer at the plasma-Ficoll-Hypaque interface, which can easily be removed with a pipette. (Reprinted with permission from Riley RS, Mahin EJ, Ross W. Clinical applications of flow cytometry. New York: Igaku-Shoin Medical Publishers, 1993:202.)

on functional differences (adherence, phagocytosis), or the presence of a particular cell surface antigen (140).

Whole blood leukocyte preparations are adequate for many purposes, including the enumeration of lymphocyte subsets by flow cytometric immunophenotypic analysis. The direct removal of red blood cells from peripheral blood by ammonium chloride lysis is being increasingly utilized for routine lymphocyte enumeration studies. This technique is efficient, rapidly performed, and minimizes specimen handling. In addition, the selective loss of certain lymphocyte subsets associated with density gradient centrifugation is avoided.

Cell density is the most common property used for the separation of mononuclear cells (lymphocytes and monocytes) from other cell types. In cell isolation procedures using differences in cell density, the unpurified cell suspension is centrifuged in a solution containing a single or multilayer density gradient. After centrifugation, cells are distributed in the solution in layers based on differences in their density. A Ficoll-Hypaque gradient is most commonly used for this purpose (140–146). Ficoll-Hypaque is composed of sodium diatroziate (3,5-*bis*-acetylamino-2,4,6-triiodobenzoic acid, hypaque, isopaque) and ficoll. Ficoll is a high–molecular weight sucrose polymer (sp. grav. = 1.076–1.078), while hypaque is a dense iodinated organic compound also used as an x-ray contrast medium. Ficoll contributes viscosity to the solution and promotes rouleaux formation of the red blood cells, while hypaque increases the viscosity of the solution. When properly prepared, a Ficoll-Hypaque solution has a specific gravity of 1.077 at room temperature, and is more dense than lymphocytes, monocytes, and platelets, but less dense than granulocytes and red blood cells.

In practice, blood for mononuclear cell isolation is collected aseptically into a heparinized container, and a buffy coat is prepared and layered over or under Ficoll-Hypaque. Mononuclear cell preparations are prepared from tissue specimens by mincing the tissue into a tissue culture media (usually RPMI containing 5% fetal calf serum, RPMI/5% FCS) or by gently forcing the tissue through nylon mesh. Wire or nylon mesh of various grades is also useful in removing cell aggregates and in removing stroma and extraneous pieces of tissue from a cell preparation. Cell suspensions prepared from lymphoid tissue usually contain few erythrocytes and can be placed directly on Ficoll-Hypaque. After a one-step centrifugation with Ficoll-Hypaque, platelets (sp. grav. = 1.040) and plasma (sp. grav. = 1.025–1.029) are located above the Ficoll-Hypaque, lymphocytes (sp. grav. = 1.070) and some platelets are found at the plasma-Ficoll-Hypaque interface, and granulocytes (sp. grav. = 1.087–1.092) and red blood cells (sp. grav. = 1.093–1.096) form a pellet at the bottom of the tube (Fig. 56.21). Residual platelets are removed by washing and a low-speed spin. Incubation of the buffy coat preparation at 37° C with carbonyl iron can also increase the purity of the final cell preparation, since neutrophils and monocytes phagocytize the carbonyl iron, thus increasing their density and allowing better gradient separation. Isolated lymphocyte preparations prepared from fresh peripheral blood by Ficoll-Hypaque isolation should provide 1 $\times 10^6$ lymphocytes/ml which are 90 to 100% viable and contain fewer than 5% granulocytes and monocytes. Granulocytes can also be obtained from a phycoerythrin to Texas red, and the emission of light at a wavelength distinct from phycoerythrin. Specifically, the PE component of the conjugate excites at 488 nm and emits light with a maximum of 575 nm. The PE emission in turn excites adjacent Texas-red molecules, which emit red light with a maximum of 618 nm. In three-color analysis, one monoclonal antibody is labeled with fluorescein isothiocyanate, a second with PE, and the third with the tandem conjugate of Texas red and PE. Unfortunately, the sensitivity of direct immunofluorescent staining is limited in circumstances where a small number of surface markers are present. In addition, cell autofluorescence can interfere with the detection of the detection of the fluorescence emission from the fluorochrome, and labeled monoclonal antibodies are not yet available for every substance of biological interest. In systems where two or more fluorochromes are simultaneously analyzed, differentiation of the separate emission signals requires more complex optical and electronic systems, and the need for additional quality control.

In indirect immunofluorescent staining procedures, an unlabeled antibody (primary antibody) is first attached to the cell and then "developed" in a second step, utilizing a fluorochrome-labeled monoclonal antibody directed against the first monoclonal antibody (secondary antibody). Polyclonal FITC-labeled goat antimouse antibody is often used as the secondary antibody (Fig. 56.24). The following steps are required:

1. Mix cell suspension with unlabeled MoAb;
2. Incubate;
3. Wash;
4. Apply FITC-labeled antimouse antibody;
5. Incubate;
6. Wash; and
7. Analyze by flow cytometry.

Indirect immunofluorescent staining is economical, since a single FITC-labeled secondary antibody can be used with many primary monoclonal antibodies. However, it is technically more complex and time-consuming than direct staining and produces a relatively higher degree of background staining. Indirect staining is primarily used when a limited quantity of a monoclonal antibody is available, to avoid the loss of antibody associated with purification and conjugation, and for the detection of cell surface antigens present at a low density. Multiparametric analysis utilizing indirect immunofluorescent staining is impractical, since it requires the use of antibodies obtained from different species.

REMOVAL OF AUTOANTIBODIES

Autoreactive antibodies are commonly present in patients with connective tissue diseases, chronic liver disease, certain renal diseases, chronic viral infections, and other diseases. In histocompatibility testing, the presence of autoantibodies (especially those that are directed against HLA Class I and Class II antigens) may interfere with the detection and analysis of alloreactive antibodies. Autoreactive antibodies are detected by the inclusion of an autocontrol (patient's serum with patient's lymphocytes) in every histocompatibility assay. If the autocontrol is positive, attempted removal of the autoreactive antibodies by absorption with lymphocytes from the same individual is attempted and the assay is repeated. Another technique (DTT treatment) is utilized when autoreactive antibodies cannot be removed by absorption.

Autoantibodies and the circulating pan-T-cell antibodies found in lupus patients are usually of the IgM class and are inactivated during treatment with dithiothreitol (DTT). The anti-HLA antibodies resulting from previous transplantation and/or multiple blood transfusions are usually of the IgG class and are not affected by DTT. DTT reduces the IgM molecule to its constituent units, while leaving the IgG molecule intact. The finding of a positive HLA crossmatch with both untreated and DTT-treated serum is consistent with the presence of anti-HLA antibodies. A positive crossmatch with untreated serum, but not with DTT-treated serum, suggests the presence of autoreactive antibodies, and is presumptive evidence for the absence of anti-HLA antibodies.

Cell Identification and Enumeration

Lymphocytes can be subdivided into stages of differentiation, and into functionally active subsets, on the basis of the cell surface antigens that are present. A revolution in immunology was brought about by the subclassification of lymphocytes into T and B cells on the basis of the cell surface antigens, and has now expanded to the analysis of other cells, such as monocytes, macrophages, myeloid stem cells, tumor cells, etc. Clinically, cell surface analysis has been useful both in the detection of abnormal cells and in the analysis of normal cells which vary in different diseases. Specific clinical applications of cell surface marker analysis (immunophenotypic analysis) include:

- Determining the origin and stage of differentiation of lymphomas and leukemias;
- Detecting early recurrence of hematological malignancies;

- Diagnosing and monitoring inherited and congenitally immunodeficient patients;
- Chemotherapeutic monitoring; and
- Pre- and posttransplantation monitoring and evaluation.

ROSETTING

Rosetting techniques were originally used in the differentiation of T and B lymphocytes (147, 148). Since T lymphocytes have a cell surface receptor (CD2) that binds sheep red blood cells, aggregates of T lymphocytes and SRBC (E-rosettes) are formed when the two cell types are incubated together. The presence of three or more SRBC adhering to a lymphocyte is considered a rosette, and evidence for the identification of the cell as a T lymphocyte. Rosettes are visualized and counted under the light microscope, with the percentage of rosetting lymphocytes taken as the percentage of T cells. B lymphocytes can be enumerated with rosetting with antibody-coated SRBCs (EA-rosette), or complement-coated SRBCs (EAC-rosette). Unfortunately, these techniques are subjective, labor-intensive, and inaccurate. In addition, the immature lymphocytes found in many types of acute leukemia and other hematologic malignancies may not possess the SRBC receptor or Fc receptors. Because of these problems, flow cytometry has became the method of choice for the quantitation of cell populations.

Assays Of Cell Function

LYMPHOCYTE TRANSFORMATION IMMUNOASSAYS

Lymphocyte transformation assays directly measure the ability of lymphocytes to respond to a stimulus. Since lymphocyte function abnormalities can occur in the absence of changes in morphology or relative or absolute cell numbers, these assays are important in the evaluation of patients with congenital immunodeficiency or acquired immune defects as a result of viral infections or immunosuppressive therapy. In addition, the principle of lymphocyte transformation is used in different ways to identify lymphokines, detect antigen sensitization, detect transplantation antigens, and in many other ways.

Principles of Lymphocyte Transformation

The basis of all lymphocyte transformation assays is the detection of metabolic changes that occur in the lymphocyte during activation. In this regard, virgin or resting lymphocytes that encounter their specific foreign antigen or a specific chemical signal are triggered to proliferate and differentiate into an "activated" form that can carry out the predestined effector or regulatory functions of the cell. During this "transformation" process T cells synthesize DNA, RNA, and protein, express Class II antigens, and synthesize and release lymphokines and other products. Morphologically, these changes are reflected by an increase in cell size, the acquisition of abundant basophilic cytoplasm, the appearance of multiple nucleoli, and changes in chromatin characteristics ("lymphoblasts"). Repeated mitotic divisions of the transformed cell occur, the progeny become progressively smaller, and the cell eventually resumes the size and appearance of the original unactivated lymphocyte.

The standard method for the quantitation of cellular proliferation incorporates tritiated thymidine (^{3}H thymidine) (160). However, technqiues utilizing fluorescent dyes have been found to provide equivalent sensitivity without the requirement for radioisotopes. In addition, flow cytometric analysis permits multiparametric quantitation of the cell populations under study and is more rapidly performed than radioisotopic determination. In one type of flow cytometric analysis, the mitogenic response of lymphoid cells, cellular activity in mixed lymphocyte cultures, and related parameters has been performed by measurement of cell cycle progression with a DNA-specific fluorochrome, such as propidium iodide (161). A fluorescent-labeled monoclonal antibody against Ki-67, a nuclear antigen that appears in proliferating cells, has been used for measuring lymphocyte proliferation (162) and the incorporation of an analog of uridine (bromodeoxyuridine, BrdUrd) (163).

Mitogen-Induced Blastogenesis

Mitogens or interleukin-2 (IL-2) are used to induce lymphocyte transformation. Of the mitogens, phytohemagglutinin (PHA) and concanavalin A (Con A) induce T blastogenesis, while pokeweed mitogen (PWM) and staphylococcal protein A (SpA) triggers B cell activation. In the past, the incorporation of tritiated thymidine has been the standard method for determining lymphocyte transformation. In this procedure, lymphocytes are isolated with Ficoll-Hypaque density gradient centrifugation and cultured for 2–4 days with a mitogen (or 5–7 days with an antigen or mixed allogeneic lymphocyte preparation) in a medium enriched with human AB serum. Tritiated thymidine is added to the culture medium, and the plates are incubated for an additional 18 hours. Cells are isolated (harvested) from the plates using a special device (cell harvester) and transferred to disks of filter paper (Fig. 56.23). The disks are placed in scintillation fluid, and counted for tritium in a liquid scintillation counter.

action. BrdUrd is an analogue of thymidine against which a monoclonal antibody is available. BrdUrd incorporation is an extremely sensitive method for the detection of cycling cells, since the incorporation of a few molecules of BrdUrd can be detected. This sensitivity permitted the detection of cell proliferation 24 to 48 hours before ^{3}H TdR incorporation.

Spontaneous Blastogenesis

Spontaneous blastogenesis (SB) assays determine the ability of cultured, unstimulated lymphocytes to undergo activation. The assay is usually performed by measuring the rate of ^{3}H thymidine incorporation. Increased spontaneous blastogenesis in transplant recipients has been associated with allograft rejection.

CYTOTOXICITY ASSAYS

Assays with cell death (cytotoxicity) as the endpoint are commonly used in cellular immunology. These assays are used in various ways to measure cell function activity and to detect cell surface antigens. In these assays, cytotoxicity may occur as the result of complement activity (complement-mediated cytotoxicity) or due to the direct effect of one cell on another (cell-mediated cytotoxicity). Until recently, target cell lysis was determined either by the release of a substance such as ^{51}chromium from the cell upon death or by the incorporation of a vital dye such as eosin or trypan blue. However, the accuracy and reproducibility of these assays has been compromised by problems such as poor uptake or nonspecific release of the marker, the length and technical complexity of the assays, or by the need for the subjective interpretation of the results. The advent of new markers, in combination with the quantitative and multiparametric abilities of the flow cytometer, may make cellular assays much more practical for routine utilization in patient care. One example of these new markers is PKH-1, a fluorochrome that emits light in the green region of the spectrum, binds avidly to the cytoplasmic membrane, and is not transferred to other cells. In one application, PKH-1 is used to label the target cells, while a second fluorochrome with a red emission signal (propidium iodide) is used to detect nonviable cells (170). This combination of markers allows statistically valid quantitation of both dead and live effectors and targets, permitting the simultaneous determination of percent target lysis, effector-to-target ratio, viability of the effector cells at the termination of the assay, and viable effector to target cell ratios. The fluorescent dyes carboxyfluorescein diacetate (CFDA) and/or propidium iodide (PI) for the determination of lymphocytotoxicity have been used and described (170–172).

Microlymphocytotoxicity Assay

One type of cytotoxicity assay, the dye exclusion lymphocytotoxicity assay, is a commonly used procedure for the detection of an antibody-antigen interaction on a cell surface. The lymphocytotoxicity assay was introduced by Terasaki and McClelland in 1964, and was later accepted as the NIH standard procedure for histocompatibility testing. In the histocompatibility laboratory, variations of the lymphocytotoxicity assay are used for HLA typing, the detection of anti-HLA antibodies, and for crossmatch testing.

In the lymphocytotoxicity procedure, viable cells (usually lymphocytes) are incubated with serum containing antisera. If a cell surface antigen is present and recognized by antibodies in the sera, an antigen-antibody complex will form on the surface. These complexes are detected by the sequential addition of rabbit complement and a vital dye, such as eosin, to the reaction mixture. The occurrence of complement fixation on the cell membrane leads to activation of the terminal complement components, and eventually to cell lysis and death. Dead cells are detected and counted by phase microscopy after differential uptake of the eosin dye and fixation with formalin. Antibody-bound lymphocytes will die, take up the eosin dye, and give a positive reaction, while unbound lymphocytes will remain viable, exclude the eosin dye, and give a negative reaction (dye exclusion) (Fig. 56.25).

Microtiter trays are read under a properly adjusted inverted phase contrast microscope in a serpentine fashion, beginning at well 1A through 1F, continuing with 2F through 2A, 3A through 3F, . . . 12F through 12A for a 72-well tray. Cells that are not injured appear small, bright and refractile, while injured cells, which have taken up the eosin dye, are larger, darker, nonrefractile, and have a slightly granular surface. The result of the analysis is expressed as an estimated percentage of cells killed, taking background killing into consideration. To facilitate and standardize the evaluation process, a standardized system approved by the NIH is used. With this system, each well is assigned a score based on the number of cells killed (Table 56.5).

HLA typing is utilized to define the HLA-A, B, C, DR, and DQ locus antigens present on human T lymphocytes. In addition to selecting donors for organ transplantation, HLA typing is important in disease association, parentage testing, and for the selection of donors for platelet or leukocyte transfusions. HLA typing is performed by lymphocytotoxicity using viable cells from the patient, and serum containing antisera of known specificity. Whole lymphocyte preparations, or purified T lymphocytes are commonly

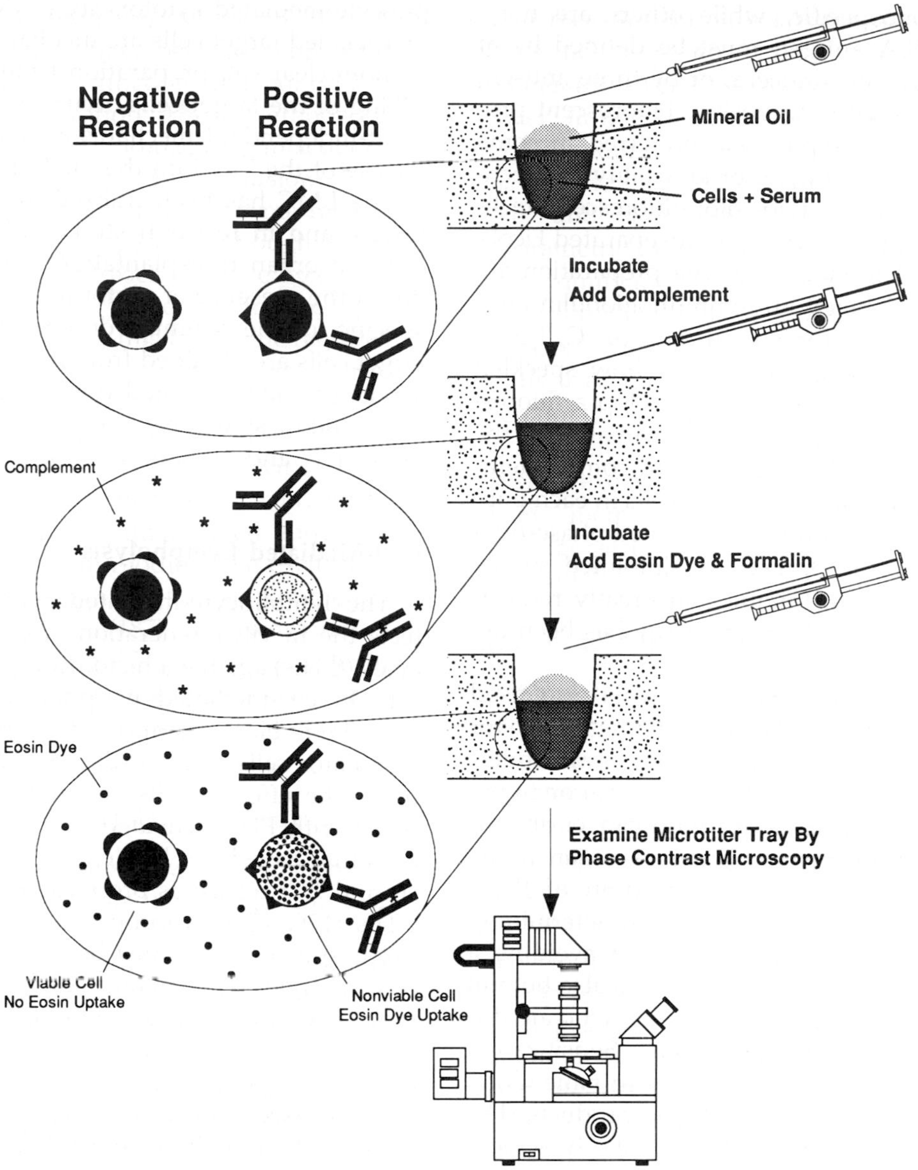

Figure 56.25. Principle of microlymphocytotoxicity by dye exclusion. Cells and serum are incubated together in the wells of a microtiter tray. Mineral oil at the top of the wells prevents fluid evaporation. Complement is added, and a second incubation is performed. The cells are washed, eosin is added, and the cells are fixed with formalin. Cells that fixed antibody and were killed through the action of complement take up eosin and appear dark and nonrefractive under a phase-contrast microscope. Living cells are refractive and easily identified by phase-contrast microscopy. Variations of the microlymphocytotoxicity assay are used for HLA typing, the HLA crossmatch, and the detection of anti-HLA antibodies. (Reprinted with permission from Riley RS, Mahin EJ, Ross W. Clinical applications of flow cytometry. New York: Igaku-Shoin Medical Publishers, 1993:639.)

Table 56.5. Scoring System for Histocompatibility Testing

Cell Death	Interpretation	Score
Unreadable well	—	0
0–10%	Negative	1
11–20%	Weak negative	2
21–50%	Weak positive	4
51–80%	Positive	6
81–100%	Strong positive	8

used for HLA class I antigen (HLA-A, B, C) determinations, while enriched B-lymphocyte suspensions are required for the determination of HLA-DR and HLA-DQ alleles. Currently, typing for HLA-DP antigens is not routinely performed by clinical laboratories since anti-HLA-DP antibodies are not generally available for microlymphocytotoxicity assays. The antisera used in HLA typing are commonly obtained from multiparous women, and are commercially available on preplated trays. Antisera are also obtained through exchanges with other laboratories, regional sharing programs, and through the National Institutes of Health (NIH) serum bank. Because some

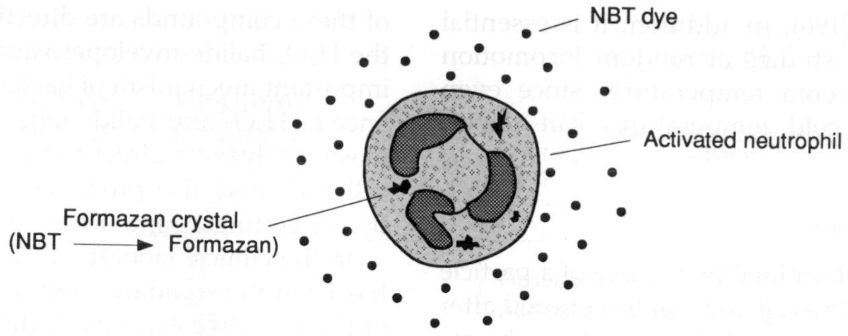

Figure 56.27. Principle of the NBT reduction assay. Neutrophils are incubated with nitroblue tetrazolium (NBT). Enzymatic action in the activated neutrophil converts NBT into an insoluble precipitate (formazan), which is visible under the microscope.

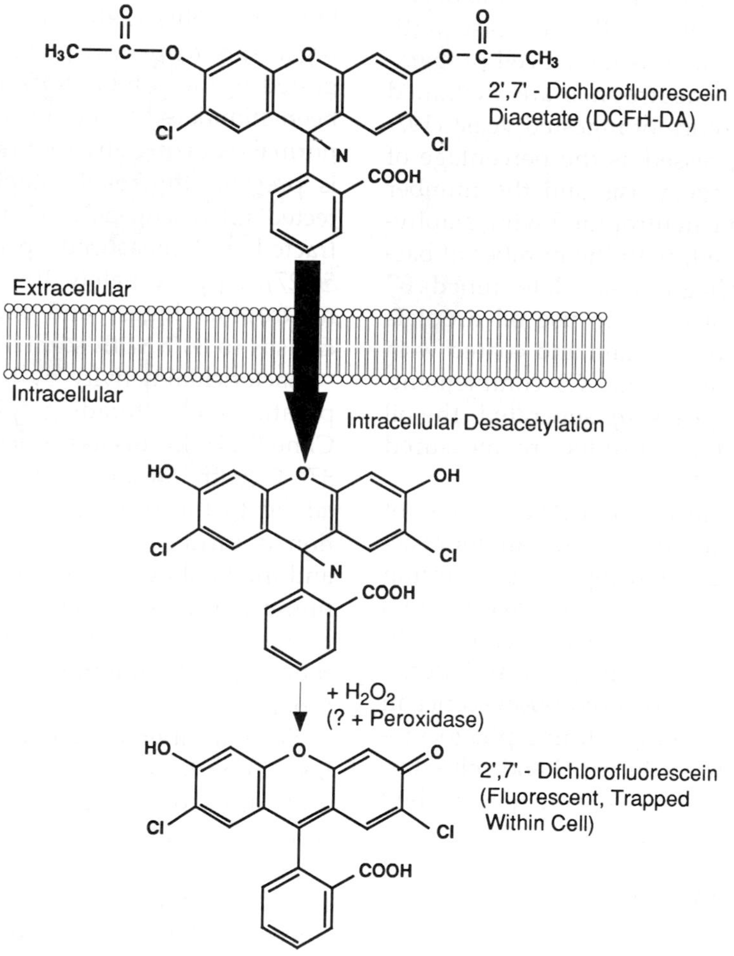

Figure 56.28. Flow cytometric analysis of the oxidative burst of polymorphonuclear leukocytes. In this assay, dichlorofluorescein-diacetate (DCFH-DA) is taken up by the cell and is trapped by deacetylation, with the formation of 2′,7′-dichlorofluorescein. During the oxidative burst, the nonfluorescent 2′,7′-dichlorofluorescein is converted into the fluorescent product dichlorofluorescein. The fluorescent intensity in the green region of the spectrum is proportional to the oxidative capacity of the cell. (Reprinted with permission from Bass et al. Flow cytometric studies of oxidative product formation by neutrophils: a graded response to membrane stimulation. J Immunol 1983;130:1910.)

Bass and other investigators have utilized this technique to study neutrophilic oxidative metabolism in normal individuals, and in patients with infectious diseases, and immunodeficiency diseases such as chronic granulomatous disease. Hydroethidine (HE) and DCFH were used by Rothe and Valet (219) to stimultaneously quantitate both H_2O_2/peroxidase and KO_2. HE is oxidized by KO_2 to ethidium bromide (EB).

Flow cytometric techniques for the simultaneous measurement of phagocytosis and intracellular killing have been reported (206, 220, 221).

Assays of Opsonization

The phagocytosis of microorganisms and other foreign bodies is greatly enhanced by the presence of certain chemical substances (opsonins) on the surface of the foreign body. Opsonization is an important function of some antibodies and is also demonstrated by certain complement breakdown products (C3b, C4b). In patients with certain immunoglobulin and complement deficiencies, an increased susceptibility to infection results in part because of decreased opsonization. Opsonins in the serum can be detected by incubating the serum with normal neutrophils and yeast particles, and visually quantitating phagocytosis of the yeast particles by normal neutrophils. In addition, flow cytometric methods have been used for the measurement of serum opsonin function (222–225). In these studies, live FITC-labeled *Neisseria meningitidis* were used to study the opsonic response in patients with serogroup B meningococcal disease. In this assay, the labeled bacteria were preopsonized by incubation with serum for 7.5 minutes, and then incubated with human polymorphonuclear neutrophilic leukocytes (PMNLs) for 5 minutes at a bacteria-to-PMNL ratio of 20:1. The results were expressed in the number of bacteria incubated per phagocyte. The opsonic response was markedly increased in acute as compared with convalescent serum, and remained elevated during the 3-year examination period. ELISA quantitation showed parallel increases in IgG1, IgG3, IgA, and IgM antibodies against type-specific group B meningococcal outer membrane proteins (223, 224).

COMPLEMENT ASSAYS

Complement is essential for the defense of the body against disease. In this regard, the complement system can eliminate target cells or organisms by direct lysis. In addition, individual complement components and fragments produced during complement activation promote immune adherence, opsonization, and chemotaxis, release histamine, and increase vascular permeability.

Complement System

The complement system consists of a series of more than 20 proteins that interact in a specific, cascade-like manner (226–238). The system is regulated by the naturally short life of the activated components and by a number of specific inhibitory compounds. There are two pathways of complement activation (classical and alternative), which are initiated by different mechanisms and may function independently or in concert. Since quantitative and functional abnormalities of the complement system have been associated with autoimmune disease and increased susceptibility to infectious disease, laboratory studies of the complement system can be of diagnostic significance (239–245). Laboratory assays for the assessment of the complement system include immunochemical quantitation of individual complement components, determinations of the functional activity of complement, and tests of complement activation. The detection of complement in tissue can be performed by immunofluorescent or immunoenzymatic staining (Table 56.6).

Table 56.6. Laboratory Evaluation of the Complement System

Functional complement assays
Hemolytic tube technique
Radial immunodiffusion technique
Quantitation of complement components
Immunonephelometry
Radial immunodiffusion
Other techniques
Complement activation assays
Immunoelectrophoresis
Immunofixation electrophoresis
Crossed immunoelectrophoresis
Electroimmunodiffusion
Radioimmunoassay
Enzyme-labeled immunoassay

Functional Complement Assays

The functional integrity of the complement system is determined by red blood cell (RBC) lysis. The principle of this assay is that the complement components, acting in concert, can lyse RBCs coated with subagglutinating amounts of an anti-RBC antibody. Since lysis occurs only when all of the complement components are functional, and present in adequate amounts, a deficiency or functional defect of a single component can prevent lysis. Therefore, the presence of complement dysfunction can be detected by this technique, but the specific nature of the defect must be determined by other methods. For this reason, these assays are usually referred to as "total hemolytic complement assays."

Hemolytic techniques for functional complement can be performed in either a liquid suspension or an agarose gel matrix. The animal source of the RBCs used in the assay determines which pathway is measured. Since the classical pathway is activated by antigen-antibody complexes, sheep RBCs sensitized with a subhemolyzing dose of rabbit antibodies to sheep RBCs are utilized in its evaluation. In the alternative pathway hemolytic assay, rabbit RBCs are used, since they selectively activate complement via the alternative pathway.

The hemolytic tube technique for functional complement utilizes a standardized suspension of RBCs

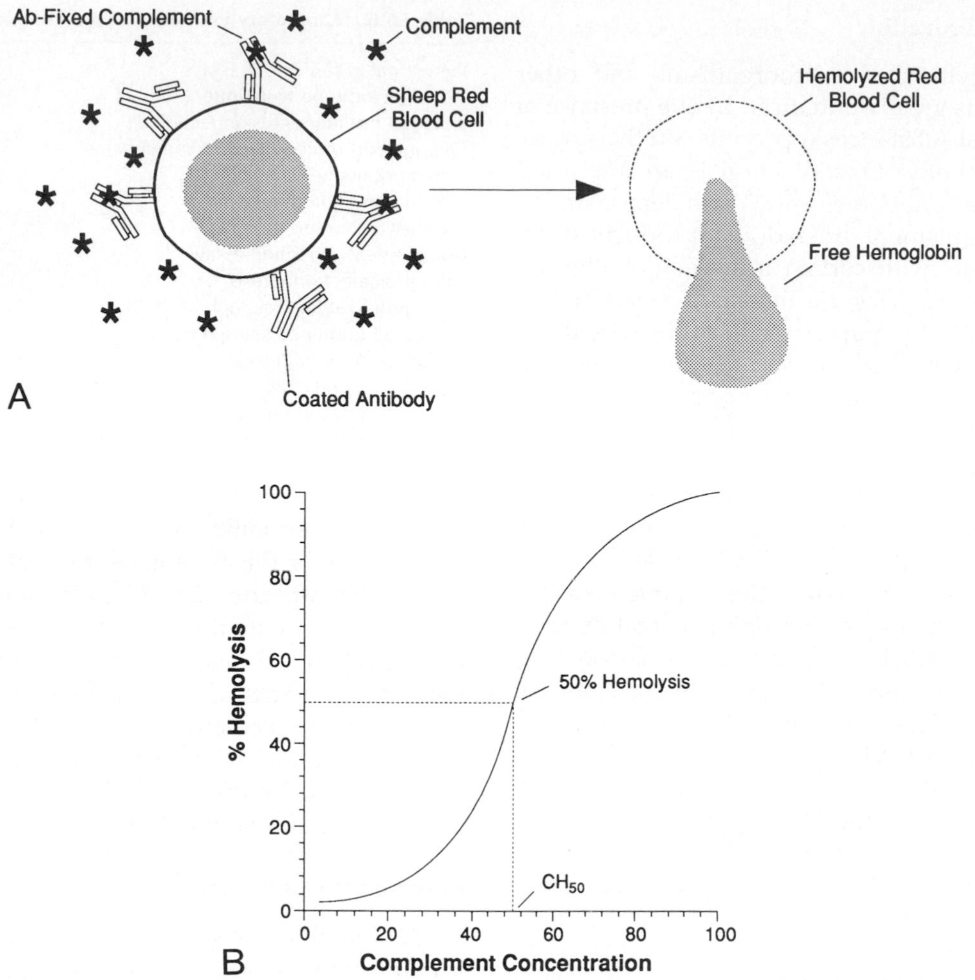

Figure 56.29. The hemolytic assay for functional complement activity. Sensitized sheep or rabbit red blood cells are the target cells in this assay. Lysis of sheep red blood cells occurs from complement activation on the surface of the red blood cell, resulting in hemolysis and the release of hemoglobin. The assay can be performed in a liquid medium (hemolytic tube assay), or in agarose gel (gel matrix or radial diffusion method). Sheep red blood cells are used to detect activation of the classical complement pathway, while rabbit red blood cells are used for the alternative pathway.

mixed with a series of dilutions of fresh serum. After an incubation period, the reaction tubes are centrifuged, and the supernatants are analyzed spectrophotometrically to determine the amount of free hemoglobin present, and the percentage of RBCs lysed. The measurement of hemolysis is most sensitive in the region where 50% of the RBCs are lysed (Fig. 56.29). Therefore, a unit of total serum hemolytic complement is the dilution of serum required to lyse 50% of a standardized amount of RBCs coated with a standard amount of antibody. The tube titration assay is usually performed in the 50% lysis area, and results expressed in CH_{50} (classical pathway) or AP_{50} units (alternative pathway). Standards can be determined by each manufacturer, or purchased by commercial sources.

In the gel matrix or radial diffusion method for the determination of functional complement, RBCs are suspended in a buffered agarose mixture, which is poured into radial diffusion plates and allowed to solidify. Wells are punched into the agarose. Complement reference sera containing known units of functional complement activity are added to the wells, together with the unknown patient's sera. After an incubation period, a cleared zone of lysed RBCs appears around each well where hemolysis has occurred. The diameter of the hemolytic zone is proportional to the functional activity of the complement in the well. Therefore, the diameter of each well is measured, and a reference graph is prepared from the known specimens. Unknowns are determined by reading from the graph.

The unit of measurement in the radial diffusion method is the dilution of serum necessary to cause 100% lysis of a standardized preparation of RBCs after activation via the classical or alternative pathway. The results are usually expressed in CH_{100} or AP_{100} units.

The results obtained by hemolytic tube titration are not directly comparable to those of hemolytic radial diffusion since the analytic techniques are different, and the endpoints of the assays are measured at different points on the complement response curve. While the 50% hemolytic units generated by tube titration assays may be considered more sensitive and quantitative than 100% hemolytic units, tube titrations are also more complicated and labor-intensive. Radial diffusion requires less elaborate laboratory equipment and is not as sensitive as tube titration to minor changes in reaction conditions. Both assays should be considered as qualitative screening tests for levels of functional complement activity, and used in conjunction with quantitative tests.

Quantitation of Individual Complement Components

The quantitation of the complement components C3 and C4 is routinely performed in the laboratory by nephelometric and other immunoassay techniques. These components are present in the highest concentration in the serum, and serve as monitors for the activation of complement. Depressed levels of C4 are usually indicative of classical pathway activation, while decreased serum C3 can result from activation of either the classical or alternative pathway. However, normal or elevated C3 and/or C4 levels do not rule out complement activation, since these substances are acute phase reactants, and their increased synthesis during acute inflammation or infection can more than compensate for consumption. Serum C1q, C2, C5, and Factor B, and other complement components can be quantitated by radial diffusion in gels or by other techniques if needed in the elevation of selected patients.

Tests of Complement Activation

Quantitative assessment of a patient sample for in vivo complement activation may be necessary when complement activation is suspected, but undetected by immunochemical or functional assays. One reason for this is the wide normal range of complement components, especially C3 and C4. If a patient's C3 or C4 level is normally near the upper range of normal, it may decrease into the lower range of normal during an illness, but still be reported as normal.

In vivo activation could also go undetected because most complement components are acute phase reactants that undergo increased synthesis during states of illness. This compensatory effect may cause normal in vitro complement levels or function, even in the presence of complement breakdown.

Testing for activation fractions can also be useful in studies of decreased complement levels, since low values may be caused by increased consumption or decreased synthesis. If activation fragments are not found in the presence of low quantitative and functional levels, the cause is decreased synthesis (240, 241, 246).

The methods utilized for the laboratory detection of complement activation fragments include (*a*) Immunoelectrophoresis; (*b*) immunofixation electrophoresis; (*c*) crossed immunoelectrophoresis; (*d*) electroimmunodiffusion; (*e*) RIA; and (*f*) ELISA. Using these techniques, it is possible to detect the smaller breakdown products of C3a, C3c, C3d, C4d, Ba, or Bb.

Immunohistochemical Staining

A new era of pathological diagnosis began with the introduction of immunochemical techniques into the histology laboratory. These techniques utilize the natural specificity of the antibody to identify and localize a variety of antigens, including immunoglobulins, cell surface markers, hormones, enzymes, oncodevelopmental antigens, viral/bacterial substances, etc., many of which were previously undetectable by cytochemical staining. Polyclonal or monoclonal antibodies labeled with a fluorescent dye were first used as immunohistochemical stains. Unfortunately, immunofluorescent staining is of limited sensitivity and requires frozen tissue sections. In addition, a fluorescent microscope is required for reading the slides. Immunoperoxidase techniques, utilizing monoclonal or polyclonal antibodies, are many times more sensitive than immunofluorescent methods and can usually be performed on fixed, paraffin-embedded tissue. Immunoperoxidase-stained sections can be examined with the ordinary light microscope and are able to withstand long storage.

Immunofluorescent Staining

Antibodies conjugated with a fluorescent dye were first used for the localization of antigens in tissue by Coons and associates in 1941. Fluorescein isothiocyanate has been the most widely used fluorescent label, since the human eye is very sensitive to its yellow-green fluorescence, and since green autofluorescence is less common in nature than red autofluorescence (117). The direct and indirect methods of tissue immunofluorescence have been used, although inhibition and complement-staining techniques have been described.

Direct immunofluorescent staining is used to detect the presence of antigen in a tissue. In this procedure, the fluorochrome-labeled antibody is directly applied to the tissue section at its optimal dilution and incubated for a short period of time. After washing to remove unbound dye, the section is mounted in a water-soluble medium (usually buffered glycerol) and visualized by light microscopy. The sensitivity of direct immunofluorescent staining is dependent upon the avidity of the antibody, the density of the antigen in the tissue, and the sensitivity of the eye.

Indirect immunofluorescent staining is primarily used to detect the presence of an antibody in body fluids, although the same procedure can also be applied for the identification of an unknown antigen in a tissue. In indirect staining, unlabeled antibody is first reacted with the antigen in the tissue. After incubation and washing to remove unlabeled antibody, a fluorochrome-labeled secondary antibody specific for the primary antibody is used. The tissue is visualized by fluorescent microscopy after a second incubation and washing. The indirect method is more sensitive than the direct technique, since the staining intensity is amplified by the second antibody. In addition, this technique is economical, since the same labeled antibody can be used with multiple primary antibodies. However, nonspecific staining can be increased relative to direct staining.

There are numerous quality control considerations in immunofluorescent staining. First, the specificity of an antibody used in immunofluorescent staining must be extensively documented and the antibody must be used at its proper dilution. For the identification of antigens in tissue, controls with and without the antigen must be available. If possible, demonstration of the specificity of binding of the antibody should be documented by inhibition or "blocking" of fluorescent staining on known positive tissue by unlabeled antigen. In addition, loss of staining should be observed in the positive control after the antisera is adsorbed with purified antigen. The dye:protein ratio is another consideration. The negative charge of a conjugate with a high dye:protein ratio can lead to increased nonspecific staining. On the other hand, the sensitivity of detection of the staining reaction is reduced by the use of a conjugate with a dye:protein ratio that is excessively low. Electrophoresis with densitometric scanning of the gel can be used to detect the presence of unlabeled fluorescein and/or protein. The total protein concentration of a conjugate is measured by the biuret reaction of similar procedure. Unlabeled dye can be removed by dialysis, while highly negatively charged conjugates can be separated by DEAE-cellulose chromatography. Nonspecific, extraneous antibodies in antisera are best detected by immunoelectrophoresis or precipitin reactions in gels (117). Documentation of the sensitivity of a conjugate is performed by gel diffusion precipitation, using serially diluted preparations of the conjugate against a solution of the antigen at a concentration of 1 mg/ml. The highest dilution of the conjugate that gives a visible line of precipitation is the unitage. Conjugates for immunofluorescent staining should have at least 4 units/1% protein (117). Although F:P ratios can be expressed as a weight ratio (micrograms of bound FITC per milligram of protein), they are usually expressed as molar ratios by multiplying the weight ratios by a factor of 0.411.

Commercial antisera and conjugates are supplied with information regarding the F:P ratio, protein concentration, and the results of assays for immunologic sensitivity and specificity. However, since the optimal working dilution will vary in each laboratory, it must be individually determined prior to using the reagent. For direct immunofluorescent staining, serial dilutions of the conjugate are used with a positive control to determine the optimal combination of bright fluorescence and low background staining. In indirect staining, where two antibodies are used, "chessboard" (or "checkerboard") titrations are performed. In this technique, serial dilutions of a primary antibody are incubated with a well-characterized positive control, and each dilution is in turn developed with serial dilutions of the fluorochrome-labeled secondary antibody. The fluorescence intensity of each combination is recorded in tabular format. For each dilution of primary antibody, the fluorescent intensity will be constant for several dilutions of conjugate (plateau titer). In general, the highest conjugate dilution (plateau endpoint) can be diluted twofold to obtain a working dilution. For fluoresceinated antibodies with an F:P ratio of 3 to 5, a plateau endpoint between 1/6 and 1/64 is expected against a high-titered primary antibody, and a working dilution of approximately 1/4 unit/ml is generally used. For conjugates employed in direct immunofluorescent staining, dilutions of 1 unit/ml to 1/4 unit/ml provide satisfactory results in most circumstances (117). Since antibody conjugates are labile, good storage conditions are critical. Generally, fresh conjugates should be ultracentrifuged, divided into small aliquots and stored in a protein-rich medium (2 mg/ml or greater) at ultracold temperatures (-80° C or the vapor phase of liquid nitrogen) for long-term storage. Conjugates should be thawed only once before use, and should be given a high-speed centrifugation before use (117). Stabilized, undiluted conjugates can usually be stored at 4° C for several weeks.

Proper preservation and sectioning of tissue is essential for the retention of immunologic reactivity and morphological detail. Needle biopsies or small pieces of tissue (approximately 3 to 5 mm) is obtained in the fresh state and placed on pieces of moistened (not soaked) gauze for transport. The tissue is then placed on a piece of a wooden tongue

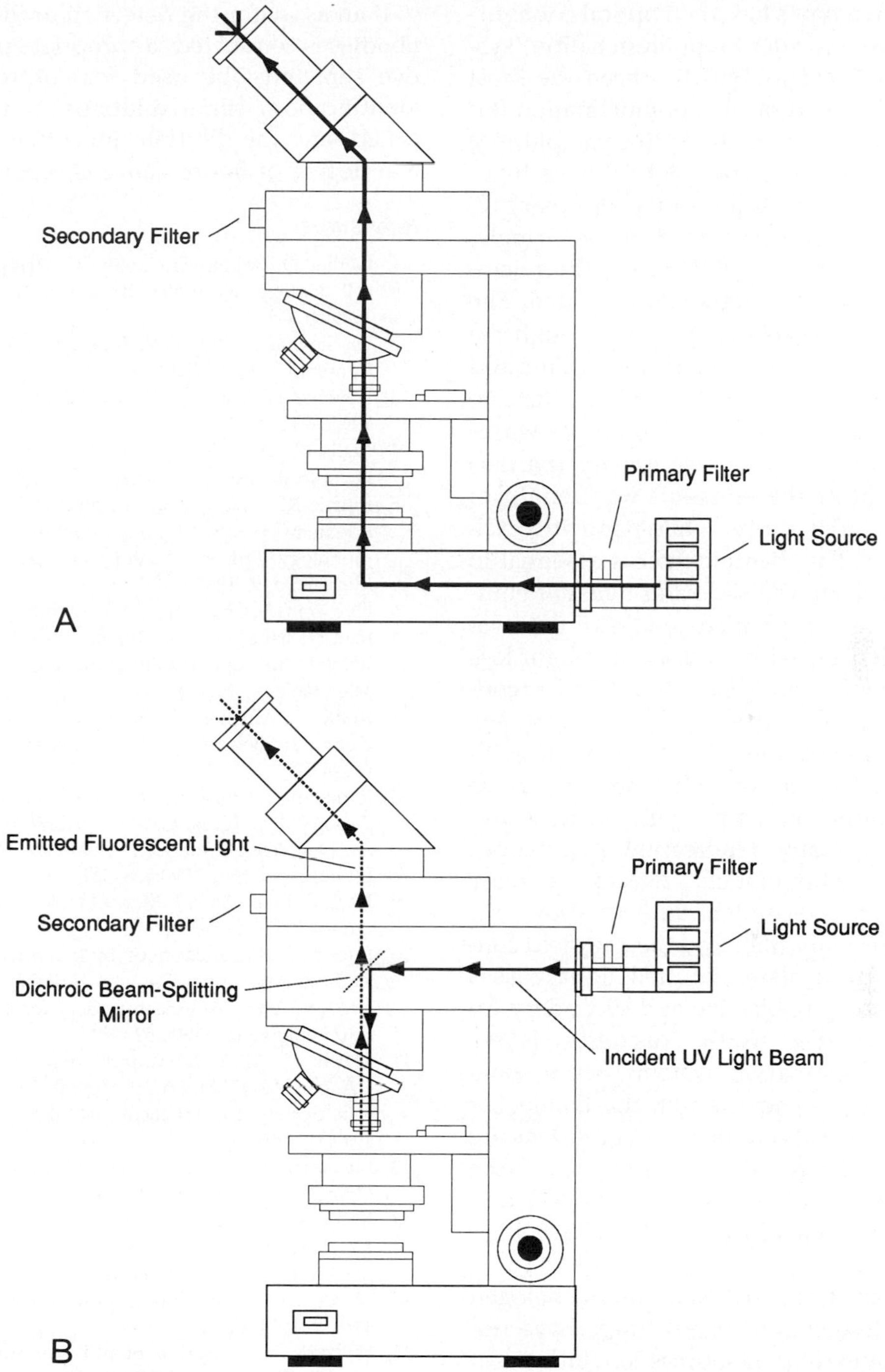

Figure 56.30. Schematic illustrations of epi-illumination (**A**) and transmitted illumination (**B**) fluorescent microscopes.

blade, sponge, or cork, embedded in OCT compound (Ames Co., Elkhart, IN), and "snap" or "flash" frozen by complete immersion in liquid nitrogen, isopentane cooled to the temperature of liquid nitrogen, or a dry ice-acetone mixture. The frozen tissue is then wrapped in aluminum foil, placed in a precooled, air-tight storage container, and stored at a temperature of −70°C or −80°C until sectioning and staining. Sections of 4 to 6 μm are cut under reduced temperature with a standard cryostat. Brief fixation of the tissue sections in acetone or absolute ethyl alcohol is sometimes employed to prevent the loss of soluble antigens or antibodies.

The fluorescent microscope provides a means of illuminating stained tissue with light of a proper wavelength under darkfield conditions, separating the excitation and emission wavelengths, and visualizing the stained tissue. Fluorescent microscopes can be classified into two types based on optical configuration. The brightfield incident (epi-illumination) system described by Ploem in 1967 has been the most widely utilized. The heart of the epi-illumination fluorescent microscope is a dichroic (beam-splitting) mirror. In this system, excitation light from a high-intensity light source is passed through a primary filter, strikes a dichroic mirror placed at a 45° angle, and is deflected through the objective of the microscope onto the slide where a darkfield is created. The light emitted from the specimen returns through the objective and passes through the dichroic filter and secondary filter to the oculars. The primary (excitation) filter is used to select light of the proper wavelength for excitation, while the secondary (barrier) filter transmits light at the emission wavelength of the fluorochrome under study, while removing excitation wavelengths. The dichroic filter is essential to reflect excitation light to the slide and transmit emitted light to the observer. One advantage of this system is that a condenser, with its associated light loss is not required, since the objective acts as a condenser. In addition, filter systems can be easily exchanged for viewing tissue sections labeled with multiple conjugated dyes, and fluorescence can be performed in conjunction with phase contrast and other types of microscopy. Fluorescent microscopes with transmitted illumination usually employ darkfield (oil immersion) condensers. Excitation light passes through a primary filter and the darkfield condenser onto the glass slide. Emitted light passes through the microscope objective and secondary filter to the ocular lens (Fig. 56.30). This design is less efficient than epi-illumination systems, since some light is diffused in passing through the condenser and barrier filter. In addition, filter configurations are more difficult to change. In all microscopes, the objectives must be nonfluorescent and collect and transmit light with high efficiency (i.e., have high numerical aperture, [NA]).

High-pressure arc (mercury, xenon) and halogen (quartz-iodine or tungsten-halogen) lamps have traditionally been the excitation sources for fluorescent microscopes. High-pressure arc lamps are the most widely used excitation sources, since they produce light of very high intensity and have relatively long life spans (approximately 200 hours). However, light intensity decreases with age, and these lamps require a protective housing since they operate at high temperature and pressure. In the near future the small, inexpensive lasers that have recently became available in flow cytometers may be incorporated into the fluorescent microscope. These have very long life spans and produce monochromatic light of very high intensity.

If an assay for the detection or identification of antibodies is conducted, appropriate positive and negative sera must be used for controls. For antibody identification, serial dilutions of the specimen are tested, and the dilution (titer) that produces a minimal degree of fluorescence is reported as positive.

References

1. Gerlier D, Rabourdin-Combe C. Antigen processing—from cell biology to molecular interactions. Immunol Today 1989;10:3–5.
2. Di Giovine F, Duff GW. Interleukin 1: the first interleukin. Immunol Today 1990;11:13–20.
3. Whicher JT, Evans SW. Cytokines in disease. Clin Chem 1990;36:1269–1281.
4. Inglis JR. Special feature on immunotechnology and industry: introduction. Immunol Today 1983;4:125–139.
5. Ritchie RF. Preparation of polyclonal antisera. In: Rose NR, Friedman H, Fahey JL, eds. Manual of clinical laboratory immunology. 3rd ed. Washington, DC: American Society for Microbiology, 1986:4–8.
6. Hudson GA. Characterization of antisera. In: Rose NR, Friedman H, Fahey JL, eds. Manual of clinical laboratory immunology. 3rd ed. Washington, DC: American Society for Microbiology, 1986:49–56.
7. Kohler G, Milstein C. Continuous cultures of fused cells secreting antibody of predefined specificity. Nature 1975;256: 445–497.
8. Johnston J. Purification of monoclonal antibodies. In: Zachary AA, Teresi GA, eds. ASHI laboratory manual. 2nd ed. New York: American Society for Histocompatibility and Immunogenetics, 1990:528–532.
9. Koch C, Bennedsen J. Monoclonal antibodies. Curr Opin Immunol 1989;2:385–391.
10. Lucero K. Production of bulk monoclonal antibodies. In: Zachary AA, Teresi GA, eds. ASHI laboratory manual. 2nd ed. New York: American Society for Histocompatibility and Immunogenetics, 1990:523–527.
11. Martin PJ. Monoclonal antibodies. In: Zachary AA, Teresi GA, eds. ASHI laboratory manual. 2nd ed. New York: American Society for Histocompatibility and Immunogenetics, 1990:519–522.
12. Melamed MD, Bradley CE. Monoclonal antibodies. Curr Opin Immunol 1989;1:929–936.
13. Milstein C. Overview: monoclonal antibodies. In: Weir DM, ed. Handbook of experimental immunology. Oxford: Blackwell Scientific Publications, 1986.
14. Moore GP. Genetically engineered antibodies. Clin Chem 1989;35:1849–1853.
15. Williams D. Purification of antigens and monoclonal antibodies. Clin Rheumatol 1987;1:43–55.
16. Zola H, Neoh SH. Monoclonal antibody purification: choice of method and assessment of purity and yield. Biotechniques 1989;7:804–808.
17. Epstein N, Epstein M. The hybridoma technology: I. Production of monoclonal antibodies. Adv Biotechnol Processes 1986;6:179–218.
18. Abrams PG, Rossio JL, Stevenson HC, Foon KA. Optimal strategies for developing human-human monoclonal antibodies. Methods Enzymol 1986;121:107–119.
19. Westerwoudt RJ. Factors affecting production of monoclonal antibodies. Methods Enzymol 1986;121:3–18.
20. Diamond BA, Yelton DE, Scharff MD. Monoclonal antibodies: a new technology for producing serologic reagents. N Engl J Med 1981;304:1344–1349.

21. Epstein N, Kobiler D, Epstein M. The hybridoma technology: II. Applications of hybrid cell products: monoclonal antibodies and lymphokines. Adv Biotechnol Processes 1986;6:219–251.
22. Fair WR. Immunodiagnosis and immunoimaging. Prog Clin Biol Res 1988;269:289–311.
23. Grossman HB. Clinical applications of monoclonal antibody technology. Urol Clin North Am 1986;13:465–474.
24. Lowder JN. The current status of monoclonal antibodies in the diagnosis and therapy of cancer. Curr Probl Cancer 1986;10:485–551.
25. Macintyre EA. The use of monoclonal antibodies for purging autologous bone marrow in the lymphoid malignancies. Clin Haematol 1986;15:249–267.
26. McCullough KC. Monoclonal antibodies: implications for virology. Brief review. Arch Virol 1986;87:1–36.
27. Miyai K, Endo Y, Ichihara K, Amino N. Application of monoclonal antibody to laboratory tests—immunoassay. Rinsho Byori 1986;34:125–132.
28. Payne WJ, Marshall DL, Shockley RK, Martin WJ. Clinical laboratory applications of monoclonal antibodies. Clin Microbiol Rev 1988;1:313–129.
29. Reading CL, Takaue Y. Monoclonal antibody applications in bone marrow transplantation. Biochim Biophys Acta 1986;865:141–170.
30. Wong JH, Irie RF, Morton DL. Human monoclonal antibodies: prospects for the therapy of cancer. Semin Surg Oncol 1989;5:448–452.
31. Mayforth RD, Quintans J. Designer and catalytic antibodies. N Engl J Med 1990;323:173–178.
32. Hedin A, Carlsson L, Berglund A. A monoclonal antibody-enzyme immunoassay for serum carcinoembryonic antigen with increased specificity for carcinomas. Proc Natl Acad Sci USA 1983;80:3470–3474.
33. Hogg N. The structure and function of Fc receptors. Immunol Today 1988;9:185–186.
34. Nichols WS, Nakamura RM. Agglutination and agglutination inhibition assays. In: Rose NR, Friedman H, Fahey JL, eds. Manual of clinical laboratory immunology. 3rd ed. Washington, DC: American Society for Microbiology, 1986:49–56.
35. Coombs RR. Harnessing the red cell for immunoassays. Med Lab Sci 1987;44:66–72.
36. Coombs RR, Scott ML, Cranage MP. Assays using red cell-labelled antibodies. J Immunol Methods 1987;101:1–14.
37. Gribnau TC, Leuvering JH, van Hell H. Particle-labelled immunoassays: a review. J Chromatography 1986;376:175–189.
38. van Hell H, Leuvering JHW, Gribnau TCJ. Particle immunoassays. In: Collins WP, ed. Alternative immunoassays. New York: John Wiley & Sons, 1985:39–58.
39. Boyden SV. The adsorption of protein on erythrocytes treated with tannic acid and subsequent hemagglutination by antiprotein sera. J Exp Med 1951;93:107–120.
40. Singer JM, Plotz CM. The latex fixation test. I. Application to the serological diagnosis of rheumatoid arthritis. Amer J Med 1956;21:888–891.
41. Hadfield SG, Lane A, McIllmurray MB. A novel cvoloured latex test for the detection and identification of more than one antigen. J Immunol Methods 1987;97:153–158.
42. Wilkins TA, Brouwers G, Mareschall JC, Limet J, Masson PL. Immunoassay by particle counting. In: Collins WP, ed. Complementary immunoassays. New York: John Wiley & Sons, 1988:227–240.
43. Collet-Cassart D, Limet JN, Van Krieken L, De Hertogh R. Turbidimetric latex immunoassay of placental lactogen on microtiter plates. Clin Chem 1989;35:141–143.
44. Johnson AM. Immunoprecipitation in gels. In: Rose NR, Friedman H, Fahey JL, eds. Manual of clinical laboratory immunology. 3rd ed. Washington, DC: American Society for Microbiology, 1986:14–24.
45. Crowe AJ. Immunodiffusion. New York: Academic Press, 1961.
46. Fahey JL, McKelvey EM. Quantitative determination of serum immunoglobulins in antibody-agar plates. J Immunol 1965;94:84–90.
47. Mancini G, Carbonara AO, Heremans JF. Immunochemical quantitation of antigens by single radial immunodiffusion. Immunochemistry 1965;2:235–254.
48. Svendsen PJ. Fused rocket immunoelectrophoresis. In: Axelsen NH, Kroll J, Weeke B, eds. A manual of quantitative immunoelectrophoresis. Oslo: Universitetsforlaget, 1973:69–70.
49. Afonso E. Quantitative immunoelectrophoresis of serum proteins. Clin Chem Acta 1964;10:114–122.
50. Clark HGM, Freeman T. Quantitative immunoelectrophoresis of human serum proteins. Clin Sci 1968;35:403–413.
51. Wilson AT. Direct immunoelectrophoresis. J Immunol 1964;92:431–434.
52. Alper CA, Johnson AM. Immunofixation electrophoresis: a technique for the study of protein polymorphism. Vox Sang 1969;17:445–452.
53. Arnaud P, Wilson GB, Koistinen J, Fudenberg HH. Immunofixation after electrofocusing: improved method for specific detection of serum proteins with determination of isoelectric points. I. Immunofixation print technique for detection of alpha-1-protease inhibitor. J Immunol Methods 1977;16:221–231.
54. Ritchie RF, Smith R. Immunofixation. I. General principles and application to agarose gel electrophoresis. Clin Chem 1976;22:1735–1737.
55. Gerson B, LaBrie J, Copeland BE. Immunofixation on thin-layer agarose. Clin Chem 1979;25:197.
56. Keshgegian AA, Peiffer P. Immunofixation as an adjunct to immunoelectrophoresis in characterization of serum monoclonal immunoglobulins. Clin Chim Acta 1981;110:337–340.
57. Pascali E, Pezzoli A, Chiarandini A. Immunofixation: application to the identification of "difficult" monoclonal components. Clin Chem 1982;28:1404–1405.
58. Pedersen NS, Axelsen NH. Detection of M-components by an easy immunofixation procedure: comparison with agarose gel electrophoresis and classical immunoelectrophoresis. J Immunol Methods 1979;30:257–262.
59. Whicher JT, Hawkins L, Higginson J. Clinical applications of immunofixation: a more sensitive method for the detection of Bence Jones protein. J Clin Pathol 1980;33:779–780.
60. Whicher JT, Price CP, Spencer K. Immunonephelometric and immunoturbidimetric assays for proteins. CRC Crit Rev Clin Lab Sci 18:213–257.
61. Sternberg JC. Rate nephelometry. In: Rose NR, Friedman H, Fahey JL, eds. Manual of clinical laboratory immunology. 3rd ed. Washington, DC: American Society for Microbiology, 1986:304–307.
62. Hellsing K, Laurent TC. The influence of dextran on the precipitin reaction. Acta Chem Scand 1964;18:1303.
63. Foster RC, Ledue TB. Turbidimetry. In: Rose NR, Friedman H, Fahey JL, eds. Manual of clinical laboratory immunology. 3rd ed. Washington, DC: American Society for Microbiology, 1986:25–32.
64. Normansell DE. Quantitation of serum immunoglobulins. CRC Crit Rev Clin Lab Sci 17:103–170.
65. Opheim KE, Glick MR, Ou C-N, et al. Particle-enhanced turbidimetric inhibition immunoassay for theophylline evaluated with the Du Pont ACA. Clin Chem 1984;30:1870–1874.
66. Gosling JP. A decade of development in immunoassay methodology. Clin Chem 1990;36:1408–1427.

67. Diamandis EP. Immunoassays with time-resolved fluorescence spectroscopy: principles and applications. Clin Biochem 1988;21:139–150.
68. Schall RF, Tenoso HF. Alternatives to radioimmunoassay: labels and methods. Clin Chem 1981;27:1157–1164.
69. Howanitz JH. Immunoassay. Innovations in label technology. Arch Pathol Lab Med 1988;112:775–779.
70. Nickoloff EL. Interference in immunoassay. CRC Crit Rev Clin Lab Sci 21:255–267.
71. Yalow RS. Practices and pitfalls in immunologic methodology. Adv. Prostaglandin Thromboxane Leukot Res 1986;16: 327–338.
72. Ekins RP. Current concepts and future developments. In: Collins WP, ed. Alternative immunoassays. New York: John Wiley & Sons, 1985:219–237.
73. Yalow RS, Berson SA. Immunological specificity of human insulin: application to immunoassay of insulin. J Clin Invest 1961;40:2190–2198.
74. Ekins RP. The estimation of thyroxine in human plasma by an electrophoretic technique. Clin Chem Acta 1960;5:453–459.
75. Larsen J, Odell WD. General principles of radioimmunoassay. In: Rose NR, Friedman H, Fahey JL, eds. Manual of clinical laboratory immunology. 3rd ed. Washington, DC: American Society for Microbiology, 1986:110–115.
76. Binoux MA, Odell WD. Use of dextran-coated charcoal to separate antibody-bound from free hormone: a critique. J Clin Endocrinol Metab 1973;36:303–310.
77. Desbuquois B, Aurbach GD. Use of polyethylene glycol to separate free and antibody-bound peptide hormones in radioimmunoassays. J Clin Endocrinol 1971;33:732–738.
78. Oellerich M. Enzyme-immunoassay: a review. J Clin Chem Clin Biochem 1984;22:895–904.
79. Johannsson A, Ellis DH, Bates DL, Plumb AM, Stanley CJ. Enzyme amplification for immunoassays. Detection limit of one hundredth of an attomole. J Immunol Methods 1986;87: 7–11.
80. Ishikawa E, Hashida S, Tanaka K, Kohno T. Development and applications of ultrasensitive enzyme immunoassays for antigens and antibodies. Clin Chim Acta 1989;185:223–230.
81. Kabakoff DS. Chemical aspects of enzyme-immunoassay. In: Maggio ET, ed. Enzyme-immunoassay. Boca Raton: CRC Press, Inc., 1980:71–104.
82. Engvall E, Perlmann P. Enzyme-linked immunosorbent assay (ELISA). Quantitative assay of immunoglobulin G. Immunochemistry 1971;8:871–874.
83. Ngo TT, Lenhoff HM. New approach to heterogenous enzyme immunoassays using tagged enzyme-ligand conjugates. Biochem Biophys Res Commun 1981;99:496–503.
84. Rowley GL, Rubenstein JE, Huisjen J, Ullman EF. Mechanism by which antibodies inhibit hapten-malate dehydrogenase conjugates. J Biol Chem 1975;250:3759–3766.
85. Ullman EF, Blakemore J, Leute RK, Eimstad W, Jaklitsch A. Homogenous enzyme immunoassay for thyroxine. Clin Chem 1075;21:1011.
86. Allain P, Turcant A, Premel-Cabic A. Automated fluoroimmunoassay of theophylline and valproic acid by flow-injection analysis with use of HPLC instruments. Clin Chem 1989;35:469–470.
87. Boguslaski RC, Li TM. Homogenous immunoassays. Appl Biochem Biotechnol 1982;7:404.
88. Carrio RJ, Christner JE, Boguslaski RC, Yeung KK. A method for monitoring specific binding reactions with cofactor labeled ligands. Anal Biochem 1976;72:271–282.
89. Schroeder HR, Carrico RJ, Boguslaski RC, Christner JE. Specific binding reactions monitored with ligand-cofactor conjugates and bacterial luciferase. Anal Biochem 1976;72:283–292.
90. Ngo TT, Lenhoff HM. Enzyme modulators as tools for the development of the homogenous enzyme immunoassays. FEBS Lettrs 1980;116:285–288.
91. Gibbons I, Hanlon TM, Skold CN, Russell ME, Ullman EF. Enzyme-enhancement immunoassay: a homogenous assay for polyvalent ligands and antibodies. Clin Chem 1981;27: 1602–1608.
92. Wei R, Reibe S. Preparation of a phospholipase C-antihuman IgG conjugate and inhibition of its enzymatic activity by human IgG. Clin Chem 1977;23:1386–1392.
93. Wilkins TA, Brouwers G, Mareschal J-C, Cambiaso CL. High sensitivity, homogenous particle-based immunoassay for thyrotropin (Multipact™). Clin Chem 1988;34:1749–1752.
94. Auditore-Hargreaves K, Houghton RL, Monji N, Priest JH, Hoffman AS, Nowinski RC. Phase-separation immunoassays. Clin Chem 1987;33:1509–1516.
95. Litchfield WJ, Freytag JW, Adamich M. Highly sensitive immunoassays based on use of liposomes without complement. Clin Chem 1984;30:1441–1445.
96. Henderson DR, Friedman SB, Harris JD, Manning WB, Zoccoli MA. CEDIA™, a new homogenous immunoassay system. Clin Chem 1986;32:1637–1641.
97. Khanna PL, Dworschack RT, Manning WB, Harris JD. A new homogenous enzyme immunoassay using recombinant enzyme fragments. Clin Chim Acta 1989;185:231–240.
98. Blum LJ, Gautier SM, Coulet PR. Design of luminescence photobiosensors. J Biolumin Chemilumin 1989;4:543–550.
99. Davis KA, Leary TR. Continuous liquid-phase piezoelectric biosensor for kinetic immunoassays. Anal Chem 1989;61: 1227–1230.
100. Green MJ. Electrochemical immunoassays. Philos Trans Roy Soc London Ser B 1987;B316:135–142.
101. Heineman WR, Halsall HB, Wehmeyer KR, Doyle MJ, Wright DS. Immunoassay with electrochemical detection. Methods Biochem Anal 1987;32:345–393.
102. Ngeh NJ, Suleiman AA, Guilbault GG. Piezoelectric crystal biosensors. Biosensors Bioelectronics 1990;5:13–26.
103. Rishpon J, Rosen I. The development of an immunosensor for the electrochemical determination of the isoenzyme LDH5. Biosensors 1989;4:61–74.
104. Stanley CJ, Cox RB, Cardosi MF, Turner APF. Amperometric enzyme-amplified immunoassays. J Immunol Methods 1988;112:153–161.
105. Tsuji I, Eguchi H, Yasukouchi K, Unoki M, Taniguchi I. Enzyme immunosensors based on electropolymerized polytyramine modified electrodes. Biosensors Bioelectronics 1990;5:87–101.
106. Yao T, Rechnitz GA. Amperometric enzyme-immunosensor based on ferrocene-mediated. Biosensors 1987;3:307–312.
107. Mayo CS, Hallock RB. Immunoassay based on surface plasmon oscillations. J Immunol Methods 1989;120:105–114.
108. Giegel JL, Brotherton MM, Cronin P, et al. Radial partition immunoassay. Clin Chem 1982;28:1894–1898.
109. Anderson RR, Lee TT, Saewart DC, Sowden KM, Valkirs GE. Internally reference ImmunoCentration™ assays. Clin Chem 1986;32:1692–1695.
110. Waggoner AS. Fluorescent probes for analysis of cell structure, function, and health by flow and imaging cytometry. In: Applications of fluorescence in the biomedical sciences. New York: Alan R. Liss, 1986:3–28.
111. Mathies RA, Stryer L. Single-molecule fluorescence detection: a feasibility study using phycoerythrin. In: Applications of fluorescence in the biomedical sciences. New York: Alan R. Liss, 1986:3–28.
112. Oi VT, Glazer AN, Stryer L. Fluorescent phycobiliprotein conjugates for analyses of cells and molecules. J Cell Biol 1982;93:981–986.

113. Glazer AN, Stryer L. Phycofluor probes. Trends Biol Sci 1984;9:423–427.
114. Kronick MN. The use of phycobiliproteins as fluorescent labels in immunoassay. J Immunol Methods 1986;92:1–13.
115. Smith DS, Al-Hakiem MHH, Landon J. A review of fluoroimmunoassay and immunofluorometric assay. Ann Clin Biochem 1981;18:253–274.
116. Hemmila I. Fluoroimmunoassays and immunofluorometric assays. Clin Chem 1985;31:359–370.
117. Nakamura RM, Tucker ES III. Antibody as reagent. In: Henry JB, ed. Clinical diagnosis and management by laboratory methods. 17th ed. Philadelphia: WB Saunders, 1984:893–923.
118. Smith DS. Enhancement fluoroimmunoassay of thyroxine. FEBS Letters 1977;77:25–27.
119. Calvin J, Burling K, Blow C, Barnes I, Price CP. Evaluation of fluorescence excitation transfer immunoassay for measurement of specific proteins. J Immunol Methods 1985;86:249–256.
120. Peterson JD, Kim JY, Melvold RW, Miller SD, Waltenbaugh C. A rapid method for quantitation of antiviral antibodies. J Immunol Methods 1989;119:83–94.
121. Dandliker WB, De Saussure VA. Fluorescence polarization in immunochemistry. Immunochemistry 1970;7:799–828.
122. Dandliker WB, Kelley RJ, Dandliker J, Farquahar J, Levin J. Fluorescence polarization immunoassay. Theory and experimental method. Immunochemistry 1973;10:219–227.
123. Jovin TM. Fluorescence polarization and energy transfer: Theory and application. In: Melamed MR, Mullaney PF, Mendelsohn ML, eds. Flow cytometry and sorting. 1st ed. New York: John Wiley & Sons, 1979:137–165.
124. Szollosi J, Trons L, Damjanoviek S, Hellewell SH, Arndt-jovin D, Jovin TM. Fluorescence energy transfer measurements on cell surfaces: a critical comparison of steady state fluorimetric and flow cytometric methods. Cytometry 1984;5:210–216.
125. Watson RAA, Landon J, Shaw EJ, Smith DS. Polarization immunoassay of gentamicin. Clin Chim Acta 1976;73:51–55.
126. McGregor AR, Crookall-Greening JO, Landon J, Smith DS. Polarization fluoroimmunoassay of phenytoin. Clin Chim Acta 1978;83:161–166.
127. Colbert DL, Galacher G, Mainwaring-Burton RW. Single-reagent polarization fluoroimmunoassay for amphetamine in urine. Clin Chem 1985;31:1193–1195.
128. Halfman CJ, Jay DW. Homogenous, micelle quenching fluoroimmunoassay for detecting amphetamines in urine. Clin Chem 1986;32:1677–1681.
129. Soini E, Hemmila I. Fluoroimmunoassay: present status and key problems. Clin Chem 1979;25:353–361.
130. Soini E, Kojola H. Time-resolved fluorometer for lanthanide chelates—a new generation of nonisotopic immunoassays. Clin Chem 1983;29:65–68.
131. Saunders GC, Jett JH, Martin JC. Amplified flow-cytometric separation-free fluorescence immunoassays. Clin Chem 1985;31:2020–2023.
132. Lindmo T, Bormer O, Ugelstad J, Nustad K. Immunometric assay by flow cytometry using mixtures of two particle types of different affinity. J Immunol Methods 1990;126:183–189.
133. Wehry EL. Molecular fluorescence, phosphorescence, and chemiluminescence spectrometry. Anal Chem 1986;58.
134. Campbell AK, Simpson JSA. Chemi- and bioluminescence as an analytical tool in biology. Tech Life Sci (Metab. Res.) 1979;B213:1–56.
135. Patel A, Morton MS, Woodhead JS, Ryall MET, Capra F, Campbell AK. A new chemiluminescent label for use in immunoassay. Biochem Soc Trans 1982;10:224–225.
136. Barnard GJ, Collins WP. The development of luminescence immunoassays. Med Lab Sci 1987;44:249–266.
137. Patel A, Campbell AK. Homogenous immunoassay based on chemiluminescence energy transfer. Clin Chem 1983;29:1604–1608.
138. Strasburger CJ, Kohen F. Two-site and competitive chemiluminescent immunoassays. Methods Enzymol 1990;184:481–496.
139. Weeks I, Sturgess ML, Woodhead JS. Chemiluminescence immunoassay: an overview. Clin Sci 1986;70:403–408.
140. Bray RA, Gebel HM. Basic concepts of cell isolation. In: Zachary AA, Teresi GA, eds. ASHI laboratory manual. 2nd ed. New York: American Society for Histocompatibility and Immunogenetics, 1990:17–22.
141. Nisperos B. Density gradient isolation of peripheral blood lymphocytes. In: Zachary AA, Teresi GA, eds. ASHI laboratory manual. 2nd ed. New York: American Society for Histocompatibility and Immunogenetics, 1990:23–27.
142. Wottawa A, Klein G, Altman H. A method for the isolation of human and animal lymphocytes with Ficoll-Urografin. Wiener Klin Wochenschr 1974;86:161–163.
143. Perer RJ, Tina WZ, Mickelson MM. Purification of lymphocytes and platelets by gradient centrifugation. J Clin Lab Med 1968;72:842–848.
144. Boyum A. Isolation of mononuclear cells and granulocytes from human blood. Scand J Clin Invest 1968;97:77–89.
145. Boyum A. Separation of lymphocytes, lymphocyte subgroups and monocytes: a review. Lymphology 1968;10:71–76.
146. Boyum A. Isolation of leukocytes from human blood. Further observations—methyl cellulose, dextran, and ficoll as erythrocyte aggregating agents. Scand J Clin Invest 1968;97:31–49.
147. Kaplan ME, Clark C. An improved rosetting assay for detection of human T lymphocytes. J Immunol Methods 1974;5:131–135.
148. Stewart D. Rosetting as a method for separating human B cells and T cells. In: Zachary AA, Teresi GA, eds. ASHI laboratory manual. 2nd ed. New York: American Society for Histocompatibility and Immunogenetics, 1990:49–64.
149. Johnson AH. Anti-Fab separation of T and B lymphocytes. In: Zachary AA, Teresi GA, eds. ASHI laboratory manual. 2nd ed. New York: American Society for Histocompatibility and Immunogenetics, 1990:71–75.
150. Grier JO, Abelson LA, Mann DL, Amos DB, Johnson AH. Enrichment of B lymphocytes using goat anti-human $F(ab')_2$. Tissue Antigens 1977;10:236.
151. Leffell MS. Assessment of purity and viability. In: Zachary AA, Teresi GA, eds. ASHI laboratory manual. 2nd ed. New York: American Society for Histocompatibility and Immunogenetics, 1990:38–48.
152. Bell RS, Bourret LA, Bell DF, et al. Evaluation of fluorescein diacetate for flow cytometric determination of cell viability in orthopaedic research. J Orthop Res 1988;6:467–474.
153. Ross DD, Joneckis CC, Ordonez JV, et al. Estimation of cell survival by flow cytometric quantification of fluorescein diacetate/propidium iodide viable cell number. Cancer Research 1989;49:3776–3782.
154. Birkland SA. The influence of different freezing procedures and different cryoprotective agents on the immunological capacity of frozen-stored lymphocytes. Cryobiology 1976;13:442–447.
155. Crowley JP, Rene A, Valeri CR. The recovery, structure and function of human blood leukocytes after freeze-preservation. Cryobiology 1974;13:442–447.
156. Gramatzki M, Strong DM, Grove SB, Bonnard GD. Cryopreserved human cultured T cells as responder cells for the qualitative measurement of interleukin-2: improvement of the assay. J Immunol Methods 1982;53:209–220.
157. Lorentzen DF. Cell preservation. In: Zachary AA, Teresi GA, eds. ASHI laboratory manual. 2nd ed. New York: American

Society for Histocompatibility and Immunogenetics, 1990: 154–157.
158. Strong DM, Sell KW. Functional properties of cryopreserved lymphocytes. Cryoimmunology 1976;62:81–92.
159. Strong DM, Ortaldo JR, Pandolfi F, Maluish A, Herberman RB. Cryopreservation of human mononuclear cells for quality control in clinical immunology. I. Correlations in recovery of K- and NK-cell functions, surface markers, and morphology. J Clin Immunol 1982;2:214–221.
160. Maluish AE, Strong DM. Lymphocyte proliferation. In: Rose NR, Friedman H. Fahey JL, ed. Manual of Clinical Laboratory Immunology. Washington, DC: American Society for Microbiology, 1986:274–281.
161. Lavergne JA, de Llano AM. Assessment of cellular activation by flow cytometric methods. Pathobiology 1990;58:107–117.
162. Palutke M, KuKuruga D, Tabaczka P. A flow cytometric method for measuring lymphocyte proliferation directly from tissue culture plates using Ki-67 and propidium iodide. J Immunol Methods 1987;105:97–105.
163. Bontadini A, Conte R, Dinota A, et al. Mixed lymphocyte reactions evaluated by means of bromodeoxyuridine incorporation. Haematologica 1990;75:7–11.
164. Dean JH, Connor R, Herberman RB, Silva J, McCoy JL, Oldham RK. The relative proliferation index as a more sensitive parameter for evaluating lymphoproliferative responses of cancer patients to mitogens and alloantigens. Int J Cancer 1977;20:359–370.
165. Cram LS, Gomez ER, Thoen CO, Forslund JC, Jett JH. Flow microfluorometric quantitation of the blastogenic response of lymphocytes. J Histochem Cytochem 1976;24:383–387.
166. Bach F, Segall M. Pooled stimulating cells as a "standard stimulator" in mixed lymphocyte culture. Transplantation 1974;22:117–135.
167. Dupont B, Hansen JA, Yunis EJ. Human mixed lymphocyte culture reactions: genetics, specificity, and biological implications. Adv Immunol 1976;23:107–202.
168. Mickelson EM, Hansen JA. The mixed lymphocyte culture (MLC) test. In: Zachary AA, Teresi GA, eds. ASHI laboratory manual. 2nd ed. New York: American Society for Histocompatibility and Immunogenetics, 1990:339–356.
169. Kanda H, Matsuura T, Akiyama T, Kurita T. A flow-cytometric DNA analysis in mixed lymphocyte reaction. Transplant Proc 1985;17:2157–2158.
170. Slezak SE, Horan PK. Cell-mediated cytotoxicity. A highly sensitive and informative flow cytometric assay. J Immunol Methods 1989;117:205–214.
171. Talbot D, Shenton BK, Givan AL, Proud G, Taylor RM. A rapid, objective method for the detection of lymphocytotoxic antibodies using flow cytometry. Clin Genet 1987;31:25–34.
172. Zarcone D, Tilden AB, Cloud G, Friedman HM, Landay A, Grossi CE. Flow cytometry evaluation of cell-mediated cytotoxicity. J Immunol Methods 1986;94:247–255.
173. Van Leeuwen A. Two color fluorescence. In: Zachary AA, Teresi GA, eds. ASHI laboratory manual. 2nd ed. New York: American Society for Histocompatibility and Immunogenetics, 1990:202–205.
174. Van Rood JJ, Van Leeuwen A, Ploem JS. Simultaneous detection of two cell populations by two-color fluorescence and application to the recognition of B-cell determinants. Nature 1976;204:998.
175. Tardif GN, LeFor WM. Single color fluorescence for HLA-Dr typing. In: Zachary AA, Teresi GA, eds. ASHI Laboratory Manual. 2nd ed. New York: American Society for Histocompatibility and Immunogenetics, 1990:206–211.
176. Carpenter CB. Lymphocyte-mediated cytotoxicity. In: Rose NR, Friedman H, Fahey JL, eds. Manual of clinical laboratory immunology. 3rd ed. Washington, DC: American Society for Microbiology, 1986:304–307.
177. Thomas FT, Lee HM, Lower RR, Thomas JM. Immunological monitoring as a guide to the management of transplant recipients. Surg Clin North Am 1979;59:253–281.
178. Beatty PG. The induction and assay of human cytotoxic T lymphocytes in vitro. In: Zachary AA, Teresi GA, eds. ASHI laboratory manual. 2nd ed. New York: American Society for Histocompatibility and Immunogenetics, 1990:399–414.
179. Dunkley M, Miller RG, Shortman K. A modified ^{51}Cr release assay for cytotoxic lymphocytes. J Immunol Methods 1974;6: 39–51.
180. Morales A, Ottenhof PC. Clinical application of a whole blood assay for human natural killer (NK) cell activity. Cancer 1983;52:667–670.
181. Moy PM, Holmes EC, Golub SH. Depression of natural killer cytotoxic activity in lymphocytes infiltrating human pulmonary tumors. Cancer Res 1985;45:57.
182. Bonavida B, Bradley TP, Grimm EA. The single cell assay in cell-mediated cytotoxicity. Immunol Today 1983;4:196–200.
183. Bradley TP, Vonavida B. Mechanism of cell-mediated cytotoxicity at the single cell level. III. Evidence that cytotoxic T lymphocytes lyse both antigen-specific and -nonspecific targets pretreated with lectins or periodate. J Immunol 1981;126:200–213.
184. Bradley TP, Vonavida B. Mechanism of cell-mediated cytotoxicity at the single cell level. IV. Natural killing and antibody-dependent cellular cytotoxicity can be mediated by the same human effector cell as determined by the two-target conjugate assay. J Immunol 1982;129:2260–2265.
185. Huttunen K, Lionen J. The determination of natural killer activity of human peripheral blood lymphocytes by measuring the DNA synthesis of proliferating target cells (K 567 cell line). Acta Pathol Microbiol Scand 1983;91:197–201.
186. McGinnes K, Chapman G, Marks R, Penny R. A fluorescence NK assay using flow cytometry. J Immunol Methods 1986;86: 7–15.
187. Shi T-X, Tong MJ, Bohman R. The application of flow cytometry in the study of natural killer cell cytotoxicity. Clin Immunol Immunopathol 1987;45:356–365.
188. Vitale M, Neri LM, Comani S, et al. Natural killer function in flow cytometry. II. Evaluation of NK lytic activity by means of target cell morphological changes detected by right angle light scatter. J Immunol Methods 1989;121:115–120.
189. Herberman RB. Natural killer cell activity and antibody-dependent cell-mediated cytotoxicity. In: Zachary AA, Teresi GA, eds. ASHI Laboratory Manual. 2nd ed. New York: American Society for Histocompatibility and Immunogenetics, 1990:308–314.
190. Stelzer GT, Robinson JP. Flow cytometric evaluation of leukocyte function. Diagn Clin Immunol 1988;5:223–231.
191. Bjerknes R, Bassoe C-F, Sjursen H, Laerum OD, Solberg CO. Flow cytometry for the study of phagocyte functions. Rev Infect Dis 1989;11:16–33.
192. Duque RE, Ward PA. Quantitative assessment of neutrophil function by flow cytometry. Anal Quant Cytol Histol 1987;9: 42–48.
193. Maderazo EG, Ward PA. Leukocyte chemotaxis. In: Rose NR, Friedman H, Fahey JL, eds. Manual of clinical laboratory immunology. 3rd ed. Washington, DC: American Society for Microbiology, 1986:290–294.
194. Nelson RD, Quie PG, Simmions RL. Chemotaxis under agarose: a new simple method for measuring chemotaxis and spontaneous migration of human polymorphonuclear leukocytes and monocytes. J Immunol 1975;115:1650–1656.

195. Glasser L, Fiederlein RL. Neutrophil migration under agarose. Quantitation and variables. Am J Clin Pathol 1979;72:956–962.
196. Glasser L, Fiederlein RL. The effect of various cell separation procedures on assays of neutrophil function. Am J Clin Pathol 1990;93:662–669.
197. Lehrer RI. Measurement of candidacidal activity of specific leukocyte types in mixed cell populations. I. Normal, myeloperoxidase-deficient, and chronic granulomatous disease neutrophils. Infect Immunol 1970;1970:42–47.
198. Lehrer RI, Cline MJ. Interaction of Candida albicans with human leukocytes and serum. J Bacteriol 1969;98:996–1004.
199. Quie PG, White JG, Holmes B, Good RA. In vitro bactericidal capacity of human polymorphonuclear leukocytes: diminished activity in chronic granulomatous disease of childhood. J Clin Invest 1967;46:668–679.
200. Southwick FS, Stossel TP. Phagocytosis. In: Rose NR, Friedman H, Fahey JL, eds. Manual of clinical laboratory immunology. 3rd ed. Washington, DC: American Society for Microbiology, 1986:326–331.
201. Bassoe CF, Solsvik J, Laerum OD. Quantitation of single cell phagocytic capacity by flow cytometry. In: Laerum OD, Lindmo T, Thorud E, eds. Flow cytometry IV. Bergen: Universitetsforlaget, 1980:170–174.
202. Bassoe C-F, Laerum OD, Solberg CO, Haneberg B. Phagocytosis of bacteria by leukocytes measured by flow cytometry. Proc Soc Exp Biol Med 1983;174:182–186.
203. Bassoe C-F, Laerum OD, Glette J, Hopen G, Haneberg B, Solberg CO. Simultaneous measurement of phagocytosis and phagosomal pH by flow cytometry: role of polymorphonuclear neutrophilic leukocyte granules in phagosome acidification. Cytometry 1983;4:254–262.
204. Bassoe C-F, Bjerknes R. Phagocytosis by human leukocytes, phagosomal pH, and degradation of seven species of bacteria measured by flow cytometry. J Med Microbiol 1985;19:115–125.
205. Bjerknes R, Bassoe C-F. Human leukocyte phagocytosis of zymosan particles measured by flow cytometry. Acta Pathol Microbiol Immune Scand 1983;91:341–348.
206. Bjerknes R. Flow cytometric assay for combined measurement of phagocytosis and intracellular killing of *Candida albicans*. J Immunol Methods 1984;72:229–241.
207. Steinkamp JA, Wilson JS, Saunders GC, Stewart CC. Phagocytosis: flow cytometric quantitation with fluorescent microspheres. Science 1982;215:64–66.
208. Ogle JD, Noel JG, Sramkoski RM, Ogle CK, Alexander JW. Phagocytosis of opsonized fluorescent microspheres by human neutrophils. A two-color flow cytometric method for the determination of attachment and ingestion. J Immunol Methods 1988;115:17–29.
209. Dunn PA, Tyrer HW. Quantitation of neutrophil phagocytosis, using fluorescent latex beads. Correlation of microscopy and flow cytometry. J Lab Clin Med 1981;98:374–381.
210. Wilson RM, Galvin AM, Robins RA, Reeves WG. A flow cytometric method for the measurement of phagocytosis by polymorphonuclear leucocytes. J Immunol Methods 1985;76:247–253.
211. Rothe G, Valet G. Phagocytosis, intracellular pH, and cell volume in the multifunctional analysis of franulocytes by flow cytometry. Cytometry 1988;9:316–324.
212. Jarstrand C, Lahnborg G, Berghem L. Human granulocyte function during dextran infusion. Acta Chir Scand 1979;489:279–285.
213. Ochs HD, Igo RP. The NBT slide test: a simple screening method for detecting chronic granulomatous disease and female carriers. J Pediatr 1973;65:77–82.
214. Cline MJ. A new white cell test which measures individual phagocyte function in a mixed leukocyte preparation. 1. A neutrophil defect in acute myelocytic leukemia. J Lab Clin Med 1973;81:311–316.
215. Hafeman DG, McConnell HM, Gray JW, Dean PN. Neutrophil activation monitored by flow cytometry: stimulation by phorbol diester is an all-or-none event. Science 1982;215:673–675.
216. Thorell B. Intracellular red-ox steady states as basis for cell characterization by flow cytofluorometry. Blood Cells 1980;6:745–751.
217. Thorell B. Flow cytometric analysis of cellular endogenous fluorescence simultaneously with emission from exogenous fluorochromes, light scatter, and absorption. Cytometry 1981;2:39–43.
218. Bass DA, Parce JW, Dechatelet LR, Szejda P, Seeds MC, Thomas M. Flow cytometric studies of oxidative product formation by neutrtophils: a graded response to membrane stimulation. J Immunol 1983;130:1910–1917.
219. Rothe G, Valet G. Flow cytometric analysis of respiratory burst activity in phagocytes with hydroethidine and 2′,7′-dichlorofluorescin. J Leukoc Biol 1990;47:440–448.
220. Trinkle LS, Wellhuasen SR, McLeish KR. A simultaneous flow cytometric measurement of neutrophil phagocytosis and oxidative burst in whole blood. Bas Appl Histochem 1987;2:5–76.
221. Fattorossi A, Nisini R, Le Moli S, De Petrillo G, D'Amelio R. Flow cytometric evaluation of nitro blue tetrazolium (NBT) reduction in human polymorphonuclear leukocytes. Cytometry 1990;11:907–912.
222. Bassoe C-F, Solberg CO. Phagocytosis of Staphyloccus aureus by human leukocytes: quantitation by a flow cytometric and a microbiological method. Acta Pathol Microbiol Immunol Scand 1984;92:43–50.
223. Sjursen H, Bjerknes R, Halstensen A, Solberg CO. Serum opsonins to group B meningococci in patients and vacinnated volunteers [abstract no. 204]. Cytometry 1987;8:38.
224. Sjursen H, Bjerknes R, Halstensen A, et al. Serum opsonins to group B meningococci. Acta Pathol Microbiol Immunol Scand 1987;95:283–289.
225. Sjursen H, Bjerknes R, Halstensen A, Naess A, Sornes S, Solberg CO. Flow cytometric assay for the measurement of serum opsonins to Neisseria meningitidis serogroup B, serotype 15. J Immunol Methods 1989;116:235–243.
226. Alper CA. Genetics of the complement system. Ann NY Acad Sci 1986;475:32–46.
227. Bentley DR. Structural superfamilies of the complement system. Exp Clin Immunogenet 1988;5:69–80.
228. Bhakdi S, Hugo F, Tranum JJ. Functions and relevance of the terminal complement sequence. Blut 1990;60:309–318.
229. Campbell RD, Law SK, Reid KB, Sim RB. Structure, organization, and regulation of the complement genes. Annu Rev Immunol 1988;6:161–195.
230. Campbell RD. The molecular genetics of components of the complement system. Baillieres Clin Rheumatol 1988;2:547–575.
231. Chakravarti DN, Kristensen T. Recent advances in the study of the molecular structure of the complement proteins. Pathol Immunopathol Res 1986;5:317–351.
232. Dalmasso AP, Falk RJ, Raij L. The pathobiology of the terminal complement complexes. Concours Med 1989;6:36–48.
233. Muller EH. The membrane attack complex of complement. Annu Rev Immunol 1986;4:503–528.
234. Mollnes TE, Lachmann PJ. Regulation of complement. Scand J Immunol 1988;27:127–142.

235. Perlmutter DH, Colten HR. Structure and expression of the complement genes. Pharmacol Ther 1987;34:247–270.
236. Reid KB. Activation and control of the complement system. Essays Biochem 1986;22:27–68.
237. Ross GD. Complement and complement receptors. Current Opinion Immunol 1989;2:50–62.
238. Volanakis JE. Structure and molecular genetics of complement proteins. An update. Year Immunol 1986;2:164–176.
239. Williams LW, Burks AW, Steele RW. Complement: function and clinical relevance. Ann Allergy 1988;60:293–300.
240. Peakman M, Senaldi G, Vergani D. Review: assessment of complement activation in clinical immunology laboratories: time for reappraisal? J Clin Pathol 1989;42:1018–1025.
241. Whaley K. Measurement of complement activation in clinical practice. Concours Med 1989;6:96–103.
242. Kay PH, Papadimitriou JM. What's new in the role of complement in diseases? Pathol Res Pract 1990;186:410–414.
243. Holme ER, Whaley K. Complement and related clinical disorders. Blood Rev 1989;3:120–129.
244. Frank MM. Complement in the pathophysiology of human disease. N Engl J Med 1987;316:1525–1530.
245. Cooper NR. Complement and infectious agents. Rev Infect Dis 1988;10 (Suppl 2):5447–5449.
246. Cooper NR. Assays for complement activation. Clin Lab Med 1986;6:139–155.

57 Flow Cytometry

J. Philip McCoy, Jr.

Flow cytometry has blossomed as a discipline over the past 2 decades due to a variety of intrinsic and extrinsic factors. Factors intrinsic to flow cytometry that have broadened its utility are the development of faster and more powerful computers and microprocessors, more sophisticated software, and relatively inexpensive and easy-to-maintain lasers. Factors extrinsic to flow cytometers per se, but that have contributed significantly to the utility of flow cytometry, include the development of monoclonal antibodies that provide exquisite specificity in fluorescence staining assays and the discovery of new fluorophores that permit simultaneous examination of multiple cellular features.

Flow cytometry is rapidly becoming far more than an automated method for enumerating cells that bear a single-color fluorescent probe. Cytometers that are now commercially available are capable of simultaneously measuring as many as eight parameters per cell. Essential to the interpretation of flow cytometric analyses is the understanding that individual cells, in suspension, are examined for each of the parameters specified in a given assay—and clumps of cells will often be misinterpreted as individual cells. It is now realized that the majority of disease processes involve the interaction of a myriad of cell types or populations and, increasingly, laboratory assays designed to assist in establishing diagnoses or in predicting disease progression or the response to therapy rely upon the evaluation of numerous features or markers relevant to the disease. Flow cytometry is virtually unique in offering the laboratory the opportunity to study several populations of cells within a specimen for multiple features or markers.

This chapter reviews the current status of flow cytometry in laboratory medicine. Only cursory mention is made of instrument design and theory of operation; several excellent texts thoroughly cover these topics (1, 2). While numerous assays are discussed in terms of methodology and interpretation, a goal of this chapter is also to convey, in a broader sense, an appreciation for the abilities, potential abilities, and limitations of flow cytometry. It is essential to bear in mind that flow cytometric analyses are adjunctive laboratory assays: clinical diagnoses must integrate the flow cytometric findings with other laboratory findings and the clinical presentation. Interpretation of data derived from flow cytometric analysis is nearly impossible without appropriate correlation of morphological and clinical parameters. Finally, flow cytometry is a single technology for which many applications have been found. The clinical applications described in this text are by no means complete; rather, they reflect those that are most commonly performed. For a more in-depth discussion of these applications, a variety of excellent texts are available (3–6).

DISEASE STATES

The primary use of the detection of cell surface markers on hematopoietic cells by flow cytometry is to identify alterations in the numbers of a particular group of cells that may correlate with a disease state or therapy. For this to be applied for routine use in the clinical laboratory, a thorough understanding of normal hematopoiesis is necessary. This is a dynamic process, as new monoclonal antibodies (as well as other probes) are constantly refining and adding to our understanding of hematology. The plethora of these reagents has led to a series of workshops designed to better classify the distribution of the antigens on hematopoietic cells. The result of these workshops is a series of cluster designations (CD), which describe the distribution of a number of antigens defined by monoclonal antibodies from a variety of sources. Representative cluster designations, their distribution, and commonly available antibodies for each CD are given in Table 57.1 (7). Armed with these tools for the understanding of hematopoiesis, one can utilize flow cytometric immunophenotyping to characterize lesions associated with disease processes.

Flow cytometric assays used in the clinical laboratory are by no means limited to immunophenotyping. Assays have been described for the quantitation of cellular DNA (for ploidy and proliferation studies), RNA (for reticulocyte maturation), cell surface receptors (e.g., estrogen), carbohydrates (by lectin binding), intracellular antigens (e.g., cytoplasmic mu

Table 57.1. CD Antigens and Cellular Distribution

Antigen	Cellular Distribution	Functional Significance/Membrane Component
CD1a	thymocytes, Langerhans dendritic dermal cells, B lymphocyte subset	gp49
CD1b	thymocytes, dendritic dermal cells, B lymphocyte subset	gp45
CD1c	thymocytes, dendritic dermal cells, B lymphocyte subset	gp43
CD2	all T lymphocytes, 95% thymocytes, natural killer cells	CD58 (LFA-3) receptor, gp50
CD2R	activated T lymphocytes	CD2 epitopes restricted to activated T cells
CD3	mature T lymphocytes	CD3 receptor complex (5 chains), gp/p26,20,16
CD4	T lymphocyte subset, helper/inducer T lymphocytes	MHC Class II/HIV receptor, gp59
CD5	all lymphocytes, some B lymphocyte subsets	gp67
CD6	mature T lymphocytes, B lymphocyte subset	gp100
CD7	all T lymphocytes	gp40
CD8	T lymphocyte subset, cytotoxic/suppressor T lymphocytes	MHC Class I receptor, gp72 heterodimer (gp30,32)
CD9	monocytes, B lymphocytes, platelets, B progenitors	p24
CD10	B lymphocytes, common acute lymphoblastic leukemia, B progenitors, granulocytes, germinal center B cells	neutral endopeptidase, gp100, CALLA
CD11a	leukocytes	LFA-1, gp180/95
CD11b	monocytes, granulocytes, natural killer cells, macrophages	C3bi receptor (CR3), gp 155/95
CD11c	monocytes, granulocytes, macrophages, natural killer cells, B lymphocyte subset	gp150/95 heterodimer
CDw12	monocytes, granulocytes, platelets	p90–120
CD13	granulocytes, monocytes	aminopeptidase N, gp150
CD14	monocytes, granulocytes, follicular dendritic reticulum cells, epidermal Langerhans cells	gp55
CD15	granulocytes, monocytes	Hapten X on granulocytes, 3-FAL
CD16	granulocyte, natural killer cells, macrophages	IgGFcRIII (low affinity), gp50–65
CDw17	granulocytes, platelets, monocytes	lactosylceramide
CD18	leukocytes, broad	β-chain to CD11a,b,c
CD19	all B lymphocytes, some myeloid progenitors	gp95
CD20	B lymphocytes, follicular dendritic reticulum cells, all peripheral B lymphocytes, some late B progenitors, some Reed-Sternberg cells	gp35, p37/32, ion channel?
CD21	B lymphocytes, B lymphocyte subset, follicular dendritic reticuium cells	C3d Epstein-Barr virus receptor, gp140, CR2 for C3d fragment
CD22	B lymphocytes, B progenitors, and most peripheral B lymphocytes; weak on germinal center B, cytoplasmic B/surface B lymphacyte subset	gp135, homology to myelin assoc. gp (MAG)
CD23	B lymphocyte subset, activated monocytes, follicular dendritic reticulum cells, eosinophil	IgE FcRiI receptor (low affinity), gp45–50
CD24	B lymphocytes, granulocytes, all B lymphocytes including progenitors, polymorphs	gp45,55,65 heterotrimer
CD25	activated T lymphocytes, B lymphocytes, monocytes	IL-2 receptor β-chain, gp55
CDw26	activated T lymphocytes	dipeptidylpeptidase IV, gp120
CD27	T lymphocytes	p55(dimer)
CD28	T lymphocyte subset	gp44
CD29	T lymphocyte subset (others)	VLA β, Integrin β-chain, platelet GPIIa, p135
CD30	activated T lymphocytes, activated B lymphocytes, activated Hodgkin's and Reed-Sternberg cells	gp120, Ki-1 prototype
CD31	monocytes, granulocytes, platelets, T lymphocytes, bone marrow cells, epithelium, B lymphocytes	gp140, platelet GPIIa
CDw32	monocytes, granulocytes, platelets, B lymphocytes	FcRII receptor, gp40
CD33	myeloid leukemia, myeloid progenitors, monocytes	gp67
CD34	myeloid and lymphoblastic leukemia, some bone marrow cells, endothelium, lymphocyte progenitor cells	gp115
CD35	granulocytes, monocytes, B lymphocytes, red blood cells, follicular dendritic reticulum cells	CR1 for C3b fragment of C3, p220
CD36	monocytes, platelets, B lymphocytes	GP90, platelet GPIV
CD37	B lymphocytes, all peripheral B lymphocytes, some late B progenitors, some leukocytes, T lymphocytes, monocytes	GP40–52
CD38	restricted multiple lineage, germinal center B lymphocytes, plasma cells, leukocyte progenitors, T lymphocyte, T blasts	p45/12 heterodimer
CD39	B lymphocytes, monocytes, vessels, some macrophages, plasma cells	gp70–100
CD40	B lymphocytes, interdigitating reticulum cells, restricted B lymphocytes, carcinomas	gp50, homology to NGF receptor
CD41a	platelets, megakaryocytes	CPIIb/IIIa complex (receptor for fibrinogen)
CD41b	platelets	GPIIb

Table 57.1.—*continued*

Antigen	Cellular Distribution	Functional Significance/Membrane Component
CD42a	platelets	GPIX, gp23
CD42b;	platelets, megakaryocytes	GPIb receptor for factor VIII antigen, gp135/25
CD43	T lymphocytes, granulocytes, brain, pre B cell lines	leukosialin, gp95
CD44	T lymphocytes, granulocytes, brain, red blood cells, epithelial cell lines	Pgp-1, pg80–95
CD45	leukocytes	leukocyte common antigen, T200
CD45R	B lymphocytes, T lymphacyte subset, granulocytes, monocytes, myeloid cells	restricted leukocyte common antigen, p205 & 220
CD45RA	T lymphocyte subset, B lymphocytes, granulocytes, monocytes, myeloid cells	restricted T200, gp220
CD45RB	T lymphocyte subset, B lymphocytes, granulcytes, monocytes	restricted T200
CD45RO	T lymphocyte subset, B lymphocytes, granulocytes, monocytes	restricted T200, gp180
CD46	leukocytes, broad	membrane cofactor protein (MCP), gp66/56
CD47	broad	gp47–52, N-linked glycan, Rh assoc.
CD48	leukocytes	gp41, PI-linked
CDw49b	platelets, cultured T lymphocytes, activated T lymphocytes, thymocytes	VLA-α2-chain, platelet GPIa
CDw49d	monocytes, T lymphocytes, B lymphocytes, epidermal Langerhans cells, thymocytes	VLA-α4-chain, gp150
CDw49f	platelets, T lymphocytes	VLA-α6-chain, gp140, platelet GPIc
CDw50	leukocytes, broad	gp180/108, PI-linked
CD51	platelets, B lymphocytes	VNR-α-chain
CDw52	leukocytes	Campath-1, gp21–28
CD53	leukocytes	gp32–40, PI-linked
CD54	broad, activated	ICAM-1
CD55	broad	decay accelerating factor (DAF)
CD56	natural killer cells, activated lymphocytes	gp220/135, NKH1, isoform of N-CAM
CD57	natural killer cells, T lymphocytes, brain, B lymphocyte subset	gp110, HNK1
CD58	leukocytes, epithelial cells	LFA-3, gp40–65
CD59	broad	gp18–20
CDw60	T lymphocyte subset	NeuAc-NeuAC-Gal-
CD61	platelets, B lymphocytes	integrin β3-, VNR β-chain, platelet GPIIIa
CD62	activated platelets	GMP-140 (PADGEM), gp140
CD63	activated platelets, monocytes, granulocytes, T lymphocytes, B lymphocytes	gp53
CD64	monocytes	FcRI, gp75
CDw65	granulocytes, monocytes	Ceramide-Dodecasaccharide 4c
CD66	granulocytes	phosphoprotein pp 180–200
CD67	granulocytes	p100, PI-linked
CD68	macrophages	gp110
CD69	activated B lymphocytes, T lymphocytes	gp32/38, AIM
CDw70	activated B lymphocytes, -T lymphocytes, Reed-Sternberg cells	Ki-24
CD71	proliferating cells, macrophages	transferrin receptor
CD72	B lymphocytes	gp43/39
CD73	B lymphocyte subset, T lymphocyte subset	ecto-5′-nucleotidase, p69
CD74	B lymphocytes, monocytes	Class II assoc. Invariant Chain, gp41/35/33
CDw75	mature B lymphocytes, T lymphocyte subset	p53
CD76	mature B lymphocytes, T lymphacyte subset	gp85/67
CD77	restricted B lymphocytes	globotriasylceramide (Gb3)
CDw78	B lymphocytes, monocytes	unknown

and Tdt), ion fluxes (such as calcium fluxes in triggering target cells), and phagocytosis, to name a few. In many instances, these parameters may be examined concomitantly with cell surface markers. This section will illustrate the application of some of these flow cytometric assays in the study of selected disease in the clinical laboratory.

Leukemia

ACUTE

While the diagnosis of acute leukemia is dependent upon clinical presentaion as well as the examination of morphology and cytochemistry, immunophenotypic analyses by flow cytometry of the abnormal cells have substantially refined our ability to classify leukemias (8–13). Primarily, these phenotypic analyses are focused on delineating cell lineage and stage of maturation. Thus, in an adjunctive manner, they provide additional diagnostic information to confirm or establish the diagnosis when standard morphology or cytochemistries provide ambiguous results. Furthermore, immunophenotyping has proven to be of prognostic significance in many instances.

A schema for surface marker expression as a function of lineage and maturation can be constructed as illustrated in Figure 57.1. Given the ease of staining

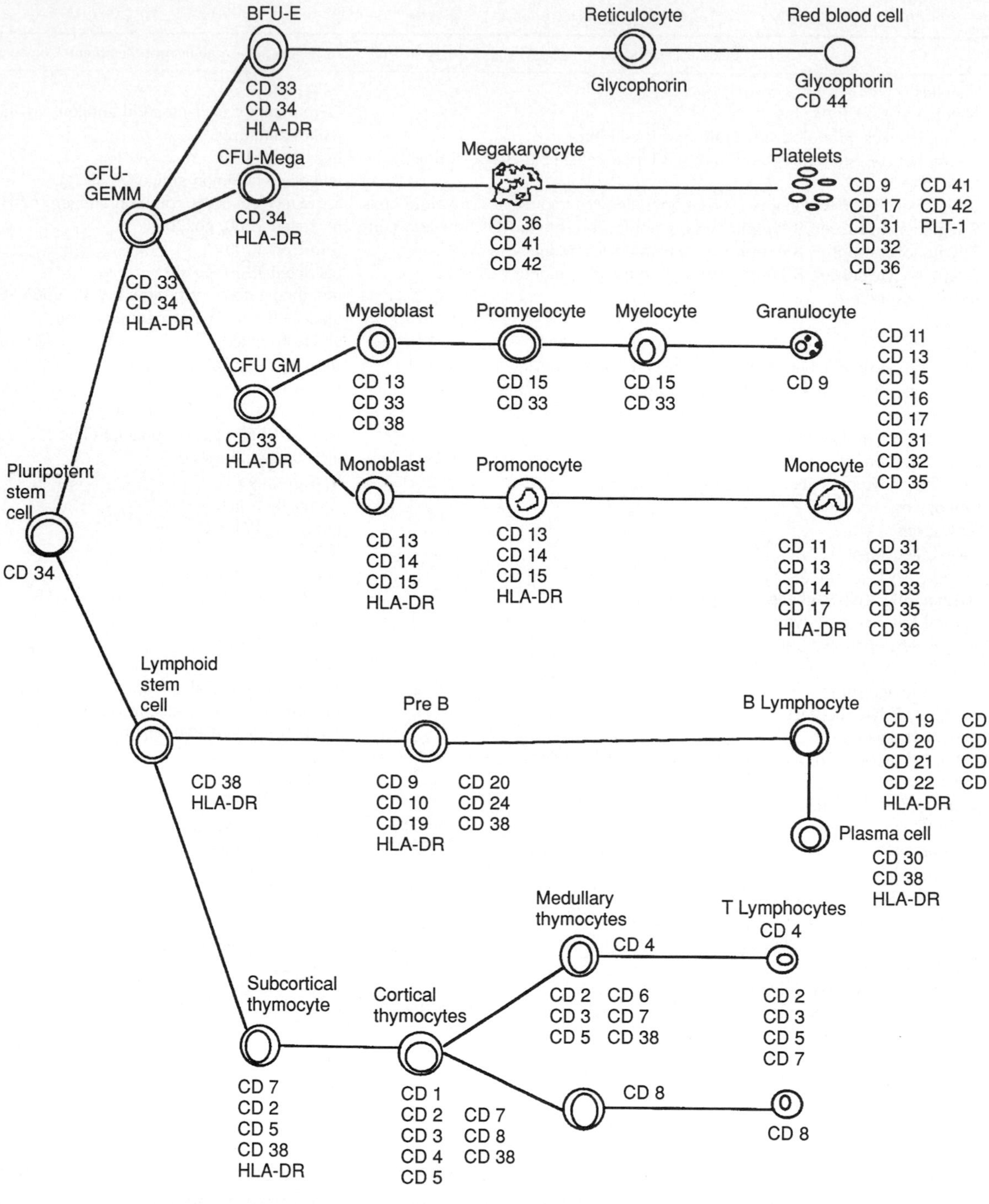

Figure 57.1. A maturation schema for hematopoietic cells in relationship to marker expression.

specimens with multiple antibodies in one assay and the short storage life of many leukemic blasts, the immunophenotyping of leukemias generally employs a rather large panel of monoclonal antibodies in one assay (as shown in Table 57.2) rather than sequential staining following a branching schema.

Because acute lymphoid leukemias (ALLs) have vastly different prognoses and responses to therapy than do acute nonlymphoid leukemias (ANLLs), a primary goal in the analysis of immunophenotyping assays of leukemias is to determine if the lesion is lymphoid in origin. While this is usually a straightforward endeavor, it is occasionally complicated by the aberrant expression of lineage markers on neoplastic cells or the presentation of a biclonal or biphenotypic lesion. In these instances, it is crucial to correlate marker expression with cell type; this will indicate whether excess expression of two divergent lineage markers is due to aberrant appearance or the presence of two concomitant neoplastic clones.

Table 57.2. A Representative Panel for Immunophenotyping Acute Leukemias and Anticipated Distribution of Antigens

	Disease State							
			ANLL					
Antibody to	T-Cell ALL	Non–T-Cell ALL	M1	M2	M3	M4	M5	M6
CD2	Yes	No	No	No	No	No	No	No
CD4	No[a]	No	No	No	No	No	No	No
CD5	Yes	No	No	No	No	No	No	No
CD8	No	No	No	No	No	No	No	No
CD10	Freq	Freq	No	No	No	No	No	No
CD11	No	No	No	No	No	Freq	Freq	No
CD13	No	No	Yes	Yes	Yes	Yes	No	No
CD14	No	No	No	No	No	Yes	Yes	No
CD19	No	Yes	No	No	No	No	No	No
CD20	No	Freq	No	No	No	No	No	No
CD33	No	No	Freq	Freq	Freq	Yes	No	No
HLA-DR	No	Yes	Yes	Yes	No	Yes	Yes	Yes

[a]Positive in leukemic phase cutaneous T-cell lymphoma.

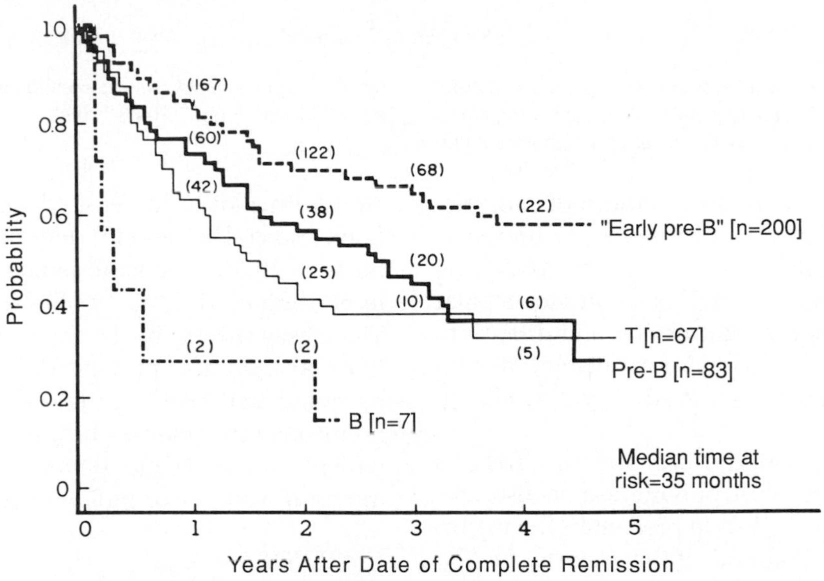

Figure 57.2. Duration of continuous complete remission in childhood acute lymphoblastic leukemia in relationship to cell phenotype. Initial relapse at any site or death while in complete remission was defined as failure. The numbers in parentheses indicate the patients remaining at risk at various time points. Approximately 10% of the patients with pre- and early pre-B-cell ALL lacked CALLA expression. (Reprinted with permission from Crist WM, Grossi CE, Pullen J et al. Immunologic markers in childhood acute lymphocytic leukemia. Sem Oncol 1985;12(2):105–121.

ALLs are usually distinguishable from ANLLs by the fact that the former bear various combinations of CALLA and markers of normal lymphoid development such as CD2, CD5, CD7, CD19, or CD20, while the latter may display combinations of markers for monocyte/granulocyte differentiation such as CD13, CD14, CD33, and HLA-DR (Table 64.2). Lymphoid leukemias may then be generally subdivided into those of T-cell linage (15 to 25% of ALLs) and those of B-cell lineage (75 to 85% of ALLs) based upon expression of T-cell markers such as CD2, CD7, and CD5 and B-cell markers such as CD19, CD20, and cell surface immunoglobulin. Both T-cell and B-cell ALLs may then be further subclassified according to stage of maturation as denoted by expression of intralineage markers of differentiation. Varying prognoses are associated with these classifications; surface immunoglobulin-negative, CALLA-positive, early pre B-All has the best prognosis, followed by T-cell and pre-B-cell ALL, and finally by the surface immunoglobulin-positive B-ALL (Fig. 57.2).

Acute nonlymphocytic (myeloblastic) leukemias (ANNLs) may similarly be subclassified using surface marker analysis. Here the degree of differentiation of the myeloblasts and the presence of monocytic, erythroid, or megakaryocytic features are characterized using monoclonal antibodies such as CD13, CD14, CD33, HLA-DR, CD41, CD42, and glycophorin A. Classically, ANNLs have been classified using the French, American, British (FAB) classification

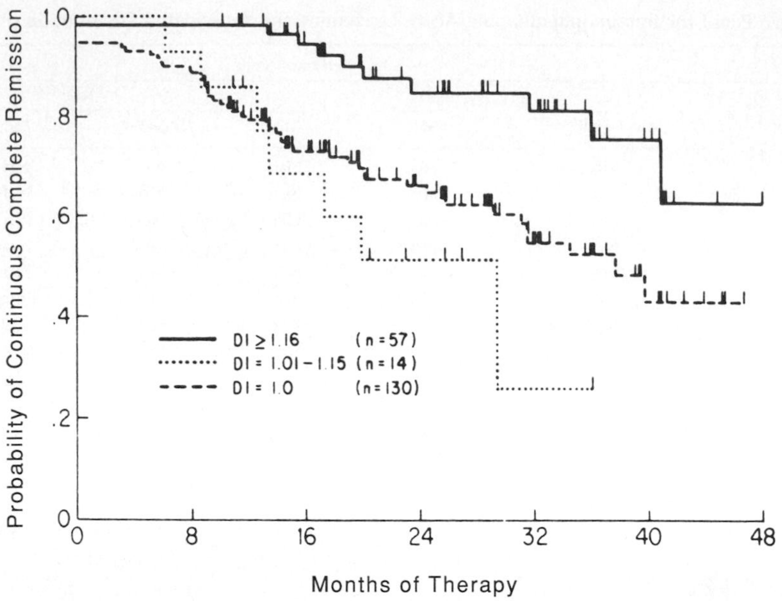

Figure 57.3. Time-to-failure in relationship to DNA index (DI) for 201 patients with childhood acute leukemia. (Reprinted with permission from Look AT, Roberson PK, Williams, et al. Prognostic importance of blast cell DNA content in childhood acute lymphoblastic leukemia. Blood 1985;65:1039–1086.)

scheme, which is based upon a variety of morphological and cytochemical characteristics. Immunophenotyping and FAB classifications of ANNL do not precisely correlate, although both provide similar assessment of the stage of maturation and differentiation of the leukemic cells. Unfortunately, neither method has been shown to be of strict prognostic significance.

Terminal deoxynucleotidyl transferase (TdT), a template-independent DNA polymerase, is also useful as a marker for ALLs. While present in the majority of ALLs, TdT is not found in the majority of ANNLs and mature non-Hodgkin's lymphomas. As part of a panel including immunophenotyping, morphological examination, and cytochemistries, TdT is a useful tool in diagnosis and in the detection of recurrent disease. While flow cytometric assays have been described for the detection of TdT, it is more commonly detected by traditional immunofluorescence assays on cells fixed on glass slides.

Measurement of cellular DNA content is often of use in the study of acute leukemias either alone or in conjunction with surface marker analysis. Measurement of DNA content serves to identify aneuploid populations of tumor (although minor DNA alterations and chromosome translocations cannot be detected) and to estimate proliferation rates. Aneuploidy is a strong indicator of malignancy and, as such, can aid in diagnosis when immunophenotypic and morphological examinations are not conclusive (14). Aneuploidy can also be used as a means to detect early recurrent disease before immunophenotyping is of much value, and prognosis has been associated with ploidy in selected diseases. For example, Look and colleagues (15) demonstrated a better prognosis in childhood acute leukemia associated with a hyperdiploid (DI >1.16) DNA content (Fig. 57.3). The observations by Look and colleagues in childhood ALL do not apply in adult ALL. Thus, it should be noted that ploidy-prognosis relationships are by no means universal; each type of lesion and group of patients must be independently assessed to determine the validity of ploidy evaluation in prognosis.

CHRONIC

Chronic lymphocytic leukemias (CLL) are monoclonal proliferations of B cells with cell surface immunoglobulins (16, 17). CLLs are immature B-cell lesions, typically identified by the expression of CD19, CD20, HLA-DR, cytoplasmic immunoglobulin heavy chain, and the weak, but monoclonal, expression of heavy and light immunoglobulin chains on the cell surface (seldom seen in B-ALLs). In contrast to B-ALLs, CLLs do not express the CALLA antigen; however, most (80%) are positive for CD5.

Chronic myelogenous leukemias (CMLs) are ubiquitous in carrying a consistent chromosomal abnormality, the Philadelphia chromosome (Ph^1). Surface marker analysis is of limited utility during the chronic phase of this disease, but it is of substantial value during the acute phase (blast crisis). The acute phase is similar to an acute leukemia, and here the cells may bear either lymphoid or myeloid characteristics. Delineation of these two forms of blast crisis is critical because each responds differently to chemotherapeutic regimens. Lymphoid variants generally bear the CD10, CD19, and HLA-DR surface markers, and the myeloid variants express CD13, CD33, and HLA-DR. Additionally, blasts can display erythroid or megakaryocytic features and thus can be identified through the use of glycophorin A or Plt-1, respectively.

Lymphoma

Non-Hodgkin's lymphomas (NHLs) are distinguished from Hodgkin's disease by methods other than immunophenotyping, such as by the presence of Reed-Sternberg or Hodgkin's cells in the latter. However, immunophenotyping is frequently of use in distinguishing lymphomas from reactive lymph nodes and, when combined with other parameters such as morphology, in the subclassifaction of non-Hodgkin's lymphomas (18, 19). A major obstacle in immunophenotyping these lesions is the presence of residual normal lymphocytes. Therefore, one must evaluate both the number of cells of a given lineage within the nodule and the clonality of these cells. For B-cell lymphomas, this is often accomplished by examination of immunogobulin light chains. For T-cell lesions, this has been a more difficult undertaking, although the recent development of antibodies to variable regions of the T-cell receptor will most likely help to establish monoclonality in many cases. This approach is currently being used in the study of cutaneous T-cell lymphomas (20, 21).

Analysis of the cellular DNA content of lymphomas is often of use when one is presented with a difficult differential diagnosis such as a reactive node (22–24). As with leukemias, aneuploidy is very strongly correlated with malignancy. High proliferation rates in lymphomas are closely associated with high-grade disease and a high frequency of an initial complete remission of short duration. These studies greatly benefit from the "two-color" approach introduced by Braylan et al. (25) to mark the malignant cells with an antibody to a surface marker and thus examine the proliferation of these cells separately from the majority of normal lymphocytes.

Immunodeficiencies

ACQUIRED IMMUNODEFICIENCY SYNDROME

Perhaps the most common application of immunophenotyping is in the diagnosis and therapy of acquired immunodeficiency syndrome (AIDS) and AIDS-related complex (ARC). The HIV virus has been shown to infect and destroy helper T (CD4+) lymphocytes (26). Thus, laboratory findings in support of a diagnosis of AIDS include a low ratio of CD4+ to CD8+ T lymphocytes due to a decrease in the absolute number of the CD4+ cells (rather than an increase in the absolute number of CD8+ cells) (27–29). Normal individuals generally have a CD4/CD8 ratio of approximately 2.0; AIDS patients most often have ratios less than 0.5. Most importantly, enumeration of CD4+ cells provides a direct indicator of disease progression in HIV-infected individuals and of survival in patients with AIDS (28, 29). Enumeration of CD4+ cells as well as other populations of lymphocytes is useful in assessing the efficacy of therapy designed to bolster or reconstitute the immune system of these patients.

PRIMARY IMMUNODEFICIENCIES

Surface marker analysis is used in conjunction with other laboratory tests, such as those for serum immunoglobulins, cell function, and enzyme deficiencies, to examine a variety of primary immunodeficiency syndromes (30). In general, surface marker analyses are used primarily to assess the immune status of the patient or the response to therapy, rather than in the diagnosis of the disorder. One example of primary immunodeficiency is severe combined immunodeficiency (SCID). Here the analyses are more complex because SCID is a heterogeneous disorder. While specific phenotypes may vary in SCID, a common finding is a lack of mature T cells and the presence of various numbers of B cells and NK cells. Immunophenotyping is of value in distinguishing SCID from other immunodeficiencies characterized by a different pattern of T-cell maturation or specific lesions in other lymphocyte subsets. Because bone marrow transplantation may be a treatment option for SCID patients, immunophenotyping is also of use in monitoring the engraftment, proliferation, and maturation of the transplanted marrow. (This is discussed in further detail later in this chapter). By contrast, DiGeorge syndrome, another T-cell immunodeficiency, displays decreased T-cell function, although mature T cells can be detected in the circulation (albeit at reduced numbers). Here the diagnosis is aided by the clinical appearance of the patient and the absence of a thymic shadow in chest x-rays.

Peripheral blood from patients with common variable immunodeficiency (CVID) demonstrates normal numbers of B lymphocytes but an inverted CD4/CD8 ratio (31). This inverted ratio may be due to an increase in CD8+ cells, a decrease in CD4+ cells, or a combination of the two. While not in itself diagnostic, the identification of an excess of suppressor T cells is predictive of a favorable response to cimetidine (32).

In addition to immunophenotyping, flow cytometry may also be used to assess various aspects of cellular immunity, such as the ability to respond to mitogens (33). Here, in response to cocultivation with certain lectins, normally functioning lymphocytes undergo rapid proliferation. This proliferation has classically been measured by the incoporation of tritiated thymidine, although recent methods have been described for assessing this proliferation using flow cytometric analysis of DNA content. Normal, responding cells display a relatively high S/G2/M fraction, but defective, nonresponding cells display little change in these fractions compared to unstimulated controls.

Various immunodeficiencies are associated with precise defects in the function of a particular cell type. Chronic granulomatous disease (CGD), for example, is classically associated with a defect in the oxidative metabolism of neutrophils, resulting in a lack of hydrogen peroxide production. This defect may be assayed by flow cytometry using dichlorofluorescein diacetate (DCF-DA)—a nonfluorogenic substrate capable of entering live cells (34). Production of hydrogen peroxide within the cell converts DCF-DA into an insoluble, fluorogenic compound, dichlorofluorescein.

Transplantation

RENAL

Flow cytometric analysis of cell surface markers has been used in the management of renal transplant recipients in a number of ways: to assist in delineating graft rejection vis à vis viral (cytomegalovirus—CMV) infection, to monitor the efficacy of cytoreductive/immunosuppressive therapy, and to detect antibodies to murine immunoglobulin during OKT3 therapy. In the study of graft rejection versus CMV infection, several studies have demonstrated an association between an increase in interleukin 2 (IL-2) receptor-positive, CD3+ T lymphocytes and graft rejection (35, 36). There is controversy concerning the value of total T-cell enumeration, CD4/CD8 ratios, and the expression of HLA-DR (Ia) on T cells in discriminating rejection from CMV infection (37, 38). Markers that further subset T-cell populations, such as 2H4, may prove to be of value in assessing long-term stability of engraftment (39).

The monoclonal antibody OKT3 is often used as antirejection therapy to block the activity of cytotoxic T lymphocytes (40). This therapy relies on the establishment of sufficient serum levels of OKT3 to bind the T cells and remove them from the circulation (at least temporarily) without the development of antimurine antibodies. Flow cytometric assays are available to monitor these parameters and, therefore, to provide an overall assessment of the likelihood of successful OKT3 therapy (41, 42).

CARDIAC

Many of the problems accompanying cardiac transplantation are the same as those encountered with renal tranplants: evaluating the efficacy and toxicity of therapeutic agents and discriminating between graft rejection and viral infection. Thus, flow cytometry is utilized in a similar matter. While the assessment of OKT3 therapy in cardiac transplant recipients parallels that in renal transplants, the analysis of lymphocyte subsets in these patients has been more controversial. There is disagreement over the value of absolute CD3 enumeration, CD4/CD8 ratios, and the quantitation of activated T cells. Given the availability of performing endomyocardial biopsies (even though these are costly, time-consuming, and potentially hazardous procedures) and the failure to arrive at a consensus for an immunophenotyping assay that has equal value in diagnosing graft rejections, most centers are reluctant to use these flow cytometric assays as anything other than ancillary procedures. Whether this will change as further studies are performed using some of the newer lymphocytes subsetting reagents, such as 2H4, remains to be seen.

BONE MARROW

Bone marrow transplantation has become an option in the treatment of several forms of leukemia and immunodeficiency. In the course of this therapy, a patient's bone marrow is eradicated and replaced with either donor (heterologous) or cleansed autologous marrow. Key clinical issues associated with the transplantation of heterologous bone marrow include assessing the engraftment of the marrow and preventing, detecting, and managing graft versus host disease. Engraftment is often assessed by bone marrow biopsies and differential counts on smears or peripheral blood. Immunophenotyping is often used as an ancillary assay to provide a more comprehensive picture of the reconstituted immune system in these patients. Flow cytometric quantitation of reticulocyte RNA has also been proposed as a method of predicting successful engraftment of bone marrow (43). Here thiazole orange is used to stain the RNA in reticulocytes, providing an index of maturity in these cells, which is thought to be an early indicator of generally functioning marrow.

Graft versus host (GVH) disease in heterologous marrow transplants is a major concern with grave consequences. Here the transplanted immune system recognizes the host as foreign. Reduction of mature T cells in the donor marrow reduces the incidence of GVH, and immunophenotyping is often of use in monitoring T-cell depletion (44).

Biological Response Modifier Therapy

Increasingly, naturally derived cytokines, products of the immune system, or agents that alter the immune status of a patient are being used therapeutically for a variety of diseases. These therapies include, but are not limited to, monoclonal antibodies (both in transplantation and oncology), IL-2, TNF, interfon, LAK cells, and TIL cells. Flow cytometry has been used in the clinical laboratory both to assess the activity or purity of the biological response modifier (BRM) prior to therapy and to evaluate the effects of the BRM of the immune system. The OKT3 therapy, previously discussed in the treatment of graft rejection, is one example of BRM therapy. Interleukin-2 therapy for various forms of cancer is another form of BRM therapy. Here IL-2 "activates" the antitumor cytolytic abilities of NK cells and induces the proliferation of these cells. The expansion in the numbers of activated NK cells is readily measured by flow cytometric immunophenotyping (45), and the effector cells can be isolated by cell sorting to evaluate their cytolytic capabilities in vitro.

Autoimmunity

ANTIBODY-MEDIATED DISEASES

There are autoimmune diseases characterized by the production of antibodies that react with, and destroy, specific cells or tissue. Included among these diseases are several forms of thrombocytopenia and neutropenia. Examples of the former are neonatal alloimmune thrombocytopenia, transfusion-induced thrombocytopenia, and autoimmune thrombocytopenia purpura; examples of the latter include transfusion-induced neutropenia and neonatal isoimmune neutropenia. In the evaluation of these diseases, it is important to establish whether the paucity of cells is due to immune-mediated destruction or lack of production or maturation. Flow cytometry is well suited for assaying peripheral blood specimens for the presence of circulating antibody or antibody bound in vivo to the cell surfaces, using indirect and direct immunofluorescence techniques, respectively (46–49). Which of these (free or cell-bound antibodies) is clinically the more relevant has yet to be definitively established, and arguments can be made for each. Some laboratories test for both and report the presence of either as a positive finding. The detection of cell-bound immunoglobulin is considered to be the more sensitive assay, although in severe cases of thrombocytopenia or neutropenia, the direct method may not always be possible. Care must be taken in interpreting the detection of platelet-binding or neutrophil-binding immunoglobulins because these may either be specific for platelets or neutrophils or nonspecific (e.g., anti-HLA antibodies). This differentiation is best accomplished by examining cells of other lineages from the same patient for the presence of bound antibody.

OTHER

Immunophenotypic studies using flow cytometry have been used extensively in the study of a variety of autoimmune diseases. Although lymphocyte subsetting is of great value in attempting to elucidate the mechanisms underlying the aberrant immune response, it is of little diagnostic value in these diseases.

Abnormal Hematopoiesis

The laboratory evaluation of anemia frequently includes reticulocyte enumeration as a measure of hematopoiesis. The normal response of bone marrow to anemia is the increased production of erythrocytes, although this is not observed when the anemia is the result of abnormal marrow function, which is often due to vitamin or iron deficiencies (hypoproliferative states). Thus, reticulocyte enumeration is often of use in determining the cause of anemia and monitoring the effect of therapy. Reticulocyte enumeration has also been proposed as a method of assessing the function of engrafted bone marrow (43). Reticulocytes are immature red blood cells that, although lacking nuclei, retain RNA in higher amounts than is found in more mature red blood cells. This residual RNA can be measured rapidly and quantitatively on a per cell basis by flow cytometry using dyes such as thiazole orange (50–52). In addition to their use for the enumeration of reticulocytes, the quantitative aspects of the flow cytometric assay have been used to devise a reticulocyte maturity index (RMI) based upon the quantity of RNA in these cells (53).

Thromboembolytic Disease

Platelet activation is associated with a variety of diseases, including adult respiratory distress syndrome (54), renal failure requiring dialysis (55), and a number of cardiovascular ailments (56, 57). Activation of platelets is generally assessed by flow cytometry using monoclonal antibodies directed against activation-related antigens, such as the S12 antibody directed against the α granule membrane protein GMP-140 (58) and the PAC1 antibody directed against the activated form of the platelet membrane glycoprotein IIb-IIIa complex (59). Flow cytometric assays of this type have several advantages over other approaches: subpopulations of platelets can be analyzed; multiple parameters may be examined simultaneously and fresh; undisturbed whole blood may be used for analysis (60, 61).

Solid Tumors

DNA ANALYSIS

The analysis of cellular DNA by flow cytometry is limited by the fact that only gross alterations in the DNA can be measured: translocations and small alterations in total DNA content escape detection. Furthermore, the need to dissociate solid tissue into monodispersed suspensions also places restrictions on this endeavor. Nonetheless, flow cytometric measurement of cellular DNA content is finding a niche in the clinical laboratory. The total G0/G1 nuclear DNA content (ploidy) and the rate of proliferation as determined by calculating the percentage of cells in each phase of the cell cycle are the two most common applications of flow cytometry in the clinical laboratory. Abnormal DNA content i.e., aneuploidy) is perhaps the single cellular feature demonstrating the strongest correlation with neoplasia (62). While many neoplastic lesions are not aneuploid, the presence of aneuploidy is virtually exclusive in its association with neoplastic or preneoplastic lesions. Thus, in specimens where morphologic or phenotypic studies are ambiguous or not available, the detection of aneuploidy can assist in arriving at a diagnosis. This use may be extended to exfoliative cytology (including bladder washes) or body cavity effusions from suspected neoplasms in which the assessment of tissue architecture is not possible and sample preparation for flow cytometry is enhanced by the more dispersed nature of the cells. DNA studies may also be conducted on paraffin-embedded tissue as well as fresh tissue, thus allowing for retrospective studies or the ploidy assessment of a specimen at a later time without the necessity of procuring extra tissue.

Numerous studies have been conducted in attempts to correlate DNA content (ploidy) with prognosis or response to therapy. How well these correlate is unique to each type of tumor as well as to the site of origin and stage; however, in general, abnormal DNA content is considered to be a poor prognostic indicator (Table 57.3). The traditional approach to DNA measurement analyzes only one cellular feature, DNA. However, many laboratories now favor multiparametric analyses that analyze cellular features such as surface markers or proliferation and tumor-associated antigens in addition to DNA content. These multiparameter assays may be used to increase the sensitivity of detection of aneuploidy by eliminating infiltrating lymphocytes from analysis (79) or to better delineate subpopulations of heterogeneous tumors (80).

The measurement of cellular DNA in solid tumors may also be used to estimate the proliferative fraction of tumor cells. Using S phase determinations, correlations between proliferation and survival have been determined for many solid tumors. For example, in astroglial tumors (81), high S-phase fractions correlate with poor patient survival. A similar correlation is observed in breast cancer (82). As discussed elsewhere (83), the high proliferative activity that portends poor survival may also indicate an increased sensitivity to selected chemotherapeutic agents.

METHODOLOGIES

Flow cytometry relies upon the intersection of a stream of cells or particles with a stable light beam of known wavelength and the subsequent detection of fluorescence or light scattering from cells. Before any specimens are analyzed on a flow cytometer, there must be assurance that the stream of cells and the light beam are intersecting at a point where the cells are optimally illuminated and the resulting signals are capable of being collected by the appropriate detectors. The process of bringing the sample stream and light beam into proper orientation is termed *alignment*. Improper alignment of an instrument can lead to weak, unusual, or even missing signals from cells. In addition to alignment, *calibration* of flow cytometers must be performed prior to the analysis of any clinical specimens to determine how reproducibly an instrument is detecting standardized signals from day to day. This is normally accomplished by analyzing standard beads or chicken erythrocytes. Fluctuations in the signal obtained with predetermined instrument settings and laser power generally are indicative of misalignment, a dirty optical path, or a failing light source, detector, or circuitry, among other causes. Reproducible calibration thus ensures standard sensitivity of a cytometer, which is particularly important in DNA studies or when studying markers that result in dim fluorescence. A third general procedure in preparing to analyze samples by flow cytometry is setting proper *compensation* for specimens stained with multiple fluorochromes. Because fluorochromes generally have wide emission spectra, they will overlap to various extents into the band of emission being collected for other fluorochromes. By using a set of standard beads with commonly used fluorochromes, this overlap can be minimized using an electronic compensation to subtract contaminating signals.

Table 57.3. Clinical Significance of DNA Measurements in Selected Solid Tumors

Tumor Site	DNA Parameter	Significance	Representative References
Ovary	Aneuploidy	Decreased survival	Friedlander et al. (63)
			Iversen (64)
Melanoma	Aneuploidy	Freq of recurrence	Von Roenn et al. (65)
Bladder	Aneuploidy	Disease progression	Frankfurt and Huben (66)
			Chin et al. (67)
		Decreased survival	Blomjous et al. (68)
Breast	Ploidy	No consensus	Cornelisse et al. (69)
			Owainati et al. (70)
			Fallenius et al. (71)
Prostate	Aneuploidy	Decreased survival	Stephenson et al. (72)
		Disease progression	McIntire et al. (73)
			Frankfurt et al. (74)
Colon	Aneuploidy	Decreased survival	Jones et al. (75)
		Disease progression	Armitage et al. (76)
			Emdin et al. (77)
Neuroblastoma stage D in infants	Hyperdiploidy	Favorable response to chemotherapy	Look et al. (78)

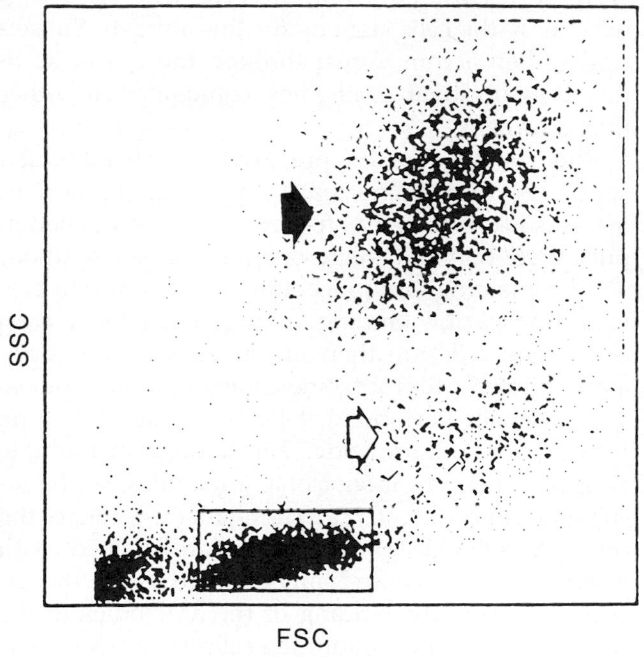

Figure 57.4. A dot density, two-parameter histogram illustrating the forward light scatter on the *x* axis and side (90°) light scatter on the *y* axis of human peripheral blood after lysis of the red blood cells. The area surrounded by the box represents the gated lymphoid cells; monocytes are indicated by the hollow arrow; the granulocytes are indicated by the solid arrow. Debris and small particles are to the left of the lymphoid cells.

Gating

Flow cytometers are intrinsically incapable of distinguishing cells from other particles that may be present in specimens submitted for analysis. Cytometers are capable of measuring (in addition to fluorescence signals) the forward and orthogonal light scatter signals eminating from cells, which are roughly indicative of particle size and granularity, respectively. Empirically, the light scatter patterns of normal peripheral blood have been determined and correlated with cell type. Armed with this knowledge, it is possible to examine only cells of interest for immunophenotyping, excluding the other cells or particles through a process referred to as *gating*. Here the cytometer is directed to ignore events (particles) whose light scatter characteristics do not fall within a predefined set of parameters. Thus, in routine lymphocyte subset analysis, peripheral blood, subsequent to the lysis of the erythrocytes, can be prepared, but by gating, only the staining on the lymphocytes is analyzed—the granulocytes and monocytes are excluded from analysis (Fig. 57.4). Failure to exclude cells of extraneous lineages from analysis can, and usually does, lead to misinterpretation of marker expression. Gating may also be performed using features other than, or in addition to, light scatter signals. For example, the identification of leukocytes in heterogeneous samples can be accomplished by gating on cells that stain with anti-CD45.

Surface Marker Staining of Lymphocyte Subsets

Flow cytometry represents more than an automated method for the enumeration of cells bearing a particular cell surface marker, although it is often used for this purpose. This technology is best used as a method for analyzing multiple cellular features in a rapid and quantitative manner. Light scatter patterns can be used to grossly resolve white blood cells of various lineages. In addition, multiple antigenic markers can also be studied to more precisely determine lineage, maturity, and/or state of activation. This is possible through the use of multiple fluoro-

Table 57.4. Commonly Used Fluorochromes for Immunophenotypic Studies

Fluorochrome	Excitation[a]	Emission[a]	Comments
	nm	*nm*	
Fluorescein isothiocyanate (FITC)	488	530	Low molecular weight, stable
Phycoerythrin (PE)	492	580	High quantum yield
Duochrome (Becton Dickinson Immunocytometry System, Inc.)	492	620	Tandem conjugate of PE and Tx Red
Allophycocyanin	633	660	Requires He, Ne, krypton, or dye laser
Texas Red	600	630	Requires dye laser

[a]The values listed for excitation and emission wavelengths are not necessarily the maximum, but rather those that are commonly used in the laboratory.

chromes that have distinct emission wavelengths. Quantitation of the emissions at prespecified wavelengths will yield a value proportional to the amount of fluorochrome-conjugated antibody bound to the cells and, ultimately, to the amount of antigen present. Examples of commonly used fluorochromes are given in Table 57.4. Staining of cells with multiple antibodies is best acccomplished using a direct immunofluorescence technique, i.e., having fluorochrome-conjugated antibodies rather than using a sandwich (indirect) technique. This is due to the fact that most antibodies to clinically relevant markers are mouse monoclonal antibodies and are likely to cross-react in many indirect techniques.

Care must be taken in sample procurement and handling to avoid the introduction of artifacts into the analysis of surface markers. Factors such as the anticoagulant used for the collection of the peripheral blood specimen and the time of day have been demonstrated to influence the enumeration of various lymphocyte subsets (84, 85). Further more, maintenance of the specimens at room temperature has been demonstrated to be a strict requirement; storage at 4°C for even short periods of time will induce capping of the antigens and alter the detection of lymphocyte subsets (86, 87).

Peripheral blood specimens are prepared for staining either by density-gradient separation of lymphocytes or by the lysis of red blood cells with agents such as ammonium chloride. Removal of erythrocytes from peripheral blood specimens is generally thought to be necessary because it allows the flow cytometer to analyze other cellular populations more quickly. The latter technique, commonly referred to as the "whole blood lysis" technique, is generally used because it is quicker, it may be performed before or after staining, and it permits the examination of monocytic and granulocytic components concomitant to the analysis of lymphocytes. The major questions regarding this approach are whether the specific antigen is altered by the lysing agent and whether there is a need for the cells of interest to be further concentrated. Phenotyping data from both methods of sample preparation are generally similar, although density-gradient procedures have been demonstrated to produce selective enrichment of certain populations of cells (88, 89). One approach to the flow cytometric analysis of lymphocyte subsets, not commonly in use, would preclude the need for removal of erythrocytes. This approach involves the use of a monoclonal antibody to the CD45 (common leukocyte) antigen to distinguish leukocytes from erythrocytes and adjusting the cytometer to "recognize" only the cells staining for this antigen. Subsetting is then accomplished through the use of additional monoclonal antibodies conjugated to other fluorochromes.

The staining of the prepared peripheral blood specimen with monoclonal antibodies to surface markers is conducted as follows: Cells are washed in phosphate-buffered saline or balanced salt solution, often containing low concentrations of serum to prevent nonspecific binding of the monoclonal antibody. The cells are then incubated with appropriately diluted fluorochrome-conjugated antibodies. This is usually performed at 4°C for 30 minutes in the presence of sodium azide. For staining of multiple antigens, different monoclonal antibodies can be incubated concomitantly to simultaneously stain the cells. Additional tubes of cells are stained with isotype-matched control antibodies to assess the extent of nonspecific binding of the antibodies to the cells. After this incubation, the cells are washed and, in most clinical laboratories, fixed with paraformaldehyde. Besides preserving the cells better for later analysis, this fixation has also been demonstrated to inactivate the human immunodeficiency virus (90). Cells prepared in this manner, if stored at 4°C and protected from light, may be stored approximately 10 to 12 days without substantial loss of staining or light scatter properties.

Other Surface Marker Staining

The technique of immunofluorescence staining, either direct or indirect, is used for the evaluation of cell surface markers. Certain specimens, such as platelets, require that special care be taken in procurement, transport, and staining. Analysis of platelet activation is highly influenced by the type of anticoagulant used, the length of time prior to analysis, and the use of aspirin or similar products by the patient. In these assays (in contrast to lymphocyte immunophenotyping), it is often desirable to fix the specimen with paraformaldehyde prior to staining to minimize the artifacts introduced after procurement of the specimen (54, 60).

The staining of platelets, neutrophils, and lymphocytes for autoantibodies against each of these cell types may be performed by using either direct or indirect immunofluorescence techniques. Direct staining, using a xenogenic antihuman immunoglobulin antibody, is used to detect antibody bound in vivo to the cells. To control for the specificity of the staining, an antibody directed against an irrelevant antigen that is derived from the same species as the anti-Ig antibody and matched for isotype and F/P ratio is used. An indirect staining method is used to detect autoantibodies in the circulation. In this approach, relevant donor cells are incubated with the serum (usually heat inactivated) from the patient with the suspected autoimmunity. After an appropriate length of incubation, the cells are washed and incubated with a fluorochrome-conjugated antihuman immunoglobulin reagent. Controls in this instance normally include identical staining with serum obtained from a normal donor. The isotype of the autoantibodies can be identified through the use of isotype-specific antihuman reagents.

DNA Staining

The staining of hematological material for DNA content is easily accomplished because the cells to be examined are predominantly in single-particle suspension. This is not the case, however, for the DNA analysis of tissue derived from solid tumors. Here the specimen must be disaggregated to obtain a monodisperse suspension. This is accomplished by mechanical dissociation and/or enzyme (e.g., pepsin) digestion, followed by filtration through a 50- to 70-μm mesh (62, 91). The yields from this procedure vary; however, cellular losses are assumed to be random, and the final suspension of cells or nuclei is felt to be representative of the original specimen. This procedure is harsh on the cell surface membrane, making it difficult to perform surface marker analyses on these preparations.

A number of fluorescent dyes that may be used to stain cellular DNA are available; however, the dye used almost exclusively for this purpose in the clinical laboratory is propidium iodide (PI). Propidium iodide intercalates into cellular DNA and yields fluorescence signals in the orange/red region proportional to the amount of DNA. It is readily excitable at 488 nm and is stable in solution, and these factors contribute to its widespread use. The staining achieved with propidium iodide is uniform and reproducible, yielding very small coefficients of variation (CVs). CVs reflect the "tightness" of a histogram peak; therefore, the tighter the CV of a G0/G1 DNA peak, the easier one can detect slight aneuploidy in a specimen (e.g., the sensitivity of an aneuploidy detection increases). A number of methods have been described for staining cellular DNA with propidium iodide (92, 93). Most of these rely upon lysis of the surface membrane of the cell, digestion of the RNA, and staining of the residual intact nuclei. Using this approach, a one-step method has been developed for DNA staining. Using a filtered solution of 10 mM Trizma base, 10 mM NaCl, 0.7 U/ml RNAse, 7×10^{-5} M PI, and 0.1% NP-40, cells can be lysed, enzyme-digested, and stained with PI concomitantly. This solution is added to the cells while vortexing, and the cells are then incubated at 4°C for 30 minutes. The stained nuclei can be analyzed immediately by flow cytometry or fixed with paraformaldehyde and stored for as long as a week until analysis. As DNA standards (discussed later), chicken or trout erythrocytes may be added to the specimen prior to staining.

Specimens stained with propidium iodide may be analyzed to determine the ploidy of the specimen and, in most instances, to assess proliferation. This is possible because PI binds proportionally to the amount of cellular DNA, and cellular DNA is increased as cells progress through S-phase and enter G2/M. In G2/M, cells have 4N DNA and yield PI fluorescence twice that observed in G0/G1 nuclei (Fig. 57.5). Proliferation may be assessed in freshly obtained specimens to determine the in vivo proliferative rate (particularly for anaplastic specimens), or specimens may be stimulated in vitro, then stained with PI to assess their proliferative response. The latter is performed in the evaluation of immunodeficiencies in which the response of peripheral blood lymphocytes to mitogen stimulation is important in pinpointing the immune defect. Patients' lymphocytes are cocultured with mitogen (e.g., phytohemagglutinin) for 72 hours, harvested, and stained with PI as described above. The percentage of cells in S-phase and G2/M is determined and compared to patient cells cultured without mitogen or to normal, resting lymphocytes stained in the same manner. This assay may also have a positive control consisting of normal lymphocytes cocultured with mitogen and responding in the predicted manner.

DNA analyses are not limited to specimens freshly obtained from the patient or in vitro cultivation. Cryopreserved specimens generally yield CVs approximating those obtained from fresh tissue. As mentioned previously, DNA assays may also be

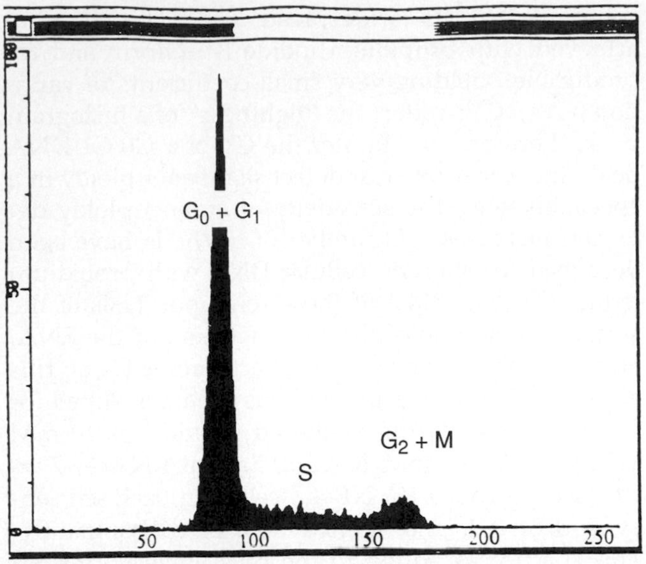

Figure 57.5. A representative one-parameter histogram of cell nuclei stained with propidiun iodide. Phases of the cell cycle are as indicated. (Note the broad, irregular S phase.) Ploidy determinations among specimens are made by comparing the position of the G0/G1 peaks.

performed on formalin-fixed, paraffin-embedded tissue (94, 95). Here sample preparation and data intepretation are more rigorous than required in DNA analysis of fresh tissue. Sample preparation concerns begin at the time of original tissue fixation and embedding. The type of fixative has a profound effect on the resulting DNA histograms, and neutral-buffered formalin has been demonstrated to be the fixative of choice (96). However, even this fixative introduces some DNA artifacts, as will be discussed later. Sections are usually processed from paraffin blocks rather than the entire tissue. This generally indicates a desire to retain tissue for any future medical or legal issues. Section thickness has a substantial effect on the resulting DNA histograms, and it is generally agreed that 50-μm sections provide the optimal results (97). The sections are deparaffinized using xylene or the equivalent and subsequently rehydrated using a series of decreasing ethanol solutions. The rehydrated tissue is now disassociated with enzymes (pepsin or trypsin) and filtered to obtain single cell suspensions. These cell suspensions are then stained with propidium iodide as described for fresh tissue.

Combined Surface Marker/DNA Staining

There are obvious advantages to being able to concomitantly examine the surface markers and DNA content of the same cells. The proliferation of neoplastic cells can be assessed much more accurately if one can gate on the relevant cells through the use of a surface marker. The detecton of aneuploidy in minimal residual disease becomes more sensitive if only cells of the pertinent lineage are examined. A technique for the dual staining of cells for surface markers and DNA was introduced by Braylan et al. (98) and remains in use with very little modification. Cells are incubated with the fluorochrome (usually FITC)-conjugated antibody against the surface marker in sodium azide at 4°C for an appropriate length of time, then are washed thoroughly. The cells, suspended in PBS or medium, are vortexed while an equal volume of 100% ethanol is added. The cells are incubated in the ethanol for 1 hour at 4°C, washed, treated with RNAse, and finally stained with propidium iodide. The only disadvantage of this procedure is the loss of resolution in the light scatter patterns.

A method has also been introduced that permits the concomitant analysis of surface markers, cytoplasmic antigens, and DNA content (99, 100). In this method, cells are stained for a specific surface marker, washed, then briefly fixed with a low concentration of paraformaldehyde and washed again. The cells are then permeabilized with 70% methanol and again washed. The cells may now be stained for the expression of intracellular antigens. If FITC was used to mark the surface antigen, a distinct fluorochrome such as allophycocyanin or Duochrome is used to stain the intracellular antigen. The cells are again washed and finally incubated with an RNAse/propidium iodide solution to stain the DNA. This method has been demonstrated to reliably stain all parameters, with a fair preservation of light scatter signals, and only minor diminution of the propidium iodide fluorescence due to the paraformaldehyde.

Reticulocyte Staining

Reticulocyte staining is dependent on the staining of residual RNA in immature erythrocytes. A number of RNA-binding dyes have been used for this purpose, including pyronin Y, acridine orange, thioflavin T, and thiazole orange. Thiazole orange (52) is a membrane-permeable dye, excited at 488 nm, that intercalates into nucleic acids and fluoresces at 533 nm. Staining of reticulocytes with this dye is easily accomplished: 5 μl of whole blood is incubated for 1 hour at room temperature with 1 ml of 0.1 μg/ml thiazole orange in PBS containing EDTA and sodium azide.

INTERPRETATION

Surface Marker Staining

Flow cytometric data are customarily displayed as histograms, or plots, of the digitized data. With digitized data, the light scatter and/or fluorescence signals eminating from individual cells are assigned to a

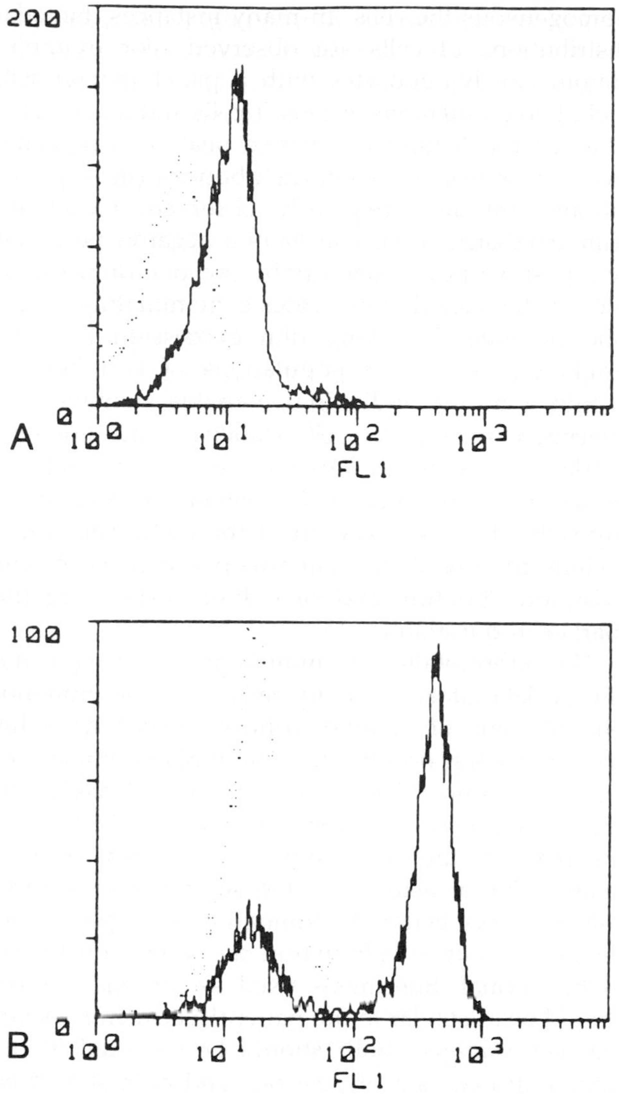

Figure 57.6. Examples of one-parameter histograms of fluorescence staining overlayed with one-parameter histograms from the isotypic controls. The *x* axis is fluorescence intensity (channel number) and the *y* axis is the number of events (cells) in each channel. The dotted lines are the isotypic controls, and the solid lines are antibodies specific for a surface marker. **A.** Dim staining of the specific antibody. Here simple integration methods will not yield an accurate estimation of the number of positive cells. In the absence of a bimodal peak (as seen in **B**), the argument can be made that all cells dimly stain with this antibody. **B.** A bimodal distribution of cells with one bright, specific staining population and a smaller population displaying background staining similar to that observed with the isotypic control. Here the number of positive cells may be readily obtained by determining the number of cells in channels beyond the peak of the control.

channel proportional to the strength of the signal. The number of channels varies from instrument to instrument but is normally 64, 256, or 1024. The stronger the signal from the cell (e.g., the more fluorescent the cell), the higher the channel number to which that cell is assigned. Various numbers of parameters may be displayed on a histogram, the most basic being a one-parameter display (Fig. 57.6). Here

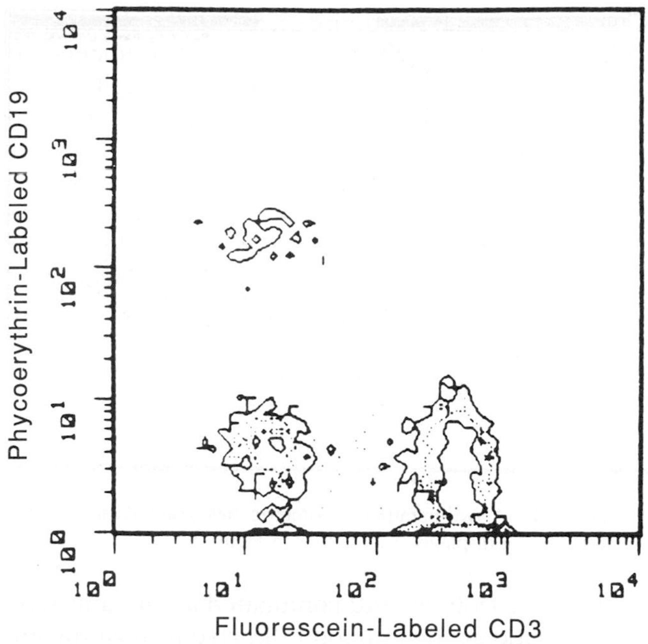

Figure 57.7. A two-parameter contour histogram illustrating the staining of peripheral blood lymphocytes with a pan B marker on the *y* axis (FL2-phycoerythrin) and a pan T marker on the *x* axis (FL1-FITC) monoclonal amtibodies. The number of cells is displayed as elevation contours.

the histogram consists of the intensity of signal (channel number) on the *x* axis (on either a log or linear scale) versus the number of particles (cells) in each channel on the *y* axis. Two-parameter histograms display the intensity of two separate signals on the *x* and *y* axes, with the number of events being displayed either by dot density (Fig. 57.4) or contours (Fig. 57.7) or in isometric form (Fig. 57.8). Three-parameter histograms are occasionally used to display multiparameter data and rely on three-dimensional (cubic) displays. The display of the number of events often requires color density graphics; therefore, the use of three-parameter histograms has been somewhat limited.

Virtually all cells will display some degree of autofluorescence if stimulated with sufficient light. This would result in nonstained cells being placed at various positions in the histogram displays. This is usually not desirable because fluorescence intensity is typically displayed on a log scale and the ability to delineate small shifts in fluorescence decreases on the upper portion of the scale. Therefore, using an unstained control, the laser power and/or voltages to the photomultiplier tubes are adjusted to bring the unstained samples near the origin of the histogram display.

Essential to assessing the specificity of antibody staining is the paired analysis of an isotypic control. This control consists of an antibody, directed against an irrelevant antigen, derived from the same species,

43. Davis BH, Bigelow N, Ball ED, Mills L, Cornwell GG. Utility of flow cytometric reticulocyte quantification as a predictor of engraftment in autologous bone marrow transplantation. Am J Hemato 1989;32:81–87.
44. Martin PJ, Hansen JA. Quantitative assays for detection of residual T cells of T-depleted human marrow. Blood 1985;65: 1134–1140.
45. Phillips JH, Gemlo BT, Myers WW, et al. In vivo and in vitro activation of natural killer cells in advanced cancer patients undergoing combined recombinant interleukin-2 and LAK cell therapy. J Clin Oncol 1987;5:1933–1941.
46. Robinson JP, Duque RE, Boxer LE, et al. Measurement of antineutrophil antibodies by flow cytometry: simultaneous detection of antibodies against monocytes and lymphocytes. Diagn Clin Immunol 1987;5:163–170.
47. Sears D, Kickler TS, Johnson RJ, Ness PM. The diagnostic usefulness of measuring antineutrophil antibodies in neutropenic patients. Acta Haematol 1986;75:65–69.
48. Ault KA. Flow cytometric measurement of platelet-associated immunoglobulin. Pathol Immunopathol Res 1988;7:395–408.
49. Rosenfeld CA, Nichols G, Bodensteiner DC. Flow cytometric measurement of antiplatelet antibodies. Am J Clin Pathol 1987;87:207–212.
50. Corash L, Rheinschmidt M, Lieu S, et al. Enumeration of reticulocytes using fluorescence-activated flow cytometry. Pathol Immunopathol Res 1988;7:381–394.
51. Tanke HJ, van Vianan PH, Emiliani FMF, et al. Changes in erythropoiesis due to radiation or chemotherapy as studied by flow cytometric determination of peripheral blood reticulocytes. Histochemistry 1986;84:544–548.
52. Lee LG, Chen CH, Chiu LA. Thiazole orange: a new dye for reticulocyte analysis. Cytometry 1986;7:508–517.
53. Davis BH, Bigelow NC. Flow cytometric reticulocyte quanification using thiazole orange provides clinically useful reticulocyte maturity index. Arch Pathol Lab Med 1989;113:684–689.
54. George JN, PIckett EB, Saucerman S, et al. Platelet surface glycoproteins. Studies on resting and activated platelets and platelet membrane microparticles in normal subjects, and observations in patients during adult respiratory distress syndrome and cardiac surgery. J Clin Invest 1986;78:340–348.
55. Hakin RM, Schafer AI. Hemodialysis-associated platelet activation and thromocytopenia. Am J Med 1985;78:575–580.
56. Fitzgerald DJ, Roy L, Catella F, et al. Platelet activation in unstable coronary artery disease. N Engl J Med 1986;315:983–989.
57. Harker LA, Malpass TW, Branson HE, et al. Mechanism of abnormal bleeding in patients undergoing cardiopulmonary bypass. Acquired transient platelet dysfunction associated with selective alpha-granule release. Blood 1980;56:824–834.
58. McEver RP, Martin MN. A monoclonal antibody to a membrane glycoprotein binds only to activated platelets. J Biol Chem 1984;259:9799–9804.
59. Shattil SJ, Hoxie JA, Cunningham M, Brass LF. Changes in the platelet membrane glycoprotein IIb-IIIa complex during platelet activation. J Biol Chem 1985;260:11107–11114.
60. Ault KA, Rinder HM, Mitchell JG, et al. Correlated measurement of platelet release and aggregation in whole blood. Cytometry 1989;10:448–455.
61. Shattil SJ, Cunningham M, Hoxie JA. Detection of activated platelets in whole blood using activation-dependent monoclonal antibodies and flow cytometry. Blood 1987;70:307–315.
62. Barlogie B, Drewinko B, Schumann J, et al. Cellular DNA content as a marker of neoplasia in man. Am J Med 1980;69: 195–203.
63. Friedlander ML, Hedley DW, Swanson C, Russell P. Prediction of long term survival by flow cytometric analysis of cellular DNA content in patients with advanced ovarian carcinoma. J Clin Oncol 1988;6:282–290.
64. Iversen OE. Prognostic value of the flow cytometric DNA index in human ovarian carcinoma. Cancer 1988;61:334–339.
65. Von Roenn JH, Kheir SM, Wolter JM, Coon JS. Significance of DNA abnormalities in primary malignant melanoma and nevi, a retrospective flow cytometric study. Cancer Res 1986;46:3192–3195.
66. Frankfurt OS, Huben RP. Clincial applications of DNA flow cytometry for human bladder tumors. Urology 1984;23:23–26.
67. Chin JL, Huben RP, Nava E, et al. Flow cytometric analysis of DNA content in human bladder tumors and irrigation fluids. Cancer 1985;56:1677–1681.
68. Blomjous CEM, Schipper NW Baak JPA, et al. Retrospective study of prognostic importance of DNA flow cytometry of urinary bladder carcinoma. J Clin Pathol 1988;41:21–25.
69. Cornelisse CJ, van de Velde CJH, Caspers RJC, et al. DNA ploidy and survival in breast cancer patients. Cytometry 1987;8:225–234.
70. Owainati AAR, Robins RA, Hinton C, et al. Tumor aneuploidy, prognostic parameters and survival in primary breast cancer. Br J Cancer 1987;55:449–454.
71. Fallenius AG, Franzen SA, Auer GA. Predictive value of nuclear DNA content in breast cancer in relation to clinical and morphological factors. Cancer 1988;62:521–530.
72. Stephenson RA, James BC, Gay H, et al. Flow cytometry of prostate cancer: relationship of DNA content of survival. Cancer Res 1987;47:2504–2509.
73. McIntire TL, Murphy WM, Coon JS, et al. The prognostic value of DNA ploidy combined with histologic substaging for incidental carcinoma of the prostate gland. Am J Clin Pathol 1988;89:370–373.
74. Frankfurt OS, Chin JL, Englander LS, et al. Relationship of DNA ploidy, clandular differentiation, and tumor spread in human prostate cancer. Cancer Res 1985;45:1418–1423.
75. Jones DJ, Moore M, Schofield PF. Refining the prognostic significance of DNA ploidy status in colorectal cancer: a prospective flow cytometric study. Int J Cancer 1988;41:206–210.
76. Armitage NC, Robias RA, Evans DF, et al. The influence of tumor cell DNA abnormalities on survival in colorectal cancer. Br J Surg 1985;72:828–830.
77. Emdin SO, Stenling R, Ross G. Prognostic value of DNA content in colorectal carcinoma. Cancer 1987;60:1282–1287.
78. Look At, Hayes FA, Nitschike R, et al. Cellular DNA content as a predictor of response to chemotherapy in infants with unresectable neuroblastoma. N Engl J Med 1984;311:213–235.
79. Park CH, Lee SH, Stephens RL, et al. Flow cytometry DNA analysis on tumor cell subpopulation of human tumor specimens by exclusion of lymphohemopoietic cells. J Histochem Cytochem 1988;36:705–709.
80. Bauer KD, Clevenger CV, Endow RK, et al. Simultaneous nuclear antigen and DNA content quantitation using paraffin-embedded colonic tissue and multiparameter flow cytometry. Cancer Res 1986;46:2428–2434.
81. Zaprianov Z, Christov K. Histological grading, DNA content, cell proliferation and survival of patients with astroglial tumors. Cytometry 1988;9:380–386.
82. Clark GM, Dressler LG, Owens MA, et al. Prediction of relapse or survival in patients with node-negative breast cancer by DNA flow cytometry. N Engl J Med 1989;320:627–630.
83. Osborne CK. DNA flow cytometry in early breast cancer: a step in the right direction. J Natl Cancer Inst 1989;81:1344–1345.
84. Bertouch JV, Roberts-Thomson PJ, Bradley J. Diurnal variation of lymphocyte subsets identified by monoclonal antibodies. Br Med J 1983;286:1171–1173.

85. Thornthwaite JT, Rosenthal PK, Vazquez DA, Seckinger D. The effects of anticoagulant and temperature on the measurements of helper and suppressor cells. Diagn Immunol 1984;2:167–174.
86. Dzik WH, Neckers L. Lymphocyte subpopulations altered during blood storage. N Engl J Med 1983;309:435–436.
87. Weiblen BJ, Debell K, Valeri CR. Acquired immunodeficiency of blood stored overnight. N Engl J Med 1983;309:793.
88. DePoali P, Rentano M, Battisin S, et al. Enumeration of human lymphocyte subsets by monoclonal antibodies and flow cytometry: a comparative study using whole blood or mononuclear cells separated by density gradient centrifugation. J Immunol Methods 1984;72:349–353.
89. Slade HB, Greenwood HJ, Hudson JL, et al. Spurious lymphocyte phenotypes by flow cytometry from mononuclear cells prepared by ficoll-hypaque. Pediatr Res 1987;21:318A.
90. Lifson JD, Sasaki DT, Engleman EG. Utility of formaldehyde fixation for flow cytometry and inactivation of the AIDS associated retrovirus. J Immunol Methods 1986;86:143–149.
91. Thornthwaite JT, Sugerbaker EV, Temple WJ. Preparation of tissues for DNA flow cytometric analysis. Cytometry 1980;1:229–237.
92. Vindelov LL, Christensen IJ, Nissen NI. A detergent-trypsin method for the preparation of nuclei for flow cytometric DNA analysis. Cytometry 1983;3:323–327.
93. Tate EH, Wilder ME, Cram LS, Wharton W. A method for staining 3T3 cell nuclei with propidium iodide in hypotonic solution. Cytometry 1983;4:211–215.
94. Hedley DW, Friedlander ML, Taylor IW, et al. Method for analysis of cellular DNA content of paraffin-embedded pathological material using flow cytometry. J Histochem Cytochem 1983;31:1333–1335.
95. Hedley DW. Flow cytometry using paraffin-embedded tissue: five years on. Cytometry 1989;10:229–241.
96. Herbert DJ, Nishiyama RH, Bagwell CB, et al. Effects of several commonly used fixatives on DNA and total nuclear protein analysis by flow cytometry. Am J Clin Pathol 1989;91:535–541.
97. Stephenson RA, Gay H, Fair WR, Melamed MR. Effect of section thickness on quality of flow cytometric DNA content determinations in paraffin-embedded tissues. Cytometry 1986;7:41–44.
98. Braylan RC, Benson NA, Nourse V, Kruth HS. Correlated analysis of cellular DNA, membrane antigens and light scatter of human lymphoid cells. Cytometry 1982;2:337–343.
99. McCoy JP, Krause JR, Hanley-Yanez K, et al. Three color analysis of surface marker, oncogene product, and DNA content in leukemia. Cytometry 1990;4(supp 1):29.
100. Shackney SE, McCoy JP, Burholt DR, et al. Sequential paraformaldehyde and methanol fixation for quantitative multiparameter cellular DNA measurement and immunofluorescence measurements of cell surface and intracellular proteins by flow cytometry (FCM). Cytometry 1990;4(supp 1):17.
101. Gratner HG. Monoclonal antibody to 5-bromo and 5-iododeoxyuridine: a new reagent for the detection of DNA replication. Science 1982;218:474–475.
102. Bagwell CB. Clinical data analysis for flow cytometry. In: Keren DF, ed. Flow cytometry in clinical diagnosis. Chicago: ASCP Press, 1989:310–330.
103. Baldetorp B, Dalberg M, Holst U, Lindgren G. Statistical Evaluation of cell kinetic data from DNA flow cytometry (FCM) by the EM algorithm. Cytometry 1989;10:695–705.
104. Horvath L. Quality control in clinical flow cytometry. Pathol Immunopathol Res 1988;7:338–344.
105. Hurley AA. Quality control in flow cytometry. Cytometry Suppl 1988;3:29–33.
106. McCoy JP, Carey JL, Krause JR. Quality control in flow cytometry for diagnostic pathology. I. Cell surface phenotyping and general laboratory procedures. Am J Clin Pathol 1990;93(suppl 1):S27–D37.
107. Green WF, Stelzer GT. Interlaboratory comparison of flow cytometric lymphocyte phenotyping analyses: implications for standardization and quality control. Cytometry 1988;3(suppl 1):23–28.

58 Immunoserology of Infectious Mononucleosis and Related Heterophil-Negative Mononucleosis-Like Illnesses

Charles A. Horwitz and Theresa A. Steeper

The designation of infectious mononucleosis (IM) classically refers to an Epstein-Barr virus (EBV)–induced illness in young adults associated with reactive blood smears, exudative pharyngitis, prominent cervical lymphadenopathy, and serologically detectable heterophil antibodies with IM-specific differential absorption traits. Similar, IM-like illnesses without heterophil antibodies can also be caused by EBV as well as cytomegalovirus (CMV), *Toxoplasma gondii*, human immunodeficiency virus (HIV), the recently described human herpes virus-6 (HHV-6), and (rarely) drugs, including halothane, hydantoin, dapasone, and Azulfidine (1-3). As a group, these illnesses have overlapping clinical and serological findings and are held together only by common, often striking, morphological findings, that is, blood smears meeting minimum morphological criteria for IM (50% or more, lymphocytes, 10 or more atypical lymphocytes per 100 white blood cells, and significant lymphocytic heterogeneity). In this chapter, we summarize the advantages and limitations of the various methodologies used for confirmation of IM or IM-like syndromes and present an algorithmic diagnostic approach that can be applied to an individual patient's illness.

DETECTION OF IM-SPECIFIC HETEROPHIL ANTIBODIES

Many transient heterophil antibody responses occur during the course of EBV-IM, including those directed against sheep, horse, or beef erythrocytes, IgG (rheumatoid factors), nuclei (ANA), intermediate filaments, cardiolipid, smooth muscle antigens (SMA), i red blood cell (RBC) antigens (cold agglutinins), and others. However, only the detection of Paul-Bunnell IM-type heterophil antibodies is specific for EBV-IM. These IgM-type antibodies are sheep or horse red-cell agglutinins that resist absorption with suspensions of guinea pig kidney (GPK), a source of Forssman antigen, but are absorbable with beef RBCs or RBC stroma. Previously, they were detected with the Paul-Bunnell-Davidsohn (PBD) test, a well-studied, highly specific, 2-hour sheep-cell differential absorption tube test (4). The PBD test is limited by its relative insensitivity when compared to recently utilized test systems that incorporate horse cells as indicators for the detection of heterophil antibodies (5). In the reference horse-cell agglutination test (HCAT), also known as the Lee-Davidsohn test, IM-specific horse-cell agglutinins are detected in test tubes following differential absorption of the test sera. Interpretation of HCAT data is simple in that positive results are recorded when the GPK-absorbed horse agglutinin titer exceeds that of a simultaneously performed beef-absorbed titer (5). If the GPK titer is less than or equal to the beef-absorbed titer, a negative result for heterophil-positive EBV-IM is recorded. Because of increased sensitivity due to the use of horse cells and retention of specificity because of pre-test differential absorption of serum, the HCAT is the reference heterophil tube test of choice. Despite its greater sensitivity, there is no evidence that a positive HCAT result is any less specific for EBV-IM than the PBD (6, 7). The HCAT is ideal for both the early diagnosis and detection of maximal numbers of heterophil-positive EBV-IM cases.

Additional heterophil reference tests include the ox cell hemolysin (OCH), immune adherence hemagglutination (IAHA), and Woellner enzyme tests. The OCH test is a well-studied, highly specific, and easily automatable test that is at least as sensitive as the PBD test. It is unclear, however, whether the OCH test is as sensitive as the HCAT in heterophil antibody detection. The IAHA test is at least as sensitive as the HCAT, but its specificity for IM-type heterophil antibodies has not been extensively evaluated. There are also technical limitations due to variable sensitivity of human erythrocytes from different donors (8). In the Woellner enzyme test, red cell receptors for the heterophil antibody are specifically removed by papain enzyme treatment, following which the absence of sheep cell agglutination implies a positive test. This test has been extensively evaluated but is seldom used today.

RAPID HETEROPHIL TESTS

Because the aforementioned reference tests (HCAT and OCH) are time-consuming (1 to 3 hours) and labor-intensive, they are impractical for routine use in most hospitals and physician offices. Thus, a variety of 1- to 2-minute agglutination heterophil slide tests have been developed. Most utilize fine suspensions of GPK and beef red-cell stroma for instantaneous differential absorption, followed by the addition of horse RBC stroma or erythrocytes for sensitive detection of IM-specific heterophil antibodies. These convenient and simple slide tests have, for the most part, replaced standard reference tube tests in screening for IM-type heterophil antibodies. They are considered to be sufficiently sensitive that a negative result implies the absence of significant levels of IM-specific heterophil antibodies. One such rapid IM slide test (Monospot, Ortho Diagnostics), which uses preserved rather than fixed indicator horse erythrocytes, is capable of detecting low levels (titer of 1:56 to 1:112) of GPK-absorbed horse agglutinins. Less sensitive tests with formalin-fixed indicator cells may require titers of 1:224 or higher before positive results are recorded. Based on experience in our laboratory, the Monospot test has a sensitivity of 98% and a false-positive rate of 2 to 3% compared with reference HCAT data (9). Results from any rapid test should always be interpreted with the knowledge of accompanying hematologic and clinical findings. A positive result with an appropriately reactive blood smear confirms the diagnosis of heterophil-positive IM, and EBV is assumed to be the cause of the patient's clinical illness. No further diagnostic tests, such as EBV-specific viral serology or the reference HCAT, are indicated. The rapid IM heterophil test should be viewed as only a qualitative test that simply determines the presence or absence of IM-specific heterophil antibodies. Because the quantitative heterophil titers do not correlate well with either the severity of acute illness or the speed of recovery, determination of the actual heterophil titer is never indicated. Thus, a patient with heterophil-negative, EBV-induced IM may have a severe illness requiring steroids, whereas another patient with minimal symptoms may have a heterophil titer of 1:100,000 or higher.

About 25% of patients with acute EBV-IM still have detectable residual IM heterophil antibodies 12 or more months following the onset of illness (6, 7). Such residual horse-cell agglutinins can lead to diagnostic problems when subsequent illnesses due to other, unrelated infectious agents occur. In a small percentage (2 to 3%) of EBV-IM cases, heterophil antibodies may arise with a delay of up to 4 to 8 weeks after the onset of clinical illness, hematologic findings, or both.

Recently, 4- to 10-minute, heterophil enzyme immunoassay (EIA) tests have been marketed. In most of these tests, the so-called "IM-specific antigen" derived from membranes of sheep or bovine erythrocytes is coated onto various solid-phase surfaces (e.g., plastic tubes, disks, membranes, or spoons) (10). The sensitized solid phase is then incubated sequentially between washing steps with serum that potentially contains IgM-specific heterophil antibodies and enzyme-labeled antihuman IgM. Finally, the substrate for the appropriate linking enzyme is added, and a colorimetric endpoint determines the heterophil test result. As a group, the heterophil EIA tests have been heavily marketed for their greater sensitivity, retention of specificity without the need for serum differential absorption, longer shelf life, and more distinctive visual endpoints. Practically, the EIA heterophil tests are more expensive than agglutination tests and have not been as extensively evaluated. Further studies will determine whether their overall accuracy warrants their substitution for the well-studied rapid IM slide agglutinin tests.

VIRUS-SPECIFIC TESTS IN IM-LIKE ILLNESSES

Various immunoassays employing different endpoint indicator systems are available for rapid viral diagnosis (11–13). The well-studied immunofluorescence assay (IFA) methods remain useful diagnostically for several virus-induced diseases. Quality control requirements, including strict criteria for interpretation of fluorescent endpoint patterns, must be maintained to avoid false-positive results. Detection of IgG, virus-specific serum antibodies by IFA can often be completed within 60 minutes, whereas tests for IgM antibodies are more time-consuming due to longer incubation periods. Overall, IFA is more sensitive than complement fixation but less sensitive than either hemagglutination inhibition (HAI) or solid-phase immunoassays like EIA. EIAs combine high sensitivity and precision with objective endpoints that can be used directly for quantitation. The test reagents are stable and inexpensive, and lend themselves to automation. Despite the obvious advantages of EIA, IFA remains the gold standard for EBV serodiagnosis and is still widely used in the serodiagnosis of active CMV infections. One can expect an increasing application for EIA in viral diagnosis, especially with the recent availability of both highly purified viral antigens and unique viral protein sequences assembled by recombinant DNA methods (13, 14).

SPECIFICITY OF IgM-SPECIFIC RESPONSES

Typically, in primary viral infections, IgM-specific antibodies appear during the acute phase of illness, peaking at 3 to 4 weeks, and then declining to undetectable levels by 4 months after onset. Their detection generally implies an active viral process. Practically, however, several limitations must be considered, including inaccuracy due to interfering substances such as rheumatoid factors (RhF) or antinuclear antibodies (ANA) (see below), heterotopic cross-reactions, and unusual persistence of IgM antibodies.

RhFs and ANAs are present transiently in 10 to 15% of patients with acute infectious diseases and are capable of inducing false positives in various IgM assays. In a standard indirect, IgM virus-specific immunoassay, RhF (IgM anti-IgG) reacts with the Fc portion of viral IgG that is attached to the solid phase by viral antigen. A false positive is recorded when labeled antihuman IgM molecules bind to attached RhFs. Such interference is often seen with intrauterine newborn infections where high levels of passively transmitted maternal virus-specific IgG interacts with RhFs. Significant levels of virus-specific IgG are also capable of producing false-negative IgM responses by competing with IgM-specific molecules for viral antigen binding sites on the solid phase. Each of these problems can be overcome to a considerable degree by separating IgM from other class-specific antibodies (IgG, IgA) prior to specific IgM testing (15, 16). A variety of separation methods have been described, including the often unsuccessful absorption of serum RhFs with IgG-coated latex particles. Other methods include the use of commercially available sucrose density-gradient columns or preabsorption of test sera with Staphylococcus protein A and streptococci (Staffinoc) to remove IgA and IgG, including IgG_3, the subtype that is notably increased in viral infections. These prior methods may be limited in application because of reported false negatives due to loss of virus-specific IgM in the separation process. An additional practical method for IgG/IgM separation involves pretreatment of serum with an anti-IgG antiserum. Briefly, a 10-μl aliquot of serum is mixed with 90 or 150 μl of a commercially available goat antihuman IgG, incubated for 30 minutes at room temperature, and centrifuged at 700g for 10 minutes. The IgM-specific test is performed on the IgG-absorbed supernate, with decreased likelihood of either false-positive or false-negative data (15).

In heterotopic cross-reactions, antigens shared by different viruses can result in false-positive data. Thus, sera from acute EBV-IM often (30%) give positive responses in the CMV IgM-specific tests (16–18). On the other hand, acute-phase samples from patients with CMV mononucleosis much less commonly cross-react in EBV-specific IgM tests. As noted, most IgM responses to infectious agents last only 3 to 4 months. An exception to this is CMV, which is frequently still detectable 12 or more months after onset. Such persistent CMV-IgM responses are commonly seen in CMV-infected patients with organ transplants or AIDS, and they are also identifiable in 25% of immunocompetent individuals 12 or more months after onset of acute CMV infection. Such persistence of IgM responses can cause interpretive problems with subsequent febrile illnesses. Finally, a positive virus-specific IgM response does not necessarily mean that the present illness is a primary viral infection because reactivated viral carrier states may also be associated with IgM-specific responses in both immunocompetent and immunocompromised patients. Practically, illnesses with positive CMV-IgM responses may be indicative of either a primary or a reactivated CMV infection, whereas positive EBV-IgM data are virtually always indicative of a primary response.

Even with serial samples, IgG viral serology by itself is limited in diagnostic usefulness. Fourfold titer increases or decreases usually indicate a recent infection. However, even such data must be evaluated with all available clinical and laboratory information. This is especially important when dealing with herpesviruses, which regularly establish lifelong latency states (19). Immunosuppressive disease states, drugs, or other infectious agents can activate the viral latency state with a fourfold anti-IgG titer increase that may be incidental to the actual cause of the patient's immediate illness. Active viral infections may also proceed without fourfold IgG titer responses. Thus, in patients undergoing primary EBV infections, peak anti-EBV IgG titers are already present in the initial sample of 80% of cases. Also, previously healthy adults with CMV-mononucleosis show significant fourfold anti-CMV IgG responses in only 50% of cases (17).

Finally, serology, including IgM as well as IgG responses, has only a limited diagnostic role in virally infected, severely immunosuppressed patients. Results are often negative or inconclusive, and when data are positive, they may lag several weeks behind the direct detection of viral antigens from various tissue specimens such as bronchoalveolar lavage, buffy coats, etc. In immunocompetent individuals with IM-like viral illnesses, standard serology remains the method of choice for definitive and rapid viral diagnosis.

DIAGNOSTIC APPROACH

Our algorithmic approach to the diagnosis of IM and IM-like syndromes is summarized in Figure 58.1 (20). This schema initially evaluates data generated from a peripheral blood smear that has been screened for significant numbers of atypical lymphocytes and from a rapid IM heterophil antibody test. It is cost-effective and practical and can be applied in doctors' offices as well as in large hospital laboratories. When a significant atypical lymphocytosis accompanies positive heterophil data, the diagnosis of heterophil-positive IM is confirmed. Over 95% of patients over the age of 5 years who are undergoing primary EBV infections develop diagnostic heterophil antibodies and require no further diagnostic workup (Table 58.1). In EBV-IM patients between the ages of 7 and 48 months, heterophil-negative presentations are common, and EBV-specific serology is required for definitive diagnosis.

When blood smears fail to fulfill IM criteria and are accompanied by positive rapid IM slide tests, false-positive results are suspected. The false-positive is confirmed when a negative result is recorded with the reference HCAT (i.e., beef-absorbed horse agglutinin titer is greater than the simultaneously performed GPK-absorbed titer). False-positive slide tests are estimated to occur in 2 to 3% of non-IM sera. Such isolated data have not been associated with any underlying disease states. Anecdotal reports associating false-positive data with lymphomas and leukemias have not been convincingly documented. It should be emphasized that, when an EBV profile is used alone to evaluate a possible false-positive rapid test, data suggesting a long-past EBV infection (M−, G+, ENA+) do not exclude the possibility that the positive rapid test was due to a silent or undiagnosed EBV infection 2 to 12 months earlier with still-circulating IM heterophil antibodies. This differential dilemma can only be solved with the HCAT. With the recent availability of even more sensitive rapid heterophil EIA tests, one can predict the occurrence of more cases where discordant data will suggest falsely positive heterophil rapid tests. As noted earlier, published clinical trials with these newer EIA tests are very limited at this time.

Table 58.1. Heterophil Antibody Status in 1517 Cases of EBV-IM[a]

Age	Positive	Negative
7–24 months	4 (16.0%)	21
25–48 months	23 (51.1%)	22
5–10 years	34 (81.0%)	8
11–15 years	90 (95.7%)	4
16–29 years	1079 (98.0%)	22
30–39 years	50 (92.8%)	4
40–76 years	47 (92.2%)	4
Unspecified	105 (100.0%)	0
Total	1432 (94.4%)	85

[a]As determined by 2-hour horse cell differential absorption of Lee-Davidsohn tube test.

The most challenging IM diagnostic problems occur when negative heterophil tests are accompanied by blood smears with atypical lymphocytosis. These data require further scrutiny of clinical findings to determine what particular serologic tests should be ordered next. Based on frequency of occurrence, patients with prominent pharyngitis and/or lymphadenopathy should be initially EBV-tested; less common causes including HHV-6, *Toxoplasma gondii* and HIV should be considered only after negative EBV studies are reported. When the clinical picture is dominated by fever and is associated with abnormal liver function studies, CMV is the most likely cause of clinical illness, and tests for CMV macroglobulins (CMV-IgM) are indicated.

EBV-Specific Tests

Table 58.2 illustrates the interpretation of representative EBV serodiagnostic profiles. The differential appearance of antibodies to various EBV-specific antigens such as viral capsid antigen (VCA) and nuclear antigens (EBNA) allows for accurate confirmation of ongoing EBV infections (21). The presence of IgM anti-VCA (1:10 or higher) responses usually indicates a current, primary EBV infection, and their absence (M−, G+, EBNA−), seen in 15% of cases, implies a recent, rather than current, primary infection. Data indicative of an old EBV infection typically have the following profile: M–, G+, EBNA+. In an individual acutely ill patient, the titration of the actual IgG anti-VCA or anti-EBNA levels is not nearly as useful as the differential appearance of VCA-M or VCA-G versus EBNA-IgG. Further confirmation of results can be obtained with convalescent specimens that show a disappearance or decline in VCA-IgM by 1 to 3 months and the emergence of anti-EBNA by 1 to 6 months. With past EBV infections, constant IgG anti-VCA and anti-EBNA titers are obtained with serial specimens.

Antibodies to EBV-specific early antigens (EA)—designated diffuse, anti-EA (D), or restrictive, anti-EA (R), depending on distinctive patterns of immunofluorescence and reactions to cell-line fixatives—become detectable in the acute phase of EBV-IM in most (80 to 90%) patients. With recovery and establishment of a latent, persistent EBV carrier state in B lymphocytes, anti-EA titers decline but may take 2 to 3 years, even in apparently healthy individuals, to reach baseline levels (1:80 or lower). Anti-EA (D) ti-

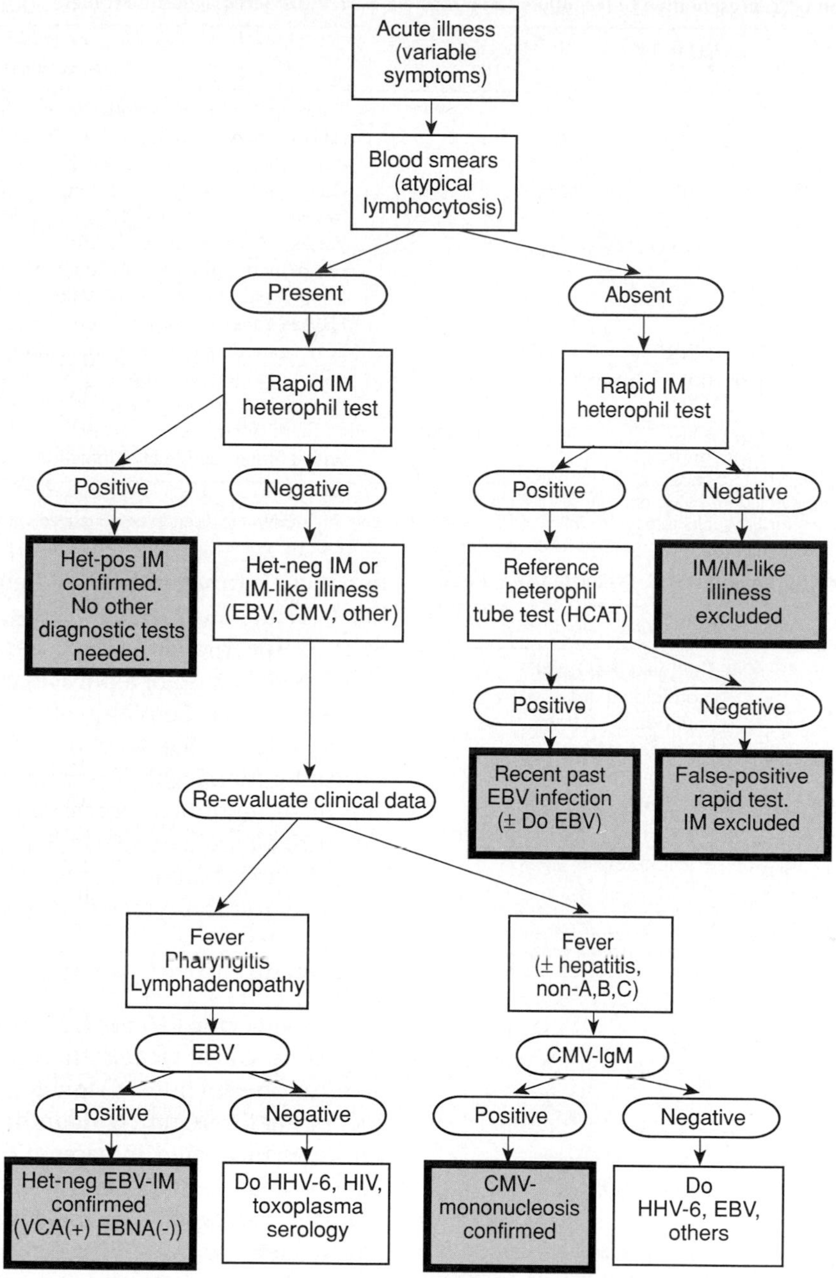

Figure 58.1. Algorithmic approach to the diagnosis of infectious mononucleosis and related heterophil-negative, mononucleosis-like syndromes. IM, infectious mononucleosis; Het-Pos, heterophil-antibody-positive; Het-Neg, heterophil-antibody negative; HCAT, horse cell differential absorption tube test; CMV, cytomegalovirus; CMV-IgM, CMV macroglobulins; EBV, Epstein-Barr virus; HHV-6, human herpsevirus-6; HIV, human immunodeficiency virus. (Modified from Steeper TA, Horwitz CA, Henle W, Henle G. Selected aspects of acute and chronic infectious mononucleosis and mononucleosis-like illnesses for the practicing allergist. Ann Allergy 1987;59:243–250.)

ters are not necessary for acute-phase diagnosis. When the EBV carrier state is reactivated, usually by poorly understood mechanisms, enhanced viral shedding in oropharyngeal secretions is associated with significant levels of anti-EA (R) (22). Thus, in the workup of patients suspected of having significant chronic, active EBV infections (e.g., lymphoproliferative processes in the immunosuppressed), titration of anti-EA as well as anti-VCA-IgG and anti-EBNA is recommended. In chronic EBV states, actual titer levels (e.g., anti-EA 1:160 or higher) are more important than they are in the acute phase. An EBV profile, including VCA-IgG, EA, and EBNA, is commonly included in the workup of patients with the chronic fatigue syndrome (CFS) (23).

CMV-Specific Tests

The available methods for confirmation of CMV-related illnesses are summarized in Table 58.3. In

Table 58.2. Interpretation of Representative Immunofluorescent Epstein-Barr Virus Serodiagnostic Profiles

VCA IgM (<1:10)	VCA IgG (<1:40)	EA IgG (D/R) (<1:10)	EBNA IgG (<1:2)	Interpretation
Neg (−)	Neg (−)	Neg (−)	Neg (−)	Still susceptible; EBV excluded as cause of illness.
Pos (+)	Pos (+)	Pos (+) (D)	Neg (−)	Diagnostic of a current, primary EBV infection; present in 85% of cases. Reactive blood smears.[c]
Neg (−)	Pos (+)	Pos (+)(D)	Neg (−)	1. Consistent with, but not diagnostic of, recent primary EBV infection; present in 15% of cases. Reactive blood smears.[a]
Neg (−)	Pos (+)	Pos (+) (R)	Neg (−)	2. Pattern also encountered in severely immunosuppressed AIDS or chemotherapy patients; nonreactive blood smears.
Neg (−)	Pos (+)	± Pos (R) (≤1:80)	Pos (+) (≥1:5)	1. Implies old, ± remote EBV infection; data generally excludes EBV as cause of present acute illness.
Neg (−)	Pos (+) (1:40 − 1:2560)	Pos (+) (R) (≤1:10 − 1:640)	Pos (+) (≥1:5)	2. Low to moderate titers; nondiagnostic data for patients with chronic fatigue syndrome (CFS); moderate titers also in nasopharyngeal carcinema and Burkitt's lymphoma.
Neg (±)	Pos (+) (≥1:5120)	Pos (+)(R) (≥1:1280)	(<1:2 − ≥1:1280)	High titers (VCA, EA), consistent with rare symptomatic patient with chronic active EBV infection.[b]

[a]Reactive blood smears of IM type noted in ≥95% of acute EBV-IM cases.
[b]Because it may take 2 to 3 years for EBV titers to baseline following a primary infection, high EBV titers need to be correlated with entire case data.

Table 58.3. Methods for Confirmation of CMV-Related Disease[a]

Serology	Virus/Viral Antigen Detection
1. IgM Anti-CMV (IFA, EIA)	4. Shell vial assay with monoclonal anti-CMV antibodies, 16 hours (BAL, blood, urine)
2. IgG Anti-CMV (latex, IFA, ACIF)	5. DNA hybridization
3. Complement fixation Anti-CMV (CMV-CF)	6. Conventional culture 7–42 days
	7. Viral inclusions (poor sensitivity)
	8. CMV-PCR

Clinical Setting	Method of Choice
A. Previously healthy, immunocompetent (IM-type blood smears)	1
B. Immunosuppressed (e.g., AIDS, chemotherapy)	4, 6, 7 (±5)
C. Selection of organ transplatation donor	2 (±8)
D. Indicator of active disease in the immunosuppressed	7, 4 (Buffy coat)

[a]CMV, cytomegalovirus; IFA, indirect immunofluorescence; EIA, enzyme immunoassays; ACIF anticomplement immunofluorescence; BAL, bronchoalveolar lavage; PCR, polymerase chain reaction.

previously healthy immunocompetent individuals undergoing active CMV infections, CMV macroglobulins (CMV-IgM) evolve in 95 to 98% of cases, with 90% of the positive results (1:32 or higher) present on the initial acute-phase sample (17). Because heterotopic cross-reactions in IgM-specific tests frequently occur between CMV and EBV, accompanying EBV profiles should be indicative of an old EBV infection (particularly anti-EBNA positivity) before accepting CMV-IgM-positive serology as confirmatory for CMV-mononucleosis. Almost all heterophil-negative, IM-like illnesses due to either CMV or EBV are associated with mild or moderate degrees of hepatic dysfunction (SGOT bewteen 41 and 999 U/liter), while normal liver function studies (SGOT, SGPT), for practical purposes, exclude EBV and CMV as the cause of a particular heterophil-negative, IM-like illness. Serology plays only a limited diagnostic role in the workup of febrile immunosuppressed patients with significant CMV infections (24–26). Such immunosuppressed patients should not be categorized as having IM-like illnesses because accompanying blood smears rarely demonstrate impressive atypical lymphocytosis.

Rapid Virus-Specific Serologic Tests

Virus-specific EIA rapid tests designed for doctors' offices have also recently become commercially available. In one such test (Monolert, Ortho Diagnostics), the patient's serum containing IgM and IgG anti-EBNA is incubated in each of two wells on a plastic paddle coated with a synthetic peptide whose sequences correspond to the EBNA-1 region of EBV-DNA. Next, enzyme-linked, anti-IgM and anti-IgG–conjugated reagents are each added to one well, followed by substrate for the particular enzymes. The relative color intensity between the IgM and IgG reactions is visually determined (M > G being equivalent to a current EBV infection and no reaction, or G > M excluding recent EBV infection). A major theoretical advantage of such a test over standard heterophil tests is the ability to detect heterophil-negative as well as heterophil-positive cases of EBV-IM. In another recently marketed test (Immune-Dot, General Biometrics), purifed antigens of EBV, CMV, and toxoplasmosis are fixed to different membranes on a single reagent strip and a modified rapid TORCH-type EIA is completed within 10 to 20 minutes. The rapid virus-specific tests will no doubt increase in number and diagnostic spectrum in the future. Presently, they do not appear to be as accurate as the standard, more time-consuming viral serologic assays.

Human Herpesvirus-6 (HHV-6)

Recently, human herpesvirus-6 (HHV-6) was identified and shown to be separable morphologically and immunologically from the other five herpes viruses (27, 28). It has been implicated causally in the short-lived, febrile exanthematous illness of infants known as infantile roseola, or exanthem subitum (29). Also, because it produces alterations of lymphocytes in cell cultures, it was not surprising when it became associated with several heterophil-negative, IM-like illnesses, including cases with persistent lymphadenopathy (30) and occasional examples of active viral hepatitis (non-A/non-B/non-C type) (31). HHV-6 may account for up to 5% of heterophil-negative, non–EBV– and non–CMV-induced IM-like illnesses. HHV-6 may also play a role in the development of the CFS.

HHV-6 antibodies of both IgM and IgG types can be detected by either the IFA or EIA method. Paired samples are often necessary for interpretation because nondiagnostic results often occur on the acute serum sample and are not sufficient to exclude HHV-6 as a causative pathogen. Discrepancies between IFA and EIA results occur in individual cases and need further resolution. It also appears that patients with EBV or CMV infections may be capable of reactivating the HHV-6 carrier or latency state, producing positive IgM-HHV-6 data and four-fold IgG HHV-6 titer changes, complicating serlogic interpretation (19, 32). Because of the latter problems, we limit the serologic diagnosis of an active HHV-6 infection to those cases where serologic studies have already excluded EBV and CMV as causes of the present illness. Antibodies to HHV-6 are found in the vast majority of children aged 4 years and older, suggesting that frequent, silent early infections are common. Thus, most HHV-6–induced illnesses in adults are probably from HHV-6 reactivation rather than primary infections in rare older patients who have escaped childhood infection, as is seen with EBV.

Other Etiologic Agents

Confirmation of *Toxoplasma gondii* as a cause of lymphadenitis is best approached serologically by detection of IgG- and IgM-specific antibodies (33). The detection of IgM-*Toxoplasma* antibodies is usually diagnostic and is mainly accompanied by moderate to high titer levels of IgG molecules detected by either Sabin dye or IFA methods. IgM-*Toxoplasma* antibodies can persist for over 12 months following onset of illness and may cause diagnostic problems when the question of recurrent toxoplasmosis lymphadenopathy arises months or years after the onset of illness (34). Acute primary HIV infections are generally diagnosable by demonstrating HIV antigenemia with or without Western blot-confirmable anti-HIV and appropriate blood smears (35). Patients undergoing HIV seroconversions, like CMV and EBV patients, often demonstrate moderate hepatic dysfunction and transient, non–IM-specific heterophil antibodies, including cold agglutinins, cryoglobulins, and antinuclear antibodies.

Table 58.4. Causes of Heterophil-Negative, Mononucleosis-like Illnesses (253 Cases)[a,b]

Age	EBV	CMV	Non-EBV/Non-CMV
1–24 months	21	0	10
25–48 months	22	0	4
5–15 years	12	2	10
16–29 years	22	77	22
30–39 years	4	14	9
40–77 years	4	15	5
Total	85	108	60[c]

[a]EBV, Epstein-Barr Virus; CMV, cytomegalovirus; IM, infectious mononucleosis; HHV-6, human herpesvirus-6; HIV, human immunodeficiency virus; HBV, hepatitis B virus; H. simplex, herpes simplex.

Spectrum of IM-like Illnesses

Table 58.4 summarizes the cause of 253 heterophil-negative, IM-like illnesses encountered in our laboratory over an 18-year period. As noted, CMV is by far the most common cause of mononucleosis-like illnesses in young adults and older patients, whereas EBV is the most frequent cause in children less than 49 months of age. We have never encountered an example of clinically apparent, CMV-induced mononucleosis in a child less than 6 years of age, despite the fact that silent CMV infections in this age group are common and congenital CMV infections are not rare. The data in Table 58.4 include a few cases in which dual pathogens may have been implicated in the disease process, and an undetermined number of cases from the unspecified non-EBV/non-CMV group where the recently described hepatitis C virus may have been responsible for the clinical illnesses.

Acknowledgment

We acknowledge with appreciation the many contributions to the authors' IM studies by Drs. Gertrude and the late Werner Henle. This work was supported by Moses Barron Fund #540 and A. M. Fiterman Fund #549, Metropolitan-Mount Sinai Medical Center.

References

1. Evans AS, IM and related syndromes. Am J Med Sci 1978;276: 325–339.

2. Penman HG,: The problem of seronegative IM. In: Carter RL, Penman HG, eds. Infectious mononucleosis. Oxford: Blackwell Scientific Publications, 1969:201–224.
3. Horwitz CA, Henle W, Henle G, et al. Heterophil-negative IM and mononucleosis-like illness. Laboratory confirmation of 43 cases. Am J Med 1977;63:947–957.
4. Davidsohn I, Nelson DA. The blood. In: Davidsohn I, Henry JB, eds. Todd-Sanford's clinical diagnosis by laboratory methods, 14th ed. Philadelphia: Saunders, 1968;280–292.
5. Lee CL, Zandrew F, Davidsohn I. Horse agglutinins in infectious mononucleosis. III. Criterion for differential diagnosis. J Clin Pathol 1968;21:631–634.
6. Evans AS, Niederman JC, Cenabre LC, et al. A prospective evaluation of heterophile and Epstein-Barr virus-specific IgM antibody tests in clinical and subclinical infectious mononucleosis. Specificity and sensitivity of the tests and persistence of antibody. J Infect Dis 1975;132:546–554.
7. Horwitz CA, Henle W, Henle G, Polesky H, Wexler H, Ward P. The specificity of heterophil antibodies in patients and healthy donors with no or minimal signs of IM. Blood 1976;47: 91–98.
8. Lennette E, Henle W, et al. Heterophil antigen in bovine sera detectable by immune adherence hemagglutination with infectious mononucleosis sera. Infect Immun 1978;19:923–927.
9. Horwitz CA, Henle W, Henle G, Penn G, Hoffman N, Ward PCJ. Persistent falsely positive rapid tests for infectious mononucleosis. Report of five cases with four-six year follow-up data. Am J Clin Pathol 1979:72:807–811.
10. Fletcher MA, Woolfolk BJ. Immunochemical studies of infectious mononucleosis. I. Isolation and characterization of heterophil antigens from hemoglobin-free stroma. J Immunol 1971;107:842–853.
11. Smith TF. Viral serology in clinical medicine. In: Homburger H, Batsaikis J, eds. Clinical laboratory annual. Norwalk, Connecticut: Appleton-Century Crofts, 1983;31–56.
12. Fuccillo DA, Shekarchi IC, Sever JL. Rapid viral diagnosis. In: Rose N, Freidman H, Fahey J, eds. Manual of clinical laboratory immunology. 3rd ed. Washington, DC: ACM, 1968:489–496.
13. Pearson GR. ELISA tests and monoclonal antibodies for EBV. J Virol Methods 1988;21:97–104.
14. Geltosky JE, Smith RS, Whalley A, Rhodes G. Use of a synthetic peptide-based ELISA for the diagnosis of IM and other diseases. J Clin Lab Anal 1987;1:153–162.
15. Smith, TF, Shelley CD. Detection of IgM antibodies to; CMV and rapid diagnosis by shell vial assay. J Virol Methods 1988;21:87–96.
16. Schmidt NJ, Update on class-specific viral antibody assay. Clin Immunol Newsletter 1984;5:81–85.
17. Horwitz C, Henly W, Henle G, et al. Clinical and laboratory evaluation of CMV-induced mononucleosis in previously healthy individuals. Report of 82 cases. Medicine 1986;65:124–134.
18. Hanshaw J, Niederman JC, Chessen LN. CMV macroglobulin in cell-associated herpesvirus infection. J. Infect Dis 1972;125: 304–306.
19. Linde A, Fridell E, Dahl H, Anderson J, Biberfeld P, Wahren B. Effect of primary EBV infection on Herpesvirus-6, CMV, measles virus—immunoglobulin G titers. J Clin Microbiol 1990;28:211–215.
20. Steeper TA, Horwitz CA, Henle W, Henle G. Selected aspects of acute and chronic infectious mononucleosis and mononucleosis-like illnesses for the practicing allergist. Ann Allergy 1987;59:243–250.
21. Henle W, Henle G, Horwitz CA. Epstein-Barr virus-specific diagnostic tests in infectious mononucleosis. Hum Pathol 1974;5:551–565.
22. Sumaya CV. Endogenous reactivation of Epstein-Barr virus infection. J Infect Dis 1977;135:374–379.
23. Straus SE, Tosato G, Armstrong G, et al. Persisting illness and fatigue in adults with evidence of Epstein-Barr virus infection. Ann Intern Med 1985;102:7–16.
24. Griffiths PD. Chronic cytomegalovirus infection. J Virol Methods 1988;21:79–86.
25. van der Bij W, Schirm J, Torensma R, et al. Comparison between viremia and antigenemia for detection of CMV in blood. J Clin Microbiol 1988;26:2531–2535.
26. Schuster EA, Beneke JS, Tegtmeier GE, et al. Monoclonal antibody for rapid laboratory detection of CMV infections: characterization and diagnostic applications. Mayo Clin Proc 1985;60: 577–585.
27. Ablashi DV, Josephs SF, Buchbinder A, et al. Human B-lymphotrophic virus (human herpesvirus-6). J Virol Methods 1988;21:29–48.
28. Krueger GRF, Koch B, Ramon A, et al. Antibody prevalence to HBLV (human herpesvirus-6, HHV-6) and suggestive pathogenicity in the general population and in patients with immune deficiency syndromes. J Virol Methods 1988;21:125–131.
29. Yamanishi K, Okuro T, Shiraki K, et al. Identification of human herpes virus 6 as a causal agent for exanthem subitum. Lancet 1988;1:1065–1067.
30. Niederman JC, Liu CR, Kaplan MH, Brown NA. Clinical and serological features of human herpesvirus-6 infection in three adults. Lancet 1988;2:817–819.
31. Horwitz CA, Krueger GRF, Steeper TA, Bertram G. HHV-6 induced mononucleosis-like illnesses. In: Ablashi DV, Krueger GRF, Salahuddin SF, eds. Human herpesvirus-6 Epidemiology, molecular biology and clinical pathology. Amsterdam: Elsevier, 1992:159–174.
32. Fox JD, Ward P, Briggs M, Irving W, Shammers TG, Tedder RS. Production of IgM antibody to HHV6 in reactivation and primary infection. Epidemiol Infect 1990;104:289–296.
33. Brooks RG, McCabe RE, Remington JS. Role of serology in toxoplasmic lymphadenopathy. J Infect Dis 1987;9:775–784.
34. Sulzer AJ, Franco EL, Takafuji E, Benenson M, Walls KW, Greenup RL. An oocyst-transmitted outbreak of toxoplasmosis: patterns of immunoglobulin G and M over one year. Am J Trop Med Hyg 1986;35:290–296.
35. Jackson JB, Balfour HH. Practical diagnostic testing for human immunodeficiency virus. Clin Microbiol Rev 1988;1:124–138.

59 Cellular and Humoral Mediators of Inflammation

Karen James

INTRODUCTION

Protective Barriers to Inflammation

The skin and mucous membrane linings of the respiratory, urinary, and gastrointestinal tracts constitute the body's first line of defense as an intact barrier of epithelial cells. The epithelial barrier cells and the biochemical defense mechanisms in the secretions serve to protect from infections. Lysozyme (muramidase) decreases the viability of susceptible bacteria by cleaving the cell wall proteoglycan between the residues of *N*-acetylglucosamine and *N*-acetylmuramic acid. Stomach gastric acids inhibit infections with *Salmonella* species, *Vibrio cholerae,* and enveloped viruses. Secretory immunoglobulins can neutralize viruses and bacterial endotoxins and prevent bacterial attachment to mucosal cells.

Nonspecific Cellular Response to Inflammation

GRANULOCYTES

Polymorphonuclear neutrophils (PMNs) are the largest population of leukocytes in the peripheral blood. These phagocytic cells contain distinct granules composed of acid hydrolases, myeloperoxidase, lysozyme, lactoferrin, and cationic proteins. These biochemicals either are bactericidal or function to degrade the organic materials that remain after bacteria are killed.

The mechanisms by which PMNs are involved in the nonspecific immune response include (*a*) attachment to the damaged epithelium; (*b*) amoeboid movement; (*c*) emigration through the blood vessels; (*d*) directed movement toward the particles to be engulfed; (*e*) ingestion of the bacteria; (*f*) increased glycolysis; (*g*) degranulation; and (*h*) digestion of the foreign material.

Adherence of PMNs to the vascular endothelial cells occurs relative to membrane changes after exposure to chemotactic factors that facilitate adherence. Locomotion or ameboid movement in conjunction with adherence to the walls of the capillaries are both necessary for diapedesis to occur. During diapedesis (emigration), the pseudopods of the PMN are inserted between the junctions of endothelial cells. This enables the leukocyte to move from the inside of the blood vessel, through the capillary walls between the endothelial cells, into surrounding tissues.

Chemotaxis is the directed migration of phagocytic cells mediated primarily by fluid phase components of the complement system, particularly C5a. Other factors known to be chemotactic include by-products of the coagulation or fibrinolytic pathways and certain bacterial products.

Phagocytosis, the ingestion of particles, occurs when the external cell wall of the PMN adheres to and completely surrounds the offending bacteria or other particle. The foreign substance becomes encapsulated with a layer of inside-out membrane, a phagosome. C3b and IgG function as opsonins because PMNs and other phagocytic cells have receptors on their surface that specifically recognize those molecules coating bacteria or other particles. These opsonins significantly increase the rate and quantity of particle uptake. During phagocytosis, O_2 and glucose are consumed, primarily through the hexose monophosphate shunt.

H_2O_2 is produced in the respiratory burst that occurs as the phagocytosed particle is digested. Digestion follows the degranulation step when the granules are fused with the vacuole containing the phagocytosed particle. The particle is then exposed to the lytic action of the enzymes. The mechanism by which many types of bacteria are killed following ingestion by phagocytes requires H_2O_2 and myeloperoxidase.

Eosinophils arise from a common progenitor with PMNs, but are less efficient at phagocytosis. Eosinophil granules are rich in acid phosphatase and peroxidase, but do not contain lysozyme. Eosinophil granules also contain a unique protein, eosinophilic basic protein, which is toxic to certain parasites. Functions attributed to eosinophils include clearance of parasites, ingestion of immune complexes, and antagonizing the effects of mediators released from basophils, mast cells, and platelets during inflammatory reactions (1). Eosinophilia is associated with parasitic infections and allergic reactions.

Basophils, mast cells, and platelets release biochemical substances (mediators) that increase both vascular permeability and smooth muscle contraction to augment the inflammatory response. Basophil granules contain histamine and several sulfidopeptide leukotrienes—potent spasmogenic agents that cause constriction of smooth muscle (2). Basophils respond to IgE-containing immune complexes that bind to their IgE receptors to stimulate degranulation. The primary function of the basophil is to amplify and disseminate the reactions that begin with mast cells at the site of the entry of antigen. No specific diseases have been associated with basophilia.

Mast cells are found in the skin and gastrointestinal tract. When injuries occur to these areas, mast cells release granules containing histamine, heparin, serotonin, hyaluronic acid, and eosinophil chemotactic factor of anaphylaxis (ECF-A). Immunologic reactions, involving IgG or IgE binding to their respective receptors on the surface of mast cells or basophils, trigger degranulation and mediator release. Nonimmunologic mechanisms such as infections of the skin and mucous membranes, surgical incisions, and certain other agents (e.g., opiates) can also stimulate mast cells to degranulate.

PLATELETS

Platelets contain serotonin and lysosomal enzymes that are released from their granules during platelet aggregation. Serotonin does not appear to have a pharmacologic role in humans, but lysosomal enzymes assist in the digestion of foreign materials.

LEUKOCYTE INTEGRINS

Integrins guide leukocyte localization during inflammation (3). The leukocyte integrins include lymphocyte function antigen-1 (LFA-1), macrophage antigen-1 (Mac-1, also called Mo-1, LKM-1, and CR3), and p150,95 (also called CR4 and LeuM5). These antigens were first defined by monoclonal antibodies (MAbs) as markers for myeloid cells and are now known to be expressed by virtually all immune cells. These leukocyte integrins are heterodimers with an α subunit noncovalently associated with the β subunit. The α subunits are unique for each molecule at 150 to 180 kd, but the β subunit (95 kd) is identical in all three proteins. The leukocyte integrins involved in cell-cell interactions are dependent on divalent cations for activity.

MONONUCLEAR PHAGOCYTES

Blood monocytes and tissue macrophages are mononuclear phagocytes that remove debris such as old or injured erythrocytes, leukocytes, platelets, bacteria, antigen-antibody complexes, and degenerated or damaged cell membranes. Tissue macrophages include Kupffer cells of the liver, pulmonary macrophages, splenic macrophages, and histiocytes of the lymph nodes, peritoneum, and other areas.

Phagocytic mechanisms described above for PMNs also occur with mononuclear phagocytes. Although PMNs are end-stage cells that die after phagocytosis and degranulation, mononuclear phagocytes are stimulated by the phagocytic processes. Following phagocytosis, monocytes and macrophages become activated secretory cells that can synthesize acute phase proteins and proliferate locally within tissues. Mononuclear phagocytes use the oxygen-dependent metabolic pathways to provide cellular energy.

Although mononuclear phagocytes can respond to chemotactic factors (e.g., C5a), they primarily respond to soluble factors released from T lymphocytes (lymphokines). Monocytes found in peripheral blood are not as efficient at phagocytosis and killing of bacteria as are PMNs, and their mechanisms of killing are not as well understood. As activated secretory cells, macrophages elicit a wide variety of biologically active factors (monokines) that influence the activities of lymphocytes.

Antigen presentation is another important function of a subset of macrophages that have Ia molecules (HLA-DR) on their surface. The complex of antigen and HLA-DR is recognized by lymphocytes as immunogenic, significantly more antigenic than an equivalent amount of free antigen.

Activated macrophages are involved in the inflammatory responses of inflammation and fever, lymphocyte activation, and tissue reorganization. These cytotoxic effector cells exhibit tumoricidal and microbicidal activity, differentiating between tumor cells and normal cells to selectively kill tumor cells while leaving normal cells unscathed. Although not dependent on recognition of major histocompatibility complex (MHC) antigens for activation, there apparently are unique tumor-specific antigens present on tumor cells that are recognized by activated macrophages. Macrophage-mediated tumor cytotoxicity is independent of any genetic factors as well as species barriers. The microbicidal activity of macrophages is similar to that of granulocytes, but significantly less potent.

MHC-UNRESTRICTED CYTOTOXIC CELLS

Cells involved in MHC-unrestricted cytotoxic responses are large granular lymphocytes (LGLs), most of which express the surface antigen phenotype: CD3− (T-cell receptor), CD2+ (E rosette receptor), CD8+/−, CD11+, CD16+ (IgG FcR), CD18+, and CD56+ (NKH1). Subsets of LGL include natural killer (NK) cells, killer (K) cells, and lymphokine-activated killer (LAK) cells. Morphologically, these cells resemble lymphocytes, but lack MHC restriction and function more like activated macrophages. These cells are termed LGL because they have azurophilic granules in their cytoplasm and have a high cytoplasm:nucleus ratio. The stages of effector function for LGL include (*a*) target cell binding, when physical contact is made between the effector cells and the target cells; (*b*) programming for lysis, during which the cytoskeletal components and Golgi apparatus of the effector cell move within the cytoplasm to the area of physical contact with the target cell; (*c*) secretion of factors by the effector cell (e.g., NK cytotoxic factor, IL-1, and granule cytolysin); (*d*) the cell-independent phase of the lytic event where soluble factors complete the killing process.

NK cells recognize and kill tumor cells in vitro. Similar to the activation of macrophages, NK cells can be activated by the cytokines interferon (IFN) and interleukin-2 (IL-2). Unlike T and B lymphocytes, activation of NK cells does not induce immunologic memory. Interleukin-1 (IL-1) triggers the proliferation of NK cells, but neither primary nor secondary responses are detectable for these cells. NK activity is suppressed by the same factors that suppress macrophage-mediated tumor cytotoxicity (e.g., prostaglandin E_2). The antitumor effects of NK cells are the first line of defense against developing tumors and metastasis, but NK activity is not effective against established solid tumors.

Killer (K) cells cannot be distinguished from NK cells by their morphological appearance or by their surface markers. K cells are characterized by their ability to bind (via their IgG Fc receptors), and subsequently lyse, antibody-coated target cells. These target cells can be erythrocytes, bacteria, parasites, or tumor cells. K cells appear to represent a particular stage of NK cell development or activation.

Lymphokine-activated killer (LAK) cells can be generated in vitro using purified or recombinant IL-2. LAK cells have many of the same cell surface markers as NK cells and apparently are previously unstimulated NK cells (4). The LAK activity reflects the potent ability of IL-2 both to stimulate cytotoxic activity and to expand the population(s) of LGL effector cells.

Nonspecific Humoral Response to Inflammation

ACUTE PHASE RESPONSE

When the body is injured, it responds by increasing the hepatic synthesis of a number of plasma proteins. The systemic acute phase response helps to ensure survival during the period immediately following injury. The systemic response must help to achieve the same goals as the localized inflammatory response; i.e., to contain or destroy infectious agents, to remove damaged tissue, and to repair the affected organ.

Fever was one of the first acute phase responses recognized. Fever may occur following many types of inflammatory stimuli, including noninfectious states. Fever results from the effects of endogenous pyrogen (IL-1), which elevates the set point of the hypothalamic center for body temperature. Another long recognized, but variable, acute phase response is an increase in the granulocyte count in the blood. This initially reflects release from the storage pool and later reflects increased production by the bone marrow. The principal reason for the leukemoid response to inflammation is to provide a source of lysosomal enzymes.

LYSOSOMAL ENZYMES

During phagocytosis and following the death of phagocytes, lysosomal contents of granules are released to enhance inflammation and provide microbicidal activity. Much of the tissue damage of inflammation is due to destruction of "innocent bystander" cells by lysosomal enzymes released during the inflammatory process.

C-REACTIVE PROTEIN

C-reactive protein (CRP) was recognized in 1930 because of its ability to precipitate with the C-polysaccharide extract of pneumococcus (5). Although CRP is distinct from antibody, many parallels between the two molecules exist. CRP will react with its substrate to cause lattice formation and precipitation. CRP can promote passive agglutination of red blood cells coated with binding substrate. An example of the similarity between CRP and immunoglobulins is the initiation of the complement cascade through C1 activation by complexed CRP (analogous to antibody-antigen complexes). Opsonization for ingestion by phagocytes can result from complement activation by CRP.

Unlike antibody, CRP is produced by hepatocytes. CRP is a pentamer with five identical, noncovalently linked subunits. The binding of CRP to

C-polysaccharide or other phosphocholine-containing compounds is calcium-dependent. Approximately one phosphate is bound to each of the five CRP subunits, requiring two Ca^{2+} ions per phosphate binding site.

CRP may be considered a primitive form of an antibody molecule, with specificity for components found in cell membranes of microorganisms (bacteria, fungi) and for damaged membranes of cells. When complexed to a binding specificity, CRP activates complement to opsonize and clear microorganisms prior to the production of specific IgM or IgG. Complexed CRP binds to LGL and to macrophages and activates these cells to be tumoricidal (6, 7). CRP is produced very early in the inflammatory response and also participates in tumor surveillance prior to the production of antibody or the activation of specific cytotoxic T cells.

ERYTHROCYTE SEDIMENTATION RATE

Measuring the erythrocyte sedimentation rate (ESR) has become a commonly used index of inflammation, most useful in assessing chronic inflammation since the ESR elevates much more slowly than does CRP. The ESR measurement is directly proportional to the plasma level of fibrinogen, haptoglobin, or other acute phase reactants (8). Immunoglobulin elevations (e.g., macroglobulinemia, myeloma) also affect rouleaux formation and cause the ESR to rise. Alterations in erythrocyte size or shape (e.g., macrocytes, microcytes, sickle cells) also influence the ESR.

COMPLEMENT

The complement system consists of 14 components involved in two separate pathways of activation. Five proteins unique to the classical pathway include the trimolecular complex of C1 (C1q, C1r, C1s), C4, and C2. Three proteins unique to the alternative pathway include factor B, factor D, and properdin (P). Six components participate in both the classical and alternative pathway: C3, C5, C6, C7, C8, and C9. Because the components were named in the order discovered, the sequence of activation is not in numerical order, but the components interact in a specific cascading sequence (Fig. 59.1). Both pathways can be divided into three units (recognition, activation, and membrane attack) to simplify the understanding of complement pathways (9).

Classical Pathway Recognition Unit

The C1q molecule contains a collagenous region with six globular head groups. When specific antibody interacts with its corresponding antigen, binding sites are exposed on the Fc region of the antibody molecule for the globular head groups of C1q. Two molecules of IgG or CRP, or one molecule of IgM, are required for the binding of C1q. In circulation and in the presence of calcium, the collagen portion of C1q is surrounded by two molecules each of C1r and C1s. When C1q binds to the Fc region of antibody or CRP, a conformational change occurs in C1q. This change in C1q causes the proenzyme C1r to become the enzymatically active C1r. The substrate for the enzyme C1r is C1s, which is then cleaved to become the serine esterase, C1s.

Classical Pathway Activation Unit

The active enzyme of C1s cleaves C4 and C2 in a magnesium-dependent reaction. C4b and C2a combine to form an active enzyme C4b2a, the classical pathway C3 convertase, with C4a and C2b as by-products. The enzymatically active C4b2a complex can cleave many molecules of C3 into C3a and C3b. The C3b then either can form a covalent bond with the antigen or with bystander surfaces (e.g., erythrocytes) in immune adherence, *or* can bind to C4b2a to form C4b2a3b, an enzyme with specificity for C5. The final enzymatic step of the classical complement pathway is the cleavage of C5 into C5a and C5b by the C5 convertase, C4b2a3b. At this point, the classical pathway and the alternative pathway converge.

Both Pathways Membrane Attack Unit

C5b binds to one molecule of C6 to form a stable bimolecular complex, C5b6. If C7 is present, the trimolecular complex C5b67 is formed which binds hydrophobically to a membrane. Once C5b67 is bound, C8 can attach to form a functional transmembrane channel. Up to six molecules of C9 then surround the lesion to prevent the channel from being resealed. C9 accelerates lysis, but is not essential for the lytic event.

Alternative Pathway Recognition Unit

Activation of the alternative pathway requires an activating surface. Substances known to provide an activation surface are bacterial cell walls, bacterial lipopolysaccharide (LPS), fungal cell walls, certain virus-infected cells, and rabbit erythrocytes. The "activating surface" is actually a *protective* surface, protecting spontaneously hydrolyzed C3 (nonenzymatically cleaved into C3a and C3b) from being inactivated by the control proteins (10). Hydrolyzed C3 becomes C3b-*like*. In the presence of factor D and Mg^{2+}, this C3b-like molecule can cleave factor B into Ba and Bb. Ba becomes a by-product, while Bb binds to the C3b to form an alternative pathway C3 convertase, C3bBb. By itself, C3bBb is a very unstable

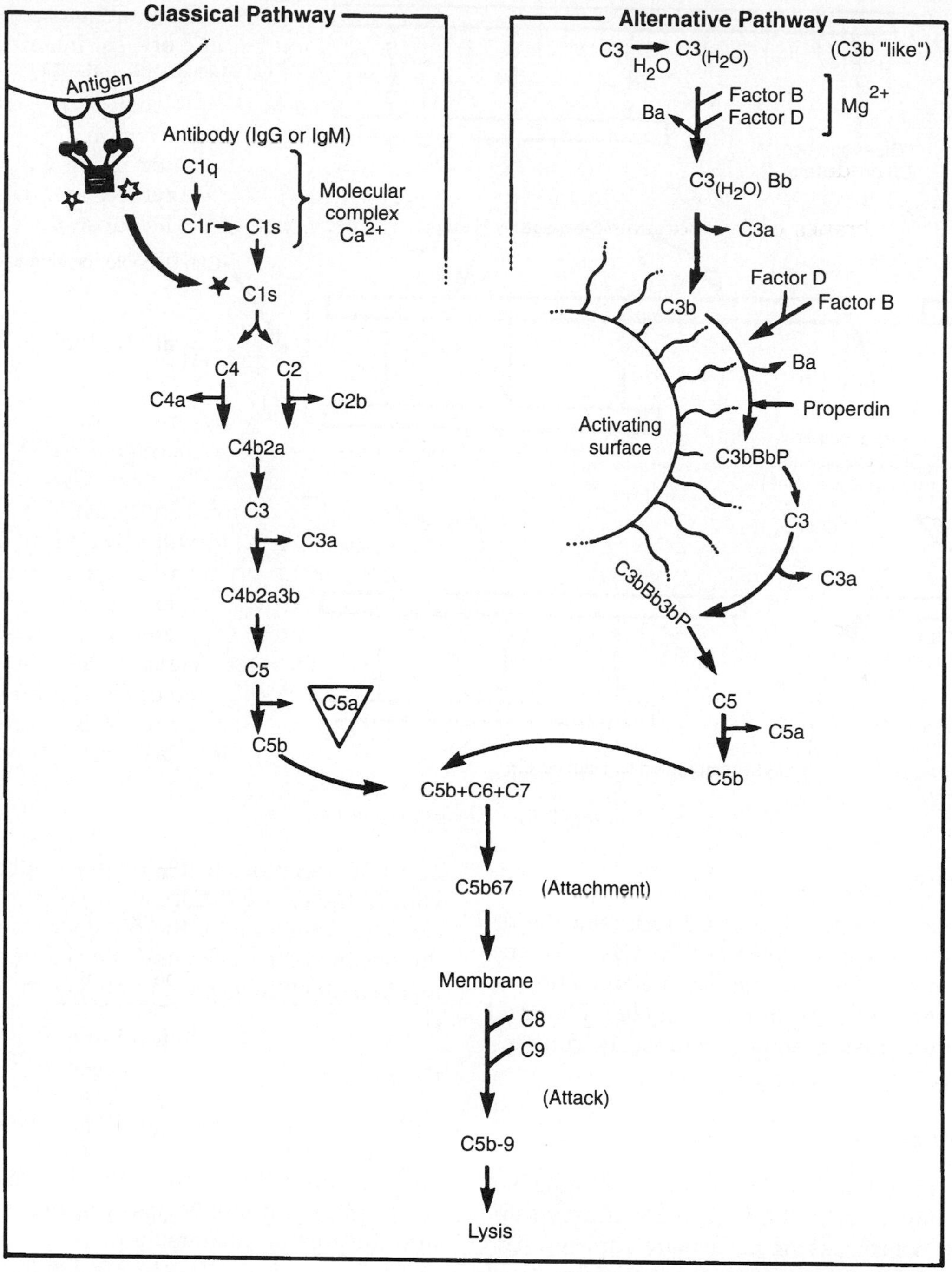

Figure 59.1. Complement pathways.

molecule and is quickly inactivated by control proteins unless it binds to an activating surface.

Alternative Pathway Activation Unit

When protected by an activating surface and stabilized by P (properdin), the C3bBbP enzymatic complex can cleave additional molecules of C3. If a second C3b molecule is inserted into the C3 convertase to become C3bBb3bP, this becomes a C5 convertase, which can cleave C5 into C5a and C5b.

BIOLOGICAL CONSEQUENCES OF COMPLEMENT ACTIVATION

Amplification

C3b can be generated by C3 convertase from either the classical pathway (C4b2a) or the alternative pathway (C3bBbP). This provides a feedback loop that uses the alternative pathway components (B, D, P) to amplify the activation of the C3 through C9 components of activation and membrane attack.

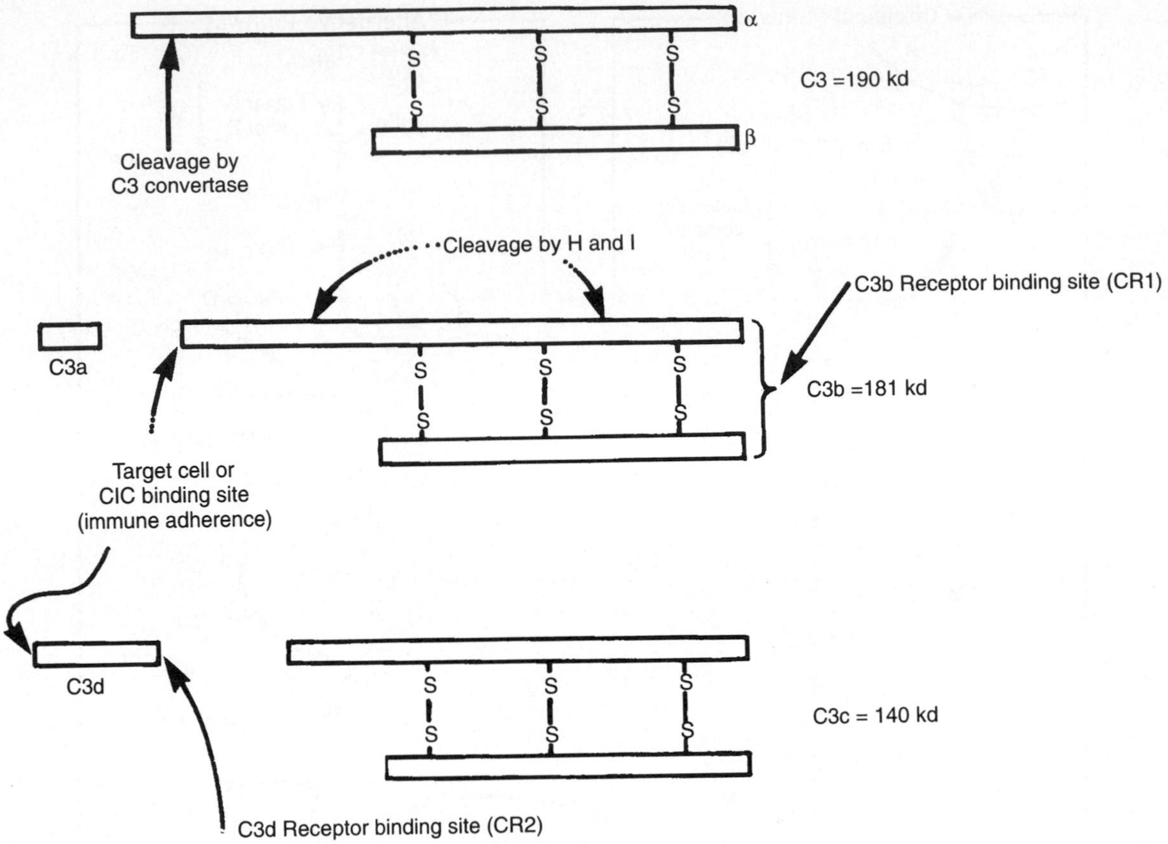

Figure 59.2. C3 Molecular structure.

Anaphylatoxin

The cleavage of C4, C3, and C5 results in the release of the biologically active peptides C4a, C3a, and C5a. These anaphylatoxins mediate inflammation by inducing the release of histamine from basophils and mast cells, by causing smooth muscle to contract, and by increasing vascular permeability.

Immune Adherence

Immune adherence is the covalent bonding between the cleaved form of C3 (C3b) and nearby soluble immune complexes or particulate surfaces. The portion of the C3b that does not adhere is exposed and available for binding to the complement receptor (CR1) for C3b or C4b on human erythrocytes. B lymphocytes and macrophages have CR2 receptors for C3d, which is formed by cleaving C3b into C3c and C3d (Fig. 59.2). One biological purpose for immune adherence would be to facilitate the removal of soluble immune complexes by the mononuclear phagocyte system.

Opsonization

Deposition of C3b opsonizes a surface, for more effective phagocytosis by PMNs and/or monocytes. The C3b receptors (CR3) on these phagocytic cells bind to the exposed C3b on the surface of the particle. The membrane of the phagocytic cell surrounds the opsonized particle, and the cell membrane fuses together, thereby enclosing/phagocytosing the particle.

Chemotaxis

The by-product resulting from the cleavage of C5 is C5a, a potent chemotactic factor as well as an anaphylotoxin. C5a induces the directed migration of neutrophils and monocytes, via their C5a receptors, into the area of inflammation.

Kinin Activation

The fragment of C2 (C2b) that is released during cleavage by C1s interacts with plasmin to produce kinin-like activity. The biological activity of C2b results in smooth muscle contraction, mucous gland secretion, increased vascular permeability, and pain.

Lysis

In the laboratory, the activity of complement is studied by measuring the degree of lysis of sheep erythrocytes (ShE) that occurs. Lysis, however, plays a relatively minor biological role. One example of lysis as the biological consequence of complement activation would be an antibody-mediated transfusion reaction. The lytic function of complement also appears to be necessary for host defense against Gram-negative bacteria, especially *Neisseria* species (11).

CONTROL MECHANISMS OF COMPLEMENT ACTIVATION

If any or all of the biological consequences of complement activation were to go uncontrolled, the effects of even minor inflammatory processes involving activation of either complement pathway would be potentially devastating. The body, however, does not leave a reaction uncontrolled.

The first means of control is the extreme lability of activated complement components. If an activated enzyme does not combine with its substrate within milliseconds, the activity is lost or markedly decayed. "Innocent bystander" cells in the vicinity of activated complement would be rapidly destroyed if the activated components were not so highly labile. There are also several inhibitors or inactivators of specific reactions or products involved in the complement cascade.

C1 Inhibitor (C1Inh)

C1Inh forms an irreversible complex with both C1r and C1s, which blocks their enzymatic activities and dissociates them from C1q. The hereditary or acquired deficiency of this protein results in uncontrolled activation of the classical pathway. Control proteins that exercise their activity at the level of C3 or later are still functioning, retarding the amplification loop and other biological consequences of C3–C9 activation. C1s, in the absence of C1Inh, continues to cleave C4 and C2 unchecked, resulting in release of C2b kinin-like activity and C4a anaphylatoxin activity.

B1H (H) and C3b Inactivator (I)

The most important biological consequence of complement activation is the feedback loop amplification mediated by C3b. Proteins H and I serve to tightly control the enzymes that cleave C3 and C5. H accelerates the decay of the alternative pathway C3 convertase by dissociating Bb from the enzyme, while I inactivates C3b and C4b. H and I are both involved in cleaving C3b into its hemolytically inactive form, C3bi, which is further cleaved into C3c and C3d (Fig. 59.2). Fluid phase C3b is rapidly inactivated by H and I. Consequently, activation of the alternative pathway is dependent upon the presence of a protective (activating) surface, which shelters C3b from these two control proteins.

C4 Binding Protein (C4BP)

C4BP can also cleave and inactivate C4, but requires an accessory protein, C3b inactivator (I). C4BP inhibits assembly and accelerates decay of C4b2a.

Anaphylatoxin Inactivator

Carboxypeptidase controls the effects of C4a, C3a, and C5a by removing a single amino acid, a carboxyterminal arginine. Cleavage of this amino acid destroys the anaphylatoxin activity of these peptides.

S Protein

The S protein binds to fluid phase C5b67, preventing attachment of this trimolecular complex to membranes (11). Lipoproteins or C8 bound to the membrane attack complex (MAC) prior to its attachment to a cell surface can also prevent that attachment.

Properdin (P)

The aforementioned control mechanisms are all inhibitors. Properdin is an *enhancer*. While not required for the activation sequence of the alternative pathway, P stabilizes the C3 and C5 convertases to prolong their activity.

C3 Nephritic Factor (NF)

NF is a *pathological* enhancing protein. NF is an IgG autoantibody with specificity for the alternative pathway C3 convertase (12). NF binds to the C3 convertase in such a way that it prevents inactivation by the control proteins H and I. When NF is present, C3 activation proceeds uncontrolled, thereby markedly depleting C3.

CYTOKINES (LYMPHOKINES AND MONOKINES)

Cytokines are one group of soluble, intercellular signaling molecules and include interleukins (ILs), interferons (IFs), colony-stimulating factors (CSFs), peptide growth factors (PGFs), and cytotoxins. Large quantities of pure cytokines, soluble low–molecular weight glycoproteins, can be synthesized by techniques now common to molecular biology. Consequently, the physiological activities of cytokines can be studied to realize how these molecules regulate the inflammatory response, and stimulate the proliferation and differentiation of specific cell types. The role of cytokines is primarily in the local environment where secretion can exert an autocrine effect, but cytokines can also generate endocrine-type systemic effects in mammals. Cytokines interact with specific receptors on multiple cell types as well as with one another. There is a great deal of redundancy in the regulatory network of cytokines. Accordingly, contradictory functions have been attributed to different molecules. The body's inflammatory response (e.g., the acute phase response and septic shock) is mediated by cytokines.

Interleukins

Most interleukins are secreted by activated T lymphocytes and had been called lymphokines. The principal source of IL-1 was monocytes/macrophages, so IL-1 and other secretory products of phagocytic mononuclear cells had been termed monokines. To date, 12 biologically potent peptides with molecular weights between 10 and 30 kd have been characterized: IL-1 (α and β), IL-2 through IL-12 (13). Many of these molecules share biological activities and are pleiotropic.

IL-1 is synthesized by activated macrophages, T and B lymphocytes, neutrophils, fibroblasts, endothelial cells, keratinocytes, smooth muscle cells, astrocytes, renal mesangial cells, and microglial cells (14). IL-1 induces fever, neutrophilia, lymphocytosis, monocytosis, release of TNF_{α} from macrophages; IL-1 also mediates the acute phase response, exudate/edema at the injury site, and angiogenesis (12, 13). The changes in endothelial cells induced by IL-1 are directly related to the pathological lesions in vascular tissues that occur during inflammation. These changes include increasing the adhesiveness of the endothelial cells, promoting leukocyte adherence to endothelial cells. IL-1 increases fibroblast proliferation and collagen synthesis and stimulates the production of IL-2 and IL-2 receptors (IL-2R) by T cells. Although $IL\text{-}1_{\alpha}$ and $IL\text{-}1_{\beta}$ have distinct amino acid sequences, the two molecules are structurally related, interact with the same receptors, are not distinguishable based on their biologic properties, and are collectively referred to as IL-1.

IL-1 receptors (IL-1R) cannot distinguish between $IL\text{-}1_{\alpha}$ and IL-1β, but do not recognize other cytokines. The IL-1R is an 80-kd glycosylated peptide with striking sequence and structural similarities to immunoglobulin light chains (15). There appear to be two forms of the IL-1R, a low-affinity, 25-kd (nonglycosylated) form and a high-affinity form of greater molecular weight. Both IL-1R forms exist on a wide variety of T cell lines and normal cells. There are only about 20,000 IL-1R per cell, in contrast to 100,000 to 200,000 receptors per cell for other cytokines.

IL-2 is synthesized and secreted by T (T_H1 cells) and B lymphocytes that have been activated in the presence of an antigen-presenting cell (macrophage) and an appropriate antigen. Once activated and producing IL-2, the T cells then develop IL-2R (induced by IL-5) for the feedback loop which promotes proliferation of the T cells. IL-2 stimulates the proliferation of B cells, induction of antibody synthesis and secretion. IL-2 also activates LGL to achieve their cytotoxic potential as NK cells or cytolytic T cells. IL-2 induces the synthesis by T cells of interferon (IFN_{γ}), IL-4, IL-5, IL-6, and granulocyte-monocyte colony stimulating factor (GM-CSF).

IL-2R exist as three classes of receptors distinguished by their ligand-binding affinities: a low affinity 55-kd polypeptide chain (the "Tac" antigen), an intermediate affinity 75-kd (p75) receptor, and a high-affinity receptor composed of an α chain (p75) and a β chain (Tac). Binding of IL-2 by both chains is required to induce a proliferative signal in T cells (15). The p75 IL-2R is found on B cells, monocytes, and resting T cells. When IL-2 interacts with the α chain IL-2R, β chain is expressed. The combination of the α (p75) and β (Tac) chain provide the high affinity receptor necessary for IL-2–induced T-cell proliferation. Activated T cells can release their IL-2R into solution, resulting in soluble IL-2R in the peripheral circulation.

IL-3 is a potent colony-stimulating factor (CSF) secreted by activated T cells (T_H1 and T_H2). This cytokine promotes the development of granulocytes, macrophages, megakaryocytes, mast cells, and normoblast erythroid cells (in conjunction with erythropoietin) from bone marrow precursors. Unlike most other cytokines, IL-3 is species-specific. IL-3 is not required for normal hemopoiesis, but sustains or amplifies the hemopoietic response during immune reactions. The principal action of IL-3 appears to be cellular ontogenesis before differentiation has taken place. There is a single high-affinity IL-3R, a 140-kd molecule with tyrosine kinase activity (12).

IL-4 is a T cell-derived B cell induction factor by up-regulating the expression of class II MHC antigens (HLA-DR), enhancing the expression of IgE FcR (CD23) on resting B cells, and stimulating IgE synthesis by isotype switching from IgG to IgE. IL-4 stimulates T cells to up-regulate the synthesis of IL-2 and induce the expression of IL-2R. IL-4 is required for the progenitor CD4 cells to mature to T_H2 cells that secrete cytokines. Unlike other cytokines, IL-4 has anti-inflammatory activity and can inhibit the actions of IFN_{γ}. IL-4R is a 140-kd glycoprotein which does not share sequence homology with immunoglobulin.

IL-5 is significantly larger (45 kd) than the other interleukins (15 to 20 kd). IL-5 induces the expression of CD23 on B cells and IL-2R on T cells. IL-5 limits B cells proliferation but enhances IgA synthesis (also requires IL-4). Recombinant IL-5 exhibits potent eosinophil generation from bone marrow precursors. The IL-5R studies are currently incomplete.

IL-6 is a major mediator of the acute phase response, acting on the liver to stimulate the production of acute phase proteins. IL-6 acts in synergy with IL-1, IL-2 and TNF_α to induce cytotoxic T-cell proliferation, cells specific for tumor cells or virally infected cells. IL-6 is 30 kd and is synthesized by activated macrophages, endothelial cells, T_H2 T cells and B cells, fibroblasts, and a number of tumor cells (e.g., myeloma cells). Plasmacytomas and plasma cells from patients with multiple myeloma produce and respond to IL-6; thus, IL-6 may be an autocrine growth factor for malignant plasma cells. IL-6R, an 80-kd glycoprotein, is a member of the Ig gene superfamily.

IL-7 is synthesized by thymic, bone marrow, and splenic stromal cells. IL-7 promotes the growth but not the differentiation of B-cell precursors, and has no effect on mature B lymphocytes. The proliferative effects of recombinant IL-7 on human bone marrow are on immature and memory T and B cells (16). Additional studies are needed to determine how IL-7 contributes to immune and inflammatory responses.

IL-8 is secreted by macrophages, endothelial cells, fibroblasts, keratinocytes and alveolar epithelial cells. IL-8 acts primarily on polymorphonuclear neutrophils (PMNs), functioning as a chemotactic factor, inducing degranulation, up-regulating receptors, promoting migration, and inhibiting adhesion to endothelium.

IL-9 is a T-cell growth factor, derived from T_H2 cells to regulate the growth of T_H cells independent of IL-2 and IL-4. IL-9 enhances the responses of mast cells to IL-3 and stimulates hematopoiesis of megakaryocytes and erythroid precursors.

IL-10 is also a T cell growth factor, secreted by T_H2 cells and B cells. IL-10 promotes the growth of cytotoxic T cells, in combination with IL-2 enhances the differentiation of antigen-specific CD8+ cells, and in synergy with IL-3 and IL-4 promotes growth of mast cells. IL-10 also markedly suppresses IFN_γ production by macrophages.

IL-11 is derived from bone marrow stromal cells and stimulates the development of IgG B cells. In conjunction with IL-3, IL-11 induces megakaryocyte development and decreases the G_0 phase of early hematopoietic precursors.

IL-12 is the most recently described interleukin, synthesized by a B lymphoblastoid cell line. IL-12 activates NK cells and T cells to grow and differentiate (17).

Interferon

Interferon (IFN) was the first cytokine to be described. There are several types of IFN (α, β, γ) as well as subtypes (α_1, α_2, α_3). There are heterogeneities within these groups, and considerable species specificity. IFNs are produced by many cell types in response to viral infections, endotoxin, and a variety of mitogenic and antigenic stimuli. IFN released from virus-infected cells, binds to receptors on other cells and prevents the virus from infecting other cells as well as inhibiting cell growth (13).

IFN_γ is a macrophage activating factor derived from T lymphocytes. IFN_γ induces class II MHC (HLA-DR) molecules on macrophages, epithelial, and endothelial cells. IFN_γ also induces NK activity and inhibits the effects of T_H2 cells.

IFN_α is the primary inhibitor of viral replication, but also has antibacterial and antifungal effects. Derived from B cells and macrophages, IFN_α stimulates macrophages to express FcR and class I MHC molecules.

IFN_β is secreted by fibroblasts and endothelial cells and also induces NK activity. IFN_β stimulates lymphocytes and monocytes to express HLA-DR, enhances the secretion of IL-1 and TNF_α by macrophages. IFN_β also modulates cytotoxic T cell activity and antibody production in synergy with other cytokines.

Colony Stimulating Factors (CSF)

One of the many activities of IL-3 is multi-CSF, capable of stimulating colony formation of several hemapoietic cells. Other CSFs include granulocyte-macrophage CSF (GM-CSF), granulocyte CSF (G-CSF), macrophage CSF (M-CSF), and eosinophil CSF (Eo-CSF) (now known as IL-5).

GM-CSF is produced by activated T cells, NK cells, monocytes, endothelial cells, and fibroblasts. GM-CSF stimulates progenitor cells to produce hemapoietic cells of multiple lineages (17). GM-CSF, like IL-3, is species specific. GM-CSF supports the proliferation of erythroid progenitors in the presence of erythropoietin and stimulates the formation of colonies composed of neutrophil, macrophage, and eosinophil lineages. GM-CSF enhances the effector function of PMNs, i.e., oxidative metabolism, chemotaxis, phagocytosis, and adhesion. Once IL-3 and GM-CSF stimulate the microenvironment, stroma cells and macrophages produce the other two CSFs (G-CSF and M-CSF) to support self-renewal and survival of stem cells. IFN_γ and tumor necrosis factor (TNF) can also induce the synthesis of M-CSF and G-CSF by macrophages.

Peptide Growth Factors

The peptide growth factor (PGF) cytokines are involved in the repair process following injury. Tissue repair and wound healing are coordinated between these cytokines and tissue components. Transforming growth factor β (TGF-β) is synthesized by platelets, macrophages, lymphocytes, bone, and most tissues with the primary role of regulating the growth and differentiation of many tissues (13).

The primary source of platelet-derived growth factor (PDGF) are the α granules of platelets, but PDGF can also be synthesized by macrophages, endothelial cells, and smooth muscle cells. PDGF functions as a potent chemotactic factor for inflammatory cells and smooth muscle cells. PDGF induces collagenase production by fibroblasts, and in general, is important in tissue repair and wound healing.

Fibroblast growth factor (FGF) and epidermal growth factor (EGF) are produced by the cells after which they were named. FGF is also secreted by macrophages and is a very potent mitogen for endothelial cells. EGF is a potent mitogen for epithelial cells and fibroblasts and accelerates the rate of wound healing. The insulin-like growth factor (Somatomedin C) increases the synthesis of proteins and functions as a mitogen for fibroblasts and endothelial cells.

Cytotoxins

Molecules cytolytic for tumor cells are produced by activated lymphocytes and macrophages. There are two main groups of these cytotoxins based on apparent differences in mechanisms of action (19). One group includes molecules with direct cytolytic activity. Subgroups under these direct mediators include molecules that form pores in target cells (analogous to complement-mediated lysis) and those that are non–pore forming. The second group of cytotoxins play an indirect role in the cytolytic pathway and include proteases, esterases, and proteoglycans. Most of the currently characterized cytotoxins are non–pore-forming direct mediators of cytolysis and include TNF, lymphotoxin (LT), and natural killer cytotoxic factor (NKCF).

Polyperferins or pore-forming proteins (PFP) have many similarities with C9, the ninth component of complement, including size (70 kd), antigenic cross-reactivity, and 27% sequence homology (18). Accessory factors for tubule polymerization are different for the two molecules, however.

TNF activity was first described as a monokine that could cause tumor cell death (necrosis). Subsequently, TNF was shown to be homologous to cachectin, the mediator of cachexia accompanying parasitic infections (20). TNF, a 17-kd protein, is now known to be produced by lymphocytes, endothelial cells, and keratinocytes as well as by activated macrophages. Some biological properties of TNF are quite similar to those of IL-1; i.e., pyrogenic, induces shock, stimulates hepatocytes to synthesize acute phase proteins, induces prostaglandin E2 and collagen synthesis. Despite the similarities, TNF and IL-1 are distinct, and receptor binding to each ligand is displaced only by the specific cytokine. TNF and IL-1 exhibit synergistic effects when used together.

Biological properties unique to TNF include activation of polymorphonuclear leukocytes for increased ADCC activity, phagocytosis, and superoxide anion production (19). These beneficial effects are most relevant as protective functions in parasitic, certain fungal, and viral infections. The detrimental effects of TNF/cachectin include induction of cachexia, a state of anorexia and wasting that occurs over a period of months. Mechanisms of action of cachectin include systemic suppression of the enzyme lipoprotein lipase (LPL) resulting in hypertriglyceridemia, antagonizing the lipogenic effects of insulin, and resorption of fat in vivo. Cachectin/TNF suppresses erythropoiesis, a contributing factor to anemia of chronic diseases. Cachectin causes the degradation of proteoglycan in cartilage, catabolizes synovial cells and dermal fibroblasts, perhaps playing an important role in local inflammatory processes involving the bones and joints (20).

TNF receptors (TNF-R) include a binding subunit (75-kd) and a second subunit (138-kd) that is required to elicit cytotoxic activity. TNF from various species can bind to heterologous receptors, but produce significantly different responses.

Lymphotoxin (LT) is 27 to 32% homologous to TNF. The two substances compete for the same cellular receptor, and are functionally indistinguishable (21). LT, TNF, and IL-1 all can stimulate bone resorption. LT can be released from myeloma cells and may be involved in the hypercalcemia and osteolytic lesions associated with multiple myeloma.

Natural killer cell cytotoxic factor (NCKF) is released from LGL after LGL bind to their susceptible target cells. NKCF then binds to the target cell, leading to target cell death. NKCF molecules from several species have been characterized as 19- to 60-kd proteins in two forms, one of which is neutralized by antibodies to TNF while the other is not (19).

IMMUNE COMPLEXES

Immune complexes are formed whenever antigen and antibody combine. In normal individuals, immune complexes are effectively and efficiently removed by PMNs and phagocytic mononuclear cells. The dynamics of immune complex formation are continuously modified relative to the concentration of antigen or antibody present. The size of the immune complexes in circulation is determined by the relative ratio of antigen to antibody and the valence of the antigen (large antigens have more antigenic determinants) and the antibody (IgG has two combining sites, IgM has 10). Antigen excess produces very small circulating immune complexes. Antibody excess produces very large immune complexes that are efficiently removed by the phagocytic system. When antigen and antibody are present in more balanced ratios (equivalence), they localize in vessels and mesangial areas. Complement is activated while the immune complexes are in circulation, depositing C3b on their surface which facilitates localization or deposition in blood vessels and renal glomeruli. C3b deposited on basement membranes provides the "activating surface" necessary to initiate the activation loop of the alternative complement pathway. Complement activation releases chemotactic factors which attract PMNs. During phagocytosis, the PMNs extrude the contents of their granules, which are cytotoxic for endothelial cells. Thus immune complexes initiate the inflammatory process.

Inflammation

The "cardinal signs" of inflammation include redness, swelling, heat, pain, and loss of function. Inflammation represents an orderly series of events that protect the host by destroying foreign invaders, eliminating the debris, and repairing any damage to host tissue. The four stages of inflammation are: increased vascular permeability, emigration of neutrophils, emigration of mononuclear cells, and cellular proliferation.

VASCULAR PERMEABILITY

The microcirculation (capillaries, arterioles, and venules) is involved in the vascular phase of the inflammatory response. When an injury occurs, blood rushes to the affected area (hyperemia), facilitated by localized dilatation of capillaries. The dilatation is a direct result of the effects of histamine released from mast cells in the skin that has been damaged. Histamine and kinins also increase vascular permeability by causing the smooth muscle of the endothelial cells to contract, creating gaps between the cells through which fluids (transudates) and cells (diapedetic PMNs) can pass. As transudation continues, the blood flow slows or stops completely (stasis), caused by hemoconcentration when fluids are lost through transudation, leaving red blood cells clumped. In contrast to thrombosis, stasis is reversible; when blood flow is restored, the clumps of red cells disperse. If the inflammation is severe, microthrombi form, and irreversible platelet aggregation occurs.

EMIGRATION OF GRANULOCYTES

Damage to the endothelial cells by the injury causes changes in the surface membranes that facilitate adherence of granulocytes, primarily polymorphonuclear leukocytes (PMNs). Chemotactic factors (C5a) attract additional PMNs until the entire area becomes pavemented by leukocytes. Emigration of PMNs into the area of inflammation results in active phagocytosis of microorganisms and any other foreign material. With phagocytosis, degranulation occurs. The contents of these granules are directly toxic to surrounding tissues.

EMIGRATION OF MONONUCLEAR PHAGOCYTES

The third stage of the inflammatory response is migration of mononuclear phagocytes into the affected area. These activated macrophages begin to synthesize cytokines, particularly IL-1, which is responsible for further inflammatory reactions such as fever, synthesis of acute phase proteins, and attraction of T and B lymphocytes to the area of inflammation.

CELLULAR PROLIFERATION AND REPAIR

Il-1 stimulates IL-2 synthesis and IL-2R generation. Interaction of IL-2 with IL-2R results in proliferation of lymphocytes and fibroblasts, which begins within 18 hours and peaks by 72 hours. During proliferation, fibroblasts produce acidic mucopolysaccharides to neutralize the effects of chemical mediators released by damaged mast cells and basophils. Resolution and repair, promulgated by PGFs, are the final stages of the normal inflammatory process.

DISEASE STATES

Loss of Protective Barriers

Most infections enter the body through epithelial or mucous membrane disruptions. When epithelial structures are damaged by punctures or destroyed by severe burns, the protective effect of the epithelial barrier has been broken. This significantly increases the danger of an infectious process. When mucous membranes are damaged by chronic inflammation, their protective barrier is broken.

Destruction of the epidermis by severe burns removes the body's protective barrier against microorganisms in the environment and eliminates the barrier to evaporation of water, which requires immediate attention to electrolyte imbalance. Burn wounds not only increase the body's susceptibility to local infections at the burn site, but also depress the humoral and cell-mediated immunity, predisposing the burn patient to invasive infections, bacteremias, metastatic infections involving the respiratory tract and urinary tract, meningitis, and endocarditis (22).

Inflammatory bowel diseases (IBD) such as ulcerative colitis and Crohn's disease are considered chronic inflammatory diseases because their inflammatory infiltrates include macrophages and lymphocytes. Both diseases also have an acute component wherein granulocytes infiltrate the inflamed mucosa, through the epithelium into the intestinal lumen. Although the etiologic agent is unknown, soluble mediators of inflammation that enhance vascular permeability and cause vasodilation appear to be responsible for the functional and histologic changes of mucosal edema and hyperemia seen in IBD (23). Epithelial cells from normal individuals do not express HLA-DR antigens, but epithelial cells from patients with IBD demonstrate marked quantities of these class II MHC antigens. The presence of HLA-DR may serve to induce direct T-cell cytotoxicity of intestinal epithelial cells, enhance antigen presentation to stimulate the production of antibodies by B cells, or otherwise cause abnormalities in the autoimmune response, resulting in IBD.

Aberrations of Cellular Responsiveness

LEUKOCYTOPENIAS

Many bacterial and viral infections induce neutropenia lasting 4 or 5 days during the bacteremic or viremic phases of the infections. During active inflammatory processes, activated chemotactic factors induce neutrophil aggregation, endothelial adherence, degranulation, and release of proteases, which lead to the sequestration of these leukocytes. In healthy young adults, the marginal pool and marrow reserves are capable of compensating and releasing 12 to 14 times the circulating neutrophil numbers. When monocytes/macrophages and lymphocytes are activated by the inflammatory process, the CSFs they synthesize cooperate in sustaining the proliferation of neutrophils and monocytes despite the demise of granulocytes at the site of inflammation. The myeloproliferative response of newborn infants, elderly patients, and myelosuppressed patients can be overwhelmed by infections.

EFFECTS OF LEUKEMIAS ON INFLAMMATORY RESPONSE

Infection is a primary presenting feature as well as the major cause of death in many types of leukemia in which leukemic cells have ablated the growth and differentiation of normal granulocytes, lymphocytes, and macrophages. The leukemia patient's susceptibility to infections increases during chemotherapeutic regimens used to eliminate leukemic cells. Supportive measures include transfusion of granulocytes from healthy donors. Marrow transplantation is the treatment of choice for acute myelogenous leukemia (AML) and adult-onset acute lymphocytic leukemia (ALL). Ablation of the recipient's marrow eradicates not only malignant cells but also residual normal stem cells. Engraftment of donor marrow takes 2 to 3 weeks, leaving the recipient with virtually no granulocyte or immunocompetent cell lines during the time required for the donor stem cells to be established and proliferate. In this immediate period post-transplantation, patients are susceptible to bacterial or fungal infections from normally nonpathogenic flora of the skin, bowel, and respiratory tract. Normal NK and neutrophil activity is not reestablished for 4 to 5 weeks, leaving the transplant recipient susceptible to viral and fungal infections, especially cytomegalovirus, *Candida albicans*, and other opportunistic infections. Prophylactic antibiotics, amphotericin B, and/or acyclovir may be required to prevent disseminated infections until successful engraftment has reconstituted the recipient's specific and nonspecific immunity.

FUNCTIONAL ANOMALIES OF LEUKOCYTES

Hereditary Stem Cell Deficiencies

Cyclic neutropenia begins in infancy and may subside in adulthood. Episodes of neutropenia last from 4 to 10 days and recur at regular intervals, usually every 3 weeks (24). Infectious complications occur during the episodes of neutropenia.

The Schwachman syndrome (neutropenia with pancreatic insufficiency) mimics cystic fibrosis (CF) with failure to thrive, growth retardation, and steatorrhea. Normal sweat chloride levels rule out CF, and the prognosis is much better for children with Schwachman syndrome than for those with CF.

Chediak-Higashi syndrome is a rare autosomal recessive disorder characterized by large inclusion bodies in leukocytes, partial albinism, recurrent infections, increased bleeding tendencies, and defective NK activity. The generalized inborn cellular dysfunction causes increased fusion of cytoplasmic granules, which apparently results in malfunctioning granules.

Drug-Induced Agranulocytosis

Diagnosis of drug-induced agranulocytosis should be considered in any patient receiving a medication who suddenly develops fever, chills, or other signs of infection (24). Antibody-mediated lysis of neutrophils results from covalent coating of the white blood cells with haptenic drugs. The antibody complexed to neutrophils not only annihilates the PMNs, but also activates complement. Drug-induced agranulocytosis subsides promptly when the drug is removed. Drugs implicated include aminopyrine, β-lactam antibiotics, phenothiazine derivatives, antidepressants, and phenylbutazone. Delayed-onset types of agranulocytosis in which marrow is suppressed either immunologically or chemically are much more protracted and eventually lethal.

Defects in Microbicidal Activity

Chronic granulomatous disease (CGD) includes a number of genetic disorders in which neutrophils and monocytes ingest, but cannot kill, catalase-positive microorganisms. Most CGD variants, either the X-linked form or the autosomal recessive form, result in life-threatening infections with *S. aureus* that begin in early childhood. Intravenous antibiotics must be given in high doses over extended periods of time, since degenerating phagocytes slowly release intracellularly proliferating microorganisms that were phagocytosed but not killed. These membrane-enclosed organisms are protected from antibiotics or antibodies, and are transported within the defective neutrophils, thereby disseminating any previously localized infection.

ALTERATIONS OF INTEGRINS

The identification of leukocyte adhesion deficiency (LAD) disease led to the characterization of the function of integrins. LAD was noted in a group of immunodeficient patients with recurrent, life-threatening bacterial and fungal infections who have neutrophils with deficient chemotactic activity and defective phagocytosis. Using MAbs to study the surfaces of the PMNs, all such patients are deficient in the common β chain of all three membrane glycoproteins: LFA-1, Mac-1, and p150,95 complex (26). Heterogeneity in this defect has been described with severely deficient patients who often die within the first 2 years of life, and moderately deficient patients who can survive to adulthood. The extent of the deficiency is related to the degree of expression of the membrane glycoproteins, with the moderately deficient group exhibiting 3 to 10% of normal and the severely deficient group less than 0.5%.

Aberrations of Humoral Responsiveness

ENZYME DEFICIENCIES OF PHAGOCYTIC CELLS

Myeloperoxidase (MPO) deficiency creates a microbicidal defect in phagocytes. The functional impairment is not severe, and infections are not generally life threatening.

Lactoferrin deficiency is a rare congenital neutrophil disorder characterized by decreased numbers of specific granules devoid of lactoferrin (24). These deficient granules cannot form adequate phagolysosome fusion and do not generate appropriate hydroxy radicals in response to ingested organisms. Impaired neutrophil reactivity is manifest as unresponsiveness to chemotactic factors, diminished adhesiveness to surfaces, and decreased release of microbicidal O_2 metabolites. Patients with lactoferrin deficiency have recurrent pyogenic skin abscesses.

ACUTE PHASE RESPONSE; CRP VERSUS ESR

Although CRP has many similarities to antibodies, deficiency states of CRP have not been found. CRP is present in microgram per liter quantities in normal humans, but elevates dramatically and rapidly in the presence of bacterial infections, where levels above 100 mg/liter are common. With resolution of those infections, the CRP levels decrease within a few days, reflecting the half-life measured in hours. Moderate CRP levels of 10 to 100 mg/liter are found in chronic inflammatory conditions such as systemic lupus erythematosus (SLE), malignancies, congestive heart failure, and pregnancy. Viral infections, by contrast, do not manifest a CRP response unless there are superimposed bacterial infections.

In contrast, the ESR elevation is slower and much more prolonged (Fig. 59.3), reflecting the significantly slower indirect stimulus of fibrinogen synthesis by hepatocytes. The magnitude of increase of fibrinogen (2- to 4-fold) is also significantly different from that of CRP (several 100-fold). Certain chronic inflammatory diseases such as SLE have very elevated ESRs, but normal to only slightly elevated CRP levels. Rheumatoid arthritis, in contrast, demonstrates elevations in both ESR and CRP (25).

COMPLEMENT DEFICIENCIES

Acquired complement deficiencies are relatively common and are frequently reversible when the underlying disease state has been treated effectively. Acquired deficiencies are classified by the responsible mechanism: consumption in immune complex diseases, vasculitis, or C3NF; synthetic in severe liver disease where production of complement components is inhibited; and catabolic breakdown of complement components at an increased rate in certain protein-losing enteropathies or nephrotic syndrome (11).

Homozygous hereditary deficiencies of most complement components are uncommon (0.03% prevalence) in the general population (11, 26). Complement components are inherited as autosomal codominant, each gene contributing half of the nor-

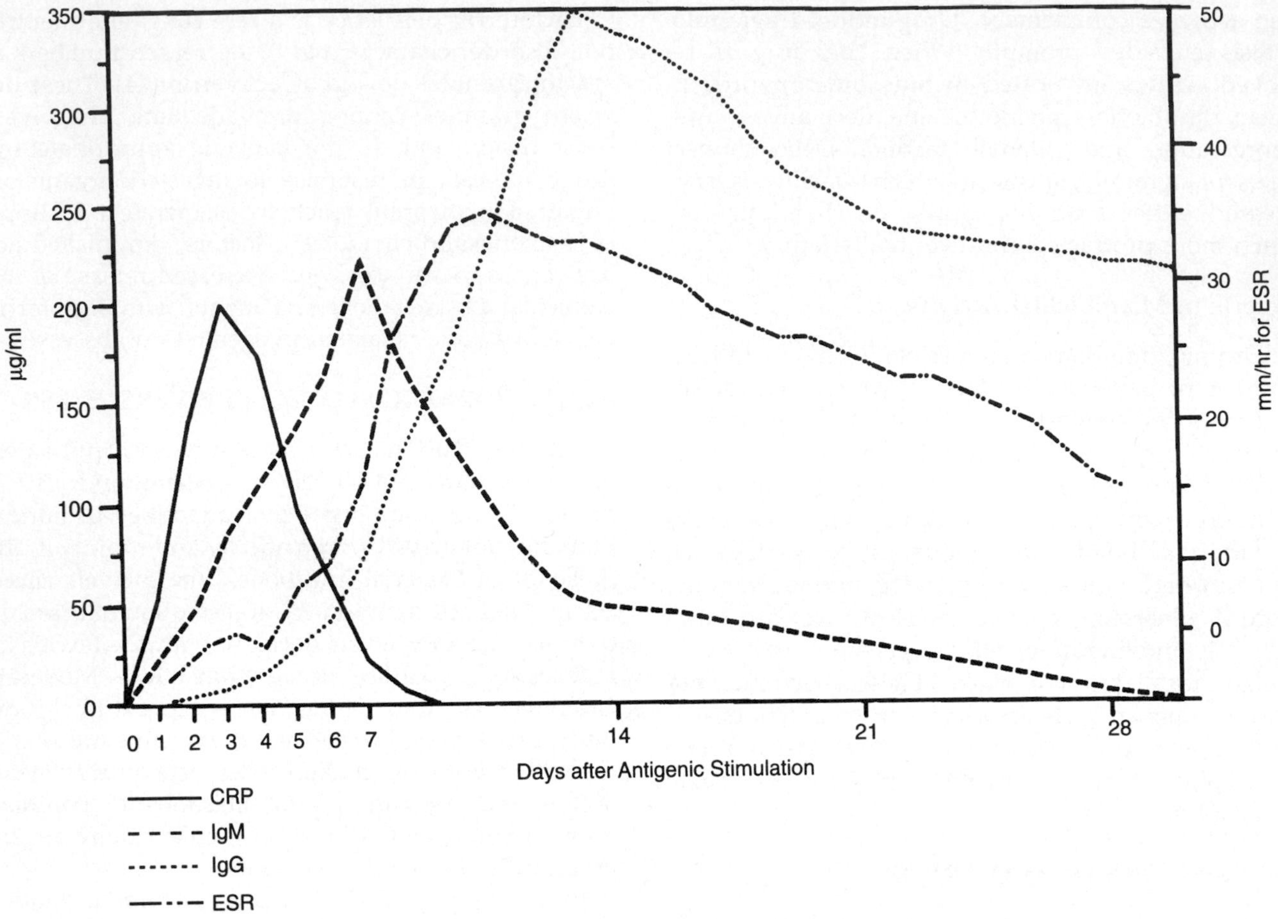

Figure 59.3. Kinetics of CRP and ESR responsiveness. (From James K. Immunoserology of infectious diseases. Clin Microbiol Rev 1990;3:135–152.)

mal protein levels. Heterozygote-deficient patients have half of the normal level, adequate amounts unless the patient is severely compromised by some other medical problem. Homozygote-deficient patients have less that 10% of the normal level of the protein, inadequate functionally as well as quantitatively.

Deficiencies of the classical pathway components C1q, C1r, C1s, C4, or C2, are associated with SLE-like diseases and glomerulonephritis. The most common complement deficiency, homogeneous C2 deficiency occurs in one in 100,000 individuals and is highly associated with the HLA haplotype A25, B18, DR2, a gene located on the short arm of the sixth chromosome. The gene for factor B appears to be closely associated with the gene for C2, since C2-deficient patients also have decreased levels of factor B. It appears that most C2-deficient subjects (some of whom are healthy) descended from a single ancestor approximately 1000 years ago (26). The gene for C4 has also been linked to the same class III histocompatibility complex, but to a number of different HLA haplotypes. Heterozygous C4 deficiency is extraordinarily common, found in approximately 25% of the Caucasian population (11). There are two phenotypes of C4, C4A and C4B variants; certain combinations of those variants result in lower than average total C4 levels that are not necessarily deficient. Homozygous deficiencies, however, are very rare.

Hereditary deficiency of C3 has been very rarely reported, suggesting that the absence of C3 is nearly incompatible with life due to its pivotal position in both the classical and alternative pathways. Deficiencies of H and I are associated with very low serum C3 levels because of the uncontrolled formation of the alternative pathway C3 convertase, resulting in rapid catabolism of C3 and Factor B. These patients are subject to recurrent bacterial infections because of poor opsonization and chemotaxis. A pathological protein, C3 nephritic factor (NF), results in markedly decreased levels of C3 due to activation or consumption. NF is an IgG antibody with specificity for the alternative pathway C3 convertase. NF binds to C3 convertase and prevents inactivation by the control proteins H and I. When NF is present, C3 activation proceeds uncontrolled, thereby markedly depleting C3. Patients with C3NF present with recurrent bacterial infections and frequently also have partial lipodystrophy (27).

Deficiencies of the terminal complement components (C5, C6, C7, or C8) result in recurrent meningococcal infections. At least 10% of patients with recurrent meningitis or systemic gonorrhea have either a late complement component, H, I, or properdin deficiency. The initial episode of meningococcal disease occurs at a median age of 3 years in the general population, but at age 17 in individuals lacking one of the terminal complement components (11). Uncommon meningococcal serogroups are more common in complement-deficient individuals; thus, the vaccines against the more common serogroups may not be effective in deficient patients. Recurrence rates for meningococcal infections in patients with terminal complement component deficiencies range between 40 and 50%.

C6 deficiencies are more common in blacks, but C7-deficient individuals are generally Caucasian. C6 and C7 are closely linked on chromosome 9 and combined C6 and C7 deficiencies occur primarily in whites. C8 is a three-chain polypeptide (α, β, γ), and deficiencies of one or two chains have been reported, including functional but not antigenic deficiencies. C9 deficiencies have an unusually high frequency in Japan, but without particular disease associations.

C1Inh deficiency is associated with angioedema. The hereditary form of the disease is transmitted as an autosomal dominant trait and occurs in approximately one in 1,000,000 individuals. Acquired forms of angioedema are much rarer and are usually associated with lymphoproliferative diseases. Uncontrolled activation of C1qrs results in perpetual cleavage of C4 and C2. C2b and C4a both stimulate smooth muscle contraction and cause increased vascular permeability, whereby fluid leaks out of blood vessels into extravascular spaces, causing edema. C2b also stimulates excess mucous membrane secretions, causing life-threatening episodes involving the respiratory and gastrointestinal tract.

ALTERATIONS OF CYTOKINES

The acute phase response to infection or tissue destruction is mediated by the cytokines IL-1, TNF, and IL-6. Fever is mediated by IL-1, an endogenous pyrogen. Neutrophilia and increase in immature granulocytes are due to IL-1, the CSFs, IL-6, and IL-8 effects on the marginal and recirculating pool of PMNs. The synthesis of acute phase proteins by the liver is stimulated primarily by IL-6. IL-1 and TNF inhibit lipoprotein lipase activity in hepatocytes, resulting in hyperlipemia. Both cytokines are also responsible for the lethargy that accompanies acute infections and the cachexia that occurs in chronic infections.

IL-1, IL-6, and TNF have also been implicated in contributing to the dysfunctions associated with septic shock, the most common cause of death in intensive care units. Most cases of septic shock are caused by endotoxin or lipopolysaccharide (LPS) that can be initiated by infection, burns, or severe trauma. The physical manifestations of septic shock include hypotension, fever, respiratory distress, tachycardia, thrombocytopenia, renal and/or hepatic failure (27). The cytokines are produced by macrophages, activated by the precipitating event. Elevated levels of TNF have been reported to have diagnostic and prognostic significance in critically ill patients (11). IL-6 and IL-8 are present in detectable levels in the serum of patients with septic shock. TNF levels correlate with the cachexia and wasting observed in cancer patients. When recombinant TNF was administered as therapy for cancer patients, IL-6 levels increased after TNF levels declined (28).

IL-2 is the primary proliferative stimulus of antigen-activated T cells, NK cells, and LAK cells. The immunosuppressive agents cyclosporine (CsA) and glucocorticoids selectively suppress the synthesis of IL-2. Elevated levels of IL-2 in plasma prior to transplant may predict which candidates for transplant will experience rejection episodes (29). Thus, measurement of IL-2 levels in patients awaiting transplant will be important in selecting the patients most likely to achieve successful engraftment. IL-2 levels also rise during acute or chronic rejection. Levels of soluble IL-2R have been reported to have prognostic significance in certain autoimmune diseases and viral infections (30).

All of the cytokines described above are available commercially as recombinant (r) cytokines, synthesized by bacteria that have had human genes for cytokines inserted. rIL-2 has been used in vitro and in vivo to generate LAK cells for cancer therapy. $rIFN_\gamma$ and rTNF have been administered to cancer patients (28). An anticipated use of rILs would be to treat immunodeficiency patients with the specific cytokine that would induce maturation of the component of their immune system that has not fully developed. Cytokine antagonists or control mechanisms are not yet fully understood, but they certainly exist. Modulation of the cytokines or their antagonists will be the emphasis of immunotherapeutics in the future.

Diseases Associated with Circulating Immune Complexes

There are three causes of immune complex-mediated diseases: chronic or persistent infections, autoimmunity, and extrinsic agents. Although many immune complexes are effectively and efficiently removed by phagocytic cells, small complexes in antigen-antibody equivalence can lead to immune complex diseases.

CHRONIC INFECTIONS

Chronic infections that can result in immune complex-mediated diseases include antigens from bacterial, parasitic, and viral microorganisms. Low-grade bacterial infections with certain streptococci can produce poststreptococcal glomerulonephritis or rheumatic fever. Staphylococcal infections can result in subacute bacterial endocarditis or infected atrial ventricular shunts. *Mycoplasma pneumoniae* is the causative agent in primary atypical pneumonia, where the antibodies cross-react with erythrocytes to cause an acute hemolytic anemia as well as induce pulmonary infiltrates. *Salmonella*, *Treponema pallidum*, and *Klebsiella* have all been implicated in infection-associated glomerulonephritis. *Plasmodium* species, *Toxoplasma gondii*, filariasis, and schistosomiasis are also associated with immune complex glomerulonephritis. Chronic viral infections with hepatitis B, measles, Epstein-Barr virus, retroviruses, and cytomegalovirus have also been associated with immune complex glomerulonephritis.

AUTOIMMUNITY

Immune complex disease is a frequent complication of autoimmune diseases. Tissue deposition in the blood vessel walls results in vasculitis or immune complex deposition in the glomeruli to precipitate glomerulonephritis. The variant of systemic lupus erythematosus (SLE) manifested by 40% of lupus patients and most often implicated in renal disease is characterized by the presence of antibodies to double-stranded (ds) DNA. Approximately 35% of SLE patients have antibodies to SS-A, which have been associated with the cutaneous manifestations of the disease, with congenital heart block in infants born to an asymptomatic mother, and with homozygous C2 and C4 complement component deficiencies (31).

Immune complex-induced glomerulonephritis is the most important demonstration of an immune complex-mediated disease. Antigen-antibody complexes in antibody excess are rapidly phagocytosed, but complexes in equivalence or slight antigen excess are deposited in the kidney. The glomerulus filters the blood from arterial capillaries through a fenestrated endothelial lining that appears to be susceptible to deposition of immune complexes. Deposition of immune complexes initiates the cycle of complement activation, chemotaxis of PMNs, and release of enzymes from the granules of phagocytic cells that cause glomerular injury. Self-antigens such as are found in autoimmunity (e.g., DNA–anti-DNA) are the primary mediators of glomerulonephritis. Exogenous or foreign antigens such as drugs or infectious agents also cause immune complex–mediated glomerulonephritis.

Rheumatoid arthritis is the prototypic *localized* immune complex disease. An (as yet unknown) antigenic stimulus results in the synthesis of an abnormal IgG by synovial lymphocytes. This abnormal IgG is recognized as foreign, which leads to increased production of rheumatoid factor (RF). When RF reacts with the abnormal IgG within the joint space, complement is activated by the classical pathway. Chemotactic factors are generated, attracting PMNs and mononuclear phagocytes. Enzymes released into the joints by these phagocytic cells amplify the inflammatory response within the synovium. At later stages of RA, extra-articular manifestations occur, including vasculitis and pneumonitis.

EXTRINSIC AGENTS

Hypersensitivity pneumonitis is an immune complex disease of the lung induced by aerosol exposure to environmental antigens. Circulating IgG antibodies (and much less frequently, IgM or IgA) are produced to those antigens. Upon repeated exposure, immune complexes are formed in the airways, resulting in an inflammatory process. Acute and chronic forms of the disease are seen with environmental antigens such as thermophilic actinomycetes (mold-infested hay, grains, mushroom compost, or contaminated water); *Alternaria* and other fungi found in sawdust and tree bark; and various isocyanates used in the production of foam, insulation, and synthetic rubber (32).

METHODOLOGIES

Leukocyte Function Assays

NEUTROPHIL

The nitroblue tetrazolium (NBT) dye reduction test is used to detect generation of H_2O_2 and superoxide radicals. Normal neutrophils phagocytize NBT dye in the presence of latex particles and reduce the yellow dye to a deep blue color. The NBT test was developed to distinguish the striking abnormality in chronic granulomatous disease (CGD) in which abnormal neutrophils do not reduce the NBT dye. A quantitative NBT method has applications in detecting patients with intraleukocyte killing defects.

The bactericidal activity of neutrophils can be measured by the ability of PMNs to kill opsonized *S. aureus*. PMNs separated from whole blood are incubated with the bacteria. After incubation extracellular bacteria are killed, and the neutrophils are lysed to liberate intracellular bacteria and are plated on media to grow *S. aureus*. The majority of bacteria are killed by normal PMNs by 2 to 3 hours, while there is virtually no killing in CGD patients. Heterozygous carriers demonstrate an intermediate level of killing. Other disorders of neutrophil function that can show defective microbicidal activity include Chediak-Higashi syndrome, myeloperoxidase deficiency, glucose-6-phosphate dehydrogenase deficiency, acute leukemias, Down's syndrome, and transient neutrophil dysfunctions such as ataxia-telangiectasia and acute infections.

Chemiluminescence (ChL) is the light energy emitted from PMNs when H_2O_2, superoxide radicals, and singlet oxygen are generated during the respiratory burst. This electromagnetic microradiation can be detected by liquid scintillation counters with sensitive photomultiplier tubes. There are direct correlations between microbicidal activity and light emissions. ChL is easier to perform than the "Staph Kill" assay since it only requires PMNs (fewer than the other assays and whole blood can be used), latex (or zymosan), a fluorescent compound to intensify the light emissions, and a scintillation counter to measure the reaction. ChL is an effective and efficient screening test for neutrophil dysfunction.

Chemotaxis is the directed movement of neutrophils toward a specific stimulus. Random motility is the indiscriminate movement of PMNs in all directions from the point of origin. Both chemotaxis and random motility are measured by a soft agar technique analogous to Ouchterlony diffusion in agar. The PMNs are placed in the center well, a chemoattractant into an outside well, and a control substance in the opposite outside well. After allowing time for migration, the distance from the center well is measured to determine directed and random motility.

MONOCYTES

Migration inhibition factor (MIF) is a lymphokine synthesized by activated T cells in response to specific antigen stimulation. If the antigen (such as a tumor extract) is recognized by the lymphocytes, MIF is elicited. MIF inhibits the normal random migration in an assay system that places macrophages into the open end of a capillary tube set into soft agar.

CYTOTOXICITY ASSAYS

Cytotoxicity assays are not routinely performed in the clinical laboratory and have no specific clinical applicability. However, cytotoxicity assays are very useful in research laboratories for characterizing and understanding the effector mechanisms that appear to have relevance in immune surveillance for tumors and to prevent metastasis of cancer cells.

Target cells for cytotoxicity assays are labeled with either ^{51}Cr or ^{3}H-thymidine. Spontaneous release must be calculated and percent cytotoxicity corrected for the spontaneous release. Because the ^{3}H-thymidine is actually incorporated into the nucleic acids of the cell nucleus, this method of labeling is considered to be more specific and sensitive than chromium labeling.

Monocyte-mediated cytotoxicity measures tumor-specific killing by monocytes/macrophages. Target cells include various tumor cell lines; control cells are nonneoplastic fibroblasts. Adherent monocytes are first incubated for several hours with or without reagents that activate phagocytic cells. Labeled target cells are then added, and incubation progresses for several more hours. In the chromium release assay, aliquots of supernatant are removed to separate tubes and counted on a gamma scintillation counter to determine the percent of chromium released from lysed target cells. In the tritiated thymidine assay, the wells are washed and residual cells lysed with NaOH. Aliquots of the lysate are placed in liquid scintillation fluid and counted in a beta scintillation counter.

Antibody-dependent cellular cytotoxicity (ADCC) uses target cells that include erythrocytes as well as nucleated cells. Although complement is not efficient at lysing nucleated cells, ADCC can effectively do so. Target cells are labeled with ^{51}Cr, and then are incubated with antibody specific for antigens on the target cell membranes. Mononuclear effector cells (monocytes and LGL) are added in effector:target (E:T) ratios ranging from 2:1 to 50:1. The antibody is bound by the Fab region to the target cell, leaving the Fc region to bind to the Fc receptors (FcR) on the effector cells. The interaction between the Fc and FcR stimulates the effector cells to become cytolytic.

Natural killer assays measure the naturally occurring (spontaneous) cytotoxic potential of LGL, which constitutes 2 to 5% of the peripheral blood lymphocytes. The most commonly used human NK target cell is K-562, a cell line derived from a patient with chronic myeloid leukemia in blast crisis. K-562 cells lack MHC Class I and Class II antigens and can be induced in vitro to differentiate into cells with myeloid, erythroid, or megakaryocyte characteristics. NK cytotoxicity can also be demonstrated using normal, virus-infected target cells. NK target cells are usually labeled with ^{51}Cr and used at several E:T ratios so that lytic units can be calculated. The use of lytic units allows the transformation of the data into a single number with standard errors. Since NK activity for normal donors remains relatively constant over an extended period of time (in the absence of infections or drugs that affect NK activity), data from patients can be normalized and compared to a pool of normal donors, allowing interlaboratory comparisons of data (33).

Lymphokine-activated killer assays are performed using "NK-resistant" target cells, particularly the Raji cell line. Evidence suggests that the potent ability of NK cells to rapidly eliminate tumor cells from circulation and to prevent metastasis to the lungs and liver is best measured by the ability of IL-2–activated NK (LAK) cells to lyse NK-resistant cells or fresh tumor cells.

PLATELET FUNCTION ASSAYS

Platelet aggregation can be measured in vitro using an aggregometer. Suspensions of platelets are treated with various aggregating agents such as low levels of adenosine diphosphate (ADP), epinephrine, collagen, or thrombin to induce the primary or "first wave" of aggregation, which is reversible. When the platelets release ADP and arachidonic acid from their granules during the primary step, these secretory products of platelets provide the feedback loop, which causes the secondary or "second wave" reaction, which is irreversible. The aggregometer measures the changes in light scatter that occur as platelets change shape, become adhesive, and aggregate.

Mediator release from platelets can be used to measure the effectiveness of these agents to aggregate patient platelets. The calcium-dependent synthesis of prostaglandins (from arachidonic acid in membrane fatty acids to thromboxane B_2 [TXB_2]) in response to the aggregating agents is necessary to effect the secondary response. ADP release by platelets during the primary and secondary waves can be measured when one of the other aggregating agents (e.g., epinephrine or collagen) is used. The byproducts of arachidonic acid metabolization (e.g., TBX_2, prostacyclin [PGI_2]), and cyclic AMP can also be measured.

Assays for Humoral Mediators

CRP QUANTITATION

A number of methods are available for measuring CRP. A widely available method uses a qualitative latex agglutination assay with a detection limit of approximately 10 mg/liter, the upper limit of normal. The results are reported as negative or positive, but the magnitude of positivity cannot be appreciated. Because CRP levels can increase so rapidly and dramatically, the latex agglutination assay is subject to false-negative reactions due to a prozone-type phenomenon in which all of the antibody combining sites on the latex particles are bound to an excess of CRP so no cross-linking (agglutination) can occur. Consequently, the qualitative test should be performed on several dilutions of serum to avoid false-negative reactions. If several dilutions are performed, the latex agglutination method can easily be converted to a semiquantitative assay so distinctions can be made between levels of positivity (e.g., less than 50 mg/liter and more than 150 mg/liter). Such semiquantitative distinctions would be very useful to the clinician trying to distinguish between bacterial (high CRP levels) and viral infections (normal to slightly elevated CRP). The latex agglutination method requires no special equipment and could be performed in clinics, urgent care centers, or on a stat basis for emergency room needs.

Radial immunodiffusion (RID) is used by many laboratories as a method for quantitating CRP. The 18- to 24-hour turnaround time (TAT) for RID is a distinct disadvantage and obviates the use of this assay for medical decision making regarding infectious processes.

Nephelometry has replaced RID for the quantitation of serum proteins in many laboratories. This technique can shorten the TAT to a few hours if the testing is performed on each shift every day. This is highly unlikely, even in a reference laboratory or a high-volume university hospital laboratory. At best, the nephelometric tests are performed on a single shift five or six days per week. Consequently, the actual TAT is not much better than RID.

Recently, instrument manufacturers have developed assay systems that allow random access assays for CRP to be performed virtually on demand with 10- to 20-minute TAT. Two types of assay systems are enzyme-multiplied immunoassay techniques (EMIT) and fluorescence polarization assays (FPA). These assay systems were originally designed to quantitate haptens (e.g., for therapeutic drug monitoring), but have been adapted to quantitate a homogeneous molecule such as CRP. These instruments and assay systems have enabled rapid TAT (STAT) with quantitative CRP results.

ERYTHROCYTE SEDIMENTATION RATE

There are three methods of measuring the ESR: Westergren, which uses blood diluted in sodium citrate; Wintrobe, which uses undiluted blood; and the zeta sedimentation rate, which requires special equipment. In older literature, a method for correcting the ESR for hematocrit was proposed, but it has been abandoned since it added no relevant information to the results. There is no evidence that any method is superior, so the simplest method (Wintrobe) should be used if the test is required (8).

COMPLEMENT ASSAYS

Assays for complement include the quantitative (RID, nephelometry) measurement of individual components or the functional evaluation of either pathway or of individual components. The components usually quantitated are C3 and C4; C3 because of its pivotal location and role in both the classical and alternative pathway, and C4 to distinguish classical from alternative pathway activation. Other complement components that can be quantitated include C1q, C1r, C1s, C2, C5, C6, C7, C8, C9, factor B, and factor D; however, these are rarely required and are best performed by research laboratories. The only reason to measure any component other than C3 and C4 would be if a component deficiency is suspected. The screening method of choice for a component deficiency is one of the hemolytic assays.

Hemolytic complement assays are measured as CH_{50} (hemolytic complement 50% lysis point), which is a fluid-phase assay, or CH_{100} (hemolytic complement 100% lysis), which is performed in agar and is quantitated similarly to RID. In both systems, either the classical pathway or the alternative pathway can be measured by varying the indicator cells. For the classical pathway hemolytic assays, sheep erythrocytes (ShE) are sensitized with antibody (ShEA). For the alternative-pathway hemolytic assays, rabbit erythrocytes (RaE) are used without antibody. In the fluid-phase assay, the ShEA (or RaE) are suspended in buffer containing the appropriate divalent cations (Ca^{2+} for the classical pathway or Mg^{2+} for the alternative pathway). Patient sera (appropriately processed and stored to optimize the functional complement activity) are prepared at several dilutions and incubated with ShE for precise times. The optical density (OD) of the hemoglobin released by lysis of the ShE is determined spectrophotometrically. The results are interpreted to yield the point at which lysis of 50% of the ShE has occurred.

The CH_{100} assay is performed by suspending the ShE (or RaE) in agarose. Patient sera or standardized control serum at various dilutions are applied to wells punched into the agarose and allowed to diffuse. The diameter of the resulting zone of hemolysis is directly proportional to the hemolytic activity of the serum and correlates relatively well with the CH_{50} values for the same sera. Because complement components are normally present in levels that exceed what is needed for lysis of either pathway, the CH_{100} would be less sensitive to half levels (heterozygous deficiencies) of certain components than the fluid-phase assay would be. Since complement deficiencies are relatively rare, and half levels are only relevant in complicated disease processes, CH_{100} can replace CH_{50} in most situations. The solid-phase assay is much easier to perform, detects consumption of components in disease states, and does detect homozygous component deficiencies. Recently a commercial company has developed a single-tube, fluid-phase classical pathway CH_{50} assay that is simple to perform and is just as precise as the laborious multiple-dilution method. Functional hemolytic assays for many of the components (C2, C3, C4, C5) are available from specialized reference laboratories. The functional component assays provide lytic units of all of the components necessary for lysis *except* the component being measured. If that component is missing from the patient sera, the indicator particles (ShE) will not be lysed. Hemolytic assays are an efficient way to detect C2 or other component deficiencies, but would not be useful to monitor C3 and C4 levels as an indicator of complement activation in an immune complex disease.

Neither CH_{50} nor CH_{100} is useful to monitor disease activity, since their endpoint (lysis) is very insensitive to changes in component levels and can occur even with significant depletion of most components. It takes very few C2 and C4 molecules to cause lysis and yield a "normal" CH_{50} level. Quantitations of C3 and C4 are much more sensitive measures of complement consumption in vivo than are the hemolytic assays.

Complement components are acute phase reactants and increase in concentration during inflammation. Consequently, the acute phase increases can offset any consumption in vivo and result in normal hemolytic and normal quantitative levels in the presence of subclinical disease. C4 is the most sensitive indicator of in vivo complement consumption, since a 50% increase in C4 (due to acute phase) represents 10 to 15 mg/dl, while the 50% acute phase response of C3 would be an increase of 75 to 100 mg/dl. It takes consumption of significantly more C3 to offset an acute phase response than it does for C4.

Unfortunately, the rheumatology literature still considers CH_{50} as the assay of choice to monitor complement activation in disease. This is at least partially attributable to a lack of understanding by commercial companies and their customers of the need to use monospecific antisera to C3c or another unique domain on the C3 molecule (Fig. 59.2). Many commercially available C3 assays use antisera that react with multiple domains on the C3 molecule and therefore detect breakdown products of C3 as well as the intact molecule, resulting in falsely elevated (or falsely normal) levels in active stages of disease. Falsely elevated levels are not as pronounced with C4, since the concentration is lower.

Specimen handling is critical for accurate measurement of complement components, and especially for the functional assays. Complement components (many of which are enzymes) are extremely labile and are easily activated in the test tube or inactivated due to adverse storage conditions. Although it is not considered a "standard of practice," specimens for quantitation of C3 and C4 *and* for functional assays should be collected as plasma with EDTA as the anticoagulant. EDTA chelates the available Ca^{2+} and Mg^{2+}, preventing activation of either pathway in vitro. The plasma should be frozen until tested to prevent breakdown by proteolytic enzymes as well as to preserve the labile complement components. The buffer systems used to test for functional activity in either the CH_{50} or the CH_{100} assay contain an excess of Ca^{2+} and Mg^{2+}, more than enough to support either the classical or alternative pathway without these divalent cations from serum. The amount of EDTA present in the plasma is insufficient to chelate the excess divalent cations provided by the buffer systems. Collection of complement specimens as EDTA plasma prevents the artificial activation of complement in vitro associated with the coagulation pathway in certain patient sera (34).

CIRCULATING IMMUNE COMPLEX ASSAYS

A multitude of methods have been developed over the years to detect circulating immune complexes (CICs) in patient sera. Unfortunately, no one method has proved to be diagnostic or prognostic in any specific disease state. CICs have been definitely implicated in certain diseases (in particular, DNA–anti-DNA complexes in SLE). However, the presence or absence of CICs in patient serum is dependent on the factors related to clearance by the mononuclear phagocyte system, which may or may not correlate to disease activity. The methods to detect CIC in the laboratory have been of four types; temperature-dependent precipitation (cryoglobulins), CICs that bind to C1q, CICs that bind to activated C3, and CICs that bind the Fc region of IgG after IgG has bound to antigen (35).

Cryoglobulins

By far the simplest and most reproducible method for detecting CICs is cold-insoluble precipitation of cryoglobulins, if present. Type I cryoglobulins are cold-insoluble monoclonal proteins, associated with B-cell or plasma cell malignancies, but not with CICs. Type II cryoglobulins are mixed monoclonal and polyclonal antibodies usually present as polyclonal IgG complexed to an unknown antigen and subsequently bound as CICs to a monoclonal IgM antibody with rheumatoid factor activity. Type III cryoglobulins are mixed polyclonal antibodies with IgG or IgA bound to unknown antigens complexed to polyclonal RF as CICs. Type II and Type III cryoglobulins are usually present in relatively low concentrations (less than 1 mg/ml).

The laboratory methods for detecting cryoglobulins are simple. Blood must be collected in prewarmed containers and kept at 37°C until clotted. Centrifugation should occur at 37°C to prevent loss of any cryoglobulins during the process of separating the serum from the cells. One aliquot of serum is stored at 4°C in an ESR tube for at least 3 days; a separate aliquot (control) is stored at 37°C for the same time. The control is necessary as a comparison to reliably detect the fine, flocculant precipitate that would indicate a Type III cryoglobulin. If cryoprecipitate is present, the specimen can be centrifuged at 4°C to determine the relative amount of cryoglobulin (cryocrit), which is expressed as a percentage. If sufficient amounts of cryoglobulin are present, the precipitate can be washed with cold buffer, resuspended, and characterized by immunofixation electrophoresis to determine which Type (I, II, or III) of cryoglobulin is present.

C1q-binding Assays

C1q-binding assays are either fluid phase or solid phase. The fluid-phase assays use purified, radiolabeled C1q added to diluted patient serum. The bound ^{125}I-C1q is then separated from the free radiolabeled C1q by ultracentrifugation or by using an aggregating agent such as polyethylene glycol.

The solid-phase C1q-binding assays use purified C1q coated to a surface (microtiter plate, test tube) under conditions of high ionic strength, which serves to maintain the hemolytic activity of C1q (36). The C1q molecule binds to the solid phase by the collagenous region, leaving the globular head group free to bind to immune complexes. Immune complexes are then detected using enzyme-conjugated anti-IgG or other immunoglobulin classes. Versions of this assay are commercially available.

C3b-binding Assays

If CICs have already bound complement and activated the classical or alternative pathway, C3b would have been bound in vivo. Such CICs would have exposed on their surface the portion of C3b that interacts with C3b receptors on cell surfaces. The assay system based on this premise was first described as the Raji cell assay. Raji cells are a B-cell line, without surface immunoglobulin. They express high-affinity C3b receptor, but sparse numbers of low-affinity IgG Fc receptors. The Raji assay was extremely difficult to standardize because the Raji cells had to be grown in culture and would change receptor characteristics. Additionally, many lupus patients have lymphocytotoxic antibodies that bind to Raji cells (a lymphoid cell line) by their Fab regions, irrespective of Fc or C3b receptors, to cause false-positive results.

A solid-phase version of the C3b binding assay was the conglutinin assay. Conglutinin is a protein unique to bovine sera that binds C3b and can be purified and used to coat surfaces. The problems with this method were that different preparations of conglutinin had different binding characteristics, so standardization was difficult.

Theoretically, monoclonal antibodies specific for the portion of C3b that binds to cell surface receptors should be an appropriate substitute for the actual cell receptors (Raji cells) or the conglutinin, but other inherent problems with CIC assays have precluded development of monoclonal C3b assays.

IgG Fc Receptor–Binding Assays

Assay systems that utilize the alteration of the IgG Fc region, which occurs when IgG binds to antigens, include platelet aggregation assays and rheumatoid factor assays. Platelets have IgG Fc receptors that facilitate their binding to immune complexes or monomeric IgG. By binding CIC, platelets participate in the clearance of soluble immune complexes from circulation by delivering CICs in particulate form to phagocytic mononuclear cells. The process of binding CICs results in platelet aggregation and can be measured using an aggregometer.

Rheumatoid factor (RF) is a naturally occurring IgM molecule with specificity for the altered Fc region of IgG bound to antigen. Two forms of RF, isolated from patient serum, have been used: polyclonal RF isolated from patients with high titers of RF associated with rheumatoid arthritis, and monoclonal RF isolated from patients with B-cell lymphoproliferative diseases (e.g., macroglobulinemia) in which these abnormal proteins exhibit RF activity in the absence of the autoimmune disease. The isolated RF can then be used as a reagent in the laboratory to bind to and detect CICs. Methods using these reagents have been similar to those described above for isolated C1q.

Standards by Which to Measure CIC

Aggregated human γ-globulin (AHGG) is the substance most often used as a standard by which to quantitate levels of CIC in patient sera. AHGG is the problem with most CIC assays, since AHGG is very difficult to standardize. AHGG is prepared by incubating a specific concentration of IgG in appropriate buffer at 63°C for precise periods of time. Minor variations in IgG concentration, buffer ionic strength, temperature, and incubation time all contribute to variability in the "standard." With time, AHGG deaggregates, so the "standard' solution cannot be stored, but must be prepared fresh with each assay. Thus, the assay systems and the standards employed in CIC assays are often not comparable between methods, between laboratories, or even between assays performed in the same laboratory (35).

In vitro prepared immune complexes was evaluated as the "standard" for use in the solid-phase C1q binding assay by adding purified bacterial DNA to patient sera containing anti-DNA antibodies (36). Although increasing levels of CICs could be detected, the magnitude of the increase was relatively small, and antigen excess resulted in loss of detectability of the CICs. The valency of the antigen and the specificity of the antibodies are limiting factors in CIC assays. Until recombinant antigens and monoclonal antibodies can be developed to truly standardize the antigen-antibody reactions, in vitro prepared CICs will not be a useful standard for CICs. But the unanswered question will remain whether artificially prepared CICs are truly equivalent to CICs in circulation in patient sera.

ASSAYS FOR CYTOKINES

Quantitative Assays for Cytokines

The ability to synthesize recombinant cytokines and several cytokine receptors has facilitated the quantitation of these molecules in patient serum. Monoclonal antibodies have been produced to virtually all of the cytokines and to the known cytokine receptors. Assay development is limited only by the picogram level of detectability of many of the cytokines in patient sera, and in determining the clinical relevance of alterations in their levels.

IL-2 is detectable in concentrations of nanograms per milliliter, so it can be quantitated with nonisotopic assays. Enzyme immunoassays (EIAs) that measure IL-2 or IL-2R in either plasma or urine are commercially available. IL-2 and IL-2R levels increase in response to rejection phenomena in transplant patients, and often precede other clinically evident measures of rejection (29).

In vitro and in vivo induction of tumor cytotoxicity by IL-2 have been studied by quantitating the levels of IFN_{γ} and TNF. Biotherapy assessment monitoring theorizes that an efficacious tumor cytotoxicity response requires normal IL-2 receptors and blastogenic responses (37). If an adequate response cannot be elicited in vitro, it is unlikely that an in vivo response will be observed. If studies support theories, monitoring cytokine responses may have a significant impact on therapeutic approaches in cancer and autoimmune diseases (particularly diabetes) as well as determining interventions necessary to overcome septic shock (38).

Cytokines were originally characterized by functional studies that detected activities in culture supernatants after certain stimuli. It took nearly a decade of study by many investigators to purify and characterize each of those activities and to synthesize recombinant forms of each cytokine. Subsequent studies with these synthetic cytokines began to demonstrate that certain combinations of cytokines were synergistic, while other combinations were antagonistic. Such studies performed in vitro as well as in inbred strains of mice are very illuminating and have helped to explain the role(s) of each cytokine. Elucidating the biological activities of the cytokines provides scientific evidence for their use as therapeutic agents in treating disease states. However, there are a multitude of other forces present in humans in vivo that have not yet been discovered, which regulate the immune responsiveness to disease states.

INTERPRETATION

Clinical Relevance of Leukocyte Abnormalities to Inflammation

LEUKOPENIAS

Most viral and rickettsial infections and certain bacterial infections cause neutropenia rather than neutrophilia. *Salmonella* infections cause a transient neutrophilia, followed by neutropenia during the bacteremic phase. Neutropenia is also found in brucellosis and tularemia. Viral and rickettsial infections cause leukopenias lasting 4 to 5 days, the duration of the viremia or rickettsemia. Myelopathic viruses (influenza, dengue fever) can also disrupt cytokinesis, leading to temporary myelosuppression (39).

Death from the severe neutropenia of overwhelming infections is most common in neonates, alcoholics, therapeutically immunosuppressed patients, immunodeficient patients, and AIDS patients. With prolonged viremias, sustained bacteremias, disseminated mycobacteremias, etc., neutrophil reserves are depleted and the production of new cells by the marrow cannot keep pace with their destruction in circulation.

LEUKEMIAS

Neoplastic proliferation of leukemic cells (acute or chronic; myelocytic or lymphocytic) leads to accumulation of incompetent, long-lived cells that eventually replace and repress normal cells (39). This results in overproduction of defective leukocytes and underproduction of normal leukocytes that participate in defending the body from invasion by pathogens. Therapeutic interventions (chemotherapy or bone marrow transplant) serve to destroy any remaining normal cells, leaving the leukemic patient extremely vulnerable to overwhelming or opportunistic infections. Treatment of such infections with broad-spectrum antibiotics or with antiviral or antifungal agents adds yet another dimension of toxicity to the already compromised patient.

FUNCTIONAL ANOMALIES

Hereditary leukocyte anomalies can be fatal to neonates or can cause lifelong increased susceptibility to infections. All leukocyte anomalies involve neutrophils, and all predispose to potentially lethal pyogenic infections (24). Treatment with antibiotics (either symptomatically or prophylactically) provides temporary control of bacterial infections, but leads to the development of antibiotic-resistant flora. Bone marrow transplantation from an HLA-identical sibling is the only rational treatment for children with any of the leukocyte anomalies to ensure any semblance of normal life.

Abnormalities of Humoral Mediators of Inflammation

CRP AND ESR IN DISEASE

CRP levels in hospitalized patients were studied by Morley and Kushner (40). Sera obtained on the day of hospital admission showed 69% had CRP levels in the normal range (less than 10 mg/liter). Only 9% of the sera tested had markedly elevated CRP levels (greater than 100 mg/liter). Uncomplicated conditions associated with marked CRP elevations included septic arthritis, bacterial meningitis, bacterial pneumonia, septicemia, deep-vein thrombophlebitis, pyelonephritis, and cellulitis. Moderate CRP elevations (greater than 10 but less than 100 mg/liter) were seen in patients with connective tissue diseases, malignancies, pancreatitis, alcoholic hepatitis, and acute cardiopulmonary disease. Conditions in which quantitative CRP levels were of substantial diagnostic value included detecting superimposed infections in SLE, leukemia, and other malignancies; neonatal or congenital infections; infections following premature rupture of membranes; and discriminating pyelonephritis from cystitis in children.

Various other investigators have found quantitative CRP levels of value in diagnosing or monitoring specific disease processes (41). Measurement of spinal fluid CRP levels has been shown to be sensitive and specific for differentiating bacterial meningitis (high CSF CRP levels) from viral meningitis (low CSF CRP levels), enabling efficient therapeutic intervention. Serum CRP levels have been used to differentiate patients with bacteremia from those with contaminated blood cultures; to monitor treatment of infective endocarditis; to monitor spinal cord–injured patients for earlier detection of urinary tract infections; to differentiate bacterial pneumonia from acute bronchitis; and to monitor for postoperative infections (especially deep-seated infections associated with complicated orthopaedic surgeries).

CRP increases more rapidly and decreases sooner with resolution of the infectious process than does the ESR (Fig. 59.3). CRP quantitation is most valuable as an early indicator of an acute disease process. ESR is a better indicator of chronic inflammatory processes. In most connective tissue diseases, both ESR and CRP are elevated on presentation. One notable exception is SLE, where even in active disease, CRP levels are not remarkable unless there is a superimposed bacterial infection (25). One possible explanation for this dichotomy is that CRP binds to DNA chromatin (42) and may be effectively removed from circulation as circulating CRP-chromatin complexes that activate complement and are phagocytosed.

COMPLEMENT LEVELS IN DISEASE

Elevated levels of complement components are of no diagnostic or prognostic significance. C1q levels tend to mimic γ-globulin levels; i.e., patients with hypergammaglobulinemia have elevated levels of C1q. C3 and several other complement components are acute phase reactants, increasing by 50% during inflammation. However, C4 does not show significantly increased levels during the acute phase and is more stable in the absence of classical pathway activation. The primary significance of elevated complement levels, quantitative or functional, is to establish a "patient-specific normal range" by which to assess complement activation during active stages of diseases such as SLE. The reference range for C3 is very wide (800 to 1600 mg/liter). Since those levels increase by 50% during an acute phase reaction, it would take *significant* amounts of activation and consumption of C3 to detect a decreased level compared with the established reference range.

Decreased levels of complement components and/or hemolytic activity are highly clinically significant. Table 59.1 lists the diseases associated with the decreased or normal patterns of reactivity seen in mild classical pathway activation, significant classical pathway activation, alternative pathway activation, and defective hemolytic function. Most complement components are present in excess of what is required to achieve the endpoint of indicator cell lysis. Exceptions are C2, C4, and factor D. Measurable hemolytic activity will be mildly impaired (50% of normal) if any of these components is present in decreased amounts. Hemolytic activity will be severely impaired (less than 10% of normal) if any component is homozygously deficient.

Table 59.1. Examples of Complement Activation

↓ CH_{50}, ↓ C3, ↓ C4
Classical Pathway Activation
Active SLE
Serum sickness
Immune complex disease
Chronic active hepatitis
Subacute bacterial endocarditis
↓ CH_{50}, ↓ C3, Normal C4
Alternate Pathway Activation
Acute streptococcal glomerulonephritis
Membranoproliferative glomerulonephritis
Severe bacteremia
C3 nephritic factor
C3, H, or I deficiency
↓ to Normal CH_{50}, Normal C3, ↓ C4
Mild Classical Pathway Activation
Cryoglobulinemia
Vasculitis
C1Inh deficiency
C4 deficiency
↓ CH_{50}, Normal C3, Normal C4
Defective Hemolytic Function
Improperly handled sera
Coagulation-associated depletion
Component deficiency (e.g., C2, C5–C8)

CIRCULATING IMMUNE COMPLEXES

Although many diseases are known to be caused or exacerbated by circulating or deposited immune complexes, detection of CICs by existing assays that detect CICs in serum are so variable and technique dependent as to be considered unreliable. If cryoglobulin is present, serial studies of the amount present in sequential samples can be used to monitor responses to therapy. This is particularly useful in essential mixed cryoglobulinemia, which responds to plasmapheresis or immunosuppression. Diseases that undoubtedly have CICs, but not cryoglobulins, are best monitored by C3 and C4 levels to detect changes in disease activity. Relatively low levels of CICs will rapidly deplete C4 from circulation, but C3 levels may be within the reference range due to the acute-phase responsiveness of C3. When both C3 and C4 are decreased, the feedback loop that initiates the alternative pathway has also been activated, resulting in more dramatic consumption of C3 as well as classical pathway consumption of C4. This can be interpreted as very active CIC-mediated disease unless some other explanation for the depletion of these complement components is present.

INTERRELATIONSHIPS OF CYTOKINES

The pathways of T- and B-cell activation and proliferation that are mediated by various cytokines are

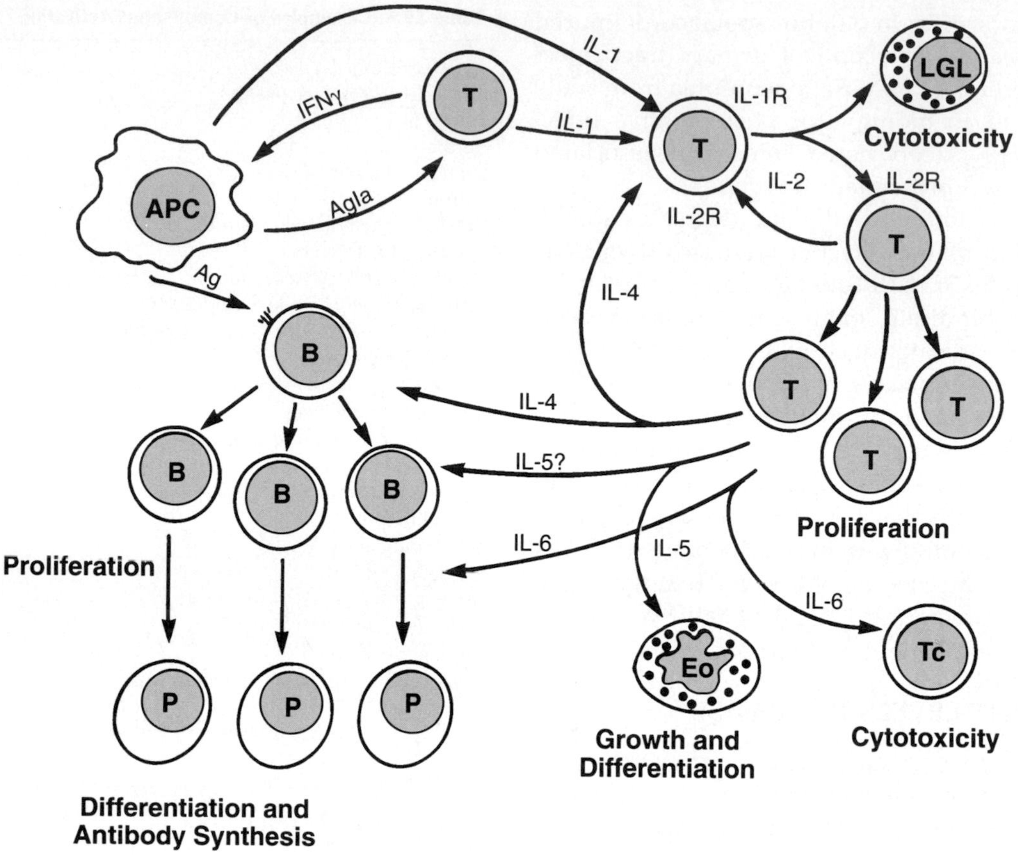

Figure 59.4. Cytokine pathways.

illustrated in Figure 59.4. These molecules exhibit autocrine-like function, stimulating the production of other cytokines in specific sequences. The mechanisms of action of cytokines on various cell types have been elucidated in vitro. The biological consequences of certain interleukins (e.g., IL-2) have been demonstrated in vivo as well as in culture. The control mechanisms are not yet well understood, but as they are revealed, cytokines will become very important in the treatment of malignancies, autoimmune diseases, and immunodeficiency states.

References

1. Gleich GJ, Adolphson CR. The eosinophilic leukocyte: structure and function. Adv Immunol 1986;177–254.
2. Lee TH, Austen R. Arachidonic acid metabolism by the 5-lipogenase pathway, and the effects of alternative dietary fatty acids. Adv Immunol 1986;39:145–175.
3. Kishimoto TK, Larson RS, Corbi AL, Dustin ML, Staunton DE, Springer TA. The leukocyte integrins. Adv Immunol 1989;46:149–182.
4. Ritz J, Schmidt RE, Michon J, Hercend T, Schlossman SF. Characterization of functional surface structures on human natural killer cells. Adv Immunol 1988;42:181–211.
5. Tillett W, Francis T. Serological reactions in pneumonia with nonprotein somatic fraction of pneumococcus. J Exp Med 1930;52:561–571.
6. James K, Baum L, Adamowski C, Gewurz H. C-reactive protein antigenicity on the surface of human lymphocytes. J Immunol 1983;131:2930–2934.
7. Deodhar SD, James K, Chiang T, et al. Inhibition of lung metastases in mice bearing a malignant fibrosarcoma by treatment with liposomes containing human C-reactive protein. Cancer Res 1982;42:5084–5088.
8. Jandl JH. Blood and bloodforming tissues. In: Blood. Boston: Little, Brown, 1987:1–48.
9. James K. Complement: activation, consequences, and control. Am J Med Technol 1982;48:735–742.
10. Pangburn MK, Schreiber RD, Muller-Eberhard HJ. Formation of the initial C3 convertase of the alternative complement pathway: acquisition of the C3b-like activities of spontaneous hydrolysis of the putative thioester in native C3. J Exp Med 1981;154:856–867.
11. Figueroa JE, Denson P. Infectious diseases associated with complement deficiencies. Clin Microbiol Rev 1991;4:359–395.
12. Davis AE, Ziegler JB, Gelf EW, et al. Heterogeneity of nephritic factor and its identification as an immunoglobulin. Proc Natl Acad Sci USA 1977;74:3980–3983.
13. Beckmann E. Cytokines in infectious disease. Clin Microbiol Newsl 1992;14:73–78.
14. Dinarello CA. Interleukin-1 and its biologically related cytokines. Adv Immunol 1989;44:153–205.
15. Mizel SB. The interleukins. FASEB J 1989;3:2379–2388.
16. Welch PA, Namen AE, Goodwin RG, Armitage R, Cooper MD. Human IL-7; a novel T cell growth factor. J Immunol 1989;143:3562–3567.
17. Stern AS, Podlaski FJ, Hulmes JD, et al. Purification to homogeneity and partial characterization of cytotoxic lymphocyte

maturation factor from human B-lymphoblastoid cells. Proc Natl Acad Sci USA 1990;6808–6812.
18. Koren HS. Proposed classification of leukocyte-associated cytolytic molecules. Immunol Today 1987;8:69–71.
19. Miyajima A, Miyatake S, Schreurs J, et al. Coordinate regulation of immune and inflammatory responses by T cell-derived lymphokines. FASEB J 1988;2:2462–2473.
20. Beutler B, Cerami A. The common mediator of shock, cachexia and tumor necrosis. Adv Immunol 1988;42:213–231.
21. Ruddle NH. Tumor necrosis factor and related cytotoxins. Immunol Today 1987;8:129–130.
22. Sherertz RJ. Management of infections in the burn patient. In: Salisbury RE, Newman NM, Dingeldein GP, eds. Manual of burn therapeutics. Boston: Little, Brown, 1983.
23. MacDermott RP, Stenson WF. Alterations in the immune system in ulcerative colitis and Crohn's disease. Adv Immunol 1988;42:285–328.
24. Jandl JH. Leukocyte anomalies. In: Jandl JH, ed. Blood. Boston: Little, Brown and Company 1987;571–588.
25. DaSilva PJA, Elkon KB, Hughes GR, Dyck RF, Pepys MB. C-reactive protein levels in systemic lupus erythematosus: a classification criterion? Arthritis Rheum 1980;23:770–771.
26. Alper CA, Rosen FS. Inherited deficiencies of complement proteins in man. Springer Semin Immunopathol 1984;7:251–261.
27. Harris RL, Musher DM, Bloom K, et al. Manifestations of sepsis. Arch Intern Med 1987;147:1895–1906.
28. Jablons DM, Mule JJ, McIntosh JK, et al. IL-6/IFN$_{\beta}$2 as a circulating hormone. Induction by cytokine administration in humans. J Immunol 1989;142:1542–1547.
29. Cornaby A, Simpson M, Madras P, Dempsey R, Clowes GHA, Monaco A. Pre-operative interleukin-2 and interleukin-2 receptor levels may predict subsequent renal allograft rejection. Transplan Proc 1989;21:1861–1862.
30. Campen DH, Horwitz DA, Quismorio FP, Ehresmann GP, Martin WJ. Serum levels of interleukin-2 receptor and activity of rheumatic diseases characterized by immune system activation. Arthritis Rheum 1988;31:1358–1364.
31. Tan EM. Antinuclear antibodies: diagnostic markers for autoimmune diseases and probes for cell biology. Adv Immunol 1989;44:93–151.
32. Richerson HB. Hypersensitivity pneumonitis: pathology and pathogenesis. Clin Rev Allergy 1983;1:469–486.
33. Trinchieri G. Biology of natural killer cells. Adv Immunol 1989;47:187–376.
34. Inai S, Kitamura H, Fujita T, et al. Differences between plasma and serum components in patients with chronic liver disease. Clin Exp Immunol 1976;25:403–409.
35. Lambert PH, Dixon FJ, Zubler RH, et al. A WHO collaborative study for the evaluation of eighteen methods for detecting immune complexes in serum. Clin Lab Immunol 1978;1:1–15.
36. James K, Vahey A, Robinson M, Marder R. A solid phase C1q enzyme assay for circulating immune complexes adapted for routine clinical laboratory testing. Am J Clin Pathol 1983;80:445–452.
37. O'Connor T, Castracane J, Lackey A, et al. Biotherapy assessment monitoring (BAM) in cancer therapy [Abstract]. 2nd Int'l Workshop on Cytokines, 1989.
38. Waage A, Halstensen A, Espevik T. Association between tumour necrosis factor in serum and fatal outcome in patients with meningococcal disease. Lancet 1987;1:355–357.
39. Jandl JH. Granulocytes. In: Jandl JH, ed. Blood. Boston: Little, Brown, 1987;441–471.
40. Morley JJ, Kushner I. Serum C-reactive protein levels in disease. Ann NY Acad Sci 1982;389:406–418.
41. James K. Immunoserology of infectious diseases. Clin Microbiol Rev 1990;3:135–152.
42. Robey FA, Jones KD, Tanaka T, Liu TY. Binding of C-reactive protein to chromatin and nucleosome core particles. J Biol Chem 1984;259:7311–7316.

60 Monoclonal Gammopathies

David F. Keren

A monoclonal gammopathy is the protein product of a single clone of plasma cells. Although the term "monoclonal gammopathy" has been often used to designate the proteins produced by the malignant cells in multiple myeloma and other B-cell lymphoproliferative lesions, such as Waldenström's macroglobulinemia, a monoclonal gammopathy may also be the product of a "regulated" cell. Patients with profound infections or considerable polyclonal autoimmune stimulation often have marked expansion of one or a few (oligo-) clones. When one clone predominates, a picture resembling a monoclonal gammopathy from a B-cell lymphoproliferative lesion may result. Thus, the presence of a monoclonal component alone does not indicate that a neoplastic process is present. Factors to consider when evaluating a monoclonal component include the quantity of the component, the fluid in which it is found (serum versus urine), and the chemical type of the component (light chains will more likely be found in the urine than in the serum). The term "M" component is used in the literature to describe the monoclonal gammopathy. It has been variously used for "monoclonal protein, myeloma protein, and macroglobulin protein" (1–3).

The clinical investigator must be able to detect even small monoclonal gammopathies. Formerly, small monoclonal gammopathies were not thought to be of clinical significance. Indeed, as discussed below, most monoclonal gammopathies less than 1000 mg/dl, are part of the monoclonal gammopathy of undetermined significance (MGUS) category. However, some of them represent the products of B-cell lymphoproliferative lesions such as chronic lymphocytic leukemia and well-differentiated lymphocytic lymphoma. Conditions often overlooked when a quantitatively small monoclonal component is detected include amyloidosis, peripheral neuropathies, and nonsecreting, or, more correctly, hyposecreting myeloma.

This chapter reviews the major disease states that result in the production of a monoclonal gammopathy. The methodologies for detecting them are evaluated and a strategy for assessing monoclonal proteins is given.

DISEASE STATES

Myeloma

Multiple myeloma is the most common malignant cause for the presence of a monoclonal gammopathy in serum or urine. This disease is due to a malignant proliferation of a clone of B lymphocytes that manifests predominantly as plasma cells. Note that multiple myeloma is often considered to be a condition of malignant plasma cells. In fact, the malignancy involves the entire B-cell lineage but manifests mainly as malignant plasma cells. When one examines the bone marrow from individuals with multiple myeloma, pre-B cells with the same idiotype as the monoclonal protein can be found. Usually, patients with multiple myeloma present with involvement of the bone marrow. The plasma cells synthesize and secrete large quantities of the monoclonal whole immunoglobulin. These plasma cells are like inefficient factories because they often produce excessive numbers of monoclonal free light chains (Bence Jones protein). Patients with multiple myeloma present with a wide variety of clinical symptoms. Bone pain is often a presenting feature because the bone marrow involvement creates lytic lesions in the ribs, vertebrae, skull, and long bones. The plasma cells produce an osteoclast-activating factor that results in recruitment of osteoclasts that dissolve the bone in these locations. Due to the destruction of the bony elements, these individuals may present with a so-called pathological fracture. These are fractures of bones resulting from relatively trivial trauma. As the cortex is weakened by the lytic lesions, it is more susceptible to breakage (4–6).

Patients with multiple myeloma also present with infectious diseases. This results from a marked suppression of the production of polyclonal immunoglobulins in these individuals. When one examines the serum protein electrophoresis, one usually finds a large "M spike" in the γ or the β region. Note, however, that a spike may occur anywhere from the α region through the γ region in monoclonal gammopathy. In multiple myeloma, the normal production of γ-globulin is suppressed so that the background of normal antibodies is markedly decreased. As a result, many patients with multiple myeloma suffer from pyogenetic bacterial infections that are normally defended by opsonizing immunoglobulins.

Other myeloma patients present with weakness due to anemia. The anemia tends to develop later in the course of the disease and is relatively nonspecific. However, examination of the peripheral blood from patients with multiple myeloma may show a blue hazy background due to the excessive amount of protein present in the serum. Other key laboratory parameters in these individuals include rouleaux formation, an increase in the serum alkaline phosphatase, and calcium due to the destruction of bone. Note that the elevated calcium usually appears relatively late in the course of this disease. Early on, one will usually not find evidence of hypercalcemia.

The excessive production of free light chains (Bence Jones protein) in these patients appears mainly in the urine. Where they occur depends on their structure. The light chains may be present as monomers, dimers, or tetramers. The monomers are small molecular weight (22,000 daltons) and are readily passed through the glomerular basement membrane into the urine. Dimers weigh approximately 44,000 daltons and pass into the glomerular filtrate less readily than monomers. Therefore, patients with dimers may have a small spike in the serum and most of the Bence Jones protein in the urine. Lastly, patients with tetramers will have virtually no Bence Jones protein in the urine, while a spike is seen in the serum. This is because the weight of the tetramer is too great to pass through a normal glomerular basement membrane. The finding of Bence Jones proteins is clinically significant for the patient. Individuals with large amounts of Bence Jones proteins tend to do worse clinically than individuals who lack Bence Jones proteins. The main reason for this is that the Bence Jones proteins are reabsorbed by the proximal convoluted tubules in the kidneys. There, depending on their immunochemical makeup, they may damage the proximal tubules. Significant damage may occur and produce myeloma kidney. In this, the proximal tubule cells form syncytia, and casts consisting of monoclonal protein are found within the tubule lumen. Renal failure is an uncommon but real cause of demise in some patients with multiple myeloma (7–14).

The classification of multiple myeloma is not merely based on finding a monoclonal protein in serum. Indeed, some investigators worry that they may not be able to detect every possible case of monoclonal gammopathy no matter how extensive a screening program they set up. Clearly, there are cases of nonsecreting or hyposecreting myelomas that will be missed. There are other unusual cases of myeloma in which a relatively small amount of the monoclonal protein is produced and hides under a normal β region component such as transferrin (simulating an iron-deficiency anemia pattern) or under C3 (simulating a subacute inflammatory response pattern). The laboratorian must be aware that serum protein electrophoresis, though an excellent screening method, is not the only criterion used for the diagnosis of multiple myeloma. These individuals need to be assessed by virtue of their clinical symptoms (bone pain, anemia, infectious disease problems, renal disease, neuropathies, etc.) (6, 15).

Some unusual variants of multiple myeloma may be more difficult to diagnose. One of these is POEMS syndrome. This stands for the 5 to 7% of cases of multiple myeloma that present mainly with a peripheral neuropathy, organomegaly (mainly the liver and spleen), endocrinopathy (often thyroid dysfunction or diabetes mellitus), monoclonal gammopathy, and skin lesions (usually increased skin pigmentation). These individuals have the interesting skeletal findings of osteosclerotic lesions rather than the usual osteolytic lesions. Note that both osteosclerotic and osteolytic lesions may be present simultaneously. Sometimes, multiple myeloma may be present with amyloidosis (amyloid AL) (16–18).

IMMUNOGLOBULIN ISOTYPES IN MULTIPLE MYELOMA

The isotypes of immunoglobulins seen in multiple myeloma largely reflect their prevalence in normal serum. IgG myeloma proteins predominate. They are almost always monomers weighing 160,000 daltons. It is rare that IgG myeloma proteins produce significant problems with hyperviscosity (see Waldenström's Macroglobulinemia, below). IgE myeloma is extremely rare and can occur as monomers or as polymers with variable molecular weight. Since IgE molecules tend to self-aggregate, they, like IgM, may cause problems with hyperviscosity symptoms. IgA myeloma may be difficult to diagnose on occasion because IgA tends to migrate in the β region. Therefore, early in its course, the IgA myeloma may be masked by the other β region bands. C3, transferrin, or fibrinogen from an inadequately clotted sample of blood or an inadvertently examined sample of plasma may obscure the presence of an IgA myeloma band. Also, IgA myeloma bands tend to be more diffuse due to the heavy glycosylation of IgA myeloma proteins. The IgD myelomas are quite uncommon, representing about 1% of the total cases of multiple myeloma. The light chain types usually reflect the percentage of κ and λ present in the serum. Two-thirds of IgG and IgA myelomas are of the κ light chain type and one-third are of the λ type. However, a marked exception occurs with IgD myeloma, for which the ratio of κ to λ chains is 1:9.

Although some anecdotal reports have illustrated minor differences in clinical course if one has κ as opposed to λ light chains, no significant difference has been documented in more extensive studies. Therefore, the typing of light chains is merely useful for classifying the patients but does not alter the prognosis.

IgD myelomas may also be missed because the amount of monoclonal component may be relatively small (19). If one is using the older five-band electrophoresis techniques, the small IgD component may be hidden by a normal α_2 or β region band. Also, as discussed later, when quantification is performed by radial immunodiffusion plates, at least two dilutions of the patient's serum must be performed to avoid antigen excess. In antigen excess, the ring of precipitation may be so small that it would go unnoticed or be washed away.

It is uncommon for multiple myeloma to occur with IgM. That is not to say that it does not occur. Sometimes one can reach that incorrect conclusion from the literature. However, only a handful of cases of multiple myeloma with IgM have been reported. This is because patients with IgM monoclonal gammopathies usually have a different clinical disease called Waldenström's macroglobulinemia. This author has seen only rare examples of multiple myeloma with IgM. One of them was a defective IgM product that contained only the CH1 and variable portion of the IgM chain together with a single light chain. It appeared mainly in the patient's urine. It is important to expect such unusual events, but overall, IgM myeloma is about as rare as IgE myeloma (20).

Heavy chain disease (usually α chain disease) is extremely uncommon in the western world. In the Middle East and Mediterranean regions, an unusual disease called α heavy chain disease occurs. The tissue distribution of the plasma cells in this lesion roughly parallels that for the normal distribution of IgA along the gastrointestinal tract and other mucosal surfaces. This disease is different from multiple myeloma. In this condition, the individuals usually have a slow progression of their disease during the early phase. Cures have been reported with antibiotic treatment at this stage. Also, the disease is particularly difficult to diagnose in the clinical laboratory. Often, serum samples do not show obvious abnormal bands on serum protein electrophoresis, although one may find a rather broad band in the β region. Since no reaction is seen with the light chain antisera, the assumption is often made that a monoclonal gammopathy is not present. Note that with IgA myeloma, light chains are often difficult to demonstrate. A technique termed immunoselection has been used to assist in this diagnosis. In this technique, antibodies against light chains are mixed into the agarose (similar to setting up a radial immunodiffusion). Then, a standard immunoelectrophoresis is carried out. Since intact immunoglobulin molecules contain either κ or λ light chains, they must precipitate with the anti-κ and anti-λ in the sample well. The only molecules to migrate from the well will be immunoglobulins that do not contain light chains (hence the α chain disease molecule). The distance from the well correlates with this concentration. Another way to determine α chain disease is always to quantify IgG, IgA, IgM, and κ and λ by nephelometry and to perform serum protein electrophoresis simultaneously. Patients with α chain disease will have increased concentrations of IgA. By subtracting the sum of the κ and λ-containing immunoglobulins from the IgG + IgA + IgM, a relatively large positive number would be obtained (normally the number should be near zero). This is because the excess α chains do not have corresponding light chains. Therefore, one would suspect the possibility of heavy chain disease from this calculation and perform an immunoselection. The diagnosis of α chain disease is likely to be missed in the western world because these cases are so rare that immunoselection technique is not a standard procedure in clinical laboratories in this country (20).

An uncommon form of heavy chain disease is Franklin's disease (γ heavy chain disease). This uncommon disease has symptoms that are reminiscent of lymphoma. The patients present with a generalized lymphadenopathy, hepatosplenomegaly, pleural effusions, and ascites. Similar to α chain disease, an immunoselection method may be optimal to confirm this diagnosis (20).

Biclonal gammopathies can be somewhat confusing. These conditions have expansion of two B lymphocyte clones rather than one. Actually, there is no special significance to this finding. Individuals who clinically have multiple myeloma have no different disease process if they have one clone or two clones. To confirm a true biclonal gammopathy, one must either demonstrate two different light chain types, which are by definition two distinct clones, or do DNA rearrangement studies to document this distinction. If one has two bonds with the same light chain, DNA studies would be the only way to determine if they were from one clone or two. Since there is no clinical significance to making this determination, it is not cost-effective. About 5% of patients with monoclonal gammopathies have a biclonal gammopathy pattern. Note that the presence of two different heavy chain types with the same light chain type does not necessarily imply a biclonal gammopathy. During maturation of B lymphocytes, there is often a stage at which a switch occurs from one heavy chain isotype to another. That is why some B lymphocytes will have both a μ chain and an α or γ chain simultaneously on their surface membrane. Therefore, the finding of two different heavy chain types with the same light chain isotype does not establish the existence of a biclonal gammopathy. As mentioned earlier, however, making the distinction is of no clinical significance (20).

Lastly, some patients with multiple myeloma present with profound hypogammaglobulinemia. Although there have been several theories as to why this profound hypogammaglobulinemia often occurs in multiple myeloma, the pathogenesis is still uncertain. Further, not all individuals with multiple myeloma will present with a hypogammaglobulinemia. Some studies have shown that peripheral blood lymphocytes from patients with multiple myeloma have a poor response to B-cell mitogens. In other studies, a marked decrease has been found in the number of normal peripheral blood B lymphocytes in patients with multiple myeloma. This implies the existence of some sort of suppressive influence on B lymphocyte maturation. However, it has not been clearly demonstrated that suppressor T lymphocytes are the cause of this change. An increase in the number of circulating T helper cells with the suppressor-inducer phenotype (CD4+, CD45R+) has been described. Patients with multiple myeloma also have an increase in the T helper cells that have the immunoglobulin-secreting helper capacity phenotype (CD4+, CD45R−). Clearly, the two helper and suppressor cells can function to effect the immunoglobulin containing cells in these patients. Patients with T helper lymphomas, for instance, will often have a polyclonal increase in γ-globulins. However, one must be careful to avoid oversimplification with these functions. For example, in individuals with acquired immunodeficiency syndrome (AIDS) the T helper (CD4+) lymphocytes have been destroyed by infection with human immunodeficiency virus (HIV). Yet a polyclonal immunoglobulin increase is consistently found in the serum of these patients. In summary, the cause of the decreased T lymphocyte helper and increased T lymphocyte suppressor function in patients with multiple myeloma remains unknown at present (20–22).

WALDENSTRÖM'S MACROGLOBULINEMIA

Patients with Waldenström's macroglobulinemia suffer from complications of hyperviscosity due to the presence of large amounts of circulating IgM. IgM almost always circulates as a pentamer (19S). Therefore, when one develops a monoclonal proliferation of cells producing IgM, the increased concentration of large proteins in the blood disturbs the normal circulation hemodynamics, resulting in the hyperviscosity syndrome. This causes a variety of neurologic complaints, cardiac insufficiency, and vascular insufficiency throughout the body. In addition to the hyperviscosity syndrome, Waldenström's macroglobulinemia differs from multiple myeloma in other respects. These patients do not develop the lytic skeletal lesions seen in multiple myeloma. They do tend to present with symptoms of weakness and fatigue because of the combination of hyperviscosity and anemia. Clinically, these patients have a more protracted course than individuals with multiple myeloma. Usually, an IgM level of greater than 20 g/liter is needed to produce the hyperviscosity syndrome. Keep in mind that IgM is not the only immunoglobulin that will produce the hyperviscosity syndrome. On occasion, IgA will also produce a hyperviscosity syndrome when secreted in large amounts. This is because IgA tends to self-aggregate and IgA can occur in serum as a multimer. IgG has rarely been reported to cause a hyperviscosity syndrome, and this author has seen one case of hyperviscosity syndrome due to κ light chain disease (20, 23).

The clinical laboratory can provide several supportive bits of information for this clinical diagnosis. On examination of the peripheral smear, rouleaux formation is characteristic of this disease. It is not pathognomonic for this condition, as it may also be seen in multiple myeloma. The bone marrow shows an infiltration by lymphoplasmacytoid cells. If one performs immunohistochemical examination, the cells would contain the monoclonal IgM component. Obviously, the serum viscosity is usually increased in these patients. Serum protein electrophoresis is an excellent screening test for this condition. The usual case of Waldenström's macroglobulinemia will show a monoclonal spike that is located close to the origin. Although this is not requisite, the bulky nature of the molecule together with the relative lack of charge at the pH 8.6 normally used for serum protein electrophoresis causes the IgM gammopathy to linger near the origin. Quantification of immunoglobulins discloses large amounts of IgM, usually greater than 20 g/liter, and normal amounts of IgG and IgA. The gammopathy can usually be identified by measuring IgG, IgA, IgM, κ and λ by nephelometry together with high-resolution electrophoresis. In occasional cases, however, it may be necessary to perform immunofixation or immunoelectrophoresis to confirm the diagnosis. Immunoelectrophoresis is a poor technique to identify these molecules since the large IgM molecule migrates poorly through the agarose, making it difficult to determine the κ and λ type. Immunofixation is preferred for this procedure (24, 25).

MONOCLONAL GAMMOPATHY OF UNDETERMINED SIGNIFICANCE

In older textbooks, the term for this section would have been "benign monoclonal gammopathies." That name is incorrect. The term benign implies that we can predict the biological behavior of the neoplasm. In pathology this means that a benign lesion will not invade further nor metastasize with potentially lethal consequences. We cannot make such a confident statement about a monoclonal gammopathy that we identify in the serum. Kyle correctly coined the term monoclonal gammopathy of undetermined significance (MGUS) to categorize these individuals until we have a better understanding of the significance of the lesions that we detect. A restricted band on serum protein electrophoresis in the γ region that is identified by immunofixation, immunoelectrophoresis, or κ and λ quantification as a monoclonal gammopathy implies that it has been the product of a single clone of plasma cells. This is correct. However, the nature (benign versus malignant) of those plasma cells and their B-lymphocyte precursors cannot be inferred from the presence of the gammopathy. Even relatively large gammopathies, up to 3000 mg/dl, may represent a product of a benign lymphoplasmacytic lesion, while some cases of multiple myeloma will produce tiny or undetectable amounts of monoclonal component (2).

In his series, Kyle found that 70% of patients with monoclonal gammopathy had MGUS as their working diagnosis. By this term, he referred to individuals who have a monoclonal component demonstrated in the serum, but who lack other key features for diagnosing a malignant monoclonal gammopathy. These patients are not anemic, they do not have lytic lesions, they do not have elevated serum calcium or serum enzymes. They do not have a prominent plasmacytosis in the bone marrow, although they may have as many as 10% plasma cells in the bone marrow. About 20% of patients with MGUS over a 10-year period will progress to develop a malignant B-cell lymphoproliferative lesion, usually multiple myeloma. Some of the other cases will develop into chronic lymphocytic leukemia, well-differentiated lymphocytic lymphoma, amyloidosis, and rarely other forms of B-cell proliferative lesions. The vast majority of patients with MGUS do not develop any other overt clinical process (2).

The majority of patients with MGUS do not have a distinctive pathological process that can be detected. Obviously, somewhere in their bodies they harbor a clone producing this gammopathy. Some may merely represent a response to a particular infection. Others may be part of an autoimmune process in which one clone against the autoantigen predominates. In many other cases, however, we have no idea if the clone is being driven by some antigen or whether it is a self-driven, neoplastic clone.

MGUS patients have quantities of monoclonal component that range from as little as 300 mg/dl to greater than 3000 mg/dl. Some of these patients have suppression of their normal immunoglobulin synthesis as shown by decrease in the normal γ-globulin component by serum protein electrophoresis. This feature alone, however, does not portend a negative prognosis. Usually, these patients do not have significant amounts of Bence Jones protein, although small amounts may be detected. Therefore, in any patients having a monoclonal gammopathy detected in serum in our laboratory, we routinely recommend that a urine sample be obtained to detect Bence Jones protein. We believe that currently, the most sensitive technique for this determination is a combination of serum protein electrophoresis and immunofixation. We also recommend that the clinician follow this patient with a serum protein electrophoresis every 6 to 12 months to determine if the process is evolving or regressing. Of course, routine hematologic and chemical analysis should be performed. If these are in the normal range, and there are no clinical symptoms of bone pain, further studies such as bone marrow examination are probably useless (2, 25a, 26).

B-CELL NEOPLASMS

A variety of B-cell neoplasms have been associated with monoclonal gammopathies. These neoplasms are discussed in detail elsewhere in this text. However, it is useful to note their association with monoclonal gammopathies, as they may provide the clinician with further evidence to do more aggressive, invasive diagnostic procedures. It used to be thought that monoclonal gammopathies were rare in cases of chronic lymphocytic leukemia or well-differentiated lymphocytic lymphoma. In fact, the majority of these patients have a monoclonal gammopathy in either their serum or their urine when high-resolution electrophoresis and immunofixation are combined to study these samples. Monoclonal gammopathies have also been demonstrated in patients with Burkitt's lymphoma and B-cell ALL. Clearly, serum protein electrophoresis is not the ideal way to diagnose these conditions. Nevertheless, the finding of a monoclonal band in the serum or urine of a patient with malaise and lymphadenopathy with splenomegaly, for example, might prompt the clinician to perform a lymph node biopsy (19, 27, 28).

AMYLOIDOSIS

About 4% patients with plasma cell proliferation will have amyloid deposition in their tissues. There are two major biochemical types of amyloid. One consists of an immunoglobulin light chain and is termed AL. The second is composed of protein A and is termed AA. AA is probably a breakdown product of the much larger normal serum molecule amyloid A-related protein. When either type of amyloid deposits in tissues, a dysfunction of the involved organs occurs, depending on the location of the amyloid deposits. For instance, in patients with AL amyloid, there is frequently deposition in the heart, gastrointestinal tract, tongue, blood vessels, tendon, skin, and peripheral nerves. The clinical picture that these individuals present with depends on which site is involved. For example, patients with amyloid deposition primarily in the tongue will present with macroglossia. Those who have deposition within the heart will present with symptoms of congestive heart failure.

Patients with amyloidosis and monoclonal gammopathy usually do not have bone pain or osteolytic lesions. They may be biopsied in the rectum, or in the involved site to determine the presence of amyloid. Tissues with extensive involvement of amyloid stain dark blue with iodine, hence the term amyloid (meaning starch-like). The definitive diagnosis of amyloidosis requires positive staining with Congo red, giving a characteristic blue-green birefringence when polarized light is used. These tinctorial qualities relate to the structural β-pleated sheet formation that occurs with either AL or AA. Monoclonal gammopathies may be found in both the serum and urine of patients with amyloidosis (18, 20).

Methodologies

IMMUNOLOGIC REACTION IN GEL DIFFUSION

The classic precipitation reaction is the basis for immunofixation and immunoelectrophoresis. As discussed earlier in this section, antibody-antigen interactions are highly concentration dependent. Therefore, when an antibody is placed in one well and diffuses toward the antigen placed in another well, a precipitation reaction occurs somewhere between the two wells. The distance from the well where the band forms depends upon the concentration and the size of the reactants. When the antigen and antibody are of approximately equal size and concentration, the band will occur midway between the two wells. These reactions are highly specific and are therefore, useful to identify the specific immunoglobulin involved in a monoclonal gammopathy (20).

SERUM PROTEIN ELECTROPHORESIS

The older five-band electrophoretic patterns have been replaced in recent years by high-resolution agarose or acetate electrophoresis patterns. These are vastly superior for evaluating serum for the presence of a monoclonal gammopathy. They permit distinction of subtle monoclonal bands that are present in the α2 and β regions, as well as the easy-to-see bands that are present in the γ region. The older five-band gel methods did not permit facile discrimination of bands in the α2 and β regions. Several versions of high-resolution electrophoresis are commercially available in both agarose and acetate form. Any of the systems is preferred over the older acetate form. The older acetate gels would be adequate screens if one were to perform immunofixation along with them. However, this is expensive, time-consuming, and redundant in most cases (20, 29).

We have developed a strategy for performing the evaluation of monoclonal gammopathy using a combination of high-resolution electrophoresis, quantification of IgG, IgA, IgM, κ, and λ by nephelometry, and occasional immunofixation. Most clinically significant monoclonal gammopathies are readily detected by high-resolution electrophoresis. They contain either a band in the γ, β or α region, a distorted band due to binding of a normal component by the monoclonal gammopathy, or hypogammaglobulinemia (the latter must *always* be evaluated with immunofixation and urine examination for Bence Jones protein) (19).

When a sample is sent for monoclonal gammopathy evaluation, a high-resolution electrophoresis together with immunoglobulin quantification (including κ and λ) is performed. The presence of any abnormal band or hypogammaglobulinemia on the high-resolution electrophoresis gel that is not explained by an obvious large increase in one light and one heavy chain (e.g., IgG κ), results in the generation of an immunofixation on that sample. If the high-resolution electrophoresis is perfectly normal, but an isolated increase in either IgA or IgM is seen, an immunofixation study will be performed. This reflects the fact that IgA and IgM may be present in the β region. The presence of transferrin, C3, and β_1 lipoprotein in this region may obscure a small band in this region. Therefore, any isolated increase in IgA or IgM should have an immunofixation evaluation. Lastly, any abnormality in the κ to λ ratio will also generate an immunofixation. In our studies on the quantification of κ and λ, with a normal sample or a polyclonal sample, the ratio is about two. Patients with subtle monoclonal gammopathies will have a distortion of this ratio. Any distortion of this ratio,

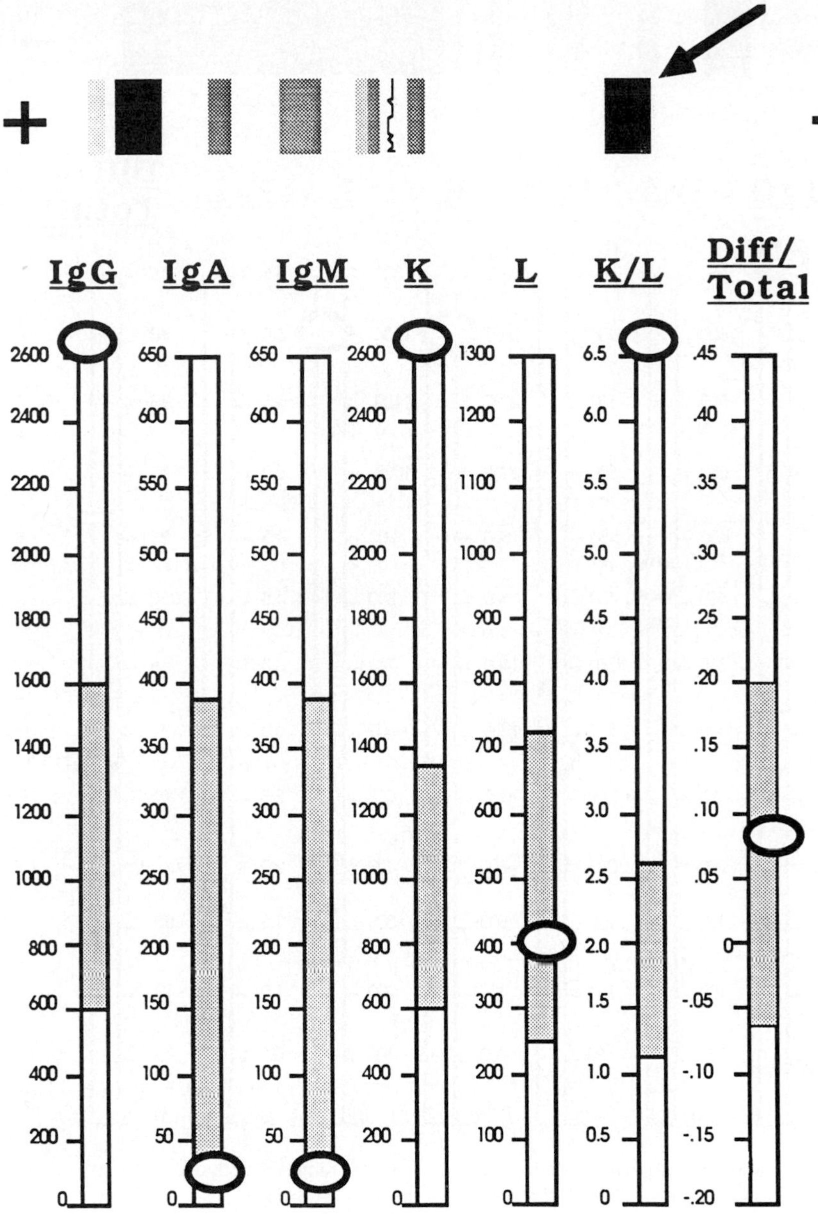

Figure 60.1. Schematic view of a monoclonal gammopathy (*arrow*) on a high-resolution electrophoresis analysis of serum. Below, the values for IgG, IgA, IgM, κ, and λ are shown (*circles*) along with the κ:λ ratio. Normal ranges are shaded. This is consistent with an IgGk monoclonal gammopathy.

even when no monoclonal band is present, will generate an immunofixation (19, 20).

Most cases can be evaluated without resorting to immunofixation if high-resolution electrophoresis is performed with quantification of IgG, IgA, IgM and κ and λ. Normal individuals with completely normal serum protein patterns and immunoglobulin quantification (including κ and λ) can be interpreted without further study. A urine study is always in order because light chain disease would be considered part of the differential diagnosis. A patient with an obvious monoclonal band (Fig. 60.1) and an obvious elevation of one heavy chain and one light chain with a distorted κ:λ ratio may have that sample signed out without further studies. A patient with a polyclonal pattern by high-resolution electrophoresis and a normal κ:λ ratio will have the sample signed out as a polyclonal increase (Fig. 60.2). No further studies are needed on such cases. Therefore, one must put the entire clinical picture together: the history that is provided, and other laboratory parameters (hematocrit, total protein, evidence of lytic lesions, serum calcium) to make the correct diagnosis (30–36).

Immunofixation is performed by repeating the serum protein electrophoresis with the patient sample run in several tracts. After the electrophoretic

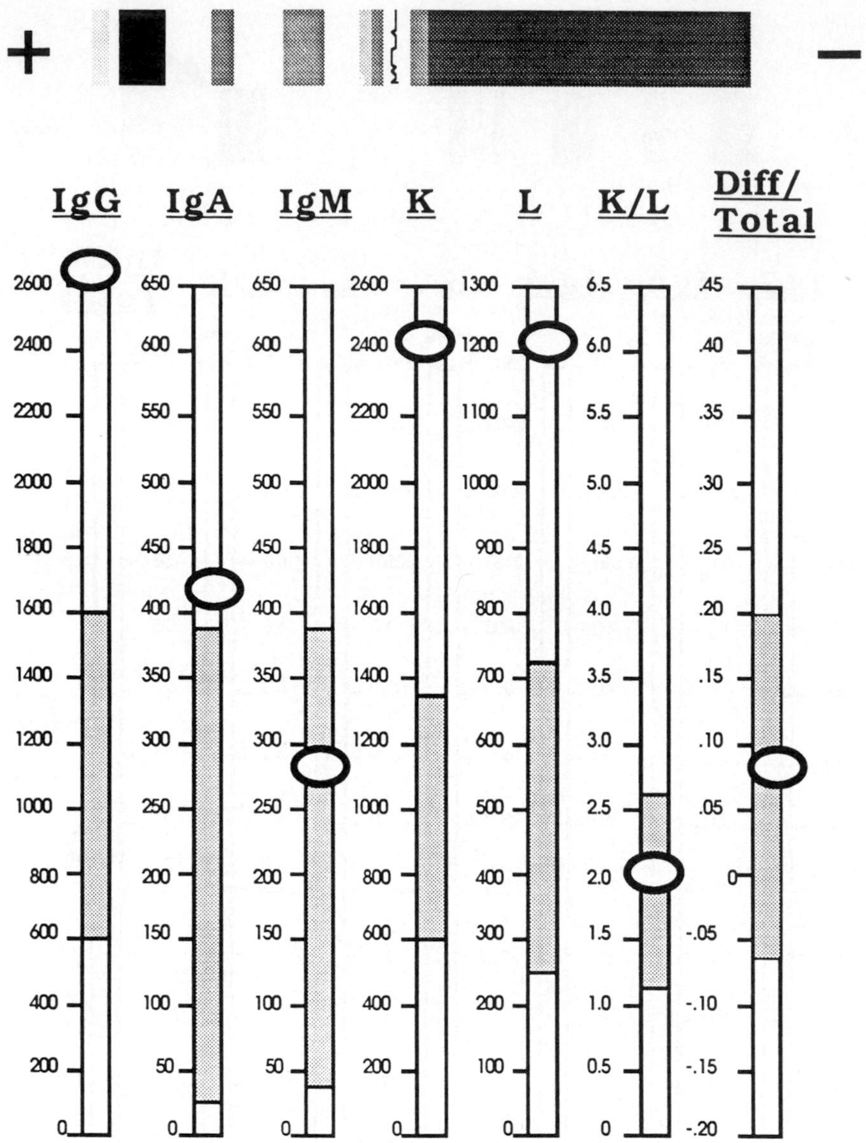

Figure 60.2. Schematic view of a polyclonal gammopathy on a high-resolution electrophoresis analysis of serum. Below, the values for IgG, IgA, IgM, κ and λ are shown (*circles*) along with the κ:λ ratio. Normal ranges are shaded. Note the increased density in the γ and β regions on the gel.

step, each tract is overlaid with a specific antiserum against IgG, IgA, IgM, κ or λ. The patient sample applied to each tract is diluted to achieve a concentration of approximately 100 mg/dl prior to electrophoresis. This optimizes the immunoprecipitation reaction. If too large a quantity of patient serum is used, an antigen excess effect will be seen. If too small a concentration is used, rarely, an antibody excess effect will be seen or the resulting reaction may be too small to be seen. Therefore, one must know the concentration of specific immunoglobulins prior to performing immunofixation in order to use the correct concentration of serum. Following electrophoresis, the specific antiserum is overlaid onto the tract and allowed to incubate for 30 minutes. After this step, the sample is washed so that unprecipitated proteins will be removed. Thereafter, the sample is stained with a sensitive dye. Coomassi blue or Crystal violet serve well in this regard. After the sample is dried, a permanent record is formed. We use only immunofixation to detect subtle gammopathies where there is not an obvious band by serum protein electrophoresis together with a marked abnormality of κ and λ by nephelometry (37–42).

IMMUNOELECTROPHORESIS

Immunoelectrophoresis is performed on an agarose medium. Symmetrical wells are cut in the agarose. Between each pair of wells, a trough is cut in the agarose. Patient samples are alternated with control samples containing human immunoglobulins in physiologic concentrations. The samples are electrophoresed to separate the major globulin components. Following electrophoresis, specific antiserum is placed in the trough between the control and patient wells. The patient's globulins diffuse radially through the agarose due to the geometry of the initial application site. As the serum proteins diffuse, the concentration of the proteins at the advancing edge decreases in a logarithmic manner. The antiserum placed in the trough diffuses in a linear manner through the agarose. Its concentration declines as it advances through the gel. When the specific antiserum meets the antigen, a specific antibody-antigen reaction occurs. Initially, the sample is likely to be in either antibody excess or antigen excess. As discussed previously, this will cause an unstable precipitation. However, as the reactants continue to diffuse, a point will be reached where the reactants are in equilibrium. Here, a stable precipitin band will form. The geometry of this band will be in the form of an arch due to the shape of the initial application well. This has a disadvantage in detecting small monoclonal gammopathies. Indeed, our laboratory no longer uses immunoelectrophoresis for any monoclonal gammopathy evaluation. However, since many laboratories continue to use this technique, this discussion is included here. The interpretation of immunoelectrophoresis is performed by comparing the reaction across the troughs. The patient and control arcs should be symmetrical and in the same location. When a patient has a monoclonal gammopathy, the patient's arc is enlarged and restricted in terms of its migration (43–49).

There are two major problems with immunoelectrophoresis. One is termed the "umbrella effect." This involves a monoclonal gammopathy of a large molecule such as IgM. IgM has a weight of approximately 1 million daltons. This bulky molecule has difficulty in diffusing through the agarose. Therefore, if the patient had a normal concentration of IgG (1,000 mg/dl), and an IgM monoclonal gammopathy of 1000 mg/dl, the IgM will not diffuse as quickly as the IgG. Therefore, the precipitin arcs seen with anti-κ and anti-λ antisera will reflect the polyclonal IgG rather than the monoclonal IgM. The antisera does not reach the larger, slower-moving IgM. Therefore, although one can see the restriction by serum protein electrophoresis and an increase in IgM by both nephelometry and by immunoelectrophoresis, one cannot make a distinction as to which type of light chain is causing the gammopathy. In the past, we would deal with this problem by either adding 2-mercaptoethanol to break the IgM molecule into smaller monomers or by separating the higher molecular weight IgM by applying it to a molecular size column. Alternatively, the IgM may be separated from most of the IgG by applying it to a charge column (usually diethylaminoethylcellulose). The immunoelectrophoresis would be repeated on this purified product, and the result obtained would usually identify the monoclonal gammopathy. This exercise is now unnecessary because a simple quantification of IgG, IgA, IgM, κ and λ by nephelometry and the obvious increase in either κ or λ will tell the observer which type of monoclonal gammopathy is present. Another way to determine which type of gammopathy is present involves using immunofixation (see previous discussion) (25, 50–53).

References

1. Killingsworth LM. Clinical applications of protein determinations in biological fluids other than blood. Clin Chem 1982;28: 1093.
2. Kyle RA. Monoclonal gammopathy of undetermined significance (MGUS): a review. Clin Haematol 1982;11:123–150.
3. Wieme RJ. Agar gel electrophoresis. Amsterdam: Elsevier, 1965.
4. Alexanian R, Barlogie B, Dixon D. Prognosis of asymptomatic multiple myeloma. Arch Intern Med 1988;148:1963–1965.
5. Clamp JR. Some aspects of the first recorded case of multiple myeloma. Lancet 1967;ii:1354–1356.
6. Shustik C, Michel R, Karsh J. Nonsecretory myeloma: a study on hypoimmunoglobulinemia. Acta Haematol 1988;80:153–158.
7. Brigden ML, Neal ED, McNeely MDD, Hoag GN. The optimum urine collections for the detection and monitoring of Bence Jones proteinuria. AJCP 1990;93:689–693.
8. Diamond J, McLaughin M. Urinary parameters to assess renal function. Clin Lab Med 1988;8:493–505.
9. Graziani MS, Lippi U. Multiple myeloma with serum IgM kappa and Bence Jones lambda biclonal gammopathy. Clin Chem 1986;32:2220–2221.
10. Graziani MS. Immunoblotting for detecting Bence Jones proteinuria. Clin Chem 1987;33:1079–1080.
11. Kim M. Proteinuria. Clin Lab Med 1988;8:527–540.
12. Kosaka M, Iishi Y, Okagawa K, Saito S, Sugihara J, Muto Y. Tetramer Bence Jones protein in the immunoproliferative diseases. Angioimmunoblastic lymphadenopathy, primary amyloidosis and multiple myeloma. Am J Clin Pathol 1989;91:639–646.
13. Norden AGW, Flynn FV, Filcher LM, Richards JDM. Renal impairment in myeloma: negative association with isoelectric point of excreted Bence Jones protein. J Clin Pathol 1989;42: 59–62.
14. Pezzoli A, Pascali E. The clinical significance of pure Bence Jones proteinuria at low concentration. Am J Clin Pathol 1989;91:473–475.
15. Smith DB, Harris M, Gowland E, Chang J, Scarffe JH. Nonsecretory multiple myeloma: a report of 13 cases with a review of the literature. Hematol Oncol 1986;4:307–313.
16. Bolling JP, Brazis PW. Optic disk swelling with peripheral neuropathy, organomegaly, endocrinopathy, monoclonal gammopathy, and skin changes (POEMS) syndrome. Am J Ophthalmol 1990;109:503–510.
17. Troussard X, de Ligny BH, Gallet B, et al. Massive systemic amyloidosis associated with light chain deposition disease. Nephron 1989;52:139–143.
18. Glenner GG. Amyloid deposits and amyloidosis. N Engl J Med 1980;302:1283–1292.

19. Keren DF, Warren JS, Lowe JB. Strategy to diagnose monoclonal gammopathies in serum: high-resolution electrophoresis, immunofixation and κ/λquantification. Clin Chem 1988;34:2196.
20. Keren DF. High-resolution electrophoresis and immunofixation: techniques and interpretation. Boston: Butterworths, 1987.
21. Danon F, Seligmann M. Transient human monoclonal immunoglobulins. Scand J Immunol 1972;1:323–328.
22. Malacrida V, De Francesco D, Banfi G, Porta FA, Riches PG. Laboratory investigation of monoclonal gammopathy during 10 years of screening in a general hospital. J Clin Pathol 1987;40:793–797.
23. Carter PW, Cohen HJ, Crawford J. Hyperviscosity syndrome in association with kappa light chain myeloma. Am J Med 1989;86:591–595.
24. Kahn SN, Bina M. Sensitivity of immunofixation electrophoresis for detecting IgM paraproteins in serum. Clin Chem 34:1633–1659, 1988.
25. Roberts RT. Usefulness of immunofixation electrophoresis in the clinical laboratory. Clin Lab Med Sci 1986;6:601–609.
25a. Crawford J, Eye MK, Cohen HJ. Evaluation of monoclonal gammopathies in the "well" elderly. Am J Med 1987;82:39–45.
26. Young VH. Transient paraproteins. Proc R Soc Med 1969;62:778–780.
27. Braunstein AH, Keren DF. Monoclonal gammopathy (IgMK) in a patient with Burkitt's lymphoma. Arch Pathol Lab Med 107:235–238, 1983.
28. Nathwani BN, Winberg CD, Berman RM. Angioimmunoblastic lymphadenopathy with dysproteinemia and its progression to malignant lymphoma. In: Jaffe ES, ed. Surgical pathology of lymph nodes and related organs. Philadelphia: WB Saunders; 1985:57–85.
29. Laurell CB. Electrophoresis, specific protein assays or both in measurement of plasma proteins. Clin Chem 1973;19:99–102.
30. Bush D, Keren DF. Over and underestimation of monoclonal gammopathies by quantification of serum kappa and lambda containing immunoglobulins. Clin Chem 1992;38:315–316.
31. Davenport RD, Keren DF. Oligoclonal bands in cerebrospinal fluids: significance of corresponding bands in serum for diagnosis of multiple sclerosis. Clin Chem 1988;34:764.
32. Dyck PJ. Intravenous immunoglobulin in chronic inflammatory demyelinating polyradiculoneuropathy and in neuropathy associated with IgM monoclonal gammopathy of unknown significance. Neurology 1990;40:327–328.
33. Fifield R, Keller I. An immunochemical evaluation for the identification and typing of monoclonal proteins. Ann Clin Biochem 1990;27:327–334.
34. Howerton DA, et al. Densitometric quantitation of high resolution electrophoresis agarose gel protein electrophoresis. Am J Clin Pathol 1986;85:213–218.
35. Keren DF, Di Sante AC, Bordine SC. Densitometric scanning of high-resolution electrophoresis of serum: methodology and clinical application. Am J Clin Pathol 1986;85:348.
36. Liu FJ, Fritsche HA, Trujillo JM. Underestimation of monoclonal proteins by serum protein electrophoresis on cellulose acetate. Clin Chem 1987;33:182–184.
37. Williamson AR, Salaman MR, Kreth HW. Microheterogeneity and allomorphism of proteins. Ann NY Acad Sci 1973;209:210–224.
38. Weiss LM, Strickler JG, Dorfman RF. Clonal T-cell population in angioimmunoblastic lymphadenopathy and angioimmunoblastic lymphadenopathy-like lymphoma. Am J Pathol 1986;122:392–397.
39. Thorner PS, Bedard YC, Fernandes BJ. l-light chain nephropathy with Fanconi's syndrome. Arch Pathol Lab Med 1983;107:654–657.
40. Stemerman D, Papadea C, Martino-Saltzman D, O'Connell CA, Demaline B, Austin GE. Precision and reliability of paraprotein determinations by high-resolution agarose gel electrophoresis. Am J Clin Pathol 1989;91:435–440.
41. Sanders PW, Herrera GA, Chen A, Booker BB, Galla JH. Differential nephrotoxicity of low molecular weight proteins including Bence Jones proteins in the perfused rat nephron in vivo. J Clin Invest 1988;82:3086–3096.
42. Rosenfeld L. Henry Bence Jones (1813–1873): the best chemical doctor in London. Clin Chem 1987;33:1687–1692.
43. DeMartino M, Sun T, York L, De Szalay H. Clinical significance of multiple monoclonal banding. AJCP 1988;89:428–429.
44. Gerard SK, Chen KH, Khayam-Bashi H. Immunofixation compared with immunoelectrophoresis for the routine characterization of paraprotein disorders. Am J Clin Pathol 1987;88:198–203.
45. Harrison HH. Fine structure of light chain ladders in urinary immunofixation studies revealed by isoDALT two dimensional electrophoresis. Clin Chem 1990;36:1526–1527.
46. Kyle RA, Greipp PR. "Idiopathic" Bence Jones proteinuria. Long-term follow-up in seven patients. N Engl J Med 1982;306:564–567.
47. Levinson SS, Keren DF. Immunoglobulins from the sera of immunologically activated persons with pairs of electrophoretic restricted bands show a greater tendency to aggregate than normal. Clin Chim Acta 1989;182:21–30.
48. McAllister HA Jr, Seger J, Bossart M, Ferrans VJ. Restrictive cardiomyopathy with κ light chain deposits in myocardium as a complication of multiple myeloma. Arch Path Lab Med 1988;112:1151–1154.
49. Mehrs PD, Patrick BA. Oligoclonal band in CSF; a diagnostic tool. Clin Immunol News 1982;3:101.
50. Cornell FN, McLachlan R. Isoelectric focusing in the investigation of gammopathies. Clin Biochm Monogr Sept 1985;31–37.
51. Radl J, Valentijn RM, Haaijman JJ, Paul LC. Monoclonal gammopathies in patients undergoing immunosuppressive treatment after renal transplantation. Clin Immunol Immunopathol 1985;37:98–1029.
52. Register LJ, Keren DF. Hazard of commercial antisera cross-reacting in monoclonal gammopathy evaluation. Clin Chem 1989;35:2016–2017.

61 Immunodeficiency Diseases

Jeffrey S. Warren

The first clinical description of an immunodeficiency disorder was published in 1952 by Colonel Ogden Bruton, a pediatrician who treated a boy with recurrent bacterial infections and agammaglobulinemia. A diagnosis of agammaglobulinemia was made possible by technical advances that allowed quantitative measurement of total serum gammaglobulins. Since 1952, many more cases of immunodeficiency diseases have been documented, and the number is growing. Again, laboratory advances have helped to provide the tools necessary to characterize defects and deficiencies in the immune system.

From a "pathogenesis of disease" standpoint it is useful to categorize immunodeficiency disorders into broad groupings based upon whether the defect is congenital or acquired and according to which arm of the immune system is defective. These systems include cell-mediated (T-cell) immunity, antibody-mediated (B-cell) immunity, and defects of phagocytes or the complement system. There is considerable overlap among these systems. For example, optimal antibody production (humoral immunity) requires intact T helper cells, and efficient phagocytosis is often dependent upon the integrity of the complement system (e.g., opsonization). Also, there are many diseases in which multiple seemingly unrelated immune defects are observed in the same patient. While specific, causative defects have been identified in only a few immunodeficiency disorders, understanding the development of the immune system provides a useful conceptual framework from which to view these diseases (Fig. 61.1).

Immunodeficiency disorders frequently present as failure to thrive, chronic or recurrent infections, unusual infections (i.e., uncommon microorganisms or atypical manifestations), and allergic disorders. Immunodeficiency patients may exhibit nonspecific manifestations such as skin rashes or eczema, chronic diarrhea, evidence of exaggerated autoimmunity, hepatosplenomegaly, lymphadenopathy, or growth failure. Certain diseases are associated with characteristic features that on the surface seem unrelated to the host defense system. For example, patients with the Chédiak-Higashi syndrome typically express partial oculocutaneous albinism, patients with the DiGeorge syndrome may exhibit structural defects related to the development of the 3rd and 4th branchial pouches (e.g., aortic anomalies or absent parathyroid glands), and patients with ataxia-telangiectasia manifest characteristic neurological and cutaneous anomalies. More common immunodeficiency disorders are sometimes

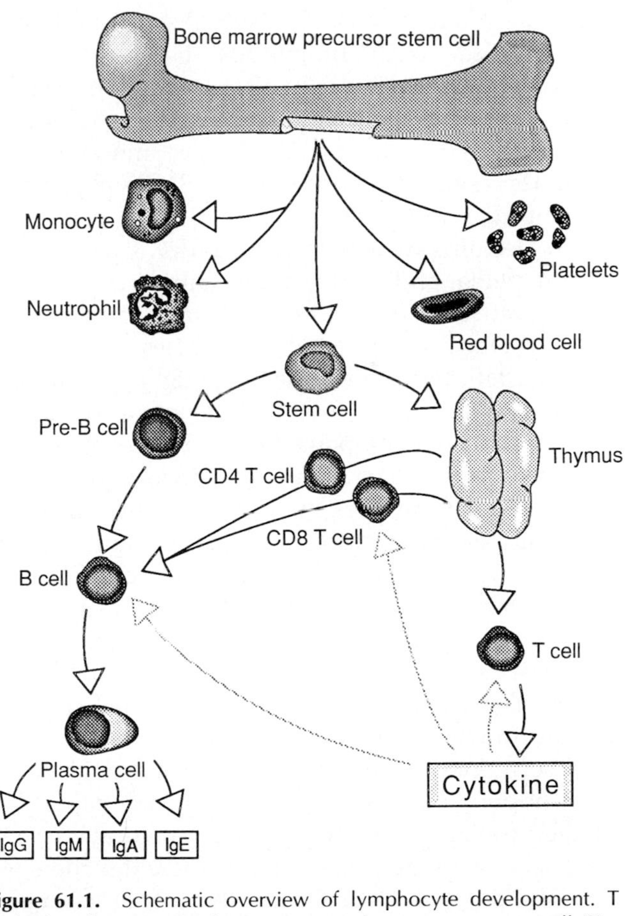

Figure 61.1. Schematic overview of lymphocyte development. T and B lymphocytes arise from a common bone marrow stem cell. Signals required for T-lymphocyte development are provided by the thymus, while those required for B-lymphocyte development are thought to be provided by the fetal liver during in utero development (not shown) and/or the bone marrow in adult development. Although most of the defects responsible for primary immunodeficiency disorders are poorly understood or have not yet been identified, this developmental scheme provides a useful conceptual framework for understanding where defects occur. (Adapted from Fireman P, Slavin RG, eds. Atlas of allergies. Philadelphia: JB Lippincott and New York: Gower Medical Publishing. 1991.)

difficult to classify because they lack such striking and characteristic findings. In general, the frequency and severity of infections observed in an immunodeficiency disease parallel the extent of the immunologic deficit. For example, patients with severe combined immunodeficiency (SCID) often live less than a year or two and suffer from overwhelming bacterial, fungal, and viral infections. In contrast, patients with isolated IgG subclass deficiencies may be asymptomatic or suffer only from a slightly increased frequency of upper respiratory infections. The types of infections that occur often provide insight into the type of immunodeficiency. Recurrent pyogenic infections such as bacterial pneumonia and otitis media are typical of hypogammaglobulinemia. Patients with cellular immune defects commonly suffer from fungal, protozoal, mycobacterial, and viral infections. In distal complement component deficiencies (C5–C8), patients are often victims of neisserial sepsis and an increased incidence of autoimmune disease.

Many immunodeficiency disorders can be classified using routinely available laboratory tests. However, such assays are often labor intensive and expensive. Clinical presentation and course of illness provide important diagnostic clues and must be considered when deciding which tests to order. Neutropenia, lymphopenia, and monocytopenia are relatively common given the large number of transplantation and chemotherapy patients. In most cases of iatrogenic immunodeficiency the cause is readily apparent. Disorders that are not primary to the immune system per se may also be accompanied by increases in susceptibility to infection. For example, patients with cystic fibrosis suffer from persistent, recalcitrant pulmonary infections secondary to *Pseudomonas* sp. and *Staphylococcus aureus*. In this case, mucous secretions are poorly cleared because of their high viscosity. Sickle cell anemia typically leads to autosplenectomy, which in turn is associated with an increased risk of bacterial sepsis. There are a variety of dysfunctional cilia syndromes in which impaired ciliary clearance of respiratory secretions results in an increased incidence of bronchopulmonary infections. Finally, the importance of the acquired immunodeficiency syndrome (AIDS) cannot be overemphasized. While these disorders will not be discussed further here, they serve to emphasize that a thorough clinical evaluation is required to successfully evaluate patients in whom immunodeficiency disorders are being considered. This chapter provides an overview of common and prototypic *primary* immunodeficiency diseases classified according to the predominantly affected arm of the host defense system. A brief survey of laboratory assays that have relevance to the diagnosis and management of immunodeficiency disorders follows.

DISEASE STATES

Disorders of the Complement System

Primary complement defects are uncommon, probably accounting for less than 1% of all immunodeficiency disorders. Complement deficiency states have been described for most of the complement components and complement regulatory proteins (Table 61.1). Deficiencies may be hereditary or acquired, and most are the result of either a deficiency of a particular protein or the presence of a nonfunctional molecule. Although the biology of the complement system is detailed elsewhere, several comments are in order. While complement activation via either the classic or alternative pathway can result in the generation of soluble mediators and the formation of surface-associated effector mechanisms, these pathways are not simply redundant. The classic pathway is most efficiently activated by pentameric IgM or multiple fixed IgG molecules and results in the generation and covalent deposition of C3b onto surfaces (microbial or host cell wall) located in close proximity to the immune deposits. Absence of complement-fixing antibody precludes complement activation via the classic pathway. The alternative pathway is maintained in a constant state of low-level activation that can be amplified when appropriate conditions are imposed. In the absence of a perturbing influence (e.g., microorganism), C3b is maintained at a low concentration by factors H and I, which prevent the binding of C3b to factor B and inactivate C3bBb complexes that are constantly being formed. When an appropriate surface (e.g., bacterial cell wall) is introduced, nascent C3bBb complexes become "protected" from the regulatory influences of H and I and then stabilized by properdin (P). Stabilized complexes (C3bBb(P)) efficiently cleave C3 into C3b, which in turn is deposited onto nearby surfaces in a nondirected manner. These comments emphasize that the alternative pathway is "less specific" (does not require specific antibody) and less efficient (requires higher concentrations of components to achieve maximum effect) than the classic pathway. The less specific, less efficient alternative pathway is presumed phylogenetically older than the classic pathway.

DEFICIENCY OF C1q, r, s, C2, or C4

Congenital deficiencies (homozygous) of C1q, C1r/s, C2, and C4 are rare. It was once believed that patients with such deficiencies were predisposed to autoimmune disorders because of the relationship between classic pathway structural genes (C2 and C4) and the major histocompatibility complex (MHC) (both on the short arm of chromosome 6), but it now

Table 61.1. Complement Components and Deficiency States[a]

Component	Major Activation Breakdown Product	Deficiency Syndrome
C1q		Yes
C1r		Yes
C1s (C1 esterase)		Yes[b]
C4	C4a, C4b	Yes
C2	C2a, C2b	Yes
C3	C3a, C3b, C3c, C3d, C3e	Yes
C5	C5a, C5b	Yes
C6		Yes
C7		Yes
C8		Yes
C9		Yes
B	Ba, Bb	No
D		No
P (properdin)		Yes
C4 binding protein		No
Protein S		Yes
C1 esterase inhibitor (C1-INH)		Yes
H		Yes
I (C3b inactivator)		Yes

[a]Table adapted from Ross SC, Denson P. Medicine 1984;63:243–273.
[b]C1s deficiency has been described only in conjunction with C1r deficiency.

appears that complement deficiency *per se* is important in the pathogenesis of the systemic lupus erythematosus (SLE) or lupus-like syndromes commonly seen in these patients. These patients infrequently suffer from serious bacterial infections. It is unclear whether infections that occur are related to the complement deficiency, associated autoimmune disease, or therapy-related immunosuppression (e.g., corticosteroids or cytotoxic agents). Patients with classic complement component deficiencies may suffer from inefficient and/or altered immune complex solubilization and clearance mechanisms, thus rendering them susceptible to the development of immune complex-mediated diseases (e.g., SLE). It has recently been discovered that as many as 50 to 80% of SLE patients are at least partially deficient (at a subclinical level) of C4. This observation lends further credence to the idea that deficiency of classic pathway components is important in the pathogenesis of autoimmune disease.

DEFICIENCY OF C3 OR FACTOR I (C3b INACTIVATOR)

C3 deficiency, either through a primary genetic defect or through absence of the regulatory protein, factor I (C3b inactivator), leads to reduced serum opsonizing capacity and an increased incidence of severe infections attributable to encapsulated pyogenic bacteria, such as *Streptococcus pneumoniae, Haemophilus influenzae,* and nonpneumococcal streptococci, as well as others, including Gram-negative enterobacteriaceae and *Staphylococcus aureus.* Patients with C3 deficiency also suffer from an increased incidence of SLE, glomerulonephritis, and vasulitis. Complete absence of C3 is inherited in an autosomal recessive pattern, while clinically normal heterozygotes possess serum C3 concentrations that approximate one-half of normal levels. In the case of factor I deficiency, C3 and factor B levels are markedly decreased or absent secondary to a state of hypercatabolism because of their unimpeded activation. Because C3b is important in both the propagation of the complement activation sequence and as an opsonin, it is difficult to know how these functional defects affect the risk of pyogenic infections. Because C3 or factor I-deficient patients tend to suffer from a spectrum of infections similar to that seen in a splenectomized person, C3b may be particularly important as an opsonin in the clearance of bacteria from the circulation.

DEFICIENCIES OF C5, C6, C7, and C8

Deficiencies of components in the lytic pathway result in impaired bacteriolysis without impairment of opsonization. Patients with C5, C6, C7, or C8 deficiencies suffer from frequent disseminated meisserial infections (*Neisseria meningitidis* and *Neisseria gonorrhoeae*), but interestingly, the clinical illness in such patients is less severe, and epidemiologically distinct from that observed in the disseminated neisserial infections seen in complement-sufficient individuals. C8-deficient patients are rare. Two defects have been described within this group: deficient C8 α-γ chain and deficient C8β chain. It appears that C8β deficiency occurs primarily in whites while C8 α-γ deficiency is more common in blacks.

DEFICIENCY OF C9

A few C9-deficient patients have been described, primarily in Japan. While C9-deficient serum contains reduced hemolytic activity, no untoward clinical consequences have been recognized to date.

DEFICIENCY OF C1 ESTERASE INHIBITOR

C1 esterase inhibitor (C1-INH) is an autosomal codominantly expressed member of the serine proteinase inhibitor ("serpin") family. Patients with C1-INH deficiency (due either to a silent C1-INH allele or an allele encoding a dysfunctional molecule) possess less than 50% of normal levels of functional protein. While some patients manifest SLE or lupus-like syndromes, virtually all C1-INH deficient patients manifest hereditary angioedema (HANE). Hereditary angioedema is an autosomal dominant disorder characterized by episodic, localized, acute attacks of painless edema typically involving the respiratory tract or face. Some patients manifest with abdominal pain due to localized involvement of gastrointestinal tract mucosa. Little is known about what triggers attacks of angioedema. Type 1 HANE (85% of cases) is characterized by low plasma levels of antigenic and functional C1-INH, normal or depressed C1 levels, depressed C4 levels, and normal C3 levels. Because intact C1-INH is catabolized more rapidly than normal, levels of intact C1-INH are often only 5 to 30% of reference concentrations. Type II HANE is less common. Type II HANE is associated with normal or elevated levels of dysfunctional mutant protein together with low levels of normal C1-INH. Therefore, these patients typically have normal to elevated antigenic C1-INH levels and depressed functional levels.

There are several acquired forms of C1-INH deficiency. These disorders are associated with increased C1-INH consumption related to benign or milignant B-cell lymphoproliferative disorders or autoimmune disorders accompanied by autoantibodies directed against C1-INH. Acquired C1-INH deficient patients typically exhibit depressed C1 and C4 levels, normal or increased antigenic C1-INH, and decreased functional C1-INH levels. Patients with acquired C1-INH deficiency almost always exhibit profoundly depressed C1q levels, while patients with HANE (type I or type II) may have depressed C1q levels, but often do not. Attenuated androgens reduce the frequency and severity of "edema attacks" in the hereditary forms and acquired forms of angioedema, but higher doses are typically required in the latter group.

Phagocytic Dysfunction Disorders

The importance of phagocyte function in host defense is perhaps best exemplified by the frequent occurrence of severe life-threatening infections in patients rendered granulocytopenic by chemotherapy. Severely granulocytopenic patients (e.g., absolute neutrophil count less than 500/μl) almost invariably suffer from episodes of bacterial sepsis. In many cases, organisms of low intrinsic pathogenicity are the culprits. Understanding the mechanisms involved in the individual steps that characterize neutrophil function in the acute inflammatory response (adhesion, chemotaxis, phagocytosis, respiratory burst, and degranulation) is helpful when classifying phagocytic cell defects. With more powerful experimental and clinical techniques (e.g., flow cytometry and molecular biology), it is much easier to recognize specific phagocytic cell defects.

LEUKOCYTE ADHESION DEFICIENCY

During the mid-1980s, several groups of investigators identified a small number of patients who suffered from recurrent bacterial infections and whose neutrophils exhibited reduced spreading on surfaces, impaired aggregation, impaired iC3b-mediated cell function, and reduced antibody-dependent cellular cytotoxicity. It was soon recognized that leukocytes from these patients lacked or were partially deficient of three surface molecules that are now known to be members of the β_2 or leukocyte integrin family. The integrins represent a superfamily of adhesion molecules each consisting of noncovalently associated α and β chains. The leukocyte integrins possess distinct α chains and a common β chain. This family includes CD11a/CD18 (also known as lymphocyte function-associated antigen (LFA-1), CD11b/CD18 (or Mac-1), and CD11c/CD18 (or p150,95). CD11b/CD18 is now known to be complement receptor 3 (CR3). CD11b/CD18 and CD11c/CD18 are expressed on the lining surfaces of specific and tertiary neutrophil granules and are thus detected by an increase in cell surface density when these lysosomes fuse with the cytoplasmic membrane following cell activation. In contrast, CD11a/CD18 is expressed only on the surface of neutrophils and is therefore not "up-regulated" upon degranulation. CD11a/CD18 (LFA-1) is found in highest density on the surfaces of T, B, and NK cells, while CD11b/CD18 (Mac-1) is found in highest density on neutrophils, eosinophils, monocytes, macrophages, and NK cells. Patients with leukocyte adhesion deficiency (LAD) possess mutations in the β chain gene resulting in variable decreases in surface β_2 integrin expression. To date, several different β chain mutations have been discovered. Most of these cases are inherited in an autosomal recessive manner. The clinical result is a heterogeneous group of patients who exhibit different degrees of adhesion defect and variable severity of problems.

Patients with LAD typically suffer from recurrent bacterial infections without much pus, periodontitis, delayed wound healing, elevated circulating leukocyte counts, and a history of delayed shedding of the umbilical cord stump. Peripheral blood neutrophil counts typically range between 15,000/μl and 60,000/μl between infections and can reach 100,000/μl or more during infections. Soft tissue infections are particularly common and are often quite severe (e.g., gangrenous). *Staphylococcus aureus, Pseudomonas sp.*, and members of the Enterobacteriaceae are the most common isolates. Perhaps the most helpful diagnostic clue is the presence of persistent neutrophilia. Diagnosis is made based on clinical data, demonstration of impaired adhesiveness and aggregation, and flow cytometric analysis. Therapy is generally supportive, although some patients with severe LAD have been successfully treated by bone marrow transplantation. In recent years intensive efforts have been made to elucidate the ligands for these molecules (Table 61.2). There is emerging evidence that β_2 integrin receptor-ligand interactions are critical deter-

Table 61.2. Ligands for Leukocyte (β_2) Integrins

Leukocyte Integrin	Ligand
CD11a/CD18 (LFA-1)	Intercellular adhesion molecule-1 (ICAM-1)
CD11b/CD18 (Mac-1; CR3)	
CD11c/CD18 (p150, 95)	
	iC3b
	iC3b
	ICAM-1
	Fibrinogen
	Zymosan
	Factor X
	Leishmania gp 63

minants of inflammatory responses. While LAD patients are rare, analysis of the molecular basis of this group of disorders has provided important insights into the mechanisms of inflammatory disease.

CHEDIAK-HIGASHI SYNDROME

The Chédiak-Higashi syndrome, described in the early 1950s, is a rare autosomal recessive disorder characterized by the presence of giant cytoplasmic granules in neutrophils, monocytes, and lymphocytes. The basic defect in this disorder is unknown, but involves multiple organ systems as evidenced by the occurrence of oculocutaneous albinism, defective platelets, and in some patients either sensory or motor neuropathies. Patients with Chédiak-Higashi syndrome typically have very light skin, photophobia, and characteristic silver-colored hair. The defects in pigmentation are the result of melanosome aggregation. Giant neutrophil granules can be seen in myeloid precursor cells. Because many myeloid series cells die before completion of maturation, Chédiak-Higashi patients are typically leukopenic (2000 to 3000 white cells/μl). Because of the neutropenia and a host of neutrophil, monocyte, and lymphocyte functional defects, patients suffer from recurrent bacterial and fungal infections. The most common infections are of the skin, mucous membranes, and respiratory tract. The platelet defect is associated with decreased storage pools of ADP and serotonin, resulting in prolonged bleeding times. Patients with Chédiak-Higashi syndrome can enter a so-called "accelerated phase" at any age. The accelerated phase is marked by local nonneoplastic lymphocytic proliferations within the liver, spleen and bone marrow as well as a progressive pancytopenia. The pancytopenia of accelerated Chédiak-Higashi syndrome is accompanied by hemorrhage and infection. Among a variety of defects described in leukocytes from Chédiak-Higashi patients are abnormally fluid cell membranes, high resting rates of cellular respiration, impaired adherence to surfaces, and reduced chemotactic responsiveness. It is thought that altered membrane fusion relates to the formation of giant cytoplasmic granules, which in the case of neutrophils, contain reduced amounts of dilute lytic enzymes. Some patients have responded to treatment with ascorbate, which decreases leukocyte membrane fluidity and augments bactericidal activity. Some patients in the accelerated phase have been successfully treated with bone marrow transplantation.

SPECIFIC GRANULE DEFICIENCY

Specific granule deficiency is somewhat of a misnomer because while such neutrophils lack specific granules, they also lack some enzymes found principally in primary and tertiary granules. Specific granule deficiency is an autosomal recessive disorder in which patients suffer from recurrent infections, especially of the skin and lungs. As in the Chédiak-Higashi syndrome, *Staphylococcus aureus* is the most commonly isolated offender. The diagnosis is based chiefly on morphology. The basic defect in specific granule deficiency is unknown, although a generalized defect in granule enzyme gene expression and/or granule packaging is suspected.

CHRONIC GRANULOMATOUS DISEASE

Chronic granulomatous disease (CGD) is a group of genetic disorders in which neutrophils and monocytes possess a defect in oxygen metabolite generation resulting in an inability to kill certain microorganisms. Normal phagocytes convert molecular oxygen, O_2, to a reduced metabolite, the superoxide anion, O_2^-. In turn, O_2^- is converted to other oxidants such as hydrogen peroxide. The clinical manifestations of CGD are variable, reflecting the heterogeneity of molecular defects that have been described. While the onset of CGD can occur at any age, it is most commonly recognized in children with recurrent and/or recalcitrant infections. Patients with CGD typically suffer from soft tissue, lymph node, and respiratory tract infections and in some cases, osteomyelitis, hepatic abscesses, and infections of the gastrointestinal tract. The most common causative organism is *Staphylococcus aureus*, although many catalase-positive agents have been isolated. Other common offenders include the Enterobacteriaceae, *Candida* sp., and *Aspergillus* sp. Infections are typically characterized by microabscesses and granuloma formation. Patients with CGD appear chronically ill, frequently suffer from anemia of chronic disease, and manifest immunologic phenomena such as arthralgias, urticaria, and costochondritis. The basic defect in CGD is in the phagocytic cell membrane-associated respiratory burst oxidase, NADPH oxidase. NADPH oxidase is a complex enzyme system that contains several subunits including cytosolic factor(s) and a membrane-associated cytochrome b, which consists of 91-kd and 22-kd subunits. Normally, NADPH oxidase catalyzes the reduction of O_2 to form O_2^-. The most common type of CGD is so-called type I, an X-linked disorder in which the 91-kd cytochrome b subunit is defective. These patients account for approximately two-thirds of cases. Type II CGD is autosomal recessive and accounts for about 30% of all CGD patients. Type II CGD neutrophils contain normal concentrations of cytochrome b but possess defective cytosolic factor(s). Thus, type I and type II CGD defects are complementary. Type II CGD, inherited as an autosomal recessive, is rare and appears to be the result of a genetic defect in the expression of the 22-kd subunit of cytochrome b. Other rare types and subtypes of CGD have also been described. Finally, patients with severe deficiencies of the hexose monophosphate shunt exzyme, glucose-6-phosphate dehydrogenase (G6PD) may manifest CGD clinically. In this case, G6PD deficiency results in low levels of intracellular NADPH, a substrate for the membrane oxidase. Unlike patients with defective NADPH oxidase, patients with severe G6PD deficiency usually also have chronic hemolytic anemia because their red blood cells are also deficient of G6PD. The histopathology and pathophysiology of CGD reflect the inability of affected phagocytes to produce normal concentrations of microbicidal oxidants. When normal neutrophils or monocytes phagocytize a microorganism, the cell undergoes a respiratory burst resulting in hydrogen peroxide formation as well as the intraphagosomal generation of hypochlorous acid. Normal cells produce enough hydrogen peroxide to exceed the capacity of microorganism-produced catalase, an enzyme that breaks down hydrogen peroxide. Chronic granulomatous disease phagocytes cannot produce enough hydrogen peroxide to counteract the microbial catalase, thus rendering such patients particularly susceptible to infection with catalase-producing organisms.

Precise diagnosis of CGD has become complicated because of all of the rare variants and the heterogeneity of the genetic lesions. Chronic granulomatous disease cells can be identified by their inability to produce superoxide anion in response to soluble or particulate stimuli. While in most cases of CGD there is no detectable respiratory burst, cells from patients with some variant forms may produce small amounts of O_2^- (typically 1 to 10% of normal controls). The nitroblue tetrazolium test (NBT) is useful in the diagnosis and classification of CGD. The NBT test is a microscopic slide test in which the capacity of individual phagocytes to produce oxidants is visually determined by the formation of insoluble blue-purple crystals (formazan) within functional cells. In most cases of CGD, no formazan crystals are present. The maternal carrier state for X-linked CGD can be detected using the NBT test since approximately one-half of the neutrophils will be positive and one-half negative. In some variant forms of CGD, the NBT test can be more difficult to interpret. For instance, most phagocytes may be weakly NBT-positive. More specialized laboratory tests include direct measurements of the cytochrome b absorption spectrum, in vitro NADPH oxidase enzyme studies, and recently, genetic analysis.

Treatment of CGD is in general supportive, that is, antibiotics and local measures such as incision and drainage of abscesses are used. Prophylactic treatment of patients with trimethoprim-sulfamethoxazole has reduced the incidence and severity of infections. Some severely affected patients have benefited from bone marrow transplantation, and very recent studies suggest that γ interferon may be useful in some CGD patients.

MYELOPEROXIDASE DEFICIENCY

Myeloperoxidase (MPO) deficiency, with a prevalence of 1:2000, is a relatively common autosomal recessive condition. Neutrophils and monocytes deficient of MPO do not generate hypohalous acid but produce supranormal concentrations of hydrogen peroxide. It is believed that the production of high concentrations of hydrogen peroxide explains the low morbidity observed in these patients. Several MPO-deficient patients who suffer from diabetes mellitus and *Candida* infections have been reported. It is unclear whether these fungal infections are attributable to the MPO deficiency or diabetes mellitus per se or the combination of these disorders.

Disorders of "Humoral" Immunity (B-Lymphocyte Defects)

As mentioned earlier, the first well-documented description of an immunodeficiency disorder was made in reference to a boy with agammaglobulinemia. Disorders of the "humoral" immune system are relatively common, considering that this group of disorders includes patients with common variable immunodeficiency (CVID) and selective IgA deficiency (Table 61.3). This classification scheme is imperfect when one considers that there are pivotal interactions between antibody-producing cells (B lymphocytes and plasma cells) and T lymphocytes, as well as between the effector molecules of the humoral system (antibodies) and phagocytes (e.g., antibody-dependent cellular cytotoxicity) or complement components (e.g., $C1_q$ binding to IgG or IgM molecules). It should be emphasized that most deficiencies of γ-globulins are not primary and that they occur in the context of many disease states (e.g., protein-losing enteropathy, nephrotic syndrome, multiple myeloma, light chain disease, and secondary to immunosuppressive therapy). In most primary humoral immune disorders the basic defect is unknown. Because trace amounts of all five isotypes of immunoglobulin can be detected in the sera of patients with "agammaglobulinemia," it appears that diseases within this group are due to regulatory defects rather than primary structural deletions or defects in immunoglobulin genes. While many patients with immunoglobulin deficiencies are recognized because they suffer from recurrent infections, individuals with some disorders experience infections no more frequently than normal (e.g., some patients with selective IgA deficiency, some patients with transient hypogammaglobulinemia of infancy).

X-LINKED AGAMMAGLOBULINEMIA

Males with X-linked agammaglobulinemia are usually well until 6 to 9 months of age, the time by which maternal antibodies acquired in utero have been largely catabolized. These patients typically suffer from recurrent respiratory tract, joint, central nervous system, and systemic infections with high-grade encapsulated pyogenic bacteria. The spectrum of infections is broad, including pneumonia, sinusitis, otitis, meningitis, and sepsis. The most common bacterial isolates include *Streptococcus pneumoniae, Haemophilus influenzae*, and *Streptococcus* sp. Patients are particularly susceptible to viral hepatitis, and a number of patients have developed paralysis after exposure to live attenuated polio vaccine. A significant number of X-linked agammaglobulinemia patients have also died as the result of chronic echovirus infections of the central nervous system. This disorder is typically accompanied by a dermatomyositis-like syndrome. A small percentage of patients with X-linked agammaglobulinemia develop neutropenia, which may be transient, cyclic, or persistent. *Pneumocystis carinii* pneumonia has been reported in neutropenic agammaglobulinemic patients. In contrast to patients with defective cellular immunity, growth retardation is uncommon as are fungal or other opportunistic infections.

Patients with X-linked agammaglobulinemia typically possess very low serum concentrations of γ-globulin (less than 100 mg/dl) and very low to undetectable concentrations of immunoglobulin in secretions. Analysis of peripheral blood typically reveals normal concentrations of total lymphocytes but very low numbers of B lymphocytes. While pre-B lymphoid series cells can be identified in the bone marrow of these patients, biopsies of lymphoid tissues reveal hypoplasia, the absence of germinal centers, and markedly diminished numbers of plasma cells. Patients with X-linked agammaglobulinemia are supported by assiduous attention to signs of infection, antibiotics, and immunoglobulin replacement therapy. The major long-term problem in patients who avoid complications like chronic viral CNS infections is the development of chronic and recurrent respiratory tract infections, which can lead to the development of bronchiectasis and pulmonary insufficiency.

SELECTIVE IgA DEFICIENCY

Selective IgA deficiency is marked by the presence of very low serum concentrations of IgA (less than 7 mg/dl) accompanied by diminished IgA concentrations in mucosal secretions. Selective IgA deficiency is the most common primary immunodeficiency, with a prevalence of between 1:350 and 1:3000. IgA deficiency is generally associated with an increased incidence and severity of respiratory, genitourinary, and gastrointestinal tract infections as well as an increased likelihood of autoimmune and lupus-like syndromes. Patients with this immunodeficiency may also develop a sprue-like malabsorption syndrome, which often responds favorably to a gluten-free diet. Interestingly, not all IgA-deficient individuals manifest such problems. It appears that many, but not all, clinically ill IgA-deficient patients suffer from concomitant deficiencies of IgG subclasses, most commonly subclasses IgG 2 and IgG 4. The most common offending organisms are pyogenic bacteria. Some IgA-deficient patients go on to develop CVID, and some IgA deficient patients have spontaneously remitted.

The basic defect responsible for selective IgA deficiency is unknown. Cell surface analysis of circulating lymphocytes reveals that IgA-bearing B lymphocytes also express IgM and IgD, an abnormal finding suggesting that such cells are maturation-arrested. Treatment of IgA-deficient patients is based on the severity of clinical illness. Antibiotics are the mainstay of therapy. Gammaglobulin replacement therapy is contraindicated. Great care to avoid sensitization of IgA deficient patients with IgA-bearing blood products should be observed because such patients can experience anaphylactic reactions following exposure to IgA-containing blood products. Unfortunately, the presence of IgE antibodies directred against IgA does not absolutely predict a predisposition to untoward reactions following receipt of blood products. If blood products are absolutely required, IgA-poor preparations should be used. Each patient must be considered at risk and observed closely when receiving blood products.

A single patient with absent secretory IgA and normal serum IgA concentrations has been de-

Table 61.3. Disorders of Humoral Immunity[a]

Disease	Deficiency/Defect	Putative Site of Defect
X-linked agammaglobulinemia	Immunoglobulin	Pre-B cell
Selective IgA deficiency	IgA	B lymphocyte (IgA)
Secretory component deficiency	Secretory IgA	Mucosal epithelium
Common variable immunodeficiency (CVID)	Immunoglobulin	B lymphocyte T lymphocyte
IgG Subclass deficiency	IgG Subclasses	?
Transient hypogammaglobulinemia of infancy	Low immunoglobulin concentration; antibodies present	?
Selective IgM deficiency	IgM	T helper cell
Immunodeficiency with elevated IgM	IgG and IgA	B lymphocyte (IgG,IgA); T helper cell
Specific antibody deficiency	Antibody	?
X-linked lymphoproliferative disease (Duncan's disease)	Anti-EBV nuclear antigen antibody	?

[a]Table adapted from Buckley RH. Textbook of Medicine, Philadelphia: WB Saunders 1988.

scribed. The abnormality in this case was due to the lack of the secretory piece needed for export of serum IgA into mucosal secretions via mucosal epithelia. This patient experienced chronic gastrointestinal candidiasis and diarrhea.

COMMON VARIABLE IMMUNODEFICIENCY

Common variable or acquired immunodeficiency is a heterogeneous group of diseases characterized by a deficiency of γ-globulins. This group of disorders manifests in a manner that is somewhat similar clinically to X-linked agammaglobulinemia except that it occurs with equal frequency in both males and females and it can present at different ages. While many patients present in infancy or early childhood, most common variable immunodeficiency patients present during later childhood or adulthood. In general the γ-globulin deficiency is less severe than that seen in X-linked agammaglobulinemia, typically on the order of 200 to 300 mg/dl of total immunoglobulins. In addition to pyogenic infections, common variable immunodeficiency disorders have been associated with a variety of autoimmune and neoplastic disorders. Patients with common variable immunodeficiency suffer from a markedly increased incidence of giardiasis and bronchiectasis. In addition to autoimmune and infectious complications, these patients suffer from an increased incidence of gastric carcinoma, lymphomas, and amyloidosis.

The defects responsible for common variability immunodeficiency appear to be heterogeneous in that various profiles of circulating B lymphocytes have been described. Patients with common variable immunodeficiency typically have normal numbers of circulating B cells but they don't differentiate normally in vivo or become immunoglobulin-producing plasma cells in vitro. Indeed, there are defects in terminal B lymphocyte maturation, a process that is now better understood in the context of interleukins 4, 5, and 6. Interestingly, first-degree relatives of CVID patients have an increased incidence of selective IgA deficiency, and vice versa, suggesting the possibility that these disorders have a related pathogenetic origin. In fact, some patients with selective IgA deficiency eventually develop CVID.

Patients with common variable immunodeficiency are treated with antibiotics and immunoglobulin replacement therapy.

IgG SUBCLASS DEFICIENCY

There are many patients with IgG subclass (IgG 1, IgG 2, IgG 3, IgG 4) deficiencies. The total serum IgG concentration may be normal or abnormal depending on which subclass is deficient and on the severity of the defect. For example, since nearly 70% of the total serum IgG is IgG 1, a marked IgG 1 subclass deficiency would be reflected in a decreased total IgG concentration. In contrast, since IgG 4 accounts for only a small percentage (less than 1 to 2%) of the total IgG, a complete absence of IgG 4 would not be reflected by measurements of total IgG concentration. Serum IgA and IgM leads are usually normal, although perhaps one-fifth of IgA-deficient patients have a concomitant IgG subclass deficiency. Some patients mount normal antibody responses following immunization while others do not. Clinically, IgG subclass-deficient patients fall within a spectrum ranging from no symptoms to recurrent pyogenic infections, typically involving the paranasal sinuses or the lower respiratory tract. The most common isolates include *Streptococcus pneumoniae, Haemophilus influenzae,* and *Staphylococcus aureus*. The diagnosis of IgG subclass deficiency is sometimes not made for years. The primary defects(s) are unknown. Therapy includes appropriate antibiotics and γ-globulin replacement therapy.

TRANSIENT HYPOGAMMAGLOBULINEMIA OF INFANCY

Transient hypogammaglobulinemia of infancy is a relatively rare disorder. As its name suggests, infants with this disorder present with recurrent infections and hypogammaglobulinemia. In contrasts to patients with common variable immunodeficiency or X-linked agammaglobulinemia, infants with this disorder possess isohemagglutinins and can respond to administered antigens such as diphtheria and tetanus toxoid. Such specific antibody responses can usually be detected before serum immunoglobulin concentrations reach normal levels. Because of the transient nature of this disorder and the potential for suppression of endogenous antibody production, replacement γ-globulin is not recommended.

SELECTIVE IgM DEFICIENCY

Only a few cases of selective IgM deficiency (IgM less than 7 mg/dl) have been reported. A variety of serious infectious, including meningococcemia, disseminated enterobacteriaceae infections, pneumoccal meningitis, staphylococcal soft tissue infections, and respiratory tract infections have been associated with IgM deficiency. The specific defect responsible for selective IgM deficiency is unknown. Treatment includes antibiotic therapy.

IMMUNODEFICIENCY WITH ELEVATED IgM

Immunodeficiency with elevated IgM is uncommon. Patients with this disorder typically present in infancy with recurrent pyogenic infections including pneumonia, sinusitis, otitis media, and tonsillitis. In contrast to patients with X-linked agammaglobulinemia, these patients have pronounced lymphadenopathy. Serum IgA and IgG concentrations are markedly depressed, and there is typically a polyclonal increase in serum IgM. Patients with immunodeficiency with elevated IgM occasionally have concomitant neutropenia and may manifest autoimmune hemolytic anemia and/or thrombocytopenia.

The specific defect(s) responsible for immunodeficiency with elevated IgM are unknown. A B-lymphocyte maturation defect is suspected in most cases because normal or nearly normal numbers of Ig-bearing B cells are present in the peripheral blood. In vitro stimulation of B lymphocytes usually results in IgM, but not IgG or IgA production. In other cases, the defect is thought to involve T cells that mediate IgM to IgG or IgA class switching. Patients with immunodeficiency with elevated IgM are treated with γ-globulin replacement therapy and antibiotics.

SPECIFIC ANTIBODY DEFICIENCY

Specific antibody deficiency, also known as "antibody deficiency with near-normal immunoglobulins," is rare. These patients have defective antibody responses to certain antigens despite normal serum immunoglobulin concentrations and normal T lymphocyte function in available laboratory assays. Selective antibody deficiency is detected as quantitatively subnormal antibody responses to various antigens, including pneumococcal polysaccharide vaccines, bacteriophage ϕX174, tetanus toxoid, and diphtheria toxoid. Most patients are also devoid of blood group antibody titers. The primary defect in selective antibody deficiency is unknown. Current therapy includes γ-globulin replacement and antibiotics.

X-LINKED LYMPHOPROLIFERATIVE DISEASE (DUNCAN'S DISEASE)

X-linked lymphoproliferative disease was initially described in a group of patients from a single kindred, the Duncan family. The syndrome is varied in its clinical manifestations but has in common an abnormal response to Epstein-Barr virus infections. Patients with X-linked lymphoproliferative disease are well until they first suffer from an EBV infection. Nearly 70% of patients die as the result of an intense lymphocyte proliferation that occurs during mononucleosis. Most survivors develop hypogammaglobulinemia, B-cell lymphoma or a combination of both.

The defect(s) responsible for this disorder remain unclear but a variety of abnormal responses have been described. For instance, most patients who survive mononucleosis do not mount a normal antibody response to EBV nuclear antigen, whereas titers to the viral capsid antigen may range from zero to markedly elevated. There is often an accompanying depression in T-cell immunity to EBV. Nonspecific immunologic defects have also been associated with Duncan's disease. Such patients may have normal numbers of circulating B and T lymphocytes with an elevated percentage of CD8+ (T-suppressor) cells. Finally, in vitro lymphocyte immunoglobulin synthesis to B-cell mitogens is also often blunted. There is currently no specific effective therapy for this disorder.

Disorders of "Cellular" Immunity (T-Lymphocyte Defects)

Disorders of cellular immunity are very uncommon. In contrast to patients with pure humoral immunodeficiency syndromes, patients with partial or complete cellular immunodeficiencies tend to suffer from opportunistic viral, fungal, or protozoal infections. Such infections tend to be more severe and less treatable than those seen in the humoral immunodeficiency syndrome patients. These patients often do not survive past childhood. Some generalizations can be made regarding cellular immunodeficiency syndromes. Patients with cellular immunodeficiency syndromes display anergic delayed-type hypersensitivity reactions, growth retardation, wasting, and diarrhea. Patients with cellular immunodeficiency disorder are susceptible to graft-versus-host disease following receipt of nonirradiated blood products or allogeneic bone marrow. Patients with cellular immunodeficiencies may suffer from fatal reactions to live vaccines. There is also an increased incidence of malignancy in these patients.

THYMIC HYPOPLASIA (DiGEORGE'S SYNDROME)

DiGeorge's syndrome is the result of defective embryogenesis involving the 3rd and 4th pharyngeal pouches. The result is hypoplasia or aplasia of the thymus and defective T-lymphocyte-dependent immunity. Patients with DiGeorge's syndrome usually suffer from defects involving other structures derived from the 3rd and 4th branchial arches including the parathyroid glands, the greatest vessels, esophagus, cardiac septa, and several facial structures. The clinical results of these defects include neonatal hypocalcemic tetany secondary to agenesis of the parathyroid glands, persistent right-sided aortic arch, esophageal atresia, atrial and ventricular septal defects, and facial defects such as hypertelorism, short philtrum, low-set ears, and mandibular hypoplasia. A minority of patients with DiGeorge's syndrome have chromosomal abnormalities.

The degree of thymic hypoplasia is variable. Some patients manifest only limited defects in cellular immunity and thus suffer from few infectious complications. At the other end of the spectrum are patients with thymic aplasia who may present like patients with severe combined immunodeficiency. These patients suffer from recurrent life-threatening viral, fungal, and protozoal infections, and frequently develop graft-versus-host disease after receipt of blood products.

Patients with DiGeorge's typically have decreased numbers of circulating T lymphocytes with normal immunoglobulin concentrations. Some patients have decreased serum IgA and may have increased serum IgE concentrations. In vitro, the response of peripheral blood lymphocytes to T-lymphocyte mitogens is usually depressed. Thymic tissue is generally atrophic, although in some cases small tissue rests containing Hassall's corpuscles, and thymocytes can be identified. Lymph nodes and splenic tissue typically show depleted T-cell-dependent areas. Therapy is supportive. Some groups have claimed benefit from fetal thymus transplantation.

CELLULAR IMMUNODEFICIENCY WITH IMMUNOGLOBULINS (NEZELOF'S SYNDROME)

Patients with Nezelof's syndrome have depressed peripheral blood lymphocyte counts, atrophic lymphoid tissue, and abnormal thymic architecture. The primary defect in Nezelof's syndrome is unknown. Thymuses from these patients are small, contain few thymocytes, and typically contain no Hassall's corpuscles. In many patients, serum immunoglobulin concentrations and the ability to form antibodies to specific antigens are normal. Patients with Nezelof's syndrome typically present with failure to thrive and diarrhea. Chronic and recurrent pulmonary infections, skin infections, Gram-negative sepsis, urinary tract infections, and varicella are relatively common. Some patients have died secondary to vaccinia, rubeola, *Pneumocystis carinii*, cytomegalovirus, and atypical mycobacterial infections. Both autosomal recessive and X-linked modes of inheritance have been reported.

Patients with Nezelof's syndrome typically exhibit cutaneous anergy and blunted in vitro responses to T cell mitogens. As noted previously, these patients have moderate to severe lymphopenia but with normal CD4/CD8 ratios. Therapy is supportive. Some patients have been treated with bone marrow transplantation.

NEZELOF'S SYNDROME WITH PURINE NUCLEOSIDE PHOSPHORYLASE DEFICIENCY

This apparent variant of Nezelof's syndrome is very uncommon. Thymuses from patients with Nezelof's syndrome with PNP deficiency possess Hassall's corpuscles. Among the few patients with this disorder, several have suffered from progressive spastic quadriplegia, and a few developed autoimmune hemolytic anemia or autoimmune thrombocytopenia. As in more typical Nezelof's patients, these patients suffer from severe generalized viral infections and graft-versus-host disease. No effective therapy has been reported.

CHRONIC MUCOCUTANEOUS CANDIDIASIS

Chronic mucocutaneous candidiasis (CMC) is a syndrome marked by chronic candidal infections of the skin and mucous membranes. In contrast to the other cellular immune disorders, CMC is rarely fatal. The cause of this disorder is unknown. In some cases no immunodeficiency cause can be identified. Some

Table 61.4. Disorders of Cellular Immunity

Disease	Deficiency/Defect	Putative Site of Defect
Thymic hypoplasia/agenesis (DiGeorge's syndrome)	T lymphocytes (thymus)	Abnormal development of 3rd and 4th brachial pouches
Cellular immunodeficiency with immunoglobulins (Nezelof's syndrome)	T lymphocytes	?
Nezelof's syndrome with purine nucleoside phosphorylase (PNP) deficiency	T lymphocytes	?
Chronic mucocutaneous candidiasis	Variable	?

patients have accompanying endocrinopathies involving the parathyroid, thyroid, parathyroid, adrenal glands or pancreas. Ketoconazole is the most efficacious therapy reported to date.

Combined Humoral and Cellular Immune Dysfunction

The combined humoral and cellular immunodeficiency disorders include syndromes that vary greatly in severity and in the spectrum of immunologic defects that constitute individual diseases (Table 61.5). For instance, patients with ataxia-telangiectasia often suffer from selective immunoglobulin deficiencies and moderately severe defects in cellular immunity, while patients with autosomal recessive severe combined immunodeficiency disease (SCID) are profoundly ill and frequently die within the first year of life. As noted for humoral and cellular immunodeficiency disorders, classification of combined disorders can be problematic. Leukocyte adhesion deficiency (see earlier discussion) affects both lymphocyte and neutrophil-mediated host defense processes and may be considered either a disorder of phagocyte function or a combined cellular and humoral defect. Except in a few disorders, the specific defect(s) responsible for combined humoral and cellular disorders are unknown. Clinically, patients with combined humoral and cellular defects may present with bacterial infections reminiscent of pure humoral deficiencies, opportunistic infections typically associated with cellular immune dysfunction, or features unique to given disorders. Examples of the latter include hemorrhage secondary to thrombocytopenia in Wiskott-Aldrich syndrome, ataxia in ataxia-telangiectasia, and dwarfism in cartilage-hair hypoplasia.

ATAXIA-TELANGIECTASIA

Ataxia-telangiectasia is an autosomal recessive disorder that most prominently involves the immune system, skin, and the central nervous system. Typical patients manifest progressive cerebellar ataxia within the first 12 to 18 months of life, and most patients suffer from recurrent bacterial sinopulmonary infections. Telangiectasias typically become apparent on the conjunctiva and skin early in childhood. In addition to disordered immune function, ataxia, and telangiectasias, patients with ataxia-telangiectasia are at risk of developing malignancies typically involving the hematopoietic system.

The defect responsible for ataxia-telangiectasia is unknown. Both patients and heterozygotic carriers of this disorder exhibit defective DNA repair accompanied by inordinate sensitivity to ionizing irradiation. The genetic lesion responsible for ataxia-telangiectasia has been localized to the long arm of chromosome 11 (11q 22-23). In vitro, B lymphocytes often exhibit an intrinsic inability to synthesize IgA.

The immunologic profile in ataxia-telangiectasia patients is variable. Most patients exhibit decreased serum IgA and IgE concentrations accompanied by variable decreases in serum IgG. Cellular immune function is usually depressed but not to the degree observed in severe combined immunodeficiency disorders or complete cases of the DiGeorge syndrome. There is no specific therapy for ataxia-telangiectasia.

WISKOTT-ALDRICH SYNDROME

Wiskott-Aldrich syndrome, also known as immunodeficiency with thrombocytopenia and eczema, is an X-linked disorder marked by immunosuppression, thrombocytopenia, and eczema. Boys with Wiskott-Aldrich syndrome sometimes present with a thrombocytopenic bleeding diathesis heralded by prolonged bleeding following circumcision. Skin lesions and recurrent infections typically occur during the first year. Early in the course of the disease patients exhibit impaired humoral responses to encapsulated high-grade bacterial pathogens, resulting in otitis media, pneumonia, meningitis, and sepsis. Later, patients suffer from herpes infections and *Pneumocystis* infections. Wiskott-Aldrich syndrome carries a grave prognosis, and most patients die during childhood. As in ataxia-telangiectasia patients, there is an increased incidence of lymphoreticular malignancy.

The primary defect responsible for Wiskott-Aldrich syndrome is unknown. Thrombocytopenia is accompanied by normal numbers of megakaryocytes in the bone marrow. Immunologic abnormalities re-

Table 61.5. Combined Humoral and Cellular Immunodeficiency Disorders

Disease	Deficiency/Defect	Putative Side of Defect
Ataxia-telangiectasia	T lymphocytes; Antibody	B lymphocyte; T lymphocyte
Wiskott-Aldrich syndrome	T lymphocytes; Antibody	?
Hyperimmunoglobulinemia E syndrome	↑ serum IgE Selective immune responses	?
Cartilage-hair hypoplasia	T lymphocytes	Cell cycle
Immunodeficiency with thymoma	T lymphocytes; antibody	B lymphocyte; T suppressor lymphocyte
T lymphocyte activation defects	T lymphocytes	T cell receptor Interleukin-2
Severe combined immunodeficiency disorders (SCID)		
Autosomal recessive	Lymphocytes; Antibody	?
Autosomal recessive with adenosine deaminase deficiency	Lymphocytes; Antibody	ADA deficiency
X-linked	Lymphocytes; Antibody	?
Major histocompatibility (MHC) antigens	Lymphocytes; some antibodies	Defective class I or II MHC expression
Reticular dysgenesis	Lymphocytes, Granulocytes	?

flect the clinical course of the disorder. Patients typically have borderline or low immunoglobulin levels with depressed serum IgM levels, low or low-normal IgG levels, and elevated serum IgA and IgE levels. Defective humoral immune responses to carbohydrate antigens and depressed isohemagglutinin levels are apparent early. Later, poor humoral responses to protein antigens become apparent. Cutaneous anergy and decreased concentrations of peripheral blood T lymphocytes are also present.

Treatment, including platelet transfusions, splenectomy, and replacement γ-globulin therapy, has generally been supportive. Some recent successes have been achieved with bone marrow transplantation.

HYPERIMMUNOGLOBULINEMIA E SYNDROME

Hyperimmunoglobulinemia E syndrome is an autosomal dominant disorder of unknown cause. Patients typically suffer from recurrent staphylococcal abscesses involving the skin, lungs, joints, and soft tissues. Some patients with hyperimmunoglobulinemia E syndrome also suffer from a generalized dermatitis. The so-called "Job syndrome" is considered to be related. The Job syndrome is characterized by recurrent skin abscesses in association with a poorly characterized neutrophil motility defect.

Patients with hyperimmunoglobulinemia E typically exhibit normal serum immunoglobulin concentrations except for IgE, which is typically markedly increased to concentrations in excess of 2000 IU/ml and as high as 20,000 to 50,000 IU/ml. In addition, peripheral blood eosinophilia is characteristic. Some patients have neutrophil and/or monocyte chemotactic defects. The mainstay of therapy is antibiotic treatment.

CARTILAGE-HAIR HYPOPLASIA

Cartilage-hair hypoplasia is an autosomal recessive disorder with variable penetrance. This disorder is particularly prevalent among the Amish and is characterized by short-limbed dwarfism accompanied by frequent, often life-threatening infections. Patients with this disorder possess fine light hair and eyebrows, hyperextensible joints of the hands and feet, and a characteristic short-limbed dwarfism that is particularly pronounced in the hands. While defective antibody immediated immunity is demonstrable in most patients, there is also defective cellular immunity and a markedly increased propensity for life-threatening infections. Progressive vaccinia and vaccine-associated poliomyelitis have been observed in some patients.

IMMUNODEFICIENCY WITH THYMOMA

Combined humoral and cellular immunodeficiency has been reported in adult patients with thymomas that are anterior mediastinal tumors of epithelial origin. Typically, patients present with thymoma, hypogammaglobulinemia, and defective cell-mediated immunity. In some patients, immune dysfunction is accompanied by hematologic abnormalities including pancytopenia, thrombocytopenia, eosinopenia, red cell hypoplasia or hemolytic anemia. The mechanism responsible for the immunodeficiency is unknown.

T-LYMPHOCYTE ACTIVATION DEFECTS

Only a few cases of defective T-lymphocyte activation have been characterized. Analyses of patients with these disorders have provided important insights into mechanisms of T-lymphocyte function. Defective interleukin 2 production, defective cell surface expression of the T-cell antigen receptor (TCR), and defective TCR-linked signal-transduction have been described. In all cases normal concentrations of circulating T lymphocytes are present, but functional responses are abnormal. Clinically, patients with defective T lymphocyte activation suffer from opportunistic viral and fungal diseases.

SEVERE COMBINED IMMUNODEFICIENCY DISORDERS (SCID)

While severe combined immunodeficiency disorders (SCID) vary in mode of inheritance, lymphoreticular histopathology, mechanism of cellular dysfunction, and to some extent, clinical characteristics, they have in common the near complete absence of cellular and humoral immune function. As a result, the patients are profoundly ill and die within a short period of time, unless they can be isolated from the environment, their immune systems can be replaced by bone marrow transplantation, or in appropriate instances, specific enzyme replacement therapy can be instituted. The severe combined immunodeficiency disorders present within the first months of life and are marked by recurrent episodes of upper respiratory, lower respiratory, and cutaneous bacterial infections. Persistent opportunistic infections caused by *Candida*, measles, varicella, cytomegalovirus, and *Pneumocystis* are also prevalent. Patients with SCID suffer extreme wasting and are at risk of developing graft-versus-host (GVH) disease.

Clinical and laboratory evaluation of immune function reveal profound abnormalities. There is a virtual absence of cellular immune function manifested by lymphopenia, cutaneous anergy, and the absence of in vitro lymphocyte proliferative responses to antigens, mitogens, or allogeneic cells. Serum immunoglobulin concentrations are usually markedly depressed, and antibody responses to immunization are difficult to detect. Varied immunophenotypic findings have been reported in SCID patients, but these have not generally provided insight into mechanisms of these disorders. A small number of autosomal recessive SCID patients in whom nearly all circulating lymphocytes appear to be natural killer (NK) cells have been reported.

The severe combined immunodeficiency disorders include several different entities including autosomal recessive SCID, autosomal recessive SCID with adenosine deaminase deficiency, X-linked recessive SCID, SCID with leukopenia, class I major histocompatibility complex (MHC) deficiency (or so-called "bare lymphocyte syndrome"), and a combined MHC class I and class II antigen deficiency.

Autosomal recessive and X-linked recessive SCID patients present with recurrent or persistent bacterial, fungal, protozoal, and viral infections accompanied by wasting. Care must be taken not to subject these patients to graft-versus-host disease. Graft-versus-host disease may develop following receipt of blood products contaminated with viable lymphocytes and can even occur as the result of maternal-fetal hemorrhage in utero. Replacement γ-globulin has not been effective in preventing the demise of SCID patients. Some patients have been immunologically reconstituted with HLA-identical or D locus-compatible bone marrow transplantation. Recent progress has also been achieved by reconstituting SCID patients with haploidentical allogeneic bone marrow purged of postthymic T lymphocytes.

Approximately one-third of autosomal recessive SCID patients are adenosine deaminase (ADA)-deficient. ADA-deficient SCID patients suffer from the same infections as other SCID patients but may also exhibit skeletal abnormalities. Deficiency of ADA, a purine salvage pathway enzyme, results in the accumulation of adenosine, 2′-deoxyadenosine, and 2′-O-methyladenosine which are toxic to lymphocytes. It appears the adenosine and deoxyadenosine inactivate the enzyme, S-adenosylhomocysteine (SAH) hydrolase, which in turn is an inhibitor of most intracellular methylation reactions. Reduction of SAH hydrolase activity leads to excessive methylation and lymphocytotoxicity. Patients with ADA-deficient SCID typically become lymphopenic within the first year of life. ADA-deficient SCID patients have been successfully treated with bone marrow from HLA-matched siblings and allogeneic haploidentical T-lymphocyte-purged bone marrow. An approach that has also been successful in some patients is ADA enzyme replacement either through infusion of irradiated adenosine deaminase-containing red blood cells or infusion of polyethylene glycol-linked bovine ADA. Autosomal recessive SCID with ADA deficiency is also a prime candidate for gene replacement therapy.

Severe combined immunodeficiency with leukopenia, also known as reticular dysgenesis, is extremely rare. This disorder is characterized by a nearly complete absence of circulating lymphocytes and granulocytes. Although a few patients have survived longer, most patients have died of disseminated infections within 6 months of birth.

Both the "bare lymphocyte syndrome" (MHC class I antigen deficiency) and combined MHC class I and class II antigen deficiency are very rare. These disorders are thought to be the result of defective cell surface expression of HLA antigens. Patients present in infancy with diarrhea, malabsorption, bacterial pneumonias, *Pheumocystis* pneumonia, sepsis, a variety of viral infections, and oral candidiasis. Both T lymphocyte and B lymphocyte functions are moderately to severely depressed. Typically, there is mod-

Table 61.6. Complement Assays[a]

Assay	Method	Clinical Utility
CH_{50}	Complement-mediated lysis of IgG (hemolysin)-coated RBCs	Functional screen of complement system
C3	Nephelometry or RID	Assess C3 level Assess complement consumption
C4	Nephelometry or RID	Assess C4 level Assess complement consumption
Component assays	Antigenic assay (nephelometry, ELISA, RIA) Functional assay (mixing studies with specific component-deficient serum)	Identify specific component deficiencies
C1-INH	Antigenic or functional assay	Evaluation of angioedema

[a]Abbreviations: RID, radial immunodiffusion; ELISA, enzyme-linked immunosorbent assay; C1-INH, C1 esterase inhibitor.

erate lymphopenia accompanied by hypoplastic lymphoid organs, anergy, and variable degrees of hypogammaglobulinemia. Most of these patients die early in childhood.

SURVEY OF USEFUL CLINICAL ASSAYS

While clinical presentation and characteristic, disease-specific manifestations (e.g., ataxia, telangiectasias, oculocutaneous albinism) may suggest a specific immunodeficiency, laboratory tests are always required to confirm the presence or absence of a given entity. The array of available laboratory tests is vast, bewildering, and expensive. Integration of clinical data and efficient, appropriate use of laboratory tests are essential to the rapid, cost-effective diagnosis and management of patients with primary immunodeficiency disorders. This section provides an overview of the laboratory assays most useful in the evaluation of primary immunodeficiency disorders.

Complement Assays

Accurate, reproducible methods are available for screening overall complement function as well as for quantifying most individual complement proteins and regulatory enzymes (e.g., C1 esterase inhibitor) (Table 61.6). While detailed analyses may be required in some immunodeficiency patients, a few basic screening tests of complement function suffice in most evaluations. If specimens are properly collected and handled, antigenic and functional complement assays are precise and sensitive.

TOTAL HEMOLYTIC COMPLEMENT; CH_{50}

Although expensive and laborious, the most widely used and arguably the most useful complement assay is a measurement of total hemolytic complement activity. Sheep red blood cells coated with rabbit antisheep red cell IgG (hemolysin) are incubated with various dilutions of serum. If the classic complement pathway is intact, the red cells will be lysed as the result of complement fixation triggered by red cell surface-bound IgG. The absence of any classic pathway complement component will result in a CH_{50} value of zero. However, CH_{50} measurements may fall within the normal range when individual components are reduced but not absent. Total hemolytic complement activity is expressed as CH_{50} units where the number of units equals the reciprocal of the serum dilution required to lyse 50% of IgG-coated sheep red blood cells. Calculation of CH_{50} units requires a mathematical transformation of the raw hemolysis data. The Von Krogh equation is used to transform a sigmoid-shaped dose-response curve into a linear relationship between serum dilution and amount of hemolysis. Hemolytic complement values are expressed as number of CH_{50} units/ml of undiluted serum. Individual complement component deficiencies can be identified by using panels of deficient sera in which all components except the component of interest are present in excess. If mixing of the test sample with the serum known to be deficient of a particular component fails to normalize the CH_{50} value, the deficient component in the test serum has been identified. Great attention to detail must be observed. For instance, the age of the sheep red blood cells, the amount of hemolysin employed, and the composition of buffers used, are absolutely critical to the provision of reproducible, accurate hemolytic complement assays.

Samples for functional complement assays must be handled properly. In most assays, including CH_{50}, fresh blood is allowed to clot at room temperature for 30 minutes and then at 4°C for 1 hour. Serum is then separated and stored in aliquots (to avoid the need to thaw and refreeze) at −70°C. The presence of cryoprecipitating antibodies can artifactually depress hemolytic complement values. In this situation complement is fixed by the antibody (at 4°C on room temperature) and thus "removed" from the serum before it can be measured. If cryoimmunoglobulins are suspected, the specimen should be maintained and processed at 37°C. Plasma samples containing EDTA can be used for CH_{50} assays if the sample is diluted enough to overcome the chelating effects of EDTA.

Table 61.7. Phagocyte Function Assays

Assay	Method	Clinical Utility
Complete blood count with differential	Coulter counter Romanowsky-stained smear	High yield screening test; several disorders can be definitely diagnosed or excluded
Nitroblue tetrazolium test	Slide or tube test (formazan dye test)	Screen for CGD[a]
Chemiluminescence	Stimulate neutrophils in presence of luminol	Screen for CGD
Hydrogen peroxide production superoxide anion production	Reduction of ferricytochrome c in presence of superoxide dismutase; flow cytometry	Screen for CGD
Bactericidal assay	Incubate isolated phagocytes with standard bacterial strains	Assess bactericidal capacity of phagocytes
Phagocytosis assay	Many; quantitation of uptake of particles by phagocytes as a function of time	Assess phagocytic capacity of cells
Chemotaxis assay	Boyden chamber Agarose gels Porous membranes	Assess cells for chemotactic defects

[a] CGD, chronic granulomatous disease.

ANTIGENIC COMPLEMENT ASSAYS; C3 and C4

The most commonly utilized antigenic complement component assays measure serum C3 and C4 concentrations by nephelometry. Nephelometry is rapid, precise, and relatively inexpensive compared with older manual methods such as radial immunodiffusion (RID). While such antigenic assays are easier to perform than functional assays, they tend to be less sensitive, and degraded, nonfunctional components may be measured. Assays of C3 and C4 concentration are particularly useful as indices of complement consumption. For example, in a patient with an active systemic immune complex disease such as systemic lupus erythematosus, the serum C3 and C4 levels may be decreased as the result of complement fixation (consumption) and catabolism. A selective decrease in C3 suggests alternative pathway activation. Obviously, isolated measurements of C3 or C4 have little value in identifying a homozygous complement component-deficient patient other than one with C3 or C4 deficiency. Specimen handling is less rigorous than for the CH_{50} assay. Serum or plasma can be used and routine −20°C storage is sufficient.

Phagocyte Function Assays

Phagocytic function testing is itself a vast and complex field. The most useful and widely available tests that are applicable to the evaluation of defective phagocyte function include a complete blood count with differential, the nitroblue tetrazolium test (NBT) or other tests of respiratory burst capacity, bactericidal assays, phagocytosis assays, and chemotaxis assays (Table 61.7). Although rare, leukocyte adhesion deficiency can be diagnosed by flow cytometry since monoclonal antibodies directed against leukocyte (β_2) integrins are commercially available. Most of these tests are time-consuming, expensive, and infrequently performed even in large laboratories.

COMPLETE BLOOD COUNT AND DIFFERENTIAL

While it is beyond the scope of this chapter to review all of the information that can be gleaned from a complete blood count (CBC) and differential, it is useful to note information that directly bears on the evaluation of primary immunodeficiency disorders. Strictly speaking, a CBC and differential are not phagocyte *function* assays. However, in any analysis of phagocyte function, a CBC plus differential is a logical starting point because of the wealth of information that it can provide. For instance, thrombocytopenia is characteristic of the Wiskott-Aldrich syndrome, and a normal platelet count essentially rules out this diagnosis. Granulocytopenia occurs in a wide variety of hematologic diseases and is the result of numerous types of iatrogenic insult. Despite the frequency and nonspecificity of this finding, granulocytopenia is characteristic of several primary immunodeficiency disorders including the Chédiak-Higashi syndrome, a subset of X-linked agammaglobulineurias, some cases of immunodeficiency with elevated IgM, reticular dysgenesis, and some patients with immunodeficiency and thymoma. In contrast, patients with LAD typically have circulating neutrophil counts ranging from 15,000/μl to 60,000/μl between infections and as high as 100,000/μl during infections. Abnormalities of peripheral blood lymphocyte count are even more commonly associated with primary immunodeficiencies. For instance, patients with X-linked lymphoproliferative disease (Duncan's disease) may transiently experience marked increases in lymphocyte count, while most patients with cellular immune disorders or combined humoral and cellular immune dysfunctions have depressed lymphocyte count. Data pertaining to red blood cell counts (and hemoglobin/hematocrit) can be useful in the evaluation of immunodeficiency disorders that may be accompanied by pancytopenia, red cell hypoplasia, or even hemolytic anemia. An example of the latter is CGD secondary to severe G6PD deficiency. In contrast to the more common CGD patients in which there is a defective NADPH oxidase, patients with CGD due to G6PD deficiency typically have a severe hemolytic anemia that is often precipitated or exacerbated by oxidant stresses introduced by various drugs or food constituents.

Examination of Romanowsky-stained blood smears can also provide invaluable clues in the evaluation of immunodeficiency patients. The Chédiak-Higashi syndrome is characterized by pathognomonic giant cytoplasmic granules in lymphocytes, monocytes, and neutrophils. Specific granule deficiency may be suspected by the appearance of neutrophils. X-linked lymphoproliferative disease that is characterized by an abnormal host response to EBV infections may be suggested on the basis of atypical lymphocytes. It should be clear from this discussion that laboratory evaluation of a suspected immunodeficiency patient begins with a CBC and differential.

NITROBLUE TETRAZOLIUM TEST AND OTHER ASSAYS OF RESPIRATORY BURST CAPACITY

The nitroblue tetrazolium test (NBT) test and other assays of respiratory burst capacity are useful in the evaluation of patients suspected of having CGD. The NBT slide test is widely available and relatively easy to perform. Activated neutrophils (or monocytes) normally undergo a respiratory burst in which molecular oxygen, O_2, is consumed and reduced to superoxide anion, O_2^-, under the catalytic influence of membrane-associated NADPH oxidase. In turn, O_2^- contributes to the generation of other oxygen-derived metabolites including hydrogen peroxide (H_2O_2), hydroxyl radical (HO•), and others. In the NBT test, the capacity of individual neutrophils (or monocytes) to reduce NBT to formazan (an insoluble blue pigment) can be visualized. In most types of CGD, no formazan is produced, indicating the absence of a respiratory burst. In some of the more obscure subtypes of CGD, the NBT test may be more difficult to interpret because there may be partial reduction of NBT, resulting in the formation of small quantities of formazan. In a typical female carrier of X-linked CGD, approximately one-half of the cells reduce NBT while the other half do not.

Chemiluminescence assays are also useful rapid screening tests for CGD. Chemiluminescence is a poorly defined by-product of oxygen radical formation. A common assay involves the detection of luminol-dependent chemiluminescence. Luminol is a compound that "amplifies" the light signal emitted by the generation of naturally occurring chemiluminescence. In this assay, isolated neutrophils are stimulated with a potent neutrophil agonist such as phorbol myristate acetate, synthetic formyl peptide, or C5a. Neutrophils from CGD patients yield little chemiluminescence. Assays must be carefully controlled with normal cells to ensure accurate results.

More direct measurements of oxygen-derived metabolites are employed in some laboratories. Superoxide anion produced by activated phagocytes reduces ferricytochrome c, resulting in an easily quantified colormetric change. Specificity of this assay is conferred by the capacity for superoxide dismutase to block cytochrome c reduction. (Superoxide dismutase is an enzyme that specifically degrades O_2^- into H_2O_2 and water.) Neutrophils from CGD patients produce little to no O_2^-. Several oxygen metabolite assays have been adapted to flow cytometry. Flow analysis of oxygen metabolite production offers the advantages of being quantitative and providing data about large numbers of individual cells.

BACTERICIDAL ASSAYS

Most in vitro bactericidal assays involve mixing isolated neutrophils with fixed numbers of a standard strain of bacteria, an incubation period, phagocyte lysis, and quantification of the residual viable bacteria. In some cases the patient's phagocytes are incubated with a bacterial isolate of special interest. In this type of assay a species or strain of bacteria to which the patient seems particularly susceptible may be employed. Such assays must be performed under standardized conditions and must be rigorously controlled. Even in large laboratories, bactericidal assays are infrequently performed. This type of testing should be employed only in very special circumstances.

PHAGOCYTOSIS ASSAYS

A large number of in vitro phagocytosis assays have been devised. The underlying principle of these assays is quantitation of uptake of particles by phagocyte cells as a function of time. Isolated neutrophils (or monocytes; macrophages) are incubated with isotope-labeled immune complexes or particulates that can be visualized under a microscope (e.g., charcoal particles, latex particles, zymosan particles). At varying times after addition of phagocytic particles, the number or percentage of material "ingested" is quantified. As in the case of other manually performed functional assays, great attention must be paid to experimental conditions and appropriate controls.

CHEMOTAXIS ASSAYS

Chemotaxis is directed cell movement up a chemical concentration gradient. Chemotaxis defects have been described in association with several primary immunodeficiency disorders. Leukocyte chemotaxis is most often examined using an adaptation of the Boyden chamber. Cell migration through agarose or through small pores in a membrane filter is quantified. In a typical membrane filter chemotaxis assay, a leukocyte suspension, most often neutrophils, is placed into a chamber that overlies a porous membrane. A solution containing the chemotactic stimulus is placed beneath the membrane. After a standard period of time the membrane is removed, the upper surface wiped clean, and the membrane fixed and stained. The number of leukocytes attached to a specified area of the undersurface is then counted under a microscope. The number of cells that migrate through the membrane is directly related to the concentration and potency of the chemotactic stimulus. Other chemotaxis assays employ similar principles. For instance, in agarose chemotaxis assays, the depth of penetration of leukocytes into the matrix material is a function of the concentration and potency of the stimulus. Again, standardization of assay conditions and the utilization of strict controls cannot be overemphasized.

Lymphocyte Function and Related Assays

"Lymphocyte function" assays, as broadly categorized here, encompass a diverse spectrum of laboratory and clinical tests that have a role in the evaluation of immunodeficiency disorders (Table 61.8). Some tests are very useful screens in the evaluation of common primary immunodeficiencies. For instance, the presence of appropriate normal serum immunoglobulin concentrations essentially excludes most of the disorders of humoral immunity and some of the combined humoral and cellular immunodeficiencies as diagnostic possibilities. Similarly, most disorders of cellular immunity can be excluded on the basis of a normal peripheral blood lymphocyte count and a normal delayed type hypersensitivity response (skin test). Not surprisingly, these tests constitute appropriate "first level" tests in a patient suspected of having an immunodeficiency disorder. As outlined in previous sections, a variety of lymphocyte functional defects have been defined in association with specific immunodeficiency states. Accordingly, the efficient utilization of more disease-specific tests must be based on sound clinical judgment. It should be emphasized that the list of assays and tests described here is not exhaustive. Likewise, in many cases there are several methods available for obtaining the same piece of data.

SERUM IMMUNOGLOBULINS

Quantitative serum immunoglobulin measurements are particularly valuable in the evaluation of patients suspected of humoral immunodeficiency disorders (see Table 61.3). Patients with severe combined immunodeficiencies and those with ataxia-telangiectasia, Wiskott-Aldrich syndrome, or hyperimmunoglobulinemia E syndrome often have characteristic patterns of immunoglobulin deficiency or excess. Serum IgG, IgA, and IgM concentrations normally increase as a function of age up to puberty, at which time they plateau at adult levels. Total γ-globulin concentration can be assessed by routine serum protein electrophoresis. While serum protein electrophoresis is essential to the diagnosis of some acquired humoral immunodeficiency states (e.g., multiple myeloma, light chain disease, monoclonal gammopathy associated with Waldenström's macroglobulinemia, or chronic lymphocytic leukemia), it should not be the determinant of humoral immune disorders. The chief problem in relying solely upon protein electrophoresis is that selective IgA or IgM deficiencies will be missed. Most laboratories quantify IgG, IgA, and IgM levels by nephelometry and IgE by enzyme-linked immunosorbent assay (ELISA). Measurements of IgD have no clinical utility except to exclude the very rare likelihood of an IgD multiple myeloma.

SPECIFIC ANTIBODY TITERS

Measurements of preexisting antibodies (e.g., anti-A and anti-B isohemagglutinins or antipolio, rubella, tetanus, or diphtheria in previously immunized individuals) can be useful in the evaluation of some patients suspected to be immunodeficient. For example, while babies with transient hypogammaglobulinemia have very low levels of IgG, IgA, and IgM, they still possess detectable isohemagglutinin titers and can respond to administered antigens such as diphtheria and tetanus toxoid. In contrast, patients with specific antibody deficiency, also known as "antibody deficiency with near-normal immunoglobulins," typically possess normal total immunoglobulin concentrations yet fail to respond to selected antigens (e.g., pneumococcal polysaccharides, tetanus, or diphtheria toxoids, or others). In this scenario, a suspected patient is immunized and pre- and postimmunization (2 weeks) titers determined. It must be remembered that patients with suspected immunodeficiency disorders should not be given a live (attenuated) vaccine. Antibody responses to this heterogeneous group of antigens is most efficiently carried out in the blood bank (isohemagglutinins) and serology laboratories. A va-

Table 61.8. Lymphocyte Function Assays[a]

Assay or Clinical Test	Method	Clinical Utility
B-Lymphocyte Tests		
Serum immunoglobulins	Nephelometry, RID, ELISA	Quantify serum IgG, IgA, IgM, IgE
Specific antibody titers	Various serologic methods	Assess performed antibody titers and specific antibody responses to protein or carbohydrate antigens
IgG subclass assays	RID, ELISA	Quantify IgG subclass concentrations
B lymphocyte enumeration	Flow cytometry (antibodies directed against B lymphocyte-specific surface antigens)	Quantity B lymphocytes
T-Lymphocyte Tests		
Skin tests (cutaneous delayed-type hypersensitivity)	Intradermal injection of tetanus toxoid, *Candida*, streptokinase-streptodornase, mumps, tuberculin, or *Trichophyton* antigens	Clinical assessment of cellular (T) immune response
T lymphocyte enumeration	Flow cytometry	Quantify T lymphocytes
T lymphocytes subset analysis	Flow cytometry	CD4/CD8 ratios (T helper; T suppressor)
Lymphocyte proliferation assays (lymphoblast transformation (LBT); mixed lymphocyte cultures (MLC))	In vitro stimulation of lymphocyte proliferation with mitogens, antigens, or allogeneic cells	Assess lymphocyte function
Enzyme assays (ADA; PNP)	Enzyme assays	Assess subtypes of SCID
Cytokine assays	Bioassays, RIA, ELISA	Quantify cytokine concentrations

[a]Abbreviations: LBT, lymphoblast transformation; MLC, mixed lymphocyte cultures; ADA, adenosine deaminase; PNP, purine nucleoside phosphorylase; RID, radial immunodiffusion; ELISA, enzyme-linked immunosorbent assay; SCID, severe combined immunodeficiency.

riety of serologic methods are employed to titer antibodies directed against vaccines.

IgG SUBCLASS ASSAYS

As noted previously, except in the case of profound IgG subclass 1 deficiency, total serum IgG measurements are not useful in the detection of IgG subclass deficiencies. The clinical significance of identifying IgG subclass deficiencies notwithstanding, most laboratories employ ELISA, RID or RIA to measure IgG subclass concentrations. Except in the rare very young patients (less than 2 years old), suspected of IgG 4 subclass deficiency, most RID assays are sensitive enough for routine clinical usage.

B-LYMPHOCYTE ENUMERATION

In antibody-deficient patients, peripheral B-lymphocyte concentration can be helpful in further clarifying the nature of the humoral immunodeficiency. Normally, 5 to 10% of peripheral blood lymphocytes are surface immunoglobulin-positive. Traditionally, B lymphocytes were enumerated by rosetting methods in which red blood cells opsonized with antibody and complement were incubated with lymphocytes. So-called "EAC" rosettes indicated that the attached lymphocytes were B lymphocytes. Most laboratories now enumerate B lymphocytes using a panel of monoclonal antisera that are directed against B lymphocyte-specific surface antigens such as immunoglobulin, HLA-DR antigens, and several B cell differentiation antigens. Flow cytometric analysis requires proper specimen collection and sample handling. It offers the advantages of rapidity, reproducibility, and the fact that many cells are examined.

SKIN TESTS

Skin testing provides a very useful and widely available means to assess cutaneous delayed-type hypersensitivity. A variety of antigens are available (see Table 61.7). It is absolutely critical that potent, standardized test antigens be utilized and that proper inoculation technique and result interpretation be employed. Too often, outdated or improperly stored test antigens are administered by inexperienced or untrained personnel. The absence of cutaneous delayed-type hypersensitivity response to a ubiquitous or previously encountered antigen is a strong indication of T-lymphocyte deficiency or dysfunction. The chief drawbacks of skin testing are that they are not specific with respect to the nature of a given T lymphocyte deficiency or defect and that babies may not have been exposed to, and may not respond to, some "ubiquitous" antigens.

T LYMPHOCYTE ENUMERATION AND SUBSET ANALYSIS

Since approximately 80% of peripheral blood lymphocytes are T cells, lymphopenia usually indicates a T-cell deficiency. Despite this, T-lymphocyte enumeration can be useful in the evaluation of immunodeficiency disorders. T-lymphocyte subset analyses, particularly CD4/CD8 ratios, are widely used in the context of the AIDS epidemic and in the era of high-volume organ transplantation and attend-

Table 61.9. Cytokines[a]

Cytokine	Comment
Tumor necrosis factor (cachectin)	Mediates septic/endotoxic shock; cachexia; acute phase response
Interleukin 1 (lymphocyte activating factor; endogenous pyrogen)	T and B lymphocyte development and activation
Interleukin 2 (T cell growth factor)	Mitogenic factor for T lymphocytes, B lymphocytes, NK cells
Interleukin 3 (multicolony stimulating factor)	Differentiation and growth of hematopoietic progenitor cells
Interleukin 4 (T cell derived B cell growth factor)	Mediates B lymphocyte proliferation
Interleukin 5 (B cell growth factor II)	Stimulation of antibody synthesis and secretion; eosinophil growth and differentiation
Interleukin 6 (B cell stimulatory factor 2)	Stimulation of antibody synthesis; mediates acute phase response
Interleukin 7	Stimulates growth of B cell precursors, T cells
Interleukin 8 (neutrophil chemotactic factor)	Neutrophil chemotaxis
Monocyte chemoattractant protein 1 (monocyte chemotactic and activating factor)	Monocyte chemotaxis; monocyte/macrophage activation

[a]This list of cytokines and associated functions is selective. Comprehensive discussions of cytokine activities can be found in the Suggested Readings list.

ant monitoring protocols. As in the case of B-lymphocyte enumeration, technology has shifted away from manual rosetting assays to flow cytometry. Traditionally, T lymphocytes have been enumerated by E-rosette formation, an assay based on the capacity of T lymphocytes to recognize and specifically bind (via CD_2) mouse red blood cells. Many laboratories enumerate T lymphocytes with panels of monoclonal antibodies directed against several T lymphocyte-specific surface molecules. In addition to T-lymphocyte enumeration and subset analysis, additional monoclonal antibodies are available to identify activated T cells and natural killer cells. Specimen handling, sample processing, and the pitfalls and advantages of flow analysis of T lymphocytes are the same as noted above.

LYMPHOCYTE PROLIFERATION ASSAYS

Lymphocyte proliferation assays are used to assess lymphocyte function in vitro. Many of the cellular and combined immunodeficiency disorders are marked by the failure of T lymphocytes to respond to proliferative stimuli including T lymphocyte mitogens (e.g., phytohemagglutinin, concanavalin A), previously encountered antigens (e.g., tuberculin, tetanus toxoid, *Candida*), and allogeneic cells. In all of these assays lymphocytes from the patient suspected to be immunodeficient are incubated with mitogen, antigen or irradiated allogeneic lymphocytes in the presence of [^{3}H]-thymidine. [^{3}H]-thymidine is incorporated into the DNA being synthesized in the proliferating cells. At the end of the assay, typically 3 to 5 days, the number of [^{3}H]-thymidine counts incorporated into the stimulated cells are determined, and a proliferation index is calculated. In recent years analogous nonisotopic assays have been developed.

ENZYME ASSAYS

Adenosine deaminase and purine nucleoside phosphorylase deficiencies are associated with autosomal recessive SCID and some patients with Nezelof's syndrome. These disorders are rare, and only a few laboratories perform the enzyme assays.

CYTOKINE ASSAYS

The clinical utilization of cytokine measurements in serum, body fluids (e.g., cerebrospinal fluid, synovial fluid, lung lavage fluid, etc.), and in vitro, holds promise for the future. In recent years, intensive investigation of cytokine function and metabolism has been carried out in experimental models of human disease and in vitro. Numerous cytokines have been identified, most of which appear to participate in immunologic and inflammatory processes (Table 61.9). While it is beyond the scope of this chapter to discuss cytokine biology in detail, it can be safely predicted that some immunodeficiency disorders are related to abnormal cytokine regulation. Most cytokines exert biological activities at picomolar to nanomolar concentrations. Currently available methods of measurement include bioassays, ELISA, and RIA.

INTERPRETATION: LABORATORY EVALUATION OF IMMUNODEFICIENCY STATES

Accurate diagnosis of immunodeficiency diseases requires complete clinical and laboratory data. Attempts to render a specific diagnosis based upon laboratory data alone will at some time result in misdiagnosis. Likewise, assiduous standardization and control measures must be applied to specimen collection, sample handling and processing, and to the assay itself. As alluded to in the preceding section, many of the assays used in the evaluation of immunodeficiency diseases are expensive, labor-intensive, and specialized. Careful selection of "first-level" screening tests based upon the patient's medical history will lead to the exclusion of many potential diagnoses. For example, a normal CH_{50} value essentially excludes nearly all of the inherited complement deficiency disorders. Antigenic or functional measurements of individual complement components do not usually provide useful data in a patient with a normal CH_{50} value. A normal complete blood count and differential will exclude numerous immunodeficiency disorders including the Chédiak-Higashi syndrome and most cellular and combined immunodeficiencies. A high leukocyte count coupled with appropriate clinical history is highly suggestive of LAD. Normal serum IgG, IgA and IgM levels exclude most humoral immunodeficiency states. Skin testing for delayed-type hypersensitivity and T- and B-lymphocyte enumeration are the most useful first-level tests. More specialized assays can be utilized when the clinical data and screening assays dictate.

The ever-broadening therapeutic armamentarium makes it increasingly important to identify patients with primary immunodeficiency disorders properly. Illnesses that were once uniformly fatal can be treated by means of immunologic reconstitution (e.g., γ-globulin replacement, bone marrow transplantation), cytokine or interferon therapy, and perhaps in the future, gene therapy.

Suggested Reading

1. Alarcon B, Regueiro JR, Arnaiz-Villena A, Terhorst C. Familial defect in the surface expression of the T-cell receptor-CD3 complex. N Engl J Med 1988;319:1203.
2. Ambrosino DM, Umetsu DT, Siber GR, et al. Selective defect in the antibody response to Haemophilus influenzae type b in children with recurrent infections and normal serum IgG subclass levels. J Allergy Clin Immunol 1988;81:1175.
3. Ammann AJ, Hong R. Disorders of the T cell system. In: Stiehm ER, ed. Immunologic disorders of infants and children. Philadelphia: WB Saunders, 1989:259–302.
4. Buckley RH, Wray BB, Belmaker EZ. Extreme hyperimmunoglobulinema E and undue susceptibility to infection. Pediatrics 1992;49:1.
5. Buckley RH. Immunodeficiency diseases. JAMA 1987;258: 2841.
6. Buckley RH. Normal and abnormal development of the immune system. In: WK Joklik, Willett HP, Amos DB, eds. Zinsser textbook of microbiology and immunology, 19th ed. New York: Appleton-Century-Crofts, 1988.
7. Buckley RH. Primary immunodeficiency disease. In: Wyngaarden JB, Smith LH, Bennett JC, eds. Textbook of medicine, 19th ed. Philadelphia: WB Saunders, 1991:1446–1453.
8. Callard RE, Shields JG, Smith SH, Lau YL, Levinsky R. Measurement of human B cell responses to growth and differentiation factors: Relevance for immunodeficiency disease. Lymphokine Res 1986;5 (suppl 1):S151.
9. Chatila T, Wong B, Young M, et al. An immunodeficiency characterized by defective signal transduction in T lymphocytes. N Engl J Med 1989;320:696.
10. Fireman P. Immunodeficiency and allergic disease. In: Fireman P, Slavin RG, eds. Atlas of allergies. New York: Gower Medical Publishing. 1991.
11. Fischer A, Lisowska-Grospierre B, Anderson DC, Springer TA. Leukocyte adhesion deficiency: molecular basis and functional consequences. Immunodef Rev 1989;1:39.
12. Geha RS. Antibody deficiency syndromes and novel immunodeficiencies. Pediatr Infect Dis J 1988;7:557.
13. Gifford RH, Malawista SE. A simple rapid micromethod for detecting chronic granulomatous disease of childhood. J Lab Clin Med 1970;75:511.
14. Hong R. Problems in host defense. In: Henry JB, ed. Clinical diagnosis and management by laboratory methods. Philadelphia: WB Saunders, 1991:1156–1178.
15. Kizai H, Sakurada T. Simple micro-assay methods for enzymes of purine metabolism. J Lab Clin Med 1977;89:1135.
16. Kniker WT, Lesourd BM, McBryde JL, Corriel RN. Cell mediated immunity assessed by multitest CMI skin testing in infants and preschool children. Am J Dis Child 1988;139:840.
17. Lawton AR, Cooper M. Ontology of immunity. In: Steihm ER, Fulginiti VA, eds. Immunologic diseases in infants and children. Philadelphia: WB Saunders, 1988.
18. Matheson DS, Green BJ. Defect in production of B cell differentiation factor-like activity by mononuclear cells from a boy with hypogammaglobulinemia. J Immunol 1987;138:2469.
19. Mayer L, Kwan SP, Thompson C, et al. Evidence for a defect in "switch" T cells in patients with immunodeficiency and hyperimmunoglobulinemia. N Engl J Med 1986;314:409.
20. Mizel SB. The interleukins. FASEB J 1989;3:2379–2388.
21. Moen RC, Oemichen SL, Kiggens AL, Hong R. ELISA detection of specific functional antibodies in human serum to E. coli, tetanus toxoid, and diphtheria-tetanus toxoids: normal values for IgG, IgA and IgM. Diag Immunol 1986;4:17.
22. Muller-Eberhard HJ. Molecular organization and function of the complement system. Annu Rev Biochem 1988;57:321.
23. Nelson RD, Quie PG, Simmons RL. Chemotaxis under agarose: a new and simple method for measuring chemotaxis and spontaneous migration of human polymorphonuclear leukocytes and monocytes. J Immunol 1975;115:1650.
24. Ochs HD, Wedgwood RJ. Disorders of the B-cell system. In: Stiehm ER, ed. Immunologic disorders in infants and children. Philadelphia: WB Saunders, 1989:214–258.
25. Oettgen HC, Terhorst C. The T-cell receptor-T3 complex and T-lymphocyte activation. Hum Immunol 1987;18:187.
26. Parry MF, Root RK, Metcalf JA, et al. Myeloperoxidase deficiency: prevalence and clinical significance. Ann Intern Med 1981;95:293.
27. Schifferli JA, Ng YC, Peters DK. The role of complement and its receptor in the elimination of immune complexes. N Engl J Med 1986;325:488.
28. Schur PH. IgG subclasses: a review. Ann Allergy 1987;58:89.
29. Stiehm ER. Immunodeficiency disorders: general considerations. In: Stiehm ER, Fulginiti VA, eds. Immunologic disorders in infants and children. Philadelphia: WB Saunders, 1988.
30. Weening RS, Corbeel L, De Boer M, et al. Cytochrome B deficiency in an autosomal form of chronic granulomatous disease. J Clin Invest 1985;75:915.
31. Winkelstein JA, Colten H. Genetically determined disorders of the complement system. In: Scriver CR, Beaudet AL, Sly WS, Valle DL, eds. The metabolic basis of inherited disease, 6th ed. New York: McGraw-Hill, 1989:2711–2737.

62 Autoimmune Disease and Serology

John L. Carey III and David F. Keren

INTRODUCTION

Immune Regulation and Natural Autoantibodies

The primary task of the immune system is to recognize the self versus the non-self. This is critical for the removal of infectious agents, the degradation of neoplastic and effete normal cells, and the development of tolerance for normal autoantigens and tissues. The two principal hypotheses of immunoregulation are Burnet's clonal deletion theory and Jerne's idiotype anti-idiotype theory. The former postulates that autoreactive T- and B-cell clones are deleted in utero when they come into contact with autoantigens. Thus, autoantibodies and autoreactive T cells should be seen only in patients with autoimmune diseases or in normal individuals immunized with "sequestered" self-antigens. In contrast, Jerne's theory postulates that autoantibodies and autoreactive T cells are normal and essential for the regulation of each other. This occurs by complementary binding of the variable regions (idiotype anti-idiotype) of anti-antibodies to autoantibodies, anti-antibodies to T- and B-cell antigen receptors, and T- and B-antigen receptors to each other.

Currently, the data from experimental animal models and from normal and autoimmune human patients support both hypotheses. These have demonstrated that (*a*) antibodies can be spontaneously produced (natural antibodies); (*b*) natural antibodies are present in humans to a large variety of normal autoantigens (natural autoantibodies—NAA); and (*c*) clonal deletion is the primary mode by which autoreactive thymocytes are deleted during development.

Thus, the cellular and humoral arms of the immune system cross-regulate each other via a combination of cell-to-cell interactions, cytokines, and idiotype/anti-idiotype reactions. These give rise to both helper and suppressor mechanisms. In the cellular arm, these are primarily mediated by T helper and suppressor cells, although B, NK, and myelomonocytic cells also play significant roles.

The NAAs are usually present in low concentrations, and have low or variable affinities for their target autoantigens. They can be found in virtually any individual, although their number and/or concentration are increased (*a*) with age, (*b*) in females, (*c*) in chronic diseases, and (*d*) in healthy first-degree relatives of patients with autoimmune disorders. The NAAs seen in normals usually will persist, but are usually of lower titer (concentration).

Etiology and Diagnosis of Autoimmune Disease

Autoimmune disease may be seen as normal autoimmunity gone awry. It probably reflects the price the organism pays for having an immune system whose baseline regulation is directed by the ongoing recognition of self by autoreactive T and B cells. Fortunately, a variety of factors must be involved for normal autoimmune processes to trigger clinical disease. Most well-defined autoimmune disorders do have a "marker" autoantibody of variable sensitivity or specificity. However, with few exceptions, these have no well-defined pathophysiological role.

The possible mechanisms of autoimmune disease may include (*a*) the failure of humoral and/or cellular suppressor mechanisms of NAAs; (*b*) the expansion of auto-B, auto-T helper and/or effector cell clones by cross-reactive activators such as infectious agents (e.g., Epstein-Barr virus; *Streptococcus*); (*c*) the enhanced presentation of autoantigens by certain HLA antigens; and (*d*) increased HLA antigen expression on damaged or immune-stimulated cells. Other predisposing factors also probably exist (e.g., hormonal, genetic, environmental).

The criteria for defining autoimmune disease similar to Koch's postulates for infectious diseases can be derived (Table 62.1). However, many autoimmune disorders fail to meet all of these criteria. Even clinically well-defined autoimmune diseases can and do have heterogeneous clinical and laboratory features and time courses. A corollary to this is that no one clinical or laboratory finding is diagnostic in and of itself for autoimmune disease.

Table 62.1. Criteria for Autoimmune Disease[a]

Defined circulating autoantibody or defined cell-mediated autoimmunity
Defined autoantigen
Passive transfer of disease by autoantibody or immune cells in experimental animals
Production of disease by immunization with autoantigen in experimental animals
Production of autoantibody or autoreactive cell-mediated immunity after immunization with autoantigen in experimental animals

[a]From Shoenfeld Y, Isenberg D. The mosaic of autoimmunity (the factors associated with autoimmune disease). Research Monographs in Immunology, Turk JL, ed. Vol. 12. Amsterdam: Elsevier, 1989:ix.

METHODOLOGY

Direct and Indirect Immunofluorescence

The most established form of testing for serum autoantibodies is incubating it with tissue substrates, then screening for bound human antibody (autoantibody) by the use of a fluorochrome-conjugated anti-human antibody. This is known as an indirect immunofluorescence assay. A similar immunofluorescence assay for the detection of autoantibody or complement bound to the patient's tissue is known as a direct assay. Both approaches can be modified to use immunoperoxidase or immunoalkaline phosphatase detection systems in place of immunofluorescence. These latter techniques allow a clearer view of the associated morphologic features, do not require a fluorescence microscope, and provide a more permanent record. However, they are probably less sensitive than immunofluorescence.

The indirect assay is more attractive because it requires only a venipuncture. However, circulating autoantibody may be absent because of extensive binding by the autoantigen. Thus, biopsy of the affected tissue and direct immunoassay for autoantibody or complement may be more sensitive in some autoimmune disorders. For most systemic and organ-specific autoimmune diseases, the direct immunoassay is not necessary for diagnosis. The major exception appears to be cutaneous autoimmune disorders.

Quantitation of the autoantibody can be done by performing serial doubling dilutions of the serum. The titer is expressed as the reciprocal of the highest dilution exhibiting specific reactivity. This quantitation is quite imprecise, with error ranges commonly in the ± 2 doubling dilution range. Thus, detection of significant alterations in titer usually require either 75% decreases or 400% increases in autoantibody concentration.

Particle Agglutination

Particle agglutination is an indirect immunoassay that measures the presence of autoantibodies to known antigens. The autoantigen must be purified, then bound to a larger structure (e.g., red blood cell, or latex). Reactivity of antigens with the autoantibody results in clumping (agglutination) of the indicator particles. The amount of autoantibody can be roughly measured by doubling or quadrupling dilutions of the serum sample until there is no significant agglutination. Agglutination is less sensitive than most other immunoassays. However, the simplicity of incubation and lack of need for instrumentation to "read" the reaction makes it very attractive in third-world and remote testing locations.

Enzyme-Linked Immunosorbent Assay

The application of enzyme-linked immunosorbent assay (ELISA) to autoimmune serology has become increasingly popular in the past decade. This is mainly because of the identification and cloning of the genes of various autoantigens (e.g., Sm, RNP, Ro/SSA, La/SSB). Usually, the purified or cloned autoantigen is used to coat the wells of the microtiter plate (solid phase). Then the patient sample is reacted with the antigen. After washing, any bound human antibody is detected by an enzyme-conjugated anti-human antibody. Most assays use a colorimetric reaction to measure the amount of bound antibody. This is usually read on a spectrophotometer modified to read the entire microtiter plate.

The attractive features of commercial ELISA assays as opposed to manual indirect immunofluorescence or agglutination are (*a*) increased simplicity of preparation; (*b*) the ability to perform both a screen and quantitation of any detectable autoantigen in one step; (*c*) increased precision; and (*d*) increased objectivity. Drawbacks include (*a*) increased sensitivity, hence increased "false" or clinically insignificant positive reactions; (*b*) often increased reagent expense; and (*c*) the need for an instrument to read and quantitate the results. ELISAs differ from radioimmunoassays because they do not use radioisotopes (hence disposal and radiation safety are not problems) and they have a relatively simple assay procedure. In addition, they do not require expensive radiation counters.

Radioimmunoassays and Enzyme Immunoassays

The radioimmunoassays (RIAs) are the gold standard for most other immunoassays. The high labeling signal, combined with monoclonal antibody specificity, sensitive detectors, and rigorous data analysis make RIA the most sensitive immunoassay, and probably one of the most specific. However, many nonisotopic assays have equivalent specificity, and their lesser sensitivity is not usually clinically significant. The development of chemoluminescence immunoassays give rise to the promise of nonisotopic procedures with sensitivity and specificity rivaling the RIA. The drawbacks of RIAs are generally related to the radioactive nature of the indicator and to the complexity of the procedure and analysis.

The enzyme immunoassay (EIA) has become increasingly attractive as a nonisotopic, sensitive assay that can be readily performed in offices, clinics, and laboratories. The qualitative assays can contain several autoantigens on a strip, allowing rapid profiling of a patient's sera.

Immunodiffusion and Immunoelectrophoresis

Classic double diffusion gel immunoprecipitation (Ouchterlony) techniques are still used to screen and specify autoantibodies. Like agglutination assays, their advantages include a relative simplicity of preparation and incubation, and the ability to read them without the need for instrumentation. The disadvantages are insensitivity and slow development time. One way to overcome these problems is to perform counterimmunoelectrophoresis (CIE). In this approach, an electric field drives the cationic serum antibody and more anionic autoantigen toward each other in a Ouchterlony gel. This allows greater speed and finer resolution of immunoreactivity.

SYSTEMIC AUTOIMMUNE DISEASES

Antinuclear Antibodies

Antinuclear antibodies (ANAs) are immunoglobulins directed against antigens normally found in the nuclei of the cells. The antigens are protein, nucleic acid, or, most commonly, nucleoprotein complexes. These biomolecules are highly conserved in evolution because of their central role in DNA and RNA metabolism. While the role of ANAs in the pathogenesis of systemic and organ-restricted autoimmune disease is variable and controversial, ANAs are quite useful as disease markers, both for diagnosis and, to a much lesser extent, to monitor the course of disease.

ANAs are found in healthy individuals. While the exact fraction has varied according to the population surveyed and the detection technique used, approximately 3.5% up to as many as 15 to 20% of normal individuals have a detectable serum ANA at a 1:40 screening titer. Usually, these ANAs are of low titer (1:40 to 1:80 or lower), and will persist over time. They are most often seen in older individuals and in females, or they may be detected during periods of active inflammatory stress (e.g., pneumonia). As demonstrated by longitudinal follow-up studies, these low-titer ANAs do not portend any increased risk of autoimmune disease.

Detection of serum ANAs by indirect immunofluorescent assay is the dominant methodology at this time. It is sensitive, screens for a wide variety of known and unknown autoantibodies, and offers insights into the probable identity of the antigen. However, because of the labor-intensive and subjective nature of the assay, other technologies (ELISA, EIA) are gaining favor.

The two primary problems with current ANA testing are the variations in substrate antigenicity and interpretation of the immunofluorescence pattern. Historically, rodent (mouse or rat) kidney sections were initially used as substrates for nuclear antigens. However, these cells occasionally lacked detectable amounts of some antigens. The ANAs to these antigens (centromeres, SSA/Ro) are significant diagnostic and prognostic markers of various systemic autoimmune disorders (scleroderma systemic lupus erythematosus).

Over the last 10 years, human carcinoma cell lines (HEp2,KB) have become the substrate of choice for ANA immunofluorescence assay, and have largely replaced mouse substrates in most clinical laboratories. The advantages of the cell lines are threefold. They possess a broader array of antigens than the rodent tissue substrates, particularly those associated with cellular proliferation. Second, the numerous dividing cells, with their histone/DNA-rich mitotic figures, serve as a useful aid in delineating the patterns (homogeneous versus speckled), and hence the general antigent specificity of the ANA. Lastly, the larger individual size of the cells further facilitates the recognition of the various ANA patterns.

Variation of antigenic expression by the substrate may not simply be due to differences in the mitotic activity or type of cell. Conditions of fixation, storage, and prewashing may cause variation in ANA reactivity of the same substrate type between different vendors or different lots from the same vendor. This is particularly germane for such antigens as SSA/Ro.

Given the subjective nature of ANA interpretation, some strict general guidelines must be followed to enhance the intraobserver and interobserver uniformity of results. A positive ANA is one in which more than 50% of the interphase nuclei have immunofluorescence greater than that of the negative control. The presence of positive mitotic figures *without* positive nuclear fluorescence is interpreted as nega-

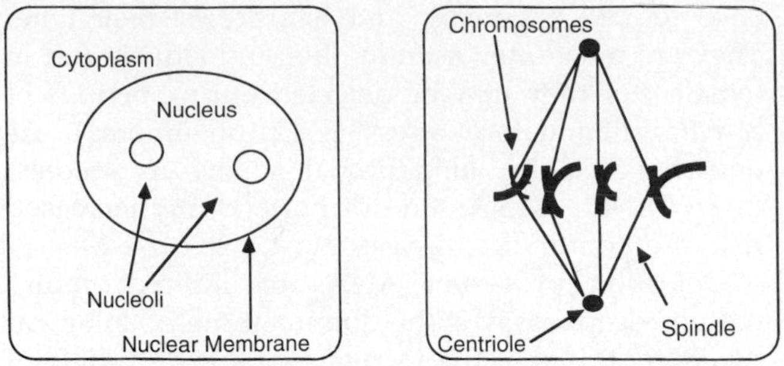

Figure 62.1. Diagram of basic HEp2 cell cytomorphology.

tive, both for screening and titering dilutions. The more concentrated and available nucleoproteins in the mitotic figure probably accounts for this last differential immunofluorescence pattern.

A general rule is to emphasize specificity in diagnosing the presence, pattern, and titer of an ANA. The primary role of the ANA screen is to detect the presence of autoantibody. Questionable screening and endpoint titer results are best interpreted as negative, given the sensitivity of the technique and the incidence of false-positive results. Most systemic autoimmune diseases have at least one high-titer autoantibody as a disease marker; hence, the ANA will usually be clearly positive on current immunofluorescence assays.

Questionable patterns are most effectively called "indeterminate." Other techniques can then be used to determine ANA specificities (e.g., anti-dsDNA/*Crithidia* immunofluorescence assay, anti-SSA and SSB/double diffusion, or CIE). Lastly, some ANA patterns may suggest the presence of two or more autoantibodies. In some instances, the patterns at a given dilution are diagnostic for both (i.e., nucleolar and anti-centromere antibody [ACA]). However, in other cases, one autoantibody pattern may partially or completely obscure the diagnostic features of the other(s) (e.g., speckled and homogeneous). In such instances, it is necessary to titrate the serum. Only if the questionable ANA is of higher titer can one see the diagnostic immunofluorescence assay pattern of the second autoantibody. When this cannot be accomplished, we indicate the definite presence of the diagnostic ANA pattern and the possible presence of the second. If need be, further confirmatory double diffusion tests may be performed to confirm or refute the presence of a second ANA.

To understand the immunofluorescence patterns seen with various ANAs, it is necessary to comprehend the distribution of their target antigens in interphase and dividing cells (Fig. 62.1). The nuclei can be divided into the diffuse nucleoplasm, nucleolus, and nuclear membrane. The nucleoplasm contains deoxynucleoproteins (DNA, histone and nonhistone proteins), along with a variety of structural and messenger RNAs with their associated proteins. The histones and DNA form a repeating nucleoprotein complex. This structure is critical to efficient packaging of DNA and formation of higher ordered structures (i.e., chromosomes).

The nonhistone proteins are also highly conserved, and play a central role in the metabolism of DNA and RNA (DNA replication and transcription, RNA processing and translation). They are highly vulnerable to leaching from suboptimally prepared substrates during washes. Thus, careful control of fixation during production of substrate slides is imperative. Double-stranded (ds) and single-stranded DNA in the immunofluorescence assay cell lines and tissues appear to be primarily available in the periphery of the nucleus. Adjacent to this is the nuclear membrane with various antigenic structures (lamins, pore protein complex).

The nucleolus shares some antigens with the non-nucleolar nucleus (ScL-70/topoisomerase), as well as a variety of structural and functional ribonucleoproteins and related enzymes (e.g., tRNA, U3 RNP, RNA polymerase I, fibrillarin). The centromeric proteins can be found in both the interphase nucleus and the mitotic figure. In the former, these appear diffusely scattered throughout the nucleus, while in the latter they are oriented along the plane of the chromosomes.

During mitosis, the nuclear membrane dissolves, and the proteins not bound to DNA (nonhistone) spill out into the cytoplasm, while the histones and centromeric proteins remain bound to the chromosomal DNA. Also present in the cytoplasm of a dividing cell is the mitotic spindle apparatus, which includes the centrioles and the associated tubulin fibers that extend to the centromeric region of each chromosome.

INDIRECT IMMUNOFLUORESCENCE ANA PATTERNS

Homogeneous

The nucleus of the interphase cell is uniformly more fluorescent than the negative control, with a smooth or finely granular pattern (Fig. 62.2). The only nonfluorescent nuclear structure may be the nucleolus. The mitotic figures seen in dividing cells will have dense uniform fluorescence, while the cytoplasm will be nonfluorescent. ANAs with a speckled pattern will have the reciprocal pattern of immunofluorescence on mitotic cells, as described later in this section.

The homogeneous ANA pattern is most commonly seen with anti-deoxynucleoprotein (DNP) and anti-histone autoantibodies. Anti-dsDNA antibodies

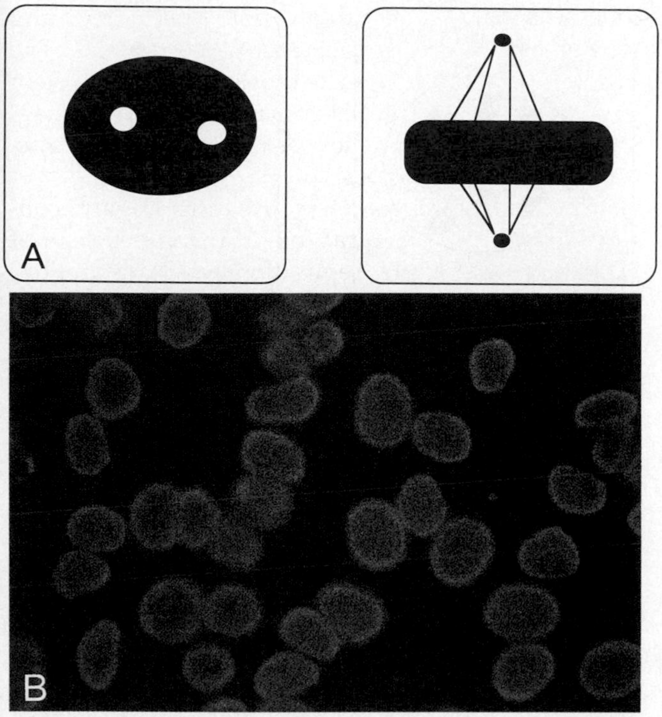

Figure 62.2. **A**, Diagram of homogeneous ANA fluorescence pattern. Black areas (compare to Fig. 62.1) are fluorescent. **B**, Homogeneous ANA immunofluorescence on HEp2 cells. 1:40 serum dilution, viewed under 400 × epifluorescence microscope.

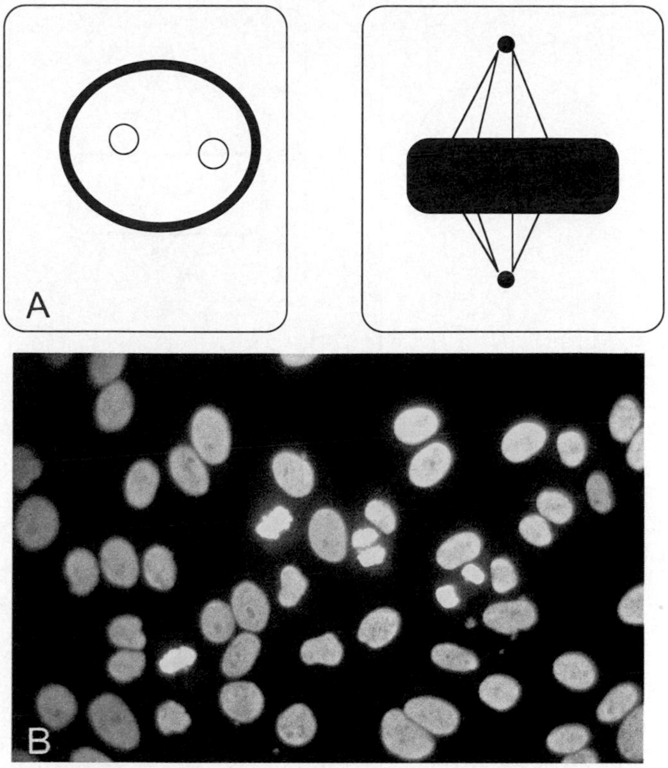

Figure 62.3. **A**, Diagram of peripheral (anti-dsDNA) ANA fluorescence pattern (see Fig. 62.2**A**). **B**, Peripheral (anti-dsDNA) ANA immunofluorescence on HEp2 cells (see Fig. 62.2**B**).

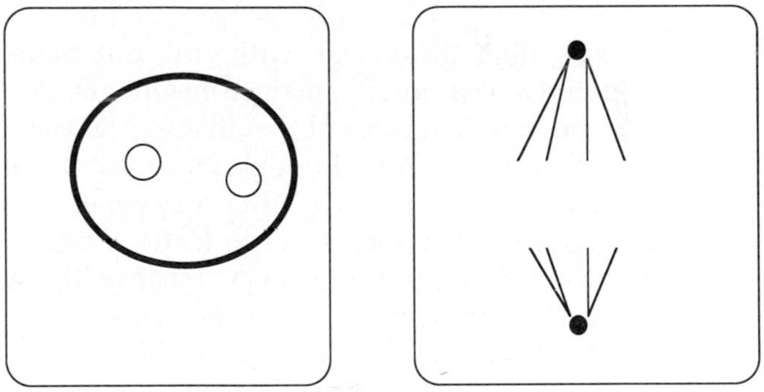

Figure 62.4. Diagram of nuclear membrane ANA fluorescence pattern (see Fig. 62.2**A**).

may also have a homogeneous appearance, although they are more often peripheral (see below). The homogeneous immunofluorescence assay pattern is most often seen with systemic lupus erythematosus (SLE), particularly if present in a high titer. High-titer anti-histone antibody may also be seen with the drug-induced lupus syndrome.

Peripheral

The rim of the nucleus has greater fluorescence than the negative control, while the dominant central nuclear area appears weakly fluorescent (Fig. 62.3). The mitotic figures are strongly and uniformly fluorescent, as is seen with a homogeneous ANA, but unlike nuclear membrane, pore, or laminin autoantibodies (see below). A pure peripheral ANA exhibits no significant cytoplasmic reactivity in either interphase or mitotic cells. The peripheral ANA pattern is due to anti–double-stranded (ds) antibodies. These are strongly associated with SLE, and the titer often correlates with the risk of SLE nephritis.

Nuclear Membrane

A nuclear "membrane" pattern may be seen with an anti-lamin or nuclear pore ANA (Fig. 62.4), and must be distinguished from a peripheral ANA pattern due to anti-dsDNA. The nuclei of interphase cells have essentially the same immunofluorescence pattern as a peripheral ANA. The key differential point is the mitotic figure in dividing cells, which is nonfluorescent (nonreactive) with the nuclear membrane antibody. A nuclear membrane ANA has been associated with clinically significant disease, and so should be reported.

Speckled Antigens

The nucleus exhibits a diffuse, finely to coarsely granular immunofluorescence, which is greater than that seen in the negative control (Fig. 62.5). These fluorescent points are much more numerous and va-

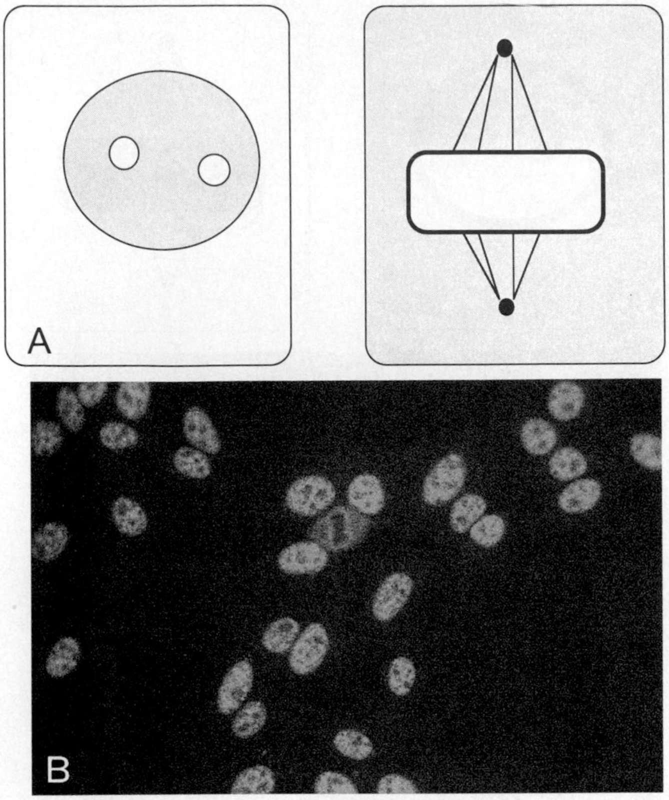

Figure 62.5. **A**, Diagram of speckled ANA fluorescence pattern (see Fig. 62.2**A**). **B**, Speckled ANA immunofluorescence on HEp2 cells (see Fig. 62.2**B**).

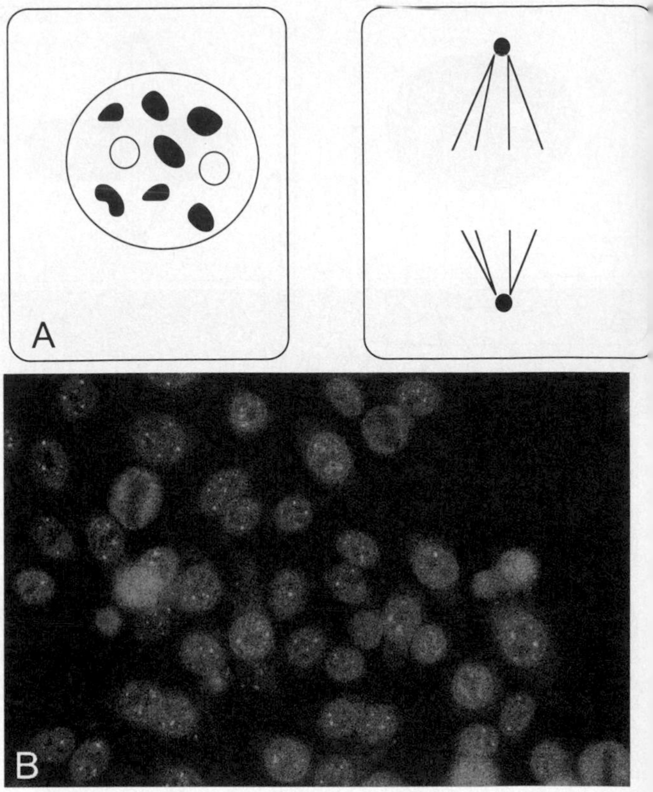

Figure 62.6. **A**, Diagram of pseudo-anti-centromere antibody (ACA) ANA fluorescence pattern (see Fig. 62.2**A**). **B**, Pseudo-ACA ANA immunofluorescence on HEp2 cells (see Fig. 62.2**B**).

riable in size than those seen with anti-centomere (ACA) antibody. The nucleoli may or may not be fluorescent. The mitotic figures of the dividing cells are essentially nonfluorescent, although there may be a perichromosomal staining. The latter may reflect increased concentration of the speckled antigens around the chromosomes. However, most of these "speckled" antigens appear to diffusely spread out into the cytoplasm after dissolution of the nucleus during mitosis. This results in enhanced immunofluorescence of the cytoplasm of the dividing cell, and is essentially the opposite picture of that seen with a homogeneous ANA. The speckled pattern may be seen with a wide variety of ANAs (anti-Sm,anti-RNP,anti-SSA,anti-SSB,anti-Scl-70). As such, its disease association is also quite broad, and includes SLE, Sjögren's syndrome, scleroderma, and mixed connective tissue disease (MCTD). Further interpretation of the speckled pattern requires more specific tests to identify the antigen(s) reacting with the ANA.

Pseudo-ACA

Three systems of pseudo–anti-centromere (ACA) autoantibodies have been identified: NSpI, NSpII, and sp-100. The NSpI and sp-100 autoantibodies have similar immunofluorescence assay patterns: a few (five to 10) coarse, large nuclear speckles, without significant cytoplasmic or mitotic staining (Fig. 62.6). Anti-NSpII has a finely speckled nucleus or more coarsely speckled mitotic immunofluorescence assay pattern. The disease associations are not well established at this time. However, anti-NSpI has been reported with chronic active hepatitis and anti-NSpII with the Sjögren's-RA syndrome. Anti-sp-100 has been reported with a variety of diseases (Wegener's, Sjögren's, primary Raynaud's, primary biliary cirrhosis) as well as undefined connective tissue diseases. However, none of these three autoantibodies has yet been reported in association with scleroderma. The most important conclusion is to distinguish them from the anti-centromere antibody ACA (see below).

Anti-centromere

The nuclei contain a finite number (ideally 46) of uniform intermediate-sized fluorescent points. These are diffusely scattered throughout the nucleus. The dividing cell will have a fluorescent mitotic figure, with a characteristic alignment of the fluorescent points (centromeres) along the long axis of the chromosomal region (Fig. 62.7). This is seen as either a

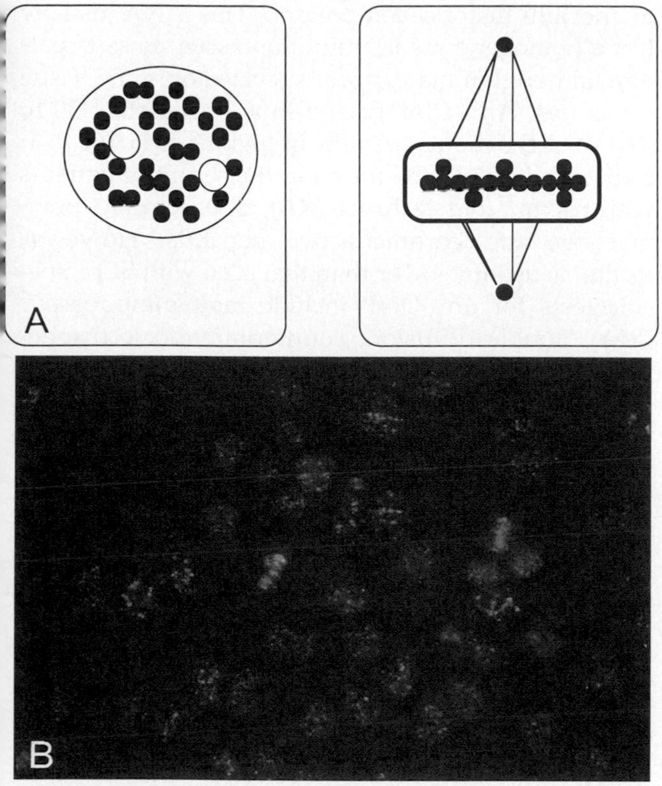

Figure 62.7. **A**, Diagram of anti-centromere (ACA) ANA fluorescence pattern (see Fig. 62.2**A**). **B**, ACA ANA immunofluorescence on HEp2 cells (see Fig. 62.2**B**).

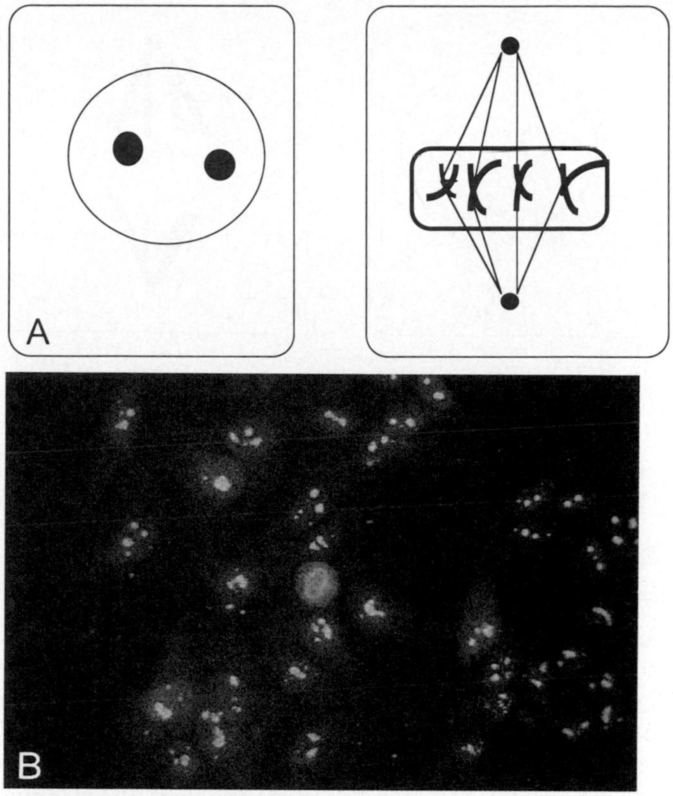

Figure 62.8. **A**, Diagram of antinucleolar ANA fluorescence pattern (see Fig. 62.2**A**). **B**, Antinucleolar ANA immunofluorescence on HEp2 cells (see Fig. 62.2**B**).

cluster of points or short, linear striations. The remainder of the mitotic figure and cytoplasm do not exhibit any significant immunofluorescence with a pure ACA antibody. The anti-ACA antibody is relatively specific for an indolent variant of scleroderma—the CREST syndrome. ACA may also be seen in a minority of diffuse scleroderma (PSS) and primary Raynaud's syndrome, and a tiny fraction of patients with SLE and MCTD.

Nucleolar

The immunofluorescence assay pattern seen with a pure antinucleolar antibody is quite distinct. The two to seven nucleoli in the cell lines are seen as large, irregular fluorescent areas within an otherwise nonfluorescent nucleus (Fig. 62.8). The mitotic figure is nonfluorescent, although there sometimes is a weak perichromosomal fluorescence with a strong antinucleolar antibody. This can be clearly distinguished from a homogeneous ANA by the lack of diffuse reactivity with the interphase nucleus. The cytoplasm of the dividing cells may be weakly immunofluorescent, due to the release of nucleolar antigens. The nucleolar ANA pattern is most often seen with PSS, particularly if the ANAs are of high titer. However, a significant minority of patients with primary Raynaud's syndrome and SLE will have nucleolar ANAs, often of lower titers than seen with PSS.

Mitotic Spindle

This pattern can be seen only on substrates with a significant mitotic rate (Fig. 62.9). Only the mitotic spindle is fluorescent in the dividing cell. Cytoplasmic staining is not seen. Most of the time, the interphase cells show no significant immunofluorescence with a pure anti–mitotic spindle autoantibody (AMSA). This autoantibody has been associated with a variety of ill-defined autoimmune disorders, as well as infectious diseases. Thus, while not diagnostically specific, AMSA should be reported as a significant positive autoantibody.

Cytoplasmic

A variety of cytoplasmic immunofluorescence assay patterns may be seen in autoimmune diseases associated with ANAs. Five major antigen-organelle structures are recognized: Golgi, intermediate filaments, mitochondria, ribosomes, and microfilaments. The antiribosomal pattern exhibits a granular cytoplasmic immunofluorescence associated with nucleolar staining. The immunofluorescence assay diagnosis of a ribosomal ANA is not definitive. If re-

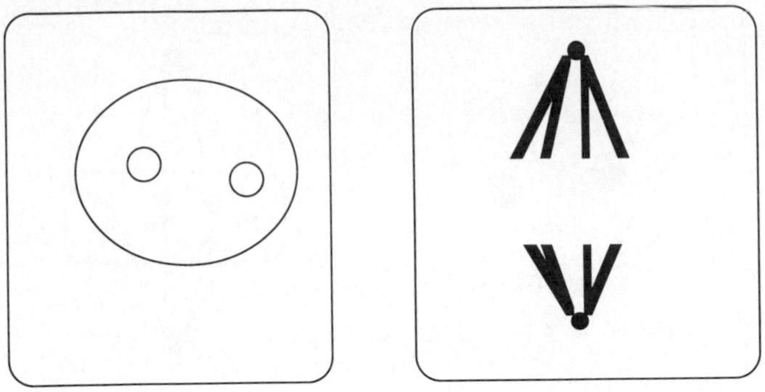

Figure 62.9. **A**, Diagram of anti–mitotic spindle (MSA) ANA fluorescence pattern (see Fig. 62.2**A**).

quired for clinical purposes, confirmatory Western immunoblotting should be done. The ribosomal pattern is seen in approximately 10% of an unselected SLE population and has been associated with SLE psychosis, although it is by no means 100% specific or sensitive for this complication.

The anti-Golgi immunofluorescence assay pattern reveals coarse prenuclear half-staining without any significant nuclear or mitotic figure fluorescence. Its overall incidence in serum from patients with autoimmune disorders is 1 in 450. Most of these have SLE, with the remainder having Sjögren's syndrome with or without lymphoma. However, anti-Golgi antibody is not sensitive for SLE and Sjögren's syndrome, being reported in only 7 of 28 and 2 of 44 cases, respectively. The autoantibody has not yet been reported with cases of MCTD, rheumatoid arthritis (RA), dermatopolymyositis, scleroderma, or autoimmune liver disease, or in normals.

Autoantibodies to cytoplasmic intermediate and microfilaments are not usually seen in other mouse tissue sections or in routinely fixed cell lines. With specially fixed HEp2 or PIK2 cell lines, anti-intermediate filaments are seen in 55 to 85% of patients with dermatomyositis/polymyositis, scleroderma, and RA, as well as in 38% of nonautoimmune disease patients and 43% of normals. Most of the latter are of low titer (1:20 or lower) compared to those seen in individuals with autoimmune disorders. Antibodies to microfilaments have a similar distribution, although at a lesser frequency. The clinical utility of such autoantibodies remains to be proved.

SPECIFIC ANAs AND AUTOANTIGENS

Antideoxynucleoprotein

Antinuclear antibodies to deoxynucleoprotein (DNP) are the ones responsible for the classic lupus erythematosus (LE) cell phenomenon (ingestion by neutrophils of anti-DNP/DNP complexes of lymphocyte nuclei). The latter appears to be specifically due to the anti-histone component. This ANA usually has a homogeneous immunofluorescence assay pattern, although it may appear speckled on some tissue substrates. Anti-DNP occurs in approximately 30 to 58% of SLE patients, usually in high titers (1:160 to 1: 640), and may also be found in the serum of patients with rheumatoid arthritis (RA), scleroderma, polymyositis, and chronic active hepatitis. However, its titer is usually lower than that seen with SLE. Specific tests for anti-DNP include radioimmunoassay (RIA), double diffusion, counterimmunoelectrophoresis (CIE), hemagglutination, and latex agglutination. The latter has relatively poor sensitivity.

Anti-Native (Double-Stranded) DNA

DNA comes in two basic forms: single-stranded (ss) and double-stranded (ds), or native, DNA. Both can be complexed with basic (histone) and nonbasic (acidic) nucleoproteins. Autoantibodies to dsDNA may be detected on routine ANA substrates, where they usually have a peripheral pattern on tissue or cell lines. Occasionally, a homogeneous pattern may be seen, although it is not always clear whether the dsDNA antibody has a homogeneous distribution, or rather the pattern is due to a concomitant anti-DNP or anti-histone antibody.

Because dsDNA is so often associated with other autoantibodies (see Systemic Lupus Erythematosus below), the definitive detection and quantitation of anti-dsDNA is performed on specific dsDNA substrates. Anti-native DNA antibodies are heterogeneous. They react with either the deoxyribose phosphate backbone or the helical structure of dsDNA. Both types of antibody can also recognize ssDNA. Because these various types of anti-DNA antibodies are often present together, the substrate used for the detection of anti-dsDNA is critical, as virtually all ssDNA must be eliminated.

A wide variety of techniques and substrates have been utilized. Currently, the Farr RIA is the "gold standard" for the detection of anti-dsDNA, and is probably the most sensitive technique. In this assay, serum is reacted with rigorously purified radiolabeled dsDNA. A popular alternative is an indirect immunofluorescence technique using the hemoflagellate *Crithidia luciliae*. The latter contains a kinetoplast near its flagella that contains circular dsDNA. It is somewhat controversial at this time whether histones or histone-like substances are also present in the kinetoplast. However, anti-histone antibodies are quite prevalent in non-SLE autoimmune disorders, yet sera from such patients only rarely react with the kinetoplast. Further, reactivity with anti-H_2A/H_2B, found in some forms of drug-induced lupus, is absent.

Autoantibodies to dsDNA are somewhat unique in that they have both a diagnostic and prognostic utility. Using assays such as the Farr radioimmunoprecipitation or the *Crithidia luciliae* indirect immunofluorescence tests, the presence of anti-dsDNA is very specific for SLE. This is particularly so if the titers are high (higher than 1:40 with the *Crithidia* or more than 50% with the Farr). High titers of anti-dsDNA are also associated with an increased risk of lupus nephritis. Low-titer anti-dsDNA may be seen in a minority of cases of MCTD, discoid lupus, RA, progressive systemic sclerosis (PSS), Sjögren's syndrome, and dermatomyositis.

Anti–Single-Stranded DNA

Autoantibodies to ssDNA are detected in a significant fraction of most systemic autoimmune disorders. Unlike the dsDNA autoantibodies, high titers of anti-ssDNA are not specific for SLE or the risk of lupus nephritis. Anti-ssDNA antibodies recognize polymers of the purine and pyrimidine bases available in ssDNA. Currently, there is no routine use in detecting or quantifying ssDNA ANAs in clinical medicine.

Anti-Histone

Autoantibodies to histones are seen most commonly in drug-induced lupus and SLE. Its ANA immunofluorescence pattern is almost always homogeneous. To differentiate between anti-histone, anti-DNP, anti-dsDNA and anti-ssDNA, an immunofluorescence assay using *Crithidia luciliae* can be utilized. The kinetoplast of the organism contains pure dsDNA. While some have questioned whether or not the kinetoplast contains histones, Konstantinov et al., have shown that the kinetoplast lacks histones H_2A and H_2B, the types to which ANAs are seen with drug-induced lupus. The most specific tests would be immunofluorescence assays using mouse tissue sections either depleted of or reconstituted with histones or an ELISA with specific histones serving as the substrate.

Anti-histone antibodies are seen in 95% of patients with drug-induced lupus, are not associated with other autoantibodies, and usually recognize the H_2A–H_2B complexes. This is in contrast to SLE and other autoimmune disorders, where the anti-histone ANA recognizes epitopes on all major histone classes and are associated with other autoantibodies. The most common etiologic agents of drug-induced lupus are procainamide and hydralazine, and, to a much lesser extent, quinidine, chlorpromazine, and acebutalol.

Anti-Smith and Anti-Ribonucleoprotein

Both anti-Smith (Sm) and anti-ribonucleoprotein (RNP) usually have a speckled immunofluorescence assay pattern on either mouse or HEp2 substrates. Direct confirmation is usually done by double diffusion or counterimmunoelectrophoresis. The Sm antigen is part of the RNP antigen, and both belong to the family of RNPs (U1, U2, U5, U4/6) that are involved in posttranslational modification of messenger RNA. Specifically, they are involved in splicing nascent mRNA into a form that can be exported from the nucleus to the cytoplasm and translated into a peptide. The core proteins of U1–6 RNPs include B, B′, D, E, F, and G. Anti-Sm recognizes epitopes on B, B′, D, and E proteins. In addition, the U1 RNP contains peptides called A and C, while U2 contains A′ and B″. The U1 RNP then associates with a nuclear matrix protein of about 70 kd. The anti-RNP ANA recognizes the 70 kd nuclear matrix and A and C U1 RNP proteins.

Anti-Sm and anti-RNP serve as disease markers for SLE and MCTD, respectively. Using immunofluorescence assays, anti-Sm is found, usually in high titers, in approximately 30% of SLE patients. Only rare cases of MCTD will have anti-Sm. This finding is important because anti-RNP is found in 95% of MCTD patients (high titer) and 26% of cases of SLE. In the latter, some cases (about 13%) have high titers of anti-RNP. The absence of anti-Sm and other autoantibodies helps to delineate MCTD serologically from SLE and other autoimmune diseases.

Anti-SSA, SSB, and SSC

Anti-SSA (Ro), SSB (La), and SSC (RAP) are significantly associated with Sjögren's syndrome. The SSA antigen is a 60-kd nuclear protein. This and a 52-kd protein are routinely recognized by anti-SSA on Western immunoblots. The SSB antigen is a 48-kd nuclear protein. Both SSA and SSB bind to small RNAs; SSA, to Y1–Y5 RNAs; and SSB, to the 3′ oligouridylate tail of small RNA polymerase III transcripts. SSA is present in only one-tenth the amount of SSB in cultured cell lines.

The SSA and SSB antibodies result in a speckled nuclear immunofluorescence assay pattern using appropriately fixed cultured cell lines. The RAP (SSC) antigen is distributed in the nucleus and cytoplasm as small round granules. All three can be definitively identified by double diffusion or CIE techniques. SSA is found in 60 to 70% of pure Sjögren's syndrome, while SSB is found in 40 to 50%, and RAP in 5%. Sjögren's syndrome associated with RA has a reciprocal pattern, with SSA and SSB present in 9% and 3% of cases, respectively, but RAP in 76%. While SSB is found only in Sjögren's syndrome and SLE,

SSA can be found in a subset of SLE, in newborns with neonatal lupus and heart block, and in some cases of primary biliary cirrhosis and chronic active hepatitis. Anti-RAP can be found in 67% of cases of RA and 7% of SLE.

Antinucleolar

The antinucleolar autoantibodies are directed to a wide variety of nucleolar antigens and have a strong association with scleroderma, particularly if of high titer. The antigenic targets for some of these nucleolar ANAs have been identified. However, it is necessary to perform immunoblotting or diffusion immunoassays to specifically identify them. Anti-RNA Pol(ymerase) I has a punctate nucleolar pattern and is found in a minor fraction (4%) of scleroderma patients. It is not seen in other autoimmune diseases. Fibrillarin, a 34-kd protein, a component of the U3 RNP nucleolar particle, is seen in 8% of scleroderma cases and has a clumpy nucleolar staining pattern. An autoantibody to PM-Scl is seen in the polymyositis-scleroderma overlap syndrome. It is a complex of 11 proteins and has a homogeneous nucleolar pattern associated with nuclear staining. Other nucleolar antigens rarely associated with autoantibodies are 7-2RNA and a 90-kd nucleolar organizer associated protein.

Anti-Centromere and Scl-70

Anti-centromere (ACA) and Scl-70 predominate in a reciprocal fashion in the major variants of scleroderma. The ACA recognizes centromeric proteins present in the trilaminar kinetochore structure, and is seen in both interphase nuclei and mitotic cells. These centromeric antigens are composed of three proteins of approximately 18 kd, 80 kd, and 140 kd. Initial biochemical analysis revealed that the antigen recognized by anti–Scl-70 has a molecular weight of 70 kd. However, further work demonstrated that this measurement reflected protease degradation of the antigen DNA topoisomerase I, which has a native molecular weight of 100 kd. This protein is involved in the relaxation of supercoiled DNA, allowing transcription and replication of the genome. The ANA immunofluorescence pattern of ACA is quite characteristic, while that of anti–Scl-70 is usually speckled (with variable nucleolar staining) and not distinctively different from other nuclear antigens with a speckled distribution, as noted earlier.

Anti-Scl-70 is present in 64 to 75% of patients with the diffuse form of scleroderma, but is only rarely seen in the calcinosis, Raynaud's syndrome, esophageal dysmotility, sclerodactyly/telangiectasia (CREST) variant. The Scl-70 antibody may also be seen in primary Raynaud's phenomenon (10%), Sjögren's syndrome (5%), and, rarely, with MCTD and SLE (1% each). The ACA is present in 96% of cases of the CREST syndrome but in only 12% of patients with diffuse scleroderma. In addition, ACA may be present in 29% of cases with primary Raynaud's phenomenon, and in a minor fraction of MCTD and SLE patients (7% and 2%, respectively). Anti-Scl-70 or ACA have not been reported to be associated with linear scleroderma, RA, SLE (Scl-70 only), or Sjögren's syndrome (ACA only).

Antinuclear Lamins

Lamins are intracellular proteins that are believed to belong to the intermediate filament class of biomolecules. The nuclear lamins (NLs) make up a network that lines the inner or nucleoplasmic surface of the inner nuclear membrane. The function of these nuclear lamins is not known. Anti-NLs are directed against lamins of 74, 68 and 60 kd. The immunofluorescence assay pattern on cultured cell substrates exhibits linear staining of the nuclear envelope of interphase cells. The mitotic figure does not stain. Anti-NLs have been seen with SLE, linear scleroderma, various peripheral cytopenias, and chronic liver disease (primary biliary cirrhosis and autoimmune chronic active hepatitis).

Anti–Proliferating Cell Nuclear Antigen

Anti–proliferating cell nuclear antigen (PCNA) is best seen in culture cell lines, as it is involved in the replication of DNA. Thus, it requires a mitotically active substrate to be seen on ANA immunofluorescence. The pattern is variable, with some cells having weak diffuse staining of the nuclei, while others show more intense nucleolar and weak nuclear membrane staining. If mouse or rat substrates are used, the nuclei of scattered interstitial cells are positive while the tubular and glomerular nuclei are negative. The antigen, a 36-kd protein, has been identified as a subunit of the DNA polymerase and is required for chain elongation during DNA synthesis. PCNA is found in 3% of SLE patients and is not detectable in the sera of normals or in other immune disorders. In addition, PCNA-positive SLE appears not to be clinically different from PCNA-negative cases.

Miscellaneous Autoantibodies

ANTI-RIBOSOMAL

Anti-ribosomal autoantibody (anti-rNP) has predominant cytoplasmic reactivity with variable nucleolar staining. The autoantibody recognizes 38; 16; and 15-kd phosphoprotein components of the large ribosomal subunit, which are responsible for the elongation step of protein synthesis. There have been reports of partial association with anti-rNP and SLE psychosis. These results have not always been reproducible, and await validation by further, larger prospective studies.

ANTI–MITOTIC SPINDLE

The anti–mitotic spindle (MSA) antibody recognizes proteins in the mitotic spindle apparatus. These proteins are not tubulin. The characteristic immunofluorescence assay pattern is best seen on cultured cell line substrates because of their greater mitotic activity. In one study, 5 of 18 anti-MSAs were seen in SLE; 2 of 18 with RA; 1 of 18 each with scleroderma or Raynaud's phenomenon, and 9 of 18 with ill-defined autoimmune/inflammatory disorders (polyarthritis, osteoarthritis, arthralgias, myalgias, urticaria). There was no correlation between anti-MSA titer and disease association. Four of the five SLE patients had one or more other ANAs in addition to the anti-MSA.

ANTI-CENTRIOLE/CENTROSOME/MIDBODY

Anti-centriole antibody recognizes the "pole" of the mitotic spindle, and can be seen in both interphase and mitotic cells. The midbody is the residual mitotic spindle that develops during cytokinesis in the cytoplasmic remnant between the two daughter cells. Antisera to one structure can recognize the other. Anti-centriole antibody has been rarely reported, usually in association with CREST, diffuse scleroderma, or Raynaud's phenomenon.

Systemic Autoimmune Diseases

SYSTEMIC LUPUS ERYTHEMATOSUS

Systemic lupus erythematosus (SLE) is an autoimmune disease with multiple organ involvement and varied immunologic and clinical manifestations. The annual incidence is estimated to be between 6.4 and 7.6 cases per 100,000. The disease, while affecting all races, age groups, and both sexes, is most frequent in young black females, primarily between the ages of 15 and 25 years. Females in general make up the vast majority of SLE cases.

Most patients present with nondeforming arthritis, and a majority have a typical "butterfly" facial skin rash and alopecia. Characteristically, patients also complain of fatigue and fever at diagnosis. A significant minority of individuals also present with photosensitivity, renal disease, pleuritis/pericarditis, discoid lupus skin lesions, mucosal ulcers, Raynaud's phenomenon, false-positive VDRL, and peripheral blood cytopenia(s). The American Rheumatism Association (ARA) has established 11 clinical and laboratory criteria for the diagnosis of SLE (Table 62.2). A patient is said to have SLE if any four or more of the 11 criteria are present, either serially or simultaneously, during any interval of observation.

Table 62.2. ARA Criteria for Classification of SLE[a]

Feature	Definition
Malar rash	Erythematous macule/papule over malar eminences
Discoid rash	Erythematous papules with adherent keratotic scaling and follicular plugging
Photosensitivity	Unusual skin rash after sun exposure
Oral ulcers	Oral or nasopharyngeal ulcers, usually painless
Arthritis	Nonerosive arthritis of two or more peripheral joints
Serositis	Pleuritis (pain, rub or effusion) or pericarditis (EKG, rub or effusion)
Renal disease	Persistent proteinuria (>0.5 g/day or 3+); cellular casts
Neurologic disease	Idiopathic seizures or psychosis
Hematologic disease	Hemolytic anemia; leukopenia (≥ 2 times); thrombocytopenia (≥ 2 times)
Autoantibody	Positive (1) LE prep.; (2) anti-dsDNA; (3) anti-Sm; (4) VDRL (false positive)
Antinuclear antibody	Positive ANA by IIF in absence of drugs associated with anti-histone antibody

Patient will be said to have SLE if 4 or more criteria are present serially or simultaneously during any interval of observation.

[a]Modified from Rothfield N. Clinical features of systemic lupus erythematosus. In: Kelly W, Harris E, Ruddy S, et al., eds. Textbook of rheumatology. 2nd ed. Philadelphia: WB Saunders, 1985:1093.

Detection of high-titer ANAs are useful in the detection and the differential diagnosis of SLE. Using cultured cell lines, approximately 95% of untreated SLE patients will have a positive ANA by immunofluorescence assay. However, while most SLE patients have multiple ANAs, the inclusion of a positive ANA only increases the combined clinical and pathological diagnostic sensitivity by 3% over that obtained by purely clinical criteria.

Most ANAs will have either a homogeneous or a speckled pattern. The average number of ANAs in an SLE patient is three, a fairly characteristic feature among the systemic autoimmune diseases. Only scleroderma appears to have nearly as many ANA specificities per patient. A majority of SLE cases will have anti-dsDNA and anti-ssDNA (50 to 60%), and anti-DNP. In addition, a significant minority will have autoantibodies to histones (25 to 30%), Sm (about 30%), RNP (25 to 30%), SSA or B (30 to 40% and 10 to 15%, respectively), ribosomal RNP, and ku (10% each). The immunologic diagnostic keys in SLE are (*a*) multiple ANAs, (*b*) the presence of anti-Sm, and (*c*) high-titer anti-dsDNA.

DRUG-INDUCED LUPUS

An SLE-like syndrome associated with long-term ingestion of several drugs (Table 62.3) has been well

Table 62.3. Agents Associated with Drug-Induced Lupus[a]

Probable	Possible
Hydralazine	Aminosalicylic acid
Oxyphenisatin	Chlorthalidone
Procainamide	D-Penicillamine
Mephenytoin	Griseofulvin
Phenylbutazone	Guanoxan
Diphenylhydantoin	Isoquinazepon
Primidone	L-Dopa
Propylthiouracil	Methyldopa
Trimethadione	Methysergide
Ethosuximide	Methythiouracil
Carbamazepine	Oral contraceptives
Phenylethylacetylurea	Penicillin
Isoniazid	Proactolol
Chlorpromazine	Quinidine
	Reserpine
	Streptomycin
	Sulfonamides
	Tetracycline
	Tolazamide

[a]Modified from Rothfield N. Clinical features of systemic lupus erythematosus. In: Kelly W, Harris E, Ruddy S, et al., eds. Textbook of rheumatology. 2nd ed. Philadelphia: WB Saunders, 1985:1092.

documented. The most common offending agents are procainamide, hydralazine, and isoniazid. Drug-induced lupus is milder than SLE, and occurs with equal frequency in both sexes. Arthritis and pleuropericardial involvement are very frequent. Rashes occur to a lesser extent in drug-induced lupus. However, discoid lupus skin lesions, Raynaud's phenomenon, and CNS or renal disease are only rarely observed. Further, a positive lupus band test is not seen in drug-induced lupus.

It is known that many patients taking these drugs will develop anti-histone antibodies, yet only a small minority will develop the SLE-like syndrome. Many patients with drug-induced lupus have been shown to be slow acetylators of drugs and other compounds by the *N*-acetyltransferase system of the liver. This characteristic is inherited in a homozygous recessive manner.

Characteristically, drug-induced lupus patients have a homogeneous ANA. This is due to anti-histone antibodies. This can be indirectly (though not absolutely) suspected when a strong homogeneous ANA is associated with an absence of anti-dsDNA and other autoantibodies in the clinical setting of a lupus-like syndrome. It is directly demonstrable by either selective depletion or repletion of histones from immunofluorescence assay tissue substrates or by ELISA or RIA assays for histones. The latter techniques have also shown that patients with the drug-induced lupus syndrome usually have high titers of IgG anti-histone, largely anti-H2A and anti-H2B. The ANAs from asymptomatic patients are of the IgM class, and recognize almost all the major histone classes. When patients with drug-induced lupus cease taking the offending drug, there is a concomitant loss of the ANA and reduction of the anti-H2A/H2B titers.

In summary, drug-induced lupus can be suspected by the association of continual ingestion of certain drugs with a slightly atypical SLE-like picture and a positive ANA with a single specificity to histones. True SLE will often present without a history of drug ingestion, may have more widely disseminated disease (renal or CNS), and will have multiple autoantibodies.

SJÖGREN'S SYNDROME

Sjögren's syndrome is best characterized by the clinical triad of keratoconjunctivitis sicca (dry eyes), xerostomia (dry mouth), and the presence of a connective tissue disease, usually RA. The first two symptoms may be associated with lacrimal and/or salivary gland enlargement. Most authors require two of the three criteria for diagnosis. Those with dry eyes and mouth only (33 to 50%) are said to have the sicca syndrome, while those associated with a systemic autoimmune disorder (50 to 67%) are described as having Sjögren's syndrome with RA, Sjögren's syndrome with SLE, etc. The disease predominates in middle-aged to elderly females.

The presence of keratoconjunctivitis or xerostomia can be difficult to assess, and they are not 100% sensitive for Sjögren's syndrome. Biopsy of minor salivary glands in the lip reveal a focal lymphoplasmacytic infiltrate associated with myoepithelial islands in approximately 70% of Sjögren's syndrome patients. However, such infiltrates may be seen in other systemic autoimmune disorders. Thus, the detection of autoantibodies is an aid to diagnosis.

The most common autoantibody seen in Sjögren's syndrome is rheumatoid factor (RF), which may be seen in the overlap cases or, less commonly, in the sicca syndrome. A variety of ANA patterns may be seen (homogeneous, speckled, nucleolar), the most common with mouse substrates being homogeneous. The speckled patterns are often associated with a set of ANAs called SSA/Ro, SSB/La, and SSC/RAP. These are found in 70%, 48%, and 3% of cases of Sjögren's syndrome *without* RA, respectively. Sjögren's syndrome *with* RA exhibits a reciprocal pattern of expression of these autoantibodies (9%, 3%, 76%). Only 3% of cases of Sjögren's syndrome have autoantibodies to dsDNA or RNP, and these are of low titer. No cases have been reported to have anti-Sm.

SCLERODERMA

Scleroderma, otherwise known as systemic sclerosis, is a multiorgan autoimmune disorder characterized by occlusive vascular lesions associated with atrophy and fibrosis. The clinical course of disease is determined by the pattern of organ involvement. In general, scleroderma is divided into a progressive diffuse form, involving many crucial visceral organs, and a more limited variety, CREST syndrome or second or third decade scleroderma. The latter, while more indolent, can progress to life-threatening disease in the second and third decades of disease, usually in the form of pulmonary fibrosis and hypertension.

Most patients are females in the fourth or fifth decades of life who present with complaints of pallor or cyanosis of the fingers (Raynaud's syndrome) and puffy facial and hand skin. Systems involved early in the course of this variant are the skin (perivascular mononuclear infiltrates with negative DFF findings; fibrosis), gastrointestinal tract (esophageal dysmotility), pulmonary (ventilation-perfusion abnormalities), and the heart (pericardial effusions; arrhythmias).

Most scleroderma patients have a positive ANA on HEp2 cell lines by immunofluorescence assay. Of the three patterns seen (speckled, homogeneous, nucleolar), the speckled is the most common in the early scleroderma patient. The most specific type of speckled pattern seen is the anti-centromere antibody (ACA; see earlier discussion). This pattern is strongly correlated with the CREST variant (96% sensitivity), being present in only 12% of diffuse cases and 29% of cases of primary Raynaud's syndrome.

Another speckled pattern is due to an autoantibody to the Scl-70/topoisomerase antigen. The speckled immunofluorescence assay pattern due to anti-Scl-70 is not specific, and its antigenic specificity must be confirmed by immunoprecipitation or Western blot methods. This antibody is found predominantly in the diffuse variant of scleroderma (sensitivity 64%), and is rarely present in the CREST variant or other systemic autoimmune disorders. Thus, the pattern of anti-ACA/Scl-70 will give insight into the diagnosis, potential extent, and time course of the disease.

In addition, an ANA to the nucleolar antigen RNA Pol I is associated with diffuse scleroderma. The nucleolar ANA pattern seen in scleroderma is seen in 54 to 70% of patients. It is usually of high titer, in contrast to those seen in other systemic autoimmune diseases. Anti-RNP and anti-dsDNA are seen in approximately 20 to 55% of scleroderma cases, respectively, but are usually of low titer. Antibodies to Sm, soluble nucleoprotein, SSA, and SSB are not seen in scleroderma or only rarely (less than 1%).

RAYNAUD'S DISEASE/SYNDROME

Raynaud's phenomenon is characterized as episodic pallor or cyanosis on cold- or stress-induced vasoconstriction with suffusion and erythema on subsequent vasodilatation. Raynaud's phenomenon can be seen as an isolated occurrence (Raynaud's *disease*), or, more commonly, in association with scleroderma, and, to a much lesser extent, with SLE, RA, MCTD, and Srögren's syndrome (Raynaud's *syndrome*). Approximately 90% of patients with scleroderma have Raynaud's syndrome. One author estimated that the incidence of scleroderma in patients presenting with Raynaud's syndrome is 5% per year. To make the diagnosis of Raynaud's disease, several years should pass with careful clinical and laboratory follow-up. ANAs commonly associated with Raynaud's phenomenon include ACA (29%) and anti-Scl-70 (10%).

MIXED CONNECTIVE TISSUE DISEASE

The mixed connective tissue disease (MCTD) is probably one of the best known of the overlap autoimmune disorders. Its incidence is slightly less than that of SLE, but it is more common than scleroderma or polymyositis. Like many autoimmune disorders, there is a marked female predominance (8:1), primarily in the second and third decades of life. The clinical appearance of MCTD includes a clustering of signs and symptoms seen in SLE, Sjögren's syndrome, scleroderma, RA, and polymyositis. Joint pain and stiffness, myalgias, pleurisy, esophageal dysmotility, and skin disease are seen in a significant majority of MCTD patients. It is more characteristic of MCTD to present with a sequence of these signs and symptoms, rather than to have several presenting at the same time. Most patients have a composite picture, suggesting either PSS or an undifferentiated RA/SLE-like autoimmune disease.

Laboratory evaluation reveals leukopenia in approximately three-quarters of MCTD patients. While a positive Coombs' test is present in a significant minority of patients, hemolytic anemia and thrombocytopenia are uncommon (in contrast to SLE). About 10% will have a false-positive VDRL. Using Hep2 cell lines, most MCTD cases have a positive ANA by immunofluorescence assay. This usually has a speckled pattern. By definition, all patients with MCTD have high-titer anti-RNP antibodies. The titers do not appear to vary much with disease activity or treatment. While about 50% of cases have a low-titer RF and 80% anti-ssDNA, the occurrence of anti-dsDNA, Sm, Scl-70, ACA, SSA, and SSB is rare.

The laboratory delineation of MCTD from SLE is best made by the absence of multiple ANAs, anti-Sm, and anti-dsDNA. Clinically, RA has much more

Table 62.4. ARA Criteria for the Diagnosis of Rheumatoid Arthritis[a]

1. Morning stiffness
2. Pain on motion or tenderness in at least one joint
3. Swelling of one joint, representing soft tissue or fluid
4. Swelling of at least one other joint with interval free of symptoms ≤ 3 months
5. Symmetrical joint swelling
6. Subcutaneous nodules over bony prominences, extensor surfaces or near joints
7. X-ray evidence including periarticular dimineralization
8. Poor mucin clot formation by synovial fluid
9. Positive Rheumatoid Factor (≥ 1:64)
10. Synovial histology consistent with rheumatoid arthritis
11. Hisotopathologic evidence of rheumatoid nodules from any site

Possible RA: Any two from criteria 1–6 and increased ESR/CRP seen for at least 3 weeks' duration; Probable RA: Any three criteria; Definite RA: Any five criteria; Classic RA: Any seven criteria.

[a]Modified from Harris E. Rheumatoid arthritis: the clinical spectrum. In: Kelly W, Harris E, Ruddy S, et al., eds. Textbook of rheumatology. 2nd ed. Philadelphia: WB Saunders, 1985:916.

Table 62.5. New York Criteria for the Diagnosis of Rheumatoid Arthritis[a]

1. History of three painful limb joints.
2. Swelling, limitation of motion, subluxation, and/or ankylosis of three limb joints (excludes DIP, 5th PIP, 1st MP and hip joints)
3. X-ray evidence of erosions
4. Positive rheumatoid factor

RA present if criteria 1 and 2 plus either 3 or 4 are present.

[a]Modified from Harris E. Rheumatoid arthritis: the clinical spectrum. In: Kelly W, Harris E, Ruddy S, et al., eds. Textbook of rheumatology. 2nd ed. Philadelphia: WB Saunders, 1985:917.

deforming arthritis associated with a significant RF, but lacks high-titer anti-RNP.

RHEUMATOID ARTHRITIS

Rheumatoid arthritis (RA) is an autoimmune disease primarily involving synovium and articular surfaces of joints. It has an overall prevalence of 0.3 to 1.5%. The incidence of RA is 0.5% in females and 0.1% in males. There is no evidence of racial predisposition. However, the evaluation of RA patients indicates that a genetic predisposition exists, with increased incidence of HLA-Dw3 and DR4 and RA patients. There is also an increased incidence of RA in first-degree relatives of RA patients.

RA is primarily diagnosed by clinical features. The American Rheumatism Association has established criteria for the diagnosis of RA (Table 62.4). An alternative is the New York classification (Table 62.5). For "classic" or "definitive" RA, seven or five criteria must be seen, respectively. "Probable" RA can be diagnosed with only three criteria. Utilizing the ARA criteria, most patients with probable or definite RA did not fulfill diagnostic criteria for RA on follow-up. These types of RA are usually relatively benign processes with a high probability of remission over several years. The more rigorous New York criteria have a much greater incidence of clinically significant disease on follow-up. Since early diagnosis of RA is not critical, there is no need to "force" the diagnosis. Rather, initial exclusion of other differential diagnoses and careful follow-up are recommended.

Typically (55 to 70%), RA has an insidious onset over weeks to months. The most characteristic signs and symptoms (each present in two-thirds of presenting patients) are (*a*) joint pain or tenderness (most frequent); (*b*) morning stiffness (least common); (*c*) pain on motion; (*d*) swelling of one other joint; and (*e*) symmetrical joint swelling. Rheumatoid nodules are present in 19% of patients at their first visit. Overall, the symmetrical nonmigratory arthritis first involving the joints of the wrists and fingers, then the larger joints, is clinically quite characteristic of RA.

The presence of rheumatoid factor (RF) is neither sensitive nor specific for the diagnosis of RA. Only 47% of RA patients will have a serum RF at their time of presentation, although RF becomes positive in 80 to 90% of definitive RA cases. There is little reason to repeat the RF test if the patient has had one positive test at a significant titer (more than 1:64). Other autoimmune (SLE, scleroderma, MCTD, Sjögren's), infectious (EBV, hepatitis B, influenza, TB, SBE), inflammatory (cryoglobulinemia, sarcoid), and treated neoplastic diseases may have RF factors in the serum, as do some normal individuals. The incidence and titers of RF in the normals will increase with age.

The RF titer is still valuable in separating a "normal" RF from the RF seen in RA. Most of the former are less than 1:64, while the latter are more commonly greater than 1:640. In addition, isotypes of the RFs seen in RA are heterogeneous (IgG, A, M) as opposed to those in non-RA (IgM). However, there is no compelling evidence to suggest that the RF isotype is of diagnostic or prognostic importance. Lastly, RFs in RA can be found in the synovium, a feature not seen with non-RA diseases with RFs.

Antinuclear antibodies may be seen in the serum of RA patients. One that appears to be relatively specific for pure RA or RA overlap syndromes is the rheumatoid arthritis precipitin (RAP), which recognizes the rheumatoid arthritis nuclear antigen (RANA). RAP is seen in approximately two-thirds of pure RA and three-quarters of Sjögren's syndrome–RA overlap disease. It is also found in a minor fraction (5 to 7%) of SLE or Sjögren's syndrome cases and in 2% of normals. Approximately 40% and 3% of RA patients will have low-titer ANAs to dsDNA and soluble nucleoprotein, respectively. While approximately 10% of RA sera will contain anti-RNP, all cases will lack anti-Sm, anti-SSA/B, ACA, and Scl-70.

SERONEGATIVE SPONDYLARTHRITIDES

The seronegative spondylarthritides include ankylosing spondylitis, Reiter's syndrome, and psoriatic arthropathy. They are characterized by chronic or relapsing arthritis that is serologically, genetically, and pathologically different from rheumatoid arthritis. They are often associated with the HLA-B27 haplotype, and, to a lesser extent, oral and/or anal-genital lesions.

Ankylosing Spondylitis

Ankylosing spondylitis is one of the most common rheumatologic diseases, affecting up to 1% of the total population. Its strong association with the HLA-B27 haplotype, familial prevalence, and association with uveitis, Reiter's syndrome, psoriatic arthropathy and/or inflammatory bowel disease all point to a probable autoimmune etiology. Pathologically, the disease is manifested by a fibrosing and ossifying process of the insertion of the ligaments and synovial capsules into the bone. This process may also involve other ligaments and tendons, such as the Achilles tendon.

Males are more commonly affected with progressive, severe ankylosing spondylitis than are females. However, women commonly have more indolent disease, with greater involvement of peripheral joints and the cervical spine. Other significant extraarticular manifestations include prostatitis (80%), conjunctivitis and iritis (25%), aortic valve disease (20% or less), and upper lobe pulmonary fibrosis. The clinical criteria for definitive diagnosis include a grade 3 to 4 bilateral sacroiliitis with limitation of lumbar spine motion or chest expansion, and a history of pain for 3 months or longer at the lumbar spine.

Laboratory documentation of HLA-B27 expression is a moderately sensitive marker in Caucasians and, to a lesser extent, in other ethnic groups. However, HLA-B27–negative ankylosing spondylitis is a well-established entity. Ultimately, the diagnosis of ankylosing spondylitis is primarily clinical and radiological. Antinuclear and rheumatoid factor serologies are not of direct diagnostic use in this disorder.

Reiter's Syndrome

Reiter's syndrome is defined as a seronegative asymmetric arthropathy associated with urethritis/cervicitis and conjunctivitis. It is a rheumatic disorder that predominates in young adult males. Like ankylosing spondylitis, it is strongly associated with the HLA-B27 haplotype in Caucasians. A significant correlation has been established between enteric (e.g., *Shigella*) and venereal infections (e.g., *Chlamydia, Mycoplasma*) and Reiter's syndrome.

Most patients have an oligoarticular arthritis, usually of the knees and ankles, along with urethritis. Back pain, Achilles tendinitis, plantar fasciitis, and prostatitis are also common complaints. Differentiation fron ankylosing spondylitis may be difficult, as approximately 20% of Reiter's syndrome patients will have a concomitant sacroiliitis. However, the sudden onset of the disease, prominent involvement of peripheral (lower-extremity) joints, and concomitant urethritis and conjunctivitis should allow confident differentiation from ankylosing spondylitis. Laboratory testing has little role in the diagnosis of Reiter's syndrome, which is clinical in nature.

Psoriatic Arthritis

Psoriatic arthritis is a peculiar form of peripheral arthritis associated with psoriasis. In contrast to rheumatoid arthritis, it has a predilection for the distal as well as the proximal interphalangeal joints. HLA-BW38 has been associated more frequently with this type of psoriatic arthritis, while HLA-B27 is found often with the form seen with sacroiliitis. As with the other seronegative spondylarthritides, laboratory testing is of little direct diagnostic utility. The serum ANA and RF factors are usually negative, and the erythrocyte sedimentation rate is only modestly elevated.

POLYMYALGIA RHEUMATICA

Polymyalgia rheumatica is a poorly understood rheumatologic disorder that is significantly associated with giant cell arteritis. The latter, along with an increased prevalance of HLA-DR4 haplotypes, support the contention that this is a form of autoimmune disease. It is almost always seen in patients older than 50 years, with a 2:1 prevalence in women. Among persons aged 50 years or older, the annual incidence ranges from 28.6 to 53.7 per 100,000 persons and the prevalence is approximately 500 per 100,000 persons.

Clinically, the patients usually present with a complaint of bilateral, symmetrical musculoskeletal pain. This is most often seen in the scapular girdle, and is often associated with similar pain in the upper extremities and/or pelvic girdle. If there is concomitant giant cell arteritis (approximately 25% of cases), complaints of headache and/or visual changes are common. However, joint deformity is not present, and pain, not muscular weakness, is the primary reason limiting joint movement.

Laboratory investigations usually reveal acute and chronic inflammatory changes (mild anemia, acute phase alterations in the serum proteins, hypergammaglobulinemia). Characteristically, the erythrocyte sedimentation rate (ESR) is markedly elevated (100 mm/hr or higher). The serum ANA and RF serologies are usually negative, and muscle enzymes (CPK, SGOT, aldolase) are usually not elevated. Electromyograms are unremarkable, and muscle biopsy usually reveals nonspecific atrophy at the most.

Most investigators require at least two of three common muscular sites to be involved for at least 1 month, along with a significantly elevated ESR in order to make the diagnosis. The concomitant diagnosis of rheumatoid arthritis, SLE, or other systemic or organ-based autoimmune disease excludes the diagnosis of polymyalgia rheumatica. Nonsteroidal drugs or corticosteroids usually suffice to treat this relatively benign disorder.

ORGAN-RESTRICTED AUTOIMMUNE DISEASE

Central and Peripheral Nervous Systems

INTRODUCTION

The diagnoses of diseases of the central nervous system (CNS) and peripheral nervous system (PNS) are among the most clinically challenging in modern medicine. While immune-mediated disorders make up only a small fraction of these disorders, they have extensive overlapping of signs and symptoms with more common, nonimmunologic etiologies. As a result, there has been an extensive effort to identify serologic markers (autoantibodies) of these CNS and PNS immune diseases.

While offering insights into the pathobiology of these disorders, many of these serologic markers have serious limitations either in their sensitivity or specificity or in the extent of clinical validation of their diagnostic and prognostic use. As a result, the diagnosis of these disorders requires careful clinical correlation with viral serologies, clinical history, imaging studies, and analysis of cerebrospinal fluid (CSF) for in situ inflammation. These factors, and the relatively high cost of screening for the autoantibodies, mandate careful consideration of the clinical differential prior to submitting serum or CSF for analysis.

MULTIPLE SCLEROSIS

The clinical diagnosis of multiple sclerosis (MS) can be very difficult, and depends on the presence of strictly defined criteria: relapsing and remitting episodes of neurological abnormalities that are referable to two or more anatomical sites in the white matter of the central nervous system. While the typical multiple sclerosis patient has a long clinical course, approximately 60 to 75% will be restricted to a wheelchair 25 years after onset. Thus, a clear diagnosis is important for prognostic and therapeutic reasons. As the clinical symptoms are quite variable and may be vague or nonspecific, confirmatory tests are useful.

These tests include physiological (evoked responses), imaging (MRI; CT), and CSF abnormalities (presence of oligoclonal bands, increased myelin basic protein, IgG index). None of these tests are 100% sensitive or specific for multiple sclerosis by themselves. The diagnosis requires close clinical and laboratory correlation. While clinical history and examination remain the gold standard, additional laboratory testing and image analysis will increase the diagnosis rate by approximately 50%. The MRI is probably the single most sensitive nonclinical diagnostic tool, particularly for more limited forms of MS (optic neuritis, chronic progressive myelopathy). However, multiple abnormal results from image, evoked response, and CSF analyses are highly specific for the diagnosis of MS in the appropriate clinical setting.

A basic differential in CNS disorders is between primary/in situ inflammatory diseases and neoplastic or metabolic processes. Based on clinical experience, in situ CNS inflammation is expected to result in both quantitative increases in and qualitative changes (clonal expansion/oligoclonal bands) in CNS immunoglobulins, as compared to serum immunoglobulins. The most widely used tests for these are the IgG index and oligoclonal banding of CSF γ-globulins, respectively.

The oligoclonal banding pattern can be seen with a wide variety of CNS inflammatory, infectious, degenerative, vascular, and neoplastic diseases. The optimal definition of oligoclonal bands is two or more γ protein bands seen in concentrated CSF (but not in the parallel, undiluted serum electrophoretigram) that are immunoglobulins (i.e., not γ trace protein or CSF transferrin).

Others have argued for a more liberal definition—i.e., any CSF γ protein band is an oligoclonal band, regardless of whether or not there is a corresponding serum γ band. The rationale here is to avoid a false-negative result for in situ CNS inflammation in general, and multiple sclerosis in particular. However, in most laboratorians' experience, the more restricted definition results in a sensitivity and specificity for multiple sclerosis of greater than 90% each. Furthermore, no matter how liberal the criteria, some 2 to 5% of patients will lack detectable oligoclonal bands by any analytic technique.

Both an elevated IgG index and an oligoclonal banding pattern have a reasonably good diagnostic sensitivity for multiple sclerosis (65 to 91% and 85 to 93%, respectively). Of the two tests, the agarose gel analysis for oligoclonal bands is probably the best. It has a diagnostic sensitivity equal to that of the IgG index for clinically definite, untreated multiple sclerosis. In addition, it retains most of its sensitivity in the face of quiescent and/or treated disease, while the IgG index will often fall into the normal range. However, approximately half of patients with more limited variants of MS will lack oligoclonal bands in the CSF. The number of bands may increase, but only very rarely will decrease, and will give the same migration in the electrophoretigram. In contrast, oligoclonal bands seen with other types of inflammatory CNS disorders will often disappear when the disease process remits or is eliminated.

From the standpoint of the clinical pathology laboratory, the IgG index and oligoclonal banding pattern are the most helpful in the diagnostic workup of multiple sclerosis. The former is roughly analogous to the renal creatinine clearance, and allows quantitative detection of in situ CNS immunoglobulin synthesis. Because the blood-brain barrier normally becomes more leaky with increasing age, the simple measurement of serum and CSF IgG is not sufficient, without correction for age. However, the ratio of IgG to albumin in the CSF and serum (IgG index) is relatively constant over age in normals. An alternative to the IgG index is the IgG synthesis rate. Some have found this to be more sensitive than the IgG index with clinically definite MS.

PROGRESSIVE MULTIFOCAL LEUKOENCEPHALOPATHY

Progressive multifocal leukoencephalopathy is a chronic active demyelinating disorder. The multifocal CNS lesions usually lead to death within a year of diagnosis, due to cerebral dysfunction. The disorder is often associated with leukemia/lymphomas, and the Jakob-Creutzfeld (JC) virus. No well-defined autoantibody markers have been identified, and the CSF IgG level is usually normal. However, oligoclonal bands may be seen in a few cases. Ultimately, the antemortem diagnosis is primarily clinical.

SUBACUTE SCLEROSING PANENCEPHALITIS

Subacute sclerosing panencephalitis (SSPE) is a progressive demyelinating disorder that develops after a measles infection. SSPE is believed to be an abnormal immune response to the measles virus. It is most often seen in children, and lasts from 1 to 3 years. In situ IgG synthesis is significantly increased in most patients, and oligoclonal bands can be seen in a minority. Characteristic histopathologic changes can be seen by biopsy, and anti–measles virus antibody is usually present in high titer in the CSF.

COGAN'S SYNDROME

Cogan's syndrome is a rare disease characterized by acute interstitial keratitis associated with auditory and vestibular symptoms (vertigo, tinnitus), usually after an upper respiratory infection. Hearing loss usually ensues within 3 months of the onset of inner ear symptoms. No specific autoantibody markers or well-characterized CSF changes have been reported, probably due to the rarity of the disease. Thus, the diagnosis is usually based on clinical criteria, with exclusion of other diagnostic considerations.

GUILLAIN-BARRÉ SYNDROME

Guillain-Barré syndrome (GBS) is a demyelinating peripheral neuropathy of probable autoimmune etiology. The incidence of GBS varies from 0.4 to 4.0 cases per 100,00, depending on the diagnostic criteria used. The latter usually include (*a*) an acute or subacute onset of bilateral, usually symmetrical weakness of the lower motor neuron type within 2 months; (*b*) cerebrospinal fluid leukocyte count of less than 100/µl; and (*c*) the absence of other conditions known to cause a polyneuropathy (SLE, neoplasia, diabetes, toxins). The incidence increases with age, and there is an approximately 2:1 male to female ratio. Many patients, both children and adults, respond dramatically to plasmapheresis. However, some individuals have a chronic, remitting/relapsing course. Indeed, some investigators do not consider the latter to be in the clinical spectrum of Guillain-Barré syndrome.

The cause of GBS is not well defined. An autoimmune etiology is supported by the association of autoantibodies to glycosphingolipids in this and other lower motor neuron disorders. In particular, IgM anti-GM1 and anti-asialo GM1 have been identified in approximately 20% of cases of GBS. However, neuropathies may develop only in a minority of individuals with these autoantibodies. Further, there is a broad spectrum of neurological diseases associated with anti-GM1, including other lower motor neuron diseases and neuropathies. Usually, the IgM anti-GM1 or asialo GM1 of high titers (more than 1:800) are more likely to be associated with GBS and these other motor neuropathies.

Antibodies to nerve sheath glycoproteins P0, P2 and myelin-associated glycoprotein have also been reported in a small minority of cases. They are insensitive and somewhat nonspecific for GBS. Thus, further study is required to assess their utility.

ANTI-MAG, ANTI-GANGLIOSIDE, AND NEUROPATHIES

Autoantibodies to components of the myelin sheath have been associated with a variety of neurological disorders, including peripheral motor and sensory neuropathies. The best studied antigen/antibody systems are myelin-associated glycoprotein (MAG) and GM1 glycospingolipids. Many of the former present as monoclonal gammopathies, and are discussed further in the following section.

The anti-GM1 antibodies are relatively nonspecific. They can be seen in low titers (less than 1:800) in the serum of normals, in nonneurologic disease, and in CNS/PNS disorders such as amyotrophic lateral sclerosis, multiple sclerosis, Alzheimer's and Parkinson's diseases, and radiculopathy. Indeed, several commercial laboratories considered anti-GM1 titers less than 1:800 to be in the normal range. However, higher titers (more than 1:800 to 1:1600) are more specifically associated with lower motor neuron and sensorimotor neuropathies. Regrettably, anti-GM1 is relatively insensitive for these latter entities, with only 14 to 33% of cases having detectable autoantibody.

ANTI-MAG AND MONOCLONAL GAMMOPATHY–ASSOCIATED POLYNEUROPATHY

A monoclonal gammopathy is seen in association with approximately 4% of all polyneuropathies, only slightly increased over that seen in the general population. However, when one excludes neuropathies due to systemic disease, approximately 10% have concomitant monoclonal proteins. Virtually all of these patients have chronic neuropathies. The autoantibodies of the IgM isotype are often composed of monoclonal proteins and may constitute a prognostically favorable subgroup of immune peripheral neuropathies. However, they are not diagnostically specific.

Indirect immunofluorescence analyses have demonstrated anti-myelin reactivity in 40 to 100% of cases. Because of these observations, a serum protein electrophoresis is recommended in the workup of individuals with idiopathic or inflammatory neuropathies. A majority of the monoclonal gammopathies seen with polyneuropathies are of uncertain significance (MGUS).

The antigenic specificity of these anti–nerve sheath antibodies is the myelin-associated glycoprotein (MAG) molecule in 35% of cases of MGUS-associated polyneuropathy. This is an antigen otherwise known as Leu7 or CD57. The disease-associated antibodies react with an epitope distinct from that bound by commercially available murine anti-CD57. Detailed clinical-pathological studies have indicated that neuropathy patients with the monoclonal IgM anti-MAG have more severe symptoms than do monoclonals with differing isotypes.

The monoclonal gammopathy–associated polyneuropathies tend to have a progressive clinical course. Small prospective studies have indicated that plasmapheresis may have a beneficial effect in such patients. If this is true, the definition of both the antigenic specificity and clonality of anti-myelin antibodies will be important both diagnostically and prognostically.

PARANEOPLASTIC SYNDROMES

Cancer patients occasionally develop central or peripheral nervous system disorders not due to invasion by the neoplasm. Rather, these are due to remote immune-mediated or so-called paraneoplastic effects. These may develop before or after the diagnosis of cancer. The two principal types of paraneoplastic syndromes are sensory neuropathy/encephalomyelitis and cerebellar degeneration. Both are characterized by cell death, with or without concomitant inflammation.

The paraneoplastic syndrome seen in patients with *small cell carcinoma of the lung* (SCLC) is usually either a sensory neuropathy or encephalomyelitis. Such cases are often (more than 95%) associated with a serum or cerebrospinal fluid autoantibody called *anti-Hu*. This is best defined by a Western immunoblot technique, which detects a 35- to 40-kd protein found in most neurons of the CNS and in the small cell carcinoma. Anti-Hu is not seen in normals, in patients with SCLC or other cancers without neurological symptoms, or in patients with neurological diseases not associated with neoplasia. However, it may be seen in approximately 17% of patients with small cell carcinoma without a paraneoplastic neuropathy.

Paraneoplastic cerebellar degeneration is characterized by rapidly progressing pancerebellar symptoms. Histologically, there is a diffuse loss of Purkinje cells, sometimes associated with inflammatory infiltrates. This is most often seen in association with non–small cell malignancies (ovarian, uterine, and breast carcinomas). Evaluations for autoantibodies have revealed up to four different anti-neuronal antibodies in approximately 50% of cases. The most commonly observed is an autoantibody to Purkinje cell cytoplasmic antigen, *Yo*. The tumor tissue often cross-reacts with anti-Yo. The anti-Hu antibody has been rarely reported with small-cell carcinomas associated with paraneoplastic cerebellar degeneration. Normal individuals, cancer patients without neurological symptoms, and patients with nonneoplastic cerebellar diseases virtually never have detectable anti-Yo in the serum or CSF.

ANTI-PHOSPHOLIPID ANTIBODIES AND STROKE

During the last decade, a great deal of research has been directed toward anti-phospholipid antibodies (anti-cardiolipin; lupus anticoagulant) and their clinical-pathological correlates. The anti-phospholipid antibodies (APLs) have been associated with an increased risk of both arterial and venous thrombosis in general, and cerebrovascular disease in particular. Most ischemic strokes associated with APLs are not large, and are in the distribution of the middle cerebral artery. While initial reports focused on female stroke patients with SLE, larger, retrospective studies have shown a nearly equal male:female incidence ratio, with an average age of 43 years. However, newer prospective studies have indicated an average age in the seventh decade of life, not unlike routine stroke patients. Similarly, cerebral angiographic studies of APL-positive stroke patients do not appear to be significantly different from the APL-negative cases. Ultimately, the diagnosis of APL thromboembolic disease is largely one of exclusion.

Currently, there is no indication for mass screening of the general population for APL to assess risk for stroke. While APLs may play a role in recurrent thrombosis with or without SLE, their use defining the risk of thrombosis or directing therapy is still unclear. Further prospective studies are necessary to define the diagnostic and prognostic implications of APLs.

STIFF-MAN SYNDROME

The stiff-man syndrome is a rare CNS disorder associated with autoantibodies to glutamic acid decarboxylase (GAD) in γ-aminobutyric acid–positive neurons. Clinically, patients exhibit a progressive rigidity and painful spasms of the musculature. Approximately two-thirds of the cases have anti-GAD in the serum and/or CSF. Interestingly, a majority of these anti-GAD-positive patients also have autoantibodies to islet cell, parietal cell, and thyroid glandular cells. A distinct minority of these patients have evidence of type I diabetes, Graves' disease, hypothyroidism, or pernicious anemia.

The GAD antigen is a 50 to 60-kd protein. Since anti-GAD immunohistochemical reactivity with CNS neurons is not distinctly different from other antineuronal antibodies, more specific biochemical confirmation is required to confirm specificity (i.e., Western immunoblotting).

These observations put the stiff-man syndrome in the spectrum of organ-specific autoimmune diseases. In the appropriate clinical setting, screening for anti-GAD may be useful in (*a*) confirming the diagnosis of the disease; and (*b*) defining the subgroup that is associated with an increase of other organ-specific autoimmune disorders.

Skeletal Muscle

MYASTHENIA GRAVIS

Myasthenia gravis (MG) is an autoimmune disease of the neuromuscular junction. Specifically, autoantibodies to the acetylcholine receptors block acetylcholine binding at the postsynaptic junction. They further damage the neuromuscular junction via complement-mediated lysis. The disease is also seen with other autoimmune disorders (SLE, thyroiditis, rheumatoid arthritis, Sjögren's syndrome), as well as with thymoma, thymic follicular lymphoid hyperplasia, and pure red-cell aplasia.

Typically, the patient is a young adult female presenting with localized muscular weakness. This may be initially limited to the ocular or pharyngeal muscles, or to the muscles of the proximal extremities. The disease spontaneously waxes and wanes, and approximately one-quarter of patients may have a spontaneous remission. Drugs are useful in both diagnosis and treatment.

A circulating anti–acetylcholine receptor antibody (AChR) is found in approximately 90% of patients, and in a variable proportion of individuals with an isolated thymoma. In a clinical setting fully consistent with myasthenia gravis, the presence of an AChR is probably diagnostic. An anti–skeletal muscle antibody is seen in some cases of myasthenia gravis.

POLYMYOSITIS/DERMATOMYOSITIS

Autoimmune inflammation of skeletal muscle may present as an isolated disorder (polymyositis, PM) or may be associated with inflammatory skin disease (dermatomyositis, DM). In addition, PM/DM may be associated with a variety of other autoimmune diseases (SLE, RA, scleroderma, polyarteritis nodosa) and/or malignancy. PM/DM has an annual incidence of two to five cases per million. Adults comprise 78 to 92% of all cases. In primary adult PM and DM, there is mild to moderate female predominance, with a mean age at presentation of approximately 50 years. Approximately 5 to 11% of adult DM patients will have an underlying malignancy. The latter is quite uncommon in childhood PM/DM, which has a significantly higher incidence of vasculitis.

Patients with PM present with signs and symptoms of proximal muscle weakness of the upper and lower extremities, and, to a lesser extent, neck flexors. This is associated with increases in serum enzymes derived from skeletal muscle (aldolase, AST, CPK) in virtually all patients. Some 90% of PM/DM patients will have partially or completely diagnostic electromyographic findings. Muscle biopsy of moderately affected tissue reveals a predominantly lymphoplasmacytic infiltrate of the muscle fibers and adjacent vascular structures. Vasculitis may be seen when the syndrome is associated with polyarteritis. This is associated with muscle cell degeneration, necrosis/phagocytosis, and regeneration. Adult patients with DM have similar findings. In addition, there is a characteristic rash, with histologic features strongly resembling lupus.

Thyroid Gland

HASHIMOTO'S THYROIDITIS (CHRONIC LYMPHOCYTIC THYROIDITIS)

Clinical

Hashimoto's thyroiditis (HT) occurs primarily in middle-aged women, with a male to female ratio of approximately 20:1. It is probably one of the most common thyroid disorders in young adults, and has an incidence of about 1.6 to 2.0% in females. Classically, HT presents in a euthyroid individual with a diffuse, nontender enlargement of the thyroid gland. Occasionally, this may be associated with sporadic releases of thyroid hormone, so-called silent thyrotoxicosis. While the intermediate stages of the untreated disease may result in a goiter with elevated serum TSH and normal to decreased T_3 and T_4, Hashimoto's thyroiditis eventually evolves into a hypothyroid atrophic thryoiditis or myxedema. There is an HLA linkage with HT, like many autoimmune disorders. The HLA-DR3 and HLA-DR5 have significant association with HT. The latter is often associated with the goitrous form, while DR3 is more often seen in the atrophic form.

Hashimoto's thyroiditis exhibits a variety of hybrid syndromes, either concomitantly or sequentially. In unusual instances, HT may evolve into a clinicopathological syndrome indistinguishable from Graves' disease ("Hashitoxicosis"), or Graves' ophthalmopathy. Hashimoto's thyroiditis may also be associated with systemic (rheumatoid arthritis) and/or other organ-specific autoimmune disorders (pernicious anemia, Addison's disease, type I diabetes).

Laboratory

The most sensitive serologic marker for HT is the auto–anti-thyroid microsomal antibody. This recognizes multiple epitopes on the thyroid peroxidase molecule. Currently, most clinical laboratories use hemagglutination or indirect immunofluorescence assays. However, the DNA for thyroid peroxidase has been cloned, and recombinant antigen has been produced. Approximately 94% of patients will have detectable anti-microsomal antibody, usually (82% of positives) of high titer (more than 1:1600). Only 29 to 55% will have anti-thyroglobulin antibodies; again, a majority being of high titer (more than 1:1600).

The anti-microsomal antibodies are not specific for HT. They may be seen in low titer in Graves' disease and in subacute (De Quervain's) thyroiditis. Further, in normal individuals, 12% of females and 1% of males will have detectable anti-thyroid antibodies, as will aproximately 15% of clinically normal individuals aged 70 years or older. Most of these (85%) will be anti-microsomal antibody, usually of low titer (less than 1:1600). It is significant that on follow-up, some 29% of these patients of all ages will develop *subclinical* thyroid abnormalities. However, in autoantithyroid-positive elderly, only 1 to 2% will progress to clinically evident hypothyroidism or hyperthyroidism over 5 years' follow-up. Overall, mass screening of the general population is not reasonable, given low clinical yield and high cost.

Some 6 to 7% of HT patients will lack detectable anti-thyroid antibodies. In such instances, a fine needle aspiration of the thyroid may be helpful, in conjunction with the clinical presentation, in rendering a diagnosis. In Hashitoxicosis, there may be a significant thyroid-stimulating antibody present in lieu of the anti-microsomal antibody. The presence of abundant lymphocytes and Askanazy cells makes the diagnosis in the appropriate clinical setting.

GRAVES' DISEASE

Clinical

Graves' disease accounts for approximately 85% of all cases of hyperthyroidism and affects slightly less than 1% of the general population. Graves' disease is associated with serum anti-TSH receptor antibodies. There is a very similar hyperthyroid syndrome lacking such autoantibodies. Supporting the contention that these are different hyperthyroid disorders is the association of HLA-B8 and HLA-DR3 haplotypes with Graves' and HLA-DR5 with the non-Graves' cases.

There is a marked female predominance (about 10:1) in Graves' disease, and it is often associated with a significant family history of hyperthyroidism and other autoimmune diseases. The patient usually presents with a gradual clinical onset of a thyrotoxic state. Typically, there is a diffuse enlargement of the thyroid gland, although up to 33% of older patients may lack a palpable enlargement. Most patients have tachycardia (with or without atrial fibrillation) and characteristic eye signs (upper eyelid retraction/widened palpebral fissue) due to increased adrenergic stimulation. However, only 33 to 50% have concomitant Graves' ophthalmopathy, an independent autoimmune process involving the periorbital soft tissue and extraocular muscles. Pretibial myxedema (infiltrative dermopathy) is observed in less than 10% of Graves' disease patients, usually those with marked hyperthyroidism. Like many organ-specific autoimmune disorders, other organ-specific autoantibodies are also found, including anti–parietal cell (20%) and acetylcholine receptor antibodies (1%).

Laboratory

Graves' disease has a very characteristic clinical presentation—so much so that extensive laboratory testing is not often necessary for diagnosis. This is fortunate, as the autoantibodies associated with this disorder are difficult to perform and are not widely available. In a clinical setting consistent with Graves' disease, the diagnosis can be most efficiently confirmed with a demonstration of either an increased serum-free T_4 and/or suppressed TSH concentration. In individuals with borderline clinical or laboratory values, a thyrotropin-releasing hormone stimulation test or radioimaging of the thyroid gland may be needed.

The autoantibodies diagnostically and etiologically associated with Graves' disease are primarily directed at the TSH receptor, although a few may not be. The original descriptor was long-acting thyroid stimulator (LATS). Later work characterized the LATS as an immunoglobulin that was directed at the TSH molecule. Based on the assay used, these autoantibodies have been called thyroid-stimulating immunoglobulin (TSIG or TSI), TSH-binding inhibitory immunoglobulin (TBII), or thyroid growth–stimulating immunoglobulin (TGI). The TSIG and TBII probably described the same type of autoantibody. The TGI often results in growth only, and is associated with euthryoid goiter in many instances. Indeed, it probably binds to non-TSH receptor molecules in these cases.

The principal clinical application of TSIG/TBII/TGI antibodies would be in (*a*) the evaluation of euthyroid goiter; (*b*) predicting the risk of neonatal hyperthyroidism in mothers with Graves' disease; and (*c*) predicting the risk of remission or relapse after antithyroid drug therapy. Lastly, about 5% of euthyroid normals with a family history of Graves' disease will have detectable TBII. Approximately two-thirds of these individuals will have a blunted TRH test and suppressed serum TSH levels. A majority of the individuals will develop clinical hyperthyroidism. Normals with an isolated TBII remain clinically euthyroid.

GRAVES' OPHTHALMOPATHY

Clinical

Graves' ophthalmopathy (GO) is an autoimmune disorder independent of Graves' disease, although 33 to 50% of cases of infiltrative ophthalmopathy are seen in association with Graves' disease. The course of the eye disease can be independent of that seen with either treated or untreated Graves' disease, and the autoantibodies associated with it are different from those in Graves' disease. Lastly, the ophthalmopathy can be seen concomitantly with approximately 10% of cases of Hashimoto's thyroiditis. It is seen with other types of thyroiditis.

The extraocular eye muscles are the primary target in GO. Histologically, the process is characterized by a lymphoplasmacytic and neutrophilic infiltrate of orbital fibroadipose and skeletal muscle tissue, associated with edema. This may eventually progress to fibrosis. Grossly, there is bilateral proptosis, and limitation of range of eye motion can result.

Laboratory

Approximately 55 to 74% of GO patients will have serum autoantibodies directed at eye muscle antigens, as determined by ELISAs of crude muscle cytosol or indirect immunofluorescence assays. Additional studies have implicated a 64-kd membrane protein found in both eye muscle and thyroid gland as the target antigen for the anti–eye muscle antibodies.

These are not specific for GO. Indeed, 20 to 26% of GD without GO, 9 to 14% of HT without GO, and 14 to 18% of subacute thyroiditis without GO have detectable titers of these autoantibodies. Furthermore, 71% of polymositis and 10% of type I diabetes will also have these autoantibodies. However, abnormally elevated levels have not been reported in normals. There is no association between titers antimicrosomal and anti-TSH receptor and autoanti–eye muscle antibodies in GO, nor is it believed that the former play any role in the pathogenesis of GO.

TRANSIENT/SUBACUTE THYROIDITIS

Clinical

Subacute and painless thyroiditis are also known as transient thyroiditis. The former is usually caused by viral infection (mumps, measles, influenza, Epstein-Barr virus, adenovirus), and is usually associated with glandular tenderness. Painless thyroiditis is believed to be an autoimmune disorder, often seen postpartum. These conditions may comprise as much as 20% of all thyrotoxic individuals. The disorders tend to predominate in young adult females, and present with an acute onset of thyrotoxic symptoms similar to but usually milder than Graves' disease.

An infiltrative ophthalmopathy is not seen in subacute thyroiditis. Histologically, a lymphocytic infiltrate is present, usually without germinal centers. Patients tend to go through a 1- to 2-month thyrotoxic state, followed by a hypothyroid period in 25 to 50%. Virtually all subacute thryoiditis eventually become euthyroid. Approximately one-third of painless thyroiditis patients will have a persistent goiter. While thyrotoxic recurrences can occur during any stage, relapse is unusual after complete resolution.

Laboratory

Transient low titers of anti-microsomal and anti-thyroglobulin antibodies are seen in both subacute and painless thyroiditis. These eventually become nondetectable as the disease resolves. TBII autoantibodies may be seen in approximately 40% of subacute thyroiditis patients, but does not indicate a better or worse prognosis. Ultimately, these diagnoses are primarily clinical and require follow-up time.

NEONATAL AND POSTPARTUM AUTOIMMUNE THYROID DYSFUNCTION

The incidence of maternal postpartum thyroid dysfunction is relatively high, ranging up to 5.5% of women with clinical thyrotoxicosis or hypothyroid states, and up to 12% with anti-thyroid antibodies. Again, while a variety of autoanti-thyroid antibodies are detected, they are usually transient. Typically, individuals present 3 to 6 months after delivery. However, most cases clinically resolve in about 1 year.

Neonatal Graves' disease can present as either (*a*) a passively acquired, self-limited thyrotoxic state seen at birth due to placental transfer of maternal TSIG autoantibodies in a mother with Graves' disease; or (*b*) a thyrotoxic state developing early in infancy without a history of maternal Graves' disease. The risk of passively acquired neonatal Graves' disease is proportional to the titer of maternal TSIG, and is one of the few indications for this type of assay. Maternal titers of anti-thyroglobulin and anti-microsomal antibodies have not been definitively demonstrated to indicate any increased risk of neonatal thryoid disease.

Other Endocrine Glands

INTRODUCTION

Endocrine-specific autoimmune diseases are most often thought to include thryoid disorders, diabetes mellitus, and, less commonly, Addison's disease. During the last 15 years, further investigations have extended this list to the pituitary gland (idiopathic diabetes insipidus; partial hypopituitarism), the parathyroid gland (idiopathic hypoparathyroidism), and the gastrointestinal tract (fundal autoimmune gastritis). All of these disorders are associated with autoantibodies, some of which clearly play a pathophysiological role. These would include antibody-mediated cytotoxicity, and receptor stimulating and blocking activities.

PANCREAS AND DIABETES MELLITUS

Diabetes mellitus is a heterogeneous disorder of glucose metabolism. It is usually classified into three pathological and physiological groups: type I or insulin-independent (IDDM), type II or noninsulin-dependent (NIDDM), and gestational diabetes. Investigators over the past 2 decades have shown that type I diabetes is almost certainly an autoimmune disorder. This includes direct demonstration of circulating anti–islet cell (ICA) and anti-insulin autoantibodies (IAA). In addition, there is a distinct familial linkage, as well as increased association with HLA-DR3, HLA-DR4, and, most strongly, with HLA-DQB1. Possible environmental triggers for type I diabetes include congenital rubella infection.

The diagnosis of diabetes mellitus is based upon a combination of clinical and biochemical abnormalities, not the presence of autoantibodies. However, there are been interest in the utility of the ICA and IAAs (*a*) to predict the risk of type I diabetes in prediabetics and in relatives of diabetics; (*b*) to confirm the diagnosis of type I diabetes; and (*c*) to monitor the response of immunotherapy in diabetics.

The antigen recognized by ICA is a glycolipid, ganglioside GT3. By indirect immunofluorescence assay, circulating ICAs are seen in approximately 74% of IDDM patients at the time of diagnosis. Further, approximately 70% of all prediabetics will have detectable ICAs. However, about 90% of IDDM patients will then lose detectable levels of ICA during the course of the overt IDDM.

About 2% of first-degree relatives of IDDM patients, 15% of persons with NIDDM, 10% gestational diabetic patients, and 0.5% of normals will also have serum ICAs. Most of the apparent NIDDM patients with ICA will develop IDDM within an average of 4 years. Evidence at this time suggests that nondiabetic individuals with ICAs usually have profoundly abnormal insulin secretion. In addition, the risk of developing overt IDDM appears high. Thus, ICA determination of first-degree relatives of an IDDM patient, along with intravenous glucose tolerance tests may be clinically useful screens in a high-risk population. This concept still remains to be definitively proved. Lastly, the response of overt IDDM patients to cyclosporine does not appear to be predicted by levels of ICA during immunosuppressive therapy.

Anti-insulin antibodies, which are measured by RIA or ELISA methods, are seen in about 30% of individuals who later develop overt IDDM. At this time, some 48% of newly diagnosed IDDM patients will have detectable IAAs, and 80% of these will have concomitant ICAs. However, unlike the latter, the IAAs will occur predominantly in prepubertal IDDMs, being present in only 20% of newly diagnosed IDDMs more than 10 years of age. A third autoantigen/autoantibody combination seen in type I diabetes is directed toward a 64-kd membrane protein of islet cells. A circulating autoantibody to this protein is seen in 60% of prediabetics. Further studies are required to confirm and extend the clinical utility of the autoanti-64-kd antibody.

AUTOIMMUNE ADRENAL DISEASE

Autoimmune Addison's disease usually presents with the signs and symptoms of adrenal failure. The disorder is most commonly seen in adult females, in the 30- to 50-year age range. Other endocrine gland–specific autoantibodies and autoimmune endocrine disease may be seen (e.g., Graves' disease, pernicious anemia). Corticosteroid replacement therapy for life is required.

Biochemically, the patients will have an increased ACTH with decreased serum and urinary cortisol. These distinguish primary/autoimmune Addison's disease from secondary (pituitary causes). Other etiologies of primary Addison's disease (e.g., tuberculosis) must be excluded. Autoantibodies to the adrenal cortical cells are seen in serum of about half of the patients with idiopathic primary Addison's disease. Some investigators have shown that these may be blocking type autoantibodies to the ACTH receptor. Anti-adrenal autoantibodies are seen in less than 5% of normals, and may indicate a predisposition to autoimmune Addison's disease in an otherwise normal individual.

Autoimmune Cushing's disease has been rarely reported. The clinical signs and symptoms appear to be essentially the same as nonimmune Cushing's disease. Interestingly, the autoantibody appears to bind to and stimulate the ACTH receptor.

Reproductive Immunology

Autoimmune disease of the reproductive organs is, not surprisingly, most often manifested by infertility. This may be due to gross destruction of the gonad, such as in autoimmune orchitis, or in more subtle failures to conceive or carry pregnancy to term. Repeated spontaneous abortion and prolonged infertility have been associated with an aberrant immunologic response in an increasing number of cells. In some instances, these may be alloantibodies; in others, autoantibodies. Many of the anti-sperm and anti-oocyte antibodies result in infertility without spontaneous abortion. Alloantibodies directed at fetal antigens of paternal origin and systemic autoimmune disease are usually associated with first-trimester losses, while the isolated anti-phospholipid syndrome more commonly results in fetal loss during the second trimester.

ANTI-SPERM

Sperm antigens are potent immunogens, as evidenced by the 70% of males with who develop anti-sperm antibodies within 1 year of vasectomy. This is not entirely unexpected, since the blood-testis barrier shields the immune system during development from testicular antigens. Thus, tolerance is not established, and inappropriate exposure can lead to autoimmune responses. High titers of such autoantibodies are often associated with postvasectomy degeneration of the testes, and may explain the 30 to 60% male infertility rate after successful vasovasotomy.

Approximately one-third of infertile couples have anti-sperm antibodies, and their titers appear to be associated with low sperm motility. Further, some investigators have found unique autoantigens on the sperm of infertile males with autoantibodies, but not on the sperm from fertile males. Antibodies to spermatozoa can either agglutinate or be cytotoxic. Isotype may also define unique blocks in fertilization. (The IgA anti-sperm antibodies to the sperm tail are particularly associated with poor motility and penetration of the cervical mucus.) IgG anti-sperm antibodies are more often associated with blockage of sperm-ovum fusion.

ANTI-PHOSPHOLIPID SYNDROME AND INFERTILITY

Recurrent first- and second-trimester spontaneous abortions can be explained by either genetic, hormonal, or anatomic etiologies in approximately half of all cases. In the remainder, an association with SLE or anti-phospholipid antibodies is often present. Interestingly, first-trimester spontaneous abortions are commonly seen in women with SLE, irrespective of the presence or absence of anti-phospholipid antibodies.

The loss seen with the anti-phospholipid syndrome occurs primarily in the second trimester. The anti-phospholipid–associated pregnancy loss in otherwise healthy women is often associated with atheromatous lesions of the uterine blood vessels. These are seen primarily at the implantation site, and presumably lead to ischemia and fetal loss.

OVARY

Autoimmune ovarian failure is often seen in conjunction with other anti-endocrine autoantibodies and autoimmune disorders (e.g., thyroid, and adrenal). The patients present with amenorrhea or early menopause. Serum autoanti-ovary antibodies are usually present, and are often directed at theca interna cells. In addition, anti-FSH antibodies have been reported with premature ovarian failure. It is very unusual to see any of these autoantibodies in nonautoimmune causes of ovarian failure.

Liver

PRIMARY BILIARY CIRRHOSIS

Clinical

Primary biliary cirrhosis (PBC) is a chronic progressive autoimmune disorder, resulting in cirrhosis and liver failure. Its prevalence has been variably estimated at approximately four to 14 per 100,000 general population, and accounts for up to 2% of the mortality from all cases of liver cirrhosis. PBC typically occurs in middle-aged to elderly females, with a female to male ratio greater than 9:1. Median survival is estimated to be 63% at 5 years. Individuals who are asymptomatic at presentation may have relatively normal life expectancies.

While some familial tendencies have been seen, no definitive HLA linkage has been demonstrated. However, HLA-B27 has been associated with PBC and rheumatoid arthritis, and HLA-B8 seen with PBC and scleroderma overlap syndromes. A related issue is the increased incidence of systemic autoimmune disorders with PBC. The most commonly reported are Sjögren's syndrome, Raynaud's syndrome, scleroderma (usually the CREST variant), or rheumatoid arthritis. Overall, approximately 17 to 34% of PBC patients will have a concomitant systemic autoimmune disorder, and this is associated with decreased survival.

In the early stages, fatigue and pruritus are the most common complaints, although concomitant jaundice is seen in 20% of patients. While the clinical and serologic data may be rather compelling, the lack of specificity of the anti-mitochondrial antibody (AMA) and the overall gravity of the diagnosis usually require that a confirmatory liver biopsy be performed. Histologically, the characteristic feature of PBC is a progressive destruction of the intrahepatic bile ducts, biliary stasis, and portal fibrosis. The former predominates in the early stages, while the latter is more marked in advanced disease. Portal granulomas, particularly if seen in the early stages of disease, are a favorable prognostic feature. However, they are not specific, as portal granulomas may be seen in primary sclerosing cholangitis.

Laboratory

The overall serum biochemistry profile is that of cholestasis. Typical alterations include a striking increase in alkaline phosphatase and γ-glutamyl transpeptidase, with relatively normal to slightly elevated aminotransferase (AST, ALT) levels. Serum albumin and bilirubin are often within normal ranges early in the disease. The serum protein electrophoretigram is unremarkable, although there is typically an elevation in polyclonal IgM. Lastly, a marked increase in serum lipids is almost always detected during all stages of disease.

The anti-mitochondrial antibody is seen in varying titers in greater than 95% of patients screened with an indirect immunofluorescence assay. More extensive work has shown that the anti-mitochondrial antibodies are heterogeneous, being directed at a diverse range of antigens. The AMA characteristic of PBC is almost always directed at the M2 antigen, the E2 component of pyruvate dehydrogenase complex on the inner membrane of the mitochondria. In addition, anti-M4 and anti-M8 are also seen if anti-M2 is present. The anti-M9 may be seen in rare PBC cases that lack anti-M2.

While the AMA is exquisitely sensitive for PBC, it lacks specificity. In a large general hospital population, 1 to 2% of all sera will be AMA positive. Of these, the majority will lack any clinical or biochemical evidence of liver disease, and only 13% will have PBC. Anti-mitochondrial antibodies are present in approximately 10% of cases of autoimmune chronic active hepatitis (CAH). Antibody titer or isotype is not able to reliably differentiate AMA-positive PBC from AMA-positive non-PBC patients. This finding is not surprising, given the heterogeneity of AMAs and the antigens. The AMAs have been seen in 8% "pure" or isolated cases of scleroderma (primarily CREST), and to a much lesser extent, in SLE. Variants may also be seen in syphilis (anti-M1) and with drug treatment (anti-M3 and anti-M6).

Other autoantibodies are often seen in PBC. Utilizing an indirect immunofluorescence assay and HEp-2 cell substrate, anti-nuclear antibodies are seen in 70% of patients. These comprise a mixture of homogeneous, speckled, anti-centromeric, and nuclear membrane patterns. The presence of the anti-centromeric antibody in PBC is often associated with concomitant scleroderma or Raynaud's syndrome. Anti-SSA and/or anti-SSB are specifically detected in approximately 8% of cases (usually with Sjögren's), while otherwise unusual anti-nuclear membrane antibodies are seen in 14% of cases of isolated PBC. Anti-asialoglycoprotein receptor, liver-kidney microsome, and anti-liver membrane antibodies are observed in a minority of cases. Lastly, anti-thyroid antibodies may also be detected.

AUTOIMMUNE CHRONIC ACTIVE HEPATITIS

Autoimmune chronic active hepatitis (CAH) has also been referred to as "lupoid" CAH. Classic autoimmune CAH is seen predominantly in adults, although one variant (anti-LKM-positive CAH) is most often observed in children. Females are disproportionately affected in all age groups, with a female to male ratio of 7:1 in adults. Evidence of a genetic/autoimmune predisposition includes an association with HLA-A1, HLA-B8, HLA-DR3, and, to a lesser extent, HLA-DR2 in all major forms. HLA-B8 and HLA-DR3 are also seen in a variety of other organ-specific autoimmune disorders.

In general, chronic hepatitis is defined as clinical, biochemical, and morphologic liver disease of greater than 6 months' duration. The division between persistent and active chronic hepatitis is based upon the morphologic examination of a liver biopsy. The morphologic examination, in addition to confirming the active inflammatory nature of the liver disorder, also defines the presence or absence of cirrhosis. The latter, in the setting of viral or autoimmune CAH, is an independently significant, adverse prognostic indicator.

A major difficulty in defining this disease has been the problem in excluding viral etiology, along with the lack of defining serologic, biochemical, or morphologic parameters, and CAH's obvious clinical and pathological heterogeneity. *Exclusionary* criteria include (*a*) the absence of serologic markers of viral hepatitis A, B, C, and D; (*b*) no evidence of α_1 antitrypsin or ceruloplasm deficiencies (Wilson's disease); and (*c*) no evidence of toxin-induced etiology (alcohol or other drugs). *Positive* criteria include biopsy-proven CAH with the presence (by no means 100% sensitive or specific) of serum anti–smooth muscle antibody (ASMA), anti–liver kidney microsome (LKM) antibody; anti–liver soluble protein (LSP), anti–liver membrane antibody (LMA), anti–asialoglycoprotein receptor (ASGP-R), and/or antinuclear antibody (ANA). Lastly, there should almost always be a polyclonal increase in serum IgG (1.5g/dl or more). A possibly more accurate, albeit operational, definition would be CAH without evidence of viral, toxic, or hereditary etiology, which responds to immunosuppressive therapy, and often relapses when this treatment is stopped.

Based on a combination of clinical and serologic profiles, three types of "autoimmune" CAH can be defined. *Type I CAH* is seen predominantly in adult females, and is the type originally called "lupoid." This type is most commonly associated with the anti–smooth muscle antibody. An ANA, anti-mitochondrial antibody, ASGP-R, and/or anti-LSP antibodies may also be present. *Type II CAH* is primarily seen in children, although it may be observed in adults. It is much less frequent than type I CAH, and is often associated with other organ-specific autoimmune disease. Type II patients tend to have a more fulminant presentation, and there is a greater incidence of cirrhosis than seen in type I. Typically, ASMA is often absent and anti–liver-kidney microsome (LKM) antibody type 1 is present. *Type III CAH* occurs primarily in adults. These patients lack both LKM and ASMA. However, most do have anti-ASGP receptor, anti–liver soluble and/or anti–liver membrane autoantibodies. Furthermore, like type I and II CAH, there is a high rate of clinical and biochemical remission with immunosuppressive therapy with type III CAH.

The distinction between hepatitis associated with systemic lupus erythematosus and organ-specific autoimmune CAH can be difficult. Both disorders have a high incidence of high-titer antinuclear antibodies, usually of the homogeneous pattern. In addition, the lupus band test is positive in a similar minority of cases in both entities. Clinically, the presence of primary renal or central nervous system disease is very unusual in the latter. However, it is quite rare to find anti-dsDNA antibodies (by *Crithidia luciliae* immunofluorescence assay) in autoimmune CAH, yet this is fairly common in SLE.

Laboratory

Much has already been said about the autoantibodies associated with CAH. In general, they have moderate to good sensitivities, but are relatively nonspecific. Their use in the differential diagnosis of chronic liver disease should follow only after a careful clinical history, physical examination, viral serologic, and serum protein studies have excluded other etiologies. Even in this setting, their presence is not absolutely diagnostic.

Anti–smooth muscle antibody (ASMA) is the most commonly recognized autoantibody in the setting of CAH. However, ASMA is only moderately sensitive for CAH, with about 70 to 80% of cases being positive. There is also a significant lack of specificity. In fact, a majority of patients with localized or systemic viral infections; some patients with carcinoma, multiple sclerosis, primary biliary cirrhosis, and *Mycoplasma* infections; and unusual cases of Wilson's disease may be associated with low titers of ASMA.

The anti–smooth muscle antibodies from various diseases are directed at differing cytoplasmic proteins. In autoimmune CAH, the target is almost always actin, a cytoskeletal protein. The antigenic specificity of the ASMA seen in viral hepatitis and in respiratory and systemic infections are directed primarily at tubulin and intermediate filaments. Unfortunately, 31 to 41% of patients with carcinoma or acute respiratory infections will have an ASMA reactive with actin.

Most CAH-associated ASMAs are of relatively high titer (1:160 or higher), in contrast to those seen with other diseases. While the titers do not appear to be predictive of prognosis or of response to therapy of CAH, there have been a few reports that children with high-titer ASMA have a greater tendency to evolve into primary sclerosing cholangitis. Lastly, most of the ASMAs associated with viral infections and multiple sclerosis are of the IgM class, while virtually all seen in autoimmune CAH are of the IgG isotype.

Anti-LKM is a recently defined autoantibody that is relatively sensitive and specific for type II CAH. At least two kinds have been defined (LKM-1 and LKM-2), both directed at variants of the cytochrome P-450 system of the smooth endoplasmic reticulum. It is LKM-1 that is most directly associated with this disease. Currently, the preferred analytic technique is indirect immunofluorescence, using a liver substrate. Anti-LKM can mimic anti-mitochondrial antibodies on stomach-kidney substrate.

Anti-LSM, anti-ASGP receptor, and *anti-LMA* are less widely recognized autoantibodies seen in the setting of CAH. These are relatively sensitive for the spectrum of autoimmune CAH, but are not specific for any one type. These autoantibodies can also be seen in acute and chronic infectious hepatitis, primary biliary cirrhosis, and primary sclerosing cholangitis. Anti-mitochondrial antibodies are detected in approximately 10% of cases of autoimmune CAH.

The principal use of anti-LSM, anti-ASGP, or anti-LMA serologic testing may be as follow-up assays in cases of "cryptogenic" CAH, in which all viral and autoimmune serologies (ASMA, AMA, LKM) have been negative. If anti-LSM, anti-ASGP receptor, or anti-LMA is positive in such a setting, then one would favor a diagnosis of type III autoimmune CAH. Lastly, monitoring their levels may allow insights into response to therapy, although this may be accomplished in a more cost-effective manner by monitoring serum transaminase levels.

PRIMARY SCLEROSING CHOLANGITIS

Clinical

Primary sclerosing cholangitis (PSC) is a chronic fibrosing inflammatory disease of the hepatobiliary tree. Its pathogenesis is controversial, although association with autoantibodies and HLA-B8 and HLA-DR3 suggest a possible autoimmune etiology. Unlike most autoimmune disorders, PSC exhibits a male predominance (the male to female ratio is approximately 2:1). The age of onset is broad, ranging from 10 to 65 years, with a mean of 34 years. The primary clinical symptoms are jaundice, pruritus, and fatigue. Approximately 70% of PSC patients have or will develop ulcerative colitis. Usually, the diagnosis of this chronic inflammatory bowel disorder precedes that of PSC by several years. The presence of HLA-B8 or HLA-DR3 in the setting of ulcerative colitis is associated with a 10-fold increase in the risk of PSC.

The diagnosis of PSC is difficult, requiring exclusion of infectious etiologies. Cholangiography is the most sensitive diagnostic modality (about 86%), while histology is confirmatory in only 36% of cases. In addition, certain morphologic features may overlap with those of chronic active hepatitis and primary biliary cirrhosis (piecemeal necrosis, loss of bile ducts). Autoantibody serology can be helpful, as most cases of PSC lack anti-mitochondrial and anti-LKM antibodies. Low-titer ANAs and ASMA are present in a minority of cases, while a variant form of peripheral anti-neutrophil antibody (P-ANCA) is present in up to 86%.

Laboratory

Serum biochemistries have a predominant "cholestatic" profile. Alkaline phosphatase, γ-glutamyl transpeptidase, and bilirubin are significantly increased in 83 to 97% of patients. Aminotransferases (AST, ALT) are also elevated, as is serum polyclonal IgM in 45% of adult cases. Interestingly, it is polyclonal IgG that is usually increased in most cases of childhood PSC, although a majority have concomitant increases in IgM.

The discovery of the association of a variant P-ANCA (anti-neutrophil nuclear antibody) in most patients with PSC and ulcerative colitis is significant from both a practical diagnostic and a pathogenetic standpoint. The autoantigen has not been well defined, although it is not a general ANA or myeloperoxidase antigen. The latter also gives a P-ANCA pattern on ethanol-fixed neutrophils, and is seen in conjunction with pauci-immune glomerulonephritis and some cases of Wegener's granulomatosis. Some trends suggest that the titer of the P-ANCA is related to disease activity of PSC, although this has not reached statistical significance.

Antinuclear antibodies are detectable in approximately one-third of patients. These are usually of low titer (less than 1:80), and are not accompanied by anti-dsDNA antibodies. Similarly, ASMA is observed in 16 to 55% of PSC cases, with titers usually less than 1:40. Anti-LMP and ASGP receptor antibodies are seen in 88 and 50% of cases of childhood PSC. Lastly, no cases of pure PSC have been reported with either anti-mitochondrial or anti–liver-kidney microsome antibodies.

GI Tract

PERNICIOUS ANEMIA

Pernicious anemia is the best defined of the variants of autoimmune gastritis. It reflects damage or blocking of vitamin B_{12} absorption by autoantibodies. No association with HLA antigens has been demonstrated. However, pernicious anemia is often seen in association with other organ-specific autoimmune disorders and autoantibodies (Graves' disease, Hashimoto's disease, type I diabetes mellitus, autoimmune Addison's disease). Further, cell-mediated immunity to intrinsic factor and parietal cell antigens has been demonstrated.

Most patients are elderly with a modest female predominance, and present with complaints of fatigue, dyspepsia, and weakness. Biopsy of the stomach usually reveals a chronic atrophic gastritis. A macrocytic anemia is classically present, and there may be a variable peripheral or central neuropathy. Examination of a peripheral blood smear, along with the CBC and serum B_{12} levels, usually serve as an adequate first screen. There is usually a significant elevation of serum LDH, due to increased intramedullary erythrocyte turnover.

Most (86%) patients have a circulating anti–parietal cell antibody, and this serves as a useful confirmatory test to the aforementioned signs and symptoms. This autoantibody can also be seen in 11% of normal individuals and in 20 to 30% of those with other types of organ-specific autoimmune diseases. It is detected by serum reactivity with gastric parietal cells and the lack of reactivity with renal tubules on mouse stomach-kidney substrate. An antimicrosomal antibody will have a nearly identical reactivity with the gastric parietal cells, but will also have strong renal tubular staining.

Anti–intrinsic factor antibody can serve as a useful confirmatory test, particularly if the anti–parietal cell antibody is absent. The anti–intrinsic factor antibodies are of two types: B_{12}-blocking (type I) and intrinsic factor binding (type II). The former prevents intrinsic factor from binding B_{12}, while the latter precludes intestinal absorption of the B_{12}–intrinsic factor complex. An alternative diagnostic procedure is the use of a functional (Schilling's) B_{12} absorbtion test with and without the addition of intrinsic factor.

CELIAC DISEASE

Celiac disease is also known as gluten-sensitive enteropathy. While the disorder is directly related to an immune response to dietary gluten, there is a strong genetic predisposition. This is manifested by family studies and an association with the HLA-DR3 antigen. These findings, a distinct female predominance, and association with the autoimmune disorder dermatitis herpetiformis indicate that celiac disease might be considered as much an autoimmune disorder as a food allergy.

The clinical presentation can be quite diverse, ranging from anemia, to aphthous oral ulcers, to growth retardation. Any combination can be seen, and some patients present without clinical GI symptoms. Most of these have malabsorption as their common etiology. While a majority of patients are diagnosed in childhood, approximately 40% present at ages above 18 years. The disorder responds to elimination of dietary gluten. Patients also have an increased risk of developing a non-Hodgkin's lymphoma in the GI tract, as well as carcinoma of the upper GI tract.

The definitive diagnostic procedure for celiac disease is a biopsy of the small intestinal mucosa, along with the exclusion of other etiologies of malabsorption and response to elimination of dietary gluten. However, screening tests that are less invasive are attractive alternatives, particularly in children presenting with growth retardation. Such alternative tests can also serve to confirm the clinical and biopsy impression of gluten-sensitive enteropathy (GSE).

Three autoantibodies have been associated with celiac disease: anti-gliadin, anti-endomysial, and anti-reticulin antibodies. The antigliadin antibody is the best single screening test. It has a high sensitivity (90%) for GSE; thus, a negative result should define the patients without clinical GI symptoms in whom biopsy is not needed. However, its specificity is not total, as 10 to 15% of normals will be positive, albeit with lower titers. Monitoring the levels of antigliadin antibody is useful in the follow-up of treatment, as they will fall with the exclusion of dietary gluten.

Anti-endomysial antibodies have sensitivities and specificities similar but not superior to anti-gliadin antibodies in the differential diagnosis of GSE. The anti-reticulin antibody has poor sensitivity (45%) and a specificity essentially the same as the anti-endomysial and anti-gliadin antibodies. Some investigators have found both enhanced sensitivity and specificity with indirect immunofluorescence assays as opposed to ELISAs. However, the former are more subjective in interpretation and require additional steps for quantitation.

ULCERATIVE COLITIS/CROHN'S DISEASE

Ulcerative colitis (UC) and Crohn's disease are chronic inflammatory bowel disorders of poorly defined etiology. The former is primarily confined to the large intestine, and presents with diarrhea and bloody stools. Its course is one of remissions and relapses, and usually ends with resection of the colon because of neoplasia or inflammatory destruction. Crohn's disease usually involves the small intestine and, to a lesser extent, the large bowel in a focal manner. There is an association between ulcerative colitis and the seronegative spondylarthritides, particularly ankylosing spondylitis.

Histologically, ulcerative colitis diffusely involves the mucosa, with a lymphoplasmacytic infiltrate with or without neutrophilic inflammation. Crohn's disease is usually focal and exhibits transmural inflammation, classically with a granulomatous component in addition to the lymphoplasmacytic infiltrate. No distinct mode of inheritance or HLA association has been shown.

Ulcerative colitis is often associated with extraintestinal complications, many of which are believed to be autoimmune diseases (e.g., primary sclerosing cholangitis, autoimmune hemolytic anemia, ankylosing spondylitis, and pyoderma gangrenosum). Thus, the lack of any other clearly defined etiology or recently defined autoantibodies suggests that ulcerative colitis may very well be an autoimmune disorder.

Serum antinuclear and anti–smooth muscle antibodies and RF are usually absent in ulcerative colitis. Anti-colonic epithelial antibodies have been detected in UC patients. However, their diagnostic specificity is limited, as they are detected in normal healthy relatives, as well as in other GI, liver, and urinary tract diseases.

A variant of the anti-neutrophil cytoplasmic antibody (ANCA) is detected in a small percentage of ulcerative colitis patients and in a majority of individuals with primary biliary sclerosis. While the indirect immunofluorescence pattern initially appears as a peripheral ANCA, it is not the myeloperoxidase antigen. The latter also gives a P-ANCA pattern on ethanol-fixed neutrophils, and is seen in conjunction with pauci-immune glomerulonephritis and some cases of Wegener's granulomatosis.

The IBD-associated P-ANCA is seen not only with UC and PSC, but also in a distinct minority of cases of nonviral (autoimmune) chronic active hepatitis, and in a few cases of Crohn's disease. Overall, while this autoantibody's sensitivity for UC and PSC is only modest, its specificity for UC appears reasonably good. If confirmed by further studies, the ANCA test may be quite helpful in supporting the diagnosis of clinically and histologically suspected ulcerative colitis.

Cardiovascular and Renal Systems

GOODPASTURE'S SYNDROME

In Goodpasture's syndrome, patients present with episodes of hemoptysis and hematuria. The disease has a variable course, with some patients developing renal failure and severe pulmonary hemorrhages leading to asphyxia, while others suffer only small amounts of bleeding. The patients may have a rapidly progressive glomerulonephritis. In all patients, a diffuse *linear* deposition of IgG is seen by immunofluorescence along the glomerular capillary walls. Sometimes the renal lesions occur in the absence of the pulmonary lesions. It is arguable whether the latter case represents true Goodpasture's disease or a variant. However, in either case, the finding of antibody to glomerular basement membrane (anti-GBM) is most helpful in the diagnosis of Goodpasture's disease.

A radioimmunoassay has been developed that is very helpful in the detection of these antibodies. In the lung, deposition of immunoglobulin may be seen; however, due to the heavy background staining seen in many normal lungs, immunofluorescence to detect such deposits is not recommended. The anti-GBM may cross-react with pulmonary basement membranes and cause the lung lesion. With the advent of dialysis, aggressive immunosuppressive therapy, and plasmapheresis to remove the autoantibodies, these patients may retain sufficient renal function, so they do not need renal transplantation. In those who have renal failure, a kidney transplant is indicated, even if some circulating anti-GBM is present.

WEGENER'S GRANULOMATOSIS

Wegener's granulomatosis (WG) is a regional systemic vasculitis in which small arteries in the kidney, lungs, and upper respiratory tract are damaged by a necrotizing inflammation. Unlike many other autoimmune diseases that occur more frequently in women, WG occurs most often in middle-aged men. The diagnosis is often difficult to make on clinical grounds alone. Patients may have several bouts of pneumonia, chronic sinusitis, and hematuria. Indeed, many cases present with confusing, less-specific complaints such as joint and muscle pain, skin rash, and polyneuritis. Necrotizing vasculitis foci are found in the upper respiratory tract and the lungs. In these lesions, plump fibroblasts with giant cells may resemble the granulomas seen in tuberculosis. The renal lesions do not have a granulomatous component. They show evidence of necrotizing crescentic glomerulonephritis.

With immunosuppressive and cytotoxic drugs, patients can have complete remission. However, without such therapy, they usually succumb to their disease within a year. Unfortunately, the aggressive immunosuppressive therapy leaves the patients susceptible to infection by microorganisms normally of relatively low virulence. The potential danger of the immunosuppressive side effects of the therapy makes the establishment of a correct diagnosis particularly important. Serologic testing now plays a key role in the diagnosis of WG and other systemic vasculitis syndromes. Most patients with WG have circulating autoantibodies against neutrophil cytoplasm, which are useful for the diagnosis.

There are two major types of patterns of ANCA reactivity. The C-ANCA pattern is highly specific for WG and gives a diffuse granular staining of the cytoplasm. This is due to antibody against proteinase 3. The titer of this antibody is useful for following the clinical course of these patients. The other major ANCA pattern is a staining of the cytoplasm surrounding the nucleus, giving a perinuclear (P-ANCA) pattern. The P-ANCA pattern is mainly due to antibodies against myeloperoxidase. However, some patients with antibodies against cathepsin and others with antibodies against elastase have been described. Although the P-ANCA pattern is found in patients with WG, it also occurs in other conditions, especially in those with microscopic polyarteritis. If a patient is suspected of having vasculitis, but the ANCA test is negative, it should be repeated during exacerbations, as the titer will fluctuate with disease.

Skin

BULLOUS PEMPHIGOID

Bullous pemphigoid is a chronic autoimmune disorder of the skin, usually seen in the elderly. The lesions are large bullae, usually distributed over the groin, abdomen, and flexor surfaces of the forearms. One-third of cases have oral lesions, and the Nikolsky sign is negative.

Biopsy specimens should be obtained from the edge of a relatively new bulla. Histologically, subepidermal bullae are formed, with vacuolization of the dermal-epidermal junction of adjacent, nonbullous skin. Noninflamed bullae contain a scant inflammatory cell infiltrate and some fibrin. The subjacent dermis also contains a minimal infiltrate.

The lesions of bullous pemphigoid are due to an autoantibody to the dermal epidermal (DEJ) basement membrane and squamous basal cells. Direct immunofluorescence assay reveals a linear and diffuse anti-IgG and anti-C3 reactivity along the dermal-epidermal junction in 87% and 100% of patients, respectively. A serum autoantibody to DEJ is detected in approximately 70% of patients, using monkey esophagus as a substrate. The antibody titers are not related to the severity of the disease.

CICATRICIAL PEMPHIGOID

Cicatricial pemphigoid is a chronic, scarring bullous disease with a predilection for the oral mucosa and conjunctiva. Skin lesions are present in only 25 to 33% of cases. The disorder more often affects women. Histologically, the bullae are subepidermal. The intensity of the chronic inflammatory cell infiltrate in the dermis is related to the risk of subsequent scarring. Corticosteroid therapy is effective in preventing scarring in general and blindness in particular.

Direct immunofluorescence reveals a diffuse, linear IgG and C3 deposits in the basement membrane of the DEJ, and, occasionally, of the sweat glands. These are primarily in the lamina lucida of the basement membrane. By indirect immunofluorescence assay, circulating autoanti-DEJ are only rarely detected.

PEMPHIGUS VULGARIS

Pemphigus vulgaris is a bullous disorder of autoimmune etiology. The autoantibody is directed at the intercellular matrix/cement between the keratinocytes of stratified squamous epithelium. Middle-aged adults tend to be most commonly affected. There is a hereditary component, evidenced by the increased prevalance of pemphigus vulgaris with HLA 10 and 13, and Mediterranean descent. The disorder is also seen in association with thymoma and myasthenia gravis. The bullae are found on the oral and anal-genital mucosa, as well as on the skin. The Nikolsky sign is present in this disorder. Corticosteroid therapy is very effective in reducing morbidity and mortality.

An early lesion should be biopsied, and it will reveal an intraepidermal bulla. Characteristically, it is suprabasal and associated with prominent acantholysis. Inflammation is usually minimal. Direct immunofluorescence of skin reveals a characteristic intercellular deposition of IgG and C3 in 80 to 100% of cases, and other immunoglobulins in approximately half. This immunofluorescence pattern may persist in skin biopsies for years after treatment and clinical resolution of the disease. A circulating autoantibody is seen on 80 to 90% of patients by indirect immunofluorescence on monkey esophagus substrate. While the titer of the serum antibody appears to parallel the clinical course of the disease, it is so variable as to preclude its use for an individual patient. The presence of such a serum autoantibody is not specific for pemphigus vulgaris. However, in such instances, the direct immunofluorescence test is almost always negative.

PEMPHIGUS FOLIACEUS AND PEMPHIGUS ERYTHEMATOSUS

Pemphigus foliaceus and pemphigus erythematosus are autoimmune bullous disorders. Similar to pemphigus vulgaris, both have autoantibodies to the intracellular matrix of stratified squamous epithelium. The Nikolsky sign is present. From a practical standpoint, pemphigus erythematosus appears to be a limited form of pemphigus foliaceus. Histologically, they appear to be the same. However, pemphigus erythematosus is more commonly associated with thymoma and myasthenia gravis, as well as having serologic (positive lupus band test) and skin manifestations of SLE ("butterfly" rash).

The biopsy should be perilesional skin. Histologically, the biopsies of pemphigus foliaceus and pemphigus erythematosus reveal acantholytic bullae in the granular layer of stratified squamous epithelium. Older lesions may show more prominent acantholysis and hyperkeratosis. The dermal inflammatory cell infiltrate is moderate, usually with a distinct number of eosinophils. By direct immunofluorescence testing, most cases reveal a deposition of IgG and C3 in an intercellular distribution in the epidermis, with IgM or IgA in about 25%. In addition, the lesions of pemphigus erythematosus often show a granular deposition of IgG and C3 at the DEJ (lupus band test positive) as well as an ANA pattern. Serum autoantibodies are detected. No clinical association with serum autoantibody titer has been demonstrated.

SYSTEMIC AND DISCOID LUPUS ERYTHEMATOSUS

The more general clinical and serologic aspects of SLE have been discussed earlier. SLE usually has significant cutaneous lesions, more often seen in sun-exposed areas (e.g., butterfly rash, alopecia). Similar lesions can be seen without the other noncutaneous manifestations of SLE. This entity is called discoid lupus erythematosus (DLE). For the optimal histologic and direct immunofluorescence differentiation among SLE, DLE, and other inflammatory lesions, the biopsies should be taken from lesional, sun-exposed normal and non–sun-exposed normal skin.

Histologically, SLE and DLE reveal epidermal atrophy with vacuolar degeneration of the basal keratinocytes. A widened eosinophilic basement membrane zone is seen, associated with a mild to moderate, perivascular lymphoid inflammatory cell infiltrate. By direct immunofluorescence analysis, a diffuse deposition of IgG, IgM, and C3 (positive lupus band test) is seen at the DEJ in SLE (90 to 95% of lesional and 80% of sun-exposed nonlesional) and DLE (90 to 95% of lesional skin). In more diffuse forms of DLE, the nonlesional sun-exposed skin may also be lupus band test positive. These deposits tend to ultrastructurally localize subjacent to the basal lamina. Approximately 50% of SLE patients will have a positive lupus band test in the non–sun-exposed normal skin; allegedly, this has been associated with greater disease activity in general. The lupus band test is usually absent in drug-induced lupus, scleroderma, dermatomyositis, and rheumatoid arthritis. Serologically, no circulating anti-DEJ antibody is seen in either DLE or SLE patients. However, the latter almost always have positive ANAs.

DERMATITIS HERPETIFORMIS

Dermatitis herpetiformis is an autoimmune papulovesicular dermatopathy. An autoimmune etiology is supported by (*a*) the presence of anti-DEJ autoantibodies; (*b*) an association with celiac disease; and (*c*) a strong linkage with HLA-B8. There is a male predominance. The disorder may present at any age, although young adults are most often affected. While most patients have histologic evidence of a small intestinal enteropathy, it is very unusual for there to be clinical evidence. The enteropathy will respond to a gluten-free diet, but there is little effect on the skin manifestations. The latter respond very well to sulfapyridine or the sulfones.

The skin lesions are very pruritic, with a symmetrical distribution of papules and/or blisters on the extensor surfaces of the extremities, shoulders, and buttocks. Oral lesions are not seen. Skin biopsies should be of both perilesional and normal skin. The classic histologic features include subepidermal clefts at the tips of dermal papillae. The clefts are filled with neutrophils, admixed with a variable fraction of eosinophils. A similar inflammatory infiltrate is seen in the subpapillary dermis.

Direct immunofluorescence testing of nonvesicular skin reveals IgA deposition at the DEJ of the dermal papillae, and, variably, throughout the remainder of DEJ. In most (85 to 90%) cases, the IgA deposits have a granular pattern, the remainder being linear. Interestingly, the latter cases usually do not have a concomitant enteropathy, nor association with HLA-B8. Deposits of other immunoglobulins and C3 may also be seen. IgA deposits will persist in clinically normal skin, without regard for disease activity or therapy. Circulating IgA anti-DEJ antibodies are seen only rarely, although more commonly with linear-type IgA anti-DEJ. Lastly, anti-gliadin antibodies are seen with dermatitis herpetiformis, and seem to correlate with the enteropathy.

Hematopoietic System

AUTOIMMUNE THROMBOCYTOPENIA

Clinical

Immune thrombocytopenias (ITPs) have a variety of etiologies. These include the classic autoimmune thrombocytopenia (AITP), those associated with particular drugs, viral infections or other autoimmune diseases, and alloimmune disorders such as post-transfusional and neonatal ITPs. These immune disorders must be separated from other pathological causes of thrombocytopenia (e.g., DIC and TTP), as well as in vitro artifacts (e.g., EDTA-induced pseudothrombocytopenia). Taken together, primary and secondary AITPs are much more common than either autoimmune hemolytic anemia or neutropenia. Usually, AITP is divided into three clinicopathological syndromes: (*a*) chronic idiopathic thrombocytopenic purpura (ITP); (*b*) secondary ITP associated with some other disease (e.g., SLE); and (*c*) acute postviral ITP.

Chronic AITP usually has a subtle onset, which is not clearly associated with any other disease. The precise delineation between acute and chronic disease is difficult. Some investigators arbitrarily use the time between the onset of symptoms and diagnosis (if more than 2 weeks, the disease is considered chronic). Like many autoimmune disorders, it predominates in young to middle-aged adult females (male to female ratio, 3:1). Splenomegaly is not usually seen with primary chronic AITP. The disorder will persist for at least 6 months, and often for many years. The course of disease can be continuous or intermittent. Spontaneous remissions are not usual. Splenectomy and immunosuppressive therapy are often required.

In contrast, acute AITP usually has an abrupt clinical onset of hemostatic disorders, and is often associated with a recent viral infection. Indeed, many investigators refer to this type as acute postviral AITP. Viral agents associated with acute AITP include Epstein-Barr, measles, and mumps viruses. It is most often seen in children and has no gender predilection. As implied by its name, acute AITP will usually remit within 6 months of onset. It must be realized that children may develop chronic AITP, and adults acute AITP. Unfortunately, it is not possible to predict at the time of diagnosis which type of AITP is present. Spontaneous remission is seen in up to 90% of acute AITPs. Immunosuppressive therapy and splenectomy should be reserved for "chronic" acute AITPs.

Secondary autoimmune ITP is often associated with autoimmune or lymphoproliferative diseases. In particular, SLE and chronic lymphocytic leukemia are the two most common diseases seen in the setting of secondary AITP. Indeed, AITP is one of the diagnostic criteria for SLE, and it may be the initial presenting symptom of the disease. Other leukemias and lymphomas, as well as autoimmune disorders such as Evans' syndrome, Hashimoto's thyroiditis, primary biliary cirrhosis, myasthenia gravis, rheumatoid arthritis, Sjögren's syndrome, and mixed connective tissue disease have also been related to AITP. Other solid tumors, and chemotherapy and bone marrow transplants have also been linked to AITP. Lastly, HIV-positive patients have a significant incidence of thrombocytopenia, particularly during the intermediate to late stages of the disease. Some of these are clearly an autoimmune type of thrombocytopenia, although the pathogenesis is complex.

Neonatal AITP is an acquired autoimmune process. Maternal IgG autoanti-platelet antibodies cross the placental barrier and react with the neonate's platelets, giving rise to the thrombocytopenia. A related entity is neonatal alloimmune thrombocytopenia. In the latter instance, the mother, who does not have ITP, is exposed to fetal platelets. She makes alloanti-platelet antibodies to unique paternal antigens on these. As with neonatal AITP, the IgG alloantibodies then cross the placenta and react with the neonate's platelets. In both instances, the disorder is short-lived, and therapy is primarily supportive. The relative risk of neonatal AITP is best predicted in mothers-to-be by either the history of AITP prior to conception, or the presence of a maternal circulating anti-platelet antibody in a mother-to-be with no prior history of ITP who is presenting with isolated thrombocytopenia during pregnancy.

Drug-induced immune thrombocytopenia must be distinguished from cytotoxic drug therapy. In the former, a drug forms neoantigens by complexing with platelet antigens and induces an immune response. The resultant autoantibody either reacts with the drug-antigen complex or cross-reacts with another platelet antigen. Drug-induced immune thrombocytopenias are most commonly seen with heparin, gold, quinine, or quinidine.

Similar to chronic AITP, drug ITP is most often seen in adult females, and the autoantibodies are not uniquely different. However, the onset is usually abrupt. The most reliable way to make the diagnosis is by a good drug history, followed by elimination of the suspected agent with subsequent rebound of platelet counts. Unfortunately, the latter may take several weeks to months after cessation of the offending drug, although it usually recovers within a few days. Treatment with IgG or steroids may offer abrupt relief, an observation somewhat unusual in AITP.

Laboratory

The sine qua non of ITP and AITP is thrombocytopenia. The peripheral blood platelet counts are usually less than 80,000/µl, and are associated with an increased mean platelet volume. In "uncomplicated" or "pure" ITP/AITP, the PT, PTT, fibrinogen, and fibrin split products are within normal limits. There are normal to increased numbers of marrow megakaryocytes. While kinetic and/or autoimmune serologic tests can serve as positive diagnostic criteria, the vast majority of cases can be defined by the aforementioned clinical and laboratory criteria.

A brief discussion of the technical approaches to anti-platelet immunoglobulin (APIG) detection is in order prior to reviewing autoimmune serology in this disease entity. Four methodologies can be used to detect platelet-bound and circulating APIG: (*a*) manual and flow cytometric immunofluorescence measurement of platelet-immunoglobulin binding; (*b*) radioimmunoassay of platelet-immunoglobulin binding; (*c*) Western immunoblotting and ELISAs of immunoglobulin-specific platelet protein binding; (*d*) antibody consumption assays; and (*e*) functional agglutination/activation assays. Because of a relatively greater technical complexity, the immunofluorescence assays and RIAs have gained favor over the consumption and functional tests for the routine screening of anti-platelet antibodies.

The platelet-immunoglobulin binding assays are quite sensitive and quantitative. However, there are difficulties with specificity, as nonspecifically bound (i.e., Fc receptor) immunoglobulin may result in a significant rate of false-positive results. ELISA and immunoblotting methods avoid this particular problem, and also may identify the autoantigen. However, these assays are currently quite time-consuming. Further, the process of isolating the antigen may result in loss of antigenicity.

A related problem is what sample to analyze. Indirect assays screen plasma or serum for circulating autoantibodies. The substrates in most instances are platelets from normal donors. A major problem here is whether any anti-platelet reactivity is due to autoantibodies or alloantibodies (e.g., HLA). In addition, the indirect assays are often negative in AITP, possibly from absorption of the circulating APIG by platelets. Direct assays, by measuring for bound APIG, usually avoid the problem of differentiating from alloantibodies (excluding neonatal alloimmune thrombocytopenia). Unfortunately, such assays require a certain minimum quantity of platelets, which may be difficult to meet in the face of severe thrombocytopenia.

Most anti-platelet antibodies in primary and secondary AITP are directed at the membrane glycoproteins (GP)IIb/IIIa or GPIb/IX. However, 20 to 30% of AITP patients will lack autoantibodies to these antigens. Using less specific radiometric or immunofluorescence binding assays, the direct, platelet-bound immunoglobulin is abnormally increased in 86% of patients, while the indirect, serum APIG is present in 66%. In chronic AITP, the APIG isotype is usually IgG, while it is mostly IgM in the "acute" postviral cases. Drug-induced immune thrombocytopenia will have an increased amount of platelet-bound IgG. If the autoantibody requires a drug-antigen complex, the demonstration of circulating APIG requires inclusion of the offending drug at all steps in the testing process.

Other autoantibodies may be seen with primary and secondary AITP. Those associated with SLE are of particular interest, as AITP can be an initial manifestation of that autoimmune disease in 3 to 16% of cases. In patients with chronic AITP, about 20% will have a positive ANA. Approximately 16 to 56% of these will develop SLE within 2 to 3 years. The remainder will fail to do so over follow-up periods of 2 to 30 years.

The presence of a high-titer ANA (1:200 or higher) is more often seen with cases evolving into SLE, although this is not absolutely specific. However, the presence of specific ANAs such as anti–double-stranded (native) DNA, anti-Sm, anti-RNP, anti-Ro/SSA and anti-La/SSB are seen in most patients with chronic AITP who develop SLE, but are essentially absent in primary chronic AITP cases. Anti-phospholipid antibodies (anti-cardiolipin) or the lupus anticoagulant is seen in approximately 40% of cases of primary and secondary AITP. They do not appear to predict an increased risk of SLE or other type of systemic autoimmune disease.

AUTOIMMUNE NEUTROPENIA

Autoimmune neutropenia (AIN) can be divided into primary (idiopathic) and secondary types. The former is more common than the latter, and is an isolated neutropenia without any other cause. The secondary cases are where neutropenias are seen with other organ-restricted or systemic autoimmune disorders, lymphoma and leukemias, viral infections, and some drugs (e.g., B-lactams). The treatment of secondary AIN is directed at the underlying disease. The correlation with anti-neutrophil serology is not well established.

Primary AIN is usually diagnosed in young children less than 3 years of age. While there is a modest female predominance, no familial or racial tendencies have been identified. The clinical presentation is usually that of recurrent pyogenic infections of the skin, respiratory tract, and middle ear. Marked splenomegaly is not seen. While spontaneous remissions typically occur in infants, these decrease in probability with age. There appears to be no increased risk of other autoimmune diseases or neoplasia.

The patients usually have markedly depressed blood neutrophil (less than 500×10^9/liter), normal lymphocyte and normal to elevated monocyte concentrations, corrected for age. Marrow myelopoiesis is quantitatively normal to increased with a significant left shift. There is no response in in vivo stimulation tests. Given the self-limited nature of primary AIN, therapy is usually supportive (i.e., antibiotics for infection; prophylactic bactrim for recurrent otitis media). The use of intravenous γ-globulin and steroids is controversial and of variable effect.

The neutropenia in primary AIN is due to phagocytosis by the reticuloendothelial system of antibody-coated neutrophils. Anti-neutrophil autoantibodies are seen in 80 to 100% of patients. These are usually directed at antigens primarily found on more mature myeloid precursors and segmented neutrophils. Where the antigen can be identified, the majority of cases have autoantibodies that are directed against the NA1 protein. Overall, this comprises approximately 10 to 55% of cases of autoimmune neutropenia. The anti-neutrophil autoantibodies are usually seen in high titers at the onset of AIN and decrease below detection thresholds as the peripheral neutrophil counts rebound.

The granulocyte agglutination test (GAT) and granulocyte immunofluorescence test (GIFT), along with a typed neutrophil panel, are currently thought to be the most sensitive methods to detect anti-neutrophil antibodies. The GIFT assay is clearly more sensitive than the GAT (97% versus 38%), with only unusual cases being GAT-positive/GIFT-negative. To enhance the specificity of these assays, anti-HLA antibodies must be excluded, as the HLA molecules are present on granulocytes.

Secondary AIN is most often seen in older, adolescent, and adult patients. These cases tend to be associated with other autoimmune cytopenias and/or systemic autoimmune diseases such as SLE and RA. A clearly defined anti-neutrophil antibody has not been reproducibly seen in several studies. In some instances, drug therapy for these latter disorders may be responsible for the granulocytopenia. Other drugs associated with immune neutropenias include β-lactams, quinidine, chlorthiazide, and chlorpromazine.

AUTOIMMUNE ANEMIAS

Autoimmune hemolytic anemias (AIHAs) are the most easily defined and well-recognized of the immune cytopenias. The autoantibody-induced destruction of the erythrocytes is due to either complement-mediated lysis or phagocytosis by the reticuloendothelial system, or both. The immunochemical qualities of these autoantibodies define the mode of red cell destruction and any therapeutic interventions.

The AIHAs and their associated autoantibodies are initially best classified by their temperature range ("warm" versus "cold"). The warm autoantibodies, which react optimally between 35° and 40°C, are usually divided into complete (detectable by the direct antiglobulin test) and incomplete (detectable by the indirect antiglobulin test). Overall, these constitute approximately 83% of red cell autoantibodies. Approximately half of the warm AIHAs are idiopathic, most of the remainder being associated with systemic autoimmune disorders (e.g., SLE, RA) or lymphomas/leukemias (e.g., CLL, NHL, Hodgkin's disease).

Most (82%) of the warm autoantibodies are of the incomplete type. These are usually of the IgG class, and react with one or more specificities in the Rh antigen system. They do not often result in complement-mediated lysis, but result in Fc-receptor binding and phagocytosis. Corticosteroid administration is a useful short-term therapy. Alternatives include high-dose intravenous γ-globulin therapy or cyclosporin. If these approaches are contraindicated and/or ineffective, then splenectomy may be effective.

Warm autohemolysins are IgM autoantibodies that lyse erythrocytes via the complement cascade and/or complement-mediated phagocytosis. Those that cause lysis in vitro usually result in severe AIHA, and require aggressive supportive and therapeutic intervention (e.g., plasma exchange, high-dose corticosteroids). Those warm autohemolysins that result in excess phagocytosis (little in vitro lysis, significant complement coating) have a much less clinically severe AIHA, and may be treated similarly to the warm incomplete autoantibodies.

Cold autoantibodies, by definition, react best below 30°C and are divided into two clinical/immunochemical classes: cold agglutinins–hemolysins and biphasic hemolysins. Overall, these comprise some 16% of red cell autoantibodies. The cold agglutinins are almost always of the IgM class and regularly have anti-I or anti-IH reactivity. They bind optimally with erythrocytes at 0° to 4°C and may cause intravascular agglutination and ischemia, or hemolysis. These autoantibodies may occur due to infection (usually EBV or mycoplasma) or a B-cell lymphoproliferative disorder (monoclonal autoantibody). Most cases are chronic.

The biphasic hemolysins are IgG antibodies, which are usually directed at the P antigen. They are usually seen as the sequelae to infections in children. These cause complement-mediated lysis in a two-step process (cold antibody binding, warm complement binding and lysis), giving the classic picture of paroxysmal cold hemoglobinuria. Acute treatment includes keeping the patient warm, and performing transfusion with compatible red cells.

Suggested Readings

Autoimmunity & Autoimmune Disease

Kelly W, Harris E, Ruddy S, et al., ed. Textbook of rheumatology. 2nd ed. Philadelphia: W.B. Saunders, 1985.

Keren DF, Warren JS. Diagnostic immunology. Baltimore: Williams & Wilkins, 1992.

Langman RE. The immune system. San Diego: Academic Press, 1989:209.

Shoenfeld Y, Isenberg D. The mosaic of autoimmunity (the factors associated with autoimmune disease). Research Monographs in Immunology, ed. Turk JL. Vol. 12. Amsterdam: Elsevier, 1989: 523.

Stites DP, Stobo JD, Wells JV, eds. Basic & clinical immunology. 6th ed. Norwalk, CT: Appleton & Lange, 1987:734.

Methodologies

Bentwich Z, Beverley PCL, Hammarstrom L, et al. Laboratory investigations in clinical immunology: methods, pitfalls, and clinical indications. Clin Immunol Immunopathol 1988;49:478–497.

Price CP, Newman DJ, eds. Principles and practice of immunoassay. New York: Macmillan, 1991:650.

Antinuclear Antibodies and Systemic Autoimmune Diseases

Courvalin JC, Lassoued K, Bartnik E, et al. The 210-kd nuclear envelope polypeptide recognized by human autoantibodies in primary biliary cirrhosis is the major glycoprotein of the nuclear pore. J Clin Invest 1990;86:279–285.

Courvalin JC, Lassoued K, Worman H, et al. Identification and characterization of autoantibodies against the nuclear envelope lamin B receptor from patients with primary biliary cirrhosis. J Exp Med 1990;172:961–967.

Fritzler M, Pauls J, Kinsella T, et al. Antinuclear, anticytoplasmic, and anti-Sjögren's syndrome antigen A (SS-A/Ro) antibodies in female blood donors. Clin Immunol Immunopathol 1985;36:120–128.

Fritzler M, Valencia D, McCarty G. Speckled pattern antinuclear antibodies resembling anticentromere antibodies. Arthritis Rheum 1984;27:92–96.

Isenberg DA, Maddison PJ. Detection of antibodies to double stranded DNA and extractable nuclear antigen. Assoc Clin Pathol Broadsheet 1987;117:1374–1381.

Konstantinov K, Russanova V. Evidence for absence of histones in the *Crithidia luciliae* kinetoplast: a study with anti-H_2A and monoclonal anti-H_3 antibodies. Br J Dermatol 1987;117:451–456.

McCarty G, Valencia D, Fritzler M. Antibodies to the mitotic spindle apparatus: immunologic characteristics and cytologic studies. J Rheumatol 1984;11:213–218.

Monier JC, Sault C, Veysseyre C, et al. Discrepancies between two procedures for Ds-DNA antibody detection: Farr test and indirect immunofluorescence on *Crithidia luciliae*. J Clin Lab Immunol 1988;25:149–152.

Nakamura R, Peebles C, Rubin R, et al. Autoantibodies to nuclear antigens. 2nd ed. Chicago: ASCP Press, 1985.

Reimer G, Steen V, Penning C, et al. Correlates between autoantibodies to nucleolar antigens and clinical features in patients with systemic sclerosis (scleroderma). Arthritis Rheum 1988;31: 525–532.

Rodrigues J, Gelpi C, Thomson R, et al. Anti-Golgi complex autoantibodies in a patient with Sjögren's syndrome and lymphoma. Clin Exp Immunol 1982;49:570–586.

Rubin R, Joslin F, Tan E. A solid-phase radioimmunoassay for anti-histone antibodies in human sera: comparison with an immunofluorescence assay. Scand J Immunol 1982;15:63–70.

Rubin R, Joslin F, Tan E. Specificity of anti-histone antibodies in systemic lupus erythematosus. Arthritis Rheum 1982;25:779–782.

Rubin R, Nusinow S, Johnson A, et al. Serologic changes during induction of lupus-like disease by procainamide. Am J Med 1986;80:999–1002.

Schmerling RH, Delbanco TL. The rheumatoid factor: an analysis of clinical utility. Am J Med 1991;91:528–534.

Steen V, Powell D, Medsger T. Clinical correlations and prognosis based on serum autoantibodies in patients with systemic sclerosis. Arthritis Rheum 1988;31:196–203.

Tan E. Antinuclear antibodies: diagnostic markers for autoimmune diseases and probes for cell biology. Adv Immunol 1989;44:93–151.

Tan E, Chan E, Sullivan K, et al. Antinuclear antibodies (ANAs): diagnostically specific immune markers and clues toward the understanding of systemic autoimmunity. Clin Immunol Immunopathol 1988;47:121–141.

CNS and PNS Autoimmunity

Alter M. The epidemiology of Guillain-Barré syndrome. Ann Neurol 1990;27(Suppl):S7–S12.

Anderson N, Rosenblum MK, Posner JB. Paraneoplastic cerebellar degeneration: clinical-immunological correlations. Ann Neurol 1988;24:559–567.

Anderson NE, Rosenblum MK, Graus F, et al. Autoantibodies in paraneoplastic syndromes associated with small-cell lung cancer. Neurology 1988;38:1391–1398.

Check IJ, Costigan DA. Polyneuropathy associated with monoclonal gammopathy of undetermined significance (MGUS). ASCP Immunopathology Check Sample Program., Vol. IP92. Chicago: ASCP Press, 1992.

Dalmau J, Furneaux HM, Gralla RJ, et al. Detection of the anti-Hu antibody in the serum of patients with small cell lung cancer—a quantitative Western blot analysis. Ann Neurol 1990;27:544–552.

Dyck PJ, Low PA, Windebank AJ, et al. Plasma exchange in polyneuropathy associated with monoclonal gammopathy of undetermined significance. N Engl J Med 1991;325:1482–1486.

Epstein MA, Sladky JT. The role of plasmapheresis in childhood Guillain-Barré syndrome. Ann Neurol 1990;28:65–69.

Farrell M, et al. Oligoclonal bands in multiple sclerosis: clinical-pathological correlation. Neurology 1985;35:212–218.

Furneaux HM, Rosenblum MK, Dalmau J, et al. Selective expression of Purkinje-cell antigens in tumor tissue from patients with paraneoplastic cerebellar degeneration. N Engl J Med 1990;322(26):1844–1851.

Gerson B, et al. Myelin basic protein, oligoclonal bands and IgG in cerebrospinal fluid as indicators of multiple sclerosis. Clin Chem 1981;27:1974–1977.

Goren H, Clinical aspects of neuroimmunologic disease. In: Barna BP, ed. Laboratory handbook of neuroimmunologic disease. Chicago: ASCP Press, 1987:27–38.

Hershey L, et al. Computerized tomography in the diagnostic evaluation of multiple sclerosis. Ann Neurol 1979;5:32–39.

Hershey L, Trotter J. The use and abuse of the cerebrospinal fluid IgG profile in the adult: a practical evaluation. Ann Neurol 1980;8:426–434.

Kelly JJ, Kyle RA, O'Brien P, et al. Prevalence of monoclonal protein in peripheral neuropathy. Neurology 1981;31:1480–1483.

Kempster P, Iansek R, Balla J, et al. Value of visual evoked response and oligoclonal bands in cerebrospinal fluid in diagnosis of spinal multiple sclerosis. Lancet 1987;1:769–771.

Levine SR, Brey RL. Antiphospholipid antibodies and ishcemic cerebrovascular disease. Semin Neurol 1991;11(4):329–338.

Marcus D. Measurement and clinical importance of antibodies to glycosphingolipids. Ann Neurol 1990;27(Suppl):S53–S55.

McDonald W, Diagnosis of multiple sclerosis. Br Med J 1989;299: 635–637.

Paty D, Oger J, Kastrukoff L, et al. MRI in the diagnosis of MS: a prospective study with comparison of clinical evaluation, evoked potentials, oligoclonal banding and CT. Neurology 1988;38:180–185.

Quarles RH, Ilyas AA, Willison HJ. Antibodies to gangliosides and myelin proteins in Guillain-Barré syndrome. Ann Neurol 1990;27(Suppl):S48–S52.

Ropper AH. The Guillain-Barré syndrome: current concepts [Review]. N Engl J Med 1992;326(17):1130–1136.

Rose A, et al. Criteria for the clinical diagnosis of multiple sclerosis. Neurology 1976;20–22.

Sadiq SA, Thomas FP, Kilidireas K, et al. The spectrum of neurologic disease associated with Anti-GM1 antibodies. Neurology 1990;40:1067–1072.

Solimena M, Folli F, Aparisi R, et al. Autoantibodies to GABA-ergic neurons and pancreatic beta cells in stiff-man syndrome. N Engl J Med 1990;322(22):1555–1560.

Staley M, et al. Oligoclonal bands are found in electrophoretigrams of serum of patients multiple sclerosis. Clin Chem 1986;32:709.

Steck AJ, Murray N, Dellagi K, et al. Peripheral neuropathy associated with monoclonal IgM autoantibody. Ann Neurol 1987;22: 764–767.

Tourtellotte W, Walsh M. Cerebrospinal fluid profile in multiple sclerosis. In: Poser C, et al, eds. The diagnosis of multiple sclerosis. New York: Thieme-Stratton, 1984:165–178.

Thyroid

Ahmann A, Baker JR Jr, Weetman AP, et al. Antibodies to porcine eye muscle in patients with Graves' ophthalmopathy: identification of serum immunoglobulins directed against unique determinants by immunoblotting and enzyme-linked immunosorbent assay. J Clin Endocrinol Metab 1987;64(3):454–460.

Betterle C, Callegari G, Presotto F, et al. Thyroid autoantibodies: a good marker for the study of symptomless autoimmune thyroiditis. Acta Endocrinol (Copenh) 1987;114:321–327.

Bottazzo GF, Doniach D. Autoimmune thyroid disease. Annu Rev Med 1986;37:353–359.

Lazarus JH, Burr ML, McGregor AM, et al. The prevalence and progression of autoimmune thyroid disease in the elderly. Acta Endocrinol, 1984;106:199–202.

Pittman CS, Menefee JK. Pathophysiology of Graves disease. Hosp Pract 1987;(May 15):147–164.

Salvi M, Miller A, Wall JR. Human orbital tissue and thyroid membranes express a 64-kDa protein which is recognized by autoantibodies in the serum of patients with thyroid-associated ophthalmopathy. FEBS Lett 1988;232(1):135–139.

Selenkow HA, Wyman P, Allweiss P. Autoimmune thyroid disease: an integreated concept of Graves' and Hashimoto's diseases. Compr Ther 1984;10(4):48–56.

Strakosch CR. Thyroiditis. Aust NZ J Med 1986;16:91–100.

Tamai H, Kasagi K, Morita T, et al. Thyroid response, especially to thyrotropin-binding inhibitory immunoglobulins, in euthyroid relatives of patients with Graves' disease: a clinical followup. J Clin Endocrinol Metab 1990;71:210–215.

Other Endocrine Glands

Bottazzo GF, Todd I, Mirakian R, et al. Organ-specific autoimmunity: a 1986 overview. Immunol Rev, 1986;94:137–169.

Eisenbarth GS. Type I diabetes mellitus: a chronic autoimmune disease. N Engl J Med 1986;314(21):1360–1368.

Gleichmann H, Bottazzo GF. Islet-cell and insulin autoantibodies in diabetes. Immunol Today 1987;8(6):163–190.

Kiechle FL, Malinski T, Moore KH. Insulin action: implications for the clinical laboratory. Lab Med 1990;21(9):565–573.

Wilkin TJ. Receptor autoimmunity in endocrine disorders. N Engl J Med 1990;323(19):1318–1324.

Reproductive Immunology

Alexander NJ. Natural and induced immunologic infertility. Curr Opin Immunol 1989;1:1125–1130.

Mowbray JF. Autoantibodies, alloantibodies and reproductive success. Curr Opin Immunol 1990;2:761–764.

Raghupathy R, Shaha C, Gupta SK. Autoimmunity to sperm antigens. Curr Opin Immunol 1990;2:757–760.

Rote NS. Pregnancy-associated immunologic disorders. Curr Opin Immunol 1989;1:1165–1172.

Vascular System

Chapman RW. Role of immune factors in the pathogenesis of primary sclerosing cholangitis. Semin Liver Dis 1991;11(1):1–4.

Goeken JA. Antineutrophil cytoplasmic antibody—a useful serological marker for vasculitis. J Clin Immunol 1991;11:161–174.

Jennette JC, Wilkman AS, Falk RJ. Anti-neutrophil cytoplasmic autoantibody-associated glomerulonephritis and vasculitis. Am J Pathol 1989;135(5):921–930.

Leatherman JW, Davies SF, Hoidal JR. Alveolar hemorrhage syndromes: diffuse microvascular lung hemorrhage in immune and idiopathic disorders. Medicine 1984;63(6):343–361.

McPhaul JJ, Dixon FJ. The presence of anti-glomerular basement membrane antibodies in peripheral blood. J Immunol 1969;103(6):1168–1175.

Pusey CD, Lockwood CM. Autoimmunity in rapidly progressive glomerulonephritis. Kidney Int. 1989;35:929–937.

Snook JA, Chapman RW, Fleming K, et al. Anti-neutrophil nuclear antibody in ulcerative colitis, Crohn's disease and primary sclerosing cholangitis. Clin Exp Immunol 1989;76:30–33.

Specks U, Sheatley CL, McDonald TJ, et al. Anticytoplasmic autoantibodies in the diagnosis and follow-up of Wegener's granulomatosis. Mayo Clin Proc 1989;64:28–36.

Tervaert JWC, Limburg PC, Elema JD, et al. Detection of autoantibodies against myeloid lysosomal enzymes: a useful adjunct to classification of patients with biopsy-proven necrotizing arteritis. Am J Med 1991;91:59–66.

Wilson CB, Dixon FJ. Anti-glomerular basement membrane antibody-induced glomerulonephritis. Kidney Int 1973;3:74–89.

Liver

Berg PA, Klein R. Autoantibodies in primary biliary cirrhosis. Springer Semin Immunopathol 1990;12:85–99.

Chapman RWG, Arborgh BAM, Rhodes JM, et al. Primary sclerosing cholangitis: a review of its clinical features, cholangiography, and hepatic histology. Gut 1980;21:870–877.

Clarke AK, Galbraith RM, Hamilton EBD, et al. Rheumatic disorders in primary biliary cirrhosis. Ann Rheum Dis 1978;37:42–47.

Fregeau DR, Leung PSC, Coppel RL, et al. Autoantibodies to mitochondria in systemic sclerosis. Arthritis Rheum 1988;31(3): 386–392.

Gurian LE, Rogoff TM, Ware AJ, et al. The immunologic diagnosis of chronic active "autoimmune" hepatitis: distinction from systemic lupus erythrematosus. Hepatology 1985;5(3):397–402.

Johnson PJ, McFarlane IG, Eddleston ALWF. The natural course and heterogeneity of autoimmune-type chronic active hepatitis. Semin Liver Dis 1991;11(3):187–196.

Kaplan MM. Primary biliary cirrhosis. In: Advances in Internal Medicine. Chicago: Year Book, 1987:359–378.

Keating JJ, O'Brien CJ, Stellon AJ, et al. Influence of aetiology, clinical and histological features on survival in chronic active hepatitis: an analysis of 204 patients. Q J Med 1987;62(237):59–66.

Kurki P, Linder E, Miettinen A, et al. Smooth muscle antibodies of actin and "non-actin" specificity. Clin Immunol Immunopathol 1978;9:443–453.

Mackay IR. Genetic aspects of immunologically mediated liver disease. Semin Liver Dis 1984;4(1):13–25.

Maggiore G, Bernard O, Hadchouel M, et al. Treatment of autoimmune chronic active hepatitis in childhood. J Pediatr 1984;104(6): 839–844.

Maggiore G, Bernard O, Homberg JC, et al. Liver disease associated with anti-liver-kidney microsome antibody in children. J Pediatr 1986;108(3):399–404.

Manns MP. Cytoplasmic autoantigens in autoimmune hepatitis: molecular analysis and clinical relevance. Semin Liver Dis 1991;11(3):205–214.

McMillan SA, Haire M. The specificity of IgG- and IgM-class smooth muscle antibody in the sera of patients with multiple sclerosis and active chronic hepatitis. Clin Immunol Immunopathol 1979;14:256–263.

Mieli-Vergani G, Lobo-Yeo A, McFarlane BM, et al. Different immune mechanisms leading to autoimmunity in primary sclerosing cholantitis and autoimmune chronic active hepatitis of childhood. Hepatology 1989;9(2):198–203.

Munoz LE, Thomas HC, Scheuer PJ, et al. Is mitochondrial antibody diagnostic of primary biliary cirrhosis? Gut 1981;22:136–140.

Mzali S, Johanet C, Chrétien P, et al. Les anticorps antinucléaires de la cirrhose biliaire primitive. Gastroenterol Clin Biol 1989;13: 690–695.

Odiévre M, Maggiore G, Homberg JC, et al. Seroimmunologic classification of chronic hepatitis in 57 children. Hepatology 1983;3(3):407–409.

Poralla T, Treichel U, Löhr H, et al. The asialoglycoprotein receptor as target structure in autoimmune liver diseases. Semin Liver Dis 1991;11(3):215–222.

Sherlock S. Pathogenesis of sclerosing cholangitis: the role of nonimmune factors. Semin Liver Dis 1991;11(1):5–10.

Storch W. Immunopathology and humoral autoimmunity in chronic active hepatitis. Scand J Gastroenterol 1988;23:513–516.

Toh BH, Smooth muscle autoantibodies and autoantigens. Clin Exp Immunol 1979;38:621–628.

Triger DR, Charlton CAC, Ward AM. What does the antimitochondrial antibody mean? Gut 1982;23:814–818.

Uddenfeldt P, Danielsson A. Evaluation of rheumatic disorders in patients with primary biliary cirrhosis. Ann Clin Res, 1985;18: 148–153.

Gastrointestinal Tract

Farré C, Ferrer I, Vilar P, et al. Evaluation of anti-gliadin and antiendomysial antibodies for the detection of coeliac disease. In: Galteau MM, Siest G, Henny J, eds. Biologie prospective. Paris: John Libbey Eurotext, 1989:337–341.

Kelly CP, Feighery CF, Gallagher RB, et al. Diagnosis and treatment of gluten-sensitive enteropathy. Adv Intern Med 1990;35: 341–364.

Trier JS. Celiac sprue. N Engl J Med 1991;325(24):1709–1717.

Skin

Hood AF, Kwan TH, Burnes DC, et al. Primer of dermatopathology. Boston: Little, Brown, 1984:378.

Lever WF, Schaumburg-Lever G. Histopathology of the skin. 6th ed. Philadelphia: J. B. Lippincott, 1983:848.

Valenzuela R, Bergfeld WF, Deodhar SD. Interpretation of immunofluorescent patterns in skin diseases. Chicago: American Society of Clinical Pathologists Press, 1984:176.

Hematopoietic System

Anderson MJ, Peebles CL, McMillan R, et al. Fluorescent antinuclear antibodies and anti-SS-A/Ro in patients with immune thrombocytopenia subsequently developing systemic lupus erythematosus. Ann Intern Med, 1985;103(4):548–550.

Berchtold P, Harris JP, Tani P, et al. Autoantibodies to platelet glycoproteins in patients with disease-related immune thrombocytopenia. Br J Haematol 1989;79:365–368.

Bux J, Mueller-Eckhardt C. Autoimmune neutropenia. Semin Hematol 1992;29(1):45–53.

Collins PW, Newland AC. Treatment modalities of autoimmune blood disorders. Semin Hematol 1992;29(1):64–74.

Engelfriet CP, Overbeeke MAM, von dem Borne EEGK. Autoimmune hemolytic anemia. Semin Hematol 1992;29(1):3–12.

Finley PR, Williams RJ, Fletcher C. Flow cytometry analysis of platelet antibodies. J Clin Lab Anal 1988;2:249–255.

Kaplan C, Morinet F, Cartron J. Virus-induced autoimmune thrombocytopenia and neutropenia. Semin Hematol 1992;29(1): 34–44.

Kiefel V, Santoso S, Weisheit M, et al. Monoclonal antibody-specific immobilization of platelet antigens (MAIPA): a new tool for the identification of platelet-reactive antibodies. Blood 1987;70(6):1722–1726.

Logue GL, Shimm DS. Autoimmune granulocytopenia. Annu Rev Med 1980;31:191–200.

McCullough J, Press C, Clay M, et al. Granulocyte serology: a clinical and laboratory guide. Chicago: American Society of Clinical Pathologists Press, 1988:265.

Nydegger UE, Kazatchkine MD, Miescher PA. Immunopathologic and clinical features of hemolytic anemia due to cold agglutinins. Semin Hematol 1991;28(1):66–77.

Panzer S, Penner E, Graninger W, et al. Antinuclear antibodies in patients with chronic idiopathic autoimmune thrombocytopenia followed 2–30 years. Am J Hematol 1989;32:100–103.

Salama A, Mueller-Eckhardt C. Immune-mediated blood cell dyscrasias related to drugs. Semin Hematol 1992;29(1):54–63.

Samuels P, Bussel JB, Braitman LE, et al. Estimation of the risk of thrombocytopenia in the offspring of pregnant women with presumed immune thrombocytopenic purpura. N Engl J Med 1990;323(4):229–235.

Schwartz KA. Platelet antibody: review of detection methods. Am J Hematol 1988;29:106–114.

Walker RW, Walker W. Idiopathic thrombocytopenia, initial illness and long term follow-up. Arch Dis Child 1984;59:316–322.

Waters AH. Autoimmune thrombocytopenia: clinical aspects. Semin Hematol 1992;29(1):18–25.

63 Allergic Conditions

Eric Brestel

INTRODUCTION

Types of Immunopathological Hypersensitivity

There are several mechanisms by which the immune response can initiate a pathological process (Table 63.1). Coombs and Gell were the first to propose this classification scheme, and it has been updated by Snyderman (1). The type I response is initiated by the reaction of allergen with IgE bound to tissue mast cells. This antigen recognition by IgE results in a transmembrane signal that initiates the release of mediators from the mast cell. These include histamine, leukotrienes, platelet-activating factor, prostaglandin D_2, and a variety of intracellular enzymes, including a specific tryptase. These mediators can result in an immediate wheal-and-flare response in the skin (within 20 minutes), rhinitis beginning within minutes of exposure, or asthma if the allergen is inhaled into the lung. IgE-mediated responses can also cause systemic anaphylaxis and gastrointestinal allergic reactions manifested by vomiting, crampy abdominal pain, and diarrhea. The IgE-mediated response occurs within several minutes following exposure to an allergen and may gradually subside over 60 minutes. A secondary exacerbation of this response, however, may occur several hours after the initial mast cell degranulation and has been called the *late response*. This late response is felt to be a key component of chronic rhinitis and asthma and can also be seen in the skin following insect sting reactions and after the injection of allergens to which the patient is sensitive.

The type II response involves antibodies, usually of the IgG or IgM class, reacting with a protein which they recognize as foreign, that is present on a cell membrane or other biological membrane. Examples of this form of immunopathology include Goodpasture disease, immune thrombocytopenic purpura, and ABO and Rh incompatibilities.

The type III response involves the reaction of antibodies, usually of the IgG class, with a soluble antigen, forming immune complexes. These react with complement and deposit on subendothelial surfaces, resulting in vasculitis.

The type IV responses involve lymphocytes in antigen recognition. Lymphocytes specific for the antigen release cytokines, which recruit more lymphocytes to the area of the antigen and further recruit monocytes and macrophages. These cells help aid in antigen processing, but they also contribute to the inflammatory response. Examples of the type IV response include the intracutaneous reaction to purified protein derivative of *Mycoplasma tuberculosis*; the type IV response is also involved in the host defense against *M. tuberculosis*. Other examples include the reaction seen with the allergic contact dermatoses, called *cutaneous basophil hypersensitivity* because of the intense basophilic infiltrate; this is the mechanism for

Table 63.1. Types of Immunopathological Hypersensitivity

Type	Cell Types Involved	Mediators	Examples
Immediate (I)	Mast cells with cooperation from basophils, eosinophils, mononuclear cells, and possibly platelets for the late response	Histamine, leukotrienes, platelet activating factor	Allergic rhinitis and asthma, insect venom hypersensitivity, penicillin hypersensitivity
Cytotoxic (II)	Macrophages and neutrophils	Complement and phagocyte-derived mediators (enzymes, oxidants, eicosanoids, etc.)	Goodpasture syndrome, ABO incompatability, thrombocytopenic purpura, myasthenia gravis
Immune complex (III)	Same as type II	Same as type II	Serum sickness, glomerulonephritis
Cell mediated (IV)	Lymphocytes, macrophages, and occasionally basophils	Cytokines	Allergic contact dermatitis, the tuberculin reaction, graft-versus-host disease, chronic allograft rejection, possibly multiple sclerosis

the inflammatory response seen in poison ivy (*Rhus*) dermatitis. In this chapter, we will primarily concentrate on type I and type IV hypersensitivities, which are IgE- and lymphocyte-mediated, respectively.

Definition of Allergy

Clinicians usually reserve the term *allergy* to apply to acquired hypersensitivities that have an immune basis. More specifically, allergy is usually reserved for conditions mediated by immunoglobulin E (IgE) and lymphocyte-mediated processes. At present, no single laboratory test or other diagnostic procedure can define a patient as being an allergic individual. Rather, the diagnosis is usually based on the accumulated evidence of the patient's history and in vivo and in vitro diagnostic procedures. Many investigators define the IgE-mediated allergic state as positivity on skin testing to one or more common aeroallergens, and perhaps an elevation of the total IgE concentration in serum. This method of defining allergy presumes the allergic individual is capable of producing exaggerated levels of specific IgE to a foreign protein. It is not uncommon for persons to have positive skin tests to allergens without exhibiting clinical sensitivity on contact with the allergen. Studies with college students, however, have indicated that individuals with positive skin tests are very likely to develop clinical symptomatology within the next 3 years.

Realm of Clinical Allergy

IgE-mediated hypersensitivity usually results in the clinical conditions of allergic rhinitis, asthma, insect sting hypersensitivity, food hypersensitivity of an immediate nature, and occasionally, urticaria and angioedema. The clinical allergist may also be asked to evaluate responses to drugs and foods that may not have a known immunopathological basis, including hypersensitivity to the nonsteroidal anti-inflammatory drugs, radiocontrast media, sulfite, and monosodium glutamate. There are nonallergic forms of rhinitis in asthma, and the amount of the IgE-mediated component of atopic dermatitis may vary from patient to patient. Likewise, occupational lung diseases may have an immune component or may have an idiopathic basis. Occasionally, the allergist is asked to evaluate a patient suspected of having a hypersensitivity pneumonitis. This is a group of conditions that is often thought to have an immunopathological basis and that is often precipitated by encounters in the workplace. With the exception of penicillin-hypersensitivity, the evaluation of adverse drug reactions is probably the most enigmatic problem facing the clinical allergist. It is rare to find a specific immunopathological mechanism for most adverse drug reactions, and clinical testing is not usually available.

Allergic contact dermatitis results when a sensitizing material is recognized as foreign by the lymphocyte. Unlike the more complex proteins that can induce IgE-mediated allergic processes, small organic compounds and inorganic ions are the usual allergens that induce allergic contact dermatitis. Some time is required for the recruitment of the cells required to mediate this type of hypersensitivity, and reactions are not usually noted for 24 to 72 hours after initial contact with the allergen. Common examples of this form of hypersensitivity include poison ivy dermatitis, dermatitis to nickel contained in jewelry and other apparel items, and the dermatitis resulting from hypersensitivity to the hair-coloring material *p*-phenylenediamine.

DISEASE STATES

Rhinitis

Allergic rhinitis. Allergic rhinitis is one of the most prevalent disease states in western civilization. Approximately 15 to 20% of the general population is allergic as defined by positive skin tests to inhaled aeroallergen(s) and clinical symptomatology that corresponds to exposure to the inhaled aeroallergen(s). The symptomatology may be seasonal, corresponding to the pollination of plants whose pollen is airborne (grasses, trees, weeds, and the spores of molds), or it may be perennial, as in the case of house dust mite and animal dander hypersensitivity, where the allergens are in the home on a perennial basis. Some patients have perennial allergic rhinitis due to house dust mite hypersensitivity with exacerbations during the pollination seasons. Clinical symptomatology of seasonal allergic rhinitis includes sneezing, watery nasal discharge, postnasal drainage of mucus, and nasal airway obstruction. Itching and swelling of the conjunctival surfaces of the lids of the eyes with increased tearing is a common accompaniment. Allergic rhinitis can be complicated by serous or infectious otitis media or sinusitis resulting from edema of the nasal airway with the occlusion of the Eustachian tubes or sinus ostia, respectively.

Nonallergic rhinitis. In some subjects who present with a history of nasal congestion and increased nasal mucus production, no evidence of an IgE-mediated disease process can be determined. This condition has often been referred to as vasomotor rhinitis, but more recently, a condition known as nonallergic rhinitis with eosinophilia has been described. It is possible that nonallergic rhinitis is actually a group of disorders with different etiologies presenting as nasal congestion with increased mucus production. The patient with vasomotor rhinitis often has the symptomatology of congestion with exacerbation of nasal symptoms on exposure to irritating vapors, bright sunlight, or the inhalation of cold, dry air. Subjects with nonallergic rhinitis with eosinophilia often have symptomatology typical of allergic rhinitis, with marked congestion and rhinorrhea; however, the symptoms often occur outside of the typical pollination seasons. This should alert the physician to look for eosinophils in the nasal mucus. It is presumed that the eosinophils are playing a role in this disorder, but the reason for their appearance in the nasal mucosa and secretions has not been determined.

Patients with disorders of immune function, such as immunoglobulin deficiency states and ciliary dyskinesia, may also present with symptoms of rhinitis. A clue to these conditions is a history of recurrent pyogenic infections of the sinuses, middle ear, and lungs.

Asthma

Asthma may be defined as a condition of reversible obstructive airways disease in which there is a high degree of airway hyperirritability to agents such as methacholine and histamine. While many asthmatics may have their obstruction completely reversed with bronchodilator therapy, there is growing evidence that poorly controlled chronic asthma may result in a condition of poorly reversible airway obstruction. Asthma is best diagnosed by performing spirometry and determining the patient's reversibility with an inhaled bronchodilating medication. Patients suspected of having asthma but having a normal spirometry can be challenged with methacholine, which can induce airways obstruction in asthmatics at a much lower concentration than normal subjects.

The prevalence of asthma in the general population is increasing in western societies, and death from asthma has been increasing in all age groups (2). The reason for these increases has not yet been determined, but it may have its basis in the nature of the life-style of western civilization.

Allergic Asthma. For many years, it was estimated that approximately 20 to 25% of all asthmatics had an allergic component to their disease. More recent data suggest that allergy may play a role in a more significant percentage of asthmatics (3). These estimates, however, are based on skin testing to common aeroallergens and elevations of total serum IgE. It remains to be determined if either of these criteria specifically indicates that a given aeroallergen, or that allergy in general, is contributing to the disease process. It is generally accepted that allergy is a common feature of the childhood asthmatic, and the severity of childhood asthma is usually proportional to the number of positive skin tests and the severity of the reaction to those skin tests (4). Allergy seems to be less frequently diagnosed in older asthmatics, especially if the onset of the asthma occurs late in life. Specific treatment of the allergic condition with allergen immunotherapy has been demonstrated to benefit allergic asthmatics and to diminish the airways' response to allergen (5).

Occupational Asthma. Asthma can result from exposure to specific agents unique to the workplace. Occupational asthma may have an allergic or nonallergic component. Allergic asthma has resulted in workers exposed to enzymes used in the manufacture of laundry detergents and in seafood processors, bakers sensitive to flours, animal handlers, grain workers sensitive to storage mites, egg processors, and workers whose jobs involve exposure to insects and insect products (6).

Asthma can also occur in response to low molecular weight chemicals on an allergic or a nonallergic basis (7). Diisocyanates are used in the production of polyurethane, adhesives, and plastics. It is possible that a small percentage of these individuals have an IgE-mediated disease, but the mechanism in the majority of individuals has not been determined. Isocyanate sensitivity can be disabling and can result in asthmatic symptoms recurring hours after the initial exposure; methacholine hypersensitivity can persist for years after removal from isocyanate exposure. Workers exposed to a variety of wood dusts can develop asthmatic symptoms. Plicatic acid is a material derived from western cedar that can cause asthma in some individuals. It is possible that some of the responses to plicatic acid are mediated by IgE. Occupational asthma has also been described in persons exposed to acid anhydrides used in the production of epoxy resins, in workers exposed to platinum salts, and to colophony present in solder fluxes. Many other occupational asthmas can result from exposure to organic compounds capable of eliciting antibody responses.

Asthma Exacerbated by Nonsteroidal Anti-inflammatory Drugs and Food Additives. Approximately 10% of all chronic asthmatics can have an exacerbation of their asthma within 30 to 60 minutes of the ingestion of a nonsteroidal anti-inflammatory drug (NSAID) (8). The mechanism of this disorder is pharmacologic, and there is no evidence of its being immune-mediated. These drugs inhibit the enzyme prostaglandin synthase, and it is presumably by this mechanism that they induce the exacerbation of asthma. There have been several proposed mechanisms, and they include the suppression of the production of prostaglandin E_2, which is a natural inhibitor of the 5-lipoxygenase, or the shunting of arachidonic acid through the 5-lipoxygenase pathway to produce bronchospastic leukotrienes. A heightened responsiveness to leukotriene E_4 has also been proposed. Asthmatics sensitive to NSAIDs often have chronic asthma that may require oral or inhaled corticosteroids for control, and they often have nasal polyposis or chronic sinusitis. Subjects identified as being sensitive to these drugs must avoid them because life-threatening adverse reactions can occur.

Chronic asthmatics also appear potentially sensitive to sulfite, which is often used as a preservative for foods, beverages, and medications (9). The mechanism in sulfite sensitivity has not been determined, but it appears the response is triggered by the inhalation of sulfer dioxide gas that is in equilibrium with sulfite and not by the gastrointestinal absorption of sulfite. Foods and beverages that commonly contain sulfite include beer, wine, dried fruits, sauerkraut, cider, fresh red meat, and processed potatoes. The use of sulfite in restaurant salads has been outlawed, but sulfite may still be applied to grapes. The flavor enhancer monosodium glutamate has also been associated with rare cases of exacerbation of asthma.

Urticaria and Angioedema

Idiopathic Urticaria and Angioedema. The specific cause of recurrent or chronic urticaria and angioedema cannot usually be determined (10). Acute urticaria (urticaria persisting for less than 6 weeks) has been associated with a variety of infectious disorders, including streptococcal pharyngitis, infectious mononucleosis, sinusitis, cholecystitis, and during the prodrome of hepatitis B infection. It is possible that the acute phase response results in the production of a compound that lowers the threshhold for mast cell degranulation. It is certainly possible that urticaria can be associated with an IgE-mediated response, as in the case of some forms of food and insect sting hypersensitivity. Most cases of angioedema are due to mast cell degranulation occurring in deeper dermal tissues; therefore, individual urticarial wheals are not visible. Many subjects with angioedema give a history of having urticaria concomitantly or on separate occasions.

In addition to IgE-mediated and idiopathic urticaria/angioedema, a number of physical factors can precipitate the disorder. Cold urticaria can occur on exposure to cold air or contact with cold objects. Cholinergic urticaria is triggered by the initiation of sweating. Delayed pressure urticaria is delayed dermal swelling (angioedema) occurring several hours after some form of pressure to a given area. Dermatographism is triggered by scratching of the skin and can be caused by the rubbing of clothing. It presents as linear streaks of urticaria and can be readily diagnosed by stroking the skin and noting the characteristic response. Urticaria pigmentosa and systemic mastocytosis can present with generalized urticaria as well as anaphylaxis.

Hereditary Angioedema. Hereditary angioedema (HAE) is a rare condition resulting from the functional absence of the C1 esterase inhibitor molecule (11). The absence of this inhibitor allows for the uninhibited activation of complement by the action of the C1 esterase on C4 and C2. This action produces a split product, which may trigger the vasular leakage and angioedema. The clinical state presents with recurrent orofacial and peripheral angioedema or with acute abdominal crises. Trauma, including surgical procedures, can trigger an attack. Plasmin, whose formation is triggered by the activation of the fibrinolytic system after thrombosis, is also inhibited by the C1 esterase inhibitor, and plasmin can activate the complement cascade and the formation of bradykinin. It is possibly through this mechanism that trauma initiates the angioedematous process.

Acquired C1 Esterase Inhibitor Deficiency. A syndrome similar to HAE can be acquired in patients with disorders associated with large levels of circulating neoantigens (12). Disorders such as autoimmune hemolytic anemia and lymphoscarcoma can be associated with the presence of antigens recognized as foreign and to which large amounts of antibodies can be produced. This large burden of immune complexes actually consumes C1 and the C1 esterase inhibitor molecule, resulting in low circulating levels. The angioedema results from the same mechanism as in patients with the hereditary form; complement kinin, and the fibrinolytic pathways are uninhibited by the C1 esterase inhibitor. Patients with the onset of angioedema after the second decade whould have an evaluation for a possible coexisting disorder that is causing the process. Angioedema may precede by many months the other signs of the process causing the decline of the C1 esterase inhibitor levels. If angioedema occurs in the setting of low serum C4 and C1 esterase inhibitor levels in a patient in the third decade or later, a careful physical examination and further laboratory screening tests should be ordered, including a complete blood count, antinuclear antibody determination, hepatocellular enzymes, or other tests helpful in the diagnosis of lymphoma.

Insect Venom Hypersensitivity

Hymenoptera venoms and venom from the imported fire ant are capable of stimulating the production of specific IgE. Reexposure to these venoms can then initiate an IgE-mediated response that can result in generalized urticaria, oropharyngeal angioedema, asthma, and anaphylactic shock. Persons with prior systemic adverse reactions are prone to potentially life-threatening reactions after future stings. One exception to this rule appears to be children who have simply had dermatologic responses to venom exposure; these children do not appear to be prone to life-threatening events on subsequent stings any more so than the general population (13).

Adverse Reactions to Foods and Food Additives

The most common manifestations of IgE-mediated hypersensitivity to food proteins are nausea, vomiting, and diarrhea within minutes after ingestion. Urticaria, angioedema, and asthma may also occur. There appear to be delayed reactions to some food substances, and food hypersensitivity has been implicated in the pathogenesis of some cases of atopic dermatitis. In this particular case, ingestion of an offending food allergen can cause an exacerbation of the eczematous dermatitis. Food hypersensitivity has been suggested as the etiologic basis for many other conditions, including hyperactivity, migraine headache, chronic fatigue, depression, and a variety of other somatic complaints not typically associated with mast cell-mediated events; definitive evidence for the involvement of IgE in these conditions is lacking.

Food protein intolerance has been associated with several other disorders for which definitive evidence of an immune-mediated mechanism is lacking. Food protein-mediated gastroenteropathy occurs in infants and young children and has been associated with intolerance to a variety of foods. The process is usually transient, but it may be associated with vomiting, diarrhea, gross and occult bleeding, and growth retardation. An immunoglobulin E-mediated hypersensitivity to cow milk has been identified in a subset of these individuals. Eosinophilic gastroenteritis can present with vomiting, diarrhea, weight loss, and abdominal pain in either adults or children. Intolerance to milk protein has been documented in several patients even though an immune-mediated hypersensitivity is often lacking. Peripheral eosinophilia and an eosinophilic infiltration in the bowel wall are characteristic features of the disorder.

A gluten-sensitive enteropathy is associated with an intolerance to the wheat protein gliadin. A definitive immune response to gliadin has not been demonstrated. The disease usually begins within the first year of life, and symptoms are episodic diarrhea and abdominal pain. Growth retardation with malabsorption of a variety of nutrients may be seen. Immunoglobulin A deficiency exists in these patients at a frequency higher than that of the general population. Dermatitis herpetiformis is a papulovesicular skin disease often associated with gluten-sensitive enteropathy. Despite this sensitivity, most patients lack a history of gastrointestinal symptoms.

Atopic Dermatitis

Atopic dermatitis is a rather common disorder occurring in up to 4% of the population. As its name implies, it is often associated with the presence of IgE-mediated hypersensitivity and is frequently associated with other IgE-mediated disease states such as allergic rhinitis and asthma. This disorder often appears in infancy, but it can have its onset at any age of life. It is associated with an eczematous dermatitis that can at times be generalized but tends to concentrate in the flexures of the neck and inguinal regions and in the popliteal and antecubital fossae. Xerosis is often found in areas of the skin that are not frankly eczematous, and skin biopsies of these areas show an infiltration of lymphocytes in the dermis. The reason that the skin is the particular shock organ in this atopic diathesis is unknown, but the frequent colonization of the skin with *Staphylococcus aureaus* and the frequent improvement of the symptomatology with antistaphylococcal antibiotics suggest that this organism may contribute to the inflammatory response. Food hypersensitivity has been associated with exacerbations of the disease; proteins from cow milk, peanut, and egg are common offenders. Double-blind, placebo-controlled food challenges have documented that such foods can exacerbate the dermatitis in patients in whom there is immediate (IgE-mediated) skin test reactivity to the food extracts (14).

Allergic Contact Dermatitis

The term *contact dermatitis* refers to any dermatologic condition that is triggered by contact with a substance. This does not necessarily imply an immune-mediated etiology. To refer to such a syndrome as *allergic* is to imply that an immune-mediated response is the cause of the inflammatory state. Allergic contact dermatitis is due to a hypersensitivity triggered by a lymphocyte recognizing the offending material as foreign (a type IV response). Because only a small percentage of circulating lymphocytes have specificity for the antigen, a considerable period of time is required for the inflammatory response to become manifest. This is because the immediate reaction of the lymphocyte with the antigen results in the release of cytokines that recruit and stimulate nonspecific lymphocytes and also recruit Langerhans' cells and monocytes to the area to participate in the inflammatory response. It takes approximately 48 hours for a significant response to appear, although reactions may appear as early as 24 hours or as late as 72 hours. The most common antigens that trigger this type of response include the urushiols, which are the contact sensitizers derived from plants of the *Rhus* genus. These include poison ivy, poison oak, and poison sumac. Nickel sensitivity, as demonstrated by an intolerance to nickel-contaminated metals found in jewelry and clothing apparel, is also very common, and its sensitivity occurs in approximately 10% of the female population in western societies. Other common contact sensitizers include chromates, the hair dye *p*-phenylenediamine, and chemicals used in the production of rubber. The eczematous dermatitis that results from allergic contact hypersensitivity may be localized to the site of initial contact, but the antigen may be spread by the fingers to other areas of the body; this is frequently the case in nickel and *Rhus* dermatitis. When allergic contact dermatitis involves the hands, a particularly severe hand eczema can result and may be very recalcitrant to medical therapy.

Drug Hypersensitivity

In the case of drug hypersensitivity, the term *hypersensitivity* is used to refer to an adverse reaction to a pharmacologic agent that is not a manifestation of the drug's normal pharmacologic action or interaction with other drugs. Drug hypersensitivities may or may not have an immune etiology. Certainly, the most common cause of drug hypersensitivity is the IgE-mediated hypersensitivity to penicillin and its semisynthetic derivatives such as ampicillin and dicloxacillin. Penicillin hypersensitivity is also associated with frequent cross-reactivity to the cephalosporins.

Drug hypersensitivity may also be manifested by erythema multiforme, which is a skin rash with lesions resembling targets and may involve the mucosal surfaces with bulla formation, erythema, and desquamation. Extreme cases may result in the desquamation of the skin as well. There is no firm evidence for an immune-mediated cause for this disorder, and it may result in some cases from an idiopathic toxic response to the drug. Other cutaneous manifestations of drug hypersensitivity include urticaria/angioedema, allergic contact sensitivity, fixed drug eruptions, and a variety of nonspecific, papular or macular eruptions.

Drugs may fix to certain elements in the blood, such as erythrocytes, platelets, and neutrophils, and act as happens to which antibodies are made. Immunoglobulins responding to the drug on the cellular surfaces can facilitate the removal of these cells, resulting in anemia, thrombocytopenia, and granulocytopenia. A number of drugs have resulted in lupus-like illnesses; these include quinidine, hydralazine, anticonvulsants, isoniazid, and procainamide. An interesting drug-induced syndrome has emerged recently in patients with the acquired immunodeficiency syndrome. Nearly 50% of these individuals will have adverse reactions to sulfonamides; the underlying mechanism for these reactions is unknown.

Immunoglobulin E hypersensitivity is a common mechanism for adverse reactions to drugs that are proteins, such as insulin, protamine, chymopapain, and heterologous antisera. If immunoglobulin G is the primary antibody produced by the host, a serum sickness can occur.

The iodinated radiocontrast media (RCM) can produce acute anaphylactoid reactions that do not appear to have an immune basis. The hyperosmolar nature of many of these preparations may contribute to their ability to initiate reactions. Persons with a history of previous RCM adverse reactions possess a greater susceptibility than the general population to react to these agents on subsequent exposure. The most common manifestations of adverse reactions to RCM are flushing, generalized urticaria, hypotension, and respiratory distress.

Hypersensitivity Pneumonitis

Hypersensitivity pneumonitis refers to a group of lung disorders having an immune etiology that are often caused by the occupational exposure to a sensitizing protein. Primary sensitization to proteins can occur through the pulmonary route, and repeat exposure to these proteins can result in an inflammatory state. There has been considerable controversy over the years as to the mechanism of the inflammatory response. Early work suggested that complement-fixing immunoglobulins were responsible for the syndrome (i.e., type III hypersensitivity), but more recent evidence suggests that antigenic stimulation of lymphocytes may be responsible for the chronic inflammatory response seen in this group of conditions. Nevertheless, the presence of precipitating (IgG) antibodies in the serum of affected individuals may assist in the diagnosis and will be discussed later in this chapter. Further evidence that delayed (type IV) hypersensitivity is instrumental in the disease process is given by the pathological finding of noncaseating granulomata containing epithelioid and giant cells.

Farmer's lung is a disorder triggered by the inhalation of spores of *Micropolyspora faeni* or thermophilic actinomycetes, which often contaminates hay used for the feeding of livestock. Pigeon breeder's disease, or bird fancier's disease, is caused by the inhalation of proteins contained in bird droppings when hobbyists or laboratory personnel enter the animal's living

Table 63.2. Examples of Hypersensitivity Pneumonitis

Disorder	Antigen Source
Farmer's lung	Thermophilic *actinomycetes* in grains and hay
Bird fancier's disease	Proteins in bird droppings
Bagassosis	Thermophilic *actinomycetes* in moldy sugar cane
Malt worker's lung	*Aspergillus* species in moldy barley
Maple bark disease	Mold in maple bark
Woodworker's lung	Wood dusts or molds in wood

facilities. Similar respiratory disorders are seen in maple bark stripper's disease, mushroom worker's lung, and many other pneumonitides resulting from the inhalation of protein antigens (15) (Table 63.2).

Clinical symptomatology often presents as fever, malaise, myalgias, and respiratory symptoms such as cough or dyspnea, occurring several hours after exposure to the offending protein. Repeated exposures over many years may result in a chronic pulmonary condition finally ending in fibrosis and irreversible pulmonary disease. Suspecting the disease process and making the diagnosis is essential so that counseling can be instituted to reduce exposure to the offending proteins and thus to prevent the end-stage lung disease that may result.

Allergic Bronchopulmonary Aspergillosis

Allergic bronchopulmonary aspergillosis (ABPA) is a complication that can occur in allergic asthmatics. It is believed that patients with IgE-mediated hypersensitivity to *Aspergillus* species may inhale spores of the organism, resulting in an acute asthmatic response associated with the increased production of tracheobronchial mucus characteristic of allergic asthma. The organism can then reside in this inflammatory material, reproducing and producing further inflammation and resulting in a chronic asthmatic state. Because of this heavy allergen exposure in the lung, the patient develops precipitating IgG antibodies to *Aspergillus* as well as very high titers of specific and nonspecific IgE. Like hypersensitivity pneumonitis, ABPA was originally thought to be caused by complement-fixing (IgG) antibodies initiating the inflammatory response, but more recent evidence suggests that this condition, too, may be associated with a significant type IV hypersensitivity component. It is also possible that a chronic late-phase response (see Introduction) exists in these individuals. If unrecognized, the condition may proceed to bronchiectasis and finally fibrosis. ABPA may also be a complication of cystic fibrosis.

Table 63.3. Methods for Evaluating Hypersensitivity

Disorder	Diagnostic Test(s)
IgE-mediated diseases:	Skin testing
Allergic rhinitis	RAST and other in vitro methods for determining allergen-specific IgE
Allergic asthma	
Atopic dermatitis	
Insect venom allergy	
Food allergy	
Penicillin and protein drug allergy	
Hypersensitivity pneumonitis	Precipitating antibody to antigen by double immunodiffusion
	Chest radiograph
Hypersensitivity to NSAID and sulfite	Oral challenge with monitoring spirometry
Allergic bronchopulmonary aspergillosis	Skin testing to *Aspergillus*
	Total serum IgE (RIST)
	Precipitating antibody to *Aspergillus* by double immunodiffusion
	Chest radiograph
Allergic contact dermatitis	Patch testing

METHODOLOGIES

IgE-mediated Disease

Skin Testing. In patients suspected of having IgE-mediated disorders, skin testing remains the most accurate and cost-effective method of diagnosis. Skin testing relies on the specific IgE-mediated release of mediators from tissue mast cells that causes a wheal-and-flare response. Skin testing should be performed by personnel trained in its application with supervision by physicians experienced in the diagnosis of IgE-mediated diseases. Extracts must be purchased from reliable suppliers, and there is a growing emphasis on the need for allergen extract standardization.

In persons suspected of having IgE-mediated hypersensitivity to inhalants or foods, the percutaneous or epicutaneous skin tests should be applied first. A 1:10 or 1:20 weight/volume (w/v) aqueous extract containing 50% glycerol is applied as a drop to the volar aspect of the forearm or to the back. The allergen is then introduced into the epidermis with a sharp device by passing the point of the device through the drop and into the epidermis. Reproducible application has been demonstrated with the Wyeth bifurcated needle (resembling the old vaccinia scarification device), the Pharmacia Lancet, and the Staller point (a variation of the Morrow Brown needle) (16, 17). In performing percutaneous tests, hypodermic needles, the standard Morrow Brown needle, and the Staller kit give slightly less reproducible skin tests than the devices previously mentioned. After the allergenic extract has been introduced into the epidermis, the extract is wiped from the skin, and the wheal-and-flare is measured 15 to 20 minutes later.

When percutaneous tests are negative, intradermal testing may be required as a more sensitive test to identify aeroallergen hypersensitivity. The intradermal test is less specific than the percutaneous test but can still be interpreted with confidence providing the proper concentrations of materials are used. A 1: 1000 w/v concentration of allergen extract is injected at a very shallow angle so that material is introduced into the dermis just beneath the epidermis. Approximately 0.02 ml of material is injected. This volume is critical because wheal size is directly proportional to the volume of the material injected. The intradermal test result is also interpreted 15 to 20 minutes after its application.

Total Serum IgE, RAST, and Other in vitro Methods. *Total serum IgE* can be determined by immunoprecipitation. An antihuman IgE precipitates the patient's IgE, which competes with a radiolabeled human myeloma IgE. A second antibody may be required to facilitate the formation of large enough complexes to be precipitated. Alternatively, the competitive binding radioimmunosorbent test (RIST), in which IgE in the test sample competes with a radiolabeled human IgE for anti-IgE covalently linked to a solid phase matrix, may be used. The most popular method for measuring total serum IgE is the noncompetitive binding RIST. In this assay, antibody to human IgE is covalently linked to a solid phase matrix. The test sample is incubated with the matrix, thoroughly washed with buffer to remove unbound protein, and finally incubated with a radiolabeled antihuman IgE. The amount of IgE in the original sample is proportionate to the amount of radiolabeled anti-IgE that eventually is bound to the matrix complex. A similar "sandwich" method for detecting IgE, developed using enzyme-linked immunoassay (ELISA) systems, covalently links the final antihuman IgE to an enzyme capable of converting a substrate to a colored or fluorescent product. Reference antiserum containing known amounts of human IgE is available for standardizing these assays.

The *radioallergosorbent test (RAST)* was developed in the late 1960s and early 1970s following the discovery of IgE as the antibody causing type I hypersensitivity reactions. While originally developed as a research laboratory method, it was rapidly translated into a commercial diagnostic procedure. Allergen is usually covalently linked to a cellulose disk, but other insoluble support systems such as agarose may be used. The patient's serum is added to the disk and incubated to allow binding of IgE specific for the allergen. The disk is washed and then incubated with a radiolabeled antibody specific for IgE. The disk is rinsed again, and the amount of bound radioactivity is quantitated to determine the amount of specific IgE directed toward the allergen in the original serum sample.

Other methods have been developed to quantitate specific IgE in vitro. The antibody binding to the allergen-affixed IgE can be labeled with an enzyme that uses a substrate that is converted to a colored product (ELISA) or produces a fluorescent product (the fluorescent allergosorbent test or FAST). One method utilizes luminescence generated by γ-rays released in the radioactive decay of ^{125}I-labeled anti-IgE (the multi-thread allergosorbent test or MAST). Each of these methodologies is available through a commercial vendor. Basically, these methods are all similar in principle to the RAST and share similar advantages and disadvantages of RAST.

Clinical States Where Skin Testing, RAST, and RIST Are Useful. Perhaps the greatest utility for skin testing and RAST lies in their ability to aid in the diagnosis of aeroallergen hypersensitivity and the resulting conditions of allergic rhinitis and asthma. Skin testing and, to a more limited extent, RAST can be used to confirm IgE-mediated hypersensitivity to *hymenoptera* and imported fire ant venoms. True IgE-mediated reactions to foods can be confirmed with skin testing to food extracts, but many adverse reactions to foods have no known immunopathological basis. The avoidance of foods to which there is skin test positivity can benefit atopic dermatitis.

Skin testing for drug hypersensitivity is much more limited in usefulness. Skin testing to drugs that are proteins, such as insulin or protamine, can be informative, but testing to smaller drugs is greatly limited. There may be several reasons for this. First, mast cell degranulation and the positive skin test depend on the reaction of at least two IgE molecules with an antigen. Most drugs are haptens, and without a "carrier" molecule with multiple drug-binding sites, IgE bridging cannot occur. Second, drug metabolites may be the sensitizing antigens. Finally, it may be that many adverse reactions to drugs do not have an IgE-dependent basis. Penicillin and local anesthetics are exceptions. Penicillin sensitivity can be determined with a polyhaptenic synthetic penicilloyl polylysine (PrePen). Skin test positivity to this so-called major determinant will predict an urticarial reaction to penicillin administration. Unfortunately, this skin test reagent will not predict all hypersensitivity reactions to penicillin, and one should also test with a fresh penicillin preparation as well as with minor determinants for which a commercial test preparation is not yet available.

RIST for the detection of the total serum IgE is not usually useful in determining whether or not a condition has an IgE-mediated basis. The test is helpful in making the diagnosis of allergic bronchopulmonary aspergillosis and can be used to monitor disease activity. RIST can also be used to aid in the diagnosis of the hyper-IgE syndrome—a condition manifested by eczema, mucocutaneous candidiasis, and recurrent cutaneous and visceral staphylococcal abscess.

In Vitro Histamine Release from Basophils. Circulating basophils possess a high-affinity receptor for IgE and contain histamine that is released when an allergen crosslinks IgE on the surface of the cell. The test is performed by first obtaining anticoagulated venous blood and removing erythrocytes by dextran sedimentation. The leukocyte and platelet-rich plasma is centrifuged slowly to sediment the leukocytes, and these cells are washed with a buffer to remove the platelets. Leukocyte suspensions are then mixed with a specific allergen and incubated at 37°C. The reaction is terminated by cooling the cells and then pelleting the cells by centrifugation. The supernatants are harvested for analysis of histamine content. Histamine is usually analyzed by one of two methods. The first method depends on the ability of histamine to react with *o*-phthalaldehyde. The resulting complex absorbs ultraviolet light and fluoresces. Histamine content of the supernatants is quantitated by the amount of fluorescence detected in the derivatized sample and compared to histamine standards. Autoanalyzers are available for this method so that large numbers of tests can be performed in a single day (18). Histamine can also be analyzed by the transfer of a radiolabelled methyl group from S-adenosyl methonine to histamine utilizing histamine-N-methyl transferase, often partially purified from rat kidney (19). The radiolabelled N-methyl histamine is extracted, and its concentration determined by liquid scintillation analysis.

Cytology. Cytologic examination of nasal secretions and lower respiratory mucus can be helpful in the diagnosis of certain pathological conditions. Nasal mucus may be obtained by scraping the inferior turbinate or by collecting nasal mucus by having the patient blow onto a waxed paper. The latter method will reveal inflammatory cells that have migrated into the mucus and will have fewer contaminating epithelial cells that are obtained when the nasal mucosa is scraped. The mucus is spread thinly on a glass slide, allowed to dry in air, fixed with methanol, and then stained with a solution that is sensitive in detecting eosinophils. Hansel's stain is popular for this purpose, but stains used for making peripheral blood smears may be adequate. The absence of eosinophils does not rule out an allergic condition because neutrophils also migrate into the nasal passages in allergic rhinitis. Furthermore, a secondary sinus infection may result in a greater percentage of neutrophils in the mucus of the allergic subject. Nasal cytology may be most helpful in confirming the diagnosis of nonallergic rhinitis with eosinophilia (NARES) and in differentiating acute viral rhinitis from allergic rhinitis. When a large percentage of the nasal inflammatory cells are eosinophils (usually greater than 50%) and all of the skin tests to common aeroallergens are negative, one should feel comfortable in making the presumptive diagnosis of NARES. It may be difficult clinically to determine the cause of acute coryza in a patient presenting during a pollination season. In such cases, nasal cytology often reveals a high percentage of eosinophils in allergic subjects, but primarily epithelial cells are seen in patients with acute viral coryza.

Lower respiratory mucus can be more difficult than nasal mucus to examine for inflammatory cells. These cells do not stain as well, and it is difficult to differentiate them. Lower respiratory mucus, however, can be examined as a wet mount preparation pressed snuggly between a cover slip and a glass slide. With a little practice, one can recognize lymphocytes, neutrophils, eosinophils, ciliated epithelial cells, erythrocytes, and alveolar macrophages at 400× magnification without the use of staining materials (Fig. 63.1). If eosinophils have been in the airway at high numbers for a fairly long period of time, Charcot-Leyden crystals, elongated, diamond-shaped bodies 15 to 50 microns in length, may be seen.

Cell-mediated Immunity (CMI)

Patch Testing. Patch testing is the preferred method for diagnosing allergic contact dermatitis that is due to a type IV hypersensitivity response. Performance of this testing requires an experienced investigator who is knowledgeable in the limitations of patch testing, who is experienced in the application of the test, and who is capable of interpreting skin reactions and counseling the patient regarding the avoidance of materials that may contain the offending allergen.

A standard tray containing 22 common contact allergens is commercially available (20). Most of the allergens used in testing are mixed in white petrolatum, but occasionally an aqueous vehicle is preferred. Only physicians well experienced in patch testing should prepare a test material that has not previously been investigated. Unstandardized materials raise the risk of irritant reactions, and marked allergic reactions can occur if the concentration of the allergen is too high. In addition to avoiding unstandardized testing materials, areas with active dermatitis must be avoided.

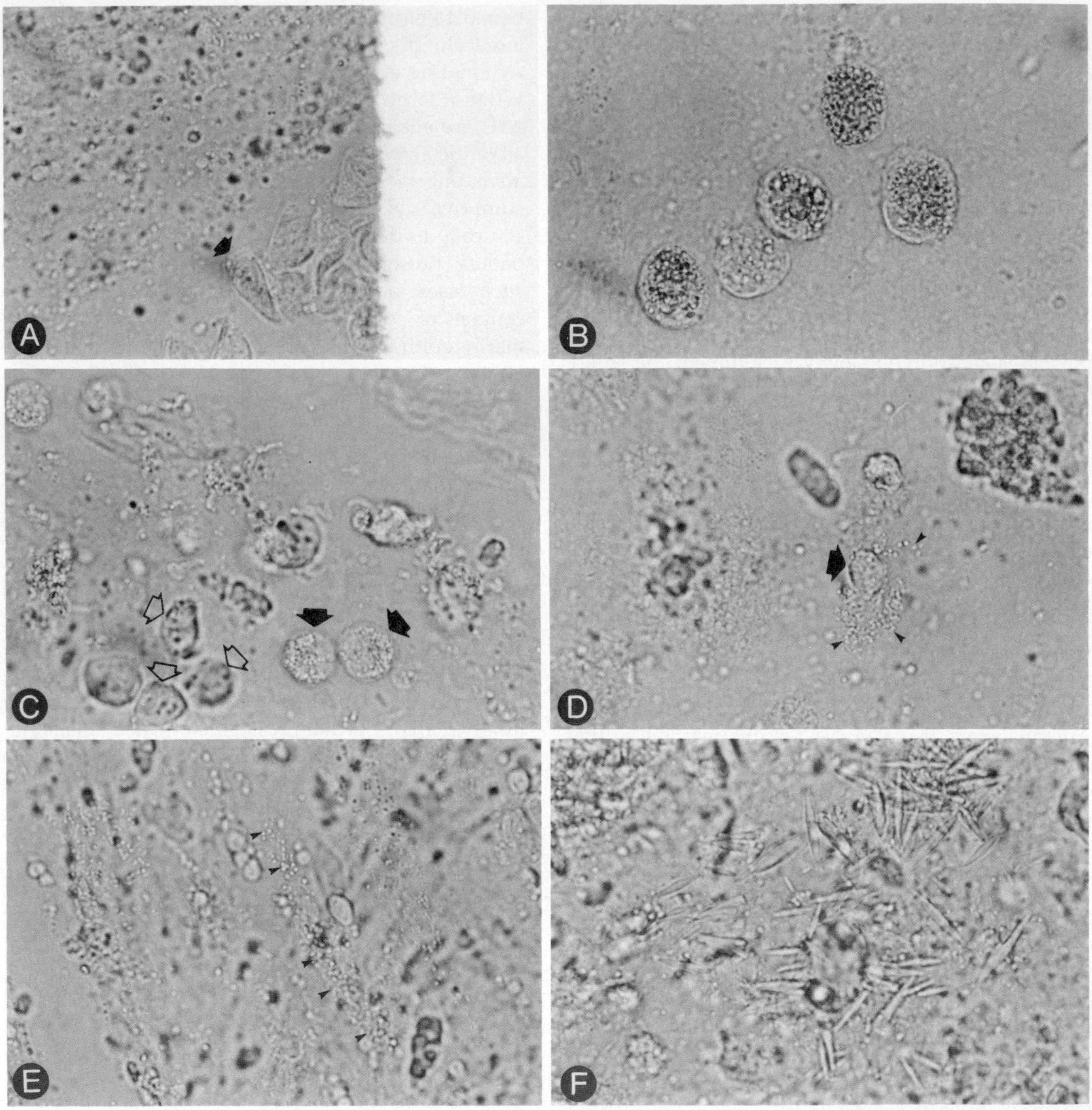

Figure 63.1. Photomicrographs of a sputum sample from an asthmatic patient. All of the micrographs were taken of unstained sputum samples pressed between a cover slip and a clear microscope slide. A sample was observed using the 40× objective and the 10× eyepiece. The final magnification of the micrographs is 1860×. **A**, The *broad arrow* points to the brush border of a ciliated epithelial cell. Note the cell's apical nucleus and its pointed tail, which serves to fix the cell to the basement membrane. These cells are often sloughed in an inflammatory condition such as asthma or bronchitis. **B**, A cluster of alveolar macrophages. Note the large intracytoplasmic inclusion bodies and granules. **C**, The *empty arrows* point to neutrophils and the *solid arrows* point to eosinophils. The eosinophils are best distinguished by their fine granules, which easily stand out, especially if one gently focuses the fine adjust knob on the microscope. The neutrophils are approximately the same size as the eosinophils, but their granules are much less distinct. **D**, The *large arrow* points to an eosinophil that is degranulating, and its granules have spilled into the extracellular space *(fine arrows)*. **E**, In sputum samples that have been allowed to stand, only eosinophil granules may be seen and intact eosinophils may be difficult to locate. The *fine arrows* point to eosinophil granules that are somewhat linearly distributed in the sputum sample. **F**, After sitting at room temperature for several hours, the granules themselves disrupt, allowing proteins to leak. Charcot-Leyden crystals form when lysophospholipase crystallizes out of solution. The presence of these crystals indicates that eosinophils have been present in the past, and it is often difficult to find intact eosinophils where Charcot-Leyden crystals are seen.

Testing material is applied from the squeeze bottle to filter paper disks spaced on an aluminized paper strip. The strip is then fixed to a hypoallergenic strip of tape and applied to the patient's back. Care must be taken to be sure that the tape is securely in place; to prevent the tape from loosening when the skin on the back is stretched, the patient should have the back bent forward while the strips are affixed. Once in place, the patient should be cautioned to keep the areas dry while bathing and to avoid situations where sweating might occur. The test should be left in place for 72 hours with the patient instructed to remove those tests where intense itching or irritation occur prior to the time when the tests are to be interpreted.

In Vitro Cytokine Production. Incubation of lymphocytes with antigen results in cytokine production with cellular proliferation. The incorporation of radiolabeled thymidine into dividing cells can be used as an index of hypersensitivity to an antigen. This method remains a laboratory tool, and reliable in vitro testing for cell-mediated immunity is not widely available at this time.

In Vivo Challenges

Food Hypersensitivity. Besides the history, the first step in diagnosing IgE-mediated food hypersensitivity is percutaneous skin testing. Foods identified as possible allergens can be confirmed by oral challenges. If a patient has had a life-threatening adverse reaction to a food to which he or she is sensitive, oral challenges should not be performed. Indeed, oral food challenges are rarely necessary in clinical practice but have been used as a research tool to prove that food hypersensitivity can exacerbate some disorders. Double-blind food challenges have been helpful in demonstrating that food hypersensitivity can contribute to atopic dermatitis; egg, peanut, and milk account for the majority of the adverse reactions. A major drawback to this testing is the difficulty in the preparation of gelatin capsules containing freeze-dried foods or food extracts.

NSAIDs. Up to 10% of all chronic asthmatics may have exacerbations of their asthma on ingesting an NSAID. This figure may rise to 70% of patients who have chronic asthma and paranasal sinusitis or nasal polyposis. Many of these individuals will not have a history of adverse reactions because pulmonary function values may not have dropped sufficiently to result in symptomatology. If, however, an asthmatic suspected of having NSAID hypersensitivity requires an NSAID for some other condition, an oral challenge may be required under close supervision. Several precautions need to be taken because adverse reactions to these compounds can be life-threatening. First, the FEV-1 (forced expiratory volume at 1 second) should be 70% of predicted or better prior to testing. It may be necessary to give a short course of corticosteroids to bring the lung functions up to an acceptable level for testing. One proposed method suggests administering a placebo at 3-hour intervals beginning at 8 AM for a total of three doses (21). The FEV-1 is recorded hourly during this time period and for 3 hours following the last dosage. On the second day of the challenge procedure, aspirin is given at 8 AM. Either a 3-mg or 30-mg dose is used initially, depending on whether or not there is a prior history of a serious adverse reaction to aspirin. Again, the FEV-1 is measured hourly or if symptoms develop. A second dose (30 mg if 3 mg was the first test dose) of aspirin may be given at 11 AM, and a final dose of 100 mg is given at 2 PM. Again, the FEV-1 is measured hourly after each dose. If no adverse reaction occurs, the patient returns to the clinic on the third day and is then given 150 mg at 8 AM, 325 mg at 11 AM, and 650 mg at 2 PM, provided that the FEV-1 has not dropped by greater than 20% at any dosage; such a drop is an indication of a positive test and hypersensitivity to NSAID.

Sulfite. The suspicion of adverse reactions to sulfite (or metabisulfite) should occur after a person has had an adverse reaction following the ingestion of a food or beverage. The adverse reaction may be due to sulfite contained in the food or beverage, to an IgE-mediated hypersensitivity reaction to a food protein, or to some other food additive, such as monosodium glutamate (MSG). It is reasonable to do a sulfite challenge in such individuals to help determine the presence or absence of sulfite sensitivity. In aqueous solutions, sulfite is in equilibrium with sulfur dioxide. Most likely, the sulfur dioxide inhaled during the ingestion of a food or beverage that contains sulfite is the cause of the adverse reaction in the lung. Therefore, sulfite is placed in acidic solutions, such as a commercial lemonade preparation. Sulfite is prepared at 100 mg/ml in water on the day of the challenge. Spirometry is performed, and the FEV-1 must be greater than 1.5 liters or 70% of predicted prior to performing the challenge. Theophylline and inhaled corticosteroids are continued. Inhaled bronchodilators are discontinued on the day of the challenge, and cromolyn is discontinued for 24 hours prior to the challenge. The patient is challenged with progressively increasing doses of sulfite (1, 5, 10, 15, 25, 50, 75, 100, 150, and 200 mg in the water solution) by adding the sulfite to 20 ml of the lemonade mixture and asking the patient to swish the solution in the mouth for 15 seconds before swallowing (22). This allows the sulfur dioxide that is in equilibrium with sulfite to effervesce and be inhaled into the lung. Increasing doses are given at 10-minute intervals with spirometry being performed just prior to the next dose. A positive test occurs when the FEV-1 drops 20% or more below the baseline value. Placebo challenges may be given periodically among the sulfite challenges to be sure that there is not a spontaneous drop of the FEV-1 occurring as the challenge progresses. Positive challenges should be repeated in a double-blind fashion.

Occupational Asthma. Asthma occurring in the workplace can be due to a type I or other immune response or may have an idiopathic etiology. Several approaches can be taken to document occupational asthma (23). The easiest way to reproduce the environmental workplace is to have the patient perform spirometry there. However, this may be time-consuming and cumbersome, and the performance of a peak expiratory flow rate (PEFR) is a practical alternative. The subject should record the PEFR prior to the work shift and at regular intervals throughout the day. Careful notation should be made of what exposures occurred prior to the drop in the PERF. The PERF should be followed after the work shift to determine if a late response occurs. Despite positive data on a drop of the PERF at the workplace, bronchoprovocation with specific materials may be required if compensation is being sought or if there may be several potential offending materials. Bronchoprovocation should be performed by clinicians familiar with the evaluation of occupational lung disease and who are aware of the test's limitations. Detailed guidelines have been published (24). Spirometry performed before and after exposure is necessary to make the diagnosis. The same precautions outlined in the sections above on sulfite and NSAID hypersensitivity should be observed while performing bronchial challenges. In some cases, a specific compound, such as toluene diisocyanate (TDI), may be suspected, and challenge may be performed with this material. For volatile compounds such as TDI, special challenge chambers that are not usually available in clinical settings are required. Challenges to proteins, however, can be performed by mixing the material in an aqueous solution and inhaling the material with a dosimeter delivery system. The protein concentration is increased serially 10-fold until the FEV-1 drops by 20% or more. If concentrations for challenge have not been standardized, it may be necessary to first perform a percutaneous skin test with the material to find a concentration that does not elicit a large response. In all cases where bronchial challenges are performed, the physician must be aware that late responses may occur 4 to 8 hours following the initial drop of the FEV-1. The patient may be at home when this occurs, and instructions must be given on the proper procedures necessary to treat the response. If severe drops in the FEV-1 occur with a challenge, it may be necessary to administer corticosteroids (such as prednisone, 1 mg/kg) at the time of the initial challenge to help prevent the late phase response from occurring. If milder reactions occur, it may be informative to monitor the patient for late phase responses, either as an inpatient or with peak expiratory flow rates monitored at home.

Hypersensitivity Pneumonitis

Hypersensitivity pneumonitis has an immune basis, but a specific hypersensitivity type cannot be ascribed to any of these conditions. A type III response has been implied because of the frequency in which IgG precipitating antibodies can be detected against a specific antigen. The clinical features of the disease, however, more closely resemble a type IV immune response with granuloma formation, and an eventual progression to pulmonary fibrosis can be seen.

Patients suspected of having hypersensitivity pneumonitis should have a radiograph of the chest. During the acute phase of the illness, a rather diffuse, small nodular appearance is noted. Occasionally, infiltrates can be seen. Eventually, the patient enters a chronic fibrotic phase, and the typical radiographic features of interstitial fibrosis are prominent. Generally, pulmonary function testing reveals a restrictive defect with impaired gas exchange. Thus, spirometry should reveal a proportionate decrease in both the FEV-1 and the forced vital capacity (FVC) with an FEV-1/FVC ratio of 0.75 or greater. In severe cases, the single breath diffusion capacity for carbon monoxide (DLco) will be impaired, and there may be a fall of the PaO_2 with exercise.

Heavy exposure to organic dust may result in the production of IgG antibodies to antigenic proteins in the dust. Commonly available antigens for screening for hypersensitivity pneumonitis include thermophilic actinomycetes (*Micropolyspora* and *Thermoactinomyces* species), and avian proteins. The presence of precipitating antibody in the patient's serum is determined by double immunodiffusion in agarose gels. Many other antigens have been implicated in causing hypersensitivity pneumonitis, and these antigens may not be readily available for testing for precipitating antibodies (15). It may be necessary to send the patient's serum to a specific research laboratory where a standardized antigen and the appropriate negative and positive control sera are available. Persons working in an environment with a heavy exposure to an organic dust may develop precipitating antibodies without the presence of clinical disease.

Allergic Bronchopulmonary Aspergillosis

Allergic bronchopulmonary aspergillosis (ABPA) occurs when *Aspergillus* species reside in the airways of allergic asthmatics. Its proteins are very antigenic, and high titers of IgE and IgG antibodies are produced. Additionally, cell-mediated hypersensitivity is likely to occur. Persons suspected of having aspergillosis should have total serum IgE and precipitins (IgG antibody) to *Aspergillus* determined, a skin test to *Aspergillus* extract, a chest radiograph, and a total eosinophil count (25). Some research laboratories are capable of measuring specific IgE and IgG antibodies to *Aspergillus fumigatus*. At present, these tests are not generally available. The majority of patients with ABPA will react on skin testing to *A. fumigatus*. A small percentage, however, may have another *Aspergillus* species responsible, and sensitivity to one of these other species should be determined if there is a high enough suspicion that aspergillosis exists and testing to *A. fumigatus* is negative. Chest radiographs are also important in following the disease process. Thick-walled bronchi, infiltrates, and mucoid impaction may be seen. If the disease is not recognized early, progression to central bronchiectasis and pulmonary fibrosis with bulla formation may occur. Response to treatment can be followed with periodic chest radiographs and total serum IgE levels. Similar syndromes have been seen with other fungi, including *Candida, Curvularia, Stemphylium,* and *Helminthosporium*.

Hereditary Angioedema

Hereditary angioedema (HAE) is due to the functional absence of the C1 esterase inhibitor.

Complement Measurements. Approximately 15% of patients with HAE will have the antigenic presence of the C1 esterase inhibitor; assays utilizing an antibody to C1 esterase will indicate normal levels and will not reflect the functional impairment of the molecule. Therefore, if the patient is suspected of having HAE and has a normal immunologic assay for the C1 esterase inhibitor, a functional C1 esterase inhibitor assay should be obtained. Because of this inhibitor deficiency, there is excessive activation of C4 and C2. For this reason, serum C4 or C2 levels are the most convenient screening tests for diagnosing this condition. The C4 level is in the low normal or below normal range between attacks and always drops to below the normal range during acute attacks. If the C4 level is low normal or below, the diagnosis should be confirmed by measuring C1 esterase levels.

Controversial Methodologies

To help diagnose allergic disorders, a number of controversial methods have arisen that have not utilized the scientific method to determine their validity. One such procedure is cytotoxic testing. This test depends on the addition of food, chemical, and inhalant extracts to peripheral blood leukocytes, which are then observed for microscopic changes. This testing procedure has been demonstrated to be invalid, and federal agencies and many insurance companies have refused to pay for this testing. As a consequence, its use has declined in recent years.

In an effort to find a lower, safer dose of allergen to be used for immunotherapy (desensitization therapy), a testing method that depended on an endpoint titration was developed. This concentration directed the clinician to a treatment dose that typically was considerably lower than the levels used in conventional immunotherapy. As a consequence, many patients on this form of therapy never reached a dosage that could benefit their symptoms. Very weakly sensitive individuals, however, could approach an effective concentration because of the higher concentration of allergen extract subsequently used for immunotherapy. Controlled studies have demonstrated the method to be ineffective in controlling symptoms of ragweed hay fever, while conventional immunotherapy resulted in improvement significantly greater than that of placebo-treated individuals.

Subcutaneous and sublingual provocation testing are currently used primarily by clinical ecologists in their treatment of allergic disorders and any of a variety of conditions that they consider to have an allergic basis, such as migraine headache or multiple somatic complaints. The therapy is based on the principle of finding a dosage of an allergen or chemical that provokes objective or subjective signs in the patient. A neutralization dose that is either slightly weaker or stronger than the provoking dose is then chosen and is injected subcutaneously in an effort to neutralize the symptoms. There are no controlled studies demonstrating the efficacy of this procedure, and a number of studies have failed to show any validity to this method. Others have proposed that sublingual solutions of chemicals or allergen extracts can also neutralize symptomatology. At present, no controlled studies have demonstrated that subcutaneous or sublingual neutralization techniques have any validity.

INTERPRETATION

IgE-mediated Disease

Skin Test Size and Scoring. Generally, a percutaneous skin test reaction is considered significant if it results in erythema (flare) greater than 20 mm in diameter and is definitely considered positive if there is an accompanying wheal. The advantages of the percutaneous (prick) test are its ease and speed of application, infrequency of false-positive reactions, sensitivity, cost, and the rapidity with which results can be obtained. Intradermal skin test reactions are generally considered positive if the erythema has a diameter of greater than 21 mm with an accompanying wheal of 5 to 10 mm. If the erythema is greater than 30 mm with an accompanying 10 mm wheal, the reaction is definitely considered to be positive.

Despite the wide degree of popularity, there are some problems with skin testing. A mild degree of discomfort is experienced, and there certainly is inter-subject variation in the skin reactivity that results in the wheal-and-flare response. Persons with dermatographism can develop erythema and wheals simply from the irritation of the skin with the test device. Patients with extensively inflamed skin, as in atopic dermatitis, may not have enough clear surface area for the test to be applied. Furthermore, patients with atopic dermatitis often have a minimal flare response to the skin test, making the results more difficult to interpret. In these cases, in vitro testing may be required. The major role for skin testing is in the determination of IgE-mediated hypersensitivity to inhaled aeroallergens, food allergens, insect venoms, pharmaceuticals that are proteins, penicillin, and local anesthetics. Most other pharmaceuticals have not been standardized as skin test reagents, thus dramatically reducing the effectiveness of the skin test in diagnosing the mechanism of possible drug hypersensitivity reactions. Furthermore, skin testing is ineffective in diagnosing hypersensitivity to radiocontrast media or to nonsteroidal anti-inflammatory drugs, and it is usually not capable of detecting persons sensitive to sulfite.

RIST Evaluation. Total serum IgE should be reported as international units (IU) per milliliter of serum. Serum from newborns may contain very low levels of IgE; therefore, two sets of standards may be required—one with the adult range and one for the range of IgE values seen in the pediatric population (26).

RAST Scoring. RAST is usually scored by arbitrarily breaking down the total radioactivity counts into classes. The interpretation of the test results should be restricted to the class designation and not to the actual total radioactivity counts. The class determination is made by comparison of the allergen-specific IgE content in test samples to strongly positive and negative controls.

The Phadebas RAST produced by Pharmacia utilizes a scoring system in which the radioactivity is compared with that produced by five reference sera. Class 0 corresponds to undetectable levels of specific IgE, and class 1 corresponds to low levels. Classes 2, 3, and 4 correspond to moderate, high, and very high levels of specific IgE, respectively, and are considered to be positive. A modified RAST scoring system with classes 0 to 5 has been developed to enhance the sensitivity of RAST by utilizing larger volumes of serum and longer periods of incubation than in the Phadebas system. In this modified system, all tubes are counted for the length of time required to generate 25,000 cpm when 25 IU of IgE/ml is incubated with an immunosorbent coated with anti-IgE. The six classes (0 to 5) are generated by breaking down these 25,000 counts into 5 zones with a class 5 being greater than 25,000 cpm.

There are several inherent problems in the RAST. First, the test may only measure specific IgE and, unlike the skin test, does not measure the patient's biological reactivity. Second, the results of RAST can be affected by the amount of specific IgG in the patient's serum that might compete with specific IgE for allergen. Third, the cost of the reagents and labor for performing RAST makes it considerably less economical than skin testing. Despite these difficulties, RAST does correlate with skin test reactivity and clinical reactivity. A sufficient number of false-positive and false-negative RAST tests occur, however, to prevent the use of RAST as an absolute indicator of IgE-mediated disease. One other problem that has occurred with RAST is its application to an allergen where there has not been sufficient research done to determine the specificity of that particular assay. Each new RAST allergen must be compared with skin testing before it can be used to interpret clinical sensitivity; unfortunately, this is often not done.

Several things can be done to improve quality control for in vitro allergen-specific IgE assays (26). A positive control serum should be included to test the binding capacity of the allergosorbent. A serum without allergen-specific IgE but with a high total IgE should be included to control for nonspecific binding to the matrix. Samples should be done in duplicate to control for technical errors, and samples may be analyzed at more than one dilution to test for "nonparallelism" as an indicator of interference in the assay by ingredients such as specific IgG antibody. The Centers for Disease Control performed a test program involving 33 laboratories and found a 10% false-positive rate among them (27).

Correlation of RAST with Skin Testing and Clinical Disease. Compared with RAST, the skin test is less likely to be negative in patients with a known history of aeroallergen hypersensitivity. In asthmatic children, bronchoprovocation results correlate better with skin tests than with RAST. While RAST may be

Table 63.4. Advantages of In Vivo and In Vitro Methods for Diagnosing Allergen-Specific Hypersensitivity

Advantages of Skin Testing	Advantages of In Vitro Testing
High specificity	Useful when skin disease (e.g., eczema or dermatographism) preclude skin testing
High sensitivity	Useful in epidemiological studies of atopy
Results with minutes of application	Useful for identifying cross-reactive allergens (RAST inhibition)
Low cost	

modified to enhance its sensitivity, this alteration often results in an unacceptably low specificity level.

In conclusion, RAST appears to be most useful in the diagnosis of IgE-mediated disease in moderately-to-highly sensitive individuals, especially if the aeroallergen is a grass or ragweed pollen. RAST is also useful in research studies on the epidemiology of certain IgE-mediated disorders. RAST is useful clinically in persons with skin disorders that preclude skin testing, provided that the limitations of RAST are understood by the physician responsible for caring for the patient. The widespread use of RAST for diagnosing IgE-mediated disorders is to be discouraged (Table 63.4).

Cell-Mediated Immunity

Patch Test Scoring. The patch test results are interpreted 72 hours after their application. Before removing the test strips, care must be taken to ensure that sites where the test materials were placed can be identified accurately. The sites must be analyzed by an experienced clinician who is adept at interpreting the differences between irritant and true allergic responses. If only mild erythema is present at the site, the reaction should be recorded as doubtful. A site with erythema and some induration and possible papule formation may be interpreted as weak. Strong reactions have erythema with papules and vesicles, and extreme reactions will have bulla formation. Irritant reactions, if strong, will have a sharply demarcated border of erythema, but in allergic reactions, the border will not be so clearly defined. It is very difficult, however, to distinguish between weak irritant and weak allergic reactions.

In Vitro Cytokine Production. In vitro analysis for cell-mediated immunity is usually directed at the assessment of T-lymphocyte responsiveness. This method of analysis is outlined in the chapter on immunodeficiency. In vitro analysis of hyperresponsiveness to contact allergens has been performed but is not commercially available. Therefore, it is unlikely to replace the patch test as a method of diagnosis.

In Vivo Challenges

Spirometry. Besides skin testing for IgE-mediated disorders, spirometry offers one of the most sensitive, objective determinations of an individual's clinical reactivity to a given allergen or other provoking substance. A positive response is usually defined as a drop in the FEV-1 by 20% below baseline values. If a positive response is found to aspirin, cross-sensitivity to other NSAIDs is implied because of the pharmacologic ability of these compounds to inhibit prostaglandin synthetase. Because some NSAIDs are more potent in this ability than others, adverse reactions may be more severe with compounds other than aspirin. Patients should be advised to avoid all aspirin and aspirin-containing compounds and be given a list of currently available NSAIDs. They should be told to avoid antiarthritic medications on the assumption that other NSAIDs may appear on the market in the future. Acetaminophen is usually tolerated but may also cause a drop in the FEV-1 when given at high doses to NSAID-sensitive individuals. Should a patient who has a positive aspirin challenge require a NSAID, a desensitization can usually be accomplished. The patient can then take the drug without adverse effects as long as the medication is taken regularly; if several days elapse between doses, sensitivity may recur, resulting in an adverse reaction. Persons found to be sensitive to sulfite and other food additives should be counseled about foods and beverages that contain the material. Accidental exposure may occur, however, and patients should have a β-adrenergic inhaler or epinephrine for subcutaneous injection should a reaction occur. Persons with adverse reactions to environmental materials in the workplace should be relocated. Retraining may be necessary for extremely sensitive individuals if avoidance in the particular environment is not possible. Persons with a hypersensitivity pneumonitis must avoid the material to which they are sensitive or face the possibility of a progressive obstructive and possibly restrictive pulmonary disease.

Reproduction of Clinical Symptoms. In some in vivo challenges, it is difficult to obtain an objective measure as sensitive as spirometry. Persons who have food challenges that result in an exacerbation of a skin disorder or who have abdominal complaints on the ingestion of the food may be difficult to interpret. For instance, exacerbations of cutaneous symptoms may require several hours to occur, and there is no clear temporal relationship between the ingestion of the food and the onset of symptoms. It is generally recommended that food challenges be repeated before concluding that the patient is definitely intolerant.

Hypersensitivity Pneumonitis

Precipitins can be found in the serum of most individuals suffering from hypersensitivity pneumonitis. However, precipitins can be detected in the serum of as many as 50% of persons with similar but asymptomatic exposure. Therefore, clinical data including chest radiographs are necessary for establishing the diagnosis. Lymphocyte transformation to antigen is seen less often (16%), but this is not a readily available laboratory test and is done only in research centers at present.

Allergic Bronchopulmonary Aspergillosis

Diagnostic criteria for allergic bronchopulmonary aspergillosis (ABPA) include the presence of asthma, a positive immediate skin test reaction to *Aspergillus*, an elevation of the total IgE, and precipitins to *Aspergillus*. Additional unessential criteria include the radiographic findings of infiltrates and central bronchiectasis. Responsiveness to therapy can be monitored by following the total serum IgE and the chest radiograph. Persons with sufficiently advanced disease may require continuous corticosteroid therapy. Remissions can be achieved in patients in whom the disease has been detected early enough.

Hereditary Angioedema

A patient with angioedema who had the onset of clinical symptoms before the age of 20 years and who has a low serum C4 should be suspected of having hereditary angioedema (HAE). If the C4 is low, an immunologic assay for the C1 esterase inhibitor should be obtained. A low level confirms the diagnosis of HAE. In 15% of individuals with HAE, however, the immunologic assay may be normal, indicating the presence of an antigenic material in plasma that is functionally inactive. In cases of angioedema where the C4 is low and the immunologic assay for the C1 esterase inhibitor is normal, a functional assay for C1 esterase inhibitor should be obtained. A low functional assay confirms the diagnosis.

In patients with antioedema beginning in the third decade or later, a C4 and C1 esterase inhibitor should be determined. If abnormal, a search for another underlying disorder should be sought, as indicated in the methodology section.

References

1. Snyderman R. Mechanisms of inflammation and tissue destruction in the rheumatic diseases. In: Wyngaarden JB, Smith LH Jr, eds. Cecil textbook of medicine. Philadelphia: WB Saunders, 1988:1984–1998.
2. Sly RM. Mortality from asthma, 1979–1984. J Allergy Clin Immunol 1988;82:705–717.
3. Kalliel JN, Goldstein BM, Braman SS, Settipane GA. High frequency of atopic asthma in a pulmonary clinic population. Chest 1989;96:1336–1340.
4. Zimmerman B, Feanny S, Reisman J, et al. Allergy in asthma. I. The dose relationship of allergy to severity of childhood asthma. J Allergy Clin Immunol 1988;81:63–70.
5. Van Bever HP, Stevens WJ. Suppression of the late asthmatic reaction by hyposensitization in asthmatic children allergic to house dust mite *(Dermatophagoides pteronyssinus)*. Clin Exp Allergy 1989;19:399–404.
6. Pepys J. Occupational allergic lung disease caused by organic agents. J Allergy Clin Immunol 1986;78:1058–1062.
7. Butcher BT, Bernstein IL, Schwartz HJ. Guidelines for the clinical evaluation of occupational asthma due to small molecular weight chemicals. J Allergy Clin Immunol 1989;84:834–838.
8. Mathison DA, Stevenson DD. Aspirin sensitivity in rhinosinusitis and asthma. Immunol Allergy Practice 1983;11:340–349.
9. Nicklas RA. Sulfites: a review with emphasis on biochemistry and clinical application. Allergy Proc 1989;10:349–356.
10. Champion RH. Urticaria: then and now. Br J Dermatol 1988;119:427–436.
11. Frank MM, Gelfand JA, Atkinson JP. Hereditary angioedema: the clinical syndrome and its management. Ann Int Med 1976;84:580–593.
12. Gelfand JA, Boss GR, Conley CL, Reinhart R, Frank MM. Acquired C1 esterase inhibitor deficiency and angioedema: a review. Medicine 1978;58:321–328.
13. Lichtenstein LM, Valentine MD, Sobotka AK. Insect allergy: the state of the art. J Allergy Clin Immunol 1979;64:5–12.
14. Sampson HA. Role of immediate food hypersensitivity in the pathogenesis of atopic dermatitis. J Allergy Clin Immunol 1983;71:473–480.
15. Richerson HB, Bernstein IL, Fink JN, et al. Guidelines for the clinical evaluation of hypersensitivity pneumonitis. J Allergy Clin Immunol 1989;84:839–844.
16. Michel FB, Skassa-Brociek W, Segalen C, Dreborg S, Bousquet J. Reproducibility of six methods of skin prick tests. J Allergy Clin Immunol 1986;77:222 (abstract).
17. Bousquet J. *In vivo* methods for study of allergy: skin tests, techniques, and interpretation. In: Middleton E Jr, Reed CE, Ellis EF, Adkinson NF Jr, Yuninger JW, eds. Allergy principles and practice. St. Louis: CV Mosby, 1988:419–436.
18. Siraganian RP, Brodsky MJ. Automated histamine analysis for *in vitro* allergy testing. J Allergy Clin Immunol 1976;57:525–540.
19. Shaff RE, Beaven MA. Increased sensitivity of the enzymatic isotopic assay of histamine: measurement of histamine in plasma and serum. Analyt Biochem 1979;94:425–430.
20. Fisher AA. Role of patch testing. In: Fisher AA, ed. Contact dermatitis. Philadelphia: Lea & Febiger, 1986;9–29.
21. Stevenson DD, Simon RA. Aspirin sensitivity: respiratory and cutaneous manifestations. In: Middleton E Jr, Reed CE, Ellis EF, Adkinson NF Jr, Yuninger JW, eds. Allergy principles and practice. St. Louis: CV Mosby, 1988:1537–1554.
22. Simon RA, Stevenson DD. Adverse reactions to sulfites. In: Middleton E Jr, Reed CE, Ellis EF, Adkinson NF Jr, Yuninger

JW, eds. Allergy principles and practice. St. Louis: CV Mosby, 1988:1555–1569.

23. Smith AB, Castellan RM, Lewis D, Matte T. Guidelines for the epidemiologic assessment of occupational asthma. J Allergy Clin Immunol 1989;84:794–805.
24. Cartier A, Bernstein IL, Burge PS, et al. Guidelines for bronchoprovocation on the investigation of occupational asthma. J Allergy Clin Immunol 1989;84:823–829.
25. Greenberger PA. Allergic bronchopulmonary aspergillosis. J Allergy Clin Immunol 1984;74:645–653.
26. Hamilton RG, Adkinson NF. Clinical laboratory methods for the assessment and management of human allergic diseases. Clin Lab Med 1986;6:117–138.
27. Przybyszewski VA, Taylor RN. Allergen-specific immunoglobulin E: performance evaluation results. U.S. Dept. of Health and Human Services, Public Health Service, Centers for Disease Control, 1983.

64 Receptor Assays of the Clinical Laboratory

Barry G. England and James B. Smart

The coordinated behavior of all cells within a multicellular organism is necessary for an organism to function normally. Intercellular communication is a prerequisite of coordinated cell behavior and must be maintained throughout the growth and development of the organism, as well as during the period of adult homeostasis. Any serious breakdown in the communication system inevitably leads to malfunction of one or more cells within the organism, perhaps leading to a disease process, or a more serious disruption that may result in death. A variety of communication or signaling mechanisms exist within the body that include nervous connections, short and long distance chemical signaling compounds that are borne by blood or lymph, and intracellular and transcellular signaling compounds that perform an autocrine or paracrine communication function. The interplay between the various signaling compounds and their respective target cells maintains normal cell growth and function. Loss of communication may lead to uncoordinated growth of a cell, or group of cells, that if not corrected may result in the uncontrolled and aggressive growth of a subset of cells (such as cancer) with resultant injury to normal tissues. A hormone is "a chemical substance, formed in one organ or part of the body and carried in the blood to another organ or part. Depending on the specificity of their effects, hormones can alter the functional activity, and sometimes the structure, of just one organ or of various numbers of them" (1). Blood-borne hormones are equally accessible to all vascularized tissues, yet it was recognized very early by Bayliss (1a) that hormone action was restricted to specific target tissues. This observation led to the concept of a recognition site in the target cells that is capable of concentrating the hormone and an effector site that elicits the specific hormone action (2). Nonresponsive tissues lack either the hormone binding or effector sites or both.

The past two decades have witnessed great advances in the knowledge of receptors and hormone-mediated receptor action in hormone responsive tissues. This chapter is devoted to the discussion of a selected few of the host of cell regulatory or signaling substances (hormones, growth factors) and their receptors, which provide for specificity in hormone/growth factor interaction with cells and tissues within the organism. In this discussion, we refer to the hormone or any other signaling substance that binds to a receptor as a ligand. Formation of a ligand-receptor complex in a cell initiates a sequence of reactions that elicits a function specific to that cell. Target cells have receptors that are specific for that cell type, although a cell may have many different receptors, each of which regulates a different process within the cell. The binding *affinity* of a receptor-ligand complex defines the strength of attraction between the ligand and the receptor, whereas binding *specificity* describes the ability of the receptor to recognize a specific ligand.

CURRENT CONCEPTS IN RECEPTOR STRUCTURE AND FUNCTION

Cell growth and differentiation are regulated by a variety of chemical regulators that act via intracellular or extracellular receptors. These include hormones that are released into the blood and act on distant targets, and growth factors and cytokines that regulate cell function through autocrine or paracrine mechanisms. Several regulators such as gonadal steroids, glucocorticoids, mineralocorticoids, vitamin D, retinoic acid, and thyroid hormones interact with intracellular receptors, which bind to hormone-dependent transcription regulatory regions (hormone response elements) on DNA and effect gene expression. However, the vast majority of regulators of cell function are hydrophilic molecules that exert their action upon the cell through their respective cell surface, or membrane-bound receptors. These include the peptide hormones that are produced by the endocrine glands, and a host of other regulatory compounds, including the growth factors, that exhibit local control of cellular growth. Among these are the peptide class of regulators, known collectively as peptide regulatory factors (PRF). PRFs are generally small molecular weight compounds, that are less than 80 kd in size and have a short or intermediate range of action. These molecules interact with specific high-affinity cell surface receptors, and through this factor/receptor interaction, form a complex that possesses the ability to regulate cellular differentiation and/or proliferation. The nomenclature used in the identification of PRF, has been based upon their biological action, or the assay system used in their original identification and isolation. Examples are the transforming growth factors (TGFα and TGFβ), which were isolated from transformed cells and shown to be capable of inducing the phenotypic transformation of untransformed cells (3). Epidermal growth factor (EGF), gonadotropin releasing hormone (GnRH), somatostatin (SS), insulin-like growth factor I (IGF-I), insulin-like growth factor II (IGF-II), and the several fibroblast growth factors, are all growth-regulating agents for which receptors have been found in normal and malignant tissue (4). Extensive investigations are currently underway to ascertain what role these molecules may play in the growth of normal and tumor tissue, and to examine their utility in determining the prognosis or treatment of endocrine responsive tumors.

As mentioned earlier, there are two major classifications of receptors based upon their location within the cell: (a) intracellular "cytosolic" receptors (e.g., steroid and thyroid hormone receptors) are located within the cell, are closely associated with the chromatin, and exert their action by turning on a specific gene response; and (b) membrane-bound receptors that possess an extracellular domain (recognition site), an intramembrane domain (transmembrane signaling), and an intracellular domain (effector or catalytic site). There are three broad classifications of membrane-bound receptors: (a) allosterically activated enzymes; (b) receptors coupled to an enzyme system via a G protein; and (c) membrane-bound receptors that form a channel by which the transport of ions and other small molecules into and out of the cell is regulated.

Intracellular Receptors

Ligands that bind to intracellular receptors alter the pattern of gene expression and are responsible for slower and longer lasting effects on the cell. They are usually molecules that have low solubility in aqueous solutions but are highly soluble in lipids, a property that facilitates their movement through the lipid-rich cell membrane. All steroid and thyroid hormone receptors, which belong to the *erb*-A superfamily, are very similar in structure, interact with DNA, and elicit their biological effect through ligand-dependent transcription regulation (5). The nature of intracellular receptors is still being clarified. It had been generally well accepted that steroid hormone receptors were present in the cytoplasm of the cell and that upon binding a steroid, the complex was rapidly translocated to the nucleus, where binding to the hormone-responsive element (HRE) regulated specific hormone-induced gene expression. The concept of rapid translocation of the hormone-receptor complex from the cytoplasm to the nucleus was based upon the well-known observation that an unoccupied receptor could be extracted from cells by treatment with low–ionic strength salt buffers and that only steroid-receptor complexes were found in the nucleus. Currently available data indicate that most unoccupied receptors are present in the nucleus in a loosely bound form and are contained in the cytosolic fraction of tissue extracts because it is easily removed from the nuclear envelope with low salt buffers. In target cells that had been previously exposed to hormone, the hormone-receptor complex is tightly bound to the nucleus and is no longer found in the soluble fraction (cytosol) of tissue extracts.

Data verifying the intracellular localization of steroid receptors awaited the development of specific monoclonal antibodies against both the estradiol and progesterone receptors. These studies yielded a wealth of information regarding the location of these receptors within the cell, as well as permitting immunoaffinity purification of these labile proteins. Immunocytochemical staining of frozen sections of human breast cancer tissue, using monoclonal antibody preparations, shows clearly that the gonadal steroid receptors, which appear in the cytosol after tissue homogenization, are localized within the nuclear compartment of the intact cell. Similar observations have been made using the technique of enucleation to minimize contamination between the cytoplasm and nucleoplasm (6). Thus, recent data using procedures capable of localizing gonadal steroid receptors within intact cells or isolated cellular components have shown that estrogen receptors (ERs) and progesterone receptors (PRs) are confined to the nucleus of responsive cells (7). The exception seems to be that unoccupied receptors for glucocorticoids and mineralocorticoids are located in the cytoplasm, and the hormone/receptor complex translocates to the nucleus.

Unoccupied cytosolic receptor has a sedimentation coefficient of about 8S (approximately 300,000 daltons) and contains the receptor molecule and a nonsteroid-binding protein of approximately 90,000 daltons. The nonsteroid-binding protein (heat shock protein (HSP) (8, 9) is released from the 8S form when hormone binds to the receptor. Loss of heat shock protein (HSP) converts the receptor to a smaller, active form (4S), which binds tightly to DNA

(10, 11). The ER has been well characterized and its DNA has been cloned and sequenced (12). It has a molecular weight of approximately 66 kd and contains domains for DNA and steroid binding (7). The proteolytic fragment containing the epitope most readily removed by mercuripapain also contains the DNA-binding domain and suggests a common evolutionary origin. Histologic studies show that the PR, like ER, is confined to the nucleus, but cellular distribution shows considerable heterogeneity throughout the tissue. Cellular production of PR requires the presence of bound ERs.

Members of this receptor superfamily are made up of a single polypeptide that contains three functional regions: (*a*) hormone-binding domain near the C-terminus, which shows specificity of binding to the respective ligand; (*b*) DNA-binding central domain that binds to specific hormone responsive element (HRE) on the chromatin; and (*c*) N-terminus domain that interacts with various factors of the transcriptional machinery as well as the hormone and DNA-binding regions of the receptor. The central domain of about 70 aa is highly conserved and forms two *fingers* (putative DNA-binding site) that are stabilized by a chelated Zn^{2+} ion (13) and interact specifically with HRE on the target genes. When the ER binds to estradiol, a conformational change is induced in the DNA-binding domain of the ER that in turn permits binding to specific regulatory regions of the DNA by the ER-hormone complex with subsequent initiation of gene transcription. Activated receptor binding to DNA is incompletely understood and is still under active investigation, although it appears to involve a hormone- and ATP-dependent phosphorylation-dephosphorylation cycle (14). Some altered proteins appear to have the ability to turn on the transcription of certain proteins, without evidence of binding to DNA (15). Another highly conserved domain of about 250 aa, the ligand-binding domain (LBD), exhibits 70 to 95% homology for the same steroid receptor when examined in different species (16). Binding affinity of the receptor to DNA increases dramatically upon formation of the hormone-receptor complex.

The vitamin D receptor (17) and the retinoic acid receptor (18) also belong to the steroid/thyroid hormone receptor superfamily. Structural changes of certain receptors within this superfamily have been described. These changes affect the ability of the receptor to regulate normal cell function; for example, the variant T_3 receptor, rat (c-*erb*-$A_\alpha 2$) binds DNA but lacks the ability to bind T_3 or to activate gene transcription (19–21). Neoplastic changes could be envisioned in which hormonal control of cell growth is lost because of the inability of an altered receptor to bind ligand, or alternatively, DNA binding may be lost and the ligand binding ability maintained. Either of these changes may prevent the hormonal signal from reaching the specific gene and eliciting its subsequent action.

Membrane-Bound Receptors

Large-protein or polypeptide hormones and PRFs occupy binding or recognition sites on the extracellular domain of membrane-bound receptors and generate an intracellular signal by eliciting a hormone-receptor response that is specific to the occupied receptor. Receptor-mediated responses include activation of any of a number of receptor-associated enzymes such as adenylate cyclase, guanylate cyclase, phosphodiesterases, GTPases, protein kinases, phospholipases, and lipid methylases. Receptors may also elicit their response by interacting with stimulatory or inhibitory G proteins that are part of a complex allosteric enzyme system associated with certain membrane-bound receptors, or they may control the transport of specific ions or selected small molecules into or out of the cell. Other receptor actions may result from an interaction with select cytoskeletal elements, membrane lipids, chromatin proteins, or the receptor enzymatic activity may be regulated by hormone-mediated phosphorylation or glycosylation. In contrast to intracellular receptors, activation of membrane receptors usually results in a rapid response by the target cell, normally within seconds or minutes.

Membrane receptors have been identified as either single membrane-spanning receptors or multiple membrane-spanning receptors. Two types of the single membrane-spanning receptors have been described—those with cytoplasmic tyrosine kinase activity (TKA), and those that lack TKA. Insulin, epidermal growth factor, and platelet-derived growth factor receptors are examples of single membrane-spanning receptors that possess TKA (22), whereas the single membrane-spanning receptors for growth hormone and prolactin lack TKA. Two groups of multiple membrane-spanning receptors have been described: Receptors with ligand-gated channels in which a number of subunits embedded within the plasma membrane make up the channel and single-chain, seven-helix receptors that may be coupled to any of the various signal transducing G proteins.

The control of receptors is usually carried out by the cell. As hormone is bound by cell surface receptors, the complex is internalized and the hormone destroyed. The receptor is either also destroyed or reexpressed on the cell surface. This process removes the hormone from circulation. The other mechanism, involving destruction or reexpression of the receptor, is also a means of self-regulation by the cell. The rate of reexpression of the receptor varies (it is never 100%). The cell also has the ability to synthesize new receptor molecules. Because the number of receptor molecules on the surface of the cell is variable, this serves as self-regulation by the cell. The more receptors available, the more chances for a hormone molecule to bind to its receptor and vice versa.

DISEASE STATES

Tissue Receptors and Cancer

Binding of a hormone to its receptor is required for receptor activation and subsequent biological action. Any molecule that can occupy the receptor binding site without activating the receptor can prevent hormone action by competitive inhibition. Attachment of a molecule, such as an antibody to an epitope or to a location on the receptor that is in close proximity to the binding site can prevent hormone action by steric hindrance. Either of these events would inhibit normal receptor function. In addition to these inhibitory actions on receptor function, any change in the molecular structure of the hormone or its receptor that prevents binding, or reduces binding affinity between the hormone and receptor, can reduce or completely prevent hormone action on the target cell. Each of these events has the potential of altering cell function. Clinical disease may result from an unwanted negative effect of receptor function, or a form of disease treatment may be realized by regulating cell growth through the use of synthetic ligands that will prevent binding and subsequent biological action of endogenous hormones or growth factors.

This type of therapy may be particularly useful in the regulation of hormone-dependent cancers. A number of clinical examples of receptor-mediated disease or treatment of disease have been described. Estrogen and progesterone receptor concentrations are widely used in the determination of prognosis and appropriate treatment regimes to be followed in several endocrine-responsive tumors, with breast cancer being the best example. Long-acting thyroid stimulator (LATS) (23–25) stimulation of the thyroid is an example of a disease process in which antibody stimulation of normal thyroid stimulating hormone (TSH) receptors results in overproduction of a thyroid hormone. Myasthenia gravis is a defect in which the acetylcholine-mediated nerve impulse transmission is impaired and is an example of the steric hindrance of the hormone binding site by endogenous anti-acetylcholine receptor antibodies (26). Testicular feminization syndrome (TFS) and familial hypercholesterolemia (FH) are two examples of disorders resulting from receptor changes; the lack of function or absence of the androgen receptor in TFS, and of the low-density lipoprotein (LD) receptor in the case of FH (27).

The first report implicating hormonal regulation of breast cancer was in 1896, when Sir George Beatson (28) reported the dramatic beneficial effect of oophorectomy in premenopausal women with advanced breast cancer. The first evidence for the existence of tissue receptors for estrogens was obtained *circa* 1960 when Jensen and Jacobson (29) and Glascock and Hoekstra (30) reported the specific uptake of ^{3}H-estrogen in target tissue after systemic administration of labeled hormone. Folca (31) administered tritiated estrogens to women with breast cancer and observed the uptake of radioactivity by the tumor. It was later shown that a significant accumulation of ^{3}H-estradiol occurred in tumors from patients who responded to hormonal therapy while those who were unresponsive to therapy lacked the receptor. The presence of progesterone receptor (PR) in human breast cancer tissue is indicative of estrogen responsiveness (32). The repertoire of prognostic cellular receptors that may be used as markers that are predictive of, or may be predictive of, tumor response to endocrine and chemotherapy treatment regimes is expanding and now includes both intracellular and membrane-bound receptors. The gonadal steroid receptors ER and PR are widely used in prognosis and treatment of breast, endometrial, vulvar, and cervical cancer, and active investigations are examining the potential role that receptors for many of the PRF may play in the prognosis and treatment of a variety of cancers. Several of the small peptides, oncogene products, growth factors, and their respective receptors currently are being examined as potential candidates for improving prognostic accuracy and possible sites of drug interdiction in cancer treatment regimes: these include: EGF, TGF-α, TGF-β, luteinizing hormone-releasing hormone, and somatostatin; the c-*erb*-B2 (a.k.a. *neu*) oncogene product, and Ki67 a nuclear proliferation antigen.

Normal endocrine responsive, or target cells, contain intracellular or membrane-bound receptor sites for each of the hormones known to influence the growth and function of the target tissue. When malignant transformation of a cell occurs, the cell may retain all or part of the normal receptor population, or undergo a structural change in the receptor that alters its function. If the cell retains intracellular receptor sites, steroid control of cell growth and function will probably be maintained as in a normal cell. However, malignant transformation that induces structural alterations may cause the receptor to lose the ability to bind the steroid, or to bind to the HRE on cellular chromatin and thereby lose its transcriptional function. These cells may then no longer recognize circulating hormones and lose endocrine-, autocrine-, or paracrine-mediated functions and fail to respond to endocrine therapy (33). The regulation of growth and function of endocrine target tissues, e.g., breast, and male and female genital tissues, and endocrine responsive tumor growth within these tissues, in many cases is dependent upon hormonal factors produced by endocrine glands, and growth factors elicited by both normal and malignant cells. The role that peptide hormones, gonadal steroids, and autocrine and paracrine growth factors play in the regulation of growth and function of normal and malignant tissue is becoming more clear, almost on a daily basis, as is the role of protein products from the increasing number of oncogenes discovered by modern molecular biology techniques. Many of these recent advances are being put to use in the clinical laboratory as aids in determining the prognosis and appropriate treatment of cancers of various endocrine-responsive tissues.

Current clinical use of receptors includes the analysis of intracellular receptors for estrogens, progestins, androgens, and glucocorticoids. Perhaps the best known example of the clinical utility of laboratory analysis of receptor function is that of estrogen and progesterone receptors in predicting patient response to adjuvant chemotherapy or endocrine therapy in breast cancer. The membrane-bound receptors for EGF, TGFα, TGF-β, and the oncogene protein product from the gene c-*erb*-B2, have also been implicated as prospective means of predicting the response to hormonal therapy and prognosis in carcinomas of the breast, prostate, uterus, ovaries, and cervix, and may be of some assistance in treating glucocorticoid-responsive leukemias. The basic molecular structures of intracellular and extracellular receptors have been determined by the work of a number of research groups, with continuing investigations to relate structure with function.

The clinical utility of tumor levels of ER is well accepted and widely used, even though only about 60% of breast cancers contain ER. Approximately two-thirds of the ER-positive tumors respond to endocrine therapy, and between 5 and 10% of ER-negative tumors also respond to endocrine therapy. Estrogen is known to regulate the production of the progesterone receptor, and the determination of both steroid receptors in breast tumors increases the prognostic value of hormone receptor measurements. Approximately 70% of PR-positive, ER-negative tumors, and 25 to 30% of PR-negative, ER-positive tumors respond to hormonal therapy. The prognosis of receptor-positive mammary tumors is better than receptor-negative carcinomas. The measurement of steroid receptors in tumor tissue does not give absolute information regarding tumor response to endocrine or adjuvent chemotherapy. Rather, it provides an imprecise indication of the response that individual tumors will display. Thus, other factors probably play a role in the regulation of malignant tumor growth. Until the putative cell regulatory factors have been identified, identification of ER or PR receptors in malignant tumors will continue to provide the best standard of care for determining which patients should receive endocrine therapy or adjuvant chemotherapy.

The protein mitogen EGF, a 6000-dalton, 53-amino acid single chain polypeptide, plays an important role in regulating the growth of many ectodermal and mesodermal derived cells and is found in significant levels in the urine, saliva, tears, bile, prostatic fluid, seminal fluid, milk and sweat. The receptor for epidermal growth factor (EGFr) has been identified in most normal cell types with an abundance of receptors in brain, thyroid, lung, liver, skin, placenta, and fetal membranes. EGFr is apparently involved in fetal growth and has been implicated in a number of developmental events, including palate and skin differentiation, growth of follicles, eye opening, tooth eruption, lung maturation, gut and liver growth, and differentiation of neurons. EGFrs are present in normal mammary epithelium (34), on the basal layer of epithelial cells, in normal urothelium, and on cervical and vulvar squamous cell surfaces (35). EGF binding sites have been identified in a variety of tumors, including breast cancer cells (36), in bladder malignancy, where EGFr were found throughout several layers of cells in the urothelium with a rich presence on the surface layer, and in psoriatic skin lesions. There appears to be increased expression of EGFr in some ectodermal-derived tumors over that found in contiguous normal tissue (37). Although it is well known that cell proliferation is the predominant response of normal cells to EGF, the relationship between increased EGFr and tumor growth has only recently come under intensive study, and at present, there is no consensus on the clinical utility and prognostic value of EGFr determination in tumor tissue. Points of consensus appear to be that approximately 45 to 50% of breast cancer patients display EGFr-positive tumors, and there is a negative correlation between the levels of EGFr and the steroid receptors ER and PR. Perhaps the wide variety of methodologies used in the determination of EGFr tissue levels, the lack of uniform measures of positivity (cutoff values) of the test, and the relatively small number of patients studied, has hampered the clinical utility of this test. Many investigators are calling for standardization of EGFr methodologies, similar to what was done with the ER and PR methods, in an attempt to make the test more useful and to facilitate interlaboratory comparisons. A wealth of information regarding EGF and EGFr (and other growth factors and their receptors) is available in a number of different reviews (38), and an abbreviated review follows in this chapter. This line of research will certainly lead to a better understanding of the endocrine, autocrine, and paracrine control of normal and malignant tissue, and may aid in the treatment of all types of cancer. If the uncontrolled growth of cells, which is characteristic of cancer, is subject to some combination of endocrine, autocrine, or paracrine control, as seems likely, then information regarding the systemic and local regulation of growth factors (GF) and growth factor receptors (GFr) may provide new treatment modalities for endocrine-responsive cancers and those cancers that appear to be independent of endocrine control.

The virus growth factor EGF-like protein also binds to the EGFr and is thought to be used for cell access by the virus. Other members of the family of small proteins that bind to EGFr are transforming growth factor α (TGF-α), platelet-derived growth factor (PDGF), and amphiregulin. While EGF and TGF-α bind with almost equal affinity, amphiregulin has a significantly lower affinity for the receptor. Amphiregulin is a weaker growth stimulator than either EGF or TGF-α except for the stimulation of keratinocyte growth, where it is equivalent to the other two proteins. Because the binding affinity of amphiregulin for the EGFr is much lower than the other two proteins, it is natural to assume that there is a primary bind for amphiregulin, but this site has not yet been found (39).

EGF and the transforming growth factors α and β (TGF-α and TGF-β) (40) are capable of enhancing or inhibiting *in vitro* cell growth in human endometrial carcinoma cell line (RL95-2) cultures, depending upon GF concentration and cell plating density. TGF-β inhibits cell proliferation at both high and low plating density and induces the appearance of large cuboidal cells that are distinct from EGF- or TGF-α–treated cells. EGF, TGF-α, and TGF-β effects appeared to be similar in hCG-producing tumors transplanted into nude mice (41). Low concentrations of EGF (5 μg) stimulated tumor growth and increased EGFr levels, whereas high EGF concentrations (50 μg) inhibited tumor growth and reduced EGFr in the tumors. TGF-α mimicked the effects of EGF and actively competed for EGFr binding sites, whereas TGF-β competed only slightly with EGF for EGFr binding sites. EGF and TGF-α levels have been compared between extracts of malignant and nonmalignant tissues (42). Approximately 30% of ovarian, endometrial, and cervical carcinomas, and 16% of breast carcinomas had elevated GF levels compared to normal tissues. In nonmalignant tissue, the mean GF concentration was 1.5 ± 0.7 ng/ml (0 to 4 ng/ml), whereas concentrations in carcinomas were significantly higher (ovarian carcinomas 4.2 ± 1.5 ng/mg (0 to 15 ng), endometrial carcinomas 4.5 ± 1.7 ng/mg (0 to 12 ng), cervical carcinomas 4.15 ± 1.1 ng/mg (0 to 8), and breast carcinomas 3.16 ± 1.1 ng/mg (0 to 10 ng). Increased levels of these growth factors (GF) may indicate autocrine or paracrine control of growth in neoplastic tissue through an autologous control of GF production by the tumor that is independent of endocrine control or perhaps loss of endocrine control of cell growth as the neoplastic process proceeds.

Distribution of EGFr appears to differ between normal and malignant urothelium. Messing showed that most (95%) normal urothelium contained EGFrs in the basal layer of the epithelial cells, whereas in patients with urothelial carcinomas there was a significant concentration of EGFrs on the surface as well as in the deeper layers, and EGFr density was correlated with tumor grade (43). Tumor growth and EGFr levels appear to be correlated. An increase in the production of EGFr may enhance the autocrine or paracrine stimulation of cell proliferation and may thus relate to tumor growth and metastatic potential. Gene amplification and overexpression of EGFr and mRNA of the *erb*-B2 oncogene have been found in mammary carcinomas. The increased EGFr levels may provide a growth advantage in cells in which overexpression of the EGFr has occurred. In contrast, EGFr concentration and prevalence is lower in endometrial adenocarcinoma than in normal endometrium (44, 45). Further, tumor grade and its relationship to EGFr is confusing. Berchuck (44) reported no correlation for these two variables, whereas Reynolds (45) showed a clear decrease in EGFr levels with advancing tumor grade. Reynolds et al. (46) have also shown that EGFr can be regulated in endometrial adenocarcinomas by estradiol and progesterone. Endometrial cells cultured with estradiol showed a decrease in EGFr in normal and malignant tissue, while progesterone treatment increased EGFr concentrations. Increasing density of EGFr sites on the cervical and vulval squamous cell carcinomas has been related to the aggressiveness of this type of tumor. In particular, it was found that levels of EGFr greater than 100 fmol/mg of protein had poor prognosis, while levels less than 100 fmol/mg of protein had more favorable outcomes (relative to recurrence and 5-year survival) (35). ER concentration was inversely correlated with EGFr in both normal and neoplastic breast and endometrial tissue (47), perhaps indicating that down-regulation of EGFr is one of the biological effects of estradiol, whereas IGF-I binding was not affected by estradiol or progesterone treatment.

Certain oncogene products show striking similarities to some GF receptors. The c-*erb*-B2 oncogene protein product is a molecule in which the transmembrane and cytoplasmic regions are homologous to the 170-kd single membrane-spanning receptor, EGFr. This glycoprotein has an extracellular domain that is highly protease resistant, heat stable, and contains the EGF binding site, an intracellular domain that contains intrinsic tyrosine kinase activity (22), and a transmembrane portion that connects these two domains. The cytoplasmic region of the EGFr is homologous to the protein product of the v-*erb*-B1 oncogene. The c-*erb*-B2 is an oncogene that has been localized to chromosome 17, and codes for a 185-kd transmembrane protein that, although structurally similar to EGFr, lacks part of the extracellular EGF recognition site.

It is noteworthy that while the capacity of the receptors increased, the affinity did not. This leads to the conclusion that it is simply an increase in the number of EGFrs and not a change in the actual receptor. In some cases, amplification of gene coding has been demonstrated. However, overexpression of this gene did not always result in increased EGFr. Other factors that might come into play here include increased transcription of the gene (over other genes); reduced degradation of the mRNA allowing more "readings" by the ribosome; and reduced receptor degradation, which might keep the cell "turned on" longer.

Growth factors with TKA stimulate cell growth and proliferation by attaching phosphates to proteins through the tyrosine or serine residues, effect cell proliferation, and may induce the phenotypic transformation of cells. The enzymatic activity is directed against several protein substrates, including the receptor itself. This latter activity includes autophosphorylation and evokes phosphorylation of a variety of cellular substrates, which is the first step in signal transduction (48). TKA is constituently active in the oncogene protein product, whereas EGFr requires the presence of EGF bound to the extracellular moiety of the receptor for kinase activity to be initiated.

Comparisons of GF receptors in normal endometrium and endometrial cancers are important because tyrosine kinase genes have the potential to mutate to an oncogene form and to produce malignant transformations. Information gained by the determination of GF receptor concentrations and their binding affinities in normal and neoplastic tissues may lead to various new treatment regimes and provide prognostic information that is not currently available. Treatments may take the form of (*a*) biologically inactive analogs of growth factors that are capable of binding to and inactivating the receptor; (*b*) receptor-specific antibodies that recognize epitopes on the extracellular domains of the receptor and sterically hinder binding of the GF to the receptor; (*c*) antibodies with attached cytotoxins that can be released into the cell following endocytosis; or (*d*) regulation of GF receptor production with estrogens, progesterones, or their biologically inactive competitive inhibitors.

METHODOLOGIES

Intracellular Receptor Analyses

In 1961, Folca (31) demonstrated that the uptake of [^{3}H]-hexestrol in vivo by breast cancer tissues was higher in four patients who responded to adrenalectomy than in 6 others who did not respond to the surgery (49). This observation led to the development of in vitro techniques using [^{3}H]-estradiol to study tissue binding in primary and metastatic breast tumors. Estrogen receptors in organs have been measured in vitro using either tissue slices or cell-free preparations. The first quantifications were performed by sucrose density gradient (SDG) analysis, which demonstrates the molecular forms of the receptor (50). While these early studies concerned themselves with ERs, the importance of understanding the role of all receptors in general has become apparent. This has led to a need to quantify and characterize receptors as a class. Over the last few years, many studies have been undertaken toward this goal. The longer history of the study of ERs has produced a body of knowledge about these receptors that is not yet accumulated for the other receptors. Thus, some of the specific comments in the methodology descriptions may only be applicable to ERs. Even though these methods have general applications, the newer receptors (e.g., EGFr) suffer from the lack of accepted standards and protocols, so quantitative comparisons are often not meaningful. Of particular importance has been the recent application of monoclonal antibodies to this endeavor, which has led to the development of techniques that are rapidly replacing the other methodologies.

In addition to new methodologies, our models are also changing. In particular, until recently, ERs were thought to reside in cytosol in the unbound state and were transferred to the nucleus when they became activated through bonding to estradiol. Studies with newer methodologies have shown us that these receptors in fact are all in or associated with the nucleus. Thus, when reviewing some of the more classic procedures, it is necessary to keep in mind that the model of intracellular ER location has evolved. Finally, it should be noted that the only receptor assays currently performed in the clinical laboratory are the dextran-coated charcoal, (DCC) assays, immunoassays, and immunocytochemical assays (ICAs).

SPECIMEN COLLECTION AND PREPARATION

Hormone receptors are heat-labile proteins. It is necessary that they be stored immediately at 4°C if the sample can be assayed within an hour. Otherwise, they should be frozen and stored in liquid nitrogen. Dry ice may be utilized for short storage (a few days) if liquid nitrogen is not available. Alternately, the cytosol can be lyophilized and stored at 4°C. The receptor is pH sensitive with maximum stability at pH 7.4. Low protein content can lead to underestimation of receptors in the DCC assay. Thus, with a low concentration of receptors, a minimum of 3 mg/ml of protein is suggested, but for higher concentrations of receptors, the protein concentration can be as low as 1 mg/ml. Miller (51) has reported that inclusion of molybdate (10 to 20 millimolar) in the extraction buffer increases the assay levels of both PR and ER. A tumor with an ER or PR concentration of 3 to 10 femtomoles of estradiol per milligram of protein or higher is usually considered estrogen receptor positive. The exact cutoff value differs among laboratories. Some laboratories have suggested that recent information shows the value of 10 fmol/mg is more clinically relevant.

Receptor inactivation can occur within intact tissues, e.g., through prolonged exposure of excised intact tumor tissue to high temperatures. Further, steroid receptors may be inactivated during the tissue handling procedures before and during the cytosol preparation through high temperatures or excess homogenization. Finally, steroid receptors may be inactivated after they have been partitioned into the cytosol fraction of the tissue during the receptor assay procedure. These cytosolic receptors may be inactivated by such agents as high temperature, high ionic strength, pH changes, exposure to active proteases or phosphatases, and oxidation of sulfhydryl groups.

PHYSICAL SEPARATIONS

Centrifugation

Dextran-Coated Charcoal Assay. Determination of receptor concentrations using dextran-coated charcoal (DCC) utilizes the adsorptive properties of charcoal to remove small and large molecular weight compounds from solution at different rates (52, 53). Low–molecular weight compounds are removed very quickly, leaving the larger compounds in solution. The procedure is very time- and temperature-dependent, with dextran being used to partially coat the charcoal particles and reduce the adsorptive properties of charcoal. This process reduces the rate and extent of adsorption of large molecular weight compounds such as proteins. The method has been widely used for the separation of free and receptor-bound radioactive ligands in the quantification of most steroid receptors. It is a sensitive and popular assay procedure and has formed the basis for most of the quality assurance, or proficiency testing programs such as the College of American Pathologists and Southwest Oncology Group. The assay is performed by using increasing concentrations of radiolabeled hormone and a concurrent range of unlabeled hormone competitor to titrate the receptor to a saturation endpoint. Specific and saturable binding can be determined by subtracting the nonspecific (nonsaturable) binding from the total binding to both specific and nonspecific sites. Specific binding can be converted to the total number of binding sites, expressed as femtomoles per milligram of protein. The dissociation constant (K_d) is a measure of the affinity of the receptor for the steroid and is approximately equal to the concentration of free steroid at which one-half the receptors are saturated. K_d is the reciprocal of K_a and can be also obtained from a Scatchard plot (54). The values obtained from the DCC method correlate well with those of the sucrose gradient methods (to follow). It is sensitive, inexpensive, and relatively easy to perform. A modification designed to hasten this assay is to use only two data points, and to assume a linear relationship. This can give workable results, but if more than one binding site is present on the receptor, the value for K_d is greatly undervalued (55).

Sucrose Density-Gradient Ultracentrifugation. This was the first ER assay applied in a routine clinical setting. The measurable quantity here is sedimentation velocity of proteins as a function of molecular weight and density. It is a long procedure because of the required centrifugation times (16 hours in a swinging bucket head). The cytosol is incubated with labeled hormone and centrifuged through a sucrose gradient. The layers are counted and compared to known markers (e.g., BSA–4.6S and IgG—6.8S). Resolution is limited, but most tumors display the presence of an 8S estrogen receptor and some also the 4S form. It has been suggested that only the 8S form of the receptor complex has predictive value for the endocrine responsiveness of a given tumor (52). The presence of molybdate in the gradient increased the amount of receptor observed in the assay. This is especially true when the progesterone receptor is being measured. This method estimates the quantity and size of the receptor molecules, but it is a slow and expensive procedure.

Precipitation. The receptor is precipitated with protamine (56) followed by incubation with excess labeled hormone. At 4°C, the receptor sites bind to the labeled hormone, leaving unbound labeled steroid in solution. The method has a very high nonspecific background and tends to give low concentrations when compared with others.

When using ammonium sulfate to precipitate the receptor fraction, Chen (57) reported that at 50% saturation, 77% of the ER and 53% of the PR precipitated. Saturation of less than 50% resulted in a significant reduction in the recovery of receptor. ERs and PRs salted out in the ammonium sulfate pellet are stable and store better than the cytosol preparation.

Chromatography

Gel Filtration and Immobilized Antisteroid Antibodies. This assay is infrequently performed and has no advantages over the other commonly performed assays. After incubation of the cytosol with labeled hormone, the mixture is passed through a Sephadex column with the receptor-hormone complex eluting in the void volume (58). Sephadex competes slightly with the receptor for E2, which can cause some dissociation of the receptor-hormone complex (about 15%) and leads to a false decrease in the amount of receptor measured. Columns packed with gels containing bound anti-E2 have been used in a similar fashion with similar results. The primary advantage of the use of this immunoaffinity method is the ability to quantify receptor levels with smaller samples.

Hydroxyapatite Assay. The hormone-receptor complex is adsorbed onto hydroxyapatite either in "batch" or column form and the free steroid and plasma contaminants are removed by washing (58). The assay is more reliable at low protein concentrations than with the DCC method. It can be performed on small samples.

Diethylaminoethyl Anion Exchange Chromatography. Steroid receptors are acidic proteins that will bind to anion exchange resins such as DEAE-cellulose (59). The major problems of this method include the tendency of free E2 and testosterone to bind to DEAE at low ionic strength and the inability of receptors to bind to the column at high ionic strength. Analysis of molecular forms of the receptor and separation from nonreceptor binding proteins is easily achieved.

Controlled Pore Glass Beads. The receptors bind strongly to controlled pore glass beads, followed by saturation with labeled hormone and elution from the column by ethanol for analysis (60).

High-Performance Liquid Chromatography. Although equipment is expensive, the required solvents are inexpensive, and good column separation usually can be obtained between the analyte and other compounds present in the sample. There are several different kinds of high-performance liquid chromatography (HPLC) analyses with the differentiation being based on the type of column used:

- High-performance size exclusion chromatography (HPSEC) utilized polyethylene glycol (PEG) gel beads to prepare columns that separate mixtures based on their molecular size and configuration. This has the ability to separate the various aggregates that the receptor displays. These columns are usually run at lower pressures and employ aqueous buffers. It gives the same type of information as obtained in the sucrose gradient method with better resolution and in less time (61).
- Reverse-phase liquid chromatography (RPLC): The elution of a receptor protein from an RP column requires high concentrations of organic solvent in the mobile phase, which may irreversibly denature the proteins (62). Affinity columns have also been employed with HPLC.
- High-performance hydrophobic interaction chromatography (HPHIC) is the mildest application of HPLC to the separation of protein molecules with retention of their biological activity. The stationary phase is nonionic and binds the hydrophobic patches present in the protein. Unlike most HPLC procedures that employ denaturing solvents, this column allows the use of physiological pH buffers (63).
- High-performance ion exchange chromatography (HPIEC). This methodology relies on the same principle as the DEAE method (described earlier). The column is packed with an anion exchange resin. The elution gradient proceeds from low to high ionic strength, which can be as high as 500 mM phosphate (63).

Electrophoresis

Agar Gel Electrophoresis. The receptor-hormone complex is separated and found on the anodal side of the well, while two peaks representing steroid hormone-binding globulin and free steroid are found on the cathodic side (64). The method compares favorably with other methods, particularly when the cytosol is treated briefly with DCC before electrophoresis to remove most of the free and albumin-bound steroid.

Isoelectric Focusing. Separation is accomplished through charge properties. In comparison with other methods, isoelectric focusing is sensitive and rapid (1.5 to 2 hours). Vollmer (65) describes an assay employing two different isotopes (^{125}I and ^{3}H) for the simultaneous determinations of ER and PR with correlations to the single isotope assay of 0.93 and 0.8, respectively.

IMMUNOASSAYS

The development of the monoclonal antibody has had a significant impact on the assay methodologies for receptors. To develop the antibody, the receptor is first isolated by affinity chromatography. The respective steroid or protein is bound to the column (usually a gel) and the homogenate containing the receptor passed through. The receptor binds to the immobilized ligand and, after washing the column, is eluted off (usually, through change in pH or ionic strength). This purified receptor is then employed to develop a monoclonal antisera using standard techniques.

Immunoradiometric Assays

A typical immunoradiometric assay (IRMA) would incorporate two monoclonal antisera that bind to different sites on the receptor (66). One of the antibodies is attached to a solid phase to serve as the capture antibody. After incubation of the solid-phase capture antibody with homogenate, the unreacted (unbound) material is washed away. Then the second monoclonal antibody, which is labeled with ^{125}I, is introduced. The solid phase is given another wash and then counted. This assay gives good correlation to earlier biochemical methods. The method is independent of binding of E2 to the receptors because the epitopes recognized by the antibodies are not hidden when the hormone binds to the receptor.

Enzyme Immunoassay

Recently, commercial monclonal-based enzyme immunoassays (EIAs) were made available (67) for both ER and PR. The assay methodology is identical to the radiometric method except that a horseradish peroxidase–labeled second antibody is employed. The assay is read by development of o-phenylenediamine (OPD). Results are consistent with other receptor assays (68, 69) but with somewhat higher values. The sensitivity of the PR EIA falls off for values below 10 fmol/mg (70, 71). The ER assay can be extended to 5 fmol/mg (69). To date, no single threshold value for the ER-EIA has won universal acceptance (72, 73).

BOUND RECEPTOR ASSAYS

The continuing studies aimed at understanding the intercellular localization of the steroid receptors have already been discussed. This had an impact on the development of ER assays. Historically, nuclear estrogen receptors were considered to be bound receptors, and those in the cytoplasm to be "free" receptors. Here, "bound" receptors means complexed to their respective steroid. For ER and PR, two receptors sites appear to be present. For the ER, the site with the higher affinity for estradiol has the characteristics (concentration, affinity, and specificity) attributed to the receptor. The second site, called type II estrogen binding site (EBS), displays the steroid and tissue specificy but it is not the true ER. It is present in higher concentration but displays a lower apparent affinity. There appears to be a close relationship between increased levels of type II receptors and true uterine growth.

The currently accepted models for depicting the intercellular location of receptor sites for the ER and PR show that both the bound and free receptors reside exclusively in the nucleus. The receptors for glucocorticoid (GR) appear to reside in both the cytoplasm and nucleoplasm. This leaves us with the task of understanding what the earlier ER assays were measuring in the cytoplasm, for both biochemical and cytochemical assays. In the biochemical assays, it is necessary to first prepare a cytosol. The preparation involves extensive homogenization of the tissue, freezing, and centrifugation. This treatment artificially separates the total cellular ER into nuclear and cytosolic fractions. Many researchers feel that the free receptors are not as tightly bound in or to the nucleus and the addition of buffer in this process causes the migration of free receptors in the cytosol. While this can explain what is biochemically measured in the cytosol, the preparation of slides may not be so destructive toward the cell and may require a different explanation. One possibility is that the type II EBS receptors are being measured here.

Biochemical assays of bound receptors are based on the principle that the receptor-estrogen complex dissociates slowly at low temperatures and rapidly at higher temperatures. The nucleus contains both bound and free receptors. To effect an exchange with the exogenous labeled estradiol, the nuclear fractions are incubated in the presence of labeled estradiol at elevated temperatures (usually 25° to 37°C). The relative quantities of free to bound receptors vary according to the hormonal milieu at the time of tumor excision. In a premenopausal or a postmenopausal tamoxifen-treated patient, the unbound receptors should be lowest and bound receptors highest, while the opposite would be true in postmenopausal women. Thus, it is sometimes desirable to evaluate both occupied and unoccupied receptor sites. In these assays, conditions are controlled (e.g., temperature) to reduce the amount of exchange.

Sucrose Pad Nuclear Exchange Assay. This approach incorporates centrifugation of tissue homogenates through 1.2 molar sucrose, which removes the large amounts of lipid present (74). This effects a reduction of the nonspecific binding from 80% to 10 to

40%. The lipid components sediment only to the buffer/sucrose interface, while the desired nuclear material continues through to the bottom of the tube. The sucrose pad nuclear exchange assay (SPA) can be modified to optimally measure the type II EBS that is thought to be related to estrogen-dependent growth. The assay is very tedious, requiring technical skill, and cannot be used as a single-point assay.

Protamine Sulfate Assay. By incubating a KCL-extracted nuclear fraction at 25° to 30°C for several hours, the previously bound hormone can be exchanged, while at 4°C only unoccupied receptor sites bind to labeled hormone (75). A major disadvantage of this method is degradation of the receptor at the higher temperature due to the proteolytic activity found in human tumor nuclear extracts.

Hydroxyapatite Exchange Procedure. Both bound and unbound receptors bind to hydroxyapatite (HAP). This is similar to the procedure with protamine sulfate, except that the labeled hormone is incubated with the (HAP) bound receptors at the requisite temperature (76). This method appears to be superior to the protamine sulfate assay.

Mersalyl Exchange Method. Exchange of bound nuclear receptor complexes may be achieved at 0° to 4°C in the presence of molybdate and mersalyl acid (77). Specific binding is subsequently measured by the hydroxyapatite procedure. This assay does not lead to receptor degradation or incomplete exchange as often occurs with temperature-dependent exchanges.

Sodium Thiocyanate (NaSCN) Exchange Assay. This assay uses NaSCN during the exchange process, which solubilizes the receptors. Exchange is carried out at 4°C in the presence of NaSCN (78).

ANALYSIS OF mRNA USING POLYMERASE CHAIN REACTION TECHNIQUES

McGuire (79) describes a simplified polymerase chain reaction (PCR) technique sensitive enough to detect ERs mRNA in breast tumor specimens from 1 μg of total RNA. In a preliminary evaluation of this method on a small series of breast tumors, the ER message was found in tumors that were positive by the DCC assay. One tumor that was ER-negative by the ligand binding assay but positive for PR was examined by the PCR method and found to contain the ER mRNA. It is known that about 2 to 11% of breast cancers are apparently ER-negative but PR-positive in the DCC assay (80). Perhaps, since PR is an end product of estrogen action, the ER in these tumors is defective in ligand binding but capable of stimulating PR.

Membrane-Bound Receptor Analyses

The need to quantitate membrane receptors is a recent one. Analysis of membrane receptors accomodates techniques employed for cytosolic receptors with the added complication that we are now dealing with tissue. Preparation of the membrane sample is critical because it is necessary to eliminate residual cytosol, which, if present, will give artificially low results. This washing also releases most of the EGF receptor trapped in the nuclear pellet. For clinical use, one washing cycle may be adequate (81). EGFr values greater than 10 fmol/mg of protein appear to be significant, and more than 100 fmol/mg of protein is significant in cervical carcinoma.

SATURATION AND DISPLACEMENT

The most common assays for membrane receptors are radiometric saturation and displacement assays employing ^{125}I-labeled ligands (82). As in the saturation assay for cytosolic receptors, increasing amounts of labeled ligand are reacted with fixed amounts of tissue sample. This also requires the determination of nonspecific binding (NSB), which requires that each of the above points be done both in the presence of a large excess of cold ligand and in the absence of the cold ligand.

A variation of this is the displacement assay. A fixed amount of tissue and labeled ligand are equilibrated with increasing amounts of cold ligand. The separation of free from bound in tissue assays is usually done by centrifugation (15,000 g for 5 minutes), with the resulting tissue pellet being counted in a gamma counter. Polyethylene glycol (PEG) has been utilized to enhance precipitation. Rapid filtration has also been utilized, with the membrane material being trapped on the filter and subsequently counted. Both the saturation and displacement assays are analyzed with Scatchard plots. Both methods give comparable binding capacities (or specific binding), but the displacement assay often understimates the association constant.

The saturating and displacement assays require multiple points. Thus, a sizable amount of tissue is necessary (100 μg of tissue for each assay tube). To reduce the tissue requirement, and to simplify the procedure, a single-point saturation assay has emerged (83). In this assay, two points are needed: (a) the tissue sample with a fixed amount of labeled ligand; and (b) the tissue with the labeled ligand plus a large excess (usually about 100-fold) unlabeled ligand. Difference in binding between these two points is the specific binding. This is converted into % of total (B/T) and multiplied by the concentration of labeled ligand. This is then converted into fmoles of receptor/mg of protein. The assay must be calibrated for each type of receptor and type of tissue to determine the optimum amount of tracer (usually the "50%" point on a Scatchard curve) and cold ligand.

IMMUNOADSORPTION

Tissue receptors can be solubilized with Triton X-100. However, for some receptors (i.e., EGFr) Triton X-100 also inactivates the receptor (84). This effect appears to be Triton X-100 concentration-dependent. Thus, utilization of this methodology requires awareness of this potential problem. EGF tissue receptors solubilized with Triton X-100 are immunoadsorbed onto microtiter wells coated with mouse anti-EGFr (85). From this point, either a radiolabel or an enzyme label can be introduced.

Use of a radiolabel requires incubating the captured EGFr with increasing concentrations of ^{125}I-EGF in the presence and absence of excess unlabeled EGF. After washing the wells and counting, a Scatchard analysis is carried out.

When an enzyme is utilized as a label, a second anti-EGFr monoclonal antibody (moAb) is incubated with the immobilized EGFr and is subsequently analyzed through bonding of this sandwich complex to a goat antimouse IgG-labeled with peroxidase. A colorimetric signal is generated through treatment of the wells with *o*-phenylenediamine. The results are compared to a standard curve from which the binding capacity can be read. Solubilized A431 cells are used to prepare the standard curve. This procedure does not yield a binding constant. However, since only a single point is needed for the unknown, the amount of sample tissue needed is greatly reduced.

WESTERN BLOT

A Western blot procedure has been developed for EGFr (86). Purified membranes are solubilized with nonionic detergent and resolved by electrophoresis. This is followed by electroblotting onto nitrocellulose and rehybridizing with ^{125}I-EGF. The receptor is identified by bands at 150 and 170 kd. The presence of 1% hemoglobin and 0.005% Tween 20 during the hybridization step optimizes the radiogram signal.

Cytochemical Analysis

In these procedures, the objective is to detect the receptors by attaching a label to the receptor that can be visualized. The cell is left intact, so the methodology is applicable to both intracellular and membrane-bound receptors. It is performed by fixing sections of the tumor tissue in graded ethanols, on uncoated glass slides, followed by incubation with the appropriate labeling material.

LIGAND-CONJUGATE LABEL

Various types of labels have been employed , the earliest being tritiated estradiol, which is then read by autoradiography (87). Conjugating steroid molecules to proteins to which fluorescent molecules or peroxidase are attached allows the direct visual identification of receptor sites in the cells. Early studies showed an accumulation of label in the cytoplasm. This finding presumably depicted the location of the receptor binding site, which was consistent with the steroid binding assays where ERs were found in the cytosolic fraction of the tissue extracts. Quantification of the binding sites is obtained by estimating the intensity of the fluorescence. Also demonstrated by this technique is the mosaic distribution of ER-positive cells in the tumor. Since there is neither uniformity of distribution of binding sites nor of intensities, a system was developed to give an "average" intensity. This was designed to provide some correlation to the DCC assay results. Using this averaging technique, the results were comparable to the reference assay (DCC).

One major problem with the cytochemical assay is that it does not supply information about the affinity of the binding site (88). Without this information, it is difficult to show that the ER sites that were being measured by the biochemical assays were the same as those visualized by the cytochemical methods. In fact, we now have strong evidence that the primary ER sites, which have the highest binding affinity, reside in the nucleus. This raises the question of what earlier cytochemical analyses were identifying in the cytoplasm. It has been suggested that the cytoplasmic estrogen binding sites represent secondary, low-affinity sites. Scatchard analysis of the data of DCC assays shows two binding sites for estradiol, with the K_d of the second site about 100-fold less than the K_d of the first.

ANTIRECEPTOR ANTIBODY METHODS

Immunocytochemical assays are performed by fixing sections in graded ethanols, on uncoated glass slides, followed by incubation with labeled monoclonal antibodies (33). The bound antibodies can be visualized by the indirect immunoperoxidase method (89) or through the use of fluorescent or chemiluminescent labels. Using this technique to localize ERs, it was observed that the staining was almost exclusively in the nucleus, as opposed to the cytoplasm, where earlier studies had placed it. (Interestingly, earlier cytochemical work using a tritium label also located the receptor in the nucleus, but apparently these data were not widely accepted.) Further, the intensity of the nuclear staining correlated to the amount of ER determined by the sucrose den-

Table 64.1 Common Sources of Error in Receptor Assays

False-Negative Results	False-Positive Results	Other Errors
Inappropriate specimen collection	Tumor heterogeneity	Choice of cold competitor, i.e., diethyl stilbestrol (DES) for E2 or cortisol for PR
Improper storage	Receptor defects	Concentration and incubation time (DCC assay)
Excess manipulation	Binding to ligand	Salt concentration
Dilution of tumor with receptor-negative fibrous tissue	Binding to DNA sites	Sites already occupied by endogenous steroid or drug—important with PR—reflective of the milieu
		Where in menstrual cycle sample is obtained
		Whether pre- or postmenopausal
		Assay of neighboring nonmalignant tissue (due to omission during pathologists exam of sample.)

sity gradient analysis, and detectable staining was always absent in the receptor-negative tumors. At present, the method is only semiquantitative, and it is usually considered as an adjunct to the biochemical assays. However, the continued development of intensity analysis will improve the quantitative aspects of this assay. As with the cytochemical analysis, ICA does not provide any quantitative information about the binding strength of the receptor.

One of the puzzling aspects of the use of steroid therapy in the treatment of breast cancer is the large number of positive ER tumors that do not respond to this therapy (20 to 40%) and, conversely, the number of ER-negative tumors that do respond to therapy (about 10%). The application of cytochemistry has highlighted one facet of this problem, which is the heterogeneity within the breast tumor. There can be within the tumor benign tissue that is ER positive while the rest of the tumor is ER negative. Conversely, an ER-positive sample might be so diluted with fibrous tissue that it gives a negative ER result.

Another interesting application combines flow cytometry and ICA to quantify PR and simultaneously perform a DNA assay (90). This allows the assignment of PR levels in subsets of cells segregated by their DNA content. In the T47D cell, PR were present throughout the cell cycle and levels doubled in G2 and mitosis.

Errors in Receptor Measurements

Receptors are thermolabile, pH and ionic strength-dependent. They can be mechanically destroyed during homogenization. Addition of reducing agents as dithiothreitol, molybdate, or glycerol to protect from oxidation can be helpful. Low values can result from too little protein in the sample. Another problem is interference by nonreceptor binders such as albumin, corticosteroid-binding globulin, and sex hormone-binding globulin (SHBG). Common sources of error are shown in Table 64.1.

INTERPRETATION

Tissue Receptors and Cancer

Clinically, endocrine-responsive tumors are assayed for receptor concentration and affinity. These include intracellular receptors for estrogens, progesterones, androgens and glucocorticoids. Recent developments have implicated the membrane-bound receptor EFGr and its related oncogene product from the gene c-*erb*-B2 in predicting the response to hormonal therapy and prognosis in breast, endometrial, prostatic, and certain renal carcinomas, and may be of some assistance in treating glucocorticoid-responsive leukemias.

BREAST CANCER

Breast cancer accounts for 30% of all cancers and 18% of all female cancer deaths. Although there is a 10% lifetime risk of breast cancer in females, there is a 90% 5-year survival rate if treatment is initiated in stage I of the disease. Survival drops to 60% if the cancer has metastasized before treatment is instituted(91). Mammography and self-examination are the best methods of early detection in risk populations. Prognosis and treatment are based on tumor size, clinical stage, histologic grade, axillary lymph node status, and the presence and binding capacity of ER and PR. More recently, growth factor receptors and oncogene protein products have been used experimentally. Generally, patients with nodal metastases have a worse prognosis than those who do not. However, about 25 to 30% of the so-called axillary node negative patients die from their disease within 10 years. A further problem using nodal status as a prognosis marker is the extensive, mutilating surgery that does not enhance survival. Patients are opting for more conservative treatment.

A good prognostic marker should provide information on the tumor cell proliferation rates and metastatic potential, and it also should indicate what therapy is appropriate. Lastly, it should be attainable with a minimum of surgical intervention. In recent years, many potential biochemical markers have been described. These included steroid hormone receptors, growth-factor receptors, activated proto-oncogenes and proteolytic enzymes (92, 93).

Estradiol and Progesterone Receptors

While receptor assays identify specific groups of patients who have a significant chance of successful estrogen treatment, the overall predictive value of the information obtained from receptor assays shows considerable disagreement in the literature. In 1977, Knight (94) showed that the absence of ER in breast tumors was associated with early recurrent disease. The role of ERs has been studied since then, and is still not clearly understood. Using the DCC assay to look for the presence of ER and PR in 4000 cases of breast cancer, Thorpe (95) described three categories: positive for ER and PR or negative ER with positive PR were hormone responsive; negative ER and PR were nonresponsive; and positive ER with negative PR gave unpredictable response (this latter category consisted mostly of postmenopausal patients).

One confusing aspect that arises when attempting to use ER content as a prognostic factor in breast cancer lies in the assays themselves. Some assays measure only unbound (to estradiol) receptor, while other assays measure total ER (see Methodologies). Thus, Syne (50) noted that there were ambiguities of response to estrogen therapy in premenopausal women whose tumors contain low levels of ER, as determined by a binding assay that primarily measures the "free" receptor. He questioned whether the low "free" receptor level in the cytoplasm was due to the influence of high levels of circulating estrogens or whether the tumor truly lacks estrogen receptor. Conversely, the high ER content of a breast tumor from an elderly postmenopausal woman may indicate a strongly ER-positive tumor or the lack of endogenous estrogen production needed to bind the usual amount of estrogen receptor to the DNA. Other studies have shown that in some so-called "false-negatives" there is a lack of unbound ER, but they do contain bound ER. Conversely, some "false-positives" (patients with ER that do not respond to estrogen therapy) show that the tumors contain "free" ER but no hormone-bound ER.

McGuire (96) has shown that for the stage I cancer patient, ER status and tumor size were the two most important prognostic factors. In stage II breast-cancer patients however, progesterone receptor (PR) status appeared to be a better prognostic marker.

Other factors have been evaluated as prognostic indicators. Hill (97) tried grouping the occurrence of ER in premenopausal patients based on body mass. He found that women with a lean body mass have a greater proportion of negative ER tumors and a higher concentration of EFGr than heavier women. In males, with the exception of a predominance of centrally located lesions and a uniquely high frequency of positive hormone receptor status, carcinoma of the breast appears biologically similar to the disease in women, and treatment should be guided by similar principles (98).

While different methodologies for receptor assays are a factor in these varied observations, there are other operative variables, which include (*a*) different cutoff points used; (*b*) different patient follow-up times; (*c*) different patient populations with respect to menopausal status, disease stage, and adjuvant treatment; (*d*) different statistical tests used to analyze the data; (*e*) small numbers of patients used in some studies; and (*f*) nonstandard criteria used to assess the date of first recurrence. Also, the comparisons of immunocytochemical and the newer receptor EIAs serve to point out the importance of cellular heterogeneity as a cause of variation (99, 100). The prognostic significance of ER values does not appear to depend on the type of tissue biopsied for assay because ER values from primary tumors or metastatic tumors predict equally well (6).

Tamoxifen, 1-(4-β-dimethylaminoethoxyphenyl)-1,2-diphenylbut-1-ene, is a synthetic nonsteroidal compound that shows varying degrees of estrogen agonist and antagonist activity. The antiestrogenic properties of this compound have led to its clinical use in the treatment of a number of human malignant tumors, especially ER-positive metastatic breast cancer. Tamoxifen exerts its effects, at least in part, via the specific estrogen receptor proteins of estrogen-responsive cells. A secondary, saturable, high-affinity tamoxifen binding site is present in ER-positive but not ER-negative tumors. Raam (101) has recently described a solid-phase EIA for this secondary binding site. This secondary site is present at an order of magnitude greater than the concentration of the high-affinity estradiol receptor site measured in the same tissue. In receptor assays, tamoxifen is bound predominately by this secondary binding site in ER-positive human mammary carcinoma cytosol, which is distinct from the classic estrogen receptor site. No saturable tamoxifen binding sites were detected in any of the ER-negative tumors studied. Elucidation of the roles, if any, of this tamoxifen binding site in mediating the antitumor activity of tamoxifen in human breast cancer awaits further experimentation (102).

Valavaara (103), in the study of 113 postmenopausal patients with advanced breast cancer that were ER-positive and treated with tamoxifen, concluded that the concentration of the ER predicts the duration of the response but not the rate of response. In this instance, PR status was not useful as a predictor of therapy response.

Growth Factor Receptors

In breast cancer, a strong inverse relationship between EGFr and ER status was found for EGFr values greater than 10 fmol/mg of protein. There appears to be an increased expression of EGFr in some ectodermal-derived tumors over that found in contiguous normal tissue. Expression of the EGFr appears to be increased in neoplastic tissue and is usually associated with increased aggressiveness of the disease. EGFr status has been used for classifying the prognosis of ER-negative tumors. ER-negative/EGFr-positive patients had a significantly worse prognosis than did patients who were negative for both receptors (104). Scatchard analysis showed that most tumors have two EGFr binding sites: a high-affinity site with K_d = 2 nM/liter and the second a low-affinity site with K_d = 9.5 nM/liter (61).

TGF-α, a peptide isolated from cultures of malignant cells stimulated the growth of malignant tissues through binding to the EGFr. There appears to be an increased expression of EGFr in some ectodermal-derived tumors over that found in contiguous normal tissue. Gene amplification and mRNA overexpression of EGFr and of the closely related *erb*-B2 oncogene have been found in mammary carcinomas. High concentrations of EGFr in breast cancer have been related to a poorer prognosis, suggesting that it might be an index of severity of the disease. One study (104) concluded that the only significant marker for disease-free survival was the absence of EGFr, but it did not correlate significantly with overall survival. Finally, EGFr status was a valid criterion for dividing ER-negative tumors into those with good and poor prognosis; i.e., ER-negative /EGFr-positive patients had a significantly worse prognosis than did patients negative for both receptors.

Amplification of the c-*erb*-B2 oncogene had a positive relationship with the number of axillary-node metastases. It was a stronger prognostic marker than PR status, tumor size, or ER status for both disease-free interval and survival (105). The presence of any of these oncogene products provides for a poor prognosis, perhaps because each is involved with the stimulation of cell growth. Further, permanent activation of TKA in the case of c-*erb*-B2 may indicate that it is involved with progression of the tumor and development of metastases. Measurement of gene amplification is relatively difficult and is currently not suitable for the routine pathology laboratory. Preliminary data suggest that other oncogenes/oncoproteins can be used to provide prognostic information in breast cancer. Clair (106) has shown that breast cancers with high concentrations of the *ras* protein have a greater likelihood of developing recurrent disease than do tumors containing low concentrations of this protein. Similarly, amplification of both the *int*-2 and c-*myc* oncogenes have been associated with aggressive breast cancer. With gene amplification, it is noteworthy that while the capacity of the receptors increased, the affinity did not. This leads to the conclusion that it is simply an increase in the number of EGFrs and not a change in the actual receptor. However, overexpression of these genes did not always result in increased EGFr. Other factors may be involved here such as increased transcription of the gene (over other genes); reduced degradation of the mRNA, allowing more "readings" by the ribosome; and reduced receptor degradation, which might keep the cell "turned on" longer.

ENDOMETRIAL, CERVICAL, AND VULVAR CANCERS

The incidence of endometrial adenocarcinoma is 11 to 12/100,000/year and rising in developed countries (American Cancer Society, 1986). The majority of endometrial cancers are adenocarcinomas (80%), with the remaining 20% comprised of adenoacanthoma, adenosquamous carcinomas, papillary, and clear cell carcinomas (107). Five-year survival of patients with treatment initiated during stage I disease varies between 70 and 94%, depending upon the histologic grade and receptor content of the tumor. Five-year survival drops to 55 to 88% with stage II disease, whereas the rates drop to 30 to 32% and 0 to 10% with stage III and stage IV disease, respectively (108–113). Cervical carcinoma occurs at the rate of about 10/100,000/year (114). Mass screening programs and early detection have been successful in reducing the incidence to about 3.6/100,000/year. Cervical carcinoma is primarily squamous, although cervical adenocarcinoma is increasing in incidence and currently makes up about 10% of invasive cervical cancers (115). The 5-year survival rate for stage I disease is 62.8 to 100%; however, if treatment is not instituted prior to metastases, survival rate drops below 10% (116). Vulvar carcinoma has an incidence of only 1 to 2/100,000/year and a 5-year survival rate of about 90% (115, 116).

Growth, development, and maintenance of the female genital tract is controlled by sex steroids, estrogen, and progesterone receptors that are found in the highly differentiated target tissues of the normal female reproductive tract and growth factor receptors, e.g., EGFr. In the endometrium, estradiol stimulates mitosis and increases progesterone receptor concentration. The progesterone-receptor complex induces differentiation of the secretory function of endometrial cells. Normal endometrium contains higher concentrations of steroid receptors than those found in endometrial carcinoma, and the malignant endometrium has a low PR to ER ratio (117). As dedifferentiation occurs in a carcinoma, it appears to be accompanied by a concomitant loss of receptors and a reduction in receptor concentration (118–121). Receptors of both types are found in highly differentiated tumors and poorly differentiated tumors, while primary tumors with metastases usually lack them (118). Taken together, these data indicate that endocrine control of endometrial cancer may be lost or reduced because of modifications that occur during the malignant process. In tumors that lack or have low concentrations of estrogen and progesterone receptors, the rate of adnexal spread of the tumor is increased and the recurrence rate of stage I cancer is higher (107). Progesterone receptor—not the estrogen receptor—appears to correlate significantly with tumor grade and histology. The greatest decline in receptor positivity occurs between grade 2 and grade 3 tumors.

The predictive value of receptors in determining the course of endometrial carcinoma is currently a topic of investigation. Distinct cutoff values have been reported by different investigators. These numbers do not reflect those obtained in breast carcinoma. This is partly due to the absence of standardized assays and reference materials. Apart from that, the presence of receptors is a predictive factor.

Creasman et al. (122) first reported that estrogen and progesterone receptor-positive endometrial tumors were less aggressive than estrogen and progesterone receptor-negative tumors, and longer survival time is associated with high levels of these receptors. Ensuing work (123, 124) indicated that the concentration of estrogen and progesterone receptors was prognostic. Palmer et al. (125), using cutoff values of 70-fmol ER/mg protein and 30-fmol PR/mg protein showed that stage, age, and each of the steroid receptors, were independently associated with survival. Recently, a number of reports confirming the utility of ER and PR levels on predicting survival time have been published (126–129). In contrast, Erlich described overall survival as superior for patients with progesterone receptor-positive tumors (P less than 0.001) but could not find any statistical relationship between estradiol receptor status and survival. In a subsequent study of 309 malignant endometrial tumors, Kleine (130) likewise observed that estrogen receptor has no significant prognostic relevance over that obtained by PR determination. In an examination of survival in early endometrial cancer, Sutton et al. (129) determined, using a Cox proportional hazards model, that tumor grade, peritoneal cytological results, PR status, and age were the most closely associated with disease-free survival. In 1989 and 1990 reviews, Kauppila (117) and Podratz (131) both concluded from an examination of a number of studies of endometrial cancer that PR is the best receptor measurement for the prognosis of survival and response to endocrine therapy. In summary, a negatve ER or PR both give similar information in identifying nonresponders, and a positive PR provides better accuracy in determining patients who will respond to endocrine therapy. However, as many as 70% of patients with endometrial cancer who have receptor levels above the cutoff limits normally used to identify candidates for endocrine therapy fail to respond to endocrine therapy. Lack of response in PR-positive tumors to endocrine therapy suggests the presence of a defect(s) in the cellular machinery distal to the steroid binding site, cellular heterogeneity within the tumor (i.e., some cells possess receptors and others do not), cellular control mechanisms that are hormone-independent, or increased hormonal metabolism (132–134).

EGF is excreted in high concentration in the urine in a biologically active form. The presence of the EGF receptors in close contact with this milieu provides the opportunity for the EGF to incubate with normal, premalignant, and malignant transitional epithelium of the bladder for long periods of time. With such favorable conditons, it is not too surprising that the density of receptor expression reflects the degree of malignancy in the bladder. It is also worthwhile noting that the expression of EGFrs on the superficial cells often precedes the standard histologic evidence for a preneoplastic state.

Attempts have been made to control the progress of malignancy through the use of toxins, radioisotopes attached to ligands or antireceptor antibody (seek out the receptor and deal a lethal dose of radiation), unconjugated antireceptor antibody (to attempt to block the receptor binding site), and anti-EGF antibody, to inactivate the EGF. None of these has proven successful. Explanations for the lack of success focus on the object of the therapy. Thus, those aimed at EGF have to deal with a large, continuous, and fresh supply of EGF (excreted in the urine). It would be very difficult to nullify this nonending influx of EGF with outside agents. The methods aimed at the EGFr need to penetrate deep into the tumor mass to get all of the receptor sites.

Another intriguing approach aimed at direct control of the EGFrs involves taking advantage of the chemistry of the receptor. As the site becomes more "acidic," it correspondingly loses its ability to bind

EGF. It was found that by decreasing the pH to 5 or 6, there was no change in the number of EGFrs, but the binding of the EGF to this site was greatly reduced. In vitro growth studies on the effect of pH validated this finding. The effects of EGF on growth were totally abrogated at pHs lower than 6. Thus, the control of urine pH offers a potential means to control of this type of carcinoma.

It appears that the increasing density of EGFr sites on the cervical and vulvar squamous cell carcinomas can be related to the biological aggressiveness of these malignancies. In particular, those neoplasms with levels of EGFr greater than 100 fmol/mg of protein show a poor prognosis, while those with levels less than 100 fmol/mg of protein had more favorable outcomes (relative to recurrence and 5-year survival) (35).

PROSTATIC CANCER

In 1983, Barkovitz (135) made the observation about carcinoma of the prostate (PC) that "an incidence of 50% is reported in 80-year-old men—but it is extremely rare before age 40." Localized PC can be cured by surgical removal or radiation therapy. When the general health and age of the patient or progress of the disease (metastases) prevents this course of treatment, hormone therapy is the next option. Treatment of PC through hormone therapy has been successful, with up to 80% favorable response. Therapy commonly consists of androgen ablation through orchiectomy or treatment with estrogen, diethylstilbestrol (DES) or luteinizing hormone-releasing hormone (LHRH) or its analogs. Orchiectomy is often combined with the administration of DES. Cyproterone acetate with DES has been used successfully (136). However, eventually the tumor becomes resistant to the hormone therapy and again progresses.

Analogous to the work in breast cancer, where receptors have been moderately successful in predicting the course of the disease, studies have been carried out to determine the utility of receptor concentrations and affinities to aid in the prognosis of PC. While receptors for androgen receptors (ARs), ERs, PRs, EGF, LHRH, and prolactin (PRL) have been quantified in PC tissue, their prognostic value has not been obvious. In fact, the presence or absence of receptors is not even a factor when PC is initially diagnosed because of the high success rate with hormone therapy.

The most studied prostate receptor is the intracellular AR. Genetically, the AR is a single unique gene product. The gene itself can be divided into eight coding exons and corresponds closely in organization to the human estrogen receptor gene. It is X-linked, and defects have been observed in males who carry only a single copy of the gene. The receptor is a 110-kd single protein chain, with three distinct regions; the ligand binding region, the nuclear interaction region (containing two zinc fingers), and a third region that modulates the protein synthesis process. The hormone and DNA binding domains are analogous to the respective domains in other steroid receptors. Much of these regions are highly conserved between the steroid receptors. In contrast to other steroid receptors, AR is present in considerably lower tissue concentrations, is extremely labile, and is susceptible to proteolytic breakdown. Consequently, it is the least well characterized of the steroid receptors. AR is capable of binding a large number of agonist molecules, but activation of the receptor appears to depend upon binding to testosterone or dihydrotestosterone (DHT). The affinity of the receptor for DHT is two-fold greater than for the unsaturated testosterone, and the dissocation rate from AR for the latter is signficantly higher than for DHT. It has been speculated the testosterone is functionally a prohormone for DHT and estrogens such as estradiol.

The AR has been found in both the epithelial and stromal cells. As with the other steroid receptors, there has been an evolution of models depicting the location of the AR. In the nucleus, the AR is present in a salt-extractable and salt-resistant form. The presence of molybdate or dithiothreitol solubilized all of the nuclear AR. It has been speculated that the molybdate interacts with the DNA binding domain of the AR. This leads to the conclusion that the salt-resistant nuclear AR is that which is associated with DNA. It has been generally assumed that the AR is also present in the cytosol. Mulder (137) describes the presence of AR aggregates in the cytosol with sedimentation coefficients of 8S and 4S. The relative populations of these two species is dependent on the presence of molybdate or salt, where the 4S is favored. Immunocytochemical studies, however, find little evidence of AR in the cytosol and locate the receptor almost exclusively in the nuclear region (138). Keep in mind that this technique depends upon the antibody recognition, and aggregates of the AR may hide or alter the antigenic site(s).

Androgens promote cellular growth, and EGF regulates the growth of both normal and tumor epithelial cells of the prostate. There is evidence that ARs also act as secondary promoters through the increased expression of EGF receptors (also found in prostate tissue) on the cellular surface membrane because the binding capacity of EGF receptors increases in the presence of androgens. Both of these receptors appear to act through enhancing the cells' sensitivity to growth factors. It is not clear whether the mechanisms follow autocrine or paracrine control. The presence of AR alone, however, is not sufficient for stimulating growth. The other condition is the ability of the tissue to convert testosterone to DHT, which is the active species.

Other receptors found in prostate tissue are estrogen, progesterone, growth hormone, hCG, and prolactin (PRL) receptors. The expression of EGF receptors in benign prostatic hyperplasia (BPH) is about twice that found in prostate carcinoma (PC) (139), while the reverse is found for AR. In PC tissue, an increase in (EGF) content appears to be associated with a corresponding decrease in AR and loss of differentiation (140). Both EGF and androgen receptors are more commonly found in highly differentiated than in poorly differentiated tumors and generally not found after prolonged estrogen therapy. Patients treated with diethylstilbestrol (DES) showed up to 50% decreases in hCG receptors after 7 days of treatment, and after 6 months of treatment with DES, levels had dropped to 25% of the original value (141). High- and low-affinity binding sites for estrogens are found in normal prostate tissues, but only the low-affinity site is present in tissue from BPH or PC (142).

Kadar (143) reports that rat PC tissue contains receptors for LHRH, somatostatin, and PRL. Treatment with either the LHRH agonist, [D-trp6]LH-RH, or the somatostatin agonist, RC160, resulted in shrinkage of the tumor mass with a corresponding decrease in the above receptor expressions. The decrease for PRL receptors was the greatest (about 50%). The authors speculate that tumor growth is inhibited by down-regulation of these receptors through binding to these agonists.

The current direction of study is toward finding prognostic indicators after therapy has been initiated. Benson et al. (144), using the initial prostate values (before treatment), observed that in a group of treated patients, 85% of those with nuclear androgen binding of greater than or equal to 26 fmol/mg did not show progression of the disease after 3 years, compared with only 40% of patients with androgen nuclear binding of less than 26 fmol/mg. However, in grade 4 lesions, androgen binding is not a useful indicator, and the PC is generally resistant to hormone therapy. They concluded that, excluding grade 4, measuring the amount of androgen bound by the nuclear AR was a gross predictor of response to endocrine therapy. But these numbers are not sufficient to make a determination to withhold therapy. In fact, the presence or complete absence of ARs does not predict the response, considering that 80% of AR-positive and 25% of AR-negative patients respond favorably to hormone therapy.

After relapses from hormone therapy, further evaluation of AR does not appear to provide any useful guidance. Here, it is of interest that the concentration of DHT present in the tumor may be a prognostic marker. Connelly (145) reports that "patients whose tumors contained more than 2 ng of DHT per gram of tissue were more likely to experience remission after endocrine treatment than those whose tumors contained lower concentrations of DHT."

There is no evident correlation between AR concentration and disease stage. The latter is best evaluated through determination of tumor size. One contributing factor to this observation is the large amount of heterogeneity of ARs in PC tissue. This may explain why response to hormone therapy and PC tissue AR concentrations are not necessarily parallel (146). This problem of heterogeneity is also dependent upon the method of obtaining samples. For example, while needle biopsy is a simple procedure, the sample is probably not representative of the whole tissue. Samples obtained by electroresection renders PC tissue unsuitable because of the heat generated.

Significant errors in current assays often invalidate correlations between the amount of AR and therapy response. In addition to the problem of heterogeneity (146), other significant problems include contamination with a plasma protein, the presence of significant amounts of sex hormone-binding globulin (SHBG), which competes for DHT, and the presence of large amounts of endogenous DHT. When there are large amounts of endogenous DHT, many of the receptor sites become bound in vivo. This requires doing an exchange assay, which is slow at low temperatures, while at elevated temperatures the receptor is unstable. The use of DHT as the label is limited because of potential metabolism of DHT during the assay procedure. More commonly, the synthetic steroid methyltrienolone (R-188) or ^{3}H-mibolerone is utilized as the ligand. They do not bind to SHBG and are not subject to metabolism during the assay procedure. The disadvantage of R-188 is that it binds to both AR and PR. This is eliminated by swamping the PR with triamcinolone acetonide.

Unfortunately, in spite of the high level of response to endocrine treatment of prostatic carcinoma, at some point all PCs progress to an androgen-resistant state, at which time the disease continues to advance. Thus, we obviously need to understand why these tumors become androgen-resistant. Perhaps the receptor becomes inactive through genetic processes that result in truncation or production of chimeric forms of the receptor.

Hormone-Resistant States

Hormone resistance disorders may be related to a defect in the hormone itself, although they are usually caused by a receptor or postreceptor defect that prevents normal functional activity of the receptor. Normal function of a receptor involves a number of intricate prereceptor, receptor, and postreceptor events that are very clearly dependent upon the structure of each of the participating molecules. The change of a single nucleotide in the genetic code can cause a structural change that if located in a strategic location in the molecule may reduce or completely inhibit receptor activity. The list of identified endocrine disorders that result from inherited receptor defects continues to increase. Gene or chromosomal deletions are responsible for many of the known receptor defects, although point mutations are much more common. In addition, the amount of genetic polymorphism present in a normal population probably accounts for at least some of the normal physiological diversity in hormone action. There are several examples of heterogeneity in the structure and function of specific receptors as a result of point mutations. This is particularly true for the low density lipoprotein (LDL) receptor, in which 10 different point mutational changes have been described (147). Nearly all of the genes that code for hormones, growth factors, and their receptors will probably show the same degree of genetic heterogeneity as has been described for the LDL receptor. Although several receptor-deficient diseases have been described, this is still a new area of research in which the analytical procedures are still largely experimental. They are performed by a relatively small number of research laboratories, and the clinical diagnosis, as a general rule, does not utilize analysis of receptor status by a clinical laboratory. Difficulties that may be encountered in the analyses of receptor characteristics in hormone-resistant disease are the procurement of appropriate specimens upon which to perform the analysis, nonuniformity of analytical procedures, the lack of standardization materials that permit interlaboratory comparisons, and the relatively low number of patients involved. However, since most of these diseases reflect genetic disorders, the mutational changes responsible for receptor or postreceptor defects will very likely be determined in the future in clinical laboratories equipped to amplify the appropriate DNA sequences by the polymerase chain reaction (PCR) and to determine polymorphisims using molecular biology procedures.

FAMILIAL HYPERCHOLESTEROLEMIA (LDL RECEPTOR)

Cholesterol plays an important role in the normal function of nearly all cells and is required by all steroid-producing cells. However, elevated plasma levels of cholesterol are responsible for coronary artery disease, and plaque formation in coronary arteries is responsible for heart attacks very early in life in patients suffering from familial hypercholesterolemia (FH). LDL contains much of the cholesterol that is found in blood and, in normal individuals, provides for the entrance of cholesterol into cells where it is used in the synthesis of membranes and serves as a precursor for the adrenal and gonadal steroids. LDL enters the cell by binding to LDL receptors located in the plasma membrane. Any one of a number of mutational changes that have been described in the LDL gene can prevent the expression of a normal LDL receptor in FH-affected patients and prevent or impede the normal uptake of LDL by target cells. About one in 500 people express one allele with a mutational change in the LDL gene. Although approximately 10 different mutations of the LDL receptor gene have been described (148), these FH patients are considered heterozygous because they have one normal and one abnormal LDL receptor gene. They express a lower than normal number of LDL receptors and show circulating cholesterol levels that are much higher than unaffected patients. Patients with two alleles for defective LDL receptors are very rare and are considered to be homozygous for LDL receptor defects. Many of these patients have no LDL receptors and exhibit very high plasma levels of cholesterol during childhood with attendant coronary artery disease. These patients usually die during adolescence of severe coronary artery plaque formation. Patients who are heterozygous for LDL receptor defects can be treated with drugs that lower cholesterol and stimulate the production of LDL receptors in liver cells. The combination of decreased liver cholesterol production, increased production of LDL receptors, and measures designed to reduce intestinal absorption of cholesterol can force circulating levels of LDL cholesterol into the normal range.

INSULIN RESISTANCE (INSULIN RECEPTOR)

Insulin is the primary hormone involved with glucose, lipid, and protein metabolism. As is the case with other hormones, insulin must bind to its receptor to produce its biological effects. The insulin receptor, which is found in a wide variety of cell types, is membrane bound, and has two α and two β chains that are derived from a single large precursor peptide. The α chains form the extracellular part of the receptor that binds insulin; the β chains form the transmembrane part of the molecule; and the tyrosine kinase activity domain in the cytosol of the cell. The actions of insulin are varied, ranging from increased glucose transport, glycogen synthesis, and antilipolysis, all of which occur within minutes of insulin binding to the receptor, to increases in protein synthesis that occur some hours after the hormone has bound to the receptor. As is the case with many membrane-bound receptors, the hormone-bound receptor is internalized through the cell membrane and the hormone removed and degraded in the lysosomes. Receptors recycle largely intact back to the cell surface where they are capable of binding additional molecules of insulin.

Diabetes is not a single disease entity because it can result from a number of environmental insults and/or genetic defects. For example, mutational changes in the insulin molecule can result in a nonfunctional hormone capable of causing diabetic changes in children or adults. The loss of pancreatic β-cell production of insulin can also cause diabetes because of the absence or scarcity of insulin; mutational changes in the insulin receptor can cause symptoms of diabetes because of the inability of insulin to effect the normal receptor-mediated biological action. Insulin resistance may result from mutational derived defects that directly affect the structure of the receptor and reduce or prevent insulin binding to the extracellular binding site, or change the transmembrane or cytosolic region of the receptor and prevent antiphosphorylation and tyrosine kinase activity. Mutational changes may also affect other postreceptor events, prevent or reduce the expression of the insulin receptor gene, or inhibit receptor recycling. Any of these structure-function changes can cause diabetes, even if the patient is heterozygous for the genetic change because of the reduced number of functional molecules. This is particularly true later in life when metabolism begins to slow down and the fat content of the body increases, increasing the level of stress on glucose metabolism.

ANDROGEN RESISTANCE; TESTICULAR FEMINIZATION (ANDROGEN RECEPTOR)

The spectrum of androgen-resistant syndromes ranges from complete testicular feminization, in which genetic males present as phenotypic females, through the incomplete form of the syndrome, in which the predominant phenotypic form is a male but characterized by any of several examples of incomplete virilization. The spectrum of partial virilization ranges from hypospadias in severely affected individuals, to gynecomastia and azoospermia in mildly affected patients (149). Some phenotypically normal men with oligospermia have been found to suffer incomplete testicular feminization with qualitative deficiencies in the androgen receptor (150). Severe cases of this syndrome are usually associated with the complete absence of the androgen receptor, whereas the incomplete forms of the disorder are associated with qualitative changes in the receptor, perhaps responding to point mutations in the androgen receptor gene.

References

1. Stedman's medical dictionary. 25th ed. Baltimore: Williams & Wilkins, 1990.

1a. Bayliss WM, Starling EH. The mechanism of pancreatic secretion. J Physiol (London) 1902;28:325.

2. Nalbandov AV. Reproductive physiology; comparative reproduction physiology of domestic animals, laboratory animals, and man. San Francisco: WH Freeman, 1958:195–197.

3. Green AR. Peptide regulatory factors: multifunctional mediators of cellular growth and differentiation. Lancet 1989;705.

4. Foekens JA, Peters HA, Portengen H, Noordegraaf E, Berns EMJJ, Klijn JGM. Cell biological prognostic factors in breast cancer: a review. Journal of Clinical Immunoassay 1991;14: 184–195.

5. Evans RM. The steroid and thyroid hormone receptor superfamily. Science 1988;240:889–895.

6. Greene GL, Sobel NB, King WJ, Jensen EV. Immunochemical studies of estrogen receptors. J Steroid Biochem 1984;20:51.

7. Green S, Gronemeyer H, Chambon P. Structure and function of steroid hormone receptors. In: Sluyser M, ed. Growth factors and oncogenes in breast cancer. England: Ellis Horwood, 1987:7–28.

8. Joab I, Radanyi C, Renoir M, et al. Common non-hormone binding component in non-transformed chick oviduct receptors of four steroid hormones. Nature 1984;308:850–853.

9. Catelli MG, Binart N, Jung-Testas I, et al., The common 90-Kd protein component of non-transformed "8S" steroid receptors is a heat-shock protein. EMBO J 1985;4:3131–3135.

10. Milgrom E, Atger M, Baulieu EE. Acidophilic activation of steroid hormone receptors. Biochemistry 1973;12:5198–5205.

11. Baulieu EE. Antibodies against highly purified B-subunit of the chick oviduct progesterone receptor. Biochem Biophys Res Commun 1984;119:433–439.

12. Walter P, Green S, Greene G, et al. Cloning of the human estrogen receptor cDNA. Proc Natl Acad Sci USA 1985;82: 7889–7893.

13. Sabbah M, Redeuilh G, Secco C, Baulieu EE. The binding activity of estrogen receptor to DNA and heat shock protein (Mr 90,000) is dependent on receptor-bound metal. J Biol Chem 1987;262:8631–8635.

14. Orti E, Bodwell JE, Munck A. Phosphorylation of steroid hormone receptors. Endocr Rev 1992;13:105–128.

15. Ruh TS, Ruh MF, Singh RK. Nuclear acceptor sites: interaction with estrogen-versus antiestrogen-receptor complexes. In: Moudgil VK, ed. Steroid receptors in health and disease. New York: Plenum Press, 1988;233–250.

16. Carson-Jurica MA, Schrader WT, O'Malley BW. Steroid receptor family: structure and functions. Endocr Rev 1990;11: 201–220.

17. Baker AR, McDonnell DP, Hughes M, et al. Cloning and expression of a full-length cDNA encoding human vitamin D receptor. Proc Natl Acad Sci USA 1988;85:3294–3298.

18. Giguere V, Ong ES, Segui P, Evans RM. Identification of a receptor for the morphogen retinoic acid. Nature 1987;330: 624–629.

19. Wang LH, Tsai SY, Cook RG, Beattle WG, Tsai MJ, O'Malley BW. COUP transcription factor is a member of the steroid receptor superfamily. Nature 1989;340:163–166.
20. Lazar MA, Hodin RA, Darling DS, Chin WW. Identification of a rat c-*erb*Aα-related protein which binds DNA but does not bind thyroid hormone. Mol Endocrinol 1988;2:893–901.
21. Mitsuhashi NT, Tennyson GE, Nikodem VM. Alternative splicing generates messages encoding rat c-*erb*Aα proteins that do not bind thyroid hormone. Proc Natl Acad Sci USA 1988;85:5804–5808.
22. Dittadi R, Gion M, Brazzale A, Bruscagnin G. Radioligand binding assay of epidermal growth factor receptor (EGFr): causes of variability and standardization of the assay. Clin Chem 1990;36:849.
23. Smith BR, Hall R. Thyroid-stimulating immunoglobulins in Graves' disease. Lancet 1974;2:427–431.
24. Zakarija M, McKenzie JM. Autoantibodies to the TSH receptor. Exp Clin Endocrinol 1991;97:165–169.
25. Zakarija M, McKenzie JM. Effects of thyrotropin and thyroid hormones in vivo on thyroid responsiveness to thyrotropin in vitro. Endocr Res Commun 1977;4:343–355.
26. Grob D. Myasthenia gravis: pathophysiology and management, retrospect and prospect. Ann NY Acad Sci 1981;377: xiii–xvi.
27. Brown MS, Goldstein JL. A receptor-mediated pathway for cholesterol homeostasis. Science 1986;232:324–47.
28. Beatson GT. On the treatment of inoperable cases of carcinoma of the mamma: suggestions for a new method of treatment, with illustrative cases. Lancet 1896;2:104–107.
29. Jensen EV, Jacobson HI, Fate of steroid estrogens in target tissues. In: Pincus G, Vollmer EP, eds. Biological activities of steroids in relation to cancer. New York: Academic Press, 1960:161–178.
30. Glascock RF, Hoekstra WG. Selective accumulation of tritium labeled hexestrol by the reproductive organs of immature female goats and sheep. Biochem J 1959;72:673–682.
31. Folca PJ, Glascock RF, Irving WJ. Studies with tritum-labeled hexestrol in advanced breast cancer. Lancet 1961;2:796–798.
32. Horwitz KB, McGuire WL. Specific progesterone receptors in human breast cancer. Steroids 1975;25:497–505.
33. Pertschuk LP. Immunocytochemistry for steroid receptors. Boca Raton, FL: CRC Press, 1990.
34. Dazzi H, Hasleton PS, Thatcher N, et al. Expression of epidermal growth factor receptor (EGF-R) in nonsmall cell lung cancer. Use of archival tissue and correlation of EGF-R with histology, tumor size, node status and survival. Br J Cancer 1989;59:746–749.
35. Pfeiffer D, Stellwag B. Pfeiffer A, Borlinghaus P, Meier W, Scheidel P. Clinical implications of EGFr in squamous cell carcinoma of the uterine cervix. Gynecol Oncol 1989;33: 146–150.
36. Hanauske AR, Osborne CK, Chamness GC, et al. Alteration of EGF-receptor binding in human breast cancer cells by antineoplastic agents. Eur J Cancer Clin Oncol 1987;23:545–551.
37. Grimaux E, Romain S, Remvikos Y, Martin PM, Magdelenat H. Prognostic value of epidermal growth factor receptor in node-positive breast cancer. Breast Cancer Res Treat 1989;14: 77–90.
38. Fernandex-Pol JA. Modulation of EGF receptor protooncogene expression by growth factors and hormones in human breast carcinoma cells. Crit Rev Oncog 1991;2: 173–185.
39. Fisher DA, Lakshmanan J. Metabolism and effects of epidermal and related growth factor in mammals. Endocr Rev 1990;11:418–442.
40. Korc M, Haussler CA, Trookman NS. Divergent effects of epidermal growth factor and transforming growth factors on a human endometrial carcinoma cell line. Cancer Res 1987;47: 4909–4914.
41. Miyachi Y, Terazono T, Nagao N, Shoji T, Irie M. Epidermal growth factor (EGF) receptors in human chorionic gonadotropin-producing tumor: transplantation in nude mice and the effect of EGF on tumor growth. J. Clin Endocrinol Metab 1990;71:329–334.
42. Bauknecht T, Kohler M, Janz I, Pfleiderer A. The occurrence of epidermal growth factor receptors and the characterization of EGF-like factors in human ovarian, endometrial, cervical and breast cancer. EGF receptors and factors in gynecological carcinomas. J Cancer Res Clin Oncol 1989;115:193–199.
43. Messing FM. Clinical implications of the expression of EGFr in human transitional cell carcinoma. Cancer Res 1990;50: 2530–2537.
44. Berchuck A, Soisson AP, Olt GJ, et al. Epidermal growth factor receptor expression in normal and malignant endometrium. Am J Obstet Gynecol 1989;161:1247–1252.
45. Reynolds RK, Talavera F, Roberts JA, Hopkins MP, Menon KM. Characterization of epidermal growth factor receptor in normal and neoplastic human endometrium. Cancer 1990;66: 1967–1974.
46. Reynolds RK, Talavera F, Roberts JA, Hopkins MP, Menon KM. Regulation of epidermal growth factor and insulin-like growth factor I receptors by estradiol and progesterone in normal and neoplastic endometrial cell cultures. Gynecol Oncol 1990;38:396–406.
47. Llorens MA, Bermejo MJ, Salcedo MC, Charro AL, Puente M. Epidermal growth factor receptors in human breast and endometrial carcinomas. J Steroid Biochem1989;34:505–509.
48. Goldschmitdt-Clermont PJ, Kim JW, Machesky LM, Rhee SG, Pollard TD. Regulation of phospholipase C-g1 by profilin and tyrosine phosphorylation. Science 1991;251:1231–1233.
49. Seibert K, Lippman ME. Hormone receptor assays in breast cancer. Journal of Clinical Immunoassay 1983;6:5.
50. Syne JS, Panko WB. New techniques for the measurement of estrogen receptors in human breast cancer. Journal of Clinical Immunoassay 1983;6:17.
51. Miller LK, Tuazon FB, Niu E. Human breast tumor estrogen receptor: effects of molybdate and electrophoretic analyses. Endocrinology 1981;108:1369–1378.
52. Valenstein SL, Voigt W, Thompsen S, Temple W. Estrogen and progesterone receptor techniques for breast cancer. In: Ashkar FS, ed. Radiobioassays, vol. II. Boca Raton, FL:CRC Press, 1983:53–64.
53. Korenman SG, Dukes BA. Specific estrogen binding by the cytoplasm of human breast carcinoma. J Clin Endocrinol Metab 1970;30:639–645.
54. Scatchard G. The attraction of proteins for small molecules and ions. Ann NY Acad Sci 1949;51:660–672.
55. Nickolson S, Sainsbury JRC, Needhan KG, Chambers P, Farndon JR, Harris AL. Quantitative assays of EGFr in human breast cancer; cut off points of clinical relevance. Int J Cancer 1988;42:36–41.
56. Steggles AW, King RJ. The use of protamine to study [6,7-^{3}H]-oestradiol-17β binding in rat uterus. Biochem J 1970;118: 695–701.
57. Chen YM, Vaughn CB. Ammonium sulfate fractionation and assay of hormone receptors. Cancer Invest 1989;7:231–235.
58. Chamness GC, McGuire WL. Methods for analyzing steroid receptors in human breast cancer. In: McGuire WL, ed. Breast cancer. 3. Advances in research and treatment. New York: Plenum Press, 1979:149–197.
59. Santine DB, Sibley CH, Perriand ER. A filter assay for steroid hormone receptors. Biochemistry 1973;12:2412–2416.
60. Jensen EV, Greene GL, Closs LE, De Sombre ER. Immunochemical probes for receptor structure and function. In:

Bresciani F, ed. Perspectives in steroid receptor research. New York: Raven Press, 1980:23–36.
61. Pavlik EJ, Nelson K, van Nagell JR Jr, et al. Steroid receptor analysis by size-exclusion liquid chromatography: considerations for the clinical laboratory. Clin Chem 1985;31:537–545.
62. Regnier FE, Gooding KM. High-performance liquid chromatography of proteins. Anal Biochem 1980;103:1–25.
63. Wittliff JL, Allegra JC, Day TG Jr., Hyder SM. Structural features and clinical significance of estrogen receptors. In: Moudgil VK, ed. Steroid receptors in health and disease. New York: Plenum Press, 1988:287–312.
64. Wagner RK, Jungblut PW. Estradiol and dihydrotestosterone receptors in normal and neoplastic mammary tissue. Acta Endrocinol 1976;82:105–120.
65. Vollmer G, Helmchen B, Knuppen R. Simultaneous quantification of oestrogen and progesterone receptors by a ligand binding assay in frozen sections. J Clin Chem Clin Biochem 1989;27:953–959.
66. Greene GL, Nolan C, Engler JP, et al. Monoclonal antibodies to human estrogen receptors. Proc Natl Acad Sci USA 1980;77:157.
67. Abbott Laboratories, Diagnostic Division, North Chicago, IL, 60064.
68. Senekjian EK, Press MF, Blough RR, Herbst AL, DeSombre ER. Comparison of the quantity of estrogen receptors in human endometrium and myometrium by steroid-binding assay and enzyme immunoassay based on monoclonal antibodies to human estrophilin. Am J Obstet Gynecol 1989;160: 592–597.
69. Andersen J, Bentzen SM, Poulsen HS. Relationship between radioligand binding assay, immunoenzyme assay and immunohistochemical assay for estrogen receptors in human breast cancer and association with tumor differentiation. Eur J Cancer Clin Oncol 1988;24:377–384.
70. Wu JT, Wilson LW. Progesterone receptor: stability studies and correlation between steroid binding assay and enzyme immunoassay. Clin Chem 1988;34:1987–1991.
71. Smyth CM, Benn DE, Reeve TS. An enzyme immunoassay compared with a ligand-binding assay for measuring progesterone receptors in cytosols from breast cancers. Clin Chem 1988;34:1116–1118.
72. Holmes FA, Fritsche HA, Loewy JW, et al. Measurement of estrogen and progesterone receptors in human breast tumors: enzyme immunoassay versus binding assay. J Clin Oncol 1990;8:1025–1035.
73. Clayton F, Wu J. The liability of estrogen receptor: correlation of estrogen binding and immunoreactivity. Clin Chem 1986;32:1774–1777.
74. Syne JS, Markaverich BM, Clark JH. Estrogen binding sites in the nucleus of normal and malignant human tissue: II. Characteristics of the multiple nuclear binding sites. Cancer Res 1982;42:4449–4454.
75. Zava DT, Harrington NY, McGuire WL. Nuclear estradiol receptor in the adult rat uterus: a new exchange assay. Biochemistry 1976;15:4292–4297.
76. Garola RE, McGuire WL. An improved assay for nuclear estrogen receptor in experimental and human breast cancer. Cancer Res 1977;37:3333–3337.
77. Traish AM, Muller RE, Wotiz HH. A new procedure for the quantitation of nuclear and cytoplasmic androgen receptors. J Biol Chem 1981;256:12028–12033.
78. Bresciani F, Sica V, Weizs HH. Effect of NaSCN on receptor-estradiol interactions and application to assay total receptor ("filled" and "unfilled" sites) in tissues and tissue fractions including nuclei, by exchange at low temperature with 17β-estradiol-^{3}H. In: Bresciani F, ed. Perspectives in steroid receptor research. New York: Raven Press, 1980:273–297.
79. Fuqua SA, Falette NF, McGuire WL. Sensitive detection of estrogen receptor RNA by polymerase chain reaction assay. J Natl Cancer Inst 1990;82:858–861.
80. Lee YTN. Variability of steroid receptors in multiple biopsies of breast cancer. Effect of systemic therapy. Breast Cancer Res Treat 1982;2:185–193.
81. Dittadi R, Gion M, Brazzale A, Bruscagnin G. Radioligand binding assay of epidermal growth factor receptor: causes of variability and standardization of the assay. Clin Chem 1990;36:849–854.
82. Nicholson S, Sainsbury JR, Needham GK, Chambers P, Farndon JR, Harris AL. Quantitative assays of epidermal growth factor receptor in human breast cancer: cut-off points of clinical relevance. Int J Cancer 1988;42:36–41.
83. Formento JL, Francoual M, Formento P, et al. Epidermal growth factor receptor assay: validation of a single point method and application to breast cancer. Breast Cancer Res Treat 1991;17:211-219.
84. Carpenter G. Binding assays for epidermal growth factor. Methods Enzymol 1985;109:101.
85. Grimaux M, Laine-Bidron C, Magdelenat H. Immunoenzymetric assay of epidermal growth factor receptor. Application to breast tumor samples. Tumour Biol 1989;10: 215–224.
86. Lin PH, Selinfreund R, Wharton W. Western blot detection of epidermal growth factor receptor from plasmalemma of culture cells using ^{125}I-labeled epidermal growth factor. Anal Biochem 1987;167:128–139.
87. Stumpf WF, Roth IJ. High resolution autoradiography with dry-mounted, freeze-dried, frozen sections. Comparative study of six methods using two different compounds [^{3}H]-estradiol and [^{3}H]-mesobilirubinogen. J Histochem Cytochem 1966;14:274.
88. Chen PZ, Mei Z, Yao XY, Meng XG. Selection of hormone-responsive advanced breast cancer with a cytoplasmic estrogen receptor assay. Analysis of 100 cases. Cancer 1989;63: 139–142.
89. King WJ, Jensen EV, Miller I, et al. Immunocytochemical detection of estrogen receptor in frozen sections of human breast tumors with monoclonal anti-receptor antibodies. San Francisco: Proceedings of the 64th Annual Meeting of the Endocrine Society, 1982.
90. Graham ML II, Bunn PA Jr, Jewett PB, Gonzalez-Aller C, Horwitz KB. Simultaneous measurement of progesterone receptors and DNA indices by flow cytometry: characterization of an assay in breast cancer cell lines. Cancer Res 1989;49: 3934-3942.
91. Hubbard EW. Tumor markers. Diagnostic Clinical Testing 1990;28:13–17.
92. Duffy MJ. Biochemical markers as prognostic indices in breast cancer. Clin Chem 1990;36:188.
93. Henry JA, Angus B, Horne CHW. Oestrogen receptor and oestrogen regulated proteins in human breast cancer: a review. Keio J Med 1989;38:241–261.
94. Knight III WA, Livingston RB, McGuire WL. Estrogen receptor as an independent prognostic factor for early recurrence in breast cancer. Cancer Res 1977;37:4669–4671.
95. Thorpe SM. Estrogen and progesterone receptor determinations in breast cancer. Technology, biology and clinical significance. Acta Oncol 1988;27:1–19.
96. McGuire WL. Prognostic factors in primary breast cancer. Cancer Surveys 1986;5:527–536.
97. Hill P. Leanness, peptide hormones and premenopausal breast cancer. Med Hypotheses 1989;28:45–50.
98. Digenis AG, Ross CB, Morrison JG, Holcomb CW 3d, Reynolds VH. Carcinoma of the male breast: a review of 41 cases. South Med J 1990;83:1162–1167.

99. Scheres HM, De Goeij AF, Rousch MJ, et al. Quantification of oestrogen receptors in breast cancer: radiochemical assay on cytosols and cryostat sections compared with semiquantitative immunocytochemical analysis. J Clin Pathol 1988;41:623–632.
100. Snijders MP, De Goeij AF, Koudstaal J, et al. Is immunohistochemical analysis of oestrogen and progesterone receptors in endometrial carcinoma superior to the radioligand binding assay? J Pathol 1990;161:129–135.
101. Raam S, Vrabel DN. Evaluation of an enzyme immunoassay kit for estrogen receptor measurement—report II. Clin Chem 1988;34:2053.
102. Sutherland RL, Murphy LC. The binding of tamoxifen to human mammary carcinoma cytosol. Europ J Cancer 1980;16:1141.
103. Valavaara R, Tuominen J, Johansson R. Predictive value of tumor estrogen and progesterone receptor levels in postmenopausal women with advanced breast cancer treated with toremifene. Cancer 1990;66:2264–2269.
104. Sainsbury J, Farndon JR, Needham GK, Malcolm AJ, Harris AL. Epidermal-growth-factor receptor status as predictor of early recurrence of death from breast cancer. Lancet 1987;1398–1402.
105. Varley JM, Swallow JE, Brammar WJ, Whittaker JL, Walker RA. Alterations to either c-erbB-2(neu) or c-myc protooncogenes in breast carcinoma correlate with poor short-term prognosis. Oncogene 1987:423–430.
106. Clair T, Miller WR, Cho-Chung YS. Prognostic signficance of the expression of a ras protein with a molecular weight of 21,000 by human breast cancer. Cancer Res 1987;47:5290–5293.
107. Ehrlich CE, Young PCM, Stehman FB, Sutton GP, Alford WM. Steroid receptors and clinical outcome in patients with adenocarcinoma of the endometrium. Am J Obstet Gynecol 1988;158:796–807.
108. Rauramo L, Gronroos M, Kyostila J. Prognosis of carcinoma corporis uteri managed by preoperative radium treatment. Acta Obstet Gynecol Scand 1968;47:517–527.
109. Gronroos M, Punnonen R, Rauramo L, Lauren P. Problems in the treatment of endometrial carcinoma. Ann Chir Gynecol 1974;63:141–145.
110. Kauppila A, Gronroos M, Nieminen U. Clinical outcome in endometrial cancer. Obstet Gynecol 1982;60:463–480.
111. Tittinen A, Forss M, Aho I, Vesterinen EE, Nieminen U. Endometrial adenocarcinoma: clinical outcome in 881 patients and analysis of 146 patients whose deaths were due to endometrial cancer. Gynecol Oncol 1986;25:11–19.
112. Podratz KC, OBrien PPPC, Malkasian GD, Decker DG, Jeffries JA, Edmonson JH. Effects of progestational agents in treatment of endometrial carcinoma. Obstet Gynecol 1985;66:106–110.
113. Aalders JG, Abeler V, Kolstad P. Recurrent adenocarcinoma of the endometrium: a clinical and histopathological study of 379 patients. Gynecol Oncol 1984;17:85–103.
114. Horm JW, Asire AJ, Young JL Jr, Pollack ES. SEER program, cancer incidence and mortality in the United States 1973-81. In: NIH Publication No. 85:1837, 1984.
115. Weiss RJ, Lucas WE. Adenocarcinoma of the uterine cervix. Cancer 1986;57:1996–2001.
116. Vesterinen E, Forss M, Nieminen U. Increase of cervical adenocarcinoma: a report of 520 cases of cervical carcinoma including 112 tumors with glandular elements. Gynecol Oncol 1989;33:49–53.
117. Kauppila A. Oestrogen and progesterone receptors as prognostic indicators in endometrial cancer. A review of the literature. Acta Oncol 1989;28:561–566.
118. Friberg LG, Kullander S, Persijn JP, Korsten CB. On receptors for estrogens (E2) and androgens (DHT) in human endometrial carcinoma and ovarian tumors. Acta Obstet Gynecol Scand 1978;57:261–264.
119. Vihko R, Janne O, Kauppila A. Steroid receptors in normal, hyperplastic and malignant human endometria. Ann Clin Res 1980;12:208–215.
120. Quinn MA, Pearce P, Fortune DW, Koh SH, Hsieh C, Cauchi M. Correlation between cytoplasmic steroid receptors and tumour differentiation and invasion in endometrial carcinoma. Br J Obstet Gynaecol 1985;92:399–406.
121. Kleine W, Maier T, Geyer H, Pfleiderer A. Estrogen and progesterone receptors in endometrial cancer and their prognostic relevance. Gynecol Oncol 1990;38:59–65.
122. Creasman WT, McCarty KS, Barton TK, McCarty KS Jr. Clinical correlates of estrogen- and progesterone-binding proteins in human endometrial adenocarcinoma. Obstet Gynecol 1980;53:363–370.
123. Kauppila A, Kujansuu E, Vihko R. Cytosol estrogen and progesterone receptors in endometrial carcinoma of patients treated with surgry, radiotherapy and progestin. Clinical correlates. Cancer 1982;50:2157–2162.
124. Chambers JT, MacLusky N, Eisenfield A, Kohorn EI, Lawrence R, Schwartz PE. Estrogen and progesterone receptor levels as prognosticators for survival in endometrial cancer. Gynecol Oncol 1988;31:65–81.
125. Palmer DC, Muir IM, Alexander AI, Cauchi M, Bennett RC, Quinn MA. The prognostic importance of steroid receptors in endometrial carcinoma. Obstet Gynecol 1988;72:388–393.
126. Martin JD, Haahnel R, McCartney AJ, Woodings TL. The effect of estrogen receptor status on survival in patients with endometrial adenocarcinomas. Am J Obstet Gynecol 1983;147:322.
127. Creasman WT, Soper JT, McCarty KS Jr, McCarty KS Sr, Hinshaw W, Clarke-Pearson DL. Influence of cytoplasmic steroid receptor content on prognosis of early stage endometrial carcinoma. Am J Obstet Gynecol 1985;151:922–932.
128. Borazjani G, Twiggs LB, Leung BS, Prem KA, Adcock LL, Carson LF. Prognostic significance of steroid receptors measured in primary metastatic and recurrent endometrial carcinoma. Am J Obstet Gynecol 1989;161:1253–1257.
129. Sutton GP, Geisler HE, Stehman FB, Young PC, Kimes TM, Ehrlich CE. Features associated with survival and disease-free survival in early endometrial cancer. Am J Obstet Gynecol 1989;160:1385–1393.
130. Kleine W, Maier T, Geyer H, Pfleiderer A. Estrogen and progesterone receptors in endometrial cancer and their prognostic relevance. Gynecol Oncol 1990;38:59–65.
131. Podratz KC. Hormonal therapy in endometrial carcinoma. Recent results. Cancer Res 1990;118:242–251.
132. Kauppila AJ, Isotalo HE, Kivinen ST, Vihko RK. Prediction of clinical outcome with estrogen and progesterone receptor concentrations and their relationships to clinical and histopathological variables in endometrial cancer. Cancer Res 1986;46:5380–5384.
133. Senler TI, Dean WL, Murray LF, Wittliff JL. Quanitification of cytochrome P-450-dependent cyclohexane hydroxylase activity in normal and neoplastic reproductive tissues. Biochem J 1985;227:379–387.
134. Kauppila AJ, Isotalo HE, Kivinen S, Stenback F, Vihko RK. Short term effects of danazol and methoxyprogesterone acetate on cytosol and nuclear estrogen and progesterone receptors, 17β-hydroxy steroid dehydrogenase activity, histopathology and ultrastructure of human endometrial adenocarcinoma. Int J Cancer 1985;35:157–163.

135. Barkovitz GD, Brown TR, Migeon CJ. Androgen receptors. Clinics in endocrinology and metabolism 1983;12:155–173.
136. Rennie PS, Bruchovsky N, Goldenberg SL. Relationship of androgen receptors to the growth and regression of the prostate. Am J Clin Oncol 1988;11(suppl 2):S13–S17.
137. Mulder D, van Loon D, de Boer W, et al. Mechanism of androgen action: recent observations on the domain structure of androgen receptors and the induction of EGF-receptors by androgens in prostate tumor cells. J Steroid Biochem 1989;32: 151–156.
138. Tilley WD, Marcelli M, McPhaul MJ. Recent studies of the androgen receptor: new insights to old questions. Mol Cell Endocrinol 1990;68:C7–C10.
139. Maddy SQ, Chisholm GD, Busuttil A, Habib FK. Epidermal growth factor receptors in human prostate cancer: correlation with histological differentiation of the tumour. Br J Cancer 1989;60:41–44.
140. Davies P, Eaton CL, France TD, Phillips ME. Growth factor receptors and oncogene expression in prostate cells. Am J Clin Oncol 1988;11(suppl 2):S1–S7.
141. Namiki M, Kitamura M, Nonomura N, et al. Effect of estrogen treatment on testicular gonadotropin receptors in prostatic cancer patients. Arch Androl 1987;19:249–252.
142. Murphy JB, Emmott RC, Hicks LL, Walsh PC. Estrogen receptors in the human prostate, seminal vesicle, epididymis, testis, and genital skin: a marker for estrogen-responsive tissues? J Clin Endocrinol Metab 1980;50:938–948.
143. Kadar T, Redding TW, Ben-David M, Schally AV. Receptors for prolactin, somatostatin, and luteinizing hormone-releasing hormone in experimental prostate cancer after treatment with analogs of luteinizing hormone–releasing hormone and somatostatin. Proc Natl Acad Sci USA 1988;85:890–894.
144. Benson RC Jr, Gormon BA, O'Brien PC, Holicky EL, Veneziale CM. Relationship between androgen receptor binding activity in human prostate cancer and clinical response to endocrine therapy. Cancer 1987;59:1599–1606.
145. Connelly JG, Mobbs BG. Clinical applications and value of receptor levels in treatment of prostate cancer. Prostate 1984;5:477–483.
146. Demura T, Kuzumaki N, Oda A, et al. Establishment of monoclonal antibody to human androgen receptor and its clinical application for prostatic cancers. Am J Clin Oncol (CCT) 1988;11(suppl 2):S23–S26.
147. Baulieu EE. Hormones: a complex communication network. In: Baulieu EE, Kelly PA, eds. Hormones: from molecules to disease. New York: Hermann, 1990:140.
148. Motulsky AG. Genetic aspects of familial hypercholesterolemia and its diagnosis. Arteriosclerosis 1989;9(suppl 1):I3–I7.
149. Griffin JE, Wilson JD. The syndromes of androgen resistance. N Engl J Med 1980;302:198–209.
150. Smallridge RC, Vigersky R, Glass AR, Griffin JE, White BJ, Eil C. Androgen receptor abnormalities in identical twins with oligospermia. Am J Med 1984;77:1049–1054.

Section XI

Section Chief: *Harold A. Oberman*

The title of this section reflects the remarkable change in this area of clinical laboratory medicine in recent years. The term blood banking is far too restrictive, and its implied scope too limited, to characterize this subspecialty. The procurement and processing of blood for transfusion is only one facet of this field, as it has been modified to include a breadth of activities unforeseen only a few decades ago. The discipline has been clearly established as one that bridges the activities of the laboratory with those of clinical medicine. The uniqueness of this practice resulted in its recognition as a medical subspecialty by the American Board of Pathology, with the creation of a certifying examination 20 years ago. Similarly, the role of the medical technologist in this area has become more sharply defined, and also has resulted in the creation of subspecialty certification.

The transfusion medicine medical specialist must translate the laboratory's results and activities to the patient's bedside. Therefore, it is insufficient for such an individual merely to be cognizant of immunohematology in a restrictive sense.

The following chapters address critical clinical activities such as apheresis procedures, blood component therapy, clinical consultation regarding adverse reactions to transfusion, the clinical significance of various blood group antibodies, and the transfusional management of various hematologic conditions. The laboratorian who assumes responsibility in this area must combine an understanding of clinical medicine with knowledge of the laboratory aspects of immunohematology.

BLOOD BANK/
RANSFUSION MEDICIN

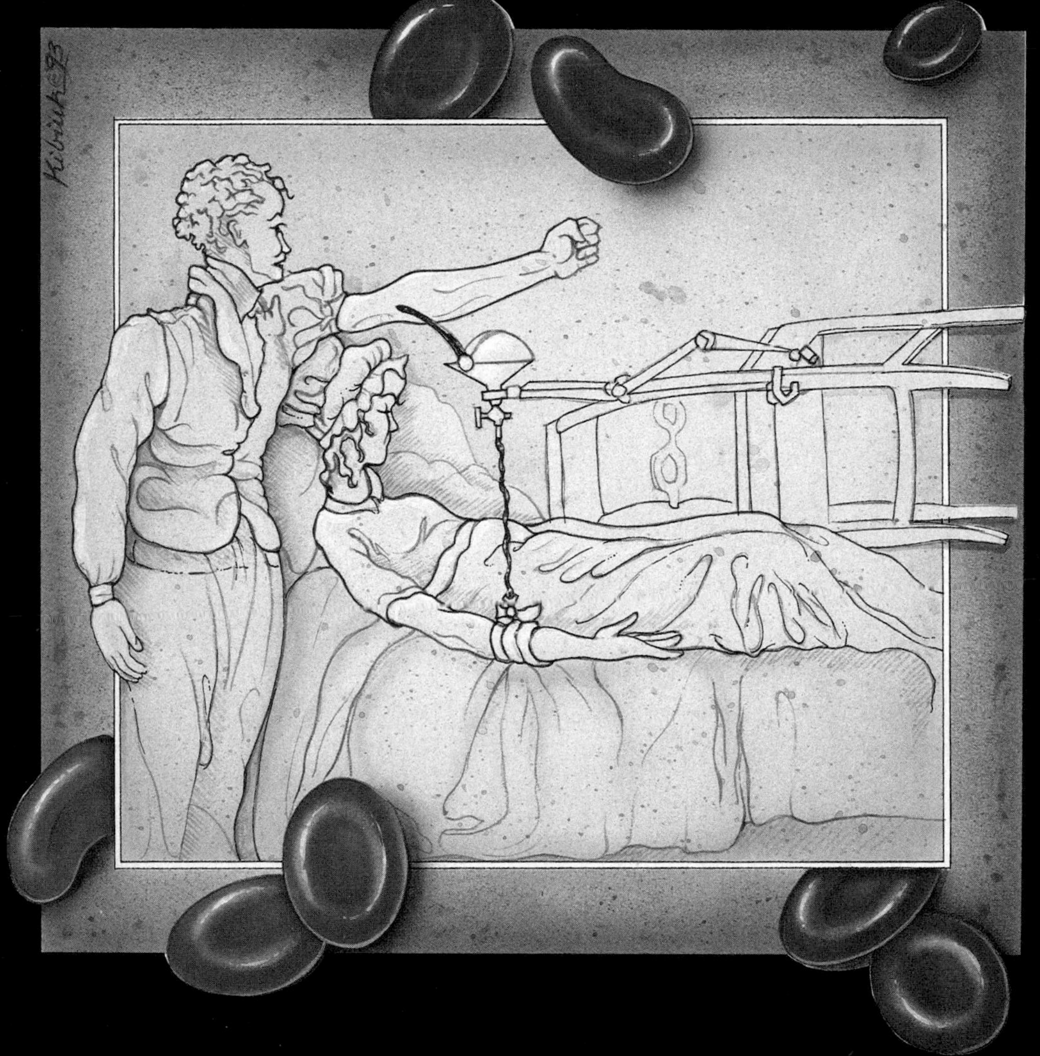

65 Organization and Legal Concerns of Blood Banks

Harold A. Oberman

THE EVOLUTION OF BLOOD TRANSFUSION

The Dawn of Blood Transfusion

Although blood has been considered a therapeutic agent since ancient times, there was little rational, scientific basis for its use, nor was there full realization of its properties or of its dangers until the present century. Among the earliest references to blood transfusion are those in the Bible and in the writings of Ovid. At several points in the Scriptures, there is admonition against transfusion (1), and this has resulted in the religious basis for the refusal of transfusion by such groups as Jehovah's Witnesses.

Ovid, in the eighth book of *The Metamorphoses*, describes restoration of youth to Aeson by the sorceress Medea through a "transfusion" of a magical potion! Unfortunately, she was unable to duplicate this remarkable feat. As other evidence of the mysticism associated with blood, Galen advised the drinking of the blood of a weasel for the cure of rabies, and Pliny described the drinking of the blood of dying gladiators as a cure for epilepsy (2).

Any rational approach to transfusion required an understanding of the circulation of the blood, and this was not available until the work of William Harvey in the early 17th century. By the middle of that century, Richard Lower in London and Jean Denys in Paris were experimenting with blood transfusion in dogs, and both subsequently transfused humans with canine blood (3). Unfortunately, in 1667, Denys transfused one of his subjects on three separate occasions, and the final transfusion resulted in the first recorded example of a fatal acute hemolytic transfusion reaction. A trial relieved Denys of guilt for this mishap because the subject was subsequently found to have been poisoned by his wife. Nevertheless, the controversy stemming from this case led to a multitude of decrees forbidding the practice; this resulted in the virtual elimination of transfusion for the next 150 years.

Blood Transfusion in the 19th Century

The reawakening of interest in transfusion in the early 19th century was led by James Blundell, one of the most prominent obstetricians in London. He looked to transfusion as the most appropriate treatment for postpartum hemorrhage, and in contrast to his 17th century forebears, reasoned that the father would be a more likely source of the blood than an animal (4). After the seemingly successful transfusion of a man dying of gastric carcinoma (5), Blundell undertook transfusions of patients with postpartum hemorrhage and consulted with other obstetricians who shared his enthusiasm for the procedure.

Transfusion during the 19th century was, at best, primitive. Among the indications cited in an 1849 publication were dyspepsia, esophageal stricture, dysentery, and prolonged fever (6). Moreover, the increased use of the technique without knowledge of blood groups or of immunology led to untoward complications. Therefore, by the last quarter of the century, the popularity of transfusion waned, and substitutes for blood were sought. Among these substitutes were milk, alcohol, and saline solution.

The Modern Era

Landsteiner's recognition of the ABO blood group system at the outset of the 20th century permitted a rational approach to blood transfusion (7). Within the subsequent few years, Ottenberg recognized the value of reacting the blood of the donor with that of the recipient before transfusion to detect incompatibility (8). At the same time, the technique of direct transfusion was popularized, initially by vascular surgeons adept at anastomosing blood vessels of donor and recipient, and subsequently through the use of a variety of mechanical devices.

The problems of anticoagulation, preservation, and storage of blood had to be solved before indirect transfusion could be accomplished. The first World War served as an impetus to the resolution of the first of these problems. At the same time, several investigators advocated citrate as an anticoagulant in 1914, and 2 years later, Rous and Turner documented the value of adding sugar to the citrate as a preservative (9). This allowed the use of preserved blood for the transfusion of casualties by 1918 (10).

Use of anticoagulated, stored blood for transfusion, so-called indirect transfusion, was slow to achieve greater popularity than direct transfusion because of the large amount of anticoagulant required in the early formulations. World War II, with the need to transport blood for long distances, hastened the development of improved preservative solutions so that, by the early 1940s, direct transfusion had all but vanished. Preservative solutions were modified initially through variations in the proportion of sodium citrate, citric acid, and dextrose (11) and more recently through the addition of sodium phosphate and adenine.

The development of organized centers for blood preservation also awaited the availability of reliable mechanical refrigeration equipment. Therefore, the first blood banks did not appear until the mid-1930s, and not until 1937 was the first blood bank organized in the United States (12). World War II provided a remarkable impetus for blood banking. Over 13 million units of blood were collected during the war, principally by the American Red Cross, although much of it was used for fractionation into dried plasma.

The number of developments in this field in the years since that war have been remarkable. One must appreciate that only the ABO, Rh, P, and MNS systems were known before 1945. Since that time, the understanding and complexity of these systems has increased, and a multitude of new systems have been identified. In 1945, the antiglobulin reaction was introduced (13), and this facilitated detection of blood group antibodies. In a contemporary development that was to have far-reaching consequences, the American Association of Blood Banks was formed in 1947. This provided a focus for educational activities in the field and led to the promulgation of standards of practice and an inspection and accreditation system that were to play a major role in enhancing the safety of blood transfusion throughout the world.

The advent of plastic transfusion equipment, an innovation of the past 30 years, circumvented such complications of transfusion from glass bottles as pyrogen-related reactions and air embolism. It also permitted separation of blood components in a closed system, thereby providing the impetus for the current emphasis on component therapy. Plamapheresis, first described in 1914 (14), was applied to large-scale plasma collection in the 1960s and, in the following decade, to the treatment of disease. The latter has resulted in the technical subspecialty of therapeutic apheresis. In another major development, the pathogenesis, treatment, and prevention of hemolytic disease of the newborn were accomplished by the end of the 1960s.

During the past 2 decades, there has been increased emphasis on infectious complications of transfusions, spurred by the development of tests for posttransfusion hepatitis and the advent of the AIDS epidemic. Finally, the breadth of this field and the multitude of clinical issues it embraces has led to the recognition of transfusion medicine as a medical specialty.

BLOOD BANKS AND TRANSFUSION SERVICES

Definitions and Functions of Blood Banks

The Standards of the American Association of Blood Banks define a blood bank as an organization that collects, stores, and processes human blood. In contrast, a transfusion service tests the blood of the intended recipient and is concerned with the transfusion of the blood and its components. While this definition may be useful in distinguishing the roles of a community blood bank and a hospital transfusion program, keep in mind that it is an arbitrary and somewhat artificial distinction.

Blood banking embraces a variety of functions, including the recruitment and selection of blood donors, collection and typing of blood, preparation of blood components, testing of the blood for transfusion-transmitted diseases, distribution of the blood to the transfusing facility, pretransfusion testing and issuance of the blood to the patient, consultation on antibody-related problems and on indications for transfusion, and investigation of adverse reactions to transfusion.

Apheresis procedures play an important role in both community and hospital blood banks. The technique is utilized in the collection of blood components and in therapeutic procedures. Many blood banks perform testing for resolution of disputed parentage, histocompatibility testing, and processing of bone marrow for autologous or allogeneic bone marrow transplantion. Finally, some institutions provide a program wherein outpatients come to the blood bank for their transfusion, or, in some instances, are responsible for a program of home transfusion.

Therefore, the scope of the specialty is broad, embracing a variety of personnel, including donor recruiters, specialized administrators, nurses, technologists, and physicians. In recent years, the medical aspects have been grouped under the rubric of transfusion medicine.

Sources of Blood

Approximately 13 million units of blood are collected annually in the United States, and the use of blood component therapy permits a much larger number of patients to be transfused. Most of this blood is collected by independent community blood banks, many of them members of the Council of Community Blood Centers, or by subsidiaries of the American Red Cross Blood Program. The latter program collects approximately half of all the blood transfused in this country; community blood banks collect 35%, and hospital blood banks supply the rest (15).

The Hospital Transfusion Service

Pretransfusion testing and issuance of the blood to the patient for transfusion are the responsibility of the hospital transfusion service. In some situations, however, they are performed by community blood banks. Removal of these roles from the hospital setting inhibits the functioning of an active transfusion medicine consultation program in the hospital.

The physician responsible for the hospital transfusion program is administratively responsible for all of the technical and medical policies and procedures of the laboratory and serves as a consultant for any related problems (16). These responsibilities include the designation of the source of the blood and components utilized in the hospital, the storage, processing, and issuance of the blood, and the provision of a consultant service to enhance patient care. This includes responsibility for the implementation of a quality control program and for compliance with the requirements of accrediting agencies. The blood bank physician also chairs the transfusion committee of the medical staff and serves as an educational resource for the hospital's physicians on the appropriate use of blood and blood components.

REGULATION OF BLOOD BANKS AND TRANSFUSION SERVICES

The Standards of the American Association of Blood Banks (AABB) form the basis for the Association's accreditation and inspection program. The Standards were first published in 1958 in an effort to improve the quality and safety of blood transfusion. Prepared by the Committee on Standards, a group of knowledgeable physicians and technologists, each specified standard is the result of a consensus decision by the committee. It is generally agreed that the Standards are the most definitive statement of minimum performance guidelines of the practice of blood banking.

The AABB inspection program is a voluntary one and is conducted every 2 years. Inspections are conducted as a prescheduled peer review undertaking, and there is an opportunity to correct deficiencies. Following the correction of deficiencies, a certificate of accreditation is issued. Therefore, the inspection should be perceived as an educational, as well as an accrediting, exercise.

Blood banks are also inspected by the College of American Pathologists (CAP) as part of their extensive biannual inspection program. This program is also prescheduled and conducted by physicians and technologists. In contrast to the AABB inspection, it covers all hospital laboratories, including the blood bank. Like the inspection of the AABB, the inspected laboratory is provided with a list of deficiencies and is given an opportunity for correction; therefore, the inspection also has a major educational component.

Federal responsibility for the regulation of blood banks is vested in the Food and Drug Administration (FDA). Whereas only blood banks engaged in the shipment of blood across state lines must be federally licensed, since 1975 all transfusion facilities have been required to register with the FDA. Regulation is based on conformity to the Code of Federal Regulations (CFR), published by the Center for Biologics Evaluation and Research of the FDA. All of the material pertaining to blood banking is contained in Title 21, Chapter 1 of the booklet. This forms the basis for the FDA inspection program, required of all licensed establishments.

In contrast to the peer-conducted AABB and CAP inspections, the annual inspections conducted by the FDA, which are necessary for maintenance of licensure, are unannounced. They are conducted by specially trained FDA personnel, who may lack any work experience in blood banking.

Similarly, the Department of Public Health of many states may conduct periodic, unannounced inspections. By law, such departments are responsible for overseeing the procurement, processing, distribution, and use of blood, its components, and its derivatives.

Finally, the Joint Commission on Accreditation of Healthcare Organizations (JCAHO) inspects all hospital laboratories, including blood banks, in the course of their annual or biannual inspections. This is a prescheduled inspection conducted by JCAHO-trained inspectors. The inspecting team includes a physician and a nurse, as well as other individuals, one of whom may be a medical technologist. Like the inspections of the AABB and the CAP, the JCAHO inspection includes a summation conference with the inspected institution and an opportunity to correct deficiencies before issuance of a final report. The type and number of deficiencies determine whether the institution will subsequently be reviewed annually or biannually.

LEGAL ISSUES IN BLOOD BANKING

While a complete review of the subject of liability of blood banks is beyond the scope of the following discussion, it is appropriate to present a summary of some of the major issues confronting blood banks and transfusion services in this area. Of all clinical laboratories, the blood bank is most subject to legal action. Moreover, the variety of activities that may result in such actions is much wider than those presenting in any other clinical laboratory.

In recent years, many claims have related to transfusion-transmitted infection, especially AIDS. Plaintiffs have sought damages on such disparate allegations as the improper screening of blood donors, failure of the transfusion to comply with clinically accepted guidelines, failure to inform the patient of the dangers of the transfusion, or failure to advise the patient of the alternatives to homologous transfusion.

The current litigious atmosphere promises increasing activity in this arena; therefore, the following comments are intended to serve as a framework to understand this important topic.

Malpractice

Malpractice is a lawsuit brought by an allegedly injured plaintiff against a defendant, in this instance a health care professional, for breach of a recognized standard of care that caused the injury. In most instances, the defendants in a transfusion-related suit will include the director of the hospital blood bank, the hospital, the blood bank that provided the blood, and very likely, the patient's physician. The independent acts of the patient's physician do not necessarily insulate the laboratory's responsibility, or vice versa (17).

A successful action requires the demonstration of negligence on the part of the defendant, wherein there has been a breach of duty that has resulted in damages to the plaintiff. The plaintiff may be either a blood donor who has been injured pursuant to the donation procedure or a patient who has suffered an adverse reaction to transfusion or has acquired a posttransfusion infection.

The basic elements of such a lawsuit embrace proof that the defendant had a duty to the plaintiff, that the duty was breached, that this breach of duty caused the injury to the plaintiff, and finally, that there were compensable damages.

The definition of the duty of the defendant to the plaintiff usually results in allegations that there was a lack of compliance with the standard of care. Definition of the standard of care may be a point of contention. In some instances, this can be established by statements in such authoritative sources as the CFR of the FDA or the Standards of the AABB. In this regard, it is important to note that the words "must" and "shall" are carefully utilized in the Standards, in contrast to "may" and "should," to distinguish mandatory practices from suggested practices, respectively. In other situations, expert witnesses are required to define and interpret this issue.

Expert witnesses also are used to determine whether or not the defendant breached the acknowledged duty and also to demonstrate that the plaintiff's injury was caused by that failure and would not have otherwise occurred. Damages are awarded on the basis of medical costs, loss of earning power, and pain and suffering; moreover, they commonly vary between jurisdictions.

Most states have legislation defining blood transfusion as a service, rather than as the sale of a product, in an attempt to protect blood banks from lawsuits based on the theory of strict liability. In the latter instance, the defendant may be held guilty even in the absence of proof of negligence. For example, a blood bank could be held liable for a transfusion-related infection acquired by a patient even if no test existed to detect that infection in the donor or in the unit of blood (18).

Consent for Transfusion

The blood donor and the patient receiving the transfusion must be informed of the risks of the procedure, and the patient must also be informed of the benefits and available alternatives. This must be done in a language that can be understood, and the subject must have an opportunity to ask questions and to refuse. Therefore, informed consent actually is a process wherein the subject, once informed, is allowed to make a choice.

In the instance of blood donation, the donor signs a form attesting that he or she understands the performance of the venipuncture and the removal of the blood or component and has provided truthful answers to questions during the screening procedure. Patient informed consent is somewhat less straightforward. The manner of obtaining and documenting consent is subject to wide variation, as discussed in a recent symposium (19). Recently, several states have mandated that written consent be obtained through the use of standardized forms before elective transfusion.

In deciding how to comply with the requirements for obtaining consent for a blood transfusion from an informed patient, one must consider when this should be done, who should be responsible for doing it, and how it should be documented. It is self-evident that the risks of transfusion must be discussed with the patient well in advance of the time the transfusion is necessary if the patient is to have an opportunity to utilize such alternative procedures as autologous transfusion.

The physician responsible for the patient's care will be the one determining the need for the transfusion. Therefore, he or she must also bear the responsibility for explaining the risks and benefits of the transfusion and for detailing alternatives. Because an elective transfusion is often necessary secondary to a surgical procedure, this explanation can best be given at the same time that the need for the surgical procedure is discussed with the patient. In most instances, the transfusion service would not be in a position to perform this function.

The explanation of the transfusion and the subsequent discussion provide the comprehending patient with an opportunity to understand the risks inherent in a potentially dangerous procedure and, if appropriate, to take an alternative action. In addition, it allows the physician to demonstrate at a later date, if necessary, that the patient agreed to accept the risk of the transfusion. Of course, there has to be some form of documentation of the consent.

Documentation is necessary only to make it easier for the patient's physician to prove at a later date that the interchange took place. In many instances, this is accomplished by a special form or a note in the patient's medical record. In some situations, a signed form or a progress note in the medical record is considered unworkable or undesirable, and the information is provided to all patients through the use of a brochure. However, it is necessary that the brochure advise the patient of a mechanism to ask questions or to clarify any areas of misunderstanding.

Refusal of Transfusion

From the foregoing discussion, it is evident that a competent patient has the right to refuse transfusion. This issue most often presents in the treatment of Jehovah's Witness patients who are unconscious and hemorrhaging or whose children require transfusion. The objection to transfusion is based on a strict interpretation of the recurrent biblical admonition against the "eating" of blood.

When there is a serious threat to a minor's life if a transfusion is not given, the court will most often order the transfusion even if this is contrary to the wishes of the parents. The court always will take into consideration the extent of the medical emergency and the extent of risk to the patient if transfusion is not performed. It is far less predictable that a court will order the transfusion of an unconscious adult in a similar situation. In this situation, the court will consider the medical need for the procedure, but it will also attempt to balance the rights of the patient with the rights of society. It may attempt to determine whether the patient had previously expressed any wishes relative to transfusion when mentally competent.

References

1. Leviticus 17:11–12.
2. Brown HM. The beginnings of intravenous medication. Ann Med Hist 1917;1:177–197.
3. Oberman HA. The evolution of blood transfusion. Univ Mich Med Ctr J 1967;33:68–74.
4. Blundell J. The after-management of floodings, and on transfusion. Lancet 1828;13:673–681.
5. Blundell J. Experiments on the transfusion of blood by the syringe. Med Chir Trans 1818;9:56–92.
6. Routh CHF. Remarks, statistical and general on transfusion of blood. Med Times 1849;20:114–117.
7. Rosenfield RE. The past and future of immunohematology. Am J Clin Pathol 1975;64:569–579.
8. Oberman HA. The crossmatch: a brief historical perspective. Transfusion 1981;21:645–651.
9. Rous P, Turner JR. The preservation of living red blood cells in vitro. J Exp Med 1916;23:219–237.
10. Robertson O. Transfusion with preserved red blood cells. Br Med J 1918;1:691–696.
11. Loutit JF, Mollison PL, Young IM. Citric acid-sodium citrate-glucose mixtures for blood storage. Q J Exp Physiol 1943;32: 183–202.
12. Fantus B. The therapy of the Cook County Hospital. JAMA 1937;109:128–131.
13. Coombs RRA, Mourant AE, Race RRA. A new test for the detection of weak and "incomplete" Rh agglutinins. Brit J Exp Path 1945;26:255–266.
14. Abel JJ, Rowntree LG, Turner BB. Plasma removal with return of corpuscles. J Pharmacol Exp Ther 1914;5:625–641.
15. Drake AW, Finkelstein SN, Sapolsky HM. The American blood supply. Cambridge, MA: MIT Press, 1982.
16. Widman FK, ed. Standards for blood banks and transfusion services. 15th ed. Bethesda MD: American Association of Blood Banks, 1993.
17. Belsey R, Greene M, Baer D. Managing liability risk in the office laboratory. JAMA 1986;256:1338–1341.
18. Rabkin B, Rabkin MS. Individual and institutional liability for transfusion-acquired diseases. JAMA 1986;256:2242–2243.
19. Widmann FK, ed. Informed consent for blood transfusion. Arlington, VA: American Association of Blood Banks, 1989.

66 Blood Collection

Alfred J. Grindon

DONOR RECRUITMENT

It has been estimated that, of an American population of approximately 250 million people, at least 100 million are eligible to be blood donors. However, only about 8 million of them actually donate, and provide an average of 1.6 units of blood every year, or a total of 12 million units of blood. Almost none of these donors receives payment, since paid donors have been shown to be more likely to be positive for markers for infectious disease and to transmit hepatitis by transfusion, even when appropriate screening tests are performed to eliminate the apparently dangerous units. Thus, donor recruiters should not offer financial incentives (including gifts or raffle tickets) as an inducement to give blood.

The most common approach to blood donor recruitment, "community responsibility," assumes that everyone who is able to give blood should do so, so that all who need it can obtain it without an implied recruitment burden on the potential or actual user of blood. Alternatively, some favor an approach using "individual responsibility," with each person responsible for provision of his or her blood needs, either by accruing blood donation "credits" against which needs can be drawn or by obtaining replacement donations from family and friends after blood has been used.

Of all eligible donors, half have given blood at some time in their lives, and half of these, or 25% of the total, have given within the last 4 years (1). These data do not suggest any lack of understanding of the donation process or of the need for blood on the part of the public at large. When former donors are asked why they no longer give, the two most common responses are the lack of a personal request, and the lack of a convenient donation site. While support of blood donation through the media is important as a reminder, without a convenient site and a personal request, blood donation is unlikely to occur.

The typical successful blood drive involves a blood center recruiter working with a designated individual in a business (or community or school) to develop a campaign, which should include (*a*) informational meetings of committees of employees; (*b*) the personal solicitation by committee members of all other employees, before the date of the drive, for pledges to donate and for a specific donation appointment time; (*c*) an informational campaign, to include a strong statement of support from the person in charge; and (*d*) a personal reminder to donors the day before or the day of the drive. In addition, those organizations that regularly have successful blood drives will have a program to recognize those who have worked to organize the blood drive, as well as the donors themselves.

From the donor's perspective, the most convenient site for blood collection is the workplace, utilizing a cafeteria or recreation facility and equipment brought by truck and set up by blood center staff. With smaller businesses that have insufficient space, a self-contained bloodmobile, typically holding four to six donor beds, can be used. Blood collections at blood centers or other fixed sites often depend upon the recruitment of individual donors by telephone.

Certain characteristics are desirable for any blood donation site: The physical environment must be pleasant, clean and uncluttered; furniture should have no sharp edges, and be capable of thorough cleaning and decontamination. Adequate space must be provided for privacy in donor interviews.

Since it is easier to retain a regular blood donor than to recruit a new one, a positive donation experience is critical. Interpersonal skills on the part of collection staff are as important as technical knowledge.

DONOR SELECTION: HISTORY

Donors are selected by history, physical examination, and laboratory testing to protect themselves and the recipient of their blood. Donor selection criteria are based upon the Code of Federal Regulations (CFR) of the Food and Drug Administration, the Standards for Blood Banks and Transfusion Services of the American Association of Blood Banks (AABB Standards) (2), state and local reglations, and internal procedures of organizations such as the American Red Cross.

Donor Safety

Since there is no tangible benefit to blood donation, it is important that the risk of the procedure be kept to an absolute minimum.

Standards require that donors be at least 17 years old. While some centers allow donation only to age 66, others have extended the age for donor eligibility to 70 or 75 years of age, with no apparent increase in adverse donor reactions. Donors are asked open-ended questions about their current state of health and previous serious illnesses, to determine that they are healthy enough to give blood. Donors with diseases of the heart, lungs, and liver, those with a convulsive disorder, a history of cancer or abnormal bleeding, and pregnant women usually are deferred. Questions are asked about medication taken by donors, to confirm the donor's general good health. While the drug itself may not represent additional donation risk or be harmful to the recipient, its use may indicate an underlying disease that would place a donor at greater risk.

Blood donation frequency has been limited to no more than once every 8 weeks, in order to maintain the iron stores of the donor. More frequent donation is acceptable where there is clear benefit to the recipient, such as with autologous donation, or with programs designed to limit donor exposure by providing several units for a given recipient from the same donor.

Recipient Safety

Most questions asked of the donor are related to recipient safety, such as the need to defer donors at risk of transmitting infectious disease. Donors are deferred if they have a history of hepatitis, a positive test for hepatitis B surface antigen, or if they were the only donor involved in a case of posttransfusion hepatitis. Since hepatitis A does not have a prolonged carrier state, and childhood hepatitis is most likely to have been hepatitis A, it is reasonable to accept for donation those prospective donors who have a history of childhood hepatitis. At this time, however, the CFR prohibits this practice.

Donors who know that they have antibody to hepatitis B surface antigen are accepted, since such individuals are immune and not infectious. Donors with known antibody to hepatitis B core antigen (anticore) are deferred, because anticore may be present without surface antigen in an infectious donor early in the course of the disease, and also because anticore may serve as a marker for the presence of other infectious sexually-transmitted diseases, such as non-A, non-B, non-C hepatitis or retroviral agents that are as yet uncharacterized. Finally, donors are deferred for 12 months if they have had recent close exposure to hepatitis, have had a blood transfusion, or have been exposed to tattooing or other potentially unsterile skin puncture.

Donors are deferred if they have engaged in practices known to increase risk of HIV-1 infection, such as intravenous drug use, male homosexual or bisexual activity, or heterosexual activity with people at such increased risk. Donors also are questioned about signs and symptoms of AIDS, AIDS-related complex, and Kaposi's sarcoma or a positive test for anti-HIV-1 (3). While the donor is asked to read a pamphlet that describes in detail the kinds of exposure leading to deferral, it is preferable to repeat this information orally, to ensure communication to the illiterate donor.

Transfusion malaria has not been seen in America with any frequency since the end of the Vietnam War. Nevertheless, it remains a cause of concern, as malaria eradication in many parts of the world has become more difficult, and therapy of malaria more of a challenge. For this reason, special criteria must be used for donors who have traveled to areas considered endemic for malaria by the Centers for Disease Control. Such donors are deferred for 6 months if they are asymptomatic and have not taken antimalarial drugs. Because antimalarial drugs may suppress the development of clinical malaria, donors having taken such drugs are deferred for 3 years after leaving the endemic area and stopping the drugs. Natives of countries endemic for malaria must be asymptomatic for 3 years after leaving before being accepted as blood donors.

Patients with tick-borne parasitic diseases, such as Lyme disease and babesiosis, may have infectious agents in the blood, but infected individuals usually are so sick during such episodes that they would be otherwise ineligible to be blood donors. Transfusion is a significant mechanism of transmission of Chagas' disease (American trypanosomiasis) in Latin American countries, but the disease is not endemic in this country. Only rare cases of transfusion-associated Chagas' disease have occurred in this country to date (4). The finding of leishmaniasis in servicemen returning from the Persian Gulf has led to the recommendation that all who have visited that area after August 1, 1990 be deferred until the risk of transfusion transmission is better defined, or until a test for the presence of this parasite is available.

Donors are permanently deferred if they have received human growth hormone, because of reports of transmission of Creutzfeldt-Jakob disease from this product. Those recently immunized with live attenuated viral preparations are deferred temporarily.

Finally, the donor is asked to indicate that he or she has read and understood the contents of provided informational pamphlets, understands the risks of blood donation, the potential for donor reactions, and consents to the process.

DONOR SELECTION: PHYSICAL EXAMINATION

As part of the donor screening process, donors' vital signs are determined and the arms are examined for evidence of intravenous drug abuse. The following types of donors are deferred: (*a*) those who are febrile (temperature above 37.5°C), to reduce the potential for transmission of infection; (*b*) those who are hypertensive (blood pressure greater than 180/100 mm Hg); (*c*) those who have abnormalities of pulse rate (below 50/min or above 100/min) or rhythm indicative of underlying heart disease; and (*d*) those who are so small (less than 50 kg) that the removal of 450 ml of blood could lead to more frequent donor reactions than with larger donors.

A hemoglobin or hematocrit determination is performed on every potential donor to ensure that donation does not cause or aggravate anemia. Both the CFR and AABB Standards have a minimum hemoglobin requirement of 12.5 g/dl; neither the FDA nor the AABB considers normal variations of hemoglobin levels with sex or height above sea level.

A sample of blood obtained from the earlobe will provide a value for hemoglobin or hematocrit somewhat higher than one obtained by fingerstick or venous sampling. Neither the AABB Standards nor the CFR specifies the sampling technique.

A copper sulfate hemoglobin screening method is frequently used today. If a drop of blood has a hemoglobin content of 12.5 g/dl or greater, it will sink in a copper sulfate solution with a specific gravity of 1.053. While this test is sensitive, it is not very specific, and blood centers often test those who fail the copper sulfate screening test with a more specific test such as a microhematocrit. This testing combination is unlikely to accept as a blood donor someone whose hemoglobin is below acceptable levels, nor will it lead to the deferral of those whose hemoglobins are truly satisfactory. Portable spectrophotometers may also be used for hemoglobin testing. All techniques used must be adequately monitored with a quality control program.

Repeated blood donation can lead to depletion of iron stores, particularly in women of childbearing age who may have marginal iron stores to begin with. Some workers have advocated protective measures, such as the use of specific tests for iron deficiency in blood donors, prolonging the acceptable period between blood donations for selected groups, and the use of oral iron supplementation for regular blood donors. Others conclude that while depletion of iron stores is common, morbidity due to iron deficiency will not occur without the development of anemia. Thus, the hemoglobin screening tests are adequate to prevent disease (5). Both groups are concerned about the safety of the donor, and both recognize that women of childbearing age are frequently deferred because of anemia. Blood donor iron supplementation may become more common in this country, particularly if oral iron in a form nontoxic to small children becomes available.

Tests required to be performed routinely on the donated blood also may be performed before donation. ALT and anti-HBc determinations each lead to the loss of a relatively high percentage of blood donors (as high as 2%). Accordingly, the cost of reagent-containing cassettes and portable spectrophotometers used for these tests could be recovered by saving the costs of collection and laboratory processing for blood that eventually will be discarded. Predonation testing has the advantage of keeping potentially infectious units out of the laboratory, and the disadvantage of requiring posttest counseling in the donor room.

COLLECTION PROCESS

Blood collection techniques must not compromise the safety and efficacy of the product obtained. These techniques include positive identification of the donor, and assigning a unique identifying number for the donation that is placed on the bag, on the donor history card, and on any pilot samples needed for laboratory testing. After finding a suitable vein, the phlebotomist prepares the skin by extensive cleansing with surgical soap in an area several inches around the site of intended venipuncture. This is followed by the application of an iodine-containing solution (typically PVP iodine, less sensitizing than tincture of iodine) to complete the process of making the skin as aseptic as possible (6). Following this skin preparation, the needle is inserted and 450 ml of blood (less if the donor weighs less than 50 kg) is collected into a bag containing an anticoagulant-preservative solution. During collection, the blood is mixed regularly, either manually or with a mechanical agitation device, to ensure adequate mixing with the anticoagulant and prevention of formation of clots. When the collection is completed, tubing from the donor to the bag is sealed, following which the needle is withdrawn. At all times, attention is paid to the need to prevent anything other than donor blood from entering the preconnected sterile plastic bags.

Pressure is applied directly to the donor's venipuncture site to ensure stoppage of the flow of blood, and the bag is prepared for transport to the testing laboratory after stripping the blood in the still-attached plastic tubing into the bag. This ensures that the blood has been adequately mixed with anticoagulant. The plastic tubing is then sealed into segments that can be used for subsequent testing in the laboratory or in the hospital.

After a few minutes, an appropriate bandage is placed on the arm, the donor sits up for brief observation by the phlebotomist, and then is escorted to a refreshment area. Here the donor is encouraged to drink several glasses of liquid, while under observation for potential reactions. Donors are given verbal or written instructions following donation regarding care of their arms, the need to drink fluids to replace lost blood volume, and permissible activity levels.

PROCESSING OF DONOR BLOOD

Each unit of donor blood must be tested for ABO group and Rh type, and blood from donors with a history of prior transfusion or pregnancy should be tested for unexpected antibodies. In addition, all donor blood is tested to determine its potential for transmission of infectious diseases. Required tests include a serologic test for syphilis, HBsAg, anti-HIV-1, anti-HIV-2, anti-HBc, ALT, anti-HTLV-I, and anti-HCV. The results of these tests would be negative or within the normal range before the blood is released for transfusion. Some severely immunodeficient patients may require blood found negative for anti-CMV.

DONOR REACTIONS

Donors may develop insignificant postphlebotomy hematomas and local pain or paresthesias. While some of these complications may require a visit to a physician for reassurance, they usually resolve within a brief interval.

The more difficult problem is the "vasovagal" reaction, seen in from 1 to 3% of blood donors. Early symptoms and signs include pallor, nausea, and diaphoresis. Some donors become apprehensive and hyperventilate, producing signs of hypocalcemia. Often these early signs are recognized and the reaction reversed, with cool compresses and leg evaluation, or for hyperventilation, rebreathing of expired air. More severe reactions proceed to a loss of consciousness, associated with a significant drop in systolic blood pressure (rarely as low as 50 mm/Hg) and a pulse rate ranging from 40 to 60 per minute. Signs of severe reactions may include convulsive movements, vomiting, and (rarely) fecal or urinary incontinence. These reactions are frightening but inconsequential in otherwise healthy donors.

While the primary cause of this vagal stimulation is felt to be psychological, it is associated with the volume of blood removed, the age and donation experience of the donor, and the ambience of the collection facility. Prevention includes assuring that underweight donors are not bled the full 450 ml, and that additional attention is paid to young and first-time donors or donors otherwise apprehensive, because early reactions often can be reversed. It is important to ensure that donors are under observation in the immediate postdonation period so that signs and symptoms are noted before fainting and injury occur.

Treatment involves keeping the donor supine, with legs elevated, to enhance blood flow to the head. Recovery usually takes 5 to 15 minutes. While some facilities are prepared to provide intravenous fluids, oxygen, or vagal-blocking medications, these interventions are almost never necessary. The donor who has had a reaction should be advised that these reactions may recur within the next several hours, and extra caution should be used in driving or operating heavy machinery. Donors with severe reactions should be discouraged from attempting to give blood again in the near future.

SPECIAL COLLECTION ISSUES

Blood Safety

Despite varied approaches to exclude those at high risk of infection from the donation process, there is serologic evidence that individuals infected with hepatitis and HIV-1 continue to donate. Continued effort must be made to reduce donation frequency by those at high risk. Adequate privacy must be provided for the donor interview, so that honest answers to personal questions can be given by the donor, without fear of being overhead by others. Information about high-risk activity should be given in verbal as well as written form, so that functionally illiterate donors are informed. Accurate donor identification must be obtained for comparison with donors who have been deferred previously, and their identification entered into a permanent donor deferral record. Sites other than the blood center must offer confidential and inexpensive infectious disease testing to prevent those at risk of infectious disease from donating blood in an attempt merely to obtain a test result. Finally, the donor should be given the opportunity to indicate confidentially after donation that his or her blood should not be used for transfusion. Opportunities for such confidential exclusion can be provided at the time of blood donation and by providing a telephone number that the donor may call afterwards.

Staff Safety

Collection staff should be protected as much as possible from exposure to blood. Sharp objects must be placed in a container that will allow disposal without fear of accidental puncture. Staff who are at risk of exposure to blood should be encouraged to be vaccinated for hepatitis B. Those preparing segments from the plastic tubing of the blood bag need to be protected from breakage and spraying of blood from these segments at the time of sealing.

"Universal precautions" (including the use of gloves by phlebotomists) are appropriate whenever dealing with patients, whether hospitalized or at the blood center for therapeutic phlebotomy or autologous donation. Collection staff is at minimal risk of infectious disease acquisition from the occasional exposure to blood of volunteer blood donors, since there is no increase in frequency in such workers for markers for highly infectious agents such as hepatitis B (7). Nevertheless, gloves should be available for those phlebotomists who wish to use them, and should be worn in every situation where a phlebotomist has broken or abraded skin.

Directed Donations

Fear of infectious disease transmission has prompted many potential recipients of transfusions to seek blood from family and friends, rather than from the general blood supply. No data exist to show greater safety of such donations. In fact, because of a higher percentage of first-time donors, directed units are likely to have a greater frequency of markers for infectious diseases. Despite concern that the availability of such blood tends to make the general blood supply less attractive in the eyes of the public, this practice is generally tolerated.

One special situation where the use of a designated donor has merit is in the attempt to limit the number of donors to whom an individual recipient is exposed. For instance, for a pediatric recipient with limited blood requirements, several donations could be obtained from one donor, thereby limiting the exposure of the recipient to blood from other homologous donors. In special situations of this sort, the benefit to the recipient may outweigh the additional risk incurred by the donor with modification of established standards for blood donors, for instance, by decreasing the interval between donations and lowering of the hemoglobin standard.

Some indications for directed donation are prompted by medical need and not patient demand. These include plateletpheresis of siblings to provide products for a bleeding patient found to be refractory to platelets from random donors, or donor-specific transfusions to facilitate renal transplantation.

Preoperative Autologous Donation

Patients may donate their own blood preoperatively for anticipated transfusion during elective surgery (8). The ideal candidate for preoperative autologous donation is someone who is otherwise in good health undergoing a procedure that is likely to require transfusion. Patients undergoing orthopaedic or plastic surgical procedures often fall into this category.

There is more controversy regarding patients who have a significant systemic disease, such as patients scheduled to undergo coronary artery bypass procedures, or patients with cerebrovascular disease. In these situations, a severe donor reaction may result in hypotension, which would be especially dangerous because of preexisting compromise of blood flow to critical organs. Nonetheless, such patients are often accepted as autologous donors (with the exception of those with significant aortic stenosis, transient ischemic attacks, and active angina pectoris). Since the risk of deleterious effect from homologous blood transfusion is low, the risk to these patients should be equally low to justify this process. In these special situations of somewhat higher donor risk, resuscitation should be available if needed, and consideration should be given to the treatment of severe vasovagal reactions with vagal blocking agents, or maintaining blood volume by saline infusion in one arm while blood is being withdrawn from the other.

Patients scheduled for operations where blood is not expected to be used are not candidates for autologous donation. Autologous donation in pregnant women is particularly controversial. There is little benefit to those in whom bleeding at the time of delivery is not expected; moreover, there is a theoretical risk related to potential compromise of the fetal blood supply.

Where preoperative autologous transfusion is indicated, it is acceptable to modify the standards set for volunteer blood donors: the increased benefit to the patient justifies some modest increase in risk to the patient as a donor, such as a minimum hemoglobin of 11 g/dl rather than 12.5 g/dl, and allowance of repeated donation at short intervals.

BLOOD COMPONENT PREPARATION AND STORAGE

General Principles

The desirability of providing patients with those elements of blood that are needed, and to the extent possible, limiting exposure to unneeded components, was recognized long before it was generally possible to utilize such an approach in practice. The widespread use of plastic bags in the late 1950s allowed centrifugal separation of the formed elements of blood on the basis of specific gravity, and separation of those elements in a closed, presterilized system without bacterial contamination. As a consequence, the often fatal septicemia resulting from introduction of bacteria into blood and blood components at the time of preparation or further manipulation have become rare. The recent availability of a sterile "docking" device provides additional flexibility, allowing the coupling of two sterile plastic containers that were not connected at the time of manufacture. If, during component preparation, the system is opened without the use of a sterile docking device, the components can be stored for no longer than 24 hours at 1 to 6°C or 4 hours at room temperature.

Red Blood Cells

CELL AGING

Red cells in the body have a life span of approximately 120 days. While minimal destruction of cells of all ages occurs normally, by far the more common pattern is the destruction of senescent red cells. This process is related in part to a loss of lipid in the red cell membrane and a loss of the ability of the membrane to maintain its shape. When red blood cells (RBCs) are stored in vitro, the process is associated with depletion of ATP. Length of storage of RBCs is related to the ability of the cells to maintain adequate levels of ATP. Energy is needed not only to drive the sodium-potassium pump, but also to support the shape of the red cell and to prevent loss of the lipid from the membrane. Ideal storage in vitro would provide red cells with a posttransfusion survival equal to, or better than, cells of a similar age remaining in the body. Since blood drawn from a normal donor contains RBCs with an average age of 60 days, it would be desirable to store those cells in vitro so that at the end of 30 days, or another 25% of the red cells' normal life span, no more than the oldest 25% of the RBC would die. In fact, it is possible to store RBCs for longer periods of time with greater survival of the remaining cells.

MEASUREMENT OF RED CELL PRESERVATION

Techniques of RBC preservation were evaluated originally with the use of a label to determine the posttransfusion survival of such stored cells. However, it is now recognized that cells circulating 24 hours after transfusion have a survival that is comparable to normal RBCs. It is therefore possible to use the more efficient 24-hour posttransfusion recovery as an index of posttransfusion survival. Seventy percent of the RBCs transfused after a period of storage should survive in the circulation 24 hours after transfusion. Because cells from one individual have poststorage survival characteristics different from those of another, the use of a 75% 24-hour survival of transfused RBCs will ensure that at the end of the allowed storage period most units of blood will have adequate recovery and survival, despite individual variation.

In the evaluation of anticoagulant-preservative solutions, posttransfusion recovery and survival are currently assessed by the transfusion of radiolabeled autologous RBC. While technically more difficult, it is probably important to utilize a double-radioisotope technique. The loss of some RBCs immediately following transfusion may lead to falsely high levels of recovery if a single-label technique is used.

RED CELL FUNCTION

The primary role of the RBC is the delivery of oxygen to tissues. Storage of RBCs in vitro leads to the depletion of 2,3-diphosphoglycerate (2,3-DPG), important for the release of oxygen from hemoglobin. While this substance is regenerated within 24 hours following transfusion in storage-depleted RBCs, it would be ideal to maintain 2,3-DPG levels during storage. Rats, resuscitated after hemorrhage to half-normal hematocrits with 2,3-DPG deplated blood, have compromised survival compared to those resuscitated with 2,3-DPG replete blood (9). However, it has not yet been possible to demonstrate in the human that absence of 2,3-DPG from transfused RBCs, even when such cells are given in massive amounts, has been associated with adverse effects, perhaps because of compensatory mechanisms such as the Bohr effect. There remain theoretical concerns. For instance, patients with underlying coronary artery insufficiency subjected to massive transfusion might benefit from provision of blood with adequate amounts of 2,3-DPG.

Transfusion of blood after the end of the allowable storage period has no apparent ill effect for the recipient, aside from a posttransfusion increase in hemoglobin catabolites, such as bilirubin. The transfusion of such outdated red cells, occasionally necessitated at times of blood shortage, has not been associated with the pathophysiological consequences of hemolytic transfusion reaction.

PRESERVATIVE SOLUTIONS

Dextrose was added to anticoagulant solutions because of the empirical recognition that it improved posttransfusion RBC recovery and survival. Buffering of the anticoagulant-sugar solution to a lower pH allowed heat sterilization without carmelization of the sugar. With greater awareness of the role of ATP and 2,3-DPG in RBC preservation and function, preservative solutions have been fashioned to optimize amounts of these materials in RBC during storage.

Citrate has long been the anticoagulant of choice. It is readily catabolized in the body upon transfusion. By chelating calcium, it inhibits several calcium-dependent steps of the coagulation sequence. It is commonly used in a sodium citrate/citric acid buffer, and is provided in substantial molar excess to calcium. Anticoagulants such as EDTA and heparin have been used from time to time, but have deleterious effects on RBC storage over all but the shortest time span.

Standard anticoagulant-preservative solutions have long included a sodium citrate/citric acid buffer, adjusted to provide an initial pH of the stored blood of 7.5 to 7.6 (at 37°C), and dextrose. Inorganic phosphate has been shown to have a minimal effect on posttransfusion recovery, but enhances maintenance of 2,3-DPG and ATP. Adenine prolongs RBC storage in vitro by serving as a substrate, allowing synthesis of ATP (10). These elements provide the basis for a commonly used solution, CPDA-1, which contains a citrate buffer with phosphate, dextrose, and adenine.

More recently, collection container techniques have allowed increased amounts of adenine to be added selectively to the red blood cells, to provide still better RBC storage. The amount of adenine added is ultimately limited by the potential for precipitation of adenine metabolites in the kidneys following massive transfusion. Some adenine-enriched solutions contain a small amount of mannitol to reduce hemolysis after extended storage. Because these newer solutions (AS-1 or AS-3) allow the separation and recovery of larger amounts of plasma, and allow RBC to be stored for a longer period, they have become the favored anticoagulant-preservative solutions.

Red Blood Cells can be prepared simply by sedimentation, followed by separation of the supernatant plasma into an attached container. Most facilities that collect blood in substantial amounts separate either Platelets, Fresh Frozen Plasma, or both, from the whole blood by centrifugation techniques shortly after collection, leaving either CPDA-1 Red Blood Cells with a volume of 250 ml, a hematocrit of 70 to 80%, and 35-day dating, or AS-1 or AS-3 red blood cells, with a volume of 350 ml, a hematocrit of 50 to 60%, and 42-day dating. Storage of RBC in vitro causes changes in plasma pH, and red cell ATP, 2,3-DPG, and potassium. The nature of these changes is shown in Table 66.1.

Table 66.1. Biochemical Changes in Blood Stored at 5°C[a]

		CPDA-1		AS-1
	WB	WB	RBC	RBCs
Days stored	0	35	35	49
% Viable cells (24-hr. posttransfusion)	100	79	71	76
pH (at 37°C)	7.6	6.98	6.71	6.6
ATP %	100	56	45	64
2,3-DPG %	100	<10	<10	<5
Plasma K^+ mmol/liter	4.2	27.3	78.5	—

[a]Modified with permission from Walker RH, ed. Technical manual. 10th ed. Arlington, VA: American Association of Blood Banks, 1990.

REJUVENATION

RBCs severely depleted of ATP and 2,3-DPG during storage can regenerate these substances with the addition of "rejuvenating" solutions, such as one containing pyruvate, inosine, phosphate, glucose, and adenine. These solutions are potentially toxic and cannot be transfused, so following rejuvenation, the RBCs are washed and transfused, or glycerolized and stored in the frozen state for subsequent transfusion.

pH

Because of continuing slow RBC metabolism of glucose to lactate during storage, the accumulation of hydrogen ions in the plasma lowers the pH over time. RBCs stored for 35 days in CPDA-1 may have pH as low as 6.7 (37°C). There is no evidence that the massive transfusion of blood with a pH at this level has any deleterious clinical effect, because of numerous in vivo mechanisms to compensate for acidosis.

POTASSIUM

Potassium is gradually lost from RBCs during storage, and it increases in the plasma overlying whole blood at a rate of approximately 1 mEq/day. The potassium concentration is higher when accumulated in smaller amounts of plasma, such as with Red Blood Cells, in either CPDA-1 or adenine-supplemented preservative solutions. The infusion of Red Blood Cells containing potassium at these high concentrations (up to 80 mEq/liter toward the end of the storage time) is of no consequence in most clinical situations, including the transfusion of massive amounts of stored blood. There are concerns, however, about potassium levels in blood used for exchange transfusion of neonatal patients and for blood given to patients with renal failure. In these situations, provision of blood that is relatively fresh (stored for less than 7 days) provides levels of potassium that although elevated are safe for clinical use.

MICROAGGREGATES

Microaggregates of white cell and platelet debris form in Red Blood Cells during storage. These aggregates are not removed by standard transfusion filters with a pore size of 170μ, designed to prevent the transfusion of visible clots. After transfusion, microaggregates may be removed from the circulation during passage through the lungs. The clinical significance of such microaggregates is unclear. They probably have little untoward effect, except in situations where the lungs are removed from the circulation, as in cardiopulmonary bypass, or perhaps in some massive transfusion situations. Early data suggesting clinical hypoxia following transfusion of microaggregates have not been substantiated, although in animal models, poor respiratory function has been seen following microaggregate transfusion. In special situations where microaggregates might represent a concern, filters designed for their removal can be used.

FROZEN RED BLOOD CELLS

Red blood cells can be stored for 10 years in the frozen state. It is possible that little additional loss of posttransfusion recoverability is seen after several decades. Such storage requires either extremely rapid freezing of RBCs and maintenance at very low temperatures (obtained with liquid nitrogen freezers that maintain a temperature below −120°C), the addition of large amounts of cryoprotective agent, or some combination of these approaches (11). The inconvenience of transport of RBCs stored in liquid nitrogen has led to the widespread use of 40% w/v glycerol as an intracellular cryoprotective agent. The glycerol must be added to the RBCs slowly with mixing to minimize hemolysis. Glycerolized RBC may be stored with mechnical refrigeration at below −65°C for up to 10 years, and they may be transported in dry ice. After thawing, most of the glycerol in the RBCs must be removed to prevent posttransfusion osmotic hemolysis. Removal of glycerol is commonly performed by washing the thawed RBCs first with a hypertonic saline solution, followed by resuspension in normal saline. RBC recovery from a freeze/thaw/wash process must be at least 80%, and the RBC viability at 24 hours posttransfusion must be at least 70%. Because of cost, this technique is not widely used, but it is valuable for storage of RBCs of rare phenotype, or for autologous transfusion situations when extended storage is needed.

LEUKOCYTE-REDUCED RED BLOOD CELLS

Buffy Coat Removal. Centrifugation allows the separation of a 50-ml leukocyte-containing buffy coat from the top of the RBC layer. With optimal techniques, buffy coat removal can eliminate up to 80% of the leukocytes from the unit, with the loss of 20% of the RBCs. This product will prevent many leukocyte-related febrile nonhemolytic transfusion reactions, but for some patients, the level of white cell removal is insufficient. Leukocyte-Reduced Red Blood Cells prepared by buffy coat removal currently are rarely used.

Leukocyte Filters. Current management of patients who have repeated febrile transfusion reactions involves the use of newer filtration techniques. Removal of most of the leukocytes, with minimal loss of RBCs, can be readily accomplished in the blood processing laboratory. One can select a unit of Red Blood Cells at least 3 weeks old, recentrifuge it to facilitate leukocyte aggregation, maintain it undisturbed for several hours at 5°C, and then transfuse it through a microaggregate filter. This approach will consistently produce a product with less than 5×10^8 leukocytes, sufficient to meet the AABB standards for prevention of febrile transfusion reactions. A better approach uses a special collection bag with in-line filtration in the laboratory shortly after collection, and subsequent storage of RBC in additive solution for 42 days. Leukocytes in this product are in the range of 10^6. This degree of leukocyte removal can also be approached at the bedside, without prior laboratory manipulation, with the use of newer adherence filters (12).

WASHED RED BLOOD CELLS

For years, a preparation of Washed Red Blood Cells has been used to treat patients whose febrile reactions persist following the administration of Leukocyte-Reduced Red Blood Cells. The washing process, using automated techniques, removes 90% of the leukocytes, with the loss of 10% of the RBCs. Although this product is adequate for treating febrile transfusion reactions, newer filters have made washing superfluous for this purpose. Washing has the advantage of removing most (99%) of the plasma, so it can be used for the treatment of patients for whom some plasma components can be deleterious. For instance, some clinicians treat patients with paroxysmal nocturnal hemoglobinuria with Washed Red Blood Cells to prevent the infusion of complement components. Washing RBCs may be sufficient to prevent reactions in patients who lack IgA and who have had reactions to blood components containing these immunoglobulins. In a few cases, however, this procedure has been insufficient to prevent such reactions, and products from donors known to be IgA deficient are preferable.

Platelets

Platelets are the lightest of the formed elements of the blood. After slow centrifugation of whole blood, platelet-rich plasma can be found at the top, and can be readily separated. Subsequent hard centrifugation of this plasma will sediment the concentrated platelets, and the platelet-poor plasma can then be removed. The collection of blood into a closed system containing several preattached plastic bags allows this manipulation without opening the bag system; therefore, platelets in concentrated form can be prepared and stored at room temperature for several days after collection without fear of growth of bacteria introduced at the time of preparation.

The techniques used to provide consistently good platelet concentrates begin with collection of blood from the donor. Blood collection should be fairly rapid and uninterrupted. The collection of blood over a prolonged period of time, or with interruptions, could lead to the initiation of coagulation on a scale too small to be detected, but sufficient to cause the initiation of platelet activation. Following collection, the temperature of whole blood is maintained above 20°C until platelets are prepared.

In the laboratory, optimal platelet recovery is best achieved by using a force as low as reasonably possible for the centrifugal preparation of the platelet-rich plasma (6). While yield can be slightly increased by extending down into the lymphocyte-rich top layer of buffy coat, this usually is unnecessary. Furthermore, the increase in white cells from such a procedure adds to the metabolic storage burden, and to a greater possibility of sensitization. The platelet-rich plasma is then recentrifuged to concentrate the platelets. This spin should be as hard as necessary to provide adequate concentration, but not so hard that platelets are damaged in the process. The platelet-poor plasma is then expressed, leaving a final product volume of between 50 and 70 ml, depending on the type of container used. The platelet-rich plasma should be separated from the unit of blood within 8 hours of the time of collection, and the platelet concentrate should be prepared within 10 hours of this time.

Platelets are stored for 5 days at room temperature, by meeting critical storage requirements in areas of pH, plastic, and agitation. The pH of the platelet concentrate must be maintained at levels above 6.0. This level will fall as a result of normal metabolic processes during storage. Newer plastics with improved gas permeability can allow development of an abnormally elevated pH; this may also be deleterious to platelets.

The type of container used for platelet storage has special requirements. Polyvinyl chloride bags have in their formulation a "plasticizer" to provide flexibility. A common plasticizer formulation, diethylhexylphthallate (DEHP), is leached from the polyvinyl into lipid-containing plasma, and from there may be transfused. Because of the possibility of toxicity from the transfusion of massive amounts of this material (13), and because of prolonged storage of DEHP in the body, manufacturers have sought formulations that would minimize its content. The plastics most often used for storage of platelets consist of polyolefin, which does not require a plasticizer; thinner polyvinyl with reduced DEHP; or polyvinyl with a different plasticizer, tri(2-ethylhexyl)trimellitate. Platelets may be stored at room temperature in these containers for 5 days. Plasticizers now in development are nontoxic in animal models and are readily catabolized in the body. Such plasticizers would eliminate the current theoretical concerns related to the infusion of DEHP. In general, plastic designed for platelet storage provides better exchange of CO_2 and O_2 across the bag, and therefore minimizes the reduction in pH in the stored platelet concentrate.

Another constant requirement for prolonged storage of platelet concentrates is agitation. Immediately after removal from the centrifuge, the concentrate should be allowed to stand undisturbed for an hour or two. Following this, the component is placed on a mechnical device for continuous agitation. Some types of agitation are particularly harsh and provide poor platelet recovery. The common types currently utilized are to-and-fro, rotary or elliptical agitation, with the bag laid flat on the rotator. The most desirable type of rotator varies to some extent with the type of bag used (14). The temperature must be controlled between 20°C and 24°C.

Plasma at room temperature is a bacterial growth medium. Donors must not be bacteremic at the time of donation, and platelets cannot be pooled in an open system, to provide a typical dose for transfusion, and then subsequently stored at room temperature. Even with these precautions, a few bacteria present at the time of collection may proliferate to unacceptable levels in platelets stored at room temperature. As a result, there is a maximum storage time of 5 days, even though survival characteristics of the platelets would permit their storage for longer periods with some containers.

Before platelets could be stored for 5 days, there was a considerable interest in their storage in the frozen state. The technique developed then, and still preferred today, uses dimethylsulfoxide (DMSO) rather than glycerol as a cryoprotective agent. However, platelets are more fragile than red blood cells, and the recovery of platelets in the recipient after freezing and thawing is poorer than that of red cells. Storage of platelets in the frozen state has little use, except when autologous platelets are obtained from patients with leukemia in remission and stored in the frozen state to provide support at the time of the next therapeutic induction. This may be especially helpful when patients are refractory to homologous platelets.

A small number of platelet concentrates prepared every month must be tested at the end of their storage time to be certain that a pH of greater that 6.0 is maintined in all units tested, and to confirm that the number of platelets present exceeds 5.5×10^{10} in 75% of the units tested. Some platelet preparation techniques result in the presence of substantial numbers of red cells in the final product, giving it a pink tinge. The presence of more than 0.5 ml of red cells is felt to be excessive. Rh-negative patients, who are given repeated transfusions of Platelets from Rh-positive donors with this level of red cell contamination, will develop Rh antibodies, although this occurs in only 8% of patients. However, it is not difficult to produce products with much less red cell contamination. Furthermore, if Rh-positive red cell-containing Platelets must be given to Rh-negative recipients, Rh immunoglobulin can be administered within 72 hours of the transfusion to prevent sensitization.

Fresh Frozen Plasma

The primary concern in the preparation of Fresh Frozen Plasma is that it be frozen quickly, before deterioration of labile clotting factors. For this reason, the time of collection should be noted. The plasma should be placed in the freezer within 8 hours of this time and frozen solid in the next 2 hours (within 10 hours of the time of collection of the whole blood). Because the time to preparation of a frozen product and the time of freezing are so important, rapid freezing techniques are used. Plasma may be immersed in an ethanol/dry ice bath or other liquid heat exchange mixture, or placed in a freezer designed for the rapid freezing of 200 to 250 ml of plasma. Once frozen, there is little deterioration of labile clotting factors in Fresh Frozen Plasma, so that it can be stored for a year below −18°C without appreciable loss of activity. Therefore, in quality control the emphasis is on the timing of the freezing process, rather than on clotting factor assays.

Liquid Plasma (Single Donor Plasma)

It is possible to transfuse the plasma remaining after the removal of cryoprecipitate, or plasma that has been separated beyond the acceptable time limits for Fresh Frozen Plasma; moreover, such plasma may be stored in the frozen state. Frozen plasma may have low levels of labile coagulation factors, and cryoprecipitate-poor plasma lacks factor VIII and fibrinogen. These plasmas can also be stored in the liquid state, again with loss of labile coagulation factors. While deficiency of stable clotting factors can be successfully treated with liquid plasma, Fresh Frozen Plasma is more commonly used, simply because it is readily available.

Plasma often is used, albeit inappropriately, for volume expansion. However, the risk of disease transmission, compared with albumin or plasma protein fraction, makes it undesirable for this purpose.

One may prepare whole blood by reconstituting the red cells with the plasma from the same unit after the removal of buffy coat, platelet concentrate, or cryoprecipitate. This preparation provides the advantage of offering the patient red cells and protein volume expander with some coagulation factors, without exposure to additional risk of disease transmission. Nevertheless, the labor-intensive preparation of these products has limited their widespread availability.

Cryoprecipitated AHF

When Fresh Frozen Plasma is thawed at 5°C, some material does not go into solution. The remaining precipitate contains much of the factor VIII (antihemophilic factor) and fibrinogen, and some of the factor XIII, of the original unit. The cold precipitation property of these proteins is important in the further manufacture of factor VIII preparations for the treatment of hemophilia. Cryoprecipitate can be separated from the precipitate-poor plasma by centrifugation of the plasma containing the cryoprecipitate. After centrifugation, the precipitate will adhere to the plastic bag sufficiently to allow transfer of the precipitate-poor plasma into another container. Between 7 and 15 ml plasma is usually left in the bag. Each cryoprecipitate is then refrozen, thawed when needed, and pooled for transfusion. In some facilities small amounts of saline are added to the cryoprecipitate to facilitate its recovery. At least 4 units are assayed each month to determine factor VIII activity. Seventy-five percent of units tested should contain at least 80 units of antihemophilic factor (AHF) activity (compared with the approximately 200 to 250 units present in the original fresh frozen plasma). Since a major use of cryoprecipitate is as a source of fibrinogen or (with an admixture of thrombin) of "fibrin glue," it may also be desirable to determine the level of fibrinogen in the product (typically between 100 and 350 mg/dl).

CYTAPHERESIS PRODUCT PREPARATION AND STORAGE

Principles

Recognizing that platelet or granulocyte products from many whole blood donors were necessary to provide an adequate dose for a single recipient, researchers created devices to allow the collection of sufficient numbers of platelets or granulocytes from a donor at one setting. The most commonly used devices utilize a continuous flow of donor blood, using principles developed in the dairy industry for separation of cream.

The donor typically is connected to a machine for a period of 1 to 2 hours, during which time blood is continuously collected, the desired component is separated by centrifugation techniques, and the unneeded components are returned to the donor through a second venous line. Both continuous and discontinuous flow devices may be used for the procedure. Early devices used for this procedure had rotating seals, which performed effectively, but represented an open system, thereby limiting the storage time of the products obtained to 24 hours. Newer approaches allow this process to be carried out in a closed system; platelets collected by such techniques can be stored with agitation for 5 days at 20 to 24°C.

Donor Selection

The historical, physical, and laboratory criteria used for the selection of apheresis donors are similar to those of whole blood donors. In addition, there are some special concerns. Since these donors can be drawn as often as every 48 hours, the cumulative loss of red cells must be less than 200 ml every 8 weeks, and of plasma, less than 1 liter (1.2 liters for persons above 80 kg) every 7 days, with a maximum of 15 liters in 12 months. Those donors who are to undergo granulocytapheresis with the use of infused rouleaux-inducing agents, such as hydroxyethyl starch, must be asked about related allergies. Since two large veins are required for most procedures, the adequacy of venous access is important. If formed elements of the blood are removed on a frequent basis, the donor's safety must be protected by measuring levels of these formed elements during the course of a series of donations. Cytapheresis donors may donate as frequently as once a day, but no more often than 24 times a year.

Plateletpheresis donors should not have taken aspirin-containing medication within the preceding 3 days, since aspirin blocks the generation of thromboxane A_2. This blockage inhibits the platelet release reaction and renders the donated platelets less effective, particularly when the donor is the sole source of platelets for the recipient.

Untoward Consequences of Cytapheresis

Lymphocytes have a density similar to that of heavier platelets, and intensive plateletpheresis will remove large numbers of lymphocytes. This will deplete long-lived T lymphocytes, and, in theory could lead, over time, to a weakening of immune function. However, while reduction in lymphocytes for immunoglobulin levels has been noted (15), no clinical change in immune response has been seen. The removal of large numbers of platelets in a plateletpheresis procedure causes a drop in the peripheral blood platelet count of perhaps 30,000/μl. It is important, therefore, that the initial platelet count be adequate to support such a loss. For sequential donors, the postprocedure count from one plateletpheresis can be used as the initial count for the subsequent procedure.

The most common donor reaction during and after a cytapheresis procedure is the reaction to infusion of the anticoagulant sodium citrate, which produces symptoms of hypocalemia. Therefore, it is desirable to reduce the amount of infused citrate as much as possible. When such a reaction occurs, it is treated by slowing the infusion rate. A donor given corticosteroid to improve granulocyte collection, particularly when the donor is used repeatedly over a short period of time, must be asked about underlying diseases that might be exacerbated by corticosteroids, such as peptic ulcer disease and infections, such as tuberculosis.

Granulocyte recovery is much improved with the intravenous administration of a rouleaux-inducing agent, such as hydroxethyl starch. However, this material has been reported to cause both anaphylactic reactions and persistent localized skin reactions. In addition, products of this type are colloid volume expanders. Consequently, when given over several days, they can cause localized edema, headache, and other symptoms of fluid retention. The total product dose given to a donor should be monitored; it may be possible to reduce the dose for a given donor from one procedure to the next.

There have been isolated reports of donor reactions related to the equipment. Kinks in tubing have been reported to cause hemolysis. Faulty rotating seals have caused particulate carbon to be found in collection containers (but without apparent ill effect for the donor). Cytapheresis devices generally have bubble detectors to guard against dangerous reactions resulting from air embolization during reinfusion.

Platelets Pheresis

INDICATIONS

Patients refractory to platelet concentrates are often responsive to platelets from donors matched at the HLA A and B loci. Adequate amounts of such platelets from a single donor can be provided only with cytapheresis techniques. Furthermore, use of cytapheresis platelets reduces the number of donors to whom a recipient is exposed with each dose of platelets from six to one, producing a similar reduction in risk of transfusion-transmitted disease and in the potential for febrile transfusion reactions.

In addition, apheresis platelets may reduce the rapidity or the frequency of development of the refractory state (16). Based on experimental data, many workers feel that if sufficient leukocytes could be removed from the platelet product (to less than 10^6), sensitization would be eliminated. Manufacturers of some machines used for cytapheresis claim the ability to produce platelet products with leukocyte depletion close to that level. Products prepared to be relatively poor in leukocytes may be subsequently filtered at the bedside to produce reduction of white cells to this desired level. Such approaches with platelets (and with similarly prepared red cells) have reduced sensitization (17).

COLLECTION TECHNIQUES

Platelet collection times vary from 1 to 2 hours. Most current techniques involve the use of a needle in each arm. Some intermittent techniques use one needle; the unused red cells and plasma are reinfused periodically through the same needle used to remove the whole blood. Each technique should be able to produce a product containing 3×10^{11} platelets in at least 75% of the units tested. Many of the products contain 10^8 leukocytes, but some newer procedures may allow reduction of this number to less than 10^7. Such platelets need not be crossmatched if they contain less than 5 ml of red cells, a level readily achieved with most techniques.

Granulocyte Pheresis

To obtain adequate amounts of granulocytes for transfusion, buffy coats from 20 to 40 units of whole blood theoretically would be required. Early techniques utilizing the adherence of granulocytes to filters produced large numbers of granulocytes, but they functioned poorly, and occasional severe complement-related donor reactions were seen.

Granulocytes are collected by procedures utilizing continuous flow techniques with differential centrifugation. Because granulocytes have densities only slightly less than red cells, it has been difficult to provide a clean centrifugal separation. Therefore, it is customary to utilize a rouleaux-inducing agent, such as hydroxethyl starch, to enhance the sedimentation of red cells with centrifugal force. Even with the use of such an agent, it is difficult to obtain adequate doses of granulocytes without pretreatment of the cytapheresis donor with corticosteroids. Prednisone has been used for this purpose because it increases the numbers of circulating granulocytes by mobilizing them from the bone marrow and by increasing the number in the circulatory pool compared with the marginal pool. Typical protocols include giving the corticosteroid in at least two doses, for instance, at 12 and 3 hours before the beginning of the cytapheresis procedure. Standards require 1×10^{10} granulocytes in 75% of the products tested.

While granulocytes may be stored at room temperature for as long as 24 hours after collection, they should be transfused as soon as possible.

Therapeutic Cytapheresis

Cytapheresis techniques may also be used therapeutically to reduce dangerously elevated levels of leukocytes (especially in myelogenous leukemia) or platelets (greater than 1,000,000/μl), before or as an adjunct to chemotherapy (18).

PLASMAPHERESIS

Plasma can be obtained from donors by withdrawal of a unit of blood, separation of the plasma by centrifugation, and reinfusion of the other components. This technique is typically repeated during one session to provide 2 units of plasma for preparation of Fresh Frozen Plasma, or to provide plasma for the manufacture of blood derivatives. A 2-unit withdrawal can be performed as often as twice weekly on an ongoing basis, with the removal of up to 1 liter of plasma per week (1.2 liters for persons weighing more than 80 kg).

The major donor concern with such a program is the potential for reinfusion of someone else's red cells; as a result, elaborate donor and product identification procedures are used. Individuals who donate plasma more frequently than every 8 weeks must have predonation serum protein determinations and periodic determinations of immunoglobulin levels.

This procedure can be performed by automated continuous flow techniques, which are quicker and avoid the possibility of reinfusion of the wrong red cells. The cost of the software has limited widespread use of automated techniques for collection of plasma for further manufacture.

Therapeutic Plasma Exchange

The availability of automated plasmapheresis equipment has facilitated the therapeutic removal of plasma and replacement with Fresh Frozen Plasma or Albumin. With adequate venous access, a 1-volume (about 3 liters) exchange can be performed in 90 minutes. This technique has been shown to be effective for patients with such conditions such as hyperviscosity syndrome, thrombotic thrombocytopenic purpura, Goodpasture's syndrome, myasthenia gravis, posttransfusion purpura, crescentic glomerulonephritis, and Guillain-Barré syndrome, among others, and in the future is likely to prove beneficial for many other diseases (19).

References

1. Drake AW. Public attitudes and decision processes with regard to blood donation: final report and executive summary. Springfield, VA: National Technical Information Service, 1978.
2. Widman FK, ed. Standards for blood banks and transfusion services. 15th ed. Bethesda, MD: American Association of Blood Banks, 1993.
3. Parkman PD. Recommendations for the prevention of human immunodeficiency virus (HIV) transmission by blood and blood products. Bethesda, MD: Center for Biologics Evaluation and Research, February 5, 1990.
4. Kirckhoff LV. Is *Trypanosoma cruzi* a new threat to our blood supply? Ann Intern Med 1989;111:773–774.
5. Garratty G. Should donor hemoglobin standards be lowered?: pro Transfusion 1989;29:261–264.
6. Walker RH, ed. Technical manual. 10th ed. Arlington, VA: American Association of Blood Banks, 1990.
7. Page PL. Risk of hepatitis B exposure in regional blood services. Transfusion 1987;27:242–244.
8. AuBuchon JP. Autologous transfusion and directed donation: current controversies and future directions. Transfusion Medicine Reviews 1989;3:290–306.
9. Collins JA. The age and hematocrit of stored blood in determining the survival of rats after exchange transfusion and hemorrhage. In: Brewer GJ, ed. Proceedings of the 4th International Conference on Red Cell Metabolism and Function, Ann Arbor, Michigan, September 14–17, 1977. New York: Alan R. Liss, 1978.
10. Beutler E. Erythrocyte metabolism and its relation to the liquid preservation of blood. In: Petz LD, Swisher SN, eds. Clinical practice of transfusion medicine. 2nd ed. New York: Churchill Livingstone, 1989:271–296.
11. Meryman HT. Frozen red cells. Transfusion Medicine Reviews 1989;3:121–127.
12. Meryman HT. Cleaning up red cells and platelets: alloimmunization, immunosuppression and disease transmission. In: McCarthy LJ, Baldwin ML, eds. Controversies of leukocyte-poor blood and components. Arlington, VA: American Association of Blood Banks, 1989:1–26.
13. Rubin RJ, Ness PM. What price progress? An update on vinyl plastic blood bags. Transfusion 1989;29:358–361.
14. Cummings E. Platelet rotaters, infusion pumps and blood warmers. Transfusion Science 1989;10:199–206.
15. Matsui Y, Martin-Alosco S, Doenges E, et al. Effects of frequent and sustained plateletapheresis on peripheral blood mononuclear cell populations and lymphocyte functions of normal volunteer donors. Transfusion 1986;26:446–452.
16. Gmür J, von Felten A, Osterwalder B, et al. Delayed alloimmunization using random single donor platelet transfusions: a prospective study in thrombocytopenic patients with acute leukemia. Blood 1983;62:473–479.
17. Saarinen UM, Kekomaki R, Siimes MA, Myllyla G. Effective prophylaxis against platelet refractoriness in multitransfused patients by use of leukocyte-free blood components. Blood 1990;75:512–517.
18. Peetoom F. Therapeutic cytapheresis. In: Westphal RG, Kasprisin DO, ed. Current status of hemapheresis: indications, technology and complications. Arlington, VA: American Association of Blood Banks, 1987:49–70.
19. Clinical Applications Committee, American Society for Apheresis. Clinical applications of therapeutic apheresis. Clin Apheresis 1986;3:1–97.

67 Pretransfusion Testing

W. John Judd

INTRODUCTION

History of Pretransfusion Testing

The scientific basis for pretransfusion testing stems from the discovery of the ABO system by Landsteiner (1). In 1907, Hektoen (2) and Weil (3) recognized the importance of Landsteiner's observations. At the urgings of Weil, Ottenberg implemented Landsteiner's work and, thus, became the first to perform both blood typing and cross-matching before transfusion (4).

In 1909, Crile (5) described a 48-hour hemolysin test for incompatibility that entailed testing donor red blood cells (RBCs) with patient serum (major cross-match) and patient RBCs with donor serum (minor cross-match). He considered agglutination of RBCs to be unimportant and, in contrast to Ottenberg (4), was of the opinion that reactions observed in the minor cross-match were more important than those seen in the major cross-match.

During World War I, compatible blood was selected for transfusion by a matching test (6) that was simpler to perform than Crile's procedure (5). It was noted that agglutination paralleled the hemolysis seen in ABO typing studies (7). Thus, ABO and cross-matching tests were done on glass slides. Both major and minor matching tests were performed, although agglutination and/or lysis of donor RBCs by recipient plasma was now considered more important than the destruction of recipient RBCs by donor plasma. Also, the use of non–cross-matched group O blood was advocated in the battlefield during World War I, and in other circumstances where adequate testing facilities were unavailable (8).

Little changed between the two World Wars. Stock reagent antisera were used for ABO typing (9). The need to perform the minor cross-match continued to be questioned (4). Some considered agglutination of donor RBCs by recipient serum to be of such importance that determination of their respective blood types was not necessary (10). By the mid-1930s, however, it became apparent that the then currently accepted pretransfusion testing practices were inadequate because hemolytic reactions occurred despite the transfusion of serologically compatible blood (11). At that time, the only other known blood group polymorphisms, in addition to ABO, were MN and P_1 (12).

What became known as the Rh antigen D was first described in 1939 (13), and the discovery of other principal Rh antigens (C, c, E, and e) soon followed (14, 15). However, it was not until 1945, when Coombs, Mourant, and Race (16) applied the antiglobulin test, described earlier by Moreschi (17), to the study of blood group antibodies, and when Diamond and Denton (18) popularized the use of albumin for enhancement of agglutination, that the science of immunohematology flourished. Subsequently, knowledge of the four then known blood group systems has expanded. At least 40 different RBC antigens are reported for both the MN and Rh blood group systems. Numerous new blood group systems were described between 1945 and 1960. By 1985, 641 different antibodies to RBC antigens had been reported (19). Many are of academic interest, while others are known to cause accelerated destruction of incompatible red cells.

Current Status

In 1958, the American Association of Blood Banks (AABB), in conjunction with the Joint Blood Council, began publishing standard codes of practice for blood banks and transfusion services (20). These minimum requirements include guidelines for pretransfusion. These have evolved (Table 67.1) to the presently acceptable practice guidelines set forth in the 15th edition of the *AABB Standards for Blood Banks Transfusion Services* (21). Practice guidelines also are promulgated by other accrediting and regulatory agencies, notably the Office of Biologics of the Food and Drug Administration (22) and the College of American Pathologists (23).

Portions of this manuscript are derived from the following sources: Walker RH, et al. Technical manual. 10th ed. Arlington, VA: American Association of Blood Banks, 1990. Judd WJ. Methods in immunohematology. Miami: Montgomery Scientific Publications, 1988. They are reproduced with permission from the publishers.

Table 67.1. Evolution of AABB Standards for Antibody Detection and Cross-matching

Required Test or Antibody Detection	1955 · 1960 · 1965 · 1970 · 1975 · 1980 · 1985 · 1990
Complete/blocking	○○○○○○○○○[a]
Coating/agglutinating	○○○○○○○○○
Hemolyzing	○○○○○○
Clinically significant	○○○○○○○
Active at 37°C	○○○○○○○○○○○
IAT for antibody detection	○○○○○○○○○○○○○○○○○
IAT cross-match	○○○○○○○○○○○○○●●●●[b]

[a] ○, required testing.
[b] ●, antiglobulin cross-match optional when clinically significant, unexpected antibodies absent, and there is no history of such antibodies.

Table 67.2. Elements of Compatibility Testing

1. ABO and Rh typing of donor blood.
2. Recognition of unexpected antibodies to RBC antigens in donor plasma.
3. Procurement of appropriate blood samples from the intended recipient.
4. ABO and Rh typing of the intended recipient's blood.
5. Recognition of unexpected antibodies to RBC antigens in the intended recipient's serum/plasma.
6. Comparison of current test results with records of previous tests.
7. Selection of RBC components that are compatible with the intended recipient's ABO group and with clinically-significant, unexpected antibodies, if present or previously detected.
8. Performance of tests to detect ABO incompatibility (and other known potential incompatibility) between selected RBC components and the intended recipient.

As currently practiced, a number of well-defined elements, not just serologic studies, define pretransfusion testing. They are designed to minimize antibody-mediated hemolysis of transfused blood. Those elements currently required by accrediting and regulatory agencies are summarized in Tables 67.2 and 67.3.

GENERAL PRINCIPLES OF IMMUNOHEMATOLOGY

An in-depth review of the physical chemistry of blood group antigen-antibody interactions is beyond the scope of this chapter, and the interested reader is referred to the excellent series of articles edited by Bell (24). What follows is only a brief review.

Direct Agglutination Tests

Blood group antigen-antibody interactions are detected either directly by agglutination or complement-mediated hemolysis, or indirectly by use of the antiglobulin test. Direct reactions occur in two phases: the first, a coating phase in which antibody attaches to corresponding antigens on RBCs; the second, an agglutination phase during which RBCs must come close enough together for antibody molecules to span intercellular distances and bind to adjacent RBCs to form an agglutination lattice.

Characteristically, IgM antibodies directly agglutinate saline-suspended RBCs; because of this, they have been called *complete* antibodies. The ability of IgM antibodies to react in this manner is a reflection of both size and valency, i.e., the number of antigen-binding sites (maximum of 10) per molecule. IgM antibodies are large enough to span the distance that exists between RBCs in suspension. Being multivalent, they can attach to antigens on adjacent RBCs.

IgG molecules do not regularly cause direct agglutination of saline-suspended RBCs, although they may do so if high molecular weight compounds or proteins (e.g., polyvinylpyrrolidone, bovine albumin) are added to the reaction medium. Because an additive is required to complete the agglutination of IgG-coated RBCs, IgG antibodies have been called *incomplete* antibodies. In simple terms, albumin neutralizes the effect of the negative charge on RBCs. This negative charge serves to keep RBCs apart in suspension. Reduction in surface charge reduces intercellular repulsion and permits RBCs to come close together so that antigen binding sites on IgG molecules can attach to adjacent RBCs. Also, IgG molecules can be converted into direct agglutinins by mild reduction with thiol reagents, such as dithiothreitol, which increases the spanning distance of the antibody molecule. This approach is used in the manufacture of some blood typing reagents (25).

Although IgG antibodies rarely cause direct agglutination of RBCs without the modifications described above, they may react directly with saline suspensions of RBCs that have been pretreated with a proteolytic enzyme (e.g., ficin, papain). Such treatment cleaves proteins carrying the sialic acid *N*-acetyl-neuraminic acid, which has a carboxyl (COO-) group that accounts for the negative charge on RBCs. However, enhancement of RBC IgG-mediated agglutination by use of enzyme techniques is not observed with all blood group antibodies because some antigens are cleaved by proteases (see Table 67.4).

Table 67.3. Pretransfusion Test Requirements[a]

Donor Bloods	
ABO	RBCs vs anti-A and anti-B; serum/plasma vs. A_1 and B RBCs
Rh	anti-D; D^u if D-negative in direct tests
Unexpected Antibodies	methods that demonstrate clinically significant antibodies
Infectious Diseases	anti-HB_sAg^a; anti-HBc; anti-HCV; alanine aminotransferase (ALT); anti-HIV; anti-HTLV-I;syphilis
Confirmatory	ABO
Testing	direct test with anti-D on units labeled Rh-negative
Recipient Bloods	
ABO	RBCs vs anti-A and anti-B; serum/plasma vs A_1 and B RBCs
Rh	direct test with anti-D and a concurrent test to detect autoagglutination
Unexpected Antibodies	methods that demonstrate clinically significant antibodies including 37°C incubation and an IAT
Major Cross-match	serologic tests for ABO incompatibility and, when unexpected antibodies are present, methods that demonstrate clinically significant antibodies, including 37°C incubation and an IAT

[a]HBsAg = hepatitis B surface antigen; HBc = hepatitis B core antigen; HCV = hepatitis C virus (non-A, non-B hepatitis); HIV = human immunodeficiency virus; HTLV = human lymphotrophic virus; IAT = indirect antiglobulin test

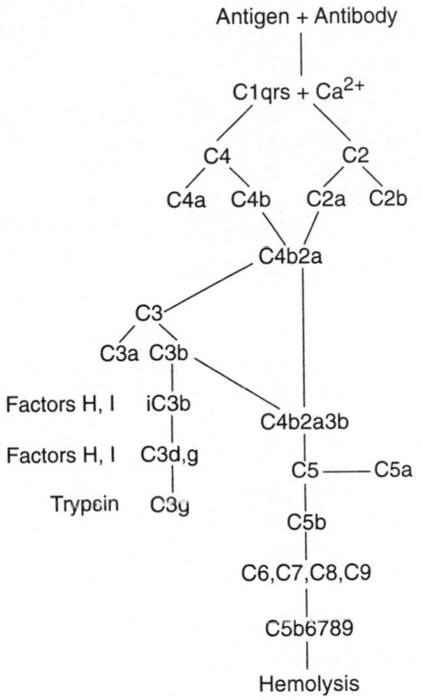

Figure 67.1. The classic pathway of the complement cascade.

Hemolysis

Antibody-mediated hemolysis is dependent upon the sequential action of a number of globulins that collectively are called complement. Figure 67.1 summarizes the classic pathway of complement activation.

Certain IgM antibodies, notably those to ABO, Lewis, and P-system antigens, bind complement to RBCs. Some IgG antibodies, especially $-Jk^a$ and $-Jk^b$, also bind complement but do so less efficiently than IgM molecules primarily because a doublet, consisting of two Fc portions of an immunoglobulin molecule in close proximity to each other, is essential for initation of the classic pathway. Such doublets exist within a single IgM molecule, but for IgG to initiate binding of C1, two immunoglobulin molecules must bind close to each other on a RBC.

Initiation of the complement cascade by the aforementioned antibodies may proceed to lysis. In other instances, complement may be bound only up to the C3 stage. Other antibodies, such as $-Fy^a$, $-K$, and $-S$, bind complement only up to the C3 stage. Bound C3 may be broken down in vivo and in vitro to C3d,g, which can be detected by the antiglobulin test (see below) when AHG reagents containing anti-C3d,g are used.

Antiglobulin Tests

Antiglobulin tests are used to detect IgG antibodies that coat RBCs but do not agglutinate them directly. Complement components that bind to RBCs also can be detected through the use of the antiglobulin test, which is based on the following simple principles:

1. Antibody molecules and complement components are globulins;
2. The injection of human globulins, either purified or in whole serum, into an animal stimulates the animal to produce antibodies against the foreign globulins (antihuman globulin, AHG). AHG can also be produced by hybridoma technology. The antibodies that are important for blood group serologic work are anti-IgG and anticomplement (anti-C3d,g);
3. AHG will react with human globulins, either bound to RBCs or free in serum. Thus, RBCs must be washed free of unbound globulins before testing with AHG. Washing of RBC before adding AHG is crucial to the avoidance of false-negative tests due to the neutralization of AHG by unbound globulins; and
4. Washed RBCs coated with human globulin are agglutinated by AHG.

Table 67.4. Serologic Characteristics of Blood Group Antibodies[a]

ANTI-	RT	37	IAT	ENZ	Ig	C3	HTR	HDN	%WCOMP	Comments
A	*	*	*	E	M,G	Y	Y	Y	56	no dosage
A$_1$	*	S	S	E	M	N	R	N	64	in 2% A$_2$, 25% A$_2$B
B	*	*	*	E	M,G	Y	Y	Y	85	no dosage
Bg			*		G	N	N	N		to HLA
C	S	S	*	E	G,M	N	Y	Y	30	
c	S	S	*	E	G,M	N	Y	Y	20	often with anti-E
Ch^a			*	D	G	N	N	N	2	HTLA; andi-C4
Cs^a			*	*	G	N	N	N	2	HTLA
C^w	S	S	*	E	G,M	N	Y	Y	98	
D	S	S	*	E	G,M	N	Y	Y	15	no dosage
E	S	S	*	E	G,M	N	Y	Y	70	often with anti-c
e		S	*	E	G,M	N	Y	Y	3	auto in WAIHA
f(ce)			*	E	G,M	N	Y	Y	36	compatible with c−
Fy^a			*	D	G	S	Y	Y	33	
Fy^b			*	D	G	N	N	R	20	
Ge	S	S	*	D	G,M			Y	R	
H	*	*	*	E	M,G	Y	Y	Y	R	allo in Oh bloods
H/IH	*	S	S	E	M	Y	N	N	36	auto in A$_1$/A$_1$B
Hy^a			*	*	G	N	Y		R	in blacks
I	*	S	S	E	M	Y	N	N		auto in 1+
I	*	*	*	E	M	Y	U	N		in CHD; allo in I−
i	*	S	S	E	M	Y	U	N		in infectious mononucleosis
Jk^a			*	E	G	*	Y	Y	25	
Jk^b			*	E	G	*	Y	Y	25	
JMH			*	D	G	N	N	N	R	HTLA
Js^a			*	V	G		Y	Y	>99	
Js^b			*	V	G		Y	Y	O	in Blacks
K	S	S	*	V	G	S	Y	Y	90	
k			*	V	G		Y	Y	R	
Kn^a			*	*	G	N	N	N	2	HTLA
Kp^a			*	V	G			Y	98	
Kp^b			*	V	G		Y	Y	R	
Lan			*		G	Y	Y	Y	R	
Le^a	*	S	*	E	M	*	R	N	78	no dosage
Le^b	*	S	*	E	M	*	R	N	28	no dosage
Lu^a		S	*	V	G,A	N			92	
Lu^b			*	V	G,A			Y	R	
M	*	S	S	D	M,G	N	R	R	22	
McC^a			*	*	G	N	N	N	1.5	HTLA
N	*	S	S	D	M,G	N	R	R	28	potent in N−U−
P$_1$	*	S	S	E	M	S	R	N	21	no dosage
PP$_1$P^k	*	*	*	E	M,G	Y	Y	Y	R	
Rg^a			*	D	G	N	N	N	3	HTLA;anti-C4
S		S	*	D	G	S	Y	Y	45	
s			*		G	S	Y	Y	11	
U			*		G	N	Y	Y	0	in Blacks
V			*	E	G	N	Y	Y	>99	
Vel		S	*	E	M,G	Y	Y	Y	R	
Wr^a		S	*	E	G		Y	Y	>99	
Xg^a			*	D	G				23	no dosage
Yk^a			*	V	G	N	N	N	8	HTLA
Yt^a			*	V	G	N	V	N	R	

[a]allo = alloantibody; auto = autoantibody; C3 = complement binding; ENZ = reactions with enzyme-treated RBCs; HDN = causes hemolytic disease of the newborn; CHD = cold hemagglutinin disease; HLA = histocompatibility antigen; HTLA = high-titer, low-avidity antibody; HTR = causes hemolytic transfusion reactions; IAT = indirect antiglobulin test; Ig = immunoglobulin class; RT = room temperature; %WCOMP = % compatible White donors; * = expected; D = depressed; E = enhanced; N = no; R = rare; S = some; U = unlikely; V = variable; Y = yes.

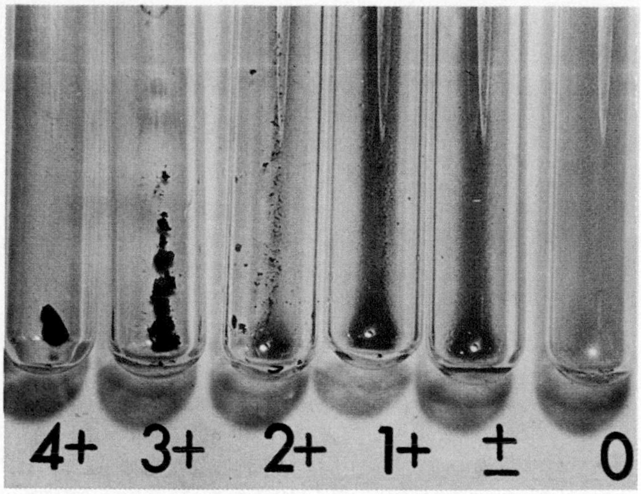

Figure 67.2. Graded strengths of hemagglutination reactions.

Antiglobulin tests can be performed either indirectly following in vitro incubation of RBCs with serum, or directly to demonstrate that RBCs have been coated with globulins in vivo. The indirect antiglobulin test (IAT) is used to detect and identify unexpected antibodies in the serum of blood donors, prospective transfusion recipients, and prenatal patients. The direct antiglobulin test (DAT) is used to detect antibodies bound to RBCs in vivo; such antibodies may be seen in patients with hemolysis due to autoantibodies and drugs, infants with hemolytic disease of the newborn (HDN), and patients manifesting an alloimmune response to a previous transfusion.

Reading for Agglutination and Hemolysis

Again, in vitro blood group antigen-antibody interactions are recognized by observation of agglutination or hemolysis. Hemolysis is best visualized by examining the supernate of centrifuged tests over a white, illuminated background. Examination for agglutination may be macroscopic, performed using an illuminated concave mirror, or microscopic. The latter is rarely necessary in routine practice; indeed, such critical examination of serologic tests can result in incorrectly recording negative tests as positive (19).

Figure 67.2 depicts a series of serologic tests manifesting varying degrees of agglutination. The strength of the observed reactions can be graded. The values given are based on a scoring system in common use (25). Reaction strength is related to antibody potency, but it is also influenced by the number of antigen sites per RBC.

RECIPIENT TESTING

Required pretransfusion testing of prospective recipient blood samples includes ABO and Rh typing, tests for unexpected antibodies, and a major crossmatch. Specific details are included in Tables 67.2 and 67.3 and are discussed more fully below.

Pretransfusion Blood Samples

The importance of the following measures cannot be overstressed because the major cause of fatal, hemolytic transfusion reactions is an ABO-incompatible transfusion resulting from patient/sample misidentification.

PATIENT IDENTITY

The collection of a properly labeled blood sample for pretransfusion testing from the correct patient is critical to safe blood transfusion (25). The person collecting the sample must positively identify the patient. This is facilitated through the use of a wristband, containing the patient's full name and unique hospital registration number, which remains attached to the patient throughout his or her hospitalization. The information on the requisition form should be compared with that on the wristband; blood samples should not be collected if there is a discrepancy. In the absence of a wristband, the nursing staff should identify the patient; this should be documented on the requisition form. The nursing staff should be reminded to attach a wristband to the patient to validate patient identity at the time of transfusion. In an emergency, a temporary identification number should be used and cross-referenced with the patient's name and hospital identification number once they are known.

LABELING

Blood samples must be drawn into correctly labeled, stoppered tubes. The tube must be clearly labeled at the bedside with the patient's first and last names, the patient's unique hospital identification number, and the date of collection. The phlebotomist should initial or sign the requisition form so that there is a means of identifying the person who collected the sample. By filing the requisition form with the patient's medical records, a permanent record is made of the phlebotomist's name.

CONFIRMATION OF SAMPLE IDENTITY

Upon receipt of blood samples for pretransfusion testing, the information on the label must be compared with that on the requisition. A new sample must be obtained whenever there are discrepancies or if there is any doubt about the identity of the sample. It is unacceptable to correct an incorrectly labeled sample.

TYPE OF SAMPLE

Either serum or plasma may be used for pretransfusion testing, but most workers use serum to avoid introducing small fibrin clots into serologic tests. Such clots may be mistaken for agglutination. Fibrin clots may also form when samples from heparinized patients are collected into nonanticoagulated tubes. These samples will clot properly following the addition of protamine sulphate (25).

Some workers prefer to use serum rather than plasma for compatibility testing, to facilitate detection of antibodies that primarily coat RBCs with the C3d,g components of complement. Bound C3d,g will not activate the lytic phase of the complement cascade, but it can be detected with AHG reagents containing anti-C3d,g. EDTA, citrate, and other commonly used anticoagulants chelate calcium ions that are essential for complement activation. However, as discussed later, the use of AHG reagents containing anti-C3d,g for compatibility testing is not mandatory.

AGE OF SPECIMEN

To ensure that the specimen used for compatibility testing is representative of a patient's current immune status, serologic studies must be performed using blood collected no more than 3 days in advance of the transfusion. This is particularly important when the patient has been transfused or pregnant within the preceding 3 months, or when such information is uncertain or unavailable (21), because both transfusion and pregnancy may stimulate alloantibody production. From a practical standpoint, it is simpler to stipulate that *all* pretransfusion samples must be collected within 3 days before RBC transfusions, rather than determine whether or not a patient has been recently transfused or is pregnant.

STORAGE

Blood samples used for compatibility testing, including donor RBCs, must be kept at 1 to 6°C for at least 1 week after each transfusion. This ensures that appropriate samples are available for investigational purposes should adverse responses to transfusion occur.

Blood Typing

ABO TYPING

Inheritance of ABO blood groups follow a straightforward Mendelian pattern for codominant genes. *A* and *B* gene products are enzymes (transferases) that attach specific carbohydrate moieties (α-*N*-acetyl-D-galactosamine for A antigen, α-D-galactose for B antigen) to H-active glycoprotein or glycolipid structures (19). Such H-active structures are formed by the *H*-gene-specified transferase, which attaches α-L-fucose to preformed glycoproteins and glycolipids. Group O RBCs lack both the *A* and *B* gene-specified sugars. AB RBCs have structures that either carry A- or B-active sugars. (See Fig. 67.3.)

ABO typing is performed using both the recipient's RBCs and serum or plasma. The RBCs are tested for the presence of A and B antigens with anti-A and anti-B; use of anti-A,B is optional, but it is generally considered unnecessary when potential transfusion recipients are ABO typed. The serum is tested for the presence of anti-A and anti-B with known A_1 and B RBCs.

Both reagent antisera and RBCs for ABO typing are available commercially. Antisera are either of human origin (polyclonal) or are prepared by hybridoma technology (monoclonal). Reagent RBCs are usually suspended in a preservative medium containing ethylenediaminetetraacetic acid (EDTA), which chelates calcium ions essential for complement activation. Lysis of the RBCs by lytic anti-A and anti-B is thereby prevented.

Specific details of the methods used for ABO typing and the expected findings for each of the four common ABO phenotypes are given in Method 67.1. When interpreting the results of such studies, it is important to note that, when either A and/or B antigens are present on the RBCs, the corresponding antibody or antibodies should not be present in the serum or plasma. This reciprocal relationship between antigens on the RBCs and antibodies in the serum is known as Landsteiner's law (26).

A and B are ubiquitous in nature, and the corresponding antibodies develop as a natural response following exposure to the antigens in the environment (e.g., bacteria). Accordingly, anti-A and anti-B are often referred to as naturally occurring antibodies. When interpreting test results, it should be remembered that, if A and/or B antigens are absent from the RBCs, the corresponding antibody or antibodies should be present in the serum or plasma. The one common exception to this is found when testing blood from newborns whose immune systems have not yet been exposed to environmental A and B.

In light of these points, and to prevent erroneous conclusions of results, any discrepancies between the reactions of RBCs with anti-A and anti-B and the anticipated antibodies in the serum must be resolved before blood is given. If this is not possible, the patient should receive group O RBCs.

RBC membrane glycoplipid

Gal(β,1-4)GlcNAc(β,1-3)Gal(β,1-3)Glc-CERAMIDE

H-active glycolipid

Gal(β,1-4)GlcNAc(β,1-3)Gal(β,1-3)Glc-CERAMIDE
|
Fuc(α,1-2)

A-active glycolipid

GalNAc(α,1-3)Gal(β,1-4)GlcNAc(β,1-3)Gal(β,1-3)Glc-CERAMIDE
|
Fuc(α,1-2)

B-active glycolipid

Gal(α,1-3)Gal(β,1-4)GlcNAc(β,1-3)Gal(β,1-3)Glc-CERAMIDE
|
Fuc(α,1-2)

Figure 67.3. Structure of ABH-active glycolipids. Gal, D-galactose; GalNAc, *N*-acetyl-D-galactosamine; Glc, D-Glucose; GlcNAc, *N*-acetyl-D-glucosamine; Fuc, L-Fucose.

Rh TYPING

Of the five major Rh antigens, only tests for D are performed routinely in pretransfusion testing. RBC samples that react in a specific manner with anti-D reagents are classified as Rh-positive; nonreactive RBC samples are classified as Rh-negative.

Unlike antibodies in the ABO system, Rh antibodies are rarely naturally occurring. Rather, they are stimulated by transfusion or pregnancy. Thus, the presence of anti-D in the serum is an unexpected finding and is not used to verify RBC Rh status.

There are two different types of reagent anti-D available for Rh typing: high-protein and low-protein (25). High-protein reagents are prepared with human IgG anti-D diluted in bovine albumin and other potentiators of agglutination. Their final protein concentration may be greater than 200 g/liter. Such a high protein level is needed to potentiate antibody reactivity so that positive and negative tests can be recognized almost instantaneously using a direct agglutination technique. Low-protein reagents (protein content about 70 g/liter) are either human IgM anti-D, human IgG anti-D that is chemically modified, or a blend of monoclonal IgM and polyclonal human IgG anti-D. Anti-D prepared from human IgM anti-D is in short supply and, consequently, exceedingly expensive; its use should be restricted to the management of problem samples. In the preparation of chemically modified anti-D, reactive antibody is treated with dithiothreitol, which increases flexibility at the hinge region of the molecule, enhancing the spanning distance of the two NH_2-terminal antigen-binding sites (27); less protein is needed to effect agglutination than when untreated IgG is used. With monoclonal-polyclonal anti-D blends, the IgM component causes direct agglutination of Rh-positive RBCs, and the IgG component permits detection of the D^u phenotype, which is essentially a weakened expression of D, by use of the IAT (see Method 67.2). Although detection of D^u is not required in studies on prospective transfusion recipients, it is done routinely in transfusion services of hospitals engaged in the care of prenatal and perinatal patients (28).

ERRONEOUS RESULTS

The importance of appropriate controls and careful technique when performing blood typing tests cannot be overstressed. Errors in ABO and Rh typing may have both clinical and legal ramifications. Of 39 deaths attributed to transfusion, 22 were associated with the transfusion of ABO-incompatible blood (29). The inadvertent transfusion of a single unit of Rh-positive blood to an Rh-negative recipient results in alloimmunization of that recipient to D antigen in 55 to 80% of cases (25). If the recipient is female and later becomes pregnant, the anti-D may cross the placenta and destroy Rh-positive fetal RBCs, resulting in HDN and its complications (30).

Most errors in blood typing are clerical in nature and are associated with misidentification of patients, mislabeled samples, or erroneous interpretation of results. Other considerations include:

Technical Factors. Improper storage of reagents, use of incorrect technique, use of wrong reagent, omission of antisera, incorrect centrifugation of tests, or use of antisera contaminated with bacteria, foreign matter, or the contents of other reagent vials may all lead to erroneous results.

IgM Autoantibodies. RBCs from patients with autoimmune hemolytic anemia due to cold-reactive antibodies (cold hemagglutinin disease, CHD) may agglutinate spontaneously at temperatures below 37°C. The IgM-mediated autoagglutination can be obviated by incubating the RBCs with thiol reagents such as dithiothreitol or 2-mercaptoethanol (31). Also, potent IgM agglutinins may mask the presence of anti-A and/or anti-B in the sera of these individuals; serum ABO typing can be done at 37°C using group O RBCs as a control for autoagglutination in addition to A_1 and B RBCs (25).

RBCs Coated with IgG. IgG-coated RBCs, such as may be found in patients with warm autoimmune hemolytic anemia (WAIHA), are prone to agglutinate spontaneously when suspended in anti-D reagents. IgM human anti-D is the least susceptible to give false-positive results with IgG-coated RBCs. An inert reagent control is available for use with high-protein anti-D and is essentially the diluent used in the formulation of the reagent antiserum. When using chemically modified or monoclonal anti-D, a negative concurrent test with anti-A and/or anti-B is considered a valid control for autoagglutination, but this has been questioned recently (32). Accordingly, an initial Rh type determination using low-protein anti-D, performed concurrently with tests with anti-A and anti-B, is suggested for all pretransfusion samples. An additional Rh typing with high-protein anti-D and an immunologically inert control is recommended when testing samples from all group AB patients and from those on whom there are no prior records of Rh typing (33).

Weak Antigen Expression, Resulting from a Disease Process or from Genetic Factors. A and B antigen expression may be depressed in leukemia or weakly expressed due to inheritance of rare alleles at the *ABO* locus or inheritance of a variant *H* gene. The latter controls the development of H substance from which A and B antigens develop (12, 19).

In some rare phenotypes, the expression of A or B may be so weak that direct tests with anti-A or anti-B are nonreactive. The absence of the corresponding antibody from the serum indicates that the RBCs carry weak A or B antigens. In phenotypes, such as A_2 and A_2B, anti-A_1 may be present in the serum and cause an apparent exception to Landsteiner's law (26) inasmuch as A antigen is present on the RBCs and anti-A is apparent in the serum. A_2 and A_2B phenotypes arise from inheritance of a variant gene (A^2) at the ABO locus or from gene interaction in which the *B* gene suppresses the expression of the *A* gene. The A antigen in A_2 and A_2B phenotypes is probably both quantitatively and qualitatively different from A antigen in the more common A_1 phenotype. Thus, Landsteiner's law is not violated; the anti-A_1 that is formed is not an antibody against a self-antigen (autoantibody).

In the Rh system, the weak expression of D antigen associated with the D^u phenotype accounts for discrepancies between test results obtained on different occasions using different reagents, and when tests are done by different facilities, one of which does not test apparent D-negatives by the D^u technique.

Missing or Weak Anti-A and Anti-B. As discussed previously, anti-A and anti-B are absent in the sera of newborns, and reliance must be placed on the results of RBC typing when concluding the results of ABO typing tests on blood from neonates. There are other conditions manifested in infancy, notably immune deficiency disorders, in which the expected anti-A and/or anti-B may be absent. Weak or missing anti-A or anti-B is also seen in elderly patients. Incubation of tests and studies with enzyme pretreated A, B, and O RBCs may be helpful in resolving discrepancies due to absent agglutinins.

The B(A) Phenotype. This is a recent finding recognized through the use of certain monoclonal anti-A (but not polyclonal reagents) that react directly with RBCs of the rare A_x phenotype (12, 34). The incidence of the B(A) phenotype may be as high as 1% of all group B samples. It occurs in individuals with a high level of *B* gene-specified transferase that is apparently capable of synthesizing trace amounts of A antigen.

Additional Antibodies in Reagent Antisera, Particularly Those to Low Incidence Antigens. Manufacturers must show absence of contaminating antibodies to antigens with an incidence of 1% or greater when tested by the stipulated method. In practice, every effort is made to exclude antibodies to a wide range of low-incidence antigens; however, the appropriate test RBCs may not always be available to exclude all such antibodies, and erroneous results occasionally can be attributed to additional specificities. Deviation from recommended procedures can also lead to false-positive reactions when contaminating antibodies are present. For example, anti-D that reacts specifically with D-positive RBCs by the stipulated method may, due to the presence of anti-G, react by enzyme techniques with C-positive, D-negative RBCs (35).

Polyagglutinable RBCs. These have abnormal membrane structures such that they are agglutinated by normal adult human sera. Causes include membrane modifications by microbial enzymes (T, Th, Tk, Tx, and acquired-B polyagglutination) and incomplete membrane carbohydrate biosynthesis resulting from somatic mutation (Tn syndrome). Occasionally, polyagglutinability can be an inherited characteristic (HEMPAS, NOR, CAD). Polyagglutinable RBCs are classified through the use of lectins, which are agglutinins derived primarily from plant seeds (36).

Naturally occurring agglutinins in human serum react with unique surface structures present on polyagglutinable RBCs. Anomalous reactions usually are seen in ABO typing tests with human source reagents, particularly with Tn and acquired-B RBCs. Tn RBCs carry A-like antigens and are, thus, agglutinated by anti-A, while acquired-B RBCs carry a B-like antigen that crossreacts with human anti-B. Monoclonal reagents vary in their ability to react with Tn and acquired-B antigens.

Abnormal Serum Proteins in the Test Sample That Promote Rouleaux. Sera with reversed albumin: globulin ratios cause RBCs to form rouleaux, which may be mistaken for agglutination. This can be obviated by washing the test RBCs.

Antibody in the Serum of a Test Sample Against a Reagent Constituent. Ingredients such as EDTA (present in reagent A_1 and B RBCs), yellow tartrazine #5 (dye added to anti-B), and sodium caprylate (once added to stabilize bovine albumin used in the formulation of anti-D) have been implicated (37).

Detection of Unexpected Antibodies

All antibodies to RBC antigens, other than naturally occurring anti-A and anti-B, are considered *unexpected.* They can either be *alloantibodies,* which are directed toward non-ABO-system antigens absent on the RBCs of the antibody producer, or *autoantibodies,* which are directed toward self-antigens. The latter may cause autoimmune hemolytic anemia (19). Unexpected antibodies in donor plasma may destroy recipient RBCs, while antibodies in the recipient may cause accelerated destruction of transfused RBCs. In pregnant women, such antibodies may cross the placenta and cause HDN (30).

Methods for detecting unexpected antibodies in the serum or plasma of prospective transfusion recipients must detect clinically significant antibodies. An IAT following 37°C incubation of patient's serum or plasma with reagent RBCs that are not pooled is specifically required. Moreover, IgG-coated RBCs should be added to all negative IATs to demonstrate that active AHG was indeed added to the tests (21).

Not all antibodies to RBC antigens are clinically significant. Those that accelerate the destruction of transfused incompatible RBCs or HDN clearly are of concern. From a practical standpoint, antibodies that do not react in vitro at body temperatures are not significant. Further, some antibodies that react at body temperatures do not cause accelerated destruction of transfused incompatible RBCs or HDN. Information regarding the potential of an antibody to cause hemolytic transfusion reactions and/or HDN is given in Table 67.4.

The technique for detecting unexpected antibodies described in Method 67.3 meets the requirements mandated by the *AABB Standards* (21). However, as discussed below, there are various options in selecting an antibody detection method.

CHOICE OF REACTION MEDIUM

A variety of RBC-suspending media or additives are used either to enhance antibody uptake or to potentiate the agglutination phase of antibody-antigen interactions. Low-ionic-strength saline (LISS) solution, normal saline, or RBC preservative (modified Alsever's solution) are used as RBC-suspending media. Bovine serum albumin (22 or 30% w/v) bovine serum albumin, LISS-additives, or polyethylene glycol are commonly added directly to serum-RBC mixtures (31). In the low-ionic Polybrene technique, serum is incubated with RBCs suspended in LISS to enhance antibody uptake. The second phase of the reaction is potentiated by aggregating RBCs with Polybrene. Aggregation is reversed with sodium citrate, but agglutinates formed by antigen-antibody are not dispersed (38).

Because of enhanced antibody uptake in a low-ionic environment, use of either LISS solution for RBC suspension or LISS-additives permits adequate detection of clinically significant antibodies following short incubation times (10 to 15 minutes). In contrast, incubation times of 30 to 60 minutes are required when albumin or saline tests are employed (25).

REAGENT RBCs

The FDA currently mandates that sets of reagent RBC samples licensed for use in pretransfusion antibody detection tests carry expression of the C, c, D, E, e, Fy^a, Fy^b, Jk^a, Jk^b, K, k, Le^a, Le^b, P_1 M, N, S, and s (22). Such RBCs must not be pooled (21).

It is impossible to find a single donor with RBCs that carry all of these antigens, for adults rarely, if ever, have strong expression of both Le^a and Le^b on their RBCs (12). Thus, reagent RBCs for antibody detection are available commercially as sets of either two or three samples. The Rh phenotypes of RBCs used in two-sample sets are R_1R_1 (C+c−D+E−e+) and R_2R_2 (C−c+D+E+e−). In three sample sets, a rr (C−c+D−E−e+) sample is provided, in addition to R_1R_1 and R_2R_2 RBCs. Use of three RBC samples facilitates the inclusion of RBCs from individuals homozygous for particular blood group genes.

DOSAGE AND ANTI-IgG

The stronger reactivity of an antibody with RBCs from homozygotes than with RBCs from individuals heterozygous for the same gene is called dosage. Use of RBCs from homozygotes (double-dose) may provide greater sensitivity for antibody detection than RBCs from heterozygotes (single-dose). However, no regulatory authority dictates that RBCs used for antibody detection must carry double-dose expression of any blood group antigen. Indeed, except for Rh antigen expression, studies undertaken in the early 1980s that led to the abbreviation of the crossmatch were done without regard for dosage (39). Moreover, in practice, the use of three RBC samples, instead of two, increases the direct costs of testing by 50% yet does not significantly permit detection of antibodies that would be missed using only two RBC samples (40).

The expression of Kidd (Jk) and Duffy (Fy) antigens on reagent RBCs warrants discussion because there are data suggesting that dosage influences detection of these antibodies when anti-IgG is used for antiglobulin testing. The data have been generated in LISS (40) and albumin studies (41) with anti-Jk^a and in albumin studies with anti-Fy^a (42). The need for double-dose antigen expression is only partly diminished when using AHG reagents containing anti-C3 (40).

Some reagent manufacturers currently market sets of R_1R_1 and R_2R_2 reagent RBC samples, one of which is Jk(a+b−). Others offer sets that include both Jk(a+b−) and Fy(a+b−) RBCs. Consumers may elect to request that both samples lack strong expression of Bg. This avoids problems due to anti-Bg, which are directed towards histocompatibility (HLA) antigens and do not cause accelerated destruction of incompatible RBCs. Anti-Bg are common among multiparous and multiply transfused patients. Their avoidance reduces the number of costly and fruitless antibody identification studies. Use of a two-reagent RBC sample set (one Jk(a+b−), both Bg-negative) in LISS tests utilizing 37°C incubation and anti-IgG provides a quick, sensitive antibody detection system that does not lead to the detection of an inordinate number of unwanted positive tests.

It is important to note that sets of two-reagent RBC samples may not include double-dose expression of Jk^b or Fy^b. Also, phenotypically Fy(a+b−) RBCs may not have double-dose expression of Fy^a, especially if the donor is black and carries the *Fy* gene (12). Moreover, reagent manufacturers will find it difficult to provide absence of Bg and double-dose expression of Jk^a in a two-reagent RBC set if requested by all consumers. Thus, to assure adequate detection of Kidd-system antibodies in the absence of a two-reagent RBC sample set that includes double-dose Kidd antigen expression on one sample, it may be necessary to use either polyspecific AHG or anti-IgG and a three-reagent RBC sample set.

UNWANTED POSITIVE TESTS AND POLYSPECIFIC ANTIHUMAN GLOBULIN

Use of polyspecific AHG reagents may yield unwanted positive reactions with sera containing complement-binding allo- and autoantibodies that are of no clinical significance. All normal adult human sera contain autoanti-I, or autoanti-HI. In certain pathological conditions, notably *Mycoplasma pneumoniae* infection, the anti-I may react at body temperature and cause CHD. Although normal anti-I/HI often can be demonstrated in vitro only at cold temperatures (4°C), it may react at room temperature; unless sera and RBCs are warmed to 37°C before testing, the RBCs may become coated with complement components, including C3d,g, that can be detected with polyspecific AHG. Some clinically insignificant alloantibodies (−P_1, −Le^a, −Le^b) that agglutinate antigen-positive RBCs below 31°C may also coat the RBCs with C3.

As indicated by data shown in Table 67.5, LISS reagents potentiate this unwanted binding of C3, but LISS tests are more sensitive than albumin tests for detecting clinically significant antibodies. Also, tests utilizing polyspecific AHG may be more sensitive than those with anti-IgG, but use of polyspecific AHG leads to the detection of an inordinate number of unwanted positive reactions (43).

Decisions relative to the aforementioned options are the responsibility of the blood bank medical director. They should be made based on the type of patient served, the causes and frequency of previous significant antibody-mediated transfusion reactions, the availability of resources, and with the realization that no one method will detect all clinically significant antibodies.

PRETRANSFUSION AUTOCONTROL

Many transfusion services routinely perform an autocontrol or DAT as part of pretransfusion testing. The autocontrol consists of testing patients' serum

Table 67.5. Sensitivity and Specificity of Different Antibody Detection Procedures

Technique	Antibodies Missed[a]	% Unwanted Positive Tests
RT-37-LISS-PS	0	1.41
37-LISS-PS	0	0.61
37-LISS-IG	5	0.1
RT-37-ALB-PS	6	0.21
37-ALB-PS	6	0.1
37-ALB-IG	10	0.1

[a]Clinically significant, unexpected antibodies; RT = incubation at room temperature; 37 = incubation at 37°C; ALB = bovine albumin; PS = polyspecific AHG; IG = anti-IgG; LISS = low-ionic strength saline.

against their own RBCs under the same conditions as those to which screening tests for unexpected antibodies are subjected. The DAT simply entails testing the patients' washed RBCs with AHG. Both the autocontrol and DAT are performed to detect globulins bound to the patients' RBCs in vivo. Such in vivo coating of RBCs occurs in patients with autoimmune hemolytic anemia or HDN and may also be seen following therapy with certain drugs or transfusion with incompatible blood (19, 25). Moreover, a positive DAT may be the earliest manifestation of an alloimmune response to a previous, recent transfusion (44).

However, inclusion of the DAT or autocontrol as part of routine pretransfusion testing is not advocated; in the absence of detectable serum antibodies, the predictive value of a positive DAT is so low (0.29%) that routine testing is not cost-effective (40, 44). It should also be noted that previous and current editions of *AABB Standards* (21) have never recommended or mandated that a DAT or autocontrol be part of pretransfusion testing. Nonetheless, the DAT/autocontrol is a good predictive test for immune-mediated hemolysis when performed on patients with clinical manifestations of hemolytic anemia (45).

Prior Records Check

The results of current ABO, Rh, and antibody detection tests should be checked against records of previous tests, if available. Any discrepancies between past and present ABO and Rh typing results must be thoroughly investigated; the most likely explanation is that the present sample is not from the same individual whose blood was tested previously.

Because of the potential for adverse consequences arising from improper patient identification and sample labeling, it is reasonable to recommend that no patient be transfused unless there are two concordant ABO and Rh typing results on file from samples obtained on different occasions. Obviously, this is not practical in an emergency situation, but it can be undertaken on elective surgical patients by requiring that samples be submitted for pretransfusion testing during a clinic visit before admission and again upon admission for surgery.

DONOR TESTING

Initial Testing

The initial ABO, Rh, and antibody detection tests on donor bloods, tests for infectious diseases, the interpretation of these tests, and the correct labeling of donor units are functions normally carried out by a regional donor center. Some hospital-based transfusion services continue to procure a portion of their blood needs from the population at large (homologous donors), and in recent years, efforts have been made for patients awaiting elective surgical procedures to predeposit their blood for later use (autologous donors). In addition, some patients request that they receive blood from relatives or friends (directed donations). Regardless of the type of donor, each unit of blood must be subjected to the serologic tests itemized in Table 67.3, which include a test for weak expression of the Rh antigen D, i.e., the D^u phenotype. Although not specifically required, most donor bloods are also tested with anti-A,B to detect bloods of the rare A_x phenotype (12). Only clinically significant, unexpected antibodies need be detected in donor plasma (21).

The antibody detection tests and the methods used to determine ABO and Rh types may be those given in the methods section. However, the volume of testing that needs to be done at major donor centers necessitates the use of automated equipment. Instrumentation currently in use is often based on microplate technology (46). The results may be interpreted electronically. Regardless of the method used, all discrepancies between RBC and serum tests must be resolved before conclusions can be made. For Rh typing, only those units that are negative with anti-D by the D^u test (see Method 67.2) or an equivalent procedure can be labeled Rh-negative. All straightforward D-positive and D^u bloods are considered Rh-positive (25).

Confirmatory Testing

The ABO type of all units of whole blood or packed RBCs and the Rh type of those labeled Rh-negative must be confirmed by the transfusion service performing the cross-match. This must be done using a sample from an attached segment after the original ABO and Rh label has been affixed. Only tests with reagent antisera and donor RBCs are required; units labeled group O can be tested with anti-A,B alone. For D-typing of units labeled Rh-negative, only direct tests with anti-D are necessary; testing for D^u is not required.

DONOR-RECIPIENT TESTING

The Cross-match

Before whole blood or packed RBCs is administered, and except in an emergency, a major cross-match must be performed using RBCs from an originally attached segment and the prospective recipient's serum or plasma sample that was used in ABO, Rh, and antibody detection tests described earlier (25). The methods used should be capable of detecting ABO incompatibility and include the IAT. However, in the absence of unexpected antibodies (and absence of records of prior detection of such antibodies) in the intended recipient's serum, only serologic testing to detect ABO incompatibility is required.

TESTING FOR ABO INCOMPATIBILITY

Only testing for ABO incompatibility is necessary when screening tests for unexpected antibodies are negative and there is no record of the patient having had such antibodies in the past. To prevent false-negative tests due to prozone by complement-fixing high-titer anti-A and anti-B, an IS cross-match between the prospective recipient's serum or plasma and donor RBCs suspended in EDTA-saline is an acceptable method for the detection of ABO incompatibility (25, 47).

The procedure, described in Method 67.4, may yield unwanted positive tests (i.e., reactions not due to ABO incompatibility) when cold-reactive autoantibodies (e.g., −HI, −I) and alloantibodies (−M, −N, $-Le^a$, $-Le^b$, $-P_1$) are present. Such antibodies may not be detected in LISS-IgG screening tests for unexpected antibodies (Method 67.3). Antibodies to low-incidence antigens may also yield positive IS tests when LISS-IgG tests are negative. When any unit gives a positive IS cross-match following a negative antibody screen, the ABO typing results of both patient and donor should be reviewed. In the absence of any errors in typing or labeling, the following protocol is suggested:

1. If an isolated unit gives a positive IS cross-match, return the unit to the stock refrigerator and select another for IS cross-matching;
2. When more than one unit gives a positive IS cross-match, retest all units with the patient's serum using the LISS-IgG procedure in Method 67.5; and
3. When both IS and LISS-IgG cross-matches are positive, repeat the screening tests for unexpected antibodies and initiate further studies, as appropriate.

An alternative approach, permissible according to section G3.100 in the 15th edition of *AABB Standards*, would be to demonstrate ABO compatibility by computer-based review of the ABO type of donor and recipient before units are released for transfusion.

ANTIGLOBULIN CROSS-MATCH

When clinically significant, unexpected antibodies are present or a patient's records indicate that such antibodies have been detected previously, blood selected for transfusion must be tested with the patient's serum or plasma by the antiglobulin cross-match (IAT) (25). The LISS-IgG procedure described in Method 67.5 is an acceptable procedure.

An IAT cross-match can also be done routinely on patients with nonreactive screening tests for unexpected antibodies (25). The IAT detects ABO incompatibility and may detect unexpected antibodies that were missed in pretransfusion screening tests. Antibodies manifesting dosage and unexpected antibodies to low-incidence antigens may be detected in this manner, as may antibodies missed in screening tests due to technical error. However, the predictive value of a positive IAT cross-match following nonreactive screening tests for unexpected antibodies is sufficiently low (7.2%) (40) that many large hospital transfusion services do not perform the IAT cross-match except when unexpected antibodies are present or there are records of such antibodies. For further discussion on the risk of eliminating the IAT cross-match, the interested reader is referred to the articles by Garratty (39) and Shulman (48).

TYPE AND SCREEN PROTOCOLS

In the late 1970s, type and screen (T&S) protocols for pretransfusion testing of surgical patients (49) and maximal surgical blood order schedules (MSBOS) (50, 51) were advocated. Under a T&S protocol, pretransfusion testing is restricted to ABO, Rh, and antibody detection tests for patients undergoing procedures that rarely require transfusion. Blood is cross-matched only if and when it is required for transfusion. Use of a MSBOS limits the number of units of blood cross-matched to that which predictably will be transfused for a particular procedure. Each institution should establish their own MSBOS from data gathered retrospectively; blood unit usage that meets the needs of 95% of patients undergoing a surgical procedure becomes the maximum order for that procedure. A portion

Table 67.6. A Partial Maximum Surgical Blood Order Schedule (MSBOS)[a]

General and Vascular Surgery			
Amputation of limb	T&S	Gastrectomy	2
Aneurysm, abdominal	5	Gastroplasty	T&S
Appendectomy	T&S	Gastrostomy	T&S
Breast		Hemorrhoidectomy	NSR
biopsy	T&S	Hepatectomy	6
mastectomy, simple	T&S	Hernia repair	T&S
mastectomy, modified	T&S	Hodgkins/lymphoma staging	T&S
mastectomy, radical	2	Laparotomy, exploratory	T&S
Neurosurgery			
Cordotomy	T&S	Peripheral nerve surgery[a]	T&S
Craninectomy for synostosis	1	Stereotactic brain biopsy	T&S
Craniotomy for:		Syringoperitoneal shunt	
		adult	2
AV malformation	6	child	1
STA/MCA/PICA bypass	2	Tarsal tunnel release	NSR
hematoma	2	Ulnar nerve transposition	NSR
tumor	3	Ventriculoarterial shunt	T&S
Hypophysectomy	2	Ventriculoperitoneal shunt	T&S
Otorhinolaryngology			
Acoustic tumor resection	T&S	Mastoidectomy	NSR
Angiofibroma resection	2	Maxillectomy	2
Branchial cleft cyst resection	T&S	Orbital exploration	NSR
Plastic Surgery			
Cleft palate repair	T&S	Mastectomy, subcutaneous	
Debridement and skin graft	2	with implants	T&S
Mammoplasty		Otoplasty	NSR
augmentation	NSR	Rhinoplasty	NSR
reduction	T&S	Skin flap	T&S
Cardiac and Thoracic Surgery			
Aneurysm, thoracic, resection	8	Hernia repair (all types)	T&S
Atrial septal defect repair	3	recurrent hiatus	2
Arterial switch operation	3	Lobectomy, pulmonary	2
Blalock-Taussig shunt	1	Patent ductus repair	1
Obstetrics/Gynecology			
Abortion, spontaneous	NSR	Examination under anesthesia	
Cervical conization	NSR	for placenta previa	2
Termination of pregnancy		High-risk labor	T&S
1st or 2nd trimester	NSR	Hysterectomy	
Cesarean section		vaginal	T&S
uncomplicated	T&S	abdominal	T&S
placenta previa	2	radical	4
Urology			
Adrenalectomy	2	Penile implant	T&S
Cystectomy	4	Prostatectomy	
Cystolithotomy	NSR	transurethal	T&S
Cystoscopy	NSR	suprapubic	2
		perineal	2
		radical	4

[a] Excluding carpal tunnel, tarsal tunnel, and ulnar nerve transposition; T&S = Type and screen; NSR = No specimen required.
Note: Each institution should establish its own MSBOS, from prior blood utilization data, for each surgical service.

of the MSBOS used at this author's institution is given in Table 67.6.

The rationale for implementing these programs is essentially threefold: (*a*) to decrease workload; (*b*) to monitor unnecessary ordering practices; and (*c*) to optimize the use of a limited blood inventory by not reserving blood for an extensive period of time for specific patients. The success of such programs can be measured by determining the ratio of units cross-matched (C) to units transfused (T). C/T ratios less than 2:1 are considered desirable (52), and many transfusion services are able to achieve ratios of 1.6:1 or less.

SELECTION OF BLOOD FOR TRANSFUSION

Selection Based on ABO and Rh Type

Two principles apply to the selection of blood for transfusion: (*a*) the donor RBCs should not carry A, B, or D antigens when those antigens are absent

Table 67.7. Selection of Blood Components Based on ABO Type

Component	Recipient	Donor	Comment
Whole blood	A	A	Identical to that of recipient
	B	B	
	AB	AB	
	O	O	
Red blood cells Granulocyte concentrates	A	A,O	Compatible with recipient plasma
	B	B,O	
	AB	A,B,O	
	O	O	
Fresh frozen plasma	A	A,AB	Compatible with recipient RBCs
	B	B,AB	
	AB	AB	
	O	A,B,AB,O	
Platelet concentrate[a] Cryoprecipitate	A	A,B,AB,O	All groups acceptable
	B	A,B,AB,O	
	AB	A,B,AB,O	
	O	A,B,AB,O	

[a]Components compatible with recipient's RBCs are preferred.

from the intended recipient's RBCs; and (*b*) the donor plasma should lack anti-A and/or anti-B when the corresponding antigens are present on the intended recipient's RBCs. However, the latter may be ignored if the total plasma volume transfused is low. Table 67.7 summarizes the selection of ABO types of blood and blood products for transfusion, based on recipient ABO type.

To prevent alloimmunization to D, Rh-negative recipients should receive Rh-negative RBC products, platelets, and granulocyte preparations. This is especially important for females of childbearing potential.

When Unexpected Alloantibodies Are Present

Unexpected antibodies detected in pretransfusion tests should be identified, if possible, before transfusion. The results of such studies facilitate the procurement of antigen-negative blood for transfusion.

In the identification of unexpected antibodies, serum or plasma is tested against a panel of eight or more group O reagent RBC samples, characterized for polymorphisms within the Rh, Duffy, Kell, Kidd, Lutheran, MN, P, and Xg blood group systems. Such panels are commercially available. Each reagent RBC panel is tested against the serum or plasma, either by the method that initially led to the detection of the unexpected antibodies or by methods more sensitive than the original procedure. The patient's own RBCs (autologous control) are tested in parallel with the reagent RBCs to help distinguish auto- from alloantibody reactivity; a negative autocontrol indicates alloantibody reactivity, while a positive autocontrol is seen with autoantibodies, alloantibodies made in response to a previous recent transfusion, or a mixture of auto- and alloantibody reactivity.

Some transfusion services have the resources to perform antibody identification tests, while others must refer such samples elsewhere. Many blood collection facilities and reagent manufacturers offer consultation services for immunohematological problems, as do many large transfusion services. For a more detailed discussion of methods and pitfalls of antibody identification, see *The AABB Technical Manual* (25) and *Methods in Immunohematology* (31).

When the specificity of antibody is known, antigen-negative blood may or may not be required, depending on what is known regarding the significance of the specific antibody. What follows is a policy for the transfusion management of patients with unexpected alloantibodies. Each antibody is placed in one of six categories, based on reported clinical significance, frequency of corresponding antigen, and availability of appropriate typing reagents. The category designation for specific antibodies is given in Table 67.8.

Category I—Potentially Clinically Significant Alloantibodies for Which Antigen-Negative Blood Can Readily Be Obtained. Antigen-negative units should be selected for transfusion regardless of current antibody strength. Units should be proven antigen-negative by testing with a "valid" reagent. *Note:* A "valid" reagent can be either an "in-date," commercially prepared typing serum or a raw serum that gives a 2+ or greater reaction with single-dose control RBCs (25).

Category II—Alloantibodies of Questionable Clinical Significance for Which Cross-match Compatible Units Can Be Obtained by Screening Available Units. Confirmation of antigen-negative status with a "valid" reagent is not required. If screening units by cross-match requires too large a quantity of patient's serum, reagent antisera may be used and antigen-negative units selected for compatibility testing. However, antigen-negative units (if available) should be given if a serum sample obtained within the previous 3 days reacted at IAT and subsequent massive transfusion diluted the antibody to undetectable levels.

Category III—Primarily High-Titer, Low Avidity (HTLA) Antibodies That, By Definition, Give Weak Reactions Both in the Undiluted State and at High Dilutions. These antibodies rarely, if ever, cause significant destruction of transfused, incompatible RBCs. The greatest hazard is that they may mask the presence of a clinically significant antibody. General cross-match directions are:

1. Issue cross-match compatible blood when possible; consider screening 20 to 30 units with the patient's serum; and

Table 67.8. Selection of Antigen-Negative Blood for Transfusion[a]

Anti-	System	Category	Anti-	System	Category
A_1	ABO	II	Kp^a	Kell	IV
Bg	Bg	V	Kp^b	Kell	VI
C	Rh	I	Lan	Langeris	VI
c	Rh	I	Le^a	Lewis	II
C^w	Rh	IV	Le^b	Lewis	II
Ch^a	Chido	III	Lu^a	Lutheran	II
Cs^a	Cost-Stirling	III	Lu^b	Lutheran	VI
D	Rh	I	M	MN	II
E	Rh	I	M_1‡	MN	II
e	Rh	I	McC^a	Knops-McCoy	III
f*	Rh	I	McC^c	Knops-McCoy	III
Fy^a	Duffy	I	N	MN	II
Fy^b	Duffy	I	N¶	MN	VI
Ge	Gerbich	VI	P_1	P	II
H/HI/Hi†	ABO/I	II	PP_1P_k	P	VI
Hy	Holley	VI	Rg^a	Rodgers	III
I/i†	I	II	S	MN	I
Jk^a	Kidd	I	s	MN	I
Jk^b	Kidd	I	Sd^a	Sid	III
JMH	JMH	III	U	MN	VI
Js^a	Kell	IV	V	Rh	IV
Js^b	Kell	VI	Vel	Vel	VI
K	Kell	I	Wr^a	Wright	VI
k	Kell	VI	Yk^a	York	III
Kn^a	Knops-McCoy	III	Vt^a	Cartwright	VI
"Kn^a-McC^a	"Knops-McCoy	III	Xg^a	Xg	II

[a]* = type for c- units; † = usually autoantibodies; ‡ = compatible units will be M-; ¶ = antibody made by N-S-s- individuals; select N-U- blood.

2. Issue least reactive units if compatible blood cannot be found.

Note: Anti-Ch^a, -Rg^a, and -JMH have not been reported to cause in vivo RBC destruction. Antibodies with Knops-McCoy related specificity, anti-Cs^a, and -Yk^a may cause a slightly shortened survival of donor RBCs, but they have not convincingly been associated with profound hemolytic transfusion reactions.

Category IV—Antibodies to Low Frequency or Private Antigens. Confirm the antigen-negative status of cross-match-compatible blood when reagent antisera are available.

Category V—Antibodies to Leukocyte-Related Antigens for Which Reagent Antisera are Not Available. Issue cross-match-compatible units.

Category VI—Potentially Clinically Significant Alloantibodies to High-Frequency Antigens. Because of the infrequent occurrence of antigen-negative donors, screening for nonreactive units should not usually be attempted. Reevaluate the need for transfusion because rare units of blood will need to be obtained. Sources for such rare blood include:

- Autologous blood—for elective surgical cases;
- Family members—in most instances, antigen-negative donors will be found only among siblings; and
- Rare donor files—the American Red Cross (ARC) and the AABB maintain files of rare donors. Some community blood centers and transfusion services in tertiary care hospitals participate in the AABB Rare Donor Program and should be consulted if the need for rare blood arises. Rare units can be obtained from national files by referral from regional ARC blood centers or immunohematology reference laboratories accredited by the AABB.

When Autoantibodies Are Present

DETECTION OF CONCOMITANT ALLOANTIBODIES

Autoantibodies may mask the presence of clinically significant alloantibodies. Thus, when a patient with autoantibodies requires transfusion, the presence of concomitant alloantibodies should be determined if time permits. If warm-reactive IgG autoantibodies are present, as in WAIHA, it may be possible to adsorb the serum at 37°C with the patient's RBCs (autologous adsorption) or donor RBCs of a phenotype similar to that of the patient (homologous adsorption). The adsorbed serum is then tested for unexpected antibodies and may also be used for cross-matching. When cold-reactive autoantibodies are present, as in CHD, autologous adsorption can be performed at 4°C, or the serum can be adsorbed with rabbit RBCs prior to testing for unexpected antibodies. Alternatively, serum and reagent or donor RBCs can be warmed to 37°C before mixing (prewarmed tests). Specific details of the procedures involved in these studies are to be found elsewhere (25, 31, 45).

TRANSFUSION MANAGEMENT IN WAIHA

Transfusion of patients with WAIHA should be avoided, if possible. Except when the autoantibody manifests clear-cut specificity, all reagent and donor RBCs will be serologically incompatible. Transfused RBCs can be expected to undergo no better fate in vivo than the autologous RBCs. When hemolysis of the patient's RBCs is brisk, yet there is active generation of new cells in the bone marrow, the sudden infusion of a large volume of incompatible blood may lead to an accelerated destruction of the transfused RBCs with clinical deterioration resulting from hemoglobinemia, hemoglobinuria, and renal failure. There is also a risk that concomitant alloantibodies may be present, necessitating that adsorption studies be performed before transfusion.

Nonetheless, it may be necessary to transfuse incompatible blood in life-threatening situations arising from severe, progressive anemia. In such circumstances, the smallest volume of RBCs required to maintain adequate oxygen transportation should be given. Although RBC survival may be abnormal, the temporary benefit may be of value until other therapies (e.g., steroids) produce a more lasting effect. Clinical judgment must be the deciding factor; the risk of transfusing incompatible blood must be weighed against the risk of withholding transfusion (53).

If the serum shows clear-cut specificity (e.g., anti-e), transfusion with antigen-negative blood (i.e., R_2R_2 blood) may have a more lasting effect than transfusion with incompatible RBCs. However, when there is relative specificity (i.e., anti-e is evident only upon dilution of the serum or R_2R_2 reagent RBCs react weaker than e-positive RBCs), there are no data demonstrating a better survival of R_2R_2 blood. Also, consideration must be given to the fact that, when selecting blood for patients with relative Rh-specific autoantibodies, it will often be necessary to transfuse blood that carries Rh antigens not present on the patient's RBCs. Provision of e-negative blood for an Rh-negative patient with autoanti-e will necessitate transfusion with Rh-positive RBCs because e-negative, D-negative donors are exceedingly rare (12).

TRANSFUSION MANAGEMENT IN CHD

Use of prewarmed tests and anti-IgG minimizes the detection of cold-reactive autoantibodies responsible for CHD, yet permits detection of clinically significant alloantibodies. Procedures that enhance the detection of C3-binding IgM antibodies (room temperature incubation, use of albumin, use of polyspecific AHG containing anti-C3) should be avoided when performing antibody detection and cross-matching.

The antibody specificity in CHD is anti-I. However, the rarity of I-negative blood precludes transfusion of such units; moreover, transfusion with I-positive blood usually produces the expected rise in hemoglobin (53). Some workers prefer to administer blood to patients with cold agglutinins through a warming device. Whether this is always necessary is debatable, albeit little harm should occur through the use of such devices, providing they are adequately maintained and monitored.

PREDICTING THE SURVIVAL OF INCOMPATIBLE BLOOD

There are no reliable methods to predict the fate of transfused RBCs. Even apparently cross-match-compatible RBCs (by IS and IAT methods) may result in an acute hemolytic reaction. However, such instances are rare, and it is generally safe to transfuse blood that is compatible using the pretransfusion testing protocols described above. In life-threatening situations, it is sometimes necessary to transfuse incompatible blood to patients with unexpected antibodies. Suffice it to say, ABO-matched blood should not be withheld from patients with unexpected antibodies who urgently require transfusion simply because IAT-compatible blood cannot be found. In less emergent situations, when antibodies to high-frequency antigens or multiple alloantibodies are present or when the specificity of the unexpected antibody is unknown, a number of predictive tests can be undertaken to assess the outcome of transfusing incompatible RBCs. These include evaluating the serologic behavior of an antibody, RBC survival tests, and mononuclear monolayer assays (MMAs).

Serologic Behavior

Antibody characteristics that affect the in vivo survival of transfused, incompatible RBCs include (*a*) thermal range; (*b*) immunoglobulin class and subclass (if IgG); (*c*) ability to activate complement; (*d*) avidity; and (*e*) concentration. Cellular (antigen) factors that influence RBC destruction include (*a*) number of antigen sites per RBC; (*b*) amount of blood transfused; (*c*) ability of antigens to dissociate from RBCs; and (*d*) presence of blood group substances in donor plasma (54).

The most relevant piece of information to be gained from serologic tests is the thermal range of an antibody. If an antibody does not agglutinate, hemolyze, or coat RBCs at 37°C, those RBCs can be transfused with anticipation of a normal RBC survival (half-life about 30 days). This has been substantiated by survival studies using ^{51}Cr-labeled RBCs (30, 55).

IgM ANTIBODIES

Numerous studies have shown that IgM agglutinins that are dubiously reactive at 37°C bring about only minor RBC destruction. Moreover, because all data have been obtained with about 1 ml of labeled RBCs, it is certain that agglutinins dubiously reactive at 37°C are incapable of causing a severe hemolytic episode when therapeutic doses of RBCs are transfused (54, 55)

When unexpected antibodies are detected in direct agglutination tests at 37°C, they have to be considered potentially significant. If they lyse RBCs in vitro, they will likely hemolyze them in vivo. However, if they only agglutinate RBCs in vitro at 37°C, they may not necessarily cause RBC destruction in vivo. For example, anti-Le^{b} that reacts at 37°C has little significance, probably because the antibody is inhibited by Lewis substances in donor plasma and because the antigens elute from donor RBCs when transfused into a Lewis-negative recipient (12, 54).

IgG ANTIBODIES

IgG antibodies detected in antiglobulin tests following incubation with RBCs at 37°C are potentially significant. However, as shown in Table 67.4, not all have been associated with hemolytic transfusion reactions or HDN. In some instances, there may be too few antigen sites present on the transfused RBCs, even though the antibody present in the recipient's plasma is of high titer, as is the case with the so-called HTLA antibodies shown in Table 67.8. With other antibodies, such as −JMH, IgG immunoglobulin class may be a factor. Anti-JMH are invariably of the subclass IgG4, for which there are no Fc receptors on macrophages to initiate removal of anti-JMH-coated RBCs (56, 57). Most alloantibodies to RBC antigens are IgG1 and IgG3 (56), but there are few data comparing the destructive ability of the two subclasses. Moreover, technical factors negate the usefulness of IgG subclass determinations for clinical use (52).

Perhaps the best predictor of the clinical significance of an unexpected antibody is prior experience. Table 67.4 was developed from the experiences of others, often anecdotal but sometimes substantiated with RBC survival studies and MMAs. Consequently, when an antibody of a specificity known to cause accelerated destruction of transfused, incompatible RBCs or HDN is encountered, efforts should be made to seek compatible donors. When there are no data or, as in the case of anti-Yt^{a}, when there are conflicting data (54) or when the specificity of the antibody is unknown, RBC survival studies and MMAs are indicated.

RBC Survival Studies

Before performing a ^{51}Cr-labeled RBC survival (see in Method 67.6), every effort should be made to identify the antibody specificity, confirm the need for transfusion, and determine if autologous donation is possible. If the antibody is of a specificity known to cause accelerated RBC destruction, compatible donors should be sought among siblings and by contacting rare donor files. When no compatible donors are available or when the specificity remains undetermined, it is worth considering how the data will be used. While the procedure is not technically difficult, it requires the cooperation of the nuclear medicine staff to ensure the validity of the analysis and the calculation of the results. The analysis of samples and the calculation of the results are subject to considerable error unless certain precautions are undertaken. Consequently, there seems little point in performing the test when the patient must be transfused, regardless of the results. Moreover, it should be noted that the data obtained and their interpretation apply only to the volume of incompatible, labeled RBCs injected into the patient. A larger volume may manifest a slower rate of destruction, while RBCs from a different donor, although incompatible in serologic tests to the same degree as those used in the ^{51}Cr survival study, may manifest a faster rate of destruction.

A 1-hour survival of 70% or more of the injected aliquot of ^{51}Cr-labeled RBCs suggests that the remainder of the donor unit can be transfused in an emergency. If values less than 70% are obtained, a decision must be made as to whether transfusion is needed to save the patient's life. If so, and time allows, an aliquot (10 to 15 ml) of donor RBCs can be injected slowly, and blood samples drawn 15 and 30 minutes postinjection. The hemoglobin levels in the pre- and postinjection plasma samples are compared to predict the outcome of transfusing the entire unit of RBCs.

Mononuclear Monolayer Assays

In the mononuclear monolayer assays (MMA), antibody is incubated with RBCs, which are then incubated with mononuclear cells harvested from peripheral blood. A smear is made and stained, and the mononuclear cells are then examined for adherent and phagocytosed RBCs.

The MMA is an indirect, noninvasive means of predicting the outcome of transfusing incompatible RBCs. A value less than 3.0 (percent adherence and/

or phagocytosis) is considered insignificant; i.e., such values correlate well with a RBC survival of 70% at 1 hour (54). Detailed procedures are given in Methods 67.7 and 67.8.

References

1. Landsteiner K. Uber Agglutinationserscheinungen normalen menschlichen Blutes. Klin Wochenschr 1901;14:1132–1134.
2. Hektoen L. Isoagglutination of human corpuscles. JAMA 1907;48:1739–1740.
3. Weil R. Sodium citrate in the transfusion of blood. JAMA 1915;64:425–426.
4. Ottenberg R. Reminiscence on the history of blood transfusion. J Mt Sinai Hosp 1937;4:264.
5. Crile GW. Hemorrhage and transfusion. New York: Appleton, 1909.
6. Rous P, Turner R. A rapid and simple method of testing donors for transfusion. JAMA 1915;64:1980–1982.
7. Moss WL. Studies on isoagglutinins and hemolysins. Bull Johns Hopkins Hosp 1910;21:63.
8. Robertson LB. Blood transfusion in war surgery. Lancet 1918;1:759–762.
9. Vincent B. A rapid macroscopic agglutination test for blood group and its value in testing donors for transfusion. JAMA 1918;70:1219–1220.
10. Riddell VH. Blood transfusion. London: Oxford University Press, 1939.
11. De Gowin EL, Baldridge CW. Fatal anemia following blood transfusions. Inadequacy of present tests for compatibility. Am J Med Sci 1934;188:555.
12. Race RR, Sanger R. Blood groups in man. 6th ed. Oxford: Blackwell Scientific Publications, 1965.
13. Levine P, Stetson RE. An unusual case of intragroup agglutination. JAMA 1939;113:126–127.
14. Weiner AS. Genetic theory of the Rh blood types. Proc Natl Exp Biol NY 1943;54:3169.
15. Mourant AE. A new rhesus antibody. Nature 1945;155:542.
16. Coombs RRA, Mourant AE, Race RR. A new test for the detection of weak and incomplete Rh agglutinins. Br J Exp Pathol 1945;26:255–266.
17. Moreschi C. Neue Tatsachen uber die Blutkorperchen Agglutinationenen. Zentralbl Bakteriol 1908;46:49–51.
18. Diamond LK, Denton RL. Rh agglutination in various media with particular reference to the value of albumin. J Lab Clin Med 1945;26:821–830.
19. Issitt PD. Applied blood group serology. 3rd ed. Miami: Montgomery Scientific Publications, 1985.
20. Strumia MM, Jennings ER, eds. Standards for a blood transfusion service. 1st ed. Washington DC: Joint Blood Council, Inc., and Chicago: American Association of Blood Banks, 1958.
21. Widmann FK, ed. Standards for blood banks and transfusion services. 15th ed. Arlington, VA: American Association of Blood Banks, 1993.
22. Code of Federal Regulations (21-CFR), parts 606 and 660. Washington, DC: U.S. Government Printing Office, 1988.
23. Commission on Laboratory Accreditation. Inspection checklist. Chicago: College of American Pathologists, 1989.
24. Bell CA, ed. Seminar on antigen antibody reactions revisited. Arlington, VA: American Association of Blood Banks, 1982.
25. Walker RH, et al. Technical manual. 11th ed. Arlington, VA: American Association of Blood Banks, 1993.
26. Huestis DW, Bove JR, Busch S. Practical blood transfusion. 3rd ed. Boston: Little, Brown, 1981.
27. Romans DG, Tilley CA, Crookston MC, Falk RE, Dorrington KJ. Conversion of incomplete antibodies to direct agglutinins by mild reduction: evidence for increased flexibility within the Fc fragment of human immunoglobulin G. Proc Natl Acad Sci, USA 1977;74:2531–2535.
28. Judd WJ, Luban NLC, Ness PM, Silberstein LE, Stroup M, Widmann FK. Prenatal and perinatal immunohematology: recommendations for management of the fetus, newborn infant and obstetric patient. Transfusion 1990;30:175–188.
29. Schmidt PJ. The mortality from incompatible transfusion. In: Sandler SG, Nusbacher G, Schanfield MS, eds. Immunobiology of the erythrocyte. New York: AR Liss, 1980;251–261.
30. Mollison PL. Blood transfusion in clinical medicine. 8th ed. Oxford: Blackwell Scientific Publications, 1987.
31. Judd WJ. Methods in immunohematology. Miami: Montgomery Scientific Publications, 1988.
32. Jones EC, Sinclair M, Unrau L, Crowe G. False-positive results with chemically modified anti-D. Transfusion 1987;27:142–144.
33. Judd WJ, Steiner EA, Oberman HA. False-positive reactions with chemically modified anti-D do not indicate the need for a separate immunologically inert Rh control reagent. Transfusion 1988;28:339–341.
34. Beck ML, Yates AD, Hardman J, Kowalski MA. Identification of a subset of group B donors reactive with monoclonal anti-A reagents. Am J Clin Pathol 1989;92:625–629.
35. Judd WJ. The Rh blood groups. Miami: American Dade, 1985.
36. Judd WJ. Lectins and polyagglutination. In: Petz LD, Swisher SN, eds. Clinical practice of blood transfusion. 2nd ed. Edinburgh: Churchill-Livingstone, 1989:137–151.
37. Pierce SR. Anomalous blood bank results. In: Dawson RB, ed. Trouble-shooting the crossmatch. Washington DC: American Association of Blood Banks, 1977:85–114.
38. Lalezari P, Jiang AF. The manual Polybrene test: a simple and rapid procedure for detection of red cell antibodies. Transfusion 1980;20:206–211.
39. Garratty G. The role of compatibility tests. Transfusion 1982;22:169–172.
40. Oberman HA, Judd WJ. In: Cash JD, ed. Progress in transfusion medicine. Vol 3. Edinburgh: Churchill-Livingsone, 1988: 145–158.
41. Shulman IA, Nelson JM, Okomoto M, Malone SA. The dependence of anti-Jk^a detection on screening cell zygosity. Lab Med 1985;16:602–604.
42. Shulman IA, Yaowasiriwatt M, Saxena S, Nelson JM. Influence of reagent red cell zygosity on anti-Fy^a detecion. Lab Med 1989;20:37–39.
43. Garratty G. The role of complement in blood group serology. CRC Crit Rev Clin Lab Sci 1985;20:25–56.
44. Judd WJ, Barnes BA, Steiner EA, et al. The evaluation of a positive direct antiglobulin test (autocontrol) revisited. Transfusion 1986;26:220–224.
45. Judd WJ. Investigation and management of immune hemolysis—autoantibodies and drugs. In: Wallace ME, Levitt J, eds. Current applications and interpretation of the direct antiglobulin test. Arlington, VA: American Association of Blood Banks, 1988;47–103.
46. Knight R, Poole G, eds. The use of microplates in blood group serology. Manchester: British Blood Transfusion Society, 1987.
47. Judd WJ, Steiner EA, O'Donnell DB, Oberman HA. Discrepancies in ABO typing due to prozone: how safe is the immediate-spin cross-match? Transfusion 1988;28:334–338.
48. Shulman IA. Controversies in red blood cell compatibility testing. In: Nance SJ, ed. immune destruction of red blood cells. Arlington, VA: American Association of Blood Banks, 1989: 171–199.
49. Boral LI, Henry JB. The type and screen: a safe alternative and supplement in selected surgical blood order schedules. Transfusion 1977;17:163–168.

50. Friedman BA, Oberman HA, Chadwick AR, Kingdon KI. The maximum surgical blood order schedule and surgical blood use in the United States. Transfusion 1976;16:380–387.
51. Mintz PD, Nordine RD, Henry JB. Expected hemotherapy in elective surgery. NY State J Med 1976;76:532–537.
52. Butch SH. Blood inventory management. Lab Med 1985;16: 17–20.
53. Petz LD, Garratty G. Acquired immune hemolytic anemias. Edinburgh: Churchill-Livingstone, 1980.
54. Garratty G. Predicting the clinical significance of alloantibodies and determining the *in vivo* survival of transfused red cells. In: Judd WJ, Barnes A, eds. Clinical and serological aspects of transfusion reactions. Arlington, VA: American Association of Blood Banks, 1982:91–119.
55. Mollison PL. Determination of red cell survival using ^{51}Cr. In: Bell CA, ed. A seminar on immune mediated cell destruction. Washington: American Association of Blood Banks, 1981: 45–69.
56. Abrahamson H, Schur PH. The IgG subclass red cell antibodies and relationship to monocyte binding. Blood 1972;40: 500–508.
57. Tregallas WM, Pierce SR, Hardman JT, Beck ML. Anti-JMH: IgG subclass composition and clinical significance [Abstract]. Transfusion 1980;20:628.

Appendix—Methods

The procedures outlined below are modified from Judd WJ. Methods in immunohematology. Miami: Montgomery Scientific Publications, 1988. They are reproduced with permission from the publisher.

Method 67.1. ABO and Rh Typing

Primary Application

Pretransfusion and prenatal testing.

Materials

1. Anti-A and anti-B.
2. Anti-D (-Rh_o): chemically modified reagent.
3. RBCs: 3 to 5% suspensions of reagent A_1 and B RBCs.
4. Test sample: clotted or anticoagulated whole blood: centrifuged at 1000 × g for 5 minutes.

Method

1. Remove approximately 0.4 ml of test serum with a Pasteur pipette and dispense 3 drops into two appropriately labeled 10 or 12 × 75-mm test tubes; discard residual serum.
2. To one tube add 1 drop of A_1 RBCs; add 1 drop of B RBCs to the other tube; gently mix the contents in each tube.
3. Dispense 1 drop of anti-A into an appropriately labeled 10 or 12 × 75-mm test tube; set up similar tubes for anti-B and anti-D.
4. Add 1 drop of a 3 to 5% suspension (in native serum or saline) of test RBCs to each tube containing antiserum; mix gently.
5. Centrifuge all tubes at 1000 × g for 15 seconds.
6. Examine the RBCs macroscopically for agglutination and hemolysis; grade and record the results.

Interpretation

The interpretation of results is as follows:

RBCs vs anti-			Serum vs RBCs		
−A	−B	−D	A_1	B	
0	0	0	4+	4+	O Rh−
4+	0	0	0	4+	A Rh−
0	4+	0	4+	0	B Rh−
4+	4+	0	0	0	AB Rh−
−A	−B	−D	A_1	B	
0	0	4+	4+	4+	O Rh+
4+	0	4+	0	4+	A Rh+
0	4+	4+	4+	0	B Rh+
4+	4	4+	0	0+	AB Rh+

Note

Resolve all discrepancies before concluding the results.

Method 67.2. D^u Testing

Primary Application

Detection of weak expression of D on donor RBCs that react weakly or not at all with anti-D in direct agglutination tests.

Materials

1. Anti-Dd (-Rh_o): suitable for D^u testing (e.g., modified-tube reagent).
2. Antihuman IgG: need not be heavy-chain specific.
3. Rh control reagent: immunologically inert diluent used for preparing anti-D, as supplied by the manufacturer.
4. Test RBCs: 3 to 5% suspension in saline or native plasma/serum.

Method

1. Dispense anti-D into an appropriately labeled 10 or 12 × 75-mm test tube, according to the manufacturer's directions.
2. Similarly, dispense the Rh control serum.
3. Add 1 drop of test RBCs to each tube.
4. Mix and incubate at 37°C, according to the manufacturer's directions.
5. Centrifuge at 1000 × g for 15 seconds.
6. Examine the RBCs macroscopically; grade and record the results. *Note:* conclude as Rh-positive when RBCs are specifically agglutinated by anti-D; in such instances, there is no need to proceed to the antiglobulin phase.
7. Wash the RBCs × 4 with saline.
8. Add anti-IgG, according to the manufacturer's directions.
9. Centrifuge at 1000 × g for 15 seconds.
10. Examine the RBCs macroscopically; grade and record the results.

Interpretation

The interpretation of results is as follows:

Anti-D	Rh Control	
+	0	Rh-positive
0	0	Rh-negative
+	+	unable to conclude; most likely due to a positive DAT

Note

D^u testing of potential blood recipients is not advocated except when Rh-negative blood is in short supply and when those patients found to be D^u will be transfused with Rh-positive blood.

Method 67.3. Screening Tests for Unexpected Antibodies

Primary Application

Detection of unexpected antibodies to RBC antigens in blood samples from potential transfusion recipients or prenatal patients.

Materials

1. Antihuman globulin (AHG): polyspecific or anti-IgG.
2. IgG-coated RBCs.
3. Low-ionic-strength saline (LISS) solution.
4. RBCs: phenotyped homologous group O R_1R_1 and R_2R_2 RBC samples, washed once with LISS and resuspended to a 2% concentration with LISS; use within 6 hours of preparation.
5. Test serum/plasma: collected within the previous 3 days if to be used for pretransfusion testing.

Method

1. Dispense 2 drops of test serum/plasma into two appropriately labeled 10 or 12 × 75-mm test tubes (see note #1).
2. To one tube, add 2 drops of 2% R_1R_1 RBCs in LISS; similarly, set up tests with the R_2R_2 RBCs.
3. Mix and incubate at 37°C for 10 minutes.
4. Centrifuge at 1000 × g for 15 seconds.
5. Examine the RBCs macroscopically for agglutination and hemolysis; grade and record the results.
6. Wash the RBCs × 4 with saline; completely decant the final wash supernatant.
7. To the dry RBC buttons thus obtained, add AHG, according to the manufacturer's directions.
8. Centrifuge at 1000 × g for 15 seconds.
9. Examine the RBCs macroscopically; grade and record the results.
10. Confirm negative reactions with IgG-coated RBCs.

Notes

1. Use uniform-bore Pasteur pipettes to dispense serum and LISS-suspended RBCs to ensure addition of equal volumes of serum/plasma and reagent RBCs.
2. Investigate the cause of all positive tests.
3. One of the reagent RBC samples should be Jk(a+b−) if anti-IgG is used.

Reference

Low B, Messeter L. Antiglobulin tests in low-ionic strength salt solutions for rapid antibody screening and cross-matching. Vox Sang 1974;26:53–61.

Method 67.4. Immediate-Spin Cross-match

Primary Application

Donor-recipient compatibility testing for patients whose sera currently lack clinically significant, unexpected antibodies and who have no prior record of having such antibodies.

Materials

1. Donor RBCs: from segments attached to the units to be transfused.
2. Test serum/plasma: collected within the previous 3 days (sample should be that previously used in tests for ABO, Rh, and unexpected antibodies).
3. EDTA-Saline (pH 6.5; 440 mOsm/ kg): NaCl, 9 g/liter; K_2EDTA, 25 g/liter; NaOH, 2 g/liter.

Method

1. For each donor unit to be tested, label a 10 or 12 ×75-mm test tube with the unit number.
2. Dispense 1 drop of each donor RBC sample into the appropriate tube; dilute each sample to a 4 to 5% RBC concentration with EDTA-saline.
3. For each donor unit to be tested, label another 10 or 12 × 75-mm test tube with the unit number and the patient's name.
4. Dispense 3 drops of test serum into each tube and add 1 drp of the appropriate RBC suspension.
5. Mix and centrifuge at 1000 × g for 15 seconds.
6. Examine the RBCs macroscopically for agglutination and hemolysis; grade and record the results.

Note

Investigate the cause of all positive tests before transfusion.

Method 67.5. Antiglobulin Cross-match

Primary Application

Donor-recipient compatibility testing for patients whose sera currently contain clinically significant, unexpected antibodies or who have prior records of having such antibodies.

Materials

1. Antihuman globulin (AHG): polyspecific or anti-IgG.
2. Donor RBCs: from segments attached to the units to be transfused.
3. IgG-coated RBCs.
4. Low-ionic-strength saline (LISS) solution: obtain commercially.
5. Test serum/plasma: collected within the previous 3 days (sample should be that previously used in tests for ABO, Rh, and unexpected antibodies).

Method

1. For each donor unit to be tested, label a 10 or 12 × 75-mm test tube with the donor unit number.
2. Dispense 1 drop of each donor RBC sample into the appropriate tube; dilute RBCs to a 4 to 5% concentration with saline.
3. For each donor unit to be tested, label another 10 or 12 × 75-mm test tube with the unit number and the patient's name.
4. Dispense 1 drop of each saline suspension of RBCs into appropriate tubes and fill the tubes with LISS solution.
5. Centrifuge at 1000 × g for 60 seconds.
6. Completely decant the supernatant fluid and blot the ends of inverted tubes with tissue paper.
7. To the dry RBC buttons thus obtained, add 2 drops of LISS solution and 2 drops of test serum/plasma.
8. Mix and incubate at 37°C for 10 minutes.
9. Centrifuge at 1000 × g for 15 seconds.
10. Examine the RBCs macroscopically for agglutination and hemolysis; grade and record the results.
11. Wash the RBCs × 4 with saline; completely decant the final wash supernatant.

12. To the dry RBC buttons thus obtained, add AHG according to the manufacturer's directions.
13. Centrifuge at 1000 × g for 15 seconds.
14. Examine the RBCs macroscopically; grade and record the results.
15. Confirm negative tests with IgG-coated RBCs.

Note

Use uniform-bore Pasteur pipettes to dispense serum and LISS-suspended RBCs to ensure addition of equal volumes of serum/plasma and reagent RBCs.

Reference

Low B, Messeter L. Antiglobulin tests in low-ionic strength salt solution for rapid antibody screening and cross-matching. Vox Sang 1974;26:53–61.

Method 67.6. ^{51}Cr-Labeled RBC Survival Studies

Theoretical Considerations

Incompatible RBCs are labeled with a radioactive isotope and injected into the patient. The percent survival of these RBCs is calculated from radioactivity measurements of postinjection blood samples.

Primary Application

Evaluating the outcome of transfusion of incompatible blood to patients for whom compatible blood cannot be obtained.

Materials

1. ^{51}Cr sodium chromate solution: $Na_2{}^{51}CrO_4$ (New England Nuclear, Boston, MA)—with a specific activity such that less than 2 g of chromium is added per ml of packed RBCs. The solution should have a minimum volume of 0.2 ml, being diluted with sterile normal saline.
2. Donor unit or heterologous blood samples for survival study: fresh, sterile anticoagulated sample (not heparinized), or a ACD/CPD/CPD-A1 anticoagulated unit, is preferred. Ensure that the results of hepatitis, HIV, and other tests for infectious agents are satisfactory.
3. Patient for study: normally, patients will be those for whom compatible blood is unobtainable due to potentially significant, unexpected serum alloantibodies (i.e., antibodies reactive at 37°C and/or by the IAT). There should be no clinical signs of bleeding. Determine the height (in meters) and weight (in kilograms) of the patient on the day of study.
4. Sterile normal saline (SNS) pyrogen-free, sterile saline NaCl, 9 g/liter).
5. Sterile tubes: 10 ml size.
6. Spinal needles: 3″ in length (for sterile aspiration of supernatant fluids).
7. Syringes: 2 ml and 10 ml sizes.

Method

1. Using sterile technique, withdraw 1 to 2 ml of whole blood (0.5 to 1.0 ml RBCs) and transfer to a sterile tube. If whole blood is used, centrifuge and remove supernatant plasma.
2. With continuous mixing, slowly add 20 μCi ^{51}Cr and incubate on a rotary mixer for 30 minutes at room temperature.
3. Using sterile technique, wash the RBCs by gently suspending them in 6 to 8 ml of SNS and centrifuging at 1000 × g for 5 minutes. Discard supernatant into radioactive waste.
4. Repeat step #3 × 1.
5. Gently suspend the RBCs in approximately 10 ml of SNS; mix well.
6. Withdraw exactly 8 ml for infusion into the patient.
7. Using a volumetric pipette, withdraw exactly 1 ml for preparation of a standard solution. Dilute, using a volumetric flask, to 250 ml with distilled water.
8. Infuse the 8 ml sample into a freely flowing antecubital vein. Aspirate a small amount of venous blood back into the syringe and reinject.
9. Collect 3 ml anticoagulated (EDTA/heparin) blood samples from the contralateral antecubital vein at 3 minutes, 7 minutes, 10 minutes, 60 minutes, and 24 hrs postinjection.

Calculations

1. Determine radioactive counts, using a γ counter, in exactly 1 ml of well-mixed whole blood. Subtract background counts and correct the 24-hour count for elution (counts × 1.03). *Note:* A minimum of 4000 counts should be recorded per sample.
2. Count 1 ml of plasma from the 3-minute sample. *Note:* Proceed if plasma counts are less than 5% of total counts in the 3-minute sample. If greater than 5%, consider very rapid hemolysis or inadequate washing of the labeled sample.
3. Predict the patient's blood volume (PBV) using the following calculations:
   MALES
   $$\text{PBV in liters} = (0.3669 \times \text{height in meters}^3) + 0.6041 + (0.03219 \times \text{weight in kilograms})$$
   FEMALES
   $$\text{PBV in liters} = (0.3561 \times \text{height in meters}^3) + 0.1833 + (0.03308 \times \text{weight in kilograms})$$
4. Calculate the patient's blood volume (CBV) from the standard solution and the 3-minute sample using the following formula:
   $$\text{CBV in liters} = \frac{\text{counts/1 ml standard} \times 8 \times 0.250}{\text{counts/1 ml 3-minute sample}}$$
5. If the CBV does not exceed the PBV by more than 10%, assume 3-minute sample equates with 100% survival. Compare subsequent sample counts to the 3-minute count to determine RBC survival.
6. If the CBV exceeds the PBV by more than 10%, suspect:
   a. inadequate mixing at 3 minutes secondary to splenomegaly, congestive heart failure, etc. Plasma counts should be low. The CBV calculated from the 7-minute sample more closely approximates the PBV. In such instances the 7-minute count can be used to represent 100% survival.
   b. extravasation at the injection site. CBVs calculated from counts on all subsequent samples are elevated

and plasma counts are low; to confirm, check site with Geiger counter.

c. very rapid hemolysis. CBV and plasma counts will be high. Extrapolate to 0 minutes.

7. Determine survival curve and percentages. In an emergency, the study may be terminated at 60 minutes. It is preferable, however, to extend the study to 24 hours, when possible. See the reference cited below for a discussion on the interpretation of results.

Reference

Davey RJ. Mechanisms of premature red cell destruction. In: Judd WJ, Barnes A, eds. Clinical and serological aspects of transfusion reactions. Arlington: American Association of Blood Banks, 1982:1–35.

Method 67.7. Mononuclear Monolayer Assay

Theoretical Considerations

Antibody-coated RBCs are incubated in vitro with mononuclear cells. The ability of mononuclear cells to adhere and phagocytose these sensitized RBCs is an index of the antibody's potential to decrease the survival of transfused RBCs.

Primary Application

In vitro prediction of the in vivo significance of antibodies to RBC antigens.

Materials

1. Anti-D: commercially prepared, modified-tube anti-D diluted 1 in 50 with human complement (see below).
2. Culture chamber: Lab-Tek tissue culture chamber slides (ICN Immuno-Biologicals, Lisle, IL).
3. Giemsa stain: SIGMA Chemicals, St. Louis, MO.
4. Human complement: freshly collected, normal human serum known to lack unexpected antibodies.
5. Mononuclear cell suspension: prepared as described in Method 67.8. *Note:* Prepare homologous mononuclear cells from normal donors and autologous mononuclear cells, if available.
6. Mounting medium: Pro-Texx (American Scientific Products, McGaw Park, IL).
7. Phosphate buffered saline (PBS) at pH 7.3.
8. Test serum: containing antibody under evaluation.
9. Tissue culture medium: RPMI 1640 medium (SIGMA Chemicals, St. Louis, MO), containing 10% (vol/vol) fetal calf serum (GIBCO Laboratories, Grand Island, NY).
10. Washed, sensitized RBCs: 5% suspensions in tissue culture medium; incubate 1 drop of 5% RBCs with 3 drops of serum for 60 minutes at 37°C; wash × 4 with saline before dilution with tissue culture medium. *Note:* Use RBCs that lack and RBCs that carry antigens to which the test serum manifests specificity; include the following reaction mixtures for RBC sensitization:
    a. test serum + antigen-positive RBCs
    b. test serum + antigen-positive RBCs + complement
    c. complement + antigen-positive RBCs
    d. PBS + antigen-positive RBCs
    e. anti-D + Rh-positive RBCs
11. Wright's stain: American Scientific Products, McGaw Park, IL.
12. Wright-Giemsa buffer: American Scientific Products, McGaw Park, IL.

Method

1. Add 0.2 ml of the mononuclear cell suspension (3 to 6 × 10^6/ml) to each well of a tissue culture slide.
2. Incubate at 37°C for 60 minutes.
3. Carefully aspirate nonadherent cells (lymphocytes) with Pasteur pipette and discard.
4. Add 0.2 ml of each sensitized RBC sample to appropriately labeled wells.
5. Incubate at 37°C for 60 minutes.
6. Aspirate the supernatant and discard.
7. Break off the plastic chambers and remove gaskets.
8. Gently rinse the slide × 3 with saline.
9. Blot the edge of the slide with a paper towel and immediately place in Wright's stain for 3 minutes.
10. Blot the edge of the slide with a paper towel and place in Giemsa stain for 20 minutes.
11. Blot the edge of the slide with a paper towel and wash in Wright-Giemsa buffer for 3 minutes.
12. Rinse with distilled water.
13. Blot the edge of the slide with a paper towel, wipe the back of the slide clean, and air dry.
14. Cover with a coverslip using Permount; allow to dry.
15. Examine microscopically for reactive mononuclear cells (RBC adherence and/or phagocytosis).
16. Count 600 mononuclear cells (200 if reactivity is greater than 20%).
17. Express the results in terms of the percent of reactive mononuclear cells.

Interpretation

Normal range is 0 to 3% reactive mononuclear cells.

Reference

Garratty G. Predicting the clinical significance of alloantibodies and determining the in vivo survival of transfused red cells. In: Judd WJ, Barnes A, eds. Clinical and serological aspects of transfusion reactions. Arlington: American Association of Blood Banks, 1982:91–119.

Method 67.8. Mononuclear Cell Separation

Primary Application

For use in mononuclear monolayer assays (see Method 67.7).

Materials

1. Whole blood sample: anticoagulated with heparin or EDTA, 20 ml.
2. Ficoll-Hypaque (F-H): Pharmacia, Piscataway, NY.
3. Phosphate-buffered saline (PBS) at pH 7.3.
4. Sterile, conical centrifuge tubes: 50 ml volume.
5. Tissue culture medium: RPMI 1640 medium (SIGMA Chemicals, St. Louis, MO), containing 10% (vol/vol) fetal calf serum (GIBCO Laboratories, Grand Island, NY).

Method

1. Allow reagents to warm to room temperature.

2. Place 15 ml of whole blood into a 50 ml sterile, conical centrifuge tube.
3. Centrifuge at 150 × g for 10 minutes.
4. Carefully remove the leukocyte/platelet-rich plasma to within ½-inch of the RBCs and dilute with 35 ml of pH 7.3 PBS.
5. Using sterile technique, place 12 ml of F-H into another 50 ml, sterile conical centrifuge tube.
6. Tilt the tube containing F-H to a 30° angle; slowly layer the diluted plasma onto the F-H with a small-bore pipette, putting it as close to the meniscus as possible but without touching the F-H.
7. Slowly tilt the tube upright and gently transfer to a centrifuge.
8. Centrifuge at 800 × g for 15 minutes. NOTE: Accelerate centrifuge gently to reach desired speed.
9. Remove supernatant plasma and PBS to within 5 ml of the leukocyte layer.
10. Carefully transfer leukocyte layer into a clean, sterile 50 ml centrifuge tube using a wide-bore Pasteur pipette. NOTE: leukocyte layer should be composed predominantly of monocytes and lymphocytes.
11. Dilute leukocytes with 40 ml of PBS; gently mix and centrifuge at 400 × g for 10 minutes.
12. Wash leukocytes × 2 with PBS; use centrifuge times of 10 minutes at 400 × g. Note: For each wash, remove PBS to within 2.5 ml, resuspend leukocytes by pipette with gentle aspiration and dilute with 40 ml of PBS; mix gently.
13. Remove final wash supernatant to within ½-inch of the leukocytes; resuspend by pipette with gentle aspiration, and add tissue culture medium to the 5.0 ml mark.
14. Determine the leukocyte concentration and adjust with tissue culture medium to 3 to 6 × 10^6/ml.
15. Use immediately in mononuclear assays as described in Method 67.7.

Reference

Garratty G. Predicting the clinical significance of alloantibodies and determining the in vivo survival of transfused red cells. In: Judd WJ, Barnes A, eds. Clinical and serological aspects of transfusion reactions. Arlington: American Association of Blood Banks, 1982:91–119.

68 Blood Component Therapy

S. Breanndan Moore

BASIC RATIONALE

The basic rationale of component therapy is the idea that a particular patient's blood cell or plasma deficiencies can be identified and precisely what is needed to correct those deficiencies can be supplied in a timely manner. This approach is logical from the standpoints of the individual patient and of those whose responsibility it is to ensure an adequate supply of blood and components for the population at large. By processing each unit of donated blood into multiple subunits containing concentrates of various cellular and noncellular products, one can benefit multiple patients from a single donation. If each recipient is transfused with only the moiety that he or she requires, then the system is truly efficient and effective.

BACKGROUND

In the opening decades of this century, medical pioneers began to use Landsteiner's seminal discovery of the ABO blood group system when choosing blood donors for a patient. In those days, their concerns were primarily the patient's desperate clinical straits, the availability of a "matchable" donor, and the ability to obtain the desired blood and infuse it without causing harm to the donor or recipient. Because of these significant concerns and the lack of standardized instruments and practices, the transfusion of blood was reserved for cases in which all routinely accepted methods of therapy had been exhausted and the patient's deteriorating condition warranted extraordinary measures. The prospect of receiving blood was often feared as much as the operation that might have created the need.

The ability to isolate a great many fractions or components from donated blood has been a major breakthrough in recent years. This process has been greatly stimulated by the increasing sophistication of both diagnostic acumen and treatment modalities.

The enormous array of complex surgical procedures, as well as the refinements in the management of medical diseases, have resulted in the successful treatment of patients who might, even a decade ago, have succumbed. These advances have been accompanied by an equivalent and concomitant increase in the quantity of blood and blood components used. Many of these surgical and medical therapeutic regimens are directly dependent on the availability of an adequate and safe supply of appropriate blood and components.

Because the demands for blood sometimes outstrip the available supply, it is important to be concerned about the ability to respond not only to current patient requirements but also to the inevitable future demands generated by medical and surgical technological advances. There is no reason to believe that the trends of increasing utilization of blood and, particularly, blood components will change in the future.

Technological Advances

When blood was first collected from donors, it was drawn into glass bottles through rubber tubing. Such bottles and tubing were still being used in this country in the 1950s. In fact, glass bottles were used in the USSR until just a few years ago. These glass bottles and rubber tubings were sterilized and reused.

The only component preparation possible from blood drawn into glass bottles was plasma separation by allowing the unit to stand immobile. The advent of disposable plastic bags and tubing created a dramatic new capability, i.e., manipulation of the donated blood in such a manner as to allow the separation of platelet-rich plasma from the red cells. This, in turn, gave us platelet concentrate and fresh frozen plasma. Subsequently, Pool discovered the antihemophilic properties of the cold-precipitated proteins from fresh-frozen plasma (1, 2). Thus was born cryoprecipitated plasma, which has revolutionized the treatment of hemophilia.

The next major advances were in the development of various anticoagulants and preservatives. These developments progressively increased the functional shelf life of blood and components by providing the necessary substances to maintain the metabolism of the preserved cells at higher levels than was previously possible. The use of newer plastics allowed better gas exchange across the bag, allowing the cells in the bag to "breathe" and thereby enhancing their function after storage.

The development of both continuous and semicontinuous apheresis machines permitted the selective separation of relatively large quantities of platelets or granulocytes (or both) from single donors. This led to the use of single-donor cellular components for patients who were septic (granulocytes) or alloimmunized (platelets). The use of HLA class I typing to match donor and recipient added another dimension to the efficacy of platelet therapy. This technique has been further modified to permit selective removal of specific plasma contents. This is accomplished by passage of the plasma over columns designed to remove specific moieties, e.g., IgG antibodies and the pruritogenic factors in biliary cirrhosis. These techniques also have been modified to produce enriched, activated, autologous lymphoid cell preparations for use in the treatment of malignant disease.

Fractionation on a commercial scale has permitted the acquisition and heat treatment of albumin from huge pools of plasma. This product has had extensive use in various situations, as will be described later.

Donor and Donation Efficiency

When the demand for blood outstrips the supply, episodic blood shortages occur, necessitating cancellation or postponement of elective surgical procedures and dependence on other geographic regions for the needed blood and components. Unfortunately, many large urban populations that have large blood needs also have inadequate donation patterns. This fact alone makes it particularly important that we achieve the maximal use of the units that are donated. Obviously, the manufacture of components from as many units as possible is the best way to achieve such efficiency. Apart from the need to respond to the transfusion needs of patients, we have an obligation not to misuse or underutilize the blood donated.

Economic Factors

The costs of obtaining a unit of blood have increased over the past few years for several reasons. Among these are: (*a*) the increased cost of donor recruitment because of personnel and advertising charges; (*b*) the cost of the ever-growing list of donor tests mandated by regulatory or accrediting agencies; and (*c*) the somewhat less clearly defined but real costs incurred as a result of blood banks' greater attention to transfusion safety. These costs include the significant time involved in the administration of autologous, directed, and minimal-exposure transfusion (MET) programs (3).

With the autologous, directed, and MET programs, a specific unit must be clearly identified (from the moment of acceptance by the blood bank) as coming from a specific donor and designated for a specific recipient. This degree of commitment requires considerably more administrative effort and computer support than does the older homologous system. These added costs are inevitably passed on to the patients, but we have an obligation to be as efficient as possible in the use of the donations to minimize these supplementary costs.

COMPONENT PREPARATION

Anticoagulants and Preservatives

Various solutions have been developed to prevent the clotting of donated blood and to preserve its functional elements. These solutions have gradually become more complex as changes have been introduced to prolong the effective shelf life of the component, to alter its flow characteristics, and to increase the yield of components from the donation. The characteristics of these various solutions are discussed in detail in Chapter 71. Suffice it to say here that the improvements in these solutions have played a major role in the burgeoning field of component therapy in the past decade.

Basic Techniques

CENTRIFUGATION

When blood was collected in glass bottles, most of it was stored and then transfused as whole blood because large-scale processing of these units could not be accomplished easily. Simple gravity separation of plasma could be performed but only by breaking the seal on the bottle. Elaborate efforts were required to carry out this separation aseptically, and although the plasma could be subsequently frozen, the residual red blood cells were often discarded or used for purposes other than infusion into patients.

The development of plastic closed-system multiple bags revolutionized blood banking and the practice of transfusion medicine. The plastic bags were malleable enough to allow centrifugal separation of plasma from red blood cells and subsequent diversion of the supernatant plasma into satellite bags while still maintaining the closed system by the connected plastic tubing. This simple technique, still widely used, permitted the easy and aseptic separation of red blood cells and plasma so that each could be safely stored and subsequently transfused. This simple change provided the ready availability of components that permitted aggressive surgical and medical therapeutic procedures.

The availability of a simple, centrifugation-based separation technique also led to experimentation with the duration and force that could be applied in either the initial centrifugation step or in a second centrifugation of the plasma. These manipulations eventually resulted in the production of platelet concentrates. For example, a "gentle" spin of a bag of freshly donated whole blood at about 2500 rpm for 3 minutes yields a supernatant platelet-rich plasma, which can be separated into a satellite bag. A second, "strong" spin of this latter bag, at about 4100 rpm for 5 minutes, packs down the platelets, allowing separation of the platelet-poor plasma into another satellite bag.

The centrifuges used for blood separation need to be maintained carefully and tested regularly so that they produce the requisite centrifugal forces in a consistent manner. Likewise, they have to be loaded carefully so that the cups are balanced. Otherwise, the rotor will shake and produce turbulence in the bags. The motors of these centrifuges are also susceptible to damage from imbalanced cup holders.

PLASMA SEPARATION

Plasma expressors are simple mechanical devices that consist of two flat, rectangular plates (metallic or hard plastic) hinged together at one end. A bag of previously centrifuged whole blood is carefully placed between the plates. A simple spring device pushes the hinged plates into apposition so that the supernatant plasma in the bag is extruded through one of the ports at the top of the bag. This port leads into one of a series of plastic satellite bags connected to one another by flexible plastic tubing. This latter tubing is an integral part of the closed, sterile, multiple-bag system. Once the requisite quantity of plasma has been expressed, the interconnecting tubing can be clamped with two small metal clips placed close together. The primary bag can then be separated by applying a scissors to the short segment of the tubing between the metal clips.

LEUKOCYTE-POOR RED BLOOD CELLS

Several techniques are available for the removal of the majority of the white blood cells from a bag of whole blood or red blood cells (3). These methods may involve simple centrifugation with subsequent separation of the buffy coat from the remaining cells or the use of various filters to accomplish the same goal. The use of machines to wash the red blood cells will also provide variable degrees of white blood cell removal. The indications and more detailed discussion of the effectiveness of these methods follow later in this chapter.

CRYOPRECIPITATION TECHNIQUES

When the plasma is separated from the red blood cells and then frozen at −18°C or lower, certain proteins precipitate. These proteins are rich in coagulation factors VIII and XIII and fibrinogen. If frozen plasma is thawed at 37°C, these precipitates go back into solution. However, Pool discovered that, if the thawing occurred between 1° and 6°C, these cold-precipitated proteins remained as a precipitate from which the rest of the plasma can be readily expressed after prompt centrifugation. This cryoprecipitated protein should be refrozen within 1 hour.

The variation of this technique used to enhance the concentration of fibrinogen in the product so that it can be used topically as a "fibrin glue" will be discussed below.

RED BLOOD CELL WASHING

Devices are available that use solutions compatible with red blood cells to suspend and centrifuge the mixture in repeated cycles to produce a suspension of red cells in the isotonic saline-based wash solution. Variable quantities of white blood cells, platelets, or plasma constituents may remain with the red blood cells, depending on the assiduousness of the procedure used, and the technique may be modified in order to decrease the level of these "contaminants." Because these washing techniques involve the rupture of the seals on the closed system, the shelf life of the washed red blood cell product is only 24 hours after washing.

FREEZING TECHNIQUES

To preserve its labile coagulation factors, plasma must be rapidly frozen within 6 hours after blood collection (4). This can be accomplished by the use of a dry ice-ethanol bath or by a mechanical freezer capable of maintaining a temperature of −30°C or lower. Once the plasma is frozen, it may be maintained at −18°C for up to 1 year. Similarly, the supernatant plasma from cryoprecipitation can be refrozen at −18°C or lower and maintained for 1 year. It is preferable to use temperatures of −30°C or lower for optimal factor activity in the product.

Freezing red blood cells is considerably more difficult because the structural integrity, viability, and function of the cells must be maintained. There are several methods described for this, including high glycerol, agglomeration, and low glycerol (4). All three methods utilize the ability of glycerol to preserve the integrity of the red blood cells during freeze/thaw processes. Glycerol, a clear, syrupy fluid, is a trihydric alcohol and is miscible with both water and alcohol. It is relatively inert pharmacologically and does not cause problems except that, if the red cells have been improperly deglycerolized prior to infusion, there may be shifts in intracellular fluids. Another cryoprotectant that is sometimes used is dimethyl sulfoxide (DMSO), a by-product of petroleum distillation. When given intravenously, it can cause nausea, vomiting, and a strong, pervasive, garlic-like taste and odor (5).

The cell injury caused by freeze/thaw seems to be a result of the formation of intracellular ice crystals. Intracellular water freezes more slowly than extracellular water if the rate of freezing is less than 10°C/min. This causes an osmotic gradient that results in the flow of water out of the cells, and damage may result from cellular dehydration (6). At much more rapid rates of freezing, there is little time for this gradient to form; therefore, very little dehydration occurs. However, because the cells do not lose their water, ice crystals tend to form and destroy intracellular organelles. Cryoprotective agents alter the tonicity of cells and thus slow the rate of freezing but not enough that severe dehydration occurs. The high-glycerol method is the one most widely used because (*a*) it does not require a controlled rate of freezing (the less expensive freezers perform satisfactorily); and (*b*) it requires only −80°C for its initial freezing as opposed to −196°C for the low-glycerol method, which also requires liquid nitrogen storage.

Multiple variations of the freezing methods have been published, but certain facts apply to all of them. Red blood cells should be frozen within 6 days after collection. Rejuvenation can be carried out several days later than this but prior to glycerolization. This rejuvenation process is designed to restore red cell ATP and 2,3-diphosphoglycerate (2,3-DPG) levels. Each method has certain limitations, but all of them yield a product of high red blood cell purity and function, minimal white blood cell and platelet contamination, and virtually no residual plasma proteins. This is important when the presence of such "contaminants" might cause adverse reactions. Frozen red cells are about twice as expensive as ordinary red cells because of the costs of freezing, storage, and thawing. In addition, the deglycerolization and washing, which are obligatory prior to transfusion, take about 45 minutes per unit. Therefore, the cells cannot be used for emergency resuscitation. The method is used to preserve rare or unusual units as well as for autologous blood stored prior to anticipated surgical use.

AVAILABLE BLOOD PRODUCTS AND INDICATIONS FOR USE

Whole Blood

A unit of whole blood has a volume of approximately 500 ml (440 ml of blood + 63 ml of anticoagulant/preservative). The hematocrit value is about 35% (12 g of hemoglobin per deciliter). Once the concept of dividing each donation of whole blood into its constituent components became widely accepted as a rational and efficient way of providing optimal transfusion care, the use of whole blood declined. In the hospital setting, the degree of sophistication of the overall medical and surgical practice was judged, at least partly, by the ratio of red blood cell use to whole blood use. Some surgeons continued to maintain that, because the patient bled whole blood, it was logical to reinfuse whole blood. Apart from the obvious need to fractionate blood so that components can be prepared, the most cogent argument to be made against the proponents of routine use of whole blood is that whole blood is not whole.

The deterioration of labile coagulation factor activity (largely factors V and VIII) and the virtual absence of platelet or granulocyte function negate claims that whole blood is "whole" in the functional sense. To make it "whole," one would have to collect it and transfuse it rapidly, i.e., within hours, which is a logistic impossibility. Cardiac surgeons sometimes have requested "fresh" whole blood for use during, and particularly after, cardiopulmonary bypass surgery. In a recent paper, Lavee et al. (7) reported that 1 unit of fresh whole blood (collected on the morning of operation) increased the platelet count to the same extent as 6 units of platelet concentrate did and restored platelet aggregation and volume comparably with 8 and 10 units of platelets, respectively. These data must be interpreted with caution because previous data (8) indicate that the use of fresh autologous blood did not decrease blood use after bypass.

Although the use of whole blood is often decried, its use does provide both oxygen delivery and volume in one product. That is precisely what is needed in the treatment of acute hemorrhagic, hypovolemic shock. However, oxygen delivery can be provided by red blood cells, and volume can be provided by giving crystalloid or colloid solution without increasing the number of donors to which a patient needs to be exposed. Blood flow rates are slower with the more viscous red blood cells than with whole blood, but this can be overcome by adding isotonic crystalloid or colloid solution directly to the bag of red blood cells prior to use. However, in acute or critical clinical situations, the latter manipulation is somewhat cumbersome and time-consuming; this has led to renewed requests for whole blood (9).

More recently, the use of storage additive solutions with anticoagulants such AS-1 or AS-3 has restored the whole blood flow characteristics to red blood cells (10), thereby facilitating their use in the operating room or the emergency room. In the absence of availability of these types of anticoagulant-preserved blood, with additives, it is reasonable and probably wise to maintain a small stock of whole blood in the blood bank or in the emergency room in an appropriate, blood bank–controlled refrigerator. Parenthetically, if blood for transfusion is stored anywhere in the medical complex outside of the blood bank, it is very important that it should be under the direct control and supervision of the blood bank personnel in order to ensure adequate quality control. It has been widely recognized that, if the blood bank abdicates this responsibility, storage probably will not be carried out properly.

If whole blood is used for emergency resuscitation, it should be used volume for volume relative to blood loss. Because it is nearly impossible to estimate acute blood loss volume in real time, the size of the loss is merely a guess and depends to some extent on the experience of those trying to make that guess. Because of this, as well as other factors, the use of whole blood in such clinical settings is not infrequently associated with volume overload. It is very difficult to judge fluid volume status in a rapidly fluctuating clinical situation unless one has the luxury of having continuous central intravascular pressure measurements. Even this approach is not necessarily foolproof.

Red Blood Cells

This component is essentially the red blood cells that remain after plasma and platelets have been separated from whole blood. The number of red blood cells in this component is the same as the number in the bag of whole blood from which it was derived. The concentration of red blood cells will vary according to the amount of residual plasma in which they are suspended or the volume of additive solution (e.g., AS-1, AS-3) added to the red blood cell bag. The volume of a bag of red blood cells is about 250 ml; that of a bag of red blood cells preserved with AS-1 is 330 ml. Other modifications, such as the removal of white blood cells or freeze/thaw/washing, may decrease the volume to as low as approximately 180 ml.

Unless platelets or white blood cells have been selectively removed from the donated whole blood, they will be contained in the final product. After 2 to 3 days of storage at 4°C, there is little, if any, remaining function in the platelets or granulocytes, and they progressively disintegrate with further storage. The degenerating granulocytes in particular contribute to the development of microaggregates in the bag.

The single indication for transfusion of red blood cells is the need for increased oxygen delivery to the tissues. In situations of acute blood loss with intravascular volume deficit, red blood cells provide the means of oxygen delivery, and crystalloid or colloid solution supplements provide the volume. When there is symptomatic chronic anemia unresponsive to various hematinics, the use of red blood cells may be reasonable and appropriate if the risks of withholding transfusion outweigh those of giving it. In other words, the mere existence of anemia or even of the symptoms attributable to it is not sufficient grounds for the transfusion of red blood cells.

The transfusion "trigger" has long been the subject of considerable controversy. For many years, perioperative transfusion practice was guided by the principle that a hemoglobin value of less than 10 g/dl was an indication for transfusion. Although this simple rule was almost universally accepted and applied, little hard evidence existed to support it other than calculations that indicated a potential for impaired oxygenation of tissues. These data usually did not take into account the appropriate calculation for cardiac output changes, oxygen extraction, or changes in the hemoglobin/oxygen affinity curve (11).

It now is generally accepted that most healthy humans do not experience a compensatory significant increase in cardiac output until the hemoglobin value is below 7 g/dl. Clearly, patients with conditions that compromise their cardiovascular or cerebral blood supply may require therapy before their hemoglobin value reaches this level. Therefore, each patient must be evaluated individually with regard to the effects of anemia before the decision to transfuse is made.

It is also important to note that there is no evidence that wound healing is impaired until a hematocrit value of 15 to 17% is reached (11, 12). Minor postoperative anemia clearly is not an indication for transfusion on the basis of wound healing or, indeed, of infection (12). On the contrary, there is some evidence that perioperative transfusions may be associated with an increased incidence of infection (13).

Patients with nonsurgical chronic anemia, such as the anemia associated with chronic renal failure, adapt remarkably well to levels of hemoglobin in the range of 5 to 7 g/dl and can perform everyday duties reasonably well at those levels. It is standard practice to transfuse these patients when the symptoms of the anemia are beginning to incapacitate them or when new or more ominous symptoms appear, such as angina pectoris or central manifestations of anoxia. It is clear that a gradual decline or long-term decrease in hemoglobin level is tolerated by patients much better than a more acute onset.

When the cause of anemia is being investigated, the blood samples for the laboratory studies should be obtained prior to transfusing the patient. The increase one expects in the hemoglobin value after the transfusion of red blood cells depends on many factors, including the patient's weight and hemodynamic stability and the presence or absence of active bleeding. In a stable, nonbleeding, 70-kg patient, one would expect to see an increase of approximately 1.5 g/dl or about 3 to 4% in hematocrit value per unit transfused. It is necessary to allow an hour or so for intravascular equilibration before the posttransfusion hemoglobin level is determined. Patients with chronic anemia often have an expanded plasma volume, which puts them at particular risk of volume overload, especially if whole blood is transfused rather than red blood cells.

Modified Red Blood Cells: Leukocyte-Poor Red Blood Cells

Red blood cells can be rendered leukocyte-poor by various techniques, including centrifugation to separate the buffy coat or filtration to remove leukocytes. Each method has its intrinsic advantages and disadvantages, and the method chosen may depend on the indication in a given patient. Meryman et al. (14) compared 13 methods of preparing this product, all based on centrifugation, automated red blood cell washing, or freeze/thaw techniques. These authors concluded that centrifugation methods removed 65 to 87% of the leukocytes, but to achieve the higher percentage, one had to use 6- to 10-day-old blood and remove 90 ml of cells, which decreased the hemoglobin content by about 30%. Automated washing or freeze/thaw techniques removed up to 96% of leukocytes and between 5 and 10% of the hemoglobin.

The two main indications for the use of leukocyte-poor red blood cells are (*a*) transfusion of patients with a history of previous febrile nonhemolytic transfusion reactions; and (*b*) prevention of the development of antileukocyte antibodies and platelet refractoriness. Over 25 years ago, Perkins and colleagues (15) first clearly demonstrated that the granulocytes were primarily responsible for febrile nonhemolytic reactions and that this reaction was dependent on both the dose and the rate of administration of the granulocytes. In that classic study, the patients responded, with a minimal degree of temperature elevation, to as few as 0.25×10^9 leukocytes. It is generally believed (16) that the majority of patients with a history of febrile nonhemolytic reactions and antileukocyte antibodies can be transfused satisfactorily with red blood cell preparations containing 0.3×10^9 leukocytes. A much greater degree of removal of contaminating granulocytes can be achieved by various filtration techniques, which also have the advantage of removing fewer red blood cells from the unit.

For a red blood cell product to be designated "leukocyte-poor," 70% of the white blood cells must be removed, and only 70% of the original red blood cells need to remain (up to 30% loss of red blood cells).

In our hands, the upright spin method yields approximately 80% red blood cell recovery and 80% removal of white blood cells; with nylon-wool filtration, the values are 90% and 95%, respectively. Looked at in another fashion, 1 unit of upright-spin, leukocyte-poor red blood cells exposes the patient to as few as 0.6 to 0.8×10^9 white blood cells, and the filtered product exposes the patient to as few as 0.06 to 0.08×10^9 such cells.

Most patients can receive upright-spin, leukocyte-poor red blood cells without subsequent reactions, but some "break through" at this dose and then require filtered red blood cells. After several years' experience with the transfusion of many hundreds of such patients, our institution has yet to see a highly sensitized patient have a febrile nonhemolytic reaction to filtered red blood cells. The patients who are most likely to have febrile nonhemolytic reactions are multiparous women or previously transfused patients (16).

Numerous studies have examined the role of antigranulocyte antibodies in these reactions; although there is a correlation, the data are not clear-cut. This probably reflects the difficulty in making the clinical diagnosis with any degree of consistency and confidence because of the confounding factors in many patients. Underlying clinical conditions such as sepsis, autoimmune disease, and medications make this a diagnosis by exclusion. A second reason for lack of clear-cut correlation is the fact that many different tests have been devised for the detection of antibodies to leukocytes, and they probably do not measure antibodies to the same antigenic targets. For instance, the following are a few of the tests that have been used: leukoagglutination (slide), leukoagglutination (microcapillary tube), lymphocytotoxin (complement-dependent dye exclusion), granulocyte membrane (fluorescence), and granulocyte membrane (radioimmunometric).

Another factor that plays a role in deciding what is the most reasonable approach is the shelf life of the product. If one uses either centrifugation or a spin/filter, closed-system method, the normal shelf life of the red blood cells is retained. On the other hand, if one uses a system that requires breaching the integrity of the system (such as washing or non-in-line filters), the subsequent shelf life becomes 24 hours. Clearly, the latter component is useful only if transfused immediately after preparation. The need to maintain an inventory of leukocyte-poor products in the blood bank with a reasonable shelf life is obvious (17).

Filtration through a white blood cell filter that can be used at the bedside (or in the blood bank immediately prior to transfusion) has been advocated. The use of such a filter resulted in 87% red blood cell recovery and 6.1×10^6 residual white blood cells (18). Problems noted by those authors were prolonged transfusion time and poor red blood cell recovery if only 1 unit was infused through the filter. Another type of filter that can be used in this setting is the microaggregate filter, originally designed for the removal of microaggregates from blood prior to massive transfusion (an indication that is highly controversial). These filters have been used successfully in the blood bank to prepare leukocyte-poor red blood cells just prior to their infusion (19).

Another recent advance in the preparation of leukocyte-poor red blood cells is the development of a closed-system method that combines centrifugation and filtration steps and the removal of microaggregates (which enhances red blood cell storage) (20). This method (Leukotrap red blood cell storage system) preserves the shelf life of 42 days for the product and apparently yields 98% white blood cell removal, i.e., 10^8 cells remaining. This approach is significant because it seems to combine efficiency of white blood cell removal with ease of operation and logistic convenience.

The second indication for the use of leukocyte-poor red blood cells is the prevention of the platelet refractory state. In their landmark paper in 1957, Brittingham and Chaplin (21) recognized the role of leukocytes in febrile nonhemolytic transfusion reactions, and subsequent studies indicated that patients with preexisting alloimmunization against HLA antigens had decreased graft survival (22). This led to a significant increase in the use of frozen/thawed red blood cells for transfusion in dialysis patients. In 1973, Opelz et al. (23) presented the apparently paradoxical data that transfused patients had better renal graft survival than untransfused patients. Opelz and Terasaki published (24) the definitive data in 1976 that indicated a previously unsuspected effect of transfusions, i.e., immunosuppression.

The fact that transfusions generally led to alloimmunization was not in dispute. Platelet refractoriness was assumed to be due to exposure of the patients to repeated doses of platelets with their abundant endowment of HLA class I antigens (HLA A, B, and C antigens). However, data began to accumulate suggesting that the platelets themselves did not evoke the immune response, but rather the "contaminating" white blood cells in the platelet infusions did. Interestingly, these data were analogous to data implicating "passenger" donor white blood cells in solid organ grafts as the culprits in evoking transplant rejection phenomena (25).

Because of the enormous strides in the past decade in the therapy of patients with hematologic malignancies, these patients achieve more remissions and survive longer. Each attempt at inducing remission usually includes transfusion support with platelets and, sometimes, red blood cells. Clinicians are increasingly faced with the specter of platelet refractoriness. It is logical to try to prevent this rather than to merely respond to its presence by using expensive, HLA-matched apheresis platelets or, occasionally, cumbersome platelet cross-matching systems.

Prevention has been achieved by the drastic reduction of the white blood cell content of red blood cell and platelet preparations used for transfusions. Again, simple centrifugal removal of the buffy coat often suffices to prevent the occurrence of febrile reactions in previously sensitized patients. Prevention of sensitization seems to require that each transfusion deliver less than 5×10^6 leukocytes. Meryman (26) has summarized the supportive data for this statement most impressively. In practical terms, to prevent alloimmunization, one must be prepared to process red blood cells (and also platelets) to remove 95 to 98% of the leukocytes to achieve the level of 5×10^6 residual cells. This requires either frozen/thawed red blood cells or the newer filtration methods, which can achieve this level of white blood cell removal with minimal red blood cell loss. Sniecinski et al. (27) showed the value of this approach in a thorough prospective study. In particular, the use of these filters permits patients to have more transfusions over a longer period before they become sensitized.

It is difficult to find hard data on the financial impact of this approach, but keep in mind that perhaps 50% of patients are destined to become refractory if one makes no special effort to prevent it. A policy of deliberately using only leukocyte-poor products for all patients with hematologic malignancies would be expensive (because of the cost of filters and labor). On the other hand, however, the cost of providing platelet support to a highly refractory patient who is consuming vast quantities of platelets (even the expensive HLA-matched variety) is enormous.

Indirectly, the transfusion of large numbers of units of blood and components exposes patients to various other complications, such as hepatitis and lem. Efforts to cross-match platelets in this situation generally are futile and may distract one from the chief problem—the underlying sepsis.

UREMIA

Patients with uremia have varying degrees of platelet dysfunction, which prolongs bleeding time. Since the 1950s, the defect in the availability of platelet factor 3 in uremia has been known, and subsequently, a defect in platelet aggregation was noted. These measurable defects were often noted to be mild and out of proportion to the prolongation of bleeding time and the degree of clinical bleeding. When dialysis was found to reverse the functional abnormalities of the platelets, various substances, including urea, phenols, and guanidinosuccinic acid, were blamed for the platelet abnormalities, but each claim was somewhat controversial (39).

More recent studies have concentrated on the role of coagulation factor VIII and, more particularly, its factor VIII:von Willebrand factor (VIII:VWF) moiety. Alteration of the platelet-membrane receptor for VIII:VWF seems to be a reasonable explanation for the prolongation in bleeding time and the platelet adhesiveness defects seen in uremia (40).

A number of clinical studies have demonstrated that the use of diamino-8-D-arginine vasopressin (DDAVP) can shorten the bleeding time in uremia (41). This seems to act by causing the secretion into the plasma of increased numbers of the large multimers of VIII:VWF, which may overcome the binding defect in uremic platelets. This property of DDAVP has led to its popularity in treating uremic patients prior to urgent surgical procedures when there may not be time for dialysis. The lack of serious side effects and the freedom from disease transmission problems have contributed to the popularity of DDAVP rather than the use of platelet transfusions for this purpose (41). The effects of DDAVP are relatively short-lived (hours), and repeated treatments can lead to tachyphylaxis.

Leukocyte-Poor Platelets

The indications for this product are essentially the same as those for leukocyte-depleted red blood cells, i.e., (*a*) to ameliorate the symptoms of febrile nonhemolytic reactions in sensitized patients; (*b*) to prevent development of the refractory state; and (*c*) to decrease exposure to certain viruses known to reside in white blood cells (e.g., CMV).

Various filtration methods have been described recently, and these have achieved a remarkable level of leukocyte removal (up to 99%). This level of removal gives a final product of pooled platelet concentrates with approximately 5×10^6 residual white blood cells per pooling bag. This degree of filtration is sufficient to prevent febrile responses in most sensitized patients. The platelet loss with these filters has been about 10% in recent years. Platelet loss greater than this leads to the need for transfusion of additional units of platelets to compensate. Cotton-wool filters remove 100% of granulocytes, 95% of monocytes, 90% of B lymphocytes, and 85% of T lymphocytes (42). Cotton-wool filtration causes almost no activation of platelets and only minimal decreases in postinfusion survival that would be of little or no consequence in a clinical setting (43).

Our own experience over several years is that cotton-wool filtration is very effective at preventing febrile reactions in patients with a history of repeated, debilitating reactions to unmodified red blood cell or platelet transfusions. This experience has been corroborated by others (44) who found such an effect when the white blood cell content was decreased to less than 10^8.

Polyester fiber filters remove almost as many white blood cells but are more expensive (45). The use of a special pooling bag for centrifugal removal of the buffy coat eliminates 93% of the white blood cells, so that febrile reactions are prevented (46). The value of this system is its ability to accomplish the white blood cell removal in a closed system shortly after the blood is obtained from the donor. This early removal should improve red blood cell and platelet storage pH while maintaining the original shelf life of all components. Whether this simple and attractive system removes enough white blood cells to prevent alloimmunization is still open to question. The immunizing dose of leukocytes is unknown, but some data suggest that 1×10^8 allogeneic leukocytes may be needed (47).

As yet, the data are insufficient to ascertain whether the use of filtered leukocyte-poor platelets will significantly diminish the occurrence of CMV or other leukocyte-borne viral infections in susceptible hosts. However, preliminary data strongly suggest that this is the case with filters capable of 3 to 4 log white cell reduction.

Other Platelet Preparations

Platelets can be washed to remove plasma proteins for patients with severe allergic reactions. A semiautomated method has been described that removes 96% of the plasma protein and yields 90% platelet recovery (48).

Platelets can be successfully frozen and then thawed for transfusion up to 3 years later with about 25% loss of platelets in the process. This is usually accomplished by using 5 to 10% dimethyl sulfoxide (DMSO) and an ultralow mechanical freezer capable of maintaining temperatures of −80° to −90°C. If storage is at −120°C, platelets can be maintained for up to 4 years. This is particularly useful for the storage of autologous platelets from alloimmunized patients who achieve leukemic remission with its attendant rebound thrombocytosis (49). It also has been used successfully to treat an infant with neonatal isoimmune thrombocytopenia with its mother's frozen platelets, which had been collected early in pregnancy (50).

Platelets in Massive Transfusion

Patients who undergo massive transfusions within a short period (e.g., 1 or more blood volumes in 12 to 24 hours) have well-documented coagulation defects resulting from the loss of blood, the inadequacy of the physiological response to the rapid replacement of the lost platelets and labile coagulation factors, and the transfusion of blood deficient in these same moieties by virtue of storage losses (51). Because the degree of deficiency is directly related to the duration of storage of the blood, such deficiencies vary among units of blood chosen randomly for transfusion. Although most blood banks generally try to transfuse their oldest units first, during massive transfusion situations, such an elective transfusion practice may be inappropriate.

There is also considerable variation in the degree of clinically significant coagulopathy seen in patients who receive massive transfusions. These factors make it difficult to establish firm correlations between the degree of coagulopathy and the quantities of blood infused. It should be recalled that the platelets may have been removed from the donated blood for processing into platelet concentrates, although this is not a realistic concern because platelets no longer function after 48 hours in stored whole blood at 4°C. Coagulation factors V and VIII are at about a 50% level after 1 week of storage. Therefore, massive infusion of stored blood is going to do little for the resultant dilutional thrombocytopenia or for depletion of labile plasma clotting factors.

Logically, one might expect that the amount of blood lost, the degree of thrombocytopenia observed, and the resultant microvascular clinical bleeding would be closely correlated. In several well-conducted studies this was not the case. Also, prophylactic platelet infusions based on a predetermined replacement formula have not proved to be effective in altering clinical bleeding patterns or in reversing prolongation of bleeding time (52, 53). The authors of these studies concluded that such indiscriminate platelet transfusion therapy is unjustified.

Table 68.1. Factors Contributing to Platelet Increment or Function after Transfusion

Platelet Factors	Patient Factors
Method of collection	Size of patient
Method and duration of storage	Medications being taken
Presence of appropriate agitation	Sepsis
pH	Splenomegaly
Number of platelets infused	Disseminated intravascular coagulopathy
Type of anticoagulent	Bleeding
Donor taking antiplatelet medication	Circulating immune complexes
	Alloimmunization

Single-Donor Platelets (Apheresis Platelets)

The American Association of Blood Banks Standards stipulate that a bag of platelets acquired by apheresis should contain a minimum of 3×10^{11} platelets in at least 75% of units tested. These platelets must be stored suspended in sufficient plasma so that the pH at the temperature of storage is 6.0 or greater at the end of the allowed storage time. In the newer plastic bags, this storage time is now up to 5 days. The collection of platelets by apheresis achieved popularity because of the recognition that platelet refractoriness was a complication of repeated exposures to random-donor platelet concentrates. This lack of responsiveness occurs in some recipients after only a few exposures; in others it is delayed or does not appear at all.

In their classic study, Howard and Perkins (54) demonstrated that about 30% of patients never became refractory despite repetitive exposures. These so-called nonresponders often have malignancies, including those of the hematopoietic or lymphoid system, and their failure to become refractory raises intriguing questions about their underlying disease, their treatment regimens, or their immunogenetics (55).

Those who do become refractory display great individual variability in both the number of platelet exposures and the time taken to become refractory. The state of platelet refractoriness is said to exist when a patient has progressively smaller increases in platelet counts following platelet transfusions. Many factors may contribute to this state, and each must be considered in the approach to a clinical problem. The most common factors are listed in Table 68.1.

A strong association has been found between the presence, in the recipient, of alloimmune lymphocytotoxic antibodies (often with HLA class I specificity) and failure to achieve the expected posttransfusion increment when other factors (such as those in Table 68.1) could be ruled out (54). There is abundant evidence that HLA class I antibodies are responsible median granulocyte count 20 hours after transfusion was decreased 30% and remained decreased for up to 4 days. These reported cases involved patients with aplastic anemia in whom the normally expected rebound granulocytosis did not occur.

Because of the prevalence of significant platelet refractoriness due to alloimmunization, various strategies have been devised to maximize the likelihood of obtaining satisfactory incremental responses to platelet transfusion. The most effective strategy is HLA matching, but a considerable body of data supports the concept of platelet cross-matching either alone or in concert with HLA matching. Virtually every type of antiplatelet antibody test has been evaluated: indirect tests such as lymphocytotoxicity tests and direct tests such as immunofluorescence, enzyme-labeled immunosorbent assays (ELISA), solid-phase red blood cell adherence, radiolabeled antiglobulin, platelet aggregometry, and others (72–76). Nearly all studies have demonstrated correlations between HLA matching and increments, between negative tests and increments, and between the degree of matching and negative tests. The data have to be viewed with some circumspection because of the obvious difficulty in finding patients who lack any of the "confounding" factors such as sepsis.

The concept of an inexpensive, predictive cross-match is appealing because it can be used instead of the expensive pool of HLA-matched donors. This is feasible only if the test can be performed on platelet aliquots stored for long periods of time (75). It could even be used to select groups of random-donor platelet concentrates on an ad hoc basis, making use of each day's supply of regular homologous donors. The solid-phase red blood cell adherence method seems to lend itself to this approach, according to early results (77).

Although ABH antigens are present in small amounts on platelet surfaces, in general they do not significantly influence the posttransfusion increments. Therefore, it is not necessary that platelets always be ABO compatible. However, ABO antigens can interfere with sensitive cross-match testing and, in alloimmunized patients, mismatching for ABO may influence increments (78). Lee and Schiffer (78) suggested that one should routinely try ABO-compatible, random-donor platelets before assuming that a patient needs HLA-matched platelets.

It has been suggested that, even though only about 50% of leukemic patients become truly alloimmunized, one should begin therapy with HLA-matched apheresis platelets in order to prevent the development of the alloimmunized state. This question was discussed lucidly by Schiffer and Slichter (79), who concluded that this approach was not cost-effective.

A different approach to the prevention of alloimmunization is the exclusive use of leukocyte-depleted blood components, including platelets. These could be filtered, random-donor platelet concentrates or apheresis products. In one study, the use of leukocyte-poor platelets was associated with platelet refractoriness in only 9% of recipients (80). In another study, 15% of recipients of filtered, leukocyte-poor platelets were alloimmunized (27). The use of UV irradiation to pretreat platelets and other blood components in an effort to render them nonimmunogenic shows some early promise (81), and the development of practical and effective radiation delivery systems probably will revolutionize the transfusion of all patients in the future.

Granulocyte Transfusions

Patients who are neutropenic are susceptible to bacterial and fungal infections, and the degree of neutropenia correlates directly with the frequency and severity of such infections (82). Combating infection with granulocytes was first reported in 1934 by Strumia, who utilized a patient with chronic myelogenous leukemia as the donor (83). It was reasoned that such patients had a greatly expanded pool of functioning, albeit abnormal, granulocytes. However, it was not until modern cell separators were developed in the 1960s that granulocyte transfusions became part of the routine armamentarium of the hematologist. At that time, it became routine to utilize healthy normal blood donors as a source of the cells, and several techniques were used to boost the yield of granulocytes from them.

Intravenous or intramuscular steroid injections increased apheresis yields by altering the extent of margination of white blood cells, thereby increasing the pool of harvestable cells. With this technique, granulocyte units from normal donors contain an average of 1×10^{10} granulocytes. Because granulocytes are essentially tissue cells and spend only a small fraction of their life span in the circulation, it is impossible to assess their effectiveness after transfusion by evaluating posttransfusion increments. The average adult produces about 1×10^{11} granulocytes per day, but only about 2×10^{10}, or 20%, circulate. During severe infections, particularly bacterial, the marrow can respond by increasing the production rate perhaps as much as 10-fold. This increased rate can be maintained for many days or even weeks. If one assumes that such numbers of granulocytes are produced because they are needed to combat microbes, the folly of trying to acquire, for transfusion, similar numbers from donors and to maintain tissue levels is evident.

This central dilemma, perhaps more than any other, has been a stumbling block to the widespread, effective use of granulocyte transfusions in infected adults. Similarly, the use of other endpoints for evaluation is plagued by problems. For instance, virtually all treated patients receive large doses of antimicrobial agents and may undergo surgical management of localized septic foci. If defervescence occurs or if local or systemic signs of infection or inflammation decrease, it is often difficult to attribute this to the granulocyte transfusions. Granulocyte transfusions have lost favor in recent years largely because of the availability of new families of effective antimicrobial agents and, perhaps, also because of improvements in the speed and accuracy of bacterial identification and antimicrobial sensitivity testing.

Because of these difficulties in evaluating efficacy, it seems reasonable to pose several practical questions and to try to provide answers. What is the ability of transfused granulocytes to migrate to sites of tissue infection? How adequate is their function? What are the indications for their use (type and duration of infection, organisms most responsive, most effective treatment regimens, matching requirements, and prophylactic use)? What collection and storage systems are best?

In nonalloimmunized patients, transfused granulocytes have normal circulation characteristics, phagocytose bacteria in vivo, and migrate to sites of infection. There seems to be a general consensus that these transfusions are indicated for severely and persistently neutropenic patients (fewer than 250 granulocytes/μl) with infection caused by Gram-negative bacteria unresponsive to adequate appropriate antimicrobial therapy for at least 48 hours (69). The data supporting these indications were presented convincingly by McCullough (84). There are no good data to support the use of granulocytes in viral or fungal infections or in patients who do not have documented Gram-negative sepsis.

Earlier studies indicated that filtration techniques gave a higher yield of granulocytes but that the granulocytes had measurable defects in function. Transfusion of filtration granulocytes ceased when, in addition to widespread severe, recurrent febrile reactions, cases of priapism were reported. The following comments deal only with granulocytes acquired by apheresis and centrifugation. The use of granulocytes tagged with indium-111 permitted elegant studies of the migration and localization of transfused cells (85) and the impact of recipients' antibodies (86) (including ABO) on these phenomena (87). The transfusion of small amounts of indium-labeled autologous granulocytes also became a useful tool in localizing sites of inflammation (85).

Granulocyte transfusions should be ABO-compatible because of the large number of contaminating red blood cells in the granulocyte bag. McCullough et al. (87) found that, although it was assumed that ABH antigens were found on the granulocyte membrane by some techniques, the intravascular recovery, survival, and tissue localization of ABO-compatible and ABO-incompatible granulocytes were the same. There is no good evidence that HLA matching is advantageous.

The presence of preformed leukocyte antibodies in the recipient of granulocyte transfusions influences the fate of these cells. The type of antibody test used may have some bearing on the correlation. Granulocyte agglutinating, but not granulocytotoxic or lymphocytotoxic, antibodies decrease granulocyte recovery and half-life of cells, increase their hepatic sequestration, and inhibit migration and localization of cells to sites of infection (86, 88). Other studies compared the clinical outcomes of alloimmunized and nonsensitized patients who received granulocytes. The data from at least one such study (89) indicated that patients with antigranulocyte antibodies, as measured by indirect immunofluorescence, had a significantly worse final outcome when treated with granulocytes. The antibodies presumably played a role in inhibiting the desired effect of the granulocytes.

Whether or not granulocytes should be used prophylactically has not been satisfactorily determined, despite several studies. Some studies were terminated because of unacceptable numbers of patients with severe reactions. From one multicenter, controlled trial of prophylactic granulocyte transfusions in patients with acute myelogenous leukemia, it was concluded that the incidence of reactions (including pulmonary infiltrates in 57%) was too great to warrant the therapy, which had not reduced the incidence of infections or improved bone marrow recovery, remission rate and duration, or survival (90). One particularly lethal pulmonary complication occurs occasionally when granulocytes are transfused to patients receiving amphotericin B, although this is controversial (91, 92).

Clift et al. (93) found substantial benefits in bone marrow transplant recipients. Others have found no obvious benefit and significant hazards; therefore, routine use cannot be recommended. If granulocyte transfusions are to be used, it seems prudent to give at least 1×10^{10} cells at least once daily for at least 5 days to ensure even minimal success.

In septic neonates, the use of even one transfusion of granulocytes has been associated with dramatic responses in those with depleted marrow neutrophil reserve (94). This topic is discussed in more detail elsewhere in this text.

Adoptive Immunotherapy

Adoptive immunotherapy can be viewed as the attempt to reconstitute immune competence (usually antitumor) by supplying surrogate lymphoid or other immune system cells.

The role of the immune system in cancer surveillance has been speculative for many years as indirect or circumstantial evidence accumulated. Such data consisted of the increased incidence of various malignancies in patients with disorders that included clinically significant depression of the immune system and similar increases in malignant disease in patients with long-term iatrogenic immunosuppression such as with organ transplants. In addition, the complexity of the various normal cell types and subtypes began to unravel with the discovery of methods to produce monoclonal antibodies to various marker epitopes on lymphoid cell subpopulations. Finally, the identification, categorization, and eventual production (by recombinant DNA methods) of various cytokines permitted further elucidation of the intricate interplay of cells and cytokines in various aspects of the immune response.

As basic knowledge of immune function grew, the prospects of replacing or augmenting specific steps in the response became more realistic. The development of automated blood cell separators gave clinicians and researchers a tool for collecting large numbers of lymphoid or other immune cells so that they could be manipulated in vitro. The transfusion of such cells with or without cytokines is adoptive immunotherapy.

LYMPHOKINE-ACTIVATED KILLER CELLS

In addition to the natural killer (NK) cells that play some role in normal antitumor activity, incubation of mouse or human lymphoid cells with interleukin 2 (IL-2) generates a population of cells capable of lysing fresh tumor cells in vitro (95). These lymphokine-activated killer cells (LAK) cells seem to differ from both NK cells and cytotoxic T cells. Subsequent studies indicated that LAK cells had a broad range of malignant cell targets, but they spared normal cells and did not seem to be MHC-restricted in their targets. LAK cells are generated after short-term (24 hours) incubation with IL-2. Prior γ-ray irradiation of the lymphoid cells inhibits LAK cell development after IL-2 incubation. This suggests that IL-2-induced proliferation is a prerequisite of LAK cell activity (96).

The origin of LAK cells is still debated, but they seem to be derived from NK cells or from NK-like cells, which are large, granular lymphocytes morphologically and produce NK cell-associated surface markers NKH1 and CD16. However, it should not be assumed that LAK activity is confined to one subtype of lymphocytes. Perhaps it should be thought of as a functional activity rather than a specific cell type.

In animal studies, LAK cells cause regression of established cancers and inhibit growth of pulmonary and hepatic metastatic lesions. These experimental studies yielded a wealth of information on the LAK phenomenon, as summarized succinctly by Klein and Leitman (97): (*a*) LAK cells alone produce little obvious benefit; (*b*) IL-2 injected alone has only a modest effect at high doses; (*c*) a mixture of LAK cells and IL-2 gives striking benefit; (*d*) for maximal effect, the cells must be cultured with IL-2 for 3 to 4 days; and (*e*) in humans, a dose of at least 10^{11} LAK cells probably would be needed. It is hypothesized that these cells migrate to sites of malignancy and, once there, expand in situ in response to endogenous IL-2. Presumably, they then destroy the adjacent malignant cells by some mechanism.

Early phase I/II studies involved patients with advanced malignancy unresponsive to conventional therapy (97). The regimen was an initial 5-day infusion of IL-2 (100,000 U/kg per 8 hours), followed by five daily leukapheresis procedures. The collected cells were incubated in IL-2 for 3 to 4 days and transfused back to the patient along with another bolus of IL-2. The results in the first group of patients gave grounds for cautious optimism; about 10% had a sustained, complete regression of tumor, and perhaps another 10% had a partial response. Renal cell carcinoma, melanoma, and non-Hodgkin lymphoma responded best (97).

A limiting factor in these early studies was the terminal status of many of the patients. Another practical limiting factor is the enormous cost because of the high doses of recombinant IL-2 needed. Finally, the severe toxicity associated with the therapy is bound to limit its usefulness. At least two treatment-associated deaths have been reported, and virtually all patients have had chills and fever. Other side effects were related to massive fluid shifts resulting in severe hypotension, interstitial pulmonary edema, and massive fluid retention (97).

Another experimental study has demonstrated that LAK cells can be used to purge bone marrow of malignant cells without decreasing or harming its normal hematopoietic cell lines (98). The processing of LAK cells has been automated in a sterilized, closed system. This shows promise because the yield of cells is excellent, and processing time and personnel requirements are decreased (99).

TUMOR-INFILTRATING LYMPHOCYTES

It is generally true that tumors showing infiltration by lymphocytes have a more favorable prognosis than those without such infiltration. It is reasonable to assume that the lymphocytes seen infiltrating the tumor are in some way responsible for the improved prognosis, and these lymphocytes may well be enriched by cells that have antitumor activity. Recently, lymphocytes that were isolated from murine tumors, expanded under the influence of IL-2, and transfused into mice showed activity against hepatic and pulmonary metastatic lesions that were unresponsive to LAK/IL-2 therapy (100). In the murine model, tumor-infiltrating lymphocytes (TIL) seem to be 50 to 100 times more potent than LAK cells (97). TIL cells from the tumor are prepared as a single-cell suspension and then incubated for up to 6 weeks with IL-2. TIL cells can be seen aggregating at tumor sites for up to 9 days after transfusion (unlike LAK cells). The long-term effects of the use of TIL are still to be determined in human subjects.

PHOTOPHERESIS

This is a technique by which a patient's lymphoid cells are removed by apheresis and photoactivated extracorporeally with UVA light. The combination of methoxsalen and UVA light causes loss of viability of nearly 90% of the lymphoid cells. These cells are reinfused. Orally administered methoxsalen transiently intercalates DNA, but when photoactivated by UVA light, it is converted to a form that reacts with the DNA to create permanent covalent cross-links. The photodestruction of these lymphoid cells over the ensuing few days and their recognition by the immune system is thought to lead to a specific immunologic reaction with the malignant clones.

This experimental therapy has been evaluated in patients with cutaneous T-cell lymphoma. In the initial study, 27 of 37 patients showed a mean decrease in cutaneous involvement of 64% after 22 weeks of therapy (101). The mechanism of the beneficial result is unknown, but it is thought to be related to the fact that the therapy is directed extracorporeally to a clone or clones of malignantly transformed cells. The prolonged response in some patients previously shown to have relentlessly progressive disease suggests that this type of T-cell cutaneous lymphoma is at least partly under the control of a specific immunologic response (101).

Early experience with this technique at the Mayo Clinic revealed a 3% patient reaction rate, consisting largely of nausea or vomiting, slight and transient hypotension, or paresthesia. The procedure was generally well tolerated and consistently produced more than 10^9 white blood cells, with a minimum of red blood cell or platelet contamination, for reinfusion (102).

Noncellular Components

FRESH FROZEN PLASMA

When plasma is separated from the red blood cells of a donor within 6 hours after donation and is then held at −18°C or lower, it is fresh frozen plasma (FFP). If these requirements are not met, it is called "liquid plasma." FFP can be stored at −18°C for up to 1 year. If possible, it is preferable to store FFP at −30°C or lower temperatures in order to maintain optimal coagulation factor VIII level. Plasma stored at −30° to −40°C retains about 90% of such activity, whereas only about 60% is retained at about −20°C (103). FFP is largely used for its content of the labile coagulation factors V and VIII, but it also contains the so-called stable factors. If properly prepared and stored, each unit contains about 200 to 250 ml of plasma and, because of some processing loss, about 180 to 200 U of the various coagulation factors.

FFP can be thawed routinely in a water bath at 30° to 37°C with slight agitation of the bag. Rapid microwave warming can be equally effective (104). Once FFP is thawed, its labile coagulation factors (V and VIII) begin to destabilize, although FFP is not usually transfused as a source of factor VIII. The unit should be transfused within 6 hours (FDA regulation) or 24 hours (AABB regulation). Some studies have detected significant alterations in plasma factors associated with microwave thawing. Luff and coworkers (105) reported decreases in factors IX, X, and XI and fibrinogen and similar changes in albumin and total protein. They noted that microwave technology does not provide uniform heating, and they were not able to distinguish between simple denaturation of protein or the presence of a "nonspecific coagulative property" of the microwave. There can be local superheating of thawed plasma immediately adjacent to still-frozen plasma, giving an unpredictable and uneven thawing cycle.

FFP corrects bleeding abnormalities in some patients with congenital (storage pool disease) or acquired (uremia) platelet abnormalities. The reasons for these responses are probably complex, but one factor may be the platelet microparticles found to "contaminate" most FFP and especially cryoprecipitate (106).

After the introduction and widespread acceptance of the principle of blood component separation and transfusion, the use of FFP increased dramatically. For example, the national use of this component increased from 180,000 units in 1971 to 1.54 million units in 1980 (107). Several studies have indicated that FFP is being used as a "volume expander" or to "reconstitute whole blood" and that objective criteria for its use are rarely documented in patients' charts.

In one such study, only 27% of the transfusions were judged to be appropriate (108). These same studies emphasized the need for the education of clinicians regarding the appropriate use of FFP, and one study (109) demonstrated the dramatic positive response to a daily survey and education program in one hospital.

There are few specific indications for FFP. They are limited to the treatment of deficiencies of coagulation factors for which specific factor concentrates are unavailable or inappropriate. The NIH Consensus Conference Summary also stated that FFP was a reasonable therapy for patients with uncontrolled bleeding and multiple coagulation protein deficiencies, even though there are few data to support the efficacy of FFP in these circumstances (110). Its use can also be justified for patients with significant hepatic dysfunction and coagulopathy and as a replacement fluid in therapeutic plasma exchange for thrombotic thrombocytopenic purpura.

For patients with specific deficiencies of factors II, V, VII, IX, X, or XI, the use of FFP may be justified although the mere presence of such demonstrable defects per se is insufficient grounds for transfusion. The levels of the factors that need to be attained for hemostasis vary considerably. For factor X, about 10% of normal is needed and can be easily achieved with FFP; patients with severe deficiency of factor IX can rarely be brought to hemostatic levels with FFP alone without incurring serious risk of volume overload (110).

Patients with severe liver disease pose a considerable challenge because of the multiplicity of their coagulation factor deficiencies. The factors differ physiologically, and coupled with the low intravascular recovery of some of these factors after transfusion, judging transfusion needs can be difficult. In a 70-kg person, 1 unit of FFP will raise the circulating levels of factors VII, IX, and V by 1 to 2%. With ascites or anasarca, the extravascular distribution may be increased, and intravascular recovery correspondingly decreased (109). Bleeding in these patients often can be controlled by as little as 10 to 12 ml of FFP/kg body weight.

Warfarin-like anticoagulants act by causing the release of dysfunctional vitamin K-dependent factors II, VII, IX, and X as well as proteins S and C. This situation is best reversed by the use of vitamin K or its analogues, but this may require 24 hours. For more rapid reversal, FFP can be used (in addition to vitamin K) in doses of about 10 ml/kg (111). Because of the different half-lives of these factors, their rates of disappearance and reemergence vary. After vitamin K administration, factor VII increases at the fastest rate, achieving 30% of normal in about 24 hours, but factors IX and X lag. Medical or surgical emergencies would dictate the concomitant use of FFP to achieve more rapid reversal.

FFP is indicated in the reversal of antithrombin III (AT III) deficiency in patients who are undergoing surgery or who need heparin for the treatment of AT III deficiency-related thrombosis.

Numerous studies of FFP use in massive transfusion settings have failed to document a significant role for this component in that setting and even have failed to demonstrate reversal of documented coagulopathy in these situations. Thus, its empiric or prophylactic use during massive transfusion episodes is not supported.

SINGLE-DONOR PLASMA

If a unit of FFP has not been utilized after a year of storage at −18°C or lower, it may be relabeled "single-donor plasma" and, as such, may be stored for 4 more years at −18°C or lower. Likewise, a unit of FFP that has been thawed at 30° to 37°C and then not transfused within 24 hours (storage at 1° to 6°C) can be relabeled "single-donor plasma." This product contains all the constituents of FFP, except for the labile coagulation factors V and VIII, at levels reasonably comparable to those in FFP. Therefore, it can be used in many of the previously discussed situations. Each unit also carries the disease transmission risks associated with any single-donor product.

CRYOPRECIPITATE-DEPLETED PLASMA

If cryoprecipitate has been removed from a unit of whole blood or FFP, the label must so state because such plasma is deficient in factors VIII and XIII, fibrinogen, and fibronectin. This component can be used for volume repletion, but it carries the risks of disease transmission common to FFP and single-donor plasma.

PLASMA PROTEIN FRACTION

This product is processed commercially to provide an isosmotic, protein-containing product; the protein is largely albumin (83 to 88%). In addition, it contains no more than 1% γ-globulin, sodium at 130 to 160 mEq/liter, and potassium at less than 2 mEq/liter. This solution is stabilized by 4 mM sodium acetyltryptophanate and 4 mM sodium caprylate. The final product is heated at 60°C for 10 hours for sterilization. The shelf life is 5 years at 5°C or 3 years if stored at between 5° and 30°C. PPF can be used as an emergency volume expander during treatment of hypovolemic shock due to burns, trauma, or even hemorrhage. In young children, it can be used as an initial therapy for shock due to dehydration or infection. The resulting increase in blood volume lasts up to 48 hours (112). Like other isosmotic protein resuscitation fluids, it must be used with caution in patients with congestive heart failure, severe anemia, high cardiac output states such as hyperthyroidism, or any other condition associated with increased plasma or blood volumes.

In patients undergoing cardiopulmonary bypass surgery, a profound hypotensive reaction has been documented when PPF was administered rapidly (faster than 10 ml/min) (113). This was subsequently shown to be caused by Hageman factor fragments, which have a potent vasodilation effect due to their generation of bradykinin in recipients (114). These reactions have been accompanied by flushing, urticaria, nausea, headache, and backache in conscious patients. There also have been reports of anaphylactic or anaphylactoid reactions to infusions of various plasma protein solutions in atopic patients. Such severe reactions were estimated by Ring and Messmer (115) to occur rarely (0.003%).

PPF and other protein-containing solutions are sometimes used to treat hypoalbuminemia or hypoproteinemia. However, such therapy is effective only in the very short term because the protein must be broken down into its constituent amino acids before it can be incorporated into new protein. This breakdown and reincorporation requires several weeks to complete, and it results in only about 45% of the infused protein becoming incorporated into the body protein pool (116).

ALBUMIN

Human serum albumin products are widely used in North America because of their relative purity, their standardization of content, and most of all, their freedom from viral contamination (as a result of heat treatment at 60°C for 10 hours). Albumin is available as a 5% solution or as a 25% solution that can be diluted at the bedside. Albumin has a molecular weight of 67,000, contains about 600 amino acids, and is conspicuously deficient in tryptophan. The viscosity of albumin solutions is remarkably low, and even 25% albumin is almost isoviscous with blood. The molecule carries a net negative charge of −19 at blood pH, a property that plays a role in the binding of albumin to a large number of compounds such as bilirubin, fatty acids, hormones, and medications. Albumin is synthesized mainly in the liver, and because the liver carries only small reserves, serious hepatic dysfunction quickly leads to hypoalbuminemia and its sequelae. Normally, about 15 g is synthesized daily in the steady state, but malnutrition or chronic hepatic disease will decrease this rate significantly.

As with other plasma proteins, albumin penetrates capillary walls more slowly than water and electrolytes, and this property confers the molecule's colloid osmotic or oncotic properties. Albumin contributes about 80% of the colloid oncotic pressure of plasma, which is about 27 mm Hg. When the total serum protein level drops to about 5.2 g/dl (the so-called control valve), the colloid oncotic pressure decreases to about 20 mm Hg, and further decreases lead to increases in the interstitial fluid compartment, resulting in ascites, edema, or anasarca.

The most common causes of hypoalbuminemia are burns, chronic hepatic disease, chronic protein-losing enteropathy, and acute nephroses. Extensive burns cause the largest acute losses of albumin from the blood. During the first 90 hours after a third- or fourth-degree burn of 50% of the body surface, albumin losses can be the equivalent of about two whole normal pools of circulating albumin. A daily loss of up to 30 g of albumin can be seen for several weeks after a major burn (117). The albumin infusions have to be carefully monitored in terms of the plasma protein levels to ensure adequate oncotic levels. The same caveat applies, to a somewhat lesser degree, to the use of albumin infusions in the other disease states mentioned previously.

Currently, one of the most frequent uses of albumin infusion is as a replacement fluid in plasma exchange procedures. These procedures are widely used for the treatment of various neurological syndromes and as therapy for the pruritus of primary biliary cirrhosis. The use of albumin infusions as a long-term treatment for malnutrition is totally inappropriate, but it may be reasonable as a short-term therapy immediately preoperatively in seriously malnourished persons or in those with severe chronic hepatic dysfunction.

CRYOPRECIPITATED ANTIHEMOPHILIC FACTOR

The late Dr. Judith Pool first described a method of concentrating coagulation factor VIII by freezing freshly obtained donor plasma and then slowly thawing the plasma at 1° to 6°C. This precipitates the cold-insoluble proteins that contain about 50% of the original factor VIII. This precipitate can then be separated aseptically from the remainder of the plasma, refrozen within 1 hour at −18°C (or preferably at −30°C), and stored for up to 1 year. This product revolutionized the therapy of classic hemophilia A.

The original source plasma from which FFP is made must be frozen within 6 hours after collection from the donor, and the cryoprecipitate must not be thawed at any time during storage except for immediate infusion. These restrictions apply because of the extreme sensitivity of factor VIII to heat. Federal regulations require that an average bag of cry-

34. National Institutes of Health Consensus Conference. Platelet transfusion therapy. Transfus Med Rev 1987;1:195–200.
35. Simon TL, Akl BF, Murphy W. Controlled trial of routine administration of platelet concentrates in cardiopulmonary bypass surgery. Ann Thorac Surg 1984;37:359–364.
36. Kelton JG, Neame PB, Gauldie J, Hirsch J. Elevated platelet-associated IgG in the thrombocytopenia of septicemia. N Engl J Med 1979;300:760–764.
37. Tate DY, Carlton GT, Johnson D, et al. Immune thrombocytopenia in severe neonatal infections. J Pediatr 1981;98:449–453.
38. van Der Lelie J, van der Plas-Van Dalen CM, von Dem Borne AEGKR. Platelet autoantibodies in septicaemia. Br J Haematol 1984;58:755–760.
39. Stewart JH, Castaldi PA. Uraemic bleeding: a reversible platelet defect corrected by dialysis. Q J Med 1967;36:409–423.
40. Carvalho ACA. Bleeding in uremia—a clinical challenge. N Engl J Med 1983;308:38–39.
41. Mannucci PM, Remuzzi G, Pusineri F, et al. Deamino-8-D-arginine vasopressin shortens the bleeding time in uremia. N Engl J Med 1983;308:8–12.
42. Sniecinski I, St. Jean J, Nowicki B. Preparation of leukocyte-poor platelets by filtration. J Clin Apheresis 1989;5:7–11.
43. Holme S, Ross D, Heaton WA. In vitro and in vivo evaluation of platelet concentrates after cotton wool filtration. Vox Sang 1989;57:112–115.
44. Stec N, Kickler TS, Ness PM, Braine HG. Effectiveness of leukocyte (WBC) depleted platelets in preventing febrile reactions in multi-transfused oncology patients (abstract). Transfusion 1986;26:569.
45. Kickler TS, Bell W, Ness PM, Drew H, Pall D. Depletion of white cells from platelet concentrates with a new adsorption filter. Transfusion 1989;29:411–414.
46. Schiffer CA, Patten E, Reilly J, Patel S. Effective leukocyte removal from platelet preparations by centrifugation in a new pooling bag. Transfusion 1987;27:162–164.
47. Ferrara GB, Tosi RM, Azzalina G, Carminati G, Kissmeyer-Nielsen F. The production of anti HLA-A cytotoxic antisera through planned immunization by intravenous injection of small aliquots of whole blood. I. Immunization of unrelated recipients. Tissue Antigens 1972;2:359–373.
48. Vesilind GW, Simpson MB, Shifman MA, Colman RE, Kao KJ. Evaluation of a centrifugal blood cell processor for washing platelet concentrates. Transfusion 1988;28:46–51.
49. Schiffer CA, Aisner J, Dutcher JP, Daly PA, Wiernik PH. A clinical program of platelet cryopreservation. Prog Clin Biol Res 1982;88:165–180.
50. McGill M, Mayhaus C, Hoff R, Carey P. Frozen maternal platelets for neonatal thrombocytopenia. Transfusion 1987;27:347–349.
51. Moore SB. Management of transfusion in the massively bleeding patient. Hum Pathol 1983;14:267–270.
52. Mannucci PM, Federici AB, Sirchia G. Hemostasis testing during massive blood replacement: a study of 172 cases. Vox Sang 1982;n.s.42:113–123.
53. Reed RL II, Ciavarella D, Heimbach DM, et al. Prophylactic platelet administration during massive transfusion. Ann Surg 1986;203:40–48.
54. Howard JE, Perkins HA. The natural history of alloimmunization to platelets. Transfusion 1978;18:496–503.
55. Holohan TV, Terasaki PI, Deisseroth AB. Suppression of transfusion-related alloimmunization in intensively treated cancer patients. Blood 1981;58:122–128.
56. Yankee RA, Grumet FC, Rogentine GN. Platelet transfusion therapy. The selection of compatible platelet donors for refractory patients by lymphocyte HL-A typing. N Engl J Med 1969;281:1208–1212.
57. Lee EJ, Schiffer CA. Serial measurement of lymphocytotoxic antibody and response to nonmatched platelet transfusions in alloimmunized patients. Blood 1987;70:1727–1729.
58. McGrath K, Wolf M, Bishop J, et al. Transient platelet and HLA antibody formation in multitransfused patients with malignancy. Br J Haematol 1988;68:345–350.
59. Murphy MF, Metcalfe P, Ord J, Lister TA, Waters AH. Disappearance of HLA and platelet-specific antibodies in acute leukaemia patients alloimmunized by multiple transfusions. Br J Haematol 1987;67:255–260.
60. Bensinger WI, Buckner CD, Clift RA, Slichter SJ, Thomas ED. Plasma exchange for platelet alloimmunization. Transplantation 1986;41:602–605.
61. Dunstan RA, Simpson MB. Stability of platelet surface antigens during storage. Transfusion 1985;25:563–566.
62. Santoso S, Mueller-Eckhardt G, Santoso S, Kiefel V, Mueller-Eckhardt C. HLA antigens on platelet membranes: in vitro and in vivo studies. Vox Sang 1986;51:327–333.
63. Daly PA, Schiffer CA, Aisner J, Wiernik PH. Platelet transfusion therapy. One-hour posttransfusion increments are valuable in predicting the need for HLA-matched preparations. JAMA 1980;243:435–438.
64. Bishop JF, McGrath K, Wolf MM, et al. Clinical factors influencing the efficacy of pooled platelet transfusions. Blood 1988;71:383–387.
65. Kotlán B, Gyódi É, Szabó T, et al. Comparative study of alloimmune reactions induced by leukocyte and platelet transfusions in humans: characteristic changes of activation markers, gamma interferon and FcR blocking antibody production. Hum Immunol 1988;22:19–29.
66. Takahashi K, Juji T, Miyazaki H. Determination of an appropriate size of unrelated donor pool to be registered for HLA-matched platelet transfusion. Transfusion 1987;27:394–398.
67. Schiffer CA, O'Connell B, Lee EJ. Platelet transfusion therapy for alloimmunized patients: selective mismatching for HLA B12, an antigen with variable expression on platelets. Blood 1989;74:1172–1176.
68. McElligott MC, Menitove JE, Duquesnoy RJ, Hunter JB, Aster RH. Effect of HLA Bw4/Bw6 compatibility on platelet transfusion responses of refractory thrombocytopenic patients. Blood 1982;59:971–975.
69. Moore SB. HLA and blood component therapy. In: Hackel E, Mallory D, eds. Theoretical aspects of HLA. Arlington, VA: American Association of Blood Banks, 1982:81–103.
70. Dahlke MB, Weiss KL. Platelet transfusion from donors mismatched for crossreactive HLA antigens. Transfusion 1984;24:299–302.
71. Herzig RH, Poplack DG, Yankee RA. Prolonged granulocytopenia from incompatible platelet transfusions. N Engl J Med 1974;290:1220–1223.
72. Kieckbusch ME, Moore SB, Koenig VA, DeGoey SR. Platelet crossmatch evaluation in refractory hematologic patients. Mayo Clin Proc 1987;62:595–600.
73. Freedman J, Garvey MB, de Friedberg ZS, Hornstein A, Blanchette V. Random donor platelet crossmatching: comparison of four platelet antibody detection methods. Am J Hematol 1988;28:1–7.
74. Heal JM, Blumberg N, Masel D. An evaluation of crossmatching, HLA and ABO matching for platelet transfusions to refractory patients. Blood 1987;70:23–30.
75. Petz LD. Platelet crossmatching (letter to the editor). Am J Clin Pathol 1988;90:114–115.
76. Welch HG, Larson EB, Slichter SJ. Providing platelets for refractory patients: prudent strategies. Transfusion 1989;29:193–195.

77. Rachel JM, Summers TC, Sinor LT, Plapp FV. Use of a solid phase red blood cell adherence method for pretransfusion platelet compatibility testing. Am J Clin Pathol 1988;90:63–68.
78. Lee EJ, Schiffer CA. ABO compatibility can influence the results of platelet transfusion: results of a randomized trial. Transfusion 1989;29:384–389.
79. Schiffer CA, Slichter SJ. Sounding board: platelet transfusions from single donors. N Engl J Med 1982;307:245–248.
80. Brand A, Claas FHJ, Voogt PJ, Wasser MNJM, Eernisse JG. Alloimmunization after leukocyte-depleted multiple random donor platelet transfusions. Vox Sang 1988;54:160–166.
81. Slichter SJ, Deeg HJ, Kennedy MS. Prevention of platelet alloimmunization in dogs with systemic cyclosporine and by UV-irradiation or cyclosporine-loading of donor platelets. Blood 1987;69:414–418.
82. Bodey GP, Buckley M, Sathe YS, Freireich EJ. Quantitative relationships between circulating leukocytes and infection in patients with acute leukemia. Ann Intern Med 1966;64:328–340.
83. Strumia MM. The effect of leukocytic cream injections in the treatment of the neutropenias. Am J Med Sci 1934;187:527–544.
84. McCullough J. Granulocyte transfusion. In: Petz LD, Swisher SN, eds. Clinical practice of transfusion medicine. 2nd ed. New York: Churchill Livingstone, 1989:469–484.
85. Dutcher JP, Schiffer CA, Johnston GS. Rapid migration of ^{111}indium-labelled granulocytes to sites of infection. N Engl J Med 1981;304:586–589.
86. McCullough J, Weiblen BJ, Clay ME, Forstrom L. Effect of leukocyte antibodies on the fate in vivo of indium-111-labelled granulocytes. Blood 1981;58:164–170.
87. McCullough J, Clay M, Loken M, Hurd D. Effect of ABO incompatibility on the fate in vivo of ^{111}indium granulocytes. Transfusion 1988;28:358–361.
88. Dutcher JP, Schiffer CA, Johnston GS, et al. Alloimmunization prevents the migration of transfused indium-111-labelled granulocytes to sites of infection. Blood 1983;62:354–360.
89. Dahlke MB, Keashen M, Alavi JB, Koch PA, Eisenstaedt R. Granulocyte transfusions and outcome of alloimmunized patients with gram-negative sepsis. Transfusion 1982;22:374–378.
90. Strauss RG, Connett JE, Gale RP, et al. A controlled trial of prophylactic granulocyte transfusions during initial induction chemotherapy for acute myelogenous leukemia. N Engl J Med 1981;305:597–603.
91. Wright DG, Robichaud KJ, Pizzo PA, Deisseroth AB. Lethal pulmonary reactions associated with the combined use of amphotericin B and leukocyte transfusions. N Engl J Med 1981;304:1185–1189.
92. Forman SJ, Robinson GV, Wolf JL, Spruce WE, Blume KG. Pulmonary reactions associated with amphotericin B and leukocyte transfusions [Letter to the editor]. N Engl J Med 1981;305:584–585.
93. Clift RA, Sanders JE, Thomas ED, Williams B, Buckner CD. Granulocyte transfusions for the prevention of infection in patients receiving bone-marrow transplants. N Engl J Med 1978;298:1052–1057.
94. Christensen RD, Anstall H, Rothstein G. Neutrophil transfusion in septic neutropenic neonates. Transfusion 1982;22:151–153.
95. Grimm EA, Mazumder A, Zhang HZ, Rosenberg SA. Lymphokine-activated killer cell phenomenon. Lysis of natural killer-resistant fresh solid tumor cells by interleukin 2-activated autologous human peripheral blood lymphocytes. J Exp Med 1982;155:1823–1841.
96. Grimm EA, Ramsey KM, Mazumder A, Wilson DJ, Djeu JY, Rosenberg SA. Lymphokine-activated killer cell phenomenon. II. Precursor phenotype is serologically distinct from peripheral T lymphocytes, memory cytotoxic thymus-derived lymphocytes and natural killer cells. J Exp Med 1983;157:884–897.
97. Klein HG, Leitman SF. Adoptive immunotherapy in the treatment of malignant disease. Transfusion 1989;29:170–178.
98. van den Brink MRM, Voogt PJ, Marijt WAF, van Luxemburg-Heys SAP, van Rood JJ, Brand A. Lymphokine-activated killer cells selectively kill tumor cells in bone marrow without compromising bone marrow stem cell function in vitro. Blood 1989;74:354–360.
99. Ryan T, Atkins MB, Mier JW, Berkman EM. Lymphokine-activated killer cell generation and recovery. Comparison of an automated cell processing device and a manual procedure. Transfusion 1989;29:491–495.
100. Rosenberg SA, Spiess P, Lafreniere R. A new approach to the adoptive immunotherapy of cancer with tumor-infiltrating lymphocytes. Science 1986;233:1318–1321.
101. Edelson R, Berger C, Gasparro F, et al. Treatment of cutaneous T-cell lymphoma by extracorporeal photochemotherapy. Preliminary results. N Engl J Med 1987;316:297–303.
102. Burgstaler EA, Pineda AA. Photopheresis: blood cell recovery and reaction incidence of 247 procedures. Transfusion 1989;29suppl:44S.
103. Rock G. Factor VIII concentrates. In: Cash JD, ed. Progress in transfusion medicine. Vol 2. New York: Churchill Livingstone, 1987:127.
104. Rock G, Tackaberry ES, Dunn JG, Kashyap S. Rapid controlled thawing of fresh-frozen plasma in a modified microwave oven. Transfusion 1984;24:60–65.
105. Luff RD, Kessler CM, Bell WR. Microwave technology for the rapid thawing of frozen blood components. Am J Clin Pathol 1985;83:59–64.
106. George JN, Pickett EB, Heinz R. Platelet membrane microparticles in blood bank fresh frozen plasma and cryoprecipitate. Blood 1986;68:307–309.
107. Snyder AJ, Gottschall JL, Menitove JE. Why is fresh-frozen plasma transfused? Transfusion 1986;26:107–112.
108. Blumberg N, Laczin J, McMican A, Heal J, Arvan D. A critical survey of fresh-frozen plasma use. Transfusion 1986;26:511–513.
109. Shanberge JN. Reduction of fresh-frozen plasma use through a daily survey and education program. Transfusion 1987;27:226–227.
110. National Institutes of Health Consensus Conference. Fresh frozen plasma: indications and risks. Transfus Med Rev 1987;1:201–204.
111. Counts RB. Acquired bleeding disorders. In: Menitove JE, McCarthy LJ, eds. Hemostatic disorders and the blood bank. Arlington VA: American Association of Blood Banks, 1984:41–47.
112. Bertrand JJ, Feichtmeir TV, Kolomeyer NK, et al. Clinical investigations with a heat-treated plasma protein fraction—Plasmanate®. Vox Sang 1959;4:385–402.
113. Bland JHL, Laver MB, Lowenstein E. Vasodilator effect of commercial 5% plasma protein fraction solutions. JAMA 1973;224:1721–1724.
114. Alving BM, Hojima Y, Pisano JJ, et al. Hypotension associated with prekallikrein activator (Hageman-factor fragments) in plasma protein fraction. N Engl J Med 1978;299:66–70.
115. Ring J, Messmer K. Incidence and severity of anaphylactoid reactions to colloid volume substitutes. Lancet 1977;1:466–469.
116. Waterhouse C, Bassett SH, Holler JW. Metabolic studies on protein-depleted patients receiving a large part of their nitrogen intake from human serum albumin administered intravenously. J Clin Invest 1949;28:245–264.
117. O'Riordan JP, Aebischer M, Darnborough J, Thoren L. The indications for the use of albumin, plasma protein solutions

patient hemodynamically to allow the laboratory time to ABO and Rh type the patient. This requires about 10 minutes after receipt of the specimen. If the clinical situation permits a 30- to 45-minute delay in transfusion, an antibody screen and/or a major cross-match with the donor unit(s) should be performed (5).

An objective clinical assessment by the patient care team followed by clear communication with the laboratory are required to optimize pretransfusion testing. The use of ABO- and Rh-identical units permits better utilization of RBC inventories. In addition, antibody screening and cross-matching lessens the possibility, already small for most patients, that the transfused RBCs will produce a hemolytic transfusion reaction. With the use of ABO-compatible units, the primary concern is the possibility that the recipient may have a non-ABO alloantibody. An estimated 0.04% of individuals will have a non-ABO alloantibody if they have not been previously transfused or pregnant. Approximately 0.3% of previously transfused, multiparous women and about 5 to 30% of chronically transfused patients, such as those with sickle cell anemia or thalassemia, have non-ABO red cell alloantibodies (6–8). Even if the recipient has a non-ABO alloantibody and receives RBCs incompatible with that antibody, it is unlikely that a life-threatening hemolytic transfusion reaction will occur. Most, though not all, clinically significant non-ABO RBC alloantibodies are IgG molecules that do not fix complement to C9. They fix complement either to C3, or not at all. Thus, they usually produce extravascular, not intravascular, hemolysis. In contrast, ABO antibodies avidly bind complement to C9, resulting in a possible acute intravascular hemolytic transfusion reaction.

If the short delay in the provision of RBCs due to the need to perform ABO and Rh typing of the recipient is life-threatening, then group O, preferably group O, Rh-negative, non–cross-matched RBCs should be transfused. For this reason, group O, Rh-negative RBCs are often available in monitored refrigerators in hospital emergency rooms and in trauma centers. These units can be given to those patients for whom the potential risk of incompatibility is small when compared with the risk of not transfusing them or of waiting for compatible blood (9–11). In general, group O, Rh-negative, non–cross-matched RBCs can be used for emergency RBC transfusion with little risk for most patients. The emergency use of group O RBC carries the risk of transfusing anti-A or anti-B antibodies into an ABO-incompatible recipient. However, a life-threatening hemolytic reaction in this setting is unlikely because the amount of plasma in a unit of RBCs is small (about 80 ml) compared with the volume of plasma present in a unit of whole blood (about 280 ml). Thus, the recipient is more likely merely to develop a positive direct antiglobulin test without significant hemolysis or a clinical reaction. The development and widespread use of additive solution RBCs has resulted in an even further decrease in the amount of plasma contained in a unit (about 40 ml) because, during component preparation, more plasma is removed from these units than from CPDA-1 RBCs. With less plasma, and accordingly fewer anti-A or anti-B antibodies, the risk of a clinically significant hemolytic transfusion reaction to ABO incompatibility is further lessened.

If RBCs are transfused prior to Rh typing of the recipient, it is preferable to use Rh-negative units, if available. About 15% of recipients will be Rh-negative and will be at significant risk of having or developing anti-D. The D antigen is the most immunogenic red cell determinant and will result in antibody formation in about 70% of Rh-negative individuals receiving 200 ml or more of D-positive RBCs (12, 13). The most significant risk is to Rh-negative women of childbearing potential. If they develop an anti-D antibody, any future Rh-positive children may be at risk for Rh hemolytic disease of the newborn. All females of childbearing potential should be assumed to be Rh-negative until they are Rh typed and should be transfused with Rh-negative RBCs if at all possible. Rh immune globulin can be used for the prevention of RH alloimmunization in Rh-negative recipients of Rh-positive RBC. However, transfusion of one unit of Rh-positive blood containing about 200 ml of RBCs would require 14 to 17 intramuscular doses of Rh immune globulin (300 μg/dose, 1 ml/dose; each dose is sufficient to neutralize 15 ml of red cells). Thus, due to the large number of painful intramuscular injections required, treatment becomes impractical when more than one unit of Rh-positive RBCs is transfused to an Rh-negative patient. An intravenous form of Rh immune globulin is not yet licensed in the United States. Since anti-D is a relatively common antibody, the use of Rh-negative RBCs also eliminates the risk of an anti-D-mediated delayed extravascular hemolytic reaction. Should a recipient of an emergency transfusion be found, subsequently, to possess an alloantibody, antigen testing should be performed retrospectively on any units transfused so that any potential hemolytic reaction can be anticipated. Despite the relative safety of an emergency transfusion, clear guidelines for its use should be established to avoid overusage in acute trauma settings.

MASSIVE TRANSFUSION

Massive transfusion is the transfusion of a volume of blood components equivalent to, or greater than, the patient's intravascular volume within a 24-hour period. Although infusion of such a large volume of RBCs in a short time period may be life-saving, it also poses hazards to the transfusion recipient that are not seen following the transfusion of smaller volumes.

Dilutional Coagulopathy

With massive hemorrhage and subsequent large-volume transfusion, platelet and coagulation factor levels may be depleted due to consumption and/or dilution (14–16). Consumption is due to activation of the coagulation cascade secondary to trauma or injury; dilution is due to replacement of blood with crystalloid, synthetic colloid, or units of stored RBCs, all of which are deficient in functional platelets and coagulation factors. Massive transfusion, per se, however, does not always result in platelet or factor deficiencies sufficient to warrant platelet or fresh frozen plasma (FFP) transfusion. Theoretical models predict that massive transfusion, i.e., loss of about 10 units of blood followed by replacement with 10 units of RBCs plus crystalloid, will leave 37% of the original blood volume (17). If starting levels of platelets and coagulation factors were normal, dilution of 37% of original levels should leave hemostatically effective amounts of platelets and coagulation factors, even assuming no further production. The liver may continue to produce sufficient coagulation factors despite the dilutional effect, and platelets may enter the circulation from extravascular sites, thus blunting the development of thrombocytopenia.

Because of the possibility of concurrent consumption of coagulation factors or platelets, the extent of platelet or coagulation factor deficiency cannot be predicted accurately from the volume of blood lost or the number of units of components transfused. Accordingly, transfusion of platelets or FFP should be based on observed clinical bleeding as well as on the laboratory measurement of platelet counts and coagulation factor levels; it should not be based on predetermined formulas linked to the number of RBC units transfused (18). Replacement formulas may lead to unnecessary transfusion, particularly if less than 1.0 to 1.5 blood volumes have been replaced. In addition, component transfusion guided by replacement formulas may be insufficient if, for example, a consumptive process such as disseminated intravascular coagulation develops. One key to appropriate replacement therapy in massive transfusion, therefore, is the timely measurement of hematocrit, platelets, and coagulation parameters. Empirical platelet and FFP transfusion should be considered only if the delays inherent in testing and reporting of laboratory results could be life-threatening due to continued and uncontrolled hemorrhage. Specimens should be sent to the laboratory as soon as possible and at appropriate intervals thereafter so that further therapy can be based on a more rational decision-making process.

Citrate Toxicity

Citrate is used as the anticoagulant in preservative solutions because of its ability to chelate calcium, which is required for coagulation factor activity. Citrate is also desirable as an anticoagulant because when infused it usually is rapidly metabolized to generate bicarbonate and does not result in systemic anticoagulation of the transfusion recipient. However, patients with normal liver function who were transfused with whole blood at a rate equivalent to, or greater than, 1 liter/10 minutes developed signs of hypocalcemia due to the lowering of levels of ionized calcium (19–22). The effects of hypocalcemia range from minor circumoral paresthesias and muscle tremors to more severe complications such as tetany and cardiac effects. The latter includes prolonged QT intervals and depression of T waves, which could potentially lead to ventricular fibrillation and cardiac arrest.

Citrate toxicity is less likely to result from RBC than from whole blood transfusion because RBCs have substantially less plasma, and thus less anticoagulant, per unit compared with whole blood. Components with high plasma content, such as FFP and pooled platelet concentrates, are usually not infused in sufficient volumes to produce citrate toxicity. Citrate toxicity does, however, remain a concern in patients with liver failure who receive rapid transfusions of large amounts of plasma-containing components such as FFP because they are unable to metabolize the citrate appropriately. It may be useful to follow ionized calcium levels in these patients and to treat them with supplemental calcium if the levels are sufficiently low or if prolonged QT intervals or signs of tetany are seen. Early mild reactions can be treated merely by slowing the rate of transfusion (22). Calcium infusion is not without risk and has been associated with the development of ventricular arrhythmias and cardiac arrest (23). Calcium must not be added to a unit of RBCs, or infused simultaneously through the same line because it would recalcify the plasma and cause clots to form. Hypomagnesemia, presumably due to chelation of magnesium by citrate, has also been reported (24). However, clinical complications have not been well documented.

Acid-Base Disturbance

Stored blood and components have an acidic pH due to citrate/citric acid buffering, and they may become more acidic due to the accumulation of lactic acid with increasing storage time (25). However, this acid load is not likely to worsen an existing acidosis even in massively transfused patients. Indeed, due to the metabolism of transfused citrate, which results in the generation of bicarbonate, massively transfused patients may develop a metabolic alkalosis (26).

Electrolyte Disturbances

Extracellular potassium levels increase in stored blood at a rate of approximately 1 mEq/day during the first 3 weeks of storage (25). The total extracellular potassium load of stored transfused RBCs may approach 20 mEq/unit. However, even massively transfused patients rarely develop more than transient hyperkalemia (27). Hypokalemia has more often been reported in massive transfusions due to the development of a metabolic alkalosis from citrate toxicity (see above) (28). The alkalosis is accompanied by a transmembrane shift of hydrogen ions into the intravascular space in an attempt by the body to lower pH. This H^+ shift is balanced by an intracellular movement of potassium ions to maintain electrical balance.

Hypothermia

The rapid transfusion of large volumes of cold (1 to 6°C) RBCs at a rate greater than 100ml/minute may lower the patient's core temperature. A drop in sinoatrial node temperature to below 30°C has been associated with the development of ventricular fibrillation (29–32). To avoid this potential complication, RBCs may be administered through a blood warmer (see below).

CHRONIC RBC TRANSFUSIONS

Patients receiving chronic RBC transfusions, such as those with thalassemia major or sickle cell anemia, are at risk for several adverse transfusion-related problems. First, as many as 30% of sickle cell patients and approximately 10% of thalassemia major patients become alloimmunized to one or more RBC antigens which, depending on the antibody specificity, can make finding compatible RBCs difficult (7). Alloimmunization could be prevented in chronically transfused patients by providing antigen-compatible RBCs. Because the frequency of many RBC surface antigens is race-dependent, it has been proposed that reduction of alloimmunization could be accomplished by transfusing RBCs from racially similar donors (7, 33). However, it is not clear that this approach is appropriate because the majority of patients do not become multiply alloimmunized (34–36). Furthermore, the social implications of such an approach are unclear. Nevertheless, it is helpful to determine, when possible, the RBC phenotype of patients who will require chronic transfusion because patients will make alloantibodies only to antigens that they lack. Thus, phenotyping may help clarify future complex serologic problems should the patient eventually become multiply alloimmunized.

Patients chronically transfused with RBCs are also at risk of developing iron overload or transfusion hemosiderosis. Every unit of RBCs contains about 200 to 250 mg of iron (1 mg of Fe^{++}/ml RBCs). By comparison, the total body iron of a normal adult male, for example, is 3 to 4 g. Because the body has no mechanism for excreting iron, the excess iron from chronic transfusions accumulates in organs such as the liver, heart, and endocrine glands. Organ damage can eventually lead to cirrhosis, congestive heart failure, or endocrine dysfunction. The toxicity apparently relates in part to the effect of iron on the mitochondria present in the target organs (37). In order to avoid iron overload, RBC should be transfused only when necessary. Iron chelation therapy with desferoxamine mobilizes and reduces iron stores, although the rate of iron removal is slow. Nevertheless, with judicious use of blood transfusion and iron chelation therapy, even chronically transfused patients can achieve negative iron balance and avoid iron overload (38, 39).

AUTOLOGOUS TRANSFUSIONS

While homologous transfusion is the transfusion of blood or blood components collected from donors other than the recipient, autologous transfusion uses the recipient's own blood or blood components for reinfusion (40–45). The goal of autologous transfusion is to eliminate the risks of homologous transfusion, including transfusion-transmitted infections and a variety of immune-mediated transfusion reactions. Autologous blood can be collected preoperatively, or it can be salvaged from blood lost in the intraoperative or postoperative periods and reinfused immediately.

Preoperative Autologous Blood Donation

Preoperative autologous blood donations can be stored in liquid form for 35 days (CPDA-1) or 42 days (AS-RBCs) prior to surgery (5). For a patient to be eligible for preoperative autologous blood donation, sufficient time must be available before surgery to permit collection of the required number of units (46). A typical collection schedule allows for donation of 1 unit/week, with the last unit being donated at least 3 days before surgery. More aggressive collection schedules can be followed as long as the patient's hematocrit remains greater than 33% at the time of each donation (5). No minimum or maximum age limits are established for autologous donation (47, 48). The amount of blood collected, 450 ml ±10%, should be less than 15% of the patient's blood volume, about 10 ml/kg for adults. Smaller volumes, as low as 300 ml, can be collected from small donors and stored in a standard bag. However, if the volume to be collected is less than 300 ml, then the amount of anticoagulant/preservative solution must be reduced proportionately (5).

Acute Normovolemic Hemodilution

Acute normovolemic hemodilution refers to the collection of units of blood immediately prior to surgery with simultaneous volume replacement using crystalloid or colloid solutions (45, 49).

Normovolemic hemodilution is used to achieve multiple goals. One is to decrease the volume of operative red cell mass loss. The lower the hematocrit of the blood lost in surgery, the smaller will be the loss of red cell mass. Moreover, the blood collected is then available for transfusion during or after surgery, when the need for the red cells may be greater. Furthermore, hemodilution decreases the viscosity of blood and therefore may increase flow rate through the microvasculature. Because oxygen transport is a function not only of the oxygen-carrying capacity but also of blood flow, this effect may help compensate for the loss in hemoglobin content of blood resulting from the blood donation (50). In addition, hemodilution can be tolerated in many patients because oxygen delivery is normally in excess of that actually required by the tissues. Lastly, blood collected immediately preoperatively contains maximum levels of coagulation factors as well as functional platelets. These hemostatic components may be useful during the operation if the patient experiences coagulation problems.

Perioperative Blood Salvage

Perioperative blood salvage refers to the collection of the patient's own blood, whether shed intraoperatively or postoperatively from surgical drainage sites (45, 51–56). After collection, the blood can be reinfused immediately without further processing, or it can be concentrated by centrifugation. The salvaged blood may also be washed with isotonic saline before reinfusion. Perioperative blood salvage is useful for patients having surgical procedures with a large anticipated blood loss (greater than 2 to 3 units). Perioperative blood salvage has the advantage of being available for many patients who cannot donate autologous blood preoperatively. It is also a useful adjunct to preoperative autologous blood donation for those patients who have not donated sufficient blood to cover their total transfusion requirements. Blood salvage should not be attempted from any operative site that is potentially contaminated with bacteria. Blood salvage should also not be performed at surgical sites involving malignancies (57, 58). This contraindication stems from the theoretical risk of promoting metastases by infusing malignant cells intravascularly. The salvage of blood shed postoperatively is also feasible and has been applied most commonly after cardiac and orthopaedic surgery.

Blood collected postoperatively, except in cases of brisk hemorrhage, usually has undergone extensive coagulation factor activation and may be defibrinated (59–61). Accordingly, coagulation factor levels and platelet numbers and activity are reduced in blood salvaged postoperatively.

PLATELETS

General Indications for Transfusion

Patients with platelet counts less than 5,000 to 10,000/µl are at significant risk of hemorrhage (62). Fortunately, most thrombocytopenic bleeding is not immediately life-threatening, and there is usually sufficient time for a platelet transfusion. However, because of the risk of intracerebral hemorrhage with its potential for irreversible morbidity and mortality, it is common practice to transfuse platelets prophylactically for platelet counts less than 10,000 to 20,000/µl. There is much controversy regarding when to transfuse platelets (63). Thrombocytopenic patients who have evidence of hemorrhage limited to skin manifestations, such as purpura or petechiae, are in a different risk category from thrombocytopenic patients who are about to undergo an invasive procedure. The latter group may benefit from raising platelet counts to at least 50,000/µl, but patients in the former group do not need to be transfused to that level.

For some patients, such as those requiring surgery, a platelet transfusion may be indicated even if the platelet count is close to 50,000/µl. Each case should be decided individually (64). Not all thrombocytopenic patients at risk for minor bleeding need to be transfused. For percutaneous solid organ biopsies such as those of the lung, liver, and kidney, or for lumbar punctures, when bleeding might not be easily detected, a transfusion to raise the platelet count to at least 50,000/µl may be indicated. For major surgical procedures, it is usually not necessary to transfuse the patient preoperatively in anticipation of bleeding as long as the platelet count is 50,000/μl. Should microvascular bleeding related to thrombocytopenia develop in the operating room, it is usually readily treatable with platelet transfusion. For hemorrhage associated with extensive vascular injuries or coexisting coagulopathies, it may be beneficial to transfuse platelets for counts less than 80,000 to 100,000/μl. Transfusion also may be indicated at this higher platelet count in a setting of massive hemorrhage accompanied by a rapid fall in platelet count due to the potential for a continued rapid fall in the platelet level. Platelet transfusions to these higher platelet count levels also may be required for patients at higher risk of bleeding secondary to platelet dysfunction related to medication or disease. Thus, clinical judgment enters into the decision to transfuse platelets as well as red cells (63).

Dose

A typical dose of platelet concentrate is 1 unit/10 kg patient body weight or 4 units of platelet concentrate/m^2 of patient body surface area. Assuming splenic sequestration of 30% in a 70-kg adult, this dose should give a theoretical platelet count increment of 70,000/μl, i. e., 10,000/μl per unit. In reality, the increment in an average adult is more likely to be 5,000/μl to 10,000/μl per unit. A useful formula for the evaluation of recipient response to platelet transfusion is the corrected count increment (CCI):

$$\text{CCI} = \frac{(\text{Postplatelet count}/\mu\text{l} - \text{Preplatelet count}/\mu\text{l}) \times (\text{Body surface area [m}^2])}{\text{Number of platelets transfused} \times 10^{-11}}$$

Because the CCI corrects for differences in intravascular volume, which is proportional to the body surface area, and for the actual number of platelets transfused, it provides a better basis for comparison of transfusion responses than platelet count increments alone. Most nonalloimmunized platelet transfusion recipients will have CCIs greater than 7500. A patient with CCIs repeatedly less than 7500 is considered refractory to platelets. In one study, patients without obvious risk factors for platelet refractoriness, such as HLA antibodies, platelet antibodies, sepsis, DIC, hemorrhage, immune thrombocytopenic purpura (ITP), or splenomegaly, had an average CCI of 14,600 (65, 66).

Massive Blood Loss

Massive blood loss (i. e., a loss of greater than, or equal to, one blood volume in a 24-hour period) can produce thrombocytopenia because of platelet consumption or platelet loss in the shed blood or because of a dilutional effect from infusion of crystalloid/colloid solutions and platelet-deficient stored blood components (14, 15). Units of stored RBCs are essentially devoid of functional platelets, and when transfused, they can contribute to dilutional thrombocytopenia. The platelet count typically may drop from normal levels to 50,000 to 60,000/μl after transfusion of 10 to 20 units of red blood cells. Platelets should not be transfused by a formula based on the number of units of RBCs transfused. Instead, platelet counts should be monitored at regular intervals after the transfusion of 10 units or more of RBCs, and a decision to transfuse platelets should be based on the nature of the hemorrhage and the measured platelet levels.

Open Heart Surgery

During cardiopulmonary bypass surgery, platelets exposed to the foreign synthetic surfaces of the extracorporeal blood circuit often undergo activation with occurrence of the release reaction. As a result, varying degrees of thrombocytopathy can develop in these patients (67–75). Despite this, the administration of platelet transfusions to all patients after cardiopulmonary bypass is not indicated because the majority do not suffer excessive postoperative bleeding. Attempts to identify that subset of patients in whom such a thrombocytopathy would contribute to excessive postoperative bleeding, and who might benefit from prophylactic platelet transfusions, have been largely unsuccessful. Preoperative bleeding times of patients, many of whom have recently been on aspirin, have not been a reliable predictor of postoperative bleeding. Aspirin often only modestly prolongs the bleeding time and does not lead to excessive bleeding in most patients (76, 77). However, those patients who have evidence of severe aspirin-induced thrombocytopathy that results in a greatly prolonged bleeding time, i.e., 15 minutes or more, are candidates for prophylactic postcardiopulmonary bypass platelet transfusion. Platelet transfusions are also indicated in patients with evidence of systemic microvascular bleeding (e. g., generalized oozing from surgical and IV sites). The decision to transfuse platelets in this setting is made on clinical grounds and should not be based solely on laboratory data. Platelet counts typically fall after cardiopulmonary bypass, but the decrease is usually not sufficient to require transfusion. However, seemingly adequate platelet counts can be misleading because platelet function can be severely impaired in some patients. Sound clinical judgment as well as proper interpretation of laboratory data are needed to treat such patients appropriately.

Immune Thrombocytopenic Purpura

Patients with immune thrombocytopenic purpura (ITP) are thrombocytopenic due to autoimmune destruction of their platelets. Transfused platelets also become affected and are destroyed rapidly. Accordingly, they are of limited benefit. In such patients, attempts to maintain platelet counts above a specific value, such as 20,000/μl, can be futile. Fortunately, the bleeding time and the tendency for hemorrhage are often not increased in proportion to the thrombocytopenia. Platelet transfusions are indicated only for those patients with life-threatening hemorrhage. Some patients with ITP can have substantial, albeit short-lived, platelet count increments immediately following platelet transfusion (78). Thus, for patients with significant bleeding, a clinical trial of platelet transfusion may be warranted (79). However, platelet transfusions usually are not indicated in ITP. There is controversy regarding the role of platelet transfusion during splenectomy for ITP. Routine prophylactic platelet transfusion is unwarranted because there is usually little operative bleeding; most often, the platelet count rises after the splenic pedicle is clamped. If the patient bleeds despite clamping of the spleen, platelet transfusion may be of temporary value. Intravenous γ-globulin therapy has also been recommended (80–82).

Thrombotic Thrombocytopenic Purpura

Thrombotic thrombocytopenic purpura (TTP) is a microvascular occlusive syndrome characterized by thrombocytopenia and fragmentational hemolysis due to the presence of platelet microthrombi in small vessels (83). The hyaline microthrombi are believed to be composed of platelet debris. The thrombocytopenia is apparently due to both abnormal platelet adhesion to blood vessel walls and accumulation of platelet aggregates. End-organ damage can occur because of microvascular occlusion and typically manifests itself as renal failure and neurological deficits. Mortality in untreated cases may be as high as 90%. Platelet transfusions are contraindicated in TTP and have been reported to worsen symptoms (84, 85). The transfused platelets may promote the formation of additional microthrombi, especially in the cardiac or cerebral circulations with potential fatal consequences. Antiplatelet therapy with inhibitory agents such as aspirin and dipyridamole are given to these patients to help minimize further platelet adhesion and/or aggregation. Patients should be treated with plasmapheresis and FFP, the current therapy of choice (86, 87). These modalities are theorized to work by removing some factors that promote platelet aggregation or by replacing some platelet inhibitory factor(s). Although the pathogenesis of TTP is obscure, these therapeutic maneuvers appear to increase the likelihood of a remission (88).

Uremia

Patients with severe renal failure are at risk for a hemorrhagic diathesis due to platelet dysfunction (89–92). Uremic patients have prolonged bleeding times and abnormal platelet aggregation that may be due to the accumulation of metabolites that are toxic to the platelets (93). Platelet transfusions are not an effective therapy in uremia because the transfused platelets presumably will also become dysfunctional when exposed to the same in vivo environment. However, several effective treatment options are available. The treatment of choice is hemo- or peritoneal dialysis. Either procedure can temporarily correct a bleeding diathesis, presumably by transiently removing the toxic metabolite that causes the uremic thrombocytopathy. Bleeding times can also be shortened in uremic patients by maintaining their hematocrits at above 30% either through the use of recombinant human erythropoietin or RBC transfusions (94–97). Desmopressin, a synthetic analogue of antidiuretic hormone, which stimulates increases in endogenous von Willebrand factor and factor VIII levels, also shortens the bleeding time in many uremic patients (98–100). Although less thoroughly evaluated, both cryoprecipitate transfusion and the intravenous infusion of conjugated estrogens have also been shown to shorten bleeding times prolonged by uremia (101–103). These maneuvers are not curative, and in some patients with a uremic thrombocytopathy, only renal transplantation offers hope for a permanent solution to the problem.

HLA Alloimmunization

Platelets carry HLA class I antigens. About 50 to 60% of patients who receive multiple transfusions become alloimmunized to HLA class I antigens and become refractory to transfusion of pooled, random donor, platelet concentrate (64, 104). Platelet alloimmunization apparently requires the infusion of donor antigen-presenting cells (APCs) such as monocytes, B cells, and dendritic cells, all of which express HLA class II antigens. It is hypothesized that alloimmunization occurs when donor HLA antigens are presented to recipient T cells by *donor* APC in the presence of a foreign class II antigen. When levels of donor APC in platelet concentrates are decreased by reducing leukocyte contamination via the use of new third-generation leukocyte depletion filters, the incidence of recipient HLA-alloimmunization is reduced

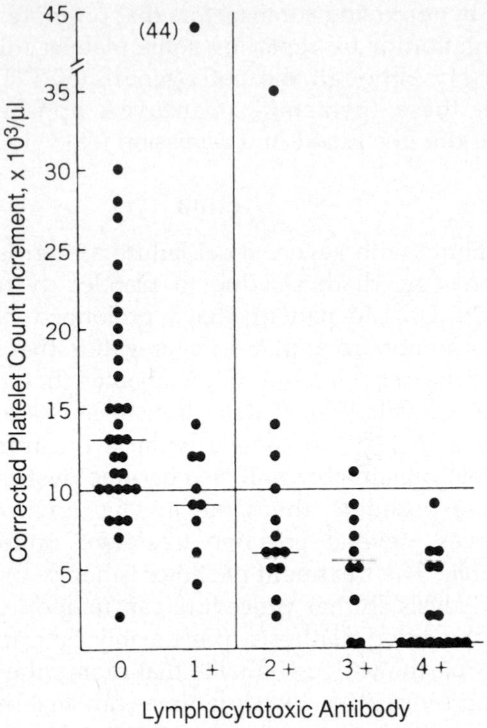

Figure 69.1 One-hour corrected count increments, CCI (see text), after the transfusion of pooled, random platelet concentrates in HLA-alloimmunized thrombocytopenic recipients. The CCI is plotted as a function of the lymphocytotoxic antibody level. Reactions 2+ to 4+ are considered positive for the presence of lymphocytotoxic antibody. Median values are indicated by horizontal bars. (From Daly PA, Schiffer CA, Aisner J. Wiernik PH. Platelet transfusion therapy; one-hour posttransfusion increments are valuable in predicting the need for HLA-matched preparations. JAMA 1980;243:435–438.)

from 60% to about 20% (104–107). Typically, patients who are HLA-alloimmunized have a poor increment in platelet count measured within 10 minutes to 4 hours after transfusion; i.e., a CCI less than 7500 (Fig. 69.1) (65, 108). However, not all patients who are refractory to platelet transfusions are HLA-alloimmunized. Other causes of platelet refractoriness include sepsis, DIC, splenomegaly, ITP, hemorrhage, fever, alloimmunization to platelet-specific antigens, circulating immune complexes, viremias, and a previous bone marrow transplantation (66). However, even patients with splenomegaly may respond to platelet transfusions (109).

If HLA alloimmunization is suspected, the presence of any HLA antibodies in the patient's serum should be identified, and if present, their antigenic specificity should be determined. The appropriate platelet component for thrombocytopenic HLA-alloimmunized patients is HLA-matched, single donor platelets (SDPs) collected by plateletapheresis from donors who are HLA-identical to the recipient, whose platelets lack the antigen(s) to which the recipient is sensitized, and/or whose platelets are cross-match-compatible with those of the recipient (110). If the results of HLA *antibody* testing on the recipient are not available, an empiric trial of several transfusions of HLA-matched SDPs using the best match available may be indicated. Table 69.1 lists the grading scale for degree of match of HLA class I antigens between the donor and the recipient. The significant antigens are coded for by two chromosomal loci, designated HLA A and B. Each individual has two alleles at each locus and can synthesize two A and two B antigens. Due to an unfortunate choice of terminology, an identical four-antigen match is called an "A" match. Donor platelets that are a "B" match have one or two antigens that are either related, i.e., cross-reactive, or unknown. "A" and "B" in this context do not refer to the A and B loci. Detection of only one antigen at a locus indicates either that the alleles are homozygous or that the other antigen was untypeable for some reason. B1U (one antigen unknown) and B2U (two antigens unknown) are potentially, but not necessarily, identical to A matches because homozygosity could explain the "unknown" antigen. A "C" match means that one of the four antigens is nonidentical and non–cross-reactive with any of the recipient's antigens. In common usage, the term "HLA-matched" usually implies that the donor and the recipient are a "C" match or better or that the donor lacks the HLA antigen(s) to which the recipient is sensitized. Paradoxically, the best response is not always obtained with the best match (Fig. 69.2). For example, a poor response could be obtained with "B"-matched single donor platelets if they express an antigen to which the recipient is sensitized. On the other hand, a "C" match may give an excellent response if the recipient is not alloimmunized to the one mismatched antigen. The most important factor in choosing the appropriate platelet donor for HLA-alloimmunized patients is the specificity of the recipient's alloantibody. Donors should be chosen who lack any antigen to which the recipient has been alloimmunized or which is cross-reactive with such an antigen. HLA-identical donors are preferred because they will usually be compatible with the recipient's alloantibody and because further alloimmunization is avoided.

Posttransfusion Purpura

Posttransfusion purpura is an immune thrombocytopenia most often seen in multiparous or previously transfused women about 1 week after a blood transfusion (111). Most commonly, the affected individual is a transfusion recipient who lacks the Pl^{A1} platelet antigen, which is present in 98% of individuals. After transfusion, the patient has an anamnestic response due to reexposure to the transfused Pl^{A1} antigen that results in the increased synthesis of a pre-

Table 69.1. HLA Matching Nomenclature[a,b]

Match Grade[c,d]	Description
A	All four donor antigens are identical to those of recipient.
B1U	Three donor antigens are identical to recipient antigens; fourth donor antigen is unknown.
B1X	Three donor antigens are identical to recipient antigens; fourth donor and recipient antigens are cross-reactive.
B2U	Two donor antigens are identical to recipient antigens; third and fourth donor antigens are unknown.
B2UX	Two donor antigens are identical to recipient antigens; third donor antigen is cross-reactive with a recipient antigen; fourth donor antigen is unknown.
B2X	Two donor antigens are identical to recipient antigens; third and fourth donor antigens are both cross-reactive with recipient antigens.
C	Three donor antigens are identical to those of recipient; fourth donor and recipient antigens are nonidentical and noncross-reactive.
D	Two donor and recipient antigens are identical; third and fourth donor antigens are nonidentical and noncross-reactive with recipient antigens.

[a]HLA matching refers to comparisons of the four HLA class I antigens coded by the HLA A and B loci of the transfusion donor and recipient.
[b]Adapted from Duquesnoy RJ, Filip DJ, Rodey GE, Rimm AA, Aster RH. Successful transfusion of platelets "mismatched" for HLA antigens to alloimmunized thrombocytopenic patients. Am J Hematol 1977;2:219–226.
[c]Match grade nomenclature (i.e., A, B, C, D) is unrelated to the similarly named HLA chromosomal loci.
[d]An unknown antigen (U) indicates either homozygosity at a locus or the presence of an antigen that is nonreactive with the typing antisera. An X denotes immunologic cross-reactivity of donor and recipient antigens. A number appearing in the match grade indicates how many donor antigens are unknown or cross-reactive.

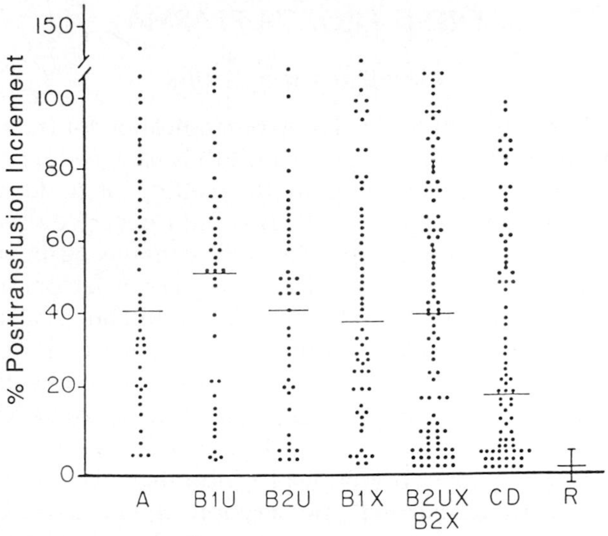

Figure 69.2 Twenty-four hour response of HLA-alloimmunized, thrombocytopenic patients to transfusion of HLA-matched, single donor platelets. See Table 69.1 for description of HLA match grades. R indicates pooled, random platelet concentrates. Median values are indicated by horizontal bars. (From Tomasulo PA. Management of the alloimmunized patient with HLA-matched platelets. In: Schiffer CJ, ed. Platelet physiology and function. Washington DC: American Association of Blood Banks, 1978:69–81.)

viously made anti-Pl^{A1} antibody. The antibody mediates destruction of any remaining transfused Pl^{A1}-positive platelets as well as, paradoxically, the patient's own Pl^{A1}-negative platelets. The mechanism of destruction of the patient's platelets is not clearly understood but may involve immune complex-mediated destruction. The resulting thrombocytopenia is often severe. While it is often a self-limiting condition, even if untreated, the thrombocytopenia may lead to significant hemorrhage, and the low platelet count may persist for more than a month if untreated. Successful therapy has included the use of steroids, intravenous immune globulin, and plasma exchange. Platelet transfusions are ineffective, and the use of platelets from Pl^{A1}-positive donors may be contraindicated, although some believe they may be therapeutic (112). In many patients, transfused Pl^{A1}-negative platelets are also rapidly destroyed as could be predicted based on the destruction of the patient's own Pl^{A1}-negative platelets. If possible, the transfusion of blood components in general should be avoided. Red cells should be washed if obtained from Pl^{A1}-positive or Pl^{A1}-untested donors in an attempt to eliminate platelet microparticles, which might exacerbate the condition. Posttransfusion purpura has been associated with the presence of HLA B8,DR3 antigens in the transfusion recipient (111). The significance of these associations is not known.

Neonatal Alloimmune Thromocytopenia

In neonatal alloimmune thrombocytopenia (NAIT), a pregnant woman becomes alloimmunized to fetal platelet antigens. As with posttransfusion purpura, the woman is commonly Pl^{A1}-negative (111, 113). The mother makes Pl^{A1} antibodies to Pl^{A1}-positive fetal platelets. The antibodies cross the placenta and mediate platelet destruction in the neonate. Thrombocytopenia may be severe and, if untreated, can last for several weeks after delivery. If platelet transfusion is required, the platelets preferentially should be obtained from the mother because her platelets will be compatible. The plasma in the platelet concentrate should be replaced by saline or with albumin-saline to avoid the infusion of additional anti-Pl^{A1}. Platelets could be obtained from a Pl^{A1}-negative donor; however, the antibody involved is not always directed against Pl^{A1}, and furthermore, the neonate will be placed at additional risk of transfusion-transmitted infection. Pl^{A1}-positive or untested platelets are not absolutely contraindicated in NAIT. An important difference from posttransfusion purpura is the fact that, in NAIT, the antibody is passively obtained and of limited quantity rather than being actively produced and replenished.

FRESH FROZEN PLASMA

General Indications

The only uniformly acceptable indication for transfusion of fresh frozen plasma (FFP) is for bleeding or prophylaxis of bleeding in the setting of a documented coagulopathy (114). It should never be used solely as a volume expander. FFP contains approximately the same levels of all coagulation factors as are present in the blood donor. By definition, 1 ml of plasma from a normal individual contains 1 unit of coagulation factor activity. Thus, a unit of FFP with an approximate volume of 200 ml contains about 200 units of each coagulation factor, as well as approximately 300 mg/dl of fibrinogen (fibrinogen is not described in units). FFP, not cryoprecipitate, is indicated for the replacement of multiple coagulation factor deficiencies and for deficiencies of specific factors for which no concentrates are available. FFP is indicated for the treatment of DIC because cryoprecipitate contains only factor VIII, von Willebrand factor, fibrinogen, and factor XIII. Cryoprecipitate does not contain clinically useful quantities of factor V, which is needed in DIC, or many of the other clotting factors. FFP is not the treatment of choice for hemophilia A (factor VIII deficiency) or hemophilia B (factor IX deficiency). The preferred treatments are commercial factor VIII or IX concentrates, respectively, which are solvent/detergent treated, heated, or monoclonal antibody purified.

Dose

FFP should be transfused with a clear understanding of its therapeutic indications. In general, the minimum level of coagulation factors required for hemostasis is 30% of normal (115). For patients with a prolonged PT and PTT who demonstrate abnormal bleeding that is not immediately life-threatening, two units of FFP can be transfused. Further therapy is based on the results of repeat coagulation testing. For immediately life-threatening bleeding in adult patients with a prolonged PT and PTT (1.5 to 1.8-fold increase relative to control), transfusion of 4 or 5 units of FFP should be followed by repeat coagulation testing (116). Four or 5 units of FFP provide about 800 to 1000 ml of plasma, which is equivalent to about 30% of the plasma volume of a 70-kg recipient. This would provide about 30% of normal levels of coagulation factors, assuming a 100% recovery in the intravascular space. Intravascular factor recovery will not be 100% for all factors, but because starting levels may be greater than 0%, 4 or 5 units remains a reasonable dose. However, a major caveat concerns the risk of fluid overload following infusion of large doses of FFP. The physician must be certain that the patient can tolerate the added intravascular fluid volume. For pediatric patients, a usual dose is 10 to 15 ml/kg.

Open Heart Surgery

Patients undergoing open heart surgery are anticoagulated with heparin during the cardiopulmonary bypass to prevent clotting in the extracorporeal circuit. Heparin inhibits coagulation by activating the natural anticoagulant molecule antithrombin III. As a result, during cardiopulmonary bypass, the patient has a prolongation of the prothrombin time, activated partial thromboplastin time, activated clotting time, and thrombin time (69, 70). At the end of cardiopulmonary bypass, the heparin effect is reversed by administering protamine, which binds and inactivates the polyanionic heparin molecule. A residual or rebound heparin effect should be considered as a possible cause of excessive bleeding or abnormal coagulation tests after cardiopulmonary bypass. A heparin effect should be ruled out prior to considering coagulation factor replacement with FFP. Controlling the coagulopathy by "neutralizing" the heparin with more protamine is preferable to the indiscriminate use of potentially biohazardous units of FFP. A heparin-prolonged PT and PTT can be corrected, in vitro, by the addition of hexadimethriene bromide (Polybrene—Aldrich Chemical Co). Similarly, a prolonged thrombin time due to heparin can be reversed in vitro by the addition of protamine or toluidine blue. Heparin characteristically will prolong the thrombin time, but not the reptilase time, whereas true coagulation factor deficiencies prolong both assays. Residual or rebound heparin should be treated in vivo with the appropriate dose of protamine; FFP transfusion in this setting is ineffective; the FFP will not inactivate the excess heparin. On the other hand, abnormal coagulation tests that are not correctable with heparin neutralization in vitro should be considered the result of true coagulation factor deficiencies, and the use of FFP is indicated.

Generally, a so-called "mixing study," in which 50% of the plasma used in the coagulation assay comes from a normal control and is mixed with 50% patient plasma, will help make a diagnosis of specific factor deficiency. A moderate reduction in clotting factor levels and corresponding prolongations in the PT and PTT are common following cardiopulmonary bypass. These changes are rarely associated with excessive bleeding. FFP transfusion should be reserved for cases of excessive bleeding, when the PT- or PTT-to-control ratios are greater than 1.5 to 1.8. This is based on the observation that PT or PTT ratios greater than or equal to 1.8 are correlated with an 80 to 85% chance of developing diffuse microvascular bleeding and are associated with a reduction in clotting factor levels to less than 20% of normal (116). One approach to treating excessive bleeding after cardiopulmonary bypass, which appears to be diffuse and microvascular, is first to transfuse platelets for presumed platelet dysfunction. While platelets are being administered, laboratory testing can proceed to detect any significant coagulopathy and if present, to determine if it is heparin-related or not. A transfusion of pooled platelet concentrates will also provide significant amounts of plasma, which may be sufficient to correct mild clotting factor deficiencies (117). For example, a pool of 8 units of platelet concentrates provides about 400 ml of plasma, a volume equivalent of 2 units of FFP. The plasma from platelet concentrates stored for 5 days contains nearly the same levels of clotting factors as FFP, with the exception of the labile coagulation factors V and VIII, which decrease by about 50% and 30%, respectively, from initial levels.

Massive Transfusion

A coagulopathy may develop in the setting of massive transfusion due to the dilutional effect of transfusing large volumes of RBCs and crystalloid/colloid solutions, which are deficient in coagulation factors. In addition, coagulation factors may be rapidly consumed due to hemorrhage or due to the development of disseminated intravascular coagulation. As with platelet transfusion in the setting of massive blood loss, FFP should not be transfused empirically or by a formula based on the number of units of RBCs transfused (18). A clotting factor deficiency should be documented in the laboratory by an elevation in the prothrombin time and/or partial thromboplastin time to a level greater than 1.5 to 1.8 times the control value. Replacement therapy should be guided by frequent monitoring of coagulation screening tests.

Hepatic Failure

Because most coagulation factors are synthesized in the liver, patients with hepatic failure can develop multiple coagulation factor deficiencies (118). FFP transfusion is indicated in a patient with liver failure for the treatment of bleeding or when preparing the patient for surgery. The dose of FFP should be calculated based on the patient's clinical status, plasma volume, and coagulation factor levels. The prophylactic transfusion of patients with hepatic failure is not recommended.

Reversal of Anticoagulant Effects

FFP transfusion can be used to reverse the anticoagulant effect of coumarin. Due to the risk of allergic or febrile reactions, as well as the risk of disease transmission, FFP transfusion is not indicated to reverse coumarin prior to *elective* surgery. The best approach to reverse the anticoagulant effect of coumarin is to simply stop the drug. In a few days, the patient's coagulation status will return to normal. The use of FFP should be reserved for those life-threatening emergencies that occur while waiting for coumarin to be metabolized or for the reversal effect of administered vitamin K_1 to begin (119). The hemostatic effects of vitamin K_1 may be observed within several hours of plasma administration, and normalization of the prothrombin time may be obtained in some patients within 12 to 14 hours of administration. However, in other patients, the effect of vitamin K_1 may not be manifest until several days after daily vitamin K_1 injections. When this delay puts the patient at risk of significant hemorrhage, FFP transfusion may be indicated. One or two units of FFP may be sufficient for reversing the coumarin effect. The in vivo effect of the FFP should be verified with posttransfusion coagulation screening tests. Larger doses of FFP may be necessary, particularly when the need for an immediate and complete coumarin reversal arises. Factor IX concentrate, which contains factors II, VII, IX, and X, can also be used to reverse coumarin effects in patients at risk of hypervolemic reactions from FFP infusion. The use of factor IX concentrates is associated with increased risks of thromboembolic events. Some believe that the use of factor IX, as well as FFP, should be avoided unless life-threatening hemorrhage, such as might occur with hemopericardium, is present.

Thrombotic Thrombocytopenic Purpura (TTP)

The basis for the therapeutic action of FFP in TTP is still unknown. In addition, the therapeutic dose of FFP has not been firmly established. Therapeutic responses have been observed with doses ranging from as little as 1 unit of FFP/day to daily plasma volume exchange with FFP via plasmapheresis. Whether the removal of the patient's plasma in plasmapheresis is, in itself, also therapeutic, or whether it serves only to facilitate the rapid transfusion of large volumes of FFP, is unclear. However, FFP transfusions alone have been shown to be therapeutic in TTP. Some researchers recommend the use of cryo-poor plasma to prevent transfusion of vWF multimers (120). A typical treatment regimen employs daily plasmapheresis, using FFP for volume replacement. Plasmapheresis and FFP infusions should continue until the clinical status of the patient improves and the platelet counts increase to normal levels (83, 86–88).

Isolated Factor Deficiencies

FFP transfusions are indicated for the replacement of documented isolated deficiencies of factors for which no concentrates exist, e.g., factors V or XI. The clotting factor deficiency should be documented by an abnormal result on the appropriate specific factor assay. Specific concentrates are the treatment of choice for factor VIII and IX deficiencies. Although FFP may be used to treat mild to moderate forms of hemophilia, advances in modern transfusion research have shown that FFP is more likely to pose an increased risk of transfusion-transmitted infections than are the heat-treated, solvent/detergent-treated or monoclonal purified factor concentrates. FFP transfusions are also indicated for the treatment of thrombotic episodes due to congenital deficiencies of antithrombin III or proteins S and C (121, 122).

CRYOPRECIPITATE

General Indications

Cryoprecipitate, properly named cryoprecipitated antihemophilic factor, contains fibrinogen, von Willebrand's factor (vWF), factor XIII, fibronectin, and some other plasma proteins in addition to factor VIII. Cryoprecipitate is not a concentrated form of FFP; it does not contain significant amounts of most of the other coagulation factors, such as factors V, VII, X, and XI. Heat-treated factor VIII concentrates with a reduced risk of hepatitis and HIV transmission have been developed, and cryoprecipitate transfusion, like FFP transfusion, is now considered by some physicians to pose a greater risk of disease transmission (123). As a result, cryoprecipitate is now more important as a source of fibrinogen and vWF than of factor VIII. A fibrinogen level greater than or equal to 50 mg/dl is necessary for efficient hemostasis (116). Fibrinogen repletion is indicated when fibrinogen levels are less than 50 to 100 mg/dl in the setting of hemorrhage or in preparation for surgery. Similarly, for patients with congenitally abnormal or absent fibrinogen, infusion of cryoprecipitate sufficient to give a fibrinogen level of greater than or equal to 50 to 100 mg/dl is indicated for control of hemorrhage or in anticipation of an invasive procedure. Fibrinogen repletion is indicated in DIC if hypofibrinogenemia contributes to serious and life-threatening hemorrhage.

Dose

Dose estimates of the amount of fibrinogen contained in 1 unit of cryoprecipitate range from 100 to 350 mg. In a 70-kg adult with a 2.8 liter blood volume, 1 unit of cryoprecipitate will theoretically raise the fibrinogen level by about 3 to 4 mg/dl, assuming 50% recovery of transfused fibrinogen in the intravascular space and an average content of 200 mg fibrinogen/unit. The appropriate number of units of cryoprecipitate to transfuse can be estimated by dividing the desired increment in fibrinogen (in mg/dl) by 4. An alternative approach is to transfuse a pool of 10 units of cryoprecipitate empirically. The fibrinogen levels should be remeasured shortly after transfusion to ensure that an appropriate level has been obtained.

A new indication for cryoprecipitate is its use in the preparation of fibrin glue (124). To make the glue, cryoprecipitate is added to bovine thrombin. The thrombin converts fibrinogen to fibrin, which forms the glue. Topical fibrin glue has found multiple uses in various surgical procedures. Whenever possible, autologous cryoprecipitate should be used to make fibrin glue.

von Willebrand's Disease

Cryoprecipitate also contains concentrated von Willebrand factor (vWF). The minimum level of vWF required for normal platelet function has not been established. Accordingly, the dose of cryoprecipitate required for vWF repletion for the treatment of hemorrhage or in preparation for surgery is determined empirically; the endpoint is achievement of normal hemostasis and/or correction of a prolonged bleeding time. Because factor VIII circulates as a complex with von Willebrand factor, factor VIII levels in the circulation are also low in von Willebrand's disease. Therefore, sufficient cryoprecipitate should also be transfused in order to maintain factor VIII at levels sufficient to stop hemorrhage, i.e., about 30 to 50% of normal for minor bleeding. A typical starting dose is 1 unit of cryoprecipitate per 10 kg of patient body weight, two to three times daily. The dose can then be adjusted according to clinical response, bleeding time correction, and factor VIII level. It is to be anticipated that, in cases of acquired rather than inherited von Willebrand's disease, required therapeutic doses may be higher, depending upon the activity of the anti-vWF antibody. Therapeutic options other than cryoprecipitate are available for treating vWD. These include use of desmopressin for type I von Willebrand's disease (100). However, desmopressin is contraindicated in type IIb and ineffective in type III vWD (125). Responses have been variable in type IIa vWD (126). Cryoprecipitate is appropriate therapy for all types of vWD. As another option, one commercial factor VIII concentrate, Humate P, which contains sufficient high molecular weight multimers of vWF to be therapeutic in von Willebrand's disease, is also available (127–129).

Hemophilia A (Factor VIII Deficiency)

At least 75% of the bags of cryoprecipitate tested should contain 80 IU of factor VIII (5). Cryoprecipitate can be used to treat bleeding due to factor VIII deficiency or for prophylaxis in a preoperative factor VIII-deficient patient. A factor VIII level of 30 to 50% of normal is required to stop minor hemorrhage. Levels 80 to 100% of normal are indicated in preparation for surgery. The half-life of factor VIII is 12 hours. Thus, doses should be given at 12-hour intervals and must be sufficient to maintain the trough levels of factor VIII in the desired therapeutic range. The dose used should be sufficient to give twice the desired trough level. A dose of cryoprecipitate is calculated as follows:

$$\text{Factor VIII dose (units)} = \frac{[\text{Plasma volume (ml)}] \times [\text{Desired \% factor VIII increment}]}{100}$$

$$\text{Number of bags of cryoprecipitate} = \frac{\text{Units of factor VIII}}{80}$$

Plasma volume can be estimated as [100% − % hematocrit] × [70 ml/kg] × [body weight × (kg)] or 40 ml/kg × body weight (kg) for a patient with a normal hematocrit.

The development of effective viral inactivation techniques has made commercial pooled factor VIII concentrates the preferred treatment for hemophilia A (123). Multiple pooled units of cryoprecipitate no longer offer a safety advantage over factor VIII concentrates, and they may pose a greater risk of HIV and hepatitis transmission. However, the safest treatment for mild-moderate hemophilia A or von Willebrand's disease from the standpoint of viral transmission is the pharmacological agent desmopressin (100).

Factor XIII Deficiency

Factor XIII is concentrated 1.5- to 4-fold in cryoprecipitate as compared to plasma. Factor XIII is a transketolase; it crosslinks fibrin monomers and stabilizes fibrin clot formation (130). Cryoprecipitate is indicated for the treatment of rare, factor XIII-deficient patients who are bleeding or who are being prepared for surgery. The hemostatic levels of factor XIII in bleeding patients are very low, and the half-life of factor XIII is long (i.e., about 12 days). A therapeutic dose for an average adult is 4 to 6 bags of cryoprecipitate every 3 weeks (131–132).

Uremia

Cryoprecipitate transfusions, at a dose of 1 bag per 10 kg of patient body weight, shorten bleeding times and control bleeding in some patients with uremic bleeding (101, 133–134). The element of cryoprecipitate responsible for this effect is unknown, but vWF or factor VIII are possible candidates. The therapeutic effect of cryoprecipitate is evident within 30 to 90 minutes of transfusion and lasts about 8 hours. Better treatments for the thrombocytopathy of uremia are dialysis, either hemo- or peritoneal, which removes the toxin(s) that may be responsible for platelet dysfunction, and RBC transfusion.

ADMINISTRATION OF BLOOD COMPONENTS

Blood Filters

Blood filters are a required part of all blood administration sets. There are three general categories of blood filters, which can be conveniently divided into generations (135, 136). A first-generation filter refers to a 170 to 260 μm clot screen that is used to remove blood clots, coagula, and other debris that form in blood during storage. A second-generation filter refers to a 20 to 40 μm blood filter that removes microaggregates that form in blood during storage. Microaggregates are composed of decaying white blood cells, platelets, and fibrin strands. Third-generation blood filters are leukocyte depletion filters that work on a principle of adsorption of blood elements to a filter (137). The media is coated with various chemical polymers, which impart surface tension characteristics to the fiber. Differences in surface tension associated with different polymer coatings permit the filters to remove different cells from filtered blood. These third-generation filters are useful for removing individual white cells and may play a role in the prevention of alloimmunization and disease transmission.

FIRST-GENERATION FILTERS

First-generation blood filters are primarily clot screens that are designed to remove clots that form in blood during storage (135). The importance of such a filter was recognized early in transfusion practice when blood was stored in glass bottles. The clots that formed were removed primarily by pouring the blood through a wire mesh screen and sterilized cotton gauze. Today, the filters are made of plastic mesh screens. The need for a 170- to 260-μm filter is universally accepted, and its use is required for administration of all blood components, including red cells, granulocytes, FFP, cryoprecipitate, and platelets, as well as factor VIII or IX concentrates. For the latter derivatives, filtration is accomplished through the use of filter needles.

SECOND-GENERATION FILTERS

Second-generation filters function by either interception or depth filtration. Second-generation microaggregate filters became popular during the 1960s when amnesia, renal failure, and visual disturbances occurred in patients after open heart surgery (135). These symptoms were attributed to microaggregate debris in the capillary beds of end organs, such as the kidney, the brain, and the retina of the eye. On investigation, this material was found to stain periodic acid–Schiff (PAS) positive as microaggregate debris was known to do. Furthermore, during the Vietnam War, soldiers receiving massive tranfusion were noted to have pulmonary dysfunction, often with development of adult respiratory distress syndrome (138–140). The cause of this pulmonary injury was attributed to microaggregate debris in the pulmonary microvasculature. Several studies purported to show that the infusion of microaggregate debris during massive transfusion was associated with respiratory distress syndrome. However, studies subsequently showed that microaggregate debris, per se, although possibly causing some degree of pulmonary dysfunction, was not the primary cause of the respiratory distress syndrome in this setting. The primary cause of this syndrome in multiply transfused patients was attributed to the nature of the trauma (141).

However, second-generation filters, by virtue of their ability to remove 1 to 2 logs of leukocytes, have been reported useful for the prevention of febrile transfusion reactions. A variety of techniques can be used to achieve this goal; the most efficient is the spin-cool filter technique (142).

THIRD-GENERATION FILTERS

Third-generation microaggregate filters were developed to permit the removal of individual white cells from units of blood components (143–146). These filters are very efficient and can remove 3 logs or more of white cells from units of blood and components. A unit of blood that contains 450 ml, collected from a patient with a white blood count (WBC) of 5000/μl, contains 2.25×10^9 white cells in the blood bag. A 3-log reduction will lower the number of white cells to 2.25×10^6. A level of 10^6 WBC is felt by some to be the threshold level of residual white cells per transfusion that will prevent, or at least delay, the onset on HLA alloimmunization (104–107).

Other studies in progress appear to show that a 3-log removal of white blood cells is also sufficient to render CMV-positive units of blood unable, or unlikely, to transmit CMV infection (147, 148). This may be of value for transfusing patients who have had bone marrow or organ transplants or for transfusing premature infants when the supply of CMV-negative blood may be insufficient to meet the demand. Although admittedly there are still 6 logs of white cells left that may contain CMV, studies have shown that the 1- to 2-log reduction in WBC achieved with frozen deglycerolized red cells will prevent the transmission of CMV infection by blood transfusion. A 3-log reduction filter, which is more efficient, would thus probably be equally as successful. Further data are necessary before filtration to prevent transmission of CMV infection is generally accepted.

Another potential use of third-generation filters is in the prevention of posttransfusion graft versus host disease (GVHD). This could occur due to the reduction in the number of white cells below the level that is felt to be necessary for the induction of GVHD, approximately 10^7 lymphocytes per kilogram body weight. However, more data are needed before conclusions can be drawn. Thus, third-generation filters will likely play a significant role in transfusions in the future (136, 149).

Blood Warmers

Warming blood became a part of transfusion practice when ventricular arrhythmias were noted in individuals undergoing major cancer surgery during rapid infusions of cold blood, approximately 1 unit/5 minutes. Warming blood to 37°C during rapid infusion prevented these adverse effects on the patient's cardiac status (29–32). Some physicians favor warming all units of blood. However, there are dangers associated with the indiscriminate warming of blood. Blood can be warmed in several ways (150). The entire bag can be immersed in warm (37°C) water. If the waterbath is not closely monitored, there is a risk of hemolysis if the blood is heated to over 40°C. In addition, there is a risk of bacterial growth and contamination if the units are put back on the shelf after warming. Finally, there is a risk of contamination of the administration outlet ports of the bag with various organisms, especially *Pseudomonas cepacia*, which can grow in the water in the waterbath. Using contaminated waterbaths to thaw or heat units of blood components can produce sepsis. One type of blood warmer is a simple plastic coil, which is designed to either remain at ambient temperature or which can be placed in a monitored waterbath. The placement of the plastic coil in a monitored waterbath is acceptable, but again, it should not be used indiscriminantly. It is imperative that the temperature of the waterbath be monitored to ensure that the temperature of the blood transfused remains below 40°C.

Another type of blood warmer heats using metal plates. The blood is circulated in a bag in close contact with metal plates that are electrically heated. This type of device, with proper quality controls at regular intervals and monitoring to ensure maintenance of the proper temperature, is safe and acceptable for use, but it should not be used indiscriminately. The temperatures of the blood warmers should be measured with mercury thermometers or some equivalent standard.

Microwave blood warmers also have been developed (151, 152). A generic problem with these devices is the development of hot-spots, which can induce hemolysis in units of red blood cells. Accordingly, a microwave warmer should not be used to warm units of RBCs or frozen RBCs. Fresh frozen plasma, however, can be thawed in a microwave. There are several models available that rotate the plasma to prevent excessive heating.

Finally, there are devices that utilize heat exchangers, in which the heat from quantities of very hot water is rapidly placed in contact with RBCs. The temperature of the cold blood mixing in the heat exchanger rapidly rises and does not exceed 40° (153). Although this temperature exceeds the 38° considered acceptable by the American Association of Blood Banks (5), it does not appear to be associated with hemolysis.

The routine use of blood warmers should be avoided because there are definite problems associated with overwarming a unit of blood. First, as previously mentioned, there is the risk of hemolysis and bacterial contamination. Second, heating blood often slows the rate of administration, which could be a problem if blood is needed rapidly (e.g., in a trauma setting). A unit of blood that has been warmed to above 10°C cannot be returned to the blood bank for storage (154). It is not acceptable to re-store a unit of blood that has been warmed. Several different organisms have been reported to grow in such units of blood (155).

Compatible IV Solutions

Only normal (0.9%) saline should be added to blood during infusion (5). Glucose solutions should not be used because the sugar easily passes the cell membrane, making the inside of the cell hyperosmotic. When these hyperosmotic units of blood are transfused, water enters the cell to restore osmotic balance. The red cells swell in response to the influx of water, and the cell mechanically hemolyzes when the red cell volume exceeds 180 fl. If lactated Ringer's solution, which contains 3 mEq/liter of calcium, is used to dilute units of red cells, the calcium could cause clots to form in the unit. Medications should never be added to a unit of blood (5). If the patient experiences a transfusion reaction and the transfusion is halted, the patient may not receive all of the needed medication. Furthermore, if the patient has a transfusion reaction during the administration of blood that contains medication, the cause of the reaction may be unclear because the reaction could be attributed to either the blood or the medication.

Blood Pumps

The infusion of blood in certain situations in which control over the rate and speed of infusion is important can be achieved with the use of blood pumps. A variety of electromechanical blood pumps that can pump from 0.9 to 999 ml an hour are available (150). Pumps work on the principle of ejecting a given volume of blood at a variable rate. Some pumps require special cassettes or software, while others will use most types of available administration tubing. The most important consideration when using any of these devices is to ensure that RBC do not hemolyze. Red cell viscosity and shear forces increase exponentially as the hematocrit increases above 55%. Accordingly, with some units of RBC with high hematocrits, the shear stress generated by a pump mechanism may be high enough to produce hemolysis. Hemolysis is less likely to occur as the hematocrit of the pumped blood falls. Shear stress-related damage does not occur when pumping platelets or fresh frozen plasma.

Reports describing the infusion of blood through several of these devices have been published (156, 157). The indiscriminant use of pumps is not encouraged, especially in trauma settings, because, like blood warmers, their use may slow the rate of infusion. However, in pediatric patients or in patients who are prone to febrile reactions, slowing the rate and time of blood administration may have a beneficial effect on transfusion outcome. Some electromechanical pumps are also acceptable for the infusion of granulocytes (158). A general rule to follow when evaluating a new pump is to have the manufacturer provide data showing that the pump is capable of handling all blood components, especially red blood cells, without adverse effect.

Transfusion Procedure

The actual infusion of a unit of blood or blood components requires great care and concentration to ensure that safe transfusion practices are being observed (2). First, a physician should discuss the need for the blood transfusion with the patient and document in the chart that informed consent has been obtained. Baseline vital signs should be obtained. Appropriate documentation, including the appropriate component, the volume desired, the duration of transfusion, and the infusion rate, should be written in the chart. The patient should be premedicated as per physician's orders. The component should be inspected for leaks and abnormal color, and the identification of both the patient and the unit should be verified by two qualified individuals and documented in the chart. No transfusion should be given unless all verifying information matches exactly. Blood should be administered through a filter and should not be transfused over longer than 4 hours. The infusion should start slowly at a rate less than or equal to 5 ml/min for the first 15 minutes. The patient should be observed closely throughout the transfusion. Symptoms of a severe transfusion reaction are usually manifested in the first 15 minutes of a transfusion. Thus, it is advisable to remain with the patient for the first few minutes after a transfusion has started. The patient's vital signs should be monitored as necessary, and the results of the transfusion should be recorded as part of the permanent record. After the tranfusion is completed, the patient should be studied to ensure that the results of the transfusion are appropriate. For example, after a platelet transfusion, a platelet count is desirable to ensure that the patient responded to the transfusion. Use of any warmers or blood filters should also be appropriately documented in the chart.

Home Transfusion

As hospital medicine shifts to the outpatient area, transfusion of the patient in the home is becoming more a part of modern transfusion practice. Home blood transfusion should follow the same practices and principles that transfusion in the hospital setting requires. A variety of patients may benefit from home transfusion (159, 160). This includes AIDS patients who are on AZT and who may require blood transfusion, thrombocytopenic oncology patients, or pediatric oncology patients. Home transfusion should never be performed because of mere convenience. There should be a sound medical indication for performing a transfusion in the home, and that indication should outweigh the risk of out-of-hospital transfusion reactions.

Patients who are fully ambulatory and could travel to the hospital transfusion service should do so, rather than have transfusions at home. In order for transfusions to occur at home, it is important that nurses or other health care providers who are trained to administer blood be available, that medications are available should a patient experience an untoward reaction, and that the providers are trained in emergency procedures. It is important that the blood product(s) be infused at an appropriate rate and that too many blood products not be infused over too short a time. The staff should be adequately trained in CPR, and physician back-up, either in an office or emergency room, must be immediately available by phone. Written protocols outlining the procedures to be followed in the event of an untoward reaction to transfusion or other emergency should be provided. The provider should never be alone in the house with the patient; there should be at least one other person present in the home who can speak English. This allows the provider to take care of the patient while the other individual can be available to call for help, if necessary. It is important that the blood samples for cross-matching be appropriately labeled and that posttransfusion laboratory tests be performed to ensure that the patient has responded appropriately to the transfusion. The local state laws regarding the infusion of medication by nonphysicians and the ability of the provider to administer a transfusion independently must be checked before a home transfusion program is established. In addition, the disposal of waste material, such as sharps and blood-soaked gauze and needles, needs to be planned to ensure compliance with all appropriate safety codes. Home blood transfusion can be a safe and convenient medical practice; however, care must be taken to ensure that the motivation for the home transfusion request is the patient's medical care and safety and not mere convenience.

References

1. NIH Consensus Conference. Perioperative red blood cell transfusion. JAMA 1988;260:2700–2703.
2. Walker RH. Blood transfusion practice. In: Technical manual. 10th ed. Arlington, VA: American Association of Blood Banks, 1990:342–375.
3. Moore FD. The effects of hemorrhage on body composition. N Engl J Med 1965;273:567–577.
4. Ebert RV, Stead EA Jr, Gibson JG. Response of normal subjects to acute blood loss. Arch Intern Med 1941;68:578–590.
5. Holland PV, ed. Standards for blood banks and transfusion services. 13th ed. Arlington, VA: American Association of Blood Banks, 1989.
6. Giblett ER. Blood group antibodies: an assessment of some laboratory practices. Transfusion 1977;17:299–308.
7. Vichinsky EP, Earles A, Johnson RA, Hoag MS, Williams A, Lubin B. Alloimmunization in sickle cell anemia and transfusion of racially unmatched blood. N Engl J Med 1990;332: 1617–1621.
8. Rosse WF, Gallagher D, Kinney TR, et al. Transfusion and alloimmunization in sickle cell disease. Blood 1990;76:1431–1437.
9. Blumberg N, Bove JR. Un-crossmatched blood for emergency transfusion: one year's experience in a civilian setting. JAMA 1978;240:2057–2059.

10. Lefebre J, McLellan B, Coovadia AS. Seven years experience with Group O, unmatched packed red blood cells in a regional trauma unit. Ann Emerg Med 1987;16:1344–1359.
11. Schwab CW, Shayne JP, Turner J. Immediate trauma resuscitation with type O uncrossmatched blood: a two-year prospective experience. J Trauma 1986;26:897–902.
12. Mollison PL, Engelfriet CP, Contreras M. The Rh blood group system. In: Blood transfusion in clinical medicine. 8th ed. London: Blackwell, 1987:330–401.
13. Issitt P. The Rh blood group system. In: Applied blood group serology. 3rd ed. Miami: Montgomery, 1985:219–277.
14. Collins JA. Problems associated with the massive transfusion of stored blood. Surgery 1974;75:274–295.
15. Counts RB, Haisch C, Simon TL, Maxwell NG, Heimbach DM, Carrico CJ. Hemostasis in massively transfused trauma patients. Ann Surg 1979;190:91–99.
16. Hewson JR, Neame PB, Kumar N, et al. Coagulopathy related to dilution and hypotension during massive transfusion. Crit Care Med 1985;13:387–391.
17. Slichter SP. Identification and management of defects in platelet hemostasis in massively transfused patients. In: Collins JA, Murawski K, Shafer AW, eds. Massive transfusion in surgery and trauma. New York: Alan R. Liss, 1982:225–258.
18. Mannucci PM, Federici AB, Sirchia G. Hemostasis testing during massive blood replacement—a study of 172 cases. Vox Sang 1982;42:113–123.
19. Dzik WH, Kirkley SA. Citrate toxicity during massive blood transfusion. Trans Med Rev 1988;2:76–94.
20. Marquez J, Martin D, Virji MA, et al. Cardiovascular depression secondary to ionic hypocalcemia during hepatic transplantation in humans. Anesthesiology 1986;65:457–461.
21. Denlinger JK, Nahrwold ML, Gibbs PS. Hypocalcemia during rapid blood transfusion in an anesthetized man. Br J Anaesth 1976;48:995–999.
22. Hester JP, McCullough J, Mishler JM, Szymanski IO. Dosage regimens for citrate anticoagulants. J. Clin Apheresis 1983;1: 149–152.
23. Wolf PL, McCarthy LJ, Hafleigh B. Extreme hypercalcemia following blood transfusion combined with intravenous calcium. Vox Sang 1970;19:544–545.
24. McLellan BA, Reid SR, Land PL. Massive blood transfusion causing hypomagnesemia. Crit Care Med 1984;12:146–147.
25. Latham JT, Bove JR, Weirich FL. Chemical and hematologic changes in stored CPDA-1 blood. Transfusion 1982;22:158–159.
26. Driscoll DF, Bistrian BR, Jenkins RL, et al. Development of metabolic alkalosis after massive transfusion during orthopedic liver transplantation. Crit Care Med 1987;15:905–908.
27. Blanchette VS, Gray E, Hardie MJ, et al. Hyperkalemia after neonatal exchange transfusion: risk eliminated by washing red cell concentrates. J Pediatr 1984;105:321–324.
28. Carmichael D, Hosty T, Kastle D, Beckman D. Hypokalemia and massive transfusion. South Med J 1984;77:315–317.
29. Boyan CP. Cold or warmed blood for massive transfusions. Ann Surg 1964;160:282–286.
30. Collins JA. Problems associated with massive transfusion of stored blood. Surgery 1974;75:274–295.
31. Boyan CP, Howland WS. Cardiac arrest and temperature of bank blood. JAMA 1963;183:58–60.
32. Boyan CP, Howland WS. Blood temperature: a critical factor in massive transfusion. Anesthesiology 1961;22:559–563.
33. Charache S. Problems in transfusion therapy [Editorial]. N Engl J Med 1990;322:166–168.
34. Blumberg N. Beyond ABO and D antigen matching: how far and for whom? [Editorial]. Transfusion 1990;30:482–484.
35. Blumberg N, Ross K, Avila E, Peck K. Should chronic transfusions be matched for antigens other than ABO and Rh_o(D)? Vox Sang 1984;47:205–208.
36. Fluit CRMG, Kunst VAJM, Drenthe-Schonk AM. Incidence of red cell antibodies after multiple blood transfusion. Transfusion 1990;30:532–535.
37. Marcus CS, Huehns ER. Transfusional iron overload. Clin Lab Haematol 1985;7:195–212.
38. Miller DR, Giardina PV. Congenital hemolytic anemias. In: Petz LD, Swisher SN, eds. Clinical practice of transfusion medicine. 2nd ed. New York: Churchill Livingstone, 1989;583–613.
39. Cohen A. Current status of iron chelation therapy with deferoxamine. Semin Hematol 1990;27:86–90.
40. The National Blood Resource Education Program Expert Panel. The use of autologous blood. JAMA 1990;263:414–417.
41. Perkins HA. Autologous transfusion. Adv Intern Med 1990;35:221–233.
42. Simon TL, Smith KJ. The issue in autologous transfusion. Hum Pathol 1989;20:3–6.
43. Toy PTCY, Strauss RG, Stehling LE, et al. Predeposited autologous blood for elective surgery. A national multicenter study. N Engl J Med 1987;316:517–520.
44. Mintz P. Autologous transfusion endorsed. JAMA 1985;254: 507.
45. Maffei LM, Thurer RL, eds. Autologous blood transfusion: current issues. Arlington, VA: American Association of Blood Banks, 1988.
46. Owings DV, Kruskall LMS, Thurer RL, Donovan LM. Autologous blood donations prior to elective cardiac surgery: safety and effect of subsequent blood use. JAMA 1989;262: 1963–1968.
47. Pindyck J, Avorn J, Kuriyan M, et al. Blood donation by the elderly. Clinical and policy considerations. JAMA 1987;257: 3403–3404.
48. McVay PA, Andrews A, Kaplan EB, et al. Donation reactions among autologous donors. Transfusion 1990;30:249–252.
49. Jobes DR, Gallagher J. Acute normovolemic hemodilution. Int Anesthesiol Clin 1982;20:59–76.
50. Shah DM, Prichard MN, Newell JC, et al. Increased cardiac output and oxygen transport after intraoperative isovolemic hemodilution. Arch Surg 1980;115:597–600.
51. AABB Autologous Transfusion Committee. Guidelines for blood salvage and reinfusion in surgery and trauma. Arlington: American Association of Blood Banks, 1990:1–12.
52. Williamson KR, Taswell HF. Indications for intraoperative blood salvage. J Clin Apheresis 1990;5:100–103.
53. Hartz RS, Smith JA, Green D. Autotransfusion after cardiac operation. J Thorac Cardiovasc Surg 1988;96:178–182.
54. Tyson GS, Sladen RN, Spainhour V, Savitt MA, Ferguson TB, Wolfe WG. Blood conservation in cardiac surgery. Ann Surg 1989;209:736–742.
55. McCarthy PM, Popovsky MA, Schaff HV, et al. Effect of blood conservation efforts in cardiac operations at the Mayo Clinic. Mayo Clin Proc 1988;63:225–229.
56. Hallett JW, Popovsky M, Ilstrup D. Minimizing blood transfusions during abdominal aortic surgery: recent advances in rapid autotransfusion. J. Vasc Surg 1987;5:601–606.
57. Dale RF, Kipling RM, Smith MF, Collier DSJ, Smith PJ. Separation of malignant cells during autotransfusion. Br J Surg 1988;75:581.
58. Stack G, Snyder EL. Alternatives to perioperative blood transfusion. Adv Anesth 1991;8:209–240.
59. Page R, Russell GN, Fox MA, et al. Hard-shell cardiotomy reservoir for reinfusion of shed mediastinal blood. Ann Surg 1989;48:514–517.

60. Duncan SE, Edwards WH, Dale WA. Caution regarding autotransfusion. Surgery 1974;76:1024.
61. Griffith LD, Billman GF, Daily PO, Lane TA. Apparent coagulopathy caused by infusion of shed mediastinal blood and its prevention by washing of the infusate. Ann Thorac Surg 1989;47:400–406.
62. Gaydos LA, Freireich EJ, Mantel N. The quantitative relation between platelet count and hemorrhage in patients with acute leukemia. N Engl J Med 1962;266:905–909.
63. NKH Consensus Conference. Platelet transfusion therapy JAMA 1987;257:1777–1780.
64. Slichter SJ. Platelet transfusion therapy. Hematol Oncl Clin North Am 1990;4:291–311.
65. Daly PA, Schiffer CA, Aisner J, Wiernik PH. Platelet transfusion therapy; one-hour posttransfusion increments are valuable in predicting the need for HLA-matched preparations. JAMA 1980;243:435–438.
66. Bishop JF, McGrath K, Wolf MM, et al. Clinical factors influencing the efficacy of pooled platelet transfusions. Blood 1988;71:383–387.
67. Ferraris VA, Gildengorin V. Predictors of excessive blood use after coronary artery bypass grafting. J. Thorac Cardiovasc Surg 1989;98:492–497.
68. Zilla P, Fasol R. Groscurth P, et al. Blood platelets in cardiopulmonary bypass operations. J Thorac Cardiovasc Surg 1989;97:379–388.
69. Mammen EF, Koets MH, Washington BC, et al. Hemostasis changes during cardiopulmonary bypass surgery. Semin Thromb Hemost 1985;11:281–292.
70. Bick RL. Hemostasis defects associated with cardiac surgery, prosthetic devices and other extracorporeal circuits. Semin Thromb Hemost 1985;11:249–280.
71. Michaelson EL, Torosian M. Morganroth J, et al. Early recognition of surgically correctable causes of excessive mediastinal bleeding after coronary artery bypass graft surgery. Am J Surg 1980;139:313–317.
72. Harker LA, Malpass TW, Branson HE, et al. Mechanism of abnormal bleeding in patients undergoing cardiopulmonary bypass: acquired transient platelet dysfunction associated with selective alpha granule release. Blood 1990;56:824–834.
73. Simon TL, Akl BF, Murphy W. Controlled trial of routine administration of platelet concentrates in cardiopulmonary bypass surgery. Ann Thorac Surg 1984;37:359–364.
74. Burns ER, Billet HH, Frater RW, Sisto DA. The preoperative bleeding time as a predictor of postoperative hemorrhage after cardiopulmonary bypass. J Thorac Cardiovasc Surg 1986;92:310–312.
75. Harding SA, Shakoor MA, Grindon AJ. Platelet support for cardiopulmonary bypass surgery. J Thorac Cardiovasc Surg 1975;70:350–353.
76. Deykin D, Janson P, McMahon L. Ethanol potentiation of aspirin-induced prolongation of the bleeding time. N Engl J Med 1982;306:852–854.
77. DeCaterina R, Giannessi D, Boem A, et al. Equal antiplatelet effects of aspirin 50 or 324 mg/day in patients after acute myocardial infarction. Thromb Haemost 1985;54:528–532.
78. Carr JM, Kruskall MS, Kaye JA, Robinson SH. Efficacy of platelet transfusions in immune thrombocytopenia. Am J Med 1986;80:1051–1054.
79. Berchtold P, McMillan R. Therapy of chronic idiopathic thrombocytopenic purpura in adults. Blood 1989;74:2309–2317.
80. Bussel JB, Saal S, Gordon B. Combined plasma exchange and intravenous gammaglobulin in the treatment of patients with refractory immune thrombocytopenic purpura. Transfusion 1988;28:38–41.
81. Baumann MA, Menitove JE, Aster RH, Anderson T. Urgent treatment of idiopathic thrombocytopenic purpura with single-dose gammaglobulin infusion followed by platelet transfusion. Ann Intern Med 1986;104:804–809.
82. Bussel JB, Pham LC. Intravenous treatment with gammaglobulin in adults with immune thrombocytopenic purpura: review of the literature. Vox Sang 1987;52:206–211.
83. Lian ECY. Thrombotic thrombocytopenic purpura. Annu Rev Med 1988;39:203–212.
84. Gordon LI, Kwaan HC, Rossi EC. Deleterious effects of platelet transfusions and recovery thrombocytosis in patients with thrombotic microangiopathy. Semin Hematol 1987;24:194–201.
85. Harkness DR, Byrnes JJ, Lian ECY, Williams WD, Hensley GT. Hazard of platelet transfusion in thrombotic thrombocytopenic purpura. JAMA 1981;246:1931–1933.
86. Shepard KV, Bukowski RM. The treatment of thrombotic thrombocytopenic purpura with exchange transfusions, plasma infusions, and plasma exchange. Semin Hematol 1987;24:178–193.
87. Lichtin AE, Schreiber AD, Hurwitz S, Willoughby TL, Silberstein LE. Efficacy of intensive plasmapheresis in thrombotic thrombocytopenic purpura. Arch Intern Med 1987;147:2122–2126.
88. Schmidt JL. Thrombotic thrombocytopenic purpura: successful treatment unlocks etiologic secrets. Mayo Clin Proc 1989;64:956–961.
89. Jubelirer SJ. Hemostatic abnormalities in renal disease. Am J Kidney Dis 1985;5:219–225.
90. Remuzzi G. Bleeding in renal failure. Lancet 1988;1:1205–1208.
91. Escolar G, Cases A, Bastida E, et al. Uremic platelets have a functional defect affecting the interaction of von Willebrand factor with glycoprotein IIb-IIIa. Blood 1990;76:1336–1340.
92. Carvalho AC. Acquired platelet dysfunction in patients with uremia. Hematol Oncol Clin North Am 1990;4:129–143.
93. Horowitz HI, Stein M, Cohen BD, White JG. Further studies on the platelet inhibitor effect of guanidinosuccinic acid and its role in uremic bleeding. Am J Med 1970;49:336–345.
94. Livio M, Marchesi D, Remuzzi G, et al. Uremic bleeding: role of anemia and beneficial effect of red cell transfusions. Lancet 1982;2:1013–1015.
95. Fernandez F, Goudable C, Sie P, et al. Low hematocrit and prolonged bleeding time in uremic patients: effect of red cell transfusions. Br J Haematol 1985;59:139–148.
96. Moia M, Mannucci PM, Vizzott L, Casati S, Cattaneo M, Ponticelli C. Improvement in the haemostatic effect of uraemia after treatment with recombinant human erythropoietin. Lancet 1987;2:1227–1229.
97. Eschbach JW, Egrie JC, Downing MR, Browne JK, Adamson JW. Correction of the anemia of end-stage renal disease with recombinant human erythropoietin. N Engl J Med 1987;316:73–78.
98. Watson AJS, Keogh JAB. Effect of 1-deamino-8-D-arginine vasopressin on the prolonged bleeding time in chronic renal failure. Nephron 1982;32:49–52.
99. Mannucci PM, Remuzzi G, Pusineri F, et al. Deamino-8-D-arginine vasopressin shortens the bleeding time in uremia. N Engl J Med 1983;308:8–12.
100. Mannucci PM. Desmopressin: a nontransfusional form of treatment for congenital and acquired bleeding disorders. Blood 1988;72:1449–1455.
101. Janson PA, Jubelirer SJ, Weinstein MJ, Deykin D. Treatment of the bleeding tendency in uremia with cryoprecipitate. N Engl J Med 1980;303:1318–1322.
102. Liu YK, Kosfeld RE, Marcum SG. Treatment of uremic bleeding with conjugated estrogen. Lancet 1984;2:887–890.

103. Livio M, Mannucci PM, Vigano G, et al. Conjugated estrogens for the management of bleeding associated with renal failure. N Engl J Med 1986;315:731–735.
104. Sniecinski I, O'Donnell MR, Nowicki B, Hill LR. Prevention of refractoriness and HLA-alloimmunization using filtered blood products. Blood 1988;71:1402–1407.
105. Andreu G, Dewailly J, Leberre C, et al. Prevention of HLA immunization with leukocyte-poor packed red cells and platelet concentrates obtained by filtration. Blood 1988;72: 964–969.
106. Meryman HT. Transfusion-induced alloimmunization and immunosuppression and the effects of leukocyte depletion. Transfusion Med Rev 1989;3:180–193.
107. Saarinen UM, Kekomaki R, Siimes MA, Myllyla G. Effective prophylaxis against platelet refractories in multitransfused patients by use of leukocyte-free blood components. Blood 1990;75:512–517.
108. O'Connell B, Lee EJ, Schiffer CA. The value of 10-minute posttransfusion platelet counts. Transfusion 1988;28:66–67.
109. Hussein MA, Lee EJ, Schiffer CA. Platelet transfusions administered to patients with splenomegaly. Transfusion 1990;30:508–510.
110. van Rood JJ. The impact of the HLA system in clinical hematology. Blutalkohol 1989;59:214–220.
111. Kunicki TJ, Beardsley DS. The alloimmune thrombocytopenias: neonatal alloimmune thrombocytopenic purpura and post-transfusion purpura. Prog Hemost Thromb 1989;9:203 232.
112. Brecher ME, Moore SB, Letendre L. Posttransfusion purpura: the therapeutic value of Pl^{A1}-negative platelets. Transfusion 1990;30:433–435.
113. Reznikoff-Etievant MF. Management of alloimmune neonatal and antenatal thrombocytopenia. Vox Sang 1988;55:192–201.
114. NIH Consensus Conference. Fresh frozen plasma: indications and risks. JAMA 1985;253:551–553.
115. Menitove JE. Preparation and clinical use of plasma and plasma fractions. In: Williams WJ, Beutler E, Erslev AJ, Lichtman MA, eds. Hematology. 4th ed. New York: McGraw-Hill 1990:1669–1673.
116. Ciavarella D, Reed RL, Counts RB, et al. Clotting factor levels and the risk of diffuse microvascular bleeding in the massively transfused patient. Br J Haematol 1987;67:365–368.
117. Simon TL, Henderson R. Coagulation factor activity in platelet concentrates. Transfusion 1979;19:186–189.
118. Friedman EW, Sussman II. Safety of invasive procedures in patients with the coagulopathy of liver disease. Clin Lab Haematol 1989;11:199–204.
119. Bolan CD, Alving BM. Pharmacologic agents in the management of bleeding disorders. Transfusion 1990;30:541–551.
120. Byrnes JJ, Moake JL, Klug P, Periman P. Effectiveness of the cryosupernatant fraction of plasma in the treatment of refractory thrombotic thrombocytopenia purpura. Am J Hematol 1990;34:169–174.
121. Esmon CT. Protein C. Prog Hemost Thromb 1984;7:25–54.
122. Hultin MA, McKay J, Abildgaard U. Antithrombin Oslo: type 1b classification of the first reported-deficient family, with a review of hereditary antithrombin variants. Thromb Haemost 1988;59:468–473.
123. Aronson DL. The development of the technology and capacity for the production of factor VIII for the treatment of hemophilia A. Transfusion 1990;30:748–758.
124. Gibble JW, Ness PM. Fibrin glue: the perfect operative sealant? Transfusion 1990;30:741–747.
125. Holmberg L, Nilsson IM, Borge L, et al. Platelet aggregation induced by 1-deamino-8-D-arginine vasopressin (DDAVP) in type IIb von Willebrand's disease. N Engl J Med 1983;309: 816–821.
126. Gralnick HR, Williams SB, McKeown LP, et al. DDAVP in type IIa von Willebrand's disease. Blood 1986;67:465–468.
127. Berntorp E, Nilsson IM. Use of a high-purity factor VIII concentrate (Humate P) in von Willebrand's disease. Vox Sang 1989;56:212–217.
128. Frick WA, Yu MY. Characterization of von Willebrand factor in factor VIII concentrates. Am J Hematol 1989;31:41–45.
129. Mazurier C, DeRoumeuf C, Parquet-Gernez A, Goudemand M. In vitro and in vivo characterization of a high-purity, solvent/detergent-treated factor VIII concentrate: evidence for its therapeutic efficacy in von Willebrand's disease. Eur J Haematol 1989;43:7–14.
130. Kitchens CS, Newcomb TF. Factor XIII. Medicine 1979;58: 413–429.
131. Amris CJ, Hilden M. Treatment of factor XIII deficiency with cryoprecipitate. Thromb Diath Haemorrh 1968;20:528–533.
132. Fisher S, Rikover M, Nady S. Factor 13 deficiency with severe hemorrhagic diathesis. Blood 1966;28:34–39.
133. Juhl A. DDAVP, cryoprecipitate, and highly "purified" factor VIII concentrate in uremia. Nephron 1986;43:305–306.
134. Triulzi DJ, Blumberg N. Variability in response to cryoprecipitate treatment for hemostatic effects in uremia. Yale J Biol Med 1990;63:1–7.
135. Snyder EL, Bookbinder M. Role of microaggregate blood filtration in clinical medicine. Transfusion 1983;23:460–470.
136. Snyder EL. Clinical use of white cell-poor blood components [Editorial]. Transfusion 1989;29:568–571.
137. Miyamoto M, Sasakawa S, Ishikawa Y, Ogawa A, Nishimura T, Kuroda T. Leukocyte-poor platelet concentrates at the bedside by filtration through Sepacell-PL. Vox Sang 1989;57:164–167.
138. Mosely RV, Doty DB. Death associated with multiple pulmonary emboli soon after battle injury. Ann Surg 1970;171:336–346.
139. McNamara JJ, Molot MD, Stremple JR. Screen filtration pressure in combat casualties. Ann Surg 1970;172:334–341.
140. Simmons RL, Heisterkamp CA III, Collins JA, et al. Respiratory insufficiency in combat casualties. IV: Hypoxemia during convalescence. Ann Surg 1969;170:53–62.
141. Collins JA, James PM, Bredenberg CE, et al. The relationship between transfusion and hypoxemia in combat casualties. Ann Surg 1978;188:513–520.
142. Parravicini A, Rebulla P, Apuzzo J, et al. The preparation of leukocyte-poor red cells for transfusion by a simple cost-effective technique. Transfusion 1984;24:508–509.
143. Sirchia G, Rebulla P, Parravicini A, et al. Leukocyte depletion of red cell units at the bedside by transfusion through a new filter. Transfusion 1987;27:402–405.
144. Kickler TS, Bell W, Ness PM, et al. Depletion of white cells from platelet concentrates with a new absorption filter. Transfusion 1989;29:411–414.
145. Domen RE, Williams L. Use of the Sepacell filter for preparing white cell-depleted red cells. Transfusion 1988;28:506–507.
146. Rydbert L, Ulfvin A, Stigendal L. White cell depletion of platelet concentrates using different filters. Transfusion 1988;28:604–605.
147. Gilbert GL, Hayes K, Hudson IL, James J. Prevention of transfusion-acquired cytomegalovirus infection in infants by blood filtration to remove leucocytes. Lancet 1989;1:1228–1231.
148. Murphy MF, Grint PCA, Hardiman AE, Lister TA, Waters AH. Use of leucocyte-poor blood components to prevent primary cytomegalovirus (CMV) infection in patients with acute leukaemia. Br J Haematol 1988;70:253–254.
149. Chambers LA. Characteristics and chemical application of blood filters. Transfusion Sci 1989;10:207–218.

150. Cummings E. Platelet rotators, infusion pumps and blood warmers. Transfusion Sci 1989;10:199–206.
151. Staples PJ, Griner PF. Extracorporeal hemolysis of blood in a microwave blood warmer. N Engl J Med 1971;285:317–319.
152. Linko K, Hynynen K. Erythrocyte damage caused by the Haemotherm microwave blood warmer. Acta Anaesth Scand 1979;23:320–328.
153. Kruskall MS, Pacini DG, Malynn ER, Button LN. Evaluation of a blood warmer that utilizes a 40°C heat exchanger. Transfusion 1990;30:7–10.
154. Hamill TR. The 30-minute rule for reissuing blood: are we needlessly discarding units? Transfusion 1990;30:58–62.
155. Scott J, Boulton FE, Govan JRW, Miles RS, McClelland DBL, Prowse CV. A fatal transfusion reaction associated with blood contaminated with *Pseudomonas fluorescens.* Vox Sang 1988;54:201–204.
156. Snyder EL, Ferri PM, Smith EO, Ezekowitz MD. Use of an electromechanical infusion pump for transfusion of platelet concentrates. Transfusion 1984;24:524–527.
157. Snyder EL, Rinder HM, Napychank P. In vitro and in vivo evaluation of platelet transfusions administered through an electromechanical infusion pump. Am J Clin Pathol 1990;94: 77–80.
158. Snyder EL, Malech HL, Ferri PM, Gardner JP, Kalish R. In vitro function of granulocyte concentrates following passage through an electromechanical infusion pump. Transfusion 1986;26:141–144.
159. Snyder E, Menitove J eds. Home transfusion therapy. Arlington: American Association of Blood Banks, 1986:61–69.
160. Crocker KS, Coker MH. Initiation of home hemotherapy program using a primary nursing model. J Intravenous Nursing 1990;13:13–19.

70 Neonatal Transfusion

Naomi L. C. Luban

The size and physiology of the neonate result in a unique set of indications for transfusion. Certain adverse effects of transfusion that would be easily overlooked or corrected by hepatic or renal clearance in the adult may become exaggerated in the asphyxiated, acidotic newborn. The infant's immune system, although not "immunologically null," responds less effectively to certain antigenic challenges. These factors require the transfusion medicine specialist to assess the needs of these infants with greater emphasis on specializing the products they receive.

HEMOLYTIC DISEASE OF THE NEWBORN

Hemolytic disease of the newborn (HDN) results from blood group incompatibilities that result in sensitization of the mother during pregnancy. The sensitization, also termed immunization, occurs because of discrepancies in the antigens of red blood cells (RBCs) between the mother and the fetus. The prevalence of HDN varies widely, depending upon the prevalence of the offending RBC antigen system in a given population. This varies widely in different races and ethnic groups. For example, the prevalence of Rh-negative genotype is 14.4% in American whites and 5.5% in American blacks (1). The most frequent causes of HDN are Rh (anti-D), ABO, other Rh antibodies (c, E, C, C^W), Kell (K, k), Duffy (Fy^a, Fy^b), and Kidd (Jk^a, Jk^b). D is very potent immunogen, and as little as 0.1 ml of Rh-positive blood may produce anti-D in an Rh-negative recipient.

The ABO group affects the likelihood of developing anti-D. Women who deliver infants who are ABO incompatible with the maternal plasma have a lower immunization rate to D than do those who are ABO compatible. This occurs because maternal ABO antibodies bind to and lyse the ABO-incompatible, Rh-positive fetal cells, reducing their circulation and immunizing potential. ABO HDN occurs in infants of group A or B who are born to mothers of blood group O with circulating anti-A or anti-B. Unlike Rh HDN, it occurs with equal frequency in first or subsequent pregnancies and has a higher incidence in blacks than in whites.

Fetal to maternal hemorrhage (FMH) occurs antepartum, increasing with each trimester, and intrapartum. Fetal RBCs are found in the maternal circulation in 50% of normal deliveries. The greater the FMH, the greater the potential for sensitization. The risk of becoming sensitized with an Rh-positive fetus is 7 to 8% with the first pregnancy and 15% with the second pregnancy. The risk for becoming sensitized with an ABO-incompatible fetus is 3%, despite the fact that 15% of the population is at potential risk based on ABO groups and types (1). Patients at risk for large FMHs include those with abruptio placenta, intrauterine manipulation, manual removal of the placenta, nonimmune hydrops, and fetal demise of unknown etiology.

The extent of FMH can be quantitated with a number of different tests. These include the rosette test, an enzyme-linked antiglobulin test (ELAT), and the Kleihauer-Betke test. Rosette and ELAT tests are based on the detection of D-positive cells in the maternal circulation. The Kleihauer-Betke test can be used to quantitate the volume of fetal RBCs and is based on the ability of fetal hemoglobin-containing cells to resist acid elution regardless of Rh status. Therefore, it provides information on FMH for other than Rh HDN. See pages 1720–1724 for methods.

The detection of FMH is critical for the prevention of Rh immunization in the Rh-negative mother. Rh immunoglobulin (RhIG) is administered at 28 weeks gestation and immediately postpartum in all Rh-negative women. This practice has dramatically reduced the incidence of Rh HDN to 0.11% (2). FMH can also occur during ectopic pregnancy and abortion. Recommendations for the administration of RhIg and for antepartum evaluation of the mother have been published (2, 3). Quantitating FMH in ABO hemolytic disease is not necessary because prophylaxis is not possible for ABO HDN.

Once it is determined that the mother has been sensitized to D antigen, one must determine whether the fetus is affected and, if so, how severely. This is done by performing paternal typing to determine homozygosity (DD) or heterozygosity (Dd) for D. Because there is no anti-d, the probability of the father being homozygous Rh-negative is calculated based on his C and E antigen phenotype. Depending upon the father's blood type, serial monitoring of the mother and fetus begins. Fetal blood sampling for direct antiglobulin testing and the determination of ABO group, Rh type, hemoglobin, and hematocrit may be performed, followed by serial amniotic fluid measurements to assess the rate of bilirubin rise (Δ OD 450) and fetal lung maturity (lecithin/sphingomyelin ratio). Alternatively, periumbilical blood sampling (PUBS) may be performed to assess fetal hemoglobin, hematocrit, ABO group, and Rh type and to permit antiglobulin testing. PUBS also allows for fetal antigen testing, which may obviate the need to perform amniocentesis. Fetal transfusion may then be performed, depending on the laboratory assessment of progression of disease. The laboratory assessment may be done via intraperitoneal or direct intravascular access (see below).

EXCHANGE TRANSFUSION

Exchange transfusion was first employed in 1948 by Diamond et al. for the treatment of hyperbilirubinemia resulting from Rh incompatibility (4). Exchange transfusion removes unconjugated bilirubin and antibody-coated RBC, increases the hematocrit, provides RBC without red cell antigens to which the infant has developed antibody, and provides some protein as albumin to allow more rapid clearance of unconjugated bilirubin. The decision to perform an exchange transfusion is based on long-established clinical indications (5, 6). In the term infant, exchange should be performed at an unconjugated serum bilirubin concentration of 18 to 20 mg/dl, a bilirubin greater than 4 mg/dl at birth, or an increase of bilirubin of 0.5 to 1 mg/dl/hr (6). At concentrations of serum bilirubin above 20 mg/dl, the secondary binding sites on albumin are filled. The binding affinity at secondary sites is lower than on primary sites, causing displacement to occur easily. Lipid-soluble free bilirubin will enter the brain and affect brain cell mitochondria, particularly in the basal ganglia and cerebellum. This results in kernicterus, or bilirubin encephalopathy.

Certain factors are known to decrease bilirubin binding and predispose to kernicterus. These include low birth weight, asphyxia, acidosis, hypoxia, hypothermia, hypoglycemia, sepsis with or without meningitis, respiratory distress, and CNS deterioration, which usually occurs from intraventricular hemorrhage. Certain drugs and the administration of free fatty acids via hyperalimentation fluids can also alter bilirubin binding (6). The need to perform an exchange transfusion would be heightened by the presence of any of these events or any combination of them. Certain formulas are used to calculate a maximum allowable bilirubin, and these are reviewed in current neonatal texts (5, 6). They all utilize the birth weight of the infant and the bilirubin-protein binding capability. In one study, the use of these formulas in 175 instances resulted in a lack of concurrence in these predictive methods. The infants most likely to fail the predictive models were sick, premature infants (7). Clinical judgment remains the most common indicator of the need to perform an exchange transfusion for the prevention of hyperbilirubinemic encephalopathy.

The efficacy of the exchange transfusion is based on the amount of bilirubin removed. A double volume exchange removes 87 to 90% of the infant's blood volume. Because of shifts in bilirubin from the tissues to the intravascular compartment, rebound hyperbilirubinemia may occur, requiring a second exchange. Also, drugs are removed during an exchange; therefore, infants on cardiotonic medications or antibiotics should have replacement doses. The amount of replacement is calculated based on drug half-life and protein binding capability (8).

Although Rh hemolytic disease and ABO incompatibility cause the vast majority of cases requiring exchange transfusion, whole blood exchange has also been advocated for neonatal sepsis, drug overdose or toxicity, acute renal failure, respiratory distress syndrome, and incompatible blood transfusion (9). However, there are few or no controlled studies to support such treatment. The rationales for these varied indications are similar to those used for hyperbilirubinemia. For example, in sepsis, exchange transfusion would remove bacteria and endotoxins, thereby removing a stimulus for disseminated intravascular coagulation (DIC) (10). In addition, exchange transfusion would correct acidosis, improve perfusion by correcting anemia, and provide some functional granulocytes and bacteria-specific antibody (11). Unless the blood that is used is fresh and unrefrigerated, it is unlikely that functional granulocytes would be provided (12, 13). However, improvement in the other physiological parameters can be accomplished with stored, banked blood. Improvement in respiratory distress syndrome (RDS) by replacement of left-shifted fetal hemoglobin by right-shifted hemoglobin A has been examined in a randomized trial (14), but improvement in the medical management of RDS infants makes this an outmoded therapy.

Exchange transfusions are most often performed through an indwelling umbilical venous line that is placed in the vena cava with its location confirmed radiologically. Techniques involving the use of dual umbilical artery (withdraw) and umbilical venous (infuse) lines (15) and the use of peripheral venous lines with large-bore intracatheters (16) have been described. Using aseptic technique, aliquots of blood are removed and infused through a temperature-controlled and alarmed blood warmer to avoid hypothermia. Aliquot volumes and the rate of removal and infusion should be adjusted to the infant's weight in kilograms and central venous pressure (CVP) and should not exceed 10 ml/kg per cycle. Because of swings in systemic blood pressure that predispose to intraventricular hemorrhage, the exchange rate should not exceed 5 ml/kg/3 min (17). The procedure was described by Fletcher and Edwards (18), and the complications of exchange transfusion were subsequently discussed in several studies (19–21). Morbidity rates of 6.7% and mortality rates from 1 to 16.3% have been reported; the smaller, sicker infants experience the greatest morbidity and mortality (18).

A major procedure-related complication of exchange transfusion is necrotizing enterocolitis, which may occur secondary to vascular spasm with secondary gut ischemia. In a piglet model, the impeding of blood flow by venous congestion during the injection phase predisposed to venous thrombosis and/or hemorrhagic infarction (22). Other complications of exchange transfusion include acidosis and citrate-induced hypocalcemia, which can be treated with sodium bicarbonate and calcium gluconate, respectively. However, these medications should not be administered routinely. Rather, the infant should be followed for these and other metabolic complications of exchange transfusion, including hypoglycemia, hyperkalemia (23), and hypernatremia (24), and these should be treated appropriately when they occur.

Severe isoimmunization to Rh or other alloantibodies has historically been treated with intraperitoneal transfusion of the fetus and early delivery. Since Rodeck's first description in 1981, such infants are now managed with fetal transfusion (25). Ultrasonic techniques permit the perinatologist direct access to the fetal umbilical circulation. This technique offers several advantages to the fetal-maternal unit. These include the quantitation of bilirubin, the assessment of the degree of anemia by direct measurement of hemoglobin, and the determination of fetal blood type (26). Either bolus transfusions or exchange transfusion (27) can be given through this route. In one study comparing the two, Ronkin et al. reviewed their experiences with 32 transfusions in eight infants. Despite a 10% overall complication rate, they suggest that bolus therapy be used as a first line of therapy; exchange transfusion is reserved for the severely hydropic infant with fluid overload and the rapid development of maternal antibody, which predisposes to further hemolysis (28). Many authors raise concern over the lack of necessary laboratory parameters to guide the timing of the transfusions. The quantitation of isoimmune antibody, reticulocyte count, or erythropoietin levels in the fetal blood, or a combination of these, has been suggested by some investigators (28). Others have developed flow cytometric analyses or rapid bedside serologic techniques to quantitate isoimmune antibody and assess hematocrit (26). The specialized RBC product used for fetal transfusion must be normokalemic, able to offload oxygen rapidly, unable to induce an immunologic response, and free of transfusion-transmitted viruses, particularly cytomegalovirus. Therefore, O-negative, washed, CMV-negative, irradiated blood, as fresh as available with current mandated testing and crossmatched against the mother's serum, is often used.

Partial exchange transfusion is used to decrease hematocrit. The incidence of polycythemia of the newborn ranges from 0.8 to 4% and is more frequent at high altitude. A hematocrit of greater than 65% is associated with poor feeding, hypoglycemia, hypoxemia, tachypnea, and central nervous system dysfunction, including seizures and hypotonia (29, 30). Black and colleagues randomized 93 infants with polycythemia to receive either partial exchange transfusion or symptomatic treatment. The infants were evaluated at 1 and 2 years for neurological abnormalities. Of the 29 infants studied at 2 years of age who did not undergo exchange transfusions, there was a higher incidence of neurological disease, including spastic diplegia, and poor fine motor skills compared with the treated group (31). This study suggests that infants with a hematocrit of greater than 65% should receive partial exchange transfusion. Partial exchange improves cerebral arterial pulsatile flow and other aspects of cerebral hemodynamics, and this may account for the differences in neurological outcome (32).

Partial exchange transfusion can be performed either by using a peripheral vein for infusion and an umbilical vein for withdrawal or by using the umbilical vein for both infusion and withdrawal. Fresh frozen plasma, albumin, and plasma protein solution have been utilized as the replacement solution. Decreased morbidity, particularly from necrotizing enterocolitis (NEC), has been reported with the use of plasma protein solution. When plasma protein solution was used for the replacement fluid, 6.5% and 204 evaluable patients had bloody stools, difficulty feeding, and/or abdominal distention. In contrast, Black et al. reported an incidence of 18.6% when fresh frozen plasma was used (33). Because NEC may be a part of the spectrum of polycythemia, it is difficult to delineate whether the NEC occurring posttransfusion is part of the syndrome or due to the procedure or the nature of the replacement fluid (34).

Table 70.1. Formulae for Transfusion of Red Cell Products

I. Calculation of hematocrit rise

$$\text{Hematocrit rise} = \frac{[0.75]\ [V_{tx}] - [(\text{EBL})\ (\text{P pre-post Hct})]}{\text{EBV}}$$

where EBL = Estimated iatrogenic loss in ml
EBV = Estimated blood volume based on 100 ml/kg
V_{tx} = Volume to be transfused
P pre-post Hct = Mean of pre- and posthematocrits

A simplified version of the above concordant with the formula described above is:

$$\text{Quantity PRBC transfused (ml)} = \frac{\text{EBV (desired hematocrit rise)}}{0.75}$$

II. Calculation of blood needed for exchange transfusion

$$\text{Volume of exchange (ml)} = \frac{\text{Body wt (kg)} \times \text{Blood volume (ml/kg)} \times \text{Desired rise in Hb}}{22\ \text{g/dl} - \text{Hbw}}$$

$$\text{Hbw} = \frac{\text{Initial hemoglobin} + \text{Desired hemoglobin}}{2}$$

Usual concentration of hemoglobin of packed cell = 22 g/dl

III. Formulas for reconstitution of blood to a specific hematocrit for exchange transfusion

$$W_{FFP} \left[\frac{Hct_{PRBC}}{Hct_{RB}} - 1 \right] W_{PRBC}$$

where
W = Weight in grams of product
Hct_{RB} = Hematocrit of red cell product
Hct_{PRBC} = Hematocrit of packed red blood cells

IV. "Rule of thumb" formula for simple transfusion
2 ml/kg of whole blood will raise hemoglobin 1 g/dl
6 ml/kg of packed cells will raise hemoglobin 1 g/dl

V. Blood volumes

Premature	~100–120 ml/kg
Full-term	~80–85 ml/kg
Adult	~70–75 ml/kg reached by 3 months of age

Fresh frozen plasma may somehow interact with hyperviscous whole blood of high hematocrit or have an effect on gastrointestinal blood flow; however, these possibilities have not been well studied to date. Albumin or plasma protein solutions should be used for partial exchange transfusion until these interactions are established.

SMALL-VOLUME TRANSFUSION

Transfusion of small volumes of blood is a necessary part of the care of the premature and full-term infant who requires intensive nursery care. In order to monitor the metabolic and cardiorespiratory status of these infants, blood sampling is necessary and results in iatrogenic anemia. In one study of 59 premature infants, a mean of 22.9 ± 10 ml of packed cells were lost during the first 6 weeks of life; 26% of these infants had blood losses that exceeded their red cell mass at birth (35). Indwelling catheters that measure PO_2, PCO_2, oxygen saturation, and calcium, and transcutaneous electrodes that measure PO_2, PCO_2, and bilirubin, have been developed, but none is sufficiently refined to replace venous blood sample measurements.

Other established indications for transfusion include the replacement of acute blood loss and the treatment of the late anemia that occurs in infants with HDN following exchange transfusion or phototherapy. Transfusion has also been used to decrease the number of episodes of apnea-bradycardia, tachypnea, and tachycardia and to improve poor feeding and promote weight gain (Table 70.1). However, its value in these cases is controversial; the few studies performed to date have provided conflicting data.

Several factors determine the systemic oxygen transport and tissue oxygen extraction of the infant. These include the cardiac output, the packed cell volume or hematocrit, and the position of the oxyhemoglobin dissociation curve. The infant has a limited ability to increase cardiac output in the presence of anemia because he or she is already functioning at the limit of the Starling curve (36, 37).

The hematocrit of the infant will be altered by the blood volume, and therefore by the red cell mass, and by clinical conditions that will alter the red cell mass (Table 70.2). The blood volume of an infant is dependent on the time of cord clamping, the infant's gestational age, and certain pre- or intrapartum events. For example, infants born following cesarean section have lower red cell mass (31.2 ± 3.6 ml/kg) than do infants born vaginally (37.5 ± 5.1 ml/kg); those born vaginally with early cord clamping have lower blood volumes (average 82 ml/kg) than those with late cord clamping (average 93 ml/kg). The preterm infant has a lower red cell mass (29.6 ± 2.9 ml/kg), regardless of the method of delivery. Intrapartum hypoxia, on the other hand, will increase the red cell mass (46.9 ± 6.3 ml/kg) in both the term and preterm infant, regardless of Apgar score (38). If the infant suffers from one of the many causes of anemia in this age group, has a limited red cell mass, or suffers from a complication of prematurity, the physiological reserve will be compromised. The presence of predominantly fetal hemoglobin at birth, rather than adult hemoglobin, further compromises peripheral oxygen delivery. Fetal hemoglobin is optimized to transport oxygen from the relatively hypoxic placental circulation and deliver it to the fetus in utero. Fetal hemoglobin has the characteristics of high affinity and poor peripheral oxygen release. These characteristics are reflected in an average p50 of 19 mm Hg in infants, compared with an average p50 of 27 mm Hg for adult hemoglobin A. Placental conditions establish a pH and 2,3-DPG content that optimize O_2 delivery in utero and at delivery (37). In the absence of hypoxia, however, the presence of large quantities of fetal hemoglobin works against the infant.

The premature infant may also suffer from the so-called physiological anemia of prematurity. This con-

Table 70.2. Pathophysiology of Fetal Erythroid Colonies and Erythropoietin in the Infant with Anemia

	As Compared with Adults
Erythropoietin	Quantitatively lower concentrations Less response to same degree of anemia Immature hypoxic threshold of EPO sensing mechanism More hepatic and less kidney-derived EPO
BFU-E[a]	Quantitatively greater Similar growth characteristics
CFU-E	Quantitatively greater in number and develop earlier in culture systems
Erythroid "burst-promoting" activity (BPA)	Quantitatively similar

[a]BFU-E, burst forming unit-erythroid; CFU-E, colony-forming unit-erythroid; BPA includes IL-3, GM-CSF, IL-6, and other cytokines.

dition is multifactorial and frequently self-limited, and its pathophysiology is slowly being uncovered. Premature infants have a lower erythropoietin response to similar degrees of anemia (36). Although peripheral blood and bone marrow progenitors (BFU-E or burst forming units—erythroid) are adequate in number (39) and are responsive to erythropoietin in vitro (40), their growth patterns are different (41). Other growth factors appear to be adequate for erythroid differentiation (42) (Table 70.2). In a preliminary study, six of seven infants with the physiological anemia of prematurity responded to recombinant erythropoietin in vivo with associated thrombocytosis, late neutropenia, and alterations in iron kinetics (43). Although this study is suggestive, transfusion will remain as the main therapy for anemia until additional clinical trials have been completed.

Two additional studies using r-Hu-EPO in infants have been reported (43a, 43b). One placebo-controlled, randomized study evaluated 20 premature infants with weights less than 1250 g who were treated with 100 units/kg of r-Hu-EPO twice per week for 6 weeks. Of all the variables studied, the volume of blood removed for laboratory tests best predicted the need to transfuse the infant. Of nine infants who had minimal phlebotomy, specifically less than 20 ml during the study period, none of four given r-Hu-EPO required transfusion, while three of five given a placebo required one transfusion. Those infants who had greater than 20 ml removed were more likely to require transfusion, regardless of r-Hu-EPO administration.

Ohls and Christensen also performed a randomized study of infants with a mean birth weight of 988g who received either r-Hu-EPO, 200 units/kg every other day for 10 doses, or transfusion to bring the hematocrit to 40%. Bone marrow aspirates to assess cellularity and hematopoietic progenitors were performed on the first six patients receiving r-Hu-EPO and on the first three transfused infants. The infants on EPO had diminishing signs of anemia, which correlated with increased reticulocyte count when compared with the transfused infants. There was a relative increase in erythroid activity, an inverse in the ratio of myeloid to erythroid cells and decreased neutrophil storage pool in the bone marrow of the EPO-treated infants. These studies further expand the work of Halperin, but use higher doses of EPO, a sensible approach because of the larger volume of distribution of the drug in neonates as compared with adults. Neither study clarifies the mechanism responsible for the neutropenia observed by two of the three groups.

The ability to summarize clear-cut indications for the simple transfusion of infants is hampered by the paucity of standardized, acceptable, and widely available laboratory parameters. These are required to demonstrate accurately the need for transfusion. In addition, there are very few adequate randomized clinical studies. Ideally, the decision to transfuse should be based upon physiological measurements, including oxygen tension, arterial oxygen saturation, central venous oxygen tension, oxyhemoglobin dissociation, cardiac output, and oxygen requirements. However, the inability to easily measure these parameters has led to the substitution of more easily measured but less complete parameters. These include measurements of red cell mass, "available oxygen," and oxygen delivery. There is poor correlation between hematocrit and red cell mass (44). Newer methods using biotin labels are promising but are not yet validated (45). Wardrop and colleagues used a formula that utilized hemoglobin, gestational age, and an estimate of fetal hemoglobin concentration to assess the amount of oxygen available for peripheral release in preterm infants. Two groups of infants were defined on the basis of normal or low "available oxygen." Those with low available oxygen had a decreased incidence of apnea and bradycardia following transfusion, while those with normal available oxygen showed no improvement (46). In a study of infants with bronchopulmonary dysplasia, oxygen consumption ($\dot{V}O_2$) and systemic oxygen transport (SOT) were measured before and 24 hours following transfusion in 10 oxygen-dependent infants. Oxygen utilization was calculated as $\dot{V}O_2$/SOT. In transfused infants with higher levels of oxygen utilization, there was a greater fall in oxygen utilization than in those with lower levels. Neither hemoglobin nor hematocrit correlated with either SOT or $\dot{V}O_2$, and neither predicted which infants would benefit from transfusion (47).

Other indications for small-volume transfusions include the replacement of iatrogenic blood loss and the treatment of apnea, tachypnea, tachycardia, and growth failure. Iatrogenic loss occurs because of the large number of laboratory tests required to monitor the sick infant, particularly the premature infant. This may account for most of the RBC transfusions that the infant receives (44, 48). In one study, 26% of infants had a cumulative blood loss that exceeded their red cell mass during the first 6 weeks of life (35). This resulted in a high rate of donor exposure (median 7) in the face of small volumes transfused (mean 16.5 ml) (49). Despite advances in the use of indwelling catheters able to monitor P_{O_2} and P_{CO_2} and transcutaneous monitoring to measure P_{O_2}, P_{CO_2}, and bilirubin, such methods are not yet routine.

Iatrogenic loss can be minimized by performing only minimal compatibility testing before transfusion. Because neonates fail to respond to many polysaccharide and glycoprotein stimuli, they are unlikely to develop antibodies to RBC transfusions (50, 51). Initial compatibility testing of the infant can be done on cord blood if it is available and should include ABO group and Rh type and an antibody screen. If the antibody screen is negative and the red cells transfused are group O or are ABO-identical or ABO-compatible with the mother, compatibility testing can be omitted during the first 4 months of life (52). The current practice is to replace iatrogenic losses when the amount of loss equals 10 ml per kilogram of body weight.

Symptomatic anemia in the infant is associated with pallor, lethargy, tachypnea, tachycardia, bradycardia, poor feeding, and inadequate weight gain. Data supporting the use of packed RBCs for weight gain are discrepant. Stockman and Clark studied 13 infants with birth weights less than 1500 g and were able to demonstrate daily weight increases associated with decreased metabolic rates as measured by oxygen consumption following transfusion (53). However, Blank et al. studied 56 low–birth weight infants, 26 of whom had received transfusion to maintain a hemoglobin concentration greater than 10 g/dl, while 30 received transfusions solely for clinical indications, and found no clinical advantage to transfusion. At discharge, as expected, the transfused group had higher hemoglobin concentrations and lower reticulocyte counts, but they did not differ from the nontransfused group in the frequency or severity of apnea, the length of hospitalization, or the number of days required to regain birth weight (54).

Hypoxemia is known to depress the respiratory center and result in transient tachypnea, often followed by apneic episodes (Table 70.3). Two studies have addressed the use of transfusion to improve apnea and bradycardia. In one study, 30 premature infants were studied during the recovery phase of their hospitalization; small-volume packed RBC transfusions resulted in decreases in heart rate, duration of periodic breathing, and the number of episodes of apnea and bradycardia. These infants were studied 6 hours before and 6 hours after transfusion (55). In another study, 33 growing premature infants were evaluated 4 hours before and 24 hours after transfusion of packed RBCs administered for unspecified indications (56). This study supported the previous findings, although a significant proportion of the infants were on methylxanthines at the time of transfusion, which might well have confounded the results.

Table 70.3. Some Conditions for Which Small-Volume Red Blood Cell Transfusions Have Been Advocated

Profound anemia—multiple causes
Symptomatic cardiovascular disease with falling hematocrit (BPD, polycythemic congenital heart disease)
"Clinical" symptomatology
Apnea/bradycardia
Poor growth/weight gain
Tiring at feeding
Iagrogenic blood loss
Anemia of prematurity
Late anemia of Rh or ABO hemolytic disease

Keyes and colleagues could not find a correlation between capillary hematocrit and either heart rate or respiratory rate over a wide range of hematocrits posttransfusion. In addition, they found that the incidence of apnea and bradycardia was unrelated to hematocrit (48). The lack of correlation of clinical findings with hematocrit and the lack of posttransfusion hematocrit increment are a striking finding. Ross and colleagues studied 16 premature infants with hematocrits less than 29% in a randomized trial in an effort to establish a series of variables that might better define criteria for transfusion. They found that a heart rate greater than 152 beats/minute, elevated blood lactate (in moles/g blood but value not specified), and frequent apnea/bradycardia episodes (number not specified) predicted which infants would benefit from transfusion (57) (Table 70.4). The lack of specificity in this study's findings do not help clarify this transfusion indication.

WHITE BLOOD CELL TRANSFUSION

Neonates are at risk for overwhelming infection from sepsis, which may result in mortality rates as high as 75%. The neonate has abnormal cell-mediated immunity, depressed antibody-mediated immunity, quantitatively low classic complement levels (58), factor B (59) and fibronectin (60) deficiencies, and quantitative and qualitative abnormalities of the neutrophil/phagocyte system (61). These all contribute to the increased risk of sepsis.

The abnormalities in the phagocyte system have been well characterized in both animal models and

Table 70.4. Some Peripartum Factors Altering Blood Volume Measurements in Infants

Factors increasing blood volume in the infant
Delayed cord clamping
Maternal hypoxemia with stress erythropoiesis
Diabetes
Anemia
Toxemia
Cesarean section—premature birth
Factors decreasing blood volume in the infant
Early cord clamping
Infant held below introitus in vaginal or cesarean section
Placenta previa or abruptio placenta
Nuchal cord
Cesarean section—term birth

human neonates (61). The neutrophil storage pool (NSP), which consists of polymorphonuclear leukocytes, band cells, and metamyelocytes, is decreased in certain infants. There is little ability to mobilize mature neutrophils by increasing marrow responsiveness in response to the stress of sepsis. This results in an exhaustion of neutrophil reserves and contributes to the neutropenia associated with sepsis. In one study where bone marrows were performed, a NSP of less than 7% was associated with death from sepsis in seven of eight infants studied (62). There are fewer myeloid progenitor colonies (CFU-C or colony forming unit–committed), and these are proliferating at a maximal rate. In addition, the precursor bone marrow progenitor, the colony forming unit–granulocyte, erythroid, monocyte, megakarocytes (CFU-GEMM), and the colony forming unit–granulocyte, macrophage (CFU-GM) are decreased in number. This further decreases the ability of the marrow to increase the proliferative pool and therefore the number of mature functioning granulocytes (62).

In some infants, adequate numbers of granulocytes may be generated, but their function is grossly abnormal. Functional abnormalities that have been reported include decreased deformability, chemotaxis, phagocytosis, bactericidal killing, and oxidative metabolism (57). These functional abnormalities, particularly hydroxyl radical generation and bactericidal killing, can be demonstrated, especially when the infant is stressed or infected (63, 64).

Term and preterm newborns have reduced quantities of γ-globulin, specifically subclasses of IgG (IgG2 and IgG4) (65); this occurs because of reduced production of immunoglobulin and poor transport of maternal IgG across the placenta. In addition, newborns respond poorly to certain antigenic stimuli, particularly polysaccharide and other carbohydrate moieties; this provides the rationale for no longer cross-matching infants to guard against alloimmunization to red cell antigens (50, 51). The presence of physiological hypogammaglobulinemia has led to the use of IV or IM immunoglobulin for certain premature infants felt to be at risk for sepsis based on low birth weight (66, 67). This practice is still experimental; therefore, recommendations on dose, frequency, and route are not firm at this time.

The presence of qualitative and quantitative abnormalities in neutrophils has led to the use of granulocytes to treat neonatal sepsis. A total of 11 studies have been published to date, using buffy coats prepared from refrigerated blood units (68, 69), granulocytes prepared by leukapheresis (62, 70–75), and whole blood exchange (13). It is difficult to compare these studies because each used different entry criteria and transfusion protocols. Some were randomized, and others were not. When evaluated in total, 79% (62/78) of neonates who received granulocytes survived versus 62% (56/90) who were treated conventionally.

Four out of six of the controlled trials demonstrated a benefit from granulocyte transfusion; the two that failed to show benefit used buffy coat-prepared neutrophils at a dose 0.3×10^9/kg, significantly less than the successful trials where 1 to 2×10^9/kg leukapheresis granulocytes were used (68, 69). The use of granulocytes to treat neonatal sepsis remains controversial (19, 61, 76–78), and the validity of using the neutrophil storage pool as a predictor of survival has come into question (76). Trials with IV immunoglobulin are underway, and this may well replace the use of granulocytes in the future (79).

PLATELET TRANSFUSIONS

Platelet transfusions may be administered to the infant for many of the same indications as in the adult. Infants may have impaired production, increased destruction, abnormal distribution, or dilution of their platelet counts. In the critically ill infant, a combination of mechanisms is most likely. The most common cause of bleeding in the neonate is disseminated intravascular coagulation (80); this may occur from any number of causes.

Two unique neonatal conditions warrant special attention. These are neonatal immune thrombocytopenia and intraventricular hemorrhage. Neonatal immune thrombocytopenia may have an alloimmune or autoimmune etiology. In autoimmune neonatal thrombocytopenia, the fetus or neonate develops thrombocytopenia in response to the transplacental passage of maternal autoantibody.

In alloimmune or isoimmune thrombocytopenia, the mother develops antibody to paternal antigens inherited by the fetus and present on his or her platelets. Thrombocytopenia develops when this antibody crosses the placenta and binds to the platelets of the infant or fetus. These antibodies are most often directed against the PL^{A1} antigen system. First-born infants are affected, and the incidence may be as high as one in 3000 births (81). Transfusion of random donor platelets frequently provides the diagnostic test needed to differentiate between alloimmune and autoimmune thrombocytopenia. Platelets are likely to be PL^{A1} positive and will not provide a sustained increase in platelet count in the infant with alloimmune thrombocytopenia because they are likely to be destroyed through antigen-antibody mediated sequestration. Maternal platelets that have been washed free of maternal antibody or PL^{A1}-negative platelets obtained from unrelated healthy donors are the therapy of choice for infants requiring such transfusion. In high-risk women with HLA-B9/DR3 phenotype and a history of a previously affected infant, intrapartum transfusion of maternal platelets has also been performed with excellent results in six of nine cases (82).

Alloimmune thrombocytopenia is more difficult to treat. The mother's platelet count does not allow for accurate prediction of risk to the fetus or neonate. Trauma through vaginal delivery puts the infant at risk for central nervous system hemorrhage. Some perinatologists advocate periumbilical blood sampling to obtain fetal platelet counts (83); others monitor maternal platelet antibody titer and count. Predelivery treatment of the mother with corticosteroids and/or IV IgG (84) and intrapartum treatment of the fetus with IV IgG (85) have been advocated.

Other clinical circumstances in which thrombocytopenia occurs without concomitant DIC include respiratory distress syndrome, persistent pulmonary hypertension, necrotizing enterocolitis, polycythemia, Rh hemolytic disease, and the use of mechanical ventilation (86). Exchange transfusion with stored blood and indwelling vascular catheters may result in thrombocytopenia because of dilution or propagating thrombi, respectively.

Platelets are usually transfused to thrombocytopenic newborns who are bleeding. At-risk newborns without bleeding may receive prophylactic platelets, although no studies have addressed the absolute levels at which to transfuse newborns. Few data have addressed the adequacy of posttransfusion platelet survival (87). Doses for infants can be calculated on a kilogram or surface area (m^2) basis. As in the adult, fever, DIC sepsis, splenomegaly, and active bleeding will result in less adequate posttransfusion-corrected increment counts. ABO-compatible platelets should be administered to the infant to avoid transfusion of the isohemagglutinins anti-A or anti-B, which might result in hemolysis (88) and decreased survival (89). Rh-negative platelets should be used, if possible, in Rh-negative female infants because the RBC contamination may result in Rh sensitization. Volume-reduced platelets may be utilized for premature infants or older infants with cardiovascular instability in whom excessive fluid might produce hypertension. Methods have been established for volume reduction from 50 to 75 to 20 to 25 ml with adequate posttransfusion survival (87).

Periventricular-intraventricular hemorrhage (PV-IVH) is a major complication of prematurity. Hypoxia-ischemic insult in the intrapartum or postpartum period produces capillary endothelial injury, resulting in rupture of the fragile vessels in the subependymal layer of the lateral ventricles. When the vascular endothelium is injured, increase in vascular flow or increase in intracranial pressure will lead to rupture of these vessels, resulting in PV-IVH. Periodic hypoxia, acidosis, intermittent hypertension, and thrombocytopenia contribute to the pathogenesis of PV-IVH (90). Andrew and colleagues compared 97 infants with platelet counts less than 100×10^9/liter with 80 nonthrombocytopenic control infants who were age, weight, and disease matched. The incidence of PV-IVH thrombocytopenic infants who weighed less than 1500 g was 78%, compared to 48% in the nonthrombocytopenic infants. Moreover, there was associated long-term neurological morbidity (91). This study further extends the work of Setzer and colleagues (92). Other studies have described reduction in platelet counts with mechanical ventilation of newborns (86), especially in the more immature infant.

ADVERSE REACTIONS TO BLOOD AND BLOOD PRODUCTS

Certain adverse reactions are unique to the newborn and have been extensively reviewed (21). Cytomegalovirus infection, graft-versus-host disease and the metabolic abnormalities are among the complications.

Cytomegalovirus

Cytomegalovirus (CMV) is a ubiquitous herpesvirus that is harbored in white blood cells and can be transmitted through transfusion of blood and some blood products. Both actively infected and latently infected donors can transmit CMV; transfusion itself may also activate latent CMV in the recipient, regardless of the CMV serostatus of the donor blood. In the neonatal setting, posttransfusion CMV (PTCMV) may be asymptomatic and only discovered because of serial serologic testing or viral culture, or it may produce significant morbidity and mortality. Clinical manifestations of CMV include cytopenias, pneumonia, hepatitis, respiratory decompensation, viral sepsis with DIC, and graft failure in organ recipients. To date, only acute infection in the seronegative infant has been reported to cause adverse effects; reactivation of latent virus and coinfection with more than one strain of virus have not been reported as posttransfusion events producing morbidity in infants. In the neonate, the incidence of PTCMV has been declining over the past several years. This may have occurred in part from increased donor screening and from changes in neonatal transfusion practice (92a).

Several factors increase the propensity of the infant to acquire PTCMV. These include birth weight less than 1500 g and receipt of more than 50 ml of blood and blood products (93). The small infant requiring transfusion in the immediate postnatal period is most likely to be immunocompromised on the basis of gestational age and degree of illness, and lacks protective maternal antibody. The fetus who requires intrauterine transfusion is at similar or increased risk as compared to the seronegative premature infant. Such fetuses and their CMV-negative mothers should receive blood and blood products processed in such a way as to prevent CMV.

There are a number of different methods that can be used to prevent or ameliorate PTCMV. These include leukodepletion by freezing and washing (94, 95), by washing alone (96, 97), and by third-generation leukodepletion filtration (96). Frozen deglycerolized red blood cells, regardless of serostatus, prevent CMV in neonates. In one study, the new leukocyte depletion filters that have been developed were effective in preventing primary CMV infection in neonates receiving serologically unscreened RBC (98). No study to date has evaluated infants receiving seropositive platelets filtered with one of these specialized leukodepletion filters. Standard leukocyte depletion and microaggregate filters do not remove a sufficient number of white blood cells to be effective.

Only cellular blood components need to be processed; FFP has not been shown to transmit CMV (99). Passive acquisition of CMV antibody is protective; this has been demonstrated by the use of IV IgG or CMV hyperimmune IV IgG in bone marrow and solid organ transplant recipients. If one is serially following neonates for PTCMV with serology alone, it is difficult to assess their CMV serostatus if they are receiving IV IgG, IM IgG, or CMV-positive plasma. In such cases, viral culture, tests for CMV early antigen, or strain-specific molecular markers of CMV by PCR would be needed to determine if the infant has acquired CMV.

There is debate as to whether seropositive infants should receive exclusively seronegative blood or blood products. The equivalent of a partial exchange transfusion effectively renders an infant seronegative, and this might put him or her at risk for CMV from a nosocomial source (100). More critically, seropositive infants receiving seropositive products do not demonstrate any sequelae of PTCMV (93).

The infant is also at risk for the acquisition of other posttransfusion viral diseases, including hepatitis and HIV. No study has ever clearly demonstrated that neonates are at any higher risk for acquiring posttransfusion diseases than are older children, although premature infants receiving HIV-positive units prior to HIV testing all appear to acquire PT HIV (101). The practice of using one unit of blood for multiple infants has, however, resulted in multiple infants being infected from a single donor. This has been reported with hepatitis A, malaria, EBV, and HIV (101).

Transfusion-associated Graft Versus Host Disease

Transfusion-associated graft versus host disease (TA-GVHD) occurs when an immunosuppressed or immunodeficient transfusion recipient receives immunologically competent donor lymphocytes. The transfused cells proliferate and engraft in the recipient who does not recognize the cells as foreign and is unable to reject them. Recent reports have focused on the similarities in HLA antigens between donor and recipient that facilitate engraftment. Although this would occur infrequently in unrelated donor-recipient pairs, it is much more likely to occur when first and second degree relatives are transfusion donors and recipients (102).

Although the incidence of TA-GVHD is unknown, it has been reported in fetuses receiving intrauterine transfusion, infants transfused postnatally following intrauterine transfusion, those with congenital T cell deficiency, and a few premature infants (103, 104). Whole blood, red blood cells, white blood cells, platelets, and fresh plasma have been implicated; however, sufficient lymphocytes may be present in frozen deglycerolized cells to induce TA-GVHD. Based on animal studies, 1×10^7 lymphocytes/kg are needed to initiate GVHD. TA-GVHD can be abrogated by either reducing the number of lymphocytes in the blood product to a critically low concentration or by irradiating the lymphocytes with 1500 to 5000 rad from a cesium or cobalt irradiation source to inhibit lymphocyte blastogenesis (102). No leukocyte depletion filter or processing has yet been shown to uniformly decrease the lymphocyte count of a product below the critical threshold. Insufficient radiation may result in a small population of lymphocytes that are mitogen responsive (105). Irradiation followed by storage is not harmful to platelets (106). However, irradiation of red blood cells followed by storage results in K^+ leakage from the stored cells with markedly elevated levels after 14 days of storage (107).

Because high K^+ levels might be detrimental to the fetus or neonate, especially those receiving exchange transfusion, special care should be taken to use red blood cell units immediately following irradiation. If units must be stored following irradiation, washing of the units prior to transfusion is effective in reducing the K^+ concentration (108). A single transfusion of small volume (10 ml/kg) is not likely to result in a significant K^+ load.

Metabolic Adverse Reactions

The physiology of the infant, including large surface area to body mass ratio, immature gluconeogenic and glycogenolytic enzyme systems, and decreased renal tubular reabsorption, put the infant at risk for the adverse effects of transfusion of red blood cells stored in anticoagulant media. During red cell storage, the ATPase-dependent sodium-potassium pump is impaired, resulting in increases in extracellular potassium, free hemoglobin, AST, and LDH. At the same time, the glycolytic intermediates 2,3-DPG and ATP, as well as glucose and pH, all decrease. Of greatest concern are electrolyte disturbances such as hyperkalemia, hypernatremia, hypophosphatemia, hypocalcemia, both hypoglycemia and hyperglycemia, and hemoglobinuria. Each of these can occur with simple transfusions but are much more exaggerated during exchange transfusion unless precautions are taken to process blood in such a way as to reduce the risks (21). However, few studies demonstrate the adverse clinical effects of high sodium or potassium in transfused blood. If clinical studies could demonstrate adequate 2,3-DPG generation, satisfactory oxygen offloading, and the absence of hyperkalemia with small volume simple transfusion of "old" packed red blood cells, then one neonate could receive blood from a single unit up to its expiration date. This practice would significantly reduce donor exposure. The new anticoagulants (Adsol, Nutricell, Optisol), which contain red cell preservative solutions, permit storage of blood for up to 42 days. Only one study, published in abstract form, has addressed the safety of one of these solutions in 11 newborns given simple transfusion (109). Another publication calculated the quantities of additives to which an infant would be exposed under different circumstances and found no potential adverse effect when transfusion of 10 ml/kg was administered (110). Investigators in Zurich quantitated albumin total protein and IgG content in nine infants and warned against the use of Adsol for exchange transfusion (111). Until the safety of these solutions is established in neonates receiving exchange transfusion or the equivalent of whole blood exchange, they should be used cautiously, especially in the premature infant.

T-Activation

T-activation is another rare but unique adverse reaction to blood in the neonate. The erythrocyte T antigen is present in all human erythrocytes, but it is not expressed unless neuraminidase acts on the membrane to express *N*-acetyl-neuraminic acid. Neuraminidase is produced by bacteria, viruses, and protozoa. Clostridial, pneumococcal, and *Bacteroides* infections have been correlated with T-activation in infants and in adults. Neonates with T antigen–activated erythrocytes are at little risk for hemolysis unless they receive blood components. Anti-T antibodies are naturally occurring in adult human plasma and are present in most plasma-containing products. Williams et al. confirmed the rarity of this phenomenon in their 3-year study of 1672 neonates, in which only 10 infants developed T-antigen activation. If this condition is suspected or confirmed, low-titer T-antigen plasma and plasma-containing products and washed red blood cells can be used to prevent hemolysis (112).

References

1. Mollison PL. Blood transfusion in clinical medicine. Oxford: Blackwell Scientific, 1983:297.
2. Grannum PAT, Chapel JA. Prevention of Rh isoimmunization and treatment of the compromised fetus. Semin Perinatol 1988;12:324–335.
3. Judd WJ, Luban NLC, Ness PM, Silberstein LE, Stroup M, Widmann FK. Prenatal and perinatal immunohematology; recommendations for serologic management of the fetus, newborn infant and obstetrical patient. Transfusion 1990;30:175–183.
4. Diamond LK, Allen FK, Thomas WO. Erythroblastosis fetalis. VII. Treatment with exchange transfusion. N Engl J Med 1951;244:39–69.
5. Oski FA. Jaundice. In: Avery ME, Taeusch HW, eds. Shaffer's disease of the newborn. Philadelphia: WB Saunders, 1984:822–832.
6. Gartner LM, Lee KS. Unconjugated hyperbilirubinemia. In: Fonaroff AA, Martin RJ, eds. Neonatal-perinatal medicine. St. Louis: CV Mosby, 1987:946–966.
7. Robertson A, Karp WB, Davis HC. Predicting the need for exchange transfusion in newborn infants: a comparison of five methods. Clin Pediatr 1983;22:533–536.
8. Lackner TE. Drug replacement following exchange transfusion. J Pediatr 1982;100:811–814.
9. Bevan HE, Weisser RW, Herman WM, Lightsey AJ, Thomas WJ. Emergency use of uncrossmatched red cells in neonatal intensive care infants. J Perinatol 1989;9:77–78.
10. Tollner U, Pohlandt F, Heinze F, Hendricks T. Treatment of sepsis. Acta Pediatr Scand 1977;66:605–610.
11. Christensen RD, MacFarlane JL, Taylor NL, Hill HR, Rothstein G. Blood and marrow neutrophils during experimental group B streptococcal infection: quantification of the stem cell, proliferative, storage and circulating pools. Pediatr Res 1982;16:549–554.
12. Lane TA. Granulocyte storage. Transfusion Med Rev 1990;4:23–34.

13. Christensen RD, Anstall H, Rothstein G. Neutrophil transfusion in septic neutropenic neonates. Transfusion 1982;22: 151–154.
14. Delivoria-Papadopoulos M, Morrow G, Oski FA. Exchange transfusion in the newborn infant with fresh and old blood. The role of storage in 2,3-diphosphoglycerate hemoglobin-oxygen affinity and oxygen release. J Pediatr 1971;79:898–903.
15. Campbell N, Stewart I. Exchange transfusion in ill newborn infants using peripheral arteries and veins. J Pediatr 1970;94: 820–822.
16. Sorella A, Gambardella P. Partial exchange transfusion using peripheral vessels in polycythemic newborn infants. Eur J Pediatr 1986;144:545–546.
17. Aranda JV, Sweet AY. Alterations in blood pressure during exchange transfusion. Arch Dis Child 1977;52:545–548.
18. Fletcher MA, Edwards MC. Exchange transfusions. In: Fletcher MA, MacDonald MG, Avery GB, eds. Atlas of procedures in neonatology. Philadelphia: JB Lippincott, 1983: 313–327.
19. Sacher RAS, Luban NLC, Strauss RG. Current practice and guidelines of cellular blood components in the newborn. Transfusion Med Rev 1989;3:39–54.
20. Keenan WJ, Novak KK, Sutherland JM, Bryla DA, Fetterly KL. Morbidity and mortality associated with exchange transfusion. Pediatrics 1985;75(suppl):417–421.
21. Luban NLC. Adverse reactions to blood and blood products. In: Kasprisin DO, Luban NLC, eds. Pediatric transfusion medicine. Boca Raton, FL: CRC Press, 1987:127–144.
22. Touloukian RJ, Kadar A, Spenser RP. The gastrointestinal complications of neonatal umbilical venous exchange transfusion: a clinical and experimental study. Pediatrics 1973;51: 36–43.
23. Scanlon JW, Krakaur R. Hyperkalemia following exchange transfusion. J Pediatr 1980;96:108–110.
24. Doyle PE, Eidelman AI, Lee K, Daum C, Gartner LM. Exchange transfusion and hypernatremia—possible role in intracranial hemorrhage in very low birth weight infants. Pediatrics 1978;92:848–849.
25. Rodeck CH, Holman CA, Karnicki J, Kemp JR, Whitmore DN, Austin MA. Direct intravascular fetal blood transfusion by fetoscopy in severe Rhesis isoimmunization. Lancet 1981;1:625–627.
26. Steiner EA, Judd WJ, Oberman HA, Hayashi RH, Nugent CE. Percutaneous umbilical vein transfusion. Transfusion 1990;30:104–108.
27. Grannum PA, Copel VA, Plaxe SC, Scioscia AL, Hobbins JC. In utero exchange transfusions by direct intravascular injection in severe erythroblastosis fetalis. N Engl J Med 1986;314: 1431–1434.
28. Ronkin S, Chayen B, Wapner RS, et al. Intravascular exchange and bolus transfusion in the severely isoimmunized fetus. Am J Obstet Gynecol 1989;160:407–411.
29. Wiswell TE, Cornish JD, Northam RS. Neonatal polycythemia: frequency of clinical manifestations and other associated findings. Pediatrics 1986;79:26–30.
30. Delaney-Black V, Camp BW, Lubchenco LO, et al. Neonatal hyperviscosity associated with lower achievement and IQ scores at school age. Pediatrics 1989;83:662–667.
31. Black VD, Lubchenco LO, Koops BL, Poland RL, Powell DF. Neonatal hyperviscosity: randomized study of effect of partial plasma exchange transfusion in long term outcome. Pediatrics 1985;75:1048–1053.
32. Bada HS, Korones SB, Kolni HW, et al. Partial plasma exchange transfusion improves cerebral hemodynamics in symptomatic neonatal polycythemia. Am J Med Sci 1986;291: 157–163.
33. Black VD, Rumack CM, Lubchenco LO, et al: Gastrointestinal injury of polycythemic term infants. Pediatrics 1985;76: 225–231.
34. Hein HA, Lathrop SS. Partial exchange transfusion in term polycythemic neonates: absence of association with severe gastrointestinal injury. Pediatrics 1987;80:75–78.
35. Nexo E, Christensen NC, Olesen J. Volume of blood removed for analytical purposes during hospitalization of low birthweight in infants. Clin Chem 1981;27:759–762.
36. Stockman JA, Graeber JE, Clark DA, McClellan K, Garcia JF, Kevey REW. Anemia of prematurity; determinants of the erythropoietin response. J Pediatr 1984;105:786–792.
37. DePalma L, Ness PM, Luban NLC. Red blood cell transfusion. In: Luban NLC, ed. Transfusion therapy in infants and children. Baltimore: Johns Hopkins University Press, 1990.
38. Linderkamp O, Versmold HT, Messow-Zahn K, Muller-Holve W, Riegel K, Betke K. The effect of intrapartum and intrauterine asphyxia on placental transfusion in premature and full term infants. Eur J Pediatr 1978;127:91–99.
39. Shannon KM, Naylor GS, Torkildson JC, et al. Circulating erythroid progenitors in the anemia of prematurity. N Engl J Med 1987;317:728–733.
40. Rhondeau SM, Christensen RD, Ross MP, Rothstein G, Simmons MA. Responsiveness of marrow erythroid progenitors from infant with "anemia of prematurity" to recombinant human erythropoeitin. J Pediatr 1988;112:935–940.
41. Holbrook ST, Christensen RD, Rothstein G. Erythroid colonies derived from fetal blood display different growth patterns from those derived from adult marrow. Pediatr Res 1988;24:605–608.
42. Ohls RX, Liechty KW, Turner MC, Kilmura RE, Christensen RD. Erythroid "burst-promoting" activity in serum of patients with the anemia of prematurity. J Pediatr 1990;116:786–789.
43. Halperin DS, Wacker P, Lacourt G, et al. The effects of recombinant human erythropoeitin in infants with the anemia of prematurity: a pilot study. J Pediatr 1990;116:779–786.
43a. Shannon KM, Mentzer WC, Abels RI, et al. Recombinant human erythropoietin in the anemia of prematurity: results of a placebo-controlled pilot study. J Pediatr 1991;118:949–955.
43b. Ohls RK, Christensen RD. Recombinant erythropoietin compared with erythrocyte transfusion in the treatment of anemia of prematurity. J Pediatr 1991;119:781–788.
44. Blanchette VS, Zipursky A. Assessment of anemia in newborn infants. Clin Perinatol 1984;11:489–510.
45. Hudson IR, Holland BR, Jones JG, Turner TL, Wardrop CAJ. First day total circulating red cell volume (RCV) predicts outcome in preterm infants [Abstract]. Pediatr Res 1990;27:209.
46. Wardrop CAJ, Holland BM, Veale KEA, Jones JG, Gray OP. Nonphysiological anemia of prematurity. Arch Dis Child 1978;53:855–860.
47. Alverson DC, Iskeu VH, Cohen RSA. Effect of booster blood transfusions on oxygen utilization in infants with bronchopulmonary dysplasia. J Pediatr 1988;113:722–726.
48. Keyes WG, Donohue PK, Spivak JL, et al. Assessing the need for transfusion of premature infants and role of hematocrit, clinical signs and erythropoietin level. Pediatrics 1989;84:412–417.
49. Donowitz LG, Turner RB, Seavey MAM, Luban NLC, Hendley JO. High rate of blood donor response for critically ill neonates. Infect Control Hosp Epidemiol 1989;10:509–510.
50. Ludvigsen CW, Swanson JL, Thompson JR, McCullough J. The failure of neonates to form red blood cell alloantibodies in response to multiple transfusions. Am J Clin Pathol 1987;87:250–251.

51. Floss AM, Strauss RG, Goeken N, Knox L. Multiple transfusions fail to provoke antibodies against blood cell antigens in human infants. Transfusion 1986;26:419–422.
52. Walker RH. Technical manual. 10th ed. Arlington, VA: American Association of Blood Banks, 1990.
53. Stockman JA, Clark DA. Weight gain: a response to transfusion in selected preterm infants. Am J Dis Child 1984;138: 828–830.
54. Blank JP, Sheagren TG, Vajaria J, et al. The role of RBC transfusion in the premature infant. Am J Dis Child 1984;138:831–833.
55. Joshi A, Gerhardt T, Shandhoff P, et al. Blood transfusion effect on the respiratory pattern of preterm infants. Pediatrics 1987;80:79–84.
56. DeMaio JG, Harris MC, Deuber C, et al. Effect of blood transfusion on apnea frequency in growing premature infants. J Pediatr 1989;114:1039–1041.
57. Ross MP, Christensen RD, Rothstein G, et al. A randomized trial to develop criteria for administering erythrocyte transfusions to anemic preterm infants 1 to 3 months of age. J Perinatol 1989;9:246–253.
58. McCracken GH Jr, Eichenwald HF. Leukocyte function and the development of opsonic and complement activity in the neonate. Am J Dis Child 1971;121:120–126.
59. Stossel TP, Alper CH, Rosen F. Opsonic activity in the newborn: role of properdin. Pediatrics 1973;52:134–137.
60. Gerdes JS, Yoder MC, Douglas SD, et al. Decreased plasma fibronectin in neonatal sepsis. Pediatrics 1983;72:877–881.
61. Strauss RG. Granulopoiesis and neutrophil function in the neonate. In: Stockman JA, Pochedly C, eds. Developmental and neonatal hematology. New York: Raven Press, 1988:88–101.
62. Christensen RD, Rothstein G, Anstall HB, Baybee B. Granulocyte transfusions in neonates with bacterial infection, neutropenia, and depletion of mature marrow neutrophils. Pediatrics 1982;70:1–6.
63. Shigeoka A, Santos J, Hill H. Functional analysis of neutrophil granulocytes from healthy, infected and stressed newborns. J Pediatr 1979;95:454–460.
64. Ambruso DR, Bentwood B, Henson PM, et al. Oxidative metabolism of cord blood neutrophils: relationship to content and degranulation of cytoplasmic granules. Pediatr Res 1984;18:1148–1153.
65. Ballow M, Cates KL, Rowe JC, et al. Development of the immune system in very low birth weight (less than 1500 g) premature infants: concentrations of plasma immunoglobulin and patterns of infection. Pediatr Res 1986;20:899–904.
66. Conway SP, Gillies DRN, Doherty A. Neonatal infection in premature infants and use of human immunoglobulin. Arch Dis Child 1987;62:1252–1256.
67. Chirico G, Rondini G, Plebani A, et al. Intravenous gammaglobulin therapy for prophylaxis of infection in high-risk neonates. J Pediatr 1987;110:437–442.
68. Baley JE, Stork EK, Warkentin PI, Shurin SB. Buffy coat transfusions in neutropenic neonates with presumed sepsis: a prospective, randomized trial. Pediatrics 1987;80:712–720.
69. Wheeler JC, Chauvenet AR, Johnson CA, et al. Buffy coat transfusions in neonates with sepsis and neutrophil storage pool depletion. Pediatrics 1987;97:422–425.
70. Laurenti F, Ferro R, Isacchi G, et al. Polymorphonuclear leukocyte transfusion for the treatment for sepsis in the newborn infant. J Pediatr 1981;98:118–123.
71. Laurenti F, LaGreca G, Ferro R, Bucci G. Transfusion of polymorphonuclear neutrophils in a premature infant with Klebsiella sepsis. Lancet 1978;2:111–112.
72. DeCurtis M, Romano G, Scarpato N, D'Antonio F, Paludetto R, Ciccimara F. Transfusions of polymorphonuclear leukocytes (PMN) in an infant with necrotizing enterocolitis (NEC) and a defect of phagocytosis. J Pediatr 1981;99:665–668.
73. Laing IA, Boulton FE, Hume R. Polymorphonuclear leucocyte transfusion in neonatal septicaemia. Arch Dis Child 1983;58:1003–1005.
74. Cairo MS, Rucker R, Bennetts GA, et al. Improved survival of newborns receiving leukocyte transfusions for sepsis. Pediatrics 1984;74:887–892.
75. Cairo MS, Worcester C, Rucker R, et al. Role of circulating complement and polymorphonuclear leukocyte transfusion in treatment and outcome in critically ill neonates with sepsis. J Pediatr 1987;110:935–941.
76. Newman RS, Waffarn F, Simmons GE, Goldsticker RD, Ocariz JA. Questionable value of saline prepared granulocytes in the treatment of neonatal septicemia. Transfusion 1988;28:196–197.
77. Engle WA, McGuire WA, Schreiner RL, Yu RL. Neutrophil storage pool depletion in neonates with sepsis and neutropenia. J Pediatr 1988;113:747–749.
78. Cairo MS. Neutrophil transfusions in the treatment of neonatal sepsis. Am J Pediatr Hematol Oncol 1989;11:227–234.
79. Baley JE. Neonatal sepsis: the potential for immunotherapy. Clin Perinatol 1988;15:755–771.
80. Castle V, Andrew M, Kelton J, et al. Frequency and mechanisms of neonatal thrombocytopenia. J Pediatr 1986;108:749–755.
81. McIntosh S, O'Brien RT, Schwartz AD, Pearson HA. Neonatal isoimmune purpura: response to platelet infusion. J Pediatr 1973;82:1020–1027.
82. Kaplan C, Deffos F, Forestier F, et al. Management of alloimmune thrombocytopenia: antenatal diagnosis and in utero transfusion of maternal platelets. Blood 1988;72:340–343.
83. Moise KJ, Carpenter RJ, Colton RB, Wasserstrum N, Kirshon DB, Canal L. Percutaneous umbilical cord blood sampling in the evaluation of fetal platelet counts in pregnant patients with autoimmune thrombocytopenia purpura. Obstet Gynecol 1988;72:346–350.
84. Sacher RA, King JC. Intravenous immunoglobulin therapy in pregnancy. Obstet Gynecol Surv 1989;44:1–9.
85. Bussel JB, Perkowitz RL, McFarland JG, Lynch L, Chitkara U. Antenatal treatment of neonatal alloimmune thrombocytopenia. N Engl J Med 1988;319:1374–1378.
86. Ballin A, Koren G, Kohelet D, et al. Reduction of platelet counts induced by mechanical ventilation in newborn infants. J Pediatr 1987;111:445–449.
87. Moroff G, Friedman A, Robkin-Klein L, et al. Reduction of the volume of stored platelet concentrated for neonatal use. Transfusion 1984;24:144–146.
88. Pierce RN, Reich LM, Mayer K. Hemolysis following platelet transfusion from ABO incompatible donors. Transfusion 1985;25:60–62.
89. Lee EJ, Schiffer CA. ABO compatibility can influence the results of platelet transfusion: results of a randomized trial. Transfusion 1989;29:284–389.
90. Bada HS, Korones SB, Perry EH, et al. Frequent handling in the neonatal intensive care unit and intraventricular hemorrhage. J Pediatr 1990;117:126–131.
91. Andrew M, Castle V, Saigal S, Carter C, Kelton K. Clinical impact of neonatal thrombocytopenia. J Pediatr 1987;110:457–464.
92. Setzer ES, Webb IB, Wassenaar JW, Reeder JD, Mehta PS, Eitzma DV. Platelet dysfunction and coagulopathy in intraventricular hemorrhage in the premature infant. J Pediatr 1982;100:599–625.
92a. Tegtmeier GE. The use of cytomegalovirus-screened blood in neonates [Editorial]. Transfusion 1988;28:201–203.

93. Yeager AS, Grumet FC, Hafleigh EB, et al. Prevention of transfusion-acquired cytomegalovirus infections in newborn infants. J Pediatr 1981;98:281–287.
94. Adler SP, Lawrence LT, Baggett J, Biro V, Sharp DE. Prevention of transfusion-associated cytomegalovirus infection in very low-birthweight infants using frozen blood and donors seronegative for cytomegalovirus. Transfusion 1985;24:333–335.
95. Brady MT, Milman JD, Anderson DC, et al. Use of deglycerolized red blood cells to prevent post-transfusion infection with cytomegalovirus in neonates. J Infect Dis 1984;150:334–339.
96. Demmler GJ, Brady MT, Bijou H, et al. Posttransfusion cytomegalovirus infection in neonates: role of saline-washed red blood cells. J Pediatr 1986;108:762–765.
97. Luban NLC, Williams AE, MacDonald MG, Mikesell GT, Williams KM, Sacher RA. Low incidence of acquired cytomegalovirus infection in neonates transfused with washed red blood cells. Am J Dis Child 1987;141:416–419.
98. Gilbert GL, Hayes K, Hudson IL, James J. Prevention of transfusion-acquired cytomegalovirus infection in infants by blood filtration to remove leukocytes. Lancet 1989;2:1228–1231.
99. Adler SP. Data that suggest that FFP does not transmit CMV [Letter]. Transfusion 1988;28:604.
100. Yeager AS, Palumbo PE, Malachowski N, et al. Sequelae of maternally derived cytomegalovirus infections in premature infants. J Pediatr 1983;102:918–922.
101. Luban NLC. Transfusion-associated infection. In: Donowitz LC, ed. Hospital acquired infection in the pediatric patient. Baltimore: Williams & Wilkins, 1988:109–139.
102. Thaler M, Shamiss A, Orgad S, et al. The role of blood from HLA-homozygous donors in fatal transfusion-associated graft-versus-host disease after open heart surgery. N Engl J Med 1989;321:25–28.
103. Holland PV. Prevention of transfusion-associated graft-versus-host disease. Arch Pathol Lab Med 1989;113:285–291.
104. Sanders MR, Graeber JE. Posttransfusion graft-versus-host disease in infancy. J Pediatr 1990;117:159–161.
105. Dobryski W, Thiboudeau S, Truitt RL, et al. Third-party-mediated graft rejection and graft-versus-host disease after T-cell-depleted bone marrow transplantation as demonstrated by hypervariable DNA probes and HLA-DR polymorphism. Blood 1989;74:2285–2294.
106. Read EJ, Kodis C, Carter CS, Leitman SF. Viability of platelets following storage in the irradiated state. Transfusion 1988;28:446–450.
107. Moore GL, Ledford ME. Effects of 4000 rad irradiation on the in vitro storage properties of packed cells. Transfusion 1985;25:583–585.
108. Rivet C, Baxter A, Rock G. Potassium levels in irradiated blood [Letter]. Transfusion 1989;29:185.
109. Gooch VM, Longhurst D, Sasich F, Laub RM. Safety of neonatal transfusions of gravity-sedimented RBC's following storage in CPDA-1 or ADSOL [Abstract]. Transfusion 1986;26:562.
110. Luban NLC, Strauss RA, Hume HA. Safety of red blood cell preserved in extended storage media for neonatal transfusion. Transfusion 1991;31:229–235.
111. Tuchschmid P, Mieth D, Burger D, Duc R. Potential hazard of hypoalbuminemia in newborn babies after exchange transfusion with Adsol red blood cell concentrates. Pediatrics 1990;85:234–235.
112. Williams RA, Brown EF, Hurst D, Franklin LC. Transfusion of infants with activation of erythrocyte T antigen. J Pediatr 1989;115:949–953.

71 Complications of Blood Transfusion

Jay E. Menitove

Blood transfusion involves the transfer of biologically active material from one human being to another. Consequences associated with transfusion include immune-mediated reactions that result from incompatibility between the donor and the recipient and the transmission of infectious diseases. Avoidance of all risk is not possible (1–3). Transfusion therapy must be reserved for situations in which there is a reasonable expectation that it will improve the well-being of the patient. Clinicians must be aware of alternatives to homologous transfusion, such as autologous blood, intraoperative cell salvage, hemodilution, hematopoietic growth factors, and pharmacologic agents that stimulate hemostasis, and they must use them whenever possible.

Complications of blood transfusions are categorized into those that occur acutely, those that occur several days or weeks following transfusion, and those involving infection.

ACUTE TRANSFUSION REACTIONS

Acute adverse effects of blood transfusion occur within minutes to hours after administering blood or blood components. These reactions may relate to red cells, white cells, platelets, or plasma. Red cell incompatibility is characterized by hemolysis, either intravascular or extravascular. Antibodies directed against white cells cause nonhemolytic chill/fever reactions. Reactions to plasma may result in a spectrum of complications ranging from hives to anaphylaxis.

The presenting signs and symptoms are not specific with regard to etiology. For example, it is not possible to distinguish patients having an acute hemolytic reaction from those suffering a febrile nonhemolytic transfusion reaction on the basis of clinical symptoms alone. Prompt laboratory investigation is required to ascertain the pathogenic mechanism and the basis for therapy (Table 71.1).

Acute Hemolytic Transfusion Reaction

Hemolytic transfusion reactions are among the most serious acute complications of blood transfusion. Fortunately, they occur uncommonly, perhaps as infrequently as 1 per 6,000 to 25,000 component infusions (4). The associated mortality is probably less than 10%.

PATHOPHYSIOLOGY

The site of red cell destruction varies according to the potency of the antibody and whether or not complement is activated. Lysis of donor red cells occurs when complement is fully activated (intravascular hemolysis). Without complement activation, red cells can be bound by antibody, but not lysed. Instead, they are removed from the circulation by macrophages in the liver and spleen (extravascular hemolysis) (Fig. 71.1).

Intravascular Hemolysis

"Naturally occurring" antibodies, such as IgM anti-A and anti-B, are found in group O individuals who have never been exposed to homologous blood. These antibodies bind complement efficiently. Hence, it is not surprising that two-thirds of the deaths due to acute hemolytic events, reported to the U.S. Food and Drug Administration over a 10-year period, occurred in group O recipients (5). In ABO mismatch situations, complement activation proceeds to completion. The C5-C9 membrane attack complex binds to the red cell and causes osmotic red cell lysis and the release into the plasma of free hemoglobin and antibody-coated red cell stroma.

Table 71.1. Complications of Blood Transfusion—Acute

	Approximate Frequency per Component
Acute hemolytic transfusion reaction	1 per 6,000 to 25,000
Febrile nonhemolytic transfusion reaction	1 per 200
Transfusion-related acute lung injury	1 per 5,000
Allergic reaction (urticaria, pruritus)	1 per 100 to 300
Anaphylactic reactions	1 per 150,000
Hypervolemia	Variable
Nonimmune hemolysis	Uncommon
Air embolism	Rare
Complications of massive transfusion	Unknown; patients require careful monitoring
Bacterial sepsis	Uncommon

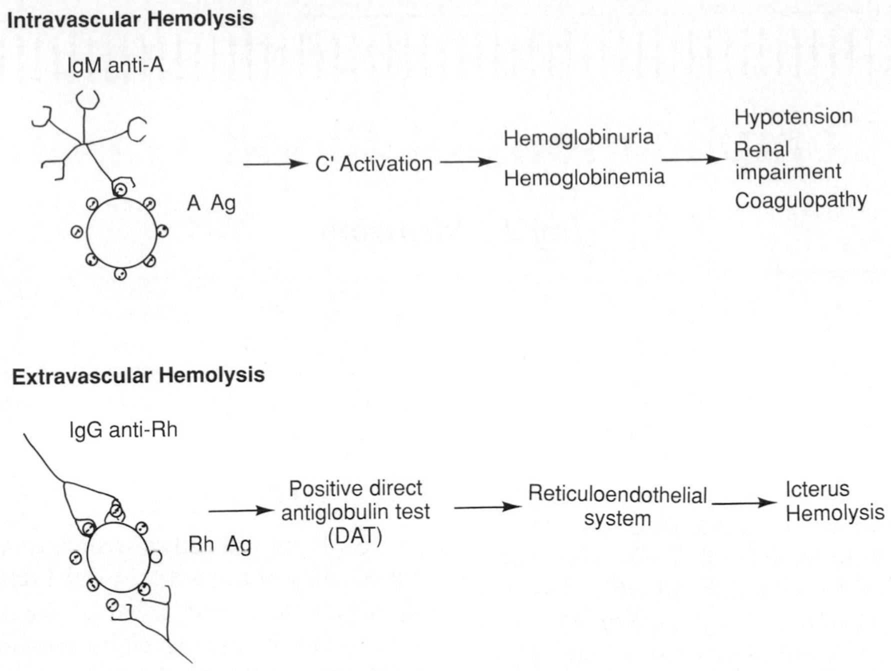

Figure 71.1. Intravascular and extravascular hemolysis are contrasted. Anti-A antibodies are usually potent and activate complement (C′) when exposed to group A red cells. Hemoglobin is released into the plasma and is excreted by the kidneys. C′ activation leads to vasomotor changes, red cell lysis with the release of thromboplastic substances, and the possibility of disseminated intravascular coagulation. Anti-Rh antibody does not activate C′. Antibody-coated cells are lysed by macrophages and killer lymphocytes. Fever, jaundice, and hemolysis result, but the clinical reaction is usually milder than that seen with ABO incompatibility.

Clinical sequelae are related to the presence of activated complement components, thromboplastic substances from erythrocyte stroma, and vasoactive compounds formed as a result of antigen-antibody interactions. In addition to anti-A and anti-B, other antibodies associated with hemolytic transfusion reactions include anti-K (Kell), anti-Jk^a (Kidd), and anti-Fy^a (Duffy).

Extravascular Hemolysis

Some antibodies, such as those directed against Rh-antigens (e.g., anti-E, anti-c, anti-D), do not activate complement. Such alloantibodies bind to red cells, but complement activation does not proceed to completion. Accordingly, these cells, coated with C3b, are removed by tissue macrophages. Hemoglobinemia and hemoglobinuria occur when plasma haptoglobin binding is exceeded. Extravascular hemolytic reactions, in general, are milder than intravascular hemolytic reactions.

CLINICAL PRESENTATION

Fever (elevation of at least 2°F or 1°C) or fever accompanied by chills occurs in almost all patients suffering a hemolytic transfusion reaction. Nausea, vomiting, and chest pain are observed less often. Pronounced facial flushing has been observed in patients having brisk intravascular hemolysis. Wheezing and dyspnea, back pain, restlessness, and discomfort at the infusion site have also been reported. Hypotension is considered a sign of a severe hemolytic reaction and may be a prelude to disseminated intravascular coagulation (DIC). In the comatose or anesthetized patient, the most important signs are hypotension, uncontrollable bleeding along surgical incisions, or hemoglobinuria (4).

SIGNIFICANT SEQUELAE

Severe symptoms may follow the transfusion of only a few milliliters of incompatible red cells in patients with potent anti-A and anti-B antibodies. However, in patients with weak, naturally occurring antibodies, the transfusion of several units of ABO-incompatible blood may cause only minor effects. Patients given Rh-incompatible blood may experience only febrile reactions, although jaundice and hemoglobinuria may develop later.

The major adverse consequences of hemolytic reactions are vasomotor instability and hypotension, bleeding diathesis characterized as DIC, and renal impairment (6).

Vasomotor Instability

Hypotension occurs when complement products C3a, C4a, and C5a are released into plasma. These peptides, with molecular weights of approximately

10,000, cause contraction of smooth muscle and degranulation of mast cells, which in turn, release vasoactive substances such as bradykinin and serotonin. Antigen-antibody complexes also activate Hageman factor (factor XII), which leads to production of bradykinin. Hypotension ensues as a result of increased capillary permeability and arteriolar dilation. The fall in blood pressure is associated with sympathetic nervous system-induced catecholamine discharge. As a result, renal, splanchnic, pulmonary, and cutaneous capillaries vasoconstrict.

Bleeding Diathesis

Antigen-antibody complexes activate the intrinsic clotting cascade through Hageman factor (factor XII) activation. Alternatively, procoagulant substances are released from red cell stromata after lysis. Activation of the clotting cascade results in thrombus formation in the microvasculature, consumption of coagulation factors, activation of the fibrinolytic system, and possible, uncontrolled bleeding.

Renal Insufficiency

Renal insufficiency and oliguria result from changes in renal blood flow that are precipitated by hypotension, vasomotor instability, and renal vasoconstriction. A direct toxic effect on renal tubular cells by free hemoglobin is unlikely. Formation of thrombi in renal vessels may also compromise the blood supply to the kidney, resulting in acute tubular necrosis.

LABORATORY DIAGNOSIS

If a hemolytic transfusion reaction is suspected, the infusion must be stopped immediately, and a posttransfusion blood specimen must be sent to the transfusion service. A clerical check to confirm the patient's name, hospital number, compatibility label, and donor unit number should be undertaken quickly. The error may involve the cross-match sample, the documentation, or the unit of blood. Because of the possibility that one or more units of blood may have been confused, mislabeled, or switched, it is important to determine immediately if another patient is at risk.

A visual determination of free hemoglobin in the postreaction serum or plasma specimens should be performed by comparing the color of the pre- and posttransfusion reaction specimens for a pink or red hue. A direct antiglobulin test should also be performed and is positive in almost all cases. A urine specimen may be examined for the presence of free hemoglobin or, subsequently, for urinary hemosiderin (Table 71.2).

Table 71.2. Transfusion Reaction Involving Febrile Episodes—Immediate Laboratory Evaluation

Check for clerical error
Compare visually for hemolysis pre- and post transfusion specimens
Direct antiglobulin test
Check urine for free hemoglobin
Further workup depends on results of above evaluation

If the clerical check, visual inspection, or result of the direct antiglobulin test supports the diagnosis of hemolytic transfusion reaction, additional testing is indicated. This includes repeating the ABO and Rh typing on pre- and posttransfusion reaction samples and on the unit of blood. If the direct antiglobulin test is positive, sensitive tests for detecting unexpected antibodies in the donor and patient sera and on the patient's cells should be pursued. A cross-match should be performed with prereaction and postreaction samples using red cells from the unit or from a stored, sealed segment. Plasma hemoglobin measurements may be evaluated. Serum haptoglobin levels on both prereaction and postreaction samples should be determined; these usually indicate a significant decline in the postreaction sample in the vast majority of patients with a hemolytic reaction. Posttransfusion hemoglobin and hematocrit results should be evaluated to determine if the expected hemoglobin or hematocrit elevation occurred: The unconjugated bilirubin level should be obtained on a specimen preferably drawn 5 to 7 hours after transfusion.

If hemolysis is suspected and an antibody-mediated etiology cannot be ascertained, a Gram stain of a blood smear from the unit of blood may be evaluated, and the unit may be cultured.

TREATMENT

Prevention is the most effective form of therapy. Identification of blood samples, donor units, and recipients is crucial.

The administration of blood to the "wrong" patient, because of a clerical error or the failure to observe procedures designed to ensure the proper identification of the donor unit and the recipient, is the most frequent underlying situation leading to acute hemolytic transfusion reactions. Conditions requiring urgent transfusion are especially conducive to error. Removal of wrist bands during an operation or the transfusion of unconscious or anesthetized patients jeopardizes proper patient identification.

As soon as a hemolytic transfusion reaction is suspected, the blood transfusion must be stopped. Therapy is directed at correction of hypotension, control of bleeding, and prevention of acute tubular necrosis. Maintenance of blood pressure is important because hypotension is a prelude to DIC and acute renal failure. Replacement of depleted coagulation factors is accomplished by the transfusion of cryoprecipitate, platelet concentrates, or fresh frozen plasma as needed.

Renal complications are prevented by maintaining renal blood flow. Systolic blood pressure should be maintained by infusion of intravenous fluids, mannitol (20 g in 100 ml infused over 5 minutes), or other diuretics, such as furosemide (40 to 120 mg IV) or ethacrynic acid (50 to 100 mg IV), to stimulate urine flow. Urine output should be maintained at 100 ml/hr. If oliguria or anuria ensues, standard measures for renal failure management must be taken.

Febrile Nonhemolytic Transfusion Reactions

Febrile nonhemolytic transfusion reactions are characterized by a posttransfusion temperature rise of 1°C or more in the absence of hemolysis or other defined cause and occur with a frequency of approximately 0.5% per component transfused.

PATHOPHYSIOLOGY

Febrile nonhemolytic transfusion reactions, or chill/fever reactions, occur predominantly in patients who have a history of pregnancy or previous transfusion. The reactions are caused by recipient cytotoxic or agglutinating antibodies that react against antigens on transfused lymphocytes, granulocytes, or platelets. On occasion, the chill/fever reaction results from the passive infusion of leukocyte antibodies contained in the plasma of infused components and the subsequent activity of these antibodies directed against the recipient's white cells.

The "threshold" leukocyte count evoking a chill/fever reaction in susceptible patients varies from 2×10^8 to 2.5×10^9 white cells per component. The majority of reactions are associated with sensitivity to granulocytes, but reactions to lymphocytes or platelets also occur. The type of antibody is less predictive of the severity of the reaction than is the amount present, the number and subset of leukocytes transfused, and the transfusion rate (7).

CLINICAL PRESENTATION

Febrile nonhemolytic transfusion reactions have three phases. The first consists of an immediate reaction, which is transient. It may start within 5 minutes of the beginning of the transfusion and is marked by a flush, palpitation, tachycardia, cough, chest discomfort, or neutropenia. The second, or latent, phase usually occurs between 15 to 60 minutes after the onset of the transfusion. During this time, the patient feels well. This is followed by a rise in diastolic blood pressure, headache, chilliness, and possible progression to rigors. Subsequently, a rapid rise in temperature occurs (Fig. 71.2). Apathy, irritability, impaired mentation, and prostration may persist for several hours. A neutrophilic leukocytosis with a marked shift to the left occurs 2 to 5 hours after the beginning of the infusion (8).

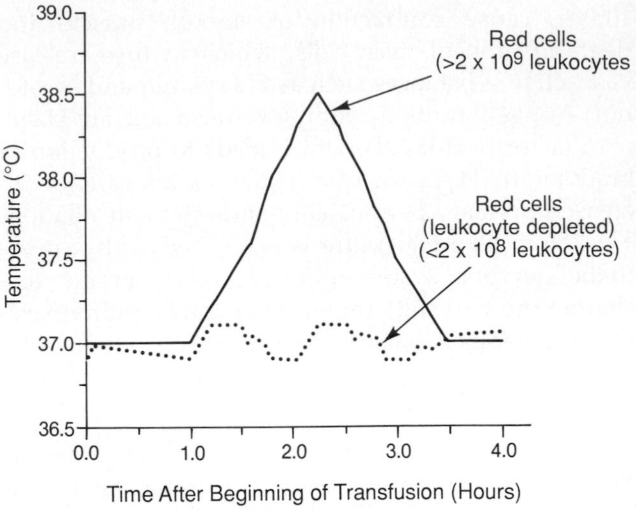

Figure 71.2. Temperature recording from a patient with a history of febrile nohemolytic transfusion reactions. One hour following the infusion of red cells containing "buffy coat" cells (greater than 2×10^9 leukocytes), a fever spike occurred. Fever was avoided with red cells, leukocytes depleted (less than 2×10^8 leukocytes). (Modified from Brittingham TE, Chaplin H Jr. Febrile transfusion reactions caused by sensitivity to donor leukocytes and platelets. JAMA 1957;165:819–825.

SIGNIFICANT SEQUELAE

Febrile nonhemolytic transfusion reactions are rarely associated with significant adverse sequelae. The signs and symptoms are usually self-limited. Although discomfort and fear occur, these reactions are not life-threatening. Because fever may be the initial manifestation of a hemolytic reaction, the presenting symptoms must be taken seriously, and laboratory evaluation undertaken as soon as possible to determine whether hemolysis has occurred.

LABORATORY DIAGNOSIS

Although alloantibodies against granulocytes, HLA antibodies, and platelet-specific antibodies can cause transfusion reactions, tests for these antibodies are not performed routinely. A single test for lymphocytotoxicity, leukoagglutination, or immunofluorescence on platelets, granulocytes, and lymphocytes is insufficient for detecting such antibodies in every patient. A combination of tests, such as lymphocytotoxicity and indirect platelet suspension immunofluorescence, will discover alloimmunization in almost all cases (9). In practice, febrile nonhemo-

Table 71.3. Febrile Nonhemolytic Transfusion Reaction—Methods for Preparing Red Blood Cells, Leukocytes Removed

	Residual Leukocytes	Leukocytes Removed	Red Cells Remaining
		%	%
Centrifugation	4–12 × 10^8	>70	>80
Filtration			
Microaggregate filters	~3–4 × 10^8	85–95+	80–90
Special leukocyte depletion filters	0.02–1.2 × 10^8	>95–99+	>90
Saline washing	1–4 × 10^8	~90	75–90
Frozen, deglycerolized red cells	0.1–1 × 10^8	95–99+	>80

lytic reactions are diagnoses of exclusion. The diagnosis is made by demonstrating no evidence of hemolysis during the routine laboratory evaluation of a transfusion reaction: The postreaction serum or plasma specimen does not have hemoglobinemia, and the direct antiglobulin test is negative.

TREATMENT

Because fever is the most frequent presenting sign of both hemolytic or nonhemolytic reactions, hemolysis cannot be distinguished on clinical grounds alone. Hence, the infusion must be stopped immediately when fever is discovered. Fortunately, most febrile nonhemolytic reactions are self-limited and can be treated with such supportive measures as orally administered antipyretics. Severe rigors may respond to meperidine.

Fewer than 15% of the patients who have a febrile reaction suffer a recurrence with subsequent transfusions. Hence, it is reasonable to make no change in transfusion practice until after a second febrile nonhemolytic transfusion reaction unless the first reaction is severe. For patients having a recurrence, future transfusions should be administered with the buffy coat removed (10). This can be accomplished by a variety of filtration techniques. Special leukocyte filters can remove approximately 99% of leukocytes while retaining more than 90% of the red cells for transfusion (Table 71.3). In patients who continue to have febrile reactions, frozen, deglycerolized red blood cells may be used.

Tranfusion-Related Acute Lung Injury

Transfusion-related acute lung injury (pulmonary infiltrates and noncardiogenic pulmonary edema) is an infrequent complication resulting from incompatibility involving leukocyte antibodies (11, 12). The incidence was 0.02% per unit and 0.16% per patient transfused in one reported study (11).

Patients develop fever, substernal chest pain, marked dyspnea, cyanosis, cough, blood-tinged sputum and hypoxemia within 4 hours (usually 1 to 2 hours) after transfusion of whole blood, red cells, fresh frozen plasma, platelet concentrates, or cryoprecipitate. The chest x-ray shows a normal heart size with bilateral diffuse, patchy pulmonary infiltrates. Left atrial and pulmonary wedge pressures are within normal limits or low. The patients appear to have pulmonary edema of noncardiac origin and require supportive therapy. On occasion, the increased fluid in the pulmonary parenchyma results in intravascular hypovolemia and hypotension. These patients require fluid replacement rather than fluid restriction. Most patients require respiratory support and mechanized ventilation, but recovery usually occurs within 48 hours. Some patients have persistence of pulmonary infiltrates and hypoxemia for up to 1 week.

At least two pathogenic models are proposed. Passive infusion of donor antibody directed against recipient leukocytes is the most widely ascribed hypothesis. Granulocyte, lymphocytotoxic, and HLA-specific antibodies are present in 65 to 89% of donors implicated in these reactions. Often, the donors are multiparous women, and there is a sharing of HLA specificity between donor antibody and recipient phenotype. Less often, the patient may have antibody directed against donor leukocytes. An alternative mechanism implicates complement activation and subsequent aggregation and trapping of white cells in the pulmonary microvasculature.

It is unknown why so few patients develop pulmonary infiltrates, in contrast to the more common chill/fever response.

Allergic Reactions

Allergic reactions, manifested by urticaria and pruritus, are among the most frequently encountered acute adverse effects of transfusion. As many as 1 to 3% of transfused patients develop these complications. Severe allergic reactions that culminate in acute anaphylaxis occur at a rate of approximately 1 per 150,000 components transfused (13).

URTICARIA

Hives and pruritus, usually without fever, occur after a plasma-containing blood component is infused. The presumed etiology is a reaction between a protein in donor plasma and a corresponding IgE antibody in the recipient. In most instances, the reaction is mild. Treatment involves stopping the transfusion, administering an antihistamine, waiting for the pruritis to subside, and continuing the transfusion. Because urticaria is not a sign of hemolysis, laboratory investigation for a transfusion reaction is unnecessary. Patients who have had urticarial reactions and require further transfusion therapy may be premedicated with an antihistamine orally prior to subsequent transfusion. If hives continue to occur, plasma should be removed from red cells and/or platelet transfusions by washing with saline solutions.

ANAPHYLACTIC TRANSFUSION REACTIONS

Anaphylactic or anaphylactoid reactions following transfusion are rare but have been associated with fatal outcomes. In general, they occur among patients who are IgA deficient (approximately one in 1000 of the normal population).

The striking clinical presentation includes apprehension and a feeling of doom, chest or lumbar pain, flushing of the face and upper body, a generalized urticarial rash with pruritus, laryngeal or facial edema with bronchospasm, wheezing and dyspnea, hypotension, loss of consciousness, vomiting, and diarrhea. Several hours after the acute reaction, chills and fever may occur.

Less dramatic presentations or anaphylactoid reactions consist of localized hives or mild, generalized urticarial rashes, headache, nausea, mild bronchospasm, or hypotension.

Pathogenesis

Anaphylactic or anaphylactoid reactions are mediated by anti-IgA antibody that is either class-specific (i.e., reacts with all human IgA) or has "limited specificity" (i.e, reactivity against a single IgA paraprotein). Class-specific IgG anti-IgA antibodies are found in patients who are congenitally deficient in IgA and who were exposed to IgA during pregnancy or through previous transfusion. Class-specific antibodies are capable of fixing complement.

Anti-IgA is detected by hemagglutination assays using panels of red cells coated with various IgA paraproteins or by radioimmunoassay methods. Although IgG anti-IgA is considered to mediate anaphylactic or anaphylactoid reactions, anti-IgA of limited specificity is found in otherwise apparently healthy individuals. However, only patients with congenital absence of IgA form class-specific anti-IgA antibodies.

Treatment and Prevention of Recurrence

Anaphylactic reactions are treated with intravenous epinephrine administration and careful clinical monitoring. Assays for IgA antibody levels and anti-IgA antibodies should be performed. If subsequent transfusions are required, cellular components should be washed to removed plasma. Components from IgA-deficient blood donors may also be used.

Hypervolemia

Patients with impaired myocardial reserve are at risk of congestive heart failure as a result of intravascular volume overexpansion. Packed red blood cell transfusions are preferred over whole blood for augmenting oxygen-carrying capacity in the elderly and others with underlying cardiac disease. An average unit of whole blood contains 56 mEq sodium, whereas a unit of red blood cells has 8 to 20 mEq sodium, and a unit of red cells with an additive solution to extend the shelf life to 42 days includes 24 to 30 mEq sodium. The plasma volume of platelet concentrates can be reduced by subjecting the concentrates to an additional centrifugation step.

Red blood cells must be transfused within 4 hours after removal from refrigerated storage conditions. If volume overload is a likely complication, the unit may be divided so that the amount tolerated can be infused during the permitted period and the remainder given at a later time.

Nonimmune Hemolysis

Transfused red cells subjected to osmotic or mechancial stress may burst and release hemoglobin into the circulation. Hypotonic solutions and medication added to blood may lead to osmotic rupture of red cells; therefore, normal saline, 5% albumin, or plasma protein fractions are the only fluids that should be added. Overheating of red cells by blood warmers may lead to red cell lysis. These devices should be monitored carefully to prevent this complication. Infusion pumps used routinely for infusion of intravenous fluids and medications do not appear to injure red cells. However, hemolysis has been reported during cell salvage procedures because of turbulence at the air/fluid interface.

In these cases, red cell destruction is suspected because of hemoglobinemia and hemoglobinuria. Often, it is not possible to distinguish nonimmune from immune causes of hemolysis until completion of the laboratory workup and investigation of the factors associated with the blood transfusion.

Air Embolism

Air embolism, a complication previously seen when vented glass bottles were used, is unlikely to occur with plastic containers. Likewise, it should not occur when cell separators are used for plasma exchange or cytoreduction procedures because reinfusion lines contain bubble detectors.

Symptoms associated with air embolism include chest pain, cough, and acute onset of dyspnea. The administration tubing should be clamped immediately and the patient placed on the left side in a head-down position to prevent obstruction of the pulmonary artery.

Complications of Massive Transfusion

Massive transfusion involves the replacement of a patient's entire blood volume in less than a 24-hour period. Patients requiring massive transfusion often have hypotension, tissue damage, and shock. Rapid restoration of circulating blood volume reduces the amount of tissue and organ damage.

INCREASED RISK OF CLERICAL ERROR

Urgent replacement of blood heightens the risk of errors in patient identification. This problem is exacerbated in situations involving multiple casualties arriving simultaneously at trauma centers. Use of group O red cells may be preferable in these circumstances until identification bands are in place.

HEMOSTATIC DEFECTS

Stored blood is devoid of functional platelets and deficient in labile coagulation factors V and VIII. Factor VIII decreases to approximately 50% of initial levels after the first day of storage and 30% after 5 days. Factor V activity falls to 50% by 14 days of storage. Other coagulation factors are stable, and their activity is maintained throughout the dating period. Standardized regimens of prescribing platelet concentrates and fresh frozen blood plasma after a predetermined number of red cell transfusions do not decrease blood component usage or augment hemostatic effectiveness. Such regimens should be avoided.

Microvascular bleeding (characterized by oozing from mucous membranes, bleeding from catheter or venipuncture sites, and generalized petechiae and enlarging ecchymoses) in these patients is likely when the platelet count is 50,000/μl or less or fibrinogen concentration is 50 mg/dl or less. It occurs infrequently when the values are above these levels. Approximately one-quarter to one-third of observed changes in platelet counts during massive transfusion are attributable to dilutional factors related to the infusion of stored blood that lacks platelets. The major factor contributing to the decrease in platelet count is platelet and/or clotting factor consumption related to the underlying condition or injury. Clotting factor deficiency, likewise, is not directly attributable to dilution. It may occur suddenly and may be associated with severe hypofibrinogenemia and thrombocytopenia.

Replacement therapy should be prescribed on the basis of measured laboratory abnormalities. Platelet transfusions are most likely to correct microvascular bleeding and should be given prophylactically if the count is less than or equal to 50,000/μl. Fresh frozen plasma or cryoprecipitate should be given if the fibrinogen concentration is less than 80 mg/dl (14, 15).

METABOLIC ABNORMALITIES

Citrate toxicity and associated hypocalcemia does not occur in the absence of liver impairment; a healthy adult can metabolize the citrate contained in stored blood despite infusion rates as rapid as 1 unit every 5 minutes. Hypocalcemia and hyperkalemia act synergistically to impair cardiac performance, especially when combined with hypothermia and acidosis. Electrocardiographic changes associated with hypocalcemia in patients receiving massive transfusions should be treated with infusions of calcium gluconate (5 ml of a 10% solution). In practice, hypokalemia occurs more frequently than hyperkalemia despite the release of potassium during red cell storage. The transfused red cells absorb potassium from plasma. Acidosis associated with hypoperfusion and tissue oxygen deprivation is ameliorated by transfusion and volume repletion. Citrate metabolism generates bicarbonate, which in turn, counteracts acidosis. Therefore, metabolic alkalosis is a more likely consequence of massive transfusion (16).

HYPOTHERMIA

Body temperature decreases in response to infusion of cold blood and intravenous fluids. Hypothermia slows citrate metabolism, potentiates the harmful myocardial depressant effects of hyperkalemia and hypocalcemia, and reduces oxygen release from red cells. Blood warmers may be useful when infusion rates exceed 1 unit/10 min. in adults (16).

ADULT RESPIRATORY DISTRESS SYNDROME

Respiratory distress syndrome occurs in the setting of a massive transfusion as a result of multiple factors related to the site of injury and the adequacy of volume repletion. (See previous discussion of transfusion-related acute lung injury.)

Bacterial Sepsis

Septicemia is a rare complication of blood transfusion therapy, but it requires rapid therapeutic intervention.

PATHOPHYSIOLOGY

Various etiologies have been proposed to explain the presence of bacteria in blood collected under sterile conditions. Bacteria may be present in the anticoagulant preservative solutions used to store blood;

they may enter tiny holes in the plastic tubing created by the heat sealers used to separate the main collection bag from the satellite containers; or they may contaminate the bag ports when frozen components are thawed in a waterbath. Alternatively, the disinfectants used in the skin preparation for phlebotomy may be tainted, or organisms may be introduced through a skin plug in the hollow port of the phlebotomy needle. The latter hypothesis is not consistent with the finding that Gram-negative bacteria are not usual skin bacteria. Several investigations of the pathogenesis of transfusion-associated bacterial sepsis cases have been inconclusive (17, 18). Recently, transfusion-associated *Yersinia enterocolitica* sepsis has been attributed to asymptomatic bacteremia in donors with resolving gastrointestinal illnesses. The red cells from these donors were stored for a minimum of 26 days at 4°C, an interval sufficient to allow initial trace amounts of bacteria to reproduce (19).

CLINICAL PRESENTATION

Following infusion of 50 to 70 ml of blood, patients develop chills or rigors, often associated with nausea, vomiting, and lethargy. On occasion, patients complain of pain in the abdominal or low back region or along the intravenous cannula site. Subsequently, fever and hypotension occur, progressing to shock and DIC.

LABORATORY DIAGNOSIS

An aliquot of the remaining blood should be examined for bacteria by Gram stain and culture. Gram-negative organisms are difficult to discern in such stains. Bacterial cultures should be obtained from the recipient. In general, culturing a segment of the attached tubing is not helpful; the source of the episode was probably a few bacteria that multipled during storage in the main container.

Profound symptoms are suggestive of the effects of endotoxin. Less dramatic clinical presentations occur when Gram-positive organisms are involved.

An increase in the number of transfusion-related sepsis cases occurred when the shelf life of room temperature-stored platelet concentrates was extended from 3 days to 7 days (20). Presumably, Gram-positive organisms gained entrance during phlebotomy. They remained at lag growth phase during the first 24 to 48 hours and then entered log-phase growth over the ensuing days. Currently, the dating period of platelet concentrates is 5 days.

TREATMENT

The symptom complex of chills occurring shortly after the onset of transfusion, associated with fever and hypotension, should raise the clinical suspicion of transfusion-related sepsis. The infusion should be stopped immediately, appropriate bacterial cultures performed, and the patient started on broad-spectrum antibiotics. Because some of the symptoms are related to bacterial endotoxin, supportive measures for maintaining blood pressure and fluid balance are essential.

Table 71.4. Complications of Blood Transfusion—Delayed

	Approximate Frequency per Component
Delayed hemolytic transfusion reaction	
Serologic	1 per 300 to 1600
Hemolytic	1 per 1500 to 8000
Alloimmunization	
Red cells	1% of hospitalized patients and 10% of multitransfused patients
Platelets	~40–50% of patients with acute leukemia
Graft versus host disease	Uncommon
Iron overload	Occurs in chronically transfused patients who receive >120 units RBC
Posttransfusion purpura	Uncommon
Immunosuppressive effects of blood transfusion	Unknown

DELAYED TRANSFUSION REACTIONS

Nonimmediate or delayed adverse consequences of blood transfusion occur days to years after the transfusion is given. Immunologic complications are characterized as hemolytic reactions, alloimmunization, graft versus host disease, and immunosuppressive effects of blood transfusion. Nonimmune complications involve iron overload and transfusion-transmitted diseases (Table 71.4).

Delayed Hemolytic Transfusion Reaction

A delayed hemolytic transfusion reaction is the result of alloantibody-mediated red cell destruction by an antibody not detected in pretransfusion testing that is present after transfusion. Antibody production usually reflects a secondary or anamnestic response. However, it is possible that some reactions are due to primary antibody formation.

The classic definition of a delayed hemolytic transfusion reaction requires three of the following five findings: (*a*) a compatible cross-match with pretransfusion serum; (*b*) a negative antibody screen on the recipient's pretransfusion serum; (*c*) an incompatible cross-match and a rising titer of the incriminated antibody in postreaction serum samples; (*d*) a history of blood transfusion, pregnancy, or both; (*e*) clinical or laboratory evidence of hemolysis demonstrated by a decrease in hemoglobin and haptoglobin levels, increased levels of indirect bilirubin, presence of hemoglobin in plasma and urine, urinary hemosiderin, or positive direct and indirect antiglobulin tests (21, 22).

Antibody may be detectable in the recipient as early as 48 hours posttransfusion. In general, clinical symptoms are seen 6 to 8 days (range 3 to 21 days) after transfusion. Serologic evidence of posttransfusion antibody not detected in pretransfusion testing may be as frequent as 1 per 300 to 1600 units transfused, and reactions may occur as frequently as 1 per 1500 to 9000 units transfused. Most patients with these serologic findings do not suffer hemolysis or clinical symptoms; therefore, most of the events are more appropriately classified as delayed serologic transfusion reactions. The term delayed hemolytic transfusion reaction should be reserved for the approximately 20% of patients with serologic findings who actually suffer clinical symptoms (21–24).

CLINICAL PRESENTATION

The triad of anemia, fever, and a recent transfusion in a patient with a history of previous tranfusion or pregnancy should raise a clinical suspicion of a delayed hemolytic transfusion reaction. A temperature elevation of at least 2°F (1°C) occurs in approximately three-quarters of patients with delayed hemolytic transfusion reactions. In one series of reported cases, anemia occured in almost 90%, jaundice developed in approximately two-thirds and 17% developed oliguria. Most of these symptoms occur approximately 1 week following transfusion (21).

LABORATORY DIAGNOSIS

Almost all patients with delayed hemolytic transfusion reactions have a positive direct antiglobulin test due to IgG sensitization. Weak complement sensitization is detected in association with antibodies known to fix complement. However, the presence of a positive direct antiglobulin reaction may be a transient finding, as may a weak mixed field reaction with IgG and, less frequently, C3d. In approximately two-third of cases, a single antibody is detected. Antibodies commonly found in delayed hemolytic transfusion reactions include anti-E, anti-Jk^a, anti-K, anti-D, anti-C, anti-c, and anti-Fy^a, alone or in combination (21, 22, 24).

The direct antiglobulin test remains positive for a prolonged period in many patients, as long as 6 months posttransfusion in some. Eluates from red cells demonstrate an alloantibody with specificity against the transfused cells or a panagglutinin. The finding of alloantibody months after transfusion suggests that autologous as well as allogeneic red cells may have been sensitized. Alternatively, these serologic results may indicate the nonspecific uptake of alloantibody in vitro. The panagglutination most likely represents autoantibodies that develop following transfusion. Because autoantibodies can mimic alloantibody specificities, it is possible that some of the "alloantibodies" represent autoantibody (24).

TREATMENT

Because there appears to be a dichotomy between serologic findings and clinical consequences, treatment rarely is needed. Supportive therapy is indicated only for serious complications, such as oliguria. Fortunately, this is uncommon.

Alloimmunization

Following exposure to homologous blood transfusion, patients may make antibodies to donor red cells, white blood cells, platelets, or serum proteins. Production of alloantibody, of itself, produces no adverse consequences. However, for patients requiring subsequent red cell transfusions, the presence of alloantibody requires selection of components that lack the corresponding antigen (25).

RED CELL ANTIBODIES

Approximately 1% of hospitalized patients have clinically significant red cell antibodies. Among multitransfused patients, approximately 10% are alloimmunized. In contrast, as many as 30% of adult patients with sickle cell anemia have red cell antibodies.

Frequently encountered antibodies have specificities within the Rh, Kell, Duffy, and Kidd systems. Historically, anti-D is the most common, clinically significant antibody detected, although anti-K is more prevalent in recent studies (presumably as a result of the use of Rh immune globulin in the perinatal setting).

Antibodies to red cell antigens usually do not appear until 3 to 4 months after transfusion.

WHITE BLOOD CELL ANTIBODIES

HLA antibodies against Class I and/or Class II antigens are the most frequently detected antibodies directed against homologous leukocytes. Approximately 30 to 60% of multitransfused patients produced cytotoxic HLA antibody.

Non-HLA granulocyte-specific alloantibody occurs as a result of transfusion or pregnancy. These antibodies have clinical significance in the pathogenesis of febrile nonhemolytic transfusion reactions and transfusion-related acute lung injury syndrome. Neonatal alloimmune granulocytopenia is the result of granulocyte-specific antibody against neutrophil antigens present in the fetus but absent in the mother.

PLATELET-RELATED ANTIBODIES

Multitransfused patients who develop anti-HLA antibody are usually refractory to platelet transfusions. In these cases, HLA-matched platelet transfusions can be beneficial. Although there appears to be no relationship between the number of platelet transfusions and the development of alloimmunization, patients with acute leukemia who are destined to become alloimmunized do so within 6 to 8 weeks of the onset of transfusion. Fewer than 5% of these patients develop platelet-specific antibody directed against platelet antigens such as PI^{A1} (26).

Although HLA-matched platelet donors are available for the majority of allommunized patients, there is substantial interest in mechanisms for reducing the occurrence of alloimmunization. Platelets prepared by apheresis from a single donor rather than from multiple random donors, or platelet and red cell transfusions depleted of leukocytes by filtration, may delay the onset of alloimmunization. Currently, studies are underway to determine whether exposure of platelet concentrates to ultraviolet-B light lessens the rate of alloimmunization (27).

Graft versus Host Disease

Graft versus host disease (GVHD) is a consequence of transfused lymphocytes recognizing and reacting against the "host" (recipient). GVHD requires the transfer of viable immunocompetent T lymphocytes that are disparate in HLA type from the patient but are sufficiently similar to permit initial engraftment (28, 29).

GVHD has been reported after transfusion of whole blood, red blood cells, platelet concentrates, granulocytes, and fresh plasma. Most of the patients who develop GVHD have severely impaired cellular immune function that is associated with severe, combined immunodeficiency disease, Wiskott-Aldrich syndrome, or bone marrow transplantation. Premature newborn babies who had received intrauterine transfusions and are now undergoing exchange transfusion for hemolytic disease of the newborn are also at increased risk for transfusion-related GVHD. A few patients undergoing therapy for Hodgkin's disease, non-Hodgkin's lymphoma, acute leukemia, and neuroblastoma, as well as immunocompetent patients undergoing cardiac surgery, have had fatal GVHD caused by transfusion. The latter cases involve transfusions from first-degree relatives who were homozygous for HLA haplotypes or occurred in Japan, where there is an increased frequency of identical HLA haplotypes within the population. Postoperative erythroderma (POE), which appears to be a GVHD-like syndrome, may occur as frequently as 1/700 patients undergoing cardiac surgery in Japan (30).

Transfusion-associated GVHD occurs between four and 30 days after transfusion. Transfusion of 10^7 lymphocytes has been shown to cause GVHD; however, the minimal dose is unknown. The condition resembles GVHD associated with bone marrow transplantation and affects the skin, liver, and gastrointestinal tract. The patients develop fever, which may be accompanied by erythema, diarrhea, liver function abnormalities, and bone marrow suppression marked by pancytopenia. The skin rash may progress to toxic epidermal necrolysis. Hepatomegaly and jaundice are common, but lymphadenopathy and splenomegaly occur less frequently.

Transfusion-associated GVHD may go unrecognized because the clinical features are not always apparent. Minor degrees or self-limiting conditions may be missed, and all of the features may not occur in every case. The diagnosis is made by performing a biopsy of the skin or GI tract. Alternatively, karyotype analysis or HLA typing of circulating lymphocytes that are not of the patient's type but, rather, are those of the donor support the diagnosis.

Treatment of transfusion-associated GVHD is usually unsuccessful; the mortality rate is approximately 90%. Hence, prevention is the most effective therapy. This is accomplished by subjecting transfusable blood and components to 2500 to 3000 rad (25 to 30 Gy). This dose of irradiation prevents lymphocyte proliferation but does not damage red cell, platelet, or granulocyte function. Gamma-irradiated red cells stored at 4°C have plasma potassium levels that are approximately twice those normally expected.

Transfusions irradiated to prevent GVHD are indicated for patients with congenital immunodeficiency syndromes, especially severe, combined immunodeficiency disease and Wiskott-Aldrich syndrome; premature neonates who had received intrauterine transfusion or exchange transfusion as birth; severely immunosuppressed patients with leukemia, lymphoma, or neuroblastoma; and, because of the recent reports of GVHD in immunocompetent patients, recipients of directed donations from first-degree relatives.

Iron Overload

Endocrine, cardiac, and liver dysfunction have been demonstrated in adults who have received 60 to 210 (mean 120) units of blood (31, 32).

Strategies for preventing or delaying the onset of iron overload in patients expected to receive multiple transfusions (e.g., those with thalassemia) include neocyte transfusions, red cell exchange transfusion, and chelation therapy with subcutaneous deferoxamine. Neocytes are young red cells that are separated from whole blood by differential centrifugation based on the progressive increase in density of red cells as they age in vivo. Neocytes have approximately 30 to 60% longer survival. However neocyte units contain approximately one-half the hemoglobin mass of normally prepared red cells.

Red cell exchange transfusions are of potential benefit for patients with impaired marrow production. Removal of patients' red cells effectively depletes older cells. This results in transfusion of donor red cells with a lower mean age. This approach can reduce overall red cell utilization by approximately 30%, but it requires twice the number of donor units.

Iron chelation therapy with deferoxamine by daily subcutaneous infusion results in the elimination of large quantities of iron in the urine and stool. Orally administered ascorbic acid increases total iron excretion.

Posttransfusion Purpura

Posttransfusion purpura (PTP) is a syndrome of profound thrombocytopenia occurring 5 to 9 days after transfusion. Most cases occur in multiparous women receiving their first blood transfusion, but PTP has been described in nulliparous, previously transfused women and in men. It has been induced by whole blood, red blood cell, and plasma transfusions. Petechiae occur in the skin and mucous membranes, and gross bleeding from the gastrointestinal and urinary tracts has been reported. In approximately one-third of cases, the inciting transfusion is accompanied by a febrile reaction (33).

The etiology is not precisely known. However, in more than 90% of cases, Pl^{A1}-negative recipients make an alloantibody specific for Pl^{A1}, an alloantigen found on the platelets of 98% of the normal population. It is unclear why a Pl^{A1}-negative person with Pl^{A1} alloantibodies becomes thrombocytopenic. Possible mechanisms include transfused platelet antigens provoking an autoantibody that binds to autologous platelets, immune complexes that are formed by alloantibody and soluble alloantigen that is released from transfused platelets, binding to autologous platelets, or soluble alloantigen binding to autologous platelets that are destroyed by subsequently formed alloantibody.

Posttransfusion purpura also occurs in association with alloantibodies directed against Pl^{A2}, Bak^{a}, Bak^{b}, and other platelet-specific antigens. There appears to be a higher frequency of anti-Pl^{A1} alloantibody production among persons who are HLA-DR3 positive.

The thrombocytopenia associated with posttransfusion purpura is profound; it is not uncommon for the patient to have a platelet count of less than 10,000/μl. Platelet-specific antibodies reactive against platelet alloantigens are usually found by indirect immunofluorescence testing and complement fixation assays. The Pl^{A1}-specific antibodies associated with PTP usually fix complement.

The diagnosis is made by recognizing that the thrombocytopenia occurred within 7 to 10 days after a blood transfusion. Drug-induced thrombocytopenia, DIC, and thrombocytopenia associated with Gram-negative sepsis must be excluded.

PTP is a self-limited condition, but it can have a fatal outcome. Treatment involves the administration of corticosteriods, plasma exchange, whole blood exchange transfusions, or intravenous γ-globulin infusion. Recurrence of PTP following a subsequent transfusion is reported, but it does not invariably occur. It is suggested that patients with a history of PTP who require transfusion should receive platelet-depleted components. Transfusion of Pl^{A1}-negative platelets to patients who have anti-Pl^{A1} alloantibodies has not resulted in satisfactory posttransfusion platelet increments.

Immunosuppressive Effects of Blood Transfusion

Anecdotal reports link patients who receive blood transfusions with an earlier recurrence of metastatic cancer and a higher incidence of postoperative infectious complications. The reported studies involve retrospective analyses rather than prospective, randomized, controlled investigations.

In experimental studies using animal models, transfusion is associated with diminished cell-mediated immunity and increased macrophage production of arachidonic acid metabolites of prostaglandin E, thromboxane, and prostacyclin. Other immunologic changes associated with blood transfusion include decreased natural killer cell function and decreased response in mixed lymphocyte cultures (34).

Although these presumed immunosuppressive effects of transfusion are tantalizing, further studies are needed to placed this potential complication in perspective.

TRANSFUSION-TRANSMITTED DISEASES

Transfusion-transmitted diseases are the most feared delayed complications of transfusion. Recent advances in the understanding of the acquired immunodeficiency syndrome (AIDS) and hepatitis have led to a significant reduction in the number of cases attributed to these infections. Improved donor

Table 71.5. Complications of Blood Transfusion—Transfusion-Transmitted Diseases

	Approximate Frequency per Component
Hepatitis A	Rare
Hepatitis B	~10% of posttransfusion hepatitis cases
Hepatitis C	? 1 per 3000–5000
Hepatitis D	Rare
HIV-1	<1 per 200,000
HIV-2	Unknown
HTLV-I/II	Rare
Cytomegalovirus	1 per 20–30 if donor is anti-CMV-positive donor
Malaria	Rare
Babesiosis	Rare
Trypanosomiasis	Rare
Syphilis	Rare

screening techniques and the introduction of highly sensitive and specific tests have made significant positive contributions to the safety of the blood supply. Nonetheless, risk remains (Table 71.5).

Hepatitis

HEPATITIS A

Transfusion-associated hepatitis A occurs only infrequently because the period of viremia is short and a carrier state does not exist. Transfusion occurs when blood is donated during the asymptomatic viremic state 7 to 28 days prior to the onset of clinical illness. Viremia occurs before alanine aminotransferase (ALT) elevation. Hence, transfusion-associated hepatitis A is not completely prevented by determining donor ALT levels (35).

HEPATITIS B

Between 6 and 10% of persons infected with hepatitis B become asymptomatic carriers. The introduction of testing for hepatitis B surface antigen in the early 1970s identified the vast majority of donors capable of transmitting hepatitis B through transfusion. Some newly infected individuals and those with HB_SAg titers below the limit of test detecton are involved in the 3 to 13% of posttransfusion hepatitis cases caused by hepatitis B reported during the past decade. Following the introduction of testing for antibody to hepatitis B core antigen (anti-HB_C) in1987, the risk decreased further because anti-HB_C is present during the convalescent stage of an asymptomatic infection, when low levels of HB_SAg are not detectable and hepatitis B surface antibody is insufficient to neutralize the virus (36) (Fig. 71.3).

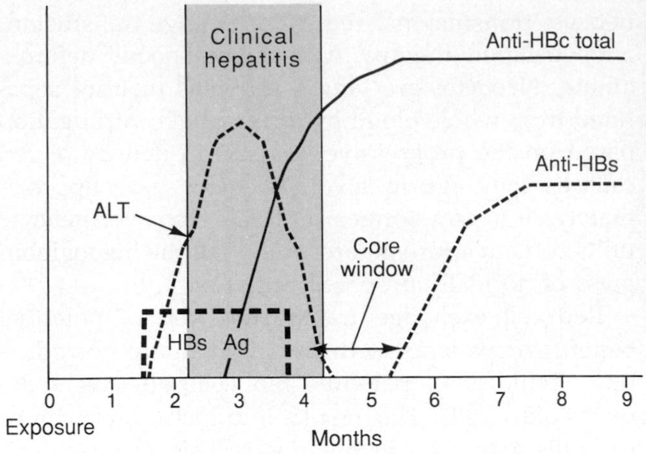

Figure 71.3. Clincial course of acute hepatitis B infection. HB_SAg is present prior to the onset of ALT elevation and clinical symptoms. Anti-HB_C occurs during the acute stage while HB_SAg is present. After HB_SAg levels become undetectable, anti-HB_S appears. However, hepatitis B may be transmitted by blood from a convalescent donor before anti-HB_S appears when anti-HB_C is the only marker for hepatitis B infection (core window).

HEPATITIS C (FORMERLY NON-A, NON-B HEPATITIS)

During the mid-1970s, approximately 90% of posttransfusion hepatitis cases were ascertained to be unrelated to hepatitis A or hepatitis B. The term "non-A, non-B hepatitis" was introduced to characterize liver dysfunction, presumably of viral origin, that occurred after transfusion but that could not be attributed to hepatitis A, hepatitis B, cytomegalovirus, or Epstein-Barr virus. Despite an inability to identify the presumed agent of non-A, non-B hepatitis, it was evident that approximately 50% of those afflicted developed evidence of chronic liver abnormalities and that 10 to 20% of these persons progressed to cirrhosis. Epidemiologic evidence indicated that approximately 50% of cases could be prevented by introducing the nonspecific or surrogate tests, ALT and anti-HB_C. These tests were introduced in 1986 and 1987 at a time when it was felt that the etiologic agent of non-A, non-B hepatitis would remain unidentified for an indefinite period of time.

In 1988, the virus that causes the majority of cases of non-A, non-B posttransfusion hepatitis was identified. The RNA molecule, approximately 10,000 nucleotides long, was termed hepatitis C and apparently is a flavivirus. Complementary DNA from nonstructural parts of the viral genome were used to prepare test kits for detecting antibody to hepatitis C. These were licensed for screening blood donors in 1990 (Fig. 71.4). Because anti-HCV seroconversion may be delayed for up to 1 year following exposure, it is anticipated that some posttransfusion hepatitis cases will continue to occur. Therefore, the use of the

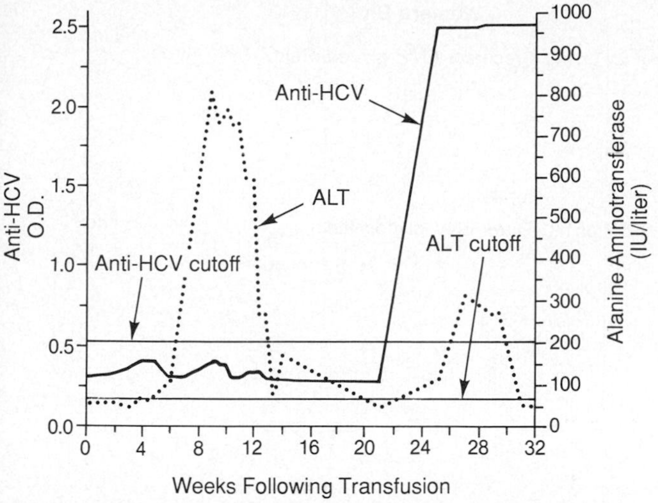

Figure 71.4 Serial alanine aminotransferase (ALT) and antibody to hepatitis C virus (HCV) in a patient with posttransfusion hepatitis C. The patient developed clinical symptoms 7 to 8 weeks after transfusion in conjunction with an elevated ALT level. Anti-HCV was not present until 14 to 16 weeks after the acute clinical episode. The fluctuating ALT values are consistent with chronic hepatitis C. (Modified from Alter HJ, Parcell RH, Shih JW, et al. Detection of antibody to hepatitis C virus in prospectively followed transfusion recipients with acute and chronic non-A, non-B hepatitis. N Engl J Med 1989;321: 1494–1500).

surrogate tests for ALT and anti-HB_C will remain in place until the role of anti-HCV testing is established (37).

HEPATITIS D (DELTA HEPATITIS)

Hepatitis delta virus is a "defective" RNA virus that requires the presence of hepatitis B virus for entry and exit from hepatocytes. Acute delta hepatitis may occur as a "coinfection" with hepatitis B, or it may occur as a "superinfection" in a patient who is a hepatitis B carrier. These illnesses are associated with a mortality rate as high as 20%. Since delta hepatitis is linked to hepatitis B, measures for preventing hepatitis B transmission are effective in preventing delta hepatitis (38).

HIV-1

HIV-1 (formerly HTLV-III) is the etiologic agent of AIDS. Approximately 3% of AIDS cases are transfusion-related, and 1% have occurred in patients treated with coagulation factor concentrates. The median latent period between transfusion with an infected unit and clinical evidence of AIDS is at least 7 years.

HIV-1 ANTIBODY TESTING

A test to detect antibody against HIV-1 was licensed as a blood screening reagent in March 1985. At that time, 0.038% of blood donors nationwide were HIV antibody-positive. Notification and deferral of these donors, more effective methods of presenting information about HIV infection to prospective donors, and better donor history questioning have reduced the rate of HIV antibody-positive blood donors to 0.01%.

Unfortunately, donors may be infectious despite testing negative for HIV antibody during the period between infection and seroconversion. In general, anti-HIV-1 antibody develops at a median interval of 2 to 3 months following infection and 95% of exposed donors seroconvert within 6 months (Fig. 71.5). However, some infected individuals have been found to remain seronegative for up to 3 years (39).

Approximately 1 per 225,000 (range 1/36,000 to 1/300,000) HIV-antibody-negative components may transmit HIV (40, 41).

Testing for HIV P24 antigen, which is present in the plasma of newly infected persons prior to the development of antibody, is not an effective screening measure for identifying blood donors capable of transmitting HIV-1 through transfusion (42). Further test improvements awaiting technological development use gene amplification techniques and polymerase chain reaction assays, recombinant protein assays, and semisynthetic peptide assays.

HIV-1 AND CLOTTING FACTOR CONCENTRATES

Approximately 80 to 90% of patients with severe hemophilia A and 40 to 50% of patients with mild or moderate hemophilia A or hemophilia B are anti-HIV-1 positive (43). AIDS has developed in 7 to 9% of these patients. Presumably, the infection was transmitted through factor VIII and IX concentrates prepared during the early 1980s from plasma pools containing up to 800 donations taken from paid donors. In an effort to reduce the risk of infectious-agent transmission, viral inactivation procedures were introduced. Initially, concentrates were heated in the lyophilized or "dry" state. Various regimens were used, including heating at 60°C for 24, 30, 72, and 144 hours; at 68°C for 72 hours; and at 80°C for 72 hours. Unfortunately, transmission of HIV occurred with concentrates prepared from anti-HIV-1-negative donors that underwent "dry heating" at 60°C for 24 and 30 hours. "Dry-heated" factor VIII concentrates are no longer available.

It is possible to "pasteurize" factor VIII in the liquid state by heating at 60°C for 10 hours. Recipients treated solely with pasteurized concentrates do not have evidence of HIV-1 infection. Factor VIII concentrates also have been prepared by immunoaffinity procedures in which VIII:C or vWf are captured on

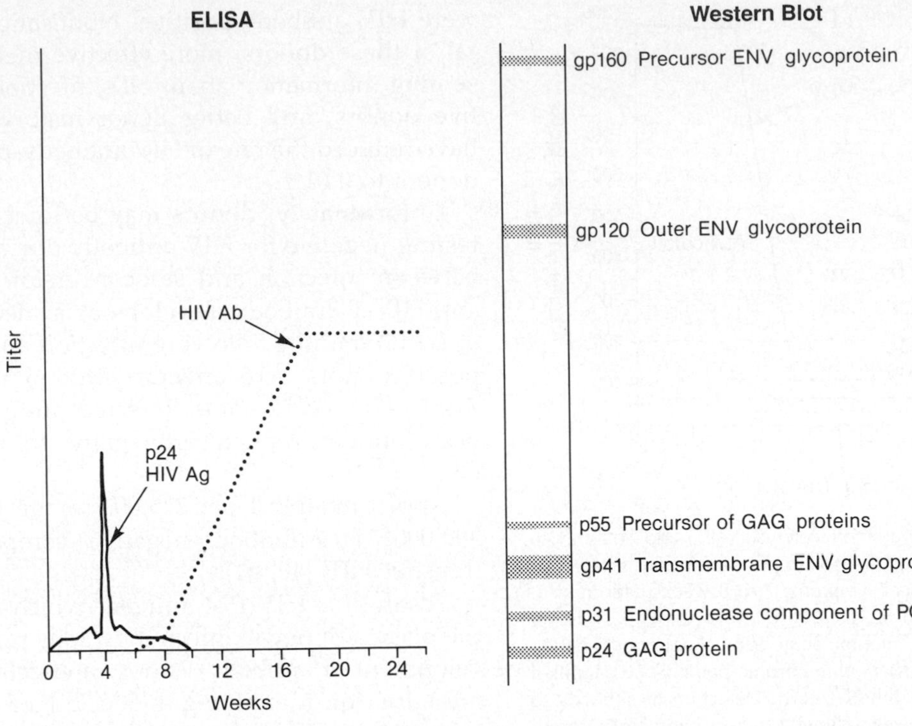

Figure 71.5 Serologic pattern of acute HIV-1 infection. ELISA: transient appearance of p24 HIV antigen occurs before anti-HIV. Western blot: Group-specific antigen (GAG) p24 and its precursor p55 are the proteins detected earliest. Antibody to the envelope (ENV) precursor, glycoprotein (Gp)160 and the final glycoproteins, Gp120 and Gp41 appear subsequently. Antibody to the polymerase (POL) gene products p31, are detected frequently in infected persons.

affinity chromatography columns with monoclonal antibody. Factor VIII subsequently is eluted from the columns and is subjected to viral inactivation procedures, either by heating at 60°C for 30 hours or by mixing with solvent detergents that inactivate HIV. Small numbers of carefully studied recipients of factor VIII concentrates subjected to pasteurization and solvent-detergent procedures indicate a lack of HIV and hepatitis C transmission by these products. Hepatitis B transmission is prevented effectively by vaccination.

HIV-2

A second human immunodeficiency virus (HIV-2) was reported in 1985. It is closely related to HIV-1 and causes illnesses similar to AIDS. Most cases occur in persons born in West Africa. Because of this, persons born in sub-Saharan Africa who have emigrated to the United States are deferred prior to a specific test for detecting HIV-2 exposure. The use of tests that combine reagents to detect anti-HIV-2 and anti-HIV-1 are under development and were implemented in 1992 for screening blood donors (44).

HTLV-I

The human T lymphotropic virus I (HTLV-I) is a transforming retrovirus that immortalizes T lymphocytes. It is associated with adult T-cell leukemia/lymphoma and tropical spastic paraparesis. It is a highly cell-associated virus that is transmitted to 60 to 70% of recipients of infected units of whole blood, red cells, or platelet concentrates but not to recipients of plasma or cryoprecipitate. A test to detect donors at risk of transmitting this infection was licensed in late 1988. However, serologic tests for anti-HTLV-I do not distinguish HTLV-I from HTLV-II infection. This requires use of polymerase chain reaction assays or peptide assays.

The lifetime risk of HTLV-I-infected people developing adult T cell leukemia is approximately 4% among those infected before the age of 20. As many as 3 to 5% of persons infected early in life develop leukemia. The latent period for tropical spastic paraparesis usually is several years, but it may be as short as a few months (45).

Cytomegalovirus

Cytomegalovirus (CMV) is a latent virus found primarily in polymorphonuclear leukocytes and lymphocytes. Most immunocompetent patients exposed to CMV become infected but rarely have symptoms. In contrast, bone marrow transplant recipients and low birth weight neonates are at risk for fever, arthralgias, enteritis, hepatitis, thrombocytopenia, leukopenia, encephalitis, and interstitial pneumonia, which may be fatal.

Blood components from donors who are anti-CMV antibody-negative do not transmit CMV. Also, red cells or platelets depleted of leukocytes by filtration that removes at least 99% of leukocytes, and frozen, deglycerolized red cells, do not transmit CMV. Saline-washed red cells and γ-irradiated components have been shown to transmit this virus by transfusion. Plasma and cryoprecipitate transfusions have not been involved in CMV transmission.

Blood and components with diminished risk of transmitting CMV are indicated for neonates weighing less than 1200 g at birth who are born of CMV-seronegative mothers and for seronegative bone marrow transplant patients who receive bone marrow from a seronegative donor. Screened units are not required for immunocompetent patients with the exception of seronegative pregnant women. Primary CMV infection during pregnancy poses a risk of intrauterine transmission and adverse outcome in the fetus. Solid organ transplant recipients who are seronegative and receive organs from seronegative donors are at risk for primary CMV infection, and CMV-screened blood reduces the incidence of these complications. However, the indication for screened components for these patients is only a relative one because improved antiviral therapy has diminished the morbidity of acute CMV infection (46).

Malaria

Malaria is caused by infection with *Plasmodium malariae, Plasmodium falciparum, Plasmodium vivax*, or *Plasmodium ovale*. Donors implicated in transfusion-associated malaria cases were born or resided in countries in which malaria is prevalent. In general, prospective donors are deferred for 3 years after departure from endemic areas and are subsequently accepted for donation if they have been asymptomatic in the interim. The incubation period following transfusion is approximately 3 weeks (range 7 to 50 days). Patients with transfusion-associated malaria should receive conventional treatment. Exchange transfusion for the treatment of malaria is controversial and should be considered experimental therapy 47).

Babesiosis

Babesiosis is caused by the parasite *Babesia microti*. It is an infection of red cells that is transmitted by the *Ixodes dammini* tick. Babesiosis is a malaria-like illness that is generally mild. However, it may be associated with hemolysis and renal failure and may be fatal in immunocompromised, asplenic, or elderly patients. Sensitive and specific tests for detecting carriers of this parasite are not available. Recommendations for decreasing the potential of transmitting this agent include deferring indefinitely those donors with a history of babesiosis and encouraging health care providers to be alert to making the diagnosis (48).

Chagas' Disease

Chagas' disease is caused by the protozoan parasite *Trypanosoma cruzi*. The organism is endemic in Mexico and Central and South America. Reduviid bugs spread infection to man, and low levels of parasitemia persist throughout life. The estimated risk of transmission is 13 to 23% for each unit of contaminated blood transfused. A few cases of transfusion-associated Chagas' disease in the U.S. have been reported among immunocompromised patients who had received transfusions from persons who emigrated from South and Central America. The incubation period between transfusion and the onset of symptoms is approximately 2 months. Currently, adequate screening tests for detecting persons at risk of transmitting this infection are not available. Epidemiologic studies to determine the prevalence of infection in the United States' donor population and the development of laboratory screening tests are in process (49).

Syphilis

Syphilis is caused by the spirochete *Treponema pallidum*. Transfusion-associated cases occur infrequently, in part, because the spirochetes remain viable in blood stored at 4°C for no more than 4 days. All donors are screened by VDRL or RPR tests, a procedure that is questioned because those positive often are not spirochetemic. It is unlikely that testing requirements will be deleted; several transfusion-transmitted diseases are also venereal infections, and screening donors for syphilis may serve as a surrogate marker for promiscuous and/or unprotected sexual contact. The period between infusion of spirochete-infected blood and symptions is 1 to 4.5 months (50).

Lyme Disease

Lyme disease, or Lyme borreliosis is caused by *Borrelia burgdorferi*, a spirochete. Transmission by blood transfusion is unlikely because the spirochetemic phase of the illness is associated with symptoms that result in deferral of persons presenting for blood donation. However, spirochetes are viable in red cells stored at 4°C, in platelet concentrates stored at room temperature, and in plasma that has been stored frozen for up to 45 days. Hence, health care workers are advised to be alert in making the diagnosis of Lyme borreliosis among those who have received transfusion (51).

CONCLUSION

The actual complications of blood transfusion, not the perceived risks, must be weighed against the potential benefits associated with transfusion when making the decision to order blood components.

Because blood transfusion will never be completely free of potential complications, it is imperative to use transfusion therapy appropriately. Alternatives to homologous transfusion should be considered and used whenever possible. These include preoperative autologous donations, autologous blood collected by intraoperative cell salvage, and use of hemodilution techniques (52). Erythropoietin administration for augmenting preoperative autologous donations and red cell production in the perioperative period is being investigated (53). GM-CSF is used to shorten the period of neutropenia in patients receiving chemotherapy. Desmopressin and aprotinin, pharmacologic agents that promote hemostasis, are effective in reducing blood loss in some surgical settings (54). For those patients requiring homologous transfusion, reduction in the number of donors to whom they are exposed (minimal exposure transfusion) may lower the risk of complications (55). For example, a single-donor apheresis platelet concentrate results in exposure to one donor, instead of six or eight, if random-donor platelets had been used. Alone or in combination, these measures present options for reducing risk while maximizing the effectiveness and safety of transfusion therapy.

References

1. Walker RH. Special report: transfusion risks. Am J Clin Pathol 1987;88:374–378.
2. Garratty G. Abbreviated pretransfusion testing [Editorial]. Transfusion 1986;26:217–219.
3. Zuck TF. Greetings—a final look back with comments about a policy of a zero-risk blood supply [Editorial]. Transfusion 1987;27:447–448.
4. Pineda AA, Brzica SM Jr, Taswell HF. Hemolytic transfusion reaction. Recent experience in a large blood bank. Mayo Clin Pro 1978;53:378–390.
5. Schmidt PJ. The algorithm and the crossmatch [Editorial]. Transfusion 1989;29:95–96.
6. Goldfinger D. Acute hemolytic transfusion reactions—a fresh look at pathogenesis and considerations regarding therapy. Transfusion 1977;17:85–98.
7. Perkins HA, Payne R, Ferguson J, Wood M. Nonhemolytic febrile transfusion reactions. Quantitative effects of blood components with emphasis on isoantigenic incompatibility of leukocytes. Vox Sang 1966;11:578–600.
8. Brittingham TE, Chaplin H Jr. Febrile transfusion reactions caused by sensitivity to donor leukocytes and platelets. JAMA 1957;165:819–825.
9. de Rie MA, van der Plas-van Dalen CM, Engelfriet CP, von dem Borne AEGKr. The serology of febrile transfusion reactions. Vox Sang 1985;49:126–134.
10. Menitove JE, McElligott MC, Aster RH. Febrile transfusion reaction: what blood component should be given next? Vox Sang 1982;42:318–321.
11. Popovsky MA, Moore SB. Diagnostic and pathogenetic considerations in transfusion-related acute lung injury. Transfusion 1985;25:573–577.
12. Van Buren NL, Stroncek DF, Clay ME, McCullough J, Dalmasso AP. Transfusion-related acute lung injury caused by an NB2 granulocyte-specific antibody in a patient with thrombotic thrombocytopenic purpura. Transfusion 1990;30:42–45.
13. Moore SB. Anaphylactic transfusion reactions—a concise review. Ir Med J 1985;78:54–56.
14. Reed RL II, Heimbach DM, Counts RB, et al. Prophylactic platelet administration during massive transfusion. A prospective, randomized, double-blind clinical study. Ann Surg 1986;203:40–48.
15. Ciavarella D, Reed RL, Counts RB, et al. Clotting factor levels and the risk of diffuse microvascular bleeding in the massively transfused patient. Br J Haematol 1987;67:365–368.
16. Waters AH and the British Committee for Standardization in Haematology Blood Transfusion Task Force. Guidelines for transfusion for massive blood loss. Clin Lab Haematol 1988;10: 265–273.
17. Khabbaz RF, Arnow PM, Highsmith AK, et al. *Pseudomonas fluorescens* bacteremia from blood transfusion. Am J Med 1984;76:62–68.
18. Murray AE, Bartzokas CA, Shepherd AJN, Roberts FM. Blood transfusion-associated *Pseudomonas fluorescens* septicemia: is this an increasing problem? J Hosp Infect 1987;9:243–248.
19. Tipple MA, Bland LA, Murphy JJ, et al. Sepsis associated with transfusion of red cells contaminated with *Yersinia enterocolitica*. Transfusion 1990;30:207–213.
20. Braine HG. Kickler TS, Charache P, et al. Bacterial sepsis secondary to platelet transfusion: an adverse effect of extended storage at room temperature. Transfusion 1986;26:391–392.
21. Pineda AA, Taswell HF, Brzica SM Jr. Delayed hemolytic transfusion reaction. An immunologic hazard of blood transfusion. Transfusion 1978;18:1–7.
22. Moore SB, Taswell HF, Pineda AA, Sonnenberg CL. Delayed hemolytic transfusion reactions. Evidence of the need for an improved pretransfusion compatibility test. Am J Clin Pathol 1980;74:94–97.
23. Hewitt PE, MacIntyre EA, Devenish A, Bowcock SJ, Contreras M. A prospective study of the incidence of delayed haemolytic transfusion reactions following perioperative blood transfusion. Br J Haematol 1988;69:541–544.
24. Ness PM, Shirey RS, Thoman SK, Buck SA. The differentiation of delayed serologic from delayed hemolytic transfusion reactions: incidence, clinical and long-term serologic findings. Transfusion 1990;30:688–693.
25. Walker RH, Lin D-T, Hartrick MB. Alloimmunization following blood transfusion. Arch Pathol Lab Med 1989;113:254–261.
26. Dutcher JP, Schiffer CA, Aisner J, Wiernick PH. Long-term follow-up of patients with leukemia receiving platelet transfusions: identification of a large group of patients who do not become alloimmunized. Blood 1981;58:1007.
27. Deeg HJ. Transfusions with a tan. Prevention of allosensitization by ultraviolet irradiation. Transfusion 1989;29:450–455.
28. Holland PV. Prevention of transfusion-associated graft-vs-host disease. Arch Pathol Lab Med 1989;113:285–291.
29. Anonymous. Transfusions and graft-versus-host disease [Letter]. Lancet 1989;1:529–530.

30. Vogelsang GB. Transfusion-associated graft-versus-host disease in nonimmunocompromised host [Editorial]. Transfusion 1990;30:101–103.
31. Schafer AI, Cheron RG, Dluhy R, et al. Clinical consequences of acquired transfusional iron overload in adults. N Engl J Med 1981;304:319–324.
32. Wolfe L, Olivieri N, Sallan D, et al. Prevention of cardiac disease by subcutaneous deferoxamine in patients with thalassemia major. N Engl J Med 1985;312:1600–1603.
33. Aster RH. Post-transfusion purpura. Baillière's Clin Immunol Allergy 1987;1:453–461.
34. Blumberg N, Heal JM. Transfusion and host defenses against cancer recurrence and infection. Transfusion 1989;29:236–245.
35. Giacoia GP, Kasprisin DO. Transfusion-acquired hepatitis A. South Med J 1989;82:1357–1360.
36. Alter MJ, Hadler SC, Margolis HS, et al. The changing epidemiology of hepatitis B in the United States. Need for alternative vaccination strategies. JAMA 1990;263:1218–1222.
37. Alter HJ, Purcell RH, Shih JW, et al. Detection of antibody to hepatitis C virus in prospectively followed transfusion recipients with acute and chronic non-A, non-B hepatitis. N Engl J Med 1989;321:1494–1500.
38. Hoofnagle JH. Type D (delta) hepatitis. JAMA 1989;261:1321–1325.
39. Horsburgh RC Jr, Ou CY, Jason J, et al. Duration of human immunodeficiency virus infection before detection of antibody. Lancet 1989;2:637–640.
40. Cumming PD, Wallace EL, Schorr JB, Dodd RY. Exposure of patients to human immunodeficiency virus through the transfusion of blood components that test antibody-negative. N Engl J Med 1989;321:941–946.
41. Menitove JE. Current risk of transfusion-associated human immunodeficiency virus infection. Arch Pathol Lab Med 1990;114:330–334.
42. Alter JH, Epstein JS, Swenson SG, et al. Prevalence of human deficiency virus Type 1 (HIV-1) p24 antigen in U.S. blood donors: assessment of efficacy for blood donor screening. N Eng J Med 1990;323:1312–1317.
43. Epstein JS, Fricke WA. Current safety of clotting factor concentrates. Arch Pathol Lab Med 1990;114:335–340.
44. Busch MP, Petersen L, Schable C, Perkins H. Monitoring blood donors for HIV-2 infection by testing for anti-HIV-1 reactive sera. Transfusion 1990;30:184–187.
45. Gout O, Baulac M, Gessain A, et al. Rapid development of myelopathy after HTLV-I infection acquired by transfusion during cardiac transplantation. N Engl J Med 1990;322:383–388.
46. Tegtmeier GE. Posttransfusion cytomegalovirus infections. Arch Pathol Lab Med 1989;113:236–245.
47. de Silva M, Contreras M, Barbara J. Two cases of transfusion-transmitted malaria (TTM) in the UK [Letter]. Transfusion 1988;28:86.
48. Popovsky MA, Lindberg LE, Syrek AL, Page PL. Prevalence of *Babesia* antibody in a selected blood donor population. Transfusion 1988;28:59–61.
49. Kirchhoff LV. Is *Trypanosoma cruzi* a new threat to our blood supply? [Editorial]. Ann Intern Med 1989;111:773–775.
50. van der Sluis JJ, Onvlee PC, Kothe FCHA, Vuzevski VD, Aelbers GMN, Menke HE. Transfusion syphilis, survival of *Treponema pallidum* in donor blood. I. Report of an orientating study. Vox Sang 1984;47:197–204.
51. Aoki SK, Holland PV. Lyme disease—another transfusion risk? Transfusion 1989;29:646–650.
52. The National Blood Resource Education Program Expert Panel. The use of autologous blood. JAMA 1990;263:414–417.
53. Goodnough LT, Rudnick S, Price TH, et al. Increased preoperative collection of autologous blood with recombinant human erythropoietin therapy. N Engl J Med 1989;321:1136–1138.
54. Bolan CD, Alving BM. Pharmacologic agents in the management of bleeding disorders. Transfusion 1990;30:541–551.
55. Brecher ME, Moore SB, Taswell HF. Minimal-exposure transfusion: a new approach to homologous blood transfusion. Mayo Clin Proc 1988;63:903–905.

Index

Page numbers followed by *f* indicate figures; those followed by *t* indicate tables.